Contents

Clinical Toxicology of Commercial Products

Fifth Edition

Clinical Toxicology of Commercial Products

Fifth Edition

ROBERT E. GOSSELIN, M.D., Ph.D.

Irene Heinz Given Professor of Pharmacology, Dartmouth Medical School, Hanover, New Hampshire

ROGER P. SMITH, Ph.D.

Professor and Chairman, Department of Pharmacology and Toxicology, Dartmouth Medical School, Hanover, New Hampshire

HAROLD C. HODGE, Ph.D., D.Sc.

Professor and Chairman Emeritus of Pharmacology and Toxicology, School of Medicine and Dentistry, The University of Rochester, Rochester, New York; Professor in Residence of Pharmacology and Oral Biology, University of California, San Francisco; of Environmental Toxicology, and of Pharmacology and Medical Therapeutics, University of California, Irvine, California

With the assistance of
JEANNETTE E. BRADDOCK

Assistant in Pharmacology, Department of Pharmacology, School of Medicine and Dentistry, The University of Rochester, Rochester, New York

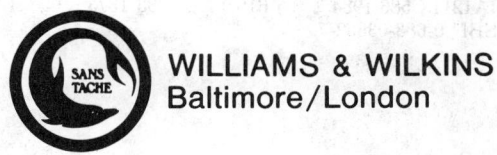

WILLIAMS & WILKINS
Baltimore/London

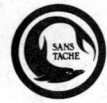

Editor: Toni M. Tracy
Copy Editor: William G. Vinck
Design: JoAnne Janowiak
Illustration Planning: Wayne Hubbel
Production: Raymond E. Reter

NOTE: The first and second editions were authored by Gleason, Gosselin, and Hodge; the third by Gleason, Gosselin, Hodge, and Smith, and the fourth by Gosselin, Hodge, Smith, and Gleason.

Copyright ©, 1984
Williams & Wilkins

Made in the United States of America

First edition, 1957
  Reprinted, 1958, 1960, 1962

Second edition, 1963

Third edition, 1969
  Reprinted, 1970, 1971, 1972, 1974

Fourth edition, 1976
  Reprinted, 1977, 1979, 1981

Library of Congress Cataloging in Publication Data

Main entry under title:
Clinical toxicology of commercial products.
  1. Toxicology. 2. Poisoning. 3. Commercial products—Toxicology. I. Gosselin, Robert E. II. Smith, Roger P. (Roger Powell), 1932–   . III. Hodge, Harold Carpenter, 1904–   . IV. Braddock, Jeanette E.
[DNLM: 1. Poisoning 2. Poisons. QV 600 G679c]
RA1211.C586 1984   615.9   83-1373
ISBN 0-683-03632-7

Preface

Concerning Poisons:

> Alcohol, hashish, prussic acid, strychnine are weak dilutions; the surest poison is time.—*Ralph Waldo Emerson*

> Cocaine isn't habit-forming, I should know—I've been using it for years.—*Tallulah Bankhead*

Concerning Consumers:

> The consumer is not a moron. She (He) is your wife (husband).—*David Oglivy*

> There is no safety in numbers, or in anything else.—*James Thurber*

Concerning Science:

> There is something fascinating about science. One gets such wholesale returns of conjecture out of such trifling investments of fact.—*Samuel Longhorne Clemens*

> Hindsight is the only exact science.—*Theo Kojak*

Concerning Truth:

> As scarce as truth is, the supply has always been in excess of the demand.—*Henry Wheeler Shaw*

Concerning Books:

> In this work, when it shall be found that much is omitted, let it not be forgotten that much likewise is performed.—*Samuel Johnson*

> Books are helpful in bed. But they are not responsive.—*Mary Hemingway*

The original purpose of this book was to assist the physician in dealing quickly and effectively with acute chemical poisonings arising through misuse of consumer products. The book provides (*a*) a list of trade name products together with their ingredients, (*b*) addresses and telephone numbers of companies for use when descriptions of products are not available, (*c*) sample formulas of many types of products with an estimate of the toxicity of each formula, (*d*) toxicological information including an appraisal of toxicity of individual ingredients, and (*e*) recommendations for treatment and supportive care.

We suggest that the physician take time to understand the organization of the material in the seven sections of the book before an emergency arises. An illustrative chart, *How to Use This Manual*, appears inside the front cover. A study of this guide, with hypothetical cases in mind, is recommended. The contents of each section are briefly described below.

Over the years a second purpose of this reference manual has received increasing emphasis, namely to acquaint therapists and others with the pathophysiological mechanisms induced by various poisons, insofar as they are understood. The book now contains detailed documentation not only of published case reports but of clinical and experimental research papers as well, which should make this compilation more useful to the professional toxicologist. Such citations are now extensive in both Sections II and III and to some extent in Section IV (see below), but with few exceptions the literature coverage in this edition does not extend beyond 1982. We have taken pains to point out areas of uncertainty or disagreement where they exist because these areas represent important gaps in knowledge and therefore opportunities for future research. Although the primary emphasis is on acute toxicity, issues of chronic toxicity and teratogenic, carcinogenic and mutagenic effects have not been totally neglected.

SECTION I. FIRST AID AND GENERAL EMERGENCY TREATMENT

As a synopsis of the physician's role in chemical poisonings from the first phone call to the final disposition, this section outlines in sequence the general emergency procedures and precautions required in all cases of acute poisoning. Included are references to relevant material in other sections.

SECTION II. INGREDIENTS INDEX

This section contains an alphabetical list of chemical substances (ingredients) commonly found in commercial products used by the consumer in and around the home and farm. Ingredients are also indexed by CAS (Chemical Abstract Service) registry numbers. The acute toxicity of each ingredient has been estimated ("toxicity rating"). Included for almost every ingredient is a brief description of toxic effects and/or cross references to more detailed information in Sections III and IV. Consult the Introduction to Section II for more information.

SECTION III. THERAPEUTICS INDEX

Section III summarizes clinical and experimental data on 85 compounds (or classes of compounds) which are named "reference congeners" in Section II because each typifies a group of related substances. This section stresses toxic signs and symptoms and recommended programs of therapy.

SECTION IV. SUPPORTIVE TREATMENT

In this section techniques of supportive treatment are discussed, with particular emphasis on those problems encountered frequently in clinical toxicology.

SECTION V. TRADE NAME INDEX

Here are listed alphabetically over 15,000 trade names of products which might be ingested accidentally or suicidally. For almost all items the category of use is indicated, e.g., rodenticide, silver polish, hair dye. In most cases the ingredients are stated, with asterisks marking those components expected to be responsible for harmful effects. With each product the manufacturer's name is given.

SECTION VI. GENERAL FORMULATIONS

This section presents formulas for the diverse types of products listed in the Trade Name Index. These formulas are believed to be "basic," "typical," or "representative" and give some guidance to physicians when the trade name of an ingested substance is not known or when information about its ingredients cannot be obtained easily. A method of estimating a toxicity rating for each product is described in the introduction to this section.

SECTION VII. MANUFACTURERS' INDEX

The names, addresses and, when available, telephone numbers of all manufacturers of products appearing in the Trade Name Index are listed for the convenience of physicians who wish to phone or write for further information.

The products listed in this book represent a wide sampling of the many thousands of items available on the market and used in homes, on farms, in small businesses, in institutions and industries—wherever toxic materials might be accessible to the public. Many of these products are relatively harmless, but are included because an attending physician needs assurance that an ingested substance is innocuous, if it is, as well as information concerning the ingredients of a product that is potentially poisonous.

Where to limit the list of trade name descriptions has been a problem. Our initial objective—to describe only products used in homes and on farms, which automatically excluded materials marketed solely for industrial use—has been modified somewhat. Many "industrial" products can now be purchased by do-it-yourself workers, hobbyists, and owners of small businesses, and so, in the absence of industrial health safeguards, become accessible to small children. On the other hand, the wide use of commercial products in institutional and industrial environments has greatly expanded the need of physicians for toxicological information about these products.

Many commercial commodities were deliberately excluded, e.g., structural materials and objects which are hazardous only because of possible physical injury, e.g., broken glass. Most poisonous plants and animal venoms have been omitted. Foods, food products, and dietary supplements are not listed unless the contents of vitamin A, vitamin D, or iron are high.

In preparing this material it was recognized that changes in formulas are frequent, that new products are marketed daily and old ones discontinued. To achieve some degree of accuracy in describing the merchandise presented in this index, contributing manufacturers were given repeated opportunities to edit descriptions of their products throughout the years between the publication of the last edition in 1976 and the appearance of the present volume. A similar procedure is planned to keep this index up to date.

The present volume represents the culmination of studies and work that have continued without interruption since the first edition was published. The authors recognize the limitations of a reference volume appearing once in five to eight years to deal with a subject that changes so rapidly. In years past we have attempted to cope with this problem by preparing monthly a bulletin with the same format as the parent volume *Clinical Toxicology of Commercial Products* (CTCP). Such a mechanism we now believe is an anachronism in this electronic and computerized age. Beginning with the 4th edition we prepared various parts of this manual in machine-readable form. These parts now include Section II, Section V and the bibliographies to each congener in Section III. This material we refer to as the *CTCP Data Base*. An earlier version of this data base constituted one of the modules of the NIH-EPA Chemical Information System (C.I.S.) which was available online nationwide and worldwide to subscribers who had access to the communications network Telenet. Other computerized versions of this data base are expected to be developed and marketed in the future.

The authors have often been told that their task is an impossible one. If the book were as all-inclusive as its title purports, i.e., if the purpose were to describe all commercial products with toxic potentialities, we would heartily agree with our critics. The coverage is admittedly incomplete. The goal has been to list the hardy perennials and the current annuals and to omit the obsolescent and evanescent thousands. For instance, hundreds of cosmetic products come on and go off the market annually. Although most of these are not included by name, the book by no means neglects them; thus the ingredients in sample or prototype formulations are listed in Section VI, together with estimates of the toxicities of the products. Because there are many similarities in the formulas of such products as perfumes and cold wave lotions, whoever the manufacturer, the General Formulations Section seems to offer the best solution to the problem of saving space while providing physicians with needed information.

Material in all sections has been extensively revised and in many places completely rewritten. Toxicity data are more extensive and more intensive than in earlier editions.

As already noted, all product information has been brought up to date; final changes were introduced during 1983. The pages of each section are numbered in sequence separately from all other sections; the appropriate section number and title appearing at the top of each page serve to designate the section. This convention was adopted to simplify the printing process and so to reduce its cost. Citations to the medical and toxicological literature are located throughout Section II with references at the end of the section. References are given throughout Section III and occasionally in Sections IV and VI. In addition, general references useful in clinical toxicology are listed in Section I (pp. 17 and 18).

Acknowledgments

To the many persons who assisted in the preparation of the four previous editions of CTCP, the authors acknowledge again their indebtedness. Many served generously and effectively in furnishing and helping to analyze material for this fifth edition. For both old and new services we are grateful.

Since the inception of this project, our efforts have brought us into contact with many informed and helpful people. Some of their names and manifold contributions to the present edition are listed in the Introductions to the various sections of this volume. It is a pleasure to acknowledge publically our gratitude to these many individuals; their contributions and collaborations were invaluable.

During the years of 1976 to 1981 this project was supported in part by a consortium of federal agencies through the mechanism of a contract administered by the Division of Poison Control, Bureau of Drugs, Food and Drug Administration. The participants in addition to the FDA included the Consumer Products Safety Commission, the Environmental Protection Agency, the National Institute of Environmental Health Sciences, the National Library of Medicine and the Occupational Safety and Health Administration. Since 1981 the FDA, EPA, CPSC and Waverly Press have provided financial assistance at various times. Royalties from the NIH-EPA Chemical Information System (see Preface) have also helped to defray operating expenses. We are particularly grateful to the many administrators in these organizations who helped us secure funds to sustain our project.

The preparation of this edition involved the collaboration of about 2300 manufacturers. With few exceptions, our many letters to manufacturers have been answered with unfailing courtesy and remarkable patience. As a rule the information we solicited was sent us, and valuable suggestions were often volunteered, such as reference sources and useful names and addresses. Especially valuable were toxicity data on products or their ingredients. Deeply appreciated were the words of commendation which appeared in hundreds of letters.

To the publisher and the printer of this complicated volume we give a special note of commendation for the vast amount of work undertaken and well done. Supervision has been ably provided by Toni M. Tracy, Vice President and Editor-in-Chief of Williams & Wilkins, who is in charge of this edition. We also acknowledge the contributions of William Vinck, Copy Editor, of Frederick Boone, Data Processing Manager, and of Raymond E. Reter, Book Production Sponsor.

Contents

SECTION I

First Aid and General Emergency Treatment

Summarized here are practical suggestions for the physician who receives an emergency call about an acute chemical poisoning. Assume that, by accident or by suicidal intent, a toxic substance has been ingested or inhaled at home or at work.

A. INSTRUCTIONS BY TELEPHONE

When alerted by phone, the therapist must first decide whether his informant is competent to give reliable information and to receive instructions. Because the person calling for help is almost always excited, the physician should speak slowly, calmly and deliberately, and give as few instructions as practical. The following nine topics in order are usually relevant to the initial telephone call:

The first alert

1. Is this a bona fide case of poisoning? With only second-hand information, this is often a hard question to answer. **If obvious physical signs and symptoms** are described, assume a toxic origin and **proceed directly to 2.**

If the victim is asymptomatic, the first requirement is a realistic prognosis; it depends upon (*a*) the amount ingested (or inhaled) and (*b*) its inherent toxicity. To characterize the toxicity of a commercial mixture by the oral route, a numerical rating has been assigned to each of the many sample formulas listed in Section VI. As indicated in Table I-1, the higher the numerical rating the greater the acute toxicity. For a specific brand that does not match any of the formulas in Section VI, a toxicity rating can often be inferred by comparing the product's composition (Section V) with the known toxicity of its separate ingredients (Section II), according to principles outlined in the Introduction to Section VI. A phone call to a regional poison center may be especially useful in this respect because center personnel can often suggest a realistic prognosis promptly.

A tentative prognosis

Although the absolute amount ingested is often unknown, approximations such as the number of swallows may sometimes be established. In a normal swallow the volume of liquid ingested (water) varies from an average of about 14 ml. for women to 21 ml. for men. Children in age group 1¼ to 3½ years average approximately 4.5 ml. (of water) per swallow or the equivalent of 1 teaspoonful. There is a relatively constant ratio of fluid volume per swallow to body weight; this ratio averages about 0.27 ml./kg. Calculations based on such estimates may be useful in prognosis (Jones and Work, 1961).

The numerical toxicity ratings in Table I-1 are really lethality ratings. A dose as small as ⅒ the lethal dose is often capable of inducing a severe and debilitating illness. If the toxicity rating implies a poor or equivocal prognosis with respect to mortality or morbidity, even the asymptomatic person should be examined as soon as possible. This is important even if the alleged exposure occurred many

Table I-1
Numerical Toxicity Rating Definitions

Toxicity Rating or Class	Probable Oral LETHAL Dose (Human)		
	Dose		For 70-kg. person (150 lb.)
6 Super toxic	Less than 5	mg./kg.	A taste (less than 7 drops)
5 Extremely toxic	5–50	mg./kg.	Between 7 drops and 1 teaspoonful (tsp)
4 Very toxic	50–500	mg./kg.	Between 1 tsp. and 1 ounce
3 Moderately toxic	0.5–5	gm./kg.	Between 1 oz. and 1 pint (or 1 lb.)
2 Slightly toxic	5–15	gm./kg.	Between 1 pt. and 1 quart
1 Practically nontoxic	Above 15	gm./kg.	More than 1 quart (2.2 lb.)

hours before. Some toxic agents produce severe sequelae after long periods of latency. A situation like this represents a challenging opportunity to the therapist.

2. Has the patient vomited? If the poison is thought to have **Induce vomiting** been ingested and if extensive vomiting has not already occurred, suggest one of the following emetic stimuli. None of these measures should be attempted if the patient is unconscious or rapidly losing consciousness, or if he is convulsing or shows pre-convulsive signs. The induction of emesis is also contraindicated if the ingested poison is thought to have been a strong alkali, corrosive acid, kerosene or a kerosene-like hydrocarbon. Severe heart disease and pregnancy are sometimes valid contraindications. Even when the induction of emesis is safe, it may be faster to inactivate a rapidly acting poison (such as bichloride of mercury) by giving activated charcoal than to remove it by provoking emesis (see instructions 3 and 4 below). If in doubt, phone a poison control center for advice. If the decision is against the induction of emesis, proceed directly to instruction 3 below.

a. If available (and it is available today in many homes), **ipecac syrup (USP)** may be administered by mouth. The conventional emetic dose is now 15 ml. in children (including toddlers) and 30 ml. in adolescents and adults. Vomiting under these circumstances is not immediate. In various clinical trials, the mean latency ranged from 14 to 25 minutes, with an average of about 15 minutes in those who vomited after the first dose (Corby *et al.*, 1968; Easom and Lovejoy, 1979; MacLean, 1973; Manoguerra and Krenzelok, 1978; Robertson, 1962). Reid (1970) and others have recommended 10 to 15 ml. ipecac syrup by mouth to young children, followed by 6 ounces of water or clear fluid (no milk). The 6 ounces of water, however, is not necessary and may or may not play a useful role. At least the latency of the emetic response is the same whether fluids are forced before or after the administration of ipecac syrup (Bukis *et al.*, 1978). All therapists recommend a second full dose of ipecac syrup to those few patients (about 10 to 15%) who fail to vomit within 20 to 30 minutes after the first dose. With this regimen about 93% of pediatric patients eventually experience emesis (Easom and Lovejoy, 1979). The same is true of adult patients, even including those who have ingested antiemetic drugs such as the phenothiazine tranquilizers, tricyclic antidepressants, etc. (Manoguerra and Krenzelok, 1978; Thoman and Verhulst, 1966). The duration and intensity of induced emesis are highly variable (MacLean, 1973), but vomiting is usually limited to 2 to 4 paroxysms over a period of 10 to 15 minutes, rarely over an hour.

b. When compared to ipecac syrup, all **other recognized emetic stimuli** are less safe, less effective or less generally available in the home. For example, sodium chloride (table salt) and copper sulfate have been employed as irritant emetics in treating accidental ingestions, but neither dependably empties the stomach and both have produced systemic poisonings and deaths (see Section II). Eliciting the gag reflex by stroking the patient's throat with a finger or other blunt object only rarely results in productive vomiting, even in children, who are believed to have a more sensitive gag reflex than adults (Dabbous *et al.*, 1965). The drug apomorphine is certainly effective (see below), but it is not available except at treatment centers. An old-fashioned emetic available in some homes is powdered black mustard (a light olive-brown powder). A teaspoonful freshly mixed in warm water and swallowed acts as a nauseant, presumably because it releases the irritant allyl isothiocyanate (see Section II). Prepared mustard is inactive. The emetic effectiveness of mustard powder, however, does not appear to have been studied adequately. Granular laundry detergents are present in most American homes, and several formulations administered by stomach tube as aqueous pastes or slurries in single doses of 40 to 75 mg./kg. caused prompt and effective vomiting in dogs (Weaver and Griffith, 1969). Episodes reported to poison centers establish that these products are also effective emetics in young children who mouth and swallow them. Until their safety is demonstrated in humans, however, laundry detergents and hand dishwashing liquids cannot be recommended as household emetics, except possibly as a last resort in poisonings with unusually grim prognoses.

c. As a useful emetic, ipecac syrup has one major rival, the drug **apomorphine.** The latter is clearly superior to ipecac in terms of its much shorter latency (Corby *et al.*, 1968; MacLean, 1973); vomiting occurs in 2 to 15 minutes with a mean latency of only 4 minutes (Hanson, 1967). In dogs (Abdallah and Tye, 1967; Corby *et al.*, 1967) and perhaps in children (Corby *et al.*, 1968), the stomach is emptied more completely in apomorphine-induced emesis than ipecac-induced emesis. In contrast to the 10 to 15% failure rate with single doses of ipecac syrup, apomorphine in the recommended dose (0.07 mg./kg. or 0.03 mg./lb., either subcutaneously or intramuscularly) induces vomiting in almost everyone. The few exceptions are individuals under the influence of centrally acting antiemetic drugs such as chlorpromazine. The major disadvantage of apomorphine is its inactivity by mouth. Parenteral routes require sterile solutions, which are usually prepared from hypodermic tablets because apomorphine solutions tend to be unstable. A second disadvantage is drowsiness and other signs of central depression that apomorphine sometimes produces (Berry and Lambdin, 1963). Apomorphine narcosis can be corrected by narcotic antagonists such as naloxone (see MORPHINE, Section III). Central depression and protracted vomiting are often mentioned as problems in using apomorphine, but except for mild drowsiness, they are seldom encountered (Corby *et al.*, 1968). Presumably all such complications could be eliminated by using smaller doses and the intravenous route of administration. For example, an intravenous dose as small as 10 to 30 μg./kg. in dogs elicits almost immediate vomiting, which lasts only 1 to 2 minutes, and is followed by no untoward reactions (Wang and Borison, 1952). Some admittedly unsatisfactory clinical evidence has been cited (Gosselin and Smith, 1966) to suggest that humans (at least adults) respond to intravenous apomorphine like the dog. We believe that clinical toxicologists at treatment centers should use apomorphine more often and more effectively, but this drug will never displace ipecac syrup as the favored household emetic.

3. As soon as productive vomiting has finished, or in about 30 minutes if it does not occur by then, administer by mouth **powdered activated charcoal in water**, if available. Small bottles of this material can now be found in some homes and in essentially all pharmacies (see Table I-3 on p. I-13). It is contraindicated in many of the same situations as syrup of ipecac (ingestion of strong acids, alkalis, kerosene and other hydrocarbon solvents), not because it is dangerous but because it is generally ineffective against these poisons (but see later with respect to kerosene). In general, activated charcoal should not be presented before ipecac syrup has had an opportunity to provoke emesis because charcoal can inactivate ipecac (Cooney, 1978); this problem does not exist with parenteral apomorphine, and so charcoal can be given immediately after (or before) apomorphine (Decker *et al.*, 1969).

Activated charcoal

The usefulness of activated charcoal as a nonspecific antidote in clinical toxicology is based on its large capacity to adsorb and retain a remarkable variety of organic and inorganic molecules and ions, including many of the common poisons (Andersen, 1946; Chin *et al.*, 1973; Corby *et al.*, 1970; Holt and Holz, 1963; Picchioni, 1970; Smith *et al.*, 1967). In the adsorbed state, a toxin produces neither local nor systemic injury, and it is eventually eliminated with the charcoal in feces. As noted in Sections II and III, however, not every poison is adsorbed to a useful degree; for example, activated charcoal is essentially useless against ethyl and methyl alcohols, strong mineral acids and alkalis, cyanide (although this 1946 observation of Andersen should be confirmed), probably most water-soluble substances (such as DDT) and others (Corby *et al.*, 1970; Decker *et al.*, 1968; Picchioni, 1970; Smith *et al.*, 1967). On the other hand, the medicinal alkaloids and many diverse synthetic drugs are well adsorbed *in vitro* and *in vivo*. In view of kerosene's low water solubility, it is surprising that kerosene blood levels were lower in charcoal-treated rats than in untreated ones (Chin *et al.*, 1969), but in general activated charcoal is not used in human cases of kerosene ingestion. Some grades of activated charcoal are superior to others (see Table I-3 on p. I-13), and charcoals that are not activated, such as burnt toast, are useless as adsorbents. As an antidote, activated charcoal is more effective the sooner it is swallowed, but it may be worthwhile to try it even several hours after the ingestion of substances which have low solubilities in gastrointestinal fluids (*e.g.*, phenytoin), which delay gastric emptying or which inhibit the propulsive activity of the gut (Easom and Lovejoy, 1979).

The optimal dose of activated charcoal cannot be stated with any useful precision; presumably it depends upon many factors that cannot be assessed in actual emergencies. In controlled studies on rats (Chin *et al.*, 1973), the most favorable outcome was achieved when the dose of charcoal exceeded the dose of test drug by a factor of 8:1. In clinical practice, one offers the patient as much activated charcoal powder as he will consume, with a minimal goal of 0.5 to 1.0 gm./kg. To assure that the full dose is delivered, the powder should be stirred more or less continuously in a few ounces of water, while the mixture is drunk. To avoid eliciting prompt emesis it may have to be consumed slowly. It is often difficult but usually possible to coax young children to swallow this slurry. The rejection is based on the unsightly black color, gritty feeling and lack of flavor, all of which make it difficult to swallow. Many attempts have been made to improve the palatability of charcoal suspensions by adding flavoring agents, thickeners, etc. (for references, see Scholtz *et al.*, 1978). In general it is not difficult to enhance acceptability, but many of the excipients in the formulas tested were partly adsorbed by the charcoal and so reduced its adsorptive capacity for poisons. Thus ice cream and other milk products are definitely contraindicated. Some promising results have been reported with suspensions of activated charcoal in sorbitol gels (Scholtz *et al.*, 1978), but more studies of the stability, acceptability and efficacy of these processed suspensions are needed. Until then, a simple slurry in water is the best way to present powdered activated charcoal for ingestion.

Once a poison in the stomach or upper bowel is fully adsorbed on the charcoal particles, it is innocuous unless desorption occurs during its transit down the alimentary canal. Apparently desorption is not a major problem under these circumstances, although more data on this point are needed (Chin *et al.*, 1969). In practice, the therapist who administers charcoal to a poison victim is not obliged to remove it by inducing emesis or by aspirating the stomach contents, although it may be safer to do so if the poison is known to be highly toxic. To minimize the time available for desorption, it is probably useful to speed transit of the charcoal-poison complex through the bowel. A saline cathartic such as sodium sulfate or magnesium citrate, administered with water by mouth or by stomach tube, is effective (see p. I-12), apparently without provoking significant desorption (Chin and Picchioni, 1979; LaPierre *et al.*, 1981).

4. If activated charcoal is not available, any of several other adsorbents may be used, although probably none is so generally effective as a good grade of charcoal. For example (Chin *et al.*, 1969; Smith *et al.*, 1967), a highly adsorptive clay known as montmorillonite is more palatable than powdered charcoal and rivals it in binding organic basic drugs (*e.g.*, amphetamine) *in vitro* and *in vivo*; it is, however, inferior to charcoal in adsorbing acidic drugs (*e.g.*, salicylic acid). Whereas highly adsorptive clays are not available in the home, one can almost always find some food protein in solution, **notably milk** or, in the absence of fresh milk, undiluted evaporated milk, gelatin solution, beaten egg whites, flour and water paste, etc. These proteins can adsorb and precipitate some poisons (*e.g.*, notably alkaloids and heavy metal ions), and they also serve to delay gastric emptying into the duodenum. In these ways the passage of poisons into the blood stream can sometimes be retarded (Chin *et al.*, 1969). Because these proteins are hydrolyzed by digestive enzymes in the stomach and duodenum, the protection is likely to be transitory. Therefore attempts should be made to remove the poison by emesis or gastric aspiration as soon as possible. Unfortunately emetine, the active constituent in syrup of ipecac, is one of the alkaloids that

Other useful adsorbents

appears to bind to milk proteins. Drinking 8 ounces of milk instead of water before syrup of ipecac delays the emetic response in adults by about 10 minutes (Varipara and Oderda, 1977).

The usual recommendation is to postpone the ingestion of all adsorbents and demulcents until syrup of ipecac has had an opportunity to empty the stomach. We believe, however, that the converse is preferable under some circumstances. Admittedly the circumstances have not been well established and may be uncommon, but with rapidly acting poisons such as bichloride of mercury, which is quickly and tightly bound to gastrointestinal mucosa, the delayed emesis produced by ipecac is likely to be futile. When toxic and corrosive heavy metals are ingested, it seems advisable to attempt first to trap them in the lumen with adsorbents such as activated charcoal, milk or any other available protein solution and to empty the stomach later by injecting apomorphine (p. I-3) or by performing gastric aspiration and lavage (p. I-10). Two concerns about milk and similar fluids as "antidotes" relate to their volume and to their fat content. The ingestion of digestible fats is widely held to increase the intestinal absorption of lipid-soluble substances. Thus milk and cream are and should be avoided after swallowing a fat-soluble poison. The issue of volume is not so clear. Whereas water and bland aqueous solutions have often been recommended as "diluents" in cases of accidental ingestion, laboratory studies with mice (Ferguson, 1962) and rats (Henderson *et al.*, 1966) demonstrate that water alone enhances the toxicity and elevates the blood levels of many orally administered systemic poisons. The relevance of these demonstrations, however, is unclear, since the dilution volumes used in these rodent studies were equivalent to 1.2 to 3.0 liters in an adult human. We believe that a glassful or two of milk is not likely to promote gastrointestinal absorption, especially if its use is restricted to water-soluble poisons that may bind to lactalbumin or other milk proteins.

5. Was any toxic material spilled in the patient's eyes, on his skin, or on his clothing? Discard any contaminated or suspected garments. Toxic liquids on the skin should be removed by blotting with any absorbent material. Then **rinse** all involved skin areas **with copious amounts of running water.** If the inhalation of a toxic gas or vapor is suspected, remove the patient (and everyone else) from the contaminated area. A chemically injured eye should be flushed immediately with water. Because of pain and spasm this seldom can be done effectively unless someone assists the victim by holding his eyelids open while a gentle stream of tap water irrigates all surfaces, preferably for several minutes. If no other facilities are available, dunk the face in a pail or pan of water while the eye is pried open.

Decontaminate skin and eyes

6. In the large majority of accidental ingestions reported by poison centers, the prognosis is so favorable that additional therapeutic measures are judged to be unnecessary. Thus, the induction of emesis, with or without the subsequent use of activated charcoal or other adsorbents, together with simple decontamination of skin, eyes, mouth and clothing, offers adequate protection to most asymptomatic persons who have inadvertently tasted or swallowed a small amount of a nonedible consumer product. If, however, toxic signs and symptoms persist or if the prognosis (p. I-1) is equivocal or unfavorable with respect to mortality or morbidity even in the absence of current symptoms, proceed immediately to **arrange transportation to the most convenient site with medical facilities.** It is usually faster and more satisfactory to have the patient brought to the hospital,

Get patient to treatment center

clinic, or office than for the doctor to speed to the home. Professional ambulance service or the police can frequently provide transportation, but a member of the family or a neighbor with a car is usually the quickest solution. This is generally a practical solution unless the victim has sustained severe physical injury as well as a toxic one, or unless he has stopped breathing.

7. Have a member of the household **collect any of the unused poison in its normal container.** A sample of any vomitus should be put in a clean bottle or jar. Insist that these **specimens are brought to the hospital or clinic** with the patient, when possible.

Bring poison and container for identification

8. If the patient can be brought for examination and treatment promptly (*e.g.*, within 15 to 30 minutes), do not delay his trip by making additional requests or suggestions. Even instructions about inducing emesis may be better omitted if these measures are expected to delay professional treatment appreciably.

Emphasize the need for speed

9. **If transportation is not immediately available** (for example, while waiting for an ambulance), it may be desirable to offer (by phone) **one or more of the following instructions:**

a. **If the patient is unconscious** and particularly if he has vomiting or retching movements while unconscious, **keep him on his side** with the trunk and head sloping slightly downward, so that the head is a few inches below the rest of the body.

b. In most neighborhoods it is possible to **locate someone with formal training in first aid.** If such a person is available, ask him to stand by. His services may become essential if the patient stops breathing before professional therapists arrive.

c. **If a convulsion occurs,** do nothing except to prevent the patient from falling or otherwise injuring himself.

d. **Do not exhaust the victim** by overzealous attempts at first aid. The use of blankets, wet compresses, and gentle massage are harmless ways to keep the family busy.

e. **Avoid home remedies** which involve the administration of drugs.

f. **Do not throw away the poison.** Keep a sample but clean up any spilled toxic material which may constitute a hazard to another member of the household (for example, a child or pet animal).

g. **If the patient becomes drowsy,** give strong tea or black coffee by mouth. Tea is probably the more useful beverage and can be given freely to children under these circumstances.

Additional first-aid suggestions for the layman (optional)

B. AWAITING THE PATIENT'S ARRIVAL

This occasion offers you (the physician) an invaluable opportunity to make necessary preparations.

1. If you were told the name of the product responsible for the poisoning, **consult this book to find the product's ingredients.** Use Section V if the brand name or trademarked name is known; use Section VI if only the general nature of the substance was revealed. With a knowledge of the exact or probable ingredients, Section II (Ingredients Index) is consulted. For each toxic ingredient Section II outlines expected toxic symptoms and recommended programs of treatment or else directs the reader to the appropriate information in Section III (Therapeutics Index). **Study carefully specific symptomatology and treatment in Sections II and III.**

If you fail to find listed in this manual the product responsible for

Use this manual
. . . to identify toxic ingredients
. . . to learn about specific symtomatology and treatment
. . . to locate manufacturer for more information

the intoxication, **a prompt telephone call to the manufacturer** may elicit valuable information about the identity and toxicity of the ingredients. The **addresses** of many manufacturers are listed **in Section VII.** Useful information or advice may also be obtained from a local or regional poison center.

2. **Alert nurses and resident physicians** at the hospital, clinic, or office. Plan to reach the hospital before the patient in order to check on preparations. If this is impractical, authority must be delegated. Leave specific instructions when possible.

Notify staff

3. **Notify the medical examiner,** police, or other representative of the law as soon as any suspicion arises that the poisoning may involve homicidal intent or criminal negligence.

Notify police

4. **Arrange for consultations** with professional colleagues if their help is expected to be necessary at any time. For example, a psychiatrist's advice may be invaluable in the management of a patient who has just attempted suicide. If the need is anticipated, an anesthesiologist, pediatrician, analytical chemist, clinical toxicologist, or some other specialist may make an essential contribution to the recovery of a severely poisoned patient. Such experts can sometimes be located by telephoning a local or regional poison center.

Consult colleagues

5. **Check preparations and equipment in the treatment room.** Special equipment and drugs that are used frequently in clinical toxicology are listed below in Tables I-2 and I-3; most, if not all, of them should be available in a well supplied emergency treatment center. An equipment checklist, like Table I-2, is desirable. In addition, many drugs should be on hand. The therapeutic agents listed in Table I-3 are particularly useful in clinical toxicology (pp. I-13–16)

Check equipment and drugs

C. GENERAL EMERGENCY TREATMENT BY THE PHYSICIAN

1. Are the signs and symptoms consistent with the history? With the presumed identity of the toxic ingredient? With the alleged dose? Try to **write at least brief notes concurrently with the examination** and treatment because all cases of poisoning are potentially medicolegal problems.

The initial physical examination

2. **Save all specimens.** Examine carefully any of the unused poison, its container and the commercial label, when available. Any specimen brought in with the patient should be properly labeled by a responsible assistant and saved for future study. Also save the first urine specimen, all vomitus, the first gastric washings, and a blood sample, when indicated. Refrigerate specimens when necessary, but never use a chemical preservative.

Collect and preserve specimens for analysis

3. **Emptying the stomach** by emesis (see p. I-2) or by gastric aspiration and lavage to remove unabsorbed poison is often the first therapeutic procedure and usually the most worthwhile one if the patient's vital signs are normal. Of course, severe respiratory distress and circulatory collapse must be corrected first (see Section IV). Emptying the stomach *per os* is generally worthwhile **any time within 3 hours after ingestion** of a poison—and perhaps even longer if large amounts of milk or cream were ingested. Intubation and the induction of emesis are impractical and **dangerous after the ingestion of strong corrosive agents** like alkali (lye, concentrated ammonia water) or mineral acids, although with appropriate caution experienced operators have performed esophageal endoscopy

Gastric lavage, indications and contraindications

Table I-2
Equipment Useful in the Treatment of Chemical Poisonings

Any approved type of respirator (*e.g.*, an anesthesia machine)	Polyethylene catheters, sterile, assorted sizes
Tank of medicinal oxygen	Sterile instrument kit for surgical cut-down on peripheral vein
Tank of compressed nitrous oxide	Sterile preparations for lumbar puncture
Assorted oronasal face masks	Restraint sheets and bedsides
Mouth gag	Chemically clean jars with air-tight covers (for excreta and other specimens)
Oropharyngeal airways (sizes No. 1, 3, 5)	
Endotracheal tubes	Ice pack
Resuscitation tubes for mouth-to-mouth breathing	Resuscitation equipment for cardiac arrest: electrical
Nasal oxygen catheter	defibrillator, artificial cardiac pacemaker, transvenous
Oxygen humidifier	catheter electrodes, assorted chest electrodes, elec-
Oxygen tents and hoods	trode paste, instrument for continuous monitoring of
Bronchoscope	ECG (see Section IV)
Tracheotomy set	Laryngoscope
Suction machine	Emesis basin
Soft rubber catheters (10–36 F)	Poison report forms
Funnels for 20 F, 24 F, 30 F, 34 F, 36 F catheters	Assorted sterile needles, hypodermic and intravenous
Large glass or metal syringes (50- and 100-ml. capacity)	Assorted syringes
Tourniquets	Spinal tray
Infusion sets	Thoracotomy tray
Transfusion equipment	Peritoneal lavage kit
	Hemodialysis or hemoperfusion apparatus

in the early hours of the injury (see Section III). Central nervous excitement with latent convulsions (*e.g.*, strychnine poisoning) also interdicts both attempted lavage and the administration of emetic drugs.

Of the two methods for emptying the stomach *per os*, aspiration with subsequent lavage has long been extolled as superior to forced emesis. During the past 15 to 20 years, many pediatricians experienced in the use of syrup of ipecac have come to the opposite conclusion. Although ipecac-induced emesis has an appreciable latency (see p. I-2), the delay in completing gastric lavage has been found to be even longer (Reid, 1970). In children, emesis after ipecac syrup appears to be more effective than lavage in removing ingested salicylate (Boxer *et al.*, 1969). Presumably the same is true of other poisons, especially if the stomach contains appreciable amounts of solid residues such as food, undissolved capsules or tablets, etc., which are difficult to remove through the usual nasogastric or orogastric tube. Because of fright, most children struggle when intubated. The result is psychological and, in a few cases, physical trauma (*e.g.*, aspiration, laryngeal spasm, gastric hemorrhage, perforation of the esophagus or stomach). In contrast, ipecac syrup is remarkably safe in children in the recommended oral dose (Shirkey, 1966). Theoretical advantages of intravenous apomorphine have been cited (Gosselin and Smith, 1966), but no adequate clinical experience has been reported.

One concludes that the availability of ipecac syrup makes **gastric lavage unwarranted in young children, unless** the ingested substance has produced coma or impending coma, or is a rapidly acting systemic poison (such as nicotine, mercuric chloride, etc.). In the latter case the procedure of choice is believed to be the prompt administration of activated charcoal and ideally its subsequent removal by gastric lavage. The rationale is discussed on p. I-6, and possible exceptions to this generalization (*e.g.*, cyanide) are indicated in Section III.

No studies in which lavage and emesis are compared in older childen and adults have been reported. Lavage, however, is probably safer and more effective in adults than in young children because the conscious adult is generally willing to cooperate with the therapist and because a wide-bore tube can be usually employed. Unless vomiting has been extensive, gastric lavage should be considered in all conscious adults who have ingested poisons other than corrosives and petroleum distillates. By using an endotracheal tube with an inflatable cuff and other precautions described below, the comatose patient can be safely lavaged. Good technique minimizes the incidence of complications such as aspiration and consequent pneumonitis.

Because it is often done inadequately, if not incorrectly, **recommended techniques of gastric lavage are summarized below.**

a. To remove unabsorbed poison, a tube is used alternately to empty and to fill the stomach with any fluid which is a satisfactory vehicle (not necessarily a solvent) for the poison. Several of these cycles are necessary for effective mechanical washing. Finally the lavage tube can be used to introduce an appropriate antidote which is allowed to remain. Questions which often arise concern the choice of tube, of intubation procedure, of lavage fluid, and of antidote. **Purpose of lavage**

b. Use as large a stomach tube as possible, so that the wash solution will flow freely and the procedure can be carried out quickly. A soft rubber tube with a diameter between ⁵⁄₁₆ and ½ inches (22 to 24 F) can usually be passed in a child, but tubes of larger diameter are desirable in adult patients. British toxicologists (Goulding and Volans, 1977; Matthew *et al.*, 1966) insist on 30 F tubes. If the stomach is expected to contain tablets or capsules, a 36 F tube should be tried. It should be inserted for a distance equal to that measured between the bridge of the nose and the tip of the xiphoid process. This distance can be measured off on the tube and marked with a small patch of adhesive tape. The tubing should be lubricated with water or a water-soluble jelly (avoid oils). It is sometimes desirable to chill the catheter. **Choice of tube**

c. In medical centers with anesthesiologists or well trained anesthetists, there seems to be a trend toward anesthetizing the patient lightly before attempting gastric lavage. Intubation and lavage become easier both for the physican and patient and probably more effective under these circumstances. At the Mary Hitchcock Memorial Hospital, small amounts of nitrous oxide or of intravenous thiopental sodium are used. In either case succinylcholine is then injected in order to make it possible to insert into the trachea an endotracheal tube with an inflatable cuff. Only then is a tube passed into the stomach. With these precautions vomiting and aspiration are minimized. As long as the endotracheal tube remains in place and an anesthesia machine or other respirator is available, resuscitation in the event of respiratory arrest is not a problem. Even patients who ingested toxic doses of sedative and hypnotic drugs have been managed successfully by this therapeutic regimen when it could be instituted in the precomatose stage, but the procedures are not recommended to physicians who lack the requisite experience. Probably in most hospitals patients are lavaged without benefit of anesthesia. **Preparation of the patient**

d. For the introduction of the lavage tube in adults and older children who will cooperate by swallowing, the oral route is preferable to the nasal route; it is also easier in infants and very young children. If nasal intubation is required, choose the nostril with the wider lumen to minimize the chance of a nosebleed. First remove dentures and any other foreign objects from the mouth. During intubation the patient is ideally positioned on his left side with his head hanging over the edge of the bed and with his face down. Particularly with a drowsy patient this precaution is important because, if reflex vomiting occurs during passage of the tube, the vomitus goes on the floor and not down the trachea. Do not force the tube; with proper technique it can be moved easily, especially if the patient swallows repeatedly. Make certain that the end of the tube lies in the stomach. If the tip enters the larynx instead of the esophagus, violent coughing and dyspnea are usually induced, but these signs may be absent in a deeply narcotized patient. Whenever in doubt, test by submerging the free end of the tube just below a water surface at the moment of expiration. (Gas from the stomach is usually expelled completely in two to three expirations, whereas air from the lungs causes bubbling at each exhalation.) In all cases **aspirate before instilling** water or antidote.

Intubation procedure

e. In most cases the composition of the wash fluid is less important than its volume or the promptness of lavage. Tap water is often as good as any vehicle, and it is never contraindicated. Isotonic saline solution is often used. In some cases solutions or solvents are known which chemically inactivate or detoxify the unabsorbed poison (*e.g.*, lime water against oxalic acid). Other examples are listed under the appropriate poison in Sections II and III. If these special reagents are not immediately available, do not delay gastric lavage but proceed promptly with tap water. Never use alcohol. With infants and small children, the lavage fluid should be warmed to prevent hypothermia.

Lavage fluid

f. In all cases the patient lies on his side with his face down or to the side. The technique of the lavage itself depends upon the diameter of the stomach tube. With relatively small-bore tubing (*viz.*, in children), a 50- or 100-ml. syringe is used to force 1 to 3 oz. of fluid down the tube. The fluid and gastric contents are then aspirated with the same syringe and the washings are saved. The procedure is repeated 10 to 15 times or until the washings are clear. If the conventional glass syringe becomes plugged with solid particles, a rubber bulb or an ear syringe may prove satisfactory. With large-bore stomach tubes (*viz.*, adult patients), the stomach is filled by gravity. Pour no more than 1 pint of water (generally 10 to 12 fl. oz.) into a funnel attached to the stomach tube and then elevate the funnel above the patient. As soon as the fluid reaches the stomach, turn the patient to promote mixing within the stomach and to wash all the mucosal surface. Promptly remove the washings by a stomach pump or by gravity siphoning. Repeat 10 to 15 times (at least 3 liters) or until the returns are clear. If a 36 F double-lumen tube is used, the lavage fluid can be introduced continuously through the small lumen while suction or gravity delivers the returns through the large lumen. Save all washings, preferably keeping the first few washings isolated from the others.

Lavage technique

g. Several choices are open at the completion of lavage. The stomach may be left empty, or an "antidote" may be instilled through the tube and allowed to remain. Section III lists an antidote appropriate for each poison, if one is known to exist. In cases of doubt a thin suspension of activated charcoal in water can be prepared, and 6 to 8 oz. of this slurry (containing at least 5 heaping teaspoonfuls of the powder) can be instilled. If the poison is thought to have no pronounced corrosive action on the stomach or bowel, a saline cathartic is often introduced. Most adult patients require about 1 oz. (*e.g.*, 4 heaping teaspoonfuls) of magnesium or sodium sulfate (Epsom and Glauber's salt, respectively) dissolved in plenty of water. Of the two, magnesium sulfate is somewhat less safe because enough Mg^{2+} is occasionally absorbed and retained to produce magnesium intoxication (central nervous depression), especially in children with impaired renal function. The average cathartic dose of sodium sulfate in a 2- or 3-year-old child is 3 to 4 gm. (1 level teaspoonful). Magnesium citrate (N.F.) is available commercially as a solution; it is said to be more pleasant tasting than the sulfate. None of these three osmotic cathartics compromises the adsorptive capacity of activated charcoal (Chin and Picchioni, 1979; Chin *et al.*, 1981; LaPierre *et al.*, 1981).

h. Remove the tube carefully to avoid the gag reflex. Pinch the tube or maintain suction while it is being withdrawn.

Antidote

4. Dependent on many circumstances, local treatment of an eye injury may or may not be postponed until systemic therapy is instituted (see **5** and **6**). To examine an eye, first apply a local anesthetic agent whenever necessary. A sterile buffered 0.5% solution of tetracaine (Pontocaine) is highly satisfactory. Use a sterile dropper; gently instill drug over the outer canthus and thereby introduce it into the conjunctival sac. Examine the eye and periorbital structures in good light and preferably with a magnifying glass. Irrigate eye, lids, etc., thoroughly with isotonic saline (0.9% NaCl) for 10 to 15 minutes. This irrigation reduces the local injury and sometimes also limits the systemic intoxication, since the cornea may serve as a persistent portal of entry for some dangerous systemic poisons which linger within the conjunctival folds. If the local ocular signs and symptoms are severe, instill a 2% buffered sterile solution of fluorescein. Greenish areas of stain mark regions where the conjunctiva, cornea, or sclera is damaged and eroded. If these areas are extensive, a dry sterile patch should be applied to the eye, and the patient should be referred to an ophthalmologist.

Emergency treatment of a chemically injured eye

5. When available, specific chemical antidotes (*e.g.*, BAL) or specific pharmacological antagonists (*e.g.*, atropine after cholinesterase poisons) **should always be administered early,** usually as soon as a diagnosis has been reached. Even the correction of shock and of respiratory insufficiency can often be delayed for a few moments while an efficient systemic antidote is given. Against most poisons, however, specific antidotes of high potency are not available. In many cases the therapeutic resources of the physician are limited to good supportive treatment. To the extent that supportive measures can be classified according to the nature of the toxic agent, programs of quasi-specific therapy can be outlined.

Specific or definitive treatment in a systemic poisoning

To employ specific (and quasi-specific) measures in therapy, the **poison must be identified;** in the case of a mixture the particular toxic ingredient must be recognized. **Sections V and VI** of this book

How treatment recommendations can be found in this manual

are designed to **furnish this information.** In Section V (Trade Name Index) each product is listed under its commercial or brand name; in Section VI (General Formulations) the common name or use serves as the basis of the compilation. For each product listed, the ingredient or ingredients of greatest toxic potential have been designated by asterisks. **To learn about the toxicities of these ingredients, Section II** (Ingredients Index) should be consulted next. Here toxic signs and symptoms are often suggested; specific treatment measures may be described, or the reader may be referred to the appropriate information in Section III (Therapeutics Index). **The recommendations about therapy found in Sections II and III** should be used to supplement and, when necessary, to modify the generalizations offered in this Section.

6. General supportive treatment is always appropriate and is usually within the resources of every physician. A well managed program of nonspecific therapy is frequently the most important element in the recovery of a poison victim. With rare exceptions, the relief of respiratory embarrassment and the correction of circulatory collapse should receive highest priority. These and other **problems of supportive treatment are discussed in Section IV.**

Problems in supportive treatment

7. In the clinical management of severely poisoned patients, there often arise detailed questions that cannot be answered in a reference manual such as this. If poison information centers are not able to help and if qualified professional specialists are unavailable, the only solution is to consult case histories in the medical literature. To aid in this endeavor, pertinent published reports are indicated at the end of almost every entry in Section II (Part D); all such references have been collected and cited fully at the end of Section II (Part E). Similarly, for each reference congener in Section III, relevant articles are cited. In all cases, clinical reports have received highest priority, but references to toxicity studies in animals are included whenever they are judged to be potentially helpful. General reference manuals, textbooks, and specialized monographs that are useful in clinical toxicology are listed on pages I-17–18.

Other sources of information

Table I-3
Drugs Useful in the Treatment of Chemical Poisonings

Drug Category	High Priority	Lower Priority
(a) Adsorbents	Powdered activated charcoal (*e.g.,* Merck, Nuchar C, Norit A)	Cholestyramine (Questran)
(b) Neutralizers	Acetic acid (5% soln.) or vinegar Milk of magnesia	Dilute hydrochloric acid (0.5% soln.) Dilute ammonia water (1% soln.) Sodium bicarbonate
(c) Emetics	Ipecac syrup, USP Apomorphine (hypo tab.)[a, b]	Dry mustard powder[b]
(d) Gastric lavage fluids	Water Sodium bicarbonate (3 to 5% soln.)[b]	Sodium thiosulfate (1% soln.) Lime water (saturated)[c] Potassium ferrocyanide (0.1% soln.)

[a] These drugs should be available in a form suitable for parenteral injection.
[b] Prepare a fresh solution just before use.
[c] These drugs should be checked for stability at 6-month intervals; all others at 12-month intervals.

Table I-3—*Continued*

Drug Category	High Priority	Lower Priority
		Potassium permanganate (1:5000) (prepared with distilled water and filtered)[c]
		Sodium or potassium iodide (1% soln.)[c]
		Calcium lactate (1–3% soln.)
		Starch soln.[b]
(e) Demulcents	Canned condensed milk	Mineral oil
	Milk of magnesia	Vegetable or cottonseed oil
	Aluminum hydroxide gel (with or without magnesium trisilicate)	Eggwhites (beaten)[b]
		Powdered milk[b]
		Starch
		Bismuth subcarbonate powder
(f) Cathartics	Magnesium sulfate (Epsom salt)	Sorbitol (70% soln.)
	Sodium sulfate (Glauber's salt)	Citrate of magnesia soln. (NF)
		Castor oil
(g) Special antidotes with systemic actions	Dimercaprol (BAL) in oil, ampuls[a]	Pilocarpine hydrochloride oral soln.[c]
	Amyl nitrate perles (0.3 ml.)[b]	Glyceryl monoacetate (monacetin)[a] not available commercially as a pharmaceutic item
	Calcium disodium edetate, ampuls[a]	
	Ethyl alcohol (not denatured)	
	Pralidoxime chloride (Protopam, 2-PAM) ampuls[a]	Levallorphan tartrate (Lorfan) 0.1% soln. in ampuls[a]
	Penicillamine (Cuprimine) caps., 250 mg.	Thioctic acid (α-lipoic acid), not available commercially as a pharmaceutic item. See Section II for source
	Sodium nitrite (3% soln. in ampuls)[a]	
	Sodium thiosulfate (25% soln. in ampuls)[a]	Neostigmine methylsulfate ampuls[a]
	Atropine sulfate hypo tab. or soln. in ampuls[a]	Leucovorin calcium injection (ampuls)[a]
	Methylene blue (1% soln. in ampuls)[a]	
	Deferoxamine (Desferal) ampuls[a]	
	Naloxone (Narcan) hydrochloride ampuls[a]	
	Pyridoxine hydrochloride[a]	
	Physostigmine (eserine) salicylate ampuls (2 mg./2 ml.)[a]	
	N-Acetylcysteine (experimental)	
(h) Analgesics	Morphine sulfate (hypo tab. or soln. in ampuls)[a]	Codeine sulfate (hypo tab. or soln. in ampuls)[a]
	Meperidine hydrochloride (Demerol) (tab. or soln. in ampuls)[a]	Acetaminophen tab. or suspension
	Aspirin tab.	
(i) Sedatives and anticonvulsants	Phenobarbital tab. and ampuls[a]	Secobarbital (Seconal) capsules and ampuls[a]
	Thiopental sodium ampuls[a, b]	Amobarbital sodium (Amytal) ampuls[a]
	Ether[c]	Pentobarbital sodium ampuls[a]
	Diazepam (Valium) tab. and ampuls[a]	Paraldehyde liquid or ampuls[c]
		Chloral hydrate soln. (0.325 gm./5 ml.)[c]
		Magnesium sulfate ampuls[a]
(j) Antiemetics	Prochlorperazine (Compazine) 0.5%	Chlorpromazine ampuls[a]

[a] These drugs should be available in a form suitable for parenteral injection.

[b] Prepare a fresh solution just before use.

[c] These drugs should be checked for stability at 6-month intervals; all others at 12-month intervals.

Table I-3—*Continued*

Drug Category	High Priority	Lower Priority
	soln. in ampuls[a]	
(k) Stimulants (analeptics)	Caffeine sodium benzoate (25% soln. in ampuls)[a] Epinephrine (1:1000, aqueous) ampuls[a, c] Aminophylline (2.5% soln. in ampuls)[a, c] Aromatic spirits of ammonia[c]	Nikethamide (Coramine) (25% soln. in ampuls)[a] Methylphenidate hydrochloride (Ritalin) tab. Doxapram (Dopram) hydrochloride (2% soln. in ampuls)[a]
(l) Antispasmodics	Atropine sulfate hypo tab. or soln. in ampuls[a] Meperidine hydrochloride (Demerol) tab. and soln. in ampuls[a] Paregoric (camphorated opium tincture)	Adiphenine hydrochloride (Trasentine) tab. Aminophylline (2.5% soln. in ampuls)[a, c] for bronchospasm
(m) Intravenous fluids	Sodium chloride (0.9% soln., 1 liter bottles)[a] Glucose (5% in water, 1 liter bottles)[a] Calcium gluconate (10% soln. in ampuls)[a] Normal human plasma[a, c] Whole blood[a, c] Sodium bicarbonate (7.5% soln. in ampuls)[a]	Glucose (5% in 0.9% NaCl soln., 1 liter bottles)[a] Ringer's solution (1 liter bottles)[a] Sodium lactate (1 M, 40-ml. bottles; M/6, 500 ml. bottles)[a] Calcium chloride (5% or 10% soln. in ampuls)[a]
(n) Intraperitoneal lavage fluids	Commercial soln.[a] with potassium (*e.g.*, Inpersol-K)	Potassium free soln.[a] Hyperosmotic soln.[a] (*e.g.*, with 7% glucose)
(o) Cardiovascular drugs	Digoxin tab. (0.25 mg.) G-Strophanthin (ouabain) ampuls[a] Glyceryl trinitrate sublingual tab.[c] Lidocaine hydrochloride (Xylocaine) 1% soln. in ampuls[a] without epinephrine Levarterenol (norepinephrine bitartrate, *l*-arterenol, Levophed) ampuls[a, c] Propranolol (Inderal) tab. and ampuls[a]	Quinidine sulfate tab. Quinidine gluconate ampuls[a] Epinephrine (1:1000, aqueous) ampuls[a, c] Ephedrine sulfate tab. Procainamide hydrochloride (Pronestyl), 10% soln. in ampuls[a] Potassium chloride, 20 mEq./10 ml. ampuls[a]
(p) Osmotic diuretics	Mannitol (25% soln. in ampuls)[a]	Urea[a] Tromethamine (THAM, 2-amino-2-hydroxymethyl-1,3-propanediol, THAM-E)[a]
(q) Vitamins and special nutrients	Ascorbic acid injection[a] Phytonadione (USP), vitamin K₁, *e.g.*, Aquamephyton, in ampuls[a, c]	Vitamin B complex concentrate, oral tab. and ampuls[a] Brewer's yeast tab. or powder Menadione bisulfite tab. or ampuls[a]
(r) Skeletal muscle relaxants	Benztropine mesylate (Cogentin) ampuls[a] Methocarbamol (Robaxin) ampuls[a]	Diphenhydramine hydrochloride (Benadryl) ampuls[a] Trihexyphenidyl hydrochloride (Artane) tab., 2 and 5 mg.

[a] These drugs should be available in a form suitable for parenteral injection.

[b] Prepare a fresh solution just before use.

[c] These drugs should be checked for stability at 6-month intervals; all others at 12-month intervals.

Table I-3—Continued

Drug Category	High Priority	Lower Priority
(s) Miscellaneous	Antibiotics[a, c] (see Section IV) Sulfonamide drug (e.g., sulfisoxazole tab. or suspension) Prednisone[a] Tetracaine soln., 0.5% sterile (ophthalmic) Injectable antihistamine (e.g., chlorpheniramine maleate ampuls)[a]	Pilocarpine Fluorescein soln., 2% sterile (ophthalmic) Hydrocortisone ointment Sodium polystyrene sulfonate (Kayexalate) 1-lb. pkg. Ammonium chloride, 0.5 and 1.0 gm. tabs.

[a] These drugs should be available in a form suitable for parenteral injection.
[b] Prepare a fresh solution just before use.
[c] These drugs should be checked for stability at 6-month intervals; all others at 12-month intervals.

REFERENCES CITED

Abdallah, A. H.; Tye, A. A comparison of the efficacy of emetic drugs and stomach lavage. Am. J. Dis. Child., 113:571–575, 1967.

Andersen, A. H. Experimental studies on the pharmacology of activated charcoal. I. Adsorption power of charcoal in aqueous solutions. Acta Pharmacol. Toxicol., 2:69–78, 1946.

Berry, F. A.; Lambdin, M. A. Apomorphine and levallorphan tartrate in acute poisonings. Am. J. Dis. Child., 105:160–163, 1963.

Boxer, L.; Anderson, F. P.; Rowe, D. S. Comparison of ipecac-induced emesis with gastric lavage in the treatment of acute salicylate ingestion. J. Pediatr., 74:800–803, 1969.

Bukis, D.; Kuwahara, L.; Robertson, W. O. Results of forcing fluids: Pre- versus post-ipecac. Vet. Human Toxicol., 20:90–91, 1978.

Chin, L.; Picchioni, A. L. Charcoal and saline laxatives for treatment of poison ingestion. Vet. Human Toxicol., 21:132, 1979.

Chin, L.; Picchioni, A. L.; Duplisse, B. R. Comparative antidotal effectiveness of activated charcoal, Arizona montmorillonite, and evaporated milk. J. Pharm. Sci., 58:1353–1355, 1969.

Chin, L.; Picchioni, A. L.; Bourn, W. M.; Laird, H. E. Optimal antidotal dose of activated charcoal. Toxicol. Appl. Pharmacol., 26:103–108, 1973.

Chin, L.; Picchioni, A. L.; Gillespie, T. Saline cathartics and saline cathartics plus activated charcoal as antidotal treatments. Clin. Toxicol., 18:865–871, 1981.

Cooney, D. O. In vitro evidence for ipecac inactivation by activated charcoal J. Pharm. Sci., 67:426–429, 1978.

Corby, D. G.; Lisciandro, R. C.; Lehman, R. H.; Decker, W. J. The efficiency of methods used to evaluate the stomach after acute ingestions. Pediatrics, 40:871–874, 1967.

Corby, D. G.; Decker, W. J.; Moran, M. J.; Payne, C. E. Clinical comparison of pharmacologic emetics in children. Pediatrics, 42:361–364, 1968.

Corby, D. G.; Fiser, R. H.; Decker, W. J. Re-evaluation of the use of activated charcoal in the treatment of acute poisoning. Pediatr. Clin. North Am., 17:545–556, 1970.

Dabbous, I. A.; Bergman, A. B.; Robertson, W. O. The ineffectiveness of mechanically induced vomiting. J. Pediatr., 66:952–954, 1965.

Decker, W. J.; Combs, H. F.; Corby, D. G. Adsorption of drugs and poisons by activated charcoal. Toxicol. Appl. Pharmacol., 13:454–460, 1968.

Decker, W. J.; Shpall, R. A.; Corby, D. G.; Combs, H. F.; Payne, C. E. Inhibition of aspirin absorption by activated charcoal and apomorphine. Clin. Pharmacol. Ther., 10:710–713, 1969.

Easom, J. M.; Lovejoy, F. H. Efficacy and safety of gastrointestinal decontamination in the treatment of oral poisoning. Pediatr. Clin. North Am., 26:827–836, 1979.

Ferguson, H. C. Dilution of dose and acute oral toxicity. Toxicol. Appl. Pharmacol., 4:759–762, 1962.

Gosselin, R. E.; Smith, R. P. Trends in therapy of acute poisonings. Clin. Pharmacol. Ther., 7:279–299, 1966.

Goulding, R.; Volans, G. N. Emergency treatment of common poisons: emptying the stomach. Proc. Roy. Soc. Med., 70:766–770, 1977.

Hanson, T. A. Apomorphine in the management of accidental ingestion of poisons. South. Med. J., 60:603–605, 1967.

Henderson, M. L.; Picchioni, A. L.; Chin, L. Evaluation of oral dilution as a first aid measure in poisoning. J. Pharm. Sci., 55:1311–1313, 1966.

Holt, L. E., Jr.; Holz, P. H. The black bottle. J. Pediatr., 63:306–314, 1963.

Jones, D. V.; Work, C. E. Volume of a swallow. Am. J. Dis. Child., 102:427, 1961.

LaPierre, G.; Algozzine, G.; Doering, P. L. Effect of magnesium citrate on the in vitro adsorption of aspirin by activated charcoal. Clin. Toxicol., 18:793–796, 1981.

MacLean, W. C., Jr. A comparison of ipecac syrup and apomorphine in the immediate treatment of ingestion of poisons. J. Pediatr., 82:121–124, 1973.

Manoguerra, A. S.; Krenzelok, E. P. Rapid emesis from high-dose ipecac syrup in adults and children intoxicated with antiemetics or other drugs. Am. J. Hosp. Pharm., 35:1360–1362, 1978.

Matthew, H.; Mackintosh, T. F.; Tompsett, S. L.; Cameron, J. C. Gastric aspiration and lavage in acute poisoning. Br. Med. J., 1:1333–1337, 1966.

Picchioni, A. L. Activated charcoal. A neglected antidote. Pediatr. Clin. North Am., 17:535–543, 1970.

Reid, D. H. S. Treatment of the poisoned child. Arch. Dis. Child., 45:428–433, 1970.

Robertson, W. O. Syrup of ipecac—a slow or fast emetic? Am. J. Dis. Child., 102:136–139, 1962.

Scholtz, E. C.; Jaffe, J. M.; Colaizzi, J. L. Evaluation of five activated charcoal formulations for inhibition of aspirin absorption and palatability in man. Am. J. Hosp. Pharm., 35:1355–1359, 1978.

Shirkey, H. C. Ipecac syrup. Its use as an emetic in poison control. J. Pediatr., 69:139–141, 1966.

Smith, R. P.; Gosselin, R. E.; Henderson, J. A.; Anderson, D. M. Comparison of the adsorptive properties of activated charcoal and Alaskan montmorillonite for some common poisons. Toxicol. Appl. Pharmacol., 10:95–104, 1967.

Thoman, M. E.; Verhulst, H. L. Ipecac syrup in antiemetic ingestion, J.A.M.A., 196:433–434, 1966.

Varipapa, R. J.; Oderda, G. M. Effect of milk on ipecac-induced emesis. N. Engl. J. Med., 296:112–113, 1977.

Wang, S. C.; Borison, H. L. A new concept of organization of the central emetic mechanism: Recent studies on the sites of action of apomorphine, copper sulfate and cardiac glycosides. Gastroenterology, 22:1–12, 1952.

Weaver, J. A.; Griffith, J. F. Induction of emesis by detergent ingredients and formulations. Toxicol. Appl. Pharmacol., 14:214–220, 1969.

GENERAL REFERENCES USEFUL IN CLINICAL TOXICOLOGY

Arena, J. M. Poisoning: Toxicology, Symptoms, Treatments, 4th ed., Charles C Thomas, Springfield, Ill., 1979.

Baker, Jr., C. E. (publisher). Physicians Desk Reference, Medical Economics Co., Oradell, N. J. (new edition annually).

Bourne, P. G. (editor). Acute Drug Emergencies. A Treatment Manual, Academic Press, New York, 1976.

Browning, E. Toxicity and Metabolism of Industrial Solvents, Elsevier, Amsterdam, 1965.

Browning, E. Toxicity of Industrial Metals, 2nd ed., Appleton-Century-Crofts, New York, 1969.

Cain, H. D. Flint's Emergency Treatment and Management, 6th ed., W. B. Saunders, Philadelphia, 1980.

Ciba Foundation Symposium 26 (New Series). The Poisoned Patient: The Role of the Laboratory, Associated Scientific Publishers, Amsterdam, 1974

Clayton, G. D.; Clayton, F. E. (editors). Patty's Industrial Hygiene and Toxicology, 3rd rev. ed., vols. 2A, 2B and 2C, Toxicology, John Wiley & Sons, New York, 1981 and 1982.

Deichmann, W. B.; Gerarde, H. W. Toxicology of Drugs and Chemicals, Academic Press, New York, 1969.

Department of the Navy. Poisonous Snakes of the World, Office of Naval Intelligence, U.S. Government Printing Office, Washington, D.C., 1965.

Doull, J.; Klaassen, C. D.; Amdur, M. O. (editors). Toxicology, The Basic Science of Poisons, 2nd ed., Macmillan, New York, 1980.

Dreisbach, R. H. *Handbook of Poisoning: Prevention, Diagnosis and Treatment*, 10th rev. ed., Lange Medical Publishers, Los Altos, Calif, 1980.

Frejaville, J.-P.; Christoforov, B; Bismuth, C.; Pebay-Peyroula, F.; Bourdon, R.; Nicaise, A.-M.; Pollet, J. *Toxicologie Clinique et Analytique*, Flammarion Médecine-Sciences, Paris, 1971.

Gerarde, H. W. *Toxicology and Biochemistry of Aromatic Hydrocarbons*, Elsevier, Amsterdam, 1960.

Gilman, A. G.; Goodman, L. S.; Gilman, A. (editors). *The Pharmacological Basis of Therapeutics*, 6th ed., Macmillan, New York, 1980.

Gorrod, J. W. (editor). *Drug Toxicity*, Taylor & Francis Ltd., London, 1979.

Grant, W. M. *Toxicology of the Eye*, 2nd. ed., Charles C Thomas, Springfield, Ill., 1974.

Hamilton, A.; Hardy, H. L. *Industrial Toxicology*, 3rd ed., Publishing Sciences Group, Inc., Acton, Mass., 1974.

Hardin, J. W.; Arena, J. M. *Human Poisoning from Native and Cultivated Plants*, 2nd ed., Duke University Press, Durham, N.C., 1974.

Hayes, W. J., Jr. *Pesticides Studied in Man*, Williams & Wilkins, Baltimore, 1982.

Kingsbury, J. M. *Poisonous Plants of the United States and Canada*, Prentice-Hall, Inc., Englewood Cliffs, N.J., 1964.

Lampe, K. F.; Fagerström, R. *Plant Toxicity and Dermatitis*, Williams & Wilkins, Baltimore, 1968.

Moeschlin, S. *Klinik und Therapie der Vergiftungen*, 4th ed., Georg Thieme Verlag, Stuttgart, 1964. Also published in 1st American ed., *Poisoning Diagnosis and Treatment*, Grune & Stratton, New York, 1965.

Polson, C. J. Tattersall, R. N. *Clinical Toxicology*, 2nd ed., J.B. Lippincott, Philadelphia, 1969.

Radeleff, R. D. *Veterinary Toxicology*, 2nd ed., Lea & Febiger, Philadelphia, 1970.

Reese, J. J. *A Manual of Toxicology*, J. B. Lippincott, Philadelphia, 1874.

Sax, N. I. *Dangerous Properties of Industrial Materials*, 4th ed., Van Nostrand Reinhold Publishing Corp., New York, 1975.

Sollmann, T. *A Manual of Pharmacology and Its Applications to Therapeutics and Toxicology*, 8th ed., W. B. Saunders, Philadelphia, 1957.

Spencer, P. S.; Schaumburg, H. H. (editors). *Experimental and Clinical Neurotoxicology*, Williams & Wilkins, Baltimore, 1980.

Thienes, C. H.; Haley, T. J. *Clinical Toxicology*, 5th ed., Lea & Febiger, Philadelphia, 1972.

von Oettingen, W. F. *Poisoning, A Guide to Clinical Diagnosis and Treatment*, 2nd ed, W. B. Saunders, Philadelphia, 1958.

Webster, R. W. *Legal Medicine and Toxicology*, W. B. Saunders, Philadelphia, 1930.

Windholz, M. (editor). *The Merck Index*, 9th ed., Merck & Co., Rahway, N.J., 1976.

Witthaus, R. A. *Manual of Toxicology*, 2nd ed., Wm. Wood and Co., New York, 1911.

Worthington, E. L.; Lunin, L. F.; Heath, M.; Catlin, F. I. *Index-Handbook of Ototoxic Agents 1966–1971*, Johns Hopkins Press, Baltimore, 1973.

SECTION II

Ingredients Index

Contents

II: A. Introduction and Explanation

Section II concerns single chemical substances (and common mixtures thereof) that constitute the ingredients in various consumer products, not the products themselves. (For information about products, consult Sections V and VI.) As noted above, Section II comprises 5 parts.

Part B is an alphabetical listing of more than 6500 ingredient names, together with Chemical Abstracts Service (CAS) registry numbers when available. CAS numbers are included here to compensate for unavoidable ambiguities in terminology. For each item in this listing, a "primary" name and a "location number" are recorded. The primary name is identical to, synonymous with, or in some other way related to the entry name. The location number is a device for finding the primary name in Part D, where toxicity data are recorded.

Part C is a compilation of CAS registry numbers, each with a corresponding location number. This numeric listing can be used as an alternative to the alphabetical listing in Part B for the purpose of locating information in Part D. Thus, if one already knows the CAS number of a substance, it is generally quicker to consult Part C than Part B. In either case one learns the location number at which relevant data can be located in Part D.

Part D consists of toxicity information concerning 1646 substances or classes of substances, listed by primary names and displayed in groups to reflect similarities in structure, toxicity, source or use. To aid in accessing this information the entries are numbered consecutively

("location numbers"). To locate the appropriate entry, Part B (or C) should always be consulted first. Most entries in Part D include a semiquantitative or categorical estimate of acute toxicity in terms of a numerical toxicity rating (see below). When possible, there is a brief description of toxic signs and programs of treatment and/or cross-references to more detailed information in Sections III and IV. A diligent but not exhaustive survey has been made to locate relevant toxicity data for each ingredient or group of ingredients listed in Part D. Sources of information are indicated by literature citations.

Part E is a bibliography of published and unpublished reports about human and animal poisonings. These references are all cited in Part D and represent some but not all of the source material upon which the toxicity statements in Part D are based. The combined bibliographies of Sections II and III contain more than 7000 entries.

More complete information about the organization and uses of Section II is offered below.

What Substances Are Included

An effort has been made to list here every compound known to be a prominent ingredient in widely used consumable products. In such a naively ambitious project, errors of commission and especially of omission are inevitable. In any case, neither the inherent toxicity nor the toxic hazard has dictated the selection of entries for this index. Innocuous materials have been included whenever it appears that medical practitioners may be unfamiliar with the compound and with its lack of significant toxicity.

In the left-hand column of Part B, each compound is listed by all of its common names, official names and at least some of its chemical synonyms. Even chemically ambiguous names are included, if widely used by manufacturers to describe their products. A few common trade names are also present (notably widely used products with only one active ingredient), but if only the brand name or trademarked name is known, Section V should be consulted first.

Many drugs and medicinal agents are listed, with particular emphasis on drugs of abuse and on nonprescription items in clinical and veterinary medicine. The drug list is incomplete, however, because we believe that considerable information on drug toxicity is readily available to most physicians. Although not available in commerce, several bacterial and mushroom toxins are listed. Only a few indigenous plants with toxic principles have been included, although the active toxic ingredient may be listed if it is commonly used in commercial formulations (*e.g.*, oil of cedar leaf from arbor vitae). With exceptions, the compilation excludes chemicals which are used only by industry in manufacturing processes and which are not found in the final consumer product. The number of industrial chemicals in the database, however, is increasing, partly because hobbyists seem to have access to them.

How to Consult This Index

To obtain toxicity information about any ingredient, one must first locate its name in the left-hand column of Part B. The position of each entry in this alphabetical compilation is determined solely by the letter sequence of its name, irrespective of the way in which these letters may be divided or interrupted by word spacings, hyphens, parentheses, numerals, etc. Not counted in the letter sequence of chemical names are abbreviated prefixes such as: *o*-, *m*-, *p*-, *O*-, *n*-, *N*-, *S*-, *α*-, *β*-, *sec*-, *tert*-, *sym*- (or *s*-,) *cis*-, *trans*-, *exo*-, *endo*-, *d*-, *l*-, *dl*-, D-, L-, etc. (Note that in industry and commerce these prefixes are commonly omitted in spite of the ambiguities that this practice sometimes produces.) On the other hand, in the case of compounds where these prefixes are commonly written out (*e.g.*, ortho, para, iso, beta, di, bis, tris, tetra, hexa, pyro, tri, mono, etc.), this index should be consulted under the first letter of the prefix. Common abbreviations have been compiled (*e.g.*, 2,4-D, DDT) and indexed under the first letter (*e.g.*, D). When an ingredient is designated in commerce by a code numeral without a single letter (*e.g.*, 1080), consult this index under

"Compound—." In looking for a particular sodium, ammonium, potassium or calcium salt, etc., it is sometimes expeditious to search under the name of the anion.

As an alternative to the above procedure, if you know the CAS Registry number of an ingredient, try to locate that number in the left-hand column of Part C, where all numbers are recorded in ascending order. Registry numbers for some recognized mixtures and polymers were formerly prefixed by the letters MX and PM, respectively. In this compilation, these prefixes have been omitted. If a known CAS registry number cannot be located in Part C, it might be worthwhile to examine the alphabetical listing in Part B to find an appropriate class name (for which no registry numbers exist) or perhaps a substance whose registry number has been missed.

Primary Names

For every entry in Part B a primary name is listed (unless identical to the entry name), as well as a location number. (In Part C the primary name is replaced by its CAS Registry number, but the location number is the same.) Location numbers designate where toxicity data are recorded in Part D.

Where entry names and primary names are not identical, they are usually synonymous. A true synonym, however, was not selected as the primary name in every case. Any one of five relationships may exist. Thus the primary name may refer to (*a*) an identical substance (*i.e.*, a genuine synonym), or (*b*) a substance so closely related that no important distinctions are recognized by clinical toxicologists, or (*c*) the active or major constituent of the entry, or (*d*) a class of substances that includes the entry, or (*e*) a specific example of, or a product (commercial or natural) containing, the entry. In many cases these distinctions are self-evident, but, to avoid ambiguities, superscripts at the end of primary names in Part B refer to explanatory footnotes.

Names serving as primary names represent arbitrary choices among the many available synonyms. Whenever practical, short and simple names were selected for the convenience of physicians who may be unfamiliar with complex chemical nomenclature, but the primary concern was to offer names that are both distinctive and well established.

Structure of Part D (Ingredient Toxicity)

Part D is a compilation of data about all substances designated by primary names. The entries are grouped under headings that reflect similarities in chemical structure, toxicity, source or use. This arrangement was designed to aid the reader who wants to compare information available about related substances.

The category headings in Part D constitute a scheme for classifying "poisons." This scheme was inspired by and is related to a classification published in the second (1963) edition of *Clincal Toxicology of Commercial Products*. Both proposals have the same fundamental defect. Because more than one independent criterion was used to establish the categories, the scheme is redundant and therefore ambiguous. For example, a substance might be listed under a heading describing its chemical structure (*e.g.*, Aliphatic Aldehydes), its source (*e.g.*, Volatile Oils), its common use (*e.g.*, Odorants and Flavoring Agents) or its dominant toxicity (*e.g.*, Lung Irritants). However, no entries are duplicated in Part D. Each substance is listed under only one of several possible headings, representing an arbitrary choice that is revealed by the location number. Accordingly, it is inappropriate to search for a substance in Part D until after one has established its location number in the index of Part B or Part C.

Under each primary name in Part D, the text generally includes a list of the more common synonyms, a numerical toxicity rating (see below for explanation) and sometimes comments on chemical structure or composition, on sources of supply and on consumer usage. The emphasis, however, is on toxicity, toxic signs and symptoms, and suggestions for therapy. In many cases, treatment is not mentioned for one of two reasons: (*a*) because the only recommended forms of therapy are symptomatic and supportive (as described in Section IV); or (*b*) because Section III is judged to provide adequate information. To locate this information in Section III, it is necessary to note the "reference congener" designated in the text. The concept of a reference congener is discussed below. For many entries in Part D, no reference congener in Section III is appropriate, and so none is listed.

The comments on ingredient toxicity in Part D are based largely on published and unpublished reports of experimental studies in animals and of accidental (and suicidal) poisonings in humans. In a few instances the remarks represent merely inferences or interpretations of obviously inadequate data. Sources of information are indicated at the end of most entries. Complete literature citations, compiled alphabetically according to the name of the senior author (or editor), can be found in Part E.

Whenever a primary name is identical to that of its reference congener, the entry in Part D may serve no purpose except to direct the reader to Section III. To be referred by the index to such an "empty" entry may be tedious, but in a project of this scope any alternative procedure might create ambiguities that could mislead the reader.

The Meaning of a Reference Congener

An attempt has been made to group toxicologically related compounds, so that each group can be typified by one of its members, designated here as a "reference congener." Ideally all substances having the same reference congener are chemically related and produce similar toxic effects by mechanisms which are biochemically akin, so that one program of treatment is appropriate to all. This ideal had to be modified in order to restrict the number of reference congeners, which were selected on largely arbitrary grounds. In practice, a compound may differ considerably from its designated congener, both in quantitative and qualitative terms. In spite of its deficiencies, the device of a reference congener is a reasonable attempt to coordinate, correlate, and record succinctly formidable masses of toxicity data.

For information about or relevant to any substance listed in Part D, its reference congener should be noted. This constitutes a reference to Section III, where the toxicology of each congener is discussed in detail. Within reasonable limits each discussion in Section III is applicable to all substances having the same reference congener; we believe that this is especially true of recommended programs of therapy.

Toxicity Ratings

Numerical toxicity ratings listed in Part D are based on Table II-1. To use toxicity ratings effectively, their many implications and limitations must be appreciated, as noted below.

1. The rating is based on mortality, not morbidity, *i.e.*, it is really a lethality rating. In general a clinically significant illness may be expected after doses of about one-tenth the probable lethal dose (as the latter is reflected in the numerical toxicity rating).

2. Unless otherwise noted, each rating is based on the acute toxicity of a single dose when taken by mouth or gavage. Other dosage regimens and other routes of administration are not represented by the rating.

3. The toxicity rating reflects an estimate of the probable or mean lethal dose, not the minimal fatal dose. Perhaps because of personal idiosyncrasy or hypersensitivity or predisposing disease, minimal lethal doses recorded in the clinical literature are usually considerably lower than those implied by the ratings.

4. With only a few compounds are clinical data adequate to establish a toxicity rating. Most of the values here are based on laboratory determinations of mean lethal doses (LD_{50}) in

Table II-1
Numerical Toxicity Rating Definitions

Toxicity Rating or Class	Probable Oral LETHAL Dose (Human)	
	Dose	For 70 kg. person (150 lb.)
6 Supertoxic	Less than 5 mg./kg.	A taste (less than 7 drops)
5 Extremely toxic	5–50 mg./kg.	Between 7 drops and 1 teaspoonful (tsp.)
4 Very toxic	50–500 mg./kg.	Between 1 tsp. and 1 ounce
3 Moderately toxic	0.5–5 gm./kg.	Between 1 oz. and 1 pint (or 1 lb.)
2 Slightly toxic	5–15 gm./kg.	Between 1 pt. and 1 quart
1 Practically nontoxic	Above 15 gm./kg.	More than 1 quart (2.2 lb.)

small laboratory mammals (rat, mouse, guinea pig, rabbit; sometimes cat, dog and monkey). Implicit in the use of such data is the conventional assumption that the mean lethal dose in man lies in the same class as does the LD_{50} for the test animals. Whenever available, however, clinical data and even clinical impressions have been given precedence.

5. Toxicity ratings followed by interrogation points are based on obviously inadequate data; some represent no more than guesses.

6. For most corrosive agents, such as mineral acids, alkalies, bleaches, etc., no toxicity rating is suggested. In these cases death is usually the result of severe local tissue injury, with secondary complications such as toxemia, shock, perforation, infection, hemorrhage and obstruction. The intensity of the local lesion and of its sequelae is often determined by the concentration of the corrosive substance, whereas the volume and "dose" are secondary considerations. For such agents no single toxicity rating is an appropriate measure of lethality, unless the concentration is also specified. No simple parameter describes this relation in a way which is thought to be clinically useful.

7. In Table II-1 common units of measure are used to describe lethal doses for an adult of average size (body weight of 150 lb. or 70 kg.). For patients who are heavier or lighter, probable lethal doses are proportionately larger or smaller, and they can be readily estimated from values of mg./kg. recorded in the table. Whereas we appreciate that infants and children are not simply small adults, reliable clinical data are so scarce that we are forced to assume that lethal doses are proportional to body weight irrespective of age. Recognized exceptions are noted in Sections II and III.

8. Although all are based on Table II-1, toxicity ratings in this section have a distinctly different meaning from those in Section VI. In Section VI each rating is an estimate of the toxicity of a complete commercial product, as it is marketed and as it is described in Section VI. Here in the Ingredients Index, each rating is a measure of the inherent toxicity of a single ingredient. In establishing the toxicity ratings listed here, each dose has been calculated in terms of a single substance (usually technical grade) and is generally based on experiments in which only an innocuous solvent or vehicle was used (such as water, corn, oil, etc.), omitting all solvents, additives, and other ingredients found in the usual commercial formulations. Because many of the ingredients listed here are unavailable to the consumer in pure or undiluted form, the toxicity ratings in Section VI are more realistic in terms of clinical exposure but are almost invariably less reliable than those in this section.

Acknowledgments

In a project such as this one, each edition builds on the accomplishments of previous editions. Accordingly, the authors are still grateful to those individuals who helped to produce earlier versions of Section II. The names of several of them were listed previously (see Section II, fourth edition, 1976).

As before, all parts of Section II except the Introduction (Part A) were computer-generated from datafiles stored in the Kiewit Computation Center at Dartmouth College. Programs written by Frederick L. Boone of the Waverley Press were used to read our magnetic tapes and to generate code for a photon typesetting machine which produced the final copy.

Since the last edition, our Section II computerized datafiles have been completely restructured. This reorganization, together with the development of new editing programs for manipulating these files, was accomplished by Harold Franklin of Hanover, N.H. He and Richard Martz of the Dartmouth Medical School have served as our consultants on all computer matters.

Dr. Sally Campbell conducted literature surveys and prepared summaries for many of the new and revised pesticide entries in Section II. At various times since the last edition, the Dartmouth staff also included Nancy Doerrer, Lynne Farnum, April Silver and Terri-Lynn Thayer, all of whom served as researchers, data processors and editorial assistants. For the talents, dedication and loyal services of all of these individuals, the authors take this opportunity to express their gratitude. In acknowledging the contributions of others, however, we in no way deny our full responsibility for the undetected errors that have inevitably crept into the material of this Section.

II: B. Alphabetical Listing of Ingredient Names

Ingredient name (CAS registry no.) *See* Primary Name *at*
location no. **XXX** *in Part D of this section*

Abalyn *See* Methyl Abietate[a] *at loc. no.* **581**
Abate (3383-96-8) *See loc. no.* **1063**
Abietic Acid (514-10-3) *See loc. no.* **580**
Abietic anhydride (8050-09-7) *See* Rosin[a] *at loc. no.* **760**
Abrin (1393-62-0) *See* Jequirity Bean[e] *at loc. no.* **677**
ABS *See* Alkyl Aryl Sodium Sulfonates[d] *at loc. no.* **943**
Abstem (8061-00-5) *See* Calcium Cyanamide[c] *at loc. no.* **1355**
Acacia (9000-01-5) *See loc. no.* **744**
Acarol (18181-80-1) *See* Bromopropylate[c] *at loc. no.* **1004**
Acenocoumarin (152-72-7) *See* Acenocoumarol[a] *at loc. no.* **1332**
Acenocoumarol (152-72-7) *See loc. no.* **1332**
Acephate (30560-19-1) *See loc. no.* **1095**
Acetal (105-57-7) *See loc. no.* **465**
Acetaldehyde (75-07-0) *See loc. no.* **480**
Acetaldehyde 2-(2-ethoxyethoxy)ethyl-3,4-(methylenedioxy)phenyl acetal (51-14-9) *See* Sesamex[a] *at loc. no.* **1154**
Acetaldehyde *N*-methyl-*N*-formylhydrazone (16568-02-8) *See* Gyromitrin[a] *at loc. no.* **816**
Acetaminophen (103-90-2) *See loc. no.* **1587**
Acetanilid(e) (103-84-4) *See loc. no.* **610**
Acetic Acid (64-19-7) *See loc. no.* **42**
Acetic aldehyde (75-07-0) *See* Acetaldehyde[a] *at loc. no.* **480**
Acetic ether (141-78-6) *See* Ethyl Acetate[a] *at loc. no.* **570**
Acetin (26446-35-5) *See* Monoacetin[a] *at loc. no.* **577**
Acetoarsenite *See* Copper Acetoarsenite[e] *at loc. no.* **200**
Acetochlor (34256-82-1) *See* Alachlor[b] *at loc. no.* **1273**
Acetone (67-64-1) *See loc. no.* **466**
Acetone chloroform (57-15-8) *See* Chlorobutanol[a] *at loc. no.* **432**
Acetone Cyanohydrin (75-86-5) *See loc. no.* **646**
Acetonitrile (75-05-8) *See loc. no.* **647**
3-(α-Acetonylbenzyl)-4-hydroxycoumarin (81-81-2) *See* Warfarin[a] *at loc. no.* **1345**
3-(α-Acetonyl-4-chlorobenzyl)-4-hydroxycoumarin (81-82-3) *See* Coumachlor[a] *at loc. no.* **1336**
3-(α-Acetonyl-4-nitrobenzyl)-4-hydroxycoumarin (152-72-7) *See* Acenocoumarol[a] *at loc. no.* **1332**
Acetophenazine (2751-68-0) *See loc. no.* **1413**
Acetophenazine maleate (5714-00-1) *See* Acetophenazine[b] *at loc. no.* **1413**
p-**Acetophenetide** (62-44-2) *See* Acetophenetidin[a] *at loc. no.* **611**
Acetophenetidin (62-44-2) *See loc. no.* **611**
p-**Acetophenetidin** (62-44-2) *See* Acetophenetidin[a] *at loc. no.* **611**
2-Acetoxybenzoic acid (50-78-2) *See* Aspirin[a] *at loc. no.* **594**
Acetoxy-triphenylstannane (900-95-8) *See* Triphenyltin Acetate[a] *at loc. no.* **295**
N-**Acetyl-*p*-aminophenol** (103-90-2) *See* Acetaminophen[a] *at loc. no.* **1587**
Acetylaniline (103-84-4) *See* Acetanilid(e)[a] *at loc. no.* **610**
Acetylated lanolin *See* Lanolin[b] *at loc. no.* **716**
Acetylcarbromal (77-66-7) *See* Carbromal[a] *at loc. no.* **1431**
N-**Acetylcysteine** (616-91-1) *See loc. no.* **1502**
Acetyldigitoxin (1111-39-3) *See* Digitoxin[b] *at loc. no.* **838**

Acetyldimethylamine (127-19-5) *See* Dimethylacetamide[a] *at loc. no.* **565**
Acetylene Dichloride (540-59-0) *See loc. no.* **361**
Acetylene tetrabromide (79-27-6) *See* 1,1,2,2-Tetrabromoethane[a] *at loc. no.* **372**
Acetylene tetrachloride (79-34-5) *See* Tetrachloroethane[a] *at loc. no.* **373**
Acetylene trichloride (79-01-6) *See* Trichloroethylene[a] *at loc. no.* **375**
Acetylenogen (75-20-7) *See* Calcium Carbide[a] *at loc. no.* **62**
Acetyl hydroperoxide (79-21-0) *See* Peroxyacetic Acid[a] *at loc. no.* **78**
3-Acetyl-6-methyl-2,4-pyrandione (520-45-6) *See* Dehydroacetic Acid[a] *at loc. no.* **1187**
N-**Acetyl-*DL*-penicillamine** (15537-71-0) *See* D-Penicillamine[b] *at loc. no.* **1507**
N¹-**Acetyl-*N⁴*-phthaloylsulfanilamide** *See* Phthalylsulfacetamide[a] *at loc. no.* **1547**
Acetylsalicylic acid (50-78-2) *See* Aspirin[a] *at loc. no.* **594**
4'-(Acetylsulfamoyl)phthalanilic acid (131-69-1) *See* Phthalylsulfacetamide[a] *at loc. no.* **1547**
N¹-**Acetyl sulfanilamide** (144-80-9) *See* Sulfacetamide[a] *at loc. no.* **1551**
Acetyl sulfisoxazole (80-74-0) *See* Sulfisoxazole[b] *at loc. no.* **1568**
N⁴-**Acetyl-*N²* - trifluoromethylsulfonyl-toluene-2,4-diamine** (47000-92-0) *See* Fluoridamid[a] *at loc. no.* **1276**
Acid *See loc. no.* **30**
Acid-citrate-dextrose solution *See* Citric Acid[b] *at loc. no.* **703**
Acintol C (8002-26-4) *See* Tall Oil[a] *at loc. no.* **723**
ACL 60 (2893-78-9) *See* Trichloroisocyanuric Acid[b] *at loc. no.* **94**
ACL 70 (2782-57-2) *See* Trichloroisocyanuric Acid[b] *at loc. no.* **94**
ACL 75 (2244-21-5) *See* Trichloroisocyanuric Acid[b] *at loc. no.* **94**
ACL 85 (87-90-1) *See* Trichloroisocyanuric Acid[a] *at loc. no.* **94**
Aconite (8063-12-5) *See* Aconitine[c] *at loc. no.* **822**
Aconitine (302-27-2) *See loc. no.* **822**
Acricid (485-31-4) *See* Dinoseb[b] *at loc. no.* **543**
Acridine (260-94-6) *See loc. no.* **1517**
Acridine Antiseptics *See loc. no.* **1518**
Acridine orange (494-38-2) *See* Acridine Antiseptics[d] *at loc. no.* **1518**
Acridine yellow (135-49-9) *See* Acridine Antiseptics[d] *at loc. no.* **1518**
Acriflavine (8048-52-0) *See* Acridine Antiseptics[d] *at loc. no.* **1518**
Acrolein (107-02-8) *See loc. no.* **481**
Acrylaldehyde (107-02-8) *See* Acrolein[a] *at loc. no.* **481**
Acrylamide (79-06-1) *See loc. no.* **1624**
Acrylic Resin Monomers *See loc. no.* **1625**
Acrylonitrile (107-13-1) *See loc. no.* **648**
Actamer (97-18-7) *See* Bithionol[a] *at loc. no.* **521**
Actidil (550-70-9) *See* Antihistaminics[d] *at loc. no.* **1487**

---

[a]A Synonym   [b]A Closely Related Substance   [c]The Active or Major Constituent   [d]A Class Name   [e]A Specific Example of or Product Containing

Ingredient name (CAS registry no.) *See* Primary Name *at*
location no. **XXX** *in Part D of this section*

Actidione (66-81-9) *See* Cycloheximide[c] *at loc. no.* **906**

Adalin (77-65-6) *See* Carbromal[c] *at loc. no.* **1431**

Adamantanamine (768-94-5) *See* Amantadine[a] *at loc. no.* **922**

Adiphenine (64-95-9) *See* Benactyzine[b] *at loc. no.* **1430**

Adrenal corticosteroids *See* Corticosteroids[d] *at loc. no.* **915**

Adrenalin (51-43-4) *See* Epinephrine[c] *at loc. no.* **1454**

Aerosol AY or IB or MA *See* Dialkyl Sodium Sulfosuccinate[c] *at loc. no.* **950**

Aerosol OT (577-11-5) *See* Dioctyl Sodium Sulfosuccinate[c] *at loc. no.* **951**

Aerosols *See loc. no.* **940**

Afalon (330-55-2) *See* Linuron[c] *at loc. no.* **1251**

African chillies *See* Capsicum[a] *at loc. no.* **659**

Afrin (2315-02-8) *See* Oxymetazoline Hydrochloride[c] *at loc. no.* **1464**

Aftate *See* Tolnaftate[c] *at loc. no.* **1532**

Agar (9002-18-0) *See* Gums (Vegetable)[d] *at loc. no.* **755**

Agene (10025-85-1) *See* Nitrogen Trichloride[a] *at loc. no.* **123**

Ague tree *See* Oil of Sassafras[c] *at loc. no.* **739**

Airbron (616-91-1) *See* N-Acetylcysteine[c] *at loc. no.* **1502**

Ajmaline (4360-12-7) *See loc. no.* **794**

Aklomix-3 (121-19-7) *See* 4-Hydroxy-3-nitrophenylarsonic Acid[a] *at loc. no.* **205**

Alachlor (15972-60-8) *See loc. no.* **1273**

Alanap (132-67-2) *See* Naptalam[b] *at loc. no.* **1279**

Alanap-1 (132-66-1) *See* Naptalam[a] *at loc. no.* **1279**

Alanap-2 (5333-99-3) *See* Naptalam[b] *at loc. no.* **1279**

Alanap-3 (132-67-2) *See* Naptalam[b] *at loc. no.* **1279**

Alar (1596-84-5) *See* Daminozide[c] *at loc. no.* **1356**

Alcloxa (1317-25-5) *See* Aluminum Dihydroxy Allantoinate[b] *at loc. no.* **179**

Alcohol ethoxylate *See* Alkyl Ethoxylate[a] *at loc. no.* **962**

Alcohol ethyl (64-17-5) *See* Ethyl Alcohol[a] *at loc. no.* **412**

Alcohol glycol ethers *See* Ethylene Glycol Alkyl (and Aryl) Ethers[a] *at loc. no.* **459**

Alcohols (Higher) *See loc. no.* **404**

Alcohol Sulfate Salts *See loc. no.* **941**

Aldicarb (116-06-3) *See loc. no.* **1112**

Aldifen (51-28-5) *See* 2,4-Dinitrophenol[c] *at loc. no.* **541**

Aldioxa (5579-81-7) *See* Aluminum Dihydroxy Allantoinate[a] *at loc. no.* **179**

Aldosterone (52-39-1) *See* Corticosteroids[d] *at loc. no.* **915**

Aldrin (309-00-2) *See loc. no.* **1017**

Algin (9005-38-3) *See loc. no.* **745**

Alginic Acid (9005-32-7) *See loc. no.* **746**

Aliphatic alcohol *See* Alcohols (Higher)[a] *at loc. no.* **404**

Aliphatic chlorinated solvents *See* Chlorinated Hydrocarbons[d] *at loc. no.* **354**

Aliphatic Hydrocarbons *See loc. no.* **303**

Aliphatic ketone *See* Acetone[e] *at loc. no.* **466**

Aliphatic naphtha *See* Petroleum Naphtha[e] *at loc. no.* **331**

Aliphatic petroleum solvent *See* Petroleum Naphtha[e] *at loc. no.* **331**

Aliphatic Thiocyanates *See loc. no.* **1034**

Alipur *See* Cycluron[c] *at loc. no.* **1244**

Aliquats *See* Dialkyl Dimethyl Ammonium Chloride[c] *at loc. no.* **989**

Aliquats 26,204,205,206,207,215,221 or H226 *See* Dialkyl Dimethyl Ammonium Chloride[c] *at loc. no.* **989**

Alizarin (72-48-0) *See loc. no.* **921**

Alkali *See* Lye[a] *at loc. no.* **51**

Alkaline phosphates and carbonates *See* Lye[b] *at loc. no.* **51**

Alkaline salts *See* Lye[e] *at loc. no.* **51**

Alkaline sulfide salts *See* Sulfide Salts[d] *at loc. no.* **118**

Alkanolamine salt of dinoseb *See* Dinoseb[b] *at loc. no.* **543**

Alkenyl *derivative. See corresponding* Alkyl *derivative in this index.*

Alkyd resin *See* Polyester Resins[a] *at loc. no.* **1634**

Alkyl amine salt of 2,4,5-T *See* Trichlorophenoxyacetic Acid[b] *at loc. no.* **1224**

Alkyl ammonium chloride (or bromide) *See* Alkyl Quaternary Ammonium Chloride (or Bromide)[a] *at loc. no.* **981**

Alkyl Aryl Ammonium Chloride (or Bromide) *See loc. no.* **975**

Alkyl aryl polyether alcohols *See* Alkyl Phenoxy Polyethoxy Ethanols[a] *at loc. no.* **963**

Alkyl Aryl Polyether Sulfates and Sulfonates *See loc. no.* **942**

Alkyl aryl polyethylene glycols *See* Alkyl Phenoxy Polyethoxy Ethanols[a] *at loc. no.* **963**

Alkyl aryl polyoxyethylene *See* Alkyl Phenoxy Polyethoxy Ethanols[a] *at loc. no.* **963**

Alkyl Aryl Sodium Sulfonates *See loc. no.* **943**

Alkyl aryl sulfonate *See* Alkyl Aryl Sodium Sulfonates[e] *at loc. no.* **943**

Alkylated aryl polyether alcohol *See* Alkyl Phenoxy Polyethoxy Ethanols[a] *at loc. no.* **963**

Alkylated Sodium Phosphates *See loc. no.* **944**

Alkyl benzene sulfonate sodium (8046-53-5) *See* Alkyl Aryl Sodium Sulfonates[d] *at loc. no.* **943**

n-Alkyl-2-cyanoacrylates *See* n-Alkyl-α-Cyanoacrylates[a] *at loc. no.* **1626**

n-Alkyl-α-Cyanoacrylates *See loc. no.* **1626**

Alkyl dimethyl benzyl ammonium chloride (or bromide) (8001-54-5) *See* Benzalkonium Chloride[a] *at loc. no.* **985**

Alkyl dimethyl cuminyl ammonium chloride *See* Cationic Surfactants[d] *at loc. no.* **974**

Alkyl Dimethyl 3,4-Dichlorobenzene Ammonium Chloride *See loc. no.* **976**

Alkyl Dimethyl Ethyl Ammonium Chloride (or Bromide) *See loc. no.* **977**

Alkyl Dimethyl Ethylbenzyl Ammonium Chloride (8045-21-4) *See loc. no.* **978**

Alkyl ester of 2,4,5-T *See* Trichlorophenoxyacetic Acid[b] *at loc. no.* **1224**

Alkyl 2-ethoxyethanol *See* Alkyl Ethoxylate[d] *at loc. no.* **962**

Alkyl Ethoxylate *See loc. no.* **962**

Alkyl ethoxylate sulfate sodium salt *See* Sodium Lauryl Trioxyethylene Sulfate[e] *at loc. no.* **955**

Alkyl Hydroxyethyl Imidazolinium Chloride (8041-00-7) *See loc. no.* **979**

Alkyl Mercuric Chloride (or Phosphate) *See loc. no.* **222**

Alkyl Naphthyl Methyl Pyridinium Chloride *See loc. no.* **980**

Alkyl oxyethylene oxide condensate *See* Alkyl Ethoxylate[a] *at loc. no.* **962**

Alkyl phenol polyglycol ethers *See* Alkyl Phenoxy Polyethoxy Ethanols[a] *at loc. no.* **963**

Alkyl Phenoxy Polyethoxy Ethanols *See loc. no.* **963**

Alkyl phosphate *See* Ethyl Phosphates[e] *at loc. no.* **1112**

Alkyl polyethoxy ethanol *See* Alkyl Ethoxylate[a] *at loc. no.* **962**

Alkyl polyethylene glycol ether *See* Alkyl Ethoxylate[a] *at loc. no.* **962**

Alkyl Quaternary Ammonium Chloride (or Bromide) *See loc. no.* **981**

Alkyl Sodium Isethionate *See loc. no.* **945**

Alkyl Sodium N-Methyltaurate *See loc. no.* **948**

Alkyl Sodium Sulfates *See loc. no.* **946**

Alkyl Sodium Sulfonates *See loc. no.* **947**

---

[a] A Synonym   [b] A Closely Related Substance   [c] The Active or Major Constituent   [d] A Class Name
[e] A Specific Example of or Product Containing

Ingredient name (CAS registry no.) *See* Primary Name *at
location no.* **XXX** *in Part D of this section*

Alkyl Tin Compounds *See loc. no.* **292**
Alkyl Tolyl Methyl Trimethyl Ammonium Chloride *See loc. no.* **982**
Alkyl Trimethyl Ammonium Chloride (or Bromide) *See loc. no.* **983**
Allantoin (97-59-6) *See loc. no.* **477**
Allantoin polygalacturonic acid *See* Allantoin[b] *at loc. no.* **477**
Allethrin (584-79-2) *See loc. no.* **884**
d-trans-Allethrin (584-79-2) *See* Allethrin[d] *at loc. no.* **884**
Allidochlor (93-71-0) *See loc. no.* **1274**
Allobarbital (52-43-7) *See loc. no.* **1373**
Allobarbitone (52-43-7) *See* Allobarbital[a] *at loc. no.* **1373**
Allyl Alcohol (107-18-6) *See loc. no.* **21**
Allyl aldehyde (107-02-8) *See* Acrolein[a] *at loc. no.* **481**
Allyl Benzene (300-57-2) *See loc. no.* **311**
Allyl Bromide (106-95-6) *See loc. no.* **379**
5-Allyl-5-sec-butyl barbituric acid (115-44-6) *See* Butalbital[b] *at loc. no.* **1368**
Allyl cinerin (584-79-2) *See* Allethrin[a] *at loc. no.* **884**
5-Allyl-5-(2-cyclohexenyl)-2-thiobarbituric acid (467-36-7) *See* Thialbarbital[a] *at loc. no.* **1388**
Allylguaiacol (97-53-0) *See* Eugenol[a] *at loc. no.* **864**
Allyl Heptylate (142-19-8) *See loc. no.* **857**
5-Allyl-5-isobutylbarbituric acid (77-26-9) *See* Butalbital[a] *at loc. no.* **1368**
5-Allyl-5-isopropylbarbituric acid (77-02-1) *See* Aprobarbital[a] *at loc. no.* **1365**
Allyl Isothiocyanate (57-06-7) *See loc. no.* **1359**
4-Allyl-2-methoxyphenol (97-53-0) *See* Eugenol[a] *at loc. no.* **864**
5-Allyl-5-(1-methylbutyl)barbituric acid sodium salt (309-43-3) *See* Secobarbital Sodium[a] *at loc. no.* **1386**
5-Allyl-5-(1-methylbutyl)-2-thiobarbituric acid sodium salt (337-47-3) *See* Thiamylal Sodium[a] *at loc. no.* **1389**
4-Allyl-1,2-methylenedioxybenzene (94-59-7) *See* Safrole[a] *at loc. no.* **872**
5-Allyl-5-phenylbarbituric Acid (115-43-5) *See loc. no.* **1363**
Allyxycarb (6392-46-7) *See loc. no.* **1121**
Aloe (8001-97-6) *See* Aloin[b] *at loc. no.* **847**
Aloe vera gel *See* Aloin[c] *at loc. no.* **847**
Aloin (8015-61-0) *See loc. no.* **847**
Alpha- *If not listed below, omit prefix and try again.*
Alphachloroacetophenone (532-27-4) *See* α-Chloroacetophenone[a] *at loc. no.* **14**
Alpha-dinitrophenol (51-28-5) *See* 2,4-Dinitrophenol[a] *at loc. no.* **541**
Alpha-naphthaleneacetic acid (86-87-3) *See* 1-Naphthaleneacetic Acid[a] *at loc. no.* **1309**
Alpha-naphthyl thiourea (86-88-4) *See* ANTU[e] *at loc. no.* **1350**
Alpha (N-phthalimido)-glutarimide (50-35-1) *See* Thalidomide[a] *at loc. no.* **1443**
Alpolygal *See* Allantoin[b] *at loc. no.* **477**
Alrosept MBC (1301-47-9) *See* Alkyl Hydroxyethyl Imidazolinium Chloride[c] *at loc. no.* **979**
Alrosept MM (1301-19-5) *See* Alkyl Hydroxyethyl Imidazolinium Chloride[c] *at loc. no.* **979**
Alseroxylon (8001-95-4) *See loc. no.* **795**
Alum (7784-24-9) *See loc. no.* **181**
Alumina hydrate (1333-84-2) *See* Aluminum Hydroxide[b] *at loc. no.* **178**
Aluminum acetate solution (8006-13-1) *See* Burow's Solution[a] *at loc. no.* **183**

Aluminum ammonium sulfate *See* Alum[b] *at loc. no.* **181**
Aluminum Chloride (7446-70-0) *See loc. no.* **182**
Aluminum chlorohydrate (12042-91-0) *See* Aluminum Chloride[b] *at loc. no.* **182**
Aluminum chlorohydrex *See* Aluminum Chloride[a] *at loc. no.* **182**
Aluminum chlorohydroxide (1327-41-9) *See* Aluminum Chloride[b] *at loc. no.* **182**
Aluminum chlorohydroxy allantoinate *See* Aluminum Dihydroxy Allantoinate[b] *at loc. no.* **179**
Aluminum Dihydroxy Allantoinate (5579-81-7) *See loc. no.* **179**
Aluminum hydrate (21645-51-2) *See* Aluminum Hydroxide[a] *at loc. no.* **178**
Aluminum Hydroxide (21645-51-2) *See loc. no.* **178**
Aluminum hydroxide gel (12040-59-4) *See* Aluminum Hydroxide[b] *at loc. no.* **178**
Aluminum oxide (1333-84-2) *See* Aluminum Hydroxide[b] *at loc. no.* **178**
Aluminum Phosphide (20859-73-8) *See loc. no.* **137**
Aluminum potassium sulfate *See* Alum[a] *at loc. no.* **181**
Aluminum Silicate (14504-95-1) *See loc. no.* **180**
Aluminum sulfate (7784-31-8) *See* Alum[b] *at loc. no.* **181**
Aluminum trihydrate *See* Aluminum Hydroxide[a] *at loc. no.* **178**
Alurate (77-02-1) *See* Aprobarbital[c] *at loc. no.* **1365**
Alvyl (9002-89-5) *See* Polyvinyl Alcohol[c] *at loc. no.* **1637**
Amanin (21150-21-0) *See* Amatoxins[d] *at loc. no.* **813**
Amanita bisporigera *See* Amatoxins[c] *at loc. no.* **813**
Amanita citrina *See* Bufotenine[c] *at loc. no.* **820**
Amanita muscaria *See* Muscimol[c] *at loc. no.* **819**
Amanita pantherina *See* Muscimol[c] *at loc. no.* **819**
Amanita phalloides *See* Amatoxins[c] *at loc. no.* **813**
Amanita toxins *See* Amatoxins[e] *at loc. no.* **813**
Amanita verna *See* Amatoxins[c] *at loc. no.* **813**
Amanita virosa *See* Amatoxins[c] *at loc. no.* **813**
α-Amanitin (23109-05-9) *See* Amatoxins[d] *at loc. no.* **813**
β-Amanitin (21150-22-1) *See* Amatoxins[d] *at loc. no.* **813**
γ-Amanitin (21150-23-2) *See* Amatoxins[d] *at loc. no.* **813**
Amantadine (768-94-5) *See loc. no.* **922**
Amatoxins *See loc. no.* **813**
Amerchol 400 *See* Lanolin[e] *at loc. no.* **716**
Amerchol BL *See* Lanolin[e] *at loc. no.* **716**
Americaine *See* Benzocaine[c] *at loc. no.* **1577**
American Mistletoe *See loc. no.* **656**
American oil of pennyroyal (8007-44-1) *See* Pennyroyal[d] *at loc. no.* **740**
American wormseed *See* Chenopodium Oil[a] *at loc. no.* **728**
Amerlate LFA *See* Lanolin[b] *at loc. no.* **716**
Amethocaine *See* Tetracaine[c] *at loc. no.* **1586**
Ametryn (834-12-8) *See* Prometon[b] *at loc. no.* **1267**
Amiben (1076-46-6) *See* Chloramben[b] *at loc. no.* **1296**
N^1-Amidinosulfanilamide (57-67-0) *See* Sulfaguanidine[a] *at loc. no.* **1556**
Amidol (137-09-7) *See* 2,4-Diaminophenol Hydrochloride[a] *at loc. no.* **620**
Amidone (76-99-3) *See* Methadone[a] *at loc. no.* **1485**
Amidopyrine (58-15-1) *See* Aminopyrine[a] *at loc. no.* **1570**
Amidosulfonic acid (5329-14-6) *See* Sulfamic Acid[a] *at loc. no.* **48**
Aminacrine (90-45-9) *See* Acridine Antiseptics[d] *at loc. no.* **1518**
Amine hardener *See* Diethylenetriamine[e] *at loc. no.* **603**
9-Aminoacridine (90-45-9) *See* Acridine Antiseptics[d] *at loc. no.* **1518**

---

[a] A Synonym   [b] A Closely Related Substance   [c] The Active or Major Constituent   [d] A Class Name
[e] A Specific Example of or Product Containing

Ingredient name (CAS registry no.) *See* Primary Name *at*
location no. **XXX** *in Part D of this section*

1-Aminoadamantan (768-94-5) *See* Amantadine[a] *at loc. no.* **922**

4-Aminoantipyrine (83-07-8) *See* Aminopyrine[b] *at loc. no.* **1570**

Aminobenzene (62-53-3) *See* Aniline[a] *at loc. no.* **612**

p-**Aminobenzenearsonic acid** (98-50-0) *See* Arsanilic Acid[a] *at loc. no.* **189**

p-**Aminobenzenesulfonacetamide** (144-80-9) *See* Sulfacetamide[a] *at loc. no.* **1551**

p-**Aminobenzene sulfonamide** (63-74-1) *See* Sulfanilamide[a] *at loc. no.* **1563**

2-(4-Aminobenzenesulfonamido)-5-methoxypyrimidine *See* Sulfameter[a] *at loc. no.* **1558**

2-*p*-Aminobenzenesulfonamidoquinoxaline *See* Sulfaquinoxaline[a] *at loc. no.* **1565**

p-**Aminobenzenesulfonyl guanidine** *See* Sulfaguanidine[a] *at loc. no.* **1556**

o-**Aminobenzoic Acid** (118-92-3) *See loc. no.* **627**

p-**Aminobenzoic Acid** (150-13-0) *See loc. no.* **628**

p-**Aminobenzoic acid propyl ester** (94-12-2) *See* Butamben[b] *at loc. no.* **1579**

Aminocarb (2032-59-9) *See loc. no.* **1122**

N-**(Aminocarbonyl)-2-bromo-2-ethyl-butanamide** (77-65-6) *See* Carbromal[a] *at loc. no.* **1431**

5-Amino-4-chloro-2-phenyl-3(2*H*)-pyridaminone *See* Pyrazon[a] *at loc. no.* **1313**

Aminocyclohexane (108-91-8) *See* Cyclohexylamine[a] *at loc. no.* **609**

1-Aminocyclopropanol *See* Coprine[b] *at loc. no.* **815**

3-Amino-2,5-dichlorobenzoic acid (133-90-4) *See* Chloramben[a] *at loc. no.* **1296**

3-Amino-1-dimethylamino-2-methyl phenazathionium chloride (92-31-9) *See* Tolonium Chloride[a] *at loc. no.* **1523**

4-Amino-6-(1,1-dimethylethyl)-3-(methylthio)-1,2,4-triazin-5(4*H*)-one (21087-64-9) *See* Metribuzin[a] *at loc. no.* **1266**

4-Aminodiphenylamine (101-54-2) *See* *p*-Aminodiphenylamine[a] *at loc. no.* **619**

p-**Aminodiphenylamine** (101-54-2) *See loc. no.* **619**

2-Aminoethanol (141-43-5) *See* Monoethanolamine (and Salts)[a] *at loc. no.* **64**

2-Aminoethyl alcohol (141-43-5) *See* Monoethanolamine (and Salts)[a] *at loc. no.* **64**

β-**Aminoethyl alcohol** (141-43-5) *See* Monoethanolamine (and Salts)[a] *at loc. no.* **64**

N-**(2-Aminoethyl)-*N'*-(2-((2-aminoethyl)amino)ethyl-1,2-ethanediamine** (112-57-2) *See* Tetraethylenepentamine[a] *at loc. no.* **605**

2-Amino-4-(ethylthio)butyric acid (55-17-4) *See* Ethionine[a] *at loc. no.* **1643**

4-Amino-1-hydroxybenzene (123-30-8) *See* *p*-Aminophenol[a] *at loc. no.* **624**

α-**Amino-3-hydroxy-5-isoxazole acetic acid** (60573-88-8) *See* Muscimol[b] *at loc. no.* **819**

2-Amino-2-hydroxymethyl-1,3-propanediol (77-86-1) *See* Tris(hydroxymethyl)aminomethane[a] *at loc. no.* **69**

3-Amino-6-hydroxynitrobenzene *See* 4-Amino-2-nitrophenol[a] *at loc. no.* **625**

Aminomercuric chloride *See* Ammoniated Mercury[a] *at loc. no.* **223**

5-(Aminomethyl)-3-isoxazolol (2763-96-4) *See* Muscimol[a] *at loc. no.* **819**

4-Amino-3-methyl-6-phenyl-1,2,4-triazin-5(4*H*)-one (41394-05-2) *See* Metamitron[a] *at loc. no.* **1265**

2-Amino-2-methyl-1,3-propanediol (115-69-5) *See loc. no.* **71**

2-Amino-2-methyl-1-propanol (124-68-5) *See loc. no.* **70**

4-Amino-2-nitrophenol (119-34-6) *See loc. no.* **625**

2-Amino-5-nitrothiazole (121-66-4) *See loc. no.* **1538**

Aminophen (62-53-3) *See* Aniline[a] *at loc. no.* **612**

Aminophenazone (58-15-1) *See* Aminopyrine[a] *at loc. no.* **1570**

p-**Aminophenol** (123-30-8) *See loc. no.* **624**

o-**Aminophenol** (95-55-6) *See p*-Aminophenol[b] *at loc. no.* **624**

m-**Aminophenol** (591-27-5) *See p*-Aminophenol[b] *at loc. no.* **624**

(4-Aminophenyl)arsonic acid (98-50-0) *See* Arsanilic Acid[a] *at loc. no.* **189**

2-Amino-5-phenyl-4(5*H*)-oxazolone *See* Pemoline[a] *at loc. no.* **1465**

2-Amino-1-phenyl-1-propanol hydrochloride (7587-43-1) *See* Phenylpropanolamine Hydrochloride[a] *at loc. no.* **1451**

p-**(5-Amino-3-phenyl-1*H*-1,2,4-triazol-1-yl)-*N,N,N',N'*-tetramethyl phosphonic diamide** (1031-47-6) *See* Triamiphos[a] *at loc. no.* **1209**

Aminophylline (317-34-0) *See loc. no.* **799**

2-Aminopyridine (504-29-0) *See loc. no.* **1320**

3-Aminopyridine (462-08-8) *See* 4-Aminopyridine[b] *at loc. no.* **1319**

4-Aminopyridine (504-24-5) *See loc. no.* **1319**

Aminopyrine (58-15-1) *See loc. no.* **1570**

p-**Aminosalicylic Acid** (65-49-6) *See loc. no.* **629**

Aminosulfonic acid (5329-14-6) *See* Sulfamic Acid[a] *at loc. no.* **48**

2-Aminothiazole (96-50-4) *See* 2-Amino-5-nitrothiazole[b] *at loc. no.* **1538**

3-Amino-1,2,4-triazole (61-82-5) *See* Amitrole[a] *at loc. no.* **1290**

4-Amino-3,5,6-trichloropicolinic acid (1918-02-1) *See* Picloram[a] *at loc. no.* **1312**

4-Amino-3,5,6-trichloro-2-pyridinecarboxylic acid (1918-02-1) *See* Picloram[a] *at loc. no.* **1312**

Aminozide (1596-84-5) *See* Daminozide[a] *at loc. no.* **1356**

Amiton (78-53-5) *See* Tetram[a] *at loc. no.* **1080**

Amitraz (33089-61-1) *See loc. no.* **1039**

Amitriptyline (50-48-6) *See loc. no.* **1470**

Amitrole (61-82-5) *See loc. no.* **1290**

Amizol (61-82-5) *See* Amitrole[c] *at loc. no.* **1290**

Ammate (7773-06-0) *See* Ammonium Sulfamate[c] *at loc. no.* **153**

Ammonia (7664-41-7) *See loc. no.* **63**

Ammonia gas (7664-41-7) *See* Ammonia[a] *at loc. no.* **63**

Ammoniated Mercury (10124-48-8) *See loc. no.* **223**

Ammonia water (8007-57-6) *See* Ammonia[b] *at loc. no.* **63**

Ammonium alum (7784-25-0) *See* Alum[b] *at loc. no.* **181**

Ammonium amidosulfate (7773-06-0) *See* Ammonium Sulfamate[a] *at loc. no.* **153**

Ammonium bifluoride (1341-49-7) *See* Fluoride[d] *at loc. no.* **100**

Ammonium bromide (12124-97-9) *See* Bromide Salts[d] *at loc. no.* **98**

Ammonium chloride (12125-02-9) *See* Ammonium Salts[d] *at loc. no.* **152**

Ammonium cyanate *See* Cyanate Salts[d] *at loc. no.* **145**

Ammonium dichromate (7789-09-5) *See* Dichromate Salts (Soluble)[d] *at loc. no.* **82**

Ammonium dimethyldithiocarbamate *See* Sodium Dimethyldithiocarbamate[b] *at loc. no.* **1163**

---

[a] A Synonym   [b] A Closely Related Substance   [c] The Active or Major Constituent   [d] A Class Name
[e] A Specific Example of or Product Containing

Ingredient name (CAS registry no.) *See* Primary Name *at*
location no. **XXX** *in Part D of this section*

Ammonium dinitro-secondary-butyl phenate (6365-83-9)
See Dinoseb[b] *at loc. no.* **543**
Ammonium dinoseb (6365-83-9) *See* Dinoseb[b] *at loc. no.*
543
Ammonium fluosilicate (16919-19-0) *See* Fluosilicate Salts[d]
at loc. no. **101**
Ammonium Glycyrrhizate (1407-03-0) *See loc. no.* **848**
Ammonium hydroxide (8007-57-6) *See* Ammonia[b] *at loc.*
no. **63**
Ammonium ichthosulfonate (8029-68-3) *See* Ichthammol[a]
at loc. no. **1528**
Ammonium lauryl sulfate (2235-54-3) *See* Alkyl Sodium
Sulfates[b] *at loc. no.* **946**
Ammonium lauryl trioxyethylene sulfate *See* Sodium
Lauryl Trioxyethylene Sulfate[b] *at loc. no.* **955**
Ammonium *N*-methyldithiocarbamate *See* Metham So-
dium[b] *at loc. no.* **1161**
Ammonium paratungstate (12501-52-9) *See* Tungsten (and
its Salts)[d] *at loc. no.* **297**
Ammonium pentachlorozincate (16485-55-5) *See* Zinc
Salts (Soluble)[d] *at loc. no.* **277**
Ammonium peroxydisulfate (7727-54-0) *See* Potassium
Monopersulfate[b] *at loc. no.* **79**
Ammonium persulfate (7727-54-0) *See* Potassium Mono-
persulfate[b] *at loc. no.* **79**
Ammonium Polysulfide (12259-92-6) *See loc. no.* **112**
Ammonium salicylate (528-94-9) *See* Salicylate[d] *at loc. no.*
600
Ammonium Salts *See loc. no.* **152**
Ammonium Sulfamate (7773-06-0) *See loc. no.* **153**
Ammonium sulfite (7783-11-1) *See* Sulfite Salts[d] *at loc. no.*
149
Ammonium sulfoichthyolate (8029-68-3) *See* Ichthammol[a]
at loc. no. **1528**
Ammonium tetrachlorozincate (14639-97-5) *See* Zinc Salts
(Soluble)[d] *at loc. no.* **277**
Ammonium thiocyanate (1762-95-4) *See* Thiocyanate Salts[d]
at loc. no. **146**
Ammonium thioglycolate (5421-46-5) *See* Thioglycolate
Salts[d] *at loc. no.* **552**
Ammonium thiosulfate (10103-43-2) *See* Thiosulfate Salts[d]
at loc. no. **161**
Ammonyx 2194 *See loc. no.* **984**
Amobam (3566-10-7) *See* Nabam[b] *at loc. no.* **1162**
Amobarbital (57-43-2) *See loc. no.* **1364**
Amobarbital sodium (64-43-7) *See* Amobarbital[b] *at loc. no.*
1364
Amodiaquin (86-42-0) *See loc. no.* **1511**
Amopyroquin (550-81-2) *See* Chloroquine[b] *at loc. no.* **1512**
Amorphous silica gel (7631-86-9) *See* Silica[b] *at loc. no.* **7**
Amosite *See* Asbestos[e] *at loc. no.* **2**
Amoxapine (14028-44-5) *See* Loxapine[b] *at loc. no.* **1476**
Amphetamine (300-62-9) *See loc. no.* **1444**
Ampicillin (69-53-4) *See* Penicillins[d] *at loc. no.* **902**
AMS (7773-06-0) *See* Ammonium Sulfamate[a] *at loc. no.* **153**
Amygdalin (29883-15-6) *See loc. no.* **846**
Amyl acetate (628-63-7) *See* Isoamyl Acetate[b] *at loc. no.* **574**
Amyl Alcohol (71-41-0) *See loc. no.* **405**
sec-**Amyl-beta-bromallyl-barbituric acid sodium salt**
See Sigmodal[b] *at loc. no.* **1387**
2-*sec*-**Amyl-4,6-dinitrophenol** (4097-36-3) *See* 4,6-Dinitro-*o*-
amylphenol[a] *at loc. no.* **538**
Amyl ester of 2,4,5-T *See* Trichlorophenoxyacetic Acid[b] *at*
loc. no. **1224**
Amyl Nitrite (463-04-7) *See loc. no.* **630**
Amylobarbitone (57-43-2) *See* Amobarbital[a] *at loc. no.* **1364**

Amyl Phenol (80-46-6) *See loc. no.* **488**
p-tert-**Amylphenol** (80-46-6) *See* Amyl Phenol[a] *at loc. no.*
488
Amylum (9005-25-8) *See* Starch[a] *at loc. no.* **707**
Amytal (57-43-2) *See* Amobarbital[a] *at loc. no.* **1364**
Anabasine (494-52-0) *See loc. no.* **773**
Anacardic acid (25377-74-6) *See* Cashew Nut[c] *at loc. no.* **661**
Anacardium *See* Cashew Nut[a] *at loc. no.* **661**
Ancylol (305-85-1) *See* 2,6-Diiodo-4-nitrophenol[c] *at loc. no.*
537
Andalusite (12183-80-1) *See* Aluminum Silicate[c] *at loc. no.*
180
Anesthesin *See* Benzocaine[c] *at loc. no.* **1577**
Anethole (104-46-1) *See loc. no.* **858**
Anhydro-*o*-sulfaminebenzoic acid (81-07-2) *See* Sacchar-
in[a] *at loc. no.* **1616**
Anhydrous- *Omit* anhydrous *and try again.*
Anilazine (101-05-3) *See loc. no.* **1170**
Anileridine hydrochloride (126-12-5) *See* Meperidine Hy-
drochloride[b] *at loc. no.* **1484**
Aniline (62-53-3) *See loc. no.* **612**
p-**Anilinearsonic acid** (98-50-0) *See* Arsanilic Acid[a] *at loc.*
no. **189**
Aniline oil (62-53-3) *See* Aniline[a] *at loc. no.* **612**
p-**Anilinesulfonamide** (63-74-1) *See* Sulfanilamide[a] *at loc.*
no. **1563**
Anilinocadmium dilactate *See* Cadmium[d] *at loc. no.* **220**
Animal fat *See* Tallow[e] *at loc. no.* **709**
Animal oil (8001-85-2) *See* Bone Oil[a] *at loc. no.* **711**
Anionic surface active agent *See* Anionic Synthetic Deter-
gents[a] *at loc. no.* **939**
Anionic surfactant *See* Anionic Synthetic Detergents[a] *at*
loc. no. **939**
Anionic Synthetic Detergents *See loc. no.* **939**
Anionic wetting agent *See* Anionic Synthetic Detergents[a]
at loc. no. **939**
Anise camphor (104-46-1) *See* Anethole[a] *at loc. no.* **858**
Anise oil (8007-70-3) *See* Oil of Anise[a] *at loc. no.* **731**
Anisindione (117-37-3) *See loc. no.* **1333**
2-*p*-**Anisyl-1,3-indandione** (117-37-3) *See* Anisindione[a] *at*
loc. no. **1333**
Ansadol (87-17-2) *See* Salicylanilide[c] *at loc. no.* **998**
Ansar 138 (75-60-5) *See* Cacodylic Acid[c] *at loc. no.* **197**
Antabuse (97-77-8) *See* Disulfiram[c] *at loc. no.* **1595**
Antak (112-30-1) *See* Decyl Alcohol[c] *at loc. no.* **411**
Anthophyllite *See* Asbestos[e] *at loc. no.* **2**
Anthracene (120-12-7) *See* Anthracene Oil[c] *at loc. no.* **341**
9,10-**Anthracenedione** (84-65-1) *See* Anthraquinone[a] *at loc.*
no. **499**
Anthracene Oil (65996-91-0) *See loc. no.* **341**
Anthracene oil chlorinated *See* Carbolineum[a] *at loc. no.*
394
Anthradione (84-65-1) *See* Anthraquinone[a] *at loc. no.* **499**
Anthranilic acid (118-92-3) *See* *o*-Aminobenzoic Acid[a] *at*
loc. no. **627**
Anthraquinone (84-65-1) *See loc. no.* **499**
Antibiotics *See loc. no.* **899**
Antihistaminics *See loc. no.* **1487**
Antimonic oxide (1314-60-9) *See* Antimony Salts[d] *at loc. no.*
212
Antimony pentoxide (1314-60-9) *See* Antimony Salts[d] *at*
loc. no. **212**
Antimony Potassium Tartrate (304-61-0) *See loc. no.* **213**
Antimony Salts *See loc. no.* **212**
Antimony sulfide (1345-04-6) *See* Antimony Salts[d] *at loc.*
no. **212**

---

[a] A Synonym   [b] A Closely Related Substance   [c] The Active or Major Constituent   [d] A Class Name
[e] A Specific Example of or Product Containing

Ingredient name (CAS registry no.) *See* Primary Name *at*
location no. **XXX** *in Part D of this section*

Antimony Trichloride (10025-91-9) *See loc. no.* **214**
Antimony trioxide (1314-60-9) *See* Antimony Salts[d] *at loc. no.* **212**
Antimony trisulfide (1345-04-6) *See* Antimony Salts[d] *at loc. no.* **212**
Antipyrine (60-80-0) *See loc. no.* **1571**
Antivert (1104-22-9) *See* Meclizine Dihydrochloride[c] *at loc. no.* **1494**
ANTU (86-88-4) *See loc. no.* **1350**
Anturane (57-96-5) *See* Sulfinpyrazone[c] *at loc. no.* **1576**
APAP (103-90-2) *See* Acetaminophen[a] *at loc. no.* **1587**
Apholate (52-46-0) *See loc. no.* **1354**
Aphoxide (545-55-1) *See* Apholate[b] *at loc. no.* **1354**
Apiol (523-80-8) *See* Essential Oils[d] *at loc. no.* **725**
Apomorphine Hydrochloride (314-19-2) *See loc. no.* **779**
Aprobarbital (77-02-1) *See loc. no.* **1365**
Aprocarb *See* Propoxur[a] *at loc. no.* **1147**
Aqua ammonia (8007-57-6) *See* Ammonia[b] *at loc. no.* **63**
Aquadene *See* Sodium Hexametaphosphate[b] *at loc. no.* **143**
Aqua fortis (7697-37-2) *See* Nitric Acid[a] *at loc. no.* **32**
Aqualin (107-02-8) *See* Acrolein[c] *at loc. no.* **481**
Aquathol (129-67-9) *See* Endothall[b] *at loc. no.* **1304**
AR-60 *See* Methyl Naphthalene[a] *at loc. no.* **320**
Arachis oil (8002-03-7) *See* Peanut Oil[a] *at loc. no.* **719**
Aracide *See* Aramite[a] *at loc. no.* **1040**
Aralen (54-05-7) *See* Chloroquine[c] *at loc. no.* **1512**
Aralkonium chloride (1329-25-5) *See* Alkyl Dimethyl 3,4-Dichlorobenzene Ammonium Chloride[d] *at loc. no.* **976**
Aramite (140-57-8) *See loc. no.* **1040**
Arasan (137-26-8) *See* Thiram[c] *at loc. no.* **1165**
Aratone *See* Prometon[b] *at loc. no.* **1267**
Arbortrine *See* Benomyl[c] *at loc. no.* **1174**
Arecoline (63-75-2) *See loc. no.* **774**
Argemone Oil *See loc. no.* **710**
Arlacels *See* Sorbitan Monostearate[c] *at loc. no.* **972**
Arnica *See loc. no.* **657**
Arochlor 1221 *See* PCB[e] *at loc. no.* **399**
Arochlor 1242 *See* PCB[e] *at loc. no.* **399**
Arochlor 1254 (27323-18-8) *See* PCB[e] *at loc. no.* **399**
Arochlor 5460 *See* PCB[e] *at loc. no.* **399**
Aromatic hydrocarbons *See* Aromatic Hydrocarbon Solvent[a] *at loc. no.* **310**
Aromatic Hydrocarbon Solvent *See loc. no.* **310**
Aromatic naphtha *See* Aromatic Solvent Naphtha[a] *at loc. no.* **342**
Aromatic petroleum derivative *See* Aromatic Hydrocarbon Solvent[a] *at loc. no.* **310**
Aromatic petroleum derivative solvent *See* Aromatic Hydrocarbon Solvent[a] *at loc. no.* **310**
Aromatic petroleum distillate *See* Aromatic Hydrocarbon Solvent[a] *at loc. no.* **310**
Aromatic petroleum hydrocarbons *See* Aromatic Hydrocarbon Solvent[a] *at loc. no.* **310**
Aromatic petroleum oil *See* Aromatic Hydrocarbon Solvent[a] *at loc. no.* **310**
Aromatic petroleum solvent *See* Aromatic Hydrocarbon Solvent[a] *at loc. no.* **310**
Aromatic Solvent Naphtha *See loc. no.* **342**
Aromatic solvents *See* Aromatic Hydrocarbon Solvent[a] *at loc. no.* **310**
Arsanilic Acid (98-50-0) *See loc. no.* **189**
Arsenates *See loc. no.* **190**
Arsenic (7440-38-2) *See loc. no.* **188**
Arsenic Acid (7778-39-4) *See loc. no.* **191**
o-Arsenic acid (7778-39-4) *See* Arsenic Acid[a] *at loc. no.* **191**
Arsenicals *See loc. no.* **192**

Arsenic pentoxide (1303-28-2) *See* Arsenic Acid[a] *at loc. no.* **191**
Arsenic sesquioxide (1327-53-3) *See* Arsenic Trioxide[a] *at loc. no.* **193**
Arsenic sulfide yellow (1303-33-9) *See* Arsenic Trisulfide[a] *at loc. no.* **194**
Arsenic trihydride (7784-42-1) *See* Arsine[a] *at loc. no.* **196**
Arsenic Trioxide (1327-53-3) *See loc. no.* **193**
Arsenic Trisulfide (1303-33-9) *See loc. no.* **194**
Arsenious acid anhydride (1327-53-3) *See* Arsenic Trioxide[a] *at loc. no.* **193**
Arsenites *See loc. no.* **195**
Arsenosobenzene (637-03-6) *See* Arsenicals[d] *at loc. no.* **192**
Arsenous oxide (1327-53-3) *See* Arsenic Trioxide[a] *at loc. no.* **193**
Arsine (7784-42-1) *See loc. no.* **196**
Artemisia plants *See* Santonic[c] *at loc. no.* **931**
Artificial essential oil of almond (100-52-7) *See* Benzaldehyde[a] *at loc. no.* **859**
Arylam (63-25-2) *See* Carbaryl[c] *at loc. no.* **1128**
ASA (50-78-2) *See* Aspirin[c] *at loc. no.* **594**
Asafetida (9000-04-8) *See loc. no.* **747**
Asafoetida (9000-04-8) *See* Asafetida[a] *at loc. no.* **747**
Asarinin (133-05-1) *See* Sesame Oil[e] *at loc. no.* **722**
Asbestos (1332-21-4) *See loc. no.* **2**
Ascaridol(e) *See* Chenopodium Oil[e] *at loc. no.* **728**
L-Ascorbic acid (50-81-7) *See* Vitamin C[a] *at loc. no.* **908**
Asendin (14028-44-5) *See* Loxapine[b] *at loc. no.* **1476**
ASP 47 (3689-24-5) *See* Sulfotepp[a] *at loc. no.* **1108**
Asphalt (8052-42-4) *See loc. no.* **343**
Aspidium (8063-11-4) *See loc. no.* **748**
Aspidosperma (1398-11-4) *See* Yohimbine[c] *at loc. no.* **834**
Aspirin (50-78-2) *See loc. no.* **594**
Aspon (3244-90-4) *See* Tetra-*n*-propyl Dithionopyrophosphate[a] *at loc. no.* **1110**
Asulam (3337-71-1) *See loc. no.* **1226**
Asulox *See* Asulam[c] *at loc. no.* **1226**
ATA (61-82-5) *See* Amitrole[a] *at loc. no.* **1290**
Atabrine (69-05-6) *See* Quinacrine Hydrochloride[c] *at loc. no.* **1515**
Atarax (2192-20-3) *See* Hydroxyzine Hydrochloride[c] *at loc. no.* **1438**
Ativan (846-49-1) *See* Lorazepam[c] *at loc. no.* **1398**
Atlas G 924 *See* Propylene Glycol Monostearate[c] *at loc. no.* **971**
Atophan (132-60-5) *See* Cinchophen[c] *at loc. no.* **1591**
Atoxyl (127-85-5) *See* Arsanilic Acid[b] *at loc. no.* **189**
Atraton (1610-17-9) *See* Prometon[b] *at loc. no.* **1267**
Atrazine (1912-24-9) *See loc. no.* **1259**
Atropa belladonna L. *See* Belladonna Leaf or Root[a] *at loc. no.* **658**
Atropine (51-55-8) *See loc. no.* **767**
Atropine sulfate (5908-99-6) *See* Atropine[b] *at loc. no.* **767**
Auralgan *See* Antipyrine[c] *at loc. no.* **1571**
Auripigment (1303-33-9) *See* Arsenic Trisulfide[a] *at loc. no.* **194**
Avadex (2303-16-4) *See* Di-allate[c] *at loc. no.* **1235**
Avadex BW (2303-17-5) *See* Di-allate[b] *at loc. no.* **1235**
Aventyl (72-69-5) *See* Nortriptyline[c] *at loc. no.* **1474**
Avitrol *See* 4-Aminopyridine[c] *at loc. no.* **1319**
Avlothane (67-72-1) *See* Hexachloroethane[c] *at loc. no.* **370**
Avogadrite *See* Potassium Fluoborate[a] *at loc. no.* **103**
10-Azaanthracene (260-94-6) *See* Acridine[a] *at loc. no.* **1517**
Azacyclonol (115-46-8) *See loc. no.* **1429**
Azacyclopropane (151-56-4) *See* Ethylenimine[a] *at loc. no.* **606**

---

[a] A Synonym   [b] A Closely Related Substance   [c] The Active or Major Constituent   [d] A Class Name
[e] A Specific Example of or Product Containing

Ingredient name (CAS registry no.) *See* Primary Name *at location no.* **XXX** *in Part D of this section*

[a] A Synonym   [b] A Closely Related Substance   [c] The Active or Major Constituent   [d] A Class Name
[e] A Specific Example of or Product Containing

Ingredient name (CAS registry no.) *See* Primary Name *at
location no.* **XXX** *in Part D of this section*

Benzoin (119-53-9) *See loc. no.* **750**

Benzoin tincture (8050-35-9) *See* Benzoin[c] *at loc. no.* **750**

Benzol (71-43-2) *See* Benzene[a] *at loc. no.* **312**

Benzophenone-3 (131-57-7) *See* Oxybenzone[a] *at loc. no.* **1537**

Benzophenone-4 (4065-45-6) *See* Oxybenzone[b] *at loc. no.* **1537**

1,4-Benzoquinone (106-51-4) *See* Quinone[a] *at loc. no.* **507**

1,4-Benzoquinone 1-benzoylhydrazone 4-oxime (495-73-8) *See* Benquinox[a] *at loc. no.* **1178**

Benzothiadiazide Diuretics *See loc. no.* **1588**

2-Benzothiazolethiol (149-30-4) *See* Mercaptobenzothiazole[a] *at loc. no.* **1198**

1-Benzothiazol-2-yl-1,1'-dimethylurea (18691-97-9) *See* Phenobenzuron[b] *at loc. no.* **1256**

4-Benzothienyl methylcarbamate (1079-33-0) *See* Mobam[e] *at loc. no.* **1142**

1-Benzoyl-1-(3,4-dichlorophenyl)-3,3-dimethylurea (3134-12-1) *See* Phenobenzuron[b] *at loc. no.* **1256**

Benzoyl Peroxide (94-36-0) *See loc. no.* **76**

Benzoylprop-ethyl (22212-55-1) *See loc. no.* **1292**

Benzoyl superoxide (94-36-0) *See* Benzoyl Peroxide[a] *at loc. no.* **76**

Benzphetamine (156-08-1) *See* Benzphetamine Hydrochloride[b] *at loc. no.* **1445**

Benzphetamine Hydrochloride (1027-30-1) *See loc. no.* **1445**

Benzthiazide (91-33-8) *See* Benzothiadiazide Diuretics[d] *at loc. no.* **1588**

Benzyl Alcohol (100-51-6) *See loc. no.* **406**

Benzyl Benzoate (120-51-4) *See loc. no.* **583**

o-Benzyl-*p*-chlorophenol (120-32-1) *See loc. no.* **520**

Benzyl cinnamate (103-41-3) *See* Cinnamic Acid Esters[d] *at loc. no.* **587**

Benzyl hexadecyl dimethyl ammonium chloride *See* Cetalkonium Chloride[a] *at loc. no.* **987**

o-Benzyl-parachlorophenol (120-32-1) *See o*-Benzyl-*p*-chlorophenol[a] *at loc. no.* **520**

Benzylpenicillin (61-33-6) *See* Penicillins[d] *at loc. no.* **902**

Berberine (2086-83-1) *See loc. no.* **823**

Beryllium Salts *See loc. no.* **169**

Beta- *If not listed below, omit prefix and try again.*

Beta-butoxy-beta-thiocyano-diethyl ether (112-56-1) *See* β-Butoxy-β-thiocyanodiethyl Ether[a] *at loc. no.* **1035**

Beta-dichloro-ethyl ether (111-44-4) *See* sym.-Dichloroethyl Ether[a] *at loc. no.* **470**

Betamethasone (378-44-9) *See* Corticosteroids[d] *at loc. no.* **915**

Betanal (13684-63-4) *See* Desmedipham[b] *at loc. no.* **1230**

Beta-naphthol (135-19-3) *See* β-Naphthol[a] *at loc. no.* **493**

Betanex *See* Desmedipham[c] *at loc. no.* **1230**

Betasan (741-58-2) *See* Bensulide[a] *at loc. no.* **1082**

Beta-thiocyanoethyl esters *See* Lethane 60[e] *at loc. no.* **1037**

Beta-Trichloroethane (79-00-5) *See* 1,1,2-Trichloroethane[a] *at loc. no.* **376**

Betula oil (119-36-8) *See* Methyl Salicylate[a] *at loc. no.* **597**

BFPO (115-26-4) *See* Dimefox[a] *at loc. no.* **1098**

BGE (2426-08-6) *See* Glycidyl Ethers[d] *at loc. no.* **1629**

BHA (25013-16-5) *See* Butylated Hydroxytoluene[b] *at loc. no.* **1614**

Bhang *See* Marihuana[a] *at loc. no.* **678**

BHC (608-73-1) *See* Benzene Hexachloride[a] *at loc. no.* **1029**

BHT (128-37-0) *See* Butylated Hydroxytoluene[a] *at loc. no.* **1614**

Bibenzene (92-52-4) *See* Diphenyl[a] *at loc. no.* **314**

Bichloride of mercury (7487-94-7) *See* Mercuric Chloride[a] *at loc. no.* **236**

Bichromate salts *See* Dichromate Salts (Soluble)[a] *at loc. no.* **82**

cis-Bicyclo-(2,2,1)-hept-5-ene-2,3-dicarboxylic acid dimethyl ester (117-24-8) *See* Dimethyl Carbate[a] *at loc. no.* **1327**

Bidrin (141-66-2) *See loc. no.* **1051**

Bifenox (42576-02-3) *See loc. no.* **1293**

"Big Chief" *See* Mescaline[a] *at loc. no.* **830**

Binapacryl (485-31-4) *See* Dinoseb[b] *at loc. no.* **543**

Bioallethrin (584-79-2) *See* Allethrin[d] *at loc. no.* **884**

Biopermethrin *See* Permethrin[d] *at loc. no.* **891**

Biophenothrin *See* Permethrin[b] *at loc. no.* **891**

Bioquin (148-24-3) *See* 8-Hydroxyquinoline[c] *at loc. no.* **1514**

Bioresmethrin *See* Resmethrin[d] *at loc. no.* **895**

Biphenyl (92-52-4) *See* Diphenyl[a] *at loc. no.* **314**

Bis- *If not listed below, substitute Di- and try again.*

Bisacodyl (603-50-9) *See* Phenolphthalein[b] *at loc. no.* **1607**

N,N'-Bis(2-aminoethyl)ethylenediamine (112-24-3) *See* Triethylenetetramine[a] *at loc. no.* **604**

Bis(bisdimethylaminophosphonous)anhydride (152-16-9) *See* Octamethyl Pyrophosphoramide[a] *at loc. no.* **1102**

2,3,4,5-Bis(Δ²-butylene)tetrahydrofurfural (126-15-8) *See loc. no.* **1321**

Bis(chloromethyl) ether (542-88-1) *See* Chloromethyl Methyl Ether[b] *at loc. no.* **467**

Bis(*p*-chlorophenoxy)methane (555-89-5) *See* Neotran[e] *at loc. no.* **1014**

1,6-Bis(4-chlorophenyldiguanido)hexane (55-56-1) *See* Chlorhexidine[a] *at loc. no.* **994**

1,1-Bis(*p*-chlorophenyl)ethanol (80-06-8) *See* DMC[a] *at loc. no.* **1011**

1,1-Bis(*p*-chlorophenyl)-2-nitrobutane (117-26-0) *See* Bulan[a] *at loc. no.* **1005**

1,1-Bis(*p*-chlorophenyl)-2-nitropropane (117-27-1) *See* Prolan[e] *at loc. no.* **1016**

α,α-Bis(4-chlorophenyl)-3-pyridinemethanol (17781-31-6) *See* Parnon[a] *at loc. no.* **1200**

α,α-Bis(*p*-chlorophenyl)-β,β,β-trichloroethane (50-29-3) *See* DDT[a] *at loc. no.* **1007**

1,1-Bis(*p*-chlorophenyl)-2,2,2-trichloroethanol (115-32-2) *See* Kelthane[e] *at loc. no.* **1012**

Bis(dialkoxyphosphinothioyl)disulfide *See* Phostex[e] *at loc. no.* **1107**

Bis(2,4-dichlorophenoxy)ethylphosphite *See* Falone[e] *at loc. no.* **1306**

Bis(1,3-dichloro-2-propyl)phosphate *See* Tris(1,3-dichloro-2-propyl)phosphate[b] *at loc. no.* **1119**

Bis(diethoxyphosphinothioylthio)methane (563-12-2) *See* Ethion[e] *at loc. no.* **1087**

Bis(diethylthiocarbamoyl)disulfide (97-77-8) *See* Disulfiram[a] *at loc. no.* **1595**

Bis(dimethylamino) fluorophosphine oxide (115-26-4) *See* Dimefox[a] *at loc. no.* **1098**

Bis(dimethylthiocarbamoyl) disulfide (137-26-8) *See* Thiram[a] *at loc. no.* **1165**

1,2-Bis(3-ethoxycarbonyl-2-thioureido)benzene (23564-06-9) *See* Thiophanate-methyl[b] *at loc. no.* **1207**

2,4-Bis(ethylamino)-6-methoxy-*s*-triazine (673-04-1) *See* Terbumeton[b] *at loc. no.* **1270**

2,4-Bis(ethylamino)-6-(methylthio)-*s*-triazine (1014-70-6) *See* Prometon[b] *at loc. no.* **1267**

Bis(2-ethylhexyl)phthalate (117-81-7) *See* Di-2-ethylhexyl Phthalate[a] *at loc. no.* **591**

---

[a] A Synonym   [b] A Closely Related Substance   [c] The Active or Major Constituent   [d] A Class Name
[e] A Specific Example of or Product Containing

Ingredient name (CAS registry no.) *See* Primary Name *at*
location no. **XXX** *in Part D of this section*

---

[a] A Synonym   [b] A Closely Related Substance   [c] The Active or Major Constituent   [d] A Class Name
[e] A Specific Example of or Product Containing

Ingredient name (CAS registry no.) *See* Primary Name *at location no.* **XXX** *in Part D of this section*

5-(2-Bromoallyl)-5-(1-methylbutyl) barbituric acid (1216-40-6) *See* Sigmodal[e] *at loc. no.* **1387**

Bromobenzene (108-86-1) *See loc. no.* **392**

5-Bromo-3-*sec*-butyl-6-methyluracil (314-40-9) *See* Bromacil[a] *at loc. no.* **1294**

3-Bromo-*d*-camphor (76-29-9) *See* Camphor[b] *at loc. no.* **875**

1-Bromo-2-chloroethane (107-04-0) *See loc. no.* **362**

Bromochloromethane (74-97-5) *See* Chlorobromomethane[a] *at loc. no.* **356**

N'-(4-Bromo-3-chlorophenyl) - N - methoxy-*N*-methylurea (13360-45-7) *See* Chlorbromuron[a] *at loc. no.* **1242**

Bromodiethylacetylcarbamide (77-65-6) *See* Carbromal[a] *at loc. no.* **1431**

Bromodiethylacetylurea (77-65-6) *See* Carbromal[a] *at loc. no.* **1431**

Bromodiphenhydramine hydrochloride *See* Diphenhydramine Hydrochloride[b] *at loc. no.* **1492**

5-Bromo-3-isopropyl-6-methyluracil (314-42-1) *See* Bromacil[b] *at loc. no.* **1294**

Bromomethane (74-83-9) *See* Methyl Bromide[a] *at loc. no.* **344**

2-Bromo-4-phenylphenol (92-03-5) *See loc. no.* **522**

3-Bromopropene (106-95-6) *See* Allyl Bromide[a] *at loc. no.* **379**

Bromopropylate (18181-80-1) *See loc. no.* **1004**

3-Bromopropylene (106-95-6) *See* Allyl Bromide[a] *at loc. no.* **379**

3-Bromopropyne (106-96-7) *See* Propargyl Bromide[a] *at loc. no.* **390**

Bromoxynil (1689-84-5) *See loc. no.* **1295**

Bromoxynil octanoate (1689-99-2) *See* Bromoxynil[b] *at loc. no.* **1295**

Brompheniramine (86-22-6) *See* Antihistaminics[d] *at loc. no.* **1487**

Bromvaletone (496-67-3) *See* Carbromal[b] *at loc. no.* **1431**

Bronze powder *See* Gold Bronze Powder[b] *at loc. no.* **260**

Brown Mixture (8030-36-2) *See loc. no.* **215**

Brucine (357-57-3) *See loc. no.* **824**

BTC (8001-54-5) *See* Benzalkonium Chloride[c] *at loc. no.* **985**

Bubartal (143-81-7) *See* Butabarbital Sodium[b] *at loc. no.* **1367**

Buclizine (82-95-1) *See loc. no.* **1488**

Bufencarb (8065-36-9) *See loc. no.* **1125**

Bufotenine (487-93-4) *See loc. no.* **820**

Builders (Detergents) *See loc. no.* **937**

Bulan (117-26-0) *See loc. no.* **1005**

Bunema (51026-28-9) *See loc. no.* **1157**

Bunker fuel oils *See* Residual Oils[a] *at loc. no.* **332**

Bupivacaine (2180-92-9) *See loc. no.* **1578**

Bupivacaine hydrochloride (14252-80-3) *See* Bupivacaine[b] *at loc. no.* **1578**

Burnt lime (1305-78-8) *See* Calcium Oxide[a] *at loc. no.* **54**

Burnt Sienna *See loc. no.* **251**

Burnt Umber (1309-37-1) *See loc. no.* **252**

Burow's Solution (8006-13-1) *See loc. no.* **183**

Busan 30A (21564-17-0) *See* 2-(Thiocyanomethylthio)-benzothiazole[c] *at loc. no.* **1206**

Busan 72A (21564-17-0) *See* 2-(Thiocyanomethylthio)-benzothiazole[c] *at loc. no.* **1206**

Busan 11-M1 (52233-42-8) *See* Barium Metaborate[c] *at loc. no.* **167**

Butabarbital (125-40-6) *See* Butabarbital Sodium[b] *at loc. no.* **1367**

Butabarbital Sodium (143-81-7) *See loc. no.* **1367**

Butabarbitone sodium (143-81-7) *See* Butabarbital Sodium[a] *at loc. no.* **1367**

Butacarb (2655-19-8) *See loc. no.* **1126**

Butachlor (23184-66-9) *See* Alachlor[b] *at loc. no.* **1273**

Butacide (51-03-6) *See* Piperonyl Butoxide[a] *at loc. no.* **1151**

Butalbital (77-26-9) *See loc. no.* **1368**

Butalgin (125-56-4) *See* Methadone[c] *at loc. no.* **1485**

Butallyonal (1142-70-7) *See loc. no.* **1369**

Butallyonal sodium (3486-86-0) *See* Butallyonal[b] *at loc. no.* **1369**

Butamben (94-25-7) *See loc. no.* **1579**

Butane (106-97-8) *See loc. no.* **306**

Butanedinitrile (110-61-2) *See* Succinonitrile[a] *at loc. no.* **654**

1,3-Butanediol (107-88-0) *See loc. no.* **444**

Butanenitrile (109-74-0) *See* n-Butyronitrile[a] *at loc. no.* **649**

Butanol (71-36-3) *See* n-Butyl Alcohol[a] *at loc. no.* **407**

n-Butanol (71-36-3) *See* n-Butyl Alcohol[a] *at loc. no.* **407**

2-Butanone (78-93-3) *See* Methyl Ethyl Ketone[a] *at loc. no.* **476**

Butazolidin (50-33-9) *See* Phenylbutazone[c] *at loc. no.* **1575**

Butesin (94-25-7) *See* Butamben[c] *at loc. no.* **1579**

Butethal (77-28-1) *See loc. no.* **1370**

Butisol sodium (143-81-7) *See* Butabarbital Sodium[c] *at loc. no.* **1367**

Butobarbital (77-28-1) *See* Butethal[a] *at loc. no.* **1370**

Butobarbitone (77-28-1) *See* Butethal[a] *at loc. no.* **1370**

Butonate (126-22-7) *See loc. no.* **1060**

Butopyronoxyl (532-34-3) *See loc. no.* **1322**

Butoxone (2758-42-1) *See* 4-(2,4-Dichlorophenoxy)butyric Acid[c] *at loc. no.* **1215**

2-Butoxy-*N*-(2-(diethylamino)ethyl)-4-quinolinecarboxamide (85-79-0) *See* Dibucaine[a] *at loc. no.* **1580**

2-Butoxyethanol (111-76-2) *See loc. no.* **453**

Butoxyethanol 4-(2,4-dichlorophenoxy)butyrate *See* 4-(2,4-Dichlorophenoxy)butyric Acid[b] *at loc. no.* **1215**

Butoxyethanol ester of 2,4,5-T (2545-59-7) *See* Trichlorophenoxyacetic Acid[b] *at loc. no.* **1224**

α-[2-(2-Butoxyethoxy)ethoxy]-4,5-methylenedioxy-2-propyl toluene (51-03-6) *See* Piperonyl Butoxide[a] *at loc. no.* **1151**

Butoxyethoxypropanol ester of 2,4,5-T *See* Trichlorophenoxyacetic Acid[b] *at loc. no.* **1224**

Butoxyethyl 2-(2,4-dichlorophenoxy)propionate *See* 2-(2,4-Dichlorophenoxy)propionic Acid[b] *at loc. no.* **1217**

Butoxyethyl ester of 2,4,5-T (2545-59-7) *See* Trichlorophenoxyacetic Acid[b] *at loc. no.* **1224**

Butoxyethyl 2 - methyl - 4 - chlorophenoxyacetate *See* MCPA[b] *at loc. no.* **1220**

Butoxy Polypropylene Glycols *See loc. no.* **454**

Butoxypropyl ester of 2,4,5-T *See* Trichlorophenoxyacetic Acid[b] *at loc. no.* **1224**

β-Butoxy-β-thiocyanodiethyl Ether (112-56-1) *See loc. no.* **1035**

Butrizol (16227-10-4) *See* Triazabutil[a] *at loc. no.* **1272**

Butter of antimony (10025-91-9) *See* Antimony Trichloride[a] *at loc. no.* **214**

"Button" *See* Peyote[a] *at loc. no.* **683**

Buturon (3766-60-7) *See loc. no.* **1241**

N-Butylacetanilide (91-49-6) *See loc. no.* **1323**

n-Butyl Acetate (123-86-4) *See loc. no.* **568**

n-Butyl acrylate (80-63-7) *See* Acrylic Resin Monomers[d] *at loc. no.* **1625**

n-Butyl Alcohol (71-36-3) *See loc. no.* **407**

Butyl *p*-aminobenzoate (94-25-7) *See* Butamben[a] *at loc. no.* **1579**

---

[a] A Synonym   [b] A Closely Related Substance   [c] The Active or Major Constituent   [d] A Class Name
[e] A Specific Example of or Product Containing

Ingredient name (CAS registry no.) *See* Primary Name *at
location no.* **XXX** *in Part D of this section*

4-(Butylamino)benzoic acid 2-(dimethylamino)ethyl ester (94-24-6) *See* Tetracaine[a] *at loc. no.* **1586**

2-(*tert*-Butylamino)-4-chloro-6-(ethylamino)-*s*-triazine (5915-41-3) *See* Atrazine[b] *at loc. no.* **1259**

2-(*sec*-Butylamino)-4-(ethylamino)-6-methoxy-*s*-triazine (26259-45-0) *See* Prometon[b] *at loc. no.* **1267**

2-(*tert*-Butylamino)-4-(ethylamino)-6-methoxy-*s*-triazine (33693-04-8) *See* Terbumeton[a] *at loc. no.* **1270**

2-(*tert*-Butylamino)-4-(ethylamino)-6-(methylthio)-*s*-triazine (886-50-0) *See* Prometon[b] *at loc. no.* **1267**

Butylate (2008-41-5) *See loc. no.* **1233**

Butylated hydroxyanisole (25013-16-5) *See* Butylated Hydroxytoluene[b] *at loc. no.* **1614**

Butylated Hydroxytoluene (128-37-0) *See loc. no.* **1614**

Butyl benzyl phthalate (85-68-7) *See* Phthalic Acid Esters[d] *at loc. no.* **589**

n-Butyl *n*-butyrate (109-21-7) *See n*-Butyl Acetate[b] *at loc. no.* **568**

Butyl Carbitol (112-34-5) *See loc. no.* **452**

n-Butyl "Carbitol" rhodanate (112-56-1) *See* β-Butoxy-β-thiocyanodiethyl Ether[a] *at loc. no.* **1035**

Butyl Carbitol thiocyanate (112-56-1) *See* β-Butoxy-β-thiocyanodiethyl Ether[a] *at loc. no.* **1035**

Butylcarbityl-(6-propylpiperonyl)ether (51-03-6) *See* Piperonyl Butoxide[a] *at loc. no.* **1151**

Butyl Cellosolve (111-76-2) *See* 2-Butoxyethanol[a] *at loc. no.* **453**

n-Butyl Chloride (109-69-3) *See loc. no.* **380**

3-*tert*-Butyl-5-chloro-6-methyluracil (5902-51-2) *See* Bromacil[b] *at loc. no.* **1294**

4-*tert*-Butyl-2-chlorophenyl methyl methylphosphoramidate (299-86-5) *See* Ruelene[e] *at loc. no.* **1104**

Butyl 4-(2,4-dichlorophenoxy)butyrate *See* 4-(2,4-Dichlorophenoxy)butyric Acid[b] *at loc. no.* **1215**

1-*n*-Butyl-3-(3,4-dichlorophenyl)-1-methylurea (555-37-3) *See* Neburon[a] *at loc. no.* **1254**

5-Butyl-2-dimethylamino-6-methyl-4-pyrimidinol (5221-53-4) *See* Dimethirimol[a] *at loc. no.* **1192**

Butyl dimethyl dihydro gamma pyrone carboxylate (532-34-3) *See* Butopyronoxyl[a] *at loc. no.* **1322**

2-*sec*-Butyl-4,6-dinitrophenol (88-85-7) *See* Dinoseb[a] *at loc. no.* **543**

4-Butyl-1,2-diphenyl-3,5-pyrazolidinedione *See* Phenylbutazone[a] *at loc. no.* **1575**

1,3-Butylene glycol (107-88-0) *See* 1,3-Butanediol[a] *at loc. no.* **444**

Butyl ester of 2,4-D (94-80-4) *See* 2,4-D Esters[d] *at loc. no.* **1213**

Butyl ester of 2,4,5-T (93-79-8) *See* Trichlorophenoxyacetic Acid[b] *at loc. no.* **1224**

5-Butyl-2-(ethylamino)-4-hydroxy-6-methylpyrimidine (23947-60-6) *See* Dimethirimol[b] *at loc. no.* **1192**

5-*sec*-Butyl-5-ethylbarbituric acid sodium salt (143-81-7) *See* Butabarbital Sodium[a] *at loc. no.* **1367**

N-Butyl-*N*-ethyl-α,α,α-trifluoro-2,6-dinitro-*p*-toluidine (1861-40-1) *See* Benefin[a] *at loc. no.* **1287**

n-Butyl formate (592-84-7) *See n*-Butyl Acetate[b] *at loc. no.* **568**

n-Butyl glycidyl ether (2426-08-6) *See* Glycidyl Ethers[d] *at loc. no.* **1629**

Butyl-*p*-hydroxybenzoate (94-26-8) *See* Paraben Esters[d] *at loc. no.* **584**

4-Butyl-1-(4-hydroxyphenyl)-2-phenyl-3,5-pyrazolidinedione (129-20-4) *See* Oxyphenbutazone[a] *at loc. no.* **1574**

6-*tert*-Butyl-4-(isobutylidine-amino)-3-(methylthio)-1,2,4-triazin-5-one (57052-04-7) *See* Isomethiozin[a] *at loc. no.* **1264**

n-Butyl isovalerate (109-19-3) *See n*-Butyl Acetate[b] *at loc. no.* **568**

Butyl mesityl oxide (oxalate) (1341-44-2) *See* Butopyronoxyl[a] *at loc. no.* **1322**

Butyl 2-methyl-4-chlorophenoxyacetate *See* MCPA[b] *at loc. no.* **1220**

N-Butyl-2-methyl-2-propyl-1,3-propanediol dicarbamate (4268-36-4) *See* Meprobamate[b] *at loc. no.* **1407**

Butyl Myristate (110-36-1) *See loc. no.* **569**

Butyl nitrite (544-16-1) *See* Amyl Nitrite[b] *at loc. no.* **630**

p-*tert*-Butyl phenol (98-54-4) *See* Amyl Phenol[b] *at loc. no.* **488**

2-(*p*-*tert*-Butylphenoxy)isopropyl 2-choroethyl sulfite (140-57-8) *See* Aramite[e] *at loc. no.* **1040**

2-*sec*-Butylphenyl *N*-methylcarbamate (3766-81-2) *See* BPMC[a] *at loc. no.* **1124**

n-Butyl Phthalate (84-74-2) *See loc. no.* **590**

1-Butyl-2′,6′-pipecoloxylidide (2180-92-9) *See* Bupivacaine[a] *at loc. no.* **1578**

4-Butyl-*s*-triazole (16227-10-4) *See* Triazabutil[a] *at loc. no.* **1272**

Butynorate (77-58-7) *See* Alkyl Tin Compounds[d] *at loc. no.* **292**

Butyrac (94-82-6) *See* 4-(2,4-Dichlorophenoxy)butyric Acid[c] *at loc. no.* **1215**

n-Butyraldehyde (123-72-8) *See* Acetaldehyde[b] *at loc. no.* **480**

n-Butyronitrile (109-74-0) *See loc. no.* **649**

Butyrum cacao *See* Theobroma Oil[a] *at loc. no.* **742**

Bux (8065-36-9) *See* Bufencarb[c] *at loc. no.* **1125**

Cacao butter (8002-31-1) *See* Theobroma Oil[a] *at loc. no.* **742**

Cacodylic Acid (75-60-5) *See loc. no.* **197**

Cade oil (8013-10-3) *See* Juniper Tar[a] *at loc. no.* **729**

Cadmium *See loc. no.* **220**

Cadmium anthranilate (7058-55-1) *See* Cadmium[d] *at loc. no.* **220**

Cadmium chloride (10108-64-2) *See* Cadmium[d] *at loc. no.* **220**

Cadmium metal (7440-43-9) *See* Cadmium[d] *at loc. no.* **220**

Cadmium oxide (1306-19-0) *See* Cadmium[d] *at loc. no.* **220**

Cadmium succinate (141-00-4) *See* Cadmium[d] *at loc. no.* **220**

Cadmium sulfate (10124-36-4) *See* Cadmium[d] *at loc. no.* **220**

Cadmium sulfide (1306-23-6) *See* Cadmium[d] *at loc. no.* **220**

Caffeine (58-08-2) *See loc. no.* **800**

Cajeputol (470-82-6) *See* Eucalyptol[a] *at loc. no.* **863**

Cake alum (7784-31-8) *See* Alum[b] *at loc. no.* **181**

Calamine (8011-96-9) *See loc. no.* **271**

Calcium acid methanearsonate (5902-95-4) *See* Disodium Methanearsonate[b] *at loc. no.* **203**

Calcium Arsenate (7778-44-1) *See loc. no.* **198**

Calcium Arsenite (1333-24-0) *See loc. no.* **199**

Calcium borate (12040-58-3) *See* Borate[d] *at loc. no.* **131**

Calcium Carbide (75-20-7) *See loc. no.* **62**

Calcium carbimide (156-62-7) *See* Calcium Cyanamide[a] *at loc. no.* **1355**

Calcium Carbonate (471-34-1) *See loc. no.* **171**

Calcium chloride (10043-52-4) *See* Calcium Salts[d] *at loc. no.* **170**

Calcium Cyanamide (156-62-7) *See loc. no.* **1355**

Calcium Cyanide (592-01-8) *See loc. no.* **107**

Calcium Disodium Edetate (62-33-9) *See* Edetate Calcium Disodium[a] *at loc. no.* **1504**

Ingredient name (CAS registry no.) *See* Primary Name *at location no.* **XXX** *in Part D of this section*

Calcium disodium ethylenediaminetetraacetate (62-33-9) *See* Edetate Calcium Disodium[a] *at loc. no.* **1504**
Calcium disodium (ethylenedinitrilo)-tetraacetate (62-33-9) *See* Edetate Calcium Disodium[a] *at loc. no.* **1504**
Calcium fluoride (7789-75-5) *See* Fluoride[d] *at loc. no.* **100**
Calcium hydroxide (1305-62-0) *See* Lime (Slaked)[a] *at loc. no.* **55**
Calcium Hypochlorite (7778-54-3) *See loc. no.* **89**
Calcium hyposulfite (10124-41-1) *See* Thiosulfate Salts[d] *at loc. no.* **161**
Calcium Oxide (1305-78-8) *See loc. no.* **54**
Calcium Polysulfide (9046-53-1) *See loc. no.* **113**
Calcium Salts *See loc. no.* **170**
Calcium sulfate (10034-76-1) *See* Plaster of Paris[a] *at loc. no.* **172**
Calcium sulfate anhydrous (7778-18-9) *See* Plaster of Paris[b] *at loc. no.* **172**
Calcium sulfide (20548-54-3) *See* Sulfide Salts[d] *at loc. no.* **118**
Calcium thioglycolate (814-71-1) *See* Thioglycolate Salts[d] *at loc. no.* **552**
Calcium thiosulfate (10124-41-1) *See* Thiosulfate Salts[d] *at loc. no.* **161**
Calgon (8012-14-4) *See* Sodium Hexametaphosphate[c] *at loc. no.* **143**
Calomel (10112-91-1) *See* Mercurous Chloride[a] *at loc. no.* **237**
Cambogia (9000-25-3) *See* Gamboge[a] *at loc. no.* **754**
2-Camphanol (507-70-0) *See* Borneol[a] *at loc. no.* **876**
2-Camphanone (76-22-2) *See* Camphor[a] *at loc. no.* **875**
Camphor (76-22-2) *See loc. no.* **875**
Camphorated Oil *See loc. no.* **726**
Camphorated tincture of opium *See* Paregoric[a] *at loc. no.* **766**
Camphor liniment (8011-47-0) *See* Camphorated Oil[b] *at loc. no.* **726**
Camphor Oil (8008-51-3) *See loc. no.* **727**
Camphor Spirit *See loc. no.* **764**
Camphor tar (91-20-3) *See* Naphthalene[a] *at loc. no.* **321**
CaNa₂EDTA (62-33-9) *See* Edetate Calcium Disodium[a] *at loc. no.* **1504**
Candelilla Wax *See loc. no.* **751**
Cannabinoids *See* Tetrahydrocannabinols[e] *at loc. no.* **933**
Cannabinol (521-35-7) *See* Tetrahydrocannabinols[b] *at loc. no.* **933**
Cannabis (8063-14-7) *See* Marihuana[a] *at loc. no.* **678**
Cantharides (8063-15-8) *See* Cantharidin[c] *at loc. no.* **924**
Cantharidin (56-25-7) *See loc. no.* **924**
Cantralax *See* Casanthranol[c] *at loc. no.* **849**
Capla (64-55-1) *See* Meprobamate[b] *at loc. no.* **1407**
Capric alcohol (112-30-1) *See* Decyl Alcohol[c] *at loc. no.* **411**
Caprylic Alcohol (111-87-5) *See loc. no.* **408**
Capsicum (8023-77-6) *See loc. no.* **659**
Captafol (2425-06-1) *See loc. no.* **1180**
Captan (133-06-2) *See loc. no.* **1179**
Captax (149-30-4) *See* Mercaptobenzothiazole[a] *at loc. no.* **1198**
Carbacryl (107-13-1) *See* Acrylonitrile[c] *at loc. no.* **648**
Carbam *See* Metham Sodium[a] *at loc. no.* **1161**
Carbamult (2631-37-0) *See* Promecarb[c] *at loc. no.* **1146**
Carbanolate (671-04-5) *See loc. no.* **1127**
Carbaryl (63-25-2) *See loc. no.* **1128**
Carbasulam *See* Asulam[b] *at loc. no.* **1226**
Carbazotic acid (88-89-1) *See* Picric Acid[a] *at loc. no.* **545**
Carbenicillin (4697-36-3) *See* Penicillins[d] *at loc. no.* **902**
Carbetamex *See* Carbetamide[c] *at loc. no.* **1228**
Carbetamide (16118-49-3) *See loc. no.* **1228**

Carbinol (67-56-1) *See* Methyl Alcohol[a] *at loc. no.* **423**
Carbitol (111-90-0) *See loc. no.* **455**
Carbitol Esters *See loc. no.* **447**
Carbocaine (96-88-8) *See* Mepivacaine[a] *at loc. no.* **1583**
Carbofuran (1563-66-2) *See loc. no.* **1129**
Carbolic acid (108-95-2) *See* Phenol[a] *at loc. no.* **494**
Carbolineum (8007-65-6) *See loc. no.* **394**
Carbomer (9003-01-4) *See* Carboxypolymethylene[a] *at loc. no.* **1627**
2-Carbomethoxy-1-methylvinyl dimethyl phosphate (7786-34-7) *See* Phosdrin[c] *at loc. no.* **1057**
Carbon bisulfide (75-15-0) *See* Carbon Disulfide[a] *at loc. no.* **125**
Carbon Disulfide (75-15-0) *See loc. no.* **125**
Carbon hexachloride (67-72-1) *See* Hexachloroethane[a] *at loc. no.* **370**
Carbon Monoxide (630-08-0) *See loc. no.* **126**
Carbonothioic dichloride (463-71-8) *See* Thiophosgene[a] *at loc. no.* **12**
Carbon oxysulfide (463-58-1) *See* Carbonyl Sulfide[a] *at loc. no.* **127**
Carbon Tetrachloride (56-23-5) *See loc. no.* **355**
Carbonyl chloride (75-44-5) *See* Phosgene[a] *at loc. no.* **11**
Carbonyl Sulfide (463-58-1) *See loc. no.* **127**
Carbophenothion (786-19-6) *See loc. no.* **1083**
Carbopol 940, 941, 960, 961 *See* Carboxypolymethylene[a] *at loc. no.* **1627**
Carbostesin (2180-92-9) *See* Bupivacaine[c] *at loc. no.* **1578**
Carbowax (25322-68-3) *See loc. no.* **441**
Carboxin (5234-68-4) *See loc. no.* **1182**
Carboxymethocel S (9000-11-7) *See* Carboxymethylcellulose[a] *at loc. no.* **853**
Carboxymethylcellulose (9000-11-7) *See loc. no.* **853**
3,3'-Carboxymethylene bis(4-hydroxycoumarin)ethyl ester (548-00-5) *See* Ethyl Biscoumacetate[a] *at loc. no.* **1340**
N-(Carboxymethyl)-N'-(2-hydroxyethyl)-N,N'-ethylene diglycine (150-39-0) *See* Ethylenediaminetetraacetic Acid (and Salts)[b] *at loc. no.* **1506**
Carboxypolymethylene (9003-01-4) *See loc. no.* **1627**
Carboxyvinyl polymer (9003-01-4) *See* Carboxypolymethylene[a] *at loc. no.* **1627**
Carbromal (77-65-6) *See loc. no.* **1431**
Carbyne (101-27-9) *See* Barban[c] *at loc. no.* **1227**
Cardiazol (54-95-5) *See* Pentylenetetrazol[c] *at loc. no.* **1606**
Cardol (25702-11-8) *See loc. no.* **925**
Carisoprodol (78-44-4) *See loc. no.* **1403**
Carnauba Wax (8015-86-9) *See loc. no.* **752**
Carphenazine maleate (2975-34-0) *See* Trifluoperazine[b] *at loc. no.* **1426**
Carrageen *See* Carrageenan[a] *at loc. no.* **753**
Carrageenan *See loc. no.* **753**
Carraghenan *See* Carrageenan[a] *at loc. no.* **753**
Cartap (15263-53-3) *See loc. no.* **1130**
Carvacrol (499-75-2) *See loc. no.* **489**
Caryophyllic acid (97-53-0) *See* Eugenol[a] *at loc. no.* **864**
Carzol (23422-53-9) *See* Formetanate[b] *at loc. no.* **1135**
Casanthranol (8024-48-4) *See loc. no.* **849**
Cascara Sagrada (8047-27-6) *See loc. no.* **660**
Cascarin *See* Cascara Sagrada[b] *at loc. no.* **660**
Cashew Nut *See loc. no.* **661**
Cassia oil (8007-80-5) *See* Cinnamaldehyde[c] *at loc. no.* **860**
Castor bean *See* Ricin[c] *at loc. no.* **930**
Castor Oil (8001-79-4) *See loc. no.* **712**
Castrix (535-89-7) *See loc. no.* **1346**
Catechol (120-80-9) *See* Pyrocatechol[a] *at loc. no.* **505**

---

[a] A Synonym [b] A Closely Related Substance [c] The Active or Major Constituent [d] A Class Name
[e] A Specific Example of or Product Containing

Ingredient name (CAS registry no.) *See* Primary Name *at
location no.* **XXX** *in Part D of this section*

Cationic emulsifier *See* Cationic Surfactants[a] *at loc. no.* **974**
Cationic softener *See* Cationic Surfactants[a] *at loc. no.* **974**
Cationic Surfactants *See loc. no.* **974**
Caustic *See* Lye[a] *at loc. no.* **51**
Caustic barley *See* Sabadilla[a] *at loc. no.* **691**
Caustic potash (1310-58-3) *See* Lye[d] *at loc. no.* **51**
Caustic soda (1310-73-2) *See* Lye[d] *at loc. no.* **51**
Cayenne pepper (8023-77-6) *See* Capsicum[a] *at loc. no.* **659**
CBP (3737-00-6) *See loc. no.* **381**
CDAA (93-71-0) *See* Allidochlor[a] *at loc. no.* **1274**
CDEA *See* Allidochlor[b] *at loc. no.* **1274**
CDEC (95-06-7) *See* Sulfallate[a] *at loc. no.* **1164**
Cedarleaf (8007-20-3) *See* Essential Oils[d] *at loc. no.* **725**
Cedar oil *See* Oil of Cedar Wood[a] *at loc. no.* **735**
Cedar wood oil (8000-27-9) *See* Oil of Cedar Wood[a] *at loc. no.* **735**
Cedilanid (17575-22-3) *See* Lanatoside(s)[d] *at loc. no.* **841**
Cedilanid D (17598-65-1) *See* Deslanoside[a] *at loc. no.* **835**
Ceepryn chloride (123-03-5) *See* Cetyl Pyridinium Chloride[a] *at loc. no.* **988**
Cellosolve (110-80-5) *See* 2-Ethoxyethanol[a] *at loc. no.* **458**
Cellosolve acetate (111-15-9) *See* 2-Ethoxyethyl Acetate (and other Esters)[a] *at loc. no.* **450**
Cellosolve esters *See* 2-Ethoxyethyl Acetate (and other Esters)[e] *at loc. no.* **450**
Cellosolves *See* Ethylene Glycol Alkyl (and Aryl) Ethers[e] *at loc. no.* **459**
Cellosolve Sulfate (34253-67-3) *See loc. no.* **456**
Cellulose nitrate (9004-70-0) *See* Collodion[e] *at loc. no.* **854**
Cement *See* Portland Cement[c] *at loc. no.* **56**
Centrax (2955-38-6) *See* Prazepam[c] *at loc. no.* **1402**
Cereclor (8029-39-8) *See* Paraffin (Chlorinated)[c] *at loc. no.* **389**
Ceredon (495-73-8) *See* Benquinox[c] *at loc. no.* **1178**
Cereline (495-73-8) *See* Benquinox[c] *at loc. no.* **1178**
Ceresan (107-27-7) *See* Ethyl Mercuric Chloride[c] *at loc. no.* **228**
Ceresan 75-100-200 *See* Ethyl Mercuri-2,3-dihydroxypropylmercaptide[c] *at loc. no.* **229**
Ceresan M (517-16-8) *See* N-(Ethylmercuri)-p-toluene Sulfonanilide[c] *at loc. no.* **230**
Cetab (57-09-0) *See* Alkyl Trimethyl Ammonium Chloride (or Bromide)[d] *at loc. no.* **983**
Cetaceum (8002-23-1) *See* Spermaceti[a] *at loc. no.* **973**
Cetalkonium Chloride (122-18-9) *See loc. no.* **987**
Cetamide *See* Sulfacetamide[c] *at loc. no.* **1551**
Cetyl *derivative. If not listed below, see corresponding* Alkyl *derivative in this index.*
Cetyl Alcohol (124-29-8) *See loc. no.* **409**
Cetylcide *See* Alkyl Dimethyl Ethyl Ammonium Chloride (or Bromide)[c] *at loc. no.* **977**
Cetyl dimethyl benzyl ammonium chloride (122-18-9) *See* Cetalkonium Chloride[a] *at loc. no.* **987**
Cetyl Pyridinium Chloride (123-03-5) *See loc. no.* **988**
Cetyl trimethyl ammonium bromide (57-09-0) *See* Alkyl Trimethyl Ammonium Chloride (or Bromide)[d] *at loc. no.* **983**
Cevadilla *See* Sabadilla[a] *at loc. no.* **691**
Cevitamic acid (50-81-7) *See* Vitamin C[a] *at loc. no.* **908**
Chalk (13397-25-6) *See* Calcium Carbonate[c] *at loc. no.* **171**
Charas *See* Marihuana[a] *at loc. no.* **678**
Chaulmoogra Oil (8001-74-9) *See loc. no.* **713**
CHE 1843 (1113-14-0) *See trans*-1,2-Bis(propylsulfonyl)ethene[a] *at loc. no.* **1175**
Chemical Mace *See* α-Chloroacetophenone[a] *at loc. no.* **14**

Chemshield *See* o-Chlorobenzylidene Malononitrile[c] *at loc. no.* **15**
Chenopodium Oil (8006-99-3) *See loc. no.* **728**
China wood oil *See* Tung Oil[a] *at loc. no.* **724**
Chinomethionate (2439-01-2) *See* Quinomethionate[a] *at loc. no.* **1205**
Chinothionat (93-75-4) *See* Eradex[a] *at loc. no.* **1044**
Chlophedianol Hydrochloride (511-13-7) *See loc. no.* **1589**
Chloral Hydrate (302-17-0) *See loc. no.* **1432**
Chloramben (133-90-4) *See loc. no.* **1296**
Chloramben-ammonium (1076-46-6) *See* Chloramben[b] *at loc. no.* **1296**
Chloramben-methyl (7286-84-2) *See* Chloramben[b] *at loc. no.* **1296**
Chlorambucil (305-03-3) *See loc. no.* **1590**
Chloramines *See loc. no.* **22**
Chloramine-T (127-65-1) *See loc. no.* **91**
Chloranil (118-75-2) *See loc. no.* **1183**
p-Chloraniline (106-47-8) *See* p-Chloroaniline[a] *at loc. no.* **613**
Chlorasol *See loc. no.* **363**
Chlorate Salts *See loc. no.* **96**
Chlorazene (127-65-1) *See* Chloramine-T[a] *at loc. no.* **91**
Chlorazine (580-48-3) *See* Atrazine[b] *at loc. no.* **1259**
Chlorazone (127-65-1) *See* Chloramine-T[a] *at loc. no.* **91**
Chlorbenside (103-17-3) *See* p-Chlorobenzyl p-Chlorophenyl Sulfide[a] *at loc. no.* **1043**
Chlorbromuron (13360-45-7) *See loc. no.* **1242**
Chlorbufam (1967-16-4) *See* Chlorpropham[b] *at loc. no.* **1229**
Chlorbutol (57-15-8) *See* Chlorobutanol[a] *at loc. no.* **432**
Chlorcosane (8029-39-8) *See* Paraffin (Chlorinated)[a] *at loc. no.* **389**
Chlorcyclizine (82-93-9) *See loc. no.* **1489**
Chlordan (57-74-9) *See* Chlordane[a] *at loc. no.* **1019**
Chlordane (57-74-9) *See loc. no.* **1019**
Chlordecone (143-50-0) *See* Kepone[a] *at loc. no.* **1032**
Chlordiazepoxide Hydrochloride (438-41-5) *See loc. no.* **1392**
Chlordimeform (6164-98-3) *See loc. no.* **1042**
Chlordimeform hydrochloride (19750-95-9) *See* Chlordimeform[b] *at loc. no.* **1042**
Chloretone (57-15-8) *See* Chlorobutanol[a] *at loc. no.* **432**
Chlorex (111-44-4) *See* sym-Dichloroethyl Ether[c] *at loc. no.* **470**
Chlorfenac *See* Fenac[a] *at loc. no.* **1219**
Chlorhexidine (55-56-1) *See loc. no.* **994**
Chlorhexidine gluconate (18472-51-0) *See* Chlorhexidine[b] *at loc. no.* **994**
Chlorhexidine hydrochloride (3697-42-5) *See* Chlorhexidine[b] *at loc. no.* **994**
Chlorhydrol (12042-91-0) *See* Aluminum Chloride[b] *at loc. no.* **182**
Chlorinated anthracene oil *See* Carbolineum[a] *at loc. no.* **394**
Chlorinated aromatic hydrocarbon *See* Chlorinated Hydrocarbons[d] *at loc. no.* **354**
Chlorinated benzene *See* Hexachlorobenzene[c] *at loc. no.* **397**
Chlorinated camphene (8001-35-2) *See* Toxaphene[a] *at loc. no.* **1030**
Chlorinated Hydrocarbons *See loc. no.* **354**
Chlorinated Lime (1332-17-8) *See loc. no.* **90**
Chlorinated naphthalenes *See* Polychlorinated Naphthalenes[a] *at loc. no.* **402**
Chlorinated paraffin (8029-39-8) *See* Paraffin (Chlorinated)[a] *at loc. no.* **389**

---

[a] A Synonym   [b] A Closely Related Substance   [c] The Active or Major Constituent   [d] A Class Name
[e] A Specific Example of or Product Containing

Ingredient name (CAS registry no.) *See* Primary Name *at
location no.* **XXX** *in Part D of this section*

Chlorinated phosphate *See* Chlorinated Trisodium Phosphate[e] *at loc. no.* **87**

Chlorinated potash solution *See* Javelle Water[a] *at loc. no.* **88**

Chlorinated propane-propylene mixture *See* D-D Mixture[a] *at loc. no.* **384**

Chlorinated quebracho *See* Yohimbine[b] *at loc. no.* **834**

Chlorinated sodium metasilicate *See* Chlorinated Trisodium Phosphate[b] *at loc. no.* **87**

Chlorinated sodium phosphate *See* Chlorinated Trisodium Phosphate[a] *at loc. no.* **87**

Chlorinated sodium tripolyphosphate *See* Chlorinated Trisodium Phosphate[b] *at loc. no.* **87**

Chlorinated solvents *See* Chlorinated Hydrocarbons[d] *at loc. no.* **354**

Chlorinated terpenes *See* Strobane[e] *at loc. no.* **1031**

Chlorinated tripolyphosphate *See* Chlorinated Trisodium Phosphate[b] *at loc. no.* **87**

Chlorinated Trisodium Phosphate *See loc. no.* **87**

Chlorine (7782-50-5) *See loc. no.* **23**

Chlorine Dioxide (10049-04-4) *See loc. no.* **24**

Chlorine oxide (10049-04-4) *See* Chlorine Dioxide[a] *at loc. no.* **24**

Chlorine peroxide (10049-04-4) *See* Chlorine Dioxide[a] *at loc. no.* **24**

Chlorine water (8012-77-9) *See* Chlorine[c] *at loc. no.* **23**

Chlormequat (7003-89-6) *See* Paraquat[b] *at loc. no.* **1286**

Chlormezanone (80-77-3) *See loc. no.* **1404**

Chloroacetic Acid (and Salts) (79-11-8) *See loc. no.* **549**

Chloroacetonitrile (107-14-2) *See* Trichloroacetonitrile[b] *at loc. no.* **655**

α-Chloroacetophenone (532-27-4) *See loc. no.* **14**

γ-Chloroallyl chloride (542-75-6) *See* 1,3-Dichloropropene[a] *at loc. no.* **386**

2-Chloroallyl diethyldithiocarbamate (95-06-7) *See* Sulfallate[a] *at loc. no.* **1164**

N-(3-Chloroallyl) methenamine (4080-31-3) *See* Dowicil 200[e] *at loc. no.* **995**

1 - (3 - Chloroallyl) - 3,5,7 - triaza - 1 - azoniaadamantane chloride (4080-31-3) *See* Dowicil 200[e] *at loc. no.* **995**

p-Chloroaniline (106-47-8) *See loc. no.* **613**

Chlorobenzene (108-90-7) *See loc. no.* **393**

Chlorobenzilate (510-15-6) *See loc. no.* **1006**

p-Chlorobenzyl p-Chlorophenyl Sulfide (103-17-3) *See loc. no.* **1043**

p-Chlorobenzyl p-fluorophenyl sulfide (405-30-1) *See* Fluorbenside[a] *at loc. no.* **1045**

o-Chlorobenzylidene Malononitrile (2698-41-1) *See loc. no.* **15**

2-Chloro-4,6-bis(diethylamino)-s-triazine (580-48-3) *See* Atrazine[b] *at loc. no.* **1259**

2-Chloro-4,6-bis(ethylamino)-s-triazine (122-34-9) *See* Simazine[a] *at loc. no.* **1269**

2-Chloro-4,6-bis(isopropylamino)-s-triazine (139-40-2) *See* Propazine[a] *at loc. no.* **1268**

Chlorobromomethane (74-97-5) *See loc. no.* **356**

1-Chloro-3-bromopropene-1 (3737-00-6) *See* CBP[a] *at loc. no.* **381**

1-Chlorobutane (109-69-3) *See* n-Butyl Chloride[a] *at loc. no.* **380**

Chlorobutanol (57-15-8) *See loc. no.* **432**

2-Chloro-N-(3-butynyl)acetanilide *See* Propachlor[b] *at loc. no.* **1282**

4-Chloro-2-butynyl m-chlorocarbanilate (101-27-9) *See* Barban[a] *at loc. no.* **1227**

4-Chloro-2-butynyl N-(3-chlorophenyl) carbamate (101-27-9) *See* Barban[a] *at loc. no.* **1227**

Chlorocamphane (464-41-5) *See* Bornyl Chloride[a] *at loc. no.* **874**

6-Chloro-m-cresol (59-50-7) *See* Chlorocresols[d] *at loc. no.* **523**

p-Chloro-m-cresol (59-50-7) *See* Chlorocresols[d] *at loc. no.* **523**

Chlorocresols *See loc. no.* **523**

4-Chloro-2-cyclopentylphenol (13347-42-7) *See loc. no.* **524**

2-Chloro-4-(cyclopropylamino)-6-(isopropylamino)-s-triazine (22936-86-3) *See* Cyprazine[a] *at loc. no.* **1262**

2-(4-Chloro-6-(cyclopropylamino)-s-triazin-2-ylamino)-2-methylpropionitrile (32889-48-8) *See* Cyanazine[b] *at loc. no.* **1260**

5-Chloro-2-(2,4-dichlorophenoxy)phenol (3380-34-5) *See* Triclosan[a] *at loc. no.* **1002**

2-Chloro-N,N-diethylacetamide (2315-36-8) *See* Allidochlor[b] *at loc. no.* **1274**

2-Chloro-4-diethylamino-6-ethylamino-s-triazine (1912-26-1) *See* Atrazine[b] *at loc. no.* **1259**

2-Chloro-4-(diethylamino)-6-(isopropylamino)-s-triazine (1912-25-0) *See* Atrazine[b] *at loc. no.* **1259**

2 - Chloro - 2′,6′ - diethyl - N - (butoxymethyl)acetanilide (23184-66-9) *See* Alachlor[b] *at loc. no.* **1273**

2-Chloro-2-diethylcarbamoyl-1-methylvinyl dimethyl phosphate (297-99-4) *See* Phosphamidon[a] *at loc. no.* **1058**

2 - Chloro - 2′,6′ - diethyl - N-(methoxymethyl)acetanilide (15972-60-8) *See* Alachlor[a] *at loc. no.* **1273**

7-Chloro-1,3-dihydro-3-hydroxy-5-phenyl-2H-1,4-benzodiazepin-2-one (604-75-1) *See* Oxazepam[a] *at loc. no.* **1401**

2-Chloro-α-[2-(dimethylamino)ethyl]-α-phenylbenzenemethanol hydrochloride (511-13-7) *See* Chlophedianol Hydrochloride[a] *at loc. no.* **1589**

2-Chloro-4-dimethylamino-6-methylpyrimidine (535-89-7) *See* Castrix[a] *at loc. no.* **1346**

4-Chloro-α,α-dimethylbenzeneethanamine hydrochloride (151-06-4) *See* Chlorphentermine Hydrochloride[a] *at loc. no.* **1446**

5 - Chloro - 3 - (1,1 - dimethylethyl) - 6 - methyl - 2,4(1H,3H) - pyrimidinedione (5902-51-2) *See* Bromacil[b] *at loc. no.* **1294**

2-Chloro-2′,6′-dimethyl-N-isobutoxymethylacetanilide (24353-58-0) *See* Alachlor[b] *at loc. no.* **1273**

6-Chloro-4,5-dimethylphenyl-N-methylcarbamate *See* Carbanolate[b] *at loc. no.* **1127**

2-Chloro-N,N-dimethylthioxanthene-propylamine (113-59-7) *See* Chlorprothixene[a] *at loc. no.* **1414**

4′-Chloro-2,2-dimethylvaleranilide (7287-36-7) *See* Propanil[b] *at loc. no.* **1283**

1-Chloro-2,4-dinitrobenzene (97-00-7) *See loc. no.* **639**

4-Chlorodiphenyl sulfone (80-00-2) *See* Sulphenone[e] *at loc. no.* **1048**

1-Chloro-2,3-epoxypropane (106-89-8) *See* Epichlorohydrin[a] *at loc. no.* **387**

Chloroethane (75-00-3) *See* Ethyl Chloride[a] *at loc. no.* **368**

Chloroethanoic acid (79-11-8) *See* Chloroacetic Acid (and Salts)[a] *at loc. no.* **549**

2-Chloroethanol (107-07-3) *See* Ethylene Chlorohydrin[a] *at loc. no.* **434**

2 - Chloro - N - (ethoxymethyl) - 6 - ethyl - o - acetotoluidide (34256-82-1) *See* Alachlor[b] *at loc. no.* **1273**

2-Chloro-4-(ethylamino)-6-(isopropylamino)-s-triazine (1912-24-9) *See* Atrazine[a] *at loc. no.* **1259**

---

[a] A Synonym   [b] A Closely Related Substance   [c] The Active or Major Constituent   [d] A Class Name
[e] A Specific Example of or Product Containing

Ingredient name (CAS registry no.) *See* Primary Name *at*
location no. **XXX** *in Part D of this section*

2-[[4-Chloro-6-(ethylamino)-*s*-triazin-2-yl]amino]-2-methylpropionitrile (21725-46-2) *See* Cyanazine[a] *at loc. no.* **1260**

N-(2-Chloroethyl)-2,6-dinitro-*N*-propyl-(4-trifluoromethylaniline) (33245-39-5) *See* Dinitramine[b] *at loc. no.* **1288**

Chloroethylene (75-01-4) *See* Vinyl Chloride[a] *at loc. no.* **378**

Chloroethylmercury (107-27-7) *See* Ethyl Mercuric Chloride[a] *at loc. no.* **228**

2-Chloro-*N*-(2-ethyl-6-methylphenyl)-*N*-(2-methoxy-1-methylethyl)acetamide (51218-45-2) *See* Alachlor[b] *at loc. no.* **1273**

1-Chloro-3-ethyl-1-penten-4-yn-3-ol (113-18-8) *See* Ethchlorvynol[a] *at loc. no.* **1434**

N-(2-Chloroethyl)-trifluoro-2,6-dinitro-*N*-propyl-*p*-toluidine (33245-39-5) *See* Dinitramine[b] *at loc. no.* **1288**

Chloroform (67-66-3) *See loc. no.* **357**

Chloroformyl chloride (75-44-5) *See* Phosgene[a] *at loc. no.* **11**

Chlorohydroquinone (615-67-8) *See loc. no.* **500**

2-Chloro-4-(hydroxymercuri)phenol (538-04-5) *See loc. no.* **224**

2-(2-Chloro-4-hydroxyphenylhydrazono)acetoacetic acid *See* Drazoxolone[a] *at loc. no.* **1194**

2-Chloro-*N*-isopropylacetanilide (1918-16-7) *See* Propachlor[a] *at loc. no.* **1282**

2-Chloro-4-(isopropylamino)-6-(methylamino)-*s*-triazine (3004-71-5) *See* Atrazine[b] *at loc. no.* **1259**

5-Chloro-2-mercaptobenzothiazole (5331-91-9) *See* Mercaptobenzothiazole[b] *at loc. no.* **1198**

Chloromethane (74-87-3) *See* Methyl Chloride[a] *at loc. no.* **345**

Chloromethapyrilene (148-65-2) *See* Chlorothen[a] *at loc. no.* **1490**

3-(3-Chloro-4-methoxyphenyl)-1,1-dimethylurea *See* Metoxuron[a] *at loc. no.* **1252**

Chloromethoxypropylmercuric Acetate (1319-86-4) *See loc. no.* **225**

4-Chloro-5-methylamino-2-(α,α,α-trifluoro-*m*-tolyl)-3(2*H*)-pyridazinone (27314-13-2) *See* Norflurazon[a] *at loc. no.* **1311**

3-Chloro-4-methylaniline (95-74-9) *See loc. no.* **614**

Chloromethyl Methyl Ether (107-30-2) *See loc. no.* **467**

N′-(4-Chloro-2-methylphenyl)-*N*,*N*-dimethylmethanimidamide (6164-98-3) *See* Chlordimeform[a] *at loc. no.* **1042**

N-(3-Chloro-4-methylphenyl)-2-methylpentanamide (2307-68-8) *See* Pentanochlor[a] *at loc. no.* **1280**

3-Chloro-2-methyl-1-propene (563-47-3) *See loc. no.* **382**

2-Chloro-*N*-(1-methyl-2-propynyl)acetanilide *See* Propachlor[b] *at loc. no.* **1282**

3′-Chloro-2-methyl-*p*-valero-toluidide (2307-68-8) *See* Pentanochlor[a] *at loc. no.* **1280**

Chloronaphthalenes *See* Polychlorinated Naphthalenes[a] *at loc. no.* **402**

Chloroneb (2675-77-6) *See loc. no.* **1184**

Chloronitroethane (30283-93-3) *See* 1-Chloro-1-nitropropane[b] *at loc. no.* **19**

1-Chloro-1-nitropropane (600-25-9) *See loc. no.* **19**

1-(Chloro-2-norbornyl)-3,3-dimethylurea (1319-96-6) *See* Phenobenzuron[b] *at loc. no.* **1256**

Chlorophacinone (3691-35-8) *See loc. no.* **1335**

Chlorophenols *See loc. no.* **525**

Chlorophenothane (50-29-3) *See* DDT[a] *at loc. no.* **1007**

p-Chlorophenoxyacetic Acid (122-88-3) *See loc. no.* **1211**

1-(4-Chlorophenoxy)-3,3-dimethyl-1-(1,2,4-triazol-1-yl)-1-butanone (43121-43-3) *See* Triadimefon[a] *at loc. no.* **1271**

3-(*p*-(*p*-Chlorophenoxy)phenyl)-1,1-dimethylurea *See* Chloroxuron[a] *at loc. no.* **1243**

2-(4-Chlorophenoxy)propionic acid (3307-39-9) *See* *p*-Chlorophenoxyacetic Acid[b] *at loc. no.* **1211**

3-(α-*p*-Chlorophenyl-β-acetylethyl)-4-hydroxy-coumarin (81-82-3) *See* Coumachlor[a] *at loc. no.* **1336**

N-[[(4-Chlorophenyl)amino]carbonyl]-2,6-difluorobenzamide (35367-38-5) *See* Diflubenzuron[a] *at loc. no.* **1246**

1-(*p*-Chloro-α-phenylbenzyl)-4-(2-hydroxyethoxyethyl)piperazine (68-88-2) *See* Hydroxyzine Hydrochloride[b] *at loc. no.* **1438**

p-Chlorophenyl-*p*-chlorobenzene sulfonate (80-33-1) *See* Ovotran[c] *at loc. no.* **1047**

p-Chlorophenyl *p*-chlorobenzyl sulfide (103-17-3) *See* *p*-Chlorobenzyl *p*-Chlorophenyl Sulfide[a] *at loc. no.* **1043**

1-(*p*-Chlorophenyl)-3-(2,6-difluorobenzoyl)urea (35367-38-5) *See* Diflubenzuron[a] *at loc. no.* **1246**

3-(*p*-Chlorophenyl)-1,1-dimethylurea (150-68-5) *See* Monuron[c] *at loc. no.* **1253**

N-(4-Chlorophenyl)-α,α-dimethylvaleramide (7287-36-7) *See* Propanil[b] *at loc. no.* **1283**

2-Chloro-1-phenylethanone (532-27-4) *See* α-Chloroacetophenone[a] *at loc. no.* **14**

4-[(*o*-Chlorophenyl)hydrazono]-3-methyl-5-isoxazolone (5707-69-7) *See* Drazoxolone[a] *at loc. no.* **1194**

4-[4-(4-Chlorophenyl)-4-hydroxy-1-piperidinyl]-1-(4-fluorophenyl)-1-butanone (52-86-8) *See* Haloperidol[a] *at loc. no.* **1437**

3-(*p*-Chlorophenyl)-1-methoxy-1-methylurea *See* Linuron[b] *at loc. no.* **1251**

2-*p*-Chlorophenyl-3-methyl-2,3-butanediol (79-93-6) *See* Phenaglycodol[a] *at loc. no.* **1410**

S-[(4-Chlorophenyl)methyl]diethylcarbamothioate (28249-77-6) *See* Thiobencarb[a] *at loc. no.* **1239**

3-(*p*-Chlorophenyl)-1-methyl-1-(1-methyl-2-propynyl)urea (3766-60-7) *See* Buturon[a] *at loc. no.* **1241**

N′-(*p*-Chlorophenyl)-*N*-methyl-*N*-(1-methyl-2-propynyl)urea (3766-60-7) *See* Buturon[a] *at loc. no.* **1241**

2-Chloro-4-phenylphenol (92-04-6) *See* Chloro-2-phenylphenol[b] *at loc. no.* **526**

Chloro-2-phenylphenol (1331-46-0) *See loc. no.* **526**

Chloro-*o*-phenylphenol (1331-46-0) *See* Chloro-2-phenylphenol[a] *at loc. no.* **526**

2-[(*p*-Chlorophenyl)phenylacetyl]-1,3-indandione (3691-35-8) *See* Chlorophacinone[a] *at loc. no.* **1335**

2-[(4-Chlorophenyl)phenylacetyl]-1,*H*-indene-1,3(2*H*)-dione (3691-35-8) *See* Chlorophacinone[a] *at loc. no.* **1335**

1-[(4-Chlorophenyl)phenylmethyl]-4-[(3-methylphenyl)methyl]piperazine dihydrochloride (1104-22-9) *See* Meclizine Dihydrochloride[a] *at loc. no.* **1494**

p-Chlorophenyl phenyl sulfone (80-00-2) *See* Sulphenone[e] *at loc. no.* **1048**

3-(*p*-Chlorophenyl)-1,1,2-trimethylisourea (3050-27-9) *See* Phenobenzuron[b] *at loc. no.* **1256**

Chlorophyll (1406-65-1) *See loc. no.* **926**

Chlorophyllin (11006-92-1) *See* Chlorophyll[b] *at loc. no.* **926**

Chlorophyllin copper complex (11006-34-1) *See* Chlorophyll[b] *at loc. no.* **926**

Chloropicrin (76-06-2) *See loc. no.* **13**

6-Chloropiperonylchrysanthemumate (70-43-9) *See* Barthrin[a] *at loc. no.* **885**

2-Chloro-2-propenyl diethylcarbamodithioate (95-06-7) *See* Sulfallate[a] *at loc. no.* **1164**

Chloropropylate (5836-10-2) *See* Bromopropylate[b] *at loc. no.* **1004**

*N*¹-(6-Chloro-3-pyridazinyl)sulfanilamide (80-32-0) *See* Sulfachlorpyridazine[a] *at loc. no.* **1552**

---

[a] A Synonym   [b] A Closely Related Substance   [c] The Active or Major Constituent   [d] A Class Name
[e] A Specific Example of or Product Containing

Ingredient name (CAS registry no.) *See* Primary Name *at location no.* **XXX** *in Part D of this section*

Chloroquine (54-05-7) *See loc. no.* **1512**

Chlorosol *See* Chloramine-T[a] *at loc. no.* **91**

N-**Chlorosuccinimide** (128-09-6) *See loc. no.* **92**

3-Chloro-6-sulfanilamidopyridazine *See* Sulfachlorpyridazine[a] *at loc. no.* **1552**

Chlorosulfonic Acid (7790-94-5) *See loc. no.* **39**

Chlorothal *See* Dimethyl-2,3,5,6-tetrachloroterephthalate[a] *at loc. no.* **1303**

Chlorothalonil (1897-45-6) *See loc. no.* **1185**

Chlorothen (148-65-2) *See loc. no.* **1490**

Chlorothene (71-55-6) *See* 1,1,1-Trichloroethane[a] *at loc. no.* **377**

Chlorothiazide (58-94-6) *See* Benzothiadiazide Diuretics[d] *at loc. no.* **1588**

Chlorothymol (89-68-9) *See loc. no.* **527**

Chlorotoloxyacetic acid (and salts) (94-74-6) *See* MCPA[a] *at loc. no.* **1220**

(*N*-**Chloro-*p*-toluenesulfonamido)sodium** (127-65-1) *See* Chloramine-T[a] *at loc. no.* **91**

3-Chloro-*p*-toluidine (95-74-9) *See* 3-Chloro-4-methylaniline[a] *at loc. no.* **614**

Chlorotoluron (15545-48-9) *See* Neburon[b] *at loc. no.* **1254**

N′-(4-**Chloro-*o*-tolyl)-*N*,*N*-dimethylformamidine** (6164-98-3) *See* Chlordimeform[a] *at loc. no.* **1042**

3-(3-Chloro-*p*-tolyl)-1,1-dimethylurea *See* Neburon[b] *at loc. no.* **1254**

Chlorotrianisene (569-57-3) *See* Estrogens (Natural and Synthetic)[d] *at loc. no.* **916**

2-Chloro-1-(2,4,5-trichlorophenyl)ethenyl phosphoric acid dimethyl ester (961-11-5) *See* Tetrachlorvinfos[a] *at loc. no.* **1061**

2-Chloro-1-(2,4,5-trichlorophenyl)vinyl dimethyl phosphate (961-11-5) *See* Tetrachlorvinfos[a] *at loc. no.* **1061**

Chlorowax *See* Paraffin (Chlorinated)[c] *at loc. no.* **389**

Chloroxifenidim *See* Chloroxuron[a] *at loc. no.* **1243**

Chloroxuron (1982-47-4) *See loc. no.* **1243**

4-Chloro-3,5-xylenol (88-04-0) *See loc. no.* **528**

Chloro-xylenol (88-04-0) *See* 4-Chloro-3,5-xylenol[e] *at loc. no.* **528**

p-**Chloro-*m*-xylenol** (88-04-0) *See* 4-Chloro-3,5-xylenol[a] *at loc. no.* **528**

6-Chloro-3,4-xylyl methylcarbamate (671-04-5) *See* Carbanolate[a] *at loc. no.* **1127**

Chlorozone (127-65-1) *See* Chloramine-T[a] *at loc. no.* **91**

Chlorparacide (103-17-3) *See* *p*-Chlorobenzyl *p*-Chlorophenyl Sulfide[c] *at loc. no.* **1043**

Chlorphenamidine (6164-98-3) *See* Chlordimeform[a] *at loc. no.* **1042**

Chlorpheniramine maleate (113-92-8) *See* Antihistaminics[d] *at loc. no.* **1487**

Chlorphentermine Hydrochloride (151-06-4) *See loc. no.* **1446**

Chlorpromazine (50-53-3) *See loc. no.* **1412**

Chlorpropham (101-21-3) *See loc. no.* **1229**

Chlorprophenpyridamine *See* Antihistaminics[d] *at loc. no.* **1487**

Chlorprophenpyridamine maleate (1102-47-2) *See* Antihistaminics[d] *at loc. no.* **1487**

Chlorprothixene (113-59-7) *See loc. no.* **1414**

Chlorpyrifos (2921-88-2) *See loc. no.* **1064**

Chlor-PZ *See* Chlorpromazine[c] *at loc. no.* **1412**

Chlorsulphacide (103-17-3) *See* *p*-Chlorobenzyl *p*-Chlorophenyl Sulfide[c] *at loc. no.* **1043**

Chlortetracycline (57-62-5) *See* Tetracyclines[d] *at loc. no.* **904**

Chlorthal dimethyl (1861-32-1) *See* Dimethyl-2,3,5,6-tetrachloroterephthalate[a] *at loc. no.* **1303**

Chlorthalidone (77-36-1) *See* Benzothiadiazide Diuretics[d] *at loc. no.* **1588**

Chlorthal methyl (887-54-7) *See* Dimethyl-2,3,5,6-tetrachloroterephthalate[b] *at loc. no.* **1303**

Chlorthiamid (1918-13-4) *See loc. no.* **1297**

Chlorthion (500-28-7) *See loc. no.* **1065**

Chlor-trimeton maleate (113-92-8) *See* Antihistaminics[d] *at loc. no.* **1487**

Choline salicylate (2016-36-6) *See* Salicylate[d] *at loc. no.* **600**

Choline theophyllinate (146-71-4) *See* Theophylline[b] *at loc. no.* **802**

Choresium *See* Chlorophyll[b] *at loc. no.* **926**

Chromate Salts *See loc. no.* **81**

Chrome alum (7788-99-0) *See* Chromium Sulfate[b] *at loc. no.* **281**

Chrome green (1308-38-9) *See* Chromium Oxide[a] *at loc. no.* **280**

Chrome red *See* Lead Chromate[b] *at loc. no.* **246**

Chrome yellow (7758-97-6) *See* Lead Chromate[a] *at loc. no.* **246**

Chromic acid (1333-82-0) *See* Chromium Trioxide[a] *at loc. no.* **80**

Chromic oxide (1308-38-9) *See* Chromium Oxide[a] *at loc. no.* **280**

Chromic sulfate (10101-53-8) *See* Chromium Sulfate[a] *at loc. no.* **281**

Chromium Oxide (1308-38-9) *See loc. no.* **280**

Chromium potassium sulfate (7788-99-0) *See* Chromium Sulfate[b] *at loc. no.* **281**

Chromium Sulfate (10101-53-8) *See loc. no.* **281**

Chromium Trioxide (1333-82-0) *See loc. no.* **80**

Chrysanthemic acid esters *See* Pyrethroids[e] *at loc. no.* **894**

Chrysanthemum cinerariaefolium *See* Pyrethrum[c] *at loc. no.* **686**

Chrysanthemumic acid esters *See* Pyrethroids[e] *at loc. no.* **894**

Chrysanthemum monocarboxylic acid esters *See* Pyrethroids[e] *at loc. no.* **894**

Chryson *See* Resmethrin[c] *at loc. no.* **895**

Chrysotile (12001-29-5) *See* Asbestos[e] *at loc. no.* **2**

Cigarette *See* Tobacco[c] *at loc. no.* **697**

Cimetidine (51481-61-9) *See loc. no.* **1491**

Cinammon wood *See* Oil of Sassafras[c] *at loc. no.* **739**

Cinchona alkaloids *See* Quinidine[e] *at loc. no.* **810**

Cinchophen (132-60-5) *See loc. no.* **1591**

Cinene (138-86-3) *See* Limonene[a] *at loc. no.* **877**

Cineol (470-82-6) *See* Eucalyptol[a] *at loc. no.* **863**

Cineole (470-82-6) *See* Eucalyptol[a] *at loc. no.* **863**

Cinerin I (97-12-1) *See* Pyrethrins[d] *at loc. no.* **893**

Cinerin II (121-20-0) *See* Pyrethrins[d] *at loc. no.* **893**

Cinnamal (104-55-2) *See* Cinnamaldehyde[a] *at loc. no.* **860**

Cinnamaldehyde (104-55-2) *See loc. no.* **860**

Cinnamein (103-41-3) *See* Cinnamic Acid Esters[d] *at loc. no.* **587**

Cinnamene (100-42-5) *See* Styrene[a] *at loc. no.* **315**

Cinnamic Acid Esters *See loc. no.* **587**

Cinnamic aldehyde (104-55-2) *See* Cinnamaldehyde[a] *at loc. no.* **860**

Cinnamon oil (8007-80-5) *See* Cinnamaldehyde[c] *at loc. no.* **860**

Ciodrin (7700-17-6) *See* Bidrin[b] *at loc. no.* **1051**

CIPC (101-21-3) *See* Chlorpropham[a] *at loc. no.* **1229**

Cismethrin *See* Resmethrin[d] *at loc. no.* **895**

Citanest *See* Prilocaine[c] *at loc. no.* **1584**

Citrated caffeine (8003-10-9) *See* Caffeine[b] *at loc. no.* **800**

Citrated calcium carbimide (8013-88-5) *See* Calcium Cyanamide[c] *at loc. no.* **1355**

---

[a] A Synonym   [b] A Closely Related Substance   [c] The Active or Major Constituent   [d] A Class Name
[e] A Specific Example of or Product Containing

Ingredient name (CAS registry no.) *See* Primary Name *at
location no.* **XXX** *in Part D of this section*

Citrated calcium cyanamide (8013-88-5) *See* Calcium Cyanamide[c] *at loc. no.* **1355**

Citric Acid (77-92-9) *See loc. no.* **703**

Citronellal (106-23-0) *See* Oil of Citronella[c] *at loc. no.* **736**

Citronella oil (8000-29-1) *See* Oil of Citronella[a] *at loc. no.* **736**

Cittrullus colocynthis *See* Colocynth[a] *at loc. no.* **663**

Claviceps purpurea *See* Ergot[a] *at loc. no.* **667**

Clay *See* Silica[c] *at loc. no.* **7**

Clioquinol (130-26-7) *See* Diiodohydroxyquin[b] *at loc. no.* **1513**

Clitocybe spp. *See* Muscarine[c] *at loc. no.* **818**

Clonazepam (1622-61-3) *See loc. no.* **1393**

Clonopin (1622-61-3) *See* Clonazepam[c] *at loc. no.* **1393**

Clorazepate Dipotassium (57109-90-7) *See loc. no.* **1394**

Clorazepate monopotassium (5991-71-9) *See* Clorazepate Dipotassium[b] *at loc. no.* **1394**

Clostridium botulinum toxins *See* Botulinal Toxins[a] *at loc. no.* **923**

Clove oil (8000-34-8) *See* Eugenol[c] *at loc. no.* **864**

CMC (9000-11-7) *See* Carboxymethylcellulose[a] *at loc. no.* **853**

CMME *See* Chloromethyl Methyl Ether[a] *at loc. no.* **467**

CMU (150-68-5) *See* Monuron[a] *at loc. no.* **1253**

CN *See* α-Chloroacetophenone[a] *at loc. no.* **14**

Coal gas *See* Gas[d] *at loc. no.* **128**

Coal oil (8002-05-9) *See* Petroleum (Crude)[a] *at loc. no.* **336**

Coal Tar (8007-45-2) *See loc. no.* **510**

Coal tar acids *See* Tars (Tar Oils and Tar Acids)[a] *at loc. no.* **519**

Coal tar aromatic solvent *See* Aromatic Solvent Naphtha[a] *at loc. no.* **342**

Coal Tar Creosote (8001-58-9) *See loc. no.* **511**

Coal tar disinfectant *See* Coal Tar Creosote[a] *at loc. no.* **511**

Coal tar distillate *See* Aromatic Hydrocarbon Solvent[d] *at loc. no.* **310**

Coal tar hydrocarbons *See* Aromatic Hydrocarbon Solvent[d] *at loc. no.* **310**

Coal tar naphtha *See* Aromatic Solvent Naphtha[a] *at loc. no.* **342**

Coal tar neutral oils *See* Coal Tar[c] *at loc. no.* **510**

Coal tar oils *See* Coal Tar[c] *at loc. no.* **510**

Coal tar phenols *See* Tars (Tar Oils and Tar Acids)[a] *at loc. no.* **519**

Cobalt alkanoate *See* Cobalt Driers[e] *at loc. no.* **283**

Cobalt carbonate (513-79-1) *See* Cobalt Salts[d] *at loc. no.* **282**

Cobalt Driers *See loc. no.* **283**

Cobaltic or cobaltous compounds *See* Cobalt Salts[a] *at loc. no.* **282**

Cobalt naphthenate (61789-51-3) *See* Cobalt Driers[e] *at loc. no.* **283**

Cobaltous acetate (71-48-7) *See* Cobalt Salts[d] *at loc. no.* **282**

Cobaltous oxide (1307-96-6) *See* Cobalt Driers[d] *at loc. no.* **283**

Cobalt Salts *See loc. no.* **282**

Cobalt sulfate (10124-43-3) *See* Cobalt Salts[d] *at loc. no.* **282**

Cocaine (50-36-2) *See loc. no.* **825**

Cocillana (1398-77-2) *See loc. no.* **662**

Cocoa butter (8002-31-1) *See* Theobroma Oil[a] *at loc. no.* **742**

Coco-Diazine *See* Sulfadiazine[c] *at loc. no.* **1553**

Coconut Oil (8001-31-8) *See loc. no.* **714**

COCS (8012-69-9) *See* Copper Oxychloride Sulfate[a] *at loc. no.* **262**

Codeine (76-57-3) *See loc. no.* **780**

Codeine phosphate (52-28-8) *See* Codeine[b] *at loc. no.* **780**

Codeine sulfate (1420-53-7) *See* Codeine[b] *at loc. no.* **780**

Colace (577-11-7) *See* Dioctyl Sodium Sulfosuccinate[c] *at loc. no.* **951**

Colchicine (64-86-8) *See loc. no.* **803**

Colistimethate sodium (8068-28-5) *See* Polymixin[b] *at loc. no.* **903**

Colistin (1066-17-7) *See* Polymixin[d] *at loc. no.* **903**

Colistin sulfate (1264-72-8) *See* Polymixin[b] *at loc. no.* **903**

Collodion (8050-69-9) *See loc. no.* **854**

Colocynth *See loc. no.* **663**

Colophony (8050-09-7) *See* Rosin[a] *at loc. no.* **760**

Colorado shale tar *See* Coal Tar[b] *at loc. no.* **510**

Compazine (58-38-8) *See* Prochlorperazine[c] *at loc. no.* **1419**

Complex Phosphates *See loc. no.* **141**

Complex polyphosphates *See* Complex Phosphates[a] *at loc. no.* **141**

Complex silicates *See* Pumice[a] *at loc. no.* **6**

Compound 42 (81-81-2) *See* Warfarin[a] *at loc. no.* **1345**

Compound 118 (309-00-2) *See* Aldrin[a] *at loc. no.* **1017**

Compound 497 (60-57-1) *See* Dieldrin[a] *at loc. no.* **1020**

Compound 6-12 (94-96-2) *See* 2-Ethyl-1,3-hexanediol[a] *at loc. no.* **1329**

Compound 1068 (57-74-9) *See* Chlordane[a] *at loc. no.* **1019**

Compound 1080 *See* Fluoroacetate[d] *at loc. no.* **548**

Compound 1081 (640-19-7) *See* Fluoroacetamide[a] *at loc. no.* **1347**

Compound 1189 (143-50-0) *See* Kepone[a] *at loc. no.* **1032**

Compound 1836 (311-47-7) *See* Diethyl 2-Chlorovinyl Phosphate[a] *at loc. no.* **1054**

Compound 3956 *See* Toxaphene[a] *at loc. no.* **1030**

Compound benzoin tincture (8050-35-9) *See* Benzoin[c] *at loc. no.* **750**

Compound mixture of opium and glycyrrhiza (8030-36-2) *See* Brown Mixture[a] *at loc. no.* **215**

Concrete *See* Portland Cement[c] *at loc. no.* **56**

Condy's crystals (7722-64-7) *See* Potassium Permanganate[a] *at loc. no.* **83**

Coniine (458-88-8) *See loc. no.* **826**

Contergan (50-35-1) *See* Thalidomide[c] *at loc. no.* **1443**

Copper (7440-50-8) *See loc. no.* **265**

Copper acetate (6046-93-1) *See* Copper[d] *at loc. no.* **265**

Copper Acetoarsenite (1299-88-3) *See loc. no.* **200**

Copper Arsenate (1327-30-6) *See loc. no.* **201**

Copper arsenite (1302-97-2) *See* Cupric Arsenite[a] *at loc. no.* **202**

Copper calcium oxychloride *See* Cupric Chloride (Basic)[b] *at loc. no.* **268**

Copper cyclopentanecarboxylate *See* Copper Naphthenates[d] *at loc. no.* **261**

Copper disodium ethylenediaminetetraacetate (12558-58-6) *See* Copper[d] *at loc. no.* **265**

Copper hydroxide (20427-59-2) *See* Copper[d] *at loc. no.* **265**

Copper Naphthenates *See loc. no.* **261**

Copper oleate (1120-44-1) *See* Copper[d] *at loc. no.* **265**

Copper oxalate (814-91-5) *See* Copper[d] *at loc. no.* **265**

Copper oxychloride (1332-65-6) *See* Cupric Chloride (Basic)[a] *at loc. no.* **268**

Copper Oxychloride Sulfate (8012-69-9) *See loc. no.* **262**

Copper 3-Phenylsalicylate (5328-04-1) *See loc. no.* **263**

Copper Quinolinolate (10380-28-6) *See loc. no.* **264**

Copper subacetate *See* Copper[d] *at loc. no.* **265**

Copper sulfate (7758-98-7) *See* Copper[d] *at loc. no.* **265**

Copper-Zinc-Chromate Complex (12001-14-8) *See loc. no.* **267**

Copra oil *See* Coconut Oil[a] *at loc. no.* **714**

Coprine *See loc. no.* **815**

Coprinus atramentarius *See* Coprine[c] *at loc. no.* **815**

---

[a] A Synonym   [b] A Closely Related Substance   [c] The Active or Major Constituent   [d] A Class Name
[e] A Specific Example of or Product Containing

Ingredient name (CAS registry no.) *See* Primary Name *at*
location no. **XXX** *in Part D of this section*

Co-Ral (56-72-4) *See* Coumaphos[e] *at loc. no.* **1066**
Cornstarch (9005-25-8) *See* Starch[a] *at loc. no.* **707**
Corrosive sublimate (7487-94-7) *See* Mercuric Chloride[a] *at loc. no.* **236**
Corticosteroids *See loc. no.* **915**
Corticosterone (50-22-6) *See* Corticosteroids[d] *at loc. no.* **915**
Corynanthe yohimbi *See* Yohimbine[c] *at loc. no.* **834**
Cotoran (2164-17-2) *See* Fluometuron[c] *at loc. no.* **1249**
Coumachlor (81-82-3) *See loc. no.* **1336**
Coumadin (81-81-2) *See* Warfarin[a] *at loc. no.* **1345**
Coumafuryl (117-52-2) *See loc. no.* **1337**
Coumaphos (56-72-4) *See loc. no.* **1066**
Coumarin (91-64-5) *See loc. no.* **861**
CPA (122-88-3) *See* p-Chlorophenoxyacetic Acid[a] *at loc. no.* **1211**
C-4 Plastic explosive *See* Cyclonite[c] *at loc. no.* **631**
4-CPP (3307-39-9) *See* p-Chlorophenoxyacetic Acid[b] *at loc. no.* **1211**
3-CPT (95-74-9) *See* 3-Chloro-4-methylaniline[a] *at loc. no.* **614**
Crab's eye *See* Jequirity Bean[a] *at loc. no.* **677**
Crag fly repellent (9007-07-2) *See* Butoxy Polypropylene Glycols[d] *at loc. no.* **454**
Crag Fruit Fungicide 341 (556-22-9) *See* Glyodin[c] *at loc. no.* **1196**
Crag Fungicide 658 (12001-14-8) *See* Copper-Zinc-Chromate Complex[a] *at loc. no.* **267**
Crag Fungicide 974 (533-74-4) *See* Dazomet[c] *at loc. no.* **1186**
Crag Herbicide 1 (136-78-7) *See* 2-(2,4-Dichlorophenoxy)ethyl Sulfate Sodium Salt[c] *at loc. no.* **1216**
Cream of tartar (868-14-4) *See* Tartaric Acid[b] *at loc. no.* **563**
Cremosuxidine *See* Succinylsulfathiazole[c] *at loc. no.* **1549**
Cremo-Thalidine *See* Phthalylsulfathiazole[c] *at loc. no.* **1548**
Creolin (12751-04-1) *See loc. no.* **512**
Creolin-Pearson (8006-47-1) *See* Creolin[a] *at loc. no.* **512**
Creosol (93-51-6) *See loc. no.* **490**
Creosote (8021-39-4) *See loc. no.* **513**
Creosote oil *See* Creosote[a] *at loc. no.* **513**
Creosotic acid (8006-63-1) *See* Cresotic Acids[a] *at loc. no.* **595**
Cresatin (122-46-3) *See* m-Cresyl Acetate[a] *at loc. no.* **491**
Cresol and Soap Solution (B.P.) *See loc. no.* **515**
Cresols (8003-33-6) *See loc. no.* **514**
Cresotic Acids *See loc. no.* **595**
Cresotinic acids *See* Cresotic Acids[a] *at loc. no.* **595**
m-Cresyl Acetate (122-46-3) *See loc. no.* **491**
Cresylic acid (8006-62-0) *See* Cresols[e] *at loc. no.* **514**
Crocidolite (12001-28-4) *See* Asbestos[e] *at loc. no.* **2**
Crocus (N.F. VII) (1317-63-1) *See* Saffron[c] *at loc. no.* **692**
Croneton *See* Ethiofencarb[c] *at loc. no.* **1134**
Crotonaldehyde (123-73-9) *See* Acrolein[b] *at loc. no.* **481**
Croton Oil (8001-28-3) *See loc. no.* **715**
Crude petroleum oil *See* Petroleum (Crude)[a] *at loc. no.* **336**
Cryolite (1344-75-8) *See loc. no.* **104**
Cryptenamine *See* Veratrum Viride Alkaloids[d] *at loc. no.* **811**
Cryptenamine tannates *See* Veratrum Viride Alkaloids[d] *at loc. no.* **811**
"Crystal" *See* Methamphetamine[a] *at loc. no.* **1459**
Crystal violet (548-62-9) *See* Gentian Violet[a] *at loc. no.* **1520**
CS (2698-41-1) *See* o-Chlorobenzylidene Malononitrile[a] *at loc. no.* **15**
Cube *See loc. no.* **664**
Cubé extract or powder or root *See* Cubé[a] *at loc. no.* **664**
Cubé resins *See* Cube[e] *at loc. no.* **664**
Cucumber dust (7778-44-1) *See* Calcium Arsenate[a] *at loc. no.* **198**
Cufraneb *See* Mancozeb[b] *at loc. no.* **1159**

Cumarin (91-64-5) *See* Coumarin[a] *at loc. no.* **861**
Cumene (98-82-8) *See loc. no.* **313**
Cumol (98-82-8) *See* Cumene[a] *at loc. no.* **313**
Cunilate (10380-28-6) *See* Copper Quinolinolate[a] *at loc. no.* **264**
Cuniphens *See* Dichlorophen(e)[c] *at loc. no.* **529**
Cupric Arsenite (1302-97-2) *See loc. no.* **202**
Cupric chloride (7447-39-4) *See* Copper[d] *at loc. no.* **265**
Cupric Chloride (Basic) (1332-65-6) *See loc. no.* **268**
Cupric compounds *See* Copper[a] *at loc. no.* **265**
Cupric-8-hydroxyquinolinate (10380-28-6) *See* Copper Quinolinolate[a] *at loc. no.* **264**
Cupric sulfate (7758-98-7) *See* Copper[d] *at loc. no.* **265**
Cuprimine (52-67-5) *See* D-Penicillamine[c] *at loc. no.* **1507**
Cuprobam *See* Sodium Dimethyldithiocarbamate[b] *at loc. no.* **1163**
Cuprous Chloride (7758-89-6) *See loc. no.* **266**
Cuprous Oxide (1317-39-1) *See loc. no.* **269**
Curatin (1229-29-4) *See* Doxepin[c] *at loc. no.* **1472**
Curitan *See* Dodine[c] *at loc. no.* **1193**
"Cyanamide" (156-62-7) *See* Calcium Cyanamide[a] *at loc. no.* **1355**
Cyanate Salts *See loc. no.* **145**
Cyanatryn (21689-84-9) *See* Prometon[b] *at loc. no.* **1267**
Cyanazine (21725-46-2) *See loc. no.* **1260**
Cyanic Acid (420-05-3) *See loc. no.* **29**
Cyanide (57-12-5) *See loc. no.* **105**
Cyanoacrylates *See* n-Alkyl-α-Cyanoacrylates[a] *at loc. no.* **1626**
α-Cyano-2,4-dichlorocinnamic acid (6013-05-4) *See* Cyanodichlorophenylacrylic Acid[a] *at loc. no.* **1298**
Cyano-dichlorophenylacrylic Acid (6013-05-4) *See loc. no.* **1298**
Cyanoethylene (107-13-1) *See* Acrylonitrile[a] *at loc. no.* **648**
Cyanogas (592-01-8) *See* Calcium Cyanide[c] *at loc. no.* **107**
Cyanomethane (75-05-8) *See* Acetonitrile[a] *at loc. no.* **647**
2-(1-Cyano-1-methylethylamino)-4-(ethylamino)-6-(methylthio)-s-triazine (21689-84-9) *See* Prometon[b] *at loc. no.* **1267**
Cyano(methylmercuri)guanidine (502-39-6) *See* Methylmercuric Dicyandiamide[a] *at loc. no.* **240**
Cyano Organic Compounds *See loc. no.* **110**
Cyano(3-phenoxyphenyl)methyl 4-chloro-alpha-(1-methylethyl)benzeneacetate (51630-58-1) *See* Fenvalerate[a] *at loc. no.* **890**
Cyanuric Acid (504-19-8) *See loc. no.* **1261**
Cyclamate sodium or calcium (139-05-9) *See* Sodium Cyclamate[a] *at loc. no.* **1617**
Cyclethrin (97-11-0) *See loc. no.* **886**
Cyclizine hydrochloride (303-25-3) *See* Meclizine Dihydrochloride[b] *at loc. no.* **1494**
Cycloate (1134-23-2) *See loc. no.* **1234**
Cyclobarbital (52-31-3) *See loc. no.* **1371**
Cyclocoumarol (518-20-7) *See loc. no.* **1338**
Cycloform (94-14-4) *See* Butamben[b] *at loc. no.* **1579**
5-Cycloheptenyl-5-ethylbarbituric acid (509-86-4) *See* Heptabarbital[a] *at loc. no.* **1374**
1,4-Cyclohexadienedione (106-51-4) *See* Quinone[a] *at loc. no.* **507**
Cyclohexane (110-82-7) *See loc. no.* **308**
Cyclohexane carboxylic acid (98-89-5) *See* Naphthenic Acids[a] *at loc. no.* **558**
Cyclohexanol (108-93-0) *See loc. no.* **410**
Cyclohexanone (108-94-1) *See loc. no.* **468**
Cyclohexanone Peroxide (78-18-2) *See loc. no.* **77**
Cyclohexatrine (71-43-2) *See* Benzene[a] *at loc. no.* **312**

---

[a] A Synonym   [b] A Closely Related Substance   [c] The Active or Major Constituent   [d] A Class Name
[e] A Specific Example of or Product Containing

Ingredient name (CAS registry no.) *See* Primary Name *at location no.* **XXX** *in Part D of this section*

5-(1-Cyclohexenyl)-1,5-dimethylbarbituric acid sodium (50-09-9) *See* Hexobarbital Sodium[a] *at loc. no.* **1376**

5-(1-Cyclohexenyl)-5-ethylbarbituric acid (52-31-3) *See* Cyclobarbital[a] *at loc. no.* **1371**

Cycloheximide (66-81-9) *See loc. no.* **906**

Cyclohexylamine (108-91-8) *See loc. no.* **609**

2-Cyclohexylcyclohexanol (6531-86-8) *See* NMRI-448[e] *at loc. no.* **425**

3-Cyclohexyl-6-(dimethylamino)-1-methyl-s-triazine-2,4-(1H,3H)-dione (51235-04-2) *See* Hexazinone[a] *at loc. no.* **1263**

2-Cyclohexyl-4,6-dinitrophenol (131-89-5) *See* 4,6-Dinitro-o-cyclohexylphenol[a] *at loc. no.* **540**

2-Cyclohexyl-4,6-dinitrophenol dicyclohexylamine (317-83-9) *See* Dicyclohexylamine 4,6-Dinitro-o-cyclohexylphenate[a] *at loc. no.* **536**

Cyclohexylmethane (108-87-2) *See* Methylcyclohexane[a] *at loc. no.* **309**

N-Cyclohexylsulfamate sodium or calcium (139-05-9) *See* Sodium Cyclamate[a] *at loc. no.* **1617**

Cyclonal sodium (50-09-9) *See* Hexobarbital Sodium[c] *at loc. no.* **1376**

Cyclonite (121-82-4) *See loc. no.* **631**

3-Cyclooctyl-1,1-dimethylurea (2163-69-1) *See* Cycluron[a] *at loc. no.* **1244**

Cyclopal (76-68-6) *See* 5-Cyclopentenyl-5-allylbarbituric Acid[c] *at loc. no.* **1372**

Cycloparaffins *See* Naphthenes[a] *at loc. no.* **339**

Cyclopen (76-68-6) *See* 5-Cyclopentenyl-5-allylbarbituric Acid[c] *at loc. no.* **1372**

5-Cyclopentenyl-5-allylbarbituric Acid (76-68-6) *See loc. no.* **1372**

dl-2-Cyclopentenyl-4-hydroxy-3-methyl-2-cyclopenten-1-one chrysanthemate (97-11-0) *See* Cyclethrin[a] *at loc. no.* **886**

Cyclopropanone hydrate *See* Coprine[b] *at loc. no.* **815**

Cyclo-tetramethylene oxide (109-99-9) *See* Tetrahydrofuran[a] *at loc. no.* **1623**

Cyclotrimethylenetrinitramine (121-82-4) *See* Cyclonite[a] *at loc. no.* **631**

Cycluron (2163-69-1) *See loc. no.* **1244**

Cydonia oblonga *See* Quince Seed[a] *at loc. no.* **687**

Cydonium *See* Quince Seed[a] *at loc. no.* **687**

Cylert *See* Pemoline[c] *at loc. no.* **1465**

Cymene (1329-98-2) *See* Xylene[b] *at loc. no.* **318**

Cymol (99-87-6) *See* Xylene[b] *at loc. no.* **318**

m-Cym-5-yl methylcarbamate (2631-37-0) *See* Promecarb[a] *at loc. no.* **1146**

Cyprazine (22936-86-3) *See loc. no.* **1262**

Cyprex (2439-10-3) *See* Dodine[c] *at loc. no.* **1193**

2,4-D (94-75-7) *See loc. no.* **1212**

D-3 (72-54-8) *See* 1,1-Dichloro-2,2-bis(p-chlorophenyl)ethane[a] *at loc. no.* **1009**

Daconil 2787 (1897-45-6) *See* Chlorothalonil[c] *at loc. no.* **1185**

Dacthal (1861-32-1) *See* Dimethyl-2,3,5,6-tetrachloroterephthalate[c] *at loc. no.* **1303**

Dactin (118-52-5) *See* 1,3-Dichloro-5,5-dimethylhydantoin[a] *at loc. no.* **93**

Dalapon (75-99-0) *See loc. no.* **1299**

Dalmane (1172-18-5) *See* Flurazepam[c] *at loc. no.* **1397**

Dalmatian insect powder *See* Pyrethrum[a] *at loc. no.* **686**

Daminozide (1596-84-5) *See loc. no.* **1356**

Danthron (117-10-2) *See* Cascara Sagrada[b] *at loc. no.* **660**

Darbid (71-81-8) *See* Isopropamide[a] *at loc. no.* **1602**

Dartal dihydrochloride (146-28-1) *See* Thiopropazate Dihydrochloride[c] *at loc. no.* **1424**

Darvon hydrochloride (1639-60-7) *See* Propoxyphene Hydrochloride[a] *at loc. no.* **1486**

Datril (103-90-2) *See* Acetaminophen[c] *at loc. no.* **1587**

Datura stramonium *See* Stramonium[a] *at loc. no.* **696**

Daturine (101-31-5) *See* Hyoscyamine[a] *at loc. no.* **770**

Dazomet (533-74-4) *See loc. no.* **1186**

2,4-DB (94-82-6) *See* 4-(2,4-Dichlorophenoxy)butyric Acid[a] *at loc. no.* **1215**

DBCP (96-12-8) *See* 1,2-Dibromo-3-chloropropane[a] *at loc. no.* **385**

DBD *See* Guthion[c] *at loc. no.* **1089**

DBNPA *See* 2,2'-Dibromo-3-nitrilopropionamide[a] *at loc. no.* **1188**

DBP *See* n-Butyl Phthalate[a] *at loc. no.* **590**

1,1-DCE (75-35-4) *See* 1,1-Dichloroethylene[a] *at loc. no.* **366**

DCP (120-83-2) *See* Chlorophenols[a] *at loc. no.* **525**

DCPC (80-06-8) *See* DMC[a] *at loc. no.* **1011**

DCPM (555-89-5) *See* Neotran[e] *at loc. no.* **1014**

DCU (116-52-9) *See* Dichloral Urea[a] *at loc. no.* **1245**

DDD (72-54-8) *See* 1,1-Dichloro-2,2-bis(p-chlorophenyl)ethane[a] *at loc. no.* **1009**

p,p'-DDD (72-54-8) *See* 1,1-Dichloro-2,2-bis(p-chlorophenyl)ethane[a] *at loc. no.* **1009**

DDH (118-52-5) *See* 1,3-Dichloro-5,5-dimethylhydantoin[a] *at loc. no.* **93**

D-D Mixture *See loc. no.* **384**

DDOA (828-00-2) *See* Dimethoxane[a] *at loc. no.* **1642**

DDT (50-29-3) *See loc. no.* **1007**

DDVP (62-73-7) *See* Dichlorvos[a] *at loc. no.* **1053**

Deacetyllanatoside C (17598-65-1) *See* Deslanoside[a] *at loc. no.* **835**

Deadly nightshade *See* Belladonna Leaf or Root[a] *at loc. no.* **658**

Deaner (3635-74-3) *See* Deanol[b] *at loc. no.* **1592**

Deanol (108-01-0) *See loc. no.* **1592**

Decachlorobis(2,4-cyclopentadiene-1-yl) (2227-17-0) *See* Dienochlor[a] *at loc. no.* **1027**

Decachloro-octahydro-1,3,4-metheno-2H-cyclobuta(cd)pentalen-2-one (143-50-0) *See* Kepone[a] *at loc. no.* **1032**

Decachloropentacyclodecan-4-one (143-50-0) *See* Kepone[a] *at loc. no.* **1032**

Decahydronaphthalene (91-17-8) *See loc. no.* **319**

Decalin (91-17-8) *See* Decahydronaphthalene[c] *at loc. no.* **319**

1-Decanol (112-30-1) *See* Decyl Alcohol[c] *at loc. no.* **411**

Decapryn succinate (562-10-7) *See* Doxylamine Succinate[a] *at loc. no.* **1493**

Decarbofuran *See* Carbofuran[b] *at loc. no.* **1129**

Dechlorane (2385-85-5) *See* Mirex[a] *at loc. no.* **1033**

Decholin (81-23-2) *See* Dehydrocholic Acid[c] *at loc. no.* **1593**

n-Decyl *derivative. See corresponding* Alkyl *derivative in this index.*

Decyl Alcohol *See loc. no.* **411**

DEET (134-62-3) *See* N,N-Diethyl-m-toluamide[a] *at loc. no.* **1326**

DEF (78-48-8) *See* S,S,S-Tributyl Phosphorotrithioate[c] *at loc. no.* **1111**

Deferoxamine (70-51-9) *See loc. no.* **1505**

Degraded carragheenan *See* Carrageenan[b] *at loc. no.* **753**

Deguelin (522-17-8) *See* Rotenoids[d] *at loc. no.* **897**

DEHP (117-81-7) *See* Di-2-ethylhexyl Phthalate[a] *at loc. no.* **591**

Dehydroabietic acid *See* Tall Oil[c] *at loc. no.* **723**

Dehydroacetic Acid (520-45-6) *See loc. no.* **1187**

Dehydrocholic Acid (81-23-2) *See loc. no.* **1593**

Dehydrorotenone (3466-09-9) *See loc. no.* **887**

---

[a] A Synonym [b] A Closely Related Substance [c] The Active or Major Constituent [d] A Class Name
[e] A Specific Example of or Product Containing

Ingredient name (CAS registry no.) *See* Primary Name *at*
location no. **XXX** *in Part D of this section*

Delachlor (24353-58-0) *See* Alachlor[b] *at loc. no.* **1273**
Delnav (78-34-2) *See* Navadel[a] *at loc. no.* **1093**
Delphene (134-62-3) *See* N,N-Diethyl-m-toluamide[c] *at loc. no.* **1326**
Delphinium *See* Larkspur Alkaloids[c] *at loc. no.* **828**
Delvinal sodium (125-44-0) *See* Vinbarbital Sodium[a] *at loc. no.* **1391**
Delysid (50-37-3) *See* Lysergic Acid Diethylamide[a] *at loc. no.* **829**
Demerol (50-13-5) *See* Meperidine Hydrochloride[c] *at loc. no.* **1484**
Demethylchlortetracycline (127-33-3) *See* Tetracyclines[d] *at loc. no.* **904**
Demeton (8000-97-3) *See loc. no.* **1067**
Demeton methyl (8022-00-2) *See* Methyl Demeton[a] *at loc. no.* **1075**
Demeton O (298-03-3) *See* Demeton[e] *at loc. no.* **1067**
Demeton S (126-75-0) *See* Demeton[e] *at loc. no.* **1067**
Demosan (2675-77-6) *See* Chloroneb[c] *at loc. no.* **1184**
Denatured alcohol *See* Ethyl Alcohol[b] *at loc. no.* **412**
Deobase (8044-51-7) *See loc. no.* **324**
Deodorized base oil *See* Deobase[e] *at loc. no.* **324**
Deodorized petroleum oil *See* Deobase[a] *at loc. no.* **324**
Deoxycorticosterone (64-85-7) *See* Corticosteroids[d] *at loc. no.* **915**
Derifil (11006-34-1) *See* Chlorophyll[b] *at loc. no.* **926**
Derris Powder *See loc. no.* **665**
Derris resins *See* Derris Powder[e] *at loc. no.* **665**
Derris root *See* Derris Powder[a] *at loc. no.* **665**
Desacetyllanatoside C *See* Deslanoside[a] *at loc. no.* **835**
Deserpidine (131-01-1) *See loc. no.* **796**
Desferal (70-51-9) *See* Deferoxamine[c] *at loc. no.* **1505**
Desipramine (50-47-5) *See loc. no.* **1471**
Deslanoside (17598-65-1) *See loc. no.* **835**
Desmedipham (13684-56-5) *See loc. no.* **1230**
11-Desmethoxyreserpine (131-01-1) *See* Deserpidine[a] *at loc. no.* **796**
Desmethylamitriptyline (72-69-5) *See* Nortriptyline[a] *at loc. no.* **1474**
Desmethylimipramine (50-47-5) *See* Desipramine[a] *at loc. no.* **1471**
Desmetryn (1014-69-3) *See* Prometon[b] *at loc. no.* **1267**
Desoxycorticosterone (64-85-7) *See* Corticosteroids[d] *at loc. no.* **915**
d-Desoxyephedrine (537-46-2) *See* Methamphetamine[a] *at loc. no.* **1459**
d-Desoxyephedrine hydrochloride (51-57-0) *See* Methamphetamine[b] *at loc. no.* **1459**
2-Desoxyphenobarbital (125-33-7) *See* Primidone[a] *at loc. no.* **1610**
2,4-D Esters *See loc. no.* **1213**
DET (134-62-3) *See* N,N-Diethyl-m-toluamide[a] *at loc. no.* **1326**
DET (61-51-8) *See* N,N-Dimethyltryptamine[b] *at loc. no.* **1448**
Detergents (Synthetic) *See loc. no.* **935**
Devil's dung *See* Asafetida[a] *at loc. no.* **747**
Devrinol *See* Napropamide[c] *at loc. no.* **1278**
Dexamethasone (50-02-2) *See* Corticosteroids[d] *at loc. no.* **915**
Dexchlorpheniramine maleate (2438-32-6) *See* Antihistaminics[d] *at loc. no.* **1487**
Dexedrine (51-64-9) *See* Amphetamine[b] *at loc. no.* **1444**
Dexon (140-56-7) *See* Fenaminosulf[c] *at loc. no.* **1195**
Dextroamphetamine (51-64-9) *See* Amphetamine[b] *at loc. no.* **1444**

Dextromethorphan Hydrobromide (125-69-9) *See loc. no.* **1594**
Dextropropoxyphene hydrochloride (1639-60-7) *See* Propoxyphene Hydrochloride[a] *at loc. no.* **1486**
DFDT (475-26-3) *See loc. no.* **1008**
DFP (55-91-4) *See* Diisopropyl Fluorophosphate[a] *at loc. no.* **1096**
DHA (520-45-6) *See* Dehydroacetic Acid[a] *at loc. no.* **1187**
Di- *If not located below, substitute* Bis- *for* Di- *and try again.*
Diacetone Alcohol (123-42-2) *See loc. no.* **469**
Diacetylmorphine (561-27-3) *See* Heroin[a] *at loc. no.* **782**
Diadol (52-43-7) *See* Allobarbital[c] *at loc. no.* **1373**
Dialkyl aniline *See* Dimethylaniline[e] *at loc. no.* **615**
Dialkyl Dimethyl Ammonium Chloride *See loc. no.* **989**
Dialkyl Sodium Sulfosuccinate *See loc. no.* **950**
Di-allate (2303-16-4) *See loc. no.* **1235**
4-(Diallylamino)-3,5-xylyl methylcarbamate (6392-46-7) *See* Allyxycarb[a] *at loc. no.* **1121**
5,5-Diallylbarbituric acid (52-43-7) *See* Allobarbital[a] *at loc. no.* **1373**
N,N-Diallyl-2-chloroacetamide (93-71-0) *See* Allidochlor[a] *at loc. no.* **1274**
N,N-Diallyl-2,2-dichloroacetamide (37764-25-3) *See* EPTC[b] *at loc. no.* **1236**
Dialog *See* Allobarbital[c] *at loc. no.* **1373**
Diamidafos (1754-58-1) *See loc. no.* **1097**
2,8-Diaminoacridine (92-62-6) *See* Acridine Antiseptics[d] *at loc. no.* **1518**
3,6-Diaminoacridinium chloride hydrochloride (531-73-7) *See* Acridine Antiseptics[d] *at loc. no.* **1518**
2,4-Diaminoanisole (615-05-4) *See* 4-Methoxy-m-phenylenediamine[a] *at loc. no.* **622**
p-Diaminobenzene (106-50-3) *See* Phenylenediamine (o- or p-)[d] *at loc. no.* **623**
2,2′-Diaminodiethylamine (111-40-0) *See* Diethylenetriamine[a] *at loc. no.* **603**
1,2-Diaminoethane (107-15-3) *See* Ethylenediamine[a] *at loc. no.* **602**
2,8-Diamino-10-methylacridinium chloride (86-40-8) *See* Acridine Antiseptics[d] *at loc. no.* **1518**
2,4-Diaminophenol Hydrochloride (137-09-7) *See loc. no.* **620**
2,6-Diamino-3-phenylazopyridine hydrochloride (136-40-3) *See* Phenazopyridine Hydrochloride[a] *at loc. no.* **1522**
2,4-Diaminotoluene (95-80-7) *See loc. no.* **621**
Diammonium ethylene bis(dithiocarbamate) (3566-10-7) *See* Nabam[b] *at loc. no.* **1162**
Diamthazole Dihydrochloride (136-96-9) *See loc. no.* **1525**
1,4:3,6-Dianhydro-D-glucitol (652-67-5) *See* Isosorbide[a] *at loc. no.* **1603**
1,4:3,6-Dianhydro-D-glucitol dinitrate (87-33-2) *See* Isosorbide Dinitrate[a] *at loc. no.* **634**
Diatomaceous earth (7631-86-9) *See* Silica[a] *at loc. no.* **7**
Diatomite *See* Silica[c] *at loc. no.* **7**
3,6-Diazaoctane-1,8-diamine (112-24-3) *See* Triethylenetetramine[a] *at loc. no.* **604**
Diazepam (439-14-5) *See loc. no.* **1395**
Diazinon (333-41-5) *See loc. no.* **1068**
Diazobenzene *See* Azobenzene[a] *at loc. no.* **1041**
1,2-Diazole (288-13-1) *See* Pyrazole[a] *at loc. no.* **1509**
Dibam (128-04-1) *See* Sodium Dimethyldithiocarbamate[c] *at loc. no.* **1163**
Dibam A (79-45-8) *See* Sodium Dimethyldithiocarbamate[b] *at loc. no.* **1163**
Dibasic lead arsenate (7784-40-9) *See* Lead Arsenate[a] *at loc. no.* **206**

---

[a] A Synonym   [b] A Closely Related Substance   [c] The Active or Major Constituent   [d] A Class Name
[e] A Specific Example of or Product Containing

Ingredient name (CAS registry no.) *See* Primary Name *at
location no.* **XXX** *in Part D of this section*

Dibasic potassium phosphate (7758-11-4) *See* Potassium Salts[d] *at loc. no.* **155**

Dibasic sodium phosphate (7558-79-4) *See* Phosphates[d] *at loc. no.* **139**

Dibrom (300-76-5) *See* Naled[c] *at loc. no.* **1055**

Dibromobenzoxyquinoline *See* Diiodohydroxyquin[b] *at loc. no.* **1513**

1,2-Dibromo-3-chloropropane (96-12-8) *See loc. no.* **385**

1,2-Dibromoethane (106-93-4) *See loc. no.* **364**

3,5-Dibromo-4-hydroxy-benzonitrile (1689-84-5) *See* Bromoxynil[a] *at loc. no.* **1295**

2,7-Dibromo-4-hydroxymercurifluorescein disodium (129-16-8) *See* Merbromin[a] *at loc. no.* **235**

Dibromohydroxyquinoline (521-74-4) *See* Diiodohydroxyquin[b] *at loc. no.* **1513**

Dibromomethane (74-95-3) *See* Methylene Bromide[a] *at loc. no.* **358**

2,2′-Dibromo-3-nitrilopropionamide *See loc. no.* **1188**

2,3-Dibromopropanol (96-13-9) *See* Tris(2,3-dibromopropyl)phosphate[b] *at loc. no.* **1118**

4′,5-Dibromosalicylanilide (87-12-7) *See* 3,4′,5-Tribromosalicylanilide[b] *at loc. no.* **1000**

Dibucaine (85-79-0) *See loc. no.* **1580**

Dibucaine hydrochloride (61-12-1) *See* Dibucaine[b] *at loc. no.* **1580**

Dibutyl Adipate (105-99-7) *See loc. no.* **1324**

2,6-Di-*tert*-butyl-*p*-cresol (128-37-0) *See* Butylated Hydroxytoluene[a] *at loc. no.* **1614**

3,5-Di-*tert*-butylphenyl-*N*-methylcarbamate (2655-19-8) *See* Butacarb[a] *at loc. no.* **1126**

Di-*n*-butyl phthalate (84-74-2) *See* n-Butyl Phthalate[a] *at loc. no.* **590**

Dibutyl phthalate (84-74-2) *See* n-Butyl Phthalate[a] *at loc. no.* **590**

Di-*n*-butyl Succinate (141-03-7) *See loc. no.* **1325**

Dibutyltin diacetate (1067-33-0) *See* Alkyl Tin Compounds[d] *at loc. no.* **292**

Dibutyltin dichloride (683-18-1) *See* Alkyl Tin Compounds[d] *at loc. no.* **292**

Dibutyltin dilaurate (77-58-7) *See* Alkyl Tin Compounds[d] *at loc. no.* **292**

2,6-Di-*tert*-butyl-*p*-tolyl-*N*-methylcarbamate (1918-11-2) *See loc. no.* **1231**

Dicamba (and Salts) (1918-00-9) *See loc. no.* **1300**

Dicamba diethanolamine salt *See* Dicamba (and Salts)[b] *at loc. no.* **1300**

Dicamba dimethylamine salt *See* Dicamba (and Salts)[b] *at loc. no.* **1300**

Dicamba monoethanolamine salt *See* Dicamba (and Salts)[b] *at loc. no.* **1300**

Dicamba potassium salt (10007-85-9) *See* Dicamba (and Salts)[b] *at loc. no.* **1300**

1,3-Di(carbamoylthio)-2-(dimethylamino)propane hydrochloride (22042-59-7) *See* Cartap[b] *at loc. no.* **1130**

S-(1,2-Dicarboethoxyethyl)-*O,O*-dimethyldithiophosphate (121-75-5) *See* Malathion[e] *at loc. no.* **1091**

Dichlofenthion (97-17-6) *See loc. no.* **1069**

Dichlofluanid (1085-98-9) *See loc. no.* **1189**

Dichlone (117-80-6) *See loc. no.* **1190**

Dichloralantipyrine (480-30-8) *See* Dichloralphenazone[a] *at loc. no.* **1572**

Dichloralphenazone (480-30-8) *See loc. no.* **1572**

Dichloral Urea (116-52-9) *See loc. no.* **1245**

Dichloramine (3400-09-7) *See* Chloramines[d] *at loc. no.* **22**

Dichloran (99-30-9) *See loc. no.* **1191**

Di-chloricide (106-46-7) *See* p-Dichlorobenzene[a] *at loc. no.* **396**

Dichloricide (106-46-7) *See* p-Dichlorobenzene[a] *at loc. no.* **396**

Dichloroacetic Acid (79-43-6) *See loc. no.* **43**

S-(2,3-Dichloroallyl)diisopropylthiocarbamate (2303-16-4) *See* Di-allate[a] *at loc. no.* **1235**

3,5-Dichloro-4-aminophenol (26271-75-0) *See* Dichloran[b] *at loc. no.* **1191**

3,4-Dichloroaniline (95-76-1) *See* Propanil[b] *at loc. no.* **1283**

3,6-Dichloro-*o*-anisic acid (1918-00-9) *See* Dicamba (and Salts)[a] *at loc. no.* **1300**

1,2-Dichlorobenzene (95-50-1) *See* o-Dichlorobenzene[a] *at loc. no.* **395**

o-Dichlorobenzene (95-50-1) *See loc. no.* **395**

p-Dichlorobenzene (106-46-7) *See loc. no.* **396**

2,6-Dichlorobenzenecarbothioamide (1918-13-4) *See* Chlorthiamid[a] *at loc. no.* **1297**

1,1-Dichloro-2,2-bis(*p*-chlorophenyl)ethane (72-54-8) *See loc. no.* **1009**

1,1-Dichloro-2,2-bis(*p*-ethylphenyl)ethane (72-56-0) *See* Perthane[e] *at loc. no.* **1015**

Dichloro-bis(*p*-ethylphenyl)ethane (72-56-0) *See* Perthane[e] *at loc. no.* **1015**

2,4-Dichloro-6-*o*-chloroanilino-*s*-triazine (101-05-3) *See* Anilazine[a] *at loc. no.* **1170**

4,6-Dichloro-*N*-(2-chlorophenyl) 1,3,5-triazin-2-amine (101-05-3) *See* Anilazine[a] *at loc. no.* **1170**

Dichlorodifluoromethane (75-71-8) *See loc. no.* **348**

5,5′-Dichloro-2,2′-dihydroxydiphenylmethane (97-23-4) *See* Dichlorophen(e)[a] *at loc. no.* **529**

1,4-Dichloro-2,5-dimethoxybenzene (2675-77-6) *See* Chloroneb[a] *at loc. no.* **1184**

1,1-Dichloro-*N*-[(dimethylamino)sulfonyl]-1-fluoro-*N*-phenyl-methanesulfenamide (1085-98-9) *See* Dichlofluanid[a] *at loc. no.* **1189**

1,3-Dichloro-5,5-dimethylhydantoin (118-52-5) *See loc. no.* **93**

3,5-Dichloro-*N*-(1,1-dimethyl-2-propynyl)benzamide (23950-58-5) *See* Pronamide[a] *at loc. no.* **1281**

Dichlorodiphenyldichloroethane (72-54-8) *See* 1,1-Dichloro-2,2-bis(p-chlorophenyl)ethane[a] *at loc. no.* **1009**

Dichloro diphenyl trichloroethane (50-29-3) *See* DDT[a] *at loc. no.* **1007**

1,1-Dichloroethane (75-34-3) *See loc. no.* **365**

1,2-Dichloroethane (107-06-2) *See* Ethylene Dichloride[a] *at loc. no.* **369**

sym-Dichloroethane (107-06-2) *See* Ethylene Dichloride[a] *at loc. no.* **369**

1,1-Dichloroethene (75-35-4) *See* 1,1-Dichloroethylene[a] *at loc. no.* **366**

1,2-Dichloroethene (540-59-0) *See* Acetylene Dichloride[a] *at loc. no.* **361**

1,1-Dichloroethylene (75-35-4) *See loc. no.* **366**

1,2-Dichloroethylene (540-59-0) *See* Acetylene Dichloride[a] *at loc. no.* **361**

sym-Dichloroethylene (540-59-0) *See* Acetylene Dichloride[a] *at loc. no.* **361**

β,β′-Dichloroethyl ether (111-44-4) *See* sym.-Dichloroethyl Ether[a] *at loc. no.* **470**

sym-Dichloroethyl Ether (111-44-4) *See loc. no.* **470**

Dichlorofluoromethane (75-43-4) *See* Dichloromonofluoromethane[a] *at loc. no.* **349**

N′-Dichlorofluoromethylthio-*N,N*-dimethyl-*N*′-phenylsulfamide (1085-98-9) *See* Dichlofluanid[a] *at loc. no.* **1189**

Dichlorohydrin (96-23-1) *See* 1,3-Dichloro-2-propanol[a] *at loc. no.* **433**

Di-(5-chloro-2-hydroxyphenyl)methane (97-23-4) *See* Dichlorophen(e)[a] *at loc. no.* **529**

---

[a] A Synonym   [b] A Closely Related Substance   [c] The Active or Major Constituent   [d] A Class Name
[e] A Specific Example of or Product Containing

Ingredient name (CAS registry no.) *See* Primary Name *at location no.* **XXX** *in Part D of this section*

Dichloroisocyanurates *See* Trichloroisocyanuric Acid[b] *at loc. no.* **94**

Dichloroisocyanuric acid (2782-57-2) *See* Trichloroisocyanuric Acid[b] *at loc. no.* **94**

Dichloroisopropyl alcohol (96-23-1) *See* 1,3-Dichloro-2-propanol[a] *at loc. no.* **433**

Dichloromethane (75-09-2) *See* Methylene Chloride[a] *at loc. no.* **359**

3,6-Dichloro-2-methoxybenzoic acid (1918-00-9) *See* Dicamba (and Salts)[a] *at loc. no.* **1300**

2,5-Dichloro-4-methoxyphenol *See* Chloroneb[b] *at loc. no.* **1184**

3′,4′-Dichloro-2-methylacrylanilide (2164-09-2) *See* Propanil[b] *at loc. no.* **1283**

Dichloromonofluoromethane (75-43-4) *See loc. no.* **349**

2,3-Dichloro-1,4-naphthoquinone (117-80-6) *See* Dichlone[a] *at loc. no.* **1190**

2,6-Dichloro-4-nitroaniline (99-30-9) *See* Dichloran[a] *at loc. no.* **1191**

1,1-Dichloro-1-nitroethane (594-72-9) *See loc. no.* **20**

Dichlorophen(e) (97-23-4) *See loc. no.* **529**

2,4-Dichlorophenol (120-83-2) *See* Chlorophenols[d] *at loc. no.* **525**

2,4-Dichlorophenol benzenesulfonate (97-16-5) *See* Genite[e] *at loc. no.* **1046**

2,4-Dichlorophenoxyacetic acid (94-75-7) *See* 2,4-D[a] *at loc. no.* **1212**

4-(2,4-Dichlorophenoxy)butyric Acid (94-82-6) *See loc. no.* **1215**

2-(2,4-Dichlorophenoxy)ethanol phosphite (94-84-8) *See* Falone[e] *at loc. no.* **1306**

2,4-Dichlorophenoxyethyl sulfate sodium (136-78-7) *See* 2-(2,4-Dichlorophenoxy)ethyl Sulfate Sodium Salt[a] *at loc. no.* **1216**

2-(2,4-Dichlorophenoxy)ethyl Sulfate Sodium Salt (136-78-7) *See loc. no.* **1216**

Di(p-chlorophenoxy)methane (555-89-5) *See* Neotran[e] *at loc. no.* **1014**

2-(4-(2′,4′-Dichlorophenoxy)-phenoxy)-methyl-propionate (51338-27-3) *See* Diclofop-methyl[a] *at loc. no.* **1301**

2-(2,4-Dichlorophenoxy)propionic Acid (120-36-5) *See loc. no.* **1217**

2,4-Dichlorophenyl benzenesulfonate (97-16-5) *See* Genite[e] *at loc. no.* **1046**

O-(2,4-Dichlorophenyl)-O,O-diethyl phosphorothioate (97-17-6) *See* Dichlofenthion[a] *at loc. no.* **1069**

3-(3,4-Dichlorophenyl)-1,1-dimethylurea (330-54-1) *See* Diuron[a] *at loc. no.* **1247**

2,6-Dichloro-p-phenylenediamine (609-20-1) *See* Dichloran[b] *at loc. no.* **1191**

Di-(p-chlorophenyl)ethanol (80-06-8) *See* DMC[a] *at loc. no.* **1011**

Di(1-chlorophenyl)ethyl carbinol *See* DMC[b] *at loc. no.* **1011**

3-(3,5-Dichlorophenyl)-N-isopropyl-2,4-dioxoimidazolidine-1-carboxamide (36734-19-7) *See* Iprodione[a] *at loc. no.* **1197**

N-(3,4-Dichlorophenyl)-methacrylamide (2164-09-2) *See* Propanil[b] *at loc. no.* **1283**

3-(3,4-Dichlorophenyl)-1-methoxy-1-methylurea *See* Linuron[a] *at loc. no.* **1251**

Di(p-chlorophenyl)methyl carbinol (80-06-8) *See* DMC[a] *at loc. no.* **1011**

O-(2,4-Dichlorophenyl)-O-methyl isopropylphosphoramidothioate (299-85-4) *See* Zytron[e] *at loc. no.* **1105**

2,4-Dichlorophenyl p-nitrophenyl ether (1836-75-5) *See* Nitrofen[a] *at loc. no.* **1310**

N-(3,4-Dichlorophenyl)propanamide (709-98-8) *See* Propanil[a] *at loc. no.* **1283**

1,2-Dichloropropane (78-87-5) *See* Propylene Dichloride[a] *at loc. no.* **391**

1,3-Dichloro-2-propanol (96-23-1) *See loc. no.* **433**

1,3-Dichloro-2-propanone (534-07-6) *See* Tris(1,3-dichloro-2-propyl)phosphate[b] *at loc. no.* **1119**

1,2-Dichloropropene *See* 1,3-Dichloropropene[b] *at loc. no.* **386**

1,3-Dichloropropene (542-75-6) *See loc. no.* **386**

Dichloropropenes *See loc. no.* **383**

3′,4′-Dichloropropionanilide (709-98-8) *See* Propanil[a] *at loc. no.* **1283**

α,α-Dichloropropionic acid (75-99-0) *See* Dalapon[a] *at loc. no.* **1299**

2,2-Dichloropropionic acid sodium salt (127-20-8) *See* Dalapon[b] *at loc. no.* **1299**

1,3-Dichloropropylene (542-75-6) *See* 1,3-Dichloropropene[a] *at loc. no.* **386**

1,2-Dichloro-1,1,2,2-tetrafluoroethane (76-14-2) *See loc. no.* **352**

2,6-Dichlorothiobenzamide (1918-13-4) *See* Chlorthiamid[a] *at loc. no.* **1297**

Dichloro-s-triazinetrione (2782-57-2) *See* Trichloroisocyanuric Acid[b] *at loc. no.* **94**

4,4′-Dichloro-α-(trichloromethyl)benzhydrol (115-32-2) *See* Kelthane[e] *at loc. no.* **1012**

2,2-Dichlorovinyldimethyl phosphate (62-73-7) *See* Dichlorvos[a] *at loc. no.* **1053**

Dichlorprop (120-36-5) *See* 2-(2,4-Dichlorophenoxy)-propionic Acid[a] *at loc. no.* **1217**

Dichlorvos (62-73-7) *See loc. no.* **1053**

Dichromate Salts (Soluble) *See loc. no.* **82**

Diclofop-methyl (51338-27-3) *See loc. no.* **1301**

Dicofol (115-32-2) *See* Kelthane[a] *at loc. no.* **1012**

Dicoumarol (66-76-2) *See* Bishydroxycoumarin[a] *at loc. no.* **1334**

Dicresyl *See* MPMC[b] *at loc. no.* **1143**

Dicryl (2164-09-2) *See* Propanil[b] *at loc. no.* **1283**

Dicumarin (66-76-2) *See* Bishydroxycoumarin[a] *at loc. no.* **1334**

Dicumarol (66-76-2) *See* Bishydroxycoumarin[c] *at loc. no.* **1334**

Dicuran (15545-48-9) *See* Neburon[b] *at loc. no.* **1254**

o-Dicyanobenzene (91-15-6) *See* Phthalonitrile[a] *at loc. no.* **651**

Dicyclohexylamine (101-83-7) *See loc. no.* **608**

Dicyclohexylamine 4,6-Dinitro-o-cyclohexylphenate (317-83-9) *See loc. no.* **536**

Dicyclohexylamine Nitrite (3129-91-7) *See loc. no.* **632**

Dicyclohexylammonium 2-cyclohexyl-4,6-dinitrophenate (317-83-9) *See* Dicyclohexylamine 4,6-Dinitro-o-cyclohexylphenate[a] *at loc. no.* **536**

Dicyclohexyl ammonium nitrate (3882-06-2) *See* Cationic Surfactants[d] *at loc. no.* **974**

Didecyl dimethyl ammonium chloride (7173-51-5) *See* Dialkyl Dimethyl Ammonium Chloride[d] *at loc. no.* **989**

Didrex (1027-30-1) *See* Benzphetamine Hydrochloride[c] *at loc. no.* **1445**

Dieldrin (60-57-1) *See loc. no.* **1020**

Dienestrol (84-17-3) *See* Estrogens (Natural and Synthetic)[d] *at loc. no.* **916**

Dienochlor (2227-17-0) *See loc. no.* **1027**

Diesel fuel *See* Diesel Oil[a] *at loc. no.* **325**

Diesel Oil *See loc. no.* **325**

Diethanolamine (and Salts) (111-42-2) *See loc. no.* **65**

Diethanolamine dinoseb *See* Dinoseb[b] *at loc. no.* **543**

---

[a] A Synonym   [b] A Closely Related Substance   [c] The Active or Major Constituent   [d] A Class Name   [e] A Specific Example of or Product Containing

Ingredient name (CAS registry no.) *See* Primary Name *at*
location no. **XXX** *in Part D of this section*

Diethanolamine hydrochloride *See* Diethanolamine (and Salts)*[d]* *at loc. no.* **65**

Diethanolamine 2-methyl-4-chlorophenoxyacetate *See* MCPA*[b]* *at loc. no.* **1220**

Diethanolamine salt of maleic hydrazide (17655-22-0) *See* Maleic Hydrazide*[c]* *at loc. no.* **1308**

1,1-Diethoxyethane (105-57-7) *See* Acetal*[a]* *at loc. no.* **465**

Diethylacetal (105-57-7) *See* Acetal*[a]* *at loc. no.* **465**

N,N-Diethylacrylamide (2675-94-7) *See* Acrylamide*[b]* *at loc. no.* **1624**

2-(Diethylamino)-*N*-(2,6-dimethylphenyl)acetamide (137-58-6) *See* Lidocaine*[a]* *at loc. no.* **1582**

6-(2-Diethylaminoethoxy)-2-dimethylaminobenzothiazole dihydrochloride (136-96-9) *See* Diamthazole Dihydrochloride*[a]* *at loc. no.* **1525**

2-Diethylaminoethyl *p*-aminobenzoate (59-46-1) *See* Procaine*[a]* *at loc. no.* **1585**

β-Diethylaminoethyl benzilate (302-40-9) *See* Benactyzine*[a]* *at loc. no.* **1430**

2-(Diethylamino)-4-(isopropylamino)-6-methoxy-*s*-triazine (3004-70-1) *See* Terbumeton*[b]* *at loc. no.* **1270**

5,5-Diethylbarbituric acid (57-44-3) *See* Barbital*[a]* *at loc. no.* **1366**

Diethylcarbamazine (90-89-1) *See loc. no.* **1539**

1-Diethylcarbamyl-4-methylpiperazine (90-89-1) *See* Diethylcarbamazine*[a]* *at loc. no.* **1539**

O,O-Diethyl *O*-3-chloro-4-methyl-2-oxo-2*H*-1-benzopyran-7-yl-phosphorothioate (56-72-4) *See* Coumaphos*[e]* *at loc. no.* **1066**

O,O-Diethyl *S*-*p*-chlorophenylthiomethyl dithiophosphate (786-19-6) *See* Carbophenothion*[a]* *at loc. no.* **1083**

O,O-Diethyl *S*-*p*-chlorophenylthiomethyl phosphorodithioate (786-19-6) *See* Carbophenothion*[a]* *at loc. no.* **1083**

Diethyl 2-Chlorovinyl Phosphate (311-47-7) *See loc. no.* **1054**

O,O-Diethyl-*S*-(β-diethylamino)ethyl phosphorothioate (78-53-5) *See* Tetram*[e]* *at loc. no.* **1080**

N³,N³-Diethyl-2,4-dinitro-6-(trifluoromethyl)-1,3-benzenediamine (29091-05-2) *See* Dinitramine*[a]* *at loc. no.* **1288**

N³,N³-Diethyl-2,4-dinitro-6-(trifluoromethyl)-*m*-phenylenediamine (29091-05-2) *See* Dinitramine*[a]* *at loc. no.* **1288**

Diethyl diphenyl dichloroethane (72-56-0) *See* Perthane*[e]* *at loc. no.* **1015**

Diethyl Dithiobis(thionoformate) (502-55-6) *See loc. no.* **1302**

Diethylenediamine (110-85-0) *See* Piperazine*[a]* *at loc. no.* **1544**

1,4-Diethylene dioxide (123-91-1) *See* Dioxane*[a]* *at loc. no.* **1621**

Diethylene dioxide (123-91-1) *See* Dioxane*[a]* *at loc. no.* **1621**

Diethylene ether (123-91-1) *See* Dioxane*[a]* *at loc. no.* **1621**

Diethylene Glycol (111-46-6) *See loc. no.* **437**

Diethylene Glycol Abietate (10107-99-0) *See loc. no.* **448**

Diethylene glycol dalapon *See* Dalapon*[b]* *at loc. no.* **1299**

Diethylene glycol dimethacrylate (2358-84-1) *See* Acrylic Resin Monomers*[d]* *at loc. no.* **1625**

Diethylene Glycol Mono- and Di- Esters *See loc. no.* **449**

Diethylene glycol monobutyl ether (112-34-5) *See* Butyl Carbitol*[a]* *at loc. no.* **452**

Diethylene glycol monoethyl ether (111-90-0) *See* Carbitol*[a]* *at loc. no.* **455**

Diethylene glycol monoethyl ether esters *See* Carbitol Esters*[e]* *at loc. no.* **447**

Diethylene glycol monomethyl ether (111-77-3) *See* Carbitol*[b]* *at loc. no.* **455**

Diethyleneimide oxide (110-91-8) *See* Morpholine*[a]* *at loc. no.* **72**

Diethylene oxide (109-99-9) *See* Tetrahydrofuran*[a]* *at loc. no.* **1623**

Diethylenetriamine (111-40-0) *See loc. no.* **603**

Diethylenetriaminepentaacetic acid (67-43-6) *See* Edetate Calcium Disodium*[b]* *at loc. no.* **1504**

Diethylethanolamine salt of 2,4,5-T *See* Trichlorophenoxyacetic Acid*[b]* *at loc. no.* **1224**

Diethyl ether (60-29-7) *See* Ethyl ether*[a]* *at loc. no.* **472**

Diethyl-*O*-(2-ethylmercaptoethyl)thiophosphate (298-03-3) *See* Demeton*[e]* *at loc. no.* **1067**

O,O-Diethyl (*S*-ethylmercaptomethyl)dithiophosphate (298-02-2) *See* Phorate*[a]* *at loc. no.* **1094**

O,O-Diethyl *S*-2-(ethylthio)ethyl phosphorodithioate (298-04-4) *See* Disulfoton*[a]* *at loc. no.* **1086**

O,O-Diethyl *O*-[2-(ethylthio)ethyl]phosphorothioate (298-03-3) *See* Demeton*[e]* *at loc. no.* **1067**

O,O-Diethyl *S*-[2-(ethylthio)ethyl]phosphorothioate (126-75-0) *See* Demeton*[e]* *at loc. no.* **1067**

O,O-Diethyl *S*-(ethylthiomethyl)phosphorodithioate (298-02-2) *See* Phorate*[a]* *at loc. no.* **1094**

Di-2-ethylhexyl Phthalate (117-81-7) *See loc. no.* **591**

O,O-Diethyl *O*-(2-isopropyl-4-methyl-6-pyrimidyl)phosphorothioate (333-41-5) *See* Diazinon*[e]* *at loc. no.* **1068**

Diethyl Isopropylthiomethyl Dithiophosphate (78-52-4) *See loc. no.* **1084**

O,O-Diethyl-*S*-(isopropylthiomethyl)phosphorodithioate (78-52-4) *See* Diethyl Isopropylthiomethyl Dithiophosphate*[a]* *at loc. no.* **1084**

Diethylmalonylurea (57-44-3) *See* Barbital*[a]* *at loc. no.* **1366**

5,5-Diethyl-1-methylbarbituric acid (50-11-3) *See* Metharbital*[a]* *at loc. no.* **1379**

3,3-Diethyl-5-methyl-2,4-piperidinedione (125-64-4) *See* Methyprylon*[a]* *at loc. no.* **1441**

O,O-Diethyl-*O*-(3-methyl-5-pyrazolyl) phosphate (108-34-9) *See* Pyrazoxon*[e]* *at loc. no.* **1059**

O,O-Diethyl-*O*-3-methyl-5-pyrazolyl phosphorothioate (108-35-0) *See* Pyrazothion*[e]* *at loc. no.* **1059**

N,N-Diethyl-2-(1-naphthalenyloxy)propionamide (15299-99-7) *See* Napropamide*[b]* *at loc. no.* **1278**

O,O-Diethyl *O*-*p*-nitrophenyl phosphate (311-45-5) *See* Paraoxon*[a]* *at loc. no.* **1056**

O,O-Diethyl *O*-*p*-nitrophenyl phosphorothioate (56-38-2) *See* Parathion*[a]* *at loc. no.* **1077**

Diethyl-*p*-nitrophenyl thiophosphate (56-38-2) *See* Parathion*[a]* *at loc. no.* **1077**

3,5-Diethylphenyl-*N*-methylcarbamate (30087-47-9) *See* Butacarb*[b]* *at loc. no.* **1126**

Diethyl phthalate (84-66-2) *See* Ethyl Phthalate*[a]* *at loc. no.* **592**

Diethylpropion (90-84-6) *See loc. no.* **1447**

O,O-Diethyl-*O*-[2-*n*-propyl-4-methyl-6-pyrimidyl] phosphorothioate (5826-91-5) *See* Diethyl Propylmethylpyrimidyl Thiophosphate*[a]* *at loc. no.* **1070**

Diethyl Propylmethylpyrimidyl Thiophosphate (5826-91-5) *See loc. no.* **1070**

O,O-Diethyl *O*-2-pyrazinyl phosphorothioate (297-97-2) *See* Thionazin*[a]* *at loc. no.* **1081**

Diethylstilbestrol (56-53-1) *See* Estrogens (Natural and Synthetic)*[d]* *at loc. no.* **916**

Diethyltin dichloride (866-55-7) *See* Alkyl Tin Compounds*[d]* *at loc. no.* **292**

N,N-Diethyl-*m*-toluamide (134-62-3) *See loc. no.* **1326**

N,N-Diethyl-*o*-toluamide *See N,N*-Diethyl-*m*-toluamide*[b]* *at loc. no.* **1326**

---

[a] A Synonym   *[b]* A Closely Related Substance   *[c]* The Active or Major Constituent   *[d]* A Class Name
[e] A Specific Example of or Product Containing

Ingredient name (CAS registry no.) *See* Primary Name *at
location no.* **XXX** *in Part D of this section*

N,N-Diethyl-*p*-toluamide *See N,N*-Diethyl-*m*-toluamide[b] *at
loc. no.* **1326**

O,O-Diethyl-*O*-(3,5,6-trichloro-2-pyridyl)phosphoro-
thioate (2921-88-2) *See* Chlorpyrifos[a] *at loc. no.* **1064**

Diethyltryptamine (61-51-8) *See N,N*-Dimethyltryptamine[b]
at loc. no. **1448**

Diethyl xanthogen disulfide (502-55-6) *See* Diethyl Di-
thiobis(thionoformate)[a] *at loc. no.* **1302**

Difenoxuron (14214-32-5) *See* Phenobenzuron[b] *at loc. no.*
1256

Difenzoquat (49866-87-7) *See* Paraquat[b] *at loc. no.* **1286**

Diflubenzuron (35367-38-5) *See loc. no.* **1246**

Difluorodichloromethane (75-71-8) *See* Dichlorodifluoromethane[a] *at loc. no.* **348**

Difluorodiphenyltrichloroethane (475-26-3) *See* DFDT[a] *at
loc. no.* **1008**

Difolatan (2425-06-1) *See* Captafol[a] *at loc. no.* **1180**

Difolatan-Botran *See* Captafol[c] *at loc. no.* **1180**

Digalen (8031-69-4) *See loc. no.* **836**

Digifolin (8001-33-0) *See loc. no.* **837**

Digilanide C (17575-22-3) *See* Lanatoside(s)[d] *at loc. no.* **841**

Digilanids *See* Lanatoside(s)[d] *at loc. no.* **841**

Digitalin (752-61-4) *See* Digitoxin[b] *at loc. no.* **838**

Digitaline *See* Digitoxin[a] *at loc. no.* **838**

Digitalis *See loc. no.* **666**

Digitalis lanata *See* Lanatoside(s)[c] *at loc. no.* **841**

Digitalis purpurea *See* Digitalis[d] *at loc. no.* **666**

Digitoxin (71-63-6) *See loc. no.* **838**

Diglycidyl ether of bisphenol A (1675-54-3) *See* Glycidyl
Ethers[d] *at loc. no.* **1629**

Diglycidyl ethers *See* Glycidyl Ethers[d] *at loc. no.* **1629**

Diglycol *derivative. See corresponding* Diethylene Glycol
derivative in this index.

Digoxin (20830-75-5) *See loc. no.* **839**

Dihydrocodeinone bitartrate (34195-34-1) *See* Hydrocodone Bitartrate[a] *at loc. no.* **783**

9,10-Dihydro-8α,10α-diazoniaphenanthrene dibromide
(85-00-7) *See* Diquat Dibromide[e] *at loc. no.* **1285**

2,3-Dihydro-2,2-dimethyl-7-benzofuranyl methylcarbamate (1563-66-2) *See* Carbofuran[a] *at loc. no.* **1129**

1,2-Dihydro-1,5-dimethyl-2-phenyl-3*H*-pyrazol-3-one
See Antipyrine[a] *at loc. no.* **1571**

Dihydroergotamine (511-12-6) *See* Ergot[d] *at loc. no.* **667**

1,2-Dihydro-6-ethoxy-2,2,4-trimethylquinoline (91-53-2)
See Ethoxyquin[a] *at loc. no.* **1615**

Dihydrohydroxycodeinone (76-42-6) *See* Oxycodone[a] *at
loc. no.* **789**

Dihydrohydroxymorphinone (76-41-5) *See* Oxymorphone[a]
at loc. no. **790**

3-((4,5-Dihydro-1*H*-imidazol-2-yl)methyl)-6-(1,1-di-
methyl ethyl)-2,4-dimethyl phenol (2315-02-8) *See* Oxymetazoline Hydrochloride[a] *at loc. no.* **1464**

2,3-Dihydro-2-methyl-7-benzofuranyl methylcarbamate *See* Carbofuran[a] *at loc. no.* **1129**

5,6-Dihydro-2-methyl-3-(phenylcarbamoyl)-4*H*-pyrane
See Pyracarbolid[a] *at loc. no.* **1204**

5,6-Dihydro-2-methyl-*N*-phenyl-1,4-oxathiin-3-carbox-
amide (5234-68-4) *See* Carboxin[a] *at loc. no.* **1182**

3,4-Dihydro-(6-methyl)-2*H*-pyran-5-carboxanilide *See*
Pyracarbolid[a] *at loc. no.* **1204**

Dihydromorphinone Hydrochloride (71-68-1) *See loc. no.*
781

2,3-Dihydro-3-oxobenzisosulfonazole (81-07-2) *See* Saccharin[a] *at loc. no.* **1616**

1,2-Dihydro-3,6-pyridazinedione (123-33-1) *See* Maleic
Hydrazide[a] *at loc. no.* **1308**

Dihydrorotenone (6659-45-6) *See loc. no.* **888**

Dihydrosafrole (94-58-6) *See loc. no.* **862**

Dihydroxyacetone (96-26-4) *See loc. no.* **471**

1,2-Dihydroxyanthraquinone (72-48-0) *See* Alizarin[a] *at loc.
no.* **921**

1,8-Dihydroxyanthraquinone (117-10-2) *See* Cascara Sagrada[b] *at loc. no.* **660**

1,4-Dihydroxybenzene (123-31-9) *See* Hydroquinone[a] *at loc.
no.* **504**

Dihydroxybenzene *See loc. no.* **501**

m-Dihydroxybenzene (108-46-3) *See* Resorcinol[a] *at loc. no.*
508

o-Dihydroxybenzene (120-80-9) *See* Pyrocatechol[a] *at loc.
no.* **505**

p-Dihydroxybenzene (123-31-9) *See* Hydroquinone[a] *at loc.
no.* **504**

Dihydroxydichlorodiphenylmethane (97-23-4) *See* Dich-
lorophen(e)[a] *at loc. no.* **529**

β,β′-Dihydroxydiethyl ether (111-46-6) *See* Diethylene Glycol[a] *at loc. no.* **437**

1,3-Dihydroxydimethyl ketone (96-26-4) *See* Dihydroxyacetone[a] *at loc. no.* **471**

7-(2,3-Dihydroxypropyl)theophylline (479-18-5) *See* Dyphylline[a] *at loc. no.* **804**

Diiodohydroxyquin (83-73-8) *See loc. no.* **1513**

Diiodohydroxyquinoline (83-73-8) *See* Diiodohydroxyquin[a]
at loc. no. **1513**

Diiodomethane (75-11-6) *See* Methylene Iodide[a] *at loc. no.*
360

2,6-Diiodo-4-nitrophenol (305-85-1) *See loc. no.* **537**

Diisobutyl cresoxy ethoxy ethyl dimethyl benzyl ammonium chloride monohydrate *See* Methylbenzethonium Chloride[a] *at loc. no.* **992**

p-Diisobutyl phenoxyethoxyethyl dimethyl benzyl ammonium chloride (121-54-0) *See* Benzethonium Chloride[a] *at loc. no.* **986**

Diisopropanolamine 2-methyl-4-chlorophenoxyacetate
See MCPA[b] *at loc. no.* **1220**

Diisopropyl ammonium nitrate *See* Cationic Surfactants[d]
at loc. no. **974**

N-(β-*O,O*-Diisopropyldithiophosphoryl-ethyl)-benzene
sulfonamide (741-58-2) *See* Bensulide[a] *at loc. no.* **1082**

Diisopropyl Fluorophosphate (55-91-4) *See loc. no.* **1096**

2,2-Diisopropyl-4-methanol-1,3-dioxolane (470-43-9) *See*
Promoxolane[a] *at loc. no.* **1411**

S(*O,O*-Diisopropyl phosphorodithioate) of *N*-(2-mercap-
toethyl) benzenesulfonamide (741-58-2) *See* Bensulide[a]
at loc. no. **1082**

Diisopropyl phosphorofluoridate (55-91-4) *See* Diisopropyl Fluorophosphate[a] *at loc. no.* **1096**

Dilan (8002-82-2) *See loc. no.* **1010**

Dilantin (57-41-0) *See* Phenytoin Sodium[e] *at loc. no.* **1609**

Dilaudid (71-68-1) *See* Dihydromorphinone Hydrochloride[c]
at loc. no. **781**

Dimecron (297-99-4) *See* Phosphamidon[c] *at loc. no.* **1058**

Dimefox (115-26-4) *See loc. no.* **1098**

Dimelone (117-24-8) *See* Dimethyl Carbate[c] *at loc. no.* **1327**

Dimenhydrinate (523-87-5) *See* Diphenhydramine Hydrochloride[b] *at loc. no.* **1492**

Di-1-*p*-menthene *See loc. no.* **878**

Dimercaprol (59-52-9) *See* BAL[a] *at loc. no.* **1503**

2,3-Dimercapto-1-propanol (59-52-9) *See* BAL[a] *at loc. no.*
1503

Dimet (144-21-8) *See* Disodium Methanearsonate[c] *at loc. no.*
203

Dimetan (122-15-6) *See loc. no.* **1131**

---

[a] A Synonym   [b] A Closely Related Substance   [c] The Active or Major Constituent   [d] A Class Name
[e] A Specific Example of or Product Containing

Ingredient name (CAS registry no.) *See* Primary Name *at location no.* **XXX** *in Part D of this section*

[a] A Synonym　　[b] A Closely Related Substance　　[c] The Active or Major Constituent　　[d] A Class Name
[e] A Specific Example of or Product Containing

Ingredient name (CAS registry no.) *See* Primary Name *at*
location no. **XXX** *in Part D of this section*

N-(3,4-Dimethyl-5-isoxazolyl)sulfanilamide *See* Sulfisoxazole[a] *at loc. no.* **1568**

Dimethyl ketone (67-64-1) *See* Acetone[a] *at loc. no.* **466**

N,*N*-Dimethyllinoleylamine salt of 2,4,5-T *See* Trichlorophenoxyacetic Acid[b] *at loc. no.* **1224**

O,*O*-Dimethyl *S*-(*N*-methylcarbamoylmethyl)phosphorodithioate (60-51-5) *See* Dimethoate[a] *at loc. no.* **1085**

N,*N*-Dimethyl-2-(*o*-methyl-α-phenylbenzyloxy)ethylamine (83-98-7) *See* Orphenadrine[a] *at loc. no.* **1496**

1,1-Dimethyl-3-(3-methylphenyl)thiourea *See* Phenobenzuron[a] *at loc. no.* **1256**

2,2-Dimethyl-3-(2-methylpropenyl)cyclopropanecarboxylic acid (10453-89-1) *See* Pyrethroids[d] *at loc. no.* **894**

O,*O*-Dimethyl *O*-(4-(methylthio)-*m*-tolyl)phosphorothioate (55-38-9) *See* Fenthion[a] *at loc. no.* **1073**

O,*O*-Dimethyl *O*-(*p*-nitrophenyl)thiophosphate (298-00-0) *See* Methyl Parathion[a] *at loc. no.* **1076**

O,*O*-Dimethyl *O*-(4-nitro-*m*-tolyl)-phosphorothioate (122-14-5) *See* Fenitrothion[a] *at loc. no.* **1072**

N,*N*-Dimethyloleylamine salt of 2,4,5-T *See* Trichlorophenoxyacetic Acid[b] *at loc. no.* **1224**

N,*N*-Dimethyl oleyl-linoleyl amine salt of 2,4,5-T *See* Trichlorophenoxyacetic Acid[b] *at loc. no.* **1224**

O,*O*-Dimethyl *S*-(4-oxobenzotriazino-3-methyl) phosphorodithioate (86-50-0) *See* Guthion[e] *at loc. no.* **1089**

5,5′-Dimethyl-3-oxo-1-cyclohexen-1-yl dimethylcarbamate (122-15-6) *See* Dimetan[e] *at loc. no.* **1131**

Dimethyl parathion (298-00-0) *See* Methyl Parathion[a] *at loc. no.* **1076**

Dimethylphenol (1300-71-6) *See* Xylenol[a] *at loc. no.* **498**

5-((3,5-Dimethylphenoxy)methyl)-2-oxazolidinone (1665-48-1) *See* Metaxalone[a] *at loc. no.* **1408**

Dimethylphenylamine (121-69-7) *See* Dimethylaniline[a] *at loc. no.* **615**

N′-(2,4-Dimethylphenyl)-*N*-(2,4-dimethylphenyl)iminomethyl-*N*-methylmethanimidamide (33089-61-1) *See* Amitraz[a] *at loc. no.* **1039**

Dimethyl 4,4′-*o*-phenylenebis(3-thioallophanate) (23564-05-8) *See* Thiophanate-methyl[a] *at loc. no.* **1207**

N-(2,6-Dimethylphenyl)-2-(ethylpropylamino) butanamide (36637-18-0) *See* Etidocaine[a] *at loc. no.* **1581**

3,4-Dimethylphenyl-*N*-methylcarbamate (2425-10-7) *See* MPMC[a] *at loc. no.* **1143**

3,4-Dimethyl-2-phenylmorpholine bitartrate (634-03-7) *See* Phenmetrazine[b] *at loc. no.* **1466**

2,3-Dimethyl-1-phenyl-3-pyrazolin-5-one (60-80-0) *See* Antipyrine[a] *at loc. no.* **1571**

1,1-Dimethyl-3-phenylurea (101-42-8) *See* Fenuron[a] *at loc. no.* **1248**

Dimethyl phosphate of alpha-methylbenzyl 3-hydroxy-*cis*-crotonate (7700-17-6) *See* Bidrin[b] *at loc. no.* **1051**

Dimethyl phosphate of 3-hydroxy-*N*,*N*-dimethyl-*cis*-crotonamide (141-66-2) *See* Bidrin[e] *at loc. no.* **1051**

Dimethyl phosphate of α-methylbenzyl 3-hydroxy-*cis*-crotonate (7700-17-6) *See* Bidrin[b] *at loc. no.* **1051**

O,*S*-Dimethyl phosphoramidothioate (10265-92-6) *See* Monitor[a] *at loc. no.* **1101**

Dimethyl phthalate (131-11-3) *See* Methyl Phthalate[a] *at loc. no.* **593**

O,*O*-Dimethyl-*S*-phthalimidomethyl phosphorodithioate (732-11-6) *See* Imidan[e] *at loc. no.* **1090**

Dimethyl polysiloxane (9006-65-9) *See* Silicone Oil[a] *at loc. no.* **1646**

N-(1,2-Dimethylpropyl)-*N*′-ethyl-6-(methylthio)-1,3,5-triazine-2,4-diamine (22936-75-0) *See* Prometon[b] *at loc. no.* **1267**

*N*¹-(4,6-Dimethyl-2-pyrimidinyl)sulfanilamide (57-68-1) *See* Sulfamethazine[a] *at loc. no.* **1559**

6,7-Dimethyl-9-*D*-ribitylisoalloxazine (83-88-5) *See* Riboflavin[a] *at loc. no.* **913**

N,*N*-Dimethylserotonin (487-93-4) *See* Bufotenine[a] *at loc. no.* **820**

3,4-Dimethyl-5-sulfanil-amidoisoxazole *See* Sulfisoxazole[a] *at loc. no.* **1568**

Dimethyl sulfide (75-18-3) *See* Methanethiol[b] *at loc. no.* **116**

Dimethyl Sulfoxide (67-68-5) *See loc. no.* **1620**

Dimethyl-2,3,5,6-tetrachloroterephthalate (1861-32-1) *See loc. no.* **1303**

3,5-Dimethyl-1,3,5,2*H*-tetrahydrothiadiazine-2-thione (533-74-4) *See* Dazomet[a] *at loc. no.* **1186**

N,*N*-Dimethyl-*N*′-(2-thenyl)-*N*′-(2-pyridyl)-ethylenediamine hydrochloride (135-23-9) *See* Methapyrilene Hydrochloride[a] *at loc. no.* **1495**

O,*O*-Dimethyl-2,2,2-trichloro-1-*n*-butyryloxyethylphosphonate (126-22-7) *See* Butonate[a] *at loc. no.* **1060**

Dimethyl trichlorohydroxyethylphosphonate (52-68-6) *See* Trichlorfon[a] *at loc. no.* **1062**

O,*O*-Dimethyl *O*-(2,4,5-trichlorophenyl) phosphorothioate (299-84-3) *See* Ronnel[a] *at loc. no.* **1079**

1,1-Dimethyl-3-(α,α,α-trifluoro-*m*-tolyl)urea *See* Fluometuron[a] *at loc. no.* **1249**

N,*N*-Dimethyltryptamine (61-50-7) *See loc. no.* **1448**

m-(3,3-Dimethylureido)phenyl *tert*-butylcarbamate (4849-32-5) *See* Karbutilate[a] *at loc. no.* **1232**

1,3-Dimethylxanthine (58-55-9) *See* Theophylline[a] *at loc. no.* **802**

3,7-Dimethylxanthine (83-67-0) *See* Theobromine[a] *at loc. no.* **801**

Dimethylyn (470-43-9) *See* Promoxolane[e] *at loc. no.* **1411**

Dimetilan (644-64-4) *See loc. no.* **1132**

Dimexano (1468-37-7) *See* Diethyl Dithiobis(thionoformate)[b] *at loc. no.* **1302**

Dimilin (35367-38-5) *See* Diflubenzuron[c] *at loc. no.* **1246**

Dimite (80-06-8) *See* DMC[c] *at loc. no.* **1011**

Dinex (131-89-5) *See* 4,6-Dinitro-*o*-cyclohexylphenol[c] *at loc. no.* **540**

Dinitolmide (148-01-6) *See loc. no.* **1540**

Dinitramine (29091-05-2) *See loc. no.* **1288**

4,6-Dinitro-2-*sec*-amyl phenol (4097-36-3) *See* 4,6-Dinitro-*o*-amylphenol[a] *at loc. no.* **538**

4,6-Dinitro-*o*-amylphenol (4097-36-3) *See loc. no.* **538**

Dinitro-*o-sec*-amyl phenol (4097-36-3) *See* 4,6-Dinitro-*o*-amylphenol[a] *at loc. no.* **538**

3,5-Dinitrobenzamide (121-81-3) *See* Dinitolmide[b] *at loc. no.* **1540**

Dinitrobenzene (25154-54-5) *See loc. no.* **640**

4,6-Dinitro-2-*sec*-butyl phenol (88-85-7) *See* Dinoseb[a] *at loc. no.* **543**

Dinitro-*o*-butyl phenol (88-85-7) *See* Dinoseb[a] *at loc. no.* **543**

Dinitrobutylphenol (88-85-7) *See* Dinoseb[a] *at loc. no.* **543**

Dinitrocellulose (50935-18-7) *See* Collodion[e] *at loc. no.* **854**

Dinitrochlorobenzene (97-00-7) *See* 1-Chloro-2,4-dinitrobenzene[a] *at loc. no.* **639**

4,6-Dinitro-*o*-cresol (534-52-1) *See loc. no.* **539**

Dinitrocresol (534-52-1) *See* 4,6-Dinitro-*o*-cresol[a] *at loc. no.* **539**

2,4-Dinitro-6-cyclohexylphenol (131-89-5) *See* 4,6-Dinitro-*o*-cyclohexylphenol[a] *at loc. no.* **540**

4,6-Dinitro-*o*-cyclohexylphenol (131-89-5) *See loc. no.* **540**

Dinitrocyclohexylphenol (131-89-5) *See* 4,6-Dinitro-*o*-cyclohexylphenol[a] *at loc. no.* **540**

---

[a] A Synonym   [b] A Closely Related Substance   [c] The Active or Major Constituent   [d] A Class Name
[e] A Specific Example of or Product Containing

Ingredient name (CAS registry no.) *See* Primary Name *at*
location no. **XXX** *in Part D of this section*

---

[a] A Synonym　　[b] A Closely Related Substance　　[c] The Active or Major Constituent　　[d] A Class Name
[e] A Specific Example of or Product Containing

Ingredient name (CAS registry no.) *See* Primary Name *at location no.* **XXX** *in Part D of this section*

Disodium tetraborate decahydrate (1303-96-4) *See* Borax[a] at loc. no. **132**

Disodium tetraborate pentahydrate *See* Borax[b] *at loc. no.* **132**

Disodium zinc ethylenediaminetetraacetate *See* Ethylenediaminetetraacetic Acid (and Salts)[b] *at loc. no.* **1506**

Disophenol (305-85-1) *See* 2,6-Diiodo-4-nitrophenol[a] *at loc. no.* **537**

Distaval (50-35-1) *See* Thalidomide[c] *at loc. no.* **1443**

Distearyl dimethyl ammonium chloride (107-64-2) *See* Cationic Surfactants[d] *at loc. no.* **974**

"Distillate" *See* Fuel Oil[a] *at loc. no.* **326**

Disulfiram (97-77-8) *See loc. no.* **1595**

Disulfoton (298-04-4) *See loc. no.* **1086**

Disulfur dichloride (10025-67-9) *See* Sulfur Chloride[a] *at loc. no.* **28**

Disul-Na (136-78-7) *See* 2-(2,4-Dichlorophenoxy)ethyl Sulfate Sodium Salt[a] *at loc. no.* **1216**

Di-syston (298-04-4) *See* Disulfoton[c] *at loc. no.* **1086**

Di-tallow dimethyl ammonium sulfate *See* Ammonyx 2194[e] *at loc. no.* **984**

Dithane A-40 (142-59-6) *See* Nabam[c] *at loc. no.* **1162**

Dithane D-14 (142-59-6) *See* Nabam[c] *at loc. no.* **1162**

Dithane M-22 (12427-38-2) *See* Maneb[c] *at loc. no.* **1160**

Dithane M-45 (8018-01-7) *See* Mancozeb[c] *at loc. no.* **1159**

Dithane M-22 Special (12427-38-2) *See* Maneb[c] *at loc. no.* **1160**

Dithane Z-78 (12122-67-7) *See* Zineb[c] *at loc. no.* **1167**

Dithiocarbonic anhydride (75-15-0) *See* Carbon Disulfide[a] *at loc. no.* **125**

β,β'-Dithiocyano diethyl ether (4617-17-8) *See* Aliphatic Thiocyanates[d] *at loc. no.* **1034**

1,2-Dithiolane-3-pentanoic acid (62-46-4) *See* Thioctic Acid[a] *at loc. no.* **1510**

Dithiosystox (298-04-4) *See* Disulfoton[c] *at loc. no.* **1086**

Diuron (330-54-1) *See loc. no.* **1247**

Dixanthogen (502-55-6) *See* Diethyl Dithiobis(thionoformate)[a] *at loc. no.* **1302**

DMA (127-19-5) *See* Dimethylacetamide[a] *at loc. no.* **565**

DMAA (75-60-5) *See* Cacodylic Acid[a] *at loc. no.* **197**

DMAC (127-19-5) *See* Dimethylacetamide[a] *at loc. no.* **565**

DMAE (108-01-0) *See* Deanol[a] *at loc. no.* **1592**

DMC (80-06-8) *See loc. no.* **1011**

DMDT (72-43-5) *See* Methoxychlor[a] *at loc. no.* **1013**

DMF (68-12-2) *See* Dimethylformamide[a] *at loc. no.* **566**

DMP (131-11-3) *See* Methyl Phthalate[a] *at loc. no.* **593**

DMPA *See* Zytron[a] *at loc. no.* **1105**

DMSO (67-68-5) *See* Dimethyl Sulfoxide[a] *at loc. no.* **1620**

DMT *See* N,N-Dimethyltryptamine[a] *at loc. no.* **1448**

DN-111 (317-83-9) *See* Dicyclohexylamine 4,6-Dinitro-o-cyclohexylphenate[c] *at loc. no.* **536**

DNAP (4097-36-3) *See* 4,6-Dinitro-o-amylphenol[a] *at loc. no.* **538**

DNBP (88-85-7) *See* Dinoseb[a] *at loc. no.* **543**

DNOC (534-52-1) *See* 4,6-Dinitro-o-cresol[a] *at loc. no.* **539**

DNOCHP (131-89-5) *See* 4,6-Dinitro-o-cyclohexylphenol[a] *at loc. no.* **540**

DNOSAP (4097-36-3) *See* 4,6-Dinitro-o-amylphenol[a] *at loc. no.* **538**

DNOSBP (88-85-7) *See* Dinoseb[a] *at loc. no.* **543**

2,4-DNP (51-28-5) *See* 2,4-Dinitrophenol[a] *at loc. no.* **541**

DNSBP (88-85-7) *See* Dinoseb[a] *at loc. no.* **543**

DNTP (56-38-2) *See* Parathion[a] *at loc. no.* **1077**

Dociton *See* Propranolol Hydrochloride[c] *at loc. no.* **1613**

Docusate sodium (577-11-7) *See* Dioctyl Sodium Sulfosuccinate[a] *at loc. no.* **951**

Dodecabonium chloride *See* Urolocide[a] *at loc. no.* **993**

Dodecachloropentacyclodecane (2385-85-5) *See* Mirex[a] *at loc. no.* **1033**

Dodecahydrodiphenylamine (101-83-7) *See* Dicyclohexylamine[a] *at loc. no.* **608**

Dodecahydrodiphenylamine nitrite (3129-91-7) *See* Dicyclohexylamine Nitrite[a] *at loc. no.* **632**

Dodecanoic acid (143-07-7) *See* Lauric Acid[a] *at loc. no.* **556**

1-Dodecanol (112-53-8) *See* Lauryl Alcohol[a] *at loc. no.* **422**

Dodecyl *derivative. If not listed below, see also corresponding* Lauryl *or* Alkyl *derivative in this index.*

Dodecyl alcohol (112-53-8) *See* Lauryl Alcohol[a] *at loc. no.* **422**

Dodecyl alcohol polyoxyethylene ether *See* Laureth 9[a] *at loc. no.* **966**

Dodecylammonium methanearsonate (7260-42-6) *See* Octyl Ammonium Metharsonate[b] *at loc. no.* **208**

Dodecyl carbamylmethyl dimethyl benzyl ammonium chloride (100-95-8) *See* Urolocide[e] *at loc. no.* **993**

Dodecyl ether of polyethylene glycol (9002-92-0) *See* Laureth 9[a] *at loc. no.* **966**

Dodecylguanidine acetate (2439-10-3) *See* Dodine[a] *at loc. no.* **1193**

Dodecyl thiocyanate (765-15-1) *See* Lauryl Thiocyanate[a] *at loc. no.* **1036**

Dodine (2439-10-3) *See loc. no.* **1193**

Dolophine (76-99-3) *See* Methadone[c] *at loc. no.* **1485**

DOM (15588-95-1) *See* 2,5-Dimethoxy-4-methyl-amphetamine[a] *at loc. no.* **1449**

Donovan's Solution (8012-54-2) *See loc. no.* **226**

DOP (117-84-0) *See* Di-2-ethylhexyl Phthalate[b] *at loc. no.* **591**

Doriden (77-21-4) *See* Glutethimide[c] *at loc. no.* **1436**

Dormison (77-75-8) *See* Methylpentynol[c] *at loc. no.* **1440**

Dosanex (19937-59-8) *See* Metoxuron[a] *at loc. no.* **1252**

Dover's powder (8013-48-7) *See* Ipecac and Opium Powder[a] *at loc. no.* **676**

Dowanol 33B (107-98-2) *See* Propylene Glycol Monomethyl Ether[c] *at loc. no.* **464**

Dowanol DB (112-34-5) *See* Butyl Carbitol[c] *at loc. no.* **452**

Dowanol DE (111-90-0) *See* Carbitol[c] *at loc. no.* **455**

Dowanol DM (111-77-3) *See* Carbitol[b] *at loc. no.* **455**

Dowanol DPM (34590-94-8) *See* Dipropylene Glycol Monomethyl Ether[c] *at loc. no.* **457**

Dowanol EB (111-76-2) *See* 2-Butoxyethanol[c] *at loc. no.* **453**

Dowanol EE (111-15-9) *See* 2-Ethoxyethyl Acetate (and other Esters)[c] *at loc. no.* **450**

Dowanol EM (109-86-4) *See* 2-Methoxyethanol[c] *at loc. no.* **461**

Dowfax 2A1 (12626-49-2) *See* Sulfonated Dodecyl Diphenyl Oxide (Sodium)[c] *at loc. no.* **957**

Dowicides *See loc. no.* **530**

Dowicide 1 (90-43-7) *See* Phenylphenol[d] *at loc. no.* **495**

Dowicide 2 (95-95-4) *See* Trichlorophenols[d] *at loc. no.* **535**

Dowicide 2S (88-06-2) *See* Trichlorophenols[d] *at loc. no.* **535**

Dowicide 4 (92-04-6) *See* Chloro-2-phenylphenol[b] *at loc. no.* **526**

Dowicide 5 *See* 2-Bromo-4-phenylphenol[c] *at loc. no.* **522**

Dowicide 6 (58-90-2) *See* 2,3,4,6-Tetrachlorophenol[c] *at loc. no.* **534**

Dowicide 7 (87-86-5) *See* Pentachlorophenol[c] *at loc. no.* **532**

Dowicide 9 *See* 4-Chloro-2-cyclopentylphenol[c] *at loc. no.* **524**

Dowicide 31 (8013-95-4) *See* Chloro-2-phenylphenol[c] *at loc. no.* **526**

Dowicide 32 (8013-95-4) *See* Chloro-2-phenylphenol[c] *at loc. no.* **526**

Dowicide A (132-27-4) *See* Phenylphenol[b] *at loc. no.* **495**

Dowicide B (136-32-3) *See* Trichlorophenols[d] *at loc. no.* **535**

Dowicide G (131-52-2) *See* Pentachlorophenol[b] *at loc. no.* **532**

---

[a] A Synonym   [b] A Closely Related Substance   [c] The Active or Major Constituent   [d] A Class Name
[e] A Specific Example of or Product Containing

Ingredient name (CAS registry no.) *See* Primary Name *at*
location no. XXX *in Part D of this section*

Dowicil 200 (4080-31-3) *See loc. no.* **995**
Doxepin (1668-19-5) *See loc. no.* **1472**
Doxinate (577-11-7) *See* Dioctyl Sodium Sulfosuccinate[c] *at loc. no.* **951**
Doxycycline (564-25-0) *See* Tetracyclines[d] *at loc. no.* **904**
Doxylamine Succinate (562-10-7) *See loc. no.* **1493**
2,4-DP (120-36-5) *See* 2-(2,4-Dichlorophenoxy)propionic Acid[a] *at loc. no.* **1217**
DPBS *See* Genite[e] *at loc. no.* **1046**
Dramamine (523-87-5) *See* Diphenhydramine Hydrochloride[b] *at loc. no.* **1492**
Drazoxolone (5707-69-7) *See loc. no.* **1194**
Dreft (151-21-3) *See* Alkyl Sodium Sulfates[d] *at loc. no.* **946**
Drene (139-96-8) *See* Alkyl Sodium Sulfates[c] *at loc. no.* **946**
Driers *See* Cobalt Driers[e] *at loc. no.* **283**
2,4-D Salts *See loc. no.* **1214**
DSMA (144-21-8) *See* Disodium Methanearsonate[a] *at loc. no.* **203**
DTMC (115-32-2) *See* Kelthane[e] *at loc. no.* **1012**
DTPA (67-43-6) *See* Edetate Calcium Disodium[b] *at loc. no.* **1504**
Dual (51218-45-2) *See* Alachlor[b] *at loc. no.* **1273**
Duboisine (8000-07-5) *See loc. no.* **768**
Duphar (116-29-0) *See* Tetradifon[c] *at loc. no.* **1049**
Duponals *See* Alkyl Sodium Sulfates[c] *at loc. no.* **946**
Duponol C (151-21-3) *See* Alkyl Sodium Sulfates[c] *at loc. no.* **946**
Dupont No. 1318 *See* Siduron[c] *at loc. no.* **1257**
Duranest *See* Etidocaine[e] *at loc. no.* **1581**
Duraset (85-72-3) *See* N-m-Tolylphthalamic Acid[c] *at loc. no.* **1284**
Dursban (2921-88-2) *See* Chlorpyrifos[c] *at loc. no.* **1064**
Dutch liquid or oil (107-06-2) *See* Ethylene Dichloride[c] *at loc. no.* **369**
Dybar (101-42-8) *See* Fenuron[c] *at loc. no.* **1248**
Dyes. *For a tabular summary of dyes and pigments, see Section VI (General Formulations).*
Dylox (52-68-6) *See* Trichlorfon[c] *at loc. no.* **1062**
Dymid (957-51-7) *See* Diphenamid[c] *at loc. no.* **1275**
Dynone II (317-83-9) *See* Dicyclohexylamine 4,6-Dinitro-o-cyclohexylphenate[c] *at loc. no.* **536**
Dyphylline (479-18-5) *See loc. no.* **804**
Dyrene (101-05-3) *See* Anilazine[c] *at loc. no.* **1170**
E-600 (311-45-5) *See* Paraoxon[c] *at loc. no.* **1056**
E-605 (56-38-2) *See* Parathion[a] *at loc. no.* **1077**
E-1059 (8000-97-3) *See* Demeton[a] *at loc. no.* **1067**
E-3314 (76-44-8) *See* Heptachlor[a] *at loc. no.* **1022**
Earthnut oil (8002-03-7) *See* Peanut Oil[a] *at loc. no.* **719**
East Indian almond *See* Cashew Nut[a] *at loc. no.* **661**
Ebimar *See* Carrageenan[b] *at loc. no.* **753**
Ecgonine methyl ester benzoate (50-36-2) *See* Cocaine[a] *at loc. no.* **825**
Ectylurea (95-04-5) *See loc. no.* **1433**
Edathamil calcium disodium (62-33-9) *See* Edetate Calcium Disodium[a] *at loc. no.* **1504**
EDB (106-93-4) *See* 1,2-Dibromoethane[a] *at loc. no.* **364**
EDC (107-06-2) *See* Ethylene Dichloride[a] *at loc. no.* **369**
EDE *See loc. no.* **367**
Edetate Calcium Disodium (62-33-9) *See loc. no.* **1504**
Edetic acid (60-00-4) *See* Ethylenediaminetetraacetic Acid (and Salts)[a] *at loc. no.* **1506**
EDTA (60-00-4) *See* Ethylenediaminetetraacetic Acid (and Salts)[a] *at loc. no.* **1506**
Edwal C.H.Q. *See* Chlorohydroquinone[c] *at loc. no.* **500**
Eichenmistel *See* European Mistletoe[b] *at loc. no.* **669**
Elavil (50-48-6) *See* Amitriptyline[a] *at loc. no.* **1470**
Elocron (6988-21-2) *See* Dioxacarb[c] *at loc. no.* **1133**

EM-923 (97-16-5) *See* Genite[a] *at loc. no.* **1046**
Emcol 888 (8034-17-1) *See* Alkyl Naphthyl Methyl Pyridinium Chloride[c] *at loc. no.* **980**
Emcol E-607 (1341-07-7) *See* Cationic Surfactants[d] *at loc. no.* **974**
Emerald green *See* Brilliant Green[a] *at loc. no.* **1519**
Emetine (483-18-1) *See loc. no.* **805**
EMMI (2597-93-5) *See loc. no.* **227**
EMP (2235-25-8) *See* Ethyl Mercury Phosphate[a] *at loc. no.* **231**
Emulsept *See* Cationic Surfactants[d] *at loc. no.* **974**
Emulsifiers *See* Surface Active Agents[d] *at loc. no.* **936**
Emulsifying agents *See* Surface Active Agents[d] *at loc. no.* **936**
Emylcamate (78-28-4) *See loc. no.* **1405**
Endosan (485-31-4) *See* Dinoseb[b] *at loc. no.* **543**
Endosulfan (115-29-7) *See* Thiodan[c] *at loc. no.* **1026**
Endothal (145-73-3) *See* Endothall[a] *at loc. no.* **1304**
Endothall (129-67-9) *See loc. no.* **1304**
3,6-Endoxohexahydrophthalic acid (145-73-3) *See* Endothall[a] *at loc. no.* **1304**
3,6-Endoxohexahydrophthalic acid disodium salt (129-67-9) *See* Endothall[b] *at loc. no.* **1304**
Endrin (72-20-8) *See loc. no.* **1021**
Enibomal (125-55-3) *See* Pronarcon[a] *at loc. no.* **1384**
Enide (957-51-7) *See* Diphenamid[c] *at loc. no.* **1275**
Enovid and Enovid-E (8015-30-3) *See* Norethynodrel with Mestranol[c] *at loc. no.* **919**
ENT-21170 (70-38-2) *See* Dimethrin[a] *at loc. no.* **889**
ENT-21557 (70-43-9) *See* Barthrin[a] *at loc. no.* **885**
Entex (55-38-9) *See* Fenthion[c] *at loc. no.* **1073**
Entramin (121-66-4) *See* 2-Amino-5-nitrothiazole[a] *at loc. no.* **1538**
Eparen (1085-98-9) *See* Dichlofluanid[a] *at loc. no.* **1189**
Ephedrine (299-42-3) *See loc. no.* **1450**
l-Ephedrine (299-42-3) *See* Ephedrine[a] *at loc. no.* **1450**
Ephedrine hydrochloride (50-98-6) *See* Ephedrine[b] *at loc. no.* **1450**
Ephedrine sulfate (134-72-5) *See* Ephedrine[b] *at loc. no.* **1450**
Epichlorohydrin (106-89-8) *See loc. no.* **387**
Epinephrine (51-43-4) *See loc. no.* **1454**
Epinephrine bitartrate (51-42-3) *See* Epinephrine[b] *at loc. no.* **1454**
Epinephrine hydrochloride (55-31-2) *See* Epinephrine[b] *at loc. no.* **1454**
EPN (2104-64-5) *See loc. no.* **1071**
4,5α-Epoxy-3,14-dihydroxy-17-methylmorphinan-6-one (76-41-5) *See* Oxymorphone[a] *at loc. no.* **790**
1,2-Epoxyethane (75-21-8) *See* Ethylene Oxide[a] *at loc. no.* **16**
2,3-Epoxy-2-ethylhexanamide (126-93-2) *See* Oxanamide[a] *at loc. no.* **1409**
4,5α-Epoxy-14-hydroxy-3-methoxy-17-methyl-morphinan-6-one (76-42-6) *See* Oxycodone[a] *at loc. no.* **789**
1,8-Epoxy-p-menthane (470-82-6) *See* Eucalyptol[a] *at loc. no.* **863**
4,5α-Epoxy-3-methoxy-17-methyl-morphinan-6-one tartrate (1:1) (34195-34-1) *See* Hydrocodone Bitartrate[a] *at loc. no.* **783**
Epoxy novolac resins *See* Epoxy Resins[d] *at loc. no.* **1628**
1,2-Epoxypropane (75-56-9) *See* Propylene Oxide[a] *at loc. no.* **17**
Epoxy Resins *See loc. no.* **1628**
6,7-Epoxytropine tropate methylbromide (155-41-9) *See* Scopolamine[b] *at loc. no.* **771**
Epson salts (7487-88-9) *See* Magnesium Salts[d] *at loc. no.* **174**
Eptam (759-94-4) *See* EPTC[c] *at loc. no.* **1236**

---

[a] A Synonym   [b] A Closely Related Substance   [c] The Active or Major Constituent   [d] A Class Name
[e] A Specific Example of or Product Containing

Ingredient name (CAS registry no.) *See* Primary Name *at*
location no. **XXX** *in Part D of this section*

Eptapur (3766-60-7) *See* Buturon[c] *at loc. no.* **1241**
EPTC (759-94-4) *See loc. no.* **1236**
Equanil (57-53-4) *See* Meprobamate[c] *at loc. no.* **1407**
Equilin (474-86-2) *See* Estrogens (Natural and Synthetic)[d] *at loc. no.* **916**
Eradex (93-75-4) *See loc. no.* **1044**
Eradicane (51990-04-6) *See* EPTC[b] *at loc. no.* **1236**
Erbon (136-25-4) *See loc. no.* **1218**
Ergonovine maleate (129-51-1) *See* Ergot[d] *at loc. no.* **667**
Ergot *See loc. no.* **667**
Ergot alkaloids (12126-57-7) *See* Ergot[e] *at loc. no.* **667**
Ergotamine tartrate (379-79-3) *See* Ergot[d] *at loc. no.* **667**
Erythrityl tetranitrate (7297-25-8) *See* Nitroglycerin(e)[b] *at loc. no.* **635**
Eserine (57-47-6) *See* Physostigmine[a] *at loc. no.* **807**
ESNN *See* Phenyl Cyclohexanol[a] *at loc. no.* **426**
Essence of mirbane (98-95-3) *See* Nitrobenzene[a] *at loc. no.* **642**
Essential oil of almond (artificial) (100-52-7) *See* Benzaldehyde[a] *at loc. no.* **859**
Essential Oils *See loc. no.* **725**
Estradiol (50-28-2) *See* Estrogens (Natural and Synthetic)[d] *at loc. no.* **916**
Estriol (50-27-1) *See* Estrogens (Natural and Synthetic)[d] *at loc. no.* **916**
Estrogens (Natural and Synthetic) *See loc. no.* **916**
Estrone (53-16-7) *See* Estrogens (Natural and Synthetic)[d] *at loc. no.* **916**
ET-14 (299-84-3) *See* Ronnel[a] *at loc. no.* **1079**
ET-15 (2591-66-4) *See loc. no.* **1099**
Etafedrine (7681-79-0) *See* *l*-*N*-Ethylephedrine[a] *at loc. no.* **1455**
Ethal (124-29-8) *See* Cetyl Alcohol[a] *at loc. no.* **409**
Ethalfluralin (55283-68-6) *See* Benefin[b] *at loc. no.* **1287**
Ethambutol Hydrochloride (1070-11-7) *See loc. no.* **1596**
Ethanal (75-07-0) *See* Acetaldehyde[a] *at loc. no.* **480**
Ethane (74-84-0) *See* Aliphatic Hydrocarbons[d] *at loc. no.* **303**
1,2-Ethanediamine (107-15-3) *See* Ethylenediamine[a] *at loc. no.* **602**
Ethanedioic acid (144-62-7) *See* Oxalic Acid[a] *at loc. no.* **47**
Ethanediol (107-21-1) *See* Ethylene Glycol[a] *at loc. no.* **436**
2,2′-[1,2-Ethanediylbis(oxy)]-bisethanol (112-27-6) *See* Triethylene Glycol[a] *at loc. no.* **439**
Ethane hexachloride *See* Hexachloroethane[a] *at loc. no.* **370**
Ethanenitrile (75-05-8) *See* Acetonitrile[a] *at loc. no.* **647**
Ethanethiol (75-08-1) *See* Methanethiol[b] *at loc. no.* **116**
Ethanol (64-17-5) *See* Ethyl Alcohol[a] *at loc. no.* **412**
Ethanolamine (141-43-5) *See* Monoethanolamine (and Salts)[a] *at loc. no.* **64**
β-Ethanolamine (141-43-5) *See* Monoethanolamine (and Salts)[a] *at loc. no.* **64**
Ethanolamine 2-methyl-4-chlorophenoxyacetate (6365-62-4) *See* MCPA[b] *at loc. no.* **1220**
Ethchlorvynol (113-18-8) *See loc. no.* **1434**
Ether (60-29-7) *See* Ethyl ether[a] *at loc. no.* **472**
Ethide (594-72-9) *See* 1,1-Dichloro-1-nitroethane[a] *at loc. no.* **20**
Ethinamate (126-52-3) *See loc. no.* **1435**
Ethinyl estradiol (57-63-6) *See* Estrogens (Natural and Synthetic)[d] *at loc. no.* **916**
Ethinyl trichloride (79-01-6) *See* Trichloroethylene[a] *at loc. no.* **375**
Ethiofencarb (29973-13-5) *See loc. no.* **1134**
Ethiolate (2941-55-1) *See* EPTC[b] *at loc. no.* **1236**
Ethion (563-12-2) *See loc. no.* **1087**
Ethionine (55-17-4) *See loc. no.* **1643**
Ethirimol (23947-60-6) *See* Dimethirimol[b] *at loc. no.* **1192**

Ethofumesate (26225-79-6) *See loc. no.* **1305**
Ethoheptazine (77-15-6) *See loc. no.* **1483**
Ethohexadiol (94-96-2) *See* 2-Ethyl-1,3-hexanediol[a] *at loc. no.* **1329**
Ethol (124-29-8) *See* Cetyl Alcohol[c] *at loc. no.* **409**
p-Ethoxyacetanilide (62-44-2) *See* Acetophenetidin[a] *at loc. no.* **611**
2-Ethoxy-2,3-dihydro-3,3-dimethyl-5-benzofuranyl methanesulfonate (26225-79-6) *See* Ethofumesate[a] *at loc. no.* **1305**
6-Ethoxy-1,2-dihydro-2,2,4-trimethylquinoline *See* Ethoxyquin[a] *at loc. no.* **1615**
2-Ethoxyethanol (110-80-5) *See loc. no.* **458**
2-Ethoxyethyl Acetate (and other Esters) (111-15-9) *See loc. no.* **450**
Ethoxylated alcohol *See* Alkyl Ethoxylate[a] *at loc. no.* **962**
Ethoxylated alkyl phenols *See* Nonionic Synthetic Detergents[d] *at loc. no.* **961**
Ethoxylated fatty alcohol *See* Alkyl Ethoxylate[a] *at loc. no.* **962**
Ethoxyquin (91-53-2) *See loc. no.* **1615**
Ethyl Acetate (141-78-6) *See loc. no.* **570**
Ethyl acrylate (140-88-5) *See* Acrylic Resin Monomers[d] *at loc. no.* **1625**
Ethyl Alcohol (64-17-5) *See loc. no.* **412**
Ethylaldehyde (75-07-0) *See* Acetaldehyde[a] *at loc. no.* **480**
Ethyl *p*-aminobenzoate (94-09-7) *See* Benzocaine[a] *at loc. no.* **1577**
2-(Ethylamino)-4-(isopropylamino)-6-methoxy-*s*-triazine (1610-17-9) *See* Prometon[b] *at loc. no.* **1267**
2-(Ethylamino)-4-(isopropylamino)-6-methylthio-*s*-triazine (834-12-8) *See* Prometon[b] *at loc. no.* **1267**
Ethylbenzene (100-41-4) *See* Xylene[b] *at loc. no.* **318**
Ethyl *N*-benzoyl-*N*-(3,4-dichlorophenyl)-2-amino propionate *See* Benzoylprop-ethyl[a] *at loc. no.* **1292**
Ethyl Biscoumacetate (548-00-5) *See loc. no.* **1340**
Ethyl bis(4-hydroxycoumarin)acetate (548-00-5) *See* Ethyl Biscoumacetate[a] *at loc. no.* **1340**
2-Ethyl-1-butanol (97-95-0) *See* Hexyl Alcohol[e] *at loc. no.* **416**
2-Ethylbutyl acrylate (3953-10-4) *See* Acrylic Resin Monomers[d] *at loc. no.* **1625**
5-Ethyl-5-*n*-butylbarbituric acid (77-28-1) *See* Butethal[a] *at loc. no.* **1370**
Ethyl *n*-butyrate (105-54-4) *See* Ethyl Acetate[b] *at loc. no.* **570**
Ethyl Cetab (124-03-8) *See* Alkyl Dimethyl Ethyl Ammonium Chloride (or Bromide)[d] *at loc. no.* **977**
Ethyl Chloride (75-00-3) *See loc. no.* **368**
Ethyl β-chlorovinyl ethynyl carbinol (113-18-8) *See* Ethchlorvynol[a] *at loc. no.* **1434**
Ethyl cinnamate (103-36-6) *See* Cinnamic Acid Esters[d] *at loc. no.* **587**
(α-Ethyl crotonyl)carbamide (95-04-5) *See* Ectylurea[a] *at loc. no.* **1433**
(2-Ethylcrotonyl)urea (95-04-5) *See* Ectylurea[a] *at loc. no.* **1433**
Ethyl cyanide (107-12-0) *See* Propionitrile[a] *at loc. no.* **653**
S-Ethyl cyclohexylethylthiocarbamate (1134-23-2) *See* Cycloate[a] *at loc. no.* **1234**
Ethyl 4,4′-dichlorobenzilate (510-15-6) *See* Chlorobenzilate[a] *at loc. no.* **1006**
Ethyl di(*p*-chlorophenyl)glycollate *See* Chlorobenzilate[a] *at loc. no.* **1006**
S-Ethyl diethylthiocarbamate (2941-55-1) *See* EPTC[b] *at loc. no.* **1236**

---

[a] A Synonym   [b] A Closely Related Substance   [c] The Active or Major Constituent   [d] A Class Name
[e] A Specific Example of or Product Containing

Ingredient name (CAS registry no.) *See* Primary Name *at*
location no. **XXX** *in Part D of this section*

S-Ethyl diisobutylthiocarbamate (2008-41-5) *See* Butylate*[a]* *at loc. no.* **1233**

O-Ethyl *S,S*-Dipropyl Phosphorodithioate (13194-48-4) *See loc. no.* **1088**

S-Ethyl dipropylthiocarbamate (759-94-4) *See* EPTC*[a]* *at loc. no.* **1236**

Ethylene aldehyde (107-02-8) *See* Acrolein*[a]* *at loc. no.* **481**

Ethylene bis(isothiocyanate sulfide) *See* Maneb*[b]* *at loc. no.* **1160**

Ethylene bromide (106-93-4) *See* 1,2-Dibromoethane*[a]* *at loc. no.* **364**

Ethylene chloride (107-06-2) *See* Ethylene Dichloride*[a]* *at loc. no.* **369**

Ethylene chlorobromide (107-04-0) *See* 1-Bromo-2-chloroethane*[a]* *at loc. no.* **362**

Ethylene Chlorohydrin (107-07-3) *See loc. no.* **434**

Ethylenediamine (107-15-3) *See loc. no.* **602**

Ethylenediamine dihydrochloride (333-18-6) *See* Ethylenediamine*[b]* *at loc. no.* **602**

Ethylenediamine dihydroiodide (5700-49-2) *See* Ethylenediamine*[b]* *at loc. no.* **602**

Ethylenediaminetetraacetic Acid (and Salts) (60-00-4) *See loc. no.* **1506**

Ethylene dibromide (106-93-4) *See* 1,2-Dibromoethane*[a]* *at loc. no.* **364**

Ethylene Dichloride (107-06-2) *See loc. no.* **369**

Ethylene dichloride emulsion *See* EDE*[a]* *at loc. no.* **367**

Ethylene dicyanide (110-61-2) *See* Succinonitrile*[a]* *at loc. no.* **654**

2,2′-(Ethylenediimino)-di-1-butanol dihydrochloride (1070-11-7) *See* Ethambutol Hydrochloride*[a]* *at loc. no.* **1596**

(Ethylene dinitrilo)tetraacetic acid tetrasodium salt (64-02-8) *See* Ethylenediaminetetraacetic Acid (and Salts)*[b]* *at loc. no.* **1506**

Ethylene dipyridylium dibromide (85-00-7) *See* Diquat Dibromide*[e]* *at loc. no.* **1285**

Ethylene Glycol (107-21-1) *See loc. no.* **436**

Ethylene Glycol Alkyl (and Aryl) Esters *See loc. no.* **451**

Ethylene Glycol Alkyl (and Aryl) Ethers *See loc. no.* **459**

Ethylene glycol-bis-(2-hydroxyethyl ether) (112-27-6) *See* Triethylene Glycol*[a]* *at loc. no.* **439**

Ethylene glycol *n*-butyl ether (111-76-2) *See* 2-Butoxyethanol*[a]* *at loc. no.* **453**

Ethylene glycol diacetate (111-55-7) *See* Ethylene Glycol Alkyl (and Aryl) Esters*[d]* *at loc. no.* **451**

Ethylene glycol diethyl ether (629-14-1) *See* Ethylene Glycol Alkyl (and Aryl) Ethers*[d]* *at loc. no.* **459**

Ethylene Glycol Dinitrate (628-96-6) *See loc. no.* **633**

Ethylene Glycol Distearate (627-83-8) *See loc. no.* **964**

Ethylene glycol mono-*n*-butyl ether (111-76-2) *See* 2-Butoxyethanol*[a]* *at loc. no.* **453**

Ethylene glycol monoether esters *See* 2-Ethoxyethyl Acetate (and other Esters)*[e]* *at loc. no.* **450**

Ethylene glycol monoethers *See* Ethylene Glycol Alkyl (and Aryl) Ethers*[e]* *at loc. no.* **459**

Ethylene glycol monoethyl ether (110-80-5) *See* 2-Ethoxyethanol*[a]* *at loc. no.* **458**

Ethylene glycol monoethyl ether acetate (111-15-9) *See* 2-Ethoxyethyl Acetate (and other Esters)*[a]* *at loc. no.* **450**

Ethylene glycol monomethyl ether (109-86-4) *See* 2-Methoxyethanol*[a]* *at loc. no.* **461**

Ethylene glycol monomethyl ether acetate (110-49-6) *See* Methyl Cellosolve Acetate*[a]* *at loc. no.* **462**

Ethylene glycol monophenyl ether (122-99-6) *See* Phenyl Cellosolve*[a]* *at loc. no.* **463**

Ethylene Oxide (75-21-8) *See loc. no.* **16**

Ethylene tetrachloride (127-18-4) *See* Tetrachloroethylene*[a]* *at loc. no.* **374**

Ethylenethiourea (96-45-7) *See loc. no.* **1169**

Ethylenimine (151-56-4) *See loc. no.* **606**

l-*N*-Ethylephedrine (7681-79-0) *See loc. no.* **1455**

Ethyl ether (60-29-7) *See loc. no.* **472**

Ethyl ether of diethylene glycol (111-90-0) *See* Carbitol*[a]* *at loc. no.* **455**

Ethylethylenimine (2549-67-9) *See* Ethylenimine*[b]* *at loc. no.* **606**

Ethyl Formate (109-94-4) *See loc. no.* **571**

Ethyl gasoline *See* Gasoline*[a]* *at loc. no.* **327**

Ethyl green (633-03-4) *See* Brilliant Green*[a]* *at loc. no.* **1519**

S-Ethyl hexahydro-1*H*-azepine-1-carbothioate (2212-67-1) *See* Molinate*[a]* *at loc. no.* **1237**

2-Ethyl-1,3-hexanediol (94-96-2) *See loc. no.* **1329**

2-Ethyl-1-hexanol (104-76-7) *See* 2-Ethylhexyl Alcohol*[a]* *at loc. no.* **413**

Ethylhexyl *compound. If not listed here, consult index under appropriate* Octyl *or* Capryl *derivative.*

2-Ethylhexyl acrylate (103-11-7) *See* Acrylic Resin Monomers*[d]* *at loc. no.* **1625**

2-Ethylhexyl Alcohol (104-76-7) *See loc. no.* **413**

2-Ethylhexyl ester of 2,4,5-T (1928-47-8) *See* Trichlorophenoxyacetic Acid*[b]* *at loc. no.* **1224**

N-(2-Ethylhexyl)-5-norbornene-2,3-dicarboximide (113-48-4) *See* MGK 264*[e]* *at loc. no.* **1150**

2-Ethylhexylsalicylate (118-60-5) *See* Isoamyl Salicylate*[b]* *at loc. no.* **596**

Ethyl-*p*-hydroxybenzoate (120-47-8) *See* Paraben Esters*[d]* *at loc. no.* **584**

Ethyl 2-hydroxy-2,2-bis(4-chlorophenyl)acetate *See* Chlorobenzilate*[a]* *at loc. no.* **1006**

Ethyl *m*-hydroxycarbanilate carbanilate (13684-56-5) *See* Desmedipham*[a]* *at loc. no.* **1230**

Ethyl α-hydroxypropionate (97-64-3) *See* Ethyl Lactate*[a]* *at loc. no.* **572**

Ethylidene chloride (75-34-3) *See* 1,1-Dichloroethane*[a]* *at loc. no.* **365**

Ethylidene dichloride (75-34-3) *See* 1,1-Dichloroethane*[a]* *at loc. no.* **365**

Ethylidene gyromitrin (16568-02-8) *See* Gyromitrin*[a]* *at loc. no.* **816**

5-Ethyl-5-isoamylbarbituric acid (57-43-2) *See* Amobarbital*[a]* *at loc. no.* **1364**

5-Ethyl-5-isopropyl barbituric acid sodium (143-82-8) *See* Probarbital Sodium*[a]* *at loc. no.* **1383**

Ethyl isovalerate (108-64-5) *See* Ethyl Acetate*[b]* *at loc. no.* **570**

N-Ethyllactamide carbanilate (16118-49-3) *See* Carbetamide*[a]* *at loc. no.* **1228**

Ethyl Lactate (97-64-3) *See loc. no.* **572**

Ethyl mercaptan (75-08-1) *See* Methanethiol*[b]* *at loc. no.* **116**

Ethyl mercuric acetate *See* Ethyl Mercury Phosphate*[b]* *at loc. no.* **231**

Ethyl Mercuric Chloride (107-27-7) *See loc. no.* **228**

Ethyl mercuric phosphate (2235-25-8) *See* Ethyl Mercury Phosphate*[a]* *at loc. no.* **231**

Ethyl Mercuri-2,3-dihydroxypropylmercaptide *See loc. no.* **229**

N-Ethylmercuri-1,2,3,6-tetrahydro-3,6-endomethano-3,4,5,6,7,7-hexachlorophthalimide (2597-93-5) *See* EMMI*[e]* *at loc. no.* **227**

N-(Ethylmercuri)-*p*-toluene Sulfonanilide (517-16-8) *See loc. no.* **230**

Ethyl Mercury Phosphate (2235-25-8) *See loc. no.* **231**

---

[a] A Synonym   *[b]* A Closely Related Substance   *[c]* The Active or Major Constituent   *[d]* A Class Name
[e] A Specific Example of or Product Containing

5-Ethyl-5-(2-methylallyl)-2-thiobarbituric acid (115-56-0) *See* Methallatal[a] *at loc. no.* **1378**

5-Ethyl-5-(1-methyl-1-butenyl)barbituric acid sodium (125-44-0) *See* Vinbarbital Sodium[a] *at loc. no.* **1391**

5-Ethyl-5-(1-methylbutyl)barbituric acid sodium (57-33-0) *See* Pentobarbital Sodium[a] *at loc. no.* **1380**

5-Ethyl-5-(1-methylbutyl)-2-thiobarbituric acid sodium (71-73-8) *See* Thiopental Sodium[a] *at loc. no.* **1390**

Ethyl 2-methyl-4-chlorophenoxyacetate *See* MCPA[b] *at loc. no.* **1220**

Ethyl methylene phosphorodithioate (563-12-2) *See* Ethion[e] *at loc. no.* **1087**

Ethyl methyl ketone (78-93-3) *See* Methyl Ethyl Ketone[a] *at loc. no.* **476**

Ethyl 3-methyl-4-(methylthio)phenyl(1-methylethyl)-phosphoramidate (22224-92-6) *See* Phenamiphos[a] *at loc. no.* **1103**

2-Ethyl-4-methylpentyl ester of 2,4,5-T *See* Trichlorophenoxyacetic Acid[b] *at loc. no.* **1224**

5-Ethyl-1-methyl-5-phenylbarbituric acid (115-38-8) *See* Mephobarbital[a] *at loc. no.* **1377**

N-Ethyl-N-(2-methyl-2-propenyl)-2,6-dinitro-4-(trifluoromethyl)benzenamine (55283-68-6) *See* Benefin[b] *at loc. no.* **1287**

1-Ethyl-1-methylpropyl carbamate (78-28-4) *See* Emylcamate[a] *at loc. no.* **1405**

N-Ethyl-α-methyl-3-(trifluoromethyl) phenylethylamine hydrochloride (458-24-2) *See* Fenfluramine[a] *at loc. no.* **1456**

Ethyl nitrite (109-95-5) *See* Amyl Nitrite[b] *at loc. no.* **630**

Ethyl p-nitrophenyl benzene thiophosphate (2104-64-5) *See* EPN[a] *at loc. no.* **1071**

O-Ethyl O-p-nitrophenyl phenylphosphonothioate (2104-64-5) *See* EPN[a] *at loc. no.* **1071**

Ethyl nitrophenyl thiobenzene phosphonate (2104-64-5) *See* EPN[a] *at loc. no.* **1071**

Ethyl p-nitrophenyl thionobenzene phosphonate (2104-64-5) *See* EPN[a] *at loc. no.* **1071**

O-Ethyl-O-paranitrophenylbenzenethiophosphate (2104-64-5) *See* EPN[a] *at loc. no.* **1071**

Ethyl 3-phenylcarbamoyloxyphenylcarbamate (13684-56-5) *See* Desmedipham[a] *at loc. no.* **1230**

α-Ethyl-α-phenylglutarimide (77-21-4) *See* Glutethimide[a] *at loc. no.* **1436**

Ethyl Phosphates *See loc. no.* **1112**

Ethyl Phthalate (84-66-2) *See loc. no.* **592**

Ethyl n-propionate (105-37-3) *See* Ethyl Acetate[b] *at loc. no.* **570**

N-(1-Ethylpropyl)-3,4-dimethyl-2,6-dinitrobenzenamine (40487-42-1) *See* Dinitramine[b] *at loc. no.* **1288**

N-(1-Ethylpropyl)-2,6-dinitro-3,4-xylidine (40487-42-1) *See* Dinitramine[b] *at loc. no.* **1288**

2-Ethyl-3-propylglycidamide (126-93-2) *See* Oxanamide[a] *at loc. no.* **1409**

3-(1-Ethylpropyl)phenyl methylcarbamate (672-04-8) *See* Bufencarb[b] *at loc. no.* **1125**

S-2-(Ethylsulfinyl)ethyl O,O-dimethyl phosphorothioate (301-12-2) *See* Meta-Systox-R[a] *at loc. no.* **1074**

N¹-(5-Ethyl-1,3,4-thiadiazole-2-yl)sulfanilamide *See* Sulfaethidole[a] *at loc. no.* **1555**

Ethyl thiocyanate (542-90-5) *See* Aliphatic Thiocyanates[d] *at loc. no.* **1034**

2-((Ethylthio)methyl)phenyl methylcarbamate (29973-13-5) *See* Ethiofencarb[a] *at loc. no.* **1134**

α-Ethylthio-o-tolyl methylcarbamate (29973-13-5) *See* Ethiofencarb[a] *at loc. no.* **1134**

Ethyl xanthogen disulfide (502-55-6) *See* Diethyl Dithiobis(thionoformate)[a] *at loc. no.* **1302**

Ethyl yohimbine *See* Yohimbine[b] *at loc. no.* **834**

Ethynodiol diacetate (297-76-7) *See* Estrogens (Natural and Synthetic)[d] *at loc. no.* **916**

Ethynodiol Diacetate with Mestranol (8056-92-6) *See loc. no.* **917**

1-Ethynylcyclohexyl carbamate (126-52-3) *See* Ethinamate[a] *at loc. no.* **1435**

Etidocaine (36637-18-0) *See loc. no.* **1581**

Etidocaine hydrochloride (36637-19-1) *See* Etidocaine[b] *at loc. no.* **1581**

Etrofolan *See* Isoprocarb[a] *at loc. no.* **1137**

ETU (96-45-7) *See* Ethylenethiourea[a] *at loc. no.* **1169**

Eucalyptol (470-82-6) *See loc. no.* **863**

Eudermol (29790-52-1) *See loc. no.* **775**

Eugenol (97-53-0) *See loc. no.* **864**

Eunarcon (125-55-3) *See* Pronarcon[a] *at loc. no.* **1384**

Euparen (1085-98-9) *See* Dichlofluanid[a] *at loc. no.* **1189**

Euparen M (731-27-1) *See* Dichlofluanid[b] *at loc. no.* **1189**

Eupatorin (855-96-9) *See* Eupatorium[e] *at loc. no.* **668**

Eupatorium *See loc. no.* **668**

Euphorbia pulcherrima *See* Poinsettia[a] *at loc. no.* **684**

European Mistletoe *See loc. no.* **669**

European oil of pennyroyal (8013-99-8) *See* Pennyroyal[d] *at loc. no.* **740**

Evik (834-12-8) *See* Prometon[b] *at loc. no.* **1267**

Evipal sodium (50-09-9) *See* Hexobarbital Sodium[c] *at loc. no.* **1376**

Evronal sodium (309-43-3) *See* Secobarbital Sodium[c] *at loc. no.* **1386**

Exhaust gas *See* Gas[d] *at loc. no.* **128**

Falone (94-84-8) *See loc. no.* **1306**

Fastin (1197-21-3) *See* Phentermine[b] *at loc. no.* **1467**

Fatty alcohols *See* Stearyl Alcohol[e] *at loc. no.* **430**

Fava Beans *See loc. no.* **670**

Fenac (85-34-7) *See loc. no.* **1219**

Fenaminosulf (140-56-7) *See loc. no.* **1195**

Fenethacarb (30087-47-9) *See* Butacarb[b] *at loc. no.* **1126**

Fenfluramine (458-24-2) *See loc. no.* **1456**

Fenfluramine hydrochloride (404-82-0) *See* Fenfluramine[b] *at loc. no.* **1456**

Fenitrooxon (2255-17-6) *See* Fenitrothion[b] *at loc. no.* **1072**

Fenitrothion (122-14-5) *See loc. no.* **1072**

Fenoprop (93-72-1) *See* Silvex[c] *at loc. no.* **1223**

Fenthion (55-38-9) *See loc. no.* **1073**

Fentin acetate (900-95-8) *See* Triphenyltin Acetate[a] *at loc. no.* **295**

Fentin hydroxide (76-87-9) *See* Triphenyltin Acetate[b] *at loc. no.* **295**

Fenuron (101-42-8) *See loc. no.* **1248**

Fenuron TCA (4482-55-7) *See* Fenuron[b] *at loc. no.* **1248**

Fenvalerate (51630-58-1) *See loc. no.* **890**

Ferbam (14484-64-1) *See loc. no.* **1158**

Fermate (14484-64-1) *See* Ferbam[a] *at loc. no.* **1158**

Fermentation amyl alcohol (123-51-3) *See* Isoamyl Alcohol[a] *at loc. no.* **417**

Fermentation butyl alcohol (78-83-1) *See* Isobutyl Alcohol[a] *at loc. no.* **418**

Ferric ammonium citrate (1333-00-2) *See* Ferric Salts[d] *at loc. no.* **253**

Ferric chloride (7705-08-0) *See* Ferric Salts[d] *at loc. no.* **253**

Ferric dimethyldithiocarbamate (14484-64-1) *See* Ferbam[a] *at loc. no.* **1158**

Ferric ferricyanide (14433-93-3) *See* Ferric Salts[d] *at loc. no.* **253**

---

[a] A Synonym   [b] A Closely Related Substance   [c] The Active or Major Constituent   [d] A Class Name
[e] A Specific Example of or Product Containing

Ingredient name (CAS registry no.) *See* Primary Name *at*
location no. **XXX** *in Part D of this section*

Ferric ferrocyanide (14638-08-5) *See* Ferrocyanide and Fer-
ricyanide Salts[d] *at loc. no.* **256**
Ferric pyrophosphate (10058-44-3) *See* Ferric Salts[d] *at loc.
no.* **253**
Ferric Salts *See loc. no.* **253**
Ferric Subsulfate (1310-45-8) *See loc. no.* **254**
Ferric sulfate (10028-22-5) *See* Ferric Salts[d] *at loc. no.* **253**
Ferrocholinate (1336-80-7) *See loc. no.* **255**
Ferrocyanide and Ferricyanide Salts *See loc. no.* **256**
Ferrolip *See* Ferrocholinate[c] *at loc. no.* **255**
Ferrous and ferric *See* Iron Salts[a] *at loc. no.* **250**
Ferrous Carbonate (563-71-9) *See loc. no.* **257**
Ferrous chloride (7758-94-3) *See* Ferrous Salts[d] *at loc. no.*
258
Ferrous fumarate (7705-12-6) *See* Ferrous Salts[d] *at loc. no.*
258
Ferrous gluconate (299-29-6) *See* Ferrous Salts[d] *at loc. no.*
258
Ferrous Salts *See loc. no.* **258**
Ferrous sulfate (7720-78-7) *See* Ferrous Salts[d] *at loc. no.*
258
Fiberglass resin *See* Polyester Resins[c] *at loc. no.* **1634**
Ficam (22781-23-5) *See* Bendiocarb[c] *at loc. no.* **1123**
Flamprop-isopropyl (52756-22-6) *See* Benzoylprop-ethyl[b] *at
loc. no.* **1292**
Flamprop-methyl (52756-25-9) *See* Benzoylprop-ethyl[b] *at
loc. no.* **1292**
Flaxseed oil *See* Linseed Oil[a] *at loc. no.* **717**
Floraltone (88-82-4) *See* 2,3,5-Tri-iodobenzoic Acid[c] *at loc.
no.* **1318**
Flowers of zinc (1314-13-2) *See* Zinc Oxide[a] *at loc. no.* **274**
Fluchloralin (33245-39-5) *See* Dinitramine[b] *at loc. no.* **1288**
Flue gas *See* Gas[d] *at loc. no.* **128**
Flunitrazepam (1622-62-4) *See loc. no.* **1396**
Fluoaluminate (sodium) (1344-75-8) *See* Cryolite[a] *at loc.
no.* **104**
Fluoboric acid (16872-11-0) *See* Potassium Fluoborate[b] *at
loc. no.* **103**
Fluocinolone acetonide (67-73-2) *See* Corticosteroids[d] *at
loc. no.* **915**
Fluohydric acid (7664-39-3) *See* Hydrofluoric Acid[a] *at loc.
no.* **36**
Fluometuron (2164-17-2) *See loc. no.* **1249**
Fluon (9002-84-0) *See* Polytetrafluoroethylene[c] *at loc. no.*
1636
Fluorbenside (405-30-1) *See loc. no.* **1045**
Fluorescent Whitening Agents *See loc. no.* **938**
Fluoridamid (47000-92-0) *See loc. no.* **1276**
Fluoride *See loc. no.* **100**
Fluoroacetamide (640-19-7) *See loc. no.* **1347**
Fluoroacetate (513-62-2) *See loc. no.* **548**
Fluoroacetate salts *See* Fluoroacetate[d] *at loc. no.* **548**
Fluoroborate salts soluble *See* Potassium Fluoborate[e] *at
loc. no.* **103**
Fluorocarbon Refrigerants and Propellants *See loc. no.*
347
Fluorocitric acid (357-89-1) *See* Fluoroacetate[b] *at loc. no.*
548
2-Fluoroethanol (371-62-0) *See* Fluoroacetate[b] *at loc. no.*
548
Fluorparacide (405-30-1) *See* Fluorbenside[c] *at loc. no.* **1045**
Fluorsulphacide (405-30-1) *See* Fluorbenside[c] *at loc. no.*
1045
Fluosilicates *See* Fluosilicate Salts[d] *at loc. no.* **101**
Fluosilicate Salts *See loc. no.* **101**
Fluosilicic Acid (1309-45-1) *See loc. no.* **37**

Fluotrimazole (31251-03-3) *See loc. no.* **1171**
Fluphenazine Hydrochloride (146-56-5) *See loc. no.* **1415**
Flurazepam (1172-18-5) *See loc. no.* **1397**
Focusan (2398-96-1) *See* Tolnaftate[c] *at loc. no.* **1532**
Folcid (2425-06-1) *See* Captafol[a] *at loc. no.* **1180**
Folex (150-50-5) *See* Tributyl Phosphorotrithioite[c] *at loc. no.*
1114
Folithion (122-14-5) *See* Fenitrothion[a] *at loc. no.* **1072**
Folpet (133-07-3) *See loc. no.* **1181**
Formaldehyde (50-00-0) *See loc. no.* **482**
Formalin (8006-07-3) *See* Formaldehyde[c] *at loc. no.* **482**
Formetanate (22259-30-9) *See loc. no.* **1135**
Formetanate hydrochloride (23422-53-9) *See* Formetanate[b]
at loc. no. **1135**
Formic Acid (and Salts) (64-18-6) *See loc. no.* **44**
Formol (8006-07-3) *See* Formaldehyde[c] *at loc. no.* **482**
Formparanate *See* Formetanate[b] *at loc. no.* **1135**
Forstan (2439-01-2) *See* Quinomethionate[c] *at loc. no.* **1205**
Fowler's Solution (8025-91-0) *See loc. no.* **204**
Foxglove (8047-05-0) *See* Digitalis[c] *at loc. no.* **666**
Frangulin *See* Cascara Sagrada[b] *at loc. no.* **660**
Frenquel (115-46-8) *See* Azacyclonol[c] *at loc. no.* **1429**
Freon (11126-05-9) *See* Fluorocarbon Refrigerants and Pro-
pellants[d] *at loc. no.* **347**
Freon 11 (75-69-4) *See* Trichloromonofluoromethane[c] *at loc.
no.* **351**
Freon 12 (75-71-8) *See* Dichlorodifluoromethane[c] *at loc. no.*
348
Freon 21 (75-43-4) *See* Dichloromonofluoromethane[c] *at loc.
no.* **349**
Freon 22 (75-45-6) *See* Monochlorodifluoromethane[c] *at loc.
no.* **350**
Freon 113 (76-13-1) *See* Trichlorofluoroethane[c] *at loc. no.*
353
Freon 114 (76-14-2) *See* 1,2-Dichloro-1,1,2,2-tetrafluoroetha-
ne[c] *at loc. no.* **352**
Fuberidazole (3878-19-1) *See loc. no.* **1176**
Fuel Oil *See loc. no.* **326**
Fuel oil no. 1 *See* Kerosene[a] *at loc. no.* **328**
Fuel oil no. 2 *See* Fuel Oil[a] *at loc. no.* **326**
Fuel oil no. 4 *See* Residual Oils[d] *at loc. no.* **332**
Fuel oil no. 5 *See* Residual Oils[d] *at loc. no.* **332**
Fulvicin (126-07-8) *See* Griseofulvin[c] *at loc. no.* **900**
Fumarin (117-52-2) *See* Coumafuryl[c] *at loc. no.* **1337**
Fumasol *See* Coumafuryl[c] *at loc. no.* **1337**
Fumazone (96-12-8) *See* 1,2-Dibromo-3-chloropropane[c] *at
loc. no.* **385**
Fuming sulfuric acid *See* Oleum[a] *at loc. no.* **34**
Furacin (59-87-0) *See* Nitrofurazone[c] *at loc. no.* **1531**
Furadan (1563-66-2) *See* Carbofuran[a] *at loc. no.* **1129**
Furadantin *See* Nitrofurantoin[c] *at loc. no.* **1530**
2-Furanmethanol (98-00-0) *See* Furfuryl Alcohol[a] *at loc. no.*
414
Furazolidone (67-45-8) *See loc. no.* **1526**
Furfural (98-01-1) *See loc. no.* **483**
Furfuraldehyde-2 (98-01-1) *See* Furfural[a] *at loc. no.* **483**
Furfuryl Alcohol (98-00-0) *See loc. no.* **414**
Furoxone (67-45-8) *See* Furazolidone[c] *at loc. no.* **1526**
2(2'-Furyl)-benzimidazole (3878-19-1) *See* Fuberidazole[a] *at
loc. no.* **1176**
Fusel oil *See* Isoamyl Alcohol[c] *at loc. no.* **417**
FWA *See* Fluorescent Whitening Agents[a] *at loc. no.* **938**
Fyrol FR2 (78-43-3) *See* Tris(1,3-dichloro-2-propyl)phos-
phate[a] *at loc. no.* **1119**
G-11 (70-30-4) *See* Hexachlorophene[a] *at loc. no.* **531**
Galerina spp. *See* Amatoxins[c] *at loc. no.* **813**

---

[a] A Synonym　　　[b] A Closely Related Substance　　　[c] The Active or Major Constituent　　　[d] A Class Name
[e] A Specific Example of or Product Containing

Ingredient name (CAS registry no.) *See* Primary Name *at
location no.* **XXX** *in Part D of this section*

Gallic Acid (149-91-7) *See loc. no.* **502**
Gallotannic acid (1401-55-4) *See* Tannic Acid[a] *at loc. no.* **852**
Gamboge (9000-25-3) *See loc. no.* **754**
Gamma benzene hexachloride (58-89-9) *See* Lindane[a] *at loc. no.* **1028**
Ganocide *See* Drazoxolone[c] *at loc. no.* **1194**
Gantanol *See* Sulfamethoxazole[c] *at loc. no.* **1561**
Gantrisin *See* Sulfisoxazole[c] *at loc. no.* **1568**
Gardinols *See* Alkyl Sodium Sulfates[c] *at loc. no.* **946**
Gardinol-type detergents (8048-56-4) *See* Alkyl Sodium Sulfates[c] *at loc. no.* **946**
Gardona (22248-79-9) *See* Tetrachlorvinfos[c] *at loc. no.* **1061**
Garrathion (786-19-6) *See* Carbophenothion[c] *at loc. no.* **1083**
Gas *See loc. no.* **128**
Gas oil *See* Fuel Oil[a] *at loc. no.* **326**
Gasoline (8006-61-9) *See loc. no.* **327**
Gaultheria oil (119-36-8) *See* Methyl Salicylate[a] *at loc. no.* **597**
GBH *See* Lindane[a] *at loc. no.* **1028**
GC-1283 (2385-85-5) *See* Mirex[a] *at loc. no.* **1033**
Gelsemium *See loc. no.* **671**
Gelsemium sempervirens L. *See* Gelsemium[a] *at loc. no.* **671**
Gemonil (50-11-3) *See* Metharbital[c] *at loc. no.* **1379**
Genetron *See* Fluorocarbon Refrigerants and Propellants[d] *at loc. no.* **347**
Genite (97-16-5) *See loc. no.* **1046**
Genitol 923 (97-16-5) *See* Genite[a] *at loc. no.* **1046**
Gentian Violet (548-62-9) *See loc. no.* **1520**
Geraniol (106-24-1) *See loc. no.* **865**
Germall 115 (39236-46-9) *See* Imidazolidinyl Urea[c] *at loc. no.* **996**
Gerovital *See* Procaine[c] *at loc. no.* **1585**
Ghatti (9000-28-6) *See* Gums (Vegetable)[d] *at loc. no.* **755**
Ghatti gum (9000-28-6) *See* Gums (Vegetable)[d] *at loc. no.* **755**
Gibberellic Acid (77-06-5) *See loc. no.* **1357**
Gibrel (potassium salt) (125-67-7) *See* Gibberellic Acid[b] *at loc. no.* **1357**
Gilurytmal *See* Ajmaline[c] *at loc. no.* **794**
Gingilli oil (8008-74-0) *See* Sesame Oil[a] *at loc. no.* **722**
Gitaligin (1405-76-1) *See* Gitalin[a] *at loc. no.* **840**
Gitalin (1405-76-1) *See loc. no.* **840**
Glacial acetic acid (64-19-7) *See* Acetic Acid[a] *at loc. no.* **42**
Glauber's salt (7727-73-3) *See* Sulfate Salts[d] *at loc. no.* **159**
D-Glucitol (50-70-4) *See* D-Sorbitol[a] *at loc. no.* **706**
2-(β-D-Glucopyranosyloxy)-2-methylpropanenitrile (554-35-8) *See* Linamarin[a] *at loc. no.* **850**
Glutamic acid (56-86-0) *See* Monosodium Glutamate[b] *at loc. no.* **1618**
Glutamic acid hydrochloride (138-15-8) *See* Monosodium Glutamate[b] *at loc. no.* **1618**
Glutaraldehyde (111-30-8) *See loc. no.* **484**
Glutethimide (77-21-4) *See loc. no.* **1436**
Glycerin (56-81-5) *See loc. no.* **704**
Glycerine (56-81-5) *See* Glycerin[a] *at loc. no.* **704**
Glyceroboric acid (279-21-0) *See* Boroglycerin[a] *at loc. no.* **134**
Glycerol (56-81-5) *See* Glycerin[a] *at loc. no.* **704**
Glycerol Esters *See loc. no.* **573**
Glycerol oleate (25496-72-4) *See* Glycerol Esters[d] *at loc. no.* **573**
Glycerol phthalate *See* Glycerol Esters[d] *at loc. no.* **573**
Glycerol trinitrate (55-63-0) *See* Nitroglycerin(e)[a] *at loc. no.* **635**

Glyceryl borate (279-21-0) *See* Boroglycerin[a] *at loc. no.* **134**
Glyceryl guaiacolate (93-14-1) *See* Guaifenesin[a] *at loc. no.* **1597**
α-Glyceryl guaicol ether (93-14-1) *See* Guaifenesin[a] *at loc. no.* **1597**
Glyceryl monoacetate (26446-35-5) *See* Monoacetin[a] *at loc. no.* **577**
Glyceryl monostearate (8050-92-8) *See* Glyceryl Stearate[a] *at loc. no.* **965**
Glyceryl Stearate (8050-92-8) *See loc. no.* **965**
Glyceryl triacetate (102-76-1) *See* Triacetin[a] *at loc. no.* **579**
Glyceryl trinitrate (55-63-0) *See* Nitroglycerin(e)[a] *at loc. no.* **635**
Glycidyl Ethers *See loc. no.* **1629**
Glycine xylidide *See* Lidocaine[b] *at loc. no.* **1582**
Glycofurol (9004-76-6) *See loc. no.* **460**
Glycol ethers *See* Ethylene Glycol Alkyl (and Aryl) Ethers[e] *at loc. no.* **459**
Glycol ethylene ether (123-91-1) *See* Dioxane[a] *at loc. no.* **1621**
Glycolic Acid (79-14-1) *See loc. no.* **45**
Glycol monosalicylate (87-28-5) *See* Methyl Salicylate[b] *at loc. no.* **597**
Glycol salicylate (87-28-5) *See* Methyl Salicylate[b] *at loc. no.* **597**
Glycolyl phthalate *See* Phthalic Acid Esters[d] *at loc. no.* **589**
Glycyrrhetinic acid (471-53-4) *See* Ammonium Glycyrrhizate[b] *at loc. no.* **848**
Glycyrrhiza *See* Ammonium Glycyrrhizate[c] *at loc. no.* **848**
Glycyrrhizic acid (1405-86-3) *See* Ammonium Glycyrrhizate[b] *at loc. no.* **848**
Glyodin (556-22-9) *See loc. no.* **1196**
Glyoxide *See* Glyodin[b] *at loc. no.* **1196**
Glyoxyldiureide (97-59-6) *See* Allantoin[a] *at loc. no.* **477**
Glysennid *See* Senna Glycosides[c] *at loc. no.* **851**
Gnoscopine (6035-40-1) *See* Noscapine[b] *at loc. no.* **788**
Gold Bronze Powder *See loc. no.* **260**
Gold Salts *See loc. no.* **284**
Gold sodium thiomalate (554-42-7) *See* Gold Salts[d] *at loc. no.* **284**
Gold sodium thiosulfate (10210-36-3) *See* Gold Salts[d] *at loc. no.* **284**
Gold trichloride (10294-30-1) *See* Gold Salts[d] *at loc. no.* **284**
Goltix (41394-05-2) *See* Metamitron[c] *at loc. no.* **1265**
Goulard's extract (8006-24-4) *See* Lead[d] *at loc. no.* **245**
Graham's salt *See* Sodium Hexametaphosphate[a] *at loc. no.* **143**
Grain alcohol (64-17-5) *See* Ethyl Alcohol[a] *at loc. no.* **412**
Gramicidin (1405-97-6) *See* Tyrothricin[e] *at loc. no.* **905**
Gramoxone (4685-14-7) *See* Paraquat[c] *at loc. no.* **1286**
Granatin (1391-79-3) *See* Pomegranate Bark[e] *at loc. no.* **685**
Granatum *See* Pomegranate Bark[a] *at loc. no.* **685**
Granosan (107-27-7) *See* Ethyl Mercuric Chloride[c] *at loc. no.* **228**
Graphite (7782-42-5) *See loc. no.* **4**
Grass *See* Marihuana[a] *at loc. no.* **678**
Grease (lubricating) *See* Lubricating Oils[a] *at loc. no.* **338**
Green potatoes *See* Solanine[c] *at loc. no.* **832**
Grey arsenic (7440-38-2) *See* Arsenic[a] *at loc. no.* **188**
Griffith's zinc white (1345-05-7) *See* Lithopone[a] *at loc. no.* **115**
Griseofulvin (126-07-8) *See loc. no.* **900**
Grotan BK (4719-04-4) *See* Hexahydro-tris(2-hydroxyethyl)-s-triazine[c] *at loc. no.* **1173**
Groundnut oil (8002-03-7) *See* Peanut Oil[a] *at loc. no.* **719**
Guaiacol (90-05-1) *See loc. no.* **492**

---

[a] A Synonym　　[b] A Closely Related Substance　　[c] The Active or Major Constituent　　[d] A Class Name
[e] A Specific Example of or Product Containing

Ingredient name (CAS registry no.) *See* Primary Name *at location no.* **XXX** *in Part D of this section*

Guaifenesin (93-14-1) *See loc. no.* **1597**
Guarea rusbyi (Britt.) *See* Cocillana[c] *at loc. no.* **662**
Gum acacia (9000-01-5) *See* Acacia[a] *at loc. no.* **744**
Gum arabic (9000-01-5) *See* Acacia[a] *at loc. no.* **744**
Gum camphor (76-22-2) *See* Camphor[a] *at loc. no.* **875**
Gum ghatti (9000-28-6) *See* Gums (Vegetable)[d] *at loc. no.* **755**
Gum karaya (9000-36-6) *See* Gums (Vegetable)[d] *at loc. no.* **755**
Gum rosin (8050-10-0) *See* Rosin[b] *at loc. no.* **760**
Gums (Vegetable) *See loc. no.* **755**
Gum tragacanth (9000-65-1) *See* Gums (Vegetable)[d] *at loc. no.* **755**
Gum turpentine *See* Turpentine[a] *at loc. no.* **763**
Guthion (86-50-0) *See loc. no.* **1089**
Gypsum (13397-24-5) *See* Plaster of Paris[b] *at loc. no.* **172**
Gyromitra spp. *See* Gyromitrin[c] *at loc. no.* **816**
Gyromitrin (16568-02-8) *See loc. no.* **816**
Halazone (80-13-7) *See* Chloramine-T[b] *at loc. no.* **91**
Haldol (52-86-8) *See* Haloperidol[a] *at loc. no.* **1437**
Halogenated hydrocarbons *See* Chlorinated Hydrocarbons[e] *at loc. no.* **354**
Halogenated salicylanilide *See* 3,3',4',5-Tetrachlorosalicylanilide[e] *at loc. no.* **999**
Haloperidol (52-86-8) *See loc. no.* **1437**
Haloprogin (777-11-7) *See loc. no.* **1527**
Halotex cream *See* Haloprogin[a] *at loc. no.* **1527**
Halowax *See* Polychlorinated Naphthalenes[c] *at loc. no.* **402**
Hamamelis *See* Witch Hazel[a] *at loc. no.* **702**
Harman (486-84-0) *See* Passiflora[e] *at loc. no.* **681**
Harmonyl (131-01-1) *See* Deserpidine[c] *at loc. no.* **796**
Hashish (8001-45-4) *See* Marihuana[e] *at loc. no.* **678**
HCA (116-16-5) *See* Hexachloroacetone[a] *at loc. no.* **1307**
HCB (118-74-1) *See* Hexachlorobenzene[a] *at loc. no.* **397**
HCCH (608-73-1) *See* Benzene Hexachloride[a] *at loc. no.* **1029**
Heavy aromatic naphtha *See* Aromatic Solvent Naphtha[a] *at loc. no.* **342**
Heavy liquid petrolatum *See* Liquid Petrolatum[a] *at loc. no.* **337**
Heliotropin (120-57-0) *See* Piperonal[a] *at loc. no.* **871**
Heliotropin acetal *See* Tropital[a] *at loc. no.* **1156**
Henbane *See* Hyoscyamus[a] *at loc. no.* **674**
HEOD (60-57-1) *See* Dieldrin[a] *at loc. no.* **1020**
Heparin Sodium (9005-49-6) *See loc. no.* **1598**
Heptabarbital (509-86-4) *See loc. no.* **1374**
Heptachlor (76-44-8) *See loc. no.* **1022**
Heptachlorocamphene *See* Strobane[e] *at loc. no.* **1031**
Heptachlorodicyclopentadiene (76-44-8) *See* Heptachlor[a] *at loc. no.* **1022**
Heptachloro-tetrahydro-4,7-endo-methanoindene (76-44-8) *See* Heptachlor[a] *at loc. no.* **1022**
2-Heptadecyl glyoxalidine acetate (556-22-9) *See* Glyodin[a] *at loc. no.* **1196**
2-Heptadecyl-2-imidazoline (105-28-2) *See* Glyodin[b] *at loc. no.* **1196**
2-Heptadecyl imidazoline acetate (556-22-9) *See* Glyodin[a] *at loc. no.* **1196**
n-Heptane (142-82-5) *See* n-Hexane[b] *at loc. no.* **307**
Heptazine (1912-25-0) *See* Atrazine[b] *at loc. no.* **1259**
Herban (18530-56-8) *See* Noruron[c] *at loc. no.* **1255**
Herbicide 273 *See* Endothall[b] *at loc. no.* **1304**
Herbisan (502-55-6) *See* Diethyl Dithiobis(thionoformate)[c] *at loc. no.* **1302**
Hercules 7531 (18530-56-8) *See* Noruron[c] *at loc. no.* **1255**
Heroin (561-27-3) *See loc. no.* **782**
Hesperidin (520-26-3) *See* Hesperidin Methyl Chalcone[b] *at loc. no.* **1599**

Hesperidin Methyl Chalcone (24292-52-2) *See loc. no.* **1599**
Hesperitin-7-rhamnoglucoside (520-26-3) *See* Hesperidin Methyl Chalcone[b] *at loc. no.* **1599**
HETP (757-58-4) *See* Hexaethyl Tetraphosphate[a] *at loc. no.* **1106**
Hetrazan (90-89-1) *See* Diethylcarbamazine[c] *at loc. no.* **1539**
Hexa-(1-aziridinyl)-triphosphatriazine (52-46-0) *See* Apholate[a] *at loc. no.* **1354**
Hexabione *See* Pyridoxine Hydrochloride[c] *at loc. no.* **912**
Hexabromobiphenyl (36355-01-8) *See* Polybrominated Biphenyls[e] *at loc. no.* **398**
Hexachloroacetone (116-16-5) *See loc. no.* **1307**
Hexachlorobenzene (118-74-1) *See loc. no.* **397**
Hexachlorocyclohexane (608-73-1) *See* Benzene Hexachloride[a] *at loc. no.* **1029**
γ-Hexachlorocyclohexane (58-89-9) *See* Lindane[a] *at loc. no.* **1028**
Hexachlorocyclopentadiene (77-47-4) *See loc. no.* **388**
Hexachlorodibenzo-p-dioxin *See* Polychlorinated Dibenzodioxins[d] *at loc. no.* **400**
Hexachloro-epoxy-octahydro-endo,endo-dimethanonaphthalene (72-20-8) *See* Endrin[e] *at loc. no.* **1021**
Hexachloro-epoxy-octahydro-endo,exo-dimethanonaphthalene (60-57-1) *See* Dieldrin[a] *at loc. no.* **1020**
Hexachloro-epoxy-octahydro-dimethanonaphthalene *See loc. no.* **1023**
Hexachloroethane (67-72-1) *See loc. no.* **370**
Hexachloroethylene (67-72-1) *See* Hexachloroethane[a] *at loc. no.* **370**
Hexachloro-hexahydro-endo,endo-dimethanonaphthalene (465-73-6) *See* Isodrin[a] *at loc. no.* **1025**
Hexachloro-hexahydro-endo,exo-dimethanonaphthalene (309-00-2) *See* Aldrin[a] *at loc. no.* **1017**
Hexachloro-hexahydro-methano-2,4,3-benzodioxathiepin oxide (115-29-7) *See* Thiodan[a] *at loc. no.* **1026**
Hexachloronaphthalene (1335-87-1) *See* Polychlorinated Naphthalenes[d] *at loc. no.* **402**
Hexachlorophene (70-30-4) *See loc. no.* **531**
Hexachloro-2-propanone (116-16-5) *See* Hexachloroacetone[a] *at loc. no.* **1307**
1-Hexadecanol (124-29-8) *See* Cetyl Alcohol[a] *at loc. no.* **409**
Hexadecyl Alcohol *See loc. no.* **415**
2,4-Hexadienoic acid (110-44-1) *See* Sorbic Acid[a] *at loc. no.* **561**
Hexaethyl Tetraphosphate (757-58-4) *See loc. no.* **1106**
Hexafluorosilicates *See* Fluosilicate Salts[d] *at loc. no.* **101**
Hexafluosilicic acid (1309-45-1) *See* Fluosilicic Acid[a] *at loc. no.* **37**
Hexahydroaniline (108-91-8) *See* Cyclohexylamine[a] *at loc. no.* **609**
Hexahydro-(1-aziridinyl)-triazaphosphorine (52-46-0) *See* Apholate[a] *at loc. no.* **1354**
Hexahydrobenzene (110-82-7) *See* Cyclohexane[a] *at loc. no.* **308**
Hexahydrobenzoic acid (98-89-5) *See* Naphthenic Acids[d] *at loc. no.* **558**
Hexahydro-3α,7α-dimethyl-4,7-epoxyisobenzofuran-1,3-dione (56-25-7) *See* Cantharidin[a] *at loc. no.* **924**
2,2,4,4,6,6-Hexahydro-2,2,4,4,6,6-hexakis(1-aziridinyl)-1,3,5,2,4,6-triazatriphosphorine (52-46-0) *See* Apholate[a] *at loc. no.* **1354**
1-[3-(Hexahydro-4,7-methanoindanyl)]-3,3-dimethylurea (28805-78-9) *See* Noruron[b] *at loc. no.* **1255**
1-[5-(Hexahydro-4,7-methanoindanyl)]-3,3-dimethylurea (18530-56-8) *See* Noruron[a] *at loc. no.* **1255**
Hexahydrophenol (108-93-0) *See* Cyclohexanol[a] *at loc. no.* **410**

---

[a] A Synonym   [b] A Closely Related Substance   [c] The Active or Major Constituent   [d] A Class Name
[e] A Specific Example of or Product Containing

Ingredient name (CAS registry no.) *See* Primary Name *at
location no.* **XXX** *in Part D of this section*

Hexahydrothymol (89-78-1) *See* Menthol[a] *at loc. no.* **868**
Hexahydrotoluene (108-87-2) *See* Methylcyclohexane[a] *at loc. no.* **309**
Hexahydro-1,3,5-triethyl-s-triazine (7779-27-3) *See loc. no.* **1172**
Hexahydro-1,3,5-trinitro-s-triazine (121-82-4) *See* Cyclonite[a] *at loc. no.* **631**
Hexahydro-tris(2-hydroxyethyl)-s-triazine (4719-04-4) *See loc. no.* **1173**
Hexakis(1-aziridinyl)-phosphonitrile (52-46-0) *See* Apholate[a] *at loc. no.* **1354**
Hexalin (108-93-0) *See* Cyclohexanol[c] *at loc. no.* **410**
Hexamethylenamine (100-97-0) *See* Methenamine[a] *at loc. no.* **486**
Hexamethylene (110-82-7) *See* Cyclohexane[a] *at loc. no.* **308**
1,1'-Hexamethylenebis(5-(p-chlorophenyl)-biguanide) *See* Chlorhexidine[a] *at loc. no.* **994**
Hexamethylenetetramine (100-97-0) *See* Methenamine[a] *at loc. no.* **486**
Hexamethylpararosaniline chloride (548-62-9) *See* Gentian Violet[a] *at loc. no.* **1520**
2,6,10,15,19,23-Hexamethyltetracosane (111-01-3) *See* Squalane[a] *at loc. no.* **932**
Hexanal N-methyl-N-formylhydrazone *See* Gyromitrin[b] *at loc. no.* **816**
n-Hexane (110-54-3) *See loc. no.* **307**
2,5-Hexanedione (110-13-4) *See* Methyl n-Butyl Ketone[b] *at loc. no.* **479**
1,2,6-Hexanetriol (106-69-4) *See loc. no.* **446**
1-Hexanol (111-27-3) *See* Hexyl Alcohol[c] *at loc. no.* **416**
2-Hexanol *See* Methyl n-Butyl Ketone[b] *at loc. no.* **479**
n-2-Hexanone (591-78-6) *See* Methyl n-Butyl Ketone[a] *at loc. no.* **479**
Hexazinone (51235-04-2) *See loc. no.* **1263**
Hexestrol (84-16-2) *See* Estrogens (Natural and Synthetic)[d] *at loc. no.* **916**
Hexethal Sodium (144-00-3) *See loc. no.* **1375**
Hexobarbital Sodium (50-09-9) *See loc. no.* **1376**
Hexogen (121-82-4) *See* Cyclonite[a] *at loc. no.* **631**
Hexyl Alcohol *See loc. no.* **416**
4-Hexyl-1,3-dihydroxybenzene (136-77-6) *See* Hexylresorcinol[a] *at loc. no.* **503**
Hexylene Glycol (107-41-5) *See loc. no.* **445**
5-n-Hexyl-5-ethylbarbituric acid sodium (144-00-3) *See* Hexethal Sodium[a] *at loc. no.* **1375**
3-Hexyl-5-(3,4-methylenedioxyphenyl)-2-cyclohexene-1-one (119-89-1) *See* Piperonyl Cyclonene[a] *at loc. no.* **1152**
n-Hexylphenol *See* Amyl Phenol[b] *at loc. no.* **488**
Hexylresorcinol (136-77-6) *See loc. no.* **503**
Hexylthiocarbam (1134-23-2) *See* Cycloate[a] *at loc. no.* **1234**
Hibiclens (18472-51-0) *See* Chlorhexidine[b] *at loc. no.* **994**
High-boiling petroleum ether *See* Petroleum Ether[b] *at loc. no.* **330**
High flash naphtha *See* Stoddard Solvent[a] *at loc. no.* **334**
High flash naphtha (aliphatic) (8032-32-4) *See* VM&P Naphthas[a] *at loc. no.* **335**
High flash naphtha (aromatic) *See* Aromatic Solvent Naphtha[a] *at loc. no.* **342**
Histadyl (135-23-9) *See* Methapyrilene Hydrochloride[c] *at loc. no.* **1495**
Histantine (82-93-9) *See* Chlorcyclizine[c] *at loc. no.* **1489**
Hoelon (51338-27-3) *See* Diclofop-methyl[a] *at loc. no.* **1301**
Holly *See loc. no.* **672**
Homatropine (87-00-3) *See loc. no.* **769**
Homatropine methylbromide (80-49-9) *See* Homatropine[b] *at loc. no.* **769**

Home heating oil no. 1 *See* Kerosene[a] *at loc. no.* **328**
Home heating oil no. 2 *See* Fuel Oil[a] *at loc. no.* **326**
Homomenthyl salicylate (118-56-9) *See* Homosalate[a] *at loc. no.* **1533**
Homosalate (118-56-9) *See loc. no.* **1533**
Homosalicylic acids *See* Cresotic Acids[a] *at loc. no.* **595**
Horse beans *See* Fava Beans[a] *at loc. no.* **670**
Hyamine 1622 (121-54-0) *See* Benzethonium Chloride[c] *at loc. no.* **986**
Hyamine 2389 (1399-80-0) *See* Alkyl Tolyl Methyl Trimethyl Ammonium Chloride[d] *at loc. no.* **982**
Hyamine 10X (25155-18-4) *See* Methylbenzethonium Chloride[a] *at loc. no.* **992**
Hydnocarpus oil (8001-74-9) *See* Chaulmoogra Oil[a] *at loc. no.* **713**
Hydrastine (118-08-1) *See loc. no.* **827**
Hydrastis *See loc. no.* **673**
Hydrastis canadensis *See* Hydrastis[a] *at loc. no.* **673**
Hydrated alumina *See* Aluminum Hydroxide[a] *at loc. no.* **178**
Hydrated aluminum silicate (13132-95-1) *See* Kaolin[b] *at loc. no.* **5**
Hydrated chromium oxide *See* Chromium Oxide[b] *at loc. no.* **280**
Hydrazine (302-01-2) *See* Monomethylhydrazine[b] *at loc. no.* **817**
Hydrazoic acid (7782-79-8) *See* Azide Salts[b] *at loc. no.* **111**
Hydrobenzthiazide (13957-38-5) *See* Benzothiadiazide Diuretics[d] *at loc. no.* **1588**
Hydrocarbons aliphatic *See* Aliphatic Hydrocarbons[a] *at loc. no.* **303**
Hydrocarbons aromatic *See* Aromatic Hydrocarbon Solvent[a] *at loc. no.* **310**
Hydrochloric Acid (7647-01-0) *See loc. no.* **31**
Hydrochlorothiazide (58-93-5) *See* Benzothiadiazide Diuretics[d] *at loc. no.* **1588**
Hydrocodone Bitartrate (34195-34-1) *See loc. no.* **783**
Hydrocortisone (50-23-7) *See* Corticosteroids[d] *at loc. no.* **915**
Hydrocortisone acetate (50-03-3) *See* Corticosteroids[d] *at loc. no.* **915**
Hydrocyanic Acid (74-90-8) *See loc. no.* **106**
Hydrofluoric Acid (7664-39-3) *See loc. no.* **36**
Hydrogen arsenide (7784-42-1) *See* Arsine[a] *at loc. no.* **196**
Hydrogen azide (7782-79-8) *See* Azide Salts[b] *at loc. no.* **111**
Hydrogen chloride (7647-01-0) *See* Hydrochloric Acid[a] *at loc. no.* **31**
Hydrogen chloride gas *See* Nitrogen Oxides[b] *at loc. no.* **9**
Hydrogen cyanate (420-05-3) *See* Cyanic Acid[a] *at loc. no.* **29**
Hydrogen cyanide (74-90-8) *See* Hydrocyanic Acid[a] *at loc. no.* **106**
Hydrogen fluoride (7664-39-3) *See* Hydrofluoric Acid[a] *at loc. no.* **36**
Hydrogen fluoride gas *See* Nitrogen Oxides[b] *at loc. no.* **9**
Hydrogen hexafluorosilicate (1309-45-1) *See* Fluosilicic Acid[a] *at loc. no.* **37**
Hydrogen Peroxide (8007-30-5) *See loc. no.* **73**
Hydrogen Sulfide (7783-06-4) *See loc. no.* **114**
Hydrogen telluride (7783-09-7) *See* Tellurium Derivatives[d] *at loc. no.* **187**
Hydrol (6392-46-7) *See* Allyxycarb[c] *at loc. no.* **1121**
Hydronol (652-67-5) *See* Isosorbide[c] *at loc. no.* **1603**
Hydrophilic petrolatum (8027-64-3) *See* Liquid Petrolatum[b] *at loc. no.* **337**
Hydroquinone (123-31-9) *See loc. no.* **504**

---

[a] A Synonym   [b] A Closely Related Substance   [c] The Active or Major Constituent   [d] A Class Name
[e] A Specific Example of or Product Containing

Ingredient name (CAS registry no.) *See* Primary Name *at*
location no. **XXX** *in Part D of this section*

Hydrosulfuric acid (7783-06-4) *See* Hydrogen Sulfide[a] *at loc. no.* **114**

Hydrothol 47 or 191 (6385-60-0) *See* Endothall[b] *at loc. no.* **1304**

Hydrous wool fat (8020-84-6) *See* Lanolin[a] *at loc. no.* **716**

Hydroxide (14280-30-9) *See* Lye[b] *at loc. no.* **51**

Hydroxide carbonate *See* Lye[a] *at loc. no.* **51**

4′-Hydroxyacetanilide (103-90-2) *See* Acetaminophen[a] *at loc. no.* **1587**

Hydroxyacetic acid (79-14-1) *See* Glycolic Acid[a] *at loc. no.* **45**

Hydroxyamphetamine (1518-86-1) *See* Hydroxyamphetamine Hydrobromide[b] *at loc. no.* **1457**

Hydroxyamphetamine Hydrobromide (140-36-3) *See loc. no.* **1457**

p-Hydroxyaniline (123-30-8) *See* p-Aminophenol[a] *at loc. no.* **624**

o-Hydroxyanisole (90-05-1) *See* Guaiacol[a] *at loc. no.* **492**

o-Hydroxybenzamide (65-45-2) *See* Salicylamide[a] *at loc. no.* **599**

Hydroxybenzene (108-95-2) *See* Phenol[a] *at loc. no.* **494**

o-Hydroxybenzoic acid (69-72-7) *See* Salicylate[d] *at loc. no.* **600**

2-Hydroxycamphane (507-70-0) *See* Borneol[a] *at loc. no.* **876**

Hydroxychloroquine (118-42-3) *See* Chloroquine[b] *at loc. no.* **1512**

7-Hydroxycoumarin (93-35-6) *See* Umbelliferone[a] *at loc. no.* **934**

3-Hydroxycrotonic acid methyl ester dimethyl phosphate (7786-34-7) *See* Phosdrin[e] *at loc. no.* **1057**

N[5]-(1-Hydroxycyclopropyl)-L-glutamine *See* Coprine[a] *at loc. no.* **815**

2-Hydroxy-p-cymene (499-75-2) *See* Carvacrol[a] *at loc. no.* **489**

3-Hydroxy-p-cymene (89-83-8) *See* Thymol[a] *at loc. no.* **497**

4-Hydroxy-N,N-dimethyltryptamine (520-53-6) *See* Psilocybin[b] *at loc. no.* **821**

5-Hydroxy-N,N-dimethyltryptamine (487-93-4) *See* Bufotenine[a] *at loc. no.* **820**

1-Hydroxy-2,4-dinitrobenzene (51-28-5) *See* 2,4-Dinitrophenol[a] *at loc. no.* **541**

2-Hydroxydiphenyl (90-43-7) *See* Phenylphenol[d] *at loc. no.* **495**

Hydroxyethanoic acid (79-14-1) *See* Glycolic Acid[a] *at loc. no.* **45**

β-Hydroxyethylamine (141-43-5) *See* Monoethanolamine (and Salts)[a] *at loc. no.* **64**

N-Hydroxy-ethyl-ethylenediaminetriacetate (150-39-0) *See* Ethylenediaminetetraacetic Acid (and Salts)[b] *at loc. no.* **1506**

N-(β-Hydroxyethyl)-2-lactamide *See loc. no.* **567**

2-Hydroxy-ethyl methacrylate (141-32-2) *See* Acrylic Resin Monomers[d] *at loc. no.* **1625**

2-Hydroxyethyl-n-octyl Sulfide (3547-33-9) *See loc. no.* **1330**

4-Hydroxy-2-keto-4-methyl pentane (123-42-2) *See* Diacetone Alcohol[a] *at loc. no.* **469**

Hydroxylamine (and Salts) (7803-49-8) *See loc. no.* **122**

Hydroxylamine hydrochloride (5470-11-1) *See* Hydroxylamine (and Salts)[d] *at loc. no.* **122**

Hydroxylamine sulfate (10039-54-0) *See* Hydroxylamine (and Salts)[d] *at loc. no.* **122**

Hydroxymercurichlorophenol (538-04-5) *See* 2-Chloro-4-(hydroxymercuri)phenol[a] *at loc. no.* **224**

Hydroxymercuricresol *See loc. no.* **232**

Hydroxymercurinitrophenol (1344-31-6) *See loc. no.* **233**

Hydroxymethoxybenzenesulfonic acid potassium salt *See* Potassium Guaiacolsulfonate[a] *at loc. no.* **496**

2-Hydroxy-4-methoxybenzophenone (131-57-7) *See* Oxybenzone[a] *at loc. no.* **1537**

2-Hydroxy-4-methoxy benzophenone-5-sulfonic acid (4065-45-6) *See* Oxybenzone[b] *at loc. no.* **1537**

N-Hydroxymethylacrylamide (924-42-5) *See* Acrylamide[b] *at loc. no.* **1624**

α-Hydroxy-β-methylaminopropylbenzene (299-42-3) *See* Ephedrine[a] *at loc. no.* **1450**

p-Hydroxymethylaniline sulfate (55-55-0) *See* p-Methylaminophenol Sulfate[a] *at loc. no.* **626**

1-Hydroxy-3-methyl-4-chloro-6-isopropylbenzene (89-68-9) *See* Chlorothymol[a] *at loc. no.* **527**

N-Hydroxymethyl N-methyldithiocarbamate of potassium (51026-28-9) *See* Bunema[a] *at loc. no.* **1157**

3-Hydroxy-17-methyl-morphinan (77-07-6) *See* Levorphanol[a] *at loc. no.* **785**

2-(Hydroxymethyl)-2-nitro-1,3-propanediol (126-11-4) *See* Tris(hydroxymethyl)nitromethane[a] *at loc. no.* **1003**

4-Hydroxy-4-methyl-2-pentanone (123-42-2) *See* Diacetone Alcohol[a] *at loc. no.* **469**

2-Hydroxy-2-methylpropanenitrile (75-86-5) *See* Acetone Cyanohydrin[a] *at loc. no.* **646**

5-Hydroxy-6-methyl-3,4-pyridine dimethanol hydrochloride (58-56-0) *See* Pyridoxine Hydrochloride[a] *at loc. no.* **912**

3-Hydroxy-2-methyl-4-pyrone (118-71-8) *See loc. no.* **866**

β-Hydroxynaphthalene (135-19-3) *See* β-Naphthol[a] *at loc. no.* **493**

4-Hydroxy-3-nitroaniline (119-34-6) *See* 4-Amino-2-nitrophenol[a] *at loc. no.* **625**

4-Hydroxynitrobenzene (100-02-7) *See* p-Nitrophenol[a] *at loc. no.* **544**

4-Hydroxy-3-nitrobenzenearsonic acid (121-19-7) *See* 4-Hydroxy-3-nitrophenylarsonic Acid[a] *at loc. no.* **205**

4-Hydroxy-3-nitrophenylarsonic Acid (121-19-7) *See loc. no.* **205**

12-Hydroxy-9-octadecenoic acid (141-22-0) *See* Ricinoleic Acid[a] *at loc. no.* **560**

2-Hydroxy-N-phenylbenzamide (87-17-2) *See* Salicylanilide[a] *at loc. no.* **998**

Hydroxyphenylmercuric chloride (90-03-9) *See* Hydroxyphenylmercurichloride[a] *at loc. no.* **234**

Hydroxyphenylmercurichloride (90-03-9) *See loc. no.* **234**

2-Hydroxy-1,2,3-propanetricarboxylic acid (77-92-9) *See* Citric Acid[a] *at loc. no.* **703**

Hydroxypropyl Methylcellulose (9004-65-3) *See loc. no.* **855**

6-Hydroxy-3(2H)-pyridazinone (10071-13-3) *See* Maleic Hydrazide[b] *at loc. no.* **1308**

5-[(α-Hydroxy-α-2-pyridyl)benzyl]-7-[α-2-(pyridylbenzyl)idine]-5-norbornene-2,3-dicarboximide (991-42-4) *See* Norbormide[a] *at loc. no.* **1349**

8-Hydroxyquinoline (148-24-3) *See loc. no.* **1514**

Hydroxyquinoline salt *See* 8-Hydroxyquinoline[e] *at loc. no.* **1514**

5-Hydroxythiabendazole *See* Thiabendazole[b] *at loc. no.* **1177**

α-Hydroxytoluene (100-51-6) *See* Benzyl Alcohol[a] *at loc. no.* **406**

Hydroxytoluenes *See* Cresols[a] *at loc. no.* **514**

Hydroxytoluic acids *See* Cresotic Acids[a] *at loc. no.* **595**

3-Hydroxy-N,N,5-trimethylpyrazole-1-carboxamide dimethylcarbamate (ester) (644-64-4) *See* Dimetilan[a] *at loc. no.* **1132**

---

[a] A Synonym   [b] A Closely Related Substance   [c] The Active or Major Constituent   [d] A Class Name
[e] A Specific Example of or Product Containing

Ingredient name (CAS registry no.) *See* Primary Name *at*
location no. **XXX** *in Part D of this section*

5-Hydroxytryptamine (50-67-9) *See* Bufotenine[b] *at loc. no.* 820

5-Hydroxytryptophan (56-69-9) *See* Bufotenine[b] *at loc. no.* 820

Hydroxyzine Hydrochloride (2192-20-3) *See loc. no.* 1438

Hyoscine (51-34-3) *See* Scopolamine[a] *at loc. no.* 771

Hyoscine hydrobromide (114-49-8) *See* Scopolamine[b] *at loc. no.* 771

Hyoscyamine (101-31-5) *See loc. no.* 770

dl-Hyoscyamine (51-55-8) *See* Atropine[a] *at loc. no.* 767

l-Hyoscyamine (101-31-5) *See* Hyoscyamine[a] *at loc. no.* 770

Hyoscyamus *See loc. no.* 674

Hypo (7772-98-7) *See* Sodium Thiosulfate[a] *at loc. no.* 163

Hypochlorite *See loc. no.* 84

Hypochlorite salts *See* Sodium Hypochlorite[e] *at loc. no.* 85

Hyposulfites *See* Thiosulfate Salts[a] *at loc. no.* 161

Hyvar X (314-40-9) *See* Bromacil[a] *at loc. no.* 1294

Ibotenic acid (60573-88-8) *See* Muscimol[b] *at loc. no.* 819

Ichthammol (8029-68-3) *See loc. no.* 1528

Ichthyol (8029-68-3) *See* Ichthammol[a] *at loc. no.* 1528

Igepals *See* Alkyl Phenoxy Polyethoxy Ethanols[c] *at loc. no.* 963

Igepons AT and AC *See* Alkyl Sodium Isethionate[c] *at loc. no.* 945

Igepons T and TK and TN and T-42 and T-51 *See* Alkyl Sodium *N*-Methyltaurate[c] *at loc. no.* 948

Ilex *See* Holly[a] *at loc. no.* 672

Illuminating gas *See* Gas[d] *at loc. no.* 128

Imidan (732-11-6) *See loc. no.* 1090

2-Imidazolidinethione (96-45-7) *See* Ethylenethiourea[a] *at loc. no.* 1169

Imidazolidinyl Urea (39236-46-9) *See loc. no.* 996

Iminodiethanol (111-42-2) *See* Diethanolamine (and Salts)[a] *at loc. no.* 65

2-Imino-5-phenyl-4-oxazolidinone *See* Pemoline[a] *at loc. no.* 1465

Imipramine (50-49-7) *See loc. no.* 1473

Imperial green (12002-03-8) *See* Copper Acetoarsenite[b] *at loc. no.* 200

Indalone *See* Butopyronoxyl[c] *at loc. no.* 1322

Indar (16227-10-4) *See* Triazabutil[c] *at loc. no.* 1272

Inderal (318-98-9) *See* Propranolol Hydrochloride[c] *at loc. no.* 1613

Indian balsam (8007-00-9) *See* Balsam Peru[a] *at loc. no.* 749

Indium (and Salts) (7440-74-6) *See loc. no.* 285

Indocin (53-86-1) *See* Indomethacin[c] *at loc. no.* 1600

Indomethacin (53-86-1) *See loc. no.* 1600

Inert Ingredients *See loc. no.* 1

Infusorial earth (7631-86-9) *See* Silica[a] *at loc. no.* 7

INH (54-85-3) *See* Isoniazid[a] *at loc. no.* 1601

Inocybe spp. *See* Muscarine[c] *at loc. no.* 818

Inorganic acid *See* Acid[d] *at loc. no.* 30

Iodate Salts *See loc. no.* 97

Iodide Salts *See loc. no.* 99

Iodine (7553-56-2) *See loc. no.* 26

Iodochlorhydroxyquin (130-26-7) *See* Diiodohydroxyquin[b] *at loc. no.* 1513

Iodoform (75-47-8) *See loc. no.* 1529

Iodomethane (74-88-4) *See* Methyl Iodide[a] *at loc. no.* 346

Iodophors (8037-86-3) *See loc. no.* 997

Iodoquinol (83-73-8) *See* Diiodohydroxyquin[a] *at loc. no.* 1513

Ionamin *See* Phentermine[c] *at loc. no.* 1467

Ipatone (3004-70-4) *See* Terbumeton[b] *at loc. no.* 1270

Ipazine (1912-25-0) *See* Atrazine[b] *at loc. no.* 1259

Ipecac (8012-96-2) *See loc. no.* 675

Ipecac and Opium Powder (8013-48-7) *See loc. no.* 676

Ipral sodium (143-82-8) *See* Probarbital Sodium[c] *at loc. no.* 1383

Iprodione (36734-19-7) *See loc. no.* 1197

Iproniazid Phosphate (305-33-9) *See loc. no.* 1475

Irgasan DP-300 (3380-34-5) *See* Triclosan[c] *at loc. no.* 1002

Irish moss *See* Carrageenan[c] *at loc. no.* 753

Iron choline citrate (1336-80-7) *See* Ferrocholinate[a] *at loc. no.* 255

Iron Salts *See loc. no.* 250

Iron sodium *N*-hydroxyethylethylenediaminetriacetate *See* Iron Salts[d] *at loc. no.* 250

Isoacetophorone (78-59-1) *See* Isophorone[a] *at loc. no.* 473

Isoamyl Acetate (123-92-2) *See loc. no.* 574

Isoamyl Alcohol (123-51-3) *See loc. no.* 417

Isoamyl formate (110-45-2) *See* Isoamyl Acetate[b] *at loc. no.* 574

Isoamyl isovalerate (659-70-1) *See* Isoamyl Acetate[b] *at loc. no.* 574

Isoamyl nitrite (110-46-3) *See* Amyl Nitrite[b] *at loc. no.* 630

Isoamyl *n*-propionate (105-68-0) *See* Isoamyl Acetate[b] *at loc. no.* 574

Isoamyl Salicylate (87-20-7) *See loc. no.* 596

Isobenzan (297-78-9) *See loc. no.* 1024

Isobornyl thiocyanoacetate (115-31-1) *See* Thanite[e] *at loc. no.* 1038

Isobutamben (94-14-4) *See* Butamben[b] *at loc. no.* 1579

Isobutane (75-28-5) *See loc. no.* 305

Isobutenyl chloride (563-47-3) *See* 3-Chloro-2-methyl-1-propene[a] *at loc. no.* 382

Isobutenyl methyl ketone (141-79-7) *See* Mesityl Oxide[a] *at loc. no.* 474

Isobutyl acetate (110-19-0) *See* *n*-Butyl Acetate[b] *at loc. no.* 568

Isobutyl Alcohol (78-83-1) *See loc. no.* 418

Isobutyl-allyl-barbituric acid *See* Butalbital[a] *at loc. no.* 1368

Isobutyl-*p*-aminobenzoate (94-14-4) *See* Butamben[b] *at loc. no.* 1579

Isobutyl *n*-butyrate (539-90-2) *See* *n*-Butyl Acetate[b] *at loc. no.* 568

Isobutyl ester of 2,4,5-T *See* Trichlorophenoxyacetic Acid[b] *at loc. no.* 1224

Isobutyl formate (542-55-2) *See* *n*-Butyl Acetate[b] *at loc. no.* 568

Isobutyl isovalerate (589-59-3) *See* *n*-Butyl Acetate[b] *at loc. no.* 568

Isobutyl 2-methyl-4-chlorophenoxyacetate *See* MCPA[b] *at loc. no.* 1220

Isobutyl nitrite (542-56-3) *See* Amyl Nitrite[b] *at loc. no.* 630

Isobutyl *n*-propionate (540-42-1) *See* *n*-Butyl Acetate[b] *at loc. no.* 568

Isobutyraldehyde (78-84-2) *See* Acetaldehyde[b] *at loc. no.* 480

Isocil (314-42-1) *See* Bromacil[b] *at loc. no.* 1294

Isocyanates (aryl) *See* Toluene-2,4-diisocyanate[e] *at loc. no.* 1641

Isocyanic acid (75-13-8) *See* Cyanic Acid[b] *at loc. no.* 29

Isocyanuric acid (504-19-8) *See* Cyanuric Acid[a] *at loc. no.* 1261

Isodrin (465-73-6) *See loc. no.* 1025

d-Isoephedrine hydrochloride (6272-89-5) *See* Pseudoephedrine Hydrochloride[a] *at loc. no.* 1453

Isoflurophate (55-91-4) *See* Diisopropyl Fluorophosphate[a] *at loc. no.* 1096

Isolan (119-38-0) *See loc. no.* 1136

Isomethiozin (57052-04-7) *See loc. no.* 1264

---

[a] A Synonym   [b] A Closely Related Substance   [c] The Active or Major Constituent   [d] A Class Name
[e] A Specific Example of or Product Containing

Ingredient name (CAS registry no.) *See* Primary Name *at location no.* **XXX** *in Part D of this section*

Isoniazid (54-85-3) *See loc. no.* **1601**
1-Isonicotinoyl-2-isopropylhydrazine phosphate (305-33-9) *See* Iproniazid Phosphate[a] *at loc. no.* **1475**
Isonicotinylhydrazine (54-85-3) *See* Isoniazid[a] *at loc. no.* **1601**
Isononyl Alcohol *See loc. no.* **419**
Isonoruron (28805-78-9) *See* Noruron[b] *at loc. no.* **1255**
Isooctyl *derivative. See corresponding* Octyl *or* Alkyl *derivative in this index.*
Isooctyl Alcohol (26952-21-6) *See loc. no.* **421**
Isooctyl 4-(2,4-dichlorophenoxy)butyrate (1320-15-6) *See* 4-(2,4-Dichlorophenoxy)butyric Acid[b] *at loc. no.* **1215**
Isooctyl 2-(2,4-dichlorophenoxy)propionate *See* 2-(2,4-Dichlorophenoxy)propionic Acid[b] *at loc. no.* **1217**
Isooctyl ester of 2,4,5-T (25168-15-4) *See* Trichlorophenoxyacetic Acid[b] *at loc. no.* **1224**
Isooctyl ester of 2-(2,4,5-trichlorophenoxy)propionic acid (32534-95-5) *See* Silvex[b] *at loc. no.* **1223**
Isooctyl 2-methyl-4-chlorophenoxyacetate *See* MCPA[b] *at loc. no.* **1220**
Isooctyl picloram (26952-20-5) *See* Picloram[b] *at loc. no.* **1312**
Isoparaffinic hydrocarbons *See* Aliphatic Hydrocarbons[d] *at loc. no.* **303**
Isopentaquine (529-73-7) *See* Primaquine[b] *at loc. no.* **1516**
Isopentyl alcohol (123-51-3) *See* Isoamyl Alcohol[a] *at loc. no.* **417**
Isopestox (371-86-8) *See* Mipafox[a] *at loc. no.* **1100**
Isophorone (78-59-1) *See loc. no.* **473**
Isopolyester resins *See* Polyester Resins[b] *at loc. no.* **1634**
Isoprocarb (2631-40-5) *See loc. no.* **1137**
Isopropalin (33820-53-0) *See* Benefin[b] *at loc. no.* **1287**
Isopropamide (7492-32-2) *See loc. no.* **1602**
Isopropanol (67-63-0) *See* Isopropyl Alcohol[a] *at loc. no.* **420**
Isopropanolamine 2-methyl-4-chlorophenoxyacetate *See* MCPA[b] *at loc. no.* **1220**
2-Isopropoxyphenyl N-methylcarbamate (114-26-1) *See* Propoxur[a] *at loc. no.* **1147**
o-Isopropoxyphenyl N-methylcarbamate (114-26-1) *See* Propoxur[a] *at loc. no.* **1147**
Isopropyl *derivative. If not listed here, see corresponding* Alkyl *derivative in this index.*
Isopropyl acetate (108-21-4) *See* Propyl Acetate[b] *at loc. no.* **578**
Isopropylacetone (108-10-1) *See* Methyl Isobutyl Ketone[a] *at loc. no.* **478**
Isopropyl Alcohol (67-63-0) *See loc. no.* **420**
2-(Isopropylamino)-4-[(3-methoxypropyl)amino]-6-(methylthio)-s-triazine (841-06-5) *See* Prometon[b] *at loc. no.* **1267**
2-(Isopropylamino)-4-(methylamino)-6-(methylthio)-s-triazine (1014-69-3) *See* Prometon[b] *at loc. no.* **1267**
1-(Isopropylamino)-3-(1-naphthyloxy)-2-propanol (318-98-9) *See* Propranolol Hydrochloride[a] *at loc. no.* **1613**
Isopropylbenzene (98-82-8) *See* Cumene[a] *at loc. no.* **313**
3-Isopropyl-(1H)-2,1,3-benzothiadiazin-4(3H)-one-2,2-dioxide (25057-89-0) *See* Bentazon[a] *at loc. no.* **1291**
5-Isopropyl-5-beta-bromallylbarbituric acid (545-93-7) *See* Propallylonal[a] *at loc. no.* **1385**
5-Isopropyl-5-β-bromallyl-N-methylbarbituric acid (125-55-3) *See* Pronarcon[a] *at loc. no.* **1384**
Isopropyl carbanilate (122-42-9) *See* Chlorpropham[b] *at loc. no.* **1229**
Isopropyl carbinol (78-83-1) *See* Isobutyl Alcohol[a] *at loc. no.* **418**
Isopropyl m-chlorocarbanilate (101-21-3) *See* Chlorpropham[a] *at loc. no.* **1229**

Isopropyl N-(3-chlorophenyl)carbamate (101-21-3) *See* Chlorpropham[a] *at loc. no.* **1229**
Isopropyl-o-cresol (499-75-2) *See* Carvacrol[a] *at loc. no.* **489**
Isopropyl-4,4'-dibromobenzilate *See* Bromopropylate[a] *at loc. no.* **1004**
Isopropyl 4,4'-dichlorobenzilate *See* Bromopropylate[b] *at loc. no.* **1004**
Isopropyl ester of 2,4-D (94-11-1) *See* 2,4-D Esters[d] *at loc. no.* **1213**
Isopropyl ester of 2,4,5-T *See* Trichlorophenoxyacetic Acid[b] *at loc. no.* **1224**
Isopropylidenacetone (141-79-7) *See* Mesityl Oxide[a] *at loc. no.* **474**
N-Isopropylmeprobamate (78-44-4) *See* Carisoprodol[a] *at loc. no.* **1403**
Isopropyl 2-methyl-4-chlorophenoxyacetate *See* MCPA[b] *at loc. no.* **1220**
N-Isopropyl-2-methyl-2-propyl-1,3-propanediol dicarbamate (78-44-4) *See* Carisoprodol[a] *at loc. no.* **1403**
1-Isopropyl-3-methylpyrazolyl-5-dimethylcarbamate (119-38-0) *See* Isolan[e] *at loc. no.* **1136**
Isopropylmethyl pyrimidyl diethyl thiophosphate (333-41-5) *See* Diazinon[e] *at loc. no.* **1068**
Isopropyl Myristate (110-27-0) *See loc. no.* **575**
Isopropyl palmitate (142-91-6) *See* Isopropyl Myristate[b] *at loc. no.* **575**
Isopropyl-N-phenylcarbamate (122-42-9) *See* Chlorpropham[b] *at loc. no.* **1229**
3-(4-Isopropylphenyl)-1,1-dimethylurea *See* Isoproturon[a] *at loc. no.* **1250**
m-Isopropylphenyl N-methylcarbamate (64-00-6) *See* Isoprocarb[b] *at loc. no.* **1137**
o-Isopropylphenyl N-methylcarbamate (2631-40-5) *See* Isoprocarb[a] *at loc. no.* **1137**
Isopropyl phosphoramidic acid 4-(methylthio)-m-tolyl ethyl ester (22224-92-6) *See* Phenamiphos[a] *at loc. no.* **1103**
Isopropylxanthic acid sodium salt (140-93-2) *See* Sodium Isopropyl Xanthate[a] *at loc. no.* **1315**
Isoproterenol (51-31-0) *See loc. no.* **1458**
Isoproturon (34123-59-6) *See loc. no.* **1250**
Isosafrole (120-58-1) *See loc. no.* **867**
Isosorbide (652-67-5) *See loc. no.* **1603**
Isosorbide Dinitrate (87-33-2) *See loc. no.* **634**
Isothan Q-15 (93-23-2) *See* Lauryl Isoquinolinium Bromide[e] *at loc. no.* **991**
Isothan Q-75 (93-23-2) *See* Lauryl Isoquinolinium Bromide[e] *at loc. no.* **991**
Isothymol (499-75-2) *See* Carvacrol[a] *at loc. no.* **489**
Isotron *See* Fluorocarbon Refrigerants and Propellants[d] *at loc. no.* **347**
Isovaleraldehyde (590-86-3) *See* Acetaldehyde[b] *at loc. no.* **480**
2-Isovaleryl-1,3-indandione (83-28-3) *See* Valone[e] *at loc. no.* **1344**
Isuprel (51-31-0) *See* Isoproterenol[c] *at loc. no.* **1458**
Jamestown weed *See* Stramonium[a] *at loc. no.* **696**
Jasmolin I (4466-14-2) *See* Pyrethrins[d] *at loc. no.* **893**
Jasmolin II (1172-63-0) *See* Pyrethrins[d] *at loc. no.* **893**
Javelle Water (8031-57-0) *See loc. no.* **88**
Jequirity Bean *See loc. no.* **677**
Jimpson or Jimson weed *See* Stramonium[a] *at loc. no.* **696**
Juniper (8012-91-7) *See* Essential Oils[d] *at loc. no.* **725**
Juniper Tar (8013-10-3) *See loc. no.* **729**
Kabam *See* Nabam[b] *at loc. no.* **1162**
Kaiser *See* Fluorocarbon Refrigerants and Propellants[d] *at loc. no.* **347**

---

[a] A Synonym   [b] A Closely Related Substance   [c] The Active or Major Constituent   [d] A Class Name
[e] A Specific Example of or Product Containing

Ingredient name (CAS registry no.) *See* Primary Name *at*
location no. XXX *in Part D of this section*

Kaolin (1332-58-7) *See loc. no.* 5
Kaopectate *See* Pectin[c] *at loc. no.* 758
Karathane (39300-45-3) *See* Dinocap[a] *at loc. no.* 542
Karbutilate (4849-32-5) *See loc. no.* 1232
Karmex (330-54-1) *See* Diuron[c] *at loc. no.* 1247
Katakar oil *See* Argemone Oil[a] *at loc. no.* 710
Katchung oil (8002-03-7) *See* Peanut Oil[a] *at loc. no.* 719
Kelthane (115-32-2) *See loc. no.* 1012
Kemate (101-05-3) *See* Anilazine[c] *at loc. no.* 1170
Kemithal (467-36-7) *See* Thialbarbital[c] *at loc. no.* 1388
Kemitrol 210 *See* Trialkyl Tin Compounds[d] *at loc. no.* 293
Kemitrol 250 *See* Trialkyl Tin Compounds[d] *at loc. no.* 293
Kepone (143-50-0) *See loc. no.* 1032
Kerb (23950-58-5) *See* Pronamide[c] *at loc. no.* 1281
Kerosene (8008-20-6) *See loc. no.* 328
Kerosine (8008-20-6) *See* Kerosene[a] *at loc. no.* 328
Ketochromin (96-26-4) *See* Dihydroxyacetone[a] *at loc. no.* 471
Ketone solvents *See* Acetone[e] *at loc. no.* 466
Kevadon (50-35-1) *See* Thalidomide[c] *at loc. no.* 1443
Kieselguhr (7631-86-9) *See* Silica[a] *at loc. no.* 7
Kola (extract) *See* Caffeine[c] *at loc. no.* 800
Kollidon (9003-39-8) *See* Polyvinylpyrrolidone[c] *at loc. no.* 1639
Korium (97-23-4) *See* Dichlorophen(e)[c] *at loc. no.* 529
Korlan (299-84-3) *See* Ronnel[c] *at loc. no.* 1079
Kuron (6047-17-2) *See* Silvex[b] *at loc. no.* 1223
Kurosal *See* Silvex[b] *at loc. no.* 1223
Kynex *See* Sulfamethoxypyridazine[c] *at loc. no.* 1562
Labarraque's Solution *See loc. no.* 86
Lac *See* Shellac[a] *at loc. no.* 761
Lacca (9000-59-3) *See* Shellac[c] *at loc. no.* 761
"Lacquer diluent" *See* Rubber Solvent[a] *at loc. no.* 333
Lactic Acid (50-21-5) *See loc. no.* 46
Lactic acid carboxamide *See* N-(β-Hydroxyethyl)-2-lac-tamide[a] *at loc. no.* 567
Lactoflavin (83-88-5) *See* Riboflavin[a] *at loc. no.* 913
Lactucarium (8001-38-5) *See* Wild Lettuce[a] *at loc. no.* 701
Laetrile (1332-94-1) *See* Amygdalin[c] *at loc. no.* 846
Lambast (845-52-3) *See* Prometon[b] *at loc. no.* 1267
Lanatoside C (17575-22-3) *See* Lanatoside(s)[d] *at loc. no.* 841
Lanatoside(s) *See loc. no.* 841
Landrin (2686-99-9) *See loc. no.* 1138
Lannate (16752-77-5) *See* Methomyl[c] *at loc. no.* 1140
Lanolin (8020-84-6) *See loc. no.* 716
Lanolin alcohols *See* Lanolin[b] *at loc. no.* 716
Lantrol *See* Lanolin[b] *at loc. no.* 716
Largon (362-29-8) *See* Propiomazine Hydrochloride[c] *at loc. no.* 1422
Larkspur Alkaloids *See loc. no.* 828
Laroxyl (50-48-6) *See* Amitriptyline[c] *at loc. no.* 1470
LAS *See* Linear Alkyl Benzene Sulfonate (Sodium)[a] *at loc. no.* 952
Lassar's Paste *See loc. no.* 272
Lasso (15972-60-8) *See* Alachlor[c] *at loc. no.* 1273
Latex (9006-04-6) *See loc. no.* 756
Laudanum *See loc. no.* 765
Laureth 9 (9002-92-0) *See loc. no.* 966
Lauric Acid (143-07-7) *See loc. no.* 556
Lauric acid 2-thiocyanatoethyl ester (301-11-1) *See* Lethane 60[e] *at loc. no.* 1037
Lauryl Alcohol (112-53-8) *See loc. no.* 422
N-(Lauryl colamino formyl methyl)pyridinium chloride *See* Cationic Surfactants[d] *at loc. no.* 974
Lauryl Isoquinolinium Bromide (93-23-2) *See loc. no.* 991
Lauryl or lauroyl *derivative. If not listed here, see corresponding* Alkyl *derivative in this index.*

Lauryl polyethylene glycol ether (9002-92-0) *See* Laureth 9[a] *at loc. no.* 966
Lauryl rhodanate (765-15-1) *See* Lauryl Thiocyanate[a] *at loc. no.* 1036
Lauryl sodium sulfate (151-21-3) *See* Alkyl Sodium Sulfates[d] *at loc. no.* 946
Lauryl sodium sulfonate *See* Alkyl Sodium Sulfonates[d] *at loc. no.* 947
Lauryl Thiocyanate (765-15-1) *See loc. no.* 1036
Lavender Oil (8000-28-0) *See loc. no.* 730
Lead (7439-92-1) *See loc. no.* 245
Lead acetate (15347-57-6) *See* Lead[d] *at loc. no.* 245
Lead acid arsenate (7784-40-9) *See* Lead Arsenate[a] *at loc. no.* 206
Lead alkyls *See* Tetraethyl Lead[e] *at loc. no.* 248
Lead Arsenate (7784-40-9) *See loc. no.* 206
Lead Arsenite (10031-13-7) *See loc. no.* 207
Lead carbonate (598-63-0) *See* Lead[d] *at loc. no.* 245
Lead Chromate (7758-97-6) *See loc. no.* 246
Lead Dioxide (1309-60-0) *See loc. no.* 247
Leaded gasoline *See* Gasoline[a] *at loc. no.* 327
Lead linoleate (1340-18-7) *See* Lead[d] *at loc. no.* 245
Lead naphthenate *See* Lead[d] *at loc. no.* 245
Lead oxide (1335-25-7) *See* Lead[d] *at loc. no.* 245
Lead peroxide (1309-60-0) *See* Lead Dioxide[a] *at loc. no.* 247
Lead sulfate (7446-14-2) *See* Lead[d] *at loc. no.* 245
Lecithin (8002-43-5) *See loc. no.* 705
Lemon-grass oil (8007-02-1) *See* Oil of Citronella[b] *at loc. no.* 736
Leopard's bane *See* Arnica[a] *at loc. no.* 657
Lethane 60 (301-11-1) *See loc. no.* 1037
Lethane 384 (112-56-1) *See* β-Butoxy-β-thiocyanodiethyl Ether[a] *at loc. no.* 1035
Lethane A-70 (4617-17-8) *See* Aliphatic Thiocyanates[d] *at loc. no.* 1034
Lethanes *See* Aliphatic Thiocyanates[d] *at loc. no.* 1034
Leukeran (305-03-3) *See* Chlorambucil[c] *at loc. no.* 1590
Levallorphan Tartrate (71-82-9) *See loc. no.* 784
Levamfetamine *See* Amphetamine[b] *at loc. no.* 1444
Levamphetamine *See* Amphetamine[b] *at loc. no.* 1444
Levanil (95-04-5) *See* Ectylurea[c] *at loc. no.* 1433
Levant wormseed (8043-43-4) *See* Santonin[c] *at loc. no.* 931
Levopropoxyphene 2-naphthalene sulfonate (55557-30-7) *See* Levopropoxyphene Napsylate[a] *at loc. no.* 1604
Levopropoxyphene Napsylate (55557-30-7) *See loc. no.* 1604
Levorphanol (77-07-6) *See loc. no.* 785
Levorphanol tartrate (125-72-4) *See* Levorphanol[b] *at loc. no.* 785
Levothyroxine sodium (55-03-8) *See* Thyroid[d] *at loc. no.* 920
Levsin (101-31-5) *See* Hyoscyamine[a] *at loc. no.* 770
Liberty bells *See* Psilocybin[c] *at loc. no.* 821
Librium hydrochloride (438-41-5) *See* Chlordiazepoxide Hydrochloride[a] *at loc. no.* 1392
Licorice *See* Ammonium Glycyrrhizate[c] *at loc. no.* 848
Lidocaine (137-58-6) *See loc. no.* 1582
Lidocaine hydrochloride (6108-05-0) *See* Lidocaine[b] *at loc. no.* 1582
Light ligroin *See* Petroleum Ether[a] *at loc. no.* 330
Light naphtha *See* VM&P Naphthas[b] *at loc. no.* 335
Lignocaine *See* Lidocaine[a] *at loc. no.* 1582
Ligroin (8032-32-4) *See* VM&P Naphthas[a] *at loc. no.* 335
Lime (1305-78-8) *See* Calcium Oxide[a] *at loc. no.* 54
Lime (Slaked) *See loc. no.* 55
Limestone (1317-65-3) *See loc. no.* 173

[a] A Synonym   [b] A Closely Related Substance   [c] The Active or Major Constituent   [d] A Class Name
[e] A Specific Example of or Product Containing

Ingredient name (CAS registry no.) *See* Primary Name *at
location no.* **XXX** *in Part D of this section*

Lime sulfur (1344-81-6) *See* Calcium Polysulfide[e] *at loc. no.* **113**

Lime water *See* Lime (Slaked)[c] *at loc. no.* **55**

Limonene (138-86-3) *See loc. no.* **877**

Linalyl acetate (115-95-7) *See* Oil of Bergamot[e] *at loc. no.* **733**

Linamarin (554-35-8) *See loc. no.* **850**

Lindane (58-89-9) *See loc. no.* **1028**

Linear alkyl *derivative. If not listed here, see corresponding* Alkyl *derivative in this index.*

Linear alkyl ammonium sulfonate *See* Alkyl Sodium Sulfonates[d] *at loc. no.* **947**

Linear alkyl aryl sulfonate *See* Linear Alkyl Benzene Sulfonate (Sodium)[e] *at loc. no.* **952**

Linear alkylate sulfonate *See* Linear Alkyl Benzene Sulfonate (Sodium)[a] *at loc. no.* **952**

Linear Alkyl Benzene Sulfonate (Sodium) *See loc. no.* **952**

Linoleic Acid (60-33-3) *See loc. no.* **555**

Linoleyl *derivative. See corresponding* Alkyl *derivative in this index.*

Linseed Oil (8001-26-1) *See loc. no.* **717**

Linuron (330-55-2) *See loc. no.* **1251**

Liothyronine sodium (55-06-1) *See* Thyroid[d] *at loc. no.* **920**

α-Lipoic acid (62-46-4) *See* Thioctic Acid[a] *at loc. no.* **1510**

Liquamar (435-97-2) *See* Phenprocoumon[c] *at loc. no.* **1342**

Liquefied hydrocarbon gas *See* Propane[c] *at loc. no.* **304**

Liquid carbonis detergent *See* Coal Tar[b] *at loc. no.* **510**

Liquid paraffin (8012-95-1) *See* Liquid Petrolatum[a] *at loc. no.* **337**

Liquid Petrolatum (8012-95-1) *See loc. no.* **337**

Liquid petroleum gas *See* Propane[c] *at loc. no.* **304**

Liquid rosin *See* Tall Oil[a] *at loc. no.* **723**

Liquiprin (103-90-2) *See* Acetaminophen[c] *at loc. no.* **1587**

Lithium (7439-93-2) *See loc. no.* **154**

Lithium carbonate (554-13-2) *See* Lithium[d] *at loc. no.* **154**

Lithium chloride (7447-41-8) *See* Lithium[d] *at loc. no.* **154**

Lithium Hydride (7580-67-8) *See loc. no.* **61**

Lithium hydroxide (1310-65-2) *See* Lye[d] *at loc. no.* **51**

Lithium hypochlorite (13840-33-0) *See* Lithium[d] *at loc. no.* **154**

Lithopone (1345-05-7) *See loc. no.* **115**

Lobelia *See* Lobeline (and Salts)[c] *at loc. no.* **776**

Lobeline (and Salts) (90-69-7) *See loc. no.* **776**

Lomotil (3810-80-8) *See* Diphenoxylate Hydrochloride[c] *at loc. no.* **1482**

Loranthus europaeus *See* European Mistletoe[b] *at loc. no.* **669**

Lorazepam (846-49-1) *See loc. no.* **1398**

Lorfan (71-82-9) *See* Levallorphan Tartrate[c] *at loc. no.* **784**

"Love Drug" *See* 3,4-Methylenedioxyamphetamine[a] *at loc. no.* **1461**

Loxapine (1977-10-2) *See loc. no.* **1476**

Loxapine hydrochloride *See* Loxapine[b] *at loc. no.* **1476**

Loxapine succinate (27833-64-3) *See* Loxapine[b] *at loc. no.* **1476**

Loxitane (1977-10-2) *See* Loxapine[c] *at loc. no.* **1476**

LPG *See* Propane[c] *at loc. no.* **304**

LSD (50-37-3) *See* Lysergic Acid Diethylamide[a] *at loc. no.* **829**

LSD-25 (50-37-3) *See* Lysergic Acid Diethylamide[a] *at loc. no.* **829**

Lubergal (115-43-5) *See* 5-Allyl-5-phenylbarbituric Acid[c] *at loc. no.* **1363**

Lubricating Oils *See loc. no.* **338**

Lucite (9011-14-7) *See* Methyl Methacrylate[b] *at loc. no.* **1630**

Lufyllin (479-18-5) *See* Dyphylline[c] *at loc. no.* **804**

Luminal (50-06-6) *See* Phenobarbital[c] *at loc. no.* **1382**

Lunar caustic (8007-31-6) *See* Silver Salts[d] *at loc. no.* **288**

Lutiomil (10262-69-8) *See* Loxapine[b] *at loc. no.* **1476**

Lye *See loc. no.* **51**

Lysergic acid butanolamide *See* Methysergide Maleate[b] *at loc. no.* **806**

Lysergic Acid Diethylamide (50-37-3) *See loc. no.* **829**

Lysergide (50-37-3) *See* Lysergic Acid Diethylamide[a] *at loc. no.* **829**

Lysol (12772-68-8) *See* Cresol and Soap Solution (B.P.)[a] *at loc. no.* **515**

Lysol Brand Disinfectant *See loc. no.* **516**

Mace *See* Nutmeg[e] *at loc. no.* **679**

Mace oil (8007-12-3) *See* Nutmeg[e] *at loc. no.* **679**

Machete (23184-66-9) *See* Alachlor[b] *at loc. no.* **1273**

Macrodantin *See* Nitrofurantoin[c] *at loc. no.* **1530**

Madribon *See* Sulfadimethoxine[c] *at loc. no.* **1554**

Magnesium aluminum silicate (1327-43-1) *See* Magnesium Silicate[b] *at loc. no.* **176**

Magnesium borate (10031-14-8) *See* Borate[d] *at loc. no.* **131**

Magnesium carbonate (546-93-0) *See* Magnesium Salts[d] *at loc. no.* **174**

Magnesium chlorate (10326-21-3) *See* Chlorate Salts[d] *at loc. no.* **96**

Magnesium chloride (7791-19-7) *See* Magnesium Salts[d] *at loc. no.* **174**

Magnesium citrate (144-23-0) *See* Magnesium Salts[d] *at loc. no.* **174**

Magnesium dalapon *See* Dalapon[b] *at loc. no.* **1299**

Magnesium fluosilicate (16949-65-8) *See* Fluosilicate Salts[d] *at loc. no.* **101**

Magnesium hydroxide (1309-42-8) *See* Milk of Magnesia[a] *at loc. no.* **175**

Magnesium lauryl sulfate (3097-08-3) *See* Alkyl Sodium Sulfates[b] *at loc. no.* **946**

Magnesium oxide (1309-48-4) *See* Magnesium Salts[d] *at loc. no.* **174**

Magnesium oxychloride *See* Magnesium Salts[d] *at loc. no.* **174**

Magnesium oxysulfate *See* Magnesium Salts[d] *at loc. no.* **174**

Magnesium phosphate (7782-75-4) *See* Magnesium Salts[d] *at loc. no.* **174**

Magnesium salicylate (18917-89-0) *See* Salicylate[d] *at loc. no.* **600**

Magnesium Salts *See loc. no.* **174**

Magnesium Silicate (1343-88-0) *See loc. no.* **176**

Magnesium silicofluoride (1310-00-5) *See* Fluosilicate Salts[d] *at loc. no.* **101**

Magnesium stearate (557-04-0) *See* Magnesium Salts[d] *at loc. no.* **174**

Magnesium sulfate (7487-88-9) *See* Magnesium Salts[d] *at loc. no.* **174**

Magnesium trisilicate (14987-04-3) *See* Magnesium Silicate[b] *at loc. no.* **176**

"Mahogany soaps" *See* Sulfonated Petroleum Oils[a] *at loc. no.* **958**

Malachite green G (633-03-4) *See* Brilliant Green[a] *at loc. no.* **1519**

Malathion (121-75-5) *See loc. no.* **1091**

Malathon (121-75-5) *See* Malathion[a] *at loc. no.* **1091**

Male fern oleoresin (8002-63-9) *See* Aspidium[e] *at loc. no.* **748**

Maleic Hydrazide (123-33-1) *See loc. no.* **1308**

Mallophene (136-40-3) *See* Phenazopyridine Hydrochloride[c] *at loc. no.* **1522**

---

[a] A Synonym   [b] A Closely Related Substance   [c] The Active or Major Constituent   [d] A Class Name   [e] A Specific Example of or Product Containing

Ingredient name (CAS registry no.) *See* Primary Name *at
location no.* **XXX** *in Part D of this section*

Malononitrile (109-77-3) *See loc. no.* **650**
Maloran (13360-45-7) *See* Chlorbromuron[c] *at loc. no.* **1242**
Maltol (118-71-8) *See* 3-Hydroxy-2-methyl-4-pyrone[c] *at loc. no.* **866**
Mancopper *See* Mancozeb[b] *at loc. no.* **1159**
Mancozeb (8018-01-7) *See loc. no.* **1159**
Mandelyltropeine (87-00-3) *See* Homatropine[a] *at loc. no.* **769**
Mandrake root *See* Podophyllum Resin[c] *at loc. no.* **759**
Mandrax *See* Methaqualone[c] *at loc. no.* **1439**
Maneb (12427-38-2) *See loc. no.* **1160**
Manganese ethylene bis(dithiocarbamate) (12427-38-2) *See* Maneb[a] *at loc. no.* **1160**
Manganese Salts *See loc. no.* **286**
Manganese sulfate (7785-87-7) *See* Manganese Salts[d] *at loc. no.* **286**
Manganic salts *See* Manganese Salts[d] *at loc. no.* **286**
Manganous dimethyldithiocarbamate (15339-36-3) *See* Sodium Dimethyldithiocarbamate[b] *at loc. no.* **1163**
Manganous salts *See* Manganese Salts[d] *at loc. no.* **286**
Mannitol hexanitrate (130-39-2) *See* Nitroglycerin(e)[b] *at loc. no.* **635**
Manufactured gas *See* Gas[d] *at loc. no.* **128**
Manzate (12427-38-2) *See* Maneb[c] *at loc. no.* **1160**
Maprotiline (10262-69-8) *See* Loxapine[b] *at loc. no.* **1476**
Marcaine (2180-92-9) *See* Bupivacaine[c] *at loc. no.* **1578**
Marevan (129-06-6) *See* Warfarin[b] *at loc. no.* **1345**
Marihuana *See loc. no.* **678**
Marsilid phosphate (305-33-9) *See* Iproniazid Phosphate[c] *at loc. no.* **1475**
Mary Jane *See* Marihuana[a] *at loc. no.* **678**
Matacil (2032-59-9) *See* Aminocarb[c] *at loc. no.* **1122**
Mataven *See* Benzoylprop-ethyl[b] *at loc. no.* **1292**
May apple *See* Podophyllum Resin[c] *at loc. no.* **759**
May pops *See* Passiflora[a] *at loc. no.* **681**
MBC *See* Benomyl[b] *at loc. no.* **1174**
MBK *See* Methyl *n*-Butyl Ketone[a] *at loc. no.* **479**
MBT (149-30-4) *See* Mercaptobenzothiazole[a] *at loc. no.* **1198**
McN-1025 (991-42-4) *See* Norbormide[a] *at loc. no.* **1349**
2M-4CP *See* Mecoprop[b] *at loc. no.* **1221**
MCP (94-74-6) *See* MCPA[a] *at loc. no.* **1220**
MCPA (94-74-6) *See loc. no.* **1220**
4-MCPB (94-81-5) *See* 4-(2-Methyl-4-chlorophenoxy)butyric Acid[a] *at loc. no.* **1222**
MCPP *See* Mecoprop[a] *at loc. no.* **1221**
MDA (300-42-5) *See* 3,4-Methylenedioxyamphetamine[a] *at loc. no.* **1461**
Mebaral (115-38-8) *See* Mephobarbital[c] *at loc. no.* **1377**
Mebenil (7055-03-0) *See* o-Toluanilide[a] *at loc. no.* **1208**
Mebutamate (64-55-1) *See* Meprobamate[b] *at loc. no.* **1407**
Meclizine (569-65-3) *See* Meclizine Dihydrochloride[b] *at loc. no.* **1494**
Meclizine Dihydrochloride (1104-22-9) *See loc. no.* **1494**
Meclizine hydrochloride (31884-77-2) *See* Meclizine Dihydrochloride[b] *at loc. no.* **1494**
Mecoprop (7085-19-0) *See loc. no.* **1221**
Mecoprop diethanolamine salt (1432-14-0) *See* Mecoprop[b] *at loc. no.* **1221**
Mecoprop dimethylamine salt *See* Mecoprop[b] *at loc. no.* **1221**
Mecoprop isooctyl ester *See* Mecoprop[b] *at loc. no.* **1221**
Mecoprop potassium salt (1929-86-8) *See* Mecoprop[b] *at loc. no.* **1221**
Mecoprop sodium salt (19095-88-6) *See* Mecoprop[b] *at loc. no.* **1221**
Medazepam Hydrochloride (2898-11-5) *See loc. no.* **1399**
Medomin (509-86-4) *See* Heptabarbital[c] *at loc. no.* **1374**

MEK (78-93-3) *See* Methyl Ethyl Ketone[a] *at loc. no.* **476**
Mellaril (50-52-2) *See* Thioridazine[c] *at loc. no.* **1425**
Melprex (2439-10-3) *See* Dodine[c] *at loc. no.* **1193**
Menadione (58-27-5) *See loc. no.* **1605**
Menadione sodium bisulfite (130-37-0) *See* Menadione[b] *at loc. no.* **1605**
3-*p*-Menthanol (89-78-1) *See* Menthol[a] *at loc. no.* **868**
p-Menth-1-en-8-ol (586-81-2) *See* Terpineol[a] *at loc. no.* **882**
Menthol (89-78-1) *See loc. no.* **868**
Menthyl Acetate (89-48-5) *See loc. no.* **869**
Menthyl *o*-aminobenzoate (134-09-8) *See* Menthyl Anthranilate[a] *at loc. no.* **1534**
Menthyl Anthranilate (134-09-8) *See loc. no.* **1534**
Menthyl Salicylate (89-46-3) *See loc. no.* **1535**
Meobal (2425-10-7) *See* MPMC[a] *at loc. no.* **1143**
Meparfynol (77-75-8) *See* Methylpentynol[a] *at loc. no.* **1440**
Mepazine (60-89-9) *See loc. no.* **1416**
Meperidine Hydrochloride (50-13-5) *See loc. no.* **1484**
Mephenesin (59-47-2) *See loc. no.* **1406**
Mephenesin carbamate (533-06-2) *See* Mephenesin[b] *at loc. no.* **1406**
Mephentermine (100-92-5) *See* Ephedrine[b] *at loc. no.* **1450**
Mephenytoin (50-12-4) *See* Phenytoin Sodium[b] *at loc. no.* **1609**
Mephobarbital (115-38-8) *See loc. no.* **1377**
Mepivacaine (96-88-8) *See loc. no.* **1583**
Mepivacaine hydrochloride (1722-62-9) *See* Mepivacaine[b] *at loc. no.* **1583**
Meprobamate (57-53-4) *See loc. no.* **1407**
Meralein sodium (4386-35-0) *See* Merodicein[a] *at loc. no.* **238**
Meratran (467-60-7) *See* Pipradrol[c] *at loc. no.* **1478**
Merbromin (129-16-8) *See loc. no.* **235**
Mercaptoacetate salts *See* Thioglycolate Salts[a] *at loc. no.* **552**
Mercaptoacetic acid (68-11-1) *See* Thioglycolic Acid[a] *at loc. no.* **49**
Mercaptobenzothiazole (149-30-4) *See loc. no.* **1198**
Mercaptodimethur (2032-65-7) *See* Methiocarb[a] *at loc. no.* **1139**
Mercaptoethane *See* Methanethiol[a] *at loc. no.* **116**
N-(2-Mercaptoethyl) benzenesulfonamide S-(0,0-diisopropyl phosphorodithioate) (741-58-2) *See* Bensulide[a] *at loc. no.* **1082**
Mercaptomethane *See* Methanethiol[a] *at loc. no.* **116**
N-(Mercaptomethyl)phthalimide S(O,O-dimethylphosphorodithioate) (732-11-6) *See* Imidan[a] *at loc. no.* **1090**
D-3-Mercaptovaline (52-67-5) *See* D-Penicillamine[a] *at loc. no.* **1507**
Mercarbolid (90-03-9) *See* Hydroxyphenylmercurichloride[c] *at loc. no.* **234**
Mercresin (8063-34-1) *See* Hydroxyphenylmercurichloride[b] *at loc. no.* **234**
Mercuric Chloride (7487-94-7) *See loc. no.* **236**
Mercuric chloride ammoniated (10124-48-8) *See* Ammoniated Mercury[a] *at loc. no.* **223**
Mercuric cyanide (592-04-1) *See* Mercury Oxycyanide[e] *at loc. no.* **108**
Mercuric iodide red (7774-29-0) *See* Mercuric Chloride[b] *at loc. no.* **236**
Mercuric oxide (21908-53-2) *See* Mercury[d] *at loc. no.* **221**
Mercurochrome (129-16-8) *See* Merbromin[a] *at loc. no.* **235**
Mercurous Chloride (10112-91-1) *See loc. no.* **237**
Mercury *See loc. no.* **221**
Mercury ammonium chloride (10124-48-8) *See* Ammoniated Mercury[a] *at loc. no.* **223**

---

[a] A Synonym   [b] A Closely Related Substance   [c] The Active or Major Constituent   [d] A Class Name
[e] A Specific Example of or Product Containing

Ingredient name (CAS registry no.) *See* Primary Name *at*
location no. **XXX** *in Part D of this section*

Mercury bichloride (7487-94-7) *See* Mercuric Chloride[a] *at loc. no.* **236**
Mercury cyanide oxide (1335-31-5) *See* Mercury Oxycyanide[a] *at loc. no.* **108**
Mercury Oxycyanide (1335-31-5) *See loc. no.* **108**
Mercury salts of polyaminopolycarboxylic acids *See* Mercury[d] *at loc. no.* **221**
Merodicein (4386-35-0) *See loc. no.* **238**
Merphenyl compounds *See* Phenylmercuric Salts of Inorganic Acids[d] *at loc. no.* **242**
Merphos (150-50-5) *See* Tributyl Phosphorotrithioite[c] *at loc. no.* **1114**
Merthiolate sodium (54-64-8) *See* Thimerosal[c] *at loc. no.* **244**
Mescaline (54-04-6) *See loc. no.* **830**
Mesityl Oxide (141-79-7) *See loc. no.* **474**
Mesoridazine besylate (32672-69-8) *See* Thioridazine[b] *at loc. no.* **1425**
Mestranol (72-33-3) *See* Estrogens (Natural and Synthetic)[d] *at loc. no.* **916**
Mesulfin *See* Sulfamethizole[c] *at loc. no.* **1560**
Mesurol (2032-65-7) *See* Methiocarb[c] *at loc. no.* **1139**
"Meta" (108-62-3) *See* Metaldehyde[c] *at loc. no.* **485**
Meta- *If not listed below, omit prefix and try again.*
Metacetaldehyde (108-62-3) *See* Metaldehyde[a] *at loc. no.* **485**
Metadihydroxybenzol (108-46-3) *See* Resorcinol[a] *at loc. no.* **508**
Metaldehyde (108-62-3) *See loc. no.* **485**
Metal Fumes *See loc. no.* **27**
Metalkamate (8065-36-9) *See* Bufencarb[a] *at loc. no.* **1125**
Metallic mercury (7439-97-6) *See* Mercury[d] *at loc. no.* **221**
Metallic sulfides *See* Sulfide Salts[d] *at loc. no.* **118**
Metal sulfides *See* Sulfide Salts[d] *at loc. no.* **118**
Metam (144-54-7) *See* Metham Sodium[b] *at loc. no.* **1161**
Metamitron (41394-05-2) *See loc. no.* **1265**
Metaphen (133-58-4) *See* Hydroxymercurinitrophenol[b] *at loc. no.* **233**
Metasilicate *See* Sodium Metasilicate[e] *at loc. no.* **57**
Meta-Systox-R (301-12-2) *See loc. no.* **1074**
Meta-systox-S (2674-91-1) *See* Meta-Systox-R[b] *at loc. no.* **1074**
Meta-toluene diisocyanate (584-84-9) *See* Toluene-2,4-diisocyanate[a] *at loc. no.* **1641**
Metaxalone (1665-48-1) *See loc. no.* **1408**
Methabenzthiazuron (18691-97-9) *See* Phenobenzuron[b] *at loc. no.* **1256**
Methacycline (914-00-1) *See* Tetracyclines[d] *at loc. no.* **904**
Methadone (76-99-3) *See loc. no.* **1485**
Methaform (57-15-8) *See* Chlorobutanol[a] *at loc. no.* **432**
Methallatal (115-56-0) *See loc. no.* **1378**
Methallenestril (517-18-0) *See* Estrogens (Natural and Synthetic)[d] *at loc. no.* **916**
Methamidophos (10265-92-6) *See* Monitor[a] *at loc. no.* **1101**
Methaminodiazepoxide hydrochloride (438-41-5) *See* Chlordiazepoxide Hydrochloride[a] *at loc. no.* **1392**
Methamphetamine (537-46-2) *See loc. no.* **1459**
Methampyrone (5907-38-0) *See* Dipyrone[a] *at loc. no.* **1573**
Metham Sodium (137-42-8) *See loc. no.* **1161**
Methane (74-82-8) *See* Aliphatic Hydrocarbons[d] *at loc. no.* **303**
Methanearsonic acid (124-58-3) *See* Disodium Methanearsonate[b] *at loc. no.* **203**
Methane Dichloride (75-09-2) *See* Methylene Chloride[a] *at loc. no.* **359**
Methanethiol (74-93-1) *See loc. no.* **116**

Methanol (67-56-1) *See* Methyl Alcohol[a] *at loc. no.* **423**
Methaphoxide (57-39-6) *See* Apholate[b] *at loc. no.* **1354**
Methapyrilene Hydrochloride (135-23-9) *See loc. no.* **1495**
Methaqualone (72-44-6) *See loc. no.* **1439**
Metharbital (50-11-3) *See loc. no.* **1379**
Methenamine (100-97-0) *See loc. no.* **486**
Methenamine hippurate (5714-73-8) *See* Methenamine[b] *at loc. no.* **486**
Methenamine mandelate (587-23-5) *See* Methenamine[b] *at loc. no.* **486**
Methergine (113-42-8) *See* Methysergide Maleate[b] *at loc. no.* **806**
Methicillin (61-32-5) *See* Penicillins[d] *at loc. no.* **902**
Methiocarb (2032-65-7) *See loc. no.* **1139**
Methionine Sulfoximine (407-40-9) *See loc. no.* **1644**
Methiuron *See* Phenobenzuron[b] *at loc. no.* **1256**
Methocarbamol (532-03-6) *See* Mephenesin[b] *at loc. no.* **1406**
Methocel (9004-67-5) *See* Methyl Cellulose[c] *at loc. no.* **856**
Methocel 60 HG (9004-65-3) *See* Hydroxypropyl Methylcellulose[c] *at loc. no.* **855**
Methocel X-2602 (9004-65-3) *See* Hydroxypropyl Methylcellulose[c] *at loc. no.* **855**
Methomyl (16752-77-5) *See loc. no.* **1140**
Methoprotryne (841-06-5) *See* Prometon[b] *at loc. no.* **1267**
D-**Methorphan** *See* Dextromethorphan Hydrobromide[b] *at loc. no.* **1594**
4-Methoxyamphetamine *See loc. no.* **1460**
p-**Methoxyamphetamine** *See* 4-Methoxyamphetamine[a] *at loc. no.* **1460**
2-Methoxy-4,6-bis(isopropylamino)-*s*-triazine (1610-18-0) *See* Prometon[a] *at loc. no.* **1267**
Methoxychlor (72-43-5) *See loc. no.* **1013**
Methoxy-DDT (72-43-5) *See* Methoxychlor[a] *at loc. no.* **1013**
2-Methoxyethanol (109-86-4) *See loc. no.* **461**
Methoxyethylmercuric acetate (151-38-2) *See* Methoxyethylmercuric Chloride[b] *at loc. no.* **239**
Methoxyethylmercuric Chloride (123-88-6) *See loc. no.* **239**
Methoxyethylmercuric oxalate *See* Methoxyethylmercuric Chloride[b] *at loc. no.* **239**
Methoxyethylmercuric silicate (19367-79-4) *See* Methoxyethylmercuric Chloride[b] *at loc. no.* **239**
Methoxyhydrastine (128-62-1) *See* Noscapine[a] *at loc. no.* **788**
3-Methoxy-4-hydroxybenzaldehyde (121-33-5) *See* Vanillin[a] *at loc. no.* **873**
2-Methoxy-4-(isopropylamino)-6-(methylamino)-*s*-triazine *See* Prometon[b] *at loc. no.* **1267**
Methoxymethane (115-10-6) *See* Methyl Ether[a] *at loc. no.* **475**
2-Methoxy-4-(methylamino)-6-(isopropylamino)-*s*-triazine *See* Prometon[b] *at loc. no.* **1267**
2-Methoxy-4-methyl phenol (93-51-6) *See* Creosol[a] *at loc. no.* **490**
o-**Methoxyphenol** (90-05-1) *See* Guaiacol[a] *at loc. no.* **492**
3-(*p*-(*p*-Methoxyphenoxy)phenyl)-1,1-dimethylurea (14214-32-5) *See* Phenobenzuron[b] *at loc. no.* **1256**
3-(*o*-Methoxyphenoxy)-1,2-propanediol (93-14-1) *See* Guaifenesin[a] *at loc. no.* **1597**
4-Methoxy-*m*-phenylenediamine (615-05-4) *See loc. no.* **622**
2-(*p*-Methoxy-phenyl)-1,3-indandione (117-37-3) *See* Anisindione[a] *at loc. no.* **1333**
Methoxypromazine (61-01-8) *See loc. no.* **1417**
Methoxy propazine (1610-18-0) *See* Prometon[a] *at loc. no.* **1267**

---

[a] A Synonym   [b] A Closely Related Substance   [c] The Active or Major Constituent   [d] A Class Name
[e] A Specific Example of or Product Containing

Ingredient name (CAS registry no.) *See* Primary Name *at
location no.* **XXX** *in Part D of this section*

1-Methoxy-4-propenylbenzene (104-46-1) *See* Anethole[a] *at loc. no.* **858**

N[1]-**(6-Methoxy-3-pyridazinyl)sulfanilamide** (80-35-3) *See* Sulfamethoxypyridazine[a] *at loc. no.* **1562**

N[1]-**(5-Methoxy-2-pyrimidinyl)sulfanilamide** *See* Sulfameter[a] *at loc. no.* **1558**

Methscopolamine bromide (155-41-9) *See* Scopolamine[b] *at loc. no.* **771**

Methscopolamine nitrate (6106-46-3) *See* Scopolamine[b] *at loc. no.* **771**

Methyl Abietate (127-25-3) *See loc. no.* **581**

Methyl acetate (79-20-9) *See* Methyl Formate[b] *at loc. no.* **576**

Methyl acetone (78-93-3) *See* Methyl Ethyl Ketone[a] *at loc. no.* **476**

Methylacetopyronone (520-45-6) *See* Dehydroacetic Acid[a] *at loc. no.* **1187**

β-**Methylacrolein** (123-73-9) *See* Acrolein[b] *at loc. no.* **481**

N-**Methylacrylamide** (1187-59-3) *See* Acrylamide[b] *at loc. no.* **1624**

Methyl acrylate (96-33-3) *See* Acrylic Resin Monomers[d] *at loc. no.* **1625**

Methyl Alcohol (67-56-1) *See loc. no.* **423**

Methyl alkyl benzyl trimethyl ammonium chloride *See* Cationic Surfactants[d] *at loc. no.* **974**

β-**Methylallyl chloride** (563-47-3) *See* 3-Chloro-2-methyl-1-propene[a] *at loc. no.* **382**

Methylaminoantipyrine methanesulfonate sodium (5907-38-0) *See* Dipyrone[a] *at loc. no.* **1573**

p-**Methylaminophenol Sulfate** (55-55-0) *See loc. no.* **626**

4-Methylaniline (106-49-0) *See* *p*-Toluidine[a] *at loc. no.* **618**

Methylarsonic acid (124-58-3) *See* Disodium Methanearsonate[b] *at loc. no.* **203**

Methylated aromatic hydrocarbons *See* Xylene[e] *at loc. no.* **318**

Methylated aromatic petroleum derivatives *See* Xylene[e] *at loc. no.* **318**

Methylated naphthalene *See* Methyl Naphthalene[a] *at loc. no.* **320**

2-Methylbenzanilide (7055-03-0) *See* *o*-Toluanilide[a] *at loc. no.* **1208**

Methyl benzene (108-88-3) *See* Toluene[a] *at loc. no.* **317**

Methylbenzethonium Chloride (25155-18-4) *See loc. no.* **992**

Methyl-2-benzimidazole carbamate *See* Benomyl[b] *at loc. no.* **1174**

Methyl 2-(*N*-benzoyl-3-chloro-4-fluoroanilino)propionate *See* Benzoylprop-ethyl[b] *at loc. no.* **1292**

α-**Methylbenzyl 3-(dimethoxyphosphinyloxy)-*cis*-crotonate** (7700-17-6) *See* Bidrin[b] *at loc. no.* **1051**

Methyl Bromide (74-83-9) *See loc. no.* **344**

1-Methyl-5-*β*-bromoallyl-5-isopropyl barbituric acid (125-55-3) *See* Pronarcon[a] *at loc. no.* **1384**

3-Methylbutanal *N*-methyl-*N*-formylhydrazone *See* Gyromitrin[b] *at loc. no.* **816**

2-Methyl-1-butanol (137-32-6) *See* Amyl Alcohol[b] *at loc. no.* **405**

3-Methyl-1-butanol (123-51-3) *See* Isoamyl Alcohol[a] *at loc. no.* **417**

Methyl 1-(butylcarbamoyl)-2-benzimidazolecarbamate (17804-35-2) *See* Benomyl[b] *at loc. no.* **1174**

2-(1-Methyl-*n*-butyl)-4,6-dinitrophenol (4097-36-3) *See* 4,6-Dinitro-*o*-amylphenol[a] *at loc. no.* **538**

Methyl *n*-Butyl Ketone (591-78-6) *See loc. no.* **479**

3-(1-Methylbutyl)phenyl methylcarbamate (2282-34-0) *See* Bufencarb[a] *at loc. no.* **1125**

Methyl *n*-butyrate (623-42-7) *See* Methyl Formate[b] *at loc. no.* **576**

Methyl carbitol (111-77-3) *See* Carbitol[b] *at loc. no.* **455**

Methylcatechol (90-05-1) *See* Guaiacol[a] *at loc. no.* **492**

Methyl Cellosolve (109-86-4) *See* 2-Methoxyethanol[a] *at loc. no.* **461**

Methyl Cellosolve Acetate (110-49-6) *See loc. no.* **462**

Methyl Cellulose (9004-67-5) *See loc. no.* **856**

Methyl Chloride (74-87-3) *See loc. no.* **345**

Methyl-*α*-chloroacrylate (868-77-9) *See* Acrylic Resin Monomers[d] *at loc. no.* **1625**

2-Methyl-4-chloroaniline (95-69-2) *See* Chlordimeform[b] *at loc. no.* **1042**

Methyl chloroform (71-55-6) *See* 1,1,1-Trichloroethane[a] *at loc. no.* **377**

Methyl chloromethyl ether (107-30-2) *See* Chloromethyl Methyl Ether[a] *at loc. no.* **467**

2-Methyl-4-chlorophenoxyacetic acid (94-74-6) *See* MCPA[a] *at loc. no.* **1220**

Methyl chlorophenoxyacetic acid (and salts) (94-74-6) *See* MCPA[a] *at loc. no.* **1220**

4-(2-Methyl-4-chlorophenoxy)butyric Acid (94-81-5) *See loc. no.* **1222**

4-(2-Methyl-4-chlorophenoxy)butyric acid sodium salt (6062-26-6) *See* 4-(2-Methyl-4-chlorophenoxy)butyric Acid[b] *at loc. no.* **1222**

2-(2-Methyl-4-chlorophenoxy)propionic acid (93-65-2) *See* Mecoprop[a] *at loc. no.* **1221**

Methylchlorothymol (1331-88-0) *See* Chlorothymol[b] *at loc. no.* **527**

Methyl cinnamate (103-26-4) *See* Cinnamic Acid Esters[d] *at loc. no.* **587**

Methylclothiazide (135-07-9) *See* Benzothiadiazide Diuretics[d] *at loc. no.* **1588**

Methyl cyanide (75-05-8) *See* Acetonitrile[a] *at loc. no.* **647**

Methyl-2-cyanoacrylate (137-05-3) *See* *n*-Alkyl-*α*-Cyanoacrylates[d] *at loc. no.* **1626**

Methylcyclohexane (108-87-2) *See loc. no.* **309**

N-**Methyl cyclohexenyl methyl barbituric acid sodium** (50-09-9) *See* Hexobarbital Sodium[a] *at loc. no.* **1376**

1-(2-Methyl cyclohexyl)-3-phenylurea (1982-49-6) *See* Siduron[a] *at loc. no.* **1257**

Methyl Demeton (8022-00-2) *See loc. no.* **1075**

Methyl 5-(2,4-dichlorophenoxy)-2-nitrobenzoate (42576-02-3) *See* Bifenox[a] *at loc. no.* **1293**

S-**Methyl-1-(dimethylcarbamoyl)-*N*-((methylcarbamoyl)oxy)thioformimidate** *See* Oxamyl[a] *at loc. no.* **1144**

1-Methyl-3-dimethylcyclohexanol-5 (116-02-9) *See* Cyclohexanol[b] *at loc. no.* **410**

Methyl *N*,*N*′-dimethyl-*N*-[(methylcarbamoyl)oxy]-1-thiooxamimidate (23135-22-0) *See* Oxamyl[a] *at loc. no.* **1144**

2-Methyl-3,5-dinitrobenzamide (148-01-6) *See* Dinitolmide[a] *at loc. no.* **1540**

4-Methyl-2,6-dinitro-*N*,*N*-dipropylbenzenamine (1918-08-7) *See* Dinitramine[b] *at loc. no.* **1288**

2-Methyl-4,6-dinitrophenol (534-52-1) *See* 4,6-Dinitro-*o*-cresol[a] *at loc. no.* **539**

N-**Methyldithiocarbamic acid** (144-54-7) *See* Metham Sodium[b] *at loc. no.* **1161**

Methyldodecylbenzyl trimethyl ammonium chloride *See* Cationic Surfactants[d] *at loc. no.* **974**

Methyldodecylxylene bis(trimethylammonium) chloride *See* Cationic Surfactants[d] *at loc. no.* **974**

---

[a] A Synonym　　[b] A Closely Related Substance　　[c] The Active or Major Constituent　　[d] A Class Name
[e] A Specific Example of or Product Containing

Ingredient name (CAS registry no.) *See* Primary Name *at
location no.* **XXX** *in Part D of this section*

2,2'-Methylenebis(4-chlorophenol) (97-23-4) *See* Dichlorophen(e)[a] *at loc. no.* **529**

3,3'-Methylenebis(4-hydroxycoumarin) (66-76-2) *See* Bishydroxycoumarin[a] *at loc. no.* **1334**

2,2'-Methylenebis(3,4,6-trichlorophenol) (70-30-4) *See* Hexachlorophene[a] *at loc. no.* **531**

Methylene Blue (61-73-4) *See loc. no.* **1521**

Methylene Bromide (74-95-3) *See loc. no.* **358**

Methylene Chloride (75-09-2) *See loc. no.* **359**

3,4-Methylenedioxyamphetamine (4764-17-4) *See loc. no.* **1461**

3,4-Methylenedioxybenzaldehyde (120-57-0) *See* Piperonal[a] *at loc. no.* **871**

Methylenedioxybenzene (274-09-9) *See loc. no.* **870**

1,2-Methylenedioxy-4-(octylsulfinylpropyl)-benzene (120-62-7) *See* Sulfoxide[a] *at loc. no.* **1155**

1,2-Methylenedioxy-4-propenylbenzene (120-58-1) *See* Isosafrole[a] *at loc. no.* **867**

1,2-Methylenedioxy-4-propylbenzene (94-58-6) *See* Dihydrosafrole[a] *at loc. no.* **862**

Methylene Iodide (75-11-6) *See loc. no.* **360**

Methylergonovine maleate *See* Methysergide Maleate[b] *at loc. no.* **806**

Methyl Ether (115-10-6) *See loc. no.* **475**

2-(1-Methylethoxy)phenol methylcarbamate (114-26-1) *See* Propoxur[a] *at loc. no.* **497**

4-(1-Methylethyl)-2,6-dinitro-N,N-dipropylbenzenamine (33820-53-0) *See* Benefin[b] *at loc. no.* **1287**

Methyl Ethyl Ketone (78-93-3) *See loc. no.* **476**

Methyl Ethyl Ketone Peroxide (and Hydroperoxides) (1338-23-4) *See loc. no.* **75**

Methyl Formate (107-31-3) *See loc. no.* **576**

N-Methyl-N-formylhydrazone of acetaldehyde (16568-02-8) *See* Gyromitrin[a] *at loc. no.* **816**

N-Methyl-N-formylhydrazone of hexanal *See* Gyromitrin[b] *at loc. no.* **816**

N-Methyl-N-formylhydrazone of 3-methylbutanal *See* Gyromitrin[b] *at loc. no.* **816**

N-Methyl-N-formylhydrazone of pentanal *See* Gyromitrin[b] *at loc. no.* **816**

Methyl-1-heptanol *See* Isooctyl Alcohol[e] *at loc. no.* **421**

2-(1-Methylheptyl)-4,6-dinitrophenyl 2-butenoate (6119-92-2) *See* Dinocap[b] *at loc. no.* **542**

Methylhexaneamine (105-41-9) *See* Ephedrine[b] *at loc. no.* **1450**

Methyl hexyl carbinol (123-96-6) *See* Caprylic Alcohol[b] *at loc. no.* **408**

Methylhydrazine (60-34-4) *See* Monomethylhydrazine[a] *at loc. no.* **817**

Methyl p-hydroxybenzoate (99-76-3) *See* Methylparaben[c] *at loc. no.* **585**

Methyl hydroxypropyl cellulose (9004-65-3) *See* Hydroxypropyl Methylcellulose[a] *at loc. no.* **855**

N,N'-(Methyliminodimethylidyne)bis-2,4-xylidine *See* Amitraz[a] *at loc. no.* **1039**

Methyl Iodide (74-88-4) *See loc. no.* **346**

Methyl Isobutyl Ketone (108-10-1) *See loc. no.* **478**

5-Methyl-2-isopropyl-1-phenol (89-83-8) *See* Thymol[a] *at loc. no.* **497**

Methyl Isothiocyanate (556-61-6) *See loc. no.* **1358**

Methyl isovalerate (556-24-1) *See* Methyl Formate[b] *at loc. no.* **576**

N¹-(5-Methyl-3-isoxazolyl)sulfanilamide (723-46-6) *See* Sulfamethoxazole[a] *at loc. no.* **1561**

1-Methyl lysergic acid butanolamide (361-37-5) *See* Methysergide Maleate[b] *at loc. no.* **806**

Methyl mercaptan (74-93-1) *See* Methanethiol[a] *at loc. no.* **116**

Methyl mercuric chloride (or phosphate) *See* Alkyl Mercuric Chloride (or Phosphate)[d] *at loc. no.* **222**

Methylmercuric cyanoguanidine (502-39-6) *See* Methylmercuric Dicyandiamide[a] *at loc. no.* **240**

Methylmercuric Dicyandiamide (502-39-6) *See loc. no.* **240**

Methyl Methacrylate (80-62-6) *See loc. no.* **1630**

α-Methyl-p-methoxyphenylamine *See* 4-Methoxyamphetamine[a] *at loc. no.* **1460**

S-Methyl-N-((methylcarbamoyl)oxy)thioacetimidate (16752-77-5) *See* Methomyl[a] *at loc. no.* **1140**

1-Methyl-2-(3,4-methylenedioxyphenyl)ethyl octyl sulfoxide (120-62-7) *See* Sulfoxide[a] *at loc. no.* **1155**

3-Methyl-5-(1-methylethyl)phenyl methylcarbamate *See* Promecarb[a] *at loc. no.* **1146**

Methyl 2-methylpropenoate (80-62-6) *See* Methyl Methacrylate[a] *at loc. no.* **1630**

2-Methyl-2-(1-methylpropyl)-1,3-propanediol dicarbamate (64-55-1) *See* Meprobamate[b] *at loc. no.* **1407**

2-Methyl-2-(methylthio)propionaldehyde O-(methylcarbamoyl)oxime (116-06-3) *See* Aldicarb[a] *at loc. no.* **1120**

Methylmetiram *See* o-Toluanilide[c] *at loc. no.* **1208**

17-Methylmorphinan-3-ol (77-07-6) *See* Levorphanol[a] *at loc. no.* **785**

Methylmorphine (76-57-3) *See* Codeine[a] *at loc. no.* **780**

Methyl mustard oil (556-61-6) *See* Methyl Isothiocyanate[a] *at loc. no.* **1358**

Methyl Naphthalene (1321-94-4) *See loc. no.* **320**

Methyl (1-naphthalene) acetate (2876-78-0) *See* 1-Naphthaleneacetic Acid[b] *at loc. no.* **1309**

2-Methyl-1,4-naphthoquinone (58-27-5) *See* Menadione[a] *at loc. no.* **1605**

Methyl-1-naphthylacetate (2876-78-0) *See* 1-Naphthaleneacetic Acid[b] *at loc. no.* **1309**

Methyl Nicotinate (93-60-7) *See loc. no.* **588**

Methylnitrophos *See* Fenitrothion[a] *at loc. no.* **1072**

Methyl-1-octanol *See* Isononyl Alcohol[e] *at loc. no.* **419**

Methyloxirane (75-56-9) *See* Propylene Oxide[a] *at loc. no.* **17**

Methylparaben (99-76-3) *See loc. no.* **585**

Methylparafynol (77-75-8) *See* Methylpentynol[a] *at loc. no.* **1440**

Methylparasept (99-76-3) *See* Methylparaben[c] *at loc. no.* **585**

Methyl Parathion (298-00-0) *See loc. no.* **1076**

2-Methyl-2,4-pentanediol (107-41-5) *See* Hexylene Glycol[a] *at loc. no.* **445**

Methyl-1-pentanol *See* Hexyl Alcohol[e] *at loc. no.* **416**

4-Methyl-2-pentanone (108-10-1) *See* Methyl Isobutyl Ketone[a] *at loc. no.* **478**

Methylpentynol (77-75-8) *See loc. no.* **1440**

α-Methylphenethylamine (300-62-9) *See* Amphetamine[a] *at loc. no.* **1444**

Methylphenidate (113-45-1) *See loc. no.* **1462**

Methylphenobarbital (115-38-8) *See* Mephobarbital[a] *at loc. no.* **1377**

Methyl phenol (8003-33-6) *See* Cresols[a] *at loc. no.* **514**

3-(2-Methylphenoxy)-1,2-propanediol (59-47-2) *See* Mephenesin[a] *at loc. no.* **1406**

2-[(3-Methylphenyl)amino]carbonyl benzoic acid (85-72-3) *See* N-m-Tolylphthalamic Acid[a] *at loc. no.* **1284**

N-Methyl-phenyl-tert-butylamine (100-92-5) *See* Ephedrine[b] *at loc. no.* **1450**

3-Methyl-5,5-phenylethylhydantoin (50-12-4) *See* Phenytoin Sodium[b] *at loc. no.* **1609**

---

[a] A Synonym   [b] A Closely Related Substance   [c] The Active or Major Constituent   [d] A Class Name
[e] A Specific Example of or Product Containing

Ingredient name (CAS registry no.) *See* Primary Name *at*
location no. **XXX** *in Part D of this section*

3-Methyl-2-phenylmorpholine hydrochloride (1707-14-8)
See Phenmetrazine[b] *at loc. no.* **1466**

3-Methyl-1-phenyl-5-pyrazolyl dimethylcarbamate (87-
47-8) *See* Pyrolan[e] *at loc. no.* **1149**

3'-Methylphthalanilic acid (85-72-3) *See* N-*m*-Tolylphthal-
amic Acid[a] *at loc. no.* **1284**

Methyl Phthalate (131-11-3) *See loc. no.* **593**

1-Methyl-2',6'-pipecoloxylidide (96-88-8) *See* Mepivacaine[a]
at loc. no. **1583**

Methylprednisolone (83-43-2) *See* Corticosteroids[d] *at loc.
no.* **915**

2-Methylpropane (75-28-5) *See* Isobutane[a] *at loc. no.* **305**

Methyl *n*-propionate (554-12-1) *See* Methyl Formate[b] *at loc.
no.* **576**

2-Methyl-2-*n*-propyl-1,3-propanediol dicarbamate (57-
53-4) *See* Meprobamate[a] *at loc. no.* **1407**

6-Methyl-2-propyl-4-pyrimidinyl-dimethylcarbamate
(2532-49-2) *See* Pyramat[e] *at loc. no.* **1148**

1-Methyl-2-propynyl *m*-chlorocarbanilate *See* Chlorpropham[b] *at loc. no.* **1229**

4-Methylpyrazole (7554-65-6) *See* Pyrazole[b] *at loc. no.* **1509**

Methyl pyrazolyldiethyl phosphate (108-34-9) *See* Pyrazoxon[e] *at loc. no.* **1059**

Methylpyrazolyldiethyl thiophosphate *See* Pyrazothion[e]
at loc. no. **1078**

1-Methyl-2-(3-pyridyl)pyrrolidine (54-11-5) *See* Nicotine[a]
at loc. no. **772**

N^1-(4-Methyl-2-pyrimidinyl)sulfanilamide (127-79-7) *See*
Sulfamerazine[a] *at loc. no.* **1557**

6-Methyl-2,3-quinoxaline dithiol *See* Quinomethionate[b] *at
loc. no.* **1205**

6-Methyl-2,3-quinoxalinedithiol cyclic S,S-dithiocar-
bonate (2439-01-2) *See* Quinomethionate[a] *at loc. no.* **1205**

Methylrosaniline chloride (548-62-9) *See* Gentian Violet[e] *at
loc. no.* **1520**

Methyl Salicylate (119-36-8) *See loc. no.* **597**

Methylsalicylic acids *See* Cresotic Acids[a] *at loc. no.* **595**

Methyl sulfanilylcarbamate (3337-71-1) *See* Asulam[a] *at
loc. no.* **1226**

Methyl sulfocyanate (556-64-9) *See* Aliphatic Thiocyanates[d]
at loc. no. **1034**

4-(Methylsulfonyl)-2,6-dinitro-N,N-dipropylaniline
(4726-14-1) *See* Benefin[b] *at loc. no.* **1287**

Methyl systox (8022-00-2) *See* Methyl Demeton[a] *at loc. no.*
1075

2-Methyl-3,4,5,6-tetrabromophenol (576-55-6) *See* Tetra-
bromo-*o*-cresol[a] *at loc. no.* **533**

Methyl-1,2,5,6-tetrahydro-1-methylnicotinate (63-75-2)
See Arecoline[a] *at loc. no.* **774**

N^1-(5-Methyl-1,3,4-thiadiazol-2-yl)sulfanilamide (144-82-
1) *See* Sulfamethizole[a] *at loc. no.* **1560**

2-Methylthio-4,6-bis(isopropylamino)-*s*-triazine (7287-
19-6) *See* Prometon[b] *at loc. no.* **1267**

Methyl thiocyanate (556-64-9) *See* Aliphatic Thiocyanates[d]
at loc. no. **1034**

2-(Methylthio)-4-(ethylamino)-6-(isopropylamino)-*s*-
triazine (834-12-8) *See* Prometon[b] *at loc. no.* **1267**

Methylthionine chloride (61-73-4) *See* Methylene Blue[a] *at
loc. no.* **1521**

4-(Methylthio)-3,5-xylyl methylcarbamate (2032-65-7)
See Methiocarb[a] *at loc. no.* **1139**

O-Methyl-O-(2,4,5-trichlorophenyl)-amidophosphoro-
thionate (2591-66-4) *See* ET-15[e] *at loc. no.* **1099**

1-Methyl-2,4,6-trinitrobenzene *See* 2,4,6-Trinitrotoluene[a]
at loc. no. **645**

Methyl Trithion (953-17-3) *See loc. no.* **1092**

Methyluracil herbicides *See* Bromacil[e] *at loc. no.* **1294**

Methyl violet (8004-87-3) *See* Gentian Violet[b] *at loc. no.* **1520**

Methyprylon (125-64-4) *See loc. no.* **1441**

Methysergide Maleate (129-49-7) *See loc. no.* **806**

Metobromuron (3060-89-7) *See* Monuron[b] *at loc. no.* **1253**

Metol (55-55-0) *See* p-Methylaminophenol Sulfate[c] *at loc. no.*
626

Metolachlor (51218-45-2) *See* Alachlor[b] *at loc. no.* **1273**

Metoxon (101-21-3) *See* Chlorpropham[a] *at loc. no.* **1229**

Metoxuron (19937-59-8) *See loc. no.* **1252**

Metrazol (54-95-5) *See* Pentylenetetrazol[c] *at loc. no.* **1606**

Metribuzin (21087-64-9) *See loc. no.* **1266**

Mevinphos (7786-34-7) *See* Phosdrin[a] *at loc. no.* **1057**

Mexacarbate (315-18-4) *See loc. no.* **1141**

Mezcaline (54-04-6) *See* Mescaline[a] *at loc. no.* **830**

MFP *See* Fluoride[b] *at loc. no.* **100**

MGK 264 (113-48-4) *See loc. no.* **1150**

MGK Repellent 11 (126-15-8) *See* 2,3,4,5-Bis(δ^2-
butylene)tetrahydrofurfural[c] *at loc. no.* **1321**

MGK Repellent 326 (136-45-8) *See* Di-*n*-propyl Isocinchomeronate[c] *at loc. no.* **1328**

MGK Repellent 874 (3547-33-9) *See* 2-Hydroxyethyl-*n*-octyl
Sulfide[c] *at loc. no.* **1330**

MH (123-33-1) *See* Maleic Hydrazide[a] *at loc. no.* **1308**

Miadone (125-56-4) *See* Methadone[c] *at loc. no.* **1485**

Midalgan (93-60-7) *See* Methyl Nicotinate[c] *at loc. no.* **588**

Midrin *See* Dichloralphenazone[c] *at loc. no.* **1572**

Milcurb (5221-53-4) *See* Dimethirimol[c] *at loc. no.* **1192**

Milk of Magnesia (1309-42-8) *See loc. no.* **175**

Miltown (57-53-4) *See* Meprobamate[c] *at loc. no.* **1407**

Mineral acid *See* Acid[d] *at loc. no.* **30**

Mineral oils (medicinal) *See* Liquid Petrolatum[e] *at loc. no.*
337

Mineral oils (unspecified) *See* Kerosene[e] *at loc. no.* **328**

Mineral pitch (8052-42-4) *See* Asphalt[b] *at loc. no.* **343**

Mineral Seal Oil *See loc. no.* **329**

Mineral spirits (8032-32-4) *See* VM&P Naphthas[a] *at loc. no.*
335

Mineral spirits no. 10 *See* Stoddard Solvent[a] *at loc. no.* **334**

Mineral turpentine *See* VM&P Naphthas[a] *at loc. no.* **335**

Minocrotophos *See* Bidrin[b] *at loc. no.* **1051**

Mipafox (371-86-8) *See loc. no.* **1100**

Miradon (117-37-3) *See* Anisindione[a] *at loc. no.* **1333**

Mirbane (essence of or oil of) (98-95-3) *See* Nitrobenzene[a]
at loc. no. **642**

Mirex (2385-85-5) *See loc. no.* **1033**

Mitox (103-17-3) *See* p-Chlorobenzyl p-Chlorophenyl Sulfide[c]
at loc. no. **1043**

MMH (60-34-4) *See* Monomethylhydrazine[a] *at loc. no.* **817**

Mobam (1079-33-0) *See loc. no.* **1142**

Mobilawn (97-17-6) *See* Dichlofenthion[c] *at loc. no.* **1069**

Mocap (13194-48-4) *See* O-Ethyl S,S-Dipropyl Phosphorodithioate[c] *at loc. no.* **1088**

Moderil (84-34-4) *See* Rescinnamine[c] *at loc. no.* **797**

Modified barium metaborate (52233-42-8) *See* Barium Metaborate[c] *at loc. no.* **167**

Mogadon (146-22-5) *See* Nitrazepam[c] *at loc. no.* **1400**

Molinate (2212-67-1) *See loc. no.* **1237**

Molybdate orange (12656-85-8) *See* Lead Chromate[c] *at loc.
no.* **246**

Molybdenum disulfide (1317-33-5) *See* Sulfide Salts[d] *at loc.
no.* **118**

Monalide (7287-36-7) *See* Propanil[b] *at loc. no.* **1283**

Monitor (10265-92-6) *See loc. no.* **1101**

Monkshood *See* Aconitine[c] *at loc. no.* **822**

Mono- *If not listed here, omit prefix and try again.*

---

[a] A Synonym   [b] A Closely Related Substance   [c] The Active or Major Constituent   [d] A Class Name
[e] A Specific Example of or Product Containing

Ingredient name (CAS registry no.) *See* Primary Name *at*
location no. **XXX** *in Part D of this section*

Monoacetin (26446-35-5) *See loc. no.* **577**
Monoammonium methanearsonate *See* Octyl Ammonium Metharsonate[b] *at loc. no.* **208**
Monobasic potassium phosphate (7778-77-0) *See* Potassium Salts[d] *at loc. no.* **155**
Monobasic sodium phosphate (7558-80-7) *See* Phosphates[d] *at loc. no.* **139**
Monobenzone (103-16-2) *See loc. no.* **1536**
Monobenzyl ether of hydroquinone (103-16-2) *See* Monobenzone[a] *at loc. no.* **1536**
Monobromomethane (74-83-9) *See* Methyl Bromide[a] *at loc. no.* **344**
Monobutyl biphenyl sodium monosulfonate (30233-81-9) *See* Alkyl Aryl Sodium Sulfonates[d] *at loc. no.* **943**
Monobutyl phenyl phenol sodium monosulfonate *See* Alkyl Aryl Sodium Sulfonates[d] *at loc. no.* **943**
Monobutyltin trichloride (1118-46-3) *See* Alkyl Tin Compounds[d] *at loc. no.* **292**
Monochloramine (10599-90-3) *See* Chloramines[d] *at loc. no.* **22**
Monochloroacetic acid (79-11-8) *See* Chloroacetic Acid (and Salts)[a] *at loc. no.* **549**
Monochlorobenzene (108-90-7) *See* Chlorobenzene[a] *at loc. no.* **393**
Monochlorodifluoromethane (75-45-6) *See loc. no.* **350**
Monochloromethane (74-87-3) *See* Methyl Chloride[a] *at loc. no.* **345**
Monochloromonobromomethane (74-97-5) *See* Chlorobromomethane[a] *at loc. no.* **356**
Mono(2,2-dimethylhydrazide)butanedioic acid (1596-84-5) *See* Daminozide[a] *at loc. no.* **1356**
Mono(2,2-dimethylhydrazide)succinic acid (1596-84-5) *See* Daminozide[a] *at loc. no.* **1356**
Monoethanolamine (and Salts) (141-43-5) *See loc. no.* **64**
Monoethanolamine thioglycolate (126-97-6) *See* Thioglycolate Salts[d] *at loc. no.* **552**
Monoethyl ether of ethylene glycol monosulfate (34253-67-3) *See* Cellosolve Sulfate[a] *at loc. no.* **456**
Mono-2-ethylhexyl phthalate *See* Di-2-ethylhexyl Phthalate[b] *at loc. no.* **591**
Monofluoroacetamide (640-19-7) *See* Fluoroacetamide[a] *at loc. no.* **1347**
Monofluoroacetate salts *See* Fluoroacetate[d] *at loc. no.* **548**
8-Monohydromirex *See* Mirex[b] *at loc. no.* **1033**
Monohydroxymercuridiiodoresorcinsulfonphthalein sodium (4386-35-0) *See* Merodicein[e] *at loc. no.* **238**
Monolinuron (1746-81-2) *See* Linuron[b] *at loc. no.* **1251**
Monometflurazon (27314-13-2) *See* Norflurazon[a] *at loc. no.* **1311**
Monomethylhydrazine (60-34-4) *See loc. no.* **817**
Monooctyltin trichloride (3091-25-6) *See* Alkyl Tin Compounds[d] *at loc. no.* **292**
Monosodium acid methanearsonate (2163-80-6) *See* Disodium Methanearsonate[b] *at loc. no.* **203**
Monosodium Glutamate (142-47-2) *See loc. no.* **1618**
Monosodium 3-nitro-4-hydroxy phenol arsonate *See* 4-Hydroxy-3-nitrophenylarsonic Acid[b] *at loc. no.* **205**
Monostearin (8050-92-8) *See* Glyceryl Stearate[a] *at loc. no.* **965**
Monsel's salt (1310-45-8) *See* Ferric Subsulfate[a] *at loc. no.* **254**
Monuron (150-68-5) *See loc. no.* **1253**
Monuron TCA (140-41-0) *See* Monuron[b] *at loc. no.* **1253**
"Moon" *See* Peyote[a] *at loc. no.* **683**
Morestan (2439-01-2) *See* Quinomethionate[c] *at loc. no.* **1205**
Morfamquat (4636-83-3) *See* Paraquat[b] *at loc. no.* **1286**

Morkit (84-65-1) *See* Anthraquinone[c] *at loc. no.* **499**
Morning glory seeds *See* Lysergic Acid Diethylamide[c] *at loc. no.* **829**
Morocide (485-31-4) *See* Dinoseb[b] *at loc. no.* **543**
Morphia (57-27-2) *See* Morphine[a] *at loc. no.* **778**
Morphine (57-27-2) *See loc. no.* **778**
Morphium (57-27-2) *See* Morphine[a] *at loc. no.* **778**
Morpholine (110-91-8) *See loc. no.* **72**
Morpholine abietate *See* Morpholine[b] *at loc. no.* **72**
Morpholine oleate (1095-66-5) *See* Morpholine[b] *at loc. no.* **72**
Mosidal (115-56-0) *See* Methallatal[c] *at loc. no.* **1378**
4-MP (7554-65-6) *See* Pyrazole[b] *at loc. no.* **1509**
MPMC (2425-10-7) *See loc. no.* **1143**
MSG (142-47-2) *See* Monosodium Glutamate[a] *at loc. no.* **1618**
MTMC (1129-41-5) *See* MPMC[b] *at loc. no.* **1143**
Mucomyst (616-91-1) *See* N-Acetylcysteine[c] *at loc. no.* **1502**
Muriatic acid (7647-01-0) *See* Hydrochloric Acid[a] *at loc. no.* **31**
Muscarine (300-54-9) *See loc. no.* **818**
Muscarone *See* Muscarine[b] *at loc. no.* **818**
Muscazone *See* Muscimol[b] *at loc. no.* **819**
Muscimol (2763-96-4) *See loc. no.* **819**
Mushroom Toxins *See loc. no.* **812**
Myanesin (59-47-2) *See* Mephenesin[c] *at loc. no.* **1406**
Myasul *See* Sulfamethoxypyridazine[c] *at loc. no.* **1562**
Mylone (533-74-4) *See* Dazomet[c] *at loc. no.* **1186**
Myrcia oil (8006-78-8) *See* Oil of Bay[a] *at loc. no.* **732**
Myristica *See* Nutmeg[a] *at loc. no.* **679**
Myristic Acid (544-63-8) *See loc. no.* **557**
Myristica fragrans *See* Nutmeg[a] *at loc. no.* **679**
Myristicin (607-91-0) *See* Nutmeg[e] *at loc. no.* **679**
Myristyl *derivative. See corresponding* Alkyl *derivative in this index.*
Myristyl Alcohol (112-72-1) *See loc. no.* **424**
Myrj 52 (9004-99-3) *See* Polyethylene Glycol Stearate[c] *at loc. no.* **968**
Mysoline (125-33-7) *See* Primidone[c] *at loc. no.* **1610**
Nabam (142-59-6) *See loc. no.* **1162**
Nacap (2492-26-4) *See* Mercaptobenzothiazole[b] *at loc. no.* **1198**
Nacconals *See* Alkyl Aryl Sodium Sulfonates[d] *at loc. no.* **943**
Nacconol DB *See* Dioctyl Sodium Sulfosuccinate[b] *at loc. no.* **951**
Nafcillin (147-52-4) *See* Penicillins[d] *at loc. no.* **902**
Naled (300-76-5) *See loc. no.* **1055**
Nalline (57-29-4) *See* Nalorphine Hydrochloride[c] *at loc. no.* **786**
Nalorphine Hydrochloride (57-29-4) *See loc. no.* **786**
Naloxone Hydrochloride (357-08-4) *See loc. no.* **787**
Naphazoline Hydrochloride (550-99-2) *See loc. no.* **1463**
Naphtha *See* Petroleum Naphtha[a] *at loc. no.* **331**
Naphthalene (91-20-3) *See loc. no.* **321**
Naphthaleneacetamide (86-86-2) *See loc. no.* **1277**
1-Naphthaleneacetic Acid (86-87-3) *See loc. no.* **1309**
Naphthalenes chlorinated *See* Polychlorinated Naphthalenes[a] *at loc. no.* **402**
Naphthalin (91-20-3) *See* Naphthalene[a] *at loc. no.* **321**
Naphtha (petroleum) (8030-31-7) *See* Petroleum Naphtha[a] *at loc. no.* **331**
Naphtha (VM&P) (8032-32-4) *See* VM&P Naphthas[a] *at loc. no.* **335**
Naphthenates *See* Naphthenic Acids[b] *at loc. no.* **558**
Naphthene (91-20-3) *See* Naphthalene[a] *at loc. no.* **321**
Naphthenes *See loc. no.* **339**
Naphthenic Acids *See loc. no.* **558**

---

[a] A Synonym   [b] A Closely Related Substance   [c] The Active or Major Constituent   [d] A Class Name
[e] A Specific Example of or Product Containing

Ingredient name (CAS registry no.) *See* Primary Name *at*
location no. **XXX** *in Part D of this section*

Naphthenic oils *See* Naphthenes[a] *at loc. no.* **339**

β-Naphthol (135-19-3) *See loc. no.* **493**

O-2-Naphthyl   m,N-dimethylthiocarbanilate (2398-96-1)
See Tolnaftate[a] *at loc. no.* **1532**

1-Naphthyl-N-methylcarbamate (63-25-2) *See* Carbaryl[a]
at loc. no. **1128**

N-1-Naphthylphthalamic acid (132-66-1) *See* Naptalam[a] *at
loc. no.* **1279**

N-1-Naphthylphthalimide (5333-99-3) *See* Naptalam[b] *at
loc. no.* **1279**

1-(1-Naphthyl)-2-thiourea (86-88-4) *See* ANTU[e] *at loc. no.*
1350

Napropamide (15299-99-7) *See loc. no.* **1278**

Naptalam (132-66-1) *See loc. no.* **1279**

Naptalam Sodium (132-67-2) *See* Naptalam[b] *at loc. no.* **1279**

Narcan (357-08-4) *See* Naloxone Hydrochloride[c] *at loc. no.*
787

Narcotine (128-62-1) *See* Noscapine[a] *at loc. no.* **788**

Nardil (156-51-4) *See* Phenelzine Sulfate[c] *at loc. no.* **1477**

Natrin (3570-61-4) *See* 2,4,5-Trichlorophenoxy Ethyl Sulfate
Sodium Salt[e] *at loc. no.* **1225**

Navadel (78-34-2) *See loc. no.* **1093**

Neatsfoot Oil (8002-64-0) *See loc. no.* **718**

Neburon (555-37-3) *See loc. no.* **1254**

Nefrosul *See* Sulfachlorpyridazine[c] *at loc. no.* **1552**

Nellite (1754-58-1) *See* Diamidafos[c] *at loc. no.* **1097**

Nemacur *See* Phenamiphos[c] *at loc. no.* **1103**

Nemafos (297-97-2) *See* Thionazin[c] *at loc. no.* **1081**

Nemagon (96-12-8) *See* 1,2-Dibromo-3-chloropropane[c] *at loc.
no.* **385**

Nembutal (76-74-4) *See* Pentobarbital Sodium[b] *at loc. no.*
1380

Nembutal sodium (57-33-0) *See* Pentobarbital Sodium[a] *at
loc. no.* **1380**

Neo-Antergan maleate (59-33-6) *See* Pyrilamine Maleate[c]
at loc. no. **1499**

Neocinchophen (485-34-7) *See* Cinchophen[b] *at loc. no.* **1591**

Neomycin (1404-04-2) *See loc. no.* **901**

Neomycin sulfate (1405-10-3) *See* Neomycin[b] *at loc. no.* **901**

Neonal (77-28-1) *See* Butethal[c] *at loc. no.* **1370**

Neonicotine (494-52-0) *See* Anabasine[a] *at loc. no.* **773**

Neo-Pynamin (7696-12-0) *See* Tetramethrin[a] *at loc. no.* **898**

Neopynamin (7696-12-0) *See* Tetramethrin[a] *at loc. no.* **898**

Neosynephrine (59-42-7) *See* Phenylephrine[c] *at loc. no.* **1468**

Neothalidine *See* Phthalylsulfathiazole[c] *at loc. no.* **1548**

Neothylline (479-18-5) *See* Dyphylline[c] *at loc. no.* **804**

Neotran (555-89-5) *See loc. no.* **1014**

Nephocarp (786-19-6) *See* Carbophenothion[c] *at loc. no.* **1083**

Nethamine *See* l-N-Ethylephedrine[c] *at loc. no.* **1455**

Neutral spirits (64-17-5) *See* Ethyl Alcohol[c] *at loc. no.* **412**

Neutronyx 600 (9002-95-3) *See* Alkyl Phenoxy Polyethoxy
Ethanols[c] *at loc. no.* **963**

Niacin (59-67-6) *See* Nicotinic Acid[a] *at loc. no.* **911**

Niacinamide (98-92-0) *See* Nicotinic Acid[b] *at loc. no.* **911**

Nialate (563-12-2) *See* Ethion[a] *at loc. no.* **1087**

Nickel carbonyl (13463-39-3) *See* Nickel Salts[b] *at loc. no.*
287

Nickel chloride (7718-54-9) *See* Nickel Salts[d] *at loc. no.* **287**

Nickel nitrate (13138-45-9) *See* Nickel Salts[d] *at loc. no.* **287**

Nickel phosphate (10381-36-9) *See* Nickel Salts[d] *at loc. no.*
287

Nickel Salts *See loc. no.* **287**

Nickel sulfate (7786-81-4) *See* Nickel Salts[d] *at loc. no.* **287**

Nicotinamide (98-92-0) *See* Nicotinic Acid[b] *at loc. no.* **911**

Nicotine (54-11-5) *See loc. no.* **772**

Nicotine bitartrate *See* Nicotine[b] *at loc. no.* **772**

Nicotine dihydrochloride (6019-02-9) *See* Nicotine[b] *at loc.
no.* **772**

Nicotine salicylate (29790-52-1) *See* Eudermol[a] *at loc. no.*
775

Nicotine sulfate (65-30-5) *See* Nicotine[b] *at loc. no.* **772**

Nicotinic Acid (59-67-6) *See loc. no.* **911**

Nicotinic acid amide (98-92-0) *See* Nicotinic Acid[b] *at loc.
no.* **911**

Nicotinic acid methyl ester (93-60-7) *See* Methyl Nicotinate[a] *at loc. no.* **588**

Nicotinyl alcohol (100-55-0) *See* Nicotinic Acid[b] *at loc. no.*
911

Nicotinyl alcohol tartrate *See* Nicotinic Acid[b] *at loc. no.*
911

Nicoumalone (152-72-7) *See* Acenocoumarol[a] *at loc. no.* **1332**

NISY (117-24-8) *See* Dimethyl Carbate[a] *at loc. no.* **1327**

Niter *See* Nitrate Salts[d] *at loc. no.* **157**

Nitralin (4726-14-1) *See* Benefin[b] *at loc. no.* **1287**

p-Nitraniline (100-01-6) *See* p-Nitroaniline[a] *at loc. no.* **617**

Nitrate of potash *See* Nitrate Salts[d] *at loc. no.* **157**

Nitrate Salts *See loc. no.* **157**

Nitrazepam (146-22-5) *See loc. no.* **1400**

Nitric Acid (7697-37-2) *See loc. no.* **32**

Nitric oxide (10102-43-9) *See* Nitrogen Oxides[d] *at loc. no.* **9**

Nitrile derivatives *See* Cyano Organic Compounds[a] *at loc.
no.* **110**

2,2',2''-Nitrilotriethanol (102-71-6) *See* Triethanolamine[a] *at
loc. no.* **66**

Nitrite *See loc. no.* **144**

o-Nitro-p-aminophenol (119-34-6) *See* 4-Amino-2-nitro-
phenol[a] *at loc. no.* **625**

4-Nitro anhydroxy mercuric orthocresol nitrocellulose
See Mercury[d] *at loc. no.* **221**

p-Nitroaniline (100-01-6) *See loc. no.* **617**

Nitrobenzene (98-95-3) *See loc. no.* **642**

Nitro-bid *See* Isosorbide Dinitrate[c] *at loc. no.* **634**

2-Nitro-1,1-bis(p-chlorophenyl)butane (117-26-0) *See* Bulan[a] *at loc. no.* **1005**

2-Nitro-1,1-bis(p-chlorophenyl)propane (117-27-1) *See*
Prolan[a] *at loc. no.* **1016**

Nitrocarbol (75-52-5) *See* Nitromethane[a] *at loc. no.* **636**

Nitrocellulose (9004-70-0) *See* Collodion[e] *at loc. no.* **854**

Nitrochlorobenzene (25167-93-5) *See loc. no.* **643**

Nitrochloroform (76-06-2) *See* Chloropicrin[c] *at loc. no.* **13**

Nitrofen (1836-75-5) *See loc. no.* **1310**

Nitroferricyanide salts *See* Nitroprusside Salts[a] *at loc. no.*
109

5-Nitro-2-furaldehyde semicarbazone (59-87-0) *See* Nitrofurazone[a] *at loc. no.* **1531**

Nitrofurantoin (67-20-9) *See loc. no.* **1530**

Nitrofurazone (59-87-0) *See loc. no.* **1531**

1-[(5-Nitro-2-furfurylidene)amino]-hydantoin (67-20-9)
See Nitrofurantoin[a] *at loc. no.* **1530**

3-(5-Nitrofurfurylideneamino)-2-oxazolidinone (67-45-8)
See Furazolidone[a] *at loc. no.* **1526**

Nitrogen dioxide (10102-44-0) *See* Nitrogen Oxides[d] *at loc.
no.* **9**

Nitrogen fluoride (7783-54-2) *See* Nitrogen Trifluoride[a] *at
loc. no.* **124**

Nitrogen Oxides *See loc. no.* **9**

Nitrogen pentoxide (10102-03-1) *See* Nitrogen Oxides[d] *at
loc. no.* **9**

Nitrogen tetroxide (10544-72-6) *See* Nitrogen Oxides[d] *at loc.
no.* **9**

Nitrogen Trichloride (10025-85-1) *See loc. no.* **123**

Nitrogen Trifluoride (7783-54-2) *See loc. no.* **124**

---

[a] A Synonym   [b] A Closely Related Substance   [c] The Active or Major Constituent   [d] A Class Name
[e] A Specific Example of or Product Containing

Nitroglycerin(e) (55-63-0) *See loc. no.* **635**
Nitroglycerol (55-63-0) *See* Nitroglycerin(e)[a] *at loc. no.* **635**
3-Nitro-4-hydroxyphenylarsonic acid (121-19-7) *See* 4-Hydroxy-3-nitrophenylarsonic Acid[a] *at loc. no.* **205**
Nitrol *See* Isosorbide Dinitrate[c] *at loc. no.* **634**
Nitromersol (133-58-4) *See* Hydroxymercurinitrophenol[b] *at loc. no.* **233**
Nitromethane (75-52-5) *See loc. no.* **636**
Nitromide (121-81-3) *See* Dinitolmide[b] *at loc. no.* **1540**
Nitrophen (1836-75-5) *See* Nitrofen[a] *at loc. no.* **1310**
Nitrophenide (537-91-7) *See loc. no.* **1541**
p-Nitrophenol (100-02-7) *See loc. no.* **544**
4-Nitrophenylarsonic acid (98-72-6) *See* Arsenicals[d] *at loc. no.* **192**
β-Nitrophenylethylene (102-96-5) *See* β-Nitrostyrene[a] *at loc. no.* **1631**
2-Nitropropane (79-46-9) *See loc. no.* **637**
Nitroprussiates *See* Nitroprusside Salts[a] *at loc. no.* **109**
Nitroprusside Salts *See loc. no.* **109**
β-Nitrostyrene (102-96-5) *See loc. no.* **1631**
Nitrous fumes *See* Nitrogen Oxides[d] *at loc. no.* **9**
Nitrous oxide (10024-97-2) *See* Nitrogen Oxides[d] *at loc. no.* **9**
NIX *See* Sodium Isopropyl Xanthate[c] *at loc. no.* **1315**
NMRI-448 (8014-87-7) *See loc. no.* **425**
Nobrium (2898-11-5) *See* Medazepam Hydrochloride[c] *at loc. no.* **1399**
Noctal (545-93-7) *See* Propallylonal[c] *at loc. no.* **1385**
Noludar (125-64-4) *See* Methyprylon[c] *at loc. no.* **1441**
Nonionic emulsifiers *See* Nonionic Synthetic Detergents[a] *at loc. no.* **961**
Nonionic surfactants *See* Nonionic Synthetic Detergents[a] *at loc. no.* **961**
Nonionic Synthetic Detergents *See loc. no.* **961**
Nonisols *See* Polyethylene Glycol Stearate[e] *at loc. no.* **968**
Nonoxynols *See* Alkyl Phenoxy Polyethoxy Ethanols[c] *at loc. no.* **963**
Nonyl *derivative. If not listed here, see corresponding* Alkyl *derivative in this index.*
Nonylcarbinol (112-30-1) *See* Decyl Alcohol[e] *at loc. no.* **411**
Nonylphenoxypolyethoxyethanol-iodine complex *See* Iodophors[d] *at loc. no.* **997**
Nonylphenyl ether of polyethylene glycoliodine complex (9006-35-3) *See* Iodophors[d] *at loc. no.* **997**
Norazine (3004-71-5) *See* Atrazine[b] *at loc. no.* **1259**
Nor-baeocystin *See* Psilocybin[b] *at loc. no.* **821**
Norbormide (991-42-4) *See loc. no.* **1349**
dl-Norephedrine hydrochloride (7587-43-1) *See* Phenylpropanolamine Hydrochloride[a] *at loc. no.* **1451**
Norethindrone with Mestranol (8015-29-0) *See loc. no.* **918**
Norethynodrel with Mestranol (8015-30-3) *See loc. no.* **919**
Norflurazon (27314-13-2) *See loc. no.* **1311**
Nornicotine (7076-23-5) *See loc. no.* **777**
Nortriptyline (72-69-5) *See loc. no.* **1474**
Nortron (26225-79-6) *See* Ethofumesate[a] *at loc. no.* **1305**
Noruron (18530-56-8) *See loc. no.* **1255**
Noscapine (128-62-1) *See loc. no.* **788**
Noscapine hydrochloride (912-60-7) *See* Noscapine[b] *at loc. no.* **788**
Nosema locustae *See loc. no.* **1645**
Nostal (545-93-7) *See* Propallylonal[c] *at loc. no.* **1385**
Nostyn (95-04-5) *See* Ectylurea[c] *at loc. no.* **1433**
Novaldin (68-89-3) *See* Dipyrone[c] *at loc. no.* **1573**
Novismuth (1304-85-4) *See* Bismuth Subnitrate[a] *at loc. no.* **218**
Novocaine (59-46-1) *See* Procaine[c] *at loc. no.* **1585**

Novon (136-25-4) *See* Erbon[c] *at loc. no.* **1218**
Novrad (55557-30-7) *See* Levopropoxyphene Napsylate[c] *at loc. no.* **1604**
NPD (3244-90-4) *See* Tetra-*n*-propyl Dithionopyrophosphate[a] *at loc. no.* **1110**
NRDC 143 (52645-53-1) *See* Permethrin[a] *at loc. no.* **891**
Numorphan (357-07-3) *See* Oxymorphone[b] *at loc. no.* **790**
Nupercainal (85-79-0) *See* Dibucaine[c] *at loc. no.* **1580**
Nupercaine (85-79-0) *See* Dibucaine[c] *at loc. no.* **1580**
Nutmeg *See loc. no.* **679**
Nux moschata *See* Nutmeg[a] *at loc. no.* **679**
Nux Vomica (8046-97-5) *See loc. no.* **680**
Oak mistletoe *See* European Mistletoe[b] *at loc. no.* **669**
Octabromobiphenyl (27858-07-7) *See* Polybrominated Biphenyls[e] *at loc. no.* **398**
Octachlorocamphene (8001-35-2) *See* Toxaphene[a] *at loc. no.* **1030**
Octachlorocyclohexenone (4024-81-1) *See loc. no.* **1199**
Octachlorodihydrodicyclopentadiene (57-74-9) *See* Chlordane[a] *at loc. no.* **1019**
Octachloro-hexahydro-methanoisobenzofuran (297-78-9) *See* Isobenzan[a] *at loc. no.* **1024**
Octachloro-4,7-methanohydroindane (57-74-9) *See* Chlordane[a] *at loc. no.* **1019**
Octachloro-4,7-methanotetrahydroindane (57-74-9) *See* Chlordane[a] *at loc. no.* **1019**
Octachloro-*endo*-methylene-tetrahydrophthalan (297-78-9) *See* Isobenzan[a] *at loc. no.* **1024**
Octacide 264 (113-48-4) *See* MGK 264[a] *at loc. no.* **1150**
9,12-Octadecadienoic acid (60-33-3) *See* Linoleic Acid[a] *at loc. no.* **555**
Octadecanoic acid (57-11-4) *See* Stearic Acid[a] *at loc. no.* **562**
9-Octadecenoic acid (112-80-1) *See* Oleic Acid[a] *at loc. no.* **559**
Octadecyl *derivative. If not listed here, see corresponding* Alkyl *derivative in this index.*
Octadecyl alcohol (112-92-5) *See* Stearyl Alcohol[a] *at loc. no.* **430**
Octadecylamine (124-30-1) *See loc. no.* **607**
Octafluoroisobutylene *See* Polytetrafluoroethylene[b] *at loc. no.* **1636**
Octalene (309-00-2) *See* Aldrin[c] *at loc. no.* **1017**
Octamethyl Pyrophosphoramide (152-16-9) *See loc. no.* **1102**
1-Octanol (111-87-5) *See* Caprylic Alcohol[a] *at loc. no.* **408**
2-Octanol (123-96-6) *See* Caprylic Alcohol[b] *at loc. no.* **408**
Octoxynol (9002-93-1) *See* Alkyl Phenoxy Polyethoxy Ethanols[c] *at loc. no.* **963**
Octyl *derivative. If not listed here, see corresponding* Alkyl *or* Ethylhexyl *derivative in this index.*
n-Octyl alcohol (111-87-5) *See* Caprylic Alcohol[a] *at loc. no.* **408**
Octyl alcohol (unspecified) *See* 2-Ethylhexyl Alcohol[e] *at loc. no.* **413**
tert-Octyl ammonium methanearsonate (6379-37-9) *See* Octyl Ammonium Metharsonate[a] *at loc. no.* **208**
Octyl Ammonium Metharsonate (6379-37-9) *See loc. no.* **208**
Octylammonium methylarsonate (6379-37-9) *See* Octyl Ammonium Metharsonate[a] *at loc. no.* **208**
N-Octyl bicycloheptene dicarboximide (113-48-4) *See* MGK 264[e] *at loc. no.* **1150**
Octyl Cresols *See loc. no.* **517**
Octyl decyl dimethyl ammonium chloride *See* Dialkyl Dimethyl Ammonium Chloride[d] *at loc. no.* **989**

---

[a] A Synonym   [b] A Closely Related Substance   [c] The Active or Major Constituent   [d] A Class Name
[e] A Specific Example of or Product Containing

Ingredient name (CAS registry no.) *See* Primary Name *at*
location no. **XXX** *in Part D of this section*

Octyl methyl phenols *See* Octyl Cresols[a] *at loc. no.* **517**
Octyl phenols *See* Octyl Cresols[b] *at loc. no.* **517**
p-tert-**Octyl phenoxyethoxyethyl dimethyl benzyl ammonium chloride** (121-54-0) *See* Benzethonium Chloride[a] *at loc. no.* **986**
p-tert-**Octyl phenoxy ethoxy ethyl dimethyl mercuric benzyl ammonium chloride** *See* Mercury[d] *at loc. no.* **221**
n-**Octyl sulfoxide of isosafrole** (120-62-7) *See* Sulfoxide[a] *at loc. no.* **1155**
Odorless base oil *See* Deobase[e] *at loc. no.* **324**
Odorless petroleum *See* Deobase[e] *at loc. no.* **324**
Off (134-62-3) *See* N,N-Diethyl-m-toluamide[c] *at loc. no.* **1326**
Oil of almond (artificial essential) (100-52-7) *See* Benzaldehyde[a] *at loc. no.* **859**
Oil of American wormseed (8006-99-3) *See* Chenopodium Oil[a] *at loc. no.* **728**
Oil of Anise (8007-70-3) *See loc. no.* **731**
Oil of apiol *See* Essential Oils[d] *at loc. no.* **725**
Oil of argemone *See* Argemone Oil[a] *at loc. no.* **710**
Oil of asafoetida *See* Essential Oils[d] *at loc. no.* **725**
Oil of Bay (8006-78-8) *See loc. no.* **732**
Oil of Bergamot (8007-75-8) *See loc. no.* **733**
Oil of Bitter Almond (8013-76-1) *See loc. no.* **734**
Oil of cade (8013-10-3) *See* Juniper Tar[a] *at loc. no.* **729**
Oil of cajeput (8008-98-8) *See* Eucalyptol[c] *at loc. no.* **863**
Oil of cajuput (8008-98-8) *See* Eucalyptol[c] *at loc. no.* **863**
Oil of cassia (8007-80-5) *See* Cinnamaldehyde[c] *at loc. no.* **860**
Oil of cedar leaf (8007-20-3) *See* Essential Oils[d] *at loc. no.* **725**
Oil of Cedar Wood (8000-27-9) *See loc. no.* **735**
Oil of chenopodium (8006-99-3) *See* Chenopodium Oil[a] *at loc. no.* **728**
Oil of cinnamon (8007-80-5) *See* Cinnamaldehyde[c] *at loc. no.* **860**
Oil of Citronella (8000-29-1) *See loc. no.* **736**
Oil of clove (8000-34-8) *See* Eugenol[c] *at loc. no.* **864**
Oil of eucalyptus (8000-48-4) *See* Eucalyptol[c] *at loc. no.* **863**
Oil of geranium (8000-46-2) *See* Essential Oils[d] *at loc. no.* **725**
Oil of ginger (8007-08-7) *See* Essential Oils[d] *at loc. no.* **725**
Oil of ginger grass *See* Oil of Citronella[b] *at loc. no.* **736**
Oil of hartshorn (8001-85-2) *See* Bone Oil[a] *at loc. no.* **711**
Oil of Hemlock (8008-10-4) *See loc. no.* **737**
Oil of juniper (8012-91-7) *See* Essential Oils[d] *at loc. no.* **725**
Oil of katakar *See* Argemone Oil[a] *at loc. no.* **710**
Oil of lavender (8000-28-0) *See* Lavender Oil[a] *at loc. no.* **730**
Oil of lemon (8008-56-8) *See* Essential Oils[d] *at loc. no.* **725**
Oil of lemon grass (8007-02-1) *See* Oil of Citronella[b] *at loc. no.* **736**
Oil of mirbane (98-95-3) *See* Nitrobenzene[a] *at loc. no.* **642**
Oil of mustard (8007-40-7) *See* Essential Oils[d] *at loc. no.* **725**
Oil of mustard (expressed) (8007-40-7) *See* Essential Oils[d] *at loc. no.* **725**
Oil of nutmeg (expressed) (8007-12-3) *See* Nutmeg[e] *at loc. no.* **679**
Oil of origanum (8007-11-2) *See* Essential Oils[d] *at loc. no.* **725**
Oil of pennyroyal (8021-41-8) *See* Pennyroyal[a] *at loc. no.* **740**
Oil of pennyroyal American (8007-44-1) *See* Pennyroyal[d] *at loc. no.* **740**
Oil of pennyroyal European (8013-99-8) *See* Pennyroyal[d] *at loc. no.* **740**
Oil of Peppermint (8006-90-4) *See loc. no.* **738**

Oil of Pycnanthemum albescens *See* Oil of Peppermint[b] *at loc. no.* **738**
Oil of rue (8014-29-7) *See* Essential Oils[d] *at loc. no.* **725**
Oil of Sassafras (8006-80-2) *See loc. no.* **739**
Oil of savin (8024-00-8) *See* Essential Oils[d] *at loc. no.* **725**
Oil of sesame (8008-74-0) *See* Sesame Oil[a] *at loc. no.* **722**
Oil of sialkata *See* Argemone Oil[a] *at loc. no.* **710**
Oil of spike (8016-78-2) *See* Essential Oils[d] *at loc. no.* **725**
Oil of sweet birch (119-36-8) *See* Methyl Salicylate[a] *at loc. no.* **597**
Oil of tansy (8016-87-3) *See* Essential Oils[d] *at loc. no.* **725**
Oil of tar *See* Tars (Tar Oils and Tar Acids)[a] *at loc. no.* **519**
Oil of thyme (8007-46-3) *See* Thyme Oil[a] *at loc. no.* **743**
Oil of turpentine (8006-64-2) *See* Turpentine[a] *at loc. no.* **763**
Oil of vitriol (7664-93-9) *See* Sulfuric Acid[a] *at loc. no.* **33**
Oil of wintergreen (119-36-8) *See* Methyl Salicylate[a] *at loc. no.* **597**
Oil of wormseed *See* Chenopodium Oil[a] *at loc. no.* **728**
Oils (lubricating) *See* Lubricating Oils[a] *at loc. no.* **338**
Oils volatile *See* Essential Oils[d] *at loc. no.* **725**
Oktane (4024-81-1) *See* Octachlorocyclohexenone[a] *at loc. no.* **1199**
Oktone (4024-81-1) *See* Octachlorocyclohexenone[a] *at loc. no.* **1199**
Oleate *See* Oleic Acid[b] *at loc. no.* **559**
Olefins *See* Petroleum Distillate[d] *at loc. no.* **323**
Oleic Acid (112-80-1) *See loc. no.* **559**
Oleoresin of capsicum (8023-77-6) *See* Capsicum[a] *at loc. no.* **659**
Oleum (8014-95-7) *See loc. no.* **34**
Oleum tiglii (8001-28-3) *See* Croton Oil[a] *at loc. no.* **715**
Oleyl *derivative. See corresponding* Alkyl *derivative in this index.*
N-**Oleyl-1,3-propylenediamine salt of 2,4,5-T** *See* Trichlorophenoxyacetic Acid[b] *at loc. no.* **1224**
Omnopon (8002-76-4) *See* Pantopon[a] *at loc. no.* **791**
OMPA (152-16-9) *See* Octamethyl Pyrophosphoramide[a] *at loc. no.* **1102**
Opacifier *See* Ethylene Glycol Distearate[c] *at loc. no.* **964**
OPI *See* Organic Phosphorus Insecticides[a] *at loc. no.* **1050**
Opium (8008-60-4) *See loc. no.* **757**
Optical brighteners *See* Fluorescent Whitening Agents[a] *at loc. no.* **938**
Ordram (2212-67-1) *See* Molinate[c] *at loc. no.* **1237**
Organic Phosphorus Insecticides *See loc. no.* **1050**
Organotin Compounds *See loc. no.* **291**
Orlon (9010-78-0) *See* Polyacrylonitrile[d] *at loc. no.* **652**
Orphenadrine (83-98-7) *See loc. no.* **1496**
Orpiment *See* Arsenic Trisulfide[a] *at loc. no.* **194**
Orsin (106-50-3) *See* Phenylenediamine (o- or p-)[d] *at loc. no.* **623**
Ortal sodium (144-00-3) *See* Hexethal Sodium[c] *at loc. no.* **1375**
Orthene *See* Acephate[c] *at loc. no.* **1095**
Ortho 4355 (300-76-5) *See* Naled[c] *at loc. no.* **1055**
Ortho 5865 (2425-06-1) *See* Captafol[c] *at loc. no.* **1180**
Orthoarsenic acid (7778-39-4) *See* Arsenic Acid[a] *at loc. no.* **191**
Ortho-benzyl-para-chlorophenol (120-32-1) *See* o-Benzyl-p-chlorophenol[a] *at loc. no.* **520**
Orthoboric acid (10043-35-3) *See* Boric Acid[a] *at loc. no.* **129**
Orthocide (133-06-2) *See* Captan[c] *at loc. no.* **1179**
Orthodichlorobenzene (95-50-1) *See* o-Dichlorobenzene[a] *at loc. no.* **395**
Ortho-Novum (8015-29-0) *See* Norethindrone with Mestranol[c] *at loc. no.* **918**

---

[a] A Synonym   [b] A Closely Related Substance   [c] The Active or Major Constituent   [d] A Class Name
[e] A Specific Example of or Product Containing

Ingredient name (CAS registry no.) *See* Primary Name *at location no.* **XXX** *in Part D of this section*

Orthophenylphenol (90-43-7) *See* Phenylphenol[d] *at loc. no.* **495**

Orthophosphoric acid (7664-38-2) *See* Phosphorus Pentoxide[b] *at loc. no.* **38**

Orvus E.S. *See* Alkyl Sodium Sulfates[d] *at loc. no.* **946**

Oryzalin (19044-88-3) *See* Benefin[b] *at loc. no.* **1287**

Osbac *See* BPMC[c] *at loc. no.* **1124**

Ouabain (630-60-4) *See loc. no.* **842**

Ovex (80-33-1) *See* Ovotran[a] *at loc. no.* **1047**

Ovotran (80-33-1) *See loc. no.* **1047**

Ovulen (8056-92-6) *See* Ethynodiol Diacetate with Mestranol[c] *at loc. no.* **917**

Oxacillin (66-79-5) *See* Penicillins[d] *at loc. no.* **902**

Oxalate *See loc. no.* **546**

Oxalic Acid (144-62-7) *See loc. no.* **47**

Oxalid (129-20-4) *See* Oxyphenbutazone[c] *at loc. no.* **1574**

Oxamyl (23135-22-0) *See loc. no.* **1144**

Oxanamide (126-93-2) *See loc. no.* **1409**

Oxazepam (604-75-1) *See loc. no.* **1401**

Oxide of iron powder *See* Iron Salts[d] *at loc. no.* **250**

Oxine (148-24-3) *See* 8-Hydroxyquinoline[a] *at loc. no.* **1514**

Oxirane (75-21-8) *See* Ethylene Oxide[c] *at loc. no.* **16**

Oxone *See* Potassium Monopersulfate[c] *at loc. no.* **79**

Oxtriphylline (146-71-4) *See* Theophylline[b] *at loc. no.* **802**

Oxybenzene (108-95-2) *See* Phenol[a] *at loc. no.* **494**

Oxybenzone (131-57-7) *See loc. no.* **1537**

Oxycarboxin (5259-88-1) *See* Carboxin[b] *at loc. no.* **1182**

Oxychloride salts *See* Sodium Hypochlorite[e] *at loc. no.* **85**

Oxycodone (76-42-6) *See loc. no.* **789**

Oxycodone hydrochloride (124-90-3) *See* Oxycodone[b] *at loc. no.* **789**

Oxycodone terephthalate *See* Oxycodone[b] *at loc. no.* **789**

Oxydemetonmethyl (301-12-2) *See* Meta-Systox-R[a] *at loc. no.* **1074**

Oxymetazoline Hydrochloride (2315-02-8) *See loc. no.* **1464**

Oxymorphone (76-41-5) *See loc. no.* **790**

Oxymorphone hydrochloride (357-07-3) *See* Oxymorphone[b] *at loc. no.* **790**

Oxyphenbutazone (129-20-4) *See loc. no.* **1574**

Oxyphenisatin acetate (115-33-3) *See* Phenolphthalein[b] *at loc. no.* **1607**

Oxyquinoline (148-24-3) *See* 8-Hydroxyquinoline[a] *at loc. no.* **1514**

Oxyquinoline salts *See* 8-Hydroxyquinoline[e] *at loc. no.* **1514**

Oxyquinoline sulfate (134-31-6) *See* 8-Hydroxyquinoline[b] *at loc. no.* **1514**

Oxytetracycline (79-57-2) *See* Tetracyclines[d] *at loc. no.* **904**

Oxythioquinox (2439-01-2) *See* Quinomethionate[a] *at loc. no.* **1205**

P-40 *See* Sodium Selenate[c] *at loc. no.* **184**

PABA (150-13-0) *See* p-Aminobenzoic Acid[a] *at loc. no.* **628**

Pacatal (60-89-9) *See* Mepazine[c] *at loc. no.* **1416**

Padan *See* Cartap[c] *at loc. no.* **1130**

Paint driers *See* Cobalt Driers[a] *at loc. no.* **283**

Pallethrine (584-79-2) *See* Allethrin[a] *at loc. no.* **884**

Palmityl derivative. *If not listed here, see corresponding* Alkyl *derivative in this index.*

Palmityl alcohol (124-29-8) *See* Cetyl Alcohol[a] *at loc. no.* **409**

2-PAM (51-15-0) *See* Pralidoxime Chloride[a] *at loc. no.* **1508**

Pamaquine (491-92-9) *See* Primaquine[b] *at loc. no.* **1516**

Panadol (103-90-2) *See* Acetaminophen[c] *at loc. no.* **1587**

Panogen 15 (502-39-6) *See* Methylmercuric Dicyandiamide[c] *at loc. no.* **240**

Pantopium *See* Pantopon[a] *at loc. no.* **791**

Pantopon (8002-76-2) *See loc. no.* **791**

Papain (9001-73-4) *See loc. no.* **927**

Papaverine (58-74-2) *See loc. no.* **793**

Papaverine hydrochloride (61-25-6) *See* Papaverine[b] *at loc. no.* **793**

Para- *If not listed below, omit prefix and try again.*

Para-aminobenzoic acid (150-13-0) *See* p-Aminobenzoic Acid[a] *at loc. no.* **628**

Paraben Esters *See loc. no.* **584**

Parabis (97-23-4) *See* Dichlorophen(e)[c] *at loc. no.* **529**

Para-*tert*-butyl meta cresol (2219-72-9) *See* Cresols[b] *at loc. no.* **514**

Paracetaldehyde (123-63-7) *See* Paraldehyde[a] *at loc. no.* **1442**

Paracetamol (103-90-2) *See* Acetaminophen[a] *at loc. no.* **1587**

Parachlorometacresol (59-50-7) *See* Chlorocresols[d] *at loc. no.* **523**

Parachlorometaxylenol (88-04-0) *See* 4-Chloro-3,5-xylenol[a] *at loc. no.* **528**

Parachlorophenyl parachlorobenzene sulfonate (80-33-1) *See* Ovotran[a] *at loc. no.* **1047**

Parachlorophenylphenyl sulfone (80-00-2) *See* Sulphenone[e] *at loc. no.* **1048**

Paradichlorobenzene (106-46-7) *See* p-Dichlorobenzene[a] *at loc. no.* **396**

Paraffin (8002-74-2) *See* Paraffin Wax(es)[a] *at loc. no.* **340**

Paraffin (Chlorinated) (8029-39-8) *See loc. no.* **389**

Paraffinic hydrocarbons *See* Aliphatic Hydrocarbons[d] *at loc. no.* **303**

Paraffin Wax(es) (8002-74-2) *See loc. no.* **340**

Paraform (9002-81-7) *See* Paraformaldehyde[a] *at loc. no.* **487**

Paraformaldehyde (9002-81-7) *See loc. no.* **487**

Paraldehyde (123-63-7) *See loc. no.* **1442**

Paramethasone (53-33-8) *See* Corticosteroids[d] *at loc. no.* **915**

Paranitrophenol (100-02-7) *See* p-Nitrophenol[a] *at loc. no.* **544**

Paraoxon (311-45-5) *See loc. no.* **1056**

Paraphenylenediamine (106-50-3) *See* Phenylenediamine (o- or p-)[d] *at loc. no.* **623**

Paraquat (1910-42-5) *See loc. no.* **1286**

Parathion (56-38-2) *See loc. no.* **1077**

Paratoluenediamine (95-80-7) *See* 2,4-Diaminotoluene[a] *at loc. no.* **621**

Paredrine *See* Hydroxyamphetamine Hydrobromide[c] *at loc. no.* **1457**

Paregoric (8029-99-0) *See loc. no.* **766**

Parinol (17781-31-6) *See* Parnon[a] *at loc. no.* **1200**

Paris green (1299-88-3) *See* Copper Acetoarsenite[a] *at loc. no.* **200**

Parnate (95-62-5) *See* Tranylcypromine[c] *at loc. no.* **1480**

Parnon (17781-31-6) *See loc. no.* **1200**

Paraffins (8002-74-2) *See* Aliphatic Hydrocarbons[d] *at loc. no.* **303**

Parvex (99-00-3) *See* Piperazine-Carbon Disulfide complex[c] *at loc. no.* **1545**

Parvex-Plus *See* Piperazine-Carbon Disulfide complex[b] *at loc. no.* **1545**

PAS (65-49-6) *See* p-Aminosalicylic Acid[a] *at loc. no.* **629**

Passiflora *See loc. no.* **681**

Passion flower or vine *See* Passiflora[a] *at loc. no.* **681**

Pavabid *See* Papaverine[c] *at loc. no.* **793**

PBB *See* Polybrominated Biphenyls[a] *at loc. no.* **398**

PBS *See* 3,4',5-Tribromosalicylanilide[e] *at loc. no.* **1000**

PCB *See loc. no.* **399**

PCH (119-89-1) *See* Piperonyl Cyclonene[a] *at loc. no.* **1152**

PCMC (59-50-7) *See* Chlorocresols[d] *at loc. no.* **523**

---

[a] A Synonym   [b] A Closely Related Substance   [c] The Active or Major Constituent   [d] A Class Name   [e] A Specific Example of or Product Containing

Ingredient name (CAS registry no.) *See* Primary Name *at
location no.* **XXX** *in Part D of this section*

PCMX (88-04-0) *See* 4-Chloro-3,5-xylenol[a] *at loc. no.* **528**
PCNB (82-68-8) *See* Pentachloronitrobenzene[a] *at loc. no.* **1201**
PCP (956-90-1)*See* Phencyclidine Hydrochloride[a] *at loc. no.* **1542**
PCP (87-86-5) *See* Pentachlorophenol[a] *at loc. no.* **532**
PCPA *See p*-Chlorophenoxyacetic Acid[a] *at loc. no.* **1211**
PDB (106-46-7) *See p*-Dichlorobenzene[a] *at loc. no.* **396**
PDU (101-42-8) *See* Fenuron[a] *at loc. no.* **1248**
Peanut Oil (8002-03-7) *See loc. no.* **719**
Peanuts *See* Peanut Oil[c] *at loc. no.* **719**
Pear oil (123-92-2) *See* Isoamyl Acetate[a] *at loc. no.* **574**
Pebulate (1114-71-2) *See loc. no.* **1238**
Pectin (9000-69-5) *See loc. no.* **758**
Pelletierine Tannate (8007-39-4) *See loc. no.* **831**
Pemoline (2152-34-3) *See loc. no.* **1465**
Pencil lead *See* Graphite[c] *at loc. no.* **4**
Penetrol *See* Sulfonated Petroleum Oils[c] *at loc. no.* **958**
D-**Penicillamine** (52-67-5) *See loc. no.* **1507**
L-**Penicillamine** (1113-41-3) *See D*-Penicillamine[b] *at loc. no.* **1507**
Penicillin G (61-33-6) *See* Penicillins[d] *at loc. no.* **902**
Penicillins *See loc. no.* **902**
Penicillin V (87-08-1) *See* Penicillins[d] *at loc. no.* **902**
Pennyroyal (8021-41-8) *See loc. no.* **740**
Penoxalin (40487-42-1) *See* Dinitramine[b] *at loc. no.* **1288**
Penta (87-86-5) *See* Pentachlorophenol[c] *at loc. no.* **532**
1,4,7,10,13-Pentaazatridecane (112-57-2) *See* Tetraethylenepentamine[a] *at loc. no.* **605**
Pentac (2227-17-0) *See* Dienochlor[c] *at loc. no.* **1027**
Pentachloroaniline (527-20-8) *See* Pentachloronitrobenzene[b] *at loc. no.* **1201**
Pentachloroethane (76-01-7) *See loc. no.* **371**
Pentachloronaphthalene (1321-64-8) *See* Polychlorinated Naphthalenes[d] *at loc. no.* **402**
Pentachloronitrobenzene (82-68-8) *See loc. no.* **1201**
Pentachlorophenol (87-86-5) *See loc. no.* **532**
Pentaerythritol Tetranitrate (78-11-5) *See loc. no.* **638**
Pentanal *N*-**methyl-***N*-**formylhydrazone** *See* Gyromitrin[b] *at loc. no.* **816**
n-**Pentane** (109-66-0) *See n*-Hexane[b] *at loc. no.* **307**
Pentanochlor (2307-68-8) *See loc. no.* **1280**
1-Pentanol (71-41-0) *See* Amyl Alcohol[a] *at loc. no.* **405**
Pentaphen (80-46-6) *See* Amyl Phenol[c] *at loc. no.* **488**
Pentaquine (86-78-2) *See* Primaquine[b] *at loc. no.* **1516**
Pentasodium triphosphate (7758-29-4) *See* Tripolyphosphate[d] *at loc. no.* **142**
Pentasodium tripolyphosphate (7758-29-4) *See* Tripolyphosphate[d] *at loc. no.* **142**
Pentazocine (359-83-1) *See loc. no.* **792**
Pentobarbital (76-74-4) *See* Pentobarbital Sodium[b] *at loc. no.* **1380**
Pentobarbital Sodium (57-33-0) *See loc. no.* **1380**
Pentothal sodium (71-73-8) *See* Thiopental Sodium[c] *at loc. no.* **1390**
Pentylenetetrazol (54-95-5) *See loc. no.* **1606**
p-tert-**Pentylphenol** (80-46-6) *See* Amyl Phenol[a] *at loc. no.* **488**
Pepper *See loc. no.* **682**
Peppermint *See* Oil of Peppermint[a] *at loc. no.* **738**
PEPS *See* Polyethylene Polysulfide[a] *at loc. no.* **1203**
Pepsin (9001-75-6) *See loc. no.* **928**
Peracetic acid (79-21-0) *See* Peroxyacetic Acid[a] *at loc. no.* **78**
Perchlorobenzene (118-74-1) *See* Hexachlorobenzene[a] *at loc. no.* **397**

Perchlorobi(cyclopenta-2,4-dienyl) (2227-17-0) *See* Dienochlor[a] *at loc. no.* **1027**
Perchloroethane (67-72-1) *See* Hexachloroethane[a] *at loc. no.* **370**
Perchloroethylene (127-18-4) *See* Tetrachloroethylene[a] *at loc. no.* **374**
Perchloromethane (56-23-5) *See* Carbon Tetrachloride[a] *at loc. no.* **355**
Percodan *See* Oxycodone[c] *at loc. no.* **789**
Perfume oils *See* Essential Oils[d] *at loc. no.* **725**
Perhydrosqualene (111-01-3) *See* Squalane[a] *at loc. no.* **932**
Peristim *See* Casanthranol[c] *at loc. no.* **849**
Peritrate (78-11-5) *See* Pentaerythritol Tetranitrate[c] *at loc. no.* **638**
Permanganate salts *See* Potassium Permanganate[e] *at loc. no.* **83**
Permethrin (52645-53-1) *See loc. no.* **891**
Permitil (146-56-5) *See* Fluphenazine Hydrochloride[c] *at loc. no.* **1415**
Pernocton *See* Butallyonal[b] *at loc. no.* **1369**
Pernoston (1142-70-7) *See* Butallyonal[c] *at loc. no.* **1369**
Pernox (52-86-8) *See* Haloperidol[a] *at loc. no.* **1437**
Peroxyacetic Acid (79-21-0) *See loc. no.* **78**
Perphenazine (58-39-9) *See loc. no.* **1418**
Persian insect powder *See* Pyrethrum[a] *at loc. no.* **686**
Perspex (9011-14-7) *See* Methyl Methacrylate[b] *at loc. no.* **1630**
Persulfate salts (inorganic) *See* Potassium Monopersulfate[e] *at loc. no.* **79**
Perthane (72-56-0) *See loc. no.* **1015**
Peruvian or Indian balsam (8007-00-9) *See* Balsam Peru[a] *at loc. no.* **749**
Pestox III (152-16-9) *See* Octamethyl Pyrophosphoramide[c] *at loc. no.* **1102**
Pethidine hydrochloride (50-13-5) *See* Meperidine Hydrochloride[a] *at loc. no.* **1484**
PETN (78-11-5) *See* Pentaerythritol Tetranitrate[a] *at loc. no.* **638**
Petrohol (67-63-0) *See* Isopropyl Alcohol[a] *at loc. no.* **420**
Petrol (8006-61-9) *See* Gasoline[a] *at loc. no.* **327**
Petrolatum (8009-03-8) *See* Liquid Petrolatum[b] *at loc. no.* **337**
Petrolatum album (8027-32-5) *See* Liquid Petrolatum[b] *at loc. no.* **337**
Petroleum asphalts *See* Asphalt[a] *at loc. no.* **343**
Petroleum base oil *See* Petroleum Distillate[d] *at loc. no.* **323**
Petroleum benzin (8030-30-6) *See* Petroleum Ether[a] *at loc. no.* **330**
Petroleum benzine (8030-30-6) *See* Petroleum Ether[a] *at loc. no.* **330**
Petroleum (Crude) (8002-05-9) *See loc. no.* **336**
Petroleum Distillate *See loc. no.* **323**
Petroleum Ether (8030-30-6) *See loc. no.* **330**
Petroleum hydrocarbon oil *See* Petroleum Distillate[d] *at loc. no.* **323**
Petroleum hydrocarbons *See* Petroleum Distillate[a] *at loc. no.* **323**
Petroleum jelly (8009-03-8) *See* Liquid Petrolatum[b] *at loc. no.* **337**
Petroleum lubricating oils *See* Lubricating Oils[a] *at loc. no.* **338**
Petroleum Naphtha (8030-31-7) *See loc. no.* **331**
Petroleum oil *See* Petroleum Distillate[d] *at loc. no.* **323**
Petroleum solvent *See* Petroleum Distillate[d] *at loc. no.* **323**
Petroleum spirits (8032-32-4) *See* VM&P Naphthas[a] *at loc. no.* **335**

[a] A Synonym   [b] A Closely Related Substance   [c] The Active or Major Constituent   [d] A Class Name
[e] A Specific Example of or Product Containing

Ingredient name (CAS registry no.) *See* Primary Name *at*
location no. **XXX** *in Part D of this section*

Petroleum sulfonate *See* Sulfonated Petroleum Oils*ᵃ at loc. no.* 958

Petroleum thinner *See* Petroleum Naphtha*ᵉ at loc. no.* 331

Peyote (11006-96-5) *See loc. no.* 683

PGE (122-60-1) *See* Glycidyl Ethers*ᵈ at loc. no.* 1629

Phallacidin (26645-35-2) *See* Phallotoxins*ᵈ at loc. no.* 814

Phallisacin *See* Phallotoxins*ᵈ at loc. no.* 814

Phalloidin (17466-45-4) *See* Phallotoxins*ᵈ at loc. no.* 814

Phallotoxins *See loc. no.* 814

Phaltan (133-07-3) *See* Folpet*ᵃ at loc. no.* 1181

Phanodorn (52-31-3) *See* Cyclobarbital*ᶜ at loc. no.* 1371

Phemerol chloride (121-54-0) *See* Benzethonium Chloride*ᵃ at loc. no.* 986

Phenacetin (62-44-2) *See* Acetophenetidin*ᵃ at loc. no.* 611

Phenacyl chloride (532-27-4) *See* α-Chloroacetophenone*ᵃ at loc. no.* 14

Phenaglycodol (79-93-6) *See loc. no.* 1410

Phenamiphos (22224-92-6) *See loc. no.* 1103

Phenanthrene (85-01-8) *See* Anthracene Oil*ᶜ at loc. no.* 341

Phenazone (60-80-0) *See* Antipyrine*ᵃ at loc. no.* 1571

Phenazopyridine Hydrochloride (136-40-3) *See loc. no.* 1522

Phencyclidine Hydrochloride (956-90-1) *See loc. no.* 1542

Phendimetrazine (634-03-7) *See* Phenmetrazine*ᵇ at loc. no.* 1466

Phenelzine Sulfate (156-51-4) *See loc. no.* 1477

Phenergan (58-33-3) *See* Promethazine*ᶜ at loc. no.* 1421

Phenethicillin (147-55-7) *See* Penicillins*ᵈ at loc. no.* 902

2-Phenethyl alcohol (60-12-8) *See* 2-Phenylethyl Alcohol*ᵃ at loc. no.* 427

Pheniramine tartrate (569-59-5) *See* Antihistaminics*ᵈ at loc. no.* 1487

Phenindione (83-12-5) *See loc. no.* 1341

Pheniramine Maleate (132-20-7) *See loc. no.* 1497

Phenisobromolate *See* Bromopropylate*ᵃ at loc. no.* 1004

Phenmedipham (13684-63-4) *See* Desmedipham*ᵇ at loc. no.* 1230

Phenmedipham-ethyl *See* Desmedipham*ᵇ at loc. no.* 1230

Phenmetrazine (134-49-6) *See loc. no.* 1466

Phenobarbital (50-06-6) *See loc. no.* 1382

Phenobenzuron (3134-12-1) *See loc. no.* 1256

Phenol (108-95-2) *See loc. no.* 494

Phenol mercuric chloride (90-03-9) *See* Hydroxyphenylmercurichloride*ᵃ at loc. no.* 234

Phenolphthalein (77-09-8) *See loc. no.* 1607

Phenolphthalin (77-09-8) *See* Phenolphthalein*ᵃ at loc. no.* 1607

Phenol red (143-74-8) *See* Phenolsulfonphthalein*ᵃ at loc. no.* 1608

Phenolsulfonphthalein (143-74-8) *See loc. no.* 1608

Phenothiazine (92-84-2) *See loc. no.* 1543

Phenothioxin (262-20-4) *See loc. no.* 1360

Phenothrin *See* Permethrin*ᵇ at loc. no.* 891

Phenoxathrin (262-20-4) *See* Phenothioxin*ᵃ at loc. no.* 1360

3-Phenoxybenzyl-3-(2,2-dichlorovinyl)-2,2-dimethylcyclopropanecarboxylate (52645-53-1) *See* Permethrin*ᵃ at loc. no.* 891

2-Phenoxyethanol (122-99-6) *See* Phenyl Cellosolve*ᵃ at loc. no.* 463

Phenprocoumon (435-97-2) *See loc. no.* 1342

Phentermine (122-09-8) *See loc. no.* 1467

Phentermine hydrochloride (1197-21-3) *See* Phentermine*ᵇ at loc. no.* 1467

N-Phenylacetamide (103-84-4) *See* Acetanilid(e)*ᵃ at loc. no.* 610

3-α-Phenyl-β-acetylethyl-4-hydroxycoumarin (81-81-2) *See* Warfarin*ᵃ at loc. no.* 1345

Phenylacrolein (104-55-2) *See* Cinnamaldehyde*ᵃ at loc. no.* 860

Phenylamine (62-53-3) *See* Aniline*ᵃ at loc. no.* 612

β-Phenylazo-α,α-diaminopyridine hydrochloride (136-40-3) *See* Phenazopyridine Hydrochloride*ᵃ at loc. no.* 1522

Phenylbenzene (92-52-4) *See* Diphenyl*ᵃ at loc. no.* 314

Phenylbutazone (50-33-9) *See loc. no.* 1575

Phenylcarbinol (100-51-6) *See* Benzyl Alcohol*ᵃ at loc. no.* 406

Phenyl Cellosolve (122-99-6) *See loc. no.* 463

2-Phenylcyclohexanol (1444-64-0) *See* Phenyl Cyclohexanol*ᵃ at loc. no.* 426

Phenyl Cyclohexanol (1444-64-0) *See loc. no.* 426

1-(1-Phenylcyclohexyl)piperidine hydrochloride (956-90-1) *See* Phencyclidine Hydrochloride*ᵃ at loc. no.* 1542

1-Phenyl-2-diethyl-1-aminopropanone (90-84-6) *See* Diethylpropion*ᵃ at loc. no.* 1447

Phenyl-N,N'-dimethyl phosphorodiamidate (1754-58-1) *See* Diamidafos*ᵃ at loc. no.* 1097

Phenyl dimethyl pyrazolone *See* Antipyrine*ᵃ at loc. no.* 1571

1-Phenyl-2,3-dimethyl-5-pyrazolone-4-methylaminomethanesulfonate sodium (50571-74-9) *See* Dipyrone*ᵃ at loc. no.* 1573

3-Phenyl-1,1-dimethylurea (101-42-8) *See* Fenuron*ᵃ at loc. no.* 1248

Phenylenediamine (*o*- or *p*-) *See loc. no.* 623

Phenylephrine (59-42-7) *See loc. no.* 1468

2-Phenylethanol (60-12-8) *See* 2-Phenylethyl Alcohol*ᵃ at loc. no.* 427

2-Phenylethyl Alcohol (60-12-8) *See loc. no.* 427

β-Phenylethyl alcohol (60-12-8) *See* 2-Phenylethyl Alcohol*ᵃ at loc. no.* 427

5-Phenyl-5-ethylbarbituric acid (50-06-6) *See* Phenobarbital*ᵃ at loc. no.* 1382

Phenylethylene (100-42-5) *See* Styrene*ᵃ at loc. no.* 315

Phenylethyl hydrazine dihydrogen sulfate (156-51-4) *See* Phenelzine Sulfate*ᵃ at loc. no.* 1477

Phenyl ethyl malonyl urea (50-06-6) *See* Phenobarbital*ᵃ at loc. no.* 1382

Phenylglycidyl ether (122-60-1) *See* Glycidyl Ethers*ᵈ at loc. no.* 1629

Phenylic acid (108-95-2) *See* Phenol*ᵃ at loc. no.* 494

2-Phenyl-1,3-indandione (83-12-5) *See* Phenindione*ᵃ at loc. no.* 1341

Phenylisohydantoin *See* Pemoline*ᵃ at loc. no.* 1465

β-Phenylisopropylamine (300-62-9) *See* Amphetamine*ᵃ at loc. no.* 1444

Phenylmercuric acetate (62-38-4) *See* Phenylmercuric Salts of Organic Acids*ᵈ at loc. no.* 241

Phenylmercuric Salts of Organic Acids *See loc. no.* 241

Phenylmercuric oleate (104-60-9) *See* Phenylmercuric Salts of Organic Acids*ᵈ at loc. no.* 241

Phenylmercuric Salts of Inorganic Acids *See loc. no.* 242

Phenylmercuric Triethanol Ammonium Lactate (4386-88-3) *See loc. no.* 243

Phenylmercurimonoethanolammonium acetate (5822-97-9) *See* Phenylmercuric Triethanol Ammonium Lactate*ᵇ at loc. no.* 243

Phenyl mercury urea (2279-64-3) *See* Mercury*ᵈ at loc. no.* 221

Phenylmethanol (100-51-6) *See* Benzyl Alcohol*ᵃ at loc. no.* 406

4-(Phenylmethoxy)phenol (103-16-2) *See* Monobenzone*ᵃ at loc. no.* 1536

5-Phenyl-5-methylbarbituric Acid (76-94-8) *See loc. no.* 1381

ᵃ A Synonym   ᵇA Closely Related Substance   ᶜThe Active or Major Constituent   ᵈA Class Name
ᵉA Specific Example of or Product Containing

Ingredient name (CAS registry no.) *See* Primary Name *at
location no.* **XXX** *in Part D of this section*

1-Phenyl-3-methyl-5-pyrazolyl dimethylcarbamate (87-47-8) *See* Pyrolan[c] *at loc. no.* **1149**

Phenylphenates *See* Phenylphenol[b] *at loc. no.* **495**

Phenylphenol (1322-20-9) *See loc. no.* **495**

N-**Phenyl-*p*-phenylenediamine** (101-54-2) *See p*-Aminodiphenylamine[a] *at loc. no.* **619**

Phenylphosphine (638-21-5) *See* Phosphine[b] *at loc. no.* **136**

2-Phenylpropane (98-82-8) *See* Cumene[a] *at loc. no.* **313**

3-Phenylpropenal (104-55-2) *See* Cinnamaldehyde[a] *at loc. no.* **860**

Phenylpropanolamine Hydrochloride (7587-43-1) *See loc. no.* **1451**

Phenylpropylene (300-57-2) *See* Allyl Benzene[a] *at loc. no.* **311**

N-**Phenylsalicylamide** (87-17-2) *See* Salicylanilide[a] *at loc. no.* **998**

Phenyl Salicylate (118-55-8) *See loc. no.* **598**

Phenylthiourea (103-85-5) *See loc. no.* **1351**

Phenyltoloxamine citrate (1176-08-5) *See* Phenyltoloxamine Dihydrogen Citrate[a] *at loc. no.* **1498**

Phenyltoloxamine Dihydrogen Citrate (1176-08-5) *See loc. no.* **1498**

Phenyral (115-43-5) *See* 5-Allyl-5-phenylbarbituric Acid[c] *at loc. no.* **1363**

Phenytoin Sodium (630-93-3) *See loc. no.* **1609**

Phloroglucinol (108-73-6) *See* Pyrogallol[b] *at loc. no.* **506**

Phobex (57-37-4) *See* Benactyzine[c] *at loc. no.* **1430**

Phoradendron flavescens *See* American Mistletoe[a] *at loc. no.* **656**

Phorate (298-02-2) *See loc. no.* **1094**

Phosdrin (7786-34-7) *See loc. no.* **1057**

Phosgene (75-44-5) *See loc. no.* **11**

Phosmet *See* Imidan[c] *at loc. no.* **1090**

Phosphamidon (297-99-4) *See loc. no.* **1058**

Phosphates *See loc. no.* **139**

Phosphatidyl choline *See* Lecithin[a] *at loc. no.* **705**

Phosphine (7803-51-2) *See loc. no.* **136**

Phosphoric acid (7664-38-2) *See* Phosphorus Pentoxide[b] *at loc. no.* **38**

Phosphoric acid anhydride (1314-56-3) *See* Phosphorus Pentoxide[a] *at loc. no.* **38**

Phosphoric sulfide (1314-80-3) *See* Phosphorus Pentasulfide[a] *at loc. no.* **117**

Phosphorus (7723-14-0) *See loc. no.* **135**

Phosphorus Pentasulfide (1314-80-3) *See loc. no.* **117**

Phosphorus Pentoxide (1314-56-3) *See loc. no.* **38**

Phosphorus persulfide (1314-80-3) *See* Phosphorus Pentasulfide[a] *at loc. no.* **117**

O-**Phosphoryl-4-hydroxy-*N,N*-dimethyltryptamine** (520-52-5) *See* Psilocybin[a] *at loc. no.* **821**

Phostex (7084-87-9) *See loc. no.* **1107**

Phostoxin (20859-73-8) *See* Aluminum Phosphide[a] *at loc. no.* **137**

Photol (55-55-0) *See p*-Methylaminophenol Sulfate[c] *at loc. no.* **626**

Photomirex *See* Mirex[b] *at loc. no.* **1033**

Phthalic Acid Esters *See loc. no.* **589**

α-(*N*-**Phthalimido)glutarimide** (50-35-1) *See* Thalidomide[a] *at loc. no.* **1443**

Phthalin (77-09-8) *See* Phenolphthalein[a] *at loc. no.* **1607**

Phthalonitrile (91-15-6) *See loc. no.* **651**

Phthalylsulfacetamide (131-69-1) *See loc. no.* **1547**

2-(*N*⁴-Phthalylsulfanilamido)thiazole *See* Phthalylsulfathiazole[a] *at loc. no.* **1548**

Phthalylsulfathiazole (85-73-4) *See loc. no.* **1548**

Phygon (117-80-6) *See* Dichlone[c] *at loc. no.* **1190**

Physeptone (76-99-3) *See* Methadone[a] *at loc. no.* **1485**

Physostigmine (57-47-6) *See loc. no.* **807**

Physostigmine salicylate (57-64-7) *See* Physostigmine[b] *at loc. no.* **807**

Picadex (99-00-3) *See* Piperazine-Carbon Disulfide complex[a] *at loc. no.* **1545**

Picloram (1918-02-1) *See loc. no.* **1312**

Picric Acid (88-89-1) *See loc. no.* **545**

Picronitric acid (88-89-1) *See* Picric Acid[a] *at loc. no.* **545**

Pigments *For a tabular summary of dyes and pigments, see Section VI (General Formulations).*

Pilocarpine (92-13-7) *See loc. no.* **808**

Pindone (83-26-1) *See* 2-Pivalyl-1,3-indandione[a] *at loc. no.* **1343**

2-Pinene (80-56-8) *See* α-Pinene[a] *at loc. no.* **879**

Pinene *See* Terpenes[d] *at loc. no.* **881**

α-**Pinene** (80-56-8) *See loc. no.* **879**

Pinene hydrochloride (464-41-5) *See* Bornyl Chloride[a] *at loc. no.* **874**

Pine Oil (8006-88-0) *See loc. no.* **741**

Pine tar (8011-48-1) *See* Creosote[b] *at loc. no.* **513**

Pine tar oil *See* Creosote[b] *at loc. no.* **513**

Pinolene (25719-60-2) *See* Di-1-*p*-menthene[c] *at loc. no.* **878**

Piperacetazine (3819-00-9) *See* Thioridazine[b] *at loc. no.* **1425**

Piperazidine (110-85-0) *See* Piperazine[a] *at loc. no.* **1544**

Piperazine (110-85-0) *See loc. no.* **1544**

1-Piperazinecarbodithioic acid (99-00-3) *See* Piperazine-Carbon Disulfide complex[a] *at loc. no.* **1545**

Piperazine-Carbon Disulfide complex (99-00-3) *See loc. no.* **1545**

α-(2-**Piperidyl)benzhydrol** (467-60-7) *See* Pipradrol[a] *at loc. no.* **1478**

α-(4-**Piperidyl)benzhydrol** (115-46-8) *See* Azacyclonol[a] *at loc. no.* **1429**

Piperonal (120-57-0) *See loc. no.* **871**

Piperonal bis(2(2'-*n*-butoxyethoxy)ethyl)acetal (5281-13-0) *See* Tropital[a] *at loc. no.* **1156**

Piperonyl Butoxide (51-03-6) *See loc. no.* **1151**

Piperonyl cyclohexenone (119-89-1) *See* Piperonyl Cyclonene[a] *at loc. no.* **1152**

Piperonyl Cyclonene (119-89-1) *See loc. no.* **1152**

Piperonyl ether butoxide (51-03-6) *See* Piperonyl Butoxide[a] *at loc. no.* **1151**

Piperonylic acid *See* Tropital[b] *at loc. no.* **1156**

Pipradrol (467-60-7) *See loc. no.* **1478**

Pirazinon (5826-91-5) *See* Diethyl Propylmethylpyrimidyl Thiophosphate[a] *at loc. no.* **1070**

Pirimicarb (23103-98-2) *See loc. no.* **1145**

Pirimor *See* Pirimicarb[a] *at loc. no.* **1145**

Pival (83-26-1) *See* 2-Pivalyl-1,3-indandione[c] *at loc. no.* **1343**

2-Pivalyl-1,3-indandione (83-26-1) *See loc. no.* **1343**

Pivalyn (132-30-9) *See* 2-Pivalyl-1,3-indandione[b] *at loc. no.* **1343**

Placidyl (113-18-8) *See* Ethchlorvynol[c] *at loc. no.* **1434**

Planofix (86-87-3) *See* 1-Naphthaleneacetic Acid[a] *at loc. no.* **1309**

Plantvax (5259-88-1) *See* Carboxin[b] *at loc. no.* **1182**

Plaquenil (118-42-3) *See* Chloroquine[b] *at loc. no.* **1512**

Plaster of Paris (10034-76-1) *See loc. no.* **172**

Plasticizers *See loc. no.* **1632**

Plexiglas *See* Methyl Methacrylate[b] *at loc. no.* **1630**

Plumbago (7782-42-5) *See* Graphite[a] *at loc. no.* **4**

Plumber's acid *See* Hydrochloric Acid[a] *at loc. no.* **31**

Pluronics *See loc. no.* **967**

PMA. *This name is used as a synonym for both* Phenylmercuric acetate *and* 4-Methoxyamphetamine, *which are unrelated. See in this index whichever is applicable.*

---

[a] A Synonym   [b] A Closely Related Substance   [c] The Active or Major Constituent   [d] A Class Name
[e] A Specific Example of or Product Containing

Ingredient name (CAS registry no.) *See* Primary Name *at location no.* **XXX** *in Part D of this section*

PMAS (62-38-4) *See* Phenylmercuric Salts of Organic Acids[d] *at loc. no.* **241**

PNU *See* Vacor[e] *at loc. no.* **1353**

Podophyllin (8050-60-0) *See* Podophyllum Resin[a] *at loc. no.* **759**

Podophyllotoxin (518-28-5) *See* Podophyllum Resin[e] *at loc. no.* **759**

Podophyllum Resin (8050-60-0) *See loc. no.* **759**

Poinsettia *See loc. no.* **684**

Polamidon (76-99-3) *See* Methadone[a] *at loc. no.* **1485**

Polyacrylonitrile (25014-41-9) *See loc. no.* **652**

Polyalkyl *derivative. See corresponding* Polyethylene Glycol *derivative in this index.*

Polybrominated Biphenyls *See loc. no.* **398**

Polybrominated salicylanilides *See* 3,4′,5-Tribromosalicylanilide[e] *at loc. no.* **1000**

Poly-1-butene (9003-28-5) *See* Polybutene[a] *at loc. no.* **1633**

Polybutene (9003-28-5) *See loc. no.* **1633**

Polychlorinated biphenyl *See* PCB[a] *at loc. no.* **399**

Polychlorinated Dibenzodioxins *See loc. no.* **400**

Polychlorinated Dibenzofurans *See loc. no.* **401**

Polychlorinated Naphthalenes *See loc. no.* **402**

Polychlorinated triphenyl *See* PCB[b] *at loc. no.* **399**

Polychlorodicyclopentadiene (8029-29-6) *See* Bandane[e] *at loc. no.* **1018**

Polydimethyl siloxane *See* Silicone Oil[a] *at loc. no.* **1646**

Polyester Resins *See loc. no.* **1634**

Polyethoxy polypropoxy ethanol iodide (9006-36-4) *See* Iodophors[d] *at loc. no.* **997**

Polyethylene (9002-88-4) *See loc. no.* **1635**

Polyethylene fatty acid ester *See* Polyethylene Glycol Stearate[e] *at loc. no.* **968**

Polyethylene glycol alkyl aryl ethers *See* Alkyl Phenoxy Polyethoxy Ethanols[a] *at loc. no.* **963**

Polyethylene glycol ether of alkylated phenol *See* Alkyl Phenoxy Polyethoxy Ethanols[a] *at loc. no.* **963**

Polyethylene glycol fatty acid ester *See* Polyethylene Glycol Stearate[e] *at loc. no.* **968**

Polyethylene Glycols *See loc. no.* **440**

Polyethylene Glycol Stearate (9004-99-3) *See loc. no.* **968**

Polyethylene Polysulfide *See loc. no.* **1203**

Polyglycol *derivative. See corresponding* Polyethylene Glycol *derivative in this index.*

Polymer fumes *See* Polytetrafluoroethylene[b] *at loc. no.* **1636**

Polymixin (1406-11-7) *See loc. no.* **903**

Polymixin A (1404-24-6) *See* Polymixin[d] *at loc. no.* **903**

Polymixin B (1404-26-8) *See* Polymixin[d] *at loc. no.* **903**

Polymixin C (1404-28-0) *See* Polymixin[d] *at loc. no.* **903**

Polymixin D (1404-29-1) *See* Polymixin[d] *at loc. no.* **903**

Polymixin E (1066-17-7) *See* Polymixin[d] *at loc. no.* **903**

Polyol *See loc. no.* **435**

Polyol esters *See* Polyol[b] *at loc. no.* **435**

Polyoxyalkylene *derivative. See corresponding* Polyethylene Glycol *derivative in this index.*

Polyoxyethylene *derivative. If not listed below, see corresponding* Polyethylene Glycol *derivative in this index.*

Polyoxyethylene dodecanol *See* Alkyl Ethoxylate[d] *at loc. no.* **962**

Polyoxyethylene fatty acid ester *See* Polyethylene Glycol Stearate[e] *at loc. no.* **968**

Polyoxyethylene (20) sorbitan mono-oleate (9005-65-6) *See* Polysorbate 80[a] *at loc. no.* **970**

Polyoxyethylene (20) Sorbitan Monostearate (9005-67-8) *See loc. no.* **969**

Polyoxyl 40 stearate (9004-99-3) *See* Polyethylene Glycol Stearate[c] *at loc. no.* **968**

Polyphenyls *See* Terphenyl[e] *at loc. no.* **316**

Polyphosphates *See* Complex Phosphates[a] *at loc. no.* **141**

Polypropylene (9003-07-0) *See* Polyethylene[b] *at loc. no.* **1635**

Polypropylene Glycols (25322-69-4) *See loc. no.* **443**

Polysiloxane substituted *See* Silicone Oil[e] *at loc. no.* **1646**

Polysorbate 60 (9005-67-8) *See* Polyoxyethylene (20) Sorbitan Monostearate[a] *at loc. no.* **969**

Polysorbate 80 (9005-65-6) *See loc. no.* **970**

Polysulfide *See* Ammonium Polysulfide[e] *at loc. no.* **112**

Polytetrafluoroethylene (9002-84-0) *See loc. no.* **1636**

Polythene (9002-88-4) *See* Polyethylene[a] *at loc. no.* **1635**

Polythiazide (346-18-9) *See* Benzothiadiazide Diuretics[d] *at loc. no.* **1588**

Polyurethane *See* Toluene-2,4-diisocyanate[b] *at loc. no.* **1641**

Polyvidone (9003-39-8) *See* Polyvinylpyrrolidone[a] *at loc. no.* **1639**

Polyvinyl acetate (9003-20-7) *See* Polyvinyl Alcohol[b] *at loc. no.* **1637**

Polyvinyl Alcohol (9002-89-5) *See loc. no.* **1637**

Polyvinyl Chloride *See loc. no.* **1638**

Polyvinylpyrrolidone (9003-39-8) *See loc. no.* **1639**

Polyviol (9002-89-5) *See* Polyvinyl Alcohol[a] *at loc. no.* **1637**

Pomegranate Bark *See loc. no.* **685**

Pondimin (404-82-0) *See* Fenfluramine[b] *at loc. no.* **1456**

Pontocaine *See* Tetracaine[c] *at loc. no.* **1586**

Portland Cement *See loc. no.* **56**

Pot *See* Marihuana[a] *at loc. no.* **678**

Potash (1310-58-3) *See* Lye[d] *at loc. no.* **51**

Potassium acid carbonate (298-14-6) *See* Potassium Bicarbonate[a] *at loc. no.* **156**

Potassium acid tartrate (868-14-4) *See* Tartaric Acid[b] *at loc. no.* **563**

Potassium alum (7784-24-9) *See* Alum[a] *at loc. no.* **181**

Potassium *p*-aminosalicylate (133-09-5) *See* *p*-Aminosalicylic Acid[b] *at loc. no.* **629**

Potassium antimonyl tartrate (304-61-0) *See* Antimony Potassium Tartrate[a] *at loc. no.* **213**

Potassium arsenite solution *See* Fowler's Solution[a] *at loc. no.* **204**

Potassium Bicarbonate (298-14-6) *See loc. no.* **156**

Potassium bichromate (7778-50-9) *See* Dichromate Salts (Soluble)[d] *at loc. no.* **82**

Potassium bitartrate (868-14-4) *See* Tartaric Acid[b] *at loc. no.* **563**

Potassium borofluoride (14075-53-7) *See* Potassium Fluoborate[a] *at loc. no.* **103**

Potassium bromate (7758-01-2) *See* Bromate[d] *at loc. no.* **95**

Potassium bromide (7758-02-3) *See* Bromide Salts[d] *at loc. no.* **98**

Potassium chlorate (3811-04-9) *See* Chlorate Salts[d] *at loc. no.* **96**

Potassium chloride (7447-40-7) *See* Potassium Salts[d] *at loc. no.* **155**

Potassium 2-chlorophenyl phenate *See* Chloro-2-phenylphenol[b] *at loc. no.* **526**

Potassium chromate (7789-00-6) *See* Chromate Salts[d] *at loc. no.* **81**

Potassium citrate (866-84-2) *See* Potassium Salts[d] *at loc. no.* **155**

Potassium cyanate (590-28-3) *See* Cyanate Salts[d] *at loc. no.* **145**

Potassium cyanide (151-50-8) *See* Cyanide[d] *at loc. no.* **105**

Potassium dichloroisocyanurate (2244-21-5) *See* Trichloroisocyanuric Acid[b] *at loc. no.* **94**

Potassium dichloro-*s*-triazinetrione (2244-21-5) *See* Trichloroisocyanuric Acid[b] *at loc. no.* **94**

Potassium dichromate (7778-50-9) *See* Dichromate Salts (Soluble)[d] *at loc. no.* **82**

---

[a] A Synonym [b] A Closely Related Substance [c] The Active or Major Constituent [d] A Class Name
[e] A Specific Example of or Product Containing

Ingredient name (CAS registry no.) *See* Primary Name *at location no.* **XXX** *in Part D of this section*

Potassium dimethyldithiocarbamate (128-03-0) *See* Sodium Dimethyldithiocarbamate[b] *at loc. no.* **1163**

Potassium ferricyanide (13746-66-2) *See* Ferrocyanide and Ferricyanide Salts[d] *at loc. no.* **256**

Potassium ferrocyanide (13943-58-3) *See* Ferrocyanide and Ferricyanide Salts[d] *at loc. no.* **256**

Potassium Fluoborate (14075-53-7) *See loc. no.* **103**

Potassium Guaiacolsulfonate (6100-07-8) *See loc. no.* **496**

Potassium hydroxide (1310-58-3) *See* Lye[d] *at loc. no.* **51**

Potassium N-hydroxymethyl-N-methyldithiocarbamate (51026-28-9) *See* Bunema[a] *at loc. no.* **1157**

Potassium hypochlorite (7778-66-7) *See* Sodium Hypochlorite[b] *at loc. no.* **85**

Potassium hyposulfite (10294-66-3) *See* Potassium Thiosulfate[a] *at loc. no.* **162**

Potassium iodate (7758-05-6) *See* Iodate Salts[d] *at loc. no.* **97**

Potassium iodide (7681-11-0) *See* Iodide Salts[d] *at loc. no.* **99**

Potassium N-methyldithiocarbamate (137-41-7) *See* Metham Sodium[b] *at loc. no.* **1161**

Potassium Monopersulfate (10361-76-9) *See loc. no.* **79**

Potassium 1-naphthaleneacetate *See* 1-Naphthaleneacetic Acid[b] *at loc. no.* **1309**

Potassium nitrate (7757-79-1) *See* Nitrate Salts[d] *at loc. no.* **157**

Potassium nitrite (7758-09-0) *See* Nitrite[d] *at loc. no.* **144**

Potassium oxalate (10043-22-8) *See* Oxalate[d] *at loc. no.* **546**

Potassium penicillin G (113-98-4) *See* Penicillins[d] *at loc. no.* **902**

Potassium Permanganate (7722-64-7) *See loc. no.* **83**

Potassium peroxymonosulfate (10361-76-9) *See* Potassium Monopersulfate[a] *at loc. no.* **79**

Potassium phenolate (100-67-4) *See* Phenol[b] *at loc. no.* **494**

Potassium phosphate *See* Potassium Salts[d] *at loc. no.* **155**

Potassium Phosphate (Tribasic) (7778-53-2) *See loc. no.* **59**

Potassium picloram (2545-60-0) *See* Picloram[b] *at loc. no.* **1312**

Potassium picrate (573-83-1) *See* Picric Acid[b] *at loc. no.* **545**

Potassium rhodanate (333-20-0) *See* Potassium Thiocyanate[a] *at loc. no.* **148**

Potassium ricinoleate (7492-30-0) *See* Ricinoleic Acid[b] *at loc. no.* **560**

Potassium salt of maleic hydrazide (28382-15-2) *See* Maleic Hydrazide[c] *at loc. no.* **1308**

Potassium Salts *See loc. no.* **155**

Potassium sodium tartrate (147-79-5) *See* Tartaric Acid[b] *at loc. no.* **563**

Potassium sulfide (1312-73-8) *See* Sulfide Salts[d] *at loc. no.* **118**

Potassium sulfite (7790-56-9) *See* Sulfite Salts[d] *at loc. no.* **149**

Potassium sulfocyanate (333-20-0) *See* Potassium Thiocyanate[a] *at loc. no.* **148**

Potassium tetraborate (1332-77-0) *See* Borate[d] *at loc. no.* **131**

Potassium tetrachlorophenate *See* 2,3,4,6-Tetrachlorophenol[b] *at loc. no.* **534**

Potassium tetrafluoroborate (14075-53-7) *See* Potassium Fluoborate[a] *at loc. no.* **103**

Potassium Thiocyanate (333-20-0) *See loc. no.* **148**

Potassium thioglycolate (34452-51-2) *See* Thioglycolate Salts[d] *at loc. no.* **552**

Potassium Thiosulfate (10294-66-3) *See loc. no.* **162**

Povidone (9003-39-8) *See* Polyvinylpyrrolidone[a] *at loc. no.* **1639**

Pralidoxime Chloride (51-15-0) *See loc. no.* **1508**

Pralidoxime methanesulfone *See* Pralidoxime Chloride[b] *at loc. no.* **1508**

Pramuscimol (60573-88-5) *See* Muscimol[b] *at loc. no.* **819**

Prayer bean *See* Jequirity Bean[a] *at loc. no.* **677**

Prazepam (2955-38-6) *See loc. no.* **1402**

Precatory bean *See* Jequirity Bean[a] *at loc. no.* **677**

Precipitated sulfur (7704-34-9) *See* Sulfur[a] *at loc. no.* **120**

Prednisolone (50-24-8) *See* Corticosteroids[d] *at loc. no.* **915**

Prednisone (53-03-2) *See* Corticosteroids[d] *at loc. no.* **915**

Prefar (741-58-2) *See* Bensulide[c] *at loc. no.* **1082**

Prefix (1918-13-4) *See* Chlorthiamid[c] *at loc. no.* **1297**

Preludin (134-49-6) *See* Phenmetrazine[c] *at loc. no.* **1466**

Premalin *See* Linuron[c] *at loc. no.* **1251**

Pre-Sate (151-06-4) *See* Chlorphentermine Hydrochloride[c] *at loc. no.* **1446**

Preventol G-D (97-23-4) *See* Dichlorophen(e)[c] *at loc. no.* **529**

Prilocaine (721-50-6) *See loc. no.* **1584**

Prilocaine hydrochloride (1786-81-8) *See* Prilocaine[b] *at loc. no.* **1584**

Primaclone (125-33-7) *See* Primidone[a] *at loc. no.* **1610**

Primaquine (90-34-6) *See loc. no.* **1516**

Primidone (125-33-7) *See loc. no.* **1610**

Princep (122-34-9) *See* Simazine[c] *at loc. no.* **1269**

Privine (835-31-4) *See* Naphazoline Hydrochloride[b] *at loc. no.* **1463**

Privine hydrochloride (550-99-2) *See* Naphazoline Hydrochloride[c] *at loc. no.* **1463**

PRN (92-12-6) *See* Phenyltoloxamine Dihydrogen Citrate[b] *at loc. no.* **1498**

Probarbital (76-76-6) *See* Probarbital Sodium[b] *at loc. no.* **1383**

Probarbital Sodium (143-82-8) *See loc. no.* **1383**

Probenecid (57-66-9) *See loc. no.* **1611**

Procainamide (51-06-9) *See loc. no.* **1612**

Procaine (59-46-1) *See loc. no.* **1585**

Prochlorperazine (58-38-8) *See loc. no.* **1419**

Procyazine (32889-48-8) *See* Cyanazine[b] *at loc. no.* **1260**

Proflavine (92-62-6) *See* Acridine Antiseptics[d] *at loc. no.* **1518**

Prolan (117-27-1) *See loc. no.* **1016**

Prolin *See* Warfarin[c] *at loc. no.* **1345**

Prolixin (146-56-5) *See* Fluphenazine Hydrochloride[c] *at loc. no.* **1415**

Promazine (58-40-2) *See loc. no.* **1420**

Promecarb (2631-37-0) *See loc. no.* **1146**

Promethazine (60-87-7) *See loc. no.* **1421**

Promethazine hydrochloride (58-33-3) *See* Promethazine[b] *at loc. no.* **1421**

Prometon (1610-18-0) *See loc. no.* **1267**

Prometone (1610-18-0) *See* Prometon[a] *at loc. no.* **1267**

Prometryn (7287-19-6) *See* Prometon[b] *at loc. no.* **1267**

Prominal (115-38-8) *See* Mephobarbital[c] *at loc. no.* **1377**

Promoxolane (470-43-9) *See loc. no.* **1411**

Pronamide (23950-58-5) *See loc. no.* **1281**

Pronarcon (125-55-3) *See loc. no.* **1384**

Pronestyl (51-06-9) *See* Procainamide[c] *at loc. no.* **1612**

Propachlor (1918-16-7) *See loc. no.* **1282**

Propadrine hydrochloride (7587-43-1) *See* Phenylpropanolamine Hydrochloride[c] *at loc. no.* **1451**

Propaesin (94-12-2) *See* Butamben[b] *at loc. no.* **1579**

Propallylonal (545-93-7) *See loc. no.* **1385**

Propane (74-98-6) *See loc. no.* **304**

1,2-Propanediol (57-55-6) *See* Propylene Glycol[a] *at loc. no.* **442**

Propanenitrile (107-12-0) *See* Propionitrile[a] *at loc. no.* **653**

1,2,3-Propanetriol (56-81-5) *See* Glycerin[a] *at loc. no.* **704**

Propanil (709-98-8) *See loc. no.* **1283**

---

[a] A Synonym   [b] A Closely Related Substance   [c] The Active or Major Constituent   [d] A Class Name
[e] A Specific Example of or Product Containing

Ingredient name (CAS registry no.) *See* Primary Name *at location no. **XXX** in Part D of this section*

Propanoic acid (79-09-4) *See* Sodium Propionate[e] *at loc. no.* **551**

1-Propanol (71-23-8) *See loc. no.* **428**

2-Propanol (67-63-0) *See* Isopropyl Alcohol[a] *at loc. no.* **420**

Propanone (67-64-1) *See* Acetone[a] *at loc. no.* **466**

Propargyl Bromide (106-96-7) *See loc. no.* **390**

Propazine (139-40-2) *See loc. no.* **1268**

Propellants *See* Fluorocarbon Refrigerants and Propellants[e] *at loc. no.* **347**

2-Propenal (107-02-8) *See* Acrolein[a] *at loc. no.* **481**

Propenamide (79-06-1) *See* Acrylamide[a] *at loc. no.* **1624**

Propenenitrile (107-13-1) *See* Acrylonitrile[a] *at loc. no.* **648**

Propene oxide (75-56-9) *See* Propylene Oxide[a] *at loc. no.* **17**

2-Propenoic acid homopolymer (9003-01-4) *See* Carboxypolymethylene[a] *at loc. no.* **1627**

1-Propenol-3 (107-18-6) *See* Allyl Alcohol[a] *at loc. no.* **21**

Propenyl alcohol *See* Allyl Alcohol[a] *at loc. no.* **21**

Propham (122-42-9) *See* Chlorpropham[b] *at loc. no.* **1229**

Prophenpyridamine (86-21-5) *See* Pheniramine Maleate[b] *at loc. no.* **1497**

Propiomazine Hydrochloride (64-89-1) *See loc. no.* **1422**

Propionaldehyde (123-38-6) *See* Acetaldehyde[b] *at loc. no.* **480**

Propionic acid (79-09-4) *See* Sodium Propionate[b] *at loc. no.* **551**

Propionitrile (107-12-0) *See loc. no.* **653**

Propoxur (114-26-1) *See loc. no.* **1147**

Propoxyphene Hydrochloride (1639-60-7) *See loc. no.* **1486**

Propoxyphene napsylate (26570-10-5) *See* Propoxyphene Hydrochloride[b] *at loc. no.* **1486**

Propranolol (525-66-6) *See* Propranolol Hydrochloride[b] *at loc. no.* **1613**

Propranolol Hydrochloride (318-98-9) *See loc. no.* **1613**

Propyl Acetate (109-60-4) *See loc. no.* **578**

n-Propyl acetate (109-60-4) *See* Propyl Acetate[a] *at loc. no.* **578**

Propyl alcohol (71-23-8) *See* 1-Propanol[a] *at loc. no.* **428**

2-(Propylamino)-o-propionotoluidide (721-50-6) *See* Prilocaine[a] *at loc. no.* **1584**

S-Propyl butylethylthiocarbamate (1114-71-2) *See* Pebulate[a] *at loc. no.* **1238**

n-Propyl n-butyrate (105-66-8) *See* Propyl Acetate[b] *at loc. no.* **578**

Propyl cinnamate (7778-83-8) *See* Cinnamic Acid Esters[d] *at loc. no.* **587**

Propyl cyanide (109-74-0) *See* n-Butyronitrile[a] *at loc. no.* **649**

Propyl Diethylsuccinamate (5834-84-4) *See loc. no.* **1331**

n-Propyl-N,N-diethylsuccinamate (5834-84-4) *See* Propyl Diethylsuccinamate[a] *at loc. no.* **1331**

S-Propyl dipropylthiocarbamate (1929-77-7) *See* Vernolate[a] *at loc. no.* **1240**

Propylene Dichloride (78-87-5) *See loc. no.* **391**

Propylene Glycol (57-55-6) *See loc. no.* **442**

Propylene glycol butyl ether ester of 2,4,5-T *See* Trichlorophenoxyacetic Acid[b] *at loc. no.* **1224**

Propylene glycol butyl ether esters of 2-(2,4,5-trichlorophenoxy)propionic acid *See* Silvex[b] *at loc. no.* **1223**

Propylene glycol isobutyl ether ester of 2,4,5-T *See* Trichlorophenoxyacetic Acid[b] *at loc. no.* **1224**

Propylene Glycol Monomethyl Ether (107-98-2) *See loc. no.* **464**

Propylene Glycol Monostearate (8028-46-4) *See loc. no.* **971**

Propylene Oxide (75-56-9) *See loc. no.* **17**

n-Propyl Gallate (121-79-9) *See loc. no.* **1619**

Propylhexedrine (101-40-6) *See loc. no.* **1452**

Propyl p-hydroxybenzoate (94-13-3) *See* Propylparaben[a] *at loc. no.* **586**

n-Propyl Isome (83-59-0) *See loc. no.* **1153**

n-Propylisome (83-59-0) *See* n-Propyl Isome[a] *at loc. no.* **1153**

n-Propyl isovalerate *See* Propyl Acetate[b] *at loc. no.* **578**

2-N-Propyl-4-methylpyrimidyl-(6)-dimethylcarbamate (2532-49-2) *See* Pyramat[e] *at loc. no.* **1148**

Propylparaben (94-13-3) *See loc. no.* **586**

Propyl parasept (94-13-3) *See* Propylparaben[a] *at loc. no.* **586**

n-Propyl n-propionate (106-36-5) *See* Propyl Acetate[b] *at loc. no.* **578**

Propyzamide (23950-58-5) *See* Pronamide[a] *at loc. no.* **1281**

Prothromadin (129-06-6) *See* Warfarin[b] *at loc. no.* **1345**

Protopam chloride (51-15-0) *See* Pralidoxime Chloride[a] *at loc. no.* **1508**

Protosol (96-26-4) *See* Dihydroxyacetone[a] *at loc. no.* **471**

Protoveratrines A and B (8053-18-7) *See* Veratrum Viride Alkaloids[d] *at loc. no.* **811**

Protriptyline Hydrochloride (1225-55-4) *See loc. no.* **1479**

Prowl (40487-42-1) *See* Dinitramine[b] *at loc. no.* **1288**

Prunasin (1300-20-5) *See* Wild Cherry[e] *at loc. no.* **700**

Prunus virginiana *See* Wild Cherry[a] *at loc. no.* **700**

Prussian blue (25869-98-1) *See* Ferrocyanide and Ferricyanide Salts[d] *at loc. no.* **256**

Prussic acid (74-90-8) *See* Hydrocyanic Acid[a] *at loc. no.* **106**

Prynachlor (21267-72-1) *See* Propachlor[b] *at loc. no.* **1282**

P2S *See* Pralidoxime Chloride[b] *at loc. no.* **1508**

Pseudoephedrine Hydrochloride (6272-89-5) *See loc. no.* **1453**

Psilocin (520-53-6) *See* Psilocybin[b] *at loc. no.* **821**

Psilocybe baeocystin *See* Psilocybin[c] *at loc. no.* **821**

Psilocybe cubensis *See* Psilocybin[c] *at loc. no.* **821**

Psilocybe semilanceata *See* Psilocybin[c] *at loc. no.* **821**

Psilocybin (520-52-5) *See loc. no.* **821**

PSP (143-74-8) *See* Phenolsulfonphthalein[a] *at loc. no.* **1608**

PTFE (9002-84-0) *See* Polytetrafluoroethylene[a] *at loc. no.* **1636**

Pulegone (89-82-7) *See* Pennyroyal[a] *at loc. no.* **740**

Pumice (1332-09-8) *See loc. no.* **6**

Punicine tannate (8007-39-4) *See* Pelletierine Tannate[a] *at loc. no.* **831**

PVA (9002-89-5) *See* Polyvinyl Alcohol[a] *at loc. no.* **1637**

PVC *See* Polyvinyl Chloride[a] *at loc. no.* **1638**

PVP (9003-39-8) *See* Polyvinylpyrrolidone[a] *at loc. no.* **1639**

Pydrin (51630-58-1) *See* Fenvalerate[a] *at loc. no.* **890**

Pydrin 2.4 EC Insecticide *See* Fenvalerate[c] *at loc. no.* **890**

Pynamin (584-79-2) *See* Allethrin[a] *at loc. no.* **884**

Pypyrethrin (97-11-0) *See* Cyclethrin[a] *at loc. no.* **886**

Pyracarbolid (24691-76-7) *See loc. no.* **1204**

Pyramat (2532-49-2) *See loc. no.* **1148**

Pyramidon (58-15-1) *See* Aminopyrine[a] *at loc. no.* **1570**

Pyramin (1698-60-8) *See* Pyrazon[c] *at loc. no.* **1313**

Pyranisamine maleate (59-33-6) *See* Pyrilamine Maleate[a] *at loc. no.* **1499**

Pyrazole (288-13-1) *See loc. no.* **1509**

Pyrazon (1698-60-8) *See loc. no.* **1313**

Pyrazothion (108-35-0) *See loc. no.* **1078**

Pyrazoxon (108-34-9) *See loc. no.* **1059**

Pyrenone (11121-38-3) *See loc. no.* **892**

Pyresin (584-79-2) *See* Allethrin[c] *at loc. no.* **884**

Pyresyn (584-79-2) *See* Allethrin[c] *at loc. no.* **884**

Pyrethrin I (121-21-1) *See* Pyrethrins[d] *at loc. no.* **893**

Pyrethrin II (121-29-9) *See* Pyrethrins[d] *at loc. no.* **893**

---

[a] A Synonym   [b] A Closely Related Substance   [c] The Active or Major Constituent   [d] A Class Name
[e] A Specific Example of or Product Containing

Ingredient name (CAS registry no.) *See* Primary Name *at
location no.* **XXX** *in Part D of this section*

Pyrethrins *See loc. no.* **893**
Pyrethroids *See loc. no.* **894**
Pyrethrum (8003-34-7) *See loc. no.* **686**
Pyrethrum flowers *See* Pyrethrum[a] *at loc. no.* **686**
Pyribenzamine hydrochloride (154-69-8) *See* Tripelennamine Hydrochloride[c] *at loc. no.* **1500**
4-Pyridinamine (504-24-5) *See* 4-Aminopyridine[a] *at loc. no.* **1319**
Pyridine (110-86-1) *See loc. no.* **1622**
2-Pyridine aldoxime methochloride (51-15-0) *See* Pralidoxime Chloride[a] *at loc. no.* **1508**
N^1-2-Pyridinylsulfanilamide (144-83-2) *See* Sulfapyridine[a] *at loc. no.* **1564**
Pyridium (136-40-3) *See* Phenazopyridine Hydrochloride[c] *at loc. no.* **1522**
Pyridoxal hydrochloride (65-22-5) *See* Pyridoxine Hydrochloride[b] *at loc. no.* **912**
Pyridoxal phosphate (54-47-7) *See* Pyridoxine Hydrochloride[b] *at loc. no.* **912**
Pyridoxine Hydrochloride (58-56-0) *See loc. no.* **912**
Pyridoxol hydrochloride (58-56-0) *See* Pyridoxine Hydrochloride[b] *at loc. no.* **912**
N-3-Pyridylmethyl-N′-p-nitrophenylurea (53558-25-1) *See* Vacor[e] *at loc. no.* **1353**
2-(3′-Pyridyl)piperidine (494-52-0) *See* Anabasine[a] *at loc. no.* **773**
2-(3′-Pyridyl)pyrrolidine (7076-23-5) *See* Nornicotine[a] *at loc. no.* **777**
Pyrilamine Maleate (59-33-6) *See loc. no.* **1499**
N^1-2-Pyrimidinylsulfanilamide (68-35-9) *See* Sulfadiazine[a] *at loc. no.* **1553**
Pyroacetic ether (67-64-1) *See* Acetone[a] *at loc. no.* **466**
Pyrocatechol (120-80-9) *See loc. no.* **505**
Pyrofax *See* Butane[a] *at loc. no.* **306**
Pyrogallic acid (87-66-1) *See* Pyrogallol[a] *at loc. no.* **506**
Pyrogallol (87-66-1) *See loc. no.* **506**
Pyrolan (87-47-8) *See loc. no.* **1149**
Pyroligneous Acid (8030-97-5) *See loc. no.* **929**
Pyroxylin (9004-70-0) *See* Collodion[e] *at loc. no.* **854**
Q-137 (72-56-0) *See* Perthane[e] *at loc. no.* **1015**
QAC *See* Cationic Surfactants[d] *at loc. no.* **974**
Quaalude (72-44-6) *See* Methaqualone[c] *at loc. no.* **1439**
Quaternary ammonium chloride *See* Cationic Surfactants[d] *at loc. no.* **974**
Quaternary ammonium compounds *See* Cationic Surfactants[d] *at loc. no.* **974**
Quaternary ammonium salt *See* Cationic Surfactants[d] *at loc. no.* **974**
Quaternary disinfectant *See* Cationic Surfactants[d] *at loc. no.* **974**
Quaternary softener *See* Cationic Surfactants[a] *at loc. no.* **974**
Quebrachine (146-48-5) *See* Yohimbine[a] *at loc. no.* **834**
Quebracho (1398-11-4) *See* Yohimbine[c] *at loc. no.* **834**
Quebracho bark *See* Yohimbine[c] *at loc. no.* **834**
Quebracho wood *See* Yohimbine[c] *at loc. no.* **834**
Quiactin (126-93-2) *See* Oxanamide[c] *at loc. no.* **1409**
Quicklime (1305-78-8) *See* Calcium Oxide[a] *at loc. no.* **54**
Quinacrine Hydrochloride (69-05-6) *See loc. no.* **1515**
Quince Seed *See loc. no.* **687**
Quinidine (56-54-2) *See loc. no.* **810**
Quinidine hydrochloride *See* Quinidine[b] *at loc. no.* **810**
Quinidine polygalacturonate *See* Quinidine[b] *at loc. no.* **810**
Quinidine sulfate (50-54-4) *See* Quinidine[b] *at loc. no.* **810**
Quinine (130-95-0) *See loc. no.* **809**
8-Quinolinol (148-24-3) *See* 8-Hydroxyquinoline[a] *at loc. no.* **1514**

Quinomethionate (2439-01-2) *See loc. no.* **1205**
Quinone (106-51-4) *See loc. no.* **507**
2,3-Quinoxalinedithiol cyclic trithiocarbonate (93-75-4) *See* Eradex[e] *at loc. no.* **1044**
N^1-2-Quinoxalinylsulfanilamide (59-40-5) *See* Sulfaquinoxaline[a] *at loc. no.* **1565**
Quintozene (82-68-8) *See* Pentachloronitrobenzene[a] *at loc. no.* **1201**
Rabon (22350-76-1) *See* Tetrachlorvinfos[c] *at loc. no.* **1061**
Racephedrine sulfate (154-45-0) *See* Ephedrine[b] *at loc. no.* **1450**
Ramrod (1918-16-7) *See* Propachlor[c] *at loc. no.* **1282**
Randox (93-71-0) *See* Allidochlor[c] *at loc. no.* **1274**
Range gas *See* Gas[d] *at loc. no.* **128**
Range oil *See* Kerosene[a] *at loc. no.* **328**
RATicate (991-42-4) *See* Norbormide[c] *at loc. no.* **1349**
Raudixin *See loc. no.* **688**
Rauwiloid *See* Alseroxylon[a] *at loc. no.* **795**
Rauwolfia (serpentina) (8063-17-0) *See* Raudixin[c] *at loc. no.* **688**
Rauwolfine (4360-12-7) *See* Ajmaline[a] *at loc. no.* **794**
RDX (121-82-4) *See* Cyclonite[a] *at loc. no.* **631**
Recanescine (131-01-1) *See* Deserpidine[a] *at loc. no.* **796**
Red amorphous phosphorus (7723-14-0) *See* Phosphorus[d] *at loc. no.* **135**
Red copper oxide (1317-39-1) *See* Cuprous Oxide[a] *at loc. no.* **269**
Red iodide of mercury (7774-29-0) *See* Mercuric Chloride[b] *at loc. no.* **236**
Red lead (1314-41-6) *See* Lead[d] *at loc. no.* **245**
Red mercuric sulfide (1344-48-5) *See* Mercury[d] *at loc. no.* **221**
Red Oil *See loc. no.* **720**
Red phosphorus (7723-14-0) *See* Phosphorus[d] *at loc. no.* **135**
Red puccoon *See* Sanguinaria[a] *at loc. no.* **693**
Red squill *See* Squill (Red or White)[a] *at loc. no.* **695**
Refined petroleum oil *See* Lubricating Oils[a] *at loc. no.* **338**
Refined solvent naphtha (8032-32-4) *See* VM&P Naphthas[a] *at loc. no.* **335**
Reglone (85-00-7) *See* Diquat Dibromide[a] *at loc. no.* **1285**
Rescinnamine (84-34-4) *See loc. no.* **797**
Reserpine (50-55-5) *See loc. no.* **798**
Reserpoid (50-55-5) *See* Reserpine[a] *at loc. no.* **798**
Residual Oils *See loc. no.* **332**
Resins soya alkyd *See* Soya Alkyd Resin[a] *at loc. no.* **1640**
Resmethrin (10453-86-8) *See loc. no.* **895**
Resorcin (108-46-3) *See* Resorcinol[a] *at loc. no.* **508**
Resorcinol (108-46-3) *See loc. no.* **508**
Resorcinol diglycidyl ether (101-90-6) *See* Glycidyl Ethers[d] *at loc. no.* **1629**
Resorcinol-epichlorohydrin epoxy resins *See* Epoxy Resins[d] *at loc. no.* **1628**
Resorcinol Monoacetate (102-29-4) *See loc. no.* **509**
Retinol (68-26-8) *See* Vitamin A[a] *at loc. no.* **907**
Rhamnus purshiana *See* Cascara Sagrada[a] *at loc. no.* **660**
Rhatany *See* Tannic Acid[b] *at loc. no.* **852**
Rhodanates *See* Thiocyanate Salts[a] *at loc. no.* **146**
Rhodanides *See* Thiocyanate Salts[a] *at loc. no.* **146**
Rhubarb (8016-55-5) *See loc. no.* **689**
Riboflavin (83-88-5) *See loc. no.* **913**
Ricin (9009-86-3) *See loc. no.* **930**
Ricine *See* Ricin[a] *at loc. no.* **930**
Ricinoleate *See* Ricinoleic Acid[b] *at loc. no.* **560**
Ricinoleic Acid (141-22-0) *See loc. no.* **560**
Ricinus oil (8001-79-4) *See* Castor Oil[a] *at loc. no.* **712**
Risocaine (94-12-2) *See* Butamben[b] *at loc. no.* **1579**
Ritalin (113-45-1) *See* Methylphenidate[c] *at loc. no.* **1462**

---

[a] A Synonym   [b] A Closely Related Substance   [c] The Active or Major Constituent   [d] A Class Name
[e] A Specific Example of or Product Containing

Ingredient name (CAS registry no.) *See Primary Name at*
location no. **XXX** *in Part D of this section*

Rivea corymbosa seeds *See* Lysergic Acid Diethylamide[c] *at loc. no.* **829**
Robane (111-01-3) *See* Squalane[c] *at loc. no.* **932**
Roccal (8001-54-5) *See* Benzalkonium Chloride[c] *at loc. no.* **985**
Rochelle salt (147-79-5) *See* Tartaric Acid[b] *at loc. no.* **563**
Rock oil (8002-05-9) *See* Petroleum (Crude)[a] *at loc. no.* **336**
Rock salt (7647-14-5) *See* Sodium Chloride[a] *at loc. no.* **165**
Rodinal (123-30-8) *See* p-Aminophenol[c] *at loc. no.* **624**
Rohypnol (1622-62-4) *See* Flunitrazepam[c] *at loc. no.* **1396**
Rolitetracycline (751-97-3) *See* Tetracyclines[d] *at loc. no.* **904**
Romilar hydrobromide (125-69-9) *See* Dextromethorphan Hydrobromide[a] *at loc. no.* **1594**
Ro-neet (1134-23-2) *See* Cycloate[c] *at loc. no.* **1234**
Ronit (1134-23-2) *See* Cycloate[c] *at loc. no.* **1234**
Ronnel (299-84-3) *See loc. no.* **1079**
Rootone (575-36-0) *See* Naphthaleneacetamide[c] *at loc. no.* **1277**
Rorasul *See* Sulfasalazine[c] *at loc. no.* **1566**
Rosary pea or bean *See* Jequirity Bean[a] *at loc. no.* **677**
Rosemary oil (8000-25-7) *See* Essential Oils[d] *at loc. no.* **725**
Rosin (8050-09-7) *See loc. no.* **760**
Rosin Oils (8002-16-2) *See loc. no.* **721**
Rosinol *See* Rosin Oils[a] *at loc. no.* **721**
Rotenoids *See loc. no.* **897**
Rotenone (83-79-4) *See loc. no.* **896**
Rovral (36734-19-7) *See* Iprodione[c] *at loc. no.* **1197**
Roxarsone (121-19-7) *See* 4-Hydroxy-3-nitrophenylarsonic Acid[a] *at loc. no.* **205**
Rozol (3691-35-8) *See* Chlorophacinone[c] *at loc. no.* **1335**
Rubber (9006-04-6) *See* Latex[b] *at loc. no.* **756**
Rubber latex *See* Latex[b] *at loc. no.* **756**
Rubber Solvent *See loc. no.* **333**
Rubber solvent naphtha *See* Rubber Solvent[a] *at loc. no.* **333**
Rue (8014-29-7) *See* Essential Oils[d] *at loc. no.* **725**
Ruelene (299-86-5) *See loc. no.* **1104**
Rusbyine *See* Cocillana[c] *at loc. no.* **662**
Rutgers 612 (94-96-2) *See* 2-Ethyl-1,3-hexanediol[c] *at loc. no.* **1329**
Rutonal (76-94-8) *See* 5-Phenyl-5-methylbarbituric Acid[c] *at loc. no.* **1381**
Ryanex (15662-33-6) *See* Ryania[c] *at loc. no.* **690**
Ryania (15662-33-6) *See loc. no.* **690**
Ryania powder (15662-33-6) *See* Ryania[a] *at loc. no.* **690**
Ryania speciosa *See* Ryania[c] *at loc. no.* **690**
Ryanicide (15662-33-6) *See* Ryania[c] *at loc. no.* **690**
Ryanodine (15662-33-6) *See* Ryania[e] *at loc. no.* **690**
Sabadilla (8028-57-7) *See loc. no.* **691**
Saccharin (81-07-2) *See loc. no.* **1616**
Saccharin sodium (128-44-9) *See* Saccharin[b] *at loc. no.* **1616**
Saccharin soluble (128-44-9) *See* Saccharin[b] *at loc. no.* **1616**
Saccharose (57-50-1) *See* Sucrose[a] *at loc. no.* **708**
Safety solvent naphtha *See* Stoddard Solvent[a] *at loc. no.* **334**
Saffron *See loc. no.* **692**
Safrol (94-59-7) *See* Safrole[a] *at loc. no.* **872**
Safrole (94-59-7) *See loc. no.* **872**
Salicylamide (65-45-2) *See loc. no.* **599**
Salicylanilide (87-17-2) *See loc. no.* **998**
Salicylate (63-36-5) *See loc. no.* **600**
Salicylazosulfapyridine (599-79-1) *See* Sulfasalazine[a] *at loc. no.* **1566**
Salicylic acid (69-72-7) *See* Salicylate[d] *at loc. no.* **600**
Salicylic acid 3,5,5-trimethylcyclohexyl ester (118-56-9) *See* Homosalate[a] *at loc. no.* **1533**
Salicyl Salicylate (552-94-3) *See loc. no.* **601**

Salicylsalicylic acid (552-94-3) *See* Salicyl Salicylate[a] *at loc. no.* **601**
Salol (118-55-8) *See* Phenyl Salicylate[a] *at loc. no.* **598**
Saloop *See* Oil of Sassafras[c] *at loc. no.* **739**
Sal soda *See* Sodium Carbonate[a] *at loc. no.* **52**
Salt (7647-14-5) *See* Sodium Chloride[a] *at loc. no.* **165**
Saltpeter *See* Nitrate Salts[d] *at loc. no.* **157**
Salysal *See* Salicyl Salicylate[c] *at loc. no.* **601**
Sandoptal (77-26-9) *See* Butalbital[c] *at loc. no.* **1368**
Sanguinaria *See loc. no.* **693**
Sanguinarine (2447-54-3) *See* Sanguinaria[e] *at loc. no.* **693**
Sansert (129-49-7) *See* Methysergide Maleate[c] *at loc. no.* **806**
Santomerse *See* Alkyl Aryl Sodium Sulfonates[c] *at loc. no.* **943**
Santonin (481-06-1) *See loc. no.* **931**
Santophen 1 (120-32-1) *See* o-Benzyl-p-chlorophenol[c] *at loc. no.* **520**
Santoquin (91-53-2) *See* Ethoxyquin[c] *at loc. no.* **1615**
Santowax OM (8013-93-2) *See* Terphenyl[c] *at loc. no.* **316**
Saprol *See loc. no.* **518**
Saran *See* 1,1-Dichloroethylene[b] *at loc. no.* **366**
Sassafras *See* Oil of Sassafras[c] *at loc. no.* **739**
Savin (8024-00-8) *See* Essential Oils[d] *at loc. no.* **725**
Sawdust *See loc. no.* **694**
Saxifrax *See* Oil of Sassafras[c] *at loc. no.* **739**
Sch 600 *See* Laureth 9[b] *at loc. no.* **966**
Scheele's green (10290-12-7) *See* Cupric Arsenite[c] *at loc. no.* **202**
Scheele's mineral (1302-97-2) *See* Cupric Arsenite[a] *at loc. no.* **202**
Schradan (152-16-9) *See* Octamethyl Pyrophosphoramide[c] *at loc. no.* **1102**
Schweinfurt green (1299-88-3) *See* Copper Acetoarsenite[a] *at loc. no.* **200**
Scilla maritima *See* Squill (Red or White)[a] *at loc. no.* **695**
Scillaren (8011-55-0) *See loc. no.* **843**
Scilliroside (8011-55-0) *See* Squill (Red or White)[e] *at loc. no.* **695**
Scopolamine (51-34-3) *See loc. no.* **771**
Scopolamine hydrobromide (114-49-8) *See* Scopolamine[b] *at loc. no.* **771**
Scopolamine methylnitrate (6106-46-3) *See* Scopolamine[b] *at loc. no.* **771**
SD alcohol 40 *See* Ethyl Alcohol[b] *at loc. no.* **412**
Sea onion *See* Squill (Red or White)[a] *at loc. no.* **695**
Secbumeton (26259-45-0) *See* Prometon[b] *at loc. no.* **1267**
Secobarbital Sodium (309-43-3) *See loc. no.* **1386**
Seconal sodium (309-43-3) *See* Secobarbital Sodium[c] *at loc. no.* **1386**
Sedaform (57-15-8) *See* Chlorobutanol[a] *at loc. no.* **432**
Seidlitz powders (8003-43-8) *See* Tartaric Acid[b] *at loc. no.* **563**
Selenate salts *See* Sodium Selenate[e] *at loc. no.* **184**
Selenic acid (7783-08-6) *See* Selenium Derivatives[d] *at loc. no.* **185**
Selenium Derivatives *See loc. no.* **185**
Selenium dioxide (7446-08-4) *See* Selenium Derivatives[d] *at loc. no.* **185**
Selenium disulfide (7488-56-4) *See* Selenium Sulfide[d] *at loc. no.* **186**
Selenium monosulfide (7446-34-6) *See* Selenium Sulfide[d] *at loc. no.* **186**
Selenium oxychloride (7791-23-3) *See* Selenium Derivatives[d] *at loc. no.* **185**
Selenium Sulfide (7446-34-6) *See loc. no.* **186**
Selsun sulfide (8012-80-4) *See* Selenium Sulfide[c] *at loc. no.* **186**
Semeron (1014-69-3) *See* Prometon[b] *at loc. no.* **1267**

---

[a] A Synonym   [b] A Closely Related Substance   [c] The Active or Major Constituent   [d] A Class Name
[e] A Specific Example of or Product Containing

Ingredient name (CAS registry no.) *See* Primary Name *at*
location no. **XXX** *in Part D of this section*

Semesan (538-04-5) *See* 2-Chloro-4-(hydroxymercuri)phenol[c] *at loc. no.* **224**

Semesan Bel (8005-50-3) *See* Hydroxymercurinitrophenol[c] *at loc. no.* **233**

Semikon hydrochloride (135-23-9) *See* Methapyrilene Hydrochloride[c] *at loc. no.* **1495**

Semoxydrine (300-42-5) *See* Amphetamine[b] *at loc. no.* **1444**

Sencor (21087-64-9) *See* Metribuzin[c] *at loc. no.* **1266**

Seneca oil (8002-05-9) *See* Petroleum (Crude)[a] *at loc. no.* **336**

Senna Glycosides *See loc. no.* **851**

Sennoside A and B (1344-35-0) *See* Senna Glycosides[d] *at loc. no.* **851**

Sequestrenes *See loc. no.* **289**

Serax (604-75-1) *See* Oxazepam[c] *at loc. no.* **1401**

Serenity-tranquility-peace *See* 2,5-Dimethoxy-4-methyl-amphetamine[a] *at loc. no.* **1449**

Serentil (5588-33-0) *See* Thioridazine[b] *at loc. no.* **1425**

Sernylan (956-90-1) *See* Phencyclidine Hydrochloride[c] *at loc. no.* **1542**

Serotonin (50-67-9) *See* Bufotenine[b] *at loc. no.* **820**

Serpasil (50-55-5) *See* Reserpine[c] *at loc. no.* **798**

SES (136-78-7) *See* 2-(2,4-Dichlorophenoxy)ethyl Sulfate Sodium Salt[a] *at loc. no.* **1216**

Sesame Oil (8008-74-0) *See loc. no.* **722**

Sesamex (51-14-9) *See loc. no.* **1154**

Sesamin (607-80-7) *See* Sesame Oil[e] *at loc. no.* **722**

Sesamolin (526-07-8) *See* Sesame Oil[e] *at loc. no.* **722**

Sesone (136-78-7) *See* 2-(2,4-Dichlorophenoxy)ethyl Sulfate Sodium Salt[a] *at loc. no.* **1216**

Sesoxane (51-14-9) *See* Sesamex[c] *at loc. no.* **1154**

Sesquicarbonate *See* Sodium Sesquicarbonate[e] *at loc. no.* **53**

Sesquicarbonate of soda (533-96-0) *See* Sodium Sesquicarbonate[a] *at loc. no.* **53**

Sethadil *See* Sulfaethidole[c] *at loc. no.* **1555**

Sevin (63-25-2) *See* Carbaryl[c] *at loc. no.* **1128**

SEX cotton defoliant *See* Sodium Ethyl Xanthate[c] *at loc. no.* **1314**

Shellac (9000-59-3) *See loc. no.* **761**

Shirlan Extra (87-17-2) *See* Salicylanilide[c] *at loc. no.* **998**

Shirlan (sodium salt) (2593-10-4) *See* Salicylanilide[c] *at loc. no.* **998**

Shoxin (991-42-4) *See* Norbormide[c] *at loc. no.* **1349**

Sialkata oil *See* Argemone Oil[a] *at loc. no.* **710**

Sicarol *See* Pyracarbolid[c] *at loc. no.* **1204**

Siduron (1982-49-6) *See loc. no.* **1257**

Sigmodal (1216-40-6) *See loc. no.* **1387**

Signal oil *See* Mineral Seal Oil[a] *at loc. no.* **329**

Silica (7631-86-9) *See loc. no.* **7**

Silica gel (1343-98-2) *See* Silica[b] *at loc. no.* **7**

Silicates *See* Magnesium Silicate[e] *at loc. no.* **176**

Silicofluoric acid (1309-45-1) *See* Fluosilicic Acid[a] *at loc. no.* **37**

Silicofluoride salts *See* Fluosilicate Salts[d] *at loc. no.* **101**

Silicone dioxide (7631-86-9) *See* Silica[a] *at loc. no.* **7**

Silicone fluid *See* Silicone Oil[a] *at loc. no.* **1646**

Silicone Oil (9006-65-9) *See loc. no.* **1646**

Silver nitrate (7761-88-8) *See* Silver Salts[d] *at loc. no.* **288**

Silver Salts (2431-21-2) *See loc. no.* **288**

Silvex (93-72-1) *See loc. no.* **1223**

Simazine (122-34-9) *See loc. no.* **1269**

Simethicone *See* Silicone Oil[a] *at loc. no.* **1646**

Simetone (673-04-1) *See* Terbumeton[b] *at loc. no.* **1270**

Simetryn (1014-70-6) *See* Prometon[b] *at loc. no.* **1267**

Sinequan *See* Doxepin[c] *at loc. no.* **1472**

Sinomin *See* Sulfamethoxazole[c] *at loc. no.* **1561**

Sinox (534-52-1) *See* 4,6-Dinitro-o-cresol[c] *at loc. no.* **539**

Sintrom (152-72-7) *See* Acenocoumarol[c] *at loc. no.* **1332**

Skelaxin (1665-48-1) *See* Metaxalone[c] *at loc. no.* **1408**

SK-Soxazole *See* Sulfisoxazole[c] *at loc. no.* **1568**

Slaked lime (1305-62-0) *See* Lime (Slaked)[a] *at loc. no.* **55**

SMDC (137-42-8) *See* Metham Sodium[c] *at loc. no.* **1161**

Snip fly band (644-64-4) *See* Dimetilan[c] *at loc. no.* **1132**

"Snow" *See* Cocaine[a] *at loc. no.* **825**

Soaps *See loc. no.* **953**

Soda ash (497-19-8) *See* Sodium Carbonate[a] *at loc. no.* **52**

Sodium acetylsalicylate (493-53-8) *See* Aspirin[b] *at loc. no.* **594**

Sodium acid fluoride *See* Fluoride[d] *at loc. no.* **100**

Sodium acid oxalate *See* Sodium Binoxalate[a] *at loc. no.* **547**

Sodium acid sulfate (7681-38-1) *See* Sodium Bisulfate[a] *at loc. no.* **40**

Sodium acid sulfite (7631-90-5) *See* Sodium Bisulfite[a] *at loc. no.* **150**

Sodium alcohol sulfate salts *See* Alkyl Sodium Sulfates[a] *at loc. no.* **946**

Sodium alginate (9005-38-3) *See* Algin[a] *at loc. no.* **745**

Sodium alkane sulfonate *See* Alkyl Sodium Sulfonates[d] *at loc. no.* **947**

Sodium alkyl aryl polyether sulfates and sulfonates *See* Alkyl Aryl Polyether Sulfates and Sulfonates[c] *at loc. no.* **942**

Sodium alkyl aryl sulfate *See* Alkyl Sodium Sulfates[d] *at loc. no.* **946**

Sodium alkyl aryl sulfonate *See* Alkyl Aryl Sodium Sulfonates[a] *at loc. no.* **943**

Sodium alkyl sulfate (8036-54-2) *See* Alkyl Sodium Sulfates[a] *at loc. no.* **946**

Sodium 5-allyl-5-(1-methylbutyl)barbiturate (309-43-3) *See* Secobarbital Sodium[a] *at loc. no.* **1386**

Sodium 5-allyl-5-(1-methylbutyl)-2-thiobarbiturate (337-47-3) *See* Thiamylal Sodium[a] *at loc. no.* **1389**

Sodium aluminum fluoride (1331-71-1) *See* Cryolite[b] *at loc. no.* **104**

Sodium aluminum silicofluoride *See* Fluosilicate Salts[d] *at loc. no.* **101**

Sodium p-aminobenzoate (555-06-6) *See* p-Aminobenzoic Acid[b] *at loc. no.* **628**

Sodium p-aminosalicylate (133-10-8) *See* p-Aminosalicylic Acid[b] *at loc. no.* **629**

Sodium p-tert-amyl phenate (31366-95-7) *See* Amyl Phenol[b] *at loc. no.* **488**

Sodium arsanilate (127-85-5) *See* Arsanilic Acid[b] *at loc. no.* **189**

Sodium Arsenate (7631-89-2) *See loc. no.* **209**

Sodium Arsenite (7784-46-5) *See loc. no.* **210**

Sodium azide (12136-89-9) *See* Azide Salts[d] *at loc. no.* **111**

Sodium benzoate (532-32-1) *See* Benzoic Acid[b] *at loc. no.* **582**

Sodium o-benzo-sulphimide (128-44-9) *See* Saccharin[b] *at loc. no.* **1616**

Sodium o-benzyl-parachlorophenol *See* o-Benzyl-p-chlorophenol[b] *at loc. no.* **520**

Sodium biborate (1303-96-4) *See* Borax[a] *at loc. no.* **132**

Sodium Bicarbonate (144-55-8) *See loc. no.* **164**

Sodium bichromate (10588-01-9) *See* Dichromate Salts (Soluble)[d] *at loc. no.* **82**

Sodium bifluoride (7783-37-1) *See* Fluoride[d] *at loc. no.* **100**

Sodium Binoxalate *See loc. no.* **547**

Sodium Bisulfate (7681-38-1) *See loc. no.* **40**

Sodium Bisulfite (7631-90-5) *See loc. no.* **150**

Sodium borate (1303-96-4) *See* Borax[a] *at loc. no.* **132**

Sodium bromate (7789-38-0) *See* Bromate[d] *at loc. no.* **95**

---

[a] A Synonym   [b] A Closely Related Substance   [c] The Active or Major Constituent   [d] A Class Name
[e] A Specific Example of or Product Containing

Ingredient name (CAS registry no.) *See* Primary Name *at location no.* **XXX** *in Part D of this section*

Sodium bromide (7647-15-6) *See* Bromide Salts[d] *at loc. no.* **98**

Sodium butalbital *See* Butalbital[b] *at loc. no.* **1368**

Sodium 5-*sec*-butyl-5-ethylbarbiturate (143-81-7) *See* Butabarbital Sodium[a] *at loc. no.* **1367**

Sodium cacodylate (124-65-2) *See* Cacodylic Acid[b] *at loc. no.* **197**

Sodium Carbonate (497-19-8) *See loc. no.* **52**

Sodium chlorate (7775-09-9) *See* Chlorate Salts[d] *at loc. no.* **96**

Sodium Chloride (7647-14-5) *See loc. no.* **165**

Sodium chlorite (7758-19-2) *See* Chlorine Dioxide[b] *at loc. no.* **24**

Sodium chlorphenylphenate *See* Chloro-2-phenylphenol[b] *at loc. no.* **526**

Sodium chromate (10034-82-9) *See* Chromate Salts[d] *at loc. no.* **81**

Sodium citrate (18996-35-5) *See* Citric Acid[b] *at loc. no.* **703**

Sodium cresylate *See* Cresols[b] *at loc. no.* **514**

Sodium cyanate (917-61-3) *See* Cyanate Salts[d] *at loc. no.* **145**

Sodium cyanide (13998-03-3) *See* Cyanide[d] *at loc. no.* **105**

Sodium cyanurate (2624-17-1) *See* Cyanuric Acid[b] *at loc. no.* **1261**

Sodium Cyclamate (139-05-9) *See loc. no.* **1617**

Sodium 5-(1-cyclohexenyl)-1,5-dimethylbarbiturate (50-09-9) *See* Hexobarbital Sodium[a] *at loc. no.* **1376**

Sodium dalapon (127-20-8) *See* Dalapon[b] *at loc. no.* **1299**

Sodium dehydroacetate (4418-26-2) *See* Dehydroacetic Acid[b] *at loc. no.* **1187**

Sodium dibasic phosphate (7558-79-4) *See* Phosphates[d] *at loc. no.* **139**

Sodium dichlorocyanurate (2893-78-9) *See* Trichloroisocyanuric Acid[b] *at loc. no.* **94**

Sodium dichloroisocyanurate (2893-78-9) *See* Trichloroisocyanuric Acid[b] *at loc. no.* **94**

Sodium dichloro-*s*-triazinetrione (2893-78-9) *See* Trichloroisocyanuric Acid[b] *at loc. no.* **94**

Sodium dichromate (7789-12-0) *See* Dichromate Salts (Soluble)[d] *at loc. no.* **82**

Sodium diethylmalonylurea (144-02-5) *See* Barbital[b] *at loc. no.* **1366**

Sodium [4-(dimethylamino)phenyl]diazenesulfonate (140-56-7) *See* Fenaminosulf[a] *at loc. no.* **1195**

Sodium dimethylarsinate (124-65-2) *See* Cacodylic Acid[b] *at loc. no.* **197**

Sodium Dimethyldithiocarbamate (128-04-1) *See loc. no.* **1163**

Sodium 4,6-dinitro-*o*-cresylate (2312-76-7) *See* 4,6-Dinitro-*o*-cresol[b] *at loc. no.* **539**

Sodium 4,6-dinitro-2-sec-butylphenate *See* Dinoseb[b] *at loc. no.* **543**

Sodium dinoseb *See* Dinoseb[b] *at loc. no.* **543**

Sodium dioctyl sulfosuccinate (577-11-7) *See* Dioctyl Sodium Sulfosuccinate[a] *at loc. no.* **951**

Sodium dithionite (7775-14-6) *See* Sodium Hydrosulfite[a] *at loc. no.* **151**

Sodium dodecyl benzene sulfonate (25155-30-0) *See* Alkyl Aryl Sodium Sulfonates[d] *at loc. no.* **943**

Sodium dodecyl benzene sulfosuccinate *See* Dioctyl Sodium Sulfosuccinate[b] *at loc. no.* **951**

Sodium ethyl hexyl sulfate (126-92-1) *See* Alkyl Sodium Sulfates[d] *at loc. no.* **946**

Sodium 5-ethyl-5-isopropylbarbiturate (143-82-8) *See* Probarbital Sodium[a] *at loc. no.* **1383**

Sodium ethylmercurithiosalicylate (54-64-8) *See* Thimerosal[a] *at loc. no.* **244**

Sodium 5-ethyl-5-(1-methylbutyl)barbiturate (57-33-0) *See* Pentobarbital Sodium[a] *at loc. no.* **1380**

Sodium 5-ethyl-5-(1-methylbutyl)-2-thiobarbiturate (71-73-8) *See* Thiopental Sodium[a] *at loc. no.* **1390**

Sodium Ethyl Xanthate (140-90-9) *See loc. no.* **1314**

Sodium ferric diethylenetriamine pentaacetate *See* Ferric Salts[d] *at loc. no.* **253**

Sodium ferric ethylenediaminetetraacetate (10346-69-7) *See* Iron Salts[d] *at loc. no.* **250**

Sodium ferricyanide (14217-21-1) *See* Ferrocyanide and Ferricyanide Salts[d] *at loc. no.* **256**

Sodium ferrocyanide (13601-19-9) *See* Ferrocyanide and Ferricyanide Salts[d] *at loc. no.* **256**

Sodium fluoride (7681-49-4) *See* Fluoride[d] *at loc. no.* **100**

Sodium fluoroacetate (62-74-8) *See* Fluoroacetate[d] *at loc. no.* **548**

Sodium fluosilicate (16893-85-9) *See* Fluosilicate Salts[d] *at loc. no.* **101**

Sodium formate (141-53-7) *See* Formic Acid (and Salts)[d] *at loc. no.* **44**

Sodium glutamate (142-47-2) *See* Monosodium Glutamate[a] *at loc. no.* **1618**

Sodium Hexametaphosphate (10124-56-8) *See loc. no.* **143**

Sodium hydrogen sulfate (7681-38-1) *See* Sodium Bisulfate[a] *at loc. no.* **40**

Sodium Hydrosulfite (7775-14-6) *See loc. no.* **151**

Sodium hydroxide (1310-73-2) *See* Lye[a] *at loc. no.* **51**

Sodium Hypochlorite (7681-52-9) *See loc. no.* **85**

Sodium hyposulfite (7772-98-7) *See* Sodium Thiosulfate[a] *at loc. no.* **163**

Sodium iodate (7681-55-2) *See* Iodate Salts[d] *at loc. no.* **97**

Sodium iodide (7681-82-5) *See* Iodide Salts[d] *at loc. no.* **99**

Sodium iodoacetate (305-53-3) *See* Fluoroacetate[b] *at loc. no.* **548**

Sodium Isopropyl Xanthate (140-93-2) *See loc. no.* **1315**

Sodium laureth sulfate (1335-72-4) *See* Sodium Lauryl Trioxyethylene Sulfate[a] *at loc. no.* **955**

Sodium Lauryl Glyceryl Ether Sulfonate (34247-28-4) *See loc. no.* **954**

Sodium lauryl sulfate (151-21-3) *See* Alkyl Sodium Sulfates[d] *at loc. no.* **946**

Sodium Lauryl Trioxyethylene Sulfate (13150-00-0) *See loc. no.* **955**

Sodium linear alkyl benzene sulfonate *See* Linear Alkyl Benzene Sulfonate (Sodium)[a] *at loc. no.* **952**

Sodium mercaptoacetate (367-51-1) *See* Sodium Thioglycolate[a] *at loc. no.* **553**

Sodium mercaptobenzothiazole (2492-26-4) *See* Mercaptobenzothiazole[b] *at loc. no.* **1198**

Sodium meta-arsenate (7631-89-2) *See* Sodium Arsenate[a] *at loc. no.* **209**

Sodium meta-arsenite (7784-46-5) *See* Sodium Arsenite[a] *at loc. no.* **210**

Sodium metaborate (7775-19-1) *See* Borate[d] *at loc. no.* **131**

Sodium Metasilicate (6834-92-0) *See loc. no.* **57**

Sodium metavanadate (13718-26-8) *See* Vanadium (and its Salts)[d] *at loc. no.* **299**

Sodium 2-methyl-4-chlorophenoxyacetate (3653-48-3) *See* MCPA[b] *at loc. no.* **1220**

Sodium N-methyldithiocarbamate (137-42-8) *See* Metham Sodium[a] *at loc. no.* **1161**

Sodium methyl oleyl taurate (7346-80-7) *See* Alkyl Sodium N-Methyltaurate[d] *at loc. no.* **948**

Sodium monobasic phosphate (7558-80-7) *See* Phosphates[d] *at loc. no.* **139**

Sodium monochloroacetate (3926-62-3) *See* Chloroacetic Acid (and Salts)[b] *at loc. no.* **549**

---

[a] A Synonym   [b] A Closely Related Substance   [c] The Active or Major Constituent   [d] A Class Name
[e] A Specific Example of or Product Containing

Ingredient name (CAS registry no.) *See* Primary Name *at*
location no. **XXX** *in Part D of this section*

Sodium monofluoroacetate (62-74-8) *See* Fluoroacetate^d *at loc. no.* **548**

Sodium monofluorophosphate (10163-15-2) *See* Fluoride^b *at loc. no.* **100**

Sodium monopersulfate *See* Potassium Monopersulfate^b *at loc. no.* **79**

Sodium 1-Naphthaleneacetate *See loc. no.* **1316**

Sodium nicotinate (54-86-4) *See* Nicotinic Acid^b *at loc. no.* **911**

Sodium nitrate (7631-99-4) *See* Nitrate Salts^d *at loc. no.* **157**

Sodium nitrite (7632-00-0) *See* Nitrite^d *at loc. no.* **144**

Sodium nitroferricyanide (14402-89-2) *See* Nitroprusside Salts^d *at loc. no.* **109**

Sodium 3-nitro-4-hydroxy phenol arsonate *See* 4-Hydroxy-3-nitrophenylarsonic Acid^b *at loc. no.* **205**

Sodium nitroprusside (14402-89-2) *See* Nitroprusside Salts^d *at loc. no.* **109**

Sodium oleate (143-19-1) *See* Soaps^d *at loc. no.* **953**

Sodium orthophosphate (7632-05-5) *See* Phosphates^d *at loc. no.* **139**

Sodium orthosilicate (13472-30-5) *See* Sodium Silicate^a *at loc. no.* **58**

Sodium oxalate (62-76-0) *See* Oxalate^d *at loc. no.* **546**

Sodium oxide (1313-59-3) *See* Lye^d *at loc. no.* **51**

Sodium palmitate (408-35-5) *See* Soaps^d *at loc. no.* **953**

Sodium pentachlorophenate (131-52-2) *See* Pentachlorophenol^b *at loc. no.* **532**

Sodium pentachlorophenolate (131-52-2) *See* Pentachlorophenol^b *at loc. no.* **532**

Sodium pentachlorophenoxide (131-52-2) *See* Pentachlorophenol^b *at loc. no.* **532**

Sodium pentobarbital (57-33-0) *See* Pentobarbital Sodium^a *at loc. no.* **1380**

Sodium Perborate (10042-94-1) *See loc. no.* **133**

Sodium Peroxide (1313-60-6) *See loc. no.* **74**

Sodium phenolate (139-02-6) *See* Phenol^b *at loc. no.* **494**

Sodium *o*-phenylphenate (132-27-4) *See* Phenylphenol^b *at loc. no.* **495**

Sodium phosphate *See* Phosphates^d *at loc. no.* **139**

Sodium phosphate tribasic (7601-54-9) *See* Trisodium Phosphate^a *at loc. no.* **60**

Sodium polymanuronate (9005-38-3) *See* Algin^a *at loc. no.* **745**

Sodium polyphosphate *See* Complex Phosphates^a *at loc. no.* **141**

Sodium Propionate (137-40-6) *See loc. no.* **551**

Sodium pyroborate (1303-96-4) *See* Borax^a *at loc. no.* **132**

Sodium pyrophosphate (7722-88-5) *See* Tetrasodium Pyrophosphate^a *at loc. no.* **140**

Sodium pyrosulfate (7681-38-1) *See* Sodium Bisulfate^a *at loc. no.* **40**

Sodium rhodanate (540-72-7) *See* Sodium Thiocyanate^a *at loc. no.* **147**

Sodium rhodanide (540-72-7) *See* Sodium Thiocyanate^a *at loc. no.* **147**

Sodium salicylanilide (2593-10-4) *See* Salicylanilide^b *at loc. no.* **998**

Sodium salicylate (54-21-7) *See* Salicylate^d *at loc. no.* **600**

Sodium salt of bentazone (50723-80-3) *See* Bentazon^b *at loc. no.* **1291**

Sodium salt of maleic hydrazide (28330-26-9) *See* Maleic Hydrazide^c *at loc. no.* **1308**

Sodium salt of 2,4,5-T (13560-99-1) *See* Trichlorophenoxyacetic Acid^b *at loc. no.* **1224**

Sodium salts. *If not listed here, consult name of anion or acid.*

Sodium salts of fatty alcohol sulfates *See* Alkyl Sodium Sulfates^d *at loc. no.* **946**

Sodium Selenate (10112-94-4) *See loc. no.* **184**

Sodium Sesquicarbonate (533-96-0) *See loc. no.* **53**

Sodium Silicate (13472-30-5) *See loc. no.* **58**

Sodium silicofluoride (16893-85-9) *See* Fluosilicate Salts^d *at loc. no.* **101**

Sodium stannous tartrate *See* Stannic and Stannous Salts^d *at loc. no.* **290**

Sodium stearate (822-16-2) *See* Soaps^d *at loc. no.* **953**

Sodium sulfacetamide (127-56-0) *See* Sulfacetamide^b *at loc. no.* **1551**

Sodium sulfadiazine (547-32-0) *See* Sulfadiazine^b *at loc. no.* **1553**

Sodium sulfamerazine (127-58-2) *See* Sulfamerazine^b *at loc. no.* **1557**

Sodium sulfamethazine (1981-58-4) *See* Sulfamethazine^b *at loc. no.* **1559**

Sodium sulfapyridine (127-57-1) *See* Sulfapyridine^b *at loc. no.* **1564**

Sodium sulfate (7757-82-6) *See* Sulfate Salts^d *at loc. no.* **159**

Sodium sulfates of fatty acid esters *See* Alkyl Sodium Sulfates^d *at loc. no.* **946**

Sodium sulfathiazole (144-74-1) *See* Sulfathiazole^b *at loc. no.* **1567**

Sodium sulfide (1313-82-2) *See* Sulfide Salts^d *at loc. no.* **118**

Sodium Sulfite (7757-83-7) *See* Sulfite Salts^d *at loc. no.* **149**

Sodium sulfocyanate (540-72-7) *See* Sodium Thiocyanate^a *at loc. no.* **147**

Sodium sulfoxylate (7775-14-6) *See* Sodium Hydrosulfite^a *at loc. no.* **151**

Sodium sulfuret *See* Sulfide Salts^d *at loc. no.* **118**

Sodium tellurate *See* Tellurium Derivatives^d *at loc. no.* **187**

Sodium tellurite (10102-20-2) *See* Tellurium Derivatives^d *at loc. no.* **187**

Sodium tetraborate (1303-96-4) *See* Borax^a *at loc. no.* **132**

Sodium tetraborate decahydrate (1344-90-7) *See* Borax^a *at loc. no.* **132**

Sodium tetrachlorophenate (131-61-3) *See* 2,3,4,6-Tetrachlorophenol^b *at loc. no.* **534**

Sodium Thiocyanate (540-72-7) *See loc. no.* **147**

Sodium Thioglycolate (367-51-1) *See loc. no.* **553**

Sodium thioglycollate (367-51-1) *See* Sodium Thioglycolate^a *at loc. no.* **553**

Sodium Thiosulfate (7772-98-7) *See loc. no.* **163**

Sodium *p*-toluenesulfonchloramide (127-65-1) *See* Chloramine-T^a *at loc. no.* **91**

Sodium tribasic phosphate (7601-54-9) *See* Trisodium Phosphate^a *at loc. no.* **60**

Sodium Trichloroacetate (650-51-1) *See loc. no.* **550**

Sodium trichlorophenate (1320-79-2) *See* Trichlorophenols^b *at loc. no.* **535**

Sodium trichlorophenolate (1320-79-2) *See* Trichlorophenols^b *at loc. no.* **535**

Sodium tripolyphosphate (13573-18-7) *See* Tripolyphosphate^d *at loc. no.* **142**

Sodium tripolyphosphate chlorinated *See* Chlorinated Trisodium Phosphate^b *at loc. no.* **87**

Sodium tungstate (13472-45-2) *See* Tungsten (and its Salts)^d *at loc. no.* **297**

Sodium warfarin (129-06-6) *See* Warfarin^b *at loc. no.* **1345**

Sodium xanthogenate (140-90-9) *See* Sodium Ethyl Xanthate^a *at loc. no.* **1314**

Sodium Zirconium Lactate (10377-98-7) *See loc. no.* **300**

Softenon (50-35-1) *See* Thalidomide^c *at loc. no.* **1443**

Softran (129-74-8) *See* Buclizine^b *at loc. no.* **1488**

Solacin (4268-36-4) *See* Meprobamate^b *at loc. no.* **1407**

---

^{a} A Synonym ^{b} A Closely Related Substance ^{c} The Active or Major Constituent ^{d} A Class Name
^{e} A Specific Example of or Product Containing

Ingredient name (CAS registry no.) *See* Primary Name *at*
location no. **XXX** *in Part D of this section*

Solan (2307-68-8) *See* Pentanochlor[a] *at loc. no.* **1280**
Solanidine *See* Solanine[e] *at loc. no.* **832**
Solanine (125-97-3) *See loc. no.* **832**
Solarcaine *See* Benzocaine[c] *at loc. no.* **1577**
Solicam *See* Norflurazon[c] *at loc. no.* **1311**
Solid polyethylene glycols *See* Carbowax[e] *at loc. no.* **441**
Solox (8046-13-7) *See loc. no.* **429**
Solvay soda *See* Sodium Carbonate[a] *at loc. no.* **52**
Solvent naphtha (8032-32-4) *See* VM&P Naphthas[a] *at loc. no.* **335**
Soma (78-44-4) *See* Carisoprodol[c] *at loc. no.* **1403**
Sonilyn *See* Sulfachlorpyridazine[c] *at loc. no.* **1552**
Sorbic Acid (110-44-1) *See loc. no.* **561**
Sorbitan Mono-oleate (5938-38-5) *See* Sorbitan Monostearate[b] *at loc. no.* **972**
Sorbitan mono-oleate polyoxyethylene (9005-65-6) *See* Polysorbate 80[a] *at loc. no.* **970**
Sorbitan Monostearate (1338-41-6) *See loc. no.* **972**
D-Sorbitol (50-70-4) *See loc. no.* **706**
Sosol *See* Sulfisoxazole[c] *at loc. no.* **1568**
Soxomide *See* Sulfisoxazole[c] *at loc. no.* **1568**
Soya Alkyd Resin *See loc. no.* **1640**
Span 60 (1338-41-6) *See* Sorbitan Monostearate[c] *at loc. no.* **972**
Span 80 (5938-38-5) *See* Sorbitan Monostearate[b] *at loc. no.* **972**
Spanish fly *See* Cantharidin[c] *at loc. no.* **924**
Sparine (58-40-2) *See* Promazine[c] *at loc. no.* **1420**
Spectracide (333-41-5) *See* Diazinon[c] *at loc. no.* **1068**
"Speed" *See* Methamphetamine[a] *at loc. no.* **1459**
Spergon (118-75-2) *See* Chloranil[c] *at loc. no.* **1183**
Spermaceti (8002-23-1) *See loc. no.* **973**
Spirit of turpentine (8006-64-2) *See* Turpentine[a] *at loc. no.* **763**
Spirits of hartshorn (8007-57-6) *See* Ammonia[b] *at loc. no.* **63**
Sporiline (2398-96-1) *See* Tolnaftate[c] *at loc. no.* **1532**
Squalane (111-01-3) *See loc. no.* **932**
Squill (Red or White) *See loc. no.* **695**
Stabisol (87-27-4) *See* Bismuth Subsalicylate[c] *at loc. no.* **219**
Stam (709-98-8) *See* Propanil[a] *at loc. no.* **1283**
Stangyl maleate *See* Trimipramine[c] *at loc. no.* **1481**
Stannic and Stannous Salts *See loc. no.* **290**
Stannous fluoride (7783-47-3) *See* Stannic and Stannous Salts[d] *at loc. no.* **290**
Stannous sulfide (1314-95-0) *See* Stannic and Stannous Salts[d] *at loc. no.* **290**
Starch (9005-25-8) *See loc. no.* **707**
Starlicide *See* 3-Chloro-4-methylaniline[c] *at loc. no.* **614**
Stauffer R-1303 (786-19-6) *See* Carbophenothion[c] *at loc. no.* **1083**
Stearalkonium chloride (122-19-0) *See* Stearyl Dimethyl Benzyl Ammonium Chloride[a] *at loc. no.* **990**
Stearate (646-29-7) *See* Stearic Acid[b] *at loc. no.* **562**
Stearic Acid (57-11-4) *See loc. no.* **562**
Stearyl *derivative. If not listed here, see corresponding* Alkyl *derivative in this index.*
Stearyl Alcohol (112-92-5) *See loc. no.* **430**
Stearyl Dimethyl Benzyl Ammonium Chloride (122-19-0) *See loc. no.* **990**
Stelazine (117-89-5) *See* Trifluoperazine[c] *at loc. no.* **1426**
Stenol (8005-44-5) *See* Stearyl Alcohol[c] *at loc. no.* **430**
"Stink damp" (7783-06-4) *See* Hydrogen Sulfide[a] *at loc. no.* **114**
Stirifos (961-11-5) *See* Tetrachlorvinfos[a] *at loc. no.* **1061**
Stoddard Solvent (8052-41-3) *See loc. no.* **334**

Storax (8023-62-9) *See loc. no.* **762**
Stove gas *See* Gas[d] *at loc. no.* **128**
STP (15588-95-1) *See* 2,5-Dimethoxy-4-methyl-amphetamine[a] *at loc. no.* **1449**
Stramonium (8063-18-1) *See loc. no.* **696**
Streptozocin (18883-66-4) *See* Vacor[b] *at loc. no.* **1353**
Striatran (78-28-4) *See* Emylcamate[c] *at loc. no.* **1405**
Strobane (8001-50-1) *See loc. no.* **1031**
Strontium bromide (7789-53-9) *See* Bromide Salts[d] *at loc. no.* **98**
Strontium chloride (10025-70-4) *See* Strontium Salts[d] *at loc. no.* **177**
Strontium hydroxide (1311-10-0) *See* Lye[d] *at loc. no.* **51**
Strontium salicylate (526-26-1) *See* Salicylate[d] *at loc. no.* **600**
Strontium Salts *See loc. no.* **177**
Strontium sulfate (7759-02-6) *See* Strontium Salts[d] *at loc. no.* **177**
Strontium Sulfide (1314-96-1) *See loc. no.* **119**
Strophanthin (8001-51-2) *See loc. no.* **844**
g-Strophanthin (630-60-4) *See* Ouabain[a] *at loc. no.* **842**
Strophanthin G (630-60-4) *See* Ouabain[a] *at loc. no.* **842**
Strophanthus kombe *See* Strophanthin[c] *at loc. no.* **844**
Strychnina *See* Strychnine[a] *at loc. no.* **833**
Strychnine (57-24-9) *See loc. no.* **833**
Strychnine nitrate (66-32-0) *See* Strychnine[b] *at loc. no.* **833**
Strychnine N^6-oxide (1300-18-1) *See* Strychnine[b] *at loc. no.* **833**
Strychnine phosphate (509-42-2) *See* Strychnine[b] *at loc. no.* **833**
Strychnine sulfate (60-41-3) *See* Strychnine[b] *at loc. no.* **833**
Strychnos nux-vomica *See* Nux Vomica[a] *at loc. no.* **680**
Styrax (8023-62-9) *See* Storax[a] *at loc. no.* **762**
Styrene (100-42-5) *See loc. no.* **315**
Styrene oxide (96-09-3) *See* Styrene[b] *at loc. no.* **315**
Suavitil (57-37-4) *See* Benactyzine[c] *at loc. no.* **1430**
Subacetate Salts *See loc. no.* **554**
Sublimed sulfur (7704-34-9) *See* Sulfur[a] *at loc. no.* **120**
Subnitrate Salts *See loc. no.* **158**
Subsulfate Salts *See loc. no.* **160**
Sucaryl sodium (139-05-9) *See* Sodium Cyclamate[a] *at loc. no.* **1617**
Succinchlorimide (128-09-6) *See* N-Chlorosuccinimide[a] *at loc. no.* **92**
Succinonitrile (110-61-2) *See loc. no.* **654**
Succinylsulfathiazole (116-43-8) *See loc. no.* **1549**
Sucrose (57-50-1) *See loc. no.* **708**
Sudafed hydrochloride (6272-89-5) *See* Pseudoephedrine Hydrochloride[c] *at loc. no.* **1453**
Suffix *See* Benzoylprop-ethyl[c] *at loc. no.* **1292**
Sugar (granulated or powdered) (57-50-1) *See* Sucrose[a] *at loc. no.* **708**
Sulcolon *See* Sulfasalazine[c] *at loc. no.* **1566**
Sulfabenzpyrazine *See* Sulfaquinoxaline[a] *at loc. no.* **1565**
Sulfabrom *See* Sulfabromethazine[c] *at loc. no.* **1550**
Sulfabromethazine (116-45-0) *See loc. no.* **1550**
Sulfacetamide (144-80-9) *See loc. no.* **1551**
Sulfacetamide sodium (127-56-0) *See* Sulfacetamide[b] *at loc. no.* **1551**
Sulfachlorpyridazine (80-32-0) *See loc. no.* **1552**
Sulfadiazine (68-35-9) *See loc. no.* **1553**
Sulfadimethoxine (122-11-2) *See loc. no.* **1554**
Sulfadimethoxydiazine *See* Sulfadimethoxine[a] *at loc. no.* **1554**
4-Sulfadimethoxypyrimidine *See* Sulfadimethoxine[a] *at loc. no.* **1554**

---

[a] A Synonym   [b] A Closely Related Substance   [c] The Active or Major Constituent   [d] A Class Name
[e] A Specific Example of or Product Containing

Ingredient name (CAS registry no.) *See* Primary Name *at*
location no. **XXX** *in Part D of this section*

Sulfadimethyldiazine *See* Sulfamethazine[a] *at loc. no.* 1559
Sulfadimethylpyrimidine *See* Sulfamethazine[a] *at loc. no.* 1559
Sulfaethidole (94-19-9) *See loc. no.* 1555
Sulfaethylthiadiazole (94-19-9) *See* Sulfaethidole[a] *at loc. no.* 1555
Sulfaguanidine (57-67-0) *See loc. no.* 1556
Sulfallate (95-06-7) *See loc. no.* 1164
Sulfamerazine (127-79-7) *See loc. no.* 1557
Sulfameter (651-06-9) *See loc. no.* 1558
Sulfamethazine (57-68-1) *See loc. no.* 1559
Sulfamethiazine *See* Sulfamethazine[a] *at loc. no.* 1559
Sulfamethizole (144-82-1) *See loc. no.* 1560
Sulfamethoxazole (723-46-6) *See loc. no.* 1561
Sulfamethoxine (651-06-9) *See* Sulfameter[a] *at loc. no.* 1558
Sulfamethoxydiazine (651-06-9) *See* Sulfameter[a] *at loc. no.* 1558
Sulfamethoxypyridazine (80-35-3) *See loc. no.* 1562
Sulfamic Acid (5329-14-6) *See loc. no.* 48
p-Sulfamidoaniline (63-74-1) *See* Sulfanilamide[a] *at loc. no.* 1563
N[1]-Sulfanilacetamide (144-80-9) *See* Sulfacetamide[a] *at loc. no.* 1551
Sulfanilamide (63-74-1) *See loc. no.* 1563
3-Sulfanilamido-6-methoxypyridazine *See* Sulfamethoxypyridazine[a] *at loc. no.* 1562
2-Sulfanilamidopyrimidine (68-35-9) *See* Sulfadiazine[a] *at loc. no.* 1553
2-Sulfanilamidoquinoxaline *See* Sulfaquinoxaline[a] *at loc. no.* 1565
2-Sulfanilamidothiazole (72-14-0) *See* Sulfathiazole[a] *at loc. no.* 1567
Sulfanilylguanidine (57-67-0) *See* Sulfaguanidine[a] *at loc. no.* 1556
Sulfapyridine (144-83-2) *See loc. no.* 1564
Sulfaquinoxaline (59-40-5) *See loc. no.* 1565
Sulfasalazine (599-79-1) *See loc. no.* 1566
Sulfasan (502-55-6) *See* Diethyl Dithiobis(thionoformate)[c] *at loc. no.* 1302
Sulfasuxidine *See* Succinylsulfathiazole[c] *at loc. no.* 1549
Sulfated Castor Oil *See loc. no.* 956
Sulfated fatty alcohols *See* Alkyl Sodium Sulfates[a] *at loc. no.* 946
Sulfated synthetic detergents *See* Alkyl Sodium Sulfates[e] *at loc. no.* 946
Sulfate Salts *See loc. no.* 159
Sulfathalidine *See* Phthalylsulfathiazole[c] *at loc. no.* 1548
Sulfathiazole (72-14-0) *See loc. no.* 1567
Sulfathiazole sodium (144-74-1) *See* Sulfathiazole[b] *at loc. no.* 1567
Sulferrous salts *See* Ferrous Salts[b] *at loc. no.* 258
Sulfide Salts (18496-25-8) *See loc. no.* 118
Sulfinpyrazone (57-96-5) *See loc. no.* 1576
Sulfisoxazole (127-69-5) *See loc. no.* 1568
Sulfisoxazole diolamine (80-74-0) *See* Sulfisoxazole[b] *at loc. no.* 1568
Sulfite Salts *See loc. no.* 149
Sulfocyanates *See* Thiocyanate Salts[a] *at loc. no.* 146
Sulfocyanates (organic) *See* Aliphatic Thiocyanates[d] *at loc. no.* 1034
Sulfoguaiacol (6100-07-8) *See* Potassium Guaiacolsulfonate[a] *at loc. no.* 496
Sulfonamides *See loc. no.* 1546
Sulfonated and saponified emulsifiers *See* Alkyl Sodium Sulfonates[d] *at loc. no.* 947
"Sulfonated" castor oil *See* Sulfated Castor Oil[a] *at loc. no.* 956

Sulfonated Dodecyl Diphenyl Oxide (Sodium) *See loc. no.* 957
Sulfonated hydrocarbons *See* Sulfonated Petroleum Oils[e] *at loc. no.* 958
Sulfonated oil *See* Sulfonated Petroleum Oils[a] *at loc. no.* 958
Sulfonated Petroleum Oils *See loc. no.* 958
Sulfonated synthetic detergents *See* Alkyl Sodium Sulfonates[e] *at loc. no.* 947
Sulfosalicylic acid (97-05-2) *See* Trichloroacetic Acid[b] *at loc. no.* 50
Sulfotepp (3689-24-5) *See loc. no.* 1108
Sulfox-cide (120-62-7) *See* Sulfoxide[c] *at loc. no.* 1155
Sulfoxide (120-62-7) *See loc. no.* 1155
Sulfoxyl (120-62-7) *See* Sulfoxide[c] *at loc. no.* 1155
Sulfur (7704-34-9) *See loc. no.* 120
Sulfurated lime (1344-81-6) *See* Calcium Polysulfide[e] *at loc. no.* 113
Sulfur Chloride (10025-67-9) *See loc. no.* 28
Sulfur Dioxide (7446-09-5) *See loc. no.* 10
Sulfureted hydrogen (7783-06-4) *See* Hydrogen Sulfide[a] *at loc. no.* 114
Sulfuric Acid (7664-93-9) *See loc. no.* 33
Sulfuric chlorohydrin (7790-94-5) *See* Chlorosulfonic Acid[a] *at loc. no.* 39
Sulfur monochloride (10025-67-9) *See* Sulfur Chloride[a] *at loc. no.* 28
Sulfurous Acid (7782-99-2) *See loc. no.* 35
Sulfurous anhydride (7446-09-5) *See* Sulfur Dioxide[a] *at loc. no.* 10
Sulfurous oxide (7446-09-5) *See* Sulfur Dioxide[a] *at loc. no.* 10
Sulfur subchloride (10025-67-9) *See* Sulfur Chloride[a] *at loc. no.* 28
Sulfuryl Fluoride (2699-79-8) *See loc. no.* 18
Sulisobenzone (4065-45-6) *See* Oxybenzone[b] *at loc. no.* 1537
Sulla *See* Sulfameter[c] *at loc. no.* 1558
Sulphenone (80-00-2) *See loc. no.* 1048
Sulquin *See* Sulfaquinoxaline[c] *at loc. no.* 1565
Sultrin *See* Sulfathiazole[c] *at loc. no.* 1567
Sumatrol (82-10-0) *See* Rotenoids[d] *at loc. no.* 897
Sumicidin *See* Fenvalerate[c] *at loc. no.* 890
Sumithion (122-14-5) *See* Fenitrothion[c] *at loc. no.* 1072
Superglue *See* n-Alkyl-α-Cyanoacrylates[a] *at loc. no.* 1626
Superphosphates *See loc. no.* 41
Surface Active Agents *See loc. no.* 936
Surfactants *See* Surface Active Agents[a] *at loc. no.* 936
Surital sodium (337-47-3) *See* Thiamylal Sodium[c] *at loc. no.* 1389
Surmontil maleate (521-78-8) *See* Trimipramine[c] *at loc. no.* 1481
Sustar (47000-92-0) *See* Fluoridamid[c] *at loc. no.* 1276
Swedish green (1302-97-2) *See* Cupric Arsenite[a] *at loc. no.* 202
Sweet birch oil (119-36-8) *See* Methyl Salicylate[a] *at loc. no.* 597
Sweet oriental gum (8023-62-9) *See* Storax[a] *at loc. no.* 762
Sweet spirits of nitre *See* Amyl Nitrite[b] *at loc. no.* 630
Sylvic acid (514-10-3) *See* Abietic Acid[a] *at loc. no.* 580
Symmetrel (665-66-7) *See* Amantadine[c] *at loc. no.* 922
Syndets *See* Detergents (Synthetic)[a] *at loc. no.* 935
Synthetic 3956 *See* Toxaphene[c] *at loc. no.* 1030
Synthetic detergents *See* Alkyl Sodium Sulfates[d] *at loc. no.* 946
Synthetic latex *See* Latex[b] *at loc. no.* 756
Synthrin *See* Resmethrin[c] *at loc. no.* 895
Systox (8000-97-3) *See* Demeton[a] *at loc. no.* 1067

---

[a] A Synonym [b] A Closely Related Substance [c] The Active or Major Constituent [d] A Class Name
[e] A Specific Example of or Product Containing

Ingredient name (CAS registry no.) *See* Primary Name *at location no.* **XXX** *in Part D of this section*

2,4,5-T (93-76-5) *See* Trichlorophenoxyacetic Acid[a] *at loc. no.* **1224**

T3 (6893-02-3) *See* Thyroid[d] *at loc. no.* **920**

T4 (51-48-9) *See* Thyroid[d] *at loc. no.* **920**

Tabasco pepper *See* Capsicum[a] *at loc. no.* **659**

Table salt (7647-14-5) *See* Sodium Chloride[a] *at loc. no.* **165**

Tabutrex (141-03-7) *See* Di-*n*-butyl Succinate[a] *at loc. no.* **1325**

Tagamet *See* Cimetidine[c] *at loc. no.* **1491**

Tagathen (148-65-2) *See* Chlorothen[c] *at loc. no.* **1490**

Talbutal (115-44-6) *See* Butalbital[b] *at loc. no.* **1368**

Talc (14807-96-6) *See loc. no.* **8**

Talcum (14807-96-6) *See* Talc[a] *at loc. no.* **8**

Talleol (8002-26-4) *See* Tall Oil[a] *at loc. no.* **723**

Tall Oil (8002-26-4) *See loc. no.* **723**

Tall oil sodium salt (65997-01-5) *See* Tall Oil[b] *at loc. no.* **723**

Tallow *derivative. If not listed here, see corresponding* Alkyl *derivative in this index.*

Tallow *See loc. no.* **709**

Tallow alcohols *See* Stearyl Alcohol[e] *at loc. no.* **430**

Talwin (359-83-1) *See* Pentazocine[c] *at loc. no.* **792**

Tandearil (129-20-4) *See* Oxyphenbutazone[c] *at loc. no.* **1574**

Tandex (4849-32-5) *See* Karbutilate[c] *at loc. no.* **1232**

Tannic Acid (1401-55-4) *See loc. no.* **852**

Tannin (1401-55-4) *See* Tannic Acid[a] *at loc. no.* **852**

Tansy (8016-87-3) *See* Essential Oils[d] *at loc. no.* **725**

Tantizon (57052-04-7) *See* Isomethiozin[c] *at loc. no.* **1264**

Taractan *See* Chlorprothixene[c] *at loc. no.* **1414**

Tar camphor (91-20-3) *See* Naphthalene[a] *at loc. no.* **321**

Tars (Tar Oils and Tar Acids) *See loc. no.* **519**

Tartar emetic (304-61-0) *See* Antimony Potassium Tartrate[a] *at loc. no.* **213**

Tartaric Acid (133-37-9) *See loc. no.* **563**

2,3,6-TBA (50-31-7) *See* Trichlorobenzoic Acid[d] *at loc. no.* **1317**

2,4,6-TBA (50-43-1) *See* Trichlorobenzoic Acid[d] *at loc. no.* **1317**

TBE (79-27-6) *See* 1,1,2,2-Tetrabromoethane[a] *at loc. no.* **372**

TBS *See* 3,4′,5-Tribromosalicylanilide[a] *at loc. no.* **1000**

TBS *See* Tetrapropylene Benzene Sulfonate (Sodium)[a] *at loc. no.* **959**

TBTO (56-35-9) *See* Bis(tri-*n*-butyltin) oxide[a] *at loc. no.* **294**

TCA (76-03-9) *See* Trichloroacetic Acid[a] *at loc. no.* **50**

TCBC (1344-32-7) *See* Trichlorobenzyl Chloride[a] *at loc. no.* **1361**

TCC (101-20-2) *See* 3,4,4′-Trichlorocarbanilide[a] *at loc. no.* **1001**

TCDD *See* Polychlorinated Dibenzodioxins[d] *at loc. no.* **400**

TCE (79-01-6) *See* Trichloroethylene[a] *at loc. no.* **375**

TCMTB (21564-17-0) *See* 2-(Thiocyanomethylthio)-benzothiazole[a] *at loc. no.* **1206**

TCP *See* Tricresyl Phosphate[a] *at loc. no.* **1115**

TDE (72-54-8) *See* 1,1-Dichloro-2,2-bis(*p*-chlorophenyl)-ethane[a] *at loc. no.* **1009**

TDI (584-84-9) *See* Toluene-2,4-diisocyanate[a] *at loc. no.* **1641**

TEA (102-71-6) *See* Triethanolamine[a] *at loc. no.* **66**

Teaberry oil (119-36-8) *See* Methyl Salicylate[a] *at loc. no.* **597**

TEA-lauryl sulfate (139-96-8) *See* Alkyl Sodium Sulfates[b] *at loc. no.* **946**

"Tear gas" *See* α-Chloroacetophenone[e] *at loc. no.* **14**

Tebulan *See* Tebuthiuron[c] *at loc. no.* **1258**

Tebuthiuron (34014-18-1) *See loc. no.* **1258**

Tedion (116-29-0) *See* Tetradifon[c] *at loc. no.* **1049**

Teel *See* Alkyl Sodium Sulfates[d] *at loc. no.* **946**

Teel oil (8008-74-0) *See* Sesame Oil[a] *at loc. no.* **722**

Teepol (1847-55-8) *See* Alkyl Sodium Sulfates[c] *at loc. no.* **946**

Teflon (9002-84-0) *See* Polytetrafluoroethylene[c] *at loc. no.* **1636**

TEG (112-27-6) *See* Triethylene Glycol[a] *at loc. no.* **439**

Tellurium (13494-80-9) *See* Tellurium Derivatives[d] *at loc. no.* **187**

Tellurium Derivatives *See loc. no.* **187**

Tellurium dioxide (7446-07-3) *See* Tellurium Derivatives[d] *at loc. no.* **187**

Telodrin (297-78-9) *See* Isobenzan[c] *at loc. no.* **1024**

Telone (542-75-6) *See* 1,3-Dichloropropene[e] *at loc. no.* **386**

Telvar (150-68-5) *See* Monuron[c] *at loc. no.* **1253**

Temaril (84-96-8) *See* Trimeprazine[c] *at loc. no.* **1428**

Temasept II (87-10-5) *See* 3,4′,5-Tribromosalicylanilide[c] *at loc. no.* **1000**

Temasept IV (87-10-5) *See* 3,4′,5-Tribromosalicylanilide[a] *at loc. no.* **1000**

Temazepam (846-50-4) *See* Oxazepam[b] *at loc. no.* **1401**

Temik (116-06-3) *See* Aldicarb[c] *at loc. no.* **1120**

Temposil (8013-88-5) *See* Calcium Cyanamide[c] *at loc. no.* **1355**

Tempra (103-90-2) *See* Acetaminophen[c] *at loc. no.* **1587**

Tenoran (1982-47-4) *See* Chloroxuron[c] *at loc. no.* **1243**

Tentone (61-01-8) *See* Methoxypromazine[c] *at loc. no.* **1417**

Tenuate (134-80-5) *See* Diethylpropion[c] *at loc. no.* **1447**

TEP (107-49-3) *See* Tetraethyl Pyrophosphate[a] *at loc. no.* **1109**

Tepanil (90-84-6) *See* Diethylpropion[c] *at loc. no.* **1447**

Tephrosin (76-80-2) *See* Rotenoids[d] *at loc. no.* **897**

TEPP (107-49-3) *See* Tetraethyl Pyrophosphate[a] *at loc. no.* **1109**

Terbacil (5902-51-2) *See* Bromacil[b] *at loc. no.* **1294**

Terbumeton (33693-04-8) *See loc. no.* **1270**

Terbuthylazine (5915-41-3) *See* Atrazine[b] *at loc. no.* **1259**

Terbutol (1918-11-2) *See* 2,6-Di-*tert*-butyl-*p*-tolyl-*N*-methyl-carbamate[a] *at loc. no.* **1231**

Terbutryn (886-50-0) *See* Prometon[b] *at loc. no.* **1267**

Terebene (8014-10-6) *See loc. no.* **880**

Tergitols *See* Alkyl Sodium Sulfates[c] *at loc. no.* **946**

Termil (1897-45-6) *See* Chlorothalonil[c] *at loc. no.* **1185**

Terpene polychlorinates (8001-50-1) *See* Strobane[e] *at loc. no.* **1031**

Terpenes *See loc. no.* **881**

Terphenyl (26140-60-3) *See loc. no.* **316**

Terpineol (586-81-2) *See loc. no.* **882**

Terpin Hydrate (2451-01-6) *See loc. no.* **883**

Terpinyl thiocyanoacetate (115-31-1) *See* Thanite[e] *at loc. no.* **1038**

Terrachlor (82-68-8) *See* Pentachloronitrobenzene[c] *at loc. no.* **1201**

Terramycin (79-57-2) *See* Tetracyclines[d] *at loc. no.* **904**

Tersan 1991 *See* Benomyl[c] *at loc. no.* **1174**

Tersan SP *See* Chloroneb[c] *at loc. no.* **1184**

2,4,5-TES (3570-61-4) *See* 2,4,5-Trichlorophenoxy Ethyl Sulfate Sodium Salt[a] *at loc. no.* **1225**

Tetrabromo-*o*-cresol (576-56-5) *See loc. no.* **533**

1,1,2,2-Tetrabromoethane (79-27-6) *See loc. no.* **372**

Tetra-*n*-butyltin (1461-25-2) *See* Alkyl Tin Compounds[d] *at loc. no.* **292**

Tetracaine (94-24-6) *See loc. no.* **1586**

Tetrachloro-1,4-benzoquinone (118-75-2) *See* Chloranil[a] *at loc. no.* **1183**

Tetrachlorobiphenyl *See* PCB[b] *at loc. no.* **399**

2,4,5,6-Tetrachloro-3-cyanobenzonitrile (1897-45-6) *See* Chlorothalonil[a] *at loc. no.* **1185**

---

[a] A Synonym   [b] A Closely Related Substance   [c] The Active or Major Constituent   [d] A Class Name
[e] A Specific Example of or Product Containing

Ingredient name (CAS registry no.) *See* Primary Name *at
location no.* **XXX** *in Part D of this section*

2,3,7,8-Tetrachlorodibenzo-*p*-dioxin *See* Polychlorinated Dibenzodioxins[d] *at loc. no.* **400**

2,3,6,7-Tetrachlorodibenzofuran *See* Polychlorinated Dibenzofurans[d] *at loc. no.* **401**

Tetrachloro diphenyl ethane (72-54-8) *See* 1,1-Dichloro-2,2-bis(*p*-chlorophenyl)ethane[a] *at loc. no.* **1009**

2,4,5,4′-Tetrachlorodiphenyl sulfone (116-29-0) *See* Tetradifon[a] *at loc. no.* **1049**

1,1,2,2-Tetrachloroethane (79-34-5) *See* Tetrachloroethane[a] *at loc. no.* **373**

Tetrachloroethane (79-34-5) *See loc. no.* **373**

sym-**Tetrachloroethane** (79-34-5) *See* Tetrachloroethane[a] *at loc. no.* **373**

Tetrachloroethylene (127-18-4) *See loc. no.* **374**

Tetrachloroisophthalonitrile (1897-45-6) *See* Chlorothalonil[a] *at loc. no.* **1185**

Tetrachloromethane (56-23-5) *See* Carbon Tetrachloride[a] *at loc. no.* **355**

Tetrachloronaphthalene *See* Polychlorinated Naphthalenes[d] *at loc. no.* **402**

2,3,4,6-Tetrachlorophenol (58-90-2) *See loc. no.* **534**

Tetrachlorophthalodinitrile (1897-45-6) *See* Chlorothalonil[a] *at loc. no.* **1185**

Tetrachloroquinone (118-75-2) *See* Chloranil[a] *at loc. no.* **1183**

3,3′,4′,5-Tetrachlorosalicylanilide (1322-37-8) *See loc. no.* **999**

Tetrachlorvinfos (961-11-5) *See loc. no.* **1061**

Tetracycline (60-54-8) *See* Tetracyclines[d] *at loc. no.* **904**

Tetracyclines *See loc. no.* **904**

Tetradecanoic acid (544-63-8) *See* Myristic Acid[a] *at loc. no.* **557**

Tetradecyl alcohol (112-72-1) *See* Myristyl Alcohol[a] *at loc. no.* **424**

Tetradifon (116-29-0) *See loc. no.* **1049**

Tetraethyl dithiopyrophosphate (3689-24-5) *See* Sulfotepp[a] *at loc. no.* **1108**

Tetraethylene glycol dimethacrylate (109-17-1) *See* Acrylic Resin Monomers[d] *at loc. no.* **1625**

Tetraethylenepentamine (112-57-2) *See loc. no.* **605**

Tetraethyl Lead (78-00-2) *See loc. no.* **248**

O,O,O′,O′-**Tetraethyl-*S,S′*-methylene bis-phosphorodithioate** (563-12-2) *See* Ethion[e] *at loc. no.* **1087**

Tetraethyl Pyrophosphate (107-49-3) *See loc. no.* **1109**

Tetraethylthiuram (97-77-8) *See* Disulfiram[a] *at loc. no.* **1595**

Tetraethylthiuram disulfide (97-77-8) *See* Disulfiram[a] *at loc. no.* **1595**

Tetraglycine hydroperiodide (7097-60-1) *See* Iodine[c] *at loc. no.* **26**

Δ⁹-**Tetrahydrocannabinol** *See* Tetrahydrocannabinols[d] *at loc. no.* **933**

Tetrahydrocannabinols (1323-34-8) *See loc. no.* **933**

Tetrahydro-3,5-dimethyl-2*H*-1,3,5-thiadiazine-2-thione (533-74-4) *See* Dazomet[a] *at loc. no.* **1186**

Tetrahydrofuran (109-99-9) *See loc. no.* **1623**

Tetrahydrofurfuryl alcohol polyethylene glycol ether (9004-76-6) *See* Glycofurol[e] *at loc. no.* **460**

Tetrahydronaphthalene (119-64-2) *See loc. no.* **322**

Tetrahydro-1,4-oxazine (110-91-8) *See* Morpholine[a] *at loc. no.* **72**

Tetrahydrozoline Hydrochloride (522-48-5) *See loc. no.* **1469**

Tetralin (119-64-2) *See* Tetrahydronaphthalene[c] *at loc. no.* **322**

Tetram (78-53-5) *See loc. no.* **1080**

Tetramethrin (7696-12-0) *See loc. no.* **898**

Tetramethylene disulphotetramine (7076-28-0) *See* Tetramine[e] *at loc. no.* **1348**

Tetramethyl lead (75-74-1) *See* Tetraethyl Lead[b] *at loc. no.* **248**

Tetramethyl-1-nonanol *See* Tridecyl Alcohol[e] *at loc. no.* **431**

Tetramethylphosphorodiamidic fluoride (115-26-4) *See* Dimefox[a] *at loc. no.* **1098**

N,N,N′,N′-**Tetramethyl phosphorodiamidic fluoride** (115-26-4) *See* Dimefox[a] *at loc. no.* **1098**

O,O,O′,O′-**Tetramethyl-*O,O*-thiodi-*p*-phenylene phosphorothioate** (3383-96-8) *See* Abate[a] *at loc. no.* **1063**

Tetramethylthionine chloride (61-73-4) *See* Methylene Blue[a] *at loc. no.* **1521**

Tetramethylthiuram disulfide (137-26-8) *See* Thiram[a] *at loc. no.* **1165**

Tetramine (7076-28-0) *See loc. no.* **1348**

Tetranap (119-64-2) *See* Tetrahydronaphthalene[c] *at loc. no.* **322**

Tetrapotassium pyrophosphate (7320-34-5) *See* Tetrasodium Pyrophosphate[b] *at loc. no.* **140**

Tetra-*n*-propyl Dithionopyrophosphate (3244-90-4) *See loc. no.* **1110**

Tetrapropylene Benzene Sulfonate (Sodium) *See loc. no.* **959**

Tetrasodium ethylenediaminetetraacetate (64-02-8) *See* Ethylenediaminetetraacetic Acid (and Salts)[b] *at loc. no.* **1506**

Tetrasodium Pyrophosphate (7722-88-5) *See loc. no.* **140**

Tetrosan (8023-53-8) *See* Alkyl Dimethyl 3,4-Dichlorobenzene Ammonium Chloride[d] *at loc. no.* **976**

Thalamyd *See* Phthalylsulfacetamide[c] *at loc. no.* **1547**

Thalidomide (50-35-1) *See loc. no.* **1443**

Thallium (7440-28-0) *See loc. no.* **249**

Thallium acetate (563-68-8) *See* Thallium[d] *at loc. no.* **249**

Thallium sulfate (7446-18-6) *See* Thallium[d] *at loc. no.* **249**

THAM (77-86-1) *See* Tris(hydroxymethyl)aminomethane[c] *at loc. no.* **69**

Thanite (115-31-1) *See loc. no.* **1038**

Thenylpyramine (91-80-5) *See* Methapyrilene Hydrochloride[b] *at loc. no.* **1495**

Thenylpyramine hydrochloride (135-23-9) *See* Methapyrilene Hydrochloride[a] *at loc. no.* **1495**

Theobroma Oil (8002-31-1) *See loc. no.* **742**

Theobromine (83-67-0) *See loc. no.* **801**

Theophylline (58-55-9) *See loc. no.* **802**

Theophylline calcium salicylate (129-98-6) *See* Theophylline[b] *at loc. no.* **802**

Theophylline ethylenediamine (317-34-0) *See* Aminophylline[a] *at loc. no.* **799**

Theophylline monoethanolamine (573-41-1) *See* Theophylline[b] *at loc. no.* **802**

Theophylline olamine (573-41-1) *See* Theophylline[b] *at loc. no.* **802**

Theophylline sodium acetate (8002-89-9) *See* Theophylline[b] *at loc. no.* **802**

Theophylline sodium glycinate (8000-10-0) *See* Theophylline[b] *at loc. no.* **802**

Thesit (1334-72-1) *See* Laureth 9[b] *at loc. no.* **966**

Thiabendazole (148-79-8) *See loc. no.* **1177**

Thiabenzole (148-79-8) *See* Thiabendazole[a] *at loc. no.* **1177**

Thiacol *See* Potassium Guaiacolsulfonate[a] *at loc. no.* **496**

Thialbarbital (467-36-7) *See loc. no.* **1388**

Thialbarbitone (467-36-7) *See* Thialbarbital[a] *at loc. no.* **1388**

Thiamine (59-43-8) *See loc. no.* **914**

---

[a] A Synonym   [b] A Closely Related Substance   [c] The Active or Major Constituent   [d] A Class Name
[e] A Specific Example of or Product Containing

Ingredient name (CAS registry no.) *See* Primary Name *at*
location no. **XXX** *in Part D of this section*

Thiamine hydrochloride (67-03-8) *See* Thiamine[b] *at loc. no.* **914**

Thiamine mononitrate (532-43-4) *See* Thiamine[b] *at loc. no.* **914**

Thiamylal Sodium (337-47-3) *See loc. no.* **1389**

2-(4-Thiazolyl)-1*H*-benzimidazole (148-79-8) *See* Thiabendazole[a] *at loc. no.* **1177**

4′-(2-Thiazolylsulfamoyl)succinanilic acid (116-43-8) *See* Succinylsulfathiazole[a] *at loc. no.* **1549**

N[1]-2-Thiazolylsulfanilamide (72-14-0) *See* Sulfathiazole[a] *at loc. no.* **1567**

Thiethylperazine (1420-55-9) *See loc. no.* **1423**

Thiethylperazine malate (52239-63-1) *See* Thiethylperazine[b] *at loc. no.* **1423**

Thiethylperazine maleate (1179-69-7) *See* Thiethylperazine[b] *at loc. no.* **1423**

Thimerosal (54-64-8) *See loc. no.* **244**

Thimet (298-02-2) *See* Phorate[c] *at loc. no.* **1094**

Thioacetamide (62-55-5) *See loc. no.* **121**

Thiobencarb (28249-77-6) *See loc. no.* **1239**

2,2-Thiobis(4,6-dichlorophenol) (97-18-7) *See* Bithionol[a] *at loc. no.* **521**

Thiocarbamide (62-56-6) *See* Thiourea[a] *at loc. no.* **1352**

Thiocarbonyl chloride (463-71-8) *See* Thiophosgene[a] *at loc. no.* **12**

Thioctic Acid (62-46-4) *See loc. no.* **1510**

Thiocyanate Salts *See loc. no.* **146**

Thiocyanates (organic) *See* Aliphatic Thiocyanates[d] *at loc. no.* **1034**

2-Thiocyanoethyl dodecanoate (301-11-1) *See* Lethane 60[e] *at loc. no.* **1037**

β-Thiocyanoethyl esters of fatty acids *See* Lethane 60[a] *at loc. no.* **1037**

β-Thiocyanoethyl laurate (301-11-1) *See* Lethane 60[e] *at loc. no.* **1037**

2-Thiocyanomethylthio)-benzothiazide (21564-17-0) *See* 2-(Thiocyanomethylthio)-benzothiazole[a] *at loc. no.* **1206**

2-(Thiocyanomethylthio)-benzothiazole (21564-17-0) *See loc. no.* **1206**

Thiodan (115-29-7) *See loc. no.* **1026**

Thiodemeton (298-04-4) *See* Disulfoton[a] *at loc. no.* **1086**

Thiodiphenylamine (92-84-2) *See* Phenothiazine[a] *at loc. no.* **1543**

Thioglycolate Salts *See loc. no.* **552**

Thioglycolic Acid (68-11-1) *See loc. no.* **49**

Thioglycollate salts *See* Thioglycolate Salts[a] *at loc. no.* **552**

Thiomersalate (54-64-8) *See* Thimerosal[a] *at loc. no.* **244**

Thiomethyl alcohol *See* Methanethiol[a] *at loc. no.* **116**

Thionazin (297-97-2) *See loc. no.* **1081**

Thiopental Sodium (71-73-8) *See loc. no.* **1390**

Thiophanate (23564-06-9) *See* Thiophanate-methyl[b] *at loc. no.* **1207**

Thiophanate-methyl (23564-05-8) *See loc. no.* **1207**

Thiophos 3422 (56-38-2) *See* Parathion[c] *at loc. no.* **1077**

Thiophosgene (463-71-8) *See loc. no.* **12**

Thiophosphoric anhydride (1314-80-3) *See* Phosphorus Pentasulfide[a] *at loc. no.* **117**

Thiopropazate Dihydrochloride (146-28-1) *See loc. no.* **1424**

Thioquinox (93-75-4) *See* Eradex[a] *at loc. no.* **1044**

Thioridazine (50-52-2) *See loc. no.* **1425**

Thioseconal (77-27-0) *See* Thiamylal Sodium[b] *at loc. no.* **1389**

Thiosulfate Salts *See loc. no.* **161**

Thiosulfil *See* Sulfamethizole[c] *at loc. no.* **1560**

Thiothixene (3313-26-6) *See* Chlorprothixene[b] *at loc. no.* **1414**

Thiourea (62-56-6) *See loc. no.* **1352**

Thiram (137-26-8) *See loc. no.* **1165**

Thiuram (137-26-8) *See* Thiram[a] *at loc. no.* **1165**

Thonzylamine (91-85-0) *See* Antihistaminics[d] *at loc. no.* **1487**

Thorazine (50-53-3) *See* Chlorpromazine[c] *at loc. no.* **1412**

Thorn apple *See* Stramonium[a] *at loc. no.* **696**

Thyme camphor (89-83-8) *See* Thymol[a] *at loc. no.* **497**

Thyme Oil (8007-46-3) *See loc. no.* **743**

Thymol (89-83-8) *See loc. no.* **497**

Thymol iodide (552-22-7) *See* Thymol[b] *at loc. no.* **497**

Thyroid *See loc. no.* **920**

Thyroxine (51-48-9) *See* Thyroid[d] *at loc. no.* **920**

2,3,5-TIBA (88-82-4) *See* 2,3,5-Tri-iodobenzoic Acid[a] *at loc. no.* **1318**

Tiguvon (55-38-9) *See* Fenthion[c] *at loc. no.* **1073**

Tillam (1114-71-2) *See* Pebulate[c] *at loc. no.* **1238**

Tinactin (2398-96-1) *See* Tolnaftate[c] *at loc. no.* **1532**

Tinaderm (2398-96-1) *See* Tolnaftate[c] *at loc. no.* **1532**

Tincture of benzoin *See* Benzoin[c] *at loc. no.* **750**

Tincture of merthiolate *See* Thimerosal[c] *at loc. no.* **244**

Tincture of opium (8013-60-3) *See* Laudanum[a] *at loc. no.* **765**

Tincture of valerian *See* Valerian[c] *at loc. no.* **699**

Tindal (5714-00-1) *See* Acetophenazine[b] *at loc. no.* **1413**

Tin salts *See* Stannic and Stannous Salts[a] *at loc. no.* **290**

Titanium dioxide (1309-63-3) *See* Titanium Oxide[a] *at loc. no.* **296**

Titanium Oxide (1309-63-3) *See loc. no.* **296**

TMA *See* 2,5-Dimethoxy-4-methyl-amphetamine[b] *at loc. no.* **1449**

TMTD (137-26-8) *See* Thiram[a] *at loc. no.* **1165**

TNT (118-96-7) *See* 2,4,6-Trinitrotoluene[a] *at loc. no.* **645**

Toadstools poisonous *See* Mushroom Toxins[c] *at loc. no.* **812**

Tobacco *See loc. no.* **697**

α-Tocopherol (59-02-9) *See* Vitamin E[a] *at loc. no.* **910**

TOCP (78-30-8) *See* Tri-*o*-cresyl Phosphate[a] *at loc. no.* **1116**

Tofranil (50-49-7) *See* Imipramine[c] *at loc. no.* **1473**

Tok (1836-75-5) *See* Nitrofen[a] *at loc. no.* **1310**

Tolnaftate (2398-96-1) *See loc. no.* **1532**

Tolonium Chloride (92-31-9) *See loc. no.* **1523**

3-*o*-Toloxy-1,2-propanediol (59-47-2) *See* Mephenesin[a] *at loc. no.* **1406**

Tolserol (59-47-2) *See* Mephenesin[c] *at loc. no.* **1406**

o-Toluanilide (7055-03-0) *See loc. no.* **1208**

Tolu balsam *See* Balsam Peru[b] *at loc. no.* **749**

Toluene (108-88-3) *See loc. no.* **317**

p-Toluenediamine (95-80-7) *See* 2,4-Diaminotoluene[a] *at loc. no.* **621**

Toluene-2,4-diisocyanate (584-84-9) *See loc. no.* **1641**

Toluene-2,6-diisocyanate (91-08-7) *See* Toluene-2,4-diisocyanate[b] *at loc. no.* **1641**

o-Toluidine (95-53-4) *See* *p*-Toluidine[b] *at loc. no.* **618**

p-Toluidine (106-49-0) *See loc. no.* **618**

Toluidine blue (92-31-9) *See* Tolonium Chloride[a] *at loc. no.* **1523**

Toluol (108-88-3) *See* Toluene[a] *at loc. no.* **317**

Tolylene diisocyanate (584-84-9) *See* Toluene-2,4-diisocyanate[a] *at loc. no.* **1641**

Tolylfluanid (731-27-1) *See* Dichlofluanid[b] *at loc. no.* **1189**

m-Tolyl-*N*-methylcarbamate (1129-41-5) *See* MPMC[b] *at loc. no.* **1143**

N-*m*-Tolylphthalamic Acid (85-72-3) *See loc. no.* **1284**

Tomaset (85-72-3) *See* *N*-*m*-Tolylphthalamic Acid[c] *at loc. no.* **1284**

---

[a] A Synonym   [b] A Closely Related Substance   [c] The Active or Major Constituent   [d] A Class Name
[e] A Specific Example of or Product Containing

Ingredient name (CAS registry no.) *See* Primary Name *at*
location no. **XXX** *in Part D of this section*

Tomatotone (122-88-3) *See* p-Chlorophenoxyacetic Acid[a] *at loc. no.* **1211**

Tomorin (81-82-3) *See* Coumachlor[c] *at loc. no.* **1336**

Tonoftal (2398-96-1) *See* Tolnaftate[c] *at loc. no.* **1532**

Tordon (1918-02-1) *See* Picloram[a] *at loc. no.* **1312**

Tordon K (2545-60-0) *See* Picloram[b] *at loc. no.* **1312**

Torecan (1420-55-9) *See* Thiethylperazine[c] *at loc. no.* **1423**

Toxaphene (8001-35-2) *See loc. no.* **1030**

Toxicarol (76-80-2) *See* Rotenoids[d] *at loc. no.* **897**

2,4,5-TP (93-72-1) *See* Silvex[a] *at loc. no.* **1223**

Tragacanth (9000-65-1) *See* Gums (Vegetable)[d] *at loc. no.* **755**

Trancopal (80-77-3) *See* Chlormezanone[c] *at loc. no.* **1404**

Tranxene (57109-90-7) *See* Clorazepate Dipotassium[c] *at loc. no.* **1394**

Tranylcypromine (95-62-5) *See loc. no.* **1480**

Trapex (556-61-6) *See* Methyl Isothiocyanate[a] *at loc. no.* **1358**

Treflan (1582-09-8) *See* Trifluralin[c] *at loc. no.* **1289**

Tremolite *See* Asbestos[e] *at loc. no.* **2**

Triacetin (102-76-1) *See loc. no.* **579**

Triadimefon (43121-43-3) *See loc. no.* **1271**

Trialkyl thiophosphate *See* Parathion[e] *at loc. no.* **1077**

Trialkyl Tin Compounds *See loc. no.* **293**

Tri-allate (2303-17-5) *See* Di-allate[b] *at loc. no.* **1235**

Triamcinolone (124-94-7) *See* Corticosteroids[d] *at loc. no.* **915**

Triamifos (1031-47-6) *See* Triamiphos[a] *at loc. no.* **1209**

Triamiphos (1031-47-6) *See loc. no.* **1209**

Triaryl phosphate *See* Tricresyl Phosphate[e] *at loc. no.* **1115**

Triazabutil (16227-10-4) *See loc. no.* **1272**

2,4,6-s-Triazinetriol (504-19-8) *See* Cyanuric Acid[a] *at loc. no.* **1261**

2,4,6(1H,3H,5H)-s-Triazinetrione (504-19-8) *See* Cyanuric Acid[a] *at loc. no.* **1261**

Tribasic Copper Sulfate (1332-03-2) *See loc. no.* **270**

Tribasic potassium phosphate (7778-53-2) *See* Potassium Phosphate (Tribasic)[a] *at loc. no.* **59**

3,4',5-Tribromosalicylanilide (87-10-5) *See loc. no.* **1000**

Tribromsalan (87-10-5) *See* 3,4',5-Tribromosalicylanilide[a] *at loc. no.* **1000**

Tributyl Phosphate (126-73-8) *See loc. no.* **1113**

S,S,S-Tributyl Phosphorotrithioate (78-48-8) *See loc. no.* **1111**

Tributyl Phosphorotrithioite (150-50-5) *See loc. no.* **1114**

Tributyltin acetate (56-36-0) *See* Trialkyl Tin Compounds[d] *at loc. no.* **293**

Tributyltin benzoate (4342-36-3) *See* Trialkyl Tin Compounds[d] *at loc. no.* **293**

Tributyltin fluoride (1983-10-4) *See* Trialkyl Tin Compounds[d] *at loc. no.* **293**

Tributyltin hydroxide (1067-97-6) *See* Trialkyl Tin Compounds[d] *at loc. no.* **293**

Tricalcium arsenate (7778-44-1) *See* Calcium Arsenate[a] *at loc. no.* **198**

Tricamba (2307-49-5) *See* Dicamba (and Salts)[b] *at loc. no.* **1300**

Trichlorfon (52-68-6) *See loc. no.* **1062**

Trichlormethiazide (133-67-5) *See* Benzothiadiazide Diuretics[d] *at loc. no.* **1588**

Trichloroacetic Acid (76-03-9) *See loc. no.* **50**

Trichloroacetonitrile (545-06-2) *See loc. no.* **655**

S-(2,3,3-Trichloroallyl)-diisopropylthiocarbamate (2303-17-5) *See* Di-allate[b] *at loc. no.* **1235**

3,5,6-Trichloro-o-anisic acid (2307-49-5) *See* Dicamba (and Salts)[b] *at loc. no.* **1300**

1,2,3-Trichlorobenzene (87-61-6) *See* Trichlorobenzenes[d] *at loc. no.* **403**

Trichlorobenzenes *See loc. no.* **403**

2,3,5-Trichlorobenzoic acid (50-73-7) *See* Trichlorobenzoic Acid[d] *at loc. no.* **1317**

2,4,6-Trichlorobenzoic acid (50-43-1) *See* Trichlorobenzoic Acid[d] *at loc. no.* **1317**

Trichlorobenzoic Acid (1319-85-3) *See loc. no.* **1317**

2,3,6-Trichlorobenzoic acid dimethylamine salt (3426-62-8) *See* Trichlorobenzoic Acid[b] *at loc. no.* **1317**

Trichlorobenzyl Chloride (1344-32-7) *See loc. no.* **1361**

1,1,1-Trichloro-2,2-bis(p-chlorophenyl)ethane (50-29-3) *See* DDT[a] *at loc. no.* **1007**

1,1,1-Trichloro-2,2-bis(p-fluorophenyl)-1-ethane (475-26-3) *See* DFDT[a] *at loc. no.* **1008**

1,1,1-Trichloro-2,2-bis(p-methoxyphenyl)ethane (72-43-5) *See* Methoxychlor[a] *at loc. no.* **1013**

β,β,β-Trichloro-tert-butyl alcohol (57-15-8) *See* Chlorobutanol[a] *at loc. no.* **432**

3,4,4'-Trichlorocarbanilide (101-20-2) *See loc. no.* **1001**

Trichlorodinitrobenzene (6379-46-0) *See loc. no.* **1202**

1,1,1-Trichloroethane (71-55-6) *See loc. no.* **377**

1,1,2-Trichloroethane (79-00-5) *See loc. no.* **376**

α-Trichloroethane (71-55-6) *See* 1,1,1-Trichloroethane[a] *at loc. no.* **377**

β-Trichloroethane (79-00-5) *See* 1,1,2-Trichloroethane[a] *at loc. no.* **376**

2,2,2-Trichloro-1,1-ethanediol (302-17-0) *See* Chloral Hydrate[a] *at loc. no.* **1432**

Trichloroethanol (115-20-8) *See* Chloral Hydrate[b] *at loc. no.* **1432**

Trichloroethene (79-01-6) *See* Trichloroethylene[a] *at loc. no.* **375**

Trichloroethylene (79-01-6) *See loc. no.* **375**

Trichlorofluoroethane *See loc. no.* **353**

2,4,4'-Trichloro-2'-hydroxydiphenyl ether (3380-34-5) *See* Triclosan[a] *at loc. no.* **1002**

Trichloroisocyanuric Acid (87-90-1) *See loc. no.* **94**

Trichloromethane (67-66-3) *See* Chloroform[a] *at loc. no.* **357**

N-Trichloromethylmercapto-4-cyclohexene-1,2-dicarboximide (133-06-2) *See* Captan[a] *at loc. no.* **1179**

Trichloromethylnitrile *See* Trichloroacetonitrile[a] *at loc. no.* **655**

1,1,1-Trichloro-2-methyl-2-propanol (57-15-8) *See* Chlorobutanol[a] *at loc. no.* **432**

N-(Trichloromethylthio)-4-cyclohexene-1,2-dicarboximide (133-06-2) *See* Captan[a] *at loc. no.* **1179**

N-(Trichloromethylthio)phthalimide (133-07-3) *See* Folpet[e] *at loc. no.* **1181**

N-Trichloromethylthio-3α,4,7,7α-tetrahydrophthalimide (133-06-2) *See* Captan[a] *at loc. no.* **1179**

Trichloromonofluoromethane (75-69-4) *See loc. no.* **351**

Trichloronaphthalenes *See* Polychlorinated Naphthalenes[d] *at loc. no.* **402**

Trichloronitromethane (76-06-2) *See* Chloropicrin[a] *at loc. no.* **13**

2,4,5-Trichlorophenol (95-95-4) *See* Trichlorophenols[d] *at loc. no.* **535**

2,4,6-Trichlorophenol (88-06-2) *See* Trichlorophenols[d] *at loc. no.* **535**

Trichlorophenols *See loc. no.* **535**

Trichlorophenoxyacetic Acid (93-76-5) *See loc. no.* **1224**

2-(2,4,5-Trichlorophenoxy)ethyl-2,2-dichloropropionate (136-25-4) *See* Erbon[a] *at loc. no.* **1218**

2,4,5-Trichlorophenoxy Ethyl Sulfate Sodium Salt (3570-61-4) *See loc. no.* **1225**

2-(2,4,5-Trichlorophenoxy)propionic acid (93-72-1) *See* Silvex[a] *at loc. no.* **1223**

---

[a] A Synonym   [b] A Closely Related Substance   [c] The Active or Major Constituent   [d] A Class Name
[e] A Specific Example of or Product Containing

Ingredient name (CAS registry no.) *See* Primary Name *at
location no.* **XXX** *in Part D of this section*

2,3,6-**Trichlorophenylacetic acid** (85-34-7) *See* Fenac[e] *at
loc. no.* **1219**

2,4,5-**Trichlorophenylacetic acid** (5393-75-9) *See* Fenac[e] *at
loc. no.* **1219**

2,3,6-**Trichlorophenylacetic acid ammonium salt** *See*
Fenac[b] *at loc. no.* **1219**

2,3,6-**Trichlorophenylacetic acid dimethylamine salt** *See*
Fenac[b] *at loc. no.* **1219**

2,3,6-**Trichlorophenylacetic acid sodium salt** (2439-00-1)
See Fenac[b] *at loc. no.* **1219**

2,4,5-**Trichlorophenylacetic acid sodium salt** *See* Fenac[b]
at loc. no. **1219**

2,4,5-**Trichlorophenyl-γ-iodopropargyl ether** (777-11-7)
See Haloprogin[a] *at loc. no.* **1527**

Trichlorotriazinetrione (87-90-1) *See* Trichloroisocyanuric
Acid[a] *at loc. no.* **94**

Triclocarban (101-20-2) *See* 3,4,4'-Trichlorocarbanilide[a] *at
loc. no.* **1001**

Triclosan (3380-34-5) *See loc. no.* **1002**

Tricresol (8003-33-6) *See* Cresols[a] *at loc. no.* **514**

Tri-o-cresyl Phosphate (78-30-8) *See loc. no.* **1116**

Tricresyl Phosphate (1330-78-5) *See loc. no.* **1115**

o-**Tricresyl phosphate** (78-30-8) *See* Tri-o-cresyl Phosphate[a]
at loc. no. **1116**

Tricyclodecan-1-amine (768-94-5) *See* Amantadine[a] *at loc.
no.* **922**

Tricyclohexyltin hydroxide (13121-70-5) *See* Trialkyl Tin
Compounds *at loc. no.* **293**

Tridecyl Alcohol *See loc. no.* **431**

n-**Tridecyl alcohol** (112-70-9) *See* Tridecyl Alcohol[e] *at loc.
no.* **431**

1-**Tridecyl-2-methyl-2-hydroxyethyl imidazolinium
chloride** (1301-19-5) *See* Alkyl Hydroxyethyl Imidazolinium Chloride[c] *at loc. no.* **979**

Trieste flowers *See* Pyrethrum[a] *at loc. no.* **686**

Trietazine (1912-26-1) *See* Atrazine[b] *at loc. no.* **1259**

Triethanolamine (102-71-6) *See loc. no.* **66**

Triethanolamine alcohol sulfate salts *See* Alkyl Sodium
Sulfates[b] *at loc. no.* **946**

Triethanolamine   2-(2,4-dichlorophenoxy)propionate
See 2-(2,4-Dichlorophenoxy)propionic Acid[b] *at loc. no.*
1217

Triethanolamine dinoseb *See* Dinoseb[b] *at loc. no.* **543**

Triethanolamine dodecylbenzenesulfonate (27323-41-7)
See Alkyl Aryl Sodium Sulfonates[d] *at loc. no.* **943**

Triethanolamine lauryl sulfate (139-96-8) *See* Alkyl Sodium Sulfates[b] *at loc. no.* **946**

Triethanolamine methanearsonate *See* Disodium Methanearsonate[b] *at loc. no.* **203**

Triethanolamine 2-methyl-4-chlorophenoxyacetate *See*
MCPA[b] *at loc. no.* **1220**

Triethanolamine Oleate (2717-15-9) *See loc. no.* **960**

Triethanolamine salicylate (2174-16-5) *See* Salicylate[d] *at
loc. no.* **600**

Triethanolamine salt of 2,4,5-T (3813-14-7) *See* Trichlorophenoxyacetic Acid[b] *at loc. no.* **1224**

Triethanolamine Salts *See loc. no.* **67**

Triethanolamine soap *See* Triethanolamine Oleate[e] *at loc.
no.* **960**

Triethanolamine stearate (4568-28-9) *See* Triethanolamine
Oleate[b] *at loc. no.* **960**

Triethylamine picloram *See* Picloram[b] *at loc. no.* **1312**

Triethylamine salt of 2,4,5-T *See* Trichlorophenoxyacetic
Acid[b] *at loc. no.* **1224**

Triethylene Glycol (112-27-6) *See loc. no.* **439**

Triethylenetetramine (112-24-3) *See loc. no.* **604**

Triethyl phosphate (78-40-0) *See* Ethyl Phosphates[d] *at loc.
no.* **1112**

Triethyltin borate *See* Trialkyl Tin Compounds[d] *at loc. no.*
293

Triethyltin chloride (994-31-0) *See* Trialkyl Tin Compounds[d] *at loc. no.* **293**

Triethyltin sulfate (57-52-3) *See* Trialkyl Tin Compounds[d]
at loc. no. **293**

Trifluomeprazine (2622-37-9) *See* Triflupromazine Hydrochloride[b] *at loc. no.* **1427**

Trifluoperazine (117-89-5) *See loc. no.* **1426**

α,α,α-**Trifluoro-2,6-dinitro-N,N-dipropyl-p-toluidine**
(1582-09-8) *See* Trifluralin[a] *at loc. no.* **1289**

1-(3-**Trifluoromethyltrityl)-1,2,4-triazole** (31251-03-3) *See*
Fluotrimazole[a] *at loc. no.* **1171**

Triflupromazine Hydrochloride (1098-60-8) *See loc. no.*
1427

Trifluralin (1582-09-8) *See loc. no.* **1289**

Triforine (26644-46-2) *See loc. no.* **1210**

Triformol (9002-81-7) *See* Paraformaldehyde[a] *at loc. no.* **487**

Trihexylphenidyl (144-11-6) *See* Benactyzine[b] *at loc. no.*
1430

Trihistan (129-71-5) *See* Chlorcyclizine[c] *at loc. no.* **1489**

1,2,3-**Trihydroxybenzene** (87-66-1) *See* Pyrogallol[a] *at loc.
no.* **506**

1,3,5-**Trihydroxybenzene** (108-73-6) *See* Pyrogallol[b] *at loc.
no.* **506**

3,4,5-**Trihydroxybenzoic acid** (149-91-7) *See* Gallic Acid[a]
at loc. no. **502**

Trihydroxycyanidine (504-19-8) *See* Cyanuric Acid[a] *at loc.
no.* **1261**

Tri(hydroxyethyl)amine (102-71-6) *See* Triethanolamine[a]
at loc. no. **66**

1,2,6-**Trihydroxyhexane** (106-69-4) *See* 1,2,6-Hexanetriol[a]
at loc. no. **446**

Trihydroxypropane (56-81-5) *See* Glycerin[a] *at loc. no.* **704**

Trihydroxytriazine (504-19-8) *See* Cyanuric Acid[a] *at loc.
no.* **1261**

Trihydroxytriethylamine (102-71-6) *See* Triethanolamine[a]
at loc. no. **66**

2,3,5-**Tri-iodobenzoic Acid** (88-82-4) *See loc. no.* **1318**

Tri-iodobenzoic acid dimethylamine salt *See* 2,3,5-Tri-
iodobenzoic Acid[b] *at loc. no.* **1318**

Tri-iodomethane (75-47-8) *See* Iodoform[a] *at loc. no.* **1529**

Triiodothyronine (6893-02-3) *See* Thyroid[d] *at loc. no.* **920**

**Triisopropanolamine   2-methyl-4-chlorophenoxyace-
tate** *See* MCPA[b] *at loc. no.* **1220**

Triisopropanolamine picloram *See* Picloram[b] *at loc. no.*
1312

Trilafon (58-39-9) *See* Perphenazine[c] *at loc. no.* **1418**

Trilene (79-01-6) *See* Trichloroethylene[c] *at loc. no.* **375**

Tri-Me *See* Methyl Trithion[a] *at loc. no.* **1092**

Trimeprazine (84-96-8) *See loc. no.* **1428**

Trimethoxyamphetamine (1082-88-8) *See* 2,5-Dimethoxy-
4-methyl-amphetamine[b] *at loc. no.* **1449**

3,4,5-**Trimethoxyphenylethylamine** (54-04-6) *See* Mescaline[a] *at loc. no.* **830**

3,5,5-**Trimethyl-2-cyclohexene-1-one** (78-59-1) *See* Isophorone[a] *at loc. no.* **473**

Trimethyl-1-heptanol *See* Decyl Alcohol[e] *at loc. no.* **411**

2,3,5-**Trimethylphenyl methylcarbamate** (2655-15-4) *See*
Landrin[b] *at loc. no.* **1138**

3,4,5-**Trimethylphenyl methylcarbamate** (2686-99-9) *See*
Landrin[a] *at loc. no.* **1138**

Trimethyltin hydroxide (56-24-6) *See* Trialkyl Tin Compounds[d] *at loc. no.* **293**

_____

[a] A Synonym   [b] A Closely Related Substance   [c] The Active or Major Constituent   [d] A Class Name
[e] A Specific Example of or Product Containing

Ingredient name (CAS registry no.) *See* Primary Name *at
location no.* **XXX** *in Part D of this section*

1,3,7-Trimethylxanthine (58-08-2) *See* Caffeine[a] *at loc. no.*
800

Trimeton (86-21-5) *See* Pheniramine Maleate[c] *at loc. no.*
1497

Trimeturon (3050-27-9) *See* Phenobenzuron[b] *at loc. no.* **1256**

Trimipramine (739-71-9) *See loc. no.* **1481**

1,3,5-Trinitrobenzene (99-35-4) *See* Trinitrobenzene[d] *at loc.
no.* **644**

Trinitrobenzene (25377-32-6) *See loc. no.* **644**

2,4,6-Trinitrophenol (88-89-1) *See* Picric Acid[a] *at loc. no.*
545

2,4,6-Trinitrotoluene (118-96-7) *See loc. no.* **645**

Triorthocresyl phosphate (78-30-8) *See* Tri-*o*-cresyl Phosphate[a] *at loc. no.* **1116**

Trioxymethylene (9002-81-7) *See* Paraformaldehyde[a] *at loc.
no.* **487**

Tripelennamine Hydrochloride (154-69-8) *See loc. no.*
1500

Triphenyl Phosphate (115-86-6) *See loc. no.* **1117**

Triphenylphosphine (603-35-0) *See* Phosphine[b] *at loc. no.*
136

Triphenyltin Acetate (900-95-8) *See loc. no.* **295**

Triphenyltin chloride (639-58-7) *See* Triphenyltin Acetate[b]
at loc. no. **295**

Triphenyltin hydroxide (76-87-9) *See* Triphenyltin Acetate[b]
at loc. no. **295**

Tripolyphosphate (14127-68-5) *See loc. no.* **142**

Triprolidine hydrochloride (550-70-9) *See* Antihistaminics[d]
at loc. no. **1487**

Tripropylene glycol isobutyl ether ester of 2,4,5-T *See*
Trichlorophenoxyacetic Acid[b] *at loc. no.* **1224**

TRIS (126-72-7) *See* Tris(2,3-dibromopropyl)phosphate[a] *at
loc. no.* **1118**

Tris (77-86-1) *See* Tris(hydroxymethyl)aminomethane[a] *at loc.
no.* **69**

Tris(1-aziridinyl)phosphine oxide (545-55-1) *See* Apholate[b] *at loc. no.* **1354**

Tris-BP (126-72-7) *See* Tris(2,3-dibromopropyl)phosphate[a] *at
loc. no.* **1118**

Tris (2,3-chloro-1-propyl)phosphate *See* Tris(1,3-dichloro-2-propyl)phosphate[b] *at loc. no.* **1119**

Tris(2,3-dibromopropyl)phosphate (126-72-7) *See loc. no.*
1118

Tris(1,3-dichloroisopropyl)phosphate (78-43-3) *See*
Tris(1,3-dichloro-2-propyl)phosphate[a] *at loc. no.* **1119**

Tris[(2,4-dichlorophenoxy)ethyl]phosphite (94-84-8) *See*
Falone[e] *at loc. no.* **1306**

Tris(1,3-dichloro-2-propyl)phosphate (78-43-3) *See loc.
no.* **1119**

Tris(hydroxymethyl)aminomethane (77-86-1) *See loc. no.*
69

Tris(hydroxymethyl)nitromethane (126-11-4) *See loc. no.*
1003

Tris(2-methyl-1-aziridinyl)phosphine oxide (57-39-6) *See*
Apholate[b] *at loc. no.* **1354**

Tris nitro *See* Tris(hydroxymethyl)nitromethane[a] *at loc. no.*
1003

Trisodium Phosphate (7601-54-9) *See loc. no.* **60**

Trisulfapyrimidines *See loc. no.* **1569**

Trithion (786-19-6) *See* Carbophenothion[c] *at loc. no.* **1083**

Tri-*o*-tolyl phosphate (78-30-8) *See* Tri-*o*-cresyl Phosphate[a]
at loc. no. **1116**

Tritolyl phosphate (1330-78-5) *See* Tricresyl Phosphate[a] *at
loc. no.* **1115**

Triton 770 (12627-37-1) *See* Alkyl Aryl Polyether Sulfates
and Sulfonates[c] *at loc. no.* **942**

Tritons X-45, X-100, X-102, X-114 (9004-88-0) *See* Alkyl
Phenoxy Polyethoxy Ethanols[d] *at loc. no.* **963**

Triton X-200 (9010-41-7) *See* Alkyl Aryl Polyether Sulfates
and Sulfonates[c] *at loc. no.* **942**

Triton X-301 (12627-38-2) *See* Alkyl Aryl Polyether Sulfates
and Sulfonates[c] *at loc. no.* **942**

Triton X-400 or K-60 (122-19-0) *See* Stearyl Dimethyl Benzyl Ammonium Chloride[c] *at loc. no.* **990**

Tritox (545-06-2) *See* Trichloroacetonitrile[c] *at loc. no.* **655**

Tromethamine (77-86-1) *See* Tris(hydroxymethyl)-aminomethane[a] *at loc. no.* **69**

Tromexan (548-00-5) *See* Ethyl Biscoumacetate[c] *at loc. no.*
1340

Tropital (5281-13-0) *See loc. no.* **1156**

Tropotox (6062-26-6) *See* 4-(2-Methyl-4-chlorophenoxy)-butyric Acid[c] *at loc. no.* **1222**

Trypan Blue (72-57-1) *See loc. no.* **1524**

Trypan red (574-64-1) *See* Trypan Blue[b] *at loc. no.* **1524**

Tryptaflavine (8048-52-0) *See* Acridine Antiseptics[d] *at loc.
no.* **1518**

"T's and Blues" *See loc. no.* **1501**

Tsumacide (1129-41-5) *See* MPMC[b] *at loc. no.* **1143**

TTD (97-77-8) *See* Disulfiram[a] *at loc. no.* **1595**

Tuads (137-26-8) *See* Thiram[a] *at loc. no.* **1165**

Tuba-root *See* Derris Powder[a] *at loc. no.* **665**

Tung nuts *See* Tung Oil[b] *at loc. no.* **724**

Tung Oil (8001-20-5) *See loc. no.* **724**

Tungsten (and its Salts) (7440-33-7) *See loc. no.* **297**

Tungsten metal (7440-33-7) *See* Tungsten (and its Salts)[a] *at
loc. no.* **297**

Tungstic anhydride (1314-35-8) *See* Tungsten (and its
Salts)[d] *at loc. no.* **297**

Tupersan (1982-49-6) *See* Siduron[c] *at loc. no.* **1257**

Turkey red oil (8002-33-3) *See* Sulfated Castor Oil[a] *at loc.
no.* **956**

Turpentine (8006-64-2) *See loc. no.* **763**

"Turpentine camphor" (464-41-5) *See* Bornyl Chloride[a] *at
loc. no.* **874**

Tusscapine (128-62-1) *See* Noscapine[c] *at loc. no.* **788**

Tween 60 (9005-67-8) *See* Polyoxyethylene (20) Sorbitan
Monostearate[a] *at loc. no.* **969**

Tween 80 (9005-65-6) *See* Polysorbate 80[c] *at loc. no.* **970**

Tybamate (4268-36-4) *See* Meprobamate[b] *at loc. no.* **1407**

Tylenol (103-90-2) *See* Acetaminophen[c] *at loc. no.* **1587**

Tyrocidine (1406-13-9) *See* Tyrothricin[e] *at loc. no.* **905**

Tyrothricin (8001-01-2) *See loc. no.* **905**

Tyzine hydrochloride (522-48-5) *See* Tetrahydrozoline Hydrochloride[c] *at loc. no.* **1469**

UCAR solvent 2LM (34590-94-8) *See* Dipropylene Glycol
Monomethyl Ether[c] *at loc. no.* **457**

Ultradiazine *See* Sulfadiazine[c] *at loc. no.* **1553**

Ultran (79-93-6) *See* Phenaglycodol[c] *at loc. no.* **1410**

Ultrawets *See* Alkyl Aryl Sodium Sulfonates[c] *at loc. no.* **943**

Umbelliferone (93-35-6) *See loc. no.* **934**

10-Undecenoic acid (112-38-9) *See* Undecylenic Acid[a] *at loc.
no.* **564**

9-Undecylenic acid (112-38-9) *See* Undecylenic Acid[a] *at loc.
no.* **564**

Undecylenic Acid (112-38-9) *See loc. no.* **564**

Unden (114-26-1) *See* Propoxur[c] *at loc. no.* **1147**

Unistat-3 *See* 4-Hydroxy-3-nitrophenylarsonic Acid[c] *at loc.
no.* **205**

Unslaked lime *See* Calcium Oxide[a] *at loc. no.* **54**

Urab (4482-55-7) *See* Fenuron[b] *at loc. no.* **1248**

Uranium salts *See* Uranyl Nitrate[e] *at loc. no.* **298**

Uranyl Nitrate (13520-83-7) *See loc. no.* **298**

---

[a] A Synonym   [b] A Closely Related Substance   [c] The Active or Major Constituent   [d] A Class Name
[e] A Specific Example of or Product Containing

Ingredient name (CAS registry no.) *See* Primary Name *at*
location no. **XXX** *in Part D of this section*

Urea hydrogen peroxide (124-43-6) *See* Hydrogen Peroxide[b] *at loc. no.* **73**

5-Ureidohydantoin (97-59-6) *See* Allantoin[a] *at loc. no.* **477**

Urginea maritima *See* Squill (Red or White)[a] *at loc. no.* **695**

Urginin (8002-35-5) *See loc. no.* **845**

Urginin A and B *See* Urginin[a] *at loc. no.* **845**

Urolocide (100-95-8) *See loc. no.* **993**

Uva Ursi (8063-21-6) *See loc. no.* **698**

Vacor (53558-25-1) *See loc. no.* **1353**

Valamin (126-52-3) *See* Ethinamate[c] *at loc. no.* **1435**

Valepotriates (18296-44-1) *See* Valerian[c] *at loc. no.* **699**

n-Valeraldehyde (110-62-3) *See* Acetaldehyde[b] *at loc. no.* **480**

Valerian (8057-49-6) *See loc. no.* **699**

Valerian oil *See* Valerian[c] *at loc. no.* **699**

Valium (439-14-5) *See* Diazepam[c] *at loc. no.* **1395**

Valmid (126-52-3) *See* Ethinamate[c] *at loc. no.* **1435**

Valmidate (126-52-3) *See* Ethinamate[a] *at loc. no.* **1435**

Valone (83-28-3) *See loc. no.* **1344**

Valtrates (18296-44-1) *See* Valerian[c] *at loc. no.* **699**

Vanadium (and its Salts) (7440-62-2) *See loc. no.* **299**

Vanadium pentoxide (1314-62-1) *See* Vanadium (and its Salts)[d] *at loc. no.* **299**

Vancide 51 (8000-96-2) *See loc. no.* **1166**

Vancide 89 (133-06-2) *See* Captan[c] *at loc. no.* **1179**

Vancide 26 and 26EC (5406-97-3) *See* Mercaptobenzothiazole[b] *at loc. no.* **1198**

Vancide PA (1113-14-0) *See* *trans*-1,2-Bis(propylsulfonyl)ethene[c] *at loc. no.* **1175**

Vancide PB (6379-46-0) *See* Trichlorodinitrobenzene[c] *at loc. no.* **1202**

Vancide 20S (5902-85-2) *See* Mercaptobenzothiazole[b] *at loc. no.* **1198**

Vancide TH (7779-27-3) *See* Hexahydro-1,3,5-triethyl-*s*-triazine[c] *at loc. no.* **1172**

Vancide 51Z *See* Vancide 51[b] *at loc. no.* **1166**

Vancide ZP (13463-41-7) *See* Zinc 2-Pyridinethiol-1-oxide[c] *at loc. no.* **276**

Vanillin (121-33-5) *See loc. no.* **873**

Vapam (137-42-8) *See* Metham Sodium[c] *at loc. no.* **1161**

Vapona (62-73-7) *See* Dichlorvos[c] *at loc. no.* **1053**

Varnish makers' and painters' naphtha (8032-32-4) *See* VM&P Naphthas[a] *at loc. no.* **335**

Vatrolite (7775-14-6) *See* Sodium Hydrosulfite[c] *at loc. no.* **151**

VC-13 Nemacide (97-17-6) *See* Dichlofenthion[c] *at loc. no.* **1069**

Vegadex (95-06-7) *See* Sulfallate[c] *at loc. no.* **1164**

Vegetable gums *See* Gums (Vegetable)[a] *at loc. no.* **755**

Vegiben (7286-84-2) *See* Chloramben[b] *at loc. no.* **1296**

Velpar (51235-04-2) *See* Hexazinone[c] *at loc. no.* **1263**

Velsicol 104 (76-44-8) *See* Heptachlor[c] *at loc. no.* **1022**

Velsicol 1068 (57-74-9) *See* Chlordane[c] *at loc. no.* **1019**

Veratrum Viride Alkaloids (8002-39-9) *See loc. no.* **811**

Veriloid (8002-39-9) *See* Veratrum Viride Alkaloids[c] *at loc. no.* **811**

Vernolate (1929-77-7) *See loc. no.* **1240**

Veronal (57-44-3) *See* Barbital[c] *at loc. no.* **1366**

Versene (64-02-8) *See* Ethylenediaminetetraacetic Acid (and Salts)[b] *at loc. no.* **1506**

Vesprin hydrochloride (1098-60-8) *See* Triflupromazine Hydrochloride[c] *at loc. no.* **1427**

Vicia faba *See* Fava Beans[a] *at loc. no.* **670**

Victawets *See* Alkylated Sodium Phosphates[c] *at loc. no.* **944**

Vikane (2699-79-8) *See* Sulfuryl Fluoride[c] *at loc. no.* **18**

Vinarol (9002-89-5) *See* Polyvinyl Alcohol[a] *at loc. no.* **1637**

Vinbarbital Sodium (125-44-0) *See loc. no.* **1391**

Vinylbenzene (100-42-5) *See* Styrene[a] *at loc. no.* **315**

Vinyl carbinol (107-18-6) *See* Allyl Alcohol[a] *at loc. no.* **21**

Vinyl Chloride (75-01-4) *See loc. no.* **378**

Vinyl cyanide (107-13-1) *See* Acrylonitrile[a] *at loc. no.* **648**

Vinylidene chloride (75-35-4) *See* 1,1-Dichloroethylene[a] *at loc. no.* **366**

Vinyl trichloride (79-00-5) *See* 1,1,2-Trichloroethane[a] *at loc. no.* **376**

Vioform (130-26-7) *See* Diiodohydroxyquin[b] *at loc. no.* **1513**

Viscum album *See* European Mistletoe[a] *at loc. no.* **669**

Vistaril (2192-20-3) *See* Hydroxyzine Hydrochloride[c] *at loc. no.* **1438**

Vitamin A (68-26-8) *See loc. no.* **907**

Vitamin B$_1$ (59-43-8) *See* Thiamine[a] *at loc. no.* **914**

Vitamin B$_2$ (83-88-5) *See* Riboflavin[a] *at loc. no.* **913**

Vitamin B$_6$ (65-22-5) *See* Pyridoxine Hydrochloride[c] *at loc. no.* **912**

Vitamin C (50-81-7) *See loc. no.* **908**

Vitamin D (1406-16-2) *See loc. no.* **909**

Vitamin E (59-02-9) *See loc. no.* **910**

Vitamin E acetate (133-80-2) *See* Vitamin E[b] *at loc. no.* **910**

Vitamin G (83-88-5) *See* Riboflavin[a] *at loc. no.* **913**

"Vitamin P" (1340-08-5) *See* Hesperidin Methyl Chalcone[e] *at loc. no.* **1599**

Vitavax (5234-68-4) *See* Carboxin[a] *at loc. no.* **1182**

Vitriolic acid (7664-93-9) *See* Sulfuric Acid[a] *at loc. no.* **33**

Vivactil (1225-55-4) *See* Protriptyline Hydrochloride[c] *at loc. no.* **1479**

Vleminckx's solution (8048-11-1) *See* Calcium Polysulfide[c] *at loc. no.* **113**

VM&P (8032-32-4) *See* VM&P Naphthas[a] *at loc. no.* **335**

VM&P Naphthas (8032-32-4) *See loc. no.* **335**

Volatile oil of mustard (57-06-7) *See* Allyl Isothiocyanate[a] *at loc. no.* **1359**

Volatile oils *See* Essential Oils[d] *at loc. no.* **725**

Voronit (39312-79-3) *See* Fuberidazole[c] *at loc. no.* **1176**

VPM (137-42-8) *See* Metham Sodium[c] *at loc. no.* **1161**

Vydate *See* Oxamyl[c] *at loc. no.* **1144**

Warfarin (81-81-2) *See loc. no.* **1345**

Warfarin sodium (129-06-6) *See* Warfarin[b] *at loc. no.* **1345**

Warf compound *See* Warfarin[a] *at loc. no.* **1345**

Washed sulfur *See* Sulfur[a] *at loc. no.* **120**

Washing soda *See* Sodium Carbonate[a] *at loc. no.* **52**

Water glass (1344-09-8) *See* Sodium Silicate[b] *at loc. no.* **58**

Weedmix *See* Sodium Isopropyl Xanthate[c] *at loc. no.* **1315**

Welldorm (480-30-8) *See* Dichloralphenazone[c] *at loc. no.* **1572**

Wepsyn (1031-47-6) *See* Triamiphos[c] *at loc. no.* **1209**

Wescodyne (8050-84-8) *See* Iodophors[c] *at loc. no.* **997**

Western red cedar dust *See* Sawdust[d] *at loc. no.* **694**

Wetting agents *See* Surface Active Agents[d] *at loc. no.* **936**

White arsenic (1327-53-3) *See* Arsenic Trioxide[a] *at loc. no.* **193**

White mercuric precipitate *See* Ammoniated Mercury[c] *at loc. no.* **223**

White mineral oil (8012-95-1) *See* Liquid Petrolatum[a] *at loc. no.* **337**

White pepper *See* Pepper[a] *at loc. no.* **682**

White petrolatum (8009-03-8) *See* Liquid Petrolatum[b] *at loc. no.* **337**

White petroleum jelly *See* Liquid Petrolatum[b] *at loc. no.* **337**

White phosphorus (7723-14-0) *See* Phosphorus[a] *at loc. no.* **135**

White spirits *See* Stoddard Solvent[a] *at loc. no.* **334**

---

[a] A Synonym   [b] A Closely Related Substance   [c] The Active or Major Constituent   [d] A Class Name
[e] A Specific Example of or Product Containing

Ingredient name (CAS registry no.) *See* Primary Name *at location no.* **XXX** *in Part D of this section*

Wild black cherry bark *See* Wild Cherry[a] *at loc. no.* **700**
Wild Cherry *See loc. no.* **700**
Wild Lettuce *See loc. no.* **701**
Wilkinite (8047-76-5) *See* Bentonite[a] *at loc. no.* **3**
Winterberry *See* Holly[b] *at loc. no.* **672**
Wintergreen oil (119-36-8) *See* Methyl Salicylate[a] *at loc. no.* **597**
Witch Hazel *See loc. no.* **702**
Wolf's bane or Wolfsbane. *These names are used as synonyms for both* Aconite *and* Arnica, *which are unrelated. See in this index whichever is applicable.*
Wood alcohol (67-56-1) *See* Methyl Alcohol[a] *at loc. no.* **423**
Wood creosote (8021-39-4) *See* Creosote[a] *at loc. no.* **513**
Wood flour *See* Sawdust[d] *at loc. no.* **694**
Wood meal *See* Sawdust[d] *at loc. no.* **694**
Wood naphtha (67-56-1) *See* Methyl Alcohol[a] *at loc. no.* **423**
Wood spirit (67-56-1) *See* Methyl Alcohol[a] *at loc. no.* **423**
Wood tar *See* Creosote[b] *at loc. no.* **513**
Wood tar creosote *See* Creosote[a] *at loc. no.* **513**
Wood turpentine *See* Turpentine[a] *at loc. no.* **763**
Wood vinegar (8030-97-5) *See* Pyroligneous Acid[a] *at loc. no.* **929**
Wool fat (8020-84-6) *See* Lanolin[a] *at loc. no.* **716**
Wormseed oil American (8006-99-3) *See* Chenopodium Oil[a] *at loc. no.* **728**
Xenene *See* Diphenyl[a] *at loc. no.* **314**
Xylene (1330-20-7) *See loc. no.* **318**
Xylenol (1300-71-6) *See loc. no.* **498**
Xylocaine (137-58-6) *See* Lidocaine[c] *at loc. no.* **1582**
Xylol (1330-20-7) *See* Xylene[a] *at loc. no.* **318**
3,4-Xylyl methylcarbamate (2425-10-7) *See* MPMC[a] *at loc. no.* **1143**
Yalan (2212-67-1) *See* Molinate[c] *at loc. no.* **1237**
Yellow cuprocide (1317-39-1) *See* Cuprous Oxide[c] *at loc. no.* **269**
Yellow jasmine *See* Gelsemium[a] *at loc. no.* **671**
Yellow phenolphthalein (8053-05-2) *See* Phenolphthalein[b] *at loc. no.* **1607**
Yellow phosphorus (7723-14-0) *See* Phosphorus[d] *at loc. no.* **135**
Yellow resin (8050-09-7) *See* Rosin[a] *at loc. no.* **760**
Yohimbine (146-48-5) *See loc. no.* **834**
Zactane (77-15-6) *See* Ethoheptazine[c] *at loc. no.* **1483**
Zactirin (8058-32-0) *See* Ethoheptazine[c] *at loc. no.* **1483**
Zactirin Compound-100 *See* Ethoheptazine[c] *at loc. no.* **1483**
Zectran (315-18-4) *See* Mexacarbate[c] *at loc. no.* **1141**
Zephiral (8001-54-5) *See* Benzalkonium Chloride[c] *at loc. no.* **985**
Zephiran chloride (8001-54-5) *See* Benzalkonium Chloride[c] *at loc. no.* **985**
Zephirol (8001-54-5) *See* Benzalkonium Chloride[c] *at loc. no.* **985**
Zerlate (137-30-4) *See* Ziram[c] *at loc. no.* **1168**
Zinc acetate (557-34-6) *See* Zinc Salts (Soluble)[d] *at loc. no.* **277**
Zinc ammonium chloride *See* Zinc Salts (Soluble)[d] *at loc. no.* **277**
Zinc ammonium compound *See* Zinc Salts (Soluble)[d] *at loc. no.* **277**
Zinc Arsenate (1303-39-5) *See loc. no.* **211**
Zinc arsenite (10326-24-6) *See* Zinc Arsenate[b] *at loc. no.* **211**
Zinc caprylate (557-09-5) *See* Zinc Stearate[b] *at loc. no.* **278**
Zinc carbonate (3486-35-9) *See* Zinc Salts (Soluble)[d] *at loc. no.* **277**
Zinc chloride (7646-85-7) *See* Zinc Salts (Soluble)[d] *at loc. no.* **277**

Zinc chromate (14018-95-2) *See* Chromate Salts[d] *at loc. no.* **81**
Zinc cyanide (557-21-1) *See* Cyanide[d] *at loc. no.* **105**
Zinc dimethyldithiocarbamate (137-30-4) *See* Ziram[a] *at loc. no.* **1168**
Zinc ethylene bis(dithiocarbamate) (12122-67-7) *See* Zineb[a] *at loc. no.* **1167**
Zinc fluoride (7783-49-5) *See* Fluoride[d] *at loc. no.* **100**
Zinc fluosilicate (1310-07-2) *See* Fluosilicate Salts[d] *at loc. no.* **101**
Zinc formate (557-41-5) *See* Zinc Salts (Soluble)[d] *at loc. no.* **277**
Zinc mercaptobenzothiazole (155-04-4) *See* Mercaptobenzothiazole[b] *at loc. no.* **1198**
Zinc Naphthenate (12001-85-3) *See loc. no.* **273**
Zinc omadine (3590-23-6) *See* Zinc 2-Pyridinethiol-1-oxide[a] *at loc. no.* **276**
Zinc Oxide (1314-13-2) *See loc. no.* **274**
Zinc oxide with 0.5% ferric oxide (8011-96-9) *See* Calamine[a] *at loc. no.* **271**
Zinc peroxide (1314-22-3) *See* Hydrogen Peroxide[b] *at loc. no.* **73**
Zinc Phenolsulfonate (127-82-2) *See loc. no.* **275**
Zinc Phosphide (1314-84-7) *See loc. no.* **138**
Zinc proprionate (557-28-8) *See* Zinc Salts (Soluble)[d] *at loc. no.* **277**
Zinc 2-Pyridinethiol-1-oxide (3590-23-6) *See loc. no.* **276**
Zinc pyridinethione (3590-23-6) *See* Zinc 2-Pyridinethiol-1-oxide[a] *at loc. no.* **276**
Zinc pyrithione (3590-23-6) *See* Zinc 2-Pyridinethiol-1-oxide[a] *at loc. no.* **276**
Zinc Salts (Soluble) *See loc. no.* **277**
Zinc Stearate (557-05-1) *See loc. no.* **278**
Zinc sulfate (7733-02-0) *See* Zinc Salts (Soluble)[d] *at loc. no.* **277**
Zinc sulfide (1314-98-3) *See* Sulfide Salts[d] *at loc. no.* **118**
Zinc sulfocarbolate (127-82-2) *See* Zinc Phenolsulfonate[a] *at loc. no.* **275**
Zinc sulfophenate (127-82-2) *See* Zinc Phenolsulfonate[a] *at loc. no.* **275**
Zinc trichlorophenate *See* Trichlorophenols[b] *at loc. no.* **535**
Zinc Undecylenate (557-08-4) *See loc. no.* **279**
Zinc white (1314-13-2) *See* Zinc Oxide[a] *at loc. no.* **274**
Zineb (12122-67-7) *See loc. no.* **1167**
Zinophos (297-97-2) *See* Thionazin[a] *at loc. no.* **1081**
Ziram (137-30-4) *See loc. no.* **1168**
Zirconia (1314-23-4) *See* Zirconium Oxide[a] *at loc. no.* **301**
Zirconium chloride (10026-11-6) *See* Zirconyl Chloride[b] *at loc. no.* **302**
Zirconium chlorohydrate (7699-43-6) *See* Zirconyl Chloride[a] *at loc. no.* **302**
Zirconium dioxide *See* Zirconium Oxide[a] *at loc. no.* **301**
Zirconium Oxide (1314-23-4) *See loc. no.* **301**
Zirconium oxychloride (7699-43-6) *See* Zirconyl Chloride[a] *at loc. no.* **302**
Zirconium tetrachloride *See* Zirconyl Chloride[b] *at loc. no.* **302**
Zirconyl Chloride (7699-43-6) *See loc. no.* **302**
Zoalene (148-01-6) *See* Dinitolmide[c] *at loc. no.* **1540**
Zorial *See* Norflurazon[c] *at loc. no.* **1311**
ZPT (3590-23-6) *See* Zinc 2-Pyridinethiol-1-oxide[a] *at loc. no.* **276**
Z.P. Tracking Powder *See* Zinc Phosphide[c] *at loc. no.* **138**
Zytron (299-85-4) *See loc. no.* **1105**

---

[a] A Synonym   [b] A Closely Related Substance   [c] The Active or Major Constituent   [d] A Class Name
[e] A Specific Example of or Product Containing

II: C. Numerical Listing of Ingredients by CAS Numbers

CAS Registry No. of Ingredient	CAS Registry No. of Primary Name	Location Number of Primary Name (See Part D)	CAS Registry No. of Ingredient	CAS Registry No. of Primary Name	Location Number of Primary Name (See Part D)	CAS Registry No. of Ingredient	CAS Registry No. of Primary Name	Location Number of Primary Name (See Part D)
35-58-5	17598-65-1	835	51-63-8	300-62-9	1444	57-15-8	←	432
35-86-9	—	841	51-64-9	300-62-9	1444	57-24-9	←	833
36-06-6	630-60-4	842				57-27-2	←	778
36-35-1	20830-75-5	839	52-28-8	76-57-3	780	57-29-4	←	786
50-00-0	←	482	52-31-3	←	1371	57-30-7	50-06-6	1382
			52-39-1	—	915			
50-02-2	—	915	52-43-7	←	1373	57-33-0	←	1380
50-03-3	—	915	52-46-0	←	1354	57-37-4	302-40-9	1430
50-06-6	←	1382				57-39-6	52-46-0	1354
50-09-9	←	1376	52-67-5	←	1507	57-41-0	630-93-3	1609
50-11-3	←	1379	52-68-6	←	1062	57-43-2	←	1364
			52-86-8	←	1437			
50-12-4	630-93-3	1609	53-03-2	—	915	57-44-3	←	1366
50-13-5	←	1484	53-16-7	—	916	57-47-6	←	807
50-14-6	1406-16-2	909				57-50-1	←	708
50-21-5	←	46	53-33-8	—	915	57-52-3	—	293
50-22-6	—	915	53-60-1	58-40-2	1420	57-53-4	←	1407
			53-86-1	←	1600			
50-23-7	—	915	54-04-6	←	830	57-55-6	←	442
50-24-8	—	915	54-05-7	←	1512	57-62-5	—	904
50-27-1	—	916				57-63-6	—	916
50-28-2	—	916	54-11-5	←	772	57-64-7	57-47-6	807
50-29-3	←	1007	54-21-7	63-36-5	600	57-66-9	←	1611
			54-47-7	58-56-0	912			
50-31-7	1319-85-3	1317	54-64-8	←	244	57-67-0	←	1556
50-33-9	←	1575	54-85-3	←	1601	57-68-1	←	1559
50-35-1	←	1443				57-74-9	←	1019
50-36-2	←	825	54-86-4	59-67-6	911	57-96-5	←	1576
50-37-3	←	829	54-95-5	←	1606	58-00-4	314-19-2	779
			54-97-7	95-62-5	1480			
50-43-1	1319-85-3	1317	55-03-8	—	920	58-08-2	←	800
50-47-5	←	1471	55-06-1	—	920	58-15-1	←	1570
50-48-6	←	1470				58-27-5	←	1605
50-49-7	←	1473	55-17-4	←	1643	58-28-6	50-47-5	1471
50-52-2	←	1425	55-31-2	51-43-4	1454	58-33-3	60-87-7	1421
			55-38-9	←	1073			
50-53-3	←	1412	55-48-1	51-55-8	767	58-38-8	←	1419
50-54-4	56-54-2	810	55-55-0	←	626	58-39-9	←	1418
50-55-5	←	798				58-40-2	←	1420
50-67-9	487-93-4	820	55-56-1	←	994	58-55-9	←	802
50-70-4	←	706	55-63-0	←	635	58-56-0	←	912
			55-91-4	←	1096			
50-73-7	1319-85-3	1317	56-23-5	←	355	58-74-2	←	793
50-78-2	←	594	56-24-6	—	293	58-89-9	←	1028
50-81-7	←	908				58-90-2	←	534
50-98-6	299-42-3	1450	56-25-7	←	924	58-93-5	—	1588
51-03-6	←	1151	56-35-9	←	294	58-94-6	—	1588
			56-36-0	—	293			
51-05-8	59-46-1	1585	56-38-2	←	1077	59-02-9	←	910
51-06-9	←	1612	56-53-1	—	916	59-33-6	←	1499
51-14-9	←	1154				59-40-5	←	1565
51-15-0	←	1508	56-54-2	←	810	59-42-7	←	1468
51-28-5	←	541	56-69-9	487-93-4	820	59-43-8	←	914
			56-72-4	←	1066			
51-30-9	51-31-0	1458	56-81-5	←	704	59-46-1	←	1585
51-31-0	←	1458	56-86-0	142-47-2	1618	59-47-2	←	1406
51-34-3	←	771				59-50-7	—	523
51-42-3	51-43-4	1454	57-06-7	←	1359	59-52-9	←	1503
51-43-4	←	1454	57-09-0	—	983	59-67-6	←	911
			57-11-4	←	562			
51-48-9	—	920	57-12-5	←	105	59-87-0	←	1531
51-55-8	←	767	57-14-7	60-34-4	817	60-00-4	←	1506
51-57-0	537-46-2	1459				60-12-8	←	427

CAS Registry No. of Ingredient	CAS Registry No. of Primary Name	Location Number of Primary Name (See Part D)	CAS Registry No. of Ingredient	CAS Registry No. of Primary Name	Location Number of Primary Name (See Part D)	CAS Registry No. of Ingredient	CAS Registry No. of Primary Name	Location Number of Primary Name (See Part D)
60-29-7	←	472	67-63-0	←	420	75-11-6	←	360
60-33-3	←	555	67-64-1	←	466	75-13-8	420-05-3	29
60-34-4	←	817	67-66-3	←	357	75-15-0	←	125
60-41-3	57-24-9	833	67-68-5	←	1620	75-18-3	74-93-1	116
60-51-5	←	1085	67-72-1	←	370	75-20-7	←	62
60-54-8	—	904	67-73-2	—	915	75-21-8	←	16
60-57-1	←	1020	67-97-0	1406-16-2	909	75-28-5	←	305
60-80-0	←	1571	68-11-1	←	49	75-34-3	←	365
60-87-7	←	1421	68-12-2	←	566	75-35-4	←	366
60-89-9	←	1416	68-26-8	←	907	75-43-4	←	349
61-01-8	←	1417	68-35-9	←	1553	75-44-5	←	11
61-12-1	85-79-0	1580	68-88-2	2192-20-3	1438	75-45-6	←	350
61-25-6	58-74-2	793	68-89-3	5907-38-0	1573	75-47-8	←	1529
61-32-5	—	902	69-05-6	←	1515	75-52-5	←	636
61-33-6	—	902	69-23-8	146-56-5	1415	75-56-9	←	17
61-50-7	←	1448	69-53-4	—	902	75-60-5	←	197
61-51-8	61-50-7	1448	69-72-7	63-36-5	600	75-69-4	←	351
61-73-4	←	1521	70-30-4	←	531	75-71-8	←	348
61-82-5	←	1290	70-38-2	←	889	75-74-1	78-00-2	248
62-33-9	←	1504	70-43-9	←	885	75-86-5	←	646
62-38-4	—	241	70-51-9	←	1505	75-99-0	←	1299
62-44-2	←	611	71-23-8	←	428	76-01-7	←	371
62-46-4	←	1510	71-36-3	←	407	76-03-9	←	50
62-53-3	←	612	71-41-0	←	405	76-06-2	←	13
62-55-5	←	121	71-43-2	←	312	76-13-1	—	353
62-56-6	←	1352	71-48-7	—	282	76-14-2	←	352
62-67-9	57-29-4	786	71-55-6	←	377	76-22-2	←	875
62-73-7	←	1053	71-63-6	←	838	76-29-9	76-22-2	875
62-74-8	513-62-2	548	71-68-1	←	781	76-41-5	←	790
62-76-0	—	546	71-73-8	←	1390	76-42-6	←	789
63-25-2	←	1128	71-81-8	7492-32-2	1602	76-44-8	←	1022
63-36-5	←	600	71-82-9	←	784	76-57-3	←	780
63-74-1	←	1563	72-14-0	←	1567	76-58-4	57-27-2	778
63-75-2	←	774	72-20-8	←	1021	76-68-6	←	1372
64-00-6	2631-40-5	1137	72-33-3	—	916	76-74-4	57-33-0	1380
64-02-8	60-00-4	1506	72-43-5	←	1013	76-76-6	143-82-8	1383
64-17-5	←	412	72-44-6	←	1439	76-80-2	—	897
64-18-6	←	44	72-48-0	←	921	76-87-9	900-95-8	295
64-19-7	←	42	72-54-8	←	1009	76-94-8	←	1381
64-43-7	57-43-2	1364	72-56-0	←	1015	76-99-3	←	1485
64-55-1	57-53-4	1407	72-57-1	←	1524	77-02-1	←	1365
64-85-7	—	915	72-69-5	←	1474	77-06-5	←	1357
64-86-8	←	803	73-48-3	—	1588	77-07-6	←	785
64-89-1	←	1422	73-78-9	137-58-6	1582	77-09-8	←	1607
64-95-9	302-40-9	1430	74-55-5	1070-11-7	1596	77-10-1	956-90-1	1542
65-22-5	58-56-0	912	74-82-8	—	303	77-15-6	←	1483
65-30-5	54-11-5	772	74-83-9	←	344	77-21-4	←	1436
65-45-2	←	599	74-84-0	—	303	77-26-9	←	1368
65-49-6	←	629	74-87-3	←	345	77-27-0	337-47-3	1389
65-61-2	—	1518	74-88-4	←	346	77-28-1	←	1370
65-85-0	←	582	74-90-8	←	106	77-36-1	—	1588
66-32-0	57-24-9	833	74-93-1	←	116	77-47-4	←	388
66-76-2	←	1334	74-95-3	←	358	77-58-7	—	292
66-79-5	—	902	74-97-5	←	356	77-65-6	←	1431
66-81-9	←	906	74-98-6	←	304	77-66-7	77-65-6	1431
67-03-8	59-43-8	914	75-00-3	←	368	77-75-8	←	1440
67-20-9	←	1530	75-01-4	←	378	77-86-1	←	69
67-21-0	55-17-4	1643	75-05-8	←	647	77-92-9	←	703
67-43-6	62-33-9	1504	75-07-0	←	480	78-00-2	←	248
67-45-8	←	1526	75-08-1	74-93-1	116	78-11-5	←	638
67-56-1	←	423	75-09-2	←	359	78-18-2	←	77

CAS Registry No. of Ingredient	CAS Registry No. of Primary Name	Location Number of Primary Name (See Part D)	CAS Registry No. of Ingredient	CAS Registry No. of Primary Name	Location Number of Primary Name (See Part D)	CAS Registry No. of Ingredient	CAS Registry No. of Primary Name	Location Number of Primary Name (See Part D)
78-28-4	←	1405	83-88-5	←	913	91-08-7	584-84-9	1641
78-30-8	←	1116	83-98-7	←	1496	91-15-6	←	651
78-34-2	←	1093	84-16-2	—	916	91-17-8	←	319
78-40-0	—	1112	84-17-3	—	916	91-20-3	←	321
78-43-3	←	1119	84-34-4	←	797	91-33-8	—	1588
78-44-4	←	1403	84-62-8	—	589	91-49-6	←	1323
78-48-8	←	1111	84-65-1	←	499	91-53-2	←	1615
78-52-4	←	1084	84-66-2	←	592	91-64-5	←	861
78-53-5	←	1080	84-74-2	←	590	91-80-5	135-23-9	1495
78-59-1	←	473	84-96-8	←	1428	91-85-0	—	1487
78-83-1	←	418	85-00-7	←	1285	92-03-5	←	522
78-84-2	75-07-0	480	85-01-8	65996-91-0	341	92-04-6	1331-46-0	526
78-87-5	←	391	85-34-7	←	1219	92-12-6	1176-08-5	1498
78-93-3	←	476	85-68-7	—	589	92-13-7	←	808
79-00-5	←	376	85-72-3	←	1284	92-31-9	←	1523
79-01-6	←	375	85-73-4	←	1548	92-52-4	←	314
79-06-1	←	1624	85-79-0	←	1580	92-62-6	—	1518
79-08-3	513-62-2	548	85-95-0	—	916	92-84-2	←	1543
79-09-4	137-40-6	551	86-21-5	132-20-7	1497	93-14-1	←	1597
79-11-8	←	549	86-22-6	—	1487	93-23-2	←	991
79-14-1	←	45	86-40-8	—	1518	93-35-6	←	934
79-20-9	107-31-3	576	86-42-0	←	1511	93-51-6	←	490
79-21-0	←	78	86-50-0	←	1089	93-60-7	←	588
79-27-6	←	372	86-78-2	90-34-6	1516	93-65-2	7085-19-0	1221
79-34-5	←	373	86-86-2	←	1277	93-71-0	←	1274
79-43-6	←	43	86-87-3	←	1309	93-72-1	←	1223
79-45-8	128-04-1	1163	86-88-4	←	1350	93-75-4	←	1044
79-46-9	←	637	87-00-3	←	769	93-76-5	←	1224
79-57-2	—	904	87-08-1	—	902	93-79-8	93-76-5	1224
79-93-6	←	1410	87-10-5	←	1000	94-09-7	←	1577
80-00-2	←	1048	87-12-7	87-10-5	1000	94-11-1	—	1213
80-06-8	←	1011	87-17-2	←	998	94-12-2	94-25-7	1579
80-13-7	127-65-1	91	87-20-7	←	596	94-13-3	←	586
80-32-0	←	1552	87-27-4	←	219	94-14-4	94-25-7	1579
80-33-1	←	1047	87-28-5	119-36-8	597	94-19-9	←	1555
80-35-3	←	1562	87-33-2	←	634	94-24-6	←	1586
80-46-6	←	488	87-47-8	←	1149	94-25-7	←	1579
80-49-9	87-00-3	769	87-61-6	—	403	94-26-8	—	584
80-56-8	←	879	87-66-1	←	506	94-36-0	←	76
80-62-6	←	1630	87-86-5	←	532	94-58-6	←	862
80-63-7	—	1625	87-90-1	←	94	94-59-7	←	872
80-74-0	127-69-5	1568	88-04-0	←	528	94-63-3	51-15-0	1508
80-77-3	←	1404	88-06-2	—	535	94-74-6	←	1220
81-07-2	←	1616	88-82-4	←	1318	94-75-7	←	1212
81-23-2	←	1593	88-85-7	←	543	94-80-4	—	1213
81-81-2	←	1345	88-89-1	←	545	94-81-5	←	1222
81-82-3	←	1336	89-46-3	←	1535	94-82-6	←	1215
82-10-0	—	897	89-48-5	←	869	94-84-8	←	1306
82-66-6	←	1339	89-68-9	←	527	94-96-2	←	1329
82-68-8	←	1201	89-78-1	←	868	95-04-5	←	1433
82-93-9	←	1489	89-82-7	—	740	95-06-7	←	1164
82-95-1	←	1488	89-83-8	←	497	95-50-1	←	395
83-07-8	58-15-1	1570	90-03-9	←	234	95-53-4	106-49-0	618
83-12-5	←	1341	90-05-1	←	492	95-55-6	123-30-8	624
83-26-1	←	1343	90-34-6	←	1516	95-62-5	←	1480
83-28-3	←	1344	90-43-7	1322-20-9	495	95-69-2	6164-98-3	1042
83-43-2	—	915	90-45-9	—	1518	95-74-9	←	614
83-59-0	←	1153	90-69-7	←	776	95-76-1	709-98-8	1283
83-67-0	←	801	90-81-3	299-42-3	1450	95-80-7	←	621
83-73-8	←	1513	90-84-6	←	1447	95-95-4	—	535
83-79-4	←	896	90-89-1	←	1539	96-09-3	100-42-5	315

CAS Registry No. of Ingredient	CAS Registry No. of Primary Name	Location Number of Primary Name (See Part D)	CAS Registry No. of Ingredient	CAS Registry No. of Primary Name	Location Number of Primary Name (See Part D)	CAS Registry No. of Ingredient	CAS Registry No. of Primary Name	Location Number of Primary Name (See Part D)
96-12-8	←	385	102-96-5	←	1631	108-35-0	←	1078
96-13-9	126-72-7	1118	103-11-7	—	1625	108-46-3	←	508
96-23-1	←	433	103-16-2	←	1536	108-62-3	←	485
96-26-4	←	471	103-17-3	←	1043	108-64-5	141-78-6	570
96-33-3	—	1625	103-26-4	—	587	108-70-3	—	403
96-45-7	←	1169	103-33-3	←	1041	108-73-6	87-66-1	506
96-50-4	121-66-4	1538	103-36-6	—	587	108-86-1	←	392
96-88-8	←	1583	103-41-3	—	587	108-87-2	←	309
97-00-7	←	639	103-84-4	←	610	108-88-3	←	317
97-05-2	76-03-9	50	103-85-5	←	1351	108-90-7	←	393
97-11-0	←	886	103-90-2	←	1587	108-91-8	←	609
97-12-1	—	893	104-46-1	←	858	108-93-0	←	410
97-16-5	←	1046	104-55-2	←	860	108-94-1	←	468
97-17-6	←	1069	104-60-9	—	241	108-95-2	←	494
97-18-7	←	521	104-76-7	←	413	109-17-1	—	1625
97-23-4	←	529	105-28-2	556-22-9	1196	109-19-3	123-86-4	568
97-53-0	←	864	105-37-3	141-78-6	570	109-21-7	123-86-4	568
97-59-6	←	477	105-41-9	299-42-3	1450	109-60-4	←	578
97-64-3	←	572	105-54-4	141-78-6	570	109-66-0	110-54-3	307
97-77-8	←	1595	105-57-7	←	465	109-69-3	←	380
97-95-0	—	416	105-66-8	109-60-4	578	109-74-0	←	649
98-00-0	←	414	105-68-0	123-92-2	574	109-77-3	←	650
98-01-1	←	483	105-99-7	←	1324	109-86-4	←	461
98-50-0	←	189	106-23-0	8000-29-1	736	109-94-4	←	571
98-54-4	80-46-6	488	106-24-1	←	865	109-95-5	463-04-7	630
98-55-5	586-81-2	882	106-36-5	109-60-4	578	109-99-9	←	1623
98-72-6	—	192	106-46-7	←	396	110-13-4	591-78-6	479
98-82-8	←	313	106-47-8	←	613	110-19-0	123-86-4	568
98-89-5	—	558	106-49-0	←	618	110-27-0	←	575
98-92-0	59-67-6	911	106-50-3	—	623	110-36-1	←	569
98-95-3	←	642	106-51-4	←	507	110-44-1	←	561
99-00-3	←	1545	106-61-6	26446-35-5	577	110-45-2	123-92-2	574
99-26-3	—	216	106-62-7	←	438	110-46-3	463-04-7	630
99-30-9	←	1191	106-69-4	←	446	110-49-6	←	462
99-35-4	25377-32-6	644	106-89-8	←	387	110-54-3	←	307
99-76-3	←	585	106-93-4	←	364	110-61-2	←	654
99-87-6	1330-20-7	318	106-95-6	←	379	110-62-3	75-07-0	480
100-01-6	←	617	106-96-7	←	390	110-80-5	←	458
100-02-7	←	544	106-97-8	←	306	110-82-7	←	308
100-41-4	1330-20-7	318	107-02-8	←	481	110-85-0	←	1544
100-42-5	←	315	107-04-0	←	362	110-86-1	←	1622
100-51-6	←	406	107-06-2	←	369	110-88-3	9002-81-7	487
100-52-7	←	859	107-07-3	←	434	110-91-8	←	72
100-55-0	59-67-6	911	107-12-0	←	653	111-01-3	←	932
100-67-4	108-95-2	494	107-13-1	←	648	111-15-9	←	450
100-92-5	299-42-3	1450	107-14-2	545-06-2	655	111-27-3	—	416
100-95-8	←	993	107-15-3	←	602	111-30-8	←	484
100-97-0	←	486	107-18-6	←	21	111-40-0	←	603
101-05-3	←	1170	107-21-1	←	436	111-42-2	←	65
101-20-2	←	1001	107-27-7	←	228	111-44-4	←	470
101-21-3	←	1229	107-30-2	←	467	111-46-6	←	437
101-27-9	←	1227	107-31-3	←	576	111-55-7	—	451
101-31-5	←	770	107-41-5	←	445	111-76-2	←	453
101-40-6	←	1452	107-49-3	←	1109	111-77-3	111-90-0	455
101-42-8	←	1248	107-64-2	—	974	111-87-5	←	408
101-54-2	←	619	107-88-0	←	444	111-90-0	←	455
101-83-7	←	608	107-98-2	←	464	112-24-3	←	604
101-90-6	—	1629	108-01-0	←	1592	112-27-6	←	439
102-29-4	←	509	108-10-1	←	478	112-30-1	—	411
102-71-6	←	66	108-21-4	109-60-4	578	112-34-5	←	452
102-76-1	←	579	108-34-9	←	1059	112-38-9	←	564

CAS Registry No. of Ingredient	CAS Registry No. of Primary Name	Location Number of Primary Name (See Part D)	CAS Registry No. of Ingredient	CAS Registry No. of Primary Name	Location Number of Primary Name (See Part D)	CAS Registry No. of Ingredient	CAS Registry No. of Primary Name	Location Number of Primary Name (See Part D)
112-53-8	←	422	119-34-6	←	625	124-29-8	←	409
112-56-1	←	1035	119-36-8	←	597	124-30-1	←	607
112-57-2	←	605	119-38-0	←	1136	124-40-3	←	68
112-70-9	—	431	119-53-9	←	750	124-43-6	8007-30-5	73
112-72-1	←	424	119-64-2	←	322	124-58-3	144-21-8	203
112-80-1	←	559	119-89-1	←	1152	124-65-2	75-60-5	197
112-92-5	←	430	120-12-7	65996-91-0	341	124-68-5	←	70
113-18-8	←	1434	120-32-1	←	520	124-90-3	76-42-6	789
113-42-8	129-49-7	806	120-36-5	←	1217	124-94-7	—	915
113-45-1	←	1462	120-47-8	—	584	125-30-4	57-27-2	778
113-48-4	←	1150	120-51-4	←	583	125-33-7	←	1610
113-52-0	50-49-7	1473	120-57-0	←	871	125-40-6	143-81-7	1367
113-59-7	←	1414	120-58-1	←	867	125-44-0	←	1391
113-92-8	—	1487	120-62-7	←	1155	125-55-3	←	1384
113-98-4	—	902	120-80-9	←	505	125-56-4	76-99-3	1485
114-26-1	←	1147	120-82-1	—	403	125-64-4	←	1441
114-49-8	51-34-3	771	120-83-2	—	525	125-67-7	77-06-5	1357
115-10-6	←	475	121-14-2	25321-14-6	641	125-69-9	←	1594
115-20-8	302-17-0	1432	121-19-7	←	205	125-72-4	77-07-6	785
115-26-4	←	1098	121-20-0	—	893	125-97-3	←	832
115-29-7	←	1026	121-21-1	—	893	126-07-8	←	900
115-31-1	←	1038	121-29-9	—	893	126-11-4	←	1003
115-32-2	←	1012	121-33-5	←	873	126-12-5	50-13-5	1484
115-33-3	77-09-8	1607	121-54-0	←	986	126-15-8	←	1321
115-38-8	←	1377	121-66-4	←	1538	126-22-7	←	1060
115-43-5	←	1363	121-69-7	←	615	126-52-3	←	1435
115-44-6	77-26-9	1368	121-75-5	←	1091	126-72-7	←	1118
115-46-8	←	1429	121-79-9	←	1619	126-73-8	←	1113
115-56-0	←	1378	121-81-3	148-01-6	1540	126-75-0	8000-97-3	1067
115-69-5	←	71	121-82-4	←	631	126-92-1	—	946
115-86-6	←	1117	122-09-8	←	1467	126-93-2	←	1409
115-95-7	8007-75-8	733	122-10-1	←	1052	126-97-6	—	552
116-02-9	108-93-0	410	122-11-2	←	1554	127-18-4	←	374
116-06-3	←	1120	122-14-5	←	1072	127-19-5	←	565
116-16-5	←	1307	122-15-6	←	1131	127-20-8	75-99-0	1299
116-29-0	←	1049	122-18-9	←	987	127-25-3	←	581
116-43-8	←	1549	122-19-0	←	990	127-33-3	—	904
116-45-0	←	1550	122-34-9	←	1269	127-56-0	144-80-9	1551
116-49-4	—	192	122-39-4	←	616	127-57-1	144-83-2	1564
116-52-9	←	1245	122-42-9	101-21-3	1229	127-58-2	127-79-7	1557
117-10-2	8047-27-6	660	122-46-3	←	491	127-65-1	←	91
117-24-8	←	1327	122-60-1	—	1629	127-69-5	←	1568
117-26-0	←	1005	122-88-3	←	1211	127-79-7	←	1557
117-27-1	←	1016	122-99-6	←	463	127-82-2	←	275
117-37-3	←	1333	123-03-5	←	988	127-85-5	98-50-0	189
117-52-2	←	1337	123-30-8	←	624	128-03-0	128-04-1	1163
117-80-6	←	1190	123-31-9	←	504	128-04-1	←	1163
117-81-7	←	591	123-33-1	←	1308	128-09-6	←	92
117-84-0	117-81-7	591	123-38-6	75-07-0	480	128-37-0	←	1614
117-89-5	←	1426	123-42-2	←	469	128-44-9	81-07-2	1616
118-08-1	←	827	123-51-3	←	417	128-62-1	←	788
118-42-3	54-05-7	1512	123-63-7	←	1442	129-06-6	81-81-2	1345
118-52-5	←	93	123-72-8	75-07-0	480	129-16-8	←	235
118-55-8	←	598	123-73-9	107-02-8	481	129-20-4	←	1574
118-56-9	←	1533	123-86-4	←	568	129-49-7	←	806
118-60-5	87-20-7	596	123-88-6	←	239	129-51-1	—	667
118-71-8	←	866	123-91-1	←	1621	129-67-9	←	1304
118-74-1	←	397	123-92-2	←	574	129-71-5	82-93-9	1489
118-75-2	←	1183	123-94-4	8050-92-8	965	129-74-8	82-95-1	1488
118-92-3	←	627	123-96-6	111-87-5	408	129-98-6	58-55-9	802
118-96-7	←	645	124-03-8	—	977	130-26-7	83-73-8	1513

CAS Registry No. of Ingredient	CAS Registry No. of Primary Name	Location Number of Primary Name (See Part D)	CAS Registry No. of Ingredient	CAS Registry No. of Primary Name	Location Number of Primary Name (See Part D)	CAS Registry No. of Ingredient	CAS Registry No. of Primary Name	Location Number of Primary Name (See Part D)
130-37-0	58-27-5	**1605**	139-96-8	—	**946**	150-50-5	←	**1114**
130-39-2	55-63-0	**635**	140-36-3	←	**1457**	150-68-5	←	**1253**
130-95-0	←	**809**	140-41-0	150-68-5	**1253**	151-06-4	←	**1446**
131-01-1	←	**796**	140-56-7	←	**1195**	151-21-3		**946**
131-11-3	←	**593**	140-57-8	←	**1040**	151-38-2	123-88-6	**239**
131-52-2	87-86-5	**532**	140-88-5	—	**1625**	151-50-8	57-12-5	**105**
131-57-7	←	**1537**	140-90-9	←	**1314**	151-56-4	←	**606**
131-61-3	58-90-2	**534**	140-93-2	←	**1315**	152-02-3	71-82-9	**784**
131-69-1	←	**1547**	141-00-4	—	**220**	152-16-9	←	**1102**
131-72-6	39300-45-3	**542**	141-03-7	←	**1325**	152-72-7	←	**1332**
131-89-5	←	**540**	141-22-0	←	**560**	154-45-0	299-42-3	**1450**
132-20-7	←	**1497**	141-32-2	—	**1625**	154-69-8	←	**1500**
132-27-4	1322-20-9	**495**	141-43-5	←	**64**	155-04-4	149-30-4	**1198**
132-30-9	83-26-1	**1343**	141-53-7	64-18-6	**44**	155-41-9	51-34-3	**771**
132-58-1	132-60-5	**1591**	141-66-2	←	**1051**	156-08-1	1027-30-1	**1445**
132-60-5	←	**1591**	141-78-6	←	**570**	156-51-4	←	**1477**
132-66-1	←	**1279**	141-79-7	←	**474**	156-62-7	←	**1355**
132-67-2	132-66-1	**1279**	142-19-8	←	**857**	260-94-6	←	**1517**
133-05-1	8008-74-0	**722**	142-47-2	←	**1618**	262-20-4	←	**1360**
133-06-2	←	**1179**	142-59-6	←	**1162**	274-09-9	←	**870**
133-07-3	←	**1181**	142-82-5	110-54-3	**307**	279-21-0	—	**134**
133-09-5	65-49-6	**629**	142-91-6	110-27-0	**575**	288-13-1	←	**1509**
133-10-8	65-49-6	**629**	143-07-7	←	**556**	297-76-7	—	**916**
133-37-9	←	**563**	143-19-1	—	**953**	297-78-9	←	**1024**
133-58-4	1344-31-6	**233**	143-33-9	57-12-5	**105**	297-88-1	76-99-3	**1485**
133-67-5	—	**1588**	143-50-0	←	**1032**	297-97-2	←	**1081**
133-80-2	59-02-9	**910**	143-71-5	34195-34-1	**783**	297-99-4	←	**1058**
133-90-4	←	**1296**	143-74-8	←	**1608**	298-00-0	←	**1076**
134-09-8	←	**1534**	143-81-7	←	**1367**	298-01-1	7786-34-7	**1057**
134-31-6	148-24-3	**1514**	143-82-8	←	**1383**	298-02-2	←	**1094**
134-49-6	←	**1466**	144-00-3	←	**1375**	298-03-3	8000-97-3	**1067**
134-62-3	←	**1326**	144-02-5	57-44-3	**1366**	298-04-4	←	**1086**
134-72-5	299-42-3	**1450**	144-11-6	302-40-9	**1430**	298-14-6	←	**156**
134-80-5	90-84-6	**1447**	144-21-8	←	**203**	299-29-6	—	**258**
135-07-9	—	**1588**	144-23-0	—	**174**	299-42-3	←	**1450**
135-19-3	←	**493**	144-49-0	513-62-2	**548**	299-84-3	←	**1079**
135-23-9	←	**1495**	144-54-7	137-42-8	**1161**	299-85-4	←	**1105**
135-49-9	—	**1518**	144-55-8	←	**164**	299-86-5	←,	**1104**
136-25-4	←	**1218**	144-62-7	←	**47**	300-42-5	300-62-9	**1444**
136-32-3	—	**535**	144-74-1	72-14-0	**1567**	300-54-9	←	**818**
136-40-3	←	**1522**	144-80-9	←	**1551**	300-57-2	←	**311**
136-45-8	←	**1328**	144-82-1	←	**1560**	300-62-9	←	**1444**
136-47-0	94-24-6	**1586**	144-83-2	←	**1564**	300-76-5	←	**1055**
136-77-6	←	**503**	145-73-3	129-67-9	**1304**	301-03-1	12427-38-2	**1160**
136-78-7	←	**1216**	146-22-5	←	**1400**	301-04-2	7439-92-1	**245**
136-96-9	←	**1525**	146-28-1	←	**1424**	301-05-3	14484-64-1	**1158**
137-05-3	—	**1626**	146-48-5	←	**834**	301-11-1	←	**1037**
137-09-7	←	**620**	146-56-5	←	**1415**	301-12-2	←	**1074**
137-26-8	←	**1165**	146-71-4	58-55-9	**802**	302-01-2	60-34-4	**817**
137-30-4	←	**1168**	147-24-0	←	**1492**	302-17-0	←	**1432**
137-32-6	71-41-0	**405**	147-52-4	—	**902**	302-27-2	←	**822**
137-40-6	←	**551**	147-55-7	—	**902**	302-40-9	←	**1430**
137-41-7	137-42-8	**1161**	147-79-5	133-37-9	**563**	303-25-3	1104-22-9	**1494**
137-42-8	←	**1161**	148-01-6	←	**1540**	304-61-0	←	**213**
137-58-6	←	**1582**	148-24-3	←	**1514**	305-03-3	←	**1590**
138-15-8	142-47-2	**1618**	148-65-2	←	**1490**	305-33-9	←	**1475**
138-86-3	←	**877**	148-79-8	←	**1177**	305-53-3	513-62-2	**548**
139-02-6	108-95-2	**494**	149-30-4	←	**1198**	305-85-1	←	**537**
139-05-9	←	**1617**	149-91-7	←	**502**	306-21-8	140-36-3	**1457**
139-33-3	62-33-9	**1504**	150-13-0	←	**628**	309-00-2	←	**1017**
139-40-2	←	**1268**	150-39-0	60-00-4	**1506**	309-43-3	←	**1386**

CAS Registry No. of Ingredient	CAS Registry No. of Primary Name	Location Number of Primary Name (See Part D)	CAS Registry No. of Ingredient	CAS Registry No. of Primary Name	Location Number of Primary Name (See Part D)	CAS Registry No. of Ingredient	CAS Registry No. of Primary Name	Location Number of Primary Name (See Part D)
311-45-5	←	1056	487-93-4	←	820	537-91-7	←	1541
311-47-7	←	1054				538-04-5	←	224
			491-92-9	90-34-6	1516	539-90-2	123-86-4	568
314-19-2	←	779	493-53-8	50-78-2	594	540-42-1	123-86-4	568
314-40-9	←	1294	494-38-2	—	1518	540-59-0	←	361
314-42-1	314-40-9	1294	494-52-0	←	773			
315-18-4	←	1141	495-73-8	←	1178	540-72-7	←	147
317-34-0	←	799				542-55-2	123-86-4	568
			496-67-3	77-65-6	1431	542-56-3	463-04-7	630
317-83-9	←	536	497-19-8	←	52	542-75-6	←	386
318-98-9	←	1613	499-75-2	←	489	542-88-1	107-30-2	467
330-54-1	←	1247	500-28-7	←	1065			
330-55-2	←	1251	502-39-6	←	240	542-90-5	—	1034
333-18-6	107-15-3	602				543-80-6	—	166
			502-55-6	←	1302	544-16-1	463-04-7	630
333-20-0	←	148	503-38-8	75-44-5	11	544-63-8	←	557
333-41-5	←	1068	504-19-8	←	1261	545-06-2	←	655
337-47-3	←	1389	504-24-5	←	1319			
346-18-9	—	1588	504-29-0	←	1320	545-55-1	52-46-0	1354
357-07-3	76-41-5	790				545-93-7	←	1385
			507-70-0	←	876	546-93-0	—	174
357-08-4	←	787	509-42-2	57-24-9	833	547-32-0	68-35-9	1553
357-57-3	←	824	509-86-4	←	1374	548-00-5	←	1340
357-89-1	513-62-2	548	510-15-6	←	1006			
359-83-1	←	792	511-12-6	—	667	548-62-9	←	1520
361-37-5	129-49-7	806				550-70-9	—	1487
			511-13-7	←	1589	550-81-2	54-05-7	1512
362-29-8	64-89-1	1422	513-62-2	←	548	550-99-2	←	1463
367-51-1	←	553	513-77-9	—	166	552-22-7	89-83-8	497
371-62-0	513-62-2	548	513-79-1	←	282			
371-86-8	←	1100	514-10-3	←	580	552-94-3	←	601
378-44-9	—	915				554-12-1	107-31-3	576
			517-16-8	←	230	554-13-2	7439-93-2	154
379-79-3	—	667	517-18-0	—	916	554-35-8	←	850
404-82-0	458-24-2	1456	518-20-7	←	1338	554-42-7	—	284
405-30-1	←	1045	518-28-5	8050-60-0	759			
407-40-9	←	1644	520-26-3	24292-52-2	1599	555-06-6	150-13-0	628
408-35-5	—	953				555-37-3	←	1254
			520-45-6	←	1187	555-89-5	←	1014
420-05-3	←	29	520-52-5	←	821	556-22-9	←	1196
435-97-2	←	1342	520-53-6	520-52-5	821	556-24-1	107-31-3	576
438-41-5	←	1392	521-35-7	1323-34-8	933			
439-14-5	←	1395	521-74-4	83-73-8	1513	556-61-6	←	1358
440-17-5	117-89-5	1426				556-64-9	—	1034
			521-78-8	739-71-9	1481	557-04-0	—	174
458-24-2	←	1456	522-17-8	—	897	557-05-1	←	278
458-88-8	←	826	522-48-5	←	1469	557-08-4	←	279
462-08-8	504-24-5	1319	523-80-8	—	725			
463-04-7	←	630	523-87-5	147-24-0	1492	557-09-5	557-05-1	278
463-58-1	←	127				557-21-1	57-12-5	105
			525-66-6	318-98-9	1613	557-28-8	—	277
463-71-8	←	12	526-07-8	8008-74-0	722	557-34-6	—	277
464-41-5	←	874	526-26-1	63-36-5	600	557-41-5	—	277
465-65-6	357-08-4	787	527-20-8	82-68-8	1201			
465-73-6	←	1025	528-94-9	63-36-5	600	561-27-3	←	782
467-36-7	←	1388				562-10-7	←	1493
			529-73-7	90-34-6	1516	563-12-2	←	1087
467-60-7	←	1478	531-73-7	—	1518	563-47-3	←	382
470-43-9	←	1411	532-03-6	59-47-2	1406	563-68-8	7440-28-0	249
470-82-6	←	863	532-27-4	←	14			
471-34-1	←	171	532-32-1	65-85-0	582	563-71-3	←	257
471-53-4	1407-03-0	848				564-25-0	—	904
			532-34-3	←	1322	569-57-3	—	916
474-86-2	—	916	532-43-4	59-43-8	914	569-59-5	—	1487
475-26-3	←	1008	533-06-2	59-47-2	1406	569-65-3	1104-22-9	1494
479-18-5	←	804	533-74-4	←	1186			
480-30-8	←	1572	533-96-0	←	53	573-41-1	58-55-9	802
481-06-1	←	931				573-83-1	88-89-1	545
			534-07-6	78-43-3	1119	574-64-1	72-57-1	1524
483-18-1	←	805	534-52-1	←	539	575-36-0	86-86-2	1277
485-31-4	88-85-7	543	535-77-3	1330-20-7	318	576-55-6	←	533
485-34-7	132-60-5	1591	535-89-7	←	1346			
486-84-0	—	681	537-46-2	←	1459	577-11-7	←	951

CAS Registry No. of Ingredient	CAS Registry No. of Primary Name	Location Number of Primary Name (See Part D)	CAS Registry No. of Ingredient	CAS Registry No. of Primary Name	Location Number of Primary Name (See Part D)	CAS Registry No. of Ingredient	CAS Registry No. of Primary Name	Location Number of Primary Name (See Part D)
580-48-3	1912-24-9	1259	739-71-9	←	1481	1113-41-3	52-67-5	1507
583-52-8	—	546	741-58-2	←	1082	1114-71-2	←	1238
584-79-2	←	884	751-97-3	—	904	1118-46-3	—	292
584-84-9	←	1641	752-61-4	71-63-6	838	1120-44-1	7440-50-8	265
586-81-2	←	882	757-58-4	←	1106	1129-41-5	2425-10-7	1143
587-23-5	100-97-0	486	759-94-4	←	1236	1134-23-2	←	1234
589-59-3	123-86-4	568	765-15-1	←	1036	1142-59-2	305-33-9	1475
590-28-3	—	145	768-94-5	←	922	1142-70-7	←	1369
590-86-3	75-07-0	480	777-11-7	←	1527	1172-18-5	←	1397
591-27-5	123-30-8	624	786-19-6	←	1083	1172-63-0	—	893
591-78-6	←	479	814-71-1	—	552	1176-08-5	←	1498
592-01-8	—	107	814-91-5	7440-50-8	265	1179-69-7	1420-55-9	1423
592-04-1	1335-31-5	108	822-16-2	—	953	1187-59-3	79-06-1	1624
592-84-7	123-86-4	568	828-00-2	—	1642	1197-21-3	122-09-8	1467
594-72-9	←	20	834-12-8	1610-18-0	1267	1216-40-6	←	1387
598-63-0	7439-92-1	245	835-31-4	550-99-2	1463	1225-55-4	←	1479
598-92-5	600-25-9	19	841-06-5	1610-18-0	1267	1229-29-4	1668-19-5	1472
599-79-1	←	1566	845-52-3	1610-18-0	1267	1240-15-9	64-89-1	1422
600-25-9	←	19	846-49-1	←	1398	1264-72-8	1406-11-7	903
603-35-0	7803-51-2	136	846-50-4	604-75-1	1401	1294-56-0	317-34-0	799
603-50-9	77-09-8	1607	855-96-9	—	668	1299-88-3	←	200
604-75-1	←	1401	866-55-7	—	292	1300-18-1	57-24-9	833
607-80-7	8008-74-0	722	866-84-2	—	155	1300-20-5	—	700
607-91-0	—	679	867-27-6	8000-97-3	1067	1300-71-6	←	498
608-73-1	←	1029	868-14-4	133-37-9	563	1301-19-5	8041-00-7	979
609-20-1	99-30-9	1191	868-77-9	—	1625	1301-47-9	8041-00-7	979
614-39-1	51-06-9	1612	870-08-6	—	292	1302-29-0	21645-51-2	178
615-05-4	←	622	886-50-0	1610-18-0	1267	1302-97-2	←	202
615-67-8	←	500	887-54-7	1861-32-1	1303	1303-28-2	7778-39-4	191
616-91-1	←	1502	900-95-8	←	295	1303-33-9	←	194
623-42-7	107-31-3	576	912-60-7	128-62-1	788	1303-39-5	←	211
627-83-8	←	964	914-00-1	—	904	1303-86-2	←	130
628-63-7	123-92-2	574	917-61-3	—	145	1303-90-8	—	131
628-96-6	←	633	919-44-8	141-66-2	1051	1303-96-4	←	132
629-14-1	—	459	919-86-8	8022-00-2	1075	1304-13-8	←	102
630-08-0	←	126	924-42-5	79-06-1	1624	1304-28-5	—	166
630-60-4	←	842	953-17-3	←	1092	1304-37-6	—	166
630-93-3	←	1609	956-90-1	←	1542	1304-85-4	—	218
633-03-4	←	1519	957-51-7	←	1275	1305-62-0	—	55
634-03-7	134-49-6	1466	961-11-5	←	1061	1305-78-8	←	54
637-03-6	—	192	991-42-4	←	1349	1306-19-0	—	220
638-21-1	7803-51-2	136	994-31-0	—	293	1306-23-6	—	220
639-58-7	900-95-8	295	1014-69-3	1610-18-0	1267	1307-96-6	—	283
640-19-7	←	1347	1014-70-6	1610-18-0	1267	1308-29-8	7758-97-6	246
641-77-0	—	915	1027-30-1	←	1445	1308-38-9	←	280
644-64-4	←	1132	1031-47-6	←	1209	1309-37-1	←	252
646-29-7	57-11-4	562	1066-17-7	1406-11-7	903	1309-42-8	←	175
650-51-1	←	550	1067-33-0	—	292	1309-45-1	←	37
651-06-9	←	1558	1067-97-6	—	293	1309-48-4	—	174
652-67-5	←	1603	1070-11-7	←	1596	1309-60-0	←	247
659-70-1	123-92-2	574	1076-46-6	133-90-4	1296	1309-63-3	←	296
665-66-7	768-94-5	922	1079-33-0	←	1142	1310-00-5	—	101
671-04-5	←	1127	1082-88-8	15588-95-1	1449	1310-07-2	—	101
672-04-8	8065-36-9	1125	1085-98-9	←	1189	1310-45-8	←	254
673-04-1	33693-04-8	1270	1095-66-5	110-91-8	72	1310-58-3	—	51
683-18-1	—	292	1095-90-5	76-99-3	1485	1310-61-8	18496-25-8	118
709-98-8	←	1283	1098-60-8	←	1427	1310-65-2	—	51
721-50-6	←	1584	1102-47-2	—	1487	1310-73-2	—	51
723-46-6	←	1561	1104-22-9	←	1494	1311-10-0	—	51
731-27-1	1085-98-9	1189	1111-39-3	71-63-6	838	1312-73-8	18496-25-8	118
732-11-6	←	1090	1113-14-0	←	1175	1312-76-1	13472-30-5	58

CAS Registry No. of Ingredient	CAS Registry No. of Primary Name	Location Number of Primary Name (See Part D)	CAS Registry No. of Ingredient	CAS Registry No. of Primary Name	Location Number of Primary Name (See Part D)	CAS Registry No. of Ingredient	CAS Registry No. of Primary Name	Location Number of Primary Name (See Part D)
1313-59-3	—	51	1333-15-9	97-23-4	529	1406-11-7	←	903
1313-60-6	←	74	1333-24-0	←	199	1406-13-9	8001-01-2	905
1313-82-2	18496-25-8	118	1333-25-1	7778-44-1	198	1406-16-2	←	909
1314-13-2	←	274	1333-28-4	112-38-9	564	1406-65-1	←	926
1314-22-3	8007-30-5	73	1333-73-9	1303-96-4	132	1407-03-0	←	848
1314-23-4	←	301	1333-82-0	←	80	1415-73-2	8015-61-0	847
1314-35-8	7440-33-7	297	1333-83-1	—	100	1420-53-7	76-57-3	780
1314-41-6	7439-92-1	245	1333-84-2	21645-51-2	178	1420-55-9	←	1423
1314-56-3	←	38	1334-72-1	9002-92-0	966	1432-14-0	7085-19-0	1221
1314-60-9	—	212	1335-25-7	7439-92-1	245	1444-64-0	←	426
1314-62-1	7440-62-2	299	1335-31-5	←	108	1461-25-2	—	292
1314-80-3	←	117	1335-69-9	548-62-9	1520	1468-37-7	502-55-6	1302
1314-84-7	←	138	1335-72-4	13150-00-0	955	1490-04-6	89-78-1	868
1314-95-0	—	290	1335-76-8	8014-10-6	880	1518-86-1	140-36-3	1457
1314-96-1	←	119	1335-85-9	534-52-1	539	1563-66-2	←	1129
1314-98-3	18496-25-8	118	1335-87-1	—	402	1582-09-8	←	1289
1317-25-5	5579-81-7	179	1336-21-6	7664-41-7	63	1596-84-5	←	1356
1317-33-5	18496-25-8	118	1336-80-7	←	255	1610-17-9	1610-18-0	1267
1317-39-1	←	269	1338-23-4	←	75	1610-18-0	←	1267
1317-63-1	—	692	1338-41-6	←	972	1622-61-3	←	1393
1317-65-3	←	173	1338-43-8	1338-41-6	972	1622-62-4	←	1396
1319-77-3	8003-33-6	514	1340-08-5	24292-52-2	1599	1639-60-7	←	1486
1319-85-3	←	1317	1340-18-7	7439-92-1	245	1639-66-3	577-11-7	951
1319-86-4	←	225	1341-07-7	—	974	1665-48-1	←	1408
1319-96-6	3134-12-1	1256	1341-44-2	532-34-3	1322	1668-19-5	←	1472
1320-15-6	94-82-6	1215	1341-49-7	—	100	1675-54-3	—	1629
1320-40-7	25155-18-4	992	1343-88-0	←	176	1689-84-5	←	1295
1320-67-8	107-98-2	464	1343-98-2	7631-86-9	7	1689-99-2	1689-84-5	1295
1320-79-2	—	535	1344-08-7	18496-25-8	118	1698-60-8	←	1313
1321-38-6	584-84-9	1641	1344-09-8	13472-30-5	58	1707-14-8	134-49-6	1466
1321-64-8	—	402	1344-28-1	21645-51-2	178	1722-62-9	96-88-8	1583
1321-94-4	←	320	1344-29-2	1309-63-3	296	1746-81-2	330-55-2	1251
1322-20-9	←	495	1344-31-6	←	233	1754-58-1	—	1097
1322-37-8	←	999	1344-32-7	←	1361	1762-95-4	—	146
1323-34-8	←	933	1344-35-0	—	851	1786-81-8	721-50-6	1584
1327-30-6	←	201	1344-45-2	—	221	1836-75-5	←	1310
1327-36-2	14504-95-1	180	1344-48-5	—	221	1847-55-8	—	946
1327-41-9	7446-70-0	182	1344-75-8	←	104	1861-32-1	←	1303
1327-43-1	1343-88-0	176	1344-81-6	9046-53-1	113	1861-40-1	←	1287
1327-52-2	7778-39-4	191	1344-90-7	1303-96-4	132	1897-45-6	←	1185
1327-53-3	←	193	1345-04-6	—	212	1910-42-5	←	1286
1329-25-5	—	976	1345-05-7	←	115	1912-24-9	←	1259
1329-98-2	1330-20-7	318	1345-11-5	18496-25-8	118	1912-25-0	1912-24-9	1259
1330-20-7	←	318	1381-00-6	—	667	1912-26-1	1912-24-9	1259
1330-78-5	←	1115	1391-75-9	1405-76-1	840	1918-00-9	←	1300
1330-82-1	—	573	1391-79-3	—	685	1918-02-1	←	1312
1331-19-7	76-03-9	50	1393-62-0	—	677	1918-08-7	29091-05-2	1288
1331-46-0	←	526	1398-11-4	146-48-5	834	1918-11-2	←	1231
1331-71-1	1344-75-8	104	1398-77-2	←	662	1918-13-4	←	1297
1331-88-0	89-68-9	527	1399-80-0	—	982	1918-16-7	—	1282
1332-03-2	←	270	1401-55-4	←	852	1928-47-8	93-76-5	1224
1332-09-8	←	6	1404-04-2	←	901	1929-77-7	←	1240
1332-17-8	←	90	1404-24-6	1406-11-7	903	1929-86-8	7085-19-0	1221
1332-21-4	←	2	1404-26-8	1406-11-7	903	1967-16-4	101-21-3	1229
1332-28-1	1303-96-4	132	1404-28-0	1406-11-7	903	1977-10-2	←	1476
1332-40-7	1332-65-6	268	1404-29-1	1406-11-7	903	1981-58-4	57-68-1	1559
1332-58-7	←	5	1404-88-2	8001-01-2	905	1982-47-4	←	1243
1332-65-6	←	268	1405-10-3	1404-04-2	901	1982-49-6	←	1257
1332-77-0	—	131	1405-76-1	←	840	1982-67-8	407-40-9	1644
1332-94-1	29883-15-6	846	1405-86-3	1407-03-0	848	1983-10-4	—	293
1333-00-2	—	253	1405-97-6	8001-01-2	905	2008-41-5	←	1233

CAS Registry No. of Ingredient	CAS Registry No. of Primary Name	Location Number of Primary Name (See Part D)	CAS Registry No. of Ingredient	CAS Registry No. of Primary Name	Location Number of Primary Name (See Part D)	CAS Registry No. of Ingredient	CAS Registry No. of Primary Name	Location Number of Primary Name (See Part D)
2016-36-6	63-36-5	600	2631-40-5	←	1137	3811-04-9	—	96
2027-47-6	112-80-1	559	2655-15-4	2686-99-9	1138	3813-14-7	93-76-5	1224
2032-59-9	←	1122	2655-19-8	←	1126	3819-00-9	50-52-2	1425
2032-65-7	←	1139	2674-91-1	301-12-2	1074	3878-19-1	←	1176
2039-46-5	94-74-6	1220	2675-77-6	←	1184	3882-06-2	—	974
2086-83-1	←	823	2675-94-7	79-06-1	1624	3926-62-3	79-11-8	549
2104-64-5	←	1071	2686-99-9	←	1138	3953-10-4	—	1625
2152-34-3	←	1465	2698-41-1	←	15	4024-81-1	—	1199
2163-69-1	←	1244	2699-79-8	←	18	4065-45-6	131-57-7	1537
2163-79-3	18530-56-8	1255	2717-15-9	←	960	4080-31-3	←	995
2163-80-6	144-21-8	203	2751-68-0	←	1413	4097-36-3	←	538
2164-09-2	709-98-8	1283	2758-42-1	94-82-6	1215	4147-51-7	1610-18-0	1267
2164-17-2	←	1249	2763-96-4	←	819	4170-30-3	107-02-8	481
2174-16-5	63-36-5	600	2764-72-9	85-00-7	1285	4268-36-4	57-53-4	1407
2180-92-9	←	1578	2782-57-2	87-90-1	94	4342-36-3	—	293
2192-20-3	←	1438	2813-95-8	88-85-7	543	4345-16-8	299-42-3	1450
2197-37-7	60-33-3	555	2876-78-0	86-87-3	1309	4360-12-7	←	794
2212-67-1	←	1237	2893-78-9	87-90-1	94	4386-35-0	←	238
2219-72-9	8003-33-6	514	2898-11-5	←	1399	4386-88-3	←	243
2227-17-0	←	1027	2921-88-2	←	1064	4418-26-2	520-45-6	1187
2235-25-8	←	231	2941-55-1	759-94-4	1236	4466-14-2	—	893
2235-54-3	—	946	2955-38-6	←	1402	4482-55-7	101-42-8	1248
2238-07-5	—	1629	2975-34-0	117-89-5	1426	4568-28-9	2717-15-9	960
2244-21-5	87-90-1	94	3004-70-4	33693-04-8	1270	4617-17-8	—	1034
2255-17-6	122-14-5	1072	3004-71-5	1912-24-9	1259	4636-83-3	1910-42-5	1286
2276-52-0	359-83-1	792	3050-27-9	3134-12-1	1256	4685-14-7	1910-42-5	1286
2279-64-3	—	221	3060-89-7	150-68-5	1253	4697-36-3	—	902
2282-34-0	8065-36-9	1125	3068-31-3	123-33-1	1308	4719-04-4	←	1173
2303-16-4	←	1235	3091-25-6	—	292	4726-14-1	1861-40-1	1287
2303-17-5	2303-16-4	1235	3097-08-3	—	946	4764-17-4	←	1461
2303-35-7	300-54-9	818	3129-91-7	←	632	4849-32-5	←	1232
2307-49-5	1918-00-9	1300	3134-12-1	←	1256	5015-89-4	—	287
2307-68-8	←	1280	3244-90-4	←	1110	5094-26-8	63-36-5	600
2312-76-7	534-52-1	539	3307-39-9	122-88-3	1211	5133-19-7	8015-61-0	847
2315-02-8	←	1464	3313-26-6	113-59-7	1414	5139-02-6	52-67-5	1507
2315-36-8	93-71-0	1274	3329-16-6	125-55-3	1384	5188-49-8	—	282
2358-84-1	—	1625	3337-71-1	←	1226	5221-53-4	←	1192
2385-85-5	←	1033	3344-18-1	—	174	5234-68-4	←	1182
2398-96-1	←	1532	3352-57-6	—	51	5259-88-1	5234-68-4	1182
2425-06-1	←	1180	3380-34-5	←	1002	5281-13-0	←	1156
2425-10-7	←	1143	3383-96-8	←	1063	5328-04-1	←	263
2426-08-6	—	1629	3400-09-7	—	22	5329-14-6	←	48
2431-21-2	←	288	3426-62-8	1319-85-3	1317	5331-91-9	149-30-4	1198
2438-32-6	—	1487	3466-09-9	←	887	5333-99-3	132-66-1	1279
2439-00-1	85-34-7	1219	3486-35-9	—	277	5393-75-9	85-34-7	1219
2439-01-2	←	1205	3486-86-0	1142-70-7	1369	5406-97-3	149-30-4	1198
2439-10-3	←	1193	3547-33-9	←	1330	5421-46-5	—	552
2440-45-1	2235-25-8	231	3566-10-7	142-59-6	1162	5470-11-1	7803-49-8	122
2447-54-3	—	693	3570-61-4	←	1225	5579-81-7	←	179
2451-01-6	←	883	3590-23-6	←	276	5588-33-0	50-52-2	1425
2492-26-4	149-30-4	1198	3635-74-3	108-01-0	1592	5635-50-7	—	916
2532-49-2	←	1148	3653-48-3	94-74-6	1220	5700-49-2	107-15-3	602
2545-59-7	93-76-5	1224	3689-24-5	←	1108	5707-69-7	←	1194
2545-60-0	1918-02-1	1312	3691-35-8	←	1335	5714-00-1	2751-68-0	1413
2549-67-9	151-56-4	606	3697-42-5	55-56-1	994	5714-73-8	100-97-0	486
2591-66-4	←	1099	3721-28-6	95-62-5	1480	5716-15-4	123-33-1	1308
2593-10-4	87-17-2	998	3737-00-6	←	381	5768-87-6	77-09-8	1607
2597-93-5	←	227	3766-60-7	←	1241	5822-97-9	4386-88-3	243
2622-37-9	1098-60-8	1427	3766-81-2	←	1124	5826-91-5	←	1070
2624-17-1	504-19-8	1261	3784-03-0	—	535	5834-84-4	←	1331
2631-37-0	←	1146	3810-80-8	←	1482	5836-10-2	18181-80-1	1004

CAS Registry No. of Ingredient	CAS Registry No. of Primary Name	Location Number of Primary Name (See Part D)	CAS Registry No. of Ingredient	CAS Registry No. of Primary Name	Location Number of Primary Name (See Part D)	CAS Registry No. of Ingredient	CAS Registry No. of Primary Name	Location Number of Primary Name (See Part D)
5892-10-4	←	217	7431-95-0	141-22-0	560	7683-59-2	51-31-0	1458
5902-51-2	314-40-9	1294	7439-92-1	←	245	7696-12-0	←	898
5902-85-2	149-30-4	1198	7439-93-2	←	154	7697-37-2	←	32
5902-95-4	144-21-8	203	7439-97-6	—	221	7699-43-6	←	302
5903-07-1	89-68-9	527	7440-28-0	←	249	7700-17-6	141-66-2	1051
5907-38-0	←	1573	7440-33-7	←	297	7704-34-9	←	120
5908-99-6	51-55-8	767	7440-38-2	←	188	7705-08-0	—	253
5915-41-3	1912-24-9	1259	7440-39-3	←	168	7705-12-6	—	258
5938-38-5	1338-41-6	972	7440-43-9	—	220	7705-14-8	138-86-3	877
5949-29-1	77-92-9	703	7440-44-0	7782-42-5	4	7718-54-9	—	287
5967-84-0	58-55-9	802	7440-50-8	←	265	7720-78-7	—	258
5989-27-5	138-86-3	877	7440-62-2	←	299	7722-64-7	←	83
5991-71-9	57109-90-7	1394	7440-74-6	←	285	7722-84-1	8007-30-5	73
6013-05-4	←	1298	7446-07-3	—	187	7722-88-5	←	140
6019-02-9	54-11-5	772	7446-08-4	—	185	7723-14-0	←	135
6035-40-1	128-62-1	788	7446-09-5	←	10	7726-95-6	←	25
6046-93-1	7440-50-8	265	7446-14-2	7439-92-1	245	7727-43-7	7440-39-3	168
6047-17-2	93-72-1	1223	7446-18-6	7440-28-0	249	7727-54-0	10361-76-9	79
6059-47-8	76-57-3	780	7446-34-6	←	186	7727-73-3	—	159
6062-26-6	94-81-5	1222	7446-70-0	←	182	7733-02-0	—	277
6100-07-8	←	496	7447-39-4	7440-50-8	265	7757-69-9	—	174
6106-46-3	51-34-3	771	7447-40-7	—	155	7757-79-1	—	157
6108-05-0	137-58-6	1582	7447-41-8	7439-93-2	154	7757-82-6	—	159
6119-92-2	39300-45-3	542	7487-88-9	—	174	7757-83-7	—	149
6164-98-3	←	1042	7487-94-7	←	236	7757-86-0	—	174
6190-38-1	34195-34-1	783	7488-56-4	7446-34-6	186	7757-87-1	—	174
6251-69-0	—	915	7488-70-2	—	920	7758-01-2	—	95
6272-89-5	←	1453	7492-30-0	141-22-0	560	7758-02-3	—	98
6365-62-4	94-74-6	1220	7492-32-2	←	1602	7758-05-6	—	97
6365-83-9	88-85-7	543	7542-12-3	497-19-8	52	7758-09-0	—	144
6369-97-7	93-76-5	1224	7546-30-7	10112-91-1	237	7758-11-4	—	155
6379-37-9	←	208	7553-56-2	←	26	7758-19-2	10049-04-4	24
6379-46-0	←	1202	7554-65-6	288-13-1	1509	7758-29-4	14127-68-5	142
6385-60-0	129-67-9	1304	7558-73-8	61-50-7	1448	7758-89-6	←	266
6392-46-7	←	1121	7558-79-4	—	139	7758-94-3	—	258
6531-86-8	8014-87-7	425	7558-80-7	—	139	7758-97-6	←	246
6586-04-5	92-31-9	1523	7580-67-8	←	61	7758-98-7	7440-50-8	265
6659-45-6	←	888	7587-43-1	←	1451	7759-02-6	—	177
6734-80-1	137-42-8	1161	7601-54-9	←	60	7761-88-8	2431-21-2	288
6834-92-0	←	57	7631-86-9	←	7	7772-98-7	←	163
6893-02-3	—	920	7631-89-2	←	209	7773-03-7	—	149
6899-05-4	142-47-2	1618	7631-90-5	←	150	7773-06-0	←	153
6914-07-4	74-90-8	106	7631-99-4	—	157	7774-29-0	7487-94-7	236
6988-21-2	←	1133	7632-00-0	—	144	7775-09-9	—	96
7003-89-6	1910-42-5	1286	7632-05-5	—	139	7775-11-3	—	81
7055-03-0	←	1208	7645-25-2	7784-40-9	206	7775-14-6	←	151
7058-55-1	—	220	7646-85-7	—	277	7775-19-1	—	131
7076-23-5	←	777	7647-01-0	←	31	7778-18-9	10034-76-1	172
7076-28-0	←	1348	7647-14-5	←	165	7778-39-4	←	191
7084-87-9	←	1107	7647-15-6	—	98	7778-43-0	7631-89-2	209
7085-19-0	←	1221	7664-38-2	1314-56-3	38	7778-44-1	←	198
7097-60-1	7553-56-2	26	7664-39-3	←	36	7778-50-9	←	82
7173-51-5	—	989	7664-41-7	←	63	7778-53-2	←	59
7260-42-6	6379-37-9	208	7664-93-9	←	33	7778-54-3	←	89
7283-42-3	68-11-1	49	7681-11-0	—	99	7778-66-7	7681-52-9	85
7286-84-2	133-90-4	1296	7681-38-1	←	40	7778-77-0	—	155
7287-19-6	1610-18-0	1267	7681-49-4	—	100	7778-83-8	—	587
7287-36-7	709-98-8	1283	7681-52-9	←	85	7779-25-1	—	174
7297-25-8	55-63-0	635	7681-55-2	—	97	7779-27-3	←	1172
7320-34-5	7722-88-5	140	7681-79-0	←	1455	7782-42-5	←	4
7346-80-7	—	948	7681-82-5	—	99	7782-50-5	←	23

CAS Registry No. of Ingredient	CAS Registry No. of Primary Name	Location Number of Primary Name (See Part D)	CAS Registry No. of Ingredient	CAS Registry No. of Primary Name	Location Number of Primary Name (See Part D)	CAS Registry No. of Ingredient	CAS Registry No. of Primary Name	Location Number of Primary Name (See Part D)
7782-75-4	—	174	8001-54-5	←	985	8007-70-3	←	731
7782-79-8	—	111	8001-58-9	←	511	8007-75-8	←	733
7782-99-2	←	35	8001-74-9	←	713	8007-80-5	104-55-2	860
7783-06-4	←	114	8001-79-4	←	712	8008-10-4	←	737
7783-08-6	←	185	8001-85-2	←	711	8008-20-6	←	328
7783-09-7	—	187	8001-95-4	←	795	8008-51-3	←	727
7783-11-1	—	149	8001-97-6	8015-61-0	847	8008-56-8	—	725
7783-37-1	—	100	8002-03-7	←	719	8008-60-4	←	757
7783-47-3	—	290	8002-05-9	←	336	8008-74-0	←	722
7783-49-5	—	100	8002-16-2	←	721	8008-98-8	470-82-6	863
7783-54-2	←	124	8002-23-1	←	973	8009-03-8	8012-95-1	337
7784-24-9	←	181	8002-26-4	←	723	8011-47-0	—	726
7784-25-0	7784-24-9	181	8002-31-1	←	742	8011-48-1	8021-39-4	513
7784-31-8	7784-24-9	181	8002-33-3	—	956	8011-55-0	—	843
7784-40-9	←	206	8002-35-5	←	845	8011-61-8	8001-01-2	905
7784-42-1	←	196	8002-39-9	←	811	8011-63-0	←	259
7784-46-5	←	210	8002-43-5	←	705	8011-78-7	1303-96-4	132
7785-87-7	—	286	8002-63-9	8063-11-4	748	8011-96-9	←	271
7786-30-3	—	174	8002-64-0	←	718	8012-14-4	10124-56-8	143
7786-34-7	←	1057	8002-74-2	←	340	8012-21-3	50-21-5	46
7786-81-4	—	287	8002-76-4	←	791	8012-45-1	80-00-2	1048
7787-32-8	—	100	8002-82-2	←	1010	8012-54-2	←	226
7787-59-9	—	216	8002-89-9	58-55-9	802	8012-69-9	←	262
7788-99-0	10101-53-8	281	8003-10-9	58-08-2	800	8012-77-9	7782-50-5	23
7789-00-6	—	81	8003-33-6	←	514	8012-80-4	7446-34-6	186
7789-09-5	—	82	8003-34-7	←	686	8012-91-7	—	725
7789-12-0	—	82	8003-43-8	133-37-9	563	8012-95-1	←	337
7789-38-0	—	95	8004-87-3	548-62-9	1520	8012-96-2	←	675
7789-53-9	—	98	8005-44-5	112-92-5	430	8013-10-3	←	729
7789-75-5	—	100	8005-49-0	94-84-8	1306	8013-48-7	←	676
7790-56-9	—	149	8005-50-3	1344-31-6	233	8013-60-3	—	765
7790-94-5	←	39	8006-07-3	50-00-0	482	8013-76-1	←	734
7791-19-7	—	174	8006-09-5	—	134	8013-88-5	156-62-7	1355
7791-23-3	—	185	8006-13-1	←	183	8013-93-2	26140-60-3	316
7791-28-8	—	166	8006-24-4	7439-92-1	245	8013-95-4	1331-46-0	526
7803-49-8	←	122	8006-47-1	12751-04-1	512	8013-99-8	8021-41-8	740
7803-51-2	←	136	8006-54-0	8020-84-6	716	8014-10-6	←	880
8000-07-5	←	768	8006-61-9	←	327	8014-16-2	8007-00-9	749
8000-10-0	58-55-9	802	8006-62-0	8003-33-6	514	8014-29-7	—	725
8000-16-6	64-17-5	412	8006-63-1	—	595	8014-87-7	←	425
8000-25-7	—	725	8006-64-2	←	763	8014-95-7	←	34
8000-27-9	←	735	8006-78-8	←	732	8015-29-0	←	918
8000-28-0	←	730	8006-80-2	←	739	8015-30-3	←	919
8000-29-1	←	736	8006-88-0	←	741	8015-61-0	←	847
8000-34-8	97-53-0	864	8006-90-4	←	738	8015-86-9	←	752
8000-41-7	586-81-2	882	8006-99-3	←	728	8016-55-5	←	689
8000-46-2	—	725	8007-00-9	←	749	8016-78-2	—	725
8000-48-4	470-82-6	863	8007-02-1	8000-29-1	736	8016-87-3	—	725
8000-96-2	←	1166	8007-08-7	—	725	8018-01-7	—	1159
8000-97-3	←	1067	8007-11-2	—	725	8018-12-0	584-79-2	884
8001-01-2	←	905	8007-12-3	—	679	8020-84-6	←	716
8001-20-5	←	724	8007-20-3	—	725	8021-39-4	←	513
8001-26-1	←	717	8007-30-5	←	73	8021-41-8	←	740
8001-28-3	←	715	8007-31-6	2431-21-2	288	8022-00-2	←	1075
8001-31-8	←	714	8007-39-4	←	831	8022-86-4	119-36-8	597
8001-33-0	←	837	8007-40-7	—	725	8023-53-8	—	976
8001-35-2	←	1030	8007-44-1	8021-41-8	740	8023-62-9	←	762
8001-38-5	—	701	8007-45-2	←	510	8023-77-6	←	659
8001-45-4	—	678	8007-46-3	←	743	8024-00-8	—	725
8001-50-1	←	1031	8007-57-6	7664-41-7	63	8024-48-4	←	849
8001-51-2	←	844	8007-65-6	←	394	8025-91-0	←	204

CAS Registry No. of Ingredient	CAS Registry No. of Primary Name	Location Number of Primary Name (See Part D)	CAS Registry No. of Ingredient	CAS Registry No. of Primary Name	Location Number of Primary Name (See Part D)	CAS Registry No. of Ingredient	CAS Registry No. of Primary Name	Location Number of Primary Name (See Part D)
8027-00-7	8002-82-2	1010	8063-21-6	←	698	9009-86-3	←	930
8027-32-5	8012-95-1	337	8063-34-1	90-03-9	234	9010-08-6	14127-68-5	142
8027-38-1	←	658	8065-36-9	←	1125	9010-41-7	—	942
8027-64-3	8012-95-1	337	8065-48-3	8000-97-3	1067	9010-78-0	25014-41-9	652
8028-32-8	8011-63-0	259	8065-67-6	8018-01-7	1159	9011-14-7	80-62-6	1630
8028-46-4	←	971	8065-95-0	12427-38-2	1160	9016-00-6	9006-65-9	1646
8028-57-7	←	691	8066-12-4	119-89-1	1152	9041-08-1	9005-49-6	1598
8028-87-3	557-05-1	278	8066-89-5	26140-60-3	316	9046-53-1	←	113
8029-29-6	←	1018	8068-28-8	1406-11-7	903	9046-54-2	12259-92-6	112
8029-39-8	←	389	9000-01-5	←	744	9046-55-3	12259-92-6	112
8029-68-3	←	1528	9000-04-8	←	747	9062-00-4	12259-92-6	112
8029-99-0	←	766	9000-11-7	←	853	9074-34-4	8001-01-2	905
8030-30-6	←	330	9000-25-3	←	754	9080-17-5	12259-92-6	112
8030-31-7	←	331	9000-28-6	—	755	10007-85-9	1918-00-9	1300
8030-35-1	563-71-3	257	9000-36-6	—	755	10022-31-8	—	166
8030-36-2	←	215	9000-59-3	←	761	10024-97-2	—	9
8030-95-3	8027-38-1	658	9000-65-1	—	755	10025-67-9	←	28
8030-97-5	←	929	9000-69-5	←	758	10025-70-4	—	177
8031-06-9	8030-30-6	330	9001-73-4	←	927	10025-85-1	←	123
8031-57-0	←	88	9001-75-6	←	928	10025-91-9	←	214
8031-69-4	←	836	9002-18-0	—	755	10026-11-6	7699-43-6	302
8032-32-4	←	335	9002-81-7	←	487	10028-16-7	—	187
8034-17-1	—	980	9002-84-0	←	1636	10028-22-5	—	253
8036-54-2	—	946	9002-88-4	←	1635	10028-24-7	—	139
8037-86-3	←	997	9002-89-5	←	1637	10031-13-7	←	207
8041-00-7	←	979	9002-90-8	—	440	10031-14-8	—	131
8043-43-4	481-06-1	931	9002-91-9	108-62-3	485	10031-37-5	10101-53-8	281
8044-51-7	←	324	9002-92-0	←	966	10031-59-1	7440-28-0	249
8044-97-1	2307-68-8	1280	9002-93-1	—	963	10034-76-1	←	172
8045-21-4	←	978	9002-95-3	—	963	10034-82-9	—	81
8046-13-7	←	429	9003-01-4	←	1627	10034-94-3	1343-88-0	176
8046-53-5	—	943	9003-03-6	9003-01-4	1627	10035-04-8	—	170
8046-97-7	←	680	9003-04-7	9003-01-4	1627	10039-54-0	7803-49-8	122
8047-05-0	—	666	9003-07-0	9002-88-4	1635	10042-91-8	7722-88-5	140
8047-27-6	←	660	9003-20-7	9002-89-5	1637	10042-94-1	←	133
8047-76-5	←	3	9003-28-5	←	1633	10043-01-3	7784-24-9	181
8048-11-1	9046-53-1	113	9003-39-8	←	1639	10043-22-8	—	546
8048-52-0	—	1518	9004-32-4	9000-11-7	853	10043-35-3	←	129
8048-56-4	—	946	9004-65-3	←	855	10043-52-4	—	170
8050-09-7	←	760	9004-67-5	←	856	10043-67-1	7784-24-9	181
8050-10-0	8050-09-7	760	9004-70-0	8050-69-9	854	10043-83-1	—	174
8050-35-9	119-53-9	750	9004-76-6	←	460	10049-04-4	←	24
8050-60-0	←	759	9004-88-0	—	963	10058-23-8	10361-76-9	79
8050-69-9	←	854	9004-99-3	←	968	10058-44-3	—	253
8050-84-8	8037-86-3	997	9005-25-8	←	707	10071-13-3	123-33-1	1308
8050-92-8	←	965	9005-32-7	←	746	10101-53-8	←	281
8052-41-3	←	334	9005-38-3	←	745	10102-03-1	—	9
8052-42-4	←	343	9005-40-7	9005-38-3	745	10102-06-4	13520-83-7	298
8053-05-2	77-09-8	1607	9005-49-6	←	1598	10102-17-7	7772-98-7	163
8053-18-7	8002-39-9	811	9005-65-6	←	970	10102-20-2	—	187
8056-92-6	←	917	9005-67-8	←	969	10102-43-9	—	9
8057-49-6	←	699	9005-80-5	9005-25-8	707	10102-44-0	—	9
8058-32-0	77-15-6	1483	9005-82-7	9005-25-8	707	10102-48-4	7784-40-9	206
8061-00-5	156-62-7	1355	9005-84-9	9005-25-8	707	10103-43-2	—	161
8061-07-2	8050-60-0	759	9006-04-6	←	756	10103-61-4	1327-30-6	201
8063-11-4	←	748	9006-35-3	8037-86-3	997	10103-62-5	7778-44-1	198
8063-12-5	302-27-2	822	9006-36-4	8037-86-3	997	10107-99-0	←	448
8063-14-7	—	678	9006-65-9	←	1646	10108-64-2	—	220
8063-15-8	56-25-7	924	9007-07-2	—	454	10112-91-1	←	237
8063-17-0	—	688	9007-16-3	9003-01-4	1627	10112-94-4	←	184
8063-18-1	←	696	9007-63-0	—	963	10117-38-1	—	149

CAS Registry No. of Ingredient	CAS Registry No. of Primary Name	Location Number of Primary Name (See Part D)	CAS Registry No. of Ingredient	CAS Registry No. of Primary Name	Location Number of Primary Name (See Part D)	CAS Registry No. of Ingredient	CAS Registry No. of Primary Name	Location Number of Primary Name (See Part D)
10124-27-3	7446-70-0	182	12002-03-8	1299-88-3	200	13717-00-5	—	174
10124-29-5	7784-24-9	181	12002-29-8	62-33-9	1504	13718-26-8	7440-62-2	299
10124-36-4	—	220	12036-23-6	1314-23-4	301	13746-66-2	—	256
10124-37-5	—	157	12040-58-3	—	131	13780-29-5	7803-51-2	136
10124-41-1	—	161	12040-59-4	21645-51-2	178	13840-33-0	7439-93-2	154
10124-43-3	—	282	12041-64-4	156-62-7	1355	13930-27-3	317-34-0	799
10124-44-4	7440-50-8	265	12042-91-0	7446-70-0	182	13943-58-3	—	256
10124-48-8	←	223	12122-67-7	←	1167	13957-38-5	—	1588
10124-55-7	—	286	12124-97-9	—	98	13998-03-3	57-12-5	105
10124-56-8	←	143	12125-02-9	—	152	14018-95-2	—	81
10163-15-2	—	100	12126-57-7	—	667	14028-44-5	1977-10-2	1476
10196-04-0	—	149	12136-89-9	—	111	14038-43-8	—	256
10210-36-3	—	284	12183-80-1	14504-95-1	180	14039-25-9	12122-67-7	1167
10233-00-8	10294-66-3	162	12244-57-4	—	284	14075-53-7	←	103
10262-69-8	1977-10-2	1476	12255-89-9	1303-33-9	194	14127-68-5	←	142
10265-92-6	←	1101	12259-92-6	←	112	14214-32-5	3134-12-1	1256
10290-12-7	1302-97-2	202	12345-57-2	7439-93-2	154	14217-21-1	—	256
10294-30-1	—	284	12379-65-6	6659-45-6	888	14252-80-3	2180-92-9	1578
10294-66-3	←	162	12427-38-2	←	1160	14280-30-9	—	51
10326-21-3	—	96	12501-52-9	7440-33-7	297	14402-89-2	—	109
10326-24-6	1303-39-5	211	12558-58-6	7440-50-8	265	14433-93-3	—	253
10346-69-7	—	250	12626-49-2	—	957	14460-20-9	137-30-4	1168
10361-37-2	—	166	12627-37-1	—	942	14480-75-2	54-05-7	1512
10361-76-9	—	79	12627-38-2	—	942	14484-64-1	←	1158
10377-37-4	7439-93-2	154	12656-85-8	7758-97-6	246	14504-95-1	←	180
10377-98-7	←	300	12671-69-1	8001-51-2	844	14550-21-1	10124-56-8	143
10378-28-6	—	286	12680-11-4	42576-02-3	1293	14638-08-5	—	256
10380-28-6	←	264	12680-48-7	—	81	14639-97-5	—	277
10381-36-9	—	287	12751-04-1	←	512	14639-98-6	—	277
10453-86-8	←	895	12770-31-9	1299-88-3	200	14762-51-7	7647-14-5	165
10453-89-1	←	894	12771-08-3	10025-67-9	28	14807-96-6	—	8
10476-81-0	—	98	12772-68-8	—	515	14987-04-3	1343-88-0	176
10476-85-4	—	177	13073-35-3	55-17-4	1643	14989-29-8	—	174
10544-72-6	—	9	13121-70-5	—	293	15015-80-2	129-16-8	235
10553-31-8	—	166	13132-95-1	1332-58-7	5	15096-52-3	1344-75-8	104
10579-83-6	—	149	13138-45-9	—	287	15124-09-1	—	159
10588-01-9	—	82	13150-00-0	←	955	15162-68-2	1918-02-1	1312
10599-90-3	—	22	13171-21-6	297-99-4	1058	15248-76-7	—	546
11003-70-6	8011-55-0	843	13194-48-4	←	1088	15263-53-3	←	1130
11006-34-1	1406-65-1	926	13281-17-9	156-62-7	1355	15299-99-7	←	1278
11006-92-1	1406-65-1	926	13347-42-7	←	524	15339-36-3	128-04-1	1163
11006-96-5	←	683	13360-45-7	←	1242	15347-57-6	7439-92-1	245
11034-77-8	—	661	13397-24-5	10034-76-1	172	15537-71-0	52-67-5	1507
11043-90-6	—	946	13397-25-6	471-34-1	171	15545-48-9	555-37-3	1254
11047-00-0	—	667	13410-01-0	10112-94-4	184	15585-90-7	57109-90-7	1394
11075-55-1	544-63-8	557	13453-07-1	—	284	15588-95-1	←	1449
11075-97-1	8015-61-0	847	13463-39-3	—	287	15662-33-6	←	690
11103-57-4	68-26-8	907	13463-41-7	3590-23-6	276	15716-02-6	25155-18-4	992
11113-50-1	10043-35-3	129	13463-67-7	1309-63-3	296	15739-80-7	7439-92-1	245
11118-57-3	1308-38-9	280	13472-30-5	←	58	15804-54-3	7758-97-6	246
11119-70-3	7758-97-6	246	13472-45-2	7440-33-7	297	15825-70-4	55-63-0	635
11120-01-7	7440-33-7	297	13494-80-9	—	187	15972-60-8	←	1273
11121-38-3	←	892	13520-83-7	—	298	16039-64-8	304-61-0	213
11126-05-9	—	347	13537-03-6	7803-51-2	136	16068-46-5	—	155
11138-47-9	10042-94-1	133	13560-99-1	93-76-5	1224	16118-49-3	←	1228
12001-14-8	←	267	13573-18-7	14127-68-5	142	16177-21-2	142-47-2	1618
12001-18-2	7446-70-0	182	13587-50-3	7803-51-2	136	16227-10-4	←	1272
12001-28-4	1332-21-4	2	13601-19-9	—	256	16409-45-3	89-48-5	869
12001-29-5	1332-21-4	2	13684-56-5	—	1230	16485-55-5	—	277
12001-44-4	89-68-9	527	13684-63-4	13684-56-5	1230	16536-89-3	51-43-4	1454
12001-85-3	←	273	13701-59-2	←	167	16568-02-8	←	816

CAS Registry No. of Ingredient	CAS Registry No. of Primary Name	Location Number of Primary Name (See Part D)	CAS Registry No. of Ingredient	CAS Registry No. of Primary Name	Location Number of Primary Name (See Part D)	CAS Registry No. of Ingredient	CAS Registry No. of Primary Name	Location Number of Primary Name (See Part D)
16690-92-9	142-47-2	1618	22350-76-1	961-11-5	1061	27833-64-3	1977-10-2	1476
16752-77-5	←	1140	22775-54-8	—	904	27858-07-7	—	398
16872-11-0	14075-53-7	103	22781-23-3	←	1123	28249-77-6	←	1239
16893-85-9	—	101	22936-75-0	1610-18-0	1267	28300-75-6	304-61-0	213
16905-00-3	—	284	22936-86-3	←	1262	28330-26-9	123-33-1	1308
16919-19-0	—	101	23103-98-2	←	1145	28382-15-2	123-33-1	1308
16949-65-8	—	101	23109-05-9	—	813	28678-26-4	106-62-7	438
17033-35-1	10034-76-1	172	23135-22-0	←	1144	28805-78-9	18530-56-8	1255
17140-70-4	7681-79-0	1455	23184-66-9	15972-60-8	1273	29091-05-2	←	1288
17146-95-1	359-83-1	792	23422-53-9	22259-30-9	1135	29348-76-3	—	957
17466-45-4	—	814	23564-05-8	←	1207	29790-52-1	←	775
17575-22-3	—	841	23564-06-9	23564-05-8	1207	29883-15-6	←	846
17598-65-1	←	835	23947-60-6	5221-53-4	1192	29973-13-5	←	1134
17655-22-0	123-33-1	1308	23950-58-5	←	1281	30087-47-9	2655-19-8	1126
17781-31-6	←	1200	24292-52-2	←	1599	30233-81-9	—	943
17804-35-2	←	1174	24353-58-0	15972-60-8	1273	30283-93-3	600-25-9	19
18010-40-7	2180-92-9	1578	24486-40-6	—	920	30402-16-5	—	402
18181-80-1	←	1004	24691-76-7	←	1204	30525-89-4	9002-81-7	487
18296-44-1	8057-49-6	699	24815-24-5	84-34-4	797	30560-19-1	←	1095
18472-51-0	55-56-1	994	25013-16-5	128-37-0	1614	31065-88-0	1335-31-5	108
18480-07-4	—	51	25014-41-9	←	652	31251-03-3	←	1171
18496-25-8	←	118	25057-89-0	←	1291	31366-95-7	80-46-6	488
18530-56-8	←	1255	25154-54-5	←	640	31884-77-2	1104-22-9	1494
18623-80-8	—	277	25155-15-1	1330-20-7	318	32534-95-5	93-72-1	1223
18642-44-9	26446-35-5	577	25155-18-4	←	992	32672-69-8	50-52-2	1425
18691-97-9	3134-12-1	1256	25155-30-0	—	943	32889-48-8	21725-46-2	1260
18883-66-4	53558-25-1	1353	25167-93-5	←	643	33089-61-1	—	1039
18917-89-0	63-36-5	600	25168-15-4	93-76-5	1224	33245-39-5	29091-05-2	1288
18933-02-3	1407-03-0	848	25265-71-8	106-62-7	438	33693-04-8	←	1270
18996-35-5	77-92-9	703	25277-93-4	1313-60-6	74	33820-53-0	1861-40-1	1287
19044-88-3	1861-40-1	1287	25321-14-6	←	641	34014-18-1	←	1258
19095-88-6	7085-19-0	1221	25322-20-7	79-34-5	373	34123-59-6	←	1250
19367-79-4	123-88-6	239	25322-68-3	←	441	34195-34-1	←	783
19750-95-9	6164-98-3	1042	25322-69-4	←	443	34247-28-4	←	954
19937-59-8	←	1252	25377-32-6	←	644	34253-67-3	←	456
20249-47-2	—	109	25377-74-6	—	661	34256-82-1	15972-60-8	1273
20285-28-3	115-31-1	1038	25482-78-4	10361-76-9	79	34363-01-4	—	878
20313-98-8	129-49-7	806	25496-72-4	—	573	34415-85-5	135-23-9	1495
20427-59-2	7440-50-8	265	25567-67-3	97-00-7	639	34452-51-2	—	552
20548-54-3	18496-25-8	118	25702-11-8	←	925	34590-94-8	←	457
20830-75-5	←	839	25719-60-2	—	878	35367-38-5	←	1246
20859-73-8	←	137	25869-98-1	—	256	35915-18-5	93-76-5	1224
21087-64-9	←	1266	26011-50-7	15588-95-1	1449	36355-01-8	—	398
21109-95-5		166	26140-60-3	←	316	36452-21-8	504-19-8	1261
21150-21-0	—	813	26225-79-6	←	1305	36478-76-9	13520-83-7	298
21150-22-1	—	813	26259-45-0	1610-18-0	1267	36637-18-0	←	1581
21150-23-2	—	813	26271-75-0	99-30-9	1191	36637-19-1	36637-18-0	1581
21267-72-1	1918-16-7	1282	26446-35-5	←	577	36653-82-4	124-29-8	409
21564-17-0	←	1206	26471-62-5	584-84-9	1641	36734-19-7	←	1197
21645-51-2	←	178	26499-65-0	10034-76-1	172	37764-25-3	759-94-4	1236
21689-84-9	1610-18-0	1267	26570-10-5	1639-60-7	1486	39236-46-9	←	996
21725-46-2	←	1260	26628-22-8	—	111	39300-45-3	←	542
21908-53-2	—	221	26644-46-2	←	1210	39312-79-3	3878-19-1	1176
22004-32-6	15588-95-1	1449	26645-35-2	—	814	39420-34-3	94-84-8	1306
22011-09-2	7803-51-2	136	26952-20-5	1918-02-1	1312	40487-42-1	29091-05-2	1288
22042-59-7	15263-53-3	1130	26952-21-6	←	421	40795-56-0	—	957
22212-55-1	←	1292	27157-85-3	149-30-4	1198	41394-05-2	←	1265
22224-92-6	←	1103	27314-13-2	←	1311	41643-35-0	15299-99-7	1278
22248-79-9	961-11-5	1061	27323-18-8	—	399	41643-36-1	15299-99-7	1278
22259-30-9	←	1135	27323-41-7	—	943	42576-02-3	←	1293
22306-05-4	154-69-8	1500	27668-50-4	156-62-7	1355	43121-43-3	←	1271

CAS Registry No. of Ingredient	CAS Registry No. of Primary Name	Location Number of Primary Name (See Part D)	CAS Registry No. of Ingredient	CAS Registry No. of Primary Name	Location Number of Primary Name (See Part D)	CAS Registry No. of Ingredient	CAS Registry No. of Primary Name	Location Number of Primary Name (See Part D)
47000-92-0	←	1276	51481-60-8	357-08-4	787	53558-25-1	←	1353
49866-87-7	1910-42-5	1286	51481-61-9	←	1491	55283-68-6	1861-40-1	1287
50571-74-9	5907-38-0	1573	51630-58-1	←	890	55557-30-7	←	1604
50723-80-3	25057-89-0	1291	51990-04-6	759-94-4	1236	57052-04-7	←	1264
50935-18-7	8050-69-9	854	52233-42-8	13701-59-2	167	57109-90-7	←	1394
51026-28-9	←	1157	52239-63-1	1420-55-9	1423	60573-88-8	2763-96-4	819
51218-45-2	15972-60-8	1273	52645-53-1	←	891	61789-51-3	—	283
51235-04-2	←	1263	52756-22-6	22212-55-1	1292	65996-91-0	←	341
51338-27-3	←	1301	52756-25-9	22212-55-1	1292	65997-01-5	8002-26-4	723

II: D. Toxicity Information about Selected Ingredients

Inorganic substances that are "inert" when ingested

1 Inert Ingredients

Ingredients labeled "inert" by the manufacturer are not necessarily inert from the viewpoint of the toxicologist and physician. For example, in many agricultural sprays the chief toxic ingredient is often the "inert" vehicle, which is usually kerosene or one of the petroleum oils. Dusts and powders often consist in large measure of such "inert ingre-dients" as hydrated lime, calcium carbonate, gypsum, calcium phosphate, magnesium carbonate, bentonite, silica, diatomaceous earth, Fuller's earth, kaolin, walnut shell powder, redwood bark dust, and talc. Some of the liquid fumigants used in agriculture contain carbon tetrachloride as the "inert" solvent.

2 Asbestos

Crocidolite, Amosite, Anthophyllite, Tremolite, Chrysotile

A fibrous material, insensitive to heat and chemical attack, widely used in textiles and insulation and as a filler in tile, reinforced cement, industrial water filters, gaskets and brake linings. The name refers to a group of naturally occurring hydrated mineral silicates of the serpentine or amphibole series. They are characterized by fibers or bundles of fine, single crystal fibrils. The commonly found serpentine asbestos is chrysotile. Anthophyllite, tremolite, amosite and crocidolite are in the amphibole series. Of these, crocidolite from South Africa ("blue" asbestos) is considered to pose the greatest health hazard. Most asbestos fiber used in the United States is chrysotile from Canada. Asbestos has a very low acute oral toxicity. Uptake of asbestos fibers from the gut is very limited. The usual and more dangerous route of exposure is respiratory. Intense exposure to asbestos fibers produces a diffuse interstitial fibrosis of the lung tissue termed "asbestosis." Although a terminal pneumoconiosis, asbestosis does not predispose to pulmonary tuberculosis or chronic bronchitis. Signs and symptoms of the condition include breathlessness, chest pain, cough, decreased lung function, basal rales, finger clubbing, cyanosis, cor pulmonale, radiographic abnormalities, and pleural effusion. High rates of lung cancer occur among persons occupationally exposed to large amounts of any type of asbestos. Shorter or less intense industrial exposures to chrysotile, crocidolite or amosite may produce pleural or peritoneal mesotheliomas. Mesotheliomas have been reported after domestic exposure to clothing worn by asbestos workers. In humans the latent period of lung cancer is about 15 to 30 years, of mesothelioma is 3.5 to 30 years. The risk of lung cancer due to asbestos is particularly high among persons who smoke. This association may be due in part to the presence of trace amounts of chromium, nickel and beryllium in the asbestos, which inhibit detoxification of benzpyrene and other carcinogenic components of smoke. Fibers of 5 to 200 μm. length lodge in the deep lung. Very short fibers (less than 5 μm.) may be engulfed by alveolar macrophages and either transported to lymph nodes or excreted via the mucociliary route. In human autopsies, asbestos fibers are found in the pleura, thoracic diaphragm and chest wall. Fibers remaining in the lungs, pleura and parenchymatous organs eventually become coated with mucopolysaccharide and hemosiderin to form "asbestos bodies" ("ferruginous bodies"). Prolonged dermal exposure may lead to asbestos warts, especially on the hands and forearms; they are of minor health significance. Wear of brake linings is a major source of asbestos in the ambient air. Chrysotile fiber concentrations near highways range from 0 to 12000 fibers per cubic meter in Los Angeles. Flaking of sprayed asbestos from ceilings and beams may lead to toxicologically significant air concentrations in buildings. The hazard resulting from exposure to asbestos fibers in food and water is apparently low. The present OSHA 8-hr. TWA air standard is 2 fibers greater than 5 microns in length per ml. of air.

Ref.: Morgan et al., 1973; National Cancer Institute, 1978p.

3 Bentonite

Toxicity Rating: 1. A hydrated aluminum silicate mineral. Biologically inert when ingested. Used as a protective colloid in suspensions. Similar to kaolin but bentonite has smaller particles.

Ref.: Osol and Farrar, 1955.

4 Graphite

Plumbago, Pencil lead, Black lead

Toxicity Rating: 1. Crystalline carbon, chemically and biologically inert, although allergic symptoms and benign pneumoconiosis have been described.

Ref.: Jaffe, 1951.

5 Kaolin

Hydrated aluminum silicate

Toxicity Rating: 1. Given by mouth in doses of 100 gm. several times a day as an absorbent for intestinal disorders. Inert except for the dangers of obstruction, perforation, and granuloma formation.

Ref.: Osol and Farrar, 1955.

Cholera patients have been fed 600 gm. of kaolin (plus water) over a 12-hr. period without ill effects. Mice have been successfully fed diets containing 80% kaolin.

6 Pumice

Complex silicates

Toxicity Rating: 1(?). Insoluble and chemically inert. Intestinal obstructions, perforations, and per-

Ref.: Osol and Farrar, 1955.

haps local granulomas are conceivable after the ingestion of large quantities.

7 Silica

Silicone dioxide

Toxicity Rating: 1. Chemically and biologically inert when ingested in any of its many physical forms, such as crystalline quartz, amorphous siliceous earth (diatomaceous earth, diatomite, kie-

Ref.: Osol and Farrar, 1955; Scheel et al., 1953.

selguhr) or colloidal silica gels. The chronic inhalation of certain samples of crystalline quartz, however, may cause a progressive pneumoconiosis commonly known as silicosis.

8 Talc

Talcum

Toxicity Rating: 1. Finely powdered native hydrous magnesium silicate. May contain various fibrous and non-fibrous accessory materials, including other silicates, such as tremolite and anthophyllite, and various serpentines. Composition varies among and within geological deposits. Commercial talc is incorporated into many industrial products and processes. A relatively pure granular form is used in cosmetics and toiletries. Harmless and inert when ingested but hazardous when inhaled, at least in large quantities. The hazard is both acute and chronic, acute in cases of massive aspiration of baby powder by infants and chronic in cases of industrial exposures in talc miners, millers and others. Infants have died from pulmonary edema and pneumonia within hours after inhaling talcum powder. The powder dries the mucous membranes of the bronchioles, thus disrupting pulmonary clearance and clogging the smaller airways. Victims usually display dyspnea, tachypnea, tachycardia, cyanosis and fever. Bronchopulmonary lavage is not effective because talc is insoluble in water. One child who survived a massive aspiration of baby powder later developed progressive diffuse pulmonary fibrosis resembling that seen in afflicted talc miners. Death rates from pneumoconiosis (talcosis) and lung cancer among miners and millers have decreased since the introduction of wet-mining and other engineering improvements which have reduced the concentration of talc dusts, especially those containing asbestiform fibers (defined as particles, even of non-asbestos materials, that are 3 or more times longer than wide). The recommended Threshold Limit Values for exposure in workroom air are 2 mg./m^3 for respirable dust containing no fibers and 2 fibers (5 μm. or longer)/cc. for fiber-containing talc dust. Workers with chronic talcosis usually present with dyspnea, productive cough and weakness. Limited chest expansion, decreased breath sounds and scattered rales are found on physical examination. Clubbing and cyanosis are symptoms of advanced disease. The major complication and cause of death is cor pulmonale. Whereas the fibrous dust is considered to be a greater respiratory hazard than granular dust, lung granulomas, regarded as an early stage of talcosis, were documented in a woman exposed to relatively pure platiform talc during the 6-7 years she was a quality control inspector of talcum powder aerosols. Her condition improved after she was treated with prednisone. Equivocal evidence has been presented linking some cervical, ovarian and gastric cancers to the presence of talc particles at these sites. However, talc administered orally to rats, mice and guinea pigs was not translocated from the gastrointestinal tract and was almost totally excreted in the feces within 4 days. Talc applied intravaginally to rabbits did not migrate to the ovaries.

Ref.: Cruthirds et al., 1977; Jacques and Benirschke, 1952; Moskowitz, 1970; Motomatsu et al., 1979.

Primary irritants and corrosives of simple chemical structure

Lung irritants (gases, vapors and fumes)

9

9　Nitrogen Oxides

Nitrous oxide, Nitric oxide, Nitrogen dioxide, Nitrogen tetroxide, Nitrogen pentoxide

See also: Nitrogen Oxides, *Reference Congener in Section III.*

10

10　Sulfur Dioxide

Sulfurous anhydride, Sulfurous oxide

A highly irritant gas, often cited as a dangerous atmospheric constituent in smog areas. Inhalation produces all grades of respiratory tract irritation, sometimes with pulmonary edema. The vapor concentration probably determines the mode of death: e.g., suffocation from reflex respiratory arrest (very high concentration), pulmonary edema (moderate concentration), or systemic acidosis (low concentration). There is some indication of individual susceptibility.

See also: Nitrogen Oxides, *Reference Congener in Section III.*
Ref.: Amer. Petroleum Institute, 1948h; Leong et al., 1961.

11

11　Phosgene

Carbonyl chloride, Chloroformyl chloride

Extreme pulmonary irritant, once used as a war gas. Even in potentially lethal exposures, however, the initial symptoms are mild and transient (burning of eyes, cough, inability to get breath), although experimental animals may show extensive emphysema and sloughing of bronchiolar mucosa immediately after gassing. The danger period is usually 6 to 24 hours after exposure with the development of peribronchial edema, pulmonary congestion and alveolar edema, all leading to death from anoxia. The delay is ascribed to slow intrapulmonary hydrolysis of phosgene to HCl and Cl_2. In massive exposures immediate death sometimes results from occlusion of the pulmonary circulation secondary to intravascular hemolysis and thrombus formation. No evidence exists for a systemic action of inhaled phosgene, but vasoconstriction of the pulmonary vasculature has been described in rabbits. Sequelae include pulmonary scarring, lobular emphysema, small irregular areas of atelectasis and bronchitis. Under special circumstances of intense heat some halogenated hydrocarbon solvents, e.g., carbon tetrachloride, trichloroethylene, methylene chloride, are said to be decomposed to phosgene; they have produced serious intoxications and death.

See also: Nitrogen Oxides, *Reference Congener in Section III.*
Ref.: Coman et al., 1947; English, 1964; Everett and Overholt, 1968; Gerritsen and Buschmann, 1960; Ivanhoe and Meyers, 1964; Spolyar et al., 1951; Tobias, 1949b.

12

12　Thiophosgene

Thiocarbonyl chloride, Carbonothioic dichloride

Toxicity Rating: 4(?). Important intermediate in chemical syntheses and a decomposition product of Captan (see latter in index). Liquid at room temperature. The vapor is a respiratory irritant and lacrimator. Toxicity may be due to phosgene generated when thiophosgene vapors are exposed to air (see Phosgene above). Liquid is irritating to skin and mucous membranes.

See also: Nitrogen Oxides, *Reference Congener in Section III.*

13

13　Chloropicrin

Trichloronitromethane

Toxicity Rating: 5. A "war gas" sometimes used as a fumigant and tracer gas. Vapor is intensely irritating to skin, eyes, mucous membrane, and stomach. Called "vomiting gas". Treatment is symptomatic with special attention to the lungs. Ingestion of liquid produces severe gastroenteritis.

See also: Nitrogen Oxides, *Reference Congener in Section III.*
Ref.: Assoc. of Amer. Pesticide Control Officials, 1966; Spencer, 1973.

14

14　α-Chloroacetophenone

"Tear gas", Phenacyl chloride, 2-Chloro-1-phenylethanone, e.g., Chemical Mace, CN

Lacrimator used in grenades and personal protective devices to repel or incapacitate would-be attackers. In very low concentrations in air it has an odor resembling apple blossoms, but an intolerable level is considered to be 0.0045 mg/l. A 10-min. exposure to 0.85 mg./l. is estimated to be lethal in man. Symptoms include tearing, burning of the eyes and difficulty in breathing, but seldom any persistent or permanent disability. High concentrations may lead to the development of acute pulmonary edema after latencies of 8 hr. to several days. First and perhaps second degree burns of the skin may occur, particularly if in contact with abraded areas. At high concentrations permanent opacification, ulceration with vascularization and perforations can be produced in the eyes of laboratory animals. Possible systemic manifestations include agitation, miosis, coma, areflexia and fatty infiltration of the liver. A potent allergic contact sensitizer. At least some devices discharge with such force that, at short range, cartridges will penetrate the human hand perhaps resulting in permanent loss of sensation in varying degrees. Thorough irrigation with tap water is recommended for eye and skin contact.

See also: Nitrogen Oxides, *Reference Congener in Section III.*
Ref.: Adams et al., 1966; Forberg and Beyers, 1969; Leopold and Lieberman, 1971; Penneys et al., 1969; Stein and Kirwan, 1964.

15 *o*-Chlorobenzylidene Malononitrile   15

CS, Chemshield

Toxicity Rating: 4. A peripheral sensory irritant, introduced in England in 1958 as a short-term incapacitant or riot control agent. CS is a white solid with a peppery odor. It is most commonly used in aerosol form to disperse crowds or as a liquid formulation in spray cannisters (e.g., Chemshield) for personal self-defense; therefore, inhalation and skin contact are the primary routes of exposure. The Threshold Limit Value (TLV) is 0.05 ppm in air. Higher concentrations result in immediate effects on eye and respiratory tract. In the eyes it causes burning pain with excessive lacrimation and blepharospasm. Burning sensations in the nose, throat and chest are accompanied by sneezing, coughing, rhinorrhea and excess salivation. Skin exposure produces mild pain and local erythema. Wash contaminated skin with soap and water and irrigate eyes with water or saline solution. Even without treatment, symptoms dissipate rapidly (usually within 30 minutes) in clean air. Systemic cyanide poisoning due to the release of HCN from one or both nitriles of the malononitrile is an important feature of lethal CS poisoning in laboratory mammals, but HCN does not appear to contribute to the relatively low-dose effects described in man. Death by inhalation is due to lung damage leading to asphyxia and circulatory failure or secondary bronchopneumonia.

Ref.: Ballantyne, 1977; Beswick et al., 1972; Frankenberg and Sorbo, 1973.

16 Ethylene Oxide   16

1,2-Epoxyethane, Oxirane

Toxicity Rating: 4. A gas at room temperature widely used as a fumigant, a sterilizer for drugs, medical devices and foodstuffs, a rocket propellant, and an intermediate in the chemical industry. Reacts with water to form ethylene glycol and with chloride ion to form ethylene chlorohydrin (see both in the Index). Forms covalent bonds with DNA. Aqueous solutions are skin vesicants and eye irritants. Vapors are irritating to the respiratory tract. The inhalation of high vapor concentrations has caused pulmonary edema, kidney damage, and death in humans. The Threshold Limit Value has been set at 10 ppm for workroom air. Acute vapor inhalation in humans has produced eye, nose and throat irritation, loss of taste and smell, headache, nausea, protracted vomiting, drowsiness, weakness, incoordination, dyspnea, cyanosis and pulmonary edema. Residues of ethylene oxide in sterilized medical devices have caused hemolysis, delayed sensitization reactions and even anaphylaxis in patients. Chronic vapor exposures reportedly lead to lymphocytosis, peripheral neuropathy and, even at levels below the OSHA standard of 50 ppm, chromosomal damage to lymphocytes. It has caused various mutations in 13 out of 14 plant and animal species tested and is suspected of being able to induce heritable mutations in humans. The incidence of leukemia among workers exposed to ethylene oxide in a Swedish industrial plant was twice that expected in the general population.

Ref.: Garry et al., 1979; Glaser, 1977; Gross et al., 1979; Hogstedt et al., 1979; Poothullil et al., 1975; Sexton and Henson, 1949; Sexton and Henson, 1950.

17 Propylene Oxide   17

1,2-Epoxypropane, Methyloxirane, Propene oxide

Toxicity Rating: 3 or 4. A low-boiling flammable liquid used as a soil fumigant, herbicide and preservative. Also important intermediate in the manufacture of oil additives, anti-oxidants and glycols. Less toxic than ethylene oxide. Usual mode of exposure is inhalation. Propylene oxide is a strong irritant to eyes, lungs and mucous membranes, a central nervous depressant, and a mild cytoplasmic poison. Symptoms of systemic intoxication include ataxia and general depression. One case of human poisoning reported in Russia resulted from vapor exposure to 1500 ppm w/v for 10 minutes. Initial symptoms included lung and eye irritation, headache, general asthenia and diarrhea. After two hours, the patient became cyanotic and collapsed. After administration of oxygen and antihistamines and treatment for shock, he regained consciousness and vomited but remained confused and weak. The pulse rate and blood pressure returned to normal in 2 hours, and recovery was complete on the following day. The authors recommended treatment with antihistamines and sodium thiosulfate (Beljaev et al., 1971). Acute inhalation exposure may be followed by secondary lung infection. Chronic feeding tests in rats resulted in mild liver damage. Even dilute solutions have caused corneal burns and necrotic skin lesions in humans, but no systemic poisoning has been observed following dermal exposure. The current OSHA Threshold Limit Value (for occupational vapor exposures) is 100 ppm, which is below the odor detection threshold.

See also: Nitrogen Oxides, *Reference Congener in Section III.*
Ref.: Beljaev et al., 1971; Patty, 1962; Pugaeva, 1967.

18   Sulfuryl Fluoride

18

Vikane

A fumigant which is a gas at ordinary temperatures. Highly irritating to respiratory tract mucosa. In laboratory animals it has proved to be about one-third as toxic as methyl bromide in single inhalation trials. Chronic exposure (35 hours weekly for 6 months) to 100 ppm resulted in no adverse effects on rabbits, rats, guinea pigs, or monkeys.

Ref.: Kenaga, 1957.

19   1-Chloro-1-nitropropane

19

Toxicity Rating: 4. Severe pulmonary edema after inhalation of vapor or ingestion of liquid. No systemic effects from skin application and no significant irritation. 1,1-Dichloro-1-nitroethane also causes pulmonary edema and generalized vascular injury.

See also: Nitrogen Oxides, *Reference Congener in Section III.*
Ref.: Machle et al., 1945.

20   1,1-Dichloro-1-nitroethane

20

Ethide

Toxicity Rating: 4. A grain fumigant. The vapor usually gives adequate warning (irritation). May produce severe pulmonary edema either by inhalation of vapor or ingestion of liquid. Also skin irritation.

See also: Nitrogen Oxides, *Reference Congener in Section III.*
Ref.: Machle et al., 1945.

21   Allyl Alcohol

21

1-Propenol-3

Toxicity Rating: 4. Vapor and liquid are intensely irritating to skin and mucous membrane. Produces lacrimation and corneal burns. Liquid may produce first or second degree burns with blistering and superficial necrosis. Penetration through intact skin is dangerous. Inhaled vapor may lead to pulmonary edema with slowly developing distress. Liver necrosis has been reported in experimental animals. Animal studies place this compound near the borderline between toxicity classes 4 and 5.

See also: Dichloropropenes, *Reference Congener in Section III.*
Ref.: Richarz and Schoetensack, 1961; Shell Chemical Co., 1956.

22   Chloramines

22

Monochloramine, Dichloramine

NH_2Cl and $NHCl_2$ are unstable water-soluble products formed when ammonium hydroxide reacts with solutions of sodium hypochlorite, as when ammonia water and household bleaches are mixed. Decompose to ammonia and hypochlorous acid. Chloramines are sometimes used as disinfectants in water purification.

See also: Ammonia, *Reference Congener in Section III.*

23   Chlorine

23

Chlorine water

Water dissolves about twice its volume of chlorine gas, forming a mixture of hydrochloric and hypochlorous acids. Corrosive because of acidity and oxidizing potential. Correct acidosis by alkali therapy. If chlorine gas has been inhaled, inhalation of the following spray (or aerosol) has been recommended: an aqueous solution of sodium hyposulfite (2%) and sodium carbonate (0.5%). A near drowning in a fresh water pool containing only 0.5 ppm chlorine resulted in fulminating pulmonary edema after aspiration. A bizarre and rare form of self-abuse is the voluntary inhalation of chlorine gas (Rafferty, 1980). (For respiratory exposures see Nitrogen Oxides; for ingestion see Hypochlorite, Reference Congeners in Section III.)

Ref.: Bloomfield, 1959; McCord, 1926b; Modell, 1963; National Safety Council, 1953; Rafferty, 1980.

24   Chlorine Dioxide   24

Chlorine peroxide, Chlorine oxide, Sodium chlorite

A strongly oxidizing, reddish-yellow gas (ClO_2) with a pungent odor similar to that of chlorine. Used for bleaching cellulose, pulp, flour, leather, fats and oils, textiles and beeswax, and for deodorizing and purifying water. It is a more severe respiratory and eye irritant than chlorine (see above). Symptoms of inhalation include coughing, wheezing, rhinitis, eye and throat irritation, dyspnea, headache, vomiting, bronchitis and pulmonary edema. It dissolves in water to form a mixture of chlorite and chlorate ions. Chlorite has been shown to produce methemoglobin in rats and cats and in isolated blood specimens of rat, cat, and man. This has prompted concern about the health effects of ClO_2-treated water especially for individuals particularly sensitive to hemolytic agents (*e.g.,* infants and those with G-6-PD deficiency). However, a study of 198 persons exposed to chlorine dioxide disinfected water (average chlorite ion level 5 ppm) for 3 months revealed no significant exposure-related effects. In another study the oral administration of 500 ml. of a chlorite solution (5 mg./L) daily over a 12-week period to healthy G-6-PD deficient adult males affirmed its safety.

See also: Nitrogen Oxides, *Reference Congener in Section III.*
Ref.: Michael et al., 1981.

25   Bromine   25

Heavy, reddish brown liquid boiling at about 59°C. Strong oxidant particularly in the presence of water. Reacts vigorously with a variety of organic compounds. Inhalation of bromine vapors may produce chemical pneumonitis. Destructive and painful burns to skin and eyes from contact with liquid or vapor. Delayed deaths were sometimes observed when mice were exposed to bromine vapors. See Nitrogen Oxides in Section III for the management of pulmonary edema. After ingestion a reaction similar to but more intense than that after iodine is predicted.

See also: Iodine *and* Nitrogen Oxides, *Reference Congeners in Section III.*
Ref.: Bitron and Aharonson, 1978.

26   Iodine   26

Toxicity Rating: 5. Clinical estimates place iodine near the borderline between toxicity classes 4 and 5.

See also: Iodine, *Reference Congener in Section III.*

27   Metal Fumes   27

Under intense heat some metals (notably zinc, copper, cadmium, lead, mercury, tin, nickel) may volatilize and burn to finely divided airborne particles of metal oxide. Inhalation of freshly formed fumes may produce an influenza-like illness called "metal fume fever" (also "brass founders' ague," etc.). Signs and symptoms include chills, fever, malaise, generalized aches, dry cough, and sometimes nausea and vomiting. Typically the disease has an acute onset and short duration; permanent damage is rare. Zinc is most commonly responsible and is probably the most benign; fumes of cadmium, lead, and mercury may cause significant systemic poisoning. Treatment is usually symptomatic, although in some cases BAL may be useful. (See Cadmium, in Section III.)

Ref.: Sayers, 1938; Swiller and Swiller, 1957; Vallee, 1959.

28   Sulfur Chloride   28

Sulfur monochloride, Sulfur subchloride, Disulfur dichloride

A fuming oily liquid used as an agricultural insecticide, wood hardener, etc. Moisture promptly decomposes it to hydrochloric acid, sulfur, hydrogen sulfide, sulfurous acid, etc.

See also: Acid, *Reference Congener in Section III.*
Ref.: Merck and Co., 1976.

29   Cyanic Acid

29

Hydrogen cyanate, Isocyanic acid

Irritant gas at body temperature. Strong, acrid odor, strong lacrimator and vesicant. Highly irritating to eyes, skin, and mucous membranes. The gas may be condensed at 0°C to form a liquid which polymerizes explosively upon warming to yield cyanuric acid and cyamelide. Cyanic acid is rapidly hydrolyzed in acid to carbon dioxide and ammonia. Inhaled gas is presumably neutralized in the respiratory tract and partly absorbed as cyanate anion. Although gas inhalation is unlikely to lead to systemic cyanate poisoning, see Cyanates (in the Index) for possible systemic effects.

See also: Nitrogen Oxides, *Reference Congener in Section III.*
Ref.: Sax, 1975.

Corrosive mineral acids

30   Acid

30

Mineral acid, i.e., hydrochloric, sulfuric

In the vernacular of the city street "Acid" refers to LSD; see latter in the index, if appropriate.

See also: Acid, *Reference Congener in Section III.*

31   Hydrochloric Acid

31

Muriatic acid

An aqueous solution of hydrogen chloride (HCl). Reagent grade concentrated hydrochloric acid contains about 38 percent HCl, but industrial muriatic acid is usually less concentrated.

See also: Acid, *Reference Congener in Section III.*

32   Nitric Acid

32

Aqua fortis

Commercial nitric acids contain 68% and 56% HNO_3 in water.

See also: Acid, *Reference Congener in Section III.*

33   Sulfuric Acid

33

Oil of vitriol

The commercial acid is 93 to 98% H_2SO_4 (the rest is water).

See also: Acid, *Reference Congener in Section III.*

34   Oleum

34

Fuming sulfuric acid

Concentrated sulfuric acid which may contain up to 80% free SO_3.

See also: Acid, *Reference Congener in Section III.*

35   Sulfurous Acid

35

Sulfur dioxide solution usually about 6% SO_2 in water. See Sulfur dioxide in the index.

See also: Acid, *Reference Congener in Section III.*

36   Hydrofluoric Acid

36

Fluohydric acid

An aqueous solution of hydrogen fluoride (HF) usually marketed in concentrations of 47 to 53 percent. Highly corrosive. The clinical management of HF burns is described in Section III under Fluoride.

See also: Fluoride, *Reference Congener in Section III.*

37   Fluosilicic Acid   **37**

Toxicity Rating: 4-5(?). H_2SiF_6 is described as a fairly strong acid (whereas hydrofluoric acid is weak). Unstable when anhydrous; marketed only as aqueous solutions. When the acid is neutralized, the fluosilicate anion gradually decomposes to yield fluoride and SiF_4. Dilute solutions of the acid (1-2%) are widely used in brewing and bottling plants to sterilize equipment. Other concentrations are employed to fluoridate municipal water supplies, to harden cement, to preserve wood and for other industrial purposes. Concentrated solutions are in- tensely corrosive on skin and mucous membranes but less corrosive than HF, probably because fluosilicic acid is more ionized and so less penetrating. Presumably both the hydrogen ion and the fluosilicic ion contribute to the local lesions, since neutral salts of the acid are also irritating and sometimes corrosive (see Fluosilicate Salts in the index). Perhaps because it decomposes to fluoride, absorbed fluosilicate is about as toxic as fluoride and produces a similar illness.

See also: Acid *and* Fluoride, *Reference Congeners in Section III.*
Ref.: Merck and Co., 1976; Lewis and Tatken, 1979.

38   Phosphorus Pentoxide   **38**

Phosphoric acid anhydride

P_2O_5 reacts with water and aqueous solutions to form phosphoric acid. Reagent-grade concentrated phophoric acid is 85-87% (w/w) H_3PO_4 (equivalent to about 17M). It appears to be as corrosive as sulfuric and hydrochloric acids. Only one report of an ingestion has come to our attention. This patient, who received four laparotomies because of recurrent abdominal hemorrhage, died on the nineteenth day with necrosis of the stomach, duodenum, jejunum and pancreas.

See also: Acid, *Reference Congener in Section III.*
Ref.: Hawkins et al., 1980; Manufacturing Chemists' Assoc., 1952a.

39   Chlorosulfonic Acid   **39**

Strong acid capable of severe local corrosive action. Contact with moisture results in the formation of sulfuric and hydrochloric acids.

See also: Acid, *Reference Congener in Section III.*
Ref.: Manufacturing Chemists' Assoc., 1949.

40   Sodium Bisulfate   **40**

Bisulfate of soda, Sodium pyrosulfate

Formula: $NaHSO_4$, sometimes as the monohydrate. Aqueous solutions are strongly acid. Corrosive to most bodily tissues.

See also: Acid, *Reference Congener in Section III.*

41   Superphosphates   **41**

Toxicity Rating: 2 or 3. Made by mixing about equal parts of "phosphate rock" and sulfuric acid producing a product containing about 1.6% phosphoric acid. The primary form of phosphate in rock is the tricalcium salt, which is insoluble in water and therefore "unavailable" to crops. The sulfuric acid treatment produces "available" forms such as mono- and di-basic calcium phosphates. Gypsum (insoluble calcium sulfate) is also formed as a by-product. Higher grades of superphosphates are produced by treating with phosphoric acid instead of sulfuric acid to produce products containing from 43 to 49% phosphoric acid; they are called "double" or "treble" superphosphates. Ammoniated superphosphate contains 16% phosphoric acid, 3% nitrogen and 2% potash, and is produced by treating normal superphosphate with an ammonia solution. Presumably any except the ammoniated preparation could produce a moderate to severe local irritation due to acidity. Some grades of superphosphates may contain appreciable quantities of calcium fluoride as an impurity (3 to 4% corresponding to 1 to 2% fluoride). Since phosphate is said to enhance the toxicity of fluoride, this could constitute an appreciable hazard.

See also: Acid *and* Fluoride, *Reference Congeners in Section III.*
Ref.: Hanna, 1958; Pallade et al., 1960.

Other corrosive acids

42   Acetic Acid

42

Vinegar and "dilute acetic acid" are about 4 to 6% acetic acid. Essence of vinegar is 14% acetic acid. Glacial acetic acid (100%) is highly corrosive, and its ingestion has produced penetrating lesions of the esophagus and later strictures of the esophagus and pylorus in man. At least the rabbit esophagus can tolerate 30 percent solutions without major damage. Vapors are capable of producing bronchial constriction with an over-all clinical picture similar to that by other irritant gases and vapors.

See also: Acid, *Reference Congener in Section III.*
Ref.: Amdur, 1961; Paar et al., 1968; Paul, 1951.

43   Dichloroacetic Acid

43

Toxicity Rating: 2 to 3. A somewhat weaker acid than trichloroacetic, although like trichloroacetic and acetic acids its toxicity may be attributed largely to its corrosive action. Does not possess the unusual metabolic actions of monochloroacetic acid. Presumably the simple salts are not hazardous. Acute oral LD_{50} in rats of 4.5 gm./kg. and in mice of 5.5 gm./kg.

See also: Acid, *Reference Congener in Section III.*
Ref.: Woodward et al., 1941.

44   Formic Acid (and Salts)

44

Sodium formate

The acid (but not its sodium salt) produces prompt burns and local necrosis, like the strong mineral acids. Concentrated aqueous solutions (75-80%) are marketed in Europe as "decalcifiers"; they have been responsible for many ingestion episodes in children and at least one death. Corrosive lesions of the lips, mouth and esophagus are described, but at least in children the esophageal lesions healed without stricture formation. Apparently dilute solutions (9% with pH 1.4) do not damage the oral mucosa. Sodium formate appears to have a low toxicity (10 gm by mouth without ill effects in man). Formate ion is extensively oxidized in vivo, but it may have direct actions on brain (cause of convulsions in poisoned animals?). Infused intravenously in male rhesus monkeys, buffered sodium formate led eventually to the same retinal lesions (and blindness) as produced by methanol ingestion, without the metabolic acidosis of the latter. In these monkeys the ocular lesions were associated with blood formate levels of 10-30 meq./l. To achieve these levels required massive intravenous doses (equivalent to about 15 gm./hr. for 10 hours in an adult man). Methemoglobinemia has also been reported in poisoned animals.

See also: Acid, *Reference Congener in Section III.*
Ref.: Fleig, 1907; Martin-Amat et al., 1978; Muhlendahl et al., 1978y; Sollmann, 1921; Sudarsky, 1965.

45   Glycolic Acid

45

Hydroxyacetic acid, Hydroxyethanoic acid

Systemic toxicity does not appear to have been described. No human poisonings known. A potential corrosive depending on its concentration.

See also: Acid, *Reference Congener in Section III.*

46   Lactic Acid

46

Toxicity Rating: 4. The official U.S.P. product is a mixture of lactic acid and lactic anhydride equivalent to 85 to 90% by weight of lactic acid. Although animal data indicate a toxicity rating of 3, clinical experience has shown that even diluted preparations have a corrosive action in the human esophagus and stomach.

See also: Acid, *Reference Congener in Section III.*

47   Oxalic Acid

47

Ethanedioic acid

Toxicity Rating: 4. A corrosive poison. Because its alkali salts are also corrosive, the acidity of this substance is probably not primarily responsible for the severe mucosal injuries that it produces.

See also: Oxalate, *Reference Congener in Section III.*

48   Sulfamic Acid

Amidosulfonic acid

Toxicity Rating: 3. Recommended for flame-proofing fabrics and wood and also sold as a swimming pool additive. Toxicity rating of 3 in rats (minimal lethal dose less than 1.6 gm./kg.). Solutions produce irritation on subcutaneous injection in rats, on the conjunctiva of rabbits and on cutaneous application to humans. Circulation and respiration were not greatly influenced after i.v. injection of 100 mg./kg. in rats. Because sulfamic acid is a strong acid, concentrated solutions may produce corrosive effects like mineral acids.

See also: Acid, *Reference Congener in Section III.*
Ref.: Ambrose, 1943.

49   Thioglycolic Acid

Mercaptoacetic acid

A stronger acid than acetic acid. Concentrated solutions on the skin produce chemical burns and blistering. An assertion that the acid releases significant amounts of hydrogen sulfide needs additional study.

See also: Acid, *Reference Congener in Section III.*
Ref.: Merck and Co., 1976.

50   Trichloroacetic Acid

TCA

A corrosive organic acid which rapidly penetrates and "fixes" tissues. Systemic effects are presumably secondary to gastrointestinal damage and to acidosis, not due to the trichloroacetate ion except after large doses; see also Sodium Trichloroacetate in the index.

See also: Acid, *Reference Congener in Section III.*
Ref.: Woodward et al., 1941.

Caustic alkalis

51   Lye

Caustic potash, Caustic soda

Any strong alkali, usually sodium or potassium hydroxide or carbonate. A corrosive poison.

See also: Lye, *Reference Congener in Section III.*

52   Sodium Carbonate

Solvay soda, Soda ash

The technical decahydrate is known as sal soda or washing soda. As with other alkaline corrosives the hazard is related more to concentration than to dose. Concentrated solutions tend to produce local necrosis of mucous membranes.

See also: Lye, *Reference Congener in Section III.*

53   Sodium Sesquicarbonate

Double salt of sodium carbonate and sodium bicarbonate. Presumably less corrosive than sodium carbonate but more alkaline than sodium bicarbonate.

See also: Lye, *Reference Congener in Section III.*

54   Calcium Oxide

Quicklime, Burnt lime, Unslaked lime

Unslaked lime (quicklime) is calcium oxide (CaO); it reacts with water with the evolution of heat, to form calcium hydroxide (Ca(OH)$_2$). This reaction on the skin or in the mouth produces both a thermal and a caustic burn. Quicklime tends to form clumps in the conjunctival sac, which are dangerous and difficult to wash out.

See also: Lye, *Reference Congener in Section III.*
Ref.: National Safety Council, Date Unknown d.

55

55   Lime (Slaked)

Calcium hydroxide

Slaked lime (calcium hydroxide) is a simple alkali; because of low solubility and apparently slow penetration into tissues, its aqueous solutions are not corrosive. Lime water, which is a saturated aqueous solution of $Ca(OH)_2$ (0.15%), has a pH of about 12.4, but unlike sodium or potassium hydroxide solutions of this pH, it usually produces only superficial opacities of the cornea, apparently because it penetrates corneal epithelium so slowly. In contrast, an aqueous suspension of lime or dried powdered lime contains particles that readily adhere to the conjunctiva; they often induce ulcerations of the corneal epithelium and stromal opacities but rarely penetrate to the iris or lens. It is difficult but essential to wash out the conjunctival sac completely. A .01-.05 M near-neutral solution of sodium edetate (EDTA) is said to be useful to loosen adherent particles. See also Calcium Salts in the index.

See also: Lye, *Reference Congener in Section III.*
Ref.: Grant, 1974; Griffith et al., 1980; National Safety Council, Date Unknown d.

56

56   Portland Cement

When any limestone that contains clay is calcined in a kiln, the resulting calcium oxide (see above) is impure because the product also contains calcium silicates, aluminates, sulfates, aluminoferrites, oxides of magnesium and manganese, and often small amounts of nickel, cobalt and chromium oxides. This mixture is sometimes called lean lime or hydraulic lime because it slakes with only a feeble heat of hydration and because it is able to "set" under water. As originally prepared in the Kent district of England, it has become generally known as Portland cement. Mixed with water, sand or pebbles, it sets in a hard mass known as concrete; cement represents only about 15% (by weight) of hardened concrete. Unhydrated Portland cement is a respirable dust, but it is not silicotogenic. Yugoslavian cement workers, however, were found to have small but significant reductions in the 1-second forced expiratory volume without any change in vital capacity (Kalacic, 1973). The principal health hazard of cement arises when water is added, and the calcium oxide is hydrated to form alkaline calcium hydroxide (slaked lime). Although many persons appear to tolerate brief skin contact with wet cement, others develop extensive skin burns with dermal necrosis requiring skin grafting.

Especially among chronically exposed workers, cement dermatitis assumes many forms: skin dryness, fissures, dystrophy of nails, eczematous rashes, etc. The causes of cement dermatitis have been widely debated. Most American authorities regard the alkalinity of wet cement (pH about 12), its abrasiveness and perhaps its hydroscopicity as the three qualities that make it hazardous to skin and mucous membranes. Several European dermatologists, however, have reported skin hypersensitivity to hexavalent chromium (see Chromium trioxide in the Index) among cement workers. Because some European cements (*e.g.*, from Switzerland) contain considerable amounts of chromates, chromium allergy has been regarded as a contributory cause of cement dermatitis (Calnan, 1960, 1973). A study in 1974 found no evidence that allergies to chromium, nickel or cobalt were importantly related to dermatitis in the American cement industry (Perone *et al.*, 1974). Because the older European evidence has not been adequately explained, the issue is not satisfactorily resolved. Acute dermal reactions to wet cement are usually treated like lye burns. Obviously gloves, impervious boots and other protective gear should be worn when pouring cement.

See also: Lye, *Reference Congener in Section III.*
Ref.: Calnan, 1960; Calnan, 1973; Greening and Tonry, 1978; Kalacic, 1973; Perone et al., 1974; Rowe and Williams, 1963.

57

57   Sodium Metasilicate

Formula Na_2SiO_3. Usually prepared as a glass by the thermal fusion of sand and soda ash. More soluble and more caustic than sodium silicate. Present as a major ingredient in some modern phosphate-free and low-phosphate household laundry detergents and dishwasher products. The most alkaline and corrosive substance in such mixtures. A 0.5 percent solution in water has a pH of about 12.5 with a relatively high buffer capacity. Dangerous on skin, in eyes and on all mucous membranes.

See also: Lye, *Reference Congener in Section III.*
Ref.: Schneider, 1970.

58

58   Sodium Silicate

Sodium orthosilicate

Toxicity Rating: 3(?). Generally a mixture of molecular species of variable composition. In commerce mole ratios of SiO_2 to Na_2O vary from 1.5 to 3.3. The mixture used as a builder in some laundry detergents usually has a mole ratio of 2.0 to 2.5. The higher the ratio (e.g., the less sodium) the lower the solubility and alkalinity. Less soluble and less caustic than sodium metasilicate, which has a mole ratio of 1:1 (see latter above). The acute oral LD_{50} in the rat varies from 1.1 to 1.6 gm./kg. Forms gelatinous mixtures with water. Except for nonspecific irritation of skin, cornea and mucous membranes, and perhaps corrosive lesions with the more alkaline mixtures, no toxic actions are recognized. Said to be partly absorbed and excreted in the urine; thus excretion during chronic exposures may contribute to the production of urinary calculi.

See also: Lye, *Reference Congener in Section III.*
Ref.: Morris, 1953; Task Force on the Health Effects of non-NTA Detergent Builders, 1981.

59 Potassium Phosphate (Tribasic) 59

Aqueous solutions are alkaline and may produce a caustic burn like Trisodium Phosphate. See also Potassium salts in the index.

See also: Lye, *Reference Congener in Section III.*

60 Trisodium Phosphate 60

Sodium phosphate tribasic

Aqueous solutions are highly alkaline and may produce a caustic burn.

See also: Lye, *Reference Congener in Section III.*
Ref.: Cann and Verhulst, 1958a.

61 Lithium Hydride 61

Lithium hydride has many uses in space and nuclear technology. It reacts vigorously when placed in water to liberate hydrogen and form lithium hydroxide. If powdered, lithium hydride may ignite spontaneously in humid air or on contact with moist mucous surfaces. The resulting tissue injury may have features of both thermal damage and strong alkali corrosion. The accidental explosion of a cylinder of lithium hydride sprayed material in the eye of a physicist and caused him to swallow a small amount of the dust. The resulting burns caused scarring of both corneas, stricture of the larynx, trachea, bronchi and esophagus. Despite intensive surgical treatment this case eventually terminated fatally.

See also: Lye, *Reference Congener in Section III.*
Ref.: Cracovaner, 1964.

62 Calcium Carbide 62

Used to generate acetylene for lighting purposes. Inert when dry, but reacts quickly with water to form acetylene and calcium hydroxide in a vigorously exothermic reaction. In contact with moist mucous membranes this reaction would probably result in a severe thermal and caustic burn. Presumably the acetylene produced would be of less toxic significance than the local lesion. Contact of calcium carbide dust with the eye or moist areas of the skin may produce marked irritation. Systemic effects do not occur.

See also: Lye, *Reference Congener in Section III.*
Ref.: Manufacturing Chemists' Assoc., 1948b.

Ammonia and amines that form strongly alkaline solutions

63 Ammonia 63

Ammonia water, Ammonium hydroxide, Ammonia gas

Most freshly opened bottles of household ammonia range from 5 to 10% (w/v) ammonia (NH_3). Dilute ammonia water (USP) is 9 to 10% (w/v) NH_3, whereas strong ammonia solution (USP) is 27 to 30% (w/v) NH_3. When ingested, any of these solutions is capable of producing a corrosive esophagitis, sometimes with an associated gastritis. The inhalation of anhydrous ammonia gas accidentally released in industrial accidents has produced acute and chronic respiratory disease. Anhydrous liquid ammonia produces second-degree burns on the skin and extensive destruction of the anterior chamber in the eye.

See also: Ammonia, *Reference Congener in Section III.*

64 Monoethanolamine (and Salts) 64

2-Aminoethanol, β-Aminoethyl alcohol, β-Hydroxyethylamine, β-Ethanolamine

Toxicity Rating: 3. A somewhat viscous, clear, hydroscopic fluid. Used to remove H_2S and CO_2 from natural gas, also as an emulsifier in polishes and hair wave solution and as a dispersing agent for various agricultural chemicals. In small amounts it is a normal constituent of human urine. Before exposure to CO_2 in air or neutralization by other acids, monoethanolamine is strongly basic; the pH of 0.1N aqueous solutions is 12.1. It is more alkaline and more toxic than di- or tri-ethanolamines. The oral LD_{50} is 2.1 and 1.5 gm./kg. in rats and mice respectively. A severe irritant in the rabbit eye, a moderate irritant on rabbit skin and a mild irritant on human skin. Percutaneous absorption is suspected. If only because of its high alkalinity, mucosal burns of the mouth and esophagus are likely after its ingestion. The vapor is also irritating to the respiratory tract, and various laboratory animals exposed subacutely to 104 ppm exhibited signs of respiratory distress, lethargy and mild degenerative changes in liver and kidneys (Treon et al., 1958, as cited by Treon, 1962). The OSHA air standard (TWA) is 3 ppm. In consumer products, monoethanolamine is usually present as a neutral salt of any one of many acids, and as such, the monoethanolamine cation is believed to lack significant toxicity (although no published evidence was located).

Ref.: Sidorov, 1968; Treon, 1962.

65   Diethanolamine (and Salts)

Iminodiethanol, Diolamine, e.g., Diethanolamine hydrochloride

Toxicity Rating: 3. A crystalline solid of low melting point (28°C). As a liquid, it is used to scrub toxic gases from smoke streams. Also employed as a cation in many water-soluble salts of drugs, pesticides and other commercial products. Moderate oral toxicity. Reported oral LD_{50}'s in experimental animals range from 0.7 (rat) to 3.5 gm./kg. (mouse). Symptoms of intoxication after large i.p. doses include sedation, ataxia, loss of righting reflex, cyanosis and death. In animals given fatal oral doses, the only gross pathology is found within the gastrointestinal tract. It has been suggested (without proof) that these deaths are due to a systemic alkalosis. Signs of transitory liver damage are seen after sublethal doses. Diethanolamine stimulates lipid phosphorylation in rat livers and causes a decrease in the oxygen uptake and respiratory quotient of hepatic tissue. The chief clinical toxicity, however, is probably moderate skin irritation and severe mucosal irritation, perhaps with corrosive lesions of mouth and esophagus. The presumptive basis of this irritancy is the high alkalinity of diethanolamine in water. A 0.1N aqueous solution has a pH of 11, which suggests that it is a stronger base than triethanolamine but weaker than monoethanolamine. As a neutral salt, cationic diethanolamine is probably innocuous, but the possibility of liver injury after ingestion needs to be investigated.

Ref.: Amer. Petroleum Institute, 1953h; Blum et al., 1972; Korsrud et al., 1973.

66   Triethanolamine

2,2',2″-Nitrilotriethanol, Trihydroxytriethylamine, Tri(hydroxyethyl)amine, TEA

Toxicity Rating: 2. A viscous hydroscopic liquid used as an emulsifier, solvent and chemical intermediate in the manufacture of textiles, waxes, herbicides, toilet goods, etc. Low toxicity (rat oral LD_{50} 8.7 gm./kg.). The ingestion of several ounces can probably be tolerated by man, but unless the liquid is partly neutralized with acid, alkali burns of the mouth, pharynx and esophagus are likely. Thus triethanolamine is a strong base (K_a 3.2×10^{-10}), and a 0.1N aqueous solution has a pH of 10.5. The principal toxic effect in animals has been ascribed to alkalinization (systemic alkalosis), but as with diethanolamine (above), functional signs of transient liver injury have been described in animals after sublethal doses. Gross pathology has been limited to the gastrointestinal tract in fatal oral poisonings in rats and guinea pigs. Percutaneous absorption is rapid, but the compound is less irritating to skin and mucous membranes than most amines.

Ref.: Amer. Petroleum Institute, 1953h; Kostrodymova et al., 1976.

67   Triethanolamine Salts

Many weak acids are used in commercial formulations as neutral salts of cationic triethanolamine. For example, triethanolamine salts of fatty acids serve as synthetic soaps (see Triethanolamine oleate in the index). As a cation triethanolamine appears to have no significant toxicity by the oral route, although the possibility of effects on liver and brain cannot be excluded (see Triethanolamine above). Consult the index for information about the corresponding sodium salt or look under the name of the acid.

Ref.: Amer. Petroleum Institute, 1953h.

68   Dimethylamine (and Salts)

Aqueous solutions of dimethylamine are highly alkaline, like ammonia (see Sec. III). Animal toxicity has been ascribed to its caustic actions and to systemic alkalosis. In contrast the amine salts (e.g., hydrochloride) are relatively benign.

Ref.: Commercial Solvents Corp., 1954.

69   Tris(hydroxymethyl)aminomethane 69

2-Amino-2-hydroxymethyl-1,3-propanediol, Tris, Tromethamine

Toxicity Rating: 3. A commercial emulsifier. Aqueous solutions are alkaline and consequently irritating. Even after neutralization, large oral doses in laboratory animals cause weakness, collapse, and coma (without convulsions). Injections of high doses in animals produce hypoglycemia, but concurrent administration of glucose does not prevent death. Solutions have been infused intravenously in human patients to correct acidosis and to promote diuresis. Doses of up to 76 grams (!) in one hour have caused hypoglycemia, but doses of 20 gm. produced no adverse effects.

Ref.: Brinkman et al., 1960; Commercial Solvents Corp., 1954; Roberts and Linn, 1961.

70   2-Amino-2-methyl-1-propanol 70

Toxicity Rating: 3. An emulsifier used in small amounts in polishes (floor, auto, shoe, etc.). Aminohydroxy compounds react with higher fatty acids to form soaps possessing good emulsifying powers. The oral toxicity of these compounds is low in rabbits and presumably in man. Prolonged skin exposure may cause irritation due to the alkalinity of the free material, but in most commercial formulas this alkalinity is neutralized. Allergic dermatitis is not described.

Ref.: Commercial Solvents Corp., 1954.

71   2-Amino-2-methyl-1,3-propanediol 71

Toxicity Rating: 3. An emulsifier used in small amounts in polishes, cleaners, cosmetic creams, etc. Aminohydroxy compounds react with higher fatty acids to form soaps possessing good emulsifying powers. The oral toxicity of these compounds is low in rabbits and presumably in man. Prolonged skin exposure may cause irritation due to the alkalinity of the free material, but in most commercial formulas this alkalinity is neutralized. Allergic dermatitis is not described.

Ref.: Commercial Solvents Corp., 1954.

72   Morpholine 72

Tetrahydro-1,4-oxazine, Diethyleneimide oxide

Toxicity Rating: 4. A secondary amine used as a corrosion inhibitor, as an antioxidant, and in the form of salts as an emulsifying agent. Strongly alkaline. Liquid and vapor are irritating to skin and mucous membranes. In rats pulmonary edema, liver necrosis, and renal tubular degeneration, but only at vapor concentrations which are intensely irritating. Moderately high percutaneous toxicity in rabbits. On the skin the liquid may produce necrosis.

Ref.: Amer. Petroleum Institute, 1948e.

Peroxides and peroxy-acids (inorganic and organic)

73   Hydrogen Peroxide 73

Official aqueous solutions are 3% with respect to H_2O_2. Said to have a low toxicity. No primary systemic effects when ingested because it is decomposed in the bowel before absorption. Decomposition may release large volumes of oxygen (10 times the volume of solution). Large doses presumably produce esophagitis and gastritis. Cases of rupture of the colon, proctitis and ulcerative colitis have been reported following hydrogen peroxide enemas. Powders and tablets that generate hydrogen peroxide, such as $KHSO_5$, have caused oral and esophageal burns when ingested.

Ref.: Abramson, 1978; Sheehan and Brynjolfsson, 1960.

74   Sodium Peroxide 74

Said to have a low toxicity. No primary systemic effects when ingested because it is decomposed in the bowel before absorption. Decomposition may release large volumes of oxygen (10 times the volume of the solution). Large doses presumably produce gastritis and esophagitis. Cases of rupture of the colon, proctitis and ulcerative colitis have been reported following hydrogen peroxide enemas.

Ref.: Sheehan and Brynjolfsson, 1960.

75   Methyl Ethyl Ketone Peroxide (and Hydroperoxides) 75

Available as a 60% solution in dimethyl phthalate (Lupersol DDM) to serve as a catalyst for polymerizing plastics. The mixture has a toxicity rating of 4 in mice (administered by mouth after diluting with oil). An unstable agent which like hydrogen peroxide releases oxygen. Concentrated solutions are corrosive to skin and mucous membrane, and

Ref.: Deisher, 1958; Floyd and Stokinger, 1958.

a human case of severe esophagitis and gastritis has been reported. Some experimental evidence for a cumulative toxicity has been presented.

76   76   Benzoyl Peroxide

Toxicity Rating: 3. Used as a catalyst for the hardening of certain Fiberglas resins. Rats have tolerated by mouth 950 mg./kg. without fatalities although death in adult mice has been reported after the intraperitoneal administration of 250 mg./kg. When placed as a dry powder on the skin of guinea pigs, only slight irritation followed, but

when dissolved as a 10% solution in propylene glycol, slight to moderate erythema and edema were observed without systemic toxicity. Has been reported as an allergen responsible for skin sensitization in man. Potentially dangerous because of inflammable and explosive properties.

Ref.: Hays, 1960; Lamson, 1931; Malten, 1958; Roudabush, 1960.

77   77   Cyclohexanone Peroxide

Toxicity Rating: 3(?). Used as a catalyst for the hardening of certain Fiberglas resins. Might be expected to have corrosive action on skin and mucous membrane. As an 85% solution in dibutyl

phthalate its parenteral LD_{50} in mice is 2 gm./kg. Has been reported as an allergen responsible for skin sensitization in man.

Ref.: National Academy of Science, Date Unknown; Malten, 1958.

78   78   Peroxyacetic Acid

Peracetic acid, Acetyl hydroperoxide

Toxicity Rating: 4(?). Commercially available as a 40% solution in acetic acid. Highly corrosive.

See also: Acid, *Reference Congener in Section III.*
Ref.: Merck and Co., 1976.

79   79   Potassium Monopersulfate

Potassium peroxymonosulfate, e.g., Oxone

Toxicity Rating: 3. Formula: $KHSO_5$. New type strong oxidizing agent used in bleaching and germicidal preparations for home laundry and bathroom (e.g., denture cleansers). Possesses the ability to oxidize chloride ion to chlorine so that the combination of monopersulfate and sodium chloride provides both oxygen and chlorine in an "activated" bleach that can be made almost odorless. Other ingredients which may be formulated with monopersulfate for special purposes are alkyl aryl sulfonates, certain nonionic detergents, some polyphosphates, carboxymethylcellulose, etc.

Since monopersulfate forms acidic solutions, an alkaline filler such as sodium carbonate (or soda ash) sufficient to provide a solution pH of 9 to 10 is necessary. The approximate lethal dose in male albino rats (presumably by mouth) is 2250 mg./kg. Aqueous solutions of 2.5 to 3.0% are not irritating on skin of the human forearm or guinea pig, but 25% solutions are strong primary irritants on guinea pigs. The ingestion of tablets and powders marketed as denture cleansers and containing both $KHSO_5$ and sodium perborate has caused corrosive injuries of the mouth and esophagus.

See also: Hypochlorite, *Reference Congener in Section III.*
Ref.: Abramson et al., 1974; Abramson, 1978; du Pont, 1961a.

Strong inorganic oxidants (exclusive of halogen compounds and peroxides)

80   80   Chromium Trioxide

Chromic acid

Toxicity Rating: 4 or 5. CrO_3 has an estimated mean lethal dose of between 1 and 10 gm. However, an adult male consumed 15 gm. as a chrome plating solution (300 gm./l, pH 0.5) and survived the subsequent vomiting, diarrhea, liver damage, hemorrhagic diathesis, and acute renal failure. Corrosive because of its oxidizing potency, not its acidity. An acute single exposure to massive concentrations of sprays or mists can severely damage deep lung

structures, but the nasal mucosa may be only mildly hyperemic. Repeated exposures to lower concentrations, however, can result in ulceration and perforation of the nasal septum. Local injuries (chrome ulcers, chrome holes) of skin and mucous membranes should be treated like acid burns. External lesions can be scrubbed with a dilute sodium hyposulfite solution (2%) or treated with calcium disodium edetate ointments. When freshly prepared and promptly applied, a 10% solution of ascorbic acid speeded healing of chrome ulcers in guinea pig skin, presumably by reducing hexavalent chromium to less toxic and less irritating trivalent chromium and by chelating the latter.

Chronic industrial exposures have also led to severe liver damage, central nervous system involvement and perhaps lung cancer. Allergic reactions are common. See also Dichromate salts below.

See also: Acid *and* Copper, *Reference Congeners in Section III.*
Ref.: Fristedt et al., 1965; Kleinfeld and Rosso, 1965; Meyers, 1950; Pascale et al., 1952; Pirozzi et al., 1968.

81   Chromate Salts   81

e.g., Sodium chromate, Potassium chromate

Toxicity Rating: 4 or 5. Corrosive because of its oxidizing potency. Treat local injuries like acid burns; also external lesions may be scrubbed with a dilute sodium hyposulfite solution (2%) or treated with calcium disodium edetate ointment. If ingested, violent gastroenteritis, severe circulatory collapse and toxic nephritis may ensue. Treat peripheral vascular shock vigorously. A less common source of poisoning than chromic acid or dichromates. See Chromium trioxide above and Dichromate salts below.

See also: Acid *and* Copper, *Reference Congeners in Section III.*

82   Dichromate Salts (Soluble)   82

e.g., Sodium dichromate, Potassium dichromate, Ammonium dichromate

Toxicity Rating: 4 or 5. The oral lethal dose in man probably lies between 1 and 10 grams. Highly corrosive to skin and mucous membranes; see Chromium trioxide above for management of local lesions, chronic poisoning, and pulmonary exposure. If ingested, violent gastroenteritis with cholera-like stools, peripheral vascular collapse, vertigo, muscle cramps, coma, hemorrhagic diathesis, fever, liver damage and acute renal failure. "Methemoglobinemia" is probably secondary to intravascular hemolysis as with chlorate salts. Extra-corporeal hemodialysis instituted for the uremia appeared in several cases to lower blood chromium levels. Perhaps dialysis should be tried earlier in the course of the intoxication. In animal experiments BAL was at least as effective against chromate as against mercury. In several clinical cases, however, BAL has been disappointing, perhaps because its administration was too late. Similarly diethylenetriamine pentaacetate was without effect in a single case, but the patient was already moribund. In neutral or alkaline solutions (pH > 6) and in dilute solutions (< .01 M), dichromate exists almost exclusively as monomeric chromate (see Chromate Salts above). A promising therapeutic stratagem is to reduce toxic hexavalent chromium (as in chromate and dichromate) to much less toxic trivalent chromium (as in chromic oxide, nitrate, etc.). A rapid and generally safe reducing agent is ascorbic acid; it does not appear to have been tested in systemic chromate poisoning, but it deserves a trial by intravenous infusion because it has proved useful in the local management of chrome ulcers (see Chromium Trioxide above). Probably large doses (5–10 gm.) of ascorbic acid should be swallowed promptly after the ingestion of a soluble chromate. If vitamin C is unavailable, activated charcoal should be swallowed, if possible. In any case do not induce emesis because chromate is a stronger oxidant in acidic media than in neutral media, and so esophageal corrosion is likely with repeated vomiting. Remove ingested chromate by gastric aspiration and lavage. Insoluble and slightly soluble chromates and dichromates appear to be carcinogenic.

See also: Copper *and* Acid, *Reference Congeners in Section III.*
Ref.: Braun et al., 1946; Connett and Wetterhahn, 1982; Cox and Wendel, 1942; Fritz et al., 1960; Goldman and Karotkin, 1935; Kaufman et al., 1970; Mosora, 1965; Norseth, 1981; Reichelderfer, 1968.

83   Potassium Permanganate   83

Condy's crystals

An oxidizing agent. Only mildly irritating in dilute solutions but concentrated solutions and dry crystals are highly corrosive. In at least three oral poisonings, death has resulted from edema of the glottis. Systemic effects are not of primary importance because of poor absorption. Treat by swallowing egg white and by gastric lavage. Preparations should be made for an emergency tracheotomy. Deaths have resulted from the use of solutions as douches in attempted abortions.

See also: Acid, *Reference Congener in Section III.*
Ref.: Jacobziner and Raybin, 1961l; Jetter and Hunter, 1949; Willimott and Freiman, 1936.

Hypochlorite and other precursors of active chlorine

84   Hypochlorite

i.e., Sodium, Potassium, Calcium

Hypochlorite salts are widely used as disinfectants, bleaches and deodorizers in home and industry. The toxicity of these salts is usually ascribed to the hypochlorite anion, to hypochlorous acid and to chlorine derived from them. Some of the common preparations are described below.

See also: Hypochlorite, *Reference Congener in Section III.*

85   Sodium Hypochlorite

The official solution (NF) contains between 4 and 6% sodium hypochlorite (NaOCl), or approximately the same concentration with respect to "available chlorine." Dilute solutions of the Carrel-Dakin type are about 0.5% NaOCl.

See also: Hypochlorite, *Reference Congener in Section III.*
Ref.: Taylor and Austin, 1918.

86   Labarraque's Solution

Toxicity Rating: 3(?). An aqueous solution: 4 to 6% sodium hypochlorite, 4% sodium chloride, and 0.1 to 1.5% sodium hydroxide or carbonate. The lye contributes to the corrosive action when swallowed. A solution of approximately half the above strength is also described as "Labarraque's solution."

See also: Hypochlorite *and* Lye, *Reference Congeners in Section III.*
Ref.: Osol and Farrar, 1955.

87   Chlorinated Trisodium Phosphate

Chlorinated sodium phosphate

As a bleaching solution this material is best described as phosphate-buffered sodium hypochlorite. It is made by adding gaseous chlorine to aqueous solutions of trisodium phosphate and then diluting to use concentrations. Related mixtures are made by chlorinating solutions of pentasodium tripolyphosphate and of sodium metasilicate. We believe that in modern consumer products these solutions are only mildly to moderately alkaline and are no more toxic than other household solutions of sodium hypochlorite. The toxicity rating depends upon the concentration of "available chlorine"; in the absence of aspiration, a rating of 2-3 is consistent with the reported oral toxicity of 5% sodium hypochlorite in man.

See also: Hypochlorite, *Reference Congener in Section III.*

88   Javelle Water

Chlorinated potash solution

Toxicity Rating: 3(?). A solution of potassium hypochlorite with an unspecified amount of unneutralized potassium hydroxide. When freshly prepared it contains about 2.5% active chlorine and is therefore about half as concentrated as the official NF solution of sodium hypochlorite.

See also: Hypochlorite, *Reference Congener in Section III.*
Ref.: Taylor and Austin, 1918.

89   Calcium Hypochlorite

The salt is the active ingredient of chlorinated lime. See latter below. As with other corrosive agents, the toxicity rating of a solution depends upon its concentration.

See also: Hypochlorite, *Reference Congener in Section III.*
Ref.: Merck and Co., 1976.

90   Chlorinated Lime

An indefinite mixture of calcium chloride, hypochlorite and hydroxide has about 35%/w active chlorine, based upon its hypochlorite content (but it may vary between 24 and 37% in commercial preparations). As with other corrosive agents, the toxicity rating of a solution depends upon its concentration.

See also: Hypochlorite, *Reference Congener in Section III.*
Ref.: Merck and Co., 1976.

91   Chloramine-T

91

Sodium *p*-toluenesulfonchloramide, Chlorosol, (*N*-Chloro-*p*-toluenesulfonamido)sodium, Chlorazone, Chlorozone, Chlorazene

Toxicity Rating: 3(?). An antibacterial agent used topically as an antiseptic. Releases active chlorine. Available chlorine is 12.6%. Not usually regarded as toxic but more so than an equivalent amount of chlorine as hypochlorite. An occasional reaction is rapid and violent, suggesting hypersensitivity. Poisoning characterized by pain, vomiting, sudden loss of consciousness, circulatory and respiratory collapse, and death. It has been suggested that Chloramine-T can react with some amino acids in the gastrointestinal tract to form toxic cyanogen compounds. Treat symptomatically.

See also: Hypochlorite, *Reference Congener in Section III.*
Ref.: Serin, 1949; Taylor and Austin, 1918.

92   *N*-Chlorosuccinimide

92

Succinchlorimide

Toxicity Rating: 3. Slowly liberates chlorine, producing gastric irritation.

See also: Hypochlorite, *Reference Congener in Section III.*
Ref.: Stohlman and Smith, 1944.

93   1,3-Dichloro-5,5-dimethylhydantoin

93

DDH, Dactin

Serves as a mild bleach by slowly releasing active chlorine. Presumably less corrosive than hypochlorite solutions with the same concentration of available chlorine. Local tissue injury is the only recognized toxic action. Similar to the chlorinated cyanuric acid derivatives such as Trichloroisocyanuric acid below.

See also: Hypochlorite, *Reference Congener in Section III.*
Ref.: Zapp, 1956.

94   Trichloroisocyanuric Acid

94

Trichlorotriazinetrione, ACL 85

Toxicity Rating: 3. Used as a source of available chlorine in "dry type" bleaches, scouring powders, dishwashing compounds, sanitizers and swimming pool disinfectants. An organic oxidant which can slowly oxidize almost its own weight of chloride ions to chlorine gas (about 90% "available chlorine"). In weak solutions it probably exists in equilibrium with mono- and di-chloro derivatives, with hypochlorous acid and with isocyanuric acid, to which it eventually decomposes (see latter in index). In strong solutions (>0.5%), it may decompose to nitrogen trichloride (see index), which is a strong lacrimator and an explosive when heated. Trichloroisocyanuric acid has an oral LD_{50} in rats of 750 mg./kg., and an oral minimal lethal dose in rabbits of 1500 to 1900 mg./kg. Related compounds with similar toxicity include dichloroisocyanuric acid (ACL 70), sodium dichloroisocyanurate (ACL 60) and potassium dichloroisocyanurate (ACL 75). In solution these salts exist in equilibrium with their enol tautomer dichlorocyanurate. The toxicity is apparently due to corrosive action on stomach lining rather than to any systemic effects. In the presence of moisture, as in the eyes, upper respiratory tract or on moist or abraded skin, it is moderately irritating. In some individuals bronchospasm may result from breathing the dust; for the management of this syndrome, see Nitrogen Oxides in Section III and appropriate parts of Section IV.

See also: Hypochlorite, *Reference Congener in Section III.*
Ref.: Canelli, 1974; Laveglia et al., 1977; Monsanto Chemical Co., 1960; Porter, 1959.

Inorganic and metallo-organic compounds

Systemically toxic halides

95   Bromate

95

e.g., Sodium bromate, Potassium bromate

Toxicity Rating: 5. The bromate anion is nephrotoxic. It has produced death due to acute renal failure in children.

See also: Bromate, *Reference Congener in Section III.*

96

96   Chlorate Salts

i.e., Sodium, magnesium

Toxicity Rating: 4. A common source of chlorate poisoning is ingested match heads. Susceptibility varies widely among men and animals, but estimated lethal dose for man is about 30 gm., representing about one-tenth the toxicity of bromate.

Produces gastritis, methemoglobinemia, and a late toxic nephritis. Less central nervous depression than bromate poisoning but perhaps more methemoglobin. Hemodialysis is recommended for removal of chlorate.

See also: Bromate, Reference Congener in Section III.

97

97   Iodate Salts

i.e., Sodium, potassium

Toxicity Rating: 4. Recommended by the World Health Organization as an additive in table salt to

prevent goiter.

See also: Bromate, Reference Congener in Section III.

98

98   Bromide Salts

i.e., Sodium, potassium, ammonium

Toxicity Rating: 3. Acute oral poisoning is rare because single doses are usually promptly rejected by vomiting, but 1 oz. has been swallowed and adsorbed sufficiently to cause death. A blood level of 125 mg./100 ml. is regarded as the minimal intoxicating level. The systemic effects of bromide ion are chiefly mental: drowsiness, irritability, ataxia, vertigo, confusion, mania, hallucinations,

and coma. Other effects include skin rashes, neurological signs, sensory disturbances, and increased spinal fluid pressures. Treatment includes hydration, the maintenance of a mild water diuresis, and sodium or, better, ammonium chloride (10 to 15 gm. daily in divided doses) with an osmotic or high-ceiling diuretic. Hemodialysis may be of value.

Ref.: Cornbleet, 1951; Dax, 1946; Hussar and Holley, 1956; Perkins, 1950; Schreiner, 1958.

99

99   Iodide Salts

i.e., Sodium, potassium

Toxicity Rating: 3(?). Iodide salts do not share the corrosive actions of free iodine, and no human fatalities are known after single oral doses of the common salts. Ten grams of NaI have been given slowly by the intravenous route without ill effects. Iodides are principally active as expectorants and diuretics. A mild toxic syndrome called "iodism" results from chronic iodide overdoses and from the repeated administration of small amounts of iodine.

Iodism is characterized by salivation, coryza, sneezing, conjunctivitis, headache, fever, laryngitis bronchitis, stomatitis, parotitis (iodine mumps) and various skin rashes (iododerma, thrombotic thrombocytopenic purpura). Edema of the glottis necessitating tracheotomy has occurred. The occasional use of iodides for asthma in pregnancy has resulted in fetal death, severe goiter and cretinoid appearance of the newborn.

Ref.: Anonymous, 1957a; Aquilina and Bissel, 1955; Barker and Wood, 1940; Carter, 1961; Ehrich and Seifter, 1949; Galina et al., 1962; Martin and Rento, 1962; Paull, 1959; Snell and Savin, 1927.

100

100   Fluoride

i.e., Sodium, barium, zinc

Toxicity Rating: 4. Clinical data indicate that the sodium salt lies near the borderline between toxicity classes 4 and 5; the rat oral LD_{50} is 80 mg./kg. Although less toxic in animals, barium fluoride may be as toxic in man as the sodium salt (or perhaps slightly more toxic). Calcium fluoride is comparatively benign (toxicity rating 3?) because

of its low solubility and low ionization. In terms of acute toxicity, most fluorides presumably lie between the sodium and calcium salts. In terms of the acute oral LD_{50} in rats (75 mg./kg.), sodium monofluorophosphate (MFP) is as toxic as sodium fluoride and can produce systemic fluoride poisoning.

See also: Fluoride, Reference Congener in Section III.
Ref.: Lewis and Tatken, 1979.

101

101   Fluosilicate Salts

i.e., Magnesium, zinc, sodium, ammonium

Toxicity Rating: 4. The sodium, ammonium and zinc salts are used in commercial laundry sours,

and the ammonium, magnesium and zinc salts have been used for mothproofing textile fabrics. Som agricultural insecticides contain the sodium, magnesium or barium salts. The sodium salt is found in various kinds of products: aluminum and stainless steel cleaners, roach and earwig poisons, insecticidal baits, etc. The zinc salt sometimes serves as a concrete hardener. Fluosilicate salts are generally more soluble than the corresponding fluoride salt (but not true in the case of sodium). Hydrolyzed to fluoride ion, especially in alkaline water. For example, Na_2SiF_6 in water yields $2NaF$ and SiF_4. In experimental animals the fluosilicates appear to be as toxic as the corresponding fluorides. Sodium fluosilicate has caused human deaths. The oral LD_{50} in rats is 125 mg./kg. After ingestion, lavage stomach with lime water (calcium hydroxide) and administer aluminum hydroxide antacid preparations (gels or tablets) to trap fluoride. On the skin (and presumably in eyes and on mucous membranes), the fluosilicates are irritants. Prolonged skin contact may lead to a pustular rash and even to ulceration. Presumably the local lesions are not due to alkalinity or acidity because they occur with all of the fluosilicates. Solutions of the sodium salt are neutral whereas those of the zinc and magnesium salts are mildly acidic (pH 3.1 for 1% solutions).

See also: Fluoride, *Reference Congener in Section III.*
Ref.: Locke, 1951; Lewis and Tatken, 1979.

102   Barium Fluosilicate   102

Barium silicofluoride

Toxicity Rating: 4. Used as an insecticide on some crops before edible parts are formed. Probably not as toxic as sodium fluoride because of low solubility in water, although reported rat oral LD_{50}'s are essentially identical (180 vs. 175 mg./kg.). Hydrolyzed by alkali to highly toxic fluoride ion. Although not described in test animals (most species being relatively resistant to barium), barium intoxication may here complicate the clinical picture of acute fluoride poisoning, but the fluosilicate is probably one of the less toxic forms of barium. See also Fluosilicate Salts above.

See also: Fluoride, *Reference Congener in Section III.*
Ref.: Locke, 1951; Lewis and Tatken, 1979.

103   Potassium Fluoborate   103

Potassium tetrafluoroborate, Potassium borofluoride, Avogadrite, Fluoroborate salts soluble

Toxicity Rating: 4. Formula: KBF_4. Found in flux for soldering and brazing. Intraperitoneal LD_{50} in rabbits 0.38 gm./kg., in rats 0.24 gm./kg., in mice 0.59 gm./kg. Does not appear to be absorbed through intact skin and doses up to 3.0 mg. in the rabbit eye produced no grossly observable reaction. Systemic toxicity probably relates to fluoride content. Boric acid and borates have been shown to protect animals from soluble fluorides presumably through the formation of fluoborates.

See also: Fluoride, *Reference Congener in Section III.*
Ref.: Blaisdell, 1955; Marcovitch and Stanley, 1942; Maynard et al., 1951.

104   Cryolite   104

Sodium aluminum fluoride

Toxicity Rating: 2(?). Formula: Na_3AlF_6 or $3NaF \cdot AlF_3$. Acute toxicity by ingestion is known to be very low (e.g., intraperitoneal lethal dose in rats is 100 times that of sodium fluoride). Much less soluble than sodium fluoride or fluosilicate and more stable than the latter with respect to hydrolysis.

See also: Fluoride, *Reference Congener in Section III.*
Ref.: Largent, 1948.

Cytochrome oxidase poisons and their precursors

105   Cyanide   105

e.g., Sodium cyanide

Toxicity Rating: 6. The soluble inorganic salts are among the fastest poisons known. To be effective, treatment must be prompt.

See also: Cyanide, *Reference Congener in Section III.*

106   Hydrocyanic Acid   106

Hydrogen cyanide, Prussic acid

Toxicity Rating: 6. Prussic acid is 2% aqueous HCN. Cyanide is one of the fastest poisons known. To be effective, therapeutic measures must be prompt!

See also: Cyanide, *Reference Congener in Section III.*

107   **107**   Calcium Cyanide

e.g., Cyanogas

Toxicity Rating: 6. All inorganic cyanide salts are toxic when ingested. If the free gastric acidity is high, toxic symptoms appear almost immediately.

See also: Cyanide, Reference Congener in Section III.

108   **108**   Mercury Oxycyanide

Mercury cyanide oxide

Toxicity Rating: 5. The commercial salt is often a mixture of the oxycyanide (1/3) and the cyanide (2/3), to reduce danger of explosion. Symptoms both of mercury and of cyanide poisoning have been described, but at least in dogs the mercury effects have proved more important. It is possible that in man cyanide poisoning appears first, especially if the free gastric acidity is high (stomach empty of food), but in one reported human poisoning by mercuric cyanide, no symptoms of cyanide poisoning were described.

See also: Mercury and Cyanide, Reference Congeners in Section III.
Ref.: Sanchez-Sicillia et al., 1963; Witthaus, 1911.

109   **109**   Nitroprusside Salts

Nitroferricyanide salts, Nitroprussiates, e.g., Sodium nitroprusside

Toxicity Rating: 4-5. Used by intravenous drip in man to control hypertension and hypertensive encephalopathy. When taken by mouth, nitroprusside is either absorbed poorly or decomposed in the gastrointestinal tract prior to absorption. By parenteral routes it is extremely toxic. Acute oral versus intraperitoneal LD_{50}'s: rats, 100 mg./kg. versus 10 mg./kg.; mice, 65 mg./kg. versus about 10 mg./kg. No sex differences noted. Single doses of nitroprusside by mouth are at least 1000 times less hypotensive in human adults than single intravenous doses. At least three humans have committed suicide by ingesting nitroprusside, but the doses were unknown, and the signs of poisoning were not observed. Decomposes on contact with biological materials to release free cyanide. Unequivocally causes cyanide poisoning in animals; it is at least 4 times more toxic than sodium cyanide on a molar basis. Death, however, is delayed for as long as an hour even after parenteral administration. Classical cyanide antidotes protect animals against death. Given chronically in therapeutic doses, nitroprusside produces toxic signs that resemble those produced by sodium thiocyanate; see latter in the index. Indeed, the long-term dosage of nitroprusside has been adjusted on the basis of blood thiocyanate levels which result from the metabolism of nitroprusside.

See also: Cyanide, Reference Congener in Section III.
Ref.: Caujolle et al., 1968; Hill, 1942; Johnson, 1929; Lazarus-Barlow and Norman, 1941; Mahaffey, 1942; Page et al., 1955; Smith, 1973b.

110   **110**   Cyano Organic Compounds

Nitrile derivatives

Many organic nitriles (i.e., cyanides) are decomposed in the body to yield highly toxic cyanide (CN- or HCN). The list includes naturally occurring cyanogenic glycosides, such as amygdalin and linamarin, and primarily industrial compounds, such as acrylonitrile and acetonitrile. Consult the index for name of specific compound.

See also: Cyanide, Reference Congener in Section III.

111   **111**   Azide Salts

Sodium azide, Hydrazoic acid

Toxicity Rating: 6. Hydrazoic acid is used in industry to prepare heavy metal azides for shell detonators. The water-soluble salts are not nearly so explosive. It is a common preservative in laboratory reagents such as diluting fluids for counting red cells (0.1%) and in buffering solutions used to screen for hepatitis antigen (4.0%). If such reagents are poured down the drain, they may accumulate in traps and form explosive copper and lead azides, which might be detonated by plumbers (LaLuna et al., 1979; Richardson et al., 1975; Roberts et al., 1974). The canister in automobile protective air bags is said to contain 3/4 pound of sodium azide (Szmant, 1980). Acute human intoxications are characterized by profound hypotension unresponsive to pressor drugs. Azide is an extremely potent, directly acting vasodilator with a hypotensive dose of 0.2 to 4.0 mcg./kg. in humans. The hypotensive response resembles that after sodium nitroprusside or sodium nitrite, but it is more prolonged (Graham, 1949). Tachycardia, tachypnea, hypothermia, acidosis, convulsions and severe headache are common in victims of acute poisoning. An adult laboratory technician who accidentally swallowed

150 mg. of sodium azide in aqueous solution experienced breathlessness and tachycardia within 5 minutes. Nausea, vomiting, headache, restlessness and diarrhea ensued within 15 minutes. Later polydipsia, ECG changes and leukocytosis occurred. Complete recovery required more than 10 days (Burger and Bauer, 1965). "Several grams" produced collapse and death within 40 minutes in another adult. Pathologic findings were limited to swelling of the brain and lungs and mild fatty degeneration of the liver (Kozlicka-Gajdzinska and Brzyski, 1966). Fifty to 60 mg. by mouth produced collapse within 5 minutes accompanied by hypotension and tachycardia lasting almost an hour, whereas in another adult 5 to 10 mg. produced only fleeting signs (Richardson et al., 1975). In experimental animals methemoglobinemia induced by sodium nitrite or by other agents confers a very small but statistically significant degree of protection against death (Abbanat and Smith, 1964). Presumably this effect is due to binding of the azide ion to the ferric heme groups of methemoglobin (Smith and Gosselin, 1966). In a single clinical case of acute azide poisoning, nitrite-induced methemoglobinemia had no discernible benefit (Emmett and Ricking, 1975). There are other similarities between azide on the one hand and cyanide and sulfide on the other (see CYANIDE and HYDROGEN SULFIDE in Section III). In each case the acid is volatile. Like the others, azide stimulates carotid body chemoreceptors (Anichkov and Belen'kii, 1963) and inhibits heme-type enzymes such as catalase, peroxidase and cytochrome oxidase (Keilin, 1936-37; Smith et al., 1977). It appears unlikely, however, that the high toxicity of azide is due to cytochrome oxidase inhibition (Smith et al., 1977). Workers exposed for many years to the volatile acid exhibited no pathological signs, although many had experienced episodes with rapid and severe falls in both systolic and diastolic blood pressure with associated headache (Graham et al., 1948). The vapors and fumes, however, are irritants of mucous membranes, and heavy exposure has caused bronchitis and pulmonary edema.

Ref.: Abbanat and Smith, 1964; Anichkov and Belen'kii, 1963; Burger and Bauer, 1965; Emmett and Ricking, 1975; Graham et al., 1948; Graham, 1949; Keilin, 1936-37; Kozlicka-Gajdzinska and Brzyski, 1966; LaLuna et al., 1979; Richardson et al., 1975; Roberts et al., 1974; Smith and Gosselin, 1966; Smith et al., 1977; Szmant, 1980.

112   Ammonium Polysulfide   112

A clear red liquid miscible with water to yield a strongly alkaline reaction. Consists of $(NH_4)_2S_3$ and other polymers. Decomposes in strong acids to hydrogen sulfide and elemental sulfur. Presumably it decomposes rapidly in the stomach.

See also: Hydrogen Sulfide, *Reference Congener in Section III.*

113   Calcium Polysulfide   113

Lime sulfur

Toxicity Rating: 4(?). Irritant and sensitizing agent. May yield hydrogen sulfide by decomposition before or after ingestion. Used in agriculture as an insecticide and fungicide.

See also: Hydrogen Sulfide, *Reference Congener in Section III.*
Ref.: Council on Pharmacy and Chemistry, 1955.

114   Hydrogen Sulfide   114

Sulfureted hydrogen, Hydrosulfuric acid, "Stink damp"
See also: Hydrogen Sulfide, *Reference Congener in Section III.*

115   Lithopone   115

Griffith's zinc white

Toxicity Rating: 3(?). Mixture of zinc sulfide, barium sulfate, and zinc oxide, used as a paint pigment. If gastric acidity is high, hydrogen sulfide may be formed.

See also: Hydrogen Sulfide, *Reference Congener in Section III.*
Ref.: Merck and Co., 1976.

116   Methanethiol   116

Methyl mercaptan, Mercaptomethane, Thiomethyl alcohol

A gas which condenses at about 6°C. Because the unpleasant odor is detectable at 1 part in 140 million, it is incorporated into natural gas to give warning of leaks. Also an important synthetic intermediate. Coma occurred in 50% of a population of rats within 15 minutes on exposure to 0.16% methanethiol, to 3.3% ethanethiol or to 9.6% dimethyl sulfide (by volume). All animals recovered consciousness within 30 minutes. These simple mercaptans potentiate the coma induced by ammonium salts in rats (see also Ammonia in Section III), and some of them have been detected in the urine and breath of patients with massive hepatic necrosis (fetor hepaticus). Animals fatally poisoned by inhalation exhibited restlessness, muscular weakness progressing to paralysis, convulsions, respiratory depression and cyanosis. Pulmonary edema was observed, but other primary systemic effects could not be ruled out. A man was found comatose within one hour after a respiratory exposure to an unknown concentration of methanethiol. Transient but severe hemolytic anemia and methemoglobinemia developed. In this victim these blood dyscrasias were ascribed to a demonstrated deficiency in red blood cell glucose-6-phosphate dehydrogenase activity. Deep coma persisted until death 28 days after exposure. Necropsy revealed a massive embolus which occluded both main pulmonary arteries. Methanethiol may be toxicologically similar to hydrogen sulfide (see latter in Section III). Both compounds reversibly inhibit rat liver mitochondrial respiration by inhibiting cytochrome c oxidase. Methanethiol also reversibly inhibits rat brain sodium- and potassium-ATPase. These inhibitions may be involved in the reversible coma observed in methanethiol intoxication.

Ref.: Shults et al., 1970; Waller, 1977; Zieve et al., 1974.

117   Phosphorus Pentasulfide

Phosphoric sulfide, Phosphorus persulfide, Thiophosphoric anhydride

Formula: P_2S_5 (or P_4S_{10}). Decomposes on contact with water to phosphoric acid, sulfur dioxide, and hydrogen sulfide. The latter is certainly the most toxic of these decomposition products.

See also: Hydrogen Sulfide, *Reference Congener in Section III.*
Ref.: Amer. Petroleum Institute, 1948g.

118   Sulfide Salts

Alkaline sulfide salts, Metal sulfides, i.e., Sodium, potassium, calcium

Toxicity Rating: 6. If free gastric acidity is high, the ingestion of these salts may result in their decomposition to hydrogen sulfide in the stomach, with subsequent systemic poisoning. In any case, the alkaline sulfides are strong local irritants to mucous membrane (and skin). Treatment: gastric lavage, demulcents, saline catharsis, plus measures outlined under hydrogen sulfide.

See also: Hydrogen Sulfide, *Reference Congener in Section III.*

119   Strontium Sulfide

Toxicity Rating: 4(?). Used in depilatories, because it is less irritating than sodium sulfide and more efficient than calcium sulfide. Cases of localized dermatitis are reported. Taken by mouth it is the sulfide moiety and not the strontium that is responsible for the high toxicity. Gastric acid decomposes it to hydrogen sulfide. Humans given 6.4 gm. of strontium lactate daily for 4 years showed no evidence of toxicity.

See also: Hydrogen Sulfide, *Reference Congener in Section III.*
Ref.: Greenberg and Lester, 1954; Loeser and Konwiser, 1929.

120   Sulfur

e.g., Precipitated sulfur, Sublimed sulfur, Washed sulfur

Toxicity Rating: 3(?). Low toxicity but may cause irritation to skin, eye, and respiratory tract. Large doses (15 gm.) by mouth may lead to hydrogen sulfide production in vivo, chiefly due to bacterial action within the colon. Small particles are more toxic than large ones. A man has survived the ingestion of 60 gm. of sulfur over a period of 24 hours.

See also: Hydrogen Sulfide, *Reference Congener in Section III.*
Ref.: Council on Pharmacy and Chemistry, 1955.

121   Thioacetamide

Toxicity Rating: 4. Relatively stable compound in neutral aqueous solutions, but on heating with acid it yields hydrogen sulfide. On heating with base, sodium sulfide is generated. Used widely as a substitute for hydrogen sulfide in heavy metal analyses. Its metabolic fate in animals has not been clarified, but the symptoms of acute poisoning do not resemble the fulminating asphyxial death produced by hydrogen sulfide. Rats receiving 100 mg./kg. by mouth showed no overt signs of toxicity, but 200 mg./kg. were invariably fatal. Death was secondary to massive hepatic necrosis involving parenchymal cells around all tributaries of the hepatic veins including the largest ones. Thus, the distribution of liver lesions resembled that produced by Bromobenzene and by Tannic acid. Decreased hepatic protein synthesis was noted early in the course of the intoxication. Massive doses (up to 2000 mg./kg.) given intraperitoneally to mice failed to produce any deaths before 9 hours, although all expired before 24 hours. These animals exhibited ataxia, loss of righting reflex, coma and death in respiratory failure. Although massive doses by mouth may react with stomach acids to release hydrogen sulfide, this phenomenon has not been established.

See also: Carbon Tetrachloride, *Reference Congener in Section III.*
Ref.: Ambrose et al., 1949; Barker et al., 1963; Fiume, 1963; Smith and Gosselin, 1963.

Inorganic trivalent nitrogen compounds (exclusive of above)

122 Hydroxylamine (and Salts)   122

Toxicity Rating: 4. Its salts are used as reducing agents in photography. The oral lethal dose for mice is about twice that for sodium nitrite, but hydroxylamine is more toxic than nitrite when given parenterally. About equipotent to nitrite as a methemoglobin former, but it has a greater tendency to produce sulfhemoglobin, Heinz bodies and other irreversible red cell damage. Methylene blue attenuates the methemoglobinemia and protects animals against death, although these effects are not so dramatic as in the case of nitrite. Arginine also protects animals against death by hydroxylamine even though the methemoglobinemic response is unchanged. Hydroxylamine elevates brain GABA levels in rats. It appears unlikely that hydroxylamine is converted to nitrite in vivo. Perhaps a more potent vasodilator than nitrite. Systemic poisoning characterized by cyanosis, convulsions, hypotension and coma. Only a slight irritant to human skin in dilute solutions.

See also: Nitrite, *Reference Congener in Section III.*
Ref.: Griffith, 1968; Riemann, 1950; Roukema et al., 1965; Smith and Layne, 1969.

123 Nitrogen Trichloride   123

Agene

Prepared by combining chlorine, ammonium chloride and water. The agene (1% NCl$_3$ in air saturated with water vapor) is aerated off and mixed intimately with flour where it acts as a bleach and "improver". This process is no longer employed in the United States because it results in the production of methionine sulfoximine, the agent responsible for canine hysteria (consult index for Methionine Sulfoximine). Agene is extremely unstable, but may be presumed to exhibit a high potential for corrosive oxidation of mucous membranes such as eyes and lungs.

See also: Nitrogen Oxides, *Reference Congener in Section III.*
Ref.: Mellanby, 1946.

124 Nitrogen Trifluoride   124

Nitrogen fluoride

Colorless gas which is insoluble in water and comparatively inert in chemical terms. Slight odor but poor warning properties in general. Moderately toxic by inhalation in single exposures. Death occurred in rats within a 4-hour exposure to 2500 ppm. Whereas 1000 ppm for 4 hours regularly produced methemoglobinemia, a 10-minute exposure to 3000 ppm failed to generate measureable amounts of methemoglobin. In lethal exposures 80 per cent of the total blood pigment may be found as methemoglobin. In non-lethal exposures the methemoglobinemia clears spontaneously over several hours. In contrast, the consequences of an intense Heinz body hemolytic reaction, i.e., decreases in hematocrit, hemoglobin, and red cell counts, may be manifested for 20 to 30 days. Nitrogen trifluoride does not seem to share the vasodilator effects of nitrite.

See also: Nitrite, *Reference Congener in Section III.*
Ref.: Dost et al., 1968; MacEwen, 1969; Torkelson et al., 1962.

Systemically toxic inorganic carbon compounds (exclusive of cyanide)

125 Carbon Disulfide   125

Carbon bisulfide

Toxicity Rating: 3. Probably this compound lies near the borderline between toxicity classes 3 and 4 in humans, but as little as 5 ml. accidentally ingested produced a severe illness in an adult woman.

See also: Carbon Disulfide, *Reference Congener in Section III.*

126 Carbon Monoxide   126

See also: Carbon Monoxide, *Reference Congener in Section III.*

127   127   Carbonyl Sulfide

Carbon oxysulfide

Formula: COS. Toxic gas encountered during petroleum refining or destructive distillation of coal. Said to be hydrolyzed by water to carbon dioxide and hydrogen sulfide. Toxic symptoms and death are ascribed to the latter. COS is said to have less prominent local irritating and olfactory warning properties than hydrogen sulfide. Two workmen have been poisoned under circumstances suggesting COS as the causative agent. The survivor (without sequelae) showed extremely labile periods of unconsciousness during exposure. The toxicity by inhalation in animals is somewhat less than that for hydrogen sulfide, but still appreciable. Concentrations of 0.1 vol. % and higher produce death in 2 hours or less. At high concentrations rapid exitus occurs in acute respiratory failure. COS is converted to hydrogen sulfide and bicarbonate by carbonic anhydrase. Pretreatment of animals with acetazolamide to inhibit carbonic anhydrase or sodium nitrite to generate methemoglobin protected them against death.

See also: Hydrogen Sulfide, *Reference Congener in Section III.*
Ref.: Chengelis and Neal, 1979; Chengelis and Neal, 1980; Thiess et al., 1968.

128   128   Gas

Carbon monoxide (CO) is the principal toxic ingredient. Exhaust or flue gases may also contain corrosive oxides of nitrogen and sulfur. Manufactured gas consists chiefly of volatile hydrocarbons of low toxicity (e.g. methane) and of hydrogen; the carbon monoxide (CO) content usually lies between 2 and 15%/v. Natural gas contains no CO (unless produced by "cracking" or some related process).

See also: Carbon Monoxide, *Reference Congener in Section III.*

Inorganic compounds of boron and phosphorus

129   129   Boric Acid

Boracic acid, Orthoboric acid

Toxicity Rating: 3-4. Oral mean lethal doses in rats and mice are reported in various studies to range from 2 and 5 gm./kg. The sodium salt appears to be slightly less toxic in animals. The clinical literature suggests that man may be more sensitive than laboratory rodents, with estimated lethal doses of less than 1 gm./kg. No major toxicological distinctions between boric acid and its salts are recognized in man.

See also: Borate, *Reference Congener in Section III.*

130   130   Boron Trioxide

Boron sesquioxide

Toxicity Rating: 4. B_2O_3, the anhydride of boric acid. Slowly reacts with water to form boric acid. Like the latter it presumably lies near the borderline between toxicity classes 3 and 4.

See also: Borate, *Reference Congener in Section III.*
Ref.: Merck and Co., 1976.

131   131   Borate

Toxicity Rating: 3. Most of the water-insoluble borates are complex or mixed salts, many of which are soluble in the dilute acid of gastric juice. Once a tetra-, di-, meta-, ortho-, or pyroborate salt dissolves in a buffered aqueous solution, one borate cannot be distinguished, on chemical or toxicological grounds, from any one of the others. In contrast perborates do not decompose immediately. Hypoborates are reducing reagents and may release hydrogen gas when they decompose. Most of these salts probably lie near the borderline between toxicity classes 3 and 4. See also Borax below.

See also: Borate, *Reference Congener in Section III.*

132   132   Borax

Sodium tetraborate, Sodium biborate, Sodium tetraborate decahydrate, Disodium tetraborate decahydrate, Sodium pyroborate

Toxicity Rating: 3. Like most sodium or potassium borates, solutions of borax are alkaline. Toxicity in animals is essentially the same as that of boric acid, best described as lying near the borderline between toxicity classes 3 and 4. There is an impression that borax and other alkali borate salts may be less toxic in man than boric acid.

See also: Borate, *Reference Congener in Section III.*
Ref.: Merck and Co., 1976.

133   Sodium Perborate   133

Toxicity Rating: 4. Can be represented by either of 2 formulas: $NaBO_3 \cdot 4H_2O$, $NaBO_2 \cdot 3H_2O \cdot H_2O_2$. Decomposes to hydrogen peroxide and sodium borate (or metaborate). Strongly alkaline and irritating. Repeated oral use as a mouthwash may cause hypertrophy of filiform papillae of tongue. Systemic effects are like those of boric acid. The ingestion of tablets and powders marketed as denture cleansers and containing both $KHSO_5$ and sodium perborate has caused corrosive injuries of the mouth and esophagus.

See also: Borate, Reference Congener in Section III.
Ref.: Abramson et al., 1974; Abramson, 1978; Merck and Co., 1976.

134   Boroglycerin   134

Glyceryl borate, Glyceroboric acid

Toxicity Rating: 3. Boric acid forms a complex with glycerin known as boroglycerin or glyceroboric acid, which is a stronger acid than boric acid alone. When 2 parts boric acid and 3 parts glycerin are mixed, heated and then diluted with more glycerin, the resulting yellow syrupy liquid is known as boroglycerin glycerite. It is 50% boroglycerin and thus a very concentrated solution of boron. Its ingestion has caused borate poisoning.

See also: Borate, Reference Congener in Section III.
Ref.: Osol and Farrar, 1955.

135   Phosphorus   135

White phosphorus, Yellow phosphorus, Red phosphorus, Black phosphorus

Toxicity Rating: 6. The toxicity rating applies only to white (also called yellow) phosphorus. Red and black phosphorus are allotropic forms that are practically insoluble in water and stable except at high temperatures. Unless contaminated with yellow phosphorus, they are judged to be essentially harmless in single-dose exposures, but chronic ingestion of red phosphorus may induce systemic phosphorus poisoning.

See also: Phosphorus, Reference Congener in Section III.

136   Phosphine   136

Toxicity Rating: 6. Phosphine, PH_3, is a highly toxic gas analogous in its chemistry to arsine, but it does not lyse erythrocytes or generate methemoglobin or methemalbumin. Slightly soluble in water and differs from NH_3 in that solutions are neutral. About 1.2 times more dense than air. The 4-hour LC_{50} value for rats was 0.44 μmol./l., whereas for phenylphosphine and triphenylphosphine it was 1.6 and 48 μmol./l. respectively; the three dose-mortality curves were parallel. The only signs noted during exposure were ascribed to mild respiratory irritation; there was no obvious histopathology post-mortem. In the experience of others, however, dyspnea, weakness, tremor, convulsions and death with pulmonary edema and hyperemia of many organs including kidney and brain occur in poisoned animals. One fatally-poisoned human experienced nausea, vomiting, diarrhea, great thirst, sensation of pressure in the chest, back pains, dyspnea, chills, stupor and fainting with marked pulmonary edema. Some of the above signs are reminiscent of acute phosphorus poisoning except that the distressing local injury of the latter is absent. Chronic phosphine poisoning is said to resemble chronic phosphorus poisoning. Very similar intoxication syndromes are produced by Aluminum Phosphide and Zinc Phosphide (below).

See also: Phosphorus and Nitrogen Oxides, Reference Congeners in Section III.
Ref.: Harger and Spolyar, 1958; Klimmer, 1969; Wartiz and Brown, 1975; Webster, 1946.

137   Aluminum Phosphide   137

Phostoxin

Toxicity Rating: 6. Although not approved at present for such use in the U.S.A., paper sachets or tablets of aluminum phosphide (3.0 gm. and 70% in combination with 30% ammonium carbonate) have been used for shipboard grain fumigation. In contact with moisture on the grain, Phosphine (above) is generated along with aluminum hydroxide in the sealed hold. At the end of the voyage, the hold is opened and the gas dissipates to the atmosphere. In two separate incidents, four small children on board ship were exposed to fumigated grain and three died. In two of the fatalities, which occurred within 18 hours of exposure, no cause of death was apparent on autopsy. In the third fatality, however, focal myocardial infiltration with necrosis, pulmonary edema and widespread small vessel injury were found. The surviving child had headache, fatigue, nausea, vomiting, cough, shortness of breath, jaundice, paresthesias, ataxia, intention tremor, diplopia, ECG and echocardiographic evidence of myocardial injury. In a bizarre incident in which aluminum phosphide was ingested in coffee, signs of respiratory, cardiac, hepatic and renal involvement occurred. The patient eventually recovered after dialysis for uremia. This clinical picture is like that for phosphine and Zinc Phosphide (below); it also resembles that of yellow phosphorus except for the distressing local injury from elemental phosphorus.

See also: Phosphorus *and* Nitrogen Oxides, *Reference Congeners in Section III.*
Ref.: Heyndrickx et al., 1976; Wilson et al., 1980; Zipe et al., 1967.

138   138   Zinc Phosphide

e.g., Z.P. Tracking Powder

Toxicity Rating: 5. Commercial material is 90 to 95% pure Zn_3P_2. Disagreeable odor. Employed as a rodenticide, particularly for Warfarin-resistant rats. Oral doses of 100 mg./kg. were lethal for dogs starved for 24 hours but not for fed ones. Human poisonings are virtually unknown in this country, but at least 25 deaths have been reported in the European literature. The ingestion of 4 to 5 gm. has produced death in human adults on at least two occasions, but doses of 25 and 50 gm. have been survived by two victims. The earliest symptoms include nausea with vomiting, abdominal pain, tightness in the chest, excitement, agitation and chills. Sometimes rapid exitus occurs with pulmonary edema. Induced emesis may produce more effective removal of the powder than gastric lavage. Early dyspnea, shock, oliguria, metabolic acidosis, hypocalcemic tetany, convulsions and coma are grave prognostic signs. In fatal cases death usually occurs after about 30 hours from peripheral vascular collapse secondary to direct toxic actions of the agent on the myocardium. In one fatality, internal hemorrhage was observed at post-mortem with focal degeneration and diffuse polymorphonuclear infiltration of the heart muscle, and hyperemia and congestion of all internal organs including the brain. Survivors are jaundiced due to extensive liver damage. Although late acute renal and hepatic failure have both caused death, most patients are considered out of danger after 3 days. Purpura preceded a fatal outcome in one child, but an asymptomatic thrombocytopenia is more common. The biochemical reactions responsible for toxic symptoms are not fully understood. Perhaps the initial reaction is due to phosphine (PH_3) released from zinc phosphide by the action of gastric acid (see also Phosphine above). Early lavage with 3 to 5% sodium bicarbonate has been suggested to minimize the conversion. Its efficacy is not well established nor are similar recommendations for 1% copper sulfate, 0.1% potassium permanganate or mineral oil. Zinc phosphide is not absorbed through intact skin but can enter blood stream through cuts. Human inhalation of the dust led to dyspnea and diarrhea, presumably resulting from the release of phosphine in the lungs. Recovery was complete. The compound does not produce irritation to eyes or skin of rabbits. Indirect poisoning due to phosphine generated extra-corporeally from acidic or neutral solutions of zinc phosphide has not occurred in recent times, but is believed to constitute a very real hazard. Some experimental evidence suggests that toxicity may be due to phosphide, but the clinical picture closely matches descriptions of human poisonings by yellow elemental phosphorus. Supplied as a tracking powder containing 10% active ingredient and in paste form.

See also: Phosphorus, *Reference Congener in Section III.*
Ref.: Curry et al., 1959; Marsh, 1979; Stephenson, 1967; Stowe et al., 1978; von Oettingen, 1947.

139   139   Phosphates

e.g., Dibasic sodium phosphate, Monobasic sodium phosphate

Toxicity Rating: 3(?). Dibasic sodium salt is sometimes used in medicine as a saline cathartic in an adult dose of 4 gm. Aqueous solutions have a pH of 9 to 10. Monobasic salt (variously called sodium acid and sodium dihydrogen phosphate) has been used to acidify the urine in doses of 0.6 gm. The pH of its aqueous solutions is 4 to 5. The pK_a of the second hydrogen is 6.8. Doses of 250 gm./kg. by mouth of the monobasic salt produced diarrhea in rats, guinea pigs and rabbits, and the intramuscular LD_{50} in rats was 250 mg./kg. The toxicity of parenteral phosphates is due to their sequestration of calcium and subsequent reduction in levels of ionized calcium. Since phosphates are slowly and incompletely absorbed, systemic reactions are unlikely when these salts are given by mouth, but they have been described. A 2.5-year old girl received 2 enemas consisting of sodium dihydrogen phosphate (3.7 gm. P each) in 67.5 ml. of water (each). She developed marked hyperphosphatemia, hypernatremia, hypocalcemia and acidosis. Symptoms, consisting of vomiting, lethargy, hyperpyrexia, diarrhea, carpal spasm and coma, began after 90 minutes and were eventually relieved by the administration of calcium gluconate. Phosphate poisoning has also resulted from the overzealous use of Fleet phosphate edema solution to lavage the stomach in iron poisoning. Trisodium Phosphate (see index) is a caustic. The "phosphates" of common household detergents are usually condensed phosphates (polyphosphates); see Tripolyphosphate below.

Ref.: Boyd and Seymour, 1946; Sotos et al., 1977.

140 Tetrasodium Pyrophosphate 140

Sodium pyrophosphate

Toxicity Rating: 3(?). Alkaline and irritating. Nausea, vomiting, and diarrhea are probable after ingestion. Presumably pyrophosphate is largely hydrolyzed to orthophosphate before absorption.

Some animal data suggest that pyrophosphate is considerably (and unaccountably) more toxic than implied by a toxicity rating of 3.

Ref.: Gosselin and Megirian, 1955; Gosselin et al., 1953; Jones, 1940.

141 Complex Phosphates 141

Complex polyphosphates, Polyphosphates, Sodium polyphosphate

Complex phosphates (also called complex polyphosphates or just polyphosphates) are the salts of polymerized phosphoric acid. See also Tripolyphosphate and Sodium Hexametaphosphate below. Usually employed as the sodium salt. Irritating because of its alkalinity and hypertoxicity. If ingested in large amounts nausea, vomiting and diarrhea are probable. Thought to be hydrolyzed to (ortho) phosphates before absorption, which may induce a metabolic acidosis. If appreciable amounts of the intact polymer are absorbed from the alimentary tract, hypocalcemic tetany may be a danger due to the binding (chelation) of ionized calcium. Hypocalcemic tetany apparently occurred in a single case of water softener poisoning.

Ref.: Cann and Verhulst, 1958a; Gosselin and Megirian, 1955; Gosselin et al., 1953.

142 Tripolyphosphate 142

Sodium tripolyphosphate

Toxicity Rating: 3(?). Usually employed as the sodium salt. Irritating because of its alkalinity and hypertonicity. A 1 percent aqueous solution has a pH of 9.8, and the pH of concentrated solutions (slurries) is about 10.5, so that there is no significant danger of corrosive injuries to eyes or esophagus as in lye poisoning involving solutions with pH's above 11 or even 12. If ingested in large amounts nausea, vomiting and diarrhea are probable. Thought to be hydrolyzed to (ortho)phosphates before absorption. If appreciable amounts of the intact polymer are absorbed from the alimentary tract, hypocalcemic tetany may be a danger due to the binding (chelation) of ionized calcium. Hypocalcemic tetany apparently occurred in one ingestion episode.

Ref.: Cann and Verhulst, 1958a; Gosselin et al., 1953; Gosselin and Megirian, 1955.

143 Sodium Hexametaphosphate 143

e.g., Calgon

Toxicity Rating: 2(?). Most preparations are neutral or only mildly alkaline. If ingested in large amounts, nausea, vomiting, and diarrhea are probable. Because this salt appears to be hydrolyzed within the bowel to phosphoric acid, a systemic acidosis may result.

Ref.: Gosselin et al., 1953; Gosselin and Megirian, 1955; Jones, 1940.

Inorganic anions of high to moderate toxicity (exclusive of above)

144 Nitrite 144

e.g., Sodium nitrite, Potassium nitrite

Toxicity Rating: 5. Toxicity rating of 4 describes animal studies, but clinical data suggest that man is more sensitive.

See also: Nitrite, *Reference Congener in Section III.*

145 Cyanate Salts 145

Sodium cyanate, Potassium cyanate, Ammonium cyanate

Toxicity Rating: 3. Non-selective herbicide. Soluble cyanate salts form the OCN⁻ ion in solution. Not converted to cyanide in toxicologically significant amounts. Indeed, 72% of an injected dose in mice was recovered as evolved CO_2 over 24 hours. Moderately low order of acute toxicity. Toxic syndrome has features in common with that elicited by Thiocyanate Salts (see below). Human volunteers took single parenteral doses up to 400 mg. sodium cyanate and experienced drowsiness followed by a short deep sleep. Miosis and mild diuresis were other signs. Mice given lethal doses exhibited tremor, hyper-reactivity, extensor rigidity and tonic-clonic convulsions. These convulsions are apparently not due to serum calcium abnormalities (Haut et al., 1975). Death appeared to be due to respiratory arrest during the tonic phase. Phenobarbital significantly protected mice against death. Survivors recovered without sequelae. Cyanate is significantly less toxic when taken with food, presumably because absorption is reduced (Cerami et al., 1973). Has been suggested as a method of managing patients with sickle cell disease, using dose levels up to 2 grams per day (33 mg./kg.). Efficacy in treatment of sickle cell anemia is due to specific carbamylation of N-terminal valine of hemoglobin, with a concomitant increase in red-cell oxygen affinity (Cerami and Manning, 1971; Kilmartin and Fogg, 1973). Therapeutic response without side-effects occurs in some patients with carbamylation levels of 0.3 to 0.6 per hemoglobin tetramer. At higher carbamylation levels, or during prolonged therapy, carbamylation of other proteins may lead to specific adverse reactions. In humans, these are weight loss, reversible cataracts, and peripheral neuropathies. The latter have been described after prolonged administration of daily doses greater than 35 mg./kg. and include hypore-

flexia, muscular weakness and nerve conduction abnormalities (Peterson et al., 1974). Fascicular biopsy indicates that the neural lesion is a result of segmental demyelination with neuronal degeneration of the distal axons. Improvement was noted after cessation of cyanate administration. Rats given daily oral doses of sodium cyanate of 200 mg./kg. for 10 days showed marked anorexia and lethargy and neuromuscular paralysis of the hind legs; they were hypoglycemic and had elevated SGOT levels. At autopsy, their livers had abnormally large glycogen deposits and significantly low glucose-6-phosphatase activity. Perinuclear vacuolization and increased mitotic activity were evident (Haut et al., 1975). Guinea pigs given daily oral doses of 200 mg./kg. became lethargic and paralyzed and died within three days. At autopsy, their livers showed patchy necrosis with infiltration of inflammatory cells and mild increase in hepatic glycogen. In mice, continuous feeding of a diet containing 1% sodium cyanate suppressed estrus. Estrus resumed and reproduction occurred after the animals were returned to a normal diet (Graziano et al., 1973).

Ref.: Balcerzak et al., 1976; Birch and Schutz, 1946; Cerami et al., 1973; Cerami and Manning, 1971; Graziano et al., 1973; Haut et al., 1975; Kilmartin and Fogg, 1973; Peterson et al., 1974; Schutz, 1949; Smith, 1973a.

146   146   Thiocyanate Salts

Sulfocyanates, Rhodanates, Rhodanides

Toxicity Rating: 4. Usually sodium, potassium or ammonium salts. The probable lethal dose in man lies between 15 and 30 gm. (when ingested at one time). Several acute fatalities have been reported, with death in 10 to 48 hours. Large overdoses induce vomiting, extreme cerebral excitement, delirium, convulsions, and spasticity of the extensor muscles (leading to opisthotonus in poisoned animals). The temperature, respirations, heart rate, and blood pressure are not directly affected. Anuria or persistent albuminuria in non-fatal cases (dogs

and cats). Other effects (which are generally restricted to subacute or chronic poisonings) may mimic iodism or bromide intoxication: coryza, skin rashes, weakness, fatigue, vertigo, nausea, vomiting, diarrhea, confusion, disorientation, aphasias, etc. The thiocyanate ion is slowly excreted in the urine; it is not decomposed to cyanide in appreciable quantities. Hemodialysis is recommended as the treatment of choice. Phenobarbital protects poisoned animals against death.

Ref.: Anderson and Chen, 1940; Danzig, 1955; Garvin, 1939; Gorman et al., 1949; Wald et al., 1939; David and Miketukova, 1967; Frohman and Klocke, 1963; Christensen and Williams, 1962; Smith, 1973a.

147   147   Sodium Thiocyanate

Sodium rhodanate, Sodium rhodanide, Sodium sulfocyanate

Toxicity Rating: 4. The probable lethal dose in man lies between 15 and 30 gm. (when ingested at one time). Several acute fatalities have been reported, with death in 10 to 48 hours. Large overdoses induce vomiting, extreme cerebral excitement, delirium, convulsions, and spasticity of the extensor muscles (leading to opisthotonus in poisoned animals). Temperature, respiration, heart rate, and blood pressure are not directly affected. Anuria or persistent albuminuria in nonfatal cases

(dogs and cats). Other toxic effects (which are generally restricted to subacute or chronic poisonings) may mimic iodism or bromide intoxication: coryza, skin rashes, weakness, fatigue, vertigo, nausea, vomiting, diarrhea, confusion, disorientation, aphasias, etc. The thiocyanate ion is slowly excreted in the urine; it is not decomposed to cyanide. Hemodialysis is recommended as the treatment of choice. See Thiocyanate salts above.

148   148   Potassium Thiocyanate

Potassium sulfocyanate, Potassium rhodanate

Toxicity Rating: 4. Theoretically more toxic than sodium thiocyanate because of possible potassium intoxication, but the major toxic effects after inges-

tion are probably due to the thiocyanate ion. See Thiocyanate salts above.

149 Sulfite Salts 149

i.e., Sodium, potassium, ammonium

Toxicity Rating: 3. Used as a preservative in food (including dehydrated fruits, vegetables and soups, as well as fruit juices, beer and wine), a skin lotion for ringworm, and a mouthwash. When ingested, solutions cause gastric irritation by the liberation of sulfurous acid. Because of rapid oxidation to sulfate by sulfite oxidase, at least in rats, sulfites are well tolerated until large doses are reached; then violent colic and diarrhea, circulatory disturbances, central nervous depression, and death are described. Treatment is symptomatic and supportive. Little information is available about the health significance of low-level chronic sulfite exposure (including endogenous production), but sulfite and bisulfite react irreversibly through free radical formation and otherwise with various endogenous substances including DNA. Some asthmatics are said to be dangerously sensitive to minute amounts of sulfites in foods.

Ref.: Fitzhugh et al., 1946; Gunnison, 1981; Lockett and Natoff, 1960.

150 Sodium Bisulfite 150

Sodium acid sulfite

$NaHSO_3$ is sometimes used as a disinfectant, bleach and antioxidant. Aqueous solutions are acidic, have an odor of sulfur dioxide and a disagreeable taste. Concentrated solutions are said to be irritating to the skin and mucous membranes. Intraperitoneal LD_{50}'s range from 244 mg./kg. in the dog to 675 mg./kg. in the mouse. Intravenous LD_{50}'s (65 mg./kg. in the rabbit to 130 mg./kg. in the mouse) also indicate that small animals are less susceptible than large ones. Given parenterally at the same dose, concentrated solutions are more toxic than dilute ones. Rabbits tolerated the intravenous administration of 0.67 LD_{50}'s every 8 hours, 5 days a week for 3 weeks. Eighty to 90 per cent of an intraperitoneal dose in rats can be accounted for as urinary sulfate in 4 hours. In fatal poisonings death occurs in 30-45 minutes; it is preceded by irritability, restlessness, clonic convulsions, variable periods of apnea and cyanosis, and terminal respiratory and cardiovascular collapse. See also Sulfite Salts above.

Ref.: Gunnison, 1981; Wilkins et al., 1968.

151 Sodium Hydrosulfite 151

Sodium dithionite, Sodium sulfoxylate

Toxicity Rating: 3(?). The name sodium hydrosulfite applies to molecular formula $Na_2S_2O_4$ and its dihydrate $Na_2S_2O_4 \cdot 2H_2O$. The compound that is used in commerce as a reducing agent, usually in dyeing and bleaching operations, contains 85-90% $Na_2S_2O_4$; it is a white or grayish crystalline powder which easily oxidizes in air, especially in the presence of moisture, to acidic sodium bisulfite or bisulfate. The pale yellow dihydrated salt is even less stable. Sodium hydrosulfite is a flammable solid and during a fire generates fumes of sulfurous acid (see in index). Confusion arises when the name "sodium hyposulfite" is sometimes used for this compound and when the name "sodium hydrosulfite" is sometimes used for $NaHSO_2$ (see also Sodium Hyposulfite in the index). Sodium hydrosulfite is a skin irritant and presumably shares the toxic potentials of bisulfite and sulfite to which it is rapidly oxidized. See also Sodium Bisulfite and Sulfite Salts above.

Neutral inorganic salts of alkali metals and of ammonia (exclusive of above)

152 Ammonium Salts 152

e.g., Ammonium chloride

If not specifically listed here, consult the index under the name of the anion, which in most cases will be responsible for any observed toxic signs or symptoms aside from diarrhea. However, with large doses of ammonium chloride, nitrate, acetate, bicarbonate, citrate, lactate, mandelate, phosphate, sulfate, etc., there arises the possibility of sufficient absorption to produce a diuresis and systemic ammonia poisoning, particularly if the material is administered parenterally.

See also: Ammonia, *Reference Congener in Section III.*

153 Ammonium Sulfamate 153

Ammate, Ammonium amidosulfate, AMS

Toxicity Rating: 3. Recommended for flameproofing fabrics and wood; also used as a weed-killer. Oral doses as high as 1.6 gm./kg. were not fatal in rats. Not irritating on subcutaneous injection in rats, on rabbit conjunctiva or on cutaneous application to humans. Circulation and respiration were not greatly influenced after i.v. injection of 100 mg./kg. in rats.

Ref.: Ambrose, 1943.

154

154   Lithium

Lithium chloride, Lithium carbonate

Toxicity Rating: 3(?). Lithium salts are toxic on chronic administration particularly with restricted salt (sodium chloride) diets. Signs and symptoms of lithium toxicity resemble those of sodium deficiency but may occur without hyponatremia; they include drowsiness, weakness, anorexia, nausea, tremors, blurring of vision, coma and death. A gastroenteritis is described in animals and man. Acute poisoning in man is reported after 4 doses of 2 gm. each of lithium chloride, causing weakness, prostration, vertigo, tinnitus.

See also: Lithium, Reference Congener in Section III.

155

155   Potassium Salts

i.e., Nitrate (saltpeter), chloride, phosphate (mono- and di-basic)

Toxicity Rating: 3. Acute potassium intoxication by mouth is rare because large single doses usually induce vomiting and because in the absence of pre-existing kidney damage potassium is rapidly excreted. Potassium chloride in a commercial dietary salt substitute, however, has produced a near-fatal poisoning in an 8-month-old infant. An 84-year-old woman with a history of many episodes of congestive failure was in an apparently controlled cardiac status when she committed suicide by ingesting her liquid potassium supplement. The estimated dose of 540 to 720 mEq of potassium (equivalent to about 40 to 50 gm. as potassium chloride) provoked neither vomiting nor diarrhea. A grand mal convulsion occurred after one hour followed by a coma in which the blood pressure was unobtainable. Intravenous metaraminol and calcium gluconate appeared to be without effect on the ECG. Terminal ventricular fibrillation was noted; death occurred 90 minutes after ingestion. This amount of potassium in divided doses over 24 hours has been taken without toxic signs. A single dose of 186 mEq by mouth as the citrate produced paresthesias of the hands and feet (regarded by some as an important and characteristic sign of intoxication by potassium) and cramps in an adult who had been on a low potassium diet for the preceding three weeks. When returned to a normal diet, however, the same dose produced no toxic effects nor did twice this dose of sodium citrate. Single doses of 170 to 175 mEq may produce a serum potassium as high as 8.8 mEq/l. Potassium poisoning disturbs the rhythm of the heart (a slow, weak pulse, heightened T waves of ECG, arrhythmias, heart block) and eventually weakens cardiac contractility (fall in blood pressure). ECG disorders may respond to sodium lactate treatment as in quinidine poisoning. Respirations are initially accelerated but skeletal muscle weakness may advance to the stage of paralysis. Orally poisoned animals died from respiratory failure sometimes following convulsions and accompanied gastroenteritis, dehydration of organs and early renal tubular necrosis. Survivors had anorexia, polydipsia, polyuria, fever, convulsive movements and gastrointestinal disturbances during the first 24 hours, but rapidly recovered thereafter. The potassium content of enteric coated mixtures of chlorothiazide-type diuretics and KCl has been associated with ulcerative lesions of the small intestine. This infrequent reaction presents with symptoms of small bowel obstructions. Occasionally perforation has occurred. The mechanism of the production of this lesion is not understood, but it is presumably associated with a sudden release of high local concentrations of potassium. If it can be instituted rapidly, extracorporeal hemodialysis may be of value in acute potassium poisoning. It is not clear whether exchange resins have sufficient capacity to be useful in acute poisoning.

See also: Quinidine, Reference Congener in Section III.
Ref.: Allen et al., 1965; Ashby et al., 1965; Bedford and Leeds, 1954; Berlyne et al., 1966; Boley et al., 1965; Boyd and Shanas, 1961; Kallen et al., 1976; Kaplan, 1969; Kieth et al., 1942; Lawrason et al., 1965; McQuarrie et al., 1936; Talbott and Schwab, 1940.

156

156   Potassium Bicarbonate

Potassium acid carbonate

Toxicity Rating: 3. Sometimes used as gastric antacid, urinary alkalizer or diuretic. No reports of human poisonings were found, and it is not clear whether the major acute hazard relates to the potassium content (see also Potassium Salts above) or the bicarbonate content (see also Sodium Bicarbonate below.)

157

157   Nitrate Salts

e.g., Sodium nitrate, Potassium nitrate, Saltpeter, Niter

Toxicity Rating: 3. Nitrate salts as such are no more toxic than other neutral salts, but if not promptly absorbed, they may be reduced to nitrites by bacteria in the bowel. Cyanosis among infants who drink well water is a frequently encountered clinical manifestation of nitrate toxicity. After an acute massive dose of saltpeter, the potassium is probably more dangerous than the nitrate; see also Potassium Salts in the index.

See also: Nitrite, Reference Congener in Section III.
Ref.: Bucklin and Myint, 1960; Goluboff and Wheaton, 1961.

158   Subnitrate Salts 158

If soluble in water or acid, the anion is present in solution as the nitrate. See Nitrate salts above.

Consult the index under the name of cation or metal.

159   Sulfate Salts 159

Soluble sulfate salts of sodium, magnesium, potassium, lithium, etc., are rather slowly absorbed from the alimentary tract. Because of their osmotic activity, they draw water into the lumen of the bowel and produce purging. The amount of sulfate anion usually absorbed has no toxicological significance, but see also Potassium salts and Lithium salts above and Magnesium salts in the index.

160   Subsulfate Salts 160

Partially hydrolyzed sulfates of metals and metalloids. If soluble in acid, the anion is present as the sulfate. Consult the index under the name of cation or metal.

161   Thiosulfate Salts 161

Hyposulfites, i.e., Sodium, potassium, calcium

Toxicity Rating: 3. Remarkably inert in vivo, except for osmotic disturbances. Poorly absorbed from the alimentary tract and so acts as an osmotic cathartic. In the treatment of cyanide poisoning, 12.5 gm. of highly purified sodium thiosulfate has been injected i.v. without ill effects. Consult index under the name of the cation.

Ref.: Bhagat and Lockett, 1960; Cardozo and Edelman, 1952; Chen and Rose, 1956.

162   Potassium Thiosulfate 162

Potassium hyposulfite

Toxicity Rating: 3. Cathartic, diuretic, and probably emetic. The thiosulfate ion is remarkably inert in vivo, but potassium is less benign. See Potassium salts above.

Ref.: Bhagat and Lockett, 1960; Cardozo and Edelman, 1952; Chen and Rose, 1956.

163   Sodium Thiosulfate 163

Sodium hyposulfite, Hypo

Toxicity Rating: 3(?). Formula: $Na_2S_2O_3$ (anhydrous or with 5 mols of water). Remarkably inert in vivo, except for osmotic disturbances. Poorly absorbed from the bowel. Acts as an osmotic cathartic. In the treatment of cyanide poisoning, 12.5 gm. has been injected intravenously without ill effects. The thiosulfate ion distributes itself in extracellular fluid.

Ref.: Bhagat and Lockett, 1960; Cardozo and Edelman, 1952; Chen and Rose, 1956.

164   Sodium Bicarbonate 164

Baking soda

Toxicity Rating: 3. Acute (14-day) oral LD_{50} in rats is about 4.3 gm./kg. when given as a 20% slurry in water, but about 6.0 gm./kg. as a 50% slurry. The common dose as an antacid is 1 to 4 gm. in adult humans. The pH of saturated aqueous solutions may range from 8 to 9. Not caustic like sodium carbonate or lye. In neutralizing gastric acid, distention and possible damage or rupture of the stomach may occur from carbon dioxide release. Large doses, particularly in patients with renal insufficiency, have produced systemic alkalosis and/or an expansion in the extracellular fluid volume with edema. Frank hypocalcemic tetany accompanied by hypoglycemia occurred in a 9-year-old girl; for the management of this complication see Oxalate in Section III.

Ref.: Griffith, 1964b; Platou, 1961; Zer et al., 1970.

165   Sodium Chloride 165

Salt, Table salt, Rock salt

Toxicity Rating: 3. Serious salt poisonings in humans have occurred from accidental ingestion, deliberate ingestion in unsuccessful attempts to induce vomiting, gastric lavage with hypertonic saline and errors in formulating infant diets. The use of salt as an emetic in poisonings should be discouraged. The acute oral LD_{50} in fasted albino rats is 3.75 ± 0.43 gm./kg., and the mean time to death is 8.6 ± 5.3 hours. Hypertonic salt solutions can produce violent inflammatory reactions in the gastrointestinal tract (lysing of columnar epithelial lining); the contact effect is diluted caudalward. Symptoms include vomiting, diarrhea, muscular twitching and rigidity, convulsions, prostration and death. Dehydration and congestion occur in most internal organs, particularly meninges and brain. Death may occur from respiratory failure secondary to an acute encephalopathy. Human infants also show vomiting, thirst, fever (but not in the neonate) and respiratory distress in the form of tachypnea and flaring nostrils. A distinctive microscopic lesion of the kidney is described; parenchymatous dehydration produces a shrinking which is most conspicuous in the convoluted tubules of the renal cortex. Some experimental evidence suggests that similar hypernatremic syndromes may be produced with normal salt diets if water intake is restricted. Good clinical responses have been obtained from peritoneal dialysis with 5% glucose in water; in severe cases 7 or 8% glucose is suggested to prevent absorption of dialysis fluid. Dialysis volumes of 15 to 50 ml./kg. have been employed; they were withdrawn after 2 hours. Potassium need not be included in the dialysis fluid, but careful monitoring of the electrolyte status is required.

Ref.: Barer et al., 1973; Boyd and Shanas, 1963b; Calvin et al., 1964; Carter and Fotheringham, 1971; DeGenaro and Nyhan, 1971; Elton et al., 1963; Finberg et al., 1963; Ward, 1963.

Alkaline earths compounds (inorganic)

166　Barium Salts (Soluble)

i.e., Oxide, chloride, nitrate, carbonate, sulfide, acetate, bromide

Toxicity Rating: 3,4 or 5. Acute toxicity varies widely with the compound, animal species, and even strain. Toxicity rating of 5 is probably the best description of clinical experience.

See also: Barium, *Reference Congener in Section III*.
Ref.: McNally, 1925.

167　Barium Metaborate

Modified barium metaborate, e.g., Busan 11-M1

Toxicity Rating: 4. A preservative, flame retardant and anti-corrosive pigment for paints, plastics and textiles. The commercial product, modified barium metaborate, is a white powder containing particles of barium metaborate which are coated with silica to reduce solubility in water, prevent caking in storage and crystal formation in water-based paints. There have been no reports of ill-effects on the health of producers and users of the product since its introduction in 1959 despite its moderately high toxicity in rats (LD_{50} 205 mg./kg.). It is not considered to be a chronic toxicant, nor is it irritating to the skin. It does not release toxic fumes when heated. If ingested, however, its solubility in water (0.3%) is probably high enough to produce symptoms of barium poisoning.

See also: Barium, *Reference Congener in Section III*.
Ref.: Buckman et al., 1973.

168　Barium

The barium ion produces violent contractions of smooth, striated and cardiac muscle. These contractions can be painful and dangerous. They can be induced by all barium compounds except for a few which are highly insoluble. For example, barium sulfate is essentially inert when ingested (toxicity rating 1), except for occasional preparations that contain soluble impurities.

See also: Barium, *Reference Congener in Section III*.
Ref.: Kay, 1954.

169　Beryllium Salts

Mixed beryllium metasilicates were used until recently as phosphors in fluorescent lamps. Very low ingestion toxicity, but inhaled dusts may produce an acute pneumonitis or a chronic progressive pulmonary granulomatosis, usually with an insidious and delayed onset. Chronic ulcers occur if soluble beryllium dusts gain entrance into superficial cuts and abrasions. Dermatitis is seen. Some promise is held for therapy with chelating agents.

Ref.: Cash et al., 1959; Hardy, 1956; Hardy and Stoeckle, 1959; van Ordstrand et al., 1945.

170　Calcium Salts

i.e., Chloride, hydroxide, carbonate

Except for gastric irritation caused in part by osmotic disturbances, calcium per se has no significant oral toxicity. For specific salts, consult this index under the name of the anion. For the toxicity of the anhydrous sulfate, see Plaster of Paris below; for the oxide, see Lime in the index. Injected subcutaneously or intramuscularly, soluble calcium salts are intensely irritating, and in infants even calcium gluconate may produce sloughing. Injected intravenously, ionized calcium salts may cause slowing of the heart rate and sinus arrhythmia; in toxic doses heart block, extrasystoles and ventricular fibrillation are described. Injected calcium may also stimulate in vivo epinephrine release.

171   Calcium Carbonate   171

Chalk

Toxicity Rating: 1. Occurs naturally as limestone, marble, coral, etc. Is an excellent antacid and a good antidote for oxalic acid. May cause alkalosis with continued use. See also Calcium salts above.

172   Plaster of Paris   172

Calcium sulfate anhydrous or with about 5% water (1/2 mol). Anhydrous calcium sulfate occurs in nature as a mineral known as anhydrite or anhydrous gypsum. Because it hardens quickly after absorbing moisture, its ingestion may result in obstruction, particularly at the pylorus. Mixed with flour (1:2), it has been used as a rodenticide. To delay "setting," drink glycerin or gelatin solutions, or large volumes of water. Surgical relief may be necessary.

Ref.: Osol and Farrar, 1955.

173   Limestone   173

Toxicity Rating: 2(?). A stone composed largely of the mineral calcite (calcium carbonate). The name is often applied to any technical or agricultural grade of calcium carbonate. See Calcium salts above.

Ref.: Merck and Co., 1976.

174   Magnesium Salts   174

i.e., Chloride, citrate, hydroxide, oxide, phosphate, sulfate, carbonate

Toxicity Rating: 3(?). Even soluble magnesium salts are generally so slowly absorbed that oral administration causes nothing more than purging. If evacuation fails (bowel obstruction or atony), mucosal irritation and absorption occur. Systemically Mg^{2+} produces central nervous depression, abolition of reflexes, and death from respiratory paralysis. Intravenous calcium chloride (10 to 20 cc. of 5% solution, diluted if desirable with isotonic saline) may counteract these toxic actions of magnesium. Provide ventilatory assistance. See also Section IV under "Disorders of Magnesium Balance."

Ref.: Fawcett and Gens, 1943; Rubenstein et al., 1945; Stevens and Wolff, 1950.

175   Milk of Magnesia   175

Magnesium hydroxide

Toxicity Rating: 2. The official U.S.P. preparation is an aqueous suspension of 7.0 to 8.5% magnesium hydroxide. Small amounts of a volatile oil may be added for flavoring. Used as an antacid and cathartic. See Magnesium salts above.

176   Magnesium Silicate   176

Toxicity Rating: 1. Occurs in various forms in nature, differing in the mol ratio of SiO_2/MgO and in the amount of associated water of hydration. Unlike comparable varieties of sodium silicate, all forms of magnesium silicate are essentially insoluble in water. No acute toxicity is recognized. Hydrated varieties are found in some antacid preparations, usually under the name magnesium trisilicate (mol ratio 3:2). Largely unabsorbed from the gastrointestinal tract. A small fraction of an oral dose, however, may be found as silicate in the urine, where it may contribute over long periods of time to the production of urinary calculi. See also Talc in the Index.

Ref.: Emerick et al., 1963; Task Force on the Health Effects of non-NTA Detergent Builders, 1981.

177   Strontium Salts   177

i.e., Chloride, sulfate, carbonate, nitrate

Toxicity Rating: 2-3(?). Such inorganic salts of strontium as the chloride, sulfate, carbonate, etc., are remarkably benign. The bromide was listed officially in the National Formulary until 1960 as a medicinal (adult oral dose 1 gm.). Like calcium, strontium salts tend to be poorly absorbed from the intestinal tract. In large oral doses they presumably exert local osmotic effects and so tend to induce vomiting and diarrhea. The oral mean lethal dose is not known, but it exceeds 5 gm./kg. in guinea pigs. The intraperitoneal LD_{50} of several strontium salts lies between 0.5 and 1.0 gm./kg. in rats. By intravenous injection in rats strontium chloride is less lethal than the chlorides of magnesium, potassium or even calcium. Apnea rather than cardiac arrest was the terminal event in mice infused with the acetate salt. Like calcium absorbed strontium tends to accumulate in teeth and bone, especially in the epiphyseal regions of rapidly growing bone. On a chronic diet high in strontium and low in calcium (ratio 3:1), young pigs developed severe bone deformities, incoordination, weakness and hindleg paralysis. Of more public health concern is the accumulation in bone of radioactive isotopes of strontium (e.g., Sr^{90}) from "fall-out".

Ref.: Bartley and Reber, 1961; Cochran et al., 1950; Cole et al., 1941; Loeser and Konwiser, 1929.

Aluminum compounds

178   Aluminum Hydroxide

Aluminum hydrate, Hydrated alumina, Aluminum hydroxide gel

Toxicity Rating: 1. This insoluble salt is essentially harmless by oral administration. It has long been employed as a gastric antacid, and its constipating side effect is well known. Aluminum oxide and some forms of finely powdered aluminum metal react slowly with water to produce aluminum hydroxide. On occasion workers chronically exposed to aluminum-containing dusts or fumes have developed severe pulmonary reactions including fibrosis, emphysema and pneumothorax. A much rarer encephalopathy has also been described. The factors which predispose to lung damage are not well characterized. Aluminum salts are much more toxic intravenously than by mouth to animals. The mechanism of this presumably systemic effect of aluminum is not known.

Ref.: Corrin, 1963; McLaughlin et al., 1962; Merck and Co., 1976; Ondreicka et al., 1966.

179   Aluminum Dihydroxy Allantoinate

Aldioxa

Toxicity Rating: 1. The above compound and the closely related aluminum chlorhydroxy allantoinate are used as astringents, keratolytics, tissue stimulants and buffers in cosmetic preparations. Both are non-sensitizing and non-irritating. Oral doses of Aldioxa as high as 23 gm./kg. were tolerated by mice.

Ref.: Mecca, 1959.

180   Aluminum Silicate

Toxicity Rating: 1. Insoluble aluminum salt. Essentially harmless by oral administration.

Ref.: Merck and Co., 1976.

181   Alum

Aluminum ammonium sulfate, Aluminum potassium sulfate, Ammonium alum, Potassium alum

Low toxicity in experimental animals (toxicity rating of 2), but on two occasions the ingestion of 30 gm. has killed an adult human. Death is probably due to the corrosive action of the sulfuric acid formed by hydrolysis of the salt. Concentrated solutions (e.g., 20%) have produced gingival necrosis and fatal hemorrhagic gastroenteritis. Also incoordination, clonic contractions, and evidence of nephritis. The only recommended treatment is supportive. Acute oral LD_{50} of aluminum sulfate in mice is about 6.1 gm./kg., but said to have a much higher toxicity by the intravenous route.

See also: Acid, *Reference Congener in Section III*.
Ref.: Ondreicka et al., 1966; Witthaus, 1911.

182   Aluminum Chloride

Toxicity Rating: 3. Acute oral LD_{50} in mice is about 3.9 gm./kg., but said to have a much higher toxicity by intravenous route. May cause allergic reactions. Irritating to abraded skin. Corrosive if anhydrous. Ingestion presumably produces the same toxic effects as alum. See Alum above.

Ref.: Ondreicka et al., 1966; Schwartz and Tulipan, 1933.

183   Burow's Solution

Toxicity Rating: 2(?). An aqueous solution of aluminum acetate (4.8 to 5.8%). When diluted 10- to 20-fold, it is used as a wet dressing in weeping skin disorders because of its astringent and antiseptic properties. Prolonged and continuous exposure can produce severe necrosis. Probably moderately irritating if ingested.

Ref.: Hertzler, 1927.

Selenium and tellurium compounds

184   Sodium Selenate   184

Toxicity Rating: 6. Formula: $Na_2SeO_4 \cdot 10H_2O$. Used as a "systemic" insecticide, i.e., accumulates in plants which are thus rendered toxic to many pests, and also to mammals. Highly toxic by all routes (probably borderline between toxicity classes 5 and 6), but slightly less toxic than sodium selenite. A general protoplasmic poison attacking sulfhydryl enzymes. Like arsenic it causes degenerative lesions in liver, kidneys, heart, spleen, stomach, bowel, and lungs. Many signs and symptoms are possible. No human fatalities have been reported. Treat like arsenic poisoning except that BAL appears to be contraindicated. Bromobenzene (oral adult dose 1 gm.) is said to increase the urinary excretion of selenium, but it may be a dangerous form of therapy because bromobenzene is a hepatic toxin. See Bromobenzene in the index.

See also: Arsenic, *Reference Congener in Section III.*
Ref.: Lemley and Merryman, 1941; Stenn, 1936.

185   Selenium Derivatives   185

e.g., Selenium oxychloride, Selenium dioxide, Selenic acid

Closely related to but more toxic than tellurium. A general tissue poison like arsenic, presumably attacking sulfhydryl enzymes. Acute toxicity of soluble selenium compounds is high. In approximate order of decreasing toxicity: soluble selenites, selenates, insoluble inorganic salts (e.g., selenium sulfide), various organic derivatives (some volatile). The oxychloride is a severe vesicant. Metallic selenium is insoluble and not toxic unless finely divided as a fume. Also see Sodium selenate above.

See also: Arsenic, *Reference Congener in Section III.*
Ref.: Greenburg, 1949; Hall et al., 1951; Lemley and Merryman, 1941; Stenn, 1936.

186   Selenium Sulfide   186

Selenium monosulfide, Selsun sulfide

A water-insoluble mixture of various molecular species, such as Se_2S_6, Se_4S_4. Unlike many selenium salts, it is not decomposed by water or dilute acid to selenic or selenious acids. Only traces are absorbed through the skin, but ingestion is hazardous. If swallowed, avoid oils or alcohol which may promote absorption. Lavage and saline catharsis are recommended. For systemic effects, see Sodium selenate above. Local irritation and sensitization are rare, but eye injuries occur.

Ref.: Cummins and Kimura, 1971; Grover, 1956; Ransone et al., 1961.

187   Tellurium Derivatives   187

e.g., Hydrogen telluride, Sodium tellurate, Sodium tellurite, Tellurium, Tellurium dioxide

Tellurium and its various derivatives are used as pigments in glass and porcelain products and are incorporated in special alloys. In general tellurium compounds are less toxic than the corresponding selenium compounds, except that tellurites appear to be more toxic than selenites. Although tellurite is more toxic than tellurate, limited data suggest that both would fall in toxicity class 5 when given by mouth. When given parenterally, however, tellurite extends into toxicity class 6. Despite this potential, ordinary industrial exposures to oxides, metallic dusts and fumes have not been associated with a high degree of toxicity. Constant findings in chronically exposed workmen include a garlic odor to breath and sweat, dryness of the mouth, metallic taste and somnolence. Given accidentally as a solution via a ureteral catheter, doses of about 2 gm. of sodium tellurite resulted in death in two adults in about 6 hours. Toxic signs preceding death included vomiting, renal pain, stupor, loss of consciousness, irregular breathing, cyanosis. Fatty degeneration of the liver was found at autopsy. Hydrogen telluride is said to be very poisonous and to resemble hydrogen selenide. Pneumonitis and hemolysis were prominent in fatally exposed animals. BAL appears to be contraindicated since it intensifies the poisoning when given before tellurium, and ascorbate had only equivocal effects in acute poisonings in animals.

Ref.: Amdur, 1958; Cerwenka and Cooper, 1961; DeMeio, 1946; Keall et al., 1946; Steinberg et al., 1942.

Arsenic, antimony and bismuth compounds

188   Arsenic   188

Grey arsenic

Toxicity Rating: 5(?). Elemental arsenic, also known as grey arsenic or metallic arsenic, is insoluble in water and dilute acids. It is less toxic than arsenous and arsenic acids and their soluble salts.

See also: Arsenic, *Reference Congener in Section III.*

189   Arsanilic Acid

(4-Aminophenyl)arsonic acid, *p*-Aminobenzenearsonic acid, *p*-Anilinearsonic acid

Toxicity Rating: 3-4. Arsanilic acid is an organic pentavalent arsenical used in the manufacture of medicinal arsenicals and as a growth promoter in animal feed. The acid and its sodium salt, both poorly absorbed from the digestive tract, are used as anthelmintics in swine and poultry. The acute oral LD_{50} of arsanilic acid in newborn rats is 216 mg./kg., while in adults it is greater than 1000 mg./kg. Pigs fed 1000 ppm arsanilic acid for 4 to 27 days exhibited a progression of effects beginning with roughening of the coat, followed by diarrhea, and finally by posterior paresis or quadraplegia due to demyelination of peripheral nerves. Sodium arsanilate may be absorbed through intact skin. The LD_{50} in mice by that route is 400 mg./kg. See also Arsenicals below.

See also: Arsenic, *Reference Congener in Section III.*
Ref.: Ledet et al., 1973.

190   Arsenates

Toxicity Rating: 5. Salts of arsenic acid (H_3AsO_4). In animals, soluble arsenates (pentavalent) are less toxic than soluble arsenites (trivalent), but the toxic syndromes are generally indistinguishable, probably because toxicity is due in both cases to arsenic trioxide, to which pentavalent arsenic may be reduced in vivo. See also sodium arsenate below.

See also: Arsenic, *Reference Congener in Section III.*

191   Arsenic Acid

o-Arsenic acid

Toxicity Rating: 5. Formula H_3AsO_4, of which 52.8% is arsenic. The anhydride of this acid is arsenic pentoxide; it dissolves freely in water to yield arsenic acid. Usually supplied as an aqueous solution containing 75 to 80% H_3AsO_4 and used as a herbicide.

See also: Arsenic, *Reference Congener in Section III.*

192   Arsenicals

Both trivalent and pentavalent arsenic occurs in organic compounds. They vary considerably in toxicity, but the final toxic syndrome is the same in qualitative terms, presumably because they all are converted in vivo, at least to a small extent, to the same biologically active form, namely trivalent organoarsenoxide.

See also: Arsenic, *Reference Congener in Section III.*

193   Arsenic Trioxide

White arsenic, Arsenious acid anhydride, Arsenic sesquioxide, Arsenous oxide

Toxicity Rating: 6. Coarse powders or pellets of As_2O_3 are much less toxic than finely dispersed powders. The acute toxic dose of the latter is said to range from 5 to 50 mg. in a human adult. The average fatal dose by mouth probably lies between 100 and 500 mg.

See also: Arsenic, *Reference Congener in Section III.*

194   Arsenic Trisulfide

Auripigment, Orpiment

Toxicity Rating: 5. The pure sulfide is said to have a relatively low acute toxicity perhaps because of low water solubility, but it gradually decomposes to arsenic trioxide (see latter above). Still found in several Chinese herbal products which are promoted for the treatment of asthma and other diseases but which cause severe chronic arsenic poisoning.

See also: Arsenic, *Reference Congener in Section III.*
Ref.: Tay and Seah, 1975.

195   Arsenites

Toxicity Rating: 6. Salts of arsenous acid (oxide). Arsenites (trivalent) are more toxic in animals than arsenates (pentavalent), but the toxic syndromes are generally indistinguishable, probably because toxicity is due in both cases to arsenic trioxide, to which pentavalent arsenic may be reduced in vivo. See also Sodium arsenite below.

See also: Arsenic, *Reference Congener in Section III.*

196 Arsine

196

Arsenic trihydride, Hydrogen arsenide

Highly toxic gas (AsH_3) with a disagreeable garlic odor. The most regularly produced untoward effect is acute renal failure secondary to severe intravas-cular hemolysis. Systemic arsenic poisoning does not seem to occur.

See also: Arsenic, *Reference Congener in Section III.*

197 Cacodylic Acid

197

Dimethylarsinic acid, DMAA

Toxicity Rating: 3-4. Organic pentavalent arsenical which is used as a non-selective herbicide. Its sodium salt (sodium dimethylarsinate) was once used medicinally in chronic skin diseases, leukemia, etc.; it is still employed in veterinary medicine as a hematinic. Sodium cacodylate is an example of the rare situation in which the safe parenteral dose (300 mg.) is significantly larger than the safe oral dose (60 mg.) because acidic gastric juice rapidly frees inorganic arsenic, presumably as arsenic acid, which is then reduced to trivalent arsenous oxide (As_2O_3). A strong garlic odor is imparted to breath, sweat and urine. Cacodylic acid is the major arsenic metabolite in the urine of man and dog after the ingestion of trivalent or pentavalent inorganic arsenic compounds.

See also: Arsenic, *Reference Congener in Section III.*
Ref.: Goodman and Gilman, 1975.

198 Calcium Arsenate

198

Tricalcium arsenate, Cucumber dust

Toxicity Rating: 5. The commercial grade is a complex molecular mixture containing 26% arsenic. It is often colored with a small amount of pink dye.

See also: Arsenic, *Reference Congener in Section III.*
Ref.: Assoc. of Amer. Pesticide Control Officials, 1966; Spencer, 1973.

199 Calcium Arsenite

199

Toxicity Rating: 5. In commerce this material has a variable composition. Significantly more toxic in man (perhaps by a factor of 2) than the pentavalent calcium arsenate. Lies near the borderline between toxicity classes 5 and 6.

See also: Arsenic, *Reference Congener in Section III.*

200 Copper Acetoarsenite

200

Paris green, Schweinfurt green

Toxicity Rating: 5. A substance of complex composition, having an arsenic trioxide equivalent of about 59%. Used as an insecticide, a wood preservative, and a paint pigment.

See also: Arsenic, *Reference Congener in Section III.*
Ref.: Lehman, 1951.

201 Copper Arsenate

201

Toxicity Rating: 5. This is usually a basic copper arsenate, i.e., a mixed salt of cupric hydroxide and cupric arsenate. One preparation used as an agricultural insecticide has an arsenic content of 41% (as arsenic pentoxide).

See also: Arsenic, *Reference Congener in Section III.*
Ref.: Assoc. of Amer. Pesticide Control Officials, 1966.

202 Cupric Arsenite

202

Scheele's green, Scheele's mineral, Swedish green

Toxicity Rating: 5. Usually 40 to 45% arsenic trioxide equivalent. Used as an insecticide.

See also: Arsenic, *Reference Congener in Section III.*
Ref.: Merck and Co., 1976.

203   Disodium Methanearsonate

DSMA, Dimet

Toxicity Rating: 3-4. The disodium salt of metha-nearsonic acid (also known as monomethylarsinic acid). Selective herbicide used for control of crabgrass in turf and cotton. Moderately high acute oral toxicity in rats (oral LD_{50} 1 to 2.8 gm./kg.), but man is probably more susceptible. Autopsy of

rats revealed severe gastroenteritis as in inorganic arsenic poisoning. The pentahydrate contains about 28% arsenic, but the commercial material usually has a purity of only 50% (14% arsenic). Also supplied as alkylammonium salts. Treat as arsenic poisoning. BAL is antidotal.

See also: Arsenic, *Reference Congener in Section III.*

204   Fowler's Solution

Potassium arsenite solution

Toxicity Rating: 4. An aqueous solution of potas-sium arsenite equivalent to 1% arsenic trioxide.

The probable lethal dose for an adult lies between 10 and 30 ml.

See also: Arsenic, *Reference Congener in Section III.*
Ref.: Osol and Farrar, 1955.

205   4-Hydroxy-3-nitrophenylarsonic Acid

4-Hydroxy-3-nitrobenzenearsonic acid, Roxarsone

Toxicity Rating: 5. A pentavalent organic arsenical. Marketed as Roxarsone, it is used as a growth promoter in animal feed and as an antibacterial agent in poultry. It has a high acute oral toxicity (oral LD_{50} 155 mg./kg. in rats and roughly 50 mg./kg. in dogs). Autopsies of rats and dogs given acute lethal doses of Roxarsone revealed gastroenteritis

with diffuse areas of hemorrhage and kidney congestion. Rats that survived a few days before succumbing displayed progressive weakness and incoordination of the hindquarters. Most rats fed 400 ppm died within 4 days. The no-effect level for rats and chickens was found to be 200 ppm in the feed. See also Arsenicals above.

See also: Arsenic, *Reference Congener in Section III.*
Ref.: Kerr et al., 1963.

206   Lead Arsenate

Toxicity Rating: 4. Lead acid arsenate or dibasic lead arsenate is approximately $PbHAsO_4$. "Basic lead arsenate" has an indefinite composition. In a single dose, arsenic is a more powerful poison than lead. Because of its low solubility this salt may be less acutely toxic than expected. A 20-yr.-old stu-dent ingested about 300 gm. (reliable estimate) as

an aqueous slurry. He vomited within 30 min. but apparently not within the first 10 min. Within 1 to 2 hrs. his stomach was lavaged, and he received both BAL and calcium disodium edetate. Essen-tially no toxic signs or symptoms developed and no serious sequellae were detected (from files of Han-over Poison Control Center).

See also: Arsenic, *Reference Congener in Section III.*
Ref.: Fairhall and Sayers, 1940; Kilgore and Rhoads, 1942; Lehman, 1951.

207   Lead Arsenite

Toxicity Rating: 5. More toxic and corrosive than lead arsenate, but see comments under latter above.

See also: Arsenic, *Reference Congener in Section III.*
Ref.: Fairhall and Sayers, 1940; Lehman, 1951.

208   Octyl Ammonium Metharsonate

tert-Octyl ammonium methanearsonate, Octylammonium methylarsonate

Toxicity Rating: 3-4. A herbicide available com-mercially as an 8% solution. Animals receiving le-thal oral doses show hyperexcitability, rapid res-piration, occasional tremors, and sometimes con-

vulsions. Autopsies reveal irritation of the intes-tinal mucosa and renal congestion. See also Arsen-icals above.

See also: Arsenic, *Reference Congener in Section III.*
Ref.: Vineland Chemical Co., 1958.

209 Sodium Arsenate 209

Sodium meta-arsenate

Toxicity Rating: 5. Contains at least 50% arsenic. Believed to lie near the borderline between toxicity classes 5 and 6. Dibasic sodium arsenate is almost as toxic; it contains 40% arsenic when anhydrous or 24% arsenic in the case of the usual hydrate.

See also: Arsenic, *Reference Congener in Section III.*

210 Sodium Arsenite 210

Sodium meta-arsenite

Toxicity Rating: 6. Approximate formula: $NaAsO_2$. Highly toxic trivalent arsenic, having an arsenic trioxide equivalent of 76.1%.

See also: Arsenic, *Reference Congener in Section III.*

211 Zinc Arsenate 211

Toxicity Rating: 5(?). Both zinc arsenate and arsenite have been used as wood preservatives. The former is also found in various agricultural insecticidal formulations. Presumably zinc has no toxic significance in this combination, poisoning being due to the arsenic content.

See also: Arsenic, *Reference Congener in Section III.*

212 Antimony Salts 212

Toxicity Rating: 5. Although it has a slightly better prognosis, antimony poisoning closely parallels arsenic poisoning, except that vomiting from antimony may be more prominent, perhaps because its compounds are less readily absorbed than arsenicals. Temporary ECG changes are reported in humans, and severe cardiac damage has been observed in animals. Trivalent antimony compounds (e.g., tartar emetic) are many times more lethal than pentavalent derivatives. However, insoluble trivalent salts, such as antimony trioxide and antimony trisulfide (also called antimony sulfide), are relatively benign (toxicity rating 3 or less). BAL appears to be effective in treating antimony poisoning, at least when it is due to trivalent forms of the metal. Tolerance to antimony is denied.

See also: Arsenic, *Reference Congener in Section III.*
Ref.: Braun et al., 1946; Brieger et al., 1954; Fairhall and Hyslop, 1947.

213 Antimony Potassium Tartrate 213

Tartar emetic

Toxicity Rating: 5. The minimum lethal dose in man is 130 mg. (although 15,000 mg. have been survived). A strong irritant and emetic, but the emetic dose (e.g., 30 mg. by mouth) is dangerously high if vomiting fails to occur. See Antimony salts above.

See also: Arsenic, *Reference Congener in Section III.*
Ref.: Fairhall and Hyslop, 1947; Schroeder et al., 1946.

214 Antimony Trichloride 214

Butter of antimony

A particularly corrosive form of trivalent antimony. See Antimony salts above.

See also: Arsenic, *Reference Congener in Section III.*
Ref.: Fairhall and Hyslop, 1947.

215 Brown Mixture 215

Compound mixture of opium and glycyrrhiza

Toxicity Rating: 2. A cough mixture and sedative. One teaspoonful contains 0.6 ml. paregoric (2.5 mg. opium), 1.2 mg. tartar emetic, and ethyl nitrite. Overdosages produce vomiting due to tartar emetic or systemic antimony poisoning. See Antimony salts above.

Ref.: Osol and Farrar, 1955.

216   Bismuth Salts (Soluble or Insoluble)

e.g., Bismuth oxychloride, Bismuth oxyiodide, Bismuth potassium tartrate, Bismuth subgallate

Toxicity Rating: 3(?). Ingestion toxicity is regarded as low. Very poor absorption from bowel. Systemic effects include ulcerative stomatitis, anorexia, headache, skin rashes, kidney tubular damage, and rarely mild jaundice. BAL may be useful if a severe renal lesion is anticipated (see BAL in Section III).

Ref.: Gryboski and Gotoff, 1961; Reekie, 1949; Gryboski et al., 961; O'Brien, 1959; Wachstein, 1944.

217   Bismuth Subcarbonate

Soluble in dilute acid; insoluble in water. See Bismuth salts above.

218   Bismuth Subnitrate

Basic bismuth nitrate, Bismuth white

Toxicity Rating: 3(?). Prepared by the partial hydrolysis of bismuth nitrate. The exact composition varies with the conditions of preparation. Especially in infants, the subnitrate may be reduced by bacteria within the bowel, to yield nitrite, which causes methemoglobinemia after absorption.

See also: Nitrite, *Reference Congener in Section III.*
Ref.: Higgins, 1916; Miller, 1945.

219   Bismuth Subsalicylate

Basic bismuth salicylate

Toxicity Rating: 3. An agricultural fungicide, consisting of 57.7% trivalent bismuth. Used medicinally as an intestinal absorbent (oral dose 1 to 2 gm.), particularly in treating traveler's diarrhea, and formerly as an antiluetic drug (i.m. dose 0.2 gm.). Practically insoluble in water but decomposed by alkali, so that salicylate poisoning is possible after ingestion. As present in Pepto-Bismol (1.75% bismuth subsalicylate), salicylate absorption from the gut was almost complete in men given doses of 60 ml. or less, whereas absorption of bismuth was not detectable. See also Bismuth salts above.

See also: Salicylate, *Reference Congener in Section III.*
Ref.: Feldman et al., 1980; Hanna, 1958; Riley, 1961.

Cadmium and mercury compounds

220   Cadmium

i.e., Chloride, oxide, sulfate

Toxicity Rating: 5(?). Inhaled as a dust or aerosol, cadmium and its salts (including even the relatively insoluble oxide) probably have a toxicity rating of 6 in man, with death from fatal pulmonary injury. When swallowed, these salts are much less lethal, in part because they induce vomiting and are not retained. Although as little as 10 mg. of cadmium salts has often produced severe toxic symptoms when ingested, a toxicity rating of 5 is probably a reasonable estimate of cadmium's lethality by the oral route.

See also: Cadmium, *Reference Congener in Section III.*

221   Mercury

e.g., Metallic mercury

In general, the toxicity of metallic mercury and of most mercury compounds depends upon in vivo release of the mercuric ion.

See also: Mercury, *Reference Congener in Section III.*

222   Alkyl Mercuric Chloride (or Phosphate)

Toxicity Rating: 5. Alkyl group is usually ethyl or methyl. Toxic by all portals. Systemic toxicity almost as high as mercuric chloride. Nervous symptoms are prominent; they include headache, vertigo, ataxia, decrease in visual fields, delirium, and paresis. No satisfactory antidote is available.

See also: Mercury, *Reference Congener in Section III.*
Ref.: Council on Pharmacy and Chemistry, 1955.

223 Ammoniated Mercury 223

Mercuric chloride ammoniated, Aminomercuric chloride

Toxicity Rating: 5. Too vigorous skin application may cause dermatitis and even systemic poisoning. Almost as toxic as the bichloride when ingested.

Said to have been responsible for many cases of acrodynia in children.

See also: Mercury, *Reference Congener in Section III.*
Ref.: Gibbs et al., 1941.

224 2-Chloro-4-(hydroxymercuri)phenol 224

Hydroxymercurichlorophenol, e.g., Semesan

Toxicity Rating: 5. Semesan contains 20% mercury, equivalent to 30% mixed hydroxymercurichlorophenols, plus diluents which promote water solubility. Less corrosive than mercuric chloride but the systemic toxicity is probably almost as great. Toxic by all portals. Nonvolatile and insoluble in water, but soluble in alkali. Oil facilitates absorp- tion from the bowel. Used in agriculture as a fungicide for treating seeds and turf diseases. Strongly irritating to the skin but not a vesicant. In its systemic actions and metabolic fate, it probably resembles phenylmercuric salts of inorganic acids; see latter below.

See also: Mercury, *Reference Congener in Section III.*
Ref.: Council on Pharmacy and Chemistry, 1955.

225 Chloromethoxypropylmercuric Acetate 225

In contrast to most phenylmercuric salts (see below), this alkoxyalkyl mercuric salt is a liquid. Used as a fungicide for treating oat and wheat seeds. No toxicity data were located, but it is probably similar to methoxyethylmercuric acetate and chloride; see latter below.

See also: Mercury, *Reference Congener in Section III.*

226 Donovan's Solution 226

Toxicity Rating: 3. An aqueous solution, each 100 ml. containing 0.9 to 1.0 gm. arsenious iodide and 1.05 gm. mercuric iodide. Since this solution contains almost equitoxic amounts of arsenic and mercury, untoward effects can be expected from both. If ingested, the first symptoms are probably due to the mercuric ion, and if vomiting is prompt, arsenic poisoning may never develop. Because of the rapid absorption of mercury, mercurialism is almost inevitable in doses of one or more ounces.

See also: Mercury, *Reference Congener in Section III.*
Ref.: Osol and Farrar, 1955.

227 EMMI 227

N-Ethylmercuri-1,2,3,6-tetrahydro-3,6-endomethano-3,4,5,6,7,7-hexachlorophthalimide

Toxicity Rating: 4. An organic mercurial fungicide with all the toxic potentialities of other mercury compounds. It can be absorbed through the gastrointestinal tract, lungs, mucous membranes, and skin with the production of systemic effects. Local application can also cause chemical dermatitis or corneal ulceration.

See also: Mercury, *Reference Congener in Section III.*
Ref.: Velsicol Chemical Corp., 1958.

228 Ethyl Mercuric Chloride 228

Chloroethylmercury, e.g., Ceresan, Granosan

Toxicity Rating: 5. A seed disinfectant which is almost as toxic as bichloride of mercury. The rat oral LD_{50} is 23 mg. (as Hg)/kg. Especially danger- ous because of its toxic vapors. See Ethyl Mercury Phosphate below.

See also: Mercury, *Reference Congener in Section III.*
Ref.: Council on Pharmacy and Chemistry, 1955.

229   Ethyl Mercuri-2,3-dihydroxypropylmercaptide

Ceresan 75-100-200

Toxicity Rating: 4–5. A seed disinfectant that probably lies near the borderline between toxicity classes 4 and 5. Lethal oral doses produce gastritis, dehydration, and marked kidney damage. Also a potent skin irritant causing erythema and blistering.

See also: Mercury, *Reference Congener in Section III.*
Ref.: Williams, 1959a.

230   *N*-(Ethylmercuri)-*p*-toluene Sulfonanilide

e.g., Ceresan M

Toxicity Rating: 4–5. A seed disinfectant which is almost as toxic as mercuric chloride. Less irritating to the skin than ethyl mercury phosphate. Symptoms are largely confined to the central nervous system and consist of deafness, ataxia, dysarthria, progressive visual deterioration, dysphagia, sphincteric incontinence, mental confusion, stupor and death. BAL is not generally useful in poisonings by alkyl mercury compounds; no effective antidote is available.

See also: Mercury, *Reference Congener in Section III.*
Ref.: Anonymous, 1957b; Jalili and Abbasi, 1961.

231   Ethyl Mercury Phosphate

Ethyl mercuric phosphate

Toxicity Rating: 4–5. A volatile fungicide which is significantly less toxic than mercuric chloride, at least in mice. The single-dose oral LD_{50} in mice is 61 mg. (as Hg)/kg. Nervous symptoms are prominent and severe, though sometimes transitory; they include headache, vertigo, ataxia, decrease in the visual fields, delirium, and paresis.

See also: Mercury, *Reference Congener in Section III.*
Ref.: Council on Pharmacy and Chemistry, 1955.

232   Hydroxymercuricresol

Toxicity Rating: 5. One of the components in some Semesan products. Similar to and often mixed with 2-Chloro-4-(hydroxymercuri)phenol. See latter above.

See also: Mercury, *Reference Congener in Section III.*
Ref.: Council on Pharmacy and Chemistry, 1955.

233   Hydroxymercurinitrophenol

Toxicity Rating: 5. Semesan Bel is 10% mercury, chiefly in the form of this compound. Similar to and often mixed with 2-Chloro-4-(hydroxymercuri)phenol. See latter above. Aqueous solutions of the sodium salt have been used in medicine as a disinfectant under the name Mercurophen. Nitromersol (Metaphen) is a closely related medicinal germicide.

See also: Mercury, *Reference Congener in Section III.*
Ref.: Taylor and Austin, 1918.

234   Hydroxyphenylmercurichloride

Phenol mercuric chloride

Contains 61% mercury. Readily soluble in water. Dilute solutions have been used in medicine as a germicide and fungicide. Less corrosive than mercuric chloride but the systemic toxicity is probably almost as great. See also Phenylmercuric salts of inorganic acids below.

See also: Mercury, *Reference Congener in Section III.*
Ref.: Merck and Co., 1976.

235   Merbromin

Mercurochrome, 2,7-Dibromo-4-hydroxymercurifluorescein disodium

Toxicity Rating: 4. Generally available in 2 to 5% aqueous solutions. Can cause mercury poisoning if taken internally, but it is less toxic than the more soluble mercury salts. Reports of skin sensitization from application of organomercurials.

See also: Mercury, *Reference Congener in Section III.*
Ref.: Gaul and Underwood, 1949.

236 Mercuric Chloride   236

Bichloride of mercury, Corrosive sublimate, Mercury bichloride

Toxicity Rating: 5–6. Very dangerous by all portals. The LD_{50} in mice is 5 to 7 mg. (as Hg)/kg. by parenteral routes and about 10 mg./kg. by mouth. Act fast!

See also: Mercury, Reference Congener in Section III.

237 Mercurous Chloride   237

Calomel

Toxicity Rating: 5. Rarely causes systemic mercury poisoning. An irritant cathartic or purgative when ingested. If retained, 30 to 40 mg./kg. may be fatal. Rarely "calomel sickness" appears after a latency of about 1 week; it is a benign reaction characterized by fever and rash (scarlatinal or urticarial).

See also: Mercury, Reference Congener in Section III.
Ref.: Cheek and Wu, 1959; Cheek et al., 1959; Cheek, 1960.

238 Merodicein   238

Monohydroxymercuridiiodoresorcinsulfonphthalein sodium, Meralein sodium

Toxicity Rating: 4. Water-soluble germicide containing about 23% organically bound mercury. Supplied as a 1:5000 aqueous solution for use in mouth and throat. Minimal lethal dose parenterally in laboratory mammals 10 mg./kg. Poorly absorbed from the mammalian gastrointestinal tract where doses of 200 mg./kg. have only a laxative effect. Systemic poisoning leads to acute renal failure.

See also: Mercury, Reference Congener in Section III.
Ref.: Macht and Cook, 1931.

239 Methoxyethylmercuric Chloride   239

Toxicity Rating: 5. One of several organic mercury compounds used in agriculture as fungicides and seed protectants. The acetate and presumably the chloride are vesicants when applied to the skin in high concentrations. The carbon-to-mercury bond is rather unstable in vivo. Within 24 hr. after dosing test animals, all of the mercury was inorganic (Hg^{+2}). The signs and symptoms of systemic poisoning are believed to resemble those induced by mercuric induced by mercuric chloride.

See also: Mercury, Reference Congener in Section III.
Ref.: Spencer, 1973.

240 Methylmercuric Dicyandiamide   240

Cyano(methylmercuri)guanidine, Panogen 15, Methylmercuric cyanoguanidine

Toxicity Rating: 5. Perhaps slightly less toxic than other methyl mercury compounds commonly used in agriculture. Because of its lower vapor pressure, less hazardous than others by inhalation. By the intraperitoneal route in mice, acute toxicity is half that of mercuric bichloride. Prolonged skin contact may produce blisters.

See also: Mercury, Reference Congener in Section III.
Ref.: Spencer, 1973.

241 Phenylmercuric Salts of Organic Acids   241

Phenylmercuric acetate, Phenylmercuric oleate, e.g., PMAS

Toxicity Rating: 5. Examples include the acetate, salicylate, oleate, benzoate, phthalate, and gluconate. (General formula is $C_6H_5HgOOCR$). An important agricultural and industrial fungicide once considered for use as a contraceptive. Acute lethal dose is perhaps twice that of mercuric chloride. Much less corrosive than the latter but prolonged cutaneous contact with the dust leads to vesication. No toxicological distinctions are recognized between organic and inorganic salts of phenylmercury; see latter below.

See also: Mercury, Reference Congener in Section III.
Ref.: McCord et al., 1941; Cotter, 1947; Eastman and Scott, 1944; Miller et al., 1960.

242 Phenylmercuric Salts of Inorganic Acids   242

i.e., Borate, nitrate, subnitrate, chloride, and hydroxide

Toxicity Rating: 5. General formula is C_6H_5HgX where X is an anionic group. These salts ionize in solution to yield the phenylmercuric ion, which is less corrosive and less toxic than the mercuric ion, perhaps in part because most of these phenylmercuric salts have a low solubility in water. The carbon-to-mercury bond is rather unstable *in vivo*; the rupture probably occurs only after the phenyl ring is hydroxylated in the para position. Except for the first few hours after dosing, most of the mercury in test animals is present as inorganic mercury. The early signs and symptoms of systemic poisoning are not well established, but no prominent central neural effects (as in methylmercury poisoning) are known. Late effects include renal tubular necrosis and, after repeated exposures, the various neurologic defects of chronic mercurialism. Used in agriculture as fungicides and in medicine as external germicides.

See also: Mercury, *Reference Congener in Section III*.
Ref.: Cotter, 1947; Eastman and Scott, 1944; Miller et al., 1960.

243 Phenylmercuric Triethanol Ammonium Lactate

Toxicity Rating: 5(?). Related compounds include phenylmercurimonoethanolammonium acetate. Used as an agricultural fungicide. Systemic toxicity is probably almost as high as mercuric chloride but less corrosive than the latter. See Phenylmercuric salts of organic acids above.

See also: Mercury, *Reference Congener in Section III*.
Ref.: Council on Pharmacy and Chemistry, 1955.

244 Thimerosal

Sodium ethylmercurithiosalicylate, Thiomersalate, e.g., Merthiolate sodium

Toxicity Rating: 4(?). Topical antiseptic containing 49% organically bound mercury. Freely soluble in water and used as an 1:1000 to 1:30,000 aqueous solutions or 1:1000 tincture. Reports of skin sensitization with serious reactions.

See also: Mercury, *Reference Congener in Section III*.
Ref.: Gaul and Underwood, 1949.

Lead and thallium compounds

245 Lead

Most lead compounds lie in toxicity classes 3 or 4.

See also: Lead, *Reference Congener in Section III*.
Ref.: Fairhall and Sayers, 1940.

246 Lead Chromate

Chrome yellow

Toxicity Rating: 4. Closely related to basic lead chromate, which is known as chrome red. One of the more insoluble lead salts both in water and acetic acid. Soluble in alkali and dilute nitric acid. The most toxic lead salts are the carbonate, monoxide and sulfate presumably because they are most soluble. Lead arsenate also belongs in this group, but its higher toxicity is due in part to its arsenic content. Lead chromate is less hazardous than any member of this group whether given parenterally, orally or by inhalation. Perhaps chromate poisoning plays a role in the acute reaction (see Chromium trioxide in the index) but signs of chronic lead poisoning may appear weeks or months after the initial insult.

See also: Lead, *Reference Congener in Section III*.
Ref.: Harrold et al., 1944; Harrold, 1949; Fairhall and Sayers, 1940.

247 Lead Dioxide

Lead peroxide

Toxicity Rating: 4. PbO_2 is used for electrodes in batteries, with amorphous phosphorus as an ignition surface for matches, and as a catalytic activator for some epoxy resins. Presumably soluble in acidic gastric juice. Approximate LD_{50} intraperitoneally in guinea pigs is 200 mg./kg. or about the same as that of several soluble lead salts.

See also: Lead, *Reference Congener in Section III*.
Ref.: Fairhall and Sayers, 1940.

248   Tetraethyl Lead   248

Motor fuels contain no more than 0.15% (3 cc./gal.) and aviation fuels no more than 0.22% (4.5 cc./gal.). Poisoning may occur through skin absorption, inhalation, or ingestion. The symptoms are referable chiefly to the nervous system: insomnia, irritability, and in severe cases an acute encephalopathy with

mania. Other symptoms are visual difficulties, gastrointestinal disturbances, weakness, tremors, muscle pains, and easy fatigability. As formulated in motor fuels, petroleum hydrocarbons are more dangerous than tetraethyl lead or other additives. See Gasoline in the index.

See also: Lead, *Reference Congener in Section III.*
Ref.: Boyd et al., 1957; Schlang, 1961; White, 1955.

249   Thallium   249

e.g., Thallium sulfate, Thallium acetate

Toxicity Rating: 5. Salts of thallium were once used as pesticides against rats, mice, ground squirrels, prairie dogs, moles and some insects, but they are

currently outlawed in pesticidal formulations in the U.S.A. Thallium is a slow but persistent systemic poison.

See also: Thallium, *Reference Congener in Section III.*

Ferric and ferrous compounds

250   Iron Salts   250

Ferrous and ferric

Toxicity Rating: 3. In large doses soluble iron salts are corrosive irritants and systemic poisons. See

ferric and ferrous salts below.

See also: Ferrous Salts, *Reference Congener in Section III.*

251   Burnt Sienna   251

Iron oxide (Fe_2O_3) plus clay. A common insoluble paint pigment. See Ferric salts below.

252   Burnt Umber   252

Toxicity Rating: 3(?). Iron oxides (Fe_2O_3 plus manganese oxide plus clay.) A common paint pigment. Both iron and manganese oxides are insoluble. See

Ferric salts below; also Manganese salts in the index.

253   Ferric Salts   253

e.g., Ferric chloride, Ferric ammonium citrate, Ferric sulfate

Toxicity Rating: 3. Given orally, ferric and ferrous salts induce essentially the same toxic syndrome.

See also: Ferrous Salts, *Reference Congener in Section III.*
Ref.: Hoppe et al., 1955.

254   Ferric Subsulfate   254

Monsel's salt, Basic ferric sulfate

Toxicity Rating: 3. Approximate formula is $Fe_4(SO_4)_5(OH)_2 \cdot H_2O$. Monsel's solution is a nearly saturated aqueous solution of this salt; it is pre-

pared by mixing and boiling ferrous sulfate with sulfuric and nitric acids. This solution, which contains 20 to 22% iron, is used externally as a styptic.

See also: Ferrous Salts, *Reference Congener in Section III.*
Ref.: Osol and Farrar, 1955.

255   Ferrocholinate   255

Iron choline citrate, e.g., Ferrolip

Toxicity Rating: 3. An iron chelate containing 12% elemental iron (by weight), used as a hematinic in an adult dose of 50 mg. three times daily. May

cause gastric distress in therapeutic doses. Minimal lethal dose for dogs and rabbits is 500 mg./kg.

See also: Ferrous Salts, *Reference Congener in Section III.*

256   **256**   Ferrocyanide and Ferricyanide Salts

i.e., Sodium, potassium, ferric

Toxicity Rating: 3(?). No adequate toxicity data were located, but apparently the sodium and potassium salts are comparatively benign. They are not decomposed to cyanide. Rapidly excreted in

Ref.: Kleeman et al., 1955.

the urine, apparently without metabolic alteration. Dogs tolerate intravenous injections of 2.5 gm./kg. For ferric ferrocyanide. see Ferric salts above.

257   **257**   Ferrous Carbonate

Blaud's mass

Toxicity Rating: 3. Each pill contains 65 mg. (1 gr.) of ferrous carbonate.

See also: Ferrous Salts, *Reference Congener in Section III.*

258   **258**   Ferrous Salts

i.e., Ferrous sulfate, chloride, carbonate, gluconate

Toxicity Rating: 3. Although iron salts differ considerably in astringency, lethal doses appear to be

closely related to the total iron content.

See also: Ferrous Salts, *Reference Congener in Section III.*

Copper and zinc compounds

259   **259**   Bordeaux Mixture

Toxicity Rating: 4. Copper sulfate and unslaked lime (sometimes slaked), freshly dissolved and then mixed in various proportions (often equal parts by weight). A gelatinous mass representing a molecular mixture of copper hydroxide and copper sulfate,

widely used as a foliage fungicide. Usually components must be freshly dissolved and then mixed, but some premixed formulations are on the market. Less astringent and presumably less toxic than copper sulfate.

See also: Copper, *Reference Congener in Section III.*
Ref.: Council on Pharmacy and Chemistry, 1955.

260   **260**   Gold Bronze Powder

Toxicity Rating: 3. Refers to bronze- or gold-colored alloys of copper and zinc, present as finely divided powders in printing inks and paint. The alloys may also contain tin, iron and aluminum. Although they are not water-soluble, partial or complete solubilization may occur in acid gastric juice, especially if the powder has been corroded by previous exposure to moisture. A 2-year-old boy inhaled and swallowed an unknown quantity used for gilding Christmas cards. Coughing and vomiting began immediately. Although "much" powder was removed by gastric lavage, he developed severe abdominal distention and watery stools containing particles of the powder. Episodes of shock and cyanosis with fever occurred on the second day, as

well as signs of renal damage. Severe pneumonia with pulmonary edema lead to dyspnea, tachypnea and tachycardia. Death occurred after 60 hours. Petechial hemorrhage of the stomach, necrosis of the proximal convoluted tubules of the kidneys and severe lung and bronchial damage were seen at autopsy (Harris and Haggerty, 1957). This bronze powder consisted of 30% zinc and 70% copper, with a small amount of stearate. The case may represent systemic copper intoxication complicated by a pneumonitis. The latter may have been induced by the metals themselves (see Metal fumes in the index) or by small amounts of zinc stearate (see latter in the index). The toxicity of bronze powder in paint is not known.

See also: Copper, *Reference Congener in Section III.*
Ref.: Harris and Haggerty, 1957.

26   **261**   Copper Naphthenates

Copper cyclopentanecarboxylate

Toxicity Rating: 3(?). Usually supplied as a viscous green solution in petroleum oil, containing 8% copper (or more). No skin irritation. Little or no cor-

rosive action when ingested. Toxicity is due chiefly to solvent or to impurities.

See also: Copper *and* Kerosene, *Reference Congeners in Section III.*
Ref.: Amer. Petroleum Institute, 1953c.

262 Copper Oxychloride Sulfate 262

COCS

Toxicity Rating: 4. An agricultural fungicide. Essentially a mixture of basic cupric chloride, cupric hydroxide and copper (cupric) sulfate. Effects similar to those of other soluble copper salts.

See also: Copper, *Reference Congener in Section III.*
Ref.: Spencer, 1973.

263 Copper 3-Phenylsalicylate 263

Toxicity Rating: 3-4. A fungicide and fungistatic agent. No skin irritation. Little or no corrosive action when ingested. Oral LD_{50} in rats is 520 mg./kg.

See also: Copper, *Reference Congener in Section III.*
Ref.: Spencer, 1973.

264 Copper Quinolinolate 264

Cupric-8-hydroxyquinolinate

Toxicity Rating: 2(?). Among copper compounds, a very low toxicity. No irritation on skin and no corrosive action when ingested.

See also: Copper, *Reference Congener in Section III.*
Ref.: Scientific Oil Compounding Co., 1950.

265 Copper 265

i.e., Sulfate, acetate, subacetate, chloride, oxychloride

Toxicity Rating: 4. The soluble salts are potent but unreliable emetics. If they fail to induce vomiting, as sometimes happens, the cupric (or cuprous) ion may induce toxic systemic reactions.

See also: Copper, *Reference Congener in Section III.*

266 Cuprous Chloride 266

Toxicity Rating: 4. Cuprous chloride is said to be more than twice as toxic as cupric chloride, but there appear to be no major toxicological distinctions between the two valence states of copper, perhaps because many cuprous salts are oxidized quickly by moist air. Other cuprous salts hydrolyze to cuprous oxide on contact with water. See Cuprous oxide below.

See also: Copper, *Reference Congener in Section III.*

267 Copper-Zinc-Chromate Complex 267

Crag Fungicide 658

Toxicity Rating: 3. A fungicide said to be composed of basic zinc chromate with a proportion of the zinc replaced by copper ions, being about 30% copper, 20% zinc, and 10% chromium. Probably because it is practically insoluble in water, it has a low oral toxicity (borderline between toxicity classes 2 and 3 in animal studies). Also low potential for causing skin irritation. (For the toxicity of soluble salts of copper, see Copper, Reference Congener in Section III.)

Ref.: Miller Chemical & Fertilizer Corp., 1958.

268 Cupric Chloride (Basic) 268

Copper oxychloride, Basic cupric chloride

Toxicity Rating: 4. An agricultural fungicide. The composition varies with the conditions of manufacture, but commercial preparations usually approach the formula $3Cu(OH)_2 \cdot CuCl_2$. Soluble in dilute acids (e.g., gastric juice). When ingested it is similar in its effects to soluble copper salts (e.g., the sulfate).

See also: Copper, *Reference Congener in Section III.*
Ref.: Spencer, 1973.

269   Cuprous Oxide

269

Red copper oxide

Toxicity Rating: 3(?). Usually red but very small particles are yellow (e.g., Yellow Cuprocide). A widely used agricultural fungicide. Presumably appreciable amounts dissolve in acidic gastric juice; if insoluble the correct toxicity rating is less than 3.

See also: Copper, *Reference Congener in Section III.*
Ref.: Council on Pharmacy and Chemistry, 1955.

270   Tribasic Copper Sulfate

270

Toxicity Rating: 4. A molecular mixture of cupric hydroxide and cupric sulfate, the exact composition of which is uncertain (about 50% copper by weight). The name is apparently applied to several commercially available powders of the premixed Bordeaux-type, used as foliage fungicides. Less astringent and presumably less toxic than copper sulfate, but the copper content may be higher than that of copper sulfate.

See also: Copper, *Reference Congener in Section III.*
Ref.: Council on Pharmacy and Chemistry, 1955.

271   Calamine

271

Toxicity Rating: 2(?). Zinc oxide with 0.5% ferric oxide. No satisfactory data. Large single doses in animals produce gastritis and vomiting like copper salts. Some calamine formulations contain significant amounts of phenol (1 to 2%); ingestion or repeated application over large areas of skin can and has caused systemic phenol poisoning.

Ref.: Osol and Farrar, 1955.

272   Lassar's Paste

272

Toxicity Rating: 2(?). A mixture of zinc oxide (1 part), starch (1 part), and petrolatum (2 parts). The ingestion toxicity of zinc oxide is not well established, but probably it is low. If the oxide is appreciably soluble in gastric juice, vomiting and gastritis may be anticipated.

Ref.: Osol and Farrar, 1955.

273   Zinc Naphthenate

273

Toxicity Rating: 2. A wood preservative of low acute oral toxicity (borderline between toxicity classes 2 and 3). Neither a primary skin irritant nor a recognized sensitizing agent. See Zinc salts below and Naphthenic acids in the index.

Ref.: Doyle, 1958.

274   Zinc Oxide

274

Flowers of zinc, Zinc white

Toxicity Rating: 3(?). The usual USP grade has a high purity, but some technical grades contain a few tenths of a percent lead. No estimates of acute oral toxicity were located, and it is assumed that no human fatalities have resulted from ingestion of the pure oxide. Because it is soluble in dilute mineral acid (presumably including gastric juice), it probably shares to a limited extent the toxic actions of water-soluble Zinc salts (see latter below). For the inhalation toxicity of freshly formed fumes of zinc oxide, see Metal Fumes in the index.

Ref.: Hegsted et al., 1945.

275   Zinc Phenolsulfonate

275

Zinc sulfocarbolate, Zinc sulfophenate

Toxicity Rating: 4(?). Formerly used as an intestinal antiseptic in doses of 60 to 200 mg. Currently found in insecticide formulations. In large doses it has emetic and astringent actions.

See also: Copper, *Reference Congener in Section III.*
Ref.: Osol and Farrar, 1955.

276 Zinc 2-Pyridinethiol-1-oxide 276

Zinc pyridinethione, Zinc pyrithione, Vancide ZP, Zinc omadine, ZPT

Toxicity Rating: 4. Oral LD_{50}'s 207 mg./kg. for male rats and 177 mg./kg. for females. Dermal LD_{50} for rabbits about 0.1 gm./kg. When given by mouth in a 2% concentration as a commercial shampoo, emesis occurred in dogs at doses above 0.05 gm. of shampoo per kg.; no other symptoms were seen with doses as high as 5 gm./kg. In rats, *Ref.*: Snyder, 1964.

rabbits and guinea pigs the commercial product has a toxicity rating of 3. Repeated administration caused hind limb paralysis in rabbits and retinal detachment in dogs. These changes do not occur in monkeys. It appears unlikely that the toxicity of this substance can be attributed solely to its zinc content.

277 Zinc Salts (Soluble) 277

i.e., Chloride, sulfate, acetate

Toxicity Rating: 3 to 4. Although no longer recommended, the sulfate has been used as an emetic drug (adult dose 0.5 to 1.0 gm.). Toxicity and toxic actions are like those of copper salts. Produces irritation or corrosion of the alimentary tract with pain, emesis, etc. The chloride appears to be more

corrosive and more toxic than the sulfate. A few grams of the chloride have killed an adult, although recovery has been reported after ingestion of 90 gm. Delayed deaths have been ascribed to inanition following severe strictures of the esophagus and pylorus.

See also: Copper *and* Acid, *Reference Congeners in Section III.*
Ref.: Cowan, 1947; Finney et al., 1960; Hegsted et al., 1945.

278 Zinc Stearate 278

Toxicity Rating: 3(?). Usually a mixture of zinc salts of stearic and palmitic acids, with an excess of zinc oxide. This zinc soap is widely used in cosmetic powders because it contributes adhesive properties to the preparation. No information about oral toxicity was located, but aspiration of the powder has

produced acute fatal pneumonitis in infants. The lesions resemble those from talc but are generally more severe. In contrast powdered zinc oxide does not produce an appreciable pulmonary reaction, although the freshly formed fume is toxic.

Ref.: Abt et al., 1925; Heiman and Aschner, 1922.

279 Zinc Undecylenate 279

Used topically as a skin fungicide. See also Zinc salts above and Undecylenic Acid in the index

because both parts of the molecule may contribute to the acute toxicity.

Other metals and their compounds

280 Chromium Oxide 280

Chrome green

Toxicity Rating: 2(?). Cr_2O_3 is insoluble in water. Used as a pigment in paints. Known to have a

comparatively low toxicity, in contrast to hexavalent chromium trioxide; see latter in index.

281 Chromium Sulfate 281

Chromic sulfate

Toxicity Rating: 3(?). Cationic chromium salts (e.g., chrome alum, chromium potassium sulfate,

etc.) are said to have a low toxicity, in contrast to chromate and dichromate salts; see latter in index.

See also: Copper, *Reference Congener in Section III.*

282 Cobalt Salts 282

Cobaltic or cobaltous compounds

Toxicity Rating: 4(?). In toxic doses soluble salts act locally on the gastrointestinal tract like copper salts (pain, vomiting, etc.). Systemic effects in man include a peculiar vasodilatation (flushing) of face and ears, mild hypotension, rash, tinnitus, and nerve deafness. Chronic administration of cobal-

tous chloride has produced a goiter, reduced thyroid activity and lowered synthesis rates and levels of cytochrome P-450 in the liver. Animals also demonstrate an increase in respiration, as well as tremors and convulsions. As with copper, a toxic nephritis may result. BAL should be tried as described in Section III. Epidemic cardiomyopathy among heavy beer drinkers in the 1960's in Canada, the United States and Belgium has been ascribed to the addition of up to 1.5 ppm of cobalt to some beers as a foam restorative and stabilizer. The amount ingested per day (up to 10 mg.) is, however, less than the amount used in the treatment of refractory anemias (up to 50 mg/day). Thus, other factors such as inadequate protein or vitamin intake and/or pre-existing cardiomyopathy due to alcohol may have rendered the heart more sensitive to injury by cobalt.

See also: Copper, *Reference Congener in Section III.*
Ref.: Jacobziner and Raybin, 1961n; Kriss et al., 1955; Saikkonen, 1959; Tephly and Hibbeln, 1971; Alexander, 1972.

283 Cobalt Driers

283

Toxicity Rating: 4(?). Small amounts of various metal oxides, salts and chelates are added to oil paints and lacquers to accelerate drying by promoting the oxidation of "drying" oils and resins. Cobalt driers usually consist of cobalt salts of fatty acids or naphthenic acids ("cobalt alkanoates"). Sometimes other metals are used with or without cobalt, notably alkanoates (also called "metallic soaps") of lead, manganese, zirconium and others. In the low concentrations present in paints, these compounds are not regarded as hazardous, but concentrated solutions of cobalt driers sold in art supply stores are highly toxic. See Cobalt salts above.

284 Gold Salts

284

e.g., Gold sodium thiosulfate, Gold trichloride, Gold sodium thiomalate

Toxicity Rating: 4(?). No information on oral toxicity was located. Given intramuscularly at weekly intervals to patients with rheumatoid arthritis, gold salts often induce toxic reactions (frequently of an allergic nature): dermatitis, nausea, vomiting, diarrhea, nephritis, blood disorders, peripheral neuritis, hepatitis, and encephalitis. Severe reactions respond well to BAL (see BAL in Section III).

Ref.: Driver and Weller, 1931; Leiper, 1946; Myerson, 1950.

285 Indium (and Salts)

285

i.e., Sulfate, citrate, chloride, sesquioxide

Toxicity Rating: 3. Poorly absorbed from the gastrointestinal tract, although demonstrated in the urine of animals given oral doses. The metal and its salts are not irritants or sensitizers and are not considered to be significant industrial hazards. When given parenterally, however, indium salts have a toxicity rating of 5 or 6. In animals the symptoms (which may be delayed several hours) include anorexia, nose bleed, hind limb paresis, rapid and spasmodic respirations. twitching, asphyxial convulsions, and perhaps alopecia. Lesions include widespread inflammation and focal hemorrhages in lungs, liver, kidney and heart. The organ most severely affected is the liver, and death may occur from hepatic necrosis, which can be prevented in animals by prophylactic ferric dextran. Incidental to their lethality is the ability of indium salts to produce localized calcification at connective tissue sites of injection.

Ref.: Anonymous, 1943; Gabbiani et al., 1962; Harrold et al., 1943; McCord et al., 1942.

286 Manganese Salts

286

Manganous salts, Manganic salts, Manganese sulfate

Toxicity Rating: 3(?). Inorganic manganese salts are poorly absorbed through lungs and gut. Acute systemic intoxication rarely occurs after oral administration, but one diabetic man consistently developed hypoglycemia after ingesting only 3 to 5 mg. of manganous chloride. Rats injected subcutaneously with 15 mg./kg. of manganese (as $MnCl_2$) showed a prompt elevation of hemoglobin and hematocrit, increased levels of serum chloride, phosphate and magnesium, and decreased levels of calcium and iron. Aside from parenteral routes, systemic poisoning may result from chronic inhalation or chronic ingestion; chronic exposure to low concentrations may lead to the accumulation of toxic concentrations in critical organs. The brain appears to sustain permanent cellular damage at exposure levels which do not otherwise affect a person. The characteristic pathological lesion in man is destruction of the ganglion cells of the basal ganglia, although symptoms appear before damage becomes discernible. Symptoms of workers exposed to manganese dusts include masklike facial expression, spastic gait, tremors, slurred speech, sometimes dystonia, fatiguability, anorexia, asthenia, apathy, and inability to concentrate. Insomnia may precede other clinical signs. Rat studies indicate that manganese gradually accumulates in brain tissue to produce a lesion similar to that of Parkinsonism. Indeed, in clinical trials with miners exposed to manganese-containing dusts, L-dopa relieved extrapyramidal symptoms in both hypokinetic and dystonic patients (Mena et al., 1970). For short periods of time, symptoms can sometimes be controlled with scopolamine or amphetamine. BAL and calcium disodium edetate are regarded as ineffective. Absorbed manganese tends to be slowly excreted in bile. Inhalation exposure to manganous oxide dust leads to a form of lobar pneumonia which is unresponsive to antibiotics. The OSHA 8-hour TWA standard for exposure to manganese in air is 5 mg./m^3. Because oral manganese intake leads to increased fecal losses of calcium and subsequent decreases in calcium blood levels, large doses of calcium salts are given by mouth. Manganese salts lend a bitter taste to water. The public health standard for drinking water is 0.05 mg./l. However, in many areas manganese ore deposits lead to metal concentrations as high as 1.3 mg./l. in natural waters. In contrast to cationic manganese, acute reactions after anionic permanganate are due to local tissue injury resulting from intense oxidation (see potassium permanganate in the index).

Ref.: Baxter et al., 1965; Chandra, 1972; Chandra et al., 1974; Cook et al., 1974; Flinn et al., 1941; Mena et al., 1970; Rubenstein et al., 1962; Tepper, 1961.

287 Nickel Salts   287

e.g., Nickel chloride, Nickel nitrate, Nickel phosphate, Nickel sulfate

Toxicity Rating: 4(?). Partly because of local astringent and irritant actions, nickel salts act as emetics when swallowed (but also by other routes). As with other irritant-emetics, the oral lethal dose is presumed to vary widely. Absorption from the bowel is poor, and systemic poisoning is rare. Systemic effects include hyperglycemia, capillary damage (especially in the brain and adrenals), renal injury, myocardial weakness, and central nervous depression. A nickel-plated water heater in a dialysis unit was believed to be responsible for contaminating dialysis fluid, which resulted in mild signs of intoxication in 23 patients. At plasma nickel levels of 3 mg./L., nausea, vomiting, weakness, headache and palpitations occurred; they regressed over 3 to 13 hours. A potent contact allergen and sensitizer. The dermatitis is known as "nickel itch". A high percentage of women with pierced ears test positively for nickel allergy because of sensitization by jewelry containing the metal. Nickel dusts and several specific compounds are carcinogenic in animals after inhalation or parenteral administration but not by ingestion or skin contact. An increased incidence of lung and nasal cavity cancers has been noted among workmen in nickel smelters and refineries. *D*-Penicillamine was the most effective of three chelating agents tested in animals in increasing the renal clearance of nickel when both the metal and the chelator were delivered continuously by implanted osmotic mini-pumps. When nickel chloride was injected intraperitoneally as a single dose, *D*-penicillamine and Na$_2$CaEDTA were the most effective of 14 chelating agents tested in preventing death. Nickel carbonyl is a colorless volatile liquid with a toxicity rating of 6. When the vapors are inhaled, pulmonary effects predominate. Severe pulmonary edema with focal hemorrhage should be anticipated within 2 to 5 days. Milder pathologic lesions are seen in many other organs. Sodium diethyldithiocarbamate (Dithiocarb) and to a lesser extent *D*-penicillamine (see in index) are effective in preventing death in nickel carbonyl poisoned animals. Dithiocarb has also been used successfully in man (Sunderman, 1979). See also Nitrogan Oxides in Section III for measures useful in the management of pulmonary edema.

See also: Copper, *Reference Congener in Section III*.
Ref.: Baselt et al., 1977; Baselt and Hanson, 1982; Basinger et al., 1980; Friberg, 1948; National Academy of Science, 1975; Prystowsky et al., 1979; Shen et al., 1979; Sunderman and Kincaid, 1954; Sunderman and Sunderman, 1958; Sunderman, 1979 Webster et al., 1980.

288 Silver Salts   288

e.g., Silver nitrate, Lunar caustic

The insoluble chloride, bromide, iodide and oxide are generally nonirritating and relatively benign. The ingestion of corrosive silver nitrate (toxicity rating 4) has been responsible for most cases of acute silver poisoning. The symptoms are those of a severe gastroenteritis and shock, with vertigo, coma, convulsions and death. Perhaps NaCl solutions (table salt) should be given by mouth to assure complete precipitation as silver chloride. The acute corrosive insult may resemble that produced by Lye or Acid; see both in Section III. Silver appears to have a very low systemic toxicity. Chronic exposure to silver salts may cause argyrism, which appears to be solely of cosmetic concern. The famous "blue man" of the Barnum and Bailey circus was said to have a total silver body burden of 90 to 100 gm. without obvious deleterious symptoms. BAL does not increase the excretion of silver in argyria, and it is of no value in acute experimental silver poisoning. In recent years 0.5% silver nitrate has been recommended topically for the management of burns. Severe and even lethal methemoglobinemia has sometimes resulted. Such a reaction presumably depends on bacterial contamination of the eschar or a systemic infection with an organism capable of reducing nitrate to nitrite, e.g., Aerobacter cloacae, Pseudomonas aeruginosa, etc. Thus, the reaction may be elicited by any soluble nitrate salt and has nothing to do with the silver moiety. See Nitrite in Section III for the management of this complication.

Ref.: Cushing and Smith, 1969; Gettler et al., 1927; Hill and Pillsbury, 1939; Strauch et al., 1969; Ternberg and Luce, 1968; Uhde, 1946.

289

289　Sequestrenes

Toxicity Rating: 3. Trade name for various organic chelates of iron, zinc, manganese and copper used in agriculture and home gardening to correct trace metal deficiencies in soils. The iron, zinc and manganese chelates have acute oral LD_{50}'s in mice and rats in the range of 5 gm./kg. and belong on the borderline between toxicity classes 2 and 3. The copper chelate is somewhat more toxic with an oral LD_{50} in rats of 1.75 gm./kg. It is presumed but not established that the toxic signs are due to metal release in vivo. See appropriate metal entries in the index.

Ref.: Geigy Agricultural Chemicals, 1964a.

290

290　Stannic and Stannous Salts

Tin salts, i.e., oxide, dioxide, chloride, sulfide, sulfate, oxalate, tartrate

The toxicology of inorganic tin salts is poorly understood, and enormous differences in acute toxicity between compounds have been observed in animals. In part these differences can be ascribed to differences in solubility and route of administration. By mouth most tin salts are relatively nontoxic and poorly absorbed from the gastrointestinal tract. In terms of human poisonings tin has a good record of safety. Tin is present in most canned foods to the extent of 20 to 50 ppm (microgm./gm.). A number of episodes of tin "food" poisoning with nausea, vomiting and diarrhea have occurred after ingestion of fruit juices, etc. with tin levels of 1400 ppm and above. There was no evidence of systemic tin toxicity and recovery was usually complete. In hearth tinners exposed to fumes of tin oxides, a benign pneumoconiosis without fibrosis or evidence of silicosis may occur. The absence of significant respiratory disability is remarkable in view of the gross radiological abnormality. When fed to rats in their diet for 4 or 13 weeks, stannous sulfide, stannous oxide or stannic oxide had no effect at levels up to 1%. Severe growth retardation and other signs of toxicity occurred with stannous chloride, orthophosphate, sulfate, oxalate and tartrate at feeding levels of 0.3%. The acute oral LD_{50} of stannous chloride in rats is 700 mg./kg., whereas by parenteral administration to mice or dogs the LD_{50} lies between 20 to 40 mg./kg. The oral LD_{50} of stannous fluoride is 112 mg./kg. in mice and between 200 and 300 mg./kg. in various strains of laboratory rats. At the concentrations present in commercial dentifrice formulations (about 1 mg. F/gm.), neither fluoride nor tin presents an appreciable toxic hazard on an acute or chronic basis. Large doses of sodium stannous tartrate injected into rabbits produced weakness and paralysis. These disparate and largely unexplained differences suggest that tin poisoning might be a fertile field for additional investigation.

Ref.: Barnes and Stoner, 1959; Benoy et al., 1971; DeGroot et al., 1973; Robertson et al., 1961; Segreto et al., 1961.

291

291　Organotin Compounds

By definition, organotins possess at least one covalent carbon-to-tin bond. Although exceptions can be cited, the general formula is $R_nSnX_{(4-n)}$, where R is an organic group, n has a range of 1 to 4, and X is an anion or acidic group. Often X is an organic acid, but it may be a halide, hydroxide, sulfide, hydride, etc. The R groups may be alkyl, alkenyl, aryl or more complex. Many organotin compounds have been synthesized. They have a wide variety of properties and of commercial uses. Similarly they vary widely in toxicity. Perhaps because of low water solubility, many of them appear to be poorly absorbed from the alimentary tract. Whereas most fall in toxicity classes 3 and 4 on the basis of the single-dose oral LD_{50}'s in mice and rats, repeated administration of very small doses over periods of a few days reveals the high intrinsic toxicities of these materials. See also Alkyl Tin Compounds below.

Ref.: NIOSH, 1976.

292

292　Alkyl Tin Compounds

e.g., Monobutyltin trichloride, Monooctyltin trichloride, Diethyltin dichloride, Dibutyltin dichloride, Dioctyltin oxide, Tetra-*n*-butyltin

Toxicity Rating: 3-5. Alkyl tin compounds have been explored for anthelmintic, fungicidal and insecticidal activities. Also employed as antioxidants or corrosion inhibitors, water-repellant coatings, thermal or electric coatings, curing agents, etc. Tetra-*n*-butyltin is a gasoline additive. Dioctyl and dibutyl derivatives are used as stabilizers for polyvinyl chloride films. Wide differences in toxicity are recognized; they depend on the number of alkyl side-chains and their length; the associated acidic group also contributes, perhaps only by influencing solubility. In general monoalkyl tin is the least and trialkyl tin the most toxic. Little is known about monoalkyl tin compounds, but the toxicity of monoethyltin trichloride is probably low. Monobutyl and mono-octyl tin fall in toxicity class 3 as judged by data on mice. Steatosis of hepatocytes and renal tubular epithelium followed toxic doses. Dialkyl tins are irritants, and undiluted dibutyl and tributyl tin chlorides have caused extensive damage in the eye and skin burns in man. In mice and rats homologues from dipropyl through dihexyl produce lesions of the common bile duct which may extend into the liver and result in hepatic failure or peritonitis. Dioctyl tin also falls in toxicity class 3 based on mouse data, but dibutyl tin as the acetate has an oral LD_{50} of only 110 mg./kg. in the mouse. Dibutyl and lower homologues are not only more toxic than dihexyl and dioctyl, but they appear to produce central neurotoxic actions like trialkyl tin. Hens and turkeys, however, are so resistant that worm control can be achieved by feeding them dibutyltin dilaurate (Butynorate). Tetraalkyl tin compounds are probably inert in the mammal until degraded to trialkyl tin by a liver enzyme. Their effects then are identical to trialkyl tins. For Trialkyltin Compounds, see below.

Ref.: Barnes and Stoner, 1958; Barnes and Stoner, 1959; Guess et al., 1968; Pelikan and Cerny, 1970a; Pelikan and Cerny, 1970b; NIOSH, 1976.

293   Trialkyl Tin Compounds   293

e.g., Trimethyltin hydroxide, Triethyltin chloride, Tributyltin acetate, Tributyltin hydroxide, Tributyltin fluoride, Tributyltin benzoate

Toxicity Rating: 3-5. These substances are used primarily as biocides to preserve wood, paper, textiles, leather, paints, etc. In general trialkyl tin compounds are more toxic than the corresponding dialkyl derivatives and certainly more toxic than monoalkyl tin. The highest acute toxicities are found among triethyl tins, especially water-soluble forms such as the chloride, but trimethyl, tripropyl and tributyl derivatives are also dangerous. Higher homologues, such as tri-octyl tin compounds, are much less toxic, at least by the oral route. After single lethal doses of the lower homologues by mouth, illness and death may be delayed several days. Whereas various mild defects of liver and kidney function have been described in rats and mice, the most distinctive and dangerous reaction is massive interstitial edema in the white matter of the brain. The mechanism is unknown, but trialkyl tins are known to impair tissue oxygen consumption and mitochondrial ATP production. In animals large intravenous doses of urea or glycerol were effective in reducing the cerebral edema, but permanent damage from trimethyltin chloride has been observed in the hippocampus, amygdaloid nuclei and neocortex. Large doses of triethyltin sulfate have also caused para- and quadraplegia in dosed animals, presumably due to intramyelenic edema in peripheral motor nerves. Triethyl tin was inferred as the toxic contaminant in an oral medication (Stalinon) once promoted in France for various skin disorders due to bacterial infection, but the principal ingredient diethyltin diiodide has much the same toxic potential as the putative contaminant. In 1954 about 100 persons died from this medication, and many more were injured, some permanently (Alajouanine *et al.,* 1958). A toxic dose of triethyl tin in an adult person is estimated to be about 70 mg., even when consumed over a week. In the France epidemic, symptoms appeared only after a latency of about 4 days: severe headache, vomiting, photophobia, various psychic disturbances and convulsions. Surgical decompression of the brain was thought to be life-saving in some cases. Aside from surgical or osmotic decompression, no forms of therapeutic intervention are known to be effective. Scanty animal data indicate that BAL may be useful against dialkyl but not trialkyl tin. *D*-penicillamine is also said to be inactive.

Ref.: Alajouanine et al., 1958; Barnes and Stoner, 1958; Barnes and Stoner, 1959; Graham et al., 1976; NIOSH, 1976.

294   Bis(tri-*n*-butyltin) oxide   294

TBTO

Toxicity Rating: 4. The formula of this water-immiscible liquid is $[(C_4H_9)_3Sn]_2O$. Used in many industrial processes to control slime, fungi or bacteria (*e.g.*, wood and textile preservative, biocide in antifouling boat paints). Acute oral LD_{50} in rats 194 mg./kg. Not significantly more toxic if given in corn oil instead of water. As a general rule trialkyltin compounds are more toxic than their dialkyl homologues and show a predilection for the central nervous system, where they produce an interstitial edema. Dosed animals were depressed and had labored respirations and ataxia. Most deaths occurred on the 2nd to 4th days and were preceded by a bloody nasal discharge, bloating and areflexia. Autopsy revealed nonspecific hyperemia of the lung, irritation of the gastrointestinal tract and congestion of the kidney and adrenals. A related compound, tributyltin acetate, produced liver damage in mice as manifested by a rise in serum glutamate-pyruvate transaminase activity and prolonged hexobarbital narcosis. The dermal LD_{50} of TBTO on rabbit skin was 11.7 gm./kg. with obvious signs of systemic intoxication. In the rabbit eye it produces necrotic and ulcerative lesions of the cornea and eyelid. May produce painless burns on human skin which heal slowly without special treatment. The mechanism of trialkyl tin poisoning is unknown and treatment should be directed toward symptomatic and supportive measures. See also Trialkyl Tin Compounds above.

Ref.: Barnes and Stoner, 1958; Calley et al., 1967; Elsea and Paynter, 1958; Pelikan, 1969.

295　Triphenyltin Acetate

Fentin acetate

Toxicity Rating: 4. This compound and the corresponding hydroxide are used as agricultural fungicides, especially in Europe. The acute oral LD_{50} of the acetate in rats is 140 mg./kg. Several human poisonings from occupational exposures have been described but no deaths. Severe headache is a common symptom, as are nausea, vomiting and epigastric pain, even in respiratory exposures. Glycosuria and hyperglycemia were encountered in several victims, as was dizziness. Transient loss of consciousness occurred in 2 farmers after spraying. Two pilots operating spray-planes reported foggy or blurred vision and were later found to have enlarged livers; in one case liver abnormalities were demonstrated by function tests and biopsy. Because other pesticides were also involved (*e.g.,* manganese dithiocarbamate), these liver injuries and similar clinical examples of mild liver dysfunction (Manzo *et al.,* 1981) cannot be ascribed unequivocally to the triphenyltin. Yugoslavian workers bagging a 20% formulation of this fungicide developed irritation of the skin and mucous membranes. The reported nausea, vomiting, headache, dizziness, transient loss of consciousness and possible convulsion all suggest central neurotoxicity, but no signs of cerebral edema have been described; in this respect triaryltin may differ importantly from trialkyl tin (see Trialkyl Tin Compounds above), but the distinction may be simply a matter of dose.

Ref.: Manzo et al., 1981; NIOSH, 1976.

296　Titanium Oxide

Titanium dioxide

Toxicity Rating: 1. A pound (16 oz.) has been ingested without apparent harm or distress. It was eliminated in feces in about 24 hours.

Ref.: Deribere, 1941; Heaton, 1929.

297　Tungsten (and its Salts)

Sodium tungstate, Tungstic anhydride, Ammonium paratungstate, Tungsten metal

Toxicity Rating: 3. Although the toxicology has been investigated on several occasions, no adequate description of the acute toxic syndrome is known. Diarrhea occurs and also respiratory arrest either of central origin or secondary to circulatory collapse. Tungsten is said to be more toxic than molybdenum, a member of the same periodic family. The tungsten salts listed above represent an approximate ranking in toxicity; the most toxic, sodium tungstate, has an oral lethal dose of 223-255 mg. in rats (66-day-old animals after 24 hours of starvation), but the mortality is markedly less in the young and after prior feeding. Given subcutaneously to rats, sodium tungstate causes a severe drop in rectal temperature. Parenteral sodium tungstate is almost completely excreted in the urine within 12 hours; given by mouth, it is found in both urine and feces. The only pathology described is enlargement of kidneys and adrenals after parenteral but not oral administration. In the latter case tungsten is deposited chiefly in the bones and spleen, with smaller amounts in kidneys and liver. Perhaps it interfers with the nutritional role of molybdenum. Industrial exposures involve chiefly dust in the milling of sheelite and wolframite. Both dimercaprol and calcium disodium edetate are said to be effective in acute experimental poisonings.

Ref.: Fairhall, 1945; Higgins et al., 1956; Kinard et al., 1940; Kinard and Van de Erve, 1941; Kinard and Van de Erve, 1943; Kinard and Aull, 1945; Lusky et al., 1949; Selle, 1942; Sivjakov and Braun, 1959.

298　Uranyl Nitrate

Toxicity Rating: 3(?). Poorly absorbed by mouth. Given parenterally it is as toxic as mercury or arsenic. Produces severe kidney tubular degeneration and renal failure. See Section IV for a discussion of general treatment in this syndrome. BAL is useless. $CaNa_2EDTA$ is recommended intravenously according to the dose schedule for lead poisoning (see Edetate calcium disodium in Section III). Other water- and acid-soluble uranyl salts such as the acetate, chloride, phosphate and sulfate share the nephrotoxicity of uranyl nitrate.

Ref.: Holman, 1941; Holman and Hewitt, 1942; Lusky et al., 1949.

299　Vanadium (and its Salts)

Sodium metavanadate, Vanadium pentoxide

Toxicity Rating: 5. This industrially important metal has a toxicity of about the same magnitude as pentavalent arsenic. Rats acutely poisoned by mouth exhibit immediate distress, a hemorrhagic exudate from the nose, marked diarrhea, hindlimb paralysis, labored respirations, convulsions (perhaps asphyxial) and death. If a critical daily level is not exceeded, rats may survive cumulative doses several times larger than the single lethal dose but they develop symptoms like those described above. Animal pathology is diffuse with acute desquamative enteritis, and congestion of many organs, including liver, kidney, lung, adrenal cortex, brain, spinal cord and bone marrow. Fatty degeneration occurs in liver and kidney and sometimes focal hemorrhage in lung and adrenal cortex. A decrease in the cystine content of animal hair has been described. Poisoning from dust inhalation is fairly common in industry; it first causes respiratory symptoms: irritation of the respiratory tract and conjunctivae, fits of dry coughing, rales, acute bronchospasm, hemoptysis and a greenish black discoloration of the tongue. Systemic symptoms may develop, such as anorexia, anemia, nausea, headache, insomnia, nervousness, dizziness, derangement of kidney function, tremor, psychic disturbances and blindness. Anionic vanadium is said to be more toxic than cationic. Humans have tolerated 150 mg. of vanadium sodium tartrate intramuscularly, and 1 to 8 mg. of sodium metavanadate by mouth. Dimercaprol (BAL) exerts no apparent therapeutic benefit in vanadium poisoning, but edetate calcium disodium and disodium catechol disulfonate are both effective antidotes in animals. The former but not the latter is available for human use (see Section III).

Ref.: Braun and Lusky, 1959; Daniel and Lillie, 1938; Mitchell, 1953; Sollmann, 1957; Thomas and Stiebris, 1956; Zenz et al., 1962.

300   Sodium Zirconium Lactate

Toxicity Rating: 3. A water soluble salt of zirconium, formerly used in deodorant sticks. The oral toxicity of the compound is believed to be low. Topical applications of these deodorant sticks to abraded skin have lead to granulomas in a few susceptible persons. These granulomas were apparently of an allergic nature. The initial sensitization required four to six weeks. Subsequent challenges with sodium zirconium lactate or other soluble zirconium salts elicited granulomas after two weeks. Such granulomas generally disappeared slowly without treatment.

Ref.: Shelley and Hurley, 1958.

301   Zirconium Oxide

Zirconium dioxide, Zirconia, Baddeleyite

Toxicity Rating: 2 or 3. Zirconium dioxide is used as a pigment for paint, as an abrasive, and in crucibles and furnace linings. Ointments containing ZrO_2 are used for the treatment of poison ivy dermatitis. Instances of persistent allergic granuloma formation have been reported following the use of the oxide on abraded skin. Zirconium was recovered from the nodules in one case. The compound is slightly soluble and poorly absorbed, and its oral toxicity is therefore low. Zirconium oxide was formerly used as a radio-opaque agent in X-ray examinations of the alimentary canal. Since pulmonary granulomas have been reported in zirconium workers, an industrial threshold limit value of 0.5 mg./m^3 has been set. The usual daily dietary intake of zirconium is about 4 mg.

Ref.: Patty, 1962; Baler, 1965.

302   Zirconyl Chloride

Zirconium oxychloride, Basic zirconium chloride

Toxicity Rating: 3. A compound prepared by crystallization from aqueous solutions of zirconium tetrachloride. Both the tetrachloride and the oxychloride are poorly absorbed and therefore have low oral toxicities (LD$_{50}$'s in rats are 0.7 gm./kg. and 3.5 gm./kg. respectively). They have appreciably greater toxicity when administered by intraperitoneal injection (LD$_{50}$ in rats is 400 mg./kg. for the oxychloride). Rats given toxic doses of soluble zirconyl compounds show progressive depression and decrease of activity until death. Granuloma formation has not been reported after topical applications of the oxychloride in 54 subjects, although other soluble compounds of zirconium are known to induce granulomas of an allergic nature (see Sodium Zirconium Lactate above).

Ref.: Cochran et al., 1950; Helton et al., 1956.

Organic compounds of simple chemical structure

Saturated hydrocarbon homologues

303   Aliphatic Hydrocarbons

Toxicity Rating: 3. Saturated hydrocarbons consisting of straight chains (paraffins), branched chains (isoparaffins) or saturated rings (cycloparaffins). Most fractions are prepared largely from crude petroleum oil. Used as fuels, solvents, vehicles, and cleaners. The lower members of the paraffinic and isoparaffinic series (e.g., methane, butane, isobutane) are gases of low anesthetic potency. The liquid fractions are also central nervous depressants when absorbed from the alimentary tract, or severe pulmonary irritants when aspirated. Narcotic potency increases with the chain length at least through octane, but very long molecules like hexadecane and above (as found in liquid petrolatum and solid paraffin) are almost inert. Kerosene is representative of the toxic liquid fractions.

See also: Kerosene, *Reference Congener in Section III*.
Ref.: von Oettingen, 1940.

304   Propane

304

e.g., Bottled gas, Liquefied hydrocarbon gas, Liquid petroleum gas, LPG

A principal ingredient of bottled gas particularly in northern states, whereas butane (below) with its considerably higher boiling and freezing points is more widely used in warmer southern states. Mixtures of the two are also common. Most bottled gas also contains ethyl mercaptan, the odor of which serves as a warning for leaks. Vapor density relative to air 1.5 to 1.6. Explosive and flammability limits in air 2 to 10% (by volume). Mildly anesthetic in cats at 93%. Principal hazards are those of fire and explosion. Alleged or suspected cases of "bottled gas intoxication" are more likely due to some overlooked source of carbon monoxide.

305   Isobutane

305

2-Methylpropane

A low-pressure aerosol propellant which, along with propane (see above), has largely replaced fluorocarbons in this capacity. Vapor density is 2 relative to air. When isobutane was inhaled by rhesus monkeys in concentrations of 10 to 20%, increased pulmonary resistance and decreased respiratory minute volume were observed. At lower concentrations, such as those found in the home and in industry, no respiratory or circulatory effects were encountered in human subjects during single and multiple inhalation exposures. Presumably very high vapor concentrations can produce central nervous depression, as with other aliphatic hydrocarbons.

Ref.: Aviado and Smith, 1975; Stewart et al., 1977.

306   Butane

306

e.g., Pyrofax

A principal ingredient of "bottled gas". A mildly anesthetic gas in high concentrations. Vapor density about twice that of air. Explosive and flammability limits in air about 2 to 8% (by volume). Reasonably good anesthetic at vapor concentrations of 22-25%. Principal hazards are those of fire and explosion. See also Propane above.

Ref.: Shugaen, 1969.

307   *n*-Hexane

307

Toxicity Rating: 3. A solvent and a mild central nervous depressant in acute exposures. Acute oral LD_{50} is 24 ml./kg. in 14-day old rats and 45 ml./kg. in adult animals. Vapor causes anesthesia of short duration without sequelae. As a low-boiling liquid (69°C) it tends to vaporize when swallowed or aspirated into the tracheobronchial tree. The result can be a rapid dilution of alveolar air and a marked fall in its oxygen content, with asphyxia and consequent brain damage or cardiac arrest. The irritative pulmonary lesions occurring after the aspiration of higher homologues (e.g., octane, nonane, decane, etc.) and of mixtures thereof (e.g., kerosene) do not appear to be a problem with pentane or hexane. Incredibly the ability of *n*-hexane to produce polyneuropathy in man and many animal species escaped notice until 1969. In that year 93 affected workers were discovered in a sandal factory in Japan. The neuropathy was of the glove-and-stocking type with both sensory and motor involvement and neurogenic atrophy of skeletal muscle. *n*-Hexane has been used as a solvent and thinner for some glues and toxic neuropathies including quadraplegia have occurred among juvenile glue sniffers. It is likely that *n*-hexane and methyl *n*-butyl ketone (see latter in index) have common neurotoxic metabolites.

See also: Tri-*o*-cresyl Phosphate, *Reference Congener in Section III*.
Ref.: Altenkirch et al., 1977; Gerarde, 1963; Herskowitz et al., 1971; Kimura et al., 1971; Korobkin et al., 1975; Paulson and Waylonis, 1976; Towfighi et al., 1976; Yamamura, 1969.

308   Cyclohexane

308

Hexahydrobenzene, Hexamethylene

Toxicity Rating: 3. Vapor causes weak anesthesia of brief duration but more potent than hexane. High vapor concentrations have produced convulsions in rabbits. Toxic oral doses in rabbits led to severe diarrhea, circulatory collapse, and death, without prominent central nervous depression or anesthesia. Autopsy revealed generalized vascular damage with degenerative lesions in brain and viscera. No effects on blood formation have been described. Mildly irritating to human skin. No systemic poisonings have been reported in man.

Ref.: Amer. Petroleum Institute, 1953d; Treon et al., 1943a; Treon et al., 1943b.

309 Methylcyclohexane 309

Hexahydrotoluene, Cyclohexylmethane

Toxicity Rating: 3(?). Vapor causes brief central nervous depression like cyclohexane. Oral doses in rabbits cause mild lethargy, severe diarrhea, and circulatory collapse. Vascular and degenerative lesions are seen in kidney and liver. Perhaps slightly more toxic than cyclohexane by mouth. No systemic poisonings reported in man.

Ref.: Amer. Petroleum Institute, 1953f; Treon et al., 1943a; Treon et al., 1943b.

Aromatic hydrocarbon homologues (exclusive of naphthalene)

310 Aromatic Hydrocarbon Solvent 310

Toxicity Rating: 4. A generic term used to designate any one or any mixture of the following substances: benzene, toluene, xylenes, cumene, ethyl benzene, mesitylene, and related compounds.

See also: Xylene, *Reference Congener in Section III.*

311 Allyl Benzene 311

Phenylpropylene

Toxicity Rating: 3. Acute oral LD_{50} is 5.54 gm./kg. in rats and 2.90 gm./kg. in mice. After 60 days of daily doses of 250 or 500 mg./kg., cumulative mortalities in mice were 21% and 29%, respectively. Central nervous system depression was noted in these studies. No liver pathology. Allyl benzene is readily metabolized by rats *via* sidechain oxidation and rearrangement to yield cinnamyl alcohol, hippuric acid and Mannich base compounds, which are excreted in urine. Ring-substituted allyl benzene derivatives are found in several foods (nutmeg, parsnips, parsnips, carrots, bananas), in various natural oils and flavoring agents and in condensed cigarette smoke.

Ref.: Hagan et al., 1965; Peele and Oswald, 1977.

312 Benzene 312

Benzol

Toxicity Rating: 4. Similar to but more hazardous than xylene. In rats, the oral lethal dose places this substance on the borderline between toxicity classes 3 and 4.

See also: Xylene, *Reference Congener in Section III.*
Ref.: Spector, 1955.

313 Cumene 313

Isopropylbenzene, 2-Phenylpropane, Cumol

Toxicity Rating: 3. An industrial solvent and a component in petroleum. A central nervous depressant like xylene. In mice cumene narcosis develops more slowly and lasts longer than the depression produced by benzene or toluene. Moderate acute oral toxicity in rodents (LD_{50} 1.4 gm./ kg.). Autopsy revealed irritation of stomach and intestine. Low dermal toxicity (LD_{50} 12.3 ml./kg. in rabbit). No human poisonings are known. Produces skin and eye irritation in rabbits. Rapidly absorbed through intact skin. In rabbit, metabolized by liver to yield 2-phenyl-1-propanol and α-phenylpropionic acid. The OSHA 8-hour TWA standard is 50 ppm.

See also: Xylene, *Reference Congener in Section III.*
Ref.: Amer. Petroleum Institute, 1948c; Robinson et al., 1955; Werner et al., 1944; Wolf et al., 1956.

314 Diphenyl 314

Bibenzene, Biphenyl, Phenylbenzene, Xenene

Toxicity Rating: 3. Used as a fungistat for oranges and as a heat transfer agent. Fungistatic action attributed to inhibition of adenosine transaminase. Almost insoluble in water. Acute oral LD_{50} 3.28 gm./kg. in rats, 2.41 gm./kg. in rabbits. After single doses experimental animals showed increased rate of respirations, lacrimation, anorexia and weight loss, muscular weakness and ataxia, with death in coma occurring between 2 hours and 18 days. Pathological findings included generalized visceral congestion, myocarditis, hepatitis, nephritis and pneumonia. Dietary levels of 0.5% fed to rats for 60 days produced polyuria and reversible kidney lesions (focal tubular dilation). In a plant manufacturing fruit-wrapping papers, 33 workers were exposed chronically to high levels of biphenyl vapors and dust. One worker exposed repeatedly to concentrations as high as 123 mg./m^3 for 10 years developed first neurological and gastric symptoms, then after several months severe ascites and massive edema in the legs. Upon admission to hospital, diffuse brain damage was demonstrated by EEG. Serum transaminase levels were high. Despite symptomatic treatment, the patient's condition gradually worsened; coma and death ensued after one month. At autopsy extensive necrosis was found in liver and kidneys, with regions of cirrhosis in the liver. Degenerative changes were present in heart muscle. The brain was edematous and degeneration of ganglion cells was seen. The bone marrow appeared hyperactive with large numbers of immature white and red blood cell precursors. Twenty-two of the remaining workers complained of headache, fatigue, abdominal pain with nausea or diarrhea and various symptoms of polyneuritis. Neurological examination revealed varying degrees of damage to the central and peripheral nervous systems (decreased conduction velocities, increased sensory thresholds and EEG and EMG abnormalities). Reexamination of seven workers after 2 years showed further neural degeneration although no further exposure to diphenyl had occurred. Diphenyl is not a local irritant but is absorbed through intact skin. It is rapidly metabolized to 4-hydroxybiphenyl, 4-phenyl-catechol and 4,4'-dihydroxyphenyl, which are excreted in urine and bile as glucuronide and mercapturic conjugates. Evidence from rat feeding experiments suggests that L-cysteine and DL-methionine may have a protective action against chronic diphenyl poisoning, perhaps by facilitating detoxication. No specific antagonists to the acute toxic effects are known.

Ref.: Booth et al., 1961; Deichmann et al., 1947; Hakkinen et al., 1973; Seppalainen and Hakkinen, 1975; West et al., 1956.

315   315   Styrene

Vinylbenzene, Phenylethylene, Cinnamene

Toxicity Rating: 3(?). Important intermediate in chemical syntheses and widely used in the manufacture of plastics, synthetic rubber and resins. Acute oral LD$_{50}$ estimated in rats to be about 5 gm./kg. Direct contact with liquid styrene produces drying and cracking of the skin. Most clinical and experimental observations have concerned respiratory exposures. Primary irritant to mucosal surfaces at vapor concentrations above 200 ppm, but pungent odor usually gives adequate warning. Exposed animals exhibit respiratory tract irritation (pulmonary edema in guinea pigs after 40 hours in 1300 ppm), central nervous depression, cardiac arrhythmias, and renal and hepatic damage. The two latter effects are said to occur also after ingestion, but if aspiration occurs, the chief hazard is probably chemical pneumonitis. "Styrene sickness" is not uncommon in industry after exposure to vapors or mists; characteristic signs and symptoms include headache, fatigue, weakness, depression and unsteadiness or feeling of drunkenness. Many patients have exhibited abnormal electroencephalograms. At least one case of toxic retrobulbar neuritis has been reported. Peripheral neuropathies (distal hypesthesia and decreased nerve conduction velocities) have been observed in chronically exposed workers. Metabolized in liver *via* styrene oxide to yield mandelic and phenylglyoxylic acids, which are excreted in urine. The acute oral toxicity of styrene oxide is about one-fourth that of the parent compound. Metabolism is suppressed by the administration of toluene. Styrene may accumulate in adipose tissue during repeated industrial exposure. No reports of hematological disturbances. The OSHA 8-hour TWA for industrial exposure is 100 ppm.

See also: Xylene, *Reference Congener in Section III.*
Ref.: Engstrom et al., 1978; Gerarde, 1960; Harkonen, 1979; Lilis et al., 1978; Lorimer et al., 1976; Pratt-Johnson, 1964; Rosen et al., 1978.

316   316   Terphenyl

Polyphenyls, e.g., Santowax OM

Toxicity Rating: 2 to 3. Used as a heat transfer agent in nuclear reactors and solar heating systems. Usually available as a mixture of the three possible isomers o-, m- and p-, where the structural designation refers to the positions of two substituent phenyl groups on a central benzene ring. Santowax OM is 64% o-terphenyl, 25% m-terphenyl, 6% p-terphenyl and 5% diphenyl (see latter above). Acute oral LD$_{50}$'s in rats: o-terphenyl 1.9, m-terphenyl 2.4 and p-terphenyl greater than 10 gm./kg. The latter appears to be poorly absorbed and largely excreted unchanged in the feces. The major metabolites of o- and m-terphenyl are free phenols and their glucuronic acid conjugates. Feeding studies in animals suggest that repeated doses decrease hemoglobin levels and produce liver and kidney damage. All were highly damaging to guinea pig skin (sensitization, necrosis) on intracutaneous injection. In laboratory animals, the inhalation of aerosols of o- and m-isomers produced death with acute tracheal necrosis, tracheobronchitis, pulmonary edema, bronchopneumonia, atelectasis and petechial hemorrhages. Workers exposed to dust and fumes at concentrations greater than 10 mg./

m³ experienced eye and respiratory tract irritation. The OSHA 8-hour TWA standard for industrial exposure is 1 ppm (9.4 mg./m³).

See also: Xylene, *Reference Congener in Section III.*
Ref.: Cornish et al., 1962; Haley et al., 1959a; Petkau and Hoogstraten, 1965.

317 Toluene   317

Methyl benzene, Toluol

Toxicity Rating: 4. Toxicity is very similar to that of xylene. High concentrations produce headache, nausea and narcosis. Metabolic acidosis has been observed. Toluene may produce a mild macrocytic anemia but no leukopenia (as benzene does). Repeated heavy exposure has led to encephalopathies (cerebellar ataxia, cognitive dysfunction) in humans. Primary urinary metabolites are hippuric acid and *o*-cresol.

See also: Xylene, *Reference Congener in Section III.*
Ref.: Boor and Hurtig, 1977; Fischman and Oster, 1979; von Oettingen, 1940.

318 Xylene   318

Xylol, Dimethylbenzene

Toxicity Rating: 4.

See also: Xylene, *Reference Congener in Section III.*

Naphthalene and its hydrocarbon derivatives

319 Decahydronaphthalene   319

Decalin

Toxicity Rating: 3(?). Dermatitis and conjunctival irritation. Systemic toxicity is not well defined but no serious industrial poisonings are known. Less toxic than tetrahydronaphthalene in rats; see latter below. Vapor exposures in guinea pigs cause cataracts and kidney lesions.

Ref.: Browning, 1953.

320 Methyl Naphthalene   320

Toxicity Rating: 3(?). Presumably less toxic than naphthalene. The only untoward effects reported in man are skin irritation and skin photosensitization.

See also: Naphthalene, *Reference Congener in Section III.*
Ref.: Gerarde, 1960.

321 Naphthalene   321

Naphthalin, Naphthene, Tar camphor

Toxicity Rating: 3 or 4. The most abundant single constituent of coal tar. Used as a moth repellent and insecticide, formerly as an intestinal anthelmintic, and as a raw material in many chemical syntheses. Moderate acute oral toxicity (rat LD_{50} 1.8 gm./kg.). Ingestion or prolonged inhalation produces nausea, vomiting, and disorientation. Delayed acute intravascular hemolysis in sensitive persons is characteristic. Liquid, vapor and dust are irritating to skin and eyes, and prolonged vapor exposure has led to cataract formation in humans. The OSHA 8-hour TWA standard for industrial exposure is 10 ppm. Naphthalene is sometimes called tar camphor, not to be confused with gum camphor or camphor.

See also: Naphthalene, *Reference Congener in Section III.*

322 Tetrahydronaphthalene   322

Tetralin, Tetranap

Toxicity Rating: 3. A degreasing agent used as a solvent for waxes, oils and fats. The oral LD_{50} in rats is 2.86 gm./kg. In man vapors are known to produce headache, nausea, vomiting, irritation of conjunctiva and of respiratory tract mucosa. High concentrations produce narcosis. Absorbed vapor is excreted by kidneys as α- and β-tetrahydronaphthols and their glucuronides, giving urine a grass-green color. Cataract formation and nephritic lesions are seen in guinea pigs after vapor exposure. Highly cytotoxic in vitro.

See also: Xylene, *Reference Congener in Section III.*
Ref.: Drayer and Reidenberg, 1973; Gerarde, 1960; Holmberg and Malmfors, 1974.

Kerosene-like hydrocarbon mixtures

323   323   Petroleum Distillate

Toxicity Rating: 3. Any one of many fractions varying from petroleum ether to lubricating oils. Major fractions of crude petroleum in order are: petroleum ether (benzine), gasoline, kerosene, fuel oil, lubricating oils (and mineral oil, etc.), paraffin wax, and asphalt or tar (pitch, coke). For more information, consult this index under name of each fraction. All fractions (when impure) tend to produce local skin irritation and rarely skin photosensitization. The latter is revealed by prickling and erythema shortly after exposure to sunlight, often followed by pigmentation.

See also: Kerosene, *Reference Congener in Section III.*
Ref.: Gerarde, 1962; von Oettingen, 1940.

324   324   Deobase

Toxicity Rating: 3. A highly purified kerosene. Deodorized but still toxic. Unsaturated and aromatic compounds have been largely removed.

See also: Kerosene, *Reference Congener in Section III.*

325   325   Diesel Oil

Diesel fuel

Toxicity Rating: 3. A complex mixture of paraffinic, olefinic, naphthenic (cycloparaffinic) and aromatic hydrocarbons (C_{11} and higher) boiling over the range 350 to 750° F (177 to 400° C). Paraffins predominate, but aromatics content can be as high as 30 to 35%.

See also: Kerosene, *Reference Congener in Section III.*
Ref.: Gerarde, 1962.

326   326   Fuel Oil

Gas oil, "Distillate", Home heating oil no. 2

Toxicity Rating: 3. A petroleum fraction consisting of a complex mixture of hydrocarbons (C_9 and higher) boiling over the range 325 to 650°F (163 to 344°C). Essentially the same as diesel oil above. Slightly less volatile and more viscous than kerosene but shares the same toxic potential.

See also: Kerosene, *Reference Congener in Section III.*
Ref.: Gerarde, 1962.

327   327   Gasoline

Toxicity Rating: 3. A mixture chiefly of C_5 to C_{12} aliphatic hydrocarbons obtained as a petroleum distillate, often after "cracking" heavy fractions. Boiling point range is approximately 40 to 225°C. Tetraethyl lead content is not of toxic significance in acute exposures by ingestion or inhalation, but persons who are careless about repeated and massive skin contact have developed lead poisoning (See Lead in Section III). No nonpetroleum additives are believed to be significantly toxic as present in commercial formulations. Appreciable amounts of aromatic hydrocarbons (e.g., xylenes) are found in commercial fuels, especially when the petroleum is from Texas and California (but not from eastern U.S. fields). A high content of aromatic hydrocarbons and a consequent high toxicity are also associated with a high "octane rating" (whenever the latter is not due to additives, such as tetraethyl lead or alcohol). Gasoline has been used by sniffers to produce euphoria.

See also: Kerosene, *Reference Congener in Section III.*
Ref.: Ainsworth, 1960; Easson, 1962; Machle, 1941; White, 1955.

328   328   Kerosene

Kerosine, Range oil, Home heating oil no. 1

Toxicity Rating: 3. Prepared by the fractional distillation of petroleum. Boiling point range is 347 to 617°F (175 to 325°C). Consists chiefly of C_{10}-C_{16} hydrocarbons of the methane series, together with a small fraction of aromatic compounds (xylenes, etc.) and of saturated rings (naphthenes). Individual compositions vary widely, depending on the source.

See also: Kerosene, *Reference Congener in Section III.*

329 Mineral Seal Oil   329

Signal oil

Toxicity Rating: 3. Constituent of many furniture polishes (especially the red ones). Light petroleum oil obtained as a fraction of distillate from crude petroleum in the range of 260 to 370°C. The unsaturated aliphatic components are largely removed so that the resulting product consists mainly of saturated aliphatic compounds of a higher molecular weight than gasoline or kerosene, with the usual proportion of cyclic and branched chain compounds. This mixture is reputed to be more toxic and more irritating to the tracheobronchial tree than kerosene. Methemoglobinemia has occurred in men who washed roller bearings in mineral seal oil and was attributed to a 0.5% concentration of 2-anilinoethanol in the oil used.

See also: Kerosene, *Reference Congener in Section III.*
Ref.: Bass et al., 1943; Griffin et al., 1954; Sax, 1957.

330 Petroleum Ether   330

Petroleum benzin, Petroleum benzine, Benzin or benzine, Light ligroin

Toxicity Rating: 3. Not to be confused with benzene. A petroleum distillate consisting principally of *n*-pentane and *n*-hexane, with a boiling point range of 35 to 80°C (95 to 176°F), although the limits are sometimes extended to 30 to 90°C. Petroleum ether (and any of its synonyms) may also refer to narrower "cuts" within the range specified above. Reference is sometimes made to a "high-boiling petroleum ether", distilling between 80 and 130°C. All of these solvents are more volatile than kerosene. Like kerosene, petroleum ether may cause central nervous depression, but it probably does not share the high liability of kerosene to induce pneumonitis when aspirated. Because of its high volatility ingested or aspirated petroleum ether is expected to vaporize quickly. In rats the result of aspiration is a rapid displacement of oxygen from the lungs and consequent profound anoxia with cardiac arrest and/or brain damage.

See also: Kerosene, *Reference Congener in Section III.*
Ref.: Gerarde, 1962; Merck and Co., 1976.

331 Petroleum Naphtha   331

Toxicity Rating: 3. A general term describing petroleum distillates that consist of various mixtures of predominately aliphatic (straight-chain or paraffinic) hydrocarbons (C_5 to C_{13}) boiling over the range 86 to 460°F (30 to 238°C). In the lower boiling range are petroleum ether and rubber solvent, in the mid-range the VM&P naphthas, and in the higher range Stoddard solvent. Thus petroleum naphtha may refer to any cut more volatile than kerosene, but the word "naphtha" alone is sometimes used as a synonym for petroleum ether; see latter above. All of these liquids are similar in toxicity to kerosene, although the most volatile fractions may induce cardiac death rather than pulmonary irritation.

See also: Kerosene, *Reference Congener in Section III.*
Ref.: Gerarde, 1962.

332 Residual Oils   332

Bunker fuel oils, Fuel oil no. 4, Fuel oil no. 5

These are generally blends of various residual oils (portion of the crude petroleum which is not vaporized by heating and is withdrawn from the still in liquid form) and lighter diluent oils from various units in a refinery, having a boiling range of about 400 degrees F (204°C) and higher. These oils contain thousands (if not millions) of hydrocarbons of varying complexity. They are available in a wide range of viscosities (e.g., fuel oils no. 4, 5, and 6). In general they are more viscous and less toxic than kerosene.

See also: Kerosene, *Reference Congener in Section III.*
Ref.: Gerarde, 1962.

333 Rubber Solvent   333

"Lacquer diluent", Rubber solvent naphtha

Toxicity Rating: 3. A name used in the petroleum industry for a petroleum "cut" distilling between 100 and 300°F (38 to 149°C) and consisting chiefly of C_5 to C_9 aliphatic (paraffinic) hydrocarbons. Somewhat less volatile than petroleum ether. One precisely characterized solvent from a major American producer distilled between 168 and 234°F; it consisted of 41% paraffins (C_6 and C_7), 54% cycloparaffins, 3.4% alkylbenzenes and 1.5% benzene (Carpenter *et al.,* 1975c). Cats were depressed but survived a 4-hour vapor exposure to 12,000 ppm.

See also: Kerosene, *Reference Congener in Section III.*
Ref.: Carpenter et al., 1975c; Gerarde, 1962.

334   334   Stoddard Solvent

White spirits, Safety solvent naphtha, Mineral spirits no. 10, High flash naphtha

Toxicity Rating: 3. One of the higher-boiling fractions of petroleum naphtha. Consists of a mixture of straight and branched chain paraffinic hydrocarbons (C_9 to C_{12}), naphthenes (cycloparaffins) and higher aromatics, boiling in the range of 305 to 410°F (152 to 210°C). Usually mineral spirits no. 10 and Stoddard solvent are considered as synonymous names, but if a distinction is made, the former has a slightly lower boiling point range than the latter within the specifications above. (When unqualified, the term mineral spirits refers to a distinctly more volatile "cut" which resembles ligroin.) These various fractions are used as dry cleaner solvents and sometimes as paint thinners. They closely resemble kerosene in toxicity. One precisely characterized solvent from a major American producer distilled between 307 and 382°F; it consisted of 48% paraffins, 38% cycloparaffins, 14% alkylbenzene and 0.1% benzene. Inhalation of 1400 ppm (substantial saturation at 25°C) killed some rats and cats within 8 hours. Only slight eye irritation in humans during 15 minutes at 150 ppm.

See also: Kerosene, *Reference Congener in Section III.*
Ref.: Carpenter et al., 1975b; Gerarde, 1962.

335   335   VM&P Naphthas

Varnish makers' and painters' naphtha, Mineral spirits, Ligroin, Refined solvent naphtha

Toxicity Rating: 3. Any of several petroleum "cuts" distilling between about 200 and 350°F (94 to 175°C), consisting chiefly of C_7 to C_{10} aliphatic (paraffinic) hydrocarbons. The terminology for these fractions is inconstant and misleading. For example, in commerce there are available at least three VM&P naphthas with different flash points and somewhat different boiling point ranges within the limits specified above. The terms ligroin and refined solvent naphtha often refer to a fraction restricted to C_8 and C_9 hydrocarbons with a boiling point range of about 265 to 310°F (130 to 155°C). Furthermore the name ligroin is sometimes used inappropriately to refer to "light ligroin", which is synonymous with petroleum ether (see latter above). All of these solvents are more volatile than kerosene but share its toxic potential. One precisely characterized solvent from a major American producer distilled between 244 and 301°F; it consisted of 55% paraffins, 33% cycloparaffins, 12% alkylbenzenes, and 0.1% benzene (Carpenter *et al.,* 1975a). Air containing saturated vapors of this product (about 15000 ppm) could not be inhaled for more than a few minutes without jeopardizing the survival of test animals. During a 15-minute inhalation period, 3 (or 4) of 7 human subjects had upper respiratory tract irritation and eye irritation at 880 ppm.

See also: Kerosene, *Reference Congener in Section III.*
Ref.: Carpenter et al., 1975a; Gerarde, 1962; Merck and Co., 1976; Sax, 1968.

Other hydrocarbon mixtures derived from petroleum and oil

336   336   Petroleum (Crude)

As taken from the ground, petroleum is a complex mixture of hydrocarbons containing mainly paraffins (saturated, straight chains), and some isoparaffins (saturated, branched chains), naphthenes (cycloparaffins) and aromatics, with molecular weights ranging from the very lightest to over 6000. Depending on the origin of the crude oil, the nature of these hydrocarbons varies over wide limits. Also present and varying with the source (but seldom exceeding 10%) are: oxygen compounds (naphthenic acids, alcohols, ketones, aromatic acids, esters and phenols, and very high molecular weight cyclic compounds of resinous or asphaltic character containing both oxygen and sulfur); sulfur compounds (elemental sulfur, H_2S, mercaptans, disulfides, thiophenes and thioethers); nitrogen compounds (basic and nonbasic nitrogen compounds present in traces and probably derived from proteins in materials from which petroleum was formed); traces of metal salts.

Ref.: Gerarde, 1962.

337   337   Liquid Petrolatum

Toxicity Rating: 1. The official USP name for a mixture of refined liquid hydrocarbons of high viscosity. Also known as white mineral oil and closely related to the semisolid hydrocarbon mixture known as white petrolatum or white petroleum jelly. All of these materials are prepared by refining cruder lubricating oils to remove unsaturated or volatile compounds, as well as resins and compounds of nitrogen and sulfur. Liquid petrolatum consists largely of saturated aliphatic (C_{14} to C_{18}) and cyclic hydrocarbons. These products vary somewhat in viscosity and other physical proper-

Ref.: Osol and Farrar, 1955.

ties (e.g., boiling point range from 400 to 1000°F). When ingested they produce a mild laxative effect. Not absorbed but may inhibit the absorption of digestible lipids.

338 Lubricating Oils

Toxicity Rating: 2(?). Mixtures of hydrocarbons which vary in chemical composition and in viscosity, all derived from crude petroleum, together with low concentrations of nonpetroleum additives. The oils are composed of straight and branched chain aliphatic (paraffinic), naphthenic (cycloparaffinic), aromatic, and polyaromatic hydrocarbons, with molecules larger than C_{16} and with boiling points ranging from about 575 to 1100 ° F. Lubricants prepared from residual oils may have fractions with

Ref.: Gerarde, 1962.

boiling points as high as 1500° F. The acute ingestion toxicity of lubricating oils and greases is believed to be low. Inhalation of dense oil mists may lead to lipoid pneumonia. Frequent and prolonged skin contact may produce acneform lesions; occasionally dermatitis due to hypersensitivity occurs. Chronic skin contact has resulted rarely in carcinoma. Under special circumstances oil additives may have toxicological significance. See *o*-Tricresyl Phosphate and Barium Sulfonate in the index.

339 Naphthenes

Naphthenic oils

Sometimes used as a synonym of naphthalene but not usually in industry or commerce. In petroleum industry "naphthenes" mean saturated (or nearly saturated) cyclic hydrocarbons like methyl-substituted cyclohexanes and larger polycyclic rings. Small quantities are found in most of the aliphatic petroleum fractions (like kerosene) but much more

Ref.: von Oettingen, 1940.

is present in aromatic fractions (like crude xylol). Because they are rarely (if ever) prepared free from benzene, etc., the toxicity of petroleum naphthenes is unknown, but cycloparaffins, in general, are central nervous depressants. See index for names of specific examples.

340 Paraffin Wax(es)

Toxicity Rating: 1. Predominately long straight-chain saturated hydrocarbons (C_{20} to C_{32}) prepared from the residue after distillation of petroleum and

Ref.: Gerarde, 1962.

subjected to varying degrees and methods of refining. Not digested and not absorbed. See also Liquid petrolatum above.

341 Anthracene Oil

Toxicity Rating: 3(?). A high boiling fraction of coal tar, consisting of anthracene, phenanthrene, and other solid hydrocarbons, as well as acridine. Anthracene and phenanthrene have low acute oral toxicities in rats but no exact estimate of the LD_{50} was located. The acute toxicity of the oil is presumably due mostly to phenolic derivatives, the amounts of which are probably small. Acridine is

also irritating to skin and mucous membranes and may lead to photosensitization. See Acridine in the index. Although pure anthracene itself is but weakly carcinogenic, the anthracene oil of commerce may contain a variety of higher molecular weight compounds having appreciable carcinogenic activity. Skin cancers in man have been ascribed to these constituents of coal tar.

342 Aromatic Solvent Naphtha

Toxicity Rating: 4. A mixture of inconstant composition prepared from the distillation of coal (sometimes from petroleum in current practice.) Contains xylenes, ethyl benzene, cumene, and perhaps toluene. Traces of benzene and of pyridine

See also: Xylene, *Reference Congener in Section III.*
Ref.: Amer. Petroleum Institute, 1953b.

derivatives may be present. Inhalation hazard is less than that of benzene or of toluene because of lower volatility. Ingestion toxicity is like that of xylene.

343   343   Asphalt

Mineral pitch, Bitumen

A complex thermoplastic mixture of high molecular weight hydrocarbons with small amounts of sulfur, nitrogen and oxygen compounds, prepared from the residue after the distillation of petroleum. Consists mainly of saturated compounds (naphthenic or cycloparaffinic), aromatic compounds (single ring structures with long side chains and other condensed ring systems averaging 3 rings with shorter side chains and dimers of these molecules connected by saturated rings or chains), and asphaltenes (high molecular weight, highly condensed ring compounds in the range of 2000 and upward).

Ref.: Gerarde, 1962.

Monohalogenated methanes

344   344   Methyl Bromide

Monobromomethane, Bromomethane

Volatile liquid (boiling point 4.6°C.) used in degreasing wool, nuts, seeds and flowers. A fumigant used for the control of insects in grain and soil. Has been used as a refrigerant and in fire extinguishers. Almost odorless; chloropicrin is sometimes added to provide a warning odor. Responsible for many human poisonings by inhalation. Produces brain, liver and kidney damage. Massive exposure may lead to pulmonary edema. The maximum short-term industrial exposure allowed under OSHA regulations is 20 ppm. Decomposes in presence of open flames with release of hydrogen bromide, a strong respiratory tract irritant (Miller et al., 1961); the latter may linger in houses improperly fumigated with methyl bromide.

See also: Methyl Bromide, *Reference Congener in Section III.*
Ref.: Miller et al., 1961.

345   345   Methyl Chloride

Monochloromethane

A gas of moderately high toxicity formerly used as a refrigerant gas and as an aerosol propellant, especially in products used in greenhouses. Its principal use currently is as an intermediate in various industrial syntheses. Practically non-odorous and non-irritating. Said to be hydrolyzed to hydrochloric acid and methyl alcohol in vivo, but this claim is disputed. In man signs and symptoms of acute intoxication by inhalation include abdominal pain, nausea and vomiting, blurred vision and nystagmus, tremors, spasticity, drowsiness, mental confusion and ataxia. Epileptiform convulsions, tachycardia and dyspnea have been reported. The level of consciousness may vary. Headache, nervousness, insomnia and intention tremor may persist during the recovery phase. Reversible kidney damage and jaundice are reported to have resulted from single or repeated toxic doses. Acute hemolysis has been described in two instances. Autopsies in human fatalities showed hyperemia of lungs, liver, kidney and brain, with petechial hemorrhage of pleura and pericardium. Chronic exposure to low concentrations of methyl chloride (8-hour TWA of 200 ppm) has lead to serious intoxication characterized by mental confusion, headache, blurred vision, memory disturbances, ataxia, anorexia and vomiting. Affected persons recover slowly after cessation of exposure. In one serious case characterized by polyuria and albuminuria, recovery followed prednisone therapy. Prolonged industrial exposures to concentrations of 7 to 70 ppm (average 34 ppm) produced EEG changes, tremor, and slightly reduced performance in cognitive tasks. Neurocirculatory dystrophy is described in Russian workers exposed to methyl chloride during the production of butyl rubber. In guinea pigs, daily 10-minute exposures to concentrations of 2% in air led to edema and necrosis of the granular cells of the cerebellum after 21 days. A concentration of 3150 ppm was lethal to mice. The OSHA standard for 8-hour exposure is 100 ppm. It has been suggested that methyl chloride is mutagenic, oncogenic and tetratogenic, but definitive studies in mammals are lacking. Methyl chloride forms toxic decomposition products, including phosgene, when exposed to open flames.

See also: Methyl Bromide, *Reference Congener in Section III.*
Ref.: Hartman et al., 1955; Kolkmann and Volk, 1975; Mackie, 1961; Repko and Lasley, 1979; Scharnweber et al., 1974; Spevak et al., 1976; von Oettingen, 1955; von Oettingen et al., 1949.

346   346   Methyl Iodide

Iodomethane

Toxicity Rating: 4. A liquid used as a methylating agent in industrial and laboratory settings. Closely related to methyl bromide and induces a similar toxic syndrome. About six human poisonings have been reported, in each instance due to inhalation of the vapor. Massive exposure has led to pulmonary edema, but prolonged or repeated exposures to smaller doses cause primarily central nervous effects. In man these effects include ataxia, slurred speech, blurred vision, Parkinsonian rigidity, and memory defects. Neuropsychiatric effects (depression, insomnia, paranoia, psychotic behavior) may be severe and long persisting. In one severe intoxication, a chemist producing methyl iodide complained of blurred vision, slurred speech, and staggering gait several hours after cessation of exposure. When hospitalized, he showed memory impairment and nystagmus and later became semistuporous. Following forced diuresis with i.v. saline and chlorthalidone to hasten excretion of inorganic iodide, he became more responsive, but iodide ex-

cretion was probably not the basis for this improvement. Neurologic disabilities, including Parkinsonian features of gait and expression, slowly resolved over a period of weeks. A late developing paranoic state gradually improved during the five months following discharge. Prolonged contact may cause skin burns. In rats, subcutaneous injections produced massive local sarcomas at the injection site. Methyl iodide reacts with sulfhydryl enzymes; BAL and cysteine have shown therapeutic value in the treatment of poisoned rodents. The OSHA 8-hour standard is 5 ppm. No warning odor; not irritating in concentrations causing intoxication. Said to be carcinogenic in laboratory rodents.

See also: Methyl Bromide, *Reference Congener in Section III*.
Ref.: Appel et al., 1975; Garland and Camps, 1945; Mizyukova et al., 1974.

Fluorocarbon refrigerants and propellants

347   Fluorocarbon Refrigerants and Propellants   347

Freon, Genetron, Isotron

A series of fluorinated, chlorinated hydrocarbons used as refrigerant gases and formerly as propellants in a wide variety of aerosol products and in devices to chill cocktail glasses, and sold under various trademarked names such as "Freon," "Genetron," "Kaiser," "Racon," "Isotron," etc. In contact with an open flame or a very hot surface fluorocarbons may decompose into highly irritant and toxic gases; chlorine, hydrogen fluoride or chloride, and even phosgene. (See also Nitrogen Oxides in Section III for the management of victims exposed to pulmonary irritants.) Early animal work and human experience indicated that high vapor concentrations (e.g., 20 percent) may cause confusion, pulmonary irritation, tremors and rarely· coma, but that these effects were generally transient and without late sequelae. In the 1960s a series of tragic deaths has accompanied the abuse of aerosol products containing fluorocarbons by thrill-seeking teenagers. Unhappily, most of these cases have been reported in the popular press instead of the medical literature. The propellant can be separated from the active ingredient of an

aerosol product by holding the can upside down and releasing the contents into a plastic bag, balloon, or other container (in one case a foot locker). Inhalation of fluorocarbons from the latter sometimes results in rapid exitus, but such exposures are not necessarily lethal or even harmful. Obviously the cause of death is in considerable doubt. Freezing of airway soft tissues can probably be eliminated as a cause of death except in cases where the product was sprayed directly into the mouth from its container or from a balloon containing some liquid. Laryngeal spasm or edema, oxygen displacement, or sensitization of the myocardium to endogenous catecholamines with subsequent ventricular fibrillation appear to be reasonable possibilities. It is of interest that Gerarde was able to induce a similar syndrome in rats when performing his aspiration hazard test with the more volatile alkanes (n-hexane, n-octane). Instead of the pulmonary edema induced by higher homologues (see also Kerosene in Section III) this rapid death was ascribed to cardiac arrest, respiratory paralysis and asphyxia.

Ref.: Baselt and Cravey, 1968; Gerarde, 1963; Lester and Greenberg, 1950; Sayers et al., 1930.

348   Dichlorodifluoromethane   348

Freon 12

A propellant in insect aerosol bombs. Not toxic except for lung irritation at very high vapor concentrations. If heated, thermal decomposition

products like HCl, Cl_2, HF, F_2 and phosgene are dangerous. See also Fluorocarbon refrigerants and propellants above.

Ref.: Lester and Greenberg, 1950; Sayers et al., 1930.

349   Dichloromonofluoromethane   349

Freon 21

In high concentrations, it may cause central nervous depression. If heated, thermal decomposition products like HCl, Cl_2, HF, F_2, and phosgene are

dangerous. See also Fluorocarbon refrigerants and propellants above.

350   **350** Monochlorodifluoromethane

Freon 22

A gas of low toxicity, but very high concentrations are not entirely inert. Possible lung injury. See also Fluorocarbon refrigerants and propellants above.

351   **351** Trichloromonofluoromethane

Freon 11

A gas of low toxicity but not entirely inert. Said to have been the most widely used aerosol propellant before that use was banned, but it has the highest degree of cardiotoxicity in monkeys. See Fluorocarbon refrigerants and propellants above.

352   **352** 1,2-Dichloro-1,1,2,2-tetrafluoroethane

Freon 114

Vapor may cause mild and usually transient central nervous depression. Perhaps slightly more toxic than methane analogue. See also Fluorocarbon refrigerants and propellants above.

353   **353** Trichlorofluoroethane

Freon 113

A gas of low toxicity but not entirely inert. See Fluorocarbon refrigerants and propellants above.

Chlorinated hydrocarbon solvents derived from methane (exclusive of above)

354   **354** Chlorinated Hydrocarbons

The chlorinated hydrocarbon solvents are best typified by carbon tetrachloride, whereas the chlorinated hydrocarbon insecticides are best exemplified by DDT. The typical toxic effects are strikingly different. The chlorinated solvents are liver and kidney poisons and central nervous depressants, whereas DDT and congeners are convulsants.

Chlorinated solvents may be of the aliphatic series (e.g., methylene chloride, chloroform, carbon tetrachloride, trichloroethylene, trichloroethanes, etc.) or of the aromatic series (chlorobenzene, o-dichlorobenzene, etc.). See index for individual entries.

See also: DDT *and* Carbon Tetrachloride, *Reference Congeners in Section III.*

355   **355** Carbon Tetrachloride

Tetrachloromethane, Perchloromethane

Toxicity Rating: 4. Man appears to be unusually susceptible to poisoning by carbon tetrachloride.

In most laboratory animals the toxicity rating is 2.

See also: Carbon Tetrachloride, *Reference Congener in Section III.*

356   **356** Chlorobromomethane

Monochloromonobromomethane, Bromochloromethane

Toxicity Rating: 4. A liquid used as a fire extinguisher. Its toxicity to man has not been evaluated, but by analogy to carbon tetrachloride, the oral toxicity of chlorobromomethane is assumed to be higher in man than in most laboratory animals. In dogs, acute exposures to high concentrations (50% in O_2) produced agitation, cardiac arrhythmias, myocardial sensitization to epinephrine, and epileptiform convulsions within 12 minutes. Three men exposed to concentrated vapors of the compound and its pyrolysis products experienced headache, nausea and stomach cramps, progressing to coma with convulsions in one and apnea in another. All survived with supportive care, although one reported daily headaches continuing for 3 months. All reported weight loss in spite of adequate food intake. No hepatic or renal damage was evident, although both liver and renal injuries have been noted in exposed laboratory animals. Like other dihalogenated methanes, a small fraction of the inhaled dose was converted in rats to carbon monoxide; during rebreathing in a closed system, a high portion of the absorbed dose was so metabolized. Precautions should also be taken to avoid inhaling the decomposition products (hydrogen chloride, hydrogen bromide and bromine gases) evolved by contact with fire. OSHA standard (8-hour TWA) 200 ppm.

See also: Carbon Tetrachloride, *Reference Congener in Section III.*
Ref.: Comstock et al., 1953; Kubic et al., 1974; Rodkey and Collison, 1977; Rutstein, 1963; Stevens et al., 1980; Van Stee and Back, 1969.

357   Chloroform

357

Trichloromethane

Toxicity Rating: 3. Several times more potent than carbon tetrachloride as a depressant of the central nervous system, but clinical experience suggests that it is less toxic than carbon tetrachloride when swallowed. Even the ingestion of 6 oz. has been survived, although as little as a teaspoonful has produced a serious illness. Mean lethal dose probably lies near 1 fl. oz. (44 gm.).

See also: Carbon Tetrachloride, *Reference Congener in Section III.*
Ref.: Fote, 1960; Heilbrunn et al., 1945; Lunt, 1953.

358   Methylene Bromide

358

Dibromomethane

Toxicity Rating: 3(?). Presumably similar to methylene chloride (below). Among the dihalomethanes known to be metabolized to carbon monoxide in rats, resulting in elevated blood carboxyhemoglobin levels.

See also: Carbon Tetrachloride, *Reference Congener in Section III.*
Ref.: Kubic et al., 1974; Rodkey and Collison, 1977; Stevens et al., 1980.

359   Methylene Chloride

359

Dichloromethane

Toxicity Rating: 3. Volatile liquid used as a paint remover, degreasing solvent, aerosol propellant, and grain fumigant. One of the least toxic of the chlorinated hydrocarbons, but it may produce central nervous depression. Human fatalities have occurred. In one case, oral ingestion of one to two pints of paint remover containing methylene chloride produced coma, hyporeflexia, gross hemoglobinuria, epiglottal edema and metabolic acidosis. The presence of intravascular hemolysis was inferred. Treatment consisted of forced diuresis with i.v. saline and hydrocortisone therapy. Subsequent investigation revealed gastrointestinal hemorrhage and ulceration of the duodenojejunal junction with eventual formation of diverticula. No cardiac, hepatic or brain damage was observed. Another patient, 24-weeks pregnant at the time of ingestion, experienced coma, shock, and metabolic acidosis, but she recovered and delivered a healthy term baby. Symptoms of intoxication in experimental animals are agitation, tremors and dyspnea, followed by narcosis and death. Autopsy revealed edema of the lungs, cloudy swelling of kidneys and incipient yellow atrophy of the liver. In humans, exposure to 2300 ppm for 30 minutes is said to cause nausea and narcosis. In rats, continuous inhalation of 44 mg./m^3 (approx. 13 ppm) led to decreased neuromuscular excitability, hypertrophy of the hepatic reticuloendothelial system and renal disturbances after 10 weeks. Exposure of Rhesus monkeys to vapor concentrations of 2.5 to 5 volumes percent caused tachycardia and hypotension. Inhalation of similar concentrations caused cardiac arrhythmias in rat, dog and monkey, especially when challenged with epinephrine. Readily absorbed through intact skin. Dermal contact for 2 minutes led to severe pain and paresthesias in the affected region. Treatment of intoxication is symptomatic. Metabolized in rats and humans to carbon monoxide with concomitant formation of carboxyhemoglobin, which in persons with an impaired cardiovascular status could prove dangerous. The OSHA standard for eight-hour industrial exposure is 500 ppm; the odor threshold is said to be 15 mg./m^3 (approx. 4.4 ppm).

See also: Carbon Tetrachloride, *Reference Congener in Section III.*
Ref.: Aviado and Smith, 1975; Belej et al., 1974; Heppel et al., 1944; Hughes, 1954; Moskowitz and Shapiro, 1952; Ratney et al., 1974; Roberts and Marshall, 1976; Stewart and Dodd, 1964; Stewart et al., 1972.

360   Methylene Iodide

360

Diiodomethane

Toxicity Rating: 3(?). Used to separate mixtures of minerals and as an intermediate in iodination reactions. Presumably similar to methylene chloride (above). Among the dihalomethanes known to be metabolized in rats to carbon monoxide resulting in elevated blood carboxyhemoglobin levels.

See also: Carbon Tetrachloride, *Reference Congener in Section III.*
Ref.: Kubic et al., 1974; Rodkey and Collison, 1977; Stevens et al., 1980.

Halogenated hydrocarbon derivatives of ethane (exclusive of above)

361   361   Acetylene Dichloride

1,2-Dichloroethylene, *sym*-Dichloroethylene, 1,2-Dichloroethene, Dioform

Toxicity Rating: 3. Industrial solvent composed of 60% cis and 40% trans isomers. The trans-isomer, being a "universal solvent", is more widely used in industry than either the cis-isomer or the mixture. Acetylene dichloride is less toxic than ethylene dichloride (see below). The acute oral rat LD_{50} is 0.60 ml./kg.; for the trans-isomer the LD_{50} is 1.0 ml./kg. Vapor exposure may produce central nervous depression or, in milder exposures, nausea, vomiting, weakness, tremor, and epigastric cramps. Recovery is usually rapid. Intravenous injection of calcium gluconate has relieved the cramps and vomiting. Reversible corneal clouding is described. In rats, single and repeated inhalation exposures to 200 ppm of the separate isomers led to temporary inhibition of the mixed-function oxidase system (MFO), fatty infiltration of the liver and morphological alterations of the lungs. At this concentration the cis-isomer, which was more readily taken up by liver tissue, was a more potent inhibitor of rat liver MFO, whereas at higher concentrations the trans-isomer was twice as strong a CNS depressant (rats and humans). The OSHA air standard for the workplace is 200 ppm.

See also: Carbon Tetrachloride, *Reference Congener in Section III*.
Ref.: Freundt et al., 1977; Freundt and Macholz, 1978; McBirney, 1955.

362   362   1-Bromo-2-chloroethane

Ethylene chlorobromide

Toxicity Rating: 4. Toxic actions inferred from those of ethylene dichloride below. Hazardous by all routes, including percutaneous absorption. May produce anesthesia and liver and kidney injuries. No human poisonings recorded.

See also: Carbon Tetrachloride, *Reference Congener in Section III*.
Ref.: von Oettingen, 1955.

363   363   Chlorasol

Toxicity Rating: 4. Said to contain 75% ethylene dichloride and 25% carbon tetrachloride. See Ethylene dichloride below.

See also: Carbon Tetrachloride, *Reference Congener in Section III*.

364   364   1,2-Dibromoethane

EDB, Ethylene dibromide, Ethylene bromide

Toxicity Rating: 4. A volatile liquid used in leaded gasoline and as a soil and grain fumigant. Also used in control of termites and pine bark beetles. Not the same as ethyl bromide. A severe irritant. Liquid on skin causes blisters if evaporation is delayed (as by clothing). Inhalation causes delayed pulmonary lesions. After short exposure to very high concentrations, drowsiness occurs, but central nervous depression is not as marked as with the dichloride. Death appears to be due to respiratory or circulatory failure, complicated by pulmonary edema. Fatal acute intoxications are rare since fume concentrations great enough to cause serious illness in short exposures have a definite and sickening odor (odor threshold: 25 ppm). In a human fatality following ingestion of 4.5 ml. of EDB, the initial toxic symptoms were vomiting and diarrhea, tachypnea and agitation. The patient became anuric after 2 days and died 4 hours after hospital admission. Autopsy revealed moderate lung congestion and edema, diffuse inflammation of gastric and intestinal mucosa, massive central lobular necrosis of the liver and patchy necrosis of the renal tubular epithelium. EDB is mutagenic (causing base-substitution errors in *Salmonella*). In intubation studies with rats and mice, it caused stomach cancer of unusually short latency in nearly all of the animals treated. Repeated inhalation of the compound has been linked to decreased fecundity and sterility in animals and man. Mixtures of EDB with carbon tetrachloride or ethylene dichloride are said to have a higher oral toxicity than EDB alone. This synergism is not seen in inhalation exposures. The OSHA standard for respiratory exposure is 20 ppm (8-hour TWA) or 30 ppm (ceiling).

See also: Carbon Tetrachloride, *Reference Congener in Section III*.
Ref.: EPA, Dec. 14, 1977; National Cancer Institute, 1978j; Olmstead, 1960; Rowe et al., 1952.

365   365   1,1-Dichloroethane

Ethylidene chloride, Ethylidene dichloride

Toxicity Rating: 3(?). A liquid used principally as a chemical intermediate and solvent. Oral LD_{50} in adult rats is about 750 mg./kg.; more toxic to immature animals. Man is presumably more sensitive. Vapor is irritating to eyes and skin. Produces narcosis in humans exposed to high vapor concentrations. In rats and dogs, repeated prolonged exposures to high concentrations (8000 to 64000 ppm) have caused pathological changes in liver and kidneys. However, 1,1-dichloroethane is significantly less potent than 1,2-dichloroethane in this regard (see Ethylene dichloride). The OSHA standard for 8-hour exposure in air is 100 ppm.

See also: Carbon Tetrachloride, *Reference Congener in Section III.*
Ref.: Hofmann et al., 1971; National Cancer Institute, 1978k.

366   1,1-Dichloroethylene   366

Vinylidene chloride, 1,1-DCE, 1,1-Dichloroethene

Toxicity Rating: 4. A liquid that serves as a monomer in the production of thermoplastics, such as Saran, and is found as a contaminant in the air of nuclear submarines and spacecraft. Narcotic at high doses. Vapor concentrations of 4000 ppm are said to induce promptly symptoms of drunkenness progressing to unconsciousness. The acute oral LD_{50} is 1550 mg./kg. in adult male rats, but man is probably more susceptible than rats to this and other chlorinated hydrocarbon solvents. Like carbon tetrachloride 1,1-DCE is hepatotoxic and nephrotoxic. After exposure to 48 ppm continuously for 90 days, liver damage was evident in monkeys, dogs and rats, and deaths occurred among monkeys and guinea pigs. In this study only rats showed evidence of renal tubular injury. Extensive hemorrhagic centrolobular liver necrosis was seen in rats 6 hours after a 4-hour exposure to 200 ppm.

The incidence and severity of liver damage were greater in fasted than fed rats and greater in female and young rats than in adult males. More hepatotoxic than other chloroethylenes to rats by inhalation or ingestion. Single oral dose of 500 mg./kg. of 1,1-DCE elicited more extensive liver enzyme changes than 1500 mg./kg. of cis- or trans- isomers of 1,2-dichloroethylene (see in index). The hepatotoxic action is similar to that of bromobenzene (see in index) in that it increases with depletion of cellular glutathione and does not involve the endoplasmic reticulum. In contrast to the related hepatotoxins vinyl chloride and carbon tetrachloride (see both in index), the extent of liver injury in rats from inhalation of 1,1-DCE is less after pretreatment with microsomal enzyme inducers. Irritating to skin and mucous membranes.

See also: Carbon Tetrachloride, *Reference Congener in Section III.*
Ref.: Andersen et al., 1980; Jenkins et al., 1972a; Reynolds et al., 1975; Short et al., 1977; Szabo et al., 1977.

367   EDE   367

Ethylene dichloride emulsion

Toxicity Rating: 3. Usually 10 to 20% emulsions with mono- and tri-ethanolamine oleates. See Ethylene dichloride below.

See also: Carbon Tetrachloride, *Reference Congener in Section III.*

368   Ethyl Chloride   368

Chloroethane

Flammable gas at room temperature. Used as topical anesthetic and refrigerant. Produces central nervous depression at high vapor concentrations (20,000 ppm). Depression is usually brief and reversible. Vapor may be irritating to mucous membranes. OSHA maximum allowable concentration for 8-hour exposures is 1000 ppm. Combustion products include phosgene, a highly toxic gas (see in this index).

See also: Carbon Tetrachloride, *Reference Congener in Section III.*
Ref.: Manufacturing Chemists' Assoc., 1953.

369   Ethylene Dichloride   369

Ethylene chloride, 1,2-Dichloroethane, EDC

Toxicity Rating: 4. A liquid used as an insecticidal fumigant in stored crops and soil. Also an intermediate in chemical synthesis, a component of leaded gasoline, a metal degreasing agent and a solvent in printing inks, adhesives, etc. The dichloroethane isomers have similar acute oral toxicities in mature rats (LD_{50}'s about 700 mg./kg.). In general the 1,2-dichloro isomer is about 5 times more toxic than the 1,1-dichloro isomer when inhaled. In man death has resulted from the ingestion of 20 to 50 ml. Ethylene dichloride is hepato- and nephro-toxic. Acute exposure also leads to central nervous depression, reduced blood pressure, and cardiac impairment. In humans, signs of intoxication are headache, nausea, vomiting, dizziness, watery stool, internal bleeding, cyanosis, weak and rapid pulse and loss of consciousness. In one human poisoning by ingestion, hypoglycemia, increased clotting time and hypercalcemia were prominent laboratory findings. Symptoms developed slowly;

death occurred after six days. Extensive necrosis of liver, kidney and adrenal glands was found at autopsy (Yodaiken and Babcock, 1973). In a second fatal ingestion, death resulted from pulmonary edema (Morozov, 1958). In survivors, recovery is slow and neurological sequelae have been described. Repeated long-term industrial inhalation exposures to concentrations of 0.05 to 0.15 mg./l. have resulted in neurological changes, anorexia, irritation of mucous membranes, liver and kidney impairments. Corneal clouding is described in poisoned dogs, and several species develop hemorrhagic necrosis of the adrenal cortex (Friedericksen-Waterhouse syndrome). In rats, radiolabeled

ethylene dichloride was excreted primarily in the urine, and the major urinary metabolites were chloroacetic acid, 5-carboxymethyl cysteine, and thiodiacetic acid. Large doses of chloroacetic acid are said to deplete liver glutathione stores, and 1,2-dichloroethane may have a similar effect. BAL and other sulfhydryl compounds (e.g., methionine) are said to have a therapeutic value in poisoned animals. Feeding studies have produced a variety of malignant tumors in experimental animals. The OSHA standard for 8-hour exposure is 50 ppm with a ceiling level of 100 ppm. The NIOSH recommended standard is 1 ppm with a 15-minute ceiling of 2 ppm. The odor threshold is 6-40 ppm.

See also: Carbon Tetrachloride, Reference Congener in Section III.
Ref.: Dorndorf et al., 1975; Heppel et al., 1945; Highman et al., 1951; Hofmann et al., 1971; Hubbs and Prusmack, 1955; Kuwabara et al., 1968; Morozov, 1958; National Cancer Institute, 1978l; National Institute for Occupational Safety and Health, 1978b; Yllner, 1971; Yodaiken and Babcock, 1973.

370   370   Hexachloroethane

Hexachloroethylene, Perchloroethane, Avlothane, Ethane hexachloride, Carbon hexachloride

Toxicity Rating: 4. A solid at room temperature, used in various industrial operations and as a veterinary anthelmintic. Prolonged oral treatment has caused kidney and liver damage in mice, rats and domestic animals. Hepatocellular carcinomas oc-

curred in rats. In humans, eye irritation and photophobia have resulted from industrial exposure to vapor; no other adverse effects were reported. The OSHA standard for occupational vapor exposure is 1 ppm (8-hour TWA).

See also: Carbon Tetrachloride, Reference Congener in Section III.
Ref.: Barsoum and Saad, 1934.

371   371   Pentachloroethane

Toxicity Rating: 4. Very hazardous. More potent central nervous effects than chloroform or even tetrachloroethane.

See also: Carbon Tetrachloride, Reference Congener in Section III.
Ref.: Wright and Schaffer, 1932.

372   372   1,1,2,2-Tetrabromoethane

Acetylene tetrabromide, TBE

Toxicity Rating: 5(?). Volatile liquid used as a solvent and in the density separation of mineral salts. Acute oral toxicity data in animals indicate that this compound may belong on the borderline between toxicity classes 3 and 4. However, a single severe human poisoning (below) suggests that man is much more sensitive, as with many other halogenated hydrocarbon solvents. It is a mild to moderate irritant in the rabbit eye and on rabbit skin. The products of heat decomposition are highly irritating to eyes and respiratory tracts. Single exposures to air saturated with TBE vapor indicate

a low acute inhalation hazard in animals. In striking contrast, a chemist working for 7.5 hours in 1 to 2 ppm TBE, with a single 10-minute exposure to about 16 ppm, was hospitalized for 9 weeks with a near-fatal liver injury which developed over several days. His initial symptoms were headache, anorexia, vomiting and stomach pains. By the fifth day after exposure, icterus, urobilinuria, bilirubinuria and monocytosis were apparent. Although animals usually exhibit prompt signs of central nervous depression, they were absent in this victim. The OSHA standard is 1 ppm (8-hour TWA).

See also: Carbon Tetrachloride, Reference Congener in Section III.
Ref.: Gray, 1950; Hollingsworth et al., 1963; van Haaften, 1969.

373   373   Tetrachloroethane

1,1,2,2-Tetrachloroethane, Acetylene tetrachloride, sym-Tetrachloroethane

Toxicity Rating: 4-5. Chemical intermediate and industrial solvent. Perhaps the most toxic of the common chlorinated hydrocarbon solvents. Readily absorbed and highly toxic by inhalation, oral and dermal routes. Acute exposure produces central nervous depression with dizziness, nervousness, incoordination, and death from respiratory

failure. Acute and chronic exposures produce jaundice, liver enlargement, fatty degeneration, hepatic necrosis, and cirrhosis. Respiratory irritation and pulmonary edema may follow inhalation exposures. Eight humans, each of whom ingested 3 ml. by mistake, became comatose and arreflexic, but recovered without sequelae. Dermal exposure leads to dryness, scaling, inflammation and purpuric rash. The compound is readily absorbed through lungs and skin. Excretion is primarily through the lungs. The current OSHA standard for industrial exposure is 5 ppm (8-hour TWA).

See also: Carbon Tetrachloride, *Reference Congener in Section III.*
Ref.: Coyer, 1944; Patty, 1962; Wilson and Brumley, 1944.

374   Tetrachloroethylene   374

Ethylene tetrachloride, Perchloroethylene

Toxicity Rating: 3. A solvent used in dry cleaning garments and degreasing metals. Widely used as an anthelmintic in veterinary medicine. Has been given by mouth therapeutically (for hookworms) to adult humans (dose 1 to 4 ml.). Less toxic than carbon tetrachloride or chloroform, but acute hepatic necrosis and oliguric uremia have followed human exposure. Vapors are irritating to skin, eyes and upper respiratory tract. The odor detection limit is said to be 50 ppm. Inhalation exposure produces giddiness, headache, inebriation, nausea and vomiting, sinus inflammation and narcosis. Massive vapor exposure may produce death by respiratory arrest. Brief immersion of hands in the liquid usually causes only mild skin irritation, but percutaneous absorption has been demonstrated in man. Low solubility in water and poorly absorbed from the gastrointestinal tract in the absence of fats or oils. Tetrachloroethylene caused a high incidence of liver cancer in mice when given by mouth at a rate of 386 mg./kg. per day for 78 weeks. The compound is stored in fatty tissue and slowly metabolized with loss of chlorine. The biological half-life of the urinary metabolites in humans is 144 hours. The current OSHA standard for occupational exposures is 100 ppm (8-hour TWA).

See also: Carbon Tetrachloride, *Reference Congener in Section III.*
Ref.: Anon., 1949; Hughes, 1954; Stewart et al., 1961; Stewart and Dodd, 1964.

375   Trichloroethylene   375

Trichloroethene, TCE, Acetylene trichloride, Ethinyl trichloride, e.g., Trilene

Toxicity Rating: 3. An important industrial degreasing agent and solvent, trichloroethylene is also used as an inhalation anesthetic in obstetrics and for short operative procedures. It has a narrower margin of safety than chloroform or halothane. Many industrial workers, operating room personnel and dentists are regularly exposed to TCE, some to large doses. The general public encounters trichloroethylene in cleaning fluids, some decaffeinated coffees and spice abstracts. Hamsters fed TCE-extracted decaffeinated coffee for 2 years showed no ill-effects. Because of the 1976 NCI bioassay implicating TCE as a cause of hepatocellular carcinoma in mice, the FDA proposed banning TCE as an additive in human food. Subsequent studies found no tumors in exposed rats. The acute oral LD$_{50}$ in rats is 4.92 gm./kg.; the estimated fatal oral dose in humans is 3-5 ml./kg. The lowest concentration to produce unconsciousness in adult humans is 16 mg./l. (3,000 ppm); the equivalent oral dose is 40-150 ml. The NIOSH standard for workroom air is 100 ppm for 8 hours; the odor threshold is 21.4 ppm. TCE produces skin irritation on prolonged contact, and it can penetrate intact human skin. Autoxidation products, such as phosgene and dichloroacetylene, added stabilizers, such as epichlorohydrin, and decomposition products, such as chlorine and HCl, may be responsible for some of the toxic and carcinogenic effects reported for TCE. Acute intoxications occur through inhalation of vapors released in industrial accidents and solvent sniffing and through accidental ingestion. The major sign of massive acute inhalation is a depressed level of consciousness, sometimes preceded by headache, nausea, incoordination and mild excitation or euphoria. Other reported effects are cardiac arrhythmias, liver and kidney lesions, hypertension, sometimes coma and death. Workers chronically exposed may exhibit CNS depression, intolerance to alcohol and increased cardiac output; symptoms abate when TCE is removed. Several cases of hepatorenal failure have been reported among such workers. Cardiac arrhythmias with secondary respiratory failure may account for deaths in acute poisonings and sudden deaths after chronic exposures; arrhythmias are documented side-effects of TCE overdose during anesthesia and after acute ingestion. TCE may sensitize the myocardium to endogenous epinephrine and stimulate secretion of adrenal medullary hormones. Autopsy findings in a 16-year old boy who died while sniffing plastic cement containing TCE indicated severe heart failure. Renal toxicity has been attributed to the passage of the toxic metabolite, trichloroethanol, through the kidney. Biopsy proved acute renal tubular degeneration in one case of spot remover sniffing; dialysis to treat renal failure was required in another. TCE has been shown to be hepatotoxic in dogs and rats. Liver failure is not the usual cause of death among solvent sniffers, but liver biopsies often reveal toxic centrilobular necrosis. Microsomal enzyme inducers increase the cardiotoxicity of TCE in experimental animals, which may be significant for workers who have pre-existing disease or drug-induced changes in drug metabolism. The metabolism of TCE in rats involves oxidation by the liver mitochondrial mixed function oxidase system to an epoxide intermediate, which binds covalently to proteins and causes centrilobular damage in the liver, a process similar to the production of tissue necrosis by the active intermediates of the metabolism of acetaminophen and indirect carcinogens. The epoxide may also bind to glutathione, but it is largely metabolized to trichloroacetic acid and trichloroethanol. The latter conjugates with glucuronide to form the major urinary metabolite. Epinephrine is contraindicated in treating TCE poisoning. Supportive treatment has been successful.

Some success has been reported in treating patients and experimental animals with propranolol, atropine, mineral oil and disulfiram.

See also: Carbon Tetrachloride, *Reference Congener in Section III.*
Ref.: Allemand et al., 1978; Aviado et al., 1976; Baerg and Kimberg, 1970; Bartonicek and Teisinger, 1962; Musclow and Awen, 1971; Waters et al., 1976; White and Carlson, 1979.

376   1,1,2-Trichloroethane

376

Beta-Trichloroethane, Vinyl trichloride

Toxicity Rating: 4. Not known to be a constituent of consumer products but used industrially as a chemical intermediate in the production of vinylidene chloride and of teflon tubing. Also used as a solvent for waxes and oils. Absorbed through lungs, intact skin, and the gastrointestinal tract. The acute oral LD_{50} in rats is 1140 mg./kg. but man is presumably much more sensitive. A central nervous depressant with a toxic potential greater than chloroform. Animals exposed to high vapor concentrations show local irritations of eyes and mucous membranes, loss of tendon reflexes, and death due to respiratory arrest. By inhalation or intraperitoneal injection, 1,1,2-trichloroethane produced liver and kidney injuries in mice and dogs. Given chronically by gavage to mice, it induced malignant hepatomas and is therefore regarded as a potential carcinogen in man.

See also: Carbon Tetrachloride, *Reference Congener in Section III.*
Ref.: Gehring, 1968; Klaassen and Plaa, 1966; Klaassen and Plaa, 1967a; National Cancer Institute, 1978m; von Oettingen, 1955.

377   1,1,1-Trichloroethane

377

Methyl chloroform, Chlorothene, α-Trichloroethane

Toxicity Rating: 3. A widely used solvent, found in various consumer products, including aerosol formulations. One of the least toxic of the liquid chlorinated hydrocarbons. Human deaths have resulted from exposures to very high vapor concentrations in unventilated tanks, drums and bags, but the concentrations normally encountered in home and industrial settings have little or no toxicological significance. High vapor concentrations cause central nervous depression leading to respiratory arrest. Decreased reaction time and impaired manual dexterity have been reported in human volunteers exposed to 350 ppm. At 500 to 1000 ppm signs and symptoms include ataxia, lightheadedness, and a positive Romberg test. Above 2000 ppm loss of consciousness may ensue. Recovery is rapid following cessation of exposure. However, transient liver and kidney dysfunctions were reported in five teenagers exposed to large concentrations of trichloroethane while "glue sniffing." Like many other solvents, 1,1,1-trichloroethane sensitizes the heart to epinephrine and may induce cardiac arrhythmias and arrest. Apparently this action has been responsible for several incidents of sudden deaths occurring among teenage sniffers of aerosol products containing the compound. In rats and dogs, the sensitization is said to be mediated by an initial drop in total peripheral resistance and decreased cardiac contractility. Pretreatment with phenylephrine (an α-agonist with only slight cardiac effects) and calcium gluconate prevented the decrease of blood pressure in acutely exposed anesthetized dogs. Pre-exposure to ethanol potentiates both cardiotoxicity and hepatotoxicity. Methyl chloroform has a moderately low acute oral toxicity in laboratory animals, but humans are probably more sensitive. In one clinical case, ingestion of one ounce of 1,1,1-trichloroethane (0.6 gm./kg.) produced nausea and diarrhea with no other signs or symptoms of intoxication. The compound is irritating to eyes. Skin contact causes only mild irritation, even on prolonged or repeated exposure. 1,1,1-Trichloroethane is absorbed through intact skin and is rapidly excreted through the lungs. Oxidation to trichloroethanol and trichloroacetic acid is not significant in man. The OSHA standard for 8-hour industrial exposure is 350 ppm; the odor threshold is 400 ppm.

See also: Carbon Tetrachloride, *Reference Congener in Section III.*
Ref.: Adams et al., 1950; Aviado et al., 1976; Bass, 1970; Eben and Kimmerle, 1974; Herd et al., 1974; Litt and Cohen, 1969; Ruotolo, 1956; Stewart, 1971; Stewart and Andrews, 1966; Stewart et al., 1969; Torkelson et al., 1958; von Oettingen, 1955.

378   Vinyl Chloride

378

Chloroethylene

A refrigerant gas and aerosol propellant, with weak depressant actions on central nervous system, like ethyl chloride. Effects from an acute exposure are usually brief. Angiosarcoma, a supposedly rare malignant tumor, has been detected in the livers of several long-time workers in plants that manufacture polyvinyl chloride plastic from vinyl chloride. A reticulated fibrosis of the liver may represent a precancerous lesion. The role of vinyl chloride in the genesis of these lesions is not known, but in the spring of 1974 the U.S Consumer Products Safety Commission banned the use of this gas as a propellant in household aerosol products.

See also: Carbon Tetrachloride, *Reference Congener in Section III.*
Ref.: Danziger, 1960; Anonymous, 1974.

Other halogenated aliphatic hydrocarbons

379   Allyl Bromide   379

3-Bromopropylene

An effective insecticidal fumigant. One of the most toxic of the halogenated hydrocarbons, causing deaths in experimental animals exposed for 4 hrs. to concentrations as low as 1 mg./liter. Extremely irritating to mucous membranes of eyes, nose, respiratory tract, and lungs. Odor, mucosal irritation, and lacrimation should provide adequate warning of exposure. Deaths in animals are apparently due to lung injury, but survivors recover without sequelae.

See also: Dichloropropenes, *Reference Congener in Section III.*
Ref.: Abreu et al., 1944; Peoples, 1934.

380   *n*-Butyl Chloride   380

1-Chlorobutane

Toxicity Rating: 3. Used as an anthelmintic in veterinary medicine. Weaker central nervous depressant actions than ethyl chloride. Dogs tolerate at least 11 ml./kg. without toxic effects. The LD_{50} in rats, however, is reported to be only 2.67 gm./kg.

See also: Carbon Tetrachloride, *Reference Congener in Section III.*
Ref.: Abreu et al., 1939; Smyth et al., 1954; Wright and Schaffer, 1932.

381   CBP   381

1-Chloro-3-bromopropene-1

Toxicity Rating: 4. Intense skin and eye irritation from vapor or liquid, abating rapidly after exposure. Percutaneous absorption is low.

See also: Dichloropropenes, *Reference Congener in Section III.*
Ref.: Hine et al., 1953a.

382   3-Chloro-2-methyl-1-propene   382

β-Methylallyl chloride, Isobutenyl chloride

Toxicity Rating: 4(?). A volatile liquid employed as an insecticidal fumigant. Liquid and vapor are irritating. Like other chlorinated hydrocarbons it is a central nervous depressant. Delayed deaths are described in laboratory animals exposed to low vapor concentrations, presumably because of severe tissue damage.

See also: Dichloropropenes, *Reference Congener in Section III.*
Ref.: von Oettingen, 1955.

383   Dichloropropenes   383

Toxicity Rating: 4. The name encompasses various isomers of 1,2-dichloropropene and of 1,3-dichloropropene. These substances and mixtures thereof are used as soil fumigants. See also D-D Mixture and 1,3-Dichloropropene below.

See also: Dichloropropenes, *Reference Congener in Section III.*

384   D-D Mixture   384

Chlorinated propane-propylene mixture

Toxicity Rating: 4. A soil fumigant consisting of a mixture of 1,2-dichloropropane and cis and trans isomers of 1,3-dichloropropene, with small amounts of various 1,2-dichloropropenes.

See also: Dichloropropenes, *Reference Congener in Section III.*

385   1,2-Dibromo-3-chloropropane   385

Nemagon, Fumazone, DBCP

Toxicity Rating: 4. A soil fumigant widely used to control nematodes. The principal constituent of Nemagon; other chlorinated C_3 compounds are also present. Very high acute and chronic toxicity by the oral, dermal and respiratory routes. Has caused human fatalities. The usual mode of exposure is inhalation. Acute one-hour LD_{50} in rats is 370 ppm, and 8-hour LD_{50} is 103 ppm. Vapor concentrations of 60 ppm caused irritation of eyes and respiratory tract, nausea, chills, central nervous depression with apathy and ataxia, and organ damage in rats. All deaths occurred within 72 hours. Degenerative kidney changes were noted in surviving animals, often leading to permanent scarring. Secondary infections occurred frequently, and recovery was slow. Repeated exposures to 12 ppm in laboratory animals (including monkeys) produced damage to liver, kidneys, sperm cells, seminiferous tubules, bronchioles, renal collecting tubules, lens, cornea and alimentary canal. Chronic exposure to vapors may lead to permanent eye damage. Pancytopenia has been reported in rats after chronic exposure (OSHA, 1978). Prolonged exposures to concentrations as low as 5 ppm produce systemic effects including organ damage. Such exposures are thought to have caused the very low sperm counts observed in production workers at several plants manufacturing DBCP. Low toxic concentrations have no strong warning odor. The acute oral LD_{50} for DBCP is about 200 mg./kg. (mice and rats). Nemagon taken by mouth causes acute gastrointestinal distress as well as pulmonary edema and organ damage described above, including disrup-tion of spermatogenesis. Daily doses of 70 mg./kg. proved fatal to mice in 20 days. Extensive organ degeneration was seen at autopsy. Nemagon is slightly irritating to skin on short single exposures. Repeated applications cause local necrosis of the dermis. Percutaneous absorption is enhanced by propylene glycol and may lead to systemic poisoning (dermal LD_{50} in rabbits is 500 mg./kg.). Daily doses of 12 mg./kg. for up to 73 weeks caused a toxic tubular nephropathy in all rats tested. The latter consisted of degenerative changes in the proximal convoluted tubules, with cloudy swelling, fatty degeneration, and frank necrosis. Affected kidneys often became fibrotic with scattered calcium deposits. Mammary tumors and squamous cell carcinoma of the stomach occurred frequently in mice and rats after repeated oral administration of technical grade DBCP at a rate of 24 mg./kg. daily for 10 weeks (Olson et al., 1973). An established carcinogen in mice and rats (National Cancer Institute, 1978). The current standard for occupational exposure is 1 ppb (8-hour average). Workers, other than pesticide applicators, who are accidentally exposed to DBCP spills must undergo immediate and late sperm counts and/or determination of serum levels of FSH, LH and testosterone (in males) and estrogen (in females) (see Fed. Reg. 43:11525, 1978 for further OSHA regulations).

See also: Dichloropropenes, *Reference Congener in Section III.*
Ref.: EPA, Sept. 22, 1977; Faidysh et al., 1970; National Cancer Institute, 1978b; Olson et al., 1973; OSHA., March 17, 1978; Shell Chemical Co., 1960c; Torkelson et al., 1961.

386   386   1,3-Dichloropropene

1,3-Dichloropropylene, Telone

Toxicity Rating: 4. Used in 95% concentrations as a soil fumigant for the control of root nematodes. When fed to rats in single doses as a 2.5% solution in corn oil, the LD_{50} was found to be between 0.25 and 0.5 gm./kg. The liver appeared to be the principal site of injury. Highly irritating to skin, eyes and all mucous membranes. Doses of 0.5 gm./kg. as a 25% solution in propylene glycol were lethal to rabbits when applied to the skin beneath a cuff for 24 hr. Death from inhalation was usually associated with severe lung injury. Present in D-D mixture.

See also: Dichloropropenes, *Reference Congener in Section III.*
Ref.: Rowe, 1960.

387   387   Epichlorohydrin

1-Chloro-2,3-epoxypropane

Toxicity Rating: 4. Liquid solvent for various gums, resins and celluloses used in varnish, paint and nail polish. Also an insect fumigant. Density at room temperature about 1.18. Oral doses of 0.5 ml./kg. killed all of a group of mice whereas half this dose was not lethal to any. Daily administration of 0.1 ml./kg. killed all mice in 10 to 20 days, indicating a cumulative potential. Daily applications of 0.5 ml./kg. to the skin killed all of a group of rats in 4 days. Thirty-minute exposures to ambient air concentrations of 8300 ppm. were lethal to mice. Va-pors produce lacrimation and coryza in man at sublethal concentrations. Poisoned animals show cyanosis, muscular relaxation or paralysis, tremor, convulsions and death in respiratory arrest. Death may be delayed as long as 2 hrs. even after parenteral administration. Although no characteristic organ pathology was observed in animals, a single human respiratory exposure was said to have resulted in chronic asthmatic bronchitis and severe diffuse fatty infiltration of the liver.

See also: Dichloropropenes, *Reference Congener in Section III.*
Ref.: Freuder and Leake, 1941; Schultz, 1964.

388 Hexachlorocyclopentadiene   388

Toxicity Rating: 4. A yellow green liquid used as an agricultural fumigant and chemical intermedi- (rabbit oral and dermal LD$_{50}$'s are about 450 mg./ kg.). In experimental animals, signs of systemic intoxication included diarrhea, lethargy and respiratory difficulty. Severe exposure by any route induced pulmonary hyperemia and edema, degenerative and necrotic changes in brain, heart and adrenal glands, and necrosis of liver and kidney tubules. In some animals given large oral doses, acute necrotizing gastritis of the proximal segment of the stomach was found at autopsy. Fumes of the compound are extremely irritating to eyes, skin and mucous membranes, causing lacrimation, ate in the manufacture of aldrin and chlordane. Very toxic by oral, dermal and inhalation exposure sneezing and salivation. In addition to the organ damage above, severe inhalation exposure produced acute bronchitis and interstitial pneumonitis with necrosis of bronchial epithelium. Diffuse degeneration of liver and kidney was observed after repeated subacute vapor exposures. Even dilute solutions of hexachlorocyclopentadiene (10%) cause inflammation, necrosis and deep burns when applied to intact skin of monkeys. No cases of human intoxication were found, but headache has been reported by investigators exposed to low concentrations of the vapor for prolonged periods.

See also: Dichloropropenes, Reference Congener in Section III.
Ref.: Treon et al., 1955.

389 Paraffin (Chlorinated)   389

Toxicity Rating: 1. No injury in test animals except when the dose was so large as to produce intestinal obstruction. The same is true of common paraffin. Do not appear to be irritants or sensitizers.

Ref.: Diamond Alkali Co., 1946.

390 Propargyl Bromide   390

3-Bromopropyne

Toxicity Rating: 6(?). A pungent and potentially explosive liquid used as a soil fumigant. Vapors and liquid are corrosive toward skin, eyes, and mucous membranes. Reported oral LD$_{50}$'s range from 29 to 67 mg./kg. in experimental rodents, but as with other halogenated hydrocarbons, man is probably more sensitive. Exposure to vapor concentrations of 200 ppm for four hours proved fatal in rats. Single and repeated lethal and sub-lethal exposures to concentrations as low as 10 ppm produced eye irritation with lung, liver and kidney damage. Releases hydrogen bromide fumes when heated.

See also: Dichloropropenes, Reference Congener in Section III.
Ref.: Dow Chemical Co., Jan. 12, 1979.

391 Propylene Dichloride   391

1,2-Dichloropropane

Toxicity Rating: 3. Volatile, flammable solvent used in dry cleaning fluids and for fumigating soil and grain. Mixtures with 1,3-dichloropropene are marketed as Telone and D-D Mixture. Moderate oral toxicity (rat oral LD$_{50}$ 1.9 gm./kg.). Irritating to skin, eyes and respiratory tract; narcotic in high concentrations. The current OSHA standard for occupational exposure is 75 ppm in air.

See also: Dichloropropenes, Reference Congener in Section III.
Ref.: Sidorenko et al., 1976; Smyth et al., 1969a; Spencer, 1973.

Halogenated aromatic hydrocarbons

392 Bromobenzene   392

Toxicity Rating: 4(?). An organic intermediate, solvent and additive to motor oils. Dogs tolerated oral doses of 3 to 5 gm. for several days before experiencing vomiting, diarrhea and eventually death. Rats given 3 gm./kg. showed toxic symptoms after 6 to 10 days. No human poisonings are known, but as with carbon tetrachloride man may be an unusually susceptible species. Absorbed through the lungs, gastrointestinal tract and intact skin. Excreted as catechol derivatives both free and conjugated with sulfate or mercapturic acid. Irritant to the skin. High vapor concentrations may be anesthetic. In rats produces widespread hepatic necrosis not only around centrolobular veins but also around all tributaries of the hepatic veins. The lesions resemble those produced by Thioacetamide and Tannic acid.

See also: Carbon Tetrachloride, Reference Congener in Section III.
Ref.: Fiume, 1963; von Oettingen, 1955.

393   Chlorobenzene

393

Monochlorobenzene

Toxicity Rating: 3(?). Sometimes used in drycleaning. Ingestion has lead, after a latency of several hours, to pallor, cyanosis (with methemoglobinemia), and collapse, strikingly similar to aniline poisoning.

See also: Aniline, *Reference Congener in Section III.*
Ref.: Cameron et al., 1937.

394   Carbolineum

394

Chlorinated anthracene oil

Toxicity Rating: 3(?). A high-boiling coal tar oil used as a wood preservative. Believed to consist chiefly of chlorinated anthracene, but it is reasonable to infer that phenolic derivatives and naphthalene are also present.

See also: Phenol *and* Naphthalene, *Reference Congeners in Section III.*

395   *o*-Dichlorobenzene

395

Orthodichlorobenzene, 1,2-Dichlorobenzene

Toxicity Rating: 4. For para isomer, see *p*-Dichlorobenzene below. Ortho isomer is more toxic: a local irritant, a strong central nervous depressant, and a liver and kidney poison. In animals liver destruction is often severe. Lens opacities have been described after known exposures in man and animals.

See also: Carbon Tetrachloride, *Reference Congener in Section III.*
Ref.: Cameron et al., 1937; Hollingsworth et al., 1958.

396   *p*-Dichlorobenzene

396

PDB, Dichloricide, Paradichlorobenzene

Toxicity Rating: 3. The least toxic active ingredient found in mothballs and related products. Sometimes used as an insecticidal fumigant. The ingestion of 20 gm. has been well tolerated in man. The vapor has caused irritation to skin, eyes, and throat, but no severe clinical poisonings are known after ingestion. Large doses in animals cause liver injury and sometimes tremors (in insects the compound is a nerve stimulant not unlike DDT). Also see *o*-Dichlorobenzene above, which appears to be much more toxic.

Ref.: Cotter, 1953; Hollingsworth et al., 1956; Weller and Crellin, 1953.

397   Hexachlorobenzene

397

Perchlorobenzene, HCB

Toxicity Rating: 3(?). Formula C_6Cl_6. Not benzene hexachloride (which refers to hexachlorocyclohexane, $C_6H_6Cl_6$). Between 1955 and 1959 about 3000 cases of porphyria cutanea tarda occurred in Turkey due to the repeated ingestion of wheat intended only for planting and so sprayed with 10% hexachlorobenzene as a fungicide. Estimated daily intakes of C_6Cl_6 ranged from 0.05 to 0.2 gm. Skin lesions were aggravated by exposure to sunlight and alcohol. In children the initial lesions resembled comedones and milia, but adults promptly developed bulbous lesions which progressed to ulceration and healed with pigmented scars containing microcysts. In severe and long standing cases permanent focal alopecia, corneal opacity, atrophic hands and hypertrichosis accompanied the dermal lesions. Hepatomegaly and porphyria were the rule; anorexia, weight loss and wasting of skeletal muscles were common findings. Recovery usually followed termination of exposure, but relapses were seen. This disease may be in part the result of contamination of the HCB by highly toxic polychlorinated dibenzodioxins which are byproducts of the manufacturing process. (See in this index.) Unlike man, rodents given toxic doses of HCB show striking neurological symptoms including tremors, paresis, ataxia, weakness, and occasionally clonic convulsions. Porphyrinuria occurs independently of nervous symptoms and is seen in both animals and man. Tracer studies indicate that HCB is bound to red blood cells in rats but not in dogs or primates. Rats also exhibit higher blood levels of HCB than do other animals, which may explain the predominance of neurological symptoms in that species. In primates, uptake of HCB occurs primarily from the small intestines, and the bulk of the compound is transported through the lymphatic system directly to fat depots. During lactation or starvation, mobilization of fat may cause toxic episodes as large concentrations of HCB enter the general circulation. Lactating animals, including humans, also excrete significant concentrations of HCB in milk. Thus, the nursing babies of porphyrinuric mothers in the Turkish episode showed a high incidence of toxic reactions known as "pinksore," which was almost uniformly fatal. In rats, the compound is also excreted in bile and very slowly metabolized by reductive dechlorination in the kidneys to form pentachlorophenol and other conjugatable compounds that are excreted in urine. Rats and monkeys given repeated doses of HCB in food showed extensive liver damage, with cytoplasmic vacuolization of cells in centrolobular zones, an increase in smooth endoplasmic reticulum, and the deposition of hemosiderin in lysosomes and on walls of vacuoles. The degree of damage was more marked in rats rendered siderotic by prior injections of iron. No drugs, other than perhaps EDTA, were found to influence the course of the disease or to relieve the symptoms.

Ref.: Cam and Nigogosyan, 1963; Cetingil and Ozen, 1960; DeMatteis et al., 1961; Iatropoulos et al., 1975; Iatropoulos et al., 1976; Ockner and Schmid, 1961; Timme et al., 1974; Villeneuve et al., 1974; Villeneuve, 1975; Yang et al., 1975.

398   Polybrominated Biphenyls   398

PBB

Flame retardants used in plastics. Mixture of brominated biphenyls with an average bromine content of six atoms per molecule. Very low acute oral toxicity; rats given single oral doses of 17 gm./kg. exhibited no toxic effects. Most poisonings are due to chronic exposure. Daily doses of 67 mg./kg. produced anorexia, diarrhea, lacrimation and salivation, dehydration, depression, and abortion in pregnant cows. Alterations in kidney, gallbladder and thymus were noted at necropsy. Extensive subcutaneous edema with petechial hemorrhages occurred in two-thirds of moribund animals. Cattle accidentally exposed to contaminated feed in Michigan exhibited the same clinical signs and, additionally, abnormal hoof growth, alopecia, decreased milk production, intramuscular hematomas and hepatic changes. Guinea pigs fed 50 ppm PBB's showed cortical atrophy of thymus, enlarged adrenals, and spleen alterations. Humans exposed in the Michigan episode reported a variety of clinical and sub-clinical symptoms and signs; increased incidence of viral and bacterial infections has been alleged. PBB's are potent inducers of rat renal mixed function oxidases and hepatic microsomal enzymes. Microsomal enzymes were also induced in suckling offspring of female rats fed PBB's. PBB is readily absorbed from the gut and stored in adipose tissue. Metabolic transformations and both kidney and biliary excretion are negligible. However, milk from exposed cows and persons may contain high concentrations of PBB. In the absence of lactation, PBB levels in humans may remain unchanged for a lifetime.

Ref.: Corbett et al., 1975; Evers et al., 1977; Moorhead et al., 1977; Waritz et al., 1977.

399   PCB   399

Polychlorinated biphenyl, e.g., Arochlor 1254

Toxicity Rating: 3(?). Non-flammable liquids formerly used in heat exchangers, electrical condensers, hydraulic and lubricating fluids and various inks, adhesives and paints. Many uses have been curtailed because of the environmental stability and chronic toxicity of the material. The article of commerce is a mixture of isomers having various numbers of chlorine atoms per molecule. In the Arochlor series, the last two digits give the percentage of chlorine in the compound. The mammalian toxicity is said to decrease as the level of chlorine increases. In rats signs and symptoms of acute intoxication include diarrhea, ataxia, lack of response to pain and central nervous depression. Hemorrhage of lungs, stomach and pancreas and alterations of liver and kidney have been found at autopsy. Hepatic microsomal activity was elevated by single large doses of Arochlor 1242. Monkeys given 300 ppm for 90 days developed alopechia, chloracne, subcutaneous edema, liver hypertrophy, and hypertrophy and hyperplasia of the gastric mucosa. Rabbits given Arochlor 1254 weekly for 14 weeks developed megalohepatocytosis followed by subcapsular midzonal necrosis and fibrotic changes. Repeated dermal applications of several technical grade PCB's produced hyperplasia and hyperkeratosis of the epidermal and follicular epithelium, liver and kidney changes, and atrophy of the thymus. Lymphopenia and increased fecal excretion of coproporphyria and protoporphyria were noted in some animals. The hepatic toxicity and chloracne observed were thought to be due, in part, to contamination with polychlorodibenzofurans. Moderate repeated doses of PCB's were said to have caused liver tumors in mice, bladder tumors in rats, and fetotoxicity in rabbits. Acute oral toxicities are generally low. Rat oral LD$_{50}$'s range from 4 gm./kg. (for Arochlor 1221) to 20 gm./m³ (for Arochlor 5460). However, Arochlor 1254 at 1000 ppm was fatal to 75% of treated rats in 43 days. In humans both dermal and oral exposures may lead to chloracne and hepatotoxicity. In Japan approximately 15,000 people consumed rice bran oil contaminated with PCB from a leaking heat exchanger. About 1000 victims of the episode have been identified. Clinical symptoms of intoxication include a persistent chloracne, skin hyperpigmentation, peripheral neuropathies (with decreased sural nerve conduction velocities), blindness, edema, nausea, vomiting and abdominal pain. Newborn infants showed skin discoloration, gingival hyperplasia, and skin changes. PCB's are readily absorbed from the gastrointestinal tract and stored in adipose tissue. The PCB's having a lower percentage of chlorine seem to be excreted more rapidly. Follow-up studies four years after the Japanese "Yusho" poisonings showed that the tetrachlorobiphenyl component had been largely excreted, but penta-and hexa-chlorobiphenyl levels in adipose tissue of the patients remained high relative to unexposed persons. Animal studies suggest that enterohepatic circulation of PCB occurs. Dietary paraffin reportedly increased PCB excretion in rats (Richter et al., 1979). Dermal exposures in industrial workers initially produce chloracne, followed by abdominal pain, vomiting and jaundice. Fatty degenerative necrosis of the liver and cirrhosis are found at autopsy.

Ref.: Allen et al., 1973; Allen and Norback, 1973; Fishbein, 1974; Grant et al., 1971; Hirayama et al., 1974; Kimbrough et al., 1972; Meigs et al., 1954; Miller, 1944; Murai and Kuroiwa, 1971; Nishizumi, 1970; Richter et al., 1979; von Oettingen, 1955; Vos and Koeman, 1970; Vos et al., 1970.

400   400 Polychlorinated Dibenzodioxins

Dioxins, e.g., 2,3,7,8-Tetrachlorodibenzo-*p*-dioxin, Hexachlorodibenzo-*p*-dioxin

Toxicity Rating: 6. Series of chlorinated derivatives of dibenzodioxin, which can range from mono- to octa-substituted. The more toxic members of the group have at least three but no more than seven halogens. Collectively referred to as dioxins, although the term is often used to designate only the most toxic member of the group, 2,3,7,8-tetrachlorodibenzo-*p*-dioxin (TCDD). For its molecular weight TCDD may be the most toxic and potent teratogen known to man. Acute oral LD_{50}'s for TCDD range from 0.6 microgm./kg. in male guinea pigs up to 115 microgm./kg. for rabbits of mixed sex. Dioxins and the related polychlorinated dibenzofurans below have been identified as impurities in 2,4,5-trichlorophenol and pentachlorophenol, where they were associated with an industrial outbreak of chloracne. Some commercial preparations of the herbicide 2,4,5-trichlorophenoxyacetic acid (See 2,4-D in Section III) have been shown to contain significant amounts of TCDD. Hexachlorodibenzo-*p*-dioxin, TCDD and related structures have been isolated from toxic fat and implicated as the chick edema factors. Presumably dioxins or their precursors accumulate in body fat of certain food species. When fat from such domestic animals was added to chicken feed, hydropericardium and ascites resulted in chicks. The association of dioxins or dibenzofurans as contaminants in polychlorinated naphthalenes and their relationship to virus x disease in cattle are speculative. Dioxins were the likely causative agent in an outbreak of porphyria cutanae tarda in a 2,4,5-T factory. Also believed to be contaminants in some polychlorinated biphenyl mixtures (above). Hepatic necrosis appears to account for death in the rat, but the proximal cause of death in other species is in doubt.

Ref.: Kimbrough, 1972; Poland and Glover, 1973a; Poland and Glover, 1973b; Schwetz et al., 1973; Sparschu et al., 1971.

401   401 Polychlorinated Dibenzofurans

e.g., 2,3,6,7-Tetrachlorodibenzofuran

Toxicity Rating: 6(?). Although not as well studied, this series of halogenated (one to eight chlorine substitutions possible) aromatic compounds appears to have toxic properties in common with the closely related polychlorinated dibenzodioxins above.

402   402 Polychlorinated Naphthalenes

e.g., Pentachloronaphthalene, Hexachloronaphthalene, Halowax

Toxicity Rating: 3(?). Series of chlorinated derivatives of naphthalene often available commercially as mixtures. Toxicity is thought to increase with the degree of chlorination, but such wide variations in toxicity have been reported that the possibility remains that the major toxic effects are due to contaminants or synthetic intermediates introduced during the manufacturing process. (See Polychlorinated biphenyls above). Tetra-, penta- and hexa-chloronaphthalene are said to be significantly more toxic than derivatives with lower degrees of halogenation. Once widely used in synthetic waxes, electrical insulating materials and as lubricants. Acneform rash (chloracne) and severe liver necrosis have occurred in humans exposed to vapors of highly halogenated derivatives. Acute ingestion toxicity is not well defined. Principal cause of hyperkeratosis (virus x disease) in cattle after repeated ingestion. Hundreds of thousands of animals were lost between 1941 and 1953 due to contamination of feed. Swine (and perhaps man) are less sensitive. As seen in cattle the disease is characterized by lacrimation, salivation, diarrhea, polyuria, anorexia, depression and weight loss. Characteristically the skin becomes dry and wrinkled and has a high keratin content. Alopecia is common and fissures may develop in the skin folds. At least part of the symptom complex is ascribed to low plasma vitamin A levels, but supplementation is not a specific cure for the disorder.

Ref.: Drinker et al., 1937; Huber and Link, 1962; McLetchie and Robertson, 1942; Sikes and Bridges, 1952; Strauss, 1944; von Oettingen, 1955.

403   Trichlorobenzenes   403

e.g., 1,2,3-Trichlorobenzene

Toxicity Rating: 3-4. Usually available as a mixture of three isomers. Has been used to combat termites. May irritate the eyes and respiratory tract. Has caused liver injury in man and animals. It is probably less toxic than o-Dichlorobenzene above.

Ref.: Cameron et al., 1937.

Simple aliphatic and aromatic alcohols

404   Alcohols (Higher)   404

i.e., Butyl, Amyl

The phrase "higher alcohols" usually refers to aliphatic alcohols of longer chain length than propyl alcohol. Several specific examples are listed below.

See also: Alcohols (Higher), *Reference Congener in Section III.*

405   Amyl Alcohol   405

1-Pentanol

Toxicity Rating: 3. When designated "*n*-amyl alcohol", pure 1-pentanol is presumably meant. In commerce, however, amyl alcohol is generally a mixture of several isomers, typically 74% (by weight) 1-pentanol, 25% 2-methyl-1-butanol, and 1% 3-methyl-1-butanol. Acute oral LD_{50} in rats is 2.7 gm./kg. Severe eye and skin irritant, and skin application results in signs of systemic toxicity. Low inhalation toxicity.

See also: Alcohols (Higher), *Reference Congener in Section III.*
Ref.: Scala and Burtis, 1973; von Oettingen, 1943.

406   Benzyl Alcohol   406

Phenylcarbinol, Phenylmethanol

Toxicity Rating: 3. Pure alcohol is irritating and corrosive but much less toxic than phenol. Aqueous concentrations up to 4% are well tolerated; they produce transient anesthesia of mucous membranes. Ingestion of large volumes is followed by vomiting, diarrhea, and central nervous depression. Converted into benzoic and hippuric acids. A human fatality has been ascribed to the rectal administration of 45 ml. In 1981 and 1982 several neonatal deaths were ascribed to benzyl alcohol present as a preservative (bactericide) in isotonic saline (9 mg./ml.), which had been used to flush catheters. Estimated daily doses ranged from 99 to 404 mg./kg. The syndrome consisted of metabolic acidosis, central neural depression, respiratory distress progressing to gasping respirations, hypotension, renal failure and sometimes convulsions. Blood and urine specimens contained high levels of benzyl alcohol, benzoic acid and hippuric acid.

Ref.: Brown et al., 1982; Gershanik et al., 1981; Graham and Kuizenga, 1945; Gruber, 1923a; Gruber, 1923b.

407   *n*-Butyl Alcohol   407

Butanol

Toxicity Rating: 3. Acute toxicity about 3 times that of ethyl alcohol. More irritating than ethyl but less so than amyl alcohol.

See also: Alcohols (Higher), *Reference Congener in Section III.*
Ref.: Tabershaw et al., 1944.

408   Caprylic Alcohol   408

1-Octanol

Toxicity Rating: 3(?). Thought to have a low ingestion toxicity. Known to be a hemolytic agent in vitro. Does it cause hemolysis when ingested?

See also: Alcohols (Higher), *Reference Congener in Section III.*
Ref.: McLain, 1940.

409   Cetyl Alcohol

1-Hexadecanol, Palmityl alcohol

Toxicity Rating: 1(?). Said to be an effective laxative when emulsified. Thought to be a metabolic product which is secreted in small amounts into the intestinal lumen.

See also: Alcohols (Higher), Reference Congener in Section III.
Ref.: Macht, 1933; Schoenheimer and Hilgetag, 1934.

410   Cyclohexanol

Hexalin, Hexahydrophenol

Toxicity Rating: 3. Human toxicity is not well defined. In animals central nervous depression without convulsions. Vomiting may occur. The vapor is irritating. In a suspected clinical poisoning due to the inhalation of vapor, nausea and tremors were prominent.

Ref.: Treon et al., 1943a; Treon et al., 1943b.

411   Decyl Alcohol

Toxicity Rating: 2-3. A synthetically prepared mixture typically containing 95% by weight trimethyl-1-heptanols and 5% other homologous primary 10-carbon alcohols. Its acute oral LD_{50} in rats is 4.7 gm./kg. A central nervous system depressant. Moderate irritant to rabbit skin, but no systemic signs of intoxication after skin application. Severe irritant in rabbit eye. Inhalation toxicity is low. The straight chain isomer has been used as a contact herbicide for sucker control in tobacco. Aspiration of 1-decanol into the tracheobronchial tree of rats results in rapid death by respiratory arrest.

See also: Alcohols (Higher), Reference Congener in Section III.
Ref.: Gerarde and Ahlstrom, 1966a; Scala and Burtis, 1973.

412   Ethyl Alcohol

Ethanol, Grain alcohol

Toxicity Rating: 2. Pure ethyl alcohol can be characterized as lying near the borderline of toxicity classes 2 and 3, on the basis of the widely accepted mean lethal dose of 1 quart of beverage alcohol (about 50% or 100 proof) in adult humans. Industrial ethyl alcohol, however, always contains a denaturant, i.e., a substance added to render it unfit or undesirable as a beverage or vehicle for any medication intended for ingestion. Denatured alcohols are designed to have objectionable odors or tastes and to provoke vomiting or to induce significant systemic toxicity. The IRS and federal regulations recognize two classes of denatured alcohol, completely denatured (CD) and specifically denatured (SD). Two CD formulas prescribe methyl isobutyl ketone and kerosene as denaturants in specified amounts. SD formulas are numerous, and each of them is designed for specific categories of use. SD formulas employ a large variety of denaturants, including gasoline, acetone, ethyl ether, formaldehyde, methyl alcohol, iodine, pine tar, bone oil, essential oils, brucine (and some other alkaloids), diethyl phthalate, etc. For example, in formula no. 40 (yielding SD alcohol 40), to each 100 gallons of ethyl alcohol are added 3 ounces of brucine or brucine sulfate and 1/8 gallon of tert-butyl alcohol. In this mixture the bitter taste of brucine is probably a more important deterrent than its central neural toxicity (see Brucine in the index). In some formulas the denaturant may induce significant untoward reactions, but in large doses ethanol itself is probably the most dangerous component in most of these mixtures.

See also: Ethyl Alcohol, Reference Congener in Section III.
Ref.: U.S. Treasury Department, 1980.

413   2-Ethylhexyl Alcohol

2-Ethyl-1-hexanol

Toxicity Rating: 3. Acute oral LD_{50} in rats is 3.7 gm./kg. Unless specified as normal (or primary) octyl or caprylic alcohol, the branched chain isomer 2-ethylhexyl alcohol is probably meant, because it is more common in commerce. Usual product is 99.5% pure. No relevant data on clinical toxicity were located.

See also: Alcohols (Higher), Reference Congener in Section III.
Ref.: Scala and Burtis, 1973.

414   Furfuryl Alcohol   **414**

2-Furanmethanol

Toxicity Rating: 4-5. Solvent and chemical intermediate in the manufacture of resins and wetting agents. Also used in acid-resistant cements and as a binder for foundry sand. Prepared from furfural obtained from corn cobs. Oil from roasted coffee bean meal contains high concentrations of furfuryl alcohol. May be metabolized in vivo to furfural (see in index) and to 2-furoic acid, but specific data are lacking. Acute oral LD_{50} in mice 40 mg./kg., in rats 275 mg./kg. (latter as a 2% aqueous solution). Poisoned laboratory animals die of respiratory arrest because of central nervous depression. Recovery from non-lethal doses is rapid and complete. Dermatitis after skin contact. Despite a relatively low vapor pressure, furfuryl alcohol induced symptoms of respiratory irritation, including severe bronchitis with spasms of coughing and chest pain, when used in confined spaces during hot weather.

Ref.: Boyland, 1940; Fine and Wills, 1950; Gajewski and Alsdorf, 1949; Mastromatteo, 1965.

415   Hexadecyl Alcohol   **415**

Toxicity Rating: 2. A white powder used as an emulsifier and emollient in cosmetics. A synthetic mixture of 2,2-dialkyl-1-ethanols, where alkyl groups are typically methyl-branched six and eight carbon chains. Overall chain length is 16-carbons, as in the related, naturally occurring cetyl alcohol (see above). Acute oral LD_{50} in rats greater than 8.4 gm./kg. A central nervous system depressant. Slight irritant on rabbit skin and in rabbit eye. Inhalation toxicity is low.

See also: Alcohols (Higher), *Reference Congener in Section III.*
Ref.: Scala and Burtis, 1973.

416   Hexyl Alcohol   **416**

Toxicity Rating: 3. Typically 44% (by weight) 1-hexanol, 53% methyl-1-pentanols and 3% 2-ethyl-1-butanol. Acute oral LD_{50} in rats is 3.7 gm./kg., whereas the LD_{50} of pure 1-hexanol is 4.9 gm./kg. Central nervous system depressant. Moderate irritant to rabbit skin with percutaneous absorption sufficient to produce systemic signs of intoxication. Inhalation toxicity is low.

See also: Alcohols (Higher), *Reference Congener in Section III.*
Ref.: Scala and Burtis, 1973; Smyth et al., 1951.

417   Isoamyl Alcohol   **417**

3-Methyl-1-butanol, Isopentyl alcohol, Fermentation amyl alcohol

Toxicity Rating: 4. The chief constituent of fusel oil, which is a by-product of carbohydrate fermentation to produce ethyl alcohol. Fusel oils vary in composition but also contain 2-methyl-1-butanol, isobutyl alcohol and others. The acute oral LD_{50} of isoamyl alcohol in rabbits is 3.4 gm./kg., but one ounce has killed adult humans.

See also: Alcohols (Higher), *Reference Congener in Section III.*
Ref.: Munch, 1972; von Oettingen, 1943.

418   Isobutyl Alcohol   **418**

Fermentation butyl alcohol, Isopropyl carbinol

Toxicity Rating: 3. Acute toxicity about three times that of ethyl alcohol. More irritating than ethyl but less so than amyl.

See also: Alcohols (Higher), *Reference Congener in Section III.*
Ref.: von Oettingen, 1943.

419   Isononyl Alcohol   **419**

Toxicity Rating: 3. Typically 75 to 85% (by weight) dimethyl-1-heptanols, 5 to 10% methyl-1-octanols, 10% to 20% other homologous primary 9-carbon alcohols. Acute oral LD_{50} in rats is 3.0 gm./kg. A central nervous system depressant. Marked irritant to rabbit skin and eyes, but no systemic signs of intoxication after skin application. Inhalation toxicity is low.

See also: Alcohols (Higher), *Reference Congener in Section III.*
Ref.: Scala and Burtis, 1973.

420   Isopropyl Alcohol

420

2-Propanol, Petrohol

Toxicity Rating: 3. Acute oral LD$_{50}$ in rabbits, 8.0 gm./kg., but clinical experience suggests that a toxicity rating of 3 is a better description of its lethality in man.

See also: Isopropyl Alcohol, *Reference Congener in Section III.*
Ref.: Munch, 1972.

421   Isooctyl Alcohol

421

Toxicity Rating: 3. Typically 70 to 80% (by weight) dimethyl-1-hexanols, 10 to 20% methyl-1-heptanols and 5 to 10% other homologous primary 8-carbon alcohols. Acute oral LD$_{50}$ in rats is 1.5 gm./kg. A central nervous system depressant. Moderate irritant to rabbit skin with percutaneous absorption sufficient to produce systemic signs of intoxication. Severe irritant in rabbit eye. Inhalation toxicity is low.

See also: Alcohols (Higher), *Reference Congener in Section III.*
Ref.: Scala and Burtis, 1973.

422   Lauryl Alcohol

422

Dodecyl alcohol, 1-Dodecanol

Toxicity Rating: 2(?). Thought to have a very low toxicity, but definitive studies were not located.

See also: Alcohols (Higher), *Reference Congener in Section III.*

423   Methyl Alcohol

423

Methanol, Wood alcohol
Toxicity Rating: 3.
See also: Methyl Alcohol, *Reference Congener in Section III.*

424   Myristyl Alcohol

424

Tetradecyl alcohol

Toxicity Rating: 2(?). Thought to have a very low toxicity, but definitive studies have not been located.

See also: Alcohols (Higher), *Reference Congener in Section III.*

425   NMRI-448

425

Toxicity Rating: 3. A mixture of 2 liquids: 2-phenyl cyclohexanol (70%) and 2-cyclohexylcyclohexanol (30%). An insect repellent for the skin. No clinical data. Symptoms in poisoned animals were not reported, but probably central nervous depression was prominent. Chronic application to rabbit skin (90 days) caused skin necrosis, bone marrow lesions, sometimes adrenal hemorrhage, and perhaps testicular atrophy.

Ref.: Draize et al., 1948.

426   Phenyl Cyclohexanol

426

2-Phenylcyclohexanol

Toxicity Rating: 3. Severe skin irritation in rabbits after repeated application. See also NMRI-448 above.

Ref.: Draize et al., 1948.

427   2-Phenylethyl Alcohol

427

2-Phenethyl alcohol, β-Phenylethyl alcohol, 2-Phenylethanol

Toxicity Rating: 3. A more potent local anesthetic than benzyl alcohol. Found in natural and synthetic oils of rose and distilled rose water. Injected in mice, it causes muscular weakness and incoordination, exophthalmos, coma, and death.

Ref.: Grote and Woods, 1955; Hjort and Eagan, 1911.

428   1-Propanol   428

Propyl alcohol

Toxicity Rating: 3. About 3 times more toxic acutely than isopropyl alcohol. Acute oral LD_{50} in rabbits is 2.8 gm./kg.

See also: Isopropyl Alcohol, *Reference Congener in Section III.*
Ref.: Mun·h, 1972; Wallgren, 1960.

429   Solox   429

Toxicity Rating: 3. This solvent mixture contains 100 parts ethyl alcohol, 5 parts methyl alcohol, 1 part gasoline, 1 part ethyl acetate and 1 part methyl isobutyl ketone. Solox intoxication and acute ethyl alcohol intoxication are similar. Coma often occurs, but mania and convulsions are also described. The conscious patient may complain of blurred vision, intense cramping abdominal pain and burning eyes. In some patients, and especially in chronic alcoholics, Solox produces a severe and unexpected hypoglycemia that may be due entirely to the ethanol. Blood glucose levels as low as 12 mg.% have been reported. A characteristic odor of the breath is described, and severe acidosis may be present. Sodium lactate solution intravenously has been used with success for the acidosis, but since high blood lactate levels have been noted during the acute phase, it may be better to use sodium bicarbonate (see Section IV). Frequent intravenous administration of dextrose is required to correct the hypoglycemia, which often recurs if treatment is not persistent. Pneumonia has arisen probably from aspiration as in kerosene intoxication.

See also: Ethyl Alcohol *and* Kerosene, *Reference Congeners in Section III.*
Ref.: Hammack, 1957.

430   Stearyl Alcohol   430

Octadecyl alcohol, e.g., Stenol

Toxicity Rating: 1(?). Stenol is a mixture of solid alcohols, principally stearyl alcohol. Used in pharmaceutical and cosmetic emulsions and as a lubri- cant and antifoaming agent. Thought to have a very low toxicity, but definitive studies were not located.

See also: Alcohols (Higher), *Reference Congener in Section III.*

431   Tridecyl Alcohol   431

Toxicity Rating: 2-3. Mainly tetramethyl-1-non- anols (13-carbon chain). Estimated acute oral LD_{50} in rats is 4.8 gm./kg. A central nervous system depressant. Moderate irritant on rabbit skin but no systemic signs of intoxication after skin application. Moderate irritant in rabbit eye. Inhalation toxicity is low.

See also: Alcohols (Higher), *Reference Congener in Section III.*
Ref.: Scala and Burtis, 1973.

Chloro-alcohols

432   Chlorobutanol   432

β,β,β-Trichloro-*tert*-butyl alcohol, Acetone chloroform, Chloretone

Toxicity Rating: 4. A central nervous depressant formerly used clinically as a hypnotic drug. Hypnotic oral dose for an adult is 0.3 to 1.0 gm. Resem- bles chloral hydrate but no gastric irritation. Has a local anesthetic action.

See also: Barbiturates, *Reference Congener in Section III.*
Ref.: Imprens, 1901.

433   1,3-Dichloro-2-propanol   433

Dichloroisopropyl alcohol

Toxicity Rating: 4(?). Similar to carbon tetrachlo- ride poisoning, but irritant actions (e.g., hemor- rhagic gastritis, pharyngitis, etc.) may be even more severe. Mutagenic in the Salmonella Ames test after activation by rat liver homogenates. A minor metabolite of the fire retardant Tris(1,3-dichloro- 2-propyl)phosphate (see latter in Index).

See also: Dichloropropenes *and* Carbon Tetrachloride, *Reference Congeners in Section III.*
Ref.: Gold et al., 1978; Lehmann and Flury, 1938.

434   **434** Ethylene Chlorohydrin

2-Chloroethanol

Toxicity Rating: 4-5. Used as a solvent and chemical intermediate and to treat sweet potatoes before planting. Vapor more toxic than that of ethylene dichloride. Signs of poisoning, such as nausea, vomiting, head and chest pains and stupefaction, have occurred after inhalation of 18 ppm. Acute oral LD_{50} of 58 mg./kg. in rats. Dangerous amounts can be absorbed through intact skin without immediate irritation to the skin. Various visceral lesions in cases of fatal inhalation of the vapors have included severe pulmonary edema and liver and kidney injury. In addition, cardiovascular damage was reported in the acute poisoning of a 24 year old Russian worker. The OSHA standard for vapor exposure in workroom air is 5 ppm.

See also: Dichloropropenes *and* Carbon Tetrachloride, *Reference Congeners in Section III.*
Ref.: Ambrose, 1950; Bush et al., 1949; Dierken and Brown, 1944; Saitanov and Kononova, 1976.

Glycols and polyglycols

435   **435** Polyol

Toxicity Rating: 1 to 3. An essentially ambiguous name used in industry to refer collectively to glycols and polyglycols. The most important members of the group are glycerol (glycerine), ethylene glycol, propylene glycol and their polymers. Glycerine and propylene glycol are practically non-toxic and are widely used in foodstuffs and pharmaceuticals. Ethylene glycol, one of the most toxic polyols, is an important industrial material widely used as an antifreeze and occasionally in cosmetics. Other polyols, including some which have appreciable toxicity, are used as solvents in consumer products and as plasticizers. Esters of the glycols may be more or less toxic than the parent compound. See individual entries below and in the index.

See also: Ethylene Glycol, *Reference Congener in Section III.*
Ref.: Rowe, 1962.

436   **436** Ethylene Glycol

Ethanediol

Toxicity Rating: 3. Toxicity rating of 3 is based on clinical data. In guinea pigs, rats, and mice, the rating is 2.

See also: Ethylene Glycol, *Reference Congener in Section III.*

437   **437** Diethylene Glycol

β,β'-Dihydroxydiethyl ether

Toxicity Rating: 3. In animals slightly less toxic than ethylene glycol, Cellosolve, or Carbitol (toxicity rating in animals 1 or 2), but probable lethal dose in man is 1 to 2 gm./kg. (toxicity rating 3). Causes central nervous depression and hydropic degenerative lesions in liver and kidney (probably without significant oxalate formation). Anuria from tubular degeneration may prove fatal within a few days.

See also: Ethylene Glycol, *Reference Congener in Section III.*
Ref.: Karel et al., 1947.

438   **438** Dipropylene Glycol

Toxicity Rating: 2. A condensation product of two moles of propylene glycol. Three linear isomers are possible and the exact composition of the commercial product is unknown. Acute oral LD_{50} in rats places this solvent on the borderline between toxicity classes 1 and 2. Low propensity for kidney and liver damage.

See also: Ethylene Glycol, *Reference Congener in Section III.*
Ref.: Hanzlik et al., 1939; Kesten et al., 1939.

439   **439** Triethylene Glycol

Ethylene glycol-bis-(2-hydroxyethyl ether), TEG, 2,2'-[1,2-Ethanediylbis(oxy)]-bisethanol

Toxicity Rating: 1-2. Used as an ingredient in fragrances and air disinfectants and to increase pliability of plastics. This compound has a lower acute toxicity than diethylene glycol but a higher toxicity than propylene glycol. The acute oral rat LD_{50} is 17 gm./kg. Blood transaminase activity increased in dogs after single i.v. doses of 4 ml./kg. Subacute and chronic exposures of dogs (i.v. injections) and rats (s.c. injections) revealed flattened epithelial cells in dog urine and elevated urea concentrations in rat blood. There is no evidence of decomposition to ethylene glycol in vivo.

See also: Ethylene Glycol, *Reference Congener in Section III.*
Ref.: Karel et al., 1947; Latven and Molitor, 1939; Lawter and Vrla, 1940; Opdyke, 1979.

440   Polyethylene Glycols   440

Toxicity Rating: 1 & 2. If a numeral is included in the name, it represents the approximate mean molecular weight. Fractions with molecular weights of 600 (and below) are liquid, of 1000 (and above) are solid. The higher the molecular weight the lower the toxicity, perhaps partly because the long polymers are so incompletely absorbed from the bowel. Very large doses are required to kill animals and deaths are renal in origin (not due to primary central nervous depression).

See also: Ethylene Glycol, *Reference Congener in Section III.*
Ref.: Carpenter and Shaffer, 1952; Smyth et al., 1950; Smyth et al., 1955.

441   Carbowax   441

Toxicity Rating: 1. Solid and semisolid polyethylene glycols. A series of waxy substances with mean molecular weights of 1000 and higher (indicated by the numeral following this trademarked name). In animals the toxicity decreases with increasing molecular weight. With massive doses some animals die from kidney injury. No human poisonings are known.

See also: Ethylene Glycol, *Reference Congener in Section III.*
Ref.: Carpenter and Shaffer, 1952; Smyth et al., 1950; Smyth et al., 1955.

442   Propylene Glycol   442

1,2-Propanediol

Toxicity Rating: 2(?). An antifreeze agent of low toxicity; also a pharmaceutical vehicle, plasticizer and industrial solvent. The oral LD_{50} in rats is 21 gm./kg. Very high doses given in feeding studies to rats and dogs have produced central nervous depression, hemolysis and minimal kidney changes. In humans partly excreted unchanged in urine and partly metabolized to lactic and pyruvic acids. Reversible symptoms of central depression have oc- curred in persons who ingested as little as 60 ml. Cases have been reported of stupor, tachypnea, tachycardia, diaphoresis and seizures in children who ingested large amounts (7.5 ml./day for 8 days in the case of a 15-month old child) as an ingredient in vitamin preparations. Alleged to be the ingredient causing skin sensitization to some topical creams used by eczema patients.

See also: Ethylene Glycol, *Reference Congener in Section III.*
Ref.: Arulanantham and Genel, 1978; Davis and Jenner, 1959; Hannuksela, 1979; Martin and Finberg, 1970; Thomas et al., 1949; Weil et al., 1971.

443   Polypropylene Glycols   443

Toxicity Rating: 3. Name is often followed by a numeral which indicates approximate mean molecular weight. Unaccountably much more toxic than propylene glycol or even ethylene glycol in laboratory animals. Polymers with molecular weights of about 1000 seem to be more toxic than longer or shorter homologues. When ingested or injected in dogs, ventricular extrasystoles result.

444   1,3-Butanediol   444

1,3-Butylene glycol

Toxicity Rating: 2(?). Said to be slightly more toxic than propylene glycol, but has been tested as a parenteral drug solvent. Subcutaneous LD_{50} 16.5 ml./kg. in mice and 20.1 ml./kg. in rats.

See also: Ethylene Glycol, *Reference Congener in Section III.*
Ref.: Spiegel and Noseworthy, 1963.

445   Hexylene Glycol   445

2-Methyl-2,4-pentanediol

Toxicity Rating: 2 or 3. Used in hydraulic brake fluids, printing inks, textile dye vehicles, and recommended as a solvent for some pharmaceuticals. Lethal doses in animals produced muscular incoordination which progressed to a narcosis lasting for several hours; death was delayed for 1 to 4 days. Evidence of slight liver and kidney damage on chronic feeding. Human subjects have ingested 5 gm. daily for 5 days without apparent ill effects or urinary abnormalities. Eliminated in urine, partly (20 to 25%) in conjugated forms. Said to constitute a negligible hazard on intact skin, but when gauze impregnated with a dressing containing 80 per cent hexylene glycol was used on 483 pediatric patients with extensive burns, 36 exhibited highly variable periods of coma (hours to weeks). Almost half of this comatose group eventually expired in renal failure.

See also: Ethylene Glycol, *Reference Congener in Section III*.
Ref.: Jacobsen, 1958; Procter, 1966; Woodward et al., 1945.

446   446   1,2,6-Hexanetriol

1,2,6-Trihydroxyhexane

Toxicity Rating: 1. Hygroscopic viscous fluid, miscible with water and used as humectant and plasticizer for hydrophilic films. Acute oral LD_{50} in male rats 16 ml./kg.; intraperitoneally as a 50 per cent solution in water, 10 gm./kg.; and intravenously as undiluted material, 5.6 ml./kg. Two ml./kg. applied to shaved rabbit skin 30 times over 6 weeks was without effect. A 30 per cent solution in 0.75 per cent saline was only slightly hemolytic in vitro. Almost 80 per cent of a large dose appeared within 24 hours in the urine of rats apparently unchanged. There was a significant increase in the urine oxalate, but it accounted for less than 0.1% of the intubated dose. It is a moderately good diuretic in rats. Fed to rats over a 2 year period a 5 per cent dietary level reduced growth, increased the relative kidney weights during the first year and produced cloudy swelling in the liver and pancreas. Although the above data indicate that hexanetriol is innocuous, great caution is advised in extrapolating animal results to man with this type of compound.

See also: Ethylene Glycol, *Reference Congener in Section III*.
Ref.: Smyth et al., 1969c.

Non-fatty esters of glycols and polyglycols

447   447   Carbitol Esters

Diethylene glycol monoethyl ether esters, i.e., acetate, citrate, laurate, phthalate, ricinoleate, stearate

Toxicity Rating: 3. These esters are apparently saponified (e.g., hydrolyzed) in the body to the glycol ether (= Carbitol) and an organic acid. Symptoms which are due to Carbitol are similar to those produced by ethylene glycol. In animals the esters are slightly less toxic than Carbitol by ingestion but more toxic by skin contact.

See also: Ethylene Glycol, *Reference Congener in Section III*.
Ref.: Karel et al., 1947; Latven and Molitor, 1939.

448   448   Diethylene Glycol Abietate

Toxicity Rating: 3(?). No specific data have been located, but in general esters of diethylene glycol are slightly more toxic than the parent glycol. See Diethylene glycol in the index.

See also: Ethylene Glycol, *Reference Congener in Section III*.

449   449   Diethylene Glycol Mono- and Di- Esters

i.e., Laurate, oleate, stearate

Toxicity Rating: 3. Believed to lie near the borderline between toxicity classes 3 and 4. In general diethylene glycol esters are slightly more toxic than the parent glycol. See Diethylene glycol in the index.

See also: Ethylene Glycol, *Reference Congener in Section III*.

450   450   2-Ethoxyethyl Acetate (and other Esters)

Ethylene glycol monoether esters, Ethylene glycol monoethyl ether acetate, Cellosolve esters, Cellosolve acetate, Dowanol EE

Toxicity Rating: 3. In general each monoether ester is somewhat less toxic (in animals) than the corresponding monoether. The esters are apparently hydrolyzed in vivo but the ether linkage is stable. Oral toxicity (and toxic actions) is similar to that of ethylene glycol, but percutaneous toxicity is probably higher.

See also: Ethylene Glycol, *Reference Congener in Section III*.
Ref.: Anonymous, 1947; Smyth et al., 1941a.

451   451   Ethylene Glycol Alkyl (and Aryl) Esters

e.g., Ethylene glycol diacetate

Toxicity Rating: 3. Generally the simple mono- and di-esters have about the same acute toxicity as ethylene glycol. They are readily saponified in the body to glycol and the corresponding organic acid.

Special problems arise where the latter is highly toxic (e.g., salicylic acid).

See also: Ethylene Glycol, *Reference Congener in Section III*.
Ref.: Anonymous, 1947; Smyth et al., 1941a.

Non-fatty ethers and ester-ethers of glycols and polyglycols

452   Butyl Carbitol 452

Diethylene glycol monobutyl ether

Toxicity Rating: 3. Probably lies near the border-line between toxicity classes 3 and 4. Slightly more toxic than the ethyl derivative (= Carbitol) but otherwise presumably like it. Both resemble ethylene glycol in toxicity and toxic actions.

See also: Ethylene Glycol, *Reference Congener in Section III*.
Ref.: Karel et al., 1947.

453   2-Butoxyethanol 453

Ethylene glycol mono-*n*-butyl ether, Ethylene glycol *n*-butyl ether, Butyl Cellosolve

Toxicity Rating: 4. A useful solvent for cellulose esters, notably nitrocellulose found in lacquers. Probably lies near the borderline between toxicity classes 3 and 4. About twice as toxic as the ethoxy analogue (= Cellosolve) but otherwise like it. Consult 2-Ethoxyethanol below.

See also: Ethylene Glycol, *Reference Congener in Section III*.
Ref.: Smyth et al., 1941a; Werner et al., 1943a; Werner et al., 1943b; Werner et al., 1943c.

454   Butoxy Polypropylene Glycols 454

e.g., Crag fly repellent

Toxicity Rating: 3. A fly repellent especially useful for live stock. No skin irritation. Very low (but significant) percutaneous toxicity. If like the monopropylene glycol ethers, these polyglycols can be expected to produce central nervous depression and kidney injury after ingestion.

See also: Ethylene Glycol, *Reference Congener in Section III*.
Ref.: Carpenter et al., 1951b; Carpenter et al., 1959.

455   Carbitol 455

Diethylene glycol monoethyl ether

Toxicity Rating: 3. About the same acute toxicity by ingestion as ethylene glycol in animals. No adequate data for human comparisons, but the mean lethal dose of ethylene glycol in man is probably 3 to 4 oz. Poisonings produce similar symptoms. Carbitol is essentially nonirritating to human skin; no skin penetration.

See also: Ethylene Glycol, *Reference Congener in Section III*.
Ref.: Karel et al., 1947; Latven and Molitor, 1939.

456   Cellosolve Sulfate 456

Monoethyl ether of ethylene glycol monosulfate

No toxicity data are known, but if the compound hydrolyzes to sulfuric acid (as ethylene glycol sulfate does spontaneously), systemic acidosis may be a serious problem after ingestion. Otherwise toxicology is probably like that of ethylene glycol ethers.

See also: Ethylene Glycol, *Reference Congener in Section III*.
Ref.: Smyth et al., 1941a; Werner et al., 1943a; Werner et al., 1943b; Werner et al., 1943c.

457   Dipropylene Glycol Monomethyl Ether 457

Toxicity Rating: 2-3. Colorless liquid with mild ethereal odor and bitter taste used in hydraulic fluids and as a high boiling solvent for nitrocellulose and synthetic resins. Oral LD_{50} in rats 5.4 ml./kg. Single exposures of rats to a vapor concentration of 500 ppm for 7 hours produced mild narcosis with rapid recovery. Daily exposures of 4 animal species, including monkeys, to 300-400 ppm for 7 hours produced mild narcosis and changes in liver and lungs. Vapor concentrations above 100 ppm, the OSHA standard for workroom air, become disagreeable to man. Eye, nose and throat irritation occur before the first signs of central nervous depression, which may appear at 1000 ppm. Said to be able to penetrate through intact skin but no skin irritation or sensitization in man.

Ref.: Rowe et al., 1954b.

458　2-Ethoxyethanol

458

Ethylene glycol monoethyl ether, Cellosolve

Toxicity Rating: 3. Acute toxicity is several times greater than that of ethylene glycol in animals (clinical data are inadequate for valid comparisons). Ether linkage is supposedly stable in vivo. Central nervous depression as with ethylene glycol, as well as kidney injury and hematuria (apparently without oxalic acid formation or crystalluria). However other monoethers of ethylene glycol (e.g., butyl cellosolve) may have somewhat more renal toxicity; see latter above. These ethers penetrate intact skin.

See also: Ethylene Glycol, *Reference Congener in Section III.*
Ref.: Smyth et al., 1941a; Werner et al., 1943a; Werner et al., 1943b; Werner et al., 1943c.

459　Ethylene Glycol Alkyl (and Aryl) Ethers

459

Cellosolves

Toxicity Rating: 3. Acute toxicities are several times greater than that of ethylene glycol in animals (clinical data are inadequate for valid comparisons). Ether linkage is supposedly stable in vivo. Central nervous depression as with ethylene glycol, but the ether derivatives produce more marked kidney injury and hematuria (apparently without oxalic acid formation or crystalluria). These ethers penetrate intact skin.

See also: Ethylene Glycol, *Reference Congener in Section III.*
Ref.: Smyth et al., 1941a; Werner et al., 1943a; Werner et al., 1943b; Werner et al., 1943c.

460　Glycofurol

460

Tetrahydrofurfuryl alcohol polyethylene glycol ether

Toxicity Rating: 3. On the average it contains 2 ethylene glycol units per molecule. Recommended as a solvent for parenteral drug administration. Unlike concentrated solutions, dilute aqueous solutions are not irritating. Intravenous LD_{50} in the mouse 3.8 gm. (3.5 ml.) per kg.

See also: Ethylene Glycol, *Reference Congener in Section III.*
Ref.: Spiegel and Noseworthy, 1963.

461　2-Methoxyethanol

461

Methyl Cellosolve, Ethylene glycol monomethyl ether

Toxicity Rating: 3. An industrial solvent, widely used in aniline dyes, printing inks, and adhesives, as a cosolvent in organic and water-based coatings, and in the manufacture of cellophane wrap and photographic film. Moderate acute toxicity by oral, dermal and inhalation routes. In rabbits and guinea pigs, the oral LD_{50} is 0.9 to 1.0 gm./kg.; the dermal LD_{50} is about 2 gm./kg. In the only human fatality reported, accidental ingestion of one-half pint of 2-methoxyethanol mixed with brandy led to coma and death within 5 hours. Autopsy revealed degeneration of kidney tubules, acute hemorrhagic gastritis, fatty degeneration of the liver, early necrosis of the pancreas, and brain edema (Young and Woolner, 1946). The total dose in this case was about 3 gm./kg. In two non-fatal cases, the initial symptoms of toxicity were muscular weakness, nausea and vomiting, leading to confusion and a profound metabolic acidosis. Partial renal failure was accompanied by oxaluria in one case. In experimental animals, however, 2-methoxyethanol is apparently not metabolized to oxalic acid. In rats, single high oral doses lead to narcosis and occasionally hematuria. Daily doses of 0.1 ml./kg. for 7 days produced tremors, exhaustion, albuminuria and hematuria in rabbits. Death was delayed and was due to kidney failure. Severe kidney damage was seen at autopsy. The usual route of human exposure is inhalation. The vapor is irritating to eyes and mucous membranes. Prolonged or chronic industrial exposure to concentrations as low as 50 ppm lead to severe neurological disabilities. In men and women exposed repeatedly to 50 to 1000 ppm, primary symptoms include headache, dizziness, lethargy, weakness, unequal pupil size, disorientation and an appearance of mental retardation. Ataxia, hyperreflexia, and disturbances in vision and hearing have been reported. The syndrome has been mistaken for schizophrenia. In some cases, macrocytic anemia is found with an excess of immature leukocytes in the circulating blood. Weight loss usually occurs. Signs and symptoms disappear several weeks after cessation of exposure; no long-term sequelae have been identified. In rabbits, repeated exposures to concentrations of 800 or 1600 ppm produced irritation of respiratory tract and lungs, hematuria, albuminuria, calcified casts in urine, and severe glomerulitis. In mice, the mean lethal vapor concentration (7-hour exposure) was found to be 1480 ppm. Death was ascribed to lung and kidney injury. The present OSHA standard for industrial exposure is 25 ppm.

See also: Ethylene Glycol, *Reference Congener in Section III.*
Ref.: Nitter-Hauge, 1970; Rowe, 1962; Smyth et al., 1941a; Stewart et al., 1970; Werner et al., 1943a; Werner et al., 1943b; Werner et al., 1943c; Young and Woolner, 1946; Zavon, 1963.

462 Methyl Cellosolve Acetate 462

Ethylene glycol monomethyl ether acetate

Toxicity Rating: 3. Slightly less toxic (in animals) than the ether itself. The ester is apparently saponified in vivo, but the ether linkage is stable. About twice as toxic as ethylene glycol but toxic effects are similar.

See also: Ethylene Glycol, *Reference Congener in Section III*.
Ref.: Smyth et al., 1941a.

463 Phenyl Cellosolve 463

Ethylene glycol monophenyl ether, 2-Phenoxyethanol

Toxicity Rating: 4. Probably lies near the borderline between toxicity classes 3 and 4. About twice as toxic as the ethyl derivative but otherwise like it. Consult 2-Ethoxyethanol above.

See also: Ethylene Glycol, *Reference Congener in Section III*.

464 Propylene Glycol Monomethyl Ether 464

e.g., Dowanol 33B

Toxicity Rating: 3(?). Both alpha and beta isomers have similar toxicities. Central nervous depression and kidney tubular necrosis are seen in experimental animals. Less toxic than ethylene glycol monomethyl ether but slightly more toxic than ethylene glycol.

See also: Ethylene Glycol, *Reference Congener in Section III*.

Aliphatic ketones and ethers

465 Acetal 465

Diethylacetal, 1,1-Diethoxyethane

Toxicity Rating: 3. Solvent and constituent of some synthetic perfumes such as jasmine. Also a central nervous depressant, similar to but less acutely toxic in rats than paraldehyde. The 14-day oral LD_{50} in rats is about 4.6 gm./kg. Dermal 15-day LD_{50} on rabbit skin is about 10 ml./kg. Exposure to 4000 ppm for 4 hours killed 2 of 6 rats over 14 days. Very mild eye and skin irritant.

Ref.: Lehmann and Flury, 1938; Smyth et al., 1949.

466 Acetone 466

Dimethyl ketone, Propanone, Pyroacetic ether

Toxicity Rating: 3. Effects similar to ethyl alcohol for equal blood levels, but the anesthetic potency is greater. Ten to 20 ml. taken by mouth without ill effect. In acute cases a latent period may be followed by restlessness and vomiting proceeding to hematemesis and progressive collapse with stupor.

See also: Ethyl Alcohol, *Reference Congener in Section III*.
Ref.: Haggard et al., 1944; Harris and Jackson, 1952.

467 Chloromethyl Methyl Ether 467

CMME, Methyl chloromethyl ether

Toxicity Rating: 3. An alkylating agent and solvent used in the manufacture of water repellents, ion-exchange resins and industrial polymers. A powerful lung irritant. In rats exposed to the vapor, death was due to pulmonary edema and hemorrhage. Acute necrotizing bronchitis was observed at autopsy. Acute oral LD_{50} in rats is 817 mg./kg. Bis(chloromethyl) ether is a closely related compound and common contaminant of CMME. It produces similar pulmonary reactions but at much lower concentrations. Rat 14-day LC_{50}'s (7-hour exposure) were 55 ppm for CMME and 9 ppm for BCME. Single exposure to 2.1 ppm BCME caused a variety of regenerative hyperplastic and metaplastic alterations in rat pulmonary tissue; repeated exposure led to carcinoma. Repeated exposure to BCME also produced symptoms of nervous irritability in rats and hamsters. Subarachnoid hemorrhage was found in some animals at autopsy. Both BCME and CMME are known to cause a high incidence of pulmonary tumors (primarily small cell carcinomas) in industrially-exposed persons. BCME but not CMME produces tumors when painted on mouse skin; however, CMME proved to be an initiating agent when followed by phorbol esters. Both compounds produced necrotic lesions at the treatment site. BCME and CMME degrade rapidly in water to yield formaldehyde and hydrochloric acid. CMME also yields methanol. Degradation products of CMME may recombine to produce BCME under physiological conditions.

See also: Nitrogen Oxides, *Reference Congener in Section III.*
Ref.: DeFonso and Kelton, 1976; Drew et al., 1975; VanDuuren et al., 1969; Weiss et al., 1979.

468   468   Cyclohexanone

Toxicity Rating: 3(?). A comparatively harmless solvent. A weak central nervous depressant and a mild or moderate irritant.

Ref.: Treon et al., 1943a; Treon et al., 1943b.

469   469   Diacetone Alcohol

4-Hydroxy-4-methyl-2-pentanone

Toxicity Rating: 3(?). A solvent, hydraulic brake fluid, and a component of some antifreeze mixtures. May cause central nervous depression and possibly renal damage. Liver injury and anemia reported in animals. More toxic than acetone.

Ref.: Smyth and Carpenter, 1948; Walton et al., 1928.

470   470   *sym.*-Dichloroethyl Ether

β,β'-Dichloroethyl ether, Chlorex

Toxicity Rating: 4. Strong irritant and lacrimator. Percutaneous toxicity can be dangerous. Possibly some late effects like carbon tetrachloride (liver and kidney injuries). We know of no fatal human poisonings.

See also: Carbon Tetrachloride, *Reference Congener in Section III.*
Ref.: Amer. Petroleum Institute, 1948b.

471   Dihydroxyacetone

1,3-Dihydroxydimethyl ketone, Protosol, Ketochromin

Toxicity Rating: 3(?). When spread as a solution over the skin, it creates a color reaction like suntan. Although found in many such commercial products, no animal toxicity data were found in the open literature. Said not to be an irritant or sensitizer even in high concentrations on the skin. Adult humans are said to tolerate by mouth 18 gm. three times a day over 2 to 3 weeks.

Ref.: Goldman, 1961.

472   472   Ethyl Ether

Diethyl ether, Ether

Toxicity Rating: 3. One or 2 oz. may be fatal when swallowed. Symptoms are similar to ethyl alcohol intoxication except that onset is more rapid and duration is shorter. Because of its volatility the stomach becomes promptly distended; this may embarrass breathing. Unlike ethanol, ether is not oxidized (or otherwise metabolized) in vivo. Ether is sometimes injected intravenously as a measure of circulation time when evaluating a patient's cardiac status. Quantities of 0.5 ml. mixed with an equal volume of saline are frequently employed, and a cough or a gasp is taken as the endpoint. In at least two cases the ether was accidentally given intra-arterially. Immediately after injection the patients experienced burning pain in their arms and hands. Over the following 24 hrs. the extremity remained painful and gradually developed massive edema, cyanosis, and ischemia. Eventual gangrene necessitated amputation.

See also: Ethyl Alcohol, *Reference Congener in Section III.*
Ref.: King and Hawtof, 1963; Manufacturing Chemists' Assoc., 1948c; National Safety Council, Date Unknown c.

473   473   Isophorone

Isoacetophorone, 3,5,5-Trimethyl-2-cyclohexene-1-one

An unsaturated cyclic ketone used as a solvent for lacquers and plastics. Has a peppermint-like odor. No report of systemic poisoning in man has been located, but the vapor is known to irritate mucous membranes. In animals this solvent has a higher acute toxicity by inhalation than does methyl butyl ketone, but it is less hazardous because less volatile. Toxic effects include mucosal irritation, occasionally pulmonary inflammation, and varying degrees of narcosis. Although reputed to produce kidney damage, death in experimental exposures is usually due to central nervous depression or occasionally to lung irritation.

Ref.: Fairhall, 1957.

474   Mesityl Oxide 474

Isobutenyl methyl ketone

An unsaturated ketone used as a solvent for many resins, oils, and fats. The vapor has produced progressive generalized central nervous depression in exposed animals. Probably less toxic than isophorone but more dangerous because much more volatile. See Isophorone above.

Ref.: Fairhall, 1957.

475   Methyl Ether 475

Dimethyl ether, Methoxymethane

Toxicity Rating: 3(?). Colorless gas at usual temperatures, but it is easily condensable. Liquid material will cause severe frostbite if spilled on the skin. Intraperitoneal doses of 5 mg./kg. produced reversible anesthesia in mice. Narcotic effects in man may be seen at concentrations of 5 to 10% in air. In animals 85% in air produced profound anesthesia with a gradual cessation of respirations. About 20 minutes were required for recovery after 50 minutes of anesthesia. No harmful effects were noted in rabbits exposed to 2000 ppm in air for 1.25 hours twice daily for 13 weeks of 5 exposure-days each. See also Ethyl ether above. Sometimes encountered as a mole-per-mole complex with boron trifluoride which is said to be a severe pulmonary irritant.

Ref.: Brown, 1924; Commerical Solvents Corp., 1969.

476   Methyl Ethyl Ketone 476

MEK, 2-Butanone

Toxicity Rating: 3. Similar to but more irritating than acetone above. Vapor is irritating to human mucous membranes and conjunctivae at 200 ppm after 15 minutes, but an odor is noticeable at 25 ppm, which presumably prevents most inadvertent exposures to hazardous concentrations. Has caused central nervous depression in laboratory animals. Potentiates the neurotoxicity of *n*-hexane and MBK (see both in index) in both inhalation exposure tests in rats and in intoxications of humans sniffing solvent thinned with MEK. May have been the agent responsible for neuropathies in shoe factory workers. Vapors in concentration of 1000 ppm or 3000 ppm were embryotoxic and fetotoxic in rats causing acaudia, imperforate anus and brachygnathia, as well as retardation of fetal development.

Ref.: Altenkirch et al., 1979; Amer. Petroleum Institute, 1948d; Dyro, 1978; Schwetz et al., 1974.

477   Allantoin 477

5-Ureidohydantoin, Glyoxyldiureide

Toxicity Rating: 1. Used topically to speed granulation of wounds and in the treatment of psoriasis and other chronic dermatoses. Said to be the wound-healing principle in comfrey. Formerly also used as a herbicide. Various allantoinate salts, e.g. aluminum dihydroxy allantoinate and aluminum chlorhydroxy allantoinate, are also used in skin creams. Neither allantoin nor its aluminum salts exhibit significant toxicity in man or laboratory animals.

Ref.: Bertolet and Mecca, 1968.

478   Methyl Isobutyl Ketone 478

Isopropylacetone

Toxicity Rating: 3(?). Used as a solvent for cellulose lacquer and a denaturant for ethyl alcohol. Similar to methyl ethyl ketone but probably more toxic. Gastroenteritis is expected to be the dominant disorder after ingestion, but central nervous depression may occur.

Ref.: Specht, 1938.

479   Methyl *n*-Butyl Ketone 479

n-2-Hexanone, MBK

Toxicity Rating: 3. Used as a solvent especially in paints and the printing of plasticized fabrics. Inhalation of high vapor concentrations has caused lethargy and narcosis in humans. May produce irritation of eyes and mucous membranes. Oral LD_{50} in rats 2590 mg./kg.; minimal lethal dose in guinea pigs 914 mg./kg. Animals of both species exhibited loss of consciousness, coma and death. In industrial workers chronic respiratory exposure to 9 to 36 ppm for as little as 5 weeks (together with undefined dermal exposure) led to symmetrical distal polyneuropathy with both motor and sensory deficits. This effect appeared to be potentiated by concurrent use of methyl ethyl ketone. Both MBK and *n*-hexane are metabolized in sensitive species to 2,5-hexanedione, which is also neurotoxic. 2-Hexanol is also a common toxic metabolite. In exposed cats lesions have also been found in the hypothalamus and optic tract. It has been suggested that the peripheral disturbance masks the central effects, but that the latter are less readily reversed on cessation of exposure. The term central-peripheral distal axonopathy has been suggested as more descriptive than polyneuropathy.

See also: Tri-*o*-cresyl Phosphate, *Reference Congener in Section III.*
Ref.: Allen et al., 1975; Billmaier et al., 1974; DiVincenzo et al., 1977; Mallov, 1976; Schaumburg and Spencer, 1978; Schrenk et al., 1935.

Aliphatic aldehydes and their precursors

480 Acetaldehyde

Ethylaldehyde, Ethanal

Toxicity Rating: 3. Less irritating but stronger central nervous depressant than formaldehyde. Vapor exposures, however, are usually limited by the intense irritation of mucous membranes and conjunctiva sometimes with pulmonary edema and albuminuria. Less toxic by inhalation than the unsaturated aldehydes (see Acrolein below) or formaldehyde. The saturated aldehydes by inhalation show decreasing toxicity with increasing chain length in the order acetaldehyde, propionaldehyde, isobutyraldehyde, *n*-butyraldehyde, *n*-valeraldehyde and isovaleraldehyde. In contrast to acrolein below, these less irritating aldehydes produced less bronchial constriction but more lung irritation. As inferred from inhalation studies ingestion of acetaldehyde or isobutyraldehyde may produce central nervous depression with symptoms like alcohol intoxication. When infused intravenously (and perhaps when ingested), acetaldehyde is sympathomimetic, as evidenced by tachycardia and hypertension. This reaction is due to norepinephrine release from adrenergic nerve endings. Pretreatment of mice and rats with sulfhydryl compounds or ascorbic acid protects them against acetaldehyde-induced loss of righting reflex and death. Acetaldehyde is rapidly metabolized. The acute circulatory collapse of the disulfiram-alcohol reaction is thought to be partly due to the metabolic accumulation of acetaldehyde. For treatment of latter, see Disulfiram in Section III.

See also: Formaldehyde, *Reference Congener in Section III.*
Ref.: Asmussen et al., 1948b; James and Bear, 1968; Manufacturing Chemists' Assoc., 1952b; O'Neill and Rahwan, 1976; Salem and Cullumbine, 1960.

481 Acrolein

2-Propenal, Acrylaldehyde

Toxicity Rating: 5. Highly reactive unsaturated aldehyde, which may polymerize with explosive violence in the presence of acid or alkali. Important synthetic intermediate, but also marketed as an aquatic herbicide. Produced in large amounts by overheated cooking oils and animal fats. Crotonaldehyde (methylacrolein), although slightly less toxic, is similar chemically and toxicologically. These unsaturated aldehydes are more toxic than their saturated homologues. Acrolein is extremely toxic by oral, inhalation, and dermal exposure (rat oral LD_{50} is 46 mg./kg.). When swallowed, it produces severe gastrointestinal distress with pulmonary congestion and edema. Inhalation has led to pneumonia and nephritis with death from cardiac failure in experimental animals. At autopsy, hyperemia and hemorrhage of the lungs and degeneration of the bronchial epithelium were found. Intense lacrimation and nasal irritation ordinarily give adequate warning of inhalation, but exposed patients should be observed for 24 hours for a slowly developing pulmonary edema. Exposure to concentrations of 1.2 ppm causes bronchial constriction relieved by atropine in experimental animals. Lungs of monkeys exposed repeatedly to low concentrations of acrolein (0.7 ppm) showed chronic inflammatory changes, including necrotizing bronchitis and emphysema. Additional nonspecific inflammation was seen in liver and kidney, with focal calcification of renal tubular epithelium occurring in some animals. Monkeys, dogs and guinea pigs exposed continuously to concentrations of 0.22 ppm for 90 days showed no overt symptoms of toxicity. At autopsy, however, many animals had emphysema and non-specific inflammatory changes in liver, lung, kidney and heart. A dose-dependent pressor effect has also been reported in anesthetized rats following doses of acrolein as low as 0.05 mg./kg. The compound is a severe skin irritant, causing vesiculation and burns. It can also be absorbed percutaneously to produce systemic intoxication (dermal LD_{50} for rabbits is 560 mg./kg.). Affected parts should be washed promptly with copious amounts of water. Recovery is usually prompt and complete. See Nitrogen Oxide in Section III for the management of pulmonary complications after inhalation, and see Formaldehyde for other routes of exposure.

See also: Nitrogen Oxides *and* Formaldehyde, *Reference Congeners in Section III.*
Ref.: Bauer et al., 1977; Egle and Hudgins, 1974; Lyon et al., 1970; Murphy et al., 1963; Salem and Cullumbine, 1960; Shell Chemical Co., 1960e.

482   Formaldehyde 482

Formalin, Formol

Toxicity Rating: 3. Commercial formaldehyde solution contains 30 to 37%/w of formaldehyde gas and 0 to 15% methyl alcohol in water. Because 1 oz. taken by mouth has caused death within 2.5 hours, the solution presumably lies near the borderline between toxicity classes 3 and 4.

See also: Formaldehyde, Reference Congener in Section III.
Ref.: Manufacturing Chemists' Assoc., 1950a.

483   Furfural 483

Furfuraldehyde-2

Toxicity Rating: 3. Said to be about one-third as toxic as formaldehyde. An irritant to mucous membranes. Central nervous depression with brain lesions in animals. Ingested furfural has produced liver cirrhosis in rats. Daily subcutaneous injections in rabbits soon induce defects in liver and kidney function and hypochromic anemia with leukopenia.

See also: Formaldehyde, Reference Congener in Section III.
Ref.: McGuigan, 1923.

484   Glutaraldehyde 484

Toxicity Rating: 3-4. Widely accepted as a tanning agent for leather and as a chemical disinfectant for cold sterilization of medical and dental equipment. Applied topically in the treatment of hyperhidrosis and onychomycosis. Employed as a 25% solution in water for an embalming fluid. Oral LD$_{50}$ of the commercial product is approximately 0.6 gm./kg. (calculated as the contained aldehyde) in male rats. Percutaneous lethal dose in rabbits 0.6 gm./kg. Powerful eye irritant in rabbits. Allergic contact dermatitis to glutaraldehyde and to glutaraldehyde-tanned leather has been described.

See also: Formaldehyde, Reference Congener in Section III.
Ref.: Jordan et al., 1972; Smyth, 1961.

485   Metaldehyde 485

Metacetaldehyde, "Meta"

Toxicity Rating: 4. Probably lies near the borderline between toxicity classes 3 and 4. Polymer of acetaldehyde similar to but more active than paraldehyde. A child has died after ingesting 3 gm. Used to kill snails and in compressed form as a dry fuel substitute for alcohol. After a time lag of 1 to 3 hr., ingestion is followed by severe abdominal pain, nausea, vomiting, diarrhea, fever, convulsions, and coma. If death is delayed, renal tubular injury and liver necrosis may appear. In one infant, signs of coarse tremor, generalized hypertonia, hyper-reflexia and irritability were delayed for 48 hours. Only symptomatic and supportive measures are available.

See also: Formaldehyde, Reference Congener in Section III.
Ref.: Goulding, 1968; Lewis et al., 1939; Miller, 1928; Romagny and Megard, 1959.

486   Methenamine 486

Hexamethylenetetramine

Toxicity Rating: 3(?). Slowly decomposes into formaldehyde, especially in an acid medium (e.g., stomach, urine). A very large oral dose (usual doses are 1 to 2 gm.) causes gastrointestinal irritation (vomiting and pain), albuminuria, gross hematuria, and dysuria, with inflammatory lesions in the renal tubules, renal pelvis, and urinary bladder. A 2.5-year old boy developed hemorrhagic cystitis and mild azotemia following the ingestion of at least 8 gm. Recovery was prompt and complete without specific treatment. Repeated use may cause sensitization with urticaria or dermatitis.

See also: Formaldehyde, Reference Congener in Section III.
Ref.: Osol and Farrar, 1955; Ross and Conway, 1970.

487   Paraformaldehyde 487

Paraform, Triformol, Trioxymethylene

Toxicity Rating: 4. Occasionally found in solid cake-type household deodorant products. Both infant and mother "tasted" such a product without incurring local burns. Same internal toxicity as formaldehyde, which it slowly releases at body temperature.

See also: Formaldehyde, Reference Congener in Section III.
Ref.: Jacobziner and Raybin, 1961d; Manufacturing Chemists' Assoc., 1950b.

Simple monohydric phenols and their esters

488   Amyl Phenol

*p-tert-*Amylphenol, *p-tert-*Pentylphenol

Toxicity Rating: 3(?). An intermediate in industrial chemical syntheses. This and various other alkyl derivatives of phenol (and of cresol) are also used as germicides, usually on non-biological surfaces. They are less corrosive than phenol and produce less skin irritation, but they may share phenol's ability to penetrate intact skin. Relevant oral toxicity data were not located, but among mono- and di-alkyl substituted phenols, water solubility and systemic toxicity decrease with increasing size of the alkyl constituents. The differences are particularly prominent in comparing *n*-amyl with *n*-hexyl phenol and in comparing 6-*n*-amyl-3-methylphenol with 6-*n*-hexyl-3-methylphenol.

See also: Phenol, *Reference Congener in Section III.*
Ref.: von Oettingen, 1949.

489   Carvacrol

Isopropyl-*o*-cresol, 2-Hydroxy-*p*-cymene, Isothymol

Toxicity Rating: 4. An isomer of thymol. Somewhat more toxic than thymol in rats and rabbits. Same symptoms and treatment as phenol.

See also: Phenol, *Reference Congener in Section III.*
Ref.: von Oettingen, 1949.

490   Creosol

2-Methoxy-4-methyl phenol

Toxicity Rating: 4. One of the active ingredients of wood creosote, not to be confused with cresol; see index. Slightly less toxic and less corrosive than phenol.

See also: Phenol, *Reference Congener in Section III.*
Ref.: von Oettingen, 1949.

491   *m*-Cresyl Acetate

Cresatin

Toxicity Rating: 4. Presumably benign until hydrolyzed in the bowel to acetic acid and *m*-cresol; see latter in the index. The latter is less corrosive and less toxic than phenol.

See also: Phenol, *Reference Congener in Section III.*
Ref.: von Oettingen, 1949.

492   Guaiacol

Methylcatechol, *o*-Hydroxyanisole, *o*-Methoxyphenol

Toxicity Rating: 4. Slightly less corrosive and less toxic than phenol. In most clinical poisonings, guaiacol was taken as wood-tar creosote. Percutaneous absorption is dangerous.

See also: Phenol, *Reference Congener in Section III.*
Ref.: von Oettingen, 1949.

493   β-Naphthol

Beta-naphthol, β-Hydroxynaphthalene

Toxicity Rating: 4. Produces crampy abdominal pain, nausea, vomiting, and sometimes convulsions. Intestinal or percutaneous absorption may lead to a severe nephritis, liver injury, and acute hemolytic anemia. Lens opacities and retinal changes have been described. Alpha isomer is said to be even more toxic.

See also: Phenol, *Reference Congener in Section III.*
Ref.: Anonymous, 1922.

494   Phenol

Carbolic acid, Phenylic acid, Hydroxybenzene, Oxybenzene
Toxicity Rating: 4.

See also: Phenol, *Reference Congener in Section III.*

495   Phenylphenol   495

Orthophenylphenol, e.g., Dowicide 1

Toxicity Rating: 3. The sodium salt is available as Dowicide A. Not absorbed in acutely toxic amounts through skin. An oil solution (5%) is well tolerated on human skin, but aqueous solutions of the sodium salt are irritating in concentrations above 0.5%. Irritating in the eye and may cause corneal injury (necrosis), especially the sodium salt. Dusts are also irritants when inhaled. In rats ingestion causes death from nervous depression, as does phenol. Single oral dose LD_{50} in rats is greater than 1.0 gm./kg. for Dowicide 1 and 0.7-0.9 gm./kg. for Dowicide A. In cats oral lethal doses of o-phenylphenol in aqueous suspensions cause hemorrhagic gastroenteritis and hemorrhages in liver, lung and myocardium.

See also: Phenol, Reference Congener in Section III.
Ref.: Dow Chemical Co., 1969a; Dow Chemical Co., 1969e; Dow Chemical Co., 1969g; Hodge et al., 1952b; MacIntosh, 1945.

496   Potassium Guaiacolsulfonate   496

Hydroxymethoxybenzenesulfonic acid potassium salt, Thiacol, Sulfoguaiacol

Toxicity Rating: 2. An expectorant of low oral toxicity used in cough syrups. The usual adult dose is 500 mg. repeated every 2 to 3 hours. Guaiacol may be released when large doses of the salt are ingested, but this assertion has not been proved. See Guaiacol above. With large doses symptoms referable to potassium poisoning should be anticipated because 6 grams of the salt contains one gram of potassium. See Potassium salts in the index.

497   Thymol   497

5-Methyl-2-isopropyl-1-phenol, 3-Hydroxy-p-cymene, Thyme camphor

Toxicity Rating: 4. A potent fungicide and anthelmintic and mild local irritant. Resembles phenol in its systemic actions but less toxic, partly because it is less soluble. Believed to lie near the borderline between toxicity classes 3 and 4. Produces gastric pain, nausea, vomiting, central hyperactivity (e.g., talkativeness), occasionally convulsions, coma, cardiac and respiratory collapse. Avoid oils and alcohol, which promote absorption.

See also: Phenol, Reference Congener in Section III.
Ref.: von Oettingen, 1949.

498   Xylenol   498

Dimethylphenol

Toxicity Rating: 4(?). Six isomers exist. A constituent of cresylic acid. See latter in the index.

See also: Phenol, Reference Congener in Section III.
Ref.: von Oettingen, 1949.

Polyhydric phenols and their esters

499   Anthraquinone   499

9,10-Anthracenedione, Anthradione, Morkit

A bird repellent used to protect planted seeds; also an important starting material in the manufacture of vat dyes. The compound is unpalatable and has a low acute oral toxicity. Mice given 5 gm./kg. by mouth showed no toxic effects. A mild skin irritant and sensitizer. It is supplied as a wettable powder containing 2.5% anthraquinone and in a mixed formulation with Voronit (2-(2'-furyl)-benzimidazole and hexachlorobenzene); see Voronit in the Index.

Ref.: Spencer, 1973.

500   Chlorohydroquinone   500

e.g., Edwal C.H.Q.

Toxicity Rating: 4(?). Used in photography. No toxicity data were located. Presumably similar in toxicity to hydroquinone. See Hydroquinone below.

501   Dihydroxybenzene   501

Toxicity Rating: 4. Three isomers (o-, m-, p-). For ortho isomer (o- or 1,2-), see Pyrocatechol below. For meta isomer (m- or 1,3-) see Resorcinol below. For para isomer (p- or 1,4-), see Hydroquinone below. In various test animals, resorcinol has usually proved to have the lowest acute toxicity, but all 3 compounds are similarly hazardous. In animals they are generally somewhat more toxic than phenol. For example, they are more potent in eliciting myoclonic jerks in mice.

Ref.: Angel and Rogers, 1972; Graham and Tisdall, 1922.

502   502 Gallic Acid

3,4,5-Trihydroxybenzoic acid

Toxicity Rating: 3(?). Apparently much less toxic than salicylic acid. Fed to men in quantities of 2 to 10 gm. without fatalities and without even severe ill effects. Readily absorbed from the gastrointestinal tract. In animals it reduces body temperature and causes progressive weakness and perhaps convulsions.

Ref.: Cameron et al., 1943; von Oettingen, 1949.

503   503 Hexylresorcinol

4-Hexyl-1,3-dihydroxybenzene

Toxicity Rating: 3. Somewhat less toxic than resorcinol or phenol. Effective by all portals including percutaneous absorption. Irritating to skin when in high concentrations. Some cutaneous reactions are due to hypersensitivity. By mouth large doses cause irritation and erosion of gastric and intestinal mucosa. Because of poor absorption, systemic symptoms are unusual but damage to liver and heart has been reported in dogs.

See also: Phenol, *Reference Congener in Section III.*
Ref.: Anderson et al., 1931b; Evans and Moore, 1942; Lamson et al., 1935.

504   504 Hydroquinone

p-Dihydroxybenzene, 1,4-Dihydroxybenzene

Toxicity Rating: 4. Irritating but not corrosive. Human poisonings have been reported from a mixture of hydroquinone and metol (see in index). Systemic actions like phenol, but in addition tremors and convulsions are prominent, plus an occasional severe hemolytic anemia (subsequent to methemoglobinemia ?). Fatal human doses have ranged from 5 to 12 gm., but 300 to 500 mg. has been ingested daily for 3 to 5 months without ill effects. Lesions of skin (especially depigmentation) and of eyes are described in man, but these effects may have been due to local contact with quinone.

See also: Phenol *and* Aniline, *Reference Congeners in Section III.*
Ref.: Amer. Petroleum Institute, 1953e; Zeidman and Deutl, 1945.

505   505 Pyrocatechol

o-Dihydroxybenzene, Catechol

Toxicity Rating: 4. As toxic as phenol. Similar to phenol, but convulsions may be more frequent, and blood dyscrasias are described. The most potent hydroxybenzene (by intraperitoneal injection) in terms of eliciting myoclonic jerks in mice.

See also: Phenol, *Reference Congener in Section III.*
Ref.: Angel and Rogers, 1972; von Oettingen, 1949.

506   506 Pyrogallol

Pyrogallic acid, 1,2,3-Trihydroxybenzene

Toxicity Rating: 4. Toxicity and toxic actions like phenol, but sometimes methemoglobinemia, hemolysis, and renal injury, as in aniline poisoning (See Resorcinol below). Delayed deaths from uremia have been reported. Percutaneous absorption is dangerous. A psoriatic patient is reported to have collapsed within 5 minutes of covering two-thirds of his body with an ointment containing pyrogallol; he died in coma 24 hours later, having absorbed an estimated 10 gm. pyrogallol. Mildly caustic to skin and mucous membranes. May potentiate endogenous epinephrine because it is an effective inhibitor in vivo of one of the enzymes which detoxifies epinephrine, namely catechol *O*-methyl-transferase. Unlike phenol and dihydroxybenzenes, pyrogallol and phloroglucinol produce somnolence in mice, not myoclonic jerks.

See also: Aniline, *Reference Congener in Section III.*
Ref.: Angel and Rogers, 1972; Pewny, 1925; von Oettingen, 1949; Wylie et al., 1960.

507   Quinone

507

1,4-Benzoquinone

Toxicity Rating: 4. An oxidizing agent. Has produced ocular and cutaneous lesions in man, but no systemic poisonings are known. In animals single oral doses are said to produce delayed deaths. Toxic effects differ from those of hydroquinone.

Ref.: Anderson and Oglesby, 1958; Woodward et al., 1949.

508   Resorcinol

508

Resorcin, *m*-Dihydroxybenzene

Toxicity Rating: 4. Used on the skin as a bactericidal and fungicidal ointment (usually 5%). About the same toxicity as phenol, but convulsions are more prominent. Perhaps slightly less toxic than catechol or hydroquinone. Sometimes associated with methemoglobinemia, Heinz bodies and hemolysis. The rarity of such reports suggests that inherited traits may have been responsible for the reactions.

See also: Phenol, *Reference Congener in Section III.*
Ref.: Angel and Rogers, 1972; Graham and Tisdall, 1922.

509   Resorcinol Monoacetate

509

Toxicity Rating: 4. Similar to resorcinol but actions are milder and more persistent. Skin ointments vary in concentration from 5 to 20%, lotions from 3 to 5%.

See also: Phenol, *Reference Congener in Section III.*
Ref.: Osol and Farrar, 1955.

Phenolic mixtures

510   Coal Tar

510

A mixture of condensible volatile products formed during the destructive distillation of bituminous coal. Composition is variable but generally it consists of: 2 to 8% light oils (chiefly benzene, toluene, xylene); 8 to 10% middle oils (chiefly phenols, cresols and naphthalene); 8 to 10% heavy oils (naphthalene and derivatives); 16 to 20% anthracene oils (mostly anthracene); and about 50% pitch. In this mixture phenol and its congeners have the highest acute toxicity. Human intoxications appear to be unknown, but epidemics of both acute and chronic poisonings have been reported in swine. Dead animals exhibit severe hemorrhagic centrilobular necrosis. See also Tars (tar oils and tar acids) below.

See also: Phenol, *Reference Congener in Section III.*
Ref.: Maclean, 1969.

511   Coal Tar Creosote

511

A black to brown oily liquid prepared by the high temperature distillation (above 200°C.) of coal tar (see latter above). It consists of the less volatile liquid and solid aromatic hydrocarbons of coal tar, together with up to 3 percent tar acids (phenolic constituents). Used as a general disinfectant, insecticide, and fungicide. Impregnated in wood it retards rot. Sometimes used as an intestinal vermicide in veterinary medicine but not prescribed for internal use in man. Probably less toxic than crude coal tar. Although present in low concentrations, phenol and phenolic derivatives of various aromatic hydrocarbons (tar acids) are the constituents most likely to be responsible for acute toxic reactions.

See also: Phenol, *Reference Congener in Section III.*
Ref.: Merck and Co., 1976.

512   Creolin

512

Creolin-Pearson

Toxicity Rating: 3(?). Said to contain cresols (about 15%), hydrocarbons (46%), and soap.

See also: Phenol, *Reference Congener in Section III.*
Ref.: von Oettingen, 1949.

513   Creosote

513

Creosote oil

Toxicity Rating: 3(?). A liquid obtained from wood tars by distillation (mostly between 203 and 220°C.). In contrast to coal tar creosote (see above), wood creosote (especially beechwood) contains lit-tle or no free phenol or cresols; it is composed chiefly of guaiacol, also creosol, etc., with toxicities similar to but less than phenol. Used externally as an antiseptic and by mouth as an expectorant.

See also: Phenol, *Reference Congener in Section III.*
Ref.: Gerarde, 1960; von Oettingen, 1949.

514   Cresols

514

Tricresol, Cresylic acid

Toxicity Rating: 4. *o*-,*m*-, and *p*-Hydroxytoluene, usually present as a mixture obtained from coal tar. About the same toxicity and toxic actions as phenol (but ortho and especially para isomers are even more toxic). Perhaps slightly more corrosive than phenol, but systemic effects may be a little milder because of slower absorption.

See also: Phenol, *Reference Congener in Section III.*
Ref.: Manufacturing Chemists' Assoc., 1952c; National Safety Council, Date Unknown b.

515   Cresol and Soap Solution (B.P.)

515

Lysol

Toxicity Rating: 4. In England, and other countries in which the British Pharmacopoeia is official, the name lysol is not a trademark, but rather it is a synonym for Cresol and Soap Solution, B.P. This toxic and corrosive germicide is a solution of cresol in a saponaceous solvent containing 50% v/v of cresol (toxicity rating 4). Generic lysol is available from several manufacturers in England and the nature of the product is as described above and as in the British Pharmacopoeia. A half pint of an English "lysol" produced serious poisoning in an adult male. The initial signs were deep coma punctuated by periods of extreme restlessness. Pharyngeal edema necessitated a tracheotomy. He was fully conscious by the third day but markedly jaundiced with elevated serum bilirubin and transaminase (SGOT) activity and a low platelet count. At one week these values were normal but difficulty in swallowing led to a jejunostomy. Eventually he recovered fully. Two adult Chinese females ingested 100 ml and 250 ml of lysol, B.P., containing 50% cresols. Besides coma, marked he-matologic changes were observed including methemoglobinemia (36% in one case), decreased red cell content of glutathione, Heinz bodies and evidence of massive intravascular hemolysis. The patient ingesting the larger dose died. The hematologic damage is not believed to depend upon red cell deficiency of glucose-6-phosphate dehydrogenase. A 6-year-old mentally retarded child severely contaminated his clothing and skin (45% of total body surface) with "undiluted lysol". Despite prompt decontamination he became comatose within one hour. Hypothermia and signs of cardiovascular weakness were observed as well as a brief period of anuria. The child eventually died from the complications of pneumonia and cardiovascular collapse. Histologic examination of the kidney suggested a direct nephrotoxic action in the proximal tubule as well as nonspecific changes due to "shock". In another case report, peritoneal dialysis was judged of no benefit in the presence of adequate renal function on the basis of results in one patient.

Ref.: Fisher, 1955; British Pharmacopoeia, 1963; Chan et al., 1971; Ferry, 1965; Herpol, 1961; McDonald, 1973; Thomas, 1969.

516   Lysol Brand Disinfectant

516

Toxicity Rating: 2. Lysol Brand Disinfectant is a registered trademark in the United States and many other countries for a popular germicide. Lysol Brand Disinfectant is a disinfectant of low toxicity; it contains soap and low concentrations of substituted phenolic compounds. Four ounces of a former but similar formulation has been swallowed by man without serious ill effects. The present formula has remained unchanged since the early 1950's. There are several Lysol Brand products; none contains cresol and some do not contain substituted phenolic compounds. For a complete list of Lysol Brand products see Section V.

Ref.: Klarmann, 1954; McDonald, 1973; Prindle, 1973.

517   Octyl Cresols

517

Octyl methyl phenols

Toxicity Rating: 3. Various isomers (*o*-, *m*-, and *p*-). Low ingestion toxicity in rats (near the borderline between toxicity classes 2 and 3), but necrosis results from cutaneous applications. No clinical data are known. Octyl phenols are assumed to be similar in toxicity, but heat is said to decompose them with the release of dangerous fumes of phenol. All of these long-chain alkyl derivatives of phenol are safer than phenol itself.

See also: Phenol, *Reference Congener in Section III.*
Ref.: von Oettingen, 1949; Sax, 1968.

518   Saprol

Toxicity Rating: 4. Said to consist of 40% cresols, 40% other coal tar derivatives, and 20% high–boiling hydrocarbons.

See also: Phenol, *Reference Congener in Section III.*
Ref.: von Oettingen, 1949.

519   Tars (Tar Oils and Tar Acids)

Toxicity Rating: 4(?). The black or dark residue remaining after the destructive distillation of coal, crude petroleum, or wood (usually pine or juniper). Tars, tar oils, and tar acids are closely related. The phrase tar acids refers to phenolic constituents in tar. Tar and tar oils vary in composition, depending upon the source and method of manufacture. In all cases, however, the principal toxic ingredients are phenol and its congeners (tar acids) and aromatic hydrocarbons (e.g., xylenes, naphthalene, etc.). Toxicity estimates are difficult because even the USP does not specify the phenol or cresol content of official preparations, but 1 oz. of most tars, if ingested, would probably jeopardize life. Most medicinal ointments are only 1 to 10% tar. See Coal tar above.

See also: Phenol, *Reference Congener in Section III.*

Chloro- and bromo- phenols

520   *o*-Benzyl-*p*-chlorophenol

Santophen 1

Toxicity Rating: 3. A germicide with a lower oral toxicity than phenol. In formulations of 10% or more, it is a primary skin irritant. Percutaneous absorption demonstrated in rabbits. Only mild skin irritation after prolonged contact with use-dilutions (0.03%). Poisoned animals exhibit diarrhea, lassitude, rapid breathing, dyspnea, collapse, and death. A cleaning woman who mixed a commercial solution of this disinfectant with hypochlorite bleach suffered a severe attack of porphyrea cutanea tarda, probably because of polychlorinated phenolic derivatives generated in the mixture (Lynch et al., 1975).

See also: Phenol, *Reference Congener in Section III.*
Ref.: Kelly, 1958; Lynch et al., 1975.

521   Bithionol

2,2-Thiobis(4,6-dichlorophenol), Actamer

Toxicity Rating: 2. A germicide of low toxicity closely related to hexachlorophene. No skin reaction when applied as a 2% ointment (in Carbowax).

See also: Phenol, *Reference Congener in Section III.*
Ref.: Osol and Farrar, 1955.

522   2-Bromo-4-phenylphenol

e.g., Dowicide 5

Toxicity Rating: 3(?). Once available as an antimicrobial agent (fungicide) but no longer marketed. Toxicity is believed to resemble that of chlorophenylphenols; see latter below.

See also: Phenol, *Reference Congener in Section III.*

523   Chlorocresols

e.g., 6-Chloro-*m*-cresol, *p*-Chloro-*m*-cresol

Toxicity Rating: 4. Used as antiseptics and disinfectants. Not irritating to skin in concentrations of 0.5 to 1.0% in alcohol. Systemic effects are presumably like phenol.

See also: Phenol, *Reference Congener in Section III.*
Ref.: von Oettingen, 1949.

524   4-Chloro-2-cyclopentylphenol

e.g., Dowicide 9

Toxicity Rating: 3-4. A germicide used on non-living surfaces. Acute oral LD_{50}'s vary from 0.42 gm./kg. in rabbits to 3.2 gm./kg. in chicks (2.5 gm./kg. in rats). Concentrated material on the skin may cause redness and moderate chemical burns. In the rabbit eye it induces conjunctival inflammation and moderate-to-severe corneal injury. Vapors and mists, may produce irritation of the respiratory tract. Believed to resemble phenol in its systemic effects.

See also: Phenol, Reference Congener in Section III.
Ref.: Dow Chemical Co., 1970d.

525   Chlorophenols

e.g., 2,4-Dichlorophenol

Toxicity Rating: 4. Many isomers; chlorine atoms vary in number from 1 to 5. Monochlorophenols are slightly less toxic than phenol but more toxic than chlorobenzene. However, they may be somewhat more potent than phenol in eliciting convulsions. The ortho isomer is more toxic than the meta or para. Additional chlorination appears to enhance toxicity. Thus pentachlorophenol is as toxic and corrosive as phenol and has the additional property of being a metabolic stimulant like dinitrophenol.

See also: Phenol, Reference Congener in Section III.
Ref.: Angel and Rogers, 1972.

526   Chloro-2-phenylphenol

e.g., Dowicide 31, Dowicide 32

Toxicity Rating: 3. Various isomers are used as antimicrobial agents on inert surfaces. Dowicides 31 and 32 are mixtures of 4-chloro-2-phenylphenol and 6-chloro-2-phenylphenol (oral LD_{50} > 3.2 gm./kg. in rats). A related substance 2-chloro-4-phenylphenol is available as Dowicide 4 (oral LD_{50} 2.6 gm./kg. in rats). The only major toxicological distinctions among these isomers concern skin and eye irritation. Concentrated preparations of Dowicides 31 and 32 on human skin may induce redness and very slight chemical burns, whereas Dowicide 4 is generally not an irritant on the skin. None of them is absorbed through rabbit skin in acutely toxic amounts and none is a skin sensitizer in man. These compounds in the eye may cause inflammation of the conjunctiva and varying degrees of corneal injury, particularly Dowicides 31 and 32. Although less toxic than simple phenol, the chlorophenylphenols presumably share some of the systemic effects of phenol.

See also: Phenol, Reference Congener in Section III.
Ref.: Dow Chemical Co., 1970b; Dow Chemical Co., 1970c.

527   Chlorothymol

1-Hydroxy-3-methyl-4-chloro-6-isopropylbenzene

Toxicity Rating: 3(?). A good germicide, but aqueous solutions are irritating to mucous membranes. Systemic effects are presumably like those of thymol and phenol, but it is probably less toxic than either.

See also: Phenol, Reference Congener in Section III.
Ref.: von Oettingen, 1949.

528   4-Chloro-3,5-xylenol

Chloro-xylenol, PCMX, p-Chloro-m-xylenol

Toxicity Rating: 3. Penetrates skin but no cutaneous irritation at concentration of 5%. Death of a 66-year-old woman resulted from the ingestion of 300 ml. of a household disinfectant (Dettol) containing 4.8% PCMX.

See also: Phenol, Reference Congener in Section III.
Ref.: von Oettingen, 1949; Meek et al., 1977.

529   Dichlorophen(e)

Di-(5-chloro-2-hydroxyphenyl)methane, 2,2'-Methylenebis(4-chlorophenol), e.g., Korium, Parabis, Di-phenthane-70, Preventol G-D

Toxicity Rating: 3. Industrial fungicide, related to hexachlorophene (see below), used for protection of textiles, leather and paper. Also used in soaps and shampoos and as a medical anthelmintic.

Acute oral LD_{50} in guinea pigs is 1.25 gm./kg. and in dogs is 2.0 gm./kg. No skin irritation (man) at

concentrations of 1% and little at 4%.

See also: Phenol, *Reference Congener in Section III.*
Ref.: Sindar Corp., Date Unknown.

530   Dowicides   530

i.e., Dowicide 1, 2, 2S, 4, 6, etc.

A series of phenolic substances used as disinfectants, including chlorinated phenols, o-phenylphenol, brominated and chlorinated o-phenylphenols, and sodium salts of these compounds. As tested

in animals the various derivatives lie in toxicity classes 3 and 4. See various individual entries in the index. Phenol is a congener common to them all.

See also: Phenol, *Reference Congener in Section III.*

531   Hexachlorophene   531

2,2′-Methylenebis(3,4,6-trichlorophenol)

Toxicity Rating: 4(?). Used in concentrations of 1 to 2% as a disinfectant in several liquid and solid soap products. Not irritating to the skin, but sensitization has been reported. Severe excoriation of skin and central nervous symptoms resulted from total body application of a 3% lotion on a newborn infant for several days. In a series of 10 cases of

accidental ingestion the gastrointestinal symptoms included anorexia, nausea, vomiting, abdominal cramps and diarrhea. Dehydration was severe in some cases and associated with shock. Water and electrolyte derangements required vigorous treatment.

See also: Phenol, *Reference Congener in Section III.*
Ref.: Beckman, 1961; Wear et al., 1962.

532   Pentachlorophenol   532

Penta, Dowicide 7, PCP

Toxicity Rating: 4. An antimicrobial agent used as a fungicide, wood preservative, molluscicide, etc. Also marketed as the sodium salt, sodium pentachlorophenate (e.g., Dowicide G). Even more toxic than simple phenol. Should be used only when wearing goggles and protective (impervious) clothing such as rubber boots, apron, and gloves. In solutions of organic solvents, the material may be absorbed through intact skin in lethal amounts. Solids and concentrated solutions may also produce skin irritation (redness) and even a skin burn, especially the sodium salt. Frequent skin contact may cause an acneform dermatitis and rarely an allergic skin response. In the eye it causes inflammation that may progress to permanent corneal

injury, especially with the sodium salt in concentrated solutions. Dusts are also irritating to the nose and pharynx. Toxic by all portals of entry. Acute oral LD_{50} is about 200 mg./kg. in rats, somewhat less in guinea pigs. When absorbed, pentachlorophenol is a metabolic stimulant like dinitrophenol. It has produced human fatalities due to hyperpyrexia. Contaminated bed linen and diapers resulted in a subacute percutaneous exposure of hospitalized infants. Nine of them became severely ill and two died. Exchange transfusions proved to be highly beneficial. Chronic exposure to a mixture of penta- and tetrachlorophenol is reported to have caused aplastic anemia in one adult.

See also: Phenol *and* 2,4-Dinitrophenol, *Reference Congeners in Section III.*
Ref.: Deichmann et al., 1942; Menon, 1958; Dow Chemical Co., 1968; Dow Chemical Co., 1969d; Roberts, 1963; Robson et al., 1969; Armstrong et al., 1969; Gordon, 1956.

533   Tetrabromo-o-cresol   533

2-Methyl-3,4,5,6-tetrabromophenol

Toxicity Rating: 3. A fungicide of low acute toxicity by mouth in guinea pigs. Concentrated solutions

are corrosive to skin. No clinical data, but presumably irritating to skin.

See also: Phenol, *Reference Congener in Section III.*

534   2,3,4,6-Tetrachlorophenol   534

Dowicide 6

Toxicity Rating: 4. An antimicrobial agent (e.g., fungicide) about as acutely lethal as phenol (oral LD_{50} in rats approx. 470 mg./kg.). The solid and 10 percent aqueous suspensions are not primary skin irritants, but repeated skin contact may result in

acneform dermatitis. Unlike aqueous suspensions, tetrachlorophenol dissolved in organic solvents may be absorbed through the skin in acutely toxic amounts. In the eye conjunctivitis and slight-to-moderate corneal injuries are described. Dust may irritate the nose and pharynx. The possibility that tetrachlorophenol shares the ability of pentachlorophenol (see latter above) to stimulate tissue oxygen metabolism and induce hyperpyrexia should be kept in mind, even though hypermetabolism has not been described in exposed animals or humans. Chronic exposure to a mixture of penta- and tetrachlorophenol is reported to have caused aplastic anemia in one adult.

See also: Phenol, *Reference Congener in Section III.*
Ref.: Dow Chemical Co., 1969c; Roberts, 1963.

535   535   Trichlorophenols

e.g., 2,4,5-Trichlorophenol, Dowicide 2, 2,4,6-Trichlorophenol, Dowicide 2S

Toxicity Rating: 3. Two technical grade isomers are marketed as antimicrobial agents: 2,4,5-trichlorophenol as Dowicide 2 and 2,4,6-trichlorophenol as Dowicide 2S. The sodium salt of Dowicide 2 is also available as Dowicide B. These materials are fungicidal and also serve as wood preservatives among their other uses. The 2 isomers are about equi-toxic (oral LD_{50} about 2.8 gm./kg. in rats), but the sodium salt (Dowicide B) is more toxic by mouth and more irritating on the skin than the two free phenols. All are less toxic than simple phenol. They appear not to penetrate intact rabbit or guinea pig skin (percutaneous absorption) in significant amounts, in contrast to phenol and its tetra- and penta-chloro derivatives (see latter above). The trichlorophenols, however, can produce redness and edema on skin contact and on prolonged exposure even mild to moderate chemical burns of the skin of man. In the eye they induce conjunctival irritation and sometimes corneal injury and iritis. The dusts are irritating to the nose and pharynx. Systemic effects are not described but presumably resemble those of phenol poisoning.

See also: Phenol, *Reference Congener in Section III.*
Ref.: Dow Chemical Co., 1969b; Dow Chemical Co., 1969f; Dow Chemical Co., 1970a; McCollister et al., 1961.

Nitro-phenols

536   536   Dicyclohexylamine 4,6-Dinitro-*o*-cyclohexylphenate

Dicyclohexylammonium 2-cyclohexyl-4,6-dinitrophenate, 2-Cyclohexyl-4,6-dinitrophenol dicyclohexylamine, DN-111, Dynone II

Toxicity Rating: 4. Selective acaricide used in the form of a 20% wettable powder. Percutaneous absorption is limited. Less toxic than 4,6-Dinitro-*o*- cyclohexylphenol (see latter below), but presumably closely resembles it.

See also: 2,4-Dinitrophenol, *Reference Congener in Section III.*
Ref.: Assoc. of Amer. Pesticide Control Officials, 1966.

537   537   2,6-Diiodo-4-nitrophenol

Disophenol, e.g., Ancylol

Toxicity Rating: 4. Anthelmintic in veterinary medicine. Vigorous exercise and high ambient temperature, combined with a therapeutic dose of disophenol, led to hyperpnea, hyperthermia and tachycardia in an Irish wolfhound.

See also: 2,4-Dinitrophenol, *Reference Congener in Section III.*
Ref.: Legendre, 1973.

538   538   4,6-Dinitro-*o*-amylphenol

4,6-Dinitro-2-*sec*-amyl phenol

Toxicity Rating: 5. Herbicide and insecticide. Skin contact may lead to local necrosis and dangerous systemic effects, like 2,4-dinitrophenol.

See also: 2,4-Dinitrophenol, *Reference Congener in Section III.*
Ref.: Hayes, 1963.

539   539   4,6-Dinitro-*o*-cresol

Dinitrocresol, 3,5-Dinitro-2-hydroxytoluene

Toxicity Rating: 5. Selective herbicide, insecticide, and plant growth regulator. More toxic than dinitrophenol, it is cumulative in man although not in laboratory animals. Skin contact may lead to local necrosis and dangerous systemic effects. The 8-hour OSHA standard for skin exposure is 200 μg./ m^3 in workroom air.

See also: 2,4-Dinitrophenol, *Reference Congener in Section III.*
Ref.: Lehman, 1951; Worthing, 1979.

540 4,6-Dinitro-*o*-cyclohexylphenol
540

2-Cyclohexyl-4,6-dinitrophenol, 2,4-Dinitro-6-cyclohexylphenol, e.g., Dinex

Toxicity Rating: 4-5. Used as an insecticide in control of citrus red mite. Very high oral toxicity in laboratory rodents (LD_{50} 50-65 mg./kg.). Observed signs of toxicity are hyperthermia, hyperpnea, excitement, and convulsions, or progressive weakness and coma. Skin contact may lead to local necrosis but rarely if ever to dangerous systemic effects (by this portal).

See also: 2,4-Dinitrophenol, *Reference Congener in Section III.*
Ref.: Hayes, 1963; Hrenoff and Leake, 1939.

541 2,4-Dinitrophenol
541

Alpha-dinitrophenol, 2,4-DNP, 1-Hydroxy-2,4-dinitrobenzene, Aldifen

Toxicity Rating: 5. Highly toxic wood preserver, insecticide, laboratory reagent and intermediate in manufacture of dyes. In rats the acute oral LD_{50} is 30 mg./kg.

See also: 2,4-Dinitrophenol, *Reference Congener in Section III.*

542 Dinocap
542

Dinitro(1-methylheptyl)phenyl crotonate, Karathane

Toxicity Rating: 4. The commercial product, once thought to be 2-(1-methylheptyl)-4,6-dinitrophenyl 2-butenoate, is a mixture of the octyl isomers of 2,4-dinitro-6-octylphenyl crotonate and 2,6-dinitro-4-octylphenyl crotonate. Used as an acaricide and fungicide on fruit and ornamental plants. In rats the acute oral LD_{50} is 980 mg./kg., but a value of 100 mg./kg. has been reported in dogs. Sold as wettable powder and emulsifiable concentrate. Irritating to the skin.

See also: 2,4-Dinitrophenol, *Reference Congener in Section III.*
Ref.: Assoc. of Amer. Pesticide Control Officials, 1966; Worthing, 1979; Spencer, 1973.

543 Dinoseb
543

4,6-Dinitro-2-*sec*-butyl phenol, Dinitrobutylphenol, Dinitro-ortho-*sec*-butyl phenol

Toxicity Rating: 5. Contact herbicide and dessicant. Very toxic in laboratory animals (rat oral LD_{50} is 58 mg./kg.). Toxicity due in part to uncoupling of oxidative phosphorylation. Symptoms of intoxication include prostration, rapid respiration, convulsions, and death. Very high percutaneous toxicity (rabbit LD_{50} 80 to 200 mg./kg.). Irritating to intact skin. Produces methemoglobinemia in ruminants, presumably because of nitro reduction to derivatives of nitroaniline. Dinoseb is teratogenic and embryotoxic in mice and rats when given by intraperitoneal injection, but not when given in sub-lethal oral doses. The compound is usually marketed as soluble sodium, ammonium or alkanolamine salts; the acetylated phenol (dinoseb acetate) and the methacrylate ester (dinoseb methacrylate, also known as binapacryl with tradenames Morocide, Acricid, Endosan, etc.) are also available.

See also: 2,4-Dinitrophenol, *Reference Congener in Section III.*
Ref.: Froslie, 1971; Gibson and Rao, 1973; Hayes, 1963.

544 *p*-Nitrophenol
544

Paranitrophenol, 4-Hydroxynitrobenzene

Toxicity Rating: 4. A fungicide and an industrially important intermediate in chemical syntheses. In mice and rats the acute oral LD_{50} is 350 and 467 mg./kg. respectively. May be absorbed through intact skin. Poisonings are assumed to resemble those due to both phenol and aniline. For example, cyanosis may arise due to the formation of methemoglobin.

See also: Phenol *and* Aniline, *Reference Congeners in Section III.*
Ref.: Monsanto Chemical Co., 1957b.

545 Picric Acid
545

2,4,6-Trinitrophenol, Carbazotic acid, Picronitric acid

A hazardous substance that may explode when heated rapidly. Used in the manufacture of explosives, fireworks, electric batteries, textiles and colored glass. Picric acid and its salts are toxic by inhalation, by ingestion and by percutaneous absorption (presumably only the free "acid"). Low-grade repeated exposures may lead to headache, pruritus, skin eruptions and yellowing of skin and conjunctiva, to vomiting and diarrhea and to oliguria. Severe human poisonings, which have occurred after the ingestion of one or two grams, may manifest themselves as severe gastroenteritis, hemorrhagic nephritis with anuria, intravascular hemolysis, acute hepatitis, progressive stupor, coma and death. Picric acid accelerates body metabolism like dinitrophenol (see Section III). The OSHA workroom air standard for skin exposure is 100 mg./m^3 (8-hour TWA).

See also: Phenol *and* 2,4-Dinitrophenol, *Reference Congeners in Section III.*
Ref.: Harris et al., 1946; National Safety Council, Date Unknown a.

Salts of aliphatic acids (exclusive of fatty acids)

546　　　　　546　Oxalate

e.g., Sodium oxalate, Potassium oxalate

Toxicity Rating: 4. Soluble salts of oxalic acid have essentially the same toxicity as the acid.
See also: Oxalate, *Reference Congener in Section III.*

547　　　　　547　Sodium Binoxalate

Sodium acid oxalate

Toxicity Rating: 4. Soluble salts of oxalic acid have essentially the same toxicity as the acid.
See also: Oxalate, *Reference Congener in Section III.*

548　　　　　548　Fluoroacetate

e.g., Sodium fluoroacetate

Toxicity Rating: 6. A delayed convulsant, with none of the toxic actions of fluorides.
See also: Fluoroacetate, *Reference Congener in Section III.*

549　　　　　549　Chloroacetic Acid (and Salts)

Chloroethanoic acid, Monochloroacetic acid, Sodium monochloroacetate

Toxicity Rating: 4. Pre-emergence herbicides and defoliants. The sodium salt is more commonly used because it is less corrosive than the acid. Both salts and acid are irritating to skin and eyes. All forms are highly toxic in laboratory rodents, more toxic than di- and tri-chloroacetates. The single dose LD$_{50}$ for monochloroacetic acid is 165 mg./kg. in mice. For the sodium salt, reported LD$_{50}$'s range from 76 mg./kg. in rats to 255 mg./kg. in guinea pigs. Like fluoroacetate, the compound is an uncompetitive inhibitor of acetate oxidation, but it also reduces the sulfhydryl content of liver and kidney by acetylating -SH residues. Signs and symptoms of intoxication include clonic and tonic convulsions, anuria, and respiratory depression. Experimental antidotes against fluoroacetate are said to be effective against chloroacetate.

See also: Fluoroacetate, *Reference Congener in Section III.*
Ref.: Hayes et al., 1973; Woodward et al., 1941.

550　　　　　550　Sodium Trichloroacetate

Toxicity Rating: 3. Di- and trichloroacetate salts have essentially the same acute toxicity in laboratory animals as sodium acetate. Animals quickly become comatose and recover within 36 hours or die in coma. Monochloroacetate is at least 20 times more toxic. See also Chloroacetic acid above.

Ref.: Woodward et al., 1941.

551　　　　　551　Sodium Propionate

Toxicity Rating: 3. The sodium salt of propanoic acid, widely used as a medical fungicide on the skin and as a preservative in commercial products, including bread. The salt occurs naturally in Swiss cheese at levels as high as 1%, and is on the GRAS list for use in foods. It is supplied as a powder and in gels and solutions containing 0.1 to 20% of the salt. Some preparations also contain calcium propionate, zinc and sodium caprylate, and propionic acid. When administered subcutaneously, sodium propionate has a molar toxicity about twice that of sodium chloride (Vincke and Never, 1944). The salt is readily absorbed through rabbit skin, and repeated applications may elicit allergic skin reactions. Rats given about 2 gm./day in food for 30 days showed no apparent ill effects (Graham et al., 1954). Toxic sequelae should be anticipated from larger doses, however. When ingested or applied topically in acidic media, the salt is converted to propionic acid. This corrosive acid is rapidly absorbed through the skin (rabbit LD$_{50}$ 0.5 gm./kg.) and penetrates gastric mucosa readily, causing desquamation and bleeding. Taken in large doses, the salt may also cause toxic symptoms referable to its sodium content (see Sodium chloride in the index).

Ref.: Davenport, 1964; Graham et al., 1954; Vincke and Never, 1944.

552   Thioglycolate Salts   552

Mercaptoacetate salts, i.e., Sodium, ammonium, potassium thioglycolates or thioglycollates

Toxicity Rating: 3(?). Commonly found in cold-wave preparations and in depilatories. Occasionally these produce a dermatitis of scalp or hands, with erythema, edema, and even subcutaneous hemorrhages. At one time available solutions were highly alkaline and produced caustic burns when ingested, but commercial solutions today are only moder- ately alkaline (pH 9-10). Serious systemic reactions are not described. Hypoglycemia has been shown experimentally to be a prominent manifestation of the toxic syndrome. Chronic exposure in animals has led to thyroid hyperplasia. Also consult index under the name of the cation.

See also: Lye, *Reference Congener in Section III.*
Ref.: Brunner, 1952; Freeman et al., 1956a; Freeman et al., 1956b; Lehman, 1949a.

553   Sodium Thioglycolate   553

Sodium thioglycollate, Sodium mercaptoacetate

Toxicity Rating: 3(?). Commonly found in cold-wave hair preparations and in depilatories. Occasionally these products cause a dermatitis of scalp or hands, with erythema, edema, and even subcu- taneous hemorrhages. When ingested, the high alkalinity of solutions causes caustic poisoning. Hy- poglycemia has been shown experimentally to be a prominent manifestation of the toxic syndrome. Chronic exposure in animals has led to thyroid hyperplasia.

See also: Lye, *Reference Congener in Section III.*
Ref.: Brunner, 1952; Freeman et al., 1956a; Freeman et al., 1956b; Lehman, 1949a.

554   Subacetate Salts   554

Partially hydrolyzed acetates of metals and metal- loids. For example, cupric subacetate is a series of hydrated complexes between cupric acetate and cupric hydroxide. If the salt is soluble in acid, the anion is present as the acetate. Consult the index under the name of cation or metal.

Aliphatic and alicyclic acids of low corrosivity (including fatty acids)

555   Linoleic Acid   555

9,12-Octadecadienoic acid

Toxicity Rating: 1. A common constituent of many vegetable oils and therefore of most normal diets. When given in large doses to rats, weight loss, progressive secondary anemia, leukopenia and pe- diculosis were observed.

Ref.: Gyorgy et al., 1942.

556   Lauric Acid   556

Dodecanoic acid

Toxicity Rating: 1. A common constituent of many vegetable oils and therefore of most normal diets.

557   Myristic Acid   557

Tetradecanoic acid

Occurs in most animal and vegetable fats (8 to 15%). Nontoxic by oral administration.

Ref.: Merck and Co., 1976.

558   Naphthenic Acids   558

In commerce this is the name of acidic petroleum fractions, consisting of cyclic carboxylic acids ex- tractable from kerosene and oil. Cyclopentane car- boxylic acid and cyclohexane carboxylic acid are included but most of the molecules are larger (e.g., methyl derivatives of the above and multiple sat- urated rings of high molecular weight). No specific toxicity information is available despite long and widespread use. Crude acids have unpleasant odors but not if purified. Cycloparaffins (like cyclopen- tanes and cyclohexanes) are central nervous de- pressants, and the potency is greater the higher the molecular weight. Perhaps the same is true of the naphthenic acids.

Ref.: Amer. Petroleum Institute, 1948f.

559   Oleic Acid

9-Octadecenoic acid

Toxicity Rating: 1. A common constituent of many animal and vegetable fats and therefore of most normal diets. The principal component of a commercial mixture known as red oil; see latter in the index.

Ref.: Jefferson and Necheles, 1948.

560   Ricinoleic Acid

12-Hydroxy-9-octadecenoic acid

Toxicity Rating: 2(?). An unsaturated fatty acid believed to be the active purgative principle in castor oil. Said to produce its cathartic effect by stimulating motor activity through a local action on the small intestinal mucosa. Also absorbed in part within the bowel and apparently metabolized. Used externally as a bland emollient. No reports of fatalities were located.

Ref.: Osol and Farrar, 1955; Paul and McCay, 1942.

561   Sorbic Acid

2,4-Hexadienoic acid

Toxicity Rating: 2. Used to protect materials against fungi. Not a primary irritant or sensitizing agent on the skin.

Ref.: Smyth and Carpenter, 1948.

562   Stearic Acid

Octadecanoic acid

Toxicity Rating: 1. A basic ingredient in vanishing creams, lotions, etc. Also a constituent of many neutral fats and therefore of most normal diets. No acute systemic ill-effects are recognized after ingestion. On intravenous injection in mice stearic acid has an LD_{50} of 23 mg./kg., the highest toxicity exhibited by any member of the homologous series from C_2 to C_{18}.

Ref.: Greenberg and Lester, 1954; Oro and Wretlind, 1961.

563   Tartaric Acid

Toxicity Rating: 3 to 4. Various salts and the free acid have been used as laxatives and diuretics and constituents of many foodstuffs. Not to be confused with the much more toxic Antimony potassium tartrate (tartar emetic); see latter in the index. Also encountered as potassium bitartrate (potassium acid tartrate, cream of tartar), potassium sodium tartrate (Rochelle salt) and Seidlitz powder (3 parts Rochelle salt and 1 part sodium bicarbonate). Surprisingly most of these substances have produced serious poisonings or death in man. The acid is said to have been fatal after an oral dose of 12 gm., whereas the lethal dose for potassium bitartrate is said to be 100 to 200 gm. Death occurred after 12 hours to 9 days. Gastrointestinal symptoms were marked (violent vomiting and diarrhea, abdominal pain, thirst) and followed by cardiovascular collapse and/or acute renal failure.

Ref.: Webster, 1930.

564   Undecylenic Acid

9-Undecylenic acid, 10-Undecenoic acid

Toxicity Rating: 3. A normal constituent of sweat. Used as a fungicide on skin. Formerly taken by mouth in the treatment of psoriasis. In daily oral doses of 6 to 14 gm., the following transient effects are described in man: gastrointestinal disturbances, headache, fever, dizziness, urticaria, folliculitis, and conjunctivitis. Lethal dose in rats about 2.5 gm./kg.

Ref.: Perlman, 1949; Perlman and Milberg, 1949.

Aliphatic amides useful as solvents

565   Dimethylacetamide

Acetyldimethylamine, DMA, DMAC

Toxicity Rating: 3. Commercial solvent tested as a parenteral drug vehicle and as an antitumor agent. Intraperitoneal LD_{50} in mice 3240 mg. (3.4 ml.) per kg. Tremors, depression, coma and delayed death were observed. Liver damage in dogs and rats occurred during chronic exposures above 0.1 ml./

kg. on the skin or 40 ppm by inhalation. When given to humans in daily doses of 400 mg./kg. for 3 or more days (route ?), depression, lethargy, confusion and disorientation ensued. In some patients there were visual and auditory hallucina- tions, perceptual distortions, delusions, emotional detachment and affective blunting, all reminiscent of the reactions induced by mescaline and by ly- sergic acid derivatives.

Ref.: Davis and Jenner, 1959; Horn, 1961; Weiss et al., 1962.

566   Dimethylformamide

DMF

Toxicity Rating: 3. Important industrial solvent also tested as a parenteral drug vehicle. Intraperi- toneal LD_{50} in mice 1120 mg./kg. (1.2 ml./kg.). Hind leg paralysis and depression were preceded by nervousness. Recommended m.a.c. for exposed workers is 20 ppm. Of several species of animals exposed to higher concentrations, only dogs ex- hibited polycythemia and cardiovascular effects: decreased pulse rate, decline in systolic pressure, and degenerative changes in heart muscle. In- creases in plasma cholesterol and liver weight were seen in other species. Losses of appetite and diges- tive disturbances have been reported in exposed industrial workers, and the possibility of liver dam- age should be investigated.

Ref.: Clayton et al., 1963; Davis and Jenner, 1959; Massmann, 1956.

567   *N*-(*β*-Hydroxyethyl)-2-lactamide

Lactic acid carboxamide

Toxicity Rating: 2. Said to be a reaction product of methyl acetate and 2-aminoethanol. Used in Eu- rope as a parenteral drug solvent. Administered as a 50% w/v aqueous solution, the acute subcuta- neous LD_{50} is 15.8 gm./kg. in mice and 16.1 gm./ kg. in rats.

Ref.: Spiegel and Noseworthy, 1963.

Simple aliphatic esters and lactones

568   *n*-Butyl Acetate

Toxicity Rating: 3. Mild irritant and central ner- vous depressant. More irritating than ethyl acetate. Except for *n*-butyl formate, all the simple esters of 1-butanol and 2-methyl-1-propanol (isobutyl alco- hol) are less acutely toxic than the parent alcohols. Acute oral LD_{50}'s in rabbits for the *n*-butanol es- ters: formate 2.6 gm./kg., acetate 7.4 gm./kg., *n*- butyrate 9.2 gm./kg. and isovalerate 8.2 gm./kg. For the isobutanol esters: formate 3.1 gm./kg., acetate 4.8 gm./kg., *n*-propionate 5.6 gm./kg., *n*- butyrate 9.5 gm./kg. and isovalerate 7.8 gm./kg. The narcotic dose for most of the esters lies very close to the lethal dose.

See also: Alcohols (Higher), *Reference Congener in Section III.*
Ref.: Munch, 1972; Sayers et al., 1936.

569   Butyl Myristate

May be hydrolyzed in vivo to myristic acid and butyl alcohol. Myristic (tetradecanoic) acid is a digestible constituent of animal and vegetable fats. See Butyl alcohol in the index.

570   Ethyl Acetate

Acetic ether

Toxicity Rating: 3. Relatively innocuous, lying on the borderline between toxicity classes 2 and 3. Mild local irritation and central nervous depres- sion. On a molar basis the simple esters of ethyl alcohol are more toxic than ethanol by 4 to 10-fold. Acute oral LD_{50}'s in rabbits: ethyl alcohol 9.9 gm./ kg., ethyl formate 2.1 gm./kg., ethyl acetate 4.9 gm./kg., ethyl *n*-propionate 5.7 gm./kg., ethyl *n*- butyrate 5.2 gm./kg. and ethyl isovalerate 7.0 gm./ kg. The ratio of the narcotic dose to the lethal dose is about 1.0 for ethyl formate and ethyl acetate, whereas it is about 2.0 for ethyl alcohol and the other esters above. Toxicity appears to be due to unhydrolyzed esters and not to ethyl alcohol.

See also: Ethyl Alcohol, *Reference Congener in Section III.*
Ref.: Munch, 1972; Spealman et al., 1945.

571   Ethyl Formate

Toxicity Rating: 3. About two-times more toxic than other simple esters of ethyl alcohol, and in rabbits the narcotic dose is the same as the lethal dose. See Ethyl Acetate above. Produces irritation and central nervous depression. A much stronger irritant than ethyl acetate, probably because of hydrolysis to formic acid.

Ref.: Munch, 1972; Schrenk et al., 1936; Smyth et al., 1954.

572   Ethyl Lactate

Ethyl α-hydroxypropionate

Toxicity Rating: 3. Industrial solvent and possible vehicle for parenteral drug administration. No industrial toxicity is recognized. Subcutaneous and intravenous LD_{50}'s in mice are 2.5 and 0.6 ml./kg., respectively. Irritating in the rabbit eye and in guinea pig skin (intradermal injection).

Ref.: Latven and Molitor, 1939.

573   Glycerol Esters

e.g., Glycerol oleate, Glycerol phthalate

If any of these esters is significantly toxic, the acid portion must be held responsible, not the glycerol. See corresponding acid in the index. Neutral fats in the diet are triglycerides of fatty acids, such as oleic and stearic acids. Monoglycerol esters of fatty acids are used as emulsifying agents in cosmetics and are produced in the body whenever fat is partially digested.

Ref.: Hine et al., 1953b; Pfeiffer and Arnove, 1937.

574   Isoamyl Acetate

Banana oil, Pear oil

Toxicity Rating: 3. Like other simple esters, an irritant and central nervous depressant. More narcotic than ethyl acetate and more irritating than butyl. Vapor has produced edema of the glottis. Secondary amyl acetate is thought to be qualitatively (and perhaps quantitatively) similar in toxicity to the more common isoamyl ester. Acute oral LD_{50}'s in rabbits: isoamyl formate 3.0 gm./kg., isoamyl acetate 7.4 gm./kg., isoamyl n-propionate, 6.9 gm./kg. and isoamyl isovalerate 14.0 gm./kg. The narcotic doses for these esters lie very close to the lethal doses.

See also: Alcohols (Higher), *Reference Congener in Section III.*
Ref.: Amer. Petroleum Institute, 1953a; Munch, 1972.

575   Isopropyl Myristate

Toxicity Rating: 2. Isopropyl ester of fatty acids derived from spermaceti. Used in cosmetics, especially alcohol-base hair lotions and after-shave preparations. No toxicity or local irritation has been reported, but if ingested, this ester would presumably be hydrolyzed in the bowel to metabolizable myristic acid and to isopropyl alcohol. See latter in the index.

Ref.: Greenberg and Lester, 1954.

576   Methyl Formate

Toxicity Rating: 3. Vapor produces irritation of mucous membranes and central nervous depression. Symptoms said to resemble methyl alcohol poisoning, but on a molar basis the simple esters of methyl alcohol are more toxic in laboratory animals by about an order of magnitude. Acute oral LD_{50}'s in rabbits: methyl alcohol 14.4 gm./kg., methyl formate 1.6 gm./kg., methyl acetate 3.7 gm./kg., methyl n-propionate 2.0 gm./kg., methyl n-butyrate 3.8 gm./kg. and methyl isovalerate 5.7 gm./kg. The ratio of the narcotic dose to the lethal dose was 2.4 for methyl alcohol and methyl isovalerate, whereas it was about 1.0 for the remaining esters. The narcotic and lethal effects of these esters appear to be related to the oil/water partition coefficient and to the intact molecules rather than the alcohols from which they were prepared.

See also: Methyl Alcohol, *Reference Congener in Section III.*
Ref.: Munch, 1972; Schrenk et al., 1936.

577   Monoacetin

Acetin, Glyceryl monoacetate

Toxicity Rating: 1. Often contaminated with glycerin. Largely (but not completely) hydrolyzed in bowel to glycerin and acetic acid. May disturb acid-base balance. Given subcutaneously or intramuscularly to laboratory animals (including monkeys), it produces vasodilation, central nervous depression, and death from respiratory failure (mean lethal dose 1 to 5 gm./kg.). Antidote of choice for fluoroacetate poisoning.

Ref.: Li et al., 1941.

578 Propyl Acetate   578

n-Propyl acetate

Toxicity Rating: 2. Like other simple esters, mild irritant and central depressant actions. Although *n*-propanol is about 3-fold more acutely toxic than isopropanol, the simple esters of each are about equi-toxic with *n*-propanol. Acute oral LD$_{50}$'s in rabbits: *n*-propyl acetate 6.6 gm./kg., isopropyl acetate 6.9 gm./kg., *n*-propyl *n*-propionate 3.9 gm./kg., *n*-propyl *n*-butyrate 5.7 gm./kg. and *n*-propyl isovalerate 8.2 gm./kg. The ratio of the narcotic to the lethal dose is smaller for the esters than for the parent alcohols.

See also: Isopropyl Alcohol, *Reference Congener in Section III*.
Ref.: Browning, 1953; Munch, 1972.

579 Triacetin   579

Glyceryl triacetate

Toxicity Rating: 1. Laboratory rats have tolerated diets consisting of 50% triacetin. If hydrolyzed, systemic acidosis is a possible consequence.

Ref.: Li et al., 1941.

Aromatic acids and their esters (exclusive of salicylates and acyl amino acids)

580 Abietic Acid   580

Sylvic acid

Toxicity Rating: 2(?). Almost no information. Low intravenous toxicity in mice (presumably low also by other routes). Central nervous paralysis in frogs.

Ref.: Fischer and Toth, 1938.

581 Methyl Abietate   581

Abalyn

An ester of low oral toxicity. The compound shows a significant *in vitro* hemolytic action at 0.5 x 10^{-5}*M* concentrations (Segal, 1972). See Abietic Acid above.

Ref.: Segal et al., 1972.

582 Benzoic Acid   582

Benzenecarboxylic acid

Toxicity Rating: 3. A 67 kg. man has ingested single doses of 50 gm. without ill effects, although the mean lethal dose in cats and dogs is 2 gm./kg. Large oral doses produce gastric pain, nausea, and vomiting. When injected in rats, tremors, convulsions, and death occur.

Ref.: Hager et al., 1942.

583 Benzyl Benzoate   583

Toxicity Rating: 3. Converted to hippuric acid in vivo. In laboratory animals ingestion causes progressive incoordination, central nervous excitation, convulsions, and death. Treat symptomatically. Has caused skin irritation in humans.

Ref.: Graham and Kuizenga, 1945; Gruber, 1923a; Gruber, 1923b.

584 Paraben Esters   584

i.e., Methyl, ethyl, propyl or butyl *p*-hydroxybenzoate

Used as preservatives in many creams, lotions, ointments and other cosmetics, foods, drugs and dentifrices. This group of compounds probably lies near the borderline between toxicity classes 2 and 3. Consult the index for specific comments about individual members of the group.

585 Methylparaben   585

Methylparasept, Methyl *p*-hydroxybenzoate

Not toxic in the small amounts found in most commercial products (0.05 to 0.2%), where it serves as a preservative and antiseptic. Said to be less toxic than salicylic acid and its derivatives.

Ref.: Osol and Farrar, 1955.

586 Propylparaben

586

Propyl p-hydroxybenzoate, Propyl parasept

Toxicity Rating: 3. Animal studies place this substance near the borderline between toxicity classes 2 and 3. All of the esters of p-hydroxybenzoic acid are less toxic than benzoic or salicylic acid. In

Ref.: Osol and Farrar, 1955.

laboratory studies dogs and rats injected with propylparaben showed no pathological changes in the liver or kidneys.

587 Cinnamic Acid Esters

587

i.e., Methyl, ethyl, benzyl propyl

Toxicity Rating: 3. In laboratory animals the propyl and isopropyl derivatives lie near the borderline between toxicity classes 2 and 3. Dermatitis has

Ref.: Powers et al., 1961; Snapper and Saltzman, 1949.

been reported. Said to be largely excreted in urine as benzoic and hippuric acids.

588 Methyl Nicotinate

588

Nicotinic acid methyl ester, Midalgan

Toxicity Rating: 3(?). No toxicity data were located. Used as a rubefacient. Presumably hydrolyzed in the body to nicotinic acid and methyl

Ref.: Merck and Co., 1976.

alcohol. The latter is not likely to be generated in toxicologically significant amounts. See also nicotinic acid.

589 Phthalic Acid Esters

589

e.g., Butyl benzyl phthalate, Diphenyl phthalate

Toxicity Rating: 2 & 3. Used as solvents, fixatives in perfumes, and plasticizers. Because of its objectionable bitter taste, the ethyl (= diethyl) ester is used as a denaturant for alcohol, especially in cosmetics. The dimethyl ester is an insect repellent. Each is an irritant on mucous membranes and a central nervous depressant if absorbed. Such plasticizers as glycolyl phthalate have been found to be extracted by blood from plastic tubing and bags

used to store blood. Similar esters have also been detected in some foodstuffs and in animal and human tissues. The degree of testicular atrophy produced in rats during feeding studies depended upon the length and structure of the esterified alcohols. In general lower molecular weight esters had more severe effects. The health significance of these findings is not yet known.

Ref.: Draize et al., 1948; Jaeger and Rubin, 1970; Lehman, 1951; Oishi and Hiraga, 1980; Smith, 1953.

590 n-Butyl Phthalate

590

Dibutyl phthalate, Di-n-butyl phthalate

Toxicity Rating: 2. An insect repellent used mainly to impregnate clothing and a plasticizer. Low toxicity in animals. Administration of 2 gm./kg. daily by gastric intubation of rats produced testicular

Ref.: Lawrence and Tuell, 1979; Smith, 1953.

atrophy and loss of testicular zinc. Said to act as an uncoupler of oxidative phosphorylation in rats. No clinical data. See also Phthalic acid esters above.

591 Di-2-ethylhexyl Phthalate

591

DEHP

Toxicity Rating: 1. Widely used as a plasticizer for polyvinyl chloride (see in Index), especially in the manufacture of medical devices. May constitute 40% by weight of final product. Soluble in blood and fluids containing lipoproteins. Leaches into food stored in PVC wrap and into blood stored in PVC bags. Has been found in tissues of patients transfused with blood stored in such bags and patients catheterized and dialyzed by PVC tubing. Lethal to chick embryo beating heart cells. Inhibits growth of human diploid cells at levels reached in

PVC stored blood after 2 days. Adult human experienced mild gastric disturbances after ingesting 10 ml. DEHP. Absorbed intact from gastrointestinal tract. When administered either i.v. or orally, it is rapidly metabolized to derivatives of mono-(2-ethylhexyl)-phthalate, which are mainly excreted in urine and bile. Feeding studies in rats produced testicular atrophy, hepatomegaly and proliferation of hepatic peroxisomes. Has become an environmental contaminant that may accumulate in the food chain. See also Phthalic Acid Esters above.

Ref.: Gray et al., 1977; Jaeger and Rubin, 1972; Lawrence and Tuell, 1979; Rubin and Schiffer, 1976.

592   Ethyl Phthalate

Diethyl phthalate

Toxicity Rating: 3. Used as a solvent, a fixative for perfume, and a denaturant for alcohol (especially in cosmetics). It serves as a denaturant because of its bitter objectionable taste. Irritating to mucous membranes. Produces central nervous depression when absorbed.

Ref.: Blickensdorfer and Templeton, 1930; Karel et al., 1947.

593   Methyl Phthalate

Dimethyl phthalate

Toxicity Rating: 2. An insect repellent. Not irritating to skin and not absorbed through skin. In eyes or on mucous membranes it is painful but not corrosive. Ingestion may produce central nervous depression. Treat symptomatically.

Ref.: Draize et al., 1948; Lehman, 1955.

Salicylic acid and derivatives

594   Aspirin

Acetylsalicylic acid, 2-Acetoxybenzoic acid

Toxicity Rating: 4.

See also: Salicylate, *Reference Congener in Section III.*

595   Cresotic Acids

Homosalicylic acids, Cresotinic acids, Hydroxytoluic acids, Creosotic acid, Methylsalicylic acids

Toxicity Rating: 4. Three isomers exist (*o-,m-,p-*). Solutions of the mixture (called creosotic acid) are sometimes used as a disinfectant. All isomers are thought to resemble salicylic acid in toxicity.

See also: Salicylate, *Reference Congener in Section III.*

596   Isoamyl Salicylate

Toxicity Rating: 4. Used in perfumery and soaps for its pleasant odor. The toxicity rating here is inferred from that of methyl salicylate. The closely related ester 2-ethylhexylsalicylate is used in skin sunscreen preparations. See Methyl salicylate below.

See also: Salicylate, *Reference Congener in Section III.*
Ref.: Greenberg and Lester, 1954.

597   Methyl Salicylate

Oil of wintergreen, Sweet birch oil, Gaultheria oil, Betula oil

Toxicity Rating: 4. A strong irritant to skin and mucous membranes. Used externally as a counterirritant. May be absorbed rapidly through intact skin. Bowel absorption is somewhat erratic, and gastric lavage may be beneficial even several hours after ingestion. Absorbed at least in part as the intact ester and small amounts are even excreted as such by the kidneys, but the compound is largely hydrolyzed. Typical systemic effects of salicylate and not of methyl alcohol are observed. Probably no more toxic than sodium salicylate.

See also: Salicylate, *Reference Congener in Section III.*
Ref.: Cann and Verhulst, 1958b; Davison et al., 1961.

598   Phenyl Salicylate

Salol

Toxicity Rating: 4. Used for enteric coating of pills, in suntan lotions and creams, and formerly as an intestinal antiseptic. Insoluble in water and gastric juice. Said to be slowly hydrolyzed to phenol (40%) and salicylic acid (60%) by intestinal alkali and enzymes, but recent evidence suggests that much hydrolysis occurs in tissues after absorption. The toxic effects are chiefly those of phenol but without phenol's marked corrosive actions on the gastrointestinal tract.

See also: Phenol *and* Salicylate, *Reference Congeners in Section III.*
Ref.: Osol and Farrar, 1955.

599   599   Salicylamide

o-Hydroxybenzamide

Toxicity Rating: 3. An analgesic with some therapeutic properties similar to aspirin and other salicylates. Rapidly absorbed from the alimentary tract, widely distributed, and quickly excreted by the kidneys. Not hydrolyzed to salicylic acid or otherwise altered. Little gastric irritation. Less toxic than other common salicylates, and unlike the latter, overdoses induce central nervous depression, hypotension, and ultimately respiratory arrest, but not excitement, convulsions, metabolic acidosis, or hypoprothrombinemia.

Ref.: Done, 1959; Hart, 1947.

600   600   Salicylate

e.g., Sodium salicylate

Toxicity Rating: 4.

See also: Salicylate, *Reference Congener in Section III.*

601   601   Salicyl Salicylate

Disalicylic acid, e.g., Salysal, Diplosal

Toxicity Rating: 4. A salicylic ester of salicylic acid which is sparingly soluble in water but gradually hydrolyzed in the intestine to two molecules of salicylic acid. This is the basis for its therapeutic use as a long-acting analgesic, antipyretic and antirheumatic. The usual dose is 0.3 to 0.6 gm. The usual toxic effects of salicylates should be anticipated, but the latency may be longer than that of other derivatives.

See also: Salicylate, *Reference Congener in Section III.*

Aliphatic and alicyclic amines

602   602   Ethylenediamine

1,2-Ethanediamine, 1,2-Diaminoethane

Toxicity Rating: 3. A very caustic liquid polyamine, hydroscopic and freely soluble in water. Useful as an industrial and pharmaceutical solvent, emulsifier and stabilizer and marketed as a hardener of epoxy resins, usually in 10% or more toluene or xylene. The acute oral LD_{50} of ethylenediamine in rats is 0.7-1.85 gm./kg., and the dermal LD_{50} in rabbits is 0.56 ml./kg. The nature and mechanism of its systemic toxicity are not defined, but like other aliphatic amines it is probably a histamine releaser in vivo. It is severely irritating to the skin and eyes of rabbits. The undiluted liquid produces necrotic patches on the skin and a 5% solution causes partial opacity of the cornea. Almost certainly alkalinity is the basis for much of the corrosiveness of its aqueous solutions. It is a strong skin sensitizer, especially when it is applied to damaged skin. Associated with severe exfoliative dermatitis when given by mouth. Humans exposed to 200 ppm of the vapors have experienced respiratory irritation and systemic reactions. Inhalation of 4000 ppm for 8 hours produced fatal kidney damage in all exposed rats, as did inhalation of 484 ppm for 30 days. Lung and liver damage were also evident. The OSHA standard for exposure of workers has been set at 10 ppm. The simple salts are safer and less irritating to the rabbit eye. The dihydrochloride has an oral LD_{50} in rats of 1.6-3.2 gm./kg. and is used in veterinary and clinical medicine as a urinary acidifier. The dihydroiodide salt has been administered to humans as a source of iodine (adult human oral dose 0.13-1.0 gm. 2 to 4 times daily). Ethylenediamine forms a mixed salt with theophylline known as aminophylline (see in Index).

Ref.: Baer et al., 1973; Beard and Noe, 1981; Nierenberg and Glazener, 1982.

603   603   Diethylenetriamine

2,2′-Diaminodiethylamine, Amine hardener

Toxicity Rating: 3. Yellow liquid with strong ammoniacal odor, hydroscopic and freely soluble in water. Marketed in xylene or toluene as a hardener for epoxy resins. Oral LD_{50} in rats is 2.33 gm./kg. Dermal LD_{50} in rabbits is 1.09 ml./kg. Classified as a strong skin sensitizer. Concentrated aqueous solutions can cause severe skin and eye burns, but 10% is not irritating on the skin. Corrosiveness is probably due to alkalinity. Breathing vapor may lead to respiratory irritation, cough, nausea and vomiting. Repeated or massive inhalation may cause an asthmatic response. The nature and mechanism of its systemic toxicity are not defined, but it is not a cumulative poison.

Ref.: Beard and Noe, 1981; Smyth, 1961.

604   Triethylenetetramine   604

N,N′-Bis(2-aminoethyl)ethylenediamine, 3,6-Diazaoctane-1,8-diamine

Toxicity Rating: 3. Triethylenetetramine is a slightly viscous liquid polyamine similar to but less volatile than diethylenetriamine (see above). A strong organic base and chelating agent used in the synthesis of detergents, softeners and dyestuffs, the manufacture of pharmaceuticals, and the vulcanization of rubber. It is moderately toxic by ingestion, percutaneous absorption and vapor inhalation with an oral LD_{50} of 4.34 gm./kg. in rats and a dermal LD_{50} of 0.82 gm./kg. in rabbits. Respiratory irritation and erythema, edema, and itching of the face have occurred in workers exposed to hot vapors. It is a primary skin irritant, slightly less active as a sensitizer and eye irritant than the lower polyamine homologues.

Ref.: Beard and Noe, 1981.

605   Tetraethylenepentamine   605

N-(2-Aminoethyl)-N′-(2-((2-aminoethyl)amino)ethyl-1,2-ethanediamine, 1,4,7,10,13-Pentaazatridecane

Toxicity Rating: 3. An aliphatic polyamine with industrial applications. Toxicity to animals is similar to that of triethylenetetramine (see above). Rat oral LD_{50} is 3.99 gm./kg. Single dose rabbit dermal LD_{50} is 0.66 gm./kg. Produces intense skin irritation and moderate eye injury in rabbits but not so severe as lower homologues (see above).

606   Ethylenimine   606

Azacyclopropane, Aziridine, Dimethylenimine

Toxicity Rating: 5. Used as an intermediate in organic syntheses, ethylenimine (and presumably N-ethylethylenimine) is a highly reactive, strongly alkaline compound with an appreciable vapor pressure. Skin contact produces painless but severely necrotizing burns. Human exposure to vapor concentrations above 100 ppm causes respiratory tract irritation and inflammation, but symptoms may be delayed several hours. Presumably severe exposures might result in an overwhelming pulmonary edema. It is a potent lacrimator and emetic. Signs and symptoms include tearing and burning of the eyes, sore throat, vomiting, coughing (which may persist for weeks or months), and a slowly healing dermatitis. Hematologic effects include transient polycythemia, leukocytosis and eosinophilia. Hemorrhagic congestion of all internal organs occurs in high level exposures of experimental animals. In man and especially in animals renal damage has been observed, including albuminuria and hematuria. For the management of chemical injuries to the lungs, see Nitrogen Oxides in Section III.

Ref.: Walpole et al., 1954; Weightman and Hoyle, 1964.

607   Octadecylamine   607

Toxicity Rating: 3. Eighteen–carbon straight–chain amine sometimes used as an anticorrosive agent in live steam lines. Toxicity rating based on studies in mice and rats. Rats have tolerated dietary levels of 500 ppm for 2 years without signs of toxicity or pathologic changes. At levels of 3000 ppm for from 89 to 209 days, anorexia, weight loss and some histologic changes in mesenteric lymph nodes, gastrointestinal mucosa and liver. Said to be a primary skin sensitizer.

Ref.: Deichmann et al., 1958; MacDonald et al., 1962.

608   Dicyclohexylamine   608

Dodecahydrodiphenylamine

Toxicity Rating: 4. In animals somewhat more toxic than cyclohexylamine, and unlike the latter it can be absorbed in dangerous amounts through skin. Rabbits which ingest it die in convulsions. The acetate is said to produce a pressor response in dogs. See Cyclohexylamine below.

Ref.: McOmie and Anderson, 1949.

609   Cyclohexylamine   609

Hexahydroaniline, Aminocyclohexane

Toxicity Rating: 4. Numerous industrial uses include the manufacture of rubber, insecticides, corrosion inhibitors, plasticizers, etc. A minor metabolite of cyclamates in man and other species. The free amine has a caustic action on skin and mucous membranes. Systemic effects in man include nausea and vomiting, anxiety, restlessness and drowsiness. Spinal-type convulsions occur in rabbits. In mice cyclohexylamine has typical sympathomimetic effects like amphetamine with hyperpnea, hyperthermia, increased metabolic rate and a degree of lethality that is dependent on ambient temperature and crowding. Chlorpromazine, reserpine and phenoxybenzamine protect mice against death.

See also: Amphetamine, Reference Congener in Section III.
Ref.: Carswell and Morrill, 1937; Lee and Dixon, 1972; Watrous and Schulz, 1950.

Aromatic amines

610

610   Acetanilid(e)

N-Phenylacetamide, Acetylaniline

Toxicity Rating: 4. Similar to but less toxic than aniline in animals, but clinical experience does not confirm this difference in man. Indeed a toxicity rating of 5 might be a better description of the recorded human fatalities. Perhaps less prominent nervous symptoms than in aniline poisoning.

See also: Acetaminophen and Aniline, Reference Congeners in Section III.
Ref.: Gross, 1946; Brodie and Axelrod, 1948; Flinn and Brodie, 1948; Hart, 1947.

611

611   Acetophenetidin

Phenacetin

Toxicity Rating: 4. Less toxic than aniline or acetanilid. Cyanosis and methemoglobinemia are less marked, but severe skin rashes may be more common. Suspected of having an addiction liability. A case is reported of a housewife who over a 5-year period ingested 77 lb. of phenacetin before succumbing to a fatal nephritis.

See also: Acetaminophen and Aniline, Reference Congeners in Section III.
Ref.: Smith, 1958; Moolten and Smith, 1960.

612

612   Aniline

Aniline oil, Aminobenzene

Toxicity Rating: 4.

See also: Aniline, Reference Congener in Section III.

613

613   p-Chloroaniline

Toxicity Rating: 5(?). Said to be more toxic than aniline. Can be absorbed through intact skin and may cause a more intense methemoglobinemia by that route than by mouth. Hematuria has been described, perhaps due to hemorrhagic cystitis.

See also: Aniline, Reference Congener in Section III.
Ref.: Linch, 1974; von Oettingen, 1941b.

614

614   3-Chloro-4-methylaniline

3-Chloro-p-toluidine, 3-CPT, Starlicide

Toxicity Rating: 3. An avicide marketed as pelleted bait for the control of starling populations. Remarkable species differences in sensitivity place this compound in toxicity class 6 for some species of birds (acute oral LD_{50} in starlings 3.8 mg./kg.) but in class 3 or 4 for some mammalian species (acute oral LD_{50} in rats 655 mg./kg.). Methemoglobinemia occurs in mice, rats and cats and should be anticipated in man, but it does not appear to be the primary cause of death. Methylene blue should be avoided. In mice methylene blue effectively attenuated the methemoglobinemia but actually increased mortality. In contrast hyperbaric oxygen intensified the methemoglobinic response without significantly affecting mortality. Hypothermia occurs in rodents and perhaps in man. In mice warming increased body temperature but did not prevent death, whereas exposure to cold significantly increased mortality. In addition to the above the following sequence of events is inferred from animal experiments. Rapid onset of a transient flaccid paralysis, probably of central origin, may result in hypoxia because of relaxation of the respiratory musculature. Apparent recovery with an asymptomatic period may follow. A slow downhill course, ending eventually in respiratory arrest, may then arise from complex centrally mediated alterations in the respiratory pattern. At the same time circulatory effects may contribute to a stagnant hypoxia and acidosis with both respiratory and metabolic components. Renal damage occurs in birds but has not been described in laboratory mammals. Treatment should be symptomatic and supportive. No effective antidotes are known. Exchange transfusion might be considered for the moribund patient.

See also: Aniline, Reference Congener in Section III.
Ref.: Apostolou and Peoples, 1971; Borison et al., 1975; Decino et al., 1966; Felsenstein et al., 1974.

615

615   Dimethylaniline

Dimethylphenylamine

Toxicity Rating: 4. Useful analytical reagent and synthetic precursor of many dyes. Recently employed as a catalytic hardener in certain Fiberglas resins. Closely resembles aniline in its toxicity with perhaps more prominent central nervous depression. Absorbed through intact skin to produce dangerous methemoglobinemia.

See also: Aniline, *Reference Congener in Section III.*
Ref.: Fairhall, 1957; von Oettingen, 1941b.

616 Diphenylamine

Toxicity Rating: 3. Used externally in cattle for the treatment of screwworm infestation. When given by mouth (oil solutions) to laboratory animals, it causes persistent anorexia, diarrhea, emaciation, hypothermia, and general debility, presumably from protracted gastroenteritis. Deaths may be delayed 2 to 3 weeks after a single lethal dose. In cats (and probably other species), transient methemoglobinemia is produced but is probably not the cause of death.

See also: Aniline, *Reference Congener in Section III.*
Ref.: Amer. Cyanamid Co., 1956.

617 *p*-Nitroaniline

p-Nitraniline

Toxicity Rating: 5(?). More toxic than aniline and probably more toxic than nitrobenzene.

See also: Aniline, *Reference Congener in Section III.*
Ref.: von Oettingen, 1941b.

618 *p*-Toluidine

4-Methylaniline

Toxicity Rating: 4(?). Like aniline, but renal injury is more likely. The ortho- and meta- isomers probably have similar acute toxicities, but *o*-toluidine has been reported to cause bladder cancer in several mammalian species. In rats all 3 isomers are metabolized to various aminomethylphenols and excreted as acid-hydrolyzable conjugates.

See also: Aniline, *Reference Congener in Section III.*
Ref.: von Oettingen, 1941b; Cheever et al., 1980.

Acyl diamines that induce little or no methemoglobinemia

619 *p*-Aminodiphenylamine

4-Aminodiphenylamine, *N*-Phenyl-*p*-phenylenediamine

Toxicity Rating: 4(?). A constituent of hair dyes which is probably of moderate toxicity. Reports of severe dermatitis from its use, but it is less irritating than the parent compound, 1,4-phenylenediamine. See Phenylenediamine below.

Ref.: Greenberg and Lester, 1954.

620 2,4-Diaminophenol Hydrochloride

Amidol

Toxicity Rating: 4. A photographic developer, sometimes used in hair dyes. No human poisonings are known. See Phenylenediamine below for effects and treatment.

Ref.: von Oettingen, 1949.

621 2,4-Diaminotoluene

p-Toluenediamine

Toxicity Rating: 4. Animal tests suggest that it is slightly less toxic but presumably similar to *p*-phenylenediamine. No human poisonings are known. See Phenylenediamine below for effects and treatment, but in addition methemoglobinemia has been reported in poisoned dogs.

Ref.: von Oettingen, 1941b.

622 4-Methoxy-*m*-phenylenediamine

2,4-Diaminoanisole

Toxicity Rating: 4. Constituent of hair dyes. Highly toxic to experimental animals (rat oral LD_{50} 460 mg./kg.). Symptoms of intoxication include lethargy, increased salivation, fine body tremors, respiratory difficulty, diuresis and diarrhea. Converted by liver enzymes to a compound which is strongly mutagenic in bacteria. Carcinogenicity in man and animals has not been established.

Ref.: Lloyd et al., 1977.

623   Phenylenediamine (*o-* or *p-*)

e.g., Orsin, Diolene

Toxicity Rating: 4. Used for dyeing hair and fur. A potent skin sensitizer. Suspected as a cause of bladder tumors in "aniline" workers. Produces severe local reactions and systemic effects from percutaneous absorption and from ingestion. Local actions include severe dermatitis and urticaria; in the eye, chemosis, lacrimation, exophthalmos, ophthalmia, and even permanent blindness. Systemic actions include asthma, gastritis (regardless of portal of entry), rise in blood pressure, transudation into serous cavities, vertigo, tremors, convulsions, and coma. Treatment is symptomatic. Whenever histamine-like effects predominate, a therapeutic trial with an antihistaminic is suggested. The ortho isomer (diolene) is less toxic than the para (orsin). Neither is believed to be capable of inducing significant methemoglobinemia.

Ref.: Erdmann and Vahlen, 1905; Tainter and James, 1930.

Aminophenols and aminobenzoic acid derivatives

624   *p*-Aminophenol

4-Amino-1-hydroxybenzene, Rodinal, *p*-Hydroxyaniline

Toxicity Rating: 4. A photographic developer. Sometimes used in hair dyes. A metabolic product of aniline, acetanilid, phenacetin, and acetaminophen. Less toxic than aniline, but the most toxic of three possible isomers. Acute oral LD_{50}'s in rats for para- 375 mg./kg., ortho- 1,300 mg./kg. and meta-isomer 1,660 mg./kg. Conversely, in mice the ortho-isomer was considerably more potent than the para-isomer in generating methemoglobin. Methemoglobinemia appears to be of limited importance in the acute or lethal reaction As with phenol, the cause of death is uncertain. The ortho- and para-isomers but not the meta-isomer are teratogenic in the Syrian golden hamster in doses that do not produce signs of maternal toxicity. In poisoned animals transient central nervous depression is described. With lethal doses cardiac and respiratory failure occurred nearly simultaneously. Aqueous solutions on the skin have produced restlessness and convulsions in man, as well as skin irritation. Dilutions used in photography do not have a significant percutaneous toxicity in most cases. Single non-lethal doses in rats produce acute proximal renal tubular necrosis. The compound appears to be activated in the kidney by microsomal enzymes to produce this nephrotoxic effect. Perhaps this is the mechanism for the nephrotoxicity (sometimes associated with hepatic necrosis) after acute acetaminophen overdosage and for the nephropathy associated with chronic phenacetin abuse.

See also: Acetaminophen *and* Aniline, *Reference Congeners in Section III.*
Ref.: Calder et al., 1979; Crowe et al., 1979; Green et al., 1969; Lester et al., 1944; Newton et al., 1982; Rutkowski and Ferm, 1982; Smith et al., 1967.

625   4-Amino-2-nitrophenol

o-Nitro-*p*-aminophenol, 4-Hydroxy-3-nitroaniline, 3-Amino-6-hydroxynitrobenzene

Toxicity Rating: 3. Constituent of hair dyes. Moderate oral toxicity (rat LD_{50} 1.5 gm./kg.). No description of toxic symptoms was found, but methemoglobinemia should be anticipated. In laboratory rats large sublethal doses (50 mg.) caused metabolic depression (decrease in oxygen consumption, in CO_2 output and in body temperature). The compound is said to color rat urine red. Has caused bladder cancer in rats but not in mice given high doses in feed.

See also: Aniline, *Reference Congener in Section III.*
Ref.: Cameron, 1958; Lloyd et al., 1977; National Cancer Institute, 1978a.

626   *p*-Methylaminophenol Sulfate

e.g., Photol, Metol

Toxicity Rating: 4. Photographic developer, sometimes used in hair dyes. Effects from ingestion by humans are not well established. Deaths from 5 to 15 gm. of mixed metol and hydroquinone, with symptoms like phenol and aniline poisonings. Question of hemolytic anemia is not clear because of possible confusion with phenolic pigments.

See also: Phenol *and* Aniline, *Reference Congeners in Section III.*
Ref.: Drew, 1942; Zeidman and Deutl, 1945.

627 o-Aminobenzoic Acid 627

Anthranilic acid

Toxicity Rating: 3. The oral LD_{50} in the rat is 4.5 gm./kg. Although it does not share the therapeutic usefulness of p-aminobenzoic acid, it is presumed to have similar toxicity. See p-Aminobenzoic Acid below.

628 p-Aminobenzoic Acid 628

PABA, Para-aminobenzoic acid

Toxicity Rating: 3. Once widely used in the chemotherapy of rickettsial diseases, in sunscreen preparations, occasionally in certain dermatoses and synergistically with salicylates in rheumatic fever. Common side reactions include nausea, vomiting, acidosis, pruritus, rash, fever, methemoglobinemia and possibly hepatitis. Oral doses of 1 gm./kg. or higher were fatal in dogs, which developed acute gastroenteritis and hemorrhage in the small intestine; acute liver necrosis was seen with doses above 2 gm./kg. Rats given lethal doses of the sodium salt showed pronounced hyperemia of the distal segment of the stomach. PABA enhanced methemoglobinemia and Heinz body formation in cats exposed to xylidine. Chronic feeding in animals has produced leukocytosis.

Ref.: Cronheim, 1951; Robin et al., 1947; Scott and Robbins, 1942; Spicer, 1949.

629 p-Aminosalicylic Acid 629

PAS

Toxicity Rating: 3. Antimetabolite useful in tuberculosis. Severe therapeutic misadventures, although rare, have included agranulocytosis, hepatitis, allergic reactions, methemoglobinemia, and crystalluria. Gastrointestinal irritation with vomiting and diarrhea is more common. Prolonged prothrombin times and some suppression of thyroid activity may be seen. Dosages up to 20 gm. a day by mouth of the sodium or potassium salts are usually well tolerated for prolonged periods.

See also: Aniline, *Reference Congener in Section III.*
Ref.: Dutta, 1961; Kneebone, 1961; Mahrer and Maret, 1955; Paine, 1958; Simmel, 1962.

Aliphatic nitro compounds (nitrites and nitrates)

630 Amyl Nitrite 630

Isoamyl nitrite

Toxicity Rating: 5(?). Amyl nitrite has long been used as a vasodilator in angina therapy, in the treatment of hydrogen cyanide and hydrogen sulfide poisonings, and as an industrial chemical and perfume scent. This volatile liquid is usually a mixture of isomers, the principal one being isoamyl nitrite. The increasing abuse of amyl nitrite "poppers" led to their restriction and to the increased popularity of butyl and isobutyl nitrites, related volatile compounds sold over-the-counter as room odorizers under such names as "RUSH" and "Locker Room". They are inhaled by enthusiasts to produce highs and to intensify sexual orgasms. They are sometimes sprayed in discotheques to stimulate dancing. Inhaling the volatile nitrites produces vasodilation and hypotension lasting about 90 seconds, occasionally accompanied by posture-related syncope. Pulsating headache, rapid flushing of the face and dizziness are common. Confusion, vertigo, motor restlessness, weakness, cyanosis, nausea and vomiting may occur in some individuals. Sniffing butyl nitrite has caused subclinical methemoglobinemia in normal subjects and still higher levels in individuals who are deficient in NADH-methemoglobin reductase activity. Chronic abuse of amyl nitrite resulted in Heinz body hemolytic anemia in two individuals without demonstrable congenital red cell defects. There are documented cases of severe and fatal methemoglobinemia following the ingestion of butyl and isobutyl nitrite room odorizers. Injection of methylene blue was sometimes effective but too late to reverse the hypoxic tissue damage in a fatal case. The methemoglobin level of a patient reached 61.7% within 1 hour of drinking a bottle of butyl nitrite in a suicide attempt. Sweet spirits of nitre, a mixture of 4 per cent ethyl nitrite in 70% ethanol, is still available without prescription in the U.S.A. Two black twins given 1 to 2 teaspoonsful in their milk bottles developed profound methemoglobinemia. Despite the reduction in the methemoglobin levels from 80 percent to 9 percent with methylene blue therapy, one twin died in respiratory arrest. The other twin recovered after reversal of his 38 percent methemoglobinemia. Heinz bodies were not observed, and methemoglobin reductase activity was normal. Laboratory mice succumbed to cardiovascular collapse after lethal i.p. injections of butyl nitrites; liver damage was seen among week-long survivors.

See also: Nitrite, *Reference Congener in Section III.*
Ref.: Chilcote et al., 1977; Crandell et al., 1931; Haley, 1980; Romeril and Concannon, 1981; Shesser et al., 1980; Smith et al., 1980; Steiner and Manoguerra, 1980; Wason et al., 1980.

631   **631** Cyclonite

Cyclotrimethylenetrinitramine, RDX, Hexahydro-1,3,5-trinitro-s-triazine, Hexogen

Used as a high explosive in World War II and employed occasionally as a rodenticide. Except for mice, which are more resistant, acute toxicity data (rats, cats) place this compound near the borderline between classes 4 and 5. Symptoms in poisoned animals range from twitching with mild hyperreflexia to severe convulsions. Industrial workers exposed to RDX have suddenly convulsed or have become unconscious without convulsions. The few premonitory signs included headache, dizziness, nausea and vomiting. When consciousness was regained (few minutes to 24 hrs.), intermittent stupor, weakness and nausea ensued. Recovery was eventually complete, although there are unsubstantiated reports of deaths in Germany. While apparently devoid of hematological effects including methemoglobin formation, at least one patient examined shortly after convulsions had cardiovascular signs like those induced by nitrite and nitroglycerin, i.e., rapid pulse, elevated systolic and depressed diastolic blood pressure.

See also: Nitrite, *Reference Congener in Section III*.
Ref.: Kaplan et al., 1965.

632   **632** Dicyclohexylamine Nitrite

Dodecahydrodiphenylamine nitrite

Toxicity Rating: 4. Used as a corrosion inhibitor. As with other nitrite salts it lowers rabbit blood pressure. The nitrite anion apparently overshadows the effect of the cation; (see Dicyclohexylamine in the index). About same level of toxicity as sodium nitrite.

See also: Nitrite, *Reference Congener in Section III*.
Ref.: McOmie and Anderson, 1949.

633   **633** Ethylene Glycol Dinitrate

Toxicity Rating: 6. Analogous structure to nitroglycerin, and also used in the explosives industry. In animals it is more rapidly absorbed through skin, lungs and gastrointestinal tract and more acutely toxic than nitroglycerin, but it produces identical cardiovascular effects. Anemia, methemoglobinemia, and Heinz body formation may be prominent in man, as in laboratory animals.

See also: Nitrite, *Reference Congener in Section III*.
Ref.: von Oettingen, 1946b.

634   **634** Isosorbide Dinitrate

1,4:3,6-Dianhydro-*D*-glucitol dinitrate, Nitrol, Nitro-bid

A "long-acting" coronary vasodilator useful in the treatment and prevention of attacks of angina pectoris. Maximal plasma levels are reached 6 minutes after sublingual administration (5 or 10 mg. is the usual dose) and are reduced by as much as 50% after first-pass through the liver. Patients may experience headache, transient light-headedness and weakness related to postural hypotension. Hypersensitivity reactions, marked by nausea, vomiting, restlessness and collapse occur in some individuals, a syndrome that may be intensified by alcohol ingestion. When swallowed, a 5 mg. dose is no more effective than a placebo but higher doses are active. High oral doses (30 mg., 4 times/day) presumably saturate the liver's capacity to denitrate the drug and provide sustained relief. Taking repeated high oral doses, however, increases the risk of developing hypotension, tachycardia, tolerance, and cross-tolerance to nitroglycerin. Most serious is the potential for developing a form of life-threatening organic nitrate dependence, as have some workers in nitroglycerin plants. Available as sublingual tablets, chewable tablets and slow-release capsules. Largely excreted in the urine as isosorbide glucuronide.

See also: Nitrite, *Reference Congener in Section III*.
Ref.: Danahy and Aronow, 1977; Gilman et al., 1980.

635   **635** Nitroglycerin(e)

Nitroglycerol, Glyceryl trinitrate

Toxicity Rating: 6. A fast-acting and much more potent drug than sodium nitrite (100-fold difference in therapeutic doses). The potency difference can be explained only partially by rates of absorption since the fatal intravenous doses in rabbits differ by a factor of at least 2 (expressed as nitrite equivalents). In man more potent when absorbed from the mouth (e.g., sublingual) than when swallowed. Can be absorbed through intact skin.

See also: Nitrite, *Reference Congener in Section III*.
Ref.: Rabinowitch, 1944; Schwartz, 1946.

636   Nitromethane   636

e.g., Nitrocarbol

Toxicity Rating: 3. Used as model aircraft engine fuel. Mildly irritating to skin and mucous mem-

Ref.: Machle and Scott, 1943; Machle et al., 1940.

brane. Less toxic than nitropropane. See 2-Nitro-propane below.

637   2-Nitropropane   637

Toxicity Rating: 3. Tested in rabbits, it lies near the borderline between toxicity classes 3 and 4. Slightly more toxic than nitromethane or nitroe-thane. Mildly irritating to mucous membranes but not skin. Reactions described in men exposed to to vapor include anorexia, nausea, vomiting, diarrhea, and severe occipital headaches. In several species

of animals, high vapor concentrations have pro-duced weakness, ataxia, dyspnea, cyanosis, coma and death (with a few terminal convulsions). In cats and probably other species, these symptoms are partially due to methemoglobinemia caused by the metabolic breakdown of nitropropane into ni-trite ions (also true of other nitroparaffins).

See also: Nitrite, *Reference Congener in Section III.*
Ref.: Machle and Scott, 1943; Machle et al., 1940; Treon and Dutra, 1952.

638   Pentaerythritol Tetranitrate   638

PETN, 2,2-[Bis(nitrooxy)-methyl]-1,3-propanediol dinitrate (ester)

Highly explosive organic compound used in the manufacture of detonators and as an orally and sublingually administered "long-acting" vasodila-tor in the management of angina pectoris. For medicinal purposes, it is diluted with an inert in-gredient, usually lactose. Absorbed slowly from intestines and lungs, not appreciably through skin. Munitions workers are likely to be exposed. Indi-viduals taking the drug may experience headache and episodes of dizziness and weakness from pos-tural hypotension, and those taking the drug orally

may develop cross-tolerance to the vasodilating effects of sublingual nitroglycerin. Rarely severe responses are encountered, consisting of nausea, vomiting, weakness, pallor, sweating and collapse, but no reports of death were found. Drug rashes, which occur occasionally with other organic nitrate drugs are especially common in patients taking pentaerythritol tetranitrate. Cross-sensitivity with nitroglycerin has been described. Available in 10, 20 and 40 mg. tablets for sublingual use and in 30, 45, 60 and 80 mg. sustained-release capsules.

See also: Nitrite, *Reference Congener in Section III.*

Aromatic nitro compounds (non-phenolic)

639   1-Chloro-2,4-dinitrobenzene   639

Dinitrochlorobenzene

Toxicity Rating: 5(?). A primary irritant; severe allergic dermatitis in almost everyone after re-peated skin contact. Systemic actions include met-

hemoglobinemia. More toxic than nitrochloroben-zene.

See also: Aniline, *Reference Congener in Section III.*
Ref.: Frey and Geleick, 1959; Landsteiner et al., 1939.

640   Dinitrobenzene   640

Toxicity Rating: 5. Probably slightly more toxic than nitrobenzene (definitely true in animals) and distinctly more toxic than dinitrotoluene. An ortho, meta and para isomer exist. The meta isomer is said to be the most important toxicologically, es-

pecially as a methemoglobin former. The principal clinical sign is cyanosis (like nitrobenzene), not liver necrosis (like dinitrotoluene). In subacute poi-soning, symptoms may be precipitated by sunlight or by the ingestion of alcohol.

See also: Aniline, *Reference Congener in Section III.*
Ref.: Rejsek, 1947; von Oettingen, 1941b.

641   Dinitrotoluene   641

Toxicity Rating: 4(?). Toxicity irregular but said to be much lower than dinitrobenzene. As in TNT poisoning, each (and all) of the following signs has been observed: methemoglobinemia, anemia, leu-

kopenia, and liver necrosis. Liver injury may be more common than cyanosis, especially if diet is deficient in protein.

See also: Aniline, *Reference Congener in Section III.*
Ref.: von Oettingen, 1941b.

642

642   Nitrobenzene

Essence of mirbane, Oil of mirbane

Toxicity Rating: 5. Toxic by all routes including skin absorption. Mean lethal dose by mouth probably lies between 1 and 5 gm. Systemic effects may be delayed a few hours. Poisoning closely resembles that due to aniline. For unknown reasons ethyl alcohol aggravates intoxication. Because of bitter almond odor, cyanide poisoning may be suspected, but cyanide acts much faster.

See also: Aniline, *Reference Congener in Section III.*
Ref.: Parkes and Neill, 1953; Wirtschafter and Wolpaw, 1944.

643

643   Nitrochlorobenzene

Toxicity Rating: 5(?). Usually a mixture of 3 isomeric forms. Severe allergic dermatitis frequent after skin contact. Less toxic than dinitrochlorobenzene. Systemic effects are like aniline (methemoglobinemia) but perhaps cardiac disorders are more severe. Avoid ingestion of ethyl alcohol, which aggravates the intoxication.

See also: Aniline, *Reference Congener in Section III.*
Ref.: Monsanto Chemical Co., 1957a; Watrous and Schulz, 1950.

644

644   Trinitrobenzene

e.g., 1,3,5-Trinitrobenzene

Toxicity Rating: 5(?). No specific toxicity data were located, but the toxic actions are probably like those of dinitrobenzene. See latter above.

See also: Aniline, *Reference Congener in Section III.*
Ref.: von Oettingen, 1941b.

645

645   2,4,6-Trinitrotoluene

TNT, 1-Methyl-2,4,6-trinitrobenzene

Toxicity Rating: 3 to 4. High explosive which requires a detonator. A young boy apparently poisoned by respiratory and/or percutaneous exposure presented with a 43% methemoglobinemia on the following day. Cyanosis, dermatitis, jaundice. anemia and purpura are signs of chronic industrial poisoning. Younger workmen (about 30 years old) tend to develop toxic hepatitis; older workmen tend to develop aplastic anemia.

See also: Aniline, *Reference Congener in Section III.*
Ref.: Crawford, 1954; Wolff and Doring, 1960.

Organonitriles

646

646   Acetone Cyanohydrin

2-Hydroxy-2-methylpropanenitrile

Toxicity Rating: 6. Important chemical intermediate, which decomposes readily to form hydrogen cyanide. In animals and in in vitro test systems, it behaves exactly as its molar equivalent in cyanide (1:1).

See also: Cyanide, *Reference Congener in Section III.*
Ref.: Willhite and Smith, 1981b.

647

647   Acetonitrile

Methyl cyanide, Cyanomethane, Ethanenitrile

Toxicity Rating: 3-4. Important chemical intermediate and solvent. Acute oral LD_{50} in adult rats about 3 gm./kg., but in young rats it was 200 mg./kg. Acute intraperitoneal LD_{50} in mice 175 mg./kg., and the LC_{50} for a 1-hour exposure in mice was about 2700 ppm. Several human deaths have been reported. The toxic syndrome included chest pains, cough, bile- or blood-stained emesis, dyspnea or tachypnea, coma and convulsions. The acute toxic effects appear to be due to the slow metabolic release of cyanide in vivo. Sodium thiosulfate antagonizes the lethal effects in mice, but the injections must be repeated at regular intervals over many hours.

See also: Cyanide, *Reference Congener in Section III.*
Ref.: Kimura et al., 1971; Willhite, 1981a; Willhite and Smith, 1981b.

648 Acrylonitrile 648

Vinyl cyanide, Carbacryl, Propenenitrile

Toxicity Rating: 5. A colorless volatile liquid with a faintly pungent odor. Chemical intermediate in production of pharmaceuticals, dyes and textile fibers. Also used as a fumigant for stored grain. Explosive and flammable, may polymerize violently in the presence of alkali. Highly toxic toward laboratory rodents: estimates of the oral LD_{50} in mice and rats range from 15 to 240 mg./kg. The most recent estimates place this compound on the borderline between toxicity classes 4 and 5. Signs of intoxication in rodents include hyperactivity, salivation, coma, convulsions, cyanosis and death from respiratory failure. Autopsy revealed edema of head, neck and lungs, extensive hemorrhage of lungs and adrenals and necrosis in the inner zones of the adrenal cortex (Szabo and Selye, 1971). The usual routes of human exposure are dermal and inhalation. Acrylonitrile spilled on human skin results in erythema and blisters. Repeated exposure may produce scaling dermatitis. Dermal absorption is rapid. Dermal or inhalation exposure leads to rapid onset of headache, sneezing, nausea, weakness, light-headedness and vomiting. Exposure to high concentrations of the vapor also produces immediate eye irritation. Recovery is rapid after cessation of exposure, but mild jaundice has been described in some severely poisoned patients. Two human fatalities have been reported. Acrylonitrile inhibits respiratory enzymes and produces death through asphyxiation. This action is due to metabolic release of cyanide. Urinary excretion of thiocyanate increases after acrylonitrile exposure, and cyanomethemoglobin has been demonstrated in animals given supralethal doses. The standard nitrite-thiosulfate therapy against cyanide poisoning is effective against acrylonitrile intoxication in laboratory animals. Because cyanide is liberated slowly the thiosulfate injections should be repeated at regular intervals (Willhite and Smith, 1981). Neither antidote is known to have been tried in human victims, probably because severe human poisonings have occurred only rarely. Acrylonitrile reacts with sulfhydryl compounds *in vitro* (Szabo and Reynolds, 1975). In guinea pigs and rabbits, large toxic doses (2 x LD_{50}) produced a significant decrease in protein and non-protein sulfhydryl groups in blood, liver and brain after one hour (Hashimoto and Kanai, 1972). A report in the Russian literature describes irritability, headaches, alcohol intolerance and tiredness in 20 workers chronically exposed to 3-20 mg./m^3 (Orusev and Popovski, 1973). In addition, acrylonitrile is said to have been responsible for an increased incidence of cancer of the colon and lung in workers at one acrylic fiber plant. The compound also caused cancer of the central nervous system in rats during chronic feeding standards. An interim emergency exposure standard now limits work place concentrations to 2 ppm (8-hr TWA) with 10 ppm ceiling concentration (29CFR 1910, FR: Jan. 17, 1978). Acrylonitrile is embryotoxic in mice, and teratogenic in hamsters (Willhite et al., 1981).

See also: Cyanide, *Reference Congener in Section III.*
Ref.: Amer. Petroleum Institute, 1948a; Bondarev et al., 1976; Brieger et al., 1952; Dinu and Klein, 1976; Graham, 1965; Hashimoto and Kanai, 1972; Lawton et al., 1943; Magos, 1962; McOmie, 1949; Orusev and Popovski, 1973; OSHA, Jan. 17, 1978; Pozzani et al., 1968; Szabo and Reynolds, 1975; Szabo and Selye, 1971; Willhite and Smith, 1981b; Willhite et al., 1981c.

649 *n*-Butyronitrile 649

Propyl cyanide, Butanenitrile

Toxicity Rating: 5. Chemical intermediate and solvent. Acute intraperitoneal LD_{50} in mice 38 mg/kg; LC_{50} for 1-hour exposure in mice 249 ppm. Acute toxicity is due to the slow metabolic release of cyanide in vivo. Standard cyanide antagonists are effective in mice, but multiple injections, particularly of the thiosulfate, may be indicated.

See also: Cyanide, *Reference Congener in Section III.*
Ref.: Willhite, 1981a; Willhite and Smith, 1981b.

650 Malononitrile 650

Toxicity Rating: 5. Synthetic intermediate. Acute intraperitoneal LD_{50} in mice 18 mg/kg. Acute toxicity is due to slow release of cyanide in vivo. Standard cyanide antagonists are effective in mice, but multiple injections, particularly of the thiosulfate, may be indicated.

See also: Cyanide, *Reference Congener in Section III.*
Ref.: Willhite and Smith, 1981b.

651 Phthalonitrile 651

o-Dicyanobenzene

Toxicity Rating: 4(?). Highly toxic stomach poison for caterpillars and dipterous larvae. As with Trichloroacetonitrile below, systemic cyanide poisoning is suspected.

See also: Cyanide, *Reference Congener in Section III.*

652   Polyacrylonitrile

652

Orlon

A synthetic fiber used in clothing (knitwear), rugs and outdoor furnishings. Has been tested as a soil conditioner. Chemically inert. Manufactured by polymerizing acrylonitrile, but unlike its monomer, polyacrylonitrile has no recognized toxicity.

653   Propionitrile

653

Propanenitrile, Ethyl cyanide

Toxicity Rating: 5. Chemical intermediate and solvent. Acute oral LD_{50} in rats 39 mg./kg. Acute intraperitoneal LD_{50} in mice 28 mg./kg.; LC_{50} for 1-hour exposure in mice 163 ppm. Teratogenic in hamsters. Acute toxicity due to slow metabolic release of cyanide in vivo. Sodium thiosulfate antagonizes the lethal effects in mice, but multiple injections may be needed.

See also: Cyanide, *Reference Congener in Section III.*
Ref.: Willhite and Smith, 1981b; Willhite et al., 1981c.

654   Succinonitrile

654

Butanedinitrile, Ethylene dicyanide

Toxicity Rating: 4-5. Synthetic intermediate. Acute intraperitoneal LD_{50} in mice 62 mg/kg. Teratogenic in hamsters. Acute toxicity due to slow metabolic release of cyanide in vivo. Sodium thiosulfate antagonizes the lethal effects in mice, but multiple injections may be needed.

See also: Cyanide, *Reference Congener in Section III.*
Ref.: Willhite and Smith, 1981b.

655   Trichloroacetonitrile

655

Trichloromethylnitrile, Tritox

Toxicity Rating: 4. Formula: CCl_3-CN. A volatile liquid used as a fumigant for treatment of stored grain and households. Inhalation produces severe damage to upper respiratory tract and bronchi which may result in prompt death. Surviving animals exhibited severe degenerative lesions of heart, liver and kidney. Lacrimation usually gives adequate warning of vapor exposure. A vesicant on the skin producing petechia and fissures. Orally 0.4 gm./kg. in rabbits produces miosis, ataxia, convulsions and death. It is unlikely that these effects in rabbits are due to cyanide released in the metabolism of trichloroacetonitrile because thiocyanate excretion is not increased after exposure, but the possibility of systemic cyanide poisoning has not been ruled out in man or other animals. Slightly less toxic than Acrylonitrile above.

Ref.: Treon et al., 1949b.

Botanicals and crude natural products

Botanicals (excluding toxic fungi)

656   American Mistletoe

656

Phoradendron flavescens

Not the same as the European mistletoe, *Viscum album* (see entry below). Contains sympathomimetic amines, probably beta-phenylethylamine and tyramine. Marked oxytocic properties but no direct cardiac toxicity. Parenteral administration of water extract of the plant produces an immediate fall in blood pressure, which is antagonized by atropine, followed by a sustained increase. Ingestion produces gastrointestinal irritation with nausea and vomiting, abdominal cramps and diarrhea, followed by transient hypertension, tachypnea and dyspnea, delirium with hallucinations, mydriasis and cardiovascular collapse. In the one reported death from the American mistletoe, a 28-year old woman drank a tea made from an unknown number of berries, thinking it to be an abortifacient. After one to two hours she developed nausea, vomiting and diarrhea, which continued until death 8 to 10 hours later. Just before death she was admitted to the hospital in severe shock, sweating profusely, and mydriatic. No cardiac arrhythmias were observed. Death was thought to be due to dehydration and electrolyte imbalances resulting from the extreme gastroenteritis.

Ref.: Hanzlick and French, 1924; Kingsbury, 1964; Lampe and Fagerstrom, 1968.

657   Arnica   657

Toxicity Rating: 3(?). Dried flower head of Arnica montana, which in the form of a tincture is used as a counter-irritant. Ingestion leads to severe gastroenteritis, nervous disturbances, tachycardia or bradycardia, and collapse. One ounce of the tincture has caused serious but not fatal symptoms. Treatment is largely supportive. The toxicity rating is presumptive and refers to the tincture.

Ref.: Jacobziner and Raybin, 1961k.

658   Belladonna Leaf or Root   658

Deadly nightshade, Atropa belladonna L.

Toxicity Rating: 3. Toxicity is based on content of atropine and related alkaloids, usually about 0.35%/w. Bellafoline is a trade name for the levo- rotatory forms of the alkaloids of belladonna as the maleate salts.

See also: Atropine, *Reference Congener in Section III.*
Ref.: Osol and Pratt, 1973.

659   Capsicum   659

Oleoresin of capsicum, Cayenne pepper, Tabasco pepper, African chillies

Toxicity Rating: 3(?). Irritating to mucous membranes. Produces severe gastritis and diarrhea. No primary systemic effects are recognized. Treat by lavage and demulcents.

Ref.: Osol and Farrar, 1955.

660   Cascara Sagrada   660

Toxicity Rating: 3(?). Dried bark of Rhammus purshiana. Active ingredients are hydroxymethyl anthroquinones. A cathartic which excites peristalsis in the colon. The adult dose is 0.6 to 2.0 gm. or 2 to 4 ml. of the fluidextract. Large doses cause enteritis, but no fatalities are known.

Ref.: Osol and Farrar, 1955.

661   Cashew Nut   661

East Indian almond, Anacardium

Nut of Anacardium occidentale L. indigenous to tropical climates particularly India, having a sweet oily kernel used as food. A black juice contained between the outer and inner shell of the nut is extremely acrid and corrosive, producing severe inflammation of the skin followed by blisters and desquamation. Cashew nuts and Jequirity Beans are encountered in primitive objet d'art and constitute a hazard to the unwary tourist. Cashew nut shell juice released by cuts into the shell contains about 90% anacardic acid (o-pentadecadienylsalicylic acid) and 10% cardol (m-pentadecadienylresorcinol). The latter is closely related to urushiol, the principal irritant of poison ivy, and is felt to be responsible for the dermatitis. Internally, cardol produces severe gastroenteritis. With heat, anacardic acid is decarboxylated to anacardol which is polymerized with formaldehyde, producing resins useful in electrical insulating varnish, brake lining dusts, moulding powders and millable rubbery compounds. Its hazard decreases in proportion to the degree of polymerization. Contact with the juice or partially cured resins should be treated like contact with poison ivy. Cases of ingestion require symptomatic and supportive care.

Ref.: Orris, 1958; Schwartz et al., 1945.

662   Cocillana   662

Toxicity Rating: 4(?). Dried bark of Guarea rusbyi (Britt.), containing a small amount of an alkaloid rusbyine. Has been used as an expectorant and nauseant. Oral doses over 1 gm. produce vomiting with prostration and purging. Dull frontal headache, sneezing and nasal discharge are described. No recognized antidote.

Ref.: Osol and Farrar, 1955.

663   Colocynth   663

Bitter apple

Toxicity Rating: 4 or 5. Dried pulp of Citrullus colocynthis. Powerful drastic, hydragogue cathartic, capable of producing violent griping, prostration, bloody discharges and dangerous inflamma- tion of bowels 2 or 3 hours after excessive oral doses. Death has followed 1-1/2 teaspoonsful of the powder. Gastric lavage with dilute tannic acid solution followed by instillation of milk is recommended, but a slurry of activated charcoal may be more effective and safer than a tannic acid solution. Morphine and atropine are usually indicated. Fluid and electrolyte balance should be maintained. Col-

Ref.: Osol and Farrar, 1955.

ocynth Extract (NF) is a fourfold concentration of the active principles. Compound colocynth extract (NF) contains ipomea, aloe and cardamon in addition to the extract.

664   664 Cube

Toxicity Rating: 4. Cube or cube' refers to several species of plants of the genus Lonchocarpus. Usually supplied as the powdered root. Insecticidal activity is due principally to the rotenone content (usually 4 to 6% in commercial preparations, although extracts may be much higher). The acute oral toxicity of powdered cube is greater than predicted from its rotenone content, perhaps because

of resins related to rotenone (see Rotenoids in the index) and perhaps because of constituents that enhance the solubility and absorbability of the rotenone. The LD_{50} in rats is similar to that of derris. In chronic feeding studies, however, cube is said to be less toxic than either derris root or rotenone.

See also: Rotenone, *Reference Congener in Section III.*
Ref.: Haag and Taliaferro, 1940; Hansen et al., 1965.

665   665 Derris Powder

Derris root

Toxicity Rating: 4. The powdered root of various species of the botanical genus Derris (tuba is the common name of one species). Used as an insecticide and to kill unwanted fish without damage to their food supply, so that game fish can be successfully introduced. The toxic principles of derris include rotenone and a variety of related rotenoids, e.g., deguelin (see Rotenoids in the index). The dried powder has a higher acute mammalian tox-

icity than would be predicted on the basis of its rotenone and rotenoid content (mouse oral LD_{50} 350 mg./kg.); however, this discrepancy may be due to the presence of other toxic or solubilizing agents in the crude powder. Absorption and toxicity are enhanced by olive oil. Derris root constituents may cause dermatitis when absorbed through abraded skin.

See also: Rotenone, *Reference Congener in Section III.*
Ref.: Dorne and Friedman, 1940; Haag, 1931; Haag et al., 1943.

666   666 Digitalis

Foxglove

Toxicity Rating: 4. Dried whole leaf of Digitalis purpurea. Clinical data place this mixture near the borderline between toxicity classes 4 and 5. The powder is available in pills, tablets, capsules, and

suppositories. One ml. of the official tincture (70% alcohol) is equivalent in digitalis content to 0.1 gm. of the standard powdered leaf or 1 USP unit.

See also: Digitalis, *Reference Congener in Section III.*

667   667 Ergot

Claviceps purpurea

Toxicity Rating: 4 or 5. A fungus which grows in the grain of cereals, particularly rye, from which several official drugs are derived. Rich source of a variety of alkaloids all of which are derivatives of lysergic acid. Consumption of grain and grain products (such as bread) contaminated with ergot has produced intoxications of epidemic proportions. Clinical intoxications also arise from excessive consumption of ergotamine tartrate used in the medical treatment of migraine. Despite insight into the etiology of ergotism and elaborate precautions to prevent grain contamination, poisonings still occur with surprising frequency. Gangrene of the extremities arising from intense peripheral vasoconstriction inspired the name "St. Anthony's fire." Semisynthetic derivatives of the natural alkaloids, such as dihydroergotamine, possess less vasoconstrictor activity and therefore are less likely to induce gangrene. Pregnant women abort or die in childbirth from the potent oxytocic activity of all ergot

alkaloids. Their lay use as abortifacients is illicit, persistent, and highly dangerous. Individual susceptibilities vary widely. Factors thought to predispose individuals toward ergotism include deficiencies of vitamins A and C, malnutrition, hepatic disease, renal disease, sepsis, and vascular disease. The primary symptoms are attributable to central stimulation and include nausea, vomiting, weakness, tremors, excitement, confusion, convulsions, tachycardia and mydriasis. Except in persons with severe vitamin A deficiency, however, the central signs are usually preceded by evidence of vascular stasis. Initial signs and symptoms of gangrenous ergotism include calf pain, cool extremities and paresthesias, usually of the distal portion of the extremities. In those with coronary insufficiency anginal pain may be elicited. Foot drop and transient monocular blindness have been described. Peripheral and coronary vasoconstriction may be antagonized by nitrites or papaverine, and short-acting barbiturates are indicated for convulsive seizures. The administration of sodium nitroprusside, anticoagulants and dextran, with continuous monitoring of the blood pressure, proved beneficial in one case of overdose due to misuse of ergotamine (Skowronski et al., 1979). Four human neonates survived accidental administration of 0.2 mg. doses of ergonovine maleate. Symptoms included cyanosis, erythema, ecchymoses of extremities, edema and pulmonary abnormalities. Treatment consisted of chloramphenicol and cortisone, and symptoms resolved in about five days (Edwards, 1971).

Ref.: Aird, 1959; Edwards, 1971; Fairbairn, 1958; Gabbai, 1951; Goldfischer, 1960; Merhoff and Porter, 1974; Skowronski et al., 1979.

668   Eupatorium   668

Eupatorin

Several species of this perennial shrub have been popular as household remedies in the form of infusions because of their diaphoretic effect. Discarded by the medical profession because of its nauseant properties, presumably due to the ingredient eupatorin. The literature concerning its toxicology is confused. One plant species is reported as causing hypoglycemia and another necrosis of the liver, tubular nephritis and glycosuria.

Ref.: Osol and Farrar, 1955.

669   European Mistletoe   669

Viscum album

Toxicity Rating: 3(?). Parasitic plant of the family Loranthaceae. Pharmacologically different from the American mistletoe (see above). Also different from the European oak mistletoe, a deciduous plant found in Central Europe, which has no pharmacologic activity. The European mistletoe has a low oral toxicity, but a specific cardiotoxicity is observed after large parenteral doses of aqueous extracts. These extracts contain choline (but not saponins), γ-aminobutyric acid and at least three toxic proteins termed "viscotoxins" (Samuelsson, 1973). The latter produce hypotension and bradycardia when given parenterally, but are destroyed by digestive proteases and thus largely ineffective when taken by mouth. Human volunteers given daily oral doses of 10 to 25 drops of a water extract (of unspecified strength) for several weeks exhibited a slight drop in blood pressure. In one individual, a mild bradycardia was also noted. Mistletoe extracts exhibit an anti-mitotic action in plants and animals. Proteinaceous fractions have been employed experimentally as antitumor drugs in humans. They are said to stimulate thymus proliferation and affect the immune system (Becker and Schwarz, 1972).

Ref.: Becker and Schwarz, 1972; Kochmann, 1931; Samuelsson, 1973.

670   Fava Beans   670

Horse beans, Vicia faba, Broad beans

Toxicity rating has no relevance since these broad beans form part of the staple diet in many areas of the Mediterranean basin. However, in certain susceptible individuals, notably Negroid and nonwhite Caucasians, ingestion of a single bean or even inhalation of the pollen from the plant can induce a severe intravascular hemolysis. The mechanism appears to be the same as that triggered by exposure to naphthalene, primaquin, and many other substances. See discussion under Naphthalene in Section III. No specific antagonists are known. Whole blood transfusions may be indicated.

Ref.: Emanuel and Schoenfeld, 1961; Hartigan and Gurnett, 1959; McPhee, 1956.

671   Gelsemium   671

Yellow jasmine

Toxicity Rating: 5(?). Dried rhizome and roots of Gelsemium sempervirens L. Has been used empirically in the treatment of neuralgias (average dose 30 mg.) Contains at least 3 potent alkaloids: gelsemine, sempervirine, and gelsemicine, each producing features reminiscent of curare, atropine, and strychnine poisonings: weakness, vertigo, tremors, ptosis, jaw drop, diplopia, mydriasis, dyspnea, anxiety, convulsions. No specific treatment has been outlined.

Ref.: Osol and Farrar, 1955.

672   Holly   672

Ilex, Winterberry, Black-alder

Toxicity Rating: 3. Three hollies are commonly found in the home at Christmas: the American holly (Ilex opaca), the English holly (Aquifolium) and the deciduous species Ilex verticellata or black-alder. Of the latter, only the berries are used for decoration. The toxicity of holly leaves is apparently low; early settlers in southeastern U.S.A. are said to have made a mild tea from the leaves of one native species. By contrast, holly berries are bitter and acrid. Their ingestion may cause vomiting, catharsis and occasionally mild narcosis. The

Ref.: Hart, 1961; Lampe and Fagerstrom, 1968.

fatal dose in children is said to be 20 to 30 berries. In the past *Aquifolium* berries were used medicinally for jaundice, gout and as a diuretic. The identity of the active ingredient is not known. In the absence of spontaneous vomiting, emesis should be induced. Further treatment is symptomatic.

673   Hydrastis

Toxicity Rating: 3(?). Dried rhizomes and roots of Hydrastis canadensis. Contains 3 active alkaloids: hydrastine (about 2%), berberine (2 to 4%), and canadine. Hydrastine (see latter in the index) in toxic doses causes strychnine-like convulsions due to hyperexcitability of the central nervous system; also relaxation of the gut; and possibly stimulation

Ref.: Osol and Farrar, 1955.

of the uterus. Berberine (see latter in the index) causes vasodilation, cardiac depression, and bronchoconstriction. Canadine has weak morphine-like effects. In toxic doses of the mixture, hydrastine's actions predominate, but the circulatory effects of berberine may also be apparent. The treatment is symptomatic and supportive.

674   Hyoscyamus

Henbane

Toxicity Rating: 3. From leaves and seeds of Hyoscyamus niger. Dried leaves contain about 0.04%

hyoscyamine alkaloids (hyoscine, hyoscyamine, etc.) See Hyoscyamine in the index.

See also: Atropine, *Reference Congener in Section III.*
Ref.: Osol and Farrar, 1955.

675   Ipecac

Toxicity varies considerably with the dosage form.

See also: Ipecac, *Reference Congener in Section III.*
Ref.: Smith and Smith, 1961.

676   Ipecac and Opium Powder

Dover's powder

Toxicity Rating: 4(?). A mixture of powdered ipecac (10%) and powdered opium (10%) in lactose. Once used as a diaphoretic and sedative. Therapeutic dose 200 to 600 mg. Presumably the chief

hazard of acute overdose would be the morphine content (1%) of the mixture, but violent emetic activity should also be anticipated.

See also: Ipecac *and* Morphine, *Reference Congeners in Section III.*

677   Jequirity Bean

Prayer bean, Rosary pea or bean, Crab's eye, Precatory bean

Toxicity Rating: 5(?). Scarlet seeds (black on lower third) of *Abrus precatorius* L. often used in primitive bead work. Importation of rosaries, voodoo dolls, jewelry, and swizzle sticks bearing decorative jequirity beans has not been officially banned, but a federally required warning label has effectively suppressed marketing of these items within the U.S.A. The plant is indigenous to tropical climates (Haiti, Florida, India, etc.). A toxic glycoprotein, abrin, is concentrated in the seeds. It consists of an acidic polypeptide chain A and a neutral chain B, joined by disulfide bridges. After attaching to the surface of mammalian cells through binding sites on the carbohydrate-containing B chain, hydrolysis appears to liberate the active A chain, which enters the cell to inhibit protein synthesis on ribosomes. Abrin is extremely toxic, but its mean lethal dose by mouth is reported to vary widely among species

of laboratory animals. If heated to 150°F, seeds are said to lose toxicity. A single seed, if thoroughly chewed, is reputedly lethal for man, but if the hard seed coat remains intact, the seed is considerably less toxic. Holes drilled by artisans expose the poisonous interior. Human symptoms are delayed 1 to 3 days; they include nausea, vomiting, severe diarrhea, colicky abdominal pain, circulatory shock, oliguria, cold perspiration, shallow and rapid pulse, drowsiness, disorientation, cyanosis, stupor, and death. Severe gastroenteritis is common in animals also. The symptomatology is reminiscent of but more severe than that induced by ricin, which has a similar mode of action (see Ricin in index). Ingested material should be removed before instituting symptomatic and supportive care. Lactose inhibits the binding of abrin to cells in vitro. Whether or not a similar phenomenon in vivo might constitute a basis for antidotal therapy remains to be explored. Immunization is regarded as a practical measure for livestock. Sometimes products with jequirity bean ornamentation also contain Cashew nuts (see latter above).

Ref.: Cann and Verhulst, 1959; Gleason et al., 1958; Muenscher, 1951; Olsnes et al., 1974; Olsnes et al., 1976; Sandvig et al., 1976.

678 Marihuana 678

Cannabis, Pot, Grass

Toxicity Rating: 1(?). Cannabis sativa (also sometimes called Cannabis indica) is the common hemp plant (also called Indian hemp). It is an annual weed, parts of which are commonly ingested or smoked to induce states of intoxication. The name marihuana generally refers to a mixture of cut, dried and ground flowers, leaves and stems of uncultivated plants. This material is known by many slang names: pot, grass, Mary Jane, tea, weed, etc. In India dried mature leaves are called bhang. In all cases the active constituents are a series of tetrahydrocannabinols, which are most prevalent in the resin produced by the flowering tops of the plant. The powdered resin is called hashish; in the form of a hard brown cake it is known in India as charas. The toxicity rating of 1 is inferred from data on the lethality of the purified ingredient Δ^9-tetrahydrocannabinol in mice and rats. No human fatalities have been documented.

See also: Marihuana, *Reference Congener in Section III.*

679 Nutmeg 679

Myristica, Nux moschata

Toxicity Rating: 3(?). Dried ripe seed of Myristica fragrans Houtt., Myristicaceae in common use since the Middle Ages as a household spice. Nutmeg has an unusual and generally unappreciated toxicity. Symptoms appear within 1 to 6 hours following the ingestion of up to three whole seeds or 5 to 15 gm. of the grated spice. Signs and symptoms are reiminiscent of atropine poisoning and include flushing of the skin, tachycardia, absence of salivation and central nervous excitation. Miosis, however, is more common than mydriasis. Bizarre central symptoms of euphoria and hallucinations have prompted the ingestion of this spice by addicts, alcoholics and others with unstable personalities. Pilocarpine is rejected as a possible antagonist because nutmeg contains no recognized anticholinergic ingredients and because pilocarpine would be ineffectual against the central symptoms. The principal ingredients are the volatile oils myristicin, eugenol, geraniol, safrol, borneol and linalool. Cats are especially sensitive to myristicin and exhibit central excitation followed by coma. On feeding large amounts fatty degeneration of the liver was seen. Appropriate and cautious barbiturate therapy is suggested to control central excitation. Myristicin bears some structural resemblance to serotonin antagonists.

Ref.: Payne, 1963.

680 Nux Vomica 680

Strychnos nux-vomica

Toxicity Rating: 4. Dried ripe seeds of Strychnos nux-vomica, containing 1.1 to 1.4% (rarely 2%) strychnine and about an equal amount of brucine. The tincture is a 10% solution in 70% alcohol (strychnine conc. 0.12%), and the probable lethal dose is 3 oz. Nux vomica fluidextract (NF) is 1.0 to 1.2% strychnine (1.5% in British Pharmacopoeia), and the dried powdered extract is 7 to 7.7% strychnine.

See also: Strychnine, *Reference Congener in Section III.*
Ref.: Osol and Farrar, 1955.

681 Passiflora 681

Passion flower or vine, May pops, Harman

The dried flowering and fruiting tops of Passiflora incarnata once used in medicine as an anodyne and sedative. All above-ground parts of the plant are utilized, including the yellow berries, which are the size of a hen's egg. Contains harman (1-methyl-9H-pyrido (3,4-b)-indole) in apparently unknown concentrations. Latter has a subcutaneous lethal dose in rabbits of 200 mg./kg. The crude drug was given to man in doses of 200-600 mg., and the fruit is said to be edible. Unknown principles in the plant produce depression in motor activity, an increase in the rate of respirations and a transient reduction in blood pressure. No human or even animal poisonings appear to have been described.

Ref.: Osol and Farrar, 1955; Merck and Co., 1976.

682   682 Pepper

Black pepper, White pepper

Toxicity Rating: 1. Dried unripe fruit of Piper nigrum L. Piperacae. White pepper is the decorticated ripe fruit of black pepper. For cayenne pepper, see Capsicum above. Used as a spice and formerly as a diaphoretic, carminative, gastric secretagogue, etc. Contains a volatile oil which is 5-9% piperine; also piperidine, chavicin, fat, proteins, and resins. The lethal dose by stomach intubation in rats is in excess of 12.5 gm./kg. In an unusual homicide a mother poured the entire contents of a pepper shaker into the mouth of her 4–year-old daughter. Death was attributed to asphyxia from occlusion of the air passages by inhaled pepper granules. No inflammatory process was described except for the presence of a brown seromucoid fluid in the stomach. Pepper removed from the stomach weighed 6.35 gm. (dry wt.). Granules were present in pharyngeal mucosa and a mass of pepper occluded the entrance to the larynx. The entire trachea, both main stem bronchi and primary intrapulmonary bronchi were completely filled.

Ref.: Adelson, 1964; Hodge and Downs, 1961; Merck and Co., 1976.

683   683 Peyote

"Button", "Moon"

Button-shaped growths of the Mexican cactus peyotl (botanically known as Lophophora williamsii), consumed for hallucinatory effects. It has long been used by Western Indians in tribal rituals. Currently it is sought by a variety of "street people". The oral route is usually employed, but the dried chopped buttons have an unpleasant gritty bitter taste and induce nausea and vomiting. Sometimes a tea is brewed and consumed, or the chopped material is swallowed in capsules or little balls. At least 10 alkaloids have been identified in the cactus, but mescaline is thought to be the chief hallucinogenic principle; see latter in the index.

See also: Marihuana, *Reference Congener in Section III.*
Ref.: Ludwig and Levine, 1965; McLain, 1968.

684   684 Poinsettia

Toxicity Rating: 2(?). Widely available ornamental plants. The most common species in the United States is *Euphorbia pulcherrima* Willd., var. Annette Hegg, Dark Red. The latexes of various *Euphorbia* species have been used medicinally as diaphoretics, emetics, expectorants and astringents. Emetic activity is due in part to saponin content. The domestic poinsettia is sometimes said to be toxic, but recent compilations of accidental ingestions by children describe only a mild emetic effect. Rats tolerated without ill effect oral doses of 25 gm./kg. of pureed leaves, stems, roots or milky juice (latex). Poinsettia derivatives were not irritating to rabbit eyes and had no anesthetic action. In humans, however, dermal applications of a water suspension of poinsettia leaves or stems caused moderate to severe skin irritation and photosensitization as manifested by erythema and blistering on exposure to ultraviolet light.

Ref.: Winek et al., 1978.

685   685 Pomegranate Bark

Granatum

Toxicity Rating: 3(?). Extracts contain a mixture of active alkaloids (0.5 to 1.0%) called pelletierine.

See Pelletierine tannate in the index.

Ref.: Osol and Farrar, 1955.

686   686 Pyrethrum

Pyrethrum flowers, Dalmatian insect powder, Persian insect powder, Trieste flowers

Toxicity Rating: 1. The dried flower heads of Chrysanthemum cinerariaefolium, containing 1 to 3% pyrethrins (see in Index), which constitute the active insecticidal principles. The powdered flowers are readily oxidized, losing 20% of their initial activity in one year. Also available are purified extracts containing 30 to 35% pyrethrins and a refined grade termed "Pale" which contains 60% pyrethrins.

See also: Pyrethrum, *Reference Congener in Section III.*

687   687 Quince Seed

Cydonium

Seed of Cydonia oblonga. Contains amygdalin, emulsin, 15% fatty oil, and 20% gum (cydonin). Emulsin is an enzyme which hydrolyzes amygdalin into benzaldehyde, hydrogen cyanide, and glucose.

The amount of available cyanide must be very small because a mucilage prepared from the seeds has long been used in medicine as a demulcent of low toxicity.

Ref.: Osol and Farrar, 1955.

688   Raudixin   688

Rauwolfia (serpentina)

Toxicity Rating: 2(?). The powdered whole dried root of Rauwolfia serpentina. It exhibits the actions of all alkaloids contained in the whole root. The toxic syndrome is presumed to resemble that due to reserpine, but Raudixin is several hundred times less potent.

See also: Reserpine, *Reference Congener in Section III.*

689   Rhubarb   689

The edible stalks of this common garden plant Rheum rhaponticum are frequently consumed in prepared dishes. The rhizomes and roots of other Rheum species indigenous to China and India contain anthraquinone glycosides and preparations of them have been used as cathartics and laxatives. American garden rhubarb is said to contain oxalate salts and under some circumstances may produce symptoms in humans which resemble oxalate poisoning. The leaves should not be eaten.

See also: Oxalate, *Reference Congener in Section III.*

690   Ryania   690

Ryania powder, Ryanicide

Toxicity Rating: 3. The ground stemwood of Ryania speciosa, a tropical shrub, used as a selective stomach poison for some insects. May be supplied in a mixture with the synergist *n*-propyl isome (see latter in the index). Ryania is moderately toxic to rats (oral LD_{50} 1.2 gm./kg.) but much more toxic to dogs (LD_{50} 150 mg./kg.). Lethality in both insects and mammals is apparently due to the alkaloid ryanodine, which is 500 to 700 times more toxic than the crude powder. Mammals given toxic doses of this alkaloid show an initial enophthalmus with subsequent vomiting, weakness, diarrhea, slow deep breathing, and profuse salivation, fol- lowed by increasing rigidity of striated muscles, depression of the central nervous system, and coma. Death is due to respiratory failure secondary to contracture of the respiratory muscles. Most anesthetized dogs, however, died from the cardiotoxicity of ryanodine, manifested by irreversible hypotension and eventual ventricular fibrillation and cardiac arrest. Single sublethal doses given i.v. produced slowly developing hypotension in various experimental animals. Artificial respiration may be helpful. Digoxin and ouabain did not protect poisoned dogs or cats.

Ref.: Merck and Co., 1947; Procita, 1958.

691   Sabadilla   691

Cevadilla, Caustic barley

Toxicity Rating: 3. The dried ripe seeds of Schoenocaulon officinate. About 0.3% alkaloids, of which crystalline veratrine (cevadine) and veratridine are the chief members. Used as an insecticide (5 to 20% dusts in lime or sulfur carrier). Not to be confused with Veratrum viride or album. Although apparently much less toxic, poisoning resembles that due to aconite: local irritation (e.g., sneezing from dust in nose), emesis, headache, giddiness, weakness, twitching, convulsions, hypothermia, drowsiness but seldom coma. Death is due to respiratory or cardiovascular collapse. As with digitalis the cardiac effects arise directly and reflexly and are often severe.

See also: Digitalis, *Reference Congener in Section III.*
Ref.: Powell, 1947.

692   Saffron   692

Crocus (N.F. VII)

Toxicity Rating: 2(?). The stigmas of Crocus sativus L., consisting of about 1% picrocrocin (a volatile oil). Used almost exclusively for coloring (yellow) and flavoring of foods, etc. No toxic effects are described. Known to be benign.

Ref.: Osol and Farrar, 1955.

693   Sanguinaria   693

Blood root, Red puccoon, Sanguinarine

The dried roots and rhizomes of Sanguinaria canadensis formerly used as an expectorant and for the treatment of chronic eczema and skin cancers. The active principle sanguinarine is related chemically to the opium alkaloids, but its ingestion causes symptoms of vomiting, diarrhea, fainting, shock and coma. No estimate of the lethal dose was located, but about 300 mg. is said to be therapeutic and 1300 mg. is emetic.

Ref.: Hardin and Arena, 1974.

694 694 Sawdust

Toxicity Rating: 1 to 3. The toxicity of sawdust varies with the species of tree. Many dusts are virtually non-toxic. For example, the finely powdered inner wood from Douglas Fir is innocuous. Known as wood flour, it is widely used as a filler in plastics, linoleum and wood putty and has been proposed for compounding pills. Sawdusts from other species, however, may contain irritants, allergens and toxins. Dusts from certain members of the pine, dogwood, beech, mahogany, mulberry, myrtle and birch families may cause asthma and contact dermatitis. There is a substantial literature reporting occupational asthma and dermatitis among workers exposed to red cedar dust. Epide-miological studies of furniture makers indicate that long term occupational exposures to wood dust may be a contributing factor in the development of cancer of the lung, tongue, larynx and nasal passages. An above-average incidence of leukemia has been reported among millwrights and lumber workers. The latter may be referable to pesticides and other toxic chemicals used to preserve harvested lumber during shipping. Sawdusts of East Indian satinwood and South African boxwood contain alkaloids which may induce systemic toxic reactions when inhaled or ingested. The symptoms include headache, anorexia, nausea, vomiting, bradycardia, dyspnea and somnolence.

Ref.: Bleumink et al., 1973; Gafafer, 1964; Ishizaki et al., 1973; Wellborn, 1977.

695 695 Squill (Red or White)

Sea onion

Toxicity Rating: 3 & 4. Consists of the cut and dried inner scales of the bulb of Scilla (or Urginea) maritima (L.). The red variety has the higher toxicity rating. Fresh squill contains a crystalline sterol glycoside (scillaren-A) and an amorphous glycoside fraction (scillaren-B). Both have cardiotonic actions like digitalis, but squill is used in medicine today only as a nauseant expectorant. Even official preparations of squill are no longer assayed for their content of cardiac glycosides, but probably scillaren-A and -B constitute less than 0.5% of dried squill. The toxic syndrome mimics that which follows digitalis overdosage. Scillarens appear to be more potent than digitoxin, but the hazard of intoxication is low because the alimentary absorption of squill is uncertain and its urinary excretion is rapid. In addition to scillaren A and B, red squill possesses a glycoside known as scilliroside; it may or may not be responsible for the convulsions seen in rats, by virtue of which red squill serves as a rodenticide. See also Scillaren in the index.

See also: Digitalis, *Reference Congener in Section III.*
Ref.: Dybing et al., 1952; Fitzpatrick, 1952; White and Viko, 1920.

696 696 Stramonium

Thorn apple, Jamestown weed, Jimpson or Jimson weed

Toxicity Rating: 3. Dried leaves and leaves and flowering tops of Datura stramonium L. Contains 0.25 to 0.45% alkaloids of the atropine-type (principally hyoscyamine). Pharmacologically and toxicologically equivalent to belladonna leaf. Has been employed as a "sensation drug". Children who eat parts of the plant, which is ubiquitously distributed in the U.S., exhibit disorientation, hallucinations and other clinical signs of atropine poisoning.

See also: Atropine, *Reference Congener in Section III.*
Ref.: Hughes and Clark, 1939; Jacobziner and Raybin, 1960b; Weintraub, 1960.

697 697 Tobacco

Toxicity Rating: 4. Dried or partially desiccated leaves of various species of the genus Nicotiana. The acute toxicity of tobacco, when eaten or inhaled as smoke, is largely ascribed to its nicotine content. Nicotine, present as salts of various organic acids, constitutes 1.0 to 2.5% (by weight) of commercial tobacco as marketed for smoking, and sometimes as high as 8% of desiccated tobacco, together with much smaller amounts of related alkaloids such as nornicotine and anabasine. Thus a modern commercial cigarette (weight approximately 1 gm.) may contain up to 25 mg. of nicotine, and 2 or 3 cigarettes may contain an amount equivalent to an adult fatal dose. In cigarette smoke, however, nicotine amounts to less than 3 mg. Although deaths have been recorded from the ingestion and rectal administration of a few grams of tobacco, even infants have survived after swallowing several cigarettes. Apparently the intestinal absorption of nicotine, as it is present in tobacco, is sometimes so slow that spontaneous vomiting eventually removes much unabsorbed alkaloid. Treat like nicotine poisoning.

See also: Nicotine, *Reference Congener in Section III.*
Ref.: Larson et al., 1961; Tso, 1972; Webster, 1930.

698 Uva Ursi   698

Bearberry

Toxicity Rating: 2(?). Dried leaves of Arctostaphy-los uva-ursi, containing volatile oil, arbutin, tannin (6-7%), gallic and malic acids, etc. Once used as a diuretic and antiseptic drug. Cleavage of arbutin, a glucoside, liberates hydroquinone, which appears in the urine after large doses. Usual dose 1 gm. three to six times a day, but no ill effects even after 20 gm.

Ref.: Osol and Farrar, 1955.

699 Valerian   699

Toxicity Rating: 3. The dried rhizome and roots of Valeriana officinalis, the perennial garden heli-otrope. The preparation contains several alkaloids; valeric, formic and malic acids (mostly esterified); the valtrates (complex esters of valeric acids); tan-nins and resin. The volatile components, consisting primarily of esters of formic, acetic, butyric and valeric acids with borneol, constitute valerian oil. It serves as a flavoring and is on the GRAS list for use in food. Valerian oil and the powdered root were formerly prescribed as sedatives. The CNS-depressant effect of the drug is apparently due to the valtrates. Since these esters are destroyed by heat, mineral acid and alkali, the actions of valerian extracts are highly variable. Valerian is moderately toxic in mice when injected i.p. (LD_{50} 360 mg./kg.), less so by mouth (LD_{50} 2.4 gm./kg.). Parenchymatous degeneration of the liver in guinea pigs was ascribed to the borneol content (Petlach, 1934). No reports of human poisonings were found. The usual oral sedative dose in man was 0.75 gm. of the root, 0.3 ml. of the oil, and 2 to 4 ml. of a tincture.

Ref.: Petlach, 1934; von Eickstedt and Rahman, 1969.

700 Wild Cherry   700

Prunus virginiana, Wild black cherry bark, Prunasin

A powder of ground wild cherry bark of the species Prunus virginiana or serotina, used to flavor cough syrups and other medications. In over-the-counter cough syrups it is referred to as a "cough sedative" but no beneficial effects were observed in con-trolled studies. Contains a cyanogenic glycoside, prunasin, and an enzyme, emulsin, which splits the glycoside into benzaldehyde, glucose and hydro-cyanic acid. Yields of the latter range from 0.05% to 0.35%. With very large doses cyanide poisoning is conceivable.

See also: Cyanide, *Reference Congener in Section III.*
Ref.: Osol and Pratt, 1973.

701 Wild Lettuce   701

Lactucarium

The juice of plants of the genus Lactuca has been used in folk medicine as a sedative. It contains a mixture of esters and bitter substances. Farm ani-mals exhibit dyspnea and weakness after ingestion of large amounts of the young plant, but dried extracts are believed to be non-toxic.

Ref.: Kingsbury, 1964; Osol and Farrar, 1955.

702 Witch Hazel   702

Hamamelis

Toxicity Rating: 2. Dried leaves of Hamamelis virginiana, containing tannin (2 to 9%). The dried leaves (or an extract thereof) are used in ointments and suppositories (dose 2 gm.). The fluidextract (prepared from leaves) has an ethyl alcohol content of 70 to 78% and significant amounts of tannin (dose 2 to 4 ml.). Witch hazel water is a saturated aqueous solution (with 15% ethanol) of volatile products distilled from dried twigs; it presumably contains small but appreciable amounts of terpenes (sesquiterpenes). All of these preparations serve as mild astringents and local sedatives. Ethyl alcohol and tannic acid are the major toxic ingredients; see both in the index.

Ref.: Osol and Farrar, 1955.

Natural products: foodstuffs

703 Citric Acid   703

2-Hydroxy-1,2,3-propanetricarboxylic acid

Toxicity Rating: 2-3. A moderately strong organic acid (first pK_a 3.1). Citrates are chelating agents found in nature. Citric acid is also added to foods, pharmaceuticals and household detergents. Esters of citric acid are used as plasticizers. The oral LD_{50} of citric acid is 11.7 gm./kg. in rats and 5.0 gm./kg.

in mice. Lethal doses in rats produce signs of metabolic acidosis and calcium deficiency. Citrate toxicity has been held responsible for the deaths of persons given rapid massive transfusions with blood containing citrate anticoagulant solutions.

When citrate accumulates faster than it can be metabolized, it reduces the plasma concentration of ionic calcium, which leads to cardiac arrhythmias, reduced cardiac output and death.

Ref.: Jennings et al., 1965; Task Force on the Health Effects of non-NTA Detergent Builders, 1981.

704   704   Glycerin

Glycerol, 1,2,3-Propanetriol, Trihydroxypropane

Toxicity Rating: 1. Glycerin is a sweet syrupy liquid with many industrial uses. In medicine it serves as an emollient and demulcent in preparations used on skin, as a vehicle for many drugs, and as an oral osmotic diuretic (in doses of 1-1.5 gm./kg.) to manage cerebral edema, reduce cerebrospinal fluid pressure and lower intraocular pressure. It absorbs water and in high concentrations is dehydrating and irritating to skin and mucous membranes (which accounts for its efficacy as a rectal suppository in promoting evacuation). While its oral toxicity in rodents is very low, large oral or parenteral doses in man may produce hemolysis, hemoglobinuria, renal failure, convulsions and paralysis.

It is rapidly metabolized and can cause hyperglycemia and glycosuria. Blood sugar levels of some normoglycemic subjects and all diabetic patients studied were raised after the ingestion of 1 gm./kg. Severe acidosis followed glycerin treatment in one 68-year-old diabetic. Two patients treated with glycerin for cerebral edema died from nonketotic hyperosmolar hyperglycemia, which can develop in maturity-onset diabetics from the combined gluconeogenic, antiketogenic and osmodiuretic effects of glycerin. Side-effects from oral doses include headache, dizziness, insomnia, nausea, vomiting, diarrhea and fever.

Ref.: Gilman et al., 1980; Hine et al., 1953b; Pfeiffer and Arnove, 1937; Sears, 1976.

705   705   Lecithin

Phosphatidyl choline

Toxicity Rating: 1. A phospholipid found in all living organisms but in especially high concentrations in nervous tissue and brain. An edible substance, it is used as an emulsifier and surfactant in chocolate, margarine and other foods. Commonly obtained from soy beans.

706   706   *D*-Sorbitol

D-Glucitol

Toxicity Rating: 1. A hexahydric sugar alcohol isomeric with mannitol. Occurs naturally in small amounts in some fruits but commercially produced by hydrogenation of glucose. As a laxative it is given by mouth in doses of 30 to 50 gm. As an osmotic diuretic it is given intravenously (50 to 100 ml. of a 50% solution). Doses of 26 gm./kg. by mouth in rats produced depression and death in 1 to 12 hours. When incorporated into peritoneal dialysis fluids in concentrations of 20 or 30 gm./l., it resulted in upper abdominal pain, hypertension, vomiting and sometimes coma in patients in chronic renal failure. With glucose in place of *D*-sorbitol, dialysis fluid was well tolerated.

Ref.: Carr and Forman, 1938; Osol and Pratt, 1973; Quellhorst et al., 1975.

707   707   Starch

Amylum, e.g., Cornstarch

Toxicity Rating: 1. Used for starching and sizing fabrics, and occasionally as an antidote in iodine poisoning. When used as a lubricant for surgical gloves, small amounts released in the course of operations have resulted in granulomas and peritonitis. Amylophagia during pregnancy is recognized as a common form of pica in certain localities. In one series the incidence was as high as 35%. Some women retain the habit for years and may ingest several pounds of starch daily. Since starch in such "addicts" accounts for the bulk of the diet, the commonly observed iron-deficiency anemia is probably a result of the practice and not its cause. Less common complications include parotid gland enlargement and partial intestinal obstruction due to starch gastroliths. Withdrawal has reversed these sequelae. Starch has such a low acute toxicity by mouth that rats given 10-20% of their total body weight showed only minimal symptoms.

Ref.: Allan and Woodruff, 1963; Blair and Blumenthal, 1964; Boyd and Liu, 1968; Kieth et al., 1968; Merkatz, 1961.

708   708   Sucrose

Sugar (granulated or powdered), Saccharose

Toxicity Rating: 1. Common household product obtained from cane or beets. Acute oral LD_{50} in rats 35.4 ± 7.0 gm./kg. in males and 29.7 ± 3.7 gm./kg. in females. While these doses may be extrapolated to the equivalent of a pound of candy in a 25-pound child, the acute gastroenteritis observed in animals would doubtless produce prompt vomiting in humans. Peppermint candy may present special problems; see Oil of Peppermint in the index. Certainly no clinical reports of acute sucrose poisoning have come to our attention. However, the intravenous use of 50% solutions (200 to 300 ml.) as a diuretic or to lower intracranial pressure carries a grave risk of damage to the kidneys. The signs and symptoms in poisoned animals include diarrhea, prostration, cyanosis, tonic-clonic convulsions, stupor and death in respiratory failure. Diffuse pathological changes included: shrinkage, swelling and necrosis of renal tubular epithelium, arteriolitis, mild hepatitis, myocarditis, congestive encephalitis and some adrenal hypertrophy.

Ref.: Boyd et al., 1965b; Hodge and Downs, 1961.

709   Tallow   709

Animal fat

Toxicity Rating: 1. In commerce tallow usually means fatty tissue of cattle and sheep. Edible grades are white or light colored. Hydrolyzed in bowel to glycerol and fatty acids. Hexadecyl, octadecyl, and especially octadecenyl groups predominate. See also Glycerol and Stearic acid in the index. Furthermore in commerce and industry the word "tallow" (also di-tallow, etc.) is sometimes used in quasi-chemical names to designate straight chain alkyl groups prepared from natural mixtures of fatty acids derived from tallow.

Ref.: Griffith, 1964a.

Natural products: fixed oils

710   Argemone Oil   710

Katakar oil, Sialkata oil

An oil derived from the seeds of Argemone mexicana L. The oil is often found as an adulterant of mustard, sesame or groundnut oil in some tropical countries. The toxic substance or substances, which may be alkaloidal, seem to be active in very low concentrations. The clinical picture after chronic ingestion of adulterated oil closely resembles dropsy. In severer cases the prominent manifestations include edema, dyspnea, hepatic enlargement and pulmonary congestion, all of which may be due to capillary dilatation. Tachycardia and minor ECG evidence of nonspecific myocarditis are described. The syndrome closely resembles congestive cardiac failure, but digitalis therapy seems to meet with only indifferent success. Sanghvi concludes that the circulatory failure is due chiefly to peripheral vascular collapse. Management requires a correct diagnosis, termination of the exposure, bed rest, measures to combat shock, and, in the presence of anemia, blood transfusions.

Ref.: Sanghvi et al., 1960.

711   Bone Oil   711

Dippel's oil, Oil of hartshorn, Animal oil, Bone tar oil

Toxicity Rating: 3. Obtained by the destructive distillation of bones in the preparation of animal charcoal. A black liquid consisting largely of nitrogenous compounds such as pyridine, aniline, methylamine, pyrrole, etc. Sometimes used as an alcohol denaturant. Rats given oral doses of 31 gm./kg. went into rapid progressive depression, terminating in about 4 min. in respiratory arrest with the heart still beating. Doses of 10 gm./kg. produced an initial weakness of the hind legs within 5 min., extreme depression within 15 min. and death in less than 2 hrs. Depression was apparent even at doses of 0.35 gm./kg. The 24-hr. oral lethal range in rats is estimated at 0.8 to 2.9 gm./kg. of undiluted material (unpublished data of H.C. Hodge, 1961).

712   Castor Oil   712

Toxicity Rating: 2(?). Chiefly the glycerides of ricinoleic and isoricinoleic acids. A purgative, often causing griping. Clinical dose 1/2 to 1 oz. Produces pelvic congestion and may induce abortions. Fatal dose unknown but presumably it is large.

Ref.: Osol and Farrar, 1955.

713   Chaulmoogra Oil   713

Hydnocarpus oil

Toxicity Rating: 2 or 3. A remedy for leprosy expressed from the seeds of Taraktogenos and Hydnocarpus species. Active ingredients (90%) are glycerides of a series of unsaturated fatty acids possessing the unusual features of optical activity and a 5-carbon ring. Representative are chaulmoogric and hydnocarpic acid. Oral doses of 5 ml./kg. of the oil produce death in rabbits as does the intravenous administration of 0.5 ml./kg. of ethyl hydnocarpate. Toxic doses produced anorexia, nausea, emesis, hemolysis, hemoglobinuria, fatty infiltration of liver. Fatal doses led to lowered blood

Ref.: Read, 1924.

calcium, convulsive retching with death from respiratory failure.

714　Coconut Oil

714

Copra oil

Toxicity Rating: 1. A white, semi-solid lard-like fat extracted from the kernels of the seeds of the coconut palm Cocus nucifera. It is used in the manufacture of soaps, candles and ointment bases, as well as chocolate and margarine. The oil is a mixture of triglycerides, including those of myristic, lauric, palmitic and stearic acids.

715　Croton Oil

715

Oleum tiglii

Toxicity Rating: 5. The fixed oil from the seed of Croton tiglium. The most drastic of all purgatives. Rarely used today. Causes hemorrhagic gastroenteritis. Death has resulted from the ingestion of 20 drops. Even on the skin, vesiculation, necrosis, and sloughing may occur.

Ref.: Ford, 1913; Osol and Farrar, 1955.

716　Lanolin

716

Wool fat

Toxicity Rating: 1. Hydrous (25 to 30% water) or anhydrous. A waxy secretion of sheep sebaceous glands found in wool. Contains cholesterol and other sterol esters of higher fatty acids and other higher alcohols (cetyl). Not absorbed from the alimentary tract. Lanolin extracts containing free sterol and cholesterol esters (e.g., Amerchol BL, C, H-9), as well as mixtures of alcohols derived from lanolin (Amerchol 400) and acetylated lanolin (Modulan), are used in pharmaceuticals and cosmetics as hypoallergenic emollients, emulsifiers and stabilizers. Mixtures of fatty acids derived from lanolin (e.g., Amerlate LFA) and their salts are also used as emulsifiers in soap emulsions such as shampoos.

Ref.: Greenberg and Lester, 1954.

717　Linseed Oil

717

Flaxseed oil

Glycerides of linoleic, oleic, stearic, palmitic, and myristic acids. A drying oil used in paints, etc. Digestible and nutritious, but it has a disagreeable taste. Large doses (over 1 oz.) are laxative. Boiled linseed oil (e.g., treated with a drier and heated to enhance the oil's ability to react with oxygen and form a hard film) is more dangerous and should never be taken internally, because lead or other toxic elements (e.g., manganese, cobalt) have usually been added.

Ref.: Osol and Farrar, 1955.

718　Neatsfoot Oil

718

Toxicity Rating: 1. Prepared by boiling ox feet, yielding the glycerides of oleic and palmitic acids. Used as a lubricant and to waterproof and soften leather. Consists of harmless and digestible fats which are found in normal diets.

Ref.: Merck and Co., 1976.

719　Peanut Oil

719

Arachis oil, Earthnut oil, Groundnut oil, Katchung oil

Toxicity Rating: 1. Peanut oil pressed from peanuts is used in foods, cosmetics and as a vehicle for intramuscular medication. Intravenous administration, however, is said to have resulted in acute rhabdomyolysis and renal failure. Innocuous by mouth, but may cause skin irritation when used in soaps. Aspirated whole peanuts have caused a severe and fatal bronchitis in small children. Experimental studies suggest that the responsible constituents are free fatty acids present in peanuts and peanut oil. Pure peanut oil has produced a similar bronchitis in rabbits with death between 24 and 72 hours after pulmonary instillation. Presumably aspiration of peanut oil could cause a similar reaction in humans.

See also: Kerosene, *Reference Congener in Section III.*
Ref.: Heatley and Clausen, 1930; Lynn, 1975.

720   Red Oil   720

Toxicity Rating: 1. A commercial mixture of fatty acids, particularly oleic acid (9-octadecenoic acid). Several grades in commerce vary in color from yellow to red-brown, depending upon the degrees of unsaturation, etc. Used to prepare soft soaps, lubricating and polishing compounds, and Turkey red oil. Unless there are unrecognized impurities, red oil is presumably as benign as any other mixture of dietary fatty acids. Sometimes the name red oil is used as a synonym for turkey red oil, which is probably more toxic; see latter in the index.

Ref.: Osol and Farrar, 1955.

721   Rosin Oils   721

Rosinol

A yellow viscous oily liquid obtained by the dry distillation of rosin. Used in lacquers, varnishes, lubricants, inks. No toxicity data were located, but the toxicity is probably low.

Ref.: Osol and Farrar, 1955.

722   Sesame Oil   722

Benne oil, Teel oil, Gingilli oil

Toxicity Rating: 1(?). Extracted from the seeds of *Sesamum indicum* L. A digestible vegetable oil consisting of glycerides of oleic, stearic, etc., acids, plus about 1% sesamin (a complex cyclic ether) and a related substance, sesamolin. The latter are potent inhibitors of hepatic microsomal enzymes. Because these enzymes act to detoxify many drugs and other exogenous chemicals, a heavy exposure to this oil might make a person temporarily vulnerable to toxic insults that would otherwise be tolerated with ease. Like other fixed oils, sesame oil is a laxative in large amounts. May cause contact dermatitis in sensitive individuals. Used as a vehicle for intramuscular medication and, because of its sesamin and sesamolin content, as a synergist for pyrethrins.

Ref.: Bruce and Tobin, 1940; Neering et al., 1975; Schiff and Hirschberger, 1937.

723   Tall Oil   723

Liquid rosin, Acintol C, Talleol

Toxicity Rating: 2(?). A mixture of rosin acids, e.g. abietic, and of fatty acids, chiefly oleic and linoleic. A byproduct of wood pulp production by the alkaline sulfate process. Tall oil is available in several grades with varying proportions of fatty and rosin acids. The resulting products are widely used in industry, e.g., in the manufacture of linoleum, soap and detergents, and printing inks. Esterified derivatives serve as core oil in metal foundries. The fatty acid components form metallic soaps that are useful drying agents. The principal toxic ingredients in the mixture are probably abietic acid and its congeners (see Abietic acid in the Index). The mixture is mildly irritating to skin and mucous membranes. One minor constituent, dehydroabietic acid, is said to be a vasodilator and partial nicotine antagonist in rabbits (Asano et al., 1973). No other evidence of mammalian toxicity was found. The effluent of sulfate pulp mills, however, is highly toxic to fish (LC_{50} 1 to 2 ppm) (Davis and Hoos, 1975). This toxicity is apparently referable to the rosin acid fraction (Leach and Thakore, 1973).

Ref.: Asano et al., 1973; Davis and Hoos, 1975; Leach and Thakore, 1973.

724   Tung Oil   724

China wood oil

Toxicity Rating: 2 or 3. The oil obtained from the kernels of the tung nut, the fruit of the tree *Aleurites cordata*. It is used as a drying oil in varnishes and linoleum and for waterproofing paper and fibers. The oil, which may be obtained by solvent extraction or pressing, consists mainly of edible fats and glycosides of fatty acids. When pure, it has a low oral toxicity (Erickson and Brown, 1942). Hypertensive rats tolerated 2 gm. doses of refined tung oil without ill effects (Grollman, 1945). The dose caused a significant reduction in blood pressure, however. This hypotensive effect is attributed to 9,14-dihydroxy-10,12-octadecadienoic acid (Lee and Nobles, 1959). Unlike the pure oil, tung nut kernel is distinctly toxic, causing severe gastroenteritis with shock, glycosuria, and respiratory depression (Balthrop et al., 1954; Kingsbury, 1964). Some preparations of the oil apparently retain appreciable amounts of the phytotoxins stored in the nuts. Rats fed 2 ml. of unrefined oil twice daily for two weeks developed a mucous diarrhea. Half of them died during a 2-week trial (McPherson, 1973). In one episode attributed to the oil, a family of five persons developed severe but transient gastroenteritis fifteen minutes after eating fish fried in an oil that appeared, upon chemical analysis, to be tung oil (Huisman and Vasbinder, 1961).

Ref.: Balthrop et al., 1954; Erickson and Brown, 1942; Grollman, 1945; Huisman and Vasbinder, 1961; Kingsbury, 1964; Lee and Nobles, 1959; McPherson, 1973.

Natural products: volatile oils

725   725   Essential Oils

e.g., Savin, Rue, Tansy, Apiol, Juniper, Cedarleaf

Toxicity Rating: 4. Most of these oils are reputed to be ecbolic but abortions cannot be induced by safe doses. Basically symptoms and treatment as after turpentine, but toxicity is greater. In most cases a teaspoonful may cause illness in an adult and less than an ounce may kill (especially if vom-iting does not occur promptly). Savin produces more renal damage than turpentine, and pennyroyal more liver degeneration. Also see Eucalyptol, Oil of Sassafras, Menthol, Pine Oil, Wintergreen Oil, Pennyroyal below or in the index.

See also: Turpentine *and* Camphor, *Reference Congeners in Section III.*
Ref.: Craig, 1953.

726   726   Camphorated Oil

Camphor liniment

Toxicity Rating: 4. Consists of 1 part camphor and 4 parts cottonseed oil. Not to be confused with camphor oil, which is a volatile oil obtained from crude natural camphor.

See also: Camphor, *Reference Congener in Section III.*
Ref.: Osol and Farrar, 1955.

727   727   Camphor Oil

Toxicity Rating: 4. A volatile oil from crude natural camphor. Constituents: safrol, acetaldehyde, 2-camphanone, orpinol, eugenol, dipentene, cadinene.

See also: Camphor, *Reference Congener in Section III.*

728   728   Chenopodium Oil

American wormseed, Oil of American wormseed

Toxicity Rating: 4. Active constituent is an organic peroxide called ascaridol (about 65% of oil). Other ingredients include cymene, camphor, and saponins. An anthelmintic with multiple toxic actions. Irritates skin and mucous membranes, inducing vomiting. Depresses bowel, causing constipation. Stimulates briefly and then depresses central nervous system, producing delirium and coma. Affects special senses, producing diplopia, blindness, tinnitus, deafness (rarely permanent). Causes circulatory collapse due to vasomotor paralysis and sometimes pulmonary edema. Late effects include liver and kidney injuries. Use saline cathartic. Treat symptomatically and vigorously. In the older literature about 70% of severe cases ended in death.

Ref.: Birnberg and Steinberg, 1939; Guyton, 1946; Sollmann, 1957; Wolf, 1935.

729   729   Juniper Tar

Oil of cade, Cade oil

Contains chiefly such derivatives of phenol as guaiacol and cresol, the sesquiterpene cadinene, aromatic hydrocarbons, and acetic acid. Used in the local treatment of skin diseases and in hair preparations and perfumes. Less corrosive than phenol.

See also: Phenol, *Reference Congener in Section III.*
Ref.: Osol and Farrar, 1955.

730   730   Lavender Oil

Oil of lavender

Alcohol extractable volatile oil of the flowers of Lavandula vera used as a perfume and flavor. Inhalation and skin absorption are said to have produced nausea, vomiting, headache and chills. May be a skin sensitizer.

Ref.: Greenberg and Lester, 1954.

731   731   Oil of Anise

Toxicity Rating: 4. Licorice-flavored volatile oil from Pimpinella anisum. Consists largely (80 to 90%) of Anethole (see latter in the index) with small amounts of methylchavicol and anisaldehyde. Widely used in cookies, candy and liqueurs. Used in some ersatz absinthes and apparently devoid of the dangerous central actions of thujone, for which it was substituted.

See also: Turpentine, *Reference Congener in Section III.*

732 Oil of Bay 732

Myrcia oil, Bay oil

Toxicity Rating: 3. Antiseptic and astringent volatile oil, which is a common ingredient in hair lotions and dressings, after-shave lotions, perfumes and flavors. Contains 40-55% eugenol and small amounts of chavicol, methyleugenol, methylchavicol, myrcene, citrol and 1-phellandrene. See also Eugenol in the index.

Ref.: Osol and Farrar, 1955.

733 Oil of Bergamot 733

Obtained from rind of fruit of bergamot tree. Contains 45% linalyl acetate. Chiefly employed as a perfume. Nervous and digestive symptoms develop from repeated skin exposure to this substance. Persons sensitive to this oil may develop photodermatitis, eczema, and pigment changes.

Ref.: Greenberg and Lester, 1954; Osol and Farrar, 1955.

734 Oil of Bitter Almond 734

Toxicity Rating: 5. Contains benzaldehyde (95%), hydrocyanic acid (2 to 4%), and amygdalin; the latter may be decomposed by digestive enzymes to form hydrocyanic acid (see also Amygdalin in the index). This oil is very rapidly poisonous when ingested, and death occurred promptly when an adult drank 7.5 cc. Dermatitis recognized in sensitive persons.

See also: Cyanide, *Reference Congener in Section III.*
Ref.: Osol and Farrar, 1955.

735 Oil of Cedar Wood 735

Cedar oil

A volatile oil obtained from the red cedar tree. Has been used to produce abortion, in some cases with a fatal outcome. Contains terpenes and a substance related to camphor.

See also: Turpentine *and* Camphor, *Reference Congeners in Section III.*
Ref.: DeNeen, 1919; McNally, 1916.

736 Oil of Citronella 736

Toxicity Rating: 3(?). Consists principally (93%) of geraniol and citronellal; also contains methyl heptanone, terpenes, etc. Used in perfumes and insect repellents (the latter property ascribed to methyl heptanone). By stomach tube in rabbits, citronellol (an alcohol derived from citronellal) produced paralysis, coma, and death in doses of about 1 to 4 ml./kg. (toxicity rating 3). Vomiting, shock, cyanosis and convulsions preceded death in a child who consumed an unknown quantity of a commercial preparation consisting largely of oil of citronella. Gastric mucosa was found to be severely damaged.

Ref.: Fischer and Bielig, 1940; Mant, 1961.

737 Oil of Hemlock 737

Volatile oil distilled from Tsuga canadensis and Abies canadensis, used in perfumery, room sprays and medicine. This material should not be confused with the poison hemlock, Conium maculatum, which contains toxic alkaloids such as coniine. See Essential Oils above.

Ref.: Greenberg and Lester, 1954.

738 Oil of Peppermint 738

Volatile oil derived from Mentha piperita L. The official product contains not less than 50% menthol, either free or as esters (not less than 5% esters calculated as menthyl acetate). Possesses pharmacological actions of Menthol; see latter in the index . Used as a carminative flavoring agent and antiseptic and local anesthetic in pharyngitis. Acute LD_{50}'s in rats: by mouth 4.4 gm./kg., intraperitoneally 0.8 gm./kg. Animals showed mild stimulation followed by depression, twitching, spastic convulsions, ataxia, hind limb paralysis and slowed respirations. Two human patients who chronically consumed large quantities of peppermint candy presented with idiopathic atrial fibrillation resist-

ant to quinidine therapy.

See also: Turpentine, *Reference Congener in Section III.*
Ref.: Eickholt and Box, 1965; Thomas, 1962.

739　Oil of Sassafras

739

Toxicity Rating: 5. One of the essential or volatile oils consisting of 80% safrole. See Safrole in the index. Thought to lie near the borderline between toxicity classes 4 and 5 with a clinical picture similar to that induced by oil of citronella (see above). Also similar to oil of eucalyptus in toxicity (see Eucalyptol in the index), except that vomiting and circulatory collapse are more common and miosis and respiratory symptoms less so. Appears to be a weak carcinogen on prolonged feeding to animals.

See also: Turpentine, *Reference Congener in Section III.*
Ref.: Abbott et al., 1961; Craig, 1953.

740　Pennyroyal

740

Oil of pennyroyal, American oil of pennyroyal, European oil of pennyroyal

Toxicity Rating: 4. American variety is derived from Hedeoma pulegioides (oil of hedeoma); European variety is derived from Mentha pulegium (oil of pulegium). Chief constituent of both varieties is pulegone, a cyclic ketone. Has been used as a carminative, abortifacient and in dysmenorrhea. Toxic encephalopathy has been reported following doses of less than 1 teaspoonful. Nausea, vomiting with eventual hematemesis, mydriasis, peripheral vasomotor collapse, confusion, restlessness, delirium and twitching of the limbs have occured. A case of frank epileptiform convulsions is reported.

See also: Camphor, *Reference Congener in Section III.*
Ref.: Braithwaite, 1906; Early, 1961; Jones, 1913.

741　Pine Oil

741

Toxicity Rating: 3. Steam-distilled pine oil is a mixture of terpene alcohols, chiefly α-terpineol, plus terpene hydrocarbons (5 to 10%), borneol (5 to 10%), and terpene ethers (5 to 10%). Irritating to eyes and mucous membranes. Produces hemor- rhagic gastritis. Systemic effects include weakness and central nervous depression, with hypothermia and respiratory failure. Consult index for names of various ingredients.

See also: Turpentine, *Reference Congener in Section III.*
Ref.: Hercules Powder Co., 1951; Schantz, 1953; Tauscher and Polich, 1959.

742　Theobroma Oil

742

Cocoa butter, Cacao butter, Butyrum cacao

Toxicity Rating: 1. An innocuous vegetable fat obtained by pressing the roasted seed of Theobroma cacao or by solvent extraction of the raw seed. It is used as a suppository base, in cosmetics, and as a skin softener. The fat consists chiefly of digestible glycerides of stearic, palmitic, oleic and lauric acids.

743　Thyme Oil

743

Toxicity Rating: 4. Volatile oil from dried leaves and flowering tops of Thymus vulgaris L. long used as a flavor, carminative, scent, rubifacient, antitussive and germicide. Major constituents are thymol (20-30%), carvacrol, cymene, pinene; minor constituents are linalool, bornyl acetate, thymene, menthene. Doses of 0.2-1.0 ml. are said to cause excitement. Extracts of fresh thyme have a smooth muscle relaxing effect and antagonize the actions of acetylcholine on the isolated guinea pig ileum, rat uterus and duodenum and guinea pig lungs. See also Thymol in the index.

Ref.: Jensen and Dyrud, 1963; Osol and Farrar, 1955.

Natural products: gums, resins and balsams

744　Acacia

744

Gum arabic, Gum acacia

Toxicity Rating: 1. Derived from gummy exudate of acacia tree. Used in various commercial preparations and cosmetics. Oral toxicity low. Proved to be a specific allergen giving rise to skin lesions and to severe asthmatic attacks in printers exposed to acacia dust. In the 1930's it was used intravenously to relieve the edema of nephrosis; reactions consisted of nausea, vomiting, dyspnea, and urticaria, all of which were controlled or prevented by epinephrine.

Ref.: Dick et al., 1935; Falkenstein and Jackson, 1940; Maytum and Magath, 1932.

745   Algin   745

Sodium alginate

Toxicity Rating: 1(?). A polymer of β-D-mannuronic acid with free carboxyl groups (sodium salt), prepared from various seaweeds (kelp), and widely used as an emulsifier and stabilizer in commercial ice cream, pharmaceuticals, etc. Apparently it is not decomposed or absorbed appreciably when ingested, and it does not swell in an acid medium. See Alginic acid below.

Ref.: Osol and Farrar, 1955.

746   Alginic Acid   746

Toxicity Rating: 1(?). A hydrophilic gum prepared from the sodium salt. It is able to absorb and chemically bind sodium and other cations when ingested, but it has proved to be less efficient than synthetic carboxylic-type resins. Various molecular weight derivatives have been shown to be effective hemostatic agents. Intraperitoneal LD_{50} in rats in the range of 2 gm./kg. Application to experimental wounds in animals produced no injury at site of application, and no retardation of healing. See Algin above.

Ref.: Osol and Farrar, 1955; Thienes et al., 1957.

747   Asafetida   747

Asafoetida, Devil's dung

Dried latex (gum oleoresin) from Ferula species (Iran, Afghanistan). Fetid odor due to apparently uncharacterized mercaptans in the volatile oil (6 to 17%). About 50% resin with free and esterified ferulic acid. No reports of poisoning are known and half an ounce is said to have been consumed without effect.

Ref.: Osol and Farrar, 1955.

748   Aspidium   748

Toxicity Rating: 4. Male fern; usually available as an ether extract of dried rhizomes, which yield not less than 6.5% of Aspidium oleoresin (USP). Active ingredients are filicic acid, filicin, and related substances. An anthelmintic. The oleoresin is a gastrointestinal irritant (nausea, vomiting, colic, bloody diarrhea). Produces central nervous excitation (dizziness, vertigo, delirium, tremors, and tonic-clonic convulsions), followed by depression (coma, respiratory or cardiac failure). Visual disturbances may culminate in temporary or permanent blindness. Mild kidney, liver and cardiac damage may appear. Intestinal absorption and toxicity are enhanced by fats and oils. Supportive treatment includes gastric lavage, saline catharsis, and control of convulsions (see Section IV).

Ref.: Hall, 1914; Osol and Farrar, 1955.

749   Balsam Peru   749

Peruvian or Indian balsam

Toxicity Rating: 3(?). It consists chiefly (50% to 60%) of esters of cinnamic and benzoic acids, especially cinnamein (benzyl cinnamate). See Cinnamein in the index. An oleoresin which is mildly antiseptic and may be mildly irritating to the skin. It has been ingested and even injected intravenously without ill effects. In man cinnamic acid is said to be largely excreted in urine as benzoic and hippuric acids.

750   Benzoin   750

Toxicity Rating: 3. Balsamic resin from Styrax benzoin, Dryand, and related species. Used internally as an expectorant and topically in various preparations as an antiseptic and protective. Common ingredient in vaporizer fluids marketed for inhalation. Consists largely of free and combined benzoic and cinnamic acids; see also Benzoic acid and Cinnamic acid esters in the index. Benzoin tincture (N.F.) is prepared with 200 gm. benzoin in a liter of ethyl alcohol; the final product is 75 to 83% ethyl alcohol by volume. Compound benzoin tincture (U.S.P.) is prepared with 100 gm. benzoin, 20 gm. aloe, 80 gm. storax and 40 gm. tolu balsam in a liter of ethyl alcohol; the final product is 74 to 80% ethyl alcohol by volume. Although additional comments concerning Aloin, Storax and Balsam peru can be found here and in the index, alcohol is expected to be responsible for the major signs and symptoms arising from the ingestion of these two tinctures.

See also: Ethyl Alcohol, *Reference Congener in Section III.*
Ref.: Osol and Farrar, 1955.

751   751   Candelilla Wax

Toxicity Rating: 1. Wax obtained mostly in Mexico from the herb *Euphorbia antisyphilitica* and *E. cerifera*. Used as a food additive in ice cream, candy and alcoholic and non-alcoholic beverages. Also used in polishes, candles, inks and as a har-

Ref.: Merck and Co., 1976.

dener of other waxes, such as Carnauba (see below). No deaths in mice fed 5 gm./kg.; larger doses could not be fed because of their bulk. Probably not absorbed from bowel.

752   752   Carnauba Wax

Brazil wax

Toxicity Rating: 1(?). Exudate from the leaves of the Brazilian wax palm tree which is used in polishing waxes and cosmetics. No reports of systemic toxicity were found, but it has caused dermatitis on

Ref.: Greenberg and Lester, 1954.

rare occasions. Probably consists of esters of high molecular weight, *n*-aliphatic primary alcohols and *n*-aliphatic acids as well as small amounts of arachidic acid, hydrocarbons, pigments and organic salts.

753   753   Carrageenan

Carrageen, Carraghenan

A sulfated polysaccharide consisting of galactose and anhydro-galactose units. It is the main constituent of the red alga, Chondrus crispus. It is used as a thickener in instant and convenience foods such as jellies and ice cream and as an emulsifier in shoe polish and cosmetics. Ebimar, a smaller polymer formed by the degradation of carrageenan with mild acids, has significant anti-peptic activity and is used in the treatment of peptic ulcer. Both the natural and degraded products are poorly absorbed from the gastrointestinal tract, and oral doses in man have induced no reported toxic reactions more

serious than watery diarrhea. The native product has a high intravenous toxicity (i.v. LD_{50} 5 mg./kg.) because it forms flocculent precipitates with blood proteins and so leads to embolism. Protein complexes of the degraded form are more soluble, hence it is less toxic by this route (i.v. LD_{50} 1 gm./kg.). Intramuscular injections of carrageenan may lead to granuloma formation at the injection site. Colonic ulcers have been reported in rats, rabbits and guinea pigs but not in dogs or squirrel monkeys after repeated oral doses of carrageenan or the degraded product.

Ref.: Anderson, 1969; Marcus and Watt, 1971; Sapeika, 1969.

754   754   Gamboge

Cambogia

Toxicity Rating: 4. A gum resin and drastic purgative, leading to severe prostration and death.

Ref.: Osol and Farrar, 1955.

The ingestion of 4 gm. has proved fatal.

755   755   Gums (Vegetable)

i.e., Gum karaya, acacia (arabic), tragacanth, ghatti, agar, and most other water-soluble gums

Toxicity Rating: 1(?). Aside from an occasional allergic reaction, these drugs can be ingested in large amounts, with little danger or distress except

Ref.: Dick et al., 1935; Maytum and Magath, 1932.

for diarrhea, flatulence, and rarely fecal impaction. They are not absorbed. See also Acacia above.

756   756   Latex

Toxicity Rating: 2 or 3. Natural latex is the milky sap of certain trees, including Hevea brasiliensis. It contains the rubber hydrocarbon $(C_5H_8)_x$, together with a number of other compounds, some of which may have appreciable toxicity. Synthetic latexes are also available; these are prepared by the polymerization of various monomers, including isoprene, butadiene, and chlorbutadiene. The pure latexes have a low oral toxicity. However, industrial

suspensions of the elastomer in water, termed "rubber latex", generally contain small amounts of the monomers and other toxic chemicals. Rubber latex is a primary skin irritant and sensitizer, and causes local irritation when ingested (Sax, 1968). Commercial products made from latex also contain plasticizers (e.g., phthalate esters) and fungicides (thiram or ziram) together with various antioxidants, activators and accelerators, the most toxic of which appears to be diphenylguanidine (rat oral LD_{50} 0.85 gm./kg.; Bourne et al., 1968). Artificial latexes may be prepared from reclaimed rubber, butyl rubber, *cis*-polyisoprene, and various terpolymers. They contain more additives than natural

Ref.: Bourne et al., 1968; Sax, 1968.

and synthetic latexes, and a higher toxicity should be anticipated. No specific oral toxicity data were found for individual latex formulations or latex products, however.

757 Opium 757

Toxicity Rating: 5. One to 3 grams of opium is considered a fatal dose in the nonaddict, as esti-

mated from its morphine content (about 10%).

See also: Morphine, *Reference Congener in Section III.*
Ref.: Osol and Farrar, 1955.

758 Pectin 758

e.g., Kaopectate

Toxicity Rating: 1. A mixture of methyl-esterified galacturonan, galactan and araban, varying in proportions depending on the source and generally thought to be harmless. Derived primarily from

fruits and fruit rinds, it is used to make jellies and similar foods. In combination with kaolin it is the popular anti-diarrheal drug, Kaopectate or kaolin-pectin mixture; see also Kaolin in the index.

759 Podophyllum Resin 759

Podophyllin

Toxicity Rating: 5. An irritant cathartic obtained from the roots of the mandrake (May apple). Contains a mixture of flavinols and lignans together with up to 20% podophyllotoxin and related compounds. Ingestion of 0.35 gm. has been fatal in an adult. The initial symptoms of overdosage are coughing, vomiting, diarrhea and abdominal pain. Cyanosis may be present. Later, respiratory stimulation, tachycardia, mental confusion, weakness and ataxia develop, progressing to flaccid paralysis and coma. Hypokalemia, glucosuria, impaired liver function, EEG changes, and a reversible granulocytopenia have also been described (Montaldi et al., 1974; Slater et al., 1978). In the case described by Slater et al. the patient was treated by charcoal hemoperfusion after five days of deepening coma. She regained consciousness after several hours but a flaccid paralysis persisted for several days. At discharge the patient showed evidence of peripheral neuropathy, including difficulty in walking and multiple areas of parasthesias and anesthesia. Such neuropathies following acute intoxication have been reported in other cases as well. Recovery is slow, extending over many months. Human fatalities, including one intrauterine death, have resulted from the topical use of podophyllum resin in the treatment of condyloma acuminata. In one such case, autopsy revealed congestion of all organs with fragmentation and swelling of the cerebral white

matter. Podophyllin has a specific toxic effect on the fetus and is a well known abortifacient. In rats the fetal LD_{50} was about one quarter of the adult LD_{50} when the compound was given by mouth to pregnant animals. One case of human phocomelia was reported after a laxative containing podophyllin was used during pregnancy. The resin is a mitotic spindle poison. Skin application causes changes in the cytonuclear pattern of the epidermis similar to those produced by colchicine. Therefore, podophyllin and several semi-synthetic derivatives have been used experimentally in the treatment of cancer. In animal studies, podophyllin is said to inhibit cellular respiration in various organs, including the brain. It is very irritating to mucous membranes, especially conjunctivae. Handling preparations of the powdered resin may lead to severe conjunctivitis, keratitis and ulcerative skin lesions. Single i.p. injections of 10 mg./kg. in rats produced severe leukopenia, transitory agranulocytosis, and aplasia of bone marrow. Damage to thymus, spleen and lymph nodes was also seen. Adrenalectomized rats showed similar tissue damage with high mortality. Only supportive treatment is available. In contrast to the root, the fruit of the May apple, occasionally eaten by children, is only slightly toxic. Catharsis may result from its ingestion.

Ref.: Balucani and Zellers, 1964; Clark and Parsonage, 1957; Kelly et al., 1952; Kingsbury, 1964; Montaldi et al., 1974; Slater et al., 1978; Sollmann, 1957.

760 Rosin 760

Abietic anhydride, Colophony, Yellow resin

The residue left after distilling away the volatile oils from pine oleoresins. Gum rosin results from distilling crude turpentine, wood rosin from distilling aged pine stumps (Pinus palustris). Both are water-insoluble. Rosin has been used in medicinal

ointments for skin and wounds. Softened with castor oil, it is the usual adhesive on sticky flypapers. No toxicity data were located, but the toxicity is probably low.

Ref.: Osol and Farrar, 1955.

761   **761 Shellac**

Lacca, Lac

A resinous excretion of certain insects feeding on appropriate host trees, usually in India. As processed for marketing, lacca may be mixed with small amounts of arsenic trisulfide (for color) and of rosin. White shellac is free of arsenic. The usual solvent is methyl alcohol. No toxicity data have been located, but the possible presence of arsenic and of methanol must be considered in suspected poisonings.

Ref.: Hirsch and Russell, 1945.

762   **762 Storax**

Styrax, Sweet oriental gum

Toxicity Rating: 3. Balsam obtained from the trunk of Liquidambar orientalis, Miller. Once used in medicine as a feeble antiseptic, expectorant and paraciticide. A constituent of compound benzoin tincture (U.S.P.); see Benzoin above. About half the drug consists of alcohol resins, but cinnamic acid both free and esterified constitutes an important part of the mixture. Also see Cinnamic acid esters in the index.

Ref.: Osol and Farrar, 1955.

763   **763 Turpentine**

Oil of turpentine, Spirit of turpentine, Gum turpentine

Toxicity Rating: 3. The oil and the spirit are synonymous. It is produced by distilling the gum (or oleoresin) from various species of pine, especially Pinus palustris. The word turpentine is used variously to designate the oil and the gum.

See also: Turpentine, *Reference Congener in Section III.*

Natural products: tinctures and fluidextracts

764   **764 Camphor Spirit**

Toxicity Rating: 4. An approximately 10% solution of camphor in 95% ethyl alcohol once used in the treatment of diarrhea and hysteria (0.5 to 1.0 ml.) and still employed on the skin for various ailments.

See also: Camphor, *Reference Congener in Section III.*

765   **765 Laudanum**

Tincture of opium

Toxicity Rating: 4. A 10% solution of opium in alcohol, equivalent to about 1% morphine. Do not confuse with the much weaker Camphorated Tincture of Opium (see Paregoric for the latter).

See also: Morphine, *Reference Congener in Section III.*
Ref.: Osol and Farrar, 1955.

766   **766 Paregoric**

Camphorated tincture of opium

Toxicity Rating: 3. A tincture of 0.4% opium (equivalent to 0.04% morphine). Based on its morphine content, it lies near the borderline between toxicity classes 2 and 3. It has been confused with tincture of opium (laudanum), which is 25 times more potent (toxicity rating 4).

See also: Morphine, *Reference Congener in Section III.*
Ref.: Osol and Farrar, 1955.

Constituents of natural products

Belladonna alkaloids and derivatives

767   **767 Atropine**

dl-Hyoscyamine

Toxicity Rating: 5(?).

See also: Atropine, *Reference Congener in Section III.*

768 Duboisine 768

Toxicity Rating: 5(?). A mixture of hyoscyamine-hyoscine alkaloids from one of the Solanaceous plants. Usually obtained as the acid salts, e.g., sulfates or hydrobromides.

See also: Atropine, Reference Congener in Section III.
Ref.: Osol and Farrar, 1955.

769 Homatropine 769

Mandelyltropeine

Toxicity Rating: 4(?). Less effective and less toxic than atropine. One-tenth as potent a parasympathomimetic blocking agent as is atropine. Used medicinally only in the eye, but reports of central nervous system involvement have appeared following use of homatropine eye drops.

See also: Atropine, Reference Congener in Section III.
Ref.: Hoefnagel, 1961.

770 Hyoscyamine 770

l-Hyoscyamine, Daturine, Levsin

Toxicity Rating: 5(?). The same toxicity to the central nervous system as atropine (equal parts of d- and l-hyoscyamine), but the l-isomer is at least twice as potent as a peripheral blocking agent.

See also: Atropine, Reference Congener in Section III.
Ref.: Cushny, 1921.

771 Scopolamine 771

Hyoscine

Toxicity Rating: 5(?). Commonly stated to be more toxic than atropine, but with either drug fatalities are rare. Idiosyncrasies, however, are definitely more common with scopolamine. Clinical doses of scopolamine commonly induce drowsiness or sleep, but large overdosages may produce excitement, hallucinations, delirium and psychotic behavior, like atropine. The scopolamine psychosis is fol-lowed by more prominent and prolonged central nervous depression. Peripheral actions mimic those of atropine. The methyl derivative of scopolamine (methscopolamine bromide or nitrate, sometimes called scopolamine methylnitrate) also shares the peripheral actions of scopolamine and atropine but lacks the central effects and is consequently much less toxic.

See also: Atropine, Reference Congener in Section III.
Ref.: Jacobziner and Raybin, 1960b.

Nicotine and related alkaloids

772 Nicotine 772

1-Methyl-2-(3-pyridyl)pyrrolidine

Toxicity Rating: 6. The probable lethal dose by ingestion is about 0.5 to 1.0 mg./kg. in man.

See also: Nicotine, Reference Congener in Section III.

773 Anabasine 773

2-(3'-Pyridyl)piperidine, Neonicotine

Toxicity Rating: 6. An alkaloid related to nicotine, present in tobacco in concentrations much lower than nicotine. Pharmacologic effects are similar to those of nicotine, but the compound is less potent. In terms of lethality, however, it may be slightly more toxic. Said to be cheaper than nicotine as an insecticide. Supplied as an aqueous solution of the sulfate salt.

See also: Nicotine, Reference Congener in Section III.
Ref.: Clark et al., 1965; Haag, 1933.

774 Arecoline 774

Methyl-1,2,5,6-tetrahydro-1-methylnicotinate

Toxicity Rating: 5(?). Often marketed as the hydrobromide salt, obtained from areca (dried seeds of Areca catechu L.). An alkaloid used in veterinary medicine against tapeworms (taeniacide). Has actions like both pilocarpine (or muscarine) and nicotine. Causes salivation, nausea, vomiting, abdominal cramps, diarrhea, clonic convulsions, and collapse. Treatment includes liberal doses of atropine.

See also: Nicotine, *Reference Congener in Section III.*
Ref.: Osol and Farrar, 1955.

775   **775**   Eudermol

Nicotine salicylate

Toxicity Rating: 6. The salts of nicotine are almost as toxic as the free alkaloidal base, except that the salts do not readily penetrate intact skin.

See also: Nicotine, *Reference Congener in Section III.*
Ref.: Merck and Co., 1976.

776   **776**   Lobeline (and Salts)

Toxicity Rating: 5(?). The chief alkaloidal constituent of the herb Lobelia inflata. Most common of the active ingredients in commercial smoking deterrents. Usually present in amounts of 1.0 mg. per unit dosage form. Subcutaneous doses of 10 mg./kg. regularly produced vomiting in dogs but at 12 mg./kg. some animals experienced excitement and convulsions. Humans have tolerated 8 mg. by mouth but some reported nausea and epigastric pain. As with nicotine, central nervous stimulation is followed by severe depression and sometimes death in respiratory paralysis.

See also: Nicotine, *Reference Congener in Section III.*
Ref.: Abdallah and Tye, 1967; Norris and Weiss, 1927; Wright and Littaur, 1937.

777   **777**   Nornicotine

2-(3′-Pyridyl)pyrrolidine

Toxicity Rating: 6. An alkaloid related to nicotine, present in tobacco in concentrations much lower than nicotine. The *l*-isomer is about as toxic as nicotine by intraperitoneal injection in rats and guinea pigs, but the *d*-isomer is about four times more toxic. Less active than nicotine in most mammalian test preparations.

See also: Nicotine, *Reference Congener in Section III.*
Ref.: Hicks and Sinclair, 1947; Larson and Haag, 1943.

Opium alkaloids and derivatives

778   **778**   Morphine

Morphia, Morphium

Toxicity Rating: 6.

See also: Morphine, *Reference Congener in Section III.*

779   **779**   Apomorphine Hydrochloride

Toxicity Rating: 5(?). This semi-synthetic opiate is a highly effective emetic drug which acts directly on the chemoreceptor trigger zone (CTZ) in the brain stem. Apomorphine is inactive by mouth and must be injected. A sterile solution is prepared from a 6-mg. hypodermic tablet at the time of use because conventional apomorphine solutions are unstable (do not use if solution is green or brown). The recommended dose is 0.07 mg./kg. or 0.03 mg./lb. either subcutaneously or intramuscularly, but a smaller dose (0.5-4 mg. in adults) may suffice if the drug is injected slowly by the i.v. route (Lindstrom and Brizzee, 1962). Vomiting occurs in almost everyone, except individuals under the influence of centrally acting anti-emetics (*e.g.,* chlorpromazine). The reaction is so fast by the intravenous route that the emetic threshold can be determined by "titrating" the patient. By s.c. and i.m. routes, the latency of the emesis is 2 to 15 minutes (mean 4 min.). In some studies the stomach was emptied more completely by apomorphine-induced emesis than ipecac-induced emesis, especially when the stomach was full. Therefore several ounces of water should be consumed before the drug is injected. Aside from speed, the major advantage of apomorphine over ipecac is that activated charcoal can be given by mouth at the same time without interference. The major complications are protracted vomiting in a few cases and significant central depression in a few others. However, apomorphine narcosis can usually be reversed by a narcotic antagonist (levallorphan 0.02 mg./kg. or naloxone 0.01 mg./kg.). Neither protracted vomiting nor depression is described in the few reports in which the drug was given intravenously in threshold doses.

See also: Morphine, *Reference Congener in Section III.*
Ref.: Lindstrom and Brizzee, 1962.

780   Codeine   780

Methylmorphine

Toxicity Rating: 5. Codeine, a naturally occurring opioid, is also produced by the methylation of morphine. One of the most effective antitussive drugs, it is commonly found in cough syrups. Less addictive than morphine, but a Schedule II drug and frequently abused. Given subcutaneously it is about one-tenth as potent as morphine in producing analgesia and respiratory depression; it retains two-thirds of its efficacy when given orally. The acute LD_{50}'s in rats are 420 mg./kg. s.c. and 600 mg./kg. orally. The lethal dose for a non-addicted person is about 0.5 to 1.0 gm. Common adverse reactions are nausea, vomiting, constipation, dizziness, palpitations, drowsiness and pruritis. As with other narcotics, overdoses produce central nervous system depression, respiratory depression, pinpoint pupils and coma. Body temperature and blood pressure may fall. Convulsions of spinal origin may occur, especially in children. Pulmonary edema, fitting the description of "heroin lung", has been reported. Deaths from codeine overdose are relatively rare. In one case a young man died shortly after he complained of a headache and collapsed, frothing at the mouth and having difficulty breathing. A history of cough syrup abuse and the presence of codeine, pheniramine and alcohol in his body were strong indications that the ingestion of several bottles of codeine cough syrup had caused his death. Among the autopsy findings were hemorrhagic bronchopneumonia and acute congestion and edema of the lungs.

See also: Morphine, Reference Congener in Section III.
Ref.: Sklar and Timms, 1977; Winek et al., 1970.

781   Dihydromorphinone Hydrochloride   781

Dilaudid

Toxicity Rating: 6. A more potent analgetic drug than morphine and correspondingly more toxic (perhaps 4 times as toxic). In clinical doses dilaudid causes less sedation and more transient analgesia than does morphine. Use nalorphine (Nalline) to combat respiratory and circulatory depression.

See also: Morphine, Reference Congener in Section III.
Ref.: Eddy, 1933; King et al., 1935.

782   Heroin   782

Diacetylmorphine

Toxicity Rating: 6. In a nontolerant adult (i.e., a nonaddict), 0.06 gm. is thought to be lethal. Not found in any legitimate product in the U.S.A.

See also: Morphine, Reference Congener in Section III.
Ref.: Strober, 1954; Walker, 1949.

783   Hydrocodone Bitartrate   783

Dihydrocodeinone bitartrate, 4,5α-Epoxy-3-methoxy-17-methyl-morphinan-6-one tartrate (1:1)

Toxicity Rating: 5. Narcotic analgesic and antitussive, available as tablets, powder and as an ingredient in combination products. Usually employed as an antitussive in adult oral doses of 3-10 mg., 3 or 4 times daily. Oral LD_{50} in rats is reported as 250 mg./kg., but humans are probably much more sensitive. About as effective as codeine for the relief of cough but more likely to be addicting. Severity of withdrawal symptoms between those of codeine and morphine. Nausea, dizziness and constipation are common side-effects. Overdoses produce the same signs and symptoms as does oxycodone (see below).

See also: Morphine, Reference Congener in Section III.

784   Levallorphan Tartrate   784

Lorfan

Toxicity Rating: 4(?). An opioid antagonist with agonistic effects. About 10 times more potent than nalorphine (below), but otherwise remarkably similar in its therapeutic utility and toxic effects. Available in injectable form at a concentration of 1 mg./ml. Intravenous LD_{50} in mice 26 mg./kg., but much less toxic by mouth because of rapid metabolic inactivation.

See also: Morphine, Reference Congener in Section III.

785   785   Levorphanol

3-Hydroxy-17-methyl-morphinan, 17-Methylmorphinan-3-ol

Toxicity Rating: 6. Narcotic analgesic with a longer duration of action than morphine and with a greater potency for inducing analgesia, respiratory depression and smooth muscle stimulation. Produces less nausea and vomiting. Therapeutic dose is 2-3 mg. subcutaneously or orally. Respiratory depression, hypotension, urinary retention and cardiac arrhythmias have been reported occasionally among surgical patients receiving levorphanol. A 41-year old woman committed suicide by ingesting an unknown amount of levorphanol, which was found in the concentration of 2.7 μg./ml. in her blood. Gross tissue examination at autopsy revealed frothy hemorrhagic fluid in the tracheobronchial tree, pulmonary edema, and vascular engorgement of liver, spleen and kidneys. Microscopic examination revealed diffuse pulmonary edema, focal pneumonia and vascular engorgement of the medulla oblongata and spinal cord.

See also: Morphine, *Reference Congener in Section III.*
Ref.: Turner and Richards, 1977.

786   786   Nalorphine Hydrochloride

Nalline

Toxicity Rating: 4(?). An opioid antagonist with agonistic activity. About 10 times less potent than levallorphan (above). Available in injectable form at concentrations of 0.2 mg./ml. for pediatric use and 5 mg./ml. for adults. Parenteral LD_{50}'s in several laboratory species 120 to 1500 mg./kg., but humans are probably much more sensitive, at least to its agonistic actions. Much less toxic by mouth presumably because of rapid metabolic inactivation. In the absence of morphine or other opioids, the agonist-antagonist drugs exhibit many of the actions of narcotics, but are far less potent. Among the effects described in normal man are nausea, giddiness, sweating, light headedness, euphoria, itching, drowsiness, crying, anxiety, postural hypotension, depression of the respiratory minute volume without a consistent change in respiratory response to carbon dioxide. High doses often induce severe dysphoric and psychotomimetic effects (*e.g.*, disturbing daydreams, frank hallucinations) that can be suppressed with high doses of naloxone. In compensated opiate addicts small doses are usually sufficient to precipitate an unequivocal withdrawal syndrome. Morphine antagonism is not always demonstrable with partial agonists, especially in patients who have received only small doses of the narcotic. Thus, a therapeutic failure does not rule out a diagnosis of morphinism. Conversely, a positive response cannot be regarded as diagnostic of morphine poisoning because these drugs are effective against a variety of opioids and opioid-like depressants including heroin, hydromorphone (dihydromorphinone, Dilaudid), Pantopan, methadone, metopon (methyldihydromorphinone), propoxyphene and meperidine (Demerol). With the possible exception of the thiobarbiturates the agonist-antagonists are ineffective against such central nervous depressants as the barbiturates, paraldehyde, nitrous oxide, pentazocine, etc. Indeed, nalorphine and levallorphan may be hazardous in compounding the respiratory compromise induced by non-opioid depressants.

See also: Morphine, *Reference Congener in Section III.*
Ref.: Buchner et al., 1972; Evans et al., 1973; Lasagna, 1954; Wikler et al., 1953; Woods, 1956.

787   787   Naloxone Hydrochloride

Narcan

Toxicity Rating: 3(?). A pure narcotic antagonist with parenteral LD_{50}'s in mice and rats ranging from 80 to 300 mg./kg. Much less toxic by mouth because of rapid hepatic biotransformation. Available in injectable form in a concentration of 0.4 mg./ml. Unlike the agonist-antagonist drugs, nalorphine and levallorphan, where the toxic effects are clearly due to the agonist activity, the acute toxic syndrome induced by naloxone in non-dependent subjects is not well defined. Oral doses in excess of 1 gm. have been tolerated in man without significant effects. Parenteral doses of 24 mg. caused only slight drowsiness. An increased rate of core temperature drop, slight miosis and reduced blood pressure occurred in humans after an intravenous dose of 1.2 mg. Because of questionable antagonism of non-opioid depressants in some species, the possibility that naloxone in massive doses may have analeptic (convulsant) activity must be considered.

See also: Morphine, *Reference Congener in Section III.*
Ref.: Zaks et al., 1971; Zilm, 1980.

788   788   Noscapine

Methoxyhydrastine, Narcotine, e.g., Tusscapine

Toxicity Rating: 3(?). An antitussive drug available as syrup or tablets. Like papaverine (see below), it belongs to the nonnarcotic isoquinoline series of alkaloids derived from opium. Usual therapeutic dose for adults should not exceed 120 mg./day because higher doses may cause nausea and drowsiness; however, patients who received doses of 3 gm. suffered only headache, nausea and vomiting.

Ref.: Empey et al., 1979; Winter and Flataker, 1961.

789 Oxycodone 789

Dihydrohydroxycodeinone, 4,5α-Epoxy-14-hydroxy-3-methoxy-17-methyl-morphinan-6-one, e.g., Percodan

Toxicity Rating: 5. A semi-synthetic analogue of codeine (see latter in Index). It is marketed in the U.S.A. as an ingredient of combination products only. Percodan, for example, contains oxycodone hydrochloride, oxycodone terephthalate and aspirin. Oxycodone is a Schedule II drug reportedly capable of inducing a morphine-like dependence greater than that of codeine. It is equivalent to morphine in its analgesic effect when given subcutaneously. By that route its LD_{50} in the mouse is 320 mg./kg., but humans are known to be far more sensitive than laboratory mammals to all opioid narcotics. It retains 50% of its effectiveness when given orally. The oral antitussive dose for adults is 3-5 mg. Signs of oxycodone overdose include respiratory depression, stupor (possibly progressing to coma), skeletal flaccidity, cold and clammy skin and sometimes bradycardia and hypotension. More severe intoxications may lead to apnea, circulatory collapse, cardiac arrest and death. Ingestion of large amounts of Percodan may result in salicylate intoxication as well.

See also: Morphine, *Reference Congener in Section III.*

790 Oxymorphone 790

4,5α-Epoxy-3,14-dihydroxy-17-methylmorphinan-6-one,   Dihydrohydroxymorphinone

Toxicity Rating: 6. Oxymorphone is a narcotic analgesic derived from oxycodone (see above) with similar adverse effects but less of a depressing action on the cough reflex. Therefore it is used chiefly for analgesia (e.g., post-surgical patients). Reported to be 10 times more potent than morphine and 1.6 times more toxic. Intraperitoneal LD_{50} is 200 mg./kg. in mice, but humans are far more sensitive than laboratory mammals to all opioid narcotics. It has about the same addicting potential as morphine.

See also: Morphine, *Reference Congener in Section III.*

791 Pantopon 791

Pantopium, Omnopon

Toxicity Rating: 6. A mixture of the hydrochlorides of the purified alkaloids of opium in the proportions which occur naturally in Turkish opium. On the basis of its morphine content (about 50%), Pantopon probably lies near the borderline between toxicity classes 5 and 6.

See also: Morphine, *Reference Congener in Section III.*
Ref.: Osol and Farrar, 1955.

792 Pentazocine 792

Talwin

Toxicity Rating: 5(?). A synthetic analgesic drug possessing some of the structural features of morphine, originally claimed to be free of addiction liability. Available as the lactate for injection and as the hydrochloride for oral administration. Rather well absorbed from the gut, but its analgesic potency by mouth is only one-third that by injection. Like other narcotic analgesics, it produces sedation and respiratory depression, but these reactions, as well as the analgesia, are not regularly intensified by raising the dose above 30-50 mg. (adult). Pentazocine does not prevent withdrawal reactions in morphine addicts; indeed it may precipitate the opiate abstinence syndrome. In nonaddicts high doses of pentazocine (60-90 mg.) often cause dysphoria, nightmares, feelings of "going crazy" and even frank hallucinations, as in nalorphine poisoning (see above). Naloxone (but not nalorphine) suppresses these unpleasant subjective reactions. Pentazocine can induce tolerance and rarely physical dependence; its abstinence syndrome is somewhat like that of morphine's. It is currently included under Schedule IV of the Controlled Substances Act. A peculiar form of abuse is the intravenous injection of a mixture of pentazocine and tripelennamine (see "T's and Blues" in the Index).

See also: Morphine, *Reference Congener in Section III.*
Ref.: Alarcon et al., 1971; Jaffe and Martin, 1980.

793   793 Papaverine

e.g., Pavabid

Toxicity Rating: 4(?). Directly acting smooth muscle relaxant found in opium, but chemically and
toxicologically unrelated to the narcotic alkaloids.
Used occasionally in medicine for treatment of
acute pulmonary and peripheral embolism. Usual
therapeutic dose 100 to 200 mg. two to three times
daily. Doses as high as 1 gm. by mouth produce
only minimal side effects. Intravenous doses of 30
and 65 mg. produced rapid demise in two adults
preceded by hyperpnea, tachypnea, and eventually
apnea. The heart sounds were not audible after the
onset of respiratory symptoms. Death may have
resulted from either a cardiac or respiratory disturbance. Arrhythmias and AV heart block are
commonly produced in both man and animals after
intravenous administration. Mild and reversible
hepatotoxicity (elevated serum alkaline phosphatase and transaminase) occurred in a series of
elderly patients following oral use of the drug. It
was ascribed to a hypersensitivity reaction.

Ref.: Ronnov-Jessen and Tjernlund, 1969; Sagall and Dorfman, 1945.

Rauwolfia alkaloids

794   794 Ajmaline

Rauwolfine, Gilurytmal

Toxicity Rating: 4(?). A pure alkaloid isolated from
Rauwolfia serpentina, recommended for the treatment of cardiac arrhythmias in a daily adult dose
of 100-150 mg. Said to lack the sedative effects of
reserpine and several other Rauwolfia alkaloids,
but coma occurs after massive overdoses. A 24-year
old man who ingested 2240 mg. was found unconscious and in circulatory shock. He eventually recovered in spite of generalized clonic convulsions,
perhaps coincident with repeated episodes of cardiac standstill and of ventricular fibrillation. Coma,
with occasional periods of tonic-clonic convulsions,
has been reported in several accidental and suicidal
poisonings. Cardiac action is compromised by severe defects in conduction, prolongation of QT and
a negative inotropic action.

See also: Reserpine *and* Quinidine, *Reference Congeners in Section III.*
Ref.: Almog et al., 1979; Ben-Shachar and Kishon, 1979; Hager et al., 1968; Jornod and Barrelet, 1965.

795   795 Alseroxylon

Rauwiloid

Toxicity Rating: 3(?). The alseroxylon fraction of
Rauwolfia serpentina. The principal useful action
is central vasomotor depression in the treatment
of hypertension. Side effects are similar to those
with reserpine, but their frequency and severity
are much less.

See also: Reserpine, *Reference Congener in Section III.*

796   796 Deserpidine

Harmonyl, Recanescine, 11-Desmethoxyreserpine

Toxicity Rating: 4. Deserpidine is an alkaloid of
Rauwolfia canescens. It resembles reserpine in its
actions, but deserpidine has a more rapid effect,
longer duration of action, and perhaps fewer side
effects. The miosis, ptosis, and catatonic states
seen after gross overdosage in animals respond
promptly to desoxyephedrine (and not quite so
markedly to caffeine and pentylenetetrazol).

See also: Reserpine, *Reference Congener in Section III.*
Ref.: Abbott Laboratories, 1957; Ferguson, 1956; Slater et al., 1955.

797   797 Rescinnamine

e.g., Moderil

Toxicity Rating: 3-4. A purified ester alkaloid of
the alseroxylon fraction of the Rauwolfia species.
Closely related chemically and pharmacologically
to reserpine. Therapeutic dosage range by mouth
0.5 to 1.0 mg. daily, although some institutionalized
patients have tolerated 12 mg. daily. Observed side
effects include behavioral toxicity, dyskinesia and
cardiovascular involvement. Autonomic reactions,
potentiation of other central depressants, extrapyramidal syndrome and hypotension should be anticipated.

See also: Reserpine, *Reference Congener in Section III.*
Ref.: Psychopharmacology Service Center, 1962.

798 Reserpine 798

Serpasil, Reserpoid

Toxicity Rating: 4(?). Reserpine is a pure alkaloid from Rauwolfia serpentina, used in the treatment of hypertension and in the control of anxiety and agitation.

See also: Reserpine, *Reference Congener in Section III*.

Miscellaneous alkaloids used in medicine

799 Aminophylline 799

Theophylline ethylenediamine

Toxicity Rating: 4. The ethylene diamine moiety has been associated with severe exfoliative der-matitis in a human patient who was not sensitive to anhydrous theophylline.

See also: Aminophylline, *Reference Congener in Section III*.
Ref.: Nierenberg and Glazener, 1982.

800 Caffeine 800

1,3,7-Trimethylxanthine

Toxicity Rating: 4. The adult mean lethal dose by mouth may be on the order of 10 gm. (Peters, 1967), but few fatalities have been reported except in recent years. An adult female was found dead after an estimated oral dose of 6.5 gm. (Alstott *et al.,* 1973). Another had a post-mortem serum level of 11.4 mg./100 ml. (Bryant, 1981), and a third had a blood level of 10.6 mg./100 ml. together with an arterial pH of 6.8 (Turner and Cravey, 1977). All three cases exhibited severe pulmonary edema on autopsy. A 19-year-old female presented with ventricular fibrillation which could not be converted to a normal rhythm. At death the stomach contained 18 gm. caffeine, and heart blood had 18 mg./100 ml. (McGee, 1980). A 5-year-old child who ingested 5.3 gm. with a blood caffeine of 16 mg./100 ml. complained of stomach cramps and chills but no convulsions were noted; severe cerebral edema was found on autopsy (Dimaio and Garriott, 1974). Various tissue levels of caffeine are reported in some of the above cases, as well as that of Parish *et al.,* (1965). In Jokela and Vartiainen's cases (1959) an intravenous preparation of caffeine was mistaken for glucose and given to two patients in insulin shock. One patient promptly developed convulsions after 3.2 gm. as the free base; death followed in a few minutes. The second patient received 0.4 gm. and had a brief convulsion before the error was discovered. Two deaths resulted from irrational, intensive and prolonged use of coffee enemas; hypokalemia was suspected as a contrib-uting cause (Eisele and Reay, 1980). A formula containing added tea concentrate produced tonic posturing and irritability in an infant (Brem *et al.,* 1977). An adult whose daily coffee consumption rose to 30 cups was eventually admitted with paroxysmal atrial tachycardia (Josephson and Stine, 1976). A positive correlation has been noted between the intensity of coffee consumption and myocardial infarction (Jick *et al.,* 1973). Full term infants given 36 to 136 mg./kg. caffeine sodium benzoate for respiratory depression after delivery developed tachypnea, tremor, opisthotonus and clonic-tonic movements before recovery (Banner and Czajka, 1980; Kulkarni and Dorand, 1979). In an unusual case a 1-year-old infant with coffee ground vomitus alternated between extreme agitation and listlessness. Her urine was 4+ for glucose with moderate acetone, and the serum glucose was 380 mg./100 ml. (Sullivan, 1977). In contrast adult subjects who consumed coffee and glucose had lower blood glucose levels at 30 and 60 minutes than when they consumed only glucose. Instead plasma free fatty acids were elevated by the combination (Feinberg *et al.,* 1968). Caffeine is extensively metabolized by man (Latini *et al.,* 1981) but human newborns are compromised greatly in their ability to carry out these reactions until after the first 7 to 9 months of life (Aldridge *et al.,* 1979). Caffeine is weakly mutagenic in non-mammalian systems and weakly teratogenic in some laboratory animal species (Thayer and Palm, 1975).

See also: Aminophylline, *Reference Congener in Section III*.
Ref.: Aldridge et al., 1979; Alstott et al., 1973; Banner and Czajka, 1980; Brem et al., 1977; Bryant, 1981; Dimaio and Garriott, 1974; Eisele and Reay, 1980; Feinberg et al., 1968; Jick et al., 1973; Jokela and Vartiainen, 1959; Josephson and Stine, 1976; Kulkarni and Dorand, 1979; Latini et al., 1981; McGee, 1980; Parish et al., 1965; Peters, 1967; Sullivan, 1977; Thayer and Palm, 1975; Turner and Cravey, 1977.

801 Theobromine 801

3,7-Dimethylxanthine

Toxicity Rating: 4. A methylxanthine closely related chemically and pharmacologically to caffeine and theophylline. Does not contain bromine despite its common name. Available as a magnesium oleoate salt for the treatment of arteriosclerosis. Found together with caffeine in cocoa and chocolate. Tea contains primarily caffeine but small amounts of theobromine and theophylline as well.

Probably there are no important distinctions among the xanthines in terms of their acute toxicity, but no reports of serious human poisonings from theobromine were found. Given by mouth to dogs single doses of 0.3 to 1.0 gm./kg. caused death. Seven of ten dogs given 75 to 150 mg./kg. per day for 3 or 4 weeks died. A degenerative, fibrotic cardiomyopathy was found in most right atrial appendages. Subacute feeding to rats produced atrophy of the thymus in both sexes and testicular atrophy in males. Mice and hamsters were much more resistant. Testicular damage in rats was also produced by caffeine and theophylline.

See also: Aminophylline, *Reference Congener in Section III.*
Ref.: Gans et al., 1980; Tarka et al., 1979; Weinberger et al., 1978.

802   802   Theophylline

1,3-Dimethylxanthine

Toxicity Rating: 4. A methylxanthine closely related chemically and pharmacologically to caffeine and theobromine (above). Uncoated tablets of anhydrous theophylline are used in the treatment of chronic asthma. More soluble salt forms, e.g., aminophylline, do not appear to offer special advantages in terms of absorption or lower incidences of gastrointestinal distress.

See also: Aminophylline, *Reference Congener in Section III.*

803   803   Colchicine

Toxicity Rating: 6. Alkaloid present in all parts of meadow saffron (Colchicum autumnale). The seeds are used to prepare tincture of colchicum. Highly effective in acute gouty arthritis. Death has resulted from single oral doses of 3 to 13 mg. of the alkaloid. The acute effects are characterized by a delayed appearance and consist of nausea, burning in throat, vomiting, intense diarrhea, abdominal pain, oliguria, delirium, convulsions and respiratory failure or coma progressing to cardiovascular collapse. A drastic fall in body temperature at death is described in animals. No known specific antidotes; treatment should be symptomatic and supportive.

Ref.: Ferguson, 1952; MacLeod and Phillips, 1947; Sternberg and Ferguson, 1954.

804   804   Dyphylline

7-(2,3-Dihydroxypropyl)theophylline, e.g., Neothylline, Lufyllin

Toxicity Rating: 4 or 3. An alkyl derivative of theophylline, used as an analeptic, bronchodilator and expectorant in the treatment of acute bronchial asthma and reversible bronchospasm associated with emphysema. Pharmacological effects are like those of theophylline and include bronchodilatation, vasodilatation, myocardial stimulation and mild diuresis, but dyphylline exhibits a lower acute oral toxicity than theophylline in experimental rodents. Also said to produce less gastric irritation than most other theophylline derivatives. Supplied as an injectable solution and in tablets. Also supplied in combination with guaifenesin and ephedrine (see in index). The latter is said to increase the toxicity but not the efficacy of dyphylline. The usual adult dose is 15 mg./kg. every six hours.

See also: Aminophylline, *Reference Congener in Section III.*
Ref.: Simons et al., 1975.

805   805   Emetine

Toxicity Rating: 5. An alkaloid extracted from the dried root of a Brazilian plant *Cephaelis ipecacuanha* and synthesized by methylation of cephaeline (another constituent of the same plant). Used in the treatment of intestinal and hepatic amebiasis. Kills amebae, apparently by inhibiting protein synthesis. Used clinically in doses of 0.5 mg./kg. (or less) twice daily for 5 days. Too irritating for oral administration. Produces inflammation at sites of injection (i.m. and s.c.). Systemic effects include nausea, vomiting and diarrhea; muscle weakness, pain and tenderness; hypotension, precordial pain, and tachycardia. In overdoses a toxic myocarditis is the most dangerous reaction. Emetine is the active emetic agent in ipecac.

See also: Ipecac, *Reference Congener in Section III.*

806   806   Methysergide Maleate

1-Methyl lysergic acid butanolamide, e.g., Sansert

Toxicity Rating: 3. A potent in vivo blocker of some of the actions of serotonin. Has been used to control diarrhea and malabsorption syndrome in patients with carcinoid and those with the postgastrectomy dumping syndrome. Said to be useful in the prevention of vascular headache but of no value against acute attacks. Adult therapeutic dose 2 to 4 tablets (2 mg. each) per day. Oral LD_{50}'s in mice and rabbits (581 and 2100 mg./kg., respectively) show this compound to be significantly less toxic than the closely related lysergic acid butanolamide (Methergine) with LD_{50}'s of 187 and 93 mg./kg., respectively. Daily doses as high as 5 mg./kg. failed to elicit major toxic signs in dogs. Significantly increased mortality of rats was not achieved until dietary levels of 150 mg./kg. per day were administered for 17 weeks. No serious human poisonings have been encountered but contraindicated in pregnancy, peripheral vascular disease and arteriosclerosis. Presumed peripheral and coronary vasoconstriction may be antagonized by nitrites or papaverine, and short–acting barbiturates may be indicated for convulsive seizures. Methysergide maleate has many actions in common with Ergot and Lysergic acid diethylamide (see both entries in the index), but it is apparently devoid of the psychic effects of the latter. In clinical doses it is only a weak vasoconstrictor or oxytocic, in contrast to the vigorous uterine contractions induced by methylergonovine.

Ref.: Sandoz Pharmaceuticals, 1962.

807 Physostigmine 807

Eserine, Physostigmine salicylate

Toxicity Rating: 6. A cholinesterase inhibitor derived from the seeds of Physostigma venenosum. Sometimes used in medicine as the salicylate salt in the treatment of poisoning by compounds with anticholinergic effects such as atropine, scopolamine and imipramine and other tricyclic anti-depressants. The usual adult dose is 0.5 to 2.0 mg. intramuscularly or intravenously. In the latter case do not exceed a dose rate of 1 mg./min. Repeat doses of 1 to 4 mg. as life-threatening signs (arrhythmias, convulsions, deep coma) occur. In ophthalmic solutions physostigmine is used in the treatment of glaucoma. The LD_{50} in mice is 3 mg./kg. by mouth and 0.23 mg./kg. intravenously. The signs and symptoms are those of cholinergic crisis. An adult male who consumed 1 gm. powdered physostigmine salicylate survived after gastric lavage with potassium permanganate, pralidoxime (P2S), mechanical ventilation and repeated bronchial aspiration. Atropine was given, but probably in inadequate amounts (1 mg.).

See also: Carbaryl, *Reference Congener in Section III.*
Ref.: Cumming et al., 1968.

808 Pilocarpine 808

Toxicity Rating: 6. Chief alkaloid obtained from the South American Pilocarpus shrubs occasionally used in clinical medicine as a parasympathomimetic drug to produce miosis, sweating, salivation, etc. Usual adult therapeutic dose 5 to 10 mg. A dangerous dose is 20 to 100 mg. by mouth in an adult. Poisoning has occurred from cutaneous absorption. Toxic actions resemble those of Muscarine; see latter in the index. Most of the effects can be suppressed with atropine.

Ref.: Moeschlin, 1965.

809 Quinine 809

Toxicity Rating: 4. Obtained from the bark of various species of the genus Cinchona. Quinine and quinidine are stereoisomers. They induce similar toxic effects at similar doses.

See also: Quinidine, *Reference Congener in Section III.*

810 Quinidine 810

i.e., Sulfate, hydrochloride, polygalacturonate

Toxicity Rating: 4. Quinidine (and quinine) are properly described as cardiac depressants. Overdoses in humans produce various toxic reactions; those on the heart are probably responsible for most of the fatalities.

See also: Quinidine, *Reference Congener in Section III.*

811 Veratrum Viride Alkaloids 811

e.g., Veriloid

Toxicity Rating: 3 or 4. An ancient galenical revived in the form of a partially purified alkaloidal extract for use in hypertensive cardiovascular disease. Believed to induce reflex peripheral vasodilatation and bradycardia producing a profound hypotension. The cardiovascular components are not fully understood but can be effectively antagonized by combined atropine-ephedrine therapy. Occasionally, reversible myotonic-like syndromes have occurred in patients during Veratrum therapy. In two cases involving infants, one of whom ingested 40 mg. of Veriloid, atropine promptly reversed the symptoms. Accidental ingestion of a related plant species (V. japonicum) has produced visual disturbances in the form of colored spots, in addition to hypotension. Because even conventional doses often produced vomiting, these alkaloids are no longer used in therapeutics.

Ref.: Connelly, 1957; Kolb and Korein, 1961; Nelson, 1954; Newman, 1952.

Alkaloids and other toxins in mushrooms

812   812 Mushroom Toxins

Mycetismus refers to any illness due to the ingestion of a toxic mushroom (also known as toadstools and fleshy fungi). Many species of wild mushrooms, representing many genera, are recognized as poisonous. In recent decades several (but not all) of the toxins have been isolated and chemically identified. Toxins differ among themselves in chemical structure and in the nature of the intoxication they induce. Poisonings range from mild and transient gastrointestinal disturbances to intense disorders of the brain, heart, liver and kidneys, terminating in death or in a slow convalescence. "Accidental" ingestions of wild mushrooms by young children are often reported, but most severe poisonings are due to the deliberate preparation and ingestion of mushrooms misidentified as edible varieties. Estimates range from 50 to 300 mushroom-related deaths per year on a worldwide basis. Some of the established mushroom toxins are described below.

See also: Mushroom Toxins, *Reference Congener in Section III.*

813   813 Amatoxins

α-Amanitin, β-Amanitin, γ-Amanitin

Toxicity Rating: 6. A group of at least 5 related cyclic polypeptides found in several species and genera of wild mushrooms, notably *Amanita phalloides, A. verna, A. virosa, A. bisporigera, Galerina autumnalis, G. marginata,* and *G. venenata.* The amatoxins possess in common a cyclic octapeptide skeleton. They are sometimes referred to as Group I mushroom toxins. All are extremely toxic by parenteral and oral routes; the estimated LD_{50} of α-amanitin in man is 0.1 mg./kg. Boiling the mushroom does not destroy these toxins. After ingestion there is a characteristic asymptomatic period of 6 to 15 hours (typically 10-12 hours), followed by a violent gastroenteritis. Absorbed toxins attack various visceral organs, notably the liver, where they may produce massive necrosis. In fatal cases death usually results from liver failure several days after the ingestion. Vigorous supportive care can influence the outcome favorably. The same is probably true of early hemoperfusion and various experimental regimens described in Section III.

See also: Mushroom Toxins, *Reference Congener in Section III.*
Ref.: Faulstich, 1979; Lampe, 1978; Wieland and Wieland, 1959; Wieland, 1968.

814   814 Phallotoxins

e.g., Phallacidin, Phalloidin, Phallisacin

A group of at least 6 related cyclic polypeptides found in several species of wild mushrooms of the genus *Amanita,* notably *A. phalloides* and *A. virosa.* They are thermostable and all possess the same cyclic heptapeptide skeleton. By parenteral routes they are extremely toxic (mouse i.p. LD_{50}'s vary from 1.5 to 4.5 mg./kg.). They attack and injure the plasma membranes of hepatocytes and of epithelial cells of the proximal convoluted tubules. Laboratory animals die of hepatic and/or renal failure. Even when injected, however, phallotoxins are only about one-tenth as acutely toxic as the amatoxins (see above), which are often found in the same mushrooms in almost the same amounts. Although the oral lethal doses of phallotoxins are not well established, they are apparently much larger than the parenteral lethal doses because, unlike amatoxins, the phallotoxins are poorly absorbed from the alimentary tract, perhaps because they are attacked by digestive proteases. At the present time it is believed that the phallotoxins do not contribute to the toxicity or lethality of mushrooms like *A. phalloides* which contain both phallotoxins and amatoxins.

See also: Mushroom Toxins, *Reference Congener in Section III.*
Ref.: Lampe, 1978.

815   815 Coprine

N^5-(1-Hydroxycyclopropyl)-L-glutamine

This water-soluble γ-glutamyl conjugate of 1-aminocyclopropanol is found in the wild mushroom *Coprinus atramentarius* and in a few other less common species of the same genus. It is hydrolyzed to 1-aminocyclopropanol in man and laboratory mammals fed the mushroom. This metabolite or a further hydrolysis product cyclopropanone hydrate inhibits the liver enzyme acetaldehyde dehydrogenase. If even small amounts of ethanol are ingested during the period of this inhibition (which probably does not begin until an hour or more after eating the mushroom and may last several days), acetaldehyde accumulates in the blood plasma, and the result is a prompt illness that mimics precisely the alcohol-disulfiram reaction (see Disulfiram in Section III). In the absence of alcohol, *C. atramentarius* is a safe, edible mushroom.

See also: Mushroom Toxins *and* Disulfiram, *Reference Congeners in Section III.*
Ref.: Hatfield and Schaumberg, 1975; Lindberg et al., 1975; Tottmar and Lindberg, 1977.

816   Gyromitrin

816

Ethylidene gyromitrin, Acetaldehyde *N*-methyl-*N*-formylhydrazone

Toxicity Rating: 5. A hydrazone of acetaldehyde found in false morels of the genus *Gyromitra*, especially *G. esculenta*; these springtime mushrooms are commonly called brain fungi or (in Europe) lorels and lorchels. One kilogram of fresh *G. esculenta* may contain (perhaps in a precursor form) 1.2-1.6 gm. gyromitrin and even larger amounts of the *N*-methyl-*N*-formylhydrazone of 3-methylbu-tanal (sometimes called 3-methylbutylidine gyromitrin), as well as related compounds. All of these hydrazones are readily hydrolyzed to mono-methylhydrazine (see below), which is believed to be responsible for the major toxicity of the gyromitrins. The oral LD_{50} of ethylidene gyromitrin in rabbits is 50 mg./kg.

See also: Mushroom Toxins, *Reference Congener in Section III*.
Ref.: Pyysalo, 1975.

817   Monomethylhydrazine

817

MMH

Toxicity Rating: 5(?). MMH is a propellant extensively used as the altitude control fuel in space craft, in contrast to hydrazine (H) and unsymmetrical dimethylhydrazine (UDMH or 1,1-dimethylhydrazine), which together are primary rocket propellants. MMH is also of toxicological interest as a decomposition product of the mushroom toxin gyromitrin; as described in Section III, MMH generated *in vivo* is believed to be responsible for the toxicity of gyromitrin (see above). All three propellants are strong convulsants as tested at high doses in laboratory animals, but in low doses at least H can cause central nervous depression. Pulmonary edema and cardiovascular collapse are other features that may contribute to deaths in acute poisonings. Animals that survive for a day or two frequently develop liver necrosis (not after UDMH) and/or renal failure. With MMH dogs are particularly sensitive to the latter injury, monkeys to the former. As judged by a few severe accidental hydrazine poisonings (Kirklin *et al.*, 1976) and by many gyromitrin poisonings, man reacts like the monkey in the sense that liver injury is much more severe than kidney damage. In animals poisoned with H or MMH, severe hypoglycemia may occur even before liver necrosis, but early hypoglycemia is apparently not described in the clinical literature. If this hypoglycemia is corrected, convulsions and other neurologic effects of H and MMH can be suppressed in animals by large parenteral doses of pyridoxine (Back and Thomas, 1970). In man H-induced hyperexcitability (Frierson, 1965) and even coma (Kirklin *et al.*, 1976) may respond to massive doses of pyridoxine, but there is no evidence that the liver necrosis can be prevented or corrected by this antidote. The recommended dose of pyridoxine to prevent MMH-induced convulsions in man is 25 mg./kg. to be repeated, if necessary, but when given with diazepam, a smaller dose may prove to be effective (George *et al.*, 1982). MMH is a low-grade carcinogen in animal assays.

See also: Mushroom Toxins, *Reference Congener in Section III*.
Ref.: Back and Thomas, 1970; Frierson, 1965; George et al., 1982; Kirklin et al., 1976.

818   Muscarine

818

Toxicity Rating: 5(?). An alkaloid isolated in 1869 from the mushroom *Amanita muscaria*, of which it is a very minor constituent (concentration in fresh fungi about .0003%). Much larger amounts, however, are present in many species of *Inocybe* and some species of *Clitocybe*; the ingestion of these mushrooms usually leads promptly to muscarine poisoning. Toxic signs and symptoms mimic those of parasympathetic nerve stimulation because muscarine, like pilocarpine, excites directly those cholinergic receptors on exocrine glands and smooth muscles that are innervated by the parasympathetic nervous system and by postganglionic cholinergic fibers of the sympathetic nervous system. The result is profuse sweating and with somewhat larger doses salivation, visual disturbances (miosis and blurring), nausea, vomiting, abdominal colic, diarrhea, headache, and bronchospasm. Very high doses may produce lacrimation, incontinence, bradycardia, hypotension and shock. The ingestion of muscarine-containing mushrooms has only rarely proven fatal, and even without treatment the symptoms usually subside in a few hours. Large doses of atropine by parenteral routes suppress all of the toxic signs and symptoms.

See also: Mushroom Toxins, *Reference Congener in Section III*.
Ref.: Jelliffe, 1937; Lampe, 1978; Lincoff and Mitchel, 1977.

819   Muscimol

819

5-(Aminomethyl)-3-isoxazolol

Toxicity Rating: 5. This water-soluble isoxazole derivative and its metabolic precursor ibotenic acid were first isolated in the early 1960's from the toxic mushrooms *Amanita muscaria* (popularly known as the "fly agaric") and *Amanita pantherina* (the "Panther mushroom"). These two compounds are now believed to be largely responsible for the toxicity of these two fungi and of a few related species.

Probably fresh mushrooms contain little or no muscimol, but drying and other manipulations cause the rapid decarboxylation of ibotenic acid to yield muscimol. Both of the pure compounds have been tested in man and animals, and muscimol appears to be 5 to 10 times more potent. The acute oral LD_{50} of muscimol in rats is 45 mg./kg. Human volunteers who ingested 7.5 to 10 mg. muscimol or 50 to 90 mg. ibotenic acid experienced within an hour symptoms that lasted 3 to 4 hours, with a few effects that lingered for about 10 hours and a hangover (headache) the next day. Subjects became inactive and experienced fatigue (the mushrooms also often cause an initial drowsiness, stupor or sleep), mild nausea and vomiting, muscle spasms in the extremities, various emotional changes (elation and excitement, or fear and withdrawal) and distorted perceptions of space and time, but only rarely hallucinations. The experience is sufficiently attractive to some that *A. pantherina* (which is more potent and more toxic than *A. muscaria*) is collected in the Pacific northwest and consumed (raw or cooked) for recreational purposes. Specimens of the fly agaric found in the eastern U.S.A (especially the yellow variety) are said to be much less psychoactive than those collected in the west. Only rarely does *A. muscaria* anywhere contain enough muscarine (see above) to produce mild muscarinic effects; unknown irritants rather than muscarine are believed to be responsible for much of the nausea and vomiting. Deaths from these mushrooms are very rare, but as with some other types of fleshy fungi, children have been known to react in unexpected and dangerous ways (*e.g.,* convulsions). Adults rarely require drug treatment for muscimol-ibotenic acid poisoning. Atropine is said to make the delirium worse, and physostigmine is ineffective.

See also: Mushroom Toxins, *Reference Congener in Section III.*
Ref.: Chilton, 1978; Waser, 1967.

820   820   Bufotenine

N,N-Dimethyl-5-hydroxytryptamine

Toxicity Rating: 4(?). First discovered as a constituent of the toxic secretion of the toad skin gland, this serotonin derivative has also been detected as a minor constituent of the wild mushroom *Amanita citrina* (which is usually classified as edible) and a few other species of *Amanita*. Similarly, serotonin itself and its metabolic precursor 5-hydroxytryptophan have been found in several species of mushrooms of the genera *Amanita* and *Panaeolus*. Although closely related in structure to the hallucinogens *N,N*-dimethyltryptamine (see in Index) and psilocin (see below), bufotenine is probably not psychoactive in man, even when injected intravenously in doses up to 20 mg. and intramuscularly in doses of up to 40 mg. One explanation is that bufotenine, like exogenous serotonin (5-hydroxytryptamine), is effectively prevented by the blood-brain barrier from entering the brain. Bufotenine shares many of the peripheral actions of serotonin, presumably by stimulating serotonin receptors on smooth muscles, glands, etc. Observed effects include intense flushing with a purplish hue, hyperventilation, salivation, slight tachycardia, mild hypertenison, abdominal distress and feelings of the need to defecate. Because bufotenine is less readily inactivated than serotonin by the enzyme monoamine oxidase, it is more effective by mouth and has a longer duration of action.

See also: Mushroom Toxins, *Reference Congener in Section III.*
Ref.: Chilton, 1978; Turner and Merlis, 1959; Tyler, 1961; Wieland et al., 1953.

821   821   Psilocybin

O-Phosphoryl-4-hydroxy-*N,N*-dimethyltryptamine

Toxicity Rating: 4. Psilocybin and its unphosphorylated analogue, psilocin, are found as natural constituents in the Mexican "magic" mushroom, *Psilocybe mexicana*, and in some other species of *Psilocybe, Panaeolus, Gymnopilus* and *Conocybe*. Also present in some of the *Panaeolus* are the monomethyl and non-alkylated analogues of psilocybin, known as baeocystin and nor-baeocystin respectively. Collecting these various small mushrooms, which are usually found growing on cow dung, and consuming them for "recreational" purposes increased rapidly during the 1960's and 1970's in various parts of North America and Europe. On the Gulf coastal region (U.S.A. and Mexico), *Psilocybe cubensis* ("blue legs") is the favorite, whereas in the Pacific northwest *P. semilanceata* ("Liberty bells") and *P. baeocystis* are commonly harvested. The Mexican mushroom has long been used in religious rituals by a few Indian tribes. Psilocybin and psilocin are hallucinogenic. They are much less potent than LSD but much more potent than mescaline; an effective oral dose of psilocybin in man is 3.5 to 12 mg. Hallucinations generally last 2 to 4 hours and are accompanied by signs of mildly increased sympathetic tone. If symptoms last more than 6 hours, one should seek another cause, such as LSD (see in Index); the latter has been used in the black market to "spike" cultivated *Agaricus*, which were then represented as specimens of *Psilocybe*. Psilocybin is said to be available also on the illicit market in the form of powders and liquids, but by analysis such materials have usually proved to be LSD or even DOM. Kits for growing *P. cubensis*, however have been sold by mail order. The psychic effects of psilocybin resemble those of LSD. Tolerance and cross-tolerance with LSD, DMT and mescaline are described. In most cases a psilocybin intoxication is so brief and mild that no treatment is required, but "bad trips" can be terminated by diazepam or by antipsychotic tranquilizers such as the phenothiazine drugs or haloperidol.

See also: Mushroom Toxins, *Reference Congener in Section III.*
Ref.: Cheek and Newell, 1970; Jacobsen, 1963; Lampe, 1978; Usdin and Efron, 1972.

Other alkaloids of natural origin

822   Aconitine   822

Toxicity Rating: 5. Aconite is the dried powdered root of monkshood or wolfsbane. Aconitine, an unstable alkaloid, is the chief active ingredient (0.4 to 0.8% of the dried powdered root). Fatal dose is 20 to 40 cc. of a 10% tincture (alcoholic). Used in some liniments and human poisoning from percutaneous absorption has been reported. In mouth and on mucous membranes, solutions produce a peculiar warm and tingling sensation with subsequent numbness. Central nervous stimulation is largely responsible for nausea, vomiting, and diarrhea; also restlessness, ataxia, vertigo, slow and dyspneic breathing, hypothermia, and convulsions. As with digitalis the cardiac effects arise directly and reflexly; they may be severe.

See also: Digitalis, *Reference Congener in Section III.*
Ref.: Fiddes, 1958; Hartung, 1930; Scherf, 1947; Solway, 1949.

823   Berberine   823

An alkaloid, usually as the sulfate; obtained from the rhizomes and roots of Hydrastis canadensis. Remarkable differences of opinion exist in regard to the toxicity of this compound, which may place it anywhere from toxicity class 2 to 5. Used as a bitter stomachic. A mild local anesthetic on mucous membrane. Toxic doses depress the heart (directly and reflexly through the vagus), relax blood vessels, depress respirations, and stimulate smooth muscle in the intestines, bronchi, and possibly uterus. Vigorous supportive treatment may be necessary for circulatory collapse.

Ref.: Jang, 1941; Keller, 1961; Seery and Bieter, 1940.

824   Brucine   824

Toxicity Rating: 5. Usually the sulfate salt. A denaturant in alcohols and oils. Probable fatal dose in an adult is estimated at 1 gm. May produce nausea, vomiting, restlessness, excitement, twitching, and rarely convulsions.

See also: Strychnine, *Reference Congener in Section III.*
Ref.: Morrison and Bliss, 1932.

825   Cocaine   825

Ecgonine methyl ester benzoate, "Snow"

Toxicity Rating: 5. As a solution of one of its acid salts (usually the hydrochloride but sometimes the nitrate or sulfate), cocaine has long served as a topical anesthetic in the eye and on mucous membranes. It is not commonly used in clinical medicine today but is still employed in veterinary medicine. Addicts prefer to inject it intravenously for the brief but intense elation that it induces. Somatic effects resemble those from amphetamine and its derivatives, but the actions of cocaine, even after a large oral dose, dissipate quickly (usually within 2 to 3 hours). Neither tolerance nor cross-tolerance with amphetamines has been established in man. Overdoses induce mania, hallucinations, and tonic-clonic convulsions. Death occurs usually in respiratory failure with or without cardiovascular collapse. The oral lethal dose is described as about 1 gram in adults, but some addicts are reported to have consumed as much as 10 grams in one day, reflecting rapid detoxification and possibly an acquired tolerance. Treatment is symptomatic, with particular emphasis on the control of convulsions with short-acting barbiturates (e.g., intravenous thiopental). Whether chlorpromazine is useful against the psychotomimetic effects, as in acute amphetamine poisoning, is not known.

See also: Cocaine, *Reference Congener in Section III.*
Ref.: Gilman et al., 1980; Webster, 1930.

826   Coniine   826

Toxicity Rating: 6. Most important of five alkaloids found in all parts of Conium maculatum (poison hemlock), an umbelliferous plant widely distributed in Europe and the United States. The whole plant in mid-summer exhudes a fetid odor reminiscent of mice to some and cat urine to others. The odor is at least in part attributable to the volatile coniine, and a narcosis is said to result from prolonged inhalation of the effluvia. The toxic potential was known in antiquity and presumably was instrumental in the death of Socrates. In man 3 mg. is said to have produced symptoms, but 150 mg. has been tolerated without discomfort. Perhaps 30-60 mg. is dangerous and death may occur with doses above 100 mg. Death occurs rapidly (less than 3 hrs.) with the most prominent signs and symptoms referable to peripheral paralysis and loss of sensation. Symptoms include drowsiness, paresthesias, weakness, ataxia, nausea, profuse salivation, and bradycardia followed by tachycardia.

Ref.: Webster, 1930; Witthaus, 1911.

Death is due to respiratory arrest from paralysis of respiratory muscles, although central depression may play a role after very large doses. Treatment is symptomatic and supportive with emphasis on artificial respiration. In non-fatal cases the effects are relatively transient.

827 Hydrastine

827

Toxicity Rating: 5(?). An alkaloid, usually as the hydrochloride; obtained from the rhizomes and roots of Hydrastis canadensis. Formerly used in the treatment of gastrointestinal inflammation and uterine hemorrhage (dose 10 mg.). Toxic doses

cause strychnine-like convulsions due to hyperexcitability of the central nervous system; also relaxation of the gut; and possibly stimulation of the uterus. Treatment as in strychnine poisoning.

See also: Strychnine, *Reference Congener in Section III.*
Ref.: Osol and Farrar, 1955.

828 Larkspur Alkaloids

828

Delphinium

Crude alkaloids are usually prepared from the seed (or roots). May be absorbed through skin when in solution, especially if skin is broken. Used since antiquity to treat body lice (ointment or fluidextract). As a poison it resembles aconite. Ingestion

produces tingling or burning pain, nausea, vomiting, salivation, bradycardia, hypotension, collapse, incontinence of urine and feces, coma and death. Treat symptomatically. Atropine may help.

Ref.: Marsh and Clawson, 1916.

829 Lysergic Acid Diethylamide

829

LSD, LSD-25, Lysergide, Delysid

Toxicity Rating: 6. Acute intravenous LD_{50} varies widely with species (46 mg./kg. for mice, 17 mg./kg. for rats and 0.3 mg./kg. for rabbits), but these doses are greatly in excess of the amount producing profound psychologic effects in man (1 microgm./kg. by mouth). No natural and no other semisynthetic ergot alkaloid containing a lysergic acid moiety exhibits so high an activity. LSD or its derivatives are said to be found in morning glory (Rivea corymbosa) seeds, and preparations of these have been ingested by amateur thrill seekers. In addition there appears to be a growing underworld traffic in LSD and similar drugs. In acute poisonings both autonomic and somatic symptoms are observed: mydriasis, tremor, piloerection, fever, salivation, vomiting, hyperreflexia, hypertension, ataxia and spastic paresis. Death results from respiratory failure. Doses of 20 micrograms/kg. have been survived, but the psychic disturbances are profound and may have permanent sequelae. The widely

recognized subjective effects of LSD are bizarre and highly variable; the following is only a partial list: intense multicolored visual (or less frequently auditory) hallucinations, synesthesias, hyperacusis, alterations of body image, aberrations of time sense, derealization, delusions, affectual changes ranging from elation to panic, complete loss of reality and total withdrawal. Tolerance develops to the psychic disturbances but physical addiction is not recognized. Instead, many LSD habitues indulge in a variety of stimulants, narcotics, sedatives, and hallucinogens. Such patients represent a supreme challenge to the therapist. The most effective antagonists to both psychic and autonomic effects of LSD are chlorpromazine and related phenothiazine tranquilizers, but only general supportive care is available for the late stages of acute poisoning. For the management of habituation, the services of an experienced psychotherapist are required.

See also: Marihuana, *Reference Congener in Section III.*
Ref.: Cohen and Ditman, 1962; Jacobsen, 1963; Rothlin, 1957.

830 Mescaline

830

3,4,5-Trimethoxyphenylethylamine

Toxicity Rating: 4(?). The active psychotomimetic (hallucinatory) constituent of peyote. The oral LD_{50} in mice is 912 mg./kg. (as the hydrochloride). The LD_{50}'s vary from 132 mg./kg. in the rat to 328 mg./kg. in the guinea pig. Intravenous LD_{50}'s in dogs and monkeys are 54 and 130 mg./kg. respectively. The oral hallucinogenic dose in man is 5-10 mg./kg., but similar doses have also been tolerated

by intravenous and other parenteral routes. Thus mescaline is less potent than LSD and most hallucinatory derivatives of tryptamine and of phenylethylamine, but its psychic effects tend to last longer (e.g., 8 to 12 hours). As with other psychotomimetic agents, frank hallucinations may be preceded or followed by distortions of sense perception in all sensory modalities, but visual distortions are most common. Psychic effects are accompanied by peripheral signs of moderately enhanced sympathetic activity: dilated pupils, tachycardia, slight elevation in blood pressure, tremor, hyperreflexia, headache, etc. Both psychic and somatic effects tend to be attenuated by therapeutic doses of chlorpromazine and presumably by other phenothiazine tranquilizers. Cross-tolerance between mescaline and LSD (but not marihuana) has been demonstrated in rats and inferred in man; see Lysergic acid diethylamide above. Material sold as mescaline on the illicit drug market is often LSD and is sometimes DOM (see latter in the index).

See also: Marihuana, Reference Congener in Section III.

Ref.: Cheek and Newell, 1970; Hardman et al., 1973; Hollister and Hartman, 1962; Jacobsen, 1963; Ludwig and Levine, 1965.

831   Pelletierine Tannate   831

Punicine tannate

Toxicity Rating: 5(?). A mixture of alkaloids as tannate salts (equivalent to not less than 20% as hydrochlorides) extracted from pomegranate bark. An anthelmintic used chiefly against tapeworm. An ordinary dose (0.3 gm.) often produces mild toxic symptoms. The alkaloids first stimulate and then depress the central nervous system; are selectively toxic to the optic nerve; have veratrine- and curare-like actions on muscle. Overdoses cause nausea, vomiting, diarrhea; twitching, cramps, weakness, and sometimes convulsions; dizziness, headache, mydriasis, partial blindness; paralysis and death. Treat by lavage, saline catharsis, supportive measures, including artificial respiration.

Ref.: Osol and Farrar, 1955.

832   Solanine   832

Toxicity Rating: 4. A generic name for a group of glycosidal alkaloids from plants of the genus Solanum, including the common potato. The isolated compounds have been used in the treatment of asthma and epilepsy. Solanine is concentrated in potato sprouts and vines and in green portions of sunscalded or blighted potatoes. Fatal poisoning from the ingestion of green or sprouting potatoes has been described, but the usual concentration of solanine in potato tubers (less than 0.01%) has no toxic significance. A toxic dose (about 0.2 gm. in an adult person according to Ruhl, 1951) induces gastrointestinal irritation and sometimes hemorrhagic gastroenteritis. Anorexia, nausea, abdominal pain, vomiting and constipation or diarrhea have been reported. These signs may be delayed as much as 48 hours. Symptomatic improvement usually occurs within 2 days of onset, even in cases that later prove fatal. The intact glyco-alkaloids are said to be responsible for the gastrointestinal irritation. By hydrolysis in the intestinal tract, the aglycones of solanine are released. These steroid alkamines (e.g. solanidine) cause cardiac and central nervous system effects, including immediate drowsiness, confusion and extreme exhaustion, dyspnea, headache, salivation, trembling and tachycardia. The symptoms may be accompanied by increased intracranial pressure (Nishie et al., 1971). Coma may ensue, followed by death from respiratory arrest. In one human poisoning characterized by severe hemorrhagic gastroenteritis, deep coma and death did not occur until fourteen days after ingestion. The glycoalkaloids also cause hyperglycemia in rats (hypoglycemia in adrenalectomized rats according to Ruhl, 1951), inhibit plasma cholinesterase in vitro, mimic the actions of cardiac glycosides on the isolated frog heart and induce intravascular hemolysis. Subtoxic doses may be teratogenic (Kirk and Mittwoch, 1975), and moderate doses (10 to 40 mg./kg. per day) given to pregnant rats in food inhibited postpartum lactation in 9 of 12 animals (Kline et al., 1961).

Ref.: Hansen, 1925; Kingsbury, 1964; Kirk and Mittwoch, 1975; Kline et al., 1961; Mun et al., 1975; Nishie, 1971; Ruhl, 1951; Satoh, 1967.

833   Strychnine   833

i.e., Sulfate, nitrate, phosphate

Toxicity Rating: 6. Strychnine and its salts are potent convulsants. The latent period after ingestion tends to be short (15 to 30 minutes).

See also: Strychnine, Reference Congener in Section III.

834   Yohimbine   834

Quebrachine

Toxicity Rating: 5. An alkaloid obtained from the bark of a West African tree (Corynanthe yohimbi Schum.) now believed to be identical with quebrachine, which is the chief alkaloid in the bark of an Argentine tree (Aspidosperma quebrachoblanco Schlecht). Also found in Rauwolfia serpentina and closely related structurally to reserpine. Chlorinated quebracho is used to control nematodes and other parasitic worms in soil. Yohimbine was once reputed to be an aphrodisiac but it has no proved therapeutic uses. It can produce a weak but specific adrenergic blockade of short duration: orthostatic hypotension, nausea, abdominal distress, miosis, weakness and fatigue. Central nervous activity is much less prominent than with the natural ergot alkaloids, and yohimbine does not block the actions of epinephrine on the heart. If hypotension becomes severe, an infusion of levarterenol or metar-

Ref.: Yonkman et al., 1944.

aminol may be helpful. Atropine, pilocarpine and angiotensin are without significant effect. Although yohimbine is the most potent alkaloid in crude preparations above, the presence of other constituents may complicate the course of intoxication.

Cardiotonic glycosides

835 Deslanoside

Deacetyllanatoside C, Cedilanid D

Toxicity Rating: 6. A cardiotonic glycoside derived from lanatoside C. More stable than the parent compound in solution. Has the same therapeutic and toxic actions as lanatoside C when given in the same way, but deslanoside is usually injected i.v.

See also: Digitalis, *Reference Congener in Section III.*

(initial dose 1.2 to 1.6 mg; daily maintenance dose i.v. about 0.4 mg.). Cardiac effects begin in 10 to 30 min., maximal in 1 to 2 hr., finished in 3 to 6 days. The lethal dose by mouth is apparently the same as that of lanatoside C.

836 Digalen

Toxicity Rating: 6. A soluble amorphous mixture of the cardiotonic glycosides from digitalis leaf (purpurea). Potency is determined by bio-assay. One USP unit is approximately equivalent, therapeutically and toxicologically, to 0.1 mg. of digi-

See also: Digitalis, *Reference Congener in Section III.*

toxin. The initial "digitalizing" dose is usually 10 to 15 USP units by mouth, 4 USP units by vein. The single fatal oral dose lies between 20 and 50 USP units in an average adult.

837 Digifolin

Toxicity Rating: 6. The natural mixture of cardiac glycosides of digitalis leaf (purpurea), separated from inert material. Potency is determined by bio-assay. One USP unit is approximately equivalent, therapeutically and toxicologically, to 0.1 mg. of

See also: Digitalis, *Reference Congener in Section III.*

digitoxin. The initial "digitalizing" dose is usually 10 to 15 USP units by mouth, 4 USP units by vein. The single fatal oral dose lies between 20 and 50 USP units in an average adult.

838 Digitoxin

Digitaline, Digitalin

Toxicity Rating: 6. A crystalline cardiac glycoside derived from the leaves of Digitalis purpurea, often contaminated with gitoxin (a related glycoside). About 1,000 times as potent as standard whole-leaf digitalis. The precursor of digitoxin in the leaf is purpurea glycoside A. Although insoluble in water, digitoxin is rapidly and completely absorbed from

See also: Digitalis, *Reference Congener in Section III.*

the bowel without irritation. A "digitalizing" dose for an average adult is 1 to 1.5 mg. orally or intravenously, and maximal cardiac effects occur in 4 to 12 hours. The action is persistent (2 to 3 wks.) and cumulative, and its maintenance usually requires only 0.1 mg. daily. An estimated single lethal dose is 3 to 10 mg.

839 Digoxin

Toxicity Rating: 6. A crystalline glycoside derived from the leaves of Digitalis lanata, specifically from its precursor lanatoside C. Has all the therapeutic and most of the toxic actions of whole-leaf digitalis. Absorbed from the bowel with little irritation. After an average oral "digitalizing" dose of 2 to 4

See also: Digitalis, *Reference Congener in Section III.*

mg. (of which about 65-90 per cent is absorbed), cardiac actions start in 5 to 60 min., are maximal in 2 to 6 hours, and are finished in 2 to 6 days. Because of its comparatively rapid dissipation, the daily maintenance dose is 0.25 to 1 mg. An estimated single lethal dose is 10 to 20 mg.

840 Gitalin

Gitaligin

Toxicity Rating: 6. An amorphous mixture of cardiotonic glycosides obtained from the leaves of

Digitalis purpurea. The chief constituent, which can be crystallized, is also named gitalin. Has all the therapeutic and toxic actions of whole-leaf digitalis, but said to have a greater margin of safety. In adults the average oral dose for rapid digitalization is about 5.7 mg. (4.5 to 9.0 mg.), whereas the daily maintenance dose is about 0.5 mg. With respect to duration of action, gitalin is faster than digitoxin and slower than digoxin. The single lethal dose in an adult probably lies between 15 and 50 mg.

See also: Digitalis, *Reference Congener in Section III.*

841   Lanatoside(s)   841

Digilanids

Toxicity Rating: 6. Glycosides from the leaves of Digitalis lanata, called lanatosides or digilanids A, B, and C. Lanatoside C is more often used as a cardiotonic drug than A or B. It has all the therapeutic and toxic actions of digitalis leaf. Its actions are less persistent than those of digitoxin but more prolonged than those of strophanthin. A "digitalizing dose" of lanatoside C is 5 to 10 mg. orally (of which about one-tenth is absorbed); the daily maintenance dose is 0.25 to 1.0 mg. The acute lethal dose by mouth is probably 5 to 10 times that of digitoxin; in an average adult this means 15 to 50 mg. of lanatoside C or somewhat less of the usual lanatoside mixture (Digilanid).

See also: Digitalis, *Reference Congener in Section III.*

842   Ouabain   842

g-Strophanthin

Toxicity Rating: 6. A crystalline glycoside obtained from the seeds of Strophanthus gratus. Given intravenously (occasionally i.m.), it has potent cardiotonic actions of brief duration (12 to 24 hours). Except for duration, poisonings resemble those of digitalis. It is poorly absorbed from the alimentary tract, where much of an oral dose appears to be destroyed. An average "digitalizing" dose intravenously (0.3 to 0.5 mg.) produces cardiac actions within 5 min., maximal in 0.5 to 2 hours, and complete in about 24 hours.

See also: Digitalis, *Reference Congener in Section III.*

843   Scillaren   843

Toxicity Rating: 6. The active cardiotonic glycosides of squill. Scillaren-A is a crystalline sterol glycoside, and scillaren-B is an amorphous glycoside fraction. Both have cardiotonic actions and toxic effects like digitalis. Unlike squill and crude extracts, scillarens are well absorbed from the alimentary tract. In terms of "cat units" they are more potent than digitoxin, but they are less toxic because of rapid excretion. A 2:1 mixture of scillarens-A and -B is given orally in a dose of 0.8 mg. one to four times daily to maintain a state of "digitalization." See also Squill in the index.

See also: Digitalis, *Reference Congener in Section III.*
Ref.: Dybing et al., 1952; Fitzpatrick, 1952; White and Viko, 1920.

844   Strophanthin   844

Toxicity Rating: 6. A glycoside (K-strophanthin-β) or mixture of glycosides obtained from the seeds of Strophanthus kombe. A cardiac glycoside with a potency officially adjusted so that 1 mg. is equivalent to 0.5 mg. of reference ouabain. Like the latter it is poorly absorbed from the alimentary tract, where much of an oral dose appears to be destroyed. Given intravenously it has potent cardiotonic actions of relatively brief duration (about 24 hours). Except for duration, poisonings resemble those due to digitalis.

See also: Digitalis, *Reference Congener in Section III.*

845   Urginin   845

Urginin A and B

Toxicity Rating: 6. A mixture of two water-insoluble glycosides from squill (Urginea maritima). Has therapeutic and toxic actions like digitalis. The usual daily maintenance dose in an adult is 0.5 to 1.0 mg. by mouth.

See also: Digitalis, *Reference Congener in Section III.*
Ref.: Merck and Co., 1960.

Glycosides that are not cardiotonic

846   846 Amygdalin

Laetrile

Toxicity Rating: 4. A chemical combination of glucose, benzaldehyde and hydrogen cyanide found in the bark, leaves, fruit and flowers of the cherry laurel and in the seeds of cherry, plum, peach, apricot and pear. In plant tissues amygdalin is hydrolyzed by a β-glucosidase to yield glucose and mandelonitrile. Cyanide is generated from the latter either by spontaneous decomposition or enzymatic action. It is not clear that β-glucosidase is found in mammalian tissues, but intestinal microflora in the rat are capable of releasing cyanide from amygdalin (Carter et al., 1980). Perhaps for this reason amygdalin is an unusual example of a compound that is more toxic (40 fold in one study) by mouth than by the intravenous route. Experimental studies in several species have established cyanide as responsible for the signs and symptoms of amygdalin poisoning whatever the route of administration (Khandekar and Edelman, 1979; Hill et al., 1980; McAnalley et al., 1980; Newton et al., 1981; Schmidt et al., 1978). On occasion kernels and seeds of the above plants have produced human poisonings (Jeannin et al., 1961; Lasch and Elshawa, 1981; Pijoan, 1942; Sayre and Kaymakcalan, 1964). Again the signs and symptoms were typical of cyanide poisoning although their appearance may have been more delayed (e.g., 0.5 to 2 hours) than after inorganic cyanide salts. The quack anti-cancer drug, laetrile, most samples of which contain amygdalin, has been the cause of accidental, iatrogenic and suicidal poisonings. An 11-month-old child died 71 hours after the ingestion of 50 to 250 mg./kg. (Braico et al., 1979). A 17-year-old died 24 hours after ingestion of approximately 210 mg./kg. (Sadoff et al., 1978). All of the reported human fatalities have involved enteral routes (per os, enemas, suppositories) of administration (Morse et al., 1979; Ortega and Creek, 1978; Vogel et al., 1981). Perhaps because the cyanide is slowly released from amygdalin, the time course of the intoxication may be protracted, necessitating repeated courses of therapy. In that event it is safer and more efficient to repeat the injections of thiosulfate and not of nitrite.

See also: Cyanide, *Reference Congener in Section III.*
Ref.: Braico et al., 1979; Carter et al., 1980; Hill et al., 1980; Jeannin et al., 1961; Khandekar and Edelman, 1979; Lasch and Elshawa, 1981; McAnalley et al., 1980; Morse et al., 1979; Newton et al., 1981; Ortega and Creek, 1978; Pijoan, 1942; Sadoff et al., 1978; Sayre and Kaymakcalan, 1964; Schmidt et al., 1978; Vogel et al., 1981.

847   847 Aloin

Toxicity Rating: 4(?). A mixture of the active principles obtained from aloe. An irritant laxative (dose 15 mg.) with bowel actions largely limited to the colon. Very irritating even in therapeutic doses, and overdosage causes abdominal pain, bloody diarrhea, hemorrhagic gastritis, and sometimes nephritis. Said to stimulate visceral smooth muscle and reputedly an abortifacient.

Ref.: Osol and Farrar, 1955; Reese, 1874.

848   848 Ammonium Glycyrrhizate

Glycyrrhiza, Licorice

Toxicity Rating: 2(?). The active constituent (about 15% by weight) and the ingredient responsible for the characteristic taste and odor of licorice extract, also called block licorice, which is prepared from the plant Glycyrrhiza glabea. In addition to this extract, confectionery or candy licorice often contains other flavoring agents, such as anise, which has a similar taste but dissimilar chemical structure (see Anethole in the index). Indeed licorice candy rarely, if ever, contains more than 2% licorice extract (Herbert Storm, Jr., personal communication, 1968). Adequate studies were not located, but the toxicity of this compound and its derivatives by mouth is presumed to be low. Glycyrrhizic acid is a glycoside of glycyrrhetic acid, a compound structurally similar to many cyclopentanophenanthrene steroids. Indeed, the only well established pharmacological actions of licorice and its active ingredients are similar to those of the natural mineralocorticoids of the adrenal cortex. A dose regimen that increased gradually from 1 to 4 gm./day over a 10-day period produced hypertension, weight increase, increase in serum sodium, decrease in serum potassium secondary to kaliuresis, and decreases in aldosterone excretion and plasma renin activity. Subjects who habitually eat large quantities of licorice candy (as little as 30-40 gm. per day) or who imbibe licorice-containing alcoholic beverages may present with some or all of the above, in addition to edema, bigeminy, extrasystoles, paresis, quadriplegia, tetany, myoglobinuria and convulsions. Withdrawal of the offending agent and potassium supplementation usually result in a rapid reversal of the signs and symptoms.

Ref.: Conn et al., 1968; Doolin, 1968; Gross et al., 1966; Cundiff, 1964; Storm, 1968.

849   Casanthranol

e.g., Peristim, Cantralax

Toxicity Rating: 3(?). The purified anthranol glycosides from cascara sagrada containing at least two active fractions, casanthranol A and B. Proprietary preparations are used as laxatives. Therapeutic dose on the order of l00 mg. See also Cascara sagrada in the index.

Ref.: Martindale, 1972.

850   Linamarin

2-(β-D-Glucopyranosyloxy)-2-methylpropanenitrile

Toxicity Rating: 4(?). A cyanogenic glycoside similar to amygdalin (above), found in the seeds, skins or embryos of flax. It evolves free cyanide when mixed with linseed meal but not with the β-glucosidase emulsin. Almost certainly linamarin causes cyanide poisoning in rats and probably also in man.

See also: Cyanide, Reference Congener in Section III.
Ref.: Philbrick et al., 1977.

851   Senna Glycosides

Sennoside A and B

Toxicity Rating: 4(?). Carthartic whose active glycosides (sennoside A and B) are of the anthraquinone type. Obtained from the dried leaflets of Cassia acutifolia or C. angustifolia. Other official preparations and their adult therapeutic doses include Senna Fluidextract (2 ml.) and Senna Syrup (8 ml.). Glysennid is a purified mixture of the calcium salts of sennosides A and B. Two-gram doses of Senna or 12-24 mg. of the purified glycosides usually produce evacuation in 6 to 10 hours. Systemic effects have not been described. Overdoses may produce purging, griping, blood in stools and abortion.

Ref.: Burrell, 1967; Osol and Farrar, 1955.

852   Tannic Acid

Tannin

Toxicity Rating: 3. Complex glucosidic polyester of gallic acid with a molecular weight of 1500 to 2000. Several chemical grades are commercially available. Found in many foods; humans may ingest as much as one gram per day. Erratically absorbed. Acute oral LD_{50} in rats about 2.3 gm./kg. with a mean time to death of 38 hours. Higher doses produce rapid demise in respiratory failure. Pathological findings included gastritis, hepatic necrosis (the usual cause of death) and nephritis. The distribution of hepatic lesions resembled that produced by Bromobenzene or by Thioacetamide; consult the index for information about these two compounds. Gallic acid does not produce liver damage, but may cause death from acute renal failure. Thus, hydrolysis of tannic acid may account for histological changes in the kidney. The astringent properties of tannic acid (due to coagulation of protein) have led to its topical use as solutions for the management of burns. Included in barium enemas in concentrations of 0.25 to 3% it improves the resolution of x-rays. In both of these uses tannic acid has resulted in human death from hepatic necrosis. Since its inclusion in barium enemas had been in vogue for many years without recognized liver damage, as yet ill-defined circumstances must play important roles: concentration of tannin, number of enemas, the retention time and the pathologic state of the colon. The reaction may be more common in children, but it is not unknown in adults.

See also: Carbon Tetrachloride, Reference Congener in Section III.
Ref.: Baker and Handler, 1943; Boyd, 1965; Cameron et al., 1943; Fiume, 1963; Hartman and Romence, 1943; Horvath et al., 1960; Lucke et al., 1963; McAlister et al., 1963; Robinson and Graessle, 1943.

Cellulose derivatives

853   Carboxymethylcellulose

Carboxymethocel S,   CMC

Toxicity Rating: 1. Usually dispensed as a water-soluble salt, e.g., Carboxymethocel S. A bulk cathartic, not absorbed from the bowel.

Ref.: Osol and Farrar, 1955.

854   Collodion

854

Pyroxylin

Toxicity Rating: 3(?). Four percent pyroxylin (chiefly nitrocellulose) in 70% ether and 24% absolute ethyl alcohol. This solvent mixture is the chief source of toxicity. See Ethyl ether in the index.

See also: Ethyl Alcohol, *Reference Congener in Section III*.
Ref.: Osol and Farrar, 1955.

855   Hydroxypropyl Methylcellulose

855

Methyl hydroxypropyl cellulose, e.g., Methocel X-2602, Methocel 60 HG

Toxicity Rating: 1. Propylene glycol ether of methyl cellulose. Similar in properties and uses to methyl cellulose, but differing in such physical properties as solubility and gelation temperature. See Methyl cellulose below.

856   Methyl Cellulose

856

e.g., Methocel

Toxicity Rating: 1. Biologically inert aside from mechanical actions. Not absorbed from the bowel. Used as an emulsifying agent, protective colloid, and bulk cathartic. Given parenterally, however, methyl cellulose produces glomerulonephritis and hypertension in rats. See also Polyvinylpyrrolidone in the index.

Ref.: Osol and Farrar, 1955; Hall and Hall, 1962.

Odorants and flavoring agents

857   Allyl Heptylate

857

Toxicity Rating: 4(?). A pineapple flavor. Acute oral LD_{50} in rats 500 mg./kg., in mice 630 mg./kg. Dogs fed 25 mg./kg. per day survived for 18 months without gross ill effects, but at 75 mg./kg. per day they died after 3 to 7 months with moderate hepatic fibrosis in the portal areas, proliferation of bile duct epithelium, diffuse focal hemorrhages and necrosis of gastric mucosa. Rats at dietary levels of 10,000 ppm for 18 weeks showed severe depression of growth, enlargement of kidneys and liver, hydropic degeneration of hepatic cells and growth of bile ducts.

Ref.: Hagan et al., 1965.

858   Anethole

858

Anise camphor, 1-Methoxy-4-propenylbenzene

Chief constituent of oil of anise. Toxicology largely unknown; intraperitoneal LD_{50}'s 70 mg./kg. in rats, 95 mg./kg. in mice. One ml. applied to mouse fur and skin produced coma in about 0.5 hr. and death in 2.5 hr. Fatty and parenchymatous degeneration of kidneys noted in animals. A case of stomatitis has been reported after use of a denture cream containing oil of anise (80-90% anethole). Applied to skin anethole causes erythema, scaling and vesiculation.

See also: Xylene *and* Phenol, *Reference Congeners in Section III*.
Ref.: Loveman, 1938; Macht, 1938; Merck and Co., 1976.

859   Benzaldehyde

859

Benzoic aldehyde, Essential oil of almond (artificial)

Toxicity Rating: 3. Subcutaneous lethal dose in rats is about 5 gm./kg., but oral fatal dose in man is estimated to be about 2 oz. Produces central nervous depression with respiratory failure. Epileptiform convulsions observed in rabbits.

Ref.: Macht, 1923.

860   Cinnamaldehyde

860

Cinnamic aldehyde, 3-Phenylpropenal, Phenylacrolein, Cinnamal

Toxicity Rating: 3(?). The chief ingredient (up to 90%) of oil of cinnamon. Both the oil and pure aldehyde are irritants; especially if undiluted, they cause inflammation and erosion of gastrointestinal mucosa. Systemic actions are probably few. Presumably oxidized in vivo to cinnamic acid, which is excreted in urine as benzoic and hippuric acids.

Ref.: Laubach et al., 1953; Powers et al., 1961.

861   Coumarin   861

Cumarin

Toxicity Rating: 4. Formerly important as a flavor and perfume in foods and pharmaceuticals. In male albino rats the acute oral LD_{50} is about 300 mg./ kg. in propylene glycol and about 500 mg./kg. in corn oil. Fatal doses quickly elicit narcosis. Prominent autopsy findings in acutely poisoned animals

Ref.: Hazleton et al., 1956.

included hyperemia of stomach and upper intestines. Prolonged feeding revealed a possible trend toward liver injury and so it is no longer used in foods. Antiprothrombin activity is not a prominent feature of coumarin toxicity.

862   Dihydrosafrole   862

1,2-Methylenedioxy-4-propylbenzene

Toxicity Rating: 3. Acute oral LD_{50}'s in mice 3.7 gm./kg., in rats 2.3 gm./kg. Given to rats as a 25% preparation in corn oil in a dose of 750 mg./kg. per day, it caused a 30% cumulative mortality in 26 days. In chronic feeding studies in rats at 10,000

Ref.: Hagan et al., 1965.

ppm the mortality at 75 wks. was 80%; at 5,000 ppm the mortality was 90% at 100 wks. At these levels benign and malignant esophageal tumors were noted, together with hepatic enlargement and moderate liver pathology. See also Safrole below.

863   Eucalyptol   863

Cajeputol, Cineol, Cineole, 1,8-Epoxy-*p*-menthane

Toxicity Rating: 4. Eucalyptol is the *dl* form. The major constituent of oil of eucalyptus and oil of cajeput. Eucalyptus oil is about 70% active eucalyptol. As little as 1 ml. has caused a transient coma. Fatalities have followed doses as small as 3.5 ml., and recovery has occurred after a dose of 20

See also: Camphor, *Reference Congener in Section III.*
Ref.: Craig, 1953; Taylor and Austin, 1918.

and even 30 ml. Symptoms include epigastric burning with nausea and usually vomiting, vertigo, ataxia, muscle weakness, stupor, pallor and sometimes cyanosis, respiratory stridor (edema), and miosis. Delirium and occasionally convulsions occur. Rarely symptoms may be delayed for 2 hrs.

864   Eugenol   864

Caryophyllic acid, 4-Allyl-2-methoxyphenol

Toxicity Rating: 3. Obtained from clove oil, which is about 80% eugenol. Acute oral LD_{50}'s 2.7 gm./ kg. in rats, 3.0 gm./kg. in mice, and 2.1 gm./kg. in guinea pigs. Possesses properties of local antisepsis and local anesthesia (used topically in control of toothache); also a rubifacient and irritant. Not corrosive like phenol but ingestion results in gastroenteritis. Systemic toxicity is similar to but less

See also: Phenol, *Reference Congener in Section III.*
Ref.: Hagan et al., 1965; Lauber and Hollander, 1950; Sober et al., 1950.

than that of phenol, perhaps because of its insolubility in water. Aqueous emulsions by mouth induce vomiting in man and dogs and promote gastric secretion of mucin. Poisoned rats exhibited paresis of hind legs and jaw with eventual prostration and coma. Death believed to be due to peripheral vascular collapse. Surviving rats showed hematuria.

865   Geraniol   865

Toxicity Rating: 3(?). One of 3 major alcohols found in rose oil (the others are citronellol and nerol). Also found in geranium oils, citronella, and others. Widely used in perfumes, soaps, and cos-

metics. No toxicity data were located, but the toxicity is probably low. See also Oil of citronella in the index.

866   3-Hydroxy-2-methyl-4-pyrone   866

Maltol

Toxicity Rating: 3. A flavoring agent which is added to some commercially processed foods in amounts of 200 to 250 parts per million. No ill effects occurred in rats fed this compound at die-

Ref.: Dow Chemical Co., 1953.

tary levels of 10,000 parts per million for 6 months. An estimated oral mean lethal dose in guinea pigs is 1.6 gm./kg.

867

867   Isosafrole

1,2-Methylenedioxy-4-propenylbenzene

Toxicity Rating: 3. Used in perfumery and in root beer and sarsaparilla flavors. Acute oral LD_{50} in rats 1.3 gm./kg. and in mice 2.5 gm./kg. Given to rats as a 25% preparation in corn oil in a dose of 500 mg./kg. per day, it caused an 80% cumulative

Ref.: Hagan et al., 1965.

mortality in 41 days. Rats fed 10,000 ppm survived less than 10 weeks, while at 5000 ppm a mortality of 56% was reached at the end of 100 weeks. Liver enlargement and moderate hepatic pathology were noted. See also Safrole below.

868

868   Menthol

Hexahydrothymol, 3-*p*-Menthanol

Toxicity Rating: 4. Obtained principally from oil of peppermint (about 50% menthol). Ingestion causes

severe abdominal pain, nausea, vomiting, vertigo, ataxia, drowsiness, and coma.

See also: Turpentine, *Reference Congener in Section III.*
Ref.: Wokes, 1932.

869

869   Menthyl Acetate

Used in perfumery. As an ester it is presumably hydrolyzed in the alimentary tract to menthol and

acetic acid. See Menthol above.

870

870   Methylenedioxybenzene

Toxicity Rating: 3. Chemically related to safrole. Acute oral LD_{50}'s 0.58 gm./kg. in rats and 1.22 gm./kg. in mice. After daily doses of 250 mg./kg. or 500 mg./kg. for 60 days, cumulative mortalities in mice

Ref.: Hagan et al., 1965.

were 73 and 81% respectively. Both central nervous system stimulation and depression were noted in these studies. Minimal liver effects were seen. See also Safrole below.

871

871   Piperonal

Heliotropin, 3,4-Methylenedioxybenzaldehyde

Toxicity Rating: 3. A constituent of vanilla and cherry flavors. Has been used as a pediculicide. Chemically related to safrole. Acute oral LD_{50} in

Ref.: Hagan et al., 1965.

rats 2.7 gm./kg. At 1000 and 10,000 ppm in the diet for 28 and 16 weeks respectively, no adverse effects were seen in rats. See also Safrole below.

872

872   Safrole

Safrol, 4-Allyl-1,2-methylenedioxybenzene

Toxicity Rating: 3. Once widely used in perfumes and as a flavoring agent but no longer allowed in foods in the U.S.A. Principal constituent of oil of sassafras (80% safrole), which has not been banned. As judged by clinical poisonings due to oil of sassafras, safrole is expected to induce vomiting, shock, cyanosis, delirium, and probably convulsions. The syndrome resembles that due to oil of eucalyptus (see Eucalyptol above), except that vomiting and circulatory collapse are more common and miosis and respiratory symptoms are less so. Acute oral LD_{50}'s in rats about 2.0 gm./kg. and in mice 2.4 gm./kg. Given to rats as a 25% preparation in corn oil in a dose of 750 mg./kg. per day, it caused a 90% cumulative mortality in 19 days. Produces more significant liver pathology in ani-

mals than isosafrole or dihydrosafrole although the same pattern has been described: hepatic cell enlargement, cystic necrosis, fatty infiltration and bile duct proliferation. Others report hepatic adenomas, testicular atrophy and bone marrow depletion in rats on deficient diets. Found to be a liver carcinogen when fed in high doses to rats and mice. Evidence exists for the transmission of carcinogenic effects in mice through the placenta and mother's milk. Carcinogenicity requires metabolic activation and bioaccumulation. Amounts of safrole usually encountered by man in food and beverages do not accumulate, and 1'-hydroxysafrole, the proximate carcinogen in mice, was not found in the urine of a human volunteer given oral doses of safrole.

See also: Phenol, *Reference Congener in Section III.*
Ref.: Benedetti et al., 1977; Hagan et al., 1965; Homburger et al., 1961; Taylor and Jones, 1961.

873 Vanillin   873

3-Methoxy-4-hydroxybenzaldehyde

Toxicity Rating: 3. Synthetic or derived from vanilla beans. Used as a flavoring agent in place of vanilla. In laboratory animals ingestion of a single toxic dose causes hyperpnea, muscular weakness, dyspnea, collapse, and death due to circulatory failure.

See also: Phenol, Reference Congener in Section III.
Ref.: Deichmann and Kitzmiller, 1940.

Terpenes and derivatives

874 Bornyl Chloride   874

Pinene hydrochloride, Chlorocamphane, "Turpentine camphor"

Toxicity Rating: 4(?). A synthetic substance resembling camphor, manufactured from turpentine.

See also: Camphor, Reference Congener in Section III.
Ref.: Osol and Farrar, 1955.

875 Camphor   875

2-Camphanone, Gum camphor

Toxicity Rating: 4. On the basis of clinical experience, man appears to be much more susceptible to camphor poisoning than other species. Toxicity rating in common laboratory animals is 2 or 3, whereas clinical data place it near the borderline between toxicity classes 4 and 5.

See also: Camphor, Reference Congener in Section III.

876 Borneol   876

Bornyl alcohol, 2-Camphanol

Toxicity Rating: 4. Toxicity is essentially indistinguishable from that of camphor. As with camphor, laboratory animals appear to be much less susceptible than man.

See also: Camphor, Reference Congener in Section III.

877 Limonene   877

Dipentene, Cinene

Toxicity Rating: 3(?). One of the terpene hydrocarbons found in turpentine. A major constituent in oils of orange, lemon, caraway, dill, bergamot, and pine needle. No toxic reactions have been described other than mild local irritation and skin sensitization, but albuminuria and hematuria are probable if ingested in sufficient quantity.

See also: Turpentine, Reference Congener in Section III.
Ref.: Hercules Powder Co., 1951.

878 Di-1-p-menthene   878

e.g., Pinolene

Organic film former used for control of pesticide residuals. A two subunit polymer of pinene, a major constituent of pine oil. Said to be non-toxic but no data were located. When deposited as a thin film on a surface, Pinolene slowly polymerizes over weeks and months to form longer chain polymers.

See also: Turpentine, Reference Congener in Section III.
Ref.: Svec, 1969.

879 α-Pinene   879

2-Pinene

Toxicity Rating: 3. The principal ingredient of turpentine, with essentially the same toxicity as turpentine.

See also: Turpentine, Reference Congener in Section III.
Ref.: Hercules Powder Co., 1951.

880 Terebene

880

Toxicity Rating: 3(?). Mixture of terpene hydrocarbons, chiefly dipentene, prepared from oil of turpentine. Used as a stimulant expectorant, and formerly for dyspepsia and for chronic urinary tract inflammation. Oral dose 0.12 to 0.5 ml. (or by inhalation). In excess it may produce albuminuria and hematuria.

See also: Turpentine, *Reference Congener in Section III.*

881 Terpenes

881

e.g., Pinene

Toxicity Rating: 3. The cyclic hydrocarbons contained in volatile oils are usually designated as terpenes (from turpentine oil).

See also: Turpentine, *Reference Congener in Section III.*
Ref.: Hercules Powder Co., 1951.

882 Terpineol

882

p-Menth-1-en-8-ol

Toxicity Rating: 3. The principal constituents of pine oil (about 75% terpineols). As judged by pine oil, terpineols are irritating to eyes and mucous membranes. Produce hemorrhagic gastritis when ingested. Systemic effects include weakness and central nervous depression, with hypothermia and respiratory failure. Acute renal failure followed an abortion induced by the vaginal instillation of 3-6 oz. of a mixture of water and a commercial preparation of steam-distilled pine oil (70%) and neutral soap (12-14%), but the role of terpineol in the genesis of the renal lesion is not known.

See also: Turpentine, *Reference Congener in Section III.*
Ref.: Hercules Powder Co., 1951; Gornel and Goldman, 1968.

883 Terpin Hydrate

883

cis-Dipenteneglycol hydrate

Toxicity Rating: 3. An expectorant said to lessen abundant sputum. Chemically related to the terpenes and terpineols. Said to be more pleasant, less irritant, and less toxic than turpentine (including the rectified oil), but no evidence was located to show that the lethal dose is greater than that of turpentine.

See also: Turpentine, *Reference Congener in Section III.*
Ref.: Osol and Farrar, 1955.

Constituents of pyrethrum and of derris and their derivatives

884 Allethrin

884

Allyl cinerin, Pallethrine

Toxicity Rating: 3. The synthetic allyl homolog of cinerin I, the latter being one of the active insecticidal ingredients of pyrethrum. Allethrin is a racemic mixture of eight isomers having a combined oral LD_{50} in the rat of 700 to 960 mg./kg. A mixture containing only the *d-trans* isomers of allethrin, termed bioallethrin, is twice as effective against flying insects and has a slightly lower oral mammalian toxicity (rat LD_{50} 1.0 gm./kg.). Both mixtures are much more toxic when given i.v. (rat LD_{50} for bioallethrin is 4 mg./kg.). Allethrin is not absorbed through the skin. Symptoms of allethrin and bioallethrin intoxication are like those from the natural pyrethrins, although reactions to oral doses of bioallethrin may be more rapid than to similar doses of other natural and synthetic pyrethrins. Allethrin and bioallethrin are supplied mainly in oil- and water-based aerosols and sprays for use in the home and restaurants against flies and mosquitoes. These are often formulated with a synergist such as piperonyl butoxide or MGK 264 (see in index).

See also: Pyrethrum, *Reference Congener in Section III.*
Ref.: Hayes, 1963; Verschoyle and Barnes, 1972.

885 Barthrin

885

6-Chloropiperonylchrysanthemumate,   ENT-21557

Toxicity Rating: 1. A synthetic pyrethrin-like insecticide of very low mammalian toxicity. Rats given a single oral dose of 20 ml./kg. of the pure oil showed no toxic symptoms. Daily doses of 10 ml./kg. per day for 3 weeks were also without effect. Rats fed 1.2 gm./kg. per day for 52 weeks showed an abnormal incidence of focal lesions within the kidney parenchyma. The substance shows no acute percutaneous toxicity, being neither an allergen nor an irritant in tests on humans. Barthrin has not been registered in the U.S.A.

See also: Pyrethrum, *Reference Congener in Section III.*
Ref.: Ambrose, 1963.

886 Cyclethrin   886

dl-2-Cyclopentenyl-4-hydroxy-3-methyl-2-cyclopenten-1-one chrysanthemate, Pypyrethrin

Toxicity Rating: 3. A synthetic cyclopentenyl analogue of allethrin. It was once used as an insecticide in aerosol and dairy sprays but is currently not produced. Its mammalian toxicity is similar to that of naturally occurring pyrethrins (rat oral LD_{50} 1.4 gm./kg.).

See also: Pyrethrum, *Reference Congener in Section III.*
Ref.: Carpenter et al., 1954; U.S. Department of Agriculture, 1966.

887 Dehydrorotenone   887

A dehydrogenated product of rotenone which is said to be much less toxic than the parent compound.

See also: Rotenone, *Reference Congener in Section III.*

888 Dihydrorotenone   888

Toxicity Rating: 4. Said to have over twice the mammalian toxicity of rotenone.

See also: Rotenone, *Reference Congener in Section III.*
Ref.: Lehman, 1951.

889 Dimethrin   889

2,4-Dimethylbenzylchrysanthemumate, ENT-21170, Dimethrine

Toxicity Rating: 1. A synthetic pyrethroid insecticide of very low oral mammalian toxicity. Because it is not readily absorbed through the skin, it can be used for control of human body lice and stable flies. The oral LD_{50} is >15 gm./kg. in rats and rabbits. Rats given 10 ml. of the pure oil 5 days per week for 3 weeks showed no signs of toxicity.

See also: Pyrethrum, *Reference Congener in Section III.*
Ref.: Ambrose, 1964.

890 Fenvalerate   890

Cyano(3-phenoxyphenyl)methyl 4-chloro-alpha-(1-methylethyl)benzeneacetate, Pydrin

Toxicity Rating: 3. A broad-spectrum insecticide for use on cotton and fruit. Said to be of the synthetic pyrethroid class but rather different chemically from pyrethrins and most other pyrethroids. Technical Pydrin, when suspended in water, has an acute oral LD_{50} in rats of 3200 mg./kg. When mixed with DMSO, it is more toxic (LD_{50} 451 mg./kg.), presumably because of better absorption from the gut. An emulsifiable concentrate, marketed as Pydrin 2.4 EC Insecticide, is comprised of 32% technical Pydrin and 68% aromatic hydrocarbon solvents and emulsifiers; its acute oral LD_{50} in rats is 1250 mg./kg. Poorly absorbed through intact rabbit skin. Exposure to fenvalerate is likely to cause central nervous system stimulation with symptoms of nervousness, anxiety, salivation, tremors and convulsions. Nerve damage was observed in rats given high doses. Fenvalerate as technical Pydrin is mildly irritating to the skin, but the emulsifiable concentrate is corrosive. Hydrogen cyanide may be formed during thermal decomposition.

See also: Pyrethrum, *Reference Congener in Section III.*
Ref.: Shell Oil Co., 1980.

891 Permethrin   891

3-Phenoxybenzyl-3-(2,2-dichlorovinyl)-2,2-dimethylcyclopropanecarboxylate, NRDC 143

Toxicity Rating: 3. Permethrin and phenothrin are semi-synthetic mixtures of insecticidal isomers closely related to pyrethrin. They are more stable to photolysis than other pyrethroids, hence longer acting in the field. Both have moderately low mammalian toxicities. For permethrin, the rat oral LD_{50} is 1.3 gm./kg. In feeding experiments in dogs, the 90-day no-effect level was 200 ppm. Permethrin may be weakly oncogenic in mice and rats. The acute oral LD_{50} of phenothrin is said to be greater than 10 gm./kg. in rats: no other toxicity data were found. Both compounds are supplied as mixtures of *cis* and *trans* isomers. They are rapidly absorbed when ingested and metabolized in the liver by hydrolysis of the ester linkage. The *trans*-isomers (designated bio-) are hydrolyzed more readily and have a significantly lower toxicity in rats than do the corresponding *cis*-isomers. The metabolites are primarily 3-phenoxybenzyl alcohol and its oxida- tion products, which are rapidly excreted in urine. The other hydrolysis products are dimethyl or dichlorovinyl acids, which are partially hydroxyl- ated and rapidly excreted. In radiolabel experi- ments, no accumulation of the parent compounds or of their metabolites was observed.

See also: Pyrethrum, *Reference Congener in Section III.*
Ref.: Elliott et al., 1976; EPA, April 25, 1979; Worthing, 1979.

892　Pyrenone

Various combinations of pyrethrins and piperonyl butoxide, used as insecticides.
See also: Pyrethrum, *Reference Congener in Section III.*

893　Pyrethrins

Toxicity Rating: 3 or 4. A group of six closely related naturally occurring compounds including pyrethrin I and II, cinerin I and II and jasmolin I and II, which are the active insecticidal compo- nents of pyrethrum. Pyrethrin I is the pyrethrolone ester of chrysanthemum monocarboxylic acid (sometimes called chrysanthemic or chrysanthe- mumic acid). The others are similar esters. Pyreth- rin II is less toxic than pyrethrin I.

See also: Pyrethrum, *Reference Congener in Section III.*

894　Pyrethroids

Toxicity Rating: 1-3. Semisynthetic derivatives of natural pyrethrins used in insecticidal mixtures. Most (if not all) are esters of chrysanthemic mono- or dicarboxylic acid. In general they are less toxic to laboratory mammals than are the natural pyr- ethrins. Examples include Allethrin, Barthrin, Cy- clethrin and Dimethrin above.

See also: Pyrethrum, *Reference Congener in Section III.*

895　Resmethrin

e.g., Synthrin, Chryson, Bioresmethrin, Cismethrin

Toxicity Rating: 3. A semi-synthetic mixture of pyrethroid isomers closely related to the natural pyrethrins. Used to control insects in homes and greenhouses. The usual mixture has a low acute oral toxicity in mammals (rat oral LD_{50} 1.5 to 4.2 gm./kg.). The *cis*-component (Cismethrin; NRDC 119) has a much higher acute toxicity (oral LD_{50} 90 to 170 mg./kg.), whereas the *trans*-component (Bioresmethrin; NRDC 107) is virtually non-toxic to rats when administered orally (LD_{50} >8 gm./ kg.). The native mixture contains about 70% *trans*- component. Resmethrin has a low dermal toxicity (rat LD_{50} 3.0 gm./kg.). The intravenous toxicity of the mixture is much greater than the oral toxicity (rat i.v. LD_{50} 7 mg./kg. for the *cis*-isomer and 340 mg./kg. for the *trans*-isomer). Toxic symptoms of resmethrin are like those of the other pyrethrins and include immediate irritability, tremors, coma and death. With bioresmethrin alone these symp- toms may be delayed. Resmethrin is supplied in a water- or oil-based syrup, often in combination with Tetramethrin (see below).

See also: Pyrethrum, *Reference Congener in Section III.*
Ref.: Verschoyle and Barnes, 1972.

896　Rotenone

Toxicity Rating: 4. Constituent of derris root.
See also: Rotenone, *Reference Congener in Section III.*

897　Rotenoids

Toxicity Rating: 4. Insecticidal alkaloids related to rotenone and, like rotenone, constituents of derris and cubé. Specific examples are deguelin, toxicarol, tephrosin and sumatrol. Most, if not all of these compounds, are less toxic to mammals than is rotenone itself.

See also: Rotenone, *Reference Congener in Section III.*

898　Tetramethrin

Neo-Pynamin, Neopynamin

Toxicity Rating: 2 or 3. A semi-synthetic pyreth- roid which is commonly supplied in combination with piperonyl butoxide or resmethrin in oil- or water-based sprays designed to control household insects. The substance has a low acute mammalian toxicity (rat oral LD_{50} >20 gm./kg.). Rats fed up to 2000 ppm in food for 3 months showed no toxic symptoms.

See also: Pyrethrum, *Reference Congener in Section III.*
Ref.: Spencer, 1973.

Antibiotics

899 Antibiotics 899

If not listed by name below, see Section IV under Miscellaneous (Infections) for a summary of the clinical toxicities of commonly used antibiotics, with emphasis on untoward reactions seen after therapeutic doses.

900 Griseofulvin 900

Fulvicin

Toxicity Rating: 3(?). Fungistatic drug derived from several penicillium strains. Used also in agriculture for control of fungal diseases of tomatoes, mushrooms and other crops. Finds medical use as a systemic antifungal in the control of superficial infection of the skin. Minor side effects after oral doses include headache, epigastric distress, nausea and diarrhea. Other untoward reactions include arthralgia, peripheral neuritis, fever, syncope, blurred vision, and proteinuria. Griseofulvin is poorly absorbed from gut but uptake is facilitated by fats and oils. Recommended adult dosage is 1 gm. daily in divided doses. In a few patients, doses of 2 gm./day have produced mental confusion. Leukopenia has also been described; it vanished promptly on cessation of therapy. Severe generalized angioneurotic edema and persistent urticaria have occurred in one subject. Griseofulvin decreases the activity of warfarin-type anticoagulants. Its efficacy is diminished by barbiturates.

The oral LD_{50} in laboratory rodents is large (more than 10 gm./kg.), probably because of poor absorption, but this may not be true of the microcrystalline preparations now used clinically. Interference with porphyrin metabolism has been reported. Rats fed 1% griseofulvin for 82 days showed extensive liver cell necrosis with bile stasis, pigmentation of Kupffer cells, extensive cellular proliferation in necrotic areas and elevation of liver transaminase. Pregnant rats given 0.5 to 1.5 gm./kg. in food daily for 10 days produced pups with a moderate to high incidence of skeletal defects and a greatly reduced survival rate. Both teratogenic effects were dose dependent. Although similar oral doses did not diminish the fertility of male dogs, male rats given 2 gm./kg. i.p. for four days showed severe damage to the intestinal and seminal epithelia. Evidence of inhibition of mitotic activity in bone marrow and intestine were also seen.

Ref.: Barich et al., 1961; Council on Drugs, 1960; Goldblatt, 1960; Klein and Beall, 1972; Paget and Walpole, 1958.

901 Neomycin 901

Toxicity Rating: 3. A broad-spectrum aminoglycoside antibiotic complex produced by a strain of *Streptomyces fradiae*. Commercial preparations now consist largely of neomycin B, one of 3 related aminoglycosides. Administered orally in the management of hepatic coma and as a pre-surgical intestinal antiseptic, parenterally in the treatment of severe and life-threatening infections. Because of systemic toxicity (see below), the parenteral use of neomycin has largely been abandoned. Acute oral LD_{50} is 2.75 gm./kg. in rats. Sensorineural deafness, respiratory depression and kidney failure have been reported following parenteral injection, pleural instillation, rectal irrigation, aerosol inhalation and oral administration. Dose-dependent cardiovascular depression has been observed in monkeys after i.v. administration. A 39-year-old woman who received a 2 gm. oral dose of neomycin sulfate and accidentally an additional 6 grams intramuscularly suffered anuria, decreased auditory acuity and azotemia. One month after hemodialysis she continued to have residual deafness. Although only 3% of an oral dose is absorbed from the gut and subsequently excreted in the urine, patients with renal insufficiency readily accumulate blood levels equivalent to the ototoxic parenteral dose (7-8 gm.) in normal patients. Neomycin acts as a nondepolarizing neuromuscular blocker, and its effect is additive with that of depolarizing blockers such as succinylcholine. Prolonged apnea (lasting 4 hours) has resulted from the use of neomycin as an intraperitoneal antiseptic in surgical patients receiving succinylcholine. Parenteral neomycin sulfate in conjunction with ether anesthesia has been implicated in the deaths of two patients. Calcium salts proved to be effective antagonists of neomycin neuromuscular blocking action in test animals. When the drug is given regularly by the oral route in doses of 3-4 gm. daily, the most important untoward reactions are intestinal malabsorption and suprainfection with yeast and other resistant microorganisms. Malabsorption is due to the precipitation of bile acids and inhibition of various intestinal enzymes. A spruelike syndrome with diarrhea and steatorrhea may result. The chief hazard with topical use is hypersensitivity reactions, usually a skin rash.

Ref.: Adams, 1975; Crawford and Teske, 1978; Foldes et al., 1963a; Krumlovsky et al., 1972; Lee et al., 1976; Pittinger et al., 1970.

902

902 Penicillins

e.g., Penicillin G, Penicillin V, Methicillin, Oxacillin, Nafcillin, Ampicillin, Carbenicillin, Phenethicillin

Data in mice, rats, rabbits, cats and dogs suggest that penicillin G lies on the borderline between toxicity classes 2 and 3 . Death from respiratory failure with or without convulsions occurred 6 to 18 hours after single oral doses. Acute gastroenteritis and cardiovascular shock were associated phenomena. This pattern was also true for guinea pigs except that a late (1 to 2 weeks) and gradually developing toxemia killed all survivors of the acute response. The 14-day LD_{50} in guinea pigs is 0.3 gm./kg., whereas the 2-day LD_{50} is on the order of 5 gm./kg. In hamsters the drug is somewhat more toxic by the oral than by the subcutaneous route when observed for 14 days after single doses. Tolerance developed to multiple dosing. Perhaps the sensitivity of guinea pigs is related to effects on intestinal microflora. The subcutaneous LD_{50} in

newborn (<72 hr.) rats was 7-fold lower than the LD_{50} in adults. Massive intravenous doses in man (20 to 60 million units/day, equivalent to approximately 12 to 36 gm.) may result in an encephalopathy with muscular hyperirritability, myoclonus, visual and auditory hallucinations and generalized convulsions. Some of these signs can be elicited in rats and cats with doses to 3 to 4 million units/kg., and the syndrome can be reversed by penicillinase. Hyperkalemia and arrhythmias may follow massive intravenous administration of potassium salts of penicillins. Allergic reactions are far more common than frank toxicity. Anaphylactic shock is rare, but can follow a one-microgram test dose. It is best managed by epinephrine. Accelerated (1 to 72 hours) and late urticarial reactions are much more common.

Ref.: Boyd and Fulford, 1961; DeSalva et al., 1969; Medical Letter, 1972; Michael and Sutherland, 1961; Raichle et al., 1971.

903

903 Polymixin

Polymixin A, Polymixin B, Polymixin C, Polymixin D, Polymixin E, Colistin, Colistimethate sodium, Colistin sulfate

The polymixins A, B, C, D, E and Colistin form a group of closely related antibiotic substances produced by various strains of *Bacillus polymyxa*. Polymixin B and Colistin (a mixture containing E) are available for clinical use (other polymixins are nephrotoxic). The polymixins are simple basic polypeptides (MW about 1000) used against gram-negative infections, especially pseudomonas, but excluding proteus species. Polymixin B is a surface-active agent containing lipophilic and lipophobic groups separated within the molecule. It is thought to destroy the molecular organization of bacterial cell membranes, and so allow the contents to escape. Poorly absorbed from the gastrointestinal tract (except in newborns), from other mucous membranes and from the surface of burns. The usual parenteral dose is 2-4 mg./kg. daily in 4 divided doses (usually i.v. or i.m.). The intravenous LD_{50} in mice is 6 mg./kg. High blood serum concentrations (in excess of 1 or 2 μgm./ml.) may cause neurotoxic effects. Principal among these are flush-

ing and dizziness, progressing to ataxia and drowsiness. Peripheral sensory disturbances, especially parasthesias of the extremities, may also occur; they disappear without sequelae after the drug is completely excreted. Parenteral doses of 2.5 mg./kg. or more may lead to proteinuria, cylindruria, hematuria and decreases in renal function. Fever and skin rash have been described. Allergic sensitization is unusual. Muscular weakness and respiratory paralysis occur rarely. They have been ascribed to abnormally low serum concentrations of ionized calcium, and injections of calcium gluconate have been helpful. In mice, apnea and convulsions produced by lethal doses of Polymixin B have been prevented by prior or subsequent injections of polyglucose sulfate and heparin sulfate. Colistimethate sodium is the salt of the sulfomethyl derivative of Colistin. It is not irritating when injected i.m. and hence is preferred over Polymixin B for this purpose.

Ref.: A.M.A. Department of Drugs., 1977; Jawetz, 1961; Mora et al., 1959.

904

904 Tetracyclines

e.g., Chlortetracycline, Demethylchlortetracycline, Doxycycline, Methacycline, Oxytetracycline, Rolitetracycline, Tetracycline, Terramycin

Toxicity Rating: 2 to 3. The broad spectrum tetracyclines appear to be less acutely toxic than antibiotics effective primarily against gram-positive bacteria. Both the acute oral and subcutaneous LD_{50}'s of tetracycline hydrochloride in hamsters over a 14-day observation period were in excess of 400 mg./kg. Rats given that dose intraperitoneally, however, developed a potentially lethal metabolic acidosis. The accompanying hyperkalemia resulted in dangerous cardiac arrhythmias. Peritoneal dialysis effectively lowered blood tetracycline levels in a poisoned infant. The most common side effects after oral administration are related to the gas-

trointestinal tract. Allergic reactions are relatively rare. Human intravenous doses on the order of 1 to 4 gm./day for 1 to 9 days may provoke an acute fatty liver. The incidence of this reaction appears to be much higher in pregnant women especially in those with renal injuries. Icterus may be noted clinically and at autopsy a large fatty liver in which fat droplets are finely dispersed in cells throughout the lobule. The mechanism of this reaction may be related in some way to the heavy metal chelating activity of tetracyclines. These drugs have been associated with at least three kinds of renal disease: acute non-oliguric renal failure in patients with pancreatitis or fatty liver, uremia in patients with previously impaired renal function, and a Fanconi-like syndrome commonly associated with outdated or degraded tetracyclines. Photosensitivity has been reported after demethylchlortetracycline and chlortetracycline. Several if not all tetracyclines tend to be deposited in bones and teeth at sites of active calcification. The long-term consequences of such deposition are not clear, but skeletal growth may be impeded.

Ref.: Davis and Kaufman, 1966; DeSalva et al., 1969; deVeber, 1962; Greenberger et al., 1967; Lew and French, 1966; Morton, 1966.

905   Tyrothricin   905

Toxicity Rating: 3(?). An antibiotic mixture of gramicidin (most active) and tyrocidine (80%) used topically against gram-positive micro-organisms. Ineffective by mouth and too toxic to be given parenterally. The toxicity rating suggested above refers to oral doses in mammals (1000 mg./kg. has been tolerated), but data on mice and rats indicate ratings of 5 and 6 by the intraperitoneal and intravenous routes respectively. Death apparently re-sults from respiratory failure. Lethal doses in dogs caused anemia, hypotension, and a fall in body temperature. Ascites, fatty degeneration of the liver and severe renal damage have occurred. Olfactory disturbances are described after its topical use as nose drops, and chemical meningitis has resulted from the irrigation of the paranasal sinuses in two patients.

Ref.: Otenasek and Fairman, 1948; Spector, 1957.

906   Cycloheximide   906

Actidione

Toxicity Rating: 5. An antibiotic fungicide of high toxicity, used in agriculture. The oral LD_{50} in monkeys and dogs is about 500 mg./kg., but LD_{50}'s vary widely among species, and that for rats is only 2 mg./kg. In all three species, toxic symptoms include excessive salivation and diarrhea. Blood-stained feces may arise from vascular lesions of the colon (monkey) or stomach and small intestines (dogs). Rat and dog show transient central nervous system excitement with tremors and in the dog perhaps meningeal irritation. Death is due to cardiovascular collapse and is preceded by coma in all species. Autopsies on rats revealed enlarged adrenals, stomach hemorrhage, liver congestion and kidney damage. Atropine, hexamethonium and sympathomimetic drugs like methoxyphenamine reduced or eliminated many symptoms in poisoned rats, but death was not prevented unless hydrocortisone or adrenal cortical extracts were also employed. Pretreatment for several days with "catatoxic" steroids such as spironolactone protected rats against the toxic effects, presumably by inducing microsomal enzyme activity. Cycloheximide is a potent inhibitor of protein synthesis in fungi and animals. It causes an increase in adrenal RNA, increased production of glucocorticoids (antagonized by hydrocortisone), and decrease in pyruvate utilization in isolated adipose tissue. Reported to be teratogenic in rats.

Ref.: Fiala and Fiala, 1965; Greig and Gibbons, 1959; Jomain-Baum and Hanson, 1975; Selye, 1970; Shepard, 1976.

Vitamins

907   Vitamin A   907

Retinol

In fish liver oils vitamin A is mostly esterified with fatty acids. A single USP or International Unit of crystalline vitamin A (actually A_1) weighs about 0.3 micrograms. Because a related substance vitamin A_2 or dehydroretinol is 60 percent less active, a single unit weighs about 0.8 micrograms. Hypervitaminosis A occurs both in young children and adults receiving more than 100,000 units daily over several months. In one adult 50,000 units/day for 18 months produced symptoms. Signs and symptoms in poisoned adults include fatigue, anorexia, bone pain, spotty alopecia, skin lesions including pigmentation and hepatomegaly. Infants may present with some of the above in addition to vomiting, increased intracranial pressure, bulging fontanels, hemorrhagic diathesis (hypoprothrombinemia) and decalcification of bones with arrest or retardation of growth. Acute poisoning is said to have occurred in man after ingestion of polar bear liver (180,000 units/gm.) with symptoms referable primarily to the central nervous system: lethargy, drowsiness, "narcolepsy", irritability, vomiting, severe headache, and a generalized peeling of the skin after 24 hours. No specific therapeutic measures are indicated, but vitamin K may be useful for bleeding if hypoprothrombinemia exists. The illness can be distinguished from hypervitaminosis D by high serum levels of vitamin A and a normal serum calcium. On withdrawal of vitamin A, derangements return spontaneously to normal within days to weeks.

Ref.: Morrice et al., 1960; Pease, 1962; Raaschou-Nielsen, 1961; Rodahl and Moore, 1943; Stimson, 1961; Woodard et al., 1961.

908

908　Vitamin C

L-Ascorbic acid, Cevitamic acid

Toxicity Rating: 1(?). Human poisonings are unknown and even reliable estimates of the lethal dose in animals are rare. Humans have consumed 40 gm./day for a month or 100 gm./day for a few days without obvious symptoms. Doses on the order of several grams on an empty stomach may provoke gastric distress and diarrhea. The therapeutic dose by mouth for deficiency states (scurvey) ranges up to 1 gm./day. Mice given 1 gm./kg. intraperitoneally each day for 3 days showed a 10-15% decrease in plasma bicarbonate and a 5-8% decrease in chloride with no change in sodium or potassium, suggesting a mild non-respiratory acidosis. Prolonged (36-48 hr.) incubations of human red cells at ascorbate concentrations 50-100 times higher than normal blood levels resulted in a decreased oxygen capacity secondary to hemoglobin denaturation.

Ref.: Bolyai et al, 1972; Langgard, 1964; Pauling, 1970.

909

909　Vitamin D

Two chemical substances are the major constituents of vitamin D preparation: D_2 or calciferol and D_3 or activated 7-dehydrocholesterol. The latter occurs in animal tissues. These two substances have about the same antirachitic activity in man, and no toxicological distinctions between them are recognized. Considerable variation appears to exist in Vitamin D tolerance. As little as 50,000 units/day produces toxicity in some patients within one month, whereas others may tolerate several hundred thousand units for prolonged periods. Hypercalcemia is said to be a constant finding in the presence of toxic symptoms. Initial symptoms usually include anorexia, nausea and vomiting, but the subsequent course often mimics hyperparathyroidism with polyuria and polydipsia, muscular weakness, nervousness and itching, Metastatic calcification in the kidneys may produce renal impairment and hypertension, whereas calcification of cerebral arteries may result in cerebellar ataxia and other dysfunctions. Withdrawal of vitamin D and low calcium diets relieve most symptoms, but kidney damage may be irreversible. Cortisone is said to alleviate the hypercalcemia, and in one case magnesium sulfate produced a dramatic fall in serum calcium and an increase in urinary calcium excretion.

Ref.: Bauer and Freyberg, 1946; Lynch et al., 1964; Skanse et al., 1959; Spaulding and Yendt, 1964; Way et al., 1958.

910

910　Vitamin E

α-Tocopherol

Toxicity Rating: 1(?). A powerful antioxidant whose role in human nutrition has not been established. Popularly believed to promote fertility. Some adults given repeated doses of 2 to 3 grams per day, in an attempt to reduce angina pectoris, developed skin rashes and mild gastrointestinal irritation with diarrhea, but 1 gram daily was consumed for months without untoward effects. Mice tolerated 50 gm./kg. per day for 2 months. No other evidence of mammalian toxicity was found. Man's dietary intake is 10 to 80 mg. daily.

Ref.: Anderson, 1974; Horwitt, 1967.

911

911　Nicotinic Acid

Niacin, Sodium nicotinate

Toxicity Rating: 3(?). One of the B vitamins specific for human pellegra, but used therapeutically for deficiency states in the form of nicotinic acid amide (nicotinamide, niacinamide) because of the unpleasant side effects of the free acid. In man 100 mg. of nicotinic acid by mouth or 10 mg. intravenously produces a transient flushing, itching and burning of the skin of the face and upper trunk without significant changes in blood pressure, pulse rate, respiration or body temperature. The reaction is alarming but usually brief and without sequelae. Although the therapeutic index of this vitamin is enormous, elevation of serum bilirubin and frank jaundice have followed large doses in man; there are several reports of severe anaphylactic reactions. One investigator reports bloody feces, convulsions and fatty metamorphosis of the liver in dogs fed 2 gm. per day for about 2 weeks; this report was not confirmed in a subsequent study. Mixtures of nicotinic acid salts and esters with ascorbate are marketed for use in meat products to preserve the bright red color; they act by apparently stabilizing heme pigments in the ferrous or red form. Several incidents of food "poisoning" from the overzealous use of these products have occurred. No serious intoxications have been reported, and no therapy is generally required even for the severe cutaneous reactions. These substances bear no pharmacological relationship to nicotine.

Ref.: Chen et al., 1938; Lyman et al., 1957; Pelner, 1947; Press and Yeager, 1962; Rivin, 1959; Unna, 1939.

912 Pyridoxine Hydrochloride 912

5-Hydroxy-6-methyl-3,4-pyridine dimethanol hydrochloride, Pyridoxol hydrochloride, Hexabione, Vitamin B_6

Toxicity Rating: 3. Pyridoxine, pyridoxal and pyridoxamine are related compounds that possess Vitamin B_6 activity. All are readily absorbed in the gastrointestinal tract and converted to pyridoxal phosphate. Excess quantities of the vitamin are rapidly excreted in the urine. The free bases and the hydrochlorides have similar toxicities. Doses of 1 gm./kg. were tolerated by rats with no ill effects, whereas oral or subcutaneous doses of 3 to 4 gm./kg. produced tonic convulsions with death in 36 to 72 hours. Autopsy showed cerebral cortical hemorrhage and enlargement of the adrenal glands. Intravenous injections of 650 mg./kg. caused immediate tonic and clonic convulsions in rats with either complete recovery or death in 5 minutes. Dilute solutions of the drug (120 ppm) caused brief inhibition of isolated rabbit intestinal motility. Adult humans have received intravenous doses of 5 gm. over 3 to 5 minutes without ill effects.

Ref.: Wiegand et al., 1940; Unna and Antopol, 1940.

913 Riboflavin 913

6,7-Dimethyl-9-*D*-ribitylisoalloxazine, Vitamin B_2, Vitamin G, Lactoflavin

Toxicity Rating: 2. Riboflavin is a sparingly soluble compound, poorly absorbed when presented orally in very large doses. The therapeutic dose is 2 to 10 mg./day. Rats fed 10 gm./kg. in aqueous suspension showed no ill effects, and rats fed 10 mg. daily showed no long-term toxicity. An oral dose of 5 gm./kg. was tolerated by 3 dogs without evidence of toxicity, with less than 1% of the administered dose appearing in the urine, indicating very poor absorption of the vitamin. The compound is absorbed slowly from subcutaneous and rapidly from intraperitoneal sites of injection. Rats injected with 560 mg./kg. intraperitoneally became listless, refused food, and showed anuria for 1 to 2 days, followed by the passage of small amounts of bright yellow urine. Death occurred in 2 to 5 days. Autopsy showed yellow crystals in the collecting tubules and pelvis of the kidneys. Urea and creatinine levels increased 3 to 10 fold in afflicted animals. Forced water intake shortened the period of anuria but did not retard concretion formation or death.

Ref.: Unna and Greslin, 1942.

914 Thiamine 914

Vitamin B_1

Toxicity Rating: 2. Water-soluble B complex vitamin. Occurs in wheat germ, whole grains, enriched breads and cereals, pork and organ meat. Recommended Daily Allowance is set at 0.5 mg./1000 kcal. In humans treated for thiamine deficiency parenteral injection of 1000 times that amount has occasionally caused anaphylactoid reactions attributed to hypersensitivity. The reactions of "thiamine shock" have ranged in severity from weakness, burning and nausea to gastrointestinal hemorrhage, pulmonary edema, collapse and sudden death. Depression of the respiratory center was the cause of death in dogs with blood thiamine levels of 7-10 mg.%. At normal physiological levels thiamine acts as a coenzyme in carbohydrate metabolism. Has been used as a neuromuscular and synaptic blocking agent.

Ref.: Reingold and Webb, 1946.

Hormones

915 Corticosteroids 915

The hormones of the adrenal cortex are classified as glucocorticoids (hydrocortisone, corticosterone) or mineralocorticoids (e.g., aldosterone, desoxycorticosterone), depending on whether the major effects are manifested on carbohydrate-protein metabolism or salt-water metabolism. Large doses of corticosteroids administered over prolonged periods of time produce intoxications which represent extensions of their therapeutic effects. Thus, both types of corticoids promote sodium retention, edema, hypokalemia and congestive heart failure. Relative to their potency as antiinflammatory agents, some synthetic glucocorticoids are much less active than others in promoting sodium retention, notably prednisone, prednisolone, methylprednisolone, triamcinalone, dexamethasone, etc. The glucocorticoids also induce a cushingoid syndrome, osteoporosis, suppression of the immune response mechanism, impairment of glucose tolerance, and euphoria, habituation, and the unmasking of latent psychiatric disorders. An acute (single dose) poisoning in man does not appear to have ever been described. Large single doses of some steroids given parenterally to animals produce sedation, whereas others induce signs of central stimulation. To some extent these phenomena may be dose-related. Thus behavioral sedation occurred in monkeys at lower doses than seizure activity (100-

200 mg./kg. of 11-deoxy-17-hydrocorticosterone). Single doses of glucocorticoids (0.5 to 8.0 gm./kg.) can suppress the immune response in mice to the extent that high mortality occurs as a result of intercurrent infections over 1 to 3 wks. Rats are 10 to 20 times more sensitive than mice to this effect. Humans ingesting massive doses of corticoids should receive symptomatic and supportive care. Vigorous therapy with broad spectrum antibiotics is indicated if infection occurs.

Ref.: Figdor et al., 1956; Good et al., 1957; Heuser et al., 1965; McCawley, 1965; Robinson, 1956; Tonelli, 1966.

916 Estrogens (Natural and Synthetic)

Toxicity Rating: 3(?). The natural and semisynthetic steroidal estrogens include estrone, estradiol, estriol, equilin and ethinyl estradiol. Synthetic nonsteroidal estrogens include diethylstilbestrol, mestranol (widely used in the progestin-estrogen combination type of oral contraceptive), chlorotrianisene, benzestrol, hexestrol, dienestrol, methallenestril, etc. Although little information appears to be available, these compounds must have a very low single dose toxicity. Side effects noted after clinical administration were headache, nausea, vomiting and sometimes vaginal bleeding. Prominent gynecomastia and other feminizing effects were produced in males occupationally exposed to estrogens. Enough material can be absorbed percutaneously or by the respiratory route to produce these effects. Breast enlargement and nodularity occurred in both male and female children after consumption of vitamin capsules contaminated with estrogens. Changes in secondary sexual characteristics are fully reversible on cessation of exposure.

Ref.: Dunn, 1940; Finkler, 1949; Goldzieher and Goldzieher, 1949; Hertz, 1958.

917 Ethynodiol Diacetate with Mestranol

e.g., Ovulen

Toxicity Rating: 3. Oral contraceptive containing 1 mg. ethynodiol diacetate and 0.1 mg. mestranol. Intraperitoneal LD$_{50}$ of former in mice 3.9 gm./kg., of latter 3.5 gm./kg. Acute toxic effects in infants and young children not known, but see Norethynodrel with Mestranol below.

Ref.: Searle, 1966.

918 Norethindrone with Mestranol

e.g., Ortho-Novum

Toxicity Rating: 3(?). Oral contraceptive available in 2 and 10 mg. tablets containing 0.1 and 0.06 mg. mestranol, respectively. Acute toxicity data not located, but probably similar to Norethynodrel with Mestranol above. No reports of serious poisonings or death from overdosage. Young children (both male and female) up to 6 years of age have tolerated accidental ingestions ranging up to 60 mg. without apparent consequence.

Ref.: Francis and Dalzeil, 1965.

919 Norethynodrel with Mestranol

e.g., Enovid and Enovid-E

Toxicity Rating: 3. Oral contraceptive product also used in amenorrhea, dysmenorrhea, habitual or threatened abortion and other gynecological disturbances. Available tablets of various sizes: 9.85, 5.0 and 2.5 mg. (Enovid-E) with mestranol content of 0.15, 0.075 and 0.1 mg., respectively. Oral LD$_{50}$ in mice 680 mg./kg., in rats 840 mg./kg. Intraperitoneal LD$_{50}$ in mice 300 mg./kg., in rats 285 mg./kg. When given in corn oil to mice or rats by stomach tube, a mixture containing 19 times more norethynodrel than mestranol (by weight) was significantly more toxic than either ingredient alone. Animals receiving a lethal dose died quietly within 18 hours. No reports of fatal overdosages or serious poisonings in humans have been encountered. In two reports of ingestions by 4-year-old girls, one took 17 five-mg. tablets and was said to be nauseated for 3 days with a pink vaginal discharge on the 9th day, but the other is said to have ingested 300 tablets without subsequent effects. A 2-year-old boy is reported to have ingested 80 tablets of Enovid-E together with 24 tablets of Valium, and an adult female is said to have ingested 220 mg., both without serious sequelae. Frequently encountered side effects include nausea, vomiting, breast engorgement, and breakthrough bleeding.

Ref.: Heibert, 1966; Searle, 1966.

920 Thyroid

Toxicity Rating: 3(?). Dried powdered thyroid gland from animals slaughtered for human food. From a therapeutic standpoint thyroxine (T4) is about 200 times and triiodothyronine (T3) 800 to 1000 times more potent than the desiccated whole gland, but the latter is probably still used more often than its purified active principles. One source ranks thyroid third among medicinal agents implicated in accidental poisonings, but clinical reports of serious intoxications are rare. Doses of 2 to 3 gm.

have been tolerated by infants, but one serious poisoning resulted from the ingestion of 3.2 gm. by a 15-month-old. Experimentally, euthyroid adults tolerated gradually increasing daily doses to levels above 1.5 gm. for extended periods; they showed only signs of mild to moderate hyperthyroidism without exophthalmos or palpable enlargement of the thyroid gland. Toxic effects after an overdose of T4 may be delayed several days because of the *in vivo* conversion of T4 to the more potent T3. Frankly toxic doses induce unpleasant but transient symptoms that resemble thyrotoxicosis (thyroid storm). Signs and symptoms include palpita-

tions, rapid and irregular pulse, headache, tremors, nervousness, insomnia, delirium, diaphoresis, hyperpyrexia, vomiting (sometimes uncontrollable), collapse and coma. Therapy should include the administration of oxygen and barbiturates and the control of hyperpyrexia. Probably antithyroid drugs are of little value, but adrenergic blocking drugs such as propranolol and phenoxybenzamine (Dibenzyline) probably deserve clinical trials. Thyroid is potentially much more dangerous in patients with pre-existing cardiac disease; digitalization may be indicated here.

See also: 2,4-Dinitrophenol, *Reference Congener in Section III.*
Ref.: Jacobziner and Raybin, 1958; Levy and Gilger, 1957; Riggs et al., 1945.

Miscellaneous constituents of natural products

921 Alizarin 921

1,2-Dihydroxyanthraquinone

Occurs in the root of madder plant. It and many derivatives are used as dyes in home and industry.

Ref.: Merck and Co., 1976.

Except for reports of allergic reactions in humans, no toxicity data were located.

922 Amantadine 922

Adamantanamine, 1-Aminoadamantan, Tricyclodecan-1-amine, e.g., Symmetrel

Toxicity Rating: 4(?). Antiviral drug. Also used in treatment of parkinsonism. Antiviral activity is apparently due to inhibition of cell penetration by some viruses (e.g., influenza A-2 virus). Anti-parkinsonian activity presumably results from enhancement of dopaminergic nerve transmission by facilitating dopamine release, inhibiting dopamine reuptake, or serving as a specific dopamine agonist. The compound is moderately toxic to man and animals (oral LD_{50} in mice is 1 gm./kg. for amantadine and 0.7 gm./kg. for the hydrochloride). It is promptly absorbed after ingestion and excreted without alteration in urine. The biological half-life in man is about 24 hours. Signs of acute intoxication in rodents include hyperactivity, tremors, convulsions, respiratory distress and death. In monkeys and most dogs, large doses (200 mg./kg.) also produced vomiting, which was life-saving (single dose of 93 mg./kg. proved fatal in one dog which did not vomit). A therapeutic course has led to rapid accumulation in persons with impaired renal function and has produced mental confusion, nightmares, ataxia, dizziness, slurred speech, blurred vision and convulsions. Prolonged hemodialysis and peritoneal dialysis reduced plasma levels in

several such patients by about 40%. In one acute poisoning, a 2–year–old girl ingested 600 mg. of amantadine HCl. Emesis ensued, but she subsequently developed agitation, hallucination, hypersensitivity to stimuli, and bizarre dystonic posturing. The CNS effects were reversed by physostigmine, in a dose of 0.5 mg. intravenously, repeated after 10 minutes. In another case, a parkinsonian patient (also receiving phenytoin) ingested 2.8 gm. of amantadine hydrochloride in a suicide attempt. The result was an acute toxic psychosis (confusion and visual hallucinations), urinary retention and a mixed acid-base disturbance. Upon admission to hospital (about 18 hours after ingestion) the patient was flushed and the pupils dilated. Body temperature and blood pressure were elevated. Treatment consisted of diuresis induced by intravenous fluids, chlorpromazine (which had a calming effect) and phenytoin. No convulsions occurred, perhaps because of the phenytoin therapy. After 3 days, the psychosis abated and signs of parkinsonism reappeared, accompanied by extreme emotional depression. Gradual introduction of imipramine, levodopa and benztropine returned the patient to a stable, non-depressed state.

Ref.: Bailey and Stone, 1975; Berkowitz, 1979; Casey, 1978; Fahn et al., 1971; Ing et al., 1979; Vernier et al., 1969.

923 Botulinal Toxins 923

Clostridium botulinum toxins

Toxicity Rating: 6. Highly toxic, globular proteins released into the culture medium by growing anaerobic bacilli of the species Clostridium botulinum. These exotoxins, which are sometimes elaborated in contaminated foods, have caused many

human deaths. After escaping destruction by gastric acid and intestinal proteases, they are absorbed from the gut and induce failure of nerve transmission at many kinds of cholinergic junctions.

See also: Botulinal Toxins, *Reference Congener in Section III.*

924 Cantharidin

Hexahydro-3α,7α-dimethyl-4,7-epoxyisobenzofuran-1,3-dione

Toxicity Rating: 6. Active ingredient (0.6 to 1%) of cantharides (Cantharis vesicatoria, Spanish fly or blister beetle and various insects of the Meloidae family such as Epicauta cinerea, E. fabricii, etc.). An extreme irritant and vesicant long falsely identified as an aphrodisiac. Adult lethal dose by mouth 65 mg. but much smaller amounts have threatened life. Man appears to be more sensitive to cantharides than most common laboratory species. Some victims who ingest cantharides experience an intolerable burning sensation of their oral cavity and throat and vomit blood-stained mucus. One lethally poisoned female had no normal mucosa left from the tongue to the pylorus. Another adult is said to have brought up his entire esophageal lining almost intact but recovered within a few weeks. Diarrhea often occurs but hemorrhagic necrosis seems limited to the upper gastrointestinal tract. Injury to the bowel does not seem to account for the excruciating abdominal pain experienced by the occasional patient. Death may occur rapidly in hypovolemic shock. This violent reaction does not always occur. Some victims who ingested pure cantharides or tinctures (the active ingredient is very insoluble in water) are unable to taste it and may have extremely mild gastrointestinal symptoms. The second stage of the intoxication is more uniform and is characterized by urinary urgency, strangury, hematuria, which may progress to the passing of pure blood, priapism, oliguria and death in renal failure secondary to acute tubular necrosis. Shock contributes to the renal damage, but cantharidin appears to be a directly acting nephrotoxin. Polycythemia cannot always be explained by hemoconcentration. A dose of 1 mg. or contact with a single insect can produce distressing symptoms which may commence immediately or be delayed for as long as 12 hours. Skin contact results in intense blister formation. Pain is relieved by morphine. For management of corrosive esophagitis see Lye in Section III; for acute renal failure see Carbon Tetrachloride in Section III.

Ref.: Lehmann et al., 1955; Andrewes, 1921; Bagatell et al., 1969; Browne, 1960; Craven and Polak, 1954; Csiky, 1958; Lecutier, 1954; Lipsitz and Cross, 1917; Nickolls and Teare, 1954; Rosin, 1967; Wertelecki et al., 1967.

925 Cardol

Irritant principle found in cashew nut shell juice. See Cashew nut in the index.

926 Chlorophyll

Toxicity Rating: 1(?). A methyl phytyl ester of tricarboxy magnesium porphyrin. This water-insoluble green pigment is extracted from plants and used to color soaps, oils, fats, waxes, confectionery, liquors, cosmetics and perfumes. Also used as an antiknock agent in gasoline, as an accelerator in the vulcanizing of rubber, and as a deodorizer. A major constituent of green leaves. As present in leafy vegetables, it is probably not absorbed from the alimentary tract. Chlorophyllins, a water-soluble derivatives, are obtained by replacing the methyl and phytyl ester groups with alkali (usually sodium but sometimes potassium). The magnesum can also be replaced with copper. The copper is so firmly bound that copper poisoning cannot arise from this complex. Taken orally, chlorophyllin allegedly helps control excretory odors, ease chronic constipation and abate excessive flatulence (said to be especially useful in colostomy and ileostomy patients). Isolated instances of stomach cramps and discomfort have been reported. Feces are commonly dark-green. Excessive ingestion of Cloret tablets (a breath deodorant containing water-soluble chlorophyll derivatives) may cause a green urine and tongue. Chlorophyll extracts soaking into the skin can sensitize sites of application to light irradiation, producing erythema.

927 Papain

No toxicity data were found. A proteolytic enzyme from the juice and leaves of Carica papaya L. used in commercial meat tenderizers. Pastes of the latter products have been recommended for pain relief after bee or jellyfish stings. Other proteolytic enzymes used in commercial detergents have caused severe asthma-like pulmonary reactions due to allergy and/or irritation in consumers and occupationally exposed workers. Inhaled papain dust may have similar effects. The intra-tracheal instillation of papain in rats has been used as an experimental model for the production of emphysema.

Ref.: Gross et al., 1965; Weill et al., 1971.

928 Pepsin

No toxicity data were found. The principal enzyme of gastric juice sometimes used to aid digestion and occasionally given with hydrochloric acid in gastric achylia. Probably harmless by mouth except for occasional allergic reactions such as rash. Other proteolytic enzymes used in commercial detergents have caused severe asthma-like pulmonary reactions due to allergy and/or irritation in consumers and occupationally exposed workers. Inhaled pepsin dust may have similar effects.

Ref.: Weill et al., 1971.

929 Pyroligneous Acid 929

Wood vinegar

Prepared by the destructive distillation of wood. Contains about 6% acetic acid in water and small concentrations of creosote, methyl alcohol, and acetone.

Ref.: Osol and Farrar, 1955.

930 Ricin 930

Ricine

Toxicity Rating: 6. A toxic glycoprotein obtained from castor beans (not present in castor oil). Powdered beans have been used as fertilizer. Low-concentration powders (0.3%) are marketed as a mole killer. Five beans have proved fatal in a child, 20 beans in an adult. Like abrin, a closely related protein from the jequirity bean (see latter in the index), ricin consists of two polypeptide chains (A and B), joined by disulfide linkages. Chain B, which contains most of the carbohydrate, is involved in the binding of ricin to the surface of mammalian cells, after which chain A appears to be liberated by hydrolysis. Chain A is the active moiety; it enters the cells and reacts with ribosomes to stop protein synthesis. Cessation of protein synthesis is the definitive biochemical lesion in ricin poisoning. After administration of ricin by any route there is a latency of many hours (sometimes several days) before symptoms appear. Ingestion results in a severe gastroenteritis, often hemorrhagic. Later the victim may become drowsy, confused, irrational, and comatose. Convulsions occur. Peripheral vascular collapse (shock) and renal failure may develop. Local inflammatory lesions result from dust in the eyes, nose, and throat. Convalescence is slow. Supportive treatment should be maintained energetically.

Ref.: Ford, 1913; Olsnes et al., 1974; Reese, 1874; Snell, 1952; Zerbst, 1944.

931 Santonin 931

Toxicity Rating: 5. The active principle of various species of Artemisia plants (Levant wormseed). A nonirritating and potent anthelmintic. Visual disturbances are common (especially color vision); sometimes disorders of hearing, taste, and smell appear. Large doses stimulate the central nervous system: headache, vomiting, abdominal pain, diarrhea, confusion, muscle twitching, tonic-clonic convulsions. There are subsequent or intermittent periods of depression: coma, fall in body temperature, circulatory or respiratory collapse. Hematuria may be prominent. Treatment is supportive and includes gastric lavage and saline catharsis. See Section IV for anticonvulsant therapy.

Ref.: Cookson and Stock, 1940; Marshall, 1927a; Marshall, 1927b.

932 Squalane 932

Robane, Perhydrosqualene, 2,6,10,15,19,23-Hexamethyltetracosane

A saturated aliphatic hydrocarbon occurring naturally in the secretions of the sebaceous glands of humans and animals. Mice have tolerated 500 mg./kg. by mouth. Used as a vehicle for cosmetics and topical pharmaceuticals. Presumably it promotes percutaneous absorption of incorporated medicinal agents.

Ref.: Clark et al., 1958; Robeco Chemicals, 1957.

933 Tetrahydrocannabinols 933

Δ^9-Tetrahydrocannabinol

Toxicity Rating: 4. The active psychotropic constituents of marihuana and hashish (from Cannabis sativa). Tetrahydrocannabinols represent one group of more than 30 "cannabinoids" found in the plant; they possess in common three 6-membered rings, a single phenolic hydroxyl group, and an amyl side-chain. Because the molecules do not contain nitrogen, they are not classified as alkaloids. The principal psychoactive components are the trans isomers of Δ^9-tetrahydrocannabinol and to a lesser extent Δ^8-tetrahydrocannabinol. By a different numbering system these components are commonly known as the Δ^1 and $\Delta^{1(6)}$ isomers respectively. The acute LD_{50} of the former is 482 mg./kg. in mice and 666 mg./kg. in rats by intragastric administration. On the other hand 9 gm./kg. by mouth as a single dose failed to kill rhesus monkeys, whereas 128 mg./kg. proved to be lethal by the intravenous route. No human fatalities have been documented, but these substances are potent hallucinogens in man.

See also: Marihuana, *Reference Congener in Section III.*

934   **934**   Umbelliferone

7-Hydroxycoumarin

In sun-screen lotions and creams. No toxicity data were located.

Ref.: Merck and Co., 1976.

Detergents, surfactants and germicides

Detergents

935   **935**   Detergents (Synthetic)

Syndets

Products used for removing dirt from soft or hard surfaces, as in washing clothes, removing wax from floors or grease from metals. Soaps are detergent materials, but in a historical sense "detergent" means a synthetic compound. All detergents are Surface Active Agents (see latter below), but the converse is not true. Three general classes are recognized on the basis of the ionization of the surface active moiety at neutral pH: Anionic, Cationic and Nonionic. Even within a given class, however, a wide range of chemical structures and toxicities is recognized.

Ref.: Calandra and Fancher, 1969; McCutcheon, 1965.

936   **936**   Surface Active Agents

Surfactants, Emulsifiers

Substances which alter energy relations at interfaces. A surfactant lowers the surface tension of a given solution, usually aqueous. According to their use surfactants may be classified as detergents (see above), emulsifiers, wetters and penetrants. The same chemical compound may find utility in any or all of these categories. Three general chemical classes are recognized on the basis of the ionization of the surface active moiety at neutral pH: anionic, cationic and nonionic. Even within a given class, however, a wide range of chemical structures and toxicities is recognized. Consult the index for information on each of these chemical classes.

Ref.: Calandra and Fancher, 1969; McCutcheon, 1965.

937   **937**   Builders (Detergents)

Those ingredients in modern detergent formulations that are designed to chelate or otherwise remove the elements responsible for water hardness (mostly calcium and magnesium) and in this way to prevent the inactivation of ingredients that serve as surface active agents (surfactants). Granular household detergent products are composed largely of builders. These builders are of two general types: those which hold calcium in solution as soluble chelates and those which precipitate it. In the first category are found polyphosphates (especially sodium tripolyphosphates) and nitrilotriacetate (NTA). The second category includes sodium carbonate, sodium bicarbonate, sodium sesquicarbonate, sodium silicate and sodium metasilicate. Consult index for specific names.

938   **938**   Fluorescent Whitening Agents

Optical brighteners, FWA

Toxicity Rating: 2. A class of dyes found in food packaging materials, detergents and soaps. Emit bluish fluorescence when exposed to UV radiation. Can be classified into 6 groups typified by the following chemical structures: stilbene; coumarin and quinolone; 1,3-diphenyl-2-pyrazoline; naphthalamide; benzoxazole and benzimidazole; combination of benzoxazole and/or benzimidazole with olefinic, aromatic or heteroaromatic constituents. FWA's that remain in detergent residues on dishes and that migrate from foodwrap into food are sources of human exposure to FWA's by ingestion. Detergent solutions containing FWA's and clothing impregnated with them are sources of skin exposure. Because of the widespread use of the compounds (estimated human daily intake from all sources is 0.004 mg./kg. body weight), the products in current use have undergone thorough toxicological testing. The acute oral LD_{50}'s in rats range from 1 to greater than 21 gm./kg. The concentration of brightener in a synthetic detergent solution varies from a few hundredths of 1% to 0.2%. The acute oral LD_{50} for a mouse (2.8 gm./kg.) is contained in 3 kg. of a typical detergent product. FWA's are considered safe for humans in the concentrations found in commercial products. FWA's have been found to have no mutagenic, teratogenic, respiratory or skin effects. All but two of the compounds tested produced little or no eye irritation; 4,4′-bis {[4-bis(2-hydroxyethyl)amino-6-methoxy-1,3,5-triazin-2-yl]amino} stilbene-2,2′disulfonic acid and 2,5-bis(5-*tert*-butylbenzoxazol-2-yl)thiophene produced marked or extreme eye irritation in test rabbits. Photocarcinogenic effects are theoretically possible because the compounds transfer energy, but reproducible data proving such effects have not been obtained.

Ref.: Buxtorf, 1975; Forbes and Urbach, 1975; Gloxhuber and Bloching, 1978; Lyman et al., 1975; Snyder et al., 1963; Thomann and Krueger, 1975.

Anionic surfactants

939   Anionic Synthetic Detergents   939

Many of these materials tend to form precipitates in the presence of calcium ions and are therefore ineffective in hard water, unless calcium is inactivated by "builders". The sulfonates are particularly calcium-sensitive. Among the more common types of synthetic anionic detergents are Alkyl sodium sulfates, Alkyl sodium sulfonates and Linear alkyl benzene sulfonate (sodium). See these entries below.

940   Aerosols   940

Toxicity Rating: 3. Trademarked name for a series of commercial surfactants. A series of anionic surface-active agents, particularly dialkyl sodium sulfosuccinate. (One exception is Aerosol C-61, which is cationic.) Irritating to eyes but not to skin at conc. of 1%.

Ref.: Benaglia et al., 1943.

941   Alcohol Sulfate Salts   941

Toxicity Rating: 3. Usually sodium or triethanolamine salt. Often a secondary or branched-chain alcohol (e.g., Tergitols, Teepol). Anionic wetting and emulsifying agents. Skin penetration suspected with some derivatives. No clinical poisonings are known. Also see Alkyl Sodium Sulfates below.

942   Alkyl Aryl Polyether Sulfates and Sulfonates   942

Triton X-200, Triton X-301, Triton 770

Toxicity Rating: 2 & 3. Anionic surfactants, marketed as sodium salts, prepared by sulfating and sulfonating compounds like alkyl phenoxy polyethoxy ethanols. Animal tests reveal no consistent difference in acute oral toxicity between the nonionic product and its anionic derivative, but the latter are always more irritating to eyes and skin, perhaps because solutions of these salts are usually alkaline.

943   Alkyl Aryl Sodium Sulfonates   943

e.g., Ultrawets, Santomerse, Nacconals

Toxicity Rating: 3. Aryl group is usually benzene, naphthalene, toluene, or xylene. This is probably the largest and most important class of anionic surfactants; they are found in many household detergent products. Prolonged skin contact with solutions may cause irritation, but sensitization or allergic reactions are rare. The mechanism of death after high oral doses in animals is not known. At low levels feeding experiments have produced no evidence of systemic toxicity in rats. For two important specific examples, see also Tetrapropylene benzene sulfonate (sodium) and Linear alkyl benzene sulfonate (sodium) below.

Ref.: Paynter and Weir, 1960; Tusing et al., 1960; Swisher, 1968.

944   Alkylated Sodium Phosphates   944

e.g., Victawets

Toxicity Rating: 3(?). When the alkyl group or groups are long-chain fatty alcohols, these phosphate esters serve as surfactants, penetrants and wetting agents. They are available both as anionic (mono- and di-alkyl) and nonionic (tri-alkyl) surfactants. Like other surface active agents these compounds are believed to have a moderately low acute toxicity and to produce no distinctive anatomical or biochemical lesions, but the only datum located is an intraperitoneal lethal dose in rats for the nonionic surfactant Victawet 12. Short-chain alkyl esters of phosphoric acid are considerably more toxic. Ethyl derivatives are believed to be weak inhibitors of cholinesterase, as is tributyl phosphate. See Ethyl phosphates and Tributyl phosphate in this index. Aryl esters of phosphoric acid such as o-tricresyl phosphate (see latter in the index) are also neurotoxic, but the lesion here is one of demyelinization.

945   Alkyl Sodium Isethionate

945

e.g., Igepons AT and AC

Toxicity Rating: 2. Anionic surfactants used as wetting agents, detergents, etc. They are fatty acid esters of sodium isethionate (HO-$(CH_2)_2$-SO_2-ONa).

946   Alkyl Sodium Sulfates

946

e.g., Sodium lauryl sulfate, Sodium alkyl aryl sulfate, Duponol C, Drene, Dreft, Teepol, Gardinols, Tergitols

Toxicity Rating: 3. Sodium salts of fatty alcohol sulfates (sometimes a secondary or branched-chain alcohol, as in Tergitols). Widely used anionic detergents of moderately low acute and chronic toxicity. A few of the branched-chain products have been shown to have significant percutaneous toxicity. Skin irritation may be encountered with any of these substances. Taken by mouth, sodium lauryl sulfate stimulates gastric mucus production and sometimes inactivates pepsin in test animals. In subacute and chronic feeding tests, even fatally poisoned animals show only diarrhea and intestinal bloating, with no gross lesions outside of the gastrointestinal tract.

Ref.: Smyth et al., 1941b.

947   Alkyl Sodium Sulfonates

947

Toxicity Rating: 3. Anionic surfactants whose structure can be expressed as RSO_3Na, where R equals C_{14} to C_{18} straight hydrocarbon chains. Acute oral LD_{50} in male albino rats 2.1 gm./kg. Acute dermal LD_{50} for rabbits is greater than 3.2 gm./kg. Moderate to marked irritant on both intact and abraded rabbit skin. Marked to severe irritant in rabbit eye. Unlike the -C-O-S- linkage of the alkyl sulfates, the sulfonates have a -C-S-bond. The sulfonates are more stable with respect to hydrolysis than the sulfates but are less soluble in hard water. Although no adequate toxicological comparison has been reported, lethal doses of alkyl sulfonates and sulfates appear to be substantially the same in laboratory animals. See Alkyl Sodium Sulfates above.

Ref.: Eckardt, 1964.

948   Alkyl Sodium *N*-Methyltaurate

948

Igepons T and TK and TN and T-42 and T-51

Toxicity Rating: 3. The alkyl group (often oleoyl) is a fatty acid attached to the nitrogen by an amide linkage. Anionic surface-active agents, some of which produce skin irritation at concs. of 5%.

Ref.: Antara Chemicals, 1955.

949   Barium Sulfonate

949

Toxicity Rating: 3. Barium salts of various alkyl aryl sulfonic acids in oil solution, prepared by sulfonating mixtures of various complex aromatic rings contained in petroleum oil. Probably the most common detergent in current lubricating oils. In 12 commercially available additives of this type, the barium content ranged from 1 to 15%. The oral LD_{50} values of the undiluted materials ranged from 2 to 10 ml/kg. in rats. Because there was no evident correlation between the barium content and the toxicity, one may suppose that this barium is not available as soluble Ba^{++} when the material is ingested. See Alkyl aryl sodium sulfonates above.

Ref.: Dooley, 1961.

950   Dialkyl Sodium Sulfosuccinate

950

e.g., Aerosol AY or IB or MA

Toxicity Rating: 3. Commercial anionic surfactants which are widely used. In Aerosol OT, the alkyl groups are octyl, in MA hexyl and in AY amyl. Toxicity rating is based on dioctyl derivative tested in rats. Irritating to eyes but human patch tests reveal no skin irritation with 1% aqueous solutions. See Dioctyl sodium sulfosuccinate below.

951   Dioctyl Sodium Sulfosuccinate

951

Docusate sodium,   Bis(2-ethylhexyl) sodium sulfosuccinate, e.g., Colace, Doxinate, Aerosol OT

Toxicity Rating: 3. A widely used anionic surfactant, one of the most powerful wetting compounds known. Dioctyl sodium sulfosuccinate (DSS) is employed as a dispersing and emulsifying agent in various dermatological preparations and as a laxative. The laxative action is said to result from enhanced penetration of water into the fecal mass in the presence of the wetting agent. Recent studies, however, indicate that an action on the intestinal mucosa may contribute to or account for the laxative effect. Water and salt accumulated in ligated colonic segments of DSS-treated rats whereas net absorption of isotonic saline solution occurred in control rats. When segments of rodent ileum, jejunum and colon were perfused with 0.5mM DSS, mucosal cells were flattened and their brush borders disappeared. DSS itself has a moderately low acute oral toxicity (rat oral LD_{50} 1.9 gm./kg.); however, the compound may increase the absorption and hence the toxicity of other drugs given concurrently. Only diarrhea and intestinal bloating are reported in animals given toxic doses. In chronic feeding tests, fatally poisoned rats showed no gross lesions outside of the gastrointestinal tract. Eye irritation may be caused by solutions containing more than 0.1% DSS. The compound is supplied in capsules containing 40 to 250 mg., as a 1% solution, and as a syrup containing 0.4% active ingredient. The usual adult dose is 50 to 250 mg. Also present in various household cleaners and waxes.

Ref.: Benaglia et al., 1943; Donowitz and Binder, 1975; Saunders et al., 1975.

952 Linear Alkyl Benzene Sulfonate (Sodium) 952

Linear alkylate sulfonate, LAS

Toxicity Rating: 3. A biodegradable anionic surfactant widely used in laundry and other household detergent products. The alkyl group, which is synthesized from petroleum raw materials, commonly consists of 12 or 13 carbon atoms in a straight chain. In the United States this material has completely replaced the poorly degradable tetrapropylene benzene sulfonate (see below). All alkyl benzene sulfonates (ABS) tested in rats have proved to have oral LD_{50}'s of 0.8 to 3 gm./kg. Because most commercial mixtures containing these surfactants induce prompt emesis, it is doubtful that the amounts absorbed have significant systemic toxicity.

Ref.: Davidsohn and Milwidsky, 1972; Swisher, 1968.

953 Soaps 953

e.g., Sodium oleate

Toxicity Rating: 2. Sodium (or potassium) salts of fatty acids, prepared from edible fats. Studies of acute oral toxicity in rats place the simple household soaps near the borderline between toxicity classes 1 and 2. They are therefore less lethal than synthetic anionic detergents and even less than most nonionic detergents. However, soaps with an appreciable content of free alkali (e.g., some laundry soaps) are less benign. By intrauterine injection (as in some criminal abortions), soaps cause hemolysis, emboli, hyperpyrexia, shock, renal damage, and often prompt death.

Ref.: Cann and Verhulst, 1958a; Cann and Verhulst, 1960b.

954 Sodium Lauryl Glyceryl Ether Sulfonate 954

Toxicity Rating: 3. Anionic surfactant suitable for use in household detergent products. Oral LD_{50} in rats is 1.82 gm./kg. Feeding experiments in rats at levels of 0.5% for 2 years produced no gross anatomical, biochemical or microscopic lesions. Twice weekly applications for 105 weeks of 5% aqueous solutions to the skin of Swiss female mice produced no skin tumors.

Ref.: Tusing et al., 1962.

955 Sodium Lauryl Trioxyethylene Sulfate 955

Toxicity Rating: 3. Anionic surfactant suitable for use in household detergent products. Oral LD_{50} in rats is 1.82 gm./kg. Feeding experiments in rats at levels of 0.5% for 2 years produced no gross anatomical, biochemical or microscopic lesions. Twice weekly applications for 105 weeks of 5% aqueous solutions to the skin of Swiss female mice produced no skin tumors.

Ref.: Tusing et al., 1962.

956 Sulfated Castor Oil 956

Turkey red oil, "Sulfonated" castor oil

Toxicity Rating: 3. True sulfated castor oil or the ammonium salt of ricinoleic sulfuric acid ester (since castor oil is 80 to 85% ricinoleic acid). One of the earliest commercially important anionic surfactants, still widely used in the textile industry and in agriculture. Has been injected to cause sclerosis of varicose veins. Toxicity rating is inferred from that of simple Alkyl sodium sulfates. See latter above.

Ref.: Osol and Farrar, 1955.

957   Sulfonated Dodecyl Diphenyl Oxide (Sodium)

Dowfax 2A1

Toxicity Rating: 3. An anionic detergent of moderate acute oral toxicity (as tested in rats). Concentrated solutions are irritating to skin and mucous membranes, but a 15% solution neither irritated nor sensitized human skin. See also Alkyl aryl polyether sulfonates above.

958   Sulfonated Petroleum Oils

"Mahogany soaps", Penetrol

Toxicity Rating: 3. Sulfonated petroleum oils are usually marketed as sodium, calcium, or barium salts, e.g., "Mahogany soaps". Anionic surfactants used as diluents and "spreaders" for agricultural sprays, detergents in lubricating oils, etc. Consist of metal salts of alkyl aryl sulfonic acids in oil solution, prepared by sulfonating mixtures of various complex aromatic rings contained in petroleum oil. See also Alkyl sodium sulfonates and Barium sulfonate above.

959   Tetrapropylene Benzene Sulfonate (Sodium)

TBS

Toxicity Rating: 3. Anionic surfactant with acute oral LD_{50} in male albino rats 2.1 gm./kg. Acute dermal LD_{50} for rabbits is greater than 3.2 gm./kg. Moderate to marked irritant on intact and abraded rabbit skin. Marked to severe irritant in the rabbit eye. From the late 1940's to about 1965 this compound was probably the most widely used anionic surfactant in household detergent products in the United States. Because of its poor biodegradability, it accumulated in some natural bodies of water in amounts that produced foaming or frothing. In the mid-1960's the U.S.A. detergent industry replaced this compound with linear alkyl substitutes that are rapidly biodegraded in the environment. See also Linear alkyl benzene sulfonate (sodium) above.

Ref.: Eckardt, 1964; Davidsohn and Milwidsky, 1972; Swisher, 1968.

960   Triethanolamine Oleate

Triethanolamine soap

Toxicity Rating: 2(?). A representative fatty acid salt of triethanolamine; these salts are synthetic soaps. They form practically neutral aqueous solutions, which are not irritating or injurious to the skin. Widely used as detergents and emulsifiers in medicine and pharmacy. Ingestion toxicity is thought to be low.

Ref.: Greenberg and Lester, 1954.

Non-ionic surfactants

961   Nonionic Synthetic Detergents

Nonionic surfactants, Nonionic emulsifiers, Ethoxylated alkyl phenols

Many types of nonionic materials are employed in commercial products. All are uncharged in aqueous solution at neutral pH. The major types are reaction products of alkylated phenols or fatty alcohols with varying amounts of ethylene oxide, e.g., Alkyl phenoxy polyethoxy ethanols (see below). See also Alkyl ethoxylate below.

962   Alkyl Ethoxylate

Alkyl polyethylene glycol ether

Toxicity Rating: 2-3. An important series of synthetic non-ionic surfactants in which a long-chain fatty alcohol is attached by a stable ether linkage to a polyethylene glycol residue of variable length. These linear molecules have one hydrophobic end (alkyl chain) and one hydrophilic end (polyglycol), and therefore they are surface-active and serve as detergents. When the alkyl chain is about 12 carbon atoms in length and the polyglycol about 6 ethylene units long, the acute oral LD_{50} is 2.2 gm./kg. in rats and 1.4 gm./kg. in mice. With 7 ethylene units in the average molecule, reported LD_{50} values are 4.1 and 1.2 gm./kg. Dogs are much less sensitive to the lethal actions, perhaps because they tend to vomit promptly (although delayed in some cases). Monkeys administered oral doses greater than 2 gm./kg. also exhibited emesis and diarrhea, and with single doses above 5 gm./kg. various signs of central nervous depression were observed (e.g., ataxia, weakness, sedation). By intraperitoneal administration alkyl ethoxylates are much more active. Several of them induce central depression followed by prolonged periods of convulsions. Because it has been on the market for decades, more information is available about a German product Thesit than about any other alkyl ethoxylate. See also Laureth 9 below.

Ref.: Grubb et al., 1960; Swisher, 1968.

963   Alkyl Phenoxy Polyethoxy Ethanols   963

e.g., Igepals, Nonoxynols

Toxicity Rating: 2 & 3. Includes Igepals and Non-oxynols, where alkyl is usually nonyl; Tritons X-45, X-100, X-102, X-114, where alkyl is octyl; Brij products where alkyl is lauryl. Alternative generic names include alkyl aryl polyether alcohols, alkyl phenol polyglycol ethers and polyethylene glycol alkyl aryl ethers. Nonionic surfactants available with a wide variety of physical properties are used as wetting agents and emulsifiers and as spermicides in vaginal jellies, creams, foams and suppositories. Even at full-strength, they rarely sensitize or irritate human skin. In topical spermicidal contraceptives, however, which in many cases contain 2 to 12.5% nonoxynol-9 (i.e., the p-nonylphenyl ether of an ethylene glycol polymer with 9 units), transient burning and irritation of the vagina and penis are not uncommon. The only symptoms (and lesions) in orally poisoned animals are related to gastrointestinal irritation (e.g., diarrhea, bloating). Little, if any, intestinal absorption or decomposition.

Ref.: Antara Chemicals, 1955; Finnegan and Dienna, 1953; Woodward and Calvery, 1945.

964   Ethylene Glycol Distearate   964

Toxicity Rating: 1. White waxy material whose insolubility and low density make it useful as an "opacifier" for imparting a milky or opaque quality to lotions, cosmetic creams, and liquid detergents.

Ref.: Griffith, 1964a.

No toxicity seen in rats given an aqueous suspension of ethylene glycol distearate in an oral dose of 15 gm./kg. See Ethylene glycol alkyl (and aryl) esters in the index.

965   Glyceryl Stearate   965

Monostearin, Glyceryl monostearate

Toxicity Rating: 1. Also mono- and di- esters of other fatty acids. These partial glycerides are widely used, often in conjunction with a little soap, as surfactants and emulsifiers in cosmetics, medicinals, and food products. Like natural fats they are well digested and assimilated.

Ref.: Greenberg and Lester, 1954.

966   Laureth 9   966

Dodecyl alcohol polyoxyethylene ether

Toxicity Rating: 3. A linear molecule consisting of a dodecyl alcohol attached by a stable ether linkage to a polyethylene glycol moiety containing 9 ethylene units on the average. In general, compounds of this type are called alkyl ethoxylates; they are highly surface-active and are present in some detergent products. Under the proprietary name Thesit, it has been marketed in Germany for incorporation into anesthetic and antipruritic ointments. The material is claimed to have analgetic, antiinflammatory and local anesthetic activity. In various concentrations Thesit and a mixture of similar alkyl ethoxylates known by the code name Sch 600 have been used in man and animals for corneal anesthesia, for mucosal anesthesia preceding endoscopy, for relief from itching (applied locally to the anus, rectum, vagina, skin lesions, etc.), for nerve blocks (by infiltration), for spermicidal activity (when instilled in the vagina), for relief of pain from peptic ulcer (when ingested). Like other local anesthetics, however, high doses (especially if administered parenterally) may induce narcosis and eventually convulsions. Laureth 9 and related materials are not employed as medicinal agents in the U.S.A. at the present time, but various alkyl ethoxylates are found in detergent formulations. See also Alkyl ethoxylate above.

Ref.: Soehring et al., 1951; Grubb et al., 1960; Schulz, 1952; Lutzenkirchen, 1952; Zipf and Kreppel, 1955; Berberian et al., 1965a; Berberian et al., 1965b.

967   Pluronics   967

Toxicity Rating: 2. Ethylene and propylene oxides chemically reacted with propylene glycol. Trademarked name for various non-ionic surfactants with a wide variety of physical forms, used in cosmetics, medicinal ointments, etc. In laboratory animals very low acute toxicity, especially Pluronic F68. No irritation or sensitization of skin or eyes.

968   Polyethylene Glycol Stearate   968

e.g., Myrj 52, Nonisols, Polyoxyl 40 stearate

Toxicity Rating: 1. This and polyethylene glycol esters of other fatty acids (e.g., oleic acid) serve as nonionic surfactants generally soluble or dispersible in water. Some of these compounds have been proposed as emulsifiers in foods (e.g., bread). These esters are hydrolyzed in the bowel. The fatty acid is absorbed and metabolized; at least the shorter polyoxyethylene residues are also absorbed, but they are excreted unchanged in the urine (no detectable metabolism to oxalic acid in man).

969   Polyoxyethylene (20) Sorbitan Monostearate

Polysorbate 60, Tween 60

Toxicity Rating: 1. A group of nonionic surfactants, generally soluble or dispersible in water. Manufactured from Span-type materials by joining polyoxyethylene chains to the unesterified hydroxyls. Small quantities are used in many foods and beverages, cosmetics, etc. No single oral dose is known to be lethal in animals, and men have been fed 15 gm. daily for several months with impunity. In the bowel the fatty acid is split off and absorbed, and the rest is eliminated in feces. See also Polysorbate 80 below.

970   Polysorbate 80

Polyoxyethylene (20) sorbitan mono-oleate, e.g., Tween 80

Toxicity Rating: 1. Unintentionally administered to a 4-month infant at a daily dose of 19.2 gm./kg. for 2 consecutive days. The patient passed 6 loose stools but showed no other evidence of intoxication. Also see Polyethylene (20) sorbitan monostearate above.

971   Propylene Glycol Monostearate

e.g., Atlas G 924

Toxicity Rating: 2(?). Slightly more toxic than propylene glycol in animals. Large doses produce central nervous depression and kidney tubular injury, as does ethylene glycol. The same is true of other fatty acid esters of propylene glycol.

See also: Ethylene Glycol, *Reference Congener in Section III.*

972   Sorbitan Monostearate

e.g., Span 60, Arlacels

Toxicity Rating: 1. Span 80 is the monooleate ester. Water-insoluble nonionic surfactants made by esterifying with digestible fatty acids various partial anhydrides of sorbitol. Added in small quantities to many foods, beverages, cosmetics, etc. When digested, both the fatty acid and the polyhydric alcohol sorbitan are absorbed, but the latter is completely excreted in urine. No single oral dose is known to be lethal in laboratory animals, and man has been fed with impunity single doses of 20 gm. or daily doses of 6 gm. for 1 month.

973   Spermaceti

Cetaceum

Toxicity Rating: 1(?). Chief constituent is cetyl palmitate; also contains free cetyl alcohol and other esters. Used as an emollient and as an ointment base. No ingestion toxicity is described.

Ref.: Greenberg and Lester, 1954.

Cationic surfactants

974   Cationic Surfactants

Toxicity Rating: 3 & 4. Alkyl- and/or aryl-substituted ammonium chloride or bromide (sometimes sulfate). Also alkyl-substituted quaternized N-heterocyclic compounds derived from pyridine, imidazole and isoquinoline. Usually one of the alkyl groups is a long hydrophobic carbon chain. A wide variety of cationic surfactants used as germicides and sanitizers. Some of them (e.g., distearyl dimethyl ammonium chloride) are also used as fabric softeners in laundry rinses.

See also: Benzalkonium Chloride, *Reference Congener in Section III.*

975   Alkyl Aryl Ammonium Chloride (or Bromide)

Toxicity Rating: 4. This is a generic name for a large number of quaternary ammonium surfactants, used chiefly as germicides and sanitizers.

See also: Benzalkonium Chloride, *Reference Congener in Section III.*

976   Alkyl Dimethyl 3,4-Dichlorobenzene Ammonium Chloride

Aralkonium chloride

Toxicity Rating: 4. A cationic surfactant used at dilutions of 1:1000 to 1:5000 as a germicide and sanitizer for clean surfaces. Based on animal studies this compound lies near the borderline between toxicity classes 3 and 4. Tetrosan also contains alkenyl groups.

See also: Benzalkonium Chloride, *Reference Congener in Section III.*

977 Alkyl Dimethyl Ethyl Ammonium Chloride (or Bromide)

e.g., Cetylcide, Ethyl Cetab

Toxicity Rating: 4. A cationic surfactant.

See also: Benzalkonium Chloride, *Reference Congener in Section III.*

978 Alkyl Dimethyl Ethylbenzyl Ammonium Chloride

e.g., BTC 471

Toxicity Rating: 4. A cationic surfactant used as a disinfectant, deodorant and fungicide.

See also: Benzalkonium Chloride, *Reference Congener in Section III.*

979 Alkyl Hydroxyethyl Imidazolinium Chloride

e.g., Alrosept MBC, Alrosept MM

Toxicity Rating: 4. A cationic surfactant.

See also: Benzalkonium Chloride, *Reference Congener in Section III.*

980 Alkyl Naphthyl Methyl Pyridinium Chloride

e.g., Emcol 888

Toxicity Rating: 4. A cationic surfactant used at concentrations of 0.1% and less as a disinfectant for clean surfaces.

See also: Benzalkonium Chloride, *Reference Congener in Section III.*

981 Alkyl Quaternary Ammonium Chloride (or Bromide)

Toxicity Rating: 4. This is a general name for the largest category of cationic surfactants. Used as germicides and sanitizers.

See also: Benzalkonium Chloride, *Reference Congener in Section III.*

982 Alkyl Tolyl Methyl Trimethyl Ammonium Chloride

e.g., Hyamine 2389

Toxicity Rating: 4. A cationic surfactant used in concs. of 1:1000 (or less) to disinfect clean surfaces. Some primary skin irritation from aqueous solutions of 10% or more.

See also: Benzalkonium Chloride, *Reference Congener in Section III.*

983 Alkyl Trimethyl Ammonium Chloride (or Bromide)

e.g., Cetab, Cetyl trimethyl ammonium bromide

Toxicity Rating: 4. A cationic surfactant. In Cetab the alkyl group is cetyl.

See also: Benzalkonium Chloride, *Reference Congener in Section III.*

984 Ammonyx 2194

Di-tallow dimethyl ammonium sulfate

Cationic fabric softener. The designation "tallow" indicates straight chain alkyl groups prepared from natural mixtures of fatty acids derived from tallow, which is animal fat. Hexadecyl, octadecyl, and octadecenyl groups predominate. Said to be non-irritating to skin in concentrations as high as 10%.

See also: Benzalkonium Chloride, *Reference Congener in Section III.*
Ref.: Hodes, 1963.

985 Benzalkonium Chloride

Alkyl dimethyl benzyl ammonium chloride (or bromide), e.g., Roccal, BTC, Zephiran chloride

Toxicity Rating: 4. Probably the most widely used cationic surfactant, employed at use concentrations of 0.1% (and less) as a germicide and sanitizer for chemically clean surfaces. Commercially available as concentrated aqueous solutions (2 to 50%). Dependent in part upon the length of the alkyl group, the toxicity rating (mice and rats) may be 3 or 4, usually the latter. The usual product contains a mixture of alkyls from C_8 to C_{18}.

See also: Benzalkonium Chloride, *Reference Congener in Section III.*
Ref.: Onyx Oil and Chemical Co., 1952a.

986   Benzethonium Chloride

p-Diisobutyl phenoxyethoxyethyl dimethyl benzylammonium chloride

Toxicity Rating: 4. A cationic surfactant used as a germicide, disinfectant and preservative.

See also: Benzalkonium Chloride, *Reference Congener in Section III.*
Ref.: Osol and Farrar, 1955.

987   Cetalkonium Chloride

Benzyl hexadecyl dimethyl ammonium chloride,   Cetyl dimethyl benzyl ammonium chloride

Toxicity Rating: 4. A quaternary ammonium germicide and fungicide closely related to benzalkonium chloride.

See also: Benzalkonium Chloride, *Reference Congener in Section III.*

988   Cetyl Pyridinium Chloride

Ceepryn chloride

Toxicity Rating: 4. A quaternary ammonium compound used as a germicide on skin and on inanimate surfaces. Available as aqueous or alcohol solutions (e.g., tinctures) in concentrations of 10% or less.

See also: Benzalkonium Chloride, *Reference Congener in Section III.*
Ref.: Warren et al., 1942.

989   Dialkyl Dimethyl Ammonium Chloride

e.g., Aliquats

Toxicity Rating: 3–4. Usually a mixture of alkyl groups, e.g., derived from coconut amines. Dilute aqueous solutions are used as germicides, deodorizers, and sanitizers on chemically clean surfaces. The dilauryl bromide salt has been used in oil emulsions for mothproofing. Aliquat 26, 204, 205, etc. refer to different alkyl groups and in some cases to the bromide rather than chloride salt. These differences are thought to have little if any toxicological significance.

See also: Benzalkonium Chloride, *Reference Congener in Section III.*

990   Stearyl Dimethyl Benzyl Ammonium Chloride

Stearalkonium chloride

A cationic surfactant used as a germicide and sanitizer. One of the molecular species in benzalkonium chloride.

See also: Benzalkonium Chloride, *Reference Congener in Section III.*

991   Lauryl Isoquinolinium Bromide

e.g., Isothan Q-15, Isothan Q-75

Toxicity Rating: 4. A cationic surfactant which has a slightly greater acute toxicity in rats than benzalkonium chloride. No skin irritation or sensitization at use concentrations of 0.1% and lower. Used as an agricultural fungicide.

See also: Benzalkonium Chloride, *Reference Congener in Section III.*
Ref.: Onyx Oil and Chemical Co., 1952b.

992   Methylbenzethonium Chloride

Toxicity Rating: 4(?). A derivative of benzethonium chloride (see above) in which a methyl radical is substituted on the benzene ring of the phenoxy group. Widely used as a germicide and disinfectant, especially in solutions and ointments against diaper rash.

See also: Benzalkonium Chloride, *Reference Congener in Section III.*
Ref.: Osol and Farrar, 1955.

993   Urolocide   993

Dodecyl carbamylmethyl dimethyl benzyl ammonium chloride,   Dodecabonium chloride

Toxicity Rating: 4. A cationic surfactant used as a disinfectant at aqueous concentrations of about 0.1%. A 5% solution is not irritating to human skin.

See also: Benzalkonium Chloride, *Reference Congener in Section III.*
Ref.: Assoc. of Amer. Pesticide Control Officials, 1966; Merck and Co., 1976.

Sanitizers and germicides (exclusive of above)

994   Chlorhexidine   994

1,6-Bis(4-chlorophenyldiguanido)hexane, 1,1′-Hexamethylenebis(5-(p-chlorophenyl)-biguanide), Chlorhexidine gluconate, Chlorhexidine hydrochloride

Toxicity Rating: 3. Broad spectrum antimicrobial compound for use in creams, gels, soaps and solutions. Very toxic when given parenterally to mice, but moderately low acute toxicity by mouth (mouse oral LD_{50} 1.8 gm./kg.). Effects observed after accidental infusions of up to a liter of 0.02% chlorhexidine solution into human patients were the same as those produced by hemodilution with water. Hepatotoxic and nephrotoxic in rats. Excretion is primarily through the bile and is slow; in radiotracer experiments in rats, 20% of the label remained in the animal for 5 days. Chlorhexidine is poorly absorbed from intact skin and does not cause skin irritation. May spontaneously decompose or be metabolized to *p*-chloroaniline.

Ref.: Chow et al., 1977; Chow et al., 1978; Honigman, 1977.

995   Dowicil 200   995

N-(3-Chloroallyl) methenamine,   1-(3-Chloroallyl)-3,5,7-triaza-1-azoniaadamantane chloride

Toxicity Rating: 3. A saturated heterocyclic compound with ring nitrogens, one of which is quaternary. Probably not strongly surface-active. Promoted as an antimicrobial agent to serve as a preservative in cosmetic formulations (liquids, powders and creams) in use concentrations of 0.05 to 0.4 percent. Even in test concentrations as high as 10 percent, it was not appreciably irritating to human skin. Also no sensitization or photosensitization. Undiluted material is slightly irritating in the eye. Not absorbed in toxic amounts through rabbit skin when applied for 21 days as a 20 percent aqueous solution. The following single-dose oral LD_{50} doses are reported in mg./kg.: 68 (rabbit), 940 (male rat), 1070 (guinea pig), 2800 (chick). The unusually high sensitivity of the rabbit is unexplained.

Ref.: Dow Chemical Co., 1971a; Dow Chemical Co., 1971b.

996   Imidazolidinyl Urea   996

Germall 115

Toxicity Rating: 2. Bactericidal preservative, widely used in such cosmetic products as shampoos, mascaras, lotions, sunscreens and facial masks. The usual concentration is 0.1 to 1%. Low acute oral toxicity in animals. In rats, single oral doses of 8 gm./kg. produced diarrhea, lethargy and weight loss but no deaths. Not irritating to skin or eyes of rabbits. Sensitization reactions have been reported in humans.

Ref.: Berke and Rosen, 1970.

997   Iodophors   997

e.g., Wescodyne

Toxicity Rating: 2. Detergent-iodine complexes used as disinfectants. Often sold as concentrates which are diluted prior to use. Wescodyne concentrate contains polyethoxy polypropoxy ethanol-iodine complex (7.75%), nonylphenylether of polyethylene glycol-iodine complex (3.75%) and inert ingredients (88.5%); it has an acute oral LD_{50} in white rats of 12 ml./kg. and in guinea pigs of 15 ml./kg. It is diluted by adding 1 to 3 oz. of concentrate to 5 gal. of water. It does not appear to be a primary irritant or a sensitizer even in the form of the concentrate.

See also: Iodine, *Reference Congener in Section III.*
Ref.: Bogash, 1955.

998   Salicylanilide   998

2-Hydroxy-*N*-phenylbenzamide,   *N*-Phenylsalicylamide, e.g., Ansadol

Toxicity Rating: 3(?). Fungicide and anti-mildew substance. Said to be of low mammalian toxicity;

rats tolerated daily doses of 1 gm./kg. for 40 days without apparent ill effect. No other toxicity data were found. Potent inhibitor of oxidative phosphorylation in rat liver mitochondria. Only slight skin irritation and no percutaneous absorption. If hydrolysis of the compound occurs in man, however, both aniline poisoning (Section III) and salicylism (Section III) might be anticipated.

Ref.: Spencer, 1973; Stetsyuk and Rotmistrov, 1971; Williamson and Metcalf, 1967.

999   999   3,3′,4′,5-Tetrachlorosalicylanilide

Halogenated salicylanilide

Toxicity Rating: 4. One of several halogenated salicylanilide derivatives with bacteriostatic and fungicidal properties. Used in soaps, textiles and petroleum products. High toxicity in rats (oral LD_{50} 240 mg./kg.), but no description of toxic symptoms was found. Addition to soaps intended for use on human skin has been restricted because of high incidence of photodermatitis in persons using such soaps.

Ref.: Calnan et al., 1961.

1000   1000   3,4′,5-Tribromosalicylanilide

Tribromsalan, TBS, e.g., Temasept II

Toxicity Rating: 4. Antiseptic and fungicide incorporated into detergents, hard surface liquid and powder cleaners, toilet soaps, creams, lotions and powders. Sometimes used in combination with 4′,5-dibromosalicylanilide; the mixture is called Temasept. Acute oral LD_{50} in rats of TBS is 500 mg./kg. Weanling rats fed 750 ppm for three months showed no growth depression. Said not to be a primary irritant or sensitizer although reports of cross-contact photosensitivity have appeared. Apparently stable to autoclaving. Although no cases of acute ingestion episodes were encountered, methemoglobinemia would appear to be a possible complication on the basis of chemical structure. See also Salicylanilide above.

Ref.: Baughman, 1964; Jillson and Baughman, 1963; Singer, 1965.

1001   1001   3,4,4′-Trichlorocarbanilide

Triclocarban, TCC

Toxicity Rating: 2. Cutaneous antiseptic used in bar soaps at concentrations of about 2%. When administered as 10% (w/v) suspension in water or corn oil, the acute oral LD_{50} was greater than 10 grams (in terms of TCC content) per kg. (body weight). TCC does not release active chlorine, and it does not appear to be a primary irritant or sensitizer on the skin. As present in soap, TCC is absorbed through the intact human skin at a barely measurable rate. By chemical assay no TCC (<25 ppb) was detected in the blood or urine of volunteers during or shortly after a 28-day intensive bathing regimen. In man, rats and Rhesus monkeys, the radioactivity of injected or absorbed C^{14}- TCC is excreted chiefly in the feces. Metabolites were largely glucuronides, either O-glucuronides formed after ring hydroxylation or N-glucuronides. In newborn monkeys, sulfate conjugates were more prevalent than O-glucuronides. All of these conjugates were excreted principally in bile. The amide bonds of TCC are not attacked *in vivo*, and so chloroanilines are not generated. Improper manufacturing practices or excessive heat (*e.g.*, autoclaving), however, may cause the formation of chloroanilines, which, if absorbed in sufficient amounts, can produce methemoglobinemia. See also *p*-chloroaniline in the index.

Ref.: Hiles et al., 1978; Howes and Black, 1976; Jeffcoat et al., 1977; Levinskas, 1972; Roman et al., 1957; Scharp et al., 1975.

1002   1002   Triclosan

2,4,4′-Trichloro-2′-hydroxydiphenyl ether,   5-Chloro-2-(2,4-dichlorophenoxy)phenol,   Irgasan DP-300

Toxicity Rating: 3. Topical disinfectant and fungicide effective against gram-positive and gram-negative organisms. Ingredient in soaps, medicated cosmetics and detergents. At use concentrations (*e.g.,* 0.5% in Ivory soap) it is not a skin irritant, sensitizer or photosensitizer. Hypoactivity, diarrhea, diuresis, and bloody nasal discharge were observed in rats given 4000 mg./kg., the approximate acute oral LD_{50} in rats and mice. In subacute studies liver damage was observed in dogs and rats which received daily oral doses of 25-200 and 125-1000 mg./kg. respectively for 13 weeks. More recent tests failed to confirm these observations at daily doses of up to 25 mg./kg. in dogs and 169 mg./kg. in rats. No illness or tissue injury was detected in baboons given by mouth (in gelatin capsules) up to 100 mg./kg. daily for 4 weeks. An observation of lung edema and necrosis in rabbits was not confirmed in a later study with daily oral doses of up to 138 mg./kg. for 13 weeks. Slightly irritating to rabbit eyes in concentrations of 1-5%; undiluted triclosan produced reversible conjunctival damage. About 9% of triclosan applied as an ointment to the forearm was absorbed by human subjects. A glucuronide of the parent compound was the major metabolite found in their urine.

Ref.: Lyman and Furia, 1969; Lyman, 1972.

1003   Tris(hydroxymethyl)nitromethane   1003

Tris nitro,   2-(Hydroxymethyl)-2-nitro-1,3-propanediol

Toxicity Rating: 3. A bactericide on non-biological surfaces and fluids. The toxicity rating is based on rat and mouse data. The nature of the toxic syndrome is not described. This substances has pro-duced no skin irritation or sensitivity among the workers who make it. Also no irritation among 25 humans subjected to exaggerated cutaneous exposures.

Ref.: Irwin, 1959; Machle et al., 1940.

Synthetic pesticides

DDT and related insecticides and acaricides

1004   Bromopropylate   1004

Isopropyl-4,4′-dibromobenzilate, Phenisobromilate, Acarol

Toxicity Rating: 2. Contact acaricide, closely related to chlorobenzilate (see below) and chloropropylate, but more resistant to enzyme detoxification.

Low acute oral toxicity in rats (LD_{50} greater than 5.0 gm./kg.). Rats tolerated 40 mg./kg. daily for four weeks without ill effect.

See also: DDT, *Reference Congener in Section III.*
Ref.: Knowles and Ahmad, 1971a; Spencer, 1973.

1005   Bulan   1005

1,1-Bis(*p*-chlorophenyl)-2-nitrobutane

Toxicity Rating: 4. Same symptoms and treatment as DDT. Can be absorbed through intact skin.

See also: DDT, *Reference Congener in Section III.*
Ref.: Lehman, 1951.

1006   Chlorobenzilate   1006

Ethyl 4,4′-dichlorobenzilate,   Ethyl di(*p*-chlorophenyl)glycollate

Toxicity Rating: 3. Miticide and acaricide for use on citrus crops. Moderately low toxicity in mice and rats. Only a slight tendency to accumulate in the body. Toxic actions are probably like those of DDT. Metabolized in dogs to yield dichlorobenzo-phenone and *p*-chlorobenzoic acid. The use of chlorobenzilate has been restricted in the United States because the compound is oncogenic in rats and mice and causes adverse testicular effects in male rats after repeated exposures.

See also: DDT, *Reference Congener in Section III.*
Ref.: EPA., July 11, 1978; Horn et al., 1955; Reuber, 1980.

1007   DDT   1007

1,1,1-Trichloro-2,2-bis(*p*-chlorophenyl)ethane, Chlorophenothane, Dichloro diphenyl trichloroethane, α,α-Bis(*p*-chlorophenyl)-β,β,β-trichloroethane

Toxicity Rating: 4.

See also: DDT, *Reference Congener in Section III.*

1008   DFDT   1008

Difluorodiphenyltrichloroethane

Toxicity Rating: 3. Similar to but less toxic than DDT. The fluorine atoms within the molecule do not appear to contribute to the symptoms.

See also: DDT, *Reference Congener in Section III.*
Ref.: Lehman, 1951.

1009   1,1-Dichloro-2,2-bis(*p*-chlorophenyl)ethane   1009

p,p′-DDD, TDE

Toxicity Rating: 3. Less toxic than DDT in animals, and poisonings are slower in onset and longer in duration. Lethargy is more prominent and convulsions are less frequent than in DDT poisoning. In chronic feeding experiments DDD, like DDT, is stored in body fat, but it is mobilized and excreted faster than DDT when a normal diet is resumed.

See also: DDT, *Reference Congener in Section III.*
Ref.: Dianol, Date Unknown.

1010   **1010 Dilan**

Toxicity Rating: 3. Mixture of Bulan (2 parts) and Prolan (1 part); see both. Same symptoms and treatment as DDT. Can be absorbed through intact skin but probably not in significant amounts.

See also: DDT, *Reference Congener in Section III.*
Ref.: Lehman, 1951.

1011   **1011 DMC**

Dimite, Di-(*p*-chlorophenyl)ethanol

Toxicity Rating: 3(?). An acaricide. Effects on humans are not known. Less toxic than DDT, but toxic actions are probably similar.

See also: DDT, *Reference Congener in Section III.*
Ref.: Grummit, 1950; Peters, 1949.

1012   **1012 Kelthane**

1,1-Bis(*p*-chlorophenyl)-2,2,2-trichloroethanol,   Dicofol

Toxicity Rating: 3. A miticide. Animal studies place compound near the borderline between toxicity classes 3 and 4. Presumably the toxic reactions resemble those in DDT poisoning.

See also: DDT, *Reference Congener in Section III.*
Ref.: Spencer, 1973; Assoc. of Amer. Pesticide Control Officials, 1966.

1013   **1013 Methoxychlor**

Methoxy-DDT,   1,1,1-Trichloro-2,2-bis(*p*-methoxyphenyl)ethane

Toxicity Rating: 3. Lower toxicity than DDT. Estimated to be one-tenth as toxic in man by ingestion, but this difference may not hold in respiratory exposures to vapor. In animals central nervous depression is more prominent than excitation, and poisonings are slower in onset and longer in duration than after DDT. A uterotrophic action has been described in rodents.

See also: DDT, *Reference Congener in Section III.*
Ref.: Hodge et al., 1950; Hodge et al., 1952a; Tullner, 1961.

1014   **1014 Neotran**

Toxicity Rating: 2. A wettable powder with 40% bis(parachlorophenoxy)methane. A miticide of very low toxicity in laboratory mammals. Only slight percutaneous absorption and no skin irritation. It has produced liver pathology in laboratory animals. No human poisonings are known.

See also: DDT, *Reference Congener in Section III.*
Ref.: Spencer et al., 1950a.

1015   **1015 Perthane**

Dichloro-bis(*p*-ethylphenyl)ethane

Toxicity Rating: 2. In animals toxic signs and symptoms are like those in DDT poisoning, but the toxicity is much lower (near the borderline between toxicity classes 2 and 3). There is little, if any, percutaneous absorption, skin irritation, or sensitization. Unlike DDT, feeding tests in rats with radioactive Perthane indicate little tendency for the material to deposit in body fat.

See also: DDT, *Reference Congener in Section III.*
Ref.: Cobey et al., 1956; Finnegan et al., 1955.

1016   **1016 Prolan**

1,1-Bis(*p*-chlorophenyl)-2-nitropropane

Toxicity Rating: 3. Same symptoms and treatment as DDT poisoning. Can be absorbed through intact skin. In rats symptoms may be prolonged for several days (unlike DDT or bulan).

See also: DDT, *Reference Congener in Section III.*
Ref.: Lehman, 1951.

Cyclodiene insecticides

1017   Aldrin   1017

Hexachloro-hexahydro-*endo,exo*-dimethanonaphthalene

Toxicity Rating: 5. Animal tests place this compound near the border line between toxicity classes 4 and 5. Similar, chemically and toxicologically, to dieldrin.

See also: Dieldrin, *Reference Congener in Section III.*
Ref.: Shell Chemical Co., 1959; Spiotta, 1951.

1018   Bandane   1018

Polychlorodicyclopentadiene

Toxicity Rating: 4. A mixture of isomers containing 60-62% chlorine used as a preemergence herbicide against crab grass and to control ants and grubs in turf. Acute oral LD_{50} in rats increases with body weight, i.e., in males with an average body weight of 92 gm. the LD_{50} was 370 mg./kg. but at 395 gm. it was 1020 mg./kg. The same trend was observed in females without significant sex differences. In acutely poisoned animals, the symptoms were like those induced by other halogenated hydrocarbon insecticides: tremor, hypersensitivity to sensory stimuli, convulsions and coma with death occurring in 6 hr. to 11 days. Liver pathology was confined to animals which died after convulsions. Mildly irritating to rabbit skin. Dermal LD_{50} of Bandane in xylol was about 12.5 gm./kg. in rats. Rats tolerated up to 500 ppm in diet for 16 weeks without significant effects on growth or food consumption, but moderate liver pathology and a few deaths occurred. Vapors have a low order of toxicity. In acutely poisoned sheep and cattle, signs were said to mimic those of tetanus.

See also: Chlordane, *Reference Congener in Section III.*
Ref.: Eisler, 1965; Palmer and Radeleff, 1964.

1019   Chlordane   1019

Chlordan,   Octachloro-4,7-methanohydroindane

Toxicity Rating: 4. Probably chlordane is best described as lying on the borderline between toxicity classes 3 and 4.

See also: Chlordane, *Reference Congener in Section III.*
Ref.: Ambrose et al., 1953.

1020   Dieldrin   1020

Hexachloro-epoxy-octahydro-*endo,exo*-dimethanonaphthalene

Toxicity Rating: 5. Believed to lie near the borderline between toxicity classes 4 and 5.

See also: Dieldrin, *Reference Congener in Section III.*

1021   Endrin   1021

Hexachloro-epoxy-octahydro-*endo,endo*-dimethanonaphthalene

Toxicity Rating: 5. A stereoisomer of dieldrin, several times more toxic than the latter but producing similar symptoms. In England over 100 people were poisoned from eating bread made from flour contaminated with endrin. Within 1 to 3 hours of eating, the more acutely ill patients were unconscious; others exhibited epileptiform convulsions, sometimes accompanied by violent muscular contractions and periods of unconsciousness. Injuries to bones and joints were sustained by falling. Those more mildly afflicted suffered from weakness, nausea, twitching and tingling of the limbs, deafness and mental confusion. All recovered without complications although some were ill for several days.

See also: Dieldrin, *Reference Congener in Section III.*
Ref.: Anonymous, 1956; Shell Chemical Co., 1960a.

1022   Heptachlor   1022

Heptachloro-tetrahydro-4,7-*endo*-methanoindene, Heptachlorodicyclopentadiene

Toxicity Rating: 4. White crystalline solid readily soluble in petroleum distillates, alcohols and ketones. Usual technical product also contains related compounds. Once widely used as an insecticide but now limited to use for underground termite control. No human fatalities have been reported, but in animals heptachlor is more toxic than chlordane (above) to which it is closely related. Acute mean lethal dose by mouth in rats and rabbits 80 to 90 mg./kg. Dangerous by ingestion, skin absorption or spray inhalation. Liver necrosis was the only pathological lesion found in acutely poisoned animals. Chronic exposures produce inanition in animals and accumulation in body fat. The storage form is the epoxide metabolite, which is apparently more toxic than the parent compound. Blood dyscrasias such as megaloblastic anemia should be anticipated. Heptachlor is a known inducer of hepatic microsomal enzymes and is carcinogenic for the liver in mice.

See also: Chlordane, *Reference Congener in Section III*.
Ref.: Davidow and Radomski, 1953; Davidson et al., 1953; Lehman, 1951; Radomski and Davidow, 1953; von Oettingen, 1955.

1023   1023 Hexachloro-epoxy-octahydro-dimethanonaphthalene

Toxicity Rating: 5. Dieldrin or its isomer endrin. Based on animal tests, endrin above lies distinctly within toxicity class 5, whereas dieldrin above lies near the borderline between classes 4 and 5. Toxic signs and symptoms are indistinguishable, however.

See also: Dieldrin, *Reference Congener in Section III*.

1024   1024 Isobenzan

Octachloro-hexahydro-methanoisobenzofuran, Octachloro-*endo*-methylene-tetrahydrophthalan, Telodrin

Toxicity Rating: 6. Halogenated hydrocarbon insecticide probably lying on the borderline between toxicity classes 5 and 6 (acute oral LD_{50} for male rats 4.8 to 5.5 mg./kg.). Very toxic by all routes; comparable to endrin. Produces hyperirritability, convulsions and frothing at the mouth in animals.

See also: Dieldrin, *Reference Congener in Section III*.
Ref.: Shell Chemical Co., 1961.

1025   1025 Isodrin

Hexachloro-hexahydro-*endo,endo*-dimethanonaphthalene

Toxicity Rating: 5. Related to Aldrin above, but at least twice as toxic in laboratory rodents.

See also: Dieldrin, *Reference Congener in Section III*.
Ref.: Assoc. of Amer. Pesticide Control Officials, 1966.

1026   1026 Thiodan

Endosulfan, Hexachloro-hexahydro-methano-2,4,3-benzodioxathiepin oxide

Toxicity Rating: 4. A heterocyclic sulfur compound serving as an agricultural insecticide. As a dust it is probably only moderately toxic by inhalation, but in solution, especially in alcohol or aromatic solvents like xylene, it is considered as toxic by ingestion and by percutaneous absorption as are dieldrin or aldrin, to which it is chemically related. Systemic poisoning causes nervousness, agitation, tremors, and convulsions. Not a cholinesterase inhibitor.

See also: Dieldrin, *Reference Congener in Section III*.
Ref.: Niagara Chemical, 1959d.

Other chlorinated hydrocarbon insecticides and acaricides

1027   1027 Dienochlor

Perchlorobi(cyclopenta-2,4-dienyl),   Pentac

Toxicity Rating: 3(?). A specific miticide with slow initial and long residual actions, it has no insecticidal activity and is non-phytotoxic. Recommended for use on indoor floral crops and nursery stocks. This tan crystalline solid is commercially available as a 50% wettable powder and as an emulsifiable concentrate (1.5 lbs./gallon). Dienochlor is a central nervous system stimulant. The toxicity rating of 3 is based on the oral, single-dose LD_{50} in rats. As judged by man's reaction to other highly chlorinated pesticides (*e.g.,* lindane, chlordane, toxaphene), a toxicity rating of 4 may be more appropriate for man, but we know of no human poisonings. The recommended treatment is the same as for other chlorinated pesticides, namely barbiturates and/or diazepam to suppress convulsions and then decontamination of the eye, skin and stomach to limit absorption.

See also: Chlordane, *Reference Congener in Section III*.

1028   1028 Lindane

γ-Hexachlorocyclohexane, Gamma benzene hexachloride, GBH

Toxicity Rating: 4. The name lindane usually refers to the gamma isomer of 1,2,3,4,5,6-hexachlorocyclohexane, but at one time it was occasionally used to mean any of 8 stereoisomers of this compound. In commerce, agriculture, and medicine, the name benzene hexachloride is synonymous with hexa-

See also: Lindane, *Reference Congener in Section III.*

chlorocyclohexane and should not be confused with hexachlorobenzene. Lindane is an insecticide, and a potent convulsant in mammals.

1029 Benzene Hexachloride   1029

Hexachlorocyclohexane, BHC, HCCH

Toxicity Rating: 4. Benzene hexachloride (more properly called 1,2,3,4,5,6-hexachlorocyclohexane) in its various forms was once a widely used insecticide, especially in the control of cotton insects. The technical mixture contained the following approximate isomeric composition: α 65-70%, β 6-8%, γ 12-15%, δ 2-5% and others 5-10%. These isomers differ qualitatively and quantitatively in biological activity. The α- and γ-isomers are central nervous stimulants; the β- and δ-isomers are depressants.

See also: Lindane, *Reference Congener in Section III.*

In such a mixture it is possible that one component may antidote another. Most of the insecticidal activity resides with the γ-isomer known as lindane. In the U.S.A. all BHC registrations have been changed administratively to lindane registrations. In commerce, agriculture and medicine, the name benzene hexachloride is synonymous with hexachlorocyclohexane and should not be confused with hexachlorobenzene.

1030 Toxaphene   1030

Chlorinated camphene, Octachlorocamphene

Toxicity Rating: 5. A complex mixture of chlorinated derivatives of camphene used as an insecticide. Induces epileptiform convulsions in poisoned

See also: Toxaphene, *Reference Congener in Section III.*

mammals. Believed to lie near the borderline between toxicity classes 4 and 5. The lethal oral dose for an adult person is estimated to be 4 to 7 gm.

1031 Strobane   1031

Chlorinated terpenes, Terpene polychlorinates, Heptachlorocamphene

Toxicity Rating: 4. Only one-third to one-quarter as acutely toxic as toxaphene in animals, but poisonings are thought to be similar in terms of symptoms and treatment. Strobane does not cause pri-

See also: Toxaphene, *Reference Congener in Section III.*
Ref.: Goodrich, 1955.

mary skin irritation or sensitization in man. Percutaneous toxicity is very low in rabbits and presumably in man too.

1032 Kepone   1032

Chlordecone, Compound 1189, Decachloro-octahydro-1,3,4-metheno-2*H*-cyclobuta(cd)pentalen-2-one, Decachloropentacyclodecan-4-one

Toxicity Rating: 4. A hydrated complex chlorinated polycyclic ketone used as an insecticide and fungicide. Available as water dispersible powder, emulsifiable concentrate and granular or dust formulations in foreign commerce but largely banned in the U.S.A. The oral LD$_{50}$ is 95.5 mg./kg. in rats and about 65 mg./kg. in rabbits. The percutaneous LD$_{50}$ in rabbits is 435 mg./kg. Typical DDT-like tremors developed, and death in the acute phase was preceded by complete prostration. Chemical workers repeatedly exposed to high concentrations of kepone dust developed nervousness and tremors, visual disturbances including rapid erratic eye movement, and occasionally ataxia, chest pain, arthralgia, erythematous skin eruption, and weight loss. Oligospermia was found in some workers. Kepone

See also: Lindane, *Reference Congener in Section III.*
Ref.: Boylan et al., 1978; Cannon et al., 1978; Cohn et al., 1978; Huber, 1965; Jaeger, 1976; Jennings, 1958.

is said to be excreted in bile and probably by nonbiliary routes as well, but it is resorbed in intestine. Oral doses of cholestyramine, an ion exchange resin, increased the rate of excretion and the recovery from exposed persons. Sensory stimulation triggered or intensified tremors, even as long as 4 weeks after the exposure. It is possible that a repository of the compound is created in cutaneous tissue or elsewhere from which it is gradually mobilized. Kepone has highly cumulative toxic effects. In rats the 3-month LD$_{50}$ is 3.2 mg./kg. per day, the 6-month LD$_{50}$ is 1.5 mg./kg. per day. Rats and mice given 40 ppm in food for 80 weeks showed a significantly increased incidence of hepatocellular carcinoma.

1033   **1033   Mirex**

Dechlorane, Dodecachloropentacyclodecane, GC-1283

Toxicity Rating: 4. A chlorinated hydrocarbon fire retardant and insecticide (especially useful against fire ants) manufactured by the dimerization of hexachloropentadiene. High acute oral toxicity (rat oral LD_{50} is 360 to 740 mg./kg.). Percutaneous LD_{50} in rabbits is 850 mg./kg. Like kepone (see above), mirex increases central excitability and causes tremors and presumably convulsions. Administration to pregnant rats and nursing dams at the rate of 5 ppm in food produced a high incidence (1% and 38% respectively) of cataracts in the pups. Repeated doses of 6 mg./kg. during organogenesis produced visceral abnormalities. Chronic feeding produced severe reproductive impairment in mice. The compound is also hepatotoxic and hepatocarcinogenic in rats. Mirex is slowly converted in the environment to kepone and other dechlorinated monohydro derivatives; the major photodecomposition product is photomirex (8-monohydromirex). Twelve years after mirex was deposited on the ground, 50% was recovered from soil samples; 10% was identified as kepone, 20% as photomirex. Both compounds are lipophilic and accumulate in the food chain. Kepone residues have been detected in human breast milk in areas treated with mirex. Photomirex may be more hepatotoxic than mirex. The cumulative oral LD_{50} in mice of photomirex is 225-250 mg./kg. In chronic feeding studies with photomirex, mottled livers and kidneys and lesions of the thyroid were found in rats; both weight loss in mice and severe liver hypertrophy in rats were found to be dose-dependent, and the mixed function oxidase system in male rats was enhanced.

See also: Lindane, *Reference Congener in Section III.*
Ref.: Allied Chemical Corp., 1965; Fujimori et al., 1980; National Research Council, 1978; Villeneuve et al., 1979; Ware and Good, 1967.

Aliphatic thiocyanate insecticides

1034   **1034   Aliphatic Thiocyanates**

e.g., Methyl thiocyanate,   Ethyl thiocyanate,   Lethanes

A series of agricultural insecticides. When tested in animals, various organic thiocyanates differ widely in toxicity.

See also: Aliphatic Thiocyanates, *Reference Congener in Section III.*

1035   **1035   β-Butoxy-β-thiocyanodiethyl Ether**

Lethane 384

Toxicity Rating: 5. Contact insecticide, highly toxic to mammals. Rat oral LD_{50} is 35 mg./kg. In experimental animals, deaths occur in 0.5 to 3 hours. Toxicity is probably due to the metabolic formation of cyanide. For symptoms and suggested treatment, see Aliphatic Thiocyanates in Section III. Toxic doses can be absorbed through intact skin. Irritating to skin and mucous membranes. The commercial preparation is 50% kerosene by volume.

See also: Aliphatic Thiocyanates, *Reference Congener in Section III.*
Ref.: Cameron et al., 1939; Draize et al., 1944b; El-Sabae and Khamis, 1975; Harrison, 1947.

1036   **1036   Lauryl Thiocyanate**

Lauryl rhodanate, Dodecyl thiocyanate

Toxicity Rating: 3. Low toxicity in animals, but a human fatality has resulted from ingesting a mixture of lauryl thiocyanate (14 gm.) and Lethane 384 (6 gm.).

See also: Aliphatic Thiocyanates, *Reference Congener in Section III.*
Ref.: Cameron et al., 1939; Harrison, 1947.

1037   **1037   Lethane 60**

Lauric acid 2-thiocyanatoethyl ester,   β-Thiocyanoethyl esters of fatty acids

Toxicity Rating: 4. Mixed with an equal volume of petroleum solvent, it is marketed as a contact insecticide. The commercial product contains a mixture of esters of fatty acids ranging from C_{10} to C_{18}, with an average composition like that of the lauric ester. The pure liquid has a high toxicity (oral rat LD_{50} about 400 mg./kg.) and is moderately irritating to skin and mucous membranes. Probably not a precursor of inorganic cyanide in vivo.

See also: Aliphatic Thiocyanates, *Reference Congener in Section III.*

1038   Thanite   1038

Isobornyl thiocyanoacetate

Toxicity Rating: 4. Refers to technical grade iso-bornyl thiocyanoacetate which is about 80% pure. Other terpenes are also present. Contact insecticide, knock-down agent, and useful as a synergist with other classes of insecticides (pyrethrum, carbamates, chlorinated hydrocarbons). May be used to control human lice. Animal studies place Thanite near the borderline between toxicity classes 3 and 4. Acute oral LD_{50} is 1.6 gm./kg. in rats and 550 mg./kg. in guinea pigs. For symptoms and treatment of intoxication, see Aliphatic Thiocyanates in Section III. Primary irritant on human skin in high concentrations but not in dilute solutions. In rabbits, percutaneous absorption is slow but systemic poisoning can be induced by repeated applications.

See also: Aliphatic Thiocyanates, *Reference Congener in Section III.*
Ref.: Lehman, 1951.

Miscellaneous acaricides (miticides)

1039   Amitraz   1039

N'-(2,4-Dimethylphenyl)-N-(2,4-dimethylphenyl)iminomethyl-N-methylmethanimidamide,
N,N'-(Methyliminodimethylidyne)bis-2,4-xylidine,   Baam

Toxicity Rating: 3. Acaricide and insecticide for control of ticks and mites on cattle and sheep; also used to control psylla infestations of pears. Moderate acute oral toxicity (rat oral LD_{50} 800 mg./kg.). Potent inhibitor of rat liver monoamine oxidase *in vitro*. Metabolic products include 2,4-dimethylaniline, which is a relatively weak methemoglobin-former in dogs and presumably in man. The no-effect level in 2-year feeding experiments in dogs was 1 mg./kg. daily.

Ref.: Aziz and Knowles, 1973.

1040   Aramite   1040

2-(p-*tert*-Butylphenoxy)isopropyl 2-choroethyl sulfite

Toxicity Rating: 3. Aramite-15W is a 15% wettable powder. Studies of acute toxicity in laboratory mammals place this acaricide near the borderline between toxicity classes 2 and 3 (rat oral LD_{50} 3.9 gm./kg.). A large oral dose causes central nervous depression of long duration. The principal autopsy finding in animals was a hemorrhagic syndrome involving particularly the lungs. Undiluted Aramite (an oil) and its concentrated solutions are irritating to the skin and conjunctiva. Chronic ingestion at high levels has induced hepatic adenomas and gall bladder adenocarcinomas in experimental animals. Production of Aramite was suspended by the Uniroyal Company, and EPA registration was voluntarily withdrawn in 1976-77 because of its high carcinogenic potential.

Ref.: Naugatuck Chemical, 1951b; Oser and Oser, 1960; Oser and Oser, 1962.

1041   Azobenzene   1041

Diphenyldiazene, Azobenzol, Benzeneazobenzene, Diazobenzene, Diphenyl diimide

Toxicity Rating: 4. A miticidal fumigant for use in greenhouses. Usually prepared as a paste (70%) which is applied to steampipes and thus vaporized. Also available in pyrotechnic form. Its toxicity is not well characterized. Dogs fed 600 ppm for 63 days suffered high mortality and liver damage. Rats tolerated 75 mg. (i.p. injection) although 100 mg. (i.p.) was often fatal. Azobenzene is reduced and cleaved in the liver and other organs; aniline, benzidine and hydrazobenzene sulfate were identified in the urine of rats given azobenzene. If the conversion to aniline is significant in man, methemoglobinemia may result. A 19-year old boy ingested 50 ml. of Azomite, a mixture of azobenzene and Aramite. Symptoms first appeared after 19 hours and included jaundice and sporadic unconsciousness. Hepatic coma occurred after 4 days and death from "cardiac insufficiency" after 6 days.

See also: Aniline, *Reference Congener in Section III.*
Ref.: Assoc. of Amer. Pesticide Control Officials, 1966; Elson and Warren, 1944; Fouts et al., 1957; Spencer, 1973; Tsunenari, 1973.

1042   Chlordimeform   1042

N'-(4-Chloro-2-methylphenyl)-N,N-dimethylmethanimidamide, N'-(4-Chloro-o-tolyl)-N,N-dimethylformamidine,   Chlorphenamidine

Toxicity Rating: 4. An ascaricide, ovicide and insecticide derived from chloroaniline. Used on cotton crops and fruit trees against many pests resistant to carbamates and organophosphates. Its mechanism of action is interference with the amine regulatory mechanisms of the target species. The acute oral LD_{50} in rats of the technical grade product is 170-340 mg./kg. and of the formulations is 220-350 mg./kg. Workers packaging chlordimeform powder developed severe hemorrhagic cystitis. The causative agent was believed to be 2-methyl-4-chloroaniline, the major metabolite of chlordimeform. Chlordimeform is known to inhibit monoamine oxidase, uncouple mitochondrial energy metabolism and produce local anesthesia in mammals, but the rapid onset of tremors and convulsions produced by lethal doses in laboratory animals cannot be fully explained by these actions. Studies with dogs, cats and isolated rabbit hearts indicate that chlordimeform has a direct depressant effect on cardiac and vascular smooth muscle, resulting in severe hypotension and death. It may also have a direct excitatory effect on neurons; lethal doses in rats have produced hyperexcitability followed by rapid death. Methemoglobinemia has not been described, but it occurs with closely related chloroanilines (see 3-chloro-4-methylaniline in the index). Chlordimeform is mildly irritating to rabbit skin and eyes. One manufacturer states that the expected early signs of poisoning by his product are nausea, vomiting and lethargy. Chlordimeform and its hydrochloride salt are available as emulsifiable concentrates, water-soluble powders, dusts and granules.

See also: Aniline, *Reference Congener in Section III.*
Ref.: Kimbrough, 1980; Lund et al., 1978.

1043   1043   *p*-Chlorobenzyl *p*-Chlorophenyl Sulfide

Mitox, Chlorbenside

Toxicity Rating: 3. A long-lasting acaricide acting primarily against eggs. Its toxicity in laboratory rodents is like that of Ovotran. See Ovotran below.

Ref.: Assoc. of Amer. Pesticide Control Officials, 1966; Spencer, 1973.

1044   1044   Eradex

2,3-Quinoxalinedithiol cyclic trithiocarbonate, Thioquinox, Chinothionat

Toxicity Rating: 3. An effective contact miticide used as dusts and wettable powders on forage and fruit crops. Acute oral LD_{50} of 2 gm./kg. in female rats and 1.8 gm./kg. in male rats; in male guinea pigs 1.0 gm./kg. Mild to moderate irritant. Apparently has a low inhalation hazard. In rats fed at levels of 100 mg./kg. per day it produced weakness, weight loss, and one death after 2 weeks. The mode of death remains to be investigated.

Ref.: Chemagro Corp., 1959; Chemagro Corp., 1961h.

1045   1045   Fluorbenside

Fluorsulphacide,   *p*-Chlorobenzyl *p*-fluorophenyl sulfide,   Fluorparacide

Toxicity Rating: 3. An acaricide with an acute mammalian toxicity higher than Chlorbenside (see latter above). Rats on a daily dose of 50 mg./kg. for 3 weeks showed slight enlargement of liver and kidneys.

Ref.: Spencer, 1973.

1046   1046   Genite

2,4-Dichlorophenol benzenesulfonate,   EM-923,   Genitol 923,   DPBS

Toxicity Rating: 3. An agricultural miticide. In acutely poisoned animals vomiting, unsteadiness, generalized weakness and fine tremors preceded death which occurred in from 1 to 4 days. Rabbits and dogs showed markedly dilated hearts and hemorrhagic areas throughout the gastrointestinal tract. It is absorbed through the intact skin of rabbits.

Ref.: Smith et al., 1959.

1047   1047   Ovotran

Toxicity Rating: 3. Parachlorophenyl parachlorobenzene sulfonate is the active ingredient (50%). An acaricide of moderately low oral toxicity in laboratory animals. Kidney and liver damage in the rat during chronic exposures. Causes skin irritation in man, but no other symptoms have been reported.

Ref.: Assoc. of Amer. Pesticide Control Officials, 1966; Spencer, 1973.

1048   1048   Sulphenone

p-Chlorophenyl phenyl sulfone,   4-Chlorodiphenyl sulfone

Toxicity Rating: 3. An acaricide of moderately low oral toxicity to laboratory mammals. No skin irritation. No significant tissue storage in chronic feeding tests.

Ref.: Assoc. of Amer. Pesticide Control Officials, 1966; Spencer, 1973.

1049   Tetradifon 1049

Tedion, 2,4,5,4'-Tetrachlorodiphenyl sulfone, Duphar

Toxicity Rating: 2. A miticide with a low mammalian toxicity. No reports of human poisonings have followed its extensive use in Europe. Dermal and corneal applications are mildly irritating to test animals.

Ref.: Niagara Chemical, 1959c.

Organophosphorus pesticides: phosphates and phosphonates

1050   Organic Phosphorus Insecticides 1050

OPI

Many alkyl phosphates, thiophosphates, and pyrophosphates are used for pest control, especially as insecticides, acaricides and nematocides. Most of them are highly toxic, but examples ranging from toxicity classes 3 to 6 are recognized. Toxic effects are referable to the central and autonomic nervous systems and are associated with cholinesterase inhibition. Many of the more important agents are listed below, including a few that are used primarily as herbicides and defoliants.

See also: Parathion, *Reference Congener in Section III.*

1051   Bidrin 1051

3-(Dimethoxyphosphinyloxy)-*N,N*-dimethyl-*cis*-crotonamide

Toxicity Rating: 5. Insecticide of the cholinesterase inhibitor type. Acute oral LD_{50} in mice 15 mg./kg., in rats 22 mg./kg. Acute dermal LD_{50} for rabbits 225 mg./kg. Closely related in structure and toxicity to Azodrin. Also related chemically to the slightly less toxic Ciodrin (α-methylbenzyl-3-(dimethoxyphosphinyloxy)-*cis*-crotonate, also known as dimethyl phosphate of alpha-methylbenzyl 3-hydroxy-*cis*-crotonate). Corresponding LD_{50}'s of the latter are 90, 125, and 385 mg./kg.

See also: Parathion, *Reference Congener in Section III.*
Ref.: Shell Chemical Co., 1962; Shell Chemical Co., 1963.

1052   Bomyl 1052

Dimethyl-1,3-di(carbomethoxy)-1-propen-2-yl-phosphate, Dimethyl 3-hydroxyglutaconate dimethyl phosphate

Toxicity Rating: 5. A phosphate insecticide insoluble in water or kerosene but soluble in acetone, alcohol, propylene glycol and xylene. Available as wettable powder and emulsifiable concentrate. Acute oral LD_{50} in albino rats is 32 mg./kg.

See also: Parathion, *Reference Congener in Section III.*
Ref.: Ram, 1965.

1053   Dichlorvos 1053

O,O-Dimethyl-*O*-2,2-dichlorovinyl phosphate, e.g., DDVP, Vapona

Toxicity Rating: 4. Chlorinated organic phosphate insecticide with an appreciable vapor pressure. Incorporated into plastic strips it slowly releases dichlorvos vapor. Such products have been approved for use in the disinfection of homes and aircraft. Acute oral LD_{50}'s in male rats 107 mg./kg., in females 75 mg./kg. Brief exposures of humans (30-60 min.) to concentrations as high as 6.9 μgm./l. did not result in clinical effects or significant depression of cholinesterase activity. As tested under use conditions a moderate decrease in plasma (but not red cell) cholinesterase activity occurred in hospitalized patients exposed 24 hours a day to airborne concentrations above 0.1 mg./m^3. No symptoms referable to cholinesterase inhibition were encountered. Dichlorvos is rapidly inactivated by mammalian liver enzymes, and patients with hepatic insufficiency may be less tolerant to its toxic effects. The antidotal effects of atropine and 2-PAM are additive in animals. Late paralysis has not been encountered in animals.

See also: Parathion, *Reference Congener in Section III.*
Ref.: Cavagna et al., 1969; Durham et al., 1957; Durham et al., 1959; Hodgson and Casida, 1962; Jaques, 1964; Laws, 1966.

1054   Diethyl 2-Chlorovinyl Phosphate 1054

Compound 1836

Toxicity Rating: 5. An organophosphate insecticide, that is almost as toxic in rats as parathion.

See also: Parathion, *Reference Congener in Section III.*
Ref.: Spencer, 1973.

1055

1055 Naled

O,O-Dimethyl O-(1,2-dibromo-2,2-dichloroethyl)phosphate, e.g., Dibrom, Ortho 4355

Toxicity Rating: 4. Organic phosphate insecticide available as emulsions, dusts and granules; considerably less toxic than parathion and some other cholinesterase inhibitors. Slightly higher toxic potential than malathion. Acute oral LD_{50} in rats 430 mg./kg. Dermal LD_{50} on rats 1,100 mg./kg.

See also: Parathion, *Reference Congener in Section III*.
Ref.: Toland, 1965.

1056

1056 Paraoxon

O,O-Diethyl O-p-nitrophenyl phosphate

Toxicity Rating: 6. One of the most toxic organic phosphate insecticides. Relatively high stability may cause residue problems. Toxic effects appear rapidly after exposure.

See also: Parathion, *Reference Congener in Section III*.
Ref.: Holtz and Westermann, 1959.

1057

1057 Phosdrin

2-Carbomethoxy-1-methylvinyl dimethyl phosphate, 3-Hydroxycrotonic acid methyl ester dimethyl phosphate, Mevinphos

Toxicity Rating: 6. Extremely dangerous by the inhalation of vapor, by skin contact, and by oral administration. About 60% of the commercial material consists of the supertoxic alpha isomer. A beta isomer is less than one-tenth as toxic.

See also: Parathion, *Reference Congener in Section III*.
Ref.: Shell Chemical Co., 1960d.

1058

1058 Phosphamidon

2-Chloro-2-diethylcarbamoyl-1-methylvinyl dimethyl phosphate,   Dimecron

Toxicity Rating: 5. An organic phosphate insecticide which is less toxic than parathion but more toxic than malathion. Toxic effects are due to cholinesterase inhibition.

See also: Parathion, *Reference Congener in Section III*.
Ref.: Assoc. of Amer. Pesticide Control Officials, 1966; Spencer, 1973.

1059

1059 Pyrazoxon

O,O-Diethyl-O-(3-methyl-5-pyrazolyl) phosphate,   Methyl pyrazolyldiethyl phosphate

Toxicity Rating: 6. An intensely toxic organic phosphate insecticide lying near the borderline between toxicity classes 5 and 6 in studies on mice.

See also: Parathion, *Reference Congener in Section III*.
Ref.: Assoc. of Amer. Pesticide Control Officials, 1966.

1060

1060 Butonate

O,O-Dimethyl-2,2,2-trichloro-1-n-butyryloxyethyl phosphonate

Toxicity Rating: 3. Organic phosphate insecticide of the cholinesterase inhibitor type. Its relatively low mammalian toxicity is attributed to rapid hydrolysis of the butyl and phosphate ester groupings. The approximate oral LD_{50} in rats is 1.1 gm./kg.; the subcutaneous and intraperitoneal LD_{50} values are both 0.7 gm./kg., and the dermal LD_{50} is about 7 gm./kg.

See also: Parathion, *Reference Congener in Section III*.
Ref.: Prentiss Drug and Chemical Co., 1960.

1061

1061 Tetrachlorvinfos

2-Chloro-1-(2,4,5-trichlorophenyl)vinyl dimethyl phosphate, 2-Chloro-1-(2,4,5-trichlorophenyl)ethenyl phosphoric acid dimethyl ester, Stirofos

Toxicity Rating: 2-3. An organophosphate insecticide used to control pests of livestock and food crops. Tetrachlorvinfos is among the least toxic of the cholinesterase inhibitors, probably because of its low solubility. The two available isomers have the same acute oral toxicity in the rat (4-5 gm./kg.). There is no record of a severe or fatal human intoxication, but the expected signs and symptoms of overexposure are increased perspiration, lacrimation and salivation, headache, blurred vision, nausea, diarrhea, pulmonary edema, respiratory embarrassment and possibly convulsions. Chronic exposures may lead to skin sensitization and gradual depletion of cholinesterase activity. Solvents used in commercial formulations may be responsible for skin irritation. Tetrachlorvinfos is available as emulsifiable concentrates, wettable powders and dust and also in a special formulation for mixing with cattle feed. In 2-year chronic feeding studies at concentrations of 8,000 to 16,000 ppm, technical grade tetrachlorvinfos was deemed carcinogenic to mice and responsible for hyperplastic thyroid lesions and adrenal cortical adenomas in rats.

See also: Parathion, *Reference Congener in Section III.*
Ref.: National Cancer Institute, 1978o; Shell Chemical Co., 1974; Whetstone et al., 1966.

1062   Trichlorfon   1062

Dimethyl trichlorohydroxyethylphosphonate

Toxicity Rating: 4. Toxicity relatively low among organic phosphate insecticides, although a potent cholinesterase inhibitor in vitro. Rapid and complete recovery from sublethal doses in laboratory animals.

See also: Parathion, *Reference Congener in Section III.*
Ref.: Chemagro Corp., 1961f; Edson and Noakes, 1960.

Organophosphorus pesticides: phosphorothioates and phosphonothioates

1063   Abate   1063

O,O,O',O'-Tetramethyl-*O,O'*-thiodi-*p*-phenylene phosphorothioate

Toxicity Rating: 3. Organophosphate of the cholinesterase inhibitor type used as a mosquito larvicide. Available as a 50% emulsifiable concentrate and as granules containing up to 5% Abate. In mammalian species it produces typical signs and symptoms of cholinesterase inhibition together with depression of plasma and red cellcholinesterase activity. Also leg weakness in chickens. Acute oral LD$_{50}$'s of pure Abate 2.0 gm./kg. in male rats and 2.3 gm./kg. in female rats. On rabbit skin LD$_{50}$'s of 1.9 gm./kg. (males) and 1.0 gm./kg. (females). Focal or diffuse necrosis of the liver occurred in some rabbits given 100 mg./kg. per day for 5 days. Mixtures of Abate and malathion are appreciably more toxic in rats than either compound alone. Human volunteers each ingested 256 mg./day for 5 days or 64 mg./day for 4 weeks without symptoms or detectable effects on plasma or red cell cholinesterase activity.

See also: Parathion, *Reference Congener in Section III.*
Ref.: Gaines et al., 1967; Golz and Shaffer, 1966; Laws et al., 1967.

1064   Chlorpyrifos   1064

O,O-Diethyl-*O*-(3,5,6-trichloro-2-pyridyl)phosphorothioate, Dursban

Toxicity Rating: 4(?). Cholinesterase inhibitor used as an insecticide. May produce delayed neurotoxicity in susceptible species. Toxicity rating for man appears in some doubt because of considerable species variations in acute oral LD$_{50}$'s: rat 163 mg./kg., guinea pig 500 mg./kg., sheep, 800 mg./kg. Dermal LD$_{50}$ in rabbits is 1.4 gm./kg. Calves sprayed with 214-428 mg./kg. showed no ill-effects. Causes skin and eye irritation.

See also: Parathion, *Reference Congener in Section III.*
Ref.: Bisultanov, 1974; Wolf, 1967.

1065   Chlorthion   1065

O,O-Dimethyl *O*-(3-chloro-4-nitrophenyl)thiophosphate

Toxicity Rating: 3. Toxic symptoms in animals resemble parathion poisoning. Conflicting reports about experimental lethal doses, but toxicity is low, in spite of high in vitro anticholinesterase potency (a distinction ascribed to slow tissue absorption). Little, if any, percutaneous toxicity (in rabbits and guinea pigs).

See also: Parathion, *Reference Congener in Section III.*
Ref.: Chemagro Corp., 1955.

1066   Coumaphos   1066

O,O-Diethyl *O*-3-chloro-4-methyl-2-oxo-2*H*-1-benzopyran-7-yl-phosphorothioate,   Co-Ral

Toxicity Rating: 4. An organic phosphate compound used as an insecticide and anthelmintic against cattle parasites. Toxic symptoms consisting of diarrhea, salivation, difficult breathing, stiffness of legs and neck are due largely if not exclusively to cholinesterase inhibition.

See also: Parathion, *Reference Congener in Section III.*
Ref.: Assoc. of Amer. Pesticide Control Officials, 1966; Spencer, 1973; Chemagro Corp., 1961b.

1067   Demeton

1067

Systox

Toxicity Rating: 5. Mixture of two active isomers: *O,O*-diethyl *O*-2-(ethylthio)ethylphosphorothioate (2 parts), also called Demeton O, and *O,O*-diethyl *S*-2-(ethylthio)ethylphosphorothioate (1 part), also called Demeton S. Demeton O has the higher acute toxicity in rats. A "systemic" insecticide, i.e., trans-located in sap to all parts of plants. Almost as toxic as parathion in animals when given orally or by inhalation. Percutaneous toxicity is higher than parathion apparently due to more rapid absorption. One human fatality has been reported.

See also: Parathion, *Reference Congener in Section III.*
Ref.: Chemagro Corp., 1961k; Hayes, 1963.

1068   Diazinon

1068

O,O-Diethyl *O*-(2-isopropyl-4-methyl-6-pyrimidyl) phosphorothioate

Toxicity Rating: 4. Introduced as an insecticide in 1952. Used for cockroach control in Hawaii. Less toxic than many organic phosphate insecticides (oral mean lethal dose in rats is 100 to 150 mg./kg.) but a potent cholinesterase inhibitor. Inappropriate indoor spraying with a 25% concentrate of diazinon (intended for use only outdoors and only after dilution) led to the poisoning of 8 members of 2 related families (Reichert *et al.,* 1977). Children who ate oatmeal and used utensils contaminated by such use became ill and were hospitalized with symptoms of profuse sweating, nausea, vomiting and abdominal cramps. All were asymptomatic 24 hours after treatment with atropine. A 54-year-old woman committed suicide by ingesting 1/2 pint of Ferti-Lome bag worm spray, calculated to have contained 22 gm. diazinon.

See also: Parathion, *Reference Congener in Section III.*
Ref.: Edson and Noakes, 1960; Geigy Chemical Corp., Date Unknown; Poklis et al., 1980; Reichert et al., 1977; Spencer, 1973.

1069   Dichlofenthion

1069

O-(2,4-Dichlorophenyl)-*O,O*-diethyl phosphorothioate

Toxicity Rating: 4. An organophosphorus insecticide and nematocide in widespread use for home gardens. Acute oral LD_{50} for rats is 270 mg./kg. Human poisonings have resulted in death with signs and symptoms of anticholinesterase poisoning. Dichlofenthion is much more fat soluble than other common organophosphorus insecticides. Percutaneous absorption is a potential danger. It is stored in and slowly released from body fat depots. As a result symptoms may be delayed hours or days after a single dose or recurrent attacks may occur. Dichlofenthion has been identified in fat biopsies, serum and urine up to 48 days after exposure. Patients respond to atropine and pralidoxime (2-PAM).

See also: Parathion, *Reference Congener in Section III.*
Ref.: Davies et al., 1975; Rowlett, 1957.

1070   Diethyl Propylmethylpyrimidyl Thiophosphate

1070

O,O-Diethyl-*O*-[2-*n*-propyl-4-methyl-6-pyrimidyl] phosphorothioate,   Pirazinon

Toxicity Rating: 4. An organic phosphorus insecticide which is somewhat less toxic in rats than its isopropyl analogue, Diazinon. Acute oral LD_{50} 260 mg./kg. in rats, 50-100 mg./kg. in mice. The acute dermal LD_{50} in rabbits is 3.5 to 11 gm./kg. A potent inhibitor of cholinesterase.

See also: Parathion, *Reference Congener in Section III.*
Ref.: Assoc. of Amer. Pesticide Control Officials, 1966.

1071   EPN

1071

Ethyl *p*-nitrophenyl thionobenzene phosphonate,   *O*-Ethyl *O*-*p*-nitrophenyl phenylphosphonothioate

A cholinesterase inhibitor which is about one-sixth to one-eighth as toxic as parathion. Skin absorption may be dangerous.

See also: Parathion, *Reference Congener in Section III.*
Ref.: Durham, 1957.

1072   Fenitrothion   1072

O,O-Dimethyl O-(4-nitro-m-tolyl)phosphorothioate,   Methylnitrophos,   Folithion,   Sumithion

Toxicity Rating: 4(?). Organophosphorus insecticide and acaricide widely used for control of chewing and sucking insects including rice stem borers, mosquitoes and sprucebud worm. Activated in animals by oxidative desulfuration to fenitrooxon, a potent cholinesterase inhibitor. Given orally, pure fenitrothion has a moderate acute toxicity (rat oral LD_{50} 1850 mg./kg.). However, technical grade fenitrothion contains the S-methyl tautomer, which is formed from fenitrothion in varying amounts in the presence of heat. This compound, which is much more toxic than the O-methyl compound, occurs in fenitrothion in concentrations ranging from 0.4 to 4%. Commercial formulations of fenitrothion are said to have an oral LD_{50} of 250 to 500 mg./kg. in rats and mice. Estimates of dermal toxicity in rodents range from 300 to 3000 mg./kg. Toxic signs are primarily those of cholinesterase inhibition. Give atropine and 2-PAM, as necessary. The major metabolites of fenitrothion in dogs, mice and rats include fenitrooxon, 4-nitro-m-cresol, and the dimethyl derivatives of fenitrothion and of fenitrooxon. Methemoglobinemia following toxic doses is described in the Russian literature.

See also: Parathion, *Reference Congener in Section III.*
Ref.: Miyamoto et al., 1976; Myatt et al., 1975.

1073   Fenthion   1073

Tiguvon,   Baytex,   Entex,   O,O-Dimethyl O-(4-(methylthio)-m-tolyl)phosphorothioate

Toxicity Rating: 4. Organic phosphorus insecticide of intermediate mammalian toxicity. Acute oral LD_{50} values: 310 mg./kg. in female rats, 190 mg./kg. in male rats and 260 mg./kg. in male guinea pigs. Acute dermal toxicity to rats (lethal dose) ranges from 330 to 500 mg./kg. Appreciably more toxic to fowl than to mammals.

See also: Parathion, *Reference Congener in Section III.*
Ref.: Chemagro Corp., 1961a.

1074   Meta-Systox-R   1074

O,O-Dimethyl S-2-(ethylsulfinyl)ethyl phosphorothioate,   Oxydemetonmethyl

Toxicity Rating: 4 or 5. Appreciably less toxic to mammals than Demeton above. Acute oral LD_{50} 52 or 75 mg./kg. in female rats, 47 or 65 mg./kg. in male rats, and 120 mg./kg. in male guinea pigs. Dermal LD_{50} 173 or 250 gm./kg. in male rats. A closely related pesticide Meta-systox-S is similar but has a higher dermal LD_{50} in rats (about 1000 mg./kg.). Both produce the typical syndrome of cholinesterase inhibition. Treat with atropine as necessary to the point of tolerance. Glucose may enhance the antidotal properties of atropine.

See also: Parathion, *Reference Congener in Section III.*
Ref.: Chemagro Corp., 1961j; Gaines, 1969.

1075   Methyl Demeton   1075

Methyl systox

Toxicity Rating: 4. An anticholinesterase insecticide that is a mixture of O,O-dimethyl-O-2(ethylthio)ethyl phosphorothioate (60-70%) and O,O-dimethyl-S-2(ethylthio)ethyl phosphorothioate (30-40%). Acute oral LD_{50} of the former in rats 180 mg./kg., of the latter 65 mg./kg.

See also: Parathion, *Reference Congener in Section III.*
Ref.: Assoc. of Amer. Pesticide Control Officials, 1966.

1076   Methyl Parathion   1076

Dimethyl parathion,   O,O-Dimethyl O-(p-nitrophenyl)thiophosphate

Toxicity Rating: 5. Slightly less toxic to rats than parathion but a much less potent cholinesterase inhibitor. Used principally in combination with parathion.

See also: Parathion, *Reference Congener in Section III.*
Ref.: Shell Chemical Co., 1960b.

1077   Parathion   1077

O,O-Diethyl O-p-nitrophenyl phosphorothioate,   Diethyl-p-nitrophenyl thiophosphate

Toxicity Rating: 6.

See also: Parathion, *Reference Congener in Section III.*

1078   **1078** Pyrazothion

Methylpyrazolyldiethyl thiophosphate,   *O,O*-Diethyl-*O*-3-methyl-5-pyrazolyl phosphorothioate

Toxicity Rating: 6. The sulfur analogue of pyrazoxon. An insecticide and acaricide of the organic

phosphorus group with an extremely high mammalian toxicity. Oral LD_{50} in mice 4 mg./kg.

See also: Parathion, *Reference Congener in Section III.*
Ref.: Merck and Co., 1976.

1079   **1079** Ronnel

O,O-Dimethyl *O*-(2,4,5-trichlorophenyl) phosphorothioate, e.g., Korlan

Toxicity Rating: 3. An anticholinesterase insecticide with a relatively low acute oral toxicity in
mammalian species. Acute oral LD_{50}'s in rats about

1.7 gm./kg., guinea pigs 1.4 to 3.1 gm./kg. and
rabbits 0.4 to 0.9 gm./kg. Dermal LD_{50} on rabbit
skin 1.6 to 2.0 gm./kg. in a 24 hour exposure.

See also: Parathion, *Reference Congener in Section III.*
Ref.: Dow Chemical Co., 1957.

1080   **1080** Tetram

Amiton, *O,O*-Diethyl-*S*-(*β*-diethylamino)ethyl phosphorothioate

Toxicity Rating: 6. Marketed as the water-soluble
oxalic acid salt (hydrogen oxalate). One of the most

toxic of the organic phosphorus insecticides. Symptoms are referable to cholinesterase inhibition.

See also: Parathion, *Reference Congener in Section III.*
Ref.: Assoc. of Amer. Pesticide Control Officials, 1966.

1081   **1081** Thionazin

O,O-Diethyl *O*-2-pyrazinyl phosphorothioate, e.g., Nemafos, Zinophos

Toxicity Rating: 5. Nematocide and soil insecticide
of the organophosphate cholinesterase inhibitor
type. Available as an emulsifiable concentrate and

as granules. Acute oral LD_{50} in male guinea pigs 10
mg./kg.

See also: Parathion, *Reference Congener in Section III.*
Ref.: Golz and Shaffer, 1966.

Organophosphorus pesticides: phosphorodithioates

1082   **1082** Bensulide

N-(*β*-*O,O*-Diisopropyldithiophosphoryl-ethyl)-benzene sulfonamide, *N*-(2-Mercaptoethyl) benzenesulfonamide *S*-(*O,O*-diisopropyl phosphorodithioate), Betasan, Prefar

Toxicity Rating: 3. Herbicide recommended for
pre-emergence control of annual grasses and
broadleaf weeds. Available as an emulsifiable liquid
(Betasan 4E, 4 lb. per gal.) and a corn cob grit
carrier formulation (Betasan 7G, 7% by weight). A
cholinesterase inhibitor; slightly less toxic than
Imidan below. Acute oral LD_{50} of technical Betasan

is 770 mg./kg., of Betasan 4E is 1910 mg./kg. (male
albino rats). Dogs fed bensulide at the 625 ppm
level for 90 days showed no ill-effects. Acute dermal
LD_{50} of technical Betasan is 3950 mg./kg. (albino
rabbits). Mild irritant in rabbit eye. Rats tolerated
1-hr. exposures to 8 mg. Betasan per liter of air.

See also: Parathion, *Reference Congener in Section III.*
Ref.: Stauffer Chemical Co., 1964a.

1083   **1083** Carbophenothion

O,O-Diethyl *S*-*p*-chlorophenylthiomethyl phosphorodithioate, e.g., Trithion, Garrathion, Nephocarp

An insecticide of the organic phosphorus group
chemically related to methyl trithion in the same
way that parathion is related to methyl parathion.
Highly toxic by the oral route. Seven members of
one family were poisoned with signs of cholinergic
crisis after eating tortillas made from contaminated
flour. Although four were comatose, all survived.

Estimates of the percutaneous LD_{50} vary widely
and the inhalation hazard is not well defined experimentally. An epidemic among 19 workers on a
sugar cane estate near Trinidad, however, occurred
under circumstances suggesting that the route of
exposure was either by inhalation or percutaneous
absorption or both.

See also: Parathion, *Reference Congener in Section III.*
Ref.: Hearn, 1961; Older and Hatcher, 1969; Williams, 1961; Williams et al., 1962.

1084   Diethyl Isopropylthiomethyl Dithiophosphate   **1084**

O,O-Diethyl-*S*-(isopropylthiomethyl)phosphorodithioate

Toxicity Rating: 5. An organic phosphorus insecticide with approximately the same mammalian toxicity as parathion. Not available commercially.

See also: Parathion, *Reference Congener in Section III.*
Ref.: Spencer, 1973.

1085   Dimethoate   **1085**

O,O-Dimethyl *S*-(*N*-methylcarbamoylmethyl)phosphorodithioate

Toxicity Rating: 4. Organic phosphate ester used as an insecticide. Relatively low vertebrate toxicity is attributed to rapid degradation by the liver (amidase?). Acute oral LD_{50} for rats 200 mg./kg. Not a primary irritant to skin or eyes, but percutaneous absorption has not been adequately evaluated. Erythrocyte cholinesterase of rats and dogs is more susceptible to dimethoate inhibition than plasma cholinesterase. Mixtures with other organic phosphates show simple additive toxicity in animals. According to animal screening tests, pralidoxime chloride (PAM) is ineffective or only marginally effective against this agent, but a clinical trial is recommended in any severe poisoning.

See also: Parathion, *Reference Congener in Section III.*
Ref.: Edson and Noakes, 1960; Uchida et al., 1964; West et al., 1961.

1086   Disulfoton   **1086**

Dithiosystox,   *O,O*-Diethyl *S*-2-(ethylthio)ethyl phosphorodithioate,   Di-syston, Thiodemeton

Toxicity Rating: 6. A super toxic organic phosphate insecticide. Chemically related to Demeton (see index) but more toxic. Toxic effects are due to cholinesterase inhibition. Used as a spray to protect seeds against various pests.

See also: Parathion, *Reference Congener in Section III.*
Ref.: Chemagro Corp., 1961e.

1087   Ethion   **1087**

Bis(diethoxyphosphinothioylthio)methane,   Ethyl methylene phosphorodithioate,   Nialate

Toxicity Rating: 4. A miticide and insecticide of the organophosphorus group. Less toxic than parathion but more toxic than malathion. Absorption can occur through all portals, including intact skin. The vapor pressure is low, but in the form of a spray it constitutes an inhalation hazard.

See also: Parathion, *Reference Congener in Section III.*
Ref.: Niagara Chemical, 1959a.

1088   *O*-Ethyl *S,S*-Dipropyl Phosphorodithioate   **1088**

e.g., Mocap

Toxicity Rating: 5. A cholinesterase inhibitor used as a nematocide-insecticide and available as a 10% granular formulation. Acute oral LD_{50} in male rats (61 mg./kg.) indicates that this compound belongs on the borderline between toxicity classes 4 and 5, but the dermal LD_{50} in rabbits (25 mg./kg.) suggests that it is more toxic by the percutaneous route.

See also: Parathion, *Reference Congener in Section III.*
Ref.: Huvar, 1969.

1089   Guthion   **1089**

Dimethoxy ester of benzotriazine dithiophosphoric acid, *O,O*-Dimethyl *S*-(4-oxobenzotriazino-3-methyl) phosphorodithioate, DBD, Azinphos methyl

Toxicity Rating: 5. An organic thiophosphate insecticide whose active metabolite is apparently the oxygen analogue. In toxicity studies on rats it is about one half as toxic as parathion. Animal experiments show that the compound is well absorbed from the gastrointestinal tract but percutaneous absorption is minimal. A potent cholinesterase inhibitor in vivo. Death is due to respiratory failure.

See also: Parathion, *Reference Congener in Section III.*
Ref.: Chemagro Corp., 1961i; DuBois et al., 1957.

1090   1090   Imidan

O,O-Dimethyl-*S*-phthalimidomethyl phosphorodithioate, *N*-(Mercaptomethyl)phthalimide *S*(*O,O*-dimethylphosphorodithioate), Phosmet

Toxicity Rating: 4. Insecticide and acaricide available as a wettable powder (50W, 50% Imidan by weight), granular formulation (10G, 10% Imidan by weight) and emulsifiable liquid (3E, 3 pounds per gallon). A cholinesterase inhibitor. Acute oral LD_{50} of technical Imidan in rats 216 mg./kg. Dermal LD_{50} in rabbits said to be in excess of 3.16 gm./kg. Mild irritant in rabbit eye.

See also: Parathion, *Reference Congener in Section III.*
Ref.: Sherman et al., 1964; Stauffer Chemical Co., 1964b.

1091   1091   Malathion

S-(1,2-Dicarboethoxyethyl)-*O,O*-dimethyldithiophosphate, *O,O*-Dimethyldithiophosphate of diethyl mercaptosuccinate, *O,O*-Dimethyl *S*-(1,2-carbethoxyethyl)phosphorodithioate, Malathon

Toxicity Rating: 4. One of few organic phosphate insecticides approved (1955) for household use. With improved synthetic methods the purity of this compound now exceeds 99 per cent. The increase in purity has resulted in a corresponding decrease in the acute toxicity so that recent oral LD_{50}'s in rats tend to cluster around 2500 mg./kg. (toxicity rating of 3). Over the years, however, a fairly extensive body of clinical experience has accumulated to suggest that man may be more susceptible to the toxic effects of malathion than rats. Reports of accidental and suicidal ingestions indicate that, at the least, this compound belongs on the borderline between toxicity classes 3 and 4. Even so, malathion is between 100 and 1000 times less toxic and less potent as a cholinesterase inhibitor than parathion. The low mammalian toxicity of malathion is due in large measure to ali-esterases that metabolize malathion to inactive products. Some species have ali-esterases in both plasma and liver, but man appears to possess only the latter enzyme. Specific inhibition of ali-esterases such as by tri-*o*-tolyl phosphate can lead to a 100-fold increase in the acute toxicity of malathion. The less dramatic but still significant potentiating effects of EPN and other insecticides on malathion toxicity are attributed to a similar mechanism. Malaoxon, the active anticholinesterase metabolite of malathion, also has aliesterase inhibiting activity. Crude or technical grade malathion may contain malaoxon as an impurity, perhaps accounting for the higher toxicity of early malathion preparations. Estimates of the total dose are available in at least 6 human intoxications and 2 deaths due to malathion ingestion. An elderly man died after 200 to 400 mg./kg. One adult survived 1 gm./kg., but was on a respirator for 2 weeks. The mean lethal dose by mouth in an untreated adult may be as low as 250 mg./kg. Two suspected poisonings in children have occurred under circumstances which indicated that percutaneous absorption was the major route of exposure. These observations are supported by the demonstration of small but significant percutaneous toxicity in rabbits. Another infant exhibited severe signs of cholinesterase inhibition after unknown conditions of exposure to an aerosol bomb containing 0.5 per cent malathion. The atropine requirements of poisoned patients may be enormous; 2-PAM has shown considerable promise, but it has only rarely been used early enough in an intoxication to effect dramatic clinical improvement. In an experimental study, malathion was found to be a weak contact sensitizer, inducing a mild cutaneous reaction in a high proportion of the subjects. Development of sensitization, however, has not been a significant problem in its widespread use.

See also: Parathion, *Reference Congener in Section III.*
Ref.: Amos and Hall, 1965; Casida, 1961; Crowley and Johns, 1966; Frawley et al., 1957; Gitelson et al., 1966; Goldin et al., 1964; Goldman and Teitel, 1958; Healy, 1959; Konig et al., 1966; Main and Braid, 1962; McLaughlin and Snyder, 1956; Milby and Epstein, 1964; Murphy et al., 1959; Murphy, 1967; Parker and Chattin, 1955; Paul, 1960; Richards, 1964; Tuthill, 1958; Walters, 1957; Wenzl and Burke, 1962.

1092   1092   Methyl Trithion

O,O-Dimethyl-*S*-(*p*-chlorophenylthiomethyl)phosphorodithioate,   Tri-Me

Toxicity Rating: 4. Insecticide-acaricide chemically related to carbophenothion above in the same way that methyl parathion is related to parathion. Much less toxic than parathion in mammals. Acute oral LD_{50}'s of technical (95%) methyl trithion 390 mg./kg. in male mice, 157 mg./kg. in male rats. Acute dermal LD_{50} on albino rabbits 2.4 to 7.5 gm./kg. The vapor concentration of an emulsifiable concentrate (methyl trithion, 48%) that killed half the exposed rats in 1 hour was 3 mg./l. Moderate eye irritant.

See also: Parathion, *Reference Congener in Section III.*
Ref.: Shafer, 1965; Sherman et al., 1964; Williams, 1961; Williams et al., 1962.

1093   1093   Navadel

Delnav,   2,3-*p*-Dioxanedithiol *S,S*-bis(*O,O*-diethyl phosphorodithioate),   Dioxathion

Toxicity Rating: 4. Given orally to laboratory animals (rats, dogs), it has caused signs of systemic intoxication that are typical of cholinesterase inhibition. At a dietary level of 100 ppm for a period of 90 days, tremor and hyperexcitability were evident in rats.

See also: Parathion, Reference Congener in Section III.
Ref.: Rosher, 1957.

1094 Phorate 1094

O,O-Diethyl (S-ethylmercaptomethyl)dithiophosphate, Thimet

Toxicity Rating: 6. A highly toxic insecticide that is a cholinesterase inhibitor and so can produce toxic reactions like parathion. Used on plants as a systemic insecticide. According to animal screening tests, pralidoxime chloride (PAM) is ineffective or only marginally effective against this agent, but a clinical trial is recommended in any severe poisoning.

See also: Parathion, Reference Congener in Section III.
Ref.: Assoc. of Amer. Pesticide Control Officials, 1966; Spencer, 1973.

Organophosphorus pesticides: amidates and fluoridates

1095 Acephate 1095

O,S-Dimethyl acetylphosphoramidothioate, e.g., Orthene

Toxicity Rating: 3 or 4. An organophosphorus insecticide of moderate persistence and relatively low mammalian toxicity. The acute oral LD_{50} is 940 mg./kg. in rats and 360 mg./kg. in mice. The acute dermal LD_{50} in rabbits exceeds 2 gm./kg. The substance is a cholinesterase inhibitor, but much less active than parathion in vivo. Atropine sulfate is antidotal. Rats fed Orthene at a dietary level of 300 ppm for 90 days showed no pathology.

See also: Parathion, Reference Congener in Section III.
Ref.: Chevron Chemical Co., 1976.

1096 Diisopropyl Fluorophosphate 1096

DFP, Isoflurophate, Diisopropyl phosphorofluoridate

Toxicity Rating: 5. A potent cholinesterase inhibitor. Seldom used today and not at all by the agriculturalist. Occasionally prescribed by physicians (ophthalmologists) for the treatment of glaucoma. Chronic topical applications in the eye may increase the incidence of cataract. Degenerative changes in peripheral and central nervous systems have resulted from chronic exposures in laboratory animals.

See also: Parathion, Reference Congener in Section III.

1097 Diamidafos 1097

Phenyl-N,N'-dimethyl phosphorodiamidate, Nellite

Toxicity Rating: 4. A soil fumigant and nematocide. The compound is readily absorbed from the gut and has a high oral toxicity (rat oral LD_{50} 140 mg./kg.). Animals given 100 ppm in food for 90 days showed depressed cholinesterase levels in brain, plasma and erythrocytes. Tracer studies indicate that diamidafos is metabolized in the liver to other phosphorodiamidates and to phenol. About 25% of an oral dose is excreted in urine unchanged. The compound is also absorbed through intact skin (dermal LD_{50} in rabbits is 100 to 200 mg./kg.).

See also: Parathion, Reference Congener in Section III.
Ref.: Sauerhoff et al., 1976.

1098 Dimefox 1098

Bis(dimethylamino) fluorophosphine oxide, BFPO, Tetramethylphosphorodiamidic fluoride

Toxicity Rating: 5. An organic phosphorus insecticide closely related to Mipafox below. Converted metabolically in the animal body to a highly toxic anticholinesterase substance. Amounts too small for chemical detection can cause blurred vision. The predominant effects are on peripheral tissues and not on the central nervous system. According to animal screening tests, pralidoxime chloride (PAM) is ineffective or only marginally effective against this agent, but a clinical trial is recommended in any severe poisoning.

See also: Parathion, Reference Congener in Section III.
Ref.: Okinaka et al., 1954.

1099

O-Methyl-*O*-(2,4,5-trichlorophenyl)amidophosphorothionate

Toxicity Rating: 3. An experimental insecticide that is presumably a cholinesterase inhibitor and so might produce toxic reactions like parathion.

Animal studies place this compound near the borderline between toxicity classes 3 and 4.

See also: Parathion, *Reference Congener in Section III.*

1100

1100 Mipafox

Bis(isopropylamino)fluorophosphine oxide, Isopestox

Toxicity Rating: 4. An insecticide and acetylcholinesterase inhibitor, like parathion. After the acute phases of the poisoning, degenerative lesions may

become apparent in the central and peripheral nervous systems.

See also: Parathion, *Reference Congener in Section III.*
Ref.: Barnes and Denz, 1953; Davies, 1952.

1101

1101 Monitor

Methamidophos, *O,S*-Dimethyl phosphoramidothioate

Toxicity Rating: 5. One of the most toxic organophosphorus insecticides, both by oral ingestion and dermal exposure. The acute oral LD_{50} in rats is 19

to 21 mg./kg., and the dermal LD_{50} in rabbits is 118 mg./kg. It is used for the control of insects in cabbage, potatoes and cotton.

See also: Parathion, *Reference Congener in Section III.*
Ref.: Chevron Chemical Co., 1973.

1102

1102 Octamethyl Pyrophosphoramide

Schradan

Toxicity Rating: 5. A "systemic" insecticide, i.e., translocated in sap to all parts of plants. Only slightly less toxic than parathion. Not a cholinesterase inhibitor in vitro, but converted to one by liver. Brain cholinesterase, however, is not in-

hibited in fatally poisoned animals. According to animal screening tests, pralidoxime chloride (PAM) is ineffective or only marginally effective against this agent, but a clinical trial is recommended in any severe poisoning.

See also: Parathion, *Reference Congener in Section III.*
Ref.: Bidstrup, 1952b; Hazleton, 1955.

1103

1103 Phenamiphos

Ethyl 3-methyl-4-(methylthio)phenyl(1-methylethyl)phosphoramidate, Isopropyl phosphoramidic acid 4-(methylthio)-*m*-tolyl ethyl ester, Nemacur

Toxicity Rating: 5. Organophosphate nematocide for use on cotton and various truck crops. Extremely toxic: oral acute LD_{50} is about 20 mg./kg. in rats and mice and 5 mg./kg. in hens. Inhibits cholinesterase. Atropine is antidotal and should be supplemented with 2-PAM. Percutaneous absorption is slow (rat dermal LD_{50} is about 500 mg./kg.). Inhalation of vapor concentrations of 100 mg./m³.

however, produces prompt systemic intoxication in rats. Not irritating to skin, eyes, or mucous membranes. No delayed neurotoxicity, as tested in hens. In rats and dogs, chronic feeding of phenamiphos for three months produced a reduction in cholinesterase activity but no biochemical, hematologic or histologic changes indicative of chronic toxicity.

See also: Parathion, *Reference Congener in Section III.*
Ref.: Loser and Kimmerle, 1971.

1104

1104 Ruelene

4-*tert.*-Butyl-2-chlorophenyl methyl methylphosphoramidate

Toxicity Rating: 4. Cholinesterase inhibitor introduced as an experimental insecticide and systemic nematocide for ruminants. Acute oral LD_{50} in rats said to be about 1 gm./kg. Single doses of 100 mg./

kg. by mouth in lambs depressed blood cholinesterase levels a maximum of 50%; signs of intoxication appeared after 200 mg./kg.

See also: Parathion, *Reference Congener in Section III.*
Ref.: Galvin et al., 1960; Weidenbach et al., 1962.

1105   Zytron   **1105**

O-(2,4-Dichlorophenyl)-*O*-methyl isopropylphosphoramidothioate,   DMPA

Toxicity Rating: 4(?). Organophosphate herbicide used against crabgrass. Acute oral LD_{50}'s 300 mg./kg. in rats; in dogs and cats greater than 1 gm./kg. Additional data suggest considerable species variation. A relatively potent inhibitor of cholinesterase in chickens when fed for 1 week, but one of the least acutely toxic compounds of a wide range of chemical types tested. Single doses in chickens produced deaths over a 7–day period with associated lethargy and ataxia. It does not appear to have been established whether or not death in mammals from Zytron can be ascribed entirely to cholinesterase inhibition. If indicated, treat symptomatically with atropine.

See also: Parathion, *Reference Congener in Section III.*
Ref.: Assoc. of Amer. Pesticide Control Officials, 1966; Spencer, 1973; Sherman et al., 1964.

Organophosphorus pesticides: others

1106   Hexaethyl Tetraphosphate   **1106**

HETP

Toxicity Rating: 6. Slightly more potent than parathion but less so than TEPP. Unstable like TEPP.

Not used currently in agriculture.

See also: Parathion, *Reference Congener in Section III.*
Ref.: Council on Pharmacy and Chemistry, 1950.

1107   Phostex   **1107**

Bis(dialkoxyphosphinothioyl)disulfide

Toxicity Rating: 3. An organic phosphorus miticide with a toxic potential similar to that of malathion. Absorption occurs principally through the oral and percutaneous routes, but inhalation in the form of dusts is also hazardous. Even though less toxic than many other organic phosphorus insecticides, chronic latent cumulative effects may occur.

See also: Parathion, *Reference Congener in Section III.*
Ref.: Niagara Chemical, 1959b.

1108   Sulfotepp   **1108**

Tetraethyl dithiopyrophosphate

Toxicity Rating: 6. Toxicity comparable to parathion in laboratory animals. Relatively resistant to hydrolysis.

See also: Parathion, *Reference Congener in Section III.*
Ref.: Lehman, 1951.

1109   Tetraethyl Pyrophosphate   **1109**

TEPP, TEP

Toxicity Rating: 6. More potent than parathion, but poisonings may be slightly more transient because TEPP is detoxified faster and because enzyme inhibition seems to be reversible in large measure.

See also: Parathion, *Reference Congener in Section III.*
Ref.: Council on Pharmacy and Chemistry, 1950.

1110   Tetra-*n*-propyl Dithionopyrophosphate   **1110**

NPD, Aspon

Toxicity Rating: 3. An organic phosphorus insecticide closely related to Tetraethyl pyrophosphate and Sulfotepp above, but with a much lower mammalian toxicity than either.
See also: Parathion, *Reference Congener in Section III.*
Ref.: Doull and DuBois, 1952.

1111   *S,S,S*-Tributyl Phosphorotrithioate   **1111**

e.g., DEF

Toxicity Rating: 4. The formula is $(C_4H_9S)_3PO$.

Used as a cotton defoliant. Acute oral LD_{50} in

female rats 325 mg./kg. and in male guinea pigs 260 mg./kg. Cutaneous application of 1000 mg./kg. produced death in female rats. A very weak cholinesterase inhibitor in vitro, but marked depression of enzymatic activity occurs in vivo. Some signs in poisoned animals, however, such as central nervous depression, cannot be ascribed to cholinesterase inhibition. Atropine was relatively ineffective in reversing or preventing the lethal course of the intoxication.

See also: Parathion, *Reference Congener in Section III*.
Ref.: Chemagro Corp., 1961c; Murphy and DuBois, 1959.

Phosphate esters that are not primarily cholinesterase inhibitors

1112   Ethyl Phosphates

e.g., Triethyl phosphate

Toxicity Rating: 3(?). Ethyl phosphate is a sedative in rats. Some ethyl phosphate derivatives (e.g., parathion) are highly toxic cholinesterase inhibitors. Triethyl phosphate is thought to be a weak enzyme inhibitor.

Ref.: Smith, 1936.

1113   Tributyl Phosphate

Toxicity Rating: 3. Formula: $(C_4H_9)_3PO_4$. Used as a plasticizer for lacquers, plastics, etc. Acute oral LD_{50} in rats is 3.0 gm./kg. An extremely weak inhibitor of cholinesterase. After mild signs of cholinesterase inhibition, poisoned rats showed weakness, dyspnea, coma and pulmonary edema. No late paralysis occurred in survivors. Primary irritant on skin.

Ref.: Carpenter and Smyth, 1946; Sabine and Hayes, 1952; Smyth and Carpenter, 1944.

1114   Tributyl Phosphorotrithioite

e.g., Folex, Merphos

Toxicity Rating: 3. Formula: $(C_4H_9S)_3P$. A cotton defoliant available as an emulsifiable concentrate. Acute oral LD_{50} in male rats 1.3 gm./kg.; percutaneous LD_{50} on rabbit skin 5 to 10 gm./kg. Mild to moderate irritant. The nature of the systemic toxic syndrome has not been described, but at least some signs in animals are consistent with cholinesterase inhibition. Not to be confused with tributyl phosphorotrithioate. Treatment should be symptomatic and supportive.

Ref.: Goyette, 1961.

1115   Tricresyl Phosphate

Tritolyl phosphate, TCP

A mixture of isomeric tricresyl phosphate which excludes the very toxic *o*-isomer as much as possible. Used as plasticizer, solvent and hydraulic fluid. No toxicity data were located but see *o*-Tricresyl phosphate below.

1116   Tri-*o*-cresyl Phosphate

Triorthocresyl phosphate, Tri-*o*-tolyl phosphate, TOCP, *o*-Tricresyl phosphate

Induces an unusual polyneuritis with flaccid paralysis, first appearing many days after the exposure ("ginger paralysis"). With large doses, however, the latent period may be very short. Recovery is slow but usually complete. None of the usual toxic effects of cresols or phenols is described in clinical poisonings. Does not produce the typical syndrome associated with cholinesterase inhibition as do phosphate esters like parathion. Meta and para isomers are relatively inactive. In 1960 approximately 10,000 persons in Morocco became ill (more than 6000 suffering paresis of the legs) following the ingestion of cooking oil which had been adulterated with turbojet engine lubricating oil containing 3% TCP.

See also: Tri-*o*-cresyl Phosphate, *Reference Congener in Section III*.
Ref.: Albertini et al., 1968; Aring, 1942; Smith and Elvove, 1930; Zeligs, 1938.

1117   Triphenyl Phosphate

Toxicity Rating: 4(?). Used as a plasticizer and a fireproofing agent. A neurotoxic substance like tri-*o*-cresyl phosphate above; more potent than the latter in cats but probably not in man. Causes a delayed peripheral neuritis involving motor neurones, resulting in a flaccid paralysis, particularly of the distal muscles. No sensory disturbances. Signs and symptoms of cholinesterase inhibition should also be anticipated and treated as in parathion poisoning (see Section III).

See also: Tri-*o*-cresyl Phosphate, *Reference Congener in Section III.*
Ref.: Hunter et al., 1944; Lehmann and Flury, 1938; Smith, 1930.

1118   Tris(2,3-dibromopropyl)phosphate   1118

TRIS, Tris-BP

Toxicity Rating: 3. TRIS was used extensively as a fire retardant additive to synthetic fibers, polyurethane foams and plastics until 1977, when TRIS-treated children's sleepware was banned in the U.S.A., and TRIS itself was banned from use in fabrics intended for children's clothing. The chemical was found to be a potent direct-acting mutagen and a carcinogen when fed to rats and mice or when painted on the skin of mice. It is slowly absorbed through the intact skin of rats, rabbits and man. A metabolite 2,3-dibromopropanol was found in the urine of children who wore even well-washed pajamas made from TRIS-treated textiles. The childhood habit of sucking on clothing increases exposure because saliva enhances the extraction of TRIS from fabric, as does urine. Testicular atrophy and sterility in rabbits have resulted from dermal applications of TRIS. Fed to rats, it has caused extensive renal tubular necrosis and subsequent renal adenomas and carcinomas. The compound is suspected to cause heritable mutations in humans: it induces sex-linked recessive lethals in *Drosophila* and unscheduled DNA synthesis and reparable DNA breaks in human cells in culture. Its mutagenic activity can be extracted from laundered fabrics. By 1977, 120 million TRIS-treated sleepware garments had been sold, and 50 million children had been exposed. Children wearing new TRIS-treated pajamas may have absorbed 180 μg. TRIS daily. The eventual incidence of TRIS-related cancer has been variously estimated at 25 to 17,000 cases of cancer per million male children exposed to TRIS-treated clothing for 1 year. TRIS is also a skin sensitizer. During the 1950's workers handling TRIS-treated acrylic fibers became sensitized to the compound. Most absorbed TRIS is excreted in the urine within one day. As with other haloalkyl phosphates, it may be a cholinesterase inhibitor. One metabolite, 2,3-dibromopropanol, is structurally related to 1,2-dibromo-3-chloropropane (see in Index), which is a minor impurity in some samples of TRIS and which is a known mutagen and animal carcinogen and an agent that has caused sterility in male factory workers and testicular atrophy in animals. TRIS may still be in use in the manufacture of cellulose insulation. With approximately 6.5 million TRIS-treated garments still in warehouses across the country and with the unscrupulous practices of some distributors, the risk of human exposure to TRIS has not ceased.

Ref.: Archer et al., 1979; Blum et al., 1978; National Cancer Institute, 1978s; Prival et al., 1977.

1119   Tris(1,3-dichloro-2-propyl)phosphate   1119

Fyrol FR2

Toxicity Rating: 3(?). A fire retardant formerly used extensively in textiles (especially polyester fabrics) and still employed in polyurethane foams, textile backcoating and adhesives. Its addition to children's sleepwear was discontinued voluntarily in 1977, when the structurally related fire retardant TRIS (see above) was banned for this purpose. Fyrol FR2 is weakly mutagenic in Ames Salmonella test after activation by rat or mouse liver homogenates. Its metabolites bis(1,3-dichloro-2-propyl)phosphate and 1,3-dichloro-2-propanol (see in Index) are also mutagenic in Salmonella in the presence of mammalian liver homogenates. One putative metabolite 1,3-dichloro-2-propanone is strongly mutagenic without activation. Fyrol FR2 and its metabolites are readily absorbed thorough the intact skin of rats and humans. Widespread exposure to Fyrol FR2 is evidenced by its presence in the seminal plasma of 34 out of 123 volunteers in a 1980 survey.

Ref.: Gold et al., 1978; Hudec et al., 1981; Nomeir et al., 1981.

Carbamate cholinesterase inhibitors used for pest control (exclusive of herbicides)

1120   Aldicarb   1120

2-Methyl-2-(methylthio)propionaldehyde *O*-(methylcarbamoyl)oxime,   Temik

Toxicity Rating: 6. A systemic insecticide, acaricide and nematocide for use in soil to control pests on cotton, tobacco, potatoes, peanuts and other crops. One of the most toxic of the carbamate insecticides. The acute oral LD_{50} in rats is 0.9 to 1 mg./kg., and the acute dermal LD_{50} in rabbits is 5 mg./kg. Reversible cholinesterase inhibitor; in humans, duration of activity is 6 to 8 hours. Atropine is antidotal; do not give 2-PAM, opiates or cholinesterase inhibiting drugs. Rats tolerated 0.3 mg./kg. daily for 2 years without ill effect. Metabolic products include sulfoxide and sulfone oxidation products of Aldicarb and of the oxime released by hydrolysis. These are found in the milk of cows given nontoxic doses of Temik. Because of its hazardous nature, Aldicarb is formulated only as 10 per cent granules (impregnated corn-cob grit). In rats, the dermal LD_{50} of the dry granules is 2 to 4 gm./kg.

The wet granules, however, are not safe.

See also: Carbaryl, *Reference Congener in Section III.*
Ref.: Dernehl, April 11, 1972; Dorough et al., 1970; Frear, 1969; Spencer, 1973.

1121   Allyxycarb

4-(Diallylamino)-3,5-xylyl methylcarbamate,   Hydrol

Toxicity Rating: 4. Carbamate insecticide, formerly used on fruit. Cholinesterase inhibitor; atropine is antidotal. Highly toxic to mammals by oral route (LD_{50} 90 mg./kg.); no significant percutaneous absorption.

See also: Carbaryl, *Reference Congener in Section III.*

1122   Aminocarb

4-Dimethylamino-*m*-tolyl methylcarbamate,   Matacil

Toxicity Rating: 5. Carbamate insecticide used to control insects in forests, fruit and vegetable crops. Very high oral mammalian toxicity (LD_{50} in rat 30 to 50 mg./kg.). Readily absorbed through intact skin (dermal LD_{50} in rats is 270 mg./kg.). Reversible cholinesterase inhibitor. Atropine is antidotal. Tissue hyperemia and dystrophic changes are described in the Russian literature. *In vitro* experiments indicate that the compound is not hydrolyzed by liver enzymes but is converted to several more toxic carbamates, including 4-amino-3-cresyl methylcarbamate, 4-methylamino-3-cresyl methylcarbamate and 4-dimethylamino-3-cresyl *N*-hydroxymethylcarbamate. However, hydrolysis is a major detoxication pathway in the intact rat. It is not known which of these pathways is dominant in humans. Supplied as wettable powders and dusts.

See also: Carbaryl, *Reference Congener in Section III.*
Ref.: Frear, 1969; Krishna and Casida, 1966; Worthing, 1979; Minina and Khomich, 1967; Spencer, 1973.

1123   Bendiocarb

2,2-Dimethyl-1,3-benzodioxol-4-yl methylcarbamate,   Ficam

Toxicity Rating: 4 or 5. Contact insecticide for use in control of crawling insects and mosquitoes in buildings, including restaurants. Very high acute oral toxicity (acute LD_{50} in laboratory mammals ranges from 34 to 64 mg./kg.). Percutaneous absorption is significant (rat LD_{50} 600 to 800 mg./kg.). Cholinesterase inhibitor; atropine is antidotal. Supplied in micropulverized form.

See also: Carbaryl, *Reference Congener in Section III.*
Ref.: Worthing, 1979.

1124   BPMC

2-*sec*-Butylphenyl *N*-methylcarbamate,   Osbac

Toxicity Rating: 4. Contact insecticide for control of hoppers on rice. Reversible cholinesterase inhibitor. High oral toxicity in mammals (rat oral LD_{50} 0.4 gm./kg.). May also be absorbed through skin. Detoxified in rats by a variety of routes, including oxidation. In domestic animals, death followed ECG changes. Autopsy findings included petechial hemorrhages of kidney, heart, thymus, urinary bladder and respiratory muscles, enlargement of lymph nodes and esophageal ulceration. BPMC is provided in solution, also in dust and granular formulations. May be combined with fenitrothion (see in this index).

See also: Carbaryl, *Reference Congener in Section III.*
Ref.: Akahori et al., 1974.

1125   Bufencarb

Bux, Metalkamate, 3-(1-Ethylpropyl)phenyl methylcarbamate, 3-(1-Methylbutyl)phenyl methylcarbamate

Toxicity Rating: 4. Insecticidal mixtures of the 1-methylbutyl phenyl and 1-ethylpropyl phenyl esters of methylcarbamic acid. Very high acute oral toxicity (rat LD_{50} is 87 mg./kg.). For use against soil and foliage insects. Cholinesterase inhibitor. Atropine is antidotal; 2-PAM is not effective. Absorbed through the skin (dermal LD_{50} is 240 mg./kg. in rat but 1400 mg./kg. in dogs). Dogs tolerated 500 ppm in food for 90 days. Very toxic to fish. Causes a variety of teratogenic effects in chick eggs when injected into the yolk sac. These effects are prevented by simultaneous injection of precursors of nicotinamide-adenine dinucleotide (NAD) and may be due to a specific effect of methylcarbamate compounds on chick embryo NAD levels.

See also: Carbaryl, *Reference Congener in Section III.*
Ref.: Worthing, 1979; Proctor et al., 1976.

1126 Butacarb 1126

3,5-Di-*tert*-butylphenyl-*N*-methylcarbamate

Toxicity Rating: 3(?). Insecticide used as a sheep dip to kill blowfly larvae. Arylesterase and cholinesterase inhibitor. In mammals, among the least toxic of the carbamate insecticides (acute oral LD$_{50}$ is 1.8 gm./kg. in rats, and 3.2 gm./kg. in mice).

Dogs given daily doses of 160 mg./kg. for 90 days showed no ill effects. Formulations do not cause skin or eye irritation. Supplied as 20% and 25% miscible oil concentrates and in combination with magnesium silicofluoride or lindane.

See also: Carbaryl, *Reference Congener in Section III*.
Ref.: Mendoza et al., 1976.

1127 Carbanolate 1127

6-Chloro-3,4-xylyl methylcarbamate, Banol

Toxicity Rating: 5. Carbamate insecticide and acaricide, formerly used to control ticks and mites on domestic animals. Very high acute oral toxicity in laboratory animals (rat LD$_{50}$ 30 mg./kg.). Cholinesterase inhibitor; atropine is antidotal. Major competing metabolic pathways are hepatic oxidation of ring substituents and hydrolysis of the carbamate linkage. Both processes are slower than with other carbamate insecticides, and thus the action of Carbanolate may have a longer duration.

See also: Carbaryl, *Reference Congener in Section III*.
Ref.: Krishna and Casida, 1966; Oonnithan and Casida, 1968.

1128 Carbaryl 1128

1-Naphthyl-*N*-methylcarbamate, Arylam, Sevin

Toxicity Rating: 4. In mammals, one of the less toxic of the carbamate insecticides (rat oral LD$_{50}$ 0.51 gm./kg.). Cholinesterase inhibitor. Said to be teratogenic in dogs. Present maximum allowed concentration in workplace atmospheres is 5 mg./m^3 (OSHA, 1974).

See also: Carbaryl, *Reference Congener in Section III*.
Ref.: OSHA., June 27, 1974.

1129 Carbofuran 1129

2,3-Dihydro-2,2-dimethyl-7-benzofuranyl methylcarbamate, e.g., Furadan

Toxicity Rating: 5. Systemic *N*-methylcarbamate insecticide, acaricide and nematocide for use on many food crops. Very toxic to mammals; acute oral LD$_{50}$ in rats is 9 to 14 mg./kg. Rapidly reversible inhibitor of cholinesterase. In humans initial signs of toxicity include sweating, nausea, and blurred vision. Toxic symptoms occur at a small fraction of the lethal dose. Recovery from a mild toxic exposure is rapid. Since the compound acts rapidly, terminating exposure as soon as initial symptoms appear may prevent a severe intoxication. Atropine is antidotal; do not give 2-PAM. Experimental animals, untreated after high nonlethal doses, return to normal activity in 4 to 6 hours. Carbofuran is rapidly detoxified in the liver and excreted in urine. Poorly absorbed from skin; the acute dermal LD$_{50}$ in rabbits is 3,400 mg./kg. Has caused teratogenic lesions in chick embryos.

See also: Carbaryl, *Reference Congener in Section III*.
Ref.: Worthing, 1979; Niagara Chemical Division, 1970; Tobin, 1970.

1130 Cartap 1130

S,S'-(2-(Dimethylamino)trimethylene)bis(thiocarbamate), Padan, 1,3-Di(carbamoylthio)-2-(dimethylamino)propane hydrochloride

Toxicity Rating: 4. A thiocarbamate insecticide, usually supplied as the hydrochloride. High acute oral toxicity in mammals (rat LD$_{50}$ 340 mg./kg.). Probably a cholinesterase inhibitor but relevant data were not located. If symptoms suggest enzyme inhibition, treat with atropine as in carbaryl poisoning.

See also: Carbaryl, *Reference Congener in Section III*.

1131 Dimetan 1131

5,5'-Dimethyldihydroresorcinol dimethylcarbamate, 5,5'-Dimethyl-3-oxo-1-cyclohexen-1-yl dimethylcarbamate

Toxicity Rating: 4. An aphicide, now little used. High acute oral toxicity (rat LD$_{50}$ 120 mg./kg.). Skin absorption is negligible. Although not described in mice and rats, toxic signs and symptoms presumably resemble those of carbaryl poisoning, since Dimetan is a reversible inhibitor of the enzyme cholinesterase and is related to physostigmine and neostigmine. No clinical data. No longer sold in the U.S.A.

See also: Carbaryl, Reference Congener in Section III.
Ref.: Ferguson and Alexander, 1953; Martin and Worthing, 1977.

1132   1132   Dimetilan

2-Dimethylcarbamyl-3-methylpyrazolyl-(5)-dimethylcarbamate, e.g., Snip fly band

Toxicity Rating: 4-5. A cholinesterase inhibitor of the carbamate type used as an insecticide. More toxic than Carbaryl (see above). Acute oral LD_{50}'s in mice, rats and guinea pigs range from 47 to 64 mg./kg. Cattle are much more susceptible; the acute LD_{50} in cows is about 5 mg./kg. When rats were given doses of 20 mg./kg. every day, no blood or organ pathology was found after 4 weeks, but at 35 mg./kg. daily half the animals died within 1 week. Cumulative effects and tolerance could not be demonstrated. The rabbit dermal LD_{50} is in excess of 2 gm./kg. Dimetilan is not irritating to rat skin or rabbit eye. The classical signs of cholinesterase inhibition are controlled in animals by atropine. 2-PAM should not be given. No longer sold in the U.S.A.

See also: Carbaryl, Reference Congener in Section III.
Ref.: Worthing, 1979; Stenger, 1962.

1133   1133   Dioxacarb

2-(1,3-Dioxolan-2-yl)phenyl methylcarbamate,   Elocron

Toxicity Rating: 4. Carbamate insecticide for use against house and garden pests. Cholinesterase inhibitor; very toxic to mammals (rat oral LD_{50} is 60-80 mg./kg.). Atropine is antidotal; do not give 2-PAM. Subacute oral administration to rats (4 mg./kg. daily for 90 days) is said to cause peridontal damage and dystrophic changes in the oral mucosa, gastrointestinal tract, liver and heart.

See also: Carbaryl, Reference Congener in Section III.
Ref.: Worthing, 1979.

1134   1134   Ethiofencarb

α-Ethylthio-o-tolyl methylcarbamate,   Croneton,   2-((Ethylthio)methyl)phenyl methylcarbamate

Toxicity Rating: 4. Systemic methylcarbamate insecticide, recommended for control of aphids on plants. High acute oral toxicity in mammals (rat LD_{50} 411 mg./kg.). Cholinesterase inhibitor. Atropine is antidotal. No percutaneous absorption. In rats, hydrolytic detoxification competes with side-chain sulfur oxidation. Although ethiofencarb disappears rapidly after oral doses, it is partially converted in tissues to the corresponding sulfoxide and sulfone, which are both highly toxic. In rats, the major urinary metabolites are the sulfoxide and conjugates of 2-ethylthiomethylphenol sulfoxide (the oxidized hydrolysis product). It is not known which pathway dominates in man.

See also: Carbaryl, Reference Congener in Section III.
Ref.: Nye et al., 1976.

1135   1135   Formetanate

3-Dimethylaminomethyleneiminophenyl methylcarbamate

Toxicity Rating: 5. Insecticide and acaricide for use on ornamentals. Extremely toxic to mammals (oral LD_{50} for rats, chicken and dog is about 20 mg./kg.). Rapidly reversible cholinesterase inhibitor; atropine is antidotal. Liver and kidney damage (with some deaths) was described in rats given 20 mg./kg. daily in food for 90 days. No percutaneous absorption, but inhalation may lead to systemic intoxication. Not irritating to intact skin. Formetanate is first converted in vitro to m-formaminophenyl-N-methylcarbamate, a weak serum cholinesterase inhibitor in man. This is subsequently decarbamylated to give acetamidophenol and ultimately aminophenol. Formetanate (a base) is unstable in basic solution; hence it is usually supplied as the hydrochloride salt (Carzol).

See also: Carbaryl, Reference Congener in Section III.
Ref.: Knowles and Ahmad, 1971; Nor-Am Agricultural Products, 1977.

1136   1136   Isolan

1-Isopropyl-3-methylpyrazolyl-5-dimethylcarbamate

Toxicity Rating: 5. Systemic aphicide closely related to Pirimicarb (see entry below) but more toxic. Reversible cholinesterase inhibitor. More toxic by cutaneous route than by oral route in rats (rat oral LD_{50} 13 mg./kg.). Dermal and inhalation exposure has caused human intoxication characterized by cool extremities, trembling, miosis, nausea and vomiting, slight cyanosis and electrocardiographic changes. Atropine is antidotal. No longer sold in U.S.A.

See also: Carbaryl, *Reference Congener in Section III.*
Ref.: Ferguson and Alexander, 1953; Tholen and Metzeler, 1955.

1137   Isoprocarb

o-Isopropylphenyl *N*-methylcarbamate,   Etrofolan

Toxicity Rating: 4. Contact insecticide with a moderate mammalian toxicity (oral LD_{50} in laboratory rodents is 500 mg./kg.). Cholinesterase inhibitor. Atropine is antidotal; do not give 2-PAM. Detoxified by hydrolysis. The meta-isomer of isoprocarb (*m*-isopropylphenyl *N*-methylcarbamate) is much more toxic to animals; its LD_{50} is about 10 mg./kg.

orally in rodents and 40 mg./kg. dermally in rabbits. Perhaps its higher toxicity is due to its metabolism by side chain oxidation to yield (1-hydroxy-1-methylethyl)phenyl methylcarbamate, which is also a cholinesterase inhibitor. It has been largely replaced by isoprocarb and other less hazardous materials.

See also: Carbaryl, *Reference Congener in Section III.*
Ref.: Oonnithan and Casida, 1968.

1138   Landrin

3,4,5-Trimethylphenyl methylcarbamate,   2,3,5-Trimethylphenyl methylcarbamate

Toxicity Rating: 4. An insecticidal mixture of isomers for use in sterilizing soil. High acute oral toxicity (rat LD_{50} 208 mg./kg.). Cholinesterase

inhibitor. Atropine is antidotal. Rapidly detoxified by side-chain oxidation and hydrolysis.

See also: Carbaryl, *Reference Congener in Section III.*
Ref.: Slade and Casida, 1970.

1139   Methiocarb

4-(Methylthio)-3,5-xylyl methylcarbamate,   Mercaptodimethur, e.g., Mesurol

Toxicity Rating: 4. Broad spectrum non-systemic insecticide, molluscicide and acaricide. High oral toxicity (LD_{50} 87 to 130 mg./kg. in rats). Cholinesterase inhibitor. Atropine is antidotal. Dermal absorption is appreciable (rat dermal LD_{50} 350 mg./kg.). Metabolized in liver by ring

hydroxylation and *N*-dealkylation to form various methylcarbamates, all of which are potent cholinesterase inhibitors. In intact animals, simultaneously detoxified by hydrolysis of carbamate linkage.

See also: Carbaryl, *Reference Congener in Section III.*
Ref.: Krishna and Casida, 1966; Strother, 1972.

1140   Methomyl

S-Methyl-*N*-((methylcarbamoyl)oxy)thioacetimidate,   Lannate

Toxicity Rating: 5. An insecticide-nematocide marketed in solid form and as aqueous solution. Used on various vegetable crops (cabbage, cauliflower, broccoli, lettuce, etc.) and as flybait. The acute oral LD_{50} in rats is 17-24 mg./kg. Reversible cholinesterase inhibitor. Atropine is antidotal; do not give morphine or 2-PAM. Three men died after ingest-

ing approximately 12 to 15 mg./kg. body weight of methomyl accidentally baked in bread. A fourth, who, like the others, displayed twitching, spasms, fasciculations and respiratory embarrassment, responded within 2 hours to atropine treatment. Percutaneous absorption is slight.

See also: Carbaryl, *Reference Congener in Section III.*
Ref.: Frear, 1969; Liddle et al., 1979; Simpson and Bermingham, 1977.

1141   Mexacarbate

4-Dimethylamino-3,5-xylyl methylcarbamate,   Zectran

Toxicity Rating: 5. Carbamate-type cholinesterase inhibitor used for the control of snails and slugs. Very high acute oral toxicity (rat oral LD_{50} 14 mg./kg.). A 17-year-old male died within 5 hours of consuming not more than 8 ounces of a 22 per cent solution which also contained 31 per cent aromatic petroleum derivatives and 47 per cent "inert ingredients." The patient was found in coma

with pinpoint pupils and intense pulmonary edema, which may have resulted from aspiration of the hydrocarbon solvent. Apparently atropine was not given. Autopsy findings and cholinesterase levels were not reported. For a discussion of aspiration pneumonitis by hydrocarbons, see Kerosene in Section III. For metabolism, see Methiocarb above. Mexacarbate may be carcinogenic.

See also: Carbaryl, *Reference Congener in Section III.*
Ref.: Meikle, 1973; Reich and Welke, 1966.

1142 Mobam

1142

4-Benzothienyl methylcarbamate

Toxicity Rating: 4. Contact insecticide related to carbaryl. High acute oral toxicity in laboratory mammals (oral LD_{50} in rat 70 mg./kg.). Reversible cholinesterase inhibitor. Atropine is antidotal; do not give 2-PAM. Rapidly detoxified by hydrolysis to 4-hydroxybenzothiophene, which is conjugated and excreted in urine. The sulfoxide of 4-hydroxybenzothiophene has been identified as a sulfate conjugate in milk from goats and cows after single sub-toxic doses of Mobam. Supplied as a 50% wettable powder and 10% granular formulation.

See also: Carbaryl, *Reference Congener in Section III*.
Ref.: Robbins et al., 1969; Robbins et al., 1970.

1143 MPMC

1143

Meobal, 3,4-Xylyl methylcarbamate

Toxicity Rating: 4. MPMC and its monomethyl analog MTMC are systemic carbamate insecticides. Both are volatile powders used for control of leaf hoppers on rice. They have high oral and inhalation toxicities (rat oral LD_{50} 380 mg./kg. for MPMC, and 270 mg./kg. for MTMC). Toxicity due to reversible cholinesterase inhibition. Atropine is antidotal; do not give 2-PAM. Detoxification is rapid. In rats, the metabolism of MPMC and MTMC is predominately by ring and side-chain oxidation. Urinary metabolic products of MTMC include 4-hydroxy MTMC, *m*-cresol (and its conjugates), *m*-hydroxybenzoic acid and *m*-carboxyphenyl *N*-methylcarbamate. Detoxification by ester hydrolysis occurs to a minor extent. Dilute aqueous emulsions are irritating to skin and eyes. Supplied as emulsifiable concentrates, powders and dusts.

See also: Carbaryl, *Reference Congener in Section III*.
Ref.: Worthing, 1979; Miyamoto et al., 1969; Ohkawa et al., 1974.

1144 Oxamyl

1144

S-Methyl-1-(dimethylcarbamoyl)-*N*-((methylcarbamoyl)oxy)thioformimidate, Methyl *N,N'*-dimethyl-*N*-[(methylcarbamoyl)oxy]-1-thiooxamimidate, e.g., Vydate

Toxicity Rating: 5 or 6. Carbamate insecticide, nematocide and acaricide. Extremely toxic; rat oral LD_{50} is about 5 mg./kg. Potent cholinesterase inhibitor. Signs of intoxication include weakness, blurred vision, nausea, abdominal cramps, constricted pupils, sweating and muscle tremors. Oral, dermal and ocular exposure may produce systemic poisoning, although dermal absorption is slow. Atropine is antidotal; do not give morphine or 2-PAM. Not irritating to skin or eyes. No cumulative toxicity was seen when rats were given twice the LD_{50} in divided doses over a 2-week period. Detoxified in rats by hydrolysis that removes carbamic acid to form methyl-*N*-hydroxy-*N'*-methyl-1-thiooxamimidate. Also converted by liver microsomal enzymes to *N,N*-dimethyloxamic acid. These compounds are all conjugated and excreted in urine and feces.

See also: Carbaryl, *Reference Congener in Section III*.
Ref.: du Pont, June 1974; Farm Chemicals Handbook, 1980; Harvey and Han, 1978; Spencer, 1973.

1145 Pirimicarb

1145

2-(Dimethylamino)-5,6-dimethyl-4-pyrimidinyl dimethylcarbamate, Pirimor

Toxicity Rating: 4. Systemic aphicide. Volatile dimethylcarbamate insecticide. High systemic toxicity in mammals (rat oral LD_{50} 147 mg./kg.) but apparently poorly absorbed through skin. A reversible cholinesterase inhibitor. Atropine is antidotal. Readily hydrolyzed in mammals. Supplied as a liquid concentrate, a 50% wettable powder and in smoke generators. Three related compounds, dimetan, Pyrolan and Pyramat, were formerly used as contact aphicides and insecticides. The toxic properties of these compounds are like those of pirimicarb.

See also: Carbaryl, *Reference Congener in Section III*.
Ref.: Krishna and Casida, 1966.

1146 Promecarb

1146

m-Cym-5-yl methylcarbamate, Carbamult, 3-Methyl-5-(1-methylethyl)phenyl methylcarbamate

Toxicity Rating: 4-5. Nonsystemic carbamate insecticide for use on potatoes, fruit and corn. A reversible cholinesterase inhibitor. Very high acute oral toxicity (LD_{50} in rat 74 mg./kg.). Absorbed through intact skin (rat dermal LD_{50} 450 mg./kg.). Atropine is antidotal. Detoxified by ester hydrolysis. In dogs given toxic doses by i.v. route, cholinesterase activity returned to normal in 6 hours. Chronic feeding tests in rats (daily doses of 50 mg./kg. for 3 months) led to liver and kidney damage with cerebral hemorrhage and elevated blood sugar, and, in some cases, death (Miyao et al., 1972).

See also: Carbaryl, *Reference Congener in Section III*.
Ref.: Worthing, 1979; Miyao et al., 1972; Plestina and Svetlicic, 1973; Van Hoof and Heyndrickx, 1975.

1147   Propoxur   1147

2-(1-Methylethoxy)phenol methylcarbamate, 2-Isopropoxyphenyl *N*-methylcarbamate, *o*-Isopropoxy-phenyl *N*-methylcarbamate, Aprocarb, e.g., Baygon, Unden

Toxicity Rating: 4 to 5. Carbamate insecticide with rapid knockdown action for use in control of flies, mosquitoes and leafhoppers. In humans, it inhibits erythrocyte cholinesterase without prominent effects on serum cholinesterase. As with other carbamate compounds, depression of cholinesterase activity is reversible and of short duration (1 hour after an oral dose of 1.5 mg./kg.). The syndrome of acute intoxication in man and laboratory animals does not appear to differ from that induced by carbaryl. Acute oral LD_{50} of the technical grade compound is 150 mg./kg. in chickens, 100 mg./kg. in rats, 40 mg./kg. in guinea pigs. Human adult volunteers have ingested single doses of 90 mg. presumably without symptoms. An unknown quantity of Unden proved lethal in an adult 6 hours after ingestion. Principal autopsy findings included brain edema, distended lungs, and marked capillary hyperemia of visceral organs. In rats, daily doses of 20 mg./kg. for 20 days (i.p.) reportedly produced hypertrophy of the intestinal epithelium. Partially hydrolyzed to 2-isopropoxyphenol and rapidly excreted in the urine. Treat intoxications with atropine.

See also: Carbaryl, *Reference Congener in Section III*.
Ref.: Dawson et al., 1964; Geldmacher-v. Mallinckrodt and Schaidt, 1971; Iverson, 1975; Nelson, 1969; Vandekar et al., 1971.

1148   Pyramat   1148

2-*N*-Propyl-4-methylpyrimidyl-(6)-dimethylcarbamate,   6-Methyl-2-propyl-4-pyrimidinyl-dimethylcar-
bamate

Toxicity Rating: 4. A liquid used as an insecticidal spray of high potency because it inhibits insect cholinesterase. Like other dimethyl carbamates (neostigmine, Pirimicarb, Pyrolan, dimetan), it is also a reversible inhibitor of mammalian cholinesterase.

See also: Carbaryl, *Reference Congener in Section III*.
Ref.: Hansens and Bartley, 1953.

1149   Pyrolan   1149

3-Methyl-1-phenyl-5-pyrazolyl dimethylcarbamate

Toxicity Rating: 5. Formerly used as an insecticide. In laboratory rodents it lies near the borderline between toxicity classes 4 and 5. Toxic signs and symptoms are not described but presumably resemble those of carbaryl poisoning, since Pyrolan is a reversible inhibitor of the enzyme cholinesterase and is related to neostigmine. No clinical data. No longer sold in U.S.A.

See also: Carbaryl, *Reference Congener in Section III*.
Ref.: Ferguson and Alexander, 1953; Hansens and Bartley, 1953.

Insecticidal synergists

1150   MGK 264   1150

N-Octyl bicycloheptene dicarboximide, Octacide 264

Toxicity Rating: 3. A synergist in pyrethrum and rotenone insecticides. The compound may act by inhibiting microsomal oxidases as does Piperonyl butoxide (see below). It has a low acute oral toxicity (rat LD_{50} 2.8 gm./kg.) but is absorbed appreciably through the skin (rabbit dermal LD_{50} 470 mg./kg.). Not irritating to human skin when applied in full strength. Systemic effects include central nervous excitation followed by depression. Treat symptomatically.

See also: Pyrethrum, *Reference Congener in Section III*.
Ref.: Gold, 1948b; Lehman, 1949b; Lehman, 1951; Spencer, 1973; Wilkinson, 1976.

1151   Piperonyl Butoxide   1151

Butacide,   Piperonyl ether butoxide,   Butylcarbityl-(6-propylpiperonyl)ether

Toxicity Rating: 2. Used as a synergist to increase the insecticidal potency of pyrethrins, rotenone, carbamates and occasionally other classes of insecticides. Formulations typically contain 5 to 20 times more synergist than insecticide. The substance has a low mammalian toxicity (rat oral LD_{50} 11.5 gm./kg.). Signs of intoxication include anorexia, vomiting, diarrhea, hemorrhagic enteritis, pulmonary hemorrhage, inanition and perhaps mild central nervous depression. Repeated contact may cause slight skin irritation. Piperonyl butoxide, like other methylenedioxybenzene synergists (e.g., sesamex, sulfoxide, n-propyl isome, piperonyl cyclonene, etc.), inhibits hepatic microsomal oxidase enzymes in laboratory rodents and by inference in man; it also inhibits a related group of enzymes in insects, apparently by serving as a competitive substrate. Because these enzymes act to detoxify many drugs and other exogenous chemicals, a heavy exposure to one of these insecticidal synergists might make a person temporarily vulnerable to a variety of toxic insults that would normally be tolerated with ease. Piperonyl butoxide is available in a technical grade which may contain up to 20% related compounds as impurities. Very little data are available on inhalation toxicity; most human exposure is by that route. Additional studies on the mutagenic and carcinogenic potential are needed.

See also: Pyrethrum, *Reference Congener in Section III.*
Ref.: Anders, 1968; Casida et al., 1966; Conney et al., 1972; Haley, 1978; Sarles et al., 1949; Wilkinson, 1976.

1152   1152   Piperonyl Cyclonene

Piperonyl cyclohexenone,   3-Hexyl-5-(3,4-methylenedioxyphenyl)-2-cyclohexene-1-one

Toxicity Rating: 3. In animals it lies on the borderline between toxicity classes 2 and 3. Used as a synergist to increase the insecticidal potency of pyrethrins and rotenone. No human poisonings are known. Caused vomiting in test animals. Only mild skin irritation but repeated skin applications (5% in dimethyl phthalate) proved fatal to rabbits. See also Piperonyl butoxide above for possible effects on detoxification reactions in laboratory mammals. Piperonyl cyclonene is no longer marketed in the U.S.A.

See also: Pyrethrum, *Reference Congener in Section III.*
Ref.: Draize et al., 1948.

1153   1153   n-Propyl Isome

n-Propylisome,   Di-n-propyl maleate isosafrole condensate

Toxicity Rating: 3. A synergist for pyrethrum and other insecticides. Closely related to piperonyl butoxide, it has a similar effect on microsomal enzyme function (see Piperonyl butoxide above). Low acute oral toxicity in mammals (rat LD_{50} 1.5 gm./kg.). Very large doses may induce central nervous system depression in laboratory animals. The compound caused no tissue damage in rats when fed at a level of 5000 ppm for 17 weeks. The manufacture of propyl isome has been discontinued.

See also: Pyrethrum, *Reference Congener in Section III.*
Ref.: Lehman, 1951; Wilkinson, 1976.

1154   1154   Sesamex

Acetaldehyde 2-(2-ethoxyethoxy)ethyl-3,4-(methylenedioxy)phenyl acetal,   Sesoxane

Toxicity Rating: 3. Employed as a synergist in insecticidal formulations of pyrethrins, allethrin and methoxychlor. Oral LD_{50} in rats is 2.0 gm./kg. Like other methylenedioxybenzene synergists (see Piperonyl butoxide above), sesamex inhibits the activity of rat hepatic microsomal enzymes both in vitro and in vivo. Because these enzymes are involved in the detoxification of many drugs and other exogenous chemicals, a heavy exposure to sesamex might make a person temporarily vulnerable to toxic insults that would normally be tolerated with ease.

Ref.: Merck and Co., 1976; Anders, 1968; Casida et al., 1966.

1155   1155   Sulfoxide

n-Octyl sulfoxide of isosafrole, 1,2-Methylenedioxy-4-(octylsulfinylpropyl)-benzene, 1-Methyl-2-(3,4-methylenedioxyphenyl)ethyl octyl sulfoxide, e.g., Sulfox-cide, Sulfoxyl

Toxicity Rating: 3. Used as a synergist to increase the insecticidal potency of pyrethrins. Commonly formulated in the ratio of 5:1 with pyrethrins and 10:1 with allethrin. The substance has a low mammalian toxicity (rat oral LD_{50} 2 gm./kg.). Toxic symptoms which may appear in 10 to 20 minutes include tremors and central nervous depression. Even surviving animals may experience prolonged coma. See also Piperonyl butoxide above.

See also: Pyrethrum, *Reference Congener in Section III.*
Ref.: Lehman, 1951; Spencer, 1973.

1156 Tropital 1156

Piperonal bis(2(2'-*n*-butoxyethoxy)ethyl)acetal, Heliotropin acetal

Toxicity Rating: 3. An insecticidal synergist, commonly used in pyrethrin and carbamate aerosols. Activity is due to inhibition of microsomal hydroxylating enzymes. Low mammalian toxicity (rat oral LD_{50} 4.4 gm./kg.). The primary metabolite, the glycine conjugate of piperonylic acid, is excreted in urine. Although Tropital is not a serious toxic hazard to man, large doses may, by inhibiting detoxification mechanisms, render a person temporarily susceptible to other chemical insults that would normally be tolerated with ease.

Ref.: Fishbein et al., 1967; Kamienski and Casida, 1970; Spencer, 1973.

Dithiocarbamate fungicides

1157 Bunema 1157

Potassium *N*-hydroxymethyl-*N*-methyldithiocarbamate, *N*-Hydroxymethyl *N*-methyldithiocarbamate of potassium

Toxicity Rating: 3. Used on foliage to control bacterial and fungal diseases and in the soil to control phytopathogenic algae, fungi and nematodes. Rat oral LD_{50}'s are 590 and 1032 mg./kg. in females and males respectively. Toxic syndrome not described, but the compound is closely related to sodium dimethyldithiocarbamate (below). If a patient has a history of alcohol ingestion concomitant with exposure to Bunema, see Disulfiram in Section III.

See also: Thiram, *Reference Congener in Section III.*

1158 Ferbam 1158

Ferric dimethyldithiocarbamate, Fermate

Toxicity Rating: 2(?). Iron salt of dimethyldithiocarbamic acid used as a fungicide. Because of the oxidizing potential of the ferric ion, this dithiocarbamate exists in equilibrium with its disulfide which is thiram. The latter can react with sulfhydryl groups *in vitro*; fungitoxicity is apparently due to reaction with a sulfhydryl coenzyme, acetyl CoA. Ferbam has a lower oral toxicity than ziram (rat LD_{50} > 17 gm./kg.). Kidney injury is described in poisoned rats. Tracer studies indicate that ferbam is largely decomposed in the gut to yield carbon disulfide (CS_2) and dimethylamine; both are absorbed together with the original compound. Both dimethylamine sulfate and the glucuronide conjugate of ferbam have been recovered in urine. When labeled ferbam was given to pregnant rats, labeled compounds were found in fetuses, in the milk of lactating dams, and in the urine of their nursing pups. Single doses of ferbam caused fetal anomalies when given to pregnant rats, mice and hamsters. Rats given 300 mg./kg. for 30 days died, whereas some given 0.25% ferbam in food for two months exhibited neurological abnormalities. At autopsy, cystic lesions were found in the cerebral cortex and cerebellum of many of these animals. No accumulation of ferbam was found in liver and kidney after two years, but the iron content of the long bones was proportional to the logarithm of the dose. May cause irritation to skin and mucous membranes and rarely skin sensitization in man. If a patient has a history of alcohol ingestion concomitant with ferbam, see Disulfiram in Section III.

See also: Thiram, *Reference Congener in Section III.*
Ref.: Council on Pharmacy and Chemistry, 1955; Fishbein, 1976; Hodge et al., 1956; Owens and Rubinstein, 1964; Periquet and Derache, 1976; Short et al., 1976.

1159 Mancozeb 1159

Dithane M-45

Toxicity Rating: 2 or 3. A fungicide closely related to maneb and zineb, being the coordination product of zinc ion with manganese ethylenebisdithiocarbamate. It has a low oral toxicity (rat LD_{50} > 8 gm./kg.). Several other mixed salts are marketed, including cufraneb and mancopper, each of which contains copper. They are appreciably more toxic than other ethylenebisdithiocarbamate preparations. Apparently none of them sensitizes to alcohol as does disulfiram. For toxic signs and symptoms, see Maneb below.

See also: Carbon Disulfide, *Reference Congener in Section III.*

1160 Maneb 1160

Manganese ethylene bis(dithiocarbamate), Manzate, Dithane M-22, Dithane M-22 Special

Toxicity Rating: 2. A widely used agricultural fungicide of low acute oral toxicity in laboratory animals. Available alone or mixed with zinc (to produce mancozeb). The oral LD_{50} in rats is 6750 mg./

kg. Under normal use conditions, maneb is generally regarded as harmless, except for occasional signs of local irritation (e.g., conjunctivitis, rhinitis, pharyngitis, bronchitis, dermatitis). However, it reportedly caused acute renal failure and ECG abnormalities in a 62-year–old man exposed while applying the compound to his garden. Symptoms resolved promptly following hemodialysis. Single toxic doses of maneb in rats induced hypotonia, bradycardia, decreased respiratory frequency, functional abnormalities of liver and thyroid, infiltrations in the lungs, bronchitis and tracheitis. Doses of 50% of the LD_{50} caused a decrease in the nonspecific immunologic reactivity of rats. Dogs given 200 mg./kg. daily for several months developed tremors, malaise, weakness, gastrointestinal disturbances, posterior incoordination, hypotonus and paresis, progressing to flaccid paraplegia. Neurotoxicity may be referable to carbon disulfide released in the acid environment of the stomach. Rats given 0.25% maneb or zineb (see below) in food for 2 years showed thyroid hyperplasia and nodular goiter, while those given single oral doses

of one-tenth the LD_{50} exhibited a decrease in ^{131}I binding rates in the thyroid. After 30 daily doses, the latter animals had thyroid cell abnormalities including numerous resorption vacuoles in follicular cells and focal epithelial hyperplasia. Single massive toxic doses of maneb (2 to 4 gm./kg.) or zineb (4 to 8 gm./kg.) produced a high proportion of fetal abnormalities in rats when given during organogenesis. Smaller doses given throughout pregnancy had no teratogenic effect. The teratogenic and goitrogenic effects may be due to ethylenethiourea (see in index), which is a contaminant and metabolic product of maneb, zineb and mancozeb. Rabbits given daily 0.05 to 0.5 gm./kg. of zineb or maneb developed leukopenia in 12 to 78 days; at autopsy they showed multiple petechial hemorrhages of the mucosa of the GI tract. Maneb is extensively metabolized in the rat, one of the primary metabolites being ethylene bis(isothiocyanate sulfide). Like other forms of ethylene bis(dithiocarbamates), maneb and zineb apparently do not sensitize to alcohol as does disulfiram.

See also: Carbon Disulfide, *Reference Congener in Section III.*
Ref.: Clayton et al., 1957; Fishbein, 1976; Gates, 1958; Ivanova-Chemishanska et al., 1971; Koizumi et al., 1979; Matokhnyuk, 1972; Petrova-Vergievo and Ivanova-Tchemishanska, 1973; Smith et al., 1953b.

1161   1161   Metham Sodium

Sodium *N*-methyldithiocarbamate, Vapam, Carbam, VPM, SMDC

Toxicity Rating: 4. A soil fungicide, nematocide and herbicide reputed to act by decomposition in moist soil to methyl isothiocyanate (see latter in the index). If true, this may be a unique property of metham, as opposed to many closely related chemicals used for much the same purposes, e.g., ferbam, nabam, ziram, zineb and maneb. Metham is usually supplied as the sodium salt, occasionally as the ammonium or potassium salt. High acute

oral toxicity (oral LD_{50} 280 mg./kg. for albino mice, 820 mg./kg. for albino rats). The salts are irritating to skin and mucous membranes; prolonged or repeated contact may cause skin burns and systemic intoxication (rat dermal LD_{50} 800 mg./kg. for metham sodium). If patient has a history of ingesting alcohol concomitantly with an exposure to metham, see Disulfiram in Section III.

See also: Thiram, *Reference Congener in Section III.*
Ref.: Assoc. of Amer. Pesticide Control Officials, 1966; Worthing, 1979; Pieroh et al., 1959.

1162   1162   Nabam

Disodium ethylene bis(dithiocarbamate), e.g., Dithane D-14, Dithane A-40

Toxicity Rating: 4. Nabam, Amobam and Kabam are the sodium, ammonium and potassium salts of ethylene bis(dithiocarbamic acid) respectively. These so-called EBDC's are fungicides produced by the reaction of CS_2 and ethylenediamine under alkaline conditions; they decompose in water to give sulfur and ethylene thiuram monosulfide. Water solutions are stabilized by the addition of zinc, iron, manganous or copper sulfate (see Zineb, Maneb, etc.). Fungitoxicity is due to inhibition of aconitase activity. These salts do not react with sulfhydryls. Their acute oral toxicity is moderately high (LD_{50} 395 mg./kg. for nabam). Experimental animals given toxic doses of nabam exhibit first stimulation, then depression of central nervous

system, bloody diarrhea, general weakness and prostration. Death is due to respiratory arrest. At necropsy, severe irritation of the gastrointestinal tract and renal necrosis are seen. These effects may be due in part to carbon disulfide released in the acid environment of the stomach. Oils increase absorption and toxicity. Protein-deficient animals are more susceptible than control animals. In chronic feeding studies, goiters were encountered, perhaps due to a metabolite of ethylene bis(dithiocarbamic acid), namely ethylenethiourea; see latter in index. Nabam causes mild skin irritation in humans. Like other EBDC's, nabam apparently does not sensitize to alcohol as does disulfiram.

See also: Carbon Disulfide, *Reference Congener in Section III.*
Ref.: Council on Pharmacy and Chemistry, 1955; Owens and Rubinstein, 1964; Periquet and Derache, 1976; Smith et al., 1953b.

1163   Sodium Dimethyldithiocarbamate   1163

Dibam,   Dibam A

Toxicity Rating: 3. Dibam and Dibam A are the sodium and ammonium salts of dimethyldithiocarbamic acid. These are stabilized for use as plant fungicides by the addition of zinc or ferrous sulfate. They have a moderate acute oral toxicity (rat LD_{50} 1 gm./kg.). Symptoms of intoxication are like those for Ziram (see below). The copper and manganous salts of dimethyldithiocarbamate are also fungicidal. Their toxicity toward animals is appreciably greater than the sodium or zinc salts, however, and they are little used. If patient has a history of alcohol ingestion concomitant with exposure to any of these compounds, see Disulfiram in Section III.

See also: Thiram, *Reference Congener in Section III.*

1164   Sulfallate   1164

2-Chloroallyl diethyldithiocarbamate,   CDEC,   Vegadex

Toxicity Rating: 3. A pre-emergence herbicide for control of grasses and weeds in vegetables, fruits and ornamentals. Absorbed and translocated by plant roots. Moderate acute toxicity in rats (oral LD_{50} 850 mg./kg.). The nature of the toxic syndrome has not been described. The technical grade material contains 90% Sulfallate. The identity of the impurities is unknown. In chronic feeding experiments, rats given 250 ppm for 6 months developed obvious eye irritation, toxic tubular nephropathy, and acanthosis and hyperkeratosis of the forestomach. Increased incidence of mammary adenocarcinoma and of squamous cell carcinomas of skin, esophagus and stomach was also observed. Hepatocellular carcinomas and lung tumors were reported in mice given 500 ppm in food. Prolonged contact with skin and eyes causes moderate irritation.

See also: Thiram, *Reference Congener in Section III.*
Ref.: National Cancer Institute, 1978c; Ploch, 1957.

1165   Thiram   1165

Bis(dimethylthiocarbamoyl) disulfide,   Tetramethylthiuram disulfide,   TMTD

Toxicity Rating: 4.

See also: Thiram, *Reference Congener in Section III.*

1166   Vancide 51   1166

Toxicity Rating: 3. A mixture of sodium dimethyldithiocarbamate and sodium 2-mercaptobenzothiazole (see ingredients in this Index). Used to control slime in pulp mills and cooling towers and in the manufacture of mildew-proof cotton, paste, and cutting oils. Animal experiments indicate that the mixture has a moderate acute oral toxicity (cat LD_{50} 2.3 gm./kg.). It is not irritating to intact human skin. It may be irritating to eyes and mucous membranes, however. Dogs given food containing 5000 ppm for one year showed no ill effects. A similar mixture of the corresponding zinc salts is marketed under the name Vancide 51Z. It has similar uses but is more toxic than the sodium mixture (rat oral LD_{50} about 1.5 gm./kg.), and it is corrosive in the eye.

See also: Thiram, *Reference Congener in Section III.*
Ref.: Vanderbilt, December 1974; Vanderbilt, August 1976a.

1167   Zineb   1167

Zinc ethylene bis(dithiocarbamate), Dithane Z-78

Toxicity Rating: 2-3. An agricultural fungicide closely related to maneb with similar toxic effects (rat oral LD_{50} > 5 gm./kg.). In rats the chief metabolite is ethylenethiourea (see in this Index). Some irritation of skin and mucous membranes has been reported in man. Sulfhemoglobinemia, Heinz body formation and acute hemolytic anemia followed contact and possible ingestion of zineb by a Persian Jew with demonstrably decreased blood levels of glucose-6-phosphate dehydrogenase, reduced glutathione and catalase. Sulfhemoglobinemia and intravascular hemolysis were considered to be independent actions of the fungicide and related to the biochemical defects inherent in this particular patient. For a discussion of the mechanism of intravascular hemolysis and the management of this syndrome, see Naphthalene in Section III. For additional toxic effects of zineb, see Maneb above.

See also: Carbon Disulfide, *Reference Congener in Section III.*
Ref.: Council on Pharmacy and Chemistry, 1955; Fishbein, 1976; Pinkhas et al., 1963; Smith et al., 1953b.

1168   **1168 Ziram**

Zinc dimethyldithiocarbamate

Toxicity Rating: 3. The zinc salt of dimethyldithio-carbamic acid, used as a rubber accelerator and fungicide. Closely related to thiram and ferbam but does not react with sulfhydryls *in vitro*. Fungitox-icity apparently due to chelation of Fe^{+2} necessary for action of aconitase. Toxic in guinea pigs and rabbits, less so in rats (rat oral LD_{50} 1.4 gm./kg.). Oral doses poorly absorbed in the absence of oils. May be absorbed through intact skin. In a fatal case of human poisoning (Buklan, 1974), brain edema and hemorrhage, *in vivo* hemolysis, "dys-

trophy" of the muscle, liver and kidney, emphy-sema, and local necrosis of the intestine were found. Prolonged human inhalation exposure is said to have produced neural and visual disturbances, der-matitis, and irritation of the upper respiratory tract. Irritating to skin and mucous membranes, especially in sensitive persons. Corrosive to eyes. Teratogenesis and oncogenesis are described in the Russian literature. If patient ingests alcohol con-comitantly with an exposure to ziram, see Disulfi-ram in Section III.

See also: Thiram, *Reference Congener in Section III.*
Ref.: Buklan, 1974; Council on Pharmacy and Chemistry, 1955; Enikeev, 1968; Hodge et al., 1956; Vanderbilt, December 1976b.

1169   **1169 Ethylenethiourea**

2-Imidazolidinethione,   ETU

Toxicity Rating: 3. Accelerator used in vulcaniza-tion of various elastomers. Also a metabolite of ethylenebisdithiocarbamate fungicides (EBCD's), found as an environmental contaminant. Produced during cooking of foods contaminated with EBCD fungicides and during their metabolism in plants and animals, including cows. Rapidly absorbed when ingested and disseminated throughout the body. Placental transfer is rapid. Strongly accu-mulated by thyroid tissue and slowly released. Excreted unchanged in urine. Moderate acute oral toxicity (rat LD_{50} 1.8 gm./kg.). In acutely poisoned rats death is due to lung edema. Repeated sublethal doses produce hypothyroidism. Single oral doses of 30 mg./kg. or more given to pregnant rats on day 15 of gestation produced prompt fetal brain damage and a high incidence of late-devel-oping hydrocephalus and microphthalmia in sur-

viving offspring. In other experiments, tail and limb defects and urogenital malformations were pro-duced by daily doses of 10 mg./kg. given during organogenesis. Single dermal applications of 50 mg./kg. produced 100% fetal abnormalities when administered to pregnant rats on days 12 or 13 of gestation. Joint administration of ETU and sodium nitrite produced dominant lethal mutations in mice, presumably by formation of N-nitroso-ethy-lenethiourea. ETU alone was ineffective. Ethyle-nethiourea is also goitrogenic and carcinogenic. Administration of a diet containing 5 ppm for 2 years produced thyroid hyperplasia in 28% of ex-posed rats, while a diet containing 125 ppm or more produced a high incidence of thyroid carcinoma. The compound is also said to have induced hepa-tomas in mice (Innes et al., 1969).

Ref.: Graham et al., 1975; Innes et al., 1969; Khera, 1973; Khera and Tryphonas, 1977; National Institute for Occupational Safety and Health, 1978a; Stula and Krauss, 1977; Teramoto et al., 1978.

Triazine-triazole fungicides

1170   **1170 Anilazine**

2,4-Dichloro-6-*o*-chloroanilino-*s*-triazine, 4,6-Dichloro-*N*-(2-chlorophenyl) 1,3,5-triazin-2-amine, Kemate, Dyrene

Toxicity Rating: 4. A protective fungicide for foli-age application. Antifungal activity is due to alkyl-ation of fungal enzymes. Animal tests place it near the borderline between toxicity classes 3 and 4. No evidence of toxic effects when fed to rats over a

period of 2 years (5000 ppm). Can cause irritation of skin with prolonged contact. Related chemically to *s*-triazine herbicides; see also Atrazine in the index.

Ref.: Chemagro Corp., 1961g.

1171   **1171 Fluotrimazole**

1-(3-Trifluoromethyltrityl)-1,2,4-triazole

Toxicity Rating: 2. Fungicide for use against pow-dery mildew. Very low acute oral toxicity in rats ($LD_{50} > 5$ gm./kg.). No description of toxic symp-

toms was found. Supplied as a 50% wettable powder and 12% emulsifiable concentrate.

Ref.: Worthing, 1979.

1172 Hexahydro-1,3,5-triethyl-s-triazine 1172

Vancide TH

Toxicity Rating: 4. Industrial fungicide and bacteriostat. Liquid is highly corrosive to skin and eyes, mummifies skin and causes permanent corneal scarring in high concentrations. Readily absorbed through intact skin (rabbit dermal LD_{50} 0.5 gm./kg.). Highly toxic when given orally (rat LD_{50} 0.3 gm./kg.). Symptoms of systemic poisoning in rats include central nervous system depression, with lethargy and ataxia, and frequently dyspnea. Rats given single fatal doses or repeated subacute doses developed fatty changes, passive congestion and severe focal necrosis of the liver. Signs of kidney toxicity including proteinuria, hemoglobinuria and glucosuria were also present. During 90-day feeding studies, some animals given 1800 ppm in food developed pulmonary edema. Dilute solutions (1000 ppm) are irritating to skin and eyes. The compound decomposes in acid media (and presumably in the stomach) to yield ethylamine and formaldehyde.

Ref.: Vanderbilt, 1978; Winek et al., 1977.

1173 Hexahydro-tris(2-hydroxyethyl)-s-triazine 1173

Grotan BK

Toxicity Rating: 3 or 4. Fungicide, used to preserve industrial cutting oils. Animal experiments place the compound on the border between toxicity classes 3 and 4. Said to cause high incidence of contact allergy in exposed workers.

Ref.: Dungemann et al., 1964; Urwin et al., 1976.

Miscellaneous agricultural and industrial fungicides

1174 Benomyl 1174

Methyl 1-(butylcarbamoyl)-2-benzimidazolecarbamate, e.g., Benlate, Tersan 1991, Arbortrine

Toxicity Rating: 2. A systemic fungistat used on orchards, field crops, turf and ornamentals. Also slows growth of mites and is used as a veterinary anthelmintic. The substance is rapidly hydrolyzed to methyl-2-benzimidazole carbamate (MBC). The latter is a potent inhibitor of DNA synthesis in fungi and is probably responsible for the fungitoxic action of the parent compound. Benomyl has a low acute oral toxicity in mammals (rat LD_{50} greater than 10 gm./kg.). Rats given ^{14}C-labeled benomyl metabolized 85% of the dose within one hour, the primary metabolite being MBC. This was subsequently converted to the glucuronide and/or sulfate of 5-hydroxy-MBC, which were readily excreted so that 99% of the radiolabel was recovered in urine and feces within 72 hours. No tissue accumulation of benomyl or of MBC could be demonstrated. Benomyl is supplied as a wettable powder. Arbortrine, a solubilized form of benomyl, has been used experimentally for control of Dutch Elm disease.

Ref.: Baude et al., 1973; Gardiner et al., 1974; Lyr, 1973; Sherman et al., 1975.

1175 *trans*-1,2-Bis(propylsulfonyl)ethene 1175

CHE 1843, Vancide PA

Toxicity Rating: 3 or 4(?). Agricultural fungicide and industrial mold inhibitor, commonly used in paints. Rat oral LD_{50} variously reported as 200 and 2070 mg./kg., but very high acute parenteral toxicity (i.p. LD_{50} is about 11 mg./kg. in rats, mice and guinea pigs). Detoxified in alkaline solution (pH greater than 9). Not irritating to intact skin. No percutaneous absorption (rabbit dermal LD_{50} greater than 10 gm./kg.).

Ref.: Vanderbilt, June 1977; Farm Chemicals Handbook, 1980.

1176 Fuberidazole 1176

2(2'-Furyl)-benzimidazole, e.g., Voronit

Toxicity Rating: 3. Related to benomyl (see above) and to thiabendazole (see below). Voronit refers to several mixtures of fuberidazole with hexachlorobenzene. Used as a seed dressing, Voronit protects against soil-borne fungal diseases of seedlings. Also used systemically for the control of vascular wilt diseases in plants. Activity is due to the inhibition of nucleotide synthesis in fungi. Fuberidazole has a moderate acute oral toxicity (rat LD_{50} 1 gm./kg.). Rapidly absorbed from the stomach and detoxified by oxidation in the liver. Excreted in bile and urine. In dogs, peak plasma and liver concentrations are seen about two hours after oral dosing. Vomiting occurs in some animals at this time. No other description of toxic symptoms was found. Not irritating to skin, but toxic doses are absorbed percutaneously by rabbits (dermal LD_{50} 1 gm./kg.).

Ref.: Bartels-Schooley and MacNeill, 1971; Frank, 1971.

1177   **1177** Thiabendazole

2-(4-Thiazolyl)-1H-benzimidazole, Thiabenzole

Toxicity Rating: 3. A systemic fungicide used to control pre- and post-harvest diseases of fruits and vegetables. Also a potent oral anthelmintic. Although the oral toxicity in experimental animals is moderately low (rat LD_{50} 3.1 gm./kg.), therapeutic doses of 150 mg./kg. can cause delayed and transitory dizziness, nausea and vomiting in humans. These effects were also seen in dogs after i.v. administration and could be suppressed by prior treatment with chlorpromazine. Single oral doses of 200 mg./kg. were eliminated by emesis in dogs and consequently no mortality was observed in that species. Laboratory rodents given fatal doses developed inanition, ataxia and narcosis, with death in coma. The compound is rapidly absorbed, metabolized and excreted. Its major metabolites in rats and humans are 5-hydroxythiabendazole and conjugates of 5-hydroxythiabendazole. In tracer experiments in humans, peak plasma concentra-tions of thiabendazole occurred 1 to 2 hours after a single oral dose, and most of the metabolites were excreted in urine and feces within 12 hours. In one reported clinical case of a delayed sensitivity re-action, small doses of the drug given several weeks apart caused a generalized allergic urticaria. How-ever, thiabendazole is neither an irritant nor a sensitizer on shaved rabbit skin. In chronic rat feeding studies, doses of 1200 mg./kg. daily were fatal in a few days. Daily doses of 200 mg./kg. for 2 years caused a mild anemia in dogs. At autopsy, moderate hypoplasia of the bone marrow was found, together with mild atrophy of lymphoid tissue and loss of colloid in the thyroid follicles. Considerable hemosiderosis was present through-out the reticuloendothelial system. The compound is a chelating agent, binding many metals, including iron, but not calcium.

Ref.: Robinson et al., 1969; Robinson et al., 1978; Tanowitz and Wittner, 1970; Tocco et al., 1966.

1178   **1178** Benquinox

1,4-Benzoquinone 1-benzoylhydrazone 4-oxime, e.g., Ceredon, Cereline

Toxicity Rating: 4. A powerful fungicide used to treat seeds for protection against fungal diseases of seedlings. Although it is very toxic (rat oral LD_{50} 100 mg./kg.), no description of its toxic effects was found. Supplied alone and in mixtures with thiram or phenylmercuric acetate for use as seed dressings.

1179   **1179** Captan

N-Trichloromethylthio-3α,4,7,7α-tetrahydrophthalimide, e.g., Orthocide

Toxicity Rating: 2(?). A fungicidal derivative of tetrahydrophthalimide widely used to protect seeds at planting. Fungitoxic effects are attributed to inhibition of protein and DNA synthesis and of acetate metabolism. Captan normally has a low acute oral toxicity due to rapid degradation in the gut (rat LD_{50} 12.6 gm./kg.). However, it is very toxic to laboratory animals maintained from wean-ing on a protein-deficient diet (rat oral LD_{50} about 100 mg./kg.). Toxic oral doses produce hypother-mia, irritability, listlessness, anorexia, hyporeflexia and oliguria, with a marked glycosuria and hema-turia on the first day. Following large doses, death is due to cardiac or respiratory failure. With smaller doses death may be delayed and is then apparently caused by infiltrative meningitis secondary to cap-illary hemorrhages. Animals dying early showed marked hemorrhagic capillary-venous congestion in the stomach, heart, lungs and highly vascular organs, including the thymus. When death was delayed, autopsy showed leukocytic invasion of the meninges, fatty degeneration of the heart and renal tubules, stress response in adrenals, spleen and thymus, and degenerative changes in pancreas, salivary glands and testes. Tracer studies show that captan is rapidly hydrolyzed in the gut, with the production of tetrahydrophthalimide and (proba-bly) thiophosgene. The latter is efficiently ab-sorbed, converted to thiazolidine-2-thione-4-car-boxylic acid through reaction with cysteine, and excreted in urine. Small amounts of dithiobis(methanesulfonic acid) and its disulfide monoxide derivative are also excreted after oral doses (DeBaun and Miaullis, 1974). When captan is given to experimental animals by intraperitoneal injection, it is very much more toxic than by mouth, reacting rapidly with cysteine to form thiophos-gene *in situ* (i.p. rat LD_{50} 50 to 100 mg./kg.). Many of the toxic effects of captan are apparently due to interactions with enzyme and membrane thiols. It increases the K^+ efflux and osmotic fra-gility of red blood cells *in vivo* (Kumar et al., 1975). It inhibits mitosis in cultured embryonic human lung cells and shows dose-dependent mutagenicity in several assay systems. This mutagenic potential is lost when captan is added to blood plasma. The latter effects and captan's fungitoxicity depend on the presence of the dichloromethylthio moiety and may be due to the release of thiophosgene. Captan induces occasional phocomelia when injected into developing chicken eggs (Verrett et al., 1969). Al-though systemic poisoning after ingestion appears unlikely (no human poisonings known), a possible antidotal action of sulfhydryl protectants such as glutathione should be investigated.

Ref.: Bridges et al., 1972; Boyd and Krijnen, 1968; Council on Pharmacy and Chemistry, 1955; DeBaun and Miaullis, 1974; Krijnen and Boyd, 1970; Kumar et al., 1975; Legator et al., 1969; Seiler, 1972; Verrett et al., 1969.

1180   Captafol   1180

Difolatan,   Ortho 5865,   Folcid,   Difolatan-Botran

Toxicity Rating: 3. The N-tetrachloroethyl analog of Captan, used as a protectant fungicide on potatoes, citrus fruit, onions, etc. The acute oral toxicity is low (rat LD_{50} 2.5 gm./kg.), probably due to rapid hydrolysis in the gut. For metabolic fate and

Ref.: Verrett et al., 1969.

possible teratogenic action, see Captan above. Available as a wettable powder (85% pure) and as a flowable seed protector containing 39% active ingredient. Also sold in combination with dichloran under the name Difolatan-Botran.

1181   Folpet   1181

N-(Trichloromethylthio)phthalimide,   Phaltan

Toxicity Rating: 2(?). A fungicide used for control of black spot and mildew on roses. Available as a 50% wettable powder. All rats tested survived the oral administration of 10 gm./kg. Male rats fed 10,000 ppm for 12 weeks showed a slight reduction

Ref.: Spencer, 1973.

in body weight; no other abnormalities were noted. May irritate mucosal surfaces. Chemically related to Captan, and like Captan it decomposes *in vivo* to thiophosgene. May also be teratogenic. See Captan above.

1182   Carboxin   1182

5,6-Dihydro-2-methyl-N-phenyl-1,4-oxathiin-3-carboxamide,   Vitavax

Toxicity Rating: 3. A systemic plant fungicide claimed to render grain crops immune to loose smut. Oxycarboxin is formed by the treatment of carboxin with hydrogen peroxide. Although carboxin is toxic only toward Basidiomycete fungi, oxycarboxin has a broad fungicidal activity. Both compounds have moderate acute oral toxicities in mammals (for oxycarboxin, the rat LD_{50} 3.2 gm./kg.). Neither is appreciably toxic when applied

Ref.: Chin et al., 1970; Lyr, 1973.

dermally. The compounds inhibit oxidative metabolism and succinic dehydrogenase in mitochondria of liver and bone. When fed to dogs, carboxin is partially oxidized to oxycarboxin. Both compounds are excreted in urine and feces. Carboxin and oxycarboxin are supplied as wettable powders and liquid concentrates. Mixtures of carboxin with thiram are also available.

1183   Chloranil   1183

Spergon,   Tetrachloro-1,4-benzoquinone,   Tetrachloroquinone

Toxicity Rating: 3. A fungicidal seed protectant. The acute oral toxicity is low (rat LD_{50} 4 gm./kg.) because it is poorly absorbed. Toxic doses produce watery diarrhea, central nervous depression, coma

Ref.: Council on Pharmacy and Chemistry, 1955; McGavack et al., 1943; Naugatuck Chemical, 1951a.

and death. Fungitoxic action is attributed to role in redox processes and to inhibition of decarboxylases. Chloranil is a skin irritant in high concentrations but is not absorbed percutaneously.

1184   Chloroneb   1184

1,4-Dichloro-2,5-dimethoxybenzene,   e.g., Demosan,   Tersan SP

Toxicity Rating: 2. Systemic fungicide for control of seedling diseases. Fungitoxicity is due to specific inhibition of DNA polymerization. Very low acute oral toxicity in mammals (rat LD_{50} > 11 gm./kg.). Rats fed 2500 ppm for 2 years showed no toxic

Ref.: Lyr, 1973; Rhodes and Pease, 1971.

effects. The primary metabolite is 2,5-dichloro-4-methoxyphenol, which is excreted in urine. Chloroneb is supplied as a wettable powder (65% pure) and in a mixture with thiram under the name Demosan T.

1185   Chlorothalonil   1185

Bravo,   Tetrachloroisophthalonitrile,   Daconil 2787,   Termil,   2,4,5,6-Tetrachloro-3-cyanobenzonitrile,   Tetrachlorophthalodinitrile

Toxicity Rating: 2. A broad spectrum fungicide used as a foliage protectant on vegetables and ornamentals, as a cotton seed protectant, and in mildew-resistant paint. Low acute oral toxicity due to poor absorption (rat oral LD_{50} > 10 gm./kg.). The compound has a very high toxicity when given i.p. (rat LD_{50} 2.5 mg./kg.). Animals given acutely

toxic doses exhibit sedation followed by increasing weakness and death. In chronic feeding studies at the 1% level, rats eventually developed ataxia, tachypnea, epistaxis, dermatitis, hematuria, hyperactivity, vaginal bleeding and bright yellow urine. Nodular masses progressing to abscesses developed in some animals. Renal tumors occurred in one-tenth of the animals. Chlorothalonil is supplied as a wettable powder and a thermal dust. The technical grade material contains about 1% pentachlorobenzonitrile and 0.5% tetrachlorodicyanobenzene isomers introduced during manufacture.

Ref.: National Cancer Institute, 1978d; Yoshikawa and Kawai, 1966.

1186   Dazomet

Tetrahydro-3,5-dimethyl-2H-1,3,5-thiadiazine-2-thione, Mylone, Crag Fungicide 974   3,5-Dimethyl-1,3,5,2H-tetrahydrothiadiazine-2-thione,

Toxicity Rating: 4. Used as a fungicide, nematocide and slimicide. Releases methyl isothiocyanate slowly in the soil and rapidly when heated. The oral LD$_{50}$ of dazomet is 180 mg./kg. in guinea pigs but higher in rats. Dazomet behaved as a sympathomimetic agent when injected intramuscularly in anesthetized dogs to produce mydriasis and elevated heart rate and blood pressure. Following single toxic oral doses, rats either died in clonic-tonic convulsions within 10 minutes or recovered completely within 24 hours. Animals fed 40 ppm for 2 years showed focal necrosis of the liver with central fatty metamorphosis. Kidneys of rats fed 10 ppm for 2 years showed focal tubular necrosis. Metabolites include carbon disulfide and perhaps formaldehyde and methylamine. The possibility that decomposition to methyl isothiocyanate (see in the Index) is responsible for the rapid lethality of dazomet should be explored. Even dilute solutions cause skin irritation and sensitization in humans.

Ref.: Assoc. of Amer. Pesticide Control Officials, 1966; Smyth et al., 1966; Spencer, 1973.

1187   Dehydroacetic Acid

3-Acetyl-6-methyl-2,4-pyrandione, DHA

Toxicity Rating: 3. The sodium salt has a similiar toxicity. A fungicide used in cosmetics and on processed fruits and vegetables. No primary or allergic skin reactions. Humans ingested 0.01 gm./kg. daily for 150 days without observable ill-effects. At high dosage levels monkeys showed anorexia, vomiting, weakness, stupor, ataxia, and convulsions. The control of convulsions by barbiturates was life-saving in experimental poisonings.

Ref.: Seevers et al., 1950; Shideman et al., 1950; Spencer et al., 1950b; Woods et al., 1950.

1188   2,2′-Dibromo-3-nitrilopropionamide

DBNPA

Toxicity Rating: 4(?). Fungicide and slimicide for use in industrial processes, cooling towers, pulp mills, etc. Stable at acid pH but rapidly hydrolyzed in alkaline media with evolution of ammonia, carbon dioxide, and dibromoacetonitrile. Radiotracer studies indicate that the compound is rapidly metabolized and eliminated when given to rats. Observations on 4 rats (personal communication, H.N. Jacoby, 1980) suggest a toxicity rating of 4, but no definitive toxicity study was located.

Ref.: Exner et al., 1973.

1189   Dichlofluanid

Euparen, Eparen, N'-Dichlorofluoromethylthio-N,N-dimethyl-N'-phenyl-sulfamide, 1,1-Dichloro-N-[(dimethylamino)sulfonyl]-1-fluoro-N-phenyl-methanesulfenamide

Toxicity Rating: 3(?). A fungicide for control of foliage diseases of fruits, vegetables and ornamentals. Low acute oral toxicity in rats (LD$_{50}$ greater than 2500 mg./kg.). Rats tolerated 1500 ppm in food daily for two years without ill effect. Tolylfluanid is a methyl derivative of dichlofluanid having similar uses and a similar oral toxicity. The compounds are supplied as 50% wettable powders and 7.5% dusts.

Ref.: Bayer, March 1978; Worthing, 1979; Spencer, 1973.

1190   Dichlone

2,3-Dichloro-1,4-naphthoquinone, Phygon

Toxicity Rating: 3. A fungicide used on food crops and textiles. Also algicidal. Moderate acute oral toxicity (rat oral LD$_{50}$ 1.3 gm./kg.). A central nervous system depressant. Reacts with enzyme thiols. Dogs vomited and survived large single doses. They tolerated 500 ppm in food for one year, showing only slight liver damage. Dichlone is irritating to skin and mucous membranes, especially when mixed with fats or oils. It is supplied as a wettable powder (50%), in dilute dusts (1 to 4%), and as a paste (55%).

Ref.: Council on Pharmacy and Chemistry, 1955; Lehman, 1965; Naugatuck Chemical, 1953.

1191 Dichloran 1191

Botran, 2,6-Dichloro-4-nitroaniline

Toxicity Rating: 3(?). A fungicide used on a wide variety of vegetable and fruit crops. Activity is due to inhibition of fungal protein synthesis. Low to moderate acute oral toxicity in rodents (LD_{50} about 8 gm./kg. in rats and 1.5 gm./kg. in mice). Rapidly converted in mammalian liver to 3,5-dichloro-4-aminophenol (DCAP) and 2,6-dichloro-p-phenylenediamine (DCPD) which are excreted in urine. Toxicity may be due in part to metabolites. Dichloran and DCAP uncouple oxidative phosphorylation in $vitro$; DCPD does not. Repeated doses of dichloran cause an induction of rat hepatic biphenyl hydroxylase and nitroreductase activities and an increase in the proportion of dichloran

excreted as the less toxic DCPD. In studies of chronic toxicity, rats survived daily oral doses of 1 gm./kg. dichloran for 3 months. In Rhesus monkeys, where dichloran does not induce hepatic enzymes and the primary metabolite is DCAP, daily doses of 160 mg./kg. were fatal within 3 months. At autopsy, monkey livers showed centrolobular fatty infiltration with swelling of mitochondria and distortion of cristae. Dogs given 24 mg./kg. of dichloran daily for 55 days developed corneal and lens opacities when exposed to natural sunlight. No information about possible methemoglobinemia was located.

See also: 2,4-Dinitrophenol, Reference Congener in Section III.
Ref.: Bernstein et al., 1970; Gallo et al., 1976; Lyr, 1973; Serrone et al., 1967.

1192 Dimethirimol 1192

5-Butyl-2-dimethylamino-6-methyl-4-pyrimidinol, Milcurb

Toxicity Rating: 3. Systemic plant fungicide for control of powdery mildew. Specific pyridoxal antagonist in fungi. Moderate acute oral toxicity in mammals (rat LD_{50} 2.3 gm./kg.). Rats given 24 mg./kg. daily for 2 years showed no ill effects. Supplied in aqueous solution as the hydrochloride

salt. Ethirimol is an ethyl analog with the same fungitoxic action and a similar oral toxicity. (Oral LD_{50} is 4.0 gm./kg. in rats but 0.5 to 1.0 gm./kg. in guinea pigs.) Neither compound is presently registered for use on crops in the U.S.A.

Ref.: Lyr, 1973; Spencer, 1973.

1193 Dodine 1193

Dodecylguanidine acetate, Cyprex, Melprex, Curitan

Toxicity Rating: 3. A cationic surfactant used as an agricultural fungicide. Moderate oral toxicity in rats (LD_{50} 0.8 gm./kg.). Dogs vomited large doses. Rats showed steadily increasing depression with diarrhea beginning after 10 to 12 hours, and death was sometimes delayed several days. The mechanism of death is unknown, but a Russian report describes significant hypoglycemia and reductions in ATP in liver and heart of acutely poisoned rats. Autopsies revealed mild irritation of the gut with adhesions of the stomach to spleen and liver (Lev-

inskas et al., 1961). Dodine is absorbed through the skin (rabbit LD_{50} 2.1 gm./kg.). Surviving rabbits showed erythema and edema of the skin with subcutaneous hemorrhage, enlarged mesenteric lymph nodes, hyperemia and thickening of the pyloric region of the stomach. Local application of strong solutions produced severe irritation of eyes but little effect at the usual spray concentrations. Dodine is supplied as a wettable dust containing 75% active ingredient and in liquid concentrates containing 20 and 24% dodine.

Ref.: Amer. Cyanamid Co., 1958; Belonozhko et al., 1973; Levinskas et al., 1961.

1194 Drazoxolone 1194

4-[(o-Chlorophenyl)hydrazono]-3-methyl-5-isoxazolone, Ganocide

Toxicity Rating: 5. A broad-spectrum lipid-soluble fungicide used against powdery mildew on apples and for seed treatment of peas and grasses. Unusually high oral toxicity (rat LD_{50} 126 mg./kg.; dog LD_{50} 17 mg./kg.). Animals given fatal doses exhibited an initial lethargy (with vomiting and salivation in dogs) followed by convulsions interspersed with periods of ataxia and then a deepening depression and coma. Death was ascribed to anoxia resulting from respiratory depression. In animals maintained by artificial respiration, a direct cardiotoxic effect was seen. Dogs given 0.5 mg./kg. daily for 90 days showed no toxic symptoms or abnormal histology, but those given daily doses of 4 mg./kg.

developed convulsions after 4 days. Tracer studies indicate that the compound is rapidly absorbed from the gut in all species and converted to 2-(2-chloro-4-hydroxyphenylhydrazono)acetoacetic acid. The latter compound also causes convulsions and may be the primary toxic agent in drazoxolone poisoning. This acid and its conjugates are rapidly excreted in urine and bile. Drazoxolone is not appreciably absorbed through intact skin. It is not irritating to the skin or eye, but is weakly sensitizing. The compound is supplied as a dispersible powder (50%) and in aqueous suspension. It is also prepared in a greasy base for use as a rubber preservative under the name Ganocide.

Ref.: Clark and McElligott, 1969; Daniel, 1969.

1195   Fenaminosulf

1195

p-Dimethylaminobenzenediazo sodium sulfonate,   Sodium [4-(dimethylamino)phenyl]diazenesulfonate, Dexon

Toxicity Rating: 5. A diazobenzene fungicide used for the protection of turf and germinating seeds and, during World War II, as a rodenticide. It forms an intense yellow solution in water which is rapidly decomposed and decolorized by light. Fungitoxicity is due to inhibition of specific mitochondrial NADH-oxidase in susceptible species. The compound has a high acute mammalian toxicity (oral LD_{50} 21 mg./kg. in mice and 25 in rats according to Herrmann and Dubois, 1949; oral LD_{50} 60 mg./kg. in female rats and 150 in male guinea pigs according to Chemagro, 1961). Toxic symptoms include lethargy followed by tremors, convulsions and death. Fenaminosulf inhibits phosphorylation and causes a marked change in glycogen metabolism. Toxic doses produced immediate hyperglycemia; after existing stores of tissue glycogen were

depleted, severe hypoglycemia ensued, resulting in convulsions and death. Insulin prevented the initial hyperglycemia and glucose prevented later convulsions, but neither prevented death in rats. At autopsy, kidney tubular degeneration and acute passive hyperemia of the liver were seen. In a study of chronic toxicity, rats fed 0.10% Fenaminosulf for 12 months developed kidney nephropathy and mineralization of the renal tubules, with a low incidence of hepatomas resembling those produced by dimethylaminoazobenzene. Fenaminosulf is readily absorbed through the skin (rat dermal LD_{50} 100 mg./kg.). The compound is supplied as a wettable powder containing 70% active ingredient and as granules containing 5% Fenaminosulf. It is also available in combination with Terrachlor (see Index).

Ref.: Chemagro Corp., 1961d; Herrmann and Dubois, 1949; Lyr, 1973; National Cancer Institute, 1978e.

1196   Glyodin

1196

2-Heptadecyl imidazoline acetate,   2-Heptadecyl glyoxalidine acetate,   Crag Fruit Fungicide 341

Toxicity Rating: 3. A fungistat used for control of fungal diseases of fruits and ornamentals. Activity attributed to destruction of fungal cell membranes. Oral LD_{50} in rats 3.8 gm./kg. Fatalities occurred in 2 to 5 days. At autopsy petechial hemorrhage and congestion of lungs, congestion of liver and kidneys, and organ adhesions were observed. Strong solutions are corrosive on human mucous membranes. Gastric lavage is contraindicated following ingestion because of probable mucosal dam-

age. Supportive treatment, including measures against circulatory shock, respiratory depression and convulsions, may be needed. Concentrated solutions may also cause eye damage and skin irritation. Glyodin is supplied as a 30% solution in combination with other fungicides. The free glyoxide (2-heptadecyl imidazoline) is also fungicidal with toxicity similar to that of glyodin. It is supplied as a 70% wettable powder.

Ref.: Carpenter et al., 1951a; Council on Pharmacy and Chemistry, 1955; Lukens, 1971.

1197   Iprodione

1197

3-(3,5-Dichlorophenyl)-*N*-isopropyl-2,4-dioxoimidazolidine-1-carboxamide, e.g., Rovral

Toxicity Rating: 3. Fungicide registered in the U.S.A. for use on turf; more extensive uses in other countries. Acute oral rat LD_{50} of 3500 mg./kg. No toxic effects observed when applied dermally to rats at 2500 mg./kg. or rabbits at 1000 mg./kg.

Feeding trials of 1000 mg./kg. and 2400 mg./kg. daily in diets of rats and dogs respectively produced no recognized effects. Available as wettable powder and in many other formulations.

1198   Mercaptobenzothiazole

1198

Captax,   2-Benzothiazolethiol,   MBT

Toxicity Rating: 3-4. A rubber vulcanization accelerator and industrial fungicide. The sodium salt (e.g., Nacap, 50% solution) is used as a corrosion inhibitor in antifreeze, coolants and other aqueous systems where corrosion is a problem, particularly with copper and brass. The monoethanolamine salt (e.g., Vancide 20S), a combination of the sodium salts of mercaptobenzothiazole and dimethyldithiocarbamic acid (e.g., Vancide 51), a combination of the zinc salts of the latter two chemicals (e.g., Vancide 51Z), and the laurylpyridinium salt of 5-chloro-2-mercaptobenzothiazole (e.g., Vancide 26 and 26EC) are marketed as commercial fungicides and bactericides. The biocidal activity of these compounds may be due to *in vivo* formation of the

corresponding dithiocarbamate (Owens, 1969). The sodium and monoethanolamine salts and the dimethyldithiocarbamate combination have acute oral LD_{50}'s in the range of 2 to 4 gm./kg. in mice, rats, cats and dogs. The combination with zinc has an acute oral LD_{50} in rats of 1.5 gm./kg. The zinc derivatives are only slightly soluble in water; see also Zinc Salts Soluble in the Index. The laurylpyridinium salt of the chloro-derivative has acute oral LD_{50}'s in rats and mice of 500 to 600 mg./kg. For information about this organic cation see also Benzalkonium Chloride, Reference Congener in Section III. The free thiol (MBT) is much more toxic than the salts (rat oral LD_{50} 0.5 gm./kg.). Rats given fatal doses exhibited increased salivation, peripheral vasodilatation and tonic and clonic convulsions; death ensued within 24 hours. In extended feeding experiments, rats given 500 mg./kg. of MBT daily for one week showed hepatic damage, with focal necrosis, profound changes in cell structures including accumulation of cytoplasmic granules, nuclear changes and ruptured bile canaliculi with bile stasis. A 2-year chronic feeding study in rats and a 1-year study in dogs at levels of 5000 ppm were completely negative. Nacap caused vesiculations and erythematous lesions in human patch tests, but other products showed no dermal effects. At least Vancide 51 is fairly alkaline (pH 10 or higher).

Ref.: Guess and O'Leary, 1969; Owens, 1969; Vanderbilt, 1955; Vanderbilt, 1956; Vanderbilt, 1958; Vanderbilt, 1961.

1199 Octachlorocyclohexenone 1199

Oktane

Oktane is a 40% solution in petroleum oil. A herbicide and fungicide. The only known toxicity data (from a preliminary screening test) indicate a mean lethal dose of about 100 mg./kg. in mice, when injected daily for 7 successive days.

Ref.: McCormick, 1955.

1200 Parnon 1200

α,α-Bis(4-chlorophenyl)-3-pyridinemethanol, Parinol

Toxicity Rating: 3. Fungicide used for control of powdery mildew on roses and fruits. Of low oral toxicity (rat oral LD_{50} is 5 gm./kg.), although animal experiments indicate much higher toxicity in newborns. No description of toxic signs was found. Parnon is supplied as a 4% liquid concentrate.

Ref.: Goldenthal, 1971.

1201 Pentachloronitrobenzene 1201

PCNB, Quintozene, Terrachlor

Toxicity Rating: 3. A soil fungicide and seed protectant. Moderately low acute oral toxicity. Better absorbed and hence more toxic when dissolved in oil (rat LD_{50} 1.7 gm./kg. for oil solution; > 16 gm./kg. for aqueous suspension). Large doses induce vomiting in dogs. In rats, daily treatment with 400 mg./kg. for eight months produced growth inhibition, polyuria and renal and hepatic lesions. The acute administration of PCNB enhanced the susceptibility of rats to poisoning by carbon tetrachloride. Skin sensitivity tests in man revealed no irritation after 48 hours contact, but a sensitivity reaction occurred in 20% of the subjects after a second skin exposure. PCNB is rapidly metabolized to pentachloroaniline (PCA) in rat, rabbit, dog and cow. The latter and its conjugates are excreted in bile. PCA has also been identified in the milk of cows fed PCNB. A second metabolite, methyl pentachlorophenyl sulfide (MPCPS), occurs in rats and dogs. In rabbits the primary urinary excretion products are PCA and *N*-acetyl-*S*-(pentachlorophenyl)-*L*-cysteine. PCNB commonly contains small amounts of pentachlorobenzene (PCB) and hexachlorobenzene (HCB) introduced during manufacture. Recent studies show that, although PCNB is not stored in animals and is readily degraded in the environment, both PCB and HCB are highly stable and fat soluble. The latter accumulate in fat stores of animals exposed to PCNB or fed plants grown on soils treated with PCNB. Technical grade PCNB is mutagenic and has induced tumors in some but not all cancer bioassays using rodents. This oncogenic activity may be in part referable to variable contamination by HCB or other compounds.

Ref.: Borzelleca et al., 1971; Clarke, 1971; EPA, October 20, 1977; Finnegan et al., 1958; Fytizas-Danielidou, 1975.

1202 Trichlorodinitrobenzene 1202

Vancide PB

Toxicity Rating: 4. A mixture of isomers, used for control of soil-borne fungi causing damping-off and stem rot. High oral toxicity (rat LD_{50} 425 mg./kg.) and even more toxic in an aromatic solvent when applied to the skin (rat LD_{50} 200 mg./kg.). No description of toxic symptoms was found.

Ref.: Spencer, 1973.

1203 Polyethylene Polysulfide 1203

PEPS

Employed as a fungicide and spray adjuvant. A brief trial in mice suggests a low acute toxicity by the oral route of administration. Not currently registered for agricultural use in the U.S.A.

Ref.: McCormick, 1955.

1204　　　　　　　　　　1204　Pyracarbolid

5,6-Dihydro-2-methyl-3-(phenylcarbamoyl)-4*H*-pyrane,　Sicarol

Toxicity Rating: 2. A systemic fungicide used to control smut in cereals. Low acute oral toxicity in mammals (rat LD_{50} 6.0 gm./kg.). Not irritating to rat skin. Rats fed a diet containing 800 ppm of the compound for 90 days showed no toxic effects.

Ref.: Spencer, 1973.

1205　　　　　　　　　　1205　Quinomethionate

Chinomethionate, 6-Methyl-2,3-quinoxalinedithiol cyclic *S,S*-dithiocarbonate, Oxythioquinox, Forstan, Morestan

Toxicity Rating: 3 or 4. An acaricide and agricultural fungicide closely related to thioquinox but more stable to oxidation. Low acute mammalian toxicity by mouth (rat oral LD_{50} is 1 to 3 gm./kg.), probably due to poor absorption from the gastrointestinal tract. Presumably metabolized to 6-methyl-2,3-quinoxaline dithiol, which is twice as toxic as the parent compound. Both quinomethionate and its metabolite are highly toxic by the i.p. route (rat LD_{50} for quinomethionate is 95 mg./kg.). Toxic doses produced inactivity and diarrhea, with death ensuing in 24 to 48 hours (sooner when the dithiol metabolite was given). In the liver inhibition of sulfhydryl enzymes and pyruvate utilization were seen, together with decreased liver glutathione levels, inhibition of glycolysis, and reduction of nitroreductase activity. The compounds have a high cumulative toxicity: daily injections greater than 25 mg./kg. invariably produced death within 60 days. Rats given 500 ppm in food for 90 days showed a decrease in body weight and liver enlargement with inhibition of acetoacetate synthesis, EPN detoxification and O-demethylation. Prolonged contact with intact skin may cause local irritation. In rats, moreover, quinomethionate is readily absorbed through the skin (acute dermal LD_{50} is 500 mg./kg.). No clinical poisonings are known.

Ref.: Carlson and Dubois, 1969; Carlson and Dubois, 1970.

1206　　　　　　　　1206　2-(Thiocyanomethylthio)-benzothiazole

TCMTB,　Busan 30A,　Busan 72A

Toxicity Rating: 3. A fungicide available as a dust and an emulsifiable liquid for the treatment of seeds (grain, flower bulbs, etc.). Acute oral LD_{50} in the rat is 1590 mg./kg. No information about the toxic syndrome was located.

Ref.: Farm Chemicals Handbook, 1980.

1207　　　　　　　　　　1207　Thiophanate-methyl

Dimethyl 4,4′-*o*-phenylenebis(3-thioallophanate)

Toxicity Rating: 3. Thiophanate-methyl and thiophanate (an ethyl homolog) are systemic fungicides used to control fungal diseases in turf and ornamentals. Activity said to result from release of methyl 2-benzimidazole carbamate (MBC) in plants and soils. The ethyl ester (thiophanate) is virtually nontoxic to rats (oral LD_{50} > 15 gm./kg.). Thiophanate-methyl is more toxic (mouse oral LD_{50} 3.4 gm./kg.; rat oral LD_{50} 7.5 gm./kg.). Signs and symptoms of thiophanate-methyl intoxication in experimental animals include tremors, tonic and clonic convulsions, a decrease in respiratory rate, lethargy and mydriasis. Fatal intravenous doses caused an abrupt drop in blood pressure leading to death. Concentrated solutions of thiophanate-methyl produced erythema in rabbits, but the compound was not appreciably toxic when applied dermally. Inhalation of the powder caused immediate gasping, wheezing and lacrimation in mice but no fatalities. In rats, mice and dogs, the major metabolite of thiophanate-methyl is MBC, although 5-hydroxymethyl bezimidazole was reportedly found in the urine of rats after doses of thiophanate-methyl. The use of thiophanate and thiophanate-methyl has been restricted in the U.S.A. because of the high mutagenic potency of MBC.

Ref.: EPA, Dec. 7, 1977; Hashimoto et al., 1972a.

1208　　　　　　　　　　1208　*o*-Toluanilide

Mebenil,　2-Methylbenzanilide,　Methylmetiram

Toxicity Rating: 2. Systemic fungicide for control of rust diseases in grains. Low acute oral toxicity in rats. No evidence of skin irritation. Mebenil is absorbed from the stomach and metabolized by *p*-hydroxylation of the aniline ring. The product is excreted free and as conjugates, primarily in urine. At least in rodents, the extent of hydrolysis to aniline is insignificant.

Ref.: Warrander and Waring, 1977.

1209 Triamiphos 1209

p-(5-Amino-3-phenyl-1*H*-1,2,4-triazol-1-yl)-*N,N,N',N'*-tetramethyl phosphonic diamide, Triamifos, Wepsyn

Toxicity Rating: 5. A fungicide used against powdery mildews. Also used as an acaricide-insecticide. Triamiphos is a cholinesterase inhibitor with a very high acute toxicity (oral LD_{50} 10 mg./kg. in mice, 20 mg./kg. in rats). The compound is slowly absorbed through intact skin. Anticholinesterase signs and symptoms indicate the need for atropine; see Parathion in Section III. Not presently produced in the United States (1977).

Ref.: Spencer, 1973.

1210 Triforine 1210

1,4-Bis(1-formamido-2,2,2-trichloroethyl)piperazine

Toxicity Rating: 2 or 1. Systemic fungicide for control of powdery mildew of fruit and vegetables. Very low acute oral toxicity in rats. Metabolism proceeds by loss of one side chain to yield trichloroethylformamide. Triforine and its metabolites are rapidly eliminated, primarily in the urine.

Ref.: Darda, 1977; Worthing, 1979.

2,4-D and related herbicides

1211 *p*-Chlorophenoxyacetic Acid 1211

CPA, PCPA, Tomatotone

Toxicity Rating: 3. A plant growth regulator used to improve tomato set. Chemically related to 2,4-D and exhibits a similar acute toxicity in laboratory animals (rat oral LD_{50} 850 mg./kg.). The toxic syndrome may be due in part to the presence of 2,4-D, which is a common impurity. The dimethylaminoethyl ester of CPA has been used clinically (at oral dose levels up to 570 mg./kg.) as a central nervous system stimulant in the treatment of consciousness disorders (stupor, coma) following neurosurgery. It is also said to raise a lowered arterial blood pressure. No myotonia was reported. The oral LD_{50} of this ester in rats is 1.7 gm./kg.

See also: 2,4-D, *Reference Congener in Section III.*
Ref.: Coirault et al., 1960; Hee and Sutherland, 1974; Hollingsworth, 1958.

1212 2,4-D 1212

2,4-Dichlorophenoxyacetic acid

Toxicity Rating: 4. A widely used herbicide of high acute oral toxicity. Usually marketed as salts and esters which are somewhat less toxic than the free acid. Has caused convulsions, peripheral neuropathies, and brain damage in large doses.

See also: 2,4-D, *Reference Congener in Section III.*

1213 2,4-D Esters 1213

i.e., Isopropyl, butyl

Toxicity Rating: 3. Lie near the borderline between toxicity classes 3 and 4. Some esters are appreciably volatile.

See also: 2,4-D, *Reference Congener in Section III.*

1214 2,4-D Salts 1214

i.e., Sodium, ammonium, alkylamine

Toxicity Rating: 3 or 4. The water-soluble salts of 2,4-D contain inorganic cations (e.g., Na^+, K^+) or amine bases (e.g., ethanolamine). See entries in this index for the appropriate cation or base.

See also: 2,4-D, *Reference Congener in Section III.*

1215 4-(2,4-Dichlorophenoxy)butyric Acid 1215

2,4-DB, Butoxone, Butyrac

Toxicity Rating: 3-4. Selective, translocated hormone-type herbicide. Converted by beta oxidation to 2,4-D in animals and susceptible plants (see 2,4-D above). Its acute oral toxicity, however, is somewhat lower than that of 2,4-D (oral LD_{50} is 700 mg./kg. in rat, but 400 in mice). Embryotoxicity is described in the Russian literature. 2,4-DB is irritating to skin and mucous membranes. The butoxyethanol, butyl and isooctyl esters, and the dimethylamine salt are also marketed.

See also: 2,4-D, *Reference Congener in Section III.*
Ref.: Sokolova, 1976; Van Petigham and Heyndrickx, 1975.

1216   1216   2-(2,4-Dichlorophenoxy)ethyl Sulfate Sodium Salt

Disul-Na,   Sesone,   Crag Herbicide 1

Toxicity Rating: 3. An herbicide of moderately low oral toxicity in laboratory animals (rat LD_{50} 1.2 gm./kg.). Converted in animals and soils to 2,4-dichlorophenoxyacetic acid (2,4-D). Absorption and hence toxicity are increased by oils and fats. A 5% solution produced necrosis of rabbit skin, but a 1% solution was not harmful. Chronic ingestion in rats caused mild lung, liver, and kidney pathology.

See also: 2,4-D, *Reference Congener in Section III.*
Ref.: Carpenter et al., 1961b; Spencer, 1973.

1217   1217   2-(2,4-Dichlorophenoxy)propionic Acid

Dichlorprop,   2,4-DP

Toxicity Rating: 3-4. Systemic herbicide, closely related to 2,4-D. Acute oral LD_{50} is similar to that of 2,4-D, but no description of toxic symptoms was found. Probably not metabolized by animals. Toxic doses may be absorbed through intact skin. Dichlorprop is supplied as sodium, potassium and organic amine salts (see entries for amines in this index) and as the isooctyl and butoxyethyl esters.

See also: 2,4-D, *Reference Congener in Section III.*

1218   1218   Erbon

2-(2,4,5-Trichlorophenoxy)ethyl-2,2-dichloropropionate,   Baron,   Novon

Toxicity Rating: 3. An herbicide related to 2,4,5-T. No appreciable percutaneous absorption. Causes irritation on contact with skin and eyes. Contaminated areas should be flushed promptly. Repeated skin contact with concentrated material has caused dermatitis. In sheep Erbon is rapidly hydrolyzed to 2-(2,4,5-trichlorophenoxy)ethanol and oxidized to 2,4,5-T.

See also: 2,4-D, *Reference Congener in Section III.*
Ref.: Rowe, 1957; Wright et al., 1970.

1219   1219   Fenac

2,3,6-Trichlorophenylacetic acid,   2,4,5-Trichlorophenylacetic acid,   Chlorfenac

Toxicity Rating: 3. An herbicidal mixture of isomeric trichlorophenylacetic acids. The 2,3,6-trichloro acid is the main component (about 70%). Closely related to silvex. Acute oral LD_{50} in rats is 1.8 gm./kg. or 2.5 to 3.0 gm./kg. for the technical grade material. No significant skin irritation or percutaneous absorption. The salts are also herbicidal; they are similar to the free acids in mammalian toxicity. The 2,3,6- isomer (and probably the 2,4,5- isomer as well) is not biologically degraded but is conjugated and excreted in urine. When fed to lactating cows, none of the compounds was detected in the milk.

See also: 2,4-D, *Reference Congener in Section III.*
Ref.: Assoc. of Amer. Pesticide Control Officials, 1966; Spencer, 1973; St. John and Lisk, 1970.

1220   1220   MCPA

2-Methyl-4-chlorophenoxyacetic acid,   MCP

Toxicity Rating: 3. MCPA, its salts and esters are postemergent herbicides, chemically related to 2,4-D. MCPA has a moderately high acute oral toxicity (LD_{50} is about 700 mg./kg. in rats, and 550 mg./kg. in mice). More toxic when given i.v. or subcutaneously. Has caused several human fatalities, one after the alleged ingestion of 250 mg./kg. For a full description of these cases, see 2,4-D, Reference Congener in Section III. The ethyl ester (MCPEE) causes teratogenic effects in rats, and the same may be true of other derivatives. In radiotracer experiments, MCPA was shown to cross the placental barrier and accumulate in the visceral yolk sac. No retention was demonstrable in either maternal or fetal tissues.

See also: 2,4-D, *Reference Congener in Section III.*
Ref.: Lindquist, 1974; Rowe, 1957; Yasuda and Maeda, 1972.

1221   Mecoprop   1221

2-(2-Methyl-4-chlorophenoxy)propionic acid,   MCPP

Toxicity Rating: 3. Herbicide for control of weeds in turf and cereal crops. Closely related to 2,4-D. Laboratory experiments place this compound near the borderline between toxicity classes 3 and 4. The no-effect level for rats in 2-month feeding experiments was 1000 ppm. Mecoprop salts have acute toxicities similar to that of the parent acid. See index for entries about the various cations. A man who attempted suicide by ingesting an un-known amount of a mixture of 2,4-D (10%) and mecoprop (20%) remained in coma for more than 3 days; arreflexia, hypertonus, metabolic acidosis, respiratory alkalosis, hypoxia and fever were noted. For a period of 2 months thereafter, he experienced muscle weakness and myotonia ascribed to dysfunction of both peripheral nerves (neuropathy) and of skeletal muscles (myopathy).

See also: 2,4-D, Reference Congener in Section III.
Ref.: Gurd et al., 1965; Park et al., 1977.

1222   4-(2-Methyl-4-chlorophenoxy)butyric Acid   1222

4-MCPB,   Tropotox

Toxicity Rating: 3. A translocated weed killer, rapidly converted by beta oxidation to MCPA in animals and susceptible plants. Toxicological effects similar to those of MCPA and 2,4-D (see above). The oral LD$_{50}$ is 700 mg./kg. in rats. Not particularly irritating to skin but can be absorbed percutaneously. Causes pain and irritation on eyes and mucous membranes. Like 2,4-D, 4-MCPB is reputed to be an uncoupler of oxidative phosphorylation in mammalian tissues.

See also: 2,4-D, Reference Congener in Section III.
Ref.: Rowe, 1957; Van Petigham and Heyndrickx, 1975.

1223   Silvex   1223

2-(2,4,5-Trichlorophenoxy)propionic acid,   2,4,5-TP

Toxicity Rating: 3. Popular herbicide for control of woody plants. Closely related to 2,4,5-T and 2,4-D. Mammalian toxicity seems to be somewhat less than that for 2,4-D, and neural effects have not been described. The compound is rapidly absorbed and excreted largely unchanged in urine, although some conversion to 2,4,5-trichlorophenol occurs. The chief toxic effects in animals are anorexia and dehydration. After administration of 50 mg./kg. to cattle daily for 90 days, erosion of the rumen mucosa and chronic enteritis were observed. Necropsy findings included enlarged and friable liver and congestion of the lower respiratory passages. The compound is irritating to skin and mucous membranes. Kuron is a non-volatile mixture of propylene glycol butyl ether esters of silvex. It has a similar toxicity in mammals, but a greater toxicity in fish and larval insect forms. It is rapidly hydrolyzed to silvex after ingestion. Both silvex and Kuron may be contaminated with small amounts of the highly toxic dioxins (see latter in the index).

See also: 2,4-D, Reference Congener in Section III.
Ref.: Assoc. of Amer. Pesticide Control Officials, 1966; Rowe and Hymas, 1954a; Spencer, 1973; St. John et al., 1964.

1224   Trichlorophenoxyacetic Acid   1224

2,4,5-T

Toxicity Rating: 3-4. A translocatable herbicide. Closely related to 2,4-D, but acute mammalian toxicity may be somewhat less. In rats the oral LD$_{50}$ is about 300 mg./kg. for the free acid and somewhat higher for the esters. Toxic doses in experimental and domestic animals produce only mild spasticity. In fatally poisoned sheep, enteritis, nephritis and hepatitis were observed at autopsy. In man the compound is absorbed rapidly and excreted unchanged in urine. This urinary excretion is probably due to the saturable renal tubular secretory process for organic anions. After large doses (100 mg./kg.) in rats, small amounts of urinary metabolites were found, including 2,4,5-trichlorophenol. 2,4,5-T is both teratogenic and oncogenic in experimental animals. These effects are probably due to contamination of the material with trace amounts of TCDD (dioxin) during manufacture (see Dioxins in the index). The compound is often supplied as a salt or ester. No specific information about the percutaneous absorption of 2,4,5-T, its salts or esters, could be located, but prolonged contact with high concentrations may cause skin burns.

See also: 2,4-D, Reference Congener in Section III.
Ref.: Berndt and Koschier, 1973; Clark and Palmer, 1971; Collins and Williams, 1971; Courtney and Moore, 1971; Drill and Hiratzka, 1953; Gehring et al., 1973; Piper et al., 1973.

1225   **1225**   2,4,5-Trichlorophenoxy Ethyl Sulfate Sodium Salt

2,4,5-TES,   Natrin

Toxicity Rating: 4. Studies in laboratory animals place this weed-killer near the borderline between toxicity classes 3 and 4. It causes moderate skin irritation and severe damage to eyes. Percutaneous

absorption is marked in rabbits and a potential hazard in man. Convulsions have been observed in acutely poisoned animals. Not presently registered in the U.S.A.

See also: 2,4-D, *Reference Congener in Section III.*
Ref.: Dernehl, 1957.

Carbamate herbicides

1226   **1226** Asulam

Methyl sulfanilylcarbamate,   Asulox

Toxicity Rating: 2. This and its acetamide derivative (generic name Carbasulam) are systemic herbicides usually supplied as sodium salts. Low acute oral toxicity (rat oral LD_{50} is greater than 5 gm./

kg.). No significant percutaneous absorption. Dogs tolerated daily doses of 500 mg./kg. for 13 weeks without adverse effects.

Ref.: Worthing, 1979.

1227   **1227** Barban

4-Chloro-2-butynyl *m*-chlorocarbanilate,   4-Chloro-2-butynyl *N*-(3-chlorophenyl) carbamate,   Carbyne

Toxicity Rating: 3. Herbicide for control of wild oats in row crops. Acute oral LD_{50} in rats is variously reported as 600 mg./kg. to 1.5 gm./kg. Weak cholinesterase inhibitor. Large doses are said to cause methemoglobinemia, which may be referable to metabolites (see below). Daily administration of 0.1 LD_{50} to guinea pigs and rabbits for 4 to 6 months is said to have caused fatty dystrophy of the liver and kidneys, hemosiderosis of the spleen and vascular hyperemia of liver, brain, kidneys, spleen, and gastric mucosa. Daily doses of 20 to 40

mg./kg. to rabbits caused a significant decrease in liver glycogen content. Systemic toxicity following prolonged dermal exposures is described. May cause allergic skin reactions in sensitive persons. Barban metabolism yields a variety of compounds, including aniline, *m*-chloroaniline, *p*-aminophenol and *p*-hydroxy barban. If methemoglobinemia is demonstrable, treat patient as for aniline poisoning; see Aniline in Section III. Also consult index for *p*-Aminophenol.

Ref.: Aleksandrova and Klisenko, 1971; Grunow et al., 1970; Gzhegotskii and Dotoshitskii, 1971; Nekrasova and Knysh, 1971; Nekrasova and Razoznaeva, 1971; Riden, 1961.

1228   **1228** Carbetamide

N-Ethyllactamide carbanilate,   Carbetamex

Toxicity Rating: 3. Persistent herbicide, for use in control of grasses and weeds in legume crops. Moderate acute oral toxicity in mammals (LD_{50} in dogs

1 gm./kg.). Dogs tolerated 13,000 ppm in food for 3 months without ill effects.

Ref.: Worthing, 1979.

1229   **1229** Chlorpropham

Isopropyl *N*-(3-chlorophenyl)carbamate,   Isopropyl *m*-chlorocarbanilate,   CIPC,   Metoxon

Toxicity Rating: 3. One of several closely related pre-emergence herbicides containing the carbamate grouping. These herbicides are frequently supplied in mixtures with other compounds such as pyrazon, diuron, endothal or fenuron (see entries in this index). A mitotic poison in plants. Used in the production of truck crops. Moderate to low oral toxicity in mammals (rat oral LD_{50} 1.5 to 5 gm./ kg. for chlorpropham, 2.5 gm./kg. for chlorbufam and 5 gm./kg. for propham). Chlorpropham (and presumably the others) was more toxic to rats on a low protein diet. Following administration of single toxic doses of chlorpropham to laboratory animals, initial symptoms included listlessness, ataxia, epistaxis, exophthalmos, hemodacryorrhea

and hemorhinorrhea. These progressed to dyspnea, prostration, anuria, glycosuria, proteinuria, hyperthermia, and death. Autopsy findings showed gastroenteritis with occasional congestion of brain, lungs and other organs. Stress response was evident in adrenal, thymus and spleen, while degenerative changes were seen in kidney and liver. Chlorpropham inhibited DNA formation in regenerating rat liver following partial hepatectomy. Chlorpropham and propham (and presumably chlorbufam) are metabolized by para-ring hydroxylation, carbamate hydrolysis, and side-chain oxidation. Chlorpropham is about 35% hydrolyzed in rats, whereas propham is hydrolyzed by a much smaller percent. The major urinary metabolites of chlorpropham are 4-hydroxychlorpropham and 4-hydroxy-3-chloroaniline. Experience with p-aminophenol (see in index) suggests that the latter metabolite may oxidize hemoglobin to methemoglobin, but the possibility of methemoglobinemia has apparently not been investigated in poisoned animals. The parent compounds may cause local skin irritation, but are not skin sensitizers. Dermal absorption is not significant. Chlorpropham and propham are said to be oncogenic. If significant methemoglobinemia is demonstrable after an acute exposure, treat as for aniline poisoning (see latter in Section III).

Ref.: Assoc. of Amer. Pesticide Control Officials, 1966; Boyd and Carsky, 1969; Fang et al., 1974; Grunow et al., 1970; Larson et al., 1960; Worthing, 1979; Ryan, 1971; Spencer, 1973.

1230   Desmedipham   1230

Ethyl *m*-hydroxycarbanilate carbanilate,   Ethyl 3-phenylcarbamoyloxyphenylcarbamate,   Betanal, Betanex

Toxicity Rating: 3. Desmedipham, phenmedipham and phenmedipham-ethyl are post-emergence herbicides for use on beets to control broad-leafed weeds. The pure compounds have low acute oral toxicity to mammals (rat LD_{50} is 9.6 gm./kg. for desmedipham). Betanex, a 16% emulsifiable concentrate of desmedipham, is more toxic (rat LD_{50} is 3.7 gm./kg. active ingredient). A single oral dose of 2.5 gm./kg. of the formulation did not produce measurable inhibition of cholinesterase in the rat. Clinical signs and symptoms in poisoned laboratory animals, however, suggest that this enzyme may be significantly inhibited in vivo. For example, signs of oral intoxication include hypoactivity, salivation and muscle weakness. After inhalation exposure, salivation, nasal discharge, muscular weakness and labored breathing may occur. In rats, dogs and humans, desmedipham and phenmedipham are readily absorbed and rapidly hydrolyzed by plasma and liver esterases, yielding the corresponding alkyl-*N*-(3-hydroxyphenyl)carbamates and aniline (see in this index) or *m*-toluidine (in the case of phenmediphan). The carbamate moiety is further cleaved, yielding *m*-aminophenol and ultimately 3'-hydroxyacetanilid. Desmedipham is mildly irritating to skin and eyes. It is rapidly hydrolyzed in basic media and decomposes at high temperatures, releasing poisonous vapors. If signs and symptoms suggest cholinesterase inhibition, treat with atropine, as in carbaryl poisoning (see latter in Section III). If significant methemoglobinemia is demonstrable, treat as for aniline poisoning (see latter in Section III).

See also: Aniline, *Reference Congener in Section III.*
Ref.: NOR-AM Agricultural Products, date unknown; Worthing, 1979; Sonawane and Knowles, 1971.

1231   2,6-Di-*tert.*-butyl-*p*-tolyl-*N*-methylcarbamate   1231

Terbutol, e.g., Azak

Toxicity Rating: 1. Pre-emergence herbicide available as an 80% wettable powder. Oral LD_{50} as a 50% suspension in corn oil is greater than 35 gm./kg. in rats and in excess of 15 gm./kg. in dogs and cats. No deaths and no frank symptoms of poisoning were observed. Emesis occurred in about half the dogs, and the rats exhibited generalized inactivity. On intact or abraded rabbit skin 10 gm./kg. was tolerated with only slight and transient erythema. Moderate irritant in rabbit eye if unwashed but flushing with water after 1-min. exposures prevented the reaction. Slight to moderate erythematous and perhaps edematous reactions on human patch tests. Mice, rats and guinea pigs exposed to dust concentrations of 2800 mg./cu. m. for 4 hours showed no untoward reactions. Although relevant data were not located, there is a possibility that this compound has weak anticholinesterase activity; see Carbaryl in the index.

Ref.: Hercules Powder Co., 1962a.

1232   Karbutilate   1232

m-(3,3-Dimethylureido)phenyl *tert.*-butylcarbamate, e.g., Tandex

Toxicity Rating: 3. Carbamate herbicide used for soil sterilization on nonfood crop areas. Acute oral LD_{50} of technical grade material 3.0 gm./kg. in rats. Data suggest that it is not well absorbed through intact skin. Mild primary irritant in rabbit eye and on skin. May be a weak cholinesterase inhibitor, but an official of Niagara Chemical Division has stated that it does not inhibit cholinesterase. Treat symptoms of cholinesterase inhibition, if any, with atropine but avoid 2-PAM.

Ref.: Niagara Chemical Division, 1969.

Thiocarbamate herbicides

1233   Butylate   1233

S-Ethyl diisobutylthiocarbamate

Toxicity Rating: 3. A thiocarbamate herbicide, used to prevent germination of grass and weeds in maize, available in solubilized and granular forms. Low acute oral toxicity (rat LD_{50} 4 to 5 gm./kg.).

Dogs and rats tolerated daily doses of 40 mg./kg. for 13 weeks. Like many carbamates and thiocarbamates, butylate can inhibit the enzyme cholinesterase by carbamylating its active site. This activity, however, is probably too weak to account for the toxicity of butylate, or else the compound is metabolized too rapidly to permit significant cholinesterase inhibition. Many thiocarbamate herbicides are detoxified by enzymatic oxidation in the liver to the corresponding sulfoxides; the latter do not react significantly with cholinesterase. Butylate undergoes such sulfoxide formation in vivo, but in contrast to other thiocarbamates tested, its sulfoxide is more toxic than the parent compound. Sulfoxides derived from thiocarbamates combine with sulfhydryl groups of glutathione in the liver and are excreted in urine as inactive mercaptides. They can also react with other tissue thiols, presumably including essential enzymes. Only symptomatic treatment can be suggested. Injections of penicillamine, BAL or other sulfhydryl drugs might be effective in butylate poisoning, but atropine is not expected to be useful.

Ref.: Casida et al., 1975; Hubbell and Casida, 1977; Worthing, 1979.

1234   1234 Cycloate

S-Ethyl cyclohexylethylthiocarbamate, Hexylthiocarbam, Ronit, Ro-neet

Toxicity Rating: 3. Selective pre-emergence herbicide for use on row crops to control grassy weeds, supplied as an emulsifiable concentrate and as granules (10%). Moderate acute oral mammalian toxicity (LD_{50} is 2 to 3 gm./kg. in rats). Possibly a weak cholinesterase poison, but relevant data were not located. Dogs given 240 mg./kg. daily for 90 days showed no ill-effects. The compound is rapidly absorbed and detoxified by various routes, including oxidation by liver enzymes. See EPTC below for description of metabolism. Irritating to skin and eyes but not absorbed percutaneously.

Ref.: Worthing, 1979; Rebrin and Aleksandrova, 1971.

1235   1235 Di-allate

S-(2,3-Dichloroallyl)diisopropylthiocarbamate, Avadex

Toxicity Rating: 3 or 4. Pre-emergence, selective, carbamate herbicide. High acute oral toxicity (rat oral LD_{50} is variously reported as 0.4 to 0.9 gm./kg.). Acute toxicity is probably due to reversible inhibition of acetylcholinesterase, as with EPTC (see entry below). Initial symptoms of intoxication in rats include tearing, salivation, panting and excitement. These are followed by depression and paralysis or clonic-tonic convulsions. In sheep, muscle spasms and a slowly developing alopecia reportedly followed three daily doses of 100 mg./kg. (Palmer, 1964). Said to cause delayed neurotoxicity in hens and pulmonary and hepatic tumors in rats and mice (EPA, 1977). Tri-allate is the tri-chloroallyl analog. Its acute toxicity is similar to that of di-allate, and it too is reported to inhibit blood cholinesterase and brain cholinesterase slightly in rabbits. Degenerative necrotic changes in liver, kidneys and reproductive organs following repeated administration of tri-allate to chickens are described in the Russian literature. Dermal absorption of di-allate may lead to systemic intoxication (rabbit dermal LD_{50} 2 to 2.5 gm./kg.). The concentrated solution is irritating to skin and eyes. May be contaminated with diisopropylamine and other (unknown) compounds introduced in the manufacturing process.

See also: Carbaryl, *Reference Congener in Section III.*
Ref.: EPA, May 31, 1977; Worthing, 1979; Palmer, 1964b; Pestova, 1966; Seleck and Kelly, 1961.

1236   1236 EPTC

S-Ethyl dipropylthiocarbamate, Eptam

Toxicity Rating: 3 or 4. A thiocarbamate herbicide, used for control of grassy and some broadleaf weeds. Moderately to highly toxic in laboratory animals. Acute oral LD_{50} values are 1.63 gm./kg. in male rats, 750 mg./kg. in mice and 112 mg./kg. in cats. Conflicting data concerning percutaneous toxicity, but known to be irritating to skin and eyes. EPTC inhibits the enzyme cholinesterase, which is probably the basis for its acute toxicity. Poisoned animals display excitement, salivation, lacrymation, blepharospasm, and finally depression. Exposed workers have complained of general malaise, headache, nausea and impaired working capacity. Like many other thiocarbamate herbicides, EPTC is detoxified by enzymatic oxidation in mouse and rat liver to its sulfoxide. The latter does not react significantly with cholinesterase but does combine with glutathione in the liver and other tissue thiols, possibly including some essential cellular enzymes. Excreted in urine, partly as mercaptides derived from glutathione. Embryotoxicity is described in the Russian literature. Ethiolate, the diethyl analog of Eptam, is somewhat more toxic to rats (oral LD_{50} 700 mg./kg.). EPTC is sometimes supplied in a mixture with *N,N*-diallyl-2,2-dichloroacetamide, which is supposed to be less toxic to maize than the thiocarbamate alone. The last compound has a low acute toxicity in mammals, although no description of toxic symptoms was found. EPTC poisoning should be treated with atropine as in carbaryl poisoning.

See also: Carbaryl, *Reference Congener in Section III*.
Ref.: Berwick, 1970; Casida et al., 1975; Chen and Casida, 1978; Hubbell and Casida, 1977; Worthing, 1979; Medved et al., 1970; Medved and Ivanova, 1971; Stauffer Chemical Co., 1961a.

1237   Molinate   1237

S-Ethyl hexahydro-1H-azepine-1-carbothioate,   Ordram,   Yalan

Toxicity Rating: 4. A thiocarbamate herbicide for use on rice to control germinating weeds. Somewhat higher oral toxicity than other thiocarbamates (rat oral LD_{50} is 500 mg./kg.). Cholinesterase inhibition may be a significant feature of the toxic syndrome but relevant data were not located. Irritating to skin and eyes but not absorbed percutaneously. Inhalation exposure may lead to systemic poisoning. Gonadotoxicity and embryotoxicity are described in the Russian literature. Said to inhibit thyroid function and decrease energy metabolism. Metabolic degradation of molinate is analogous to that of EPTC (see entry above). If symptoms suggest cholinesterase inhibition, treat with atropine as in carbaryl poisoning.

Ref.: Anina et al., 1975; Casida et al., 1975; Dyadicheva, 1969; Hubbell and Casida, 1977; Voitenko and Medved, 1973.

1238   Pebulate   1238

S-Propyl butylethylthiocarbamate,   Tillam

Toxicity Rating: 3 or 4. Translocatable thiocarbamate herbicide for use on truck crops to control grassy and broadleaf weeds. Moderate acute oral toxicity (rat LD_{50} 1.1 gm./kg.). Perhaps a cholinesterase inhibitor, but relevant data have not been located. Cows given repeated doses of 100 mg./kg. died after 6 days. Necropsy findings included congestion of thyroid, spleen, adrenal and lung parenchyma, acute toxic tubular nephritis with hemorrhaging, and coagulative necrosis of the liver. Metabolism is rapid and analogous to that of EPTC (see latter above). Large doses are said to increase susceptibility to infection in experimental animals. Decreases in oxidative metabolism are described in medium-term (16 week) feeding experiments in rats (Proklina-Kaminskaya, 1969). Pebulate is irritating to eyes. No significant cutaneous irritation or percutaneous absorption. If symptoms suggest cholinesterase inhibition, treat with atropine as in carbaryl poisoning.

Ref.: Casida et al., 1975; Hubbell and Casida, 1977; Olefir, 1973; Proklina-Kaminskaya, 1969.

1239   Thiobencarb   1239

S-[(4-Chlorophenyl)methyl]diethylcarbamothioate,   Benthiocarb,   Bolero

Toxicity Rating: 3. A thiocarbamate herbicide, used for control of sedges and grasses in paddy fields, supplied as granules (5 and 10%) and in combination with simetryne. Moderate acute oral toxicity in mammals (oral LD_{50} 1.3 gm./kg. in rats, 0.6 mg./kg. in mice). Probably a weak cholinesterase inhibitor, but relevant data were not located. Percutaneous absorption is significant (rat dermal LD_{50} 2.9 gm./kg.). Thiobencarb is readily absorbed from the stomach. Like EPTC (see above), it is rapidly detoxified in the liver by oxidation to the sulfoxide, followed by cleavage of the sulfur-carbon bond by the soluble glutathione system. Ester cleavage without sulfoxide formation and N-dealkylation reactions may also occur in the liver and other tissues. Ultimate metabolites in urine include 4-chlorohippuric acid, 4-chlorobenzoic acid, and various mercaptides. If symptoms suggest cholinesterase inhibition, treat with atropine as in carbaryl poisoning.

Ref.: Casida et al., 1975; Hubbell and Casida, 1977; Worthing, 1979.

1240   Vernolate   1240

S-Propyl dipropylthiocarbamate

Toxicity Rating: 3. Selective thiocarbamate herbicide for use on sweet potatoes, peanuts and soybeans to control broadleaf weeds. Moderate acute oral toxicity (LD_{50} in rats 1.5 gm./kg.). Like some but not all thiocarbamate herbicides, vernolate may be a cholinesterase inhibitor, but relevant data were not located. No skin irritation or percutaneous absorption, but irritating to eyes. Metabolism is analogous to that of EPTC (see latter above).

Ref.: Casida et al., 1975; Worthing, 1979.

Urea herbicides

1241   Buturon   1241

3-(p-Chlorophenyl)-1-methyl-1-(1-methyl-2-propynyl)urea,   Eptapur

Toxicity Rating: 3. Pre- and post-emergence herbicide. Low mammalian toxicity (acute oral LD_{50}

3 gm./kg. in rats). Rats tolerated 500 ppm in food for 120 days without ill effects. Slightly irritating to intact skin. Supplied as a 50% wettable powder.

1242   Chlorbromuron

N'-(4-Bromo-3-chlorophenyl)-N-methoxy-N-methylurea,   Maloran

Toxicity Rating: 2. Urea herbicide for control of weeds in row crops. Low acute oral and dermal toxicity (rat $LD_{50} > 5$ gm./kg.). The no-effect level in 3-month feeding studies of rats and dogs was 320 ppm. Dermal absorption is not significant.

1243   Chloroxuron

3-(p-(p-Chlorophenoxy)phenyl)-1,1-dimethylurea,   Tenoran,   Chloroxifenidim

Toxicity Rating: 3. Post-emergence herbicide for control of broad-leafed weeds in soybeans, celery and strawberries. Moderate acute oral toxicity in rats (LD_{50} 3.7 gm./kg.). No significant percutaneous absorption. In 90-day feeding studies, daily doses of 15 mg./kg. produced no toxicity in rats and dogs.

Ref.: Worthing, 1979.

1244   Cycluron

3-Cyclooctyl-1,1-dimethylurea,   Alipur

Toxicity Rating: 3. Pre-emergence herbicide, often used in a mixture with Chlorbufam. Moderate acute oral toxicity (rat LD_{50} 2.6 gm./kg.). Not irritating to rabbit skin.

Ref.: Worthing, 1979.

1245   Dichloral Urea

1,3-Bis(1-hydroxy-2,2,2-trichloroethyl)urea,   DCU

Toxicity Rating: 2. An herbicide used formerly for the control of weeds in field crops. Low acute oral toxicity (LD_{50} 6.8 gm./kg. in rats). Low skin irritancy. Chronic feeding in rats caused functional alterations in blood, liver and kidney.

1246   Diflubenzuron

N-[[(4-Chlorophenyl)amino]carbonyl]-2,6-difluorobenzamide,   1-(p-Chlorophenyl)-3-(2,6-difluorobenzoyl)urea, Dimilin

Toxicity Rating: 2. Insecticide used in controlling larvae of leaf feeders. Insecticidal activity is due to inhibition of chitin synthesis. Low acute oral toxicity in mammals ($LD_{50} > 4.0$ gm./kg. in rats, > 4.6 in mice). Said to cause methemoglobinemia and sulfhemoglobinemia in laboratory animals and perhaps in man, presumably due to p-chloroaniline released by enzymatic hydrolysis. See p-Chloroaniline in the index. Depression of testosterone in maturing rats and possible oncogenicity have been reported. In a two-year rat feeding test, the "no-effect" level was 40 ppm. In cows large oral doses are not completely absorbed, but absorbed material appears to be rapidly and completely metabolized by ring hydroxylation and hydrolysis.

Ref.: EPA, May 1, 1979; Ivie, 1978.

1247   Diuron

3-(3,4-Dichlorophenyl)-1,1-dimethylurea,   Karmex

Toxicity Rating: 3. A general herbicide chemically related to Monuron (see latter below). Acute oral LD_{50} in rats 3400 mg./kg. More toxic to rats previously fed protein-deficient diets. Toxic syndrome same as for monuron. In one human poisoning, a 39-year-old woman ingested 20 mg./kg. with aminotriazole with no ill-effects. Analysis of urine suggested that the diuron was partially metabolized in the liver by N-dealkylation and ring hydroxylation. Only trace amounts of 3,4-dichloroaniline were found. No unaltered diuron was detected. One Russian study reports gastric carcinomas, hepatomas and pancreatic tumors in rats after repeated doses of 450 mg./kg. per day for 22 months. Nonirritating to intact guinea pig skin and mildly irritating to broken skin. Not a skin sensitizer. Repeated doses produce anemia in rats. Methemoglobinemia may be anticipated if significant amounts of the compound are hydrolyzed to dichloroaniline.

Ref.: Boehme and Ernst, 1965; Boyd and Krupa, 1970; du Pont, 1961b; Geldmacher-v. Mallinckrodt and Schuessler, 1971; Hodge et al., 1967b; Rubenchik et al., 1973.

1248 Fenuron 1248

1,1-Dimethyl-3-phenylurea, 3-Phenyl-1,1-dimethylurea, PDU, Dybar

Toxicity Rating: 2 to 3. A brush and weed killer of high persistency in the environment. Stable at neutral pH but hydrolyzed in acid and basic media. Lower acute toxicity than Monuron below. Acute oral LD_{50} in rats is 6400 mg./kg. Rats given 500 ppm in food for 90 days showed no ill-effects. However, in guinea pigs daily oral doses of 15 to 150 mg./kg. for 10 months produced anemia, hypothyroidism and structural alterations in liver, kidney, spleen and myocardium. Cows and sheep receiving 2 to 5 daily doses of 500 mg./kg. showed anorexia and incoordination progressing to death. In surviving animals, recovery was extremely slow. Necropsy revealed congestion of lungs and myocardial hemorrhages. Practically nonirritating to intact skin of guinea pigs and only moderately irritating to abraded skin. Not a skin sensitizer. Methemoglobinemia is possible if the compound is hydrolyzed in vivo to aniline. May be supplied in combination with other herbicides such as chlorpropham or propham. Also supplied as the salt of trichloroacetic acid.

Ref.: du Pont, 1961c; Palmer and Radeleff, 1964; Vrochinskii et al., 1974.

1249 Fluometuron 1249

1,1-Dimethyl-3-(α,α,α-trifluoro-*m*-tolyl)urea, Cotoran

Toxicity Rating: 3(?). Herbicide for pre- and postemergence control of annual grasses and weeds in food crops. Very low acute oral toxicity in rats (LD_{50} 8 gm./kg.) but reportedly much more toxic to mice and guinea pigs (LD_{50} about 800 mg./kg.). Closely related to Diuron. Said to be a mild cholinesterase inhibitor and to cause an increased leukocyte count in circulating blood in exposed agricultural workers. Metabolized in plants and animals by oxidative N-demethylation and hydrolysis to yield 3-trifluoromethylaniline. Carcinogenesis is described in the Russian literature, with gastric carcinomas and hepatomas appearing in rats given 450 mg./kg. daily for 22 months.

Ref.: Rubenchik et al., 1973; Plakhova et al., 1974.

1250 Isoproturon 1250

3-(4-Isopropylphenyl)-1,1-dimethylurea

Toxicity Rating: 3. Herbicide for control of annual grasses in cereal grains. Closely related to Monuron (see below). Moderate acute oral toxicity in rats (LD_{50} 1.8 gm./kg.). Rats given 500 ppm for 30 days showed no ill-effects.

1251 Linuron 1251

3-(3,4-Dichlorophenyl)-1-methoxy-1-methylurea, Premalin, Afalon

Toxicity Rating: 3. Selective, translocatable herbicide for pre- or post-emergence control of weeds in corn and soybeans, and row crops. Closely related to Monuron and Diuron and somewhat more toxic. Herbicidal action due to inhibition of photosynthesis. Low acute oral toxicity in rats (LD_{50} 3 to 4 gm./kg.), but more toxic toward dogs (LD_{50} 500 mg./kg.). The toxic syndrome is presumably like that from Monuron. Chronic administration of 4 mg./kg. per day in rats caused hypochromic anemia, decreased cholinesterase and peroxidase activities in blood, and ultrastructural changes in the liver. Dogs given 125 ppm for 2 years and rats given 400 ppm for 90 days experienced anemia and an abnormal hemoglobin thought to be sulfhemoglobin. Increased erythrogenesis was seen in spleen and bone marrow, and haemosiderin deposits were found in spleen and Kupffer cells of liver. In rats linuron is metabolized by demethoxylation followed by hydroxylation of the benzene ring. Major urinary metabolites are urea derivatives; no unchanged linuron could be demonstrated. Only trace amounts of 3,4-dichloroaniline were found. If metabolism to dichloroaniline is a major pathway in humans, however, methemoglobinemia should be anticipated after toxic doses.

Ref.: Boehme and Ernst, 1965; Hodge et al., 1968; Mironenko, 1975.

1252 Metoxuron 1252

3-(3-Chloro-4-methoxyphenyl)-1,1-dimethylurea, Dosanex

Toxicity Rating: 3. Pre- and post-emergence herbicide and defoliant, closely related to Monuron (see below). Moderate acute oral toxicity in mice (LD_{50} 3.2 gm./kg.). No significant percutaneous absorption. Not irritating to skin. Dogs fed 2500 ppm and rats fed 1250 ppm for 90 days showed no toxic symptoms.

Ref.: Martin and Worthing, 1977.

1253   1253 Monuron

3-(p-Chlorophenyl)-1,1-dimethylurea,   CMU,   Telvar

Toxicity Rating: 3. A herbicide for soil application. Acute oral LD_{50} in rats 1.5 to 3.6 gm./kg. Toxic doses caused ataxia, drowsiness, hyporeflexia, pallor and tachypnea, progressing to dacryorrhea, aciduria, diarrhea, epistaxis, hyperreflexia and irritability. Fatally poisoned animals exhibited adipsia, dyspnea, hypothermia and anuria. Death occurred within two days and was due to cardiac or respiratory failure. In survivors, recovery was accompanied by diuresis, alkalinuria and sometimes hematuria, glycosuria or proteinuria. Clinical signs of poisoning disappeared in 3 to 4 days. Autopsies of fatally poisoned rats revealed gastroenteritis, fatty necrosis of the liver, renal and splenic pallor, and degenerative changes in kidneys, muscle, salivary glands and testes. Capillary-venous congestion in brain, heart and lungs accompanied signs of a stress reaction in adrenal, spleen and thymus. Monuron shows increased toxicity toward rats previously fed a protein-deficient diet. No skin irritation or sensitization. Repeated doses in rats produce anemia, liver damage and methemoglobinemia. The latter is due to the formation of p-chloroaniline by metabolic hydrolysis. In another chronic feeding study, the presence of an abnormal pigment, thought to be sulfhemoglobin, correlated with the extent of hemolysis and hemosiderin deposits. Russian authors describe pulmonary tumors and hepatomas in rats and mice fed monuron for many months. The use of monuron in the U.S.A. has been curtailed because of its high oncogenic potential. Also supplied as the trichloroacetic acid salt. The latter has a somewhat higher oral toxicity. Metobromuron is the bromophenyl analog of Monuron.

Ref.: Boyd and Dobos, 1969; du Pont, 1961d; Hodge et al., 1958; Nezefi, 1974.

1254   1254 Neburon

1-n-Butyl-3-(3,4-dichlorophenyl)-1-methylurea

Toxicity Rating: 2. Pre-emergence herbicide available as a wettable powder. Oral lethal dose for rats greater than 11 gm./kg. Mild irritant to intact skin; no sensitization. Less toxic than the related Monuron or Diuron. Methemoglobinemia is possible if the compound is hydrolyzed in vivo to dichloroaniline.

Ref.: du Pont, 1961e.

1255   1255 Noruron

1-[5-(Hexahydro-4,7-methanoindanyl)]-3,3-dimethylurea, Herban

Toxicity Rating: 3. Herbicide used for control of grasses and broad-leafed weeds. Acute oral LD_{50} as a 10% suspension in mice 4.6 gm./kg., in rats 4.1 gm./kg. and in dogs 3.7 gm./kg. Somewhat more toxic in rats as a 4% solution in corn oil; LD_{50}'s 1.5 to 2.5 gm./kg. Poisoned animals showed symptoms of central depression such as sedation, ataxia, loss of righting reflex, dyspnea, coma and convulsions. Blood and brain cholinesterase levels were not depressed. No significant pathological lesions were observed. Acute dermal LD_{50} on intact or abraded rabbit skin greater than 23 gm./kg. Non-irritating to rabbit eye. About 50% of a group of mice died after 6-hour respiratory exposure to 60 mg./l., but rats and guinea pigs tolerated this exposure without symptoms. At 90-day feeding levels of 3000 ppm and above, mild ischemia of the kidneys was noted in rats, and moderate damage was apparent histologically.

Ref.: Hercules Powder Co., 1962b.

1256   1256 Phenobenzuron

1,1-Dimethyl-3-(3-methylphenyl)thiourea

Toxicity Rating: 3. One of a group of urea herbicides having moderate to low acute oral toxicities. No description of toxic signs and symptoms was found. However, signs of central nervous depression commonly occur after toxic doses of other urea herbicides and may be anticipated with this group as well. Percutaneous absorption is insignificant, but skin irritation may occur. Largely superseded by other herbicides.

Ref.: Martin and Worthing, 1977.

1257   1257 Siduron

1-(2-Methyl cyclohexyl)-3-phenylurea,   Dupont No. 1318,   Tupersan

Toxicity Rating: 2. Siduron is a selective pre-emergence herbicide belonging to the family of substituted ureas. Tupersan is a wettable powder containing 50% active ingredient. The acute oral LD_{50} of siduron for rats is greater than 5 gm./kg., and 5.5 gm./kg. applied to intact or abraded skin of rabbits caused no signs of toxicity. Label states powder may irritate eyes, nose, throat and skin.

Ref.: Belasco and Rusir, 1969.

1258 Tebuthiuron 1258

N-[5-(1,1-Dimethylethyl)-1,3,4-thiadiazol-2-yl]-N,N'-dimethylurea, Tebulan

Toxicity Rating: 3. Wide spectrum herbicide for control of woody and herbaceous plants in grasslands and sugar cane. High acute oral toxicity in experimental animals (rat LD_{50} 640 mg./kg.). In rodents, toxic doses produced hypoactivity, anorexia, ataxia and death. Emesis occurred in cats and dogs. Rats fed 2500 ppm for 3 months showed decreased gain in body weight. Diffuse vacuolization of pancreatic acinar cells, accompanied by a decrease in zymogen granules, was attributed to an inhibition of protein synthesis in these cells. In skin tests on rabbits, applications of 200 mg./kg. produced neither skin irritation nor signs of systemic intoxication. Metabolism of tebuthiuron proceeds by oxidative demethylation of the urea nitrogens. In tests using material in which the ring was labelled with C^{14}, virtually all of the radiolabel was excreted in 72 hours, primarily in a variety of urinary metabolites.

Ref.: Griffing and Todd, 1974; Morton and Hoffman, 1976; Todd et al., 1974.

Triazine and triazole herbicides

1259 Atrazine 1259

2-Chloro-4-(ethylamino)-6-(isopropylamino)-s-triazine

Toxicity Rating: 3. One of several closely related chloro-substituted triazine herbicides. Closely related to Simazine (see below). This class of herbicide is very insoluble and quite persistent in the soil. Used on corn and sugar cane and, at higher levels, for nonspecific weed control. For description of herbicidal action see Prometon below. Moderately low acute oral toxicity (reported rat oral LD_{50}'s for the group range from 1.2 to 3.7 gm./kg.). Daily oral doses of atrazine at 400 mg./kg. for 6 weeks killed half of a test group of rats. Acutely poisoned sheep and cattle exhibited muscular spasms, fasciculations, stiff gait and increased respiratory rates. Adrenal degeneration and congestion of lungs, liver and kidneys were observed. Large doses given by injection to pregnant rats proved fetotoxic. Inhalation hazard from aerosols is apparently low. No reports of skin irritation or other toxic injuries in man. Rapidly absorbed when ingested; metabolism proceeds via side-chain oxidation and amine dealkylation. Metabolites are excreted in urine and feces. In radiolabel experiments, about 20% of a dose appeared in the feces, 64% appeared in urine, and 16% remained in the carcass after 3 days.

Ref.: Bakke et al., 1972; Dalgaard-Mikkelsen and Poulsen, 1962; Olney, 1956; Palmer and Radeleff, 1964; Peters and Cook, 1973.

1260 Cyanazine 1260

2-[[4-Chloro-6-(ethylamino)-s-triazin-2-yl]amino]-2-methylpropionitrile, Bladex

Toxicity Rating: 4. Cyanazine and procyazine are cyano-substituted triazine herbicides used to control weeds in corn and wheat. Herbicidal activity is due to inhibition of plant respiration (see Prometon below). Highly toxic in rats (acute oral LD_{50} 180 to 334 mg./kg.). Symptoms of intoxication included lethargy, labored breathing, and blood-stained saliva. Vasodilation of ear veins and engorgement of fundus oculi were observed in intoxicated rabbits. So strongly emetic in dogs that no other immediate effects could be elicited by the oral route. Delayed deaths associated with inanition occurred, however, in some dosed dogs. Not irritating to rabbit skin or eyes when applied as a 5 percent solution in DMSO; dermal absorption not significant. The major metabolic residues of cyanazine in plants (and probably in mammals) are the 2-hydroxy and 6-dealkyl derivatives. These metabolites have no significant toxicity in test animals.

Ref.: EPA, July 14, 1978; Walker et al., 1974.

1261 Cyanuric Acid 1261

2,4,6-s-Triazinetriol, Trihydroxytriazine, Trihydroxycyanidine

Toxicity Rating: 2. Selective herbicide and chemical intermediate used in the manufacture of dry bleaches and of melamine, sponge rubber and other plastics. Cyanuric acid and its salts (sodium) are also used in swimming pools to lower the rate of photochemical reduction of chlorine, hypochlorous acid and hypochlorite ion, probably by forming reversible mono- and perhaps di-chloro derivatives (chloramines) in dilute solutions containing chlorine. Exists in solution in equilibrium with its keto tautomer known as isocyanuric acid. (See also Trichloroisocyanuric acid in the index.) The dry material decomposes at high temperatures (above $330°$ C) to yield cyanic acid (see latter in index). Rats survived single oral doses of 10 gm./kg., and the compound was excreted in urine largely unchanged. When fed chronically to mice, rats and dogs at dietary levels of 1 to 8%, sodium cyanurate induced chronic renal disease characterized by various tubular lesions and calcium concretions in the renal tubules and pelvis and in the urinary bladder. A paste of the acid produced mild irritation of the rabbit eye, but daily instillations into the conjunctival sac of a suspension of the monosodium salt caused no ocular damage or irritation. No skin irritation. No convincing evidence of teratogenicity or mutagenicity, but perhaps cyanuric acid is weakly carcinogenic in animals.

Ref.: Canelli, 1974; Hodge et al., 1965; Laveglia et al., 1977; Monsanto Chemical Company., May 1962.

1262   1262   Cyprazine

2-Chloro-4-(cyclopropylamino)-6-(isopropylamino)-*s*-triazine

Toxicity Rating: 3. A triazine used as a post-emergence herbicide on corn. Cyprazine is rapidly absorbed and metabolized by side-chain dealkylation. Metabolites are rapidly excreted in urine and feces. In one radiotracer experiment, 84% of the label was recovered in the first 24 hours. Cyprazine is not irritating to skin. The compounds were supplied as wettable powders and emulsifiable concentrates and in herbicidal mixtures with other triazines, but it has been largely superseded by other agents.

Ref.: Larsen and Bakke, 1975; Martin and Worthing, 1977.

1263   1263   Hexazinone

3-Cyclohexyl-6-(dimethylamino)-1-methyl-*s*-triazine-2,4-(1H,3H)-dione,   Velpar

Toxicity Rating: 3. Contact herbicide. Moderately toxic toward rodents (oral LD_{50} 1.7 gm./kg. in rat, 0.9 gm./kg. in guinea pig). No significant percutaneous absorption. An eye irritant in rabbits. Supplied as a soluble powder of 90 percent active agent.

Ref.: du Pont, January 1976.

1264   1264   Isomethiozin

6-*tert*-Butyl-4-(isobutylidine-amino)-3-(methylthio)-1,2,4-triazin-5-one,   Tantizon

Toxicity Rating: 2(?). Selective pre-emergence herbicide for control of grassy weeds in wheat. No significant acute toxicity towards rodents or birds. In rats the no-effect level in chronic feeding experiments was 100 ppm. Supplied as a 70% wettable powder.

Ref.: Worthing, 1979.

1265   1265   Metamitron

4-Amino-3-methyl-6-phenyl-1,2,4-triazin-5(4H)-one,   Goltix

Toxicity Rating: 3. Selective herbicide for control of weeds in sugar beets. Moderate acute oral toxicity (oral LD_{50}'s in rodents range from 1.4 to 3.3 gm./kg.). Female rats are more susceptible than male rats. Dogs tolerated 500 ppm in feed for 3 months without ill effect. Supplied as a 70% wettable powder.

Ref.: Worthing, 1979.

1266   1266   Metribuzin

4-Amino-6-(1,1-dimethylethyl)-3-(methylthio)-1,2,4-triazin-5(4H)-one,   Sencor

Toxicity Rating: 3. Triazole herbicide. Moderate acute oral toxicity (oral LD_{50} 2 gm./kg. in rats and 700 mg./kg. in mice). Poisoned rats exhibited sedation and labored breathing. Deaths occurred within 24 hours; survivors recovered slowly without permanent effects. No organ changes were found in either group. Dogs tolerated 500 ppm in feed for 3 months without ill effects. Inhalation of 885 mg./m^3 for four hours proved fatal to half of a group of exposed rats. Metribuzin was not irritating to the skin of rabbits or human volunteers, and dermal application did not produce skin sensitization or systemic intoxication.

Ref.: Loser and Kimmerle, 1972.

1267   1267   Prometon

2-Methoxy-4,6-bis(isopropylamino)-*s*-triazine,   Prometone,   Methoxy propazine

Toxicity Rating: 3. One of a series of methoxy or methylthio-substituted triazine herbicides. Used for pre- and post-emergence control of weeds in cereal and vegetable crops. Herbicidal action is due to inhibition of Hill reaction necessary for plant respiration. The resistance of a plant to a particular triazine depends on its ability to detoxify the compound under field conditions. Triazine herbicides may persist in soils for a year. The pure compounds have moderately low acute oral toxicities in laboratory animals; rat LD_{50}'s range from 1.4 to 5.0 gm./kg. except for 6-methoxy-*s*-triazines (see Terbumeton below). Technical grade material has a somewhat greater toxicity, however. No reports of human poisonings were found. All of these herbicides are rapidly absorbed and metabolized when ingested; amine dealkylation and side-chain oxidation are the predominant detoxification reactions (Boehme and Baer, 1967). The mercapto derivatives of triazine may also undergo sulfoxidation followed by reaction with hepatic glutathione to yield mercapturic acid derivatives (Bedford et al., 1975). Metabolites of most compounds are excreted in urine and feces within 72 hours. Symptoms of acute intoxication in experimental rodents include ataxia, dyspnea and convulsions. One of the more toxic of this group of triazines is Lambast, a superseded compound. In sheep, a single oral dose of 250 mg./kg. produced immediate ataxia, uncoordination and lameness, followed after 2 hours by extreme depression. Improvement occurred later the same day. Recovery extended over five weeks (Palmer, 1964). As an emulsifiable concentrate, Lambast has an oral LD_{50} of 1.4 gm./kg. in rats. In feeding experiments, no-effect levels of triazines are about 10 mg./kg. per day in rats and 40 mg./kg. per day in dogs. Some compounds may cause skin irritation. Dermal exposure may also lead to systemic intoxication with prometon, but not with prometryn, ametryn, or desmetryn. Repeated large doses of prometryn caused destruction of spermatocytes and spermatogenic testicular epithelium (Shtabskii, 1976). Ametryn doses of 100 mg./kg. daily for 90 days produced slight liver changes in rats. In chickens, dietary administration of ametryn is said to have inhibited hepatic gluconeogenic enzymes with accumulation of pyruvate and decrease in hepatic glucose (Srebocan et al., 1975). Increased pyruvic acid levels in liver and adrenals were also reported after administration of propazine and prometryn (Dinerman and Lavrent'eva, 1969). Plant metabolites of triazine herbicides have very low toxicities toward mammals. Prometon and the other compounds have low water solubilities and are supplied as emulsifiable concentrates and wettable powders (usually 25 to 80%). Triazines are also sold in herbicidal mixtures.

Ref.: Bedford et al., 1975; Boehme and Baer, 1967; Ciba-Geigy Corp.., Oct. 1972a; Dinerman and Lavrent'eva, 1969; Geigy Agricultural Chemicals, 1964b; Palmer, 1964b; Shtabskii, 1976; Srebocan et al., 1975.

1268 Propazine 1268

2-Chloro-4,6-bis(isopropylamino)-*s*-triazine

Toxicity Rating: 3. Herbicide of the triazine group, closely related to Atrazine. The acute mean lethal dose in rats indicates that this compound belongs on the borderline between toxicity classes 2 and 3. Poisoned cattle and sheep exhibited progressive anorexia and depression. Propazine given orally to rabbits for 1 to 4 months (500 mg./kg. daily) was reported to have caused macrocytic anemia. Doses of 2500 mg./kg. in rats decreased hepatic DNA synthesis and content; both effects were reportedly reversed by the administration of thymidine (Semencheva et al., 1972; Kuznetsova and Okunev, 1970). Propazine is readily absorbed and metabolized by amine-dealkylation and side-chain oxidation. See also Atrazine above.

Ref.: Kuznetsova and Okunev, 1970; Palmer and Radeleff, 1964; Semencheva et al., 1972.

1269 Simazine 1269

2-Chloro-4,6-bis(ethylamino)-*s*-triazine, Princep

Toxicity Rating: 3(?). Herbicide of the triazine group; used as a selective pre-emergent herbicide or, at higher application rates, as a soil sterilant. Slowly degraded in the environment. Very low acute oral toxicity in experimental rodents (rat LD_{50} is greater than 5 gm./kg.). Intoxicated rats exhibit drowsiness and irregular respiration. Acutely poisoned sheep and cattle exhibit muscular spasms, fasciculations, stiff gait, and increased respiratory rate. A single oral dose of Simazine of 500 mg./kg. is said to kill sheep. In this case, the onset of neurological symptoms (paralysis, ataxia and polydipsia) was delayed by 10 to 20 days. Oral doses are absorbed rapidly and completely. Urinary excretion of simazine is slower than with other triazine herbicides. In sheep, maximal urinary excretion occurred 2-6 days after a single toxic dose. Simazine is neither a primary irritant nor a skin sensitizer in humans.

Ref.: Ciba-Geigy Corp.., Oct. 1972b; Dalgaard-Mikkelsen and Poulsen, 1962; Hapke, 1968; Palmer and Radeleff, 1964.

1270 Terbumeton 1270

2-(*tert*-Butylamino)-4-(ethylamino)-6-methoxy-*s*-triazine

Toxicity Rating: 3 or 4. One of a group of 6-methoxy-*s*-triazine herbicides used for weed control in orchards and forests. Closely related to Prometon but said to be more toxic by oral route (rat oral LD_{50} 485 mg./kg. for terbumeton, 535 mg./kg. for simetone, 880 mg./kg. for ipatone). Not absorbed through skin. No description of toxic syndrome was found but see Prometon above.

Ref.: Worthing, 1979.

1271   1271   Triadimefon

1-(4-Chlorophenoxy)-3,3-dimethyl-1-(1,2,4-triazol-1-yl)-1-butanone,   Bayleton

Toxicity Rating: 3(?). Systemic fungicide. Animal experiments place this compound on the border between toxicity classes 3 and 4. In a three-month feeding study, the no-effect level for dogs was 600 ppm. The compound is supplied as a 5% and 25% wettable powder, a 10% emulsifiable concentrate, and as a 10% dust.

Ref.: Worthing, 1979.

1272   1272   Triazabutil

4-Butyl–*s*-triazole,   Butrizol,   Indar

Toxicity Rating: 4. Experimental systemic fungicide used for control of wheat leaf rust. High acute oral and dermal toxicities (rat oral LD_{50} 90 mg./kg.; dermal LD_{50} 310 mg./kg.). No description of toxic symptoms was found.

Substituted-amide herbicides

1273   1273   Alachlor

2-Chloro-2′,6′-diethyl-*N*-(methoxymethyl)acetanilide,   Lasso

Toxicity Rating: 3. Alachlor, delachlor, butachlor and metolachlor are four of several pre-emergence herbicides, which are closely related to propachlor (see below) but less toxic by oral and dermal routes (rat oral LD_{50} 1.2 to 1.8 gm./kg. for alachlor, delachlor and metolachlor, and 3.1 gm./kg. for butachlor). The toxic syndrome was not described but is probably similar to that of propachlor. Alachlor (and butachlor) has similar oral and dermal toxicities, indicating that percutaneous absorption is efficient. Both compounds are irritating to skin and eyes. Allergic skin reactions have been reported in humans. Inhalation exposure to alachlor at 32.6 mg./l. and to metolachlor at 0.96 mg./l. proved fatal to rats. The compounds are supplied as emulsifiable concentrates and in various mixed formulations.

Ref.: EPA, March, 1980; Worthing, 1979; Monsanto Chemical Co., Nov. 1969.

1274   1274   Allidochlor

N,N-Diallyl-2-chloroacetamide,   CDAA,   Randox

Toxicity Rating: 3. A pre-emergence herbicide used to control grasses in vegetable crops and ornamentals. Moderate acute oral toxicity in mammals (rat LD_{50} 700 mg./kg.); more toxic in rabbits when applied percutaneously (LD_{50} 350 mg./kg.). Causes severe irritation of skin and temporary sensitivity to cold (for 4 to 6 hrs.). Undiluted material in the eye has caused serious ocular damage. The nature of the toxic syndrome after oral administration has not been described. In rats, the primary metabolite of allidochlor is the mercapturic acid derivative, which is excreted in urine.

Ref.: Hamm and Speziale, 1956; Lamoureux and Davison, 1975; Ploch, 1957.

1275   1275   Diphenamid

N,N-Dimethyl-2,2-diphenylacetamide, e.g., Dymid, Enide

Toxicity Rating: 3 to 4. Pre-emergence herbicide. Acute oral LD_{50}'s of 80% material in adult rats is 970 mg./kg., but in weanling or newborn rats is 270 to 290 mg./kg. Produces emesis in monkeys and dogs. In mice, an initial central nervous depression was followed by clonic-tonic spasms. Poisoned rats exhibited ataxia and increased excitability. When given orally diphenamid is rapidly absorbed and extensively metabolized by microsomal oxidation and demethylation. Metabolic products, principally nor-diphenamid and *p*-hydroxydiphenamid, are rapidly conjugated and excreted in urine. Diphenamid does not appear to be a primary irritant or sensitizer. Dermal LD_{50} on normal or abraded rabbit skin greater than 6 gm./kg. with 24-hour contact. Dilute (0.1%) suspensions are not irritant to rabbit eye.

Ref.: McMahon and Sullivan, 1965; Weed Society of America, 1967; Vishnevskaya, 1966.

1276   1276   Fluoridamid

N^4-Acetyl-N^2-trifluoromethylsulfonyl–toluene-2,4-diamine,   Sustar

Toxicity Rating: 3. Plant growth regulator and retardant. Moderate acute oral toxicity (rat oral LD_{50} 2.6 gm./kg.). Not irritating to rabbit skin or eyes. Supplied as a 25% solution of the diethanolamine salt.

Ref.: Carboni, 1975.

1277 Naphthaleneacetamide

e.g., Rootone

Toxicity Rating: 3. Herbicide related to naphthaleneacetic acid (see index). Has superseded the latter as a fruit thinning material because of lessened foliage damage. Less soluble than the free acid. Acute oral LD_{50} in mammals reported to be 1000 mg./kg.

Ref.: Farm Chemicals Handbook, 1980; Kirchoff, 1961.

1278 Napropamide

N,N-Diethyl-2-(1-naphthalenyloxy)propionamide, Devrinol

Toxicity Rating: 2. Selective herbicide. No significant acute toxicity in rodents by oral or dermal routes. In chronic feeding experiments with rats, histological changes in liver and kidney were observed at the 2000 ppm level and increased alkaline phosphatase levels in liver and kidney at the 7000 ppm level. Not irritating to skin and eyes.

Ref.: Kawada et al., 1973.

1279 Naptalam

N-1-Naphthylphthalamic acid, Alanap-1

Toxicity Rating: 2. A pre-emergence herbicide of low acute toxicity in rats; oral LD_{50} greater than 8.5 gm./kg. No skin irritation described in man or animals. The sodium salt is somewhat more toxic with an LD_{50} of 2.0 gm./kg. In rats and dogs, the no-effect level for naptalam sodium in 90-day feeding experiments was 1000 ppm. Alanap-2 is *N*-1-naphthylphthalimide. No toxicity data were located for the latter. Alanap-3 is variously described as the sodium salt or as the free acid.

Ref.: Assoc. of Amer. Pesticide Control Officials, 1966; Spencer, 1973.

1280 Pentanochlor

N-(3-Chloro-4-methylphenyl)-2-methylpentanamide, 3′-Chloro-2-methyl-*p*-valero-toluidide, Solan

Toxicity Rating: 3. Post-emergence herbicide used on tomato fields. Available as an emulsifiable concentrate (Solan 4 EC, 4 lbs./gal.). Chemically related to propanil (see below) but less toxic by the oral route. Acute LD_{50}'s in male rats exceed 10 gm./kg. orally and 3.2 gm./kg. intraperitoneally. Signs of intoxication in rats included immediate ptosis, labored respiration and ataxia, followed in four hours by salivation and central nervous depression (e.g., loss of righting reflex). Coma and death occurred within 72 hours. Autopsy revealed congestion of lungs, kidneys and adrenals. No gross pathology was observed in the survivors. The LD_{50} of the emulsifiable concentrate is 5.6 ml./kg. by mouth. Mild irritant on rabbit skin with acute dermal LD_{50} in excess of 10 gm./kg. After 140 days at a dietary level of 2%, rats showed growth retardation. Red cell counts, hemoglobin levels and hematocrits were all depressed, and an abnormal blood pigment seemed to be present in trace amounts. Livers were enlarged.

Ref.: Holsing, 1965.

1281 Pronamide

3,5-Dichloro-*N*-(1,1-dimethyl-2-propynyl)benzamide, Propyzamide, Kerb

Toxicity Rating: 2. Pre-emergence herbicide for use on lettuce and alfalfa. Low acute oral toxicity. Reported LD_{50} values are 8.3 gm./kg. for male and 5.6 gm./kg. for female rats. Use of pronamide in the United States has been restricted because of reported oncogenic activity in mice. Produced slight local irritation but no systemic intoxication when applied to skin and eyes of rabbits. Poorly absorbed from the gastrointestinal tract of rats and cows; metabolized by side-chain oxidation and excreted in urine and feces.

Ref.: EPA, May 20, 1977; Rohm and Haas Co., date unknown.

1282 Propachlor

2-Chloro-*N*-isopropylacetanilide, Ramrod

Toxicity Rating: 3 or 4. Pre-emergence herbicide for control of grasses. Highly toxic in experimental animals. Acute oral LD_{50}'s reportedly range from 230 mg./kg. in mice to 970 mg./kg. in rats. Signs of intoxication include muscle weakness, salivation, tremors, collapse, coma and death. Dystrophic changes in visceral organs were observed in rats, rabbits and mice (Strateva, 1974). Dogs survived daily doses of 133 mg./kg. for 90 days without ill effects. Propachlor has caused severe skin irritation in man. Well absorbed through skin; the dermal LD_{50} in rabbits is 320 mg./kg. Repeated daily skin applications to rats (200 mg./kg. for 3 weeks) caused anemia and reduced tissue cytochrome oxidase activity. Dermal applications of 50 mg./kg. for 90 days inhibited blood catalase and serum transaminase activity and produced a decrease in sulfhydryl content of brain (Bainova et al., 1977). Embryotoxicity and teratogenesis have been described in rats given 5 to 20% of the LD_{50} by mouth during the first 20 days of pregnancy (Mirkova,

1975). Propachlor is readily absorbed after ingestion and rapidly excreted in feces and, as the mercapturic acid derivative, in urine (Lamoureux and Davison, 1975). Prynachlor is a closely related compound having a similar oral toxicity in laboratory animals but less readily absorbed through skin.

Ref.: Bainova et al., 1977; Hunt, 1969; Lamoureux and Davison, 1975; Mirkova, 1975; Strateva, 1974.

1283   1283   Propanil

3',4'-Dichloropropionanilide,   *N*-(3,4-Dichlorophenyl)propanamide, e.g., Stam

Toxicity Rating: 3. Selective, post-emergence contact herbicide, related to Dicryl and recommended for use on rice and potatoes. Moderately toxic; acute oral LD_{50} in rats is 1.5 gm./kg. Symptoms of intoxication in laboratory animals are central nervous depression, loss of righting reflex, cyanosis and death. Propanil is hydrolyzed to yield dichloroaniline by an acylamidase found in liver and kidneys of rats, mice and guinea pigs. Dichloroaniline produces methemoglobinemia in rats and mice (see Aniline in Section III). Inhibition of the acylamidase by pretreatment with triorthotolylphosphate prevents methemoglobin formation but not the central nervous depression or death resulting

from large doses of propanil. In long-term feeding experiments (330 ppm in the diet), rats showed marked polychromatophilia and evidence of hemolytic anemia after 13 weeks. Mild liver changes and "bile nephrosis" were observed in some female rats fed 10,000 ppm. The no-effect level in dogs was 600 ppm for 4 weeks. Workers in a propanil plant have experienced chloracne, and the herbicide produces mild hyperkeratosis in the rabbit ear; these effects are apparently due to contaminants in one of the starting materials for the synthesis, namely 3,4-dichloroaniline. The contaminants are 3,4,3',4'-tetrachloroazobenzene and its oxy derivative, both strongly chloracnegenic.

See also: Aniline, *Reference Congener in Section III.*
Ref.: Ambrose et al., 1972; Kimbrough, 1980; Marrese, 1961; Singleton and Murphy, 1973.

1284   1284   *N-m*-Tolylphthalamic Acid

3'-Methylphthalanilic acid, e.g.,   Duraset,   Tomaset

Toxicity Rating: 3. Plant growth regulator, used to set fruit and to prevent shock due to transplanting. Acute toxicity in rats places this compound near the borderline between toxicity classes 2 and 3 (oral LD_{50} 5.2 gm./kg.). However, chemical data indicate that gastric acid (pH 3) and intestinal

alkali (pH 10) may hydrolyze this amide to phthalamic acid (low toxicity) and to *m*-toluidine (high toxicity in man). See *p*-Toluidine in the index. Not irritating to mucous membranes and eyes of rabbits.

See also: Aniline, *Reference Congener in Section III.*
Ref.: Naugatuck Chemical, 1957.

Bipyridylium herbicides

1285   1285   Diquat Dibromide

Ethylene dipyridylium dibromide, 9,10-Dihydro-8α,10α-diazoniaphenanthrene dibromide, e.g., Reglone, Diquat

Toxicity Rating: 4. Pre-emergent non-selective herbicide used also to produce desiccation and defoliation. Closely related to Paraquat. Acute oral LD_{50} in rats 400-440 mg./kg.; subcutaneous LD_{50} 20 mg./kg. with death in 5 to 7 days. Ninety to 97% of an oral dose can be recovered from the feces in 48 hours, suggesting minimal absorption from the gas-

trointestinal tract. Distension and irritation of the gastrointestinal tract and thickening of the pulmonary alveolar walls are seen after large doses. Rats given 500 mg./kg. intraperitoneally exhibit cyanosis and convulsions culminating in death within 2 hours. Not carcinogenic.

See also: Paraquat, *Reference Congener in Section III.*
Ref.: Dalgaard-Mikkelsen and Poulsen, 1962.

1286   1286   Paraquat

1,1'-Dimethyl-4,4'-dipyridylium dichloride, e.g., Gramoxone

Toxicity Rating: 5. Bipyridylium type herbicide structurally related to diquat and widely used in the British Commonwealth. Symmetrical mole-

cule, each half containing a quaternary nitrogen which is positively charged at physiologic pH's. Marked species differences in acute oral toxicity;

approximate LD_{50}'s: hens, 260 mg./kg.; rats, 130 mg./kg.; cats and guinea pigs, 35-30 mg./kg. Intra-

peritoneally, LD_{50} for rats, 18 mg./kg.; and guinea pigs, 3 mg./kg.

See also: Paraquat, *Reference Congener in Section III.*
Ref.: Clark et al., 1966.

Substituted dinitroaniline herbicides

1287   Benefin   1287

N-Butyl-N-ethyl-α,α,α-trifluoro-2,6-dinitro-p-toluidine,   Balan,   Benfluralin

Toxicity Rating: 2. One of a group of substituted dinitroaniline herbicides with very low acute oral toxicity, used to control grasses and weeds in cotton, fruit trees, and other food crops. Rat oral LD_{50}'s for members of the group are greater than 10 gm./kg., except nitralin and isopropalin for

which the LD_{50}'s are reportedly greater than 5 gm./kg. Newborn animals are more sensitive than adults to benefin (oral LD_{50} 0.8 gm./kg.). Benefin and related compounds may cause skin and eye irritation but no sensitization.

Ref.: Goldenthal, 1971.

1288   Dinitramine   1288

N^3,N^3-Diethyl-2,4-dinitro-6-(trifluoromethyl)-1,3-benzenediamine, N^3,N^3-Diethyl-2,4-dinitro-6-(trifluoromethyl)-m-phenylenediamine

Toxicity Rating: 3. Dinitramine, fluchloralin, dipropalin, and Prowl are herbicides closely related to benefin (see above) but having greater acute oral toxicities. Oral LD_{50}'s in rats are 3.0 gm./kg. for dinitramine, 3.6 gm./kg. for dipropalin, 1.6 gm./kg. for fluchloralin, and 1.2 gm./kg. for Prowl. All of

the compounds except Prowl are irritating to skin and eyes. The compounds are rapidly metabolized in liver microsomes by side-chain oxidation and amine-dealkylation to yield a variety of polar and non-polar metabolites which are excreted equally in feces and urine.

Ref.: Kennedy et al., 1975; Nelson et al., 1977.

1289   Trifluralin   1289

α,α,α-Trifluoro-2,6-dinitro-N,N-dipropyl-p-toluidine, e.g., Treflan

Toxicity Rating: 2. Selective pre-emergence herbicide available in granular formulations and as an emulsive concentrate. Used on a variety of food and ornamental plants. Benefin is a structurally related herbicide which also has a very low toxicity. Acute oral LD_{50} is greater than 5 gm./kg. in mice and rats. The compound is poorly absorbed from the gastrointestinal tract, and 80 per cent of an oral dose in rats and dogs is excreted in the feces.

Several recognized metabolites also have a low order of toxicity. Female mice given 2740 ppm in food for 78 weeks showed a 28 per cent incidence of hepatocellular carcinoma and a smaller incidence of alveolar/bronchiolar adenomas. This carcinogenic activity may have been due to N-nitroso-di-n-propylamine, said to be present as a contaminant in the technical grade product.

Ref.: Emmerson and Anderson, 1966; Hotchkiss et al., 1978; National Cancer Institute., 1978f; Worth, 1970; Worth and Anderson, 1965.

Miscellaneous herbicides

1290   Amitrole   1290

3-Amino-1,2,4-triazole,   ATA,   Amizol

Toxicity Rating: 2. A herbicide used against poison ivy and poison oak. The toxic hazard to man is not yet established, but the acute oral LD_{50} (14.7 gm./kg.) in rats places this substance on the borderline between toxicity classes 1 and 2. Ingestion of 20 mg./kg. of Amitrole produced no symptoms of intoxication in a 39-year old woman; much of the dose was recovered unchanged in urine within 24 hours. Liver catalase depression, fatty degeneration of the liver, and hepatomas were found in rats given large doses in food. Chronic feeding also

produced depression of thyroid peroxidase activity with goiter formation, and possible thyroid tumorogenesis. Amitrole exhibited fetotoxicity but not teratogenesis when fed at 500 or 1000 ppm to female rats during mating, gestation and nursing. Daily doses of 20 or 100 mg./kg. given on days 7 to 15 of pregnancy produced no abnormalities in the offspring. Radiolabeled amitrole given to pregnant dams was found to cross the placenta and concentrate in rapidly dividing fetal tissues.

Ref.: Gaines et al., 1973; Geldmacher-v. Mallinckrodt and Schmidt, 1970; Heim et al., 1955; Spencer, 1973; Strum and Karnovsky, 1971; Tjalve, 1974.

1291　Bentazon

3-Isopropyl-(1*H*)-2,1,3-benzothiadiazin-4(3*H*)-one-2,2-dioxide,　Bendioxide

Toxicity Rating: 3. Post-emergence herbicide for control of broadleaf weeds in mint and truck crops. Moderately high acute oral toxicity. Reported LD_{50}'s range from 500 mg./kg. in cats to 1.1 gm./ kg. in rats. The compound is rapidly absorbed and readily excreted unchanged in urine. Irritating to eyes and mucous membranes. Usually supplied as the soluble sodium salt.

Ref.: Chasseaud et al., 1972.

1292　Benzoylprop-ethyl

Ethyl *N*-benzoyl-*N*-(3,4-dichlorophenyl)-2-amino propionate,　Suffix

Toxicity Rating: 3. One of a group of herbicides used to control wild oats in wheat and barley fields. Activity due to inhibition of plant cell elongation. Moderate mammalian toxicity; the oral LD_{50} is 1.5 gm./kg. in rats but 0.7 gm./kg. in mice. No description of toxic signs and symptoms was found. Flamprop-methyl and Flamprop-isopropyl are esters of the acid derived from benzoylprop by the substi- tution of fluorine for one of the chlorine atoms. The methyl and isopropyl esters in the flamprop series are less acutely toxic in rats than Benzoyl- prop-ethyl. All three compounds are rapidly ab- sorbed, de-esterified and excreted in rats, cows and pigs. No accumulation could be demonstrated. Rats given 1000 ppm Benzoylprop-ethyl in food for 13 weeks showed no toxic symptoms.

Ref.: Crayford et al., 1976; Hutson et al., 1977; Worthing, 1979.

1293　Bifenox

Methyl 5-(2,4-dichlorophenoxy)-2-nitrobenzoate

Toxicity Rating: 2. Pre-emergence herbicide for use in small grains. Low acute oral toxicity in rats (LD_{50} greater than 6.4 gm./kg.). Dogs and rats given bifenox in food for 90 days at the 500 ppm level showed no ill-effects.

Ref.: Mobil Chemical Co., 1977.

1294　Bromacil

5-Bromo-3-*sec*-butyl-6-methyluracil, e.g., Hyvar X

Toxicity Rating: 3. Herbicide of the substituted methyluracil type used for weed control in non-cropland areas. Activity is due to inhibition of photosynthesis. The closely related compounds, isocil (5-bromo-3-isopropyl-6-methyluracil) and terbacil (3-*tert*-butyl-5-chloro-6-methyluracil) have similar toxicity. Bromacil is available as an 80% wettable powder (Hyvar X) and a 50% water-soluble powder (Hyvar X-WS). Acute oral LD_{50} in rats is 5.2 gm./kg. Said to be an irritant on guinea pig skin, but not a sensitizer. Slight transient conjunctival irritation without corneal injury was produced in the rabbit eye. As little as 100 mg./kg. caused vomiting, salivation, muscular weakness, excitability, diarrhea and mydriasis in dogs. One dog survived a single dose of 5 gm./kg. Rats given repeated doses of 1500 mg./kg. daily died after 5 days. Autopsy revealed focal liver cell hypertrophy and hyperplasia. Sheep given 250 mg./kg. of either bromacil or isocil showed tympany and stilted gait within 4 hours. After administration on 4 successive days the sheep given bromacil died in prostration. Pathologic findings included gastroenteritis, liver enlargement and congestion, a friable appearance of the adrenals, hemorrhages in the heart and swollen and hemorrhagic lymph nodes. Bromacil and terbacil are metabolized in rodents by side-chain oxidation. Excretion in urine and feces is rapid and complete. Small amounts of bromacil and terbacil (0.03 ppm) were found in milk from lactating cows given 5 ppm in food.

Ref.: Gutenmann and Lisk, 1969; Krister, 1965; Palmer, 1964a; Rhodes et al., 1969.

1295　Bromoxynil

3,5-Dibromo-4-hydroxy-benzonitrile

Toxicity Rating: 4. Selective herbicide. Highly toxic in rats (oral LD_{50} 190 mg./kg.). Dermal LD_{50} is about 2 gm./kg. Dogs fed 25 mg./kg. in food daily for 13 weeks showed no ill-effects. Supplied as potassium salt or as the octanoate ester. Usually used in mixtures with phenoxyalkanoic acids such as mecoprop. If ingested, induce vomiting.

1296　Chloramben

3-Amino-2,5-dichlorobenzoic acid

Toxicity Rating: 2-3. Selective pre-emergence her-bicide used on vegetables and some ornamentals. Aqueous solutions and granular formulations of the ammonium salt and the emulsifiable concentrate of the methyl ester are commercially available. On the borderline between toxicity classes 2 and 3. A National Cancer Institute bioassay found chloramben to be carcinogenic to mice fed about 1.3 gm./kg. per day for 80 weeks. In other feeding trials no adverse effects were seen in rats fed 10 mg./kg. per day for 2 years.

1297 Chlorthiamid

2,6-Dichlorothiobenzamide, Prefix, 2,6-Dichlorobenzenecarbothioamide

Toxicity Rating: 3 or 4. Herbicide for control of woody perennials. High acute oral toxicity in laboratory animals. Acute oral LD_{50}'s range from 100 to 200 mg./kg. in sheep to 1 gm./kg. in dogs. In rats toxic doses produce sedation and narcosis by both oral and dermal routes. In dogs, large doses cause vomiting, which may be life-saving. In rat feeding experiments at the 100 ppm level, chlorthiamid produced reversible hepatocellular alterations. The compound is rapidly absorbed and metabolized. The initial metabolic product is said to be 2,6-dichlorobenzonitrile, which is subsequently hydroxylated at the 3- and 4-ring positions. Products are eliminated largely in urine. Chlorthiamid is supplied as a 75% wettable powder and in a low concentration granular form.

Ref.: Brown et al., 1967b; Griffiths et al., 1966.

1298 Cyano-dichlorophenylacrylic Acid

α-Cyano-2,4-dichlorocinnamic acid

Toxicity Rating: 4 to 5. A plant growth regulating substance whose inhibitory action on plants resembles that of maleic hydrazide. Very high acute oral toxicity in rats (oral LD_{50} 50 mg./kg.). Apparently not readily absorbed through skin because rabbits are able to tolerate a 24-hr. skin application of 250 mg./kg.

Ref.: Spencer, 1973.

1299 Dalapon

α,α-Dichloropropionic acid

Toxicity Rating: 3. Studies in laboratory animals place this herbicide near the borderline between toxicity classes 2 and 3. Long term feeding tests in dogs and rats produced no lesions except increased kidney weights in animals fed very high daily doses (up to 50 mg./kg. daily). Undiluted material causes irritation of skin and conjunctivae. Contaminated areas should be flushed promptly with water. Percutaneous absorption is negligible.

Ref.: Rowe, 1957.

1300 Dicamba (and Salts)

3,6-Dichloro-2-methoxybenzoic acid, 3,6-Dichloro-o-anisic acid, Dicamba dimethylamine salt, Dicamba monoethanolamine salt, Dicamba potassium salt, Dicamba diethanolamine salt

Toxicity Rating: 3. Herbicides used for brush control along highways and utility lines. Toxicities of salts are similar to that of parent compound, but see entries in this index for information about the various cations. Moderately high acute oral toxicity (rat LD_{50} is 760 to 1190 mg./kg., but 500 mg./kg. was fatal in sheep). Poisoned rats exhibited myotonic muscular spasms, urinary incontinence, dyspnea, exhaustion, cyanosis, and death. Minor lung hemorrhages were found in some animals. Subcutaneous application produced necrosis at injection site. Adhesions occurred after intraperitoneal injection. In cows and rats, the bulk of the compound is excreted unchanged in urine. Small amounts of 3,6-dichlorosalicylic acid may also be formed. Irritating to skin, eyes, and mucous membranes. Usually supplied as a salt.

Ref.: Edson and Sanderson, 1965; Tye and Engel, 1967.

1301 Diclofop-methyl

2-(4-(2′,4′-Dichlorophenoxy)–phenoxy)-methyl–propionate

Toxicity Rating: 3 to 4. Selective herbicide for postemergence control of annual grasses. Moderately high acute oral toxicity in rats (LD_{50} 580 mg./kg.). Toxic doses produced vomiting in dogs which was life-saving. Not irritating to skin. Formulated product produced corneal opacities and conjunctival irritation in rabbits.

Ref.: Lawatsch, 1979.

1302   1302   Diethyl Dithiobis(thionoformate)

Bisethylxanthogen, Bis(ethylxanthic)disulfide, Herbisan

Toxicity Rating: 4 or 3. A herbicide and insecticide of moderately high acute oral toxicity in laboratory animals. Reported oral LD_{50}'s range from 480 mg./kg. in rats to 770 mg./kg. in rabbits. Undiluted material applied to human skin has led to primary irritation and sensitization. Systemic poisoning has not been described, but the ingestion of alcohol should be prohibited after known exposures because this material is related chemically to disulfiram (Antabuse). Dimexano is the dimethyl analog and has similar uses but a somewhat higher toxicity in rats (oral LD_{50} 240 mg./kg.).

See also: Disulfiram, *Reference Congener in Section III.*
Ref.: Fike, 1958.

1303   1303   Dimethyl-2,3,5,6-tetrachloroterephthalate

Chlorthal dimethyl, Chlorthal methyl, Chlorothal, e.g., Dacthal

Toxicity Rating: 3. An insoluble powder used as a pre-emergence herbicide on a variety of turfs, ornamental and edible plants. Acute oral LD_{50} of the pure compound is greater than 3 gm./kg. in male albino rats. Mild skin irritation, but no evidence of systemic toxicity from percutaneous absorption after application of 10 gm./kg. on albino rabbit skin. Single applications of 3 mg. to rabbit eyes produced mild irritation which subsided in 24 hours. Tolerated without gross or histopathologic effects in the diets of rats and dogs for 2 years at dosages up to 10,000 ppm. Human volunteers have ingested 50 mg. without detectable effects. Metabolism studies in man and dog indicate that substantial hydrolysis of the ester bonds occurs in vivo, resulting in the urinary excretion of mono- or dicarboxylic acid derivatives. Remainder excreted unchanged in the feces. No appreciable storage in body tissue has been demonstrated.

Ref.: Utter, 1965.

1304   1304   Endothall

3,6-Endoxohexahydrophthalic acid

Toxicity Rating: 4 to 5. A herbicide available as the free acid and also as the disodium salt (Aquathol), dipotassium salt (Herbicide 273), and as various amine salts (Hydrothol 47 and 191). The free acid has a high oral toxicity in rats (acute LD_{50} 38 to 51 mg./kg.) with delayed deaths. The salts are somewhat less acutely toxic (LD_{50}'s range from 180 to 200 mg./kg.). Closely related chemically to cantharidin. Systemic effects are obscure and debated. One group reports that rabbits and dogs given lethal doses intravenously died after several hours in respiratory failure. Cats and dogs showed a drop in blood pressure up to the point of death. Others, however, suggest that the heart is the target organ and report cardiac failure in dogs without neurological signs. Solutions (1:20,000) depress isolated frog ventricles and rabbit auricles. Feeding tests in rats produced disorders of gait and convulsions. Moderate skin irritation and marked irritation of abraded skin, eyes and mucous membranes without sensitization. Death from systemic absorption occurred in those animals with most severe skin lesions. Severe gastrointestinal inflammation with erosion, especially if endothall is undiluted or unmixed with food. Cold milk or aluminum hydroxide gel (1 oz.) is recommended instead of emetics.

Ref.: Goldstein, 1952; Pennsylvania Salt Manufacturing Co., 1955; Srensek and Woodward, 1951.

1305   1305   Ethofumesate

2-Ethoxy-2,3-dihydro-3,3-dimethyl-5-benzofuranyl methanesulfonate, Nortron

Toxicity Rating: 2. Selective herbicide used for control of weeds in sugar beets. Low acute oral toxicity (rat LD_{50} greater than 6400 mg./kg.). Supplied as an emulsifiable concentrate containing about 20 per cent active ingredient.

1306   1306   Falone

2-(2,4-Dichlorophenoxy)ethanol phosphite, Bis[(2,4-dichlorophenoxy)ethyl]phosphite

Toxicity Rating: 3. Falone is a 3:1 mixture of the two compounds listed here. A herbicide which is moderately toxic to laboratory animals. Oral administration to rats causes abdominal pain, diarrhea, urinary incontinence, nasal irritation, and prostration. A 25% solution in xylene is very irritating to skin and mucous membranes, and there is some evidence of skin absorption in rabbits. No information of the effect of this mixture on cholinesterase has been located, but the toxic signs listed above suggest the possibility that it is able to inhibit cholinesterase at least weakly. See also Parathion in Section III.

Ref.: Naugatuck Chemical, 1959.

1307 Hexachloroacetone 1307

Hexachloro-2-propanone, HCA

Toxicity Rating: 3. Pre- and post-emergence herbicide. Moderately low acute toxicity by oral and dermal routes (acute oral LD_{50} in rats is 1.3 gm./kg., dermal LD_{50} is 3 gm./kg.). In animals toxic doses produced moderate to severe central nervous depression persisting for several days. No clinical poisonings known. Irritating to mucous membranes and skin, slight lacrimatory action. Inhalation exposure caused pulmonary edema, hemorrhage and congestion in laboratory rats. Only slight repair of lung tissue was noted in these animals 15 days after exposure. Chronic feeding studies in rats revealed hypertrophy of liver and kidneys and slight growth depression. Usually supplied in mixtures with other weed killers such as bromacil.

Ref.: Borzelleca and Lester, 1965; Cox, 1957.

1308 Maleic Hydrazide 1308

1,2-Dihydro-3,6-pyridazinedione, MH

Toxicity Rating: 3. A growth inhibitor of plants. Moderately low acute toxicity in mammals (rat oral LD_{50} 3.8 gm./kg.). In animals it causes tremors and muscle spasms. In female rats, toxicity is enhanced four-fold by prior exposure to a mixture of DDT, dieldrin and diazinon. No recognized effect on human skin. Said to have caused liver tumors in mice fed maximally tolerated doses for a prolonged period. The compound is readily absorbed and excreted in urine largely unchanged. In one radio-label experiment in rats, 77% of the administered radioactivity was recovered in urine within 6 days. Ninety per cent of the activity was found to be unaltered maleic hydrazide. The remainder was present as a conjugate of MH.

Ref.: EPA, Oct. 28, 1977; Luckens, 1969; Mays et al., 1968; Naugatuck Chemical, 1954.

1309 1-Naphthaleneacetic Acid 1309

Alpha-naphthaleneacetic acid, Planofix

Toxicity Rating: 3. A synthetic plant hormone. In animals it produces gastroenteritis and central nervous depression. Slight to moderate irritation of rabbit skin after prolonged contact (not so the methyl ester). The dust may cause nasal irritation.

1310 Nitrofen 1310

2,4-Dichlorophenyl *p*-nitrophenyl ether, Nitrophen, Tok

Toxicity Rating: 3. Pre- and post-emergence herbicide for control of weeds in cereal crops. Moderate acute oral toxicity (LD_{50} of the technical grade in rats is about 2.6 gm./kg.). Agricultural workers exposed to nitrofen for prolonged periods show reductions in hemoglobin and leukocyte counts and reduced serum cholinesterase and erythrocyte catalase activities. Male rats given a diet containing 4600 ppm for 80 weeks developed massive hemorrhages of the pelvic cavity involving the genitalia. Massive centrilobular necrosis of the liver, presumably secondary to hypoxia, was observed in the affected animals. Female rats showed an increased incidence of carcinoma of the pancreas and various tumors of the reproductive system. Prolonged feeding of maximally-tolerated doses produces a high incidence (96%) of hepatocellular carcinoma in mice. Nitrofen is fetotoxic in rats. Pups were stillborn or died shortly after birth. Autopsy of pups showed extensive fibrotic changes in lungs with an inflammatory exudate and squamous metaplasia. Alveolar cells were cuboidal with a granular cytoplasm and gave an impression of immaturity. Not irritating to skin and eyes, but prolonged skin contact with the concentrated product produced skin necrosis in rabbits. Nitrofen is readily absorbed from the gut. It accumulates in adipose tissue, muscle and kidney. About 10% of single doses in sheep and repeated doses in rats is excreted unchanged in the feces. The remainder is metabolized to yield 2,4-dichlorophenol and 4-nitrophenol and 2,4-dichlorophenyl 4-aminophenyl ether.

Ref.: Ambrose et al., 1971; Hunt et al., 1977; Kimbrough et al., 1974; National Cancer Institute, 1978g.

1311 Norflurazon 1311

4-Chloro-5-methylamino-2-(α,α,α-trifluoro-*m*-tolyl)-3(2*H*)-pyridazinone, Monometflurazon, Solicam, Zorial

Toxicity Rating: 2. Selective pre-emergence herbicide for use on cotton, nuts and fruits. Activity due to inhibition of carotenoid biosynthesis. Very low acute oral toxicity (rat LD_{50} greater than 8 gm./kg.). No appreciable dermal toxicity. Supplied as wettable powder and granular formulations.

1312

1312   Picloram

4-Amino-3,5,6-trichloropicolinic acid,   4-Amino-3,5,6-trichloro-2-pyridinecarboxylic acid,   Tordon

Toxicity Rating: 3. Herbicide and growth regulator. Low acute oral toxicity in mammals (LD_{50} is about 2 gm./kg. for rabbits and 8 gm./kg. for rats). Prolonged feeding of rats and mice at 7,400 ppm or 14,900 ppm for 80 weeks produced an increased incidence of dermatitis, alopecia, tachypnea, diar-rhea and vaginal bleeding. Follicular hyperplasia, C-cell hyperplasia, and C-cell adenoma of the thyroid and neoplastic nodules and focal alterations of the liver were observed at autopsy. Picloram salts may be irritating to skin and eyes.

Ref.: Worthing, 1979; National Cancer Institute, 1978h.

1313

1313   Pyrazon

5-Amino-4-chloro-2-phenyl-3(2*H*)-pyridaminone,   Pyramin

Toxicity Rating: 3. Pre- and post-emergence herbicide for control of annual broad-leafed weeds. Moderately low acute oral toxicity (rat LD_{50} 2.3 gm./kg.). Rapidly absorbed and excreted by exper-imental animals. Slightly irritating to skin. Blood alterations following dermal applications have been described in the Russian literature.

Ref.: Gzhegotskii and Dotoshitskii, 1971; Worthing, 1979.

1314

1314   Sodium Ethyl Xanthate

Sodium xanthogenate,   SEX cotton defoliant

Toxicity Rating: 3 to 4. Defoliant and herbicide. Oral mean lethal dose in mice is 0.73 gm./kg. (about the same in guinea pigs). Concentrated solutions (and presumably dusts) are irritating to rabbit skin and eyes, and percutaneous toxicity is comparatively high (lethal dose less than 1 gm./kg.). Poi-soned animals show salivation, loss of righting reflex, pulmonary congestion, pleural effusion, and death. Mild dermatitis is the only lesion observed to date in man. Related to Diethyl dithiobis(thionoformate) above.

Ref.: Rowe, 1956.

1315

1315   Sodium Isopropyl Xanthate

Isopropylxanthic acid sodium salt

Toxicity Rating: 3 to 4. A herbicide and defoliant. Toxic properties are like those of sodium ethyl xanthate. See latter above.

Ref.: McCormick, 1955.

1316

1316   Sodium 1-Naphthaleneacetate

Toxicity Rating: 3. A plant growth regulator of moderate oral toxicity in laboratory animals (rat oral LD_{50} 1 gm./kg.), causing gastroenteritis and central nervous depression. Prolonged application to rabbit skin (as a 10% solution in propylene glycol) produces local irritation. Heavy dust concentrations induce moderate nasal irritation in man. See also 1-Naphthaleneacetic acid above.

Ref.: Hollingsworth, 1958.

1317

1317   Trichlorobenzoic Acid

e.g., 2,4,6-Trichlorobenzoic acid,   2,4,6-TBA, 2,3,5-Trichlorobenzoic acid,   2,3,6-TBA

Toxicity Rating: 3. Mixed isomers of trichlorobenzoic acid, used as a weed killer for industrial and non-crop applications. Moderate acute oral toxicity (rat LD_{50} 1.4 gm./kg.; mouse LD_{50} 615 mg./kg.). Poisoned sheep and cattle showed salivation, tremor, depression and tympanites. Autopsy findings included lung congestion, hemorrhages and kidney inflammation. Rabbits developed erythema and edema after a second skin application of either pure 2,3,6-TBA or the isomer mixture. The compound has been withdrawn from commerce in the U.S.A. because of oncogenic activity evidently referable to nitrosamine contamination of the technical-grade product.

Ref.: Girard, 1957; Palmer and Radeleff, 1964.

1318

1318   2,3,5-Tri-iodobenzoic Acid

2,3,5-TIBA

Toxicity Rating: 3. Plant hormone used to stimulate flowering of fruit trees and increase soybean yield. Moderate acute oral toxicity (rat LD_{50} 813 mg./kg.). No significant dermal toxicity. Readily absorbed from the gut. In rats, goats and cows, it is metabolized with loss of iodine to yield 2,5- and 2,3-diiodobenzoic acids. Excreted primarily in urine. Iodine appears in milk of lactating animals. Supplied as the dimethylamine salt.

Repellents against insects and other pests

1319   4-Aminopyridine

4-Pyridinamine, e.g., Avitrol

Toxicity Rating: 5-6. A bird repellent. In poisoned birds, small doses cause involuntary contractions, resulting in distress calls which frighten away others. The oral LD_{50} is about 20 mg./kg. in rats, less in dogs and birds. In rats, dogs and horses the symptoms of intoxication include hyperexcitability, salivation, and tremors progressing to clonic and tonic convulsions. Death is due to respiratory or cardiac arrest. 4-Aminopyridine has a strong excitatory effect on the central nervous system, probably by enhancing cholinergic transmission. It causes contraction of isolated rat ileum, and has a vasoconstrictor action that is enhanced by ergotoxine. 4-Aminopyridine is excreted in urine and rapidly detoxified in the liver, so that the flesh of dead birds is not toxic to predatory animals. Two other isomers, 3-aminopyridine and 2-aminopyridine, have similar pharmacological effects on experimental animals. The latter (see entry below) has resulted in a human fatality following dermal exposure. The 3-amino isomer is less basic and somewhat less toxic than the others. Percutaneous exposure to any of the isomers may lead to systemic intoxication.

Ref.: Fastier and McDowell, 1958; Lemeignan, 1973; Schafer et al., 1973.

1320   2-Aminopyridine

Toxicity Rating: 5. Important intermediate in chemical synthesis. Closely related to 4-aminopyridine (see above) with similar effects on experimental animals. Three cases of human intoxication have been reported. In one case, prolonged exposure to the dust resulted in a severe headache, nausea, flushing of the extremities and elevated blood pressure. The patient recovered fully within one day. Another worker developed headache, weakness and convulsions followed by a stuporous state lasting several days. In the last instance, a chemical operator worked for 1.5 hours in clothes contaminated with the chemical. Two hours later he developed dizziness, headache, respiratory distress, and convulsions. Death followed respiratory failure.

Ref.: Patty, 1962; Watrous and Schulz, 1950.

1321   2,3,4,5-Bis(Δ^2-butylene)tetrahydrofurfural

MGK Repellent 11

The active ingredient in water emulsion or oil sprays used as insect repellents (final recommended conc. 0.2 to 0.4%). Reported to be less toxic than pyrethrins in mammals. In warm-blooded animals (presumably rats were used) it has an acute oral LD_{50} of 2 gm./kg.

Ref.: McLaughlin Gormley King Co., 1958a.

1322   Butopyronoxyl

Indalone,   Butyl mesityl oxide (oxalate)

Toxicity Rating: 2. Insect repellent. May be mildly irritating to skin on repeated application. Mild focal necrosis in liver and kidneys of rabbits after repeated cutaneous exposures. No human poisonings are known.

Ref.: Draize et al., 1948.

1323   *N*-Butylacetanilide

Toxicity Rating: 4. An insect repellent used to impregnate clothing. Moderate acute oral toxicity in mice (LD_{50} 800 mg./kg.); reportedly more toxic in guinea pigs. Because this compound is somewhat more toxic in laboratory animals than is the parent compound acetanilide and because man appears to be peculiarly sensitive to the latter, *N*-butylacetanilide may be particularly toxic in man. If deacetylation occurs at an appreciable rate, methemoglobinemia is probable after large doses. Not analgesic. In mice, toxic doses given orally produced central nervous depression which was maximal at 30 minutes after ingestion. Survivors recovered rapidly; no late mortality was observed.

See also: Aniline, *Reference Congener in Section III.*
Ref.: Starmer et al., 1971.

1324

1324   Dibutyl Adipate

Toxicity Rating: 2. A repellent against chiggers and ticks. Used on dogs and clothing. Very low acute toxicity in laboratory rodents.

Ref.: Spencer, 1973.

1325

1325   Di-*n*-butyl Succinate

Tabutrex

Toxicity Rating: 2. A liquid insect repellent of low acute oral toxicity in laboratory animals. Not irritating to skin or mucous membranes.

Ref.: Glenn Chemical Co., 1958.

1326

1326   *N,N*-Diethyl-*m*-toluamide

Delphene, DEET, DET, e.g., Off

Toxicity Rating: 3. An insect repellent. Some commercial preparations contain several isomers although the meta- form has been found to be most useful. On gastric intubation in rats the ortho-isomer is most toxic and the para-isomer least toxic. Acute oral LD_{50} of *m*-DET is 2.0 gm./kg. in rats. Toxic doses in rats and rabbits have produced lacrimation, chromodacryorrhea, depression, loss of righting reflexes, labored respiration, tremors, coma and terminal convulsions. Survivors recovered rapidly without sequelae. A child exposed to a product containing *m*-DET experienced disorientation, staggering gait, slurred speech and episodes consisting of stiffening into a sitting position, crying out, extending the extremities, flexing the fingers and dorsiflexing the toes. General supportive treatment led to eventual recovery. A 5-year old girl, sprayed with DET nightly for three months, developed headaches and slurred speech, progressing to athetosis, shaking, screaming and convulsions. She died 24 days after hospitalization. At autopsy the brain showed generalized edema with intense congestion of meninges. There was no demyelination and no evidence of meningitis. An 18-month old child who ingested an unknown quantity of a liquid preparation of DET exhibited similar signs and symptoms but eventually recovered. Both intoxications were thought to represent sensitization to the compound. In chronic feeding experiments, rats tolerated a diet containing 1% DET for 29 weeks. The compound is much more toxic when given parenterally (rat i.v. LD_{50} 50 mg./kg.). After intravenous injection, DET is rapidly distributed through the body and quickly eliminated by the kidneys, 98% of a small dose being recovered in urine within the first eight hours. The compound is selectively concentrated within the lacrimal glands, nasal mucosa and mouse yolk sac. Undiluted material is a moderate-to-severe irritant in the eye. Dermal application of undiluted material and 50% solutions caused no primary irritation or skin sensitization in man, but in rabbits erythema and desquamation are described as well as percutaneous intoxication. Repeated dermal applications of the *o*- and *p*- isomers produced slight renal tubular necrosis in rats and mild interstitial nephritis in rabbits. Embryotoxicity following dermal applications of large amounts of DET to rabbits is described in the Russian literature.

Ref.: Ambrose, 1959; Blomquist et al., 1975; Gleiberman et al., 1976; Gryboski et al., 961; Zadikoff, 1979.

1327

1327   Dimethyl Carbate

Dimethyl *cis*-bicyclo(2,2,1)-5-heptene-2,3-dicarboxylate, NISY, Dimelone

Toxicity Rating: 3. Repellent used in mixtures against some species of mosquitoes. Perhaps the toxic syndrome resembles that due to MGK 264, which is an insecticide that produces hyperexcitability followed by central nervous depression in acutely poisoned animals. See latter in the index.

Ref.: Lehman, 1955.

1328

1328   Di-*n*-propyl Isocinchomeronate

MGK Repellent 326

Toxicity Rating: 2. Used either in emulsifiable or oil-base sprays as a fly repellent. Reported to have an acute oral LD_{50} of 6.2 ± 1.0 gm./kg. in white rats; an intravenous LD_{50} of 2.5 gm./kg. Produced red, wrinkled skin on shaved rabbit at 9.4 ml./kg. after 18 days. No differences detected between control rats and those fed 20,000 ppm in daily diet for 90 days.

Ref.: McLaughlin Gormley King Co., 1958b.

1329   2-Ethyl-1,3-hexanediol   1329

Ethohexadiol,   Rutgers 612

Toxicity Rating: 3. Insect repellent. Little or no skin absorption. Ingestion causes central nervous depression. Death in rats is accompanied by severe kidney and liver damage. Treat with lavage, artificial respiration, and supportive measures.

Ref.: Draize et al., 1948.

1330   2-Hydroxyethyl-*n*-octyl Sulfide   1330

e.g., MGK Repellent 874

Toxicity Rating: 2. Roach repellent available in a wide range of strengths in oil bases and as emulsifiable concentrates. Acute LD_{50}'s of MGK Repellent 874 (95% 2-hydroxyethyl-*n*-octyl sulfide, 5% related compounds) for albino rabbits are 8.5 gm./kg. by stomach tube and 15 ml./kg. by skin application. Inhalation hazard appears to be low. Produces erythema on shaved rabbit skin and corneal necrosis in the eye. A dietary level of 2% was tolerated by rats for 90 days without apparent effect.

Ref.: Shocket, 1964.

1331   Propyl Diethylsuccinamate   1331

n-Propyl-*N,N*-diethylsuccinamate

Toxicity Rating: 2. Effective repellent against certain species of mosquitoes. Acute lethal dose in rats indicates that this compound belongs near the borderline between toxicity classes 2 and 3.

Ref.: Draize et al., 1948.

Anticoagulant rodenticides (and drugs)

1332   Acenocoumarol   1332

3-(α-Acetonyl-4-nitrobenzyl)-4-hydroxycoumarin,   Acenocoumarin,   Nicoumalone,   Sintrom

Most potent anticoagulant in coumarin-class.

See also: Warfarin, *Reference Congener in Section III.*

1333   Anisindione   1333

Miradon,   2-*p*-Anisyl-1,3-indandione,   2-(*p*-Methoxy-phenyl)-1,3-indandione

Toxicity Rating: 4(?). A long acting orally effective anticoagulant drug with a half-life in man of 4 days. Said to be less toxic than pheninindione, to which it is related. May produce dermatitis and color alkaline urine orange. It is available in 50 mg. tablets (Miradon).

See also: Warfarin, *Reference Congener in Section III.*

1334   Bishydroxycoumarin   1334

3,3'-Methylenebis(4-hydroxycoumarin),   Dicoumarol,   Dicumarol

Anticoagulant drug related to warfarin. Single therapeutic dose in man is 200 to 300 mg. Single-dose toxicity is not well established but is probably low relative to the cumulative multiple–dose toxicity.

See also: Warfarin, *Reference Congener in Section III.*
Ref.: Duff and Shull, 1949; Eisenberg, 1959; Pearson and MacKenzie, 1958.

1335   Chlorophacinone   1335

2-[(*p*-Chlorophenyl)phenyl]acetyl-1,3-indandione

Toxicity Rating: 5-6. Anticoagulant rodenticide with an acute oral LD_{50} of 1.06 and 3.58 mg./kg. in female mice and 2.1 mg./kg. in laboratory rats, but some wild rats (*e.g.*, Rattus norvegicus) are much more resistant. Apparently man is also because human volunteers tolerated single 20 mg. doses (presumably by mouth) with uneventful recoveries. Application of a solution of 5 mg. in 2 ml. of liquid paraffin to shaved rabbit skin produced only a slight reduction of prothrombin level. After single lethal doses in rodents death tends to be delayed for 5-8 days and is presumably due to internal hemorrhages. Vitamin K_1 is an antidote by antagonizing the inhibition of prothrombin synthesis, but chlorophacinone is said also to uncouple oxidative phosphorylation. Commercially available as

See also: Warfarin, *Reference Congener in Section III.*
Ref.: Webb et al., 1973; Worthing, 1979.

oil concentrate for impregnating bait material and as dust concentrate for incorporation into paraffin blocks, into poisons for rat drinking water and in tracking powders.

1336   Coumachlor

Tomorin,   3-(α-Acetonyl-4-chlorobenzyl)-4-hydroxycoumarin

A rodenticide like warfarin, with delayed actions on prothrombin level and blood clotting, resulting in death by hemorrhage.

See also: Warfarin, *Reference Congener in Section III.*
Ref.: Wanntorp, 1959.

1337   Coumafuryl

Fumarin,   Fumasol

An anticoagulant related to warfarin and used as a rodenticide. Highly toxic by continuous feeding over 8 to 10 days (oral LD_{50} 25 mg./kg. in rats). Single-dose toxicity is not established.

See also: Warfarin, *Reference Congener in Section III.*

1338   Cyclocoumarol

Anticoagulant closely related to bishydroxycoumarin.
See also: Warfarin, *Reference Congener in Section III.*

1339   Diphenadione

2-Diphenylacetyl-1,3-inandione,   Diphacinone

Toxicity Rating: 5. A rodenticide with delayed effects on the prothrombin level and consequent disturbances in blood coagulation, resulting in death by hemorrhage. More potent than warfarin in multiple dose experiments and especially after single dose exposures. Commercial baits, e.g., Diphacin, contain 0.005% active ingredient.

See also: Warfarin, *Reference Congener in Section III.*
Ref.: Saunders et al., 1955.

1340   Ethyl Biscoumacetate

3,3'-Carboxymethylene bis(4-hydroxycoumarin)ethyl ester,   Tromexan

Anticoagulant closely related to bishydroxycoumarin.
See also: Warfarin, *Reference Congener in Section III.*

1341   Phenindione

2-Phenyl-1,3-indandione

Anticoagulant similar in action to warfarin but chemically unrelated. Fatal agranulocytosis, hepatitis, febrile episodes and hypersensitivity reactions have occurred.

See also: Warfarin, *Reference Congener in Section III.*
Ref.: Mather and Riley, 1960.

1342   Phenprocoumon

Liquamar

Anticoagulant closely related to bishydroxycoumarin.
See also: Warfarin, *Reference Congener in Section III.*

1343   2-Pivalyl-1,3-indandione

Pindone, Pival

Toxicity Rating: 4(?). A water-soluble sodium salt of this compound is known as Pivalyn. A rodenticide with delayed effects on the prothrombin level and consequent disturbances in blood coagulation, producing death by hemorrhage. When tested in rats (single intraperitoneal injections), pindone proved to be more toxic than warfarin, but it is apparently less potent than warfarin by multiple daily doses.

See also: Warfarin, Reference Congener in Section III.
Ref.: Beauregard et al., 1955; Saunders et al., 1955.

1344   Valone   1344

2-Isovaleryl-1,3-indandione

Toxicity Rating: 4. Used as a rodenticide and in insecticidal mixtures. Toxicity rating is based on single oral doses dissolved in olive oil and given to rats and rabbits. Even more toxic by multiple doses over periods of several days because of hemorrhages due to severe hypoprothrombinemia. Single lethal doses in rats led to muscle weakness, hyperexcitability, pulmonary congestion and death with heart in systolic standstill after 1 or 2 hours; prothrombin levels were low but hemorrhages were not usually encountered and vitamin K was not protective. Try vitamin K_1.

See also: Warfarin, Reference Congener in Section III.
Ref.: Kabat et al., 1944.

1345   Warfarin   1345

3-(α-Acetonylbenzyl)-4-hydroxycoumarin

Toxicity Rating: 4. Single-dose toxicity is not well defined in man, but it is probably low relative to the cumulative multiple-dose toxicity. An effective rodenticide. Practically insoluble in water but freely soluble in NaOH solution, where it forms a sodium salt. Warfarin sodium is used in clinical medicine as an anticoagulant. Strains of laboratory rats vary considerably in sensitivity to warfarin. In male Sprague-Dawley rats the single-dose LD_{50} of sodium warfarin is about 100 mg./kg., with the highest mortality rates between the fourth and tenth post-treatment days. Extensive internal hemorrhages were found at autopsy. Commercial ready-to-use warfarin baits may also contain sulfaquinoxaline to suppress vitamin K producing bacteria in target rodents and so to increase the effectiveness of the warfarin. See Sulfaquinoxaline in the index.

See also: Warfarin, Reference Congener in Section III.
Ref.: Back et al., 1978.

Miscellaneous synthetic rodenticides

1346   Castrix   1346

2-Chloro-4-dimethylamino-6-methylpyrimidine

Toxicity Rating: 6. A rodenticide causing fatal convulsions. In laboratory animals symptoms begin 30 to 50 min. after ingestion. Compound is not chemically related to strychnine, but recommended treatment is the same.

See also: Strychnine, Reference Congener in Section III.
Ref.: Lehman, 1951.

1347   Fluoroacetamide   1347

Compound 1081,   Monofluoroacetamide

Toxicity Rating: 4 to 5. Rodenticide, closely related to sodium fluoroacetate (see Fluoroacetate in the index) but slower acting and somewhat less toxic. Highly toxic in rodents (oral LD_{50} 80 mg./kg.). As with fluoroacetate, fluoroacetamide's toxicity is due to its in vivo conversion to fluorocitrate, which inhibits the essential enzyme aconitase. Acetamide is said to be antidotal. Sublethal oral doses of fluoroacetamide in mice reduced fertility, increased pre-natal mortality, and slowed neonatal development when given during pregnancy.

See also: Fluoroacetate, Reference Congener in Section III.
Ref.: Tokareva et al., 1971; Lotspeich et al., 1952.

1348   Tetramine   1348

Tetramethylene disulphotetramine

Toxicity Rating: 6. An experimental rodenticide which may be too toxic to be marketed. It is a powerful convulsant poison, even more potent than strychnine.

See also: Strychnine, Reference Congener in Section III.
Ref.: Assoc. of Amer. Pesticide Control Officials, 1966.

1349   **1349**   Norbormide

5-[(α-Hydroxy-α-2-pyridyl)benzyl]-7-[α-2-(pyridylbenzyl)idine]-5-norbornene-2,3-dicarboximide, McN-1025, Shoxin, e.g., RATicate

Toxicity Rating: 2–5. A highly selective rat toxicant; LD_{50} by mouth 5 to 15 mg./kg. in genus Rattus. Mice, cotton rats, guinea pigs, hamsters and nutria were killed by oral doses between 100 and 1000 mg./kg. but most test animals tolerated 1000 mg./kg. without apparent effect. Humans ingesting doses up to 300 mg. showed slight transient decreases in body temperature and blood pressure. Intradermal injections (0.1 ml. of 0.1% solution) produced no skin reactions or lesions in man. Tolerated by animal primates in single oral doses of 300 to 1000 mg./kg. Apparently toxic to rats by virtue of an intense, direct, generalized constriction of small peripheral vessels, leading to local ischemic organ damage and death. The vasoconstriction could not be reversed in rats by a variety of drugs including direct vasodilators such as sodium nitrite. Signs in poisoned rats include an initial increase in motor activity accompanied by incoordination and a generalized weakening of hind extremities. This may be followed by dyspnea and a marked blanching of ears, eyes, feet and tail. Convulsions apparently of anoxic origin precede death. No specific gross or histopathologic tissue changes were observed. Although some signs and symptoms and the species selectivity of norbormide are reminiscent of ANTU poisoning (see Section III), the characteristic pleural effusions of the latter do not occur with norbormide.

Ref.: Roszkowski et al., 1964; Roszkowski, 1965.

1350   **1350**   ANTU

Alpha-naphthyl thiourea,   1-(1-Naphthyl)-2-thiourea

Toxicity Rating: 3(?).

See also: ANTU, *Reference Congener in Section III.*

1351   **1351**   Phenylthiourea

Toxicity Rating: 5(?). Used occasionally as a rodenticide and as a test substance in medical genetics. The ability to taste phenylthiourea (PTU) is an inherited trait. Considerable species differences in acute toxicity. Acute oral LD_{50} in wild Norway rats 8.6 mg./kg., domestic rats 3.1 mg./kg., and rabbits 40 mg./kg. Poisoned rats exhibited pleural effusions and pulmonary edema. Extensively metabolized in rabbits and 86% excreted in the urine over 2 days with an additional 10% in the feces. Desulfuration of the molecule is extensive, and the sulfur label is excreted more slowly. Eventually 60% is recovered as urinary sulfate. Pretreatment of animals with 1-methyl-1-phenylthiourea prevents desulfuration and reduces the toxicity of PTU. Because the LD_{50} of PTU is about the same as the LD_{50} for intravenous hydrogen sulfide solutions, the suggestion has been made that the toxicity of PTU is due to sulfide release in vivo. This suggestion seems unlikely on several grounds. Hydrogen sulfide by any route produces an acute fulminating asphyxia within minutes. Mice given massive doses of PTU (100 mg./kg.) intraperitoneally survived at least 8 hours although all had died by 22 hours. Similarly, rats given 25 mg./kg. intraperitoneally survived many hours. Because animals and man have a very large capacity to detoxify sulfides, a lethal dose presented slowly (as by the metabolism of PTU) would have to be many times larger than the intravenous lethal dose.

See also: ANTU, *Reference Congener in Section III.*
Ref.: Dieke et al., 1947; Scheline et al., 1961; Smith and Williams, 1961; Smith and Gosselin, 1963.

1352   **1352**   Thiourea

Thiocarbamide

Toxicity Rating: 3-4. Found in silver polishes, usually acidified with hydrochloric acid. Rat oral LD_{50} differs from strain to strain: 0.125-0.640 gm./kg. in the "domestic rat", 1.86 in the Norway rat. The nature of the toxic reaction is not described but α-naphthyl thiourea induces pulmonary edema. Repeated exposure may induce agranulocytosis and thrombopenia. Thiourea is rapidly excreted unchanged in urine. Fed chronically to rats, it induced hepatic tumors, bone marrow depression and goiters.

See also: ANTU, *Reference Congener in Section III.*
Ref.: Dieke and Richter, 1945; Dieke et al., 1947; Newcomb and Deane, 1944.

1353   **1353**   Vacor

N-3-Pyridylmethyl-*N'*-*p*-nitrophenylurea,   PNU

Marketed between 1975 and 1979 as a specific poison for rats and mice. Sales were discontinued after reports of many severe human poisonings, including at least seven fatalities. Signs and symptoms of intoxication in dogs and humans include abdominal pain, nausea and vomiting, central nervous depression, visual disturbances, anorexia, painful paresthesias, autonomic nervous system dysfunction with dystonia, and orthostatic hypotension. Ataxia, hyporeflexia, tremors and muscular weakness develop later. Death may be delayed for several days. Human survivors regularly develop an insulin-deficient, ketosis-prone form of diabetes mellitus associated with severe toxic neu-

ropathies. This disease evidently results from a specific toxic action of Vacor on pancreatic beta-cells (as with streptozocin and alloxan). Immediate niacinamide administration prevents death in rats and may prove useful in preventing beta-cell destruction in human poisonings. Delayed administration of niacinamide appears to be ineffective. By analogy with streptozocin, a closely related compound, pancreatic tumor formation may be anticipated in survivors of severe Vacor intoxication.

Ref.: Johnson et al., 1980; Pont et al., 1979; Prosser and Karam, 1978.

Miscellaneous agricultural chemicals

1354   Apholate   1354

2,2,4,4,6,6-Hexahydro-2,2,4,4,6,6-hexakis(1-aziridinyl)-1,3,5,2,4,6-triazatriphosphorine,   Hexakis(1-aziridinyl)-phosphonitrile,   1-Aziridinyl-phosphonitrile trimer

Toxicity Rating: 6. A representative experimental insect chemosterilant active against both sexes of the common house fly and other economically important species. Closely related compounds include aphoxide and methaphoxide. The high toxicity of these compounds limits their present use to laboratories in which sterile populations of insects are raised and released to compete for fertile mates. Said to be alkylating agents with effects on genetic material similar to ionizing radiation. Single intramuscular doses of apholate of 2.5 mg./kg. killed calves in 5-7 days. Single oral doses of 50 mg./kg. of all these compounds were lethal to sheep in 1 to 6 days. Cumulative toxicity was apparent in sheep

at daily oral doses above 1 mg./kg. With all 3 compounds the pattern of intoxication included depression, anorexia, and diarrhea, appearing 2-3 days before death, followed by terminal dyspnea, incoordination, epistaxis, salivation, prostration and cyanosis. Convulsions were not observed. Marked leukopenia characterized by lymphocytopenia occurred within 24 hrs. of apholate injection. Pathologic changes were widespread but most consistently in the liver with congestion of hepatic sinusoids, cloudy swelling, fatty degeneration and necrosis. Only symptomatic and supportive measures are available.

Ref.: Khan, 1963; Younger and Radeleff, 1964.

1355   Calcium Cyanamide   1355

"Cyanamide"

Toxicity Rating: 3. Reacts with acid to liberate HN=C=NH, a solid with an appreciable vapor pressure. A synthetic agricultural fertilizer. Contains no free cyanide and apparently is not metabolized to cyanide. When absorbed, the cyanamide ion $(CN_2)^{-2}$ causes intense cutaneous and mucosal flushing (congestive hyperemia), headache, vertigo, rapid breathing, hypotension, and profound shock. The primary vascular reaction is not correctable by atropine or any known antidote. An attack after a single oral dose is usually transient (1/2 to 2 hr.), and the fatal dose in man is estimated

at 40 to 50 gm. The vapor is intensely irritating and may produce both pulmonary and systemic signs. After mild exposures, symptoms may be precipitated or intensified by the ingestion of alcohol. Citrated calcium cyanamide is marketed as a drug (Abstem, Temposil) for the aversion therapy of alcoholism. The symptoms of the alcohol-induced reaction are said to be milder than with disulfiram, but a death has occurred. For a discussion of the management of this syndrome see Disulfiram in Section III.

Ref.: Barnard, 1943; Rodger, 1962.

1356   Daminozide   1356

Mono(2,2-dimethylhydrazide)succinic acid,   Aminozide,   Alar

Toxicity Rating: 2. A plant growth regulating agent used in orchard crops and ornamentals. Only slightly toxic to mammals when given orally. Re-

ports in Russian literature describe alterations in liver function of experimental animals given very large doses. Sold as an 85% water-soluble powder.

Ref.: Grabliauskiene, 1974; Spencer, 1973.

1357   Gibberellic Acid   1357

Gibrel (potassium salt)

Toxicity Rating: 1. Metabolic product of fungus Gibberella fujikuroi. It produces acceleration of growth in plants. In rats and mice it is relatively harmless when administered orally, parenterally,

by inhalation, or by topical application. No deaths observed in mice given single oral doses of 25 gm./kg.

Ref.: Albertini et al., 1960; Peck et al., 1957.

1358   **1358** Methyl Isothiocyanate

Methyl mustard oil, e.g., Trapex

Toxicity Rating: 4. A highly irritating volatile solid, slightly soluble in water. Said to have potential as a chemical warfare agent. Oral LD_{50} in rats 97 mg./ kg. Said to be slowly liberated as the active constituent of certain soil fungicides and nematocides; see Vapam in the index.

Ref.: Pieroh et al., 1959.

1359   **1359** Allyl Isothiocyanate

Volatile oil of mustard

Occurs naturally in black mustard seed and in raw cabbage where it is a weak goitrogen. Used as a counter-irritant in medicine, a fungicide, an insecticidal fumigant and a repellent for cats and dogs. Included in some model airplane cements to deter "glue sniffers" at concentrations (0.25 to 0.5%) that probably have no toxicological significance. A violent irritant unless diluted. Used externally as a rubefacient (0.1 to 0.2% in 50% ethanol). Aqueous suspensions are more irritating than oil solutions and may produce blisters. Acute oral LD_{50} of 10% solution in corn oil is 339 mg./kg. in rats. Death occurred between 4 hr. and 15 days, and the animals had a scrawny appearance with rough fur and a porphyrin-like deposit around the eyes and nose.

Ref.: Jenner et al., 1964; Langer, 1964; Osol and Farrar, 1955.

1360   **1360** Phenothioxin

Phenoxathrin

Toxicity Rating: 4. Used as an insecticide. In rats and guinea pigs it lies near the borderline between toxicity classes 3 and 4. Liver pathology described in chronic feeding tests with rats. Moderate to marked irritation of rabbit skin after prolonged contact. No human data.

Ref.: Smith et al., 1936.

1361   **1361** Trichlorobenzyl Chloride

TCBC

Toxicity Rating: 3. Used as an adjunct in some insecticides. Approximate oral LD_{50} in rats 3075 mg./kg. No apparent pulmonary complications from vapor exposure, but it produces moderate nasal inflammation and is a moderately strong lacrimator. Lethal doses in animals caused gastrointestinal irritation, salivation, pulmonary hemorrhage, general irritability and death in 24 to 48 hours.

Ref.: Seleck and Kelly, 1961.

Synthetic drugs

Barbiturates

1362   **1362** Barbiturates

Dozens of dialkyl and alkyl-aryl substituted barbituric acids and their salts have been employed in clinical medicine as sedative and hypnotic agents. They are responsible for many accidental and suicidal poisonings. On the basis of clinical reports most of them lie in toxicity class 5. Some of the more common examples are described below.

See also: Barbiturates, *Reference Congener in Section III*.

1363   **1363** 5-Allyl-5-phenylbarbituric Acid

Lubergal,   Phenyral

Toxicity Rating: 4. Barbiturate drug of the long-acting class. Adult therapeutic dose by mouth 0.1 to 0.3 gm.

See also: Barbiturates, *Reference Congener in Section III*.

1364 Amobarbital

Amylobarbitone, 5-Ethyl-5-isoamylbarbituric acid, Amytal, Barbamil

Toxicity Rating: 5. A sedative and hypnotic drug with an intermediate duration of action. Detoxified by the liver. Fatal blood level is 3 to 6 mg./100 ml., although one patient who ingested 7 grams survived in spite of a reported blood concentration of 8 mg./100 ml. The drug binds to human albumin.

In dogs peritoneal dialysis with a 4% solution of albumin is said to have reduced very high plasma concentrations promptly. Adult hypnotic dose: 100 to 300 mg. (oral). Fatal dose: 2 to 3 gm. (30 to 40 mg./kg.). Treatment after overdose is largely supportive.

See also: Barbiturates, *Reference Congener in Section III.*
Ref.: Campion and North, 1965; Setter et al., 1966.

1365 Aprobarbital

5-Allyl-5-isopropylbarbituric acid, Alurate

Toxicity Rating: 5. A sedative and hypnotic drug. Longer acting than amobarbital; shorter acting

than barbital. Slowly eliminated; detoxified by the liver. Adult hypnotic dose: 60 to 130 mg.(oral).

See also: Barbiturates, *Reference Congener in Section III.*

1366 Barbital

5,5-Diethylbarbituric acid, Barbitone, Diethylmalonylurea, Veronal

Toxicity Rating: 4. Prepared in 1882; used medicinally as a sedative and hypnotic since 1904. The first commercially important derivative of barbituric acid. Now used only in the preparation of laboratory buffers. Long duration of action. Following the ingestion of a toxic dose, the concentrations in blood may be an order of magnitude higher than are seen with similar doses of other barbiturates. Binding to plasma proteins is negligible. Major portion is excreted unchanged in urine; elimination

may require several days. A 68–year–old woman is known to have survived after ingesting 18 grams of barbital (sodium salt). A peak blood concentration of 60 mg./100 ml. was observed. Hemodialysis is said to speed elimination of the drug and shorten drug-induced coma (Balme et al., 1962). Barbital is teratogenic in mice. Adult hypnotic dose: 300 to 600 mg. (oral). Fatal dose: 5 to 20 gm. (70 to 290 mg./kg.).

See also: Barbiturates, *Reference Congener in Section III.*
Ref.: Bailey and Jatlow, 1975; Balme et al., 1962; Shepard, 1976.

1367 Butabarbital Sodium

Sodium 5-*sec*-butyl-5-ethylbarbiturate, Butisol sodium, Butabarbitone sodium

Toxicity Rating: 5(?). A sedative and hypnotic drug with an intermediate duration of action. Usually destroyed rapidly in the body by side chain oxidation, probably in the liver. Found in the urine only after excessive doses. In one reported human poisoning, a 30-year-old man ingested an unknown number of butabarbitone sleeping tablets. The maximal plasma concentration was 12 mg./100 ml.

Recovery was aided by hemodialysis, which removed 1.5 grams of the drug in seven hours. Only 0.63 grams were excreted in urine during the preceding 4.5 days. In other instances, forced diuresis resulted in greatly enhanced urinary excretion. Adult hypnotic dose: 50 to 200 mg. (average 100 mg. by mouth).

See also: Barbiturates, *Reference Congener in Section III.*
Ref.: Honey and Jackson, 1959; Linton et al., 1967; Maynert and Losin, 1955.

1368 Butalbital

5-Allyl-5-isobutylbarbituric acid, Sandoptal

Toxicity Rating: 4(?). A sedative and hypnotic drug possessing an intermediate duration of action. Metabolized in liver. Adult hypnotic dose 100 to 200 mg. (oral). A component of an anti-migraine prep-

aration known as Fiorinal, each capsule and tablet of which contains 50 mg. butalbital, along with aspirin (200 mg.), phenacetin (130 mg.) and caffeine (40 mg.).

See also: Barbiturates, *Reference Congener in Section III.*

1369 Butallyonal

5-(2-Bromoallyl)-5-*sec*-butylbarbituric acid, Pernoston

Toxicity Rating: 5(?). A sedative and hypnotic drug having an intermediate duration of action. Essen-

tially completely metabolized. In duration and indications for use, it is similar to amobarbital. Adult hypnotic dose: 200 mg. (oral). Fatal dose: more than 1 gm. (more than 14 mg./kg.).

See also: Barbiturates, Reference Congener in Section III.

1370   1370   Butethal

Butobarbitone,   5-Ethyl-5-n-butylbarbituric acid,   Neonal,   Butobarbital

Toxicity Rating: 5(?). A sedative and hypnotic drug with intermediate duration of action. Similar to amobarbital in duration of action and indications for use, but substantially more potent. Almost com- pletely destroyed in the body by side chain oxida- tion, probably in the liver. Adult hypnotic dose: 50 to 100 mg. (oral).

See also: Barbiturates, Reference Congener in Section III.

1371   1371   Cyclobarbital

5-(1-Cyclohexenyl)-5-ethylbarbituric acid,   Phanodorn

Toxicity Rating: 4. A sedative and hypnotic drug with an intermediate duration of action. Destroyed in the body; detoxified by liver and kidneys. Said to be more readily removed by diuresis and dialysis than other intermediate acting barbiturates. A 16-year-old girl survived the ingestion of 8 grams of cyclobarbital; the peak serum barbiturate concen- tration was 14.8 mg./100 ml. Vigorous supportive treatment was supplemented by forced diuresis, peritoneal dialysis and hemodialysis. Adult hyp- notic dose: 100 to 200 mg. (orally). Fatal dose is reputed to be more than 10 grams.

See also: Barbiturates, Reference Congener in Section III.
Ref.: Kennedy et al., 1969.

1372   1372   5-Cyclopentenyl-5-allylbarbituric Acid

Cyclopal,   Cyclopen

Toxicity Rating: 5(?). A sedative and hypnotic drug possessing a short to moderate duration of action. Adult hypnotic dose 50 to 150 mg. (oral).

See also: Barbiturates, Reference Congener in Section III.

1373   1373   Allobarbital

Allobarbitone,   5,5-Diallylbarbituric acid,   Diadol,   Dialog

Toxicity Rating: 5(?). A sedative and hypnotic drug. Onset of action is relatively slow (orally) and effects are well sustained. Symptoms of intoxica- tion are like those for other intermediate-acting barbiturates. Detoxified by liver and kidney; 30 to 40% is excreted in 2 to 11 days. Hemodialysis is recommended in severe intoxications. Adult hyp- notic dose: 100 to 300 mg. (oral). Fatal dose: more than 2.5 gm. (35 mg./kg.). Supplied in a mixture with acetaminophen under the name Dialog for use in relieving headache and muscular pain.

See also: Barbiturates, Reference Congener in Section III.

1374   1374   Heptabarbital

5-Cycloheptenyl-5-ethylbarbituric acid,   Medomin

Toxicity Rating: 4. A sedative and hypnotic drug having a short to intermediate duration of action. Readily absorbed orally. Rapidly destroyed by the liver. Adult hypnotic dose: 200 to 400 mg. (oral).

See also: Barbiturates, Reference Congener in Section III.

1375   1375   Hexethal Sodium

5-n-Hexyl-5-ethylbarbituric acid sodium,   Ortal sodium

Toxicity Rating: 5(?). A sedative and hypnotic drug having intermediate duration of action. Detoxified by the liver. Toxicity is similar to that of amobar- bital; duration of action is somewhat less (about one-third in one study). Adult hypnotic dose: 60 to 200 mg. (oral).

See also: Barbiturates, Reference Congener in Section III.

1376   1376   Hexobarbital Sodium

Cyclonal sodium,   Sodium 5-(1-cyclohexenyl)-1,5-dimethylbarbiturate,   Evipal sodium

Toxicity Rating: 4. Used intravenously as an an- esthetic agent in surgery. Rapid and ultrashort duration of action. Unlike the thiobarbiturates, it is also active by mouth, but large doses are required. The adult oral sedative dose is 250 to 400 mg.

See also: Barbiturates, *Reference Congener in Section III.*

1377 Mephobarbital 1377

5-Ethyl-1-methyl-5-phenylbarbituric acid, Mebaral, Prominal, Methylphenobarbital

Toxicity Rating: 4(?). Used as a sedative and an anticonvulsant drug, especially in the treatment of epilepsy. Partly demethylated, presumably in the liver, to yield phenobarbital; only traces of unme- tabolized drug are excreted in the urine. Relatively long duration of action. Average total daily adult dose is 400 to 600 mg.

See also: Barbiturates, *Reference Congener in Section III.*

1378 Methallatal 1378

Mosidal, 5-Ethyl-5-(2-methylallyl)-2-thiobarbituric acid

Related to thiopental but said to be effective by mouth in the control of vertigo and motion sick- ness. Sedative action appears to be weak. Adult therapeutic dose: 150 mg. (oral).

See also: Barbiturates, *Reference Congener in Section III.*

1379 Metharbital 1379

Gemonil, 5,5-Diethyl-1-methylbarbituric acid

Toxicity Rating: 4. A sedative and anticonvulsant drug, believed to have a relatively long duration of action. In mice, less toxic and lighter sedative effect than phenobarbital. Demethylated in liver to bar- bital (see above). Birth defects have been reported in children of women given metharbital during pregnancy for control of epilepsy.

See also: Barbiturates, *Reference Congener in Section III.*
Ref.: Physicians' Desk Reference, 1981.

1380 Pentobarbital Sodium 1380

Sodium 5-ethyl-5-(1-methylbutyl)barbiturate, Nembutal sodium

Toxicity Rating: 5. A sedative and hypnotic drug with intermediate to short duration of action. Well and rapidly absorbed. Metabolized by liver. Treat- ment of overdose is largely supportive. Diuresis and dialysis are of little value, although hemodi- alysis may be indicated if liver disease is present. Alkalinization of urine does not speed excretion. Pentobarbital may be teratogenic. Adult hypnotic dose: 100 mg. (oral). Doses greater than 2 grams (30 mg./kg.) are often fatal, but several reports of recovery after doses of more than five grams were found. In one fatality, after the ingestion of pen- tobarbital with propylene glycol, unusually high blood concentrations and rapid death were attrib- uted to enhanced absorption.

See also: Barbiturates, *Reference Congener in Section III.*
Ref.: Poklis and Hameli, 1975; Shepard, 1976.

1381 5-Phenyl-5-methylbarbituric Acid 1381

Rutonal

Toxicity Rating: 4(?). A sedative, hypnotic and anticonvulsant drug with a long duration of action. Probably less potent than phenobarbital.

See also: Barbiturates, *Reference Congener in Section III.*

1382 Phenobarbital 1382

5-Phenyl-5-ethylbarbituric acid, Luminal

Toxicity Rating: 4. One of the oldest and most useful of the barbiturate drugs. A sedative-hyp- notic with specific anticonvulsant activity. Well absorbed orally. Action is slow in onset, sustained, and more powerful than barbital. Partially detoxi- fied in the liver. Slowly excreted by kidneys over a period of 2 to 8 days. Adult hypnotic dose is 100 to 200 mg. (oral). Doses of 6 to 9 grams (80 to 130 mg./kg.) often prove fatal, although one person was reported to have survived the ingestion of 25 grams. Only general supportive measures are indi- cated in mild poisonings. In severe intoxications, forced diuresis, peritoneal dialysis and hemodi- alysis may shorten the period of coma and prove life-saving. Phenobarbital, unlike other barbitu- rates, is excreted significantly faster following al- kalinization of the urine. May be teratogenic. Spon- taneous abortion, presumably because of fetal death, occurred in one case of severe human intoxication.

See also: Barbiturates, *Reference Congener in Section III.*
Ref.: Parke, 1971; Plum and Swanson, 1957; Setter et al., 1966; Waddell and Butler, 1957.

1383   1383   Probarbital Sodium

Sodium 5-ethyl-5-isopropylbarbiturate,   Ipral sodium

Toxicity Rating: 5(?). A sedative and hypnotic drug related to amobarbital and like it possessing an intermediate duration of action. Largely detoxified, presumably in the liver, but also excreted by the kidneys. Adult hypnotic dose: 250 mg. (oral).

See also: Barbiturates, *Reference Congener in Section III.*

1384   1384   Pronarcon

Eunarcon,   5-Isopropyl-5-β-bromallyl-N-methylbarbituric acid

The sodium salt is a European drug used intravenously for surgical anesthesia (5 to 10 ml. 10% sol.). Like hexobarbital sodium (above), it produces rapid anesthesia of short duration. Presumably it is also active by mouth.

See also: Barbiturates, *Reference Congener in Section III.*

1385   1385   Propallylonal

5-Isopropyl-5-beta-bromallylbarbituric acid,   Noctal,   Nostal

A sedative and hypnotic drug possessing an intermediate duration of action, apparently no longer available in U.S.A. Adult hypnotic dose is 100 to 300 mg. (oral). Said to have caused delayed death in some rats with degenerative changes in liver and kidneys and pulmonary edema. Eunarcon (see above) is a closely related compound with a short duration of action which is used to induce anesthesia. This compound, and presumably propallylonal as well, are metabolized in man by side chain oxidation with hydrolytic release of bromine. The products are excreted in urine over a period of several days.

See also: Barbiturates, *Reference Congener in Section III.*
Ref.: Holck and Cannon, 1936; Ravn-Jonsen, 1970.

1386   1386   Secobarbital Sodium

Sodium 5-allyl-5-(1-methylbutyl)barbiturate,   Evronal sodium,   Seconal sodium

Toxicity Rating: 4-5. A hypnotic and sedative drug. Rapid onset and short duration of action (perhaps somewhat longer than that of pentobarbital). Also supplied in a delayed-release preparation that may cause toxic effects only after several hours. Detoxified by liver. Adult hypnotic dose is 100 to 200 mg. (oral). A dose of 3 grams may prove fatal, but survival after ingestion of 8 grams has been reported. Treatment is largely supportive. Dialysis and forced diuresis are of little value. Secobarbital binds to human albumin.

See also: Barbiturates, *Reference Congener in Section III.*
Ref.: Campion and North, 1965; Michelson et al., 1954.

1387   1387   Sigmodal

Toxicity Rating: 4. A sedative and hypnotic drug marketed in Europe only as a 10% solution for rectal instillation.

See also: Barbiturates, *Reference Congener in Section III.*

1388   1388   Thialbarbital

Thialbarbitone,   5-Allyl-5-(2-cyclohexenyl)-2-thiobarbituric acid,   Kemithal

A British drug used intravenously for the induction of anesthesia. Perhaps half as potent as thiopental and less depressing to respiration. Said to inhibit and possibly uncouple oxidative phosphorylation in rat liver mitochondria. Almost completely destroyed in the body. Possesses an ultrashort duration of action, probably due to rapid deposition in body fat which reduces the amount of circulating drug. Presumably inactive by mouth.

See also: Barbiturates, *Reference Congener in Section III.*
Ref.: Aldridge and Parker, 1960.

1389 Thiamylal Sodium

Sodium 5-allyl-5-(1-methylbutyl)-2-thiobarbiturate, Surital sodium

Marketed only as a sterile powder. Used as a solution for the intravenous induction of anesthesia. Ultrashort duration of action. Rapidly distributed in fat depots and ultimately detoxified by the liver. Optically active; in mice the S(-) isomer has twice the therapeutic potency and is twice as toxic as the racemic mixture. Slightly more potent and less stable than thiopental.

See also: Barbiturates, Reference Congener in Section III.
Ref.: Christensen and Lee, 1973.

1390 Thiopental Sodium

Pentothal sodium, Sodium 5-ethyl-5-(1-methylbutyl)-2-thiobarbiturate

Widely employed as an intravenous anesthetic agent. Possesses an ultrashort duration of action due to rapid redistribution into fat storage depots. Detoxified by all body tissues; converted to pentobarbital by rat liver enzymes. Strongly bound to plasma protein. Said to be inactive by mouth. Has been used rectally for basal anesthesia.

See also: Barbiturates, Reference Congener in Section III.
Ref.: Anderson and Magee, 1956; Dundee, 1974; Winters et al., 1955.

1391 Vinbarbital Sodium

5-Ethyl-5-(1-methyl-1-butenyl)barbituric acid sodium, Delvinal sodium

Toxicity Rating: 5(?). A sedative and hypnotic drug. Described as possessing a short to moderate duration of action in man. Rapidly absorbed. Detoxified by liver and kidneys. Adult hypnotic dose 100 to 200 mg. (oral).

See also: Barbiturates, Reference Congener in Section III.

Benzodiazepines

1392 Chlordiazepoxide Hydrochloride

Librium hydrochloride, Methaminodiazepoxide hydrochloride

Toxicity Rating: 3-4. A tranquilizer related in chemical structure to diazepam and oxazepam (see below), which are antidepressant drugs. It can be described as a useful ataractic, a potent muscle relaxant, an effective anticonvulsant, and a weak analgesic. In high doses it produces ataxia, emesis, and diarrhea. With usual doses (up to 40 mg. daily) side effects are not common. Drowsiness and ataxia may be seen with doses up to 100 mg. daily. No extrapyramidal tract disorders and no damage to vital organs. The margin of safety is much greater than for meprobamate. In most adult subjects doses greater than 600 mg. (2,250 mg. in one case) produce no serious effects. No deaths appear to have been reported after chlordiazepoxide alone. Occasionally smaller doses result in sleep or coma; in one case an 11-year-old boy was involved. Hypotension and respiratory depression are generally not found. Hemodialysis has been employed, but its efficacy is not well established. Physical dependence is recognized, but the withdrawal syndrome is slower to develop and less severe than for meprobamate or barbiturates. In rats the oral LD_{50} is 540 mg./kg.

See also: Diazepam, Reference Congener in Section III.
Ref.: Brophy, 1967; Cruz et al., 1967; Essig, 1964; Davis et al., 1968; Zbinden et al., 1961.

1393 Clonazepam

e.g., Clonopin

Toxicity Rating: 2. Clonazepam is the only benzodiazepine presently approved for the chronic treatment of petit mal and myoclonic seizures in children. Unlike most other benzodiazepines, it produces muscle relaxation in man in non-sedative doses. The usual daily anticonvulsant oral dose is 1.2 mg. for adults, 0.01-0.03 mg./kg. for children. The acute oral LD_{50} in the mouse is greater than 4000 mg./kg. The peak plasma concentration is reached within 2 to 4 hours of oral administration; the plasma half-life is 1 to 2 days. Intravenous administration may produce cardiovascular and respiratory depression, especially if the patient is also being treated with other anticonvulsants or central depressants. The usual features of overdosage by ingestion are somnolence, confusion, coma and diminished reflexes. In one unusual case intermittent coma persisted in a 4-year-old boy for 24 hours after he ingested 14-32 mg. of clonazepam. After gastric lavage he was treated with magnesium sulfate and activated charcoal, but shifting levels of consciousness continued for 16 hours after charcoal appeared in the stools. Ingestions of 60 mg. by a small child and 100 mg. by an adult were treated by gastric lavage and supportive measures and resulted in no permanent sequelae. Commonly reported adverse effects from therapeutic doses are muscular incoordination, ataxia, hypotonia, dysarthria, and dizziness; they often disappear as treatment continues. Less frequently occurring effects are behavior disorders in children, anorexia or hyperphagia, and increased salivary and bronchial secretions in children. Abrupt withdrawal of the drug after chronic use may exacerbate seizures and precipitate status.

See also: Diazepam, *Reference Congener in Section III.*
Ref.: Gilman et al., 1980; Welch et al., 1977.

1394   1394   Clorazepate Dipotassium

e.g., Tranxene

Toxicity Rating: 3. Tranxene is a benzodiazepine recommended for the management of anxiety disorders and the symptomatic relief of acute alcohol withdrawal. The usual oral therapeutic dose for an adult is 30 mg. per day in divided doses (in extreme cases, 90 mg. per day). A slow-release tablet is also available. The acute oral rat LD_{50} is 1320 mg./kg. Individuals reportedly survived single doses of 450 and 675 mg., and daily doses of 120 mg. produced no toxic effects in healthy volunteers participating in clinical trials. The primary feature of overdosage is central nervous depression, varying in degree from mild sedation to coma, although in reported cases of deep coma other drugs had also been taken. Abrupt withdrawal of Tranxene, after several months of therapeutic doses, has induced nervousness, insomnia, irritability, diarrhea, muscle aches and memory impairment. After the ingestion of clorazepate, the active metabolites desmethyldiazepam and nordiazepam are produced quickly and nonenzymatically in the stomach. Clorazepate itself is not found in the bloodstream.

See also: Diazepam, *Reference Congener in Section III.*
Ref.: Gilman et al., 1980; Physicians' Desk Reference, 1981.

1395   1395   Diazepam

e.g., Valium

Toxicity Rating: 3. A tranquilizing agent with anticonvulsant and muscle relaxant properties. Used therapeutically in doses of 2 to 10 mg. three or four times a day. Chemically related to chlordiazepoxide (see latter above). In its pharmacological actions diazepam is more like meprobamate than chlorpromazine. Acute LD_{50}'s in mice: 720 mg./kg. by mouth, 300 mg./kg. subcutaneously and 220 mg./kg. intraperitoneally. Acute oral LD_{50} in rats is 1.5 gm./kg. Rats fed dietary mixtures of 1 gm./kg. (per day ?) for 6 weeks showed reductions in growth and food consumption. No hematologic abnormalities or histologic tissue changes were observed. Maximal single dose in man (suicide attempt) reported to be 300-400 mg.; this patient was drowsy and ataxic for 8 hours but recovered without treatment. Common side effects include drowsiness, fatigue, dizziness and ataxia. Children have recovered rapidly from doses of 20 to 60 mg. with general supportive care. Diazepam may potentiate the respiratory depressant effects of opiates and barbiturate-like sedatives.

See also: Diazepam, *Reference Congener in Section III.*
Ref.: Doughty, 1970; Herzka and Haber, 1965; Spark and Goldman, 1965; Thearle and Hailey, 1973.

1396   1396   Flunitrazepam

e.g., Rohypnol

Toxicity Rating: 4. More potent and more toxic than most benzodiazepine drugs (acute oral LD_{50} in rats is 485 mg./kg.). The therapeutic hypnotic oral dose for an adult human is only 1-2 mg./day. The effects last for 10-24 hours, which makes it potentially a good choice for patients who need the drug effect for the duration of sleep. Flunitrazepam probably accumulates during daily administration. It is not yet available in the U.S.A.

See also: Diazepam, *Reference Congener in Section III.*

1397   1397   Flurazepam

e.g., Dalmane

Toxicity Rating: 3 to 4. A benzodiazepine similar to diazepam and chlordiazepoxide but promoted as a hypnotic rather than a tranquilizer. Acute oral LD_{50} in rats 1200 mg./kg., in mice 870 mg./kg. Usual adult therapeutic dose is 30 mg. at bed time. Serious poisonings following even large overdosage with benzodiazepines alone are extremely rare, but these drugs probably have additive effects with alcohol, barbiturates and other central nervous system depressants.

See also: Diazepam, *Reference Congener in Section III.*

1398 Lorazepam 1398

e.g., Ativan

Toxicity Rating: 2. Of the benzodiazepines used to treat the symptoms of anxiety, lorazepam is considered one of the safest for use in the elderly and in patients with impaired hepatic function. It has a shorter duration of action than most (plasma half-life 12 hours), and its metabolism to the inactive lorazepam glucuronide does not rely solely on the action of hepatic microsomes. There is a wide margin between the acute lethal dose in rats (oral LD_{50} greater than 5000 mg./kg.) and the usual therapeutic oral dose in adult humans (2-6 mg./day in divided doses). Leukopenia has developed in some patients taking lorazepam, and an elevation of LDH has occurred in some others. The

cardiovascular effects of anesthetic doses are like those of diazepam (see above). Given as a preanesthetic (in doses of 0.05 mg./kg. i.m. or 0.044 mg./kg. i.v.), lorazepam produces sedation, relief from anxiety and mild amnesia. Partial airway obstruction may result from overdoses, as well as a depressed response to CO_2. Patients over the age of 50 years may experience more intense and prolonged sedation than younger individuals. In France a few cases of restlessness and visual hallucinations have been reported in overdosed children. Inadvertent intra-arterial injection may cause arteriospasm and consequent gangrene.

See also: Diazepam, Reference Congener in Section III.
Ref.: Physicians' Desk Reference, 1981.

1399 Medazepam Hydrochloride 1399

e.g., Nobrium hydrochloride

Toxicity Rating: 3. Medazepam is a benzodiazepine used in the treatment of anxiety. It has an acute oral LD_{50} in the rat of 900 mg./kg. It is metabolized

to at least 11 nonconjugated metabolites, 5 of which are known to be biologically active, including diazepam, oxazepam, and temazepam.

See also: Diazepam, Reference Congener in Section III.

1400 Nitrazepam 1400

e.g., Mogadon

Toxicity Rating: 3. Nitrazepam is not yet available in the U.S.A., but it is used in Europe as a hypnotic. The usual oral dose for an adult is 5-10 mg. The acute oral LD_{50} in the rat is 825 mg./kg. The drug accumulates during nightly administration, and effects may last for nearly 20 hours (longer if alcohol is also ingested). Nitrazepam increases the inci-

dence of nightmares. Because of its respiratory depressant properties, it is not a good choice for patients with sleep apnea. After an overdose of nitrazepam a 41-year–old man lapsed into "alpha coma." His respiration was depressed, but he was not hypoxic, and he recovered fully.

See also: Diazepam, Reference Congener in Section III.
Ref.: Carroll and Mastaglia, 1979.

1401 Oxazepam 1401

e.g., Serax

Toxicity Rating: 3. One of the benzodiazepine group of drugs used in the management of anxiety-tension states. The acute oral LD_{50} in rats (5 gm./kg.) places oxazepam on the borderline between toxicity classes 2 and 3 and makes it significantly less toxic than its relatives Chlordiazepoxide and Diazepam above. A poisoned infant (dose unknown) exhibited lethargy, ataxia, paradoxical excitation, depressed reflexes and facial edema. These signs persisted several days after blood

levels of the drug became undetectable and much longer than the usual sedation seen in adult patients. One adult (again after an unknown dose) was in a deep coma for 3 days. He was subjected to an exchange transfusion with 2250 ml. whole blood and felt well on the fourth day. Oxazepam gives a false positive reaction in the Somogyi blood glucose procedure (1680 mg. "glucose"/100 ml. in the case above) but not with the glucose oxidase procedure.

See also: Diazepam, Reference Congener in Section III.
Ref.: Owen et al., 1970; Shimkin and Shaivitz, 1966; Zileli et al., 1972.

1402 Prazepam 1402

e.g., Centrax

Toxicity Rating: 2-3. Prazepam is an antianxiety drug with an acute oral LD_{50} in dogs of more than 4000 mg./kg. and a therapeutic oral dosage range in humans of 10-60 mg./day. The adverse reactions

experienced by users of other benzodiazepines are also seen in prazepam users. Central nervous depression and rarely hypotension are the expected reactions to overdose. The chief active metabolite, norprazepam, reaches its peak plasma level after 6 hours; its half-life is 24-200 hours.

See also: Diazepam, *Reference Congener in Section III.*

Sedative muscle relaxants

1403

1403 Carisoprodol

Soma, *N*-Isopropylmeprobamate, *N*-Isopropyl-2-methyl-2-propyl-1,3-propanediol dicarbamate

Toxicity Rating: 3. Agent intended to relieve pain, stiffness, and spasm associated with muscle and joint disorders with minimal tranquilization. The intraperitoneal LD_{50} in mice is 790 ± 75 mg./kg.

Unlike meprobamate, carisoprodol has only slight anticonvulsant activity. Side effects in clinical trials were sleepiness, dizziness, and occasional nausea.

See also: Meprobamate, *Reference Congener in Section III.*
Ref.: Wallace Laboratories, 1958.

1404

1404 Chlormezanone

Trancopal

Toxicity Rating: 3. A potent muscle relaxant with an oral toxicity less than meprobamate, zoxazolamine, or methocarbamol. Blocks polysynaptic reflex arcs but not related in chemical structure to meprobamate. In chronic laboratory studies the only adverse effect noted was ataxia, at a high dosage level. In clinical trials only 2.3% of 4653 patients

has side effects, mainly nausea, drowsiness, dizziness, weakness and flushing. Overdosage up to 10 gm. has not caused death. Even large amounts produce only mild side effects (slight confusion, vertigo, nausea, drowsiness). Recommended clinical dose in adults 100 mg. t.i.d.

Ref.: Roth, 1961; Winthrop Laboratories, 1959.

1405

1405 Emylcamate

1-Ethyl-1-methylpropyl carbamate

Toxicity Rating: 3. Can be regarded as the carbamate ester of 3-methyl-3-pentanol. A tranquilizer, muscle relaxant, and anticonvulsant. About twice as active as meprobamate, to which it is related. In acute toxicity studies the oral LD_{50} in mice and rats lay between 800 and 1000 mg./kg., and death appeared to be due to respiratory paralysis. The

usual adult dose is 200 mg. t.i.d. or q.i.d. Side effects are generally mild; gastrointestinal distress (nausea), headache, dry mouth, dizziness, palpitations, anxiety, insomnia are occasionally noted. Drowsiness occurs at high doses. Euphoria and habituation may be a problem.

See also: Meprobamate, *Reference Congener in Section III.*
Ref.: Martens, 1960; Merck Sharp and Dohme, 1961.

1406

1406 Mephenesin

3-(2-Methylphenoxy)-1,2-propanediol, 3-*o*-Toloxy-1,2-propanediol, Myanesin, Tolserol

Toxicity Rating: 3 or 4. Antispasmodic, sedative and muscle relaxant. Overdosages may produce nystagmus, diplopia, lassitude, weakness, muscular incoordination, syncope, sedation and respiratory depression, usually of short duration. An adult

woman who ingested between 5.5 and 11 gm. was comatose with intercostal paralysis and evident cyanosis. The usual adult dose is 1 to 2 gm. 3 to 5 times daily.

See also: Meprobamate, *Reference Congener in Section III.*
Ref.: Barron and Milliken, 1960.

1407

1407 Meprobamate

Equanil, Miltown, 2-Methyl-2-*n*-propyl-1,3-propanediol dicarbamate

Toxicity Rating: 3.

See also: Meprobamate, *Reference Congener in Section III.*

1408

1408 Metaxalone

5-((3,5-Dimethylphenoxy)methyl)-2-oxazolidinone, e.g., Skelaxin

Toxicity Rating: 3. Skeletal muscle relaxant, which probably acts as a central nervous depressant to

relieve discomfort from acute musculoskeletal conditions. Usual therapeutic dose in adults is 800 mg.

Common adverse effects are nausea, vomiting, gastrointestinal upset, drowsiness, dizziness, headache and nervousness. Hypersensitivity reactions, in the form of a light rash, have occurred, as have leukopenia, hemolytic anemia and jaundice. Rats who succumbed to the LD_{50} displayed progressive sedation, hypnosis and finally respiratory failure.

1409   Oxanamide   1409

Quiactin,   2-Ethyl-3-propylglycidamide,   2,3-Epoxy-2-ethylhexanamide

Toxicity Rating: 3. A tranquilizing drug not related chemically to those in general use at the present time. In its central depressing actions it resembles a short acting barbiturate, but is much less potent (average tranquilizing dose 0.4 gm. several times daily). Side effects and cumulative toxicity are not established. A 19-month-old child who ingested about 6 gm. was subjected to gastric lavage within 0.5 hr.; only drowsiness (without sequelae) was noted. An animal study indicated that pentylenetetrazol (Metrazol) may be a potent antidote in acute poisonings, but clinical experience has contradicted similar findings in experimental poisonings produced by several other depressant drugs.

See also: Barbiturates, *Reference Congener in Section III.*
Ref.: Feuss and Gragg, 1957; Warren et al., 1949.

1410   Phenaglycodol   1410

Ultran,   2-*p*-Chlorophenyl-3-methyl-2,3-butanediol

Toxicity Rating: 3. A butanediol with tranquilizing and anticonvulsive actions. Drowsiness occurs as a side effect with high doses (300 mg.). In animal experiments death is caused by respiratory arrest. No reports of human fatalities from Ultran were located. The ingestion of as much as 15 gm. has led to coma with recovery after several days. Animal tests place this compound near the borderline between toxicity classes 3 and 4. As far as is known, phenaglycodol does not potentiate the effects of other drugs. It is related chemically to meprobamate and presumably shares its toxicity. The drug has not been marketed in the U.S.A. since the late 1970's.

See also: Meprobamate, *Reference Congener in Section III.*
Ref.: Lilly, Date Unknown; Slater et al., 1956.

1411   Promoxolane   1411

Dimethylane,   2,2-Diisopropyl-4-methanol-1,3-dioxolane,   Dimethylyn

Toxicity Rating: 3. A tranquilizing drug of the diphenyl methane group. No clinical data describing the toxic reactions to this drug have been located. The suggested adult dose is 500 mg. q.i.d., but the drug is no longer marketed, at least not in the U.S.A.

Ref.: Merck and Co., 1976.

Phenothiazine tranquilizers

1412   Chlorpromazine   1412

Thorazine

Toxicity Rating: 4.

See also: Chlorpromazine, *Reference Congener in Section III.*

1413   Acetophenazine   1413

Acetophenazine maleate,   Tindal

Toxicity Rating: 4. An antipsychotic piperazine phenothiazine derivative. More potent than chlorpromazine (20 mg. of acetophenazine is therapeutically equivalent to 100 mg. of chlorpromazine). Produces moderate sedation and low level alpha-adrenergic blocking and anticholinergic effects. There is a high incidence of extrapyramidal reactions, such as dystonia, akathisia, tardive dyskinesia and a parkinsonian syndrome. It potentiates the action of other CNS depressants. The usual adult outpatient oral dose is 40 to 80 mg./day, with hospitalized patients receiving 60-120 mg./day. Some patients with severe schizophrenia have received as much as 600 mg./day. The drug has a prolonged half-life in elderly patients. The rat LD_{50} is 415 mg./kg. by mouth.

See also: Chlorpromazine, *Reference Congener in Section III.*

1414 Chlorprothixene

2-Chloro-*N,N*-dimethylthioxanthene-propylamine,   Taractan

Toxicity Rating: 4. A tranquilizer related chemically and pharmacologically to the phenothiazines. The acute oral LD_{50} is 380 mg./kg. in rats, 140 mg./kg. in mice. Oral therapeutic doses are usually 50-400 mg./day. Although 2.5 grams has proved lethal, complete recovery without sequelae has occurred following a single dose of 1075 mg. in a child and up to 12 gm. in adults. Initial signs of intoxication include tremor, drowsiness, coma, respiratory depression, hypotension, tachycardia, and constricted pupils, followed by tonic-clonic convulsions and kidney disorders (hematuria, aminoaciduria and oliguria). Although extrapyramidal reactions are said to be rare, at least one such case has been reported. Treatment should include early gastric lavage, maintenance of airway, i.v. fluids, levarterenol for hypotension (avoid epinephrine), diazepam for convulsions and diphenhydramine for extrapyramidal signs.

See also: Chlorpromazine, Reference Congener in Section III.
Ref.: Dietze, 1963; Baker, 1982; Plumb and Joseph, 1964.

1415 Fluphenazine Hydrochloride

Permitil,   Prolixin

Toxicity Rating: 4. A phenothiazine derivative used as a tranquilizer. More potent and more toxic than chlorpromazine. Chief side-effect of therapeutic doses (less than 2 mg. daily) is akathisia, usually reparable by reducing the amount of drug. Hyperpyrexia contributed to death in one patient taking conventional doses.

See also: Chlorpromazine, Reference Congener in Section III.
Ref.: Duggan, 1960; Zelman and Guillan, 1970.

1416 Mepazine

Pacatal

Toxicity Rating: 4(?). A tranquilizing drug of the phenothiazine type. It possesses atropine-like actions (e.g., dryness of the mouth, paralysis of visual accommodation, bladder atony, paralytic ileus). Side effects of the hypersensitivity type include granulocytopenia, jaundice, dermatitis, and toxic psychosis. Overdosage leads to coma probably resembling that in chlorpromazine poisoning. A single dose of 10 gm. has proved fatal in a psychotic patient. Hyperpyrexia (heat stroke) has occurred in 25 patients on conventional doses during extremely hot weather.

See also: Chlorpromazine, Reference Congener in Section III.
Ref.: Feldman, 1957; Sherman et al., 1958.

1417 Methoxypromazine

Tentone

Toxicity Rating: 4. A phenothiazine tranquilizer differing from chlorpromazine by the substitution of a methoxy group for the chlorine. The pharmacologic activities and all toxicities of these two compounds are quite similar. Drowsiness is the most common side effect; with high doses (over 200 mg. daily) dry mouth, slurred speech and blurred vision have been noted. No reports of agranulocytosis or liver damage and Parkinson-like symptoms are rare. One case of drug overdosage (1500 mg.) resulted in no ill effects following a sleep of 8 hours.

See also: Chlorpromazine, Reference Congener in Section III.
Ref.: Lederle Laboratories, 1959; Psychopharmacology Service Center, 1962; Sylbert, 1961.

1418 Perphenazine

Trilafon

Toxicity Rating: 4. This tranquilizing and antiemetic drug is several times more potent than chlorpromazine but only about two-thirds as acutely toxic (in laboratory animals). In its structure and actions it resembles chlorpromazine. No human fatalities have been described and no cases of agranulocytosis, but side effects such as blurred vision and a Parkinson-like syndrome (evidenced by muscle spasm especially of the face and neck) have occurred even after therapeutic doses. As with many other phenothiazine tranquilizers, ECG abnormalities, particularly disorders of repolarization, are common.

See also: Chlorpromazine, Reference Congener in Section III.
Ref.: Chouinard and Annable, 1977; Irwin et al., 1959; Robinson, 1960; Roth et al., 1959.

1419   Prochlorperazine   1419

Compazine

Toxicity Rating: 3. A tranquilizer similar to but more potent and considerably less toxic than chlorpromazine. Side effects are infrequent, but on very high doses (100 to 900 mg./day) there have been reports of somnolence, postural hypotension, convulsions, and extrapyramidal signs especially involving the face and shoulder muscles. Most of these effects are reversed by reducing the dose. Leukopenia and/or agranulocytosis have been ascribed to this drug; the true incidence is not known.

See also: Chlorpromazine, Reference Congener in Section III.
Ref.: Scime and Tallant, 1959; Solomon and Champagna, 1959.

1420   Promazine   1420

Sparine

Toxicity Rating: 4. This tranquilizing drug has the same chemical structure as chlorpromazine except that it lacks the chlorine atom. It is also similar to chlorpromazine in its actions, but its potency and toxicity are lower. Severe side effects have occurred in a few patients on therapeutic doses, of which the most serious are agranulocytosis and convulsions. An adult patient is said to have survived after ingesting 2500 mg., but doses of 400 to 800 mg. have proved fatal to a few children (3 to 7 years old).

See also: Chlorpromazine, Reference Congener in Section III.
Ref.: Glaser and Adams, 1958; Kaplan, 1959; Wyeth Laboratories, 1956; Zelman and Guillan, 1970.

1421   Promethazine   1421

10-(2-Dimethylaminopropyl)phenothiazine,   Phenergan

Toxicity Rating: 3(?). Like chlorpromazine, promethazine is a phenothiazine derivative. It was promoted originally for the treatment of allergic conditions, motion sickness, and nausea, but more recently its sedative action has been utilized in psychiatric disorders. There are few severe side effects even with large therapeutic doses (e.g., 25 mg.), but leukopenia and/or agranulocytosis have been reported. Drowsiness is the most common complaint. A case is reported of a 2-year-old child who ingested 250 mg. with resulting confusion, convulsions, and stupor, but eventual recovery. Phenergan potentiates the action of central nervous system depressants.

See also: Antihistaminics and Chlorpromazine, Reference Congeners in Section III.
Ref.: Erwin, 1957; Silbert, 1952; Wyeth Laboratories, 1958b.

1422   Propiomazine Hydrochloride   1422

Largon

Toxicity Rating: 4(?). A phenothiazine derivative which is used parenterally in preanesthetic management of surgical and obstetrical patients. It enhances the actions of central nervous system depressants such as barbiturates, analgesics, and anesthetics. Largon also has an antiemetic action. Side effects include hypotension and respiratory depression. Its toxicity compares with promethazine, but the effective dose is only one-sixth of the latter. No information on oral toxicity was located.

See also: Chlorpromazine, Reference Congener in Section III.
Ref.: Wyeth Laboratories, 1960.

1423   Thiethylperazine   1423

Torecan

Toxicity Rating: 3. A phenothiazine antiemetic with a substituted thioethyl group in the phenothiazine nucleus and a piperazine side-chain. In animal experiments it was found to act directly on both the chemoreceptor trigger zone (CTZ) and on the emetic center. Thiethylperazine is used to treat nausea and vomiting associated with the administration of cytotoxic drugs, general anesthetics, radiation sickness and toxins. It is "possibly effective" for the treatment of vertigo. The usual human dose is 10 to 30 mg./day, and the rat oral LD_{50} is 1260 mg./kg. It can potentiate the effects of other CNS depressants, atropine and organophosphorus insecticides; it may produce epinephrine "reversal" because of alpha-adrenergic blocking activity. Adverse reactions noted occasionally include drowsiness, dizziness, dryness of the mouth, tachycardia, moderate hypotension and anorexia. Thiethylperazine may produce extrapyramidal reactions characteristic of the piperazine phenothiazines. Acute dystonic reactions in children have occurred at therapeutic doses. A 7-year-old girl with acute lymphocytic leukemia was given two 10 mg. doses of thiethylperazine i.v. (separated by 8 hours) for nausea and vomiting due to chemotherapy. Twenty minutes after the second dose she experienced a dystonic reaction (involuntary tongue spasm, facial rigidity and oculogyric crisis). Complete reversal of symptoms occurred following i.v. administration of 25 mg. diphenhydramine.

See also: Chlorpromazine, *Reference Congener in Section III.*
Ref.: Lacouture et al., 1979.

1424   Thiopropazate Dihydrochloride

Dartal dihydrochloride

Toxicity Rating: 4. A tranquilizer related to chlorpromazine, now infrequently used. Like the latter it potentiates the actions of barbiturates. Side effects sometimes encountered in therapy include Parkinson-like symptoms and parasympathomimetic reactions such as nasal stuffiness, blurring of vision, and hypotension.

See also: Chlorpromazine, *Reference Congener in Section III.*
Ref.: Robinson, 1960; Searle, 1957.

1425   Thioridazine

Mellaril

Toxicity Rating: 4. A phenothiazine derivative of the piperidine type used as a tranquilizing drug. Similar in action to chlorpromazine except that it does not produce catalepsy and has no antiemetic activity. Side-effects include weakness, dizziness, drowsiness, some dryness of the mouth and orthostatic hypotension. In 4 of 5 patients receiving cumulative total doses in excess of 85 gm., pigmentary retinopathy occurred. In an attempted suicide a young man ingested 5 to 8 gm. of Mellaril at one time. Aside from lethargy there were no abnormal findings and recovery was prompt following lavage. Several deaths due to overdoses, however, have been recorded. In poisonings, heart block and arrhythmias are often encountered.

See also: Chlorpromazine, *Reference Congener in Section III.*
Ref.: Donlon and Tupin, 1977; Gimpel, 1960; Haley et al., 1959b; Kinnoss-Wright, 1959; May et al., 1960; Weiss, 1981.

1426   Trifluoperazine

Stelazine

Toxicity Rating: 3-4. A phenothiazine tranquilizer effective at a dose level (5 to 10 mg. b.i.d.) about one tenth that required of chlorpromazine. The oral mean lethal dose is about one-fourth that of chlorpromazine. In rats the acute oral LD_{50} is 543 mg./kg. Neurologic side effects are the most troublesome and occur in about 35% of patients, especially a Parkinson-like syndrome involving facial muscles and shoulder girdle. These symptoms respond readily to antispasmodic drugs and a reduction in the dose. Two deaths have been attributed to trifluoperazine (although both patients also received paraldehyde); in each case respiratory failure preceded death. In animal experiments no toxic effects on the liver, kidney and blood-forming organs have been demonstrated. No clinical reports of jaundice or agranulocytosis. Carphenazine maleate, a related but less effective tranquilizer, is no longer commonly used; its acute oral LD_{50} in rats of 162 mg./kg. puts it in toxicity class 4.

See also: Chlorpromazine, *Reference Congener in Section III.*
Ref.: Brill, 1958; Weisdorf et al., 1978.

1427   Triflupromazine Hydrochloride

Vesprin hydrochloride

Toxicity Rating: 4. A phenothiazine tranquilizing drug similar to but more potent and slightly less toxic than chlorpromazine. Side effects sometimes encountered in therapy include a Parkinsonian syndrome, hypotension, skin rash (including photosensitivity) and leukopenia or agranulocytosis. Overdoses are believed to induce the same toxic reactions as chlorpromazine.

See also: Chlorpromazine, *Reference Congener in Section III.*
Ref.: Freed, 1957; Piala et al., 1959.

1428   Trimeprazine

Temaril

Toxicity Rating: 4(?). A phenothiazine derivative alleged to have specific antipruritic activity (adult dose 2.5 to 5 mg.). Sedation and mild tranquilization also occur. Symptoms of overdosage are dizziness, drowsiness, gastrointestinal disturbances, and central depression leading to coma. Depression can be treated with dextroamphetamine and, if indicated, levarterenol (but not epinephrine). Has been implicated in a case of agranulocytosis.

See also: Chlorpromazine, *Reference Congener in Section III.*
Ref.: Brachman et al., 1959; Callaway and Olansky, 1957.

Other sedatives and tranquilizers (exclusive of antihistamines)

1429 Azacyclonol 1429

Frenquel, α-(4-Piperidyl)benzhydrol

Toxicity Rating: 3. Chemically related to pipradrol but with markedly different effects. A very mild sedative, it is usually described as an "anti-hallucinatory" drug. The maximal recommended single dose is 100 mg. Even in overdosage, overt effects are usually insignificant. A patient who took 8.8 gm. exhibited signs of kidney irritation, but recovery was prompt and complete.

Ref.: Allin and Pogge, 1956; Brown et al., 1956b; Pogge, 1957.

1430 Benactyzine 1430

Suavitil

Toxicity Rating: 4. Benactyzine, an anticholinergic agent, is alleged to be capable of "normalizing" stress-induced behavior in man and animals. The liver and kidneys rapidly metabolize this compound by hydrolysis. Psychoses and hallucinations have been precipitated in humans by doses of 50- 200 mg. Large doses in laboratory animals induce excitement, ataxia, tremors, mydriasis, dryness of the mouth, and clonic convulsions. Conservative treatment is advised because benactyzine potentiates the sedative actions of barbiturates.

See also: Atropine, *Reference Congener in Section III.*
Ref.: MacLean, 1957; Vojtechovsky et al., 1958.

1431 Carbromal 1431

Bromodiethylacetylurea, *N*-(Aminocarbonyl)-2-bromo-2-ethyl-butanamide, Bromodiethylacetyl-carbamide, Adalin

Toxicity Rating: 4. Mild sedative and hypnotic drug. Contains 34% combined bromide. Doses of 2 gm. caused toxic symptoms in adults. Toxic doses produce mental confusion, ataxia, arreflexia, loss of pupillary response, cyanosis and coma. Immediate deaths occur rarely, but because recovery from carbromal-induced coma is slow, fatal complications frequently supervene. Carbromal appears in the plasma soon after ingestion, but significant amounts of the drug have reportedly been recovered through gastric lavage even several days afterwards. Metabolism proceeds rapidly with the formation of bromoethylbutyramide, ethyl butyrylurea, and inorganic bromide. Serum concentrations of carbromal and its organic metabolites decline rapidly after single oral doses, but serum bromide may remain high for days or weeks. It is probable that the more serious toxic effects in both acute and chronic poisoning are due to the accumulation of bromide ion. Treatment of intoxication is largely supportive, as for barbituate intoxication. Sodium chloride administration and forced diuresis have proved useful in speeding excretion of bromide ion and reducing the duration of coma. Characteristic purpuric skin reactions have been described in patients taking large therapeutic courses of carbromal over long periods. Chronic abuse of carbromal may also lead to bromism (see Bromide Salts in this index). The usual adult dose of Adalin is 0.3 to 1 gm. daily in divided doses.

See also: Barbiturates, *Reference Congener in Section III.*
Ref.: Siang, 1960; Thomas, 1958; Vohland et al., 1976.

1432 Chloral Hydrate 1432

2,2,2-Trichloro-1,1-ethanediol

Toxicity Rating: 4. A central nervous depressant used as a hypnotic drug. Rapidly reduced in vivo to trichloroethanol, which is itself a depressant and which is probably responsible for the hypnotic effect of the parent drug. Overdoses produce coma with severe respiratory depression and hypotension. Ventricular tachycardia and cardiac arrest have been described. Extracorporeal hemodialysis yielded whole-blood extraction ratios of more than 0.5 for trichloroethanol in 2 severely ill patients and may have contributed to their survival. Mean lethal dose in man is about 10 gm., but 17.5 and 35 grams have been survived with vigorous treatment. Large doses or concentrated solutions act like corrosive agents, producing hemorrhagic gastritis and enteritis and rarely gastric necrosis.

See also: Barbiturates, *Reference Congener in Section III.*
Ref.: Finnegan et al., 1951; Franklin, 1931; Sollmann and Hatcher, 1908; Stalker et al., 1978; Vaziri et al., 1977.

1433 Ectylurea

1433

(2-Ethylcrotonyl)urea, (α-Ethyl crotonyl)carbamide, Levanil, Nostyn

Toxicity Rating: 3. This sedative drug of the tranquilizing type is rapidly absorbed and metabolized. Chronic feeding to rats (0.6 gm./kg. daily) caused no alteration in growth and no recognized lesions. A woman ingested 5 gm. (usual dose 0.3 gm. t.i.d.) resulting in a 72-hr. sleep from which she could be aroused. There were no changes in blood pressure, pulse, or respirations; recovery was uneventful. Treat like barbiturate poisoning.

See also: Barbiturates, *Reference Congener in Section III.*
Ref.: Ames Co., 1953; Ferguson and Linn, 1956; Hochman and Robbins, 1958.

1434 Ethchlorvynol

1434

Ethyl β-chlorovinyl ethynyl carbinol, Placidyl

Toxicity Rating: 4. A hypnotic-sedative drug differing chemically from barbiturates and other common hypnotics, sold in capsules containing a polyethylene glycol solution of the drug. The recommended hypnotic dose for adults is 500 mg. Considerable tolerance is acquired by chronic users. An oral dose as small as 2.5 gm. (taken with alcohol) has killed an adult, but a dose as large as 80-120 grams has been survived. These accidental and suicidal ingestions have resulted in coma of long duration (usually 3-6 days, but as long as 17 days). In the absence of intercurrent infections, the vital signs are remarkably well maintained in many of these comatose patients, but hypoventilation, hypotension and bradycardia are not uncommon. In the presence of alcohol or barbiturates, the depressant effects are considerably intensified. One form of abuse of Placidyl is to inject the capsular solution intravenously; pulmonary edema, hemolysis and liver injury have resulted from this practice. Ethchlorvynol is rapidly absorbed from the gastrointestinal tract; it is extensively stored in body fat and eventually metabolized by the liver. Treatment consists of prompt lavage and supportive therapy as in barbiturate poisoning. Hemoperfusion through Amberlite XAD-4 cartridges appears to be a promising mode of therapy for severe ethchlorvynol poisoning. Both psychic and physical dependence occur in chronic users, and withdrawal symptoms of the alcohol-barbiturate type have been described during recovery from acute intoxications.

See also: Barbiturates, *Reference Congener in Section III.*
Ref.: Cahn, 1959; Flemenbaum and Gunby, 1971; Lynn et al., 1979; Teehan et al., 1970; Tozer et al., 1974.

1435 Ethinamate

1435

1-Ethynylcyclohexyl carbamate, e.g., Valmid, Valamin, Valmidate

Toxicity Rating: 4. Non-barbiturate sedative drug with a duration of action about one-half that of pentobarbital, but with an equivalent margin of safety (lethal dose/hypnotic dose). The therapeutic dose is 1 (0.5 gm.) or 2 capsules before retiring. As much as 28 gm. has been survived. In one patient 16 gm. produced coma, but recovery was apparently complete 6 hours after ingestion. In at least two other adults, however, 15 gm. produced profound coma, and one victim expired from supervening pulmonary edema. It is extensively metabolized, but preliminary experience indicates appreciable quantities can be removed by extracorporeal hemodialysis. In view of the high lipid solubility of the drug, a trial with mannitol or some other osmotic diuretic would appear to be warranted in victims of dangerous overdose. Habituation, tolerance and dependence are recognized. One patient consumed 13 to 15 gm./day for extended periods. The abstinence syndrome is similar to that seen after barbiturate withdrawal.

See also: Barbiturates, *Reference Congener in Section III.*
Ref.: Anonymous, 1957; Davis et al., 1959; Ellingwood et al., 1962; Gruber, 1956; Siang, 1960.

1436 Glutethimide

1436

Doriden, α-Ethyl-α-phenylglutarimide

Toxicity Rating: 4. A nonbarbiturate sedative drug. Average hypnotic dose 0.25 to 0.5 gm. Adults have died after the ingestion of 10 to 20 gm. Overdoses lead to coma, arreflexia, mydriasis, hypotension, respiratory depression and the accumulation of respiratory tract secretions. General supportive treatment is required. Because glutethimide can be removed from blood by dialysis, an artificial kidney has been employed, but higher clearance values are possible by hemoperfusion.

See also: Barbiturates, *Reference Congener in Section III.*
Ref.: Algeri and Katsas, 1960; McBay and Katsas, 1957; Rosenbaum et al., 1976; Schreiner et al., 1958.

1437 Haloperidol

1437

4-[4-(4-Chlorophenyl)-4-hydroxy-1-piperidinyl]-1-(4-fluorophenyl)-1-butanone, Haldol, Pernox

Toxicity Rating: 3(?). Haloperidol is a highly potent antipsychotic drug. Like other butyrophenones it has strong neuroleptic effects. With a wide margin of safety between lethal doses in animals and therapeutic doses in humans (the rat oral LD$_{50}$ is 850 mg./kg. whereas the maximum recommended daily therapeutic dose for adult humans is 0.3 mg./kg.), haloperidol has been considered to be a safe drug. However, three cases of unexplained sudden death have been reported in patients receiving only haloperidol in doses of 20 to 140 mg. daily for one to four days. Severe hypoglycemia resulting in coma occurred in a 77-year-old woman who had been treated with haloperidol for six days; this hypoglycemia ceased 48 hours after the drug was withdrawn. Acute intoxications among children have been cited. Three children who ingested unknown amounts of haloperidol suffered from delayed onset of acute dystonia, akathisia and extrapyramidal symptoms, all of which abated after treatment with biperiden hydrochloride. Tachycardia and hypotension are expected side-effects of haloperidol therapy, but two young children who, between them, had consumed 265 mg. haloperidol presented with hypothermia and bradycardia. And a 2-year-old child who had eaten 15 or 20 mg. haloperidol required five days of antihypertensive therapy to bring her blood pressure to normal; her systolic pressure had risen as high as 180 mm. Hg. Rarely hyperpyrexia has occurred after even conventional doses (see "malignant neuroleptic syndrome" under Chlorpromazine in Section III). It is recommended that children who ingest overdoses of haloperidol be hospitalized and observed for at least two days because of the delayed onset and severity of hypertension and problems with cardiac and thermal regulation. Haloperidol raises prolactin levels and the elevation persists during chronic administration. The rate of fetal development was decreased and delivery was delayed in rats given 2 to 20 times the maximum human dose. No teratogenic effects were seen in the offspring. Two women who were taking haloperidol along with other suspected teratogenic drugs during the first trimester gave birth to children with malformed limbs.

See also: Chlorpromazine, *Reference Congener in Section III.*
Ref.: Cummingham and Challapalli, 1979; Ketai et al., 1979; Kojak et al., 1969; Scialli and Thornton, 1978; Sinaniotis et al., 1978.

1438 Hydroxyzine Hydrochloride 1438

e.g., Atarax, Vistaril

Toxicity Rating: 4. A tranquilizing drug closely related to the antihistamine chlorcyclizine. In recommended doses (25 mg. t.i.d.) minor side-effects, such as mild drowsiness and dry mouth, commonly occur. Overdoses (1000 to 2000 mg. in adults) have led to drowsiness and coma with rapid recovery without recognized sequelae. Increased motor activity, central nervous irritability, tremor and generalized seizures are rarely reported. Convulsions, sinus tachycardia, mydriasis and peripheral vasodilatation occurred in a 13-month-old child two and a half hours after she ingested 500-625 mg. Atarax. Careful management with physostigmine and diazepam led to her complete recovery. High doses in geriatric patients have produced delays in cardiac repolarization, which may be associated with an increased risk of sudden death. A similar ECG abnormality is produced by thioridazine and tricyclic antidepressants; co-administration of these drugs with hydroxyzine may enhance a patient's vulnerability to a cardiac death.

Ref.: Hollister, 1975; Magera et al., 1981.

1439 Methaqualone 1439

e.g., Quaalude

Toxicity Rating: 4. Hypnotic-sedative similar in its effects to the barbiturates with intermediate durations of action. Supplied as tablets in the recommended therapeutic dose of 150 or 300 mg. Early clinical experience, however, involved European products, *e.g.,* Mandrax with 250 mg. methaqualone and 25 mg. diphenhydramine hydrochloride. The contribution of the latter to the toxic syndrome is not clear, but methaqualone alone is capable of inducing the same kind of coma, which is characterized by increased tendon reflexes, myoclonia and hypertonia, sometimes progressing to convulsions. In non-tolerant adults, a single dose of about 2.4 gm. is likely to cause coma. In two fatal cases adults ingested the equivalent of 8 and 14 gm. methaqualone. With intensive care a patient who ingested 100 tablets of Mandrax survived. His plasma level of methaqualone was 23 mg./100 ml. and he was treated intermittently with both peritoneal dialysis (estimated clearance 7.5 ml./min.) and extra-corporeal hemodialysis (estimated clearance of 29 ml./min.). Hemoperfusion, however, has yielded far higher clearances (Chang, 1980). Methaqualone is said to be sparingly soluble in water and apparently ionizes as a weak base. Tolerance and a withdrawal syndrome have been described. One addict who consumed sixty 150 mg. tablets daily experienced severe delirium tremens on abrupt withdrawal. Most abusers, however, limit their daily dose to less than 2 gm. (average about 725 mg.). Pulmonary edema and aspiration pneumonitis are common complications of acute overdose, but many patients have recovered with only supportive care. It is a common clinical impression that the respiratory depression and hypotension are less severe than in most barbiturate poisonings. Analeptics should be avoided.

See also: Barbiturates, *Reference Congener in Section III.*
Ref.: Burston, 1967; Caridis et al., 1967; Chang, 1980; Ewart and Priest, 1967; Ibe, 1965; Ibe, 1966a; Ibe, 1966b; Lawson and Brown, 1967; Mathew et al., 1968; Proudfoot et al., 1968; Sanderson et al., 1966.

1440 Methylpentynol

1440

Dormison, Methylparafynol, Meparfynol

Toxicity Rating: 3. A sedative related to chloral hydrate. Rapidly inactivated, hence short duration of action. The recommended adult hypnotic dose is 0.25 to 0.75 gm. Toxicity rating is based on rodent data, but it may be more toxic in man. Case report of patient who recovered after ingesting 8.75 gm., but a 45-year-old woman who took about 5 gm. died within 3 hours from cardiac arrest following a period of coma. Other clinical reports of exfoliative dermatitis, toxic psychosis, and altered liver function.

See also: Barbiturates, *Reference Congener in Section III*.
Ref.: Cares et al., 1953; De Lamater, 1952; Lemere, 1952; Marley, 1955.

1441 Methyprylon

1441

Noludar, 3,3-Diethyl-5-methyl-2,4-piperidinedione

Toxicity Rating: 4. A central nervous system depressant. Overdosage leads to coma. Death has resulted from 6 gm., but 9 gm. have been survived. At the usual adult hypnotic dose (0.2 to 0.4 gm.) its actions are similar to secobarbital but with less tendency to depress respiration. Dehydrogenated in vivo to a tetrahydropyridine compound, which appears in the bile and urine. No reports of toxic effects on kidney, liver or blood. Mild side-effects include nausea, vomiting and vertigo. Hemoperfusion, particularly with a column containing activated charcoal coated with albumin and cellulose nitrate, appears to be a promising mode of therapy for severe methyprylon poisoning.

See also: Barbiturates, *Reference Congener in Section III*.
Ref.: Chang, 1980; Jacobziner and Raybin, 1961j; Schallek et al., 1956.

1442 Paraldehyde

1442

Paracetaldehyde

Toxicity Rating: 3. Liquid hypnotic-sedative drug with a specific gravity of about 1.0. Therapeutic dose by mouth or rectum 1 to 30 ml. Also given parenterally in doses of 2 to 8 ml. in saline; the intravenous route, however, is hazardous and may produce acute failure of the right heart. Decomposes on prolonged storage to acetaldehyde and acetic acid. One deteriorated product (40% acetic acid by analysis) produced sudden death with intense corrosion of the buccal mucosa and upper air passages, whereas rectal administration was attended in another victim by great pain and sloughing of rectal mucosa (see also Acid in Section III). Considerable variation is recognized in the adult lethal dose. Less than 1 ounce by mouth has caused death but 4 ounces has been survived on several occasions. Death presumably from respiratory failure is usually preceded by prolonged and profound coma. Interactions between paraldehyde and ethyl alcohol are not well understood, probably because the metabolism of paraldehyde in man has not been studied in recent times. Doses of 1 to 2 ounces in alcoholics sometimes kill within 0.5 to 4 hours. In animals ethanol and paraldehyde are synergistic but less than additive in terms of lethality; under some dosage schedules, however, experimental data suggest that these drugs are antagonistic. Habituation is recognized, but acquired tolerance appears to be of a low grade, perhaps because intense metabolic acidosis frequently attends continuous use of the drug. The acidosis has not been correlated with blood acetate, lactate or ketone acid levels. Some acidotic patients also exhibit azotemia, oliguria, albuminuria and other signs of acute renal insufficiency. Although detailed recovery studies appear to be lacking, paraldehyde is probably dialyzable. Peritoneal or extracorporeal hemodialysis could, therefore, be used to supplement renal function, decrease the body burden of drug and perhaps correct the acidosis. The latter, however, is better controlled by systemic administration of bicarbonate. Similarly, hyperventilation has been suggested as a means of ridding the body of paraldehyde because appreciable quantities of unchanged drug are excreted via the lungs. The use of osmotic diuretics does not appear to have been explored. For the comatose patient in normal acid-base status, see Barbiturates in Section III. For the management of metabolic acidosis, see Ethylene Glycol in Section III.

Ref.: Anonymous, 1954; Beier et al., 1963; Burstein, 1943; Elkinton et al., 1957; Hayward and Boshell, 1957; Hutchinson, 1930; Kaye and Haag, 1964; Kotz et al., 1938; Lang and Borgstedt, 1968; Waterhouse and Stern, 1957; Weatherby and Clements, 1960.

1443 Thalidomide

1443

Contergan, Softenon, Distaval, Kevadon, α-(*N*-Phthalimido)glutarimide

Any assessment of the acute ingestion hazard of this sedative drug is perhaps facetious since it has been totally withdrawn from the U.S. market. Worldwide attention was focused on it in late 1961 when it was first suspected as the causative agent in the German outbreak of phocomelia. The critical exposure occurs in utero when as little as 100 mg. are ingested by a woman in the 4th to 6th week of pregnancy. At least 8000 victims of this teratogenic substance have been born. Although the severity varies, the pattern is remarkably specific for abnormalities of the long bones of the extremities. Hemangioma of the face is the most characteristic but unfortunately the most benign sign. In addition to phocomelia and amelia, alimentary abnormalities such as atresia, stenosis and malrotation are frequent. Structures developing from the mesenchyme are most profoundly affected. With the possible exception of the virus of German measles and adrenocorticotropic hormones, thalidomide represents the most specific agent encountered to date for exerting a selective toxicity on the human foetus (attempts to produce this syndrome in experimental animals have been largely unsuccessful). The structure of thalidomide is notable in that it contains two imide groups. Original reports on its pharmacological investigations are not readily available, but among its pecularities is a virtual absence of sedative activity in experimental animals. Apparently there have been no successful suicides in almost 200 attempts. In one of these episodes the patient ingested 144 times the usual therapeutic dose without depression of respiration or heart action. An LD_{50} in animals could not be established because of its low toxicity. Early in its clinical use thalidomide was shown to induce peripheral neuritis in a few individuals. In addition to numbness and paresthesias in the extremities, signs of upper motor neuron disease were occasionally encountered.

Ref.: Fullerton and Kremer, 1961; Rodin et al., 1962; Taussig, 1962a; Taussig, 1962b; Getnam, 1962.

Sympathomimetic amines

1444   Amphetamine

β-Phenylisopropylamine,   Benzedrine,   α-Methylphenethylamine

Toxicity Rating: 5.

See also: Amphetamine, *Reference Congener in Section III.*

1445   Benzphetamine Hydrochloride

e.g., Didrex

Toxicity Rating: 4. The usual adult dose prescribed for this anorectic drug is 25-50 mg., 3 times daily. Tachyphylaxis and tolerance have been described.

Adverse reactions like those reported for other amphetamine-related anorectics; see Phentermine below.

See also: Amphetamine, *Reference Congener in Section III.*

1446   Chlorphentermine Hydrochloride

4-Chloro-α,α-dimethylbenzeneethanamine hydrochloride,   Pre-Sate

Toxicity Rating: 5(?). An anorectic drug with milder central nervous system stimulant effects than amphetamine. Excitement and signs of sympathetic stimulation have been seen in cases of accidental overdosage. Acute oral LD_{50} in rats is 180 mg./kg. Recommended dose for adult humans in a weight-loss program is 65 mg. daily. Dry mouth and dyspepsia are reported side-effects. One of several drugs which induce what has been called a phospholipidosis in laboratory animals on chronic doses. The condition reveals itself principally by accumulations of foam cells (modified alveolar macrophages) in the lungs. The health significance of these microscopic and submicroscopic lesions is unclear.

See also: Amphetamine, *Reference Congener in Section III.*
Ref.: Lullmann-Rauch and Reil, 1974.

1447   Diethylpropion

Tenuate,   Tepanil,   1-Phenyl-2-diethyl-1-aminopropanone

Toxicity Rating: 4(?). A sympathomimetic drug related pharmacologically to amphetamine and used chiefly as an anorexigenic in recommended oral doses of 25 mg. three times daily. Said to have fewer side effects than amphetamine. Habituation has been reported in a 27-year-old woman who consumed at first 10 and later 100 times the usual therapeutic dose without major ill effects. Whether or not she had an unusual tolerance was not established.

See also: Amphetamine, *Reference Congener in Section III.*
Ref.: Caplan, 1963.

1448   *N,N*-Dimethyltryptamine

DMT

Toxicity Rating: 4. A synthetic psychotomimetic (hallucinogenic) substance, also identified as a natural constituent of a South American plant (Piptadenia peregrina or Prestonia amazonica), from which a snuff is prepared. Available on the illicit market in the U.S.A., as are the diethyl and perhaps the dipropyl analogues, which have similar biological activities. The intraperitoneal LD$_{50}$ of DMT is 110 mg./kg. in mice. Essentially inactive by mouth. Usually self-administered by needle (e.g., intramuscular injection). In a dose of about 1 mg./kg., the result in man is a prompt but brief (1 to 2 hour) period of hallucinations, accompanied by signs of enhanced sympathetic tone (e.g., mydriasis, slight hypertension, tachycardia or sometimes reflex bradycardia secondary to the hypertension, mild elevation of body temperature, etc.). Sympathetic effects are said to be more prominent than after LSD, but the somatic and psychic reactions are of much shorter duration. The victim should be protected from the consequences of a possible panic reaction. Presumably chlorpromazine is effective in suppressing the hallucinations, but because of the brevity of the disorder, drug therapy is seldom required. For a current hypothesis concerning the genesis of the hallucinations after DMT and many other hallucinogens, see Psilocybin in the index.

See also: Marihuana, *Reference Congener in Section III.*
Ref.: Jacobsen, 1963; Szara, 1957; Usdin and Efron, 1972.

1449   2,5-Dimethoxy-4-methyl-amphetamine

STP,   DOM

Toxicity Rating: 6(?). A highly potent, illicit amphetamine derivative used as a drug of abuse. Pills on the black market have been found to contain 10 mg. Doses of more than 3 mg. in man cause pronounced hallucinations lasting over 8 hours. The hallucinations are said to resemble those produced by LSD, mescaline and psilocybin. In spite of claims to the contrary, the psychic effects and associated behavior appear to be attenuated by therapeutic doses of chlorpromazine and presumably by other phenothiazine tranquilizers. STP is a very dangerous agent sometimes misrepresented to be mescaline.

See also: Amphetamine, *Reference Congener in Section III.*
Ref.: Snyder et al., 1967b.

1450   Ephedrine

l-Ephedrine, α-Hydroxy-β-methylaminopropylbenzene

Toxicity Rating: 5. The probable lethal dose in man is 50 mg./kg. Poisoning is characterized by restlessness, anxiety, sweating, tremor, rapid pulse, extrasystoles, confusion, and delirium. Treatment is symptomatic with emphasis on sedatives (e.g., barbiturates) or tranquilizers (e.g., chlorpromazine).

See also: Amphetamine, *Reference Congener in Section III.*
Ref.: Chen and Schmidt, 1930.

1451   Phenylpropanolamine Hydrochloride

2-Amino-1-phenyl-1-propanol hydrochloride

Toxicity Rating: 5(?). A widely used ingredient in over-the-counter diet pills and in bronchodilators, nasal decongestants and cold remedies. Subject to abuse because of its amphetamine-like effects. Severe hypertensive episodes have followed doses as small as 1 to 6 unit doses of 50 to 85 mg. each. Acute psychosis without physical findings occurred in a young housewife who consumed excessive amounts. Commonly misrepresented on the street as authentic speed (methamphetamine). The hypertensive effects are said to be potentiated by indomethacin and perhaps other similar non-steroid anti-inflammatory inhibitors of prostaglandin synthesis.

See also: Amphetamine, *Reference Congener in Section III.*
Ref.: Frewin et al., 1978; Horowitz et al., 1979; Lee et al., 1979; Ostern and Dodson, 1965; Schaffer and Pauli, 1980.

1452   Propylhexedrine

N,α-Dimethylcyclohexaneethanamine

Toxicity Rating: 5(?). A cotton plug inside the Benzedrex inhaler used for nasal decongestion contains 250 mg. propylhexedrine, together with menthol and other aromatics. Propylhexedrine is also marketed in Europe as an anorectic drug. Less potent as a pressor agent and as a central nervous stimulant than amphetamine, but abused in the same manner either by ingestion or intravenously. Implicated in a number of deaths. After intravenous abuse death is sudden with postmortem findings of pulmonary edema, foreign body granulomas, fibrosis and right ventricular hypertrophy suggestive of pulmonary hypertension. Other deaths were suicides or homocides apparently secondary to drug-induced psychosis. Exercise and perhaps elevated ambient temperatures potentiate toxicity.

See also: Amphetamine, *Reference Congener in Section III.*
Ref.: Anderson et al., 1979a.

1453 Pseudoephedrine Hydrochloride 1453

d-Isoephedrine hydrochloride, e.g., Sudafed hydrochloride

Toxicity Rating: 4 to 5. An isomer of ephedrine that occurs naturally as *d*-pseudoephedrine in various species of Ephedra plants. Used orally as a nasal decongestant and bronchodilator where it is about as effective as ephedrine. Weaker pressor agent and not as cardiotoxic in large doses as ephedrine. Available on prescription and over-the-counter. Usual adult therapeutic dose, 30 mg. three times daily. Overdoses may cause nervousness, dizziness and other signs of hyperexcitability, especially in children.

See also: Amphetamine, *Reference Congener in Section III.*

1454 Epinephrine 1454

Epinephrine bitartrate,   Epinephrine hydrochloride,   Adrenalin

It is commonly believed that pharmacologically active concentrations of epinephrine cannot be achieved in man by oral administration because of the many mechanisms available for rapid inactivation. The oral ingestion of labelled epinephrine by normal volunteers has shown that 60 to 70% of the total radioactivity is excreted in the urine within 72 hours. Phenolic amines make up 80 to 85% of the urinary metabolites while 15 to 20% are phenolic acids. In these studies as much as 4 mg. of *dl*-epinephrine *d*-bitartrate was ingested by adults with essentially no evidence of biological activity except for one subject who showed facial flushing 20 to 30 min. after ingestion. Iatrogenic overdoses, accidental intravenous administration and the injection of solutions intended for nebulization, however, have produced serious intoxications and death. The chief hazards include cerebrovascular hemorrhage from elevated arterial pressure, pulmonary edema from pulmonary arterial hypertension and ventricular fibrillation. Some of these effects may be counteracted by the administration of nitrites or other rapidly acting vasodilators, but α and β adrenergic blocking drugs (such as phentolamine and propranolol) may also be useful if injected promptly.

See also: Amphetamine, *Reference Congener in Section III.*
Ref.: Curry, 1962; Resnick, 1963.

1455 *l*-*N*-Ethylephedrine 1455

Etafedrine, e.g., Nethamine

Toxicity Rating: 4. Used orally as a bronchodilator (adult dose 25-50 mg.). Similar to *l*-ephedrine in toxicity but said to have less prominent cardiovascular and central excitatory actions. Minimal lethal dose in rabbits is 50 mg./kg. i.v., 550 mg./kg. by mouth. See also Ephedrine above.

Ref.: Becker et al., 1942.

1456 Fenfluramine 1456

N-Ethyl-α-methyl-3-(trifluoromethyl) phenylethylamine hydrochloride

Toxicity Rating: 5. Anorexigenic drug. Structurally similar to amphetamines, but in small doses it produces central nervous depression rather than excitation. Has caused many human poisonings. Toxic doses in adults range from 300 to 2,000 mg. with fatal blood levels ranging from 6.5 to 28 $\mu g./$ ml. Signs and symptoms of toxicity include mydriasis, rotary nystagmus, hyperreflexia, muscle twitching, shivering and either agitation or drowsiness. Opisthotonos, trismus, hypersalivation and facial flushing are described. Chief cardiac signs are tachycardia and occasionally arrhythmias. Convulsions and coma follow large doses; hyperpyrexia is a grave prognostic sign. Epigastric pain and vomiting have been reported by some patients. Neurologic and cardiac signs develop within 2 hours. In each of nine fatal cases, death occurred within 4 hours of ingestion and was attributed to cardiac arrest (asystole or ventricular fibrillation). Cardiopulmonary resuscitation has proven ineffective in fenfluramine poisoning. In children, doses of 28 to 33 mg./kg. have proven fatal. However, two children, age 3 and 3 1/2, recovered after ingesting 30 and 70 mg./kg. (plasma concentrations were 630 and 1140 ng./ml.). Treatment in these cases consisted of gastric lavage and charcoal, followed by 5 mg. doses of diazepam given i.v. as needed to control convulsions. The older child received 45 mg. of diazepam in eight hours. Both patients were semi-conscious with tachycardia and hypertension during the first hours after admission, but showed rapid improvement thereafter. Nystagmus continued for 24 hours. Both patients were drowsy and had difficulty passing urine but were otherwise normal on the third day. Fenfluramine is rapidly absorbed from the gut and distributed to fat and muscle tissues. In man, metabolism proceeds through de-ethylation, deamination, and oxidation. The chief metabolite is *m*-trifluoro-methyl benzoic acid. Fenfluramine and its metabolites are excreted, primarily in urine. Treatment of overdosed patients consists of immediate gastric lavage with installation of activated charcoal. Convulsions may be controlled by diazepam; propanolol may be used to moderate extreme tachycardia. No specific antidote is known. Forced diuresis with acidification of urine may be beneficial in hastening the excretion of the drug. Fenfluramine is usually supplied as a 20 mg. tablet.

See also: Amphetamine, *Reference Congener in Section III.*
Ref.: Darmady, 1974; Muhlendahl and Krienke, 1978z; von Muhlendahl and Krienke, 1979; Veltri and Temple, 1975.

1457   Hydroxyamphetamine Hydrobromide

e.g., Paredrine

The only current medical use for hydroxyamphetamine is the induction of mydriasis. As a mydriatic it is less effective than phenylephrine. It is supplied as 15 ml. of a 1% solution with 2% boric acid, preserved with thimerosal. Except for the almost total lack of central stimulant activity, the actions of hydroxyamphetamine are like those of ephedrine (see above). Accidental ingestion of the ophthalmic solution may result in a rise in blood pressure, palpitations, cardiac arrhythmias, headache, sweating, nausea, vomiting, and gastrointestinal irritation. Intense mydriasis may cause increased intraocular pressure, photophobia and blurred vision, which can be counteracted by 1% pilocarpine instilled onto the conjunctiva.

See also: Amphetamine, *Reference Congener in Section III.*

1458   Isoproterenol

e.g., Isuprel

Sympathomimetic amine that acts almost exclusively on beta-adrenergic receptors. Used therapeutically as a bronchodilator in respiratory disorders and as a cardiac stimulant in heart block. Usually administered by inhalation, injection or sublingual tablets (10 and 15 mg.). As with epinephrine (above), it is probably difficult to achieve pharmacologically active concentrations of isoproterenol by oral administration because of the many mechanisms available for rapid inactivation. No serious human intoxications are known, but patients often experience tachycardia, headache and flush. Serious arrhythmias, myocardial necrosis and cardiac arrest can occur with large or repeated doses, particularly in the presence of cardiac fatigue. Although cardiac lesions are produced in animals by many sympathomimetic amines, isoproterenol causes an apparently unique parenchymal cell necrosis. Cardiotoxicity in rats is dramatically related to the whole body fat content. Propranolol is a specific pharmacological antagonist to the short term cardiovascular effects.

Ref.: Balazs et al., 1962; Lockett, 1965; Rosenblum et al., 1965.

1459   Methamphetamine

"Speed", "Crystal", *d*-Desoxyephedrine

Toxicity Rating: 5(?). An amphetamine derivative widely abused as a psychotropic agent in the U.S.A., Western Europe and Japan since World War II. Like other amphetamines it elevates mood, allays fatigue, increases motor activity, and suppresses appetite. Injected intravenous, it induces intense euphoria (a "rush"). Overdoses may produce confusion, hallucinations, convulsions, mania, and acts of self-destruction. Its psychic and motor effects resemble those of cocaine but last longer.

See also: Amphetamine, *Reference Congener in Section III.*

1460   4-Methoxyamphetamine

α-Methyl-*p*-methoxyphenylamine

Toxicity Rating: 5(?). An illicit hallucinogen. Lethal effects in mice antagonized by pretreatment with phentolamine, 6-hydroxydopamine and methysergide but not by 4-chloroamphetamine, practolol or haloperidol. Haloperidol is also ineffective against amphetamine poisoning in mice, but it is useful in human intoxications by amphetamine and presumably by 4-methoxyamphetamine.

See also: Amphetamine, *Reference Congener in Section III.*
Ref.: Lopatka et al., 1976.

1461   3,4-Methylenedioxyamphetamine

MDA, "Love Drug"

Toxicity Rating: 5(?). An amphetamine derivative that serves as a drug of abuse, usually sold on the illicit market in capsules. The agent produces a "high" reputedly like that of methamphetamine. Human fatalities have been described. A near-fatality has been ascribed to the ingestion of about 500 mg.

See also: Amphetamine, *Reference Congener in Section III.*
Ref.: Reed et al., 1972; Richards and Borgstedt, 1971; Hardman et al., 1973.

1462 Methylphenidate

1462

Ritalin

Toxicity Rating: 4. A central nervous stimulant with actions between those of amphetamine and caffeine, but with less sympathomimetic effects than either. It is often used during reserpine therapy to counteract depression. Side effects are not prominent: nervousness, insomnia, palpitations, headache, and sometimes changes in blood pressure and pulse rate. Overdoses in animals and presumably man lead to extreme excitement, motor restlessness, ataxia, and tonic and clonic convulsions. Treatment is symptomatic and supportive, with special emphasis on sedation (e.g., barbiturates).

See also: Amphetamine, *Reference Congener in Section III.*
Ref.: Chernoff et al., 1962; Pollack, 1964.

1463 Naphazoline Hydrochloride

1463

e.g., Privine hydrochloride

A sympathomimetic amine closely related to tetrahydrozoline and producing the same disturbing side effect in the occasional infant or young child, namely an unexplained sedation. See also Tetrahydrozoline below. The systemic effects following either oral or nasal administration also appear to include most of the common sympathetic actions such as prolonged hypertension with peripheral vasoconstriction, mild cortical stimulation followed by psychic depression and depression of basal centers. Only symptomatic and supportive treatment is recommended.

Ref.: Greenblatt, 1947; Hainsworth, 1948; House and Carey, 1948; Waring, 1945.

1464 Oxymetazoline Hydrochloride

1464

3-((4,5-Dihydro-1H-imidazol-2-yl)methyl)-6-(1,1-dimethyl ethyl)-2,4-dimethyl phenol, e.g., Afrin

Toxicity Rating: 5-6. A potent vasoconstrictor due to α-adrenergic activity and a central nervous system depressant. Used in nose drops, it is supplied as a 0.05% solution in water and the usual adult dose is 0.2 ml. The compound has a high oral toxicity (rat oral LD$_{50}$ 10 mg./kg.) and is readily absorbed through the nasal mucosa. Toxic symptoms include drowsiness, respiratory distress and elevated blood pressure. An infant of 1 month given accidentally about five times the recommended adult dose became unresponsive, with gasping respiration and a blood pressure of 140 mm Hg systolic; he recovered with supportive care (Greenstein, 1955). Following a therapeutic dose, a girl of 22 months suffered vasomotor collapse with loss of consciousness and arreflexia. After treatment with epinephrine and caffeine, the patient recovered consciousness briefly but relapsed into coma. After about five hours, vomiting, defecation and urination occurred. Skin color returned after seven hours, and twelve hours after the original dose she was sufficiently recovered to eat (Friedman, 1955). Several other instances were reported in which infants and toddlers fell asleep and could not be roused for several hours following a therapeutic dose of the compound. Oxymetazoline hydrochloride is no longer recommended for children under six. No reports of toxicity to adults were found, although hypertensive crises should be anticipated in individuals receiving MAO inhibitors.

Ref.: Friedman, 1955; Greenstein, 1955.

1465 Pemoline

1465

2-Amino-5-phenyl-4(5H)-oxazolone, 2-Imino-5-phenyl-4-oxazolidinone, Phenylisohydantoin, Cylert

Toxicity Rating: 3. Central nervous stimulant, chemically dissimilar to amphetamines and methylphenidate. Used in treatment of children with minimal brain dysfunction; the recommended starting dose is 37.5 mg. in school-aged children. Adverse effects of therapeutic doses include insomnia, stomachache, rash, irritability, depression, nausea, dizziness, headache, drowsiness and hallucinations. Acute overdosage produces agitation, restlessness, dyskinetic movements and tachycardia. Vomiting should be induced. Subsequent management is symptomatic. Extracorporeal hemodialysis may be helpful. In fatally poisoned rats death is due to severe circulatory shock. Autopsy revealed congestion of abdominal organs, hemorrhagic areas in lungs and thymus and generalized tissue damage resulting from anoxia. In one reported childhood poisoning, a 35-month–old boy ingested an unknown quantity of his brother's pemoline. Four hours later, he became hyperactive with dilated pupils, and was hospitalized on the following day after vomiting and choreiform movements of trunk and extremities developed. Phenobarbital had a calming effect, but symptoms persisted until the third hospital day. Pemoline is readily absorbed and metabolized to yield pemolinedione and mandelic acid. Pemoline, its conjugates and metabolite, are excreted by the kidneys, mostly within 24 hours of oral administration.

Ref.: McCall and Rice, 1962; McNeil, 1979; Physicians' Desk Reference, 1981.

1466   **1466** Phenmetrazine

Preludin

Toxicity Rating: 5. A sympathomimetic drug related pharmacologically to amphetamine and used chiefly as an anorexigenic in recommended oral doses of 25 mg. three times daily. Said to be less effective as a central nervous stimulant than amphetamine. No reports of dangerous toxic reactions. Like amphetamine it can produce psychic dependence and occasionally a state of "addiction" with a withdrawal reaction manifested by EEG abnormalities during sleep. A common drug of abuse, as is also the closely related drug phendimetrazine.

See also: Amphetamine, Reference Congener in Section III.
Ref.: Oswald and Thacore, 1963.

1467   **1467** Phentermine

e.g., Ionamin

Toxicity Rating: 5(?). An anorectic drug supplied as a cationic resin complex (acute oral LD_{50} in rats 450 mg./kg.) and as the hydrochloride salt. Acute oral LD_{50} in rats for the free base is 151 mg./kg. (a 30 mg. capsule of the hydrochloride contains the equivalent of 24 mg. of the free base). Both formulations are about equal to dextroamphetamine as anorectics. The usual daily dose for adults is 15-30 mg. The product is not recommended for children under 12. Acutely intoxicated patients exhibit tremor, hyperreflexia, rapid respiration, confusion, assaultive behavior, hallucinations, panic, nausea, vomiting, diarrhea and abdominal cramps. Death may occur in convulsions and coma. A 26-year-old schizophrenic woman developed an acute psychotic disorganization with mydriasis, tachycardia and restlessness after 240 mg. phentermine. Lavage, sedation with hypnotic drugs and symptomatic treatment are the usual therapeutic regimen. Intravenous phentolamine has been suggested in cases complicated by severe hypertension. Tolerance to the anorectic effect develops within a few weeks. Psychic and possibly physical dependence occur after long-term use. Signs of chronic intoxication are severe dermatoses, marked insomnia, irritability, hyperactivity and, in the severe cases, a psychosis resembling schizophrenia. Extreme fatigue, mental depression and changes in the sleep EEG have been observed after abrupt cessation of long-term usage.

See also: Amphetamine, Reference Congener in Section III.
Ref.: Becker, 1961; Physicians' Desk Reference, 1981; Rubin, 1964.

1468   **1468** Phenylephrine

e.g., Neosynephrine

Toxicity Rating: 5(?). Sympathomimetic drug intermediate in activity between epinephrine and ephedrine. Used for the relief of nasal congestion, to delay absorption of local anesthetic, as a mydriatic, to prevent hypotension in spinal anesthesia and shock and for the control of bradycardia in heart block. Effective by mouth but apparently poorly absorbed since recommended oral doses are at least 10 times the usual hypodermic doses. Single oral doses as large as 250 mg. have been used in the management of hypotension. Overdoses may produce ventricular premature beats and short paroxysms of ventricular tachycardia. Perhaps less active as a central stimulant than is ephedrine.

See also: Amphetamine, Reference Congener in Section III.
Ref.: Sollmann, 1957.

1469   **1469** Tetrahydrozoline Hydrochloride

e.g., Tyzine hydrochloride

A peripheral vasoconstrictor commonly used as a nasal decongestant in the form of an aerosol or drops (0.1%). In a few cases of apparent idiosyncracy in infants and young children, symptoms have ranged from drowsiness through coma, with marked respiratory embarrassment and complete vasomotor collapse. Said to have a higher toxicity than its homologue Naphazoline (see above). Toxic by both the intranasal and oral routes. The recommended treatment is symptomatic and supportive; oxygen may be indicated.

Ref.: Brainerd and Olmsted, 1956; Friedman, 1955; Greenstein, 1955.

Antidepressant drugs (exclusive of above)

1470   **1470** Amitriptyline

e.g., Elavil, Laroxyl

Toxicity Rating: 5. One of the tricyclic antidepressant drugs with pronounced tranquilizing and anticholinergic activity. In vitro amitriptyline weakly blocks histamine and 5-hydroxytryptamine. Usual starting dose is 75 mg./day which in some patients may be gradually increased to as much as 300 mg./day. The drug appears to be at least an order of magnitude more toxic to man than to laboratory rodents. Acute oral LD_{50} in mice 280 mg./kg. The mean lethal dose by mouth in man appears to be in the range of 1000 mg. for an adult. Only 4 mg./ kg. produced mild signs of intoxication in a child. Acutely poisoned victims present with deep coma which may alternate with periods of restlessness or excitability. A cardinal feature of the intoxication, however, is a bewildering array of disturbances in the cardiac mechanism reminiscent of the gamut of arrhythmias and conduction defects seen in digitalis poisoning.

See also: Imipramine, *Reference Congener in Section III.*

1471 Desipramine   1471

Desmethylimipramine

Toxicity Rating: 5. One of the tricyclic antidepressant drugs with pronounced tranquilizing and anticholinergic activity. A two-year-old child died after ingestion of 2500 mg. Doses on the order of 1 to 2.5 gm. have produced severe poisonings in adults. Desipramine is a major metabolite of imipramine after monodemethylation; it appears to resemble the parent compound in all important toxicological respects.

See also: Imipramine, *Reference Congener in Section III.*

1472 Doxepin   1472

e.g., Sinequan, Curatin

Toxicity Rating: 4 or 5. A dibenzoxepine with both antidepressant and tranquilizing properties. Chemical structure is similar to that of amitriptyline. Acute toxic signs suggest similarities with the tricyclic antidepressants.

See also: Imipramine, *Reference Congener in Section III.*

1473 Imipramine   1473

Tofranil

Toxicity Rating: 4. A phenothiazine-like molecule in which a 2-carbon chain replaces the sulfur atom of the phenothiazine nucleus. Usually referred to as a tricyclic antidepressive drug. The oral LD_{50} is 682 mg. in rats, 175 mg. in dogs.

See also: Imipramine, *Reference Congener in Section III.*

1474 Nortriptyline   1474

Desmethylamitriptyline, e.g., Aventyl

Toxicity Rating: 5. One of the tricyclic antidepressant drugs with pronounced tranquilizing and anticholinergic activity. A severe intoxication in an adult occurred after ingestion of 600 mg. but more than three times this dose has been survived. Nortriptyline is a major metabolite of Amitriptyline after monodemethylation; it appears to resemble the parent compound in all important toxicological respects.

See also: Imipramine, *Reference Congener in Section III.*

1475 Iproniazid Phosphate   1475

Marsilid phosphate,   1-Isonicotinoyl-2-isopropylhydrazine phosphate

The isopropyl derivative of isoniazid. Effective as a tuberculostatic agent and as a "psychic energizer." A central nervous stimulant and potent inhibitor of monoamine oxidase, which is thought to be the basis for its ability to potentiate other centrally acting drugs, particularly alcohol, ether, barbiturates, meperidine, cocaine, procaine, and phenylephrine. Its action is cumulative and the effect is prolonged. Man seems to be more susceptible than laboratory animals to side effects. Toxic actions are numerous and may be serious, so that the drug should be administered with caution. Psychological effects ranging from mild behavioral imbalance to frank psychoses subside on discontinuing the drug. Autonomic effects are many: postural hypotension is particularly frequent and is not relieved by the pressor amines. Neurological disturbances include tremors, paresthesias, peripheral neuropathies, syncope. But the most ominous sign is jaundice, which may herald a rapidly fatal hepatitis. Only symptomatic and supportive therapy is available. No longer commercially available.

Ref.: Frantz, 1958; Zetzel and Kaplan, 1958.

1476 Loxapine

Loxitane

Toxicity Rating: 5. One of the newer tricyclic antidepressants. As with imipramine, overdoses produce coma and convulsions, but cardiac disorders are less common than with imipramine or amitriptyline.

See also: Imipramine, *Reference Congener in Section III.*

1477 Phenelzine Sulfate

Nardil, Phenylethyl hydrazine dihydrogen sulfate

Toxicity Rating: 5. A substituted hydrazine which acts as an inhibitor of monoamine oxidase and is employed as an antidepressive drug. Side effects have been frequent and varied: hypotension, agitation, occasionally convulsions, cholestasis with jaundice, and skin eruptions. Nine successful suicides have been ascribed to doses ranging from 39 to 100 tablets (25 to 30 mg./kg.). Death in most cases was due to peripheral circulatory failure. In one case a very low blood sugar was demonstrated.

Ref.: Lutz, 1960.

1478 Pipradrol

Meratran, α-(2-Piperidyl)benzhydrol

Toxicity Rating: 5(?). Central nervous stimulant without prominent autonomic effects. It appears to be mildly depressant in small doses. The rat oral LD_{50} is 180 mg./kg., but man appears to be much more sensitive. The maximal recommended single dose is 2 mg. (6 mg. daily) in an adult. Heavy overdosage causes severe hyperkinesis, marked agitation, abdominal pain, and insomnia. One patient on a daily oral dose of 35 mg. developed a paranoid psychosis. Meratran is rapidly metabolized; 4 hours after an oral dose, no drug was demonstrable in any tissue. Barbiturates have been employed in treating acute poisonings.

Ref.: Allin and Pogge, 1956; Brown and Werner, 1954.

1479 Protriptyline Hydrochloride

e.g., Vivactil

Toxicity Rating: 5. One of the tricyclic antidepressant drugs. Available in 5 and 10 mg. tablets. Dangerous neurologic and cardiovascular symptoms should be anticipated on overdosage.

See also: Imipramine, *Reference Congener in Section III.*

1480 Tranylcypromine

Parnate

Toxicity Rating: 5. An antidepressant drug with actions resembling both dextroamphetamine and iproniazid. A potent monoamine oxidase inhibitor in vitro and in vivo but not a hydrazine derivative. Recommended daily adult dose 10 to 60 mg. In animals it produces irritability, restlessness, hyperreflexia, hypertonia, salivation, lacrimation, mydriasis, and mild elevations in blood pressure. It suppresses appetite and in high doses shows anticonvulsant activity. Hexobarbital sleeping time is prolonged by Parnate, indicating its ability to potentiate other drugs presumably by interferring with their detoxification. In two clinical poisonings due to massive overdoses (300 to 1400 mg.), confusion, dizziness, somnolence, and hypotension were noted. Do not use epinephrine in treating this hypotension, because it may cause a fall in blood pressure in the presence of tranylcypromine.

Ref.: Baker, 1961.

1481 Trimipramine

e.g., Stangyl maleate, Surmontil maleate

Toxicity Rating: 5(?). An antidepressant-tranquilizer of the tricyclic group.

See also: Imipramine, *Reference Congener in Section III.*

Synthetic narcotic analgesics

1482 Diphenoxylate Hydrochloride

e.g., Lomotil

Toxicity Rating: 5. Synthetic narcotic analgesic chemically related to meperidine. Possesses both cholinergic blocking properties and direct spasmolytic effects on smooth muscle. Used as an antidiarrheal agent. One product (Lomotil) contains 2.5 mg. diphenoxylate and a "sub-therapeutic" amount (0.025 mg.) of atropine. The latter is present to discourage addiction since the addiction liability of diphenoxylate is said to be similar to that of codeine. The adult therapeutic dose is 15 to 20 mg./day. Although the dose recommended for a 2-year-old child is 5 mg./day, a severe poisoning has resulted from the accidental ingestion of only 4 times this dose. Even after vomiting with some recovery of tablets, the boy became drowsy and irritable within 2 hours. Mild respiratory difficulty seen in 5 to 6 hours progressed to apnea and cyanosis after 8 hours. A rapid respiratory response and recovery occurred after nalorphine. Other derangements, e.g., loss of bladder tone and diminution of light reflex, resembled the side effects of atropine.

See also: Morphine *and* Atropine, *Reference Congeners in Section III.*
Ref.: Canby, 1965.

1483   Ethoheptazine   1483

e.g., Zactane,   Zactirin,   Zactirin Compound-100

Toxicity Rating: 5(?). Narcotic analgesic structurally related to meperidine (see latter). Said to have a low abuse potential. Therapeutic dose by mouth 75 to 150 mg. Available as ethoheptazine citrate in 75 mg. tablets. Also generally available in multiple layered tablets as Zactirin (containing 75 mg. ethoheptazine and 325 mg. aspirin) and Zactirin Compound-100 (containing 100 mg. ethoheptazine, 227 mg. aspirin, 162 mg. phenacetin, and 32.4 mg. caffeine).

Ref.: Gilman et al., 1980.

1484   Meperidine Hydrochloride   1484

Pethidine hydrochloride,   Demerol

Toxicity Rating: 5. Believed to lie near the borderline between toxicity classes 4 and 5; this rating is based on poisonings in nonaddicts (i.e., no drug tolerance). A synthetic narcotic analgetic drug. Side effects after therapeutic doses are similar to those after equianalgetic doses of morphine, except that constipation and urinary retention are less common. In toxic doses, however, meperidine causes central nervous excitation: subjective vertigo, apprehension, tremors, ataxia, confusion, hallucinations, and convulsions. These signs and symptoms resemble atropine poisoning, as does mydriasis, tachycardia, and dryness of mouth. Hyperpyrexia, however, is rare. Unlike morphine poisoning, severe respiratory depression occurs only terminally, but naloxone is useful in the treatment of severe meperidine poisoning; sometimes it even suppresses meperidine convulsions. Otherwise symptomatic treatment as in atropine poisoning.

See also: Atropine *and* Morphine, *Reference Congeners in Section III.*
Ref.: Gruber et al., 1941; Mather and Tucker, 1976; Polonio, 1947; Zuck, 1951.

1485   Methadone   1485

Dolophine,   Amidone,   Physeptone,   Miadone,   Butalgin

Narcotic analgesic structurally unrelated to morphine but possessing qualitatively similar pharmacological actions. Methadone effects, like those of morphine, can be antagonized by naloxone.

See also: Morphine, *Reference Congener in Section III.*

1486   Propoxyphene Hydrochloride   1486

Dextropropoxyphene hydrochloride, e.g., Darvon hydrochloride

Toxicity Rating: 5. A synthetic non-narcotic drug, roughly equivalent in analgesic potency to codeine. Well tolerated by adults in therapeutic doses of 32-65 mg., 3 or 4 times daily. Said to be non-addicting but classical withdrawal signs and perhaps low grade tolerance are described in one patient. Data in rats and mice suggest a toxicity rating of 4, but clearly humans are more susceptible. Single doses in the range of 200 mg. in infants and young children have regularly produced near-fatal poisonings and at least one death (640 mg.). Doses above 800 mg. in adults have produced severe intoxications and one death (1280 mg.). A common pattern in poisonings includes ataxia, coma, convulsions, cyanosis and death in respiratory arrest. The symptoms are rapid in onset, and the patient may become comatose in less than an hour. Miosis is not seen. ECG changes (bigeminy, prolongation of QRS, etc.) are probably associated with myocardial hypoxia. Cerebral edema may be a complication. Nalorphine is an impressive antagonist in animals and, where given in adequately large doses, has produced favorable results in humans, but naloxone is safer and generally more effective.

See also: Morphine, *Reference Congener in Section III.*
Ref.: Cann and Verhulst, 1960a; Elson and Domino, 1963; Frasier et al., 1963; Hyatt, 1962; McCarthy and Keenan, 1964; Qureshi, 1964; Swarts, 1964.

Antihistaminics

1487   **1487**   Antihistaminics

e.g., Thonzylamine,   Phenindamine tartrate,   Chlorpheniramine maleate,   Dexchlorpheniramine maleate

Toxicity Rating: 5.

See also: Antihistaminics, *Reference Congener in Section III.*

1488   **1488**   Buclizine

Softran

Toxicity Rating: 4(?). A piperazine derivative with antihistaminic, antiemetic, and tranquilizing effects. There is a low incidence of side effects consisting of drowsiness, headache, and jitters. Said to have a limited potential for lowering the systolic blood pressure. Demonstrated to be effective against seasickness.

See also: Antihistaminics, *Reference Congener in Section III.*
Ref.: Gaillard, 1955; P'an et al., 1954; Stuart Co., 1960.

1489   **1489**   Chlorcyclizine

e.g., Histantine,   Trihistan

Toxicity Rating: 4. Fairly long acting antihistaminic with minimal sedative effects. Adult therapeutic dose by mouth is 50 mg.

See also: Antihistaminics, *Reference Congener in Section III.*

1490   **1490**   Chlorothen

Chloromethapyrilene,   Tagathen

Toxicity Rating: 4. An antihistaminic more effective and less toxic than tripelennamine (see below). Produces slightly more sedation. Side effects occur in about 25% of those who use it.

See also: Antihistaminics, *Reference Congener in Section III.*
Ref.: Castillo et al., 1949.

1491   **1491**   Cimetidine

Tagamet

Toxicity Rating: 3. An antihistaminic drug which blocks H_2 receptors, in contrast to the classical antihistaminics which block H_1 receptors. Useful in the management of peptic ulcer. Acute oral LD_{50}'s in rats 5.0 gm./kg.; mouse 2.6 gm./kg.; and in dogs approximately 2.6 gm./kg. Considerably more toxic i.v.: rat 106 mg./kg.; mouse 150 mg./kg. No sex differences noted. None of the poisoned rodents died after 24 hours. In dogs death occurred within 4 hours and was preceded by clonic convulsions. Chronic studies in rats and dogs failed to produce evidence for renal or hematologic changes. Four adult humans, each consuming doses from 5 to almost 20 gm. (about 100 tablets), presented only with dry mouth and slight drowsiness. The highest plasma concentration was 57 mg./L. as compared with a plasma concentration of 1 mg./L. after a therapeutic dose of 200 mg. On rare occasions overdoses and even therapeutic doses produce a toxic psychosis within a few hours of ingestion, with confusion, disorientation, agitation and hallucinations. The sensorium clears within 24 hours without sequelae.

See also: Antihistaminics, *Reference Congener in Section III.*
Ref.: Barnhart and Bowden, 1979; Brimblecombe et al., 1975; Illingworth and Jarvic, 1979.

1492   **1492**   Diphenhydramine Hydrochloride

Benadryl hydrochloride

Toxicity Rating: 5. According to clinical experience, this antihistaminic drug is probably best described as lying near the borderline between toxicity classes 4 and 5.

See also: Antihistaminics, *Reference Congener in Section III.*
Ref.: Aaron, 1953; Davis and Hunt, 1949.

1493   **1493**   Doxylamine Succinate

e.g., Decapryn succinate

Toxicity Rating: 4. Antihistaminic closely related to diphenhydramine. Oral LD_{50} in mice is 470 mg./

kg. Said to produce a high incidence of sedation. The adult single therapeutic dose is 12 to 25 mg.

See also: Antihistaminics, *Reference Congener in Section III.*
Ref.: Merck and Co., 1976.

1494   Meclizine Dihydrochloride   1494

1-[(4-Chlorophenyl)phenylmethyl]-4-[(3-methylphenyl)methyl]piperazine dihydrochloride, e.g., Bonine, Antivert

Toxicity Rating: 4(?). Antihistaminic of the piperazine type, useful in the treatment of the nausea and vomiting of motion sickness, vertigo and radiation sickness. Available over-the-counter in 12.5 and 25 mg. tablets. Usual adult dose is 25-50 mg. once daily; effects last 24 to 48 hours. Mouse oral LD_{50} is 1600 mg./kg. Drowsiness is the most common side-effect with clinical doses. Dizziness, blurred vision, dryness of mouth and urinary retention sometimes occur. Metabolized to norchlorcy-clizine, buclizine (see above) and hydroxyzine (see in index). Cleft palate was found among offspring of rats given 500 mg./kg. meclizine and its congeners during pregnancy. Epidemiological studies of pregnant women revealed no unusual occurrence of abnormalities in children of mothers who took meclizine. The FDA ruled that the product label no longer must contain a warning against use during pregnancy.

See also: Antihistaminics, *Reference Congener in Section III.*
Ref.: FDA, July 13, 1979.

1495   Methapyrilene Hydrochloride   1495

Histadyl,   Semikon hydrochloride,   Thenylpyramine hydrochloride

Toxicity Rating: 5. An antihistaminic now being promoted as an "over-the-counter" hypnotic drug. Similar to other antihistaminics in acute toxicity. Overdoses produce excitement, convulsions, hyperpyrexia, cerebral edema, depression, and occasionally renal tubular necrosis. A death has been reported from an oral dose as small as 12 mg./kg., but others have survived after 80 mg./kg. Only supportive treatment is available. Animal studies at the National Cancer Institute indicate that methapyrilene is a potent animal carcinogen, and its sale may be banned.

See also: Antihistaminics, *Reference Congener in Section III.*

1496   Orphenadrine   1496

N,N-Dimethyl-2-(*o*-methyl-α-phenylbenzyloxy)ethylamine, e.g., Disipal

Toxicity Rating: 5. A close chemical relative of diphenhydramine used in parkinsonism to decrease muscle spasm. Weak antihistaminic and sedative effects. Centrally acting cholinergic blocking drug with minimal peripheral atropine-like side effects. Initial dose regimen is one 50 mg. tablet three times daily. Acute oral LD_{50} in mice 219 mg./kg. In young children doses as low as 600-800 mg. have produced severe intoxications and death. At least two adults expired after ingestion of 1 to 1.5 gm., but with supportive care one adult survived the severe symptoms precipitated by ingestion of 7.5 gm. Signs and symptoms in human poisonings include cyanosis, mydriasis with absent light reflex, deep coma, clonic convulsions, respiratory arrest and alarming disturbances in cardiac mechanisms. Because convulsing patients did not respond to paraldehyde or phenytoin, some victims have been managed by curarization and artificial ventilation. The quinidine-like arrhythmias and conduction defects are probably due to direct effects of the drug on the myocardium; however, correction of electrolyte disturbances and acid-base disorders may be beneficial. In mice both neostigmine and physostigmine increased the toxicity of orphenadrine, but arecoline (because it penetrates the central nervous system?) provided significant protection against the acute lethal effects. Extracorporeal hemodialysis attempted at least once was felt not to result in clinical improvement, and the presence of the drug could not be detected in the dialysis fluid.

See also: Antihistaminics *and* Quinidine, *Reference Congeners in Section III.*
Ref.: Bosche and Mallach, 1969; Heinonen et al., 1968; Stoddart et al., 1968.

1497   Pheniramine Maleate   1497

e.g., Trimeton

Toxicity Rating: 5(?). Antihistaminic used in oral adult doses of 25-50 mg. Overdoses produce inability to concentrate, lassitude, sedation, dizziness, palpitations, muscle weakness, and toxic psychosis; also dryness of mouth, gastrointestinal disturbances, and dermatitis.

See also: Antihistaminics, *Reference Congener in Section III.*
Ref.: Merck and Co., 1960.

1498   Phenyltoloxamine Dihydrogen Citrate

Phenyltoloxamine citrate

Toxicity Rating: 3. An antihistaminic of moderately low toxicity. Adult single dose 100 to 200 mg. Has useful sedative and tranquilizing properties. Prolongs barbiturate-induced sleep. Toxic doses in animals cause central nervous depression, ataxia, emesis, convulsions, and death due to respiratory depression.

See also: Antihistaminics, Reference Congener in Section III.
Ref.: Cronk and Naumann, 1955; Hoekstra et al., 1953.

1499   Pyrilamine Maleate

Neo-Antergan maleate

Toxicity Rating: 5. A potent antihistaminic drug. It probably lies near the borderline between toxicity classes 4 and 5.

See also: Antihistaminics, Reference Congener in Section III.
Ref.: Castillo et al., 1949; Sherrod et al., 1947.

1500   Tripelennamine Hydrochloride

Pyribenzamine hydrochloride

Toxicity Rating: 5(?). A popular antihistamine available in regular and sustained-release tablets. In conventional doses it commonly causes drowsiness, dryness of the mouth and throat and nose, thickening of bronchial secretions, disturbances of coordination and epigastric distress. Overdoses tend to produce coma in adults (except when injected i.v.), whereas CNS stimulation predominates in children. The latter is manifest by excitement, ataxia, incoordination, hallucinations, athetosis, and convulsions, followed by severe post-ictal depression. Mixed with pentazocine, it is injected intravenously by ex-heroin addicts who seek a heroin-like "rush" (see "T's and Blues" below).

See also: Antihistaminics, Reference Congener in Section III.
Ref.: Physicians' Desk Reference, 1981; Towers and Giuffra, 1950.

1501   "T's and Blues"

The common name of an illicit "street drug" widely procured, mixed and consumed by ex-heroin addicts. "T's" refers to the 50-mg. tablet of pentazocine hydrochloride (see in Index) and "Blues" to the blue, 50-mg. tablet of tripelennamine hydrochloride (see above). The mixture (preferably in the ratio of 2 pentazocines to 1 tripelennamine) is commonly dissolved in water, filtered through cotton to remove some of the excipients and injected intravenously. The result is an immediate "rush" (euphoria) lasting 5 to 10 minutes, said to be indistinguishable from the heroin rush. Other effects may also occur: nausea, vomiting, dizziness, tachycardia, tightness in the chest, shortness of breath, muscle spasm and, especially with 1:1 mixtures, tonic-clonic convulsions. The latter are usually ascribed to the tripelennamine. Other complications include pulmonary talc granuloma, pulmonary angiothrombosis, pulmonary hypertension, septicemia, endocarditis, etc. This form of compulsive drug abuse appears to have begun in Chicago in 1976, when heroin addicts became dissatisfied with the poor quality of illicit heroin. The practice is now widespread in major American metropolitan areas. It appears to have replaced an earlier practice of injecting intravenously a mixture of tripelennamine and heroin (or morphine) known in the street as "Blue velvet". Aside from the septic and pulmonary complications listed above, the major therapeutic problem is the underlying narcotic addiction.

See also: Morphine and Antihistaminics, Reference Congeners in Section III.
Ref.: Butch et al., 1979; Showalter, 1980.

Systemic antidotes

1502   N-Acetylcysteine

Mucomyst, Airbron

Toxicity Rating: 2. Originally intended for mucolysis in patients with bronchopulmonary disease, who inhale aerosols of sterile solutions of Mucomyst. It apparently decreases the viscosity of mucoprotein solutions by cleaving disulfide bonds in the macromolecules. Now the investigational drug of choice in the management of acetaminophen poisoning (see Section III), where it apparently functions as a scavenger for the reactive metabolite responsible for hepatic necrosis. The LD_{50} by mouth in the dog is greater than 1 gm./kg., in the mouse greater than 3 gm./kg. and in the rat greater than 6 gm./kg. With intravenous or intraperitoneal administration to the same three species, as well as the guinea pig, LD_{50}'s ranged from 700 mg./kg. in the dog to 2650 mg./kg. in the rat. No serious adverse effects have been reported in the 15 years that it has been in use as a mucolytic agent. Human adults can tolerate 5 gm./day by mouth for 3

Ref.: Anonymous, 1979; McKinney and Sisson, 1979.

months or intravenous doses of 9 gm./day. Vomiting is common after large oral doses, and it occurs sometimes with intravenous administration. A transient maculopapular rash has also been observed.

1503 BAL 1503

Dimercaprol, 2,3-Dimercapto-1-propanol, British Anti-Lewisite

Toxicity Rating: 4(?).

See also: BAL, *Reference Congener in Section III.*

1504 Edetate Calcium Disodium 1504

Calcium Disodium Edetate, Calcium disodium ethylenediaminetetraacetate, Edathamil calcium disodium, Calcium disodium (ethylenedinitrilo)-tetraacetate, $CaNa_2EDTA$

Toxicity Rating: 2.

See also: Edetate Calcium Disodium, *Reference Congener in Section III.*

1505 Deferoxamine 1505

e.g., Desferal

Chelating agent used as an adjunct to the clinical management of acute iron poisoning. Said to be poorly (erratically?) absorbed from the gastrointestinal tract. Oral toxicity data were not located. The intravenous LD_{50}'s in the mouse and rat were about 300 mg./kg. Dogs tolerate single intravenous doses up to 100 mg./kg. with signs suggesting transient hypotension. For patients not in shock from iron poisoning, give 1 gm. intramuscularly, followed by 0.5 gm. every 4 hours for 2 doses. Subsequent

doses of 0.5 gm. may be given every 4 to 12 hours, although the total dose should not exceed 6 gm. in 24 hours. For patients in cardiovascular collapse the drug may be given intravenously in the same doses as above except that the rate of administration should not exceed 15 mg./kg. per hour. Flush, urticaria, hypotension and shock have followed rapid intravenous administration. Deferoxamine is contraindicated in renal failure.

1506 Ethylenediaminetetraacetic Acid (and Salts) 1506

EDTA, Edetic acid

This acid and many of its salts bind metal cations tightly and so render them essentially innocuous. The calcium-disodium salt of this acid is a drug used intravenously to detoxify and enhance the renal excretion of lead and some other heavy metals. This calcium derivative (chelate) has a low

toxicity in experimental animals (toxicity rating of 2 in rats and mice), in contrast to the sodium salts which may cause hypocalcemic tetany and a negative calcium balance. The disodium salt has an oral LD_{50} in mice greater than 1 gm./kg. (toxicity rating of 3?).

See also: Edetate Calcium Disodium, *Reference Congener in Section III.*
Ref.: Wolf, 1976.

1507 *D*-Penicillamine 1507

D-3-Mercaptovaline, β,β-Dimethylcysteine, e.g., Cuprimine

Toxicity Rating: 4. A metabolic product of penicillin that catalyzes disulfide-sulfhydryl exchange reactions. Only the *D*-isomer is used therapeutically. Penicillamine is a metal chelating agent of low oral toxicity. Used to hasten excretion of copper in Wilson's hepatolenticular degeneration. Also promotes the excretion of lead, mercury, arsenic, zinc and probably some other metals. Penicillamine decreases the excretion of cystine and promotes dissolution of cystine calculi. It has been used experimentally in treatment of cystinuria. Also used in treatment of rheumatoid arthritis, where its effectiveness may be due to inhibition of collagen cross-linking reactions. Therapeutic doses may cause fever, drowsiness, stupor, headache, anorexia, nausea and muscle pains. Frequent adverse

reactions to therapeutic courses include nephrotic syndrome and hypersensitivity responses such as rash, fever, and transient blood dyscrasias including leukopenia, thrombocytopenia and eosinophilia. Life-threatening reactions, including aplastic anemia and neutrophilic agranulocytosis, as well as autoimmune diseases such as Goodpasture's syndrome and a lupus-like syndrome, have also been reported. In rheumatoid arthritis patients, both rash and bone marrow suppression may be more common among those who have had similar adverse reactions to gold treatment. Penicillamine treatment during pregnancy is said to have caused a rapidly fatal congenital connective tissue defect in one newborn (Mjolnerod et al., 1971). The *L*-isomer and the racemic mixture are more toxic than the D-isomer: the acute oral LD_{50} of the latter in rats is 365 mg./kg. Rats given toxic doses of the racemic mixture exhibited running fits, excessive salivation and severe convulsions. Deaths generally occurred within 3 to 12 hours. Similar doses of the D-isomer or of the N-acetyl derivative of the mixed isomers were inactive. The higher toxicity of the L-isomer may be referable to a specific inhibitory effect on pyridoxine metabolism in mammals (Du Vigneaud et al., 1957). Repeated doses of the racemic mixture were said to have caused optic neuritis in one patient with Wilson's disease. Vision returned to normal after treatment with pyridoxine hydrochloride (Tu et al., 1963). The N-acetyl derivative is less toxic than the free amine. The adult dose of D-penicillamine is 1-4 gm. per day in divided doses by mouth (usually 0.25 to 0.5 gm. every 6 hours). In chronic lead poisoning (see Section III), adults may receive 250 mg. three or four times daily for many months; with children the usual single dose is 10 mg./kg. or 30-40 mg./kg. per day (but not to exceed 1 gram per day), also given for many months. In mercury poisoning (see Section III) the N-acetyl derivative has often been prescribed in the same doses. In acute arsenic poisoning in children, higher doses of D-penicillamine have been recommended (see Section III). Because cross-sensitivity may exist, D-penicillamine should be used cautiously, if at all, in patients known to be allergic to penicillin.

Ref.: Adams et al., 1964; Aposhian and Aposhian, 1959; Chenoweth, 1968; Du Vigneaud et al., 1957; Jaffe et al., 1964; Mjolnerod et al., 1971; Rosenberg and Hayslett, 1967; Stein and Smythe, 1968; Tu et al., 1963; Weiss et al., 1978a.

1508   1508   Pralidoxime Chloride

2-PAM,   Protopam chloride,   2-Pyridine aldoxime methochloride

An anticholinesterase antagonist found to be of value in the treatment of poisoning due to organophosphorus insecticides and to certain chemical warfare agents (nerve gases). Presumably causes regeneration of cholinesterase that has been inhibited by organic phosphorus compounds. It also reacts chemically with some cholinesterase inhibitors and has certain pharmacological actions of its own. In doses approaching 2.0 gm. in normal subjects common side-effects were dizziness, blurred vision, diplopia, and transient tachycardia. Effective when given with atropine in poisonings by all classes of organophosphorus anticholinesterases, but ineffective or only marginally effective against dimefox, dimethoate, OMPA and phorate according to animal screening tests. It is only moderately effective alone or with atropine against carbamates such as neostigmine and may enhance the toxicity of carbaryl. For more information, see also Parathion and Carbaryl in Section III.

Ref.: Campbell Pharmaceuticals, 1961.

1509   1509   Pyrazole

1,2-Diazole

Toxicity Rating: 3. Pyrazole and 4-methylpyrazole are potent inhibitors of alcohol dehydrogenase and are potentially valuable tools for studying the effects and metabolism of various alcohols. 4-Methylpyrazole (4-MP) in particular may become useful in the management of methyl alcohol and ethylene glycol poisonings. Acute oral LD_{50}'s in rats: pyrazole 1.0 gm./kg., 4-methylpyrazole 534 mg./kg. Livers of rats dying 6 to 11 days after lethal doses of pyrazole showed extensive centrolobular necrosis with inflammatory reactions in the parenchyma and fatty changes in surviving cells. Feeding rats for 24 days retarded growth, increased liver weight, produced mitochondrial and smooth endoplasmic reticulum changes, and induced hyperbilirubinemia and hypoglycemia. Pyrazole is teratogenic in rats, producing a high incidence of ocular and urinary bladder anomalies. Besides its higher acute toxicity, 4-methylpyrazole is a more potent inhibitor of alcohol dehydrogenase than pyrazole. Therefore, it is less toxic in doses that are effective in blocking alcohol metabolism. More importantly the subacute and chronic toxicities of 4-MP are much less than those for pyrazole. Chronic feeding to rats in doses producing a 60% inhibition of alcohol dehydrogenase resulted in no detectable adverse effects.

Ref.: Blomstrand et al., 1980; McMartin et al., 1980; Varma and Persaud, 1979.

1510   1510   Thioctic Acid

α-Lipoic acid,   1,2-Dithiolane-3-pentanoic acid

A growth factor for many bacteria and protozoa and a coenzyme or substrate in plants and animal tissues, it is sometimes regarded as one of the B vitamins. It is possibly effective in protecting the liver against toxic insults and in promoting its regeneration. Kubicka (in 1963) may have been the first to assert its effectiveness in poisonings due to lethal mushrooms of the genus *Amanita*. Many others also claimed successes, but more recent reports have been less enthusiastic. As an experimental antidote against amatoxins (see in Index), it is currently available in ampoules from Dr. Frederic C. Bartter of San Antonio, Texas (phone 512-696-9660, extension 6463). Under his IND no. 9957, the protocol calls for a continuous slow intravenous infusion of 5 percent dextrose (D-glucose) in saline. During the first day of treatment, 25 mg. thioctic acid is added to the infusion 4 times (total dose 100 mg.). Thereafter, the dosage may be increased to 75 mg. four times a day (300 mg. daily). The inclusion of glucose is important because both amatoxins and thioctic acid tend to induce hypoglycemia.

See also: Mushroom Toxins, *Reference Congener in Section III.*
Ref.: Bartter et al., 1980; Kubicka and Alder, 1968.

Synthetic antimalarials and amebicides

1511 Amodiaquin 1511

Toxicity Rating: 4. Synthetic antimalarial and amebicide. Large doses may cause sialorrhea, nausea, vomiting, diarrhea, insomnia, palpitations, syncopé, incoordination, spasticity and convulsions.

See also: Quinidine, *Reference Congener in Section III.*

1512 Chloroquine 1512

e.g., Aralen

Toxicity Rating: 5. One of the 4-aminoquinoline group of suppressant antimalarials also used in discoid and disseminated lupus erythematosus and extra-intestinal amebiasis. Doses of 1 gm. have regularly produced a fulminating cardiorespiratory arrest in children and 3 gm. killed at least one adult. Death may occur in less than 2 hours. Perform gastric lavage and/or give activated charcoal.

See also: Quinidine, *Reference Congener in Section III.*

1513 Diiodohydroxyquin 1513

Diiodohydroxyquinoline, Diodoquin, Iodoquinol

Toxicity Rating: 4(?). Used orally as an amebicide (adult dose 650 mg. 3 times a day) and intravaginally as a trichomonacide. Representative of a large group of similar compounds except that its toxicity is unpredictable. For example, the acute oral LD_{50} of iodochlorhydroxyquin (Vioform) in guinea pigs is 175 mg./kg. and in kittens, 400 mg./kg. In contrast, diiodohydroxyquin in either species was occasionally fatal at doses which ranged from 50 to 2000 mg./kg. Its low solubility must contribute to a highly erratic absorption. Both drugs produced elevated iodine levels in blood, which may interfere for months with some thyroid function tests. Liver damage has been observed in animals. In humans toxic effects may be reminiscent of the effects of iodide salts (see latter). The halogenated derivatives as a group produce frequent allergic reactions in humans with sensitization and cross-sensitization. In one case, ingestion of 1 gm. of dibromohydroxyquinoline and 100 mg. of dibromobenzoxyquinoline by a 68-year–old man produced prompt thrombocytopenia with hemorrhages and subsequent polyneuropathy.

Ref.: David et al., 1944; Liefer and Steiner, 1951; Reinhardt, 1979.

1514 8-Hydroxyquinoline 1514

8-Quinolinol, Oxyquinoline, Oxine

Toxicity Rating: 3(?). A metal chelating agent used as a fungistat and bactericide on textiles and in farm buildings, often as a water-soluble salt such as the sulfate or benzoate. At one time used in clinical medicine as a topical antiseptic. For the treatment of dysentery, men have received oral doses of 3 gm. in solution four times daily, without apparent ill-effects. Rabbits tolerated single doses of 3.7 gm./kg. (as the sulfate, mixed with potassium sulfate). Various halogenated derivatives used in treating amebiasis in man are also comparatively benign except for frequent allergic reactions (see Diiodohydroxyquin above). Hydroxyquinoline is moderately toxic in rats (oral LD_{50} 1.2 gm./kg.). When injected, it is distinctly toxic (rat i.p. LD_{50} 50 mg./kg.) and causes marked stimulation of the central nervous system. Mice given large doses exhibited confusion, respiratory difficulty, hind leg paralysis and violent convulsions, with death within two hours. After smaller fatal doses, death was delayed several days. Toxic symptoms then included anorexia, malaise, and a general indifference to sound and light. After lethal intramuscular doses in mice (30 mg./kg.), injected *D*-penicillamine (1 gm./kg.) prevented symptoms and death but not transient hyperglycemia. Federal registration for use of 8-hydroxyquinoline benzoate in food production was withdrawn in 1969 because repeated doses of the compound caused cancer in laboratory animals.

Ref.: Anderson et al., 1931a; Bernstein et al., 1965; Matsuda and Makino, 1961.

1515 Quinacrine Hydrochloride

Atabrine

Toxicity Rating: 4. Suppressive and alleviative antimalarial also used in amebiasis, atrial fibrillation, rheumatoid arthritis and lupus erythematosus. Acute oral toxicity in rats and monkeys about the same as that of chloroquine. Nausea, vomiting, and diarrhea occur after overdoses or even therapeutic doses when taken on an empty stomach. The skin is turned a peculiar shade of yellow, which is often mistaken for jaundice. Psychic symptoms such as restlessness, excitement, confusion, and delirium are sometimes seen. Aplastic anemia has caused death. Dermatologic disorders are not uncommon. In gross overdoses death is probably due to its quinidine-like actions on the heart.

See also: Quinidine, *Reference Congener in Section III.*
Ref.: Bass et al., 1972; Loeb, 1946; Custer, 1946; Shamberg, 1951.

1516 Primaquine

Toxicity Rating: 5(?). An 8-aminoquinoline antimalarial effective against the exo-erythrocytic forms of the parasite. These drugs are known to produce an intravascular hemolysis sometimes of severe proportions in certain non-Caucasian individuals. This susceptibility is due to the sex-linked inheritance of a deficiency of glucose-6-phosphate dehydrogenase activity in red blood cells, and it is precipitated in these individuals by ordinary therapeutic doses (15 mg./day for 14 days). See Naphthalene in Section III for the management of this reaction. More rarely the drug can provoke methemoglobinemia without hemolysis in individuals deficient in methemoglobin reductase activity. Based on cardiac anti-arrhythmic activity in mice, the drug is predicted to have a toxicity like that of quinidine.

See also: Naphthalene *and* Quinidine, *Reference Congeners in Section III.*
Ref.: Bass et al., 1972; Beutler, 1959; Cohen et al., 1968.

Antiseptic basic dyes

1517 Acridine

10-Azaanthracene

Toxicity Rating: 3. Originally derived from high-boiling tar oils. An intermediate in the synthesis of dyes and antiseptics. See also Acridine antiseptics below. Strongly irritating to skin and mucous membranes. Acute oral LD_{50} in rats 2.14 gm./kg.

Ref.: Fairhall, 1957.

1518 Acridine Antiseptics

e.g.,   Acriflavine, Tryptaflavine, Proflavine, 9-Aminoacridine, 2,8-Diaminoacridine, 3,6-Diaminoacridinium chloride hydrochloride,   2,8-Diamino-10-methylacridinium chloride

Toxicity Rating: 3 to 4. The parent compound of this series is acridine. Trypanocidal activity of acridines was discovered by Ehrlich, and a large number of derivatives have been screened for biological activity. Few, however, have found utility in modern medicine. Some derivatives are useful dyes (acridine orange, acridine yellow). At least one is a systemic chemotherapeutic agent (quinacrine, see index), but most, if used at all, are topical antiseptics. Acriflavine is a mixture of 2,8-diamino-10-methylacridinium chloride and 2,8-diaminoacridine. Proflavine is 3,6-diaminoacridinium chloride hydrochloride. In a large series of derivatives given subcutaneously to mice the acute toxicity was related to the degree of ionization as a cation. Derivatives having pK_a's less than 7.6 (pK_a acridine 4.8) were about three times less toxic than those with pK_a's above 7.6 (pK_a proflavine 10, acriflavine 12). All are irritant to gastrointestinal mucosa and cause nausea and vomiting. Some derivatives are powerful skin photosensitizers. Acriflavine (0.1 to 0.5%) solutions have been used intravenously in humans in doses of 200 mg. without evidence of toxicity. With somewhat higher or repeated doses, however, there are several reports of jaundice and acute toxic (and even fatal) hepatitis. Rabbits exhibit both hepatic and renal damage and some species show profound intravascular hemolysis.

Ref.: Martin, 1944; Rubbo, 1947.

1519 Brilliant Green

Malachite green G,   Ethyl green,   Emerald green

Toxicity Rating: 4. A highly colored substance which has been employed medicinally as an intestinal anthelmintic, a wound antiseptic, and in the treatment of mycotic infections. It has also found use as an agricultural fungicide. Chemically related to gentian violet below. Ingestion causes diarrhea and abdominal pain. Oral doses of 75 mg./kg. in rabbits have caused death. Primary lesions in experimental animals seem to be renal. Note that the name Emerald Green is sometimes used to mean Copper acetoarsenite; if appropriate, see latter in the index.

Ref.: Deschiens and Bablet, 1944; Taylor and Austin, 1918.

1520   Gentian Violet   1520

Toxicity Rating: 4(?). Various isomers of methyl rosaniline chloride; crystal violet is relatively pure hexamethyl-*p*-rosaniline chloride. Occasionally used as an intestinal anthelmintic or topically as an antiseptic or antifungal agent. Prior to about 1950 gentian violet was found in most copying or indelible pencils. They were the cause of many serious ocular injuries. Accidents in which small bits of the writing tip became imbedded in the cornea led frequently to necrosis and permanent opacification. In more recent years pencil manufacturers have replaced gentian violet with acidic (anionic) dyes which are not recognized to produce such damage. Ingestion of gentian violet causes nausea, vomiting, diarrhea and abdominal pain even in therapeutic doses (0.06 gm. three times a day for adults). Severe systemic poisonings have not been reported in man. Intravenous administration to animals produces a sudden, transient rise in blood pressure and death in respiratory failure. In dogs and cattle 10 to 40 ml. i.v. of 1% aqueous solutions of either crystal violet or methyl violet induce numerous dye-protein emboli resulting in thrombosis and infarction of the lungs. The coagulation of heparinized plasma or serum can be produced in vitro by these dyes.

Ref.: Cutlip and Monlux, 1967; Grant, 1962; Pindar and Donnelly, 1925; Sutton, 1938; Wright and Brady, 1940.

1521   Methylene Blue   1521

Methylthionine chloride,   Tetramethylthionine chloride

Toxicity Rating: 4. Used as a bacteriological stain, redox indicator, antiseptic dye and antidote for acquired methemoglobinemia. Well absorbed in man after oral administration. Intraperitoneal LD_{50} in mice 67 mg./kg., with most deaths occurring 2 to 4 days after administration. Although methylene blue is a potent and paradoxical generator of methemoglobin in solutions of hemoglobin at low oxygen tensions, this activity in vivo is so weak that it usually escapes detection. Instead, Heinz bodies and hemolysis occur after large doses in several species. Hemolytic anemia has occurred in man a week after excessive doses of methylene blue. In adults intravenous doses in the range of 500 mg. have produced nausea, abdominal and precordial pain, dizziness, headache, profuse sweating and mental confusion. Additional effects noted after parenteral administration to animals include hemoconcentration, hypothermia, acidosis and hypercapnia, hypoxia, increased blood pressure and increased frequency and amplitude of respiration. For therapeutic doses see Aniline in Section III.

Ref.: Felsenstein et al., 1974; Goluboff and Wheaton, 1961; Macht and Harden, 1933; Nadler et al., 1934; Spicer and Thompson, 1949; Stossel, 1968.

1522   Phenazopyridine Hydrochloride   1522

2,6-Diamino-3-phenylazopyridine hydrochloride, β-Phenylazo-α,α-diaminopyridine hydrochloride, e.g., Pyridium,   Mallophene

Toxicity Rating: 4. A brick-red azo dye once widely used as a urinary antiseptic but now only occasionally employed as a urinary tract analgesic. Animal toxicity data indicate that this compound belongs on the borderline between toxicity classes 3 and 4. Rats given a large intraperitoneal dose exhibited rapid onset of dyspnea, coma, and death. Survivors regained the righting reflex in 4 to 6 hours. Some rats, however, died over the next four days. Methemoglobin accumulation did not account for either early or late deaths. Said to be an irritant and oral doses in dogs produced emesis. Dogs tolerated intravenous doses up to 100 mg./kg. without gross cardiac irregularities, but methemoglobinemia and hemolytic anemia were noted. Chronically treated dogs exhibited anemia and evidence of mild kidney and liver damage. Methemoglobinemia with or without a Heinz body hemolytic component constituted the key feature in at least seven human intoxications. The drug is said to generate methemoglobin in vitro, and at least one attempt to demonstrate antibody formation involving phenazopyridine was unsuccessful. It produces Heinz body anemia in patients whose red cells have normal glucose-6-phosphate dehydrogenase activity, but the reaction is more intense in erythrocytes deficient in this enzyme. Patients with methemoglobinemia, but a clear serum, respond favorably to methylene blue. Exchange transfusion has been successfully employed. A 15-month-old girl survived the ingestion of 8 gm., but exhibited hepatic enlargement and transiently abnormal renal function before complete recovery. Vomitus and urine are deeply stained. Large doses of phenazopyridine hydrochloride have caused adenocarcinomas of the colon of rats.

See also: Aniline *and* Naphthalene, *Reference Congeners in Section III.*
Ref.: Bruton, 1958; Crawford et al., 1951; Gabor et al., 1964; Greenberg and Wong, 1964; National Cancer Institute, 1978q; Sand and Edelmann, 1961; Walton and Lawson, 1934; Wander and Pascoe, 1965.

1523

1523   Tolonium Chloride

Toluidine blue,   3-Amino-1-dimethylamino-2-methyl phenazathionium chloride, e.g., Blutene chloride

Toxicity Rating: 4(?). Basic cationic dye similar in structure to azure A and methylene blue. Used intravenously (100 mg.) or orally (200 to 300 mg./day) for menorrhagia. Antihemorrhagic effects are presumably due to heparin inhibition. Side effects in humans include nausea, vomiting, tenesmus, burning on urination, diarrhea, abdominal pain and hematuria. A 39-year-old nurse in her first trimes-ter of pregnancy may have ingested as much as 8.8 gm. in an effort to arrest vaginal bleeding. Vomiting of deep bluish-purple material was extensive. She complained of chest pain and difficulty in breathing but made an uneventful recovery. Many of the above toxic signs and symptoms have also been elicited by methylene blue (see above). See also discussion under Aniline in Section III.

Ref.: Winek et al., 1969.

1524

1524   Trypan Blue

Toxicity Rating: 3. Trypan blue and the closely-related trypan red are complex derivatives of benzidine once investigated for use in trypanosomiasis. Rats tolerated 1 gm./kg. trypan blue by mouth, whereas parenteral doses in the range of 200-400 mg./kg. produced death, apparently in central nervous depression. Thyroiditis has been described in rats with repeated doses.

Ref.: Anderson et al., 1934; Reuber, 1969; Sollmann, 1957.

Topical and other synthetic anti-infective drugs

1525

1525   Diamthazole Dihydrochloride

6-(2-Diethylaminoethoxy)-2-dimethylaminobenzothiazole dihydrochloride

Toxicity Rating: 4. An antifungal agent used topically in ringworm of the scalp, infections of Candida albicans, and athlete's foot. In mice the oral LD_{50} is 0.5 gm./kg. and the subcutaneous LD_{50} is 0.375 gm./kg. A toxic encephalopathy characterized by ataxia, tremors, convulsions, hallucinations and behavior changes has been reported in infants and very young children after topical use. Contraindi-cated in children under 2 years; it should be used only in reduced amounts in children between 2 and 10. Because of its apparent neurotoxicity it should never be used over extensive areas of the skin. Drug is usually employed in 5% concentrations in tinctures, ointments and powders. No specific treatment is known.

Ref.: Dittmer, 1959; Featherstone, 1952; Hitch, 1952; Wilson et al., 1952.

1526

1526   Furazolidone

3-(5-Nitrofurfurylideneamino)-2-oxazolidinone, e.g., Furoxone

Toxicity Rating: 3. Used in vaginal preparations for trichomonas or other infections. Also in oral tablets and liquids as a bactericide in enteritis. LD_{50} (presumably oral) 4.6 gm./kg. in mice. Toxic doses in animals produced ataxia, weakness, tremors, and convulsions.

Ref.: Eaton Laboratories, 1959.

1527

1527   Haloprogin

2,4,5-Trichlorophenyl-γ-iodopropargyl ether, e.g., Halotex cream

Toxicity Rating: 2(?). A synthetic antifungal recommended for fungal infections of the skin. Its oral toxicity is low (oral doses of 5 gm./kg. produced no toxic symptoms in rats), but it may cause minor skin irritation. The substance is much more toxic when given i.v. (rat LD_{50} 150 mg./kg.), and it penetrates rabbit skin rapidly. However, massive doses of Halotex cream applied dermally induced no signs of toxicity in rabbits. Apparently the compound is rapidly detoxified *in vivo*. Tracer studies indicate that the major metabolic products are 2,4,5-trichlorophenol and its sulfate conjugate, both of which are excreted rapidly in the urine. See Trichlorophenol in the Index. Haloprogin is supplied as a 1% solution in a neutral cream base.

Ref.: Weikel and Bartek, 1972.

1528

1528   Ichthammol

Ichthyol, Ammonium ichthosulfonate

Toxicity Rating: 3(?). Obtained by sulfonating the distillate of certain bituminous schists and neutralizing with ammonia. Contains about 10% sulfur as alkyl derivatives, notably sulfides and mercaptans (half the sulfur), sulfones, and sulfonates. A feeble skin irritant and antiseptic. Formerly prescribed by mouth (200 mg.) as an expectorant. Large doses cause gastrointestinal irritation and diarrhea. No systemic effects are recognized.

Ref.: Osol and Farrar, 1955.

1529 Iodoform 1529

Tri-iodomethane

Toxicity Rating: 4. Best described as lying near the borderline between toxicity classes 4 and 5. Poisoning is often due to absorption through wounds when iodoform dressings are applied (no more than 2 gm. iodoform should be so used). May cause dermatitis. Systemic effects include vomiting and all degrees of cerebral depression or excitation, including delirium, hallucinations, coma and death. A very rapid pulse is characteristic, with or without a slight fever. In rats, iodoform produces severe hepatic degeneration like that observed with carbon tetrachloride. Administration of sulfhydryl compounds may be prophylactic. Iodoform is converted to carbon monoxide in vitro and in vivo. This conversion, if significant in man, could result in the production of carboxyhemoglobin concentrations hazardous to those with impaired cardiovascular status. No useful antidote is recognized, but a trial with *N*-acetylcysteine might prove to be helpful. The odor threshold for iodoform in air is said to be 0.4 ppb.

See also: Carbon Tetrachloride, *Reference Congener in Section III.*
Ref.: Morgenstern, 1963; Sell and Reynolds, 1969; von Oettingen, 1955.

1530 Nitrofurantoin 1530

1-[(5-Nitro-2-furfurylidene)amino]-hydantoin, e.g., Furadantin, Macrodantin

Toxicity Rating: 4. An antibacterial drug used primarily to treat urinary tract infections in oral doses of 50 to 100 mg. four times daily. Common side-effects include nausea, vomiting, diarrhea. Sometimes hypersensitivity reactions are noted such as chills, fever, leukopenia, granulocytopenia, hemolytic anemia (in persons with glucose-6-phosphate dehydrogenase deficiency), cholestatic jaundice and hepatocellular damage. Chronic active hepatitis has occurred in a few patients after 1 to 3 years of continued nitrofurantoin treatment. Elderly patients sometimes exhibit allergic pneumonitis and interstitial pulmonary fibrosis after prolonged use. Vitamin E deficient rats are especially sensitive to severe lung damage by nitrofurantoin. Mild to severe neurologic disorders including irreversible polyneuropathy have been reported. Minimal lethal dose by mouth in mice is 100 mg./kg.

Ref.: Boyd et al., 1979; Gilman et al., 1980; Iwarson et al., 1979.

1531 Nitrofurazone 1531

5-Nitro-2-furaldehyde semicarbazone, e.g., Furacin

Topical antiseptic agent. Oral LD_{50} in mice 1.3 gm./kg. Dogs on high dosage schedules manifested convulsions and paralysis. No specific antidote is known. Has produced contact dermatitis in man.

Ref.: Eaton Laboratories, 1959; George, 1954.

1532 Tolnaftate 1532

O-2-Naphthyl *m,N*-dimethylthiocarbanilate, e.g., Tinactin, Focusan, Sporiline, Tinaderm, Tonoftal, Aftate

Toxicity Rating: 2(?). A topical fungicide for medical use. Very low oral toxicity. Neither single oral doses of 14 gm./kg. nor repeated doses of 0.5 gm./kg. for 30 days induced toxic symptoms in mature dogs. It may cause sensitization or irritation in susceptible persons. Tolnaftate is available in creams, solution, powder and aerosol powder forms, each containing 1% active ingredient.

Ref.: Hashimoto et al., 1966.

Other dermatologic agents

1533 Homosalate 1533

Homomenthyl salicylate, Salicylic acid 3,3,5-trimethylcyclohexyl ester

Toxicity Rating: 3-4(?). Ingredient in over-the-counter sun-screen products. Absorbs ultraviolet light and prevents skin tanning at 15% concentrations. Considered safe in appropriate concentrations by the FDA OTC Panel on Topical Analgesics, Antirheumatic, Otic, Burn, Sunburn Treatment and Prevention Drugs. If the pure liquid were available on the consumer market, probably enough could be ingested to induce symptoms from its hydrolysis products, salicylic acid and homo-

menthol. See also Menthyl Salicylate below.

1534   Menthyl Anthranilate

Menthyl o-aminobenzoate

Toxicity Rating: 3-4(?). Found in some sunscreen preparations intended to be applied to the skin to absorb UV rays that induce sunburn. No toxicity

data were located, but if ingested, this ester is likely to be hydrolyzed in the bowel to menthol and o-aminobenzoic acid (see both in the Index).

1535   Menthyl Salicylate

Toxicity Rating: 3-4(?). Used as a "sun screen" to absorb ultraviolet light in preparations used to prevent sunburn. As an ester it is presumably

hydrolyzed in the alimentary tract to menthol and salicylic acid. See Menthol and Salicylic acid in the index.

1536   Monobenzone

Monobenzyl ether of hydroquinone, 4-(Phenylmethoxy)phenol

Toxicity Rating: 2(?). A more potent depigmentor than hydroquinone no longer marketed in the U.S.A. Applied to the skin, it produced leukoderma, which was sometimes irreversible. Contact dermatitis occurred in 13% of persons using monobenzone ointment, and semipermanent hyperpigmentation occurred in some of them. The use of

monobenzone sometimes resulted in severe dermatitis and bizarre hypo- and hyper-pigmentary changes in the skin even at sites distant from application. Low acute toxicity by mouth. Oral doses of 16 gm./kg. given intermittently for 78 weeks and single subcutaneous doses of 1000 mg./kg. produced neoplasms in mice.

1537   Oxybenzone

Benzophenone-3, 2-Hydroxy-4-methoxybenzophenone

Toxicity Rating: 3(?). A substituted benzophenone used as a chemical sunscreen. The 5-sulfonic acid derivative (sulisobenzone) is used for similar purposes. Topical formulations of .5 to 2% oxybenzone are used on the skin to prevent sunburn and premature aging and to protect against photosensitivity caused by certain drugs. It controls U.V. light at 320 to 400 nm. and absorbs the major portion at 280 to 320 nm. This wide absorption spectrum accounts for the use of benzophenones in many industries. They are often incorporated in textiles

and plastics and are put into transparent shades to protect window displays from U.V. light. They are commonly found in paints and varnishes to preserve color and have widespread use in cosmetics such as hair dyes and soap bars. Although sensitization reactions are rare, both contact dermatitis and urticaria have been noted. No information about the systemic toxicity was found, except for the intraperitoneal LD_{50} of 300 mg./kg. in the mouse.

Ref.: Ramsay et al., 1972.

Synthetic drugs used chiefly in veterinary medicine

1538   2-Amino-5-nitrothiazole

Toxicity Rating: 4(?). Used for treatment of blackhead disease (histomoniasis, a protozoan enterohepatitis) in poultry. No toxicity data were located, but a related compound, 2-aminothiazole, has a

rating of 4 for several laboratory mammals, and single oral doses produce hyperpnea, dyspnea, weakness, hypotension, mild clonic-tonic and asphyxial convulsions, and death in 6 to 24 hours.

Ref.: Osol and Farrar, 1955.

1539   Diethylcarbamazine

1-Diethylcarbamyl-4-methylpiperazine, Hetrazan

Toxicity Rating: 3(?). Used against filariasis in man and animals. Especially popular in veterinary medicine. The average adult man tolerates a single dose of 1.5 gm. without ill effects. Untoward reactions include nausea, vomiting, headache, weak-

ness, and (as seen in dogs) muscle tremors and convulsions. Intravenous injection in dogs produces transient rise in blood pressure and heart rate.

Ref.: Harned et al., 1948.

1540   Dinitolmide   1540

Zoalene, 3,5-Dinitro-*o*-toluamide, 2-Methyl-3,5-dinitrobenzamide

Toxicity Rating: 4(?). Coccidiostat for poultry, used as a feed additive. High oral toxicity in rats. Single oral doses of 150 mg./kg. caused methemoglobin formation in rats. Metabolized in chickens by reduction of either nitro group, followed by partial amide hydrolysis. Primary products are 3-amino-5-nitro-*o*-toluamide, 5-amino-3-nitro-*o*-toluamide and 3-amino-5-nitrotoluic acid. The parent compound and its metabolites are rapidly eliminated in feces.

1541   Nitrophenide   1541

Bis(*m*-nitrophenyl)disulfide, *m,m*-Dinitrophenyl disulfide

An anticoccidial agent used in veterinary medicine. No human poisonings are known, but dogs which were unintentionally fed nitrophenide in cereal developed a nonfatal illness lasting 1 week and characterized by ataxia, vertigo, nystagmus, mydriasis, and opisthotonus.

Ref.: Osol and Farrar, 1955.

1542   Phencyclidine Hydrochloride   1542

1-(1-Phenylcyclohexyl)piperidine hydrochloride, PCP, Sernylan

Toxicity Rating: 6 One of a group of structurally related compounds including ketamine known as the phencyclidines; they possess unique activity in animals and man. Still used as an intravenous or intramuscular anesthetic in veterinary medicine, but discarded for human use because of frequent adverse emergence reactions including confusion, excitement, delirium and hallucinations. Catatonia accompanies states of analgesic-anesthesia in laboratory animals, and catatonic states have been observed in man. The drug is also active by mouth, by inhalation of fine powders and when smoked (often mixed with parsley or marihuana). Perhaps the most commonly encountered hallucinogenic drug of abuse in the United States, but it is often misrepresented as tetrahydrocannabinol, mescaline or LSD. Known by dozens of street names, such as elephant tranquilizer, angel dust, hog, sheets, rocket fuel, etc. Because the effects of PCP as used recreationally differ somewhat from the early clinical experience, pre-existing psychopathology, the dose, the "set" and perhaps the route of administration probably influence the response. PCP has both excitatory and depressant effects that are both somatic and psychic. Intravenous doses of as little as 1 mg. produced subjective effects in human volunteers. Oral doses up to 7.5 mg. have induced drunkenness, blurred vision, visual hallucinations and delusions that mimic schizophrenia. The drug is so potent that intoxications have resulted from "passive smoking" (Welch and Correa, 1980), the inhalation of fumes from illicit laboratories and the handling of confiscated material (Aniline *et al.*, 1980). The more common physical signs include "burst-like" horizontal, vertical and/or rotatory nystagmus, hypertension and agitation or coma. Abusers are often hostile, aggressive and dangerous. Instead of "talking down", the intoxicated individual should be isolated from sensory stimuli, and precautions should be taken to protect against violent and self-destructive acts. PCP has been responsible for several deaths; the mechanism of death was often unclear. The most common serious medical complication may be rhabdomyolysis, sometimes with severe hyperkalemia and acute renal failure (Barton *et al.*, 1980). Cerebrovascular hemorrhages, presumably secondary to hypertension have been reported (Bessen and Torrance, 1982), as also has extreme or "malignant" hyperpyrexia (Jan *et al.*, 1978). Aside from trauma, the most common cause of death is respiratory arrest with or without seizures (Burns and Lerner, 1978). Most of the measures useful in amphetamine poisoning (see Section III) are applicable also in PCP intoxication. Exceptions are that barbiturates are probably best avoided and that butyrophenones may be preferable to phenothiazines to control the psychosis (Khantzian and McKenna, 1979). Even with therapy, psychotic symptoms may persist for weeks (Allen and Young, 1978). Forced diuresis with acidification of the urine, continuous gastric aspiration and activated charcoal with saline catharsis may prevent futher absorption and hasten excretion. As yet untried in humans are calcium blockers, such as verapamil, which prevent and reverse PCP-induced cerebral artery vasospasm *in vitro* (Altura and Altura, 1981). Blood levels of PCP correlate poorly with the intensity of the clinical presentation because the drug is metobolized to active forms and is intensively and even covalently bound in many tissues (Bailey et al., 1978a). Traces may be found in the urine for months after exposure. As if the drug itself were not hazardous enough, some street samples have been found to be contaminated with significant amounts of an intermediate which releases cyanide *in vivo* (Davis *et al.*, 1980).

See also: Amphetamine, *Reference Congener in Section III.*
Ref.: Allen and Young, 1978; Altura and Altura, 1981; Aniline et al., 1980; Bailey et al., 1978a; Barton et al., 1980; Bessen and Torrance, 1982; Burns and Lerner, 1978; Davis et al., 1980; Domino, 1964; Jan et al., 1978; Khantzian and McKenna, 1979; Welch and Correa, 1980.

1543　　　　　　　　1543　Phenothiazine

Thiodiphenylamine

Toxicity Rating: 3. Probably lies near the border-line between toxicity classes 3 and 4. Used as an insecticide and in pharmaceutical manufacturing. At one time employed in human medicine as an anthelmintic and urinary antiseptic. Cumulative therapeutic dose should be kept below 20 gm. Overdosage (and accidental exposures) have caused hemolytic anemia, toxic hepatitis, skin photosensitization, and intense pruritus but apparently not central nervous depression.

See also: Chlorpromazine, *Reference Congener in Section III.*
Ref.: Hubble, 1941.

1544　　　　　　　　1544　Piperazine

Piperazidine,　Diethylenediamine

Toxicity Rating: 2. Used for the treatment of oxyuriasis in man and animals. Especially popular in veterinary medicine. In clinical medicine several of its salts (*e.g.,* citrate, phosphate, adipate, tartrate) are given by mouth, usually to children, in doses up to 150 mg./kg. daily for 2 to 7 days. They are generally well tolerated and excreted in the urine. Lethal doses (in animals) produce convulsions and respiratory depression.

Ref.: Brown et al., 1956a.

1545　　　　　　1545　Piperazine-Carbon Disulfide complex

1-Piperazinecarbodithioic acid,　Picadex,　Parvex

Toxicity Rating: 3(?). Anthelmintic (common brand name Parvex) given orally to horses and ponies in doses of 7.5 gm. (1 fl. oz.)/100 lb. body weight. Also available in 20 gm. boluses. Acute oral LD_{50} in rats is 6 gm./kg. Also marketed as a mixture with phenothiazine called Parvex-Plus, which has a similar toxicity in the rat and contains 5 gm. Parvex and 0.83 gm. phenothiazine in each fluid ounce of suspension. These products are not intended for human consumption, and there have been no reports of symptoms in persons who have handled them in the course of deworming horses. In weak acids, such as those found in the stomach, the complex dissociates into its components piperazine and CS_2; the latter (47% by weight) is the more toxic component. Phenothiazine (see above) in Parvex-Plus might cause hemolytic anemia, skin reactions including photosensitization, and possibly drug fever if that product were ingested by humans.

See also: Carbon Disulfide, *Reference Congener in Section III.*
Ref.: Upjohn Co., 1971.

Sulfonamide drugs

1546　　　　　　　　1546　Sulfonamides

A class of drugs derived from *p*-aminobenzenesulfonamide (sulfanilamide). Although the degree of oral toxicity of the individual drugs depends upon the extent and speed with which they are absorbed and excreted, symptoms of overdose are generally similar. Experimental animals given single toxic doses exhibit salivation, hyperpnea, excitement, muscular weakness, ataxia, athetotic movements, clonic convulsions, paralysis and death from respiratory failure (Lehr, 1940). An overdose of sulfanilamide may lead to acidosis resulting from an interference with carbonic anhydrase activity. In one case of sulfameter overdosage, hypoglycemia was reported with mental confusion and coma. Methemoglobinemia, sulfhemoglobinemia and cyanosis develop occasionally during therapeutic courses. Crystalluria, hematuria and even anuria should be anticipated when large doses of absorbable sulfanilamides are ingested; some of the drugs impair renal function even in the absence of crystalluria. Rarely signs of liver injury, including jaundice and hypoprothrombinemia, are described (see sulfamethoxazole and sulfaquinoxaline below). The long-acting sulfonamides are known to induce Stevens-Johnson syndrome (severe erythema multiforme) during a therapeutic course. Hypersensitivity reactions include rash, urticaria, photosensitivity, drug fever, vasculitis, and serum sickness. Sulfonamide drugs may cause congenital anomalies (e.g., cleft palate and other skeletal defects). Given in late pregnancy or during lactation, they may cause kernicterus in the newborn. Blood dyscrasias such as leukopenia, thrombocytopenic purpura and aplastic anemia have been reported. Persons deficient in glucose-6-phosphate dehydrogenase may develop hemolytic anemia. Sodium salts of the sulfonamides are more readily absorbed and therefore more toxic than the free acids. Their solutions are also generally very alkaline and so may produce mucosal injuries and possibly systemic alkalosis after repeated doses. Treatment of overdosage is primarily symptomatic. Charcoal is a useful antidote if given early. Sodium bicarbonate may be given to raise the pH of the urine and reduce the danger of crystalluria. The sulfonamides are generally dialyzable, and dialysis may be considered in

Ref.: Lehr et al., 1940.

cases of acute poisoning by long-acting sulfonamides or in the presence of renal shutdown.

1547   Phthalylsulfacetamide   1547

4'-(Acetylsulfamoyl)phthalanilic acid, N^1-Acetyl-N^4-phthaloylsulfanilamide, e.g., Thalamyd

Toxicity Rating: 2. A sulfonamide used as an intestinal antimicrobial drug. Although poorly absorbed, its absorption is greater and more variable than that of phthalylsulfathiazole, and side effects

Ref.: Lehr, 1949.

are seen more frequently. Significant blood levels are seldom encountered, but the substance is said to penetrate deeply into the intestinal wall. The usual single therapeutic dose in adults is 2 gm.

1548   Phthalylsulfathiazole   1548

2-(N^4-Phthalylsulfanilamido)thiazole, e.g., Sulfathalidine, Neothalidine, Cremo-Thalidine

Toxicity Rating: 2. A drug used in medical and veterinary practice as an intestinal antibacterial agent. The oral toxicity is limited by poor absorption, but allergic reactions typical of sulfonamides may be seen in sensitized persons. The drug may

cause suppression of vitamin K formation in the intestine, and the Stevens-Johnson syndrome has been reported in patients after a therapeutic course. The usual oral therapeutic dose in adults is 1 to 2 gm. See Sulfonamides above.

1549   Succinylsulfathiazole   1549

4'-(2-Thiazolylsulfamoyl)succinanilic acid, e.g., Cremosuxidine, Sulfasuxidine

Toxicity Rating: 2 or 3. One of the sulfonamides finding medical and veterinary uses as an intestinal antiseptic and in infections of the urinary tract. The oral toxicity of the drug is relatively low because very little is absorbed. Side effects common

to the sulfonamides may be seen in sensitive persons, however. The usual adult therapeutic dose is 1 to 3 gm. For the general symptoms and treatment of sulfonamide toxicity, see Sulfonamides above.

1550   Sulfabromethazine   1550

e.g., Sulfabrom

Toxicity Rating: 3. A long-acting sulfonamide used only in veterinary practice. General signs and treatment of sulfonamide intoxication are given under Sulfonamides above. This compound is excreted

slowly, and consequently there is a greater likelihood of serious side effects such as blood dyscrasias. Crystalluria, however, is unlikely.

1551   Sulfacetamide   1551

N^1-Acetyl sulfanilamide, N^1-Sulfanilacetamide, *p*-Aminobenzenesulfonacetamide

Toxicity Rating: 3. A drug now used primarily in veterinary practice. Sodium sulfacetamide is the only sulfonamide sodium salt which is not strongly alkaline. It is therefore used in a 30% solution in the treatment of infections of the skin and cornea. The drug and its salt are readily absorbed in the

gastrointestinal tract but not reabsorbed after glomerular filtration. They are less likely to lead to urinary concretions than the pyridine derivatives of sulfanilamide. For general symptoms and treatment of overdose, see Sulfonamides above.

1552   Sulfachlorpyridazine   1552

N^1-(6-Chloro-3-pyridazinyl)sulfanilamide, 3-Chloro-6-sulfanilamidopyridazine, e.g., Sonilyn, Nefrosul

Toxicity Rating: 3. A sulfonamide closely related to sulfamethoxypyridazine, this drug is readily absorbed and excreted, and finds medical use in the treatment of urinary tract infections. The usual

adult dose is 1 gm. The symptoms and treatment of sulfachlorpyridazine overdose are similar to those of other sulfonamides (see latter above).

1553   Sulfadiazine   1553

N^1-2-Pyrimidinylsulfanilamide, 2-Sulfanilamidopyrimidine, e.g., Ultradiazine, Coco-Diazine

Toxicity Rating: 3. One of the sulfonamides that is rapidly absorbed and excreted, sulfadiazine is

somewhat less toxic than the sulfapyridines. The sodium salt is supplied as a 5% solution suitable for intravenous use. Sulfadiazine and its salts are more likely to induce leukopenia and crystalluria than most other sulfonamides. In one case of overdose, a 3-year-old girl given a therapeutic course of 450 mg./kg. daily for 3 days developed severe hypoglycemia accompanied by an elevated plasma insulin level and acute renal failure with crystalluria. Following the administration of glucose and interperitoneal dialysis, the child regained consciousness

Ref.: Craft et al., 1977; Kutscher et al., 1954.

but remained anuric. Sulfonamide crystals blocking the ureteral orifices were dissolved by infusing sodium bicarbonate solution into the renal pelvis. The child then made a full and uneventful recovery. The usual adult therapeutic dose of sulfadiazine is 1 to 4 gm. of the acid by mouth or 4 gm. of the sodium salt i.v. Sulfadiazine is present in trisulfapyrimidine preparations.

1554   1554   Sulfadimethoxine

N^1-(2,6-Dimethoxy-4-pyrimidinyl)sulfanilamide, 4-Sulfadimethoxypyrimidine, Sulfadimethoxydiazine, e.g., Madribon

Toxicity Rating: 3. A long-acting drug, now used primarily in veterinary practice. Its administration to humans was discontinued in the U.S.A. because of a high incidence of severe exudative erythema multiforme (the Stevens-Johnson syndrome) resulting from its use. The compound is well ab-

sorbed and slowly excreted, and its toxicity is expected to be similar to that of Sulfameter below. For the more general symptoms and treatment of sulfonamide overdose, see Sulfonamides above. The normal adult dose is 1 to 2 gm. by mouth.

1555   1555   Sulfaethidole

N^1-(5-Ethyl-1,3,4-thiadiazole-2-yl)sulfanilamide, Sulfaethylthiadiazole, e.g., Sethadil

Toxicity Rating: 3. Sulfaethidole is rapidly absorbed and excreted, and is available in a sustained release form. Because of its high solubility in body fluids, the dangers of crystalluria and hematuria are minimal, but the drug has been linked to toxic

hepatitis and thrombocytopenia. For signs and treatment of overdose, see Sulfonamides above. The usual adult oral therapeutic dose is 1.3 gm. every 12 hours.

Ref.: Smith, Kline and French Laboratories, 1963.

1556   1556   Sulfaguanidine

N^1-Amidinosulfanilamide,   p-Aminobenzenesulfonyl guanidine,   Sulfanilylguanidine

Toxicity Rating: 3. A poorly absorbed sulfonamide used now only in veterinary practice. Although blood levels are low because of poor gastrointestinal absorption, side effects are more likely than with phthalylsulfathiazole, which has now largely

replaced it in medical use. The usual adult oral therapeutic dose was 2 gm. For the general symptoms and treatment of sulfonamide toxicity, see Sulfonamides above.

Ref.: Marshall et al., 1940.

1557   1557   Sulfamerazine

N^1-(4-Methyl-2-pyrimidinyl)sulfanilamide

Toxicity Rating: 3. This drug is used primarily in veterinary practice. Clinical use is restricted to trisulfapyrimidine preparations in which it is a component (see latter below). The absorption, excretion and toxicity of sulfamerazine are similar to

those of sulfadiazine. The drug has been implicated in peripheral neuritis. For expected symptoms and recommended treatment of sulfamerazine poisoning, see Sulfonamides above. The usual adult dose is 1 to 4 gm. by mouth.

1558   1558   Sulfameter

Sulfamethoxine, N^1-(5-Methoxy-2-pyrimidinyl)sulfanilamide, 2-(4-Aminobenzenesulfonamido)-5-methoxypyrimidine, Sulfamethoxydiazine, e.g., Sulla

Toxicity Rating: 3. This antibacterial drug is readily absorbed and slowly excreted. In one case of accidental overdose extending over several days, a 7-month-old infant developed oliguria and anuria and extreme hypoglycemia with coma. A transitory thrombocytopenia developed with a normal bone

marrow. The drug has also been associated with Stevens-Johnson syndrome, especially in children. For general symptoms and treatment of overdose, see Sulfonamides above. The normal adult dose is 0.5 gm. daily, after an initial loading dose of 1.5 gm.

Ref.: Robins, 1972.

1559   Sulfamethazine   1559

N^1-(4,6-Dimethyl-2-pyrimidinyl)sulfanilamide, Sulfamethiazine, Sulfadimethylpyrimidine, Sulfadimethyldiazine

Toxicity Rating: 3. This sulfonamide is a component of trisulfapyrimidine preparations. It is rapidly absorbed and excreted and has a toxicity similar to that of sulfadiazine. The sodium salt may induce alkalosis. For other symptoms and treatment of overdosage, see Sulfonamides above.

1560   Sulfamethizole   1560

N^1-(5-Methyl-1,3,4-thiadiazol-2-yl)sulfanilamide, e.g., Thiosulfil, Mesulfin

Toxicity Rating: 3. One of the sulfonamides that is rapidly absorbed and excreted. Its toxicity is similar to that of other sulfonamides. Because it is readily soluble in urine, however, the danger of crystalluria is small. Methenamine should not be given because formaldehyde precipitates may form with sulfamethizole. The normal therapeutic dose is 0.25 to 0.5 gm. For general signs and treatment of overdose, see Sulfonamides above.

1561   Sulfamethoxazole   1561

N^1-(5-Methyl-3-isoxazolyl)sulfanilamide, e.g., Gantanol, Sinomin

Toxicity Rating: 3. A congener of sulfisoxazole, this antibacterial drug is more slowly absorbed and excreted and therefore of longer action. It is more likely to cause crystalluria than sulfisoxazole, although its toxicity is similar. Two cases of hepatitis have been ascribed to administration of this drug for periods of 3 weeks, but serum hepatitis was not adequately ruled out (Macoul, 1966). See Sulfonamides above for a general description of the signs and treatment of overdose. The adult therapeutic dose 1 to 2 gm. daily.

Ref.: Macoul, 1966; Roche Laboratories., 1964.

1562   Sulfamethoxypyridazine   1562

N^1-(6-Methoxy-3-pyridazinyl)sulfanilamide, 3-Sulfanilamido-6-methoxypyridazine, e.g., Kynex, Myasul

Toxicity Rating: 3. This drug, a long-acting sulfonamide, is readily absorbed and slowly excreted. Its toxicology is similar to that of sulfameter (see above). It has been withdrawn from medical use in the U.S.A. because of a high incidence of severe exudative erythema multiforme (the Stevens-Johnson syndrome) resulting from its use. It has a low incidence of side effects in therapeutic doses, and crystalluria is unlikely. Thrombocytopenia has been reported, however.

Ref.: Janovsky, 1960.

1563   Sulfanilamide   1563

p-Aminobenzene sulfonamide

Toxicity Rating: 3. Once the sulfonamide of choice in clinical medicine, now limited largely to veterinary practice. In contrast to many other sulfonamides it rarely produces urinary tract injury by precipitating within the kidney. Its higher water solubility, however, is reflected in a higher acute toxicity. Lethal doses in animals produce ataxia, clonic convulsions, paralysis and death from respiratory failure. Side effects in man include nausea, vomiting, fever, cyanosis, dizziness, dermatitis, acidosis, hepatitis, and psychosis. The acidosis has been traced to the inhibition of carbonic anhydrase. Certain blood dyscrasias such as leukopenia, agranulocytosis, hemolytic anemia and altered blood pigments (methemoglobinemia) are frequently seen. The latter two conditions are believed to involve the same mechanisms as in the Heinz body anemia induced by naphthalene and primaquin. See Naphthalene in Section III. No specific antagonists are known.

Ref.: Beutler, 1959; Fisher and Haag, 1942; Harris and Michel, 1939; Long et al., 1940b; Molitor and Robinson, 1939.

1564   Sulfapyridine   1564

N^1-2-Pyridinylsulfanilamide

Toxicity Rating: 3. One of the earliest sulfonamides to be used therapeutically but now largely replaced by related compounds that are less toxic and more effective. The drug is absorbed poorly in the stomach but somewhat more readily in the intestine. It is likely to induce crystalluria. Large doses caused vomiting in dogs, with a temporary decrease in renal clearance seen after a dose of only 0.25 gm./

kg. All twelve monkeys fed 0.5 gm. daily died within 10 days. Autopsies showed pyelonephritis with concretions in the urinary bladder and kidneys. The sodium salt is strongly basic; it is more soluble and more readily absorbed than the free acid. Large doses of the sodium salt caused excitement, rigidity, auditory and tactile hyperesthesia, dyspnea and running convulsions in 10 to 15 minutes in mice. Death followed in 0.5 to 6 hours. For the treatment of overdoses, see Sulfonamides above.

Ref.: Marshall and Litchfield, 1939; Toomey et al., 1940.

1565 Sulfaquinoxaline

N^1-2-Quinoxalinylsulfanilamide, 2-*p*-Aminobenzenesulfonamidoquinoxaline, 2-Sulfanilamidoquinoxaline, Sulfabenzpyrazine, e.g., Sulquin

Toxicity Rating: 2. A drug used only in veterinary practice, often as a feed additive to treat intestinal coccidiosis in fowl. It is among the least soluble of the sulfonamides. Although it is quite toxic when given subcutaneously, poor absorption limits its oral toxicity. Sulfaquinoxaline is unique among the sulfonamides in that it induces in rats and dogs prompt hypoprothrombinemia which may lead to fatal hemorrhages but which may be counteracted by vitamin K_1 therapy. No human data known. Crystalluria is somewhat less likely than with other congeners. For general symptoms and treatment of overdoses, see Sulfonamides above. For management of hypoprothrombinemia, see Warfarin in Section III.

Ref.: Seeler et al., 1944; Mushett and Seeler, 1947.

1566 Sulfasalazine

Salicylazosulfapyridine, e.g., Azulfidine, Rorasul, Sulcolon

A diazotization product formed from sulfapyridine and salicylic acid and recommended for the treatment of ulcerative colitis. The drug is partially absorbed from the intestine. The remainder is hydrolyzed in the colon where the sulfapyridine and 5-aminosalicylic acid are absorbed. The drug is capable of producing oxidative (Heinz-body) hemolytic anemia. Transient reticulocytosis, cyanosis, leukopenia and agranulocytosis, neurotoxicity and pancreatitis have also been reported in patients receiving therapeutic doses.

Ref.: Das et al., 1973; Gabor, 1973.

1567 Sulfathiazole

N^1-2-Thiazolylsulfanilamide, 2-Sulfanilamidothiazole, e.g., Sultrin

Toxicity Rating: 3. One of the oldest of the sulfonamides, now used primarily in veterinary practice. The drug is readily absorbed and excreted. The incidence of serious side effects is the highest seen among the sulfonamides. See Sulfonamides above for a full discussion of side effects and of the signs and treatment of overdose.

Ref.: Long et al., 1940a; Long et al., 1940b.

1568 Sulfisoxazole

N-(3,4-Dimethyl-5-isoxazolyl)sulfanilamide, 3,4-Dimethyl-5-sulfanil-amidoisoxazole, e.g., Gantrisin, SK-Soxazole, Sosol, Soxomide

Toxicity Rating: 2. A sulfonamide drug that is well absorbed, readily excreted and usually well tolerated. Because of its high solubility in body fluids, the compound is less likely to cause crystalluria than other sulfonamides. Furthermore, sulfisoxazole, unlike other sulfonamide drugs, is confined to extracellular fluids. Implicated in several cases of agranulocytosis, including a case of congenital agranulocytosis seen after treatment of the mother in late pregnancy. Leukopenia has also been reported, as well as thrombocytopenic purpura. Sulfisoxazole is alleged to have reactivated lupus erythematosus and has been implicated in pancreatitis. The acetyl derivative of sulfisoxazole (Lipo-Gantrisin) is tasteless and therefore preferred by children. It is slowly deacetylated in the small intestine and absorbed. The diethanolamine salt is supplied as a 40% solution suitable for slow intravenous injection. The usual daily dose in adults is 4 to 12 gm. of sulfisoxazole or 4 to 5 gm. of the acetyl derivative. The diethanolamine derivative is given i.v. in a dose of 4 gm. two or three times per day.

Ref.: Roche Laboratories., 1964.

1569 Trisulfapyrimidines

A mixture of equal amounts of Sulfadiazine, Sulfamerazine and Sulfamethazine. The therapeutic efficacy of the combination is said to equal the sum of the efficacies of its components, but the tendency toward crystalluria is greatly reduced because the concentration of each component is only one-third of that normally employed. See above for comments about each component. For general

signs and symptoms of sulfonamide overdose, see Sulfonamides above.

Anti-inflammatory and related pyrazones

1570 Aminopyrine 1570

4-(Dimethylamino)-1,2-dihydro-1,5-dimethyl-2-phenyl-3*H*-pyrazol-3-one, Dimethylaminoantipyrine, Pyramidon, Amidopyrine, Aminophenazone

Toxicity Rating: 4. Analgesic, antipyretic and antiinflammatory drug now used only in veterinary medicine. Moderate oral toxicity in mammals (rat oral LD_{50} 600 mg./kg.). Dose response in humans is highly variable, and some untoward reactions appear to be allergic. In a 2-year-old child, 0.25 gm. has proven fatal. More rapidly absorbed and hence more toxic when given rectally. Aminopyrine has an initial excitatory effect on the central nervous system and a strong spasmolytic effect on smooth muscle of peripheral blood vessels. In human poisonings, the initial toxic symptoms are irritability, vomiting and copious sweating, progressing rapidly to epileptiform or tetanic convulsions, cyanosis, and coma. Pupils are dilated. Death is due to circulatory failure following cardiovascular collapse. After large doses, symptoms appear in minutes and death occurs promptly. Sublethal doses may also induce palsy, sharp drop and then rise in body temperature, sweating, tinnitus, dysuria, dyspnea and anxiety. Recovery is usually rapid, but in one case convalescence was slow and complicated by tenesmus, urinary frequency and intermittent fever. At autopsy, severe congestion, edema and perivascular hemorrhage in meninges, brain, lungs, spleen, kidney and liver are described. Necrotic lesions are found in ganglion cells of the motor cortex and brain stem. Fatty infiltration of liver and focal parenchymal degeneration of heart muscle and kidneys have been reported. Subendocardial hemorrhage in the left chamber is often seen. Aminopyrine has no effect on red blood cells or hemoglobin. In humans, the primary metabolites are 4-aminoantipyrine, *N*-acetyl-4-aminoantipyrine and 4-hydroxyantipyrine. They are rapidly excreted in urine. In cows, symptoms of intoxication following intravenous injections of 4-aminoantipyrine were similar to those following toxic doses of aminopyrine. The parent compound and all of the metabolites were found in milk from cows receiving aminopyrine therapy. Medical use of aminopyrine has been discontinued because of a high incidence of agranulocytosis in persons taking the drug for extended periods.

Ref.: Banerjee et al., 1967a; Banerjee et al., 1967b; Brodie and Axelrod, 1950; Fazekas, 1957; Gossner, 1952; Jansch and Wolkart, 1954.

1571 Antipyrine 1571

1,2-Dihydro-1,5-dimethyl-2-phenyl-3*H*-pyrazol-3-one, Phenazone, Phenyl dimethyl pyrazolone, e.g., Auralgan

Toxicity Rating: 4. Analgesic and antipyretic drug now used only topically in otic drugs for its antiinflammatory effect. Internal use was discontinued because of the high incidence of agranulocytosis in patients given therapeutic courses. Signs and symptoms of intoxication are like those for aminopyrine, but acute oral toxicity is somewhat less

(rat oral LD_{50} 1.8 gm./kg.). Antipyrine, but not other pyrazones, may cause methemoglobinemia. For management of methemoglobinemia, see Aniline in Section III. Skin rashes which are common after repeated exposures may persist for several weeks; they may resemble the erythematous macules seen after phenolphthalein.

Ref.: McCulloch and Zeligman, 1951.

1572 Dichloralphenazone 1572

Dichloralantipyrine, e.g., Midrin, Welldorm

Mild sedative and hypnotic, also used in headache preparations for relief of associated anxiety. A complex of chloral hydrate (see in index) and phenylbutazone (see below). Dissociates in water or alcohol and therefore may produce toxic effects of either compound. An overdose usually induces vomiting. A 65-year-old man who took 39 to 65 gm. of the compound with four ounces of rum went

into coma and died within three hours. At autopsy marked edema of the lungs and intense congestion of the stomach mucosa were observed. Continued use may induce dependency and renal damage. Because of phenylbutazone content, ingestion of the drug may cause serious complications in persons undergoing MAO inhibitor therapy and in those with hypotension, liver or kidney diseases.

Ref.: Curry, 1962; Physicians' Desk Reference, 1981.

1573 Dipyrone 1573

Methylaminoantipyrine methanesulfonate sodium, 1-Phenyl-2,3-dimethyl-5-pyrazolone-4-methylaminomethanesulfonate sodium, e.g., Novaldin

Toxicity Rating: 4(?). Antipyretic drug usually available as the monohydrate and closely related

to antipyrine (see above). Previously called methampyrone. Same activity, including serious side-effects, as antipyrine. More soluble, hence more readily absorbed and more toxic than antipyrine. Has caused agranulocytosis, thrombocytopenic purpura and aplastic anemia. May accentuate hypoprothrombinemia. The usual adult dose is 500 mg. Allergic reactions, including asthma and angioedema, have been reported.

Ref.: A.M.A. Department of Drugs., 1977; Huguley, 1964.

1574　　1574　Oxyphenbutazone

4-Butyl-1-(4-hydroxyphenyl)-2-phenyl-3,5-pyrazolidinedione, e.g., Oxalid, Tandearil

Toxicity Rating: 4. Antiinflammatory drug used in treatment of gout and arthritis. The primary metabolite of phenylbutazone (see entry below). Identical to phenylbutazone in mode of action, therapeutic uses and adverse reactions. Acute oral toxicity is somewhat greater than that of the parent compound in experimental animals, but oxyphenbutazone may cause less gastric irritation. The drug is also used in ointment form to suppress ocular inflammation. It is absorbed through the cornea and distributed throughout the tissues of the eye, but cannot be detected in the bloodstream. The ointment may cause conjunctival irritation in sensitized persons.

Ref.: A.M.A. Department of Drugs., 1977; Domenjoz, 1960; Murphy, 1973; Physicians' Desk Reference, 1981.

1575　　1575　Phenylbutazone

4-Butyl-1,2-diphenyl-3,5-pyrazolidinedione, e.g., Azolid, Butazolidin

Toxicity Rating: 4. Antiinflammatory drug used in the treatment of gout and arthritis. The acute oral toxicity is very high. In humans large single doses induce nausea, vomiting, epigastric pain, excessive perspiring, tinnitus, cyanosis, respiratory depression, agitation, hallucinations, convulsions followed by stupor and coma. Sodium retention may lead to edema and hypertension. Ulceration of the buccal and gastrointestinal mucosa may occur, and reactivation of pre-existing peptic ulcers should be anticipated. Even therapeutic courses have occasionally produced serious side-effects, especially in older people. They include (in addition to the above) ulcerative esophagitis, hepatic necrosis and renal damage, including glomerulonephritis, renal cortical necrosis and renal stones, progressing to renal failure. Cardiac toxicity is revealed by pericarditis, diffuse interstitial myocarditis with muscle necrosis, and perivascular granulomata. Blood dyscrasias, especially agranulocytosis, aplastic anemia, hemolytic anemia, thrombocytopenic purpura, pancytopenia, leukopenia and leukemia occur occasionally. Both phenylbutazone and its metabolite, oxyphenhydrazone, suppress incorporation of tritiated thymidine by human bone marrow cells in tissue culture. Reported allergic reactions include rash, urticaria, arthralgia, exfoliative dermatitis, Lyell's syndrome, Steven-Johnson syndrome, erythema multiforme, and anaphylactic shock. Phenylbutazone may induce an optic neuritis causing blurred vision. Toxic amblyopia and detached retina have been reported. The drug inhibits iodine uptake by the thyroid and potentiates the action of coumarin anticoagulants and insulin. In man phenylbutazone is rapidly and completely absorbed and slowly excreted. Radiotracer experiments indicate that the primary metabolites are oxyphenbutazone (see above), ψ-hydroxyphenylbutazone, and several dihydroxy derivatives, all excreted as glucuronide conjugates. In cases of acute intoxication only supportive therapy is available, but respiratory stimulants should not be used. The usual adult dose is 100 mg. 3 to 4 times daily.

Ref.: A.M.A. Department of Drugs., 1977; Dewse and Potter, 1975; Dieterle et al., 1976; Domenjoz, 1960; McCarthy and Chalmers, 1964; Physicians' Desk Reference, 1981; Tubaro et al., 1970.

1576　　1576　Sulfinpyrazone

1,2-Diphenyl-4-(2-(phenylsulfinyl)ethyl)-3,5-pyrazolidinedione, e.g., Anturane

Toxicity Rating: 4. Uricosuric drug used in treatment of gout. Closely related to oxyphenbutazone and phenylbutazone (see above). Symptoms of acute intoxication are the same as those from phenylbutazone, but the lethality is greater because sulfinpyrazone is more rapidly absorbed from the gut. Hydroxylation and excretion of the drug is also rapid. Serious side-effects, including allergic reactions, occur less frequently than with other pyrazone compounds, although anemia, leukopenia, agranulocytosis and thrombocytopenia have been reported. The drug may reactivate or exacerbate peptic ulcer and potentiate the action of insulin. Unlike other pyrazones, sulfinpyrazone may aggravate renal calculi and can precipitate attacks of gout in asymptomatic persons with high serum uric acid levels. In animal feeding experiments, the compound induced hyperemia of the stomach, petechial bleeding and ulceration of the gastric mucosa. Sulfinpyrazone, but not other pyrazones, produced a moderate retardation of renal tubular function (PSP clearance). In man, the drug is 98% bound to plasma protein. The usual adult dose is 200 mg. twice daily.

Ref.: A.M.A. Department of Drugs., 1977; Dayton et al., 1961; Domenjoz, 1960; Physicians' Desk Reference, 1981.

Local anesthetics

1577 Benzocaine 1577

Ethyl p-aminobenzoate

Toxicity Rating: 3(?). A local anesthetic of low acute toxicity found in many proprietary products. Other aminobenzoate esters are also used as local anesthetic agents, e.g., butyl, isobutyl, diethyl-aminoethyl, etc. Despite its low water solubility and poor absorption from most sites, a number of instances of severe acquired methemoglobinemia have occurred in both children and adults. Such reactions have followed topical application of ben-zocaine in ointments, the use of rectal suppositories and ingestion. In at least some of these cases sys-temic absorption may have been enhanced by in-flamed skin, rectal fissures or gastritis. Oral doses of 150 to 300 mg. produced cyanosis in four adults within four hours. The relative rarity of these episodes suggest a genetic predisposition to this reaction, but in at least one patient a normal eryth-rocytic methemoglobin reductase activity was found. The methemoglobinemia responds dramat-ically to methylene blue. Acute human poisonings with other prominent systemic effects do not ap-pear to have been reported, but central nervous excitement is predicted.

See also: Aniline and Cocaine, Reference Congeners in Section III.
Ref.: Bernstein, 1950; Block, 1965; Goluboff and MacFadyen, 1955; Goluboff, 1958; Haggerty, 1962; Hughes, 1965; Peterson, 1960; Steinberg and Zeppernick, 1962; Wolff, 1957.

1578 Bupivacaine 1578

1-Butyl-2′,6′-pipecoloxylidide, Marcaine

Toxicity Rating: 4. Amide-type local anesthetic related to mepivacaine and lidocaine (see below) but with a much longer duration of action. Used for infiltration, nerve block and epidural anesthe-sia, but not currently used for spinal anesthesia. Should not be injected intravenously. Inadvertent intravascular administration has resulted in almost simultaneous seizures and cardiovascular collapse without antecedent hypoxia. Prolonged block of more than 60 hours followed extradural injection of 90 mg. of bupivacaine (0.5% plain) in a 26-year-old woman in labor. The scalp of a 23-year-old epileptic was infiltrated with 750 mg. of bupiva-caine (4 times the usual recommended dose). Six minutes later she began convulsing. Diazepam was effective in controlling the seizures. Unusual in this case was the administration of lidocaine (see below) to aid in the conversion of ventricular tachycardia. The patient's recovery was uneventful. The mouse i.p. CD_{50} (median convulsant dose) and LD_{50} were 57.7 and 58.7 mg./kg. respectively. The hydrochlo-ride is available in solutions for injection (0.25, 0.5 and 0.75% with or without epinephrine 1:200,000).

See also: Cocaine, Reference Congener in Section III.
Ref.: Davis and De Jong, 1982; De Jong and Bonin, 1980; Pathy and Rosen, 1975.

1579 Butamben 1579

Butyl p-aminobenzoate, Butesin

Toxicity Rating: 3(?). One of several related esters of p-aminobenzoic acid used as topical local anes-thetics. Because of its low water solubility, it pro-duces a prolonged anesthetic effect and only rarely systemic toxicity. However, local hypersensitivity reactions (rash, erythema, pruritis) do occur occa-sionally. If absorbed, it is probably hydrolyzed to p-aminobenzoic acid (see in Index). The intraperi-toneal LD_{50} in the mouse is 67 mg./kg.

See also: Cocaine, Reference Congener in Section III.

1580 Dibucaine 1580

2-Butoxy-N-(2-(diethylamino)ethyl)-4-quinolinecarboxamide, Nupercaine, Nupercainal

Toxicity Rating: 5(?). This amide-type local anes-thetic is a quinoline derivative. One of the most potent, toxic and longest-acting of the common local anesthetics, it is used for surface and spinal anesthesia. Isobaric, hypobaric (light) and hyper-baric (heavy) solutions are available for subarach-noid anesthesia. Topical preparations include cream, ointment, suppositories and throat lozenges. A 3-year-old child ingested 8 lozenges each con-taining 1 mg.(?) of dibucaine hydrochloride. Gastric lavage was started twenty minutes after ingestion. Hypotension, reduced pulse rate, anoxia and a generalized nonpitting edema of the whole body developed, but no convulsions. The child died in coma 8 hours later in spite of supportive measures. A 13-year-old girl developed a photosensitivity re-action to dibucaine which was used as a local anesthetic for her dental treatment.

See also: Cocaine, Reference Congener in Section III.
Ref.: Deichmann and Gerarde, 1969; Horio, 1979.

1581　Etidocaine

1581

N-(2,6-Dimethylphenyl)-2-(ethylpropylamino) butanamide,　Duranest

Toxicity Rating: 4. A long-acting (5-10 hours) local anesthetic of the amide type related to lidocaine and similar to bupivacaine. Indicated for epidural and all types of regional and infiltration anesthesia (not for spinal anesthesia). Produces a profound degree of motor blockade. The maximal dose as a single injection should not exceed 5.5 mg./kg. with epinephrine 1:200,000 or 4 mg./kg. without epinephrine. For symptoms and treatment of overdosage see Lidocaine (below).

See also: Cocaine, *Reference Congener in Section III.*

1582　Lidocaine

1582

2-(Diethylamino)-*N*-(2,6-dimethylphenyl)acetamide,　Xylocaine

Toxicity Rating: 4. This substituted amide is widely used as a local anesthetic and as an antiarrhythmic agent. More prompt, intense, long-lasting and toxic than procaine. The oral mouse LD_{50} is 457 mg./kg. Quickly absorbed from mucous membranes including the G.I. tract. Because it undergoes extensive and rapid hepatic metabolism, only about one-third of an oral dose reaches the systemic circulation. However, two of the metabolites (monoethylglycylxylidide and glycine xylidide) have some anesthetic and toxic activity. Overdoses produce CNS and cardiovascular effects, including drowsiness, dizziness, paresthesias, muscle twitching, dysarthria, blurred vision, vomiting, hypotension, bradycardia, respiratory arrest, convulsions and death. Methemoglobinemia has also been reported. Deaths have occurred from overdoses of intravenous lidocaine and from several accidental ingestions of topical lidocaine preparations. A 22-month-old girl ingested about 50 mg./kg. of Xylocaine 2% Viscous (lidocaine hydrochloride). Convulsions, cyanosis, hypertension, tachycardia and respiratory arrest followed. She was successfully resuscitated, and her seizures were controlled with i.v. diazepam. In a similar case an 18-month-old girl swallowed 80 ml. of an orange-flavored preparation of lidocaine hydrochloride jelly 2% (calculated ingested dose 1.6 gm.). Thirty minutes later she began convulsing; cyanosis and respiratory arrest followed. Diazepam (i.v.) eliminated the seizures and gastric lavage recovered approximately 30 ml. of the product. The child's condition, however, continued to deteriorate (cold perspiration, dilated pupils unresponsive to light, muscle twitching, hypotension and extreme bradycardia). She was given i.v. pancuronium bromide, and an endotracheal tube was inserted. Several hours later her condition was good and she recovered. A 74-year-old woman who accidentally swallowed 1200 mg. (38.7 mg./kg.) of 4% topical lidocaine became agitated, combative and disoriented. Sinus tachycardia was present. The plasma lidocaine concentration was 10 μg./ml. (therapeutic level 1-5 μg./ml.). The symptoms of delirium were completely resolved in about 4 hours, at which time the lidocaine level was 6.3 μg./ml. A 27-year-old woman died after swallowing 10 gm. lidocaine hydrochloride (119 mg./kg.). Treatment should include respiratory support and i.v. diazepam to control convulsions. Cardiac massage or extracorporeal pump assistance may be required to sustain blood flow and arterial pressure. As long as hepatic blood flow is maintained, lidocaine is cleared by metabolism at a rate of 900-1000 ml./min., which is much higher than can ever be achieved with hemoperfusion or hemodialysis.

See also: Cocaine, *Reference Congener in Section III.*
Ref.: Fruncillo et al., 1982; Rahde, 1979; Sakai and Lattin, 1980; Stadler et al., 1979.

1583　Mepivacaine

1583

1-Methyl-2′,6′-pipecoloxylidide,　Carbocaine,　Mepivacaine hydrochloride

Toxicity Rating: 4. Synthetic local anesthetic drug of the amide type. Similar chemically and pharmacologically to lidocaine (see above), but it has a more rapid onset and longer duration of action without the drowsiness seen with lidocaine. The oral mouse LD_{50} is 310 mg./kg. Used for all types of infiltration, nerve block, epidural and intravenous regional anesthesias, but not effective topically except in large doses and therefore not used for that purpose. Its popularity as a caudal anesthetic in obstetrics has resulted in several cases of accidental intoxication of the fetus. The triad of apnea, bradycardia (persisting despite oxygenation) and convulsions is commonly observed in poisoned newborns. Treatment includes diazepam for convulsions and positive-pressure ventilation. Since this drug is believed to be concentrated in gastric juice, some of these infants have been treated by repeated gastric lavage and exchange transfusions. The hydrochloride is marketed in solutions for injection (2% with levonordefrin and 1.0, 2.0 and 3.0% without vasoconstrictor).

See also: Cocaine, *Reference Congener in Section III.*
Ref.: Gilman et al., 1980; Sinclair et al., 1965.

1584　Prilocaine

1584

2-(Propylamino)-*o*-propionotoluidide,　Citanest

Toxicity Rating: 4(?). An amide-type local anesthetic pharmacologically similar to lidocaine (see above), but with a longer duration of action. Used for all types of infiltration and regional anesthesia.

Like lidocaine it may cause drowsiness. Found to produce methemoglobinemia both *in vitro* and *in vivo*, and its use is declining for this reason. A dose-response relationship seems to exist between the amount of prilocaine injected and the incidence and degree of methemoglobin formed. The methemoglobinemia responds to treatment with methylene blue, as in aniline poisoning.

See also: Cocaine *and* Aniline, *Reference Congeners in Section III.*
Ref.: Bridenbaugh et al., 1969; Daly et al., 1964.

1585 Procaine   1585

2-Diethylaminoethyl *p*-aminobenzoate, e.g., Novocaine, Gerovital

Toxicity Rating: 3(?). This aminobenzoate ester is a short-acting local anesthetic used for infiltration, epidural and subarachnoid anesthesia (not used topically). Toxicity rating is based on scanty data from oral administration to mice. The possibility of poisoning from ingestion would appear remote; we know of no cases. Indeed, it is a matter of conjecture as to whether enough unhydrolyzed procaine could be absorbed by this route to produce toxic signs. Rapidly hydrolyzed (mainly by plasma cholinesterase but to a small extent by liver esterase) to *p*-aminobenzoic acid and diethylaminoethanol, which have low toxicities. However, *p*-aminobenzoic acid inhibits the action of sulfonamides. Following absorption from parenteral routes, procaine is a central nervous stimulant, producing restlessness and tremors proceeding to clonic convulsions. Stimulation is followed by depression, and death is usually due to respiratory failure. Artificial respiration is a useful measure, but respiratory stimulants are ineffective and irrational. Procaine acts on the myocardium to reduce excitability, slow conduction and weaken the force of contraction. On rare occasions small doses have produced cardiovascular collapse and death. In contrast, an adult pretreated with thiopental, hexafluorenium and succinylcholine survived the accidental intravenous administration of 4 grams of procaine (43 mg./kg.). The time-honored treatment is aimed at controlling procaine convulsions with barbiturates, but benzodiazepines (*e.g.*, diazepam) are now preferred. Hypersensitivity to ester-type local anesthetics has been reported. The systemic administration of procaine (Gerovital) is claimed to delay the aging process and favorably alter the course of common chronic diseases of middle and later life. However, an extensive review of the literature by Ostfeld *et al.*, 1977 suggests that aside from an antidepressant effect these claims are unsubstantiated.

See also: Cocaine, *Reference Congener in Section III.*
Ref.: Gilman et al., 1980; Moore and Bridenbaugh, 1960; Ostfeld et al., 1977; Wikinski et al., 1970.

1586 Tetracaine   1586

4-(Butylamino)benzoic acid 2-(dimethylamino)ethyl ester, Pontocaine

Toxicity Rating: 5(?). This ester of *p*-aminobenzoic acid is used for surface, subarachnoid and epidural anesthesia. Available in ophthalmic solutions (0.5%) and creams, 2% solutions for topical use on mucous membranes, and ampuls containing 20 mg. of the hydrochloride. A dose of 10 to 20 mg. is usually sufficient for spinal anesthesia in adults. It has a comparatively slow onset and long duration of action, but it can be rapidly absorbed from mucous membranes. Like other local anesthetics it behaves as a convulsant when it reaches the brain. If a solution were swallowed, it is unlikely that appreciable amounts of unhydrolyzed drug could reach the systemic circulation from the stomach or bowel; under these circumstances, however, absorption from the mucous membranes of the mouth, pharynx and esophagus might deliver critical amounts to the brain. A 48-year-old woman received 3 ml. of 2% tetracaine hydrochloride (60 mg.) through a nasal catheter in preparation for bronchoscopy (no premedication). She quickly became comatose, convulsed repeatedly and died 30 minutes later despite parenteral phenobarbital. A 63-year-old man survived a pharyngeal-laryngeal spraying with 20 ml. of 5% tetracaine hydrochloride (1000 mg.), but heroic measures were required to control his convulsions. Tetracaine's slow rate of ester hydrolysis in plasma and in the liver presumably contributes to its high toxicity. Ewert (1967) demonstrated that tetracaine arrested mucus flow and ciliary activity in the cat trachea and mucus flow in the human nose. Hypersensitivity reactions are not uncommon (asthmatic crisis, contact dermatitis and anaphylactoid reaction).

See also: Cocaine, *Reference Congener in Section III.*
Ref.: Balamoutsos and Alevizou-Christophoridou, 1979; Ewert, 1967.

Miscellaneous synthetic drugs

1587 Acetaminophen   1587

4′-Hydroxyacetanilide, *N*-Acetyl-*p*-aminophenol, APAP, Paracetamol

Toxicity Rating: 4. An antipyretic-analgesic drug. A potentially toxic dose by mouth in an adult person is 10 gm. It is essential that treatment begin as soon as possible after ingestion to prevent the development of hepatic necrosis.

See also: Acetaminophen, *Reference Congener in Section III.*
Ref.: Done, 1959; MacLean et al., 1968.

1588

1588 Benzothiadiazide Diuretics

Benzthiazide, Hydrochlorothiazide, Hydrobenzthiazide, Chlorthalidone, Chlorothiazide, Trichlormethiazide, Polythiazide, Bendroflumethiazide, Methylclothiazide

Toxicity Rating: 3. A large group of therapeutic agents which includes chlorothiazide, hydrochlorothiazide, benzthiazide, hydrobenzthiazide, polythiazide, trichlormethiazide, chlorthalidone and many others. Their dominant action is to increase the renal excretion of sodium and chloride with an accompanying volume of water. Potassium excretion may also be increased to a degree that results in hypokalemia. Enteric coated potassium supplements given in combination with benzothiadiazides may lead to ulceration of the small bowel. See Potassium Salts in the index. These drugs are widely used in the management of edema secondary to congestive heart failure or other causes and sometimes in hypertensive disease without overt edema. The margin of safety between therapeutically effective and frankly toxic doses is large, but a number of hypersensitivity reactions has been reported - pancreatitis, depression of the formed elements of the blood, purpura, photosensitive dermatitis, necrotizing vasculitis, hyperglycemia, aggravation of diabetes mellitus and exacerbation of renal and/or hepatic insufficiency. The symptoms of acute poisoning in man are usually presumed to reflect fluid and electrolyte derangements as above. Two small children, however, who ingested a total dose of 15 gm. chlorothiazide between them, presented with lethargy which progressed to deep coma within 12 hours. Both recovered without sequelae, and neither child exhibited objective evidence of a fluid or electrolyte disorder. In a separate case a 22-month-old child who ingested 3 gm. exhibited lethargy. Attempts to duplicate this syndrome in monkeys were not entirely successful. Doses of up to 5 gm./kg. by gavage produced only a transient lethargy of a moderate degree.

Ref.: Bass and Beisel, 1963; Bjornberg and Gisslen, 1965; Gelfand et al., 1964; Harber et al., 1959; Jones and Caldwell, 1962; Rougraff, 1959; Schifrin and Little, 1969; Schotland and Grumbach, 1963; Sherlock et al., 1966; Wolff et al., 1963.

1589

1589 Chlophedianol Hydrochloride

2-Chloro-α-[2-(dimethylamino)ethyl]-α-phenylbenzenemethanol hydrochloride

Toxicity Rating: 4. A non-narcotic antitussive ingredient in cough syrup. The usual adult dose of 25 mg. is as effective as 15 mg. of codeine. The oral acute LD_{50} in the rat is 422 mg./kg. Reported adverse reactions in man are urticaria, dry mouth, nausea, vomiting, vertigo, visual disturbances, drowsiness, excitability, nightmares and hallucinations.

1590

1590 Chlorambucil

e.g., Leukeran

Toxicity Rating: 5. A slow acting and relatively safe nitrogen mustard used in chronic lymphocytic leukemia, Hodgkin's disease, etc. Available in 2 mg. tablets for oral administration; a common therapeutic dose schedule is 0.1 to 0.2 mg./kg. per day. Single doses of 20 mg. regularly produce nausea and vomiting, whereas 6.5 mg./kg. may be associated with irreversible bone marrow depression. Additional cytotoxic effects may be manifested in lymphoid organs and epithelial tissue as well. In two accidentally poisoned children (2 and 2.5 yr. old), however, the major signs were of central nervous excitation. A dose of about 1.5 mg./kg. produced vomiting, ataxia and jerky movements without frank seizures. Recovery was complete after a moderate pancytopenia. Grand mal convulsions occurred 5 hours after 5 mg./kg. The seizures were controlled with barbiturates and paraldehyde (see Section IV), and no toxic effects were present on the second day. This child recovered without hematologic, hepatic or renal sequelae.

Ref.: Green and Naiman, 1968; Wolfson and Olney, 1957.

1591

1591 Cinchophen

Atophan

Toxicity Rating: 3. Once used as an analgesic, uricosuric and anti-inflammatory drug. The occurrence of jaundice with cinchophen and its various derivatives was observed with such frequency and heralded such severe degenerative and necrotizing changes in the liver that these drugs have been largely abandoned. The most frequent hepatic reaction is an acute or subacute yellow atrophy or cirrhosis, which may have a fatal outcome. The suggestion has been made, however, that cinchophen jaundice may often have been due to intercurrent viral hepatitis. Doses of 1 gm./kg. by mouth are lethal to rabbits; neocinchophen may be somewhat more toxic. The lethal dose range of cinchophen for frogs, mice, rats and guinea pigs by a variety of routes lies between 0.5 and 1.0 gm./kg. Death appears to result from respiratory paralysis.

Ref.: Hueper, 1948.

1592   Deanol

1592 1592

2-Dimethylaminoethanol, DMAE

A unique type of nervous system stimulant. A normal constituent of brain and perhaps a precursor of brain acetylcholine. Doses as high as 1200 mg. daily produce no serious side effects, and a single 2500 mg. dose taken in a suicide attempt had no adverse effects. Experimentally deanol is shown to antagonize the depressant effects of barbiturates. In high daily doses it is able to produce epileptic seizures in mice and rats. The principal contraindication to its use is grand mal epilepsy.

Ref.: Heatley, 1960; Moriarty and Mebane, 1959; Murphree et al., 1959.

1593   Dehydrocholic Acid

e.g., Decholin

Toxicity Rating: 3. A choleretic which is also used (as the sodium salt) to measure arm-to-tongue circulation time. By far the least toxic of the common bile acids. Intravenous lethal dose in rabbits 1.1 gm./kg. Produces death after 7 days when given by mouth (rabbits?) at a dose of 2 gm./kg. Less hemolytic than other bile acids, but kidney damage has been described. A digitalis-like action on the heart should be anticipated.

Ref.: de Haen, 1944.

1594   Dextromethorphan Hydrobromide

e.g., Romilar hydrobromide

Toxicity Rating: 4. Specific anti-tussive drug with about the same therapeutic potency as codeine, but perhaps less toxic (oral LD_{50}'s in mice 165 mg./kg., in rats 350 mg./kg.). Virtually devoid of analgesic activity. Side effects from therapeutic doses include nausea, vomiting and dizziness. Tolerance and addiction are not recognized. Although clinical reports of acute intoxication have not been encountered, dextromethorphan, like codeine, may produce central excitement rather than coma. The antidotal efficacy of morphine antagonists such as nalorphine is not established.

See also: Morphine, *Reference Congener in Section III.*
Ref.: Benson et al., 1953; Ralph, 1954.

1595   Disulfiram

Antabuse, Tetraethylthiuram disulfide

Toxicity Rating: 3. Toxicity rating based on animal tests in which no alcohol was given.

See also: Disulfiram *and* Thiram, *Reference Congeners in Section III.*

1596   Ethambutol Hydrochloride

2,2′-(Ethylenediimino)-di-1-butanol dihydrochloride

Toxicity Rating: 2. Oral antitubercular drug. Low acute oral toxicity in experimental animals (rat LD_{50} 6.8 gm./kg.). In humans it has induced allergic reactions, including anaphylaxis. The compound is rapidly absorbed and excreted. About 30% of the dose is metabolized to the dicarboxylic acid derivative before urinary excretion. Prolonged therapeutic administration may produce central nervous system effects such as dizziness, headache, mental confusion, and occasionally hallucinations. Peripheral neuritis occurs occasionally. Reversible visual disturbances, including loss in visual acuity, is reported in some patients. Retrobulbar neuritis is described. Elevated serum uric acid levels may lead to acute attacks of gout. No heart abnormalities in man have been ascribed to this drug, but dogs given large daily doses for several months developed cardiac pathology, including ECG changes and occasionally fatal heart attacks. The cardiac disorders apparently followed reductions in myocardial cytochrome-c oxidase activity resulting from an organ-specific loss of copper. In these dogs the tapetum lucidum of the eye was depigmented by a local zinc deficiency. Increased zinc excretion has been demonstrated in ethambutol-treated dogs following single oral doses. In monkeys given large doses of the drug for 6 months both copper and zinc levels in the eye tissues were reduced to 10% of normal levels. Both single acute and chronic doses produced lesions of the monkey optic tract, especially in the optic chiasma. The usual daily adult dose of ethambutol hydrochloride is 25 mg./kg.

Ref.: Physicians' Desk Reference, 1981.

1597   **1597**   Guaifenesin

α-Glyceryl guaicol ether, Glyceryl guaiacolate, 3-(*o*-Methoxyphenoxy)-1,2-propanediol

Toxicity Rating: 2(?). Used in cough remedies as an expectorant because of its ability to increase the production of respiratory tract secretions. Administered by stomach tube to test animals in doses up to 5 gm./kg., it produced no signs of toxicity. It is excreted in urine principally as glucuronates and sulfonates.

Ref.: Jackson, 1958.

1598   **1598**   Heparin Sodium

Biogenic mucopolysaccharide used in clinical medicine as an anticoagulant drug. Inactive after oral administration. Single dose toxicity is not well established. Furthermore, variations in potency are still seen among different preparations, and all therapeutic doses should be individualized. Common adult doses range from about 50 mg. (5000 U.S.P. units) as a single intravenous dose up to 200 to 400 mg. intramuscularly in a repository form. Although the actions of heparin are evanescent, iatrogenic intoxications have produced serious hemorrhage. Unlike the coumarin anticoagulants, heparin does not block prothrombin synthesis in the liver. Vitamin K is therefore not a useful antagonist. Heparin overdoses can be inactivated by the administration of protamine sulfate (U.S.P.), which avidly complexes with heparin to form a stable salt with decreased anticoagulant activity. Protamine itself, however, also possesses anticoagulant activity, and so care must be taken through the use of frequent coagulation time determinations not to overtitrate the patient. The protamine–to–heparin ratio (doses expressed in mg. administered) should not exceed one, and if protamine treatment is delayed a half-hour after heparin, a ratio of only 0.5 may be required.

Ref.: Pachman, 1965.

1599   **1599**   Hesperidin Methyl Chalcone

Toxicity Rating: 1. Hesperidin and hesperidin chalcone are the predominant flavanoids in lemons and sweet oranges; also found in paprika. The methyl derivative is available in purified form for use as a drug in conditions of increased capillary permeability. No toxicity in humans has been noted with oral doses up to 15 gm./day or 5 gm./day for longer periods of time. Intravenous administration resulted in an abrupt but transient decline in blood pressure and a fleeting bitter taste. No reports of allergic reactions were found in the literature.

Ref.: Kirtley and Peck, 1948.

1600   **1600**   Indomethacin

Indocin

Toxicity Rating: 4(?). Analgesic, antipyretic, anti-inflammatory drug. Maximal recommended adult oral dose 200 mg./day in divided doses. Acute oral LD_{50}'s range from as low as 12 mg./kg. in rats to as high as 540 mg./kg. in guinea pigs. Signs in poisoned animals include decreased activity, moderate decrease in respiratory rate (all species except dogs) and ulceration of the gastrointestinal tract. Dogs showed blanching of the gums, diarrhea, emesis and occult blood in feces. Acute human poisonings include one adult who ingested 31 capsules (size unknown; total amount either 775 or 1550 mg.). On examination at 4 hours the patient was lethargic, stuporous and mildly confused but could be aroused. Vital signs were all normal. Complete recovery at 24 hours. As many as 20 capsules have been consumed by an adult without symptoms. Gastrointestinal ulceration and hemorrhage are possible consequences of a single massive oral dose but they have not been described in man. Antacids may be helpful.

Ref.: Press, 1969.

1601   **1601**   Isoniazid

Isonicotinylhydrazine

Toxicity Rating: 4. Accidental and suicidal overdoses (often 6-10 gm. in adults) and even therapeutic doses (300 mg. daily) of this tuberculostatic drug have produced many severe poisonings, especially among American Indians and Eskimos. In conventional doses (5 mg./kg. in adults), peripheral neuropathy is the commonest adverse effect, but toxic psychoses and other CNS reactions occur occasionally, as well as liver and bone marrow damage. After the acute ingestion of a toxic amount (20 or more 300-mg. tablets), the victim is often asymptomatic for 0.5 to 2 hours. This latent period is followed by the appearance of nausea, vomiting, dizziness, slurring of speech and atropinic signs (mydriasis, brightly colored lights and other visual hallucinations, tachycardia, urinary retention). Very large overdoses may produce stupor and coma. The most definitive and dangerous reaction, however, consists of violent and persistent tonic-clonic convulsions, usually beginning about 1.5 to 3 hours after ingestion; they lead to intense metabolic acidosis, exhaustion and ultimately death (mean lethal dose probably 100-300 mg./kg.). These convulsions are difficult to control with conventional anticonvulsants. Short-acting barbiturates, diazepam and phenytoin sodium have all been used, but intravenous diazepam is probably superior (see Section IV). Isoniazid convulsions are said to be due to the inhibition of brain L-glutamic acid decarboxylase and the consequent fall in GABA levels in the brain. This enzyme inhibition is antagonized by pyridoxine, which in large doses is antidotal. The recommended dose is 1 gm. for each gram of isoniazid believed to have been ingested. In the absence of specific information, an initial adult dose of pyridoxine hydrochloride is 5 gm. (50 ml. of 10% solution) injected intravenously over 3 to 5 minutes, even if no seizures have occurred. This injection may be repeated every 5 to 20 minutes until the dose exceeds that of the isoniazid or until the convulsions cease. Intravenous sodium bicarbonate is used to control the acidosis, and forced diuresis with mannitol promotes the excretion of the poison (see Section IV). Hemodialysis or hemoperfusion may be useful in severe cases, but these procedures complicate the pyridoxine therapy.

Ref.: Brown, 1972; Miller et al., 1980; Sievers and Herrier, 1975; Wason et al., 1981.

1602   Isopropamide   1602

Darbid

An anticholinergic, antispasmodic drug with actions like atropine.

See also: Atropine, *Reference Congener in Section III.*

1603   Isosorbide   1603

1,4:3,6-Dianhydro-D-glucitol, Hydronol

Toxicity Rating: 1. A non-toxic dihydric polyol derived from sorbitol. The single-dose oral LD_{50} is said to be 24 and 28 gm./kg. in female and male rats respectively. Like glycerine (see in Index), it is given orally as an osmotic diuretic to reduce intraocular pressure during ophthalmological procedures. The usual dose (1.5 gm./kg. in solution) is rapidly absorbed and excreted unchanged in urine with a half-life of about 8 hours. It has a slower onset of action and produces a smaller degree of diuresis than parenterally administered diuretics. Unlike glycerine it does not cause hyperglycemia. Usual side-effects are headache, nausea and vomiting. As with any diuretic, the systemic effects of dehydration are potential hazards. The manufacturer suggests using isosorbide in industry as a humectant and plasticizer in paper, tobacco, textiles, glue, cork products and pharmaceuticals.

Ref.: Nodine et al., 1973.

1604   Levopropoxyphene Napsylate   1604

Levopropoxyphene 2-naphthalene sulfonate, Novrad

Toxicity Rating: 3. A non-opioid antitussive agent which was found in an objective study to be no more effective than a placebo. Its acute oral LD_{50} in rats is 1450 mg./kg. Usual adult dose is 50-100 mg. every 4 hours; usual pediatric dose is 6 mg./kg. body wt. in divided doses every 24 hours. Its side effects are minor and include drowsiness, nervousness, dizziness, nausea, vomiting, urinary frequency and urgency, rash and urticaria. Available in 100 mg. capsules and 50 mg./ml. suspension. No information on overdoses was found, but see also the dextroisomer listed in the index as Propoxyphene Hydrochloride.

1605   Menadione   1605

2-Methyl-1,4-naphthoquinone

Toxicity Rating: 3. A synthetic naphthoquinone derivative having physiologic properties of vitamin K. Newborns exhibit a marked sensitivity characterized by hyperbilirubinemia and possible fatal kernicterus.

Ref.: Anonymous, 1961.

1606   Pentylenetetrazol   1606

Metrazol, Cardiazol

Toxicity Rating: 4. Central nervous and cardiovascular stimulant sometimes used as an analeptic in the therapy of poisoning by central depressants. Death has followed the ingestion of 10 gm. Typical symptoms of higher motor and spinal cord stimulation include muscle tremor, spontaneous clonic and tonic convulsions followed by profound depression. Death is a result of anoxia, medullary depression, and respiratory arrest. Since it is rapidly detoxified, its therapeutic actions can be well controlled.

See also: Amphetamine *and* Strychnine, *Reference Congeners in Section III.*
Ref.: Gilman et al., 1980.

1607

1607   Phenolphthalein

Phenolphthalin, Phthalin

A laxative widely used since 1902, often in preparations flavored with chocolate. No systemic toxicity after oral doses has been established except for occasional reactions that are probably allergic. Children have tolerated without distress single oral doses as high as 8 gm. No prophylactic treatment is regarded as necessary, except perhaps the ingestion of activated charcoal. If urine or feces is alkaline, it may acquire a red color; this is not blood. Several cases of acute reactions to oral doses of the drug have been reported. Various types of skin rashes have been described, in some cases followed by persistent pigmentation. Signs of systemic lupus erythematosus have been ascribed to phenolphthalein. In one fatal case (Sarcinelli, 1970) a 3-year-old child developed cerebral and pulmonary edema and became comatose after the ingestion of 600 mg. of the drug in chocolate. In another case (Buchanan et al., 1976), a 35-year-old man developed hypothermia, hypotension, severe acidosis, pulmonary edema and oliguria after ingesting 2 gm. of the drug in chocolate.

Ref.: Abramowitz, 1950; Blatt et al., 1943; Buchanan et al., 1976; Fantus and Dyniewicz, 1938; Sarcinelli et al., 1970.

1608

1608   Phenolsulfonphthalein

Phenol red, PSP

Toxicity Rating: 3(?). Closely related chemically to phenolphthalein above, it is available as the monosodium salt. Excreted in the urine chiefly by tubular secretion and used as an index of renal function. Six mg. is given by the intravenous or intramuscular route, and urine is collected at suitable intervals thereafter for analysis. After i.v. administration 65 to 80% of the dye is excreted in the first hour by normal humans. No human poisonings are known. The subcutaneous LD_{50} in rats is in excess of 600 mg./kg. Given twice weekly for a year to rats in doses of 1 mg./kg. no dye-related mortality was detected, and there were no effects on weight gain or drug-related organ pathology.

Ref.: Mason et al., 1971b.

1609

1609   Phenytoin Sodium

Diphenylhydantoin sodium, e.g., Dilantin

Toxicity Rating: 3-4. An anticonvulsant drug notably lacking in sedative properties and widely used in the control of epilepsy. Toxic doses in animals produce mydriasis, nystagmus, salivation, incoordination and ataxia. Muscular spasticity and rigidity, tremors, convulsive movements and opisthotonus may precede death from respiratory failure. Most of the toxic effects in man are similarly referable to the central nervous system. Despite the widespread use of this drug, relatively few cases of severe acute intoxication have been reported. Ingestions of 4.5 gm. by an adult and of 0.6 to 0.9 gm. by children between 3 and 4 years of age have produced transient coma with motor restlessness; 2 gm. has killed a 7-yr.-old child, but 25 gm. has been tolerated by an adult without serious central depression. As an instrument of suicide, phenytoin is commonly ingested in combination with phenobarbital, provoking central depression to a degree not usually seen with phenytoin alone. In contrast to acute poisonings, allergic and other untoward effects of phenytoin are common. They include gastric distress, rash, gingival hypertrophy, hirsutism and blood dyscrasias.

See also: Barbiturates, *Reference Congener in Section III*.
Ref.: Theil et al., 1961.

1610

1610   Primidone

Primaclone, 2-Desoxyphenobarbital, e.g., Mysoline

Toxicity Rating: 4. Non-barbiturate anticonvulsant drug related chemically to phenobarbital. Indeed, as much as 15 per cent of an ingested dose of primidone is said to be metabolically converted to phenobarbital. Used in the management of grand mal seizures and focal motor and psychomotor epilepsy. The mean lethal dose in adults appears to be on the order of 20 to 30 gm. Usual adult therapeutic dose is 0.25 to 2.0 gm./day. At least two children have survived doses of 12.5 gm., but were comatose for 24 hours and required up to 5 days for complete recovery. A primidone crystalluria has been described without renal sequelae. Alkalinization of the urine, osmotic diuresis, peritoneal dialysis, extracorporeal hemodialysis and other measures appropriate for phenobarbital poisoning would be expected to benefit the primidone-intoxicated patient.

See also: Barbiturates, *Reference Congener in Section III*.
Ref.: Ajax, 1966; Arnold and Ceranke-Hofermayer, 1953; Blair et al., 1968; Del Greco and Arieff, 1962; Dotevall and Herner, 1957; Fazekas and Rengei, 1960; Kappy and Buckley, 1969; Morley and Wynne, 1957; Plaa et al., 1958.

1611   Probenecid   **1611**

e.g., Benemid

Toxicity Rating: 3(?). This effective and safe uricosuric agent has been tolerated in daily doses of 2 gm. for as long as four years. No fatalities from its use were reported in a review of 2,502 patients published in 1955. Gastrointestinal upsets occurred in about 3% of the patients. Since then a single fatality has been attributed to hypersensitivity to probenecid. In this patient jaundice, asthma, skin rash and eosinophilia preceded a massive hepatic necrosis. The pathology resembled the few reported cases of hepatic necrosis from sulfonamides.

Ref.: Boger and Strickland, 1955; Reynolds et al., 1957.

1612   Procainamide   **1612**

Pronestyl

Toxicity Rating: 4(?). Drug useful in controlling ventricular tachycardia, premature contractions and some atrial arrhythmias. Available in a 250-mg. capsule in addition to various parenteral formulations. It lacks the central nervous stimulant actions of procaine, but is capable of inducing the same types of cardiac arrhythmia against which it is useful. Profound but transitory drops in blood pressure are seen after intravenous administration. Ventricular fibrillation and standstill are also hazards of its intravenous use. Said to be less toxic than quinidine, but this has not been established in man. Mild allergic manifestations have followed oral therapy with this drug. ECG disorders respond to treatment with sodium lactate as in quinidine poisoning.

See also: Quinidine, *Reference Congener in Section III.*
Ref.: Bakos and Askey, 1952; Denney et al., 1952; Epstein, 1953; Mark et al., 1951; Read, 1952.

1613   Propranolol Hydrochloride   **1613**

1-(Isopropylamino)-3-(1-naphthyloxy)-2-propanol, e.g., Inderal

Toxicity Rating: 4. A β-adrenergic receptor blocking drug useful in relieving cardiac arrhythmias, hypertension and angina pectoris. In very large doses it exerts a quinidine-like or anesthetic-like membrane action which affects the cardiac action potential and depresses cardiac function; transient intraventricular conduction blocks are sometimes seen in overdosed patients (Buiumsohn *et al.,* 1979). The drug is readily absorbed from the gastrointestinal tract. Much of it is extracted by and metabolized by the liver during its first passage through the portal circulation. Its biological half-life is about 3 hours but may be much longer after massive doses (Halloran and Phillips, 1981). Overdoses commonly induce bradycardia, heart failure, hypotension and sometimes bronchospasm. Atropine and isoproterenol may be used to reduce bradycardia, but glucagon, epinephrine and even levarterenol have proved to be superior in several cases, especially in the presence of severe hypotension. Asthmatics are particularly sensitive to bronchospasm induced by propranolol, which may be relieved by isoproterenol or epinephrine. Less serious or less common effects include lightheadedness, nausea, vomiting, mild diarrhea, lassitude, weakness, insomnia, nightmares, and even hallucinations, confusion, and paranoia. Patients with massive overdoses commonly present in coma and shock, with intermittent epileptiform seizures. The drug has been implicated in rashes, agranulocytosis and thrombocytopenic purpura. Mice given lethal doses developed convulsions, a marked increase in respiratory rate and exhaustion; smaller doses produced significant CNS depression. The drug increases the lethality of morphine sulfate (Winter, 1974). In one attempted suicide (Lagerfelt and Matell, 1976), a 41-year-old man took 5.1 grams of propranolol in tablet form. Within 100 minutes he was comatose and cyanotic with a weak pulse of 50 beats per minute. Generalized intermittent convulsions occurred. The bradycardia progressed to asystole, but he recovered after prolonged administration of isoproterenol and epinephrine and the introduction of a transvenous pacemaker. Intermittent clonic convulsions are frequently observed in massive overdoses. Allegedly they are not due to cerebral ischemia. Whatever the mechanism, they are said to be resistant to diazepam and barbiturates (Laake *et al.,* 1981). Several successful suicides have been reported.

Ref.: Buiumsohn et al., 1979; Halloran and Phillips, 1981; Kosinski and Malindzak, 1973; Laake et al., 1981; Lagerfelt and Matell, 1976; Winter, 1974.

Miscellaneous synthetic substances

Synthetic food additives

1614   Butylated Hydroxytoluene   **1614**

BHT, 2,6-Di-*tert*-butyl-*p*-cresol

Toxicity Rating: 3. BHT is a commonly used and Generally Recognized As Safe (GRAS) antioxidant allowed in foods in amounts up to 0.02% of the weight of fat present. It is also used as a stabilizer in pesticides, gasolines and lubricants, soaps and cosmetics, and as an antiskinning agent in paints and inks. Although the average person consumes no more than 0.5 mg./kg. per day, the vast amounts added annually to foodstuffs (600,000 lbs. in 1970) have prompted thorough investigations into its toxic potential. Various morphological and biochemical changes have been observed in experimental animals fed doses 100-1000 times higher than those used for human consumption. Prominent among these changes are dose-dependent reductions in growth rate and body weight of rodents; damage to the alveolar epithelium of mice within 24 hours of exposure (progressing to fibrosis if pure oxygen follows closely the exposure to BHT); dose-dependent fatalities from massive hemorrhages into the pleural and peritoneal cavities of rodents and hemorrhages of the epididymis, testis, nasal cavity and pancreas even in survivors; hyperfunctional liver enlargement, induction of microsomal enzymes, increased synthesis of hepatic smooth endoplasmic reticulum in rats and male mice and to a lesser degree in monkeys. Another commonly used and closely related antioxidant, BHA or bu-

tylated hydroxyanisole, also induces hemorrhages and similar liver lesions in rats and monkeys. Hepatic nucleolar changes, possibly related to inhibition of RNA synthesis, were also seen in monkeys. The hepatic lesions are not necessarily pathogenic, but it is difficult to draw the line between adaptation and disease. A hydroperoxide metabolite of BHT, produced by rat liver microsomes and also nonenzymatically in the presence of oxygen, was found to be 18 times more potent than the parent compound in causing hemorrhage and liver lesions. Infant rodents and infant monkeys are more resistant than adults to the effects of BHT. BHT has complex cocarcinogenic actions in mice. Given in multiple doses before a carcinogen, it inhibited tumorigenesis, but given afterwards it augmented the number of hepatomas induced by 2-acetylaminofluorene and the number of pulmonary adenomas induced by urethane. The NCI bioassay for carcinogenic effects of BHT alone in rats and mice was negative. A reported teratogenic effect of anophthalmia in rats has not been duplicated in other laboratories. BHT is mildly irritating to human skin and severely irritating to rabbit eyes.

See also: Phenol, *Reference Congener in Section III.*
Ref.: Allen and Engblom, 1972; National Cancer Institute, 1979a; Yamamoto et al., 1980.

1615   1615   Ethoxyquin

6-Ethoxy-1,2-dihydro-2,2,4-trimethylquinoline, Santoquin

Toxicity Rating: 3. Antioxidant, used as a postharvest fruit-dip to prevent common scald of apples and pears in storage. Formerly added to poultry feeds and forage crops. Moderate toxicity in laboratory animals (rat LD_{50} 1 gm./kg.). Toxic oral doses produce a slowly developing depression lasting 4 to 6 days. Parenteral administration produces convulsions, coma, and prompt death. Single subcutaneous doses of 5 to 10 mg. led to nearly

100% mortality in treated groups of neonatal mice. A skin irritant. May produce reversible liver changes. The compound is readily absorbed, metabolized, and excreted in urine and feces. Repeated doses induce and inhibit phenobarbital-type cytochrome P450 in rat liver microsomes. Slight inhibitory effect on aryl hydrocarbon hydroxylase activity. Said to protect animals against tumor formation following exposure to benzpyrene.

Ref.: Epstein et al., 1970; Kahl and Netter, 1977; Kelly, 1961.

1616   1616   Saccharin

2,3-Dihydro-3-oxobenzisosulfonazole, Anhydro-*o*-sulfaminebenzoic acid

Toxicity Rating: 2. Often marketed as its sodium salt. A sweetening agent or sugar substitute, excreted almost quantitatively without metabolic alteration (75 to 90% in urine). Oral doses of 5 to 25 gm. daily or single doses of 100 gm. may cause anorexia, nausea, vomiting, and diarrhea. Large

daily doses may also produce gastric hyperacidity. Rabbits are killed by oral doses of 8 to 10 gm./kg., presumably as a result of gastroenteritis. Sometimes used in combination with sodium cyclamate; see latter below.

Ref.: Food Protection Committee of the Food and Nutrition Board, 1955; Taylor et al., 1968.

1617   1617   Sodium Cyclamate

Cyclamate sodium or calcium, *N*-Cyclohexylsulfamate sodium or calcium, e.g., Sucaryl sodium

Toxicity Rating: 2. Non-caloric sweetening agent used alone or in combination with saccharin (see also latter above). Ten parts cyclamate to one part saccharin is a common combination; its toxicity does not appear to differ significantly from either ingredient given alone. Some non-nutritive soft drinks contain 0.125% cyclamate. Acute oral LD_{50}'s in mice and rats place this compound on the borderline between toxicity classes 1 and 2 (10 to 17 gm./kg.). After such doses mice show only intes-

tinal fluid accumulation and slight cardiac distension with death occurring in 1 to 24 hours. The intravenous administration of 4 to 5 gm./kg. produces rapid exitus apparently in respiratory failure. Vomiting occurs in dogs and cats after large oral doses. Human subjects have consumed 5 to 12 gm./day for several weeks; the only noted effect was a change in stools to a mushy consistency. Not all subjects had increased frequency of bowel movements, but in some, cathartic action may be due to osmotic fluid retention by unabsorbed cyclamate. Rats and dogs excrete 98-99% unchanged cyclamate in urine and feces. It has been alleged that some but not all humans metabolize cyclamate to cyclohexylamine to an extent that might lead to significant chromosomal breakage; see cyclohexylamine in the index. Experimental studies in mammals and in bacterial assay systems, however, indicate that neither cyclamate nor cyclohexylamine is mutagenic or carcinogenic or teratogenic (Cattanach, 1976). Cyclamates are currently banned as food additives in many countries (U.S.A., U.K., Canada, Sweden, Finland, etc.).

Ref.: Cattanach, 1976; Food Protection Committee of the Food and Nutrition Board, 1955; Hwang, 1966; Miller et al., 1966; Richards et al., 1951; Schoenberger et al., 1953; Taylor et al., 1968.

1618   Monosodium Glutamate   1618

MSG, Disodium glutamate, Glutamic acid hydrochloride, Glutamic acid, Sodium glutamate

Toxicity Rating: 1. MSG is a common ingredient in products used to impart a meat flavor to foods or to enhance other natural food flavors. Despite assertions to the contrary, no good evidence exists that the glutamates listed here differ in any important pharmacological respects. The hydrochloride has been given by mouth to epileptics in divided doses up to 20 gm./day without untoward effects. Elderly patients have ingested 15 to 45 gm. daily for 3 months with impunity. The intravenous administration of glutamic acid (8 gm.) produced vomiting in 11 to 17 subjects. Although adverse reactions may be less common with parenteral mixtures than with single amino acids, large intravenous doses of many amino acids given alone induce occasionally abdominal pain, flushing, hypotension, chills and fever (see also Section IV). Such a reaction is therefore not specific for glutamate. At various times glutamate has been said to terminate hypoglycemic coma, stimulate intellectual activity in mental deficiency and alleviate convulsive disorders. Most of these claims have been disputed, and none has been adequately explained. A rash of correspondence in medical journals describes an alleged link between MSG and a distress syndrome after consuming Chinese food. Whereas a sincere concern may have motivated some of these communications, others are regarded as hoaxes, provoking more mirth than anxiety. The syndrome is suggestive of that which occurs in subjects treated with monoamine oxidase inhibitors when challenged by foods rich in tyramine. Subjective symptoms of burning sensation, facial pressure and chest pains have been provoked in human subjects by large oral doses of MSG (18/36 subjects responded to 4 gm. or less).

Ref.: Anonymous, 1968; Floyd et al., 1966; Price et al., 1943; Schaumburg et al., 1969; Smyth et al., 1947.

1619   *n*-Propyl Gallate   1619

Toxicity Rating: 3. Used as an antioxidant to preserve edible fats in processed foods and cosmetics. Usually present only in very low concentrations in such products. Acute oral LD_{50} in rats 2.5 to 4.0 gm./kg. and in mice 2.5 to 3.1 gm./kg. Terminal signs included gasping respirations and convulsions. Presumably hydrolyzed in part within the bowel to Gallic acid; see also latter in the index.

See also: Phenol, *Reference Congener in Section III*.
Ref.: Orten et al., 1948.

Miscellaneous laboratory and commercial solvents

1620   Dimethyl Sulfoxide   1620

DMSO

Toxicity Rating: 1. Water-miscible liquid used as antifreeze, hydraulic fluid, paint and varnish remover and potentially as a pharmaceutical solvent. Several clinical uses have been proposed, including bladder instillation for the treatment of interstitial cystitis. The mean lethal dose by mouth is about 17 gm. (20 ml.) per kg. in rats and mice and about 14 gm./kg. in chickens. Even by the intravenous and intraperitoneal routes, the LD_{50} in mice, rats and dogs exceeds 15 gm./kg. After massive single doses, rapid breathing, restlessness and then coma are described in experimental animals, leading to hypothermia and death within a few hours. In high concentrations (e.g., 50%), DMSO induces intravascular hemolysis, with hemoglobinuria, renal tubular injury, and death after several days, presumably because of renal failure. Repeated oral doses (1-5 gm./kg. daily) result in liver necrosis as well as renal lesions. Rapidly absorbed through skin and mucous membranes. After topical applications, an immediate garlic-like taste and odor may develop on the breath and skin. Transient disturbances of color vision, photophobia, headache, diarrhea, and dermatitis are also said to have resulted from dermal applications. Enhances dermal absorption (hence effectiveness) of many other chemicals, including drugs and allergens of moderate molecular weight (<3000 daltons). Compounds such as sunscreens, steroids, insecticides, or procaine, when applied with DMSO to the skin, form depots within the stratum corneum which are resistant to soap and water and from which the compounds are slowly released to the body. Additional pharmacological actions of moderate doses of DMSO include an antiinflammatory effect, nerve blockade, bacteriostasis, diuresis, mild cholinesterase inhibition, some reduction in fibrotic masses, and vasodilatation. In humans, topical applications of concentrated solutions of DMSO induce immediate histamine release with wheal and flare formation. Repeated applications caused a mild erythematous, scaling dermatitis in some subjects. Repeated oral (and topical) treatments with large doses of DMSO have caused lens alterations in rats, rabbits and pigs but not in monkeys or humans. Rabbits inhaling 25 to 50 ml./hr. of DMSO mist for five months developed chemical pneumonia, cloudy swelling in the liver, and signs of renal toxicity. In man and experimental animals, the primary route of excretion of DMSO is the urine. Partially metabolized to dimethylsulfone, dimethyl sulfide and possibly formaldehyde. Dimethyl sulfoxide appeared to be teratogenic in some but not all trials with experimental animals.

Ref.: Brown et al., 1963; Caujolle et al., 1964; David, 1972; DiStefano and Borgstedt, 1964; Jacob and Wood, 1967; Klein et al., 1980; Shepard, 1976.

1621 Dioxane

1621

Diethylene dioxide, Glycol ethylene ether, Diethylene ether

Toxicity Rating: 3. A cyclic diether, used in industry as a solvent for cellulose acetate, resins, oils and other organic and inorganic compounds. The substance is readily absorbed through intact skin, but its acute toxicity by any route is low (rat oral LD_{50} 8.0 gm./kg.) (Smyth et al., 1941a). Inhalation of concentrated vapors has caused anesthesia, renal and hepatic damage and death due to acute renal failure in five humans. Pathological findings included hemorrhagic nephritis and central necrosis of the liver (Barber, 1934). Since the odor of dioxane is not irritating, atmospheric concentrations high enough to produce anesthesia and organ damage may not provoke alarm. Symptoms of subacute exposures include gastric distress, drowsiness, vertigo, dyspnea, and tenderness in the lumbar and abdominal regions. Dioxane is metabolically converted to β-hydroxyethoxyacetic acid (HEAA) in man and rats (Braun and Young, 1977). Oxalic acid is not a metabolite or at least not a significant one. Rats excreted as dioxane only about 5% of a small i.v. dose (0.01 gm./kg.) but about 38% of a large dose (1 gm./kg.). If man oxidizes dioxane as rapidly as the rat, a sublethal dose may induce a severe metabolic acidosis. Workers exposed to atmospheric concentrations of 1 to 2 ppm dioxane in a chemical plant converted virtually all of the absorbed dioxane to HEAA (Young et al., 1976). Dioxane may also be tumorigenic. Rats given repeated oral doses developed liver and kidney damage and ulceration of the stomach at low dose rates (90 to 200 mg./kg. per day for 2 years). Higher doses, 1200 mg./kg. per day for 13 months, resulted also in hepatomas and carcinoma of the nasal cavity. It is not known whether single large doses can lead to tumor formation in man.

See also: Ethylene Glycol, *Reference Congener in Section III.*
Ref.: Barber, 1934; Braun and Young, 1977; Karel et al., 1947; National Cancer Institute, 1978n; Schrenk and Yant, 1936; Smyth et al., 1941a; Young et al., 1976.

1622 Pyridine

1622

Toxicity Rating: 3. Absorbed from the respiratory and gastrointestinal tracts, but probably not significantly from the skin (although a dermatitis may result). In animals central nervous depression; also in man after vapor inhalation. Small oral dose (2 to 3 ml.) in man produce mild anorexia, nausea, fatigue, and mental depression, and after prolonged daily administration hepatorenal damage (in rats prevented by methionine). The ingestion of several ounces has produced severe vomiting, diarrhea, hyperpyrexia, delirium, and death in 43 hours; autopsy revealed pulmonary edema and membranous tracheobronchitis (due to aspiration?).

Ref.: Amer. Petroleum Institute, 1953g.

1623 Tetrahydrofuran

1623

Cyclo-tetramethylene oxide, Diethylene oxide

Toxicity Rating: 4. Used industrially as a solvent for various polymers and resins. Liquid with an acetone odor; boils at 66°C. Tends to form peroxides with an explosive potential. Oral lethal dose of a 20% solution in rabbits 2.5 gm./kg. Strong irritant to skin and mucous membranes but not a sensitizer. No toxic effects from industrial use on record, but severe occipital headache reported in investigators testing its pharmacological properties. Produces general anesthesia in animals. A vapor concentration of 2.2 vol. % killed 50% of exposed mice in less than 2 hours. Anesthesia marked by prolonged induction, profuse salivation, poor muscular relaxation, marked fall in blood pressure, respiratory stimulation and a narrow margin of safety. Although more recent studies failed to find evidence of liver or kidney damage in intensely exposed rats, both have been reported in earlier work.

Ref.: Browning, 1965; Stoughton and Robbins, 1936; Zeller et al., 1964.

Synthetic polymers (plastics) and related substances

1624   Acrylamide   1624

Propenamide

Toxicity Rating: 4. A water-soluble crystalline material that can be polymerized to various forms some of which are also water-soluble. The monomer is widely used as a chemical grout in which a solution with catalysts (ammonium persulfate, β-dimethylaminopropionitrile) is pumped into the dirt or stone walls of excavations to form a water-tight shield. Acute oral LD_{50}'s of the monomer in rats, guinea pigs and rabbits range from 150 to 180 mg./kg. Moderate irritant to eyes and skin. Readily absorbed through the intact skin from aqueous solutions. In animals the same effects are produced with large single doses or repeated small doses, namely a progressive stiffness and/or weakness of the hindquarters, urinary retention, ataxia and

eventually an inability to stand. The syndrome develops over days to weeks. A similar neuropathy has been reported after somewhat larger doses of N-methylacrylamide, N-hydroxymethylacrylamide and N,N-diethylacrylamide, but the issue is somewhat clouded by the possibility that acrylamide may have been present as an impurity in all of these derivatives. Humans exposed to the monomer have developed peripheral neuropathies with mid-brain disturbances and numbness, paresthesias and weakness particularly in the lower limbs. Bluish cold hands which dripped sweat and erythema and peeling of the palms have been described.

See also: Tri-o-cresyl Phosphate, Reference Congener in Section III.
Ref.: Auld and Bedwell, 1967; Barnes, 1970; Edwards, 1975; Garland and Patterson, 1968; McCollister et al., 1964.

1625   Acrylic Resin Monomers   1625

e.g., Methyl acrylate, Ethyl acrylate, 2-Hydroxy-ethyl methacrylate, n-Butyl acrylate

Toxicity Rating: 2-4. Esters of acrylic and methacrylic acid are liquids that polymerize to form thermo-plastic resins (see also methyl methacrylate and acrylonitrile in this index) which are used in latex paints, metal coatings, adhesives, plastic panels and textile finishes. The lower molecular weight monomeric esters are highly reactive and are stabilized for storage by adding hydroquinone (see in this index) or the monomethyl ether of hydroquinone. Except for occasional allergic skin reactions, which may be due to unpolymerized monomers, the resins are inert and essentially non-toxic. The acrylic monomers, however, are moderately toxic. Rat oral LD_{50}'s range from 300 mg./kg. for methyl acrylate to 18,000 mg./kg. for butyl methacrylate. Methyl and ethyl acrylates are strong lacrimators and irritating to the respiratory tract, skin, mucous membranes and eyes, in some cases causing burns of the cornea. Methyl-a-chlo-

roacrylate is a strong vesicant; a trace on the skin causes large blisters. 2-Hydroxy-ethyl methacrylate and di- and tetra-ethylene glycol dimethacrylates have produced contact sensitization in workers in the printing industry. Cutaneous absorption of methyl and ethyl acrylates may lead to systemic effects (rabbit acute percutaneous LD_{50} 1300 mg./kg.). Damage to lungs, kidneys and liver has been observed in animals subjected to repeated skin applications of small doses of methyl acrylate. Inhalation of high vapor concentrations of methyl and ethyl acrylates may cause rapid breathing, headache, nausea, lethargy, pulmonary edema, convulsions and death. The OSHA standard for 8-hour vapor exposure to methyl acrylate is 10 ppm, to ethyl acrylate 25 ppm. Both can form explosive mixtures with air. The higher weight monomers (e.g., butyl, 2-ethylbutyl, etc.) are much less irritating.

Ref.: Lefaux, 1968; Malten and Bende, 1979; Rohm and Haas Co., 1963; Union Carbide and Carbon Corp., 1955.

1626   n-Alkyl-α-Cyanoacrylates   1626

n-Alkyl-2-cyanoacrylates, e.g., Methyl-2-cyanoacrylate

A group of rapidly polymerizing clear, colorless liquids often found in household "super glues" (e.g., Krazy Glue, Wonder Bond). The ability to wet and polymerize rapidly on the surface of living tissue has led to their use as biological tissue adhesives, especially to arrest bleeding and to close wounds without sutures. Monomeric homologues from methyl to octyl undergo an exothermic reaction upon polymerization. The higher monomers polymerize (and degrade) more slowly, produce less heat of polymerization, are less histotoxic and adhere better to moist tissue than the lower homo-

logues. In the process of healing, the adhesive barrier is thought to break down and to be replaced by the body's own tissue. The heat of polymerization and the release of toxic metabolites upon degradation (presumably formaldehyde and cyanoacetate) probably account for the histotoxicity. Formaldehyde may be partly responsible for the self-sterilizing properties of the adhesives. Skin, eye or mouth contact may result in almost immediate tissue-to-tissue bonding. To pull or pry adherent skin surfaces apart commonly causes evulsion of epidermis. If exposed areas are flushed immediately with warm water and if eyelids are kept separated, tissue-to-tissue bonding may be prevented. In the absence of tissue-to-tissue bonding, do not attempt to peel off the adhesive; sweat or other secretions will eventually accumulate under the adhesive film and cause it to lift off. If fingers or other skin surfaces are stuck together, a gentle rolling motion may sometimes safely separate them. If not, acetone or nitromethane (model aircraft engine fluid) may dissolve or weaken the bonding so that the surfaces separate safely and painlessly. Acetone should not be used in the eye, and the same is probably true of nitromethane. Most bonded eyelids release spontaneously in 1 to 4 days. An outbreak of irritant dermatitis among electronic assembly workers was caused by the vaporization of a monomer under conditions of low relative humidity. When the humidity was raised above 55%, the skin complaints ceased.

Ref.: Calnan, 1979; De Fonseka, 1976a; De Fonseka, 1976b; Margo and Trobe, 1982.

1627 Carboxypolymethylene

Carbomer, Carbopol (*940, 941, 960, 961*)

Toxicity Rating: 1(?). A synthetic high molecular weight cross-linked polymer of acrylic acid, marketed as sodium and ammonium salts. Dilute aqueous solutions have a high viscosity. An anionic polymer in water because of many free carboxyl groups. These groups react with fatty amines to form thick stable emulsions of oil in water. Carboxypolymethylene is used as an emulsifier, thickener, disperser and spreader in printing inks, cosmetics and pharmaceuticals. It is believed to be stable and unabsorbed in the gastrointestinal tract and therefore essentially non-toxic.

1628 Epoxy Resins

Toxicity Rating: 2. Epoxy resins are highly viscous liquid or solid thermosetting polyethers produced by polymerization of the condensation products of epichlorohydrin and a dihydroxy compound, such as bisphenol A (2,2-bis[4-hydroxyphenyl]propane), novolacs (products of phenolic compounds and formaldehyde), resorcinol or glycerin. The resins find application as anti-corrosive coatings, high-strength adhesives for home and industry, caulking compounds, castings, encapsulators and sealers for electrical equipment and as binders for laminates of fiber glass, polyester cloth and paper. A commercial mixtures of epoxy resin and concrete is used for grouting and anchoring machinery. Uncured resin oligomers, especially epoxy fatty acids of vegetable oils and glycidyl ethers of bisphenol A, are used as plasticizers and stabilizers for polyvinyl chloride, polyvinyl acetate, ethyl cellulose and synthetic rubbers. An epoxy resin is usually supplied as two components to be mixed together at the time of use. The first contains uncured resin oligomers, such as the diglycidyl ether of bisphenol A or resorcinol diglycidyl ether sometimes in combination with an epoxy monomer such as a monoglycidyl ether. The second contains a curing agent, which may be (and for home use often is) a free aliphatic amine, such as diethylenetriamine (see in index), or it may be an organic acid anhydride, such as phthalic or maleic anhydride, a polyamine or, least frequently, an organic acid, such as oxalic acid. Small amounts of accelerator, such as phenol or resorcinol, may be added to this component. The aliphatic amines are "cold-curing" agents, meaning they set at room temperature. However, the reaction is an exothermic one and may produce fumes of unreacted caustic amines and phenols, which are irritating to skin, eyes and the respiratory tract. The epoxy oligomers and final resins have low oral toxicities; the oral rat LD_{50} ranges from 2 to 19 gm./kg. They are poorly absorbed from the gastrointestinal tract. The lethal dose in the rat depresses the respiratory center. The most common ill-effects in humans from exposure to epoxy resins are dermatitis, including skin and asthma-like sensitization reactions, and eye and respiratory tract irritation. The incompletely cured resins, vapors from the curing agents and reactive diluents, and dusts produced by machining operations performed on hardened resins are all known to produce these effects. Heat and mechanical disruption can release the components and cause irritation. Dermatitis may occur immediately or months after exposure. People have become sensitized to epoxy resins from exposure to uncured resin plasticizers in household items made of PVC. Pipe-coating plant workers inhaling fumes or powder from a bisphenol epoxy resin cured with tri-mellitic anhydride had symptoms of chemical pneumonitis. Workers exposed to dust while airhammering epoxy-cement grouting cured with amines suffered upper respiratory irritation. Xylene, which had been the liquid vehicle for the original uncured resin component, was thought to be the causative agent of the nephrotoxic effects observed in a few of the workers. See also Glycidyl Ethers below.

Ref.: Borgstedt, 1963; Hine et al., 1981.

1629 Glycidyl Ethers

Phenylglycidyl ether, Diglycidyl ethers, Diglycidyl ether of bisphenol A

Toxicity Rating: 3(?). All glycidyl ethers consist of a three-carbon chain with a 2,3-epoxy ring and a terminal ether linkage to an alkyl or aryl residue. The latter may serve as a bridge to a second glycidyl group, to yield a diglycidyl ether. Because of the two epoxy rings on the same molecule, diglycidyl ethers are called bifunctional epoxy resins, sometimes referred to as uncured resin oligomers. In the presence of so-called curing agents, they, like other epoxides, polymerize at room temperature to form hard epoxy resins (see latter above). Most glycidyl ethers and some diglycidyl ethers are viscous liquids, usually with low vapor pressures. Epoxy monomers, such as styrene oxide (see in index) and n-butyl glycidyl ether, are sometimes added to these liquids as "reactive diluents" to reduce viscosity. The rat oral LD_{50} of resorcinal diglycidyl ether is 2.57 gm./kg., but most glycidyl ethers are probably less toxic. Dermal contact is the usual mode of exposure, but droplets in mist can also attack the eyes and respiratory tract. Glycidyl and diglycidyl ethers tend to be irritants

Ref.: Hine et al., 1981; NIOSH, 1978.

and sensitizing agents. In this respect they are more active than the final epoxy resin (see above) but less active than many of the common curing agents (e.g., polyfunctional aliphatic amines). On the skin or in the eye, phenylglycidyl ether and the diglycidyl ether(s) of bisphenol A tend to be mild irritants (in the absence of sensitization), whereas resorcinol diglycidyl ether is a severe irritant. All glycidyl ethers tested have shown mutagenic activity in bacteria, but only n-butyl glycidyl ether was mutagenic in a dominant lethal test in mice. The issue of carcinogenicity is not yet resolved, but these compounds do not appear to be strongly carcinogenic.

1630   Methyl Methacrylate   1630

Methyl 2-methylpropenoate

Toxicity Rating: 2. This substance readily polymerizes to a clear plastic known variously as Lucite, Plexiglas and Perspex. The polymeric form is essentially inert and nontoxic. The liquid monomer (methyl methacrylate) is reportedly lethal at oral doses of from 6 to 9 gm./kg. in laboratory animals. Poisoned animals exhibit respiratory depression and coma; also irritation of skin, eyes and respiratory tract. Inhalation of vapor at concentrations of 150 mg./m^3 is said to produce central nervous effects in humans. A rhesus monkey who died in coma after an accidental 22-hour exposure to the vapor was found to have pulmonary edema and

centrilobular necrosis of the liver (Kessler *et al.*, 1977). Hypotension during hip replacement operations has been ascribed to contact with the monomer. Both the monomer and the polymerizing catalyst, benzoyl peroxide, may cause contact dermatitis. Such cases have been reported among dental technicians who make dentures from the resins and among surgeons who use methyl methacrylate as orthopedic cement. The skin and oral mucosa of some denture wearers have become sensitized. The OSHA 8-hour TWA standard for industrial vapor exposure is 100 ppm.

Ref.: Anonymous, 1972a; Deichmann, 1941; Kessler et al., 1977; Pegum and Medhurst, 1971; Schwartz, 1957; Spealman et al., 1945; Tansy and Kendall, 1979.

1631   β-Nitrostyrene   1631

β-Nitrophenylethylene, BNS

Toxicity Rating: 4(?). Useful intermediate in polymerization reactions. Usually supplied as a 30% solution in styrene. β-Nitrostyrene in propylene glycol at intravenous doses of 80 to 110 mg./kg. produced no deaths in mice. It possesses anti-fun-

Ref.: Kithil, 1962; Schales and Graefe, 1952.

gal, anti-bacterial, and insecticidal activities and has been recommended for repelling rodents, particularly bats. It is a primary irritant to the skin and eyes and a moderate fire hazard. See also Styrene in the index.

1632   Plasticizers   1632

The capacity of a solid material to suffer permanent deformation is called plasticity. Many high molecular weight polymers, or plastics, exhibit this property. Plasticity is enhanced by heat which increases the degree of separation of the macromolecular constituents, weakens their forces of interaction and permits displacement or sliding of the molecules relative to each other. Besides heat certain chemical substances called plasticizers can be added to achieve the same result. Plasticizers increase the degree of separation of macromolecules by reacting chemically with them or by simply fitting between them. The molding temperature of the plastic is then lowered and the material

Ref.: Lefaux, 1968.

becomes more flexible and less fragile. Most plasticizers are organic liquids but some are solids at room temperature, e.g., camphor, diphenylphthalate, triphenylphosphate, waxes, etc. An enormous diversity of chemical compounds are used as plasticizers, including esters of phosphoric acid, phthalic acid, glycolic acid, and aliphatic acids; aromatic chlorinated compounds; glycols and their derivatives; amides; ketones. In addition to obviously plastic products, plasticizers are found in paints, floor finishes, resins, glues and rubber products. For available toxicity information consult the index under specific chemical names.

1633   1633   Polybutene

Poly-1-butene

A linear polymer, relatively stiff and very resistant to cracking. It is used in films, as a coating for wire, and in pipes used for domestic plumbing. The pure substance is chemically and biologically inert. Rats

fed a diet containing 10% polybutene powder for 6 months showed no evidence of toxicity and reproduced normally.

Ref.: Bornmann and Loeser, 1968.

1634   1634   Polyester Resins

Alkyd resin, Isopolyester resins, Fiberglass resin

A term applied collectively to the mixtures of esters formed by polymerizing anhydrides of dicarboxylic acids (phthalic, maleic, etc.) with dihydric alcohols (glycerol, ethylene glycol, sorbitol, etc.). The polymerization occurs in the presence of suitable catalysts to form various plastic sheets and fibers. Among the common types of polyester resins are the alkyd resins; they are saturated, partially polymerized mixtures composed primarily of phthalic acid esterified with either glycerol or fatty acid adducts of glycerol. They are soluble in organic solvents and are widely used in decorative paints. The polymerization process (curing) is completed by air drying, during which volatile constituents are lost. The unsaturated polyester resins, often supplied in styrene solutions, are used in the production of molded fiberglass materials and other

formed products. During curing the resins react with styrene in the presence of various catalysts and promotors, including methyl ethyl ketone peroxide, to form insoluble films. Isopolyesters are unsaturated polyesters derived from isophthalic acid. All of the monomers used to produce polyester resins and low molecular weight polymers, as well as the partially cured resins, may cause skin reactions. Many monomers and partially condensed resins are primary irritants as well as sensitizers. Fully cured resins, however, seldom cause dermatitis (Schwartz, 1957). The oral toxicity of the resins is not known. In the case of unsaturated resins dissolved in styrene solutions, such as those used in fiberglass construction, the styrene is probably the primary hazard. See Styrene in the index.

Ref.: Malten, 1964; Schwartz, 1957.

1635   1635   Polyethylene

Polythene

Toxicity Rating: 1(?). A waxy, translucent plastic consisting of high molecular weight mostly linear hydrocarbons. Both high and low density forms are available. The latter contains more branched chains and is softer. The plastic is chemically unreactive (although strong oxidizing agents may eventually make it brittle), and no solvent for it is known. Polyethylene gradually decomposes when exposed to ultraviolet light. Although a small percentage (less than 1%) of the mass of powdered

polymer can be removed by water extraction, no evidence was found that polyethylene produces toxic symptoms when inhaled or ingested. Rats fed 8 gm./kg. daily showed no toxic reactions and gained weight normally (Lefaux, p.51). Thin polyethylene implants have induced neoplasms in animals, perhaps because impervious films can isolate cells and so release them from normal growth controls.

Ref.: Bering and Handler, 1957; Lambke, 1958; Lefaux, 1968.

1636   1636   Polytetrafluoroethylene

Teflon, Polymer fumes, PTFE, Fluon

Teflon, a thermoplastic resin which is a polymer of tetrafluoroethylene, has a number of highly desirable properties and its inertness under physiological conditions makes it useful in prosthetic devices. In most homes it is found as a non-stick coating on frying pans and other cooking utensils. It is more thermostable than most plastics and can be used safely from temperatures as low as that of liquid nitrogen to over 250°C. Above 250°C, however, Teflon slowly decomposes to release minute amounts of pyrolysis products. When inhaled, they can give rise to an influenza-like illness similar to that induced by metal fumes (see index). The symptoms include dizziness, headache, nausea,

chills, weakness, cough, "tightness" in the chest, sore throat and pyrexia. The most common source of exposure is the smoking of cigarettes contaminated with Teflon dust. No serious sequelae have been noted, and one women suffered 40 attacks in a nine-month period. Above 400°C the quantity of pyrolysis products increase rapidly and so does their toxic nature. Small amounts of hydrogen fluoride have been identified, as well as octafluoroisobutylene, which causes pulmonary edema in animals. Frank pulmonary edema did occur in one workman exposed to Teflon heated to very high temperatures, but again recovery was complete.

See also: Nitrogen Oxides, *Reference Congener in Section III.*
Ref.: Lewis and Kerby, 1965; Nuttall et al., 1964; Robbins and Ware, 1964; Williams and Smith, 1972.

1637   Polyvinyl Alcohol   1637

Polyviol, PVA, Vinarol, Alvyl

A polymer with the structure (-CH$_2$-CHOH-)$_x$. Usually creamy white odorless powders, many of which are soluble in water. Widely used in the plastics industry and once proposed as a substitute for blood plasma. Prepared by the alkaline hydrolysis of polyvinyl acetate, which is not water-soluble. Varying degrees of residual acetylation impart differing viscosities. Acute oral toxicity data were not located. As with polyvinylpyrrolidone (see below), however, PVA's are probably not absorbed from the gastrointestinal tract. The single dose toxicity is presumably low. When given chronically to rats (1 ml. 5% solution subcutaneously each day for 49 days), widely variant toxic syndromes were

produced. Six different PVA's were tested with molecular weights ranging from 35,000 to 240,000. All caused anemia and infiltrated various organs and tissues. Four caused hepatosplenomegaly, and the other two resulted in striking histologic changes. All caused thymus involution. Only two resulted in hypertension, widespread vascular lesions, hypertrophy of the heart and kidney, extensive renal pathology and increased thyroid weight. One of the two caused edema, ascites, high mortality and changes reminiscent of eclamptogenic toxemia. High toxicity appeared to correlate with relatively poor cold water solubility rather than with molecular weight.

Ref.: Hall and Hall, 1963; Lefaux, 1968.

1638   Polyvinyl Chloride   1638

PVC

A solid plastic of low chemical reactivity, insoluble in water and non-flammable, manufactured by the polymerization of vinyl chloride, and employed as a rubber substitute (e.g., electrical insulation, raincoats, shoe soles, etc.). Presumably the polymer cannot be absorbed through skin or gastrointestinal mucosa. Some fresh samples of PVC, however, are said to contain small amounts of unpolymerized vinyl chloride. High temperatures may cause thermal decomposition (pyrolysis) to poten-

tially toxic gases such as hydrogen chloride, ethyl chloride, etc. Several cases of angiosarcoma of the liver have been detected among long-time workers in plants that make PVC from monomeric vinyl chloride. Whether the polymer or monomer is involved in the genesis of this malignancy is not known. See also Vinyl chloride (monomer) and Di(ethylhexyl) phthalate (plasticizer used in PVC) in the index.

1639   Polyvinylpyrrolidone   1639

Povidone, PVP

Toxicity Rating: 1. A variable molecular weight polymer of the monomer *N*-vinylpyrrolidone. The polymer is widely employed in the pharmaceutical, chemical, food and cosmetic industries. Used as a binder and coating on tablets, a dispersant, solubilizer and emulsion stabilizer. Found in some shampoos and hair care preparations, in lipsticks, skin lotions, dentifrices, in textiles, detergents and even fruit beverages. As a colloid in salt solutions it has been used to increase the blood volume in shock. Renal excretion is governed by the molecular weight of the particles not metabolized. Similar non-metabolized macromolecules include natural gums such as gum arabic and synthetics such as methylcellulose, carboxymethylcellulose and polyvinyl alcohol. The kidney is impermeable to such substances if the molecular weight of the particle exceeds 60- to 70,000; up to molecular weights of 10- to 20,000 excretion is fairly prompt. Intermediate molecular weight particles may be slowly excreted over several months to a year. These substances are not absorbed from the gastrointestinal tract and may produce bulk catharsis, flatulence and fecal impaction. In conventional acute and chronic toxicity tests, PVP is remarkably benign. When given parenterally, the unexcreted particles are phagocytized by the cells of the reticuloendothelial system and deposited in storage sites in the liver, spleen, lung, bone marrow, etc. (thesaurosis). The severity and clinical symptomatology of the resulting thesaurosis depend on the

storage site and the nature of the macromolecule. It is not necessarily associated with pathologic changes, but in some cases an inflammatory or granulomatous reaction may be incited. Such lesions have occurred in human liver following parenteral PVP, and glomerulonephritis has been produced in animals with parenteral methylcellulose. Contrary to preliminary evidence, parenteral PVP does not appear to be a carcinogen in mice or rats (Hueper, 1961). Toxicologic interest in PVP stems from its inclusion as a constituent in many hairsprays. Strong circumstantial evidence seems to indicate that lung thesaurosis may be produced in susceptible individuals from continued exposures to these hairsprays (Bergmann *et al.*, 1958, 1962). Presumably PVP is the responsible etiologic agent. The lungs in such cases may exhibit a diffuse interstitial fibrosis while lymph node changes may be reminiscent of sarcoidosis. The only distinctive feature of the syndrome appears to be the presence of large numbers of macrophages in the lungs and lymph nodes containing PAS-positive granules. Termination of exposure has resulted in regression of the lesions, but permanent pathologic changes are a possibility. Many investigators were (and presumably still are) unconvinced that hairspray thesaurosis exists. Sarcoidosis has been held responsible for the pulmonary lesions. The disease cannot be induced in any laboratory animals by exposure to any hairspray constituent. Repeated epidemiological studies of hairspray users have failed to demonstrate an excess prevalence of lung disease (Discher, 1977). The heated controversy of the mid-1960's seems to have subsided. We know of no recent clinical reports of hairspray thesaurosis.

Ref.: Bergmann et al., 1958; Bergmann et al., 1962; Discher, 1977; Edelston, 1959; Hall and Hall, 1962; Hueper, 1961; Jasmin and Bois, 1961.

1640   1640   Soya Alkyd Resin

Toxicity Rating: 2(?). A glycerol polyester alkyd resin modified by esterification with fatty acids obtained from soy oil. These solids are widely used in paints. Skin rashes have been reported from topical exposure to uncured polyester resins. The incidence of dermatitis decreases as polymerization (curing) becomes complete during air-drying. The fully cured film is virtually non-irritating. No specific oral toxicity data were found, but gastrointestinal obstruction is a possible hazard after ingestion of paint containing these resins. Trace amounts of the chemicals used in forming the resin may be present in both the partially polymerized and fully cured products. See Polyester resin above.

Ref.: Schwartz, 1957.

1641   1641   Toluene-2,4-diisocyanate

TDI, Meta-toluene diisocyanate, Tolylene diisocyanate

Toxicity Rating: 2. One of the essential ingredients for polyurethane "foamed-in-place" plastics. The ultimate polymer, which may vary in consistency from soft and sponge-like to hard and porous, is biologically inert. The 2,6-isomer is also encountered; no important toxicological distinctions are recognized. Toxicity rating of 2 is based on data in rats. When ingested, solutions are irritating to the gastrointestinal tract. As a vapor TDI is a powerful irritant to the eyes, skin, respiratory tract. Industrial exposures to surprisingly low concentrations have produced respiratory systems: a sensation of constriction of the chest, cough and dyspnea. The similarity to asthmatic attack with severe bronchospasm has been mentioned. X-rays were uniformly negative. Eosinophilia was noted. Removal from exposure has resulted in sequelae-free recovery, but on re-exposure there may be increased sensitivity.

Ref.: Fahy, 1958; Johnstone, 1957b; Woodbury, 1956; Zapp, 1957.

Unclassified

1642   1642   Dimethoxane

2,6-Dimethyl-*m*-dioxan-4-ol acetate, DDOA

Toxicity Rating: 3(?). A broad-spectrum antimicrobial of low acute oral toxicity, used as a preservative in cutting oils, paints and cosmetics. The compound is a carcinogen. Fourteen tumors were found in 25 rats fed 1.2 gm./kg. per day for 213 days. The tumors included hepatomas that resembled those found in rats exposed to dioxane. It is not known whether a single sublethal exposure to dimethoxane can lead to tumor formation.

Ref.: Hoch-Ligeti et al., 1974.

1643   1643   Ethionine

2-Amino-4-(ethylthio)butyric acid

Toxicity Rating: 3(?). Methionine analogue once proposed as an antineoplastic agent. Inhibits the incorporation of methionine and glycine into rat protein in vivo and the conversion of methionine into cysteine. Ethionine is deethylated, and the ethyl group appears in analogues of metabolites known to participate in transmethylation reactions, e.g., ethyl choline. In the rat it is itself incorporated into abnormal proteins competitively, but its affinity is only 1/600 that of methionine. When given orally to small series of patients with far advanced neoplasias in doses of 0.67 to 45 gm. per day (total doses of 9.7 to 55 gm.), ethionine produced the following symptoms when the diet was deficient in methionine: impairment of liver function, proteinuria, hematuria, dermatitis, leukopenia, thrombocytopenia and diarrhea. Deterioration of mental status and frank toxic psychosis (reminiscent of symptoms seen with Methionine sulfoximine; see below) also occurred. These signs and symptoms were reversed or prevented by methionine.

Ref.: White and Shimkin, 1954.

1644   Methionine Sulfoximine   1644

Toxicity Rating: 3(?). Methionine analogue produced in wheat flour during the agenizing process in vogue between 1920 and 1950. Agene is about 1% nitrogen trichloride (NCl_3) in air saturated with water vapor; on mixing intimately with flour it bleaches and "improves" the flour, but converts some of the methionine to methionine sulfoximine. The latter compound has been shown to be responsible for the syndrome known variously as running fits, canine hysteria, and fright disease in dogs. Methionine sulfoxime inhibits the synthesis of glutamine from glutamate, the metabolic transfer of glutamyl groups and the incorporation of amino acids into protein. It enhances the antineoplastic capacity of certain agents against mouse sarcoma, and the synthetic material has been given a limited clinical trial in far advanced carcinomas. While it exhibited no antineoplastic activity of its own, in doses of 100 to 400 mg. per day (total doses of 500 to 5,800 mg.), it produced for the first time an apparent human counterpart of canine hysteria, notably anxiousness, restlessness, agitation, disorientation, hallucinations, and EEG changes. Methionine appears to be a specific antagonist to these symptoms although the amount of methionine required varies widely with the species (high in dogs, low in monkeys). It is not clear whether or not these changes represent simple methionine deficiency. Other therapy is supportive and symptomatic.

Ref.: Krakoffs, 1961; Mellanby, 1946.

1645   Nosema locustae   1645

A protozoan of the class Sporozoa. Spores are now registered for control of grasshoppers in rangelands. Intracellular parasite of low virility which infests fat bodies of grasshoppers and kills by competing for energy reserves. Effective in applications of 2.5×10^9 spores per acre. Single oral or inhalation exposure to 229×10^6 spores produced no signs of toxicity in rats. A concentrated suspension of spores in water was not irritating to skin of rabbits or guinea pigs. Spores do not germinate in cow rumen or rat stomach, and infective spores could not be isolated from rats given oral doses of infective spores. No data on human toxicity or allergic reactions were found.

Ref.: Hazleton Laboratories, 1973a; Hazleton Laboratories, 1973b; Hazleton Laboratories, 1973c; Henry, 1973; Henry et al., 1973.

1646   Silicone Oil   1646

Dimethyl polysiloxane

No unequivocal toxic effects are recognized. A large dose of hexamethyl disiloxane by mouth is said to have caused mild inebriation and subsequent transient central nervous depression.

Ref.: Rowe et al., 1948.

II: E. Bibliography of Source Materials

A. M. A. Department of Drugs. A. M. A. Drug Evaluations, 3rd ed. Publishing Sciences Group, Inc., Littleton, Mass, 1977.

Aaron, F. E. A case of acute diphenhydramine hydrochloride poisoning. Br. Med. J., 2:24, 1953.

Abbanat, R. A.; Smith, R. P. The influence of methemoglobinemia on the lethality of some toxic anions I. Azide. Toxicol. Appl. Pharmacol., 6:576-583, 1964.

Abbott Laboratories. Brochure (Unique new Rauwolfia derivative, Harmonyl). North Chicago, Illinois, 1957.

Abbott, D. D.; Packman, E. W.; Wagner, B. M.; Harrisson, J. W. E. Chronic oral toxicity of oil of sassafras and safrol. Pharmacologist, 3:62, 1961.

Abdallah, A. H.; Tye, A. A comparison of the efficacy of emetic drugs and stomach lavage. Am. J. Dis. Child., 113:571-575, 1967.

Abramowitz, E. W. Phenolphthalein today. A critical review. Am. J. Dig. Dis., 17:79-82, 1950.

Abramson, A. L. Corrosive injury of the esophagus. Result of ingesting some denture cleanser tablets and powder. Arch. Otolaryngol., 104:514-516, 1978.

Abramson, A. L.; Eason, R. L.; Pryor, W. H., Jr.; Messer, E. J. Corrosive injury of the oral cavity and esophagus caused by some denture cleanser powders. Ann. Otol. Rhinol. Laryngol., 83:714-719, 1974.

Abreu, B. E.; Auerbach, S. H.; Thuringer, J. M.; Peoples, S. A. Chronic and delayed toxic effects of certain saturated and unsaturated halogenated hydrocarbons on white rats and white mice. J. Pharmacol. Exp. Ther., 80:139-143, 1944.

Abreu, B. E.; Peoples, S. A.; Emerson, G. A. Preliminary survey of anesthetic properties of certain halogenated hydrocarbons. Anesth. Analg., 18:156-161, 1939.

Abt, I. A.; Woodward, W. C.; Leech, P. N. Accidents from zinc stearate. J. A. M. A., 84:750-751, 1925.

Adams, D. E.; Goldman, R.; Maxwell, M. H.; Latta, H. Nephrotic syndrome associated with penicillamine therapy of Wilson's disease. Am. J. Med., 36:330-336, 1964.

Adams, E. M.; Spencer, H. C.; Rowe, V. K.; Irish, D. D. Vapor toxicity of 1,1,1-trichloroethane (methyl chloroform) determined by experiments on laboratory animals. Arch. Ind. Hyg. Occup. Med., 1:225-236, 1950.

Adams, H. R. Cardiovascular depressant effects of neomycin and gentamicin in rhesus monkeys. Br. J. Pharmacol., 54:453-462, 1975.

Adams, J. P.; Fee, N.; Kenmore, P. I. Tear-gas injuries. A clinical study of hand injuries and an experimental study of its effects on peripheral nerves and skeletal muscles in rabbits. J. Bone Joint Surg., 48. A:436-442, 1966.

Adelson, L. Homicide by pepper. J. Forensic Sci., 9:391-395, 1964.

Ainsworth, R. W. Petrol-vapour poisoning. Br. Med. J., 1:1547-1548, 1960.

Aird, D. C. Ergot poisoning. Case report and review of literature. J. Obstet. Gynaecol. Br. Commonw., 66:86-90, 1959.

Ajax, E. T. An unusual case of primidone intoxication. Dis. Nerv. Syst., 27:660-661, 1966.

Akahori, F.; Masaoka, T.; Arai, K. Basic studies on toxicity assay of agricultural chemicals. I. Short-term toxicity test of the carbamate insecticide BPMC (2-sec-butylphenyl N-methylcarbamate) on goats, sheep and miniature pigs. Azabu Juika Daigaku Kenkyu Hokoko 28:135-156, 1974.

Alajouanine, T.; Derobert, L.; Thieffry, S. Etude clinique d'ensemble de 210 cas d'intoxication par les sels organiques d'etain. Rev. Neurol., 98:85, 1958.

Alarcon, R. D.; Gelfond, S. D.; Alarcon, G. S. Parenteral and oral pentazocine abuse. Johns Hopkins Med. J., 129:311-318, 1971.

Albertini, A. V.; Gross, D.; Zinn, W. M. *Triaryl-phosphate Poisoning in Morocco 1959.* . Georg Thieme Verlag, Stuttgart, 1968.

Albertini, E.; Volpe, R. D.; Rezzesi, F. Biological action of gibberellic acid on laboratory animals. Med. Ex., 2083 2:344, 1960.

Aldridge, A.; Aranda, J. V.; Neims, A. H. Caffeine metabolism in the newborn. Clin. Pharmacol. Ther., 25:447-453, 1979.

Aldridge, W. N.; Parker, V. H. Barbiturates and oxidative phosphorylation. Biochem. J. 76:47-56, 1960.

Aleksandrova, L. G.; Klisenko, M. A. Metabolism of N-phenylcarbamic acid derivatives in warm-blooded animals. Gig. Sanit. 36:108-109, 1971.

Alexander, C. S. Cobalt-beer cardiomyopathy. A clinical and pathologic study of twenty-eight cases. Am. J. Med., 53:395-417, 1972.

Algeri, E. J.; Katsas, G. G. Toxicology of glutethimide. J. Forensic Sci., 5:217-225, 1960.

Allan, J. D.; Woodruff, J. Starch gastrolith. Report of a case of obstruction. N. Engl. J. Med., 268:776-778, 1963.

Allemand, H.; Pessayre, D.; Descatoire, V.; Degott, C.; Feldmann, G.; Benhamou, J. -P. Metabolic activation of trichloroethylene into a chemically reactive metabolite toxic to the liver. J. Pharmacol. Exp. Ther., 204:714-723, 1978.

Allen, A. C.; Boley, S. J.; Schultz, L.; Schwartz, S. Potassium-induced lesions of the small bowel. II. Pathology and pathogenesis. J. A. M. A., 193:1001-1006, 1965.

Allen, J. R.; Abrahamson, L. J.; Norback, D. H. Biological effects of polychlorinated biphenyls and triphenyls on the subhuman primate. Environ. Res., 6:344-354, 1973.

Allen, J. R.; Engblom, J. F. Ultrastructural and biochemical changes in the liver of monkeys given butylated hydroxytoluene and butylated hydroxyanisole. Food Cosmet. Toxicol., 10:769, 1972.

Allen, J. R.; Norback, D. H. Polychlorinated biphenyl- and triphenyl-induced gastric mucosal hyperplasia in primates. Science, 179:498-499, 1973.

Allen, N.; Mendell, J. R.; Billmaier, D. J.; Fontaine, R. E.; O'Neill, J. Toxic polyneuropathy due to methyl n-butyl ketone: an industrial outbreak. Arch. Neurol. 32:209-218, 1975.

Allen, R. M.; Young, S. J. Phencyclidine-induced psychosis. Am. J. Psychiat. 135:1081–1084, 1978.

Allied Chemical Corporation. Technical Bulletin 1283-02-1005, Morex. General Chemical Division, Morristown, New Jersey, 1965.

Allin, T. G., Jr.; Pogge, R. C. The use of azacyclonal and pipradrol in general practice. Intern. Record Med. & Gen. Pract. Clins., 169:222-230, 1956.

Almog, C.; Maidan, A.; Pik, A.; Schlesinger, Z. Acute intoxication with ajmaline. Isr. J. Med. Sci., 15:570-572, 1979.

Alstott, R. L.; Miller, A. J.; Forney, R. B. Report of a human fatality due to caffeine. J. Forensic Sci., 18:135-137, 1973.

Altenkirch, H.; Mager, J.; Stoltenburg, G.; Helmbrecht, J. Toxic polyneuropathies after sniffing a glue thinner. J. Neurol. 214:137-152, 1977.

Altenkirch, H.; Stoltenburgdidinger, H.; Wagner, H. M. Experimental data on the neurotoxicity of methyl-ethyl-ketone (MEK). Experientia, 35:503-504, 1979.

Altura, B. T.; Altura, B. M. Phencyclidine, lysergic acid diethylamide, and mescaline: cerebral artery spasms and hallucinogenic activity. Science 212:1051–1052, 1981.

Ambrose, A. M. Studies on the physiological effects of sulfamic acid and ammonium sulfamate. J. Ind. Hyg. Toxicol., 25:26, 1943.

Ambrose, A. M. Toxicological studies of compounds investigated for use as inhibitors of biological processes. II. Toxicity of ethylene chlorohydrin. Arch. Ind. Hyg. Occup. Med., 2:591-597, 1950.

Ambrose, A. M. Pharmacologic and toxicologic studies on N, N-diethyltoluamide. I. N, N-diethyl-m-toluamide. Toxicol. Appl. Pharmacol., 1:97-115, 1959.

Ambrose, A. M. Toxicologic studies on pyrethrin-type esters of chrysanthemumic acid. I. Chrysanthemumic acid, 6-chloropiperonyl ester (Barthrin). Toxicol. Appl. Pharmacol. 5:414-426, 1963.

Ambrose, A. M. Toxicologic studies on pyrethrin-type esters of chrysanthemumic acid. II. Chrysanthemumic acid, 2, 4-dimethyl benzyl ester. Toxicol. Appl. Pharmacol. 6:112-120, 1964.

Ambrose, A. M.; Christensen, H. E.; Robbins, D. J.; Rather, L. J. Toxicological and pharmacological studies on chlordane. Arch. Ind. Hyg. Occup. Med. 7:197-210, 1953.

Ambrose, A. M.; DeEds, F.; Rather, L. J. Toxicity of thioacetamide in rats. J. Ind. Hyg. Toxicol., 31:158-161, 1949.

Ambrose, A. M.; Larson, P. S.; Borzelleca, J. F.; Hennigar, G. R., Jr. Toxicologic studies on 3',4'-dichloropropionanilide. Toxicol. Appl. Pharmacol., 23:650-659, 1972.

Ambrose, A. M.; Larson, P. S.; Borzelleca, J. F.; Smith, R. B., Jr.; Hennigar, G. R., Jr. Toxicologic studies on 2,4-dichlorophenyl p-nitrophenyl ether. Toxicol. Appl. Pharmacol. 19:263-276, 1971.

Amdur, M. L. Tellurium oxide, an animal study in acute toxicity. Arch. Ind. Health, 17:665-667, 1958.

Amdur, M. O. The respiratory response of guinea pigs to the inhalation of acetic acid vapor. Am. Ind. Hyg. Assoc. J., 22:1-5, 1961.

American Cyanamid Co. Report on limited release toxicity studies (Diphenylamine). New York, Jan, 1956.

American Cyanamid Co. Report CL 7521 (Dodecyl guanidine acetate, Cyprex). New York, 1958.

American Petroleum Institute. API Toxicological Review (Acrylonitrile). New York, 1948a.

American Petroleum Institute. API toxicological review (beta, beta'-Dichloroethylether, Chlorex). New York, 1948b.

American Petroleum Institute. API toxicological review (Cumene). New York, 1948c.

American Petroleum Institute. API toxicological review (Methyl ethyl ketone). New York, 1948d.

American Petroleum Institute. API toxicological review (Morpholine). New York, 1948e.

American Petroleum Institute. API toxicological review (Naphthenic acids). New York, 1948f.

American Petroleum Institute. API toxicological review (Phosphorus pentasulfide). New York, 1948g.

American Petroleum Institute. API toxicological review (Sulfur dioxide). New York, 1948h.

American Petroleum Institute. API toxicological review (Amyl acetate). New York, 1953a.

American Petroleum Institute. API toxicological review (Aromatic solvent naphtha). New York, 1953b.

American Petroleum Institute. API toxicological review (Copper naphthenate). New York, 1953c.

American Petroleum Institute. API toxicological review (Cyclohexane). New York, 1953d.

American Petroleum Institute. API toxicological review (Hydroquinone). New York, 1953e.

American Petroleum Institute. API toxicological review (Methylcyclohexane). New York, 1953f.

American Petroleum Institute. API toxicological review (Pyridine). New York, 1953g.

American Petroleum Institute. API toxicological review (Triethanolamine). New York, 1953h.

Ames Company. Brochure (The Nostyn Conference). Elkhart, Ind, 1953.

Amos, W. C., Jr.; Hall, A. Malathion poisoning treated with Protopam. Ann. Intern. Med., 62:1013-1016, 1965.

Anders, M. W. Inhibition of microsomal drug metabolism by methylenedioxybenzenes. Biochem. Pharmacol., 17:2367-2370, 1968.

Andersen, M. E.; Thomas, O. E.; Gargas, M. L.; Jones, R. A.; Jenkins, L. J., Jr. The significance of multiple detoxication pathways for reactive metabolites on the toxicity of 1,1-dichloroethylene. Toxicol. Appl. Pharmacol., 52:422-432, 1980.

Anderson, B.; Oglesby, F. Corneal changes from quinone-hydroquinone exposure. Am. J. Ophthalmol., 59:495-501, 1958.

Anderson, E. G.; Magee, D. F. A study of the mechanism of the effect of dietary fat in decreasing thiopental sleeping time. J. Pharmacol. Exp. Ther. 117:281-286, 1956.

Anderson, H. H.; David, N. A.; Koch, D. A. Effects of the halogenation of oxyquinoline on biological activity. Proc. Soc. Exp. Biol. Med., 28:484-485, 1931a.

Anderson, H. H.; David, N. A.; Leake, C. D. Oral toxicity of certain alkyl resorcinols in guinea pigs and rabbits. Proc. Soc. Exp. Biol. Med., 28:609-612, 1931b.

Anderson, H. H.; Emerson, G. A.; Fisher, B. H. Acute toxicity of trypan blue, gentian violet and brilliant green. Proc. Soc. Exp. Biol. Med., 31:825-828, 1934.

Anderson, R. C.; Chen, K. K. Absorption and toxicity of sodium and potassium thiocyanates. J. Pharm. Sci., 29:152-161, 1940.

Anderson, R. J.; Garza, H. R.; Garriott, J. C.; Dimaio, V. Intravenous propylhexedrine (Benzedrex) abuse and sudden death. Am. J. Med., 67:15-20, 1979a.

Anderson, T. W. Vitamin E in angina pectoris. Can. Med. Assoc. J. 110:401-406, 1974.

Anderson, W. Pharmacological aspects of carrageenans. Proc. Int. Seaweed Symp. 6, 627-635, 1969.

Andrewes, C. H. A case of poisoning by cantharidin. Lancet, 2:654-655, 1921.

Angel, A.; Rogers, K. J. An analysis of the convulsant activity of substituted benzenes in the mouse. Toxicol. Appl. Pharmacol., 21:214-229, 1972.

Anichkov, S. V.; Belen'kii, M. L. Pharmacology of the Carotid Body Chemoreceptors. The Macmillan Co., New York, 1963.

Aniline, O.; Pitts, F. E.; Allen, R. E.; Burgoyne, R. Incidental intoxication with phencyclidine. J. Clin. Psych. 41:393–394, 1980.

Anina, I. A.; Medved, I. L.; Proklina, T. L. Gonadotoxic action of pesticidal thiocarbamic acid derivatives. Farmakol. Toksikol. (Moscow) 38:90-93, 1975.

Anon. Toxicity of tetrachloroethylene. J. A. M. A., 141:426, 1949.

Anonymous. Fatal poisoning with naphthol salve. J. A. M. A., 79:51, 1922.

Anonymous. Toxic properties of indium. Br. Med. J., 1:793, 1943.

Anonymous. Cellosolve acetate. J. A. M. A., 134:1057, 1947.

Anonymous. Death from decomposed paraldehyde. Br. Med. J., 2:1114-1115, 1954.

Anonymous. Flour contaminated with insecticide. J. A. M. A., 161:1582, 1956.

Anonymous. Current concepts in Therapy. Sedative-hyponotic drugs. V. Non-barbiturates. N. Engl. J. Med., 256:314-316, 1957.

Anonymous. Effects of prolonged iodine administration. J. A. M. A., 164:975, 1957a.

Anonymous. Toxicity of mercury. J. A. M. A., 165:1769, 1957b.

Anonymous. Toxicity of vitamin K substitutes in premature infants. Nutr. Rev., 19:75-77, 1961.

Anonymous. Post-Sino-cibal syndrome. N. Engl. J. Med., 278:1122, 1968.

Anonymous. How surgeon's probe led to vinyl hazard findings. American Medical News, May 27, 1974.

Anonymous. Acetylcysteine for acetaminophen overdose. Medical Letter, 21:98-100, 1979.

Anonymous. Hand in glove with dermatitis. Med. World News, p. 67-68, Mar. 17, 1972a.

Antara Chemicals. Report. Division of General Dyestuff Corp., New York, 1955.

Aposhian, H. V.; Aposhian, M. M. N-Acetyl-DL-penicillamine, a new oral protective agent against the lethal effects of mercuric chloride. J. Pharmacol. Exp. Ther., 126:131-135, 1959.

Apostolou, A.; Peoples, S. A. Toxicity of the avicide 2-chloro-4-acetotoluidide in rats: a comparison with its nonacetylated form 3-chloro-p-toluidine. Toxicol. Appl. Pharmacol. 18:517-521, 1971.

Appel, G. B.; Galen, R.; O'Brien, J.; Schoenfeldt, R. Methyl iodide intoxication. A case report. Ann. Intern. Med. 82:534-536, 1975.

Aquilina, J. T.; Bissel, G. B. Fungating iododerma treated with hydrocortisone. J. A. M. A., 158:727-730, 1955.

Archer, S. R.; Blackwood, T. R.; Murin, P. J. Status assessment of toxic chemicals: tris(2, 3-dibromopropyl)phosphate. Report EPA-600/2-79-210N: Order No. PB80-146434, 1979.

Aring, C. D. The systemic nervous affinity of triorthocresyl phosphate (Jamaica ginger palsy). Brain, 65:34-47, 1942.

Armstrong, R. W.; Eichner, E. R.; Klein, D. E.; Barthel, W. F.; Bennett, J. V.; Jonsson, V.; Bruce, H.; Loveless, L. E. Pentachlorophenol poisoning in a nursery for newborn infants. II. Epidemiologic and toxicologic studies. J. Pediatr., 75: 317-325, 1969.

Arnold, O. H.; Ceranke-Hofermayer, S. Ein Fall von Suicidversuch mit Mysoline. Wein. Med. Wochenschr., 103:692, 1953.

Arulanantham, K.; Genel, M. Central nervous system toxicity associated with ingestion of propylene glycol. J. Pediatr., 93:515-516, 1978.

Asano, M.; Ohkubo, C.; Suzuki, A.; Tamura, S. Biological activities of D-pimaric acid and dehydroabietic acid from pine oleoresin as antinicotinic substance. I. Effects of their intravascular application. Koshu Eiseiin Kenkyu Hokoku 22:1-8, 1973.

Ashby, W. B.; Humphreys, J.; Smith, S. J. Small bowel ulceration induced by potassium chloride. Br. Med. J., 2:1409-1412, 1965.

Asmussen, E.; Hald, J.; Larsen, V. The pharmacological action of acetaldehyde on the human organism. Acta Pharmacol. Toxicol., 4:311-320, 1948, 1948b.

Association of American Pesticide Control Officials, Inc. Pesticide chemicals official compendium. College Park, Maryland, 1966.

Auld, R. B.; Bedwell, S. F. Peripheral neuropathy with sympathetic overactivity from industrial contact with acrylamide. Can. Med. Assoc. J. 96:652-654, 1967.

Aviado, D. M.; Smith, D. G. Toxicity of aerosol propellants in the respiratory and circulatory systems. VIII. Respiration and circulation in primates. Toxicology 3:241-252, 1975.

Aviado, D. M.; Zakhari, S.; Simaan, J. A.; Ulsamer, A. G. Methyl Chloroform and Trichloroethylene in the Environment. CRC Press, Cleveland, Ohio, 1976.

Aziz, S. A.; Knowles, C. O. Inhibition of monoamine oxidase by the pesticide chlordimeform and related compounds. Nature 242:417-418, 1973.

Back, K. C.; Thomas, A. A. Aerospace problems in pharmacology and toxicology. Ann. Rev. Pharmacol., 10:399, 1970.

Back, N.; Steger, R.; Glassman, J. M. Comparative acute oral toxicity of sodium warfarin and microcrystalline warfarin in the Sprague-Dawley rat. Pharmacol. Res. Commun., 10:445-452, 1978.

Baer, R. L.; Ramsey, D. L.; Biondi, E. The most common contact allergens. Arch. Dermatol., 108:74, 1973.

Baerg, R. D.; Kimberg, D. V. Centrilobular hepatic necrosis and acute renal failure in "solvent sniffers." Ann. Intern. Med., 73:713-720, 1970.

Bagatell, F. K.; Dugan, K.; Wilgram, G. F. Structural and biochemical changes in tissues isolated from the cantharidin-poisoned rat with special emphasis upon hepatic subcellular particles. Toxicol. Appl. Pharmacol., 15:249-261, 1969.

Bailey, D. N.; Jatlow, P. I. Barbital overdose and abuse. A new problem. Am. J. Clin. Pathol. 64:291-296, 1975.

Bailey, D. N.; Shaw, R. F.; Guba, J. J. Phencyclidine abuse: plasma levels and clinical findings in casual users and in phencyclidine-related deaths. J. Anal. Toxicol. 2:233-237, 1978a.

Bailey, E. V.; Stone, T. W. Mechanism of action of amantadine in parkinsonism. Review. Arch. Int. Pharmacodyn. Ther. 216:246-262, 1975.

Bainova, A.; Burkova, T.; Mikhailova, A. Determination of dermal toxicity of Ramrod. Khig. Zdraveopaz. 20:234-240, 1977.

Baker, C. E., Jr. (publisher). Physicians' Desk Reference., 36th ed. Medical Economics Co., Oradell, N. J, 1982.

Baker, G. S. Personal communication. Smith, Kline and French Laboratories, Philadelphia, 1961.

Baker, R. D.; Handler, P. Animal experiments with tannic acid suggested by the tannic acid treatment of burns. Ann. Surg., 118-417-426, 1943.

Bakke, J. E.; Larson, J. D.; Price, C. E. Metabolism of atrazine and 2-hydroxyatrazine by the rat. J. Agric. Food Chem. 20:602-607, 1972.

Bakos, A. C. P.; Askey, J. M. Fever due to procaine amide hydrochloride therapy. J. A. M. A., 149:1393, 1952.

Balamoutsos, N. G.; Alevizou-Christophoridou, F. Survival following 1000 mg. of Amethocaine. Br. J. Anaesth. 51:469-470, 1979.

Balazs, T.; Sahasrabudhe, M. R.; Grice, H. C. The influence of excess body fat on the cardiotoxicity of isoproterenol in rats. Toxicol. Appl. Pharmacol., 4:613-620, 1962.

Balcerzak, S. P.; Melaragno, A.; Flanigan, P. W.; Bromberg, P. A. Impaired tissue oxygenation in cyanate-treated animals. J. Pharmacol. Exp. Ther., 197:229-234, 1976.

Baler, G. R. Granulomas from topical zirconium in poison ivy dermatitis. Arch. Dermatol. 91:145-148, 1965.

Ballantyne, B. Riot control agents; biomedical and health aspects of the use of chemicals in civil disturbances. Medical Annual, 1977.

Balme, R. H.; Lloyd-Thomas, H. G.; Shead, G. V. Severe barbitone poisoning treated by haemodialysis. Br. Med. J. 1:231-232, 1962.

Balthrop, E.; Gallagher, W. B.; McDonald, T. F.; Camariotes, S. Tung nut poisoning. J. Florida Med. Assoc. 40:813-820, 1954.

Balucani, M.; Zellers, D. D. Podophyllum resin poisoning with complete recovery. J. A. M. A. 189:639-640, 1964.

Banerjee, N. C.; Miller, G. E.; Stowe, C. M. Metabolism and excretion of aminopyrine by cows. Toxicol. Appl. Pharmacol. 10:596-603, 1967a.

Banerjee, N. C.; Miller, G. E.; Stowe, C. M. Excretion of aminopyrine and its metabolites into cows' milk. Toxicol. Appl. Pharmacol. 10:604-612, 1967b.

Banner, W.; Czajka, P. A. Acute caffeine overdose in the neonate. Am. J. Dis. Child., 134:495-498, 1980.

Barber, H. Haemorrhagic nephritis and necrosis of liver from dioxan poisoning. Guys Hosp. Rep., 84:267-280, 1934.

Barer, J.; Hill, L. L.; Hill, R. M.; Martinez, W. M. Fatal poisoning from salt used as an emetic. Am. J. Dis. Child., 125:889-890, 1973.

Barich, L. L.; Schwarz, J.; Barich, D. J.; Horowitz, M. G. Toxic liver damage in mice after prolonged intake of elevated doses of griseofulvin. Antibiotics Chemother. 11:566-571, 1961.

Barker, E. A.; Smuckler, E. A.; Benditt, E. P. Effects of thioacetamide and yellow phosphorus poisoning on protein synthesis in vivo. Lab. Invest., 12: 955-960, 1963.

Barker, W. H.; Wood, W. B., Jr. Severe febrile iodism during the treatment of hyperthyroidism. J. A. M. A., 114:1029-1038, 1940.

Barnard, R. D. Cholinergic porphyrin lacrymation and paradoxical mydriasis in the rat. Possible heme nature of choline esterase. Proc. Soc. Exp. Biol. Med., 54:254-258, 1943.

Barnes, J. M. Observations on the effects on rats of compounds related to acrylamide. Br. J. Ind. Med. 27:147-149, 1970.

Barnes, J. M.; Denz, F. A. Experimental demyelination with organo-phosphorus compounds. J. Pathol. Bacteriol., 65:597-605, 1953.

Barnes, J. M.; Stoner, H. B. Toxic properties of some dialkyl and trialkyl tin salts. Br. J. Ind. Med., 15:15-22, 1958.

Barnes, J. M.; Stoner, H. B. The toxicology of tin compounds. Pharmacol. Rev., 11:211-231, 1959.

Barnhart, C. C.; Bowden, C. L. Toxic psychosis with cimetidine. Am. J. Psychiatry 136:725-726, 1979.

Barron, D. W.; Milliken, T. G. Mephenesin poisoning. Lancet, 1:262, 1960.

Barsoum, G. S.; Saad, K. Relative toxicity of certain chlorine derivatives of aliphatic series. Q. J. Pharm. Pharmacol., 7:205-214, 1934.

Bartels-Schooley, J.; MacNeill, B. H. Comparison of the modes of action of three benzimidazoles. Phytopathology

61:816-819, 1971.

Bartley, J. C.; Reber, E. F. Toxic effects of stable strontium in young pigs. J. Nutr., *75*:21-28, 1961.

Barton, C. H.; Sterling, M. L.; Vaziri, N. D. Rhabdomyolysis and acute renal failure associated with phencyclidine intoxication. Arch. Intern. Med. *140*:568-569, 1980.

Bartonicek, V.; Teisinger, J. Effect of tetraethyl thiuram disulfide (Disulfiram) on metabolism of trichloroethylene in man. Br. J. Ind. Med., *19*:216-221, 1962.

Bartter, F. C.; Berkson, B.; Gallelli, J.; Hiranaka, P. Thioctic acid in the treatment of poisoning with alpha-amanitin. In *Amanita Toxins and Poisoning*. H. Faulstich, B. Kommerell and T. Wieland (editors). Verlag Gerhard Witzstrock, New York, pp. 197-202, 1980.

Baselt, R. C.; Cravey, R. H. A fatal case involving trichloromonofluoromethane and dichlorodifluoromethane. J. Forensic Sci., *13*:407-410, 1968.

Baselt, R. C.; Sunderman, F. W., Jr.; Mitchell, J.; Horak, E. Comparison of antidotal efficacy of sodium diethyldithiocarbamate, *D*-penicillamine and triethylenetetramine upon acute toxicity of nickel carbonyl in rats. Res. Commun. Chem. Pathol. Pharmacol. *18*:677–688, 1977.

Baselt, R. C.; Hanson, V. W. Effect of orally administered chelating agents for nickel carbonyl toxicity in rats. Res. Commun. Chem. Pathol. Pharmacol. *38*:113–123, 1982.

Basinger, M. A.; Jones, M. M.; Tarka, M. P. Relative efficacy of chelating agents as antidotes for acute nickel (II) acetate intoxication. Res. Commun. Chem. Pathol. Pharmacol. *30*:133–141, 1980.

Bass, A. C.; Frost, L. H.; Salter, W. T. 2-Anilinoethanol, industrial hazard; production of methemoglobinemia. J. A. M. A., *123*:761-763, 1943.

Bass, J. W.; Beisel, W. R. Coma due to acute chlorothiazide intoxication. Am. J. Dis. Child., *106*:620-623, 1963.

Bass, M. Sudden sniffing death. J. A. M. A. *212*:2075-2079, 1970.

Bass, S. W.; Ramirez, M. A.; Aviado, D. M. Cardiopulmonary effects of antimalarial drugs. Toxicol. Appl. Pharmacol., *21*:464-481, 1972.

Baude, F. J.; Gardiner, J. A.; Han, J. C. Y. Characterization of residues on plants following foliar spray applications of benomyl. J. Agric. Food Chem. *21*:1084-1090, 1973.

Bauer, J. M.; Freyberg, R. H. Vitamin D intoxication with metastatic calcification. J. A. M. A., *130*:1208-1215, 1946.

Bauer, K; Czech, K.; Porter, A. Severe accidental acrolein intoxication in the home. Wien. Klin. Wochenschr. *89*:243-244, 1977.

Baughman, R. D. Contact photodermatitis from bithionol II. Cross-sensitivities to hexachlorophene and salicylanilides. Arch. Dermatol., *90*:153-157, 1964.

Baxter, D. J.; Smith, W. O.; Klein, G. C. Some effects of acute manganese excess in rats. Soc. Exp. Biol. Med. *119*:966-970, 1965.

Bayer, Plant Protection Division. Personal communication. Federal Republic of Germany, March 1978.

Beard, R. R.; Noe, J. T. Aliphatic and alicyclic amines. Chapter 44 In *Patty's Industrial Hygiene and Toxicology*, Vol. 2B, 3rd ed. (G. D. Clayton and F. E. Clayton, editors). Wiley-Interscience, New York, 1981.

Beauregard, J. R.; Tusing, T. W.; Hanzal, R. F. Toxicity and antidotal studies on 2-pivalyl-1,3-indandione (Pival), an anticoagulant rodenticide. J. Agric. Food Chem., *3*:124-127, 1955.

Becker, B. A. Pharmacologic activity of phentermine (phenyl-t-butylamine). Toxicol. Appl. Pharmacol., *3*:256-259, 1961.

Becker, H.; Schwarz, G. Die Mistel (Viscum album L.) als Krebstherapeutikum. Deut. Apoth. -Ztg. *112*:1462-1465, 1972.

Becker, T. J.; Warren, M. R.; Marsh, D. G.; Thompson, C. R.; Shelton, R. S. Pharmacological and toxicological studies on 1-N-ethylephedrine hydrochloride. J. Pharmacol. Exp. Therap., *75*:289-298, 1942.

Beckman, H. Pharmacology, the Nature, Action and Use of Drugs. 2nd Ed., W. B. Saunders Co., Philadelphia, 1961.

Bedford, C. T.; Crawford, M. J.; Hutson, D. H. Sulfoxidation of cyanatryn, a 2-mercapto-sym-triazine herbicide, by rat liver microsomes. Chemosphere *4*:311-316, 1975.

Bedford, P. D.; Leeds, M. D. Acute potassium intoxication. Lancet, *2*:268-270, 1954.

Beier, L. S.; Pitts, W. A.; Gonick, H. C. Metabolic acidosis occurring during paraldehyde intoxication. Ann. Intern. Med., *58*:155-158, 1963.

Belasco, I. J.; Rusir, R. W. Metabolic fate of siduron in the animal. J. Agric. Food Chem. *17*:1000-1003, 1969.

Belej, M. A.; Smith, D. G.; Aviado, D. M. Toxicity of aerosol propellants in the respiratory and circulatory systems. IV. Cardiotoxicity in the monkey. Toxicology *2*:381-395, 1974.

Beljaev, V. A.; Politykin, A. Ja.; Cernyseva, L. A. Acute poisoning by propylene oxide. Gig. Truda Prof. Zabol. *15*:48-49, 1971.

Belonozhko, G. A.; Tovstenko, A. I.; Shevchenko, N. F. Mechanism of action of dodecylguanidine acetate (dodine). (As cited in Chem. Abstracts, *80*:128988, 1971) Farmakol. Toksikol. (Kiev), No. 8, pp. 134-137, 1973.

Ben-Shachar, G.; Kishon, Y. Intoxication with ajmaline in an infant. Chest, *76*:97-98, 1979.

Benaglia, A. E.; Robinson, E. J.; Utley, E.; Cleverdon, M. A. The chronic toxicity of Aerosol-OT. J. Ind. Hyg. Toxicol., *25*:175, 1943.

Benedetti, M. S.; Malnoe, A.; Broillet, A. L. Absorption, metabolism and excretion of safrole in the rat and man. Toxicology, *7*:69-83, 1977.

Benoy, C. J.; Hooper, P. A.; Schneider, R. The toxicity of tin in canned juices and solid foods. Food Cosmet. Toxicol., *9*:645-656, 1971.

Benson, W. M.; Stefko, P. L.; Randall, L. O. Comparative pharmacology of levorphan, racemorphan and dextrorphan and related methyl esters. J. Pharmacol. Exp. Therap., *109*:189-200, 1953.

Berberian, D. A.; Gorman, W. G.; Drobeck, H. P.; Coulston, F.; Slighter, R. G. Jr. Toxicology and spermicidal activity of a new contraceptive cream containingchlorindanol and laureth 9. Toxicol. Appl. Pharmacol., *7*:215-226, 1965b.

Berberian, D. A.; Gorman, W. G.; Drobeck, H. P.; Coulston, F.; Slighter, R. G., Jr. The toxicology and biological properties of laureth 9 (a polyoxyethylenelauryl ether), a new spermicidal agent. Toxicol. Appl. Pharmacol., *7*:206-214, 1965a.

Berg, G. L. (editor). *Farm Chemicals Handbook*. Meister Publishing Co., Willowughby, Ohio, 1980.

Bergmann, M.; Flance, I. J.; Blumenthal, H. T. Thesaurosis following inhalation of hair spray. N. Engl. J. Med., *258*:471-476, 1958.

Bergmann, M.; Flance, I. J.; Craz, P. T.; Klam, N.; Aronson, P. R.; Joshi, R. A.; Blumenthal, H. T. Thesaurosis due to inhalation of hair spray, report of twelve new cases including three autopsies. N. Engl. J. Med., *266*:750-755, 1962.

Bering, E. A.; Handler, A. H. The production of tumors in hamsters by implantation of polyethylene film. Cancer *10*:414-415, 1957.

Berke, P. A.; Rosen, W. E. Germall, a new family of antimicrobial preservatives for cosmetics. Amer. Perfum. Cosmet. *85*:55-59, 1970.

Berkowitz, C. D. Treatment of acute amantadine toxicity with physostigmine. J. Pediatr. *95*:144-145, 1979.

Berlyne, G. M.; Janabi, K.; Shaw, A. B.; Hocken, A. G. Treatment of hyperkalemia with a calcium resin. Lancet, *1*:169-172, 1966.

Berndt, W. O.; Koschier, F. *In vitro* uptake of 2,4-dichlorophenoxyacetic acid (2,4-D) and 2,4,5-trichlorophenoxyacetic acid (2,4,5-T) by renal cortical tissue of rabbits and rats. Toxicol. Appl. Pharmacol. *26*:559-570, 1973.

Bernstein, B. M. Cyanosis following use of anesthesin (ethylamino-benzoate). Rev. Gastroenterol., *17*:123-124, 1950.

Bernstein, E. H.; Pienta, P. W.; Gershon, H. Acute toxicity studies on 8-quinolinol and some derivatives. Toxicol. Appl. Pharmacol. *5*:599-604, 1965.

Bernstein, H. N.; Curtis, J.; Earl, F. L.; Kawabara, T. Phototoxic corneal and lens opacities in dogs receiving a fungicide, 2,6-dichloro-4-nitroaniline. Arch. Ophthalmol. *83*:336-348, 1970.

Bertolet, R. DeB.; Mecca, S. B. Allantoin and the aluminum

allantoinates. Soap, Perfum., Cosmet. 41:569-572, 1968.

Berwick, P. 2,4-Dichlorophenoxyacetic acid poisoning in man. J. A. M. A., 214:1114-1117, 1970.

Bessen, H. A.; Torrance, M. D. Intracranial hemorrhage associated with phencyclidine abuse. J.A.M.A. 248:585–586, 1982.

Beswick, F. W.; Holland, P.; Kemp, K. H. Acute effects of exposure to orthochlorobenzylidene malononitrile (CS) and the development of tolerance. Br. J. Ind. Med., 29:298-306, 1972.

Beutler, E. The hemolytic effect of primaquine and related compounds, A review. Blood, 14:103-139, 1959.

Bhagat, B.; Lockett, M. F. The absorption and elimination of metabisulfite and thiosulfate by rats. J. Pharm. Pharmacol., 12:690-694, 1960.

Bidstrup, P. L. Clinical aspects of poisoning by organic phosphorus insecticides. Proc. R. Soc. Med., 45:572-573, 1952b.

Billmaier, D.; Yee, H. T.; Allen, N.; Craft, E.; Williams, N.; Epstein, S.; Fontaine, R. Peripheral neuropathy in a coated fabrics plant. J. Occup. Med. 16:665-671, 1974.

Birch, K. M.; Schutz, F. Actions of cyanate. Br. J. Pharmacol., 1:186-193, 1946.

Birnberg, T. L.; Steinberg, C. L. Case of oil of chenopodium poisoning: Treatment with forced perivascular (spinal) drainage. Arch. Pediatr., 56:304-310, 1939.

Bisultanov, A. B. Toxicity of Dursban to sheep following its internal administration. (As cited in Chem. Abstracts, 86:84430b), Tr., Vses. Nauchno-Issled. Inst. Vet. Sanit., No. 49:162-166, 1974.

Bitron, M. D.; Ahronson, E. F. Delayed mortality of mice following inhalation of acute doses of CH_2O, SO_2, Cl_2, and Br_2. Am. Ind. Hyg. Assoc. J., 39:129-138, 1978.

Bjornberg, A.; Gisslen, H. Thiazides: A cause of necrotizing vasculitis?. Lancet, 2:982-983, 1965.

Blair, A. A. D.; Hallpike, J. F.; Lascelles, P. T.; Wingate, D. L. Acute diphenylhydantoin and primidone poisoning treated by peritoneal dialysis. J. Neurol. Neurosurg. Psychiatry, 31:520-523, 1968.

Blair, C. R.; Blumenthal, J. Starch peritonitis. N. Y. State J. Med., 64:1202-1204, 1964.

Blaisdell, C. T. Toxicity of sodium borohydride, trimethyl borate, lithium borohydride, potassium fluoborate and sodium hydride. Chemical Corps Med. Lab., Army Chemical Center, Report MLRR-351, 1955.

Blatt, M. L.; Steigmann, F.; Dyniewicz, J. M. Phenolphthalein tolerance in childhood. J. Pediatr., 22:719-725, 1943.

Bleumink, E.; Mitchell, J. C.; Nater, J. P. Allergic contact dermatitis from cedar wood. J. Dermatol. 88:499-504, 1973.

Blickensdorfer, P.; Templeton, L. A study of the toxic properties of diethyl phthalate. J. Am. Pharm. Assoc. Sci. Ed., 19:1179-1181, 1930.

Block, A. More on infantile methemoglobinemia due to benzocaine suppository. J. Pediatr., 67:509-570, 1965.

Blomquist, L.; Stroman, L.; Thorsell, W. Distribution and fate of the insect repellent ^{14}C-N,N- excretion after injection into mice. Acta Pharmacol. Toxicol. 37:121-133, 1975.

Blomstrand, R.; Ellin, A.; Lof, A.; Ostlung-Wintzell, H. Biological effects and metabolic interactions after chronic and acute administration of 4-methylpyrazole and ethanol to rats. Arch. Biochem. Biophys. 199:591-505, 1980.

Bloomfield, A. F. Domestic chlorine poisoning. Br. Med. J., 2:1332, 1959.

Blum, A.; Gold, M. D.; Ames, B. N.; Kenyon, C.; Jones, F. R.; Hett, E. A.; Doherty, R. C.; Horning, E. C. Dzidic, I.; Carroll, D. I.; Stillwell, R. N.; Thenot, J. P. Children absorb tris-BP flame retardant from sleepwear: Urine contains the mutagenic metabolite, 2, 3-dibromopropanol. Science, 201:1020-1023, 1978.

Blum, K.; Huizenga, C. G.; Ryback, R. S.; Johnson, D. K.; Geller, I. Toxicity of diethanolamine in mice. Toxicol. Appl. Pharmacol. 22:175-185, 1972.

Boehme, C.; Baer, F. The transformation of triazine herbicides in the animal. Food Cosmet. Toxicol. 5:23-28, 1967.

Boehme, C.; Ernst, W. Metabolism of urea herbicides in the rat. II. Diuron and afalon. Food Cosmet. Toxicol. 3:797-802, 1965.

Bogash, R. C. A new iodophor disinfectant. Survey and evaluation. Bull. Am. Soc. Hosp. Pharmacists, 12:135-136, 1955.

Boger, W. P.; Strickland, S. C. Probenecid (benemid): Its use and side effects in 2,502 patients. Arch. Intern. Med., 95:83-92, 1955.

Boley, S. J.; Allen, A. C.; Schultz, L.; Schwartz, S. Potassium-induced lesions of the small bowel. I. Clinical aspects. J. A. M. A., 193:997-1000, 1965.

Bolyai, J. Z., Smith, R. P.; Gray, C. T. Ascorbic acid and chemically induced methemoglobinemia. Toxicol. Appl. Pharmacol., 21:176-185, 1972.

Bondarev, G. I.; Stasenkova, K. P.; Vissarionova, V. Ya. Protective effect of sulfur-containing compounds in acrylonitrile poisoning. Vopr. Pitan. No. 4, p. 55-58, 1976.

Boor, J. W.; Hurtig, H. I. Persistent cerebellar ataxia after exposure to toluene. Ann. Neurol. 2:440-442, 1977.

Booth, A. N.; Ambrose, A. M.; DeEds, F.; Cox, A. J., Jr. The reversible nephrotoxic effects of biphenyl. Toxicol. Appl. Pharmacol., 3:560-567, 1961.

Bordstedt, H. H. The toxic hazards of epoxy resins. Indust. Med. & Surg., 32:426-429, 1963.

Borison, H. L.; Snow, S. R.; Longnecker, D. S.; Smith R. P. 3-Chloro-p-toluidine: effects of lethal doses in rats and cats. Toxicol. Appl. Pharmacol. 31:403-412, 1975.

Bornmann, G.; Loeser, A. Zur toxikologie von polybuten-(1). Arch. Toxikol. 23:240-244, 1968.

Borzelleca, J. F.; Larson, P. S.; Crawford, E. M.; Hennigar, G. R.; Kuchar, E. J.; Klein, H. H. Toxicologic and metabolic studies on pentachloronitrobenzene. Toxicol. Appl. Pharmacol. 18:522-534, 1971.

Borzelleca, J. F.; Lester, D. Acute toxicity of some perhalogenated acetones. Toxicol. Appl. Pharmacol. 7:592-597, 1965.

Bosche, J.; Mallach, H. J. Uber anatomische und chemisch-toxikologische Befunde bei einer todlichen Vergiftung durch Orphenadrin. Arch. Toxikol., 25:76-82, 1969.

Bourne, H. G.; Yee, H. T.; Seferian, S. The toxicity of rubber additives. Arch. Environ. Health 16:700-705, 1968.

Boyd, E. M. The acute toxicity of tannic acid administered intragastrically. Can. Med. Assoc. J., 92:1292-1297, 1965.

Boyd, E. M.; Carsky, E. The acute oral toxicity of the herbicide chlorpropham in albino rats. Effect of diets containing varying amounts of protein. Arch. Environ. Health 19:621-627, 1969.

Boyd, E. M.; Dobos, I. Acute oral toxicity of monuron in albino rats fed from weaning on different diets. J. Agric. Food Chem. 17:1213-1216, 1969.

Boyd, E. M.; Fulford, R. A. The acute oral toxicity of benzyl penicillin potassium in guinea pigs. Antibiot. Chemother., 11:276-283, 1961.

Boyd, E. M.; Godi, I.; Abel, M. Acute oral toxicity of sucrose. Toxicol. Appl. Pharmacol., 7:609-618, 1965b.

Boyd, E. M.; Krijnen, C. J. Toxicity of captan and protein-deficient diet. J. Clin. Pharm. 8:225-234, 1968.

Boyd, E. M.; Krupa, V. Protein-deficient diet and diuron toxicity. J. Agric. Food Chem. 18:1104-1107, 1970.

Boyd, E. M.; Liu, S. J. Toxicity of starch administered by mouth. Can. Med. Assoc. J., 98:492-499, 1968.

Boyd, E. M.; Seymour, K. G. W. Ethylenediamine dihydrochloride or "chlor-ethamine". II. Untoward and toxic reactions. Exp. Med. Surg., 4:223-227, 1946.

Boyd, E. M.; Shanas, M. N. The acute oral toxicity of potassium chloride. Arch. Int. Pharmacodyn. Ther., 133:275-283, 1961.

Boyd, E. M.; Shanas, M. N. The acute oral toxicity of sodium chloride. Arch. Int. Pharmacodyn. Ther., 144:86-96, 1963b.

Boyd, M. R.; Catignani, G. L.; Sasame, H. A.; Mitchell, J. R.; Stiko, A. W. Acute pulmonary injury in rats by nitrofurantoin. Am. Rev. Respir. Dis., 120:93-99, 1979.

Boyd, P. R.; Walker, G.; Henderson, I. N. The treatment of tetraethyl lead poisoning. Lancet, 1:181-185, 1957.

Boylan, J. J.; Egle, J. L.; Guzelian, P. S. Cholestyramine: use as a new therapeutic approach for chlordecone (kepone) poisoning. Science, 199:893-895, 1978.

Boyland, E. Experiments on the chemotherapy of cancer 4. Further experiments with aldehydes and their derivatives.

Biochem. J. *34*:1196-1201, 1940.

Brachman, P. S.; McCreary, T. W.; Florence, R. Agranulocytosis induced by trimeprazine. N. Engl. J. Med., *260*:378-380, 1959.

Braico, K. T.; Humbert, J. R.; Terplan, K. L.; Lehotay, J. M. Laetrile intoxication - report of a fatal case. N. Engl. J. Med., *300*:238-240, 1979.

Brainerd, W. K.; Olmsted, R. W. Toxicity due to the use of Tyzine hydrochloride. J. Pediatr., *48*:157-160, 1956.

Braithwaite, P. F. A case of poisoning by pennyroyal. Recovery. Br. Med. J., *2*:865, 1906.

Braun, H. A.; Lusky, L. M. The protective action of disodium catechol disulfonate in experimental vanadium poisoning. Toxicol. Appl. Pharmacol., *1*:38-41, 1959.

Braun, H. A.; Lusky, L. M.; Calvery, H. O. The efficacy of 2, 3-dimercaptopropanol (BAL) in the therapy of poisoning by compounds of antimony, bismuth, chromium, mercury and nickel. J. Pharmacol. Exp. Ther., (Suppl.)*87*:119-125, 1946.

Braun, W. H.; Young, J. D. Identification of β-hydroxy-ethoxyacetic acid as the major urinary metabolite of 1, 4-dioxane in the rat. Toxicol. Appl. Pharmacol. *39*:33-38, 1977.

Brem, A. S.; Martin, H.; Stern, L. Toxicity from tea ingestion in an infant - computer simulation analysis. Clin. Biochem., *10*:148-149, 1977.

Bridenbaugh, P. O.; Bridenbaugh, L. D.; Moore, D. C. Methemoglobinemia and infant response to lidocaine and prilocaine in continuous caudal anesthesia: A double blind study. Anesth. Analg., *48*:824-830, 1969.

Bridges, B. A.; Mottershead, R. P.; Rothwell, M. A.; Green, M. H. L. Repair-deficient bacterial strains suitable for mutagenicity screening. Tests with the fungicide captan. Chem. -Biol. Interact. *5*:77-84, 1972.

Brieger, H.; Rieders, F.; Hodes, W. A. Acrylonitrile: Spectrophotometric determination, acute toxicity, and mechanism of action. Arch. Ind. Hyg. Occupat. Med., *6*:128-140, 1952.

Brieger, H.; Semisch, C. W.; Stasney, J.; Piatnek, D. A. Industrial antimony poisoning. Ind. Med. Surg., *23*:521-523, 1954.

Brill, H. Trifluoperazine, Clinical and Pharmacological Aspects. Lea & Febiger, Philadelphia, 1958.

Brimblecombe, R. W.; Duncan, W. A. M.; Durant, G. J.; Emmett, J. C.; Ganellus, C. R.; Parsons, M. D. Cimetidine--a non-thiourea H$_2$-receptor antagonist. J. Int. Med. Res. *3*:86-92, 1975.

Brinkman, G. L.; Remp, D. G.; Coates, E. O.; Priest, E. M. The treatment of respiratory acidosis with THAM. Am. J. Med. Sci., *239*:341-346, 1960.

British Pharmacopia. Great Britain General Council of Medical Education and Registration, British Pharmacopia. General Medical Council, 1963.

Brodie, B. B.; Axelrod, J. The fate of acetanilide in man. J. Pharmacol. Exp. Ther., *94*:29-38, 1948.

Brodie, B. B.; Axelrod, J. The fate of aminopyrine (Pyramidon) in man and methods for the estimation of aminopyrine and its metabolites in biological material. J. Pharmacol. Exp. Ther. *99*:171-184, 1950.

Brophy, J. J. Suicide attempts with psychotherapeutic drugs. Arch. Gen. Psychiatry, *17*:652-657, 1967.

Brown, B. B.; Braun, D. L.; Feldman, R. G. The pharmacologic activity of alpha(4-piperidyl)-benzhydrol hydrochloride (azacyclonal hydrochloride): An ataractive agent. J. Pharmacol. Exp. Ther., *118*:153-161, 1956b.

Brown, B. B.; Werner, H. W. Pharmacologic studies on a new central stimulant, alpha-(2-piperidyl)-benzhydrol hydrochloride (MRD-108). J. Pharmacol. Exp. Ther., *110*:180-187, 1954.

Brown, C. V. Acute isoniazid poisoning. Am. Rev. Respir. Dis., *105*:206-216, 1972.

Brown, H. W.; Chan, K. F.; Hussey, K. L. Treatment of enterobiasis and ascariasis with piperazine. J. A. M. A., *161*:515-520, 1956a.

Brown, V. K.; Robinson, J.; Stevenson, D. E. A note on the toxicity and solvent properties of dimethyl sulphoxide. J. Pharm. Pharmacol., *15*:688-692, 1963.

Brown, V. K. H.; Chambers, P. L.; Ferrigan, L. W.; Stevenson, D. E.; Williams, D. A. Toxicological studies with the her-bicide 2,6-dichlorothiobenzamide (chlorthiamid, Prefix). Arch. Toxicol., *23*:42-51, 1967b.

Brown, W. E. Experiments with anesthetic gases propylene, methane, dimethyl ether. J. Pharmacol. Exp. Ther., *23*:485-496, 1924.

Brown, W. J.; Buist, N. R. M.; Gipson, H. T. C.; Hutson, R. K.; Kennaway, N. G. Fatal benzyl alcohol poisoning in a neonatal intensive care unit. Lancet *1*:1250, 1982.

Browne, S. G. Cantharidin poisoning due to a "blister beetle". Br. Med. J., *2*:1290-1291, 1960.

Browning, E. Toxicity of Industrial Organic Solvents. Chemical Publishing Co., Inc., New York, 1953.

Browning, E. Toxicity and metabolism of industrial solvents. Elsevier Publishing Co., Amsterdam, 2nd ed, 1965.

Bruce, R. A.; Tobin, C. E. The effects of sesame oil and fractions of sesame oil on adrenalectomized and other experimental rats. Endocrinology, *27*:956-970, 1940.

Brunner, M. J. Medical aspects of home cold waving. Arch. Dermatol., *65*:316-326, 1952.

Bruton, O. C. Exchange transfusion for acute poisoning in children. U. S. Armed Forces Med. J., *9*:1128-1131, 1958.

Bryant, J. Suicide by ingestion of caffeine. Arch. Pathol. Lab. Med., *105*:685-686, 1981.

Buchanan, N.; Cane, R. D.; Glantz, R.; Hunt, J. A. Phenolphthalein poisoning: a case report. S. Afr. Med. J. *50*:1060-1061, 1976.

Buchner, L. H.; Cimino, J. A.; Raybin, H. W.; Stewart, B. Naloxone reversal of methadone poisoning. N. Y. State J. Med. *72*:2305-2309, 1972.

Bucklin, R.; Myint, M. K. Fatal methemoglobinemia due to well water nitrates. Ann. Intern. Med., *52*:703-705, 1960.

Buckman, S. J.; Ross, R. T.; Wienert, L. A. Modified barium metaborate. In *Pigment Handbook*., T. C. Patton (editor). Wiley, N. Y., pp. 935-946, 1973.

Buiumsohn, A.; Eisenberg, E. S.; Jacob, J.; Rosen, N.; Bock, J.; Frishman, W. H. Seizures and intraventricular conduction defect in propranolol poisoning - report of 2 cases. Ann. Intern. Med., *91*:860-862, 1979.

Buklan, A. I. Acute poisoning with ziram. (as cited in Chem. Abstracts *82*:133715b) Sud. -Med. Ekopert. 17:51, 1974.

Burger, E.; Bauer, H. M. Akuter Vergiftungsfall durch versehentliches Trinken von Natriumazidlosung. Arch. Toxikol. *20*:279-283, 1965.

Burns, R. S.; Lerner, S. E. Causes of phencyclidine-related deaths. Clin. Toxicol. *12*:463–481, 1978.

Burrell, C. D. Personal communication. Sandoz Pharmaceuticals, Hanover, N. J, 1967.

Burstein, C. L. The hazard of paraldehyde administration. Clinical and laboratory studies. J. A. M. A., *121*:187-190, 1943.

Burston, G. R. Self-poisoning with Mandrax. Practitioner, *199*:340-344, 1967.

Bush, A. F.; Abrams, H. K.; Brown, H. V. Fatality and illness caused by ethylene chlorohydrin in an agricultural occupation. J. Ind. Hyg. Toxicol., *31*:352-358, 1949.

Butch, A. J.; Yokel, R. A.; Sigell, L. T.; Hanenson, I. B.; Nelson, E. D. Abuse and pulmonary complications of injecting pentazocine and tripelennamine tablets. Clin. Toxicol., *14*:301-306, 1979.

Buxtorf, A. Toxicological investigations with fluorescent whitening agents. Environ. Qual. Saf., Suppl. 4(Fluoresc. Whitening Agents):191-193, 1975.

Cahn, C. H. Intoxication by ethchlorvynol (Placidyl): Report of four cases. Can. Med. Assoc. J., *81*:733-734, 1959.

Calandra, J. C.; Fancher, O. E. Cleaning Products and Their Accidental Ingestion. Soap and Detergent Assoc. Scientific and Technical Report No. 5R, New York, 1969.

Calder, I. C.; Yong, A. C.; Woods, R. A.; Crowe, C. A.; Ham, K. N.; Tange, J. D. The nephrotoxicity of *p*-aminophenol. II. The effect of metabolic inhibitors and inducers. Chem. Biol. Interact. *27*:245–254, 1979.

Callaway, J. L.; Olansky, S. Trimeprazine. An adjuvant in the management of itching dermatoses. N. C. Med. J., *18*:320-321, 1957.

Calley, D. J.; Guess, W. L.; Autian, J. Hepatotoxicity of a series of organotin esters. J. Pharm. Sci., *56*:240-243, 1967.

Calnan, C. D. Cement dermatitis. J. Occup. Med., 2:15-22, 1960.

Calnan, C. D. Cutaneous hazards for construction workers. Chem. Indus., 2:1019-1026, 1973.

Calnan, C. D. Cyanoacrylate dermatitis. Contact Dermatitis, 5:165-167, 1979.

Calnan, C. D.; Harman, R. R. M.; Wells, G. C. Photodermatitis from soaps. Br. Med. J. 2:1266-1268, 1961.

Calvin, M. E.; Knepper, R.; Robertson, W. O. Salt poisoning. N. Engl. J. Med., 270:625-626, 1964.

Cam, C.; Nigogosyan, G. Acquired toxic porphyria cutanea tarda due to hexachlorobenzene. J. A. M. A., 183:88-91, 1963.

Cameron, G. R.; Doniger, C. R.; Hughes, A. W. M. The toxicity of lauryl thiocyanate and N-butyl-carbitolthiocyanate (lethane 384). J. Pathol. Bacteriol., 49:363-379, 1939.

Cameron, G. R.; Milton, R. F.; Allen, J. W. Toxicity of tannic acid. An experimental investigation. Lancet, 2:179-186, 1943.

Cameron, G. R.; Thomas, J. C.; Ashmore, S. A.; Buchan, J. L.; Warren, E. H.; Hughes, A. W. M. The toxicity of certain chlorine derivatives of benzene with special reference to o-dichlorobenzene. J. Pathol. Bacteriol., 44:281-296, 1937.

Cameron, M. A. M. The action of nitrophenols on the metabolic rate of rats. Br. J. Pharmacol. 13:25-29, 1958.

Campbell Pharmaceuticals, Inc. Brochure (Protopam chloride). New York, 1961.

Campion, D. S.; North, J. D. K. Effect of protein binding of barbiturates on their rate of removal during peritoneal dialysis. J. Lab. Clin. Med. 66:549-563, 1965.

Canby, J. R. Antidiarrheal agent poisoning in a child. J. A. M. A., 192:920-921, 1965.

Canelli, E. Chemical, bacteriological and toxicological properties of cyanuric acid and chlorinated isocyanurates as applied to swimming pool disinfection. Am. J. Public Health 64:155-162, 1974.

Cann, H. M.; Verhulst, H. L. Esophageal stricture following ingestion of detergent. Bull. National Clearinghouse for Poison Control Centers, 1958a.

Cann, H. M.; Verhulst, H. L. The salicylate problem with special reference to methyl salicylate. J. Pediatr., 53:271-276, 1958b.

Cann, H. M.; Verhulst, H. L. Voodoo dolls have hex. Bull. National Clearinghouse for Poison Control Centers, 1959.

Cann, H. M.; Verhulst, H. L. Convulsions as a manifestation of acute dextro propoxyphene intoxication. A. M. A. J. Dis. Child., 99:380-382, 1960a.

Cann, H. M.; Verhulst, H. L. Treatment of household soap and detergent ingestion. Bull. National Clearinghouse for Poison Control Centers, 1960b.

Cannon, S. B.; Veazey, J. M., Jr.; Jackson, B. S.; Burse, V. W.; Hayes, C.; Straub, W.; Landrigan, P. J.; Liddle, J. A. Epidemic kepone poisoning in chemical workers. Am. J. Epidemiol. 107:529-537, 1978.

Caplan, J. Habituation to diethyl-propion (Tenuate). Can. Med. Assoc. J., 88:943-944, 1963.

Carboni, G. Sustar 2-S: Un nouvel regulateur de croissance. Notiziario sulle malattii delle piante, p. 273-275, 1975.

Cardozo, R. H.; Edelman, I. S. The volume distribution of sodium thiosulfate as a measure of the extracellular fluid space. J. Clin. Invest., 31:280-290, 1952.

Cares, R.; Newman, B.; Mauceri, J. Poisoning by Dormison, fatal suicidal overdose. Am. J. Clin. Pathol., 23:129-132, 1953.

Caridis, D. T.; McAndrew; Matheson, N. A. Haemodialysis in poisoning with methaqualone and diphenhydramine. Lancet, 1:51-52, 1967.

Carlson, G. P.; Dubois, K. P. Studies on the toxicity and mode of action of Morestan. Toxicol. Appl. Pharmacol. 14:632-633, 1969.

Carlson, G. P.; Dubois, K. P. Studies on the toxicity and biochemical mechanism of action of 6-methyl-2,3-quinoxalinedithiol cyclic carbonate (Morestan). J. Pharmacol. Exp. Ther. 173:60-70, 1970.

Carpenter, C. P.; Critchfield, F. H.; Nair, J. H., III; Shaffer, C. B. Toxicology of two butoxypolypropylene glycol fly repellents. Arch. Inc. Hyg. Occup. Med., 4:261-269, 1951b.

Carpenter, C. P.; Kinkead, E. R.; Geary, D. L., Jr.; Sullivan, L. J.; King, J. M. Petroleum hydrocarbon toxicity studies II. Animal and human response to vapors of varnish maker's and painter's naphtha. Toxicol. Appl. Pharmacol., 32:263-281, 1975a.

Carpenter, C. P.; Kinkead, E. R.; Geary, D. L., Jr.; Sullivan, L. J.; King, J. M. Petroleum hydrocarbon toxicity studies III. Animal and human response to vapors of stoddard solvent. Toxicol. Appl. Pharmacol., 32:282-297, 1975b.

Carpenter, C. P.; Kinkead, E. R.; Geary, D. L., Jr.; Sullivan, L. J.; King, J. M. Petroleum hydrocarbon toxicity studies IV. Animal and human response to vapors of rubber solvent. Toxicol. Appl. Pharmacol., 33:526-542, 1975c.

Carpenter, C. P.; Shaffer, C. B. A study of the polyethylene glycols as vehicles for intramuscular and subcutaneous injection. J. Am. Pharm. Assoc., Sci. Ed., 41:27-29, 1952.

Carpenter, C. P.; Smyth, H. F., Jr. Chemical burns of the rabbit cornea. Am. J. Ophthalmol., 29:1363-1372, 1946.

Carpenter, C. P.; Weil, C. S.; Palm, P. E.; Woodside, M. D.; Smyth, H. F., Jr. The toxicology of butoxypolypropylene glycol 800 (Crag fly repellent). J. Agric. Food Chem., 7:763-769, 1959.

Carpenter, C. P.; Weil, C. S.; Pozzani, U. C.; Smyth, H. F., Jr. Acute and subacute toxicity of cyclethrin. Arch. Ind. Hyg. Occup. Med., 10:162-168, 1954.

Carpenter, C. P.; Weil, C. S.; Smyth, H. F., Jr. Toxicity of an imidazoline (or glyoxalidine) fungicide. Arch. Ind. Hyg. Occup. Med., 4:494-503, 1951a.

Carpenter, C. P.; Weil, C. S.; Smyth, H. F., Jr. Mammalian toxicity of sesone herbicide. J. Agric. Food Chem., 9:382-385, 1961b.

Carr, C. J.; Forman, S. E. Sugar alcohols XX. The fate of d-sorbitol, styracitol and l-sorbose in the animal body. J. Biol. Chem. 128:425-430, 1938.

Carroll, W. M.; Mastaglia, F. L. Alpha and beta coma in drug intoxication uncomplicated by cerebral hypoxia. Electroencephal. Clin. Neurophysiol., 46:95-105, 1979.

Carswell, T. S.; Morrill, H. L. Cyclohexylamine and dicyclohexylamine-properties and uses. Ind. Eng. Chem., 11:1247-1251, 1937.

Carter, J. E. Iodide "mumps". N. Engl. J. Med., 264:987-988, 1961.

Carter, J. H.; McLafferty, M. A.; Goldman, P. Role of the gastrointestinal microflora in amygdalin (Laetrile)-induced cyanide toxicity. Biochem. Pharmacol., 29:301-304, 1980.

Carter, R. F.; Fotheringham, B. J. Fatal salt poisoning due to gastric lavage with hypertonic saline. Med. J. Aust., 1:539-541, 1971.

Casey, D. E. Amantadine intoxication reversed by physostigmine. New Engl. J. Med. 298:516, 1978.

Cash, R.; Shapiro, R. I.; Levy, S. H.; Hopkins, S. M. Chelating agents in the therapy of beryllium poisoning. N. Engl. J. Med., 260:683-686, 1959.

Casida, J. E. Specificity of substituted phenyl phosphorus compounds for esterase inhibition in mice. Biochem. Pharmacol., 5:332-342, 1961.

Casida, J. E.; Engle, J. L.; Essac, E. G.; Kamienski, F. X.; Kuwatsuka, S. Methylene-C¹⁴-dioxyphenyl compounds: Metabolism in relation to their synergistic action. Science, 153:1130-1133, 1966.

Casida, J. E.; Kimmel, E. C.; Ohkawa, H.; Ohkawa, R. Sulfoxidation of thiocarbamate herbicides and metabolism of thiocarbamate sulfoxides in living mice and liver enzyme systems. Pestic. Biochem. Physiol. 5:1-11, 1975.

Castillo, J. C.; De Beer, E. J.; Jaros, S. H. A pharmacological study of N-methyl-N'-(4-chlorobenzhydryl) piperazine dihydrochloride - a new antihistaminic. J. Pharmacol. Exp. Ther., 96:388-395, 1949.

Cattanach, B. M. The mutagenicity of cyclamates and their metabolites. Mutation Res. 39:1-28, 1976.

Caujolle, F.; Caujolle, D.; Bouyssou, H.; Calvet, M. M. Toxicite et aptitudes pharmacologiques du dimethylsulfoxyde. C. R. Acad. Soc. (Paris), 258:2224-2226, 1964.

Caujolle, F.; Chanh, P. H.; Lecointe, P. Pharmacologie du nitrosopentacyanoferrate$_{III}$ de cobalt. Arch. Int. Pharmacodyn. 172:487-495, 1968.

Cavagna, G.; Locati, G.; Vigliani, E. C. Clinical effects of exposure to DDVP (Vapona) insecticide in hospital wards. Arch. Environ. Health, 19:112-123, 1969.

Cerami, A.; Manning, J. M. Potassium cyanate as an inhibitor of the sickling of erythrocytes in vitro. Proc. Natl. Acad. Sci. U. S. A., 68:1180-1183, 1971.

Cerami, A. P.; Allen, T. A.; Graziano, J. H.; DeFuria, F. G.; Manning, J. M.; Gillette, D. N. Pharmacology of cyanate. I. General effects on experimental animals. J. Pharmacol. Exp. Ther., 185:653-666, 1973.

Cerwenka, E. A. Jr.; Cooper, W. C. Toxicology of selenium and tellurium and their compounds. Arch. Environ. Health, 3:189-200, 1961.

Cetingil, A. I.; Ozen, M. A. Toxic porphyria. Blood, 16:1002-1011, 1960.

Chan, T.; Ki, L.; Mak, N.; Ng, R. P. Methemoglobinemia, Heinz bodies and acute massive intravascular hemolysis in Lysol poisoning. Blood, 38:739-744, 1971.

Chandra, S.; Seth, P. K.; Mankeshwar, J. K. Manganese poisoning: clinical and biochemical observations. Environ. Res. 7:374-380, 1974.

Chandra, S. V. Histological and histochemical changes in experimental manganese encephalopathy in rabbits. Arch. Toxicol. 29:29-38, 1972.

Chang, T. M. S. Clinical experience with ACAC coated charcoal hemoperfusion in acute intoxication. Clin. Toxicol., 17:529-542, 1980.

Chasseaud, L. F.; Hawkins, D. R.; Cameron, B. D.; Fry, B. J.; Saggers, V. H. Metabolic fate of bentazon in the rat. Xenobiotica 2:269-276, 1972.

Cheek, D. B. On the nature of pink disease. Med. J. Aust., 1:153-155, 1960.

Cheek, D. B.; Bondy, R. K.; Johnson, L. R. The effect of mercurous chloride (calomel) and epinephrine (sympathetic stimulation) on rats. The importance of the findings to mechanisms in infantile acrodynia (pink disease). Pediatrics, 23:302-313, 1959.

Cheek, D. B.; Wu, F. The effect of calomel on plasma epinephrine in the rat and the relationship to mechanisms in pink disease. Arch. Dis. Child., 34:501-504, 1959.

Cheek, F. E.; Newell, S. Deceptions in the illicit drug market. Science, 167:1276, 1970.

Cheever, K. L.; Richards, D. E.; Plotnick, H. B. Metabolism of ortho-, meta-, and para-toluidine in the adult male rat. Toxicol. Appl. Pharmacol., 56:361-369, 1980.

Chemagro Corp. Brochure (Chlorthion). New York, 1955.

Chemagro Corp. Brochure (Bayer 30686 and Bayer 28589, Miticides). Kansas City, Mo, 1959.

Chemagro Corp. Brochure (Bayer 29493, Insecticide). Kansas City, Mo, 1961a.

Chemagro Corp. Brochure (Co-Ral Insecticide and Anthelmintic (Bayer 21/199)). Kansas City, Mo, 1961b.

Chemagro Corp. Brochure (DEF Defoliant). Kansas City, Mo, 1961c.

Chemagro Corp. Brochure (Dexon Seed and Soil Fungicide (Bayer 22555)). Kansas City, Mo, 1961d.

Chemagro Corp. Brochure (Di-Syston Insecticide (Bayer 19639)). Kansas City, Mo, 1961e.

Chemagro Corp. Brochure (Dylox Insecticide (Bayer L 13/59)). Kansas City, Mo, 1961f.

Chemagro Corp. Brochure (Dyrene Fungicide). Kansas City, Mo, 1961g.

Chemagro Corp. Brochure (Eradex Miticide (Bayer 30686)). Kansas City, Mo, 1961h.

Chemagro Corp. Brochure (Guthion Insecticide (Bayer 17147)). Kansas City, Mo, 1961i.

Chemagro Corp. Brochure (Meta-Systox-R Insecticide (Bayer 21097)). Kansas City, Mo, 1961j.

Chemagro Corp. Brochure (Systox Insecticide). Kansas City, Mo, 1961k.

Chen, K. K.; Rose, C. L. Treatment of acute cyanide poisoning. J. A. M. A., 162:1154-1155, 1956.

Chen, K. K.; Rose, C. L.; Robbins, E. B. Toxicity of nicotinic acid. Proc. Soc. Exp. Biol. Med., 38:241-245, 1938.

Chen, K. K.; Schmidt, C. F. Ephedrine and related substances. Medicine, 9:1-117, 1930.

Chen, Y. S.; Casida, J. E. Thiocarbamate herbicide metabolism: microsomal oxygenase metabolism of EPTC involving mono- and dioxygenation at the sulfur and hydroxylation at each alkyl carbon. J. Agric. Food Chem. 26:263-267, 1978.

Chengelis, C. P.; Neal, R. A. Hepatic carbonyl sulfide metabolism. Biochem. Biophys. Res. Commun. 90:995-999, 1979.

Chengelis, C. P.; Neal, R. A. Studies of carbonyl sulfide toxicity; metabolism by carbonic anhydrase. Toxicol. Appl. Pharmacol., 55:198-202, 1980.

Chenoweth, M. B. Clinical uses of metal-binding drugs. Clin. Pharmacol. Ther., 9:365-387, 1968.

Chernoff, R. W.; Wallen, M. H.; Miller, O. F. Cardiac toxicity of methylphenidate. New Engl. J. Med., 266:400-401, 1962.

Chevron Chemical Co., Ortho Division. Experimental Data Sheet (Monitor Insecticide). Chevron Chemical Co., Ortho Division, Richmond, CA, 1973.

Chevron Chemical Co., Ortho Division. Experimental Data Sheet (Orthene Insecticide). Chevron Chemical Co., Ortho Division, Richmond, CA, 1976.

Chilcote, R. R.; Williams, B.; Wolff, L. J.; Baehner, R. L. Sudden death in an infant from methemoglobinemia after administration of sweet spirits of nitre. Pediatrics, 59:280-282, 1977.

Chilton, W. S. Chemistry and mode of action of mushroom toxins. In *Mushroom Poisoning: Diagnosis and Treatment.*, B. H. Rumack and E. Salzman (editors). CRC Press, Inc, 1978.

Chin, W. T.; Stone, G. M.; Smith, A. E.; Von Schmeling, B. Fate of carboxin in soil, plants and animals. Proc. Brit. Insectic. Fungic. Conf., 5th, 1969, 2:322-327, Publ. 1970.

Chouinard, G.; Annable, L. Phenothiazine-induced ECG abnormalities: effect of a glucose load. Arch. Gen. Psychiatry, 34:951-954, 1977.

Chow, A. Y. K.; Husch, G. H.; Buttar, H. S. Nephrotoxic and hepatotoxic effects of triclosan and chlorhexidine in rats. Toxicol. Appl. Pharmacol. 42:1-10, 1977.

Chow, C. P.; Buttar, H. S.; Downie, R. H. Percutaneous absorption of chlorhexidine in rats. Toxicol. Lett. 1:213-216, 1978.

Christensen, H. D.; Lee, I. S. Anesthetic potency and acute toxicity of optically active disubstituted barbituric acids. Toxicol. Appl. Pharmacol. 26:495-503, 1973.

Christensen, J.; Williams, B. J. Thiocyanate psychosis treated by extracorporeal hemodialysis. J. A. M. A., 181:340-342, 1962.

Ciba-Geigy Corporation. Caparol-Brand of Prometryne herbicide. Ardsley, New York, Oct. 1972a.

Ciba-Geigy Corporation. Toxicology data sheet (Simazine). Ardsley, New York, Oct. 1972b.

Clark, A. N. G.; Parsonage, M. J. A case of podophyllum poisoning with involvement of the nervous system. Br. Med. J., 2:1155-1157, 1957.

Clark, D. E.; Palmer, J. S. Residual aspects of 2,4,5-T and an ester in sheep and cattle with observations on concomitant toxicological effects. J. Agric. Food Chem. 19:761-764, 1971.

Clark, D. G.; McElligott, T. F. Acute and short-term toxicity of drazoxolon (4-(2-chlorophenylhydrazone-3-methyl-5-isoxazolone). Food Cosmet. Toxicol. 7:481-491, 1969.

Clark, D. G.; McElligott, T. F.; Hurst, E. W. The toxicity of paraquat. Br. J. Ind. Med., 23:126-132, 1966.

Clark, G. L. (Ed.); Hawley, G. G.; Hamor, W. A. Robane. Robane, in The Encyclopedia of Chemistry-Supplement, Reinhold Publishing Corp., New York, p. 283, 1958, 1958.

Clark, M. S. G.; Rand, M. J.; Vanov, S. Comparison of pharmacological activity of nicotine and related alkaloids occurring in cigarette smoke. Arch. Int. Pharmacodyn. Ther. 156:363-379, 1965.

Clarke, C. H. Mutagenic specificities of pentachloronitrobenzene and captan, two environmental mutagens. Mut. Res. 11:247-248, 1971.

Clayton, J. W., Jr.; Barnes, J. R.; Hood, D. B.; Schepers, G. W. H. The inhalation toxicity of dimethyl formamide (DMF). Am. Ind. . Hyg. Assoc. J., 24:144-154, 1963.

Clayton, J. W.; Hood, D. B.; Barnes, J. R.; Borgmann, A. R. Chronic oral toxicity of manganese ethylene bis dithiocarbamate. Am. Ind. Hyg. Assoc. J. (Abstracts 1 and 2), p. 96,

1957.

Cobey, F. A.; Taliaferro, I.; Haag, H. B. Effect of DDD and some of its derivatives on plasma 17-OH-corticosteroids in the dog. Science, 123:140, 1956.

Cochran, K. W.; Doull, J.; Mazur, M.; DuBois, K. P. Acute toxicity of zirconium, columbium, strontium, lanthanum, cesium, tantalum and yttrium. Arch. Ind. Health, 1:637-650, 1950.

Cohen, R. J.; Sachs, J. R.; Wicker, D. J.; Conrad, M. E. Methemoglobinemia provoked by malarial chemoprophylaxis in Viet Nam. N. Engl. J. Med., 279:1127-1131, 1968.

Cohen, S.; Ditman, K. S. Complications associated with lysergic acid diethylamide (LSD-25). J. A. M. A., 181:161-162, 1962.

Cohn, W. J.; Boylan, J. J.; Blanke, R. V.; Fariss, M. W.; Howell, J. R.; Guzelian, P. S. Treatment of chlordecone (kepone) toxicity with cholestyramine. N. Engl. J. Med., 298:243-248, 1978.

Coirault, R.; Pourpre, H.; Damasio, R.; Rouif, G.; Deligne, P.; David, M.; Talairach, J. The treatment of consciousness disorders in neurosurgery by the dimethylaminoethyl ester of p-chlorophenoxyacetic acid (ANP-235). Presse Med. 68:215-216, 1960.

Cole, V. V.; Harned, B. K.; Hafkesbring, R. Toxicity of strontium and calcium. J. Pharmacol. Exp. Ther., 71:1-3, 1941.

Collins, T. F. X.; Williams, C. H. Teratogenic studies with 2,4,5-T and 2,4-D in the hamster. Bull. Environ. Contam. Toxicol. 6:559-567, 1971.

Coman, D. R.; Bruner, H. D.; Horn, R. C., Jr.; Friedman, M.; Boche, R. D.; McCarthy, M. D.; Gibbon, M. H.; Schultz, J. Studies on experimental phosgene poisoning. I. The pathologic anatomy of phosgene poisoning with special reference to the early and late phases. Am. J. Path., 23:1037-1073, 1947.

Commercial Solvents Corp. Industrial chemicals catalog. 24s Park Avenue, New york, N. Y. 10017, 1954.

Commerical Solvents Corp. Technical Data Sheet No. 32 Dimethyl Ether. Commercial Solvents Corp., 245 Park Avenue, New York, N. Y. 10017, 1969.

Comstock, C. C.; Fogleman, R. W.; Oberst, F. W. Acute narcotic effects of monochloromonobromomethane vapor in rats. Arch Ind. Hyg. Occup. Med. 7:526-528, 1953.

Conn, J. W.; Rovner, D. R.; Cohen, E. L. Licorice-induced pseudoaldosteronism. J. A. M. A., 205:492-496, 1968.

Connelly, J. P. Accidental ingestion of a veratrum alkaloid. N. Engl. J. Med., 257:577-578, 1957.

Connett, P. H.; Wetterhahn, K. E. Metabolism of the carcinogen chromate by cellular constituents. In Structure and Bonding (M. J. Clarke, editor) Springer-Verlag Berlin Heidelberg, In Press, 1982.

Conney, A. H.; Chang, R.; Levin, W. M.; Garbut, A.; Munro-Faure, A. D.; Peck, A. W.; Bye, A. Effects of piperonyl butoxide on drug metabolism in rodents and man. Arch. Environ. Health 24:97-106, 1972.

Cook, D. G.; Fahn, S.; Brait, K. A. Chronic manganese intoxication. Arch. Neurol. 30:59-64, 1974.

Cookson, H. A.; Stock, C. J. H. Santonin poisoning; a fatal case. Lancet, 2:745, 1940.

Corbett, T. H.; Beaudoin, A. R.; Cornell, R. G.; Anver, M. R.; Schumacher, R.; Endres, J.; Szwabowska, M. Toxicity of polybrominated biphenyls (Firemaster BP-6) in rodents. Environ. Res. 10:390-396, 1975.

Cornbleet, T. Bromide intoxication treated with ammonium chloride. J. A. M. A., 146:1116-1119, 1951.

Cornish, H. H.; Bahor, R. E.; Ryan, R. C. Toxicity and metabolism of ortho-, meta- and para-terphenyls. Am. Ind. Hyg. Assoc. J., 23:372-378, 1962.

Corrin, B. Aluminum pneumoconiosis. II. Effect on the rat lung of intratracheal injections of stamped aluminum powders containing different lubricating agents and of a granular aluminum powder. Br. J. Ind. Med., 20:268-276, 1963.

Cotter, L. H. Hazard of phenylmercuric salts. Occupational Med., 4:305-309, 1947.

Cotter, L. H. Paradichlorobenzene poisoning from insecticides. New York State J. Med., 53:1690-1692, 1953.

Council on Drugs, A. M. A. Monograph (Griseofulvin), 1960.

Council on Pharmacy and Chemistry, A. M. A. Pharmacology and toxicology of certain organic phosphorus insecticides. J. A. M. A., 144:104-108, 1950.

Council on Pharmacy and Chemistry, A. M. A. Outlines of information on pesticides. Part 1, Agricultural fungicides. J. A. M. A., 157:237-241, 1955.

Courtney, K. D.; Moore, J. A. Teratology studies with 2,4,5-trichlorophenoxyacetic acid and 2,3,7,8-tetrachlorodibenzo-P-dioxin. Toxicol. Appl. Pharmacol. 20:396-403, 1971.

Cowan, G. A. B. Unusual case of poisoning by zinc sulfate. Br. Med. J., 1:451-452, 1947.

Cox, W. T., Chemical Co. Personal communication. Kansas City, Mo, 1957.

Cox, W. W.; Wendel, W. B. The normal rate of reduction of methemoglobin in dogs. J. Biol. Chem., 143:331-340, 1942.

Coyer, H. A. Tetrachloroethane poisoning. Seven cases: Review of several treated. Ind. Med. Surg. 13:230-233, 1944.

Cracovaner, A. J. Stenosis after explosion of lithium hydride. Arch. Otolaryngol., 80:87-92, 1964.

Craft, A. W.; Brocklebank, J. T.; Jackson, R. H. Acute renal failure and hypoglycaemia due to sulphadiazine poisoning. Postgrad. Med. J. 53:103-104, 1977.

Craig, J. O. Poisoning by the volatile oils in childhood. Arch. Dis. Child., 28:475-483, 1953.

Crandell, L. A.; Leake, C. D.; Lovenhart, A. S.; Muehlberger, C. W. Acquired tolerance to and cross tolerance between the nitrous and nitric acid esters and sodium nitrite in man. J. Pharmacol. Exp. Ther. 41:103-119, 1931.

Craven, J. D.; Polak, A. Cantharidin poisoning. Br. Med. J., 2:1386-1388, 1954.

Crawford, L. M.; Teske, R. H. Urinary calcium excretion by neomycin-treated dogs. Toxicol. Appl. Pharmacol., 44:567-570, 1978.

Crawford, M. A. D. Aplastic anemia due to trinitrotoluene. Br. Med. J., 2:430-437, 1954.

Crawford, S. E.; Moon, A. E.; Panos, T. C.; Hooks, C. A. Methemoglobinemia associated with Pyridium administration: Report of a case. J. A. M. A., 146:24-25, 1951.

Crayford, J. V.; Harthoorn, P. A.; Hutson, D. H. Excretion and residues of the herbicides benzoylprop-ethyl, flamprop-isopropyl and flamprop-methyl in cows, pigs and hens. Pestic. Sci. 1:559-70, 1976.

Cronheim, G. Acute toxicity of salicylic, p-aminobenzoic and p-aminosalicylic acid alone and in combination. Fed. Proc., 10:289-290, 1951.

Cronk, G. A.; Naumann, D. E. Phenyltoloxamine-dosage, toxicity, and clinical application. N. Y. State J. Med., 55:1465-1467, 1955.

Crowe, C. A.; Yong, A. C.; Calder, I. C.; Ham, K. N.; Tange, J. D. The nephrotoxicity of p-aminophenol. I. The effect of microsomal cytochromes, glutathione and covalent binding in kidney and liver. Chem. Biol. Interact. 27:235–243, 1979.

Crowley, W. J., Jr.; Johns, T. R. Accidental malathion poisoning. Arch. Neurol., 14:611-616, 1966.

Cruthirds, T. P.; Cole, F. H.; Paul, R. N. Pulmonary talcosis as a result of massive aspiration of baby powder. South. Med. J., 70:626-628, 1977.

Cruz, H. A.; Cramer, N. C.; Parrish, A. E. Hemodialysis in chlordiazepoxide toxicity. J. A. M. A., 202:438-440, 1967.

Csiky, P. Intoxikationsfalle durch das pulver der spanischen Fluge, beziehungsweise durch Cantharidin. Arch. Toxikol., 17:27-31, 1958.

Cumming, G.; Harding, L. K.; Prowse, K. Treatment and recovery after massive overdose of physostigmine. Lancet 2, 147-149, 1968.

Cummingham, D. G.; Challapalli, M. Hypertension in acute haloperidol poisoning. J. Pediatr., 95:489-490, 1979.

Cummins, L. M.; Kimura, E. T. Safety evaluation of selenium sulfide antidandruff shampoos. Toxicol. Appl. Pharmacol., 20:89-96, 1971.

Cundiff, R. H. Spectophotometric determination of glycyrrhizic acid in licorice extract. Anal. Chem., 36:1871-1873, 1964.

Curry, A. S. Twenty-one uncommon cases of poisoning. Br. Med. J., 1:687-689, 1962.

Curry, A. S.; Price, D. E.; Tryhorn, F. G. Absorption of zinc phosphide particles. Nature, 184:642-643, 1959.

Cushing, A. H.; Smith, S. Methemoglobinemia with silver nitrate therapy of a burn. Pediatrics, 74:613-615, 1969.

Cushny, A. R. Optical isomers. VII. Hyoscines and hyoscyamines. J. Pharmacol. Exp. Ther., 17:41-61, 1921.

Custer, R. P. Aplastic anemia in soldiers treated with atabrine (Quinacrine). Am. J. Med. Sci., 212:211-224, 1946.

Cutlip, R. C.; Monlux, W. S. Experimental crystal violet and methyl violet poisoning in dogs and cattle. Can. J. Comp. Med. Vet. Sci., 31:80-84, 1967.

Dalgaard-Mikkelsen, S.; Poulsen, E. Toxicology of herbicides. Pharmacol. Rev., 14:225-250, 1962.

Daly, D. J.; Davenport, J.; Newland, M. C. Methaemoglobinaemia following the use of prilocaine ("Citanest"). Brit. J. Anaesth., 36:737-739, 1964.

Danahy, D. T.; Aronow, W. S. Hemodynamics and antianginal effects of high dose oral isosorbide dinitrate after chronic use. Circulation, 56:205-212, 1977.

Daniel, E. P.; Lillie, R. D. Experimental vanadium poisoning in the white rat. Pub. Health Rep., 53:765-777, 1938.

Daniel, J. W. Metabolism of arylazoisoxazolones by rats and dogs. Biochem. J. 111:695-702, 1969.

Danzig, L. E. Dynamics of thiocyanate dialyses, the artificial kidney in the therapy of thiocyanate intoxication. N. Engl. J. Med., 252:49-57, 1955.

Danziger, H. Accidental poisoning by vinyl chloride. Report of two cases. Can. Med. Assoc. J., 82:828-830, 1960.

Darda, S. Absorption, metabolism and excretion of the fungicide triforine in the rat. Pestic. Sci. 8:193-202, 1977.

Darmady, J. M. Diazepam for fenfluramine intoxication. Arch. Dis. Child. 49:328-330, 1974.

Das, K. M.; Eastwood, M. A.; McManus, J. P. A.; Sircus, W. The metabolism of salicylazosulphapyridine in ulcerative colitis. I. The relationship between metabolites and the response to treatment in inpatients. Gut 14:631-641, 1973.

Davenport, H. W. Gastric mucosal injury by fatty and acetylsalicylic acids. Gastroenterology 46:245-253, 1964.

David, A.; Miketukova, V. Akute Kaliumthiozyanatvergiftung. Arch. Toxikol., 23:66-72, 1967.

David, N. A. The pharmacology of dimethyl sulfoxide. Ann. Rev. Pharmacol. 12:353-374, 1972.

David, N. A.; Phatak, N. M.; Zener, F. B. Iodochlorhydroxyquinoline and diiodohydroxyquinoline: Animal toxicity and absorption in man. Am. J. Trop. Med. Hyg., 24:29-33, 1944.

Davidow, B.; Radomski, J. L. Isolation of an epoxide metabolite from fat tissues of dogs fed heptachlor. J. Pharmacol. Exp. Ther. 107:259-265, 1953.

Davidsohn, A.; Milwidsky, B. M. Synthetic Detergents. 5th ed., Chemical Rubber Company Press, Cleveland, Ohio, 1972.

Davidson, B.; Radomski, J. L.; Elay, R. Excretion of heptachlor epoxide in milk of a dairy cow fed heptachlor. Science 118:383-384, 1953.

Davies, D. R. The effect of organo-phosphorus insecticides on enzymes. Proc. R. Soc. Med., 45:570-571, 1952.

Davies, J. E.; Barquet, A.; Freed, V. H.; Haque, R.; Morgade, C.; Sonneborn, R. E.; Vaclavek, C. Human pesticide poisonings by a fat-soluble organophosphate insecticide. Arch. Environ. Health 30:608-613, 1975.

Davis, J. C.; Hoos, R. A. W. Use of sodium pentachlorophenate and dehydroabietic acid as reference toxicants for salmonid bioassays. J. Fish. Res. Board Can. 32:411-416, 1975.

Davis, J. H.; Hunt, H. H. Accidental Benadryl poisoning. Report of a fatal case. J. Pediatr., 34:358-361, 1949.

Davis, J. M.; Bartlett, E.; Termini, B. A. Overdosage of psychotropic drugs: A review. Dis. Nerv. Syst., 29:157-164 and 246-256, 1968.

Davis, J. S.; Kaufman, R. H. Tetracycline toxicity. Am. J. Obstet. Gynecol., 95:523-529, 1966.

Davis, K. J.; Jenner, P. M. Toxicity of three drug solvents. Toxicol. Appl. Pharmacol., 1:576-578, 1959.

Davis, N. L.; De Jong, R. H. Successful resuscitation following massive bupivacaine overdose. Anesth. Analg., 61:62-64, 1982.

Davis, R. P.; Blythe, W. B.; Newton, M.; Welt, L. G. Treatment of intoxication with ethynylcyclohexyl carbamate (Valmid)

by extracorporeal hemodialysis: Case report. Yale J. Biol. Med., 32:192-196, 1959.

Davis, W. M.; Borne, R. F.; Hackett, R. B.; Waters, I. W. Lethal synergism of phencyclidine with a precursor and contaminant, 1-piperidinocyclohexanecarbonitrile. Life Sci. 26:2105–2111, 1980.

Davison, C.; Zimmerman, E. F.; Smith, P. K. On the metabolism and toxicity of methyl salicylate. J. Pharmacol. Exp. Ther., 132:207-211, 1961.

Dawson, J. A.; Heath, D. F.; Rose, J. A.; Thain, E. M.; Ward, J. B. The excretion by humans of the phenol derived in vivo from 2-isopropoxyphenyl N-methylcarbamate. Bull. W. H. O., 30:127-134, 1964.

Dax, E. C. Overdosage with bromides. A report on 59 cases. Br. Med. J., 2:226-227, 1946.

Dayton, P. G.; Sicam, L. E.; Landrau, M.; Burns, J. J. Metabolism of sulfinpyrazone (Anturane) and other thio analogues of phenylbutazone in man. J. Pharmacol. Exp. Ther. 132:287-290, 1961.

De Fonseka, C. P. Danger of instant adhesives. Br. Med. J., 2:234, 1976a.

De Fonseka, C. P. Danger of instant adhesives. Br. Med. J., 2:1447, 1976b.

de Haen, P. Recent progress in pharmacologic studies on bile acids. J. Am. Pharm. Assoc. (Sci. Ed.) 33:161-169, 1944.

De Jong, R. H.; Bonin, J. D. Deaths from local anesthetic-induced convulsions in mice. Anesth. Analg., 59:401-405, 1980.

De Lamater, J. N. Acute exfoliative dermatitis due to Dormison. Calif. Med., 77:339-340, 1952.

DeBaun, J.; Miaullis, J. B. Fate of N-trichloro-¹⁴C-methylthio-4-cyclohexene-1,2-dicarboxamide (¹⁴C-captan) in the rat. Xenobiotica 4:101-119, 1974.

Decino, T. J.; Cunningham, D. J.; Schafer, E. W. Toxicity of DRC-1339 to starlings. J. Wildlife Manag. 30:249-253, 1966.

DeFonso, L. R.; Kelton, S. C., Jr. Lung cancer following exposure to chloromethyl methyl ether. Arch. Environ. Health 31:125-130, 1976.

DeGenaro, F.; Nyhan, W. L. Salt - a dangerous "antidote". J. Pediatr., 78:1048-1049, 1971.

DeGroot, A. P.; Feron, V.; Til, H. Short-term toxicity studies on some salts and oxides of tin in rats. Food Cosmet. Toxicol., 11:19-30, 1973.

Deichmann, W. B. Toxicity of methyl, ethyl and n-butyl methacrylate. J. Ind. Hyg. Toxicol., 23:343-351, 1941.

Deichmann, W. B.; Gerarde, H. W. Toxicology of Drugs and Chemicals. Academic Press, N. Y, 1969.

Deichmann, W. B.; Kitzmiller, K. V. On the toxicity of vanillin and ethyl vanillin for rabbits and rats. J. Pharm. Sci., 29:425-428, 1940.

Deichmann, W. B.; Kitzmiller, K. V.; Dierker, M.; Witherup, S. Observations on the effects of diphenyl, o- and p-aminodiphenyl, o- and p-nitrodiphenyl and dihydroxyoctachlorodiphenyl upon experimental animals. J. Ind. Hyg. Toxicol., 29:1-13, 1947.

Deichmann, W. B.; Machle, W.; Kitzmiller, K. V.; Thomas, G. Acute and chronic effects of pentachlorophenol and sodium pentachlorophenate upon experimental animals. J. Pharmacol. Exp. Ther., 76:104-117, 1942.

Deichmann, W. B.; Radomski, J. L.; MacDonald, W. E.; Kascht, R. L.; Erdman, R. L. The chronic toxicity of octadecylamine. Arch. Indust. Health, 18:483-487, 1958.

Deisher, J. B. Poisoning with a liquid plastic catalyst; report of a case. Northwest Med., 57:46-47, 1958.

Del Greco, F.; Arieff, A. J. Primidone (Mysoline) and glutethimide (Doriden) intoxication (biotransformation to a barbiturate). Arch. Neurol., 7:244, 1962.

DeMatteis, F.; Prior, B. E.; Rimington, C. Nervous and biochemical disturbances following hexachlorobenzene intoxication. Nature, 191:363-366, 1961.

DeMeio, R. H. Tellurium. I. The toxicity of ingested elementary tellurium for rats and rat tissues. J. Ind. Hyg. Toxicol., 28:229-232, 1946.

DeNeen, D. D. A case of cedar oil poisoning in a pregnant woman. Am. J. Surg., 33:277, 1919.

Denney, J. L.; Miller, H.; Griffith, G. C.; Nathanson, M. N.

Ventricular acceleration following procaine amide hydrochloride therapy. J. A. M. A., *149*:1391-1392, 1952.

Deribere, M. Titanium compounds and hygiene. Ann. Hyg. Publ. Ind. et Sociale, *18*:133-137, 1941.

Dernehl, C. U. Personal communication. Union Carbide Corp., New York, 1957.

Dernehl, C. U. Information for poison control centers - Temik 10G. Union Carbide Corp. Technical Data Sheet, Union Carbide Corp., New York, April 11, 1972.

DeSalva, S. J.; Evans, R. A.; Marcussen, H. W. Lethal effects of antibiotics in hamsters. Toxicol. Appl. Pharmacol., *14*:510-514, 1969.

Deschiens, R.; Bablet, J. Recherches sur la toxicite des derives triphenylmethaniques anthelminthiques. C. Rend. Soc. Biol., *138*:838-839, 1944.

deVeber, L. L. Photosensitivity, loosening of the nails, and discolouration of the nails and teeth in association with demethylchlortetracycline (Declomycin): Report of a case with review of other reported cases. Can. Med. Assoc. J., *86*:168-172, 1962.

Dewse, C. D.; Potter, C. G. Inhibitory effect of phenylbutazone and oxyphenbutazone on DNA synthesis in normal human bone marrow cells in vitro. J. Pharm. Pharmacol. *27*:523-526, 1975.

Diamond Alkali Co. Chlorowax toxicity report. Cleveland, Ohio, 1946.

Dianol, Inc. Brochure (resume of Toxicological Investigations Rhothane D-3), Date Unknown.

Dick, M. W.; Warweg, E.; Andersch, M. Acacia in the treatment of nephrosis. J. A. M. A., *105*:654-657, 1935.

Dieke, S. H.; Allen, G. S.; Richter, C. P. The acute toxicity of thioureas and related compounds to wild and domestic Norway rats. J. Pharmacol. Exp. Ther., *90*:260-270, 1947.

Dieke, S. H.; Richter, C. P. Acute toxicity of thiourea to rats in relation to age, diet, strain and species variation. J. Pharmacol. Exp. Ther., *83*:195-202, 1945.

Dierken, H.; Brown, P. G. Study of a fatal case of ethylene chlorohydrin poisoning. J. Ind. Hyg. Toxicol., *26*:277, 1944.

Dieterle, W.; Faigle, J. W.; Frueh, F.; Mory, H.; Theobald, W.; Alt, K. O.; Richter, W. J. Metabolism of phenylbutazone in man. Arzneim. -Forsch. *26*:572-577, 1976.

Dietze, H. J. Dyskinetic syndrome associated with chloroprothixene. Am. J. Psychiatry, *120*:450-451, 1963.

Dimaio, V. J. M.; Garriott, J. C. Lethal caffeine poisoning in a child. Forensic Sci., *3*:275-278, 1974.

Dinerman, A. A.; Lavrent'eva, N. A. Toxicity of the herbicides, propazine and prometryn. Gig. Sanit. *34*:94-96, 1969.

Dinu, V.; Klein, R. Catalase activity and glutathione and lactic acid concentrations in rats acutely poisoned by acrylonitrile. J. Pharmacol. 7:223-226, 1976.

Discher, D. P. Inhalation of hairspray resin - Does it cause pulmonary disease? Proceedings of the National Technical Conference, "Safety and Health with Plastics", Society of Plastics Engineers., Nov. 8-10, 1977.

DiStefano, V.; Borgstedt, H. H. Reduction of dimethylsulfoxide to dimethylsulfide in the cat. Science, *144*:1137-1138, 1964.

Dittmer, D. S. (Ed.). Handbook of Toxicology, Volume V, Fungicides. W. B. Saunders Co., Philadelphia, 1959.

DiVincenzo, G. D.; Hamilton, M. L.; Kaplan, C. J.; Dedinas, J. Metabolic fate and disposition of ^{14}C-labelled methyl n-butyl ketone in the rat. Toxicol. Appl. Pharmacol. *41*:547-560, 1977.

Domenjoz, R. The pharmacology of phenylbutazone analogues. Ann. N. Y. Acad. Sci. *86*:263-291, 1960.

Domino, E. F. Phencyclidine. Int. Rev. Neurobiol., *6*:303-347, 1964.

Done, A. K. Uses and abuses of antipyretic therapy. Pediatrics, *23*:774-780, 1959.

Donlon, P. T.; Tupin, J. P. Successful suicides with thioridazine and mesoridazine. Arch. Gen. Psychiatry, *34*:955-957, 1977.

Donowitz, M.; Binder, H. J. Effect of dioctyl sodium sulfosuccinate on colonic fluid and electrolyte movement. Gastroenterology *69*:941-950, 1975.

Dooley, A. E. Personal communication. Texaco, Inc., New York, 1961.

Doolin, G. S. Personal Communication. National Confectioners Association, Inc., Chicago, Illinois, 1968.

Dorndorf, W.; Kresse, M.; Christian, W.; Katritzki, G. Dichloroethane poisoning with myoclonic syndrome, seizures and irreversible cerebral defects. Arch. Psychiatr. Nervenkr. *220*:373-379, 1975.

Dorne, M.; Friedman, T. B. Derris root dermatitis. J. A. M. A., *115*:1268-1270, 1940.

Dorough, H. W.; Davis, R. B.; Ivie, G. W. Fate of Temik-carbon-14 in lactating cows during a 14-day feeding period. J. Agric. Food Chem. *18*:135-142, 1970.

Dost, F. N.; Reed, D. J.; Wang, C. H. The mechanism of methemoglobin formation in nitrogen fluoride intoxication. Fed. Prod., *27*:466, 1968.

Dotevall, G.; Herner, B. Treatment of acute primidone poisoning with bemegride and amiphenazole. Br. Med. J., 2:451-452, 1957.

Doughty, A. G. Unexpected danger of diazepam. Br. Med. J., 2:239, 1970.

Doull, J.; DuBois, K. P. Toxicity and anticholinesterase action of tetra-n-propyl dithionopyrophosphate. J. Pharmacol. Exp. Ther., *106*:382, 1952.

Dow Chemical Co. Communication (3-hydroxy-2-methyl-1, 4-pyrone (Palatone)). Midland, Mich., July 15, 1953.

Dow Chemical Co. ACD information bulletin no. 109 (Korlan). Midland, Mich, 1957.

Dow Chemical Co. Antimicrobial Agents, Section IV-I (General Handling Information). Midland, Michigan, 1968.

Dow Chemical Co. Antimicrobial Agents, Section IV-2 (Dowicide 1). Midland Michigan, 1969a.

Dow Chemical Co. Antimicrobial Agents, Section IV-3 (Dowicide 2). Midland, Michigan, 1969b.

Dow Chemical Co. Antimicrobial Agents, Section IV-6 (Dowicide 6). Midland, Michigan, 1969c.

Dow Chemical Co. Antimicrobial Agents, Section IV-7 (Dowicide 7). Midland, Michigan, 1969d.

Dow Chemical Co. Antimicrobial Agents, Section IV-10 (Dowicide A). Midland, Michigan, 1969e.

Dow Chemical Co. Antimicrobial Agents, Section IV-11 (Dowicide B). Midland, Michigan, 1969f.

Dow Chemical Co. Antimicrobial Agents, Section IV-12 (Dowicide G). Midland, Michigan, 1969g.

Dow Chemical Co. Antimicrobial Agents, Section IV-4 (Dowicide 2S). Midland, Michigan, 1970a.

Dow Chemical Co. Antimicrobial Agents, Section IV-5 (Dowicide 4). Midland, Michigan, 1970b.

Dow Chemical Co. Antimicrobial Agents, Section IV-8 (Dowicide 31 and 32). Midland, Michigan, 1970c.

Dow Chemical Co. Antimicrobial Agents, Section IV-9 (Dowicide 9). Midland, Michigan, 1970d.

Dow Chemical Co. Personal communication. Midland, Michigan, Jan. 12, 1979.

Dow Chemical Company. Antimicrobial Agents, Section I-13 (Dowicil 200). Midland, Michigan, 1971a.

Dow Chemical Company. Problems keeping cosmetics fresh? Try Dowicil 200. Midland, Michigan, 1971b.

Doyle, H. W. Personal communication. Darworth, Inc., Simsbury, Conn, 1958.

Draize, J. H.; Alvarez, E.; Whitesell, M. F. Toxicological investigations of compounds proposed for use as insect repellents. J. Pharmacol. Exp. Ther., *93*:26-39, 1948.

Draize, J. H.; Woodard, G.; Calvery, H. O. Methods for the study of irritation and toxicity of substances applied topically to the skin and mucous membranes. J. Pharmacol. Exp. Ther., *82*:377-390, 1944b.

Drayer, D. E.; Reidenberg, M. Metabolism of tetralin and toxicity of cuprex in man. Drug. Metab. Dispos. *1*:577-579, 1973.

Drew, E. C. Some notes on metol dermatitis. Radiography, 8:103, 1942.

Drew, R. T.; Laskin, S.; Kuschner, M.; Nelson, N. Inhalation carcinogenicity of alpha halo ethers: I. The acute inhalation toxicity of chloromethyl methyl ether and bis(chloromethyl) ether. Arch. Environ. Health *30*:61-69, 1975.

Drill, V. A.; Hiratzka, T. Toxicity of 2,4-dichlorophenoxy-acetic acid and 2,4,5-trichlorophenoxyacetic acid. Arch. Ind. Hyg. Occup. Med., 7:61-67, 1953.

Drinker, C. K.; Warren, M. F.; Bennett, G. A. The problem of possible systemic effects from certain chlorinated hydrocarbons. J. Ind. Hyg. Toxicol., 9:283-299, 1937.

Driver, J. R.; Weller, J. N. Untoward results from the use of gold compounds; Report of a fatal case. Arch. Dermatol., 23:87-109, 1931.

du Pont, E. I., de Nemours and Co. Brochure (Oxone monopersulfate compound). Inc. Wilmington, Del, 1961a.

du Pont, E. I., de Nemours and Co. Condensed technical information (Diuron). Inc., Wilmington, Del, 1961b.

du Pont, E. I., de Nemours and Co. Condensed technical information (Fenuron). Inc., Wilmington, Del, 1961c.

du Pont, E. I., de Nemours and Co. Condensed technical information (Monuron). Inc., Wilmington, Del, 1961d.

du Pont, E. I., de Nemours and Co. Condensed technical information (Neburon). Inc., Wilmington, Del, 1961e.

du Pont, E. I., de Nemours and Co. Technical data sheet ("Velpar" Weed Killer). Wilmington, Del, January 1976.

du Pont, E. I., de Nemours and Co. Technical Data Sheet (Oxamyl). Wilmington, Del, June 1974.

Du Vigneaud, V.; Kuchinskas, E. J.; Horvath, A. L-Penicillamine and rat liver transaminase activity. Arch. Biochem. Biophys. 69:130-137, 1957.

DuBois, K. P.; Thrush, D. R.; Murphy, S. D. Studies on the toxicity and pharmacologic actions of the dimethoxyester of benzotriazine dithiophosphoric acid (DBD, Guthion). J. Pharmacol. Exp. Ther., 119:208-218, 1957.

Duff, I. F.; Shull, W. H. Fatal hemorrhage in Dicumarol poisoning, with report of necropsy. J. A. M. A., 139:762-766, 1949.

Duggan, M. Personal communication. White Laboratories, Kenilworth, N. J, 1960.

Dundee, J. W. Biotransformation of thiopental and other thiobarbiturates. Int. Anesthesiol. Clin. 12:121-133, 1974.

Dungemann, V. H.; Borelli, S.; Reber, E. Kontaktallergien gegen eine Gruppe neuer Desinfektionsmittel. Substanzen zur technischen Anwendung in Kuhlmitteln der metallverarbeitenden Industrie. Med. Klin. 59:170-175, 1964.

Dunn, C. W. Stilbesterol-induced gynecomastia in the male. J. A. M. A., 115:2263-2264, 1940.

Durham, W. F. The toxicity of chemicals used in mosquito control. Proc. 44th Annual Meeting N. J., Mosquito Extermination Assoc, 1957.

Durham, W. F.; Gaines, T. B.; McCauley, R. H., Jr.; Sedlak, V. A.; Mattson, A. M.; Hayes, W. J., Jr. Studies on the toxicity of 0,0-dimethyl-2,2-dichlorovinyl phosphate (DDVP). Arch. Ind. Health, 15:340-349, 1957.

Durham, W. F.; Hayes, W. J., Jr.; Mattson, A. M. Toxicological studies of 0,0-dimethyl-2,2-dichlorovinyl phosphate (DDVP) in tobacco warehouses. Arch. Ind. Health, 20:202-210, 1959.

Dutta, J. C. Fatal reaction following PAS. J. Indian Med. Assoc., 37:30-31, 1961.

Dyadicheva, T. V. Toxicity of the herbicide yolan (S-ethyl hexamethylenethiocarbamate). Vrach Delo, No. 1, p. 119-121, 1969.

Dybing, F.; Dybing, D.; Stormorken, H. The toxicity of red squill and scilliroside to rats and mice. Acta Pharmacol. Toxicol., 8:391-399, 1952.

Dyro, F. M. Methyl ethyl ketone polyneuropathy in shoe factory workers. Clin. Toxicol., 13:371-376, 1978.

Early, D. F. Pennyroyal: A rare cause of epilepsy. Lancet, 2:580-581, 1961.

Easson, W. M. Gasoline addiction in children. Pediatrics, 29:250-254, 1962.

Eastman, N. J.; Scott, A. B. Phenylmercuric acetate as a contraceptive. Human Fertility, 9:33, 1944.

Eaton Laboratories. Brochure (Acute Toxicity Data). Division of Norwich Pharmacal Co., Norwich, N. Y, 1959.

Eben, A.; Kimmerle, G. Metabolism, excretion and toxicology of methylchloroform in acute and subacute exposed rats. Arch. Toxikol. 31:233-242, 1974.

Eckardt, R. E. Personal communication. Esso Research and Engineering Co., Linden, N. J, 1964.

Eddy, N. B. Dilaudid (dihydromorphinone hydrochloride). J. A. M. A., 100:1032-1035, 1933.

Edelston, B. G. Thesaurosis following inhalation of hair spray. Lancet, 2:112-113, 1959.

Edson, E. F.; Noakes, D. N. The comparative toxicity of six organophosphorus insecticides in the rat. Toxicol. Appl. Pharmacol., 2:523-539, 1960.

Edson, E. F.; Sanderson, D. M. Toxicity of the herbicides, 2-methoxy-3,6-dichlorobenzoic acid (dicamba) and 2-methoxy-3,5,6-trichlorobenzoic acid (tricamba). Food Cosmet. Toxicol. 3:299-304, 1965.

Edwards, P. M. Neurotoxicity of acrylamide and its analogs and effects of these analogs and other agents on acrylamide neuropathy. Br. J. Ind. Med. 32:31-38, 1975.

Edwards, W. M. Accidental poisoning of newborn infants with ergonovine maleate. A lesson applicable to all delivery rooms. Clin. Pediatr. 10:257-260, 1971.

Egle, J. L., Jr.; Hudgins, P. M. Dose-dependent sympathomimetic and cardioinhibitory effects of acrolein and formaldehyde in the anesthetized rat. Toxicol. Appl. Pharmacol. 28:358-366, 1974.

Ehrich, W. E.; Seifter, J. Thrombotic thrombocytopenic purpura caused by iodine. Report of a case. Arch. Pathol., 47:446-449, 1949.

Eickholt, T. H.; Box, R. H. Toxicities of peppermint and Pycnanthemum albescens oils, fam. Labiateae. J. Pharm. Sci., 54:1071-1072, 1965.

Eisele, J. W.; Reay, D. T. Deaths related to coffee enemas. J. A. M. A., 244:1608-1609, 1980.

Eisenberg, M. M. Bishydroxycoumarin toxicity; some physiological aspects and report of a death from spontaneous subdural hematoma. J. A. M. A., 170:2181-2184, 1959.

Eisler, M. Personal communication. Velsicol Chem. Corp., Chicago, 1965.

El-Sabae, A. H.; Khamis, A. E. Organic thiocyanates as insecticidal synergists. Alexandria J. Agric. Res. 23:333-336, 1975.

Elkinton, J. R.; Huth, E. J.; Clark, J. K.; Barker, E. S.; Seligson, D. Renal tubular acidosis with organic aciduria during paraldehyde ingestion. Six-year study of an unusual case. Am. J. Med., 23:977-986, 1957.

Ellingwood, E. H., Jr.; Ewing, J. A.; Hoaken, P. C. S. Habituation to ethinamatc. N. Engl. J. Med., 266:185-186, 1962.

Elliott, M.; Janes, N. F.; Pulman, D. A.; Gaughan, L. C.; Unai, T.; Casida, J. E. Radiosynthesis and metabolism in rats of the 1R isomers of the insecticide permethrin. J. Agric. Food Chem. 24:270-276, 1976.

Elsea, J. R.; Paynter, O. E. Toxicological studies on bis(tri-n-butyltin)oxide. Arch. Ind. Health, 18:214-217, 1958.

Elson, E.; Domino, E. F. Dextropropoxyphene addiction. J. A. M. A. 183:482-485, 1963.

Elson, L. A.; Warren, F. L. The metabolism of azo compounds: 1. Azobenzene. Biochem. J. 38:217-220, 1944.

Elton, N. W.; Elton, W. J.; Nazareno, J. P. Pathology of acute salt poisoning in infants. Am. J. Clin. Pathol., 39:252-264, 1963.

Emanuel, B.; Schoenfeld, A. Favism in a nursing infant. J. Pediatr., 58:263-266, 1961.

Emerick, R. J.; Kugel, E. E.; Wallace, V. Urinary excretion of silicon and the production of siliceous urinary calculi in rats. Am. J. Vet. Res., 24:610, 1963.

Emmerson, J. L.; Anderson, R. C. Metabolism of trifluralin in the rat and dog. Toxicol. Appl. Pharmacol., 9:84-97, 1966.

Emmett, E. A.; Ricking, J. A. Fatal self-administration of sodium azide. Ann. Intern. Med., 83:224-226, 1975.

Empey, D. W.; Laitinen, L. A.; Young, G. A.; Bye, C. E.; Hughes, D. T. B. Comparison of the antitussive effects of codeine phosphate 20 mg, dextromethorphan 30 mg and noscapine 30 mg using citric acid-induced cough in normal subjects. Eur. J. Calin. Pharmacol., 16:393-397, 1979.

English, J. M. A case of probable phosgene poisoning. Br. Med. J., 1:38, 1964.

Engstrom, J.; Astrand, I.; Wigaeus, E. Exposure to styrene in a polymerization plant. Uptake in the organism and concentration in subcutaneous adipose tissue. (as cited in Chem. Abs. 90:156384x) Scand. J. Work, Environ. Health

4:324-329, 1978.

Enikeev, V. Kh. Problems of industrial hygiene in the production of ziram - a poisonous chemical substance. Gig. Truda Prof. Zabol. 12:12-16, 1968.

EPA. Rebuttable presumption against registration and continued registration of pesticide products containing ethylene dibromide (EDB). Federal Register 42:63134-63136, Dec. 14, 1977.

EPA. Rebuttable presumption against registration and continued registration of pesticide products containing thiophanate-methyl. Federal Register 42:61970-61975, Dec. 7, 1977.

EPA. Notice of determination pursuant to 40CFR 162. 11(a)(5) concluding the chlorobenzilate RPAR. Federal Register 43:29824-29828, July 11, 1978.

EPA. Proposed tolerances for 2-4-chloro-6-(ethylamino)-s-triazin-2-ylamino-2-methylpropionitrile. Federal Register 43:30314-30315, July 14, 1978.

EPA. Rebuttable presumption against registration and continued registration of pesticide products containing diallate. Federal Register 42:27669-27674, May 31, 1977.

EPA. Rebuttable presumption against registration and continued registration of pesticide products containing maleic hydrazide. Federal Register 42:56920-56935, Oct. 28, 1977.

EPA. Rebuttable presumption against registration and continued registration of pesticide products containing pentachloronitrobenzene (PCNB). Federal Register 42:56072-56100, October 20, 1977.

EPA. Rebuttable presumption against registration and continued registration of pesticide products containing dibromochloropropane (DBCP). Federal Register 42:48026-48045, Sept. 22, 1977.

EPA. Tolerances and exemptions from tolerances for pesticide chemicals in or on raw agricultural commodities; Permethrin. Federal Register 44:24287-24288, April 25, 1979.

EPA. Metolachlor pesticide registration standard. Office of Pesticides and Toxic Substances, Environmental Protection Agency, Washington, D. C., Mar., 1980.

EPA. Tolerances and exemptions from tolerances for pesticide chemicals in or on raw agricultural commodities; difluben-zuron. Federal Register 44:25452-25454, May 1, 1979.

EPA. Rebuttable presumption against registration and continued registration of pesticide products containing pronamide. Federal Register 42:25906-25911, May 20, 1977.

Epstein, M. A. Ventricular standstill during the intravenous procaine amide treatment of ventricular tachycardia. Am. Heart J., 45:898-908, 1953.

Epstein, S. S.; Fujii, K.; Andrea, J.; Mantel, N. Carcinogenicity testing of selected food additives by parenteral administration to infant Swiss mice. Toxicol. Appl. Pharmacol. 16:321-334, 1970.

Erdmann, E.; Vahlen, E. Ueber die Wirkungen des p-Phenylendiamins und Chinondiimines. Nauyn. Schmiedebeigs Arch., 53:401-418, 1905.

Erickson, J. L. E.; Brown, J. H. A study of the toxic properties of tung nuts. J. Pharmacol. Exp. Ther. 74:114-117, 1942.

Erwin, H. J. Clinical observations on the use of promethazine hydrochloride in psychiatric disorders. Am. J. Psychiatry., 113:783-787, 1957.

Essig, C. F. Addiction to nonbarbiturate sedative and tranquilizing drugs. Clin. Pharmacol. Ther., 5:334-343, 1964.

Evans, H. L.; Moore, H. A comparison of gentian violet and hexylresorcinol in the treatment of pinworm infestation. J. Pediatr., 20:627-631, 1942.

Evans, L. E. J.; Roscoe, P.; Swanson, C. P.; Prescott, L. F. Treatment of drug overdosage with naloxone, a specific narcotic antagonist. Lancet 1:452-455, 1973.

Everett, E. D.; Overholt, E. L. Phosgene poisoning. J. A. M. A., 205:243-245, 1968.

Evers, W. D.; Hook, J. B.; Bond, J. T. Effect of polybrominated biphenyls on renal tubular transport of organic ions. J. Toxicol. Environ. Health 3:759-767, 1977.

Ewart, R. B. L.; Priest, R. G. Methaqualone addiction and delirium tremens. Br. Med. J., 3:92-93, 1967.

Ewert, G. The effect of two topical anesthetic drugs on the mucus flow in the respiratory tract. Ann. Oto. Rhino. Laryng., 76:359-367, 1967.

Exner, J. H.; Burk, G. A.; Kyriacou, D. Rates and products of decomposition of 2,2-dibromo-3-nitrilopropionamide. J. Agric. Food Chem. 21:838-842, 1973.

Fahn, S.; Craddock, G; Kumin, G. Acute toxic psychosis from suicidal overdosage of amantadine. Arch. Neurol. 25:45-48, 1971.

Fahy, J. P. Toluene-2,4-diisocyanate (TDI). N. Engl. J. Med., 259:404-405, 1958.

Faidysh, E. V.; Rakhmatullaev, N. N.; Varshavskii, V. A. Cytotoxic action of Nemagon in a subacute experiment. Med. Zh. Uzb. 1:64-65, 1970.

Fairbairn, J. F. II. Severe arteriospastic disease secondary to use of ergot preparations. Med. Clin. North. Am., 42:971-974, 1958.

Fairhall, L. T. Inorganic industrial hazards. Physiol. Rev., 25:182-202, 1945.

Fairhall, L. T. Industrial Toxicology. The Williams & Wilkins Co., Baltimore, 1957.

Fairhall, L. T.; Hyslop, F. The toxicology of antimony. Public Health Repts., Suppl. No. 195, 1947.

Fairhall, L. T.; Sayers, R. R. The relative toxicity of lead and some of its common compounds. Public Health Bull. No. 253, 1940.

Falkenstein, D. F.; Jackson, R. L. Acacia therapy in a child with nephrosis. J. Pediatr., 16:700-703, 1940.

Fang, S. C.; Fallin, E.; Montgomery, M. L.; Freed, V. H. Metabolic studies of carbon-14-labeled propham and chlorpropham in the female rat. Pestic. Biochem. Physiol. 4:1-11, 1974.

Fantus, B.; Dyniewicz, J. M. Phenolphthalein studies. The therapy of overdosage. J. A. M. A., 110:1656-1658, 1938.

Fastier, F. N.; McDowell, M. A. A comparison of the pharmacological properties of the three isomeric aminopyridines. Austral. J. Exp. Biol. 36:365-372, 1958.

Faulstich, H. New aspects of amanita poisoning. Klin. Wochenschr., 57:1143-1152, 1979.

Fawcett, D. W.; Gens, J. P. Magnesium poisoning following an enema of epsom salt solution. J. A. M. A., 123:1028-1029, 1943.

Fazekas, I. G.; Rengei, B. Todliche Vergiftung (Selbstmord) Mit Mysoline und Phenobarkiturat. Arch. Toxikol., 18:213-223, 1960.

Fazekas, I. Gy. Todliche Pyramidonvergiftung bei einem Saugling mit besonderer Berucksichtigung der histologischen Veranderungen. Deutsche Zeitschrift fur gerichtliche Medizin, Bd. 46:374-396, 1957.

Featherstone, W. M. Convulsions following use of asterol dihydrochloride. J. A. M. A., 150:1006, 1952.

Feinberg, L. J.; Sandberg, H.; DeCastro, O.; Bellet, S. Effects of coffee ingestion on oral glucose tolerance curves in normal human subjects. Metabolism, 17:916-922, 1968.

Feldman, P. E. Clinical evaluation of Pacatal. Am. J. Psychiatry, 114:143-146, 1957.

Feldman, S.; Chen, S. -L.; Pickering, L. K.; Cleary, T. G.; Ericsson, C. D.; Hulse, M. Absorption of salicylate from a bismuth subsalicylate antidiarrheal preparation (Pepto-Bismol). Clin. Pharmacol. Ther. 27:252 (abstract), 1980.

Felsenstein, W. C.; Smith, R. P.; Gosselin, R. E. Toxicological studies on the avicide 3-chloro-p-toluidine. Toxicol. Appl. Pharmacol., 28:110-125, 1974.

Ferguson, F. C., Jr. Colchicine. I. General pharmacology. J. Pharmacol. Exp. Ther., 106:261-270, 1952.

Ferguson, G. R.; Alexander, C. C. Heterocyclic carbamates having systemic insecticidal action. J. Agric. Food Chem., 1:888-889, 1953.

Ferguson, J. T. Comparison of Reserpine and Harmonyl in psychiatric patients; preliminary report. J. Lancet, 76:389-390, 1956.

Ferguson, J. T.; Linn, F. V. Z. A new compound for the symptomatic treatment of tension and anxiety; 2-ethylcrotonyl urea (Nostyn). Antibiotic Med. Clin. Ther., 3:329-333, 1956.

Ferry, M. M. A case of acute lysol poisoning. Nurs. Times, 61:123-124, 1965.

Feuss, C. D.; Gragg, L., Jr. Quiactin: An adjunct in the treatment of chronic psychoses. Dis. Nerv. Syst., 18:29-33, 1957.

Fiala, S.; Fiala, E. Hormonal dependence of Actidione (cyclo-heximide) action. Biochim. Biophys. Acta 103:699-701, 1965.

Fiddes, F. S. Poisoning by aconitine; report of two cases. Br. Med. J., 2:779-780, 1958.

Figdor, S. K.; Kodet, M. J.; Bloom, B. M.; Agnells, E. J.; P'An, S. Y.; Laubach, G. D. Central activity and structure in a series of water-soluble steroids. J. Pharmacol. Exp. Ther., 119:299-309, 1956.

Fike, E. A. Personal communication. Roberts Chemical Co., Nitro, W. Va, 1958.

Finberg, L.; Kiley, J.; Luttrell, C. Mass accidental salt poisoning in infancy. J. A. M. A., 184:187-190, 1963.

Fine, E. A.; Wills, J. H. Pharmacologic studies of furfuryl alcohol. Arch. Ind. Hyg. Occup. Med. 1:625-632, 1950.

Finkler, R. S. Toxic Effects of estrogens. J. A. M. A., 141:738, 1949.

Finnegan, J. K.; Dienna, J. B. Toxicological observations in certain surface-active agents. Proc. Sci. Sect. Toilet Goods Assoc., No. 20, 1953.

Finnegan, J. K.; Hennigar, G. R.; Smith, R. B., Jr.; Larson, P. S.; Haag, H. B. Acute and chronic toxicity studies on 2,2-bis-(p-ethylphenyl)-1,1-dichloroethane (Perthane). Arch. Int. Pharmacodyn. Ther., 103:404-418, 1955.

Finnegan, J. K.; Larson, P. S.; Haag, H. B.; Page, S. G., Jr. Sedative and toxic effects of several chloral derivatives. Fed. Proc., 10:294, 951.

Finnegan, J. K.; Larson, P. S.; Smith, R. B., Jr.; Haag, H. B.; Hennigar, G. R. Acute and chronic toxicity studies on pentachloronitrobenzene. Arch. Int. Pharmacodyn. Ther., 114:38-52, 1958.

Finney, D. C. W.; Schnaufer, L.; Stafford, E. S. Total gastrectomy in an infant made necessary by ingestion of tinning paint. Am. Surg., 151:891-895, 1960.

Fischer, F. G.; Bielig. H. J. Uber die Hydrierung ungesattigter Stoffe im Tierkorper. Z. Physiol. Chem., 266: 73-98, 1940.

Fischer, R.; Toth, D. Uber einige Wirkungen der Agaricin-saure, Abietinsaure und Lichesterinsaure. Nauyn. Schon-iedebergs Arch. Pharmakol., 190:500-509, 1938.

Fischman, C. M.; Oster, J. R. Toxic effects of toluene. J. A. M. A. 241:1713-1715, 1979.

Fishbein, L. Toxicity of chlorinated biphenyls. Ann. Rev. Pharmacol., 14:139-156, 1974.

Fishbein, L. Environmental health aspects of fungicides. I. Dithiocarbamates. J. Toxicol. Environ. Health 1:713-735, 1976.

Fishbein, L.; Fawkes, J.; Falk, H. L.; Thompson, S. Thin-layer chromatography of rat bile and urine following intravenous administration of Tropital-methylene-^{14}C. J. Chromatogr. 31:102-108, 1967.

Fisher, B. The significance of Heinz bodies in anemia of obsure etiology. Am. J. Med. Sci., 230:143-146, 1955.

Fisher, R. S.; Haag, H. B. Studies of the comparative toxicity, absorption and elimination of sulfacetimide and sulfanil-amide. J. Urol., 47:183-195, 1942.

Fitzhugh, O. G.; Knudsen, L. F.; Nelson, A. A. The chronic toxicity of sulfites. J. Pharmacol. Exp. Ther., 86:37, 1946.

Fitzpatrick, R. J. The toxicity of red squill raticide to domesticated animals. J. Comp. Pathol. Ther., 62:23-40, 1952.

Fiume, L. Topographic distribution of hepatic necrosis in bromobenzene, thioacetamide, tannic acid poisoning, and inhibition by aminoacetonitrile of the necrosis induced by bromobenzene. Nature, 197:394-395, 1963.

Fleig, M. C. Etude physiologigue de quelques composes for-miques. Arch. Int. Pharmacodyn. Ther., 17:147-230, 1907.

Flemenbaum, A.; Gunby, B. Ethchlorvynol (Placidyl) abuse and withdrawal. Dis. Nerv. Syst., 32:188-192, 1971.

Flinn, F. B.; Brodie, B. B. The effect on the pain threshold on N-acetyl-p-aminophenol, a product derived in the body from acetanilide. J. Pharmacol. Exp. Ther., 94:76-77, 1948.

Flinn, R. H.; Neal, P. A.; Fulton, W. B. Industrial manganese poisoning. J. Ind. Hyg. Toxicol., 23:374, 1941.

Floyd, E. P.; Stokinger, H. E. Toxicity studies of certain organic peroxides and hydroperoxides. Am. Ind. Hyg. Assoc. J., 19:205-212, 1958.

Floyd, J. C., Jr.; Fajans, S. S.; Conn, J. W.; Knopf, R. F.; Rall, J. Stimulation of insulin secretion by amino acids. J. Clin.

Invest., 45:1987-1502, 1966.

Foldes, F. F.; Lunn, J. N.; Benz, H. G. Prolonged respiratory depression caused by drug combinations. J. A. M. A., 183:146-147, 1963a.

Food and Drug Administration. Antiemetic drug products for over-the-counter human use. Fed. Red., 44:41063-41073, July 13, 1979.

Food Protection Committee of the Food and Nutrition Board. Publ. No. 386 (The safety of artificial sweeteners for use in foods). Natl. Acad. Sci. Natl. Research Council, 1955.

Forberg, P. K.; Beyers, W. L. Chemical Mace: A nonlethal weapon. J. Trauma, 9:339-342, 1969.

Forbes, P. D.; Urbach, F. Experimental modification of pho-tocarcinogenesis. II. Fluorescent whitening agents and sim-ulated solar UVR UV radiation. Food Cosmet. Toxicol. 13:339-342, 1975.

Ford, W. W. Plant poisons and their antibodies. Zentralbl. Bakteriol., 58:129-162 and 193-222, 1913.

Fote, F. A. Hepatic effects of chloroform anesthesia in obstet-rics. Am. J. Obstet. Gynecol., 79:1142-1148, 1960.

Fouts, J. R.; Kamm, J. J.; Brodie, B. B. Enzymatic reduction of Prontosil and other azodyes. J. Pharmacol. Exp. Ther. 120:291-300, 1957.

Francis, W. G.; Dalzeil, D. Accidental ingestion of oral contra-ceptives by children. Canad. Med. Assoc. J., 92:191, 1965.

Frank, A. Metabolism of 2-(2-(furyl)benzimidazole in certain mammals. Acta Pharmacol. Toxicol., Suppl. 29, 124 pp, 1971.

Frankenberg, L.; Sorbo, B. Formation of cyanide from o-chlorobenzylidene malononitrile and its toxicological signif-icance. Arch. Toxikol., 31:99-108, 1973.

Franklin, K. J. The pharmacology of some compounds allied to chloral and to urethane. J. Pharmacol. Exp. Ther., 42:1-7, 1931.

Frantz, A. G. Fatal jaundice associated with iproniazid (Mar-silid) therapy. J. A. M. A., 167:987-988, 1958.

Frasier, S. D.; Crudo, F. S., Jr.; Johnson, D. H. Dextropropox-yphene hydrochloride poisoning in two children. J. Pediatr., 63:158-159, 1963.

Frawley, J. P.; Fuyat, H. N.; Hogan, E. C.; Blake, J. R.; Fitzhugh, O. G. Marked potentiation in mammalian toxicity from simultaneous administration of two anticholinesterase compounds. J. Pharmacol. Exp. Ther., 121:96-106, 1957.

Frear, D. E. H. Pesticide Index. 4th ed., College Science Publ., College Park, Pa, 1969.

Freed, H. Some preliminary observations on the use of Vesprin in children and adults. Monographs on Therapy (Squibb), 2:197-202, 1957.

Freeman, M. V.; Draize, J. H.; Smith, P. K. Some aspects of the mechanism of toxicity of thioglycolate. J. Pharmacol. Exp. Ther., 118:296-303, 1956a.

Freeman, M. V.; Draize, J. H.; Smith, P. K. Some aspects of the absorption, distribution and excretion of sodium thio-glycolate. J. Pharmacol. Exp. Ther., 118:304-308, 1956b.

Freuder, E.; Leake, C. D. The toxicity of epichlorohydrin. Univ. Calif. Publ. Pharmacol., 2:69-78, 1941.

Freundt, K. J.; Liebaldt, G. P.; Lieberwirth, E. Toxicity studies on trans-1,2-dichloroethylene. Toxicology 7:141-153, 1977.

Freundt, K. J.; Macholz, J. Inhibition of mixed function oxi-dases in rat liver by trans- and cis-1,2-dichloroethylene. Toxicology, 10:131-139, 1978.

Frewin, D. B.; Leonello, P. P.; Frewin, M. E. Hypertenison after ingestion of trimolets. Med. J. Aust., 2:497-498, 1978.

Frey, von J. R.; Geleick, H. Experimentelles Kontaktekzem durch Dinitrochlorbenzol an Ratten und Kaninchen. Der-matologica, 119:294-300, 1959.

Friberg, L. Proteinuria and kidney injury among workmen exposed to cadmium and nickel dust. J. Ind. Hyg. Toxicol., 30:32-36, 1948.

Friedman, H. T. Reactions following use of nasal deconges-tants. J. A. M. A., 157:1153, 1955.

Frierson, W. B. Use of pyridoxine HCl in acute hydrazine and UDMH intoxication. Indus. Med. Surg., 34:650-651, 1965.

Fristedt, B.; Lindqvist, B.; Schutz, A.; Ovrum, P. Survival in a case of acute oral chromic acid poisoning with acute renal failure treated by haemodialysis. Acta Med. Scand.,

177:153-159, 1965.

Fritz, K. W.; Bohm, P.; Buntru, G.; Lowen, C. H. Die akute gewerbliche Dichromatvergiftung und ihre Behandlung. Klin. Wochenschr., 17:856-861, 1960.

Frohman, L. A.; Klocke, F. J. Recurrent thiocyanate intoxication with pancytopenia, hypothyroidism and psychosis. N. Engl. J. Med., 268:701-705, 1963.

Froslie, A. Methaemoglobin formation in vitro by 6-amino metabolites of DNOC and DNBP. Acta Pharmacol. Toxicol. 29:490-498, 1971.

Fruncillo, R. J.; Gibbons, W.; Bowman, S. M. CNS toxicity after ingestion of topical lidocaine. N. Engl. J. Med., 306:426-427, 1982.

Fujimori, K.; Ho, I. K.; Mehendale, H. M. Assessment of photomirex toxicity in the mouse. J. Toxicol. Environ. Health, 6:869-876, 1980.

Fullerton, P. M.; Kremer, M. Neuropathy after intake of thalidimide (Distaval). Br. Med. J., 2:855-858, 1961.

Fytizas-Danielidou, R. Some aspects of the chronic toxicity of quintozene (pentachloronitrobenzene) in rats. Meded. Fac. Landbouwwet. Rijksuniv. Gent. 40:1175-1185, 1975.

Gabbai, Lisbonne, Pourquier. Ergot poisoning at Pont St. Espirit. Br. Med. J., 2:650-651, 1951.

Gabbiani, G.; Selye, H.; Tuchweber, B. Prevention of indium intoxication by ferric dextran. Br. J. Pharmacol. Chemother., 19:508-512, 1962.

Gabor, E. P. Hemolytic anaemia as adverse reaction to salicylazosulfapyridine. N. Engl. J. Med. 289:1372, 1973.

Gabor, E. P.; Lowenstèin, L.; De Leeuw, N. K. M. Hemolytic anemia induced by phenylazo-diamino-pyridine. Can. Med. Assoc. J., 91:756-759, 1964.

Gafafer, W. K. Occupational Diseases. U. S. Dept. HEW, Publ. No. 1097, U. S. Government Printing Office, 1964.

Gaillard, G. E. Clinical evaluation of a new antihistamine, buclizine hydrochloride (Vibazine). J. Allergy, 26, 1962:373-376, 1955.

Gaines, T. B. Acute toxicity of pesticides. Toxicol. Appl. Pharmacol. 14:515-534, 1969.

Gaines, T. B.; Kimbrough, R.; Laws, E. R., Jr. Toxicology of Abate in laboratory animals. Arch. Environ. Health, 14:283-288, 1967.

Gaines, T. B.; Kimbrough, R. D.; Linder, R. E. The toxicity of amitrole in the rat. Toxicol. Appl. Pharmacol. 26:118-129, 1973.

Gajewski, J. E.; Alsdorf, W. R. Studies on furan compounds: toxicity and pharmacological actions of furfuryl alcohols. Fed. Proc. 8:294 (abstract), 1949.

Galina, M. P.; Avnet, N. L.; Einhorn, A. Iodides during pregnancy. An apparent cause of neonatal death. New Engl. J. Med., 267:1124-1127, 1962.

Gallo, M. A.; Bachman, E.; Golberg, L. Mitochondrial effects of 2,6-dichloro-4-nitroaniline and its metabolites. Toxicol. Appl. Pharmacol. 35:51-61, 1976.

Galvin, T. J.; Bell, R. R.; Turk, R. D. Anthelmintics for ruminants. II. Anthelmintic activity and toxicity of Ruelene in sheep. Am. J. Vet. Res., 21:1058-1061, 1960.

Gans, J. H.; Korson, R.; Cater, M. R.; Ackerly, C. C. Effects of short-term and long-term theobromine administration to male dogs. Toxicol. Appl. Pharmacol., 53:481-496, 1980.

Gardiner, J. A.; Kirkland, J. J.; Klopping, H. L.; Sherman, H. Fate of benomyl in animals. J. Agric. Food Chem. 22:419-427, 1974.

Garland, A.; Camps, F. E. Methyl iodide poisoning. Br. J. Ind. Med., 2:209-211, 1945.

Garland, T. O.; Patterson, M. W. H. Six cases of acrylamide poisoning. Food Cosmet. Toxicol. 6:105, 1968.

Garry, V. F.; Hozier, J.; Jacobs, D.; Wade, R. L.; Gray, D. G. Ethylene oxide: evidence of human chromosomal effects. Environ. Mutagen., 1:375-382, 1979.

Garvin, C. F. The fatal toxic manifestations of the thiocyanates. J. A. M. A., 112:1125-1127, 1939.

Gates, R. L. Personal communication. Niagara Chemical Div., Food Machinery and Chemical Corp., Middleport, N. Y, 1958.

Gaul, L. E.; Underwood, G. B. Dermatitis venenata from organomercurial compounds, with a comparison of their

pharmacologic action on normal and injured skin. J. A. M. A., 140:860-865, 1949.

Gehring, P. J. Hepatotoxic potency of various chlorinated hydrocarbon vapors relative to their narcotic and lethal potencies in mice. Toxicol. Appl. Pharmacol. 13:287-298, 1968.

Gehring, P. J.; Kramer, C. G.; Schwetz, B. A.; Rose, J. Q.; Rowe, V. K. The fate of 2,4,5-trichlorophenoxyacetic acid (2,4,5-T) following oral administration to man. Toxicol. Appl. Pharmacol. 26:352-361, 1973.

Geigy Agricultural Chemicals, Geigy Chemical Corp. Toxicology data (Sequestrene metal chelates). Geigy Agricultural Chemicals, Geigy Chemical Corp., Dept. of Industrial Medicine, Yonkers, New York, July, 1964a.

Geigy Agricultural Chemicals, Geigy Chemical Corp. Toxicology data (Prometryne). Dept. of Industrial Medicine, Yonkers, New York, July, 1964b.

Geigy Chemical Corp. Brochure (Diazinon). Ardsley, N. Y, Date Unknown.

Geldmacher-v. Mallinckrodt, M.; Schaidt, G. Lethal poisoning by Unden. Mitteilungsblatt der GDCh-Fachgruppe Lebensmittelchemie und gerichtliche Chemie 25:349-353, 1971.

Geldmacher-v. Mallinckrodt, M.; Schmidt, H. P. Zur Toxicitat und Stoffwechsel von Aminotriazol beim Menschen. Arch. Toxikol., 27:13-18, 1970.

Geldmacher-v. Mallinckrodt, M.; Schuessler, F. Toxicity of diuron and its metabolism in man. Arch. Toxicol. 27:187-192, 1971.

Gelfand, M. L.; Garren, M. G.; Rowan, R. L. Acute anuria associated with chlorothiazide and hydrochlorothiazide therapy: Recovery. N. Y. State J. Med., 64:1865-1870, 1964.

George, C. Nitrofurazone dermatitis following coitus. J. A. M. A., 156:247-248, 1954.

George, M. E.; Pinkerton, M. K.; Back, K. C. Therapeutics of monomethylhydrazine intoxication. Toxicol. Appl. Pharmacol., 63:201-208, 1982.

Gerarde, H. W. Toxicology and Biochemistry of Aromatic Hydrocarbons. Elsevier, Amsterdam, 1960.

Gerarde, H. W. Personal communication. Esso Co., New York, May, 1962.

Gerarde, H. W. Toxicological studies on hydrocarbons. IX. The aspiration hazard and toxicity of hydrocarbons and hydrocarbon mixtures. Arch. Environ. Health, 6:329-341, 1963.

Gerarde, H. W.; Ahlstrom, D. B. The aspiration hazard and toxicity of a homologous series of alcohols. Arch. Environ. Health, 13:457-461, 1966a.

Gerritsen, W. B.; Buschmann, C. H. Phosgene poisoning caused by the use of chemical paint removers containing methylene chloride in ill-ventilated rooms heated by kerosene stoves. Br. J. Ind. Med., 17:187-189, 1960.

Gershanik, J. J.; Boecler, B.; George, W.; Sola, A.; Leitner, M.; Kapadia, C. The gasping syndrome: benzyl alcohol (BA) poisoning? Clin. Res. 29:895A, 1981.

Getnam, F. N. Personal communication. William S. Merrell Co., Cincinnati, Ohio, 1962.

Gettler, A. O.; Rhoads, C. P.; Weiss, S. A contribution to the pathology of argyria with a discussion of the fate of silver in the human body. Am. J. Pathol., 3:631-651, 1927.

Gibbs, O. S.; Pond, H.; Hansmann, G. A. Toxicological studies on ammoniated mercury. J. Pharmacol. Exp. Ther., 72:16-17, 1941.

Gibson, J. E.; Rao, K. S. Disposition of 2-sec-butyl-4,6-dinitrophenol (Dinoseb) in pregnant mice. Food Cosmet. Toxicol. 11:45-52, 1973.

Gilman, A. G.; Goodman, L. S.; Gilman, A. Goodman and Gilman's Pharmacological Basis of Therapeutics, 6th ed. The MacMillan Publishing Co., Inc., New York, 1980.

Gimpel, S. Personal communication. Sandoz Pharmaceuticals Div., Hanover, N. J, 1960.

Girard, T. A. Personal communication. Heyden Newport Chemical Corp., Garfield, N. J, 1957.

Gitelson, S.; Aladjemoff, L.; Ben-Hador, S.; Katznelson, R. Poisoning by a malathion-xylene mixture. J. A. M. A., 197:819-821, 1966.

Glaser, G. L.; Adams, D. A. Agranulocytosis associated with

promazine administration; report of three cases. Ann. Intern. Med., 48:872-879, 1958.

Glaser, Z. R. Special occupational hazard review and control recommendations for the use of ethylene oxide as a sterilant in medical facilities. U. S. DHEW, Public Health Service, NIOSH, Rockville M. D, 1977.

Gleason, M. N.; Gosselin, R. E.; Hodge, H. C. Abrin, lethal jewelry. Bull. of Supplementary Material, Clinical Toxicology of Commercial Products, Vol. II, No. 3, July, 1958.

Gleiberman, S. E.; Volkova, A. P.; Nikolaev, G. M.; Zukova, E. V. Study of long-range consequences of using repellants. Communication I. Experimental study of the consequences of the long-term effect of the repellant diethyl-toluamide (DETA). (as cited in Chem. Abs. 85:104911u) Med. Parazitol. Parazit. Bolezni 45:65-69, 1976.

Glenn Chemical Co. Bulletin No. I (Tabutrex (Di-n-butyl succinate)). Chicago, Ill, 1958.

Gloxhuber, C. H.; Bloching, H. Toxicologic properties of fluorescent whitening agents. Clin. Toxicol. 13:171-203, 1978.

Gold, H. Personal communication (Summary of Experiments on Local Irritant Action of Pyrdone (MGK 264)). McLaughlin Gormley King Co., Minneapolis, Minn., July 9, 1948, 1948b.

Gold, M. D.; Blum, A.; Ames, B. N. Another flame retardant tris-(1,3-dichloro-2-propyl)phosphate and its expected metabolites are mutagens. Science, 200:785-787, 1978.

Goldblatt, S. Severe reaction to griseofulvin. J. A. M. A., 172:1643-1644, 1960.

Goldenthal, E. I. A compilation of LD50 values in newborn and adult animals. Toxicol. Appl. Pharmacol. 18:185-207, 1971.

Goldfischer, J. D. Acute myocardial infarction secondary to ergot therapy. N. Engl. J. Med., 262:860-863, 1960.

Goldin, A. R.; Rubenstein, A. H.; Bradlow, B. A.; Elliot, G. A. Malathion poisoning with special reference to the effect of cholinesterase inhibition on erythrocyte survival. N. Engl. J. Med., 271:1289-1293, 1964.

Goldman, H.; Teitel, M. Malathion poisoning in a 34-month-old child following accidental ingestion. J. Pediatr., 52:76-81, 1958.

Goldman, L. Some toxicologic and clinical investigative studies with dihydroxyacetone. J. Soc. Cosmet. Chem., 12:163-167, 1961.

Goldman, M.; Karotkin, R. H. Acute potassium bichromate poisoning. Am. J. Med. Sci., 189:400-403, 1935.

Goldstein, F. Cutaneous and intravenous toxicity of 'endothal' (disodium 3,6-endoxohexahydrophthalic acid). Fed. Proc., 11:349, 1952.

Goldzieher, M. A.; Goldzieher, J. W. Toxic effects of percutaneously absorbed estrogens. J. A. M. A., 140:1156, 1949.

Goluboff, N. Methemoglobinemia due to benzocaine. Pediatrics, 21:340, 1958.

Goluboff, N.; MacFadyen, D. J. Methemoglobinemia in infants associated with application of tar-benzocaine ointment. J. Pediatr., 47:222, 1955.

Goluboff, N.; Wheaton, R. Methylene blue induced cyanosis and acute hemolytic anemia complicating the treatment of methemoglobinemia. J. Pediatr., 58:86-89, 1961.

Golz, H. H.; Shaffer, C. B. Toxicological information on Cyanamid insecticides. American Cyanamid Co., Wayne, N. J, 1966.

Good, R. A.; Vernier, R. L.; Smith, R. T. Serious untoward reactions to therapy with cortisone and adrenocorticotropin. Pediatrics, 19:95-118, 1957.

Goodman, L. S.; Gilman, A. The Pharmacological Basis of Therapeutics. 5th ed., The Macmillan Co., New York, 1975.

Goodrich, B. F., Chemical Co. Technical Data Sheet (Strobane). Akron, Ohio, 1955.

Gordon, D. How dangerous is pentachlorophenol? Med. J. Aust., 2:485-488, 1956.

Gorman, W. F.; Messinger, E.; Herman, M. Toxicity of thiocyanates used in treatment of hypertension. Ann. Intern. Med., 30:1054-1059, 1949.

Gornel, D. L.; Goldman, R. Acute renal failure following hexol-induced abortion. J. A. M. A., 203:146-149, 1968.

Gosselin, R. E.; Megirian, R. The influence of chain length on the metabolic fate of condensed phosphate. J. Pharmacol. Exp. Ther., 115:402-407, 1955.

Gosselin, R. E.; Tidball, C. S.; Megirian, R.; Maynard, E. A.; Downs, W. L.; Hodge, H. C. Metabolic acidosis and hypocalcemia as toxic manifestations of polymeric phosphates. J. Pharmacol. Exp. Ther., 108:117-127, 1953.

Gossner, W. Todliche Pyramidonvergiftung bei einem Kinde. Arch. Toxikol. 14:36-40, 1952.

Goulding, R. Toxicological case records. Practitioner 200:319-320, 1968.

Goyette, L. E. Personal communication. Virginia-Carolina Chemical Corp., Richmond, Va, 1961.

Grabliauskiene, M. On the toxicity of the preparations alar and ethrel. Primen. Fiziol. Akt. Veshchestv. Sadovod. Mater. Simp. 2:145-151, 1974.

Graham, B. E.; Kuizenga, M. H. Toxicity studies on benzyl benzoate and related benzyl compounds. J. Pharmacol. Exp. Ther., 84:358-362, 1945.

Graham, D.; Teed, H.; Grice, H. C. Chronic toxicity of bread additives to rats. J. Pharm. Pharmacol. 6:534-545, 1954.

Graham, D. I.; de Jesus, P. V.; Pleasure, D. E.; Gonatas, N. K. Triethyltin sulfate-induced neuropathy in rats. Arch. Neurol., 33:40-48, 1976.

Graham, J. D. P. Actions of sodium azide. Br. J. Pharmacol., 4:1-6, 1949.

Graham, J. D. P. Hydroxycobalamin as an antidote to acrylonitrile. Toxicol. Appl. Pharmacol., 7:367-372, 1965.

Graham, J. D. P.; Rogan, J. M.; Robertson, D. G. Observations on hydrazoic acid. J. Ind. Hyg. Toxicol. 30:98-102, 1948.

Graham, S. G.; Tisdall, F. F. Poisoning from external use of resorcin. Can. Med. Assoc. J., 12:730-732, 1922.

Graham, S. L.; Davis, K. J.; Hansen, W. H.; Graham, C. H. Effects of prolonged ethylene thiourea ingestion on the thyroid of the rat. Food Cosmet. Toxicol. 13:493-499, 1975.

Grant, D. L.; Phillips, W. E. J.; Villeneuve, D. C. Metabolism of a polychlorinated biphenyl (Aroclor 1254) mixture in the rat. Bull. Environ. Contam. Toxicol., 6:102-112, 1971.

Grant, W. M. Toxicology of the Eye. Charles C. Thomas, Springfield, Ill, 1962.

Grant, W. M. Toxicology of the Eye. 2nd ed. Charles C Thomas, Springfield, Ill, 1974.

Gray, M. G. Effect of exposure to the vapors of tetrabromoethane (acetylene tetrabromide). Arch. Ind. Hyg. Occup. Med., 2:407-419, 1950.

Gray, T. J. B.; Butterworth, K. R.; Gaunt, I. F.; Grasso, P.; Gangolli, S. D. Short-term toxicity study of Di-(2-ethylhexyl)phthalate in rats. Fd. Cosmet. Toxicol., 15:389-399, 1977.

Graziano, J. H.; Thornton, Y. S.; Leong, J. K.; Cerami, A. Pharmacology of cyanate. II. Effects on the endocrine system. J. Pharmacol. Exp. Ther., 185:667-675, 1973.

Green, A. A.; Naiman, J. L. Chlorambacil poisoning. Am. J. Dis. Child., 116:190-191, 1968.

Green, C. R.; Ham, K. N.; Tange, J. D. Kidney lesions induced in rats by p-aminophenol. Br. Med. J. 1:162-164, 1969.

Greenberg, L.; Lester, D. Handbook of Cosmetic Materials, Their Properties, Uses and Toxic and Dermatologic Actions. Interscience Publishers, Inc., New York, 1954.

Greenberg, M. S.; Wong, H. Methemoglobinemia and Heinz body hemolytic anemia due to phenazopyridine hydrochloride. N. Engl. J. Med., 271:431-435, 1964.

Greenberger, N. J.; Perkins, R. L.; Cuppage, F. E.; Ruppert, R. D. Severe metabolic acidosis in the rat induced by toxic doses of tetracycline. Proc. Soc. Exp. Biol. Med., 125:1194-1197, 1967.

Greenblatt, J. Hypersensitivity to Privine. J. Pediatr., 31:355-359, 1947.

Greenburg, L. Diagnosis and treatment of occupational metal poisoning. J. A. M. A., 139:815-818, 1949.

Greening, N. R.; Tonry, J. R. Burn hazard with cement. Brit. Med. J., 2:1370, 1978.

Greenstein, N. M. Reactions following the use of nasal decongestants. J. A. M. A., 157:1153-1154, 1955.

Greig, M. E.; Gibbons, A. J. An antidote to cycloheximide (Acti-dione) poisoning. Toxicology Appl. Pharmacol., 1:598, 1959.

Griffin, J. W.; Daeschner, C. W.; Collins, V. P.; Eaton, W. L. Hydrocarbon pneumonitis following furniture polish ingestion. J. Pediatr., 45:13, 1954.

Griffing, W. J.; Todd, G. C. Development and reversibility of pancreatic acinar cell changes in the rat produced by tebuthiuron (1-(5-tert-butyl-1,3,4-thiadiazol-2-yl)-1,3-dimethylurea). Food Cosmet. Toxicol. 12:665-669, 1974.

Griffith, J. F. Personal communication. Procter and Gamble Co., Cincinnati, Feb, 1964a.

Griffith, J. F. Interlaboratory variations in the determination of acute oral LD50. Toxicol. Appl. Pharmacol., 6:726-730, 1964b.

Griffith, J. F. Personal communication. Procter and Gamble Co., Cincinnati, July, 1968.

Griffith, J. F.; Nixon, G. A.; Bruce, R. D.; Reer, P. J.; Bannan, E. A. Dose-response with chemical irritants in the albino rabbit eye as a basis for selecting optimum testing conditions for predicting hazard to the human eye. Toxicol. Appl. Pharmacol., 55:501-513, 1980.

Griffiths, M. H.; Moss, J. A.; Rose, J. A.; Hathway, D. E. The comparative metabolism of 2,6-dichlorothiobenzamide (Prefix) and 2,6-dichlorobenzonitrile in the dog and rat. Biochem. J. 98:770-781, 1966.

Grollman, A. The preparation of extracts from oxidized marine and other oils for reducing the blood pressure in experimental and human chronic hypertension. J. Pharmacol. Exp. Ther. 84:128-135, 1945.

Gross, E. G.; Dexter, J. D.; Roth, R. G. Hypokalemic myopathy with myoglobinuria associated with licorice ingestion. N. Engl. J. Med., 274:602-606, 1966.

Gross, J. A.; Haas, M. L.; Swift, T. R. Ethylene oxide neurotoxicity: report of four cases and review of the literature. Neurology, 29:978-983, 1979.

Gross, M. Acetanilid, A Critical Bibliographic Review. Hillhouse Press, New Haven, 1946.

Gross, P.; Pfitzer, E. A.; Tolker, E.; Babyak, M. A.; Kaschak, M. Experimental emphysema, its production with papain in normal and silicotic rats. Arch. Environ. Health 11:50-58, 1965.

Grote, I. W.; Woods, M. Beta-phenylethyl alcohol as a preservative for ophthalmic solutions. J. Am. Pharm. Assoc., Sci. Ed., 44:9-11, 1955.

Grover, R. W. Diffuse hair loss associated with selenium (Selsun) sulfide shampoo. J. A. M. A., 160:1397-1398, 1956.

Grubb, T. C.; Dick, L. C.; Oser, M. Studies on the toxicity of polyoxyethylene dodecanol. Toxicol. Appl. Pharmacol., 2:133-143, 1960.

Gruber, C. M. Pharmacology of benzyl alcohol and its esters. I. The effect of benzyl alcohol, benzyl acetate and benzyl benzoate when given by mouth upon the blood pressure, pulse and alimentary canal. J. Lab. Clin. Med., 9:15-33, 1923a.

Gruber, C. M. The pharmacology of benzyl alcohol and its esters. II. Some of the effects of benzyl alcohol, benzyl benzoate and benzyl acetate when injected intravenously upon the respiratory and circulatory systems. J. Lab. Clin. Med., 9:92-112, 1923b.

Gruber, C. M. Treatment of insomnia with special reference to Valmid. J. Indiana Med. Assoc., 49:35-37, 1956.

Gruber, C. M.; Hart, E. R.; Gruber, C. M., Jr. The pharmacology and toxicology of the ethyl ester of 1-methyl-4-phenylpiperidine-4-carboxylic acid (Demerol). J. Pharmacol. Exp. Ther., 73:319-334, 1941.

Grummit, O. Di-(p-chlorophenyl) methyl carbinol, a new miticide. Science, 111:361-362, 1950.

Grunow, W.; Boehme, C.; Budczies, B. Metabolism of carbamate herbicides in the rat. 2. Metabolism of chlorpropham and barban. Food Cosmet. Toxicol. 8:277-288, 1970.

Gryboski, J.; Weinstein, D.; Ordway, N. K. Toxic encephalopathy apparently related to the use of an insect repellent. N. Engl. J. Med., 264:289-291, 961.

Gryboski, J. D.; Gotoff, S. P. Bismuth nephrotoxicity; report of a case. N. Engl. J. Med., 265:1289-1291, 1961.

Guess, W. L.; O'Leary, R.; Calley, D.; Autian, J. Parenteral toxicity of a series of commercially available dioctyl and dibutyl tin stabilizers used in PVC formulations. Fd. Cos-

met. Toxicol. 6:102, 1968.

Guess, W. L.; O'Leary, R. K. Toxicity of a rubber accelerator. Toxicol. Appl. Pharmacol. 14:221-231, 1969.

Gunnison, A. F. Sulphite toxicity: a critical review of in vitro and in vivo data. Fd. Cosmet. Toxicol., 19:667-682, 1981.

Gurd, M. R.; Harmer, G. L. M.; Lessel, B. Acute toxicity and 7-month feeding studies with mecoprop and MCPA. Food Cosmet. Toxicol. 3:883-885, 1965.

Gutenmann, W. H.; Lisk, D. J. Excretory pathway of terbacil (Sinbar) in lactating cows. J. Agric. Food Chem. 17:1011-1013, 1969.

Guyton, W. L. Poisoning due to oil of chenopodium. J. A. M. A., 132:330-331, 1946.

Gyorgy, P.; Tomarelli, R.; Ostergard, R. P.; Brown, J. B. Unsaturated fatty acids in the dietary destruction of N, N-dimethylaminobenzene (Butter Yellow) and in the production of anemia in rat. J. Exp. Med., 76:413-420, 1942.

Gzhegotskii, M. I.; Dotoshitskii, S. L. Skin resorption effect of herbicides. (as cited in Chem. Abstracts 77:29945n) Vrach. Delo, No. 11, p. 133-134, 1971.

Haag, H. B. Toxicological studies of Derris elliptica and its constituents. I. Rotenone. J. Pharmacol. Exp. Ther., 43:193-208, 1931.

Haag, H. B. A contribution to the pharmacology of anabasine. J. Pharmacol. Exp. Ther., 48:95-104, 1933.

Haag, H. B.; Taliaferro, I. Toxicological studies on cube. J. Pharmacol. Exp. Ther., 69:13-20, 1940.

Haag, H. B.; Taliaferro, I.; Goodhue, L. D. Toxicity of extracts of derris root for mice. Proc. Soc. Exp. Biol. Med. 54:140, 1943.

Hagan, E. C.; Jenner, P. M.; Jones, W. I.; Fitzhugh, O. G.; Long, E. L.; Brouwer, J. C.; Webb, W. K. Toxic properties of compounds related to safrole. Toxicol. Appl. Pharmacol., 7:18-24, 1965.

Hager, G. P.; Chapman, C. W.; Starkey, E. B. The toxicity of benzoic acid for white rats. J. Am. Pharm. Assoc., Sci. Ed., 31:253-255, 1942.

Hager, W.; Friedrich, K. H.; Wink, K.; Wegehaupt, R. Suizidversuch mit Ajmalin. Deutsche Medizinische Wochenschrift, 93:1809-1812, 1968.

Haggard, H. W.; Greenberg, L. A.; Turner, J. M. The physiological principles governing the action of acetone together with determination of toxicity. J. Ind. Hyg. Toxicol., 26:133-151, 1944.

Haggerty, R. J. Blue baby due to methemoglobinemia. N. Engl. J. Med., 267:1303, 1962.

Hainsworth, W. C. Accidental poisoning with naphazoline (Privine) HCl. Am. J. Dis. Child., 75:76-79, 1948.

Hakkinen, I.; Siltanen, E.; Hernberg, S.; Seppalainen, A. M.; Karli, P.; Vikkula, E. Diphenyl poisoning in fruit paper production. Arch. Environ. Health 26:70-74, 1973.

Haley, J. H.; Detrick, L. E.; Komesu, N.; Williams, P.; Upham, H.; Baurmash, L. Toxicologic studies of polyphenyl compounds used as atomic reactor moderator-coolants. Toxicol. Appl. Pharmacol., 1:515-523, 1959a.

Haley, T. J. Piperonyl butoxide, α2-(2-Butoxyethoxy)ethoxy-4, 5-methylenedioxy-2-propyltoluene: a review of the literature. Ecotoxicol. Environ. Safety, 2:9-31, 1978.

Haley, T. J. Review of the physiological effects of amyl, butyl, and isobutyl nitrites. Clin. Toxicol., 16:317-329, 1980.

Haley, T. J.; Flesher, A. M.; Raymond, K.; Konesu, N.; Williams, P. A pharmacologic study of mellaril, 2-methyl-mer-capto-10-(2-(N-methyl-2-piperidyl)-ethyl)-phenothiazine hydrochloride. Toxicol. Appl. Pharmacol., 1:377-383, 1959b.

Hall, C. E.; Hall, O. Glomerulonephritis and hypertension produced by parenteral administration of methylcellulose. Am. J. Pathol., 40:167-183, 1962.

Hall, C. E.; Hall, O. Polyvinyl alcohol: Relationship of physicochemical properties to hypertension and other pathophysiologic sequelae. Lab. Invest., 12:721-736, 1963.

Hall, M. C. Unusual case of fatal poisoning from the administration of male-fern as a vermifuge. J. A. M. A., 63:242-243, 1914.

Hall, R. H.; Laskin, S.; Frank, P.; Maynard, E. A.; Hodge, H. C. Preliminary observations on toxicity of elemental selenium. Arch. Ind. Hyg. Occup. Med., 4:458-464, 1951.

Halloran, T. J. .; Phillips, C. E. Propranolol intoxication: a severe case responding to norepinephrine therapy. Arch. Intern. Med., 141:810-811, 1981.

Hamm, P. C.; Speziale, A. J. Relation of herbicidal activity to the amide moiety of N-substituted alpha-chloro-acetamides. J. Agric. Food Chem., 4:518-522, 1956.

Hammack, W. J. Solox intoxication. J. A. M. A., 165:24, 1957.

Hanna, L. W. Hanna's Handbook of Agricultural Chemicals. 2nd Ed., The New-Times Publishing Co., Forest Grove, Ore., 1958, p. 115, 1958.

Hannuksela, M. Allergic and toxic reactions caused by cream bases in dermatological patients. Int. J. Cosmet. Sci., 1:257-263, 1979.

Hansen, A. A. Two fatal cases of potato poisoning. Science 61:340-341, 1925.

Hansen, W. H.; Davis, K. J.; Fitzhugh, O. G. Chronic toxicity of cube. Toxicol. Appl. Pharmacol. 7:535-542, 1965.

Hansens, E. J.; Bartley, C. E. Three new insecticides for house fly control in barns. J. Econ. Entomol., 46:372-374, 1953.

Hanzlick, P. J.; French, W. O. The pharmacology of Phoradinadron flavescens (American mistletoe). J. Pharmacol. Exp. Ther. 23:269-306, 1924.

Hanzlik, P. G.; Newman, H. W.; Van Winkle, W., Jr.; Lehman, A. J.; Kennedy, N. K. Toxicity, fate and excretion of propylene glycol and some other glycols. J. Pharmacol. Exp. Ther., 67:101-113, 1939.

Hapke, H. J. Toxicology of the herbicide simazine. Berlin Muenchen. T. W. 81:301-303, 1968.

Harber, L. C.; Lashinsky, A. M.; Baer, R. L. Photosensitivity due to chlorothiazide and hydrochlorothiazide. N. Engl. J. Med., 261:1378-1381, 1959.

Hardin, J. W.; Arena, J. M. Human Poisoning from Native and Cultivated Plants. 2nd ed., Duke University Press, Durham, North Carolina, 1974.

Hardman, H. F.; Haavik, C. O.; Seevers, M. H. Relationship of the structure of mescaline and seven analogs to toxicity and behavior in five species of laboratory animals. Toxicol. Appl. Pharmacol., 25:299-309, 1973.

Hardy, H. L. Differential diagnosis between beryllium poisoning and sarcoidosis. Am. Rev. Tuberc. Pulmonary Dis., 74:885-896, 1956.

Hardy, H. L.; Stoeckle, J. D. Beryllium disease. J. Chronic Dis., 9:152-160, 1959.

Harger, R. N.; Spolyar, L. W. Toxicity of phosphine with a possible fatality from this poison. Arch. Ind. Health 18:497-504, 1958.

Harkonen, H. Styrene, its experimental and clinical toxicology. A review. Scand. J. Work Environ. Health 4:104-113, 1979.

Harned, B. K.; Cunningham, R. W.; Halliday, J.; Vessey, R. E.; Yuda, N. N.; Clark, M. C.; Subbarow, Y. Some toxicological and pharmacological properties of 1-diethylcarbamyl-4-methylpiperazine hydrochloride, Hetrazan. Ann. NY Acad. Sci., 50:141-160, 1948.

Harris, A. H.; Binkley, O. F.; Chenoweth, B. M. Hematuria due to picric acid poisoning at a naval anchorage in Japan. Am. J. Pub. Health 36:727-733, 1946.

Harris, G. B. C.; Haggerty, R. J. Toxic hazards - bronze powder inhalation. N. Engl. J. Med. 256:40-41, 1957.

Harris, J. S.; Michel, H. O. The formation of methemoglobin and sulfhemoglobin during sulfanilamide therapy. J. Clin. Invest., 18:507-519, 1939.

Harris, L. C.; Jackson, R. H. Acute acetone poisoning caused by setting fluid for immobilizing casts. Br. Med. J., 2:1024-1026, 1952.

Harrison, C. V. Fatal poisoning by "Lethane" insecticide. Br. Med. J., 1:722, 1947.

Harrold, G. C. Solubility of lead compounds in human pleural fluid and blood serum. J. Ind. Hyg. Toxicol., 31:327-335, 1949.

Harrold, G. C.; Meek, S. F.; Collins, G. R.; Markell, T. F. Toxicity of lead chromate. J. Ind. Hyg. Toxicol., 26:47, 1944.

Harrold, G. C.; Meek, S. F.; Whitman, N.; McCord, C. P. The physiologic properties of indium and its compounds. J. Ind. Hyg. Toxicol., 25:233-237, 1943.

Hart, E. R. The toxicity and analgetic potency of salicylamide and certain of its derivatives as compared with established analgetic-antipyretic drugs. J. Pharmacol. Exp. Ther., 89:205-209, 1947.

Hart, R. C. Toxicity of traditional Christmas greens. Ind. Med. Surg. 30:522-525, 1961.

Hartigan, J. D.; Gurnett, T. J. Favism; report of a case. J. A. M. A., 171:299-300, 1959.

Hartman, F. W.; Romence, H. L. Liver necrosis in burns. Ann. Surg., 118:402-416, 1943.

Hartman, T. L.; Wacker, W.; Roll, R. M. Methyl chloride intoxication: report of two cases, one complicating pregnancy. N. Engl. J. Med., 253:552-554, 1955.

Hartung, E. F. A case of aconitine poisoning causing cardiac collapse. J. A. M. A., 95:1265, 1930.

Harvey, J., Jr.; Han, J. C. -Y. Metabolism of oxamyl and selected metabolites in the rat. J. Agric. Food Chem. 26:902-910, 1978.

Hashimoto, K.; Kanai, R. Effect of acrylonitrile on sulfhydryls and pyruvate metabolism in tissues. Biochem. Pharmacol. 21:635-640, 1972.

Hashimoto, Y.; Makita, T.; Ohnuma, N.; Noguchi, T. Acute toxicity on dimethyl 4,4'-o-phenylene bis(3-thioallophanate), Thiophanate-methyl fungicide. Toxicol. Appl. Pharmacol. 23:606-615, 1972a.

Hashimoto, Y.; Noguchi, T.; Kitagawa, H.; Ohta, G. Toxicologic and pharmacologic properties of tolnaftate, an antitrichophyton agent. Toxicol. Appl. Pharmacol. 8:380-385, 1966.

Hatfield, G. M.; Schaumberg, J. P. Isolation and structural studies of coprine, the disulfiram-like constituent of Coprinus atramentarius. Lloydia, 38:489-496, 1975.

Haut, M. J.; Toskes, P. P.; Hildebrandt, P. K.; Glader, B. E.; Conrad, M. E. In vivo hepatic and intestinal toxicity of sodium cyanate in rats: cyanate-induced alterations in hepatic glycogen metabolism. J. Lab. Clin. Med., 85:140-154, 1975.

Hawkins, D. B.; Demeter, M. J.; Barnett, T. E. Caustic ingestion-controversies in management - review of 214 cases. Laryngoscope, 90:98-109, 1980.

Hayes, F.; Short, R.; Gibson, J. Differential toxicity of monochloroacetate, monofluoroacetate and monoiodoacetate in rats. Toxicol. Appl. Pharmacol. 26:93-102, 1973.

Hayes, W. J., Jr. Clinical Handbook on Economic Poisons. USPHS Publication No. 476. U. S. Government Printing Office, Washington, D. C, 1963.

Hays, H. W. Personal communication. Advisory Center on Toxicology, National Academy of Sciences, Washington, D. C., 1960.

Hayward, J. N.; Boshell, B. R. Paraldehyde intoxication with metabolic acidosis. Report of two cases, experimental data and a critical review of the literature. Am. J. Med., 23:965-976, 1957.

Hazleton Laboratories, Inc. Acute dermal toxicity - guinea pigs Nosema locustae. Report to U. S. Dept. of Agriculture. Vienna, Va, March 21, 1973a.

Hazleton Laboratories, Inc. Acute inhalation toxicity - rats Nosema locustae. Report to U. S. Dept. of Agriculture. Vienna, Va, May 18, 1973b.

Hazleton Laboratories, Inc. 13-Week dietary administration - rats Nosema locustae. Report to U. S. Dept. of Agriculture. Vienna, Va, Nov. 2, 1973c.

Hazleton, L. W. Review of current knowledge of toxicity of cholinesterase inhibitor insecticides. J. Agric. Food Chem., 3:312-319, 1955.

Hazleton, L. W.; Tusing, T. W.; Zeitlin, B. R.; Thiessen, R., Jr.; Murer, H. K. Toxicity of coumarin. J. Pharmacol. Exp. Ther., 118:348-358, 1956.

Healy, J. K. Ascending paralysis following malathion intoxication: a case report. Med. J. Aust., 1:765-767, 1959.

Hearn, C. E. D. Trithion poisoning. Br. J. Ind. Med., 18:231-233, 1961.

Heatley, C. A.; Clausen, S. W. Experimental studies in peanut bronchitis. Arch. Otolaryngol. 11:569-579, 1930.

Heatley, W. G. Personal communication. Riker Laboratories, Northridge, Calif, 1960.

Heaton, N. Titanium oxide pigments - their development and possibilities. Chem. Trade J., 85:439, 1929.

Hee, S. S. Q.; Sutherland, R. G. Purity of reagent grade p- and o-chlorophenoxyacetic acids and its biological implications. J. Agric. Food Chem. 22:726-727, 1974.

Hegsted, D. M.; McKibbin, J. M.; Drinker, C. K. The biological, hygienic, and medical properties of zinc and zinc compounds. Public Health Rpts. No. 179, 1945.

Heibert, T. G. Personal communication. Searle, G. D. and Co., Chicago, Ill, 1966.

Heilbrunn, G.; Liebert, E.; Szanto, P. B. Chronic chloroform poisoning. Clinical and pathologic report of a case. Arch. Neurol. Psychiat., 53:68-72, 1945.

Heim, W. G.; Appleman, D.; Pyfrom, H. T. Production of catalase changes in animals with 3-amino-1,2,4-triazole. Science, 122:693, 1955.

Heiman, H.; Aschner, P. W. The aspiration of stearate of zinc in infancy. Am. J. Dis. Child., 23:503-510, 1922.

Heinonen, J.; Heikkila, J.; Mattila, M. J.; Takki, S. Orphenadrine poisoning. A case report supplemented with animal experiments. Arch. Toxikol., 23:264-272, 1968.

Helton, E. G.; Daley, E. W.; Ervin, J. C. Zirconium oxychloride; a new ingredient for antiperspirants. Proc. Scientific Section Toilet Goods Assoc. 26:27-31, 1956.

Henry, J. E. Tests on the viability of spores in ruminant animals. Report to U. S. Dept. of Agriculture. Agricultural Research Service, Bozeman, Montana, 1973.

Henry, J. E.; Oma, E. A.; Billeb, B. Special report G-260. Safety of Nosema locustae: Bioassay of tissues from rats treated with spores. U. S. Dept. of Agriculture, Agricultural Research Service, Bozeman, Montana, 1973.

Heppel, L. A.; Neal, P. A.; Perrin, T. L.; Endicott, K. M.; Porterfield, V. T. The toxicology of 1,2-dichloroethane. III. Its acute toxicity and the effect of protective agents. J. Pharmacol. Exp. Ther., 84:53-63, 1945.

Heppel, L. A.; Neal, P. A.; Perrin, T. L.; Orr, M. L.; Porterfield, V. T. Toxicology of dichloromethane (methylene chloride). I. Studies on effects of daily inhalation. J. Ind. Hyg. Toxicol. 26:8-16, 1944.

Hercules Powder Co. Brochure (Terpenes and related materials). Wilmington, Del., Revised Ed, 1951.

Hercules Powder Co. Toxicological Data Sheet, Bull. T-111, (Azak). Wilmington, Del., 1962a.

Hercules Powder Co. Toxicological Data Sheet, Bull. T-109, (Herban). Wilmington, Del, 1962b.

Herd, P. A.; Lipsky, M.; Martin, H. F. Cardiovascular effects of 1,1,1-trichloroethane. Arch. Environ. Health 28:227-233, 1974.

Herpol, J. Acute uremic door lysolvergiftiging bij een kind van 6 jaar. Anatomische en fysiopathologische studie. Maandschr. Kindergeneesk, 19:401-413, 1961; Through Toxic Episodes in Child., 3:26, 1961.

Herrmann, R. G.; Dubois, K. P. Studies on the toxicity and pharmacological action of p-dimethylaminobenzenediazo sodium sulfonate (DSS). J. Pharmacol. Exp. Ther. 95:262-271, 1949.

Herskowitz, A.; Ishii, N.; Schaumburg, H. n-Hexane neuropathy, a syndrome occurring as a result of industrial exposure. N. Engl. J. Med. 285:82-85, 1971.

Hertz, R. Accidental ingestion of estrogens by children. Pediatrics, 21:203-206, 1958.

Hertzler, A. E. Dangers in the use of aluminum acetate solution as a wet dressing. Am. J. Surg., 2:573-574, 1927.

Herzka, H.; Haber, J. Klinische Mitteilung uber die Wirksamkeit von Daptazole (Amiphenazol) in einem Fall von Vergiftung mit Valium. Schweiz. Med. Wochenschr., 95:365-366, 1965.

Heuser, G.; Ling, G. M.; Buchwald, N. A. Sedation or seizures as dose dependent effects of steroids. Arch. Neurol., 13:195-203, 1965.

Heyndrickx, A.; Van Petigham, C.; Van den Heede, M.; Lauwaert, R. A double fatality with children due to fumigated wheat. Eur. J. Toxicol. Environ. Hyg. 9:113-118, 1976.

Hicks, C. S.; Sinclair, D. A. Toxicities of optical isomers of nicotine and nornicotine. Aust. J. Exp. Biol. Med. Sci. 25:83-86, 1947.

Higgins, E. S.; Richert, D. A.; Westerfield, W. W. Competitive role of tungsten in molybdenum nutrition. Fed. Proc., 15:274-275, 1956.

Higgins, W. H. Systemic poisoning with bismuth. J. A. M. A., 66:648-650, 1916.

Highman, B.; Heppel, L. A.; Lamprey, R. J. The toxicology of 1, 2-dichloroethane. V. Effect of protective agents in visceral fatty changes in exposed rats. Arch. Pathol., 51:346-350, 1951.

Hiles, R. A.; Caudill, D.; Birch, C. G.; Eichhold, T. The metabolism and disposition of 3,4,4'-trichlorocarbanilide in the intact and bile duct-cannulated adult and in the newborn rhesus monkey (M. mulatta). Toxicol. Appl. Pharmacol., 46:593-608, 1978.

Hill, H. E. A contribution to the toxicology of sodium nitroprusside I. The decomposition and determination of sodium nitroprusside. Aust. Chem. Inst. J. Proc., 9:89-93, 1942.

Hill, H. Z.; Backer, R.; Hill, G. J. Blood cyanide levels in mice after administration of amygdalin. Biopharm. Drug Dispos., 1:211-220, 1980.

Hill, W. R.; Pillsbury, D. M. Argyria. The Pharmacology of Silver. Williams and Wilkins Co., Baltimore, 1939.

Hine, C.; Rowe, V. K.; White, E. R.; Darmer, K. I., Jr.; Youngblood, G. T. Epoxy compounds. In Patty's Industrial Hygiene and Toxicology, 3rd Ed., (Clayton, G. D. and F. E. Clayton, editors). John Wiley and Sons, N. Y. pp. 2141-2257, 1981.

Hine, C. H.; Anderson, H. H.; Moon, H. D.; Dunlap, M. K.; Morse, M. S. Comparative toxicity of synthetic and natural glycerin. Arch. Ind. Hyg. Occup. Med., 7:282-291, 1953b.

Hine, C. H.; Anderson, H. H.; Moon, H. D.; Kodama, J. K.; Morse, M.; Jacobsen, N. W. Toxicology and safe handling of CBP-55 (Technical 1-chloro-3-bromopropene-1). Arch. Ind. Hyg. Occup. Med., 7:118-136, 1953a.

Hirayama, C.; Okumura, M.; Nagai, J.; Masuda, Y. Hypobilirubinemia in patients with polychlorinated biphenyls poisoning. Clin. Chim. Acta, 55:97-100, 1974.

Hirsch, E. F.; Russell, H. B. Chronic exudative and indurative pneumonia due to inhalation of shellac. Arch. Pathol., 39:281-286, 1945.

Hitch, J. M. Neurotoxic symptoms following use of asterol dihydrochloride. J. A. M. A., 150:1004-1005, 1952.

Hjort, A. M.; Eagan, J. T. Benzyl carbinol; a local anesthetic. J. Pharmacol. Exp. Ther., 14:211-219, 1911.

Hoch-Ligeti, C.; Argus, M. F.; Arcos, J. C. Oncogenic activity of an M-dioxane derivative, 2,6-dimethyl-m-dioxan-4-ol-acetate (dimethoxane). J. Natl. Cancer Inst., 53:791-794, 1974.

Hochman, R.; Robbins, J. J. Jaundice due to ectylurea. N. Engl. J. Med., 259:583-585, 1958.

Hodes, L. J. Personal communication. Onyx Chemical Corp., Jersey City, N. J, 1963.

Hodge, H. C.; Downs, W. L. The approximate oral toxicity in rats of selected household products. Toxicol. Appl. Pharmacol., 3:689-695, 1961.

Hodge, H. C.; Downs, W. L.; Panner, B. S.; Smith, D. W.; Maynard, E. A.; Clayton, J. W.; Rhodes, R. C. Oral toxicity and metabolism of diuron (N-(3,4-dichlorophenyl)-N',-N'-dimethylurea) in rats and dogs. Food Cosmet. Toxicol., 5:513-531, 1967b.

Hodge, H. C.; Downs, W. L.; Smith, D. W.; Maynard, E. A.; Clayton, J. W., Jr.; Pease, H. L. Oral toxicity of linuron 3-(3,4-dichlorophenyl)-1-methoxy-1-methylurea in rats and dogs. Food Cosmet. Toxicol. 6:171-183, 1968.

Hodge, H. C.; Maynard, E. A.; Blanchet, H. J., Jr. Chronic oral toxicity tests of methoxychlor (2,2-di-(p-methoxyphenyl)-1,1,1-trichloroethane) in rats and dogs. J. Pharmacol. Exp. Ther., 104:60-66, 1952a.

Hodge, H. C.; Maynard, E. A.; Blanchet, H. J., Jr.; Spencer, H. C.; Rowe, V. K. Toxicological studies of orthophenylphenol (Dowicide-1). J. Pharmacol. Exp. Ther., 104:202-210, 1952b.

Hodge, H. C.; Maynard, E. A.; Downs, W. L.; Coye, R. D., Jr.; Steadman, L. T. Chronic oral toxicity of ferric dimethyldithiocarbamate (Ferbam) and zinc dimethyldithiocarbamate (Ziram). J. Pharmacol. Exp. Ther., 118:174-181, 1956.

Hodge, H. C.; Maynard, E. A.; Downs, W. L.; Coye, R. D. Chronic toxicity of 3-(p-chlorophenyl)-1,1-dimethylurea

(Monuron). Arch. Ind. Health 17:45-47, 1958.

Hodge, H. C.; Maynard, E. A.; Thomas, J. F.; Blanchet, H. J., Jr.; Wilt, W. G., Jr.; Mason, K. E. Short-term oral toxicity tests of methoxychlor (2,2-di-(p-methoxphenyl)-1,1,1-trichloroethane) in rats and dogs. J. Pharmacol. Exp. Ther., 99:140-148, 1950.

Hodge, H. C.; Panner, B. J.; Downs, W. L.; Maynard, E. A. Toxicity of sodium cyanurate. Toxicol. Appl. Pharmacol. 7:667-674, 1965.

Hodgson, E.; Casida, J. E. Mammalian enzymes involved in the degradation of 2,2-dichlorovinyl dimethyl phosphate. Agric. Food Chem., 10:208-214, 1962.

Hoefnagel, D. Toxic effects of atropine and homatropine eye drops in children. N. Engl. J. Med., 264:168-171, 1961.

Hoekstra, J. B.; Tisch, D. E.; Rakieten, N.; Dickison, H. L. Pharmacological properties of new antihistaminic agent, phenyltoloxamine (Bristamin). J. Am. Pharm. Assoc., Sci. Ed., 42:587-593, 1953.

Hofmann, H. Th.; Birnstiel, H.; Jobst, P. Inhalation toxicity of 1,1- and 1,2-dichloroethane. (as cited in Chem. Abstracts 75:61562e) Arch. Toxicol. 27:248-265, 1971.

Hogstedt, C.; Malmqvist, N.; Wadman, B. Leukemia in workers exposed to ethylene oxide. J. A. M. A., 214:1132-1133, 1979.

Holck, H. G. O.; Cannon, P. R. On the cause of the delayed death in the rat by isopropyl betabromallyl barbituric acid (Nostal) and some related barbiturates. J. Pharmacol. Exp. Ther. 57:289-309, 1936.

Hollingsworth, R. L. Personal communication. Dow Chemical Co., Midland, Mich, 1958.

Hollingsworth, R. L.; Rowe, V. K.; Oyen, F. Toxicity of acetylene tetrabromide determined on experimental animals. Am. Ind. Hyg. Assoc. J., 24:28-35, 1963.

Hollingsworth, R. L.; Rowe, V. K.; Oyen, F.; Hoyle, H. R.; Spencer, H. C. Toxicity of paradichlorobenzene; determinations on experimental animals and human subjects. Arch. Ind. Health, 14:138-147, 1956.

Hollingsworth, R. L.; Rowe, V. K.; Oyen, F.; Torkelson, T. R.; Adams, E. M. Toxicity of O-dichlorobenzene; studies on animals and industrial experience. Arch. Ind. Health, 17:180-187, 1958.

Hollister, L. E. Hydroxyzine hydrochloride: possible adverse cardiac interactions. Psychopharmacol. Commun., 1:61-65, 1975.

Hollister, L. E.; Hartman, A. M. Mescaline, lysergic acid diethylamide and psilocybin: comparison of clinical syndromes, effects on color perception and biochemical measures. Comp. Psychiatr., 3:235, 1962.

Holman, R. L. Acute necrotizing arteritis, aortitis, and auriculitis following uranium nitrate injury in dogs with altered plasma proteins. Am. J. Pathol., 17:359-375, 1941.

Holman, R. L.; Hewitt, W. C. Experimental necrotizing arteritis; II. Mercuric chloride as effective as uranium nitrate in its production. Proc. Soc. Exp. Biol. Med., 49:58-62, 1942.

Holmberg, B.; Malmfors, T. The cytotoxicity of some organic solvents. Environ. Res. 7:183-192, 1974.

Holsing, G. C. Personal communication. FMC Corp., Niagara Chemical Division, Middleport, N. Y., Aug, 1965.

Holtz, P.; Westermann, E. Giftung und Entgiftung von Parathion und Paraoxon. Nauyn. Schmiedebergs Arch. Pharmakol., 237:211-221, 1959.

Homburger, F.; Kelley, T., Jr.; Friedler, G.; Russfield, A. B. Toxic and possible carcinogenic effects of 4-allyl-1, 2-methylenedioxybenzene (Safrole) in rats on deficient diets. Med. Exp., 4:1-11, 1961.

Honey, G. E.; Jackson, R. C. Artificial respiration and an artificial kidney for severe barbiturate poisoning. Br. Med. J. 2:1134-1137, 1959.

Honigman, J. L. Desinfexation og klohexidins symposium. Danmarks Apotekerforening, Kobenhaven, 1977.

Hoppe, J. O.; Marcell, G. M. A.; Tainter, M. L. A review of the toxicity of iron compounds. Am. J. Med. Sci., 230:558-571, 1955.

Horio, T. Photosensitivity reaction to dibucaine. Case report and experimental induction. Arch. Dermatol., 115:986-987, 1979.

Horn, H. J. Toxicology of dimethylacetamide. Toxicol. Appl. Pharmacol., 3:12-24, 1961.

Horn, H. J.; Bruce, R. B.; Paynter, O. E. Toxicology of chlorobenzilate. J. Agric. Food Chem., 3:752-756, 1955.

Horowitz, J. D.; McNeil, J. J.; Sweet, B.; Mendelsohn, F. A. O.; Louis, W. J. Med. J. Aust., 1:175-176, 1979.

Horvath, E.; Solyom, A.; Korpassy, B. Histochemical and biochemical studies in acute poisoning with tannic acid. Br. J. Exp. Pathol., 41:298-304, 1960.

Horwitt, M. K. and Mason, K. E. The Vitamins, vol. 5 (series edited by Sebrell and Harris). 2nd. ed., Academic Press, New York, 1967.

Hotchkiss, J. H.; Barbour, J. F.; Libbey, L. M.; Scanlan, R. A. Nitramines as thermal energy analyzer positive non-nitroso compounds for certain herbicides. J. Agric. Food Chem. 26:884-887, 1978.

House, L. R.; Carey, W. C. Constitutional effects from the use of sympathomimetic drugs as nasal medication in children. Report of a case of privine toxicity. Laryngoscope, 58:1294-1297, 1948.

Howes, D.; Black, J. G. Percutaneous absorption of triclocarban in rat and man. Toxicology, 6:67-76, 1976.

Hrenoff, A. K.; Leake, C. D. Toxicity studies on 2, 4-dinitro-6-cyclohexyl-pheriol, a new insecticide. Univ. Calif. Pub. Pharmacol. 1:151-160, 1939.

Hubbell, J. P.; Casida, J. E. Metabolic fate of the N, N-dialkylcarbamoyl moiety of thiocarbamate herbicides in rats and corn. J. Agric. Food Chem. 25:404-413, 1977.

Hubble, D. Toxicity of phenothiazine. Lancet, 2:600, 1941.

Hubbs, R. S.; Prusmack, J. J. Ethylene dichloride poisoning. J. A. M. A., 159:673-675, 1955.

Huber, J. J. Some physiological effects of the insecticide kepone on the laboratory mouse. Toxicol. Appl. Pharmacol., 7:516-524, 1965.

Huber, W. G.; Link, R. P. Toxic effects of hexachloronaphthalene in swine. Toxicol. Appl. Pharmacol., 4:257-262, 1962.

Hudec, T.; Thean, J.; Kuchl, D.; Dougherty, R. C. Tris (dichloropropyl)phosphate a mutagenic flame retardant: frequent occurrence in human seminal plasma. Science, 211:951-952, 1981.

Hueper, W. C. Cinchophen (Atophan), a critical review. Medicine, 27:43-103, 1948.

Hueper, W. C. Bioassay of polyvinylpyrrolidones with limited molecular weight range. J. National Cancer Instit., 26:229-238, 1961.

Hughes, J. D.; Clark, J. A., Jr. Stramonium poisoning; a report of two cases. J. A. M. A., 112:2500-2502, 1939.

Hughes, J. P. Hazardous exposure to some so-called safe solvents. J. A. M. A., 156:234, 1954.

Hughes, J. R. Infantile methemoglobinemia due to benzocaine suppository. J. Pediatr., 66:797-799, 1965.

Huguley, C. M., Jr. Agranulocytosis induced by dipyrone, a hazardous antipyretic and analgesic. J. A. M. A. 189:938-941, 1964.

Huisman, J. and Vasbinder, H. A case of food poisoning caused by Chinese wood oil. Trop. Geogr. Med. 13:183-185, 1961.

Hunt, L. M.; Chamberlain, W. F.; Gilbert, B. N.; Hopkins, D. E. Absorption, excretion, and metabolism of nitrofen by a sheep. J. Agric. Food Chem. 25:1062-1065, 1977.

Hunt, W. H. Personal communication. Monsanto Company, St. Louis, 1969.

Hunter, D.; Perry, K. M. A.; Evans, R. B. Toxic polyneuritis arising from manufacture of tricresyl phosphate. Br. J. Ind. Med., 1:227-231, 1944.

Hussar, A. E.; Holley, H. L. Treatment of bromide intoxication with mercurial diuretics. Am. J. Med., 20:100-106, 1956.

Hutchinson, R. A danger from paraldehyde. Br. Med. J., 1:718, 1930.

Hutson, D. H.; Crayford, J. V.; Hoadley, E. C. The fate of the herbicide flamprop-isopropyl (Barnon) in rats and dogs. Xenobiotica 7:279-300, 1977.

Huvar, A. J. Personal communication. Mobil Chemical Co., Ashland, Virginia, 1969.

Hwang, K. Mechanism of the laxative effect of sodium sulfate, sodium cyclamate and calcium cyclamate. Arch. Int. Pharmacodyn. Ther., 163:302-340, 1966.

Hyatt, H. W. Near fatal poisoning due to accidental ingestion of an overdose of dextropropoxyphene hydrochloride by a two-year-old child. N. Engl. J. Med., 267:710, 1962.

Iatropoulos, M. J.; Hobson, W.; Knauf, V.; Adams, H. P. Morphological effects of hexachlorobenzene toxicity in female rhesus monkeys. Toxicol. Appl. Pharmacol 37:433-444, 1976.

Iatropoulos, M. J.; Milling, A.; Muller, W. F.; Nohynek, G.; Rozman, K.; Coulston, F.; Korte, F. Absorption, transport and organotropism of dichlorobiphenyl (DCB), dieldrin, and hexachlorobenzene (HCB) in rats. Environ. Res. 10:384-389, 1975.

Ibe, K. Die akute Methaqualong-Vergiftung. I. Statistik Literaturubersicht and Kasauistik. Arch. Toxikol., 21:179-198, 1965.

Ibe, K. Die akute Methaqualon-Vergiftung. II. Mitteilung Klink, Pathophysiologie and Therapie. Arch. Toxikol., 21:289-309, 1966a.

Ibe, K. Die akute Methaqualon-Vergiftung. Mitteilung Klinisch-chemisch-toxikologische Untersuchungen. III. Arch. Toxikol., 22:16-23, 1966b.

Illingworth, R. N.; Jarvic, D. R. Absence of toxicity in cimetidine overdosage. Br. Med. J. 1:453-454, 1979.

Imprens, E. Le Chloretone. Arch. Int. Pharmacodyn. Ther., 8:77-100, 1901.

Ing, T. S.; Daugirdas, J. T.; Soung, L. S.; Klawans, H. L.; Mahurkar, S. D.; Hayashi, J. A.; Geis, W. P.; Hano, J. E. Toxic effects of amantadine in patients with renal failure. CMA J. 120:695-697, 1979.

Innes, J. R. M.; Valerio, M.; Ulland, B. M.; Pallotta, A. J.; Petrucelli, L.; Fishbein, L.; Hart, E. R.; Falk, H. L.; Klein, M.; Peters, A. J. Bioassay of pesticides and industrial chemicals for tumorigenicity in mice. J. Natl. Cancer Inst. 42:1101-1109, 1969.

Irwin, C. M. Personal communication. Irwin-Willert Co., St. Louis, Mo, 1959.

Irwin, S.; Slabock, M.; Debiase, P. L.; Govier, W. M. Perphenazine (Trilafon), a new potent tranquilizer and antiemetic. I. Behavior profile, acute toxicity and behavioral mode of action. Arch. Int. Pharmacodyn. Ther., 118:358-374, 1959.

Ishizaki, T.; Shida, T.; Miyamoto, T.; Matsumara, Y.; Mizuno, K.; Tomaru, M. Occupational asthma from western red cedar dust (Thuja plicata) in furniture factory workers. J. Occup. Med. 15:580-585, 1973.

Ivanhoe, F.; Meyers, F. H. Phosgene poisoning as an example of neuroparalytic acute pulmonary edema: The sympathetic vaso motor reflex involved. Dis. Chest, 46:211-218, 1964.

Ivanova-Chemishanska, L.; Markov, D. V.; Dashev, G. Light and electron microscopic observations on rat thyroid after administration of some dithiocarbamates. Environ. Res. 4:201-212, 1971.

Iverson, F. Affinity and carbamylation rate constants of propoxur in reaction with erythrocyte and serum cholinesterase. Biochem. Pharmacol. 24:1537-1538, 1975.

Ivie, G. W. Fate of diflubenzuron in cattle and sheep. J. Agric. Food Chem. 26:81-89, 1978.

Iwarson, S.; Lindberg, J.; Lundin, P. Nitrofurantoin-induced chronic liver disease. Scand. J. Gastroent., 14:497-502, 1979.

Jackson, E. L. Personal communication. A. H. Robins Co., Inc., Richmond, Va, 1958.

Jacob, S. W.; Wood, D. C. Dimethyl sulfoxide (DMSO). Toxicology, pharmacology, and clinical experience. Am. J. Surg. 114:414-426, 1967.

Jacobsen, E. The excretion of hexylene glycol (2-methyl-2, 4-pentanediol) in man. Acta Pharmacol. Toxicol., 14:207-213, 1958.

Jacobsen, E. The clinical pharmacology of the hallucinogens. Clin. Pharmacol. Ther., 4:480-503, 1963.

Jacobziner, H.; Raybin, H. W. Thyroid intoxication. N. Y. State J. Med., 58:408-409, 1958.

Jacobziner, H.; Raybin, H. W. Briefs on accidental chemical poisonings in New York City. N. Y. State J. Med., 60:3139-3142, 1960b.

Jacobziner, H.; Raybin, H. W. Trioxymethylene (deodorant) poisoning. Arch. Pediatr. 78:330-334, 1961d.

Jacobziner, H.; Raybin, H. W. Briefs on accidental chemical poisonings in New York City. N. Y. State J. Med., 61:1935-1938, 1961j.

Jacobziner, H.; Raybin, H. W. Poison control. Dexedrine, metallic mercury, arsenic and arnica intoxications. Arch. Pediatr., 78:19-22, 1961k.

Jacobziner, H.; Raybin, H. W. Potassium permanganate poisoning. Arch. Pediatr., 78:120-124, 1961l.

Jacobziner, H.; Raybin, H. W. Accidental cobalt poisoning. Arch. Pediatr. 78:200-205, 1961n.

Jacques, W. E.; Benirschke, K. Pulmonary talcosis with involvement of the stomach and heart; report of a case. Arch. Ind. Hyg., 5:451-463, 1952.

Jaeger, R. J. Kepone chronology. Science 193:94-96, 1976.

Jaeger, R. J.; Rubin, R. J. Plasticizers from plastic devices; extraction, metabolism and accumulation by biological systems. Science, 170:460-461, 1970.

Jaeger, R. J.; Rubin, R. J. Migration of a phthalate ester plasticizer from polyvinyl chloride blood bags into stored human blood and its localization in human tissues. N. Engl. J. Med., 287:1114-1118, 1972.

Jaffe, F. A. Graphite pneumoconiosis. Am. J. Pathol., 27:909-923, 1951.

Jaffe, I. A.; Altman, K.; Merryman, P. The antipyridoxine effect of penicillamine in man. J. Clin. Invest., 43:1869-1873, 1964.

Jaffe, J. H.; Martin, W. R. Opioid analgesics and antagonists. In The Pharmacological Basis of Therapeutics. (Gilman, A. G.; Goodman, L. S.; Gilman, A., editors). Macmillan Publishing Co., Inc., pp. 494-534, 1980.

Jalili, M. A.; Abbasi, A. H. Poisoning by ethyl mercury toluene sulphonanilide. Br. J. Ind. Med., 18:303-308, 1961.

James, T. N.; Bear, E. S. Cardiac effects of some simple aliphatic aldehydes. J. Pharmacol. Exp. Ther., 163:300-308, 1968.

Jan, K. M.; Dorsey, S.; Bornstein, A. Hot hog: hyperthermia from phencyclidine. N. Engl. J. Med. 299:722, 1978.

Jang, C. The action of berberine on mammalian hearts. J. Pharmacol. Exp. Ther., 71:178-186, 1941.

Janovsky, R. C. Fatal thrombocytopenic purpura after administration of sulfamethoxypyridazine. J. Am. Med. Assoc. 172:155-157, 1960.

Jansch, H.; Wolkart, N. Zur todlichen Pyramidonvergiftung beim Kleinkind. (Chemischer Nachweis an der faulen Leiche.). Arch. Toxikol. 15:1-10, 1954.

Jaques, R. The protective effect of pyridine-2-aldoxime methiodide (P(2)AM), bis-(4-hydroxyiminomethyl pyridinium-1-methyl)ether dichloride (Toxogonin) and atropine in experimental DDVP poisoning. Helv. Physiol. Acta., 22:174-183, 1964.

Jasmin, G.; Bois, P. Storage and tissue disposal of carboxymethylcellulose injected into rats. Rev. Can. Biol., 20:819-822, 1961.

Jawetz, E. Polymyxin, Colistin and Bacitracin. Ped. Clin. North Amer. 8:1057-1071, 1961.

Jeannin, J.; Berrod, R.; Lemaire; Bazin. Severe poisoning in a child from swallowing peach kernels. Lyon. Med. 205:785-793; Abstract in Toxic Episodes in Child. 2:42, 1961.

Jeffcoat, A. R.; Handy, R. W.; Francis, M. T.; Willis, S.; Wall, M. E. Birch, C. G.; Hiles, R. A. The metabolism and toxicity of halogenated carbanilides: biliary metabolites of 3,4,4′-trichlorocarbanilide and 3-trifluoromethyl-4,4′-dichlorocarbanilide in the rat. Drug Metab. Dis., 5:157-166, 1977.

Jefferson, N. C.; Necheles, H. Oleic acid toxicity and fat embolism. Proc. Soc. Exp. Biol. Med., 68:248-250, 1948.

Jelliffe, S. E. Some notes on poisoning by Clitocybe dealbata (Sow.) var. sudorifica (Peck). N. Y. State J. Med. 37:1357-1361, 1937.

Jenkins, L. J., Jr.; Trabulus, M. J.; Murphy, S. D. Biochemical effects of 1,1-dichloroethylene in rats: comparison with carbon tetrachloride and 1,2-dichloroethylene. Toxicol. Appl. Pharmacol., 23:501-510, 1972a.

Jenner, P. M.; Hagan, E. C.; Taylor, J. M.; Cook, E. L.; Fitzhugh, O. G. Food flavorings and compounds of related structure. I. Acute Oral Toxicity. Food Cosmet. Toxicol., 2:327-343, 1964.

Jennings, C. C. Personal communication. Allied Chemical and

Dye Corp., New York, 1958.

Jennings, E. R.; Beland, A. J.; Cope, J. A.; Ellestad, M. H.; Monroe, C.; Shadle, O. W. Citrate toxicity and the use of anticoagulant acid citrate dextrose blood for extracoporeal circulation. Surgery, 120:997-1008, 1965.

Jensen, K. B.; Dyrud, O. K. The smooth muscle relaxing effect of thyme (Thymus vulgaris L.). Acta Pharmacol. Toxicol., 19:345-355, 1963.

Jetter, W. W.; Hunter, F. T. Death from attempted abortion with a potassium permanganate douche. N. Engl. J. Med., 240:794-798, 1949.

Jick, H.; Miettinen, O. S.; Neff, R. K.; Shapiro, S.; Heinonen, O. P.; Slone, D. Coffee and myocardial infarction. N. Engl. J. Med., 289:63-67, 1973.

Jillson, O. F.; Baughman, R. D. Contact photodermatistis from bithionol. Arch. Dermatol., 88:409-418, 1963.

Johnson, C. C. The actions and toxicity of sodium nitroprusside. Arch. Int. Pharmacodyn. Ther., 35:480-496, 1929.

Johnson, D.; Kubic, P.; Levitt, C. Accidental ingestion of vacor rodenticide. Am. J. Dis. Child. 134:161-164, 1980.

Johnstone, R. T. Toluene-2,4-diisocyanate: clinical features. Ind. Med. Surg., 26:33-34, 1957b.

Jokela, S.; Vartiainen, A. Caffeine poisoning. Acta Pharmacol. Toxicol. 15:331-334, 1959.

Jomain-Baum, M.; Hanson, R. W. Inhibition by cycloheximide of lipid metabolism by rat adipose tissue in vitro. Life Sci. 16:345-351, 1975.

Jones, C. O. A case of poisoning by pennyroyal. Br. Med. J., 2:746, 1913.

Jones, K. K. The physiology of sodium hexametaphosphate. J. Am. Water Works Assoc., 32; 1471-1483, 1940.

Jones, M. F.; Caldwell, J. R. Acute hemorrhagic pancreatitis associated with administration of chlorothalidone. N. Engl. J. Med., 267:1029-1031, 1962.

Jordan, W. P., Jr.; Dahl, M. V.; Albert, H. L. Contact dermatitis from glutaraldehyde. Arch. Derm. 105:94-95, 1972.

Jornod, J. C.; Barrelet, J. A. Suicidal attempt by overdosage of ajmaline. Am. Heart J., 70:719-720, 1965.

Josephson, G. W.; Stine, R. J. Caffeine intoxication: a case of paroxysmal atrial tachycardia. J. Am. Coll. Emerg. Phys., 5:776-778, 1976.

Kabat, H.; Stohlman, E. F.; Smith, M. I. Hypoprothrombinemia induced by administration of indandione derivatives. J. Pharmacol. Exp. Ther., 80:160-170, 1944.

Kahl, R.; Netter, K. J. Ethoxyquin as an inducer and inhibitor of phenobarbital-type P-450 in rat liver microsomes. Toxicol. Appl. Pharmacol. 40:473-483, 1977.

Kalacic, I. Ventilatory lung function in cement workers. Arch. Environ. Health, 26:84-85, 1973.

Kallen, R. J.; Rieger, C. H. L.; Cohen, H. S.; Sutter, M. A.; Ong, R. T. Near-fatal hyperkalemia due to ingestion of salt substitute by an infant. J. A. M. A., 235:2125-2126, 1976.

Kamienski, F. X.; Casida, J. E. Importance of dimethylenation in the metabolism in vivo and in vitro of methylenedioxyphenyl synergists and related compounds in mammals. Biochem. Pharmacol. 19:91-112, 1970.

Kaplan, A. S.; Berghout, C. F.; Peczenik, A. Human intoxication from RDX. Arch. Environ. Health, 10:877-883, 1965.

Kaplan, M. Suicide by oral ingestion of a potassium preparation. Ann. Intern. Med., 71:363-364, 1969.

Kaplan, N. M. Hypotension as a complication of promazine therapy. Arch. Intern. Med., 103:219-223, 1959.

Kappy, M. S.; Buckley, J. Primidone intoxication in a child. Arch. Dis. Child. 44:282-284, 1969.

Karel, L.; Landing, B. H.; Harvey, T. S. The intraperitoneal toxicity of some glycols, glycol ethers, glycol esters and phthalates in mice. Fed. Proc., 6:342, 1947.

Kaufman, D. B.; Dinicola, W.; McIntosh, R. Acute potassium dichromate poisoning. Am. J. Dis. Child., 119:374-376, 1970.

Kawada, T.; Sakurai, H.; Ikarashi, A.; Imai, S. Acute and subacute toxicities of napropamide in rats. (as cited in Chem. Abs. 80:56257h) Niigata Igakkai Zasshi 87:289-296, 1973.

Kay, S. Tissue reaction to barium sulfate contrast medium. Arch. Pathol., 57:279-284, 1954.

Kaye, S.; Haag, H. B. Study of death due to combined action

of alcohol and paraldehyde in man. Toxicol. Appl. Pharmacol., 6:316-320, 1964.

Keall, J. H. H.; Martin, N. H.; Tunbridge, R. E. A report of three cases of accidental poisoning by sodium tellurite. Br. J. Ind. Med., 3:175-176, 1946.

Keilin, D. The action of sodium azide on cellular repiration and in some catalytic oxidation reactions. Proc. Roy. Soc. Lond. B 121:165-173, 1936-37.

Keller, J. G. Personal communication. Hazelton Laboratories, Falls Church, Va, 1961.

Kelly, M. G.; Leiter, J.; Ghosh, O. Role of the adrenal glands in the hematopoietic and thymicolymphatic response of the rat to podophyllotoxin. J. Natl. Cancer Inst. 12:1177-1201, 1952.

Kelly, R. E. Personal communication. Monsanto Chemical Co., St. Louis, Mo, 1958.

Kelly, R. E. Personal communication. Monsanto Chemical Co., St. Louis, Mo, 1961.

Kenaga, E. E. Some biological, chemical and physical properties of sulfuryl fluoride as an insecticidal fumigant. J. Econ. Entomol., 50:1-6, 1957.

Kennedy, A. C.; Lindsay, R. M.; Briggs, J. D.; Luke, R. G.; Young, N.; Campbell, D. Successful treatment of three cases of very severe barbiturate poisoning. Lancet 1:995-998, 1969.

Kennedy, G. L., Jr.; Keplinger, M. L.; Fancher, O. E.; Stone, J. D.; Calandra, J. C. Metabolic studies with dinitroamine. Toxicol. Appl. Pharmacol. 33:341-349, 1975.

Kerr, K. B.; Cavett, J. W.; Thompson, O. L. The toxicity of an organic arsenical, 3-nitro-4-hydroxyphenylarsonic acid. 1. Acute and subacute toxicity. Toxicol. Appl. Pharmacol., 5:507-525, 1963.

Kessler, M. J.; Kupper, J. L.; Brown, R. Accidental methyl methacrylate inhalation toxicity in a rhesus monkey (Macaca mulatta). Lab. Animal Sci. 27:388–390, 1977.

Kesten, H. D.; Mulinos, N. G.; Pomerantz, L. Pathologic effects of certain glycols and related compounds. Arch. Pathol., 27:447-465, 1939.

Ketai, R.; Matthews, J.; Mozdzen, J. J. Sudden death in a patient taking haloperidol. Am. J. Psychiatr., 136:112-113, 1979.

Khan, M. A. Toxicity of apholate to cattle. Can. J. Comp. Med. Vet. Sci., 27:233-236, 1963.

Khandekar, J. D.; Edelman, H. Studies of amygdalin (laetrile) toxicity in rodents. J. A. M. A., 242:169-171, 1979.

Khantzian, E. J.; McKenna, G. J. Acute toxic and withdrawal reaction associated with drug use and abuse. Ann. Intern. Med. 90:361–372, 1979.

Khera, K. S. Teratogenic effects of ethylenethiourea in rats and rabbits (Abstract). Toxicol. Appl. Pharmacol. 25:455-456, 1973.

Khera, K. S.; Tryphonas, L. Ethylenethiourea-induced hydrocephalus: pre- and postnatal pathogenesis in offspring from rats given a single oral dose during pregnancy. Toxicol. Appl. Pharmacol. 42:85-97, 1977.

Kieth, L.; Evenhouse, H.; Webster, A. Amylophagia during pregnancy. Obstet. Gynecol., 32:415-418, 1968.

Kieth, N. M.; Osterberg, A. E.; Burchell, H. B. Some effects of potassium salts in man. Ann. Intern. Med., 16:879-892, 1942.

Kilgore, H. H.; Rhoads, P. S. A case of lead arsenate poisoning with recovery. J. A. M. A., 120:1125, 1942.

Kilmartin, J. V.; Fogg, J. Role of the α-amino groups of the α and β chains of human hemoglobin in oxygen-linked binding of carbon dioxide. J. Biol. Chem., 248:7039-7043, 1973.

Kimbrough, R. D. Toxicity of chlorinated hydrocarbons and related compounds. Arch. Pathol., 125:125-131, 1972.

Kimbrough, R. D. Human health effects of selected pesticides, chloroaniline derivatives. J. Environ. Sci. Health, Part B, B15:977-992, 1980.

Kimbrough, R. D.; Gaines, T. B.; Linder, R. E. 2, 4-Dichlorophenyl p-nitrophenyl ether (TOK) effects on the lung maturation of rat fetus. Arch. Environ. Health. 28:316-320, 1974.

Kimbrough, R. D.; Linder, R. E.; Gaines, T. B. Morphological changes in livers of rats fed polychlorinated biphenyls. Arch. Environ. Health, 25:354-364, 1972.

Kimura, E. T.; Ebert, D. M.; Dodge, P. W. Acute toxicity and limits of solvent residue for sixteen organic solvents. Toxicol. Appl. Pharmacol. 19:699-704, 1971.

Kinard, F. W.; Aull, J. C. Distribution of tungsten in the rat following ingestion of tungsten compounds. J. Pharmacol. Exp. Ther., 83:53-55, 1945.

Kinard, F. W.; Van de Erve, J. The toxicity of orally ingested tungsten compounds in the rat. J. Pharmacol. Exp. Ther., 72:196-201, 1941.

Kinard, F. W.; Van de Erve, J. Effect of tungsten metal diets in the rat. J. Lab. Clin. Med., 28:1541-1543, 1943.

Kinard, F. W.; Van de Erve, J.; Voight, D. Rat mortality following sodium tungstate injection. Am. J. Med. Sci., 199:668-670, 1940.

King, H.; Hawtof, D. B. Accidental intra-arterial injection of ether. J. A. M. A., 184:241-242, 1963.

King, M. R.; Himmelsbach, C. K.; Saunders, B. S. Dilaudid (Dihydromorphinone); a review of the literature and a study of its addictive properties. Public Health Repts. Suppl. No. 113, 1935.

Kingsbury, J. M. Poisonous Plants of the United States and Canada. Prentice-Hall, Inc., Englewood Cliffs, N. J, 1964.

Kinnoss-Wright, J. Newer phenothiazine drugs in treatment of nervous disorders. J. A. M. A., 170:1283-1288, 1959.

Kirchoff, T. F. Personal communication. Amchem Products Inc, 1961.

Kirk, D.; Mittwoch, U. Changes in mitotic cycle induced by α-solanine. Humangenetik 26:105-111, 1975.

Kirklin, J. K.; Watson, M.; Bondoc, C. C.; Burke, J. F. Treatment of hydrazine-induced coma with pyridoxine. N. Engl. J. Med., 294:938-939, 1976.

Kirtley, W. R.; Peck, F. B. Administration of massive doses of vitamin P, hesperidin methyl chalcone. Am. J. Med. Sci. 216:64-70, 1948.

Kithil, R. Personal communication. Carwin Company, North Haven, Conn, 1962.

Klaassen, C. D.; Plaa, G. L. The relative effects of various chlorinated hydrocarbons on liver and kidney function in mice. Toxicol. Appl. Pharmacol. 9:139-151, 1966.

Klaassen, C. D.; Plaa, G. L. Relative effects of various chlorinated hydrocarbons on liver and kidney function in dogs. Toxicol. Appl. Pharmacol. 10:119-131, 1967a.

Klarmann, E. G. Personal communication. Lehn and Fink, Inc., New York, Nov. 1954, 1954.

Kleeman, C. R.; Epstein, F. H.; Rubini, M. E.; Lamdin, E. Initial distribution and fate of ferrocyanide in dogs. Am. J. Physiol., 182:548-552, 1955.

Klein, M. F.; Beall, J. R. Griseofulvin: a teratogenic study. Science 175:1483-1484, 1972.

Klein, S. M.; Cohen, G.; Cederbaum, A. I. The interaction of hydroxyl radicals with dimethyl sulfoxide produces formaldehyde. FEBS Lett., 116:220-222, 1980.

Kleinfeld, M.; Rosso, A. Ulceration of the nasal septum due to inhalation of chromic acid mist. Ind. Med. Surg., 34:242-243, 1965.

Klimmer, O. R. Beitrag zur Wirkung des Phosphorwasserstoffes (PH₃) Zur Frage der sog. chronischen Phosphorwasserstoffvergiftung. Arch. Toxikol., 24:164-187, 1969.

Kline, B. E.; von Elbe, H.; Dahle, N. A.; Kupchan, S. M. Toxic effects of potato sprouts and of solanine fed to pregnant rats. Proc. Soc. Exp. Biol. Med. 107:807-809, 1961.

Kneebone, G. M. A case of hypersensitivity to paraaminosalicyclic acid in a child. J. Pediatr., 59:90-92, 1961.

Knowles, C. O.; Ahmad, S. Mode of action studies wtih formetanate and formparanate acaricides. Pestic. Biochem. Physiol. 1:445-452, 1971.

Knowles, C. O.; Ahmad, S. Comparative metabolism of chlorobenzilate, chloropropylate, and bromopropylate acaricides by rat hepatic enzymes. Can. J. Physiol. Pharmacol. 49:590-597, 1971a.

Kochmann, M. Zur Pharmakologie der Mistel. Arch. Exp. Pathol. Pharmacol. 161:553-561, 1931.

Koizumi, A.; Shiojima, S.; Omiya, M.; Nakano, S.; Sato, N.; Ikeda, M. Acute renal failure and maneb (manganous ethylenebisdithiocarbamate) exposure. J. A. M. A. 242:2583-2585, 1979.

Kojak, G.; Barry, M. J.; Gastineau, C. F. Severe hypoglycemic

reaction with haloperidol: report of a case. Am. J. Psychiatry, 126:573-576, 1969.

Kolb, E. J.; Korein, J. Neuromuscular toxicity of Veratrum alkaloids. Neurology, 11:159-163, 1961.

Kolkmann, F. W.; Volk, B. Necroses in the granular cell layer of the cerebellum due to methylchloride intoxication in guinea pigs. Exp. Pathol. 10:298-308, 1975.

Konig, J.; Hynie, I.; Kacl, K. Todliche suicidale malathionvergiftung. Arch. Toxikol., 22:129-136, 1966.

Korobkin, R.; Asbury, A. K.; Summer, A. J.; Nielsen, S. L. Glue-sniffing neuropathy. Arch. Neurol. 32:158-162, 1975.

Korsrud, G. O.; Grice, H. G.; Goodman, T. K.; Knipfel, J. E.; McLaughlin, J. M. Sensitivity of several serum enzymes for the detection of thioacetamide-, dimethylnitrosamine-, and diethanolamine-induced liver damage in rats. Toxicol. Appl. Pharmacol. 26:299-313, 1973.

Kosinski, E. J.; Malindzak, G. S., Jr. Glucagon and isoproterenol in reversing propranolol toxicity. Arch. Intern. Med., 132:840-843, 1973.

Kostrodymova, G. M.; Voronin, V. M.; Kostrodymova, N. N. Toxicity during complex action and possibility of carcinogenic and cocarcinogenic properties of triethanolamines. Gig. Sanit. No. 3, 20-25, 1976.

Kotz, J.; Roth, G. B.; Ryon, W. A. Idiosyncrasy to paraldehyde. J. A. M. A., 110:2145-2148, 1938.

Kozlicka-Gajdzinska, H.; Brzyski, J. A case of fatal intoxication with sodium azide. Arch. Toxikol. 22:160-163, 1966.

Krakoffs, I. H. Effect of methionine sulfoximine in man. Clin. Pharmacol. Ther., 2:599-604, 1961.

Krijnen, C. J.; Boyd, E. M. Susceptibility to captan pesticide of albino rats fed from weaning on diets containing various levels of protein. Food Cosmet. Toxicol. 8:35-42, 1970.

Krishna, J. G.; Casida, J. E. Fate in rats of the radiocarbon from ten variously labeled methyl- and dimethylcarbamate-¹⁴C insecticide chemicals and their hydrolysis products. J. Agric. Food Chem. 14:98-105, 1966.

Kriss, J. P.; Carnes, W. H.; Gross, R. T. Hypothyroidism and thyroid hyperplasia in patients treated with cobalt. J. A. M. A., 157:117-121, 1955.

Krister, C. J. Personal communication. du Pont, E. I. de Nemours and Co., Wilmington, Del, 1965.

Krumlovsky, F. A.; Emmerman, J.; Parker, R. H.; Wisgerhof, M.; Del Greco, F. Dialysis in treatment of neomycin overdosage. Ann. Intern. Med., 76:443-446, 1972.

Kubic, V. L.; Anders, M. W.; Engel, R. R.; Barlow, C. H.; Caughey, W. S. Metabolism of dihalomethanes to carbon monoxide. I. in vivo studies. Drug Metab. Dispos., 2:53-57, 1974.

Kubicka, J.; Alder, A. E. Ueber eine neuere Behandlungsmethode der Vergiftung durch den Knollenblatterpilz. Praxis 57:1304-1306, 1968.

Kulkarni P. B.; Dorand, R. D. Caffeine toxicity in a neonate. Pediatrics, 64:254-255, 1979.

Kumar, S. S.; Sikka, H. C.; Saxena, J.; Zweig, G. Membrane damage in human erythrocytes caused by captan and captafol. Pestic. Biochem. Physiol. 5:338-347, 1975.

Kutscher, A. H.; Lane, S. L.; Segall, R. The clinical toxicity of antibiotics and sulfonamides. J. Allerg. 25:135-150, 1954.

Kuwabara, T.; Quevedo, A. R.; Cogan, D. G. An experimental study of dichloroethane poisoning. Arch. Ophthal. 79:321-330, 1968.

Kuznetsova, L. I.; Okunev, V. N. Effect of 4,6-diamino-s-triazines on nucleic acids of rat liver and kidneys. Ukr. Biokhim. Zh. 42:617-620, 1970.

Laake, K.; Kittang, E.; Refstad, S. O.; Holm, H. A. Convulsions and possible spasm of the lower oesophageal sphincter in a fatal case of propranolol intoxication. Acta Medica Scand. 210:137-138, 1981.

Lacouture, P. G.; Mitchell, A. A.; Lovejoy, F. H. Thiethylperazine (Torecan)-associated dystonic reactions in children. Pediatrics, 64:954-955, 1979.

Lagerfelt, J.; Matell, G. Attempted suicide with propranolol. Acta Med. Scand., 199:517-518, 1976.

LaLuna, F. J.; Wright, R. E.; Heim, W. J. Explosive hazard of blood diluents containing sodium azide. N. Engl. J. Med., 301:382-383, 1979.

Lambke, A. On the hygienic suitability of plastics for the dairy industry. Kieler Milchwirtschaftliche Forschungsberichte 10:227-232, 1958.

Lamoureux, G. L.; Davison, K. L. Mercapturic acid formation in the metabolism of propachlor, CDAA, and fluorodifen in the rat. Pestic. Biochem. Physiol. 5:497-506, 1975.

Lampe, K. F. Pharmacology and therapy of mushroom intoxications. In Mushroom Poisoning: Diagnosis and Treatment. B. H. Rumack and E. Salzman (editors). CRC Press, Inc, 1978.

Lampe, K. F.; Fagerstrom, R. Plant Toxicity and Dermatitis. The Williams and Wilkins Co., Baltimore, 1968.

Lamson, P. D. Benzoyl peroxide - an apology. J. A. M. A., 97:1225, 1931.

Lamson, P. D.; Brown, H. W.; Ward, C. B. Anthelmintic studies on alkylhydroxybenzenes. I. Alkyl polyhydroxybenzenes. J. Pharmacol. Exp. Ther., 53:198-217, 1935.

Landsteiner, K.; Rostenberg, A.; Sulzberger, M. S. Individual differences in susceptibility to eczematous sensitization with simple chemical substances. J. Invest. Dermatol., 2:25-29, 1939.

Lang, D. W.; Borgstedt, H. H. Rate of pulmonary excretion of paraldehyde in cats. Toxicol. Appl. Pharmacol., 13:24-29, 1968.

Langer, P. Study of chemical representatives of the goitrogenic activity of raw cabbage. Physiol. Bohemoslov., 13:542-549, 1964.

Langgard, H. Effects of ascorbic acid on electrolyte composition of the skin of mice. Acta Pharmacol. Toxicol., 21:371-380, 1964.

Largent, E. J. The comparative toxicity of cryclite for rats and for rabbits. J. Ind. Hyg. Toxicol., 30:92-97, 1948.

Larsen, G. L.; Bakke, J. E. Metabolism of 2-chloro-4-cyclopropylamino-6-isopropylamino-s-triazine (Cyprazine) in the rat. J. Agric. Food Chem. 23:388-392, 1975.

Larson, P. S.; Crawford, E. M.; Smith, R. B., Jr.; Hennigar, G. R.; Haag, H. B.; Finnegan, J. K. Chronic toxicologic studies on isopropyl N-(3-chlorophenyl) carbamate (CIPC). Toxicol. Appl. Pharmacol., 2:659-673, 1960.

Larson, P. S.; Haag, H. B. Studies on the fate of nicotine in the body. III. On the pharmacology of some methylated and demethylated derivatives of nicotine. J. Pharmacol. Exp. Ther., 77:343-349, 1943.

Larson, P. S.; Haag, H. B.; Silvette, H. Tobacco. Experimental and Clinical Studies. Williams and Wilkins Co., Baltimore, Md, 1961.

Lasagna, L. Nalorphine (N-allylnormorphine). Practical and theoretical considerations. Arch. Intern. Med. 94:532-558, 1954.

Lasch, E. E.; Elshawa, R. Multiple cases of cyanide poisoning by apricot kernels in children from Gaza. Pediatrics, 68:5-7, 1981.

Latini, R.; Bonati, M.; Marzi, E.; Garattini, S. Urinary excretion of uracilic metabolite of caffeine by rats, monkeys and man. Toxicol. Lett., 7:267-272, 1981.

Latven, A. R.; Molitor, H. Comparison of the toxic, hypnotic and irritating properties of eight organic solvents. J. Pharmacol. Exp. Ther., 65:89-94, 1939.

Laubach, J. L.; Malkinson, F. D.; Ringrose, E. J. Cheilitis caused by cinnamon (Cassia) oil in tooth paste. J. A. M. A., 152:404-405, 1953.

Lauber, F. U.; Hollander, F. Toxicity of the mucigogue, eugenol, administered by stomach tube in dogs. Gastroenterology, 15:481-486, 1950.

Laveglia, J.; MacKellar, D. G.; Wedig, J. H.; Keplinger, M. L.; Wright, P. L.; Levinskas, G. J. Chlorinated-s-triazine trione compounds: acute and chronic toxicity studies. Toxicol. Appl. Pharmacol. 41:131, 1977.

Lawatsch, D. J. Personal communication. American Hoechst Corp., Somerville, N. J, 1979.

Lawrason, F. D.; Alpert, A.; Mohr, F. L.; McMahon, F. G. Ulcerative-obstructive lesions of the small intestine. J. A. M. A., 191:641-644, 1965.

Lawrence, W. H.; Tuell, S. F. Phthalate esters. The question of safety - an update. Clin. Toxicol., 15:447-466, 1979.

Laws, E. R., Jr. Route of absorption of DDVP after oral administration to rats. Toxicol. Appl. Pharmacol., 8:193-196, 1966.

Laws, E. R., Jr.; Morales, F. R.; Hayes, W. J., Jr.; Josephs, C. R. Toxicology of abate in volunteers. Arch. Environ. Health, 14:289-291, 1967.

Lawson, A. A. H.; Brown, S. S. Acute methaqualone (Mandrax) poisoning. Scott. Med. J., 12:63-68, 1967.

Lawter, W. M.; Vrla, V. L. Toxicity of triethylene glycol and the effect of para-amino-benzene-sulfonamide upon the toxicity of this glycol. J. Pharm. Sci., 29:5-8, 1940.

Lawton, A. H.; Sweeny, T. R.; Dudley, H. C. Toxicology of acrylonitrile (vinyl cyanide). III. Determination of thiocyanates in blood and urine. J. Ind. Hyg. Toxicol., 25:13-19, 1943.

Lazarus-Barlow, P.; Norman, G. M. Fatal cases of poisoning with sodium nitroprusside. Br. Med. J., 2:407, 1941.

Leach, J. M.; Thakore, A. N. Identification of the constituents of the Kraft pulping effluent that are toxic to juvenile coho salmon (Oncorhynchus kisutch). J. Fish. Res. Board Can. 30:479-484, 1973.

Lecutier, M. A. A case of cantharidin poisoning. Br. Med. J., 2:1399-1400, 1954.

Lederle Laboratories. Brochure (Tentone). Pearl River, N. Y, 1959.

Ledet, A. E.; Duncan, J. R.; Buck, W. B.; Ramsey, F. K. Clinical toxicological and pathological aspects of arsanilic acid poisoning in swine. Clin. Toxicol., 6:439-457, 1973.

Lee, C.; Chen, D.; Barnes, A.; Katz, R. L. Neuromuscular block by neomycin in the cat. Can. Anaesth. Soc. J., 23:527-533, 1976.

Lee, I. P.; Dixon, R. L. Various factors affecting the lethality of cyclohexylamine. Toxicol. Appl. Pharm., 22:465-473, 1972.

Lee, K. Y.; Beilin, L. J.; Vandongen, R. Severe hypertension after ingestion of an appetite suppressant with indomethacin. Lancet, 1:1110-1111, 1979.

Lee, Y. C.; Nobles, W. L. A chemical study of American tung oil. Amer. Pharmaceut. Assoc. Sci. Ed. 48:162-165, 1959.

Lefaux, R. Practical Toxicology of Plastics. Chemical Rubber Co. Press., Cleveland, Ohio, 1968.

Legator, M. S.; Kelley, F. J.; Green, S.; Oswald, E. J. Mutagenic effects of captan. Ann. N. Y. Acad. Sci. 160:344-351, 1969.

Legendre, A. M. Disophenol toxicosis in a dog. J. Am. Vet. Med. Assoc. 163:149-150, 1973.

Lehman, A. J. Health aspects of common chemicals used in hair waving preparations. J. A. M. A., 141:842-844, 1949a.

Lehman, A. J. Untitled. Abstract of a paper presented to Agricultural and Food Chemistry Section of ACS March 28 to April 1, San Francisco, Calif, 1949b.

Lehman, A. J. Chemicals in foods: a report to the Association of Food and Drug Officials in Current Developments, Part II. Pesticides. Assoc. Food & Drug Officials U. S. Quart. Bull. 15:122-125, 1951.

Lehman, A. J. Insect repellents. Assoc. Food & Drug Officials U. S. Quart. Bull. 19:87-99, 1955.

Lehman, A. J. Summaries of Pesticide Toxicity. The Association of Food and Drug Officials of the U. S., Topeka, 1965.

Lehmann, C. F.; Pipkin, J. L.; Ressmann, A. C. Blister beetle dermatosis. Arch. Dermatol., 71:36-38, 1955.

Lehmann, K. B.; Flury, F. Toxicology and Hygiene of Industrial Solvents. The Williams & Wilkins Co., Baltimore, 1938.

Lehr, D. Sodium phthalyl sulfacetimide: a new gastrointestinal antiseptic. Fed Proc. 8:315, 1949.

Lehr, D.; Antopol, W.; Churg, J.; Sprinz, H. Acute toxicity of sodium salts of sulfapyridine, sulfathiazole and sulfamethizole. Proc. Soc. Exp. Biol. Med. 45:15-20, 1940.

Leiper, E. J. R. A case of polyneuritis due to gold. Br. Med. J., 2:119-120, 1946.

Lemeignan, M. Analysis of the effects of 4-aminopyridine on the lumbar spinal cord of the cat. II. Modification of certain spinal inhibitory phenomena, post-tetanic potentiation, and dorsal root potentials. Neuropharmacology 12:641-651, 1973.

Lemere, F. Dormison overdose. Northwest Med., 51:778, 1952.

Lemley, R. E.; Merryman, M. P. Selenium poisoning in the human. J. Lancet, 61:435-438, 1941.

Leong, K. J.; MacFarland, H. N.; Sellers, E. A. Acute sulfur dioxide toxicity. Arch. Environ. Health, 3:668-675, 1961.

Leopold, I. H.; Lieberman, T. W. Chemical injuries of the cornea. Fed. Proc., 30:(1), 92-95, 1971.

Lester, D.; Greenberg, L. A. Acute and chronic toxicity of some halogenated derivatives of methane and ethane. Arch. Ind. Hyg. Occup. Med., 2:335-344, 1950.

Lester, D.; Greenberg, L. A.; Shukovsky, E. Formation of methemoglobin IV. Limited importance of methemoglobinemia in the toxocity of certain aniline derivatives. J. Pharmacol. Exp. Ther. 80:78-80, 1944.

Levinskas, G. J. personal communication. Monsanto Co, 1972.

Levinskas, G. J.; Vidone, L. B.; O'Grady, J. J.; Shaffer, C. B. Acute and chronic toxicity of dodine (n-dodecylguanidine acetate). Toxicol. Appl. Pharmacol. 3:127-142, 1961.

Levy, R. P.; Gilger, W. G. Acute thyroid poisoning, report of a case. N. Engl. J. Med., 256:459-460, 1957.

Lew, H. T.; French, S. W. Tetracycline nephrotoxicity and nonoliguric acute renal failure. Arch. Intern. Med., 118:123-128, 1966.

Lewis, C. E.; Kerby, G. R. An epidemic of polymer-fume fever. J. A. M. A., 191:375-378, 1965.

Lewis, D. R.; Madel, G. A.; Drury, J. Fatal poisoning by 'meta fuel' tablets. Br. Med. J., 1:1283-1284, 1939.

Lewis, R. J., Sr.; Tatken, R. L. Registry of Toxic Effects of Chemical Substances. NIOSH, Volumes 1 & 2, 1979.

Li, R. C.; San, P. P. T.; Anderson, H. H. Acute toxicity of monacetin, diacetin and triacetin. Proc. Soc. Exp. Biol. Med., 46:26-28, 1941.

Liddle, J. A.; Kimbrough, R. D.; Needham, L. L.; Cline, R. E.; Smrek, A. L.; Yert, L. W.; Bayse, D. D. A fatal episode of accidental methomyl poisoning. Clin. Toxicol., 15:159-167, 1979.

Liefer, W.; Steiner, K. Studies in sensitization to halogenated hydroxyquinolines and related compounds. J. Invest. Dermatol., 17:233-240, 1951.

Lilis, R.; Lorimer, W. V.; Diamond, S.; Selikoff, I. J. Neurotoxicity of styrene in production and polymerization workers. Environ. Res. 15:133-138, 1978.

Lilly, Eli, and Co. Brochure (Ultran). Indianapolis, Ind, Date Unknown.

Linch, A. L. Biological monitoring for industrial exposure to cyanogenic aromatic nitro and amino compounds. Am. Ind. Hyg. Ass. J., 7:426-432, 1974.

Lincoff, G.; Mitchel, D. H. Toxic and Hallucinogenic Mushroom Poisoning. Van Nostrand Reinhold Co, 1977.

Lindberg, P.; Bergman, R.; Wickberg, B. Isolation and structure of coprine, a novel physiologically active cyclopropanone derivative from Coprinus atramentarius and its synthesis via 1-aminocyclopropanol. J. Chem. Soc. Chem. Commun., 23:946-947, 1975.

Lindquist, N. G. Autoradiographic study on the distribution of the herbicide 4-chloro-2-methylphenoxyacetic acid in pregnant mice. Toxicol. Appl. Pharmacol. 30:227-236, 1974.

Lindstrom, P. A.; Brizzee, K. R. Relief of intractable vomiting from surgical lesions in the area postrema. J. Neurosurg., 19:228-236, 1962.

Linton, A. L.; Luke, R. G.; Briggs, J. D. Methods of forced diuresis and its application in barbiturate poisoning. Lancet 2:377-380, 1967.

Lipsitz, S. T.; Cross, S. J. A case of cantharides poisoning with special reference to the blood picture. Arch. Intern. Med., 20:889-891, 1917.

Litt, I. F.; Cohen, M. I. "Danger. . . vapor harmful": spot-remover sniffing. N. Engl. J. Med. 281:543-544, 1969.

Lloyd, G. K.; Liggett, M. P.; Kynoch, S. R.; Davies, R. E. Assessment of the acute toxicity and potential irritancy of hairdye constituents. Food Cosmet. Toxicol. 15:607-610, 1977.

Locke, A. Personal communication. Zonite Products Corp., New Brunswick, N. J, 1951.

Lockett, M. Dangerous effects of isoprenaline in myocardial failure. Lancet, 2:104-106, 1965.

Lockett, M. F.; Natoff, I. L. A study of the toxicity of sulfide. J. Pharm. and Pharmacol., 12:488, 1960.

Loeb, R. F. Activity of a new antimalarial agent, chloroquine (SN 7618). J. A. M. A., 130:1069-1070, 1946.

Loeser, D.; Konwiser, A. L. A study of the toxicity of strontium and comparison with other cations employed in therapeutics. J. Lab. Clin. Med., 15:35-41, 1929.

Long, P. H.; Haviland, J. W.; Edwards, L. B. Acute toxicity, absorption and excretion of sulfathiazole and certain of its derivatives. Proc. Soc. Exp. Biol. Med., 43:328-332, 1940a.

Long, P. H.; Haviland, J. W.; Edwards, L. B.; Bliss, E. A. The toxic manifestations of sulfanilamide and its derivatives. J. A. M. A., 115:364-368, 1940b.

Lopatka, J. E.; Brewerton, C. N.; Brooks, D. S.; Cook, D. A.; Paton, D. M. The protective effects of methysergide, 6-hydroxydopamine and other agents on the toxicity of amphetamine, phetermine, MDA, PMA and STP in mice. Res. Commun. Chem. Pathol. Pharmacol., 14:677-687, 1976.

Lorimer, W. V.; Lilis, R.; Nicholson, W. J.; Anderson, H.; Fischbein, A.; Daum, S.; Rom, W.; Rice, C.; Selekoff, I. J. Clinical studies of styrene workers: initial findings. Environ. Health Perspect. 17:171-181, 1976.

Loser, E.; Kimmerle, G. Acute and subchronic toxicity of nemacur active ingredient. Pflazenshutz Nachr. 'Bayer' 24:69-113, 1971.

Loser, E.; Kimmerle, G. Acute and subchronic toxicity of Sencor active ingredient. Pflanzenschutz-Nachrichten 25:186-209, 1972.

Lotspeich, W. D.; Peters, R. A.; Wilson, T. H. The inhibition of aconitase by inhibitor fraction isolated from tissues poisoned with fluoracetate. Biochem. J. 51:20-25, 1952.

Loveman, A. Stomatitis venenata. Report of a case of sensitivity of mucous membranes and skin to oil of anise. Arch. Dermatol., 37:70-81, 1938.

Lucke, H. H.; Hodge, K. E.; Patt, N. L. Fatal liver damage after barium enemas containing tannic acid. Can. Med. Assoc. J., 89:1111-1114, 1963.

Luckens, M. M. Acute toxicity of combinations of maleic hydrazide diethanolamine and selected insecticides. Exp. Med. Surg. 27:245-255, 1969.

Ludwig, A. M.; Levine, J. Patterns of hallucinogenic drug abuse. J. A. M. A., 191:92-96, 1965.

Lukens, R. J. Chemistry of Fungicidal Action. Springer-Verlag, Berlin, 1971.

Lullmann-Rauch, R.; Reil, G. H. Chlorphetermine-induced lipidosislike ultrastructural alterations in lungs and adrenal glands of several species. Toxicol. Appl. Pharmacol., 30:408-421, 1974.

Lund, A. E.; Shanklance, D. L.; Chinn, C.; Yim, G. K. W. Similar cardiovascular toxicity of the pesticide chlordimeform and lidocaine. Toxicol. Appl. Pharmacol., 44:357-365, 1978.

Lunt, R. L. Delayed chloroform poisoning in obstetric practice. Br. Med. J., 1:489-490, 1953.

Lusky, L. M.; Braun, H. A.; Laug, E. P. The effect of BAL on experimental lead, tungsten, vanadium, uranium, copper and copper-arsenic poisoning. J. Ind. Hyg. Toxicol., 31:301-305, 1949.

Lutz, W. H. Personal communication. Warner-Chilcott Laboratories, Morris Plains, N. J, 1960.

Lutzenkirchen, A. Klinische Erfahrungen mit einem neuen Oberfachenanastheticum in der Dermatologie. Med. Klin., 47:618-620, 1952.

Lyman, E. D.; Potthoff, C. J.; Jacobi, H. P. Food poisoning due to nicotinic acid in meat, report of an outbreak. Nebraska Med. J., 42:243-245, 1957.

Lyman, F. L. Personal Communication. Ciba-Geigy Corporation, N. Y, 1972.

Lyman, F. L.; Furia, T. Toxicology of 2,4,4'-trichloro-2'-hydroxydiphenyl ether. Ind. Med. Surg., 38:64-71, 1969.

Lyman, F. L.; Schulze, J.; Ganz, C. R.; Stensby, P. S.; Keplinger, M. L.; Calandra, J. C. Long-term toxicity of four fluorescent whitening agents. Food Cosmet. Toxicol. 13:521-527, 1975.

Lynch, H. T.; Lemon, H. M.; Henn, M. J.; Ellingson, R. J.; Grissom, R. L. Vitamin D intoxicated patient with hypoparathyroidism. Arch. Intern. Med., 114:375-380, 1964.

Lynch, R. E.; Lee, G. R.; Kushner, J. P. Porphyria cutanea tarda associated with disinfectant misuse. Arch. Intern.

Med. *135*:549-552, 1975.

Lynn, K. L. Acute rhabdomyolysis and acute renal failure after intravenous self-administration of peanut oil. Br. Med. J. *4*:385-386, 1975.

Lynn, R. I.; Honig, C. L.; Jatlow, P. I.; Kliger, A. S. Resin hemoperfusion for treatment of ethchlorvynol overdose. Ann. Internal Med., *91*:549-553, 1979.

Lyon, J. P.; Jenkins, L. J., Jr.; Jones, R. A.; Coon, R. A.; Siegel, J. Repeated and continuous exposure of laboratory animals to acrolein. Toxicol. Appl. Pharmacol. *17*:726-732, 1970.

Lyr, V. H. Uber den Wirkungsmechanismus neuer Fungizide. Biol. Rundsch. *11*:156-166, 1973.

MacDonald, W. E.; Deichmann, W. B.; Radomski, J. L.; Austin, B. S. The chronic toxicity of octadecylamine in the rat - A supplemental report. Toxicol. Appl. Pharmacol., *4*:610-612, 1962.

MacEwen, J. D. Personal communication. Wright-Patterson Air Force Base, Ohio, 1969.

Machle, W. Gasoline intoxication. J. A. M. A., *117*:1965-1971, 1941.

Machle, W.; Scott, E. W. Effects of mononitroparaffins and related compounds on blood pressure and respiration of rabbits. Proc. Soc. Exp. Biol. Med., *53*:42-43, 1943.

Machle, W.; Scott, E. W.; Treon, J. F. The physiological response of animals to some simple mononitroparaffins and to certain derivatives of these compounds. J. Ind. Hyg. Toxicol., *22*:315-322, 1940.

Machle, W.; Scott, E. W.; Treon, J. F.; Heyroth, F. F.; Kitzmiller, K. V. The physiological response of animals to certain chlorinated mononitroparaffins. J. Ind. Hyg. Toxicol., *27*:95-102, 1945.

Macht, D. I. A pharmacological examination of benzaldehyde and mandelic acid. Arch. Int. Pharmacodyn. Ther., *27*:163-174, 1923.

Macht, D. I. Purgative effect of some aliphatic alcohols. Proc. Soc. Exp. Biol. Med., *30*:1272-1273, 1933.

Macht, D. I. The absorption of drugs and poisons through the skin and mucous membranes. Arch. Int. Pharmacodyn. Ther., *58*:1-26, 1938.

Macht, D. I.; Cook, H. M. Pharmacology and toxicology of monohydroxy-mercuri-di-iodo-resorcin-sulphonphthalein. J. Pharmacol. Exp. Ther., *43*:571-605, 1931.

Macht, D. I.; Harden, W. C. Toxicology and assay of methylene blue. Ann. Intern. Med., *7*:738-745, 1933.

MacIntosh, F. C. The toxicity of diphenyl and o-phenylphenol. Analyst, 70: 334-335, 1945.

Mackie, I. J. Methyl chloride intoxication. Med. J. Aust. *1*:203-205, 1961.

Maclean, C. W. Observations on coal for poisoning in pigs. Vet. Rec., 594-598, 1969.

Maclean, D.; Peters, T. J.; Brown, R. A. G.; McCathie, M.; Baines, G. F.; Robertson, P. G. C. Treatment of acute paracetamol poisoning. Lancet 2:849-852, 1968.

MacLean, R. E. G. Benactyzine hydrochloride (Suavitil) in out-patient psychiatric treatment; preliminary study. Med. J. Aust., *1*:67-70, 1957.

MacLeod, J. G.; Phillips, L. Hypersensitivity to colchicine. Ann. Rheum. Dis., *6*:224-229, 1947.

Macoul, K. L. Hepatitis attributed to sulfamethoxazole. N. Engl. J. Med. 275:39, 1966.

Magera, B. E.; Betlech, C. J.; Sweatt, A. P.; Derrick, C. W., Jr. Hydroxyzine intoxication in a 13-month-old child. Pediatrics, *67*:280-283, 1981.

Magos, L. A study of acrylonitrile poisoning in relation to methaemoglobin-CN complex formation. Br. J. Ind. Med., *19*:283-286, 1962.

Mahaffey, L. W. A contribution to the toxicology of sodium nitroprusside. II. Toxicity of sodium nitroprusside for guinea pigs. Aust. Chem. Inst. J. Proc., *9*:93-94, 1942.

Mahrer, R. A.; Maret, R. Agranulocytosis complicating PAS and streptomycin therapy. U. S. Armed Forces Med. J., *6*:1193-1198, 1955.

Main, A. R.; Braid, P. E. Hydrolysis of malathion by aliesterases in vitro and in vivo. Biochem. J., *84*:255-263, 1962.

Mallov, J. S. MBK neuropathy among spray painters. J. A. M. A. 235:1455-1457, 1976.

Malten, K. E. and Zielhaus, R. L. Industrial Toxicology and Dermatology in the Production and Processing of Plastics. Elsevier, New York, 1964.

Malten, K. E. Eczema caused by plastics (Eng. summary of original). Arch. Ind. Health, *18*:71, 1958.

Malten, K. E.; Bende, W. J. M. 2-Hydroxy-ethyl-methacrylate and di and tetraethylene glycol dimethacrylate: contact sensitizers in a photoprepolymer printing plate procedure. Contact Dermatitis, *5*:214-220, 1979.

Mant, A. K. VI. A cast of poisoning by oil of citronella. Toxic Episodes in Child., *2*:18, 1961.

Manufacturing Chemists' Association, Inc. Chemical safety data sheet, SD-23 (Calcium carbide). Washington, D. C., 1948b.

Manufacturing Chemists' Association, Inc. Chemical safety data sheet, SD-29 (Ethyl Ether). Washington, D. C., 1948c.

Manufacturing Chemists' Association, Inc. Chemical Safety Data Sheet, Chlorosulfonic Acid. Washington, D. C., 1949.

Manufacturing Chemists' Association, Inc. Chemical safety data sheet, SD-1 (Formaldehyde). Washington, D. C., 1950a.

Manufacturing Chemists' Association, Inc. Chemical safety data sheet, SD-6 (Paraformaldehyde). Washington, D. C., 1950b.

Manufacturing Chemists' Association, Inc. Chemical safety data sheet, SD-28 (Phosphoric anhydride). Washington, D. C., 1952a.

Manufacturing Chemists' Association, Inc. Chemical safety data sheet, SD-43 (Acetaldehyde). Washington, D. C., 1952b.

Manufacturing Chemists' Association, Inc. Chemical safety data sheet, SD-48 (Cresol). Washington, D. C., 1952c.

Manufacturing Chemists' Association, Inc. Chemical safety data sheet, SD-50 (Ethyl chloride). Washington, D. C., 1953.

Manzo, L.; Richelmi, P.; Sabbioni, E.; Pietra, R.; Guardia, L.; Bono, F. Poisoning by triphenyltin acetate. Report of two cases and determination of tin in blood and urine by neutron activation analysis. Clin. Toxicol., *18*:1343-1353, 1981.

Marcovitch, S.; Stanley, W. W. A study of antidotes for fluorine. J. Pharmacol. Exp. Ther., *74*:235-238, 1942.

Marcus, R.; Watt, J. Colonic ulceration in young rats fed degraded carrageenan. Lancet *1*:765-767, 1971.

Margo, C. E.; Trobe, J. D. Tarsorrhaphy from accidental instillation of cyanoacrylate adhesive in the eye. J. A. M. A., *247*:660-661, 1982.

Mark, L. C.; Kayden, H. J.; Steele, J. M.; Cooper, J. R.; Berlin, I.; Rovenstine, E. A.; Brodie, B. B. The physiological disposition and cardiac effects of procaine amide. J. Pharmacol. Exp. Ther., *102*:5-15, 1951.

Marley, E. Toxic psychosis with neurological features due to methylpentynal. Lancet, *2*:535, 1955.

Marrese, R. J. Personal communication. Diamond Alkali Co., Cleveland, 1961.

Marsh, C. D.; Clawson, A. B. Larkspur poisoning of livestock. U. S. Dept. Agr. Bull. No. 365, 1916.

Marsh, R. E. Tracking powders--a research report. Freedom of Information Request RIN-1096-78. U. S. EPA, Washington, D. C., 1979.

Marshall, E. K.; Bratton, A. C.; White, H. J.; Litchfield, J. T. Sulfanylylguanidine, a chemotherapeutic agent for intestinal infections. Bull J. Hop. Hosp. *67*:163-188, 1940.

Marshall, E. K.; Litchfield, J. T. Some aspects of the pharmacology of sulfapyridine. J. Pharmacol. Exp. Ther. *67*:454-475, 1939.

Marshall, W. A study of santonin xanthopsia. J. Pharmacol. Exp. Ther., *30*:361-388, 1927a.

Marshall, W. Santonin excretion and its relation to santonin xanthopsia. J. Pharmacol. Exp. Ther., *30*:389-405, 1927b.

Martens, S. Clinical trial of emylcamate, a new internuncial blocking tranquilizer. Q. J. Stud. Alcohol, *21*:223-232, 1960.

Martin, G.; Finberg, L. Propylene glycol: a potentially toxic vehicle in liquid dosage form. J. Pediatr., *77*:877-878, 1970.

Martin, G. J. Acridine antiseptics, a review. Medicine, *23*:79-103, 1944.

Martin, H.; Worthing, C. R. Pesticide Manual, 5th ed. British Crop Protection Council, Worcestershire, England, 1977.

Martin, M. M.; Rento, R. D. Exogenous iodide goiter in infants. J. Pediatr., 61:94-99, 1962.

Martin-Amat, G.; McMartin, K. E.; Hayreh, S. S.; Hayreh, M. D.; Tephly, T. R. Methanol poisoning: ocular toxicity produced by formate. Toxicol. Appl. Pharmacol. 45:201-208, 1978.

Martindale, W. The Extra Pharmacopoeia. 26th ed., The Pharmaceutical Press, London, 1972.

Mason, M. M.; Cate, C. C.; Baker, J. Toxicology and carcinogenesis of various chemicals used in the preparation of vaccines. Clin. Toxicol., 4:185-204, 1971b.

Massmann, W. Toxicological investigations in dimethylformamide. Br. J. Ind. Med., 13:51-59, 1956.

Mastromatteo, E. Recent occupational health experiences in Ontario. J. Occup. Med. 7:502-511, 1965.

Mather, G.; Riley, C. Idiosyncrasy to phenindione. Br. Med. J., 2:506-507, 1960.

Mather, L. E.; Tucker, G. T. Systemic availability of orally administered meperidine. Clin. Pharmacol. Ther., 20:535-540, 1976.

Mathew, H.; Proudfoot, A. T.; Brown, S. S.; Smith, A. C. A. Mandrax poisonings: Conservative management of 116 patients. Br. Med. J., 2:101-102, 1968.

Matokhnyuk, L. A. Change in the blood pressure and the electrocardiogram in carbamine pesticide poisoning. Farmakol. Toksikol. No. 7, p. 143-145, 1972.

Matsuda, M.; Makino, K. D-Penicillamine as an antidote to 8-hydroxyquinoline and alloxan. Nature, 192:261-262, 1961.

May, R. H.; Selymes, P.; Weekley, R. D.; Potts, A. M. Thioridazine therapy; results and complications. J. Nerv. Ment. Dis., 130:230-234, 1960.

Maynard, E. A.; Downs, W. L.; LeSher, M. F. Toxicity of some fluoride compounds. A. E. C. Q. Tech. Report UR-164:73-77, 1951.

Maynert, E. W.; Losin, L. The metabolism of butabarbital (butisol) in the dog. J. Pharmacol. Exp. Ther. 115:275-282, 1955.

Mays, D. L.; Born, G. S.; Christian, J. E.; Liska, B. J. Fate of ^{14}C-labeled maleic hydrazide in rats. J. Agric. Food Chem. 16:356-357, 1968.

Maytum, C. K.; Magath, T. B. Sensitivity to acacia. J. A. M. A., 99:2251-2252, 1932.

McAlister, W. H.; Anderson, M. S.; Bloomberg, G. R.; Margulis, A. R. Lethal effects of tannic acid in the barium enema. Report of three fatalities and experimental studies. Radiology, 80:765-773, 1963.

McAnalley, B. H.; Gardiner, T. H.; Garriott, J. C. Cyanide concentrations in blood after amygdalin (laetrile) administration in rats. Vet. Human Toxicol., 22:400-402, 1980.

McBay, A. J.; Katsas, G. C. Glutethimide poisoning; a report of four fatal cases. N. Engl. J. Med., 257:97-100, 1957.

McBirney, R. S. Trichloroethylene and dichloroethylene poisoning. (Reprinted from Arch. Ind. Hyg. Occupational Med., 10:130, 1954.) N. Y. Dept. Lab. Monthly Rev., 34:5-7, 1955.

McCall, J. D.; Rice, W. B. Pharmacology of pemoline. Can. J. Biochem. Physiol. 40:501-509, 1962.

McCarthy, D. D.; Chalmers, T. M. Hematological complications of phenylbutazone therapy: review of the literature and report of two cases. Can. Med. Assoc. J. 90:1061-1067, 1964.

McCarthy, W. H.; Keenan, R. L. Propoxyphene hydrochloride poisoning. Report of the first fatality. J. A. M. A., 187:460-461, 1964.

McCawley, A. Cortisone habituation - a clinical note. N. Engl. J. Med., 273:976, 1965.

McCollister, D. D.; Lockwood, D. T.; Rowe, V. K. Toxicologic information on 2,4,5-trichlorophenol. Toxicol. Appl. Pharmacol., 3:63-70, 1961.

McCollister, D. D.; Ogen, F.; Rowe, V. K. Toxicology of acrylamide. Toxicol. Appl. Pharmacol. 6:172-181, 1964.

McCord, C. P. Industrial poisoning from low concentrations of chlorine gas. J. A. M. A., 86:1687-1688, 1926b.

McCord, C. P.; Meek, S. F.; Harrold, G. C.; Heussner, C. E. The physiological properties of indium and its compounds. J. Ind. Hyg. Toxicol., 24:243-254, 1942.

McCord, C. P.; Meek, S. F.; Neal, T. A. Phenyl mercuric oleate; skin irritant properties. J. Ind. Hyg. Toxicol., 23:466, 1941.

McCormick, W. E. Personal communication. B. F. Goodrich Co., Akron, Ohio, 1955.

McCulloch, H.; Zeligman, I. Fixed drug eruption and epididymitis due to antipyrine. Arch. Dermatol., 64:198-199, 1951.

McCutcheon, J. W., Inc. Annual Report (Detergents and Emulsifiers). Morristown, N. J, 1965.

McDonald, J. C. Personal communication. Sterling Drug Inc., New York, 1973.

McGavack, T. H.; Boyd, L. J.; Terranova, R.; Lehr, D. Toxicity studies with the fungicide tetrachloro-p-benzoquinone (Spergon). J. Ind. Hyg. Toxicol., 25:98, 1943.

McGee, M. B. Caffeine poisoning in a 19-year-old female. J. Forensic Sci., 25:29-32, 1980.

McGuigan, H. The action of furfural. J. Pharmacol. Exp. Ther., 21:65-75, 1923.

McKinney, G. R.; Sisson, G. M. Acetylcysteine. In *Pharmacological and Biochemical Properties of Drug Substances*, Vol. 2, M. E. Goldberg (editor), Am. Pharm. Assoc., pp. 479-488, 1979.

McLain, L. A study of peyote. Clin. Toxicol., 1:81-85, 1968.

McLain, P. L. Hemolytic effects of ethyl and caprylic alcohol. J. Lab. Clin. Med., 25:531-534, 1940.

McLaughlin Gormley King Co. Brochure (MGK 11). Minneapolis, 1958a.

McLaughlin Gormley King Co. Brochure (MGK 326). Minneapolis, 1958b.

McLaughlin, A. I. G.; Kazantyis, G.; King, E.; Teare, D.; Porter, R. J.; Owen, R. Pulmonary fibrosis and encephalopathy associated with the inhalation of aluminum dust. Br. J. Ind. Med., 19:253-263, 1962.

McLaughlin, L. A., Jr.; Snyder, C. H. Encephalopathy in a child following exposure to malathion. Ochsner Clin. Rep., 2:37, 1956.

McLetchie, N. G. B.; Robertson, D. Chlorinated naphthalene poisoning. Br. Med. J., 1:691-692, 1942.

McMahon, R. E.; Sullivan, H. R. The metabolism of the herbicide diphenamid in rats. Biochem. Pharmacol. 14:1085-1092, 1965.

McMartin, K. E.; Ambre, J. J.; Tephly, T. R. Methanol poisoning in human subjects. Role for formic acid accumulation in the metabolic acidosis. Am. J. Med. 68:414-418, 1980.

McNally, W. D. A fatal case of cedar oil poisoning. Med. Record, 89:330-331, 1916.

McNally, W. D. Two deaths from the administration of barium salts. J. A. M. A., 84:1805-1807, 1925.

McNeil, J. R. Accidental ingestion of pemoline. Clin. Pediatr. 18:761-762, 1979.

McOmie, W. A. Comparative toxicity of methacrylonitrile and acrylonitrile. J. Ind. Hyg. Toxicol., 31:113-116, 1949.

McOmie, W. A.; Anderson, H. H. The toxicity of dicyclohexylamine nitrite. Univ. Calif. Publ. Pharmacol., 2:231-240, 1949.

McPhee, W. R. Acquired hemolytic anemia caused by ingestion of fava beans. Am. J. Clin. Pathol., 26:1287-1302, 1956.

McPherson, J. C. Suppression of food intake in the rat by tung oil. Can. J. Physiol. Pharmacol. 51:733-736, 1973.

McQuarrie, I.; Thompson, W. H.; Anderson, J. A. Effects of excessive ingestion of sodium and potassium salts on carbohydrate metabolism and blood pressure in diabetic children. J. Nutr., 11:77-101, 1936.

Mecca, S. B. Allantoin and the newer aluminum allantoinates. Proc. Sci. Sect. Toilet Goods Assoc., No. 31, 1959.

Medical Letter. Handbook of Antimicrobial Therapy. Medical Letter, Inc., New Rochelle, N. Y. Issue No. 340, 21 Jan, 1972.

Medved, I. L.; Ivanova, Z. V. Hygienic assessment of working conditions in the use of Eptam in agriculture. Gig. Sanit. 36:29-32, 1971.

Medved, I. L.; Vinogradova, V. Kh.; Olefir, A. I. Embryotoxic action of Eptam. Vrach. Delo, No. 5, p. 140-143, 1970.

Meek, D.; Gabriel, R.; Piercy, D. M. Fatal self-poisoning with Dettol. Postgrad. Med. J., 53:229-231, 1977.

Meigs, J. W.; Albim, J. J.; Kartin, B. L. Chloracne from an

unusual exposure to Arochlor. J. A. M. A., *154*:1417-1418, 1954.

Meikle, R. W. Metabolism of 4-dimethylamino-3,5-xylyl methylcarbamate (Mexacarbate, active ingredient of Zectran insecticide): A unified picture. Bull. Environ. Contam. Toxicol. *10*:29-36, 1973.

Mellanby, E. Diet and canine hysteria, experimental production by treated flour. Br. Med. J., *2*:885-887, 1946.

Mena, I.; Court, J.; Fuenzalida, S.; Papavasiliou, P. S.; Cotzias, G. C. Modification of chronic manganese poisoning. Treatment with L-dopa or 5-OH tryptophane. N. Engl. J. Med. *282*:5-10, 1970.

Mendoza, C. E.; Augustinsson, K. B.; Axenfors, B. Some properties of isolated pig plasma esterases sensitive to 3,5-di-tert-butylphenyl methylcarbamate (butacarb). Biochem. Pharmacol. *25*:701-705, 1976.

Menon, J. A. Tropical hazards associated with the use of pentachlorophenol. Br. Med. J., *1*:1156-1157, 1958.

Merck and Co., Inc. Ryania Insecticides. Rahway, N. J, 1947.

Merck and Co., Inc. The Merck Index of Chemicals and Drugs. Merck and Co., Inc., Rahway, N. J., 7th ed, 1960.

Merck and Co., Inc. The Merck Index, 9th ed. Merck and Co., Inc., Rahway, N. J, 1976.

Merck Sharp and Dohme. Brochure (Striatran). Rahway, N. J, 1961.

Merhoff, G. C.; Porter, J. M. Ergot intoxication: historical review and description of unusual clinical manifestations. Ann. Surg. *180*:773-779, 1974.

Merkatz, I. R. Parotid enlargement resulting from excessive ingestion of starch. N. Engl. J. Med., *265*:1304-1306, 1961.

Meyers, J. B. Acute pulmonary complications following inhalation of chromic acid mist. Arch. Ind. Health, *2*:742-747, 1950.

Michael, A. F.; Sutherland, J. M. Antibiotic toxicity in newborn and adult rats. Am. J. Dis. Child., *101*:442-446, 1961.

Michael, G. E.; Miday, R. K.; Bercz, J. P.; Miller, R. G.; Greathouse, D. G.; Kraemer, D. F.; Lucas, J. B. Chlorine dioxide water disinfection: a prospective epidemiology study. Arch. Environ. Health, *36*:20-27, 1981.

Michelson, A. L.; Frahm, C. J.; Katz, K. H. Delayed barbiturate intoxication. J. A. M. A. *155*:440-441, 1954.

Milby, T. H.; Epstein, W. L. Allergic contact sensitivity to malathion. Arch. Environ. Health, *9*:434-437, 1964.

Miller Chemical & Fertilizer Corp. Technical bulletin (Copper-zinc-chromate complex). Oct, 1958.

Miller, B. H.; Navone, R.; Ota, M. Irritation from residual bromides after methyl bromide fumigation. Public Health Rep. (U. S.) *76*:216-218, 1961.

Miller, G. E. Bismuth subnitrate poisoning with methemoglobinemia. Gastroenterology, *4*:430-434, 1945.

Miller, J.; Robinson, A.; Percy, A. K. Acute isoniazid poisoning in childhood. Am. J. Dis. Child., *134*:290-292, 1980.

Miller, J. P.; Crawford, L. E. M.; Sonders, R. C.; Cardinal, E. V. Distribution and excretion of 14C-cyclamate sodium in animals. Biochem. Biophys. Res. Commun., *25*:153-157, 1966.

Miller, J. W. Pathologic changes in animals exposed to a commercial chlorinated diphenyl. Public Health Rep., *59*:1085-1093, 1944.

Miller, R. Poisoning by "metal fuel" tablets (metacetaldehyde). Arch. Dis. Child., *3*:292-295, 1928.

Miller, V. L.; Klavano, P. A.; Csonka, E. Absorption, distribution and excretion of phenylmercuric acetate. Toxicol. Appl Pharmacol., *2*:344-352, 1960.

Minina, N. G.; Khomich, N. V. Toxicity of Matacil, Zectran, and Mesurol, insecticidal derivatives of carbamic acid. Zdravookhr. Beloruss. No. 12, pp. 47-49, 1967.

Mirkova, E. Effect of the herbicide Ramrod on the embryogenesis of white rats. Probl. Khig. *1*:57-60, 1975.

Mironenko, N. N. Safe levels of the herbicide linuron and dichlorophenylhydroxyurea in reservoir water. Gig. Sanit. No. 7, p. 46-49, 1975.

Mitchell, W. G. Antagonism of toxicity of vanadium by ethylene diamine-tetraacetic acid in mice. Proc. Soc. Exp. Biol. Med., *83*:346-348, 1953.

Miyamoto, J.; Mihara, K.; Hosokawa, S. Comparative metabolism of sumithion-m-methyl-^{14}C in several species of mammals in vivo. Nippon Noyaku Gakkaishi *1*:9-21, 1976.

Miyamoto, J.; Yamamoto, K.; Matsumoto, T. Metabolism of 3, 4-dimethylphenyl N-methylcarbamate in white rats. Agr. Biol. Chem. *33*:1060-1073, 1969.

Miyao, N.; Ishiguro, S.; Kono, I.; Yasuda, N. Toxicity of carbamate compounds. I. Subchronic toxicity of 3-methyl-5-isopropylphenyl N-methylcarbamate. Kagoshima Daigaku Nogakuba Gakujutsu Hokoku No. 22, pp. 131-144, 1972.

Mizyukova, I. G.; Petrun'kin, V. E.; Bakhishev, G. N.; Vasil'eva, Z. A.; Krivenchuk, V. E.; Kruchatov, G. V. Tezisy Dokl. Nauchn. Sess. Khim. Tekhnol. Org. Soidin Sery. Sernistykh Neftei, 13th, p. 60-61, 1974.

Mjolnerod, O. K.; Rasmussen, K.; Dommerud, S. A.; Gjeruldsen, S. T. Congenital connective-tissue defect probably due to D-penicillamine treatment in pregnancy. Lancet *1*:673-675, 1971.

Mobil Chemical Company. Technical Bulletin. Modown Herbicide. Richmond, Va, 1977.

Modell, J. H. Resuscitation after aspiration of chlorinated fresh water. J. A. M. A., *185*:651-655, 1963.

Moeschlin, S. Poisoning, Diagnosis and Treatment. 1st Amer. Ed., Grune and Stratton, New York, 1965.

Molitor, H.; Robinson, H. Some pharmacological and toxicological properties of sulfanilamide and benzylsulfanilamide. J. Pharmacol. Exp. Ther., *65*:405-423, 1939.

Monsanto Chemical Co. Technical data sheet (o-Nitrochlorobenzene). St. Louis, Mo, 1957a.

Monsanto Chemical Co. Technical data sheet (p-Nitrophenol). St. Louis, Mo, 1957b.

Monsanto Chemical Co. Technical bulletin 1-177 (Monsanto ACL). St. Louis, Mo, 1960.

Monsanto Chemical Company. Technical data sheet (Cyanuric acid). St. Louis, Mo, May 1962.

Monsanto Chemical Company. Technical data sheets (Ramrod and Lasso). St. Louis, Mo, Nov. 1969.

Montaldi, D. H.; Giambrone, J. P.; Courey, N. G.; Taefi, P. Podophyllin poisoning associated with the treatment of condyloma acuminatum: a case report. Am. J. Obstet. Gynecol. *119*:1130-1131, 1974.

Moolten, S. E.; Smith, I. B. Fatal nephritis in chronic phenacetin poisoning. Am. J. Med., *28*:127, 1960.

Moore, D. C.; Bridenbaugh, L. D. Oxygen: The antidote for systemic toxic reaction from local anesthetic drug. J. A. M. A., *174*:842-847, 1960.

Moorhead, P. D.; Willett, L. B.; Brumm, C. J.; Mercer, H. D. Pathology of experimentally induced polybrominated biphenyl toxicosis in pregnant heifers. J. Am. Vet. Med. Assoc. *170*:307-313, 1977.

Mora, P. T.; Young, B. G.; Shear, M. J. Reduction of toxicity of cationic macromolecules by complexing with anionic derivatives of synthetic polyglucoses. Nature *184*:431-432, 1959.

Morgan, A.; Lally, A. E.; Holmes, A. Some observations on the distribution of trace metals in chrysotile asbestos. Ann. Occup. Hyg., *16*:231-240, 1973.

Morgenstern, A. L. Toxic psychosis due to iodoform. Am. J. Psychiatr. *119*:1180-1181, 1963.

Moriarty, J. D.; Mebane, J. C. Clinical uses of Deanol (Deaner); a new type of psychotropic drug. Am. J. Psychiatry, *115*:941-942, 1959.

Morley, D.; Wynne, N. A. Acute primidone poisoning in a child. Br. Med. J., *1*:90, 1957.

Morozov, G. N. On acute dichloroethane poisoning. Pharmacol. Toxicol. *21*:80-83, 1958.

Morrice, G., Jr.; Havener, W. H.; Kapetansky, F. Vitamin A intoxication as a cause of pseudotremor cerebri. J. A. M. A., *173*:1802-1805, 1960.

Morris, G. E. Dermatitis from water glass. Arch. Ind. Hyg. Occup. Med., *7*:411-412, 1953.

Morrison, R. W.; Bliss, A. R., Jr. The strychnine-brucine ratio of nux vomica and the relative potency of the alkaloids. J. Am. Pharm. Assoc., Sci. Ed., *21*:648-658 and 753-760, 1932.

Morse, D. L.; Boros, L.; Findley, P. A. More on cyanide poisoning from laetrile. N. Engl. J. Med., *301*:892, 1979.

Morton, D. M.; Hoffman, D. G. Metabolism of a new herbicide, tebuthiuron 1-5-(1,1-dimethylethyl)-1,3,4-thiadiazol-2-yl-1, 3-dimethylurea, in mouse, rat, rabbit, dog, duck, and fish. J. Toxicol. Environ. Health 1:757-768, 1976.

Morton, K. C. Peritoneal dialysis in acute poisoning. Successful treatment of a 15-month old child ingesting 30 times the adult dose of Achrocidin. Clin. Pediatr., 5:565-566, 1966.

Moskowitz, R. L. Talc pneumoconiosis: a treated case. Chest, 58:37-41, 1970.

Moskowitz, S.; Shapiro, H. Fatal exposure to methylene chloride vapor. Arch. Ind. Hyg. Occup. Med., 6:116-123, 1952.

Mosora, N. Akute todliche Vergiftung mit Kaliumbichromat. Arch. Toxikol., 20:334-336, 1965.

Motomatsu, K.; Adachi, H.; Uno, T. 2 Infant deaths after inhaling baby powder. Chest, 75:448-450, 1979.

Muenscher, W. C. Poisonous plants of the United States. The Macmillan Co., New York, 1951.

Muhlendahl, K. E. v.; Krienke, E. G. Vergiftungen mit Fenfluramin (Ponderax) bei Kindern. Mschr. Kinderheik., 126:631-635, 1978z.

Muhlendahl, K. E. v.; Oberdisse, U.; Krienke, E. G. Local injuries by accidental ingestion of corrosive substances by children. Arch. Toxicol., 39:299-324, 1978y.

Mun, A. M.; Barden, E. S.; Wilson, J. M.; Hogan, J. M. Teratogenic effects in early chick embryos of solanine and glycoalkaloids from potatoes infected with late-blight, Phytophthora infestans. Teratology 11:73-77, 1975.

Munch, J. C. Aliphatic alcohols and alkyl ester: narcotic and lethal potencies to tadpoles and to rabbits. IMS, 41:31-33, 1972.

Murai, Y.; Kuroiwa, Y. Peripheral neuropathy in chlorobiphenyl poisoning. Neurology, 21:1173-1176, 1971.

Murphree, H. B.; Jenney, E. H.; Pfeiffer, C. C. 2-Dimethyleminoethanol as a central nervous system stimulant; one aspect of the pharmacology of reserpine. (Braceland, F. J.), Association for Research in Nervous and Mental Diseases, Proceedings, p. 204-217, Vol. 37, The Williams & Wilkins Co., Baltimore, 1959.

Murphy, J. E. Drug profile. Tanderil eye ointment. J. Int. Med. Res. 1:136-140, 1973.

Murphy, S. D. Malathion inhibition of esterases as a determinant of malathion toxicity. J. Pharmacol. Exp. Ther., 156:352-365, 1967.

Murphy, S. D.; Anderson, R. L.; DuBois, K. P. Potentiation of toxicity of malathion by tri-ortho-tolyl phosphate. Proc. Soc. Exp. Biol. Med., 100:483-487, 1959.

Murphy, S. D.; DuBois, K. P. Toxicity and anticholinesterase activity of tributyl phosphorotrithioate (DEF). Arch. Indust. Health, 20:161-166, 1959.

Murphy, S. D.; Klingshirn, D. A.; Ulrich, C. E. Respiratory response of guinea pigs during acrolein inhalation and its modification by drugs. J. Pharmacol. Exp. Ther. 141:79-83, 1963.

Musclow, C. E.; Awen, C. F. Glue sniffing: report of a fatal case. Can. Med. Assoc. J., 104:315-319, 1971.

Mushett, C. W.; Seeler, A. O. Hypoprothrombinemia resulting from the administration of sulfaquinoxaline. J. Pharmacol. Exp. Ther., 91:84-91, 1947.

Myatt, G. L.; Ecobichon, D. J.; Greenhalgh, R. Fenitrooxon and S-methyl fenitrothion: acute toxicity and hydrolysis in mammals. Environ. Res. 10:407-414, 1975.

Myerson, R. M. Meningitis during gold therapy. J. A. M. A., 143:1336-1337, 1950.

Nadler, J. E.; Green, H.; Rosenbaum, A. Intravenous injection of methylene blue in man with reference to its toxic symptoms and effect on electrocardiogram. Am. J. Med. Sci., 188:15-21, 1934.

National Academy of Science. CBCC screening file. National Research Council, Washington, D. C., Date Unknown.

National Academy of Science. Nickel. Committee on Medical and Biological Effects of Environmental Pollutants. Washington, D. C., 1975.

National Cancer Institute. Bioassay of 4-amino-2-nitrophenol for possible carcinogenicity. U. S. DHEW, Public Health Service. Technical Report Series No. 94, Publication No. 78-1344, 1978a.

National Cancer Institute, National Institutes of Health. Bioassay of dibromochloropropane for possible carcinogenicity. Technical Report Series No. 28. DHEW Publication No. 78-828, 1978b.

National Cancer Institute. Bioassay of sulfallate for possible carcinogenicity. U. S. DHEW, Public Health Service. Technical Report Series No. 115, Publication No. 78-1370, 1978c.

National Cancer Institute. Bioassay of chlorothalonil for possible carcinogenicity. U. S. DHEW, Public Health Service, Technical Report Series No. 41, Publication No. 78-841, 1978d.

National Cancer Institute. Bioassay of formulated fenaminosulf for possible carcinogenicity. U. S. DHEW, Public Health Service. Technical Report Series No. 101, Publication No. 78-1351, 1978e.

National Cancer Institute. Bioassay of trifluralin for possible carcinogenicity. U. S. DHEW, Public Health Service. Technical Report Series No. 34, Publication No. 78-834, 1978f.

National Cancer Institute. Bioassay of nitrofen for possible carcinogenicity. U. S. DHEW, Public Health Service. Technical Report Series No. 26, Publication No. 78-826, 1978g.

National Cancer Institute. Bioassay of picloram for possible carcinogenicity. U. S. DHEW, Public Health Service, Technical Report Series No. 23, Publication No. 78-823, 1978h.

National Cancer Institute. Bioassay of 1, 2-Dibromoethane for possible carcinogenicity. U. S. DHEW, Public Health Service. Technical Report Series No. 86, Publication No. 78-1336, 1978j.

National Cancer Institute. Bioassay of 1,1-dichloroethane for possible carcinogenicity. U. S. DHEW, Public Health Service. Technical Report Series No. 66, Publication No. 78-1316, 1978k.

National Cancer Institute. Bioassay of 1,2-dichloroethane for possible carcinogenicity. U. S. DHEW, Public Health Service. Technical Report Series No. 55, Publication No. 78-1361, 1978l.

National Cancer Institute. Bioassay of 1,1,2-trichloroethane for possible carcinogenicity. U. S. DHEW, Public Health Service. Technical Report Series No. 74, Publication No. 78-1324, 1978m.

National Cancer Institute. Bioassay of 1,4-dioxane for possible carcinogenicity. U. S. DHEW, Public Health Service, Technical Report Series No. 80, Publication No. 78-1330, 1978n.

National Cancer Institute. Bioassay of tris(2,3-dibromopropyl)phosphate for possible carcinogenicity. U. S. DHEW, Public Health Service, Technical Report Series No. 76, Publication No. 78-1326, 1978s.

National Cancer Institute. Bioassay of tetrachlorvinfos for possible carcinogenicity. U. S. DHEW, Public Health Service. Technical Report Series No. 33, Publication No. 78-833, 1978o.

National Cancer Institute. Bioassay of phanazopyridine hydrochloride for possible carcinogenicity. U. S. DHEW, Public Health Service. Technical Report Series No. 99, Publication No. 78-1349, 1978q.

National Cancer Institute. Bioassay of butylated hydroxytoluene (BHT) for possible carcinogenicity. U. S. DHEW, Public Health Service, Technical Report Series No. 150 Publication no. 79-1706, 1979a.

National Cancer Institute. Asbestos: an information resource. U. S. DHEW, Public Health Service. Publication No. 78-1681, May, 1978p.

National Institute for Occupational Safety and Health. Ethylene dichloride. U. S. DHEW, Public Health Service. Current Intelligence Bulletin 25, Publication No. 78-149, 1978b.

National Institute for Occupational Safety and Health. Special occupational hazard review with control recommendations for ethylene thiourea. U. S. DHEW, Public Health Service Center for Disease Control, DHEW (NIOSH) Publication No. 79-109, 1978a.

National Research Council Coordinating Committee for Scientific and Technical Assessments of Environmental Pollutants. Kepone/Mirex/Hexachlorocyclopentadiene: an environmental assessment. National Academy of Sciences, Washington, D. C., 1978.

National Safety Council. Data sheet d-207 (Chlorine). Chicago, 1953.

National Safety Council. Data sheet d-351, d-chem. 28 (Picric acid). Chicago, Date Unknown a.

National Safety Council. Data sheet d-chem. 36 (Cresols). Chicago, Date Unknown b.

National Safety Council. Data sheet d-chem. 7 (Ethyl Ether (Diethyl Oxide)). Chicago, Date Unknown c.

National Safety Council. Data sheet d-241 d-chem. 19 (Lime). Chicago, Date Unknown d.

Naugatuck Chemical, Div. U. S. Rubber Co. Report (Spergon toxicology). Naugatuck, Conn, 1951a.

Naugatuck Chemical, Div. U. S. Rubber Co. Report (Toxicology of aramite). Naugatuck, Conn, 1951b.

Naugatuck Chemical, Div. U. S. Rubber Co. Bethany information sheet #44 (Phygon animal toxicity report). Naugatuck, Conn, 1953.

Naugatuck Chemical, Div. U. S. Rubber Co. Brochure (Maleic hydrazide). Naugatuck, Conn, 1954.

Naugatuck Chemical, Div. U. S. Rubber Co. Brochure (Technical summary on anacet). Naugatuck, Conn, 1957.

Naugatuck Chemical, Div. U. S. Rubber Co. Technical summary (Falone). Naugatuck, Conn, 1959.

Neering, H.; Vitanyi, B. E. J.; Malten, K. E.; Van Ketel, W. G.; Van Dijk, E. Allergens in sesame oil contact dermatitis. Acta Derm. Venereol. (Stockholm) 55:31-34, 1975.

Nekrasova, A. S.; Knysh, V. S. Change in the content of glycogen in the liver and kidneys of rabbits during long-term administration of small carbine doses. Tr. Nauch. -Issled. Inst. Kraev. Patol., Alma-Ata, No. 22, p. 83-84, 1971.

Nekrasova, A. S.; Razoznaeva, O. N. Pathomorphology of the organs of guinea pigs and rabbits during peroral administration of carbine. Tr. Nauch. -Issled. Inst. Kraev. Patol., Alma-Ata, No. 22, p. 77-83, 1971.

Nelson, D. A. Accidental poisoning by Veratrum japonicum. J. A. M. A., 156:33-35, 1954.

Nelson, D. L. Personal communication. Chemagro Corp., Kansas City, Mo, 1969.

Nelson, J. O.; Kearney, P. C.; Plimmer, J. R.; Menger, R. E. Metabolism of trifluralin, profluralin, and fluchloralin by rat liver microsomes. Pestic. Biochem. Physiol. 7:73-82, 1977.

Newcomb, P. B.; Deane, E. W. Thiourea causing granulopenia and thrombopenia. Lancet, 1:179, 1944.

Newman, A. J. Intoxication with Veratrum viride. J. Pediatr., 40:233-234, 1952.

Newton, G. W.; Schmidt, E. S.; Lewis, J. P.; Conn, E.; Lawrence, R. Amygdalin toxicity studies in rats predict chronic cyanide poisoning in humans. West. J. Med., 134:97-103, 1981.

Newton, J. F.; Kuo, C. H.; Gemborys, M. W.; Mudge, G. H.; Hook, J. B. Nephrotoxicity of p-aminophenol, a metabolite of acetaminophen in the Fischer 344 rat. Toxicol. Appl. Pharmacol. 65:336-344, 1982.

Nezefi, T. A. Morphological changes in white rat organs under the influences of some herbicides. (as cited in Chem. Abs. 81:164295y) Zdravookhr. Turkm. 18:24-25, 1974.

Niagara Chemical Division, Food Machinery and Chemical Corp. Tandex data sheet. Middleport, N. Y, 1969.

Niagara Chemical Division, Food Machinery and Chemical Corp. Brochure (Toxicity and Safe Handling of Furadan Insecticide). Middleport, N. Y, 1970.

Niagara Chemical, Division, Food Machinery and Chemical Corp. Data sheet (Ethion). Middleport, N. Y., June, 1959a.

Niagara Chemical, Division, Food Machinery and Chemical Corp. Data sheet (Phostex). Middleport, N. Y, 1959b.

Niagara Chemical, Division, Food Machinery and Chemical Corp. Data sheet (Tedion). Middleport, N. Y., June, 1959c.

Niagara Chemical, Division, Food Machinery and Chemical Corp. Data sheet (Thiodan). Middleport, N. Y., June, 1959d.

Nickolls, L. C.; Teare, D. Poisoning by cantharidin. Br. Med. J., 2:1384-1386, 1954.

Nierenberg, D. W.; Glazener, F. S. Aminophylline-induced exfoliative dermatitis: etiology and implications. West. J. Med., 137:328-331, 1982.

NIOSH. Criteria for a recommended standard . . . occupational exposure to organotin compounds. U. S. DHEW, Public Health Service, Publication No. 77-115, 1976.

NIOSH. Criteria for a recommended standard. . . occupational exposure to glycidyl ethers. DHEW (NIOSH) Publication No. 78-166, 1978.

Nishie, K. Pharmacology of solanine. Toxicol. Appl. Pharmacol. 19:81-92, 1971.

Nishizumi, M. Light and electron microscope study of chlorobiphenyl poisoning. Arch. Environ. Health, 21:620-632, 1970.

Nitter-Hauge, S. Poisoning with ethylene glycol monomethyl ether. Acta Med. Scand. 188:277-280, 1970.

Nodine, J. H.; Modi, K. N.; Rhodes, M.; Paz-Martinez, V.; Ibarra, L.; Santos, R. J. Pharmacodynamics and pharmacokinetics of isosorbide in man. Clin. Pharmacol. Therap., 14:196-203, 1973.

Nomeir, A. A.; Kato, S.; Mathews, H. B. The metabolism and disposition of tris (1,3-dichloro-2-propyl)phosphate (Fyrol FR-2) in the rat. Toxicol. Appl. Pharmacol., 57:401-413, 1981.

Nor-Am Agricultural Products, Inc. Technical Information Sheet (Carzol SP). Chicago, Illinois, 1977.

NOR-AM Agricultural Products, Inc. Technical Information Sheet (Betanex). Chicago, Ill, date unknown.

Norris, V. H.; Weiss, S. The pharmacological and therapeutic properties of alpha-lobelin, a comparison of its action on the respiratory center with that of other respiratory stimulants. J. Pharmacol. Exptl. Therap., 31:43-63, 1927.

Norseth, T. The carcinogenicity of chromium. Environ. Health Perspect. 40:121-130, 1981.

Nuttall, J. B.; Kelley, R. J.; Smith, B. S.; Whiteside, C. K., Jr. In flight toxic reactions resulting from fluorocarbon resin pyrolysis. Aerosp. Med., 35:676-683, 1964.

Nye, D. E.; Hurst, H. E.; Dorough, H. W. Fate of Croneton (2-ethylthiomethylphenyl N-methylcarbamate) in rats. J. Agric. Food Chem. 24:371-377, 1976.

O'Brien, D. Anuria due to bismuth thioglycollate. Am. J. Dis. Child., 97:384-386, 1959.

O'Neill, P. J.; Rahwan, R. G. Protection against acute toxicity of acetaldehyde in mice. Res. Comm. Chem. Pathol. Pharmacol. 13:125-128, 1976.

Ockner, R. K.; Schmid, R. Acquired porphyria in man and rat due to hexachlorobenzene intoxication. Nature, 189:499, 1961.

Ohkawa, H.; Yoshihara, R.; Kohara, T.; Miyamoto, J. Metabolism of m-tolyl N-methylcarbamate (Tsumacide) in rats, houseflies and bean plants. Agr. Biol. Chem. 38:1035-1044, 1974.

Oishi, S.; Hiraga, K. Testicular atrophy induced by phthalic acid esters: Effect on testosterone and zinc concentrations. Toxicol. Appl. Pharmacol., 53:35-41, 1980.

Okinaka, A. J.; Doull, J.; Coon, J. M.; DuBois, K. P. Studies on the toxicity and pharmacological actions of bis (dimethylamido) fluorophosphate (BFP). J. Pharmacol. Exp. Ther., 112:231-245, 1954.

Older, J. J.; Hatcher, R. L. Food poisoning caused by carbophenothion. J. A. M. A., 209:1328-1330, 1969.

Olefir, A. I. Effect of acute poisoning with carbamine pesticides on immunological reactivity. Vrach Delo, No. 4, p. 138-141, 1973.

Olmstead, E. V. Pathological changes in ethylene dibromide poisoning. A. M. A. Arch. Ind. Health 21:525-529, 1960.

Olney, V. W. Geigy 444. Proc. 15th Western Weed Control Conf., p. 79-80, 1956.

Olsnes, S.; Refsnes, K.; Pihl, A. Mechanism of action of the toxic lectins abrin and ricin. Nature 249:627-631, 1974.

Olsnes, S.; Sandvig, K.; Refsnes, K.; Pihl, A. Rates of different steps involved in the inhibition of protein synthesis by the toxic lectins abrin and ricin. J. Biol. Chem. 257:3985-3992, 1976.

Olson, W. M.; Habermann, R. T.; Weisberger, E. K.; Ward, J. M.; Weisberger, J. H. Induction of stomach cancer in rats and mice by halogenated aliphatic fumigants. J. Natl. Cancer Inst. 51:1993-1995, 1973.

Ondreicka, R.; Ginter, E.; Kortus, J. Chronic toxicity of aluminum in rats and mice and its effects on phosphorus metabolism. Br. J. Ind. Med., 23:305-312, 1966.

Onyx Oil and Chemical Co. Technical data sheet (BTC 50%). Jersey City, N. J, 1952a.

Onyx Oil and Chemical Co. Personal communication. Jersey City, N. J, 1952b.

Oonnithan, E. S.; Casida, J. E. Oxidation of methyl- and dimethylcarbamate insecticide chemicals by microsomal enzymes and anticholinesterase activity of the metabolites. J. Agric. Food Chem. 16:28-44, 1968.

Opdyke, D. L. J. Triethylene glycol. Food Cosmet. Toxicol., 17(Suppl.):913-916, 1979.

Oro, L.; Wretlind, A. Pharmacological effects of fatty acids, triolein and cottonseed oil. Acta Pharmacol. Toxicol., 18:141-152, 1961.

Orris, L. Cashew nut dermatitis. N. Y. State J. Med., 58:2799, 1958.

Ortega, J. A.; Creek, J. E. Acute cyanide poisoning following administration of laetrile enemas. J. Pediatr., 93:1059-1067, 1978.

Orten, J. M.; Kuyper, A. A.; Smith, A. H. Studies on the toxicity of propylgallate and of antioxidant mixtures containing propylgallate. Food Technol. 2:308-316, 1948.

Orusev, T.; Popovski, P. Symptoms of chronic occupational acrylonitrile poisoning. God. Zb. Med. Fak. Skopji 19:187-192, 1973.

Oser, B. L.; Oser, M. 2-(p-tert-Butylphenoxy) isopropyl-2-chloroethyl sulfite (Aramite). I. Acute, subacute and chronic oral toxicity. Toxicol. Appl. Pharmacol., 2:441-457, 1960.

Oser, B. L.; Oser, M. 2-(p-tert-Butylphenoxy) isopropyl-2-chloroethyl sulfite (Aramite). II. Carcinogenicity. Toxicol. Appl. Pharmacol., 4:70-88, 1962.

OSHA. Occupational health and environmental control. Air contaminants. Federal Register 39:23540, June 27, 1974.

OSHA. Occupational exposure to 1, 2-dibromo-3-chloropropane (DBCP). Federal Register 43:11514-11533, March 17, 1978.

OSHA. Occupational exposure to acrylonitrile (vinyl chloride). Federal Register 43:2608-2621, Jan. 17, 1978.

Osol, A.; Farrar, G. E., Jr. The Dispensatory of the United States of America. 25th Ed., J. B. Lippincott, Co., Philadelphia, 1955.

Osol, A.; Pratt, R. The United States Dispensatory. 27th ed., J. B. Lippincott Co., Philadelphia, 1973.

Ostern, S.; Dodson, W. H. Hypertension following Ornade ingestion. J. A. M. A., 194:472, 1965.

Ostfeld, A.; Smith, C. M.; Stotsky, B. A. The systemic use of procaine in the treatment of the elderly: A review. J. Am. Geriat. Soc., 25:1-19, 1977.

Oswald, I.; Thacore, V. A. Amphetamine and phenmetrazine addiction. Br. Med. J., 2:427-431, 1963.

Otenasek, F. J.; Fairman, D. Chemical meningitis following use of tyrothyricin. Arch. Otolaryngol, 47:21-28, 1948.

Owen, G.; Smith, T. H. F.; Agersborg, H. P. K., Jr. Toxicity of some benzodiazepine compounds with CNS activity. Toxicol. Appl. Pharmacol., 16:556-570, 1970.

Owens, R. Metabolism of fungicides and related compounds. Ann. N. Y. Acad. Sci. 160:114-131, 1969.

Owens, R. G.; Rubinstein, J. H. Chemistry of the fungicidal action of tetramethylthiuram disulfide (thiram) and ferbam. Contrib. Boyce Thompson Inst. 22:241-258, 1964.

P'an, S. Y.; Gardocki, J. F.; Reilly, J. C. Pharmacological properties of two new antihistaminics of prolonged action. J. Am. Pharm. Assoc. Sci. Ed., 43:653-656, 1954.

Paar, D.; Heimsoth, V.; Werner, M.; Bock, K. D. Verbrauchskoagulopathie als Ursache hamorrhagischer Diathese bei akuter Essigsaure-Intoxikation. Dtsch. Med. Wochenschr. 93:206-209, 1968.

Pachman, D. J. Accidental heparin poisoning in an infant. Am. J. Dis. Child., 110:210-212, 1965.

Page, I. H.; Corcoran, A. C.; Dustan, H. P.; Koppanyi, T. Cardiovascular actions of sodium nitroprusside in animals and hypertensive patients. Circulation, 11:188-198, 1955.

Paget, G. E.; Walpole, A. L. Some cytological effects of griseofulvin. Nature 82:1320, 1958.

Paine, D. Fetal hepatic necrosis associated with aminosalicylic acid. J. A. M. A., 167:285-289, 1958.

Pallade, S.; London, M.; Roventa, A.; Popovici, C. Toxicity of a largely used agricultural fertilizer: superphosphate. Med. lavoro, 51:49-58, 1960; English Abstract from Exerpta Medica, Sect. II, 13:1370, 1960.

Palmer, J. S. Toxicity of methyluracil and substituted urea and phenol compounds to sheep. J. Am. Vet. Med. Assoc., 145:787-789, 1964A.

Palmer, J. S. Toxicity of carbamate, triazine, dichloropropionanilide, and diallylacetamide compounds to sheep. J. Am. Vet. Med. Assoc. 145:917-920, 1964b.

Palmer, J. S.; Radeleff, R. D. The toxicologic effects of certain fungicides and herbicides on sheep and cattle. Ann. N. Y. Acad. Sci., 111: Art. 2, p. 729-736, 1964.

Parish, R. F.; Frick, C.; Richards, A. B.; Forney, R. B. Human caffeine fatality. Toxicol. Appl. Pharmacol. 7:494, 1965.

Park, J.; Darrien, I.; Prescott, L. F. Pharmacokinetic studies and severe intoxication with 2,4-D and mecoprop. Proc. Eur. Soc. Toxicol., 18:154-155, 1977.

Parke, D. V. Biochemistry of the barbiturates. In Acute Barbiturate Poisoning, edited by H. Matthew. Excerpta Medica, Amsterdam, 1971.

Parker, G. F., Jr.; Chattin, W. R. A case of malathion intoxication in a ten-year-old girl. J. Indiana State Med. Assoc., 48:491-492, 1955.

Parkes, W. E.; Neill, D. W. Acute nitrobenzene poisoning with transient aminoaciduria. Br. Med. J. 1:653-655, 1953.

Pascale, L. R.; Waldstein, S. S.; Engbring, G.; Dubin, A.; Szanto, P. B. Chromium intoxication with special reference to hepatic injury. J. A. M. A., 149:1385-1389, 1952.

Pathy, G. V.; Rosen, M. Prolonged block with recovery after extradural analgesia for labour. Br. J. Anaesth., 47:520-522, 1975.

Patty, F. A. Industrial Hygiene and Toxicology, Vol. II. Interscience Publishers, New York, 1962.

Paul, A. H. Poisoning by organo-phosphorus insecticide (malathion): Report of case. N. Z. Med. J., 59:346, 1960.

Paul, H.; McCay, C. M. The utilization of fats by herbivora. Arch. Biochem. Biophys., 1:247-253, 1942.

Paul, M. Gastric obstruction from swallowing a corrosive poison. Lancet 2:1064-1066, 1951.

Pauling, L. Vitamin C and the Common Cold. W. H. Freeman and Co., San Francisco, 1970.

Paull, A. M. Toxic reactions to iodine. R. I. Med. J., 42:96-99, 1959.

Paulson, G. W.; Waylonis, G. W. Polyneuropathy due to n-hexane. Arch. Intern. Med. 136:880-882, 1976.

Payne, R. B. Nutmeg intoxication. N. Engl. J. Med., 269:36-38, 1963.

Paynter, O. E.; Weir, R. J., Jr. Chronic toxicity of santomerse no. 3 from Olefin (dodecyl benzene sodium sulfonate). Toxicol. Appl. Pharmacol., 2:641, 1960.

Pearson, S. C.; MacKenzie, R. J. Intestinal obstruction due to bishydroxycoumarin poisoning. J. A. M. A., 167:455-456, 1958.

Pease, C. N. Focal retardation and arrestment of growth of bones due to vitamin A intoxication. J. A. M. A., 182:980-985, 1962.

Peck, H. M.; McKinney, S. E.; Tytell, A.; Byham, B. B. Toxicologic evaluation of gibberellic acid. Science, 126:1064, 1957.

Peele, J. D., Jr.; Oswald, E. O. Metabolism of naturally occurring propenylbenzene derivatives III. Allylbenzene, propenyl benzene, and related metabolic products. Biochim. Biophys. Acta 497:598-607, 1977.

Pegum, J. S.; Medhurst, F. A. Contact dermatitis from penetration of rubber gloves by acrylic monomer. Br. Med. J., 2:141-143, 1971.

Pelikan, Z. Effects of bis(tri-n-butyltin)oxide on the eyes of rabbits. Br. J. Ind. Med., 26:165-170, 1969.

Pelikan, Z.; Cerny, E. The toxic effects of some di- and mono-n-octyl tin compounds in white mice. Arch. Toxikol., 26:196-202, 1970a.

Pelikan, Z.; Cerny, E. Toxic effects of some mono-n-butyl tin compounds on white mice. Arch. Toxikol., 27:79-84, 1970b.

Pelner, L. Anaphylaxis to injection of nicotinic acid (niacin); successful treatment with epinephrine. Ann. Intern. Med.,

26:290-294, 1947.

Penneys, N. S.; Israel, R. M.; Indgin, S. M. Contact dermatitis due to 1-chloroacetophenone and Chemical Mace. N. Engl. J. Med., *281*:413-415, 1969.

Pennsylvania Salt Manufacturing Co. Brochure. Wyndmoor, Penna, 1955.

Peoples, S. A. The anesthetic action of brominated propane derivatives. J. Pharmacol. Exp. Ther., *51*:129-130, 1934.

Periquet, A.; Derache, R. Influence D'un Regime Alimentaire Hypoproteique sur la Toxicite Aigue D'un Pesticide: Le Nabame. Ann. Nutr. Aliment. *30*:29-44, 1976.

Perkins, H. A. Bromide intoxication. Analysis of cases from a general hospital. Arch. Intern. Med., *85*:783-794, 1950.

Perlman, H. H. Undecylenic acid given orally in psoriasis and neurodermatitis; a preliminary report. J. A. M. A., *139*:444-447, 1949.

Perlman, H. H.; Milberg, I. L. Peroral administration of undecylenic acid in psoriasis. J. A. M. A., *140*:865-868, 1949.

Perone, V. B.; Moffitt, A. E.; Possick, P. A.; Key, M. M.; Danzinger, S. J.; Gellin, G. A. The chromium, cobalt, and nickel contents of American cement and their relationship to cement dermatitis. Am. Indust. Hyg. Assoc. J., *35*:301-306, 1974.

Pestova, A. G. Toxicity of diptal and avadex. Gig. Toksikol. Pestits. Klin. Otravtenii, No. 4, p. 166-169, 1966.

Peters, J. M. Factors affecting caffeine toxicity. J. Clin. Pharmacol. *1*:131-141, 1967.

Peters, J. W.; Cook, R. M. Effects of atrazine on reproduction in rats. Bull. Environ. Contam. Toxicol. *9*:301-304, 1973.

Peters, L. Oral toxicity of a new miticide, di-(p-chlorophenyl) methyl carbinol. Proc. Soc. Exp. Biol. Med., *72*:304-305, 1949.

Peterson, C. M.; Tsairis, P.; Ohnishi, A.; Lu, Y. S.; Grady, R.; Cerami, A.; Dyck, P. J. Sodium cyanate induced polyneuropathy in patients with sickle-cell disease. Ann. Intern. Med., *81*:152-158, 1974.

Peterson, H. de C. Acquired methemoglobinemia in an infant due to benzocaine suppository. N. Engl. J. Med., *263*:454, 1960.

Petkau, A.; Hoogstraten, J. Chronic toxicity of polyphenyl mixtures. Am. Ind. Hyg. Assoc. J., *26*:380-387, 1965.

Petlach, S. The toxicology of valerian. Biol. Abst. 8:110, 1934.

Petrova-Vergievo, T.; Ivanova-Tchemishanska, L. Assessment of the teratogenic activity of dithiocarbamate fungicides. Food Cosmet. Toxicol. *11*:239-244, 1973.

Pewny, R. Fatal poisoning with pyrogallol. J. A. M. A., *85*:555, 1925.

Pfeiffer, C.; Arnove, I. Glycerol toxicity and hemoglobinuria in relation to vitamin C. Proc. Soc. Exp. Biol. Med., *37*:467-469, 1937.

Philbrick, D. J.; Hill, D. C.; Alexander, J. C. Physiological and biochemical changes associated with linamarin administration to rats. Toxicol. Appl. Pharmacol., *42*:539-551, 1977.

Physicians' Desk Reference, 35th ed. C. E. Baker, Jr. (Publisher). Medical Economics Co., Oradell, N. J, 1981.

Piala, J. J.; High, J. P.; Hassert, G. L., Jr.; Burke, J. C.; Craver, B. N. Pharmacological and acute toxicological comparisons of triflupromazine and chlorpromazine. J. Pharmacol. Exp. Ther., *127*:55-65, 1959.

Pieroh, E. A.; Werres, H.; Rasche, K. Trapex, ein neues Nematizid zur Bodenentseuchung. Anz. Schadlingsk, *32*:183-189, 1959.

Pijoan, M. Cyanide poisoning from choke cherry seed. Am. J. Med. Sci. *204*:550-553, 1942.

Pindar, A. W.; Donnelly, I. C. The pharmacological action of gentian violet. J. Pharmacol. Exp. Ther., *25*:163-165, 1925.

Pinkhas, J.; Djaldetti, M.; Joshua, H.; Resnick, C.; de Vries, A. Sulfhemoglobinemia and acute hemolytic anemia with Heinz bodies following contact with a fungicide - zinc ethylene bisdithiocarbamate - in a subject with glucose-6-phosphate dehydrogenase deficiency andhypocatalasemia. Blood, *21*:484-494, 1963.

Piper, W. N.; Rose, J. Q.; Leng, M. L.; Gehring, P. J. The fate of 2,4,5-trichlorophenoxyacetic acid (2,4,5-T) following oral administration to rats and dogs. Toxicol. Appl. Pharmacol. *26*:339-351, 1973.

Pirozzi, D. J.; Gross, P. R.; Samitz, M. H. The effect of ascorbic acid on chrome ulcers in guinea pigs. Arch. Environ. Health *17*:178-180, 1968.

Pittinger, C. B.; Eryasa, Y.; Adamson, R. Antibiotic-induced paralysis. Anesth. Analg., *49*:487-501, 1970.

Plaa, G. L.; Fujimoto, J. M.; Hine, C. H. Intoxication from primidone due to its biotransformation to phenobarbital. J. A. M. A., *168*:1769-1770, 1958.

Plakhova, A. G.; Vengerskaya, Kh. Ya.; Maisrova, T. N. Hygienic features of labor conditions and prophylactic measures for work with cotoran. (as cited in Chem. Abs. *81*:81901s) Med. Zh. Uzb. No. 2, p. 17-20, 1974.

Platou, R. V. Poisonings in children. Lancet, *81*:548-551, 1961.

Plestina, R.; Svetlicic, B. Toxic effects of two carbamate insecticides in dogs. Arh. Hig. Rada Toksikol. *24*:217-225, 1973.

Ploch, H. J. Personal communication. Monsanto Chemical Co., St. Louis, 1957.

Plum, F.; Swanson, A. G. Barbiturate poisoning treated by physiological methods. J. A. M. A. *163*:827-835, 1957.

Plumb, R. L.; Joseph, S. W. Ingestion of a toxic overdose of chlorprothixene by a 3-year-old. J. Pediatr., *65*:458-461, 1964.

Pogge, R. C. Personal communication. Wm. S. Merrell Co., Cincinnati, 1957.

Poklis, A.; Hameli, A. Z. Two unusual barbiturate deaths. Arch. Toxicol. *34*:77-80, 1975.

Poklis, A.; Kutz, F. W.; Sperling, J. F.; Morgan, D. P. A fatal diazinon poisoning. Forensic Sci. Int., *15*:135-140, 1980.

Poland, A; Glover, E. Studies in the mechanism of toxicity of the chlorinated dibenzo-*p*-dioxins. Environ. Health Perspect., Expt. Issue No. *5*:245-251, 1973b.

Poland, A; Glover. E. 2,3,7,8-Tetrachloro-dibenzo-*p*-dioxin: A potent inducer of δ-aminolevulinic acid synthetase. Science, *179*:476-477, 1973a.

Pollack, B. Report of an unusually large dosage of methylphenidate hydrochloride. Am. J. Psychiatry, *121*:189-190, 1964.

Polonio, P. Pethidine addiction. Lancet, *1*:592-594, 1947.

Pont, A.; Rubino, J. M.; Bishop, D.; Peal, R. Diabetes mellitus and neuropathy following vacor ingestion in man. Arch. Intern. Med. *139*:185-187, 1979.

Poothullil, J.; Shimizu, A.; Day, R. P.; Dolovich, J. Anaphylaxis from the product(s) of ethylene oxide gas. Ann. Intern. Med., *82*:58-60, 1975.

Porter, D. C. Personal communication. Los Angeles Soap Co., Los Angeles, Calif, 1959.

Powell, John and Co. Technical Bulletin (Sabadilla, an outline of its use as an insecticide). Inc, 1947.

Powers, M. F.; Darby, T. D.; Schueler, F. W. A study of the toxic effects of cinnamon oil. Pharmacologist, *3*:62, 1961.

Pozzani, U. C.; Kinkead, E. R.; King, J. M. The mammalian toxicity of methacrylonitrile. Am. Ind. Hyg. Assoc. J., *29*:202-210, 1968.

Pratt-Johnson, J. A. Retrobulbar neuritis following exposure to vinyl benzene. Can. Med. Assoc. J., *90*:975-977, 1964.

Prentiss Drug and Chemical Co. Brochure (butonate). Inc., New York, 1960.

Press, E.; Yeager, L. Food "poisoning" due to sodium nicotinate, report of an outbreak and review of literature. Am. J. Public Health, *52*:1720-1728, 1962.

Press, H. A. Personal communication. Merck, Sharp and Dohme, West Point, Pa, 1969.

Price, J. C.; Waelsch, H.; Putnam, T. J. dl-Glutamic acid hydrochloride in treatment of petit mal and psycho motor seizures. J. A. M. A., *122*:1153-1156, 1943.

Prindle, R. F. Personal communication. Lehn and Fink Products Co., New Jersey, 1973.

Prival, M. J.; McCoy, E. C.; Gutter, B.; Rosenkranz, H. S. Tris (2,3-dibromropyl)phosphate: mutagenicity of a widely used flame retardant. Science, *195*:76-78, 1977.

Procita, L. Some pharmacological actions of ryanodine in the mammal. J. Pharmacol. Exp. Ther. *123*:296-305, 1958.

Procter, D. S. C. Coma in burns - the cause traced to dressings. S. Afr. Med. J., *40*:1116-1120, 1966.

Proctor, N. H.; Moscioni, A. D.; Casida, J. E. Chicken embryo

NAD levels lowered by teratogenic organophosphorus and methylcarbamate insecticides. Biochem. Pharmacol. 25:757-762, 1976.

Proklina-Kaminskaya, T. L. Effect of continuous exposure to pesticides (carbamates, thiocarbamates, and dithiocarbamates) on oxidative processes in animals. Gig. Tr., No. 1, p. 91-94, 1969.

Prosser, P. R.; Karam, J. H. Diabetes following rodenticide ingestion in man. J. A. M. A. 239:1148-1150, 1978.

Proudfoot, A. T.; Noble, J.; Nimmo, J.; Brown, S. S.; Cameron, J. C. Peritoneal dialysis and haemodialysis in methaqualone (Mandrax) poisoning. Scott. Med. J., 13:232-236, 1968.

Prystowsky, S. D.; Allen, A. M.; Smith, R. W.; Nonomura, J. H.; Odom, R. B.; Akers, W. A. Allergic contact hypersensitivity to nickel, neomycin, ethylenediamine, and benzocaine. Arch. Dermatol. 115:959–962, 1979.

Psychopharmacology Service Center. Bull. 2:no. 1 (a selective list of drugs used in psychiatry). Bethesda, Md, 1962.

Pugaeva, V. P. Pathogenesis of propylene oxide intoxication. Mater. Nauch. -Prakt. Konf. Molodykh Gig. Sanit. Vrachei, 11th, p. 207-208, 1967.

Pyysalo, H. Some new toxic compounds in false morels, Gyromitra esculenta. Nataswissenshoften, 8:395, 1975.

Quellhorst, E.; Mietzsch, G.; Doht, B.; Fernandez-Redo, E.; Kubosch, J.; Leititis, U.; Volles, E.; Thorwirt, V.; Scheler, F. Sorbithaltige Spullosung als Ursache schwerer Unvertraglichkeitserscheinungen bei der Peritonealdialyse. Dtsch. Med. Wschr. 100:1431-1435, 1975.

Qureshi, E. H. Propoxyphene hydrochloride poisoning. J. A. M. A., 188:470-471, 1964.

Raaschou-Nielsen, W. Chronic intoxication with Vitamin A in adults. Dermatologica, 123:293-300, 1961.

Rabinowitch, I. M. Acute nitroglycerine poisoning. Can. Med. Assoc. J., 50:199-202, 1944.

Radomski, J. L.; Davidow, B. The metabolite of heptachlor, its estimation, storage, and toxicity. J. Pharmacol. Exp. Ther. 107:266-272, 1953.

Rafferty, P. Voluntary chlorine inhalation: a new form of self abuse. Br. Med. J., 281:1178-1179, 1980.

Rahde, A. F. Personal Communication. Centro De Informacao Toxicologiga, Brazil, 1979.

Raichle, M. E.; Kutt, H.; Louis, S.; McDowell, F. Neurotoxicity of intravenously administered penicillin G. Arch. Neurol., 25:232-239, 1971.

Ralph, N. Evaluation of a new cough suppressant. Am. J. Med. Sci., 227:297-303, 1954.

Ram, A. F., Jr. Personal communication. Allied Chemical Corp., Morristown, N. J, 1965.

Ramsay, D. L.; Cohen, H. J.; Baer, R. L. Allergic reaction to benzophenone. Arch. Derm., 105:906-908, 1972.

Ransone, J. W.; Scott, N. M.; Knoblock, E. C. Selenium sulfide intoxication. N. Engl. J. Med., 264:384-385, 1961.

Ratney, R. S.; Wegman, D. H.; Elkins, H. B. In vivo conversion of methylene chloride to carbon monoxide. Arch. Environ. Health 28:223-226, 1974.

Ravn-Jonsen, A. The urinary excretion of Enibomalum (NFN) in man after administration of anaesthetic doses. Acta Pharmacol. Toxicol. 28:484-492, 1970.

Read, B. E. The toxicity of chaulmoogra oil (oleum hydnocarpi). J. Pharmacol. Exp. Ther., 24:221-258, 1924.

Read, J. M. Fatal ventricular fibrillation following procaine amide hydrochloride therapy. J. A. M. A., 149:1390-1391, 1952.

Rebrin, V. G.; Aleksandrova, L. G. Toxicological-hygienic characteristics of the new herbicide ronit. (as cited in Chem. Abstracts 76:108896e) Vrach Delo, No. 12, p. 118-121, 1971.

Reed, D. R.; Cravey, H.; Sedgwick, R. R. A fatal case involving methylenedioxyamphetamine. Clin. Toxicol., 5:3-6, 1972.

Reekie, A. A. M. Treatment of bismuth stomatitis with BAL (British anti-lewisite). Br. Med. J., 2:1213, 1949.

Reese, J. J. A Manual of Toxicology. J. B. Lippincott Co., Philadelphia, 1874.

Reich, G. A.; Welke, J. O. Death due to a pesticide. N. Engl. J. Med., 274:1432, 1966.

Reichelderfer, T. E. Accidental death of an infant caused by ingestion of ammonium dichromate. South. Med. J., 61:96-

97, 1968.

Reichert, E. R.; Yauger, W. L., Jr.; Rashad, M. N.; Klemmer, H. W. Diazinon poisoning in eight members of related households. Clin. Toxicol., 11:5-11, 1977.

Reingold, I. M.; Webb, F. R. Sudden death following intravenous injection of thiamine hydrochloride. J. A. M. A., 130:491-492, 1946.

Reinhardt, P. Akute toxische Polyneuropathie nach kurzzeitiger Hydroxychinolin-Medikation. Dtsch. Med. Wochenschr. 29:1047-1048, 1979.

Rejsek, K. m-Dinitrobenzene poisoning. Mobilization by alcohol and sunlight. Acta Med. Scand., 127:179-191, 1947.

Repko, J. D.; Lasley, S. M. Behavioral, neurological, and toxic effects of methyl chloride: a review of the literature. CRC Crit. Rev. Toxicol. 6:283-302, 1979.

Resnick, O. The metabolism of orally ingested epinephrine in man. Life Sciences, 2:629-636, 1963.

Reuber, M. D. Thyroiditis in rats given subcutaneous injections of trypan blue. Toxicol. Appl. Pharmacol., 14:108-113, 1969.

Reuber, M. D. Carcinogenicity of chlorobenzilate in mice, rats, and dogs. Clin. Toxicol. 16:67-98, 1980.

Reynolds, E. S.; Moslen, M. T.; Szabo, S.; Jaeger, R. J.; Murphy, S. Hepatotoxicity of vinyl chloride and 1, 1-dichloroethylene. Role of mixed function oxidase system. Am. J. Pathol., 85:219-236, 1975.

Reynolds, E. S.; Schlant, R. C.; Gonick, H. C.; Dammin, G. J. Fatal massive necrosis of the liver as a manifestation of hypersensitivity to probenecid. N. Engl. J. Med., 256:592-596, 1957.

Rhodes, R. C.; Pease, H. L. Fate of chloroneb in animals. J. Agric. Food Chem. 19:750-753, 1971.

Rhodes, R. C.; Reiser, R. W.; Gardiner, J. A.; Sherman, H. Identification of the metabolites of terbacil in dog urine. J. Agric. Food Chem. 17:974-979, 1969.

Richards, A. G. Malathion poisoning successfully treated with large doses of atropine. Can. Med. Assoc. J., 91:82-83, 1964.

Richards, K. C.; Borgstedt, H. H. Near fatal reaction to ingestion of the hallucinogenic drug MDA. J. A. M. A., 218:826-827, 1971.

Richards, R. K.; Taylor, J. D.; O'Brien, J. L.; Duescher, H. O. Studies in cyclamate sodium (Sucaryl sodium), a new noncaloric sweetening agent. J. A. Pharm. Sci., 40:1-6, 1951.

Richardson, S. G. N.; Giles, C.; Swan, C. H. J. Two cases of sodium azide poisoning by accidental ingestion of Isotin. J. Clin. Pathol., 28:350-351, 1975.

Richarz, G.; Schoetensack, W. Lebernekrosen, Serumtransaminase und Bromsulphthalein-retention bei der Ratte nach Allylalkohol-Vergiftung. Nauyn. Schmiedebergs Arch. Pharmakol., 241:153, 1961.

Richter, E.; Lay, J. P.; Klein, W.; Korti, F. Paraffin-stimulated excretion of 2,4,6,2',4'-pentachlorobi[14]Cphenyl by rats. Toxicol. Appl. Pharmacol., 50:17-23, 1979.

Riden, J. R. Personal communication. Spencer Chemical Co, 1961.

Riemann, H. On the toxicity of hydroxylamine. Acta Pharmacol. Toxicol., 6:285-292, 1950.

Riggs, D. S.; Man, E. B.; Winkler, A. W. Serum iodine of euthyroid subjects treated with desiccated thyroid. J. Clin. Invest., 24:722-731, 1945.

Riley, P. Toxicity of bismuth subsalicylate. The New Physician, 10:30, 1961.

Rivin, A. V. Jaundice occurring during nicotinic acid therapy for hypercholesteremia. J. A. M. A., 170:2088-2089, 1959.

Robbins, J. D.; Bakke, J. E.; Feil, V. J. Metabolism of benzo(b)thien-4-yl methylcarbamate (Mobam) in rats. Balance study and urinary metabolite separation. J. Agric. Food Chem. 17:236-242, 1969.

Robbins, J. D.; Bakke, J. E.; Feil, V. J. Metabolism of benzo(b)thien-4-yl methylcarbamate (Mobam) in dairy goats and a lactating cow. J. Agric. Food Chem. 18:130-134, 1970.

Robbins, J. J.; Ware, R. L. Pulmonary edema from Teflon fumes. N. Engl. J. Med., 271:360-361, 1964.

Robeco Chemicals, Inc. Personal communication, 1957.

Roberts, C. J. C.; Marshall, F. P. F. Recovery after "lethal" quantity of paint remover. Br. Med. J. 1:20-21, 1976.

Roberts, H. J. Aplastic anemia due to pentachlorophenol and tetrachlorophenol. South. Med. J., 56: 632-635, 1963.

Roberts, M.; Linn, S. Acute and subchronic toxicity of 2-amino-2-hydroxymethyl-1-3-propanediol. Ann. N. Y. Acad. Sci., 92:724-734, 1961.

Roberts, R. J.; Simmons, A.; Barrett, D. Accidental exposures to sodium azide. Am. J. Clin. Pathol., 61:879-880, 1974.

Robertson, A. J.; Rivers, D.; Nagelschmidt, G.; Duncumb, P. Stannosis: Benign pneumoconiosis due to tin oxide. Lancet, 1:1089-1093, 1961.

Robin, E. D.; Tabor, C. W.; Smith, P. K. Studies on the toxicity of para-aminobenzoic acid in rats. Fed. Proc., 6:366, 1947.

Robins, A. H., Co., Inc. Poison control information on A. H. Robins preparations. 1407 Cummings Drive, Richmond, VA 23220, 1972.

Robinson, A. S. "Neck-face syndrome" related to phenothiazine drugs. J. A. M. A., 173:504-506, 1960.

Robinson, D.; Smith, J. N.; Williams, R. T. Studies in detoxication; metabolism of alkylbenzenes. Isopropylbenzene (cumene) and derivatives of hydratropic acid. Biochem. J. 59:153-159, 1955.

Robinson, H. J.; Graessle, O. E. Toxicity of tannic acid. J. Pharmacol. Exp. Ther., 77:63-69, 1943.

Robinson, H. J.; Phares, H. F.; Graessle, O. E. The toxicological and antifungal properties of thiabendazole. Ecotoxicol. Environ. Safety 1:471-476, 1978.

Robinson, H. J.; Silber, R. H.; Graessle, O. E. Thiabendazole: Toxicological, pharmacological and antifungal properties. Texas Rep. Biol. Med. 27(Suppl. 2):537-560, 1969.

Robinson, W. D.; Bunim, J. J.; Clark, W. S.; Crain, D. C.; Engelman, E. P.; Graham, D. C.; Montgomery, M. M.; Norcross, B. M.; Raggan, C.; Ropes, M. W.; Rosenberg, E. F.; Smith, C. J. Rheumatism and arthritis. Ann. Intern. Med., 45:831-945 and 1059-1210, l956, 1956.

Robson, A. M.; Kissane, J. M.; Elvick, N. H.; Pundavela, L. Pentachlorophenol poisoning in a nursery for newborn infants. I. Clinical features and treatment. J. Pediatr. 75: 309-316, 1969.

Roche Laboratories. Product reference manual (including treatment of overdosage). Roche Laboratories, Nutley, NJ, 1964.

Rodahl, K.; Moore, T. Vitamin A content and toxicity of bear and seal liver. Biochem. J., 37:166-168, 1943.

Rodger, W. Hazards of calcium carbimide (Absten). Br. Med. J., 2:989, 1962.

Rodin, A. E.; Koller, L. A.; Taylor, J. D. Association of thalidomide (Kevadon) with congenital anomalies. Can. Med. Assoc. J., 86:744-746, 1962.

Rodkey, F. L.; Collison, H. A. Effect of dihalogenated methanes on the in vivo production of carbon monoxide and methane by rats. Toxicol. Appl. Pharmacol. 40:39-47, 1977.

Rohm and Haas Co. Storage and handling of acrylic and methacrylic esters and acids. Rohm and Haas Co., Philadelphia, Pa, 1963.

Rohm and Haas Company. Summary of toxicity reports on technical Kerb, Kerb 75WP, or Kerb 50W. Philadelphia, Pa, date unknown.

Romagny, G.; Megard, M. Retentissement penal d'une intoxication par le "Meta." Essai d'interpretation pathogenique. J. Med. Lyon 40:237-241, 1959.

Roman, D. P.; Barnett, E. H.; Balske, R. J. Cutaneous antiseptic activity of 3,4,4'-trichlorocarbanilide. Proc. Sci. Sect. Toilet Goods Assoc., No. 28:12-13, 1957.

Romeril, K. R.; Concannon, A. J. Heinz body haemolytic anaemia after sniffing volatile nitrites. Med. J. Aust., 1:302-303, 1981.

Ronnov-Jessen, V.; Tjernlund, A. Hepatotoxicity due to treatment with papaverine. N. Engl. J. Med., 281:1333-1335, 1969.

Rosen, I.; Haeger-Aronsen, S.; Rehnstrom, S.; Welinder, H. Neurophysiological observation after chronic styrene exposure. Scand. J. Work Environ. Health 4(Suppl. 2):184-194, 1978.

Rosenbaum, J. L.; Kramer, M. S.; Raja, R. Resin hemoperfu-

sion for acute drug intoxication. Arch. Internal Med., 136:263-266, 1976.

Rosenberg, L. E.; Hayslett, J. P. Nephrotoxic effects of penicillamine in cystinuria. J. A. M. A., 201:698-699, 1967.

Rosenblum, I.; Wohl, A.; Stein, A. A. Studies in cardiac necrosis. I. Production of cardiac lesions with sympathomimetic amines. Toxicol. Appl. Pharmacol., 7:1-8, 1965.

Rosher, R. Personal communication. Hercules Powder Co., Wilmington, Del, 1957.

Rosin, R. D. Cantharides intoxication. Br. Med. J., 4:33, 1967.

Ross, R. R., Jr.; Conway, G. F. Hemorrhagic cystitis following accidental overdose of methenamine mandelate. Am. J. Dis. Child 119:86-87, 1970.

Roszkowski, A. P. The pharmacological properties, a selective rat toxicant. J. Pharmacol. Exp. Ther., 149:288-299, 1965.

Roszkowski, A. P.; Poos, G. I.; Mohrbacher, R. J. Selective rat toxicant. Science, 144:412-413, 1964.

Roth, C. H. Personal communication. Winthrop Laboratories, New York, 1961.

Roth, F. E.; Irwin, S.; Eckhardt, E.; Tabachnick, I. I. A.; Govier, W. M. Perphenazine (trilafon), a new potent tranquilizer and antiemetic. II. General pharmacology. Arch. Int. Pharmacodyn. Ther., 118:375-383, 1959.

Rothlin, E. Pharmacology of lysergic acid diethylamide and some of its related compounds. J. Pharm. Pharmacol., 9:569-587, 1957.

Roudabush, R. L. Personal communication. Eastman Kodak Co., Rochester, N. Y, 1960.

Rougraff, M. E. Chlorothiazide overdosage effects in a two-year-old child. Pa. Med., 62:694-695, 1959.

Roukema, P. A.; Kafoe, W. F.; Roozemond, R. C. The effects of some hydroxylamine compounds on γ-aminobutyric acid-α-ketoglutaric acid transaminase and glutamic acid decarboxylase activities in rat brain. Arch. Int. Pharmacodyn. Ther., 158:429-438, 1965.

Rowe, R. J.; Williams, G. H. Severe reaction to cement. Arch. Environ. Health, 7:709-711, 1963.

Rowe, V. K. Personal communication. Dow Chemical Co., Midland, Mich, 1956.

Rowe, V. K. Personal communication. Dow Chemical Co., Midland, Mich, 1957.

Rowe, V. K. Personal communication. Dow Chemical Co., Midland, Mich, 1960.

Rowe, V. K. Glycols and derivatives of glycols. In Industrial Hygiene and Toxicology, Edited by F. A. Patty, Vol. II. Toxicology. 2nd ed. Edited by D. W. Fassett and D. D. Irish. Interscience Publishers, Inc., New York, 1962.

Rowe, V. K.; Hymas, T. A. Summary of toxicological information on 2,4-D and 2,4,5-T type herbicides and an evaluation of the hazards to livestock associated with their use. Am. J. Vet. Res. 15:622-629, 1954a.

Rowe, V. K.; McCollister, D. D.; Spencer, H. C.; Oyen, F.; Hollingworth, R. L.; Drill, V. A. Toxicology of mono-, di-, and tri-propylene glycol methyl ethers. A. M. A. Arch. Ind. Hyg. Occup. Med., 9:509-525, 1954b.

Rowe, V. K.; Spencer, H. C.; Bass, S. L. Toxicological studies on certain commercial silicones and hydrolyzable silane intermediates. J. Ind. Hyg. Toxicol., 30:332-352, 1948.

Rowe, V. K.; Spencer, H. C.; McCollister, D. D.; Hollingsworth, R. L.; Adams, E. M. Toxicity of ethylene dibromide determined on experimental animals. Arch. Ind. Hyg. Occup. Med., 6:158-173, 1952.

Rowlett, R. J., Jr. Personal communication. Virginia-Carolina Chemical Co., Richmond, Va, 1957.

Rubbo, S. D. The influence of chemical constitution on toxicity. Part I. A general survey of the acridine series. Br. J. Exp. Pathol., 28:1-11, 1947.

Rubenchik, B. L.; Botsman, N. E.; Gorban, G. P.; Loevskaya, L. I. Relation between the chemical structure and carcinogenic activity of urea derivatives. Onkologiya (Kiev) 4:10-16, 1973.

Rubenstein, A. D.; Tabershaw, I. R.; Daniels, J. Pseudo-gas gangrene of the hand. J. A. M. A., 129:659-662, 1945.

Rubenstein, A. H.; Levin, N. W.; Elliot, G. A. Hypoglycemia induced by manganese. Nature, 194:188-189 (1962), 1962.

Rubin, R. J.; Schiffer, C. A. Fate in humans of plasticizer, di-

2-ethylhexyl phthalate, arising from transfusion of platelets stored in vinyl plastic bags. Transfusion, *16*:330-335, 1976.

Rubin, R. T. Acute psychotic reaction following ingestion of phentermine. Am. J. Psychiatry, *120*:1124-1125, 1964.

Ruhl, R. Beitrag zur Pathologie und Toxikologie des Solanins. Arch. Pharm. Berichte Deutsch. Pharm. Gesellsch. *284*:67-74, 1951.

Ruotolo, B. P. W. Toxic hazards, methyl chloroform. N. Engl. J. Med., *255*:1105-1106, 1956.

Rutkowski, J. V.; Ferm, V. H. Comparison of the teratogenic effects of the isomeric forms of aminophenol in the Syrian golden hamster. Toxicol. Appl. Pharmacol. *63*:264-269, 1982.

Rutstein, H. R. Acute chlorobromomethane toxicity. Arch. Environ. Health *7*:440-444, 1963.

Ryan, A. J. The metabolism of carbamate pesticides. C. R. C. Critical Rev. Toxicol. *1*:33-54, 1971.

Sabine, J. C.; Hayes, F. N. Anticholinesterase activity of tributyl phosphate. Arch. Ind. Hyg. Occup. Med., *6*:174-177, 1952.

Sadoff, L.; Fuchs, K.; Hollander, J. Rapid death associated with laetrile ingestion. J. A. M. A., *239*:1532-1533, 1978.

Sagall, E. L.; Dorfman, A. Death following the intravenous administration of papaverine hydrochloride. N. Engl. J. Med., *233*:590-591, 1945.

Saikkonen, J. Cobalt as a producer of porphyrinuria and polycythemia. J. Lab. Clin. Med., *54*:860-866, 1959.

Saitanov, A. O.; Kononova, A. M. Acute ethylene chlorohydrin poisoning. (As cited in Chem. Abstracts, *84*:145550y) Gig. Tr. Prof. Zabrol., No. 2:49-50, 1976.

Sakai, R. I.; Lattin, J. E. Lidocaine ingestion. Am. J. Dis. Child., *134*:323, 1980.

Salem, H.; Cullumbine, H. Inhalation toxicities of some aldehydes. Toxicol. Appl. Pharmacol. *2*:183-187, 1960.

Samuelsson, G. Mistletoe toxins. Syst. Zool. *22*:566-569, 1973.

Sanchez-Sicillia, L.; Seto, D. S.; Nakamoto, S.; Kolff, W. J. Acute mercurial intoxication treated by hemodialysis. Ann. Intern. Med. *59*:692-706, 1963.

Sand, R. E.; Edelmann, C. M., Jr. Pyridium-induced methemoglobinemia. Report of a case. J. Pediatr., *58*:845-848, 1961.

Sanderson, J. H.; Cowdell, R. H.; Higgins, G. Fatal poisoning with methaqualone and diphenhydramine. Lancet., *2*:803-804, 1966.

Sandoz Pharmaceuticals. Brochure (Sansert). Hanover, N. J., Jan, 1962.

Sandvig, K.; Olsnes, S.; Pihl, A. Kinetics of binding of the toxic lectins abrin and ricin to surface receptors of human cells. J. Biol. Chem. *251*:3977-3984, 1976.

Sanghvi, L. M.; Misra, S. N.; Bose, T. K. Cardiovascular manifestations in Argemone mexicana poisoning (epidemic dropsy). Circulation, *21*:1096, 1960.

Sapeika, N. Food Pharmacology. Charles C. Thomas, Springfield, Illinois, 1969.

Sarcinelli, L.; Signore, L.; Malizia, E. Lethal phenolphthalein poisoning in a child. Eur. Soc. for Study of Drug Toxicity *11*:261-262, 1970.

Sarles, M. P.; Dove, W. E.; Moore, D. H. Acute toxicity and irritation tests on animals with the new insecticide, piperonyl butoxide. Am. J. Trop. Med. Hyg., *29*:151-166, 1949.

Satoh, T. Glycemic effects of solanine in rats. Jap. J. Pharmacol. *17*:652-658, 1967.

Sauerhoff, M. W.; Heeschen, J. P.; Nyquist, R. A.; Braun, W. H. Pharmacokinetic profile of diamidfos in rats. Food Cosmet. Toxicol. *14*:401-408, 1976.

Saunders, D. R.; Sillery, J.; Rachmilewitz, D. The effect of dioctyl sodium sulfosuccinate on structure and function of rodent and human intestine. Gastroenterology *69*:380-386, 1975.

Saunders, J. P.; Heisey, S. R.; Goldstone, A. D.; Bay, E. C. Comparative toxicities of warfarin and some 2-acyl-1, 3-indandiones in rats. J. Agric. Food. Chem., *3*:762-765, 1955.

Sax, N. I. Dangerous Properties of Industrial Materials. Reinhold Publishing Corp., New York, 1957.

Sax, N. I. Dangerous Properties of Industrial Materials. 3rd ed., Reinhold Book Corp., New York, 1968.

Sax, N. I. *Dangerous Properties of Industrial Materials*, 4th ed. Van Nostrand Reinhold Co., New York, 1975.

Sayers, R. R. Metal fume fever and its prevention. Public Health Repts., No. *53*:1080-1086, 1938.

Sayers, R. R.; Schrenk, H. H.; Patty, F. A. Acute response of guinea pigs to vapors of some new commercial organic compounds. III. Normal butyl acetate. Public Health Repts., No. *51*:1229-1236 (1936), 1936.

Sayers, R. R.; Yant, W. P.; Chornyak, J.; Shoaf, H. W. Toxicity of dichlorodifluoromethane: A new refrigerant. U. S. Bur. Mines, Rept. Invest. No. 3013, 1930.

Sayre, J. W.; Kaymakcalan, S. Cyanide poisoning from apricot seeds among children in central Turkey. N. Engl. J. Med. *270*:1113-1115, 1964.

Scala, R. A.; Burtis, E. G. Acute toxicity of a homologous series of branched-chain primary alcohols. Am. Ind. Hyg. Assoc. J. *34*:493-499, 1973.

Schafer, E. W., Jr.; Brunton, R. B.; Cunningham, D. J. Summary of the acute toxicity of 4-aminopyridine to birds and mammals. Toxicol. Appl. Pharmacol. *26*:532-538, 1973.

Schaffer, C. B.; Pauli, M. W. Psychotic reaction caused by proprietary oral diet agents. Am. J. Psychiatry, *137*:1256-1257, 1980.

Schales, D.; Graefe, H. A. Arylnitroalkenes: A new group of antibacterial agents. J. Am. Chem. Soc., *74*:4486-4490, 1952.

Schallek, W.; Kuehn, A.; Seppelin, D. K. Central depressant effects of methyprylon. J. Pharmacol. Exp. Ther., *118*:139-147, 1956.

Schantz, J. M. Personal communication. Hercules Powder Co., Wilmington, Del., 1953.

Scharnweber, H. C.; Spears, G. N.; Cowles, S. R. Chronic methyl chloride intoxication in six industrial workers. J. Occup. Med. *16*:112-113, 1974.

Scharp, L. G., Jr.; Hill, I. D.; Maibach, H. I. Percutaneous penetration and disposition of triclocarban in man. Arch. Environ. Health, *30*:7-14, 1975.

Schaumburg, H. H.; Byck, R.; Gestl, R.; Mashman, J. H. Monosodium L-glutamate: Its pharmacology and role in the Chinese restaurant syndrome. Science, *163*:826-828, 1969.

Schaumburg, H. H.; Spencer, P. S. Environmental hydrocarbons produce degeneration in cat hypothalamus and optic tract. Science *199*:199-200, 1978.

Scheel, L. D.; Fleisher, E.; Klemperer, F. W. Toxicity of silica. I. Silica solutions. Arch. Ind. Hyg. Occup. Med., *8*:564-573, 1953.

Scheline, R. R.; Smith, R. L.; Williams, R. T. The metabolism of aryl thioureas. II. The metabolism of 14C- and 35S-labelled 1-phenyl-2-thiourea and its derivatives. J. Med. Chem., *4*:109-135, 1961.

Scherf, D. Studies on auricular tachycardia caused by aconitine administration. Proc. Soc. Exp. Biol. Med., *64*:233-239, 1947.

Schiff, E.; Hirschberger, C. Thrombocytosis produced by a hitherto unknown substance - the "Fat-soluble T factor". Am. J. Dis. Child., *53*:32-38, 1937.

Schifrin, B. S.; Spellacy, W. N.; Little, W. A. Maternal death associated with excessive ingestion of a chlorothiazide diuretic. Obstet. Gynecol., *34*:215-220, 1969.

Schlang, H. A. Poisoning caused by tetraethyl lead. Aerosp. Med., *32*:333-335, 1961.

Schmidt, E. S.; Newton, G. W.; Sanders, S. M.; Lewis, J. P. Laetrile toxicity studies in dogs. J. A. M. A., *239*:943-947, 1978.

Schneider, C. J., Jr. The ingestion hazard of dishwasher detergents and liquid waxes and polishes. Cornell Aeronautical Laboratory, Inc. Report No. VZ2926-D-7 prepared for the National Commission on Product Safety, 1970.

Schoenberger, J. A.; Rix, D. M.; Sakamoto, A.; Taylor, J. D.; Kark, R. M. Metabolic effects, toxicity and excretion of calcium N-cyclohexyl sulfamate (Sucaryl) in man. Am. J. Med. Sci., *225*:551-559, 1953.

Schoenheimer, R.; Hilgetag, G. The occurrence and secretion mechanism of cetyl alcohol in the animal organism. J. Biol. Chem., *105*:73-77, 1934.

Schotland, M. G.; Grumbach, M. M. Neutropenia in an infant secondary to hydrochlorothiazide therapy with a review of hematologic reactions to 'thiazide' drugs. Pediatrics, 31:751-757, 1963.

Schreiner, G. E. The role of hemodialysis (artificial kidney) in acute poisoning. Arch. Intern. Med., 102:896-913, 1958.

Schreiner, G. E.; Berman, L. B.; Kovach, R.; Bloomer, H. A. Acute glutethimide (Doriden) poisoning. The use of bemegride (Megimide) and hemodialysis. Arch. Intern. Med., 101:899-911, 1958.

Schrenk, H. H.; Yant, W. P. Toxicity of dioxan. J. Ind. Hyg. Toxicol., 18:448-460, 1936.

Schrenk, H. H.; Yant, W. P.; Chornyak, J.; Patty, F. A. Acute response of guinea pigs to vapors of some new commercial organic compounds. XIII. Methyl formate. Pub. Health Rep. 51:1329-1337, 1936.

Schrenk, H. H.; Yant, W. P.; Patty, F. A. Acute response of guinea pigs to vapors of some new commercial organic compounds. X. Hexanone methyl butyl ketone. Pub. Health Rep. 51:624-631, 1935.

Schroeder, E. F.; Rose, F. A.; Most, H. Effect of antimony on the electrocardiogram. Am. J. Med. Sci., 212:697-706, 1946.

Schultz, C. Bronchitis nach Inhalation eines Farbenlosungsmittels (Epichlorhydrin). Dtsch. Med. Wochenschr., 89:1342-1344, 1964.

Schulz, K. H. Uber die Verwendung von Alkyl-Polyathylenoxyd-Derivaten als Oberflachenanaesthetica. Dermatol. Wochenschr., 126:657-662, 1952.

Schutz, F. Cyanate. Experimentia, 5:133-141, 1949.

Schwartz, A. M. The cause, relief and prevention of headaches arising from contact with dynamite. N. Engl. J. Med., 235:541-544, 1946.

Schwartz, L. Dermatitis from synthetic resins. Arch. Indust. Health 15:239-255, 1957.

Schwartz, L.; Birmingham, D. J.; Campbell, P. C., Jr.; Mason, H. S. Skin hazards in the manufacture and use of cashew nut shell liquid-formaldehyde resins. Ind. Med. Sug., 14:500-506, 1945.

Schwartz, L.; Tulipan, L. Dermatitis from chemicals used in removing velvet pile. Public Health Repts., No. 48:872-875, 1933.

Schwetz, B. A.; Leong, B. K. J.; Gehring, P. J. Embryo- and fetotoxicity of inhaled carbon tetrachloride, 1,1-dichloroethane and methyl ethyl ketone in rats. Toxicol. Appl. Pharmacol., 23:452-464, 1974.

Schwetz, B. A.; Norris, J. M.; Sparschu, G. L.; Rowe, V. K.; Gehring, P. J.; Emmerson, J. L.; Gerbig, C. G. Toxicology of chlorinated dibenzo-p-dioxins. Environ. Health Perspect., Expt. Issue No. 5:245-251, 1973.

Scialli, J. V. K.; Thornton, W. E. Toxic reactions from a haloperidol overdose in two children. Thermal and cardiac manifestations. J. A. M. A., 239:48-49, 1978.

Scientific Oil Compounding Co. Brochure, 2nd Ed. (Cunilates). Jan, 1950.

Scime, I. A.; Tallant, E. J. Tetanus-like reactions to prochlorperazine (Compazine); report of eight cases exhibiting extrapyramidal disturbances after small doses. J. A. M. A., 171:1813-1817, 1959.

Scott, C. C.; Robbins, E. B. Toxicity of p-aminobenzoic acid. Proc. Soc. Exp. Biol. Med., 49:184-186, 1942.

Searle, G. D., and Co. Reference manual no. 78 (Dartal dihydrochloride). Chicago, 1957.

Searle, G. D., and Co. Manual for treatment of overdosage with Searle products. Chicago, Ill, 1966.

Sears, E. S. Nonketotic hyperosmolar hyperglycemia during glycerol therapy for cerebral edema. Neurology, 26:89-94, 1976.

Seeler, A. O.; Mushett, C. W.; Graessle, O.; Silber, R. H. Pharmacological studies on sulfaquinoxaline. J. Pharmacol. Exp. Ther., 82:357-363, 1944.

Seery, T. M.; Bieter, R. N. A contribution to the pharmacology of berberine. J. Pharmacol. Exp. Ther., 69:64-67, 1940.

Seevers, M. H.; Shideman, F. E.; Woods, L. A.; Weeks, J. R.; Kruse, W. T. Dehydroacetic acid (DHA)., II. General pharmacology and mechanism of action. J. Pharmacol. Exp. Ther., 99:69-83, 1950.

Segal, R.; Milo-Goldzweig, I.; Seiffe, M. Hemolytic properties of nonionic hemolysins. Life Sci. 11:61-70, 1972.

Segreto, V. A.; Yeary, R. A.; Brooks, R.; Harns, N. O. Toxicity study of stannous fluoride in Swiss strain mice. J. Dent. Res., 40:623, 1961.

Seiler, J. P. The mutagenicity of benzimidazole and benzimidazole derivatives. I. Forward and reverse mutations in Salmonella typhimurium caused by benzimidazole and some of its derivatives. Mutation Res. 15:273-276, 1972.

Seleck, C. W.; Kelly, R. E. Personal communication. Monsanto Chemical Co., St. Louis, Mo, 1961.

Sell, D. A.; Reynolds, E. S. Liver parenchymal cell injury. VIII. Lesions of membranous cellular components following iodoform. J. Cell. Biol. 41:736-752, 1969.

Selle, S. R. Effects of subcutaneous injections of sodium tungstate on the rat. Fed. Proc., 1:165, 1942.

Selye, H. Protection by catatoxic steroids against cycloheximide intoxication. Toxicol. Appl. Pharmacol. 17:721-725, 1970.

Semencheva, E. M.; Rodionov, G. A.; Kuznetsova, L. I.; Bebeshko, V. G. Action mechanism of propazine, a symmetrical triazine group compound, on rabbits. Byull. Eksp. Biol. Med. 73:47-51, 1972.

Seppalainen, A. M.; Hakkinen, I. Electrophysiological findings in diphenyl poisoning. J. Neurol. Neurosurg. Psychiatr. 38:248-252, 1975.

Serin, F. Formation of cyanogen compounds from amino acids as a factor in chloramine T poisoning. Acta Pharmacol. Toxicol. 5:Suppl. 1, 1949.

Serrone, D. M.; Pakdaman, P.; Stein, A. A.; Coulston, F. Comparative toxicity of 2,6-dichloro-4-nitroaniline in rats and Rhesus monkeys. Toxicol. Appl. Pharmacol. 10:404, 1967.

Setter, J. G.; Maher, J. F.; Schreiner, G. E. Barbiturate intoxication. Arch. Intern. Med. 117:224-236, 1966.

Sexton, R. J.; Henson, E. V. Dermatological injuries by ethylene oxide. J. Ind. Hyg. Toxicol., 31:297-300, 1949.

Sexton, R. J.; Henson, E. V. Experimental ethylene oxide human skin injuries. Arch. Ind. Hyg. Occup. Med., 2:549-564, 1950.

Shafer, W. B. Personal communication. Stauffer Chemical Co., New York, 1965.

Shamberg, I. L. Studies on Atabrine dermatitis. I. Long term observations of veterans with permanent atrophic residua of the disease. J. Invest. Dermatol., 17:85-98, 1951.

Sheehan, J. F.; Brynjolfsson, G. Ulcerative colitis following hydrogen peroxide enema; case report and experimental production with transient emphysema of colonic wall and gas embolism. Lab. Invest., 9:150, 1960.

Shell Chemical Co. Summary of basic data (Allyl alcohol). New York, 1956.

Shell Chemical Co. Technical bulletin sc:59-45 (Technical aldrin). New York, 1959.

Shell Chemical Co. Technical bulletin, sc 60-103 (Technical endrin). New York, 1960a.

Shell Chemical Co. Technical bull, sc 60-105 (Shell methyl parathion). New York, 1960b.

Shell Chemical Co. Technical bull. sc 60-106 (Nemagon soil fumigant). New York, 1960c.

Shell Chemical Co. Technical Bull. sc:60-104 (Phosdrin insecticide). New York, 1960d.

Shell Chemical Co. Summary of Basic Data (Aqualin herbicide). New York, NY, May, 1960, 1960e.

Shell Chemical Co. Summary of basic data (Telodrin insecticide). New York, 1961.

Shell Chemical Co. Summary of basic data (Technical Ciodrin insecticide). New York, 1962.

Shell Chemical Co. Summary of basic data (Technical Bidrin insecticide). New York, 1963.

Shell Chemical Co. Safety Guide for Rabon Insecticide. Shell Chemical Co., San Ramon, Calif, 1974.

Shell Oil Co. Material Safety Data Sheet (Pydrin). Shell Oil Co., Houston, Texas, 1980.

Shelley, W. B.; Hurley, H. J. The allergic origin of zirconium deodorant granulomas. Brit. J. Dermatol. 70:75-101, 1958.

Shen, S. K.; Williams, S.; Onkelinx, C.; Sunderman, F. W., Jr. Use of implanted minipumps to study the effects of chelating drugs on renal [63]Ni clearance in rats. Toxicol. Appl.

Pharmacol. *51*:209–217, 1979.

Shepard, T. H. Catalog of Teratogenic Agents, 2nd ed. The Johns Hopkins University Press, Baltimore, 1976.

Sherlock, S.; Walker, J. G.; Senewiratne, B.; Scott, A. The complications of diuretic therapy in patients with cirrhosis. Ann. N. Y. Acad. Sci., *139*:497-505, 1966.

Sherman, H.; Culik, R.; Jackson, R. A. Reproduction, teratogenic and mutagenic studies with benomyl. Toxicol. Appl. Pharmacol. 32:305-315, 1975.

Sherman, M.; Ross, E.; Chang, M. T. Y. Acute and subacute toxicity of several organophosphorus insecticides to chicks. Toxicol. Appl. Pharmacol., *6*:147-153, 1964.

Sherman, S.; Baur, E.; Klahre, H.; Lever, P. G. Agranulocytosis after 10-(N-methylpiperdyl-3-methyl) phenothiazine, with recovery. N. Engl. J. Med., *258*:287, 1958.

Sherrod, T. R.; Loew, E. R.; Schloemer, H. F. Pharmacological properties of antihistamine drugs, Benadryl, Pyribenzamine and Neoantergan. J. Pharmacol. Exp. Ther. *89*:247-255, 1947.

Shesser, R.; Dixon, D.; Allen, Y.; Mitchell, J.; Edelstein, S. Fatal methemoglobinemia from butyl nitrite ingestion. Ann. Intern. Med., *92*:131-132, 1980.

Shideman, F. E.; Woods, L. A.; Seevers, M. H. Dehydroacetic acid (DNA). IV. Detoxification and effects on renal function. J. Pharmacol. Exp. Ther., *99*:98-111, 1950.

Shimkin, P. M.; Shaivitz, S. A. Oxazepam poisoning in a child. J. A. M. A., *196*:662-663, 1966.

Shocket, J. L. Personal communication. Fumol Corp., Long Island City, N. Y, 1964.

Short, R. D., Jr.; Russel, J. Q.; Minor, J. L.; Lee, C. -C. Developmental toxicity of ferric dimethyldithiocarbamate and bis(dimethyl- thiocarbamoyl)disulfide in rats and mice. Toxicol. Appl. Pharmacol. 35:83-94, 1976.

Short, R. D.; Winston, J. M.; Minor, J. L.; Seifter, J.; Lee, C. -C. Effect of various treatments on toxicity of inhaled vinylidene chloride. Environ. Health Perspect., *21*:125-129, 1977.

Showalter, C. V. T's and Blues. J. A. M. A., *244*:1224-1225, 1980.

Shtabskii, B. M. Cumulative properties and gonadotoxic action of chemical substances. Gig. Sanit. *1*:82-84, 1976.

Shugaen, B. B. Concentrations of hydrocarbons in tissues as a measure of toxicity. Arch. Environ. Health, *18*:878-882, 1969.

Shults, W. T.; Fountain, E. N.; Lynch, E. C. Methanethiol poisoning; irreversible coma and hemolytic anemia following inhalation. J. Am Med. Assoc. 211:2153-2154, 1970.

Siang, S. C. Acute poisoning with ethinamate and with carbromal. Br. Med. J., *1*:1412, 1960.

Sidorenko, G. I.; Tsulaya, V. R.; Korenevskaya, E. I.; Bonashevskaya, T. I. Methodological approaches to the study of the combined effect of atmospheric pollutants as illustrated by chlorinated hydrocarbons. Environ. Health Perspect. *13*:111-116, 1976.

Sidorov, K. K. Comparative toxicity of mono-, di-, and triethanolamines. (As cited in Chem. Abstracts, 73:118618t) Mater. Nauch. -Prakt. Konf. Molodykh Gig. Sanit. Vrachei, 11th, pp. 217-219, 1986.

Sievers, M. L.; Herrier, R. N. Treatment of acute isoniazid toxicity. Am. J. Hosp. Pharmacy, 32:202-206, 1975.

Sikes, D.; Bridges, M. E. Experimental production of hyperkeratosis (X-disease) of cattle with a chlorinated naphthalene. Science, *116*:506-507, 1952.

Silbert, N. E. Phenergan hydrochloride; a new antihistamine. Ann. Allergy, *10*:328-334, 1952.

Simmel, E. R. Methemoglobinemia due to aminosalicylic acid (PAS). Am. Rev. Resp. Dis. *85*:105-109, 1962.

Simons, F. E. R.; Simons, K. J.; Bierman, C. W. Pharmacokinetics of dihydroxypropyltheophylline. Basis for rational therapy. J. Allergy Clin. Immunol. *56*:347-355, 1975.

Simpson, G. R.; Bermingham, S. Poisoning by carbamate insecticides. Med. J. Aust., *2*:148-149, 1977.

Sinaniotis, C. A.; Spyrides, P.; Vlachos, P.; Papadatos, C. Acute haloperidol poisoning in children. J. Pediatr., *93*:1038-1039, 1978.

Sinclair, J. C.; Fox, H. A.; Lentz, J. F.; Fuld, G. L.; Murphy, J.

Intoxication of the fetus by a local anesthetic. A newly recognized complication of maternal caudal anesthesia. N. Engl. J. Med. *273*:1173-1177, 1965.

Sindar Corp. Technical bulletin 48-3 (Compound 6-4). New York, Date Unknown.

Singer, E. J. Personal communication. Lever Brothers Co., Edgewater, N. J, 1965.

Singleton, S. D.; Murphy, S. D. Propanil (3, 4-Dichloropropionanilide0-induced methemoglobin formation in mice in relation to acylamidase activity. Toxicol. Appl. Pharmacol., *25*:20-29, 1973.

Sivjakov, K. I.; Braun, H. A. The treatment of acute selenium, cadmium and tungsten intoxication in rats with calcium disodium ethylenediaminetetraacetate. Toxicol. Appl. Pharmacol., *1*:602-608, 1959.

Skanse, B.; Nyman, G. E.; Tornegren, L. Electroencephalographic abnormalities in Vitamin D intoxication and the effect of cortisone. Acta Endocrinol., *31*:282-290, 1959.

Sklar, J.; Timms, R. M. Codeine-induced pulmonary edema. Chest, 72:230-231, 1977.

Skowronski, G. A.; Tronson, M. D.; Parkin, W. G. Successful treatment of ergotamine poisoning with sodium nitroprusside. Med. J. Aust. 2:8-9, 1979.

Slade, M.; Casida, J. E. Metabolic fate of 3,4,5- and 2,3,5-trimethylphenyl methylcarbamates, the major constituents in landrin insecticide. J. Agric. Food Chem. *18*:467-474, 1970.

Slater, G. E.; Rumack, B. H.; Peterson, R. G. Podophyllin poisoning. Systemic toxicity following cutaneous application. Obstet. Gynecol. *52*:94-96, 1978.

Slater, I. H.; Jones, G. T.; Young, W. K. Mode of action of phenaglycodol, a new neurosedative agent. Proc. Soc. Exp. Biol. Med., *93*:528-531, 1956.

Slater, I. H.; Rathbun, R. C.; Henderson, F. G.; Neuss, R. Pharmacological properties of recanescine, a new sedative alkaloid from Rauwolfia canescens linn. Proc. Soc. Exp. Biol. Med., *88*:293-295, 1955.

Smith, C. C. Toxicity of butyl stearate, dibutyl sebacate, dibutyl phthalate, and methoxyethyl oleate. Arch. Ind. Hyg. Occup. Med., 7:310-318, 1953.

Smith, Kline and French Laboratories. Product and overdosage information. Smith, Kline and French Laboratories, Philadelphia, PA, 1963.

Smith, L.; Kruszyna, H.; Smith, R. P. The effect of methemoglobin on the inhibition of cytochrome c oxidase by cyanide, sulfide or azide. Biochem. Pharmacol., 26:2247-2250, 1977.

Smith, L. E.; Siegler, E. H.; Munger, F. Potential new insecticides. J. Econ. Entomol., *29*:1027, 1936.

Smith, M.; Stair, T.; Rolnick, M. A. Butyl nitrite and a suicide attempt. Ann. Intern. Med., *92*:719-720, 1980.

Smith, M. I. The pharmacological action of certain phenol esters, with special reference to the etiology of so-called ginger paralysis. Public Health Repts., No. *45*:2509-2524, 1930.

Smith, M. I. The pharmacologic action of some alcoholic phosphoric esters. Natl. Inst. Health Bull. No. 165 (Part II), 1936.

Smith, M. I.; Elvove, E. Pharmacological and chemical studies of the course of so-called ginger paralysis. Public Health Repts. No. *45*:1703-1716, 1930.

Smith, P. K. Acetophenetidin, A Critical Bibliographic Review. Interscience Publishers, New York, 1958.

Smith, R. B., Jr.; Deichmann, W. B.; Hennigar, G. R.; Finnegan, J. K.; Haag, H. B.; Larson, P. S. Toxicity studies on dichlorophenylbenzene sulfonate. Arch. Int. Pharmacodyn. Ther., *121*:306-317, 1959.

Smith, R. B., Jr.; Finnegan, J. K.; Larson, P. S.; Sahyoun, P. F.; Dreyfuss, M. L.; Haag, H. B. Toxicologic studies on zinc and disodium ethylene bisdithiocarbamates. J. Pharmacol. Exp. Ther., *109*:159-166, 1953b.

Smith, R. L.; Williams, R. T. The metabolism of aryl thioureas. III. (a) The toxicity of hydrogen sulfide in relation to that of phenylthiourea. (b) The protection of rats against the toxic effects of phenylthiourea with 1-methyl-1-phenylthiourea. J. Med. Chem., *4*:137-146, 1961.

Smith, R. P. Cyanate and thiocyanate: Acute toxicity. Proc. Soc. Exp. Biol. Med., 142:1041-1044, 1973a.

Smith, R. P. Toxicology of sodium nitroferricyanide. Pharmacologist, 15:227, 1973b.

Smith, R. P.; Alkaitis, A. A.; Shafer, P. R. Chemically induced methemoglobinemias in the mouse. Biochem. Pharmacol. 16:317–328, 1967.

Smith, R. P.; Gosselin, R. E. Unpublished observations. Dartmouth Medical School, Hanover, N. H., 1963.

Smith, R. P.; Gosselin, R. E. On the mechanism of sulfide inactivation by methemoglobin. Toxicol. Appl. Pharmacol. 8:159-172, 1966.

Smith, R. P.; Layne, W. R. A comparison of the lethal effects of nitrite and hydroxylamine in the mouse. J. Pharmacol. Exp. Ther., 165:30-35, 1969.

Smith, R. P.; Smith, D. M. Acute ipecac poisoning, report of a fatal case and review of the literature. N. Engl. J. Med., 265:523-525, 1961.

Smyth, C. J.; Levey, S.; Lasichak, A. G. The relationship of glutamic and aspartic acids to the production of nausea and vomiting in man. Am. J. Med. Sci., 214:281-285, 1947.

Smyth, H. F., Jr. Personal communication. Mellon Institute, Pittsburgh, 1961.

Smyth, H. F., Jr.; Carpenter, C. P. The place of the range finding test in the industrial toxicology laboratory. J. Ind. Hyg. Toxicol., 26:269-273, 1944.

Smyth, H. F., Jr.; Carpenter, C. P. Further experience with range finding test in industrial toxicology laboratory. J. Ind. Hyg. Toxicol., 30:63-68, 1948.

Smyth, H. F., Jr.; Carpenter, C. P.; Weil, C. S. Range finding toxicity data. List III. J. Ind. Hyg. Toxicol. 31:60-62, 1949.

Smyth, H. F., Jr.; Carpenter, C. P.; Weil, C. S. The toxicology of the polyethylene glycols. J. Am. Pharm. Assoc., Sci. Ed., 39:349-354, 1950.

Smyth, H. F., Jr.; Carpenter, C. P.; Weil, C. S. Range-finding toxicity data: list IV. Arch. Ind. Hyg. Occup. Med., 4:119-122, 1951.

Smyth, H. F., Jr.; Carpenter, C. P.; Weil, C. S. The chronic oral toxicology of the polyethylene glycols. J. Am. Pharm. Assoc. Sci. Ed., 44:27-30, 1955.

Smyth, H. F., Jr.; Carpenter, C. P.; Weil, C. S.; Pozzani, U. C.; Striegel, J. A.; Nycum, J. S. Range-finding toxicity data. VII. Am. Ind. Hyg. Assoc. J. 30:470-476, 1969a.

Smyth, H. F., Jr.; Pozzani, U. C.; Weil, C. S.; Tallant, M. J.; Carpenter, C. P. Experimental toxicity and metabolism of 1,2,6-hexanetriol. Toxicol. Appl. Pharmacol., 15:282-286, 1969c.

Smyth, H. F., Jr.; Seaton, J.; Fischer, L. The single dose toxicity of some glycols and derivatives. J. Ind. Hyg. Toxicol., 23:259-268, 1941a.

Smyth, H. F., Jr.; Seaton, J.; Fischer, L. Some pharmacological properties of the "Tergitol" penetrants. J. Ind. Hyg. Toxicol., 23:478-483, 1941b.

Smyth, H. F., Jr; Carpenter, C. P.; Weil, C. S.; Pozzani, U. C. Range-finding toxicity data; list V. Arch. Ind. Hyg. Occup. Med., 10:61-68, 1954.

Smyth, H. F.; Carpenter, C. P.; Weil, C. S. Toxicologic studies on 3,5-dimethyltetrahydro-1,3,5,2H-thiadiazine-2-thione, a soil fungicide and slimicide. Toxicol. Appl. Pharmacol. 9:521-527, 1966.

Snapper, I.; Saltzman, A. Hippuric acid, cinnamoylglucuronic acid and benzoylglucuronic acid in the urine of normal individuals and in patients with hepatic dysfunction after ingestion of sodium cinnamate. Arch. Biochem., 24:1-8, 1949.

Snell, M. A. Castor bean pomace exposure. Arch. Ind. Hyg. Occup. Med., 6:113-115, 1952.

Snell, N. W.; Savin, L. H. Iodism in which edema glottitis necessitated tracheotomy. Lancet, 1:759-760, 1927.

Snyder, F. H. Personal communication. Procter and Gamble Co., Cincinnati, Ohio, 1964.

Snyder, F. H.; Opdyke, D. L.; Rubenkoenig, H. L. Toxicologic studies on brighteners. Toxicol. Appl. Pharmacol. 5:176-183, 1963.

Snyder, S. H.; Faillace, L.; Hollister, L. 2,5-Dimethoxy-4-methylamphetamine (STP): A new hallucinogenic drug. Science, 158:669-670, 1967b.

Sober, H. A.; Hollander, F.; Sober, E. K. Toxicity of eugenol; determination of LD50 on rats. Proc. Soc. Exp. Biol. Med., 73:148-151, 1950.

Soehring, K.; Scriba, K.; Frahm, M.; Zoellner, G. Beitrage zur Pharmacologie der Alkylpolyathylenoxydderivate. 1. Untersuchungen uber die akute und subchronische Toxizitat bei verschiedenenTierarten. Arch. Int. Pharmacodyn., 87:301-320, 1951.

Sokolova, L. A. Study of the effect of the herbicide 2,4-DM on pregnancy, embryonic development, and gonadal function in white rats. Gig. Sanit. No. 2, 20-23, 1976.

Sollmann, T. Studies of chronic intoxication on albino rats. III. Acetic and formic acids. J. Pharmacol. Exp. Ther., 16:463-474, 1921.

Sollmann, T. A Manual of Pharmacology. 8th Ed., W. B. Saunders Co., Philadelphia, 1957.

Sollmann, T.; Hatcher, R. A. A comparative study of the dosage and effects of chloral hydrate, isopral and bromural on cats. J. A. M. A., 51:487-492, 1908.

Solomon, F. A.; Champagna, F. A. Jaundice due to prochlorperazine (Compazine). Am. J. Med., 27:840-843, 1959.

Solway, R. I. H. Aconite intoxication and myocardial infarction. Conn. State Med. J., 13:727-728, 1949.

Sonawane, B. R.; Knowles, C. O. Comparative metabolism of two carbanilate herbicides (EP-475 and phenmedipham) in rats. Pestic. Biochem. Physiol. 1:472-482, 1971.

Sotos, J. F.; Cutler, E. A.; Finkel, M. A.; Doody, D. Hypocalcemic coma following two pediatric phosphate enemas. Pediatrics, 60:305-307, 1977.

Spark, R.; Goldman, A. S. Diazepam intoxication in a child. Am. J. Dis. Child., 109:128-129, 1965.

Sparschu, G. L.; Dunn, F. L.; Rowe, V. K. Study of the teratogenicity of 2,3,7,8-tetrachloro-dibenzo-p-dioxin in the rat. Food Cosmet. Toxicol., 9:405-412, 1971.

Spaulding, W. B.; Yendt, E. R. Prolonged Vitamin D intoxication in a patient with hypoparathyroidism. Can. Med. J., 90:1049-1054, 1964.

Spealman, C. R.; Main, R. J.; Haag, H. B.; Larson, P. S. Monomeric methyl methacrylate; studies on toxicity. Ind. Med. Surg., 14:292-298, 1945.

Specht, H. Acute response of guinea pigs to inhalation of methyl isobutyl ketone. Public Health Repts., No. 53:292-300, 1938.

Spector, W. S. Handbook of Toxicology. Vol. I, W. B. Saunders Co., Philadelphia, 1955.

Spector, W. S. Handbook of Toxicology. Vol. II. Antibiotics. W. B. Saunders Co., Philadelphia, 1957.

Spencer, E. Y. Guide to the Chemicals Used in Crop Protection. 6th ed., Information Canada, Ottawa, Canada, 1973.

Spencer, H.; Rowe, V.; Adams, E.; Irish, D. Toxicologic studies on the new miticide bis(parachlorophenoxy)methane. Arch. Ind. Hyg. Occup. Med. 1:341, 1950a.

Spencer, H. C.; Rowe, V. K.; McCollister, D. D. Dehydroacetic acid (DHA). I. Acute and chronic toxicity. J. Pharmacol. Exp. Ther., 99:57-68, 1950b.

Spevak, L.; Nadj, V.; Felle, D. Methyl chloride poisoning in four members of a family. Br. J. Ind. Med. 33:272-274, 1976.

Spicer, S. S. Effect of para-aminobenzoic acid in the in vivo oxidation of hemoglobin. J. Ind. Hyg. Toxicol., 31:204-205, 1949.

Spicer, S. S.; Thompson, E. C. Heinz body formation in vivo, a property of methylene blue. J. Ind. Hyg. Toxicol., 31:206-208, 1949.

Spiegel, A. J.; Noseworthy, M. M. Use of nonaqueous solvents in parenteral products. J. Pharm. Sci., 52:917-927, 1963.

Spiotta, E. J. Aldrin poisoning in man. Arch. Ind. Hyg. Occup. Med., 4:560-566, 1951.

Spolyar, L. W.; Harger, R. N.; Keppler, J. F.; Bumsted, H. E. Generation of phosgene during operation of trichloroethylene degreaser. Arch. Ind. Hyg., 4:156-160, 1951.

Srebocan, V.; Plazonic, M.; Pompe-Gotal, J.; Brmalj, V. Biochemical mechanism of the toxicity of triazine herbicides: effect on the gluconeogenic activity in chick liver. Vet. Arh. 45:273-287, 1975.

Srensek, S. E.; Woodward, G. Pharmacological actions of

'endothal' (disodium 3,6-endoxohexahydrophthalic acid). Fed. Prod., 10:337, 1951.

St. John, L. E., Jr.; Lisk, D. J. Metabolism of fenac herbicide in a lactating cow. J. Dairy Sci. 53:161-164, 1970.

St. John, L. E., Jr.; Wagner, D. G.; Lisk, D. J. Fate of atrazine, Kuron, silvex, and 2,4,5-T in the dairy cow. J. Dairy Sci. 47:1267-1270, 1964.

Stadler, F. X.; Herold, R.; Kistler, H. J. Lidocain-Intoxikation. Schweiz. Med. Wochenschr., 109:1941-1945, 1979.

Stalker, N. E.; Gambertoglio, J. G.; Fukumitsu, C. J.; Naughton, J. L.; Benet, L. Z. Acute massive chloral hydrate intoxication treated with hemodialysis: A clinical pharmacokinetic analysis. J. Clin. Pharmacol., 18:136-142, 1978.

Starmer, G. A.; McLean, S.; Thomas, J. Analgesic potency and acute toxicity of substituted anilides and benzamides. Toxicol. Appl. Pharmacol. 19:20-28, 1971.

Stauffer Chemical Co. Technical information sheet (Eptam). New York, 1961a.

Stauffer Chemical Co. Technical information (Betasan). New York, 1964a.

Stauffer Chemical Co. Technical information (Imidan). New York, 1964b.

Stein, A. A.; Kirwan, W. E. Chloracetophenone (tear gas) poisoning: A clinico-pathologic report. J. Forensic Sci., 9:374-382, 1964.

Stein, J.; Smythe, H. A. Nephrotic syndrome induced by penicillamine. Can. Med. Assoc. J., 98:505-507, 1968.

Steinberg, H. H.; Massari, S. C.; Miner, A. C.; Rink, R. Industrial exposure to tellurium: Atmospheric studies and clinical evaluation. J. Ind. Hyg. Toxicol., 24:183-192, 1942.

Steinberg, J. B.; Zeppernick, R. G. Methemoglobinemia during anesthesia. J. Pediatr., 61:885-886, 1962.

Steiner, R. W.; Manoguerra, A. S. Butyl nitrite and methemoglobinemia. Ann. Intern. Med., 92:570, 1980.

Stenger, E. G. Zur Toxikologie des Dimetilan (Dimethylcarbamylmethyl-pyrazolyl-(5)-dimethylcarbamate). Med. Exp., 6:331-338, 1962.

Stenn, F. Alkali disease - selenium poisoning. Arch. Pathol., 22:398-412, 1936.

Stephenson, J. B. P. Zinc phosphide poisoning. Arch. Environ. Health, 15:83-88, 1967.

Sternberg, S. S.; Ferguson, F. C. Colchicine. III. Pathology and hematology in cats and rats. Cancer, 7:607-616, 1954.

Stetsyuk, V. G.; Rotmistrov, M. M. Effect of salicylanilide on the peripheral blood picture in rats. (as cited in Chem. Abs. 75:33609g) Farm. Zh. (Kiev) 26:73-76, 1971.

Stevens, A. R., Jr.; Wolff, H. G. Magnesium intoxication; absorption from the intact gastrointestinal tract. Arch. Neurol. Psychiatr., 63:749-759, 1950.

Stevens, J. L.; Reitnayake, J. H.; Anders, M. W. Metabolism of dihalomethanes to carbon monoxide. IV. Studies in isolated rat hepatocytes. Toxicol. Appl. Pharmacol., 55:484-489, 1980.

Stewart, D. J.; Inaba, T.; Tang, B. K.; Kalew, W. Hydrolysis of cocaine in human plasma by cholinesterase. Life Sci. 20:1557-1564, 1977.

Stewart, R. D. Methyl chloroform intoxication. Diagnosis and treatment. J. A. M. A. 215:1789-1792, 1971.

Stewart, R. D.; Andrews, J. T. Acute intoxication with methylchloroform. J. A. M. A. 195:904-906, 1966.

Stewart, R. D.; Baretta, E. D.; Dodd, H. C.; Torkelson, T. R. Experimental human exposure to vapor of propylene glycol monomethyl ether. Arch. Environ. Health 20:218-223, 1970.

Stewart, R. D.; Dodd, H. C. Absorption of carbon tetrachloride, trichloroethylene, methylene chloride and 1, 1, 1-trichloroethane through the human skin. Am. Ind. Hyg. Assoc. J. 25:439-446, 1964.

Stewart, R. D.; Fisher, T. N.; Hosko, M. J.; Peterson, J. E.; Baretta, E. D.; Dodd, H. C. Experimental human exposure to methylene chloride. Arch. Environ. Health, 25:342-348, 1972.

Stewart, R. D.; Gay, H. H.; Erley, D. S.; Hake, C. L.; Schaffer, A. W. Human exposure to tetrachloroethylene vapor. Arch. Environ. Health, 2:516-522, 1961.

Stewart, R. D.; Gay, H. H.; Schaffer, A. W.; Erley, D. S.; Rowe, V. K. Experimental human exposure to methyl chloroform

vapor. Arch. Environ. Health. 19:467-472, 1969.

Stimson, W. H. Vitamin A intoxication in adults, report of a case with a summary of the literature. N. Engl. J. Med., 265:369-373, 1961.

Stoddart, J. C.; Parkin, J. H.; Wynne, N. A. Orphenadrine poisoning, a case report. Br. J. Anaesth., 40:789-790, 1968.

Stohlman, E. F.; Smith, M. I. Experiments on the pharmacologic action of succinchlorimide. Public Health Rept. No. 59:541-546, 1944.

Storm, H., Jr. Personal communication. Mafco Company, Camden, N. J., November, 1968.

Stossel, T. P. Effect of methylene blue in blood pH, oxygen and carbon dioxide content. Proc. Soc. Exp. Biol. Med., 128:96-97, 1968.

Stoughton, R. W.; Robbins, B. H. The anesthetic properties of tetrahydrofurane. J. Pharmacol. Exp. Ther., 58:171-173, 1936.

Stowe, C. M.; Nelson, R.; Werdin, R.; Fangmann, G.; Fredrick, P.; Weaver, G.; Arendt, T. D. Zinc phosphide poisoning in dogs. J. Am. Vet. Med. Assoc. 173:270, 1978.

Strateva, A. Amide preparations with herbicidal effect. Acute oral poisoning of propachlor. Eksp. Med. Morfol. 13:123-129, 1974.

Strauch, B.; Buch, W.; Grey, W.; Laub, D. Successful treatment of methemoglobinemia secondary to silver nitrate therapy. N. Engl. J. Med., 281:257-258, 1969.

Strauss, N. Hepatotoxic effects following occupational exposure to halowax. Rev. Gastroenterol., 11:381-439, 1944.

Strober, M. Treatment of acute heroin intoxication with nalorphine (Nalline) hydrochloride. J. A. M. A., 154:327-328, 1954.

Strother, A. In vitro metabolism of methylcarbamate insecticides by human and rat liver fraction. Toxicol. Appl. Pharmacol. 21:112-129, 1972.

Strum, J. M.; Karnovsky, M. J. Aminotriazole goiter. Fine structure and localization of thyroid peroxidase activity. Lab. Invest. 24:1-12, 1971.

Stuart Co. Brochure (Softran). Pasadena, Calif, 1960.

Stula, E. F.; Krauss, W. C. Embryotoxicity in rats and rabbits from cutaneous application of amide-type solvents and substituted ureas. Toxicol. Appl. Pharmacol. 41:35-55, 1977.

Sudarsky, R. D. Ocular injury due to formic acid. Arch. Ophthalmol., 74:805-806, 1965.

Sullivan, J. L. Caffeine poisoning in an infant. J. Pediatr., 90:1022-1023, 1977.

Sunderman, F. W., Sr. Efficacy of sodium diethyldithiocarbamate (dithiocarb) in acute nickel carbonyl poisoning. Ann. Clin. Lab. Sci. 9:1-10, 1979.

Sunderman, F. W.; Kincaid, J. F. Nickel poisoning. II. Studies on patients suffering from acute exposure to vapors of nickel carbonyl. J. A. M. A., 155:889-894, 1954.

Sunderman, F. W.; Sunderman, F. W., Jr. Nickel poisoning. VIII. Dithiocarb: a new therapeutic agent for persons exposed to nickel carbonyl. Am. J. Med. Sci., 236:26-31, 1958.

Sutton, R. L. Gentian violet as a therapeutic agent, with notes on a case of gentian violet tatoo. J. A. M. A., 110:1733-1738, 1938.

Svec, C. H. Personal communication. Miller Chemical and Fertilizer Corporation, Hanover, Pa, 1969.

Swarts, C. L. Propoxyphene (Darvon) poisoning. Am. J. Dis. Child., 107:177-179, 1964.

Swiller, A. I.; Swiller, H. E. Metal fume fever. Am. J. Med., 22:173-174, 1957.

Swisher, R. D. Exposure levels and oral toxicity of surfactants. Arch. Environ. Health, 17:232-246, 1968.

Sylbert, P. Personal communication. Lederle Laboratories, Pearl River, NY, 1961.

Szabo, S.; Jaeger, J.; Moslen, M. T.; Reynolds, E. S. Modification of 1, 1-dichloroethylene hepatotoxicity by hypothyroidism. Toxicol. Appl. Pharmacol., 42:367-376, 1977.

Szabo, S.; Reynolds, E. S. Structure-activity relations for ulcerogenic and adrenocorticolytic effects of alkyl nitriles, amines, and thiols. Environ. Health Perspect. 11:135-140, 1975.

Szabo, S.; Selye, H. Adrenal apoplexy and necrosis produced by acrylonitrile. Endokrinologie 57:405-408, 1971.

Szara, S. The comparison of the psychotic effect of tryptamine derivatives with the effects of mescaline and LSD in self-experiments. Psychotropic Drugs, Garattini, S. and Ghetti, V., Ed., pp. 460-467. Elsevier, Amsterdam, 1957, 1957.

Szmant, H. H. Sodium azide in air bags. C & EN., 58:2, 1980.

Tabershaw, I. R.; Fahy, J. P.; Skinner, J. B. Industrial exposure to butanol. J. Ind. Hyg. Toxicol., 26:328, 1944.

Tainter, M. L.; James, M. The pharmacological activity of orthophenylenediamine. Arch. Int. Pharmacodyn. Ther., 36:140-151, 1930.

Talbott, J. H.; Schwab, R. S. Recent advances in the biochemistry and therapeusis of potassium salts. N. Engl. J. Med., 222:585-590, 1940.

Tanowitz, H. B.; Wittner, M. Probable thiabendazole allergy after repeated administration. J. Trop. Med. Hyg. 73:141-142, 1970.

Tansy, M. F.; Kendall, F. M. Update on the toxicity of inhaled methyl methacrylate vapor. Drug Chem. Toxicol. 2:315-330, 1979.

Tarka, S. M.; Zoumas, B. L.; Gans, J. H. Short-term effects of graded levels of theobromine in laboratory rodents. Toxicol. Appl. Pharmacol., 49:127-149, 1979.

Task Force on the Health Effects of non-NTA Detergent Builders. Report to the Great Lakes Science Advisory Board of the International Joint Commission on the Health Implications of non-NTA Detergent Builders. Great Lakes Science Advisory Board, Ontario, Canada, 1981.

Tauscher, J. W.; Polich, J. J. Treatment of pine oil poisoning by exchange transfusion. J. Pediatr., 55:511-515, 1959.

Taussig, H. B. A study of the German outbreak of phocomelia. J. A. M. A., 180:1106-1114, 1962a.

Taussig, H. B. The thalidomide syndrome. Sci. Am., 207:No. 2, 1962b.

Tay, C. -H.; Seah, C. -S. Arsenic poisoning from anti-asthmatic herbal preparations. Med. J. Aust. 2:424-428, 1975.

Taylor, H. D.; Austin, J. H. Toxicity of certain widely used antiseptics. J. Exp. Med., 27:635-646, 1918.

Taylor, J. D.; Richards, R. K.; Wiegand, R. G.; Weinberg, M. S. Toxicological studies with sodium cyclamate and saccharin. Food Cosmet. Toxicol., 6:313-327, 1968.

Taylor, J. M.; Jones, W. I. Metabolism of safrole in the rat. Fed. Proc., 20:432, 1961.

Teehan, B. P.; Maher, J. F.; Carey, J. J. H.; Flynn, P. D.; Schreiner, G. E. Acute ethchlorvynol (Placidyl) intoxication. Ann. Intern. Med., 72:875-882, 1970.

Tephly, T. R.; Hibbeln, P. The effect of cobalt chloride administration on the synthesis of hepatic microsomal cytochrome P-450. Biochem. Biophys. Res. Commun., 42:589-595, 1971.

Tepper, L. B. Manganese. N. Engl. J. Med., 264:347-348, 1961.

Teramoto, S.; Shingu, A.; Shirasu, Y. Induction of dominant-lethal mutations after administration of ethylenethiourea in combination with nitrite or of N-nitroso-ethylenethiourea in mice. Mutat. Res. 56:335-340, 1978.

Ternberg, J. L.; Luce, E. Methemoglobinemia: A complication of the silver nitrate treatment of burns. Surgery, 63:328-330, 1968.

Thayer, P. S.; Palm, P. E. A current assessment of the mutagenic and teratogenic effects of caffeine. CRC Crit. Rev. Toxicol., 3:345-369, 1975.

Thearle, M. H.; Hailey, D. M. Exchange transfusion for diazepam intoxication at birth followed by jejunal stenosis. Proc. Roy. Soc. Med., 66:349-350, 1973.

Theil, G. B.; Richter, R. W.; Powell, M. R.; Doolan, P. D. Acute Dilantin poisoning. Neurology, 11:138-142, 1961.

Thienes, C. H.; Skillen, R. G.; Meredith, O. M.; Fairchild, M. D.; McCandless, R. S.; Thienes, R. P. The hemostatic, laxative and toxic effects of alginic acid preparations. Arch. Int. Pharmacodyn. Ther., 111:167-181, 1957.

Thiess, A. M.; Hey, W.; Hofmann, H. T.; Oettel, H. Zur Toxicitat des Kohlenoxysulfids dargestellt an einer todlich verlaufenen Vergiftung. Arch. Toxikol., 23:253-263, 1968.

Tholen, H.; Metzeler, E. Poisoning with insecticides. Schweiz. Med. Wochenschr. 85:296-299, 1955.

Thomann, P.; Krueger, L. Acute, oral, dermal and inhalation studies. Environ. Qual. Saf., Suppl. 4(Fluoresc. Whitening Agents):193-198, 1975.

Thomas, B. B. Peritoneal dialysis and lysol poisoning. Br. Med. J., 3:720, 1969.

Thomas, D. L. G.; Stiebris, K. Vanadium poisoning in industry. Med. J. Aust., 1:607-609, 1956.

Thomas, E. W. P. Purpuric eruption due to carbromal. Lancet 1:1024, 1958.

Thomas, J. F.; Kesel, R.; Hodge, H. C. Range-finding toxicity tests on propylene glycol in the rat. J. Ind. Hyg. Toxicol., 31:256-257, 1949.

Thomas, J. G. Peppermint fibrillation. Lancet, 1: 222, 1962.

Timme, A. H.; Taljaard, J. J. F.; Shanley, B. C.; Joubert, S. M. Symptomatic porphyria. Part II. Hepatic changes with hexachlorobenzene. S. Afr. Med. J. 48:1833-1836, 1974.

Tjalve, H. Fetal uptake and embryogenetic effects of amino-triazole in mice. Arch. Toxicol. 33:41-48, 1974.

Tobias, J. M. Localization of the site of action of a pulmonary irritant, diphosgene. Am. J. Physiol., 158:173-183, 1949b.

Tobin, J. S. Carbofuran: a new carbamate insecticide. J. Occup. Med. 12:16-19, 1970.

Tocco, D. J.; Rosenblum, C.; Martin, C. M.; Robinson, H. J. Absorption, metabolism, and excretion of thiabendazole in man and laboratory animals. Toxicol. Appl. Pharmacol. 9:31-39, 1966.

Todd, G. C.; Gibson, W. R.; Kehr, C. C. Oral toxicity of tebuthiuron (1-(5-tert-butyl-1,3,4-thiadiazol-2-yl)-1,-3-dimethylurea) in experimental animals. Food Cosmet. Toxicol. 12:461-470, 1974.

Tokareva, T. G.; Turov, I. S.; Allkseev, A. N. Effect of fluoroacetamide on albino mouse fecundity. Zh. Mikrobiol., Epidemiol. Immunobiol. 48:24-26, 1971.

Toland, W. G. Personal communication. Chevron Chemical Company; Richmond, Calif, 1965.

Tonelli, G. Acute toxicity of cortocoids in the mouse. Steroids, 8:857-863, 1966.

Toomey, J. A.; Reichle, H. S.; Takacs, W. S. Effects upon monkeys of sulfapyridine in doses comparable with those used for infants. J. Pediatr. 16:179-190, 1940.

Torkelson, T. R.; Oyen, F.; McCollister, D. D.; Rowe, V. K. Toxicity of 1,1,1-trichloroethane as determined on laboratory animals and human subjects. Am. Ind. Hyg. Assoc. J., 19:353-362, 1958.

Torkelson, T. R.; Oyen, F.; Sadek, S. E.; Rowe, V. K. Preliminary toxicologic studies on nitrogen trifluoride. Toxicol. Appl. Pharmacol., 4:770-781, 1962.

Torkelson, T. R.; Sadek, S. E.; Rowe, V. K.; Kodama, J. K.; Anderson, H. H.; Loquvam, G. S.; Hine, C. H. Toxicologic investigations of 1,2-dibromo-3-chloropropane. Toxicol. Appl. Pharmacol., 3:545-559, 1961.

Tottmar, O.; Lindberg, P. Effects on rat liver acetaldehyde dehydrogenases in vitro and in vivo by coprine, the disulfiram-like constituent of Coprinus atramentarius. Acta Pharmacol. Toxicol., 40:476-481, 1977.

Towers, P. A.; Giuffra, L. J. An unusual reaction following the use of pyribenzamine. N. Y. State J. Med., 50:214-215, 1950.

Towfighi, J.; Gonatas, N. K.; Pleasure, D.; Cooper, H. S.; McCree, L. Glue sniffer's neuropathy. Neurology 26:238-243, 1976.

Tozer, T. N.; Witt, L. D.; Tong, T. G. Evaluation of hemodialysis for ethchlorvynol (Placidyl) overdose. Amer. J. Hosp. Pharm., 31:986-989, 1974.

Treon, J. F. Alcohols. Chap. XXXIV in Patty's Industrial Hygiene and Toxicology, Vol. II, edited by D. D. Irish and D. W. Fassett. 2nd edition, Interscience Publ., New York, 1962.

Treon, J. F.; Cleveland, F. P.; Cappel, J. The toxicity of hexachlorocyclopentadiene. A. M. A. Arch. Ind. Health 11:459-472, 1955.

Treon, J. F.; Crutchfield, W. E., Jr.; Kitzmiller, K. V. The physiological response of rabbits to cyclohexane, methylcyclohexane and certain derivatives of these compounds. I. Oral administration and cutaneous application. J. Ind. Hyg. Toxicol., 25:199, 1943a.

Treon, J. F.; Crutchfield, W. E., Jr.; Kitzmiller, K. V. The physiological response of animals to cyclohexane, methyl cyclohexane and certain derivatives of these compounds. II.

Inhalation. J. Ind. Hyg. Toxicol., *25*:323, 1943b.

Treon, J. F.; Dutra, F. R. Physiological response of experimental animals to the vapor of 2-nitropropane. Arch. Ind. Hyg. Occup. Med., *5*:52-61, 1952.

Treon, J. F.; Kitzmiller, K. V.; Sigmon, H.; Dutra, F. R.; Younkers, W. The physiological response of animals to trichloroacetonitrile administered orally, applied on the skin or inhaled as a vapor in air. J. Ind. Hyg. Toxicol., *31*:235-250, 1949b.

Tso, T. C. Physiology and Biochemistry of Tobacco Plants. Dowden, Hutchinson and Ross, Inc., Stroudsburg, Pa, 1972.

Tsunenari, S. Studies on an organic miticide, Azomite, from forensic toxicological aspects. Nippon Hoigaku Zasshi (Jap. J. Legal Med.) *27*:123-133, 1973.

Tu, J. -B.; Blackwell, R. Q.; Lee, P. -F. DL-Penicillamine as a cause of optic axial neuritis. NAMRU-2 Res. Rep., pp. 1-6, Jan. 8, 1963.

Tubaro, E.; Bulgini, M. J.; Del Grande, P.; Monal, A. Some toxicological aspects of a nicotinamidomethylaminopyrazolone (Ra 101). Arzneim. -Forsch. *20*:1024, 1970.

Tullner, W. W. Uterotrophic action of the insecticide, methoxychlor. Science, *133*:647-648, 1961.

Turner, J. E.; Cravey, R. H. A fatal ingestion of caffeine. Clin. Toxicol., *10*:341-344, 1977.

Turner, J. E.; Richards, R. G. A fatal case involving levorphanol. J. Analyt. Toxicol., *1*:103-104, 1977.

Turner, W. J.; Merlis, S. Effect of some indolealkylamines on man. AMA Arch. Neurol. Psychiatry, *81*:121-129, 1959.

Tusing, T. W.; Paynter, O. E.; Opdyke, D. L. The chronic toxicity of sodium alkylbenzene-sulfonate by food and water administration to rats. Toxicol. Appl. Pharmacol., *2*:464, 1960.

Tusing, T. W.; Paynter, O. E.; Opdyke, D. L.; Snyder, F. H. Toxicologic studies on sodium lauryl glyceryl ether sulfonate and sodium lauryl trioxyethylene sulfate. Toxicol. Appl. Pharmacol., *4*:402-409, 1962.

Tuthill, J. W. G. Malathion poisoning. N. Engl. J. Med., *258*:1018-1019, 1958.

Tye, R.; Engel, D. Distribution and excretion of dicamba by rats as determined by radiotracer technique. J. Agric. Food Chem. *15*:837-840, 1967.

Tyler, V. E., Jr. Indole derivatives in certain North American mushrooms. Lloydia *24*:71-74, 1961.

U. S. Department of Agriculture, Agricultural Research Service. U. S. D. A. Information Memorandum, No. 20. Beltsville, Md, 1966.

U. S. Treasury Department. Formulas for Denatured Alcohol, Part 212 of Title 26, Code of Federal Regulations. Internal Revenue Service Publication 368. Office of the Federal Register, Washington, D. C., 1980.

Uchida, T.; Dauterman, W. C.; O'Brien, R. D. The metabolism of dimethoate by vertebrate tissues. Agric. Food Chem., *12*:48-62, 1964.

Uhde, G. I. Chemical burns of the esophagus. Ann. Otol. Rhinol. Laryngol., *55*:795-820, 1946.

Union Carbide and Carbon Corp. Technical Information. Acrylic Esters. Union Carbide and Carbon Corp., New York, 1955.

Unna, K. Studies on the toxicity and pharmacology of nicotinic acid. J. Pharmacol. Exp. Ther., *65*:95-103, 1939.

Unna, K.; Antopol, W. Toxicity of vitamin B₆. Proc. Soc. Exp. Biol. Med. *43*:116-117, 1940.

Unna, K.; Greslin, J. G. Studies on the toxicity and pharmacology of riboflavin. J. Pharmacol. Exp. Ther. *76*:75-80, 1942.

Upjohn Co., Medical Division. Parvex. Symptoms of and treatment for overdosage of selected Upjohn products. The Upjohn Co., Kalamazoo, Michigan, 1971.

Urwin, C.; Richardson, J. C.; Palmer, A. K. An evaluation of the mutagenicity of the cutting oil preservative Grotan BK. Mutat. Res. *40*:43-46, 1976.

Usdin, E.; Efron, D. H. Psychotropic Drugs and Related Compounds. 2nd ed., DHEW Publ. no. 72-9074, U. S. Gov. Printing Office, Washington, 1972.

Utter, L. G. Personal communication. Diamond Alkali Co., Cleveland, Ohio, 1965.

Vallee, B. L. Biochemistry, physiology and pathology of zinc. Physiol. Rev., *39*:443-490, 1959.

van Haaften, A. B. Acute tetrabromoethane (acetylene tetrabromide) intoxication in man. Amer. Ind. Hyg. Assoc. J. *30*:251-256, 1969.

Van Hoof, F.; Heyndrickx, A. Excretion in urine of four insecticidal carbamates and their phenolic metabolites after oral administration to rats. Arch. Toxicol. *34*:81-88, 1975.

van Ordstrand, H. S.; Hughes, R.; de Nardi, J. M.; Carmody, M. G. Beryllium poisoning. J. Am. Med. Assoc. *129*:1084-1090, 1945.

Van Petigham, C. H.; Heyndrickx, A. M. The β-oxidation of chlorophenoxybutyric acid herbicides in guinea pigs. Bull. Environ. Contam. Toxicol. *14*:632-640, 1975.

Van Stee, E. W.; Back, K. C. Short-term inhalation exposure to bromotrifluoromethane. Toxicol. Appl. Pharmacol., *15*:164-174, 1969.

Vandekar, M.; Plestina, R.; Wilhelm, K. Toxicity of carbamates for mammals. Bull. W. H. O. *44*:241-249, 1971.

Vanderbilt, R. T., Co., Inc. Technical data sheets (Vancide 26 and Vancide 26EC). New York, 1955.

Vanderbilt, R. T., Co., Inc. Technical data sheet (Vancide 20s). New York, 1956.

Vanderbilt, R. T., Co., Inc. Technical data sheets (Vancide 51 and Vancide 51z). New York, 1958.

Vanderbilt, R. T., Co., Inc. Technical data sheet (Nacap). New York, 1961.

Vanderbilt, R. T., Co., Inc. Technical data sheet (Vancide TH). New York, 1978.

Vanderbilt, R. T., Co., Inc. Technical data sheet (Vancide 51Z Dispersion). Norwalk, Ct, August 1976a.

Vanderbilt, R. T., Co., Inc. Technical data sheet (Vancide 51). Norwalk, Ct, December 1974.

Vanderbilt, R. T., Co., Inc. Technical data sheet (Vancide MZ-96). Norwalk, Ct, December 1976b.

Vanderbilt, R. T., Co., Inc. Technical Data Sheet (Vancide PA). Norwalk, Ct, June 1977.

VanDuuren, B. L.; Sivak, A.; Goldschmidt, B. M.; Katz, C.; Melchionne, S. Carcinogenicity of halo-ethers. J. Natl. Cancer Inst. *43*:481-486, 1969.

Varma, P. K.; Persaud, T. V. N. Influence of pyrazole, an inhibitor of alcohol dehydrogenase on the prenatal toxicity of ethanol in the rat. Res. Comm. Chem. Pathol. Pharmacol. *26*:65-73, 1979.

Vaziri, N. D.; Kumar, K. P.; Mirahmadi, K.; Rosen, S. M. Hemodialysis in treatment of acute chloral hydrate poisoning. South. Med. J., *70*:377-378, 1977.

Velsicol Chemical Corp. Information manual 515-1 (EMMI (N-Ethylmercuri-1,2,3,6-tetrahydro-3,6-methano-3,4,5,6,7-hexachlorophthalimide)). Chicago, 1958.

Veltri, J. C.; Temple, A. R. Fenfluramine poisoning. J. Pediatr. *87*:119-121, 1975.

Vernier, V. G.; Harmon, J. B.; Stump, J. M.; Lynes, T. E.; Marvel, J. P.; Smith, D. H. The toxicologic and pharmacologic properties of amantadine hydrochloride. Toxicol. Appl. Pharmacol. *15*:642-665, 1969.

Verrett, M. J.; Mutchler, M. K.; Scott, W. F.; Reynaldo, E. F.; McLaughlin, J. Teratogenic effects of captan and related compounds in the developing chicken embryo. Ann. N. Y. Acad. Sci. *160*:334-343, 1969.

Verschoyle, R. D.; Barnes, J. M. Toxicity of natural and synthetic pyrethrins in rats. Pest. Biochem. Physiol. *2*:308-311, 1972.

Villeneuve, D. The effect of food restriction on the redistribution of HCB in the rat. Toxicol. Appl. Pharmacol. *31*:313-319, 1975.

Villeneuve, D. C.; Panopio. L. G.; Grant, D. L. Placental transfer of hexachlorobenzene in the rabbit. Environ. Physiol. Biochem. *4*:112-115, 1974.

Villeneuve, D. C.; Ritter, L.; Felsky, G.; Norstrom, R. J.; Marino, I. A.; Valli, V. E.; Chu, I.; Becking, G. C. Short-term toxicity of photomirex in the rat. Toxicol. Appl. Pharmacol., *47*:105-114, 1979.

Vincke, E.; Never, H. E. Untersuchungen uber Thromboseprophylaxe mit organischen Salzen seltener Erden. z. f. d. Gesamte Exp. Med. (Heidelberg) *113*:536, 1944.

Vineland Chemical Co. Report from Hazelton Laboratories (Octyl ammonium metharsonate). Vineland, N. J, 1958.

Vishnevskaya, G. I. Toxicity of diphenamid. Gig. Toksikol. Pestits. Klin. Otravlenii. No. 4, p. 247-248, 1966.

Vogel, S. N.; Sultan, T. R.; Ten Eyck, R. P. Cyanide poisoning. Clin. Toxicol., 18:367-383, 1981.

Vohland, H. -W.; Hadisoemarto, S.; Wanke, B. Zur Toxikologie von Carbromal. Arch. Toxicol. 36:31-42, 1976.

Voitenko, G. A.; Medved, I. L. Effect of some thiocarbamates on the generative function. Gig. Sanit., No. 7, p. 111-114, 1973.

Vojtechovsky, M.; Vitek, V.; Rysanek, K.; Bultasova, H. Psychotogenic and hallucinogenic properties of large doses of benactyzine. Experientia 14:422, 1958.

von Eickstedt, K. W.; Rahman, S. Psychopharmakologische wirkung von valepotriaten. Arzneim. -Forsch. 19:316-319, 1969.

von Muhlendahl, K. E.; Krienke, E. G. Fenfluramine poisoning. Clin. Toxicol., 14:97-106, 1979.

von Oettingen, W. F. Toxicity and potential dangers of aliphatic and aromatic hydrocarbons. Public Health Bull. No. 255, 1940.

von Oettingen, W. F. The aromatic amino and nitro compounds, their toxicity and potential dangers. U. S. Public Health Serv. Public Health Bull. No. 271, 1941b.

von Oettingen, W. F. Aliphatic alcohols: their toxicity and potential dangers in relation to their constitution and their fate in metabolism. Public Health Bull. No. 281, 1943.

von Oettingen, W. F. Effects of aliphatic nitrous and nitric acid esters on the physiological functions with special reference to their chemical constitution. Natl. Insts. Health Bull. No. 186, 1946b.

von Oettingen, W. F. The toxicity and potential dangers of zinc phosphide and of hydrogen phosphide. Public Health Repts. Suppl. No. 203, 1947.

von Oettingen, W. F. Phenol and its derivatives: the relation between their chemical constitution and their effect on the organism. Natl. Insts. Health Bull. No. 190, 1949.

von Oettingen, W. F. The Halogenated Hydrocarbons, Toxicity and Potential Dangers. Public Health Service Publication No. 414, U. S. Government Printing Office, Washington, D. C, 1955.

von Oettingen, W. F.; Powell, C. C.; Sharpless, N. E.; Alford, W. C.; Pecora, L. J. Relation between the toxic action of chlorinated methanes and their chemical and physiochemical properties. Natl. Insts. Health Bull. No. 191, 1949.

Vos, J. G.; Koeman, J. H. Comparative toxicologic study with polychlorinated biphenyls in chickens with special reference to porphyria, edema formation, liver necrosis and tissue residues. Toxicol. Appl. Pharmacol., 17:656-668, 1970.

Vos, J. G.; Koeman, J. H.; Van Der Maas, H. G.; Ten Noever De Braun, M. C.; De Vos, R. H. Identification and toxicological evaluation of chlorinated dibenzofuran and chlorinated naphthalene in two commercial polychlorinated biphenyls. Food Cosmet. Toxicol., 8:625-633, 1970.

Vrochinskii, K. K.; Perlovskaya, E. D.; Kazachuk, Yu. S. Functional and morphological alterations occurring in warm-blooded animals in fenuron poisoning. Farmakol. Toksikol. (Moscow) 37:604-607, 1974.

Wachstein, M. Fatal bismuth poisoning in the course of antisyphilitic treatment. Am. J. Clin. Pathol., 14:392-398, 1944.

Waddell, W. J.; Butler, T. C. The distribution and excretion phenobarbital. J. Clin. Invest. 36:1217-1226, 1957.

Wald, M. H.; Lindberg, H. A.; Barker, M. H. The toxic manifestations of the thiocyanates. J. A. M. A., 112:1120-1124, 1939.

Walker, A. I. T.; Brown, V. K. H.; Kodama, J. K.; Thorpe, E.; Wilson, A. B. Toxicological studies with the 1, 3, 5-triazine herbicide cyanazine. Pestic. Sci. 5:153-159, 1974.

Walker, C. Dangerous symptoms after injections of heroin (diamorphine). Br. Med. J., 1:619, 1949.

Wallace Laboratories. Brochure (Soma, pharmacology and toxicity). New Brunswick, N. J, 1958.

Waller, R. L. Methanethiol inhibition of mitochondrial respiration. Toxicol. Appl. Physiol., 42:111-117, 1977.

Wallgren, H. Relative intoxicating effects on rats of ethyl, propyl and butyl alcohols. Acta Pharmacol. Toxicol., 16:217-222, 1960.

Walpole, A. L.; Roberts, D. C.; Rose, F. L.; Hendry, J. A.; Homer, R. F. Cytotoxic agents. IV. The carcinogenic actions of some monofunctional ethyleneimine derivatives. Br. J. Pharmacol., 9:306-323, 1954.

Walters, M. N. I. Malathion intoxication. Med. J. Aust., 1:876-877, 1957.

Walton, D. C.; Kehr, E. F.; Loevenhart, A. S. A comparison of the pharmacological action of diacetone alcohol and acetone. J. Pharmacol. Exp. Ther., 33:175-183, 1928.

Walton, R.; Lawson, E. H. Pharmacology and toxicology of the azo dye, phenyl-azo-alpha, alpha-diaminopyridine. J. Pharmacol. Exp. Ther., 51:200, 1934.

Wander, H. J.; Pascoe, D. J. Phenylazopyridine hydrochloride poisoning, report of case and review of literature. Am. J. Dis. Child., 110:105-107, 1965.

Wanntorp, H. Studies on chemical determination of warfarin and coumachlor and their toxicity for dog and swine. Acta Pharmacol. Toxicol., 16:Suppl. 2, 1959.

Ward, D. J. Fatal hypernatraemia after a saline emetic. Br. Med. J., 2:432, 1963.

Ware, G. W.; Good, E. E. Effects of insecticides in reproduction in the laboratory mouse. II. Mirex, telodrin and DDT. Toxicol. Appl. Pharmacol., 10:54-61, 1967.

Waring, J. I. Sedation as an unexpected systemic effect of Privine. J. A. M. A., 129:129-130, 1945.

Waritz, R. S.; Aftosmis, J. G.; Culik, R.; Dashiell, O. L.; Faunce, M. M.; Griffith, F. D.; Hornberger, C. S.; Lee, K. P.; Sherman, H.; Tayfun, F. O. Toxicological evaluations of some brominated biphenyls. Am. Ind. Hyg. Assoc. J. 38:307-322, 1977.

Warrander, A.; Waring, R. H. The metabolism of mebenil in rats, rabbits and guinea pigs. Pestic. Sci. 8:54-58, 1977.

Warren, M. R.; Becker, T. J.; Marsh, D. G.; Shelton, R. S. Pharmacological and toxicological studies on cetylpyridinium chloride, a new germicide. J. Pharmacol. Exp. Ther., 74:401-408, 1942.

Warren, M. R.; Thompson, C. R.; Werner, H. W. Pharmacological studies on the hypnotic, 2-ethyl-3-propylglycidamide. J. Pharmacol. Exp. Ther., 96:209-212, 1949.

Wartiz, R. S.; Brown, R. M. Acute and subacute inhalation toxicities of phosphine, phenylphosphine and triphenylphosphine. Am. Ind. Hyg. Assoc. J., 36:452-458, 1975.

Waser, P. G. The pharmacology of Amanita muscaria. In: Ethnopharmacologic Search for Psychoactive Drugs, edited by D. Efron, B. Holmstedt and N. Kline. Proceedings of symposium held in San Francisco, 1967, pp. 419-439, 1967.

Wason, S.; Detsky, A. S.; Platt, O. S.; Lovejoy, F. H. Isobutyl nitrite toxicity by ingestion. Ann. Intern. Med., 92:637-639, 1980.

Wason, S.; Lacouture, P. G.; Lovejoy, F. H. Single high-dose pyridoxine treatment for isoniazid overdose. J. A. M. A., 246:1102-1104, 1981.

Waterhouse, C.; Stern, E. A. Metabolic-acidosis occurring during administration of paraldehyde. Am. J. Med., 23:987-989, 1957.

Waters, E. M.; Gerstner, H. B.; Huff, J. E. Trichloroethylene I. An impact overview. National Technical Information Service, Document No. ORNL/TIRC-7612. U. S. Dept. of Commerce, Springfield, Virginia, 1976.

Watrous, R. M.; Schulz, H. N. Cyclohexylamine, p-chloronitrobenzene, 2-aminopyridine: Toxic effects in industrial use. Ind. Med. Surg., 19:317-320, 1950.

Way, W. G.; Morgan, D. L.; Sutton, L. E. Hypertension and hypercalcemic nephropathy due to vitamin D intoxication. Pediatrics, 21:59-69, 1958.

Wear, J. B., Jr.; Shanahan, R.; Ratliff, R. K. Toxicity of ingested hexachlorophene. J. A. M. A., 181:587-589, 1962.

Weatherby, J. H.; Clements, E. L. Concerning synergism between paraldehyde and ethyl alcohol. Q. J. Stud. Alcohol, 21:394-399, 1960.

Webb, R. E.; Hartgrove, R. W.; Randolph, W. C.; Petrella, V. J.; Horsfall, F., Jr. Toxicity studies in endrin-susceptible and resistant strains of pine mice. Toxicol. Appl. Pharmacol., 25:42-47, 1973.

Webster, J. D.; Parker, T. F.; Alfrey, A. C.; Smythe, W. R.; Kubo, H.; Neal, G.; Hull, A. R. Acute nickel intoxication by dialysis. Ann. Intern. Med. 92:631-633, 1980.

Webster, R. W. Legal Medicine and Toxicology. W. B. Saunders Co., Philadelphia, 1930.

Webster, S. H. Volatile hydrides of toxicological importance. J. Ind. Hyg. Toxicol. 28:167-182, 1946.

Weed Society of America. Herbicide Handbook. W. F. Humphrey Press, Inc., Geneva, NY, 1967.

Weidenbach, C. P.; Radeleff, R. D.; Buck, W. B. Toxicologic studies of Ruelene. J. Am. Vet. Med. Assoc., 140:460-463, 1962.

Weightman, J.; Hoyle, J. P. Accidental exposure to ethylenimine and N-ethylethylenimine vapors. J. A. M. A., 189:543-545, 1964.

Weikel, J. H.; Bartek, M. J. Toxicologic properties and metabolic fate of haloprogin, an antifungal agent. Toxicol. Appl. Pharmacol. 22:375-386, 1972.

Weil, C. S.; Woodside, M. D.; Smyth, H. F., Jr.; Carpenter, C. P. Results of feeding propylene glycol in the diet to dogs for two years. Fd. Cosmet. Toxicol., 9:479-490, 1971.

Weill, H.; Waddell, L. C.; Ziskind, M. A study of workers exposed to detergent enzymes. J. A. M. A. 217:425-433, 1971.

Weinberger, M. A.; Friedman, L.; Farber, T. M.; Moreland, F. M.; Peters, E. L.; Gilmore, C. E.; Khan, M. A. Testicular atrophy and impaired spermatogenesis in rats fed high levels of the methylxanthines caffeine, theobromine, or theophylline. J. Environ. Pathol. Toxicol., 1:669-688, 1978.

Weintraub, S. Stramonium poisoning. Postgrad. Med., 28:364-366, 1960.

Weisdorf, D.; Kramer, J.; Goldborg, A.; Klawans, H. L. Physostigmine for cardiac and neurologic manifestations of phenothiazine poisoning. Clin. Pharmacol. Ther., 24:663-667, 1978.

Weiss, A. J.; Mancall, E. L.; Koltes, J. A.; White, J. C.; Jackson, L. G. Dimethylacetamide: A hitherto unrecognized hallucinogenic agent. Science 136:151-152, 1962.

Weiss, A. S.; Markenson, J. A.; Weiss, M. S.; Kammerer, W. H. Toxicity of D-penicillamine in rheumatoid arthritis. A report of 63 patients including two with aplastic anemia and one with the nephrotic syndrome. Am. J. Med. 64:114-120, 1978a.

Weiss, L. R. The cardiotoxicity of neuroleptic and tricyclic antidepressant drugs. In Cardiac Toxicology., Vol. II (Tibor Balazs, ed.). CRC Press Inc. Boca Raton, Florida, pp. 125-143, 1981.

Weiss, W.; Moser, R. L.; Auerbach, O. Lung cancer in chloromethyl ether workers. Am. Rev. Respir. Dis. 120:1031-1037, 1979.

Welch, M. J.; Correa, G. A. PCP intoxication in young children and infants. Clin. Pediatr. 19:510-514, 1980.

Welch, T. R.; Rumack, B. H.; Hammond, K. Clonazepam overdose resulting in cyclic coma. Clin. Toxicol., 10:433-436, 1977.

Wellborn, S. N. Health hazards in woodworking. Simple precautions minimize risks. Fine Woodworking, 4 pp, Winter 1977.

Weller, R. W.; Crellin, A. J. Pulmonary granulomatosis following extensive use of paradichlorobenzene. Arch. Intern. Med., 91:408-413, 1953.

Wenzl, J. E.; Burke, E. C. Poisoning from a malathion aerosol mixture. J. A. M. A., 182:495-507, 1962.

Werner, H. W.; Dunn, R. C.; von Oettingen, W. F. The acute effects of cumene vapors in mice. J. Ind. Hyg. Toxicol., 26:264, 1944.

Werner, H. W.; Mitchell, J. L.; Miller, J. W.; von Oettingen, W. F. The acute toxicity of vapors of several monoalkyl ethers of ethylene glycol. J. Ind. Hyg. Toxicol., 25:157-163, 1943a.

Werner, H. W.; Mitchell, J. L.; Miller, J. W.; von Oettingen, W. F. Effects of repeated exposure of dogs to monoalkyl ethylene glycol ether vapors. J. Ind. Hyg. Toxicol., 25:409-414, 1943c.

Werner, H. W.; Nawrocki, C. Z.; Mitchell, J. L.; Miller, J. W.; von Oettingen, W. F. Effects of repeated exposures of rats

to vapors or monoalkyl ethylene glycol ethers. J. Ind. Hyg. Toxicol., 25:374-379, 1943b.

Wertelecki, W.; Vietti, T. J.; Kulapongs, P. Cantharidin poisoning from ingestion of a "blister beetle". Pediatrics, 39:287-289, 1967.

West, B.; Vidone, L. B.; Shaffer, C. B. Acute and subacute toxicity of dimethoate. Toxicol. Appl. Pharmacol., 3:210-223, 1961.

West, H. D.; Lawson, J. R.; Miller, I. H.; Mathura, G. R. The fate of diphenyl in the rat. Arch. Biochem. Biophys. 60:14, 1956.

Whetsonte, R. R.; Phillips, D. D.; Sun, Y. P.; Ward, L. F., Jr.; Shellenberger, T. E. 2-Chloro-1-(2,4,5-trichlorophenyl)vinyl dimethyl phosphate, a new insecticide with low toxicity to mammals. J. Agric. Food Chem., 14:352, 1966.

White, J. F.; Carlson, G. P. Influence of alterations in drug metabolism on spontaneous and epinephrine-induced cardiac arrhythmias in animals exposed to trichloroethylene. Toxicol. Appl. Pharmacol., 47:515-527, 1979.

White, L. P.; Shimkin, M. B. Effects of D, L-ethionine in six patients with neoplastic disease. Cancer, 7:867-872, 1954.

White, N. G. Personal communication. Shell Oil Co., New York, 1955.

White, P. D.; Balboni, G. M.; Viko, L. E. Clinical observations on the digitalis-like action of squill. J. A. M. A., 75:971-976, 1920.

Wiegand, C. G.; Eckler, C. R.; Chen, K. K. Action and toxicity of vitamin B_6 hydrochloride. Proc. Soc. Exp. Biol. Med. 44:147-151, 1940.

Wieland, T. Poisonous principles of mushrooms of the genus Amanita. Science 159:946-952, 1968.

Wieland, T.; Motzel, W.; Merz, H. Uber das Vorkommen von Bufotenine im gelben Knollenblatterpilz. Ann. Chem. 581:10-16, 1953.

Wieland, T.; Wieland, O. Chemistry and toxicology of Amanita phalloides. Pharmacol. Rev. 11:87-107, 1959.

Wikinski, J. A.; Usubiaga, J. E.; Wikinski, R. W. Cardiovascular and neurological effects of 4,000 mg of procaine. J. A. M. A. 213:621-623, 1970.

Wikler, A.; Fraser, H. F.; Isbell, H. N-Allylnormorphine. Effects of single doses and precipitation of acute "abstinence syndromes" during addiction to morphine, methadone or heroin in man (post addicts). J. Pharmacol. Exp. Ther. 109:8-20, 1953.

Wilkins, J. W., Jr.; Greene, J. A., Jr.; Weller, J. M. Toxicity of intraperitoneal bisulfite. Clin. Pharmacol. Ther., 9:328-332, 1968.

Wilkinson, C. F. Insecticide Biochemistry and Physiology. Plenum Press, New York, 1976.

Willhite, C. C. Inhalation toxicology of acute exposure to aliphatic nitriles. Clin. Toxicol., 18:991-1003, 1981a.

Willhite, C. C.; Ferm, V. H.; Smith, R. P. Teratogenic effects of aliphatic nitriles. Teratology, 23:317-323, 1981c.

Willhite, C. C.; Smith, R. P. The role of cyanide liberation in the acute toxicity of aliphatic nitriles. Toxicol. Appl. Pharm., 59:589-602, 1981b.

Williams, J. W. Personal communication. du Pont Chemical Co., Wilmington, Del, 1959a.

Williams, M. W. Acute and subacute toxicity of trithion and the dimethyl homolog. Toxicol. Appl. Pharmacol., 3:500-508, 1961.

Williams, M. W.; Baker, R. D.; Couill, R. W. Blood cholinesterase inhibition after dermal absorption of two organophosphorus agents. Toxicol. Appl. Pharmacol., 4:271-275, 1962.

Williams, N.; Smith, F. K. Polymer-fume fever. J. A. M. A., 219:1587-1589, 1972.

Williamson, R. L.; Metcalf, R. L. Salicylanilides; a new group of active uncouplers of oxidative phosphorylation. Science 158:1694-1695, 1967.

Willimott, S. G.; Freiman, M. Potassium permanganate poisoning. Br. Med. J., 1:58-59, 1936.

Wilson, J. W.; Levitt, H.; Harris, T. L.; Heiligman, E. M. Toxic encephalopathy occuring during topical therapy with asterol. J. A. M. A., 150:1002-1004, 1952.

Wilson, R.; Lovejoy, F. H., Jr.; Jaeger, R. J.; Landrigan, P. L.

Acute phosphine poisoning aboard a grain freighter. J. A. M. A., *244*:148-150, 1980.

Wilson, R. H.; Brumley, D. R. Health hazards in the use of tetrachloroethane. Ind. Med. Surg., *13*:233-234, 1944.

Winek, C. L.; Butala, J.; Shanor, S. P.; Fochtman, F. W. Toxicology of poinsettia. Clin. Toxicol. *13*:27-45, 1978.

Winek, C. L.; Collom, W. D.; Wecht, C. H. Codeine fatality from cough syrup. Clin. Toxicol., *3*:97-100, 1970.

Winek, C. L.; Collum, W. D.; Martineau, P. Toluidine blue intoxication. Clin. Toxicol., 2:1-3, 1969.

Winek, C. L.; Fochtman, F. W.; Shanor, S. P.; McClain, R. M.; Davis, E. R. Acute and subacute toxicology and safety evaluation of hexahydro-1,3,5-triethyl-s-triazine. Drug Chem. Toxicol. *1*:1-18, 1977.

Winter, C. A.; Flataker, L. Toxicity studies on noscapine. Toxicol. Appl. Pharmacol., *3*:96-106, 1961.

Winter, J. C. Propranolol and morphine: a lethal interaction. Arch. Intern. Pharm. Ther., *212*:195-198, 1974.

Winters, W. D.; Spector, E.; Wallach, D. P.; Shideman, F. E. Metabolism of thiopental-S^{35} and thiopental-2-C^{14} by a rat liver mince and identification of pentobarbital as a major metabolite. J. Pharmacol. Exp. Ther. *114*:343-357, 1955.

Winthrop Laboratories. Brochure (Trancopal). New York, 1959.

Wirtschafter, Z. T.; Wolpaw, R. A case of nitrobenzene poisoning. Ann. Intern. Med., *21*:135-140, 1944.

Witthaus, R. A. Manual of Toxicology. Wm. Wood & Co., New York, 1911.

Wokes, F. Antiseptic value and toxicity of menthol isomers. Q. J. Pharm. Pharmacol., *5*:233-244, 1932.

Wolf, I. J. Fatal poisoning with oil of chenopodium in a negro child with sickle cell anemia. Arch. Pediatr., *52*:126-130, 1935.

Wolf, M. Personal communication. Dow Chemical Co., Midland, Mich, 1976.

Wolf, M. A. Personal communication. Dow Chemical Co., Midland, Mich, 1967.

Wolf, M. A.; Rowe, V. K.; McCollister, D. D.; Hollingsworth, R. L.; Ogen, F. Toxicological studies of certain alkylated benzenes and benzene. Arch. Ind. Health *14*:387-398, 1956.

Wolff, F. W.; Parmley, W. W.; White, K.; Okun, R. Drug-induced diabetes. J. A. M. A., *185*:568-574, 1963.

Wolff, H.; Doring, G. Methamoglobinamie durch Vergiftung mit aromatischen Nitroverbindungen. Arch. Kinderheilk., *163*:166-170, 1960.

Wolff, J. A. Methemoglobinemia due to benzocaine. Pediatrics, *20*:915, 1957.

Wolfson, S.; Olney, M. B. Accidental ingestion of a toxic dose of chlorambucil, report of a case in a child. J. A. M. A., *165*:239-240, 1957.

Woodard, W. K.; Miller, L. J.; Legant, O. Acute and chronic hypervitaminosis in a 4-month-old infant. J. Pediatr., *59*:260-264, 1961.

Woodbury, J. W. Asthmatic syndrome following exposure to tolylene diisocyanate. In. . Med. Surg., *25*:540-543, 1956.

Woods, L. A. The pharmacology of nalorphine (*N*-allylnormorphine). Pharmacol. Rev. *8*:175-198, 1956.

Woods, L. A.; Shideman, F. E.; Seevers, M. H., ; Weeks, J. R.; Kruse, W. T. Dehydroacetic acid (DHA)., III. Estimation, absorption and distribution. J. Pharmacol. Exp. Ther., *99*:84-97, 1950.

Woodward, G.; Calvery, H. O. Toxicological properties of surface-active agents. Proc. Sci. Sect. Toilet Goods Assoc., No. 3, 1945.

Woodward, G.; Hagan, E. C.; Radomski, J. L. Toxicity of hydroquinone for laboratory animals. Fed. Proc., *8*:348, 1949.

Woodward, G.; Johnson, V. D.; Nelson, A. A. Acute toxicity of 2-methyl-2, 4-pentanediol. Fed. Proc., *4*:142-143, 1945.

Woodward, G.; Lange, S. W.; Nelson, K. W.; Calvery, H. O. The acute oral toxicity of acetic, chloracetic, dichloracetic and trichloracetic acids. J. Ind. Hyg. Toxicol., *23*:78-81, 1941.

Worth, H. M. Toxicologic evaluation of benefin and trifluralin. Pestic. Symp., Collect. Pap. Inter-Amer. Conf. Toxicol. Occup. Med., 6th, 7th 1968-1970, p. 263-267, 1970.

Worth, H. M.; Anderson, R. C. Toxicological studies with trifluralin and metabolites. Pharmacologist, 7:150, 1965.

Worthing, C. R. Pesticide Manual, 6th ed. British Crop Protection Council, Worcestershire, England, 1979.

Wright, F. C.; Riner, J. C.; Palmer, J. S.; Schlinke, J. C. Metabolic and residue studies with 2-(2,4,5-trichlorophenoxy)ethyl 2, 2-dichloropropionate (erbon) herbicide in sheep. J. Agric. Food Chem. *18*:845-847, 1970.

Wright, I. S.; Littaur, D. Lobeline sulfate. Its pharmacology and use in the treatment of the tobacco habit. J. A. M. A., *109*:649-654, 1937.

Wright, W. H.; Brady, F. J. Studies on oxyuriasis. XXII. The efficacy of gentian violet in the treatment of pinworm infestation. J. A. M. A., *114*:861-866, 1940.

Wright, W. H.; Schaffer, J. M. Critical anthelmintic tests of chlorinated alkyl hydrocarbons and a correlation between the anthelmintic efficacy, chemical structure and physical properties. Am. J. Hyg., *16*:325-428, 1932.

Wyeth Laboratories. Brochure (Management of overdoses of promazine). Philadelphia, 1956.

Wyeth Laboratories. Brochure (Phenergan hydrochloride). Wyeth Laboratories, Philadelphia, 1958b.

Wyeth Laboratories. Brochure (Largon). Philadelphia, 1960.

Wylie, D. W.; Archer, S.; Arnold, A. Augmentation of pharmacological properties of catecholamines by O-methyl transferase inhibitors. J. Pharmacol. Exp. Ther., *130*:239-244, 1960.

Yamamoto, K.; Tajima, K.; Mizutani, T. The acute toxicity of butylated hydroxytoluene and its metabolites in mice. Toxicol. Lett., *6*:173-175, 1980.

Yamamura, Y. *n*-Hexane polyneuropathy. Folia Psychiatr. Neurol. Jpn. *23*:45-57, 1969.

Yang, R. S. H.; Coulston, F.; Golberg, L. Binding of hexachlorobenzene to erythrocytes: species variation. Life Sci. *17*:545-550, 1975.

Yasuda, M.; Maeda, H. Teratogenic effects of 4-chloro-2-methylphenoxyacetic acid ethylester (MCPEE) in rats. Toxicol. Appl. Pharmacol. *23*:326-333, 1972.

Yllner, S. Metabolism of 1, 2-dichloroethane-^{14}C in the mouse. Acta Pharmacol. Toxicol. *30*:257-265, 1971.

Yodaiken, R. E.; Babcock, J. R. 1, 2-Dichloroethane poisoning. Arch. Environ. Health *26*:281-284, 1973.

Yonkman, F. F.; Stilwell, D.; Jeremias, R. The adrenolytic and sympatholytic actions of yohimbine and ethyl yohimbine. J. Pharmacol. Exp. Ther., *81*:111-115, 1944.

Yoshikawa, H.; Kawai, K. Toxicity of phthalodinitrile and tetrachlorophthalodinitrile. Ind. Health 4:11-15, 1966.

Young, E. G.; Woolner, L. B. A case of fatal poisoning from 2-methoxy ethanol. J. Ind. Hyg. Toxicol. *28*:267-268, 1946.

Young, J. D.; Braun, W. H.; Gehring, P. J.; Horvath, B. S.; Daniel, R. L. 1,4-Dioxane and β-hydroxyethoxyacetic acid excretion in urine of humans exposed to dioxane vapors. Toxicol. Appl. Pharmacol. *38*:643-646, 1976.

Younger, R. L.; Radeleff, R. D. The toxicologic and pathologic effects of three insect chemosterilants in sheep. Ann. N. Y. Acad. Sci., 111:Art. 2, p. 715-728, 1964.

Zadikoff, C. M. Toxic encephalopathy associated with the use of insect repellant. J. Pediatr. *95*:140-142, 1979.

Zaks, A.; Jones, T.; Fink, M.; Freedman, A. Treatment of opiate dependence with high dose oral naloxone. J. A. M. A., *215*:2108-2110, 1971.

Zapp, J. A., Jr. Hazards of isocyanates in polyurethane foam plastic production. Arch. Ind. Med., *15*:324-330, 1957.

Zapp, J. A. Personal communication. E. I. du Pont de Nemours Co., Wilmington, Del, 1956.

Zavon, M. R. Methylcellosolve intoxication. Am. Ind. Hyg. Assoc. J. *24*:36-41, 1963.

Zbinden, G.; Bagdon, R. E.; Keith, E. F.; Phillips, R. D.; Randall, L. O. Experimental and clinical toxicology of chlordiazepoxide (Librium). Toxicol. Appl. Pharmacol., *3*:619-637, 1961.

Zeidman, I.; Deutl, R. Poisoning by hydroquinone and monomethylparaaminophenol sulfate; report of 2 cases of autopsy findings. Am. J. Med. Sci., *210*:328-333, 1945.

Zeligs, M. A. Upper motor neuron sequelae in "Jake" paralysis; a clinical followup study. J. Ner. Mental Dis., *87*:464-470,

1938.

Zeller, H.; Hofmann, H. T.; Meinecke, K. H.; Oettel, H. Zur Toxicitat von Tetrahydrofuran. Nauyn. Schmiedebergs Arch. Pharmakol., *247*:359-360, 1964.

Zelman, S.; Guillan, R. Heat stroke in phenothiazine-treated patients: A report of three fatalities. Am. J. Psychiatry, *126*:1787-1790, 1970.

Zenz, C.; Bartlett, J. P.; Thiede, W. H. Acute vanadium pentoxide intoxication. Arch. Environ. Health, *5*:542-546, 1962.

Zer, M.; Chaimoff, C.; Dintsman, M. Spontaneous rupture of the stomach following ingestion of sodium bicarbonate. Arch. Surg., *101*:532-533, 1970.

Zerbst, G. H. Unusual hazard in a fertilizer factory. Ind. Med. Surg., *13*:552, 1944.

Zetzel, L.; Kaplan, H. Liver damage concurrent with iproniazid administration. N. Engl. J. Med., *258*:1209-1211, 1958.

Zieve, L.; Doizaki, W. M.; Zieve, F. J. Synergism between mercaptans and ammonia or fatty acids in the production of coma: a possible role for mercaptans in the pathogenesis of hepatic coma. J. Lab. Clin. Med. *83*:16-28, 1974.

Zileli, M. S.; Teletar, F.; Deniz, S.; Ilter, E.; Adalar, N. Pseudohyperosmolar non-ketoacedotic coma due to oxazepam intoxication. Clin. Toxicol., *5*:337-341, 1972.

Zilm, D. H. Naloxone response in non-dependent man: effect on six physiological variables. Neuropharmacology, *19*:591-595, 1980.

Zipe, K. E.; Arndt, T.; Heintz, R. Klinische Beobactungen bei einer Phostoxin-Vergiftung. Arch. Toxicol. *22*:209-222, 1967.

Zipf, H. F.; Kreppel, E. Langanhaltende Endoanaesthesie durch Dodecyl polyathylenoxydather. Arch. exper. Path. u. Pharmakol. *226*:340-347, 1955.

Zuck, D. Case of pethidine sensitivity. Brit. Med. J. *1*:125, 1951.

SECTION III
Therapeutics Index

CONTENTS

INTRODUCTION AND EXPLANATION

Section III summarizes clinical and experimental data on 85 compounds (or classes of compounds) which in Section II are named "reference congeners" because each typifies toxicologically a group of related substances. This section stresses toxic signs and symptoms ("Symptomatology") and recommended programs of therapy ("Treatment"). That the identity of the offending toxic agent is established is implicit here.

As elsewhere, the emphasis is on acute poisonings of nonindustrial origin; in some instances subacute and chronic intoxications are described. Allergic reactions receive only casual mention, although they constitute a large and important class of clinical cases. With medicinal chemicals no attempt is made here to record the numerous minor "untoward reactions" encountered when drugs are used in the customary doses. Section III concerns primarily syndromes of frank overdosage, as revealed in accidental, willful, suicidal, and homicidal poisonings. Within these restrictions, parenteral routes of administration are seldom involved. Ingestion, inhalation, and percutaneous absorption are the usual modes of poisoning described here.

Under "Symptomatology" toxic signs and symptoms are grouped into convenient categories and arranged in a sequence. The order is intended to describe approximately the succession of clinical events during progressive intoxication. Since only the severest poisonings reach terminal stages, these lists are useful as scales of reference and as guides for prognosis. In an analogous way, the order of listing under "Treatment" implies a system of priorities which is believed to be appropriate for cases of severe poisoning.

Unless specified otherwise, all doses (both toxic and therapeutic) refer to an adult of average size (70 kg. or 150 lb). When scaled to the correct body weight, most of these doses are believed to be appropriate to the very young and the very old. Recognized exceptions are specified in the text. Physicians with experience in pediatrics and in geriatrics are probably aware of other exceptions to the body weight rule and may prefer other empirical methods for translating doses. For details of supportive treatment, Section IV should be consulted (see specific page references in the text).

At the conclusion of each congener summary, useful references are listed. Many of the literature citations are intended for the physician who seeks more detailed clinical information. Case histories reported in the recent medical literature are well represented. Earlier clinical experience is summarized by various standard reference manuals which are also listed. Some of the references are concerned exclusively with observations on experimental animals; these are invaluable sources of toxicity data where clinical experience is inadequate or nonexistent. In many cases laboratory reports are also the only sources of information about the mechanism of poisoning and therefore the rationale of treatment. Although no attempt was made to provide an exhaustive compilation of the toxicological literature or to document every statement in the text, the increasing use of this reference book by professional toxicologists and allied scientists has led us to expand the bibliography considerably.

ACETAMINOPHEN

Acetaminophen (N-acetyl-p-aminophenol, APAP, paracetamol) is a popular analgesic-antipyretic drug, which is available without prescription in many countries including the United States. It is essentially devoid of anti-inflammatory and uricosuric activity, but it is otherwise similar to aspirin in its potency and therapeutic indications. Acetaminophen is available in liquid formulations (Liquiprin, Tempra, etc.), which are used primarily for infants and young children, as well as solid dosage forms (Tylenol, Datril, etc.). The drug is marketed in the United States under at least 50 brand names and in about 200 combination products with other drugs (Ameer and Greenblatt, 1977). The usual adult therapeutic dose is 325 to 650 mg. every 4

hours. Regular tablets or capsules contain 325 mg. each, whereas "extra-strength" tablets or capsules contain 500 mg. each. The therapeutic dose in young children is 60 to 120 mg. depending on age and weight.

Acetaminophen is also the major metabolite of both phenacetin and acetanilid in man, and it has almost completely replaced both of its predecessors on the American drug market. At least in therapeutic doses, acetaminophen is less toxic than either parent drug.

Toxicology: A single toxic dose of acetaminophen by mouth in an adult is about 10 gm. (Koch-Weser, 1976). Fatalities are rare with single ingestions of under 15 gm. (McNeil, 1980), except in individuals chronically exposed to alcohol or other drugs that induce hepatic microsomal mixed function oxidase activity (Barker et al., 1977; Emby and Fraser, 1977; Goldfinger et al., 1978; Licht et al., 1980; McClain et al., 1980; Wilson et al., 1978). One 16-year-old girl, however, died after the alleged ingestion of 5.8 gm. (Fernandez and Fernandez-Brito, 1977). Serious intoxications in children under the age of 11 years are uncommon (Meredith et al., 1978). In one large-scale study, children under age 5 years had the mildest clinical courses of any age group with a known or suspected acute ingestion of 7.5 gm. or more (Rumack and Peterson, 1978). If young children are more resistant than adults to the toxic effects of acetaminophen, the physiologic basis for this difference is unknown. At least one experimental study found younger mice and rats to be more susceptible to the lethal effects than older animals (Tanihata et al., 1979). A 3.5-year-old child was fatally poisoned by 5 gm. given in divided doses over 24 hours (Nogen and Bremner, 1978).

The clinical course of the overdosed patient may have three distinct phases (Peterson and Rumack, 1978a; Rumack and Matthew, 1975). The initial phase, consisting of nonspecific features such as nausea, malaise and diaphoresis, may begin shortly after ingestion and last for 12 to 24 hours. It often belies the potential severity of the illness as well as confounding the diagnosis. Indeed, the initial signs and symptoms may abate in intensity over the subsequent 24 hours to lull the unwary into a false sense of confidence. In mildly poisoned patients, however, this quiescent period may progress to complete recovery. Two to 6 days may elapse after ingestion before clinical evidence of the critical lesion, namely hepatic necrosis, appears in the severely poisoned patient. By then it is too late for any meaningful therapeutic intervention (Ameer and Greenblatt, 1977).

Signs of hepatotoxicity include sharp elevations in serum hepatic enzyme activities such as glutamic-oxaloacetic transaminase (SGOT, also known as aspartate aminotransferase, AST), glutamic-pyruvic transaminase (SGPT, also known as alanine aminotransferase, ALT) and lactic dehydrogenase (LDH). A 3-year-old child presenting 3 days after the ingestion of 11.4 gm. had the highest levels of these enzymes ever recorded at Duke Hospital: SGOT 20,376 IU, SGPT 13,303 IU and LDH 11,640 IU. Despite these grave prognostic signs, she had only a moderate illness and was discharged on the 7th day in good condition (Arena et al., 1978).

Eastham et al. (1976) believe that the serum ferritin level correlates more closely with the severity of liver injury in biopsy specimens and is a more sensitive index of hepatic damage than are the transaminases. Serum alkaline phosphatase is often elevated as well as bilirubin, some-

times to the point of frank jaundice. Hyperglycemia and hypoglycemia with or without coma have occurred (Koch-Weser, 1976). Mild acidosis and prolongation of the prothrombin time are common findings. In spite of prothrombin deficits in one group of 22 poisoned patients, two-thirds exhibited disseminated intravascular coagulation, presumably secondary to hepatic necrosis (Gazzard et al., 1974a). In a series of 18 patients, the 12 who died each had serum bilirubin concentrations greater than 4 mg./100 ml. and prothrombin ratios (prothrombin time of patient/prothrombin time of control) greater than 2.2 (Clark et al., 1973). Despite the apparent severity of the clotting defect, significant bleeding occurs in only a small proportion of patients, perhaps because the hepatic necrosis is only of short duration.

These indices of liver damage gradually return to normal in moderately poisoned patients who experience full recovery. At least one follow-up study on 30 patients found no evidence of longlasting hepatic damage (Hamlyn et al., 1977). Others (Clark et al., 1973) found severe centrilobular necrosis and collapse in liver biopsy specimens from recovered patients but no progression to cirrhosis. An increased sensitivity to drugs inactivated by hepatic microsomal enzymes should be anticipated for a week or two after the acute insult (Forrest et al., 1974).

Fatally poisoned patients exhibit the familiar progression in hepatic encephalopathy from confusion to stupor to coma and death (Clark et al., 1973; Hamlyn et al., 1978; Peterson and Rumack, 1978a). Although the extent of the centrilobular necrosis is the primary determinant of survival, sometimes other visceral organs are involved as well. In Hamlyn's (1978) series of 200 patients, only 2 went into renal failure of sufficient severity to require dialysis. Others have reported a somewhat higher incidence of acute renal failure among severely poisoned patients (Prescott et al., 1976a, b; Smith et al., 1978). Renal tubular necrosis has been found postmortem (Kleinman et al., 1980; McJunken et al., 1976; Wilson et al., 1978).

In a series of 200 patients admitted with a history of acetaminophen overdose, the serum amylase was elevated in 22% (Hamlyn et al., 1978). Gilmore and Tourvas (1977) have described one case in which acute pancreatitis appeared to dominate the clinical picture because of guarding, rebound tenderness, severe upper abdominal pain that radiated into the back and a serum amylase of 1440 IU/L. Histologic evidence of pancreatitis, however, has not been reported to our knowledge.

Elevated serum myocardial lactic dehydrogenase activity with or without an abnormal ECG is suggestive of myocardial damage. One or the other or both were found in 12% of a large series of patients, although no other evidence for a toxic myocarditis was seen (Hamlyn *et al.*, 1978). The ECG changes included nonspecific T-wave alterations, bundle branch block, delayed onset sinus bradycardia and ST segment depression. In one case involving what may be the highest plasma level of acetaminophen ever recorded (1082 μg./ml.), an adult woman spontaneously developed ventricular fibrillation, and the ECG after resuscitation suggested myocardial damage. Small hemorrhages in the visceral pericardium were found postmortem (Jones and Thomas, 1977). Other cases involving myocardial damage have been reviewed by Rumack and Matthew (1975).

Acetaminophen is quickly absorbed from the gastrointestinal tract. As with many drugs the rate of absorption is influenced by the gastric emptying time. Peak concentrations in plasma are generally reached within two hours after an oral dose. Perhaps absorption is slightly more rapid with liquid dosage forms (Peterson and Rumack, 1978b). As evaluated in newborn full-term infants, the plasma half-life of acetaminophen was 3.5 ± 0.8 hours following oral doses in the therapeutic range (Levy *et al.*, 1975). Several studies in adults indicated a plasma half-life of 1.9 to 2.2 hours. Older children had values intermediate between these two age groups, but no striking age-related differences in overall elimination rate constants were observed (Miller *et al.*, 1976; Peterson and Rumack, 1978b). The apparent biologic half-life of acetaminophen is longer in severely poisoned patients either because of developing hepatotoxicity or because capacity-limited metabolic pathways become saturated (Slattery and Levy, 1979). The drug is widely distributed in body fluids with an apparent volume of distribution of 850 ml./kg. (Prescott and Wright, 1973). The drug is not extensively bound in any tissue or to plasma proteins (Koch-Weser, 1976).

The determination of acetaminophen plasma levels assumes a special importance because the benign nature of the initial course may mask a life-threatening intoxication and because estimates of the dose ingested are often unreliable (Ambre and Alexander, 1977). The drawing of the blood specimen for assay, however, should be delayed until at least 4 hours after ingestion to assure that peak plasma concentrations have been achieved. The preferred technique for analysis is high-pressure liquid chromatography (Duffy and Byhers, 1979). Colorimetric methods are also available but are less satisfactory (Glynn and Kendal, 1975; McNeil, 1980). The nomogram shown as Fig. III-1 indicates blood levels at which hepatotoxicity may occur and at which active treatment is recommended (Rumack and Matthew, 1975).

Perhaps as much as 80% of the drug is conju-

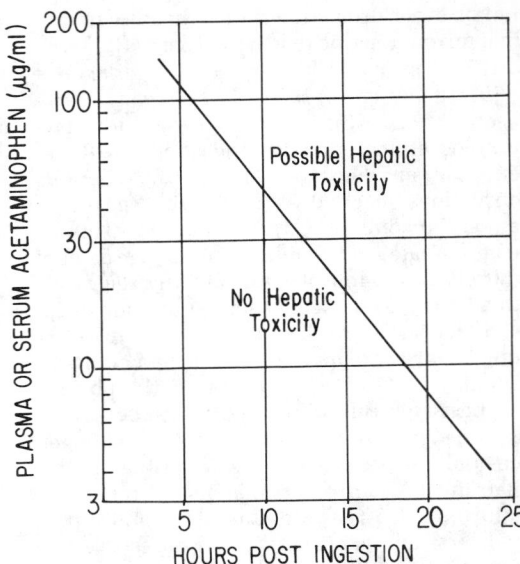

Figure III-1. Plasma or serum acetaminophen concentrations at which hepatotoxicity may occur and at which active treatment is recommended. (Modified from Rumack and Matthew, Pediatrics *55*:871–876, 1975, with permission. Copyright American Academy of Pediatrics, 1975.)

gated, predominately with glucuronic acid but also with sulfate and to a much lesser extent with cysteine and mercapturic acid. Only a very small fraction (<4%) is excreted unchanged in the urine. In human volunteers the fraction excreted as the sulfate conjugate reached a plateau as the dose was increased throughout the usual therapeutic range. In poisoned patients and especially those with liver damage, the renal excretion of the glucuronide conjugate also reached a plateau, whereas at that point the urinary excretion of cysteine and mercapturic acid conjugates showed a striking increase (Davis *et al.*, 1976). Thus, the major conjugation pathways leading to inactive products are saturable. Neonates appear to compensate for a lesser capacity for glucuronidation by a greater capacity for sulfation relative to adults (Levy *et al.*, 1975).

A small fraction of an ingested dose appears to be metabolically activated in the liver (Mitchell *et al.*, 1973a), and perhaps in the kidney as well (Duggin and Mudge, 1976), to a form which reacts covalently with tissue nucleophiles (Mitchell *et al.*, 1974; Jollow *et al.*, 1973). This active metabolite is presumably detoxified *in vivo* by conjugation with reduced glutathione. When the dose of acetaminophen reaches a critical threshold, however, the active metabolite is generated in amounts sufficient to deplete liver stores of reduced glutathione, and the excess arylating agent is free to react with essential tissue macromolecules, resulting in cell death and necrosis (Mitchell *et al.*, 1973b, 1974). Extensive experimental evidence with hepatic microsomal enzyme inducers and inhibitors indicates that the activation is mediated by mixed function oxidase or the cytochrome P450 system (Potter *et al.*, 1973). Agents which inhibit hepatic microsomal enzymes have protective and sometimes antidotal effects in experimental animals. These include piperonyl butoxide (Mitchell *et al.*, 1973a), 2-dimethylaminoethanol (Siegers, and Younes, 1979) and metyrapone (Goldstein and Nelson, 1979), but this approach has not been tried in man.

Potter *et al.* (1973) suggested that the toxic metabolite of acetaminophen is the *N*-hydroxy derivative. When synthesized, *N*-hydroxyacetaminophen was found to be moderately unstable in aqueous solutions at physiological pH and temperature (Gemborys *et al.*, 1978, 1980). One of the products of the spontaneous decomposition of *N*-hydroxyacetaminophen, which is also formed from acetaminophen in microsomal enzyme preparations, is *N*-acetyl-*p*-benzoquinoneimine; it is most likely the active arylating intermediate (Corcoran *et al.*, 1980). Oxidation of acetaminophen to an arylating intermediate by fetal liver proceeded at a rate that was 10-fold slower than that of adult human liver, but there was a decided increase with fetal age toward adult levels (Rollins *et al.*, 1979).

Therapy: Elucidation of the pharmacokinetics of acetaminophen suggested several therapeutic interventions which might benefit the acutely poisoned patient. The prompt administration of activated charcoal partially prevents acetaminophen absorption from the gastrointestinal tract (Levy and Houston, 1976). Administration of osmotic cathartics may also limit absorption (Koch-Weser, 1976). In mice the administration of sodium sulfate concurrent with intraperitoneal acetaminophen protects against death; presumably the extra sulfate prevents saturation of the capacity-limited sulfate conjugation pathway (Slattery and Levy, 1977). Attempts at forced diuresis, hemodialysis and charcoal resin hemoperfusion have not proved to be of benefit to most patients (Farid *et al.*, 1972; Gazzard *et al.*, 1947b; Rigby *et al.*, 1978; Rose, 1969; Winchester *et al.*, 1975).

The major therapeutic effort has been directed toward finding a safe, effective scavenging agent to compete with cellular nucleophiles for the active arylating metabolite. Such an agent would supplement the autoprotective role of endogenous reduced glutathione. Administration of glutathione *per se* is ineffective because it does not penetrate into the hepatocyte (Mitchell *et al.*, 1974). Cysteine was originally tried as an antagonist because it is one of the precursors of glutathione, but it is now believed to be effec-

tive as such without incorporation into glutathione (Mitchell *et al.*, 1973b). Other agents which are effective in poisoned animals, presumably because they scavenge the reactive metabolite, include α-tocopherol (Kelleher *et al.*, 1974) and ascorbic acid (Raghuram *et al.*, 1978). The following agents have been tried in man as well as animals with varying degrees of success: cysteamine (Chiu and Bhakthan, 1978; Dougles *et al.*, 1976; Prescott *et al.*, 1974), parenteral amino acid mixtures containing cysteine and methionine (Solomon *et al.*, 1977), dimercaprol (Hughes *et al.*, 1977), penicillamine (Prescott *et al.*, 1976a; Zera and Nagasawa, 1980), and methionine (Crome *et al.*, 1976; McLean, 1974; Smith *et al.*, 1978).

The agent of choice at present, however, for the management of acute acetaminophen overdose is *N*-acetylcysteine (Piperno and Berssenbruegge, 1976; Prescott *et al.*, 1977; St. Omer and McKnight, 1980; Rumack and Peterson, 1978). *N*-Acetylcysteine is available as a 10 or 20% sterile solution in 4-, 10- and 30-ml. vials for inhalation therapy as a mucolytic agent in patients with bronchopulmonary diseases (Mucomyst by Mead Johnson or Airbron by A&H in Canada). It is nontoxic (see Section II) and effective by mouth if treatment is started within 16 hours of ingestion. It should be withheld, however, if more than 24 hours have elapsed since acetaminophen ingestion. Since the FDA has not yet approved of Mucomyst for use as an antidote, except as an investigational drug, supervision must be obtained by calling the Rocky Mountain Poison Center's toll-free number 800-525-6115.

Activated charcoal definitely adsorbs acetaminophen; allegedly it also adsorbs *N*-acetylcysteine. In human volunteers, however, there was no difference in the area under the time-blood concentration curve of *N*-acetylcysteine in those who did and those who did not receive activated charcoal (Krenzelok and Peterson, 1980). Similarly, charcoal did not interfere with *N*-acetylcysteine protection of acetaminophen-poisoned mice. In dogs given acetaminophen by mouth, the area under the time-plasma concentration curve was reduced 93% by oral charcoal and 15 to 30% by oral castor oil or mannitol or sorbitol. These osmotic cathartics, however, also reduced somewhat the effectiveness of activated charcoal in limiting acetaminophen gastrointestinal absorption (Van de Graaff *et al.*, 1982).

Symptomatology:
1. Anorexia, nausea, vomiting, epigastric pain and sweating shortly after ingestion. Generalized malaise and pallor. Less commonly, paresthesias of distal extremities (Krenzelok *et al.*, 1977), muscular aching,

weakness and dizziness (Ferguson *et al.*, 1977).

2. Coma or other signs of central nervous system depression are rare within the first few hours after ingestion. Their appearance suggests the probable ingestion of other drugs.
3. Initial signs and symptoms may abate in intensity but continue for 48 hours.
4. Pain in the right upper quadrant and an enlarged and tender liver after 2 to 6 days.
5. Oliguria and sometimes anuria requiring dialysis.
6. Jaundice, coagulation defects, hepatic encephalopathy.
7. Myocardiopathy characterized by ST segment abnormalities, T-wave flattening and pericarditis.
8. Death in hepatic failure.

Treatment:
1. If bowel sounds are not audible, perform gastric lavage or give syrup of ipecac (p.I-2) regardless of interval after ingestion. If bowel sounds are audible, these procedures are also apt to be of value within 12 hours post ingestion but perhaps not thereafter.
2. After emptying the stomach, administer activated charcoal (p. I-4).
3. Saline catharsis with sodium sulfate (15 to 30 gm. in water) may be useful. High colonic enemas may help to stimulate prompt evacuation.
4. Dilute 20% *N*-acetylcysteine (Mucomyst) 1:3 in Coca-Cola, Pepsi-Cola, Fresca or grapefruit juice to disguise the taste and give 140 mg./kg. (about 3 ml./kg. of the diluted solution) as a loading dose if not more than 24 hours have elapsed since ingestion.
5. Draw a blood sample for plasma assay of acetaminophen at 4 hours or more after ingestion. Base further treatment on results of plasma assay and Fig. III-1.
6. If dictated by assay results, continue maintenance doses of *N*-acetylcysteine, 70 mg./kg. every 4 hours for 17 doses. If vomiting occurs within 1 hour of the administration of any dose, repeat that dose. For the occasional patient unable to retain *N*-acetylcysteine, it may be necessary to give it by duodenal intubation.
7. Treat early signs of central depression or coma due to other drugs, *e.g.*, morphine, ethyl alcohol, barbiturates, tranquilizers (chlorpromazine, diazepam, meprobamate, etc.)
8. Maintain fluid and electrolyte balance (p. IV-64). Treat as necessary for hypoglycemia (p. IV-61). Give vitamin K_1, fresh frozen plasma or clotting factor concentrate as necessary (p. IV-62).
9. Avoid diuretics, forced fluid diuresis and dialysis.
10. Follow hepatic function for at least 96 hours and be prepared for the management of hepatic failure (p. IV-61).

Laboratory:
1. Serial determinations of serum hepatic enzyme activities SGOT, SGPT and LDH.
2. Elevations of serum alkaline phosphatase, serum amylase, bilirubin and prothrombin times, as well as a mild acidosis, are common. Baseline determinations of glucose, creatinine and electrolytes (Na, K, Cl, CO_2) should be made.
3. Colorimetric methods for serum acetaminophen levels sensitive to 1 mg./L. are available (Frings and Soloom, 1979; Glynn and Kendall, 1975; McNeil, 1980).
4. Methemoglobinemia has been reported in animals but not in man. Intense cyanosis may indicate a rare acute intravascular hemolysis by an immune mechanism (Manor *et al.*, 1976).

References:

Ambre, J.; Alexander, M. Liver toxicity after acetaminophen ingestion. Inadequacy of the dose estimate as an index of risk. J. A. M. A. *238*:500-501, 1977.

Ameer, B.; Greenblatt, D. J. Acetaminophen. Ann. Intern. Med. *87*:202-209, 1977.

Arena, J. M.; Rourk, M. H., Jr.; Sibrack, C. D. Acetaminophen: report of an unusual poisoning. Pediatrics *61*:68-72, 1978.

Barker, J. D., Jr.; de Carle, D. J.; Anuras, S. Chronic excessive acetaminophen use and liver damage. Ann. Intern. Med. *87*:299-301, 1977.

Chiu, S.; Bhakthan, N. M. G. Experimental acetaminophen-induced hepatic necrosis: biochemical and electron microscopic study of cysteamine protection. Lab. Invest. *39*:193-203, 1978.

Clark, R.; Borirakchanyavat, V.; Davidson, A. R.; Thompson, R. P. H.; Widdop, B.; Goulding, R.; Williams, R. Lancet *1*:66-69, 1973.

Corcoran, G. B.; Mitchell, J. R.; Vaishnav, Y. N.; Horning, E. C. Evidence that acetaminophen and N-hydroxyacetaminophen form a common arylating intermediate, N-acetyl-p-benzoquinoneimine. Mol. Pharmacol., *18*:536-542, 1980.

Crome, P.; Vale, J. A.; Volans, G. N.; Widdop, B.; Goulding, R. Oral methionine in the treatment of severe paracetamol (acetaminophen) overdose. Lancet *2*:829-830, 1976.

Davis, M.; Simmons, C. J.; Harrisson, N. G.; Williams, R. Paracetamol overdose in man: relationship between pattern of urinary metabolites and severity of liver damage. Q. J. Med. *45*:181-191, 1976.

Douglas, A. P.; Hamlyn, A. N.; James, O. Controlled trial of cysteamine in treatment of acute paracetamol (acetaminophen) poisoning. Lancet *1*:111-118, 1976.

Duffy, J. P.; Byhers, J. Acetaminophen assay: the clinical consequences of a colorimetric vs. a high-pressure liquid chromatography determination in the assessment of two potentially poisoned patients. Clin. Toxicol. *15*:427-435, 1979.

Duggin, G. G.; Mudge, G. H. Analgesic neuropathy: renal distribution of acetaminophen and its conjugates. J. Pharmacol. Exp. Ther. *199*:1-9, 1976.

Eastham, E. J.; Bell, J. I.; Douglas, A. P. Sodium ferritin levels in acute hepatocellular damage from paracetamol overdosage. Br. Med. J. *1*:750-751, 1976.

Emby, D. J.; Fraser, B. N. Hepatotoxicity of paracetamol enhanced by ingestion of alcohol: report of two cases. S. Afr. Med. J. *51*:208-209, 1977.

Farid, N. R.; Glynn, J. P.; Kerr, D. N. S. Haemodialysis in paracetamol self-poisoning. Lancet *2*:396-398, 1972.

Ferguson, D. R.; Snyder, S. K.; Cameron, A. J. Hepatotoxicity in acetaminophen poisoning. Mayo Clinic Proc. *52*:246-248, 1977.

Fernandez, E.; Fernandez-Brito, A. C. Acetaminophen toxicity. N. Engl. J. Med. *296*:577, 1977.

Forrest, J. A. H.; Roscoe, P.; Prescott, L. F.; Stevenson, I. H. Abnormal drug metabolism after barbiturate and paracetamol overdose. Br. Med. J. *4*:499-502, 1974.

Frings, C. S.; Soloom, J. M. Colorimetric method for the quantitative determination of acetaminophen in serum. Clin. Toxicol. *15*:67-73, 1979.

Gazzard, B. G.; Clark, R.; Borirakchanyavat, V.; Williams, R. A controlled trial of heparin therapy in the coagulation defect of paracetamol-induced hepatic necrosis. Gut *15*:89-93, 1974a.

Gazzard, B. G.; Portmann, B.; Weston, M. J.; Langley, P. G.; Murray-Lyon, I. M.; Dunlop, E. H.; Flax, H.; Mellon, P. J.; Record, C. O.; Ward, M. B.; Williams, R. Charcoal haemoperfusion in the treatment of fulminant hepatic failure. Lancet *1*:1303-1307, 1974b.

Gemborys, M. W.; Gribble, G. W.; Mudge, G. H. Synthesis of N-hydroxyacetaminophen, a postulated toxic metabolite of acetaminophen, and its phenolic sulfate conjugate. J. Med. Chem. *21*:649-652, 1978.

Gemborys, M. W.; Mudge, G. H.; Gribble, G. W. Mechanism of decomposition of N-hydroxyacetaminophen, a postulated toxic metabolite of acetaminophen. J. Med. Chem. *23*:304-308, 1980.

Gilmore, I. T.; Tourvas, E. Paracetamol-induced acute pancreatitis. Br. Med. J. *1*:753-754, 1977.

Glynn, J. P.; Kendal, S. E. Paracetamol measurement. Lancet *1*:1147-1148, 1975.

Goldfinger, R.; Ahmed, K. S.; Pitchumoni, C. S.; Weseley, S. A. Concomitant alcohol and drug abuse enhancing acetaminophen toxicity. Am. J. Gastroenterol. *70*:385-388, 1978.

Goldfrank, L.; Kirstein, R. The un-aspirin: a bigger headache? Hosp. Physician, Sept., pp. 22-25, 1976.

Goldstein, M.; Nelson, E. B. Metyrapone as a treatment for acetaminophen (paracetamol) toxicity in mice. Res. Commun. Chem. Pathol. Pharmacol. *23*:203-206, 1979.

Hamlyn, A. N.; Douglas, A. P.; James, O. F. W.; Lesha, M.; Watson, A. J. Liver function and structure in survivors of acetaminophen poisoning: a follow-up study of serum bile acids and liver histology. Am. J. Dig. Dis. *22*:605-610, 1977.

Hamlyn, A. N.; James, O.; Douglas, A. P. Spectrum of paracetamol (acetaminophen) overdose -- clinical and epidemiological studies. Postgrad. Med. J. *54*:400-404, 1978.

Hughes, R. D.; Gazzard, B. G.; Hanid, M. A.; Trewby, P. N.; Murray-Lyon, I. M.; Davis, M.; Williams, R.; Bennett, J. R. Controlled trial of cysteamine and dimercaprol after paracetamol overdose. Br. Med. J. *2*:1395, 1977.

Jollow, D. J.; Mitchell, J. R.; Potter, W. Z.; Davis, D. C.; Gillette, J. R.; Brodie, B. B. Acetaminophen-induced hepatic necrosis. II. Role of covalent binding in vivo. J. Pharmacol. Exp. Ther. *187*:195-202, 1973.

Jones, G.; Thomas, P. Treatment of acute paracetamol poisoning. (Letter to the editor). Br. Med. J. *2*:1224, 1977.

Kelleher, J.; Walker, B. E.; Dixon, M. F.; Losowsky, M. S. Treatment of paracetamol poisoning. Lancet *1*:865, 1974.

Kleinman, J. G.; Breitenfield, R. V.; Roth, D. A. Acute renal failure associated with acetaminophen ingestion: report of a case and review of the literature. Clin. Nephrol. *14*:201-205, 1980.

Koch-Weser, J. Drug therapy: acetaminophen. N. Engl. J. Med. *295*:1297-1300, 1976.

Krenzelok, E. P.; Best, L.; Manoguerra, A. S. Acetaminophen toxicity. Am. J. Hosp. Pharm. *34*:391-394, 1977.

Krenzelok, E. P.; Peterson, R. G. The effect of activated charcoal administration on N-acetylcysteine serum levels in human subjects. Vet. Hum. Toxicol. *22*(Suppl. 2):56-58, 1980.

Levy, G.; Houston, J. B. Effect of activated charcoal on acetaminophen absorption. Pediatrics *58*:432-435, 1976.

Levy, G.; Khanna, N. N.; Soda, D. M.; Tsuzuki, O.; Stern, L. Pharmacokinetics of acetaminophen in the human neonate: formation of acetaminophen glucuronide and sulfate in relation to plasma bilirubin concentration and d-glucaric acid excretion. Pediatrics *55*:818-825, 1975.

Licht, H.; Seeff, L. B.; Zimmerman, H. J. Apparent potentiation of acetaminophen hepatotoxicity by alcohol. Ann. Intern. Med. *92*:511, 1980.

Manor, E.; Marmor, A.; Kaufman, S.; Leiba, H.; Ya'acov, B. Massive hemolysis caused by acetaminophen. J. A. M. A. *236*:2777-2778, 1976.

McClain, C. J.; Kromhout, J. P.; Peterson, F. J.; Holtzman, J. L. Potentiation of acetaminophen hepatotoxicity by alcohol. J. A. M. A. *244*:251-253, 1980.

McJunkin, B.; Barwick, K. W.; Little, W. C.; Winfield, J. B. Fatal massive hepatic necrosis following acetaminophen overdose. J. A. M. A. *236*:1874-1875, 1976.

McLean, A. E. M. Prevention of paracetamol poisoning (letter). Lancet *1*:729, 1974.

McNeil Consumer Products Company. Management of acetaminophen overdose with N-acetylcysteine. McNeil Consumer Products Company, Fort Washington, Pa, 1980.

Meredith, T. J.; Newman, B.; Goulding, R. Paracetamol poisoning in children. Br. Med. J. *2*:478-479, 1978.

Miller, R. P.; Roberts, R. J.; Fischer, L. J. Acetaminophen elimination kinetics in neonates, children and adults. Clin. Pharmacol. Ther. *19*:284-294, 1976a.

Mitchell, J. R.; Jollow, D. J.; Potter, W. Z.; Davis, D. C.; Gillette, J. R.; Brodie, B. B. Acetaminophen-induced hepatic necrosis. I. Role of drug metabolism. J. Pharmacol. Exp. Ther. *187*:185-194, 1973a.

Mitchell, J. R.; Jollow, D. J.; Potter, W. Z.; Gillette, J. R.; Brodie, B. B. Acetaminophen-induced hepatic necrosis. IV. Protective role of glutathione. J. Pharmacol. Exp. Ther. *187*:211-217, 1973b.

Mitchell, J. R.; Thorgeirsson, S. S.; Potter, W. Z.; Jollow, D. J.; Keiser, H. Acetaminophen-induced hepatic injury: protective role of glutathione in man and rationale for therapy. Clin. Pharmacol. Ther. *16*:676-684, 1974.

Nogen, A. G.; Bremner, J. E. Fatal acetaminophen overdosage in a young child. J. Pediatr. *92*:832-833, 1978.

Peterson, R. G.; Rumack, B. H. Toxicity of acetaminophen overdose. J. Am. Coll. Emer. Physicians *1*:202-205, 1978a.

Peterson, R. G.; Rumack, B. H. Pharmacokinetics of acetaminophen in children. Pediatrics *62*(Suppl.):877-879, 1978b.

Piperno, E.; Berssenbruegge, D. A. Reversal of experimental paracetamol toxicosis with N-acetylcysteine (letter). Lancet *2*:738-739, 1976.

Potter, W. Z.; Davis, D. C.; Mitchell, J. R.; Jollow, D. J.; Gillette, J. R.; Brodie, B. B. Acetaminophen-induced hepatic necrosis. III. Cytochrome P-450-mediated covalent binding in vitro. J. Pharmacol. Exp. Ther. *187*:203-210, 1973.

Prescott, L. F.; Newton, R. W.; Swainson, C. P.; Wright, N.; Forrest, A. R. W.; Matthew, H. Successful treatment of severe paracetamol overdosage with cysteamine. Lancet *1*:588-592, 1974.

Prescott, L. F.; Park, J.; Ballantyne, A.; Adriaenssens, P.; Proudfoot, A. T. Treatment of paracetamol (acetaminophen) poisoning with N-acetylcysteine. Lancet *2*:432-434, 1977.

Prescott, L. F.; Park, J.; Sutherland, G. R.; Smith, I. J.; Proudfoot, A. T. Cysteamine, methionine and penicillamine in the treatment of paracetamol poisoning. Lancet *2*:109-114, 1976a.

Prescott, L. F.; Park, J.; Proudfoot, A. T. Cysteamine, L-methionine and D-penicillamine in paracetamol poisoning. J. Int. Med. Res. *4*(Suppl. 4):112-117, 1976b.

Prescott, L. F.; Wright, N. The effects of hepatic and renal damage on paracetamol metabolism and excretion following overdosage. A pharmacokinetic study. Br. J. Pharmacol. *49*:602-613, 1973.

Raghuram, T. C.; Krishnamurthi, D.; Kalamegham, R. Effect of Vitamin C on paracetamol hepatotoxicity. Toxicol. Lett. 2:175-178, 1978.

Rigby, R. J.; Thomson, N. M.; Parkin, G. W.; Cheung, T. P. F. The treatment of paracetamol overdose with charcoal haemoperfusion and cysteamine. Med. J. Aust. 1:396-399, 1978.

Rollins, D. E.; Von Bahr, C.; Glaumann, H.; Moldeus, P.; Rane, A. Acetaminophen: potentially toxic metabolite formed by human fetal and adult liver microsomes and isolated fetal liver cells. Science 205:1414-1416, 1979.

Rose, P. G. Paracetamol overdose and liver damage (letter). Br. Med. J. 1:381-382, 1969.

Rumack, B. H.; Matthew, H. Acetaminophen poisoning and toxicity. Pediatrics 55:871-876, 1975.

Rumack, B. H.; Peterson, R. G. Acetaminophen overdose -- incidence, diagnosis, and management in 416 patients. Pediatrics 62(Suppl.):898-903, 1978.

Siegers, V. C. -P.; Younes, M. Einfluss von 2-Dimethylaminoethanol auf die hepatotoxischen Wirkungen von Paracetamol bei Ratten und Mausen. Arzneim. Forsch. 29:520-523, 1979.

Slattery, J. T.; Levy, G. Reduction of acetaminophen toxicity by sodium sulfate in mice. Res. Commun. Chem. Pathol. Pharmacol. 18:167-170, 1977.

Slattery, J. T.; Levy, G. Acetaminophen kinetics in acutely poisoned patients. Clin. Pharmacol. Ther. 25:184-195, 1979.

Smith, J. M.; Roberts, W. O.; Hall, S. M.; White, T. A.;

Gilbertson, A. A. Late treatment of paracetamol poisoning with mercaptamine. Br. Med. J. 1:331-333, 1978.

Solomon, A. E.; Briggs, J. D.; Knepil, J.; Henry, D. A.; Winchester, J. F.; Birrell, R. Therapeutic comparison of thiol compounds in severe paracetamol poisoning. Ann. Clin. Chem. 14:200-202, 1977.

St. Omer, V. V.; McKnight, E. D., III. Acetylcysteine for treatment of acetaminophen toxicosis in the cat. J. Am. Vet. Med. Assoc. 176:911-913, 1980.

Tanihata, T.; Matsuura, S.; Matsuura, M.; Kajiwara, S.; Kuwamura, T.; Ito, R. Comparison of LD_{50} of acetaminophen between infant and adult rats and mice. Toho Igakkai Zasshi 26:223-229, 1979.

Van de Graaff, W. B.; Thompson, W. L.; Sunshine, I.; Fretthold, D.; Leickly, F.; Dayton, H. Adsorbent and cathartic inhibition of enteral drug absorption. J. Pharmacol. Exp. Ther. 221:656-663, 1982.

Wilson, J. T.; Kasantikul, V.; Harbison, R.; Martin, D. Death in an adolescent following an overdose of acetaminophen and phenobarbital. Am. J. Dis. Child. 132:466-473, 1978.

Winchester, J. F.; Edwards, R. O.; Tilstone, W. J.; Woodcock, B. G. Activated charcoal hemoperfusion and experimental acetaminophen poisoning. Toxicol. Appl. Pharmacol. 31:120-127, 1975.

Zera, R. T.; Nagasawa, H. T. N-Acetyl-DL-penicillamine and acetaminophen toxicity in mice. J. Pharm. Sci. 69:1005-1006, 1980.

ACID

Corrosive mineral acids such as hydrochloric (muriatic), sulfuric, nitric and phosphoric are found in many homes in a variety of forms. Automobile battery acid is usually about 28% sulfuric acid (Degenhardt and Henderson, 1942). Toilet bowl cleaners frequently contain sodium bisulfate, which forms sulfuric acid in water (Bovill et al., 1951); similar products containing hydrochloric (Berry et al., 1965) or phosphoric acids are also marketed. Soldering fluxes are often solutions or pastes of zinc chloride and hydrochloric acid. Gun barrel cleaning fluid may contain about 5% nitric acid.

Some low molecular weight organic acids present a similar hazard, including formic, acetic, lactic and trichloroacetic acids. Ingestion of these materials leads to features in common with corrosive mineral acids (Meyer and Steigmann, 1944; Steigmann and Dolehide, 1956).

Aqueous solutions of free halogens such as iodine or bromine are also intensely corrosive (see IODINE, p. III-213). For ingestion of bleach products, which may contain active chlorine, see HYPOCHLORITE, p. III-202). Alkaline corrosives are discussed either under AMMONIA, p. III-21 or LYE, p. III-245. The following acidic compounds have important systemic effects and are discussed elsewhere: boric acid (see BORATE, p. III-66), carbolic acid (see PHENOL, p. III-344), hydrocyanic acid (see CYANIDE, p. III-123), hydrofluoric acid (see FLUORIDE, p. III-185), oxalic acid (see OXALATE, p. III-326), salicylic acid (see SALICYLATE, p. III-368).

Toxicology: Corrosive burns may result from the inhalation of acid fumes and from skin contact with or the ingestion of strong acids. Chemical pneumonitis is to be expected after respiratory exposure to acid vapors or after the tracheobronchial aspiration of ingested acid. For management of this complication, which occurs more commonly with fuming acid vapors (e.g., HCl, SO_2, Cl_2, etc.), see NITROGEN OXIDES, p. III-319.

Because of immediate pain when taken into the mouth, strong mineral acids are probably less often swallowed than are solutions of corrosive alkalis. Spasm from the first swallow tends to prevent further ingestion; yet, determined or inebriated individuals have consumed 4 to 8 oz. of concentrated hydrochloric acid and survived with medical treatment (Latraverse, 1955; Poteshman, 1967).

The lethal dose and the interval before death are difficult to predict with any useful degree of accuracy. Perhaps the impression that sulfuric acid is the most hazardous (Gray and Holmes, 1948) is based on the concentrations of mineral acids as they are commonly produced: 95% sulfuric acid is about 18 M, 85% phosphoric acid about 17 M, 69% nitric acid about 15 M, 36% hydrochloric acid about 12 M. As with most corrosive solutions, concentration appears to be more critical than volume. A reasonable estimate of the lethal dose in an adult is 1 oz. of mineral acid in the above concentrations (Polson and Tattersall, 1959). However, a few milliliters (less than a teaspoonful) has killed (Gonzales et al., 1954), and even a few drops present a serious hazard if aspirated into the larynx. The intratracheal instillation of 2 to 3 ml./kg. of 0.1 N hydrochloric acid in dogs produced deaths with pulmonary consolidation (Greenfield et al., 1969).

It has been asserted (Latraverse, 1955; Uhde, 1946) that hydrochloric acid produces more esophageal injury than either sulfuric or nitric acid, but a recent survey (Hawkins et al., 1980) suggests that sulfuric acid has the highest liability in this respect. According to most reports, cases of sulfuric acid ingestion (Boikan and Singer, 1930: Bovill et al., 1951; Bruce, 1930; Degenhardt and Henderson, 1942; Karon, 1962; Stewart-Harrison, 1934) and of nitric acid ingestion (Boikan and Singer, 1930; O'Donnell et al., 1949; Paul, 1951) resemble in all important clinical aspects the more frequently documented cases of hydrochloric acid ingestion. Only one report of a phosphoric acid ingestion has come to our attention (Hawkins et al., 1980).

Mineral acids usually produce a more fulminating illness than do corrosive alkalis, and death is commonly ascribed to one or more of the following complications: circulatory shock, asphyxia due to glottic or laryngeal edema, perforation of the stomach with peritonitis, gastric hemorrhage, intercurrent infections or inanition from late stricture formation.

It is clear that esophageal involvement occurs much less frequently with acids than with alkalis. The incidence of esophageal involvement in acute acid ingestion episodes has been estimated at 6 to 20% (Boikan and Singer, 1930; Gray and Holmes, 1948), and with rare exception (e.g., Thomas and Dedo, 1977), significant esophageal lesions are reported only in those patients with major gastric damage (Hawkins et al., 1980; Penner, 1980). In contrast, esophageal necrosis is the rule in lye ingestion (see pp. III-246–247). The reason for this striking difference between corrosive acids and alkalis is not clear. In general, mineral acids penetrate mucosae more slowly than strong alkalis, and so acid lesions tend to be shallower. Apparently acids usually have only a superficial effect on the squamous epithelium as they pass rapidly down the esophagus (Strode and Dean, 1950). If, however, contact with acid is sustained for more than a few seconds, as in disorders of esophageal motility, mucosal and submucosal corrosion of the esophagus may occur (Ashcraft and Padula, 1974), and even esophageal strictures are described (Hawkins et al., 1980). Based on x-ray findings in women who ingested 27% hydrochloric acid, corrosive esophagitis may be more common than generally recognized (Muhletaler et al., 1980), but acid-induced esophageal lesions usually heal promptly with only conservative treatment.

Once in the stomach, acids and alkalis behave similarly (except that alkalis are neutralized to some extent by stomach acids). They tend to flow along the magenstrasse in the lesser curvature, causing prompt necrosis. On reaching the pyloric sphincter and antrum, they induce pylorospasm, entrapping the agent at this site where it causes the greatest damage (Boikan and Singer, 1930; Meyer and Steigmann, 1944; Steigmann and Dolehide, 1956). The damage may be more diffuse if the corrosive is ingested when the stomach is full (Palmer and Scott, 1949; Steigmann and Dolehide, 1956). In 20% of reported cases reviewed by Penner (1980), the small bowel was also injured, presumably indicating that the pyloric sphincter sometimes relaxes enough to permit passage of acid into the duodenum.

Concentrated mineral acids can induce rapid full-thickness necrosis of the stomach wall, with perforation within a few days, often in the region of the antrum. Obviously aggressive surgical intervention is then required. Whereas it is clearly preferable to anticipate this complication and to perform a gastrectomy before perforation and peritonitis, no general agreement exists about methods of distinguishing viable from necrotizing stomach in the early phases of the illness or about the success of early surgery. Probably proponents of early surgery (e.g., Berry et al., 1965; Chodak and Passaro, 1978) are outnumbered by those who favor waiting until the extent of injury and the need for operative intervention are clearly recognized (e.g., Di Costanzo et al., 1980; Marks et al., 1963; Penner, 1980). Similarly, opinions differ about the safety and efficacy of nasogastric and orogastric intubation to keep the acid-burned stomach decompressed in the acute phase of the illness (compare Di Costanzo et al. (1980) with Hawkins et al. (1980)). Published case reports, however, describe no adverse experience with indwelling nasogastric tubes in these patients (Penner, 1980). When and if surgery becomes necessary because of extensive gastric necrosis, the commonest operation is partial (distal) gastrectomy with a Billroth I anastomosis (Chong et al., 1974; Maull et al., 1979).

Pyloric stenosis is undoubtedly the most frequent and characteristic complication among patients who survive the acute episode (Baker and Spellberg, 1952; Berry et al., 1965; Herrington, 1964; Hodgson, 1958–59; Maggi and Meeroff, 1953; Nevin et al., 1959; Tucker and Gerrish, 1960). Symptomatic evidence of pyloric obstruction is usually manifested after several weeks (Boikan and Singer, 1930), but sometimes only after 5 or 6 years (Gray and Holmes, 1948). The incidence is said to approach 80% (Karon, 1962). In contrast to the strictures of lye poisoning, there is no convincing evidence that early or vigorous steroid therapy prevents or lessens acid-induced strictures (Chong *et al.*, 1974; Hawkins *et al.*, 1980; Chodak and Passaro, 1978), but perhaps a course of penicillamine should be tried (see p. III-250).

Less commonly seen lesions include antral stenosis, hourglass deformity or linitis plastica (Boikan and Singer, 1930). Corrosive-induced obstruction is easily mistaken for gastric carcinomas (Karon and Wall, 1951; Steward-Harrison, 1934, Strode and Dean, 1950); indeed, one patient did develop an ulcerating adenocarcinoma following gastroenterostomy (O'Donnell *et al.*, 1949). Other rarely reported complications include hepatitis (Baker and Spellberg, 1952), achlorhydria (Karon, 1962), low serum albumin (Marks *et al.*, 1963), and chronic discoid lupus erythematosus after skin contact (Spencer, 1951).

Low molecular weight organic acids such as acetic are strong irritants but somewhat less corrosive than concentrated mineral acids. They may, however, be more penetrating and injurious than dilute mineral acid solutions of the same pH (*e.g.*, Muhlendahl *et al.*, 1978). Of three reported cases of acetic acid ingestion two developed esophageal strictures. One of these cases, together with the third case, developed late pyloric stenosis (Fox, 1948; Paul, 1951). In one case of acetic acid ingestion a hemorrhagic diathesis and intravascular coagulation were managed with exchange transfusions and infusions of heparin (Paar *et al.*, 1968). Trichloroacetic acid resembles acetic acid in its toxicity to experimental animals (Woodward *et al.*, 1941). Lactic acid (even when diluted with milk!) is corrosive and also has a tendency to produce both esophageal and gastric damage (Delph, 1937; Trainer *et al.*, 1945; Young and Smith, 1944). Concentrated formic acid solutions (75 to 80%) produce burns of the mouth and esophagus, but at least in children the esophageal lesions healed without stricture formation (Muhlendahl *et al.*, 1978).

Serious theoretical objections exist to the administration of diluents (such as water or milk) and antacids (such as milk of magnesia) after the ingestion of concentrated acid solutions. Thus, by rapidly releasing the unavoidable heats of dilution and of neutralization, high temperatures may be produced in the esophagus and stomach with consequent thermal as well as chemical burns (Penner, 1980). Because the heat is removed continuously and rapidly by the mucosal blood flow, it is not possible to calculate by the techniques of Penner (1980) and others the tissue temperatures that are attained, and so it is impossible to evaluate the relative risk of thermal versus chemical (corrosive) injury. The issue warrants more study, but perhaps a slurry of chipped ice or snow is the ideal diluent when the stomach contains unneutralized concentrated acid.

Concentrated mineral acids are also painful and corrosive when spilled on human skin, but the reaction can usually be terminated promptly by flushing the affected area with water. Because acids tend to penetrate the skin more slowly than strong lye solutions, acids are usually easier to remove by washing than are corrosive alkalis. Moderate concentrations of mineral acids are surprisingly well tolerated on the skin. In a controlled test on persons with normal and abraded skin (Nixon *et al.*, 1975), irritation from 10% sulfuric acid was judged to be negligible, whereas that from 10% acetic acid was slight.

The surface of the eye, however, is much more susceptible to acid injury than is the skin (Grant, 1974). Concentrated mineral acids cause extensive necrosis of the conjunctiva and corneal epithelium. They penetrate and injure the stroma of the cornea, with resulting perforation or with permanent opaque scar formation. Only rarely is the lens or iris injured. Dilute acids, including 4 to 6% acetic acid as present in ordinary vinegar, cause immediate pain, conjunctival hyperemia and sometimes injury of the corneal epithelium, but the latter regenerates promptly and corneal opacities are uncommon (Grant, 1974). With more concentrated acid solutions in the eye, the outcome depends largely on how soon and how effectively the conjunctival sac can be irrigated with clean water to remove the poison. Because they penetrate more slowly, acids are easier to remove than strong alkalis, but eye irrigation should usually be continued for 10 to 15 minutes in any symptomatic exposure.

Symptomatology (after ingestion or skin contact):

1. Corrosion of mucous membranes of mouth, throat, and esophagus, with immediate pain and dysphagia. The necrotic areas are at first grayish white but soon acquire a blackish discoloration (yellow in the case of nitric acid) and sometimes a shrunken or wrinkled texture (eschar); the process is described as a "coagulation necrosis."

2. Epigastric pain, which may be associated with nausea and the vomiting of mucoid and "coffee-ground" material. At times, gastric hemorrhage may be intense, and the vomitus then contains fresh blood. Profound thirst.

3. Ulceration of all membranes and tissues with which the acid comes in contact. After the ingestion of concentrated mineral acid, this corrosion may lead within a few hours or a few days to gastric perforation and peritonitis.

4. Circulatory collapse with clammy skin, weak and rapid pulse, shallow respirations, and scanty urine. Circulatory shock is often the immediate cause of death.
5. Asphyxial death due to glottic edema.
6. Late esophageal, gastric and pyloric strictures and stenoses, which may require major surgical repair, should be anticipated. Signs of obstruction commonly appear within a few weeks but may be delayed for months and even years. Permanent scars may also appear in the cornea, skin and oropharynx.
7. Uncorrected circulatory collapse of several hours' duration may lead to renal failure and ischemic lesions in the liver and heart.

Treatment:

1. Avoid gastric lavage or emetics. If spontaneous vomiting or retching persists, administer parenterally an antiemetic drug such as prochlorperazine (p. IV-49).
2. If the ingested acid solution was not concentrated acid, drink immediately, if possible, copious amounts of cold water or milk as a diluent and administer by mouth a neutralizer such as magnesium oxide, milk of magnesia, calcium hydroxide (lime water), or aluminum hydroxide gel (2 fl. oz.). Avoid carbonates and bicarbonates, because they release carbon dioxide, which produces gastric distention and sometimes rupture.
3. If a concentrated acid solution (mineral or organic) was ingested, it may be dangerous to administer water or antacids, as noted in the text above. In any case, these patients often cannot swallow anything.
4. Opiates for the control of pain (p. IV-32).
5. Correct circulatory shock with intravenous replacement fluids, such as isotonic saline, serum albumin and whole blood (p. IV-18). Keep the patient warm.
6. If dilute or weak acid is ingested, the quantity may be sufficiently large to induce a derangement in the systemic acid-base balance that warrants attention.
7. As soon as shock and pain are controlled, esophagoscopy and even gastroscopy may be attempted to evaluate the extent and depth of mucosal lesions. As noted under LYE (pp. III-249–250), flexible fiberoptic endoscopy is relatively safe in experienced hands.
8. If the esophagus is not deeply burned, a soft nasogastric (or orogastric) tube may be passed and left in place. Gentle continuous suction is useful in keeping the stomach decompressed.
9. Prompt surgical intervention in cases of respiratory obstruction, perforation, and stricture formation. (see text above).
10. Give nothing by mouth (except perhaps a nasogastric tube) after the initial administration of diluents, neutralizers, and demulcents. Parenteral alimentation (p. IV-76) should be continued until mucosal repair is essentially complete (usually about 1 week). Then try liquids, soft foods, and finally a regular diet (p. IV-77).
11. Antibiotic therapy (p. IV-86) if an infection occurs.
12. Cortisone therapy has been recommended, but it appears to be ineffective in preventing acid-induced strictures. Perhaps parenteral penicillamine should be tested; see LYE, p. III-250.
13. For skin burns, wash with large amounts of water and then apply a paste of sodium bicarbonate. As long as the contaminated surface can be irrigated continuously with water, the heats of dilution and of neutralization are not a problem.
14. For eye burns hold the lids open and flush immediately with a slow stream of water; continue this procedure for 10 to 15 minutes. A few drops of a topical anesthetic such as butacaine sulfate (2%) or tetracaine hydrochloride (0.5%) will relieve lid spasm and facilitate irrigation. For the treatment of severe eye burns, an ophthalmologist should be consulted (Grant, 1974).

Laboratory:

1. Albuminuria, hematuria, and casts may be observed. Leukocytosis is common.
2. Blood chemical analyses are important to assess acid-base and electrolyte disturbances.

References:

Ashcraft, K. W.; Padula, R. T. The effect of dilute corrosives on the esophagus. Pediatrics 53:226-232, 1974.
Baker, L.; Spellberg, M. A. Pyloric stenosis secondary to hydrochloric acid ingestion. Report of two cases in which hepatitis developed. J. A. M. A. 150:442-446, 1952.
Berry, W. B.; Hall, R. A.; Jordan, G. L., Jr. Necrosis of the entire stomach secondary to ingestion of a corrosive acid. Am. J. Surg. 109:652-655, 1965b.
Boikan, W. S.; Singer, H. A. Gastric sequelae of corrosive poisoning. Arch. Intern. Med. 46:342-357, 1930.
Bovill, E. G.; Bulawa, F. A.; Olivetti, R. G. Severe corrosive gastritis with antral stenosis following ingestion of Sani-Flush. Gastroenterology 17:436-441, 1951.
Bruce, H. A. Pyloric occlusion from sulfuric acid. Ann. Surg. 92:897-899, 1930.
Chodak, G. W.; Passaro, E., Jr. Acid ingestion. Need for gastric resection. J. A. M. A. 239:225-226, 1978.
Chong, G. C.; Beahrs, O. H.; Payne, W. S. Management of corrosive gastritis due to ingested acid. Mayo Clin. Proc. 49:861-865, 1974.
Degenhardt, D. P.; Henderson, R. G. Corrosive pyloric stenosis without esophageal involvement. Lancet 2, 425, 1942.
Delph, J. F. Chemical burns of the oral cavity and esophagus. Surg. Clin. North Am. 17:585-592, 1937.
Di Costanzo, J.; Noirclerc, M.; Jouglard, J.; Escoffier, J. M.;

Cano, N.; Martin, J.; Gauthier, A. New therapeutic approach to corrosive burns of the upper gastrointestinal tract. Gut *21*:370-375, 1980.

Fox, J. R. Chemical burn of the esophagus. U. S. Naval Med. Bull. *48*:118-120, 1948.

Gonzales, T. A.; Vance, M.; Helpern, M.; Umberger, C. J. *Legal Medicine, Pathology and Toxicology,* 2nd ed. Appleton-Century-Crofts, New York, 1954.

Grant, W. M. *Toxicology of the Eye.* 2nd ed. Charles C Thomas, Springfield, Ill, 1974.

Gray, H. K.; Holmes, C. L. Pyloric stenosis caused by ingestion of corrosive substances. Report of a case. Surg. Clin. North Am. *28*:1041-1056, 1948.

Greenfield, L. J.; Singleton, R. F.; McCaffree, D. R.; Coalson, J. J. Pulmonary effects of experimental graded aspiration of hydrochloric acid. Ann. Surg. *170*:74-86, 1969.

Hawkins, D. B.; Demeter, M. J.; Barnett, T. E. Caustic ingestion-controversies in management - review of 214 cases. Laryngoscope *90*:98-109, 1980.

Herrington, J. L., Jr. Stenosis of the gastric antrum and proximal duodenum resulting from ingestion of a corrosive agent. Am. J. Surg. *107*:580-585, 1964.

Hodgson, J. H. Corrosive stricture of the stomach. Case report and review of the literature. Br. J. Surg. *46*:358-361, 1958-59.

Karon, A. B. The delayed gastric syndrome with pyloric stenosis and achlorhydria following the ingestion of acid - a definite clinical entity. Am. J. Dig. Dis. *7*:1041-1046, 1962.

Karon, A. B.; Wall, H. C. Pyloric stenosis caused by ingestion of corrosive acid, simulating gastric carcinoma; Report of a case. Gastroenterology *17*:445-449, 1951.

Latraverse, V. Acute acid esophagitis. Can. Med. Assoc. J. *73*:293-294, 1955.

Maggi, A. L. C.; Meeroff, M. Stenosis of the stomach caused by corrosive gastritis. Gastroenterology *24*:573-578, 1953.

Marks, I. N.; Bank, S.; Werbeloff, L.; Farman, J.; Louw, J. H. The natural history of corrosive gastritis. Report of five cases. Am. J. Dig. Dis. *8*:509-524, 1963.

Maull, K. I.; Scher, L. A.; Greenfield, L. J. Surgical implications of acid ingestion. Surg. Gynecol. Obstet. *148*:895-898, 1979.

Meyer, K. A.; Steigmann, F. The surgical treatment of corrosive gastritis. Surg. Gynecol. Obstet. *79*:306-310, 1944.

Muhlendahl, K. E. V.; Oberdisse, U.; Krienke, E. G. Local injuries by accidental ingestion of corrosive substances by children. Arch. Toxicol. *39*:299-324, 1978.

Muhletaler, C. A.; Gerlock, A. J.; Soto, L. D.; Halter, S. A. Acid corrosive esophagitis - radiographic findings. Am. J. Roentgenol. Radium Ther. Nucl. Med. *134*:1137-1140, 1980.

Nevin, I. N.; Turner, W. W.; Gardner, H. T. Early and late roentgenographic findings in corrosive gastritis. Report of a case. Am. J. Roentgenol. Radium Ther. Nucl. Med. *81*:603-608, 1959.

Nixon, G. A.; Tyson, C. A.; Wertz, W. C. Interspecies comparisons of skin irritancy. Toxicol. Appl. Pharmacol. *31*:481-490, 1975.

O'Donnell, C. H.; Abbott, W. E.; Hirshfeld, J. W. Surgical treatment of corrosive gastritis. Am. J. Surg. *78*:251-255, 1949.

Paar, D.; Heimsoth, V.; Werner, M.; Bock, K. D. Verbrauchskoagulopathie als Ursache hamorrhagischer Diathese bei akuter Essigsaure-Intoxikation. Dtsch. Med. Wochenschr. *93*:206-209, 1968.

Palmer, E. D.; Scott, M. N. Acute corrosive gastritis: Observations on the gastric mucosa following ingestion of concentrated hydrochloric acid. Gastroenterology *12*:879-883, 1949.

Paul, M. Gastric obstruction from swallowing a corrosive poison. Lancet *2*: 1064-1066, 1951.

Penner, G. E. Acid ingestion: toxicology and treatment. Ann. Emer. Med. *9*:374-379, 1980.

Polson, C. J.; Tattersall, R. N. *Clinical Toxicology.* J. B. Lippincott Co., Philadelphia, 1959.

Poteshman, N. L. Corrosive gastritis due to hydrochloric acid ingestion. Report of a case. Am. J. Roentgenol. Radium Ther. Nucl. Med. *99*:182-185, 1967.

Spencer, G. A. Lupus erythematosus following burns from hydrochloric acid. Arch. Dermatol. *64*:215-217, 1951.

Steigmann, F.; Dolehide, R. A. Corrosive (acid) gastritis, management of early and late cases. N. Engl. J. Med. *254*:981-986, 1956.

Stewart-Harrison, R. Pyloric stenosis due to sulphuric acid. Br. J. Radiol. *7*:48, 1934.

Strode, E. C.; Dean, M. L. Acid burns of the stomach. Report of 2 cases. Ann. Surg. *131*:801-811, 1950.

Thomas, A. N.; Dedo, H. H. Pharyngogastrostomy for treatment of severe caustic stricture of the pharynx and esophagus. J. Thorac. Cardiovasc. Surg. *73*:817-822, 1977.

Trainer, J. B.; Krippaehne, W. W.; Hunter, W. C.; Lagozzino, D. A. Esophageal stenosis due to lactic acid. Am. J. Dis. Child. *69*:173-175, 1945.

Tucker, A. S.; Gerrish, E. W. Hydrochloric acid burns of the stomach. J. A. M. A. *174*:890-893, 1960.

Uhde, G. I. Chemical burns of the esophagus. Ann. Otol. Rhinol. Laryngol. *55*:795-820, 1946.

Woodward, G.; Lange, S. W.; Nelson, K. W.; Calvery, H. O. The acute oral toxicity of acetic, chloracetic, dichloracetic and trichloracetic acids. J. Ind. Hyg. Toxicol. *23*:78-81, 1941.

Young, E. G.; Smith, R. P. Lactic acid: A corrosive poison. Report of three fatal cases with experimental confirmation. J. A. M. A. *125*:1179-1181, 1944.

ALCOHOLS, HIGHER

The "higher" saturated aliphatic alcohols are defined here to exclude methyl alcohol (p. III-275), ethyl alcohol (p. III-166), ethylene glycol (p. III-172) and isopropyl alcohol (together with *n*-propyl alcohol, p. III-217).

Included here are such liquid alcohols as butyl, amyl, isoamyl, ethylhexyl, etc., which are used principally as solvents. Isoamyl alcohol is the chief constituent of "fusel oil" in fermentative distillates (Webster, 1930). Higher homologues include the solid fatty alcohols, such as lauryl, myristyl, cetyl, and stearyl; they are important as emulsifiers and emollients in cosmetics (Greenberg and Lester, 1954). In some cases additional information about the individual alcohols can be found in Section II.

Toxicology: With the exception of methanol, the toxicity of primary aliphatic alcohols is greater the longer the chain length at least through amyl alcohol, and within this homologous series narcotic potency may increase even faster than lethality (Munch and Schwartze, 1925). In terms of the intraperitoneal dose to produce pronounced impairment of gait in rats, the straight chain primary alcohols increased in potency by almost 2 orders of magnitude from methanol to 1-hexanol. With further increases in chain length the potency decreased in a perfectly symmetrical fashion at least through 1-decanol (McCreery and Hunt, 1978).

In general the secondary alcohols are less toxic than the corresponding primary isomers (Macht, 1920). In the rat (Spector, 1955; Treon, 1962) the order of increasing lethality by single-dose oral administration is as follows: ethyl, isopropyl (and *sec*-butyl), *n*-butyl, *tert*-butyl, isobutyl, and amyl alcohols. Primary or normal propyl alcohol may belong anomalously late in this list (between isobutyl and amyl), but the comparative toxicities of the various butyl and amyl isomers have not been adequately defined.

The butyl alcohols are generally less irritating and less potent as central nervous depressants than are amyl alcohols, but they are 2 to 5 times more toxic than ethanol when tested acutely in the rat (Treon, 1962); reported oral LD_{50} values vary from 2.5 to 6.5 gm./kg. Toxic symptoms from butyl and amyl alcohol are usually more severe and more prolonged than those in ethanol intoxication. Vapor exposures in man (Treon, 1962) have caused marked irritation of the eyes, nose and throat, as well as headache, vertigo and drowsiness. Eye inflammation (Tabershaw *et al.*, 1944) and keratitis characterized by translucent vacuoles in the superficial layers of otherwise normal corneas have followed exposure to *n*-butyl alcohol vapors (Cogan and Grant, 1945).

Most liquid alcohols appear to act as primary skin irritants in human subjects. Significant percutaneous absorption occurs in the rabbit but has not been described in man. As inferred from experiments in which lightly anesthetized rats were induced to aspirate test substances placed in the mouth (Gerarde and Ahlstrom, 1966), all of these alcohols are especially toxic if aspirated. Apparently liquids with low viscosities and low surface tensions are able to penetrate deeply into the lung. Whatever pulmonary injury may be sustained, undiluted aliphatic alcohols ranging from ethyl to decyl are believed to be rapidly absorbed from the lungs. The result is a high blood level and prompt death at doses that would be tolerated if swallowed without aspiration.

No reports of human intoxication from the ingestion of butyl alcohols were located, but *n*-butyl alcohol has been administered to patients for the control of postoperative pain in otolaryngeal surgery (Welt, 1950) and for an unexplained anti-hemorrhagic effect (due to hypotension?) in those with far advanced cancer (Revici and Ravich, 1953). Doses of 5 to 10 ml. of isotonic saline saturated with 1-butanol were administered by the oral, intramuscular and intravenous routes. No ill effects were described after intravenous infusions of 500 ml. of a 7% solution of *n*-butyl alcohol in saline (Welt, 1950), and as much as 1500 ml. of a 7% solution in water is said to have been tolerated by mouth every day for 10 days. As extrapolated from rat data, however, 3 to 7 oz. represents a reasonable estimate of the single oral mean lethal dose of any butyl alcohol in man.

The amyl alcohols are even more toxic (LD_{50} values in rats, 1 to 3 gm./kg.), and the ingestion and rectal instillation of about 30 ml. of tertiary amyl alcohol (amylene hydrate) have proved lethal in human adults (von Oettingen, 1943). Human fatalities have also been ascribed to amyl alcohol vapors during industrial exposures.

Older reports (cited by Treon (1962)) ascribed such bizarre effects as glycosuria and methemoglobinemia to the ingestion of isoamyl alcohol in fermentative fusel oil, but these isolated assertions should be regarded with skepticism.

It is difficult to find clinically useful generalizations about the relative toxicities of the various butyl and amyl alcohols. Four isomers of butanol and eight isomers of pentanol (amyl alcohol) exist, and several of them can be readily purchased. Among the primary alcohols isobutyl and isoamyl are undeniably more toxic and more hazardous than the corresponding straight chain isomers. In general, secondary alcohols are less toxic and tertiary alcohols more toxic than the corresponding "normal" alcohols (see list above), but the order changes with any change in the test conditions, such as the route of administration. It also differs for different operational criteria of potency, such as the LD_{50} (Treon, 1962), dose to induce ataxia (McCreery and Hunt, 1978; Wallgren, 1960) and blood level at the time of respiratory arrest (Haggard *et al.*, 1945). For example, in terms of body content at death the tertiary alcohol 2-methylbutanol-2 is definitely less toxic in mice than are any of the three primary amyl alcohols (Haggard *et al.*, 1945). To further confound comparisons, the cytotoxicity of alcohols up to three carbons in chain length increased progressively in tissue cultures of neuroblastoma cells, but the corresponding aldehyde metabolites showed a decreasing toxicity with increasing chain length (Koerker *et al.*, 1976).

Only scanty toxicity information is available about higher homologues of the aliphatic alcohol series, but animal data establish that the lethality does not continue to increase with increasing chain length. Methylamyl and 2-ethylbutyl alcohols (as summarized by Treon, 1962) are similar to amyl alcohols in terms of acute oral LD_{50} values in rats. Aliphatic alcohols with 8 carbons (octanols) are less toxic. Thus caprylic alcohol (octanol-2) and the important industrial solvent 2-ethylhexyl alcohol (2-ethylhexanol-2) resemble the butyl alcohols in acute toxicity, as do at least a few nonyl alcohols (Treon, 1962). Many of the longer branched-chain primary alcohols of commerce, especially the "oxo" alcohols, are mixtures (Scala and Burtis, 1973; see also Section II).

Still longer chain primary aliphatic alcohols are apparently less toxic in rats. A mixture of 7- to 9-carbon alcohols had an acute oral LD_{50} of about 11 gm./kg. (Brown *et al.*, 1970). The 10-carbon homologue *n*-decyl alcohol also has a very low acute toxicity (LD_{50} greater than 10 gm./kg. in rats), as do the solid fatty alcohols (*e.g.*, lauryl, myristyl, cetyl and stearyl). However, the rat aspiration test (Gerarde and Ahlstrom, 1966) suggests that decyl and melted dodecyl (lauryl) alcohols are dangerous if they enter the trachea. In the rat even a small quantity (0.2 ml.) behaves like the hydrocarbon solvents (*e.g.*, kerosene) in causing death from pulmonary edema.

Toxicity comparisons are difficult because the various isomeric alcohols are metabolized at different rates and by different mechanisms. Primary alcohols are oxidized rather rapidly to the corresponding aldehydes and acids. A significant metabolic acidosis may result. Secondary alcohols are converted to ketones, which are also central nervous depressants and which in the case of higher homologues persist in the blood and tissues for many hours (Haggard *et al.*, 1945). Tertiary alcohols are metabolized slowly and incompletely, so that their toxic effects are especially persistent (*e.g.*, Wallgren, 1960; Haggard *et al.*, 1945); at least in part they are excreted in the urine as glucuronides.

Although some evidence suggests that higher alcohols may be metabolized at least in part by hepatic microsomal enzymes (Cohen and Cederbaum, 1980), pyrazole, a known inhibitor of alcohol dehydrogenase, blocks the metabolism of *n*-butanol and isobutyl alcohol in rats (Lester and Benson, 1970). *n*-Butanol is metabolized extensively in rats, 83% of an oral dose being converted to carbon dioxide within 24 hours; 4% was excreted in the urine and 12% remained in the carcass (DiVincenzo and Hamilton, 1979).

Although liver injury has not been described in man, it has been reported occasionally in exposed laboratory animals. Given daily by mouth for 4 months, 2.5 ml./kg. of grain alcohol fusel oils produced hepatic necrosis in rats (Gibel *et al.*, 1969). Liver damage was inferred in late deaths (up to 6 days) after single doses of *n*-butyl, *sec*-butyl, *tert*-butyl and isobutyl alcohols in rats (Maickel and McFadden, 1979), but daily administration of 1 gm./kg. of *n*-amyl alcohol in corn oil to rats for 13 weeks was found to be a "no untoward effect level" (Butterworth *et al.*, 1978).

Only symptomatic and supportive therapy is available in managing patients poisoned by higher alcohols. In the absence of effective treatment, respiratory arrest is the usual cause of death in acutely poisoned animals and presumably in man. If gas exchange is maintained by artificial respiration, larger doses can be survived, but high blood levels of ethanol, propanol-1 and butanol-1 eventually induce serious cardiac toxicity in dogs (MacGregor *et al.*, 1964). It may be manifest by atrial standstill, AV block and/or distortions of the QRS complex in the ECG. Probably all of the toxic aliphatic alcohols share this ability to depress the myocardium (Loomis, 1952).

In the presence of deep and persistent coma, hemodialysis should be considered as a possible way to remove the unmetabolized alcohol or its toxic metabolic products. This procedure may be especially useful with secondary and tertiary butyl alcohols, which are excreted only slowly by the kidneys (Wallgren, 1960).

Symptomatology:
1. Central nervous system: headache, muscle weakness, giddiness, ataxia, confusion, delirium, coma.
2. Gastrointestinal: nausea, vomiting, diarrhea (odor of the alcohol in excreta).
3. Irritation of skin, eyes, throat—from vapor or liquid. Cough and dyspnea.
4. Death from respiratory failure.
5. Disturbances of cardiac rhythm.
6. Occasional complications:
   a. Gastrointestinal hemorrhage
   b. Renal damage with glycosuria
   c. Liver damage
   d. Cardiac failure
   e. Pulmonary edema
   f. Methemoglobin formation reportedly from amyl alcohols.

Treatment:
1. Gastric lavage with copious amounts of water.
2. It may be beneficial to instill 60 ml. of mineral oil into the stomach.
3. Oxygen and artificial respiration as needed (pp. IV-12 and 7).
4. Electrolyte balance: it may be useful to start 500 ml. M/6 sodium bicarbonate intravenously but maintain a cautious and conservative attitude toward electrolyte replacement unless shock or severe acidosis threatens.
5. To protect the liver, maintain carbohydrate intake by intravenous infusions of glucose. See also pp. IV-61 and 76.
6. Hemodialysis if coma is deep and persistent (see text above and also pp. IV-55–57)

Laboratory: Not generally relevant, but information about blood levels of the alcohols and of their metabolites will be of great interest. Repeated electrocardiograms and liver function tests may prove to be helpful.

References:

Brown, V. K. H.; Muir, C. M. C.; Thorpe, E. A contribution to the toxicology of some alcohol mixtures containing 7 to 9 and 9 to 11 carbon atoms and the corresponding phthalate esters. Arch. Toxikol. 26:84-90, 1970.

Butterworth, K. R.; Gaunt, I. F.; Heading, C. E.; Grasso, D.; Gangnolli S. D. Short-term toxicity of *n*-amyl alcohol in rats. Food Cosmet. Toxicol. 16:203-207, 1978.

Cogan, D. G.; Grant, W. M. An unusual type of keratitis associated with exposure to *n*-butyl alcohol (butanol). Arch. Ophthalmol. 33:106-109, 1945.

Cohen, G.; Cederbaum, A. I. Microsomal metabolism of hydroxyl radical scavenging agents: relationship to the microsomal oxidation of alcohols. Arch. Biochem. Biophys. 199:438-447, 1980.

DiVincenzo, G. D.; Hamilton, M. L. Fate of n-butanol in rats after oral administration and its uptake by dogs after inhalation or skin absorbtion. Toxicol. Appl. Pharmacol. 48:317-325, 1979.

Gerarde, H. W.; Ahlstrom, D. B. The aspiration hazard and toxicity of a homologous series of alcohols. Arch. Environ. Health 13:457-461, 1966a.

Gibel, W.; Wildner, G. P.; Los, K. H. Experimentelle Untersuchungen uber die hepatotoxische Wirkung von hoheren Alkoholen (Fuselol). I. Mitteilung. Z. Gastroenterol. 7:108-113, 1969.

Greenberg, L.; Lester, D. Handbook of Cosmetic Materials, Their Properties, Uses and Toxic and Dermatologic Actions. Interscience Publishers, Inc., New York, 1954.

Haggard, H. W.; Miller, D. P.; Greenberg, L. A. The amyl alcohols and their ketones: their metabolic fates and comparative toxicities. J. Ind. Hyg. Toxicol. 27:1-14, 1945.

Koerker, R. L.; Berlin, A. J.; Schneider, F. H. The cytotoxicity of short-chain alcohols and aldehydes in cultured neuroblastoma cells. Toxicol. Appl. Pharmacol. 37:281-288, 1976.

Lester, D.; Benson, G. O. Alcohol oxidation in rats inhibited by pyrazole, oximes and amides. Science 169:282-283, 1970.

Loomis, T. A. The effect of alcohol on myocardial and respiratory function. Q. J. Stud. Alcohol 13:561-570, 1952.

MacGregor, D. C.; Schonbaum, E.; Bigelow, W. G. Acute toxicity studies on ethanol, propanol and butanol. Can. J. Physiol. Pharmacol. 42:689-696, 1964.

Macht, D. I. A toxicological study of some alcohols with especial reference to isomers. J. Pharmacol. Exp. Ther. 16:1-10, 1920.

Maickel, R. P.; McFadden, D. P. Acute toxicity of butyl nitrites and butyl alcohols. Res. Commun. Chem. Pathol.

Pharmacol. 26:75-83, 1979.

McCreery, M. J.; Hunt, W. A. Physico-chemical correlates of alcohol intoxication. Neuropharmacology 17:451-461, 1978.

Munch, J. C. Aliphatic alcohols and alkyl ester: narcotic and lethal potencies to tadpoles and to rabbits. IMS 41:31-33, 1972.

Munch, J. C.; Schwartze, E. W. Narcotic and toxic potency of aliphatic alcohols upon rabbits. J. Lab. Clin. Med. 10:985-996, 1925.

Revici, E.; Ravich, R. A. Antihemorrhagic action of n-butanol in advanced cancer. Angiology 4:510-515, 1953.

Scala, R. A.; Burtis, E. G. Acute toxicity of a homologous series of branched-chain primary alcohols. Am. Ind. Hyg. Assoc. J. 34:493-499, 1973.

Spector, W. S. Handbook of Toxicology. Vol. I, W. B. Saunders Co., Philadelphia, 1955.

Tabershaw, I. R.; Fahy, J. P.; Skinner, J. B. Industrial exposure to butanol. J. Ind. Hyg. Toxicol. 26:328, 1944.

Treon, J. F. Alcohols. Chap. XXXIV in Patty's Industrial Hygiene and Toxicology, Vol. II, edited by D. D. Irish and D. W. Fassett. 2nd edition, Interscience Publ., New York, 1962.

von Oettingen, W. F. Aliphatic alcohols: their toxicity and potential dangers in relation to their constitution and their fate in metabolism. Public Health Bull. No. 281, 1943.

Wallgren, H. Relative intoxicating effects on rats of ethyl, propyl and butyl alcohols. Acta Pharmacol. Toxicol., 16:217-222, 1960.

Webster, R. W. Legal Medicine and Toxicology. W. B. Saunders Co., Philadelphia, 1930.

Welt, B. n-Butanol: Its use in control of post-operative pain in otorhinolaryngological surgery. Arch. Otolaryngol. 52:549-564, 1950.

ALIPHATIC THIOCYANATES

Various synthetic aliphatic thiocyanates (rhodanates) have been widely used as contact insecticides since the 1930s. They were the first truly synthetic insecticides. Low molecular weight homologues, such as methyl, ethyl, and isopropyl thiocyanates, are volatile liquids sometimes employed as insecticidal fumigants. Long-chain derivatives, such as lauryl thiocyanate and certain ester and ether derivatives are oily liquids marketed as dusting powders and as kerosene-base sprays, often in combination with pyrethrum and rotenone, for use in fields, gardens and homes. The thiocyanates have synergistic insecticidal effects in combination with DDT, carbaryl and organophosphates like parathion. They have also been used on the skin as delousing preparations and as livestock sprays.

The following insecticide products are available commercially: Thanite (isobornyl thiocyanoacetate), Lethane 384 (β-butoxy-β-thiocyanodiethyl ether in an equal volume of petroleum solvent), and Lethane 60 (β-thiocyanoethyl esters of C_{10}–C_{18} fatty acids in an equal volume of petroleum solvent). Lethane 384 Special can be described as a diluted mixture of Lethane 384 and Lethane 60.

Toxicology: As observed in laboratory animals, aliphatic thiocyanates differ widely among themselves in oral and parenteral toxicity (Ohkawa et al., 1972; Taubmann, 1930; Yokoi, 1954).

The only human fatalities known to us involved an adult who drank a mixture containing no more than 3.5 gm. of Lethane 384 and 10 gm. of lauryl thiocyanate (Harrison, 1947) and a 2-year-old boy who swallowed a small quantity of a mixture of Lethane 384 (conc. about 6%) and Lethane 60 (conc. about 18%) in a petroleum solvent (Coulter and Creery, 1953). Another 2-year-old boy ingested 1 to 2 tsp. of 50% Lethane 384 in mineral oil (Guy, 1951); he eventually recovered after a severe bronchopneumonia probably due to aspiration.

Of the common thiocyanate insecticides, Lethane 384 has the highest acute toxicity; based on various animal species, the lethal oral dose in an adult person may lie anywhere between 1 teaspoonful and 1 oz. of the concentrated commercial solution (50% active ingredient). Lauryl thiocyanate appears to be considerably less toxic (Cameron et al., 1939), whereas Lethane 60 and Thanite possess intermediary toxicities. None of these compounds is as toxic as ethyl or methyl thiocyanate (Ohkawa et al., 1972; von Oettingen et al., 1936; Yokoi, 1954).

All derivatives have an appreciable percutaneous toxicity, although this is not regarded as an important hazard with the concentrations usually employed in agriculture (Main and Haag, 1942). Primary irritation of skin and eyes due to local contact, however, is not a negligible hazard, and the undiluted liquids may produce very severe cutaneous reactions, particularly lauryl thiocyanate and isobornyl thiocyanoacetate (Cameron et al., 1939).

Besides these quantitative differences, important qualitative distinctions are recognized among the various organic thiocyanates. For example, methyl, ethyl, and isopropyl thiocyanates and Lethane 384 are rapidly acting poisons of high potency; the oral mean lethal dose of methyl thiocyanate is less than 20 mg./kg. in rats (von Oettingen et al., 1936). They produce central nervous depression, usually with a transient period of respiratory stimulation, progressing promptly to death from respiratory failure. Enzymes in the liver and perhaps other organs are known to liberate cyanide ion from methyl, ethyl, and other thiocyanates including Lethane 384 (von Oettingen et al., 1936). Glutathione S-transferase catalyzes the attack of reduced glutathione at the thiocyanate sulfur, resulting in the liberation of HCN, oxidized glutathione and the mercaptan moiety of the organothiocyanate. Although it is less toxic, Thanite reacts readily with glutathione to liberate HCN even in the absence of the enzyme (Ohkawa et al., 1972).

Because cyanide is probably largely responsible for poisonings due to methyl, ethyl, and isopropyl thiocyanates and to Lethane 384 and Thanite, antidotal measures against cyanide should be instituted promptly (see p. III-127). Because the cyanide is liberated slowly, the thiosulfate injections should be repeated at regular intervals. Butyl thiocyanate and higher homologues (e.g., octyl and lauryl) do not furnish significant amounts of cyanide in vivo (Ohkawa et al., 1972; von Oettingen et al., 1936). The mechanism of action of the higher thiocyanates is unknown.

No toxicological connection between aliphatic and inorganic thiocyanates has been demonstrated. On the basis of SCN content, sodium thiocyanate probably has a lower acute toxicity than any thiocyanate insecticide. In contrast to the hyperexcitability induced by overdoses of the inorganic salts, the principal systemic action of organic thiocyanates is central nervous depression, intense dyspnea, cyanosis, and sometimes convulsions which are probably asphyxial in origin. In some instances, however, tremors, paralysis, spasticity, and even opisthotonos have been described, notably in rabbits given Lethane 384 by various routes (Cameron et al., 1939; Main and Haag, 1942).

Some toxic effects reported in laboratory studies must be ascribed to the petroleum vehicle (purified kerosene in the case of the Lethanes). Especially with the dilute formulations commonly used in the home (e.g., 4% active ingredient), kerosene is expected to contribute appreciably to any poisonings which may arise from accidental ingestion or other misuse (Guy, 1951).

Symptomatology (largely inferred from animal tests):

1. The ingestion of concentrated solutions may lead to vomiting because of mucosal irritation.
2. The principal systemic reaction is probably one of central nervous depression, interrupted by periods of restlessness, hyperpnea, and tonic convulsions. As judged by animal tests, depression may last for many days.
3. The signs and symptoms of kerosene poisoning are often dominant after ingestions of dilute solutions of thiocyanate insecticides (see p. III-223).
4. In the absence of aspiration, death is usually due to respiratory arrest from paralysis of the medullary centers.
5. Massive skin contamination with organic thiocyanate solutions may produce systemic poisoning as described above and in addition local irritation and dermatitis.
6. In nonfatal cases evidence of injuries to the liver and kidneys may appear.

Treatment:

1. In poisonings due to methyl, ethyl, or isopropyl thiocyanate, Lethane 384 and Thanite, proceed immediately as with cyanide poisoning (p. III-127). Because cyanide is released slowly, the thiosulfate injections should be repeated at regular intervals, but do not give more than the recommended number of injections of nitrite.
2. For long-chain aliphatic derivatives such as octyl or lauryl thiocyanates, proceed as follows. Cautious gastric lavage with copious amounts of water, unless spontaneous vomiting is judged to have removed most of the ingested material. Observe all precautions to avoid aspiration (p. I-10).
3. At the conclusion of lavage, instill 20 to 60 ml. of mineral oil in the stomach, as well as a saline cathartic (e.g., sodium sulfate 15 to 30 gm. in water). Avoid digestible fats, oils, and alcohol, which may promote absorption from the bowel.
4. Symptomatic and supportive measures for central nervous depression (see p. IV-39).
5. If severe or persistent, convulsions should be controlled by the intravenous administration of a short-acting barbiturate drug or diazepam (p. IV 35–39).
6. Positive pressure oxygen therapy (p. IV-15) is advisable if pulmonary edema arises as a toxic response to the petroleum solvent (kerosene). See also KEROSENE, p. III-224.

Laboratory:

1. Function tests should be used to detect and evaluate incipient renal and liver injuries.
2. The concentrations of inorganic (ionic) thiocyanate and cyanide in blood plasma are elevated in acute poisonings due to some thiocyanate insecticides in animals. Appropriate analyses in clinical poisonings would be highly desirable to confirm this observation in man.

References:

Cameron, G. R.; Doniger, C. R.; Hughes, A. W. M. The toxicity of lauryl thiocyanate and N-butyl-carbitolthiocyanate (lethane 384). J. Pathol. Bacteriol. 49:363-379, 1939.

Coulter, E.; Creery, R. D. G. "Lethane" poisoning. Report of a fatal case. Br. Med. J. 1:379, 1953.

Guy, A. Aspiration pneumonia due to "Lethane" hair-oil. Br. Med. J. 2:94-95, 1951.

Harrison, C. V. Fatal poisoning by "Lethane" insecticide. Br. Med. J. 1:722, 1947.

Main, R. J.; Haag, H. B. Toxicity of two organic thiocyanate insecticides. Ind. Med. Surg. 11:531-533, 1942.

Ohkawa, H.; Ohkawa, R.; Yamamoto, I.; Casida, J. E. Enzymatic mechanisms and toxicological significance of hydrogen cyanide liberation from various organo thiocyanates and organonitriles in mice and houseflies. Pesticide Biochem. Physiol. 2:95-112, 1972.

Taubmann, G. Untersuchungen uber die Wirkungen organischer Rhodanide. Naunyn-Schmiedebergs Arch. Pharmakol. 150:257-284, 1930.

von Oettingen, W. F.; Hueper, W. C.; Deichmann-Grubler, W. The pharmacologic action and pathologic effects of alkyl thiocyanates in relation to their chemical constitution and physical chemical properties. J. Ind. Hyg. Toxicol. 18:310-336, 1936.

Yokoi, Y. Pharmacological studies of some organic thiocyanates. Jap. J. Pharmacol. 3:99-111, 1954.

AMINOPHYLLINE

The most popular nonalcoholic stimulant beverages of the world are prepared from plants containing derivatives of xanthine. Coffee and many soft drinks contain caffeine, tea contains theophylline as well, whereas cocoa contains both caffeine and theobromine. The latter term is perhaps misleading since none of these compounds contains bromine; all are methyl derivatives of xanthine.

Certain physical mixtures and chemical combinations (double salts) of xanthines with other substances were introduced originally because they are more soluble than are the free bases. Notable among them are aminophylline (theophylline ethylenediamine), theophylline sodium acetate or glycinate, caffeine sodium benzoate, citrated caffeine, theobromine calcium salicylate, theobromine sodium acetate or salicylate, and choline theophyllinate (oxtriphylline). Hydroalcoholic solutions of theophylline, however, are more rapidly absorbed from the human stomach than either the choline or the ethylenediamine salts (Schluger et al., 1957).

Presumably the major pharmacological activity and toxicity of each of these mixtures are attributable to the xanthine moiety, with the possible exception of those combinations containing salicylate. The ethylenediamine moiety of aminophylline, however, has been specifically associated with severe exfoliative dermatitis in two patients who were not sensitive to theophylline (Elias and Levinson, 1981; Nierenberg and Glazener, 1982).

Indeed, in recent years there has been a trend back to the use of anhydrous theophylline in the treatment of chronic asthma; it is efficiently absorbed when ingested. Some of these products are sustained-release preparations. Overdoses of the latter are particularly dangerous because the slow onset of symptoms causes therapists to misjudge the seriousness of the ingestion (Olson et al., 1982).

Toxicology: The available acute toxicity data (Table III-1) in animals indicate that the methyl xanthines fall within toxicity class 4. Theophylline and caffeine are said to be equally toxic in rats (Poe and Johnson, 1953). Humans do not appear to be more sensitive to the lethal effects of caffeine than are other species, but man may be more sensitive to nonlethal effects (Peters, 1967). Tolerance to some of the effects of caffeine (Colton et al., 1968) and cross-tolerance to other xanthines are widely recognized; however, tolerance did not develop to the lethal effects of caffeine in rats (Boyd et al., 1965a).

Although the methylated xanthines have been used since antiquity, only recently have fatalities from acute intoxications been reported in the medical literature. We are not aware of any published accounts of fatal intoxications from theobromine, and reported fatalities due to caffeine are uncommon (but see Section II).

There is probably a wide range in the adult

Table III-1.

Experimental Acute Toxicity Studies with Methyl Xanthines

Drug	Route	Species	LD$_{50}$
			mg./kg.
Caffeine	Oral	Rat	233[a]
Caffeine	Intravenous	Rat	105[a]
Caffeine	Intravenous	Mouse	101[a]
Aminophylline	Oral	Mouse	540[b]
Aminophylline	Intravenous	Rabbit	150[b]

[a] Scott and Chen (1944).

[b] Thompson and Warren (1946).

human lethal dose by mouth. A serious poisoning in a teen-ager followed the ingestion of 1.6 gm. theophylline (Jefferys et al., 1980), but an adult woman survived after swallowing 21 gm. oxtriphylline (64% theophylline) perhaps because explosive diarrhea and extensive vomiting limited absorption (Iberti and Hammond, 1978). Blood plasma or serum levels also tend to vary widely among individuals. In a large-scale study with adult humans on oral multiple-dose aminophylline, the "trough" levels in serum varied from 3 to 38 μg./ml. Nausea, vomiting and anorexia were regularly associated with trough levels greater than 20 μg./ml. and were not seen below 13 μg./ml., whereas the maximal bronchodilator effect occurred between 8 and 20 μg./ml. (Jenne et al., 1972). An adult female who consumed 10 gm. oxtriphylline in a suicidal gesture had a peak serum level of 127 μg./ml. and was said to be "asymptomatic" (Snodgrass et al., 1980). A premature infant who accidentally received a total intravenous dose of 380 mg./kg. over 18 hours exhibited only "jitteriness" with a serum level of 300 μg./ml. (Wells and Ferlauto, 1979). Two other infants with serum levels of 48 and 79 μg./ml. exhibited only a sustained tachycardia (Cole and Davies, 1980) whereas a 70-year-old man died in cardiopulmonary arrest with a serum level of 33 μg./ml. (Vincent, 1978). In dictating management the clinical findings in any given patient should take precedence over estimates of the dose or values of the serum level. We know of no physiological basis for the clinical impression that theophylline toxicity is more common in patients over the age of 50 (Helliwell and Berry, 1979).

Therapeutic misadventures have occurred with single conventional doses of aminophylline. Cardiac palpitations, syncope, extreme dilatation of the pupils, and sudden death were prominent features of three poisonings arising from the intravenous injection of aminophylline to patients in status asthmaticus (Merrill, 1943, 1944). In three other adult patients with histories of coronary disease or myocardial damage, Bresnick et al. (1948) suggested cardiac arrest or ventricular fibrillation as a cause of death during the rapid intravenous administration of aminophylline and emphasized the threat of adverse cardiac actions in such patients.

A large series of poisonings arising from the use of aminophylline suppositories led to several fatalities (e.g., Frazier, 1954; Pioppi, 1954) before it was pointed out that the unit dose in commercial preparations was too large for infants. Commercial aminophylline suppositories were available in two sizes, 0.5 gm. for adults and a "half-strength" size for children. Although perhaps appropriate for a child of 75 to 100 lb., a dose of 250 mg. is recognized to be dangerously high for infants (Rounds, 1954). Before a 125-mg. suppository was marketed, the 250-mg. "pediatric" preparation had gained great popularity and was responsible for a large number of poisonings (Love and Corrado, 1955; Veum and Schwartz, 1956; White and Daeschner, 1956; Nolke, 1956). Rectal doses as low as 9 mg./kg. have produced toxic symptoms in children (Cohen, 1958). As generally safe but effective individual doses in children, 3.5 mg./kg. intravenously or intramuscularly, 5 mg./kg. orally, and 7 mg./kg. rectally, repeated at intervals of 6 to 12 hours, have been recommended (White and Daeschner, 1956). Clinical experience suggests that children may be more susceptible to the lethal effects of aminophylline than are common laboratory animals.

Besides the suppository, theophylline as a solution of the monoethanolamine salt can be administered rectally in the form of an enema, and a severe poisoning has been reported from this practice (Jacobziner and Raybin, 1960a). In the hopes of obviating the severe gastrointestinal irritation which often results from its oral administration, aminophylline is frequently prescribed as enteric coated tablets. Two fatalities have resulted from the accidental ingestion of this dosage form (Tindall et al., 1957; Couch et al., 1958). Probably the first reported fatality from oral administration of a xanthine involved an antiasthmatic preparation containing ephedrine, theophylline, and phenobarbital (Gardner et al., 1950). Theophylline synergism with ephedrine is now well recognized (Bacal et al., 1959).

Whatever the route of administration, the first sign of aminophylline overdosage appears to be restlessness. The only regular exception is cardiac standstill or ventricular fibrillation in patients with preexisting heart disease who receive intravenous aminophylline. Restlessness and irritability are signs of the stimulatory actions of theophylline on all parts of the central nervous system, actions which may progress to extreme agitation, tremors, delirium, maniacal behavior, convulsions, and coma. Periods of intense emotional lability alternating with withdrawal were associated with toxic blood levels in one patient (Wasser et al., 1981). Perhaps some of these effects are due to or exaggerated by brain anoxia, since at least caffeine has been shown to produce marked constriction of cerebral blood vessels (Wechsler et al., 1950). About half of the reported cases of aminophylline poisoning had clonic-tonic convulsions, usually alternating with periods of stupor, during which extensor rigidity sometimes persisted. Seizures are a grave prognostic sign and may be difficult to control (Helliwell and Berry, 1979). Residual neurologic deficits, including paraparesis, have been reported (Ehlers et al., 1978).

If restlessness is commonly the first sign of

intoxication, vomiting is the most constant one (Soifer, 1957). It occurs whatever the route of administration and is a reflection of medullary stimulation. It is generally violent and persistent but may be slight or absent in poisonings due to slow-release preparations of theophylline (Olson et al., 1982). Usually the vomitus is initially clear, but signs of bleeding develop promptly and the vomitus has been variously described as bloody and syrup-like, brown and thick, and "coffee grounds." Presumably this blood arises from multiple mucosal erosions, particularly of the gastric mucous membrane, ascribed to the excessive gastric acid secretion stimulated by the drug. Hypersecretion and persistent vomiting may lead to extensive ulceration and in one case to esophageal perforation (Couch et al., 1958). What appeared to be chemical burns on the lips and cheeks have been described in several poisoned children and ascribed to the high acidity of vomitus (McKee and Haggerty, 1957).

The diuretic action of theophylline leads to large water losses as does the persistent vomiting. The result is severe dehydration and intense thirst. The fever which is frequently encountered may arise from this dehydration as well as from motor restlessness. Tachycardia and premature beats are often noted, but except in patients with preexisting heart disease circulatory disorders are not a prominent feature of theophylline toxicity, perhaps because the central and peripheral actions of methyl xanthines on the cardiovascular system are generally antagonistic and so lead to variable and unpredictable responses (Bacal et al., 1959; Colton et al., 1968; Sollmann and Pilcher, 1911). We are aware, however, of one unreported case of cardiac arrest in a young adult without known heart disease, presumably as a result of too frequent intravenous infusions of aminophylline.

The terminal event appears to consist of both respiratory and cardiovascular collapse, presumably due in large measure to medullary exhaustion. Although no specific antidotes are known, an opportunity for effective supportive therapy is afforded by the long interval between the first toxic sign and final collapse. Furthermore a long latency may precede the appearance of toxicity (in Tindall's case more than 18 hours), particularly after the administration of suppositories and of enteric coated tablets. Peak drug levels in the blood plasma are said to be obtained almost immediately after intravenous and intramuscular administration, about 1 hour after plain tablets taken by mouth, 5 hours after enteric coated tablets, and 3 to 5 hours after rectal administration (Waxler and Schack, 1950), but absorption from all parts of the gastrointestinal tract tends to be rather uncertain and unpredictable.

Failure to appreciate the persistence of aminophylline in the body is perhaps in part responsible for the large number of iatrogenic poisonings that can now be cited in the literature (van Heyst and Oort, 1966). As estimated by blood levels, its biological half-life even after intravenous administration is 3 to 4 hours (Truitt et al., 1950). With toxic doses the effective half-life is considerably longer, especially in infants (Buchanan et al., 1979; Kadlec et al., 1978; Miceli et al., 1980; Vaucher et al., 1977). At least 7 hours are required to clear the blood completely in normal adult subjects after 300 to 500 mg. intravenously (Brodwall, 1953; Truitt et al., 1950). Lower peak blood levels are attained after oral or rectal administration, but 10 hours or more are required before the drug disappears entirely from the blood. A cumulative effect on blood theophylline levels was observed in normal subjects taking theophylline sodium glycinate (650 mg.) by mouth at 4-hour intervals for 4 doses (Truitt et al., 1950). It would appear unnecessary and dangerous to administer aminophylline at more frequent intervals than 6 to 8 hours. The drug should be withheld immediately if vomiting occurs.

Theophylline is extensively metabolized by the liver to a variety of oxidized products and to a limited extent to caffeine (Baltassat et al., 1979). The latter pathway may be of significance in premature infants since toxic signs were more prominent when the plasma caffeine levels were elevated as a result of theophylline biotransformation (Boutroy et al., 1979). An inverse relationship is said to exist between theophylline blood levels and age over 4 to 18 months (Rosen et al., 1979). Considerable variation, however, is recognized. Some infants eliminate theophylline in accord with the usual first-order kinetics (half-life 8 to 9 hours) even at very high serum levels (Buchanan et al., 1979; Vaucher et al., 1977), whereas others clearly exhibit an initial phase of saturation (zero-order) followed by a late phase of first-order kinetics (Kadlec et al., 1978). A similar pattern has been observed in severely poisoned adults (Miceli et al., 1980; Snodgrass et al., 1980). An occasional individual may be found with unexplained but markedly impaired ability to clear the drug. In a 64-year-old man the blood theophylline half-life was 18 hours and caffeine half-life was also prolonged (Gotz et al., 1979). It has been suggested that abrupt changes in hepatic metabolism may occur in some but not all patients during acute viral illnesses with consequent sudden increases to toxic blood levels (Woo et al., 1980).

Occasionally infants present with hyperglycemia, glycosuria and ketoacidosis (Larcher et al., 1978; Vaucher et al., 1977). Perhaps this reaction is secondary to a generalized increase in the activity of the sympathetic nervous system. In weanling mice aminophylline increased the cerebral metabolic rate 3-fold and significantly decreased the incidence of anoxic survival (Thurston *et al.*, 1978). Therefore extreme caution should be exercised in the use of this drug in hypoxic human newborns. Hypokalemia probably resulting from fluid and electrolyte loss by vomiting and diarrhea may be a significant complication (Helliwell and Berry, 1979; Jefferys *et al.*, 1980).

Although theophylline is a weak base, it does not reaccumulate in gastric fluid, and there is probably little to be gained by acidification of the urine to hasten excretion (Done, 1980). Exchange transfusion failed to alter the blood concentration in one massively overdosed premature infant (Wells and Ferlauto, 1979). Theophylline is not intensively bound to plasma proteins (Vallner *et al.*, 1979) and it is distributed in total body water.

Peritoneal dialysis has been studied experimentally in rats where 27% of the total dose was recovered in 4 hours (Emonds and Driessen, 1978). Favorable results have also been obtained in poisoned infants (Miceli *et al.*, 1979, 1980). In one case the peritoneal clearance was about 5 ml./min. when the renal clearance was 2 ml./min. (Miceli *et al.*, 1980). Extracorporeal hemodialysis in two adults increased clearance rates 2- to 3-fold (Levy *et al.*, 1977a; Snodgrass *et al.*, 1980). Even higher clearance rates (up to 160 ml./min.) were obtained by hemoperfusion over charcoal (Ehlers *et al.*, 1978; Jefferys *et al.*, 1980; Russo, 1979) or resin columns (Lawyer *et al.*, 1978). Activated charcoal by mouth is also highly effective in preventing theophylline absorption (Sintek *et al.*, 1979).

Symptomatology:
1. Wakefulness, restlessness, tinnitus, mild excitement or irritability alternating with drowsiness.
2. Anorexia, nausea, emesis usually beginning early.
3. As with caffeine, mild tachycardia with or without premature beats sometimes occurs even before dehydration, hypotension or hypokalemia.
4. Fever, increased vomiting, diuresis, dehydration, extreme thirst.
5. Eventual bloody, syrup-like or "coffee-ground" vomitus (even when the route of administration is not oral).
6. Tremors, delirium, tonic extensor spasm interrupted by clonic convulsions, apathy, stupor, coma.
7. After a fairly long course, cardiovascular and respiratory collapse, leading to shock, cyanosis and death.

Treatment:
1. If the patient is asymptomatic shortly after ingesting a massive overdose, induce emesis or perform gastric lavage.
2. Leave 15 to 30 gm. sodium sulfate (in solution) in the stomach and at least 30 gm. of activated charcoal (see Section I).
3. Supportive and symptomatic treatment with special emphasis on sedative drugs such as barbiturates or diazepam to control convulsions (see p. IV-36).
4. Parenteral fluids and electrolytes (see p. IV-64), as necessary. Check serum electrolyte levels, and correct any hypokalemia (p. IV-73). A ketoacidosis, especially in infants, may require attention (p. IV-71).
5. Oxygen and shock therapy, including blood transfusion, as indicated (see pp. IV-12 and 17). Hypotension can usually be avoided if dehydration and electrolyte disturbances are corrected promptly.
6. In severe poisonings, peritoneal dialysis, hemodialysis or hemoperfusion may be important in shortening the critical period of the illness.

Laboratory: Electrocardiographic changes may be seen. A reversible proteinuria and leukocytosis have been described. Reductions of prothrombin time and of coagulation time have been reported but presumably are not of clinical significance (Scherf and Schlachman, 1946). Hyperglycemia, glycosuria and ketoacidosis have been described in poisoned infants.

References:

Bacal, H. L.; Linegar, K.; Denton, R. L.; Gourdeau, G. Aminophylline poisoning in children. Can. Med. Assoc. J. *80*:6-9, 1959.

Baltassat, P.; Hartmann, E.; Bory, C.; Frederich, A. Theophylline acute poisoning in a child: Evidence for biotransformation of theophylline into caffeine. Vet. Human Toxicol. *21*:Suppl., 211-213, 1979.

Boutroy, M. J.; Vert, P.; Monin, P.; Royer, R. J.; Royer-Morrot, M. J. Methylation of theophylline to caffeine in premature infants. Lancet *1*:830, 1979.

Boyd, E. M.; Dolman, M.; Knight, L. M.; Sheppard, E. P. The chronic oral toxicity of caffeine. Can. J. Physiol. Pharmacol. *43*:995-1007, 1965a.

Bresnick, E.; Woodward, W. K.; Sageman, C. B. Fatal reactions to intravenous administration of aminophylline. J. A. M. A. *136*:397-398, 1948.

Brodwall, E. K. The resorption of theophyllamine (theophylline ethylenediamine). Blood concentrations after intravenous, peroral, rectal and intramuscular administration. Acta Med. Scand. *146*:123-126, 1953.

Buchanan, N.; Wainwright, L.; de Villiers, F. Theophylline poisoning in an infant: a case report. S. Afr. Med. J. *56*:811-812, 1979.

Cohen, N. J. Aminophylline poisoning. Ann. Pediatr. *191*:16-26, 1958.

Cole, G. F.; Davies, D. P. Theophylline poisoning. Br. Med. J. *280*:52, 1980.

Colton, T.; Gosselin, R. E.; Smith, R. P. The tolerance of coffee drinkers to caffeine. Clin. Pharmacol. Ther. *9*:31-39, 1968.

Couch, R. D.; Franz, M.; Forney, R. B. Aminophylline poisoning. Report of a case with complete pathologic and toxicologic findings. Am. J. Clin. Pathol. *30*:435-438, 1958.

Done, A. K. Ion trapping in the pathogenesis and treatment of poisoning. Vet. Human Toxicol. *22*:Suppl. 2, 2-9, 1980.

Ehlers, S. M.; Zaske, D. E.; Sawchuck, R. J. Massive theophylline overdose. Rapid elimination by charcoal hemoperfusion. J. A. M. A. *240*:474-475, 1978.

Elias, J. A.; Levinson, A. I. Hypersensitivity reactions to ethylenediamine in aminophylline. Am. Rev. Respir. Dis. 123:550-552, 1981.

Emonds, A. J. G.; Driessen, O. M. J. Treatment of theophylline intoxication: A model study utilizing peritoneal dialysis. Clin. Toxicol. 13:505-571, 1978.

Frazier, C. A. Toxicity of aminophylline. J. A. M. A. 155:222, 1954.

Gardner, R. A.; Hansen, A. E.; Ewing, P. L.; Emerson, G. A. Unexpected fatality in a child from accidental consumption of antiasthmatic preparation containing ephedrine, theophylline, and phenobarbital. Tex. Med. 46:516-520, 1950.

Gotz, V. P.; Drayer, D. E.; Schmed, E. S.; Reidenberg, M. M. Unusual case of theophylline toxicity. N. Y. State J. Med. 79:1232-1234, 1979.

Helliwell, M.; Berry, D. Theophylline poisoning in adults. Br. Med. J. 2:1114, 1979.

Iberti, T. J.; Hammond, R. S. Massive oral theophylline poisoning. South. Med. J. 71:965-966, 1978.

Jacobziner, H.; Raybin, H. W. Aminophylline and other severe poisonings. N. Y. State J. Med. 60:3300-3303, 1960a.

Jefferys, D. B.; Raper, S. M.; Helliwell, M.; Berry, D. J.; Crome, P. Haemoperfusion for the theophylline overdose. Br. Med. J. 280:1167, 1980.

Jenne, J. W.; Wyze, E.; Rood, F. S.; MacDonald, F. M. Pharmacokinetics of theophylline. Clin. Pharmacol. Ther. 13:349-360, 1972.

Kadlec, G. J.; Jarboe, C. H.; Pollard, S. J.; Sublett, J. L. Acute theophylline intoxication. Biphasic first order elimination kinetics in a child. Ann. Allergy 41:337-339, 1978.

Larcher, V. F.; Gamser, H. R.; Sanderson, M. C.; Drayton, M. R.; Sandhu, B. Theophylline toxicity in a neonate. Arch. Dis. Child. 53:757-759, 1978.

Lawyer, C.; Aitchison, J.; Sutton, J.; Bennett, W. Treatment of theophylline neurotoxicity with resin hemoperfusion. Ann. Intern. Med. 88:516-517, 1978.

Levy, G.; Gibson, T. P.; Whitman, W.; Procknal, J. Hemodialysis clearance of theophylline. J. A. M. A. 237:1466-1467, 1977a.

Love, F. M.; Corrado, A. G. Aminophylline overdosage in children. Am. J. Dis. Child. 89:468-471, 1955.

McKee, M.; Haggerty, R. J. Aminophylline poisoning. N. Engl. J. Med. 256:956-957, 1957.

Merrill, G. A. Aminophylline death. J. A. M. A. 123:1115, 1943.

Merrill, G. A. Aminophylline deaths. J. A. M. A. 124:250, 1944.

Miceli, J. N.; Bidani, A.; Aronow, R. Peritoneal dialysis of theophylline. Clin. Toxicol. 14:539-544, 1979.

Miceli, J. N.; Clay, B.; Fleischmann, L. E.; Sarnaik, A. P.; Aronow, R.; Done, A. K. Pharmacokinetics of severe theophylline intoxication managed by peritoneal dialysis. Dev. Pharmacol. Ther. 1:16-25, 1980.

Nierenberg, D. W.; Glazener, F. S. Aminophylline-induced exfoliative dermatitis: etiology and implications. West. J. Med. 137:328-331, 1982.

Nolke, A. C. Severe toxic effects from aminophylline and theophylline suppositories in children. J. A. M. A. 161:693-697, 1956.

Olson, K.; Benowitz, N.; Pentel, P. Survey of causes and conseuqences of seizures during drug intoxication. Vet. Human Toxicol. 24:280, 1982.

Peters, J. M. Factors affecting caffeine toxicity. J. Clin. Pharmacol. 1:131-141, 1967.

Pioppi, N. W. Toxicity of aminophylline. J. A. M. A. 154:543, 1954.

Poe, C. F.; Johnson, C. C. Toxicity of caffeine, theobromine and theophylline. Acta Pharmacol. Toxicol. 9:267-274, 1953.

Rosen, J. P.; Danish, M.; Ragni, M. C.; Lopez Saccar, C.; Yaffe, S. J.; Lecks, H. I. Theophylline pharmacokinetics in the young infant. Pediatrics 64:248-251, 1979.

Rounds, V. J. Aminophylline poisoning. Pediatrics 14:528-532, 1954.

Russo, M. E. Management of theophylline intoxication with charcoal-column hemoperfusion. N. Engl. J. Med. 300:24-26, 1979.

Scherf, D.; Schlachman, M. The effect of methylxanthines on the prothrombin time and the coagulation of the blood. Am. J. Med. 212:83-89, 1946.

Schluger, J.; McGinn, J. T.; Hennessy, D. J. Comparative theophylline blood levels following the oral administration of three different theophylline preparations. Am. J. Med. Sci. 233:296-302, 1957.

Scott, C. C.; Chen, K. K. Comparison of the action of l-ethyltheobromine and caffeine in animals and man. J. Pharmacol. Exp. Ther. 82:89-97, 1944.

Sintek, C.; Hendeles, L.; Weinberger, M. Inhibition of theophylline absorption by activated charcoal. J. Pediatr. 94:314-316, 1979.

Snodgrass, W.; Sawyer, D.; Conner, C. S.; Rumack, B. H.; Peterson, P. G.; Sullivan, J. B. Asymptomatic theophylline overdose. Drug Intell. Clin. Pharmacol. 14:783-785, 1980.

Soifer, H. Aminophylline toxicity. J. Pediatr. 50:657-669, 1957.

Sollmann, T.; Pilcher, J. D. The actions of caffeine on the mammalian circulation. J. Pharmacol. Exp. Ther. 3:19-92, 1911.

Thompson, C. R.; Warren, M. R. Acute and chronic toxicity studies on theophylline aminoisobutanol and theophylline ethylenediamine. J. Lab. Clin. Med. 31:1337-1343, 1946.

Thurston, J. H.; Hauhart, R. E.; Dugo, J. A. Aminophylline increases cerebral metabolic rate and decreases anoxic survival in young mice. Science 201:649-651, 1978.

Tindall, H. L.; Clayton, T. D.; Winfield, A. C. Fatal accidental poisoning by aminophylline in a child. Am. J. Dis. Child. 94:80-82, 1957.

Truitt, E. B., Jr.; McKusick, V. A.; Krantz, J. C., Jr. Theophylline blood levels after oral, rectal and intravenous administration, and correlation with diuretic action. J. Pharmacol. Exp. Ther. 100:309-315, 1950.

Vallner, J. J.; Speir, W. A., Jr.; Kolbeck, R. C.; Harrison, G. N.; Bransome, E. D., Jr. Effect of pH on the binding of theophylline to serum proteins. Respir. Dis. 120:83-86, 1979.

van Heyst, A. N. P.; Oort, M. Theofyllinevergiftiging bij een kind. Ned. Tijdschr. Geneeskd. 110:1603-1605, 1966.

Vaucher, Y.; Lightner, E. S.; Walson, P. D. Theophylline poisoning. J. Pediatr. 90:827-830, 1977.

Veum, J.; Schwartz, A. B. Toxic effects of half-strength aminophylline suppositories in asthmatic children. J. Pediatr. 49:703-707, 1956.

Vincent, F. M. Case Report: Fatal theophylline-induced seizures. Postgrad. Med. 63:76-77, 1978.

Wasser, W. G.; Bronheim, H. E.; Richardson, B. K. Theophylline madness. Ann. Intern. Med. 95:191, 1981.

Waxler, S. H.; Schack, J. A. Administration of aminophylline (theophylene ethylenediamine). J. A. M. A. 143:736-739, 1950.

Wechsler, R. L.; Kleiss, L. M.; Kety, S. S. The effects of intravenously administered aminophylline on cerebral circulation and metabolism in man. J. Clin. Invest. 29:28-30, 1950.

Wells, D. H.; Ferlauto, J. J. Survival after massive aminophylline overdose in a premature infant. Pediatrics 64:252-253, 1979.

White, B. H.; Daeschner, C. W. Aminophylline (theophylline ethylenediamine) poisoning in children. J. Pediatr. 49:262-271, 1956.

Woo, O. F.; Koup, J. R.; Kraemer, M.; Robertson, W. O. Acute intoxication with theophylline while in chronic therapy. Vet. Human Toxicol. 22:Suppl. 2, 48-51, 1980.

AMMONIA

Ammonia in solution (ammonia water, ammonium hydroxide) in varying concentrations is used in a variety of products such as cleaning agents, liniments and aromatic spirits. Fresh household ammonia ranges in concentration from 5 to 10% (w/v) NH_3 (3 to 6 M), but a 27 to 30% solution (Spirits of Hartshorn) is also available commercially.

Ammonia solutions are sometimes used as fertilizers. Anhydrous ammonia gas, liquefied under pressure, is also applied directly to the soil or mixed with irrigation waters as a fertilizer. Furthermore liquid ammonia is encountered as an industrial refrigerant. Because of highway accidents involving tank trucks, tank car derailments and other industrial catastrophes, mass poisonings with ammonia gas have occurred (*e.g.*, Caplin, 1941; Close *et al.*, 1980; Montague and Macneil, 1980; Walton, 1973). Ammonia is also released in the combustion of wool, silk, nylon and melamine, but its concentration is low in most ordinary building fires (Terrill *et al.*, 1978). Ammonia gas has an odor threshold of about 5 ppm (in air) in most individuals; 20 ppm and above are often annoying (Subcommittee on Ammonia, 1979).

When an ammonia solution is partially or wholly neutralized by an acid such as vinegar, ammonia gas in solution is converted to nonvolatile ammonium ion, whose toxicity is also reviewed below. The addition to ammonia water of a strong alkali, *e.g.*, lye or sodium hydroxide, tends to promote the evolution of ammonia gas. Mixing ammonia with household bleach preparations containing HYPOCHLORITE (see p. III-202) leads to the formation of chloramines. Monochloramine (NH_2Cl) and dichloramine ($NHCl_2$) are soluble in water and decompose to ammonia and hypochlorous acid (Gleason *et al.*, 1964). Choramines are sometimes used as disinfectants in water purification. The toxicology of chloramines has not been thoroughly investigated, but exposure to these acrid fumes produces lacrimation, irritation of membranes of the respiratory passages and nausea. Available case reports indicate that victims suffer no serious sequelae (Dunn and Ozere, 1966; Faigel, 1964).

Toxicology of ammonia and ammonia water: Ammonium hydroxide differs from other alkalis in its volatility; the vapor (NH_3) even in low concentrations is extremely irritating to skin, eyes and respiratory passages (Boyd *et al.*, 1944; Caplin, 1941; Clinton, 1948; Silverman *et al.*, 1949; Slot, 1938). The most dangerous consequence of exposure to high concentrations of ammonia gas is pulmonary edema, often appearing 6 or more hours after exposure (Caplin, 1941; Levy *et al.*, 1964). Occasionally victims die as a result of this lung edema or later secondary bronchopneumonia (Caplin, 1941). Whereas eventual recovery without residual pulmonary damage is the rule (Levy *et al.*, 1964; Montague and Macneil, 1980), chronic airway dysfunction (*e.g.*, bronchitis) and even alveolar disease (emphysema, bronchiectasis) have been ascribed to ammonia gassing (Close *et al.*, 1980; Taplin *et al.*, 1976; Walton, 1973). In a gassed population, perhaps those individuals who are likely to develop chronic respiratory disease can be identified by demonstrating hydroxylysine metabolites in the urine, presumably indicating the breakdown of lung collagen (Hatton *et al.*, 1979). For the management of these inhalation episodes, see NITROGEN OXIDES, p. III-323.

One teaspoonful (3 to 5 ml.) of strong (28%) ammonia solution has been recorded as a fatal oral dose, but recovery has followed as much as 1 fl. oz. on several occasions (Webster, 1930). Although the oral ingestion of 3 to 4 oz. of household ammonia (5 to 10%) has been tolerated (Chassin and Slattery, 1953), the exact nature and intensity of the toxic syndrome are unpredictable, and so recorded values of the lethal dose can be very misleading. Probably the most acceptable view is that any amount of ammonia can be dangerous.

The ingestion of ammonia solutions produces effects similar to other corrosive alkalis (see also LYE, p. III-241), notably corrosive esophagitis and gastritis (Cardona and Daly, 1964; Chassin and Slattery, 1953; Ernst *et al.*, 1963; Gonzales *et al.*, 1962; Jacobziner and Raybin, 1959b; Leegaard, 1945; Norton, 1960; O'Donnell *et al.*, 1949). In addition, respiratory signs and symptoms should be anticipated after ingestion episodes as a consequence of aspiration of the solution or inhalation of its fumes (Ernst *et al.*, 1963; Norton, 1960; Pollack, 1945). Three swallows of a 10% "ammonical solution" (presumably meaning ammonia water) resulted in both esophageal corrosion and necrosis of the stomach with perforation and peritonitis (Poelman *et al.*, 1977). As with other strong alkalis, ulcerative esophagitis from ammonia ingestion produces a high incidence of late strictures (Cardona and Daly, 1964; Yarington, 1965). Gastric, duodenal and jejunal stenosis have also resulted (Chassin and Slattery, 1953; Ernst *et al.*, 1963; Gonzales *et al.*, 1962; Norton, 1960; O'Donnell *et al.*, 1949). Unrecognized late strictures may be confused with malignant growths (O'Donnell *et al.*, 1949). Ammonia-induced injuries of the alimentary tract are managed by the same medical and surgical techniques (Ernst *et al.*, 1963) used in lye poisoning (see pp. III-247 and 249-250).

Although the eye is able to tolerate higher concentrations of ammonia gas than the respiratory tract can (Grant, 1974), a splash of anhydrous liquid ammonia or of a strong ammonia solution can severely injure the eyes, as well as produce first and second degree burns of the skin (Levy *et al.*, 1964). Indeed ammonium hydroxide has a greater tendency than other alkalis to penetrate the cornea and to damage it and deeper structures within the eye, such as the iris and lens. The resulting uveitis may lead to iris atrophy and to cataracts, both lesions occurring only late in the course of the illness. The prompt eye effects include blepharospasm, corneal edema, cornea anesthesia, a fixed semidilated pupil and acute glaucoma with high intraocular tensions (Grant, 1974; Highman, 1969). A few weeks later, angle closure or obstruction of the pupil may produce secondary glaucoma.

Corneal ulcers may perforate or heal as opaque scars. The stroma of the alkali-burned cornea release collagenase, and collagenase inhibitors such as acetylcysteine have been applied topically to prevent perforation (Subcommittee on Ammonia, 1979). In experimental studies (Nirankari et al., 1981), superoxide radical scavenging agents, such as superoxide dismutase and ascorbic acid, have been used for the same purpose. The usefulness of these treatments is not yet established. At least all forms of ammonia injury to the eye can be minimized by washing the contaminated eye promptly with clean water. Speed is essential.

Although a rare exception can be cited (Anon., 1945), the inhalation or ingestion of ammonia does not produce signs of systemic intoxication. Experimental evidence indicates no significant cumulative effects of chronic ammonia exposure (Weatherby, 1952). Perhaps inhalation or ingestion does not permit absorption of toxicologically significant amounts.

In the absence of metabolic disease, the human body has a high capacity to buffer ammonia base, generating the ammonium ion, which is subsequently used in the synthesis of urea. Whether or not the small concentration of ammonia base which can exist at physiologic pH has a unique toxic action is unknown, but the parenteral (and perhaps oral) administration of ammonium salts produces a systemic intoxication which is apparently distinct from the hyperchloremic acidosis produced by ammonium chloride (Relman et al., 1961).

Toxicology of ammonium salts: Normal human subjects infused with ammonium acetate exhibit flaccidity of the facial muscles, tremor, generalized discomfort, anxiety, and impairment of motor performance, of recognition and of critical flicker fusion (Eichler, 1964). This description of acute intoxication by ammonium ion resembles the clinical picture of terminal liver failure, which is characterized by confusion, tremor, slurred speech, ataxia, stupor and coma. Elevated levels of blood ammonia (present as NH_4^+) are found regularly in advanced liver disease (Bessman and Bessman, 1955; Martini, 1961; Vanamee and Poppell, 1960) and sometimes in renal failure (Cobb et al., 1964).

Both central nervous depression and blood ammonia levels in liver failure can be reduced by hemodialysis (Kiley et al., 1958). Surgical exclusion of the colon (Dienst, 1964), purges, enemas, administration of broad spectrum antibiotics (Manning and Delp, 1958) and restriction of dietary protein (Summerskill et al., 1959)

have led to clinical improvement attributed to a decrease in ammonia synthesis by bacterial flora. Blood ammonia levels in Eck-fistula animals gavaged with blood can be reduced by whole body hypothermia (Zuidema et al., 1963b) or by the oral administration of cation exchange resins (Zuidema et al., 1962). Finally, the administration of urea cycle intermediates, such as arginine, to accelerate ammonia detoxication is said to result in some clinical improvement (Manning and Delp, 1958). Patients with far advanced liver disease, however, might be expected to respond less favorably, since the liver is the primary site of urea synthesis. For a more detailed discussion of the management of hepatic coma, see p. IV-62.

Systemic poisoning induced by the parenteral administration of ammonium salts or urease (e.g., purified jackbean urease) has been extensively studied in laboratory animals. Urease hydrolyzes endogenous urea to produce ammonia, which is in turn utilized to resynthesize urea. This self-perpetuating cyclic release results in a sustained (24 to 48 hours) elevation of blood ammonia. The resulting disease differs in various respects from that induced by the acute administration of ammonium salts (Dang and Visek, 1966, Hanford, 1961). Early experimental work is further confused by the circumstance that some investigators selected acidifying ammonium salts instead of those which are totally metabolized and excreted, such as ammonium acetate. After injection of either urease or ammonium salts, coma is preceded by signs of neural excitation.

In mice the intravenous administration of ammonium chloride resulted in hyperventilation and clonic movements, which were followed sometimes by tonic extensor convulsions, but usually by profound coma; death was preceded by convulsions, but survivors made a complete and rapid recovery. This syndrome, which was strikingly potentiated by short periods of hypoxia, occurred so promptly that the ammonium ion itself was believed to be responsible for the signs and symptoms and not the later hypochloremic acidosis (Warren and Schenker, 1960). Similarly, rats injected intraperitoneally with ammonium acetate (Navazio et al., 1961) and dogs given urease intravenously (Hanford, 1961) developed spasticity and convulsions coincident with high concentrations of ammonia in blood and brain.

Although the precise mechanism of systemic ammonia intoxication remains to be elucidated, evidence exists to suggest that an interference with cerebral oxidative energy metabolism is involved (Baraona et al., 1965; McKhann and Towers, 1961; Schenker and Warren, 1962). In rats made comatose with ammonium acetate, samples of basilar brain structures showed significant decreases in glycogen, glucose, ATP, and especially in phosphocreatine (Schenker *et al.*, 1967). These changes could not be mimicked by anesthesia, psychomotor stimulation or moderate hypoxia. Contrary evidence, however, can be cited. Hawkins *et al.*(1973) believe that ammonia stimulates oxidative metabolism in rat brain. Brain concentrations of most glycolytic intermediates were elevated, and adenine nucleotide levels were sustained (Hawkins *et al.*, 1973; Hindfelt *et al.*, 1977). It seems unlikely that cerebral dysfunction in ammonia intoxication is due to a primary energy failure (Hindfelt *et al.*, 1977). A poor correlation between blood or brain ammonia levels and the severity of symptoms in poisoned animals has been noted. (Navazio *et al.*, 1961; Salvatore *et al.*, 1963; Villarreal *et al.*, 1962).

Ornithine-arginine cycle intermediates including aspartate, glutamate and arginine at least partially block increases in blood ammonia and protect animals against death from ammonium salts or urease (Barnes *et al.*, 1964; Dang and Visek, 1966; Rosen *et al.*, 1963). Ammonia metabolism in neural tissues is less well understood. Although it has been asserted that glutamine synthesis may be an important metabolic route (Bessman and Bessman, 1955; Hanford, 1961), methionine sulfoximine, a competitive inhibitor of glutamine synthetase, protected mice against death by ammonium chloride in the face of an increased brain ammonia concentration (Warren and Schenker, 1964). Although the protective effect of each agent below has been at least partially explained, it is still difficult to fit them all into a comprehensive explanation of systemic ammonia poisoning: γ-aminobutyric acid (Manning *et al.*, 1964), carbamyl aspartate (Cittadini *et al.*, 1966), α-methylglutamic acid (Lamar, 1970), phenobarbital and alloxan (Dang and Visek, 1966), carbonic anhydrase inhibitors (Lange *et al.*, 1964), monoamine oxidase inhibitors (Zuidema *et al.*, 1963a) and diphenhydramine (Kirsch *et al.*, 1965).

In summary, a distinct syndrome of systemic ammonia intoxication is recognized in both man and laboratory animals in an experimental context. Only a remote possibility exists, however, that it might occur in man as the result of ingesting ammonia solutions or ammonium salts, except in the person with preexisting liver disease. Of course, abuse of ammonium chloride can produce a profound and life-threatening acidosis even in normal healthy individuals (Relman *et al.*, 1961). For a discussion of the management of acid-base disturbances, see pp. IV-69–72.

Symptomatology (ammonia gas and ammonia water only):

1. Vapors cause irritation of eyes and respiratory tract. High concentrations may cause conjunctivitis, laryngitis, tracheitis, and pulmonary edema or pneumonitis. Cough, dyspnea and pleuritic chest pain are common symptoms. A sensation of suffocation may be induced by spasm of the glottis or by laryngeal edema.
2. Contact with skin can cause burns with vesication. If squirted into the eyes, an early rise in intraocular pressure may mimick narrow-angle glaucoma. Corneal edema and oval semidilated fixed pupils are typical (Highman, 1969). Late injuries include obstructive glaucoma, opaque corneal scars, iris atrophy and cataracts.
3. Ingestion can lead to all the signs and symptoms, pathological lesions, and complications induced by other corrosive alkalis (see p. III-245).
4. If systemic absorption becomes extensive (which is extremely unlikely), coma may arise, perhaps preceded by a period of hypertonus and convulsions.

Treatment:

1. Lavage and emetics are contraindicated.
2. If ammonia water is swallowed, the victim should try to drink immediately large quantities of water or milk. The ingestion of weak acids such as diluted vinegar is no longer advised, but the issue has not been adequately resolved.
3. Administer a demulcent (egg white, olive oil, milk, etc.).
4. Control pain with injections of opiates or meperidine (Demerol).
5. Treat shock (p. IV-17). Keep the patient warm.
6. Contaminated eyes and skin should be washed immediately with copious amounts of tap water. Probably the irrigation should continue for 10 to 15 minutes. Pilocarpine eye drops may reduce a high intraocular tension, but they should not be used routinely because of the danger of promoting posterior synechiae. For the definitive treatment of most chemical burns of the eye, an ophthalmologist should be consulted.
7. Dyspnea due to partial airway obstruction may respond to intravenous aminophylline or aerosolized salbutamol.
8. Tracheotomy is indicated if signs of upper tract obstruction develop (p. IV-6).
9. For the management of pulmonary edema encountered after respiratory exposures to gaseous ammonia, see p. IV-14.
10. In ingestion cases, attempts to establish the presence or absence of esophageal and/or gastric injury should be initiated as soon as pain and shock are controlled. The techniques are the same as in lye poisoning; see p. III-249.
11. Prompt and aggressive surgical interven-

tion is indicated in the presence of mucosal lesions that are judged likely to perforate. An emergency esophagogastectomy may be required if the necrosis is deep and diffuse (see p. III-249).

12. In the presence of penetrating mucosal burns of the esophagus that are considered unlikely to perforate, nonsurgical treatment is appropriate. A steroid-antibiotic regimen is outlined on p. III-250; it should be initiated promptly and pursued vigorously.

Laboratory: Not generally relevant. Chest x-rays may reveal generalized pulmonary edema or localized consolidation, but a normal chest film shortly after the exposure does not preclude eventual chronic pulmonary dysfunction.

References:

Anon. (Queries and minor notes.) Ammonia and the nervous system. J. A. M. A. *127*:620, 1945.

Baraona, E.; Salinas, A.; Navia, E.; Orrego, H. Alterations of ammonia metabolism in the cerebral cortex of rats with hepatic damage induced by carbon tetrachloride. Clin. Sci. *28*:201-208, 1965.

Barnes, R. H.; Labadan, B. A.; Siyamoglu, B.; Bradfield, R. B. Effect of exercise and administration of aspartic acid on blood ammonia in the rat. Am. J. Physiol. *207*:1242-1246, 1964.

Bessman, S. P.; Bessman, A. N. The cerebral and peripheral uptake of ammonia in liver disease with a hypothesis for the mechanism of hepatic coma. J. Clin. Invest. *34*:622-628, 1955.

Boyd, E. M.; MacLachlan, M. L.; Perry, W. F. Experimental ammonia gas poisoning in rabbits and cats. J. Ind. Hyg. Toxicol. *26*:29-34, 1944.

Caplin, M. Ammonia-gas poisoning. Forty-seven cases in a London shelter. Lancet *2*:95-96, 1941.

Cardona, J. C.; Daly, J. F. Management of corrosive esophagitis. Analysis of treatment, methods, and results. N. Y. State J. Med. *64*:2307-2313, 1964.

Chassin, J. L.; Slattery, L. R. Jejunal stricture due to ingestion of ammonia. J. A. M. A. *152*:134-136, 1953.

Cittadini, E.; De Cristofaro, D.; Balestrieri, C.; Cimino, F. Carbamyl-aspartate, a new agent against acute ammonia intoxication. Biochem. Pharmacol. *15*:992-994, 1966.

Clinton, M. Toxic effects of gases and vapors; Mechanism of poisoning by volatile solvents. N. Engl. J. Med. *238*:51-54, 1948.

Close, L. G.; Catlin, F. I.; Cohn, A. M. Acute and chronic effects of ammonia burns of the respiratory tract. Arch. Otolaryngol. *106*:151-158, 1980.

Cobb, F. R.; Aldridge, J. E.; Johnson, B. B. Uremic symptoms and cerebrospinal fluid levels of ammonia, pH and other electrolytes. Clin. Research *12*:197, 1964.

Dang, H. C.; Visek, W. J. Antagonism of urease toxicity by chemical agents and antisera. Toxicol. Appl. Pharmacol. *8*:318-324, 1966.

Dienst, S. G. Treatment of progressive ammonia intoxication by exclusion of the colon. N. Engl. J. Med. *270*:555-556, 1964.

Dunn, S.; Ozere, R. L. Ammonia inhalation poisoning - household variety. Can. Med. Assoc. J. *94*:401, 1966.

Eichler, M. Psychological changes associated with induced hyperammonemia. Science *144*:886-888, 1964.

Ernst, R. W.; Leventhal, M.; Luna, R.; Martinez, H. Total esophagogastric replacement after ingestion of household ammonia. N. Engl. J. Med. *268*:815-818, 1963.

Faigel, H. C. Mixtures of household cleaning agents. N. Engl. J. Med. *271*:618, 1964.

Gleason, M. N.; Gosselin, R. E.; Hodge, H. C. Mixing of chlorine bleach with other household cleaning agents. Bull. Supplementary Materials, Clinical Toxicology of Commercial Products 8(No. 5):8-11, 1964.

Gonzales, L. L.; Zinninger, M. J.; Altemeier, W. A. Cicatricial gastric stenosis caused by ingestion of corrosive substances. Ann. Surg. *156*:84-89, 1962.

Grant, W. M. *Toxicology of the Eye*. 2nd ed. Charles C Thomas, Springfield, Ill, 1974.

Handford, S. W. Urease poisoning in the dog. Am. J. Physiol. *201*:71-73, 1961.

Hatton, D. V.; Leach, C. S.; Beaudet, A. L.; Dillman, R. O.; Di Ferrante, N. Collagen breakdown and ammonia inhalation. Arch. Environ. Health *34*:83-87, 1979.

Hawkins, R. A.; Miller, A. L.; Nielsen, R. C.; Veech, R. L. The acute action of ammonia on rat brain metabolism in vivo. Biochem. J. *134*:1001-1008, 1973.

Highman, V. N. Early rise in intra-ocular pressure after ammonia burns. Br. Med. J. *1*:359-360, 1969.

Hindfelt, B.; Plum, F.; Duffy, T. E. Effect of acute ammonia intoxication on cerebral metabolism in rats with portacaval shunts. J. Clin. Invest. *59*:386-396, 1977.

Jacobziner, H.; Raybin, H. W. Briefs on accidental chemical poisonings in New York City. N. Y. State J. Med. *59*:2223-2227, 1959b.

Kiley, J. E.; Pender, J. C.; Welch, H. F.; Welch, C. S. Ammonia intoxication treated by hemodialysis. N. Engl. J. Med. *259*:1156-1161, 1958.

Kirsh, M. M.; Abrams, B.; Coon, W.; Zuidema, G. Diphenhydramine (Benadryl) hydrochloride in the treatment of ammonia intoxication. Arch. Surg. *91*:466-467, 1965.

Lamar, C., Jr. Ammonia toxicity in rats: Protection by ɴ-methylglutamic acid. Toxicol. Appl. Pharmacol. *17*:795-803, 1970.

Lange, P.; Blazejewski, D.; Gores, E.; Jung, F. Untersuchung uber die Beeinflussung der Ammoniumtoxizitat durch Hemmstoffe der Carbonhydratase am Gunztier. Acta Biol. Med. Ger. *13*:369-377, 1964.

Leegaard, T. Corrosive injuries of the oesophagus, with particular reference to the treatment of acute corrosive oesophagitis. J. Laryngol. Otol. *60*:389-414, 1945.

Levy, D. M.; Divertie, M. B.; Litzow, T. J.; Henderson, J. W. Ammonia burns of the face and respiratory tract. J. A. M. A. *190*:873-876, 1964.

Manning, R. T.; Delp, M. Management of hepatocerebral intoxication. N. Engl. J. Med. *258*:55-66, 1958.

Manning, R. T.; Thorning, D.; Falleta, J. Protective effect of gamma-aminobutyric acid in experimental ammonia intoxication. Nature *202*:89-90, 1964.

Martini, G. A. The role of blood ammonia in the aetiology of hepatic coma. Ger. Med. Mon. *6*:369-372, 1961.

McKhann, G. M.; Towers, D. B. Ammonia toxicity and cerebral oxidative metabolism. Am. J. Physiol. *200*:420-424, 1961.

Montague, T. J.; Macneil, A. R. Mass ammonia inhalation. Chest *77*:496-498, 1980.

Navazio, F.; Gerritsen, T.; Wright, G. J. Relationship of ammonia intoxication to convulsions and coma in rats. J. Neurochem. *8*:146-151, 1961.

Nirankari, V. S.; Varma, S. D.; Lakhanpal, V.; Richards, R. D. Superoxide radical scavenging agents in treatment of alkali burns. An experimental study. Arch. Ophthalmol. *99*:886-887, 1981.

Norton, R. A. Esophageal and antral strictures due to ingestion of household ammonia. N. Engl. J. Med. *262*:10-12, 1960.

O'Donnell, C. H.; Abbott, W. E.; Hirshfeld, J. W. Surgical treatment of corrosive gastritis. Am. J. Surg. *78*:251-255, 1949.

Poelman, J. R.; Hausman, R. H.; Hoitsma, H. F. W. Endoscopy in lye burns of oesophagus and stomach. Endoscopy *9*:172-177, 1977.

Pollak, O. J. Ammonia poisoning and hemolytic anemia with bone marrow heterotopia. Am. J. Clin. Pathol. *15*:481-486, 1945.

Relman, A. S.; Shelborne, P. F.; Talman, A. Profound acidosis resulting from excessive ammonium chloride in previously healthy subjects. N. Engl. J. Med. *264*:848-852, 1961.

Rosen, H.; Blumenthal, A.; Consalvi, A. Effects of the potassium and magnesium salts of aspartic acid on ammonia intoxication in the rat. Acta Pharmacol. Toxicol. 20:115-120, 1963.

Salvatore, F.; Bocchini, V.; Cimino, F. Ammonia intoxication, and its effects on brain and blood ammonia levels. Biochem. Pharmacol. 12:1-6, 1963.

Schenker, S.; McCandless, D. W.; Brophy, E.; Lewis, M. S. Studies on the intracerebral toxicity of ammonia. J. Clin. Invest. 46:838-848, 1967.

Schenker, S.; Warren, K. S. Effect of temperature variation on toxicity and metabolism of ammonia in mice. J. Lab. Clin. Med. 60:291-301, 1962.

Silverman, L.; Whittenberger, J. L.; Muller, J. Physiological response of man to ammonia in low concentrations. J. Ind. Hyg. Toxicol. 31:74-78, 1949.

Slot, G. M. J. Ammonia gas burns. An account of six cases. Lancet 2:1356-1357, 1938.

Subcommittee on Ammonia, Committee on Medical and Biologic Effects of Environmental Pollutants, Division of Medical Sciences, Assembly of Life Sciences, NRC. Ammonia. University Park Press, Baltimore, 1979.

Summerskill, W. H. J.; Wolfe, S. J.; Davidson, C. S. The management of hepatic coma in relation to protein withdrawal and certain specific measures. Am. J. Med. 23:59-76, 1959.

Taplin, G. V.; Chopra, S.; Yanada, R. L.; Elam, D. Radionuclidic lung-imaging procedures in the assesment of injury due to ammonia inhalation. Chest 69:582-586, 1976.

Terrill, J. B.; Montgomery, R. R.; Reinhardt, C. F. Toxic gases from fires. Science, 200:1343-1347, 1978.

Vanamee, P.; Poppell, J. W. Hepatic coma. Med. Clin. North Am. 44:765-778, 1960.

Villarreal, H.; Ronces, R.; Sanchez, V.; Arcila, H. Failure of l-arginine to protect in ammonia intoxication: Its role in urea source. Am. J. Physiol. 202:364-366, 1962.

Walton, M. Industrial ammonia gassing. Br. J. Ind. Med. 30:78-86, 1973.

Warren, K. S.; Schenker, S. Hypoxia and ammonia toxicity. Am. J. Physiol. 199:1105-1108, 1960.

Warren, K. S.; Schenker, S. Effect of an inhibitor of glutamine synthesis (methionine sulfoximine) on ammonia toxicity and metabolism. J. Lab. Clin. Med. 64:442-449, 1964.

Weatherby, J. H. Chronic toxicity of ammonia fumes by inhalation. Proc. Soc. Exp. Biol. Med. 81:300-301, 1952.

Webster, R. W. Legal Medicine and Toxicology. W. B. Saunders Co., Philadelphia, 1930.

Yarington, C. T., Jr. Ingestion of caustic: A pediatric problem. J. Pediatr. 67:674-677, 1965.

Zuidema, G. D.; Fletcher, M. M.; Burton, W. D.; Child, C. G., III. Oral cation exchange resin therapy for ammonia intoxication in dogs. Surgery 52:117-126, 1962.

Zuidema, G. D.; Kirsh, M. M.; Cares, H.; Kowalczyk, R. S.; Coon, W. W. Effect of a monoamine oxidase inhibitor in experimental ammonia intoxication. Ann. Surg. 158:363-369, 1963a.

Zuidema, G. D.; Gaisford, W. D.; Kowalczyk, R. S.; Wolfman, E. F., Jr. Whole-body hypothermia in ammonia intoxication. Arch. Surg. 87:578-582, 1963b.

AMPHETAMINE

Amphetamine and its congeners are drugs that are widely misused (see below). The sulfate salt of racemic amphetamine is sold under the familiar trade name of Benzedrine Sulfate, whereas the *dextro*-isomer is marketed under the name Dexedrine. The *levo*-isomer has not found use in medical practice. N-Methyl-substituted *dextro*-amphetamine (*d*-desoxyephedrine or Methedrine) has some limited uses. Methamphetamine ("speed") is a derivative with a particularly high abuse potential (see below). Phenmetrazine, methylphenidate and pipradrol are some examples of pharmacologically related drugs (see Section II).

Interest in the properties of amphetamine arose in the early 1930s when its vasopressor activity was first observed and described in detail (Alles, 1933). The amphetamines have many properties in common with other sympathomimetic agents, but they possess strong central stimulatory activity in doses that do not produce peripheral reactions. These central effects have been described as a lessening of fatigue, increased energy and work capacity, exhilaration, euphoria, and an allaying of hunger (Nathanson, 1937). Like ephedrine, the amphetamines resist destruction in the gastrointestinal tract and so can be administered by mouth.

When amphetamine was found to be more satisfactory than ephedrine for the treatment of narcolepsy (Prinzmetal and Bloomberg, 1935), the first specific use for its central stimulating action was discovered. It was then employed in many different depressed states, including neurotic and psychotic depressions, parkinsonism, epilepsy, barbiturate intoxication, alcoholism, drug addiction, geriatric depression, postoperative depression and behavioral problems in children, but the most important use at the peak of its popularity was in the control of obesity (Leake, 1958). In almost all these situations dextroamphetamine sulfate has been found to offer some advantages over the racemic mixture. The medical use of the other amphetamines has dwindled to the point that the term amphetamine today is usually taken to mean the *dextro*-isomer.

Today amphetamines are properly used only for narcolepsy and hyperkinesis in children and under very limited circumstances for the control of appetite in obesity; they are regulated under Schedule II of the Controlled Substances Act.

Toxicology: Animal data (Ehrich *et al.*, 1939) place amphetamine well within toxicity class 5. Whether or not it is more toxic to the young of several animal species, toxic effects are at least more variable than in adult members of the same species. It has been suggested that man may be more sensitive to amphetamine than are most animals (Apfelberg, 1938). That 100 to 200 mg. is sometimes lethal to nontolerant adult persons (see below) suggests that toxicity class 6 is the appropriate descriptor of amphetamine's lethality in humans. In spite of its high toxicity and wide distribution, death occurs rarely in clinical poisonings (Greenwood and Peachey,

1957). The saving grace may be the relatively large margin of safety between the amount of drug incorporated in unit therapeutic doses and the lethal dose (Schulte *et al.*, 1941), but high degrees of tolerance also protect chronic users.

The poisoned child usually presents a striking picture. There may be constant twisting and turning, purposeless movements and mumbling. Hyperirritability may increase until the child throws his body wildly about, waves his arms and legs and screams (Keiter and Arnold, 1955; Ong, 1962). In adults the initial symptoms are cardiovascular in origin, with flushing or pallor, palpitation, labile pulse rate and blood pressure, extrasystoles, heart block, chest pains, and eventual collapse (Greenwood and Peachey, 1957). Both adults and children may show confusion, delirium, hallucinations, panic states, and other acute psychotic syndromes (Norman and Shea, 1945; Rosenbaum, 1943). Convulsions and coma are terminal events.

Also ominous are reports of vascular lesions in the brain, certainly in animals (Ehrich *et al.*, 1939) and circumstantially in man because of observed hemiplegia (Goodman and Becker, 1970; Kane *et al.*, 1969; Poteliakhoff and Roughton, 1956) and autopsy findings of petechial hemorrhages (Bernheim and Cox, 1960) and hemorrhage of the temporal cortex (Gericke, 1945). Severe intracranial hypertension in a known amphetamine abuser occurred during anesthesia for a neurosurgical procedure (Michel and Adams, 1979). Marked increases in cerebral regional blood flow (left hemisphere and frontal) were noted during acute intoxication in a young addict (Berglund and Risberg, 1980). Among other severe reactions reportedly due to amphetamine are pancytopenia (Mitchell and Denton, 1950) and aplastic anemia (Davies, 1937).

The acute toxicity of amphetamine is strongly influenced by certain environmental factors. For example, crowding or aggregation markedly increases the toxicity to mice (Chance, 1946). In an acute poisoning in a child described by Patuck (1956), external stimuli precipitated increased hyperactivity.

Elevated environmental temperatures are also associated with increased acute toxicity in animals (Alles, 1933). Hyperpyrexia, perhaps secondary to a hypermetabolic state produced by release of endogenous catecholamines, is a prominent feature of amphetamine poisoning in many species (Askew, 1961; Clark *et al.*, 1967; Zalis *et al.*, 1967). Although comparable clinical data are lacking, hyperpyrexia has been noted as a frequent and prominent sign in acute human intoxication (Jordan and Hampson, 1960). During a grueling bicycle race a cyclist collapsed with symptoms closely resembling heat exhaustion, and, despite vigorous treatment, he died in cardiovascular collapse; it was learned subsequently that he had consumed 105 mg. of amphetamine during the race (Bernheim and Cox, 1960). Dehydration has been found to increase amphetamine toxicity in animals (Ewing *et al.*, 1951), as does forced exercise (Hardinge and Peterson, 1964), various stresses including cold (Chance, 1947; Goldberg and Salama, 1969) and high altitude (Robinson and Milberg, 1970).

Tolerance to amphetamines, when it occurs, develops rapidly (Isbell and White, 1953; Knapp, 1952). During prolonged courses of therapy occasional reports of decreasing drug effectiveness have appeared. However, no clear-cut physical disability such as hypertension has been ascribed to long courses of treatment. Undoubtedly tolerance is an important consideration in acute poisonings.

In view of the many variables enumerated above it is not surprising that acute amphetamine intoxication has occurred over a striking range of dosage. A toxic reaction was induced in a 2-year-old child by 40 to 50 mg. of dextroamphetamine even when 60 to 75 mg. of phenobarbital was ingested at the same time (Fletcher, 1953). In another case (Patuck, 1956) a slightly older child survived 115 mg. with vigorous treatment. Although 55 mg. has precipitated an acute psychotic syndrome in an adult (Wallis *et al.*, 1949), this may have been due to an idiosyncrasy. In addition to Bernheim's case above, death in an adult has resulted from as little as 120 mg. (Gericke, 1945) and a severe intoxication from 140 mg. of racemic amphetamine (Apfelberg, 1938). Yet a woman who had been using dextroamphetamine to lose weight and who was not known to have developed tolerance showed only mild signs of peripheral sympathomimetic activity and hostile behavior 12 hours after ingesting 200 mg. (Greenwood and Peachey, 1957).

The toxic effects of amphetamines can be blocked nonspecifically by anesthetic doses of many central nervous system depressants, *e.g.*, barbiturates, meprobamate (Esplin and Done, 1968; Gardocki *et al.*, 1966a, b; Lasagna and McCann, 1957). Barbiturates and amphetamines have each been used to antagonize toxic effects of the others (Freireich and Landsberg, 1946; Greenwood and Peachey, 1957). As indicated below, newer antagonists to amphetamine are effective clinically in nondepressant doses.

Amphetamine effects involve actions in both the central and the peripheral nervous systems. In the periphery its sympathomimetic effects are both direct at the level of adrenergic receptors and indirect by virtue of the release of norepinephrine from adrenergic nerve terminals. The effects of amphetamine in the central nervous system are more intense than those of most other sympathomimetics. With increasing doses it first releases norepinephrine (Moore, 1963, 1964), then dopamine and finally 5-hydroxytryptamine (serotonin) from their respective brain neurons (Nwanze and Jonsson, 1981; Trulson and Jacobs, 1979). These freed transmitter substances in the brain may be responsible for most if not all of the central effects initiated by amphetamine.

Since phenothiazines, such as chlorpromazine, and butyrophenones, such as haloperidol, block both α-adrenergic receptors and dopaminergic receptors (Peroutka *et al.*, 1977), their efficacy in acute amphetamine poisoning is almost certainly related to that mechanism. Chlorpromazine reverses the hyperthermia, convulsions and EEG activation produced by amphetamine (Esplin and Done, 1968). Excessive sedation after chlorpromazine was seen only in children poisoned with an amphetamine-sedative combination, and it could be avoided by decreasing the chlorpromazine dose. Both haloperidol and chlorpromazine reversed many of the signs of amphetamine poisoning in dogs and prevented death (Catravas *et al.*, 1977a), but haloperidol did not protect poisoned mice (Lopatka *et al.*, 1976). Practolol also did not affect the lethality of amphetamine in mice (Lopatka *et al.*, 1976), nor did propranolol in dogs (Catravas *et al.*, 1977a). On the other hand propranolol did protect rats but haloperidol was clearly superior, and the combination was less effective than haloperidol alone (Davis *et al.*, 1974). Droperidol infusion was effective in calming one tolerant patient who had recently ingested an alleged 1.4 gm. methamphetamine (Gary and Saidi, 1978).

In mice pretreatment with 6-hydroxydopamine, which destroys adrenergic nerve terminals, protected them against death by amphetamine. Phentolamine, an α-adrenergic blocker also protected against death. Finally, methysergide, which blocks 5-hydroxytryptamine receptors, was also effective (Lopatka *et al.*, 1976). Pretreatment of animals with monamine oxidase inhibitors increases amphetamine toxicity presumably by prolonging the biological half-life of the catecholamines or indoleamines released (Brittain *et al.*, 1964).

Important species differences are recognized with respect to amphetamine metabolism (Dring *et al.*, 1970). After a wide range of oral doses in man, a relatively constant one-third of the drug is excreted in the urine unchanged (Alles and Wisegarver, 1961; Dring *et al.*, 1970). Formation of *p*-hydroxyamphetamine, which is an active pressor agent (Axelrod, 1954), although important in the rat, is a minor route of biotransformation in man (Dring *et al.*, 1970). Instead, oxidative deamination and eventual excretion as benzoic or hippuric acid are more important in primates (Dring *et al.*, 1970; Ellison *et al.*, 1966). More than half of the drug is excreted within 24 hours following an oral dose (Dring *et al.*, 1970). Methamphetamine is metabolized by a process involving demethylation (Cartoni and DeStefano, 1963).

Amphetamine abuse: Publicity about the central excitatory actions of amphetamine shortly after its introduction led promptly to a tragic series of abuses of the drug, which continues in various forms even today. Because of its ability to lessen fatigue, it finds surreptitious use by persons in situations that require extremes of endurance. It has often been employed by students who want to stay awake and alert for long hours in preparing for examinations; probably the first authenticated fatality from amphetamine occurred under such circumstances (Smith, 1939). At various times it has been suggested that some athletes use it in an effort to attain superior performances. Truck drivers as a group have been widely accused of the misuse of amphetamines.

These early abuses arose because amphetamine at one time was readily available to the public in an economical form, namely as an inhaler. Monroe and Drell (1947) have reported in detail the techniques employed for the consumption of amphetamine obtained from inhalers. Such inhalers are no longer marketed in the United States, but it is possible that they are still used in some foreign countries. Acute psychotic reactions were encountered frequently among those who misused the amphetamine inhalers (Herman and Nagler, 1954). It is not clear what role if any the aromatic principles, notably menthol, played in the precipitation of these states, but similar reactions have occurred from the ingestion of tablets (Wallis *et al.*, 1949).

Although the term "addict" is commonly employed in reference to habitual users of amphetamine, the state is perhaps best described as a psychic dependence. Records of use for periods up to 15 years at dosages of 100 to 700 mg. daily have appeared (Knapp, 1952), and some addicts are known to take as much as 2 gm. daily (Isbell and White, 1953; Kalant, 1966). Except for somnolence, which might be accounted for by overcompensation, and an occasional psychotic reaction, no clear-cut withdrawal syndrome seems to exist (Knapp, 1952). In certain aspects these individuals resemble cocaine users. Amphetamine may be used alone, but the drug is also taken concurrently or alternately with alcohol or barbiturates (Isbell and White, 1953).

By 1967 a particularly malignant pattern of amphetamine abuse became dominant in the Haight-Ashbury district of San Francisco. This pattern involved the intravenous use of high doses of methamphetamine (crystal, flash, meth, speed, splash). The initial choice of methamphetamine may have been governed by the circumstance that it was the only derivative commercially available in a parenteral form. It was eventually synthesized in illicit laboratories because the doses used were far in excess of those available for legitimate therapeutic purposes.

The pattern of methamphetamine abuse is somewhat unique in that the habitué is often totally absorbed and preoccupied with his drug habit. "Speed freaks" simply have no time for meaningful social activity even when the financial burden of the habit is not a consideration. During the early stages, 20- to 40-mg. doses may be injected 3 to 4 times a day, but tolerance builds rapidly. A well established habit may require 100- to 300-mg. doses, which are taken every few hours around the clock for 3 to 6 days in the so-called "run." In some cases, 15 gm. per day have been tolerated (Kramer *et al.*, 1967).

The initial "rush" is felt instantaneously on intravenous administration and it is described as an intensely pleasurable experience like an orgasm. This reaction can be reduced or blocked in man by pretreatment with α-methyl-*p*-tyrosine (Jönsson *et al.*, 1971). The rush may be followed by bustling, purposeful activity, but later in the run the performance degenerates into pointless, repetitive, stereotyped activities. At this time psychosis with prominent paranoia may appear. Opinions differ as to whether auditory and visual hallucinations are experienced, but violent behavior is more common than with most other drugs of abuse (Cox and Smart, 1970; Kramer *et al.*, 1967; Smith and Fischer, 1970).

During a run the user is continually awake and often avoids food. At the termination of a run the excitement phase is rapidly replaced by profound depression (the "crash"). The subject may sleep for as long as 48 hours and awaken with a voracious appetite. Once these needs have been met, the cycle may begin again. In many ways the syndrome resembles that of the cocaine habitué (see pp. III-114–120).

The slogan "Speed Kills" has little basis in current documentation, but few data are available on the long-term consequences. Surprisingly few deaths have been ascribed to the drug itself although there have been a number of deaths due to self-destructive acts secondary to the drug-induced psychosis. Fatal intracerebral hemorrhage has occurred at least once (Hall *et al.*, 1973). Mild to moderate withdrawal reactions have been described (Smith and Fischer, 1970). A major associated medical problem is hepatitis probably due to poor sanitation, but direct hepatotoxic effects have not been ruled out (Lee and Wiebe, 1979).

Various substituted amphetamine derivatives with few, if any, legitimate therapeutic uses have appeared on the illicit drug market. They include 2,5-dimethoxy-4-methylamphetamine (STP, serenity-tranquility-peace, DOM), 3,4,5-trimethoxyamphetamine (TMA), 3-methoxy-4,5-methylenedioxyphenyl isopropylamine (MDA) and others; see Section II. The efficacy of the treatment recommendations below is not well established for these more obscure derivatives.

Symptomatology:
1. Increased awareness and activity—lessening of fatigue, exhilaration, talkativeness, restlessness, insomnia, irritability, tremors, dizziness, exaggerated reflexes, sweating, mydriasis, flushing or pallor.
2. Anorexia, dry mouth, nausea, vomiting, diarrhea.
3. Fever, chilliness, dehydration.
4. Hyperactivity, purposeless motions, confusion.
5. Tachycardia or sometimes bradycardia, extrasystoles and other arrhythmias, palpitations, heart block, anginal chest pain, marked hypertension, tachypnea.
6. Anxiety, headache, hallucinations, paranoid hostile behavior, delirium, mania, self-injury.
7. Convulsions, coma, circulatory collapse and death.

Treatment:
1. Delayed gastric emptying makes lavage or induced emesis worthwhile for long periods of time after ingestion.
2. After emptying the stomach, give a slurry of activated charcoal (Section I).
3. Chlorpromazine produces dramatic relief of symptoms even in cases refractory to barbiturates. The intramuscular route is preferred, with adults receiving an initial dose of 50 mg. and young children 1 mg./kg. Half these doses are recommended in cases where amphetamine-sedative combinations were ingested. A butyrophenone such as haloperidol or droperidol is probably as effective as chlorpromazine and may be used in its place. See p. IV-35.
4. Chlorpromazine and other phenothiazines and butyrophenones should be avoided if the drug psychosis is due to anticholinergics (atropine, scopolamine, etc.) or to unknown psychotomimetic agents. In the latter case a short-acting barbiturate or diazepam may be the best choice (p. IV-35). Note: an abnormally high tolerance to barbiturate effects will usually be observed.
5. Isolate the patient and avoid all unnecessary external stimuli. See pp. IV-33–35. A "talk-down" may help to control anxiety but probably not so successfully as in cocaine poisoning, which has a much shorter duration than amphetamine intoxication.
6. A hypertensive crisis may require the injection of a short-acting α-adrenergic blocking drug such as phentolamine (Regitine) or the use of a direct vasodepressor

drug such as sublingual glyceryl trinitrate. Avoid propranolol and other β-blockers.

7. Hypothermic measures (p. IV-84) to reduce a high fever.

8. If the intracranial pressure rises, institute measures (pp. IV-43–46) to combat cerebral edema and congestion.

9. Aside from terminal events, convulsions are not often described in amphetamine poisoning, but they do occur. Chlorpromazine is not an anticonvulsant. To control convulsions, give i.v. diazepam (p. IV-37).

10. Acidification of the urine by administering ammonium chloride and a diuresis induced by mannitol (p. IV-52) are almost always worthwhile to promote excretion and hasten recovery (Gary and Saidi, 1978).

11. Appreciable quantities of amphetamine have been recovered by peritoneal dialysis (p. IV-56) in poisoned patients (Wallace *et al.*, 1964; Zalis and Parmley, 1963). Hemodialysis or hemoperfusion (p. IV-57) is presumably even more efficient. None of these measures, however, is likely to be necessary if renal function is not impaired.

Laboratory: Significant increases in both red and white blood cell counts, presumably due to dehydration and to constriction of the spleen and other blood reservoirs (Myerson *et al.*, 1936). Monitor blood electrolytes and urine pH.

References:

Alles, G. A. The comparative physiological actions of *dl*-beta-phenylisopropylamines. I. Pressor effect and toxicity. J. Pharmacol. Exp. Ther. *47*:339-354, 1933.

Alles, G. A.; Wisegarver, B. B. Amphetamine excretion studies in man. Toxicol. Appl. Pharmacol. *3*:678-688, 1961.

Apfelberg, B. A case of Benzedrine sulfate poisoning. J. A. M. A. *110*:575-576, 1938.

Askew, B. M. Amphetamine toxicity in aggregated mice. J. Pharm. Pharmacol. *13*:701-703, 1961.

Axelrod, J. Studies on sympathomimetic amines. II. The biotransformation and physiological disposition of *d*-amphetamine, *d*-para-hydroxyamphetamine and *d*-metamphetamine. J. Pharmacol. Exp. Ther. *110*:315-326, 1954.

Berglund, M.; Risberg, J. Regional cerebral blood flow in a case of amphetamine intoxication. Psychopharmacol. *70*:219-221, 1980.

Bernheim, J.; Cox, J. N. Amphetamine overdosage in an athlete. Schweiz. med. Wochenschr. *90*:322 (1960). Abstracted in Br. Med. J. 2:590 (1960), 1960.

Brittain, R. T.; Jack, D.; Spencer, P. S. J. Mechanism of monoamine oxidase inhibitors in enhancing amphetamine toxicity. J. Pharm. Pharmacol. *16*:565-567, 1964.

Cartoni, G. P.; DeStefano, F. Determination of amphetamine by gas chromatography. Urinary excretion of amphetamines in rat and man. Ital. J. Biochem. *12*:296-309, 1963.

Catravas, J. D.; Waters, I. W.; Hickenbottom, J. P.; Davis, W. M. The effects of haloperidol, chlorpromazine, and propranolol on amphetamine poisoning in the conscious dog. J. Pharmacol. Exp. Ther. *202*:230-243, 1977a.

Chance, M. R. A. Aggregation as a factor influencing the toxicity of sympathomimetic amines in mice. J. Pharmacol. Exp. Ther. *87*:214-219, 1946.

Chance, M. R. A. Factors influencing the toxicity of sympathomimetic amines to solitary mice. J. Pharmacol. Exp. Ther. *89*:289-296, 1947.

Clark, W. C.; Blackman, H. J.; Peterson, J. E. Certain factors in aggregated mice *d*-amphetamine toxicity. Arch. Int. Pharmacodyn. Ther. *170*:350-363, 1967.

Cox, C.; Smart, R. G. The nature and extent of speed use in North America. Can. Med. Assoc. J. *102*:724-729, 1970.

Davies, I. J. Benzedrine. A review of its toxic effects with the report of a severe case of anaemia following its use. Br. Med. J. *2*:615-617, 1937.

Davis, W. M.; Logston, D. G.; Hickenbottom, J. P. Antagonism of acute amphetamine intoxication by haloperidol and propranolol. Toxicol. Appl. Pharmacol. *29*:397-403, 1974.

Dring, L. G.; Smith, R. L.; Williams, R. T. The fate of amphetamine in men and other species. Biochem. J. *116*:425-435, 1970.

Ehrich, W. E.; Lewy, F. H.; Krumbhaar, E. B. Experimental studies upon the toxicity of Benzedrine sulfate in various animals. Am. J. Med. Sci. *198*:785-803, 1939.

Ellison, T.; Gutzait, L.; Van Loon, E. J. The comparative metabolism of *d*-amphetamine-C^{14} in the rat, dog and monkey. J. Pharmacol. Exp. Ther. *152*:383-387, 1966.

Esplin, D. E.; Done, A. K. Amphetamine poisoning, effectiveness of chlorpromazine. N. Engl. J. Med. *278*:1361-1365, 1968.

Ewing, P. L.; Moore, W. T.; Doucet, B. M. Dehydration and hydration as factors in amphetamine toxicity. J. Pharmacol. Exp. Ther. *101*:10-11, 1951.

Fletcher, T. F. Acute dextroamphetamine sulfate poisoning. Am. J. Dis. Child. *86*:777-779, 1953.

Freireich, A. W.; Landsberg, J. W. Amphetamine (Benzedrine) sulfate for acute barbiturate poisoning. J. A. M. A. *131*:661-663, 1946.

Gardocki, J. F.; Schaler, M. E.; Goldstein, L. Reconsideration of the central nervous system pharmacology of amphetamine. I. Toxicity in grouped and isolated mice. Toxicol. Appl. Pharmacol. *8*:550-557, 1966a.

Gardocki, J. F.; Schaler, M. E.; Goldstein, L. Reconsideration of the central nervous system pharmacology of amphetamine. II. Influence of pharmacologic agents on cumulative and total lethality in grouped and isolated mice. Toxicol. Appl. Pharmacol. *9*:536-554, 1966b.

Gary, N. E.; Saidi, P. Methamphetamine intoxication. A speedy new treatment. Am. J. Med. *64*:537-540, 1978.

Gericke, O. L. Suicide by ingestion of amphetamine sulphate. J. A. M. A. *128*:1098-1099, 1945.

Goldberg, M. E.; Salama, A. I. Amphetamine toxicity and brain monoamines in three models of stress. Toxicol. Appl. Pharmacol. *14*:447-456, 1969.

Goodman, S. J.; Becker, D. P. Intracranial hemorrhage and amphetamine. J. A. M. A. *212*:480, 1970.

Greenwood, R.; Peachey, R. S. Acute amphetamine poisoning, an account of 3 cases. Br. Med. J. *1*:742-744, 1957.

Hall, C. D.; Blanton, D. E.; Scatliff, J. H.; Morris, C. E. Speed kills: Fatality from the self-administration of methamphetamine intravenously. South. Med. J. *66*:650-652, 1973.

Hardinge, M. G.; Peterson, D. I. The effect of forced exercise on body temperature and amphetamine toxicity. J. Pharmacol. Exp. Ther. *145*:47-51, 1964.

Herman, M.; Nagler, S. H. Psychosis due to amphetamine. J. Nerv. Ment. Dis. *120*:268-272, 1954.

Isbell, H.; White, W. M. Clinical characteristics of addictions. Am. J. Med. *14*:558-565, 1953.

Jonsson, L. E.; Anggard, E.; Gunne, L. M. Blockade of intravenous amphetamine euphoria in man. Clin. Pharmacol. Ther. *12*:889-896, 1971.

Jordan, S. C.; Hampson, F. Amphetamine poisoning associated with hyperpyrexia. Br. Med. J. *2*:844, 1960.

Kalant, O. J. The Amphetamines, Toxicity and Addiction. Charles C Thomas, Springfield, Ill, 1966.

Kane, F. J., Jr.; Keeler, M. H.; Reifler, C. B. Neurologic crises following methamphetamine. J. A. M. A. *210*:556-557, 1969.

Keiter, W. E.; Arnold, J. H. Acute dexedrine intoxication in children. Arch. Pediatr. 72:126-128, 1955.

Knapp, P. H. Amphetamine and addiction. J. Nerv. Ment. Dis. *115*:406-432, 1952.

Kramer, J. C.; Fischman, V. S.; Littlefield, D. C. Amphetamine abuse, pattern and effects of high doses taken intravenously. J. A. M. A. *201*:305-309, 1967.

Lasagna, L.; McCann, W. Effect of tranquilizing drugs on amphetamine toxicity in aggregated mice. Science *125*:1241-1242, 1957.

Leake, C. D. The Amphetamines. Charles C Thomas, Springfield, Ill, 1958.

Lee, Y. W.; Wiebe, L. I. Amphetamine metabolism in mice exposed chronically to phenobarbital and to phenobarbital with carbon tetrachloride. Clin. Biochem. *12*:56-58, 1979.

Lopatka, J. E.; Brewerton, C. N.; Brooks, D. S.; Cook, D. A.; Paton, D. M. The protective effects of methysergide, 6-hydroxydopamine and other agents on the toxicity of amphetamine, phetermine, MDA, PMA and STP in mice. Res. Commun. Chem. Pathol. Pharmacol. *14*:677-687, 1976.

Michel, R.; Adams, A. P. Acute amphetamine abuse - problems during general anaesthesia for neurosurgery. Anaesthesia *34*:1016-1019, 1979.

Mitchell, H. S.; Denton, R. L. Overdosage with Dexedrine. Can. Med. Assoc. J. *62*:594-595, 1950.

Monroe, R. R.; Drell, H. J. Oral use of stimulants obtained from inhalers. J. A. M. A. *135*:909-915, 1947.

Moore, K. E. Toxicity and catecholamine releasing actions of *d*- and *l*-amphetamine in isolated and aggregated mice. J. Pharmacol. Exp. Ther. *142*:6-12, 1963.

Moore, K. E. The role of endogenous norepinephrine in the toxicity of *d*-amphetamine in aggregated mice. J. Pharmacol. Exp. Ther. *144*:45-51, 1964.

Myerson, A.; Loman, J.; Dameshek, W. Physiologic effects of Benzedrine and its relationship to other drugs affecting the autonomic nervous system. Am. J. Med. Sci. *192*:560-574, 1936.

Nathanson, M. H. The central action on beta-amino-propylbenzene (Benzedrine). J. A. M. A. *108*:528-531, 1937.

Norman, J.; Shea, J. T. Acute hallucinosis as a complication of addiction to amphetamine sulfate. N. Engl. J. Med. *233*:270-271, 1945.

Nwanze, E.; Jonsson, G. Amphetamine neurotoxicity on dopamine nerve terminals in the caudate nucleus of mice. Neurosci. Lett. *26*:163-168, 1981.

Ong, B. H. Dextro-amphetamine poisonings. N. Engl. J. Med. *266*:1321-1322, 1962.

Patuck, D. Acute dextroamphetamine sulfate poisoning in a child. Br. Med. J. *1*:670-671, 1956.

Peroutka, S. J.; U'Prichard, D. C.; Greenberg, D. A.; Snyder, S. H. Neuroleptic drug interactions with norepinephrine alpha receptor binding sites in rat brain. Neuropharmacology *16*:549-556, 1977.

Poteliakhoff, A.; Roughton, B. C. Two cases of amphetamine poisoning. Br. Med. J. *1*:26-27, 1956.

Prinzmetal, M.; Bloomberg, W. The use of Benzedrine for the treatment of narcolepsy. J. A. M. A. *105*:2051-2054, 1935.

Robinson, S. M.; Milberg, J. Alterations of *d*-amphetamine lethality and body temperature in mice during altitude exposure. Toxicol. Appl. Pharmacol. *16*:540-546, 1970.

Rosenbaum, H. A. Amphetamine poisoning in a child of twenty months. J. A. M. A. *122*:1011, 1943.

Schulte, J. W.; Reif, E. C.; Bacher, J. A., Jr.; Lawrence, W. S.; Tainter, M. L. Further study of central stimulation from sympathomimetic amines. J. Pharmacol. Exp. Ther. *71*:62-74, 1941.

Smith, D. E.; Fischer, C. M. An analysis of 310 cases of acute high-dose methamphetamine toxicity in Haight-Ashbury. Clin. Toxicol. *3*:117-124, 1970.

Smith, L. C. Collapse with death following the use of amphetamine sulfate. J. A. M. A. *113*:1022-1023, 1939.

Trulson, M. E.; Jacobs, B. L. Long-term amphetamine treatment decreases brain serotonin metabolism: Implications for theories of schizophrenia. Science *205*:1295-1297, 1979.

Wallace, H. E.; Neumayen, F.; Gutch, C. F. Amphetamine poisoning and peritoneal dialysis. Am. J. Dis. Child. *108*:657-661, 1964.

Wallis, G. G.; McHarg, J. F.; Scott, O. C. A. Acute psychosis caused by dextroamphetamine. Br. Med. J. *2*:1394, 1949.

Zalis, E. G.; Parmley, L. F., Jr. Fatal amphetamine poisoning. Arch. Intern. Med. *112*:822-826, 1963.

Zalis, E. G.; Lundberg, G. D.; Knutson, R. A. The pathophysiology of acute amphetamine poisoning with pathologic correlation. J. Pharmacol. Exp. Ther. *158*:115-127, 1967.

ANILINE

Aniline is widely used in industry as an intermediate in chemical syntheses. Most knowledge about its effects in man has resulted from industrial exposures (Halsted, 1960; Hamblin, 1962; Hunter, 1943; Mangelsdorff, 1956; Wetherhold *et al.*, 1960; Wuertz *et al.*, 1964). Aniline and its derivatives, however, also occur in various products found in the home, such as paints, varnishes, marking inks, stove polishes and shoe polishes. For information on the composition of modern products of these types, see Section VI, General Formulations.

The medical literature contains innumerable reports of toxic episodes in which only circumstantial evidence implicates aniline or nitrobenzene (Banning *et al.*, 1965; Donovan, 1920; Leinoff, 1936; Parks and Neill, 1953; Scott and Hanzlik, 1920; Steele and Spink, 1933; Stevens, 1928; Stevenson and Forbes, 1942). In addition, at least three types of consumer products (indelible ink, shoe dye, wax crayons) have produced many intoxications as indicated below. Except in the chemical industry, poisoning by pure aniline or nitrobenzene is a rare occurrence; ingestion of the pure liquid is almost unknown.

As described below, aniline induces methemoglobinemia. The extensive literature concerning classifications of methemoglobin-generating compounds, hereditary and acquired toxic methemoglobinemias, and the metabolic and chemical processes involved in the formation and reduction of methemoglobin has been summarized in several reviews (Kiese, 1974; Smith and Olson, 1973; Smith, 1980). Additional information may be found under NITRITE, p. III-314. The discussion below has been limited primarily to toxic reactions encountered in aniline and nitrobenzene intoxications, although the remarks may be germane to poisonings by structurally similar compounds. See also Section II for comments on specific compounds.

Toxicology: Since aniline and nitrobenzene are volatile liquids, they gain access to the body by inhalation as well as by skin penetration and ingestion. Aniline crosses the placental barrier and poisons the fetus (Harley and Celermajer,

1970). Minute quantities of these substances have produced severe methemoglobinemia in man. As little as 6 gm. has been suggested as a lethal dose, but much larger amounts have been tolerated (Webster, 1930). The mean lethal dose may be between 15 and 30 gm. (ml.) of pure aniline. Technical aniline as found in many commercial products may be even more dangerous because of unknown toxic impurities or decomposition products of aniline (Treon et al., 1949a, 1950; von Oettingen, 1941b).

The outstanding feature of aniline (and nitrobenzene) poisoning in man is cyanosis due to methemoglobin and sometimes to low levels of "sulfhemoglobin" and Heinz bodies (Hughes and Treon, 1954; Healy, 1932; Lubash et al., 1964). The result is a functional anemia since these abnormal pigments are incapable of binding oxygen for normal gas transport. A given circulating level of methemoglobin, however, produces a more severe impairment of peripheral oxygen transport than an equivalent true anemia, because the shape of the dissociation curve of residual oxyhemoglobin is altered so that a smaller proportion of blood oxygen is released in tissue capillaries (Darling and Roughton, 1942).

It is characteristic that oxygen therapy fails to relieve the cyanosis of methemoglobinemia and that blood specimens retain their abnormal brown-black discoloration even when aerated. Occasionally blood stored overnight for analyses has been found to have reverted to a normal color (Casciano, 1952), a result of the spontaneous activity of methemoglobin reductase, a red cell enzyme which reduces methemoglobin to normal hemoglobin even at 5° C. Clinical cyanosis is evident when the methemoglobin level exceeds 15% of the total circulating blood pigment. Lethargy and semistupor are associated with blood levels of about 60% and the lethal range may be 70 to 85% (Bodansky, 1951; Mangelsdorff, 1952). A moderately good correlation seems to exist between the severity of the intoxication and the methemoglobin level (Hamblin and Mangelsdorff, 1938).

Aniline in a single oral dose of 20 mg./kg. caused no methemoglobinemia or Heinz bodies or splenic enlargement in rats. The corresponding no-effect dose in normal human volunteers was 5 to 15 mg. (0.07 to 0.21 mg./kg.), and doses ranging from 25 to 65 mg. significantly elevated methemoglobin levels (Jenkins et al., 1972b). By mechanisms that are not clear, alcohol is said to intensify the methemoglobinemia induced by aniline and nitrobenzene (Jung, 1939).

In 1964 Lubash et al. described the events following the ingestion of 80 ml. of reagent grade aniline by a psychotic adult. The victim was found in coma and shock. The skin, mucous membranes and retinal blood vessels were a deep slate-blue. Therapy included gastric lavage,

endotracheal intubation, injections of methylene blue and partial exchange transfusion. Metaraminol produced a favorable cardiovascular response. In spite of the treatment the patient experienced a generalized seizure. Acting on the suggestion of Schreiner and Maher (1960), the therapists instituted prolonged hemodialysis with the recovery of significant quantities of aniline. The patient eventually recovered after a severe, late intravascular hemolytic episode.

In two milder poisonings by aniline (Casciano, 1952; Stening, 1951) the toxin apparently penetrated the intact skin. Symptoms were delayed 2 to 4 hours after initial skin contact; they included weakness, headache, deep cyanosis and collapse with stupor. Except for the additional feature of vomiting, this clinical picture matches that of two confirmed cases of nitrobenzene ingestion (Leader, 1932; Nabarro, 1948).

A young male chemistry student accidentally ingested 5 to 10 ml. of a mixture of aniline and nitrobenzene in unknown proportions. The compounds were identified in gastric aspirates. When admitted to a hospital 2 hours later, he was unconscious but responded to painful stimuli. The pupils were widely dilated but reactive. The lips, tongue and mucous membranes were navy-blue to black, and the skin was slate grey. Tachypnea, dyspnea and tachycardia were evident, and there was vomitus in the pharynx. The methemoglobin level was 65%. He was exchange transfused with what was estimated to be twice his total blood volume, and he was given 3.3 mg./kg. methylene blue, with a reduction in methemoglobin to 25% at 12 hours. Seven days after admission he experienced a hemolytic crisis (hemoglobin 4.5 gm./dl., bilirubin 2.9 mg./dl., reticulocytes 25%), but eventually he recovered fully (Harrison, 1977).

Studies of chemically induced methemoglobinemia in laboratory animals have been inappropriately extrapolated to man. The relative resistance of rodents (mice, rats, rabbits) to methemoglobin formation must be ascribed in part to greater methemoglobin reductase activity in the red cells of these species than in the red cells of dogs, cats and humans (Stolk and Smith, 1966).

Because aniline and its derivatives are incapable of generating methemoglobin in vitro, it is apparent that they require biotransformation to active forms. Convincing evidence indicates that the activation of nitrobenzene is mediated exclusively by intestinal microflora in the rat (Reddy et al., 1976). Aniline is in part metabolized by gut mucosa (Irons et al., 1980), but several studies show that it is also a substrate for hepatic microsomal enzymes as well (Ikeda et al., 1972; Hlavica and Kehl, 1976; Wisniewska-Knypl et al., 1975). Aminophenols or N-hydroxylamines have been suggested as the active metabolites (von Oettingen, 1941b; Kiese *et al.,* 1972). Differences in metabolic pathways and in the rates of formation and detoxication of active compounds must account for some of the species variation in susceptibility to aniline (Bodansky, 1951). The high reactivity of the cat to various aromatic amines may be due to inadequate mechanisms for detoxifying them (Welch *et al.,* 1966). Other species such as mice apparently metabolize aniline and nitrobenzene to active forms only slowly, if at all, even in lethal doses (Smith *et al.,* 1967). In such species methemoglobinemia cannot account for death, but probably it does in man since measures that reduce methemoglobin levels have been life-saving.

About 80 to 100% of an oral dose of aniline in sheep and rats was eliminated in the urine in 24 hours, whereas pigs eliminated only 56% by that route. Fecal excretion was only 2% of the total dose in all three species. N-Acetyl metabolites in all three species accounted for about 80% of the dose. The double conjugate N-acetyl-p-glucuronide amounted to about 63% of the N-acetyl metabolites in sheep and pigs, whereas the N-acetyl-p-sulfate was 56% of the N-acetyl form in the rat (Kao *et al.,* 1978). Aniline is a weak inducer of hepatic microsomal enzymes, but nitrobenzene is even less effective (Wisniewska-Knypl *et al.,* 1975).

In the rat intravenous aniline is concentrated in the stomach and jejunum and subsequently reabsorbed from the small intestine in an enterogastric cycle (Irons *et al.,* 1980). Perhaps aniline accumulates in the stomach in accord with the principle of non-ionic diffusion of weak bases. Repeated or continuous gastric lavage with acidic fluids may constitute an effective means for removing aniline from the body.

The agent of choice for accelerating the reduction of methemoglobin is methylene blue. Ascorbic acid, although used in hereditary methemoglobinemia, has no place in the treatment of an acute toxic episode (Bodansky and Gutmann, 1947; Halsted, 1960). Moreover, ascorbate tends to produce large numbers of Heinz bodies (Gajdos and Tiprez, 1945; Magos and Sziza, 1962). Depending on the offending substances, differences are recognized in the degree to which methylene blue accelerates methemoglobin reduction (Smith *et al.,* 1967), but significant effects are almost always demonstrable, except perhaps in the case of unsubstituted hydroxylamine (Layne and Smith, 1969). Laboratory determinations of the blood methemoglobin levels are helpful in deciding if and when to institute therapy. Some authorities maintain that methylene blue administration is unwarranted unless the methemoglobin level is above 40% (Mangelsdorff, 1956). Patients with alarming cyanosis have recovered with only supportive care (Casciano, 1952; Graubarth *et al.,* 1945; Ross and

Cicarelli, 1962; Stifel, 1919a). Toluidine blue is said to act more rapidly and is better tolerated by humans than methylene blue, but it has not been approved for use in the United States (Kiese *et al.,* 1972).

In severe methemoglobinemia as induced by aniline or nitrobenzene, oxygen deficits undoubtedly arise in many tissues. Thus, central nervous and cardiac disorders are predicted on the basis of hypoxia alone. Prominent and even lethal effects on these organs are also demonstrable in species resistant to the methemoglobin-producing actions of aniline, *e.g.,* mice, rats (Clark *et al.,* 1943; Smith *et al.,* 1967; Young, 1926; Young *et al.,* 1926). If the histotoxic effects in man are not due exclusively to hypoxia, oxygen lack must at least intensify them. Intravascular hemolysis and anemia with mild renal involvement may occur a week after poisoning by aniline and its derivatives, whether or not methylene blue was given (Graubarth *et al.,* 1945; Hunter, 1943; Wuertz *et al.,* 1964). Death in acute renal failure is unknown or very rare. Jaundice is uncommon except after an acute hemolytic event (Graubarth *et al.,* 1945; Harrison, 1977; Hunter, 1943). Liver disease is recognized after nitrobenzene (Stone, 1904; Wirtschafter and Wolpaw, 1944) but not after aniline (Webster, 1930). Adrenal hyperplasia has been described in rats given aniline daily for 1 to 2 weeks (Kovacs *et al.,* 1971).

In years past numerous severe intoxications manifested by methemoglobinemia have occurred after skin contact or ingestion of commercial products said to contain "aniline dyes." Indelible marking ink (laundry ink) has been a frequent source of exposure. The black pigment is variously described as nigrosin, aniline black or induline (see Section VI). Because these dyes are extremely insoluble in water, they were often dissolved in aniline or nitrobenzene. Thus, it appears likely in retrospect that the major signs and symptoms of poisoning produced by inks were due to the vehicles rather than the colorants. The clinical picture of such poisoning matches in all important respects the available case histories of "pure" nitrobenzene or aniline intoxication.

In 1886 Rayner reported a "wimberry cyanosis" in 10 infants on a maternity ward. No other objective signs were present, and in all cases the cyanosis cleared spontaneously within a week. In a second such outbreak black stains were noted on the buttocks of some affected infants. These stains came from diapers which had been freshly stamped with an identifying mark of the hospital. It was the usual practice to launder napkins after marking them with ink and before issuing them for use. An urgent demand, however, had pressed these into service before washing. Rayner (1886) was able to duplicate the cyanotic syndrome by dressing a healthy infant in a freshly marked napkin. Thus, it appeared probably that percutaneous absorption of a toxin from the ink was responsible for the cyanosis, although respiratory exposure in the confined space of the bassinette could not be eliminated. This century-old episode with only minor variations has been repeated with astonishing regularity through modern times (Etteldorf, 1951; Graubarth et al., 1945; Holczabek, 1963; Howarth, 1951; Kagan et al., 1949; MacMath and Apley, 1954; Pickup and Eeles, 1953; Ramsay and Harvey, 1959; Scott et al., 1946; Weinberg, 1931; Zeligs, 1929). According to these reports (many others could be cited) the overall infant mortality was between 5 and 10%.

Several factors which predispose the neonate to methemoglobinemia are listed under NITRITE (p. III-316). In addition, infant skin may be particularly permeable to aniline congeners, and hepatic detoxication mechanisms are known to be immature or absent in the newborn. However, percutaneous absorption of marking ink constituents has produced poisonings in adults (Greenberg, 1964). Ingestion of similar products resulted in identical syndromes (Fistler and Krienke, 1965; Wirtschafter and Wolpaw, 1944).

A second type of product involved in many cases of methemoglobinemia is shoe dye. Most frequently shoes with canvas upper portions or puttees were dyed black or russet and then worn while the dye was still wet. As in the case of the laundry ink above, most shoe dyes of that era contained high concentrations of aniline or nitrobenzene as the solvent and vehicle (Miner, 1919; Maehlberger, 1925). Except that many of these incidents involved adults as well as children, the clinical syndrome was similar to that produced by the laundry inks (Graves, 1928; Levin, 1927, 1931; Patek, 1926; Sanders, 1920; Stifel, 1919a, b; Stone, 1904). Intoxications under these circumstances have not been reported in recent times, but ingestions of modern shoe dyes have also resulted in severe methemoglobinemia (Joly et al., 1966; MacDonald, 1951).

Finally, intense methemoglobinemia and Heinz body formation have occurred in young children after the ingestion of wax crayons (Clark, 1947; Jones and Brieger, 1947; Murphy et al., 1948). Only low levels of methemoglobin could be induced in cats fed these red or orange crayons (Spicer et al., 1948), and none was detectable in the blood of dogs or rabbits fed para-red, the principal colorant (Brieger, 1949). Some samples of para-red dye, however, and some red wax crayons were said to contain free p-nitroaniline, one of the reactants used to produce the dye (Rieders and Brieger, 1953). Modern crayons, especially those marketed for children, are regarded as safe (see Section VI).

Symptomatology:

1. Lips, tongue and mucous membranes navy blue to black; skin slate gray, all without signs of cardiac or pulmonary insufficiency.
2. Severe headache, nausea, sometimes vomiting, dryness of throat.
3. Central nervous symptoms: confusion, ataxia, vertigo, tinnitus, weakness, disorientation, lethargy, drowsiness, and finally coma. Convulsions may occur but appear to be uncommon.
4. Cardiac effects: heart blocks, arrhythmias, and shock.
5. Death, although uncommon, is usually due to cardiovascular collapse and not respiratory paralysis.
6. Urinary signs and symptoms may include painful micturition, hematuria, hemoglobinuria (and methemoglobinuria), oliguria, and renal insufficiency (usually mild).
7. A late acute hemolytic episode should be anticipated at 6 to 8 days after ingestion.

Treatment:

1. Gastric lavage with water. Alternatively, repeated or continuous lavage with acidic fluids (e.g., 0.1 M HCl) to remove aniline, which may be reconcentrated in the stomach.
2. Leave a solution of magnesium or sodium sulfate in the stomach (15 to 30 gm. in water).
3. Administer oxygen (p. IV-12) and use artificial respiration as indicated (p. IV-7). Do not use hyperbaric oxygen because it prolonged the methemoglobinemia of an aniline derivative in rats (Goldstein and Doull, 1973).
4. Treat shock cautiously because of the uncertain cardiac status (p. IV-17).
5. Transfusions with whole blood or washed red cells (in saline) may be necessary.
6. Methylene blue (1% solution) 1 to 2 mg./kg. intravenously or, in less severe cases of methemoglobinemia, 5 mg./kg. orally.
7. Extracorporeal hemodialysis (p. IV-55) may be useful to remove absorbed aniline in severe systemic poisonings.
8. If aniline is spilled on clothing, remove immediately and discard. Any contaminated area of skin should be washed for 10 to 15 minutes with soap and running water. A rinse with vinegar (5% acetic acid) may be helpful.
9. The late hemolytic episode (see above) does not usually require therapeutic intervention, but if it becomes intense, treat as for NAPHTHALENE hemolysis (p. III-310).

Laboratory:

1. Techniques exist for quantifying a variety of aniline metabolites in biological fluids (Sternson and DeWitte, 1977).
2. Simple spectrophotometric methods for the determination of methemoglobin and oxyhemoglobin, even in the presence of methylene blue, are available and can be used to monitor levels well below that at which cyanosis is clinically evident (Smith, 1971). The "hemoglobin" level is typically normal, whereas the blood oxygen-carrying capacity is measurably low in the absence of effective treatment. This difference is also a sensitive index of methemoglobinemia. Visual comparison of drops of control and methemoglobinemic blood on filter paper can be used by most individuals to detect levels above 10% (Harley and Celermajer, 1970).
3. An acute intravascular hemolysis may occur late (6 to 8 days), when methemoglobin levels have returned to normal (less than 2%).
4. The urinary findings are often compatible with intravascular hemolysis, methemoglobinuria, and kidney injury. The urine is almost always dark.

References:

Banning, A.; Harley, J. D.; Hughes, D. W. O.; Beveridge, J. Prolonged methemoglobinemia after eating a toy-shaped deodorant. Med. J. Aust. 2:922-924, 1965.

Bodansky, O. Methemoglobinemia and methemoglobin-producing compounds. Pharm. Rev. 3:144-196, 1951.

Bodansky, O.; Gutmann, H. Treatment of methemoglobinemia. J. Pharmacol. Exp. Ther. 90:46-56, 1947.

Brieger, H. Poisoning due to ingestion of wax crayons. Am. J. Public Health 39:1023-1024, 1949.

Casciano, A. D. Acute methemoglobinemia due to aniline. J. Med. Soc. N. J. 49:141-142, 1952.

Clark, B. B.; VanLoon, E. J.; Morrissey, R. W. Acute experimental aniline intoxication. J. Ind. Hyg. Toxicol. 25:1-12, 1943.

Clark, E. B. Poisoning due to ingestion of wax crayons. J. A. M. A. 135:917-918, 1947.

Darling, R. C.; Roughton, F. J. W. The effect of methemoglobin on the equilibrium between oxygen and hemoglobin. Am. J. Physiol. 137:56-58, 1942.

Donovan, W. M. The toxicity of nitrobenzene with report of a fatal case. J. A. M. A. 74:1647, 1920.

Etteldorf, J. N. Methylene blue in treatment of methemoglobinemia in premature infants caused by marking ink, 8 cases reported. J. Pediatr. 38:24-27, 1951.

Fistler, I.; Krienke, E. G. Die Behandlung einer Anilinvergiftung durch Austauschtransfusion. Dtsch. Med. J. 16:35-38, 1965.

Gajdos, A.; Tiprez, G. La signification biologique des corpuscules de Heinz. C. R. Soc. Biol. 139:545-546, 1945.

Goldstein, G. M.; Doull, J. The use of hyperbaric oxygen in the treatment of p-aminopropiophenone-induced methemoglobinemia. Toxicol. Appl. Pharmacol. 26:247-252, 1973.

Graubarth, J.; Bloom, C. J.; Coleman, F. C.; Solomon, H. N. Dye poisoning in the nursery. J. A. M. A. 128:1155-1157, 1945.

Graves, G. W. Shoe-dye poisoning. Med. Clin. North Am. 12:673-677, 1928.

Greenburg, H. B. Syncope and shock due to methemoglobinemia. Arch. Environ. Health 9:762-764, 1964.

Halstead, H. C. Industrial methemoglobinemia. J. Occup. Med. 2:591-596, 1960.

Hamblin, D. O. Aromatic nitro and amino compounds. In Industrial Hygiene and Toxicology. Edited by F. A. Patty. Vol. II. Toxicology. 2nd ed., pp. 2105-2169. Edited by D. W. Fassett and D. D. Irish. Interscience Publishers, Inc., New York, 1962.

Hamblin, D. O.; Mangelsdorff, A. F. Methemoglobinemia and its measurement. J. Ind. Hyg. Toxicol. 20:523-530, 1938.

Harley, J. D.; Celermajer, J. M. Neonatal methemoglobinemia and the "red-brown" screening test. Lancet 2:1223-1225, 1970.

Harrison, M. R. Toxic methaemoglobinaemia. A case of acute nitrobenzene and aniline poisoning treated by exchange transfusion. Anaesthesia 32:270-272, 1977.

Healy, J. C. Sulphemoglobinemia. J. Lab. Clin. Med. 18:348-354, 1932.

Hlavica, P.; Kehl, M. Comparative studies on the N-oxidation of aniline and N, N-dimethylaniline by rabbit liver microsomes. Xenobiotica 6:679-689, 1976.

Holczabek, W. Methamoglobinvergiftungen durch frisch mit Anilinfarben gestempelte Windeln. Wein. Med. Wochenschr. 113:230-232, 1963.

Howarth, B. E. Epidemic of aniline methemoglobinemia in newborn babies. Lancet 1:934-935, 1951.

Hughes, J. P.; Treon, J. F. Erythrocytic inclusion bodies in the blood of chemical workers. Arch. Ind. Health 10:192-202, 1954.

Hunter, D. Industrial toxicology. Q. J. Med. 12:185-258, 1943.

Ikeda, M.; Ohtsuji, H.; Imamura, T. Comparative studies on aniline hydroxylation and p-nitrotoluene hydroxylation by the liver. Jpn. J. Pharmacol. 22:479-491, 1972.

Irons, R. D.; Gross, E. A.; White, E. L. Aniline: evidence for an enterogastric cycle in the rat. Fd. Cosmet. Toxicol. 18:393-397, 1980.

Jenkins, F. P.; Robinson, J. A.; Gellatly, J. B. M.; Salmond, G. W. A. The no-effect dose of aniline in human subjects and a comparison of aniline toxicity in man and the rat. Food Cosmet. Toxicol. 10:671-679, 1972b.

Joly, J. B.; Huault, G.; Fabiani, P.; Thieffry, S. Traitement de six cas de methemoglobinemie toxique de l'enfant. Bull. Soc. Med. Hop., Paris 117:1177-1190, 1966.

Jones, J. A.; Brieger, H. Poisoning due to ingestion of wax crayons. Report of a case. J. Pediatr. 30:422-427, 1947.

Jung, F. Studien uber Methamoglobinbildung XIV. Mitteilung: Uber die Ruckbildung des Methamoglobins bei Gegenwart von Alkohol. Arch. Exptl. Path. Pharmakol. 192:464-471, 1939.

Kagan, B. M.; Mirman, B.; Calvin, J.; Lundeen, E. Cyanosis in premature infants due to aniline dye intoxication. J. Pediatr. 34:574-578, 1949.

Kao, J.; Faulkner, J.; Bridges, J. W. Metabolism of aniline in rats, pigs, and sheep. Drug Metab. Dispos. 6:549-555, 1978.

Kiese, M. Methemoglobinemia: A Comprehensive Treatise. CRC Press, Inc., Cleveland, 1974.

Kiese, M.; Lorcher, W.; Weger, N.; Zierer, A. Comparative studies on the effects of toluidine blue and methylene blue on the reduction of ferrihaemoglobin in man and dog. Eur. J. Clin. Pharmacol. 4:115-118, 1972.

Kovacs, K.; Blascheck, J. A.; Yeghiayan, B.; Hatakeyama, S.; Gardell, C. Adrenocortical lipid hyperplasia induced in rats by aniline: A histologic and electron microscopic study. Am. J. Pathol. 62:17-30, 1971.

Layne, W. R.; Smith, R. P. Methylene blue uptake and the reversal of chemically induced methemoglobinemias in human erythrocytes. J. Pharmacol. Exp. Ther. 165:36-44, 1969.

Leader, S. D. Nitrobenzene poisoning. Report of an unusual case in a child. Arch. Pediatr. 49:245-250, 1932.

Leinoff, H. D. Methylene blue therapy in nitrobenzene poisoning with case report. N. Engl. J. Med. 215:191-193, 1936.

Levin, S. J. Shoe dye poisoning—relation to methemoglobin formation, report of a case in a two-year-old child. J. A. M.

A. 89:2178-2180, 1927.

Levin, S. J. Shoe dye poisoning: Report of a case in an eight-months-old infant. J. A. M. A. 96:681, 1931.

Lubash, G. D.; Phillips, R. E.; Shields, J. D.; Bonsnes, R. W. Acute aniline poisoning treated by hemodialysis. Arch. Intern. Med. 114:530-532, 1964.

MacDonald, W. B. Methaemoglobinaemia resulting from poisoning in children. Med. J. Aust. 1:145-147, 1951.

MacMath, I. F.; Apley, J. Cyanosis from absorption of marking ink in newborn babies. Lancet 2:895-896, 1954.

Maehlberger, C. W. Shoe dye poisoning. J. A. M. A. 84:1987-1991, 1925.

Magos, L.; Sziza, M. Effect of ascorbic acid in aniline poisoning. Nature 194:1084, 1962.

Mangelsdorff, A. F. Methemoglobinemia-Recognition, treatment and prevention. Ind. Med. Surg. 21:395-398, 1952.

Mangelsdorff, A. F. Treatment of methemoglobinemia. Arch. Ind. Health 14:148-153, 1956.

Miner, C. S. Methemoglobinemia due to poisoning by shoe dyes. J. A. M. A. 72:593, 1919.

Murphy, F. J.; Zinzi, F. L.; Murphy, L. Methemoglobinemia, case report no. 91. Clin. Proc. Child. Hosp., Wash., D. C. 3:105-108, 1948.

Nabarro, J. D. N. A case of acute mononitrobenzene poisoning. Br. Med. J. 1:929-931, 1948.

Parkes, W. E.; Neill, D. W. Acute nitrobenzene poisoning with transient aminoaciduria. Br. Med. J. 1:653-655, 1953.

Patek, A. J. Aniline shoe dye poisoning, report of 3 cases. J. A. M. A. 86:944-945, 1926.

Pickup, J. D.; Eeles, J. Cyanosis in newborn babies caused by aniline-dye poisoning. Lancet 2:118, 1953.

Ramsay, D. H. E.; Harvey, C. C. Marking ink poisoning. An outbreak of methemoglobinemia cyanosis in newborn babies. Lancet 1:910-912, 1959.

Rayner, W. Cyanosis in newly born children caused by aniline marking ink. Br. Med. J. 1:294, 1886.

Reddy, B. G.; Pohl, L. R.; Krishna, G. The requirement of the gut flora in nitrobenzene-induced methemoglobinemia in rats. Biochem. Pharmacol. 25:1119-1122, 1976.

Rieders, F.; Brieger, H. Mechanism of poisoning from wax crayons. J. A. M. A. 151:1490/-80, 1953.

Ross, J. D.; Cicarelli, R. F. Acquired methemoglobinemia due to ingestion of acetophenetidin. N. Engl. J. Med. 266:1202-1204, 1962.

Sanders, F. G. Nitrobenzene poisoning with cyanosis. J. A. M. A. 74:1518-1519, 1920.

Schreiner, G. E.; Maher, J. F. Dialysis of poisons. Bull. N. J. Acad. Med. 6:310-324, 1960.

Scott, E. P.; Prince, G. E.; Rotondo, C. C. Dye poisoning in infancy. J. Pediatr. 28:713-718, 1946.

Scott, R. W.; Hanzlik, J. P. Poisoning by alcohol "denatured" with nitrobenzene. J. A. M. A. 74:1000, 1920.

Smith, R. P. Spectrophotometric determination of methemoglobin and oxyhemoglobin in the presence of methylene blue. Clin. Toxicol. 4:273-285, 1971.

Smith, R. P. Toxic responses of the blood. in Toxicology, the Basic Science of Poisons, 2nd ed. (J. Doull, C. D. Klaassen and M. O. Andur, Ed.) Macmillan, N. Y, 1980.

Smith, R. P.; Alkaitis, A. A.; Shafer, P. R. Chemically induced methemoglobinemias in the mouse. Biochem. Pharmacol. 16:317-328, 1967.

Smith, R. P.; Olson, M. V. Drug-induced methemoglobinemia. Semin. Hematol. 10:253-268, 1973.

Spicer, S. S.; Hanna, C. H.; Neal, P. A. A note on methemoglobinemia and Heinz body formation in cats fed commercial crayons. J. Pediatr. 33:739-741, 1948.

Steele, C. W.; Spink, W. W. Methylene blue in the treatment of poisonings associated with methemoglobinemia (Report

of two cases). N. Engl. J. Med. 208:1152-1153, 1933.

Stening, S. E. L. Methemoglobinemia due to aniline. Med. J. Aust. 1:578-579, 1951.

Sternson, L. A.; DeWitte, W. J. High-pressure liquid chromatographic analysis of aniline and its metabolites. J. Chromatogr. 137:305-314, 1977.

Stevens, A. M. Cyanosis in infants from nitrobenzene. J. A. M. A. 90:116, 1928.

Stevenson, A.; Forbes, R. P. Nitrobenzene poisoning. Report of a case due to exterminator spray. J. Pediatr. 21:224-228, 1942.

Stifel, R. E. Methemoglobinemia due to poisoning by shoe dye. Report of a series of cases at an Army camp. J. A. M. A. 72:395-396, 1919a.

Stifel, R. E. Report of a case of cyanosis at Camp Jackson, S. C. due to poisoning from shoe dye. J. A. M. A. 72:592-593, 1919b.

Stolk, J. M.; Smith, R. P. Species differences in methemoglobin reductase activity. Biochem. Pharmacol. 15:343-351, 1966.

Stone, W. J. Fatal poisoning due to skin absorption of liquid shoe blacking (Nitrobenzol) with autopsy report. J. A. M. A. 43:977-980, 1904.

Treon, J. F.; Deichmann, W. B.; Sigmon, H. E.; Wright, H.; Witherup, S. O.; Heyroth, F. F.; Kitzmiller, K. V.; Keeman, C. The toxic properties of xylidene and monomethylaniline. J. Ind. Hyg. Toxicol. 31:1-20, 1949a.

Treon, J. F.; Deichmann, W. B.; Sigmon, H. E.; Wright, H.; Witherup, S. O.; Heyroth, F. F.; Kitzmiller, K. V.; Keeman, C. The toxic properties of xylidene and monomethylaniline. J. Ind. Hyg. Toxicol. 31:1-20, 1949a.

Treon, J. F.; Sigmon, H. E.; Wright, H.; Heyroth, F. F.; Kitzmiller, K. V. The toxic properties of xylidine and monomethylaniline. Arch. Ind. Hyg. Occup. Med. 1:506-524, 1950.

von Oettingen, W. F. The aromatic amino and nitro compounds, their toxicity and potential dangers. U. S. Public Health Serv. Public Health Bull. No. 271, 1941b.

Webster, R. W. Legal Medicine and Toxicology. W. B. Saunders Co., Philadelphia, 1930.

Weinberg, A. A. Anitone poisoning in the newborn with a report of thirteen cases. Am. J. Obstet. Gynecol. 21:104-108, 1931.

Welch, R. M.; Conney, A. H.; Burns, J. J. The metabolism of acetophenetidin and N-acetyl-p-aminophenol in the cat. Biochem. Pharmacol. 15:521-531, 1966.

Wetherhold, J. M.; Linch, A. L.; Charsha, R. C. Chemical cyanosis; Causes, effects and prevention. Arch. Environ. Health 1:353-361, 1960.

Wirtschafter, Z. T.; Wolpaw, R. A case of nitrobenzene poisoning. Ann. Intern. Med. 21:135-140, 1944.

Wisniewska-Knypl, J. M.; Jablonska, J. K.; Piotrowski, J. K. Effect of repeated exposure to aniline, nitrobenzene, and benzene on liver microsomal metabolism in the rat. Br. J. Ind. Med. 32:42-48, 1975.

Wuertz, R. L.; Frazee, W. H., Jr.; Hume, W. G.; Linch, A. L.; Wetherhold, J. M. Chemical cyanosis-anemia syndrome. Arch. Environ. Health 9:478-491, 1964.

Young, A. G. Toxicological studies of anilin and anilin compounds. II. Hematological studies of anilin poisoning. J. Pharmacol Exp. Ther. 27:125-131, 1926.

Young, A. G.; Muehlberger, C. W.; Meek, W. J. Toxicological studies of acute anilin poisoning. I. Experimental studies of acute anilin poisoning. J. Pharmacol. Exp. Ther. 27:101-123, 1926.

Zeligs, M. Aniline and nitrobenzene poisoning in infants. Arch. Pediatr. 46:502-506, 1929.

ANTIHISTAMINICS

The enthusiastic reception of the early antihistaminic drugs (around 1942) promoted a search for new histamine antagonists; many of these efforts were successful. The number of antihistaminics now available through commercial channels is legion. Their toxicity is not widely recognized by the layman, and so they are often used indiscriminately.

The discussion and recommendations below are relevant to the so-called H_1 receptor blocking drugs, which are the classical antihistaminics. For a description of the newer H_2 receptor blockers such as cimetidine, consult Section II. The classical antihistaminics resemble several other drugs which possess antihistaminic actions but which are used primarily for other purposes, e.g., promethazine, orphenadrine, hydroxyzine, etc. The latter find utility as anti-motion sickness remedies, skeletal muscle relaxants, preanesthetic medications, mild antianxiety drugs and anticholinergics.

"Over-the-counter" sedative preparations (e.g., Sominex, Nytol) owe their effectiveness in large measure to their content of antihistaminic drugs. Most of them in years past contained methapyrilene but this is now being replaced by pyrilamine (Allen et al., 1979; Johnson, 1981). Some of them contain other ingredients, notably scopolamine and salicylamide, so that overdoses often lead to confusing symptomatology (Jacobziner and Raybin, 1961h). Because these proprietaries are readily available to the public, they are often involved in accidental poisonings and serve as important instruments of suicide.

In addition to an antihistaminic, many over-the-counter cold remedies may contain a cough suppressant and/or a sympathomimetic nasal decongestant in sufficient amounts to contribute to the toxic syndrome arising from overdoses. It is small wonder that confusing and conflicting reports about poisonings by these products are abundant in the medical literature.

Toxicology: Although the incidence of side reactions varies from one preparation to another, 20 to 50% of persons receiving antihistaminic drugs complain of some kind of untoward effects (Michelson and Lowell, 1958). With conventional doses the most common side effect is sedation in varying degrees, particularly marked with diphenhydramine (Benadryl) (Loveless, 1947). Although sedation may be an asset in night-time medication, it is often a hazard in the ambulatory patient.

Other untoward reactions referable to the central nervous system are dizziness, tinnitus, fatigue, ataxia, and blurred vision. Sometimes clinical doses precipitate central excitation evidenced by euphoria, nervousness, tremors, and insomnia. Anorexia and other gastrointestinal symptoms are not uncommon. Miscellaneous complaints include dryness of the mouth, headache, tingling and weakness of the hands, hypotension, palpitations and dysuria (Loew, 1947; Loveless, 1947). The paradox of allergic reactions to these antiallergic drugs is well estab-

lished. Allergic and allergic-like manifestations include dermatitis and rarely leukopenia or agranulocytosis, especially after tripelennamine (Adams and Perry, 1958; Michelson and Lowell, 1958; Norris, 1959).

When an antihistaminic drug is ingested in an amount distinctly greater than the customary dose, any one of many toxic syndromes may result. Frequently these reactions represent extensions of the common side effects listed above. In terms of the clinical picture significant differences are recognized among the various groups of antihistaminics and among patients of different age ranges.

In young children central stimulation, convulsions, and high fever appear to be the dominant signs, followed by a profound cardiorespiratory depression with death in vascular collapse (Brody and Tobin, 1957; Broadfoot, 1953; Reyes-Jacang and Wenzel, 1969; Snyderman, 1949; Tobias, 1949a). The latent period is characteristically short (½ to 2 hours following ingestion) unless a delayed release preparation is involved (Meadows and Leeson, 1979), and mild signs of depression may be observed before the onset of convulsions (Aaron, 1953; Gill-Carey, 1954; Judge and Dumars, 1953; Oberst, 1955; Slade, 1952; Wyngaarden and Seevers, 1951).

In adults, central nervous depression is more prominent, and convulsions are the exception (O'Dea and Liss, 1953) but do occur. Occasionally a case is encountered that also presents atropine-like symptoms; this has been observed with diphenhydramine and pheniramine maleate (Brody and Tobin, 1957; Nigro, 1968; Waldman and Pelner, 1950). A toxic psychosis occurred in a 16-year-old girl after 500 mg. of diphenhydramine (Nigro, 1968); a normal mental state was observed 29 hours after ingestion.

Indeed, few important distinctions can be made between ATROPINE poisoning (p. III-47) and poisoning by many antihistaminics. Coma and seizures are more common with the latter but not unknown with the former. Antihistaminic-induced deaths are usually the result of respiratory arrest during coma. Most severe poisonings have been due to the accidental ingestion of these drugs by young children.

Antihistaminics that are phenothiazine derivatives (e.g., promethazine) and several others may produce poisonings with features similar to CHLORPROMAZINE intoxication; see p. III-112. These features include prominent anticholinergic and sedative effects, which are also characteristic of the ethanolamine derivatives, e.g., diphenhydramine. The alkylamines like chlorpheniramine are more prone to produce central excitation. The ethylenediamines (pyrilamine) and the piperazines (chlorcyclizine) lie between these two extremes. Facial dyskinesias including intermittent bilateral trismus, tongue protrusion and spasms of the platysma were the major signs in an infant who ingested 24 mg. dexbromphen-iramine and 480 mg. pseudoephedrine (Barone and Raniola, 1980). Similar reactions in adults have followed the prolonged use of chlorpheni-ramine, brompheniramine and phenindamine. The blepharospasm, grimacing and tic-like bob-bing of the head resembled late-onset drug-in-duced tardive dyskinesias associated with L-dopa and the antipsychotic phenothiazines and butyrophenones (Thach et al., 1975).

A considerable margin of safety separates the therapeutic dose from the usual lethal one. How-ever, because the convulsant dose lies near the lethal dose, convulsions indicate a poor prog-nosis (Geiringer, 1952). Adults have survived single doses of 2.5 to 5.0 gm. (Siegler et al., 1962; Wyngaarden and Seevers, 1951). Children may be disproportionately more susceptible; 30 to 60 mg./kg. has produced serious poisonings and death in toddlers (Duerfeldt, 1947; Hardmeier and Schmidlin-Mészáros, 1965; Matsuoka et al., 1962), and in two fatal cases the dose was only about 10 mg./kg. (Fatteh and Dudley, 1972; Wyngaarden and Seevers, 1951). Increased sen-sitivity of the young to antihistamines is also recognized in animals, and cannot be explained on the basis of different rates of metabolism (Lee, 1966).

Almost all clinical reports of antihistamine intoxication involve ingestion of the drug. An unusual poisoning followed the percutaneous ap-plication of 2.14 gm. of Pyribenzamine as an aerosol spray on an 8-year-old boy with severe poison ivy of the trunk and extremities (Schi-pior, 1967).

Antihistaminics have not only complex effects of their own but also unpredictable interactions with a variety of other drugs. A pentazocine-tripelennamine combination known by the street name of "T's and blues" is used by narcotic addicts for its heroin-like effects. In addition to problems associated with talc granulomata aris-ing from intravenous injections, tonic-clonic sei-zures are common. These two drugs potentiate each other's lethality in mice (Waller et al., 1980). Also in mice various dose ratios of ethyl alcohol and chlorpheniramine showed either an antagonism of lethality or an independence of effects (Smith et al., 1974). Clinical experience, however, suggests that ethanol and antihista-minics reinforce each other's central depressant actions. Several antihistamines appear to poten-tiate the toxicity of some organophosphate cho-linesterase inhibitors by unknown mechanisms (Fernandez et al., 1975).

Treatment is strictly symptomatic and sup-portive, and the proper measures change with each stage of the poisoning. Analeptic drugs are inadvisable because of the danger of precipitat-ing convulsions. The use of central nervous de-pressants such as diazepam or short-acting bar-biturates to control the convulsive stage must be attended with caution to avoid hastening or deepening postconvulsive respiratory depres-sion. Animal studies on the antagonism of anti-histamine poisoning by drugs, e.g., chlorproma-zine, barbiturates, have led to conflicting conclu-sions (Maël and Bester, 1963; Müller and Fuller, 1965). The depression which follows the excit-atory phase is rarely responsive to the analep-tics.

Fortunately the vital signs are usually well maintained even without support from any arousal drug. Indeed tachycardia and arterial hypertension are often described. One severely poisoned infant, however, exhibited multifocal premature ventricular contractions followed by complete left bundle branch block (Hestand and Teske, 1977). Cardiac arrhythmias are apt to be prominent when products containing both an antihistaminic and a sympathomimetic are taken (Rumack et al., 1974a). Nonspecific local anesthetic properties may contribute to a QUIN-IDINE-like effect on myocardial conduction (p. III-356).

The role of cerebral edema in the genesis of the nervous symptoms has not been adequately explored (Reyes-Jacang and Wenzel, 1969; Wyn-gaarden and Seevers, 1951). The victim with a high spinal fluid pressure may benefit from measures that decompress brain, but in three poisoned children lumbar punctures showed normal pressures, cell counts, protein and sugar (Reyes-Jacang and Wenzel, 1969). In no instance does histamine have any place in the treatment of antihistaminic poisoning (Geiringer, 1951; Wyngaarden and Seevers, 1951).

Exchange transfusion has been successfully employed in severe diphenhydramine (Huxtable and Landworth, 1963) and pheniramine (Diek-mann et al., 1972) poisonings. Peritoneal dialysis was judged to be ineffective in Diekmann's (1972) case, but forced diuresis and purgatives were thought to be helpful. Purgation may be particularly useful with delay-release products; tablet fragments have been recovered in colonic washouts (Meadows and Leeson, 1979). Serial gastric lavages may be worthwhile since these weak bases tend to reaccumulate in the stomach (Winek et al., 1977a).

Physostigmine is said to be effective against both the atropine-like delirium and the seizure-coma state (Lee et al., 1975; Magera et al., 1981; Rumack et al., 1974a; Snyder, 1976). It has not, however, been uniformly effective (Bayley et al., 1975). With the over-the-counter sleep-aids the toxic psychosis is often benign and of short du-ration, so that physostigmine may not be indi-cated (Allen et al., 1979). Remarkable differ-ences in sensitivity must exist. One 5-year-old had "hallucinations" for a week following only twice the recommended dose of tripelennamine (Hays *et al.*, 1980).

Symptomatology:

1. Central nervous depression is usually the dominant reaction in adults; it is evidenced by drowsiness, lethargy, fatigue, hypnosis, and coma. Related nervous symptoms include vertigo, ataxia, tinnitus and blurred vision.
2. Central nervous hyperexcitability often follows initial sedation; in children excitement is often the first evidence of poisoning. The stimulant phase brings tremors, anxiety, insomnia, excitement, hallucinations, delirium, toxic psychosis and convulsions (Towers and Giuffra, 1950).
3. Dangerous hyperpyrexia may occur in poisoned children (Davis and Hunt, 1949; Reichelderfer *et al.*, 1955; Rives *et al.*, 1949).
4. Gastrointestinal reactions include a dry mouth, anorexia, nausea, vomiting, abdominal distress, constipation and/or diarrhea.
5. Pulmonary edema is an infrequent complication (Backer *et al.*, 1977; Reed, 1981), as are cardiac arrhythmias.
6. The terminal phase is one of severe central nervous depression, with death from respiratory arrest or cardiovascular collapse.

Treatment:

1. Repeated gastric lavage (p. I-8) with warm tap water, diluted vinegar or charcoal slurries. Leave 15 to 30 gm. sodium sulfate in solution in the stomach. These interventions should take place in the presymptomatic stage. If given promptly after the ingestion, syrup of ipecac may obviate the need for gastric lavage (see p. I-2-4), but do not use an emetic drug after symptoms of intoxication appear.
2. Cautious use of diazepam or a short-acting barbiturate for the control of central nervous stimulation (p. IV-37).
3. Forced diuresis with acidification of the urine; see p. IV-52.
4. Cold water packs, alcohol sponge baths, etc. (p. IV-84), for the control of hyperpyrexia. Probably salicylates should be avoided here.
5. Artificial respiration and oxygen therapy as necessary (pp. IV-7 and 12). Do *not* use analeptic drugs in these comatose patients.
6. If cerebral edema is present as evidenced by high cerebrospinal fluid pressure, measures to decompress the brain may be worthwhile. See pp. IV-43-46.
7. Cautious trial with physostigmine (p. III-49 and 210) in the severely delirious patient.
8. Symptomatic and supportive measures as indicated.

Laboratory:

1. Elevations of serum transaminase and creatinine phosphokinase have been reported. In one infant poisoned by diphenhydramine the serum lactic dehydrogenase activity was elevated for 10 weeks (Hestand and Teske, 1977).
2. A wide range of lethal blood levels has been reported: diphenhydramine 3 mg./dl.; chlorpheniramine 0.1 mg./dl.; methapyrilene 0.4 to 38 mg./dl. (Ainsworth and Biggs, 1977; Backer *et al.*, 1977; Reed, 1981).

References:

Aaron, F. E. A case of acute diphenhydramine hydrochloride poisoning. Br. Med. J. *2*:24, 1953.

Adams, D. A.; Perry, S. Agranulocytosis associated with thenalidine (Sandostene) tartrate therapy. J. A. M. A. *167*:1207-1210, 1958.

Ainsworth, C. A., III.; Biggs, J. D. A fatality involving methapyrilene. Clin. Toxicol. *11*:281-286, 1977.

Allen, M. D.; Greenblatt, D. J.; Noel, B. J. Self-poisoning with over-the-counter hypnotics. Clin. Toxicol. *15*:151-158, 1979.

Backer, R. C.; Pisano, R. V.; Sopher, I. M. Diphenhydramine suicide - case report. J. Anal. Toxicol. *1*:227-228, 1977.

Barone, D. A.; Raniolo, J. Facial dyskinesia from an overdose of an antihistamine. N. Engl. J. Med. *303*:107, 1980.

Bayley, M.; Walsh, F. M.; Valaske, M. J. Fatal overdose from bendectin. Clin. Pediatr. *14*:507-514, 1975.

Broadfoot, E. M. A case of "Anthisan" poisoning. Med. J. Aust. *1*:189-190, 1953.

Brody, J. I.; Tobin, J. L. Apnea due to Benadryl. Ann. Intern. Med. *47*:172-177, 1957.

Davis, J. H.; Hunt, H. H. Accidental Benadryl poisoning. Report of a fatal case. J. Pediatr. *34*:358-361, 1949.

Diekmann, L.; Hosemann, R.; Dibbern, H. W. Pheniramin (Avil)-Intoxikation bei einem Kleinkind. Arch. Toxikol. *29*:317-324, 1972.

Duerfeldt, T. H. Acute "Benadryl" poisoning. Northwest Med. *46*:781, 1947.

Fatteh, A.; Dudley, J. B. Fatal poisoning involving methapyrilene. J. A. M. A. *219*:756, 1972.

Fernandez, G.; Diaz Gomez, M. I.; Castro, J. A. Cholinesterase inhibition by phenothiazine and nonphenothiazine antihistaminics: Analysis of its postulated role in synergizing organophosphate toxicity. Toxicol. Appl. Pharmacol. *31*:179-190, 1975.

Geiringer, E. Treatment of anthisan poisoning. Br. Med. J. *1*:163, 1952.

Gill-Carey, M. C. Chlorcyclizine hydrochloride poisoning in an infant. Br. Med. J. *1*:687-688, 1954.

Hardmeier, E.; Schmidlin-Meszaros, J. Todliche Vergiftung eines Kleinkindes mit dem Antiallergicum Plimasm. Arch. Toxikol. *21*:131-141, 1965.

Hays, D. P.; Johnson, B. F.; Perry, R. Prolonged hallucinations following a modest overdose of tripelennamine. Clin. Toxicol. *16*:331-333, 1980.

Hestand, H. E.; Teske, D. W. Diphenhydramine hydrochloride intoxication. J. Pediatr. *90*:1017-1018, 1977.

Huxtable, R. F.; Landworth, J. Diphenhydramine poisoning treated by exchange transfusion. Am. J. Dis. Child. *106*:496-500, 1963.

Jacobziner, H.; Raybin, H. W. Thallium and methapyrilene poisonings. N. Y. State J. Med. *61*:1345-1347, 1961h.

Johnson, G. R. A fatal case involving pyrilamine. Clin. Toxicol. *18*:907-909, 1981.

Judge, D. J.; Dumars, K. W., Jr. Diphenhydramine (Benadryl) and tripelennamine (Pyribenzamine) intoxication in children. Am. J. Dis. Child. 85:545-550, 1953.

Lee, C. C. Comparative pharmacologic responses to antihistamines in newborn and young rats. Toxicol. Appl. Pharmacol. 8:210-217, 1966.

Lee, J. H.; Turndorf, H.; Poppers, P. J. Physostigmine reversal of antihistamine-induced excitement and depression. Anesthesiology 43:683-684, 1975.

Loew, E. R. Pharmacology of antihistamine compounds. Physiol. Rev. 27:542-573, 1947.

Loveless, M. H. Therapeutic and side effects of Pyribenzamine and Benadryl. Am. J. Med. 3:296-308, 1947.

Mael, I. H.; Bester, J. F. Chlorpromazine and dextro-amphetamine as antidotes in acute antihistamine toxicity in rats. J. Pharm. Sci. 52:451-453, 1963.

Magera, B. E.; Betlech, C. J.; Sweatt, A. P.; Derrick, C. W., Jr. Hydroxyzine intoxication in a 13-month-old child. Pediatrics 67:280-283, 1981.

Matusuoka, S.; Sadanaga, Y.; Nishi, Y.; Takano, M.; Kinjo, K. A case of Chlortrimeton (chlorpheniramine) intoxication. Clin. Neurol. 2:159-162, 1962.

Meadows, S. R.; Leeson, G. A. Poisoning with delayed release tablets. Treatment of Debendox poisoning with purgation and dialysis. Arch. Dis. Child. 49:310-312, 1979.

Michelson, A. L.; Lowell, F. C. Antihistamic drugs. N. Engl. J. Med. 258:994-1000, 1958.

Muller, M.; Fuller, H. Zur Beurteilung und Therapie der AH-3 Vergiftung bei Kindern. Dtsch. Gesundheitsw. 20:769-772, 1965.

Nigro, S. A. Toxic psychosis due to diphenhydramine hydrochloride. J. A. M. A. 203:301-302, 1968.

Norris, B. F. Agranulocytosis following antihistamine therapy. Report of a fatal case. N. Y. State J. Med. 59:2606-2608, 1959.

O'Dea, A. E.; Liss, M. Suicidal poisoning by methapyrilene hydrochloride with documentation by paper chromatography. N. Engl. J. Med. 249:566-567, 1953.

Oberst, B. B. Accidental fatal dibistine poisoning. J. Pediatr. 46:451-452, 1955.

Reed, D. A fatal case involving chlorpheniramine. Clin. Toxicol. 18:941-943, 1981.

Reichelderfer, T. E.; Livingston, S.; Auld, R. M. G.; Peck, J. L.

Treatment of acute Benadryl (diphenhydramine hydrochloride) intoxication with severe central nervous system changes and recovery. J. Pediatr. 46:303-307, 1955.

Reyes-Jacang, A.; Wenzel, J. E. Antihistamine toxicity in children. Clin. Pediatr. 8:297-299, 1969.

Rives, H. F.; Ward, B. B.; Hicks, M. L. A fatal reaction to methapyrilene (Thenylene). J. A. M. A. 140:1022-1024, 1949.

Rumack, B. H.; Anderson, R. J.; Wolfe, R.; Fletcher, E. C.; Vestal, B. K. Ornade and anticholinergic toxicity: Hypertenison, hallucinations, and arrhythmias. Clin. Toxicol. 7:573-581, 1974a.

Schipior, P. G. An unusual case of antihistamine poisoning. J. Pediatr. 71:589-591, 1967.

Siegler, P. E.; Bodi, T.; Mapp, Y.; Nodine, J. H. Antihistamines and their side effects. G. P. 26:116-119, 1962.

Slade, D. A. Fatal poisonings in children from aspirin, quinine and Anthisan. Lancet 2:809-810, 1952.

Smith, R. B.; Rossi, G. V.; Orzechowski, R. F. Interactions of chlorpheniramine ethanol combinations: Acute toxicity and antihistaminic activity. Toxicol. Appl. Pharmacol. 28:240-247, 1974.

Snyder, B. D. Orphenadrine overdose treated with physostigmine. N. Engl. J. Med., 295:1435, 1976.

Snyderman, H. S. Accidental Thenylene hydrochloride poisoning. J. Pediatr. 35:376-377, 1949.

Thach, B. T.; Chase, T. N.; Bosma, J. F. Oral facial dyskinesia associated with prolonged use of antihistaminic decongestants. N. Engl. J. Med., 293:486-487, 1975.

Tobias, M. Anthisan poisoning. Br. Med. J., 1:1098, 1949a.

Towers, P. A.; Giuffra, L. J. An unusual reaction following the use of pyribenzamine. N. Y. State J. Med., 50:214-215, 1950.

Waldman, S.; Pelner, L. Toxic psychosis due to overdosage with prophenpyridamine (Trimeton). J. A. M. A. 143:1334-1335, 1950.

Waller, D. P.; Katz, N. L.; Morris, R. W. Potentiation of lethality in mice by combination of pentazocine and tripelennamine. Clin. Toxicol., 16:17-23, 1980.

Winek, C. L.; Fochtman, F. W.; Trogus, W. J., Jr.; Fusia, E. P.; Shanor, S. P. Methapyrilene toxicity. Clin. Toxicol., 11:287-294, 1977a.

Wyngaarden, J. B.; Seevers, M. H. The toxic effects of antihistaminic drugs. J. A. M. A. 145:277-282, 1951.

ANTU

Alpha-naphthylthiourea (ANTU) was developed as an outgrowth of the observation that phenylthiourea kills rats but is not toxic to man (Richter and Clisby, 1942). Many derivatives were prepared before one was found which had the same high toxicity to rodents without the bitter taste of phenylthiourea. ANTU proved to be the most effective (Richter, 1945). Some species of rats, however, are not sensitive to it, and others develop resistance rapidly (Dieke and Richter, 1946a). ANTU is a stable bluish-gray powder, highly insoluble in water, without perceptible odor, and with only a transient bitter taste. It is used in baits in concentrations of 1 to 3% (Emlen, 1947).

Toxicology: ANTU is probably not toxic to man except in large amounts; the mean lethal dose by mouth is 4 gm./kg. in monkeys and presumably much the same in man (Brewer and Haggerty, 1958).

In the only human intoxication known to us, 80 gm. of a rat poison consisting of 30% ANTU was ingested by a suicidal adult man, together with considerable alcohol (Cimbal, 1952). He vomited promptly. The amount of ANTU retained was estimated as 15 gm. Examined within 1.25 hours, he exhibited drunkenness, restlessness, horizontal nystagmus, mild conjunctivitis and an irritated throat, all of which might be ascribed to the alcohol. ANTU, however, was presumably responsible for the transient vomiting, obvious dyspnea, distinct cyanosis and coarse pulmonary rates. No pleural effusion occurred. The pulmonary signs cleared gradually. Presumably he would have recovered even without therapy, which consisted here of codeine and 5 to 10 ml. of 10% calcium thiosulfate intravenously. The rationale of this therapy was unexplained.

Observations on experimental animals (*e.g.*, rats, dogs) indicate that the principal organ affected is the lungs; fibrin-rich pulmonary edema and pleural effusion develop due to the action of ANTU on pulmonary capillaries (Lillie, 1945; McClosky and Smith, 1945); pericardial effusion is less marked. Dogs are quite susceptible to

ANTU but are usually protected by prompt vomiting unless the stomach contains food (McClosky and Smith, 1945). In forensic examinations of poisoned dogs, lung edema and hydrothorax were always found in cases where ANTU could be identified in the stomach or intestinal contents (Wanntorp, 1953). Pulmonary edema due to high pressure oxygen, convulsants or pressor agents is not accompanied by pleural effusion, tends to be hemorrhagic and is not influenced by various pretreatments (below) which modify the response to ANTU (Van den Brenk et al., 1976).

In a review of experimental work DuBois (1948) noted that lethal doses of ANTU in poisoned rats produce marked hyperglycemia, depletion of liver glycogen and inhibition of glycogen synthesis. The changes could be blocked by adrenal demedullation, but survival time of poisoned animals and the edemagenic process were not altered. Iodine or iodide given to animals 6 hours prior to ANTU affords significant protection, but neither is effective after the exposure. Thyroidectomy blocks the protective effect of iodine pretreatment, but neither thyroxin nor diiodotyrosine mimicks the iodine effect. ANTU may possess antithyroid activity in chronic sublethal exposures (Fitzhugh and Nelson, 1947).

Poisoned rats have also been noted to develop oliguria or anuria concomitantly with the onset of pleural effusion (Baker, 1954; Richter, 1952). Glomerular lesions were detected 8 hours after an acute exposure (Patil and Radhakrishnamurty, 1978). Capillary tufts became sclerosed and infiltrated with inflammatory cells and eventually red blood cells.

ANTU is said to be a sulfhydryl group blocking agent, and cysteine and thiosorbitol are effective antidotes in rats under some conditions (DuBois et al., 1946; Koch and Schwarze, 1955). 1-Ethyl-1-phenylthiourea (EPTU) is also effective in protecting rats (Saunders and Spaulding, 1951).

Rats up to 4 weeks of age are highly resistant to ANTU, but susceptibility appears rapidly over the next 2 weeks (Van den Brenk et al., 1976). Tolerance to the acute effects has been induced in rats by administering progressively increasing doses. Pleural effusions are not observed in tolerant animals dying from large doses (McClosky and Smith, 1945). Since pulmonary edema is observed only in those species that are most susceptible (Dieke and Richter, 1946a), it is apparent that ANTU can cause death by other undefined mechanisms. Perhaps man can be classified as one of the more resistant species, but the evidence is obviously inadequate. Some of the miscellaneous visceral lesions that developed in poisoned laboratory mammals are described by Lillie (1945). ANTU is not irritating to the human skin.

Metabolism of ANTU by hepatic microsomal enzyme preparations (mixed function oxidation) gives rise to mutagenic and perhaps carcinogenic metabolites (Kawalek et al., 1979). Similarly, ANTU is activated by both lung and liver microsomes to metabolites that bind to macromolecules in those organs. The process requires NADPH and it results in a decrease in mixed function oxidase activity and in the cytochrome P450 content of the microsomal fractions. If macromolecular binding in the lungs is responsible for the toxic effects of ANTU, a decrease in the ability to metabolize ANTU may account for the marked tolerance that develops when animals are pretreated with small doses of ANTU before challenge with a potentially lethal dose (Boyd and Neal, 1976). α-Naphthylurea is a known metabolite of ANTU. Atomic sulfur has been proposed as another metabolite, which is postulated to bind covalently by reacting with cysteine side chains of proteins to form hydrodisulfides (Lee et al., 1980). However, the desulfuration reaction that leads to α-naphthylurea may generate H_2S as a metabolite of ANTU. Hydrogen sulfide is known to bind covalently to proteins by opening disulfide bridges to produce hydrodisulfides (Smith and Abbanat, 1966).

Symptomatology (as observed in animals):
1. Vomiting.
2. Dyspnea, rales, cyanosis (due to severe pulmonary edema and sometimes pleural effusion).
3. Lowered body temperature (hypothermia).
4. Death from asphyxia.
5. In nonlethal poisonings glomerular injury may lead to oliguria and anuria.

Treatment:
1. Emetics or prompt gastric lavage with tap water (see Section I).
2. Saline catharsis with 15 to 30 gm. sodium sulfate in water.
3. Positive-pressure oxygen (see p. IV-15). Postural drainage. Absolute rest.
4. Avoid fat ingestion, since ANTU may be more readily absorbed in its presence.
5. Use caution in giving oral or intravenous fluids because of the danger of precipitating pulmonary edema.
6. Measure and record the intake of fluid and the urine flow to detect incipient renal damage (see p. IV-52).

Laboratory: Not known to be relevant. A marked rise in blood sugar has been reported in ANTU-poisoned rats (DuBois et al. 1946), as well as hemorrhagic glomerular nephritis (Patil and Radhakrishnamurty, 1978).

References:

Baker, S. P. Anuria produced by alpha-naphthylthiourea. Am. J. Physiol. *179*:457-461, 1954.

Boyd, M. R.; Neal, R. A. Studies on the mechanism of toxicity and of development of tolerance to the pulmonary toxin γ-naphthylthiourea (ANTU). Drug Metab. Dispos. *4*:314-322, 1976.

Brewer, E.; Haggerty, R. J. Rat poisons. III. Thallium, strychnine and ANTU. N. Engl. J. Med. *259*:1038-1040, 1958.

Cimbal, G. Alpha-Naphthylthioharnstoff-Vergiftung beim Menschen. Arch. Toxikol. *14*:2-6, 1952.

Dieke, S. H.; Richter, C. P. Age and species variation in the acute toxicity of alpha-naphthylthiourea. Proc. Soc. Exp. Biol. Med. *62*:22-25, 1946a.

DuBois, K. P. New rodenticidal compounds. J. Pharm. Sci. *37*:307-310, 1948.

DuBois, K. P.; Holm, L. W.; Doyle, W. L. Biochemical changes following poisoning of rats by alpha-naphthylthiourea. Proc. Soc. Exp. Biol. Med. *61*:102-104, 1946.

Emlen, J. T. Baltimore's community rat control program. Am. J. Public Health *37*:721-727, 1947.

Fitzhugh, O. G.; Nelson, A. A. Chronic oral toxicity of alpha-naphthylthiourea. Proc. Soc. Exp. Biol. Med. *64*:305-310, 1947.

Kawalek, J. C.; Andrews, A. W.; Peinta, R. J. 1-Naphthylthiourea: a mutagenic rodenticide that transforms hamster embryo cells. Mol. Pharmacol. *15*:678-684, 1979.

Koch, R.; Schwarze, W. Die Hemmung der α-Naphthylthioharnstoffvergiftung durch Cysteamin und seine Derivate (Zugleich ein Beitrag zur Toxikologie und Strahlenschutzwirkung dieser Sulfhydrylkorper). Naunyn-Schmiedebergs Arch. Pharmakol. *225*:428-441, 1955.

Lee, P. W.; Arnau, T.; Neal, R. A. Metabolism of α-naphthyl-thiourea by rat liver and rat lung microsomes. Toxicol. Appl. Pharmacol. *53*:164-173, 1980.

Lillie, R. D. Studies on the pharmacologic action and the pathology of alpha-naphthylthiourea . II. Pathology. Public Health Repts. (U. S.) *60*:1108-1113, 1945.

McClosky, W. T.; Smith, M. I. Studies of the pharmacologic action and the pathology of alpha-naphthylthiourea. I. Pharmacology. Public Health Repts. (U. S.) *60*:1101-1108, 1945.

Patil, T. N.; Radhakrishnamurty, R. Biochemical changes induced by α-naphthylthiourea in albino rats. Pest. Biochem. Physiol. *8*:217-224, 1978.

Richter, C. P. The development and use of alpha-naphthylthiourea (ANTU) as a rat poison. J. A. M. A. *129*:927-931, 1945.

Richter, C. P. The physiology and cytology of pulmonary edema and pleural effusions produced in rats by alpha-naphthylthiourea (ANTU). J. Thorac. Cardiovasc. Surg. *23*:66-91, 1952.

Richter, C. P.; Clisby, K. H. Toxic effects of the bitter tasting phenylthiocarbamines. Arch. Pathol. *33*:46-57, 1942.

Saunders, J. P.; Spaulding, R. C. Effects of some substituted thioureas on alpha-naphthylthiourea (ANTU). Proc. Soc. Exp. Biol. Med. *76*:84-85, 1951.

Smith, R. P.; Abbanat, R. A. Protective effects of oxidized glutathione in acute sulfide poisoning. Toxicol. Appl. Pharmacol. *9*:209-217, 1966.

Van den Brenk, H. A. S.; Kelly, H.; Stone, M. G. Innate and drug-induced resistance to acute lung damage caused in rats by naphthyl thiourea (ANTU) and related compounds. Br. J. Exp. Pathol. *57*:621-636, 1976.

Wanntorp, H. α-Naphthylthiourea (ANTU) as a cause of poisoning in dogs and its chemical identification in material of animal origin. Acta Pharmacol. Toxicol. *9*:313-321, 1953.

ARSENIC

Arsenic is encountered as an occasional ingredient of rodenticides, insecticides, herbicides, paints and other products. Several organic arsenic compounds are employed as therapeutic agents in clinical and veterinary medicine (Buchanan, 1962; Valee *et al.*, 1960). Arsenic sulfide is still found in several Chinese herbal products promoted for asthma (Tay and Seah, 1975).

Toxicology of inorganic salts of arsenic: Arsenic was formerly used extensively as a "criminal poison" because it is odorless and nearly tasteless. Accidental poisoning is still rather common because arsenic compounds are widely used and readily available. The mortality in acute poisoning is high (50 to 75%); death usually occurs within 48 hours. The lethal dose varies with the compound, but if finely dispersed, 0.2 to 0.3 gm. of the trioxide ("white arsenic") is usually fatal in an adult person (Sollmann, 1957), and the single toxic dose is said to range from 5 to 50 mg. Coarsely powdered or granular arsenic trioxide (As_2O_3) is significantly less toxic than finely powdered material, since appreciable amounts of the latter may be eliminated in feces without dissolving (Schwartze, 1923). Before it was banned in 1977, As_2O_3 in pre-emergence herbicidal formulations was coarsely divided.

The soluble arsenic acids and their salts represent a much greater acute toxic hazard than do the relatively insoluble arsenic trioxide and lead arsenate. For example, in rats the oral lethal dose of coarsely ground arsenic trioxide is 385 mg./kg. (equivalent to 293 mg. As), whereas that of soluble sodium arsenite is only 42 mg./kg. (equivalent to 24 mg. As) (Done and Peart, 1971). Among soluble salts, trivalent arsenic (arsenites) is generally regarded as more lethal than pentavalent arsenates. When doses are computed on the basis of equal arsenic contents, the organic alkane arsonates used as herbicides resemble arsenic trioxide in acute lethality (Done and Peart, 1971). Systemic poisoning is the principal concern with all arsenic compounds, but arsenic trichloride and some organic derivatives (*e.g.*, Lewisite) are also strong local irritants; they may penetrate intact skin and act as vesicants.

Acute arsenic poisoning is now more common than chronic intoxication (see below). Whatever the route of exposure, the presenting symptoms in most cases are those of a severe gastritis or gastroenteritis. Because the lesions are usually due not to local corrosion but to vascular damage from absorbed arsenic (Hanna and McHugo, 1960; Sollmann, 1957), the first symptoms may be delayed for several hours. Eventually a violent hemorrhagic gastroenteritis leads to profound losses of fluid and electrolytes, resulting in collapse, shock, and death. Occasionally the alimentary symptoms are mild or absent, in which case the presenting complaints are usually referable to the central nervous system: headache, vertigo, muscle spasm or convulsions, delirium, and sometimes mania (Buchanan, 1962; Webster, 1930).

Because of vigorous replacement therapy, patients who previously would have died from the effects of fluid loss during the acute phase now often survive only to develop late neuropathies and other disorders seen formerly in only those with chronic exposures. For example, in a series of 57 patients, 37 had peripheral neuropathy and 5 encephalopathy. The motor system appears to be spared only in the mildest cases, and severe crippling is common (Jenkins, 1966), unless therapy with BAL (dimercaprol) is prompt (see below). Cardiac complications (ventricular fibrillation, asystole) have also been reported in some of these cases (St. Petery et al., 1970; Wang and Mazzia, 1969). Cardiopulmonary resuscitation has generally been unsuccessful. However, one survivor of the acute phase of arsenic poisoning developed ventricular fibrillation during general anesthesia on two occasions 19 and 21 days following an ingestion with suicidal intent and was resuscitated successfully both times.

Subacute and chronic exposures may reveal themselves in these and many other ways. Among the protean manifestations of chronic poisoning are anorexia, mild gastrointestinal disturbances, low-grade fever, persistent headache, pallor, weakness, and a catarrhal inflammation of nose, throat, conjunctivae and larynx—simulating an infectious coryza. Stomatitis and salivation are common (Cannon, 1936; Greenberg, 1949; Sollmann, 1957). Skin afflictions are many and varied: erythema, eczema, pigmentation (arsenic melanosis), diffuse alopecia, keratosis (especially of palms and soles), scaling and desquamation, brittle nails, white lines or bands in the nails (Mees lines), loss of hair and nails, and localized subcutaneous edema (especially of the eyelids) (Ayres and Anderson, 1934; Carleton et al., 1948; Holmquist, 1951; Mees, 1919; Tay and Seah, 1975).

Signs of renal damage develop after acute and chronic exposures. Hepatomegaly with jaundice (and sometimes pruritus) may evolve into cirrhosis with ascites (Franklin et al., 1950; Wade and Frazer, 1953). Idiopathic portal hypertension accompanied by bleeding esophageal varices has been described in chronic poisonings (Chainuvati and Viranuvatti, 1979; Szuler et al., 1979). An even rarer reaction is a protein-losing enteropathy (Kobayashi and Ohbe, 1971). Arsenic crosses the placental barrier and has been incriminated in neonatal death (Lugo et al., 1969).

Severe blood dyscrasias result from depression of any and all cellular elements in bone marrow (Eagle and Magnuson, 1946; Kjeldsberg and Ward, 1972; Kyle and Pease, 1965). Megaloblastic anemia reportedly followed a single prolonged exposure to an arsenical weed spray (Westhoff et al., 1975). These effects may be related to inhibition of folic acid metabolism (Van Tongeren et al., 1965). Lymphocyte chromosomal aberrations were found in a group of persons chronically exposed to arsenic (Petres et al., 1970).

In advanced poisoning, nervous symptoms are prominent; encephalopathies have been described (Eagle and Magnuson, 1946; Prickman and Millikan, 1953), but peripheral neuritis is more common (Heyman et al., 1956). Sensation is involved first (paresthesia, hypesthesia, pain), but eventually paralysis and muscular atrophy appear, usually in the legs. "Glove and stocking" distribution of sensory loss may be prominent (Dreifuss et al., 1972). Reduced nerve conduction velocities were demonstrated in copper smelter workers following prolonged industrial exposure to arsenic trioxide (Feldman et al., 1979). If therapy with BAL is begun within 18 hours of single acute exposures, it may protect against the subsequent development of these neuropathies (Jenkins, 1966).

Treatment of psoriasis with Fowler's solution (potassium arsenite) is said to have caused skin and visceral cancers (Currie, 1947; Jackson and Grainge, 1975). Occupational exposures to arsenical dusts have also lead to various skin lesions, including keratoses and cancer, as well as perforations of the nasal septum. Prolonged inhalation of arsenical dusts and fumes has also been implicated in lung cancer. Vineyard workers repeatedly exposed to arsenical insecticides in the Moselle wine district of Germany showed an incidence of lung cancer as high as 56%. Likewise, populations exposed to arsenical fumes from nonferrous smelters experienced a higher than normal incidence of lung cancer (Lee and Fraumeri, 1969). Taiwanese exposed to arsenic in well water have experienced skin cancer. Thus inorganic and organic compounds of arsenic are established carcinogens in man (Committee, 1977).

In all cases the toxic moiety is presumably trivalent arsenic, in the form of inorganic arsenious acid (arsenite) or an organic arsenoxide, rather than the element itself. Pentavalent arsenicals are believed to be reduced to a small extent in vivo to the active trivalent form, but the issue is not entirely settled (Committee, 1977). This in vivo conversion may explain why all chemical forms of arsenic eventually produce the same toxic syndrome. As arsenite, but not as arsenate, the element is an active enzyme inhibitor, presumably because of its attachment to sulfhydryl groups of essential proteins (Stocken and Thompson, 1949; Voegtlin et al., 1923, 1925).

Trivalent organic arsenicals such as phenylarsenoxide are even more potent inhibitors of certain sulfhydryl enzymes than are inorganic arsenites (Barron et al., 1947; Peters et al., 1946). Arsenate (but not arsenite) appears to compete with phosphate in some biochemical systems, and it has been shown to uncouple oxidative phosphorylation (Committee, 1977).

Absorbed arsenic is excreted largely by the kidneys, but feces, skin and hair sometimes contain appreciable amounts (Webster, 1941). In three patients, 45% of the absorbed dose of inhaled radio-arsenic was eliminated in urine within 3 days, and another 2.5% was excreted in feces (Holland et al., 1959). After a single oral dose, excretion is essentially complete within 2 weeks. Following oral ingestion of inorganic arsenic by man, much arsenic in the urine is present as two metabolites: methylarsinic acid and dimethylarsinic acid (DMAA), especially the latter (Crecelius, 1977), but the proportions vary with time. For example, after ingesting arsenic trioxide, five humans excreted mostly inorganic arsenic during the first 2 to 3 days and mostly the methyl metabolites thereafter, with 90% of the urinary arsenic present as methylated derivatives by the 6th day (Mahieu et al., 1981). Thus inorganic trivalent arsenic tends to be extensively oxidized in vivo to pentavalent arsenic, presumably before methylation. Because the methylated metabolites are relatively innocuous, their generation constitutes a detoxification reaction.

Urinary excretion is markedly enhanced, without damage to the excretory organs, by the administration of BAL (dimercaprol). If prompt, this treatment suppresses most signs and symptoms of acute poisoning (Woody and Kometani, 1948), but recurrence of symptoms may require additional courses of BAL therapy. With BAL the biologic half-life of arsenic in blood is about 60 hours (Mahieu et al., 1981). In case of arsenic-induced renal failure, hemodialysis may be lifesaving by removing arsenic and its BAL-complex (Giberson et al., 1976). Intraperitoneal dialysis, however, is apparently not effective (Gillies and Taylor, 1979). The oral chelating agent D-penicillamine also appears to promote the urinary excretion of arsenic in both acute (Kuruvilla et al., 1975; Peterson and Rumack, 1977) and chronic (Kjeldsberg and Ward, 1972) poisonings. Although D-penicillamine is often well tolerated, untoward reactions are sometimes severe and even life-threatening (see Section II). If only for this reason, BAL remains the chelating agent of choice in arsenic poisoning.

Toxicology of arsine: An exceptional arsenic compound is gaseous AsH_3 or arsine, which may be found whenever hydrogen is generated in the presence of arsenic (Vallee et al., 1960). Arsine is the most dangerous compound of arsenic, and it produces a unique intoxication syndrome. Even among modern industrial workers intoxication is surprisingly common (Buchanan, 1962; Elkins and Fahy, 1967; Nielson, 1969; Uldall et al., 1970).

The major clinical feature is an acute, self-limiting, intravascular hemolysis, commonly followed by acute renal failure (Kensler et al., 1946; McKinstry and Hickes, 1957; Pinto et al., 1950; Neuwirtova et al., 1961). Nausea and vomiting, headache, and neurologic signs and symptoms (parasthesias, delirium) may also be present (Parish et al., 1979). A transient pulmonary edema is sometimes seen; it has been ascribed to a local irritant action of the gas (Hocken and Bradshaw, 1970; Wills, 1948). Electrocardiographic changes such as heightened T waves may simply reflect elevated plasma potassium levels secondary to hemolysis (Josephson et al., 1951). Bronze skin pigmentation may be confused with jaundice (Hocken and Bradshaw, 1970; Jenkins et al., 1965; Levinsky et al., 1970). Delayed neurotoxicity, including a reversible toxic polyneuropathy and a mild psycho-organic syndrome, occurred in six survivors of acute arsine poisoning after a latency of 1 to 6 months (Frank, 1976).

BAL, even when given soon after exposure, does not protect against the subsequent development of arsine hemolysis (Coles et al., 1964; Pinto et al., 1950; Teitelbaum and Kies, 1969). Both the symptomatology and therapy recommendations outlined below for inorganic salts of arsenic are, therefore, inappropriate for arsine. Exchange transfusions may be helpful (Levinsky et al., 1970; Teitelbaum and Kies, 1969), as well as peritoneal or extracorporeal hemodialysis for the usual indications (Coles et al., 1964; Teitelbaum and Kies, 1969). Symptoms and treatment relevant to the hemolytic episode and its consequences are described under NAPHTHALENE, p. III-309.

Symptomatology (acute poisoning only; exclusive of arsine above):

1. Symptoms usually appear ½ to 1 hour after ingestion but may be delayed many hours, especially when arsenic is taken with food.
2. Sweetish metallic taste; garlicky odor of breath and feces.
3. Constriction in the throat and difficulty in swallowing. Burning and colicky pains in esophagus, stomach and bowel.
4. Vomiting and profuse painful diarrhea. Often the excreta resemble the "rice water" stools of cholera; later the feces become bloody.
5. Dehydration with intense thirst and muscular cramps.

6. Hematuria, albuminuria, glycosuria. Elevation of liver enzymes in the plasma.
7. Initial sinus tachycardia and occasionally ventricular arrhythmias, followed by cyanosis, feeble pulse and cold extremities.
8. Vertigo, frontal headache. In some cases ("cerebral type") vertigo, stupor, delirium and even mania develop without prominent gastrointestinal signs.
9. Syncope, coma, occasionally convulsions, general paralysis, ventricular fibrillation, and death.
10. If the acute phase is survived, peripheral neuritis with sensory and motor involvement is not uncommon.
11. Various skin eruptions and colorations, more often as a late manifestation or in chronic poisoning (see above).
12. During recovery, weakness and diarrhea may persist for weeks, and occasionally a syndrome indistinguishable from chronic poisoning evolves (see above).

Treatment (acute poisoning only):

1. If the patient is seen soon after the ingestion, is alert and has not already vomited, induce emesis with syrup of ipecac (see p. I-2) or else perform gastric lavage with 1 to 2 liters of tap water (pp. I-8–11).
2. At the beginning and again at the end of the lavage, it may be helpful to drink or to introduce through the lavage tube a demulcent-adsorbent. A glassful of milk is often recommended, but a slurry of 30 to 100 gm. of powdered activated charcoal in water (p. I-4) is probably more effective. A cathartic such as magnesium sulfate is usually unnecessary and potentially dangerous in acute arsenic poisoning.
3. Administer BAL intramuscularly as a 10% solution in oil. The dosage schedule recommended in Table III-2 (p. III-52) is thought to be adequate for patients of all ages. All doses are expressed as milligrams of BAL (*not* of solution). For the clinical toxicity of BAL and the basis for these dosage recommendations, see p. III-51.
4. If the patient does not tolerate BAL or if symptoms recur following a full course of BAL therapy (5 to 10 days), oral D-penicillamine may be substituted. Although arsenic poisoning is not a currently approved indication for this drug, it appears to be efficacious in suppressing symptoms and in promoting arsenic excretion (see above). Do not use until the alimentary tract has been cleared of ingested arsenic (as evidenced by the appearance of the charcoal marker in feces). A recommended course of D-penicillamine in children (Peterson and Rumack, 1977) consists of a daily intake of 100 mg./kg. (not to exceed 1 gm. per day), divided into 4 doses and administered by mouth every 6 hours (0.5 to 1 hour before meals) for about 5 days. Probably the daily dose in adults should not exceed 2 gm. (500 mg. every 6 hours), although higher doses have been used in cystinuria. These doses are 2 to 3 times larger than the doses usually employed in lead and mercury poisoning. See Section II for a summary of the clinical toxicity of D-penicillamine.
5. Counteract dehydration by intravenous fluids as needed and correct electrolyte deficiencies. See pp. IV-64–73.
6. Treat shock vigorously; use intravenous fluids, blood transfusions, oxygen, and pressor agents as necessary (pp. IV-18 and 17).
7. Morphine may be necessary to control abdominal pain, but do not use so extensively that colonic contents containing arsenic are retained.
8. If renal failure intervenes, hemodialysis may be essential to remove absorbed arsenic and its BAL-complex (pp. IV-55–57).

Laboratory:

1. Save the initial gastric washings and a urine specimen (100 ml.) for arsenic analysis.
2. Urine output is usually diminished. Albuminuria and hematuria may be prominent.
3. Liver function tests may reveal subclinical hepatic injury.
4. Arsenic trioxide and presumably other insoluble arsenic compounds may sometimes be detected as radiopaque materials in x-rays of the gastrointestinal tract (Hilfer and Mandel, 1962).
5. Blood levels above 1 ppm and urine levels above 0.4 ppm suggest exposures greater than that encountered by the general population. The same is true of concentrations above 1 or 2 ppm in hair (Hayes, 1982).

References:

Ayres, S., Jr.; Anderson, N. P. Cutaneous manifestations of arsenic poisoning. Arch. Dermatol. *30*:33-43, 1934.

Barron, E. S. G.; Miller, Z. B.; Bartlett, G. B.; Meyer, J. J.; Singer, T. P. Reactivation by dithiols of enzymes inhibited by Lewisite. Biochem. J. *41*:69-74, 1947.

Buchanan, W. D. *Toxicity of Arsenic Compounds.* Elsevier Publishing Co., New York, 1962.

Cannon, A. B. Chronic arsenical poisoning, symptoms and sources. N. Y. State J. Med. *36*:219-241, 1936.

Carleton, A. B.; Peters, R. A.; Thompson, R. H. S. The treatment of arsenical dermatitis with dimercaptopropanol (BAL). Q. J. Med. *17*:49-79, 1948.

Chainuvati, T.; Viranuvatti, V. Idiopathic portal hypertension and chronic arsenic poisoning. Report of a case. Am. J. Dig. Dis. *24*:70-73, 1979.

Coles, G. A.; Daley, D.; Davies, H. J.; Malick, N. P. Acute

intravascular hemolysis and renal failure due to arsine poisoning. Postgrad. Med. J. 45:170-172, 1964.

Committee on Medical and Biological Effects of Environmental Pollutants, Division of Medical Sciences, Assembly of Life Sciences, National Research Council. *Arsenic.* Medical and Biological Effects of Environmental Pollutants Series, National Academy of Sciences, Washington, D. C., 1977.

Crecelius, E. A. Changes in the chemical speciation of arsenic following ingestion by man. Environ. Health Perspect. 19:147-150,1977.

Currie, A. N. The role of arsenic in carcinogenesis. Br. Med. Bull. 4:402-405, 1947.

Done, A. K.; Peart, A. J. Acute toxicities of arsenical herbicides. Clin. Toxicol. 4:343-355, 1971.

Dreifuss, F. E.; Stewart, L. F.; Joseph, B.; Feibel, J. An epidemic of arsenic poisoning. Va. Med. Mon. 99:746-748, 1972.

Eagle, H.; Magnuson, H. J. The systemic treatment of 227 cases of arsenic poisoning (encephalitis, dermatitis, blood dyscrasias, jaundice, fever) with 2, 3-dimercaptopropanol (BAL). Am. J. Syphilis Neurol. 30:420-441, 1946.

Elkins, H. B.; Fahy, J. P. Arsine poisoning from aluminum tank cleaning. Ind. Med. Surg. 36:747-749, 1967.

Feldman, R. G.; Niles, C. A.; Kelly-Hayes, M.; Sax, D. S.; Dixon, W. J.; Thompson, D. J.; Landau, E. Peripheral neuropathy in arsenic smelter workers. Neurology 29:939-944, 1979.

Frank, G. Neurological and psychiatric disorders following acute arsine poisoning. J. Neurol. 213:59-70, 1976.

Franklin, M.; Bean, W. B.; Hardin, R. C. Fowler's solution as an etiologic agent in cirrhosis. Am. J. Med. Sci. 219:589-596, 1950.

Giberson, A.; Vaziri, N. D.; Mirahamadi, K.; Rosen, S. M. Hemodialysis of acute arsenic intoxication with transient renal failure. Arch. Intern. Med. 136:1303-1304, 1976.

Gillies, A. J. D.; Taylor, A. J. Acute arsenical poisoning in Dunedin. NZ Med. J. 89:379-381, 1979.

Greenberg, L. Diagnosis and treatment of occupational metal poisoning. J. A. M. A. 139:815-818, 1949.

Hanna, C.; McHugo, P. B. Studies on the capillary and cardiovascular actions of intravenous sodium arsenate and arsenite. Toxicol. Appl. Pharmacol. 2:674-682, 1960.

Hayes, W. J., Jr. *Pesticides Studied In Man.* Williams & Wilkins, Baltimore, Md, 1982.

Heyman, A.; Pfeiffer, J. B., Jr.; Willet, R. W.; Taylor, H. M. Peripheral neuropathy caused by arsenical intoxication. A study of 41 cases with observations on the effects of BAL (2, 3-dimercaptopropanol). N. Engl. J. Med. 254:401-409, 1956.

Hilfer, R. J.; Mandel, A. Acute arsenic intoxication diagnosed by roentgenograms. N. Engl. J. Med. 266:663-664, 1962.

Hocken, A. G.; Bradshaw, G. Arsine poisoning. Br. J. Ind. Med. 27:56-60, 1970.

Holland, R. H.; McCall, M. S.; Lanz, H. C. A study of inhaled arsenic-74 in man. Cancer Res. 19:1154-1156, 1959.

Holmquist, I. Occupational arsenical dermatitis. A study among employees at a copper ore smelting work including investigations of skin reactions to contact with arsenic compounds. Acta Derm. Venereol. 31(Suppl. 26), 1951.

Jackson, R.; Grainge, J. W. Arsenic and cancer. CMA J. 113:396-399, 1975.

Jenkins, G. C.; Ind, J. E.; Kazantzis, G.; Owen, R. Arsine poisoning: Massive haemolysis with minimal impairment of renal function. Br. Med. J. 2:78-80, 1965.

Jenkins, R. B. Inorganic arsenic and the nervous system. Brain 89:479-498, 1966.

Josephson, C. J.; Pinto, S. S.; Petronella, S. J. Arsine: Electrocardiographic changes produced in acute human poisoning. Arch. Ind. Hyg. Occup. Med. 4:43-52, 1951.

Kensler, C. J.; Abels, J. C.; Rhoads, C. P. Arsine poisoning, mode of action and treatment. J. Pharmacol. Exp. Ther. 88:99-108, 1946.

Kjeldsberg, C. R.; Ward, H. P. Leukemia in arsenic poisoning. Ann. Intern. Med. 77:935-937, 1972.

Kobayashi, A.; Ohbe, Y. Protein-losing enteropathy associated with arsenic poisoning. Am. J. Dis. Child. 121:515-517, 1971.

Kuruvilla, A.; Bergeson, P. S.; Done, A. K. Arsenic poisoning in childhood. Clin. Toxicol. 8:535-540, 1975.

Kyle, K. A.; Pease, G. L. Hematologic aspects of arsenic intoxication. N. Engl. J. Med. 273:18-23, 1965.

Lee, A. M.; Fraumeni, J. F. Arsenic and respiratory cancer in man: an occupational study. J. Natl. Cancer Inst. 42:1045-1052, 1969.

Levinsky, W. J.; Shalley, R. V.; Hillyer, P. N.; Shindler, R. L. Arsine hemolysis . Arch. Environ. Health 20:436-440, 1970.

Lugo, G.; Cassady, G.; Palmisano, P. Acute maternal arsenic intoxication with neonatal death. Am. J. Dis. Child. 117:328-330, 1969.

Mahieu, P.; Buchet, J. P.; Roels, H. A.; Lauwerys, R. The metabolism of arsenic in humans acutely intoxicated by As$_2$O$_3$. Its significance for the duration of BAL therapy. Clin. Toxicol. 18:1067-1075, 1981.

McKinstry, W. J.; Hickes, J. M. Emergency-arsenic poisoning. Arch. Intern. Med. 100:34-43, 1957.

Mees, R. A. Nails with arsenical polyneuritis. J. A. M. A. 72:1337, 1919.

Neuwirtova, R.; Chytil, M.; Valek, A.; Daum, S.; Valach, V. Acute renal failure following an occupational intoxication with arsine (AsH$_3$) treated by the artificial kidney. Acta Med. Scand. 170:535-546, 1961.

Nielson, B. Arsine poisoning in metal refining plant, fourteen simultaneous cases. Acta Med. Scand. 185:(Suppl. 496), 1969.

Parish, G. G.; Glass, R.; Kimbrough, R. Acute arsine poisoning in two workers cleaning a clogged drain. Arch. Environ. Health 34:224-227, 1979.

Peters, R. A.; Sinclair, H. M.; Thompson, R. H. S. An analysis of the inhibition of pyruvate oxidation by arsenicals in relation to the enzyme theory of vesication. Biochem. J. 40:516-524, 1946.

Peterson, R. G.; Rumack, B. H. D-Penicillamine therapy of acute arsenic poisoning. J. Pediatr. 91:661-666, 1977.

Petres, J.; Schmid-Ullrich, K.; Wolf, U. Chromosomenaberrationen an menschlichen Lymphozyten bei Chronischen Arsenschaden. Dtsch. Med. Wochenschr. 95:79-80, 1970.

Pinto, S. S.; Petronella, S. J.; Johns, D. R.; Arnold, M. F. Arsine poisoning, a study of thirteen cases. Arch. Ind. Hyg. Occup. Med. 1:437-451, 1950.

Prickman, L. E.; Millikan, H. Hemorrhagic encephalopathy during arsenic therapy for asthma. J. A. M. A. 152:1710-1713, 1953.

Schwartze, E. W. The so-called habituation to "arsenic". Variation in the toxicity of arsenious oxide. J. Pharmacol. Exp. Ther. 20:181-203, 1923.

Sollmann, T. *A Manual of Pharmacology.* 8th Ed., W. B. Saunders Co., Philadelphia, 1957.

St. Petery, J.; Gross, C.; Victoria, B. E. Ventricular fibrillation caused by arsenic poisoning. Am. J. Dis. Child. 120:367-371, 1970.

Stocken, L. A.; Thompson, R. H. S. Reactions of British Anti-Lewisite with arsenic and other metals in living systems. Physiol. Rev. 29:168-194, 1949.

Szuler, I. M.; Williams, N.; Hindmarsh, J. T.; Park-Dincsoy, H. Massive variceal hemorrhage secondary to presinusoidal portal hypertension due to arsenic poisoning. CMA J. 120:168-171, 1979.

Tay, C. -H.; Seah, C. -S. Arsenic poisoning from anti-asthmatic herbal preparations. Med. J. Aust. 2:424-428, 1975.

Teitelbaum, D. T.; Kies, L. C. Arsine poisoning. Arch. Environ. Health 19:133-143, 1969.

Uldall, P. R.; Khan, H. A.; Ennis, J. E.; McCallum, R. I.; Grimson, T. A. Renal damage from industrial arsine poisoning. Br. J. Ind. Med. 27:372-377, 1970.

Vallee, B. L.; Ulmer, D. D.; Wacker, W. E. C. Arsenic toxicology and biochemistry. Arch. Ind. Health 21:132-151, 1960.

Van Tongeren, J. H. M.; Kunst, A.; Majoor, C. L. H.; Schillings, P. H. M. Folic acid deficiency in chronic arsenic poisoning. Lancet 1:784-786, 1965.

Voegtlin, C.; Dyer, H. A.; Leonard, C. S. Mechanism of action of arsenic upon protoplasm. Public Health Repts. (U. S.) 38:1882-1912, 1923.

Voegtlin, C.; Dyer, H. A.; Leonard, C. S. Specificity of the so-called arsenic receptor in higher animals. J. Pharmacol. Exp. Ther. 25:297-307, 1925.

Wade, H. J.; Frazier, E. S. Toxipathic hepatitis due to Fowler's solution, a case treated with dimercaprol. Lancet 1:269-271, 1953.

Wang, B. C.; Mazzia, V. D. B. Arsenic poisoning as an anesthetic risk. N. Y. State J. Med. 69:2911-2912, 1969.

Webster, R. W. Legal Medicine and Toxicology. W. B. Saunders Co., Philadelphia, 1930.

Webster, S. H. Lead and arsenic ingestion and excretion in man. Public Health Repts. (U. S.) 56:1359-1368, 1941.

Westhoff, D. D.; Samaha, R. J.; Barnes, A., Jr. Arsenic intoxication as a cause of megaloblastic anemia. Blood 45:241-246, 1975.

Wills, R. A. Arsine gas poisoning - report of a case. Ind. Med. Surg. 17:208, 1948.

Woody, N. C.; Kometani, J. T. BAL in the treatment of arsenic ingestion of children. Pediatrics 1:372-378, 1948.

ATROPINE

Atropine (dl-hyoscyamine) is an alkaloid widely used in clinical medicine for its ability to block the effects of parasympathetic nerve stimulation. It is prepared by extraction of the powdered roots of Atropa belladonna, Datura stramonium, and other solanaceous plants (where it occurs naturally as the l-isomer). Active alkaloids related to atropine have been obtained from natural and synthetic sources. Indigenous plants are frequently responsible for cases of poisoning, particularly jimpson weed or D. stramonium (Arena, 1963; Blattner, 1962; Jennings, 1935; Rosen and Lechner, 1962; Schumacher, 1965). Similar syndromes are induced by ingestion of various parts of D. sanguinea, D. cornigera, D. aurea, D. sauveolens and D. rosei (Belton and Gibbons, 1979; Hall, 1977; Hudson, 1973).

Common over-the-counter sedative preparations may contain scopolamine in amounts of 0.15 to 0.5 mg./unit dose, but this ingredient seems to be included less commonly now than formerly. Many attempted suicides with these products demonstrate that atropine-like signs and symptoms are prominent in the intoxication syndrome (Beach et al., 1964; Bernstein and Leff, 1967; Thakkar and Lasser, 1972; Ullman and Groh, 1972). The Asthmador line of products (powders, cigarettes, etc.) contain mixtures of belladonna alkaloids. They are intended for burning with inhalation of the fumes by asthmatics, but they have been abused for their hallucinogenic effects. These materials, called "splugie," are also taken by mouth or as "teas" to increase the dose (Cummins et al., 1968; Dean, 1963; DiGiacomo, 1968; Gowdy, 1972; Teitelbaum, 1968). Abuse of atropine-like drugs by religious cults dates from the Middle Ages, and a recurrence of these practices has occurred among thrill-seeking adolescents in recent years (Shervette et al., 1979). As instruments for homicide, these alkaloids are seldom effective, since they produce obscure illnesses but only rarely cause death. Given surreptitiously, they have proved to be an effective means of immobilizing victims for robbery (Kaplan et al., 1974).

Toxicology: The use of massive doses of atropine in anticholinesterase poisoning (see p. III-339) and in the management of certain psychiatric states (Wada et al., 1960) has led to a realization that the margin of safety of this drug (and of related alkaloids) is much higher than formerly appreciated (Gordon and Frye, 1955). Although 10 mg. of atropine usually produce severe distress, many adult persons have recovered from single doses of 100 mg. and more. Recovery after the ingestion of 1000 mg. has been reported in an adult male (Alexander et al., 1946). Indeed, in the absence of predisposing disease, deaths from atropine poisoning are thought to be rare in adults, and the mean lethal dose is not known. Children are more susceptible than adults to this and related alkaloids (Unna et al., 1950), but young children are probably more tolerant than implied by the commonly stated lethal estimate of 10 mg. (Gold, 1949). Death followed 20 hours after the ingestion of 100 mg. by a 3-year-old (Legroux, 1962).

Neither the fatal dose nor the nature of the toxic syndrome is significantly determined by the route of administration. Severe symptoms have followed application to apparently intact skin (Doland, 1906). Poisoning from intranasal administration has resulted from confusing an ophthalmic solution with nose drops (Hoffman and Gay, 1959). Systemic intoxication from the conventional use of ophthalmic ointments and drops of atropine occurs with high frequency in both children and adults (Baker and Farley, 1958; Gamboa and Gamble, 1959; Heath, 1950; Hoefnagel, 1961). Such cases have led to the suggestion that atropine has no place in pediatric therapeutics (Joos, 1950).

Although many of the untoward signs and symptoms can be related to paralysis of the glands and smooth muscles innervated by the parasympathetic nervous system, the most dangerous and spectacular manifestations of poisoning arise from intense excitation of the central nervous system (Hoefnagel, 1961; Morton, 1939; Welbourne and Buxton, 1948). The combination of parasympathetic blockade and central stimulation can produce a clinical picture described in the following mnemonic: blind as a bat, dry as a bone, red as a beet, hot as a hare, and mad as a hatter.

The nervous syndrome has been confused with botulism (Eichner et al., 1967), schizophrenia (Ullman and Groh, 1972) and other affective disorders (Sportsman, 1946). A similar toxic syndrome has been induced by ANTIHISTA-MINICS, some of which have marked anticholinergic activity (p. III-37), and by tricyclic antidepressants (see IMIPRAMINE, p. III-207). Some patients have abused trihexyphenidyl and benztropine for similar psychotropic effects (Rubinstein, 1978).

Recovery from psychotic states is concomitant with return of peripheral parasympathetic function (Alexander et al., 1946). During the acute phase the EEG may show slow-wave activity and bizarre rhythmic bursts of high-voltage sharp-wave activity, which subside along with other signs (Mikolich et al., 1975). States of idiosyncrasy and hypersensitivity have also been described. One such case with induced psychotic behavior and unusual changes in T waves and ST segments of the ECG has been reported (Baker and Farley, 1958). Tachycardia is common because of the blockade of vagal influences; an increase in systolic blood pressure is presumably secondary to an increased cardiac output (Belton and Gibbons, 1979; Rumack, 1973; Shervette et al., 1979).

Convulsions, possible secondary to hyperpyrexia, are uncommon but have been observed (Hall, 1977). Status opisthotonus occurred in one infant recovering from surgery (Gillick, 1974), and hyperreflexia, bilateral dorsiflexor Babinski responses and decerebrate posturing have occurred in adults (Mikolich et al., 1975).

Studies with radiocarbon-labeled atropine have established marked differences between man and various laboratory animals in their capacities to metabolize this alkaloid. The amounts of intact atropine recovered in urine after its parenteral administration were as follows: 39% in rats, 25% in mice (Gosselin et al., 1955), one-third in dogs, about the same in kittens, somewhat less in guinea pigs (Kalser et al., 1957), and essentially none in many (but not all) rabbits. In contrast, each of two men who received 2 mg. of atropine by deep intramuscular injection excreted about 50% of the radioactive label in the form of unmodified atropine in a 24-hour urine specimen (Gosselin et al., 1960).

With the ^{14}C restricted to the α-carbon atom on the tropic acid portion of the molecule, 10 radioactive excretion products were detected in mouse and rat urine; the principal metabolites were glucuronide conjugates of hydroxyatropines formed in vivo by metabolic hydroxylation of the aromatic ring (Gabourel and Gosselin, 1958). Whereas glucuronides of atropine could not be detected in human urine by using a bacterial β-glucuronidase (Gosselin et al., 1960), bovine β-glucuronidase served to reveal substantial amounts of a labeled glucuronide in the urine of two humans given atropines labeled with ^{14}C in the tropine ring (Kalser and McLain, 1970). Like the rat, man appears to N-demethy-late atropine (Kalser and McLain, 1970). Like rats and mice but unlike guinea pigs and rabbits (Kalser et al., 1957; Godeaux and Tønnesen, 1949), man fails to hydrolyze the ester bond of atropine (Gosselin et al., 1960).

The presence of an atropinase in rabbit serum has led to the speculation that pooled rabbit sera may be of value in treating atropine poisoning in man. Preliminary studies by Shirkey et al. (1962) indicated that commercially available rabbit antipertussis serum was not so active as sterile rabbit plasma in hydrolyzing hyoscyamine and atropine in vitro. Clinical trials with antipertussis serum have given equivocal results. It is not yet clear to what degree anaphylaxis constitutes a hazard in such therapy, but heroic and potentially dangerous regimens of therapy are rarely if ever justified in atropine poisoning. Forced diuresis with urea led to the excretion of significant quantities of atropine in one poisoned adult and perhaps hastened his recovery (Groden and Williams, 1964).

Fairly extensive experience has accumulated in the use of physostigmine to reverse the signs and symptoms of muscarinic blockade. Physostigmine is probably more effective against the central nervous system effects of atropine-like drugs than against the peripheral manifestations (Temple and English, 1979). In some institutions it is common practice to give physostigmine to postoperative and obstetric patients to reverse either somnolence or delirium due to premedication with scopolamine (Holzgrafe et al., 1973; Smiler et al., 1973). It has also been recommended for similar syndromes induced by antihistaminics and by amitriptyline (Rumack, 1973; Ullman et al., 1970). Physostigmine has been given by the subcutaneous (Young et al., 1971), intramuscular (Caine, 1979) and intravenous (Rumack, 1973) routes. There has been rather limited experience in small children (Hudson, 1973; Rumack, 1973). In at least one infant, wheezing, hypersalivation, hyperperistalsis and bradycardia were interpreted as indicative of an overtitration with physostigmine, and glycopyrrolate was given to reverse the signs (Gillick, 1974).

Chronic atropine poisoning has evidently not been encountered as a clinical entity, but the parenteral administration of large doses (16 mg./kg. daily) for periods of 1 to 3 weeks produces in young puppies a syndrome clinically similar to advanced fibrocystic disease of the pancreas. The only points of dissimilarity between the two states were referable to inhibition of peripheral parasympathetic function in the atropinized animals (Boyd and Jarzylo, 1960). Again without clinical parallel is the observation that the parenteral administration of lethal doses of atropine to young rabbits produces two distinctly different types of death. About half the animals died promptly in a convulsive state perhaps comparable to the commonly encountered clinical syndrome of central excitement, but a smaller group suffered delayed deaths in about 2 weeks with endarteritis obliterans in the distal portions of the injected limbs (Boyd and Boyd, 1961).

Symptomatology:

1. Dryness of mucous membranes, burning pain in the throat, difficulty in swallowing, and intense thirst.
2. Dilatation of pupils, which become unreactive to light; blurred vision and photophobia.
3. The skin becomes hot, dry, and flushed. A scarlatiniform or maculopapular rash may appear over the face, neck, and upper trunk, especially in infants and children, and desquamation may follow.
4. Hyperpyrexia.
5. Sinus tachycardia, palpitations, elevated blood pressure.
6. Uncommonly nausea, vomiting, and (in infants) abdominal distension. Urinary urgency and hesitancy. Inability to void.
7. Restlessness, fatigue, excitement, and confusion, progressing to mania and delirium, which may persist for many hours and even several days. Hallucinations, particularly of the visual type. Patients must be watched carefully to prevent self-destructive acts.
8. True convulsions are rare, but seizure-like activity and decerebrate posturing may occur, as well as bilateral dorsiflexor Babinski responses.
9. In rare instances, coma, depression of medullary centers, circulatory collapse, and death from respiratory failure.

Treatment:

1. If any doubt exists as to the diagnosis of poisoning by atropine-like drugs, one may inject subcutaneously 10 to 30 mg. of methacholine. The failure to elicit the characteristic responses of perspiration, salivation, lacrimation and rhinorrhea serves as presumptive evidence for atropine-like intoxication (Dameshek and Feinsilver, 1937).
2. Gastric lavage with water, or empty the stomach by inducing emesis with syrup of ipecac (p. I-2) if it can be administered promptly after the toxic ingestion.
3. The most effective antagonist to the central nervous system manifestations is physostigmine salicylate in doses of 1 to 2 mg. by any parenteral route (Crowell and Ketchum, 1967; Duvoisin and Katz, 1968; Forrer and Miller, 1958; Ullman and Groh, 1972). For details of dosage, see p. III-210. Physostigmine treatment is not necessary

or desirable in mild poisonings. Avoid the phenothiazines, which potentiate anticholinergic effects, and avoid systemic pilocarpine because of its high toxicity. Caution is indicated in cases of obvious drug abuse where other psychoactive principles may have been consumed at the same time (Taylor et al., 1970).

4. Short-acting barbiturates administered cautiously may control excitement. Avoid large doses. Chloral hydrate, paraldehyde or diazepam (MacKenzie and Pigott, 1971) may be substituted for barbiturate drugs.
5. Artificial respiration and oxygen therapy in cases of respiratory depression (pp. IV-7–14).
6. Check for urinary retention and catheterize if necessary (p. IV-51). Bladder paralysis with retention is common even among young victims.
7. Antipyretic therapy—alcohol sponges (p. IV-84). Aspirin and other salicylates are probably best avoided.
8. A miotic drug (e.g., pilocarpine nitrate 0.5%) in the conjunctival sac may be used to counteract mydriasis. Because of photophobia, a darkened room may add to the patient's comfort.
9. In experimental atropine poisoning in some animal species, pronethalol reduces the mortality, apparently by reducing the tachycardia (Lendle et al., 1966). Except perhaps in elderly patients or those with preexisting heart disease, sinus tachycardia is not believed to be dangerous in man.

Laboratory:

1. A leukocytosis may be observed.
2. Elevations in serum glutamic-oxaloacetic transaminase and lactic dehydrogenase, together with an increase in prothrombin time, may be secondary to hyperthermia (Mikolich et al., 1975).

References:

Alexander, E., Jr.; Morris, D. P.; Eslick, R. L. Atropine poisoning. Report of a case with recovery after the ingestion of one gram. N. Engl. J. Med. 234:258-259, 1946.

Arena, J. M. Atropine poisoning. A report of two cases from Jimson weed. Clin. Pediatr. 2:182-184, 1963.

Baker, J. P.; Farley, J. D. Toxic psychosis following atropine eye drops. Br. Med. J. 2:1390-1392, 1958.

Beach, G. O.; Fitzgerald, R. P.; Holmes, R.; Phibbs, B.; Stockenhoff, H. Scopolamine poisoning. N. Engl. J. Med. 270:1354-1355, 1964.

Belton, P. A.; Gibbons, D. O. Datura intoxication in West Cornwall. Br. Med. J. 1:585-586, 1979.

Bernstein, S.; Leff, R. Toxic psychosis from sleeping medicines containing scopolamine. N. Engl. J. Med. 277:638-639, 1967.

Blattner, R. J. Jimson weed poisoning: Stramonium intoxication. J. Pediatr. 61:941-943, 1962.

Boyd, C. E.; Boyd, E. M. The acute toxicity of atropine sulfate. Can. Med. Assoc. J. 85:1241-1244, 1961.

Boyd, E. M.; Jarzylo, S. Chronic atropinization and fibrocystic disease of the pancreas. Can. Med. Assoc. J. 82:821-824, 1960.

Caine, E. L. Anticholinergic toxicity. N. Engl. J. Med. 300:1278, 1979.

Crowell, E. G.; Ketchum, J. S. The treatment of scopolamine-induced delirium with physostigmine. Clin. Pharmacol. Ther. 8:409-414, 1967.

Cummins, B. M.; Obetz, S. W.; Wilson, M. R. Belladonna poisoning as a facet of psychodelia. J. A. M. A. 204:1011, 1968.

Dameshek, W.; Feinsilver, O. Human autonomic pharmacology. XIV. Use of acetyl-beta-methyl choline (Mecholyl) as a diagnostic test for poisoning by the atropine series of drugs. J. A. M. A. 109:561-564, 1937.

Dean, E. S. Self-induced strammonium intoxication. J. A. M. A. 185:882, 1963.

DiGiacomo, J. N. Toxic effect of strammonium simulating LSD trip. J. A. M. A. 204:173-174, 1968.

Doland, C. M. Belladonna poisoning due to belladonna plasters. Am. J. Med. Sci. 131:623-625, 1906.

Duvoisin, R.; Katz, R. Reversal of central anticholinergic syndrome in man by physostigmine. J. A. M. A. 206:1963-1965, 1968.

Eichner, E. R.; Gunsolus, J. M.; Powers, T. F. "Belladonna" poisoning confused with botulism. J. A. M. A. 201:695-696, 1967.

Forrer, G. R.; Miller, J. J. Atropine coma: A somatic therapy in psychiatry. Am. J. Psychiatry 115:455-458, 1958.

Gabourel, J. D.; Gosselin, R. E. The mechanism of atropine detoxication in mice and rats. Arch. Int. Pharmacodyn. Ther. 115:416-432, 1958.

Gamboa, M. E.; Gamble, E. W., III. Atropine poisoning with psychosis. Am. J. Dis. Child. 97:342-344, 1959.

Gillick, J. S. Atropine toxicity in a neonate. Br. J. Anaesthesia 46:793-794, 1974.

Godeaux, J.; Tonnesen, M. Investigations into atropine metabolism in the animal organism. Acta Pharmacol. Toxicol. 5:95-109, 1949.

Gold, H. Conference on therapy. Household poisonings. Am. J. Med. 6:237-246, 1949.

Gordon, A. S.; Frye, C. W. Large doses of atropine, low toxicity and effectiveness in anticholinesterase intoxication. J. A. M. A. 159:1181-1184, 1955.

Gosselin, R. E.; Gabourel, J. D.; Kalser, S. C.; Wills, J. H. The metabolism of C14 labelled atropine and tropic acid in mice. J. Pharmacol. Exp. Ther. 115:217-229, 1955.

Gosselin, R. E.; Gabourel, J. D.; Wills, J. H. The fate of atropine in man. Clin. Pharmacol. Ther. 1:597-603, 1960.

Gowdy, J. M. Strammonium intoxication. J. A. M. A. 221:585-587, 1972.

Groden, B. M.; Williams, W. D. Atropine poisoning treated by forced diuresis. Postgrad. Med. J. 40:28-29, 1964.

Hall, R. C. W. Angel's trumpet psychosis: a central nervous system anticholinergic syndrome. Am. J. Psychiatry 134:312-314, 1977.

Heath, W. E. Death from atropine poisoning. Br. Med. J. 2:608, 1950.

Hoefnagel, D. Toxic effects of atropine and homatropine eye drops in children. N. Engl. J. Med. 264:168-171, 1961.

Hoffman, G. M.; Gay, J. R. Atropine in an unusual case of poisoning. Pa. Med. 62:1340-1341, 1959.

Holzgrafe, R. E.; Vondrell, J. J.; Mintz, S. M. Reversal of postoperative reactions to scopolamine with physostigmine. Anesth. Analg. 52:921-925, 1973.

Hudson, M. J. Acute atropine poisoning from ingestion of Datura rosei. N. Z. Med. J. 77:245-248, 1973.

Jennings, R. Strammonium poisoning: Review of literature and report of 2 cases. J. Pediatr. 6:657-664, 1935.

Joos, H. A. Atropine intoxication in infancy. Am. J. Dis. Child. 79:855-861, 1950.

Kalser, S. C.; McLain, P. L. Atropine metabolism in man. Clin. Pharmacol. Ther. 11:214-227, 1970.

Kalser, S. C.; Wills, J. H.; Gabrourel, J. D.; Gosselin, R. E.; Epes, C. F. Further studies of the excretion of atropine-alpha-C14. J. Pharmacol. Exp. Ther. 121:449-456, 1957.

Kaplan, M. M.; Register, D. C.; Bierman, A. H.; Risacher, R. L. A nonfatal case of intentional scopolamine poisoning. Clin. Toxicol. 7:509-512, 1974.

Legroux, R. A propos d'un cas d'intoxication mortelle par un collyre a l'atropine. Ann. Ocul. 195:48-52, 1962.

Lendle, L.; dal Ri, H.; Schmidt, G. Zur Verwendung von β-Rezeptorenhemmstoffen bei Atropinvergiftungen. Dtsch. Med. Wochenschr. 91:1299-1302, 1966.

MacKenzie, A. L.; Pigott, J. F. G. Atropine overdose in three children. Br. J. Anaesth. 43:1088-1090, 1971.

Mikolich, J. R.; Paulson, G. W.; Cross, C. J. Acute anticholinergic syndrome due to Jimson seed ingestion. Ann. Intern. Med. 83:321-325, 1975.

Morton, G. H. Atropine intoxication, its manifestations in infants and children. J. Pediatr. 14:755-760, 1939.

Rosen, C. S.; Lechner, M. Jimson-weed intoxication. N. Engl. J. Med. 267:448-450, 1962.

Rubinstein, J. S. Abuse of anticholinergic drugs. N. Engl. J. Med. 299:834, 1978.

Rumack, B. H. Anticholinergic poisoning: Treatment with physostigmine. Pediatrics 52:449-451, 1973.

Schumacher, M. A case of atropine alkaloid poisoning. Med. J. Aust. 1:547-548, 1965.

Shervette, R. E.; Schydlower, M.; Lampe, R. M.; Fearnow, R. G. Jimson loco weed abuse in adolescents. Pediatrics 63:520-523, 1979.

Shirkey, H. C.; Miller, R. G.; Hinkump, L.; Flamm, G. Animal sera and specific enzymes in the treatment of poisoning. J. Pediatr. 60:711-715, 1962.

Smiler, B. G.; Bartholomew, E. G.; Sivak, B. J.; Alexander, G. D.; Brown, E. M. Physostigmine reversal of scopolamine delirium in obstetric patients. Am. J. Obstet. Gynecol. 116:326-329, 1973.

Sportsman, L. M. Strammonium poisoning, a diagnostic problem with psychiatric implications. J. Pediatr. 29:345-349, 1946.

Taylor, R. L.; Maurer, J. I.; Tinklenberg, J. R. Management of "bad trips" in an evolving drug scene. J. A. M. A. 213:422-425, 1970.

Teitelbaum, D. T. Strammonium poisoning in "teeny-boppers". Ann. Intern. Med. 68:174-175, 1968.

Temple, A. R.; English, P. H. Treatment of methapyrilene toxicity with physostigmine. Vet. Human Toxicol. 21:84-86, 1979.

Thakker, M. K.; Lasser, R. P. Scopolamine intoxication from nonprescription sleeping pill. N. Y. State J. Med. 72:725-726, 1972.

Ullman, K.; Groh, R. Identification and treatment of acute psychotic states secondary to the usage of over-the-counter sleeping preparations. Am. J. Psychiatry 128:1244-1248, 1972.

Ullman, K. C.; Groh, R. H.; Wolf, F. W. Treatment of scopolamine-induced delirium. Lancet 1:252, 1970.

Unna, K. R.; Glaser, K.; Lipton, E.; Patterson, P. R. Dosage of drugs in infants and children. I. Atropine. Pediatrics 6:197-207, 1950.

Wada, T.; Horigome, S.; Sakurada, T. Clinical experience of the so called "Atropine toxicity therapy (Forrer)". Tohoku J. Exp. Med. 72:398-404, 1960.

Welbourne, R. B.; Buxton, J. D. Acute atropine poisoning. Review of eight cases. Lancet 2:211-213, 1948.

Young, S. E.; Ruiz, R. S.; Falletta, J. Reversal of systemic toxic effects of scopolamine with physostigmine salicylate. Am. J. Ophthal. 72:1136-1139, 1971.

BAL

BAL (2,3-dimercapto-1-propanol or dimercaprol) has been shown to be of value (often life-saving) in acute poisoning due to arsenicals of any type (except arsine) and soluble inorganic mercury compounds. It is also the drug of choice for the treatment of chronic arsenic or gold poisoning. Its value has been challenged in chronic mercurialism and in experimental poisoning by several organic mercury compounds, e.g., phenylmercuric acetate, methylmercuric chloride; in both of these situations central nervous system involvement predominates over the risk of acute renal failure (Berlin and Rylander, 1964; Berlin and Lewander, 1965); see also p. III-268 for a fuller discussion of BAL in mercury poisoning. Further clinical evaluation is necessary to prove its efficacy in poisoning from antimony, bismuth, copper, chromium, cobalt, nickel, and zinc. It appears to be ineffective against tellurium, thallium, and vanadium, and it may enhance the toxicity of uranium, iron, selenium, and cadmium (Braun et al., 1946; Edström, 1950; Lusky et al., 1949; Neuman and Allen, 1949; Woody and Kometani, 1948). Although BAL is valueless in the treatment of experimental lead poisoning in animals, it has been reported to be effective in the treatment of lead encephalopathy in children. See also LEAD, p. III-230–234.

BAL exerts its beneficial effect in heavy metal poisonings by displacing the metal from its combination with sulfhydryl groups of enzyme proteins and by forming a nontoxic metal-BAL complex which is excreted. A metal ion is more firmly bound by 2 molecules of BAL (2:1 chelate) than by 1 molecule (1:1 chelate), but because both types of union are reversible and the complex may dissociate, doses of BAL must be repeated for several days (Waters and Stock, 1945). The rapid metabolism of BAL also dictates frequent dosage over prolonged periods (Tamboline et al., 1955).

BAL is available commercially as a 10% preparation (w/v) in peanut oil, containing 20% benzyl benzoate; it is suitable for intramuscular injection only.

Toxicology: The administration of BAL in therapeutic doses may produce transient side effects. A dose of 8 mg./kg. will almost always cause untoward symptoms. Doses of 5 mg./kg. repeated every 3 hours for 24 hours usually produce no significant cumulative toxicity (Modell et al., 1946). Perhaps this is due to the rapid breakdown of BAL (Tamboline et al., 1955). The intraperitoneal LD_{50} in mice is 100 mg./kg., and death occurs in convulsions (Graham and Hood, 1948). Mortality in rats increases at ambient temperatures above and below 17° C. (McDonald, 1948).

The most consistent objective response to BAL in therapeutic doses is a rise in systolic and diastolic blood pressures, accompanied by tachycardia. This rise, which is roughly proportional to the dose, begins promptly and is usually complete within 2 hours (Sulzberger et al., 1946a, b). Children react like adults, except that a persist-

ent fever is frequently observed in children after the second or third injection. Large overdoses in children (e.g., 10, 25, and 40.5 mg./kg.) have caused convulsions and coma, from which recovery was prompt. There is evidence that BAL is less toxic in patients with heavy metal poisoning than in normal subjects (Gold, 1948a). In glucose-6-phosphate dehydrogenase deficient individuals, BAL is one of the many drugs that is apt to provoke hemolysis (Janakiraman et al., 1978).

All commercial samples of BAL are said to be contaminated with 1,2,3-trimercaptopropane (Zvirblis and Ellin, 1976), although concentrations were not specified. Trimercaptopropane is about 5 times more acutely toxic than BAL when injected in mice and rats. Moreover, injections of the isolated impurity were much more painful and produced more severe convulsions than pure BAL. Eventually such derivatives as 2,3-dimercaptopropane-1-sulfonate (Gabard and Walser, 1979) or N-(2,3-dimercaptopropyl)-phthalamidic acid (Yonaga and Morita, 1981) may prove to be superior to BAL in the treatment of metal poisoning.

Symptomatology (in approximate order of frequency) (Longcope and Luetscher, 1950):

1. Nausea and sometimes vomiting.
2. Headache.
3. Burning sensation of lips and mouth.
4. Feeling of constriction in throat, chest and hands.
5. Conjunctivitis, tearing, and salivation.
6. Tingling of hands.
7. Burning sensation in the penis.
8. Sweating of forehead and hands.
9. Abdominal pain.
10. Tremors.
11. Lower back pain.
12. Anxiety, weakness and restlessness may accompany any of these symptoms.
13. Objective signs often encountered include tachycardia and elevation of the arterial blood pressure.
14. Persistent fever is common in children.
15. Positive Chvostek and Trousseau signs occasionally.
16. Occasionally painful sterile abesses at injection sites.
17. Coma and convulsions at very high dose.

Treatment for BAL poisoning: Since reports indicate that the symptoms of BAL poisoning subside in 30 to 90 minutes, no emergency measures are usually required. To relieve unpleasant symptoms, however, some authorities advocate intramuscular use of a 1:1000 solution of epinephrine hydrochloride (0.1 to 0.5 ml.) or an oral dose of ephedrine sulfate (25 to 50 mg.). The latter may also be used prophylactically ½ hour before the injection of BAL. Antihistamine

Table III-2.
Recommended Dosage of BAL (Dimercaprol) in Metal Poisoning

	Arsenic or Gold Severe Poisoning	Arsenic or Gold Mild Poisoning	Mercury Poisoning
1st day	3.0 mg./kg. q4h (6 inj.)	2.5 mg./kg. q6h (4 inj.)	5.0 mg./kg. once 2.5 mg./kg. q8–12h
2nd day	3.0 mg./kg. q4h (6 inj.)	2.5 mg./kg. q6h (4 inj.)	2.5 mg./kg. q12–24h (1–2 inj.)
3rd day	3.0 mg./kg. q6h (4 inj.)	2.5 mg./kg. q12h (2 inj.)	2.5 mg./kg. q12–24h (1–2 inj.)
Each of the following 10 days or until recovery	3.0 mg./kg. q12h (2 inj.)	2.5 mg./kg. qd (1 inj.)	2.5 mg./kg. q12–24h (1–2 inj.)

drugs are said to provide symptomatic relief also.

Laboratory: A transient reduction in the polymorphonuclear leukocyte count is sometimes observed as a toxic effect of BAL.

Dosage schedule of BAL in heavy metal poisoning: The above schedule (Table III-2) incorporates the recommendations of the manufacturer (Hyson, Wescott and Dunning, Inc., Baltimore, Maryland), as approved by the FDA.

The dose schedules shown in Table III-2 have been used in both adults and children, and they are probably appropriate for infants as well. All doses are expressed as milligrams of BAL (*not* of solution), and all injections should be intramuscular. In cases of arsenical dermatitis, avoid injection through inflamed skin areas, as infection may be carried into deeper tissues.

For the dosage of BAL in conjunction with edetate calcium disodium against lead encephalopathy in children, see EDETATE CALCIUM DISODIUM (p. III-165).

References:

Berlin, M.; Lewander, T. Increased brain uptake of mercury caused by 2,3-dimercaptopropanol (BAL) in mice given mercuric chloride. Acta Pharmacol. Toxicol. 22:1-7, 1965.

Berlin, M.; Rylander, R. Increased brain uptake of mercury induced by 2, 3-dimercaptopropanol (BAL) in mice exposed to phenylmercuric acetate. J. Pharmacol. Exp. Ther. 146:236-240, 1964.

Braun, H. A.; Lusky, L. M.; Calvery, H. O. The efficacy of 2, 3-dimercaptopropanol (BAL) in the therapy of poisoning by compounds of antimony, bismuth, chromium, mercury and nickel. J. Pharmacol. Exp. Ther. (Suppl.)87:119-125, 1946.

Edstrom, G. The effects of 2,3-dimercaptopropanol (BAL) on gold reactions. Ann. Rheum. Dis. 9:109-115, 1950.

Gabard, B.; Walser, R. A note on the metabolism of the mercury chelating agent, sodium 2,3-dimercaptopropane-1-sulfonate. J. Toxicol. Environ. Health 5:759-764, 1979.

Gold, H. BAL (British Anti-Lewisite). Am. J. Med. 4:1-2, 1948a.

Graham, J. D. P, ; Hood, J. Actions of British anti-lewisite (2, 3-dimercaptopropanol). Br. J. Pharmacol. 3:84-90, 1948.

Janakiraman, N.; Seeler, R. A.; Royal, J. E.; Chen, M. F. Hemolysis during BAL chelation therapy for high blood lead levels in two G6PD deficient children. Clin. Pediatr. 17:485-487, 1978.

Longcope, W. T.; Luetscher, J. A., Jr. The treatment of acute mercury bichloride poisoning with BAL (2,3-dimercaptopropanol). Med. Clin. North Am. 34:469-484, 1950.

Lusky, L. M.; Braun, H. A.; Laug, E. P. The effect of BAL on experimental lead, tungsten, vanadium, uranium, copper and copper-arsenic poisoning. J. Ind. Hyg. Toxicol. 31:301-305, 1949.

McDonald, F. F. The effect of environmental temperature on the toxicity of BAL. Br. J. Pharmacol. 3:116-117, 1948.

Modell, W.; Gold, H.; Cattell, M. Clinical use of 2, 3-dimercaptopropanol (BAL). IV. Pharmacologic observations on BAL by intramuscular injection in man. J. Clin. Invest. 25:480-487, 1946.

Neuman, W. F.; Allen, R. P. The failure of 2,3-dithiopropanol (BAL) to affect acute systemic uranium poisoning. J. Pharmacol. Exp. Ther. 96:95-98, 1949.

Sulzberger, M. B.; Baer, R. L.; Kanof, A. Clinical uses of 2,3-dimercaptopropanol (BAL) III. Studies on the toxicity of BAL on percutaneous and parenteral administration. J. Clin. Invest. 25:474-479, 1946a.

Sulzberger, M. B.; Baer, R. L.; Kanof, A. Clinical uses of 2,3-dimercaptopropanol (BAL). V. Skin sensitization to BAL. J. Clin. Invest. 25:488-496, 1946b.

Tamboline, G.; Matheson, A. T.; Zbarsky, S. H. Radioactive compounds excreted by rats treated with S[35]-labelled British Anti-Lewisite. Preliminary studies. Biochem. J. 61:651-657, 1955.

Waters, L. L.; Stock, C. BAL (British Anti-Lewisite). Science 102:604-606, 1945.

Woody, N. C.; Kometani, J. T. BAL in the treatment of arsenic ingestion of children. Pediatrics 1:372-378, 1948.

Yonaga, R.; Morita, K. Comparison of the effect of N(2,3-dimercaptopropyl) phthalamidic acid DL-penicillamine, and dimercaprol on the excretion of tissue retention of mercury in mice. Toxicol. Appl. Pharmacol. 57:197-207, 1981.

Zvirblis, P.; Ellin, R. I. Acute systemic toxicity of pure dimercaprol and trimercaptopropane. Toxicol. Appl. Pharmacol. 36:297-300, 1976.

BARBITURATES

Many dialkyl and alkyl-aryl substituted malonylureas are employed in clinical medicine as sedative and hypnotic agents. The oldest of these barbiturates is the diethyl derivative, barbital, first introduced as a drug in 1903. Since then hundreds of derivatives have been synthesized and tested, and several dozen are in current clinical use. Some serve as potent anticonvulsants, others as intravenous anesthetic agents. Unsubstituted malonylurea (barbituric acid) is widely used by the chemical industry in the manufacture of plastics, etc. At one point the

annual consumption of barbiturates in the
United States exceeded 400 tons, and acute barbiturate intoxication accounted for about 1500
deaths annually.

With the introduction of the various benzodiazepines into clinical medicine (see DIAZE-
PAM, p. III-138) for many of the same therapeutic indications, the number of barbiturate
prescriptions written declined steadily throughout the 1970s. This decreasing legitimate use
was paralleled by a decreasing incidence of acute
poisonings both in the United States and abroad.
In most surveys, however, barbiturates still account for a high proportion of the successful
suicide attempts by drug ingestion, so that acute
overdoses continue to represent a serious medical problem (Johns, 1977; McGuire, 1976; Ninet
et al., 1981).

Chronic barbiturate intoxication is an important social and medical problem; together with
the treatment of the withdrawal syndrome, however, it is beyond the scope of this manual. The
interested reader is directed to the following
papers and reviews on barbiturate addiction and
chronic poisoning: Allgulander (1978), Fraser *et*
al. (1954), Isbell and Fraser (1950), Isbell *et al.*
(1950), Kornetsky (1951), Smith *et al.* (1970).
Acute barbiturate poisoning has also been reviewed extensively; for detailed information see
specialized treatises (*e.g.,* Loennecken, 1967;
Matthew, 1971a).

Toxicology: Derivatives of barbituric acid
differ from one another in latency of onset, duration of action, and metabolic fate. Differences
of potency are comparatively minor (2- to 3-
fold). In Table III-3, some of the popular drugs
are classified according to the duration of the

Table III-3.
Classification of Barbiturate Drugs

   A. *Long-acting:*
      Barbital (Veronal)
      Phenobarbital (Luminal)
      Mephobarbital (Mebaral)
      Diallylbarbituric acid (Dial)
   B. *Intermediate duration of action:*
      Amobarbital (Amytal)
      Aprobarbital (Alurate)
      Butabarbital (Butisol)
      Butethal (Neonal)
      Cyclobarbital (Phanodorn)
      Hexethal (Ortal)
      Vinbarbital (Delvinal)
   C. *Short-acting:*
      Pentobarbital (Nembutal)
      Secobarbital (Seconal)
   D. *Ultrashort-acting:*
      Hexobarbital sodium (Evipal)
      Thiamylal sodium (Surital)
      Thiopental sodium (Pentothal)

hypnosis which they induce. Speed of onset (latency) follows the same classes. Differences in
metabolic fate can be represented by similar
groupings. Specifically, short- and ultrashort-
acting barbiturates are almost exclusively detoxified *in vivo* (chiefly in the liver), whereas long-
acting congeners are largely excreted in the urine
as pharmacologically active molecules. Spontaneous recovery from poisoning depends ultimately on the liver in the first instance and on
the kidneys in the second. With drugs of intermediate durations of action, both detoxification
and excretion are generally important disposal
mechanisms.

Thiobarbiturates, like thiopental (Pentothal)
and thiamylal (Surital), differ from oxyderivatives in many respects; besides an ultrashort
duration of action, they are inactive by mouth
and can be administered only by the intravenous
or rectal routes. They are also extremely lipophilic, so much so that redistribution into body
fat is an important determinant of their duration
of action. Unlike most barbiturates, phenobarbital and mephobarbital (Mebaral) have specific
anticonvulsant properties. With the exceptions
noted above, the barbiturate drugs closely resemble one another.

Most acute barbiturate poisonings arise from
attempted suicide. Some poisonings arise in the
course of normal clinical practice and are due to
natural or acquired hypersensitivity. Although
the various derivatives differ somewhat in degree of toxicity, an oral dose of 1 gm. of most
barbiturates produces serious poisoning in an
adult, and death commonly occurs after 2 to 10
gm. The lethal dose of phenobarbital is believed
to be 5 gm., whereas barbital is considerably less
toxic. Lethal doses for pentobarbital, amobarbital and secobarbital are in the range of 3 gm.
(Berman *et al.,* 1956). Presumably the lethal
dose is smaller by parenteral routes of administration. It has long been felt that even mild liver
insufficiency enhances markedly the toxicity of
all common barbiturates except barbital and
phenobarbital, but careful clinical evaluation
has failed to substantiate this opinion with respect to pentobarbital (Sessions *et al.,* 1954).
Low doses of barbiturates may lead to deep
depression when the clinical status is complicated by shock, anoxia, additive effects of other
depressants, senility and possibly parkinsonism
(Wright, 1955). Long-acting barbiturates have
been responsible for most fatal poisonings, although in terms of lethal dose they are no more
toxic and may be less potent than shorter acting
derivatives. At least some authorities believe
that the short-acting drugs produce a deeper
coma and more complications than the long-
acting ones (Setter *et al.,* 1966).

Although sodium salts of rapidly acting congeners have produced death within 1 hour after

massive oral doses, most barbiturate deaths are delayed for several hours or several days. Fatalities have been reported on the 4th and 5th days, but the prognosis is usually favorable if the patient survives the first 24 or 36 hours. In a poisoning arising from the ingestion of a delayed disintegration preparation of secobarbital, the patient showed no evidence of depression during the first 9 hours after ingestion and yet was comatose 4 hours later (Michelson et al., 1954). In a limited study, poisoned patients were found to regain consciousness when the drug concentration in blood fell to 5 to 9 mg./100 ml. with long-acting barbiturates, 2 to 4 mg./100 ml. with drugs of intermediate action, and 1 to 2 mg./100 ml. with short-acting congeners (Broughton et al., 1956). The highest blood levels from which recoveries have ensued are 58 mg./100 ml. for phenobarbital, 68 mg./100 ml. for barbital and 16 mg./100 ml. for butethal and cyclobarbital (Kennedy et al., 1969; Raeburn et al., 1969).

An overdose of a barbiturate drug induces the classical picture of progressive central nervous depression. In its severest form this syndrome leads to respiratory arrest as a result of general reflex paralysis; in its milder forms, it may mimic any stage of clinical anesthesia (Eckenhoff and Dam, 1956). Except for a rapid (and weak) pulse, vital signs are characteristically reduced. In addition to direct inhibition of the cardiac contractile mechanism with consequent hypotension (see also below), circulatory insufficiency may be aggravated by hypoxia from inadequate pulmonary ventilation. Besides the well-known suppression of central respiratory drive, some evidence suggests that barbiturates also induce substantial impairment in the mechanical properties of the respiratory apparatus (Sybrecht et al., 1979). Early deaths are usually due to respiratory arrest, but delayed fatalities may arise from one or any combination of the following complications: hypostatic pneumonia, bronchopneumonia, lung abscess, pulmonary edema, cerebral edema, circulatory collapse, and irreversible renal shutdown (Plum and Swanson, 1957). The mortality rate in acute barbiturate poisoning lies between 1 and 10%.

Occasionally, a patient who survives severe and prolonged hypoxia during the acute phase may suffer residual neurological lesions, but recovery is usually complete. The world literature was said to contain examples of less than a score of patients who survived a barbiturate coma for 4 days or longer, and half of them acquired significant neurological deficits (Slager et al., 1966). Abnormal sleep patterns in survivors may require several months to resolve (Haider and Oswald, 1970).

Management of the poisoned patient: Some studies suggest that gastric lavage is of little value unless performed within 4 hours of ingestion (Matthew et al., 1966), but large amounts of barbiturates were recovered at autopsy from the gastric contents of two patients who died in coma 36 and 60 hours after hospital admission (Victor et al., 1968). In another case a mass resulting from the ingestion of 1000 tablets of phenobarbital (16 mg. each) was clearly visible in the stomach on routine x-ray of the chest. Over the ensuing 12 hours vigorous measures resulted in the removal of 200 intact tablets (Johanson, 1967). If gastric lavage is unproductive, a slurry of activated charcoal by mouth or by stomach tube may be worthwhile. Given 30 minutes after hypnotic doses of secobarbital, phenobarbital or glutethimide, activated charcoal resulted in plasma drug concentrations at least 50% lower in treated dogs than in untreated dogs, even when the charcoal was allowed to pass through the entire gastrointestinal tract; these reductions in hypnotic blood levels persisted for 24 hours (Fiser et al., 1971).

The only recognized treatment of barbiturate poisoning is supportive and symptomatic, with the highest priority going to the correction of anoxia. Any one or combination of the following measures may be necessary: the removal of airway obstruction, oxygen administration and artificial respiration. If anoxia can be minimized, the danger of cardiovascular collapse (below) is largely averted. In animal tests, however, hyperbaric oxygen was no more efficient than 100% oxygen at 1 atmosphere, and the former may carry some risk of compounding neurological complications (Meyerowitz, 1965).

Since the challenge to the former popularity of analeptic drug therapy by Scandinavian and other investigators (Böttiger and Ostman, 1959; Clemmesen and Nilsson, 1961; Dobos et al., 1961; Eckenhoff and Dam, 1956; Ferguson and Grace, 1961; Nilsson, 1951), this potential adjunct to the correction of anoxia has been virtually abandoned. There may, however, be a legitimate role for analeptic drugs in situations where intensive hospital care is unavailable or where the vital signs cannot be monitored continuously. If so, the milder agents caffeine and nikethamide are probably preferable to the convulsant drugs picrotoxin and pentylenetetrazol. Although the rationale is unknown, some but not all barbiturate-poisoned patients seemed to respond to physostigmine by a dramatic decrease in the depth of coma. Physostigmine has been recommended for coma due to drugs with anticholinergic activity. Perhaps its injection may become a useful diagnostic procedure because patients poisoned with anticholinergics responded by a decrease in mean arterial pressure and heart rate with no change in pupil size, whereas patients in coma due to barbiturates or benzodiazepines responded with an increase in mean arterial pressure, heart rate and pupil size (Nattel et al., 1979).

A major threat to the survival of anyone in

barbiturate coma is circulatory shock, evidenced by severe arterial hypotension and cyanosis, developing gradually or precipitously. Indeed, the systolic blood pressure is the best single prognosticator of survival in barbiturate poisoning (Afifi *et al.*, 1971). The pathophysiology of this form of circulatory collapse has been studied intensively. In intoxications due to barbiturates and perhaps other central depressant drugs, hypotension is accompanied by a normal or high peripheral vascular resistance (Shubin and Weil, 1965), indicating that the vasomotor center, sympathetic vasoconstrictor nerves and arteriolar smooth muscle are not paralyzed. Accordingly, treatment with a drug that constricts primarily arterioles, such as methoxamine, is neither rational nor effective in raising the blood pressure.

Sometimes infusions of epinephrine or norepinephrine are helpful, but the benefits if any are probably due to cardiac stimulation, not vasoconstriction (Hulting and Thorstand, 1972). Barbiturates depress the contractile mechanism of the heart and reduce the cardiac output (Bevegard and Thorstrand, 1972; Shubin and Weil, 1965). Arrhythmias and other disorders in the mechanism of the heart beat may contribute to the poor cardiac output, but they can usually be prevented by assuring adequate oxygenation (Shubin and Weil, 1971) and correcting hypothermia (Linton and Ledingham, 1966). The negative inotropic effect of the drug, however, tends to persist.

In most barbiturate-poisoned patients, however, circulatory collapse is not primarily cardiogenic, as evidenced by normal or low pressures in the pulmonary artery and great veins (Hulting and Thorstrand, 1972; Shubin and Weil, 1965). Any elevation of the central venous pressure is a bad prognostic sign (Afifi *et al.*, 1971). Severe hypotension in barbiturate poisoning is usually an expression of oligemic shock (see p. IV-17). Hypovolemia may be either relative or absolute. Relative hypovolemia arises from paralytic venodilatation, which causes the volume of these capacitance vessels to increase markedly. A normal blood volume is then insufficient to fill the venous channels or to sustain an adequate venous pressure and venous return (Shubin and Weil, 1965). Venodilatation is not dependably corrected by drugs. Absolute hypovolemia in barbiturate poisoning arises from a loss in blood volume due to excessive extravasation of plasma into tissues. The mechanism is unknown, but capillary hyperpermeability has been inferred (Frick *et al.*, 1962) because hemoglobin levels were found to be high in circulating blood whereas plasma protein levels were normal.

Relative and absolute hypovolemia demand parenteral fluid therapy, specifically intravenous infusions of plasma or serum albumin and of isotonic saline. Fluid administration without vasoconstrictor drugs is usually adequate to correct severe hypotension in barbiturate poisoning (Arieff and Friedman, 1973). With other depressants, vasoconstrictors may also be required. Fluid, however, must be infused slowly to avoid precipitating pulmonary edema by overloading the hypodynamic heart.

Severe hypothermia in neglected cases of barbiturate poisoning may induce ventricular fibrillation and cardiac arrest. Hypothermia alone induces ECG changes, but an elevated ST segment localized to the inferior limb leads may be specific for barbiturate intoxication (Edwards and Epps, 1978). Recovery has occurred after body temperatures as low as 70° F., but extreme measures of therapy have been required. In two cases fibrillation was arrested only after thoracotomy followed by rewarming of the mediastinum directly (Linton and Ledingham, 1966) or indirectly via a cardiopulmonary bypass (Fell *et al.*, 1968). A less drastic rewarming procedure was employed successfully by Lash *et al.* (1967), who heated dialysis fluid to 98.6° F. before placing it in the peritoneal cavity.

Conversely, cooling dialysis fluids may be helpful in the rare cases of hyperpyrexia secondary to barbiturate intoxication. In connection with this paradoxical febrile reaction, it is of interest that barbiturate hypnosis has been potentiated in animals by agents that uncoupled oxidative phosphorylation, such as dinitrophenol, chlortetracycline and 2,4-D (Killam *et al.*, 1958). Sweat gland necrosis and other skin lesions may play a role in body temperature variations in barbiturate poisoning (Leavell, 1969). The oxyderivatives (phenobarbital, amobarbital, hexobarbital) inhibit but do not uncouple oxidative phosphorylation, whereas the thiobarbiturates both inhibit and uncouple (Aldridge and Parker, 1960). One might predict, therefore, that fever would be more common with the latter.

Hastening barbiturate elimination: The lack of effective antidotes has inspired considerable research on ways to hasten the elimination of barbiturates from the body. Attention has focused on forced diuresis, alkalinization of the urine, peritoneal dialysis, extracorporeal hemodialysis, hemoperfusion and various combinations of these procedures. It is sometimes difficult to compare these various maneuvers (Gosselin and Smith, 1966), but some generalities can be cited.

The therapeutic and toxic actions of barbiturates are normally terminated by metabolic inactivation and by renal excretion. For most agents listed in Table III-3, metabolism is the more rapid process, but the converse is true of barbital (Lous, 1954a). Nevertheless, urinary excretion plays a significant role in removing several barbiturates. For example, the fraction of an oral overdose ultimately recovered unchanged in the urine of untreated subjects is 35 to 70% for barbital, 35 to 70% for aprobarbital, 25 to 30% for diallylbarbituric acid and 14 to 27% for phenobarbital (Lous, 1954a, b). With the possible exception of cyclobarbital (Linton *et al.*, 1967), renal excretion is believed to be considerably less important with other barbiturates, especially the short-acting ones (Table III-3); it is entirely negligible with the ultrashort-acting derivatives. Even with those drugs extensively eliminated in urine, excretory rates tend to be inherently slow. For example, the unassisted kidneys require several days to remove half the body burden of barbital (Lous, 1954a). Attempts to speed the excretory process have attracted much attention.

Ohlsson first reported in 1949 (Ohlsson and Fristedt, 1962) that several barbiturates can be recovered in the urine of poisoned patients much faster if a brisk diuresis is produced by intensive parenteral fluid therapy ("blood lavage"). For long-acting barbiturates and for at least some congeners of intermediate duration (Table III-3), renal clearances increase significantly with increasing rates of urine flow. The relationship has been described as linear (Bunn and Lubash, 1965; Linton *et al.*, 1967), but the expected trend toward a plateau at high urine volumes has also been observed (Lous, 1954a). To achieve high urine flows while minimizing the risk of overhydration and cardiac decompensation, "blood lavage" was superseded by diuretic drug regimens in which parenteral fluid administration was limited to amounts required to correct any preexisting hypovolemia (see above) and to replace continuously urinary losses of water and electrolytes (Lassen, 1960; Myschetzky and Lassen, 1963; Strickler, 1965).

Many diuretic drugs appear to have been used successfully. When compared at the same rates of urine flow, furosemide, chlorothiazide and mannitol were equally effective in accelerating excretion of phenobarbital and butethal in poisoned patients (Linton *et al.*, 1967). Most clinical experience, however, has concerned osmotic agents, primarily mannitol (Cirksena *et al.*, 1964) but also tromethamine (tris, THAM) and urea (Balagot *et al.*, 1961; Myschetzky and Lassen, 1963). The amine buffer tris has not become popular, even though it may have a special advantage in the presence of systemic acidosis. The chief hazard of administering large volumes of fluid with or without osmotic diuretics is iatrogenic pulmonary edema (Morgan *et al.*, 1968). To avoid overrepletion or underrepletion during intensive fluid therapy, the therapist should monitor input and output volumes, the composition of the blood and the central venous pressure (Shubin and Weil, 1971).

Alkalinization of the urine is often used in conjunction with forced diuresis. Because bar-

biturates are weak acids, advantage can be taken of the principles of nonionic diffusion to maximize their urinary excretion. Both from theoretical considerations and a large body of practical experience, the benefits of raising the urinary pH above 7.5 are more pronounced with barbiturates of low pK_a (*e.g.*, phenobarbital at 7.2) than those of higher pK_a (*e.g.*, pentobarbital and secobarbital at 7.9 to 8.0). Thus alkalinization of the urine with or without diuresis has been disappointing in the case of the short-acting drugs (Bloomer, 1965, 1966; Hawer and Lee, 1968). It does, however, produce an appreciable increase in phenobarbital clearance, which is independent of and additive to the increase in clearance due to diuresis alone (Bloomer, 1966; Hawer and Lee, 1968; Henderson and Merrill, 1966; Linton *et al.*, 1967). One potentially fatal case of phenobarbital ingestion was successfully managed by forced alkaline diuresis with dopamine. Only after the patient regained consciousness and apparently began inappropriate antidiuretic hormone secretion was a conventional diuretic required (Costello and Poklis, 1981).

Peritoneal dialysis has also been explored intensively in barbiturate poisoning, but in practice barbiturate clearances by ordinary peritoneal dialysis are similar to those obtained by forced diuresis (Bloomer, 1965; Setter *et al.*, 1966). Again, attempts have been made to exploit the principles of nonionic diffusion. In experiments on dogs a dialysis fluid containing TRIS buffer at pH 10 sustained faster peritoneal clearances of secobarbital and phenobarbital than did ordinary dialysis fluid at a pH of 5 (Knochel *et al.*, 1964, 1965). In both cases, however, only a disappointingly small fraction (less than 5%) of the total dose was removed.

Alternatively, a ligand such as albumin can be added to the dialysis fluid to trap barbiturate and prevent back-diffusion. In four human poisonings with pentobarbital, secobarbital or phenobarbital, the inclusion of 5% human serum albumin in the dialysis fluid doubled the rate of barbiturate removal (Berman and Vogelsang, 1964). This effect depends of course on the extent to which any barbiturate is protein-bound. Binding characteristics of human serum albumin for secobarbital, amobarbital and phenobarbital have been measured (Campion and North, 1965). As judged by experiments in dogs, the protein-binding effect (4 gm. albumin/100 ml. dialysis fluid) was independent of and greater in magnitude than that of a pH change from 5.3 to 7.3. The two-unit pH change increased peritoneal clearances 10 to 15%, whereas the combined pH change and protein binding increased the clearance of phenobarbital by 25% and the clearances of secobarbital and amobarbital by 55 to 60% (Campion and North, 1965).

In terms of speed of elimination, none of the

above modifications alone or in combination is so effective as extracorporeal hemodialysis (Berman *et al.*, 1956; Honey and Jackson, 1959; Kyle *et al.*, 1953; Setter *et al.*, 1966; Walsh *et al.*, 1952). Hemodialysis has been employed successfully in infants under 1 year of age (Fine *et al.*, 1968) and for prolonged periods of time, *i.e.*, 68 of 80 consecutive hours (Hudson *et al.*, 1969). It has been used together with forced diuresis, alkalinization and peritoneal dialysis in various combinations (Kennedy *et al.*, 1969; Lee and Ames, 1965; Linton *et al.*, 1964). The complications of hemodialysis and the fact that it was usually reserved for moribund patients may have been responsible for a higher mortality rate than in more conservative programs of management (Henderson and Merrill, 1966). Dialysis was judged helpful in deep comas due to phenobarbital and barbital and perhaps in cases involving other barbiturates when the plasma level was above 10 mg./100 ml. (Balme *et al.*, 1962); probably most therapists today would not require such high levels.

In addition to machines for extracorporeal hemodialysis, considerable interest has been generated in extracorporeal devices for hemoperfusion. In these devices, shunted blood is allowed to come into intimate contact with a bed of adsorbent material, such as activated charcoal, an anion exchange resin or an uncharged resin which has a selective affinity for high-molecular-weight, lipid-soluble substances (Nealon *et al.*, 1966; Rosenbaum *et al.*, 1971). In many patients with life-threatening intoxications by barbiturates having various durations of action, plasma clearances by hemoperfusion were higher than published values by hemodialysis (Hennemann *et al.*, 1976; Iversen *et al.*, 1979; Rosenbaum *et al.*, 1976, 1980). Perhaps the highest barbital clearances are those achieved with columns of the uncharged resin Amberlite XAD-4 (Trafford *et al.*, 1980). All these devices produce some fall in blood platelet counts. The decrease in platelet counts was often transient and considered acceptable (Keusch-Beck *et al.*, 1980; Winchester *et al.*, 1978). See Section IV (pp. 57–58) for a more detailed discussion of this technique.

In summary, opinions vary widely about the proper roles of forced diuresis, peritoneal dialysis, hemodialysis and hemoperfusion in barbiturate poisoning. Forced diuresis is probably the least complicated procedure; it is generally safe and unquestionably effective in removing significant amounts of barbital and other long-acting derivatives (Table III-3). Only with phenobarbital is alkalinization of the urine also useful. Forced diuresis has been employed with apparent success in poisonings by several barbiturates with intermediate duration of actions, notably aprobarbital (Myschetzky and Lassen,

1963), butethal (Hawer and Lee, 1968) and cyclobarbital (Linton *et al.*, 1967). With short-acting congeners, however, forced diuresis is probably not worthwhile. Although it does elevate the renal clearances of pentobarbital and secobarbital (Bloomer, 1966; Linton *et al.*, 1967), the gains are small. For example, in one patient the rate of pentobarbital excretion during peak diuresis with mannitol was only 20% of the rate of metabolic inactivation (Bloomer, 1965). The results of peritoneal dialysis are similar to those of diuretic therapy. Although peritoneal clearances may be somewhat higher than renal clearances during forced diuresis (Setter *et al.*, 1966), neither procedure is judged to be useful in secobarbital or pentobarbital poisoning (Bloomer, 1965) and probably not with amobarbital (Hadden *et al.*, 1969). In one series of 50 patients in deep barbiturate coma, mostly from short-acting agents, a regimen of supportive care alone gave results that were not significantly different from those obtained with either forced diuresis or peritoneal dialysis (Hadden *et al.*, 1969). Extracorporeal hemodialysis is reserved for the most seriously ill patients; the procedure can benefit victims both of long-acting and short-acting barbiturates (Lee and Ames, 1965).

Hemoperfusion now has many vigorous proponents. It may prove to be a more useful measure in chemical toxicology than hemodialysis. Probably hemoperfusion has been used in barbiturate poisoning more often than in any other kind of intoxication. The most dramatic clinical improvement is said to be that observed in patients with phenobarbital overdoses (Koffler *et al.*, 1978). The procedure, however, should probably be reserved for patients in profound coma requiring cardiac or respiratory support, in whom the plasma drug level exceeds 50 mg./L. in the case of short- and intermediate-acting barbiturates or 80 to 100 mg./L. in the case of phenobarbital or barbital (Trafford *et al.*, 1980).

Symptomatology (based in part on the classification of Reed *et al.*, 1952):

1. Drowsiness is usually the first symptom. A transient period of confusion, excitement, delirium, and perhaps hallucinations is not uncommon.
2. Ataxia, vertigo, slurred speech, headache, paresthesias, and subjective visual disturbances.
3. A stupor progressing through deepening states of coma, with inhibition or absence of superficial and deep reflexes. Responses to painful stimuli gradually cease. The Babinski toe sign may become positive.
4. Respirations may be rapid and shallow or slow and labored, but the minute volume (pulmonary ventilation) is always reduced.

5. Mild but progressive cardiovascular collapse, evidenced by cyanosis, hypotension, a weak rapid pulse, and cold and clammy skin. Circulatory insufficiency may or may not be the result of hypoxia from respiratory depression. Transient electrocardiographic changes may be seen (Kirkegaard and Nörregaard, 1951).
6. The pupils are usually slightly constricted but react to light; they may dilate during terminal asphyxia.
7. Urine formation is slowed or suppressed completely.
8. The body temperature is usually reduced. If a fever develops, it usually signals bronchopneumonia, but paradoxical hyperpyrexia is recognized as a rare complication.
9. Respirations become irregular, sometimes Cheyne-Stokes in character, and eventually cease.
10. Although death is usually due to respiratory arrest, circulatory shock may be the proximal cause. Occasionally severe grades of pulmonary edema are encountered (especially in poisonings with ultrashort-acting barbiturates). Hypostatic or aspiration pneumonia late in the course of the illness may prove lethal. Renal shutdown due to circulatory collapse can complicate the illness but is rarely irreversible.
11. Among survivors, residual damage is rare, but occasionally a patient who has suffered prolonged and severe hypoxia during the acute phase may exhibit permanent neurological damage.
12. Irregular erythematous cutaneous lesions and bullae containing a clear fluid are seen in many patients.
13. Sometimes barbiturate poisoning is due to or complicated by natural or acquired idiosyncrasy. Allergic reactions from acquired hypersensitivity are of the usual types: asthma, urticaria, angioneurotic edema, dermatitis, fever, delirium, liver necrosis. Natural idiosyncrasy commonly expresses itself as an excitement reaction, a prolonged hangover, and a pain syndrome. The latter consists of paroxysms of localized or diffuse pain of a myalgic, neuralgic, or arthralgic character.

Treatment:
1. If the patient is awake and loss of consciousness is not imminent, give by mouth syrup of ipecac (p. I-2) or a slurry of activated charcoal (p. I-4).
2. Gastric lavage with warm water or saline as soon as practical. Especially if the patient is comatose, precautions against aspiration are essential (p. I-8).
3. Leave in the stomach 15 to 30 gm. of sodium sulfate in water as a saline cathartic.
4. If sensory stimuli (*e.g.*, pinching) arouse the patient even briefly from his coma and if his respirations are full and regular, further treatment may not be required, but he should be kept under observation until fully conscious.
5. Monitor (continuously if possible) the ECG and the following vital signs: respiratory rate, pulse rate, blood pressure and body temperature. Observe frequently and record the skin color, pupillary size and light reflex, corneal and gag reflexes, response to pain, and tendon reflexes.
6. Correct airway obstruction. The insertion of an oropharyngeal airway is usually advisable in a comatose patient who has no gag reflex. Suction frequently to remove saliva and mucus. See p. IV-4.
7. At the slightest suspicion of hypoxia, continuous or intermittent oxygen therapy is warranted (p. IV-12).
8. Sometimes the inhalation of oxygen causes an arrest of spontaneous breathing. Artificial respiration is then essential. Do not wait for respiratory arrest; give mechanical assistance whenever the rate or depth of breathing is clearly inadequate. See pp. IV-7–12.
9. The threat of cardiovascular collapse often disappears when hypoxia is corrected. If not, an infusion of plasma or of human serum albumin is useful to expand the blood volume and raise the blood pressure. Vasoconstrictor drugs are generally not helpful. A rapidly acting cardiac glycoside (*e.g.*, ouabain) is recommended only if the central venous pressure is elevated.
10. Correct dehydration by the cautious administration of replacement fluids. In the treatment of barbital and phenobarbital poisoning, diuretic drugs have a legitimate role (see above), but diuresis is not beneficial in pentobarbital or secobarbital poisoning. Except in phenobarbital poisoning, alkalinization of the urine does not speed excretion significantly. Perhaps the urinary bladder should be catheterized to prevent retention. Measure and record urine output.
11. In the rare patient with signs of elevated intracranial pressure (Mousel, 1953), treat brain edema as outlined on pp. IV-43–46.
12. In severe poisonings hemodialysis or hemoperfusion, by speeding the removal of the drug, may prove life-saving in that the duration of coma is shortened and so lethal complications are prevented. These

measures are normally reserved for massive poisonings by those barbiturates that are only slowly detoxified (*e.g.,* barbital, phenobarbital), but they may be helpful with short-acting agents, if begun promptly. See criteria in text above. See also pp. IV-55–58.

13. Good nursing is essential (p. IV-105). The normal body temperature should be maintained if possible. Antibiotic therapy is necessary if pneumonia or other infections arise. By repeatedly changing the patient's posture, hypostatic pneumonia, thrombophlebitis and decubitis ulcers are avoided. See pp. IV-83–84.

Laboratory:

1. Qualitative and quantitative analyses for barbiturates are desirable in the management of severe poisonings (Wright, 1955). Measurements of the plasma level are widely available.

2. Periodic analyses of blood gases and blood electrolytes are helpful. The latter data are essential to manage forced diuresis.

3. Electroencephalographic recordings may be useful in prognosis (Cohn *et al.,* 1950; Edwards and Epps, 1978).

4. Activity patterns of serum glutamic oxaloacetic and pyruvic transaminases, lactic dehydrogenase, and maleic dehydrogenase similar to those seen in acute hepatitis have been reported. Muscle necrosis is suggested as the cause (Fahlgren *et al.,* 1958).

References:

Afifi, A. A.; Sacks, S. T.; Liu, V. Y.; Weil, M. H.; Shubin, H. Accumulative prognostic index for patients with barbiturate, glutethimide and meprobamate intoxication. N. Engl. J. Med. *285*:1447-1502, 1971.

Aldridge, W. N.; Parker, V. H. Barbiturates and oxidative phosphorylation. Biochem. J. *76*:47-56, 1960.

Allgulander, C. Dependence on sedative and hypnotic drugs. Acta Psychiatr. Scand., Suppl. *270*:1-120, 1978.

Arieff, A. I.; Friedman, E. A. Coma following nonnarcotic drug overdosage. Management of 208 adult patients. Am. J. Med. Sci. *266*:405-426, 1973.

Balagot, R. C.; Tsuji, H.; Sadove, M. S. Use of an osmotic diuretic - THAM - in treatment of barbiturate poisoning. J. A. M. A. *178*:1000-1004, 1961.

Balme, R. H.; Lloyd-Thomas, H. G.; Shead, G. V. Severe barbitone poisoning treated by haemodialysis. Br. Med. J. *1*:231-232, 1962.

Berman, L. B.; Jeghers, H. J.; Schreiner, G. E.; Pallotta, A. J. Hemodialysis, an effective therapy for acute barbiturate poisoning. J. A. M. A. *161*:820-827, 1956.

Berman, L. B.; Vogelsang, P. Removal rates for barbiturates using two types of peritoneal dialysis. N. Engl. J. Med. *270*:77-80, 1964.

Bevegard, S.; Thorstand, C. Central hemodynamics in severe poisoning by hypnotic drugs. Acta Med. Scand. *191*:325-331, 1972.

Bloomer, H. A. Limited usefulness of alkaline diuresis and peritoneal dialysis in phenobarbital intoxication. N. Engl. J. Med. *272*:1309-1313, 1965.

Bloomer, H. A. A critical evaluation of diuresis on the treatment of barbiturate intoxication. J. Lab. Clin. Med. *67*:898-905, 1966.

Bottiger, L. E.; Ostman, J. On the treatment of barbiturate intoxication with a survey of 311 cases. Acta Med. Scand. *165*:437-444, 1959.

Broughton, P. M. G.; Higgins, G.; O'Brien, J. R. P. Acute barbiturate poisoning. Lancet *1*:180-184, 1956.

Bunn, H. G.; Lubash, G. D. A controlled study of induced diuresis in barbiturate intoxication. Ann. Intern. Med. *62*:246-251, 1965.

Campion, D. S.; North, J. D. K. Effect of protein binding of barbiturates on their rate of removal during peritoneal dialysis. J. Lab. Clin. Med. *66*:549-563, 1965.

Cirksena, W. J.; Bastian, R. C.; Malloy, J. P.; Barry, K. G. Use of mannitol in exogenous and endogenous intoxications. N. Engl. J. Med. *270*:161-166, 1964.

Clemmesen, C.; Nilsson, E. Therapeutic trends in the treatment of barbiturate poisoning. Clin. Pharmacol. Ther. *2*:220-229, 1961.

Cohn, R.; Savage, C.; Raines, G. N. Barbiturate intoxication. A clinical electroencephalographic study. Ann. Intern. Med. *32*:1049-1065, 1950.

Costello, J. B.; Poklis, A. Treatment of massive phenobarbital overdose with dopamine diuresis. Arch. Intern. Med. *141*:938-940, 1981.

Dobos, J. K.; Phillips, J.; Covo, F. A. Acute barbiturate intoxication. J. A. M. A. *176*:268-272, 1961.

Eckenhoff, J. E.; Dam, W. The treatment of barbiturate poisoning with or without analeptics. Am. J. Med. *20*:912-918, 1956.

Edwards, R. C.; Epps, R. G. Electrocardiographic changes associated with hypothermia due to acute barbiturate intoxication. Aust. N. Z. J. Med. *8*:86-88, 1978.

Fahlgren, H.; Hed, R.; Ordell, R. Studies on serum transaminase activity in barbiturate intoxication. Acta Med. Scand. *160*:215-219, 1958.

Fell, R. H.; Gunning, A. J.; Bardhan, K. D.; Triger, D. R. Severe hypothermia as a result of barbiturate overdose complicated by cardiac arrest. Lancet *1*:392-394, 1968.

Ferguson, M. J.; Grace, W. J. The conservative management of barbiturate intoxication. Experience with 96 unconscious patients. Ann. Intern. Med. *54*:726-733, 1961.

Fine, R. N.; Stiles, Q.; DePalma, J. R.; Donnell, G. N. Hemodialysis in infants under 1 year of age for acute poisoning. Am. J. Dis. Child. *116*:657-661, 1968.

Fiser, R. H.; Maetz, H. M.; Treuting, J. J.; Decker, W. J. Activated charcoal in barbiturate and glutethimide poisoning of the dog. J. Pediatr. *78*:1045-1047, 1971.

Fraser, H. F.; Isbell, H.; Eisenman, A. J.; Wikler, A.; Pescor, F. T. Chronic barbiturate intoxication, further studies. Arch. Intern. Med. *94*:34-41, 1954.

Frick, P. G.; Reutter, F.; Rechenberg, H. K. Hypovolemic shock following extravasation of plasma into interstitial space in poisoning with sedatives. Schweiz. Med. Wochenschr. *92*:1061-1065, 1962.

Gosselin, R. E.; Smith, R. P. Trends in the therapy of acute poisonings. Clin. Pharmacol. Ther. *1*:279-299, 1966.

Hadden, J.; Johnson, K.; Smith, S.; Price, L.; Giardina, E. Acute barbiturate intoxication. J. A. M. A. *209*:893-900, 1969.

Haider, I.; Oswald, I. Late brain recovery processes after drug overdose. Br. Med. J. *2*:318-322, 1970.

Hawer, G. E.; Lee, H. A. Value of forced diuresis in acute barbiturate poisoning. Br. Med. J. *3*:790-793, 1968.

Henderson, L. W.; Merrill, J. P. Treatment of barbiturate intoxication. Ann. Intern. Med. *64*:876-891, 1966.

Hennemann, H.; Naujoks, R.; Gattenlohner, W.; Rockel, A.; Kassler, G.; Reiners, W.; Heidland, A. Charcoal hemoperfusion in the treatment of sleeping drug intoxication. Deut. Med. Wochenschr. *101*:155-158, 1976.

Honey, G. E.; Jackson, R. C. Artificial respiration and an artificial kidney for severe barbiturate poisoning. Br. Med. J. *2*:1134-1137, 1959.

Hudson, J. B.; Dennis, A. J., Jr.; Hobbs, D. R.; Sussman, H. C.

Extended hemodialysis in short acting barbiturate poisoning. South. Med. J. 62:457-460, 1969.

Hulting, J.; Thorstrand, C. Hemodynamic effects of norepinephrine in severe hypnotic drug poisoning with arterial hypotension. Acta Med. Scand. 192:447-453, 1972.

Isbell, H.; Altschul, S.; Kornetsky, C. H.; Eisenman, A. J.; Flanary, H. G.; Fraser, H. F. Chronic barbiturate intoxication, an experimental study. Arch. Neurol. 64:1-28, 1950.

Isbell, H.; Fraser, H. F. Addiction to analgesics and barbiturates. Pharmacol. Rev. 2:355-397, 1950.

Iversen, B. M.; Willassen, Y.; Bakke, O. M.; Wallem, G. Assessment of barbiturate removal by charcoal hemoperfusion in overdose cases. Clin. Toxicol. 15:139-149, 1979.

Johanson, W. G., Jr. Massive phenobarbital ingestion with survival. J. A. M. A. 202:1106-1107, 1967.

Johns, M. W. Self-poisoning with barbiturates in England and Wales during 1959-1974. Brit. J. 1:1128-1130, 1977.

Kennedy, A. C.; Lindsay, R. M.; Briggs, J. D.; Luke, R. G.; Young, N.; Campbell, D. Successful treatment of three cases of very severe barbiturate poisoning. Lancet 1:995-998, 1969.

Keusch-Beck, M.; Keusch, G.; Bammatter, F.; Schiffl, H.; Baumann, P. C.; Binswanger, U. Hemoperfusion with activated charcoal for the treatment of poisoning. Schweiz. Med. Wochenschr. 110:1566-1577, 1980.

Killam, K. F.; Brody, T. M.; Bain, J. A. Potentiation of barbiturate hypnosis by certain uncoupling agents. Proc. Soc. Exp. Biol. Med. 97:744-748, 1958.

Kirkegaard, A.; Norregaard, S. Electrocardiogram in severe acute barbiturate poisoning. Acta Med. Scand. 140:119-126, 1951.

Knochel, J. P.; Barry, K. G. THAM dialysis: An experimental method to study diffusion of certain weak acids in vivo. II. Secobarbital. J. Lab. Clin. Med. 65:361-369, 1965.

Knochel, J. P.; Clayton, L. E.; Smith, W. L.; Barry, K. G. Intraperitoneal THAM: An effective method to enhance phenobarbital removal during peritoneal dialysis. J. Lab. Clin. Med. 64:361-369, 1964.

Koffler, A.; Bernstein, M.; LaSette, A.; Massry, S. G. Fixed-bed charcoal hemoperfusion. Treatment of drug overdose. Arch. Intern. Med. 138:1691-1694, 1978.

Kornetsky, C. H. Psychological effect of chronic barbiturate intoxication. Arch. Neurol. Psychiat. 65:557-567, 1951.

Kyle, L. H.; Jeghers, H.; Walsh, W. P.; Doolan, P. D.; Wishinsky, H.; Pallotta, A. The application of hemodialysis to the treatment of barbiturate poisoning. J. Clin. Invest. 32:364-371, 1953.

Lash, R. F.; Burdette, J. A.; Ozdil, T. Accidental profound hypothermia and barbiturate intoxication. A report of rapid "core" rewarming by peritoneal dialysis. J. A. M. A. 201:269-270, 1967.

Lassen, N. A. Treatment of severe acute barbiturate poisoning by forced diuresis and alkalinisation of the urine. Lancet 2:338-342, 1960.

Leavell, V. W. Sweat gland necrosis in barbiturate poisoning. Arch. Dermatol. 100:218-221, 1969.

Lee, H. A.; Ames, A. C. Haemodialysis in severe barbiturate poisoning. Br. Med. J. 1:1217-1219, 1965.

Linton, A. L.; Ledingham, I. M. Severe hypothermia with barbiturate intoxication. Lancet 1:24-26, 1966.

Linton, A. L.; Luke, R. G.; Briggs, J. D. Methods of forced diuresis and its application in barbiturate poisoning. Lancet 2:377-380, 1967.

Linton, A. L.; Luke, R. G.; Speirs, I.; Kennedy, A. C. Forced diuresis and haemodialysis in severe barbiturate intoxication. Lancet 1:1008-1010, 1964.

Loennecken, S. J. Acute Barbiturate Poisoning. John Wright and Sons Ltd., Bristol, 1967.

Lous, P. Plasma levels and urinary excretion of three barbituric acids after oral administration to man. Acta Pharmacol. Toxicol. 10:147-165, 1954a.

Lous, P. Barbituric acid concentration in serum from patients with severe acute poisoning. Acta Pharmacol. Toxicol. 10:261-280, 1954b.

Matthew, H. Acute Barbiturate Poisoning. Excerpta Medica, Amsterdam, 1971a.

Matthew, H.; Mackintosh, T. F.; Tompsett, S. L.; Cameron, J. C. Gastric aspiration and lavage in acute poisoning. Br. Med. J. 1:1333-1337, 1966.

McGuire, F. L. A comparison of suicide and non-suicide deaths involving psychotropic drugs in four major U. S. Cities. Am. J. Public Health 66:1058-1061, 1976.

Meyerowitz, B. R. Present status of hyperbaric oxygenation. Am. J. Surg. 109:611-619, 1965.

Michelson, A. L.; Frahm, C. J.; Katz, K. H. Delayed barbiturate intoxication. J. A. M. A. 155:440-441, 1954.

Morgan, A. G.; Bennett, J. M.; Polak, A. Mannitol retention during diuretic treatment of barbiturate and salicylate overdosage. Q. J. Med. 37:589-606, 1968.

Mousel, L. H. Cerebral edema and its relation to barbituric acid poisoning. J. A. M. A. 153:459-462, 1953.

Myschetzky, A.; Lassen, N. A. Urea-induced, osmotic diuresis and alkalinization of urine in acute barbiturate intoxication. J. A. M. A. 185:936-942, 1963.

Nattel, S.; Bayne, L.; Ruedy, J. Physostigmine in coma due to drug overdose. Clin. Pharmacol. Ther. 25:96-102, 1979.

Nealon, T. F., Jr.; Sugerman, H.; Shea, W.; Fleegler, E. An extracorporeal device to treat barbiturate poisoning. J. A. M. A. 197:118-120, 1966.

Nilsson, E. On treatment of barbiturate poisoning. Acta Med. Scand. 139(Suppl. 253) 1-127, 1951.

Ninet, J.; Polidori, M.; Bouletreau, P.; Ducluzeau, R.; Rouzioux, J. M. Modifications de l'intoxication barbiturique aigue volontaire au cours des dix dernieres annees. Etude comparative de deux series cliniques. Nouv. Presse Med. 10:893-896, 1981.

Ohlsson, W. T. L.; Fristedt, B. I. Blood lavage in acute barbiturate poisoning. Lancet 2:12-16, 1962.

Plum, F.; Swanson, A. G. Barbiturate poisoning treated by physiological methods. J. A. M. A. 163:827-835, 1957.

Raeburn, J. A.; Cameron, J. C.; Matthew, H. Severe barbiturate poisoning contrasts in management. Clin. Toxicol. 2:133-142, 1969.

Reed, C. E.; Driggs, M. F.; Foote, C. C. Acute barbiturate intoxication. A study of 300 cases based on a physiologic system of classification of the severity of the intoxication. Ann. Intern. Med. 37:290-303, 1952.

Rosenbaum, J. L. Hemoperfusion for acute drug intoxication. Kidney Int. 18(Suppl. 10):s106-s108, 1980.

Rosenbaum, J. L.; Kramer, M. S.; Raja, R. Resin hemoperfusion for acute drug intoxication. Arch. Internal Med. 136:263-266, 1976.

Rosenbaum, J. L.; Kramer, M. S.; Raja, R.; Boreyko, C. Resin hemoperfusion: A new treatment for acute drug intoxication. N. Engl. J. Med. 284:874-877, 1971.

Sessions, J. T., Jr.; Minkel, H. D.; Bullard, J. C.; Ingelfinger, F. J. The effect of barbiturates in patients with liver disease. J. Clin. Invest. 33:1116-1127, 1954.

Setter, J. G.; Maher, J. F.; Schreiner, G. E. Barbiturate intoxication. Arch. Intern. Med. 117:224-236, 1966.

Shubin, H.; Weil, M. H. The mechanism of shock following suicidal doses of barbiturates, narcotics and tranquilizer drugs, with observations on the effects of treatment. Am. J. Med. 38:853-863, 1965.

Shubin, H.; Weil, M. H. Shock associated with barbiturate intoxication. J. A. M. A. 215:263-268, 1971.

Slager, U. T.; Reilly, E. B.; Brandt, R. A. The neuropathology of barbiturate intoxication. J. Neuropathol. Exp. Neurol. 25:237-243, 1966.

Smith, D. E.; Wesson, D. R.; Lannon, R. A. New developments in barbiturate abuse. Clin. Toxicol. 3:57-65, 1970.

Strickler, J. C. Forced diuresis in the management of barbiturate intoxication. Clin. Pharmacol. Ther. 6:693-699, 1965.

Sybrecht, G. W.; Taubner, E. M.; Bohm, M. M.; Fabel, H. Mechanical properties of the respiratory system and mouth-occlusion pressure in patients acutely intoxicated with hypnotics. Lung 156:49-62, 1979.

Trafford, A.; Horn, C.; Sharpstone, P.; O'Neal, H.; Evans, R. Hemoperfusion in acute drug toxicity. Clin. Toxicol. 17:547-556, 1980.

Victor, L. B.; Gordon, E. L.; Greendyke, R. M. Therapeutic implications of autopsy findings in acute barbiturate intox-

ication. N. Y. State J. Med. 68:2090-2092, 1968.
Walsh, W. P.; Kyle, L. H.; Doolan, P. D.; Jeghers, H. J. Treatment of barbiturate poisoning by hemodialysis. Am. J. Med. 13:104-105, 1952.
Winchester, J. F.; Gelfand, M. C.; Tilstone, W. J. Hemoper-

fusion in drug intoxication: clinical and laboratory aspects. Drug Metab. Rev. 8:69-104, 1978.
Wright, J. T. The value of barbiturate estimations in the diagnosis and treatment of barbiturate intoxication. Q. J. Med. 24:95-108, 1955.

BARIUM

Barium salts are contained in some rodenticides, depilatories, and fireworks. In any of these forms barium may become available accidentally to children. Whereas human poisonings by soluble barium salts are uncommon, isolated accidental and suicidal ingestions are reported with surprising frequency (e.g., Berning, 1975; Gould et al., 1973). Epidemics have also been described. In the early 1940s an endemic state of barium intoxication arose in a Chinese province due to the contamination of table salt with barium chloride (Allen, 1943; Du and Dung, 1943). Flour containing barium carbonate poisoned 85 British soldiers in India (Morton, 1945). An outbreak of severe food poisoning in Israel was traced to sausage contaminated with barium carbonate. Nineteen of 100 patients involved were admitted to hospitals. No children appear to have been affected, although many were known to have eaten the sausage (Lewi and Bar-Khayim, 1964).

Various barium salts have been mistaken for the sulfate and administered by clinical radiologists, sometimes with fatal results (Dean, 1950; McNally, 1925). A series of cases of fatal fulminating liver disease following barium sulfate enemas have been ascribed to the tannic acid content (up to 2%) of the mixture (e.g., Lucke et al., 1963), which is said to improve the definition of the mucosal pattern. See also tannic acid in Section II.

Toxicology: The acid-soluble barium salts (carbonate, chloride, hydroxide, nitrate, acetate, sulfide) are highly toxic, whereas the insoluble barium sulfate is quite benign (Boyd and Abel, 1966). Barium polysulfide (Neopol) and barium sulfide produce symptoms of HYDROGEN SULFIDE poisoning, as well as barium effects; see p. III-198 (Jobba and Rengei, 1971). The lethal oral dose of barium chloride can be as low as 1.0 gm., but much larger doses have been tolerated (Graham, 1934; McNally, 1925). For most of the acid-soluble salts of barium the lethal dose for adults appears to lie between 1 and 15 gm. (Webster, 1930). Death occurs within a few hours or a few days. A 26-year-old man survived the ingestion of 15.8 gm. of barium sulfide (Gould et al., 1973). Severe reactions have also been reported from the inhalation of barium carbonate and peroxide dusts (Anon., 1941), whereas the inhalation of barium sulfate particles produces a benign pneumoconiosis (Pendergrass and Greening, 1953).

Barium ion stimulates smooth, striated, and cardiac muscle; the result is violent peristalsis, arterial hypertension, muscle twitching, and disturbances in cardiac action. Motor disorders include stiffness and immobility of the limbs and sometimes of the trunk, leg cramps, twitching of facial muscles, and paralysis of the tongue and pharynx with attendant loss or impairment of speech and deglutition (Witthaus, 1911). The central nervous system may be first stimulated and then depressed (Morton, 1945). Small amounts in cerebrospinal fluid induce convulsions (Chou and Chin, 1943). Ventricular tachyarrhythmias (including ventricular fibrillation) and transient asystole have been observed (Habicht et al., 1970). Kidney damage has been described as a late complication, presumably a result of circulatory insufficiency (McNally, 1925). Probably the most distinctive effect of barium in large doses, however, is skeletal muscle weakness and eventually flaccid paralysis involving extremities and respiratory muscles (Allen, 1943; Du and Dung, 1943; Morton, 1945; Huang, 1943).

In an experimental study in rats, Schott and McArdle (1974) demonstrated that barium-induced paralysis was due to a defect in muscle itself. During intravenous infusions of $BaCl_2$ (cumulative doses of about 20 mg./kg.), curarized rat leg muscles stimulated electrically produced twitches with amplitudes that were transiently increased and then greatly attenuated. At the same time the plasma level of potassium fell rapidly to about 2 mEq./L. The partial paralysis correlated with the hypokalemia much better than with the plasma barium concentration. The plasma sodium level was unaffected.

Hypokalemia in barium-poisoned humans was probably first described by Diengott et al. (1964). Two severely poisoned patients, one of whom had experienced no vomiting or diarrhea, were found to have plasma K^+ levels of 2.0 and 2.4 mEq./L. Both responded clinically to intravenous KCl, although one eventually died from severe pulmonary edema and hemorrhagic gastritis and duodenitis. This episode confirms the dramatic relief of symptoms described by Huang (1943) in two victims of barium poisoning treated with intravenous potassium citrate. In a victim of acute barium sulfide poisoning, hypokalemia and flaccid paralysis responded to intensive potassium therapy and a saline diuresis augmented by furosemide (Gould et al., 1973). Huang (1943) was impressed with similarities between barium intoxication and the rare disorder known as familial periodic paralysis. Features of the two states have been compared (Schott and McArdle, 1974).

The mechanism of barium-induced hypokalemia has not been completely clarified. Enhanced renal excretion does not appear to be responsible (Roza and Berman, 1971). The rapidity of the fall in plasma potassium suggests that K^+ migrates into tissue cells. Presumably muscle cells are involved, but the phenomenon has been demonstrated *in vivo* only with dog red blood cells (Roza and Berman, 1971). Whereas epinephrine secretion from the adrenal medulla is provoked by barium (Douglas and Rubin, 1964) and this hormone can promote an accumulation of K^+ in cells (Vick *et al.*, 1972), barium-induced hypokalemia cannot be ascribed to epinephrine because it cannot be prevented by adrenergic blockers, such as phentolamine (Roza and Berman, 1971) or propranolol (Schott and McArdle, 1974). A direct action of barium on muscle is inferred. Perhaps it activates Na^+-K^+-stimulated ATPase at cell surfaces to promote K^+ entry at the expense of the extracellular stores (Henn and Sperelakis, 1968). In isolated frog muscle, however, it did not modify the K^+ content, but it did decrease inward and outward K^+ permeability constants equally (Henderson and Volle, 1972). Barium's ability to induce hypokalemia and paralysis is not shared by strontium or any other alkaline earth element.

In poisoned rats, infusions of K^+ (but not of Ca^{2+}) corrected promptly both the hypokalemia and muscle weakness (Schott and McArdle, 1974). In dogs (Roza and Berman, 1971), all signs and symptoms of barium poisoning except hypertension were responsive to the administration of K^+; specifically, muscle weakness, diarrhea, and cardiac arrhythmias were alleviated. Whatever the mechanism of the hypertension, neither K^+ nor adrenergic blocking drugs suppressed it. As noted above, clinical experience with potassium therapy has also been favorable (Huang, 1943; Lewi and Bar-Khayim, 1964), and at times the benefits have been spectacular. Large parenteral doses, however, may be required; in recent reports of acute barium poisoning in three adults (Berning, 1975; Gould *et al.*, 1973; Habicht *et al.*, 1970), the cumulative dose of K^+ administered over the first 24 hours was 420, 260, and 250 mEq., respectively.

Thus, potassium administration is judged to be a rational and effective form of treatment for barium poisoning. Although the recommendation is over 30 years old, it apparently is not widely recognized by clinical toxicologists.

Symptomatology:
1. Excessive salivation, vomiting, severe abdominal pain, and violent purging with watery and bloody stools.

2. A slow and often irregular pulse due to ventricular premature contractions and a transient elevation in arterial blood pressure.
3. Tinnitus, giddiness and vertigo.
4. Muscle twitchings, progressing to convulsions and/or paralysis.
5. Dilated pupils with impaired accommodation.
6. Confusion and increasing somnolence, without coma.
7. Collapse and death from respiratory failure, apparently due to flaccid paralysis of the respiratory muscles.
8. Cardiac arrest after periods of ventricular tachycardia and fibrillation.

Treatment:
1. Rapid oral administration of a soluble sulfate in water, such as magnesium or sodium sulfate (2 oz.). These agents precipitate barium as the insoluble sulfate.
2. Gastric lavage or induced emesis (p. I-2) unless spontaneous vomiting is intensive.
3. Atropine sulfate (0.5 to 1.0 mg.) to alleviate colic. In severe cases morphine (10 to 15 mg.) may be necessary to relieve abdominal pain.
4. Blood pressure may be reduced, if elevated, by sublingual tablets of nitroglycerin (0.6 to 1.3 mg.).
5. In the presence of demonstrated hypokalemia, potassium salts should be administered. If vomiting is present, cautious intravenous therapy is indicated. For techniques see p. IV-73. Large doses may be required. Two adult victims of barium were given 260 and 420 mEq. K^+ in 24 hours (Gould *et al.*, 1973; Habicht *et al.*, 1970).
6. Cardiac arrhythmias, flaccid skeletal muscle paralysis and diarrhea in barium poisoning appear to be responsive to potassium therapy. Even if hypokalemia cannot be demonstrated, K^+ administration (p. IV-73) is recommended for the control of ventricular tachycardia and other tachyarrhythmias.
7. Ventilatory assistance (p. IV-7) in the phase of respiratory muscle weakness or paralysis.
8. Ringer solution intravenously (one or more liters) to combat dehydration from vomiting and diarrhea (pp. IV-66–67) and to promote the renal excretion of barium.
9. To supplement the saline diuresis, give furosemide parenterally (20 to 40 mg. intramuscularly or slowly intravenously). Perhaps the addition of a potassium-sparing diuretic such as triamterene (100 mg. orally) would be advisable.

Laboratory: Severe hypokalemia has been described in several cases. Serial determinations of serum K^+ are essential for the proper management of barium poisoning. The ECG should be recorded at frequent intervals, if not continuously.

References:

Allen, A. S. Pa ping or kiating paralysis. Chinese Med. J. 61:296-301, 1943.

Anon. (Queries and Minor Notes). Effect of barium carbonate fumes on the respiratory tract. J. A. M. A. 117:1221, 1941.

Berning, J. Hypokalaemia of barium poisoning. Lancet 1:110, 1975.

Boyd, E. M.; Abel, M. The acute toxicity of barium sulfate administered intragastrically. Can. Med. Assoc. J. 94:849-853, 1966.

Chou, C.; Chin, Y. C. The absorption, fate, and concentration in serum of barium in acute experimental poisoning. Chinese Med. J. 61:313-322, 1943.

Dean, G. Seven cases of barium carbonate poisoning. Br. Med. J. 2:817-818, 1950.

Diengott, D.; Rozsa, O.; Levy, N.; Maummar, S. Hypokalaemia in barium poisoning. Lancet 2:343-344, 1964.

Douglas, W. W.; Rubin, R. P. Stimulant action of barium on the adrenal medulla. Nature (London) 203:305-307, 1964.

Du, K. T.; Dung, C. L. "Pa" disease. Chinese Med. J. 61:302, 1943.

Gould, D. B.; Sorrell, M. R.; Lupariello, A. D. Barium sulfide poisoning. Arch. Intern. Med. 132:891-894, 1973.

Graham, C. F. Barium chloride poisoning. J. A. M. A. 102:1471, 1934.

Habicht, W.; v. Smekal, P.; Etzrodt, H. Verlauf und Behandlung einer Barium-vergiftung. Med. Welt 28:1292-1295, 1970.

Henderson, E. G.; Volle, R. L. Ion exchange in frog sartorius muscle treated with 9-aminoacridine or barium. J. Pharmacol. Exp. Ther. 183:356-369, 1972.

Henn, F. A.; Sperelakis, N. Stimulative and protective action of Sr^{2+} and Ba^{2+} on (Na^+-K^+)-ATPase from cultured heart cells. Biochim. Biophys. Acta 163:415-417, 1968.

Huang, K. Pa ping (transient paralysis simulating family periodic paralysis). Chinese Med. J. 61:305-312, 1943.

Jobba, G.; Rengei, B. Uber die Neopol-Vergiftung. Arch. Toxikol. 27:106-110, 1971.

Ku, D. Y.; Yen, C. K.; Li, C. C. Acute poisoning by common salt containing barium chloride. An experimental study. Chinese Med. J. 61:303-304, 1943.

Lewi, Z.; Bar-Khayim, Y. Food poisoning from barium carbonate. Lancet 2:342-343, 1964.

Lucke, H. H.; Hodge, K. E.; Patt, N. L. Fatal liver damage after barium enemas containing tannic acid. Can. Med. Assoc. J. 89:1111-1114, 1963.

McNally, W. D. Two deaths from the administration of barium salts. J. A. M. A. 84:1805-1807, 1925.

Morton, W. Poisoning by barium carbonate. Lancet 2:738-739, 1945.

Pendergrass, E. P.; Greening, R. R. Baritosis, report of a case. Arch. Ind. Hyg. Occup. Med. 7:44-48, 1953.

Roza, O.; Berman, L. B. The pathophysiology of barium: hypokalemia and cardiovascular effects. J. Pharmacol. Exp. Ther. 177:433-439, 1971.

Schott, G. D.; McArdle, B. Barium-induced skeletal muscle paralysis in the rat, and its relationship to human familial periodic paralysis. J. Neurol. Neurosurg. Psychiatry 37:32-39, 1974.

Vick, R. L.; Todd, E. P.; Luedke, D. W. Epinephrine-induced hypokalemia: Relation to liver and skeletal muscle. J. Pharmacol. Exp. Ther. 181:139-146, 1972.

Webster, R. W. Legal Medicine and Toxicology. W. B. Saunders Co., Philadelphia, 1930.

Witthaus, R. A. Manual of Toxicology. Wm. Wood & Co., New York, 1911.

BENZALKONIUM CHLORIDE

Many modern germicides are synthetic derivatives of ammonium chloride, in which the four hydrogens of the ammonium cation have been replaced by organic groups, at least one of which is a long-chain aliphatic residue. One popular compound of this type is alkyldimethylbenzylammonium chloride (benzalkonium chloride), where the alkyl group represents a mixture of linear saturated hydrocarbon residues from C_8 to C_{16} (chiefly C_{12} and C_{14}).

In a related group of substances, the nitrogen atom is included in a heterocyclic ring. Thus, there are quaternary pyridinium germicides, such as cetylpyridinium chloride, and imidazoline derivatives. Although most of these substances are marketed as chloride salts, some are available as bromides, iodides, nitrates, etc. These salts are often called cationic surfactants or cationic detergents because their aqueous solutions have low surface tensions. Collectively they are sometimes referred to as "quaternary ammonium compounds" or QAC.

Dozens of quaternary ammonium germicides are available commercially as powders, ointments, jellies, aqueous solutions and tinctures. At concentrations between 0.01 and 1.0%, they are used as antiseptics, bactericides, fungicides, sanitizers and deodorants. In restaurants, dairies, food plants, laundries and operating rooms, they are popular disinfectants for utensils, containers, instruments, etc. Because they react with soap and most proteins, their maximal germicidal effectiveness is attained only on chemically clean surfaces. With proteins the reaction occurs only on the alkaline side of their isoelectric points (Putnam, 1948).

Dilute solutions have been employed in medicine to sterilize the skin, conjunctivae, and mucous membranes and, rarely, to irrigate the urinary bladder and other body cavities. They have been used to keep bodies of water free of slime mold, algae, fish pathogens, and certain mollusks. Some derivatives have served as mothproofing agents, oil preservatives, soil pathogen eradicators and foliage sprays. For a detailed review of these compounds including their toxicity, see Cutler and Drobeck (1970).

Toxicology: The mammalian toxicity of quaternary ammonium germicides is not well established, although several human fatalities have been ascribed to them (Adelson and Sunshine, 1952; Tiess and Nagel, 1967). Probably all common derivatives produce similar toxic reactions, but as tested in laboratory mammals the oral mean lethal dose varies with the compound between the approximate limits of 100 and 700 mg./kg. (Finnegan and Dienna, 1953; Gloxhuber, 1974; Shelanski, 1949; Woodward and Calvary, 1945). The oral LD_{50} of benzalkonium chloride in rats is 445 mg./kg. (Shelanski, 1949). Some of these substances are several hundred times more toxic by the intravenous route than by the oral route, whereas the oral and parenteral toxicities of other congeners differ only slightly (Arnold and Krefft, 1952; Ing, 1946; Hohensee, 1951; Hopper et al., 1949). At least some quaternary compounds are significantly more toxic in 50% dimethyl sulfoxide than in plain water when given by mouth to rodents (Rosen et al., 1965).

Concentrated aqueous solutions (10% and sometimes less) are primary skin irritants and concentrations as low as 0.1 to 0.5% are often irritating to conjunctivae and mucous membranes (Draize and Kelley, 1952; Finnegan and Dienna, 1953). Whereas benzalkonium chloride is said to be well tolerated at these lower concentrations, occasional cases of allergic contact-dermatitis and conjunctivitis continue to be reported (e.g., Fisher and Stillman, 1972; Schmunes and Levy, 1972). In one of these cases (Gasset, 1977) a soft contact lens apparently acted as a reservoir for the slow release onto the cornea. Asthma due to occupational exposure has been reported at least once (Innocenti, 1978).

Percutaneous absorption is probably insignificant (Finnegan and Dienna, 1953). A rough correlation has been noted between the acute oral toxicity in mice and the irritation produced in the rabbit eye (Hopper et al., 1949). Surface activity per se is not predictably related to toxicity (Food Protection Committee, 1956). In general it appears that quaternary ammonium compounds with two long-chain alkyl groups, which are sometimes used as fabric softeners, are much less toxic and less irritating than those with a single such substitution (personal communication from J. F. Griffith, Proctor and Gamble Company, 1961). Only the latter are useful as germicides.

In reviewing 10 human fatalities (all adults except for a 2-year-old child) in which quaternary ammonium compounds were implicated, Tiess and Nagel (1967) concluded that the nature of the human toxic response varies widely with the dose and concentration of the product as well as with the rate of administration and survival time of the victim. Only two aqueous solutions of alkyldimethylbenzylammonium chloride are represented in this series: a 10% solution of "Zephirol" where the alkyl group ranges from 8 to 18 carbons in length and a 15% solution of "C₄" where the alkyl chain ranges from 15 to 18 carbons. After intramuscular or intravenous administration (Spann, 1955; Wagner, 1965) as well as intrauterine instillation (Arnold and Krefft, 1952), 5 to 15 mg. of these salts per kg. of body weight produced death in 5 victims. In 5 additional cases 100 to 400 mg./kg. by mouth produced rapid demise within a few minutes to 3 hours (Stoye and Bittersohl, 1968; Tiess and Nagel, 1967; Wolff, 1961). Three patients who received intravenous injections of what was probably "Zephirol" died in 21 to 46 hours (Wagner, 1965). In Spann's (1955) case the victim survived 15 days, and the clinical course included a confirmed myocardial infarction as well as a severe terminal uremia. The site of intramuscular injection was marked by necrotic and thrombotic changes. No emboli were found in the circulation, but many mural thrombi were present in the heart. Severe degenerative changes were present in the kidney as well as patchy hepatic necrosis.

Strong aqueous solutions (10 to 20%) commonly produce superficial necrosis of mucous membranes with which they come in contact. Severe corrosion of the upper alimentary tract was the rule in the series of Tiess and Nagel (1967) but was apparently absent in an isolated case in this country (Adelson and Sunshine, 1952). Erosion, ulceration and petechial hemorrhages may be found throughout the small intestine. In one case the fundus of the stomach was said to be completely devoid of mucosa (Wolff, 1961). Glottic edema and pulmonary edema have been reported. Even in prompt death, cloudy swelling, patchy necrosis and fatty infiltration occur in such visceral organs as heart, liver and kidneys (Tiess and Nagel, 1967). Brain edema and hemorrhage have been described (Stoye and Bittersohl, 1968).

Fatal poisonings in animals can be induced by feeding concentrations which create no recognized pathological lesions except visceral congestion, cloudy swelling, mild pulmonary edema, and varying degrees of gastrointestinal irritation (Alfredson et al., 1951; Woodward and Calvary, 1945). Even in chronic exposures of several weeks, the only lesion found in fatally ill rats was focal hemorrhagic necrosis of the gastric mucosa, and these animals apparently died of inanition associated with chronic diarrhea (Alfredson et al., 1951; Coulston et al., 1961; Fitzhugh and Nelson, 1948).

Although a definitive biochemical and pharmacological effect is probably responsible for systemic poisoning by quaternary ammonium germicides, the nature of this specific disorder is not established. On highly circumstantial evidence, the suggestion has been made that the ingestion of methyl dodecyl benzyl trimethyl ammonium chloride (Hyamine 2389) may cause a fatal inhibition of the enzyme cholinesterase (Adelson and Sunshine, 1952). Inhibition of this enzyme has been produced in vitro by several quaternary ammonium surfactants (Huidobro and Atria, 1949), but presumably many other protein precipitants would serve as well. Indeed these compounds inhibit bacterial glycolysis and respiration (Baker *et al.*, 1941; Knox *et al.*, 1949; Sevag and Ross, 1944) in a manner suggestive of a nonspecific mechanism.

In isolated observations in our laboratory, no inhibition of plasma cholinesterase was found in rats sacrificed *in extremis* after an intraperitoneal injection of benzalkonium chloride or cetylpyridinium chloride. A 50% inhibition of the red cell cholinesterase was noted, but such a depression is not expected to produce untoward reactions. It is improbable that toxic signs and symptoms arising from quaternary ammonium compounds can be attributed to cholinesterase inhibition.

A curare-like paralysis of skeletal muscles has been ascribed to quaternary ammonium salts, specifically to cetylpyridinium chloride (Warren *et al.*, 1942) and benzalkonium chloride. Parenteral injections in rats, rabbits and dogs have resulted in prompt but transient limb paralysis and sometimes fatal paresis of the respiratory muscles (Arnold and Krefft, 1952). This effect appears to be highly transient, and to our knowledge it has not been demonstrated after oral administration.

In human poisonings, however, paralysis is not a well-established phenomenon. In 3 fatal cases allegedly resulting from the intravenous administration of Zephirol (Wagner, 1965), cardiovascular collapse appeared to be responsible for most of the signs and symptoms, which consisted of shortness of breath, cyanosis, chills, vomiting, tachycardia, arrhythmias, profound hypotension, oliguria, confusion and coma. Curariform signs were also absent in Spann's case (1955).

Although detailed clinical descriptions of quaternary ammonium compound poisoning are not available, a curariform paralysis is consistent with the signs and symptoms reported in two fatally poisoned women, of whom one drank Hyamine 2389 and the other received benzalkonium chloride by vaginal instillation in the course of an abortion (Adelson and Sunshine, 1952; Arnold and Krefft, 1952). It is also compatible with the symptoms produced in a child poisoned by the ingestion of benzalkonium chloride (Wolff, 1961). Besides a curare-like paralysis of the motor end plates in skeletal muscle, severe central nervous depression, sometimes preceded by excitement and convulsions, has been reported in poisoned animals (Adelson and Sunshine, 1952; Lehman, 1954). These multiple actions are reminiscent of nicotine poisoning (p. III-311). The impressions and inferences outlined above receive support from the structural analogy between quaternary ammonium germicides and decamethonium (a recognized neuro-muscular blocking agent) and hexamethonium (an established ganglionic blocking agent).

Symptomatology (partly inferred from animal studies):

1. The ingestion of a concentrated solution leads to immediate burning pain in the mouth, throat, and abdomen, with profuse salivation. Exposed areas of mucous membranes may ulcerate. Emesis and hematemesis may occur.
2. Hypotension and other signs and symptoms of circulatory shock.
3. Rapidly developing apprehension, restlessness, confusion, and weakness.
4. Specific muscle weakness, perhaps associated with a transient period of muscle fasciculation, is a possibility that requires confirmation.
5. Central nervous depression may or may not be preceded by weak convulsive movements and may or may not be due to cerebral ischemia.
6. Labored breathing and cyanosis due to weakness of the respiratory muscles or to circulatory shock.
7. An asphyxial death, with or without a terminal convulsion, due to paralysis of the muscles of respiration or to cardiovascular collapse. In fatal cases, death is expected to occur promptly, *i.e.*, within 1 or 2 hours after ingestion.
8. If the patient survives a period of severe hypotension, renal failure may develop.

Treatment:

1. If a concentrated solution (10% or higher) has been ingested, swallow promptly a large quantity of milk, egg whites, or gelatin solution. If these or other protein solutions are not readily available, a slurry of activated charcoal (see p. I-4) may be useful. Avoid alcohol, which has been shown to increase the oral toxicity of at least one quaternary ammonium germicide (cetylpyridinium chloride), presumably by promoting absorption. Because of probable mucosal damage, omit gastric lavage and emetic drugs.
2. If a dilute solution (usually 2% or less) has been ingested and little or no emesis appears spontaneously, administer syrup of ipecac (p. I-2) or perform gastric lavage (p. I-8).
3. If hypotension becomes severe, institute measure against circulatory shock (pp. IV-17-20).
4. Skeletal muscle weakness or paralysis can be detected by a loss in grip strength, inability to stand, perhaps ptosis, and diminution or absence of tendon reflexes. Cur-

are antagonists, such as neostigmine and edrophonium (Tensilon), are probably of no value and may enhance the paralysis (as in decamethonium poisoning). Presumably, central nervous stimulants are also ineffective.

5. If respirations become labored, administer oxygen (p. IV-12) and support breathing mechanically by any approved method of artificial respiration (p. IV-7–12). In the absence of a gag reflex, an oropharyngeal airway should be inserted (p. IV-3). Epiglottic or laryngeal edema may necessitate a tracheotomy (p. IV-6).

6. If persistent, convulsions may be controlled by the cautious intravenous injection of diazepam or a short-acting barbiturate drug (p. IV-37).

7. As in lye ingestions (p. III-249), cautious endoscopy may be required to evaluate corrosive injuries of the esophagus and stomach.

8. If a quaternary ammonium drug is spilled on the skin, wash promptly with soap and water.

Laboratory: Probably irrelevant.

References:

Adelson, L.; Sunshine, I. Fatal poisoning due to a cationic detergent of the quaternary ammonium compound type. Am. J. Clin. Pathol. 22:656-661, 1952.

Alfredson, B. V.; Stiefel, J. R.; Thorp, F., Jr.; Baten, W. D.; Gray, M. L. Toxicity studies on alkyldimethylbenzylammonium chloride in rats and dogs. J. Pharm. Sci. 40:263-267, 1951.

Arnold, W.; Krefft, S. The toxicity of Zephiran. Z. Rechtsmed. 41:297-310, 1952.

Baker, Z.; Harrison, R. W.; Miller, B. F. Inhibition by phospholipids of the action of synthetic detergents on bacteria. J. Exp. Med. 74:621-637, 1941.

Coulston, F.; Drobeck, H. P.; Mielens, Z. E.; Garvin, P. J., Jr. Toxicology of benzalkonium chloride given orally in milk or water to rats and dogs. Toxicol. Appl. Pharmacol. 3:584-594, 1961.

Cutler, R. A.; Drobeck, H. P. Toxicology of cationic surfactants. In Cationic Surfactants (E. Jungermann, Ed.). Dekker, N. Y, 1970.

Draize, J. H.; Kelley, E. A. Toxicity to eye mucosa of certain cosmetic preparations containing surface-active agents. Proc. Sci. Sect., Toilet Goods Assoc. No. 17 (May), 1952.

Finnegan, J. K.; Dienna, J. B. Toxicological observations in certain surface-active agents. Proc. Sci. Sect. Toilet Goods Assoc., No. 20, 1953.

Fisher, A. A.; Stillman, M. A. Allergic contact sensitivity to benzalkonium chloride: cutaneous, ophthalmic and general medical implications. Arch. Dermatol. 106:169-171, 1972.

Fitzhugh, O. G.; Nelson, A. A. Chronic oral toxicities of surface-active agents. J. Pharm. Sci. 37:29-32, 1948.

Food Protection Committee of the Food and Nutrition Board, NAS-NRC. The relation of surface activity to the safety of surfactants in foods. Publication No. 463 (Oct.), 1956.

Gasset, A. R. Benzalkonium chloride toxicity to the human cornea. Am. J. Ophthalmol. 84:169-171, 1977.

Gloxhuber, C. Toxicological properties of surfactants. Arch. Toxicol. 32:245-270, 1974.

Hohensee, F. Curare-like effect of invert soaps. Z. Gesamte Inn. Med. 6:219-223, 1951.

Hopper, S. S.; Hulpieu, H. R.; Cole, V. V. Some toxicological properties of surface-active agents. J. Pharm. Sci. 38:428-432, 1949.

Huidobro, E.; Atria, P. Effect of detergents on various structures with special reference to muscle and ganglion. J. Pharmacol. Exp. Ther. 96:438-444, 1969.

Ing, H. R. Curariform action of onium salts. Physiol. Rev. 16:527-544, 1946.

Innocenti, A. Occupational asthma due to benzalkonium chloride. Med. Lav. 69:713-715, 1978.

Knox, W. E.; Auerbach, V. H.; Zarudnaya, K.; Spirites, M. Action of cationic detergents on bacteria and bacterial enzymes. J. Bacteriol. 58:443-452, 1949.

Lehman, A. J. Quaternary ammonium surfactants. Acute and chronic toxicity. Assoc. Food and Drug Officials U. S. Quart. Bull. 18:43-66, 1954.

Putnam, F. W. Interactions of proteins and synthetic detergents. In Advances in Protein Chemistry, Vol. IV. Edited by M. L. Anson and J. T. Edsall. Academic Press, Inc., New York, 1948.

Rosen, H.; Blumenthal, A.; Panasevich, R.; McCallum, J. Dimethylsulfoxide (DMSO) as a solvent in acute toxicity determinations. Proc. Soc. Exp. Biol. Med. 120:511-514, 1965.

Schmunes, E.; Levy, E. J. Quaternary ammonium compound contact dermatitis from a deodorant. Arch. Dermatol. 105:91-93, 1972.

Sevag, M. G.; Ross, O. A. Studies on the mechanism of the inhibitory action of Zephiran on yeast cells. J. Bacteriol. 48:677-681, 1944.

Shelanski, H. A. Toxicity of quaternaries. Soap Sanit. Chemicals 25:125-129 and 153, 1949.

Spann, W. Uber die toxische Wirkung von Zephirol auf den menschlichen Organismus. Arch. Toxikol. 15:196-201, 1955.

Stoye, H.; Bittersohl, G. Todliche Vergiftung durch das Desinfektionsmittel C4 bei einem Kleinkind. Z. Aerztl. Fortbild. 62:436-438, 1968.

Tiess, D.; Nagel, K. H. Beitrag zur Morphologie und Analytik der Invertseifenintoxikation. Zwei akut-todliche Vergiftungen durch perorale Aufnahme des Desinfektionmittels D4. Arch. Toxikol. 22:333-348, 1967.

Wagner, H. -J. 3 Todesfalle durch Intoxikation (Invertseife) oder durch anaphylaktische Schock (Rosskastanienextrakt)? Arch. Toxikol. 21:83-88, 1965.

Warren, M. R.; Becker, T. J.; Marsh, D. G.; Shelton, R. S. Pharmacological and toxicological studies on cetylpyridinium chloride, a new germicide. J. Pharmacol. Exp. Ther. 74:401-408, 1942.

Wolff, F. Todliche Vergiftung durch Trinken des Desinfektionsmittels "C₄". Arch. Toxikol. 19:8-14, 1961.

Woodward, G.; Calvery, H. O. Toxicological properties of surface-active agents. Proc. Sci. Sect. Toilet Goods Assoc., No. 3, 1945.

BORATE

Borates are still encountered as antiseptic agents despite their limited effectiveness. Powders, ointments, and solutions containing boric acid have long been prescribed for dermatological disorders, eye washes, gargles, urinary antiseptics, and diaper rinses. Borates have also been used as food preservatives, but they are now largely supplanted by safer agents (Ross and Conway, 1943). Sodium borate (borax) is used in cleaning compounds, wood preservatives, and herbicides. When dissolved in buffered aqueous solution, the various complex salts, such as meta-, di-, tetra-, pyro-, and orthoborate, cannot be differentiated from one another chemically or toxicologically (Kingma, 1958; Sciarra, 1958).

Toxicology: The reputation of borates is so firmly entrenched that they are still readily available despite toxic reactions reported as early as 1883 (Bumbalo, 1952). Acute poisonings have followed ingestion, parenteral injection, enemas, lavage of serous cavities, irrigation of the bladder and application of powders and ointments to burned and abraded skin. Ironically, many of these incidents have occurred in hospitals through ignorance or error (Brooke and Boggs, 1951; Connelly et al., 1958; Ducey and Williams, 1953; Johnstone et al., 1955; Jordan and Crissey, 1957; McIntyre and Burke, 1937; Rosen and Haggerty, 1956; Schmid et al., 1972; Wong et al., 1964; Young et al., 1949).

The biochemical mechanism of borate poisoning is unknown. Clinical and pathological findings relate principally to the central nervous system, gastrointestinal tract, kidneys, liver, and skin, and the highest concentrations of boron are found at these sites (McNally and Rust, 1928). Chronic feeding to rats and dogs leads to accumulation in the testes, germ cell depletion and testicular atrophy (Lee et al., 1978; Weir and Fisher, 1972). On several occasions (e.g., Valdes-Dapena and Arey, 1962), pancreatic acinar cell cytoplasmic inclusions have been described in fatal cases.

Borates are rapidly absorbed from mucous membranes and abraded skin but not from intact or unbroken skin (Sciarra, 1958). Toxic symptoms may be delayed for several hours. Borate excretion occurs mainly through the kidneys; about half is excreted in the first 12 hours, and the remainder is eliminated over a period of 5 to 7 days (Locksley and Sweet, 1954). The renal clearance observed in eight patients given sodium pentaborate for neutron capture therapy of intracranial tumors was 39.1 ml./min. per 1.7 square meters of body surface (Farr and Konikowski, 1963).

Clinical findings commonly consist of gastrointestinal disturbances (hemorrhagic gastroenteritis), erythematous skin eruptions, and signs of central nervous stimulation followed by depression (Pfeiffer et al., 1945). In an adult the mean lethal dose of boric acid and sodium borate probably exceeds 30 gm. As one phase of treatment for brain tumor, each of 10 adults was injected intravenously with about 20 gm. of borax ($Na_2B_4O_7 \cdot 10H_2O$); no deaths resulted, but severe untoward reactions included nausea, vomiting, diarrhea, mild peripheral vascular collapse, mental confusion with subsequent drowsiness, rash, and intermittent retching for several days; renal dysfunction was not observed (Farr et al., 1954; Locksley and Farr, 1955). In severe

and fatal poisonings, however, oliguria, anuria and tubular necrosis are recognized (Baker and Wilson, 1963; Hauck and Henn, 1969; Skipworth et al., 1967; von Schulthess et al., 1969). Even total anuria for 14 hours, however, is not incompatible with complete recovery of renal function (Stolpmann and Hopmann, 1975).

Infants and young children are thought to be more susceptible to borate intoxication than are adults. In a series of 11 newborns fed boric acid in their formulae, the 5 who each received 4.6 to 14 gm. died within 2 to 3 days, whereas the 6 who each consumed 4.5 gm. or less (2 to 4.5 gm.) survived (Wong et al., 1964). In a study of over 100 cases of accidental poisoning, the overall fatality rate was 55%, but in infants under 1 year of age, 70% of the cases ended fatally (Goldbloom and Goldbloom, 1953). Death may occur in a few hours but is usually delayed several days.

In a remarkable case of chronic intoxication an adult male allegedly consumed 25 gm. of undefined "boric tartrate" daily for 20 years. All signs and symptoms (cachexia, dermatitis, alopecia, hypoplastic anemia, gastric ulcer) disappeared on withdrawal (Herren and Wyss, 1964). Hair loss in a young woman with obscure diffuse alopecia was traced to the chronic ingestion of boric acid-containing mouth washes (Stein et al., 1973). In two infants who ingested 2 and 10 gm. of borax per week for 5 and 10 weeks, respectively, the presenting complaint was generalized seizures, although one child developed a profound anemia as well (Gordon et al., 1973).

The lack of an effective antidote for borate has led to trials with a variety of therapeutic measures in severe poisonings. Exchange transfusion (Boggs and Anrode, 1955) and peritoneal dialysis (Baliah et al., 1969; Martin, 1971; Segar, 1960) have both been employed to advantage to promote the removal of borate. Hemodialysis with an artificial kidney was employed in one case in combination with forced diuresis; the two interventions appeared to be about equally effective (Stolpmann and Hopmann, 1975). Although relatively small amounts of borate were recovered (100 to 500 mg.) in a series of 9 poisoned newborns, peritoneal dialysis was extolled as the most successful therapeutic measure tested when judged by the improved clinical status (Wong et al., 1964).

Symptomatology:
1. Nausea, vomiting, diarrhea, epigastric pain. Vomiting is often persistent, and the vomitus and feces may contain blood. Hemorrhagic gastroenteritis may develop irrespective of the route of administration.
2. Weakness, lethargy, headache, restlessness, tremors, and intermittent convulsions—with subsequent central nervous depression.

3. Erythematous skin eruptions (giving rise to a boiled lobster appearance) followed by extensive exfoliation. The skin lesions resemble scarlet fever (Baker and Wilson, 1963) and Ritter's disease (Rubenstein and Musher, 1970). Typical sites of this rash are the palms, soles, buttocks, and scrotum, but no skin surface is immune. The pharynx and tympanic membranes may also be involved.
4. Shock syndrome—cold clammy skin, cyanosis, thready pulse, and low blood pressure.
5. Occasionally kidney injury (oliguria, albuminuria, anuria) and rarely liver damage (hepatomegaly, jaundice) have been reported; the former may be a cause of death. Circulatory shock with hypoperfusion does not appear to be fully responsible for these visceral lesions.
6. Metabolic acidosis and signs of intravascular coagulation have been described (Rosenkranz and Weissenbacher, 1965; von Schulthess et al., 1969).
7. The body temperature is usually normal (or even low), but fevers are described in the absence of recognized intercurrent infection.
8. Death is due to vascular collapse in the early stages or to central nervous depression later in the course of poisoning. Bronchopneumonia, meningitis, and other terminal infections have been described.

Treatment:
1. In ingestion cases, administer syrup of ipecac unless spontaneous emesis is extensive.
2. Gastric lavage with warm tap water if the vomitus is of scanty volume.
3. Saline catharsis with 15 to 30 gm. of sodium sulfate in water.
4. Replace water and electrolytes lost through vomiting and diarrhea. Parenteral administration is usually necessary (pp. IV-66–67, 72–73).
5. Treat shock with oxygen, intravenous plasma or blood (pp. IV-12 and 17).
6. Control convulsions with a short-acting barbiturate or diazepam (p. IV-37).
7. Peritoneal dialysis (p. IV-56) or hemodialysis in cases with severe systemic reactions.
8. Sodium bicarbonate for any metabolic acidosis. See p. IV-72.
9. Antibiotics (pp. IV-86–91) in the presence of infection.
10. Symptomatic treatment for skin lesions, but the antiinflammatory action of topical corticosteroids, such as 0.04% dexamethasone cream, may be required. Severe generalized skin eruptions, especially with exfoliation, may warrant a short but intense course of systemic steroid therapy.
11. Because borates induce riboflavin depletion in several animal species (Roe et al., 1972), supplementation with this vitamin may be desirable.

Laboratory:
1. Boron is detectable in urine and sometimes in cerebrospinal fluid by the turmeric paper test (Boggs and Anrode, 1955), but quantitative techniques have been used to measure boron in blood.
2. Urinalysis may reveal albumin.
3. Biochemical tests of liver function are useful and appropriate.
4. Hyperchloremic acidosis has been described (Wong et al., 1964).

References:

Baker, D. H.; Wilson, R. E. The lethality of boric acid in the treatment of burns. J. A. M. A. 186:1169-1170, 1963.

Baliah, T.; MacLeish, H.; Drummond, K. N. Acute boric acid poisoning; report of an infant successfully treated by peritoneal dialysis. Can. Med. Assoc. J. 101:166-168, 1969.

Boggs, T. R., Jr.; Anrode, H. G. Boric acid poisoning treated by exchange transfusion. Report of a case. Pediatrics 16:109-114, 1955.

Brooke, C.; Boggs, T. Boric acid poisoning. Report of a case and review of the literature. Am. J. Dis. Child. 82:465-472, 1951.

Bumbalo, T. S. Boric acid poisoning. N. Y. State J. Med. 52:1913-1914, 1952.

Connelly, J. P.; Crawford, J. D.; Soloway, A. H. Boric acid poisoning in an infant. N. Engl. J. Med. 259:1123-1125, 1958.

Ducey, J.; Williams, D. B. Transcutaneous absorption of boric acid. J. Pediatr. 43:644-651, 1953.

Farr, L. E.; Konikowski, T. The renal clearance of sodium pentaborate in mice and men. Clin. Chem. 9:717-726, 1963.

Farr, L. E.; Sweet, W. H.; Robertson, J. S.; Foster, C. G.; Locksley, H. B.; Sutherland, D. L.; Mendelsohn, M. L.; Stickley, E. E. Neutron capture therapy with boron in the treatment of glioblastoma multiforme. Am. J. Roentgenol. Radium Ther. Nucl. Med. 71:279-293, 1954.

Goldbloom, R. B.; Goldbloom, A. Boric acid poisoning. Report of four cases and a review of 109 cases from the world literature. J. Pediatr. 43:631-643, 1953.

Gordon, A. S.; Prichard, J. S.; Freedman, M. H. Seizure disorders and anemia associated with chronic borax intoxication. Can. Med. Assoc. J. 108:719-722, 1973.

Hauck, G.; Henn, R. Histopathologische and chemisch-toxikologische Befunde bei einer akuten todlichen Borsaurevergiftung. Arch. Toxikol. 25:83-88, 1969.

Herren, C.; Wyss, F. Chronische Borsaurevergiftung. Schweiz. Med. Wochenschr. 94:1815-1818, 1964.

Johnstone, D. E.; Basila, N.; Glaser, J. Study of boric acid absorption in infants from use of baby powders. J. Pediatr. 46:160-167, 1955.

Jordan, J. W.; Crissey, J. T. Boric acid poisoning. A report of a fatal adult case from cutaneous use. A critical evaluation of the use of this drug in dermatologic practice. Arch. Dermatol. 75:720-728, 1957.

Kingma, H. The pharmacology and toxicology of boron compounds. Can. Med. Assoc. J. 78:620-622, 1958.

Lee, I. P.; Sherins, R. J.; Dixin, R. L. Evidence for induction of germinal aplasia in male rats by environmental exposure to boron. Toxicol. Appl. Pharmacol. 45:577-590, 1978.

Locksley, H. B.; Farr, L. E. Tolerance of large doses of sodium borate intravenously by patients receiving neutron capture therapy. J. Pharmacol. Exp. Ther. 114:484-489, 1955.

Locksley, H. B.; Sweet, W. H. Tissue distribution of boron compounds in relation to neutron-capture therapy of cancer. Proc. Soc. Exp. Biol. Med. 86:56-63, 1954.

Martin, G. J. Asymptomatic boric acid intoxication; value of peritoneal dialysis. N. Y. State J. Med. 71:1842-1844, 1971.

McIntyre, A. R.; Burke, J. C. Intravenous boric acid poisoning in man. J. Pharmacol. Exp. Ther. 60:112-113, 1937.

McNally, W. D.; Rust, C. A. The distribution of boric acid in human organs in six deaths due to boric acid poisoning. J. A. M. A. 90:382-383, 1928.

Pfeiffer, C. C.; Hallman, L. F.; Gersh, I. Boric acid ointment. A study of possible intoxication in the treatment of burns. J. A. M. A. 128:266-274, 1945.

Roe, D. A.; McCormick, D. B.; Lin, R. T. Effects of riboflavin on boric acid toxicity. J. Pharm. Sci. 61:1081-1085, 1972.

Rosen, F. S.; Haggerty, R. J. Fatal poisoning from topical use of boric acid powder. N. Engl. J. Med. 255:530-531, 1956.

Rosenkranz, A.; Weissenbacher, G. Borsaurevergiftung beim Neugeborenen. Wien. Klin. Wochenschr. 77:46-50, 1965.

Ross, C. A.; Conway, J. F. The dangers of boric acid. Its use as an irrigant and report of a case. Am. J. Surg. 60:386-395, 1943.

Rubenstein, A. D.; Musher, D. M. Epidemic boric acid poisoning simulating staphylococcal toxic epidermal necrolysis of the newborn infant: Ritter's disease. J. Pediatr. 77:884-887, 1970.

Schmid, R.; Zbinden, J.; Schlatter, C. Zwei Falle von letaler Borsaurevergiftung nach Blasenspulung. Schweiz. Med.

Wschr. 102:83-88, 1972.

Sciarra, J. J. A selective review of boric acid toxicity. J. Am. Pharm. Assoc. 19:494-495, 1958.

Segar, W. E. Peritoneal dialysis in the treatment of boric acid poisoning. N. Engl. J. Med. 262:798-800, 1960.

Skipworth, G. B.; Goldstein, N.; McBride, W. P. Boric acid intoxication from medicated "talcum powder". Arch. Dermatol. 95:83-86, 1967.

Stein, K. M.; Odom, R. B.; Justice, G. R.; Martin, G. C. Toxic alopecia from ingestion of boric acid. Arch. Dermatol. 108:95-97, 1973.

Stolpmann, R.; Hopmann, G. Hamodialyse behandlung einer akuten Borsaurevergiftung. Dtsch. Med. Wochenstr. 100:899-901, 1975.

Valdes-Dapena, M. A.; Arey, J. B. Boric acid poisoning, three fatal cases with pancreatic inclusions and a review of the literature. J. Pediatr. 61:531-546, 1962.

von Schulthess, F. P.; Straub, P. W.; Kistler, H. J. Akute letale Borsaurevergiftung durch Blasenspulung nach Prostatektomie. Schweiz. Med. Wochenschr. 99:1688-1689, 1969.

Weir, R. J.; Fisher, R. S. Toxicologic studies on borax and boric acid. Toxicol. Pharmacol. 23:351-364, 1972.

Wong, L. C.; Heimbach, M. D.; Truscott, D. R.; Duncan, B. D. Boric acid poisoning, report of 11 cases. Can. Med. Assoc. J. 90:1018-1023, 1964.

Young, E. G.; Smith, R. P.; MacIntosh, O. C. Boric acid as a poison. Report of six accidental deaths in infants. Can. Med. Assoc. J. 61:447-450, 1949.

BOTULINAL TOXINS

Botulinal toxins are highly toxic globular proteins elaborated by *Clostridium botulinum*, an anaerobic, spore-forming, Gram-positive rod-shaped bacterium. Ingestion of foodstuffs contaminated with these exotoxins can lead to an acute and often fatal illness called botulism. Prior to ingestion by a susceptible host, the usual sequence of events includes contamination of the food by viable bacilli or more commonly by spores, adequate time and proper conditions for germination of the spores, growth of the organism and production of toxin. Spores survive several months at temperatures as low as 6° C., and even toxin production by the bacteria can occur at 6° C. Spores are destroyed by heating to 120° C. for 30 minutes, whereas the more heat-labile toxin is inactivated at 80° C. for 30 minutes (also 100° C. for 10 minutes). Caution is indicated at high altitude where the boiling temperature of water may be too low to destroy the toxin promptly (Cherington, 1974).

Because about half the known human cases have ended fatally, it is fortunate that botulism is a rare disease and that its incidence in the United States has declined steadily since 1940. In a survey of 659 outbreaks between 1899 and 1969, almost 90% of the cases in which the etiology could be defined involved home-preserved foods (Gangarosa et al., 1971). Since spore germination is inhibited at low pH, acidic foods are less frequently involved. Because strictly anaerobic conditions are not necessary for toxin production, foods other than canned or vacuum-packed varieties may serve as the vector. In the late 1700s and early 1800s the disease was first recognized and associated with the consumption of spoiled sausage (*botulus* is Latin for sausage) in the kingdom of Würtemberg. A raw ham was involved in an 1895 incident in Belgium, which led to the discovery of the cause of botulism (*e.g.*, Rogers, 1963). Various commercially processed foods continue to be implicated in sporadic outbreaks, *e.g.*, smoked fish (Foster et al., 1965), mushroom sauce (Geiger, 1941), soft cheese (Jenzer et al., 1975), liver pate (Reed et al., 1965) and vichyssoise. A history of failure to heat or boil food before consumption is a useful diagnostic clue, but botulinal toxins are not revealed by and not usually associated with an odd or peculiar taste in commercially preserved foods (Werner and Chin, 1973).

Toxicology: Different strains of *C. botulinum* produce six antigenically distinct exotoxins: A, B, C, D, E and F. Types A, B and E have been involved most frequently in human disease, but at least two outbreaks due to type F have been documented. Types C and D are probably capable of causing human disease, but they have been recognized only in birds and nonhuman mammals. Mixed poisonings have been recognized in man, *e.g.*, type A and B together (Dolman, 1974), though a given strain of the organism produces only one toxin type. Type A and B spores are widely distributed in soils throughout the world. In the United States, type A outbreaks tend to occur west of the Mississippi

River and type B outbreaks to the east. Type E disease is found around the Great Lakes and north to Alaska. Type F spores have been identified in marine sediments 100 km. off the Pacific coast (Eklund and Poysky, 1965). Only minor differences are recognized among the syndromes produced in man by the various toxins, and the basic mechanism of poisoning is believed to be the same for all (Lamanna and Carr, 1967).

Bona fide botulism is a true medical emergency, and each hour following ingestion of the toxin is critical to survival. Signs and symptoms can appear as soon as 6 hours after consumption of contaminated food or as late as 8 days, but the usual time lapse is 18 to 36 hours. In general, the shorter the incubation period the more severe and protracted the intoxication (Donadio *et al.*, 1971). The first manifestations are gastrointestinal, particularly in type E poisoning and often in types A or B as well; they include nausea, vomiting, substernal burning or pain, abdominal distension, decreased bowel sounds and sometimes diarrhea followed by constipation. A variety of eye signs may be early features, including blurred vision, diplopia, photophobia, ptosis and mydriasis. Ataxia, generalized weakness and respiratory impairment may signal the onset of a relentlessly progressive bulbar and skeletal muscle paralysis which can lead ultimately to respiratory arrest and death. An important diagnostic triad is the presence of dilated nonreactive pupils, marked dryness of the mouth and tongue and respiratory difficulty (Koenig *et al.*, 1964).

The most common cause of death is paralysis of the muscles of respiration, but occasionally victims succumb to sudden laryngeal obstruction (Whittaker *et al.*, 1964) or unexpected cardiac arrest (Tyler, 1963a). Changes in T waves in patients poisoned by type B toxin support other evidence that the toxin has direct cardiac actions (Koenig *et al.*, 1967). There are strong indications that the toxins can cross the blood-brain barrier and exert direct effects on the central nervous system (Tyler, 1963b). Somnolence was noted in some patients (Koenig *et al.*, 1967), but "excitatory" phenomena were described in another (Tyler, 1963a). Peculiar cyclic changes in the EEG of monkeys that appeared to be independent of dose or time have been observed (Polley *et al.*, 1965).

Despite uncertainties about the molecular weights of the various toxins and the nature of the essential toxophore, it is still probably true that they are "the most poisonous poisons" known to man (Lamanna, 1959). Types A and B toxin furnish about 200×10^6 mouse intraperitoneal lethal doses per mg. of nitrogen. Man is believed to be among the most sensitive of species. The mean lethal dose in man by parenteral routes is estimated to equal 7 mouse lethal doses,

whereas the oral human dose is said to be equivalent to 7000 mouse (intraperitoneal) lethal doses. Such estimates, however, are not helpful to the physician confronting a suspected case of poisoning. Lamanna and Carr (1967) were skeptical of claims that human cases of botulism have resulted from the mere tasting of tainted food, but they admitted that the ingestion of as little as 0.1 ml. of heavily contaminated food might cause the disease. Type A toxin, the first bacterial protein ever to be crystallized, has been described with macabre humor as a "white odorless protein of high molecular weight and unknown taste" (Lamanna, 1959). Even so, investigators have not always used sufficient caution, since at least one human case of botulism is said to have resulted from inhalation of powdered toxin (Holzer, 1962).

Wide individual differences in susceptibility to the toxin add to the uncertainties in estimating the mean lethal dose for man. A common observation in outbreaks is that the disease does not develop in everyone known to have eaten the same contaminated food. Inhomogeneous distribution of toxin within the food or unequal amounts of food consumed might account for some of the differences in susceptibility, but it seems likely that some individuals are inherently more resistant than others. Whatever the basis of that resistance, it clearly is not due to high preexisting titers of antibodies to the toxin (Koenig *et al.*, 1967).

Elegant pharmacological studies have localized the site of action of botulinal toxins to the terminals of cholinergic nerves. In order of decreasing importance in generating clinical signs and symptoms in poisoned humans, cholinergic junctions are found at the ends of motor nerves, of postganglionic parasympathetic fibers within visceral organs, of preganglionic fibers within all autonomic ganglia and of cholinergic neurones in the central nervous system. The central effects of the toxins cannot be related unequivocally to effects on cholinergic nerves. Ganglionic actions *in vivo* appear to be minor; *e.g.*, the arterial blood pressure is usually well sustained in clinical poisonings. Dry mouth, mydriasis, decreased salivary and lacrimal secretions (Jenzer *et al.*, 1975), constipation (or absence of bowel sounds) and urinary retention (Carpenter, 1967; Koenig *et al.*, 1964) are probably due to a blockade of transmission in postganglionic parasympathetic nerves. The eye signs and blockade of secretions are often among the last effects of the toxin to disappear during recovery from poisoning.

In the isolated rat phrenic nerve-diaphragm preparation, Burgen *et al.* (1949) showed that nerve axonal conduction was unaffected by botulinal toxin and that the muscle responded to both direct electrical stimulation and the application of acetylcholine to the region of the motor end-plates. The amount of acetylcholine released by nerve stimulation, however, was greatly reduced, although no alteration in the ultrastructure of the nerve terminal was demonstrable (Thesleff, 1960). Brooks (1956) noted that the toxin causes a reduction in the frequency of miniature end-plate potentials but no change in their amplitude. Shortly after its onset, this effect was partially reversible on repetitive stimulation of the nerve trunk (posttetanic potentiation). Thus the effects of botulinal toxin in some ways resemble those of curare, except that the toxin acts presynaptically and its effects are only occasionally reversed by cholinesterase inhibitors, such as edrophonium or neostigmine (Masland and Gammon, 1949; Ryan and Cherington, 1971). The current view is that the toxin interferes with acetylcholine release from nerve terminals by blocking exocytosis at release sites (Kao et al., 1976).

Because botulism is rare but potentially fatal and because more common but perhaps less life-threatening conditions resemble it, a severe problem in differential diagnosis exists. Diseases likely to be confused with botulism include myasthenia gravis, certain cerebrovascular accidents, tick paralysis, Guillain-Barré syndrome, a variety of chemical intoxications, trichinosis, Eaton-Lambert syndrome, some psychiatric disorders, diphtheritic polyneuritis, acute poliomyelitis and paralytic shellfish poisoning. The dry, red and painful mucous membranes of the mouth, tongue and pharynx are often taken as signs of an upper respiratory infection (Donadio et al., 1971; Werner and Chin, 1973). Important confirmatory tests, such as those for the toxin or the organism and electromyography, are mentioned below under Laboratory.

The toxic infection theory of botulism asserts that in some cases the disease is due to infection of the bowel by C. botulinum and elaboration of the toxin in situ (e.g., Petty, 1965). Most modern authorities have given little credence to this theory (Lamanna and Carr, 1967), but it now appears that the theory has relevance in two special circumstances, namely infant botulism and wound botulism.

Although only a handful of documented cases of botulism in infancy can be found in the recent medical literature (Arnon et al., 1978; McKee et al., 1977; Midura and Arnon, 1976; Pickett et al., 1976; Turner et al., 1978) and infants have long been thought to be less at risk because of their diet, it has been suggested that infant botulism often goes unrecognized and that it may constitute one cause of the sudden infant death syndrome (Arnon et al., 1978). The organism may survive passage through the infant stomach because of its relatively high pH and its relative lack of protease activity (Midura and Arnon,

1976). By food exposure history, honey has been implicated in type B infant botulism, and it should not be fed to infants (Arnon et al., 1979).

Similarly, in a small number of cases of so-called wound botulism, the evidence for infection and endogenous intoxication is quite strong (de Jesus et al., 1973; Merson and Dowell, 1973; Wapen and Gutman, 1974). As noted above, the spores of the organism are widely distributed in soil, and they are potential contaminants of most traumatic wounds. The presence of the organism and/or its toxin have been demonstrated unequivocally in several cases showing the clinical features of botulism, but the conditions necessary for growth and toxin production by the bacillus in wounds have not been defined.

Very little is known about the absorption, distribution and elimination of botulinal toxins in man or animals. Because they are sensitive to tryptic digestion and perhaps to other proteases, the fatal oral dose for man is estimated to be at least 1000 times the fatal parenteral dose (Lamanna and Carr, 1967). For that fraction of ingested toxin that escapes enzymatic hydrolysis, the intestinal mucosa presents a formidable permeability barrier. Even the smallest unit claimed to possess the characteristic toxic effect has a molecular weight of 3,800 (which is still large enough to be called a protein), and one estimate of the molecular weight of type A toxin is 900,000. It would be unusual for molecules of that size to be transported across the intestinal mucosa by ordinary diffusion. In laboratory animals it is known that one route for intestinal absorption of toxin is the lymphatics. Absorbed toxins have very long biological half-lives. They can be detected in blood serum and feces many days after exposure. In one case, fecal specimens contained toxin 32 days after the onset of the disease (Dowell et al., 1977). The possibility that an enterohepatic circulation of toxin may exist does not appear to have been explored. Besides crossing the blood-brain barrier, the toxin crosses the placenta in mice (Hart et al., 1965).

Several adjunctive drugs have been tried in attempts to break through the toxin blockade of cholinergic transmission, but none has been unequivocally successful. As noted above, cholinesterase inhibitors do not always result in improvement, although they have been administered often when the condition was confused with myasthenia gravis (Horwitz et al., 1976). Because guanidine increases the quantity of acetylcholine released at nerve endings by an action potential (Otsuka and Endo, 1960), it was tested as an antagonist to botulinal toxin. In human cases, guanidine has resulted in only mild and transient improvement, if it has been effective at all, but it has no intolerable side effects (Cherington and Ryan, 1970; Faich et al., 1971; Oh et al., 1975; Scaer et al., 1969). Germine diacetate is said to have a veratrinic effect on skeletal muscle. It appears to act postsynaptically, so that a single nerve action potential gives rise to multiple muscle action potentials (repetitive firings). Its effects in clinical botulism have been disappointing, as also were the effects of high parenteral doses of corticosteroids (Cherington and Schultz, 1977) and intravenous calcium salts (Cherington and Ginsberg, 1971).

The treatment of choice is the use of type-specific or polyvalent antitoxin, but even here the antitoxin must be given as soon as possible after diagnosis, and its use should be combined with good supportive care, of which respiratory support is the most important (Oberst et al., 1968; Merson et al., 1974). Modern treatment has reduced the fatality rate to 25 to 40% for adults and 10% for children and teenagers. Enormous amounts of the horse serum antitoxin have been given without toxic effects (Sutherland, 1960), but serum sickness and other reactions should always be anticipated. Toxoids for active immunization have been prepared for the protection of laboratory workers exposed to toxins, but the disease in the general population is so rare that its indiscriminate use cannot be justified (Lamanna and Carr, 1967).

Other bacterial food poisonings: The three most common types of bacterial food poisoning are due to *Staphylococcus*, *Clostridium perfringens* (formerly *C. welchii*) and *Salmonella*. *Salmonella* species give rise to the infectious type of food poisoning, which requires the ingestion of large numbers of living organisms and their subsequent multiplication in the gastrointestinal tract. Some species of *Shigella* induce a similar syndrome, but they are less frequently associated with food or water as the vehicle. The incubation period is 24 to 48 hours, and the cardinal signs and symptoms are headache, nausea, vomiting and abdominal pain. Since the process is infective, fever is a helpful finding. Positive diagnosis depends on isolation and identification of the organism, and fecal specimens should be cultured before antibiotic therapy is started (Taylor and McCoy, 1969).

In the toxin type of bacterial food poisoning, such as that associated with *Staphylococcus*, the period between ingestion and illness is only 1 to 6 hours. The syndrome is characterized by abdominal cramping pain with violent and often repeated vomiting. Diarrhea is variable, and although the syndrome is violent, it is usually short-lived, subsiding in 6 to 8 hours and rarely lasting more than 24. Staphylococcal food poisoning is the most common type in the United States. It is occasionally life-threatening in the elderly or those suffering from other serious disease (*e.g.*, Currier *et al.*, 1973). Staphylococcal toxins are heat-stable, and a period of slow cooling or holding at ambient temperatures may provide an opportunity for growth of the organism and elaboration of toxin. In severe cases treatment is directed toward relieving shock, replacing fluid and electrolyte losses and controlling the vomiting and diarrhea (Angelotti, 1969).

Perhaps a third of all reported cases of food poisoning in the United States and England are due to *C. perfringens*. The incubation period is 8 to 12 hours after ingestion, and the main feature is diarrhea and griping abdominal pain. Nausea and vomiting are inconstant findings, and fever is absent. The illness is not severe and rarely lasts longer than 24 hours. It usually involves a meat or poultry product that was originally cooked but then inadequately refrigerated or reheated prior to serving (Loewenstein, 1972). *Bacillus cereus* produces a very similar illness (Hobbs, 1969; Terranova and Blake, 1978).

Outbreaks due to *Vibrio parahaemolyticus* are common in Japan and have been recently reported in the United States in the summer months. These have been associated with raw fish or shellfish. As with staphylococcal and perfringens food poisonings, the disease is rarely fatal (Sakazaki, 1969). The "turista" or "Montezuma's revenge" is a well-known diarrhea experienced by travelers in Mexico. This syndrome has been ascribed recently to a heat-labile enterotoxin secreted by some strains of *Escherichia coli* often found on raw vegetables (Merson *et al.*, 1976).

Chemical food poisonings: Storage of acidic foods in galvanized or enameled metal containers sometimes leads to acute gastric irritation, nausea, vomiting and diarrhea due to contamination of the food or drink with such metals as CADMIUM (p. III-77), COPPER (p. III-120) or zinc or antimony (see Section II).

Symptomatology (of botulism):
1. Nausea, vomiting, substernal burning or pain, abdominal distension, decreased bowel sounds and sometimes diarrhea followed by constipation.
2. Blurred vision, diplopia, photophobia, mydriasis, ptosis, nystagmus, loss of light reflex.
3. Lassitude, dizziness, vertigo, ataxia, generalized weakness and respiratory difficulty.
4. Decreased lacrimal and salivary secretions; dry, red and painful mucous membranes of mouth, tongue and pharynx.
5. Difficulty in swallowing, difficulty in speech, paralysis of pharyngeal muscles and muscles of the neck.
6. Urinary retention, particularly in type E poisoning.
7. Death due to paralysis of the muscles of respiration.
8. If infection can be avoided and if artificial ventilation can be sustained, recovery can

be expected, but disabling symptoms may persist for weeks or months.

Treatment:

1. At the first signs of involvement of the bulbar muscles, the patient should be hospitalized in an intensive care unit with arrangements made for respiratory assistance. A tracheostomy may become necessary and should be prepared for (p. IV-6). In the presence of hypoventilation, mechanical assistance in breathing is imperative (pp. IV-7-12).

2. If food was recently ingested, give by mouth syrup of ipecac (p. I-2), or if signs of abdominal wall paresis or esophageal dysfunction have developed, a nasogastric tube may be passed for lavage.

3. Unless paralytic ileus is present, give sodium sulfate by mouth to purge the colon of unabsorbed toxin. High colonic enemas are also recommended. Fecal specimens should be saved for analysis for toxin or identification of organism.

4. After the risks of giving equine antitoxin have been carefully weighed, sensitivity tests should be conducted. Epinephrine should be available to counteract a sensitivity reaction. Trivalent ABE antitoxin is given in cases where the toxin type is unknown. Monovalent type E antitoxin should be reserved for proved outbreaks of the E type. Bivalent AB antitoxin should be used if either type A or B or both have been established as the cause. The USPHS Communicable Disease Center in Atlanta can be phoned for advice on sources of the antitoxin.

5. Guanidine hydrochloride (15 to 40 mg./day by mouth) has been recommended. Failure to observe beneficial effects does not rule out a diagnosis of botulism. Improvement is more notable in ocular muscles than in respiratory muscles (Puggiari and Cherington, 1978).

6. Because toxin is known to exist in the alimentary tract for long periods, possibly because of its enterohepatic circulation, repeated doses of activated charcoal or possibly cholestyramine by mouth unless paralytic ileus is severe.

7. Because the block at neuromuscular junctions is delayed experimentally by cold, a therapeutic trial with hypothermia should be considered.

8. Antibiotics at the earliest sign of infection. Pneumonia is frequently the proximal cause of death in botulism. See p. IV-86.

9. Fluids and electrolytes as indicated.

Laboratory:

1. Plasma and fecal samples should be collected for analysis by the Communicable Disease Center in Atlanta, Georgia, or by any closer laboratory with the capability of assaying botulinal toxins or detecting *C. botulinum* by growing them in culture (Boroff and Fleck, 1965).

2. Electromyography is said to be helpful in the diagnosis (Gutman and Pratt, 1976).

References:

Angelotti, R. Staphylococcal intoxications. In *Food-borne Infections and Intoxications.* Edited by H. Riemann. Academic Press, New York, 1969.

Arnon, S. S.; Midura, T. F.; Damus, K.; Thompson, B.; Wood, R. M.; Chin, T. Honey and other environmental risk factors for infant botulism. J. Pediatr. *94*:331-338, 1979.

Arnon, S. S.; Midura, T. F.; Damus, K.; Wood, R. M.; Chin, J. Intestinal infection and toxin production by *Clostridium botulinum* as one cause of sudden infant death syndrome. Lancet *1*:1273-1277, 1978.

Boroff, D. A.; Fleck, U. Studies of the toxin *Clostridium botulinum.* Int. Arch. Allergy *27*:1-5, 1965.

Brooks, V. B. An intracellular study of the action of repetitive nerve volleys and of botulism toxin on miniature end plate potentials. J. Physiol. *134*:264-277, 1956.

Burgen, A. S. V.; Dickens, F.; Zatman, L. J. The action of botulinum toxin on the neuromuscular junction. J. Physiol. *109*:10-24, 1949.

Carpenter, F. G. Motor responses of the urinary bladder and skeletal muscle in botulinum intoxicated rats. J. Physiol. *188*:1-11, 1967.

Cherington, M. Botulism, ten-year experience. Arch. Neurol. *30*:432-437, 1974.

Cherington, M.; Ginsberg, S. Type B botulism: Neurophysiologic studies. Neurology *21*:43-46, 1971.

Cherington, M.; Ryan, D. W. Treatment of botulism with guanidine: Early neurophysiologic studies. N. Engl. J. Med. *282*:195-197, 1970.

Cherington, M.; Schultz, D. Effect of guanidine, germine and steroids in a case of botulism. Clin. Toxicol. *11*:19-25, 1977.

Currier, R. W.; Taylor, A., Jr.; Wolf, F. S.; Warr, M. Fatal staphylococcal food poisoning. South. Med. J. *66*:703-705, 1973.

de Jesus, P. V.; Slater, R.; Spitz, L. K.; Penn, A. S. Neuromuscular physiology of wound botulism. Arch. Neurol. *29*:425-431, 1973.

Dolman, C. E. Human botulism in Canada (1919-1973). Can. Med. Assoc. J. *110*:191-197, 1974.

Donadio, J. A.; Gangarosa, E. J.; Faich, G. A. Diagnosis and treatment of botulism. J. Infect. Dis. *124*:108-112, 1971.

Dowell, V. R.; McCroskey, L. M.; Hatheway, C. L.; Lombard, G. L.; Hughes, J. M.; Merson, M. H. Coproexamination for botulinal toxin and *Clostridium botulinum,* a new procedure for laboratory diagnosis of botulism. J. A. M. A. *238*:1829-1832, 1977.

Eklund, M. W.; Poysky, F. *Clostridium botulinum* Type F from marine sediments. Science *149*:306, 1965.

Faich, G. A.; Graebner, R. W.; Sato, S. Failure of guanidine therapy in botulism A. N. Engl. J. Med. *285*:773-776, 1971.

Foster, E. M.; Deffner, J. S.; Bott, T. L.; McCoy, E. *Clostridium botulinum* food poisoning. J. Milk Food Technol. *28*:86-91, 1965.

Gangarosa, E. J.; Donadio, J. A.; Armstrong, R. W.; Meyer, K. F.; Brachman, P. S.; Dowell, V. R. Botulism in the United States, 1899-1969. Am. J. Epidemiol. *93*:93-101, 1971.

Geiger, J. C. An outbreak of botulism. J. A. M. A. *117*:22, 1941.

Gutman, L.; Pratt, L. Pathophysiologic aspects of human botulism. Arch. Neurol. *33*:175-179, 1976.

Hart, L. G.; Dixson, R. L.; Long, J. P.; Mackay, B. Studies using *Clostridium botulinum* toxin Type A. Toxicol. Appl. Pharmacol. *7*:84-89, 1965.

Hobbs, B. C. *Clostridium perfringens* and *Bacillus cereus* infections. In *Food-borne Infections and Intoxications.* Edited by H. Riemann. Academic Press, New York, 1969.

Holzer, E. Botulismus durch Inhalation. Med. Klin. *41*:1735-1740, 1962.

Horwitz, M. A.; Hatheway, C. L.; Dowell, V. R. Laboratory confirmation of botulism complicated by pyridostigmine treatment of patient. Am. J. Clin. Pathol. 66:737-742, 1976.

Jenzer, G.; Mumenthaler, M.; Ludin, H. P.; Robert, F. Autonomic dysfunction in botulism B: A clinical report. Neurology 25:150-153, 1975.

Kao, I.; Prachman, D. B.; Price, D. L. Botulinum toxin: Mechanism of presynaptic blockade. Science 193:1256-1258, 1976.

Koenig, M. G.; Drutz, D. J.; Muchlin, A. I.; Schaffner, W.; Rogers, D. E. Type B botulism in man. Am. J. Med. 42:208-219, 1967.

Koenig, M. G.; Spickard, A.; Cardella, M. A.; Rogers, D. E. Clinical and laboratory observations on type E botulism in man. Medicine 43:517-545, 1964.

Lamanna, C. The most poisonous poison. Science 130:763-772, 1959.

Lamanna, C.; Carr, C. J. The botulinal, tetanal and enterostaphylococcal toxins: A review. Clin. Pharmacol. Ther. 8:286-332, 1967.

Loewenstein, M. S. Epidemiology of Clostridium perfringens food poisoning. N. Engl. J. Med. 286:1006-1008, 1972.

Masland, R. L.; Gammon, G. D. The effect of botulinus toxin on the electromyogram. J. Pharmacol. Exp. Ther. 97:499-506, 1949.

McKee, K. T.; Kilroy, A. W.; Harrison, W. W.; Schaffner, W. Botulism in infancy - Report of a case. Am. J. Dis. Child. 131:857-859, 1977.

Merson, M. H.; Dowell, V. R. Epidemiologic, clinical and laboratory aspects of wound botulism. N. Engl. J. Med. 289:3-8, 1973.

Merson, M. H.; Hughes, J. M.; Dowell, V. R.; Taylor, A.; Barker, W. H.; Gangarosa, E. J. Current trends in botulism in the United States. J. A. M. A. 229:1305-1308, 1974.

Merson, M. H.; Morris, G. R.; Sack, D. A.; Wells, J. G.; Feeley, J. C.; Sack, R. B.; Creech, W. B.; Kapikian, A. Z.; Gangarosa, E. J. Travelers' diarrhea in Mexico. A prospective study of physicians and family members attending a Congress. N. Engl. J. Med. 294:1299-1305, 1976.

Midura, T. F.; Arnon, S. S. Infant botulism: Identification of Clostridium botulinum and its toxins in faeces. Lancet 3:934-936, 1976.

Oberst, F. W.; Crook, J. W.; Cresthull, P.; House, M. J. Evaluation of botulinum antitoxin, supportive therapy, and artificial respiration in monkeys with experimental botulism. Clin. Pharmacol. Ther. 9:209-214, 1968.

Oh, S. J.; Halsey, J. H., Jr.; Briggs, D. D. Guanidine in type B botulism. Arch. Intern. Med. 135:726-728, 1975.

Otsuka, M.; Endo, M. The effect of guanidine on neuromuscular transmission. J. Pharmacol. Exp. Ther. 128:273-282, 1960.

Petty, C. S. Botulism: The disease and the toxin. Am. J. Med. Sci. 249:345-359, 1965.

Pickett, J.; Berg, B.; Chaplin, E.; Brunstetter-Shafer, M. -A. Botulism in infancy: Clinical and electrophysiologic study. N. Engl. J. Med. 295:770-772, 1976.

Polley, E. H.; Vick, J. A.; Ciuchta, H. P.; Fischetti, D. A.; Macchitelli, F. J.; Montanarelli, N. Botulinum toxin, type A: Effects on central nervous system. Science 147:1036-1037, 1965.

Puggiari, M.; Cherington, M. Botulism and guanidine, ten years later. J. A. M. A. 240:2276-2277, 1978.

Reed, R. W.; Butas, C. A.; Gall, R. J. Human botulism due to commercial products. Can. Med. Assoc. J. 93:244-247, 1965.

Rogers, D. E. Botulism, vintage 1963 (Editorial). Ann. Intern. Med. 61:581-588, 1963.

Ryan, D. W.; Cherington, M. Human type A botulism. J. A. M. A. 216:513-514, 1971.

Sakazaki, R. Halophilic Vibrio infections. In Food-borne Infections and Intoxications. Edited by H. Riemann. Academic Press, New York, 1969.

Scaer, R. C.; Tooker, J.; Cherington, M. Effect of guanidine on the neuromuscular block of botulism. Neurology 19:1107-1110, 1969.

Sutherland, H. P. Report of a case of botulinus poisoning. J. A. M. A. 172:1266-1269, 1960.

Taylor, J.; McCoy, J. H. Salmonella and Arizona infections. In Food-borne Infections and Intoxications. Edited by H. Riemann. Academic Press, New York, 1969.

Terranova, W.; Blake, P. A. Bacillus cereus food poisoning. N. Engl. J. Med. 298:143-144, 1978.

Thesleff, S. Supersensitivity of skeletal muscle produced by botulinum toxin. J. Physiol. 151:598-607, 1960.

Turner, H. D.; Brett, E. M.; Gilbert, R. J.; Ghosh, A. C. Infant botulism in England. Lancet 1:1277-1278, 1978.

Tyler, H. R. Botulism. Arch. Neurol. 9:652-660, 1963a.

Tyler, H. R. Physiological observations in human botulism. Arch. Neurol. 9:661-670, 1963b.

Wapen, B. D.; Gutman, L. Wound botulism. A case report. J. A. M. A. 227:1416-1417, 1974.

Werner, S. B.; Chin, J. Botulism - diagnosis, management and public health considerations. Calif. Med. 118:84-88, 1973.

Whittaker, R. L.; Gilbertson, R. B.; Garrett, A. S., Jr. Botulism, Type E. Report of eight simultaneous cases. Ann. Intern. Med. 61:448-454, 1964.

BROMATE

Bromate poisoning was formerly a clinical rarity, but in the 1940s and 1950s potassium (and less often sodium) bromate was marketed as a "neutralizer" in home permanent cold wave hair kits (Anon., 1950). Several cases of accidental poisoning in children resulted from the ingestion of these clear, odorless, and reputedly tasteless bromate solutions. Manufacturers have since substituted less toxic substances as neutralizers (e.g., sodium perborate and sodium hexametaphosphate). Potassium bromate is sometimes used as a bread improver; sugar contaminated with it was the source of an outbreak of mild food poisoning in New Zealand (Paul, 1966).

Chlorates are less toxic than bromates but produce somewhat similar poisonings. Potassium chlorate has been used in throat gargles, some dentrifices (Bernstein, 1930; Oliver et al., 1951), in match heads (Vahlqvist, 1961) and

fireworks. The latter attests to the flammability of chlorates. Clothing contaminated with sodium chlorate when sprayed as a herbicide caused death when it was accidentally ignited (Dalgaard-Mikkelsen and Poulsen, 1962). It is still encountered today as a weed killer (Helliwell and Nunn, 1979).

Toxicology of bromate salts: The mean lethal dose of potassium bromate ($KBrO_3$) has not been definitely established, but a few ounces (2 to 4) of a 2% solution have caused serious poisonings in children ranging in age from 1½ to 3 years (Kitto and Dumars, 1949; Thompson and Westfall, 1949; Parker and Barr, 1951). A 19-month-old boy died after consuming an unknown amount (Dunsky, 1947), but a 14-year-old girl survived after ingesting what may have been all (14.2 gm.) of the potassium bromate in one commercial cold wave kit (Robertson et al.,

1950). Rabbits died about 12 hours after the oral administration of 0.5 gm./kg. of sodium bromate (Santesson and Wickberg, 1913).

Death in man (Dunsky, 1947) and in animals (Santesson and Wickberg, 1913) is apparently due to acute renal failure resulting from the nephrotoxic action of the bromate ion. Renal tubular necrosis with flattening of the proximal convoluted tubular epithelium and interstitial edema has been noted. In Dunsky's case (1947) the liver was also involved with cloudy swelling and karyolysis, and histological evidence of a mild toxic myocarditis was reported. In most severe poisonings in children, oliguria or anuria was noted on the 1st or 2nd day, but urine formation reappeared spontaneously on the 3rd or 4th day (Kitto and Dumars, 1949; Parker and Barr, 1951; Thompson and Westfall, 1949). Albuminuria and other evidence of impaired renal function, however, persisted for days or weeks, and convalescence was slow.

Nausea and vomiting were almost always noted, usually with epigastric pain. Diarrhea occurred sometimes and hematemesis was reported once (Parker and Barr, 1951). These effects have been ascribed to the caustic actions of bromic acid and bromine produced by stomach acid acting on the bromate ion (Santesson and Wickberg, 1913). When potassium bromate was incubated at 38° C. in normal gastric juice, however, Parker and Barr (1951) failed to find either bromine or bromide ion unless the pH was reduced below 1.

A third category of toxic responses to the bromate ion involves the central nervous system. In poisoned animals, Santesson and Wickberg (1913) described various states of central nervous depression. Until the stage of azotemia was reached, however, most poisoned children showed little more than transient restlessness and then apathy or mild lethargy. The exception was Thompson and Westfall's case (1949) of a 2½-year-old boy who was comatose and flaccid 4 hours after swallowing half a glass of potassium bromate solution. Generalized convulsions have been described but only during the stage of severe renal failure (Thompson and Westfall, 1949; Dunsky, 1947).

Like chlorates, bromates are surprisingly stable in the body and are excreted as such by the kidneys. The only hint of extensive reduction *in vivo* is the single observation by Kitto and Dumars (1949) of a high bromide level in the blood of a boy who had consumed potassium bromate. Because bromate is present and relatively stable in blood plasma, hemodialysis and peritoneal lavage may constitute useful treatment measures, as is probably true in chlorate poisoning in man (Jackson *et al.*, 1961; Pringle and Smith, 1964; Schreiner, 1958). Exchange transfusion has been successfully employed in combination with dialysis for treatment of chlorate poisoning (Klendshoj *et al.*, 1962; Knight *et al.*, 1967).

To reduce the highly toxic bromate ion to the relatively innocuous bromide ion, the intravenous administration of sodium thiosulfate has been recommended. Thiosulfate has also been used as a lavage fluid, but Parker and Barr (1951) believe that, when it reacts with bromate in the presence of stomach acid, highly toxic hydrogen sulfide is formed. For this reason it is probably inadvisable to leave a thiosulfate solution in the stomach after gastric lavage for the removal of ingested chlorate or bromate salts.

At various times methemoglobin formation has also been ascribed to bromates (Sollmann, 1957), but Santesson and Wickberg (1913) were unable to detect methemoglobinemia in bromate-poisoned dogs, rabbits, or guinea pigs, although discolorations at the injection site and in certain tissues suggested the local formation of abnormal blood pigments. In more than half a dozen cases of bromate poisoning reported in the clinical literature, methemoglobinemia was not encountered, although it was sought in at least a cursory way in most of these cases. Robertson *et al.*, (1950), however, reported a moderate degree of sickling and vacuolization of red blood cells in one case. Until more sophisticated studies of blood pigments and red cell injuries have been performed, the danger of methemoglobinemia and hemolysis cannot be properly evaluated in bromate-poisoned patients.

Toxicology of chlorate salts: The mean lethal dose of a chlorate salt by mouth has been established to be 20 to 30 gm. in human adults (Witthaus, 1911), but others would place this figure at 8 gm. (Ansbacher, 1931; Bernstein, 1930). Witthaus (1911) believed that children and infants were more sensitive than adults. A serious illness was incurred by one teenager who ingested a minute amount (Stavrou *et al.*, 1978). Mortality in one series of untreated cases was 80%, with death occurring generally on the 4th day after ingestion (Witthaus, 1911). Even in a more modern series of cases (Helliwell and Nunn, 1979), mortality was 64%. Death occurred with doses above 100 gm. irrespective of treatment. Supportive care alone was successful in only one case, in which the amount ingested was well below the lethal dose.

Chlorate salts induce most if not all the toxic reactions of bromate salts (Dérot *et al.*, 1948), but central nervous depression may be less intense in chlorate poisoning. In addition, severe intravascular hemolysis and "methemoglobinemia" are prominent features of chlorate poisoning, although they may not become apparent until several hours after ingestion (Ansbacher, 1931; Cochrane and Smith, 1940; Davies, 1956;

Ehrhardt, 1952; Gettler and St. George, 1935; Jackson *et al.*, 1961; Klendshoj *et al.*, 1962; Knight *et al.*, 1967).

Methemoglobinemia may be delayed because hemolysis is a prerequisite to hemoglobin oxidation. At least lysed human red cells *in vitro* showed much more methemoglobin formation with chlorate than did intact erythrocytes; indeed, the latter mixture contained methemoglobin only after hemolysis was prominent (Richardson, 1937). Gordon and Brown (1947) noted that washed red cells from their patient contained mostly oxyhemoglobin, whereas the plasma pigment was almost all methemoglobin. Because the "methemoglobin" is largely extracorpuscular, methylene blue has little or no effect in promoting its conversion to hemoglobin (Lee *et al.*, 1970). Indeed, methylene blue may intensify oxidative hemolysis. Many patients have received the drug without notable benefit (Bloxham *et al.*, 1979; Helliwell and Nunn, 1979).

Methemalbumin and Heinz bodies also contribute to the abnormal appearance of the blood (Davies, 1956; Knight *et al.*, 1967; Trincao *et al.*, 1952). Ulrich and Shertnor (1928) found that the *in vitro* methemoglobin-forming activity of a series of chlorate salts increased in the following order: potassium, sodium, calcium, magnesium.

In both man and animals, systemic signs of toxicity precede the blood changes, which are usually incidental to the major cause of death, acute renal failure. Probably bromate, chlorate and iodate (see below) are all direct nephrotoxins, but the renal lesion is undoubtedly aggravated by intravascular hemolysis in the case of chlorate. Acidosis has been inferred in some poisoned animals (Richardson, 1937); it intensifies the renal damage which can be induced by high levels of plasma methemoglobin (Bing, 1943).

Toxicology of iodate salts: No human ingestions of iodate salts can be cited, but animal experiments suggest that these compounds share the nephrotoxic and hemolytic potential of chlorate and bromate. Large doses by mouth regularly produced emesis in fasted dogs, but when this action was blocked by morphine pretreatment, the minimal lethal dose was estimated as 200 to 250 mg./kg. (Webster *et al.*, 1966). Nonspecific fatty changes were noted in the viscera, together with necrotic lesions in the liver, kidney, gastrointestinal mucosa and urinary bladder. Irreversible retinal degeneration also occurred.

When fed to dogs for several months, potassium iodate in doses up to 60 to 90 mg./kg. per day were tolerated, and pathological findings were confined to hemosiderin deposits in the spleen, liver and kidneys. There was no evidence of methemoglobin formation (Webster *et al.*, 1966). Iodate salts are 3 to 6 times more acutely toxic to mice than iodide salts. Potassium and

sodium iodate have about the same LD_{50} and produce death in acute renal failure. Sometimes hemoglobinuria preceded renal shutdown (Webster *et al.*, 1957). Mice were found to tolerate each day more than the LD_{50} when administered in divided doses (Webster *et al.*, 1959). Parenteral administration had no effect on gastric pH, but oral administration to mice increased the pH of gastric contents (Webster *et al.*, 1957).

Symptomatology:

1. Nausea, vomiting, diarrhea, abdominal or gastric pain, dyspnea. Mucosal irritation by bromate and chlorate does not usually lead to ulceration.
2. Restlessness and later apathy. Severe central nervous depression is common in poisoned animals but is not prominent in clinical poisonings until uremia is advanced.
3. Methemoglobin formation and hemolysis, which develop slowly at first, are prominent features of chlorate poisoning; they may or may not occur in bromate poisoning (see above). Cyanosis and later icterus, yielding a greenish hue to skin and mucous membranes.
4. Lumbar pain, oliguria, and albuminuria, progressing to anuria and azotemia within a few hours or a few days.
5. Death from renal failure, usually within 1 to 2 weeks.

Treatment:

1. Syrup of ipecac or gastric lavage with tap water or perhaps with a 1% solution of sodium thiosulfate.
2. Administer a demulcent and an analgesic like meperidine (Demerol). Avoid morphine.
3. If readily available, the prompt use of hemodialysis or peritoneal lavage may serve to remove absorbed but unreacted bromate in significant amounts. See pp. IV-55–57.
4. Administer oxygen. If methemoglobinemia becomes severe, a replacement transfusion with whole blood may become essential.
5. Do not attempt to correct methemoglobinemia with methylene blue because this dye may enhance the toxicity.
6. Sodium thiosulfate solution (100 to 500 ml. of 1%) by intravenous drip has been recommended; see text above.
7. Correct dehydration by infusing intravenously a glucose solution (5% in water). Avoid electrolytes (except as above) unless acid-base imbalance or shock becomes severe.
8. Supportive treatment of acute renal failure (see p. IV-53).

Laboratory:

1. Bromate may be detected in blood and urine. If this test is impractical, an analysis

for the presence of bromide may help to establish the diagnosis (Kitto and Dumars, 1949).

2. Periodic measurements of the oxygen-carrying capacity of blood are desirable, as well as a spectroscopic search for abnormal blood pigments. Neutrophils may contain basic staining material, perhaps due to phagocytized red cells. (Bloxham *et al.*, 1979).

3. Repeated urinalysis may reveal albumin, hemoglobin, red blood cells, and cellular casts.

4. Hyperkalemia due to massive hemolysis.

References:

Anon. (Editorials and Comments.). Neutralizers in home permanent waving kits. J. A. M. A. *144*:397, 1950.

Ansbacher, S. A case of poisoning by potassium chlorate. J. A. M. A. *96*:1681, 1931.

Bernstein, R. Kaliumklorat Vergiftung. Arch. Toxikol. *1*:15, 1930.

Bing, R. J. Etiology of renal failure following crush injuries. Proc. Soc. Exp. Biol. Med. *53*:29-30, 1943.

Bloxham, C. A.; Wright, N.; Hoult, J. G. Self-poisoning by sodium-chlorate - some unusual features. Clin. Toxicol. *15*:185-188, 1979.

Cochrane, W. J.; Smith, R. P. A fatal case of accidental poisoning by chlorate of potassium, with a review of the literature. Can. Med. Assoc. J. *42*:23-26, 1940.

Dalgaard-Mikkelsen, S.; Poulsen, E. Toxicology of herbicides. Pharmacol. Rev. *14*:225-250, 1962.

Davies, P. Potassium chlorate poisoning with oliguria treated by the Bull regime. Lancet *1*:612-613, 1956.

Derot, M.; Derobert, L.; Girard, M.; Dupeyron, T.; Menager, M. J. L'intoxication par le chlorate de sodium. Sem. Hop. Paris *24*:719-730, 1948.

Dunsky, I. Potassium bromate poisoning. Am. J. Dis. Child. *74*:730-734, 1947.

Ehrhardt, L. Todliche Natriumchloratvergiftung zweier Saugelinge. Zentralbl. Gesamte Rechtsmed. *41*:96-104, 1952.

Gettler, A. O.; St. George, A. V. Toxicology in children. Am. J. Clin. Pathol. *5*:466-488, 1935.

Gordon, S.; Brown, J. A. H. Potassium chlorate poisoning, report of a case. Lancet *2*:503-504, 1947.

Helliwell, M.; Nunn, J. Mortality in sodium chlorate poisoning. Br. Med. J. *169*:1119-1121, 1979.

Jackson, R. C.; Elder, W. J.; McDonnell, H. Sodium chlorate poisoning. Lancet *2*:1381-1383, 1961.

Kitto, W.; Dumars, K. W. Potassium bromate poisoning. J. Pediatr. *35*:197-200, 1949.

Klendshoj, N. C.; Burke, W. J.; Anthone, R.; Anthone, S. Chlorate poisoning. J. A. M. A. *180*:1133-1134, 1962.

Knight, R. K.; Trounce, J. R.; Cameron, J. S. Suicidal chlorate poisoning treated with peritoneal dialysis. Br. Med. J. *2*:601-602, 1967.

Lee, D. B. N.; Brown, D. L.; Baker, L. R. I. Haematological complications of chlorate poisoning. Br. Med. J. *2*:31-32, 1970.

Oliver, J.; MacDowell, M.; Tracy, A. The pathogenesis of acute renal failure associated with traumatic and toxic injury. Renal ischemia, nephrotoxic damage and the ischemic episode. J. Clin. Invest. *30*:1306-1351, 1951.

Parker, W. A.; Barr, J. R. Potassium bromate poisoning. Br. Med. J. *1*:1363-1364, 1951.

Paul, A. H. Chemical food poisoning by potassium bromate. N. Z. Med. J. *65*:33-36, 1966.

Pringle, A.; Smith, E. K. M. Daily peritoneal dialysis in renal failure. Br. J. Urol. *36*:493-500, 1964.

Richardson, A. P. Toxic potentialities of continued administration of chlorate for blood and tissues. J. Pharmacol. Exp. Ther. *59*:101-113, 1937.

Robertson, H. F.; Flothow, M. W., Jr.; Kissen, M. D. Potassium bromate poisoning. Report of a case. J. Pediatr. *36*:241-243, 1950.

Santesson, C. G.; Wickberg, G. Uber Wirkungen von Natriumbromat. Skand. Arch. Physiol. *30*:337-374, 1913.

Schreiner, G. E. The role of hemodialysis (artificial kidney) in acute poisoning. Arch. Intern. Med. *102*:896-913, 1958.

Sollmann, T. *A Manual of Pharmacology*. 8th Ed., W. B. Saunders Co., Philadelphia, 1957.

Stavrou, A.; Butcher, R.; Sakula, A. Accidental self-poisoning by sodium chlorate weed-killer. Practitioner *221*:397-399, 1978.

Thompson, H. C.; Westfall, S. W. Potassium bromate poisoning. Report of a case due to ingestion of a "cold wave" neutralizer. J. Pediatr. *34*:362-364, 1949.

Trincao, C.; Madeira, F.; Parreira, R.; Goncalves, E.; Diniz, J. T. Etude hematologique d'un cas d'intoxication aigue par le chlorate de potassium. Sang *23*:81-86, 1952.

Ulrich, R.; Shertnor, S. T. The action of chlorates, in particular potassium chlorate, on blood in animals. J. Pharmacol. Exp. Ther. *34*:391-406, 1928.

Vahlquist, B. PicA of matches. Acta Paediatr. Scand. *50*:319, 1961.

Webster, S. H.; Rice, M. E.; Highman, B.; Stohlman, E. F. The toxicology of potassium and sodium iodates. II. Subacute toxicity of potassium iodate in mice and guinea pigs. Toxicol. Appl. Pharmacol. *1*:87-96, 1959.

Webster, S. H.; Rice, M. E.; Highman, B.; von Oettingen, W. F. The toxicology of potassium and sodium iodates: Acute toxicity in mice. J. Pharmacol. Exp. Ther. *120*:171-178, 1957.

Webster, S. H.; Stohlman, E. F.; Highman, B. The toxicology of potassium and sodium iodates. III. Acute and subacute oral toxicity of potassium iodate in dogs. Toxicol. Appl. Pharmacol. *8*:185-192, 1966.

Witthaus, R. A. *Manual of Toxicology*. Wm. Wood & Co., New York, 1911.

CADMIUM

Cadmium is primarily produced as a by-product of zinc-smelting operations. Metallic cadmium is used as a rustproof plating for iron, as a constituent of various alloys, in the production of phosphors and pigments, as a plastic stabilizer, in nickel-cadmium batteries and in a variety of metallurgical processes (Tierney *et al.*, 1980). The use of cadmium-lined containers for food and beverage is banned in several states because of the tendency of the metal to dissolve when in contact with acid foods, with the production of poisonous concentrations of cadmium salts. Many nonfatal cases of "food poisoning" have followed the ingestion of such foods kept even for brief periods in coated containers, such as ice cube trays and metal pitchers (Baker and Hafner, 1961; Frant and Kleeman, 1941; Schifter and Mahler, 1943).

Welding (or cutting as with an acetylene torch) cadmium-plated or cadmium-containing metal objects constitutes a very significant and potentially lethal hazard after even short exposures (see below). The same is true for brazing or silver-soldering with cadmium-containing rods or wires. Some silver solders contain more than 20% cadmium (Lucas *et al.*, 1980). In its early stages this syndrome may be confused with a much more benign illness caused by exposure to the fumes of zinc and some other metals (see Metal Fumes in Section II).

Cadmium constitutes a significant environmental pollutant, and humans are exposed through food, water, air and, especially, heavy smoking (Adamsson *et al.*, 1979; Friberg *et al.*, 1971).

Toxicology: Acute poisoning may result from the inhalation of cadmium dusts and fumes (usually cadmium oxide) and from the ingestion of cadmium salts. When swallowed, cadmium compounds are much less lethal than when inhaled, in part because they induce vomiting and so are not retained. Although as little as 10 to 20 mg. of soluble cadmium salts have produced severe toxic symptoms when ingested, death probably requires several hundred milligrams by the oral route (Schwartze and Alsberg, 1923).

The dangerous actions following acute inhalation of dust or fumes are limited initially to the lungs and respiratory mucosa. Edema and necrosis of the pulmonary epithelium are described, and in the dog three clinical stages are recognized: (1) acute pulmonary edema developing within 24 hours and reaching its maximum within 3 days, (2) proliferative interstitial pneumonitis lasting from approximately the 3rd to the 10th day, and (3) permanent lung damage consisting of perivascular and peribronchial fibrosis (Paterson, 1947). Except for the latter, a similar sequence is inferred from clinical observations and human autopsy material (Beton *et al.*, 1966; Blejer *et al.*, 1966; Patwardhan and Finckh, 1976; Spolyar *et al.*, 1944; Zavon and Meadow, 1970). The inhalation of 40 mg. of cadmium with the pulmonary retention of 4 mg. has been estimated to be fatal in man (Barrett *et al.*, 1947; Barrett and Card, 1947). Fumes may be anticipated to be more toxic than dusts or aerosols, but all are highly dangerous. Finely divided metallic cadmium of a critical particle size is flammable, and its ignition may generate lethal fumes of cadmium oxide (Ross, 1944).

Animals that survive acute cadmium pneumonitis later develop pulmonary fibrosis, but that reaction has not been described in man (Townsend, 1968). On the other hand, chronic respiratory exposure to cadmium can produce a severely disabling emphysema sometimes without clinical or histological evidence of chronic bronchitis (Kazantzis *et al.*, 1963; Smith *et al.*, 1960b). In rats, pulmonary fibrotic changes can also be induced by the chronic ingestion of cadmium chloride in drinking water (Miller *et al.*, 1974).

Cadmium is absorbed much more efficiently from the respiratory tract than from the gastrointestinal tract. Following absorption, cadmium accumulates in the liver and kidneys, perhaps because these two organs contain low-molecular-weight (about 10,000 daltons) proteins called metallothioneins (MTNs). MTNs avidly bind such metals as cadmium, zinc and mercury, and these metals are also able to induce MTN synthesis. The induction process occurs in many tissues but most dramatically in the liver (Probst *et al.*, 1977a). Induction is believed to account for the observation that pretreatment of animals with small doses of zinc or cadmium protects them against a toxic or lethal dose of cadmium administered subsequently (Leber and Miya 1976). Induction is maximal at 24 to 48 hours after predosing. Above a threshold dose of cadmium, the degree of induction is dose-dependent and is accompanied by a proportional increase in tolerance to cadmium (Probst *et al.*, 1977b) Even without predosing, however, injected cadmium shifts from binding sites on non-MTN proteins at 1 and 3 hours to MTN binding exclusively at 5 hours, presumably as a consequence of induction (Squibb *et al.*, 1976).

Cadmium pretreatment 24 hours prior to a toxic oral dose resulted in increased cadmium uptake by liver, kidney and testes. Induction o intestinal MTN also occurred, which may have implications for cadmium absorption (Squibb *et al.*, 1976). Induction and cadmium binding have been demonstrated in human cervical carcinoma cells maintained in culture (Rudd and Herschman, 1979) and in fetal rabbit liver following maternal cadmium dosing (Waalkes *et al.*, 1982) Human lymphocytes in culture accumulate cadmium bound to MTN to a level of 3000 times the concentration in the medium; perhaps this accumulation is responsible for reports of altered immunocompetence (Hildebrand and Cram 1979). Cadmium-MTN can be released from hepatic stores by a challenge dose of carbon tetrachloride. Dose-related decreases in hepatic cadmium-MTN are accompanied by proportional increases in the metalloprotein in plasma kidney and urine (Tanaka *et al.*, 1981). In the kidney, cadmium-MTN is reabsorbed by two processes, only one of which is saturated at low plasma concentrations of cadmium-MTN. The latter process is greatly depressed in cadmium pretreated animals, leading to enhanced excretion (Nimiyama and Foulkes, 1977). At least in rats during postnatal development, factors other than MTN appear to play important roles in the distribution and retention of cadmium (Wing and Klaassen, 1980).

MTN transport of cadmium to the kidneys may play a role in the renal toxicity of the metal Single intravenous doses of the cadmium-MTN complex produced necrosis and sloughing o renal tubular cells in rabbits (Fowler and Nordberg, 1978). Kidney damage in rabbits can also be produced by long-term parenteral (Axelsson and Piscator, 1966) or oral (Stowe et al., 1972) administration of cadmium salts. Renal injuries are also common among workers in cadmium industries, whether the exposure is acute (Beton et al., 1966) or chronic over may years (Adams et al., 1969; Clarkson and Kench, 1956; Dalhamn and Friberg, 1957; Kazantzis et al., 1963). In such industrial exposures, both inhalation and ingestion are believed to be involved (Lauwerys et al., 1979).

Acute massive exposures may result in acute renal necrosis (Beton et al., 1966), whereas prolonged low-level exposures commonly produce renal tubular dysfunction evidenced by a characteristic type of low-grade proteinuria due to an elevated clearance of β_2-microglobulin (Bernard et al., 1979; Friberg et al., 1971). The elevation is said to reflect an impaired tubular resorption of the filtered microglobulin (Bernard et al., 1979). Its detection has been employed in industry to identify workers with renal involvement (Friberg et al., 1971; Piscator, 1978). With heavier exposures or those that persist for periods of many years, glomerular injury may also appear, as evidenced by a more intense proteinuria with the excretion of some of the high-molecular-weight plasma proteins, decreased creatinine excretion, and elevations in plasma levels of creatinine and of β_2-microglobulin (Bernard et al., 1979; Friberg et al., 1971; Kazantzis, 1979). Some industrial toxicologists (e.g., Bernard et al., 1979) believe that cadmium-induced glomerular and tubular damage may occur either separately or together and that the two separate lesions are about equally common. Renal tubular dysfunction may occur at levels that correspond to as little as 10 μmol. Cd/mol. creatinine in the urine (Welinder et al., 1977), presumably reflecting a critical tissue threshold variously reported as 100 to 300, 200 to 250 and 300 to 400 ppm in the renal cortex (Ellis et al., 1981).

In chronic cadmium poisoning osteomalacia, radiological decreases in bone density, hypercalcinuria and renal stones reflect disturbances in calcium metabolism (Adams et al., 1969; Itokawa et al., 1974; Kennedy, 1966). The alteration in calcium metabolism has often been ascribed to the cadmium-induced renal tubular injury (Kazantzis, 1979). Recent evidence in rats suggests that under some circumstances the calcium disorders may arise from cadmium actions directly on bone (Yoshiki et al., 1975). Demineralization (Ando et al., 1978) is believed to reflect cadmium actions on bone collagen, leading to accelerated collagen catabolism (Nagai et al., 1982; Takashima et al., 1980). Cadmium produces more profound elevations in the urinary excretion of amino acids than do lead or mercury; urinary concentrations of hydroxyamino

acids are particularly elevated (Clarkson and Kench, 1956).

In Japan an extreme form of osteomalacia has been encountered which in combination with the renal disorder is known as itai-itai byo (literally the ouch-ouch disease) because of the pain accompanying the skeletal deformities. Contamination of food supplies, such as shellfish and rice, with cadmium is believed to be responsible for this syndrome. Other factors must play a role, however, because many patients with renal dysfunction do not exhibit osteomalacia, and the severity of the osteomalacia in other patients appears out of proportion to the estimated exposure to cadmium (Friberg et al., 1971). Because of evidence that at least some cases have been caused by nutritional and environmental factors, such as insufficient exposure to ultraviolet light, it is still possible that cadmium acts only as a promoting agent for itai-itai disease (Tsuchiya, 1976).

Liver damage and a microcytic hypochromic anemia refractory to iron therapy have been observed on feeding cadmium to rabbits (Berlin et al., 1961; Stowe et al., 1972), and both are recognized sequelae to acute or chronic human respiratory exposure. Neither lesion in man appears to have been life-threatening. Another significant finding from a diagnostic standpoint may be the formation of a yellow ring as a part of the tooth structure in chronically exposed humans (Princi, 1947).

Soluble cadmium salts given parenterally to rats, mice, or calves (Kumar et al., 1978) induced a temporary castration phenomenon, which progressed with larger doses to irreversible damage to the seminiferous tubules, necrosis of the germinal epithelium and complete loss of fertility. In proper dosage this action of cadmium is apparently selective; comparable amounts in female rats produced no detectable lesions in any organs. The concomitant injection of zinc salts with the cadmium protected the testes completely. The protection afforded was related to the zinc-cadmium molar ratio; an amount of zinc 80 to 200 times that of cadmium was effective. Barring toxicity from zinc, this protective treatment could presumably have been maintained for long periods of time (Gunn et al., 1961, 1968; Parizek, 1957). Damage to seminiferous tubules has not been observed in chronically exposed men, but in four workers who died from cadmium-related emphysema the testes contained few spermatids or mature spermatozoa, probably indicating an impairment of maturation (Smith et al., 1960b).

Laboratory animals sometimes show a significant hypertension after single parenteral doses of cadmium salts or after chronic exposure to cadmium in drinking water (Schroeder et al., 1970; Thind et al., 1970). Epidemiological studies suggest a relationship between cadmium levels in air and human cardiovascular disease (Carroll, 1966), but a causal association has not been proved.

Clearly the major target organs for parenteral or oral cadmium are the kidney and the liver. Particularly after chronic administration, however, functional changes in a wide variety of tissues and organs have been described in animals. They include disturbances in glucose homeostasis, *i.e.*, depletion of liver glycogen, increases in blood glucose, increased gluconeogenic potential in the liver and decreases in insulin secretion by the pancreas. In the adrenal glands, hypertrophy and increased catecholamine synthesis have also been reported (Singhal *et al.*, 1976). Many of these effects of cadmium are blocked by selenium in doses which have no effect when given alone (Merali and Singhal, 1975). Changes in biogenic amines in the central nervous system may be responsible for the hyperactivity of poisoned rats but histological lesions have been observed as well (Rastogi *et al.*, 1977; Wing and Klaassen, 1982). Effects on myocardial contractility and excitability have also been observed in laboratory studies (Kopp *et al.*, 1978; Pilati *et al.*, 1982).

Single doses of cadmium acetate (2 mg./kg.) inhibit oxidative hepatic drug-metabolizing activity in male rats. The inhibitory effect also occurs *in vitro* and is accompanied by a decrease in the cytochrome P450 content of the microsomal fractions of liver homogenates (Hadley *et al.*, 1974). Tolerance develops to this effect of cadmium as well as to lethality, testicular necrosis and inhibition of insulin secretion. Although the induction of MTN synthesis could account for tolerance to all these effects, other factors appear to play important roles with respect to cadmium inhibition of drug metabolism (Roberts and Schnell, 1982). Short exposures to cadmium oxide fumes also appear to destroy cytochrome P450 in rat lung microsomes, leading to alterations in their drug-metabolizing activity (Boisset and Boudene, 1981). Pretreatment of rats with phenobarbital reduces the lethality of subsequent parenteral doses of cadmium salts (Yoshikawa and Ohsawa, 1975). Although this pretreatment induced hepatic microsomal enzymes, the protection against cadmium was probably due instead to enhanced biliary excretion of cadmium (Klaassen and Kotsonis, 1977).

Chelating agents: Clinical experience in treating cadmium poisoning with chelating agents has been extremely limited. Cotter (1958) used oral edetate calcium disodium (CaNa$_2$EDTA) in three cases of chronic intoxication resulting from industrial exposures of several months to several years duration. Recoveries were said to be complete after a few weeks, and in one case marked mental irritability disappeared. In an acute suicidal ingestion episode (Wisniewska-Knypyl *et al.*, 1971), the administration of CaNa$_2$EDTA increased the urinary excretion of cadmium, but it did not prevent death. No cases in which BAL was used to treat human cadmium poisoning have come to our attention.

Although there is an abundance of experimental reports on chelation therapy in cadmium-poisoned animals, no generally satisfactory therapeutic regimen has been described. The experimental literature indicates that critical differences exist with respect to acute and chronic poisoning, the type of chelating agent, the route of exposure (whether oral or respiratory) and the route of elimination of the cadmium chelates (whether urinary or biliary).

Parenteral dimercaprol (BAL), given together with cadmium to rabbits daily for 10 weeks, was thought to intensify the weight loss, proteinuria and anemia, as compared to the effects of cadmium given alone (Dalhamn and Friberg, 1955). Treatment of rabbits with CaNa$_2$EDTA after prolonged exposure to cadmium resulted in severe degenerative renal changes (Friberg, 1956). Thus, in contrast to the clinical experience above, the experimental work to date suggests that chelation therapy in general may be ill-advised in chronic cadmium poisoning.

Among the sulfhydryl-type chelators, BAL ameliorated the acute signs of intoxication after single parenteral doses of cadmium in rabbits, but it did not prevent mortality due to late renal failure (Gilman *et al.*, 1946). Similarly, L-cysteine appeared to intensify the renal damage after single doses of cadmium in rats (Kennedy, 1968) and to increase mortality in mice (Gunn *et al.*, 1968). Given immediately after intravenous cadmium in mice, a single intraperitoneal dose of BAL failed to reduce mortality or to increase the urinary excretion of cadmium (Cantilena and Klaassen, 1981). These results suggest that BAL may facilitate the delivery of cadmium to the kidney where a fraction of the metal-chelate may release free cadmium to produce epithelial damage. Indeed, treatment with BAL did result in large increases in the kidney content of cadmium, a phenomenon that did not occur in similar experiments with BAL-glucoside (Tepperman, 1947). Both chelators accelerated cadmium excretion, but BAL increased both urinary and fecal excretion, whereas BAL-glucoside increased urinary excretion almost exclusively.

When given to rats at various times from 30 minutes to 14 days after intravenous cadmium chloride, BAL was effective in mobilizing cadmium into bile at those times (24 hr. or more) when it was preferentially bound to hepatic MTN. Structurally similar dithiols, such as 1,3-dimercaptopropanol or 2,3-dimercapto-1-propane sulfonic acid (DMPS), were not effective.

Biliary excretion of cadmium increased with increasing doses of BAL without concomitant increases in urinary excretion. BAL was most effective when given 30 minutes after the CdCl$_2$ injection, but significant effects were still apparent as late as 14 days after the cadmium (Cherian, 1980). BAL may be unique in increasing biliary excretion of cadmium.

Neither BAL nor D-penicillamine, however, prevented death in mice when given intraperitoneally immediately after intravenous cadmium chloride (Cantilena and Klaassen, 1981), although a small degree of protection was achieved with BAL given parenterally immediately after a subcutaneous injection of CdCl$_2$ (Eybl and Sykora, 1966; Gunn et al., 1968). In contrast, DMPS given orally in three doses at 20, 90 and 210 minutes after intraperitoneal cadmium acetate significantly reduced mortality in mice; it was a more effective antidote than 2,3-dimercaptosuccinic acid (DMSA) or N-acetyl-DL-penicillamine (Jones et al., 1978). Thus the sulfhydryl-type chelators have received mixed reviews in terms of preventing mortality due to injected cadmium.

Zinc acetate injected subcutaneously protected mice against death from subcutaneous cadmium chloride (Gunn et al., 1968), and orally administered trisodium nitrilotriacetate (NTA) protected rats against death from oral CdCl$_2$ (Scharpe et al., 1972). In mice, however, neither NTA nor diethyldithiocarbamate (DDC) decreased mortality when given intraperitoneally immediately after intravenous cadmium chloride (Cantilena and Klaassen, 1981). DDC greatly increased the cerebral extraction of cadmium from blood in rats, suggesting that the cadmium chelate readily crossed the blood-brain barrier (Cantilena et al., 1982). Despite the above, when DDC treatment of mice was delayed for at least 30 minutes or for as long as 8 hours, it was effective in reducing mortality (Gale et al., 1981). The reasons behind these apparently contradictory reports are not clear.

The aminopolycarboxylic acid-type chelating agents, e.g., edetate calcium disodium (CaNa$_2$EDTA), protect experimental animals against acute poisoning by parenterally administered cadmium salts whether the results are based on early deaths or late deaths in renal failure (Eybl and Sykora, 1966; Sivjakov and Braun, 1959). The most effective in a series of such agents was penthanil (diethylenetriaminepentaacetic acid, DTPA), even though its cadmium chelate was neither the most stable nor the least toxic in the series. A similar conclusion was reached by Cantilena and Klaassen (1981), who also found DTPA to be the most effective, followed by CaNa$_2$EDTA and DMSA. If given immediately after the metal, all three increased the urinary excretion of cadmium and decreased tissue concentrations. When these agents were delayed even for as little as 2 hours, however, the effects were of much smaller magnitude (Cantilena and Klaassen, 1982). Thus, the aminopolycarboxylic acid-type chelators appear to increase preferentially the urinary excretion of cadmium without affecting the biliary excretion, and they are effective in reducing mortality at least when given very soon after the cadmium.

In contrast to cadmium administered parenterally or orally, cadmium inhaled in the form of dusts, fumes or aerosols almost always leads to acute (and sometimes chronic) lung reactions associated with the pulmonary retention of the metal. Experimental therapy has focused on attempts to remove cadmium from the lungs. In mice and dogs, BAL proved effective when given about 30 minutes after an acute inhalation exposure to CdCl$_2$, but paradoxically, when given beforehand, BAL tended to increase the lung retention of cadmium and to enhance mortality. When used as a therapeutic agent after the exposure, BAL in large doses lowered the mortality significantly, presumably by moving cadmium from the lungs to the liver and kidneys (Harrison et al., 1947; Potts et al., 1950; Tobias et al., 1946). Late kidney damage was not observed, perhaps because the amount of cadmium mobilized was insufficient to injure those organs. These results, however, may not hold for long-term or chronic respiratory exposures where the experimental evidence indicates that the risk of a serious renal insult during BAL therapy is greater (Friberg et al., 1971). The aminopolycarboxylic acid-type chelating agents are presumably efficacious in acute respiratory exposures, perhaps without the risk of inducing a cadmium-related renal injury.

Although DMSA and DMPS would appear superficially to incorporate structural features of both the dithiol and the carboxylic acid-type chelators, it is not clear that they actually fulfill both attributes in the case of cadmium. In any event they are not generally available or approved for that purpose; the same is true of DPTA. If administered promptly in acute cadmium poisoning, CaNa$_2$EDTA is probably the best single agent available for this purpose in the United States (see pp. III-163–166), but perhaps a cautious trial using both BAL and CaNa$_2$EDTA, as recommended for LEAD (p. III-233) encephalopathy, is warranted when the pulmonary reaction is both acute and severe.

Symptomatology:

A. Inhalation (an asymptomatic period of 4 to 8 hours may precede the clinical illness).
   1. Metallic taste in the mouth, and headache.
   2. Shortness of breath, chest pain, cough with foamy or bloody sputum. Pulmo-

nary rales and related physical signs. These signs and symptoms mimic "the flu."

3. Weakness, leg pains.
4. An asphyxial death from intense pulmonary edema, or 5.
5. Gradual resolution of pulmonary edema (over a period of a few days) and development of fever, with persistence of cough, chest pain, and dyspnea for one or more weeks. Physical signs of pneumonic consolidation.
6. Late kidney and/or liver damage has followed respiratory exposures in industry.

B. Ingestion (an asymptomatic period of ½ to 1 hour may precede the clinical illness).
1. Severe nausea, vomiting, diarrhea and abdominal cramps, and salivation.
2. Headache, muscular cramps, vertigo, and perhaps convulsions (rarely).
3. Exhaustion, collapse, shock, and death, usually within a period of 24 hours.
4. The gradual evolution of signs and symptoms of liver and kidney damage should be anticipated but are rarely seen in man.

Treatment:
A. Inhalation
1. Terminate exposure and remove patient to fresh air.
2. Codeine sulfate for cough and chest pain.
3. Treat the adult respiratory distress syndrome (ARDS) by the several measures described on pp. IV-14–16, including oxygen with continuous positive airway pressure.
4. Edetate calcium disodium intravenously according to the dosage schedules on p. III-165.
5. If the inhalation exposure was an acute one and the pulmonary reaction is especially severe, a cautious trial with both BAL and edetate calcium disodium, as recommended for lead encephalopathy (p. III-165), may be warranted.
6. Penicillin as prophylaxis against secondary infection and bacterial pneumonia, but see pp. IV-85–86.
7. Prophylactic and supportive measures for possible kidney and/or liver injury (pp. IV-52 and 60).

B. Ingestion
1. Allay gastrointestinal irritation by swallowing milk or beaten egg whites at frequent intervals.
2. Gastric lavage with water, milk, or albumin solution if vomiting is not prompt and intensive.
3. Administer by mouth sodium or magnesium sulfate in water (15 to 30 gm.).
4. Avoid dimercaprol (BAL), since its administration might convert a gastroenteritis into a severe toxic nephritis (see above).
5. After the gastrointestinal tract has been emptied by emesis and catharsis, intravenous edetate calcium disodium may be useful; see p. III-165 for dosage.
6. Parenteral fluids and electrolytes, given cautiously to maintain hydration and acid-base balance.
7. Supportive measures for acute renal failure as outlined on p. IV-53.
8. Prophylactic and supportive measures for possible liver injury (p. IV-60).

Laboratory:
1. X-ray findings in the chest after inhalation exposures are consistent with diffuse pulmonary edema; later findings are like those of bronchopneumonia (proliferative interstitial pneumonitis).
2. Function tests may demonstrate subclinical kidney and liver injuries (Cotter and Cotter, 1951).
3. Analytic methods are available for the quantitative analysis of cadmium in blood and urine. Tubular-type proteinuria among industrial workers occurs mainly in those with blood cadmium levels above 1 μg./dl. and urine cadmium levels above 10 μg./gm. creatinine (Bernard et al., 1979; Lauwerys et al., 1979).

References:

Adams, R. G.; Harrison, J. F.; Scott, P. The development of cadmium-induced proteinuria, impaired renal function and osteomalacia in alkaline battery workers. Q. J. Med. 38:425-443, 1969.

Adamsson, E.; Piscator, M.; Nogawa, K. Pulmonary and gastrointestinal exposure to cadmium oxide dust in a battery factory. Environ. Health Perspect. 28:219-222, 1979.

Ando, M.; Sayato, Y.; Osawa, T. Studies on the disposition of calcium in bones of rats after continuous oral administration of cadmium. Toxicol. Appl. Pharmacol. 46:625-632, 1978.

Axelsson, B.; Piscator, M. Renal damage after prolonged exposure to cadmium, an experimental study. Arch. Environ. Health 12:360-373, 1966.

Baker, T. D.; Hafner, W. G. Cadmium poisoning from a refrigerator shelf used as an improvised barbecue grill. Public Health Repts. (U. S.) 76:543-554, 1961.

Barrett, H. M.; Card, B. Y. Studies on the toxicity of inhaled cadmium. II. The acute lethal dose of cadmium oxide for man. J. Ind. Hyg. Toxicol. 29:286-293, 1947.

Barrett, H. M.; Irwin, D. A.; Semmons, E. Studies on the toxicity of inhaled cadmium. I. The acute toxicity of cadmium oxide by inhalation. J. Ind. Hyg. Toxicol. 29:279-285, 1947.

Berlin, M.; Fredricsson, B.; Linge, G. Bone marrow changes in chronic cadmium poisoning in rabbits. Arch. Environ. Health 3:176-184, 1961.

Bernard, A.; Buchet, J. P.; Roels, H.; Masson, P.; Lauwerys, R. Renal excretion of proteins and enzymes in workers exposed to cadmium. Eur. J. Clin. Invest. 9:11-22, 1979.

Beton, D. C.; Andrews, G. S.; Davies, H. J.; Howells, L.; Smith, G. F. Acute cadmium fume poisoning, five cases with one death from renal necrosis. Br. J. Ind. Med. 23:292-301, 1966.

Blejer, H. P.; Caplan, P. E.; Alcocer, A. E. Acute cadmium fume poisoning in welders - a fatal and a nonfatal case in California. Calif. Med. 105:290-296, 1966.

Boisset, M.; Boudene, C. Effect of a single exposure to cadmium oxide fumes on rat lung microsomal enzymes. Toxicol. Appl. Pharmacol. 57:335-345, 1981.

Cantilena, L. R., Jr.; Irwin, G.; Preskorn, S.; Klaassen, C. D. The effect of diethyldithiocarbamate on brain uptake of cadmium. Toxicol. Appl. Pharmacol. 63:338-343, 1982.

Cantilena, L. R., Jr.; Klaassen, C. D. Comparison of the effectiveness of several chelators after single administration on the toxicity, excretion and distribution of cadmium. Toxicol. Appl. Pharmacol. 58:452-460, 1981.

Cantilena, L. R., Jr.; Klaassen, C. D. Decreased effectiveness of chelation therapy with time after acute cadmium poisoning. Toxicol. Appl. Pharmacol. 63:173-180, 1982.

Carroll, R. E. The relationship of cadmium in the air to cardiovascular disease death rates. J. A. M. A. 198:267-269, 1966.

Cherian, M. G. Biliary excretion of cadmium in rat. IV. Mobilization of cadmium from metallothionein by 2, 3-dimercaptopropanol. J. Toxicol. Environ. Health 6:393-401, 1980.

Clarkson, T. W.; Kench, J. E. Urinary excretion of amino acids by men absorbing heavy metals. Biochem. J. 62:361-372, 1956.

Cotter, L. H. Treatment of cadmium poisoning with edathamil calcium disodium. J. A. M. A. 166:735-736, 1958.

Cotter, L. H.; Cotter, B. H. Cadmium poisoning. Arch. Ind. Health 3:495-504, 1951.

Dalhamn, T.; Friberg, L. Dimercaprol (2, 3-dimercaptopropanol) in chronic cadmium poisoning. Acta Pharmacol. Toxicol. 11:68-71, 1955.

Dalhamn, T.; Friberg, L. Morphologic investigations on kidney damage in chronic cadmium poisoning. Acta Pathol. Microbiol. Scand. 40:475-479, 1957.

Ellis, K. J.; Morgan, W. D.; Zanzi, I.; Yasumura, S.; Vartsky, D.; Cohn, S. H. Critical concentrations of cadmium in human renal cortex: dose-effect studies in cadmium smelter workers. J. Toxicol. Environ. Health 7:691-703, 1981.

Eybl, V.; Sykora, J. Die Schutzwirkung von Chelatbildnern bei der akuten Kadmiumchloridvergiftung. Acta Biol. Med. Ger. 16:61-64, 1966.

Fowler, B. A.; Nordberg, G. F. The renal toxicity of cadmium metallothionein: Morphometric and X-ray microanalytical studies. Toxicol. Appl. Pharmacol. 46:609-623, 1978.

Frant, S.; Kleeman, I. Cadmium "food poisoning". J. A. M. A. 117:86-89, 1941.

Friberg, L. Edathamil calcium-disodium in cadmium poisoning. Arch. Ind. Health 13:13-23, 1956.

Friberg, L.; Piscator, M.; Nordberg, G. Cadmium in the Environment. Chemical Rubber Company Press, Cleveland, 1971.

Gale, G. R.; Smith, A. B.; Walker, E. M. Diethyldithiocarbamate in the treatment of acute cadmium poisoning. Ann. Clin. Lab. Sci. 2:476-483, 1981.

Gilman, A.; Phillips, F. S.; Allen, R. P.; Koelle, E. S. The treatment of acute cadmium intoxication in rabbits with 2, 3-dimercaptopropanol (BAL) and other mercaptans. J. Pharmacol. Exp. Ther. 87(Suppl.):85-101, 1946.

Gunn, S. A.; Gould, T. C.; Anderson, W. A. Zinc protection against cadmium injury to rat testis. Arch. Pathol. 71:274-281, 1961.

Gunn, S. A.; Gould, T. C.; Anderson, W. A. D. Specificity in protection against lethality and testicular toxicity from cadmium. Proc. Soc. Exp. Biol. Med. 128:591-595, 1968.

Hadley, W. M.; Miya, T. S.; Bousquet, W. F. Cadmium inhibition of hepatic drug metabolism in the rat. Toxicol. Appl. Pharmacol. 28:284-291, 1974.

Harrison, H. E.; Bunting, H.; Ordway, N. K.; Albrink, W. S. The effects and treatment of inhalation of cadmium chloride aerosols in the dog. J. Ind. Hyg. Toxicol. 29:302-314, 1947.

Hildebrand, C. E.; Cram, L. S. Distribution of cadmium in human blood cultured in low levels of CdCl$_2$: Accumulation of Cd in lymphocytes and preferential binding to metallo-

thionein. Proc. Soc. Exp. Biol. Med. 161:438-443, 1979.

Itokawa, Y.; Abe, T.; Tabei, R.; Tanaka, S. Renal and skeletal lesions in experimental cadmium poisoning. Histological and biochemical approaches. Arch. Environ. Health 28:149-154, 1974.

Jones, M. M.; Weaver, A. D.; Weller, W. L. The relative effectiveness of some chelating agents as antidotes in acute cadmium poisoning. Res. Comm. Chem. Pathol. Pharmacol. 22:581-588, 1978.

Kazantzis, G. Renal tubular dysfunction and abnormalities of calcium metabolism in cadmium workers. Environ. Health Perspect. 28:155-159, 1979.

Kazantzis, G.; Flynn, F. V.; Spowage, J.; Trott, D. G. Renal tubular malfunction and pulmonary emphysema in cadmium pigment workers. Q. J. Med. 32:165-192, 1963.

Kennedy, A. Hypocalcemia in experimental cadmium poisoning. Br. J. Ind. Med. 23:313-317, 1966.

Kennedy, A. The effects of L-cysteine on the toxicity of cadmium. Br. J. Exp. Pathol. 49:360-364, 1968.

Klaassen, C. D.; Kotsonis, F. N. Biliary excretion of cadmium in the rat, rabbit and dog. Toxicol. Appl. Pharmacol. 41:101-112, 1977.

Kopp, S. J.; Fischer, V. W.; Erlanger, M.; Perry, E. F.; Perry, H. M., Jr. Electrocardiographical, biochemical and morphological effects of chronic low level cadmium feeding on the rat heart. Proc. Soc. Exp. Biol. Med. 159:339-345, 1978.

Kumar, B. A.; Vijayasarthi, S. K.; Kailas, M. M.; Setty, S. V. S. Cadmium induced chemical sterilization of male calves. Curr. Res. 7:131-133, 1978.

Lauwerys, R.; Roels, H.; Regniers, M.; Buchet, J. P.; Bernard, A.; Goret, A. Significance of cadmium concentration in blood and in urine in workers exposed to cadmium. Environ. Res. 20:375-391, 1979.

Leber, A. P.; Miya, T. S. A mechanism for cadmium- and zinc-induced tolerance to cadmium toxicity: Involvement of metallothionein. Toxicol. Appl. Pharmacol. 37:403-414, 1976.

Lucas, P. A.; Jariwalla, A. G.; Jones, J. H.; Gough, J.; Vale, P. T. Fatal cadmium fume inhalation. Lancet 2:205, 1980.

Merali, Z.; Singhal, R. L. Protective effect of selenium on certain hepatotoxic and pancreotoxic manifestations of subacute cadmium administration. J. Pharmacol. Exp. Ther. 195:58-66, 1975.

Miller, M. L.; Murthy, L.; Sorenson, J. R. J. Fine structure of connective tissue after ingestion of cadmium. Observations on interstitium of male rat lung. Arch. Pathol. 98:386-392, 1974.

Nagai, Y.; Sato, M.; Sasaki, M. Effect of cadmium administration upon urinary excretion of hyroxylysine and hydroxyproline in the rat. Toxicol. Appl. Pharmacol. 63:188-193, 1982.

Nimiyama, K.; Foulkes, E. C. Reabsorption of filtered cadmium-metallothionein in the rabbit kidney. Proc. Soc. Exp. Biol. Med. 156:97-99, 1977.

Parizek, J. The destructive effect of cadmium ion on testicular tissue and its prevention by zinc. J. Endocrinol. 15:56-63, 1957.

Paterson, J. C. Studies on the toxicity of inhaled cadmium. III. The pathology of cadmium smoke poisoning in man and in experimental animals. J. Ind. Hyg. Toxicol. 29:294-301, 1947.

Patwardhan, J. R.; Finckh, E. S. Fatal cadmium-fume pneumonitis. Med. J. Aust. 1:962-966, 1976.

Pilati, C. F.; Ewing, K. L.; Paradise, N. F. Effects of cadmium on contractility and calcium concentration in isolated heart muscle. Proc. Soc. Exp. Biol. Med. 169:480-486, 1982.

Piscator, M. Serum β_2-microglobulin in cadmium exposed workers. Pathol. Biol. 26:321-323, 1978.

Potts, A. M.; Simon, F. P.; Tobias, J. M.; Postel, S.; Swift, M. N.; Patt, H. M.; Gerard, R. W. Distribution and fate of cadmium in the animal body. Arch. Ind. Hyg. Occup. Med. 2:175-188, 1950.

Princi, F. A study of industrial exposures to cadmium. J. Ind. Hyg. Toxicol. 29:315-320, 1947.

Probst, G. S.; Bousquet, W. F.; Miya, T. S. Kinetics of cadmium-induced hepatic and renal metallothionein synthesis in the mouse. Toxicol. Appl. Pharmacol. *39*:51-60, 1977a.

Probst, G. S.; Bousquet, W. F.; Miya, T. S. Correlation of hepatic metallothionein concentrations with acute cadmium toxicity in the mouse. Toxicol. Appl. Pharmacol. *39*:61-69, 1977b.

Rastogi, R. B.; Merali, Z.; Singhal, R. L. Cadmium alters behaviour and the biosynthetic capacity for catecholamines and serotonin in neonatal rat brain. J. Neurochem. *28*:789-794, 1977.

Roberts, S. A.; Schnell, R. C. Cadmium-induced inhibition of hepatic drug oxidation in the rat: Time dependency of tolerance development and metallothionein synthesis. Toxicol. Appl. Pharmacol. *64*:42-51, 1982.

Ross, P. Cadmium poisoning. Br. Med. J. *1*:252-253, 1944.

Rudd, C. J.; Herschman, H. R. Metallothionein in a human cell line: the response of HeLa cells to cadmium and zinc. Toxicol. Appl. Pharmacol. *47*:273-278, 1979.

Scharpe, L. G.; Kamos, F. J.; Hill, J. D. Influence of nitrilotriacetate (NTA) on the toxicity, excretion and distribution of cadmium in female rats. Toxicol. Appl. Pharmacol. *22*:186-192, 1972.

Schifter, J. J.; Mahler, H. Illness caused by cadmium. Am. J. Public Health *33*:1224-1226, 1943.

Schroeder, H. A.; Baker, J. T.; Hansen, N. M., Jr.; Size, J. G.; Wise, R. A. Vascular reactivity of rats altered by cadmium and a zinc chelate. Arch. Environ. Health *21*:609-614, 1970.

Schwartze, E. W.; Alsberg, C. L. Studies on the pharmacology of cadmium and zinc with particular reference to emesis. J. Pharmacol. Exp. Ther. *21*:1-22, 1923.

Singhal, R. L.; Merali, Z.; Hrdina, P. D. Aspects of the biochemical toxicology of cadmium. Fed. Proc. *35*:75-80, 1976.

Sivjakov, K. I.; Braun, H. A. The treatment of acute selenium, cadmium and tungsten intoxication in rats with calcium disodium ethylenediaminetetraacetate. Toxicol. Appl. Pharmacol. *1*:602-608, 1959.

Smith, J. P.; Smith, J. C.; McCall, A. J. Chronic poisoning from cadmium fume. J. Pathol. Bacteriol. *80*:287-296, 1960b.

Spolyar, L. W.; Keppler, J. F.; Porter, H. G. Cadmium poisoning in industry. Report of five cases, including one death. J. Ind. Hyg. Toxicol. *26*:232-237, 1944.

Squibb, K. S.; Cousins, R. J.; Silbon, B. L.; Levin, S. Liver and intestinal metallothionein: Function in acute cadmium toxicity. Exp. Mol. Pathol. *25*:163-171, 1976.

Stowe, H. D.; Wilson, M.; Goyer, R. A. Clinical and morphologic effects of oral cadmium toxicity in rabbits. Arch. Pathol. *94*:389-405, 1972.

Takashima, M.; Moriwaki, S.; Itokawa, Y. Osteomalacic change induced by long-term administration of cadmium to rats. Toxicol. Appl. Pharmacol. *54*:223-228, 1980.

Tanaka, K.; Nomura, H.; Onosaka, S.; Min, K. S. Release of hepatic cadmium by carbon tetrachloride treatment. Toxicol. Appl. Pharmacol. *59*:535-539, 1981.

Tepperman, H. M. The effect of BAL and BAL-glucoside therapy on the excretion and distribution of injected cadmium. J. Pharmacol. Exp. Ther. *89*:343-349, 1947.

Thind, G. S.; Darreman, G.; Stephan, K. F.; Blakemore, W. S. Vascular reactivity and mechanical properties of normal and cadmium hypertensive rabbits. J. Lab. Clin. Med. *76*:560-568, 1970.

Tierney, D. R.; Blackwood, T. R.; Wilson, R. D. Status assessment of toxic chemicals: cadmium. Gov. Rep. Announce. Index *80*:1928, 1980.

Tobias, J. M.; Lushbaugh, C. C.; Patt, H. M.; Postel, S.; Swift, M. N.; Gerard, R. W. The pathology and therapy with 2, 3-dimercaptopropanol (BAL) of experimental Cd poisoning. J. Pharmacol. Exp. Ther. *87*(Suppl.):102-118, 1946.

Townsend, R. H. A case of acute cadmium pneumonitis: Lung function tests during a four year follow-up. Br. J. Ind. Med. *25*:68-71, 1968.

Tsuchiya, K. Epidemiological studies on cadmium in the environment in Japan: etiology of itai-itai disease. Fed. Proc. *35*:2412-2418, 1976.

Waalkes, M. P.; Thomas, J. A.; Bell, J. U. Induction of hepatic metallothionein in the rabbit fetus following maternal cadmium exposure. Toxicol. Appl. Pharmacol. *62*:211-218, 1982.

Welinder, H.; Skerfving, S.; Henriksen, O. Cadmium metabolism in man. Br. J. Ind. Med. *34*:221-228, 1977.

Wing, K. L.; Klaassen, C. D. Tissue distribution and retention of cadmium in rats during postnatal development: minimal role of hepatic metallothionein. Toxicol. Appl. Pharmacol. *53*:343-353, 1980.

Wing, K. L.; Klaassen, C. D. Neurotoxic effect of cadmium in young rats. Toxicol. Appl. Pharmacol. *63*:330-337, 1982.

Wisniewska-Knypyl, J. M.; Jablonska, J.; Myslak, Z. Binding of cadmium on metallothionein in man; An analysis of a fatal poisoning by cadmium iodide. Arch. Toxikol. *28*:46-55, 1971.

Yoshikawa, H.; Ohsawa, M. Protective effect of phenobarbital on cadmium toxicity in mice. Toxicol. Appl. Pharmacol. *34*:517-520, 1975.

Yoshiki, S.; Yanagisawa, T.; Kimura, M.; Otaki, N.; Suzuki, M.; Suda, T. Bone and kidney lesions in experimental cadmium intoxication. Arch. Environ. Health *30*:559-562, 1975.

Zavon, M. R.; Meadow, C. D. Vascular sequelae to cadmium fume exposure. Am. Ind. Hyg. Assoc. J. *31*:180-182, 1970.

CAMPHOR

Camphor (2-camphanone) and camphorated oils are no longer used as stimulants in clinical medicine. Neither is permitted as an internal medication (except in paregoric), and camphorated oil has been banned on the American market. Camphor, however, is still a common ingredient in liniments, salves and ointments used as analgesic skin rubs and nasal decongestants and promoted for treating fever blisters and diaper rash. A bromo derivative, 3-bromo-*d*-camphor, is also used as a topical counterirritant. Paregoric (see Section II) contains camphor, but the main hazard of paregoric overdose probably relates to its content of MORPHINE (p. III-284).

Camphor is still employed in "camphor ball" moth repellents and flakes, but NAPHTHALENE (p. III-307) and *p*-dichlorobenzene (see Section II) are probably more commonly encountered in such products. In some lay circles, camphor has been worn as protection against infection (usually in a bag suspended from the neck).

Toxicology: Most cases of camphor intoxication have arisen from the accidental ingestion of camphor liniment (camphorated oil), which is 20% camphor in cottonseed oil (Jacobziner and Raybin, 1959a, 1962a; Rübin *et al.*, 1949; Verhulst *et al.*, 1961). Camphorated oil has been confused with castor oil, cod liver oil, Castoria, and cough and colic remedies (Aronow and Spigiel, 1976). Camphor spirit, which is 10% camphor in alcohol (Jacobziner and Raybin, 1959a), and other common official and proprietary liniments, salves and ointments have been responsible for clinical camphor poisonings (Krueger, 1967; Phelan, 1976; Rübin *et al.*, 1949; Seife and

Leon, 1954). The ingestion of solid camphor "moth balls" has also produced symptoms and death (Barker, 1910; Davies, 1887).

Camphor is readily absorbed from all sites of administration. It produces a feeling of coolness on the skin and in the respiratory tract. In contrast, a small oral dose causes a sensation of warmth in the stomach; large doses may induce nausea and vomiting (Craig, 1953; Rübin et al., 1949; Verhulst et al., 1961). Camphor is a central nervous stimulant. Agitation and hallucinations may be the presenting complaints (Köppel et al., 1982a), but systemic poisoning is characterized by epileptiform convulsions (Craig, 1953; Rübin et al., 1949; Verhulst et al., 1961) which may be punctuated by periods of apnea and asystole (Laurie, 1950; Riggs et al., 1965). Postconvulsive depression of the central nervous system follows stimulation. In one case, coma lasted for 29 hours (Benz, 1919). Neuronal necrosis has been reported in human fatalities (Riggs et al., 1965; Smith and Margolis, 1954), and similar lesions have been produced experimentally in mice by the administration of multiple doses (Smith and Margolis, 1954).

Man appears to be much more susceptible to camphor poisoning than the common laboratory mammals. The ingestion of 2 gm. generally produces dangerous effects in an adult person, although 1.5 oz. have been ingested with recovery (Haft, 1925), and 0.7 to 1.0 gm. (1 teaspoonful of liniment or camphorated oil) has proved fatal in children (Haas, 1916; Smith and Margolis, 1954). With such doses, expired air, eructations, urine and other excreta smell strongly of camphor (Webster, 1930).

A camphor-containing spray product, used both as an air freshener and as a decongestant, produced pneumonitis in an infant when sprayed directly in his face by a mentally retarded relative (Krueger, 1967). Although camphor is a recognized irritant, its role in this reaction is uncertain, since the product also contained thymol, menthol, eucalyptol, glycol solvents and a Freon propellant. In another child, exposure to a vaporized decongestant containing camphor resulted in the more typical syndrome of seizures (Skoglund et al., 1977). By a bizarre coincidence the latter patient had suffered a severe intoxication 5 years previously when he had crawled through spilled spirits of camphor.

Camphor has been used occasionally in attempts to induce abortion. In two cases, healthy infants were born after camphor ingestion by the mothers (Blackmon and Curry, 1957; Weiss and Catalano, 1973), but fetal death has resulted under similar circumstances (Riggs et al., 1965). In the Riggs case (1965), camphor was detectable in maternal blood 15 minutes after ingestion but not after 8 hours. At delivery 36 hours later, however, it was present in amnionic fluid, cord and fetal blood and fetal brain, liver and kidneys. Perhaps this distribution reflects immaturity of the fetal liver in its capacity to form glucuronic acid conjugates, a major detoxication process for camphor in adults (Klingensmith, 1934; Köppel et al., 1982a; Riggs et al., 1965; Smith and Margolis, 1954). This infant appeared viable at birth but failed to initiate respirations. Postmortem examination revealed severe atelectasis and central neuronal necrosis (Riggs et al., 1965).

Urinary retention, albuminuria and anuria are sometimes described in nonfatal cases (Smith and Margolis, 1954), but kidney lesions in fatal poisonings are not always prominent (Clark, 1924; Rübsamen, 1912). Mild and transient hepatic derangements may occur (Antman et al., 1978; Riggs et al., 1965; Trestrail and Spartz, 1977), and widespread hemorrhages (skin, stomach, bowel, kidney) are described in one fatal case (Clark, 1924).

Extracorporeal hemodialysis against soybean oil (lipid dialysis) resulted in recovery of more than half of a total ingested dose of 12 gm. in one case (Ginn et al., 1968) and clinical improvement in another (Antman et al., 1978). One severely poisoned adult, who may have ingested 18 gm., was subjected to both resin hemoperfusion and lipid hemodialysis with the equipment arranged in series. Blood samples taken before and after entering each apparatus suggested that resin hemoperfusion was the superior procedure (Kopelman et al., 1979). Hemoperfusion through Amberlite XAD-4 is superior to that through charcoal (Köppel et al., 1982a).

Symptomatology (within 5 to 90 minutes after ingestion):

1. Nausea and vomiting, sometimes projectile.
2. Feeling of warmth. Headache.
3. Confusion, vertigo, excitement, restlessness, delirium, and hallucinations.
4. Increased muscular excitability, tremors, and jerky movement.
5. Epileptiform convulsions, followed by depression. Convulsions sometimes occur early in the syndrome and may be severe, but they do not have the generally grave prognosis of strychnine convulsions.
6. Coma. Central nervous depression may at times be the primary clinical response.
7. Death results from respiratory failure or from status epilepticus.
8. Slow convalesence (days or weeks), often with persistent gastric distress.

Treatment:

1. Treatment is aimed at preventing convulsions. Intravenous sodium thiopental, pentobarbital or amobarbital (Amytal) is effective. The drug should be injected *slowly* until the desired condition is reached, namely a degree of depression sufficient to

prevent or stop convulsions and to keep the patient asleep, but not deep enough to depress respirations or blood pressure. Intramuscular sodium phenobarbital may also be helpful. Of course these same drugs, as well as diazepam, can also be used to terminate camphor convulsions. For details of anticonvulsant therapy, see pp. IV-35–39.

2. The patient should be kept under careful observation for many hours and protected from all possible stimuli. Wakefulness, muscular twitchings, and increased reflex excitability are signs that warn of need for additional barbiturate.

3. Oxygen therapy, artificial respiration (pp. IV-7–12), as indicated.

4. Gastric lavage (with warm water) may be performed when the patient is asleep or well premedicated. In the presymptomatic stage, lavage or the induction of emesis should take precedence over all measures. Because of its low water solubility, pieces of camphor may remain in the stomach unless a large tube is used for lavage.

5. After the stomach is emptied, a slurry of activated charcoal and/or a saline cathartic may be administered by mouth. See Section I for details (p. I-4 and 12).

6. Avoid the ingestion of oils or alcohol which may promote intestinal absorption of camphor.

7. Extracorporeal hemodialysis with a lipid dialysate (p. IV-55) or resin hemoperfusion (p. IV-57) may be indicated.

Laboratory: Laboratory data are not usually relevant, but liver and kidney function tests may be advisable. Camphor has been detected in sera of intoxicated patients at levels of 0.3 to 1.8 μgm./ml. (Köppel *et al.*, 1982a; Kopelman *et al.*, 1979).

References:

Antman, E.; Jacob, G.; Volpe, B.; Finkel, S.; Savona, M. Camphor overdosage. Therapeutic considerations. N. Y. State J. Med. *78*:896-897, 1978.

Aronow R.; Spigiel, R. W. Implications of camphor poisoning. Drug Intell. Clin. Pharm. *10*:631-634, 1976.

Barker, F. A case of poisoning by camphorated oil. Br. Med. J. *1*:921, 1910.

Benz, R. W. Camphorated oil poisoning with no mortality, report of twenty cases. J. A. M. A. *72*:1217-1218, 1919.

Blackmon, W. P.; Curry, H. B. Camphor poisoning. Report of case occurring during pregnancy. J. Fl. Med. Assoc. *43*:999-1000, 1957.

Clark, T. L. Fatal case of camphor poisoning. Br. Med. J. *1*:467, 1924.

Craig, J. O. Poisoning by the volatile oils in childhood. Arch. Dis. Child. *28*:475-483, 1953.

Davies, R. A fatal case of camphor poisoning. Br. Med. J. *1*:726, 1887.

Ginn, H. E.; Anderson, K. E.; Mercier, R. K.; Stevens, T. W.; Matter, B. J. Camphor intoxication treated by lipid dialysis. J. A. M. A. *203*:230-231, 1968.

Haas, S. V. Death following ingestion of 1 dram of camphorated oil. Am. J. Obstet. Dis. Women Child. *73*:1153-1154, 1916.

Haft, H. H. Camphor liniment poisoning. J. A. M. A. *84*:1571, 1925.

Jacobziner, H.; Raybin, H. W. Briefs on accidental chemical poisonings in New York City. N. Y. State J. Med. *59*:115-118, 1959a.

Jacobziner, H.; Raybin, H. W. Camphor poisoning. Arch. Pediatr. *79*:28-30, 1962a.

Klingensmith, W. R. Poisoning by camphor. J. A. M. A. *102*:2182-2183, 1934.

Köppel, C.; Tenczer, J.; Schirop, T.; Ibe, K. Camphor poisoning. Abuse of camphor as a stimulant. Arch. Toxicol. *51*:101-106, 1982a.

Kopelman, R.; Miller, S.; Kelly, R.; Sunshine, I. Camphor intoxication treated by resin hemoperfusion. J. A. M. A. *241*:727-728, 1979.

Krueger, R. P. Chemical pneumonitis from medicated vapor aerosol spraying. Clin. Pediatr. *6*:465-467, 1967.

Laurie, M. M. Camphorated oil asphyxia. Can. Med. Assoc. J. *63*:298, 1950.

Phelan, W. J. Camphor poisoning. Over counter dangers. Pediatrics *57*:428-431, 1976.

Riggs, J.; Hamilton, R.; Homel, S.; McCabe, J. Camphorated oil intoxication in pregnancy. Obstet. Gynecol. *25*:255-258, 1965.

Rubin, M. B.; Recinos, A, Jr.; Washington, J. A.; Koppanyi, T. Ingestion of poisons in children: A survey of 250 admissions to Children's Hospital. A special report. Clin. Proc. Child. Hosp., Wash. *5*:57-73, 1949.

Rubsamen, W. Todliche Kampervergiftung nach Anwendung von offizinellem Kampferol zur postoperativen Peritonitisprophylaxe. Zentralbl. Gynaekol. *36*:1009-1015, 1912.

Seife, M.; Leon, J. L. Camphor poisoning following ingestion of nose drops. J. A. M. A. *155*:1059, 1954.

Skoglund, R. R.; Ware, L. L., Jr.; Schanberger, J. E. Prolonged seizures due to contact and inhalation exposure to camphol. A case report. Clin. Pediatr. *16*:901-902, 1977.

Smith, A.; Margolis, G. Camphor poisoning, anatomical and pharmacological study, report of a fatal case, experimental investigation of protective action of barbiturate. Am. J. Pathol. *30*:857-869, 1954.

Trestrail, J. H.; Spartz, E. M. Camphorated and castor oil confusion and its toxic results. Clin. Toxicol. *11*:151-158, 1977.

Verhulst, H. L.; Page, L. A.; Crotty, J. J. Camphor. Am. J. Dis. Child. *101*:536-537, 1961.

Webster, R. W. *Legal Medicine and Toxicology*. W. B. Saunders Co., Philadelphia, 1930.

Weiss, J.; Catalano, P. Camphorated oil intoxication during pregnancy. Pediatrics *52*:713-714, 1973.

CARBARYL

Derivatives of carbamic acid (H_2N-COOH) are used as herbicides, insecticides and medicinal agents. The herbicidal carbamates usually have a phenyl substituent on the nitrogen. In general this group does not include potent inhibitors of acetylcholinesterase, but relevant data are often lacking. See Section II for comments about the toxicity of specific herbicidal carbamates (*e.g.*, chlorpropham).

The insecticidal carbamates including carbaryl are usually mono-*N*-methyl substituted and are often aryl esters as well. These compounds are insecticidal by virtue of an ability to inhibit cholinesterase. Presumably cholinesterase inhibition also accounts for their major toxic effects in mammals, but because of important differences in absorption, distribution, metabolism, excretion and inherent "side effects," no general correlation can be drawn between toxicity and anticholinesterase activity (Ryan, 1971).

The drug physostigmine also fits the chemical pattern of carbamate insecticides, but neostigmine is exceptional in that it is di-N-methyl substituted. These and similar drugs are used therapeutically as cholinesterase inhibitors in treating myasthenia gravis and certain exogenous intoxications.

Toxicology: Literature estimates of the acute oral LD_{50} of carbaryl in rats range from 250 mg./kg. (Vandekar et al., 1971) up to 400 to 850 mg./kg. (Desi et al., 1974). Nine other monomethyl carbamates with advanced status in a World Health Organization insecticide evaluation program have oral LD_{50} values in rats that range from 40 to 1000 mg./kg. (Vandekar et al., 1971). Most insecticidal carbamates appear to lie in toxicity class 4, but at least one qualifies for toxicity class 6 (see also Section II).

Clinical experience with carbaryl poisoning has not been extensive. In one confirmed case of carbaryl ingestion, miosis, salivation and muscular incoordination occurred in a 19-month-old child. The dose was not known, but the symptoms were promptly relieved by 0.3 mg. of atropine (Best and Murray, 1962). A moderately severe poisoning in an adult male followed the ingestion of only 250 mg. (2.8 mg./kg.). Violent epigastric pain, profuse sweating and lassitude were relieved after a cumulative atropine dose of 3 mg. (Hayes, 1963). An adult male suicide victim expired in terminal acute pulmonary edema 6 hours after ingesting an unknown dose (Farago, 1969). In one reported series of 50 alleged poisonings, however, there were no deaths. Indeed, less than a dozen victims had signs or symptoms referable to cholinesterase inhibition, and these effects were transient (Back, 1965). Male volunteers who consumed doses up to 0.13 mg./kg. per day for 6 weeks had no subjective effects that could be related to carbaryl, although they exhibited a slight, transient decrease in the ability of their kidneys to reabsorb amino acids (Wills et al., 1968).

Carbaryl may be a weak sensitizer, but it is not a primary irritant to the skin (Carpenter et al., 1961a). When applied to the ventral forearm of humans, ^{14}C-labeled carbaryl (label position unspecified) was slowly but almost completely absorbed. Given intravenously in trace amounts, only 8.2% of the ^{14}C was excreted in the urine after 120 hours; the estimated half-life was 9 hours (Feldmann and Maibach, 1974). When, however, human subjects were given 2 mg./kg. by mouth, about 27% of the dose was accounted for by identified metabolites in a 24-hour urine collection (Knaak et al., 1968). In most laboratory mammals, 65 to 75% of the radiolabel in an orally administerd dose of ^{14}C-ring-labeled carbaryl is found in the urine in the first 24 hours (Kuhr and Dorough, 1976). Almost no unchanged carbaryl is excreted. At least in rats, enterohepatic recycling prolongs the biological half-life of carbaryl metabolites (Houston et al., 1974). Although the whole-body half-life of ^{14}C derived from ingested or injected carbaryl appears to exceed 4 hours in rats (Krishna and Casida, 1966; Kuhr and Dorough, 1976), a half-life of only 77 minutes characterizes the slower of two components in the plasma clearance of unchanged carbaryl (Houston et al., 1974).

The intoxication syndrome induced by carbamate cholinesterase inhibitors differs dramatically from that induced by organophosphorus insecticides, such as parathion, in terms of duration. An adult volunteer who ingested 1.5 mg./kg. of isopropoxyphenyl-N-methylcarbamate (propoxur) experienced a prompt fall in red cell cholinesterase activity that reached a minimum of 27% of normal in 15 minutes. This was quickly followed by blurred vision, nausea, pallor, sweating, tachycardia and vomiting. All symptoms had abated, and enzyme levels were back to normal by 2 hours (Vandekar et al., 1971). Carbaryl, however, is a longer acting compound, and cholinergic signs and symptoms may persist for 6 to 8 hours. Symptoms in parathion poisoning tend to last much longer. Even the newer generation of highly toxic and supertoxic carbamates have short-lasting effects (Simpson and Bermingham, 1977).

Another difference between carbamates and organophosphates relates to their penetrability into the central nervous system. Although exceptions clearly exist (e.g., physostigmine), carbamates appear to enter the brain poorly if at all and/or produce only minimal effects on brain cholinesterase activity (Baron et al., 1964; Carpenter et al., 1961a). Thus, the prominent central nervous system effects of some organophosphorus compounds are minimal or nonexistent with carbamates.

A third difference between carbaryl and parathion apparently relates to effects other than cholinesterase inhibition, although at present these are incompletely defined. Carbamate pesticides on the average are more toxic by an order of magnitude when given intravenously than when administered orally. By the intravenous route, carbaryl and some (but by no means all) carbamates produce a transient but deep "anesthesia" with severe dyspnea and rapid onset of respiratory arrest. When dosed rats were maintained on artificial respiration for only a few minutes, spontaneous respirations resumed and were followed by typical cholinergic signs.

The mechanism is unknown, but the effect is considerably less after intraperitoneal administration and is not seen at all after oral administration (Vandekar et al., 1971). Perhaps the high first-pass effect (see below) plays a role in these observations. It is tempting to speculate that the ability of sedative doses of reserpine, chlordiazepoxide and phenobarbital to enhance the intraperitoneal toxicity of carbaryl is related to this phenomenon, but the same interaction with sedatives was seen with parathion, with which "anesthetic" effects have not been described (Weiss and Orzel, 1967).

Carbaryl does not produce the demyelination reaction exhibited by some organophosphates in chickens, but poisoned fowl did have fat droplets in the epithelial cells of their proximal renal tubules (Carpenter et al., 1961a). Desi et al. (1974) documented permanent behavioral aberrations in rats which received carbaryl or propoxur repeatedly, although the authors did not consider either carbamate to be a dangerous neurotoxin. After more than 4 weeks of 150 mg./ kg. carbaryl per day, swine exhibited progressive myasthenia, incoordination, ataxia, tremors, clonic muscular contractions, paraplegia, prostration and death. Pathological lesions in the central nervous system appeared to be due to vasogenic edema (Smalley et al., 1969).

As judged by in vitro studies with human and rat liver preparations (Chin et al., 1974; Strother, 1972), carbaryl and several other carbamates are metabolized by ring hydroxylation and N-dealkylation. The products retain the functional ester grouping necessary for cholinesterase inhibition. Indeed, the resistance of carbamates to hydrolysis in vivo is surprisingly high, especially in monkeys and pigs (Knaak et al., 1968), which accounts for the variety of oxidized metabolites. The resistance to hydrolysis, however, is far from complete in rats (Krishna and Casida, 1966), dogs and humans (Knaak et al., 1968).

Based on identified urinary metabolites excreted by two men who each swallowed 2 mg./ kg. in gelatin capsules (Knaak et al., 1968), carbaryl is hydrolyzed to 1-naphthol and excreted as conjugates of glucuronic and sulfuric acids, together with smaller amounts of conjugated 4-hydroxycarbaryl. In the isolated, perfused rabbit lung, carbaryl is metabolized to 4-hydroxycarbaryl, α-naphthol and several unidentified products (Blase and Loomis, 1976). In rat urine the major metabolic products are the glucuronide or sulfate conjugates of 5,6-dihydro-5,6-dihydroxycarbaryl and of N-hydroxymethylcarbaryl (Chen and Dorough, 1979). The ultimate metabolism of carbaryl is complex (see review by Kuhr and Dorough, 1976), but it is unlikely that the acute toxicity of carbamates depends on any of their metabolites (Ryan, 1971).

The reaction between organophosphates and cholinesterase is essentially irreversible, and the product, a phosphorylated enzyme, is stable in water. The carbamates inhibit cholinesterase by carbamylating the active site. Unlike the phosphorylated enzyme the carbamylated enzyme undergoes spontaneous hydrolysis to reactivate the enzyme. The classical antidote against a cholinesterase inhibitor is atropine, which blocks muscarinic cholinergic receptors in all tissues. Tetraethylammonium, a ganglionic blocking agent, was inferior to atropine as an antidote against a series of carbamate insecticides (Kimmerle, 1971).

In poisonings by organophosphates it is a common practice to administer (in addition to atropine) pralidoxime chloride (2-PAM) or some other oxime that reacts with the phosphorylated enzyme to regenerate the active site. Whether an analogous benefit accrues with the carbamylated enzyme in carbamate poisoning is unclear. The monomethylcarbamylated cholinesterase of bovine erythrocytes has an in vitro recovery half-time (at pH 7) of 19 minutes whether 2-PAM (or a related oxime) is present or not (O'Brien, 1968; Wilson et al., 1960).

Toxicity data, however, suggest that 2-PAM and other oximes may be effective at motor end plates (or perhaps some other critical sites) in accelerating the recovery of acetylcholinesterase inhibited by various methylcarbamate insecticides. For example, atropine alone was found to be an effective antidote in rats against eight carbamates including carbaryl. When either of two oximes was given together with atropine, the antidotal effects were generally enhanced, except in the case of carbaryl where the oximes reduced the efficacy of atropine. Used alone, the oximes were effective against seven carbamates in varying degrees, except again in the case of carbaryl, whose toxicity was markedly increased (Natoff and Reiff, 1973). This remarkable difference was also reflected in the profiles of cholinesterase activity, and its basis remains unexplained.

One concludes that, although 2-PAM appears to be an optional adjunct to atropine in carbamate poisoning generally, it is contraindicated in the case of carbaryl. Even against other carbamate insecticides, it is probably of very limited usefulness because of the rapid spontaneous reactivation of cholinesterase inhibited by monomethylcarbamates.

Several carbamates (carbofuran, aldicarb, pirimicarb) cross the rat placenta and inhibit acetylcholinesterase in fetal tissues to a greater extent than in corresponding maternal tissues (Cambon et al., 1979). Carbaryl was not teratogenic in dogs or rhesus monkeys, nor was it oncogenic in mice (EPA, September 15, 1978).

Symptomatology: Except for diminished intensity and duration, particularly of the central nervous signs and symptoms, carbamate poisoning resembles parathion intoxication in its clinical manifestations.

1. Nausea, vomiting, abdominal cramps, diarrhea and excessive salivation (sialorrhea) and sweating.
2. Lassitude and weakness.
3. Rhinorrhea and a sensation of tightness in the chest may occur with respiratory exposures.
4. Blurring or dimness of vision, miosis (with fixed pinpoint pupils), tearing, ciliary muscle spasm, loss of accommodation, and ocular pain. None of these eye signs, however, is dependable for diagnosis. Mydriasis may be seen secondary to sympathoadrenal discharge.
5. Loss of muscle coordination, slurring of speech, fasciculations and twitching of muscles.
6. Difficulty in breathing, excessive secretions of saliva and of respiratory tract mucus, oronasal frothing, cyanosis, pulmonary rales and rhonchi, and hypertension (presumably due to asphyxia).
7. Random jerky movements, incontinence, convulsions and coma.
8. Death primarily due to respiratory arrest of central origin, paralysis of the respiratory muscles, intense bronchoconstriction or all three.

Treatment:

1. Atropinize the patient immediately. In an adult the usual dose is 1 to 4 mg. of the sulfate (or other salt) given intramuscularly or, better, intravenously (if there is no cyanosis). The maintenance of full atropinization may require 2-mg. doses at intervals of 10 to 60 minutes for several hours. Because of their high tolerance, poisoned patients commonly receive too little atropine, rarely too much. The need for more atropine can be recognized by the continuation or recurrence of those toxic symptoms described above; excessive salivation is a particularly useful criterion (but not eye signs). It is said that atropine is dangerous in the presence of anoxia and that cyanosis should be corrected before atropinization, if possible.
2. Relieve upper airway obstruction (see p. IV-2). Mucus and other respiratory tract secretions may have to be aspirated continuously. Endotracheal intubation or tracheostomy may become necessary (see pp. IV-4–6).
3. Give oxygen and artificial respiration as needed (see p. IV-7). In addition to upper tract obstruction (p. IV-3), pulmonary edema may occur and may require treatment (p. IV-14).
4. Gastric lavage or syrup of ipecac may be warranted if spontaneous vomiting is not prompt and profuse. See Section I for details.
5. Wash any contaminated areas of the skin with soap and water or, perhaps better, with 95% ethyl alcohol. Irrigate the eyes with water or saline.
6. Administer continuously by the intravenous route isotonic saline to correct dehydration and electrolyte imbalances.
7. Avoid pralidoxime chloride (2-PAM) in the case of carbaryl poisoning. With other carbamates, 2-PAM is in general unnecessary even in severe intoxications, although with atropine it has been shown in animals to have a higher antidotal effectiveness than atropine alone. See p. III-340 for dosage schedules.
8. Avoid central nervous system depressants, such as reserpine, chlordiazepoxide, phenobarbital, etc., which potentiate carbaryl poisoning in animals.
9. Keep the patient under constant observation for at least 24 hours.

Laboratory: Assays for cholinesterase activity may or may not aid in the diagnosis or prognosis. Any depression of activity can be expected to be transitory. It is often difficult to demonstrate a clear-cut inhibition of cholinesterase activity by standard laboratory techniques. At least with some carbamates, red cell cholinesterase may be significantly depressed at times when the plasma activity is normal. A favorable response to atropine is a more reliable diagnostic aid than any cholinesterase assay.

References:

Back, R. C. Significant developments in eight years with Sevin insecticide. J. Agric. Food Chem. *13*:198-199, 1965.

Baron, R. L.; Casterline, J. L., Jr.; Fitzhugh, O. G. Specificity of carbamate-induced esterase inhibition in mice. Toxicol. Appl. Pharmacol. *6*:402-410, 1964.

Best, E. M., Jr.; Murray, B. L. Observations on workers exposed to Sevin insecticide: a preliminary report. J. Occup. Med. *4*:507-517, 1962.

Blase, B. W.; Loomis, T. A. The uptake and metabolism of carbaryl by isolated perfused rabbit lung. Toxicol. Appl. Pharmacol. *37*:481-490, 1976.

Cambon, C.; Declume, C.; Derache, R. Effect of the insecticidal carbamate derivatives (carbofuran, pirimicarb, aldicarb) on the activity of acetylcholinesterase in tissues from pregnant rats and fetuses. Toxicol. Appl. Pharmacol. *49*:203-208, 1979.

Carpenter, C. P.; Weil, C. S.; Palm, P. E.; Woodside, M. W.; Nair, J. H., III; Smyth, H. F., Jr. Mammalian toxicity of 1-naphthyl-N-methyl carbamate (sevin insecticide). J. Agric. Food Chem. *9*:30-39, 1961a.

Chen, K. C.; Dorough, H. W. Glutathione and mercapturic acid conjugations in the metabolism of naphthalene and 1-naphthyl N-methylcarbamate (carbaryl). Drug Chem. Toxicol. *2*:331-354, 1979.

Chin, B. H.; Eldridge, J. M.; Sullivan, L. J. Metabolism of carbaryl by selected human tissues using an organ maintenance technique. Clin. Toxicol. *7*:37-56, 1974.

Desi, I.; Gonczi, L.; Simon, G.; Farkas, I.; Kneffel, Z. Neurotoxicologic studies of two carbamate perticides in subacute animal experiments. Toxicol. Appl. Pharmacol. *27*:465-476, 1974.

EPA. Tolerances and exemptions from tolerances for pesticide chemicals in or on raw agricultural commodities: Proposed tolerances for the pesticide chemical carbaryl. Federal Register 43:41240, September 15, 1978.

Farago, A. Suicidale, todliche Sevin-(1-Naphthyl-N-methylkarbamat) Vergiftung. Arch. Toxikol. 24:309-315, 1969.

Feldmann, R. J.; Maibach, H. I. Percutaneous penetration of some pesticides and herbicides in man. Toxicol. Appl. Pharmacol. 28:126-132, 1974.

Hayes, W. J., Jr. Clinical Handbook on Economic Poisons. USPHS Publication No. 476. U. S. Government Printing Office, Washington, D. C., 1963.

Houston, J. B.; Upshall, D. G.; Bridges, J. W. Pharmacokinetics and metabolism of two carbamate insecticides, carbaryl and landrin in the rat. Xenobiotica 5:637-648, 1974.

Kimmerle, G. Comparison of the antidotal actions of tetraethylammonium chloride and atropine in acute poisoning of carbamate insecticides in rats. Arch. Toxikol. 27:311-314, 1971.

Knaak, J. B.; Tallant, M. J.; Kozbelt, S. J.; Sullivan, L. J. The metabolism of carbaryl in man, monkey, pig and sheep. J. Agr. Food Chem. 16:465-470, 1968.

Krishna, J. G.; Casida, J. E. Fate in rats of the radiocarbon from ten variously labeled methyl- and dimethylcarbamate-^{14}C insecticide chemicals and their hydrolysis products. J. Agric. Food Chem. 14:98-105, 1966.

Kuhr, R. J.; Dorough, H. W. Carbamate Insecticides: Chemistry, Biochemistry and Toxicology. CRC Press Inc., Cleveland, Ohio, 1976.

Natoff, I.; Reiff, B. Effect of oximes on the acute toxicity of anticholinesterase carbamates. Toxicol. Appl. Pharmacol. 25:569-575, 1973.

O'Brien, R. D. Kinetics of the carbamylation of cholinesterase. Mol. Pharmacol. 4:121-130, 1968.

Ryan, A. J. The metabolism of carbamate pesticides. C. R. C. Critical Rev. Toxicol. 1:33-54, 1971.

Simpson, G. R.; Bermingham, S. Poisoning by carbamate insecticides. Med. J. Aust. 2:148-149, 1977.

Smalley, H. E.; O'Hara, P. J.; Bridges, C. H.; Radeleff, R. D. The effects of chronic carbaryl administration on the neuromuscular system of swine. Toxicol. Appl. Pharmacol. 14:409-419, 1969.

Strother, A. In vitro metabolism of methylcarbamate insecticides by human and rat liver fraction. Toxicol. Appl. Pharmacol. 21:112-129, 1972.

Vandekar, M.; Plestina, R.; Wilhelm, K. Toxicity of carbamates for mammals. Bull. W. H. O. 44:241-249, 1971.

Weiss, L. R.; Orzel, R. A. Enhancement of toxicity of anticholinesterases by central depressant drugs in rats. Toxicol. Appl. Pharmacol. 10:334-339, 1967.

Wills, J. H.; Jameson, E.; Coulston, F. Effect of oral doses of carbaryl on man. Clin. Toxicol. 1:265-271, 1968.

Wilson, I. B.; Hatch, M. A.; Ginsburg, S. Carbamylation of acetylcholinesterase. J. Biol. Chem. 235:2312-2315, 1960.

CARBON DISULFIDE

Carbon disulfide (or bisulfide) (CS_2) is a clear, colorless liquid which, in its pure state, smells like ether or chloroform and in a commercial grade has an offensive odor like decaying cabbage. It is used as a solvent for waxes and resins, as a cleaner for removing grease, and, in vapor form, as a disinfectant and insecticide. Most cases of poisoning have arisen from industrial exposures, formerly in the vulcanization of rubber and more recently in the production of viscose rayon and other artificial fibers. Workers in these industries are often exposed concomitantly to HYDROGEN SULFIDE (p. III-198), an extremely dangerous gas but one which lacks a cumulative toxicity. A useful source book and guide to the voluminous foreign literature on the toxicology of carbon disulfide is edited by Brieger and Teisinger (1967).

Toxicology: Carbon disulfide is hazardous as a liquid and as a vapor. Absorption occurs through all portals including the intact skin (Brieger, 1967; Cohen et al., 1958). First-hand accounts of carbon disulfide ingestion episodes are extremely rare. Half an ounce has killed on at least three occasions (Foreman, 1886; Gonzales et al., 1954; citation in Moeschlin, 1965). Victims exhibited spasmodic tremor, prostration, dyspnea, cyanosis, peripheral vascular collapse, hypothermia, mydriasis, convulsions, coma and death in a few hours from respiratory paralysis (Davidson and Feinleib, 1972). Only mild gastrointestinal irritation and visceral congestion were noted at autopsy (Foreman, 1886; Gonzales et al., 1954).

Two ounces have failed to kill when ingested with suicidal intent (as cited in Foreman, 1886), but 5 ml. ingested accidentally by a 42-year-old woman induced an illness that lasted more than a week (Yamada, 1977). She experienced numbness of the lips, nausea and vomiting and within about 12 hours hyperesthesia and agitation. Her tendon reflexes were hyperactive, and the Babinski sign was positive. Illusions, delusions and memory impairment were noted. Abnormal brain waves persisted throughout the sixth day.

A vapor concentration of 15 mg./L. (4800 ppm) may cause death within an hour, whereas 3 to 5 mg./L. may be tolerated for the same time without serious sequelae (Division of Industrial Hygiene, NIH, 1941). Such acute massive exposures produce symptoms not unlike those seen in the available reports of ingestions: severe narcosis followed or preceded by delirium, areflexia, mydriasis, coma, paralysis and death in respiratory failure or sometimes permanent neurological disorders in survivors (see below). Again, however, such reports are rare (Division of Industrial Hygiene, NIH, 1941; Harmsen, 1905).

In contrast, a rich literature of clinical reports and experimental studies exists on chronic carbon disulfide poisoning. Severe intoxications have resulted from prolonged vapor exposures to concentrations as low as 30 ppm (Division of Industrial Hygiene, NIH, 1941). Unlike the chlorinated hydrocarbon solvents, carbon disulfide is not principally a hepatic or renal toxin (but see below); it is, however, a dangerous nerve poison (Cohen et al., 1959; Lewey, 1941b) that attacks both the central and peripheral nervous systems. To protect industrial workers, the current OSHA threshold limit value (TLV) is 20 ppm (TWA) in air, but a TLV of 1 ppm was recommended in 1977 (NIOSH, 1977). The maximal permissible limit in the Soviet Union is said to be 0.33 ppm.

Industrially exposed workers have exhibited a fantastic variety of neurological signs and symptoms. The outstanding sequelae are neuropsychiatric disorders ranging from irritability to a manic-depressive psychosis, especially of the manical type, with or without evidence of organic nervous disease of pyramidal and extrapyramidal tracts, basal ganglia and peripheral nerves. Among the reported clinical manifestations of neuronal damage are all grades of emotional and mental disorders, weakness and paralysis, hypesthesias, blindness, and the signs of parkinsonism (Gordy and Trumper, 1938, 1940; Kleinfeld and Tabershaw, 1955; Lewey, 1941a; Paluch, 1948; Vigliani, 1946, 1950). Women appear to be more sensitive than men to the neurotoxic effects of carbon disulfide (Ehrhardt, 1967).

Carbon disulfide peripheral neuritis affects both motor and sensory nerves. Nerves in the legs are particularly susceptible, but even the cranial nerves may be injured (optic, auditory). The initial symptom is apt to be a sensation of crawling over the skin (formication), progressing to constant or paroxysmal pain in the distribution of one or more peripheral nerves. Eventually, weakness and paralysis occur. The peripheral neuritis of carbon disulfide may resolve slowly over a period of 6 to 8 months; any residual disability at that time is likely to be permanent (Hamilton and Hardy, 1974).

Perhaps because of improved measures of industrial hygiene, the above classical picture of carbon disulfide intoxication (encephalopathy, psychosis, polyneuritis) appears to be a vanishing phenomenon (Toyama and Sakurai, 1967). Intoxications seen in modern times develop slowly over many years of exposure and tend to be milder in form. With reductions in the incidence of flagrant neurological disease, derangements in other organ systems have attracted increasing attention.

Abnormally high serum levels of cholesterol (but not cholesterol esters) and of β-lipoprotein are common findings in chronically exposed workers (Gavrilescu and Lilis, 1967; Toyama and Sakurai, 1967). These findings are presumably related to the high incidence of early arteriosclerosis and hypertension (von Rechenberg, 1957; Vigliani, 1954). By biopsy, autopsy and angiography, arterial lesions have been found in skeletal muscles (notably in the major arteries to leg muscles), kidneys, heart, and especially the brain. In neurological victims, marked cerebral vascular damage has been described, involving pyramidal, extrapyramidal and pseudobulbar tracts. Atherosclerosis and ischemia, however, are probably not the principal cause of neural damage in carbon disulfide poisoning because not all neurological patients show evidence of vascular lesions or of hypertension (von Rechenberg, 1957). Epidemiological studies strongly suggest that carbon disulfide is an etiological factor in coronary artery disease with angina pectoris (Gavrilescu and Lilis, 1967; Hernberg et al., 1970; Tiller et al., 1968).

Chronically exposed workers also have an increased incidence of retinal microaneurysms that correlates with the duration of exposure. That these lesions may be related to similar ones seen in diabetes mellitus is suggested by increased blood glucose levels during prednisolone oral glucose tolerance tests (Goto et al., 1971). The existence of subclinical defects in carbohydrate metabolism among viscose rayon workers has been confirmed many times (e.g., Franco et al., 1979). One group of Czech investigators has reported that frank diabetes was 3 times more prevalent in an exposed group than in a control group (Balcarova et al., 1980). This latent or overt diabetes has been ascribed (Franco et al., 1979) to CS_2-induced alterations in zinc metabolism (see below). Speculation has suggested that the peripheral polyneuritis of carbon disulfide poisoning and that of diabetes may have an unknown pathogenesis in common. Renal biopsies of exposed patients have revealed glomerulosclerotic lesions remarkably like those seen in diabetes mellitus (Kusunoki, cited by Toyama and Sakurai, 1967). Chronic renal dysfunction with impaired creatinine clearances may become one of the more important manifestations of long-term CS_2 poisoning among workers whose exposure is not intense enough to elicit neurological deficits (Toyama and Sakurai, 1967).

Many other functional derangements are described in chronic poisoning by carbon disulfide vapor. The incidence of chronic gastritis with dyspepsia is high; both hyperacidity and hypoacidity are encountered (Hassman et al., 1967). Perhaps vascular lesions (see above) are responsible for the gastritis and occasionally enteritis (Lysina, 1967). Exposed male workers show a significant decrease in 17-ketosteroids and hydroxycorticosteroids (Cavalleri et al., 1967). Loss of libido is a common complaint (Gordy and Trumper, 1940), as are menstrual disorders. The fibrinolytic activity of blood serum is said to be significantly reduced (Visconti et al., 1967).

Liver damage is not a prominent feature of acute or chronic carbon disulfide poisoning in man. Among exposed Russian workers, however, Lysina (1967) reports a 20.6% incidence of palpable, tender livers and frequent, although minor, derangements of liver function (low albumin-to-globulin plasma ratios). There is no doubt that carbon disulfide can damage the liver, at least in the rat. Rats surviving a single oral dose of CS_2 showed liver enlargement and depression of hepatic drug-metabolizing enzyme activity but not liver necrosis. When hepatic microsomal enzyme activity was induced by phenobarbital pretreatment, the LD_{50} of CS_2 remained the same, but liver necrosis became evident (Bond et al., 1969). This phenomenon has attracted much experimental work (e.g., Torres et al., 1980), but its relevance to human toxicology is not clear.

Carbon disulfide vapor is rapidly absorbed when inhaled; an approximate equilibrium between blood and inhaled vapor is reached in 1 to 2 hours. At the termination of exposure, some absorbed carbon disulfide is excreted in the expired air, but opinions vary about the proportion of the absorbed dose that is eliminated in this way (Brieger, 1967). Although traces have been detected in the blood 80 hours after termination of exposure, about 70% of an inhaled dose is excreted or metabolized within a few hours. The remaining 30% is slowly excreted in the urine as such or as metabolites (as cited in Brieger, 1967; McKee et al., 1943; Teisinger and Souček, 1949). A small amount of the absorbed carbon disulfide is apparently converted to hydrogen sulfide (Brieger, 1967), which is rapidly oxidized to sulfate and excreted in the urine (McKee et al., 1943; Strittmatter et al., 1950). It appears most unlikely that hydrogen sulfide plays any role in the acute or chronic toxicity of carbon disulfide.

Carbon disulfide reacts with a variety of nucleophilic functional groups: (1) amino, to form dithiocarbamic acids; (2) mercapto, to form trithiocarbonic acids; (3) hydroxyl, to form xanthogenic acids; (4) compounds with two such groups to form heterocycles (Souček and Madlo, 1956; Vašák and Kopecký, 1967). This type of direct chemical inactivation appears to be the major means of disposal of retained carbon disulfide (Brieger, 1967). Based on animal studies, administration of glutamic acid or urea has been recommended as a means of inactivating free carbon disulfide and in this way protecting key endogenous substances (Abramova, 1967).

Some thiocarbamates as formed by carbon disulfide above are able to chelate polyvalent cations tightly, particularly copper and to a lesser degree zinc. In animals exposed to carbon disulfide the copper content of the brain and spinal cord was significantly lowered; at the same time, marked degenerative changes were observed in axons of the spinal cord and the Purkinje cells of the cerebrum (Cohen et al., 1959). Carbon disulfide workers were found to have low serum levels of zinc with increased rates of urinary zinc excretion (El-Gazzar et al., 1973).

Dopamine-β-oxidase, a key copper-containing enzyme of neural tissue, has been suggested as a possible site for the crucial biochemical lesion in carbon disulfide poisoning (Scheel, 1967). The hypothesis has been largely confirmed in rats (McKenna and DiStefano, 1977). However, carbon disulfide is also recognized as an inhibitor of brain monoamine oxidase (Magistretti and Peirone, 1961; Melson and Weigelt, 1967), and signs of carbon disulfide poisoning in animals are intensified by reserpine, iproniazid and amphetamine (Abramova, 1967). Monoamine oxidase also contains copper and utilizes pyridoxal phosphate (a form of vitamin B_6) as a coenzyme. Since carbon disulfide can react with pyridoxamine to form pyridoxaminedithiocarbamic acid (which in turn can be oxidized by iodine in vitro to an analogue of disulfiram; see p. III-159), it is possible that this reaction in vivo leads to a functional vitamin B_6 deficiency (Vašák and Kopecký, 1967). Thus two possible mechanisms exist for inhibition of monoamine oxidase in CS_2-exposed individuals. Transaminases also require pyridoxal phosphate, and in vitamin B_6 deficiency these enzymes are also inhibited. As judged by the increased urinary excretion of xanthurenic acid in a tryptophan loading test, the transaminases involved in tryptophan metabolism are impaired in chronic CS_2 poisoning (Vašák and Kopecký, 1967).

Pyridoxine has also been recommended for the therapy of carbon disulfide poisoning (Abramova, 1967), but differences are recognized between vitamin B_6 deficiency and carbon disulfide intoxication (Vašák and Kopecký, 1967). A decrease in urinary catecholamine excretion was observed in exposed rabbits (Vašák and Kopecký, 1967), a finding that is more consistent with inhibition of dopamine-β-oxidase than of monoamine oxidase. Perhaps a lesion also occurs in serotonin metabolism since a tryptophan-enriched diet increases the toxicity of carbon disulfide (Abramova, 1967).

Symptomatology:

A. Acute

1. Mild to moderate irritation of skin, eyes, and mucous membranes from liquid or concentrated vapors. If its evaporation is prevented, the liquid acts as a skin vesicant (Hueper, 1936). Percutaneous absorption occurs.

2. Headache.

3. Garlicky breath, nausea, vomiting, diarrhea (even after vapor exposures), and occasionally abdominal pain.

4. Weak pulse, palpitations.

5. Fatigue, weakness in the legs, unsteady gait, vertigo.
6. Hyperesthesia, agitation, mania, hallucinations of sight, hearing, taste, and smell in acute, massive vapor exposures and sometimes in ingestion episodes.
7. Central nervous depression with respiratory paralysis.
8. Death may occur during coma or after a convulsion.

B. Chronic
1. Headache, fatigue, inability to concentrate, insomnia, dyspepsia, tremor, giddiness or vertigo.
2. Peripheral polyneuritis is often encountered: formication, pain, weakness, paralysis. The absence of a corneal reflex is highly characteristic according to Lewey (1941a).
3. Emotional instability of all grades ranging from mild neurasthenia and depression to frank psychosis with psychomotor excitement, delirium and hallucinations.
4. Chronic, low-grade exposures of many years duration are associated with a high incidence of hypertension, atherosclerosis, renal and other parenchymal lesions (e.g., stomach and perhaps liver).
5. Recovery may occur within a few months or perhaps a few years, but paralyses may be permanent.

Treatment:
1. Remove patient to fresh air.
2. Artificial respiration (p. IV-7) and oxygen therapy (p. IV-12), as necessary.
3. Gastric lavage with warm water (if intoxication is due to ingestion).
4. If the patient is comatose, respiratory support may be required (p. IV-10). Avoid analeptic drugs. Because monoamine oxidase may be inhibited, catecholamines and catecholamine-releasing agents, like reserpine and amphetamine, should also be avoided or used only cautiously.
5. For severe excitement (delirium), see discussion on pp. IV-33–35.
6. A trial with large parenteral doses of vitamin B_6. Pyridoxine hydrochloride can be injected or tablets can be administered by mouth in daily doses as high as 25 mg./kg. Whereas these doses are well tolerated (but see p. III-295), their efficacy in CS_2 poisoning is not established.
7. An intravenous infusion of urea may also serve to trap chemically any absorbed carbon disulfide. Doses of 0.5 to 1.5 gm./kg. have been injected in man, but the efficacy of this treatment is unproven.

Laboratory:
1. Blood may show a slight increase in lymphocytes, a marked increase in monocytes, and occasionally an eosinophilia.
2. Serum cholinesterase activity is said to be reduced in poisoned patients, but this enzyme inhibition is apparently insufficient to produce characteristic symptoms.
3. Elevated serum levels of cholesterol and of β-lipoprotein after chronic exposures, probably correctable by large daily doses of vitamin B_6 (see above).
4. Specific chemical tests (e.g., iodine azide test) are available to evaluate exposure by measuring urinary metabolites (Djurić et al., 1965).

References:

Abramova, J. I. The questions of pathogenesis specific prevention, and therapy of carbon disulphide intoxication. In *Toxicology of Carbon Disulphide*, edited by H. Brieger and J. Teisinger. Excerpta Medica Foundation, Amsterdam, pp. 32-34, 1967.

Balcarova, O.; David, A.; Valnickova, J.; Stepanova, I.; Svandova, E.; Hromadka, M.; Lambl, V. Epidemiological study of ischemic heart disease in workers exposed to carbon disulfide. Prac. Lek. *32*:338-344, 1980.

Bond, E. J.; Butler, W. H.; DeMatteis, F.; Barnes, J. M. Effect of carbon disulfide on the liver of rats. Br. J. Ind. Med. *26*:335-337, 1969.

Brieger, H. Carbon disulfide in the living organism, retention, biotransformation and pathophysiological effects. In *Toxicology of Carbon Disulphide*, edited by H. Brieger and J. Teisinger. Excerpta Medica Foundation, Amsterdam, pp. 27-31, 1967.

Brieger, H.; Teisinger, J.; editors. *Toxicology of Carbon Disulphide.* . Excerpta Medica Foundation, Amsterdam, 1967.

Cavalleri, A.; Djuric, D.; Maugeri, U.; Brankovic, D.; Viscenti, E.; Rezman, I. 17-Ketosteroids and 17-hydroxycorticosteroids in the urine of young workers exposed to carbon disulfide. In *Toxicology of Carbon Disulphide*, edited by H. Brieger and J. Teisinger. Excerpta Medica Foundation, Amsterdam, pp. 86-91, 1967.

Cohen, A. E.; Paulus, H. J.; Keenan, R. G.; Scheel, L. D. Skin absorption of carbon disulfide vapor in rabbits. Arch. Ind. Health *17*:164-169, 1958.

Cohen, A. E.; Scheel, L. D.; Kopp, J. F.; Stockwell, F. R., Jr.; Keenan, R. G.; Moutain, J. T.; Paulus, H. J. Biochemical mechanisms in chronic carbon disulfide poisoning. Am. Ind. Hyg. Assoc. J. *20*:303-323, 1959.

Davidson, M.; Feinleib, M. Carbon disulfide poisoning; a review. Am. Heart J. *53*:100-114, 1972.

Division of Industrial Hygiene. National Institutes of Health. Carbon disulfide, its toxicity and potential dangers. Public Health Repts. (U. S.) *56*:574-581, 1941.

Djuric, D.; Surducki, N.; Berkes, I. Iodine-azide test on urine of persons exposed to carbon disulfide. Br. J. Ind. Med. *22*:321-323, 1965.

Ehrhardt, W. Experiences with the employment of woman exposed to carbon disulfide. In *Toxicology of Carbon Disulphide*, edited by H. Brieger and J. Teisinger. Excerpta Medica Foundation, Amsterdam, pp. 240-244, 1967.

El-Gazzar, R.; El-Sadik, Y. M.; Hussein, M. Changes in zinc and serum proteins due to carbon disulphide exposure. Br. J. Ind. Med. *30*:284-288, 1973.

Foreman, W. Notes of a fatal case of poisoning by bisulphide of carbon with post-mortem appearances and remarks. Lancet *2*:118-119, 1886.

Franco, G.; Malamani, T.; Piazza, A.; Candura, F. Subclinical defect of carbohydrate metabolism in viscose rayon workers exposed to carbon disulfide. G. Ital. Med. Lav. 1:75-78, 1979.

Gavrilescu, N.; Lilis, R. Cardiovascular effects of extended carbon disulphide exposure. In Toxicology of Carbon Disulphide, edited by H. Brieger and J. Teisinger. Excerpta Medica Foundation, Amsterdam, pp. 165-167, 1967.

Gonzales, T. A.; Vance, M.; Helpern, M.; Umberger, C. J. Legal Medicine, Pathology and Toxicology, 2nd ed. Appleton-Century-Crofts, New York, 1954.

Gordy, S. T.; Trumper, M. Carbon disulfide poisoning with a report of six cases. J. A. M. A. 110:1543-1549, 1938.

Gordy, S. T.; Trumper, M. Carbon disulfide poisoning. Report of 21 cases. Ind. Med. Surg. 9:231-234, 1940.

Goto, S.; Hotta, R.; Sugimoto, K. Studies on chronic carbon disulfide poisoning. Int. Arch. Arbeitsmed. 28:115-126, 1971.

Hamilton, A.; Hardy, H. L. Industrial Toxicology. 3rd ed. Publishing Sciences Group, Inc., (Acton, Massachusetts), 1974.

Harmsen, E. Die Schwefelkohlenstoff-Vergiftung im Fabrikbetriebe und ihre Verhutung. Z. gerichtl. Med. 30:149, 1905.

Hassman, P.; Simko, A.; Jindrichova, J.; Herout, V.; Hradsky, M. The problem of chronic gastritis in workers in the artificial fibres industry. In Toxicology of Carbon Disulphide, edited by H. Brieger and J. Teisinger. Excerpta Medica Foundation, Amsterdam, pp. 182-189, 1967.

Hernberg, S.; Partanen, T.; Nordman, C. H.; Sumari, P. Coronary heart disease among workers exposed to carbon disulfide. Br. J. Ind. Med. 27:313-325, 1970.

Hueper, W. C. Etiologic studies on the formation of skin blisters in viscose workers. J. Ind. Hyg. Toxicol. 18:432-447, 1936.

Kleinfeld, M.; Tabershaw, I. R. Carbon disulfide poisoning. Report of two cases. J. A. M. A. 159:677-680, 1955.

Lewey, F. W. Neurological, medical and biochemical signs and symptoms indicating chronic industrial carbon disulfide absorption. Ann. Intern. Med. 15:869-883, 1941a.

Lewey, F. W. Experimental chronic carbon disulfide poisoning in dogs, a clinical, biochemical and pathological study. J. Ind. Hyg. Toxicol. 23:415-420, 1941b.

Lysina, G. G. Some changes in the internal organs due to the effects of carbon disulphide. In Toxicology of Carbon Disulphide, edited by H. Brieger and J. Teisinger. Excerpta Medica Foundation, Amsterdam, pp. 179-181, 1967.

Magistretti, M.; Peirone, E. The action of carbon disulfide on cerebral monoamine oxidase. Med. Lav. 52:1-10, 1961.

McKee, R. W.; Kiper, C.; Fountain, J. H.; Riskin, A. M.; Drinker, P. A solvent vapor, carbon disulfide: absorption, elimination, metabolism and mode of action. J. A. M. A. 122:217-222, 1943.

McKenna, M. J.; DiStefano, V. Carbon disulfide. II. A proposed mechanism for the action of carbon disulfide on dopamine β-hydroxylase. J. Pharmacol. Exp. Ther. 202:253-266, 1977.

Melson, F.; Weigelt, H. The influence of tetramethyl thiuram and carbon disulfide on the enzymes monoaminoxidase and

alcoholdehydrogenase. In Toxicology of Carbon Disulphide, edited by H. Brieger and J. Teisinger. Excerpta Medica Foundation, Amsterdam, pp. 100-103, 1967.

Moeschlin, S. Poisoning, Diagnosis and Treatment. 1st Amer. Ed., Grune and Stratton, New York, 1965.

NIOSH. Occupational exposure to carbon disulfide. Criteria for a recommended standard. U. S. DHEW, Public Health Service, Publication No. 77-156, 1977.

Paluch, E. A. Two outbreaks of carbon disulfide poisoning in rayon staple fiber plants in Poland. J. Ind. Hyg. Toxicol. 30:37-40, 1948.

Scheel, L. D. Experimental carbon disulphide poisoning in rabbits - its mechanism and similarities with human case reports. In Toxicology of Carbon Disulphide, edited by H. Brieger and J. Teisinger. Excerpta Medica Foundation, Amsterdam, pp. 107-117, 1967.

Souček, B.; Maldo, Z. Dithiocarbamincarbonsauren als Abbauprodukte des Schwefelkohlenstoffs. Arch. Gewerbepath. u. Gewerbehyg. 14:511-521, 1956.

Strittmatter, C. F.; Peters, T.; McKee, R. W. Metabolism of labeled carbon disulfide in guinea pigs and mice. Arch. Ind. Hyg. Occup. Med. 1:54-64, 1950.

Teisinger, J.; Soucek, B. Absorption and elimination of carbon disulfide in man. J. Ind. Hyg. Toxicol. 31:67-73, 1949.

Tiller, J. R.; Schilling, R. S. F.; Morris, J. N. Occupational toxic factor in mortality from coronary heart disease. Br. Med. J. 4:407-411, 1968.

Torres, M.; Feldmann, G.; Perrault, M. A.; Jarvisalo, J.; Hakim, J. Morphological and biochemical effects of carbon disulfide on rat liver. Exp. Mol. Pathol. 33:333-344, 1980.

Toyama, T.; Sakurai, H. Ten-year changes in exposure level and toxicological manifestations in carbon disulfide workers. In Toxicology of Carbon Disulphide, edited by H. Brieger and J. Teisinger. Excerpta Medica Foundation, Amsterdam, pp. 197-204, 1967.

Vašák, V.; Kopecký, J. On the role of pyridoxamine in the mechanism of the toxic action of carbon disulphide. In Toxicology of Carbon Disulphide, edited by H. Brieger and J. Teisinger. Excerpta Medica Foundation, Amsterdam, pp. 35-41, 1967.

Vigliani, E. C. l'Intossicazione cronica du Sulfuro du Carbino. Med. Lav. 37:165-193, 1946.

Vigliani, E. C. Clinical observations on carbon disulfide intoxication in Italy. Ind. Med. Surg. 19:240-242, 1950.

Vigliani, E. C. CS₂ poisoning in viscose rayon factories. Br. J. Ind. Med. 11:235-244, 1954.

Visconti, E.; Vidakovic, A.; Cavalleri, A.; Rezman, I.; Maugeri, U.; Visnjic, V. Fibrinolytic activity in young workers exposed to carbon disulphide. In Toxicology of Carbon Disulphide, edited by H. Brieger and J. Teisinger. Excerpta Medica Foundation, Amsterdam, pp. 128-132, 1967.

von Rechenberg, H. K. Das vasculare Spatsyndrom der chronischen Schwefelkohlenstoffvergiftung. Helv. Med. Acta 24:510-513, 1957.

Yamada, Y. A case of acute carbon disulfide poisoning by accidental ingestion. Jpn. J. Ind. Health 19:140-141, 1977.

CARBON MONOXIDE

Carbon monoxide (CO) is a combustible, nonirritating, colorless, tasteless and essentially odorless gas. It readily mixes with air without stratification because it has about the same density. It may be found wherever organic material is burned under conditions of incomplete combustion (e.g., dynamite explosions), and it is a prominent constituent of flue gas from furnaces and exhaust gas from internal combustion engines. Concentrations as high as 30% have been measured in automobile exhaust gas, although 7% is more common (von Oettingen, 1944). Py-

rolysis of some vinyl plastics results in the production of appreciable concentrations of carbon monoxide (Cornish and Abar, 1969). Perhaps these or other plastics are also responsible for elevations of blood cyanide in victims of smoke inhalation (Clark et al., 1981).

Natural gas associated with petroleum deposits has no carbon monoxide, but in processing natural gas (e.g., cracking), carbon monoxide may be produced. As distributed, manufactured gas commonly has a carbon monoxide content between 2 and 15% (by volume). Occasionally, natural and manufactured gases are mixed prior to distribution, resulting in an intermediate carbon monoxide concentration (Bell, 1961).

Carbon monoxide is a hazard in many industrial processes. Among nonindustrial workers, firemen, cooks, bakers, chauffeurs, garage mechanics, linotypists, and furnace repairmen bear the greatest risk. An unusual emission source is represented by propane-fueled ice-surfacing machines in indoor skating rinks (Johnson et al., 1975). Smoking, however, constitutes a far more important source of exposure than ambient metropolitan atmospheres or common industrial occupations. The mean carboxyhemoglobin concentrations in smokers have been reported variously as 5 (Kahn et al., 1974) to 12% (Smith and Landaw, 1978). A summary of the voluminous early literature is provided by Drinker (1938).

Toxicology: Carbon monoxide is responsible for a larger number of severe chemical poisonings than any other single agent. Carbon monoxide acts primarily by depriving body cells of necessary oxygen (Haldane, 1895), although recent evidence summarized below suggests that there are subtle differences between hypoxic hypoxia and carbon monoxide poisoning. Oxygen is effectively excluded from the tissues by the formation of a reversible complex between carbon monoxide and the hemoglobin molecule; this complex, known as carboxyhemoglobin, is unable to transport as much oxygen as normal hemoglobin. Not only is the oxygen-carrying capacity of blood markedly reduced, but also the shape of the dissociation curve of oxyhemoglobin is altered so that a smaller portion of blood oxygen is released in tissue capillaries (Roughton and Darling, 1944). Tolerance sometimes encountered in chronically exposed animals or men may be due to polycythemia (Brieger, 1944; Smith and Landaw, 1978; Wilks et al., 1959), but a tolerance to the lethal effects that develops in as little as 24 hours has been observed in rats (Winston and Roberts, 1975).

The reduction in the oxygen-carrying capacity of blood is proportional to the amount of carboxyhemoglobin formed. The latter depends in turn upon the concentrations of carbon monoxide and of oxygen in inspired air and on the relative affinities of the hemoglobin molecule for these two gases. Because the affinity for carbon monoxide is 245 times that for oxygen (Lilienthal et al., 1946), a small concentration of CO in inspired air can tie up a large proportion of circulating hemoglobin. For example, CO concentrations of 0.01, 0.02, 0.1, and 1.0% should eventually saturate 11, 19, 54, and 92% of the hemoglobin, respectively; similar values have been cited elsewhere (Forbes et al., 1945; Sayers and Davenport, 1930). To reach any of these levels of carboxyhemoglobin requires exposures of appreciable duration; blood-gas equilibrium is nearly attained in 1 to 5 hours in the average adult (Forbes et al., 1945), but dangerous levels can be reached in a few minutes if the inspired CO concentration is very high (e.g., above 0.5%). All factors which speed respiration and circulation accelerate this process and so shorten the latent period before toxic signs and symptoms. Thus exercise, fever, and anemia increase the hazard of collapse from carbon monoxide. The hypoxic effects of altitude also summate with those of carboxyhemoglobin (Lilienthal and Pine, 1946; Pitts and Pace, 1947).

The nature and intensity of toxic signs and symptoms can be correlated, under certain circumstances, with the blood level of carboxyhemoglobin; see Symptomatology below (Sayers and Davenport, 1930). Any such correlation is clearly impossible when the blood concentration is changing rapidly. In massive exposures, consciousness may be lost with few or no premonitory signs or symptoms.

As with other chemical asphyxiants, the critical organ is that which is most sensitive to oxygen lack, notably the brain. Most signs and symptoms are referable to disturbed cerebral function, but cardiac abnormalities (see below) are also common. Both should be anticipated with carboxyhemoglobin concentrations above 20% (Winter and Miller, 1976).

The characteristic cherry-red color of the skin in carbon monoxide poisoning is due to a low concentration of reduced hemoglobin and a high concentration of carboxyhemoglobin in circulating blood. It is not, however, a regular or reliable sign, particularly in long exposures to low concentrations where victims are more apt to exhibit pallor or cyanosis (Binet and Conte, 1946; Dutra, 1958; Meigs and Hughes, 1952). Matthew (1971b) insists that the cherry-red skin color is characteristic at autopsy but rare in the living patient.

Until very high blood levels of carboxyhemoglobin are attained, little or no hyperpnea is observed at rest. The absence of significant chemoreceptor drive from the carotid body (Joels and Neil, 1962) is explained by the fact that the arterial oxygen tension (P_{O_2}) is normal, or only slightly reduced (Ayres et al., 1965) when the blood oxygen content is lowered by CO. In carbon monoxide poisoning, the breathlessness that is commonly observed with even mild exercise may arise solely from the metabolic acidosis that occurs because of generalized tissue hypoxia (see below). In part, however, the breathlessness of these patients during exercise may reflect carotid body activation due to obscure changes in the blood flow or metabolism of the receptor itself, in spite of the essentially normal arterial P_{O_2}. Hyperventilation may lead to respiratory alkalosis.

In severe carbon monoxide poisoning, tissue

oxygen tensions are very low, as evidenced by the low oxygen content of central venous blood (Ginsberg and Myers, 1974). In anoxic states, those tissues like skeletal muscle which can sustain high rates of anaerobic metabolism generate and release lactic and other organic acids into the blood stream. The resulting metabolic acidosis can be recognized by low values of pH, P_{CO_2} and bicarbonate in arterial blood. Moderately severe acidosis of this sort has been reported in clinical carbon monoxide poisoning (e.g., Neufeld et al., 1981; Zimmerman and Truxal, 1981), but such reports are surprisingly uncommon, perhaps in part because metabolic acidosis is obscured by the respiratory alkalosis arising from hyperventilation (Larkin et al., 1976). Rhesus monkeys exposed for over 3 hours to 0.2% CO, with resulting carboxyhemoglobin of 76%, had arterial anion gaps of 10 to 15 mEq./ L., but the average arterial pH remained above 7.3 (Ginsberg and Myers, 1974).

If the patient is still breathing, biochemical repair begins as soon as he is exposed to fresh air. Carboxyhemoglobin is a completely reversible complex, and essentially all absorbed CO is eventually exhaled; only trace amounts are oxidized to CO_2 (Clark, 1950; Tobias et al., 1945). Normal human blood may contain up to 5% carboxyhemoglobin, part of which comes from endogenous CO production, but a major factor in producing the "normal" blood level is cigarette smoking, whether active or passive (Coburn et al., 1965; Hackney et al., 1962; Ringold et al., 1962). The hemoglobin recovered from carboxyhemoglobin is in every way normal, as are the red blood cells which contained it. Carbon monoxide excretion is always fast at first but slows down as the body content of CO decreases.

Good therapy is designed to accelerate the dissociation and exhalation of carbon monoxide. If the patient is breathing adequately, the administration of pure oxygen is the most important element in therapy (Killick and Marchant, 1959). Oxygen at greater than atmospheric pressure is more efficient as an antidote, since advantage can be taken of the principle of mass action to reverse the carboxyhemoglobin complex. The optimal range of pressures is 2 to 2.5 atmospheres, but these high pressures may induce O_2 poisoning within a few hours (Ledingham, 1964; Smith et al., 1962). Also, at hyperbaric pressures, small but perhaps significant amounts of oxygen may be transported by simple solution in the blood. One requires a compression chamber to utilize oxygen at these pressures (Kokame and Schuler, 1968; Lawson et al., 1961; Smith and Sharp, 1960).

For a resting adult, half-recovery time (in terms of carboxyhemoglobin) is about 4 hours breathing air and 40 minutes breathing pure oxygen (Roughton and Root, 1945). If respira-

tions have ceased or are inadequate, artificial ventilation is essential. Anything which speeds respiration and circulation enhances the rate at which active hemoglobin is regenerated. Analeptic drugs, however, are neither effective nor safe because of the tissue hypoxia which inevitably accompanies carbon monoxide poisoning. Even the addition of CO_2 to oxygen, to serve as a respiratory stimulant, is now regarded as more hazardous than beneficial. Although the addition of 5 to 7% CO_2 together with precautions against rebreathing does hasten the pulmonary excretion of CO (Apthorp et al., 1958; Douglas et al., 1961, 1962), it is much less effective than oxygen alone at 2 atmospheres. The use of CO_2 entails some risk of intensifying the usually mild metabolic acidosis that arises from tissue hypoxia. The patient should be kept strictly at rest.

In severe CO poisonings, myocardial anoxia sometimes becomes sufficient to produce untoward reactions (Anderson et al., 1967; Beck and Suter, 1938; Cosby and Bergeron, 1963; Hayes and Hall, 1964; Middleton et al., 1961; Shafer et al., 1965; Stearns et al., 1938), and myocardial infarction with or without coronary thrombosis may be precipitated (Anderson et al., 1967; Cosby and Bergeron, 1963; Hayes and Hall, 1964). Myocardial lesions are seen frequently at autopsy in fatal cases. Echocardiographic findings in 3 of 5 acute nonfatal cases showed evidence of abnormal left ventricular wall motion. Also, 3 of these 5 had mitral valve prolapse, which might have preexisted, but the high incidence of lesions in papillary muscles in fatal cases suggests a causal relationship (Corya et al., 1976). Breathing 50 ppm carbon monoxide to produce 2.7% carboxyhemoglobin at 2 hours (vs. 0.8% in control subjects breathing air) resulted in a significant decrease in the time to onset of exercise-induced angina (Aronow and Isbell, 1973). Dogs breathing 100 ppm for 2 hours to 6.5% carboxyhemoglobin (vs. 1.0% in controls breathing air) showed a significant decrease in the threshold current necessary to cause ventricular fibrillation (Aronow et al., 1979). In monkeys the effect of induced myocardial infarctions was additive to the effect of carbon monoxide in terms of the threshold for electrically induced ventricular fibrillation (DeBias et al., 1976). In very severely poisoned rhesus monkeys, dangerous hypoventilation occurred only rarely, whereas arterial hypotension and ventricular fibrillation constituted the major risks to life (Ginsberg and Myers, 1974).

In severe human exposures, however, death is usually due to respiratory arrest from central nervous depression. This may be associated with acute cerebral edema and increased intracranial pressure because of excessive transudation from anoxic brain capillaries (Dutra, 1952). Occasionally, pulmonary complications are the proximal cause of death, *e.g.*, hypostatic or aspiration pneumonia, pulmonary edema. Abnormal chest films were found in 18 of 62 acutely poisoned patients. A "ground glass" appearance was the most common initial change, followed by perihilar haze and peribronchial and perivascular cuffing (Sone *et al.*, 1974).

Permanent or slowly resolving psychiatric sequelae and central or peripheral neurological defects may first become evident days or weeks after an acute exposure with apparent recovery (Ginsburg and Romano, 1976; Smith and Brandon, 1973). A similar phenomenon may result from mild, recurring, acute toxic episodes (Breysse, 1961a; Zorn and Kruger, 1960). Although carbon monoxide is not a cumulative poison and all of the inhaled gas can be ventilated out of the blood, repeated bouts of oxygen deprivation may summate in persistent manifestations, such as anorexia, headache, lassitude, dizziness, ataxia, etc. (Beck, 1936; Gilbert and Glazer, 1959; Katz, 1958; Lewey and Drabkin, 1944; Pfrender, 1962; Lindgren, 1960), perhaps inappropriately referred to as "chronic" intoxications. Neuropsychiatric sequelae such as depression were once thought to be rare (Shillito *et al.*, 1936); they now appear to be more common, at least in severe intoxications (Jefferson, 1976; Lacey, 1981; Remick and Miles, 1977; Smith and Mellick, 1975). Lateralized epileptiform discharges in the EEG were noted in one patient within hours of exposure (Neufeld *et al.*, 1981).

Perhaps improved methods of resuscitation after severe poisoning have contributed to the impression that late myocardial and central nervous lesions are more common now than in years past (Bokonjic, 1963; Bour and Ledingham, 1967; Gordon, 1965). Hearing loss (Baker and Lilly, 1977) and peripheral neuropathy (Snyder, 1970) are rarer complications, although decreases in motor nerve conduction velocity and histopathological changes in peripheral nerves have been well characterized in laboratory animals (Grunnet and Petajan, 1976; Pankow *et al.*, 1976; Petajan *et al.*, 1976).

Skeletal muscle necrosis may be precipitated by histotoxic anoxia in conjunction with the weight of the body on itself during prolonged coma (Bessoudo and Gray, 1978; Finley *et al.*, 1977; House and Seddon, 1966). The resulting myoglobinuria may lead to acute renal failure with terminal hyperkalemia. Hemodialysis is of value in this syndrome (Jackson *et al.*, 1959; Loughridge *et al.*, 1958), although it may be presumed to be of little or no benefit in the usual clinical case. Exchange transfusion should be effective, and the recirculation of the patient's blood through an artificial oxygenator has been successfully performed (Pokorny and Simko, 1961). Experimentally this procedure has been

used in combination with exposure of the column of blood to a mercury vapor lamp, the emissions of which are said to accelerate the dissociation of carboxyhemoglobin (Linder *et al.*, 1963).

Infants and young children are generally believed to be more susceptible to carbon monoxide than are adults, but this question has received relatively little attention in the pediatric literature. The acute manifestations are qualitatively similar to those in adults, and such complications as long-term neurological sequelae and renal failure secondary to myonecrosis have been reported (Binder and Roberts, 1980; Zimmerman and Truxal, 1981). On the other hand, a 1-month-old child survived an exposure that killed both young adult parents (Cretney *et al.*, 1979). The elderly are also said to be more susceptible to carbon monoxide than are younger adults (Bogusz *et al.*, 1975).

Carbon monoxide can be transported across the placental barrier, and cases of high blood saturation have been reported in fetuses *in utero* (Goldstein, 1965; Woodruff, 1961). Exposures of neonatal laboratory animals to carbon monoxide have produced effects lasting weeks to months (Binder and Roberts, 1980). Rats exposed prenatally to levels of carbon monoxide that resulted in carboxyhemoglobin concentrations equivalent to those in human cigarette smokers showed reduced birth weight and weight gain as well as behavioral effects which might have been related to altered catecholamine activity in the central nervous system (Fechter and Annau, 1977). Because normal fetal oxygen tensions are only 20 to 30% of those in adults (at least in sheep) and because the oxygen tension in fetal blood decreases in proportion to the carboxyhemoglobin concentration in fetal and maternal blood, exposure *in utero* may constitute a special risk (Longo, 1976).

Because carbon monoxide binds to and inhibits cytochrome P450 and its isozymes, it is commonly employed in *in vitro* systems to study xenobiotic metabolism. Effects on drug metabolism have also been described in intact laboratory animals (Montgomery and Rubin, 1973). These effects, however, appear to be secondary to tissue hypoxia and not to direct inhibition of drug metabolism via binding of carbon monoxide to cytochrome P450 (Roth and Rubin, 1976a, b).

On the other hand, some evidence has accumulated to suggest that factors other than a simple hypoxia contribute to carbon monoxide lethality. Pretreatment of mice with phenobarbital had no effect on carbon monoxide lethality, but it increased the lethality of exposure to low oxygen tensions (Winston *et al.*, 1974). Preexposure of mice to nonlethal concentrations of carbon monoxide protected them against carbon monoxide lethality 24 hours later but not against low oxygen tensions or injection of cyanide. Preexposure to low oxygen protected against both carbon monoxide and low oxygen tensions but not cyanide, whereas pretreated with cyanide did not protect against any of these challenges (Winston and Roberts, 1975). Pretreatment of mice with potassium cyanate increased the affinity of their hemoglobin for oxygen and protected them against low oxygen lethality but not against carbon monoxide (Winston and Roberts, 1977). Carbon monoxide exposure results in altered patterns of glucose metabolism that are not mimicked by exposure to low oxygen (Winston and Roberts, 1978). Carbon monoxide decreases dopamine turnover in the caudate nucleus in a manner different from hypoxia, and the effect outlasts the time of exposure (Newby et al., 1978). Perhaps these differences between hypoxic hypoxia and carbon monoxide exposure can be accounted for on the basis of subtle alterations in tissue blood flow.

Symptomatology: In the following discussion the symbol COHb refers to carboxyhemoglobin, and the numeral represents the percentage of circulating hemoglobin which is so modified (Sayers and Davenport, 1930):

1. No symptoms or shortness of breath during vigorous muscular exercise (0 to 10% COHb).
2. A mild headache ("tightness across the forehead") and breathlessness on moderate exertion (10 to 20% COHb).
3. Throbbing headache, irritability, emotional instability, impaired judgment, defective memory, and rapid fatigue (20 to 30% COHb).
4. Severe headache, weakness, nausea and vomiting, dizziness, dimness of vision, confusion (30 to 40% COHb).
5. Increasing confusion, sometimes hallucinations, severe ataxia, acclerated respirations, and collapse with attempts at exertion (40 to 50% COHb).
6. Syncope or coma, with intermittent convulsions, accelerated respirations, tachycardia with a weak pulse, and a pink or red discoloration of the skin due to the presence (in blood) of carboxyhemoglobin (50 to 60% COHb). This sign, however, is more common at autopsy than in living patients, who may exhibit pallor or cyanosis instead.
7. Increasing depth of coma with incontinence of urine and feces (60 to 70% COHb).
8. Profound coma with depressed or absent reflexes, a weak thready pulse, shallow and irregular respiration, and complete quiescence (70 to 80% COHb).
9. Rapid death from respiratory arrest (above 80% COHb).
10. Miscellaneous and atypical reactions include various skin lesions (Dutra, 1958; Leavell et al., 1969), sweating, hepatomegaly, hyperpyrexia, albuminuria, oliguria, anginal pain, and congestive heart failure (Meigs and Hughes, 1952). Prolonged delirium occurred in 20% of one series of cases (Smith and Branden, 1970).
11. During convalescence a bronchopneumonia may develop because of the aspiration of saliva or vomitus. Even in the absence of frank infection, varying grades of pulmonary edema are reported occasionally.
12. Myocardial infarction, with or without coronary thrombosis, may appear at any time up to 1 week following an acute poisoning.
13. After an uneventful convalescence, signs of nerve or brain injury may appear at any time within 3 weeks after an acute exposure. Among the permanent sequelae are neuropathies, various motor and mental defects, some of which mimic multiple sclerosis or parkinsonism, and death. Neuropsychiatric syndromes involving anorexia, headache, lassitude, ataxia, emotional depression and many other symptoms may persist. Such permanent or long-term injuries, however, are encountered only occasionally even after severe poisonings; usually there are no sequelae (e.g., Abbott, 1972; Garland and Pearce, 1967; Townsend and Stetson, 1968).

Treatment:

1. Terminate exposure immediately.
2. Administer pure oxygen by the best method available. An oronasal mask is usually best (p. IV-13). Artificial ventilation is necessary whenever breathing is inadequate. Apneic patients have often been saved by efficient and persistent artificial ventilation (p. IV-7). As always, a patent airway must be carefully maintained (p. IV-2). Patients with 40% carboxyhemoglobin or more and an uncompensated metabolic acidosis (arterial pH less than 7.4) should be managed aggressively with ventilatory support or hyperbaric oxygenation (Larkin et al., 1976). See pp. IV-10-14.
3. Gastric aspiration and lavage early in the course of therapy may prevent aspiration pneumonitis and reveal the presence of ingested intoxicants.
4. Avoid stimulant drugs, including carbon dioxide. Do not inject methylene blue.
5. Hypothermia has been employed to reduce the patient's oxygen requirement (Craig et al., 1959; Lorhan and Brookler, 1961).
6. Consider antibiotics as prophylaxis against pulmonary infection, but see pp. IV-85-86.
7. A whole blood transfusion may be useful

if it can be given early in the treatment program.

8. Infuse sodium bicarbonate and balanced electrolyte solutions if blood analyses indicate a significant metabolic acidosis (see text above and pp. IV-69–72).

9. Ancillary therapy for brain edema may be necessary if hypoxia has been severe (Winter and Miller, 1976); see pp. IV-43–46.

10. Ensure absolute rest in bed for at least 48 hours; in severe poisonings, 2 to 4 weeks in bed may prevent sequelae.

11. Watch for late neurological, psychiatric and cardiac complications.

Laboratory:

1. Carbon monoxide analyses of blood are useful for diagnosis and prognosis. Colorimetric methods have the advantages of simplicity and speed, combined with sufficient accuracy for the clinical situation (Berninger and Smith, 1959). Gasometric methods are more accurate but cumbersome (Scholander and Roughton, 1943). Several modern devices are available for rapid, precise measurements. If a victim succumbs in an atmosphere containing carbon monoxide, a postmortem blood sample usually shows at least 60% carboxyhemoglobin (Gettler and Freimuth, 1940), but it may be virtually devoid of COHb if resuscitation was attempted.

2. Repeated electrocardiograms are desirable, and a chest film may reveal pulmonary complications. Bilateral areas of low density in the globus pallidus seen on CAT scans were associated with late sequelae (Sawada et al., 1980; Sawa et al., 1981).

3. Arterial blood samples should be analyzed for oxygen content, pH and electrolyte levels (Na^+, K^+, Cl^-, bicarbonate), and the anion gap should be computed as an index of possible metabolic acidosis.

4. A decrease in plasma volume may be secondary to endothelial damage and increased capillary permeability (Stonesifer, 1978).

5. In laboratory animals, serum creatine phosphokinase and lactate dehydrogenase were elevated following exposure (Penney and Maziarka, 1976).

6. Elevated carboxyhemoglobin concentrations are sometimes used as evidence that decedents were alive in a fire. Victims of flash fires, however, are exceptions to this rule (Hirsch et al., 1977).

References:

Abbott, D. F. Slow recovery from carbon monoxide poisoning. Postgrad. Med. J. 48:639-642, 1972.

Anderson, R. F.; Allensworth, D. C.; DeGroot, W. J. Myocardial toxicity from carbon monoxide poisoning. Ann. Intern. Med. 67:1172-1182, 1967.

Apthorp, G. H.; Bates, D. V.; Marshall, R.; Mendel, D. Effect of acute carbon monoxide poisoning on work capacity. Influence of 5% CO_2 on rate of recovery. Br. Med. J. 2:476-478, 1958.

Aronow, W. S.; Isbell, M. W. Carbon monoxide effect on exercise-induced angina pectoris. Ann. Intern. Med. 79:392-395, 1973.

Aronow, W. S.; Stemmer, E. A.; Zweig, S. Carbon monoxide and ventricular fibrillation threshold in normal dogs. Arch. Environ. Health 34:184-186, 1979.

Ayres, S. M.; Giannelli, S., Jr.; Armstrong, R. G. Carboxyhemoglobin: Hemodynamic and respiratory responses to small concentrations. Science 149:193-194, 1965.

Baker, S. R.; Lilly, D. J. Hearing loss from acute carbon monoxide intoxication. Ann. Otol. Rhinol. Laryngol. 86:323, 1977.

Beck, H. G. Slow carbon monoxide asphyxiation: A neglected clinical problem. J. A. M. A. 107:1025-1029, 1936.

Beck, H. G.; Suter, G. M. Role of carbon monoxide in the causation of myocardial disease. J. A. M. A. 110:1982-1986, 1938.

Bell, M. A. Subacute carbon monoxide poisoning. Arch. Environ. Health 3:594-596, 1961.

Berninger, H.; Smith, R. A modification of the spectrophotometric determination of carbon monoxide in blood enabling direct determination of per cent hemoglobin saturation. Clin. Chem. 5:127-134, 1959.

Bessoudo, R.; Gray, J. Carbon monoxide poisoning and nonoliguric acute renal failure. Can. Med. Assoc. J. 119:41-44, 1978.

Binder, J. W.; Roberts, R. J. Carbon monoxide intoxication in children. Clin. Toxicol. 16:287-295, 1980.

Binet, L.; Conte, M. Etude de 136 cas d'intoxication oxycarbonee aigue. Sem. Hop. Paris 22:1938-1945, 1946.

Bogusz, M.; Cholewa, L.; Pach, J.; Mlodkowska, K. A comparison of two types of acute carbon monoxide poisoning. Arch. Toxicol. 33:141-149, 1975.

Bokonjic, N. Stagnant anoxia and carbon monoxide poisoning. Electroencephalogr. Clin. Neurophysiol. Suppl. No. 21, 1963.

Bour, H.; Ledingham, I. M. Carbon monoxide poisoning. Vol. 24, Progress in Brain Research. Elsevier Publishing Col, Amsterdam, 1967.

Breysse, P. A. Chronic carbon monoxide poisoning. Ind. Med. Surg. 30:20-22, 1961a.

Brieger, H. Carbon monoxide polycythemia. J. Ind. Hyg. Toxicol. 26:321-327, 1944.

Clark, C. J.; Campbell, D.; Reid, W. H. Blood carboxyhaemoglobin and cyanide levels in fire survivors. Lancet 1:1332-1335, 1981.

Clark, R. T., Jr. Evidence for conversion of carbon monoxide to carbon dioxide by the intact animal. Am. J. Physiol. 162:560-564, 1950.

Coburn, R. F.; Forster, R. E.; Kane, P. B. Considerations of the physiological variables that, determine the blooc carboxyhemoglobin concentration in man. J. Clin. Invest. 44:1899-1910, 1965.

Cornish, H. H.; Abar, E. L. Toxicity of pyrolysis products of vinyl plastics. Arch. Environ. Health 19:15-21, 1969.

Corya, B. C.; Black, M. J.; McHenry, P. L. Echocardiographic findings after acute carbon monoxide poisoning. Br. Heart J. 38:712-717, 1976.

Cosby, R. S.; Bergeron, M. Electrocardiographic changes in carbon monoxide poisoning. Am. J. Cardiol. 11:93-96, 1963.

Craig, T. V.; Hunt, W.; Atkinson, R. Hypothermia - its use in severe carbon monoxide poisoning. N. Engl. J. Med. 261:854-856, 1959.

Cretney, M. J.; Ginger, R. C.; Bullivant, C. M. Some unusual toxicological aspects of two carbon monoxide deaths. J. Forensic Sci. Soc. 19:211-218, 1979.

DeBias, D. A.; Banerjee, C. M.; Birkhead, N. C.; Greene, C. H.; Scott, S. D.; Harrer, W. V. Effect of carbon monoxide inhalation on ventricular fibrillation. Arch. Environ. Health 31:42-46, 1976.

Douglas, T. A.; Lawson, D. D.; Ledingham, I. M.; Norman, J. N.; Sharp, G. R.; Smith, G. Carbogen in experimental carbon monoxide poisoning. Br. Med. J. 2:1673-1675, 1961.

Douglas, T. A.; Lawson, D. D.; Ledingham, I. M.; Norman, J. N.; Sharp, G. R.; Smith, G. Carbon monoxide poisoning, a comparison between the efficiencies of oxygen at one atmosphere pressure, at two atmospheres pressure and of 5 and 7% carbon dioxide in oxygen. Lancet 1:68-69, 1962.

Drinker, C. K. Carbon Monoxide Asphyxia. Oxford University Press, New York, 1938.

Dutra, F. R. Cerebral residue of acute carbon monoxide poisoning. Am. J. Clin. Pathol. 22:925-935, 1952.

Dutra, F. R. The skin in carbon monoxide poisoning, report of two cases. Lab. Invest. 7:328-335, 1958.

Fechter, L. D.; Annau, Z. Toxicity of mild prenatal carbon monoxide exposure. Science 197:680-682, 1977.

Finley, J.; VanBeek, A.; Glover, J. L. Myonecrosis complicating carbon monoxide poisoning. J. Trauma 17:536-540, 1977.

Forbes, W. H.; Sargent, F.; Roughton, F. J. W. The rate of carbon monoxide uptake by normal men. Am. J. Physiol. 143:594-608, 1945.

Garland, H.; Pearce, J. Neurological complications of carbon monoxide poisoning. Q. J. Med. 36:445-455, 1967.

Gettler, A. O.; Freimuth, H. C. The carbon monoxide content of the blood under various conditions. Am. J. Clin. Path. 11:603-616, 1940.

Gilbert, G. J.; Glazer, G. H. Neurologic manifestations of chronic carbon monoxide poisoning. N. Engl. J. Med. 261:1217-1220, 1959.

Ginsberg, M. D.; Myers, R. E. Experimental carbon monoxide encephalopathy in the primate. I. Physiologic and metabolic aspects. Arch. Neurol. 30:202-208, 1974.

Ginsburg, R.; Romano, J. Carbon monoxide encephalopathy: need for appropriate treatment. Am. J. Psychiatry 133:317-320, 1976.

Goldstein, D. P. Carbon monoxide poisoning in pregnancy. Am. J. Obstet. Gynecol. 92:526-528, 1965.

Gordon, E. B. Carbon monoxide encephalopathy. Br. Med. J. 1:1232, 1965.

Grunnet, M. L.; Petajan, J. H. Carbon monoxide-induced neuropathy in the rat. Arch. Neurol. 33:158-163, 1976.

Hackney, J. D.; Kaufman, G. A.; Lashier, H.; Lyon, K. Rebreathing estimate of carbon monoxide hemoglobin. Arch. Environ. Health 5:300-307, 1962.

Haldane, J. The relation of the action of carbonic oxide to oxygen tension. J. Physiol. 18:201-217, 1895.

Hayes, J. M.; Hall, G. V. The myocardial toxicity of carbon monoxide. Med. J. Aust. 1:865-868, 1964.

Hirsch, C. S.; Bost, R. D.; Gerber, S. R.; Cowan, M. E.; Adelson, L.; Sunshine, I. Carboxyhemoglobin concentrations in flash fire victims. Report of six simultaneous fire fatalities without elevated carboxyhemoglobin. Am. J. Clin. Pathol. 68:317-320, 1977.

House, A. J. G.; Seddon, H. Ischemic contracture of muscle associated with carbon monoxide and barbiturate poisoning. Br. Med. J. 1:192-195, 1966.

Jackson, R. C.; Bunker, N. V.; Elder, W. J.; O'Conner, P. J. Case of carbon monoxide poisoning with complications, successful treatment with an artificial kidney. Br. Med. J. 2:1130-1134, 1959.

Jefferson, J. W. Subtle neuropsychiatric sequelae of carbon monoxide intoxication - 2 case reports. Am. J. Psychiatry 133:961-964, 1976.

Joels, N.; Neil, E. The action of high tensions of carbon monoxide on the carotid chemoreceptors. Arch. Int. Pharmacodyn. Ther. 139:528-534, 1962.

Johnson, C. J.; Moran, J. C.; Paine, S. C.; Anderson, H. W.; Breysse, P. A. Abatement of toxic levels of carbon monoxide in Seattle ice-skating rinks. Am. J. Public Health 65:1087-1090, 1975.

Kahn, A.; Rutledge, R. B.; Davis, G. L.; Altes, J. A.; Ganter, G. E. Thornton, C. A.; Wallace, N. D. Carboxyhemoglobin sources in the metropolitan St. Louis population. Arch. Environ. Health 29:127-135, 1974.

Katz, M. Carbon monoxide asphyxia. A common clinical entity. Can. Med. Assoc. J. 78:182-186, 1958.

Killick, E. M.; Marchant, J. V. Resuscitation of dogs from severe acute carbon monoxide poisoning. J. Physiol. 147:274-298, 1959.

Kokame, G. M.; Shuler, S. E. Carbon monoxide poisoning, treatment by hyperbaric oxygenation. Arch. Surg. 96:211-215, 1968.

Lacey, D. J. Neurologic sequelae of acute carbon monoxide intoxication. Am. J. Dis. Child. 135:145-147, 1981.

Larkin, J. M.; Brahos, G. J.; Moylan, J. A. Treatment of carbon monoxide poisoning: prognostic factors. J. Trauma 16:111-114, 1976.

Lawson, D. D.; McAllister, R. A.; Smith, G. Treatment of acute experimental carbon monoxide poisoning with oxygen under pressure. Lancet 1:800-802, 1961.

Leavell, U. W.; Farley, C. H.; McIntyre, J. S. Cutaneous changes in a patient with carbon monoxide poisoning. Arch. Dermatol. 99:429-433, 1969.

Ledingham, I. M. Hyperbaric oxygenation. Proc. R. Soc. Med. 57:807-809, 1964.

Lewey, F. H.; Drabkin, D. L. Experimental chronic carbon monoxide poisoning of dogs. Am. J. Med. Sci. 208:502-571, 1944.

Lilienthal, J. L., Jr.; Pine, M. B. The effect of oxygen pressure on the uptake of carbon monoxide at sea level and at altitude. Am. J. Physiol. 145:346-350, 1946.

Lilienthal, J. L., Jr.; Riley, R. L.; Proemmel, D. D.; Franke, R. E. The relationships between carbon monoxide, oxygen and hemoglobin in the blood of man at altitude. Am. J. Physiol. 145:351-358, 1946.

Linder, E.; Sakai, Y.; Paton, B. C. Experimental treatment of carbon monoxide poisoning by extracorporeal circulation. Sur. Forum 14:277-279, 1963.

Lindgren, S. A. A study of the effect of protracted occupational exposure to carbon monoxide. Acta Med. Scand. 167 (Suppl. 356), 1960.

Longo, L. D. Carbon monoxide: Effects on oxygenation of the fetus in utero. Science 194:523-525, 1976.

Lorhan, P. H.; Brookler, H. A. Carbon monoxide poisoning. Management with hypothermia. Anesth. Analg. 40:504-504, 1961.

Loughridge, L. W.; Leader, L. P.; Bowen, D. A. L. Acute renal failure due to muscle necrosis in carbon monoxide poisoning. Lancet 2:349-351, 1958.

Matthew, H. Acute poisoning; some myths and misconceptions. Br. Med. J. 1:519-522, 1971b.

Meigs, J. W.; Hughes, J. P. W. Acute carbon monoxide poisoning, an analysis of one hundred five cases. Arch. Ind. Hyg. Occup. Med. 6:344-356, 1952.

Middleton, G. D.; Ashby, D. W.; Clark, F. Delayed and long-lasting electrocardiographic changes in carbon monoxide poisoning. Lancet 1:12-14, 1961.

Montgomery, M. R.; Rubin, R. Adaptation to the inhibitory effect of carbon monoxide inhalation on drug metabolism. J. Appl. Physiol. 35:601-607, 1973.

Neufeld, M. Y.; Swanson, J. W.; Klass, D. W. Localized EEG abnormalities in acute carbon monoxide poisoning. Arch. Neurol. 38:524-527, 1981.

Newby, M. B.; Roberts, R. J.; Bhatnagar, R. K. Carbon monoxide- and hypoxia-induced effects on catecholamines in the mature and developing rat brain. J. Pharmacol. Exp. Ther. 206:61-68, 1978.

Pankow, D.; Glatzel, W.; Tietze, K.; Ponsold, W. Motor nerve conduction velocity after carbon monoxide or m-dinitrobenzene poisoning following elimination of poisons. Arch. Toxikol. 34:325-330, 1976.

Penney, D.; Maziarka, T. Effect of acute carbon monoxide poisoning on serum lactate dehydrogenase and creatine phosphokinase. J. Toxicol. Environ. Health 1:1017-1021, 1976.

Petajan, J. H.; Packham, S. C.; Frens, D. B.; Dinger, B. G. Sequelae of carbon monoxide-induced hypoxia in the rat. Arch. Neurol. 33:152-157, 1976.

Pfrender, R. E. Chronic carbon monoxide poisoning. A critical resume. Ind. Med. Surg. 31:99-103, 1962.

Pitts, G. C.; Pace, N. The effect of blood carboxyhemoglobin concentration on hypoxia tolerance. Am. J. Physiol.

148:139-151, 1947.

Pokorny, J.; Simko, S. Treatment of carbon monoxide poisoning with oxygen under pressure. Lancet *1*:57, 1961.

Remick, R. A.; Miles, J. E. Carbon monoxide poisoning: neurologic and psychiatric seuqelae. Can. Med. Assoc. J. *117*:654-655, 1977.

Ringold, A.; Goldsmith, J. R.; Helwig, H. L.; Finn, R.; Schuette, F. Estimating recent carbon monoxide exposures. Arch. Environ. Health *5*:308-318, 1962.

Roth, R. A., Jr.; Rubin, R. J. Comparison of the effect of carbon monoxide and of hypoxic hypoxia. I. *In vivo* metabolism, distribution and action of hexobarbital. J. Pharmacol. Exp. Ther. *199*:53-60, 1976a.

Roth, R. A., Jr.; Rubin, R. J. Comparison of the effect of carbon monoxide and of hypoxic hypoxia. II. Hexobarbital metabolism in the isolated, perfused rat liver. J. Pharmacol. Exp. Ther. *199*:61-66, 1976b.

Roughton, F. J. W.; Darling, R. C. The effect of carbon monoxide on the oxyhemoglobin dissociation curve. Am. J. Physiol. *141*:17-31, 1944.

Roughton, F. J. W.; Root, N. S. The fate of CO in the body during recovery from mild carbon monoxide poisoning in man. Am. J. Physiol. *145*:239-252, 1945.

Sawa, G. M.; Watson, C. P. N.; Terbrugge, K.; Chiu, M. Delayed encephalopathy following carbon monoxide intoxication. Can. J. Neurol. Sci. *8*:77-79, 1981.

Sawada, Y.; Takahashi, M.; Ohashi, N.; Fusamoto, H.; Maemura, K.; Kobayashi, H.; Yoshioka, T.; Sugimoto, T. Computerized tomography as an indication of long-term outcome after acute carbon monoxide poisoning. Lancet *1*:783-784, 1980.

Sayers, P. R.; Davenport, S. J. Review of carbon monoxide poisoning. U. S. Public Health Serv., Public Health Bull. No. 195, 1930.

Scholander, P. F.; Roughton, F. J. W. Microgasometric estimation of the blood gases. II. Carbon monoxide. J. Biol. Chem. *148*:551-560, 1943.

Shafer, N.; Smilay, M.; MacMillan, F. P. Primary myocardial disease in man resulting from acute carbon monoxide poisoning. Am. J. Med. *38*:316-320, 1965.

Shillito, F. H.; Drinker, C. K.; Shaughnessy, T. J. The problem of nervous and mental sequelae in carbon monoxide poisoning. J. A. M. A. *106*:669-674, 1936.

Smith, G.; Ledingham, J. M.; Sharp, G. R.; Norman, J. N.; Bates, E. H. Treatment of coal-gas poisoning with oxygen at 2 atmospheres pressure. Lancet *1*:816-819, 1962.

Smith, G.; Sharp, G. R. Treatment of carbon monoxide poisoning with oxygen under pressure. Lancet *2*:905-906, 1960.

Smith, J. R.; Landaw, S. A. Smokers' polycythemia. N. Engl. J. Med. *298*:6-10, 1978.

Smith, J. S.; Brandon, S. Acute carbon monoxide poisoning - 3 years experience in a defined population. Postgrad. Med. J. *46*:65-70, 1970.

Smith, J. S.; Brandon, S. Morbidity from acute carbon monoxide poisoning at three-year follow-up. Br. Med. J. *1*:318-321, 1973.

Smith, J. S.; Mellick, R. S. Neuropsychiatric release following acute carbon monoxide poisoning - the contribution of electroconvulsive therapy. Med. J. Aust. *1*:465-468, 1975.

Snyder, R. D. Carbon monoxide intoxication with peripheral neuropathy. Neurology *20*:177-180, 1970.

Sone, S.; Higashihara, T.; Kotake, T.; Morimoto, S.; Miura, T. Ogawa, M.; Sugimoto, T. Pulmonary manifestations in acute carbon monoxide poisoning. Am. J. Roentgenol. Radium Ther. & Nucl. Med. *120*:865-871, 1974.

Stearns, W. H.; Drinker, C. K.; Shaughnessy, T. J. The electrocardiographic changes found in 2 cases of carbon monoxide (illuminating gas) poisoning. Am. Heart. J. *15*:434-447, 1938.

Stonesifer, L. D. How carbon monoxide reduces plasma volume. N. Engl. J. Med. *299*:311-312, 1978.

Tobias, C. A.; Lawrence, J. H.; Roughton, F. J. W.; Root, W. S.; Gregersen, M. J. The elimination of carbon monoxide from the human body with reference to the possible conversion of CO to CO_2. Am. J. Physiol. *195*:253-263, 1945.

Townsend, G. L.; Stetson, J. B. Treatment of carbon monoxide poisoning by mechanical ventilation. Can. Anesth. Soc. J. *15*:184-195, 1968.

von Oettingen, W. F. Carbon monoxide; its hazards and the mechanism of its action. U. S. Public Health Serv., Public Health Bull. No. 290, 1944.

Wilks, S. S.; Tomashefski, J. F.; Clark, R. T., Jr. Physiological effects of chronic exposure to carbon monoxide. J. Appl. Physiol. *14*:305-310, 1959.

Winston, J. M.; Creighton, J. M.; Roberts, R. J. Alteration of carbon monoxide- and hypoxic hypoxia-induced lethality following phenobarbital, chlorpromazine, or alcohol pretreatment. Toxicol. Appl. Pharmacol. *30*:458-465, 1974.

Winston, J. M.; Roberts, R. J. Influence of carbon monoxide, hypoxic hypoxia or potassium cyanide pretreatment on acute carbon monoxide and hypoxic hypoxia lethality. J. Pharmacol. Exp. Ther. *193*:713-719, 1975.

Winston, J. M.; Roberts, R. J. Effect of potassium cyanate on carbon monoxide- and hypoxic hypoxia-induced lethality. J. Toxicol. Environ. Health *2*:625-631, 1977.

Winston, J. M.; Roberts, R. J. Glucose catabolism following carbon monoxide or hypoxic hypoxia exposure. Biochem. Pharmacol. *27*:377-380, 1978.

Winter, P. M.; Miller, J. N. Carbon monoxide poisoning. J. A. M. A. *236*:1502-1504, 1976.

Woodruff, R. S. Carbon monoxide in fetal blood, report of a case. J. Forensic Sci. *6*:249-254, 1961.

Zimmerman, S. S.; Truxal, B. Carbon monoxide poisoning. Pediatrics *68*:215-224, 1981.

Zorn, O.; Kruger, P. D. The problem of chronic carbon monoxide poisoning. Ind. Med. Surg. *29*:580-581, 1960.

CARBON TETRACHLORIDE

Because of its excellent solvent properties and noninflammability, carbon tetrachloride (CCl_4) had been in common use for many decades in such commercial products as cleaners, grease solvents and fire extinguishers. Its notoriously poor record of safety, however, led in November 1970 to an FDA regulation that placed an outright ban on the sale of carbon tetrachloride or any mixture containing it for use in the home. The FDA classified it as a substance so hazardous that no warning label could be devised that would be adequate to protect the householder and his family. It appears likely that carbon tetrachloride poisoning in future years will be encountered chiefly after occupational exposures. For example, it is still widely used as a liquid grain fumigant. Although uniquely potent, carbon tetrachloride is in many respects representative of a large class of related chlorinated hydrocarbon solvents.

Toxicology: Adult humans exhibit an astonishingly wide variation in their sensitivity to carbon tetrachloride. As little as 2 ml. by mouth has killed on several occasions (Lamson *et al.*, 1928; Phelps and Hu, 1924). In years past when it was used as an ascaricide, however, thousands of adults received doses of 4 to 5 ml. without serious toxicity (Lamson *et al.*, 1928). One condemned murderer volunteered to drink 6 ml. after a meal, and he repeated the same dose 13 days later on an empty stomach. He experienced only giddiness and drowsiness. After his execution a week later, a postmortem examination failed to reveal evidence of visceral damage (Nicholls and Hampton, 1922). Doses of four (Kennaugh, 1975), eight (Truss and Killenberg, 1982) and even twelve ounces (Bagnasco et al., 1978) produced serious poisonings, but each of these patients survived with supportive care. An adult mean lethal dose may, therefore, defy estimation. Perhaps any amount should be considered dangerous, but hope for survival should not be abandoned after even massive doses.

Susceptibility to CCl_4 poisoning is enhanced by the contemporaneous use of alcohol, by a poor nutritional status and perhaps by a calcium deficiency (Drill, 1952; Friedman and Eales, 1962; Hammes, 1941; New et al., 1962; Stevens and Forster, 1953). The influence of alcohol has been confirmed many times in experimental animals. Fourteen workers in an isopropyl alcohol packaging plant became ill after exposure to carbon tetrachloride. In four of them renal failure or hepatitis developed. These workers had elevated levels of acetone in their alveolar air, confirming experimental reports (below) that ketogenic substances also potentiate carbon tetrachloride toxicity (Folland et al., 1976). Children, adolescents and persons with preexisting liver disease are said to be especially sensitive to the hepatotoxic action. On the other hand, prior exposure of animals to sublethal doses of CCl_4 confers a remarkable protection against an ordinarily lethal dose administered subsequently (Ugazio et al., 1972).

Carbon tetrachloride is toxic when ingested as a liquid and when inhaled as a vapor (Quadland, 1943; von Oettingen, 1964). It is absorbed more slowly through intact skin than several similar halogenated hydrocarbon solvents, but its much higher toxicity made it the only one tested likely to be absorbed through skin in toxicologically significant quantities (Stewart and Dodd, 1964). A clear-cut case of acute human poisoning arising from percutaneous absorption, however, has not yet been reported. Repeated skin applications are required to cause systemic poisoning in animals (von Oettingen, 1964). If not removed promptly, local application of carbon tetrachloride to human skin produces distinct pain with erythema, hyperemia and wheal formation followed by vesication (von Oettingen, 1964).

The principal toxic actions of carbon tetrachloride are central nervous depression and cellular necrosis in the kidneys, liver or both. Death may be due to any one of these lesions, but in nonfatal cases recovery is eventually complete. Occasionally, ventricular fibrillation and cardiac arrest are responsible for sudden death in CCl_4 poisoning. Prominent histopathological changes in brain are sometimes seen after massive inhalation exposures (Korenke and Pribilla, 1969; Luse and Wood, 1967). Many other visceral lesions have been described as primary responses to carbon tetrachloride, but except for occasional cases of hemorrhagic necrosis of the adrenal cortex (Dvorackova, 1963; Phelps and Hu, 1924), pancreatitis (Dume et al., 1969) and optic neuritis (Smith, 1950), these claims require further substantiation. Much of the edema and hemorrhage described in various tissues (Guild et al., 1958; New et al., 1962) is undoubtedly secondary to severe kidney and liver injuries.

Carbon tetrachloride rarely produces primary pulmonary edema, but this complication may occur as a result of tracheobronchial aspiration of ingested solvent (Dillenberg and Thompson, 1945; Friedberg, 1950) or as a result of uremia and overzealous fluid therapy in anuric patients (Farrier and Smith, 1950; Myatt and Salmons, 1952). As with other chlorinated hydrocarbons, intense heat (open flame or very hot metal surface) may cause decomposition into such notorious pulmonary irritants as hydrogen chloride (HCl), chlorine gas (Cl_2) and phosgene ($COCl_2$) (Luse and Wood, 1967; Noweir et al., 1972; Seidelin, 1961; Webster, 1930).

Although there are many exceptions, nervous symptoms are said to predominate in inhalation exposures, whereas gastrointestinal and hepatorenal injuries are more prominent after ingestion (Adams et al., 1952; Guild et al., 1958; Hardin, 1954; Lamson et al., 1928). Whether or not such a generalization is valid, central nervous depression and coma may occur without evidence of visceral injury, and renal failure may develop in cases without nervous involvement. With the exception of nausea and vomiting, symptoms develop more slowly after ingestion (latency 24 to 36 hours) than after inhalation (latency usually a few minutes). Intestinal absorption is aided by fats, oils and alcohol (Lamson et al., 1928). Much of the absorbed material is eliminated through the lungs (Robbins, 1929).

The principal liver lesion is necrosis of the hepatic cells (especially those in the central portion of each lobule), together with fatty infiltration. In the kidneys, fatty degeneration and necrosis of the renal tubular epithelium may be extensive. Although liver injury probably begins first, the kidney lesion is more prominent and more often recognized clinically (Alston, 1970; Joron et al., 1957; New et al., 1962; Sirota, 1949; Smetana, 1939).

Three patients developed fatal aplastic anemia after chronic exposure to carbon tetrachloride (Straus, 1954). A prominent peripheral eosinophilia and an increase in eosinophils in the splenic pulp were observed in a fatal illness resulting from a single oral dose (Dvorackova, 1963). Cancer may be another long-term hazard of CCl_4 exposure. At least in chronic feeding tests in male and female rats and mice, it proved to increase significantly the incidence of hepatocellular carcinoma (National Cancer Institute, 1976).

Studies of mechanism: Experimental studies on the toxic mechanism of action of carbon tetrachloride typify much of modern toxicology (Plaa and Larson, 1964). The hepatic damage, which in many animal species predominates over renal injury, has been investigated most intensively. It has been suggested that the liver injury represents a composite of three separate lesions: (1) necrosis, (2) dilatation of the endoplasmic reticulum (balloon cell formation), and (3) steatosis (Popp et al., 1978). It is now well established that the key lesion responsible for CCl₄-induced fat accumulation in the liver is a blockade in the exit of hepatic triglycerides to plasma (Recknagel, 1967). Propyl gallate relieves this blockade of triglyceride secretion without preventing other hepatotoxic effects of CCl₄ (Torrielli and Ugazio, 1975). Recknagel (1967) has suggested that CCl₄ may block the coupling reaction between triglyceride and acceptor protein to prevent formation of lipoprotein, the form actually released to the plasma.

Ultrastructural studies have revealed early dilatation, vesiculation and disorganization of the hepatocyte endoplasmic reticulum. Ribosomes are detached, and the Golgi cisterna and sometimes the perinuclear membrane are dilated (Bernacchi et al., 1980). Similar morphological abnormalities including balloon cell formation have been observed in vitro with cultured rat hepatocytes. These changes are believed to be responsible for the leakage of intracellular enzymes, which gives rise to common laboratory measures of the degree of the hepatic insult, namely elevations of serum levels of liver enzyme activities (Chenery et al., 1981). A role for extracellular calcium in this leakage has been disputed (Smith et al., 1981).

The key to understanding the mechanism of the necrotic changes was the observation that the allegedly stable carbon tetrachloride molecule actually undergoes a small degree of metabolism in vivo (Butler, 1961; McCollister et al., 1951). The homolytic cleavage of the carbon-chlorine bond gives rise to highly reactive free radical products and constitutes an example of a lethal synthesis or the inverse of a detoxication reaction (Recknagel and Glende, 1973). It is generally believed that this cleavage is mediated by the hepatic microsomal enzyme system. Indeed, cytochrome P450 appears to be the sole site of CCl₄ reduction (Wolf et al., 1980). Pretreatment of rats with microsomal enzyme-inducing agents, such as phenobarbital and chlordane, potentiates the hepatotoxicity of CCl₄ presumably by increasing the rate or extent of toxic metabolite formation (Stenger et al., 1975;

Suarez et al., 1975). At the same time, CCl₄ activation actually leads to destruction of hepatocyte cytochrome P450, particularly in the induced liver (Stenger et al., 1975). Presumably, this destruction of cytochrome P450, which occurs even in noninduced livers, accounts for the protective effect of a small dose of CCl₄ against a normally lethal dose administered subsequently.

Homolytic cleavage of the carbon-chlorine bond gives rise to a trichlorocarbon free radical species, ·CCl₃. In addition, the known metabolites of CCl₄ in rats include trace amounts of chloroform, carbon monoxide, carbon dioxide and phosgene (Harris and Anders, 1981). The biochemical events associated with the necrotic process include covalent binding of CCl₄ fragments to liver DNA, nuclear proteins and especially phospholipids. Chemically generated ·CCl₃ showed similar binding patterns to these cellular macromolecules in vitro (Diaz Gomez and Castro, 1980). Covalent binding is greater in anaerobic mixtures than in aerobic ones, but it is completely inhibited in vitro by carbon monoxide, which blocks the activation process by cytochrome P450 (Villarruel et al., 1975). Covalent binding of reactive metabolites to hepatocyte macromolecules in vitro can be blocked by pyrazole with an accompanying decrease in the ultrastructural damage (Bernacchi et al., 1980). Feeding rats cholestyramine for 5 days or giving dipyridamole also decreased the extent of necrosis induced by subsequent CCl₄ but not the steatosis, further indicating the independence of these two toxic effects (Bioulac et al., 1981; Kast et al., 1982).

Unlike other hepatotoxic agents whose effects depend on reactive metabolite formation (e.g., ACETAMINOPHEN, p. III-2), CCl₄ is alleged not to deplete the liver of reduced glutathione. On the other hand, chloroform produced necrosis only at doses that did deplete glutathione (Docks and Krishna, 1976). Indeed, pretreatment of rats with diethylmaleate (DEM) to first deplete liver glutathione actually protected against CCl₄ necrosis. Presumably this phenomenon reflected a concomitant effect of DEM in inhibiting CCl₄ activation by cytochrome P450 (Suarez et al., 1981). In contrast, pretreatment of mice with DEM to decrease the kidney content of glutathione increased the nephrotoxicity of chloroform. The microsomal enzyme inhibitor piperonyl butoxide protected against chloroform nephrotoxicity (Kluwe and Hook, 1981). Others (Harris and Anders, 1980), however, have reported that both DEM and fasting potentiate CCl₄ hepatotoxicity by depleting the liver of glutathione.

Formerly it was believed (Recknagel and Glende, 1973) that free radical attack on polyenoic fatty acids (lipid peroxidation) in the vicinity of the endoplasmic reticulum was the critical lesion in initiating necrotic changes. It is now widely held that the covalent binding phenomenon is more important. Pyrazole, which blocked covalent binding and necrosis, did not modify the extent of lipid peroxidation (Bernacchi et al., 1980). Species differences between the extent of covalent binding of CCl$_4$-fragments and the degree of lipid peroxidation also suggested that necrosis is better correlated with the former than with the latter (Diaz Gomez et al., 1975). It is still possible, however, that endogenous decomposition products of peroxidized lipids with prostaglandin-like activity may modulate the hepatotoxic response (Willis, 1980).

Although it is still not possible to explain satisfactorily the potentiation of CCl$_4$ hepatotoxicity by ethanol in terms of the above mechanisms (Harris and Anders, 1980), there has been considerable recent interest in the potentiating effects of ketones and ketogenic substances. Astonishingly varied chemical structures having in common only a carbonyl moiety or the potential for metabolic transformation to a ketone are known to potentiate CCl$_4$ hepatotoxicity in mice; they include acetone, 2-butanone, methyl n-butyl ketone, 2,5-hexanedione, kepone, isopropyl alcohol, 2-butanol, n-hexanone and even metabolic ketosis as in alloxan-induced diabetes or after 1,3-butanediol administration (Hewitt et al., 1980). The effects of these ketones and potential ketones appear to differ from those of ethyl alcohol (Maling et al., 1975). The latter may be in some way related to an inhibition of aldehyde dehydrogenase by CCl$_4$ (Hjelle and Petersen, 1981). Perhaps the potentiating effect of ketones on CCl$_4$ hepatotoxicity is related to the observation that pretreatment with alcohol but not with phenobarbital increases the metabolism of CCl$_4$ selectively to phosgene (Harris and Anders, 1981). Methyl n-butyl ketone also potentiates the hepatotoxicity of chloroform in rats (Branchflower and Pohl, 1981). Thus, at least two toxic metabolites appear to be involved in CCl$_4$ hepatic necrosis, and the suggestion has been made that cleavage of the carbon-hydrogen bond in chloroform may be specifically involved in its nephrotoxicity (Branchflower and Pohl, 1981).

Studies of therapy: In animals studies, liver injury can be prevented or minimized by the prompt administration of antioxidants such as α-tocopherol acetate or N,N-diphenyl-p-phenylenediamine (DiLuzio and Costales, 1965; Gallagher, 1962). In rats, cystamine, cysteine and SKF 525A were effective even as late as 12 hours after CCl$_4$ in limiting the extent of liver damage at 24 hours (Ferreyra et al., 1977). Others (Siegers et al., 1978) found diethyldithiocarbamate to be superior to cysteine, cysteamine and other thio compounds. Few of these substances except

α-tocopherol have been tried in human carbon tetrachloride poisoning. Perhaps a cautious trial with N-acetylcysteine is warranted (see also ACETAMINOPHEN, p. III–6).

Induced hypothermia in animals also protects against liver damage, presumably by delaying the metabolic activation of CCl$_4$ to free radicals (Plaa and Larson, 1964; Larson and Plaa, 1965). Hypothermia in combination with α-tocopherol has been tried in at least one human case, but the favorable outcome was ascribed to concomitant therapy with hyperbaric oxygen (Truss and Killenberg, 1982).

One human adult who drank 80 to 100 ml. of pure carbon tetrachloride and subsequently developed severe signs and symptoms was successfully treated by extracorporeal hemoperfusion through activated charcoal. In vitro clearance studies confirmed the efficacy of this form of treatment in removing CCl$_4$ from blood (Schwarzbeck and Kosters, 1976).

Other chlorinated hydrocarbon solvents: It is singularly difficult to characterize toxicologically simple chlorinated hydrocarbons as a group because they can and do produce death by a variety of mechanisms. Thus, a congener's propensity to produce visceral lesions does not necessarily parallel its acute toxicity. Moreover, many authorities believe that the molecular basis for CCl$_4$-induced visceral damage will prove eventually to be either unique or limited to a very small number of closely related compounds.

Gehring (1968) exposed mice to a series of compounds at vapor concentrations such that each would produce 50% mortality over 9 to 12 hours of continuous exposure. Under these conditions, carbon tetrachloride and chloroform (CHCl$_3$) produced significant hepatic damage in terms of increased serum glutamic-pyruvate transaminase activity at subanesthetic vapor concentrations. Tetrachloroethylene, trichloroethylene, methylene chloride and 1,1,1-trichloroethane required exposure to concentrations high enough to produce death by anesthesia before evidence of hepatic damage could be obtained. 1,1,2-Trichlorethane was intermediate in that liver damage could be produced at sublethal anesthetic levels of exposure.

Klaassen and Plaa (1966) compared exactly the same series of compounds in terms of LD$_{50}$ and effects on liver and kidney function when given intraperitoneally to mice. Under these conditions, 1,1,2-trichloroethane was clearly the most toxic by factors of 4 to 10. In terms of the median effective doses for inducing organ dysfunction (BSP, SGPT, PSP, glucose and protein excretion), moderate to severe hepatic damage was encountered with carbon tetrachloride and chloroform, and moderate dysfunction was seen with 1,1,2-trichloroethane. Only mild hepatic damage was observed with the remaining compounds, and renal dysfunction was detected only with chloroform and 1,1,2-trichloroethane. Rather similar results were obtained in dogs except that $CHCl_3$ was somewhat less hepatotoxic than in mice (Klaassen and Plaa, 1967a). As induced by chloroform and 1,1,2-trichloroethane, renal dysfunction in mice showed a remarkable sex difference in that females were resistant, but both males and females were susceptible to the hepatotoxic effects (Klaassen and Plaa, 1967b).

Dihalogenated derivatives of methane (*e.g.*, methylene chloride and bromochloromethane) are apparently unique in that they are appreciably metabolized to carbon monoxide (Ratney *et al.*, 1974; Stewart *et al.*, 1972). Appreciable levels of carboxyhemoglobin have been detected in men exposed to methylene chloride vapor. These levels are not likely to be dangerous except in persons with preexisting coronary artery disease. More detailed information about individual halogenated hydrocarbons can be found in Section II and in von Oettingen (1964).

Symptomatology:

1. Prompt nausea, vomiting, and abdominal pain. Sometimes the pain becomes intense enough to mimic an acute surgical complication (Kirkpatrick and Sutherland, 1956). After ingestion, hematemesis and diarrhea.
2. Headache, dizziness, confusion, drowsiness, and occasionally convulsions.
3. Visual disturbances, sometimes consisting of a concentric restriction of the color fields without central scotomata (toxic amblyopia).
4. Rapid progression of central nervous depression with deepening coma and death from respiratory arrest or circulatory collapse.
5. Occasionally, sudden death due to ventricular fibrillation. Presumably this event may be heralded by frequent ventricular premature systoles.
6. In massive exposures the above symptoms merge with those outlined below, but central nervous depression may subside without sequelae (especially after a short vapor exposure), or an essentially asymptomatic interval of a few days may precede hepatorenal decompensation.
7. Kidney and/or liver injury, symptomatic or subclinical. Either may occur insidiously after an otherwise unrecognized exposure. The kidney lesion usually produces the more severe disturbance in human carbon tetrachloride poisoning.
8. Oliguria, albuminuria, anuria, gradual weight gain, edema. Death may occur within 1 week in the absence of effective supportive treatment.
9. Anorexia, jaundice, and right upper quadrant pain due to an enlarged and tender liver.
10. Carpopedal spasm that was relieved by calcium gluconate appears to be a very rare reaction (Weir, 1969).

Treatment:

1. Restore patient to fresh air and remove any contaminated clothing.
2. Oxygen and artificial ventilation as needed (pp. IV-7–14). Check for signs of impending pulmonary edema.
3. If CCl_4 was swallowed and if the patient is not drowsy, comatose or in respiratory difficulty, empty the stomach by giving syrup of ipecac to induce vomiting. A slurry of activated charcoal may be swallowed after the emesis. See pp. I-2–5.
4. As an alternative to 3, remove CCl_4 from the stomach by gastric lavage with water or saline solution and instill a saline cathartic, such as sodium or magnesium sulfate in water (15 to 30 gm.).
5. Do not administer fats, oils, alcohol, epinephrine, or ephedrine.
6. Respiratory stimulants, such as doxapram or nikethamide, may be given a trial if central nervous depression is severe (pp. IV-41–42).
7. Any time before severe kidney damage becomes apparent, treatment with an osmotic diuretic, such as mannitol, may be useful. If no diuresis ensues, fluids and electrolytes should be administered only cautiously, if at all. See pp. IV-52–55.
8. Extracorporeal hemoperfusion through a canister containing activated charcoal is alleged to be useful (Schwarzbeck and Kosters, 1976).
9. Adopt prophylactic measures for possible liver injury, as outlined on p. IV-60.
10. As soon as acute nervous symptoms subside and before the appearance of visceral lesions, a clinical trial of induced hypothermia might be considered in an attempt to prevent hepatic and perhaps renal damage. See discussion above.
11. As an alternative but clinically unproven way to prevent or minimize CCl_4-induced visceral lesions, administer a free-radical "scavenger," such as tocopherol (vitamin E). Either α-tocopherol or mixed tocopherols can be given by mouth in doses of several hundred milligrams. Possibly a more effective "scavenger" would be *N*-acetylcysteine (see p. III-6).
12. At least two case reports and some experimental evidence suggest that 100% oxygen at 1 atmosphere or at 2 atmospheres

for 2 hours twice daily may reduce the extent of hepatic necrosis (Truss and Killenberg, 1982).

13. For the management of acute renal failure, see pp. IV-53–55.

Laboratory: Carbon tetrachloride has a radiographic density equivalent to ordinary contrast media. Abdominal films may be used to confirm its presence in the gastrointestinal tract and to evaluate the efficacy of lavage (Bagnasco *et al.*, 1978). Repeated function tests are desirable to detect and evaluate kidney and liver injuries. Although nonspecific in their indications, serum glutamic-pyruvic and glutamic-oxaloacetic transaminase activities are elevated following carbon tetrachloride exposure. Decreases in these enzyme activities may parallel clinical recovery and serve as a useful tool in prognosis (Dawborn *et al.*, 1961; Fleisher and Wakin, 1956; Frankl *et al.*, 1957).

References:

Adams, E. M.; Spencer, H. C.; Rowe, V. K.; McCollister, D.D.; Irish, D. D. Vapor toxicity of carbon tetrachloride determined by experiments on laboratory animals. Arch. Ind. Hyg. Occup. Med. 6:50-65, 1952.

Alston, W. C. Hepatic and renal complications arising from accidental carbon tetrachloride poisoning in the human subject. J. Clin. Pathol. 23:249-253, 1970.

Bagnasco, F. M.; Stringer, B.; Muslim, A. M. Carbon tetrachloride poisoning: radiographic findings. N. Y. State J. Med. 78:646-647, 1978.

Bernacchi, A. S.; de Castro, C. R.; de Toranzo, E. G. D.; Marzi, A.; de Ferreyra, E. C.; de Fenos, O. M.; Castro, J. A. Pyrazole prevention of CCl₄-induced ultrastructural changes in rat liver. Br. J. Exp. Pathol. 61:505-511, 1980.

Bioulac, P.; Despuyoos, L.; Bedin, C.; Iron, A.; Saric, J.; Balabaud, C. Decreased acute hepatotoxicity of carbon tetrachloride and bromobenzene by cholestyramine in the rat. Gastroenterology 81:520-526, 1981.

Branchflower, R. V.; Pohl, L. R. Investigation of the mechanism of the potentiation of chloroform-induced hepatotoxicity and nephrotoxicity by methyl *n*-butyl ketone. Toxicol. Appl. Pharmacol. 61:407-413, 1981.

Butler, T. C. Reduction of carbon tetrachloride in vivo and reduction of carbon tetrachloride and chloroform in vitro by tissues and tissue constituents. J. Pharmacol. Exp. Ther. 134:311-319, 1961.

Chenery, R.; George, M.; Krishna, G. The effect of ionophore A23187 and calcium on carbon tetrachloride-induced toxicity in cultured rat hepatocytes. Toxicol. Appl. Pharmacol. 60:241-252, 1981.

Dawborn, J. K.; Ralston, M.; Weiden, S. Acute carbon tetrachloride poisoning. Transaminase and biopsy studies. Br. Med. J. 2:493-494, 1961.

Diaz Gomez, M. I.; Castro, J. A. Covalent binding of carbon tetrachloride metabolites to liver nuclear DNA, proteins and lipids. Toxicol. Appl. Pharmacol. 56:199-206, 1980.

Diaz Gomez, M. I.; de Castro, C. R.; D'Acosta, N.; de Fenos, O. M.; de Ferreyra, E. C.; Castro, J. A. Species differences in carbon tetrachloride-induced hepatotoxicity: The role of CCl₄ activation and of lipid peroxidation. Toxicol. Appl. Pharmacol. 34:102-114, 1975.

Dillenberg, S. M.; Thompson, C. M. Carbon tetrachloride poisoning. A report of twenty cases with one death. Milit. Surg. 97:39-44, 1945.

DiLuzio, N. R.; Costales, F. Inhibition of the ethanol and carbon tetrachloride induced fatty liver by antioxidants.

Exp. Mol. Pathol. 4:141-154, 1965.

Docks, E. L.; Krishna, G. The role of glutathione in chloroform-induced hepatotoxicity. Exp. Mol. Pathol. 24:13-22, 1976.

Drill, V. A. Hepatotoxic agents. Mechanism of action and dietary interrelationships. Pharmacol. Rev. 4:1-42, 1952.

Dume, T.; Herms, W.; Shroder, E.; Wetzels, E. Klinik und Therapie der Tetrachlorkohlenstuffvergiftung. Dtsch. Med. Wochenschr. 94:1646-1651, 1969.

Dvorackova, I. Ein Fall von todlicher oraler Tetrachlorkohlenstoffvergiftung. Arch. Toxikol. 20:72-78, 1963.

Farrier, R. M.; Smith, R. H. Carbon tetrachloride nephrosis, a frequently undiagnosed cause of death. J. A. M. A. 143:965-967, 1950.

Ferreyra, E. C.; de Fenos, O. M.; Bernacchi, A. S.; de Castro, C. R.; Castro, J. A. Treatment of carbon tetrachloride-induced liver necrosis with chemical compounds. Toxicol. Appl. Pharmacol. 42:513-521, 1977.

Fleisher, G. A.; Wakin, K. G. Transaminase in canine serum and cerebrospinal fluid after carbon tetrachloride poisoning and injection of transaminase concentrates. Proc. Mayo Clin. 31:640-648, 1956.

Folland, D. S.; Schaffner, W.; Ginn, H. E.; Crofford, O. B.; McMurray, D. R. Carbon tetrachloride toxicity potentiated by isopropyl alcohol. J. A. M. A. 236:1853-1856, 1976.

Frankl, H. D.; Gaertner, P. L.; Kossuth, L. C.; Milch, L. J. Toxic vapor inhalation and serum enzyme levels. Texas Repts. Biol. Med. 15:868-873, 1957.

Friedberg, C. K. Congestive heart failure of renal origin. Pathogenesis and treatment in four cases of carbon tetrachloride nephrosis. Am. J. Med. 9:164-174, 1950.

Friedman, R.; Eales, L. Carbon tetrachloride poisoning, a report of three cases with commentaries. S. Afr. Med. J. 36:1067-1071, 1962.

Gallagher, C. H. The effect of antioxidants in poisoning by carbon tetrachloride. Aust. J. Exp. Biol. 40:241-254, 1962.

Gehring, P. J. Hepatotoxic potency of various chlorinated hydrocarbon vapors relative to their narcotic and lethal potencies in mice. Toxicol. Appl. Pharmacol. 13:287-298, 1968.

Guild, W. R.; Young, J. V.; Merrill, J. P. Anuria due to carbon tetrachloride intoxication. Ann. Intern. Med. 48:1221-1227, 1958.

Hammes, E. M. Carbon tetrachloride as an industrial hazard. A report of two cases. J. Ind. Hyg. Toxicol. 23:112-117, 1941.

Hardin, B. L. Carbon tetrachloride poisoning - a review. Ind. Med. Surg. 32:93-105, 1954.

Harris, R. N.; Anders, M. W. Effect of fasting, diethylmaleate and alcohols on carbon tetrachloride-induced hepatotoxicity. Toxicol. Appl. Pharmacol. 56:191-198, 1980.

Harris, R. N.; Anders, M. W. 2-Propanol treatment induces selectively the metabolism of carbon tetrachloride to phosgene - implications for carbon tetrachloride hepatotoxicity. Drug Metab. Dis. 9:551-556, 1981.

Hewitt, W. R.; Miyajuna, H.; Cote, M. G.; Plaa, G. L. Modification of haloalkane-induced hepatotoxicity by exogenous ketones and metabolic ketosis. Fed. Proc. 39:3118-3123, 1980.

Hjelle, J. J.; Petersen, D. R. Decreased *in vivo* acetaldehyde oxidation and hepatic aldehyde dehydrogenase inhibition in C57BL and DBA mice treated with carbon tetrachloride. Toxicol. Appl. Pharmacol. 59:15-24, 1981.

Joron, G. E.; Hollenberg, C. H.; Bensley, E. H. Carbon tetrachloride - an underrated hazard. Can. Med. Assoc. J. 76:173-175, 1957.

Kast, A.; Nishikawa, J.; Yabe, T. Decrease of carbon tetrachloride liver toxicity in rats given dipyridamole. Exp. Pathol. 21:123-133, 1982.

Kennaugh, R. C. Carbon tetrachloride overdosage: A case report. S. Afr. Med. J. 49:635-636, 1975.

Kirkpatrick, H. J. R.; Sutherland, J. M. A fatal case of poisoning with carbon tetrachloride. J. Clin. Pathol. 9:242-247, 1956.

Klaassen, C. D.; Plaa, G. L. The relative effects of various chlorinated hydrocarbons on liver and kidney function in mice. Toxicol. Appl. Pharmacol. 9:139-151, 1966.

Klaassen, C. D.; Plaa, G. L. Relative effects of various chlorinated hydrocarbons on liver and kidney function in dogs. Toxicol. Appl. Pharmacol. 10:119-131, 1967a.

Klaassen, C. D.; Plaa, G. L. Susceptibility of male and female mice to the nephrotoxic and hepatotoxic properties of chlorinated hydrocarbons. Proc. Soc. Exp. Biol. Med. 124:1163-1166, 1967b.

Kluwe, W. M.; Hook, J. B. Potentiation of acute chloroform nephrotoxicity by the glutathione depletor diethyl maleate and protection by the microsomal enzyme inhibitor piperonyl butoxide. Toxicol. Appl. Pharmacol. 59:457-466, 1981.

Korenke, H. D.; Pribilla, O. Suicid durch einmalige Inhalation von Tetrachlorkohlenstoff (CCl₄) mit Leukoencephalopathie. Arch. Toxikol. 25:109-126, 1969.

Lamson, P. D.; Minot, A. S.; Robbins, B. H. The prevention and treatment of carbon tetrachloride intoxication. J. A. M. A. 90:345-349, 1928.

Larson, R. E.; Plaa, G. L. A correlation of the effects of cervical cordotomy, hypothermia and catecholamines on carbon tetrachloride-induced hepatic necrosis. J. Pharmacol. Exp. Ther. 147:103-111, 1965.

Luse, S. A.; Wood, W. G. The brain in fatal carbon tetrachloride poisoning. Arch. Neurol. 17:304-312, 1967.

Maling, H. M.; Stripp, B.; Sipes, I. G.; Highman, B.; Saul, W.; Williams, M. A. Enhanced hepatotoxicity of carbon tetrachloride, thioacetamide, and dimethylnitrosamine by pretreatment of rats with ethanol and some comparisions with potentiation by isopropanol. Toxicol. Appl. Pharmacol. 33:291-308, 1975.

McCollister, D. D.; Beamer, W. H.; Atchison, G. J.; Spencer, H. C. The absorption, distribution and elimination of radioactive carbon tetrachloride by monkeys upon exposure to low vapor concentration. J. Pharmacol. Exp. Ther. 102:112-124, 1951.

Myatt, A. V.; Salmons, J. A. Carbon tetrachloride poisoning. Arch. Ind. Hyg. Occup. Med. 6:74-82, 1952.

National Cancer Institute. Carcinogenesis bioassay of trichloroethylene. U. S. DHEW, Public Health Service, Technical Report Series No. 2, Publication No. 76-802, 1976.

New, P. S.; Lubash, G. D.; Scherr, L.; Rubin, A. L. Acute renal failure associated with carbon tetrachloride intoxication. J. A. M. A. 181:903-906, 1962.

Nicholls, L.; Hampton, G. G. Treatment of human hookworm infection with carbon tetrachloride. Br. Med. J. 2:8-11, 1922.

Noweir, H.; Pfitzer, E. A.; Hatch, T. F. Decomposition of chlorinated hydrocarbons. A review. Am. Ind. Hyg. Assoc. J. 33:454-460, 1972.

Phelps, B. M.; Hu, C. H. Carbon tetrachloride poisoning; report of 2 fatal cases and a series of animal experiments. J. A. M. A. 82:1254-1256, 1924.

Plaa, G. L.; Larson, R. E. CCl₄-induced liver damage. Arch. Environ. Health 9:536-543, 1964.

Popp, J. A.; Shinozaka, H.; Farber, E. The protective effects of diethyl dithiocarbamate and cycloheximide in the multiple hepatic lesions induced by carbon tetrachloride in the rat. Toxicol. Appl. Pharmacol. 45:549-564, 1978.

Quadland, H. P. Carbon tetrachloride. Part II of a literature study of reports of occupational injuries attributed to volatile solvents. Ind. Med. Surg. 12:821-829, 1943.

Ratney, R. S.; Wegman, D. H.; Elkins, H. B. In vivo conversion of methylene chloride to carbon monoxide. Arch. Environ. Health 28:223-226, 1974.

Recknagel, R. O. Carbon tetrachloride hepatotoxicity. Pharm. Rev. 19:145-208, 1967.

Recknagel, R. O.; Glende, E. A., Jr. Carbon tetrachloride hepatotoxicity: An example of lethal cleavage. C. R. C. Critical Rev. Toxicol. 2:263-297, 1973.

Robbins, B. H. The absorption, distribution and excretion of carbon tetrachloride in dogs under various conditions. J. Pharmacol. Exp. Ther. 37:203-216, 1929.

Schwarzbeck, A.; Kosters, W. Extrakorporale Hamoperfusion

bei akuter Tetrachlorkohenstoff-Vergiftung. Arch. Toxicol. 35:207-211, 1976.

Seidelin, R. The inhalation of phosgene in a fire extinguisher accident. Thorax 16:91-93, 1961.

Siegers, C. P.; Strubelt, O.; Volpel, M. The antihepatotoxic activity of dithiocarb as compared with 6 other thio compounds in mice. Arch. Toxicol. 41:79-88, 1978.

Sirota, J. H. Carbon tetrachloride poisoning in man. I. The mechanism of renal failure and recovery. J. Clin. Invest. 28:1412-1422, 1949.

Smetana, H. Nephrosis due to carbon tetrachloride. Arch. Intern. Med. 63:760-777, 1939.

Smith, A. R. Optic atrophy following inhalation of carbon tetrachloride. Arch. Ind. Hyg. Occup. Med. 1:348-351, 1950.

Smith, M. T.; Thor, H.; Orrenias, S. Toxic injury to isolated hepatocytes is not dependent on extracellular calcium. Science 213:1257-1259, 1981.

Stenger, R. J.; Porway, M.; Johnson, E. A.; Dalta, R. K. Effect of chlordane pretreatment on the hepatotoxicity of carbon tetrachloride. Exp. Mol. Pathol. 23:144-153, 1975.

Stevens, H.; Forster, F. M. Effects of carbon tetrachloride on the nervous system. Arch. Neurol. 70:635-649, 1953.

Stewart, R. D.; Dodd, H. C. Absorption of carbon tetrachloride, trichloroethylene, methylene chloride and 1, 1, 1-trichloroethane through the human skin. Am. Ind. Hyg. Assoc. J. 25:439-446, 1964.

Stewart, R. D.; Fisher, T. N.; Hosko, M. J.; Peterson, J. E.; Baretta, E. D.; Dodd, H. C. Experimental human exposure to methylene chloride. Arch. Environ. Health 25:342-348, 1972.

Straus, B. Aplastic anemia following exposure to carbon tetrachloride. J. A. M. A. 155:737-739, 1954.

Suarez, K. A.; Carlson, G. P.; Fuller, G. C. Effect of phenobarbital or 3-methylcholanthrene pretreatment on carbon tetrachloride-induced lipid peroxidation in rat liver. Toxicol. Appl. Pharmacol. 34:314-319, 1975.

Suarez, K. A.; Griffin, K.; Kopplin, R. P.; Bhonsle, P. Protective effect of diethylmaleate pretreatment on carbon tetrachloride hepatotoxicity. Toxicol. Appl. Pharmacol. 57:318-324, 1981.

Torrielli, M. W.; Ugazio, G. Biochemical aspects of the protective action of propyl gallate on liver injury in rats poisoned with carbon tetrachloride. Toxicol. Appl. Pharmacol. 34:151-169, 1975.

Truss, C. D.; Killenberg, P. G. Treatment of carbon tetrachloride poisoning with hyperbaric oxygen. Gastroenterology 82:767-769, 1982.

Ugazio, G.; Koch, P. R.; Recknagel, R. O. Mechanism of protection against carbon tetrachloride by prior carbon tetrachloride administration. Exp. Mol. Pathol. 16:281-285, 1972.

Villarruel, M. C.; Diaz Gomez, M. I.; Castro, J. A. The nature of the in vitro irreversible binding of carbon tetrachloride to microsomal lipids. Toxicol. Appl. Pharmacol. 33:106-114, 1975.

von Oettingen, W. F. The Halogenated Hydrocarbons of Industrial and Toxicological Importance. Elsevier Publishing Co., New York, 1964.

Webster, R. W. Legal Medicine and Toxicology. W. B. Saunders Co., Philadelphia, 1930.

Weir, R. J. Carbon tetrachloride poisoning as a hazard of wig cleaning. Br. Med. J. 1:487, 1969.

Willis, R. J. Possible role of endogenous toxigenic lipids in the carbon tetrachloride poisoned hepatocyte. Fed. Proc. 39:3134-3137, 1980.

Wolf, C. R.; Harrelson, W. G., Jr.; Nastainczyk, W. M.; Philpot, R. M. Kalyanaraman, B.; Mason, R. P. Metabolism of carbon tetrachloride in hepatic microsomes and reconstituted monooxygenase systems and its relationship to lipid peroxidation. Mol. Pharmacol. 18:553-558, 1980.

CHLORDANE

Chlordane, a mixture of various isomers of octachloro-4,7-methanohydroindane and related compounds, is an amber viscous liquid that is soluble in practically all petroleum solvents. It was once widely used as an insecticide (Ingle, 1965), but currently it is limited to underground applications for termite control. Human chlordane poisonings were never common, but even though the agent is no longer available to amateur gardeners, accidental poisonings still occur. The transient contamination of part of the municipal water supply of Chattanooga, Tennessee, exposed 105 persons, of whom 13 reported mild symptoms of poisoning (Harrington et al., 1978). See also DIELDRIN, p. III-143.

Toxicology: In animals, chlordane is less toxic than heptachlor, to which it is closely related. The acute oral LD_{50} in rats has been reported variously as 250 and 590 mg./kg. (Stohlman et al., 1950; Ambrose et al., 1953). It is rapidly absorbed through the integument (Barnes, 1967; Derbes et al., 1955) and may be even more toxic by this route than by oral administration. Chlordane is probably also hazardous by inhalation of sprays or mists.

Like other halogenated hydrocarbon insecticides, chlordane is a stimulant of the central nervous system. Even in subconvulsant doses, characteristic changes occur in the spontaneous electrocortical activity in rats. In fatal poisonings, EEG patterns suggest that death is due to respiratory arrest between or during convulsive episodes (Hyde and Falkenberg, 1976). The signs and symptoms are said to be of longer duration than those from DDT, and at least in animals, death after oral poisoning may be delayed for several days (Stohlman et al., 1950).

It has been estimated that the fatal oral dose for an adult human lies somewhere between 6 and 60 gm., with onset of symptoms within 45 minutes to several hours after ingestion (Aldrich and Holmes, 1969; Curley and Garrettson, 1969; Derbes et al., 1955). On occasion, however, "inordinately small amounts" have apparently caused severe poisoning in children (Jacobziner and Raybin, 1961a; Lensky and Evans, 1952), and in one adult the estimated lethal dose retained after vomiting was only 10 mg./kg. (Dadey and Kammer, 1953). Once absorbed, chlordane is an extremely persistent poison. The serum half-life in one child was 88 days (Aldrich and Holmes, 1969). In another toddler the fat concentrations of chlordane after a single dose continued to rise through the 8th postingestion day, and after 3 months the fat:serum partition was about 1500:1 (Curley and Garrettson, 1969).

Large differences have also been reported in the time to death in poisoned adults; one died within "minutes" after accidentally spilling a suspension of chlordane on her dress, and another survived 10 days after the ingestion of 6 gm. (Derbes et al., 1955). Perhaps because of the unusually long survival, the latter victim exhibited unusual complications, such as severe hemorrhagic gastritis, shock, anuria and confluent bronchopneumonia, as well as the more characteristic sign of convulsions. In a case in which an overnight stay in an apartment freshly sprayed with chlordane resulted only in severe cough and vomiting (Lemmon and Pierce, 1952), one cannot be certain that the signs were in fact due to chlordane (Heyroth, 1952). In a patient exposed to both chlordane and an organophosphate cholinesterase inhibitor insecticide like PARATHION (p. III-336), the administration of 2-PAM produced rapid restoration of blood cholinesterase activity to normal levels, but signs of central nervous stimulation ascribed to the chlordane persisted (Dinman, 1964).

Chronic exposure to related insecticides, particularly LINDANE (p. III-239), has been associated with the appearance of blood dyscrasias. In one patient extensively exposed to chlordane over 3 to 5 months, the bone marrow showed evidence of dyserythropoiesis, eosinophilia and megaloblastosis. Recovery was complete 4 months after termination of the exposure (Furie and Trubowitz, 1976). Infante et al. (1978) reported three cases of aplastic anemia associated with chlordane exposure.

Chronic poisoning in animals produces inanition and degenerative changes in the liver, renal tubules, lungs, intestinal submucosa and heart (Ingle, 1952; Stohlman et al., 1950). Like most halogenated hydrocarbon insecticides, chlordane is very slowly metabolized (Brimfield et al., 1978) and is excreted primarily in the feces (Poonawalla and Korte, 1964). Because of its storage in body fat, chlordane has a high degree of persistence and also a high potential for cumulative neurotoxicity. Starvation leads to chlordane mobilization and an intensification of the toxic effects in exposed animals (Hyde and Falkenberg, 1976). It is a potent inducer of hepatic microsomal enzymes (Hart et al., 1963; Fouts and Rogers, 1965). These effects may result in alterations in the rate of metabolism and toxicity of other drugs or pesticides administered concurrently (Conney et al., 1967; Williams et al., 1967) and perhaps to hormonal disturbances because of accelerated metabolism of endogenous steroids (Street et al., 1969; Talamantes and Jang, 1977; Welch et al., 1971).

Chlordane is an established carcinogen in mouse liver. Exposure to chlordane formulations have been implicated in the development of three human cases of leukemia and of five cases of neuroblastoma in children (Infante *et al.*, 1978).

Symptomatology:

1. Earliest signs of poisoning are increased sensitivity to stimuli due to hyperexcitability of the central nervous system, generalized hyperactive reflexes, muscle twitching, tremor, incoordination, ataxia, and clonic convulsions with or without coma. Cycles of excitement and depression may be repeated several times.
2. Liver damage as a possible late manifestation.
3. Anorexia and weight loss.
4. Severe gastroenteritis has been described in one of the fatal human poisonings (Derbes *et al.*, 1955).

Treatment:

1. Administer syrup of ipecac or perform gastric lavage with warm tap water (unless convulsions are imminent).
2. Sodium sulfate catharsis (30 gm. in 6 to 8 oz. of water). Avoid oil laxatives.
3. A rapidly acting barbiturate or diazepam may aid in controlling convulsions, but care must be taken not to augment any respiratory depression. See pp. IV-35–39.
4. Oxygen therapy and artificial ventilation may be necessary (pp. IV-12 and 7).
5. Avoid epinephrine.
6. Since no specific antidotes are known, symptomatic therapy must be accompanied by complete rest.
7. Use soap and water in adequate quantities to wash off any compound spilled on the skin. If spilled in eyes, wash repeatedly with water.

Laboratory: Function tests to detect and evaluate possible liver and kidney disturbances. Electroencephalography (EEG) may be helpful in revealing the persistency of cortical dysfunction. Hematological studies of blood and bone marrow may be appropriate in chronic exposures.

References:

Aldrich, F. D.; Holmes, J. H. Acute chlordane intoxication in a child. Arch. Environ. Health *19*:129-132, 1969.

Ambrose, A. M.; Christensen, H. E.; Robbins, D. J.; Rather, L. J. Toxicological and pharmacological studies on chlordane. Arch. Ind. Hyg. Occup. Med. *7*:197-210, 1953.

Barnes, R. Poisoning by the insecticide chlordane. Med. J. Aust. *1*:972-973, 1967.

Brimfield, A. A.; Street, J. C.; Futrell, J.; Chatfield, D. A. Identification of products arising from the metabolism of *cis-* and *trans-*chlordane in rat liver microsomes *in vitro*: Outline of a possible metabolic pathway. Pest. Biochem. Physiol. *9*:84-95, 1978.

Conney, A. H.; Welch, R. M.; Kuntzman, R.; Burns, J. J. Effects of pesticides on drug and steroid metabolism. Clin. Pharmacol. Ther. *8*:2-10, 1967.

Curley, A.; Garrettson, L. K. Acute chlordane poisoning. Arch. Environ. Health *18*:211-215, 1969.

Dadey, J. L.; Kammer, A. G. Chlordane intoxication. Report of a case. J. A. M. A. *153*:723-725, 1953.

Derbes, V. J.; Dent, J. H.; Forrest, W. W.; Johnson, M. F. Fatal chlordane poisoning. J. A. M. A. *158*:1367-1369, 1955.

Dinman, B. D. Acute combined toxicity due to DDVP and chlordane. Arch. Environ. Health *9*:765-769, 1964.

Fouts, J. R.; Rogers, L. A. Morphological changes in the liver accompanying stimulation of microsomal drug metabolizing enzyme activity by phenobarbital, chlordane, benzpyrene or methylcholanthrene in rats. J. Pharmacol. Exp. Ther. *147*:112-114, 1965.

Furie, B.; Trubowitz, S. Insecticides and blood dyscrasias. Chlordane exposure and self-limited refractory megaloblastic anemia. J. A. M. A. *235*:1720-1722, 1976.

Harrington, J. M.; Baker, E. L., Jr.; Folland, D. S.; Saucier, J. W.; Sandifer, S. H. Chlordane contamination of a municipal water supply. Environ. Res. *15*:155-159, 1978.

Hart, L. G.; Shultice, R. W.; Fouts, J. R. Stimulatory effects of chlordane on hepatic microsomal drug metabolism in the rat. Toxicol. Appl. Pharmacol. *5*:371-386, 1963.

Heyroth, F. F. Chlordane poisoning. J. A. M. A. *150*:715, 1952.

Hyde, K. M.; Falkenberg, R. L. Neuroelectrical disturbance as indicator of chronic chlordane toxicity. Toxicol. Appl. Pharmacol. *37*:499-515, 1976.

Infante, P. F.; Epstein, S. S.; Newton, W. A. Blood dyscrasias and childhood tumors and exposure to chlordane and heptachlor. Scand. J. Work Environ. Health *4*:137-150, 1978.

Ingle, L. Chronic oral toxicity of chlordan to rats. Arch. Ind. Hyg. Occup. Med. *6*:357-367, 1952.

Ingle, L. A Monograph on Chlordane, Toxicological and Pharmacological Properties. Privately published, 1965.

Jacobziner, H.; Raybin, H. W. Plant and insecticide poisonings. N. Y. State J. Med. *61*:2463-2466, 1961a.

Lemmon, G. B., Jr.; Pierce, W. F. Intoxication due to chlordane. Report of a case. J. A. M. A. *149*:1314-1316, 1952.

Lensky, P.; Evans, H. L. Human poisoning by chlordane. Report of a case. J. A. M. A. *149*:1394-1395, 1952.

Poonawalla, N. H.; Korte, F. Metabolism of insecticides VIII (1): Excretion, distribution and metabolism of α-chlordan-C^{14} by rats. Life Sci. *3*:1497-1500, 1964.

Stohlman, E. F.; Thorp, W. T. S.; Smith, M. I. Toxic actions of chlordan. Arch. Ind. Hyg. Occup. Med. *1*:13-19, 1950.

Street, J. C.; Mayer, F. L.; Wagstaff, D. J. Ecological significance of pesticide interactions. Ind. Med. Surg. *38*:409-414, 1969.

Talamantes, F.; Jang, H. Effects of chlordane isomers administered to female mice during the neonatal period. J. Toxicol. Environ. Health *3*:713-720, 1977.

Welch, R. M.; Levin, W.; Kuntzman, R.; Jacobson, M.; Conney, A. H. Effect of halogenated hydrocarbon insecticides on the metabolism and uterotropic action of estrogens in rats and mice. Toxicol. Appl. Pharmacol. *19*:234-246, 1971.

Williams, C. H.; Casterline, J. L., Jr.; Jacobson, K. H. Studies of toxicity and enzyme activity resulting from interaction between chlorinated hydrocarbon and carbamate insecticides. Toxicol. Appl. Pharmacol. *11*:302-307, 1967.

CHLORPROMAZINE

Among the many therapeutic agents that have risen to prominence over the past 3 decades, perhaps none has equaled chlorpromazine in the rapidity with which it was widely adopted. Virtually unknown in 1953, chlorpromazine was renowned throughout the United States by 1955. In view of its phenomenal popularity, it was perhaps inevitable that it would serve as the prototype for many derivatives varying in toxicity and also in therapeutic usefulness. Derivatives of phenothiazine include not only tranquilizers but antihistaminics, antiemetics and adjuncts to anesthesia as well. It is apparent that a broad toxicological spectrum is presented by the group as a whole.

Chemically, phenothiazine drugs may be classified according to the nature of the substituent on the phenothiazine ring nitrogen. The principal types of N-side chains are aliphatic groups (chlorpromazine, promazine, triflupromazine, methoxypromazine), piperidine derivatives (mepazine, thioridazine) and piperazine derivatives (prochlorperazine, trifluoperazine, fluphenazine, thiopropazate) (Hollister, 1961a). The presence of a pyrrolidine ring (methdilazine, pyrathiazine) in this side chain apparently imparts more prominent antihistaminic and parasympatholytic properties to the drug. The substituent on the number 2 carbon of the phenothiazine ring provides yet another means of chemical classification. It may be a hydrogen atom (promethazine, trimeprazine), a chlorine atom (chlorpromazine, pipamazine), a trifluoromethyl group (triflupromazine, fluphenazine), a methoxy group (methoxypromazine) or a methylmercapto group (thioridazine). Hydrogen appears at this location in all phenothiazines which are employed as antihistaminics and parasympatholytics.

Chlorpromazine is effective as a central nervous depressant in a wide range of psychiatric disturbances, but it is of particular value in the management of psychotics (Vogt, 1958). It suppresses hallucinations and delusion induced by various psychotomimetic drugs of abuse (exclusive of anticholinergic agents, where the toxicity appears to be enhanced by phenothiazines). It has a broad antiemetic effectiveness against agents acting on the chemoreceptor trigger zone (Cross, 1959); in particular it is capable of suppressing vomiting due to apomorphine (Moyer et al., 1954).

Toxicology: Chlorpromazine is readily absorbed by any route and exhibits local anesthetic properties, like cocaine, on mucous membranes (Moyer, 1955). It is weakly sympatholytic, hypotensive, hypometabolic and hypothermic (Azima and Ogle, 1954). Apparently both the liver and kidneys are involved in the metabolism of the drug. The principal metabolite in both urine and feces is the sulfoxide, whose pharmacological properties closely resemble the parent compound except for decreased sedative activity (Moran and Butler, 1956). A potentially danger-

ous drug interaction between chlorpromazine and meperidine may result from an interference with metabolic biotransformation (Stambaugh and Wainer, 1981).

Acute animal toxicity studies (Table III-4) indicate that chlorpromazine falls into toxicity class 4 (Piala et al., 1959). Because it is available to large numbers of emotionally disturbed people, poisoning due to overdosage occurs frequently. Although successful suicides due to congeners of chlorpromazine are occasionally encountered (Donlon and Tupin, 1977; Joubert and Olivier, 1974), published reports of human fatalities from chlorpromazine are remarkably rare (Brophy, 1967; Davis et al., 1968). A 13-month-old girl died following the ingestion of 750 mg. or about 75 mg./kg. (Haggerty, 1957); a 4-year-old girl died after 350 mg. (Wallman, 1957); and a 3-year-old boy, after 800 mg. (Dilworth et al., 1963). A 40-year-old woman was found dead after an estimated total dose of 2 gm. (Algeri et al., 1959).

On the evidence offered by so few cases, one should not conclude that chlorpromazine is more toxic in man than in experimental animals. Given medical care, adults have recovered from 10 to 30 gm. (Brophy, 1967; Douglas and Bates, 1957; Samuels, 1957). In an unpublished case seen by one of us (R. E. G.) in consultation with Drs. L. Lambert and J. McKenna, a 19-year-old male patient recovered after a single dose of 17.5 gm. In clinical psychiatry it is not unusual to treat severe manic or schizophrenic patients with doses of 2 to 3 gm./day (Davis et al., 1968).

The prominent manifestations of acute intoxication reflect varying degrees of central nervous depression as evidenced by coma, hypotension, hypothermia, suppression of tendon reflexes and miosis (Algeri et al., 1959; Cann and Verhulst, 1960c). Respiratory difficulties have been ascribed to partial obstruction from a relaxed pharyngeal wall and weak respiratory movements (Ferguson, 1957). Pulmonary edema has been observed in at least three fatal cases of thioridazine ingestion. Aspiration of vomitus seems the most likely cause for this complication, but an interference with pulmonary surfactant pro-

Table III-4.

Experimental Acute Toxicity Studies with Chlorpromazine

Species	LD$_{50}$		
	Oral	Intra-peritoneal	Intravenous
	mg./kg.	mg./kg.	mg./kg.
Mouse	375	115	31
Rat	–	58	–
Dog	–	–	37

duction could not be ruled out (Joubert and Olivier, 1974). In contrast to the flaccidity seen in severe barbiturate poisoning, coma due to chlorpromazine is often punctuated by periods of motor restlessness, tremors, spasms, and other signs ascribed to extrapyramidal tract activity. In one child, thought not to be a latent diabetic, a prolonged quiet sleep occurred with hyperglycemia and acetonemia (Strauss, 1968).

Tonic and clonic convulsions were described in an 18-year-old girl 18 hours after the ingestion of a huge amount (Samuels, 1957). EEG patterns in patients receiving therapeutic doses of chlorpromazine resemble those seen after many other sedatives (e.g., accentuation of the α-rhythm), but some epileptics do not tolerate chlorpromazine because of an increased incidence of focal spikes and of overt convulsions. In at least one poison victim (Mauceri and Strauss, 1956), diffuse spikes resembling those seen after pentylenetetrazol (Metrazol) were prominent in the EEG in the absence of clinical convulsions or a history of convulsions. A necrosing encephalopathy with neuronal, glial, myelinic and vascular lesions developed in one infant weeks after apparent recovery from an accidental overdose (Arseni et al., 1976).

An important group of neurological signs and symptoms after overdoses and after daily medication with therapeutic doses arises from dysfunction of the extrapyramidal system. Although induced by chlorpromazine, extrapyramidal signs are more prominent with phenothiazine tranquilizers that have a piperazine side chain (Cohen, 1959), such as fluphenazine, and with haloperidol. At least four neurological syndromes are recognized. An early reaction (typically during the first 5 days of therapy or after a single massive overdose) consists of acute dystonias, including grimacing, torticollis, oculogyric crises, and sometimes trismus, tongue protrusion, dysphagia, dysphonia, carpopedal spasm, opisthotonus and even epileptiform convulsions (Shaw et al., 1959; Sobel, 1960). These effects are said to be more common among children and among those who are convulsion-prone (Bellman, 1974; Fazekas et al., 1957). After 5 to 30 days of phenothiazine medication a syndrome clinically indistinguishable from idiopathic parkinsonism may appear (Goldman, 1955; Hall et al., 1956), with the usual rigidity, mask-like facial expression, shuffling gait and variable tremor. A third syndrome, which appears typically after the first week but before the third month of medication, is characterized by akathisia, i.e., motor restlessness without anxiety or agitation. A fourth syndrome, known as tardive dyskinesia, tends to arise only after long-term medication (months and years) and is more common in females, in the elderly and in those with organic brain damage. The neurological signs consist of involuntary orofacial dyskinesias (lip smacking and sucking, etc.) and of widespread choreoathetotic movements (Crane, 1968).

Tardive dyskinesia is sometimes a permanent disability, but most of the extrapyramidal syndromes induced by tranquilizers disappear spontaneously when the drug is discontinued or the dose reduced. The acute dystonia and the pseudoparkinsonism tend to be intensified by administering l-dopa (Gerlach et al., 1974) and relieved by caffeine and by such antiparkinsonian drugs as benztropine and diphenhydramine, which is evidence that they are not epileptic equivalents (Duffy, 1971; Goldsmith, 1959; Gupta and Lovejoy, 1967). Tardive dyskinesia may worsen under the influence of these drugs, whereas akathisia is usually resistant to all drug therapy.

The phenothiazines are chemically related to the so-called tricyclic antidepressants (see IMIPRAMINE, p. III-205) and have some pharmacological properties in common with them. Poisoning by imipramine, however, is a more serious threat to life than a comparable overdose of chlorpromazine because of the cardiac arrhythmias and conduction defects associated with the former. Except in patients with preexisting heart disease, cardiotoxicity is infrequently described in phenothiazine intoxications, but ECG changes, arrhythmias, conduction disturbances, myocardial failure and coronary complications are occasionally recognized and resemble their counterparts produced by tricyclic antidepressants (Alexander and Nino, 1969; Moccetti et al., 1971; Weiss, 1981). As adverse drug reactions with therapeutic doses, disorders of the cardiac mechanism are more commonly encountered with piperazine- and piperidine-type phenothiazine tranquilizers than with chlorpromazine (Weiss, 1981).

Perhaps because of a greater hypotensive effect, especially in the elderly, and a high degree of anticholinergic activity, thioridazine may carry a particular risk for inducing cardiotoxicity (Kelly et al., 1963; Weiss, 1981). In a series of 6 suicide attempts involving thioridazine or mesoridazine, the only survivor exhibited reversible total heart block (Donlon and Tupin, 1977). In a patient who had consumed 6 gm. chlorpromazine and 6 gm. thioridazine, the ventricular tachycardia did not respond to conventional drug therapy, and a transvenous pacemaker had to be inserted (Lumpkin et al., 1979). A glucose load seemed to increase repolarization abnormalities in patients chronically treated with perphenazine (Chouinard and Annable, 1977).

Perhaps cardiotoxicity is involved in sudden, unexplained deaths among patients being treated with phenothiazines (Hollister and Kosek, 1965; Reinert and Hermann, 1960). In one of these cases, irreversible ventricular fibrillation was demonstrated. Central respiratory failure, however, has also been suspected in sudden autopsy-negative deaths (Whyman, 1976).

Chlorpromazine and the other phenothiazine tranquilizers may cause a failure of thermoregulation and lead to serious deviations in the deep body temperature. Among comatose patients in a cool or temperate environment, impaired body heat conservation and the absence of shivering often result in at least a small drop in deep body temperature; in some cases the hypothermia is intense. In a warm or hot environment, overdoses or even conventional doses sometimes lead to severe hyperpyrexia (heat stroke); several deaths have been ascribed to this complication (Ayd, 1956; Zelman and Guillan, 1970).

Phenothiazine hyperthermia is not always associated with hot weather. An unusual syndrome encountered in France has been named the "malignant neuroleptic syndrome." It occurs with conventional doses of tranquilizers of both the phenothiazine and butyrophenone types and consists of the gradual onset of hyperpyrexia, hypertonus, rhabdomyolysis, metabolic acidosis, hyperkalemia and respiratory distress. The incidence is said to be about 40 cases annually in France, and the mortality rate in untreated cases is 30 to 50%. There is no known genetic predisposition as in malignant hyperpyrexia, but like the latter disease, the malignant neuroleptic syndrome may be responsive to treatment by intravenous sodium dantrolene (Bismuth et al., 1982).

Much attention has been paid to chlorpromazine-induced jaundice. The incidence is about 1% and is higher in women (Isaacs et al., 1955). The nature of the liver injury has been disputed. Portal inflammation with intrahepatic cholestasis is widely recognized, but hepatocellular necrosis also occurs (Zelman, 1959). Death from this cause has been reported (Boardman, 1954; Rodin and Robertson, 1958). Hemorrhage and coagulation defects have been associated with clinical jaundice (Floch and Leibowitz, 1959; McHardy et al., 1955). The cholestatic effects of chlorpromazine are enhanced by delays in its metabolism (Tavoloni and Boyer, 1980). Comprehensive review articles on this subject are available (Plaa and Priestly, 1976; Zelman, 1959; Shay and Siplet, 1957).

A more grave reaction to chlorpromazine is agranulocytosis, the incidence of which has been estimated at 0.001 to 0.002% (Platzer and Glaser, 1957) with a fatal outcome in about 40% of afflicted patients within a few days (Fiore and Noonan, 1959). It too is seen more frequently in women (Pisciotta et al., 1958) and perhaps is an expression of a preexisting low reserve in the marrow proliferative capacity (Pisciotta, 1978). There are indications that many if not all of the phenothiazines present this hazard, and cross-

sensitization appears likely (Korst, 1959). The concomitant occurrence of jaundice is said to be highly fatal (Fiore and Noonan, 1959). A profound neutropenia was observed 45 hours after the acute ingestion of chlorpromazine by a 5-year-old girl. A 3-year-old male sibling who apparently ingested a similar dose and had a similar clinical course did not become neutropenic (Burckart et al., 1981).

Miscellaneous hazards associated with chlorpromazine include contact dermatitis (Levan, 1957), urticaria, abnormal skin pigmentation and photosensitivity characterized by an exaggerated cutaneous response to ultraviolet light with resulting erythema and edema (Epstein et al., 1957). With large daily doses, particularly of thioridazine, pigmentary retinopathy has been encountered rarely. Chlorpromazine augments the central depressant activity of anesthetics, sedatives, narcotics and alcohol, and therefore these agents should be employed with extreme caution (Moyer, 1955; Zirkle et al., 1959). Because the vasoconstrictor but not the vasodilator activity of epinephrine may be blocked by chlorpromazine, epinephrine may lower instead of raise the blood pressure. Levarterenol is a safer drug under these circumstances.

Since gastric motility is usually inhibited by chlorpromazine, lavage is indicated even several hours after its ingestion (Beal, 1955). On the other hand, because of the high degree of protein binding of the drug in the blood, hemodialysis appears to be of little value (Avram and McGinn, 1966) and the same is probably true of hemoperfusion. In cases in which the condition of the patient appears to warrant it, exchange transfusions may be helpful (Haggerty, 1957). The remainder of the therapeutic regimen should be directed toward alleviating the signs and symptoms of central depression and hypotension. Fluid therapy, pressor drugs, oxygen, and artificial respiration may be indicated (Cann and Verhulst, 1960c). Physostigmine was said to be effective in a 2½-year-old male child in reversing the coma. The intravenous dose of 0.5 mg. was repeated 3 times at lengthening intervals (Wang and Marlowe, 1977). In an adult who had consumed 300 mg. trifluoperazine, physostigmine both restored consciousness and improved ECG changes which included an idioventricular rhythm with marked conduction delay (Weisdorf et al., 1978). More experience is necessary, however, before physostigmine can be recommended as an analeptic in chlorpromazine poisoning.

Symptomatology:

1. Central nervous depression progressing from drowsiness to somnolence to stupor to coma, ultimately with arreflexia. In early or mild intoxications, some patients experience restlessness, confusion and ex-

citement.

2. Hypotension, tachycardia, miosis.
3. Restlessness, tremor or muscular twitching, spasm, rigidity, convulsions.
4. Extrapyramidal signs of overdoses occasionally include dystonia, torticollis, oculogyric crises and opisthotonus.
5. Either hypothermia or hyperthermia may be encountered.
6. Muscular hypotonia, difficulty in swallowing and breathing, cyanosis.
7. Respiratory and/or vasomotor collapse. Sudden apnea has been described.
8. Sometimes cardiac arrhythmias, conduction defects, ventricular fibrillation or cardiac arrest.
9. Side effects of therapeutic doses, as described in the text above, are occasionally encountered after single overdoses.

Treatment:

1. Although ipecac syrup is said to be effective in promoting vomiting even after overdoses of phenothiazine tranquilizers (Manoguerra and Krenzelok, 1978), it should not be administered if the patient is already drowsy.
2. Gastric lavage is indicated even many hours after ingestion because gastric motility is greatly reduced. Use precautions against aspiration (p. I-10). Leave 30 gm. sodium sulfate in water in the stomach and/or a slurry of 50–100 gm. activated charcoal (p. I-12).
3. In severe shock, phenylephrine or, better, levarterenol by intravenous infusion. Avoid epinephrine because of its vasodepressor action (see above). Ephedrine and dextroamphetamine may be helpful occasionally, but convulsant stimulants must be avoided. See pp. IV-16–17.
4. Fluid and electrolyte therapy (see pp. IV-64–69).
5. Oxygen and artificial respiration as indicated (pp. IV-12 and 7–12).
6. Hypothermia is common and sometimes difficult to control. Both blankets and heat lamps may be required. Caution is indicated, however, because fever may also occur (see below).
7. In hot weather, even the comatose patient may present with dangerous hyperpyrexia requiring prompt intervention; see p. IV-84 for appropriate measures. As noted above, sodium dantrolene may be helpful in the malignant neuroleptic syndrome.
8. In extreme cases, exchange transfusion may be useful, but hemodialysis and hemoperfusion are probably of little value because the drug binds intensely to plasma proteins.
9. Continuously monitor the ECG. In the event of irregularities in rhythm or conduction, follow the recommendations for treatment of IMIPRAMINE poisoning, p. III-210.
10. Although parenteral physostigmine may have some analeptic value (see text above), it is potentially dangerous and is not recommended at the present time.
11. Diphenhydramine (10 to 50 mg.) intravenously will provide relief from extrapyramidal signs. The maximal 24-hour dose is 400 mg. in adults and 5 mg./kg. in children.

Laboratory: Most clinical laboratories are capable of conducting a quantitative analysis by colorimetry.

References:

Alexander, C. S.; Nino, A. Cardiovascular complications in young patients taking psychotropic drugs. Am. Heart J. 78:757-769, 1969.

Algeri, E. J.; Katsas, G. G.; McBay, A. J. Toxicology of some new drugs. Glutethimide, meprobamate, and chlorpromazine. J. Forensic Sci. 4:111-134, 1959.

Arseni, C.; Nereantiu, F.; Nicolescu, P.; Horvath, L. Encephalopathy subsequent to accidental poisoning with chlorpromazine. Europ. Neurol. 14:29-38, 1976.

Avram, M. M.; McGinn, J. T. Extracorporeal hemodialysis in phenothiazine overdosage. J. A. M. A. 197:142-143, 1966.

Ayd, F. J., Jr. Fatal hyperpyrexia during chlorpromazine therapy. J. Clin. Exp. Psychopath. 17:189-192, 1956.

Azima, H.; Ogle, W. Effects of Largactil in mental syndromes. Can. Med. Assoc. J. 71:116-121, 1954.

Beal, J. A. Chlorpromazine poisoning. Br. Med. J. 2:1620, 1955.

Bellman, M. H. Treatment of phenothiazine drug intoxication with benztropine. Arch. Dis. Child. 49:664, 1974.

Bismuth, C.; De Rohan-Chabot, P.; Conso, F.; Elkharat, D. Theoretic indication of dantrolene in malignant neuroleptic syndroma. Efficiency in 3 cases. Vet. Human Toxicol. 24:280, 1982.

Boardman, R. H. Fatal case of toxic hepatitis implicating chlorpromazine. Br. Med. J. 2:579, 1954.

Brophy, J. J. Suicide attempts with psychotherapeutic drugs. Arch. Gen. Psychiatry 17:652-657, 1967.

Burckart, G. J.; Snidow, J.; Bruce, W. Neutropenia following acute chlorpromazine ingestion. Clin. Toxicol. 18:797-801, 1981.

Cann, H. M.; Verhulst, H. L. Accidental ingestion and overdosage involving psychopharmacologic drugs. N. Engl. J. Med. 263:719-724, 1960c.

Chouinard, G.; Annable, L. Phenothiazine-induced ECG abnormalities: effect of a glucose load. Arch. Gen. Psychiatry 34:951-954, 1977.

Cohen, S. Clonic convulsions. J. A. M. A. 169:2066, 1959.

Crane, G. E. Tardive dyskinesias in patients treated with major neuroleptics; a review of the literature. Am. J. Psychiatry 124 (Suppl):40-48, 1968.

Cross, R. J. Tranquilizing drugs. Am. J. Med. 27:767-780, 1959.

Davis, J. M.; Bartlett, E.; Termini, B. A. Overdosage of psychotropic drugs: A review. Dis. Nerv. Syst. 29:157-164 and 246-256, 1968.

Dilworth, N. M.; Dagdale, A. E.; Hillen, H. B. Acute poisoning with chlorpromazine. Lancet 1:137-138, 1963.

Donlon, P. T.; Tupin, J. P. Successful suicides with thioridazine and mesoridazine. Arch. Gen. Psychiatry 34:955-957, 1977.

Douglas, A. D. M.; Bates, T. J. N. Chlorpromazine as a suicidal agent. Br. Med. J. 1:1514, 1957.

Duffy, B. Acute phenothiazine intoxication in children. Med. J. Aust. 1:676-678, 1971.

Epstein, J. H.; Brunsting, L. A.; Petersen, M. C.; Schwarz, B. E. A study of photosensitivity occurring with chlorpromazine therapy. J. Invest. Dermatol. 28:329-338, 1957.

Fazekas, J. F.; Shea, J. G.; Ehrmantraut, W. R.; Alman, R. W. Convulsant action of phenothiazine derivatives. J. A. M. A. 165:1241-1245, 1957.

Ferguson, J. T. Neuropharmacological agents in rehabilitation of patients with chronic mental illness. J. A. M. A. 165:1677-1682, 1957.

Fiore, J. M.; Noonan, F. M. Agranulocytosis due to Mepazine (phenothiazine). Report of 3 cases. N. Engl. J. Med. 260:375-378, 1959.

Floch, M.; Leibowitz, S. Hemorrhage from multiple sites associated with chlorpromazine-induced jaundice. J. A. M. A. 170:2060-2064, 1959.

Gerlach, J.; Reisby, N.; Randrup, A. Dopamine hypersensitivity and cholinergic hypofunction in the pathophysiology of tardive dyskinesia. Psychopharmacologia 34:21-35, 1974.

Goldman, D. Treatment of psychotic states with chlorpromazine. J. A. M. A. 157:1274-1278, 1955.

Goldsmith, R. W. Toxicity of phenothiazine compounds. Pediatrics 23:1015-1016, 1959.

Gupta, J. M.; Lovejoy, F. H., Jr. . Acute phenothiazine toxicity in childhood; a five-year survey. Pediatrics 39:771-776, 1967.

Haggerty, R. J. Fatal chlorpromazine poisoning. N. Engl. J. Med. 256:527-528, 1957.

Hall, R. A.; Jackson, R. B.; Swain, J. M. Neurotoxic reactions resulting from chlorpromazine administration. J. A. M. A. 161:214-218, 1956.

Hollister, L. E. Current concepts in therapy. Complications from psychotherapeutic drugs. N. Engl. J. Med. 264:291-293, 1961a.

Hollister, L. E.; Kosek, J. C. Sudden death during treatment with phenothiazine derivatives. J. A. M. A. 192:1035-1038, 1965.

Isaacs, B.; MacArthur, J. G.; Taylor, R. M. Jaundice in relation to chlorpromazine therapy. Br. Med. J. 2:1122-1124, 1955.

Joubert, P. H.; Olivier, J. A. Fatal suicidal ingestion of thioridazine. Clin. Toxicol. 7:133-138, 1974.

Kelly, H. G.; Fay, J. E.; Laverty, S. G. Thioridazine hydrochloride (Mellaril): Its effect on the electrocardiogram and a report of two fatalities with electrocardiographic abnormalities. Can. Med. Assoc. J. 89:546-554, 1963.

Korst, D. R. Agranulocytosis caused by phenothiazine derivatives. J. A. M. A. 170:2076-2081, 1959.

Levan, N. E. Chlorpromazine dermatitis, occupational and immunochemical aspects. N. Engl. J. Med. 256:651-652, 1957.

Lumpkin, J.; Watanabe, A. S.; Rumack, B. H.; Peterson, R. G. Phenothiazine-induced ventricular tachycardia following acute overdose. J. Am. Coll. Emerg. Phys. 8:476-478, 1979.

Manoguerra, A. S.; Krenzelok, E. P. Rapid emesis from high-dose ipecac syrup in adults and children intoxicated with antiemetics or other drugs. Am. J. Hosp. Pharm. 35:1360-1362, 1978.

Mauceri, J.; Strauss, H. Effects of chlorpromazine on electroencephalogram with report of case of chlorpromazine intoxication. Electroencephalogr. Clin. Neurophysiol. 8:671-675, 1956.

McHardy, G.; McHardy, R.; Canale, S. Chlorpromazine (Thorazine) hepatitis. Gastroenterology 29:184-188, 1955.

Moccetti, T.; Lichtlen, P.; Albert, H.; Meier, E.; Imbach, P. Kardiotoxizitat der trizyklischen Antidepressiva. Schweiz. Med. Wochenschr. 101:1-10, 1971.

Moran, N. C.; Butler, W. M., Jr. The pharmacological properties of chlorpromazine sulfoxide, a major metabolite of chlorpromazine; a comparison with chlorpromazine. J. Pharmacol. Exp. Ther. 118:328-337, 1956.

Moyer, J. H. Pharmacology of chlorpromazine. Int. Rec. Med. 168:301-311, 1955.

Moyer, J. H.; Kent, B.; Knight, R. W.; Morris, G.; Dizon, M.; Rogers, S.; Spurr, C. Clinical studies of an antiemetic agent, chlorpromazine. Am. J. Med. Sci. 228:174-189, 1954.

Piala, J. J.; High, J. P.; Hassert, G. L., Jr.; Burke, J. C.; Craver, B. N. Pharmacological and acute toxicological comparisons of triflupromazine and chlorpromazine. J. Pharmacol. Exp. Ther. 127:55-65, 1959.

Pisciotta, A. V. Drug-induced agranulocytosis. Drugs 15:132-143, 1978.

Pisciotta, A. V.; Ebbe, S.; Lennon, E. J.; Metzger, G. O.; Madison, F. W. Agranulocytosis following administration of phenothiazine derivatives. Am. J. Med. 25:210-223, 1958.

Plaa, G. L.; Priestly, B. G. Intrahepatic cholestasis induced by drugs and chemicals. Pharmacol. Rev. 28:207-273, 1976.

Platzer, R. F.; Glaser, G. L. Agranulocytosis due to chlorpromazine. N. Y. State J. Med. 57:1424-1426, 1957.

Reinert, R. E.; Hermann, C. G. Unexplained deaths during chlorpromazine therapy. J. Nerv. Ment. Dis. 131:435-442, 1960.

Rodin, A. E.; Robertson, D. M. Fatal toxic hepatitis following chlorpromazine therapy; report of a case with autopsy findings. Arch. Pathol. 66:170-175, 1958.

Samuels, A. S. Acute chlorpromazine poisoning. Am. J. Psychiatry 113:746-748, 1957.

Shaw, E. B.; Dermott, R. V.; Lee, R.; Burbridge, T. N. Phenothiazine tranquilizers as a cause of severe seizures. Pediatrics 23:485-492, 1959.

Shay, H.; Siplet, H. Study of chlorpromazine jaundice, its mechanism and prevention; special reference to serum alkaline phosphatase and glutamic oxalacetic transaminase. Gastroenterology 32:571-591, 1957.

Sobel, A. M. Treatment of extrapyramidal reactions to phenothiazine derivatives. U. S. Armed Forces Med. J. 11:1447-1450, 1960.

Stambaugh, J. E., Jr.; Wainer, I. W. Drug interaction: meperidine and chlorpromazine, a toxic combination. J. Clin. Pharmacol. 21:140-146, 1981.

Strauss, A. J. Coma from accidental phenothiazine ingestion, an unusual metabolic effect. Clin. Pediatr. 7:59-60, 1968.

Tavoloni, N.; Boyer, J. L. Relationship between hepatic metabolism of chlorpromazine and cholestatic effects in the isolated perfused rat liver. J. Pharmacol. Exp. Ther. 214:269-274, 1980.

Vogt, M. Pharmacology of tranquilizing drugs. Br. Med. J. 2:965-967, 1958.

Wallman, I. S. Death from chlorpromazine poisoning. Med. J. Aust. 2:903-904, 1957.

Wang, S. F.; Marlowe, C. L. Treatment of phenothiazine overdosage with physostigmine. Pediatrics 59:301-303, 1977.

Weisdorf, D.; Kramer, J.; Goldborg, A.; Klawans, H. L. Physostigmine for cardiac and neurologic manifestations of phenothiazine poisoning. Clin. Pharmacol. Ther. 24:663-667, 1978.

Weiss, L. R. The cardiotoxicity of neuroleptic and tricyclic antidepressant drugs. In Cardiac Toxicology., Vol. II (Tibor Balazs, ed.). CRC Press Inc. Boca Raton, Florida, pp. 125-143, 1981.

Whyman, A. Phenothiazine death: an unusual case report. J. Nerv. Ment. Dis. 163:214-217, 1976.

Zelman, S. Liver cell necrosis in chlorpromazine jaundice (allergic cholangiolitis). Am. J. Med. 27:708-729, 1959.

Zelman, S.; Guillan, R. Heat stroke in phenothiazine-treated patients: A report of three fatalities. Am. J. Psychiatry 126:1787-1790, 1970.

Zirkle, G. A.; King, P. D.; McAtee, O. B.; Van Dyke, R. Effects of chlorpromazine and alcohol on coordination and judgment. J. A. M. A. 171:1496-1499, 1959.

COCAINE

Cocaine is a plant alkaloid that has been employed in therapeutics for almost a century, but it is now of interest chiefly as a stimulant drug of abuse. The active principle is obtained from the leaves of a shrub, *Erythroxylon coca* and related species, which grow in the mountains of Peru, Bolivia, Columbia, Mexico, West Indies and Indonesia (Java). The drug makes up about

0.5 to 1.0% of the dry weight of the leaves. Although modern studies have failed to produce a physical explanation for the practice (Hanna, 1970), coca leaves have been chewed by South American Indians to allay hunger and fatigue since the dawn of recorded history.

In the 16th century the conquistadores brought coca leaves back to Europe, where at first they attracted little attention. Cocaine was among the last of the major drug plant alkaloids to be isolated in the 19th century. In 1884, Sigmund Freud published the first of a celebrated series of cocaine papers (Byck, 1975) and launched the drug on a frenzied wave of popularity. At Freud's request a young Viennese physician, Dr. Carl Koller, experimented with cocaine and became the first to describe its local anesthetic effects. Dr. William Halsted exploited this action in several surgical procedures at Johns Hopkins University.

The fame of the drug was spread by Sir Arthur Conan Doyle, who inserted references to cocaine as a "seven per cent solution" in accounts of the mythical life of Sherlock Holmes. Robert Louis Stevenson is said to have been receiving cocaine when he wrote the first drafts of Dr. Jekyll and Mr. Hyde. The greatest promoter of cocaine, however, was Angelo Mariani, whose coca-leaf Bordeaux wine, Vin Mariani, became the most avidly endorsed tonic in the world. Testimonials to its powers were contributed by royalty, physicians, authors, performers, artists, statesmen and scientists. In 1885, John S. Pemberton, a patent medicine manufacturer in Atlanta, Georgia, introduced the American public to Coca Cola, which quickly inspired hordes of imitators.

Eventually, reports of abuse by some of the same luminaries who had spread its reputation, a scathing series of films, plays and novels, and fear of drug-crazed habitués swung public opinion strongly against cocaine. In 1906, the Federal Pure Food and Drug Act classified cocaine legally, but unscientifically, as a narcotic. Now it is regulated under Schedule II of the Controlled Substances Act. The use of cocaine as an illicit stimulant, however, has continued, and claims have been made that the drug experienced a dramatic revival among the intelligentsia in the 1970s. Cocaine is generally acknowledged to be second only to alcohol as a drug abuse problem among all socioeconomic classes in the U.S. today. A series of monographs give additional details of the fascinating history of cocaine (Ashley, 1975; Ellinwood and Kilbey, 1977; Mulé, 1976; Petersen and Stillman, 1977).

Toxicology: Acute animal experiments involving parenteral routes of administration place cocaine and its common salts (hydrochloride, nitrate, sulfate) in toxicity class 4 for mice and rats and in toxicity class 5 for larger mammalian species, e.g., rabbit, dog, cat (Evans and Harbison, 1978; Paeile et al., 1965; Tatum et al., 1925).

Reliable estimates of the acute LD_{50} by mouth in any animal species are essentially nonexistent. Although some past authorities have insisted that the acute toxicity is critically dependent on the route of administration, more recent work suggests that cocaine is absorbed efficiently when given by a variety of routes. For example, the "approximate LD_{50}" in the rabbit was 15 mg./kg. intravenously, 30 mg./kg. intratracheally and 50 mg./kg. intranasally (Åström and Persson, 1961).

Cocaine deaths in man are uncommon, and few reports of well-documented poisonings can be found in the modern clinical literature (Finkle and McCloskey, 1977). Webster (1930) has cited estimates of 1.0 to 1.2 gm. as the mean lethal dose in man, whether given orally or parenterally. At the same time he noted that doses as small as 20 mg. given subdurally produced death on two occasions. Many writers allude to wide variations in the lethal dose. An impression that epinephrine increases the toxicity of cocaine was noted as early as 1923 (Webster, 1930).

The paucity of human case reports may relate in part to the fact that acute cocaine poisoning runs a rapid course. Death may occur within minutes and without warning. Five victims died between 2 and 6 minutes after injection or instillation of cocaine solutions. After oral administration, the latency is somewhat longer, but deaths beyond 3 hours are rare (Webster, 1930). The longer the period of survival, the better the chances for ultimate recovery. We have encountered no reports of sequelae to cocaine poisoning.

The local anesthetic effects of cocaine and of many synthetic drugs classified as local anesthetics are due to blockade of conduction in sensory nerves. Conduction blocks can also occur in other types of excitable tissues, such as mixed peripheral nerves and heart. Cocaine and many of its derivatives produce anesthesia when applied topically to mucous membranes.

In the central nervous system, cocaine and its congeners behave as stimulants. The initial effects are cortical, but the excitation moves progressively downward through the brain. Medullary and hypothalamic centers are stimulated, as evidenced by marked increases in the rate and depth of breathing, elevated oxygen consumption, a rise in body temperature and various signs of excessive output in the sympathetic nervous system. Eventually, tonic-clonic convulsions may occur. Presumably some, if not most, of these excitatory actions result from depression of central inhibitory pathways (Caldwell and Sever, 1974). By analogy with poisonings due to other convulsants, cocaine is presumed to kill eventually by inducing central respiratory failure during or between periods of convulsions, but cardiovascular collapse is also a possibility (Mulé, 1976). To some extent all local anesthetics can produce decreases in the electrical excitability of the heart, its conduction rate and force of contraction (see QUINIDINE, p. III-355). Thus cardiac standstill may occur as the terminal event in cocaine poisoning (Steinhaus and Tatum, 1950). Whether cardiac arrest is primary or secondary to respiratory failure is not clear (Catravas et al., 1978).

Cocaine blocks catecholamine reuptake by adrenergic nerve endings, an effect that occurs at concentrations of the alkaloid that do not result in local anesthesia. The result is the accumulation of endogenous norepinephrine in synaptic spaces outside of adrenergic nerve endings and the consequent excitation of adrenergic receptors on the postsynaptic cell surface. This mechanism explains why cocaine is the only local anesthetic to produce dose-related increases in blood pressure and heart rate (Fischman et al., 1976). Diastolic and systolic arterial pressures, heart rate, stroke volume, and cardiac output are all elevated. At least in the conscious, acutely poisoned dog (Catravas et al., 1978), the total peripheral vascular resistance is reduced, presumably as a reflex response to the excessive cardiac stimulation. The combination of direct and reflex effects on the heart may induce a variety of arrhythmias. Ventricular fibrillation has been reported in cocaine poisoning, whereas the synthetic local anesthetics are sometimes used therapeutically to terminate this condition in noncocainized subjects.

Blockade of catecholamine reuptake at adrenergic junctions in the central nervous system may be responsible for the intense euphoria characteristic of cocaine but not of other local anesthetics. That this euphoria is unrelated to a general increase in the level of central excitability produced by all local anesthetics is suggested by the results of various pharmacological manipulations. For example, pretreatment of rats with α-methyl-p-tyrosine to deplete the brain of catecholamines failed to alter the convulsant activity or the mean lethal dose of cocaine (Wilson and Holbrook, 1978). Patients being treated with lithium, which accelerates catecholamine reuptake at adrenergic nerve endings (an effect opposite to that of cocaine), report no euphoria after cocaine in doses that made others "high" (Cronson and Flemenbaum, 1978).

In addition to the above, the subject acutely poisoned with cocaine exhibits mydriasis, excitement (usually euphoric but sometimes dysphoric), restlessness, anxiety and confusion. The subjective effects of cocaine are said to be very similar to those of amphetamine (Fischman et al., 1976). The affective disturbance can progress to delirium with hallucinations or a violent maniacal behavior. For example, "snow lights" are visions likened to the twinkling of sunlight on snow crystals. "Cocaine bugs" or formication is a sensation like that which might be elicited by insects crawling under the skin (Siegel, 1978). Only rarely do victims appear calm, and they are never drowsy. Vomiting may occur, presumably as a result of central stimulation. Respirations are at first accelerated, but later they are reduced in both rate and depth. A chill may signal the onset of a dangerous hyperpyrexia.

It is now clear that several of these physiological and subjective effects of cocaine can be correlated with the plasma concentration of the drug and with the dose (Javaid et al., 1978). A mystique associated with the illicit use of cocaine dictates the intranasal route of administration ("sniffing" or "snorting"), although it has been shown that at a dose of 2 mg./kg. in humans the oral route is equally effective in terms of subjective effects and peak plasma concentrations (Van Dyke et al., 1978). Absorption from the nasal mucosa appears to be more rapid at first, but the detection of residual cocaine in the mucosa 3 hours after its application suggests that the local vasoconstrictor action eventually slows absorption and extends the plasma half-life (Van Dyke et al., 1976). A dose of 10 mg. by vein in man produced all of the same effects elicited by the intranasal administration of 100 mg. (Resnick et al., 1977).

The cocaine molecule is a diester, ecgonine methyl ester benzoate (Fig. III-2), and esterases play an important role in cocaine metabolism in man. Hydrolysis of the benzoyl ester bond yields ecgonine methyl ester, a reaction catalyzed by plasma cholinesterase (Stewart et al., 1977). In two humans the methyl ester amounted to 32 and 49% of the total radioactivity in urine, which in turn accounted for 65 to 75% of the given dose. Since ecgonine methyl ester is much less toxic than cocaine (Misra et al., 1975), cholinesterase inhibitors might potentiate cocaine toxicity in man, and individuals deficient in plasma cholinesterase might be unusually sensitive to the drug. In a single habitual user of cocaine, 1 to 9% unchanged drug was excreted in the urine, and the cumulative excretion was dependent on urine pH (Fish and Wilson, 1969). Norcocaine, the N-demethylated diester, is a minor metabolite of cocaine; it retains the pharmacological activity of the parent alkaloid (Misra et al.,

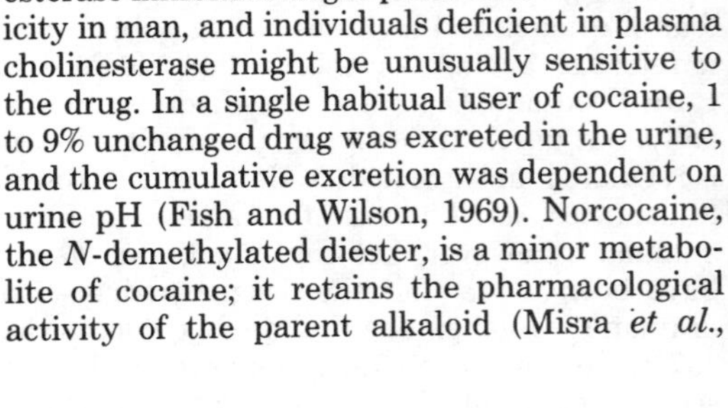

Figure III-2. Cocaine molecule.

1975). In man, metabolism to norcocaine accounts for 2 to 6% of an administered dose of cocaine (Inaba *et al.*, 1978).

In contrast to the benzoyl ester bond, the methyl ester bond of cocaine is stable in human plasma (Stewart *et al.*, 1977). Nevertheless, benzoyl ecgonine, the product of methyl ester hydrolysis, appears to be a major metabolite in the brains of several laboratory species (Misra *et al.*, 1976; 1977; Nayak *et al.*, 1976). Benzoyl ecgonine and benzoyl norecgonine both produce signs of central nervous excitation in rats, although those effects are said to be distinctly different from those of cocaine or norcocaine. Ecgonine and ecgonine methyl ester are essentially inactive (Misra *et al.*, 1975). The metabolism of cocaine promises to be quite complex; several metabolites remain to be identified, and the role of an enterohepatic circulation is still undefined. In mice (but not rats), pretreatment with phenobarbital to induce hepatic microsomal enzymes protected against acute cocaine lethality, but the animals subsequently developed hepatic necrosis (Evans and Harbison, 1978).

Cocaine abuse: The euphoria produced by cocaine is highly sought after and may be more intense than that induced in man by any other drug. Unlike the narcotic analgesics and the barbiturate-alcohol group of drugs, cocaine is nonaddicting in the sense that a true abstinence syndrome does not occur after drug withdrawal (Isbell and White, 1953). Thus cocaine dependence appears to be psychological and not physical. Occasionally a user, however, may experience emotional depression, somnolence and fatigue after a period of heavy usage. Rarely, delusions that continue for some time after withdrawal have been described (Eddy *et al.*, 1965). Perhaps polar metabolites of cocaine, such as benzoyl ecgonine and benzoyl norecgonine, persist in the brains of some users, as they do in treated dogs (Misra *et al.*, 1976).

The continued use of many psychotropic drugs results in the development of tolerance, which may promote increased consumption and sometimes physical dependence. The possibility of acquired tolerance to the toxic or the euphoric actions of cocaine is an important issue and needs more study. Woolverton and Schuster (1978) were unable to demonstrate the development of tolerance to the lethal effects of cocaine in rats. That finding is disputed by Wilson and Holbrook (1978), but only half of their animals survived the pretreatment regimen. In monkeys, distinct tolerance to the convulsant activity and to cardiorespiratory stimulation has been shown, together with a possible drug-induced reduction in the plasma half-life (Matsuzaki *et al.*, 1976). In general, however, attempts to find metabolic or dispositional differences between animals treated acutely and those treated chronically with cocaine have been unsuccessful (Misra *et al.*, 1976; 1977; Nayak *et al.*, 1976). At present, no basis is known for the clinical impression that increased sensitivity to the excitatory effects of cocaine occurs in man with continued use (Isbell and White, 1953), but a similar phenomenon of reverse tolerance has been demonstrated in chronically treated dogs (reviewed by Kosman and Unna, 1968).

In many respects the cocaine habitué resembles that of the compulsive user of amphetamines (see AMPHETAMINE, p. III-28). Continued high dose abuse may lead to nervousness, depression, sleeplessness, irrationality, paranoia, antisocial behavior, violence and a true toxic psychosis (Gay *et al.*, 1975). The difficulty of obtaining legal cocaine has resulted in an illicit market with extraordinarily high prices and a flood of adulterants. Half of 270 street samples of cocaine showed the presence of some other drug, usually a synthetic local anesthetic such as lidocaine, in addition to or instead of cocaine. Amphetamine and phencyclidine are sometimes misrepresented as "cocaine." Adverse reactions were more frequent with adulterated samples than with "pure" cocaine (Olivares *et al.*, 1977).

In past years, cocaine abusers seemed to prefer the intravenous route, but the modern recreational user inhales the drug into the nose through a straw or a rolled bank bill of large denomination. The latter custom symbolizes the exalted social and monetary status of the habitué. Reactive hyperemia results in a chronically stuffy nose, for which the cocaine sniffer frequently uses nasal vasoconstrictor sprays or drops. Sneezing and coryza-like symptoms are common, as well as frequent infections of the nasal mucosa and upper respiratory tract. Perforation of the nasal septum may occur because of the frequent and intense vasoconstriction (Gay *et al.*, 1976). Cocaine is also active by mouth, and the alkaloidal base can be smoked in pipes or cigarettes. Many habitués prefer the intravenous route, injecting cocaine alone or in combination with heroin ("speed balls"). "Free basing" involves the inhalation of heat-vaporized cocaine in special pipes, again either alone or in combination with heroin or alcohol.

Although opportunities to intervene therapeutically in acute cocaine poisoning are uncommon, possible measures of therapy continue to attract attention. Early studies (Tatum *et al.*, 1925) suggested that artificial respiration alone elevated significantly the lethal dose of cocaine in the rabbit but not in the dog or cat. Barbiturates and paraldehyde were effective in terminating cocaine convulsions in monkeys, but they seemed also to increase the risk of respiratory failure or cardiac arrest (Tatum and Collins, 1926; Steinhaus and Tatum, 1950). In rats, diazepam was clearly superior to barbiturates and other agents in preventing convulsions and death (Aldrete and Daniel, 1971). In 50 human cases, propranolol is said to have been effective against cocaine hypertension, tachycardia and tachypnea (Rappolt et al., 1977). In a study in dogs, however, propranolol did not delay death or elevate the lethal dose of cocaine. Both pretreated and control dogs exhibited hyperpyrexia, acidemia and hyperpnea. In contrast, dogs given chlorpromazine (12 mg./kg. intravenously) one hour prior to cocaine survived a dose twice that which killed all control animals. Chlorpromazine also prevented the cocaine-induced changes in cardiovascular function, hyperpyrexia and acidosis (Catravas et al., 1977).

Synthetic local anesthetics: The synthetic drugs can be divided into two chemical classes: (1) esters of benzoic or aminobenzoic acid, and (2) substituted amides, such as lidocaine (Xylocaine), dibucaine (Nupercaine), mepivacaine (Carbocaine), prilocaine (Citanest) and bupivacaine (Marcaine). This distinction has toxicological significance because in general the esters are susceptible to hydrolysis by plasma cholinesterase, and the amides are not. Rates of hydrolysis, however, are also influenced by other features of the chemical structure. The drugs which are more rapidly hydrolyzed (e.g., procaine, chloroprocaine, piperocaine) tend to be less toxic. Exceptions, such as isobucaine, may represent drugs that penetrate the blood-brain barrier with unusual rapidity. Genetic or acquired reductions in plasma cholinesterase activity increase the toxicity of drugs like procaine (Foldes et al., 1965). The hydrolysis products of the ester-type local anesthetics are inactive.

The amide-type drugs are metabolized by the liver. Lidocaine, for example, is successively N-dealkylated to the monoethyl derivative and then to the unsubstituted amide. These reactions are mediated by the mixed-function oxidases of the hepatic endoplasmic reticulum. Both metabolites have local anesthetic activity and are presumed to contribute to the central nervous system toxicity, which in the case of lidocaine is said to produce somnolence occasionally, instead of excitement (Nevins, 1973). An alternative metabolic pathway is mediated by a liver amidase which yields inactive products (Strong et al., 1973). The two local anesthetics regularly associated with a mild methemoglobinemia (prilocaine and benzocaine) are also activated by hepatic microsomal enzymes (Smith and Olson, 1973).

Local anesthetics are employed in a variety of clinical situations that dictate various routes of administration. For nerve block by infiltration the drugs used most commonly are procaine, chloroprocaine and lidocaine. Epinephrine is frequently added to solutions intended for infiltration to delay systemic absorption of the drug. Sometimes, however, the epinephrine escapes from the local depot to produce generalized vasoconstriction and tachycardia. Local anesthetics in general tend to induce the opposite effects, namely vasodilation and bradycardia. The single exception is cocaine, and the systemic cardiovascular effects of epinephrine are easily confused with those of cocaine.

Lidocaine (and formerly procaine) is injected intravenously to terminate dangerous cardiac arrhythmias. Benzocaine, benoxinate, butamben and cocaine are used almost exclusively by topical application for surface anesthesia. Tetracaine is the most commonly employed spinal anesthetic. Lidocaine, prilocaine and mepivacaine are frequently used for caudal or epidural anesthesia. The increased use of caudal anesthesia in obstetrics has resulted in several tragic accidents due to accidental injection of the fetus (Dodson, 1976). The triad of apnea, bradycardia persisting despite oxygenation and convulsions is commonly observed in poisoned newborns. Since the drugs are believed to be concentrated in gastric juice, some of these infants have been treated by repeated gastric lavage with or without exchange transfusions (Finster et al., 1965; Sinclair et al., 1965).

The toxicity of a given local anesthetic tends to parallel its potency. For example, because tetracaine is allegedly 10 times more potent than procaine, toxicity should be expected at 10-fold lower doses. Bupivacaine is about as potent and toxic as tetracaine. The medical literature is replete with accounts of toxic or lethal reactions to small doses of local anesthetics. Usually these episodes are ascribed to allergy, to idiosyncrasy or to decreased tolerance. Some authorities believe that most such cases are really due to frank overdoses, whereas others postulate accidental injections into a blood vessel (Grimes and Cates, 1976). In most cases the true explanation is not known (Covino, 1978). In contrast to small dose effects, very large doses have been tolerated under special circumstances. One adult who had been pretreated with thiopental and succinylcholine survived the accidental administration of 4 gm. of procaine (Wikinski et al., 1970).

Symptomatology (primarily for cocaine, but some signs and symptoms listed under 1, 4, 5, 6 and 8 may arise from overdoses of synthetic local anesthetic agents):

1. Talkativeness, restlessness, euphoric excitement or apprehension, grandiose feelings, strong sexual arousal.
2. Sympathomimetic effects include tachycardia, palpitations, hypertension, mydriasis, exophthalmos, tachypnea, salivation and sweating. After local anesthetics other than cocaine, hypotension is more common than hypertension.

3. Confusion, disorientation, hallucinations (visual, auditory, tactile), paranoid delusions, violent acts.

4. Dizziness or light-headedness, tinnitus, vomiting, and hyperpyrexia, which may be heralded by a chill.

5. Fine skeletal muscle twitchings of face and digits, widespread tremor, hyperreflexia culminating in generalized tonic-clonic convulsions. Intense central nervous stimulation leading to convulsions and to postictal depression is the chief threat to survival (Fink, 1973).

6. Unconsciousness, irregular and shallow breathing leading to apnea and death, usually within 1 hour (if at all) and rarely beyond 3 hours.

7. Early sudden death may be due to cardiac arrhythmias (*e.g.*, ventricular fibrillation), but presumably serious disturbances in the mechanism of the heart beat usually follow rather than precede the anoxia of respiratory depression.

8. Cyanosis may be due to methemoglobinemia, at least in poisonings by synthetic local anesthetics, especially prilocaine and benzocaine.

Treatment:

1. In spite of the rapidity with which cocaine is detoxified, efforts to reduce rates of absorption may be worthwhile after massive overdoses. Swallowing a slurry of activated charcoal (p. I-4) is appropriate in poisonings by ingestion. Gastric lavage is not of proved benefit in such cases and is probably hazardous if convulsions are imminent. After intramuscular injections a tourniquet is sometimes a practical way to slow absorption.

2. A hypomanic patient who is not paranoid or delusional and who displays no preconvulsive signs (see above) may require no active treatment, but he should be kept under careful observation. Isolate the victim as much as possible, and avoid all extraneous stimuli (see p. IV-34).

3. Severe anxiety, delirium, frightening hallucinations and maniacal behavior respond well to injections of phenothiazine tranquilizers, such as chlorpromazine. The intramuscular route is preferred, with adults receiving an initial dose of 50 mg. (total) and young children 1 mg./kg. Chlorpromazine and its congeners, however, should be avoided whenever the poisoning might be due to anticholinergics (*e.g.*, atropine, scopolamine, etc.) or to unknown psychotomimetics. See pp. IV-33–35.

4. Convulsions or rapidly intensifying preconvulsive signs (see above) warrant anticonvulsive therapy. Intravenous diazepam (Valium) is probably the most satisfactory agent (see p. IV-36). If it is not available, thiopental sodium (p. IV-37) may be the next best choice, but all depressant drugs carry some risk of compounding postictal depression.

5. Propranolol is effective in correcting cocaine-induced tachycardia, palpitations, hypertension and hyperpnea and perhaps in forestalling cardiac arrhythmias. Except in victims with preexisting cardiac disease, however, these derangements are seldom disabling or life-threatening and so can usually be neglected. Avoid all sympathomimetics in the excitatory phase of the poisoning.

6. A rapidly rising fever warrants vigorous hypothermic measures (p. IV-84).

7. Correct anoxia by mechanically supporting ventilation and by administering oxygen (see pp. IV-7–14) when indicated in the late depressive phase of the intoxication.

8. Late hypotension may require circulatory support. Dopamine has been used as a pressor agent (p. IV-21), but intravenous fluids should be administered first to correct dehydration and acidosis. See pp. IV-71–72.

Laboratory:

1. Acute cocaine poisoning rarely lasts long enough to compromise severely body water and electrolyte balances, but multiple high doses over periods of one or more days may induce metabolic disturbances that require attention. Particularly with hyperpyrexia, metabolic acidosis may be encountered.

2. Chemical assays have been used to detect local anesthetics in autopsy material for forensic purposes (Sunshine and Fike, 1964).

References:

Aldrete, J. A.; Daniel, W. Evaluation of premedicants as protective agents against convulsive (LD$_{50}$) doses of local anesthetic agents in rats. Anesth. Anal. *50*:127-130, 1971.

Ashley, R. *Cocaine: Its History, Uses and Effects*. St. Martins Press, New York, 1975.

Astrom, A.; Persson, N. H. The toxicity of some local anesthetics after application on different mucous membranes and its relation to anesthetic action on the nasal mucosa of the rabbit. J. Pharmacol. Exp. Ther. *132*:87-90, 1961.

Byck, R. *Cocaine Papers: Sigmund Freud*. Stonehill, New York, 1975.

Caldwell, J.; Sever, P. S. The biochemical pharmacology of abused drugs. I. Amphetamines, cocaine and LSD. Clin. Pharmacol. Ther. *16*:625-638, 1974.

Catravas, J. D.; Waters, I. W.; Walz, M. A.; Davis, W. M. Antidotes for cocaine poisoning. N. Engl. J. Med. *297*:1238, 1977.

Catravas, J. D.; Waters, I. W.; Walz, M. A.; Davis, W. M. Acute cocaine intoxication in the conscious dog: Pathophysiologic profile of acute lethality. Arch. Int. Pharmacodyn. Ther. *235*:328-340, 1978.

Covino, B. G. Systemic toxicity of local anesthetic agents. Anesth. Anal. *57*:387-388, 1978.

Cronson, A. J.; Flemenbaum, A. Antagonism of cocaine highs

by lithium. Am. J. Psychiatr. 135:856-857, 1978.

Dodson, W. E. Neonatal drug intoxication: Local anesthetics. Pediatr. Clin. North Amer. 23:399-411, 1976.

Eddy, N. B.; Halback, H.; Isbell, H.; Seevers, M. H. Drug dependence: its significance and characteristics. Bull. W. H. O. 32:721-733, 1965.

Ellinwood, E. H.; Kilbey, M. M. Cocaine and Other Stimulants. Plenum Press, New York, 1977.

Evans, M. A.; Harbison, R. D. Cocaine-induced hepatotoxicity in mice. Toxicol. Appl. Pharmacol. 45:739-754, 1978.

Fink, B. R. Acute and chronic toxicity of local anesthetics. Can. Anaesth. Soc. J. 20:5-16, 1973.

Finkle, B. S.; McCloskey, K. L. The forensic toxicology of cocaine. In Cocaine: 1977. Edited by R. C. Petersen and R. C. Stillman. U. S. Government Printing Office, Washington, D. C., 1977.

Finster, M.; Poppers, P. J.; Sinclair, J. C.; Morishima, H. O.; Daniel, S. S. Accidental intoxication of the fetus with local anesthetic drug during caudal anesthesia. Am. J. Obstet. Gynecol. 92:922-924, 1965.

Fischman, M. W.; Schuster, C. R.; Resnekov, L.; Shick, J. F. E.; Krasnegor, N. A.; Fennell, W.; Freedman, D. X. Cardiovascular and subjective effects of intravenous cocaine administration in humans. Arch. Gen. Psychiatr. 33:983-989, 1976.

Fish, F.; Wilson, W. D. C. Excretion of cocaine and its metabolites in man. J. Pharm. Pharmacol. 21:135S-138S, 1969.

Foldes, F. F.; Davidson, G. M.; Duncalf, D.; Kuwabara, S. The intravenous toxicity of local anesthetic agents in man. Clin. Pharmacol. Ther. 6:328-335, 1965.

Gay, G. R.; Inaba, D. S.; Rappolt, R. T.; Gushue, G. F.; Perkner, J. J. "An' ho, ho, baby, take a whiff on me:" La dama blanca. Cocaine in current perspective. Anesth. Anal. 55:582-587, 1976.

Gay, G. R.; Inaba, D. S.; Sheppard, C. W.; Newmeyer, J. A.; Rappolt, R. T. Cocaine: History, epidemiology, human pharmacology, and treatment. A perspective on a new debut for an old girl. Clin. Toxicol. 8:149-178, 1975.

Grimes, D. A.; Cates, W., Jr. Deaths from paracervical anesthesia used for first-trimester abortion 1972-1975. N. Engl. J. Med. 295:1397-1399, 1976.

Hanna, J. M. The effects of coca chewing on exercise in the Quechua of Peru. Human Biol. 42:1-11, 1970.

Inaba, T.; Stewart, D. J.; Kalew, W. Metabolism of cocaine in man. Clin. Pharmacol. Ther. 23:547-552, 1978.

Isbell, H.; White, W. M. Clinical characteristics of addictions. Am. J. Med. 14:558-565, 1953.

Javaid, J. I.; Fischman, M. W.; Schuster, C. R.; Dekirmenjian, H.; Davis, J. M. Cocaine plasma concentrations: Relation to physiological and subjective effects in humans. Science 202:227-228, 1978.

Kosman, M. E.; Unna, K. K. Effects of chronic administration of the amphetamines and other stimulants on behavior. Clin. Pharmacol. Ther. 9:240-254, 1968.

Matsuzaki, M.; Spingler, P. J.; Misra, A. L.; Mule, S. J. Cocaine: Tolerance to its convulsant and cardiorespiratory stimulating effects in the monkey. Life Sci. 19:193-204, 1976.

Misra, A. L.; Giri, V. V.; Patel, M. N.; Alluri, V. R.; Mule, S. J. Disposition and metabolism of [³H]cocaine in acutely and chronically treated monkeys. Drug Alcohol Depend. 2:261-272, 1977.

Misra, A. L.; Nayak, P. K.; Bloch, R.; Mule, S. J. Estimation and disposition of [³H]benzoylecgonine and pharmacological activity of some cocaine metabolites. J. Pharm. Pharmacol. 27:784-786, 1975.

Misra, A. L.; Patel, M. N.; Alluri, V. R.; Mule, S. J.; Nayak, P. K. Disposition and metabolism of [³H]cocaine in acutely and chronically treated dogs. Xenobiotica 6:537-552, 1976.

Mule, S. J. Cocaine: Chemical, Biological, Clinical, Social

and Treatment Aspects. CRC Press, Inc., Cleveland, Ohio, 1976.

Nayak, P. K.; Misra, A. L.; Mule, S. J. Physiological disposition and biotransformation of ³Hcocaine in acutely and chronically treated rats. J. Pharmacol. Exp. Ther. 196:556-569, 1976.

Nevins, M. A. Reevaluating the use of lidocaine: Toxic and metabolic effects, sinus node depression and paradoxical cardiac influences are potential hazards and limitations. Geriatrics 28:48-51, 1973.

Olivares, G. -J.; Gupta, R. C.; Landberg, G. D.; Montgomery, S. H. Street cocaine 1971-1975: Nature, costs and effects. Vet. Human Toxicol. 19:169-172, 1977.

Paeile, C.; Tampier, L.; Munoz, C. Comparacion de la sensibilidad a los efectos toxicos de la procaina en machos y hembras de diversas especies. Arch. Biol. Med. Exper. 2:38-41, 1965.

Petersen, R. C.; Stillman, R. C. Cocaine: 1977. NIDA Research Monograph #13. U. S. Government Printing Office, Washington, D. C., 1977.

Rappolt, R. T., Sr.; Gay, G. R.; Inaba, D. S. Propranolol: A specific antagonist to cocaine. Clin. Toxicol. 10:265-271, 1977.

Resnick, R. B.; Kestenbaum, R. S.; Schwartz, L. K. Acute systemic effects of cocaine in man: A controlled study by intranasal and intravenous routes. Science 195:696-698, 1977.

Siegel, R. K. Cocaine hallucinations. Am. J. Psychiatr. 135:309-314, 1978.

Sinclair, J. C.; Fox, H. A.; Lentz, J. F.; Fuld, G. L.; Murphy, J. Intoxication of the fetus by a local anesthetic. A newly recognized complication of maternal caudal anesthesia. N. Engl. J. Med. 273:1173-1177, 1965.

Smith, R. P.; Olson, M. V. Drug-induced methemoglobinemia. Semin. Hematol. 10:253-268, 1973.

Steinhaus, J. E.; Tatum, A. L. An experimental study of cocaine intoxication and its treatment. J. Pharmacol. Exp. Ther. 100:351-361, 1950.

Stewart, D. J.; Inaba, T.; Tang, B. K.; Kalew, W. Hydrolysis of cocaine in human plasma by cholinesterase. Life Sci. 20:1557-1564, 1977.

Strong, J. M.; Parker, M.; Atkinson, A. J. Identification of glycinexylidide in patients treated with intravenous lidocaine. Clin. Pharmacol. Ther. 14:67-72, 1973.

Sunshine, I.; Fike, W. W. Value of thin-layer chromatography in two fatal cases of intoxication due to lidocaine and mepivacaine. N. Engl. J. Med. 271:487-490, 1964.

Tatum, A. L.; Atkinson, A. J.; Collins, K. H. Acute cocaine poisoning, its prophylaxis and treatment in laboratory animals. J. Pharmacol. Ther. 26:325-335, 1925.

Tatum, A. L.; Collins, K. H. Acute cocaine poisoning and its treatment in monkeys (Macacus rhesus). Arch. Int. Med. 38:405-409, 1926.

Van Dyke, C.; Barash, P. G.; Jatlow, P.; Byck, R. Cocaine: Plasma concentrations after intranasal application in man. Science 191:859-861, 1976.

Van Dyke, C.; Jatlow, P.; Ungerer, J.; Barash, P. G.; Byck, R. Oral cocaine: Plasma concentrations and central effects. Science 200:211-213, 1978.

Webster, R. W. Legal Medicine and Toxicology. W. B. Saunders Co., Philadelphia, 1930.

Wikinski, J. A.; Usubiaga, J. E.; Wikinski, R. W. Cardiovascular and neurological effects of 4,000 mg of procaine. J. A. M. A. 213:621-623, 1970.

Wilson, M. C.; Holbrook, J. M. Intravenous cocaine lethality in the rat. Pharmacol. Res. Comm. 10:243-256, 1978.

Woolverton, W. L.; Schuster, C. R. The effects of daily cocaine administration on cocaine-induced mortality. Res. Comm. Psychol. Psychiatr. Behavior 3:257-265, 1978.

COPPER

Copper is an essential trace element in animals and plants. Its distribution, effects and toxicity have been extensively reviewed (NRC-NAS, 1977). Soluble and insoluble copper salts are used widely in agriculture as fungicides and insecticides. Copper arsenates and arsenites (e.g., copper acetoarsenite or paris green) are dangerous principally for their arsenic content; consult ARSENIC poisoning (p. III-42). Copper sulfate (cupric sulfate) is still occasionally used in clinical medicine as an emetic drug; the adult dose is 0.25 to 0.5 gm. in water repeated no more than once (after an interval of 15 minutes) if necessary. This use must be vigorously discouraged because toxic effects and death may occur if vomiting does not (Stein et al., 1976). Even when vomiting was successfully induced, significant elevations in serum copper were observed (Holtzman and Haslam, 1968).

Many cases of poisoning result from the use of copper containers for food or drink (Hopper and Adams, 1958; LeVan and Perry, 1961; Nicholas, 1968; Semple et al., 1960; Wyllie, 1957). In recent years extracorporeal hemodialysis has been a source of copper poisoning (see below). Accidental and suicidal ingestions of copper sulfate are not uncommon in India (Chugh et al., 1977).

Toxicology: Acute poisoning from the ingestion of copper salts is rarely severe, if the metal is removed promptly by emesis. Vomiting is provoked chiefly by the local irritant and astringent action of ionic copper on stomach and bowel. Emesis usually begins within 5 to 10 minutes, but if the stomach is full of food, it may be delayed for half an hour or more (Hopper and Adams, 1958; LeVan and Perry, 1961; Semple et al., 1960; Wyllie, 1957). If vomiting fails to occur or is delayed, gradual absorption from the bowel may cause systemic copper poisoning. Death is delayed for several days, and apparent recovery may be followed by a fatal relapse (Witthaus, 1911).

Copper resembles many other heavy metals in its systemic toxic effects: widespread capillary damage, kidney and liver injury, and central nervous excitation followed by depression. Jaundice and pain over the liver have been reported in acute human poisonings (Webster, 1930; Chuttani et al., 1965). Hemolytic anemias are also described in acute poisonings in man (Chuttani et al., 1965; Fairbanks, 1967; Holtzman et al., 1966) and are prominent in chronic poisonings in sheep and cattle. Circulatory shock and intravascular hemolysis, singly or together, may lead to renal tubular injury and death in renal failure (Chugh et al., 1977). Signs and symptoms resulting from the ingestion of copper sulfate by Indians have been well described by Chuttani et al. (1965) and by Chugh et al. (1977).

In general the soluble ionized salts of copper are much more toxic than the insoluble or slightly dissociated compounds. Probably the most poisonous salts are the chloride and the subacetate. Cuprous chloride is said to be twice as toxic as the more common cupric salt, but no major toxicological distinctions are recognized between the two valence states of copper. As with other irritant emetics, the lethal dose of any copper salt varies widely (from less than 1 gm. to several ounces in adults); the mean lethal dose of the sulfate probably lies near 15 gm. (Webster, 1930).

Treatment is largely symptomatic. Further clinical trials are required to evaluate BAL (Lusky et al., 1949) and penicillamine in both acute and chronic copper poisoning. BAL shows particular promise in systemic poisonings in which the effects are not exclusively the result of severe gastroenteritis. At times it has been called life-saving (Moeschlin, 1965). The combination of BAL and edetate calcium disodium was more effective in hastening urinary copper excretion in a poisoned infant than was penicillamine, when it was subsequently substituted (Walsh et al., 1977). In an experimental study in mice, however, sodium 2,3-dimercapto-1-propane sulfonate was far more effective in reducing copper lethality than any of eight other chelating agents tested. Penicillamine was a poor second (Jones et al., 1980).

Exchange transfusion may be of value if symptoms appear to warrant intensive therapy (Chowdhury et al., 1961). In one severely poisoned infant the addition of salt-poor albumin to the peritoneal dialysis fluid resulted in a 15-fold increase in the dialysate-to-serum ratio of copper concentrations. Although the amount of copper recovered by this procedure was small relative to the total dose, the child made a full recovery (Cole and Lirenman, 1978). Extracorporeal hemodialysis without ligands to bind copper in the dialysis fluid was judged totally ineffective when instituted within 13 hours of the ingestion (Argarwal et al., 1975).

Paradoxically, hemodialysis for other indications has been the cause of severe and even fatal copper poisoning (Klein et al., 1972; Manzler and Schreiner, 1970; Matter et al., 1969). In these cases, exhausted deionization systems allowed water of a low pH to come in contact with copper components of the dialysis unit, resulting eventually in high copper levels in the dialysis fluid (Bloomfield et al., 1971; Ivanovich et al., 1969). By this bizarre route of exposure the hematological manifestations of copper poisoning appear to be particularly prominent (methemoglobinemia, Heinz body formation, hemolysis), together with a significant metabolic acidosis. This hemolytic reaction resembles that produced by primaquine and many other chemicals in glucose–6-phosphate dehydrogenase (G-6-PD) deficiency (see p. III-308). Like NAPHTHALENE (p. III-307), copper hemolysis would be predicted to be more severe in a G-6-PD deficiency, but the reaction can be precipitated in normal red cells by appropriate concentrations of the metal (Fairbanks, 1967). An individual with G-6-PD-deficient red cells developed intense methemoglobinemia and intravascular hemolysis after ingesting 50 gm. of copper sulfate (Chugh *et al.*, 1975). In poisoned sheep, significant concentrations of intraerythrocytic methemoglobin also accumulated prior to hemolysis (Soli and Froslie, 1977).

Extensive tissue damage may follow chronic exposure of skin or mucous membranes (Barsky, 1937; Cole, 1924). Systemic copper poisoning followed repeated debridement of burned skin with copper sulfate solutions (Holtzman *et al.*, 1966).

Copper appears to be less deleterious than most heavy metals when ingested continuously in small amounts, but chronic feeding to animals results in a pigmentary cirrhosis of the liver (Mallory and Parker, 1931; Wiederanders *et al.*, 1968). Electron microscopic changes have been described in the livers of exposed rats (Barka *et al.*, 1964). In isolated rat hepatocytes, copper caused a time- and concentration-dependent decrease in cell viability and reduced glutathione. Potassium and aspartate aminotransferases were lost to the media. Although lipid peroxidation occurred, it was judged not to be the cause of the injury (Stacey and Klaassen, 1981).

Chronic copper poisoning due to excessive intake is rarely recognized in man. In at least one documented case (Salmon and Wright, 1971), however, the clinical picture was that of infantile acrodynia (pink disease), which is more commonly associated with mercurialism; see p. III-265.

A type of chronic copper poisoning in man is recognized in the form of a metabolic disease called hereditary hepatolenticular degeneration (Wilson's disease). Tissue copper levels are elevated in Wilson's disease, and this accumulation has been noted to precede the development of liver pathology, which may ultimately prove fatal. Episodes of intravascular hemolysis are also recognized (Deiss *et al.*, 1970). If dietary copper intake is reduced and urinary excretion promoted, the neurological signs and symptoms associated with Wilson's disease are alleviated (Scheinberg, 1961).

BAL, edetate calcium disodium and sulfur-containing amino acids can mobilize tissue copper stores for excretion in Wilson's disease. In laboratory animals, however, the Cu-EDTA complex has a higher toxicity than cupric ion or the calcium disodium salt of EDTA (Fiedler, 1969). At least BAL has been shown to produce some clinical improvement, but repeated injections are painful and frequently give rise to undesirable side effects (Walsche, 1956a). In isolated cases, penicillamine in a regimen of 0.3 gm. by mouth 3 times a day half an hour before meals was believed to promote copper excretion better than either BAL or edetate (Fister *et al.*, 1958; Walsche, 1956b). Indeed it is at present the drug of choice for the oral treatment of Wilson's disease (Walsche, 1956b; Aposhian, 1961).

Symptomatology:
1. Prompt emesis (usually within 5 to 10 minutes). The vomitus is often green. Vomiting may persist.
2. Burning pain in mouth, esophagus, and stomach.
3. Metallic taste in mouth.
4. Diarrhea with or without colicky abdominal pain may be delayed several hours or may not appear until the 2nd day. Melena or occult blood in the feces.
5. Severe headache, cold sweat, weak pulse, and other signs of circulatory shock usually occur early.
6. Jaundice is not infrequent on the 2nd or 3rd day. When severe, it is usually due to hepatic necrosis with a swollen and painful liver. Sometimes the hepatic lesion is progressive.
7. Mild to moderately severe jaundice may evidence an acute hemolytic crisis without liver injury. Methemoglobinemia with intense cyanosis occasionally precedes the hemolysis.
8. Anuria and other signs of renal tubular necrosis may appear after 24 to 48 hours, even in patients whose blood pressure has been well maintained. Intravascular hemolysis is probably the usual antecedent of renal failure in copper poisoning.
9. Death may be preceded by convulsions, paralysis, or coma. Early deaths are usually associated with shock. Late deaths occur in hepatic or renal failure.

Treatment:
1. Unless extensive vomiting has occurred, empty the stomach by lavage with water, milk, sodium bicarbonate solution or a 0.1% solution of potassium ferrocyanide (the resulting copper ferrocyanide is insoluble).
2. Administer egg white and other demulcents.
3. Maintain electrolyte and fluid balances (see pp. IV-64–67, 72–73).
4. Morphine or meperidine (Demerol) may be necessary for the control of pain (p. IV-32).
5. If symptoms persist or intensify (especially circulatory collapse or cerebral disturbances), try BAL intramuscularly according to the arsenic dosage schedule in Table III-2 (p. III-52) or penicillamine in accordance with the supplier's recommendations.
6. Treat shock vigorously with blood transfusions and perhaps vasopressor amines (pp. IV-16–20).
7. If intravascular hemolysis becomes evident, protect the kidneys as in naphthalene poi-

soning (p. III-310) by maintaining a diuresis with mannitol and perhaps by alkalinizing the urine with sodium bicarbonate.

8. It is unlikely that a dose of methylene blue would be effective against the occasional methemoglobinemia, and it might exacerbate the subsequent hemolytic episode.

9. Institute measures for impending renal (pp. IV-52-53) and hepatic (pp. IV-60-62) failure.

Laboratory:

1. Liver and kidney function tests may be indicated.

2. Whole blood (but not plasma or serum) copper levels may aid in prognosis (Chuttani *et al.*, 1965).

3. Hematological signs may occur (methemoglobinemia, Heinz body formation, hemolysis).

References:

Agarwal, B. N.; Bray, S. H.; Bercz, P.; Plotzker, R.; Labovitz, E. Ineffectiveness of hemodialysis in copper sulphate poisoning. Nephron *15*:74-77, 1975.

Aposhian, H. V. Biochemical and pharmacological properties of the metal-binding agent penicillamine. Fed. Proc. 20 (Part II, Suppl. 10):185-190, 1961.

Barka, T.; Scheuer, P. J.; Schaffner, F.; Popper, H. Structural changes of liver cells in copper intoxication. Arch. Pathol. *78*:331-349, 1964.

Barsky, M. H. Ulcerations of the nasal membranes and perforation of the septum in a copperplating factory. N. Y. State J. Med. *37*:1031-1034, 1937.

Bloomfield, J. S.; Dixon, R.; McCredie, D. A. Potential hepatotoxicity of copper in recurrent hemodialysis. Arch. Intern. Med. *128*:555-560, 1971.

Chowdhury, A. K. R.; Ghosh, S.; Pal, D. Acute copper sulfate poisoning. J. Indian Med. Assoc. *36*:330-336, 1961.

Chugh, K. S.; Singhal, P. C.; Sharma, B. K. Methemoglobinemia in acute copper sulfate poisoning. Ann. Intern. Med. *82*:226-227, 1975.

Chugh, K. S.; Singhal, P. C.; Sharma, B. K.; Das, K. C.; Datta, B. N. Acute renal failure following copper sulphate intoxication. Postgrad. Med. J. *53*:18-23, 1977.

Chuttani, H. K.; Gupta, P. S.; Gulati, S.; Gupta, D. N. Acute copper sulfate poisoning. Am. J. Med. *39*:849-854, 1965.

Cole, D. E. C.; Lirenman, D. S. Role of albumin-enriched peritoneal dialysate in acute copper poisoning. J. Pediatr. *92*:955-957, 1978.

Cole, H. N. Extensive copper sulfate necrosis. Arch. Dermatol. *9*:589-593, 1924.

Deiss, A.; Lee, G. R.; Cartwright, G. E. Hemolytic anemia in Wilson's disease. Ann. Intern. Med. *73*:413-418, 1970.

Fairbanks, U. F. Copper sulfate-induced hemolytic anemia, inhibition of glucose-6-phosphate dehydrogenase and other possible etiologic mechanisms. Arch. Intern. Med. *120*:428-432, 1967.

Fiedler, H. Untersuchungen uber die Toxicitat des Kupferdinatrium-athylendiamintetraacetats. Arch. Toxikol. *25*: 140-149, 1969.

Fister, W. P.; Boulding, J. E.; Barker, R. A. The treatment of hepatolenticular degeneration with penicillamine, with report of two cases. Can. Med. Assoc. J. *78*:99-102, 1958.

Holtzman, N. A.; Elliott, D. A.; Heller, R. H. Copper intoxication, report of a case with observations on ceruloplasmin. N. Engl. J. Med. *275*:347-352, 1966.

Holtzman, N. A.; Haslam, H. A. Elevation of serum copper following copper sulfate as an emetic. Pediatrics *42*:189-193, 1968.

Hopper, S. H.; Adams, H. S. Copper poisoning from vending machines. Public Health Rep. (U. S.) *73*:910-914, 1958.

Ivanovich, P.; Manzler, P.; Drake, R. Acute hemolysis following hemodialysis. Trans. Am. Soc. Artif. Intern. Organs *15*:316-320, 1969.

Jones, M. M.; Basinger, M. A.; Tarka, M. P. The relative effectiveness of some chelating agents in acute copper intoxication in the mouse. Res. Commun. Chem. Pathol. Pharmacol. *27*:571-577, 1980.

Klein, W. J., Jr.; Metz, E. N.; Price, A. R. Acute copper intoxication, a hazard of hemodialysis. Arch. Intern. Med. *129*:578-582, 1972.

LeVan, J. H.; Perry, E. L. Copper poisoning on shipboard. Public Health Rep. (U. S.) *76*:334, 1961.

Lusky, L. M.; Braun, H. A.; Laug, E. P. The effect of BAL on experimental lead, tungsten, vanadium, uranium, copper and copper-arsenic poisoning. J. Ind. Hyg. Toxicol. *31*:301-305, 1949.

Mallory, F. B.; Parker, F., Jr. Experimental copper poisoning. Am. J. Pathol. *7*:351-363, 1931.

Manzler, A. D.; Schreiner, A. W. Copper-induced acute hemolytic anemia; a new complication of hemodialysis. Ann. Intern. Med. *73*:409-412, 1970.

Matter, B. J.; Pederson, J.; Psimenos, G.; Lindeman, R. D. Lethal copper intoxication in hemodialysis. Trans. Am. Soc. Artif. Intern. Organs *15*:309-315, 1969.

Moeschlin, S. *Poisoning, Diagnosis and Treatment.* 1st Amer. Ed., Grune and Stratton, New York, 1965.

Nicholas, P. O. Food poisoning due to copper in the morning tea. Lancet *2*:40-42, 1968.

NRC-NAS, Committee on Medical and Biological Effects of Environmental Pollutants. *Copper.* Washington, D. C, 1977.

Salmon, M. A.; Wright, T. Chronic copper poisoning presenting as pink disease. Arch. Dis. Child. *46*:108-110, 1971.

Scheinberg, I. H. Copper metabolism. Fed. Proc. 20 (Part II, Suppl. 10):179-185, 1961.

Semple, A. B.; Parry, W. H.; Phillips, D. E. Acute copper poisoning. Lancet *2*:700-701, 1960.

Soli, N. E.; Froslie, A. Chronic copper poisoning in sheep. I. The relationship of methaemoglobinemia to Heinz body formation and haemolysis during the terminal crisis. Acta Pharmacol. Toxicol. *40*:169-177, 1977.

Stacey, N. H.; Klaassen, C. D. Copper toxicity in isolated rat hepatocytes. Toxicol. Appl. Pharmacol. *58*:211-220, 1981.

Stein, R. S.; Jenkins, D.; Korns, M. E. Death after use of cupric sulfate as emetic. J. A. M. A. *235*:801, 1976.

Walsche, J. M. Wilson's disease, new oral therapy. Lancet *1*:25-26, 1956a.

Walsche, J. M. Penicillamine, new oral therapy for Wilson's disease. Am. J. Med. *21*:487-495, 1956b.

Walsh, F. M.; Crosson, F. J.; Bayley, M.; McReynolds, J.; Pearson, B. J. Acute copper intoxication - pathophysiology and therapy with a case report. Am. J. Dis. Child. *131*:149-151, 1977.

Webster, R. W. *Legal Medicine and Toxicology.* W. B. Saunders Co., Philadelphia, 1930.

Wiederanders, R. E.; Evans, G. W.; Wasdahl, W. W. Acute and chronic copper poisoning in the rat. J. Lancet. *88*:286-291, 1968.

Witthaus, R. A. *Manual of Toxicology.* Wm. Wood & Co., New York, 1911.

Wyllie, J. Copper poisoning at a cocktail party. Am. J. Public Health *47*:617, 1957.

CYANIDE

Hydrocyanic acid (prussic acid) and alkali salts like sodium and potassium cyanide are found in vermicidal fumigants, insecticides, rodenticides, metal polishes (especially silver polish), electroplating solutions, and in various metallurgical and photographic processes. As a fumigant, particularly for such structures as greenhouses, ships, mills, and warehouses, hydrogen cyanide (HCN) is applied directly as a solution (hydrocyanic acid), or the gas is generated from one of the cyanide salts by the action of dilute mineral acid. Cyanogen chloride (CNCl) can produce systemic cyanide poisoning but it also can induce pulmonary edema, especially on chronic exposure (Jandorf and Bodansky, 1946; Reed, 1920-21). These fumigations should be performed only by expert exterminators. Organically bound cyanides (*e.g.*, acrylonitrile) are sometimes used as fumigant gases, especially for grains.

Cyanogenic glycosides (*e.g.*, amygdalin, linamarin) are found naturally in many plants. In addition to these natural products, industrial intermediates, such as aliphatic nitriles (*e.g.*, acrylonitrile, acetonitrile), and the antihypertensive drug sodium nitroprusside are all capable of causing acute cyanide poisoning (see Section II). Street samples of phencyclidine (see Section II) have been found to be contaminated with high concentrations of 1-piperidinocyclohexanecarbonitrile, a cyanide-generating compound, but no human victims of cyanide poisoning from this source have been reported (Soine *et al.*, 1979). Hydrogen cyanide may be generated during the pyrolysis of wool, polyamides, polyurethanes, polyacrylonitriles and other substances. Carbon monoxide poisoning among firemen is probably more common than cyanide poisoning, but with low-temperature smoldering fires involving plastics, the possibility of cyanide intoxication should be considered (Clark *et al.*, 1981; Daunderer, 1979).

Most recognized poisonings have been traced to the accidental, suicidal or homicidal ingestion of hydrocyanic acid or one of its alkali salts. Cyanide poisoning appears to be less prevalent now than in the past (Chen and Rose, 1952); in the early decades of the 20th century, it was a major cause of chemical intoxication, particularly in Europe.

Toxicology: Poisoning may arise from any substance which releases the cyanide ion. For example, mercuric cyanide (Rose *et al.*, 1964) can produce signs of both cyanide and mercury intoxication, and these signs can be reversed on administration of the respective antidotes (see also MERCURY, p. III-262). Other chemicals that release or generate cyanide are mentioned above and are listed in Section II.

Cyanide is a potent and rapidly acting chemical asphyxiant; it prevents tissue utilization of oxygen by inhibiting the tissue enzyme cytochrome oxidase (Stotz *et al.*, 1938). Because oxygen cannot be utilized, venous blood may retain the bright red color of oxyhemoglobin. Cyanide does not react with oxyhemoglobin or reduced (deoxy) hemoglobin.

As with other chemical asphyxiants, the critical organs are those which are most sensitive to oxygen lack, notably the brain and the heart. A transient stage of central nervous stimulation is followed by central nervous depression and, finally, hypoxic convulsions and death due to respiratory arrest (Ward and Wheatley, 1947). Cardiac irregularities are commonly observed, particularly bradycardia (Lee-Jones *et al.*, 1970), but the heart beat invariably outlasts breathing movements (Wexler *et al.*, 1947).

Few poisons are more rapidly lethal than cyanide. Time to the appearance of toxic signs is largely determined by the rate of absorption (Ward, 1947). The inhalation of hydrogen cyanide commonly produces reactions within a few seconds and death within minutes. With the ingestion of cyanide salts death may be delayed as long as an hour. The prognosis is fairly good if the patient is still alive 1 hour after swallowing a dose of cyanide, but fatal relapses have been described after periods as long as 4 hours. If the stomach is empty and the free gastric acidity is high, poisoning is especially fast. After large doses some victims have had time only for a warning cry before sudden loss of consciousness.

Hydrogen cyanide in aqueous solution (hydrocyanic acid) is readily absorbed from the skin (Potter, 1950; Tovo, 1955) and from all mucous membranes (such as the rectum and vagina), but the alkali salts are usually toxic only when ingested. The average lethal dose of HCN taken by mouth is believed to lie between 60 and 90 mg. (1 to 1½ grains); this corresponds to about 1 teaspoonful of a 2% solution of hydrocyanic acid and to about 200 mg. of potassium cyanide (Gettler and St. George, 1934; Gettler and Baine, 1938). Prompt treatment, however, has saved people who swallowed 4 to 6 gm. of KCN (De Busk and Seidl, 1969; Miller and Toops, 1951), and some people who have swallowed 3 to 5 gm. have survived without specific therapy (Liebowitz and Schwartz, 1948). The lethality of most derivatives is regarded as proportional to the content of readily available cyanide. The mortality rate is high, but in nonfatal cases recovery is generally complete. Rarely, neuropsychiatric sequelae are observed as in carbon monoxide poisoning (p. III-97).

Absorbed cyanide is in small measure excreted unchanged by the lungs. About 15% of an administered dose apparently reacts with cysteine in the rat and is ultimately excreted as 2-iminothiazolidone-4-carboxylic acid (Wood and Cooley, 1956). Other minor routes of detoxication include trapping as the cyano group of vitamin B_{12} (see below), oxidation to formate and carbon dioxide, and incorporation into methyl groups of choline and methionine (Boxer and Rickards, 1952).

The major mechanism of detoxication, however, is conversion to the relatively harmless thiocyanate ion by an enzymatic reaction which is mediated by the enzyme rhodanese (thiosulfate:cyanide sulfurtransferase). This enzyme is widely distributed in tissues, but the greatest activity is found in the liver (Himwich and Saunders, 1948). The body has a large capacity to detoxify cyanide, but the rhodanese system responds sluggishly to a cyanide challenge (Clemedson et al., 1955). The rate of the rhodanese reaction can be accelerated by supplying an exogenous source of sulfur; clinically, this is best accomplished by the injection of sodium thiosulfate (Chen and Rose, 1952; Saunders and Himwich, 1950). Thiosulfate alone is effective against cyanide. Despite its slow onset of action, its many advantages (e.g., nontoxic, high water solubility, economical, high capacity, essentially irreversible inactivation of cyanide) make it the best single antidote (Ivankovich et al., 1980).

To protect tissue cells until the cyanide ion is detoxified, however, the therapist usually first converts a portion of the circulating hemoglobin into methemoglobin because the latter can compete effectively and rapidly with cytochrome oxidase for cyanide (Albaum et al., 1946). Each of the four ferric heme groups on a molecule of methemoglobin can trap a molecule of cyanide, and the binding is so tenacious that complete saturation of available ferric heme groups occurs in vivo at very low free cyanide concentrations (Smith and Gosselin, 1966). Cyanmethemoglobin, however, is a dissociable complex. As cyanide is released in response to a decreasing plasma concentration, it becomes available for metabolic detoxication. Thus, cyanmethemoglobin represents a potentially lethal depot of cyanide and one that can lead to a recurrence of signs and symptoms if other measures, e.g., thiosulfate, are not instituted. The methemoglobin is eventually reconverted spontaneously to oxyhemoglobin by intraerythrocytic enzymes.

It is customary to recommend amyl nitrite as an emergency means of inducing methemoglobinemia. Probably this recommendation is based more upon its common availability and the speed with which it can be administered and absorbed than upon the velocity with which it generates methemoglobin (Bastian and Mercker, 1959). When given by the pulmonary route, amyl nitrite is a weak methemoglobin-generating agent (see Section II). Even sodium nitrite has been criticized for its slow onset of action. As tested in the mouse, sodium nitrite was the slowest of a series of common methemoglobin-generating compounds to produce peak circulating levels of methemoglobin (Smith et al., 1967). Some aminophenols are more rapidly acting and perhaps safer (Kiese and Weger, 1969; Schwarzkopf and Friedberg, 1971), but they are not yet available for general use in this country. p-Aminopropiophenone has been used successfully in the resuscitation of poisoned dogs (Rose et al., 1947), but it is commonly held to generate methemoglobin too slowly in man to be of value (Tepperman et al., 1946).

When combined with artificial respiration and general supportive treatment, the nitrite-thiosulfate regimen has saved the lives of cyanide victims even after the onset of apnea (Chen et al., 1944; Hirsch, 1964; Proudfoot and Brown, 1967; Wolfsie, 1951).

In years past, methylene blue was used in human cyanide poisoning, and most experimental reports agree that it has weak anticyanide effects (Chen et al., 1933, 1934; Rentsch and Wittekind, 1967; Smith, 1969a). The same is true of the related ethyl methylene blue (Levine, 1977). Several reports agree that methemoglobin does not accumulate in animals or red cells injected with or exposed to methylene blue (Rentsch and Wittekind, 1967; Smith and Thron, 1972; Stossel and Jennings, 1966). Indeed, in modern times the only accepted use of methylene blue is to accelerate methemoglobin reduction (see ANILINE, p. III-31, and NITRITE, p. III-314). Certainly the combination of methylene blue and nitrite is irrational as an anticyanide regimen (Chen and Rose, 1956). An explanation of the anticyanide effects of methylene blue came with the realization that its potent methemoglobin-reducing action masked a weaker methemoglobin-generating capability. Although methemoglobin does not accumulate, methylene blue increases the rate of hemoglobin-methemoglobin turnover (Smith and Thron, 1972). Thus, over a period of time more methemoglobin is made available to react with cyanide, even though the concentration at any specific instant is not significantly increased. It is possible, however, that methylene blue may also have other cyanide antagonistic effects unrelated to methemoglobin (Smith, 1969a).

Several salts and chelates of cobalt have been tested as potential cyanide antagonists. The effects of sodium cobaltinitrite, $Na_3Co(NO_2)_6$, have been attributed in large measure to methemoglobin formation by dissociable nitrite (Rose et al., 1965b). As tested in mice, however, only about half the cyanide detoxified in vivo could be ascribed to cyanmethemoglobin formation (Smith, 1969b). Apparently cobalt can react directly with cyanide, and both cobalt and strongly bound cyanide have been identified in the urine of treated animals (Frankenberg and Sorbo, 1975).

Cobalt gluconate (Estler, 1966), acetate (Evans, 1964) and chloride (Isom and Way, 1973; Smith, 1969b) have been reported to have significant antidotal effects. As in the case of oxygen (see below), the antidotal effects of cobaltous chloride are dramatically potentiated by thiosulfate (Isom and Way, 1973). Cobalt histidine is rapidly acting but has the disadvantage common to this group of having only a limited capacity for cyanide detoxication (Schwarzkopf and Friedberg, 1971).

Although the monocobalt chelate of ethylenediaminetetraacetic acid is said to be inactive (Paulet, 1958), the dimetal chelate (Co₂-EDTA) is efficacious (Bartelheimer, 1962; Friedberg et al., 1966; Mercker and Bastian, 1959; Paulet et al., 1963; Weber et al., 1962). In animals, side effects of Co₂-EDTA (circulatory depression, hyperventilation, metabolic acidosis) were judged to be more serious than those of other cyanide antagonists (Klimmek et al., 1979a, b). This type of chelate has been employed successfully in human cyanide intoxication (Bain and Knowles, 1967; Bourrelier and Paulet, 1971), but the clinical experience is not encouraging. Among the side effects reported are anaphylactoid reactions, crushing retrosternal pain, sinus tachycardia, ventricular tachycardia and facial and palpebral edema (Hillman et al., 1974; McKiernan, 1980; Nagler et al., 1978).

Hydroxocobalamin (aquacobalamin, vitamin B₁₂ₐ) contains a central cobalt atom in a porphyrin-like ring structure; it avidly reacts with cyanide to form vitamin B₁₂ or cyanocobalamin in a manner analogous to methemoglobin (Mushett et al., 1952; Posner et al., 1976). This reaction inactivates 1 mole of cyanide per mole of hydroxocobalamin, and because the resultant complex is extremely stable, there is a high degree of antidote utilization in vivo (Friedberg et al., 1965). Poor solubility characteristics impose some practical limits on dose, so that hydroxocobalamin is not particularly suited for the inactivation of multiple lethal doses of cyanide (Rose et al., 1965a). Moreover, the compound is unstable and extremely expensive. With cobalt preparations as with nitrite, thiosulfate and other antidotal adjuncts are useful (Delga et al., 1961; Friedberg and Shukla, 1975).

Although the mechanism of its action is not clear, oxygen has often been recommended as a therapeutic adjunct in cyanide poisoning (Dall and Hannah, 1964; Gordh and Norberg, 1947). This impression now has a basis in experimental findings. Way et al. (1966, 1972) noted that although oxygen alone even at hyperbaric pressures had only a slight protective effect against cyanide in mice, it potentiated the protective effects of thiosulfate alone or a nitrite-thiosulfate combination (Sheehy and Way, 1968). As tested in dogs, however, oxygen did not have dramatic effects even in combination with thiosulfate in reversing the cardiovascular and respiratory changes induced by cyanide (Burrows et al., 1973). Oxygen at 1 atmosphere is presumably safe and may be worthwhile for patients receiving the nitrite-thiosulfate regimen.

Several adrenergic agonists and blockers have cyanide antagonist activity that appears to be unrelated to methemoglobin formation, cyanide metabolism or changes in cardiovascular status (Maeda and Furukawa, 1977). Pyruvate has dose-related cyanide antagonistic effects in mice (Cettadini et al., 1972).

Given in daily doses to rats, cyanide produced no mortality due to cumulative actions (Hayes, 1967; Hertting et al., 1960). So-called human cases of "chronic" cyanide poisoning (e.g., Sandberg, 1967; Smith, 1964a) probably represent persistent neuropsychiatric sequelae from one or more acute exposure episodes. The clinical syndrome of delayed neurological deterioration sometimes follows hypoxia irrespective of its cause.

Demyelinating lesions in brain after experimental cyanide intoxication are well known (Hirano et al., 1968; Ibrahim et al., 1963; Levine and Stypulkowski, 1959). They do not appear to be specific for cyanide but are similar to those produced by azide and by hypoxia (Bass, 1968; Hurst, 1942). The lesions after cyanide, however, have been produced by doses that caused no overt signs of hypoxia (Smith et al., 1963a). When cyanide was infused into monkeys and rats, neuronal damage was thought to be secondary to changes in circulation or respiration (Brierley et al., 1976, 1977). Remyelination after cyanide occurs in the central nervous system, but the process is incomplete and slow in comparison to that in the peripheral nervous system (Hirano et al., 1968). Ultrastructural lesions have also been described in heart muscle after delayed death by cyanide (Suzuki, 1968).

Thyroid changes including frank goiter have been reported following long-term exposure to cyanides (El Ghawabi et al., 1975). Perhaps they are attributable to the thiocyanate arising from the continuous detoxication of minute quantities of cyanide (Hardy et al., 1950). Even single doses of cyanide produce alterations in the pattern of brain metabolites consistent with a decrease in oxidative metabolism and an increase in glycolysis (Estler, 1965). Decreases in brain γ-aminobutyric acid that are not duplicated by asphyxia in nitrogen or carbon dioxide have been ascribed to a cyanide inhibition of glutamic acid decarboxylase (Tursky and Sajter, 1962).

Symptomatology:

1. Massive doses may produce, without warning, sudden loss of consciousness and prompt death from respiratory arrest.

With smaller but still lethal doses, the illness may be prolonged for 1 or more hours.

2. Upon ingestion, a bitter, acrid, burning taste is sometimes noted, followed by a feeling of constriction or numbness in the throat. Salivation, nausea and vomiting are not unusual. Solutions of sodium and potassium cyanide are corrosive because of their high alkalinity. Other symptoms follow in rapid progression.

3. Anxiety, confusion, vertigo, giddiness, and often a sensation of stiffness in the lower jaw.

4. Hypernea and dyspnea. Respirations become very rapid and then slow and irregular. Inspiration is characteristically short while expiration is greatly prolonged.

5. The odor of bitter almonds may be noted on the breath or vomitus. This characteristic is sometimes a diagnostic help, but as many as 20 to 40% of all persons are said to be congenitally insensitive to the odor of HCN (e.g., De Busk and Seidl, 1969).

6. In the early phases of poisoning, an increase in vasoconstrictor tone causes a rise in blood pressure and reflex slowing of the heart rate. Thereafter the pulse becomes rapid, weak, and sometimes irregular. The victim notes palpitations and a sensation of constriction in the chest. A bright pink coloration of the skin due to high concentrations of oxyhemoglobin in the venous return may be confused with that of carbon monoxide poisoning.

7. Unconsciousness, followed promptly by violent convulsions, epileptiform or tonic, sometimes localized but usually generalized. Opisthotonus and trismus may develop. Involuntary micturition and defecation occur.

8. Paralysis follows the convulsive stage. The skin is covered with sweat. The eyeballs protrude, and the pupils are dilated and unreactive. The mouth is covered with foam, which is sometimes blood-stained, indicative of pulmonary edema (Graham et al., 1977; Stewart, 1974). The skin color may be brick red. Cyanosis is not prominent in spite of weak and irregular gasping. In the unconscious patient, bradycardia (above) and the absence of cyanosis may be key diagnostic signs.

9. Death from respiratory arrest. As long as the heart beat continues, prompt and vigorous treatment offers some promise of survival.

Treatment (must be prompt):

1. If the patient is asymptomatic administer syrup of ipecac and/or perform gastric lavage. Do not use activated charcoal because it is said to be ineffective in trapping cyanide (Andersen, 1946). See also 9, below.

2. If the patient is apneic, start artificial respiration immediately. Keep the airway clear. See pp. IV-2–12 for techniques.

3. Administer amyl nitrite (amyl nitrite perles) by inhalation for 15 to 30 seconds of every minute, while a sodium nitrite solution is being prepared. Check perles for date of expiration and use the freshest product available. Perles in storage should be replaced on an annual basis.

4. Discontinue amyl nitrite and immediately inject 10 ml. of a 3% solution of sodium nitrite intravenously over a period of 2 to 4 minutes. If necessary, inject a nonsterile solution. Do not remove the needle. Caution: this dose of nitrite may be lethal to young children and appropriate adjustments in dose should be made on a body weight basis (Berlin, 1970).

5. Through the same needle infuse intravenously 50 ml. of a 25% aqueous solution of sodium thiosulfate. The injection should take about 10 minutes. Other concentrations (5 to 50%) are permissible if the total dose is held at approximately 12 gm. Injectable forms of nitrite and thiosulfate have expiration datings of 5 years.

6. Oxygen therapy (p. IV-12) may be of value in combination with nitrite and sodium thiosulfate therapy.

7. In the event of cardiac asystole, external massage (p. IV-26) and artificial pacemakers (p. IV-30) are indicated.

8. If symptoms recur, the injections of nitrite and thiosulfate may be repeated at half the above doses. In very severe poisonings it is safer and perhaps more efficient to keep repeating the thiosulfate injections instead of the nitrite.

9. Because of the speed of absorption and the rapidity with which symptoms appear, gastric lavage is seldom a practical procedure and should be postponed at least until after procedures 2 to 5. Perhaps the best lavage fluid is a dilute solution of potassium permanganate (1:5000), but tap water or dilute sodium bicarbonate solution are likely to be more quickly available.

10. Oxygen therapy and a whole blood transfusion may become necessary if nitrite-induced methemoglobinemia becomes too severe (but see 3 under Laboratory). In laboratory animals, exchange transfusions alone increased survival (Tauberger et al., 1974).

Laboratory:

1. In cyanide poisoning, laboratory tests are

seldom useful in prognosis or treatment, but specimens (*e.g.*, gastric contents) should be saved in case of legal need for a chemical analysis (Curry *et al.*, 1967; Halstrom and Moller, 1945). If the reagents have been prepared in advance, however, a simple chemical test for cyanide can be performed on a gastric aspirate to confirm the diagnosis in less than 10 minutes (Lee-Jones *et al.*, 1970).

2. Quantitative analyses for cyanide are available. In dogs the total plasma concentration of cyanide at the moment of respiratory arrest was about 40 μM, and it was about 60% protein-bound (Christel *et al.*, 1977). Cyanide is said to be concentrated in red cells (Ballantyne *et al.*, 1973), even in the absence of induced methemoglobinemia. Whole blood cyanide levels in fatal human cases are said to exceed 0.5 mM (>3 μgm./ml.) (Graham *et al.*, 1977).

3. Laboratory determinations of methemoglobin as an index of the adequacy of nitrite treatment are meaningless because some or all of the methemoglobin will complex cyanide *in vivo* and will not be measured *in vitro*.

4. Severe metabolic acidosis (lactic acidemia, ketosis) and anion gap (Graham *et al.*, 1977; Vogel *et al.*, 1981).

References:

Albaum, H. G.; Tepperman, J.; Bodansky, O. A spectrophotometric study of the competition of methemoglobin and cytochrome oxidase for cyanide *in vitro*. J. Biol. Chem. *163*:641-647, 1946.

Andersen, A. H. Experimental studies on the pharmacology of activated charcoal; I. Adsorption power of charcoal in aqueous solutions. Acta Pharmacol. *2*:69-78, 1946.

Bain, J. T. B.; Knowles, E. L. Successful treatment of cyanide poisoning. Br. Med. J. *1*:763, 1967.

Ballantyne, B.; Bright, J.; Williams, P. An experimental assessment of decreases in measurable cyanide levels in biological fluids. J. Forensic Sci. Soc. *13*:111-117, 1973.

Bartelheimer, E. W. Unterschiede der toxischen und cyanidantagonistischen Wirksamkeit von Kobaltchelat-Verbindungen (Co-Histidin und Co$_2$-EDTA). Nauyn Schmiedebergs Arch. Pharmakol. *243*:254-268, 1962.

Bass, N. H. Pathogenesis of myelin lesions in experimental cyanide encephalopathy. Neurology *18*:167-177, 1968.

Bastian, G.; Mercker, H. Zur Frage der Zweckmassigkeit der Inhalation von Amylnitrit in der Behandlung der Cyanidvergiftung. Nauyn Schmiedebergs Arch. Pharmakol. *237*:285-295, 1959.

Berlin, C. M., Jr. The treatment of cyanide poisoning in children. Pediatrics *46*:793-796, 1970.

Bourrelier, J.; Paulet, G. Intoxication cyanhydrique consecutive a des brulures graves par cyanure de sodium fondu. Presse Med. *79*:1013-1014, 1971.

Boxer, G. E.; Rickards, J. C. Studies on the metabolism of the carbon of cyanide and thiocyanate. Arch. Biochem. Biophys. *39*:7-29, 1952.

Brierley, J. B.; Brown, A. W.; Calverley, J. Cyanide intoxication in the rat: physiological and neuropathological aspects. J. Neurol. Neurosurg. Psychiatry *39*:129-140, 1976.

Brierley, J. B.; Prior, P. F.; Calverley, J.; Brown, A. W. Cyanide

intoxication in *Macaca mulatta* - physiological and neuropathological aspects. J. Neurolog. Sci. *31*:133-157, 1977.

Burrows, G. E.; Liu, D. H.; Way, J. Effect of oxygen on cyanide intoxication. J. Pharmacol. Exp. Ther. *184*:739-747, 1973.

Cettadini, A.; Caprino, L.; Terranova, T. Effect of pyruvate in the acute cyanide poisoning in mice. Experientia *28*:943-944, 1972.

Chen, K. K.; Rose, C. L. Nitrite and thiosulfate therapy in cyanide poisoning. J. A. M. A. *149*:113-119, 1952.

Chen, K. K.; Rose, C. L. Treatment of acute cyanide poisoning. J. A. M. A. *162*:1154-1155, 1956.

Chen, K. K.; Rose, C. L.; Clowes, G. H. A. Amyl nitrite and cyanide poisoning. J. A. M. A. *100*:1920-1922, 1933.

Chen, K. K.; Rose, C. L.; Clowes, G. H. A. Comparative values of several antidotes in cyanide poisoning. Am. J. Med. Sci. *188*:767-781, 1934.

Chen, K. K.; Rose, C. L.; Clowes, G. H. A. The modern treatment of cyanide poisoning. J. Indiana State Med. Assoc. *37*:344-350, 1944.

Christel, D.; Eyer, P.; Hegemann, M.; Kiese, M.; Lorcher, W.; Weger, N. Pharmacokinetics of cyanide in poisoning of dogs, and the effect of 4-dimethylaminophenol or thiosulfate. Arch. Toxicol. *38*:177-189, 1977.

Clark, C. J.; Campbell, D.; Reid, W. H. Blood carboxyhaemoglobin and cyanide levels in fire survivors. Lancet *1*:1332-1335, 1981.

Clemedson, C.; Hultman, H.; Sorbo, B. A combination of rhodanese and ethanethiosulfonate as an antidote in experimental cyanide poisoning. Acta. Physiol. Scand. *35*:31-35, 1955.

Curry, A. S.; Price, D. E.; Rutter, E. R. The production of cyanide in post mortem material. Acta Pharmacol. Toxicol. *25*:339-344, 1967.

Dall, J. L. C.; Hannah, W. M. Oxygen therapy in cyanide poisoning. Br. Med. J. *2*:33-34, 1964.

Daunderer, M. Lethal smoke poisoning with hydrocyanic acid from low temperature smoldering fires. Fortschr. Med. *97*:1401-1405, 1979.

De Busk, R. F.; Seidl, L. G. Attempted suicide by cyanide. Calif. Med. *110*:394-396, 1969.

Delga, J.; Mizoule, J.; Veverka, B. Sur la valeur de l'hydroxocobalamine dans le traitement de l'intoxication cyanhydrique. C. R. Soc. Biol. (Paris) *155*:1016-1019, 1961.

El Ghawabi, S. H.; Gaafar, M. A.; El Sahartz, A. A.; Ahmed, S. H., Malash, K. K.; Fares, R. Chronic cyanide exposure: a clinical, radioisotope, and laboratory study. Br. J. Ind. Med. *32*:215-219, 1975.

Estler, C. -J. Stoffwechselveranderungen des Gehirns im Verlauf der nicht letalen Kaliumcyanidvergiftung und ihre Beeinflussung durch Cyanidantagonisten. Nauyn Schmiedebergs Arch. Pharmakol. *251*:413-432, 1965.

Estler, C. -J. Der Einfluss von Kobaltgluconat und des Dikobaltsalzes der Athylendiamintetraessigsaure (Co$_2$-EDTA) auf den Hirnstoffwechsel normaler und cyanidvergifteten Mause. Nauyn Schmeidebergs Arch. Pharmakol. *252*:305-313, 1966.

Evans, C. L. Cobalt compounds as antidotes for hydrocyanic acid. Br. J. Pharmacol. *23*:455-475, 1964.

Frankenberg, L.; Sorbo, B. Effect of cyanide antidotes on the metabolic conversion of cyanide to thiocyanate. Arch. Toxicol. *33*:81-89, 1975.

Friedberg, K. D.; Grutzmacher, J.; Lendle, L. Aquocobalamin (Vitamin B$_{12a}$) als spezifisches Blausaureantidot. Arch. Int. Pharmacodyn. Ther. *154*:327-350, 1965.

Friedberg, K. D.; Grutzmacher, J.; Lendle, L. Die Bedeutung der Wirkungsgeschwindigkeit von Antidoten bei der Behandlung der Blausaurevergiftung. Arch. Toxikol. *22*:176-191, 1966.

Friedberg, K. D.; Shukla, U. R. The efficiency of aquocobalamine as an antidote in cyanide poisoning when given alone or combined with sodium thiosulfate. Arch. Toxicol. *33*:103-113, 1975.

Gettler, A. O.; Baine, J. O. The toxicology of cyanide. Am. J. Med. Sci. *195*:182-198, 1938.

Gettler, A. O.; St. George, A. V. Cyanide poisoning. Am. J.

Clin. Pathol. 4:429-437, 1934.

Gordh, T.; Norberg, B. Studies on oxygen treatment in connection with experimental hydrocyanic acid poisoning. Acta. Physiol. Scand. 13:26-34, 1947.

Graham, D. L.; Laman, D.; Theodore, J.; Robin, E. D. Acute cyanide poisoning complicated by lactic acidosis and pulmonary edema. Arch. Intern. Med. 137:1051-1055, 1977.

Halstrom, F.; Moller, K. The content of cyanide in human organs from cases of poisoning with cyanide taken by mouth, with a contribution to the toxicology of cyanides. Acta Pharmacol. Toxicol. 1:18-28, 1945.

Hardy, H. L.; Jeffries, W. M.; Wasserman, M. M.; Waddel, W. R. Thiocyanate effect following industrial cyanide exposure. N. Engl. J. Med. 242:968-972, 1950.

Hayes, W. J., Jr. The 90-dose LD_{50} and a chronicity factor as measures of toxicity. Toxicol. Appl. Pharmacol. 11:327-335, 1967.

Hertting, G.; Kraupp, O.; Schnetz, E.; Wuketich, St. Untersuchungen uber die Folgen einer chronischen Verabreichung akut toxischer Dosen von Natriumcyanid an Hunden. Acta Pharmacol. Toxicol. 17:27-43, 1960.

Hillman, B.; Bardhan, K. D.; Bain, J. T. B. The use of dicobalt edetate (Kelocyanor) in cyanide poisoning. Postgrad. Med. J. 50:171-174, 1974.

Himwich, W. A.; Saunders, J. P. Enzymatic conversion of cyanide to thiocyanate. Am. J. Physiol. 153:348-354, 1948.

Hirano, A.; Levine, S.; Zimmerman, H. M. Remyelination in the central nervous system after cyanide intoxication. J. Neuropathol. Exp. Neurol. 27:234-245, 1968.

Hirsch, F. G. Cyanide poisoning. Arch. Environ. Health 8:622-624, 1964.

Hurst, E. W. Experimental demyelination of the central nervous system. 3. Poisoning with potassium cyanide, sodium azide, hydroxylamine, narcotics, carbon monoxide, etc. with some considerations of bilateral necrosis occurring in the basal nuclie. Aust. J. Exp. Biol. Med. Sci. 20:297-305, 1942.

Ibrahim, M. Z. M.; Briscoe, P. B., Jr.; Bayliss, O. B.; Adams, C. W. M. The relationship between enzyme activity and neuroglia in the prodomal and demyelination stages of cyanide encephalopathy in the rat. J. Neurol. Neurosurg. Psychiatry 26:479-486, 1963.

Isom, G.; Way, J. Cyanide intoxication; protection with cobaltous chloride. Toxicol. Appl. Pharmacol. 24:449-456, 1973.

Ivankovich, A. D.; Braverman, B.; Kanuru, R. P.; Heyman, H. J.; Paulissian, R. Cyanide antidotes and methods of their administration in dogs - comparative study. Anesthesiology 52:210-216, 1980.

Jandorf, B. J.; Bodansky, O. Therapeutic and prophylactic effect of methemoglobinemia in inhalation poisoning by hydrogen cyanide and cyanogen chloride. J. Ind. Hyg. Toxicol. 28:125-132, 1946.

Kiese, M.; Weger, N. Formation of ferrihaemoglobin with aminophenols in the human for the treatment of cyanide poisoning. Eur. J. Pharmacol. 7:97-105, 1969.

Klimmek, R.; Fladerer, H.; Sziniez, L.; Weger, N.; Kiese, M. Effects of 4-dimethylaminophenol and CO_2EDTA on circulation, respiration, and blood homeostasis in dogs. Arch. Toxicol. 42:75-84, 1979a.

Klimmek, R.; Fladerer, H.; Weger, N. Circulation, respiration, and blood homeostasis in cyanide-poisoned dogs after treatment with 4-dimethylaminophenol or cobalt compounds. Arch. Toxicol. 43:121-133, 1979b.

Lee-Jones, M.; Bennett, M. A.; Sherwell, J. M. Cyanide self-poisoning. Br. Med. J. 4:780-781, 1970.

Levine, S. Interaction between ethyl methylene blue and cyanide-induced increases in blood lactate. J. Lab. Clin. Med. 89:632-639, 1977.

Levine, S.; Stypulkowski, W. Experimental cyanide encephalopathy. Arch. Pathol. 67:306-323, 1959.

Liebowitz, D.; Schwartz, H. Cyanide poisoning. Report of a case with recovery. Am. J. Clin. Pathol. 18:965-970, 1948.

Maeda, Y.; Furukawa, T. Alpha-adrenergic blocking and beta-adrenergic agents - antidotes for cyanide toxicity. Jpn. J. Pharmacol. 27:470-473, 1977.

McKiernan, M. J. Emergency treatment of cyanide poisoning.

Lancet 2:86, 1980.

Mercker, H.; Bastian, G. Kobaltverbindungen zur Entgiftung von Blausaure. Nauyn Schmiedebergs Arch. Pharmakol. 236:449-458, 1959.

Miller, M. H.; Toops, T. C. Acute cyanide poisoning. Recovery with sodium thiosulfate therapy. J. Indiana State Med. Assoc. 44:1164, 1951.

Mushett, C. W.; Kelley, K. L.; Boxer, G. E.; Rickards, J. C. Antidotal efficacy of vitamin B_{12a} (hydroxocobalamin) in experimental cyanide poisoning. Proc. Soc. Exp. Biol. Med. 81:234-237, 1952.

Nagler, J.; Provoost, R. A.; Parizel, G. Hydrogen cyanide poisoning treatment with cobalt EDTA. J. Occup. Med. 20:414-416, 1978.

Paulet, G. Intoxication cyanhydrique et chelates de cobalt. J. Physiol. (Paris) 50:438-442, 1958.

Paulet, G.; Bernard, J. P.; Olivier, M. L'hydroxocobalamine dans le traitement de l'intoxication cyanhydrique. C. R. Soc. Biol. (Paris) 156:1867-1869, 1963.

Posner, M. A.; Tobey, R. E.; McElroy, H. Hydroxocobalamin therapy of cyanide intoxication in guinea pigs. Anesthesiology 44:157-160, 1976.

Potter, A. L. The successful treatment of two recent cases of cyanide poisoning. Br. J. Ind. Med. 7:125-130, 1950.

Proudfoot, A. T.; Brown, S. S. Successful treatment of cyanide poisoning. Br. Med. J. 2:112, 1967.

Reed, C. Chronic poisoning from cyanogen chloride. J. Ind. Hyg. Toxicol. 2:140-143, 1920-21.

Rentsch, G.; Wittekind, D. Methylene blue and erythrocytes in the living animal. Contribution to the toxicology of methylene blue and formation of Heinz bodies. Toxicol. Appl. Pharmacol. 11:81-87, 1967.

Rose, C. L.; Chen, K. K.; Harris, P. N. Mercuric cyanide poisoning and its treatment in dogs. Proc. Soc. Exp. Biol. Med. 116:371-373, 1964.

Rose, C. L.; Welles, J. S.; Fink, R. D.; Chen, K. K. The antidotal action of p-aminopropiophenone with or without sodium thiosulfate in cyanide poisoning. J. Pharmacol. Exp. Ther. 89:109-114, 1947.

Rose, C. L.; Worth, R. M.; Chen, K. K. Hydroxocobalamine and acute cyanide poisoning in dogs. Life Sci. 4:1785-1789, 1965a.

Rose, C. L.; Worth, R. M.; Kikuchi, K.; Chen, K. K. Cobalt salts in acute cyanide poisoning. Proc. Soc. Exp. Biol. Med. 120:780-783, 1965b.

Sandberg, C. G. A case of chronic poisoning with potassium cyanide? Acta Med. Scand. 181:233-236, 1967.

Saunders, J. P.; Himwich, W. A. Properties of transulfurase responsible for conversion of cyanide to thiocyanate. Am. J. Physiol. 163:404-409, 1950.

Schwarzkopf, H. A.; Friedberg, K. D. Zur Beurteilung der Blausaure-Antidote. Arch. Toxikol. 27:111-123, 1971.

Sheehy, M.; Way, J. L. Effect of oxygen on cyanide intoxication; II. Mithridate. J. Pharmacol. Exp. Ther. 161:163-168, 1968.

Smith, A. D. M. Cyanide encephalopathy in man?. Lancet 2:668-671, 1964a.

Smith, A. D. M.; Dirckett, S.; Waters, A. H. Neuropathological changes in chronic cyanide intoxication. Nature 200:179-181, 1963a.

Smith, R. P. The significance of methemoglobinemia in toxicology. in Essays in Toxicology, Vol. I (F. R. Blood, Ed.), Academic Press, N. Y., pp. 83-113, 1969a.

Smith, R. P. Cobalt salts; effects on cyanide and sulphide poisoning and on methemoglobinemia. Toxicol. Appl. Pharmacol. 15:505-516, 1969b.

Smith, R. P.; Alkaitis, A. A.; Shafer, P. R. Chemically induced methemoglobinemias in the mouse. Biochem. Pharmacol. 16:317-328, 1967.

Smith, R. P.; Gosselin, R. E. On the mechanism of sulfide inactivation by methemoglobin. Toxicol. Appl. Pharmacol. 8:159-172, 1966.

Smith, R. P.; Thron, C. D. Hemoglobin, methylene blue and oxygen interactions in human red cells. J. Pharmacol. Exp. Ther. 183:549-558, 1972.

Soine, W. H.; Vincek, W. C.; Agee, D. T. Phencyclidine contaminant generates cyanide. N. Engl. J. Med. *301*:438, 1979.

Stewart, R. Cyanide poisoning. Clin. Toxicol., *7*:561-564, 1974.

Stossel, T. P.; Jennings, R. B. Failure of methylene blue to produce methemoglobinemia *in vivo*. Am. J. Clin. Pathol. *45*:600-604, 1966.

Stotz, E.; Altschul, A. M.; Hogness, T. R. The cytochrome c-cytochrome oxidase complex. J. Biol. Chem. *124*:745-754, 1938.

Suzuki, T. Ultrastructural changes of heart muscle in cyanide poisoning. Tohoku J. Exp. Med. *95*:271-287, 1968.

Tauberger, G.; Karzel, K.; Roezel, V. Versuche zur Cyanidentgiftung mit Blut-Austauschtransfusionerr. Arch. Toxicol. *32*:189-197, 1974.

Tepperman, J.; Bodansky, O.; Jandorf, B. J. The effect of *p*-aminopropiophenone-induced methemoglobinemia on oxygenation of working muscle in human subjects. Am. J. Physiol. *146*:702-709, 1946.

Tovo, S. Avvelenamento con cianuro di potassio da assorbimento percutaneo. Minerva Medicoleg. *75*:158-161, 1955.

Tursky, T.; Sajter, V. The influence of potassium cyanide poisoning on the γ-aminobutyric acid level in rat brain. J. Neurochem. *9*:519-523, 1962.

Vogel, S. N.; Sultan, T. R.; Ten Eyck, R. P. Cyanide poisoning. Clin. Toxicol. *18*:367-383, 1981.

Ward, A. A., Jr. Sodium cyanide: time of appearance of signs as a function of the rate of injection. Proc. Soc. Exp. Biol. Med. *64*:190-193, 1947.

Ward, A. A., Jr.; Wheatley, M. D. Sodium cyanide. Sequence of changes of activity induced at various levels of the central nervous system. J. Neuropathol. Exp. Neurol. *6*:292-294, 1947.

Way, J. L.; End, E.; Sheeny, M. H.; DeMiranda, P.; Feitknecht, U. F.; Bachand, R.; Gibbon, S. L.; Burrows, G. E. Effect of oxygen on cyanide intoxication; IV. Hyperbaric oxygen. Toxicol. Appl. Pharmacol. *22*:415-421, 1972.

Way, J. L.; Gibbon, S. L.; Sheehy, M. Effect of oxygen on cyanide intoxication. I. Prophylactic protection. J. Pharmacol. Exp. Ther. *153*:381-385, 1966.

Weber, D.; Friedberg, K. D.; Lendle, L. Beurteilung therapeutischer Massnahmen bei der Blausaurevergiftung unter konstanter Cyanid-Infusion. Nauyn Schmiederbergs Arch. Pharmakol. *244*:1-16, 1962.

Wexler, J.; Whittenberger, J. L.; Dumke, P. R. The effect of cyanide on the electrocardiogram of man. Am. Heart J. *34*:163-173, 1947.

Wolfsie, J. H. Treatment of cyanide poisoning in industry. Arch. Ind. Hyg. *4*:417-425, 1951.

Wood, J. L.; Cooley, S. L. Detoxification of cyanide by cystine. J. Biol. Chem. *218*:449-457, 1956.

2,4-D

2,4-Dichlorophenoxyacetic acid, commonly known as 2,4-D, and its derivatives are among the most widely used substances in weed control. They are particularly effective in weeding grain crops because of their selective action on broadleafed plants. Millions of pounds are consumed each year. At present the acid itself is not used as a herbicide, but it serves as the basic material from which soluble esters and salts are produced, such as sodium 2,4-dichlorophenoxyacetate (Audus, 1964; Dalgaard-Mikkelsen and Poulsen, 1962). The K_a of 2,4-D is 2.3×10^{-3} M; thus it is a stronger acid than aspirin, acetic acid or lactic acid.

Toxicology: The mammalian pharmacology is not well characterized. Both acute and chronic toxicities in laboratory mammals are low. All species which have been tested react similarly, and there seems to be only minor differences in potency between various salts and esters of 2,4-D, either as pure chemicals or as commercial preparations (Hill and Carlisle, 1947). As a general rule the LD_{50} values of these preparations range from around 300 to 700 mg./kg. by mouth in all species tested, with the possible exception of the dog, which may be more susceptible (Drill and Hiratzka, 1953; Rowe and Hymas, 1954a). The free acid has a somewhat higher toxicity than the sodium salt, the amine salts or the esters.

These materials penetrate the intact skin of laboratory mammals and man. Percutaneous absorption, however, does not appear to be extensive in man (Feldmann and Maibach, 1974) or to present a large hazard. In rats the dermal LD_{50} is about 1500 mg./kg. Subacute applications of 2,4-D esters and of the dimethylamine

salt to rabbit skin produced only local skin irritation, probably due to the oil vehicle (Kay *et al.*, 1965), but aqueous preparations have also caused skin rashes.

The syndrome of systemic intoxication is characteristic except perhaps in man and has been studied particularly in dogs (Bucher, 1946; Drill and Hiratzka, 1953). In several species, early deaths after massive doses have been ascribed to ventricular fibrillation (Hill and Carlisle, 1947). If death is delayed, motor disturbances become evident. A disinclination to move progresses to rigidity of skeletal muscles (myotonia) and ataxia. During this period the animal may improve temporarily with movement. Severe cases show progressive apathy, depression, muscular weakness of the hind limbs, periodic clonic spasms and finally coma. The myotonia, like that induced by veratrum alkaloids, occurs even in curarized muscle (Eyzaguirre *et al.*, 1948).

In subacute poisonings in laboratory animals, anorexia is marked, and irritation of the nose and eyes may be accompanied by epistaxis or bleeding from the mouth. Diarrhea with occult blood has also occurred. Mild pathological lesions have been described in the kidneys and liver of animals (Rowe and Hymas, 1954a) and man (Curry, 1962).

Clinical reports of 2,4-D poisoning are rare, and no consistent pattern is discernible except in scattered cases of protracted peripheral neuritis with myopathies (see below). A young farm worker ingested not less than 6500 mg. of 2,4-D and apparently experienced violent convulsions (they were not actually observed). Postmortem findings were limited to nonspecific hyperemia of the lungs, liver and brain (Nielsen *et al.*, 1965). An elderly man with senile dementia died 6 days after consuming a "large" amount of 2,4-D in a kerosene-like base. Death was apparently due to cardiac failure, but widespread plaques of acute demyelination were found in all parts of the brain (Dudley and Thapar, 1972). The case reported by Berwick (1970) involved the ingestion of a commercial mixture containing 49% Eptam (a carbamate-type herbicide), 36% isooctyl ester of 2,4-D, 9% kerosene, and other minor ingredients. In part the signs in this patient were consistent with cholinesterase inhibition perhaps caused by Eptam, but there was also evidence of generalized skeletal muscle damage, *e.g.*, elevated serum enzymes, myoglobinuria.

Additional fatalities have resulted from ingestions of the ethyl ester of 2,4-D (Curry, 1962) and the closely related herbicide 2-methyl-4-chlorophenoxyacetic acid (Johnson and Koumides, 1965; Popham and Davies, 1964). Although all these compounds are thought to act in the same manner, convulsions did not occur in Curry's case (1962) or that of Johnson and Koumides (1965), whereas they were either inferred (Nielsen *et al.*, 1965) or observed (Popham and Davies, 1964) in two other fatal poisonings. Popham and Davies (1964) report epileptiform, grand mal seizures with extreme opisthotonus. Although only one convulsed, the two patients examined before death (Johnson and Koumides, 1965; Popham and Davies, 1964) exhibited many similarities: both victims had a prior history of incapacitating respiratory disease; the estimated doses ingested were 250 and 440 mg./kg.; the terminal events were associated with a slow, steady intractable decline in blood pressure; and both died in about 20 hours. In Curry's case (1962) the dose was estimated at 1.2 to 1.8 gm./kg., but the peripheral blood concentration was 26 mg./100 ml., as compared with 23 mg./100 ml. in the case of Popham and Davies (1964). In an unsuccessful suicide by ingestion (Park *et al.*, 1977), a plasma 2,4-D level of 40 mg./100 ml. was measured.

Significant cumulative toxicity is not recognized. One individual consumed 500 mg. daily for 3 weeks with no perceptible effect (Assouly, 1951). In general, 2,4-D and most of its congeners are not metabolized. They do not accumulate in body fat or in the food chain. Urinary excretion, however, is rather slow. The plasma half-life of 2,4-D in man is said to be about 33 hours (Kohli *et al.*, 1974). On the other hand, in a comatose man with metabolic acidosis and an acid urine due to the ingestion of a mixture of the amine salts of 2,4-D and mecoprop (Park *et al.*, 1977), the plasma half-life of 2,4-D was estimated to be over 200 hours until an alkaline diuresis forced the urine pH above 8.0, when the plasma half-life fell to 4.7 hours. When a tracer dose of labeled 2,4-D was injected intravenously in a normal man, all of the ^{14}C was recovered in the urine, with a half-life of 13 hours (Feldmann and Maibach, 1974).

Seabury (1963) used herbicides to treat two patients with disseminated coccidioidomycosis. One patient received a total of 12.7 gm. of the sodium salt of 2,4-D over a period of 34 days. A single dose of 2 gm. intravenously was tolerated without incident, but after a 2-day rest, a single dose of 3.6 gm. produced stupor, hyporeflexia, fibrillary movements about the mouth and of the hands and forearms, and urinary incontinence. Recovery from those effects required 48 hours. Both patients eventually succumbed to the underlying disease (Seabury, 1963).

Goldstein and his associates (1959) described three cases of severe peripheral neuropathy in elderly patients apparently caused by the percutaneous absorption of a spilled 2,4-D ester. The initial signs and symptoms beginning some hours after exposure included fatigue, nausea, vomiting, anorexia, diarrhea, swelling and aching of the extremities, and muscle fasciculations. These symptoms progressed over a period of days until pain, paresthesias and limb paralysis were severe. Disability was protracted, and recovery was incomplete even after several years. Electromyographic examination supported the diagnosis of peripheral neuropathy. No elevation of body temperature was noted. Since the report of Goldstein *et al.* (1959), reports of similar cases have substantiated these observations (Berkley and Magee, 1963; Monarca and DiVito, 1961; Todd, 1962), but some of the muscle symptoms probably reflect an accompanying myopathy (Park *et al.*, 1977).

Desi *et al.* (1962) described experiments in which the parenteral administration of 2,4-D both acutely and chronically produced in animals reversible inhibition of cerebral electrical activity characterized by failure of EEG desynchronization in response to a sound stimulus. Studies of conditioned reflexes were interpreted as demonstrating a severe disturbance of higher nervous activity. The reticular formation was postulated as the point of attack. These changes were seen as early as 24 hours following exposure. The only suggestion of a cerebral action of 2,4-D in man is memory loss and temporary disorder of color vision reported in one acutely poisoned person (Brandt, 1971).

Fasting rats became distinctly poikilothermic for a period as long as 7 hours after a subcutaneous injection (200 to 300 mg./kg.) of 2,4-D or of 2,4,5-T (Sudak *et al.*, 1957, 1958; also C. L. Claff, personal communication, 1962). In a cold environment the metabolic rate rose only slightly, and the deep body temperature fell. Perhaps of more toxicological significance is the hypermetabolism and hyperthermia which occurred when injected rats were kept in a warm room (35° C.); apparently the death of these animals was due to hyperpyrexia. The phenomenon deserves more study, but one is reminded of the toxic syndrome that is recognized after exposure to 2,4-dinitrophenol or pentachlorophenol, both of which have produced human fatalities on hot days. Intoxication by these two substituted phenols is characterized by an uncoupling of tissue oxidative phosphorylation, and a similar lesion has been produced by 2,4-D in rat and fish liver mitochondria in phosphate-deficient media (Brody, 1952; Kuhn and Stein, 1965). The result is hypermetabolism, metabolic heat accumulation, and death from hyperpyrexia. For the clinical management of this syndrome, see pp. III-158 and IV-84. At least mild pyrexia has been reported in one human who ingested 2,4-D (Park et al., 1977).

Effects on thyroid function in the rat have also been noted. 2,4-D can effect a decrease in the serum level of PBI, apparently by competing for plasma protein-binding sites with thyroxin (Florsheim et al., 1963). It also increases the rate of ^{131}I uptake by rat thyroid in vivo by some unexplained mechanism (Florsheim and Velcoff, 1962).

2,4,5-T: The 2,4,5-trichloro derivative of phenoxyacetic acid (2,4,5-T) resembles 2,4-D but appears to be more irritating on skin and mucous membranes. For example, mucosal ulcers in the mouth, inflammation and stasis of the rumen, and enteritis have been described in cattle and sheep (e.g., Rowe and Hymas, 1954a; Palmer and Radeleff, 1964). Similar reactions have occurred with related trichlorophenoxy herbicides, such as silvex and Kuron. Three children who ate blackberries contaminated with 2,4,5-T experienced nausea and severe abdominal pain (Robert Lash, personal communication, 1960). Severe erythema and edema of skin and mucous membranes developed in two young girls exposed to a 2,4,5-T spray and to poison oak (Flint, 1959). These inflammatory lesions may have been due to dioxins (see Section II), which were and, to a lesser extent, still are present as impurities in commercial preparations of the trichlorophenoxy herbicides. Dioxins, however, are not found in 2,4-D or other dichlorophenoxy derivatives. The teratogenicity of 2,4,5-T may also be due to its dioxin content (Courtney and Moore, 1971).

Unlike 2,4-D and related disubstituted phenoxy herbicides, such as MCPA, the trichlorophenoxy compounds appear to generate few neural or neuromuscular disorders. Frank myotonia has not been reported, although mild spasticity has been observed in dogs (Drill and Hiratzka, 1953).

Like 2,4-D, 2,4,5-T is not extensively degraded in mammals. The plasma clearance in rats is markedly dependent on the size of the oral dose. The plasma half-life increased from 5 hours after 5 mg./kg. to 25 hours after 200 mg./kg. The apparent volume of distribution also increased with the dose, and a minor metabolite was found at the higher dose level. In contrast, the plasma half-life in dogs given 5 mg./kg. by mouth was 77 hours, suggesting why 2,4,5-T is more toxic to dogs than to rats (Piper et al., 1973). Human volunteers who consumed 5 mg./kg. of 2,4,5-T by mouth excreted essentially all the compound unchanged in urine; the plasma half-life was 23 hours (Gehring et al., 1973). In rats and rabbits, both 2,4,5-T and 2,4-D are transported by the renal tubular secretory mechanism for organic anions (Berndt and Koschier, 1973).

Symptomatology (partly inferential):
1. Fatigue, weakness, anorexia; perhaps nausea, vomiting and diarrhea.
2. Hyporeflexia and lethargy progressing to coma, with constricted pupils (miosis).
3. Flaccid paralysis has been described in one comatose patient, grand mal convulsions with opisthotonus in another, hypertonia with areflexia in a third, and twitching and jerking in a fourth (Jones et al., 1967).
4. At least in poisoned animals, sudden death has been ascribed to ventricular fibrillation and subsequent cardiac arrest.
5. Progressive decline in blood pressure with death in deep coma. The possibility that hyperpyrexia and hypermetabolism may have contributed to the fatal outcome does not appear to have been ruled out (one comatose patient was described as sweating profusely). A terminal pneumonia is likely.
6. Disturbances in body temperature regulation may be encountered. Perhaps severe reduction of body temperature in cool or cold environments. More probably, febrile responses in warm environments or during exercise.
7. Progressive hypotension with death in peripheral vascular collapse, perhaps associated with acidosis due to lactic acidemia and other products of hypermetabolism.
8. In nonfatal poisonings, severe and protracted neuritis with pain, paresthesias and weakness. Poisoned animals display muscle rigidity (myotonia), and humans have experienced muscle fasciculations as well as myotonia. Chronic exposure may lead to central nervous system defects in the control of motor function.

Treatment:
1. Gastric lavage if there are no signs of impending convulsions.
2. Cautious administration of a short-acting

anticonvulsant drug if convulsions appear to be imminent (pp. IV-35–39).

3. General supportive measures for central nervous depression (pp. IV-39–43).

4. If hypotension appears, search vigorously for a contributing cause (*e.g.*, dehydration, electrolyte imbalance, acidosis, myocardial disturbance, hyperpyrexia).

5. As appropriate, treat dehydration (p. IV-64), electrolyte disturbances (p. IV-66), acidosis (p. IV-69) and hyperpyrexia (p. IV-84).

6. To promote excretion of 2,4-D, initiate alkaline diuresis, as in salicylate poisoning (p. III-372), by injecting sodium bicarbonate intravenously (p. IV-72) until the urine pH exceeds 7.5, and then infuse mannitol (p. IV-52). The renal clearance rises sharply as urine pH rises above 7.5; above pH 8.0 it is said to be about 100-fold greater than at pH 6 (Park *et al.*, 1977).

7. If cardiac disturbances are suspected, monitor the ECG continuously when possible. Prepare to deliver defibrillating shocks in the event of ventricular fibrillation. See pp. IV-26–31.

8. If hypotension intensifies, a trial with a vasopressor drug may be appropriate (pp. IV-16–17). Epinephrine should be avoided because of possible ventricular fibrillation.

9. If myotonia appears, a trial with quinidine may be helpful (Eyzaguirre *et al.*, 1948).

10. Physiotherapy may be necessary for motor disorders associated with peripheral neuritis, myopathy or brain stem dysfunction.

Laboratory:

1. Repeated ECGs might prove helpful.
2. Albuminuria and increased protein levels in the cerebrospinal fluid are described.
3. EEGs to detect and monitor cerebral dysfunction. Nerve conduction tests and electromyograms to detect and monitor peripheral neuropathies and myopathies.
4. Test for elevated transaminase activities in serum and for occult blood in feces.
5. Muscle damage may be detected by elevations in serum creatine phosphokinase (Park *et al.*, 1977).

References:

Assouly, M. Desherbants selectifs et substances de croissance. Apercu technique. Effet pathologique sur l'homme au cours de la fabrication de l'ester du 2, 4-D. Arch Mal. Prof. *12*:26-30, 1951.

Audus, L. J. *The Physiology and Biochemistry of Herbicides.* Academic Press, New York, 1964.

Berkley, M. C.; Magee, K. R. Neuropathy following exposure to a dimethylamine salt of 2,4-D. Arch. Intern. Med. *111*:351-352, 1963.

Berndt, W. O.; Koschier, F. *In vitro* uptake of 2,4-dichloro.phenoxyacetic acid (2,4-D) and 2,4,5-trichloro-phenoxyacetic acid (2,4,5-T) by renal cortical tissue of rabbits and rats. Toxicol. Appl. Pharmacol. *26*:559-570, 1973.

Berwick, P. 2,4-Dichlorophenoxyacetic acid poisoning in man. J. A. M. A. *214*:1114-1117, 1970.

Brandt, M. R. Herbatoxforgiftning En kort oversigt og et nyt tilfaelde. Ugeskr. Laeger *133*:500-503, 1971.

Brody, T. M. Effect of certain plant growth substances on oxidative phosphorylation in rat liver mitochondria. Proc. Soc. Exp. Biol. Med. *80*:533-536, 1952.

Bucher, N. L. R. Toxicity of 2,4-dichlorophenoxyacetic acid on experimental animals. Proc. Soc. Exp. Biol. Med. *63*:204-205, 1946.

Courtney, K. D.; Moore, J. A. Teratology studies with 2, 4, 5-trichlorophenoxyacetic acid and 2,3,7,8-tetrachlorodibenzo-P-dioxin. Toxicol. Appl. Pharmacol. *20*:396-403, 1971.

Curry, A. S. Twenty-one uncommon cases of poisoning. Br. Med. J. *1*:687-689, 1962.

Dalgaard-Mikkelsen, S.; Poulsen, E. Toxicology of herbicides. Pharmacol. Rev. *14*:225-250, 1962.

Desi, I.; Sos, J.; Olasz, J.; Sule, F.; Markus, V. Nervous system effects of a chemical herbicide. Arch. Environ. Health *4*:95-102, 1962.

Drill, V. A.; Hiratzka, T. Toxicity of 2, 4-dichlorophenoxyacetic acid and 2,4,5-trichlorophenoxyacetic acid. Arch. Ind. Hyg. Occup. Med. *7*:61-67, 1953.

Dudley, A. W.; Thapar, N. T. Fatal human ingestion of 2,4-D, a common herbicide. Arch. Pathol. *94*:270-275, 1972.

Eyzaguirre, C.; Folk, B. D.; Zierler, K. L.; Lilienthal, J. L., Jr. Experimental myotonia and repetitive phenomena; the veratrinic effects of 2, 4-dichlorophenoxyacetate (2, 4-D) in the rat. Am. J. Physiol. *155*:69-77, 1948.

Feldmann, R. J.; Maibach, H. I. Percutaneous penetration of some pesticides and herbicides in man. Toxicol. Appl. Pharmacol. *28*:126-132, 1974.

Flint, T., Jr. Dermatitis and kidney damage ascribed to the weedkiller 2,4,5-T. Informal report written for the Bull. of Supplementary Material, Clinical Toxicology of Commercial Products. (Edited by M. N. Gleason, R. E. Gosselin and H. C. Hodge). *III*:No. 2, 1959.

Florsheim, W. H.; Velcoff, S. M. Some effects of 2,4-dichlorophenoxyacetic acid on thyroid function in the rat: Effects on iodine accumulation. Endocrinology *71*:1-6, 1962.

Florsheim, W. H.; Velcoff, S. M.; Williams, A. D. Some effects of 2,4-dichlorophenoxyacetic acid on thyroid function in the rat: Effects on peripheral thyroxine. Endocrinology *72*:327-333, 1963.

Gehring, P. J.; Kramer, C. G.; Schwetz, B. A.; Rose, J. Q.; Rowe, V. K. The fate of 2,4,5-trichlorophenoxyacetic acid (2,4,5-T) following oral administration to man. Toxicol. Appl. Pharmacol. *26*:352-361, 1973.

Goldstein, N. P.; Jones, P. H.; Brown, J. R. Peripheral neuropathy after exposure to an ester of dichlorophenoxyacetic acid. J. A. M. A. *171*:1306-1309, 1959.

Hill, E. C.; Carlisle, H. Toxicity of 2,4-dichlorophenoxyacetic acid for experimental animals. J. Ind. Hyg. Toxicol. *29*:85-95, 1947.

Johnson, H. R. M.; Koumides, O. A further case of MCPA poisoning. Br. Med. J. *2*:629-630, 1965.

Jones, D. I. R.; Knight, A. G.; Smith, A. J. Attempted suicide with herbicide containing MCPA. Arch. Environ. Health *14*:363-366, 1967.

Kay, J. H.; Palazzolo, R. J.; Calandra, J. C. Subacute dermal toxicity of 2,4-D. Arch. Environ. Health *11*:648-651, 1965.

Kohli, J. D.; Khanna, R. N.; Gupta, B. N.; Dhar, M. M.; Tandon, J. S.; Sircar, K. P. Absorption and excretion of 2, 4-dichlorophenoxyacetic acid in man. Xenobiotica *4*:97-100, 1974.

Kuhn, E.; Stein, W. Modellmyotonie nach 2,4-Dichlorphenoxyacetat (2,4-D) bei der Ratte. Klin. Wochensch. *12*:673-677, 1965.

Monarca, G.; DiVito, G. Akute Vergiftung durch 2,4-Dichlorophenoxyessigsaure. Folia Med. (Napoli) *44*:480-485, 1961.

Nielsen, K.; Kaempe, B.; Jensen-Holm, J. Fatal poisoning in man by 2,4-dichlorophenoxyacetic acid (2,4-D); determination of the agent in forensic materials. Acta Pharmacol.

Toxicol. 22:224-234, 1965.

Palmer, J. S.; Radeleff, R. D. The toxicologic effects of certain fungicides and herbicides on sheep and cattle. Ann. N. Y. Acad. Sci. 111: Art. 2, p. 729-736, 1964.

Park, J.; Darrien, I.; Prescott, L. F. Pharmacokinetic studies and severe intoxication with 2,4-D and mecoprop. Proc. Eur. Soc. Toxicol. 18:154-155, 1977.

Piper, W. N.; Rose, J. Q.; Leng, M. L.; Gehring, P. J. The fate of 2,4,5-trichlorophenoxyacetic acid (2,4,5-T) following oral administration to rats and dogs. Toxicol. Appl. Pharmacol. 26:339-351, 1973.

Popham, R. D.; Davies, D. M. A case of MCPA poisoning. Br. Med. J. 1:677-678, 1964.

Rowe, V. K.; Hymas, T. A. Summary of toxicological infor-

mation on 2,4-D and 2,4,5-T type herbicides and an evaluation of the hazards to livestock associated with their use. Am. J. Vet. Res. 15:622-629, 1954a.

Seabury, J. H. Toxicity of 2,4-dichlorophenoxyacetic acid for man and dog. Arch. Environ. Health 7:202-209, 1963.

Sudak, F. N.; Claff, C. L.; Cantor, M. H. Metabolic responses of albino rats treated with 2,4-dichlorophenoxyacetic acid to changes in ambient temperature. Biol. Bull. 113:357, 1957.

Sudak, F. N.; Claff, C. L.; Greenberg, A. Relation of halogen position to physiological properties of mono-, di-, and trichlorophenoxyacetic acid. Biol. Bull. 115:368, 1958.

Todd, R. L. A case of 2,4-D intoxication. J. Iowa Med. Soc. 52:663-664, 1962.

DDT

Since 1972, DDT has been virtually banned for domestic use, but a few exemptions or waivers have been granted. Prior to 1972, DDT played important roles in many phases of agriculture, in the control of insects of public health significance, and in the eradication of household pests. Technical DDT, which has 48 to 51% organic chlorine by weight, contains various isomers, of which two-thirds to three-quarters (by weight) is 1,1,1-trichloro-2,2-bis(p-chlorophenyl)ethane, or p,p'-DDT. The major contaminant is o,p'-DDT. A minor contaminant, o,p'-DDD, is used in the chemotherapy of adrenal tumors (mitotane).

DDT has been formulated as wettable powders, solutions, emulsions, aerosols, and dusts, in concentrations varying from 1 to 75%. At one time most common household insecticidal sprays consisted of a 5% solution of DDT in purified kerosene (e.g., Deobase). These commercial preparations are still found in and around many homes.

Useful sources of information on DDT and related pesticides include: Davies and Edmundson, 1972; Edwards, 1970; Müller, 1955 and 1959.

Toxicology: DDT has a wide margin of safety when used judiciously, and few if any adequately documented cases of DDT poisoning in man have ended fatally. The dry powder and aqueous suspensions are poorly absorbed from the gastrointestinal and respiratory tracts, and they do not penetrate the skin appreciably. Oils, fats, and lipid solvents (such as acetone, diethyl phthalate, etc.), however, enhance the absorption of DDT from all sites, including intact skin (Draize et al., 1944a; Taylor, 1945). Given by stomach tube to rats, a digestible vegetable oil significantly promoted the intestinal absorption of DDT, whereas mineral oil did not (Keller and Yeary, 1980). Both DDT and DDE (2,2-bis(p-chlorophenyl)-1,1-dichloroethylene) are extensively bound to human plasma proteins (Morgan et al., 1972).

The single oral dose of DDT necessary to produce untoward symptoms in man is about 10 mg./kg. After a dose of 16 mg./kg. or more, there are sometimes convulsions in the absence of effective treatment. Amounts at least as high as 285 mg./kg. have been ingested without fatalities, but since these doses lead promptly to vomiting, the amount actually retained is not known (Hayes, 1963, 1982). Although considerable individual variation is recognized, the value generally accepted as an acute mean lethal dose (LD_{50}) in rats is 250 mg./kg. (Woodward et al., 1944); it is perhaps a reasonable estimate for man. Fats and oils enhance toxicity by promoting absorption. In many instances of alleged poisoning the principal symptoms have been due to the commercial vehicle (usually kerosene), not to DDT (Hill and Robinson, 1945; Reingold and Lasky, 1947); but see also the report by Biden-Steele and Stuckey (1946).

In mice the acute toxicity of technical DDT mixture appeared to be due almost exclusively to p,p'-DDT. The toxicity of such mixtures decreased in proportion to their content of o,p'-DDT. Perhaps because of intensive redistribution and storage, the acute toxicity of DDT is less the larger the amount of body fat (Okey and Page, 1974). Wide species differences in acute lethal doses may be related to differences in the permeability of the blood-brain barrier (Gingell and Wallcave, 1974).

DDT acts primarily on the central nervous system; the cerebellum and higher motor cortex appear to be the chief sites of action. Abnormal EEG patterns have been observed in occupationally exposed workmen even in the absence of abnormal neurological findings (Mayersdorf and Israeli, 1974). In rats a good correlation has been demonstrated between brain levels of DDT and toxic signs and symptoms (Dale et al., 1963).

Clinical manifestations include paresthesias, tremors, and convulsions (Campbell, 1949; Cunningham and Hill, 1952; Hsieh, 1954). In addition, peripheral neuropathy has been rarely ascribed to DDT, usually to a chronic occupational exposure; one syndrome consists of numbness and paresthesias, hypotonia, and asymmetric weakness or paralysis, with a slow spontaneous recovery when the exposure is terminated (Jenkins and Toole, 1964; Mackerras and West, 1946; Onifer and Whisnant, 1957). Effects on the mechanical characteristics of skeletal muscle in rats result in significant decreases in tension (Santolucito and Whitcomb, 1971).

In isolated nerve axons, DDT results in a prolongation of action potentials, repetitive firing after a single stimulus and spontaneous trains of action potentials (Narahashi and Hass, 1967), but the relationship of these peripheral effects to the established site of action of DDT in the central nervous system is not known (Joy, 1973). In toxic doses in mice and rats, DDT myoclonus was aggravated by serotonin (5-HT) antagonists and decreased by drugs that increased serotonergic activity, suggesting that the seizures were due to central blockade of 5-HT receptors or to decreased 5-HT release (Hwang and Van Woert, 1978). Others, however, have reported changes in brain levels of norepinephrine, acetylcholine and ammonia (Hrdina et al., 1975).

Most pathologists deny the existence of histopathological lesions in the brain of DDT-poisoned animals, with the exception of small petechial hemorrhages resulting from convulsions. Only in animals given large and/or repeated doses of DDT is it possible to find consistent pathological lesions, namely liver cell necrosis and mild degeneration of kidney tubular epithelium (Ortega et al., 1956). In the rat a characteristic hepatic lesion is described (Ortega, 1966). Liver and kidney dysfunctions have not been described in human poisonings (with perhaps one exception: Smith, 1948). Workers exposed for more than 20 years to levels equivalent to a daily intake of 4 to 18 mg. showed no signs of hepatic disease or liver function abnormality (Laws et al., 1973).

Primary skin irritation is rarely if ever due to DDT, and allergic dermatitis has been reported only occasionally (Higgens and Kindel, 1949). Purpura with marked thrombocytopenia has occurred in exposed children (Karpinski, 1950). An isolated case of agranulocytosis (Wright et al., 1946) and postmortem findings resembling periarteritis nodosa (Hill and Damiani, 1946) suggest more serious allergic manifestations. Indeed, an impressive body of circumstantial evidence has gradually accumulated to implicate DDT as a cause of aplastic anemia and thrombocytopenia (Sánchez-Medal et al., 1963).

Perhaps uniquely in dogs, DDT appears to sensitize the heart to endogenous catecholamines, with sudden death in ventricular fibrillation (Philips and Gilman, 1946; Philips et al., 1946). When rats and rabbits were fed DDT, however, and then given vasopressin to induce myocardial ischemia, no increase in the incidence of arrhythmias was noted. The hearts were not more sensitive to norepinephrine, and isolated heart muscle behaved like that from control animals despite a tissue DDT content that was 100-fold higher (Jeyaratnam and Forshaw, 1974). With respect to humans, the issue is not clear, but if not DDT, the hydrocarbon solvents in which it has been marketed are known to sensitize the heart to catecholamines with the occasional production of arrhythmias.

In acute exposures, recovery is usually complete or well advanced in 24 hours. Aside from rare peripheral neuropathies and aplastic anemia (see above), no clinical syndrome of chronic intoxication is recognized in man (Hayes et al., 1956, 1971). After a single dose or small repeated doses, however, DDT and some metabolic degradation products accumulate in body fat, where they remain in a largely inactive form for long periods of time. The principal stored metabolite is DDE.

Biopsy specimens of human subcutaneous fat and other adipose tissue have been analyzed for DDT residues. There has been no progressive increase in human fat levels of DDT in this country since 1951, and the general population is assumed to have reached or perhaps passed a state of dynamic equilibrium with respect to environmental exposure (Hoffman et al., 1964; Quimby et al., 1965). Concentrations in human fat often correlate with dietary patterns or geographical location, but the major differences among individuals probably relate to occupational exposure (Durham et al., 1961; Hayes et al., 1958; Read and McKinley, 1961). In a community downstream of a defunct DDT factory, the major determinant of body burden was age, followed by fish consumption (Kreiss et al., 1981).

Some ingested DDT is metabolized in a slow series of dehydrohalogenation reactions and eventually excreted in the urine and feces as DDA, which is bis(p-chlorophenyl)acetic acid (Peterson and Robison, 1964; Pinto et al., 1965). This process is apparently accelerated in individuals on chronic drug therapy with phenobarbital and/or phenytoin, presumably because of induction of hepatic microsomal enzymes (Watson et al., 1972). Thus, a mechanism exists for decreasing the total body burden of DDT and derived materials, but since these stores have not yet been associated with harmful effects, there is no reason for instituting such measures. DDT and DDE are excreted in human breast milk (Wilson et al., 1973), but again this phenomenon has not been demonstrated as a clear-cut health hazard to nursing infants (Rogan et al., 1980).

Other phenomena related to the fat storage of halogenated hydrocarbon insecticides are still being evaluated for their significance to man. Interactions among different kinds of insecticides are recognized. Some of these interactions relate to mutual influences on metabolism and may be manifested in unpredictable ways (Street and Blau, 1966). Possible effects of starvation on body stores of DDT have been examined. At storage levels considerably higher than those in the human population, starvation has precipitated symptoms of acute DDT poisoning in rats because of the sudden mobilization of these stores (Dale *et al.*, 1962). Finally, DDT and related compounds are known to induce hepatic microsomal enzyme activity, and effects on the metabolism of both endogenous and exogenous substrates can be demonstrated in animals at fat levels equivalent to those of the present human population (Conney *et al.*, 1967).

A long-lasting decrease in glucose tolerance without concomitant effects on basal blood glucose has been described in mice. Apparently, DDT can decrease insulin secretion by the pancreas (You and Mennear, 1977). Others, however, have reported that DDT alters glucose homeostasis by activating adenylate cyclase in the liver and kidney cortex, resulting in hyperglycemia, glycosuria and decreases in liver glycogen (Singhal and Kacew, 1976).

DDT interferes with the metabolism and function of steroid hormones by at least two known mechanisms. The induction of hepatic microsomal enzymes results in an increased conversion of estrogens, androgens and glucocorticoids to more polar metabolites. The increased urinary excretion of the latter is usually compensated for by increased steroid biosynthesis. The *o,p'*-DDT contaminant acts like estradiol and bonds to a uterine cytosolic receptor to induce uterine enzymes, especially ornithine decarboxylase. An alleged antiandrogenic activity has not been satisfactorily explained (Kupfer, 1975; Kupfer and Bulger, 1976). DDT is not carcinogenic in mice or rats, but DDE is carcinogenic in both sexes of mice (National Cancer Institute, 1978r).

Symptomatology (onset is usually 2 to 3 hours after ingestion):

1. Very large doses are followed promptly by vomiting due to local gastric irritation. Delayed emesis and/or diarrhea may occur (the mechanism is not understood).
2. Numbness and paresthesias, usually first of lips, tongue, and face.
3. Malaise, headache, sore throat, fatigue, weakness.
4. Coarse tremors (usually first of the neck and head and particularly of the eyelids), apprehension, ataxia, and confusion.
5. Convulsions, both clonic and tonic. Convulsions may alternate with periods of coma and paresis.
6. In the absence of convulsions, the vital signs are essentially normal, but in severe poisoning the pulse may be irregular and abnormally slow. Whether DDT, the solvent or the convulsions are responsible for occasional disorders in the cardiac mechanism is not clear.
7. Hyperthermia and signs of sympathetic discharge have been described in animals (Hrdina *et al.*, 1973; Philips and Gilman, 1946).
8. If pulmonary edema supervenes, it is probably an expression of solvent intoxication (see kerosene poisoning, p. III-220).
9. Death is usually due to respiratory failure from medullary paralysis.
10. In acute exposures, recovery is usually complete within 1 to 3 days, but sometimes weakness or paralysis and ataxia may persist for weeks.

Treatment:

1. In any ingestion episode not involving a hydrocarbon solvent, induce vomiting by administering syrup of ipecac (see Section I) or empty the stomach by gastric aspiration and lavage with tap water (if convulsions are not imminent).
2. Saline cathartic, *e.g.*, sodium sulfate (15 to 30 gm.) left in the stomach (although this treatment did not significantly reduce absorption in rats, according to Keller and Yeary, 1980).
3. Phenobarbital (0.1 gm.) prophylactically in the absence of central nervous signs and symptoms. Parenteral diazepam or barbiturate therapy if tremors or convulsions develop. See pp. IV-35–39.
4. Calcium gluconate (10 cc. of 10% solution given slowly by intravenous injection) is useful (in addition to sedation) to control DDT convulsions in experimental animals and perhaps in man.
5. Avoid fats, oils, and fat solvents, epinephrine, sudden strong external stimuli.
6. Rest and observation for at least 24 hours.
7. Give parenteral fluids as needed.

Laboratory:

1. When the diagnosis is uncertain, the urine can be examined for the presence of DDA (bis(*p*-chlorophenyl)acetic acid).
2. Biochemical tests to detect liver and kidney dysfunction should be performed, although the results are expected to be negative. See pp. IV-59 and 52.
3. Hyperlipoproteinemia has been observed in men chronically exposed to DDT and lindane (Carlson and Kolmodin-Hedman, 1972).
4. Determinations of blood sugar and of sugar tolerance are desirable.

References:

Biden-Steele, K.; Stuckey, R. E. Poisoning by DDT emulsion. Lancet 2:235-236, 1946.

Campbell, A. M. G. A suspected case of DDT poisoning in man. Lancet 2:1178, 1949.

Carlson, L. A.; Kolmodin-Hedman, B. Hyper-α-lipoproteinemia in men exposed to chlorinated hydrocarbon pesticides. Acta. Med. Scand. 192:29-32, 1972.

Conney, A. H.; Welch, R. M.; Kuntzman, R.; Burns, J. J. Effects of pesticides on drug and steroid metabolism. Clin. Pharmacol. Ther. 8:2-10, 1967.

Cunningham, R. E.; Hill, F. S. Convulsions and deafness following ingestion of DDT. Pediatrics 9:745-747, 1952.

Dale, W. E.; Gaines, T. B.; Hayes, W. J., Jr. Storage and excretion of DDT in starved rats. Toxicol. Appl. Pharmacol. 4:89-106, 1962.

Dale, W. E.; Gaines, T. B.; Hayes, W. J., Jr.; Pearce, G. W. Poisoning by DDT: Relation between clinical signs and concentration in rat brain. Science 142:1474-1476, 1963.

Davies, J. E.; Edmundson, W. F. Epidemiology of DDT. Futura Publishing Co., New York, 1972.

Draize, J. H.; Nelson, A. A.; Calvery, H. L. The percutaneous absorption of DDT (2, 2-bis(p-chlorophenyl)-1,1,1-trichloroethane) in laboratory animals. J. Pharmacol. Exp. Ther. 82:159-166, 1944a.

Durham, W. F.; Armstrong, J. F.; Upholt, W. M.; Heller, C. Insecticide content of diet and body fat of Alaskan natives. Science 134:1880-1881, 1961.

Edwards, C. A. Persistent Pesticides in the Environment. Chemical Rubber Co., Cleveland, 1970.

Gingell, R.; Wallcave, L. Species differences in the acute toxicity and tissue distribution of DDT in mice and hamsters. Toxicol. Appl. Pharmacol. 28:385-394, 1974.

Hayes, W. J., Jr. Clinical Handbook on Economic Poisons. USPHS Publication No. 476. U. S. Government Printing Office, Washington, D. C., 1963.

Hayes, W. J., Jr. Pesticides Studied in Man. Williams & Wilkins, Baltimore, Md, 1982.

Hayes, W. J., Jr.; Dale, W. E.; Pirkle, C. I. Evidence of safety of long term, high oral doses of DDT for man. Arch. Environ. Health 22:119-135, 1971.

Hayes, W. J., Jr.; Durham, W. F.; Cueto, C., Jr. The effect of known repeated oral doses of chlorophenothane (DDT) in man. J. A. M. A. 162:890-897, 1956.

Hayes, W. J., Jr.; Quimby, G. E.; Walker, K. C.; Elliot, J. W.; Upholt, W. M. Storage of DDT and DDE in people with different degrees of exposure to DDT. Arch. Ind. Health 18:398-403, 1958.

Higgins, E. L.; Kindel, D. J. Exfoliative dermatitis from contact with DDT. J. Invest. Dermatol. 12:207-209, 1949.

Hill, K. R.; Robinson, G. A fatal case of DDT poisoning in a child, with an account of two accidental deaths in dogs. Br. Med. J. 2:845-847, 1945.

Hill, W. R.; Damiani, C. R. Death following exposure to DDT. Report of a case. N. Engl. J. Med. 235:897-899, 1946.

Hoffman, W. S.; Fishbein, W. I.; Andelman, M. B. Pesticide storage in human fat tissue. J. A. M. A. 188:819, 1964.

Hrdina, P. D.; Singhal, R. L.; Ling, G. M. DDT and related chlorinated hydrocarbon insecticides: Pharmacological basis of their toxicity in mammals. Adv. Pharmacol. Chemother. 12:31-83, 1975.

Hrdina, P. D.; Singhal, R. L.; Peters, D. A. V.; Ling, G. M. Some neurochemical alterations during acute DDT poisoning. Toxicol. Appl. Pharmacol. 25:276-288, 1973.

Hsieh, H. C. DDT intoxication in a family of southern Taiwan. Arch. Ind. Hyg. Occup. Med. 10:344-346, 1954.

Hwang, E. C.; Van Woert, M. H. p,p'-DDT-induced neurotoxic syndrome: Experimental myoclonus. Neurol. 28:1020-1025, 1978.

Jenkins, R. B.; Toole, J. F. Polyneuropathy following exposure to insecticides. Arch. Intern. Med. 113:691-695, 1964.

Jeyaratnam, J.; Forshaw, P. J. A study of the cardiac effects of DDT in laboratory animals. Bull. W. H. O. 51:531-535,

1974.

Joy, R. M. Electrical correlates of preconvulsive and convulsive doses of chlorinated hydrocarbon in the CNS. Neuropharmacology 12:63-76, 1973.

Karpinski, F. E., Jr. Purpura following exposure to DDT. J. Pediatr. 37:373-379, 1950.

Keller, W. C.; Yeary, R. A. A comparison of the effects of mineral oil, vegetable oil, and sodium sulfate on the intestinal absorption of DDT in rodents. Clin. Toxicol. 16:223-231, 1980.

Kreiss, K.; Zack, M. M.; Kimbrough, R. D.; Needham, L. L.; Smrek, A. L.; Jones, B. T. Cross-sectional study of a community with exceptional exposure to DDT. J. A. M. A. 245:1926-1930, 1981.

Kupfer, D. Effects of pesticides and related compounds on steroid metabolism and function. CRC Crit. Rev. Toxicol. 4:83-124, 1975.

Kupfer, D.; Bulger, W. H. Interactions of chlorinated hydrocarbons with steroid hormones. Fed. Proc. 35:2603-2608, 1976.

Laws, E. R.; Maddrey, W. C.; Curley, A.; Burse, V. W. Long-term occupational exposure to DDT. Arch. Environ. Health 27:318-321, 1973.

Mackerras, I. M.; West, R. F. K. "DDT" poisoning in man. Med. J. Aust. 1:400-401, 1946.

Mayersdorf, A.; Israeli, R. Toxic effects of chlorinated hydrocarbon insecticides on the human electroencephalogram. Arch. Environ. Health 28:159-163, 1974.

Morgan, D. P.; Roan, C. C.; Paschal, E. H. Transport of DDT, DDE and dieldrin in human blood. Bull. Environ. Contam. Toxicol. 8:321-325, 1972.

Muller, P. Das Insektizid Dichlordiphenyltrichlorathan und seine Bedeutung. Vol. I and II. Berkhauser Verlag, Basel, 1955 and 1959.

Narahashi, T.; Hass, H. G. DDT: Interaction with nerve membrane conductance changes. Science 157:1438-1440, 1967.

National Cancer Institute, U. S. DHEW, Public Health Service. Bioassays of DDT, TDE, and p,p'-DDE for possible carcinogenicity. Technical Report Series no. 131, Publication no. 78-1386, 1978r.

Okey, A. B.; Page, D. J. Acute toxicity of o,p'-DDT to mice. Bull. Environ. Contam. Toxicol. 11:359-363, 1974.

Onifer, T. M.; Whisnant, J. P. Cerebellar ataxia and neuronitis after exposure to DDT and lindane. Proc. Mayo Clin. 32:67-72, 1957.

Ortega, P. Light and electron microscopy of dichlorodiphenyltrichloroethane (DDT) poisoning in the rat liver. Lab. Invest. 15:657-679, 1966.

Ortega, P.; Hayes, W. J., Jr.; Durham, W. F.; Mattson, A. DDT in the diet of the rat. U. S. Public Health Serv. Public Health Monograph No. 43, 1956.

Peterson, J. E.; Robison, W. H. Metabolic products of p,p'-DDT in the rat. Toxicol. Appl. Pharmacol. 6:321-327, 1964.

Philips, F. S.; Gilman, A. Studies on the pharmacology of DDT (2,2-bis-(parachlorophenyl)-1,1,1-trichloroethane); I. The acute toxicity of DDT following intravenous injection in mammals with observations on the treatment of acute DDT poisoning. J. Pharmacol. Exp. Ther. 86:213-221, 1946.

Philips, F. S.; Gilman, A.; Crescitelli, F. N. Studies on the pharmacology of DDT (2,2-bis(parachlorophenyl)-1,1,1-trichloroethane); II. The sensitization of the myocardium to sympathetic stimulation during acute DDT intoxication. J. Pharmacol. Exp. Ther. 86:222-228, 1946.

Pinto, J. D.; Camien, M. N.; Dunn, M. S. Metabolic fate of p,p'-DDT (1,1,1-trichloro-2,2-bis(p-chlorophenyl)ethane) in rats. J. Biol. Chem. 240:2148-2154, 1965.

Quimby, G. E.; Hayes, W. J., Jr.; Armstrong, J. F.; Durham, W. F. DDT storage in the U. S. population. J. A. M. A. 191:175-179, 1965.

Read, S. I.; McKinley, W. P. DDT and DDE content of human fat. A survey. Arch. Environ. Health 3:209-211, 1961.

Reingold, I. M.; Lasky, I. I. Acute fatal poisoning following ingestion of a solution of DDT. Ann. Intern. Med. 26:945-

947, 1947.

Rogan, W. J.; Bagniewska, A.; Damstra, T. Pollutants in breast milk. N. Engl. J. Med. *302*:1450-1453, 1980.

Sanchez-Medal, L.; Castanedo, J. P.; Garcia-Rojas, F. Insecticides and aplastic anemia. N. Engl. J. Med. *269*:1365-1367, 1963.

Santolucito, J. A.; Whitcomb, E. Mechanical response of skeletal muscle following oral administration of pesticides. Toxicol. Appl. Pharmacol. *20*:66-72, 1971.

Singhal, R. L.; Kacew, S. The role of cyclic AMP in chlorinated hydrocarbon-induced toxicity. Fed. Proc. *35*:2618-2623, 1976.

Smith, N. J. Death following accidental ingestion of DDT. J. A. M. A. *136*:469-471, 1948.

Street, J. C.; Blau, A. D. Insecticide interactions affecting residue accumulation in animal tissues. Toxicol. Appl. Pharmacol. *8*:497-504, 1966.

Taylor, E. L. Danger of inunction with DDT. Lancet *2*:320, 1945.

Watson, M.; Gabica, J.; Benson, W. W. Serum organochlorine pesticides in mentally retarded patients on differing drug regimens. Clin. Pharmacol. Ther. *13*:186-192, 1972.

Wilson, D. J.; Locker, D. J.; Ritzen, C. A.; Watson, J. T.; Schaffner, W. DDT concentrations in human milk. Am. J. Dis. Child. *125*:814-817, 1973.

Woodward, G.; Nelson, A. A.; Calvery, H. O. Acute and subacute toxicity of DDT (2, 2-bis(*p*-chlorophenyl)-1, 1, 1-trichloroethane) to laboratory animals. J. Pharmacol. Exp. Ther. *82*:152-158, 1944.

Wright, C.; Doan, C. A.; Haynie, H. C. Agranulocytosis occurring after exposure to a DDT pyrethrum bomb. Am. J. Med. *1*:562-567, 1946.

You, E. T.; Mennear, J. H. The inhibitory effect of DDT on insulin secretion in mice. Toxicol. Appl. Pharmacol. *39*:81-88, 1977.

DIAZEPAM

Diazepam is one of a rapidly growing group of benzodiazepine derivatives used as hypnotics, sedatives, antianxiety agents, anticonvulsants, muscle relaxants, anesthetics and preanesthetics. The first to be introduced was chlordiazepoxide. At present it and diazepam may be the two most widely prescribed drugs in the United States. Table III-5 lists other members of the group, some of which are not yet available in the United States.

Diazepam and chlordiazepoxide are sold in injectable forms as well as in tablets and capsules. Table III-5 indicates the usual adult daily therapeutic doses, but considerably larger doses are sometimes employed in selected patients. The daily dose may be taken once at night as with flurazepam or in divided amounts 2 to 4 times a day as with diazepam and chlordiazepoxide.

Toxicology: The safety record of the benzodiazepines is remarkably good in view of the enormous volume of their use and the highly suicidal population for which they are often prescribed. Overdosage is frequent, but severe poisonings are rare, and deaths are almost unknown. In the few fatal cases the dose was unknown, and other complicating factors may have contributed to the demise (Cardauns and Iffland, 1973; McBay, 1966). It is difficult to estimate the adult mean lethal dose by mouth for any of the benzodiazepines. Laboratory animal data (Table III-5) suggest that most derivatives are in toxicity class 3 or even borderline class 2. Chlordiazepoxide and flunitrazepam are the most toxic to rats, and they lie only on the borderline between classes 3 and 4.

Among the more severe poisonings reported in adults is the case of a 54-year-old diabetic who consumed 4.3 gm. of oxazepam. He was comatose for 12 days and was resuscitated from respiratory arrest before making a complete recovery (Ayd, 1975). A 16-year-old male was comatose for 24 hours after ingesting 900 mg. oxazepam (Ayd, 1975). At least 5 patients were in coma after oral doses of chlordiazepoxide ranging from 300 to 600 mg., but all recovered fully (Essig, 1964; Schaefer, 1962; Zbinden *et al.*, 1961). Doses of 400 to 2000 mg. of diazepam have produced moderately deep coma, but some of these patients were discharged after as little as 48 hours of hospitalization (Greenblatt *et al.*, 1978b; Varma *et al.*, 1977). In Varma's case (1977), bullae and eccrine sweat gland necrosis occurred like that described in barbiturate and carbon monoxide coma.

In contrast to the above cases, ingestions of massive amounts of benzodiazepines have been reported without the occurrence of coma, hypotension or respiratory depression. This disparity suggests considerable variation in individual sensitivity. At least 8 adults have consumed single doses of chlordiazepoxide ranging from 875 to 2,250 mg. without serious complications. Their poisonings were characterized by such mild signs as drowsiness, ataxia, dysarthria, bilateral nystagmus, and moderate incoordination of the upper extremities (Clarke *et al.*, 1961; Davis *et al.*, 1968; Essig, 1964; Jenner and Parkin, 1961; Smith, 1961b).

In one study, patients who had consumed flurazepam were significantly more drowsy on arrival at the emergency room than were those who had consumed other benzodiazepines. Only 2.6% of individuals overdosed exclusively with benzodiazepines were unconscious on arrival at a treatment center, whereas 15 to 16% of those who had taken other depressant drugs, with or without benzodiazepines, were comatose (Busto *et al.*, 1980). One group has concluded that if the patient cannot be aroused, another drug or another cause for the coma should be sought (Cate and Jatlow, 1973; Gjerros, 1966; Greenblatt *et al.*, 1977).

A few severe poisonings with benzodiazepines have occurred among young children, but as a general rule the experience with children accords

Table III-5.
Acute Toxicity of Benzodiazepines

Generic Name	Trade Name	Daily Adult Therapeutic Dose by Mouth (mg.)	Acute Oral LD$_{50}$ (mg./kg.)	Species	Reference
Chlordiazepoxide	Librium	15–60	540	Rat	Owen et al., 1970
Clonazepam	Clonapin	1.5	>4000	Mouse	
Clorazepate	Tranxene	30	1320	Rat	Physicians' Desk Reference, 1981
Diazepam	Valium	4–40	1520	Rat	Owen et al., 1970
Flunitrazepam	Rohypnol	1–2	485	Rat	Garattini et al., 1973
Flurazepam	Dalmane	15–30	1300	Rat	Goldenthal, 1971
Lorazepam	Ativan	2–6	>5000	Rat	Merck, 9th ed., 1976
Medazepam	Nobrium		900	Rat	Goldenthal, 1971
Nitrazepam	Mogadon		825	Rat	Goldenthal, 1971
Oxazepam	Serax	30–60	>5000	Rat	Owen et al., 1970
Prazepam	Centrax	20–60	>4000	Dog	Kakishita et al., 1978b

with that in adults. After ingesting 70 mg. of diazepam, one 2-year-old had repeated episodes of cardiac arrest from which she was successfully resuscitated (Berger et al., 1975). Drowsiness, ataxia, hyporeflexia, muscular weakness and coma have occurred in children aged 2 through 5 after doses of 20 to 200 mg. diazepam (Bell, 1975; Berger et al., 1975; DiLiberti et al., 1975; Spark and Goldman, 1965) or 90 mg. oxazepam (Ayd, 1975). Most made a full and rapid recovery.

Rarely, after doses similar to those above, young children exhibit a paradoxical excitement phase which may then be followed by a depressant phase (Herzka and Haber, 1965). In one such case the signs persisted for several days after the blood concentration of oxazepam had fallen to zero. In addition, an unusual facial edema was described (Shimkin and Shaivitz, 1966). Lorazepam-induced delirium occurred in 2 patients postoperatively (Blitt and Petty, 1975).

An intravenous dose of 120 mg. diazepam given just prior to delivery was held responsible for apneic attacks in the newborn infant. The infant had 34 such episodes in the first 23 hours after birth. Previously an infant with a similar history had been lost after 5 days of assisted ventilation (Thearle and Hailey, 1973).

In addition to low intrinsic toxicity, benzodiazepines exhibit few clinically significant drug interactions when taken in therapeutic doses (Shader et al., 1975). An interaction between chlordiazepoxide and ethyl alcohol, resulting in greater than additive effects, has been shown in mice (Gebhart et al., 1969), and a prolongation of the biological half-life of diazepam by alcohol has been shown in human subjects (Sellers et al., 1980). Cimetidine also decreased the plasma clearance of diazepam in humans, probably by inhibiting its metabolism by hepatic microsomal enzymes (Klotz et al., 1979).

Exchange transfusions in a severely poisoned infant (Thearle and Hailey, 1973) and in an adult who had been comatose for 3 days (Zileli et al., 1972) apparently were effective in decreasing the time course of the intoxication. Forced saline diuresis in dogs, however, did little to enhance the renal excretion of chlordiazepoxide (Rice et al., 1972). It is difficult to evaluate limited experience with hemodialysis in benzodiazepine poisoning (Cruz et al., 1967).

Physostigmine was said to reverse rapidly a coma induced in an adult by an overdose of thioridazine and diazepam (Bernards, 1973) and a coma in an infant caused by diazepam (DiLiberti et al., 1975). It was also said to have been effective in lorazepam delirium (Blitt and Petty, 1975). Experimental studies have produced contradictory data on the effects of physostigmine in benzodiazepine poisoning. It was reported to be ineffective in reversing diazepam-induced loss of righting reflex in mice and rats (Walz and Davis, 1979). Others, however, found a surprisingly strong antidotal effect against diazepam in rabbits, cats and rats. The EEGs were restored to normal, behavior was normalized, and mortality was significantly decreased (Nagy and Decsi, 1978). Naloxone was said to reverse quickly a diazepam-induced coma in an infant (Bell, 1975). Similarly in mice and rats it reversed the loss of righting reflex but without decreasing mortality (Walz and Davis, 1979). No rationale can be offered at present for the use of either agent in poisonings by benzodiazepines.

Benzodiazepines are absorbed at varying rates, which are said to be slow for oxazepam and lorazepam and fast for chlordiazepoxide, diazepam and flurazepam. They are extensively bound to plasma proteins and are metabolized in complex patterns by hepatic microsomal enzymes. Many have active metabolites, but oxazepam and lorazepam apparently do not.

Tolerance, physical dependence and a withdrawal syndrome are now recognized as possible sequelae to long-term, high-dose therapy with benzodiazepines. This dependence is of the type described variously as "barbiturate" or "alcohol-barbiturate." Reports of agitation, insomnia, grand mal seizures, organic brain syndrome, and paradoxical extended coma have appeared (DeBard, 1979; Hollister et al., 1961c). Other studies, however, indicate that the physical dependence is slower to develop and less threatening than that with meprobamate or barbiturates and that its hazards may have been exaggerated (Essig, 1964; Greenblatt and Shader, 1978a).

Several benzodiazepines are teratogenic in laboratory animals (Jurand, 1980; Shah et al., 1979). These drugs tend to be weak inducers of hepatic microsomal enzymes.

Symptomatology:

1. Occasionally, paradoxical excitement, delirium, hallucinations and even convulsions, as described in animals and young children.
2. When the excitement phase occurs, it may be followed by the more usual signs of nausea, vomiting, drowsiness, lethargy, ataxia, hyporeflexia, muscular weakness, dysarthria, nystagmus and coma.
3. Hypotension and respiratory failure are uncommon but should be anticipated in massive overdoses.
4. Death in respiratory or cardiac arrest, or progression to complete recovery.

Treatment:

1. If the patient is awake and neither loss of consciousness nor convulsions are imminent, give by mouth syrup of ipecac (p. I-2) or a slurry of activated charcoal (p. I-4).
2. Gastric lavage with warm water or saline as soon as practical if productive vomiting is not produced by syrup of ipecac or if ipecac cannot be used. Precautions against aspiration are essential (I-10), especially in the comatose patient.
3. After lavage, leave in the stomach 15 to 30 gm. of sodium sulfate in water as an osmotic cathartic and a slurry of activated charcoal (p. I-12).
4. If sensory stimuli arouse the comatose patient even briefly and if respirations are full and regular, further treatment may not be required, but he should be kept under observation until fully conscious.
5. Monitor vital signs and be prepared to administer cardiopulmonary resuscitation (pp. IV-26–31).
6. Correct airway obstruction and give oxygen if warranted (p. IV-2).
7. Correct dehydration. Practice good nursing care.
8. More vigorous measures are rarely warranted, and such techniques as hemodialysis are not of proven value in benzodiazepine poisoning.

Laboratory:

1. Poor correlations have been noted between the severity of the intoxication and plasma concentrations of benzodiazepines.
2. Oxazepam gives a false positive reaction in the Somogyi blood glucose determination but not with the glucose oxidase technique (Zileli et al., 1972).

References:

Ayd, F. J., Jr. Oxazepam: an overview. Dis. Nervous System 36:14-16, 1975.

Bell, E. F. Use of naloxone in treatment of diazepam poisoning. J. Pediatr. 87:803-804, 1975.

Berger, R.; Green, G.; Meinick, A. Cardiac arrest caused by oral diazepam intoxication. Clin. Pediatr. 14:842-844, 1975.

Bernards, W. Reversal of phenothiazine-induced coma with physostigmine. Anesth. Analg. 52:938-941, 1973.

Blitt, C. D.; Petty, W. C. Reversal of lorazepam delirium by physostigmine. Anesth. Analg. 54:607-608, 1975.

Busto, U.; Kaplan, H. L.; Sellers, E. M. Benzodiazepine-associated emergencies in Toronto. Am. J. Psychiatr. 137:224-227, 1980.

Cardauns, H.; Iffland, R. Fatal intoxication of a young drug addict with diazepam. Arch. Toxikol. 31:147-151, 1973.

Cate, J. C.; Jatlow, I. Chlordiazepoxide overdose: interpretation of serum drug concentrations. Clin. Toxicol. 6:553-561, 1973.

Clarke, T. P.; Simpson, T. R.; Wise, S. P., III. Two unsuccessful suicidal attempts with a new drug: methaminodiazepoxide (librium). Texas State J. Med. 57:24-26, 1961.

Cruz, H. A.; Cramer, N. C.; Parrish, A. E. Hemodialysis in chlordiazepoxide toxicity. J. A. M. A. 202:438-440, 1967.

Davis, J. M.; Bartlett, E.; Termini, B. A. Overdosage of psychotropic drugs: A review. Dis. Nerv. Syst. 29:157-164 and 246-256, 1968.

DeBard, M. L. Diazepam withdrawal syndrome - case with psychosis, seizure, and coma. Am. J. Psychiatr. 136:104-105, 1979.

DiLiberti, J.; O'Brien, M. L.; Tainer, T. Use of physostigmine as an antidote in accidental diazepam intoxication. J. Pediatr. 86:106-107, 1975.

Essig, C. F. Addiction to nonbarbiturate sedative and tranquilizing drugs. Clin. Pharmacol. Ther. 5:334-343, 1964.

Garattini, S.; Mussini, E.; Randall, L. O. (editors). The Benzodiazepines. Raven Press, N. Y., 1973.

Gebhart, G. F.; Plaa, G. L.; Mitchell, C. L. The effects of ethanol alone and in combination with phenobarbital, chlorpromazine, or chlordiazepoxide. Toxicol. Appl. Pharmacol. 15:405-414, 1969.

Gjerros, F. Poisoning with chlordiazepoxide (librium). Danish Med. Bull. 13:170-172, 1966.

Goldenthal, E. I. A compilation of LD50 values in newborn and adult animals. Toxicol. Appl. Pharmacol. 18:185-207, 1971.

Greenblatt, D. J.; Allen, M. D.; Noel, B. J.; Shader, R. I. Acute overdosage with benzodiazepine derivatives. Clin. Pharmacol. Ther. 21:497-514, 1977.

Greenblatt, D. J.; Shader, R. I. Dependence, tolerance, and addiction to benzodiazepines: clinical and pharmacokinetic considerations. Drug Metab. Rev. 8:13-28, 1978a.

Greenblatt, D. J.; Woo, E.; Allen, M. D.; Orsulak, P. J.; Shader, R. I. Rapid recovery from massive diazepam overdose. J. A. M. A. 240:1872-1874, 1978b.

Herzka, H.; Haber, J. Klinische Mitteilung uber die Wirksamkeit von Daptazole (Amiphenazol) in einem Fall von Vergiftung mit Valium. Schweiz. Med. Wochenschr. 95:365-366, 1965.

Hollister, L. E.; Motzenbecker, F. P.; Degan, R. O. Withdrawal reactions from chlordiazepoxide ("librium"). Psychopharmacologia 2:63-68, 1961c.

Jenner, F. A.; Parkin, D. A large overdose of chlordiazepoxide. Lancet 2:322-323, 1961.

Jurand, A. Malformations of the central nervous system induced by neurotropic drugs in mouse embryos. Develop. Growth Differ. 22:61-78, 1980.

Kakishita, T.; Aoki, Y.; Ota, T.; Tanaka, M.; Kato, Y.; Otani, G. Safety studies of prazepam (K-373). IV. Acute and subacute toxicity studies of prazepam in dogs. Oyo Yakuri 15:759-775, 1978a.

Kakishita, T.; Aoki, Y.; Ota, T.; Tanaka, M.; Saito, N.; Otani, G. Safety studies of prazepam (K-373). V. Chronic toxicity study of prazepam in dogs. Oyo Yakuri 15:777-795, 1978b.

Klotz, V.; Anttila, V. -J.; Reimann, I. Cimetidine diazepam interaction. Lancet 2:699, 1979.

McBay, A. J. Law-medicine notes, chemical findings in poisonings. N. Engl. J. Med. 274:1257-1258, 1966.

Merck and Co., Inc. The Merck Index, 9th ed. Merck and Co., Inc., Rahway, N. J., 1976.

Nagy, J.; Decsi, L. Physostigmine, a highly potent antidote for acute experimental diazepam intoxication. Neuropharmacol. 17:469-475, 1978.

Owen, G.; Smith, T. H. F.; Agersborg, H. P. K., Jr. Toxicity of some benzodiazepine compounds with CNS activity. Toxicol. Appl. Pharmacol. 16:556-570, 1970.

Physicians' Desk Reference, 35th ed. C. E. Baker, Jr. (Publisher). Medical Economics Co., Oradell, N. J, 1981.

Rice, A. J.; Gruhn, S. W.; Gibson, T. P.; Delle, M.; DiBona, G. F. Effect of saline infusion on the renal excretion of secobarbital, glutethimide, meprobamate, and chlordiazepoxide. J. Lab. Clin. Med. 80:56-62, 1972.

Schaefer, S. Toxicity from drug overdosage in an eleven-year-old boy. Case report. Clin. Pediatr. 1:103-104, 1962.

Sellers, E. M.; Naranjo, C. A.; Giles, H. G.; Frecker, R. C.; Beeching, M. Intravenous diazepam and oral ethanol interaction. Clin. Pharmacol. Ther. 28:638-645, 1980.

Shader, R. I.; Greenblatt, D. J.; Salzman, C.; Kochansky, G. E.; Harmatz, J. S. Benzodiazepines: safety and toxicity. Dis. Nervous System 36:23-26, 1975.

Shah, R.; Donaldson, D.; Burdett, D. Teratogenic effects of diazepam in the hamster. Can. J. Physiol. Pharmacol. 57:556-561, 1979.

Shimkin, P. M.; Shaivitz, S. A. Oxazepam poisoning in a child. J. A. M. A. 196:662-663, 1966.

Smith, M. E. Suicidal attempt by oral ingestion of chlordiazepoxide (librium). Clin. Med. 8:72-74, 1961b.

Spark, H.; Goldman, A. S. Diazepam intoxication in a child. Am. J. Dis. Child. 109:128-129, 1965.

Thearle, M. H.; Hailey, D. M. Exchange transfusion for diazepam intoxication at birth followed by jejunal stenosis. Proc. Roy. Soc. Med. 66:349-350, 1973.

Varma, A. J.; Fisher, B. K.; Sarin, M. K. Diazepam-induced coma with bullae and eccrine sweat gland necrosis. Arch. Intern. Med. 137:1207-1210, 1977.

Walz, M. A.; Davis, W. M. Experimental diazepam intoxication in rodents: physostigmine and naloxone as potential antagonists. Drug Chem. Toxicol. 2:257-267, 1979.

Zbinden, G.; Bagdon, R. E.; Keith, E. F.; Phillips, R. D.; Randall, L. O. Experimental and clinical toxicology of chlordiazepoxide (Librium). Toxicol. Appl. Pharmacol. 3:619-637, 1961.

Zileli, M. S.; Teletar, F.; Deniz, S.; Ilter, E.; Adalar, N. Pseudohyperosmolar non-ketoacedotic coma due to oxazepam intoxication. Clin. Toxicol. 5:337-341, 1972.

DICHLOROPROPENES

Various mixtures of dichloropropenes are used as fumigants applied to the soil before crops are planted. For example, a mixture which the USDA has officially designated by the common name D-D consists of many chlorinated C_3 hydrocarbons, chiefly 1,2-dichloropropane (propylene dichloride) and the cis and trans isomers of 1,3-dichloropropene. The mixture has a dark-brown to amber color and a pungent garlic-like odor. It is soluble in most organic solvents but only slightly in water. As a soil fumigant, D-D is used at full strength by injection into the soil (Shell Chemical Company, 1960f).

Toxicology: Dichloropropenes are highly toxic to mammals by ingestion and inhalation and moderately toxic by skin absorption. Odor and intense irritation of eyes, skin, and respiratory mucosa warn of danger and reduce the exposure hazard. The mean lethal dose of D-D in rats is about 140 mg./kg. by ingestion. A mixture of dichloropropenes dissolved in propylene glycol proved lethal when applied for 24 hours under a cuff on intact rabbit skin at a dose of 0.5 gm./kg. (V. K. Rowe, personal communication, 1960). In continued exposures, inhalation is the chief hazard (Heppel et al., 1946a, b). The symptoms abate promptly after a respiratory exposure ceases (Shell Chemical Company, 1960f).

In animals, visceral lesions of the liver, heart and kidney have been described (Highman and

Heppel, 1946; Hjermstad and Berg, 1977; Wright and Schaffer, 1932). Unsaturation of aliphatic propyl derivatives predisposes to greater hepatic damage and higher acute toxicity (Taylor et al., 1964). Whereas these visceral lesions have not yet been described in man, an exposed victim should probably receive all of the prophylactic and supportive measures recommended for impending hepatic and renal failure (see pp. IV-58–62; also pp. IV-52–55).

The only known human fatality occurred a few hours after the accidental ingestion of D-D (J. M. Arena, personal communication, 1961). The victim experienced abdominal pain and vomiting. When seen in the hospital, he was semicomatose and exhibited muscle twitching. Death occurred in spite of gastric lavage and therapy for pulmonary edema.

In a remarkable accident in Philadelphia (Conner et al., 1962), a somewhat similar product, DOW 421 (4 parts o-dichlorobenzene, 2 parts propylene dichloride, 1 part ethylene dichloride) was involved in a mass poisoning. Three thousand gallons of DOW 421 were liberated into a narrow courtyard containing 45 men when a tank car exploded. Seven men were either killed in the blast or died within 24 hours in various hospitals, but 6 men who developed severe respiratory complications were treated as one group. Although coughing and choking were initial symptoms, these subsided on termination of exposure and were replaced by a period of quiescence (4 to 6 hours). During this period much of the lining of the entire upper and lower respiratory tracts was apparently destroyed without distress to the patient. Over the succeeding 2 to 3 days, pulmonary edema, atelectasis, emphysema and bronchopneumonia were all present, as was tachycardia and occasional atrial premature beats. Three patients died with various attendant complications. Only 1 of the 3 survivors showed residual impairment of respiratory tract function.

A truck collision in Yuba City, California, resulted in the release of about 1200 gallons of 1,3-dichloropropene (Flessel *et al.*, 1978). About 80 persons were estimated to have been exposed to the vapor. None died but 3 lost consciousness. Several of these victims reported long-persisting symptoms of headache, fatigue, irritability and chest or abdominal discomfort.

It is unlikely that dichloropropenes or dichloropropanes are cumulative poisons. At least rats excrete these materials rapidly. When ^{14}C-labeled materials (1,2-dichloropropane, *cis*- and *trans*-1,3-dichloro-2-propene) were administered by stomach tube, 90% of the label appeared in urine, feces and expired air within 24 hours (Hutson *et al.*, 1971). The urine was the major route of excretion, but expired air was also important, especially with 1,2-dichloropropane, which is partly metabolized to CO_2, and partly excreted unchanged. The major urinary metabolite in rats given 1,3-dichloro-2-propene was a mercapturic acid. Apparently the chlorine in the 1-position is removed prior to conjugation with cysteine. Formation of a glutathione conjugate was shown in an *in vitro* system (Climie *et al.*, 1979). Although this conjugation appears to require the enzyme hepatic glutathione transferase, many other molecules with electrophilic centers also form glutathione conjugates nonenzymatically. Some of them, such as methyl bromide (see p. III-280), are also known to S-alkylate cysteine residues in various enzymes and other proteins. Perhaps alkylation of critical proteins is the molecular basis of the widespread visceral lesions in D-D poisoning. A therapeutic trial with BAL, *N*-acetylcysteine or some other sulfhydryl antidote should prove informative.

D-D, Telone and various ingredients (*cis*- and *trans*-1,3-dichloropropene) are mutagenic by the Ames assay (de Lorenzo *et al.*, 1977).

Symptomatology:

1. A. Inhalation, high vapor concentrations: gasping, refusal to breathe, coughing, substernal pain, and extreme respiratory distress at vapor concentrations over 1500 ppm. Irritation of eyes and upper respiratory mucosa appears promptly after exposure to concen-

trated vapors. Lacrimation and headache are prominent. Coma may occur rapidly.

   B. Inhalation, low vapor concentrations: central nervous depression and moderate irritation of respiratory system. Headache is frequent.

2. Dermal: severe skin irritation with marked inflammatory response of epidermis and underlying tissues.

3. Oral: acute gastrointestinal distress with pulmonary congestion and edema. Central nervous depression, perhaps even in the absence of impaired oxygen uptake.

4. By any route, possible late injuries to liver, kidneys and heart.

5. After inhalation exposures, malaise, headache, chest and abdominal discomfort and irritability have been reported to persist for several weeks and perhaps for several years (Flessel *et al.*, 1978).

Treatment:

1. Remove ingested material by gastric aspiration and lavage. Use water as a lavage fluid.

2. Demulcents like alumina gels, but no fats or oils.

3. Opiates and atropine for the control of pain and intestinal spasm.

4. Aminophylline (theophylline-ethylenediamine) intravenously slowly to correct bronchospasm. See p. IV-15.

5. Oxygen and other measures described on pp. IV-14–16 for management of the adult respiratory distress syndrome.

6. Digitalis and/or lidocaine in the event of cardiac disturbances (pp. IV-22–26).

7. Wash extensively any contaminated areas of skin with soap and water. Discard contaminated clothing.

8. As noted in the text above, a therapeutic trial with BAL (p. III-52) or *N*-acetylcysteine (p. III-6) might be useful if instituted promptly after the exposure.

9. For the management of liver insufficiency, see p. IV-62; for renal failure, see p. IV-53.

Laboratory: Repeated function tests are desirable to detect and evaluate possible liver and kidney injuries (pp. IV-51 and 59).

References:

Climie, I. J. G.; Hutson, D. H.; Morrison, B. J.; Stoydin, G. Glutathione conjugation in the detoxication of (2)-1, 3-dichloropropene (a component of the nematocide D-D) in the rat. Xenobiotica 9:149-156, 1979.

Conner, E. H.; DuBois, A. B.; Comroe, J. H., Jr. Acute chemical injury of the airway and lungs. Experience with six cases. Anesthesiology 23:538-547, 1962.

de Lorenzo, F.; Degl'Innocenti, S.; Ruocco, A.; Silengo, L.; Cortese, R. Mutagenicity of pesticides containing 1, 3-dichloropropene. Cancer Res. 37:1915-1917, 1977.

Flessel, P.; Goldsmith, J. R.; Kahn, E.; Wesolowski, J. J. Acute and possible long-term effects of 1, 3-dichloropropene -

California. Morbidity and Mortality Weekly Report, 27:50, 1978.

Heppel, L. A.; Highman, B.; Porterfield, V. T. Toxicology of 1, 2-dichloropropane (propylene dichloride); II. Influence of dietary factors on the toxicity of dichloropropane. J. Pharmacol. Exp. Ther. 87:11-17, 1946b.

Heppel, L. A.; Neal, P. A.; Highman, B.; Porterfield, V. T. Toxicology of 1, 2-dichloropropane (propylene dichloride); I. Studies on the effects of daily inhalations. J. Ind. Hyg. Toxicol. 28:1-8, 1946a.

Highman, B.; Heppel, L. A. Toxicology of 1, 2-dichloropropane (propylene dichloride); III. Pathologic changes produced by a short series of daily exposures. Arch. Pathol. 42:525-534, 1946.

Hjermstad, H. P.; Berg, R. The toxicity of 1, 3-dichloropropene

as determined by repeated exposure of laboratory animals. Am. Ind. Hyg. Assoc. J. 38:217-223, 1977.

Hutson, D. H.; Moss, J. A.; Pickering, B. A. The excretion and retention of components of the soil fumigant D-D and their metabolites in the rat. Food Cosmet. Toxicol. 9:677-680, 1971.

Shell Chemical Co. Summary of basic data (D-D soil fumigant). New York, 1960f.

Taylor, J. M.; Jenner, P. M.; Jones, W. I. A comparison of the toxicity of some allyl, propenyl and propyl compounds in the rat. Toxicol. Appl. Pharmacol. 6:378-387, 1964.

Wright, W. H.; Schaffer, J. M. Critical anthelmintic tests of chlorinated alkyl hydrocarbons and a correlation between the anthelmintic efficacy, chemical structure and physical properties. Am. J. Hyg. 16:325-428, 1932.

DIELDRIN

Technical dieldrin (hexachloro-epoxy-octahydro-endo,exo-dimethanonaphthalene or HEOD) has a minimal purity of 85%. Alone or in combination with other insecticides, it has been used widely to eradicate insect pests. In this role, its chemical stability and persistence in the environment are advantageous. It is effective in the control of a wide variety of economic pests, but its use on edible leaf crops or where residues might appear in foods for man or animals has long been prohibited. It has been formulated and marketed as powders for dusting, wettable powders for emulsion sprays, oil solutions, aerosols, and granules for bait (Jager, 1970).

Dieldrin and the closely related compounds, aldrin, endrin, isobenzan, isodrin, heptachlor, chlordane, etc., form a group known as cyclodiene insecticides. Their persistency has attracted the serious attention of environmentalists and others. At present, dieldrin and aldrin are virtually banned by federal regulation for use in the United States, except for a few restricted and specialized uses. Furthermore, almost all of the EPA registrations of the other cyclodiene insecticides have been canceled or suspended. Laws in many states also prohibit use of these compounds. In several cases, manufacturers have discontinued production and withdrawn their products from the market. The cyclodiene insecticides, however, are still used in some foreign countries, and products containing them are still harbored in many American homes and farms. See also CHLORDANE (p. III-108).

Toxicology: Dieldrin, particularly in oil solution, is absorbed very readily through the skin, the respiratory mucosa and the gastrointestinal tract. Untoward symptoms are known to occur in man after oral doses as small as 10 mg./kg. The acute mean lethal dose by the oral route lies between 20 and 70 mg./kg. in various birds and mammals (Hodge et al., 1967a). Man presumably lies in the same range (Committee on Toxicology, 1960; Hodge et al., 1967a).

Several human deaths have been ascribed to the ingestion of dieldrin, but little reliable information about doses is available (Hayes, 1975 and 1982; Pribilla, 1963; Weinig et al., 1966). Several suicide attempts have resulted in very severe poisonings; in each case, intensive medical care was probably responsible for the survival (Black, 1974; Jacobs and Lurie, 1967). Fry (1964) described two very severe but nonfatal poisonings in "senior boys," each of whom ingested a cupful of hot water with one heaping teaspoonful of a wettable powder containing 50% dieldrin. Endrin-contaminated flour was responsible for four explosive outbreaks of acute poisoning in Saudi Arabia, resulting in 26 deaths and 874 hospitalizations (Curley et al., 1970; Weeks, 1967). A large outbreak in Mali in 1977 was caused by dieldrin-contaminated rice (Hayes, 1982).

In animals the percutaneous toxicity of dieldrin is almost as high as its oral toxicity (much higher according to one laboratory). Even undissolved dieldrin is said to penetrate intact skin. Dermal exposures result in systemic poisoning without skin irritation or local sensitization, except secondary to the solvent or vehicle, which is usually kerosene or xylene (Bundren et al., 1952). In six volunteers, about 7.7% of a tracer dose of ^{14}C-dieldrin applied to the skin of the forearm was absorbed (Feldmann and Maibach, 1974). Skin disease, such as scleroderma, may facilitate cutaneous absorption (Starr and Clifford, 1971).

The actions of dieldrin and other cyclodiene insecticides are similar both qualitatively and quantitatively in animals and apparently also in man. In all cases the principal site of action is the central nervous system, and the principal sign is a series of convulsions. The convulsions are self-remitting but recur with increasing severity; they characteristically alternate with periods of severe depression (Hayes et al., 1951).

Convulsions induced by the cyclodiene insecticides may be preceded by subjective complaints, but frequently they occur with no forewarning or prodromal signs or symptoms (Hoogendam et al., 1962). Abnormalities of the EEG, such as bilateral synchronous θ-wave activity and occasional bilateral synchronous spike and wave complexes, are seen in patients without clinical symptoms both before and after convulsions (Kazantzis et al., 1964). Myoclonia indicates that a convulsive episode is imminent. Prodromal signs that have been reported include headache, visual disturbances, dizziness, sweating, insomnia, nausea, and malaise (Jacobs and Lurie, 1967; Klemmer et al., 1977). Convulsions are accompanied by loss of consciousness and "frothing at the mouth" but not incontinence (Cobel et al., 1967; Hayes, 1957).

An extensive literature on occupational poisonings by dieldrin has been summarized by Hayes (1982). In contrast to acute poisonings, after repeated exposures several spraymen developed a syndrome indistinguishable from idiopathic epilepsy, except that it ceased when the exposure was terminated (Hayes, 1957). A motor polyneuropathy resembling the Guillain-Barré syndrome is a rare complication of exposure (Jenkins and Toole, 1964). In the usual acute intoxication, recovery is complete or well advanced within 24 to 48 hours, but animal experiments and clinical experience (Hayes, 1957; Patel and Rao, 1958) indicate the possibility of seizures for many days after a single dose or repeated doses. In rhesus monkeys a single symptomatic dose of dieldrin or a series of subclinical doses altered the frequency spectrum of the spontaneous EEG for a year (Burchfiel et al., 1976).

Several signs of intoxication in rats and dogs suggest an enhancement of sympathetic tone and/or adrenal discharge in acute poisonings by dieldrin congeners: increase in blood glucose (Bhatia et al., 1972), hypertension, fever, leukocytosis, acidosis, salivation, hemoconcentration (Emerson et al., 1964), and an increase in blood catecholamines (Hinshaw et al., 1966). Bradycardia, persistent decrease in peripheral vascular resistance and left heart failure, however, indicate that the cardiovascular effects are more complicated.

Absorption of dieldrin from the rat gastrointestinal tract is rapid. Transportation to the liver occurs mainly via the portal vein. Dieldrin is partly metabolized in the liver and partly redistributed (Iatropoulos et al., 1975). Like DDT, dieldrin is stored in body fat (Dale and Quimby, 1963; Hunter and Robinson, 1968). Aldrin is epoxidized to dieldrin in humans and therefore can contribute to dieldrin fat stores. Unchanged dieldrin is not excreted in human urine (Cueto and Hayes, 1962), although it may be found in feces. Many metabolites are eliminated by both excretory routes, but in rats urinary excretion of total labeled material was much greater than fecal excretion, i.e., 90% vs. 10% (Heath and Vandekar, 1964).

In human adult volunteers who ingested dieldrin chronically, the half-life in blood was estimated after withdrawal to be 140 to 600 days (Hunter et al., 1969), but in one acutely poisoned child the half-life appeared to be only 50 days (Garrettson and Curley, 1969).

Dieldrin, endrin and aldrin are directly toxic to the mammalian central nervous system (Joy, 1976), but three mammalian metabolites of endrin were all more acutely toxic to rats than the parent compound (Bedford et al., 1975b). Endrin and isobenzan are more acutely toxic to animals than dieldrin or aldrin (Jager, 1970), but endrin is cleared much more rapidly from plasma than is dieldrin because of more rapid biliary excretion (Cole et al., 1970; Curley et al., 1970). Although the distribution of dieldrin is eventually weighted heavily toward fat, studies on one acutely poisoned child suggested that short-term redistribution from brain to skeletal muscle may be more important in terminating convulsions (Garrettson and Curley, 1969). Although this clinical impression could not be confirmed by an experimental study in rats (Hayes, 1974), an intensification of toxic signs and symptoms in one chronically exposed sprayman was ascribed to extreme weight loss and mobilization of dieldrin from fat stores (Glass, 1975). Dieldrin and presumably its congeners cross the placenta (Selby et al., 1969).

Miscellaneous toxic effects produced by repeated doses or chronic feeding include chromosomal aberrations in rats (Dikshith and Datta, 1973), hepatic vein thrombosis resulting in liver infarcts, and hepatocellular carcinomas in mice (Reuber, 1977). Mild and transient injuries of kidney (edema of tubular epithelium) and liver (small foci of central lobular necrosis) have been described in man (Committee on Toxicology, 1960). In one case, evidence of liver damage persisted for more than 1 year (Garrettson and Curley, 1969). Chronic exposures to related insecticides, particularly LINDANE (p. III-239) and CHLORDANE (p. III-108), have been associated with the appearance of blood dyscrasias.

Symptomatology (onset of symptoms between 20 minutes and 12 hours after ingestion):
1. Malaise, headache, nausea, vomiting, dizziness, and tremors.
2. Clonic and tonic convulsions, sometimes without premonitory symptoms.
3. Convulsive episodes may alternate with periods of severe central nervous depression. Death from respiratory arrest may

occur during coma, which commonly outlasts the convulsive phase and may persist for a few days.

4. During the acute phase, leukocytosis, rise in blood pressure, tachycardia, arrhythmias, metabolic acidosis, and fever have been described; presumably they represent the consequences of hyperactivity of the sympathetic nervous system.

5. Disturbances of sleep, memory and behavior may persist for several days or weeks after the acute phase of dieldrin poisoning (Fry, 1964).

6. Generalized cerebral dysrhythmia (EEG evidence) persisting for months, and both hematuria and albuminuria of about 2 weeks duration have been described in one aldrin poisoning in man (Spiotta, 1951). Transient hematuria occurred on the second day of an acute dieldrin poisoning (Jacobs and Lurie, 1967).

Treatment:

1. Decontaminate any suspicious areas of skin promptly by blotting with an absorbent material and then washing extensively with soap and running water. If skin and clothing are obviously contaminated, the therapist should protect himself by wearing gloves of Neoprene or artificial rubber.

2. After ingestion, evacuate and lavage stomach with warm water (unless convulsions are imminent).

3. Administer a saline cathartic. Avoid oils or oil laxatives.

4. Barbiturates are said to be the treatment of choice in the prevention and control of tremors and convulsions (p. IV-37). Presumably diazepam is also effective, but no reports of its use in dieldrin poisoning are known to us. Large doses of barbiturates are surprisingly well tolerated. Phenobarbital is preferable as a prophylactic measure, but a short-acting drug (e.g., thiopental, pentobarbital, Seconal) is preferable after convulsions have begun. As soon as the intensity of the postconvulsive depression can be judged, the patient should be continued on adequate maintenance doses of a barbiturate drug. Anticonvulsive therapy may have to be continued for 1 or more weeks. See pp. IV-35–39.

5. Avoid sudden physical stimuli which may precipitate convulsions during periods of central hyperirritability.

6. Oxygen therapy and artificial ventilation if needed during periods of depression (pp. IV-12 and 7–12).

7. Based on observations in dogs, it has been suggested that forced feeding of high caloric foods may have a place in the overall management of the poisoned patient (Keane et al., 1969).

8. Any patient who experiences a convulsion should be observed carefully for at least 1 week.

Laboratory: In severe intoxications, laboratory tests may reveal kidney and liver injuries, which according to present evidence remit spontaneously during recovery. See pp. IV-52 and 59. Repeated EEGs are useful to detect prolonged cortical dysfunction. Severe acidosis has been reported in animals.

References:

Bedford, C. T.; Hutson, D. H.; Natoff, I. L. The accute toxicity of endrin and its metabolites to rats. Toxicol. Appl. Pharmacol. 33:115-121, 1975b.

Bhatia, S. C.; Sharma, S. C.; Venkitasubramanian, T. A. Acute dieldrin toxicity; biochemical changes in the blood. Arch. Environ. Health 24:369-372, 1972.

Black, A. M. S. Self poisoning with dieldrin: A case report and pharmacokinetic discussion. Anaesth. Intensive Care 2:369-374, 1974.

Bundren, J.; Howell, D. E.; Heller, V. G. Absorption and toxicity of dieldrin. Proc. Soc. Exp. Biol. Med. 79:236-238, 1952.

Burchfiel, J. L.; Duffy, F. H.; Sim, V. M. Persistent effects of sarin and dieldrin upon the primate encephalogram. Toxicol. Appl. Pharmacol. 35:365-379, 1976.

Cobel, Y.; Hildebrandt, P.; Davis, J.; Raasch, F.; Curley, A. Acute endrin poisoning. J. A. M. A. 202:489-493, 1967.

Cole, J. F.; Klevay, L. M.; Zavon, M. R. Endrin and dieldrin; a comparison of hepatic excretion in the rat. Toxicol. Appl. Pharmacol. 16:547-555, 1970.

Committee on Toxicology, A. M. A. Occupational dieldrin poisoning. J. A. M. A. 172:2077-2080, 1960.

Cueto, C., Jr.; Hayes, W. J., Jr. The detection of dieldrin metabolites in human urine. J. Agric. Food Chem. 10:366-369, 1962.

Curley, A.; Jennings, R. W.; Mann, H. T.; Sediak, V. Measurement of endrin following epidemics of poisoning. Bull. Environ. Contam. Toxicol. 5:24-29, 1970.

Dale, W. E.; Quimby, G. E. Chlorinated insecticides in the body fat of people in the United States. Science 142:593-595, 1963.

Dikshith, T. S. S.; Datta, K. A. Endrin induced cytological changes in albino rats. Bull. Endrin. Contam. Toxicol. 9:65-69, 1973.

Emerson, T. E., Jr.; Brake, C. M.; Hinshaw, L. B. Cardiovascular effects of the insecticide endrin. Can. J. Physiol. Pharmacol. 42:41-51, 1964.

Feldmann, R. J.; Maibach, H. I. Percutaneous penetration of some pesticides and herbicides in man. Toxicol. Appl. Pharmacol. 28:126-132, 1974.

Fry, D. R. Human dieldrin poisoning. Lancet 1:764, 1964.

Garrettson, L. K.; Curley, A. Dieldrin, studies in a poisoned child. Arch. Environ. Health 19:814-822, 1969.

Glass, W. I. Dieldrin poisoning: case report. NZ Med. J. 81:202-203, 1975.

Hayes, W. J., Jr. Dieldrin poisoning in man. Public Health Rep. (U. S.) 72:1087-1091, 1957.

Hayes, W. J., Jr. Distribution of dieldrin following a single oral dose. Toxicol. Appl. Pharmacol. 28:485-492, 1974.

Hayes, W. J., Jr. Toxicology of Pesticides. Williams and Wilkins Co., Baltimore, Md, 1975.

Hayes, W. J., Jr. Pesticides Studied In Man. Williams & Wilkins, Baltimore, Md, 1982.

Hayes, W. J., Jr.; Ferguson, F. F.; Cass, J. S. The toxicology of dieldrin and its bearing on field use of the compound. Am. J. Trop. Med. 31:519-522, 1951.

Heath, D. F.; Vandekar, M. Toxicity and metabolism of dieldrin in rats. Br. J. Ind. Med. *21*:269-279, 1964.

Hinshaw, L. B.; Soloman, L. A.; Reins, D. A.; Fiorica, V.; Emerson, T. E., Jr. Effects of the insecticide endrin on the cardiovascular system of the dog. J. Pharmacol. Exp. Ther. *153*:225-236, 1966.

Hodge, H. C.; Boyce, A. M.; Deichmann, W. B.; Kraybill, H. F. Toxicology and no effect levels of aldrin and dieldrin. Toxicol. Appl. Pharmacol. *10*:613-675, 1967a.

Hoogendam, L.; Versteeg, J. P. J.; DeVlieger, M. Electroencephalograms in insecticide toxicity. Arch. Environ. Health *4*:86-94, 1962.

Hunter, C. G.; Robinson, J. Aldrin, dieldrin and man. Food Cosmet. Toxicol. *6*:253-260, 1968.

Hunter, C. G.; Robinson, J.; Roberts, M. Pharmacodynamics of dieldrin (HEOD). Arch. Environ. Health *18*:12-21, 1969.

Iatropoulos, M. J.; Milling, A.; Muller, W. F.; Nohynek, G.; Rozman, K.; Coulston, F.; Korte, F. Absorption, transport and organotropism of dichlorobiphenyl (DCB), dieldrin, and hexachlorobenzene (HCB) in rats. Environ. Res. *10*:384-389, 1975.

Jacobs, P.; Lurie, J. B. Acute toxicity of the chlorinated hydrocarbon insecticides. S. Afr. Med. J. *41*:1147-1150, 1967.

Jager, K. W. *Aldrin, Dieldrin, Endrin and Telodrin. An Epidemiological and Toxicological Study of Long-term Occupational Exposure.* Elsevier, Amsterdam, 1970.

Jenkins, R. B.; Toole, J. F. Polyneuropathy following exposure to insecticides. Arch. Intern. Med. *113*:691-695, 1964.

Joy, R. M. Convulsive properties of chlorinated hydrocarbon insecticides in the cat central nervous system. Toxicol. Appl. Pharmacol. *35*:95-106, 1976.

Kazantzis, G.; McLaughlin, A. I. G.; Prior, P. F. Poisoning in industrial workers by the insecticide aldrin. Br. J. Ind. Med. *21*:46-51, 1964.

Keane, W. T.; Zavon, M. R.; Witherup, S. H. Dieldrin poisoning in dogs; relation to obesity and treatment. Br. J. Ind. Med. *26*:338-341, 1969.

Klemmer, H. W.; Budy, A. M.; Takahashi, W.; Haley, T. J. Human tissue distribution of cyclodiene pesticides--Hawaii 1964-1973. Clin. Toxicol. *11*:71-82, 1977.

Patel, T. B.; Rao, V. N. "Dieldrin" poisoning in man. A report of 20 cases observed in Bombay State. Br. Med. J. *1*:919-921, 1958.

Pribilla, O. Akute todliche Dieldrinvergiftung. Arch. Toxikol. *20*:61-71, 1963.

Reuber, M. D. Hepatic vein thrombosis in mice ingesting chlorinated hydrocarbons. Arch. Toxicol. *38*:163-168, 1977.

Selby, L. A.; Newell, K. W.; Hauser, G. A.; Junker, G. Comparison of chlorinated hydrocarbon pesticides in maternal blood and placental tissue. Environ. Res. *2*:247-255, 1969.

Spiotta, E. J. Aldrin poisoning in man. Arch. Ind. Hyg. Occup. Med. *4*:560-566, 1951.

Starr, H. G., Jr.; Clifford, N. J. Absorption of pesticides in a chronic skin disease. Arch. Environ. Health *22*:396-400, 1971.

Weeks, D. E. Endrin food poisoning, a report on four outbreaks caused by two separate shipments of endrin-contaminated flour. Bull. WHO *37*:499-512, 1967.

Weinig, E.; Machbert, G.; Zink, P. Uber den Nachweis des Dieldrins bei einer Dieldrinvergiftung. Arch. Toxikol. *22*:115-124, 1966.

DIGITALIS

Digitoxin and other so-called cardiac glycosides constitute a group of chemically and pharmacologically related substances derived from various plants, notably of the genus *Digitalis;* each consists of a characteristic steroid (known as the aglycone or genin) coupled with one or more types of sugar molecules. Single crystalline glycosides and mixtures are available from many botanical sources and in many physical forms (Hoch, 1961). In clinical medicine "digitalis" is often used as a generic name for any of these active glycosides. They are widely used in clinical medicine because of their inotropic and chronotropic actions on the diseased heart. Formerly, extracardiac actions were sometimes sought, such as the use of squill as a nauseant expectorant. A nonmedicinal variety of squill, known as red squill, is used in the form of the powdered dry bulb as a potent rodenticide. Accidental and suicidal ingestions of red squill and of other digitalis preparations have caused fatal poisonings in man, but most poisonings are due to overdosage in therapy.

Toxicology: Among hospitalized patients receiving digitalis in one form or another, the incidence of toxic reactions has been estimated to range from 8 to 35%, and the mortality rate attributable to its cardiotoxicity lies between 3 and 21% (Rodensky and Wasserman, 1961; Smith and Haber, 1973). In accidental or suicidal ingestions by adults without preexisting heart disease, the fatality rate tends to be lower in spite of the high doses consumed (Bergy *et al.*, 1957; Hansteen *et al.*, 1981). A mortality of only 6% has been reported in children who "accidentally" ingested large numbers of tablets (Fowler *et al.*, 1964).

The therapeutic and toxic actions of the various cardiac glycosides are basically similar; the differences relate principally to potency, latency, and persistency (Chung, 1969). These distinctions imply that the various drugs differ from one another in stability, absorbability, penetrability, tissue fixation, metabolic degradation, and excretion. Because the chief actions of the cardiac glycosides are common to them all, the toxicities of these compounds are additive (Cohen, 1952). This discussion concerns principally digoxin and whole-leaf digitalis (powdered leaves of *Digitalis purpurea*) or digitoxin (a pure glycoside derived from the latter). Quantitative distinctions between digoxin, digitoxin and several other cardiac glycosides are outlined in Section II.

Irrespective of the route of administration, a cardiac glycoside must be fixed to the myocardium before its cardiac effects begin. With digitoxin and digitalis leaf, the latency varies between 1 and 2 hours; the cardiac actions are maximal in 4 to 12 hours and disappear only after 2 to 3 weeks. With oral digoxin latency, peak and duration are 0.5 hours, 3 to 6 hours and 3 to 6 days, respectively (Chung, 1969). In most poisonings the danger period lasts for several days. About 20% of the glycosides in an oral dose of whole-leaf digitalis is absorbed (whether given as the powder or tincture), in contrast to the essentially complete absorption of digitoxin and 65 to 90% absorption of digoxin in most individuals (Henderson, 1969). In about 10% of the subjects tested, however, 40% or more of an oral dose of digoxin was degraded by bacteria in the gut (Lindenbaum *et al.*, 1981).

The biological fate of cardiac glycosides is not well understood. With digitoxin, only about 10% of a dose is excreted unchanged, but an appreciable fraction (perhaps 30%) is found in the urine as biologically active metabolites (including digoxin). Much of the excretion occurs within the first 48 hours, but small amounts can be detected in the urine for several weeks, and the biological half-life is 4 to 6 days. By contrast, digoxin is excreted largely unchanged; less than 10% of a dose appears as metabolites in the urine. Its biological half-life is usually only 1.8 to 1.9 days (Chung, 1969; Henderson, 1969). After massive doses, however, digoxin half-lives as short as 13 to 15 hours have been reported (Hobson and Zettner, 1973; Rumack *et al.*, 1974). Both glycosides are excreted in bile and partly resorbed (enterohepatic circulation). Transplacental neonatal digitalis intoxication may represent a hazard in pregnancy (Sherman and Locke, 1960).

In toxic doses, digitalis produces nervous and mental disturbances (Batterman and Gutner, 1948) including persistent nausea and vomiting of reflex origin (Borison and Wang, 1953), but the most definitive and most dangerous actions concern the rate and rhythm of the heart and the mechanism of the heart beat. Much experimental work suggests that both cardiac and extracardiac sites of digitalis action are involved in the genesis of these cardiac disorders. Because of the known neuroexcitatory actions of digitalis, the extracardiac loci that have attracted the most attention are all in the central and peripheral nervous systems. Digitalis increases afferent discharges from chemoreceptors and baroreceptors, modifies central neuronal activity, alters activity in preganglionic autonomic neurones, affects transmission in autonomic ganglia and enhances the adrenal medullary secretion of epinephrine. The evidence for these phenomena and their relationship to disorders of the cardiac mechanism in digitalis poisoning have been reviewed (Gillis and Quest, 1979; Lathers and Roberts, 1980). A centrally mediated rise in vagal tone undoubtedly contributes to digitalis-induced sinus bradycardia, nodal rhythms and atrioventricular (AV) blocks, but direct actions on the Purkinje apparatus are probably far more important after overdoses. Even more controversial is the possibility that the ventricular tachyarrhythmias of digitalis poisoning are due to enhanced and/or nonuniform activity in sympathetic postganglionic fibers of the cardiac plexus. Many neurotropic drugs have been shown to raise the threshold to digitalis poisoning in one or more experimental animals, but aside from atropine in an occasional patient, no success can be claimed yet for any of these measures in clinical digitalis intoxications.

Digitalis-induced disorders in the mechanism of the beat, which in part are extensions of therapeutic actions, are best detected and analyzed with the aid of an electrocardiogram (ECG). Digitalis has been held responsible for the production of every known type of cardiac dysrhythmia (Cohen, 1952; Rodensky and Wasserman, 1961), but some disorders, such as an intraventricular block evidenced by a wide QRS, which is a frequent finding in quinidine poisoning, are only rarely associated with digitalis (Chung, 1969; Levine and Somlyo, 1962). No dysrhythmia is unique to digitalis poisoning, but cardiotonic glycosides are by far the most likely cause of nonparoxysmal nodal tachycardia (Soffer, 1961), atrial tachycardia with AV dissociation and bidirectional ventricular tachycardia (Lyon and DeGraff, 1967).

The more common toxic disturbances revealed by the ECG are listed in Fig. III-3; *arrows* indicate some of the recognized sequences of events during progressive digitalis poisoning. Serial ECGs are usually necessary for the intelligent management of these patients. Whenever a cardiac glycoside is responsible for any of the disturbances listed at the bottom of Fig. III-3 (*TOXIC ZONE*), the drug should be immediately discontinued; at least a reduction in dosage is warranted whenever the *BORDER ZONE* is reached. When these same derangements in mechanism of beat are due to causes other than cardiac glycosides, digitalis is not necessarily contraindicated. For example, digitalis may be administered in the presence of a complete heart block from causes other than drug; in contrast, ventricular bigeminy and ventricular tachycardia are probably valid contraindications to digitalis under all cirumstances, although not everyone agrees (Somlyo, 1960). In all cases the ECG should be regarded only as a diagnostic and prognostic aid. It is the patient, not the ECG, who needs treatment, but the ECG is emphasized because it may reveal signs of severe intoxication in patients who are almost asymptomatic (in borderline poisonings the converse may be true, *i.e.*, symptoms may precede ECG signs) (Soffer, 1961; Somlyo, 1960).

The toxic dose is subject to a wide range of variation, but toxicity is often encountered when the therapeutic dose is exceeded even slightly (Soffer, 1961). An unannounced "improvement" in digoxin tablets that enhanced slightly the bioavailability of the glycoside produced a mini-

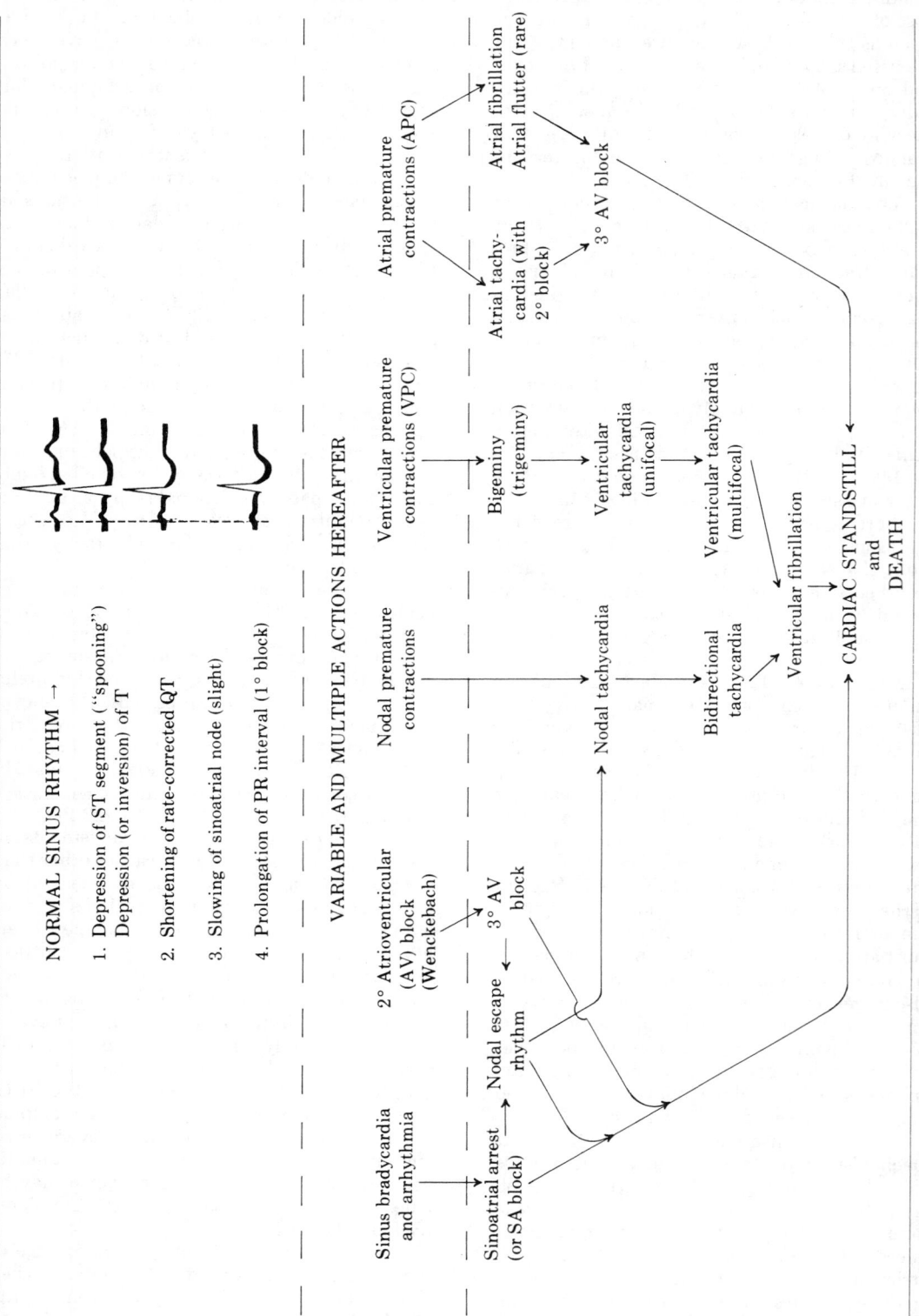

Figure III-3. Progessive effects of digitalis on ECG and on mechanism of heart beat

epidemic of poisonings (Danon *et al.*, 1977). In spite of frequent claims that one or another of the cardiac glycosides has a greater margin of safety, only small differences in this respect exist among the common drugs (Hoch, 1961). Most deaths have followed multiple doses in patients on digitalis therapy. The single oral lethal dose, as inferred from accidental and suicidal ingestions, probably lies between 20 and 50 times the usual daily maintenance dose (Drevets, 1958; Joos and Johnson, 1957), but adults have survived single doses of more than 20 mg. of digoxin (Hobson and Zettner, 1973; Smith and Willerson, 1971) or digitoxin (Bismuth *et al.*, 1973). With other things being equal, a drug of long persistency is a greater toxic hazard than a drug with a rapid rate of dissipation; digitoxin and whole-leaf digitalis are among the worst offenders in this respect.

Many factors are believed to contribute to the wide range of toxic and lethal doses observed in clinical practice (Chung, 1969). Impaired renal excretion is undoubtedly a major factor predisposing to iatrogenic poisonings. Digitalis dose schedules should be lowered in patients with known or suspected renal disease. Perhaps because of slower excretion, elderly patients are comparatively intolerant of cardiac glycosides and are prone to manifest toxic reactions with supposedly safe doses (Somlyo, 1960). The same is true of persons with hypothyroidism. In contrast, patients with atrial fibrillation or flutter appear to tolerate digitalis doses that are toxic in the presence of a sinus rhythm (Gilbert and Cuddy, 1965). Changes in absorption may also precipitate digitalis poisoning. For example, antibacterial chemotherapy may enhance the absorption of oral digoxin by reducing the gut flora of organisms that inactivate digoxin; such a flora has been found in about 10% of patients tested (Lindenbaum *et al.*, 1981).

Because experimental and clinical data suggest that the glycosides and calcium may have additive or synergistic actions on the heart, the intravenous use of calcium salts is regarded as unwise in a digitalized patient (Cohen, 1952; Eliot and Blount, 1961; Shrager, 1957). Perhaps ephedrine also enhances the toxicity of digitalis. Diuretic therapy sometimes precipitates digitalis poisoning, probably by depleting tissues of potassium and so inducing hypokalemia (Lown *et al.*, 1953; Rodensky and Wasserman, 1961), although hypomagnesemia may contribute under these circumstances (Seller *et al.*, 1970). When patients with impaired renal function are subjected to hemodialysis, a dangerous loss in extracellular potassium and gain in calcium may result (Kohn and Kiley, 1953). (The glycosides *per se* are only slowly removed by dialysis.) Drug allergy or hypersensitivity is rarely implicated in the genesis of digitalis poisoning (Somlyo, 1960; Wolfe and Geiger, 1953).

Two of the most significant determinants of susceptibility to digitalis poisoning are the age of the patient and the presence or absence of preexisting heart disease. Except for premature infants (Levine and Somlyo, 1962) and neonates (Krasula *et al.*, 1974), infants and children are more tolerant than adults to the therapeutic and toxic actions of cardiac glycosides (Neill, 1965). Similarly, young adults are probably more tolerant than old adults. Unquestionably preexisting heart disease of any type is a special liability in the presence of an excessive dose of digitalis (Chung, 1969). Thus, the diseased heart is particularly likely to develop ectopic rhythms, especially ventricular premature beats, ventricular tachycardia and, ultimately, ventricular fibrillation (Hansteen *et al.*, 1981; Somlyo, 1960; Smith and Willerson, 1971), although severe bradycardia and eventual cardiac standstill have also been described (Asplund *et al.*, 1971).

In contrast, bradycardia with various degrees of entrance and exit blocks at the AV junction are the rule in the digitalis-poisoned child (Drevets, 1958; Fowler *et al.*, 1964; Joos and Johnson, 1957) and young adult without heart disease (Asplund *et al.*, 1971; Reza *et al.*, 1974; Rumack *et al.*, 1974). The same is probably true of older persons who have structurally sound hearts (Bergy *et al.*, 1957; Navab and Honey, 1967). An exaggerated sinus arrhythmia is particularly prominent in poisoned infants. In the few fatalities reported in young individuals (*e.g.*, Fowler *et al.*, 1964; Smith and Willerson, 1971), cardiac standstill and not ventricular fibrillation was the usual terminal event. Thus a typical poisoning in a patient without heart disease progresses according to one of the pathways on the left in Fig. III-3. When and if ectopic beats and tachycardia do appear, they are more commonly supraventricular than ventricular (Krasula *et al.*, 1974; Levine and Somlyo, 1962).

The ingestion of large doses of powdered whole-leaf digitalis often produces prompt vomiting due to local irritation, but with digitoxin and other purified glycosides, emesis is delayed because it arises only from actions on the central nervous system (Borison and Wang, 1953). Many other toxic signs and symptoms are also referable to the nervous system (Batterman and Gutner, 1948). Because they may appear when cardiac output is uncompromised, the mental and emotional disorders of digitalis poisoning probably do not have a circulatory origin. Drowsiness, usually without coma, is common, particularly in poisoned children (Fowler *et al.*, 1964). Other complaints include extreme fatigue, weakness, neuritic pain, confusion, delirium, and rarely convulsions or coma (Church and Marriott, 1959).

A wide range of visual disturbances has been described, including transient amblyopia, scotoma, photophobia, colored haloes and other aberrations of color vision (Carroll, 1945; Sykowski, 1949). In a large-scale subacute poisoning over a period of more than 3 weeks (Lely and Van Enter, 1970), 119 of 125 patients experienced significant visual disturbances, which were thought to reflect transient retrobulbar optic neuritis (Sykowski, 1949), although functional derangements of the retina were more likely responsible in view of the high concentrations of digoxin that accumulate in the choroid-retina (Binnion and Frazer, 1980). Color vision is the most sensitive process, with 80% of intoxicated patients showing generalized color vision deficits (Rietbrock and Alken, 1980).

Although degenerative and necrotic myocardial and extracardiac (e.g., cerebral, adrenal, hepatic and renal) lesions have been observed in animals receiving lethal or chronic sublethal doses of digitalis (Hueper and Ichniowski, 1941), such changes have not been reported in humans. Acute hemorrhage and necrosis of the intestine, however, has accompanied frank digitalis intoxication in man (Gazes et al., 1961; Muggia, 1967). Rarely, petechial hemorrhages are reported in the myocardium (Asplund et al., 1971; Hansteen et al., 1981).

Many experimental studies have sought to explain the therapeutic and toxic actions of digitalis in the heart. Electrophysiological effects of cardiac glycosides have been well described (e.g., Fisch and Surawicz, 1969). The genesis of some of the common rhythm disorders can be understood in terms of digitalis effects on the excitability, automaticity, refractory period and conduction velocity of myocardial and Purkinje fibers. What remains obscure is the chemical bases for these chronotropic and inotropic actions of digitalis. An ability to inhibit potassium- and sodium-activated ATP phosphohydrolase (ATPase) in cell surface membranes is common to all cardiotonic glycosides. Presumably this biochemical lesion is responsible for many (if not all) of the electrophysiological expressions of the digitalis effect. Because this ATPase appears essential to couple metabolic energy to the active cation transport mechanism at the cell surface, the digitalis-poisoned myocardium cannot extrude the sodium gained or recover the potassium lost during each action potential. The result is a gradual intracellular K^+ loss and gain in Na^+ and Ca^{++} at rates that depend on the respective electrochemical gradients. A low extracellular concentration of K^+ promotes potassium efflux. Hypokalemia also accelerates the appearance of digitalis poisoning in test animals (Chung, 1969; Lown et al., 1953), and hyperkalemia delays it but does not raise the cumulative lethal dose in dogs (Zelis et al., 1970). Life-threatening tachyarrhythmias were found to be more common among digitalis-poisoned patients with hypokalemia than among those with nor-mokalemia (Lehmann et al., 1978), and the death rate was higher (13.1 vs. 4.2%). These observations underlie the use of potassium chloride as an antiarrhythmic agent in digitalis poisoning (see below).

The efflux of intracellular K^+ may also account for the hyperkalemia often encountered in victims of severe digitalis poisoning (Asplund et al., 1971; Reza et al., 1974; Rumack et al., 1974; Smith and Willerson, 1971), although dehydration and anuria undoubtedly contribute in many cases. Hyperkalemia is a bad prognostic sign in digitalis poisoning. In a series of 91 accidental or suicidal ingestions (Bismuth et al., 1973), survival correlated better with the serum K^+ level than with the dose.

Management of digitalis poisoning: If membrane ATPase inhibition is truly the primary chemical lesion in digitalis poisoning, a regenerator of this enzyme should prove to be an ideal antidote. Ionic strontium or barium reactivates the poisoned enzyme and induces hyperpolarization in monolayers of cultured embryonic chick ventricles (Henn and Sperelakis, 1968). Perhaps the same is true of Mg^{++}, because in anesthetized dogs an infusion of magnesium sulfate prevented acetylstrophanthidin-induced myocardial efflux of K^+ (Neff et al., 1972). Diuretic drugs are also known to affect cation transport mechanisms at cell surfaces. Whereas ethacrynic acid inhibits cation pumps in red blood cells and smooth muscle, it does not act on the myocardium to affect the cardiotoxicity of digitalis (Mason et al., 1971a). Triamterene, however, suppressed K^+ and Mg^{++} effluxes from the myocardium and converted ventricular tachycardia to a sinus rhythm in ouabain-poisoned dogs (Weber, 1972). Aside from the occasional use of magnesium sulfate as an antiarrhythmic agent (see below), these substances have not been adequately tested in clinical digitalis poisoning.

Established therapy assumes many forms, depending on the pattern of cardiotoxicity. In patients with slow supraventricular rhythms and/or varying degrees of AV block, which is the dominant pattern in patients with structurally sound hearts (see above), useful measures include continuous monitoring of the ECG, injection of vagolytic drugs, and electrical pacing of the ventricles. To block the inhibitory effects of enhanced vagal tone on sinoatrial (SA) node rhythmicity and on conduction through the AV node, atropine is often administered (Duke, 1972; Smith and Willerson, 1971). Sometimes the heart rate and circulation are benefited dramatically (Navab and Honey, 1967). The depressant actions of digitalis, however, are mediated only in part through the vagus; the direct effects, which may predominate at high doses, are more difficult to manage.

The ability of phenytoin to improve conduction through a depressed AV node has been utilized successfully to sustain the ventricular rate in digoxin poisoning (Rumack et al., 1974). More commonly a transvenous bipolar electrode catheter is inserted into the right ventricle, and pulses from an external standby pacemaker are delivered to sustain the ventricular rate (Asplund et al., 1971). Ventricular standstill unresponsive to pacing has been described (Reza et al., 1974; Smith and Willerson, 1971). Among 68 seriously ill patients with acute self-induced digitoxin poisoning in whom endocardial pacing was performed, 16 died, 1 from asystole refractory to pacing and 5 from ventricular fibrillation that interrupted apparently successful pacing (Bismuth et al., 1977).

When digitalis toxicity is manifested by tachycardia, many stratagems are available. If the ECG reveals only a sinus tachycardia, occasional premature beats, a modest nodal (or supraventricular) tachycardia (rate below 90) or perhaps atrial fibrillation with a ventricular rate not much above 100, continued surveillance may be all that is required. In order to interrupt, however, any sequence of events that might lead to ventricular fibrillation (Fig. III-3), active treatment is probably warranted in the presence of frequent ventricular premature beats, any ventricular tachycardia and most nodal tachycardias.

Many so-called antiarrhythmic or antifibrillatory drugs are available for this purpose. Currently popular are potassium salts, phenytoin sodium and perhaps lidocaine. Infrequent trials are reported with propranolol, edetate trisodium (EDTA) and magnesium sulfate. Perhaps procainamide and quinidine should now be regarded as obsolete in the treatment of digitalis poisoning, because in suppressing ventricular ectopic rhythms they tend also to intensify digitalis-induced conduction blockade at the AV node and so provoke fatal cardiac arrest (Smith and Haber, 1973).

Until recently the most widely used antiarrhythmic agent in digitalis poisoning was undoubtedly potassium. It was and is usually administered as KCl, by mouth when practical or by slow intravenous infusion. The rationale for this treatment is the presumed deficit of intracellular potassium in the overdigitalized heart (see above). When seen, the beneficial effects appear within 40 minutes and last up to 8 hours; they consist principally of a suppression of ectopic rhythms, including ventricular tachycardia and extrasystoles of all kinds. Atrial flutter and fibrillation are rarely modified, and most conduction disturbances are intensified by this treatment. Potassium therapy may be effective without producing a measurable rise in the level of plasma potassium, but it is contraindicated in patients with impaired renal function (Cohen, 1952) or with preexisting hyperkalemia. During the past decade it has become recognized that severe hyperkalemia is not uncommon in untreated victims of digitalis overdoses (see above). Accordingly, recommendations for potassium therapy are more restricted than formerly.

As noted above, hypokalemia from any cause is a distinct liability in the presence of a digitalis overdose, and K^+ is a rational and effective agent for controlling ectopic rhythms under these circumstances (Smith and Haber, 1973). Furthermore, chronically digitalized patients on diuretic therapy are apt to develop potassium deficits and concurrent signs of digitalis toxicity (Rodensky and Wasserman 1961; Somlyo, 1960). After single acute massive overdoses, however, hypokalemia is unusual. No consensus appears to exist concerning the role of potassium therapy in the normokalemic victim of digitalis poisoning. Except in the presence of 2° or 3° AV heart block, it is generally safe and usually effective, particularly with atrial tachyarrhythmias. The more dangerous ventricular ectopic rhythms, however, appear to be less sensitive to potassium. It has been suggested (Lyon and DeGraff, 1967) that potassium therapy is apt to delay the use of more effective agents.

At the present time, phenytoin sodium appears to be the most popular antiarrhythmic drug in digitalis poisoning. It is particularly effective against ventricular and nodal (junctional) tachycardias. Atrial tachycardia is sometimes suppressed but not digitalis-provoked atrial fibrillation or flutter (Mason et al., 1971a). Phenytoin is active in the presence of abnormal plasma K^+ levels and severe disturbances in acid-base balance (Bashour et al., 1968; Rumack et al., 1974). Like K^+, it suppresses ectopic rhythms without compromising the capacity of cardiac glycosides to enhance myocardial contractility. Lidocaine is somewhat similar but has essentially no effect on atrial rhythms and lacks the capacity of phenytoin to improve digitalis-inhibited conduction through the AV node (Mason et al., 1971a). If phenytoin and/or lidocaine are ineffective or contraindicated, propranolol is often tried. It is said to be particularly effective against digitalis-induced ventricular ectopic beats and atrial tachycardia with a regular 2° block (Irons et al., 1967). Compared with the other two drugs, however, it is more likely to compromise transmission through the AV node and to induce bradycardia (Mason et al., 1971a).

With respect to the other antiarrhythmic agents, very few generalizations can be offered that are both valid and useful. Procainamide remains a valuable drug, but in digitalis poisoning it should probably be reserved for tachyarrhythmias refractory to other agents. Various sodium salts of ethylenediaminetetraacetic acid

(EDTA), particularly the trisodium salt, have been infused intravenously to suppress digitalis-induced tachyarrhythmias (Eliot and Blount, 1961). The mechanism is evidently a transient reduction in the extracellular concentration of ionized calcium. Beneficial responses, however, are neither well sustained nor specific for digitalis rhythm disorders. In digitalis poisoning, Mg^{++} shows some of the same actions as K^+. Rarely, magnesium sulfate is given intravenously in doses of 10 to 20 ml. of a 20% aqueous solution. Even when an ectopic rhythm is suppressed by this treatment, the original disorder is likely to recur within a few minutes. The theoretician rather than the practitioner tends to maintain a continuing interest in calcium chelation and in magnesium therapy because of the many unexplained interactions between digitalis, Ca^{++} and Mg^{++}.

Studies by Zelis et al. (1970) have demonstrated the feasibility of capturing control of the ventricles by simple electrical pacing in the presence of ventricular or nodal tachycardia, but as a therapeutic measure this procedure is still experimental. Interruption of ectopic rhythms by synchronized countershock applied to the precordium is generally regarded as very hazardous because of the high incidence of ventricular fibrillation induced by countershock in the presence of a digitalis overdose (Mason et al., 1971a). If the procedure becomes mandatory, initial shocks should be at low energy levels (5, 20, then 40 watt-sec.); see p. IV-26.

Promoting digitalis elimination: Because all of the above measures represent empirical attempts to control the rate and rhythm of the heart ("mechanism of the beat") until the body can eliminate the offending glycoside and because they are not uniformly successful or safe, any technique for accelerating excretion deserves serious attention. Digoxin and presumably other cardiotonic glycosides are removed only slowly by peritoneal dialysis or hemodialysis (Ackerman et al., 1967). Hemoperfusion is far more efficient in removing digoxin. Indeed, its plasma clearance in dogs exceeded the plasma flow rate through an Amberlite XAD-4 resin column, demonstrating that the column also removed digoxin bound to blood cells (Gibson et al., 1978; Risler et al., 1979). Patients with digoxin poisoning have also been subjected to hemoperfusions through XAD-4 and through coated and uncoated charcoal (reviewed by Gibson, 1980). In general, blood and plasma clearance values were high, but because cardiotonic glycosides have large volumes of distribution due to extensive binding to tissue cells, high clearances did not yield large recoveries, at least not large in terms of the ingested dose (Clerckx-Braun et al., 1979; Gibson, 1980). Except perhaps in those with severe renal disease, it seems unlikely that hemoperfusion is a worthwhile procedure in digitalis poisoning (Clerckx-Braun et al., 1979; Gibson, 1980; Risler et al., 1979).

A more promising approach is the administration by mouth or stomach tube of an insoluble sterol-binding material to trap digitalis in the alimentary tract and so promote its fecal excretion. Given soon after the ingestion of a glycoside, such an adsorbent might prevent the gastrointestinal absorption of a toxic dose. Given later in the course of an intoxication, it might interrupt the enterohepatic circulation and so shorten the duration of the illness.

Both expectations have been realized with cholestyramine (Caldwell and Greenberger, 1971; Saral and Spratt, 1967). This anionic exchange resin is available commercially in the chloride form, but presumably only nonionic forces are involved in binding cardiac glycosides (Saral and Spratt, 1967). It binds more digitoxin than digoxin and appears to hold it more tightly (Caldwell and Greenberger, 1971). In normal human subjects who ingested 4-gm. doses of cholestyramine 4 times daily beginning 8 hours after swallowing a solution with 1.2 mg. of $[^3H]$-digitoxin, the resin treatment accelerated the elimination of the tritium and abbreviated the cardiac response (Caldwell et al., 1971). In normal subjects a reduction in the plasma half-life of digitoxin from 142 to 84 hours was produced (Carruthers and Dujovne, 1980). The resin has been used with apparent benefit in human intoxications from digoxin (Fresard et al., 1979) and from digitoxin (Cady et al., 1979; Pieroni and Fisher, 1981).

Colestipol, a related synthetic resin, is said to bind slightly more digitoxin and digoxin than cholestyramine in the presence of duodenal juice (Bazzano and Bazzano, 1972). Given by mouth to 4 patients poisoned with digitoxin, colestipol shortened the plasma half-life of the drug from 9.3 days (in a single untreated patient) to a mean of 2.75 days (Bazzano and Bazzano, 1972).

Whereas more information about the use of these resins in digitalis poisoning is desirable, there appears to be little reason for withholding them, at least in digitoxin poisoning, after vomiting is controlled. One group, however, has reported that intense diarrhea forced discontinuance of cholestyramine treatment in 4 of 5 toxic patients (Hansteen et al., 1981). The suggestion was made that activated charcoal is preferable because it is better tolerated. A critical comparison of charcoal and cholestyramine in digitalis poisoning is needed.

An area of current investigation that may contribute importantly to future therapeutic regimens is the development and characterization of antibodies to specific cardiac glycosides (Schmidt and Butler, 1971). Digoxin-specific antibodies of high affinity and specificity were elicited by immunizing sheep with digoxin covalently linked to serum albumin. Similar antibodies to ouabain have been prepared. To reduce the threat of anaphylactic reactions and to allow prompt renal excretion, these sheep antibodies were digested with papain, and the Fab fragments were purified by affinity chromatography. The intact antibodies and the Fab fragments have been shown to reverse many digoxin effects in isolated cells, tissues, laboratory animals and man (reviewed by Smith and Haber, 1973). Furthermore, when these Fab fragments were infused intravenously in patients with severe digoxin poisoning, they caused prompt and dramatic reductions in the cardiac signs of toxicity (Hess *et al.*, 1979; Smith *et al.*, 1976a). Although methods of preparing these antibodies have been carefully described, no commercial source is known, and preparations do not appear to be widely available at the present time.

Symptomatology:

1. An asymptomatic period of several minutes to several hours follows a single oral toxic dose.
2. Anorexia is often the first complaint. Nausea, salivation, and vomiting follow. Sometimes abdominal pain or discomfort accompanies these symptoms. Diarrhea is occasionally observed.
3. Nausea and vomiting occur irrespective of the route of administration; they are often persistent.
4. Early electrocardiographic changes are illustrated in Fig. III-3 (*1* through *4*); taken together they are diagnostic of a "digitalis action" on the heart. In severe intoxications, however, these subtle ECG changes can seldom be recognized because of gross disturbances in the rhythmicity and location of the pacemaker and in the conduction pathway. The disorders listed in the diagram (Fig. III-3) are not mutually exclusive and do not exhaust all the known possibilities. Thus an intoxication may progress along more than one sequence in Fig. III-3 at the same time. Associated with these disturbances in rate and rhythm of the pulse, the patient may experience palpitations.
5. Headache, malaise, fatigue, weakness, and drowsiness without coma. Drowsiness appears to be particularly common in poisoned children. Neuritic pain, especially that resembling trigeminal neuralgia, is described. Paresthesias are not uncommon.
6. Mental and emotional disorders include drowsiness, confusion, disorientation, aphasia, paranoia, delirium, hallucinations and, rarely, convulsions.
7. Visual disturbances include all grades of transient amblyopia, photophobia, blurring, halos, scotoma and aberrations of color vision.
8. Skin rashes of various types are noted rarely (Wolfe and Geiger, 1953); they are usually accompanied by eosinophilia. Other rare complications of digitalis poisoning include hypertension, stroke, heart failure and nonocclusive mesenteric infarction (Hess and Stucki, 1975), all of which are thought to indicate increased arterial vascular tone.
9. Death is due often to ventricular fibrillation or to cardiac standstill.

Treatment:

1. If overdosage is recognized promptly, the use of an emetic drug and/or gastric lavage is advisable. In most cases these measures are pointless once toxic signs and symptoms appear.
2. Nausea and vomiting are difficult, if not impossible, to suppress in digitalis poisoning, but sedation is sometimes useful in this regard.
3. When vomiting subsides, administer by mouth or stomach tube a slurry of powdered cholestyramine in water in a dose of 4 to 8 gm. (one or two 4-gm. packages of Questran). Repeat with a single 4-gm. dose (1 package) every 6 hours. The efficacy of this regimen is reasonably well established in digitoxin poisoning, less well in digoxin poisoning.
4. Monitor the ECG continuously if possible. In severe poisonings be prepared to deliver defibrillating shocks and/or to insert pacemaker electrodes in the event of ventricular fibrillation or cardiac arrest, respectively. See pp. IV-30–31.
5. If the ECG indicates severe and/or intensifying sinus bradycardia or if the ventricular rate is slow because of 2° AV block, initiate the following measures.
   A. Inject (intramuscularly or slowly intravenously) atropine sulfate in a dose of at least 0.6 mg. (0.01 mg./kg.). Probably twice this dose is preferable. A beneficial but transient increase in the heart rate indicates a need for additional doses, often at hourly intervals for many hours.
   B. If atropine is unsuccessful, small intravenous doses of phenytoin sodium may improve AV conduction and so prevent asystole.
   C. If the above measures are unsuccessful in sustaining a ventricular rate of 40 to 50 beats/min. (or higher), a slow intravenous infusion of isoproterenol hydrochloride or sublingual isoprotere-

nol (p. IV-24) may be tried, although the risk of inducing an ectopic ventricular rhythm is considerable. An alternative option is electrical pacing.

D. Insert a transvenous bipolar catheter electrode into the right ventricle and deliver pulses from an external pacemaker adjusted to sustain the ventricular rate at 60 to 80/min. (p. IV-30).

E. In the presence of asystole unresponsive to electrical pacing, cardiac massage (p. IV-26) is the only remaining option in most emergencies.

6. If the ECG indicates tachycardia from one or more ectopic foci at or below the AV node (e.g., frequent ventricular premature contractions, nodal tachycardia over 90/min., ventricular tachycardia at any rate), administer (while monitoring the ECG) one or more antiarrhythmic drugs as described below (see also text above).

A. In the patient with demonstrated hypokalemia, potassium chloride therapy may be sufficient to correct the dysrhythmia. See pp. IV-72–73 for techniques of administering KCl. This agent may or may not be useful in the normokalemic victim of digitalis poisoning. It is definitely contraindicated in hyperkalemia (K^+ concentration above 5 mEq./L.).

B. In the absence of hypokalemia or if no information is available about the plasma K^+ level, administer intravenously phenytoin sodium by techniques described on pp. IV-25–26.

C. If phenytoin sodium is ineffective or contraindicated, try intravenous lidocaine hydrochloride (p. IV-25) or perhaps propranolol hydrochloride (1 to 3 mg. at a rate not to exceed 1 mg./min., repeated once if necessary after 2 minutes).

D. If other measures fail, try procainamide (p. IV-25) with great caution.

7. If the ECG indicates tachycardia from an ectopic atrial focus (e.g., many atrial premature contractions, atrial tachycardia with 2° block, atrial fibrillation or flutter).

A. Correct hypokalemia if present.

B. Administer propranolol (as above) if the atrial pacemaker is driving the ventricles at a dangerously high rate.

C. Otherwise withhold therapy and maintain surveillance.

8. Mental and emotional signs and symptoms tend to be unpredictable and inconstant in digitalis poisoning. Because they are rarely life-threatening, supportive measures are all that is generally required.

9. Dehydration and ionic imbalances (due to vomiting and diarrhea) should be corrected cautiously by the parenteral administration of water, glucose, and the appropriate mixture of electrolytes. See pp. IV-64–73. As noted above, hypokalemia is particularly dangerous in the presence of excessive amounts of digitalis. Life-threatening levels of hyperkalemia are also encountered in digitalis poisoning and may require emergency measures, such as peritoneal dialysis or hemodialysis.

10. Hemoperfusion through Amberlite XAD-4 or through coated charcoal may be of some small benefit, particularly in digoxin-poisoned patients with severe renal disease.

11. Although not described in man, lesions suggestive of myocardial ischemia have been observed in fatally poisoned animals. Anginal pain is a rare manifestation of digitalis poisoning in man. When it occurs, a therapeutic trial with a recognized coronary vasodilator is recommended (e.g., sublingual nitroglycerin or isosorbide dinitrate).

Laboratory:

1. Serial ECGs are essential for proper diagnosis, prognosis, and treatment evaluation. A high inverse correlation exists between the serum level of digoxin and the corrected QT interval (Erbel et al., 1979).

2. An occasional eosinophilia is the only abnormality described in routine laboratory tests.

3. The serum level of potassium should be checked repeatedly in order that hypokalemia can be corrected by replacement therapy or that hyperkalemia can receive proper attention. Hypomagnesemia (less than 1.5 mEq./L.) has also been described; it may both predispose to and arise from digitalis poisoning.

4. Even in patients with normal serum electrolyte levels, salivary levels of Ca^{++} and Mg^{++} (and sometimes K^+) are significantly higher in toxic than nontoxic patients receiving digitalis. Electrolyte analyses of saliva have been suggested as a way of detecting digitalis poisoning (Wotman et al., 1971), especially because the rise in Ca^{++} concentration may precede and outlast clinical manifestations of the intoxication (Avissar et al., 1975). A low calcium content in platelets has also been suggested as a good correlate of digitalis poisoning (Tishler et al., 1979). The same appears to be true of rises in the sodium-to-potassium ratio in red cells of children (Loes et al., 1978).

5. Radioimmunoassay and other techniques

are now available for determining plasma levels of digitoxin, digoxin, etc. Highly diverse opinions are still held about the usefulness of these data in diagnosing and treating cases of digitalis intoxication (Fogelman et al., 1971; Grahame-Smith and Everest, 1969; Ingelfinger and Goldman, 1976; Smith and Haber, 1970; Tishler et al., 1979). A serum digoxin level of 1.5 ng./ml. and above is often considered in the toxic range, but a few patients are asymptomatic at twice this level. A value of 52 ng./ml. was detected in a suicide victim (Reza et al., 1974).

References:

Ackerman, G. L.; Doherty, J. E.; Flanigan, W. J. Peritoneal dialysis and hemodialysis of tritiated digoxin. Ann. Intern. Med. 67:718-723, 1967.

Asplund, J.; Edhag, O.; Mogensen, L.; Nyquist, O.; Orinius, E.; Sjogren, A. Four cases of massive digitalis poisoning. Acta Med. Scand. 189:293-297, 1971.

Avissar, R.; Merrache, R.; Mandel, E. M.; Rubinstein, I.; Djaldetti, M. Increased salivary calcium levels as an indicator of digoxin intoxication. Arch. Intern. Med. 135:1029-1032, 1975.

Bashour, F. A.; Edmonson, R. E.; Prati, R. Treatment of digitalis toxicity by diphenylhydantoin (Dilantin). Dis. Chest 53:263-270, 1968.

Batterman, R. C.; Gutner, L. B. Hitherto undescribed neurological manifestations of digitalis toxicity. Am. Heart J. 36:582-586, 1948.

Bazzano, G.; Bazzano, G. Digitalis intoxication; treatment with a new steroid-binding resin. J. A. M. A. 220:828-830, 1972.

Bergy, G. G.; Fergus, E. B.; Bruce, R. A. Acute massive digitoxin poisoning; report of a case and review of the literature. Ann. Intern. Med. 46:964-976, 1957.

Binnion, P. F.; Frazer, G. ³H-digoxin in the optic tract in digoxin intoxication. J. Cardiovasc. Pharmacol. 2:699-706, 1980.

Bismuth, C.; Gaultier, M.; Conso, F.; Efthymiou, M. L. Hyperkalemia in acute digitalis poisoning; prognostic significance and therapeutic implications. Clin. Toxicol. 6:153-162, 1973.

Bismuth, C.; Motte, G.; Conso, F.; Chauvin, M.; Gaultier, M. Acute digitoxin intoxication treated by intracardiac pacemaker: Experience in sixty-eight patients. Clin. Toxicol. 10:443-456, 1977.

Borison, H. L.; Wang, S. C. Physiology and pharmacology of vomiting. Pharmacol. Rev. 5:193-230, 1953.

Cady, W. J.; Rehder, T. L.; Campbell, J. Use of cholestyramine resin in the treatment of digitoxin toxicity. Am. J. Hosp. Pharm. 36:92-94, 1979.

Caldwell, J. H.; Bush, C. A.; Greenberger, N. J. Interruption of the enterohepatic circulation of digitoxin by cholestyramine; II. Effect on metabolic disposition of tritium labeled digitoxin and cardiac systolic intervals in man. J. Clin. Invest. 50:2638-2644, 1971.

Caldwell, J. H.; Greenberger, N. J. Interruption of the enterohepatic circulation of digitoxin by cholestyramine; I. Protection against lethal digitoxin intoxication. J. Clin. Invest. 50:2626-2637, 1971.

Carroll, F. D. Visual symptoms caused by digitalis. Am. J. Ophthalmol. 28:373-376, 1945.

Carruthers, S. G.; Dujovne, C. A. Cholestyramine and spironolactone and their combination in digitoxin elimination. Clin. Pharmacol. Ther. 27:184-187, 1980.

Chung, E. K. Digitalis Intoxication. Williams & Wilkins, Baltimore, 1969.

Church, G.; Marriott, H. J. Digitalis delirium. Circulation 20:549-553, 1959.

Clerckx-Braun, R.; Kadima, N. T.; Lesne, M.; Mahieu, P.; Vandenbroucke, J. M. Digoxin acute intoxication: Evaluation of the efficiency of charcoal hemoperfusion. Clin. Toxicol. 15:437-446, 1979.

Cohen, B. M. Digitalis poisoning and its treatment. N. Engl. J. Med. 246:225-230 and 254-259, 1952.

Danon, A.; Horowitz, J.; Ben-Zvi, Z.; Kaplanski, J.; Glick, S. An outbreak of digoxin intoxication. Clin. Pharmacol. Ther. 21:643-646, 1977.

Drevets, C. C. Accidental digitoxin poisoning in children; report of a case and review of the literature. J. Pediatr. 52:577-583, 1958.

Duke, M. Atrioventricular block due to accidental digoxin ingestion treated with atropine. Am. J. Dis. Child. 124:754-756, 1972.

Eliot, R. S.; Blount, S. G., Jr. Calcium chelates and digitalis. A clinical study. Am. Heart J. 62:7-22, 1961.

Erbel, R.; Kraemer, R.; Kleesiek, K.; Schweizer, P.; Pop, T.; Effert, S. Suizidale Digitalisintoxikation: Beziehung zwischen der Digitalis-Serumkonzentration und den elektrokardiographischen Befunden. Pharmacodynamic studies in suicidal digoxin poisoning. Z. Kardiol. 68:590-598, 1979.

Fisch, C.; Surawicz, B. Digitalis. Grune & Stratton, New York, 1969.

Fogelman, A. M.; LaMont, J. T.; Finkelstein, S.; Rado, E.; Pearce, L. Fallibility of plasma-digoxin in differentiating toxic from non-toxic patients. Lancet 2:727-729, 1971.

Fowler, R. S.; Rathi, L.; Kieth, J. D. Accidental digitalis intoxication in children. J. Pediatr. 64:188-200, 1964.

Fresard, F.; Balant, L.; Noble, J.; Garcia, B.; Muller, A. F. Cholestyramine et intoxication a la digoxine: efficacite therapeutique?. Schweiz. Med. Wochenschr. 109:431-436, 1979.

Gazes, P. C.; Holmes, C. R.; Moseley, V.; Pratt-Thomas, H. R. Acute hemorrhage and necrosis of the intestines associated with digitalization. Circulation 23:358-364, 1961.

Gibson, T. P. Hemoperfusion of digoxin intoxication. Clin. Toxicol. 17:501-513, 1980.

Gibson, T. P.; Lucas, S. V.; Nelson, H. A.; Atkinson, A. J., Jr.; Okita, G. T.; Ivanovich, P. Hemoperfusion removal of digoxin from dogs. J. Lab. Clin. Med. 91:673-682, 1978.

Gilbert, R.; Cuddy, R. P. Digitalis intoxication following conversion to sinus rhythm. Circulation 32:58-64, 1965.

Gillis, R. A.; Quest, J. A. The role of the nervous system in the cardiovascular effects of digitalis. Pharmacol. Rev. 31:19-97, 1979.

Grahame-Smith, D. G.; Everest, M. S. Measurement of digoxin in plasma and its use in diagnosis of digoxin intoxication. Br. Med. J. 1:286-289, 1969.

Hansteen, V.; Jacobsen, D.; Knudsen, K.; Reikvam, A.; Skuterud, B. Acute, massive poisoning with digitoxin: Report of seven cases and discussion of treatment. Clin. Toxicol. 18:679-692, 1981.

Henderson, F. G. Chemistry and biological activity of cardiac glycosides. In Digitalis (C. Fisch and B. Surawicz, Eds.), pp. 3-26. Grune & Stratton, New York, 1969.

Henn, F. A.; Sperelakis, N. Stimulative and protective action of Sr^{2+} and Ba^{2+} on (Na^+-K^+)-ATPase from cultured heart cells. Biochim. Biophys. Acta 163:415-417, 1968.

Hess, T.; Stucki, P. Mesenterialinfarkt bei Digitalisintoxikation. Schweiz. Med. Wochenschr. 105:1237-1240, 1975.

Hess, T.; Stucki, P.; Barandun, S.; Scholtysik, G.; Riesen, W. Antikorperbehandlung einer Digoxin-Intoxikation bei einem Patienten mit Niereninsuffizienz. Deutsche Med. Wochenschr. 104:1273-1277, 1979.

Hobson, J. D.; Zettner, A. Digoxin serum half-life following suicidal digoxin poisoning. J. A. M. A. 223:147-149, 1973.

Hoch, J. H. A Survey of Cardiac Glycosides and Genins. University of South Carolina Press, Columbia, S. C, 1961.

Hueper, W. C.; Ichniowski, C. T. Pathologic lesions in organs of cats, guinea pigs and frogs produced by digitalis poisoning. J. Lab. Clin. Med. 26:1565-1574, 1941.

Ingelfinger, J. A.; Goldman, P. The serum digitalis concentration - does it diagnose digitalis toxicity? N. Engl. J. Med. 294:867-870, 1976.

Irons, G. V., Jr.; Ginn, W. N.; Orgain, E. S. Use of a beta adrenergic receptor blocking drug (propanolol) in the treatment of cardiac arrhythmias. Am. J. Med. 43:161-170, 1967.

Joos, H. A.; Johnson, J. L. Digitalis intoxication in infancy and childhood. Pediatrics 20:866-876, 1957.

Kohn, R. M.; Kiley, J. E. Electrocardiographic changes during hemodialysis with observations on contribution of electrolyte disturbances to digitalis toxicity. Ann. Intern. Med. 39:38-50, 1953.

Krasula, R.; Yanagi, R.; Hastreiter, A.; Levitsky, S.; Soyka, L. Digoxin intoxication in infants and children; correlation with serum levels. J. Pediatr. 84:265-269, 1974.

Lathers, C. M.; Roberts, J. Digitalis cardiotoxicity revisited. Life Sci. 27:1713-1733, 1980.

Lehmann, H. U.; Witt, E.; Temmen, L.; Hochrein, H. Lebensbedrohliche Digitalisintoxikationen mit und ohne saluretische Zusatztherapie. Deutsche Med. Wochenschr. 103:1566-1571, 1978.

Lely, A. H.; Van Enter, C. H. Large-scale digitoxin intoxication. Br. Med. J. 3:737-740, 1970.

Levine, O. R.; Somlyo, A. P. Digitalis intoxication in premature infants. J. Pediatr. 61:70-78, 1962.

Lindenbaum, J.; Rund, D. G.; Butler, V. D., Jr.; Tse-Eng, D.; Saha, J. R. Inactivation of digoxin by the gut flora: Reversal by antibiotic therapy. N. Engl. J. Med. 305:789-794, 1981.

Loes, M. W.; Singh, S.; Lock, J. E.; Mirkin, B. L. Relation between plasma and red-cell electrolyte concentrations and digoxin levels in children. N. Engl. J. Med. 299:501-504, 1978.

Lown, B.; Wyatt, N. F.; Crocker, A. T.; Goodale, W. T.; Levine, S. A. Interrelationship of digitalis and potassium in auricular tachycardia with block. Am. Heart J. 45:589-601, 1953.

Lyon, A. F.; DeGraff, A. C. Reappraisal of digitalis. Am. Heart J. 73:710-712 and 835-837, 1967.

Mason, D. T.; Zelis, R.; Lee, G.; Hughes, J.; Spann, J.; Amsterdam, E. Current concepts and treatment of digitalis toxicity. Am. J. Cardiol. 27:546-559, 1971a.

Muggia, F. M. Digitalis intoxication. Hemorrhagic necrosis of the intestine; its occurrence with digitalis intoxication. Am. J. Med. Sci. 253:263-271, 1967.

Navab, F.; Honey, M. Self-poisoning with digoxin; successful treatment with atropine. Br. Med. J. 3:660-661, 1967.

Neff, M. S.; Mendelssohn, S.; Kim, K. E.; Banach, S.; Swartz, C.; Seller, R. H. Magnesium sulfate in digitalis toxicity. Am. J. Cardiol. 29:377-382, 1972.

Neill, C. A. The use of digitalis in infants and children. Progr. Cardiovasc. Dis. 7:399-416, 1965.

Pieroni, R. E.; Fisher, J. G. Use of cholestyramine resin in digitoxin toxicity. J. A. M. A. 245:1939-1940, 1981.

Reza, M. J.; Kovick, R. B.; Shine, K. I.; Pearce, M. L. Massive intravenous digoxin overdosage. N. Engl. J. Med. 291:777-778, 1974.

Rietbrock, N.; Alken, R. G. Color vision deficiencies: a common sign of intoxication in chronically digoxin-treated patients. J. Cardiovasc. Pharmacol. 2:93-99, 1980.

Risler, T.; Arnold, G.; Grabensee, B.; Krokou, J. Ist die Ham-

operfusion zur Behandlung der Digoxin-Intoxikation geeignet? Is hemoperfusion effective in the treatment of digoxin intoxication?. Z. Kardiol. 68:313-319, 1979.

Rodensky, P. L.; Wasserman, F. Observations on digitalis intoxication. Arch. Intern. Med. 108:171-178, 1961.

Rumack, B. H.; Wolfe, R. R.; Gilfrich, H. Phenytoin (diphenylhydantoin) treatment of massive digoxin overdose. Br. Heart J. 36:405-408, 1974.

Saral, R.; Spratt, J. L. Alteration of oral digitoxin toxicity and its in vitro binding to cholestyramine. Arch. Int. Pharmacodyn. Ther. 167:10-18, 1967.

Schmidt, D. H.; Butler, V. P., Jr. Reversal of digoxin toxicity with specific antibodies. J. Clin. Invest. 50:1738-1744, 1971.

Seller, R. H.; Cangiano, J.; Kim, K. E.; Mendelssohn, S.; Brest, A.; Swartz, C. Digitalis toxicity and hypomagnesemia. Am. Heart J. 79:57-68, 1970.

Sherman, J. L.; Locke, R. V. Transplacental neonatal digitalis intoxication. Am. J. Cardiol. 6:834-837, 1960.

Shrager, M. W. Digitalis intoxication. Arch. Intern. Med. 100:881-893, 1957.

Smith, T. W.; Haber, E. Digoxin intoxication; the relationship of clinical presentation to serum digoxin concentration. J. Clin. Invest. 49:2377-2386, 1970.

Smith, T. W.; Haber, E. Medical progress. Digitalis (fourth of four parts). N. Engl. J. Med. 289:1125-1129, 1973.

Smith, T. W.; Haber, E.; Yeatman, L.; Butler, V. P., Jr. Reversal of advanced digoxin intoxication with Fab fragments of digoxin-specific antibodies. N. Engl. J. Med. 294:797-800, 1976a.

Smith, T. W.; Willerson, J. T. Suicidal and accidental digoxin ingestion; report of five cases with serum digoxin level correlations. Circulation 44:29-36, 1971.

Soffer, A. The changing clinical picture of digitalis intoxication. Arch. Intern. Med. 107:681-688, 1961.

Somlyo, A. P. The toxicology of digitalis. Am. J. Cardiol. 5:523-533, 1960.

Sykowski, P. Digitoxin intoxication resulting in retrobulbar optic neuritis. Am. J. Ophthalmol. 32:572-574, 1949.

Tishler, M.; Creter, D.; Djaldetti, M. Decreased calcium content in patients with digoxin intoxication. Biomed. Express 31:12-13, 1979.

Weber, D. J. Intravenous triamterene in the treatment of acute digitalis intoxication. Clin. Pharmacol. Ther. 13:868-874, 1972.

Wolfe, L. S.; Geiger, A. J. Urticaria due to drugs of the digitalis series. N. Engl. J. Med. 248:148-149, 1953.

Wotman, S.; Bigger, J.; Mandel, I.; Bartelstone, H. Salivary electrolytes in the detection of digitalis toxicity. N. Engl. J. Med. 285:871-876, 1971.

Zelis, R.; Mason, D. T.; Spann, J. F.; Braunwald, E. Effects of ventricular stimulation and potassium administration on digitalis-induced arrhythmias. Am. J. Cardiol. 25:428-433, 1970.

DINITROPHENOL

α-Dinitrophenol (2,4-dinitrophenol) has been and occasionally still is used as a spray against aphids and mites, as a fungicide and wood preservative against various molds and mildews, and sometimes as a weed killer. Various substituted derivatives, e.g., 4,6-dinitro-o-cresol, 4,6-dinitro-2-isobutylphenol (Cann and Verhulst, 1960e), and 2,6-diiodo-4-nitrophenol (Kaiser, 1964) and many others have similar uses and similar toxicities (Ambrose, 1942). All (except the last) have produced human poisonings. These compounds are available as oil solutions, wettable powders, and salts of aliphatic amines and sodium. At one time dinitrophenol was used

as a weight-reducing drug, especially in nostrums of secret composition, but this use has been abandoned because of its toxicity (Cutting et al., 1933).

Original observations on the human toxicity of dinitrophenol stem from exposures in the French munitions industry in World War I (Perkins, 1919). Early animal experimentation was reported or reviewed by Cutting et al. (1933), Heymans and Casier (1935), Magne et al. (1932), Tainter and Cutting (1933a, b), Tainter (1934) and Tainter et al. (1935a).

Toxicology: Dinitrophenol is rapidly absorbed from all portals (gastrointestinal tract, respiratory tract, and intact skin). The fatal dose in adults is about 1 to 3 gm. by mouth, and 3 gm. has proved fatal even in divided doses over a period of 5 days (MacBryde and Taussig, 1935). Unlike rats (Eiseman et al., 1972) and rabbits, man does not detoxify or eliminate dinitrophenol rapidly (Harvey et al., 1951; Smith et al., 1953a).

The metabolism of all body cells is stimulated by contact with dinitrophenol, which appears to act by uncoupling oxidative phosphorylation (Loomis and Lipmann, 1948). In a poisoned person, the result is an almost immediate increase in oxygen consumption, body temperature, breathing rate, and heart rate. Because circulation and respiration do not accelerate in proportion to the metabolic demand, anoxia and acidosis develop. Body fat is the major, if not the exclusive fuel for this extra metabolism (Shils and Goldwater, 1953; Tainter et al., 1935b).

In addition to this metabolic action, dinitrophenol shares many of phenol's toxic properties: it is a milder corrosive to skin and mucous membrane than phenol (Spencer et al., 1948), but concentrated solutions have produced corrosion of the oropharyngeal, esophageal and gastric mucous membranes (Swamy, 1953); it exerts direct actions on the cerebrum and lower brain centers consisting of stimulation followed by depression (Simon, 1953); it may produce a necrotizing tubular injury of the kidneys (Cann and Verhulst, 1960e). If the acute phase of poisoning is survived, the patient usually tolerates successfully the later complications, which may include renal insufficiency and a toxic hepatitis.

The fulminating type of poisoning is characterized by sudden onset, severe symptoms, and prompt death (within 24 hours). Death is due to respiratory or circulatory collapse, especially the former. Many factors undoubtedly contribute to this collapse, notably hyperpyrexia, anoxia, acidosis, dehydration, muscle rigor (due to heat and/or lactic acid), and occasionally pulmonary edema. Rigor mortis may appear promptly after death. Alcohol does not potentiate the toxic syndrome in animals (Bidstrup and Payne, 1951; Cann and Verhulst, 1960e; Parker et al., 1951; Steer, 1951).

In subacute poisoning due to repeated daily exposures, some individuals complain of lassitude, headache, and malaise, while others experience a disarming sense of well-being, energy, and drive (Bidstrup, 1952a; Pollard and Filbee, 1951). Termination of the exposure and the administration of small doses of phenobarbital usually constitute adequate therapy in these cases (Edson, 1955). All patients should be warned against overheating, since the metabolic actions and consequent toxicity of dinitrophenol and most of its congeners are exaggerated by heat (Harvey, 1959). Indeed at low ambient air temperatures (below 16°C.), hypermetabolism cannot be produced in animals by this compound (Tainter, 1934). Most clinical poisonings have occurred on hot days.

Miscellaneous hazards in the use of dinitrophenol include neutropenia, agranulocytosis and cataract formation (Bidstrup and Payne, 1951). Species differences in cataractogenic activity may be related to differences in the permeability of a blood-aqueous humor barrier (Gehring and Buerge, 1969).

Dinitrophenol appears to act by interfering with the intracellular synthesis of high energy phosphate esters and not by hydrolyzing or otherwise inactivating them (Eisenhardt and Rosenthal, 1964; Pinchot, 1967). Uncoupling of oxidative phosphorylation occurs with many types of compounds. Pentachlorophenol is an important example (Stohlman, 1951). Brody (1955) has classified uncouplers into two groups: (1) agents which stimulate oxygen consumption and are insensitive to changes in magnesium ion concentration (e.g., dinitrophenol, salicylate) and (2) agents which do not stimulate oxygen consumption while depressing phosphorylation and whose action is reversed by magnesium ions (e.g., tetracyclines). More recent evidence, however, suggests that salicylates may act by a somewhat different mechanism from that of dinitrophenol (Sproull, 1957). 2,4-D (see p. III-130) and thyroid hormone are other examples of uncouplers of oxidative phosphorylation. Dinitrophenol does not act by stimulating thyroid activity. Indeed, in vitro dinitrophenol appears to block further iodination of monoiodotyrosine (Hart et al., 1961), and thyroid hypofunction occurs on repeated administration to animals (Lagerspety and Tarkkonen, 1961).

The most important therapeutic measures may be those directed at preventing body heat accumulation and even inducing mild hypothermia (Bidstrup and Payne, 1951; Edson, 1955). An apparently high degree of binding to plasma proteins (Edson, 1955) would appear to preclude the successful use of hemodialysis in cases of poisoning by these compounds.

Symptomatology:
1. Marked fatigue, tremendous thirst, profuse sweating, flushing of face.
2. Nausea, vomiting, abdominal pain, and occasionally diarrhea.
3. Restlessness, anxiety, excitement, occasionally leading to convulsions.
4. A rise in body temperature, which is roughly proportional to the toxic dose, may culminate in severe hyperpyrexia (e.g., 110° F.).
5. Tachycardia, hyperpnea, dyspnea, cyanosis, and sometimes muscle cramps.
6. Loss of consciousness, cessation of breathing, and death.

7. Late complications:
   A. Decreased urine output with albumin-uria, casts, pigment, and sometimes blood cells, due to toxic nephritis.
   B. Jaundice and tenderness in liver region due to toxic hepatitis.
8. Occasional hypersensitivity reactions after repeated exposures (or in chronic poisoning) include agranulocytic angina, skin rashes, peripheral neuritis, and late cataract formation.

Treatment:

1. Gastric lavage with large quantities of 5% sodium bicarbonate solution, leaving 1 to 2 pints in the stomach.
2. Saline cathartics, *e.g.*, 15 to 30 gm. sodium or magnesium sulfate in water.
3. Cold packs and alcohol sponges to reduce body temperature. Antipyretic drugs are ineffective here. Cold water enemas have been used. Intensive efforts to correct a dinitrophenol fever are justified. If it can be accomplished, mild hypothermia (rectal temperature between 92° and 97° F.) is probably desirable because dinitrophenol appears to lose much of its metabolic activity at these reduced temperatures.
4. Fluids, orally or intravenously (*e.g.*, 5% glucose in saline, 1000 ml.), to correct dehydration and acidosis (pp. IV-64–67, 69–72).
5. Because dinitrophenol is actively transported by the renal organic acid transport process in some species (Berndt and Grote, 1968), a trial of forced diuresis with alkalinization of the urine is warranted (Young and Haley, 1978).
6. Oxygen therapy. Artificial ventilation as needed (see pp. IV-7–14).
7. Prophylactic measures in anticipation of kidney and liver insufficiencies (see pp. IV-52 and 59, respectively).

Laboratory:

1. The urine may contain albumin, casts, bile pigment, sometimes blood. It darkens rapidly on contact with the air. Dinitrophenol and 2-amino-4-nitrophenol may be present in urine.
2. Repeated tests are desirable to detect and evaluate possible disturbances of kidney and liver function.
3. Methods are available for following blood levels of 4,6-dinitro-*o*-cresol (Harvey, 1952). Intoxications are associated with blood levels above 20 μg./ml. whole blood (Bidstrup *et al.*, 1952a; Edson, 1955).

References:

Ambrose, A. M. Some toxicological and pharmacological studies on 3, 5-dinitro-*o*-cresol. J. Pharmacol. Exp. Ther. 76:245-251, 1942.

Berndt, W. O.; Grote, D. The accumulation of ^{14}C-dinitrophenol by slices of rabbit kidney cortex. J. Pharmacol. Exp.

Ther. 164:223-231, 1968.

Bidstrup, P. L. Clinical aspects of poisoning by dinitro-*ortho*-cresol. Proc. R. Soc. Med. 45:574-575, 1952a.

Bidstrup, P. L.; Bonnell, J. A. L.; Harvey, D. G. Prevention of acute dinitro-ortho-cresol (DNOC) poisoning. Lancet 1:794-795, 1952.

Bidstrup, P. L.; Payne, D. J. H. Poisoning by dinitro-o-cresol. Report of eight fatal cases occurring in Great Britain. Br. Med. J. 2:16-19, 1951.

Brody, T. M. The uncoupling of oxidative phosphorylation as a mechanism of drug action. Pharmacol. Rev. 7:335-363, 1955.

Cann, H. M.; Verhulst, H. L. Fatality from dinitrophenol derivative poisoning. Bull. National Clearinghouse for Poison Control Centers, June, 1960e.

Cutting, W. C.; Mehrtens, H. G.; Tainter, M. L. Actions and uses of dinitrophenol. J. A. M. A. 101:193-195, 1933.

Edson, E. F. Emergencies in general practice. Agricultural poisons. Br. Med. J. 1:841-844, 1955.

Eiseman, J. L.; Gehring, P. J.; Gibson, J. E. The *in vitro* metabolism of 2, 4-dinitrophenol by rat liver homogenates. Toxicol. Appl. Pharmacol. 21:275-285, 1972.

Eisenhardt, R. H.; Rosenthal, O. 2, 4-Dinitrophenol: Lack of interaction wth high energy intermediates of oxidative phosphorylation. Science 143:476-477, 1964.

Gehring, P. J.; Buerge, J. F. The distribution of 2, 4-dinitrophenol relative to its cataractogenic activity in ducklings and rabbits. Toxicol. Appl. Pharmacol. 15:579-592, 1969.

Hart, K. T.; Bauer, M. A.; Druet, D.; Mack, R. E. The effect of 2, 4-dinitrophenol on iodine metabolism. J. Pharmacol. Exp. Ther. 134:227-232, 1961.

Harvey, D. G. Estimation of dinitro-*ortho*-cresol in blood. Lancet 1:796-797, 1952.

Harvey, D. G. On the metabolism of some aromatic nitro compounds by different species of animal; III. The toxicity of the dinitrophenols, with a note on the effects of high environmental temperatures. J. Pharm. Pharmacol. 11:462-474, 1959.

Harvey, D. G.; Bidstrup, P. L.; Payne, J. A. L. Poisoning by dinitro-*ortho*-cresol. Some observations on the effects of dinitro-*ortho*-cresol administered by mouth to human volunteers. Br. Med. J. 2:13-16, 1951.

Heymans, C.; Casier, H. Recherches sur l'action de differents nitroderives sur le metabolisme et sur la temparature. Arch. Int. Pharmacodyn. Ther. 50:20-64, 1935.

Kaiser, J. A. Studies on the toxicity of disophenol (2, 6-diiodo-4-nitrophenol) to dogs and rodents plus some comparisons with 2, 4-dinitrophenol. Toxicol. Appl. Pharmacol. 6:232-244, 1964.

Lagerspety, K.; Tarkkonen, H. Metabolic and antithyroid effects of prolonged administration of dinitrophenol in mice. Ann. Med. Exp. Biol. Fenn. 39:287-296, 1961.

Loomis, W. F.; Lipmann, F. Reversible inhibition of the coupling between phosphorylation and oxidation. J. Biol. Chem. 173:807-808, 1948.

MacBryde, C. M.; Taussig, B. L. Functional changes in liver, heart and muscles and loss of dextrose tolerance resulting from dinitrophenol. J. A. M. A. 105:13-17, 1935.

Magne, H.; Mayer, A.; Plantefol, L. Action pharmacodynamique des phenols nitres. Un agent augmentant les oxydations cellulaires. Le dinitrophenol 1-2-4 (thermol); caracteres generaux de l'intoxication par le dinitrophenol 1-2-4. Ann. de Physiol. 8:1-61, 70-91, and 157-175, 1932.

Parker, V. H.; Barnes, J. M.; Denz, F. A. Some observations on the toxic properties of 3, 5-dinitro-*ortho*-cresol. Br. J. Ind. Med. 8:226-235, 1951.

Perkins, R. G. A study of the munitions intoxications in France. Public Health Rep. (U. S.) 34:2335-2374, 1919.

Pinchot, G. B. The mechanism of uncoupling of oxidative phosphorylation by 2,4-dinitrophenol. J. Biol. Chem. 242:4577-4583, 1967.

Pollard, A. B.; Filbee, J. F. Recovery after poisoning with dinitro-*ortho*-cresol. Lancet 2:618-619, 1951.

Shils, M. E.; Goldwater, L. J. Effect of diet on the susceptibility of the rat to poisoning by 2, 4-dinitrotoluene. Arch. Environ. Health 8:262-267, 1953.

Simon, E. W. Mechanisms of dinitrophenol toxicity. Biol. Rev.

28:453-479, 1953.

Smith, J. N.; Smithies, R. H.; Williams, R. T. Studies in detoxication. 48. Urinary metabolites of 4, 6-dinitro-o-cresol in the rabbit. Biochem. J. 54:225-230, 1953a.

Spencer, H. C.; Rowe, V. K.; Adams, E. M.; Irish, D. D. Toxicological studies on laboratory animals of certain alkyl dinitrophenols used in agriculture. J. Ind. Hyg. Toxicol. 30:10-25, 1948.

Sproull, D. H. A comparison of sodium salicylate and 2, 4-dinitrophenol as metabolic stimulants in vitro. Biochem. J. 66:527-532, 1957.

Steer, C. Death from dinitro-o-cresol. Lancet 1:1419, 1951.

Stohlman, E. F. The toxicity of some related halogenated derivatives of phenol. Public Health Rep. 66:1303-1313, 1951.

Swamy, S. A. Suicidal poisoning by dinitrophenol. J. Indian Med. Assoc. 22:504-505, 1953.

Tainter, M. L. Low oxygen tensions and temperatures on the actions and toxicity of dinitrophenol. J. Pharmacol. Exp. Ther. 51:45-58, 1934.

Tainter, M. L.; Bergstrom, F. W.; Cutting, W. C. Metabolic activity of compounds related to dinitrophenol. J. Pharmacol. Exp. Ther. 53:58-66, 1935a.

Tainter, M. L.; Cutting, W. C. Febrile, respiratory and some other actions of dinitrophenol. J. Pharmacol. Exp. Ther. 48:410-429, 1933a.

Tainter, M. L.; Cutting, W. C. Miscellaneous actions of dinitrophenol. Repeated administrations, antidotes, fatal doses, antiseptic tests and action of some isomers. J. Pharmacol. Exp. Ther. 49:187-208, 1933b.

Tainter, M. L.; Cutting, W. C.; Hines, E. Effects of moderate doses of dinitrophenol on the energy exchange and nitrogen metabolism of patients under conditions of restricted dietary. J. Pharmacol. Exp. Ther. 55:326-353, 1935b.

Young, J. F.; Haley, T. J. A pharmacokinetic study of pentachlorophenol poisoning and the effect of forced diuresis. Clin. Toxicol. 12:41-48, 1978.

DISULFIRAM

Disulfiram (tetraethylthiuram disulfide or Antabuse) is used in clinical medicine to establish and reinforce a conditioned reflex by which many chronic alcoholics are able to refuse alcoholic beverages. The drug acts by interfering with alcohol metabolism so that the ingestion of alcohol is followed by distressing and occasionally dangerous symptoms. Several hundred thousand abstinent patients are said to take the drug every day.

Toxicology: Neither disulfiram nor its congeners appear to have a high inherent toxicity in either acute or chronic exposures; most of them are moderately or slightly toxic. The smallest fatal oral dose of disulfiram has been reported as 3 gm./kg. in rabbits; thiram (see below) proved to be about 10 times more toxic (Hanzlik and Irvine, 1921). Rats are more resistant to disulfiram than rabbits, the acute oral LD_{50} being 8.6 gm./kg. (Child and Cramp, 1952).

The most frequent complication of disulfiram (Antabuse) therapy is the reaction which comparatively small doses of ethyl alcohol induce in persons who are on disulfiram therapy. The primary toxicity of disulfiram in the absence of alcohol is a different problem in all respects. In clinical doses (500 mg./day for 1 to 2 weeks, followed by a maintenance dose of 125 to 250 mg. daily), disulfiram is usually well tolerated if alcohol is avoided; the commonest side effects are slight drowsiness, an unpleasant taste, mild gastrointestinal disturbances and orthostatic hypotension. Occasionally, psychotic reactions (Bennett et al., 1951; Heath et al., 1965; Liddon and Satran, 1967), catatonia (Weddington et al., 1980), depressed confusional states (Rathod, 1958) and severe peripheral sensorimotor neuropathies (Hayman and Wilkins, 1956) have been reported as side reactions to therapeutic doses in patients who had no access to ethyl alcohol. In almost all clinical reports of frank disulfiram overdosage, however, the possibility that alcohol was also consumed has not been convincingly excluded. The psychological makeup of patients in whom this drug is commonly used is such that reports of toxic states due to disulfiram alone must be viewed with circumspection.

For a further discussion of the inherent toxicity of disulfiram, see THIRAM on p. III-383. The following discussion is restricted to ethanol-disulfiram interactions and to the symptom complex precipitated by ethyl alcohol in those who have taken otherwise insignificant amounts of disulfiram.

The disulfiram-alcohol reaction is apparently due to a drug-induced disturbance in alcohol metabolism and is not a simple intensification of alcoholic intoxication, although this may also play a role. Chevens (1953) described a group of patients who sought disulfiram as a means of achieving a state of inebriation without consuming much alcohol. The acute drug-alcohol reaction, however, is usually considered unpleasant, at times alarmingly so. It consists of flushing, headache, vasodilatation, tachycardia, hypotension (after a transient rise in systolic pressure), nausea, vomiting, hyperpnea, chest pain, sweating, restlessness, confusion and many other signs and symptoms. The syndrome is reminiscent of a massive release of endogenous histamine. Indeed, alcohol ingestion particularly after disulfiram results in degranulation of mast cells in guinea pig lung and a reduction of lung histamine content (Berg et al., 1977). No increase in blood histamine, however, was detected (Hald et al., 1948), and the respiratory effects did not entirely match those of histamine in normal human subjects (Asmussen et al., 1948a). Antihistaminic therapy is said to be ineffective against the disulfiram-alcohol reaction, but we know of no controlled study.

The disulfiram-alcohol reaction appears at the same time as excessive concentrations of acetaldehyde in the blood (Hald and Jacobsen, 1948). The enzyme alcohol dehydrogenase generates acetaldehyde from ethanol. Acetaldehyde accumulates presumably because disulfiram inhibits aldehyde dehydrogenase, the enzyme which normally oxidizes this intermediary product of alcohol metabolism to "active" acetate (Hald et al., 1948; Hald and Jacobsen, 1948). This inhibition has been demonstrated in vitro with NAD-dependent isozymes of this liver enzyme (Lindahl, 1980). Acetaldehyde, when infused into normal human subjects to achieve blood levels of 0.2 to 0.7 mg./100 ml., is said to produce some of the same responses as in the disulfiram-alcohol reaction (Asmussen et al., 1948a, b). The hypothesis that endogenous acetaldehyde is responsible for the disulfiram-ethanol reaction was quickly accepted.

Additional investigations, however, were inspired by observed differences between responses to acetaldehyde infusion into laboratory animals and the disulfiram-alcohol reaction (Perman, 1962). When infused into animals, acetaldehyde, propionaldehyde and butyraldehyde all have sympathomimetic effects. The rise in blood pressure resembles that seen after tyramine, and as with tyramine, it has been ascribed to a release of norepinephrine from adrenergic nerve terminals but not from the adrenal medulla (Eade, 1959). This prominent effect of acetaldehyde, however, is inconsistent with the hypotensive crisis of the disulfiram-ethanol reaction (Hine et al., 1952).

Further elucidation came with the discovery that disulfiram is a potent inhibitor of dopamine β-oxidase. This enzyme requires copper, which disulfiram apparently removes by chelation. Dopamine β-oxidase is an essential enzyme in the norepinephrine biosynthetic pathway (Goldstein et al., 1965). Daily treatment with disulfiram leads to depletion of norepinephrine at adrenergic nerve terminals, as with reserpine (Goldstein and Nakajima, 1966; Hashimoto et al., 1965a). Indeed, mild postural hypotension is a recognized side effect of disulfiram even in patients abstaining from alcohol, although blood pressures in the supine position may be slightly and unaccountably elevated (Rogers et al., 1979). With the sympathomimetic effects of acetaldehyde blocked by disulfiram depletion of the adrenergic transmitter, the direct vasodilator effect of acetaldehyde is unmasked. The latter is presumably responsible for the fall in blood pressure in the disulfiram-alcohol reaction.

Pyrazole is an experimental compound that is a potent inhibitor of alcohol dehydrogenase. It has been suggested that pyrazole may find application in the management of the disulfiram-alcohol reaction. By inhibiting alcohol dehydrogenase it prevents the further accumulation of acetaldehyde (Lester and Benson, 1970). However, disulfiram itself and its metabolite diethyldithiocarbamate inhibit alcohol dehydroge-

nase in rat and mouse liver (Sharkawi, 1980). After ethanol administration, higher ethanol blood levels and slower ethanol elimination rates have been demonstrated in disulfiram-pretreated mice, rats, rabbits and dogs than in disulfiram-free animals. This phenomenon, however, is not recognized in man, and controlled clinical trials failed to demonstrate effects on blood alcohol levels with disulfiram-ethanol doses that greatly elevated acetaldehyde levels in the blood (Sauter et al., 1977).

About 0.5 to 1 gm. of disulfiram daily for a few days sensitizes an adult of average size to as little as half an ounce of whiskey or any other alcoholic beverage. Even a teaspoonful may lead to mildly unpleasant symptoms. With less safety, a large single dose of disulfiram can establish this reactive state, which may persist for more than 1 week. The greater the doses of drug and of alcohol, the more violent is the reaction. In mild cases the effects last only 1 hour, in severe cases several hours (McCabe and Wilson, 1954; Woolley et al., 1980). In persons receiving disulfiram, deaths have occurred following the ingestion of alcoholic beverages (Alha et al., 1957; Becker and Sugarman, 1952; Jones, 1949). Indeed, the secretive administration of disulfiram has been implicated in a homicide. Autopsy revealed multiple hemorrhagic necrosis of the cerebral cortex, the thalamus, the medulla and the myocardium (Althoff, 1968). The reaction has been accidentally triggered by commercial cough mixtures, mouthwashes and other medicinals, some of which are 50 to 70 proof in ethanol (Koff et al., 1971; Petroni and Cardoni, 1979).

That the state of alcohol intolerance commonly persists for 7 to 10 days (rarely even 14 days) after discontinuing disulfiram therapy is difficult to reconcile with the rapid metabolism of the drug. Added to shed blood, disulfiram is quickly and quantitatively reduced (Cobby et al., 1977), probably by glutathione reductase in red cells (Strömme, 1963). The reaction is essentially complete within 4 minutes. The reduction product is the monomer diethyldithiocarbamate (DDC), which has a half-life of only 70 minutes in shed blood (Cobby et al., 1977). In rats, DDC is metabolized by several pathways, including glucuronide formation, oxidation to sulfate, and decomposition to carbon disulfide and diethylamine (Faiman et al., 1980; Strömme, 1965). In man as well as animals, disulfiram is essentially undetectable in blood after ingestion of the drug; DDC is the principal chemical species found (e.g., Strömme, 1965). On the other hand, the dimer disulfiram, not the monomer DDC, appears to be the active inhibitor of acetaldehyde dehydrogenase (Lindahl, 1980), probably because it readily forms mixed disulfides with thiol groups on enzymes, whereas the monomer does not (Strömme, 1965). Enzyme inhibition may persist because of the slow reoxidation of small amounts of DDC to disulfiram and the promp and long-lasting sulfhydryl exchange reactions of the latter (Strömme, 1963, 1965).

Other chemicals with disulfiram-like effects: Similar states of alcohol intolerance can be elicited by exposure to a variety of compounds related to disulfiram and to some unrelated chemicals. For example, coprine is effective; it occurs as a natural constituent of some species of poisonous mushrooms of the genus *Coprinus*; see MUSHROOM TOXINS, p. III-295. Citrated calcium carbimide (see Calcium Cyanamide in Section II) has been used therapeutically in the management of alcoholism. The methyl analogue of disulfiram (tetramethylthiuram disulfide or thiram) has been used as a rubber accelerator (Thuads) and as an important agricultural fungicide. Also, thiram and similar compounds have served as successful insecticides and are marketed as repellents against the Japanese beetle (see also THIRAM, p. III-383). Accidental exposure to any one of these substances might escape detection or even suspicion until the ingestion of alcohol. For example, a gardener experienced a typical reaction after exposure to a thiram fungicide (Reinl, 1966), and a woman who bathed with a bactericidal soap containing thiram experienced scarlet flushing whenever she drank a cocktail (Welsh, 1961).

Indeed, in tests on rabbits, thiram was even more potent than disulfiram in promoting acetaldehyde accumulation during ethanol metabolism, but the propyl and butyl analogues were inactive (Hald *et al.*, 1952). The monosulfides (*e.g.*, tetraethylthiuram monosulfide) showed marked and prolonged effects. They also possess fungicidal and insecticidal properties; the monosulfide analogue of disulfiram has been incorporated into a medicinal soap for the treatment of human scabies.

Soluble diethyl and dimethyl dithiocarbamates (*e.g.*, sodium and potassium salts) have a potent but transient capacity to sensitize to alcohol, whereas the insoluble salts (*e.g.*, ferric, zinc, manganese) were not tested (Hald *et al.*, 1952). Both groups have been widely used as agricultural fungicides (Hodge *et al.*, 1956).

The hypoglycemic sulfonylurea drugs, carbutamide, tolbutamide and chlorpropamide, produce a somewhat milder intolerance to alcohol (Truitt *et al.*, 1962). An antitrichomonas drug metronidazole also evokes a disulfiram-like response to alcohol and has produced an acute psychosis in combination with disulfiram (Rothstein and Clancy, 1969).

The transient cutaneous vasodilatation (degreasers' flush) seen after repeated exposure to trichloroethylene on challenge with alcohol is a similar phenomenon (Müller *et al.*, 1975; Stewart *et al.*, 1974). Coincidentally, disulfiram is a potent inhibitor of trichloroethylene metabolism to trichloroethanol and trichloroacetic acid (Bartonicek and Teisinger, 1962; Müller *et al.*, 1975).

Symptomatology (the alcohol-induced reaction only):

1. The reaction begins within 15 minutes (usually 5 to 10 minutes) after ingesting alcohol and is usually finished in 1 to 3 hours.
2. Sensation of heat, flushing, restlessness, anxiety.
3. Vasodilatation with fall in systolic and diastolic blood pressures, tachycardia, palpitations, orthostatic syncope. A pressor rather than a depressor reaction is possible in those who have taken disulfiram for only a few days (see text above).
4. Severe pulsating headache, nausea and vomiting.
5. Hyperventilation and sensation of constriction in the neck, chest pain, dyspnea but apparently not bronchospasm.
6. Sweating, thirst, weakness, vertigo and confusion. Even visual hallucinations have been described (Cockburn, 1964).
7. Circulatory collapse, coma and death.
8. Severe atypical reactions include myocardial infarction, acute congestive heart failure, cardiac arrhythmias, marked respiratory depression and convulsions.

Treatment:

1. Hypotension and shock are the derangements that usually require the most vigorous measures. Put patient in the Trendelenburg position (legs high, head low). Infuse rapidly by the intravenous route isotonic saline and/or 5% glucose in water (pp. IV-16–20).
2. Ephedrine sulfate (30 mg.) intramuscularly or an intravenous infusion of levarterenol if the hypotension is severe (p. IV-17).
3. Oxygen inhalation may or may not relieve any of the distressing symptoms (p. IV-12).
4. With the intent of reversing any disulfiram-induced inhibition of cell oxidative metabolism, 1 gm. ascorbic acid has been given intravenously (slowly), but the effectiveness of this measure has not been established, and its need has not been demonstrated.
5. In severe cases the slow and cautious intravenous injection of saccharated iron has been recommended (100 mg. in 5 ml.). The basis of this proposal is a 1950 observation that a Finnish medication ("Ferroscorbin") consisting of ascorbic acid and ferrous chloride delayed or ameliorated the symptoms

if injected promptly (Jokivartio, 1950). However, the effectiveness and safety of intravenous iron have not been adequately established.

6. The possibility that antihistaminic therapy may offer some symptomatic benefit should be explored but only under controlled conditions.

7. Administer potassium cautiously if the clinical signs, ECG or serum analysis indicates significant hypokalemia (p. IV-73).

8. The rigorous prohibition of any ethyl alcohol for at least 10 days after the last dose of disulfiram.

Laboratory: Blood analyses for acetaldehyde or disulfiram (as its metabolite DDC) may aid in the diagnosis (Alha *et al.*, 1957). Presumably because of hyperventilation, blood pH tends to be elevated, whereas blood pCO_2 and potassium are lowered (Asmussen *et al.*, 1948a; Sauter *et al.*, 1977).

References:

Alha, A. R.; Hjelt, E.; Tamminen, V. Disulfiram-alcohol intoxication. Investigation of five fatal cases and the chemical determination of disulfiram and blood acetaldehyde. Acta Pharmacol. Toxicol. *13*:277-288, 1957.

Althoff, H. Multiple hemorrhagic necroses of the brain as a complication of disulfiram (Antabuse) therapy. Ger. Med. Mon. *13*:180-183, 1968.

Asmussen, E.; Hald, J.; Jacobsen, E.; Jorgensen, G. Studies on the effect of tetraethylthiuram-disulfide (Antabuse) and alcohol or respiration and circulation in normal human subjects. Acta Pharmacol. Toxicol. *4*:297-304, 1948a.

Asmussen, E.; Hald, J.; Larsen, V. The pharmacological action of acetaldehyde on the human organism. Acta Pharmacol. Toxicol. *4*:311-320, 1948, 1948b.

Bartonicek, V.; Teisinger, J. Effect of tetraethyl thiuram disulfide (Disulfiram) on metabolism of trichloroethylene in man. Br. J. Ind. Med. *19*:216-221, 1962.

Becker, M. C.; Sugarman, G. Death following "test drink" of alcohol in patients receiving Antabuse. J. A. M. A. *149*:568-571, 1952.

Bennett, A. E.; McKeever, L. G.; Turk, R. E. Psychotic reaction during tetraethylthiuram disulfide (Antabuse) therapy. J. A. M. A. *145*:483-484, 1951.

Berg, S.; Garbe, G.; Hirtz, J. Die Wirkung von Athanol und Antabus-Alkohol-Reaktion auf den Histamin-und Mastzellgehalt der Lunge. Z. Rechtsmed. *79*:115-123, 1977.

Chevens, L. C. F. Antabuse addiction. Br. Med. J. *1*:1450-1451, 1953.

Child, G. P.; Cramp, M. The toxicity of tetraethylthiuram disulfide (Antabuse) to mouse, rat, rabbit and dog. Acta Pharmacol. Toxicol. *8*:305-314, 1952.

Cobby, J.; Mayersohn, M.; Selliah, S. The rapid reduction of disulfiram in blood and plasma. J. Pharmacol. Exp. Ther. *202*:724-731, 1977.

Cockburn, J. J. Abnormal reaction to disulfiram. Br. Med. J. *1*:770, 1964.

Eade, N. R. Mechanism of sympathomimetic action of aldehydes. J. Pharmacol. Exp. Ther. *127*:29-34, 1959.

Faiman, M. D.; Artman, L.; Haya, K. Disulfiram distribution and elimination in the rat after oral and intraperitoneal administration. Alcohol. Clin. Exp. Res. *4*:412-419, 1980.

Goldstein, M.; Lauber, E.; McKereghan, M. R. Studies in the purification and characterization of 3,4-dihydroxyphenylethylamine β-hydroxylase. J. Biol. Chem. *24*:2066-2072, 1965.

Goldstein, M.; Nakajima, K. The effects of disulfiram on the repletion of brain catecholamine stores. Life Sci. *5*:1133-1138, 1966.

Hald, J.; Jacobsen, E. The formation of acetaldehyde in the organism after ingestion of Antabuse (tetraethylthiuramdisulphide) and alcohol. Acta Pharmacol. Toxicol. *4*:305-310, 1948.

Hald, J.; Jacobsen, E.; Larsen, V. The formation of acetaldehyde in the organism after ingestion of Antabuse (tetraethylthiuram disulfide) and alcohol. Acta Pharmacol. Toxicol. *4*:285-296, 1948.

Hald, J.; Jacobsen, E.; Larsen, V. The Antabuse effect of some compounds related to Antabuse and cyanamide. Acta Pharmacol. Toxicol. *8*:329-337, 1952.

Hanzlik, P. J.; Irvine, A. The toxicity of some thioureas and thiuram disulfides. J. Pharmacol. Exp. Ther. *17*:349-355, 1921.

Hashimoto, J.; Ohi, Y.; Imaizumi, R. Inhibition of brain dopamine-β-oxidase in vivo by disulfiram. Jap. J. Pharmacol. *15*:445-446, 1965a.

Hayman, M.; Wilkins, P. A. Polyneuropathy as a complication of disulfiram therapy of alcoholism. Q. J. Stud. Alcohol *17*:601-607, 1956.

Heath, R. G.; Nesselhof, W.; Bishop, M. P.; Byers, L. W. Behavioral and metabolic changes associated with administration of tetraethylthiuram disulfide (Antabuse). Dis. Nerv. Syst. *26*:99-104, 1965.

Hine, C. H.; Burbridge, T. N.; Macklin, E. A.; Anderson, H.; Simon, A. Some aspects of the human pharmacology of tetraethylthiuram disulfide (Antabuse)-alcohol reactions. J. Clin. Invest. *31*:317-325, 1952.

Hodge, H. C.; Maynard, E. A.; Downs, W. L.; Coye, R. D., Jr.; Steadman, L. T. Chronic oral toxicity of ferric dimethyldithiocarbamate (Ferbam) and zinc dimethyldithiocarbamate (Ziram). J. Pharmacol. Exp. Ther. *118*:174-181, 1956.

Jokivartio, E. Effect of iron preparations on "Antabuse"-alcohol toxicosis. Q. J. Stud. Alcohol *11*:183-189, 1950.

Jones, R. O. Death following ingestion of alcohol in Antabuse treated patient. Can. Med. Assoc. J. *60*:609-612, 1949.

Koff, R. S.; Papadimas, I.; Honig, E. G. Alcohol in cough mixture, a hazard to disulfiram user. J. A. M. A. *215*:1988-1989, 1971.

Lester, D.; Benson, G. O. Alcohol oxidation in rats inhibited by pyrazole, oximes and amides. Science *169*:282-283, 1970.

Liddon, S. C.; Satran, R. Disulfiram (Antabuse) psychosis. Am. J. Psychiatry *123*:1284-1289, 1967.

Lindahl, R. Differentiation of normal and inducible rat liver aldehyde dehydrogenases by disulfiram inhibition *in vitro*. Biochem. Pharmacol. *29*:3026-3029, 1980.

McCabe, E. S.; Wilson, W. W. Dangerous cardiac effects of tetraethylthiuram disulfide (Antabuse) therapy in alcoholism. Arch. Inter. Med. *94*:259-263, 1954.

Muller, G.; Spassowski, M.; Henschler, D. Metabolism of trichloroethylene in man. III. Interaction of trichloroethylene and ethanol. Arch. Toxicol. *33*:173-189, 1975.

Perman, E. S. Studies on the Antabuse-alcohol reaction in rabbits. Acta Physiol. Scand. 55:Suppl. No. 196, 1962.

Petroni, N. C.; Cardoni, A. A. Alcohol content of liquid medicinals. Clin. Toxicol. *14*:407-432, 1979.

Rathod, N. H. Toxic effects of disulfiram therapy, with two case reports. Q. J. Stud. Alcohol *19*:418-427, 1958.

Reinl, W. Alkoholuberempfindlichkeit nach Umgang mit dem Fungicid Tetramethylthiuramdisulfid (TMTD). Arch. Toxikol. *22*:12-15, 1966.

Rogers, W. K.; Benowitz, N. L.; Wilson, K. M.; Abbott, J. A. Effect of disulfiram on adrenergic function. Clin. Pharmacol. Ther. *25*:469-477, 1979.

Rothstein, E.; Clancy, D. D. Toxicity of disulfiram combined with metronidazole. N. Engl. J. Med. *280*:1006, 1969.

Sauter, A. M.; Boss, D.; von Wartburg, J. -P. Reevaluation of the disulfiram-alcohol reaction in man. J. Stud. Alcohol *38*:1680-1695, 1977.

Sharkawi, M. Inhibition of alcohol dehydrogenase by disulfiram; possible relation to the disulfiram-ethanol reaction. Life Sci., *27*:1939-1945, 1980.

Stewart, R. D.; Hake, C. L.; Peterson, J. E. "Degreasers' flush," dermal response to trichloroethylene and ethanol. Arch. Environ. Health 29:1-5, 1974.

Stromme, J. H. Effects of diethyldithiocarbamate and disulfiram on glucose metabolism and glutathione content of human erythrocytes. Biochem. Pharmacol. 12:705-715, 1963.

Stromme, J. H. Metabolism of disulfiram and diethyldithiocarbamate in rats with demonstration of an in vivo ethanol-induced inhibition of the glucuronic acid conjugation of the thiol. Biochem. Pharmacol. 14:393-410, 1965.

Truitt, E. B., Jr.; Puritz, G.; Morgan, A. M.; Prouty, R. W. Disulfiram-like actions produced by hypoglycemic sulfurylurea compounds. Q. J. Stud. Alcohol 23:197-207, 1962.

Weddington, W. W.; Marks, R. C.; Verghese, J. P. Disulfiram encephalopathy as a cause of the catatonia syndrome. Am. J. Psychiatry 137:1217-1219, 1980.

Welch, A. L. Fixed Eruptions. Charles C Thomas, Springfield, Ill, 1961.

Woolley, B.; Devenyi, P. Acute disulfiram overdose. J. Stud. Alcohol 41:740-743, 1980.

EDETATE CALCIUM DISODIUM

Edetate calcium disodium is the calcium disodium salt of ethylenediaminetetraacetic acid, hereafter referred to as CaNa$_2$EDTA. It and many of its derivatives are widely recognized by the trade name Versenes. Extensively used as tools in analytical chemistry, these substances are called "chelating agents" because of their ability to combine with polyvalent metallic ions (cations) in solution to form soluble ring structures or chelates. This property has been exploited in the treatment of heavy metal intoxications, notably lead poisoning.

To chelate lead in vivo with CaNa$_2$EDTA is to render it unavailable for its usual biochemical reactions. The ability to sequester selectively any particular cation depends on the stability of the cation-chelating agent complex, the nature, concentration, and tissue distribution of the cation, and the degree to which other systems are available to compete for the cation. Rapid intravenous administration of various sodium salts of EDTA may produce precipitous drops in the serum level of ionized calcium and symptoms of hypocalcemia in man (Popovici et al., 1950; Spencer et al., 1956).

The severity of the hypocalcemic syndrome is related to the speed of injection and the dose (Done, 1961b; Foreman, 1963; Meltzer et al., 1961); frank tetany would appear to be rare. Moreover, the hypocalcemia after a single dose is surprisingly transient because it triggers a prompt release of calcium due to resorption of bone (Holland et al., 1953; Spencer et al., 1956). However, the possibility of a hypocalcemic reaction led to the development of CaNa$_2$EDTA (Popovici et al., 1950), from which calcium becomes displaced in vivo by any available Pb^{++}.

CaNa$_2$EDTA is now generally acknowledged as the agent of choice in hastening the urinary excretion of lead. It is probably useful in acute cadmium poisoning (see p. III-80). Further experimental and clinical trials are indicated to demonstrate its value in poisonings due to americium, chromium, cobalt, copper, iron, manganese, nickel, plutonium, radium, selenium, thorium, tungsten, uranium, vanadium, yttrium and zinc. It is apparently not effective in strontium or thallium poisonings (Done, 1961b). Gold, mercury, and arsenic are probably best antidoted by BAL (see p. III-52).

CaNa$_2$EDTA is available commercially as a 20% solution which is diluted prior to injection. Although there are serious reservations about its effectiveness when given by mouth (Byers, 1959; Selander, 1967; Sidbury et al., 1953), it was at one time also available as 500-mg. tablets.

Toxicology: The intravenous administration of CaNa$_2$EDTA may lead to thrombophlebitis proximal to the site of injection. This reaction appears to be related to the concentration of the drug, and it is rarely seen at concentrations below 0.5% (Seven, 1960).

Although some believe that the hazard has been overemphasized (Chenoweth, 1968), the most serious objection to the uncontrolled use of CaNa$_2$EDTA and related compounds is their predilection to cause severe renal damage (Moeschlin, 1957; Vogt and Cottier, 1957). Dudley et al. (1955) reported two fatal cases in which sodium EDTA was used in the therapy of hypercalcemia. Severe damage to the renal tubular epithelium, engorgement of reticuloendothelial cells with coarse eosinophilic granules, and hemorrhagic manifestations were seen postmortem. Others (Holland et al., 1953) have noted renal tubular vacuolization; as induced in rats, this lesion has been ascribed to the induction of pinocytosis (Schwartz et al., 1970). Signs of transient renal dysfunction in a patient receiving CaNa$_2$EDTA to lower the body plutonium burden prompted Foreman and his associates (1956) to investigate the problem in rats. With moderately high doses they regularly observed severe hydropic degeneration of the proximal tubules. During initial stages the lesion was reversible, which affords a means of using the drug safely. The ED$_{50}$ (amount of drug required to produce minimal histological evidence of damage in 50% of the animals treated daily for 16 days) was 203 mg./kg. per day by the intraperitoneal route.

Reubner and Bradley (1960) reported a case in which a 1-year-old child being treated for lead poisoning died from uremic complications after receiving 125 mg./kg. of CaNa$_2$EDTA daily for 3 days. The mechanism of renal damage is poorly understood. In clinical situations the tubular cells are undoubtedly being presented with a variety of metallic ions, but it is not necessary to postulate cleavage of the metal chelate since examples of enzyme inhibition by intact chelates are known (Seven, 1960).

A lesion, induced in experimental animals by CaNa₂EDTA and similar compounds, which at present appears to be without a clinical parallel, is damage to the gastrointestinal mucosa (Weber, 1969). Intravenous infusion of toxic doses into dogs resulted in hemorrhage and necrosis of the intestinal epithelium with loss of villous structure, as well as renal lesions. Since a stable chromium chelate of EDTA was nontoxic, the CaNa₂EDTA-induced damage appears to be related to chelation activity (Ahrens and Aronson, 1971). In rats a marked increase in the permeability of the intestine to normally nonpermeating solutes was associated with an increase in the urinary excretion of hydroxyproline. Thus, the intestinal effects may be related to collagen degradation induced by CaNa₂EDTA (Aronson and Rogerson, 1972). If this lesion occurs in man, it may be responsible for the increased lead absorption from gastrointestinal depots observed after oral CaNa₂EDTA (Byers, 1959; Selander, 1967). An inhibition of DNA synthesis in rat intestine, which is reversed by zinc, has also been described, although it was not thought to constitute a direct cause of death (Rosenblatt and Aronson, 1978; Rosenblatt et al., 1978).

An occasionally encountered systemic reaction known as the "excessive chelation syndrome" consists of malaise, fatigue, thirst, and paresthesias, followed by sudden chills and fever. Then myalgia, headache, anorexia, nausea, and occasionally marked urinary frequency and urgency occur (Done, 1961b; Foreman, 1963; Seven, 1960). Minor reactions resembling those produced by histamine or the common cold are sometimes seen. Glycosuria (Seven, 1960) and potassium diuresis (Batchelor et al., 1964) have occurred. Anemia and hypotension of mild proportions are described (Seven, 1960). Reversible hydropic changes of hepatic parenchymal cells were observed in young rats given the calcium chelate repeatedly (Reuber, 1967).

Diuresis and excessive thirst may be anticipated as sequelae of CaNa₂EDTA administration, particularly if the drug is given in physiological saline rather than 5% glucose. Abdominal cramps and diarrhea are occasionally noted (Seven, 1960). No significant effect on the clotting mechanism has been observed (Seven, 1960), and in therapeutic doses, cardiovascular changes do not occur (Foreman, 1960) except for transient orthostatic hypotension during the infusion (Meltzer et al., 1961). Excretion following parenteral administration is virtually complete in 24 hours (Foreman, 1960).

CaNa₂EDTA is poorly absorbed from the gastrointestinal tract (maximum of 5%) and not at all through the skin (Foreman, 1960). The acute oral LD₅₀ in rats is 10 gm./kg. (Oser et al., 1963). After parenteral administration to rats 95 to 98% is excreted unchanged in the urine in 6 hours. Less than 0.1% is oxidized to carbon dioxide (Foreman et al., 1953). The mechanism for renal excretion appears to be exclusively that of glomerular filtration (Aronson and Ahrens, 1971).

The use of CaNa₂EDTA for the prophylaxis of lead poisoning has been termed rash and irresponsible (Kehoe, 1955; Lilis and Fischbein, 1976). Its use by mouth in lead-burdened patients may be dangerous (Byers, 1959). Pretreatment with cathartics or cleansing enemas to remove intestinal lead depots may be a wise precaution even prior to parenteral use, but dehydration should be avoided and therapy should not be delayed. Parenteral CaNa₂EDTA is sometimes used as a diagnostic tool in an attempt to provoke lead excretion in patients suspected of having an unusually high body burden of this metal (Emmerson, 1963; Whitaker et al., 1962). See below for recommended doses.

Symptomatology (following intravenous administration):
1. Thrombophlebitis proximal to site of administration.
2. Mild signs of hypocalcemia as numbness and tingling in fingers and perioral areas, more rarely an increase in reflex activity and a positive Trousseau sign.
3. Hypotension with lightheadedness, dizziness and vertigo.
4. Sneezing, nasal congestion, lacrimation and other minor histamine-like responses.
5. Abdominal cramps, diarrhea.
6. Sudden fever preceded or followed by chills, severe myalgia, frontal headache, anorexia, nausea, urinary frequency and urgency.
7. After several days, transient polyuria, albuminuria, cylindruria, anuria and eventual death associated with azotemia.

Treatment of CaNa₂EDTA overdosage:
1. Symptomatic and supportive treatment is indicated. No specific antagonists are known. The administration of any type of metallic cation is not warranted.
2. Hemodialysis or other therapy for renal failure may become necessary (p. IV-55).
3. Mucocutaneous lesions (including a sore, magenta-colored tongue) resulting from prolonged therapy have responded to vitamin B complex, especially B₆.
4. Presumably corticosteroids should be avoided because cortisone intensified the renal lesions of CaNa₂EDTA overdosage in

rats (Perry and Schroeder, 1957; Reuber, 1963).

Laboratory: The word "hypocalcemia" as used above refers to functional hypocalcemia, *i.e.*, a reduction in the plasma concentration of ionized calcium, which normally amounts to 42 to 45% of the total. Acute signs and symptoms of hypocalcemia are due to deficits of this component only. Such deficits commonly arise from infusions of sodium EDTA. However, the total amount of plasma calcium (ionized plus nonionized) is not reduced acutely and may even be elevated, as after infusions of CaNa₂EDTA. Although electrometric methods for estimating ionic calcium concentrations are recognized, most clinical chemistry laboratories measure and report only total plasma calcium or perhaps the total exclusive of that bound to EDTA. Such determinations are more apt to confuse than to help the therapist.

Repeated urinalyses are highly desirable. Determination of α-aminoacid nitrogen has been suggested as a method of evaluating proximal renal tubular function (Andrews, 1961), but the more common renal function tests are also helpful. Symptomatic hypokalemia and increased potassium excretion are described after edetate calcium disodium (Batchelor *et al.*, 1964).

Dosage schedule for CaNa₂EDTA in the treatment of lead poisoning: The *AMA Drug Evaluations* (1980) recommends the following schedules for edetate calcium disodium, which is supplied as a 20% sterile solution in ampuls (1 gm. in 5 ml.). In adults the intravenous or intramuscular routes of administration may be used. In either case the dose is 1.5 gm./sq. meter of surface area (not to exceed 50 mg./kg.) daily in 2 divided doses for 3 to 5 days. For intramuscular administration a 20% solution is used, often containing 0.5 to 1.5% procaine to reduce pain. For intravenous administration, each dose is diluted with 250 or 500 ml. isotonic saline or 5% dextrose in water and infused over a period of 8 hours (others say "at least 1 hour" or not faster than 20 mg./kg. per hour).

In children the intramuscular route is preferred. Severe local reactions appear to be rare (Chisolm and Harrison, 1957). The usual dose (12.5 mg./kg. 3 or 4 times daily) is equivalent to that in adults (per square meter of surface area), but the maximum 24-hour dose in children can be increased from 50 to 75 mg./kg. in very severe poisonings, and the fluid volume used with intravenous administration should be limited. For combined therapy with dimercaprol, see below.

If necessary, a second course of therapy can be employed, to begin not sooner than 2 days after the first course and preferably 2 weeks later. Children may require several courses of therapy. The goal is to reduce the blood lead level to less than 50 μg./dl. Oral D-penicillamine can be substituted for the second course of Ca₂NaEDTA; see p. III-271.

Dose schedule for combined BAL and CaNa₂EDTA therapy in lead encephalopathy: Lead encephalopathy in children demands vigorous treatment. The following regimen is recommended by the *AMA Drug Evaluations* (1980). Therapy begins with an intramuscular injection of dimercaprol (BAL) at a dose of 4 mg./kg. The injection is repeated every 4 hours, but subsequent doses can be reduced to 3 mg./kg. in less severe poisonings. After the first injection, CaNa₂EDTA is administered at the same time as the dimercaprol but at a different injection site. The intramuscular dose of CaNa₂EDTA is 12.5 mg./kg. 4 to 6 times daily. This regimen is continued for 5 to 7 days. For additional treatment, see p. III-233.

Dose schedule for CaNa₂EDTA in the diagnosis of lead poisoning: The *AMA Drug Evaluations* (1980) recommends the following mobilization test in suspected lead poisoning. In adults, 500 mg./sq. meter (to a maximum of 1 gm.) is diluted in 500 ml. 5% dextrose and infused intravenously over a period of not less than 1 hour. Urine is collected for 24 hours before and after the start of the infusion. The test is considered positive if the second urine specimen has a lead concentration at least 3 times the control and a total lead content of 50 μg. or more. In children the intramuscular route is preferred. The adult dose rate (500 mg./sq. meter) is appropriate, but it is administered as two divided doses 12 hours apart.

References:

A. M. A. Department of Drugs. *A. M. A. Drug Evaluations.* 4th ed., Publishing Sciences Group, Inc., Acton, Mass, 1980.

Ahrens, F. A.; Aronson, A. L. A comparative study of the toxic effects of calcium and chromium chelates of ethylenediaminetetraacetate in the dog. Toxicol. Appl. Pharmacol. *18*:10-25, 1971.

Andrews, B. F. Calcium disodium edathamil therapy of lead intoxication. Arch. Environ. Health *3*:563-567, 1961.

Aronson, A. L.; Ahrens, F. A. The mechanism of renal transport and excretion of ethylenediaminetetraacetate with interspecies comparisons. Toxicol. Appl. Pharmacol. *18*:1-9, 1971.

Aronson, A. L.; Rogerson, K. M. Effect of calcium and chromium chelates of ethylene diaminetetraacetate in intestinal permeability and collagen metabolism in the rat. Toxicol. Appl. Pharmacol. *21*:440-453, 1972.

Batchelor, T. M.; McCall, M.; Mosher, R. E. Potassium diuresis induced by edathamil disodium. J. A. M. A. *187*:305-306, 1964.

Byers, R. K. Lead poisoning: review of the literature and report on 45 cases. Pediatrics *23*:585-603, 1959.

Chenoweth, M. B. Clinical uses of metal-binding drugs. Clin. Pharmacol. Ther. *9*:365-387, 1968.

Chisolm, J. J., Jr.; Harrison, H. E. The treatment of acute lead encephalopathy in children. Pediatrics *19*:2-20, 1957.

Done, A. K. Clinical pharmacology of systemic antidotes. Clin. Pharmacol. Ther. *2*:750-793, 1961b.

Dudley, H. R.; Ritchie, A. C.; Shilling, A.; Baker, W. H. Pathologic changes associated with use of sodium ethylenediaminetetraacetate in treatment of hypercalcemia. Report of two cases with autopsy findings. N. Engl. J. Med. *252*:331-337, 1955.

Emmerson, B. T. Chronic lead nephropathy. The diagnostic use of calcium EDTA and the association with gout. Aust. N. Z. J. Med. *12*:310-324, 1963.

Foreman, H. The pharmacology of some useful chelating agents. In *Metal-Binding in Medicine*, edited by M. J. Seven. J. B. Lippincott Co., Philadelphia, 1960.

Foreman, H. Toxic side effects of ethylenediaminetetraacetic acid. J. Chronic Dis. *16*:319-323, 1963.

Foreman, H.; Finnegan, C.; Lushbaugh, C. C. Nephrotoxic hazard from uncontrolled edathamil calcium-disodium therapy. J. A. M. A. *160*:1042-1046, 1956.

Foreman, H.; Vier, M.; Magee, M. The metabolism of C[14]-labelled ethylenediaminetetraacetic acid in the rat. J. Biol. Chem. *203*:1045-1053, 1953.

Holland, J. F.; Danielson, F.; Sahagian-Edwards, A. Use of ethylenediaminetetraacetic acid in hypercalcemic patients. Proc. Soc. Exp. Biol. Med. *84*:359-364, 1953.

Kehoe, R. A. Misuse of edathamil calcium-disodium for prophylaxis of lead poisoning. J. A. M. A. *157*:341-342, 1955.

Lilis, R.; Fischbein, A. Chelation therapy in workers exposed to lead: a critical review. J.A.M.A. *235*:2823-2824, 1976.

Meltzer, L. E.; Kitchell, J. R.; Palmon, F., Jr. The long term use, side effects, and toxicity of disodium ethylenediaminetetraacetic acid (EDTA). Am. J. Med. Sci. *242*:11-17, 1961.

Moeschlin, S. Zur Klinik und Therapie der Bleivergiftung mit Bericht uber eine todliche toxische Nephrose durch Ca-EDTA (Calciumversenat). Schweiz. Med. Wochenschr. *87*:1091-1096, 1957.

Oser, B. L.; Oser, M.; Spencer, H. C. Safety evaluation studies of calcium EDTA. Toxicol. Appl. Pharmacol. *5*:142-162, 1963.

Perry, H. M.; Schroeder, H. A. Lesions resembling vitamin B complex deficiency and urinary loss of zinc produced by ethylenediaminetetraacetate. Am. J. Med. *22*:168-174, 1957.

Popovici, A.; Geschickter, C. F.; Reinovsky, A.; Rubin, M. Experimental control of serum calcium levels in vivo. Proc. Soc. Exp. Biol. Med. *74*:415-419, 1950.

Reuber, M. D. Accentuation of Ca edetate nephrosis by cortisone. Arch. Pathol. *76*:382-386, 1963.

Reuber, M. D. Hepatic lesions in young rats given calcium disodium edetate. Toxicol. Appl. Pharmacol. *11*:321-326, 1967.

Reuber, M. D.; Bradley, J. E. Acute Versenate nephrosis occurring as the result of treatment for lead intoxication. J. A. M. A. *174*:263-269, 1960.

Rosenblatt, D. E.; Aronson, A. L. Calcium ethylenediaminetetraacetate (CaEDTA) Toxicity: time- and dose- response studies on intestinal DNA synthesis in the rat. Exp. Mol. Pathol. *28*:202-214, 1978.

Rosenblatt, D. E.; Doyle, D. G.; Aronson, A. L. Calcium ethylenediaminetetraacetate (CaEDTA) Toxicity: time- and dose- response studies on intestinal morphology in the rat. Exp. Mol. Pathol. *28*:215-226, 1978.

Schwartz, S. L.; Johnson, C. B.; Doolan, P. D. Study of the mechanism of renal vacuologenesis induced in the rat by ethylenediaminetetraacetate. Mol. Pharmacol. *6*:54-60, 1970.

Selander, S. Treatment of lead poisoning, a comparison between the effects of sodium calcium edetate and penicillamine administered orally and intravenously. Br. J. Ind. Med. *24*:272-282, 1967.

Seven, M. J. Observations on the toxicity of intravenous chelating agents. In *Metal-Binding in Medicine*, edited by M. J. Seven. J. B. Lippincott Co., Philadelphia, 1960.

Sidbury, J. B.; Bynum, J. C.; Fetz, L. L. Effect of chelating agent on urinary lead excretion. Comparison of oral and intravenous administration. Proc. Soc. Exp. Biol. Med. *82*:226-228, 1953.

Spencer, H.; Greenberg, J.; Berger, E.; Perrone, M.; Laszlo, D. Studies on the effect of ethylenediaminetetraacetic acid in hypercalcemia. J. Lab. Clin. Med. *47*:29-35, 1956.

Vogt, W.; Cottier, H. Nephrotisierende Nephrose nach Behandlung einer subakutchronischen Bleivergiftung mit Versenat in hohen Dosen. Schweiz. Med. Wochenschr. *87*:665-667, 1957.

Weber, K. M. Die Wirkung von Na₃(Ca-DPTA) auf den Glykogengehalt von Niere und Leber der Ratte. Experientia *25*:509-511, 1969.

Whitaker, J. A.; Austin, W.; Nelson, J. D. Edathamil calcium disodium (Versenate) diagnostic test for lead poisoning. Pediatrics *29*:384-388, 1962.

ETHYL ALCOHOL

Ethyl alcohol (ethanol, grain alcohol, neutral spirits) in concentrations up to 50% (100 proof) is often available in the home in drug formulations (*e.g.*, tinctures, elixirs, spirits), cosmetic preparations, rubbing alcohol, and intoxicating beverages. All except the latter are commonly "denatured" by the addition of substances intended to induce prompt vomiting (*e.g.*, brucine) or to discourage consumption by a bitter and objectionable taste or odor (*e.g.*, diethylphthalate, pyridine). These denaturants are not found in products such as mouthwashes, which may contain surprisingly high concentrations of alcohol (Varma and Cincotta, 1978).

Denatured alcohol seldom presents special problems in therapy unless the denaturant is methyl alcohol in high concentrations. Denaturation or contamination with small amounts of methanol does not necessarily constitute a hazard, since ethanol obviates the most dangerous features of methanol poisoning by inhibiting methanol's metabolism. One should, however, be alert to possible complications arising from the concomitant ingestion of METHYL ALCOHOL; see discussion (p. III-275).

Much "moonshine" or "white lightning" encountered in this country is contaminated with lead salts because automobile radiators and other metal parts of illicit stills are repaired with solder containing high concentrations of LEAD (see p. III-226). Frank lead poisoning has followed repeated consumption of such products (Eskew *et al.*, 1961). Another metallic element found at one time in an alcoholic beverage (beer) is cobalt; see also Cobalt Salts in Section II.

For the symptoms and treatment induced by alcohol in a person premedicated with Antabuse (disulfiram), see discussion of DISULFIRAM (p. III-159).

Only acute ethanol intoxication is considered below. Chronic alcoholism presents many special and perplexing problems to the therapist, who should consult standard textbooks in medicine and psychiatry. A useful source book on the biochemistry of alcohol is that by Kisson and Begleiter (1971).

Toxicology: As a classical example of a central nervous depressant, ethanol can induce all stages of anesthesia. If ingested within a period of a few minutes, the fatal dose in an average adult is considered to be 1½ to 2 pints of whiskey or gin (Webster, 1930). The same is true of any other distilled beverage that contains 40 to 55% ethyl alcohol (*e.g.*, rum, vodka, brandy, etc.). Such a dose is about the maximal amount that can be metabolized by a surviving adult in 24 hours (Newman *et al.*, 1952).

Intoxication with alcohol may be simulated by many pathological conditions, including diabetic acidosis, the postconvulsive depression of epilepsy, uremia, head injuries, hepatic coma, hypoglycemia and poisonings by any other central nervous depressant and by some stimulants (*e.g.*, atropine). A diagnosis of acute alcoholism should not be made casually; a chemical test of blood, urine, or expired air is always desirable.

Although a general relationship between symptoms and blood alcohol concentrations cannot be stated with precision, even a drinker with tolerance is unequivocally intoxicated when his blood alcohol level reaches 0.15% (150 mg./100 ml., 150 mg.%, 1.5 mg./ml.). The most common legal limit for operation of a motor vehicle is 0.10%. A blood concentration between 0.3 and 0.4% is commonly associated with stupor or coma, and 0.5% is often fatal (Greenberg, 1955; Himwich, 1957; Jetter, 1938a, b; Kaye and Haag, 1957). Death, however, has occurred at 0.4%, and survival after 0.7 to 0.8% (Hammond *et al.*, 1973; Poklis and Pearson, 1977). When coma is present at 0.4%, the patient should be carefully examined for other pathological conditions noted above (Sellers and Kalant, 1976).

Every patient in an alcoholic coma should be considered critically ill. The prognosis is especially poor if coma persists for more than 12 hours. In the absence of effective treatment, respiratory arrest is the usual cause of death. In one study, however, abnormalities of arterial blood gases were seen only at blood alcohol concentrations above 0.35% (Johnstone and Witt, 1972). In doses producing moderate to severe intoxication in man, alcohol is a weak respiratory depressant when compared with other sedative and narcotic drugs (Johnstone and Reier, 1973). If gas exchange is maintained by artificial respiration, larger doses of ethanol can be survived, but higher blood levels eventually induce serious cardiac toxicity in dogs (MacGregor *et al.*, 1964) and presumably in man. Because alcohol impairs thermoregulation even during recovery from cold exposure (Graham and Baulk, 1980), hypothermia is sometimes a fatal complication of alcoholic coma.

Ethyl alcohol is rapidly absorbed through gastric and intestinal mucosae, and its absorption is complete when the peak in blood alcohol concentration is reached (Harger and Forney, 1963). On rare occasions, inebriation has been ascribed to the inhalation of vapor (Lehman and Flury, 1938; Moss, 1970), but ingestion is the widely preferred route. Percutaneous absorption is said to be negligible, but severe intoxications have been reported in young children from the practice of tucking alcohol-soaked cloths under rubber pants (Gimenez *et al.*, 1968). In all cases, central nervous depression is ascribed to alcohol itself and not importantly to its metabolites.

Ethanol is distributed throughout the body water, and over 90% of a dose is metabolized in the liver by oxidation to acetaldehyde, to acetate, and to carbon dioxide and water, in that order. The first two steps in the sequence are mediated by alcohol and acetaldehyde dehydrogenases, respectively; both enzymes require oxidized nicotinamide adenine dinucleotide (NAD) as a cofactor. Alcohol dehydrogenase is found in the cytosol, whereas aldehyde dehydrogenase is a mitochondrial enzyme. A presumably minor, alternative pathway of oxidative metabolism is described below.

The rate of metabolic degradation is unexpectedly constant in a given individual. Within wide limits it is independent of the amount consumed; an average adult is said to be able to oxidize each hour the equivalent of ⅔ oz. of 100-proof whiskey (*e.g.*, Forney and Hughes, 1963). Most authorities no longer hold that the rate of alcohol metabolism can be materially increased by the administration of hormones, glucose, cofactors, or vitamins (Loomis, 1950; Jacobsen, 1952). Fructose is not only without value for increasing the rate of alcohol metabolism, but it produces hyperuricemia and lacticacidemia as undesired effects (Levy *et al.*, 1977).

Sizable differences in the rate of alcohol metabolism are recognized among various ethnic and racial groups. These individual differences must be ascribed to both acquired and inborn traits. No distinctions were found between American Indians and Caucasians in terms of alcohol metabolism (Bennion and Li, 1976), but some Chinese volunteers converted alcohol to acetaldehyde more rapidly than did Caucasians. An inherited atypical alcohol dehydrogenase was held responsible. The presence of higher blood acetaldehyde levels in these Orientals was associated with aversive symptoms, such as flushing, tachycardia and nausea (Zeiner *et al.*, 1979).

Less than 10% of the absorbed alcohol is excreted, chiefly in urine, measurably in expired air, and detectably in sweat (Haggard and Greenberg, 1934a, b). Excretion cannot be accelerated to a beneficial degree by diuretic drugs, by hyperventilation, or by the induction of sweating.

Hemodialysis has been employed in acute

ethyl alcohol intoxications. In one case it was said to have decreased the plasma half-life over natural processes of elimination by a factor of 11 (Jorgensen and Wieth, 1963). Marc-Aurele and Schreiner (1960) have estimated that the dialysance of ethyl alcohol in a commercial hemodialysis unit tested on dogs is about 200 ml./min. Although this represents a high value of dialysance in comparison with other drugs, at a blood alcohol concentration of 3 mg./ml., hemodialysis would be predicted to remove alcohol somewhat more slowly than oxidative metabolism does, so that the combined elimination rate would be less than doubled. This expectation was substantiated in one child subjected to peritoneal dialysis (Dickerman et al., 1968). Thus hemodialysis may be justifiable with potentially lethal blood alcohol concentrations (e.g., Elliot and Hunter, 1974), but its use should certainly be reserved for such life-threatening cases. Curiously, six patients detoxified acutely by hemodialysis did not develop delirium tremens, even though some of them had previously experienced that syndrome on spontaneous detoxication (Walder et al., 1969).

Severe hypoglycemia following a heavy drinking bout is now well established in some individuals (Fredericks and Lazor, 1963; Gumpel and Kaufman, 1964; Steer et al., 1969). Although severe hypoglycemia was originally reported to result from ingestion of denatured alcohols ("smoke") or Solox (Brown and Harvey, 1941; Tucker and Porter, 1942), ethanol, and not the other ingredients, is now recognized as the major precipitant of the reaction. Because hypoglycemia with convulsions has occurred in children after ingestion of alcoholic beverages, mouthwash and cologne (Cummins, 1961; Neame and Joubert, 1961; Varma and Cincotta, 1978), chronic alcohol intake is not necessary for this reaction.

Hypoglycemic reactions, however, appear to be more frequent in states of fasting and malnutrition with low carbohydrate reserves (Freinkel et al., 1965). Hypoglycemia may occur within 12 to 16 hours of drinking and at blood alcohol levels associated with mild intoxication. Thus, an inebriated patient may lapse into a fatal hypoglycemic coma. This effect is apparently due to an inhibition of gluconeogenesis associated with alcohol metabolism and not with alcohol itself. (Freinkel et al., 1965). Perhaps alcohol-hypoglycemia is more common in infants and children than in adults. This could account for the clinical impression that children are more susceptible to alcohol than adults and that the syndrome differs somewhat in character in that the coma in children is sometimes punctuated by severe convulsions (Turai et al., 1961; Verron, 1969).

Acute transplacental intoxication should be anticipated if a woman consumes alcohol just prior to delivery (Cook et al., 1975; Kim and Hodgkinson, 1976). In Cook et al. (1975), the blood alcohol level in the newborn was 0.15% at a time when it was only 0.1% in the mother. Chronic maternal consumption of alcohol during gestation may result in a teratogenic mental deficiency known as the fetal alcohol syndrome (Clarren and Smith, 1978).

Alcohol-drug interactions and tolerance: The subject of the interactions between alcohol and other drugs has received an enormous amount of attention, as attested to in a separate monograph (Forney and Hughes, 1968). Certain general principles are beginning to emerge. For example, although the "knock out" effect is now regarded as myth, there can be little doubt that the depressant effects of alcohol are synergistic with those of chloral hydrate. In vivo chloral hydrate is reduced to the more potent central depressant, trichloroethanol. Trichloroethanol is a competitive inhibitor of alcohol dehydrogenase, so that peak blood concentrations of ethanol are reached sooner and persist longer. In turn, the alcohol that is metabolized stimulates the production of NADH, which increases chloral hydrate reduction to trichloroethanol (Sellers et al., 1972).

Other known inhibitors of alcohol dehydrogenase which potentiate or are synergistic with the central nervous system depression induced by ethyl alcohol include chlorpromazine (Mezey, 1976), dimethyl formamide and dimethyl sulfoxide (Sharkawi, 1979), diethyldithiocarbamate (Sharkawi and Caille, 1979) and especially pyrazole and 4-methylpyrazole (e.g., Blomstrand et al., 1980). Diethyldithiocarbamate is an active metabolite of DISULFIRAM, which is a known inhibitor of aldehyde dehydrogenase. For a discussion of the alcohol-disulfiram reaction, and a list of other inhibitors of aldehyde dehydrogenase, see p. III-159.

An alleged interaction between paraldehyde and alcohol that can result in sudden death is not well understood (Kaye and Haag, 1964). Alcohol increases blood levels of diazepam and mephenytoin either by increasing absorption or by blocking the so-called first-pass metabolism by the liver (Hayes et al., 1977; Zysset et al., 1980).

Alternative pathways of ethanol metabolism (other than via alcohol dehydrogenase) have been demonstrated in man and other species. In rats, alternative pathways are said to account for 20 to 25% of the total alcohol metabolism (Lieber and DeCarli, 1972). The importance of these pathways in man, however, has been disputed, particularly the hepatic microsomal drug-metabolizing pathway involving cytochrome P450 (also called mixed function oxidase). Oxidation of alcohol to acetaldehyde can be demonstrated *in vitro* with microsomal enzyme preparations (Lieber and DeCarli, 1968; Rubin *et al.*, 1970; Rubin and Lieber, 1971). It is not clear, however, that this so-called microsomal ethanol-oxidizing system (MEOS) plays a role at low to moderate blood alcohol concentrations in man. On the other hand, there can be no doubt that chronic exposure to ethanol leads to induction of hepatic microsomal enzymes, although some evidence suggests that the mechanism differs from that by other known inducers (Tobon and Mezey, 1971). Induction is accompanied by unequivocal increases in the rates of disappearance from plasma of many drugs, including pentobarbital, meprobamate, isoniazid, warfarin, phenytoin, *etc.* (Misra *et al.*, 1971; Mezey, 1976; Rubin *et al.*, 1970), so long as ethanol is not consumed at the same time.

The above mechanism explains the tolerance of alcoholics to drugs inactivated by microsomal metabolism when the subject has been withdrawn from alcohol. However, if alcohol and pentobarbital, for example, are present concomitantly, they may interfere with each other's metabolism and a potentiation of the depressant effects may be seen instead of tolerance (Rubin and Lieber, 1968). This inhibitory effect of ethanol on drug metabolism by hepatic microsomal enzymes is believed to be an indirect rather than a direct competition at the level of cytochrome P450. Although ethanol binds to cytochrome P450, its K_i is in the range of lethal blood alcohol concentrations for man (Reinke *et al.*, 1980).

A true neuronal tolerance must be evoked to explain the common impression that alcoholics are tolerant to the depressant effects of drugs that are not metabolized, *e.g.*, ether, chloroform, barbital. The consequence of neuronal tolerance is that the individual must reach a higher blood alcohol concentration to achieve the same subjective (pharmacological) effects. In addition, a metabolic tolerance to alcohol itself is believed to occur, although alcohol dehydrogenase is only weakly inducible. The consequence of metabolic tolerance is that the individual must consume more alcohol to achieve the same blood concentration as in his nontolerant state. Both types of tolerance lead to increased consumption and a higher risk of incurring physical dependence. The relative magnitudes of these various phenomena remain to be evaluated. Presumably both "metabolic" and "tissue" tolerances are lost during abstinence from alcohol.

Physical dependence, withdrawal and cross-tolerance: Acute withdrawal of alcohol from a physically dependent individual may precipitate a life-threatening abstinence syndrome. Patients with mild signs and symptoms (insomnia, irritability, tremor), however, do not need hospitalization. Early treatment with benzodi-azepines (*e.g.*, diazepam, chlordiazepoxide) will usually prevent progression to more serious manifestations of withdrawal (seizures, anxiety, agitation, diaphoresis, delirium). Phenytoin should be added to the regimen in patients with a history of seizure disorders. Other drugs, such as phenothiazines, barbiturates, paraldehyde, antihistamines, and alcohol itself, may be effective but are more toxic (Sellers and Kalant, 1976).

The acute effects of alcohol are probably not due to actions on specific tissue receptors. Modern concepts about the acute effects speak of a transient and reversible "fluidization" of neuronal membranes (*e.g.*, von Wartburg, 1978). The behavioral effects of acute alcohol intoxication can be mimicked by a wide variety of simple organic molecules, including monohydric, dihydric and cyclic alcohols. At least 60 different compounds showed a high inverse correlation between the dose to produce ataxia in rats and the membrane/buffer partition coefficient (McCreery and Hunt, 1978).

The membrane hypothesis further states that with continued ethanol exposure and the onset of tolerance and physical dependence, the altered state of the neuronal membrane becomes less readily reversible (*e.g.*, Goldstein, 1976; von Wartburg, 1978). Decreased reversibility of neuronal membrane changes may be a paradigm of physical dependence. The slow return of the membrane to its pre-alcohol state may be related to the abstinence syndrome. When artificial membranes were prepared from synaptosomal extracts from mice tolerant to alcohol, the ability of ethanol to increase "lipid thermal motions" was less than in similar preparations from mice not exposed to ethanol or from mice withdrawn from chronic access to alcohol. The effect exhibited "cross-tolerance" with pentobarbital but not with morphine (Johnson *et al.*, 1980a).

The lack of specificity with respect to the acute behavioral effects of ethanol (above) extends also to cross-tolerance and suppression of the abstinence syndrome in laboratory animals. Rats or mice tolerant to alcohol are also cross-tolerant to nitrous oxide (Koblin *et al.*, 1980), *n*-propanol, isopropyl alcohol, *n*-butanol, *tert*-butanol (LeBlanc and Kalant, 1975), a wide variety of aliphatic diols and even two halogenated hydrocarbons (Hunt and Majchrowicz, 1980). The lack of specificity in these processes and the membrane hypothesis (as opposed to the receptor hypothesis) suggests that the search for specific antagonists to the effects of alcohol may be futile.

Symptomatology (acute intoxication):
1. Early emotional lability: exhilaration, boastfulness, talkativeness, remorse, and belligerency.

2. Impaired motor coordination: slowed re-action time, slurred speech, ataxia.
3. Sensory disturbances: diplopia, vertigo.
4. Flushing of face, rapid pulse, sweating.
5. Nausea and vomiting. Eventual incontinence of urine and feces.
6. Drowsiness, stupor and finally coma, with impaired or absent tendon reflexes. Convulsive episodes may indicate hypoglycemia.
7. Pupils dilated or normal.
8. Peripheral vascular collapse (shock): hypotension, tachycardia, cold pale skin, hypothermia.
9. Slow stertorous respirations.
10. Death from respiratory or circulatory failure or from aspiration pneumonitis.
11. During convalescence: postalcoholic headache and gastritis; infections (*e.g.*, pneumonia, septicemia); alcoholic psychoses (*e.g.*, delirium tremens).

Treatment:
1. Gastric lavage with warm water or sodium bicarbonate solution (3 to 5%)—unless more than 2 hours have elapsed since alcohol was ingested. Do not use apomorphine. Syrup of ipecac may be a safe way to empty the stomach if given promptly after the ingestion (p. I-2).
2. Oxygen and artificial respiration as needed for hypoventilation (pp. IV-7–14).
3. Treat circulatory collapse, dehydration and acidosis by intravenous infusions of isotonic sodium chloride or sodium bicarbonate. See pp. IV-17, 71 and 72.
4. Administer intravenous glucose if laboratory reports hypoglycemia. Poisoned children should receive glucose prophylactically.
5. Multivitamin preparations, especially B complex, are widely used parenterally in the treatment of acute alcoholism; the practice is harmless but not unequivocally beneficial or relevant.
6. Keep patient warm. Avoid the aspiration of vomitus. Good nursing care (p. IV-105) minimizes the incidence of pneumonia.
7. Indications for hemodialysis include a blood alcohol concentration of 0.60% or more, an arterial pH of 7.0 or lower in the presence of a blood alcohol concentration of 0.40% or more, the demonstrated presence of other dialyzable drugs, or severe intoxication in small children (Sellers and Kalant, 1976).

Laboratory:
1. Quantitative analyses for ethyl alcohol on samples of blood are useful. Highly specific methods based on gas chromatography or the use of purified alcohol dehy-

drogenase eliminate troublesome false positive reactions (Lundquist, 1959).
2. In contrast to other alcoholic beverages, beer causes a diminution in the fibrinolytic activity of the blood. The effect is presumably due to a fermentation product other than ethyl alcohol. No clinical significance is attached to this phenomenon, but abnormal clotting times are frequently observed in habitual beer drinkers (Fearnley *et al.*, 1960).
3. Monitor blood glucose because severe hypoglycemia may intervene (see above).

References:

Bennion, L. J.; Li, T. -K. Alcohol metabolism in American Indians and Whites. Lack of racial differences in metabolic rate and liver alcohol dehydrogenase. N. Engl. J. Med. 294:9-13, 1976.

Blomstrand, R.; Ellin, A.; Lof, A.; Ostlung-Wintzell, H. Biological effects and metabolic interactions after chronic and acute administration of 4-methylpyrazole and ethanol to rats. Arch. Biochem. Biophys. 199:591-505, 1980.

Brown, T. M.; Harvey, A. M. Spontaneous hypoglycemia in "smoke" drinkers. J. A. M. A. 117:12-15, 1941.

Clarren, S. K.; Smith, D. W. The fetal alcohol syndrome. N. Engl. J. Med. 198:1063-1067, 1978.

Cook, L. N.; Shott, R. J.; Andrews, B. F. Acute transplacental ethanol intoxication. Am. J. Dis. Child. 129:1075-1076, 1975.

Cummins, L. H. Hypoglycemia and convulsions in children following alcohol ingestion. J. Pediatr. 58:23-26, 1961.

Dickerman, J. D.; Bishop, W.; Marks, J. F. Acute ethanol intoxication in a child. Pediatrics 42:837-840, 1968.

Elliott, R. W.; Hunter, P. R. Acute ethanol poisoning treated by haemodialysis. Postgrad. Med. J. 50:515-517, 1974.

Eskew, A. E.; Crutcher, J. C.; Zimmerman, S. L.; Johnston, G. W.; Butz, W. C. Lead poisoning resulting from illicit alcohol consumption. J. Forensic Sci. 6:337-350, 1961.

Fearnley, G. R.; Ferguson, J.; Chakrabarti, R.; Vincent, C. T. Effect of beer on blood fibrinolytic activity. Lancet 1:184-186, 1960.

Forney, R. B.; Hughes, F. W. Alcohol accumulation in humans after prolonged drinking. Clin. Pharmacol. Ther. 4:619-621, 1963.

Forney, R. B.; Hughes, F. W. Combined Effect of Alcohol and Other Drugs. Charles C Thomas, Springfield, Ill, 1968.

Fredericks, E. J.; Lazor, M. Z. Recurrent hypoglycemia associated with acute alcoholism. Ann. Intern. Med. 59:90-94, 1963.

Freinkel, N.; Arky, R. A.; Singer, D. L.; Cotten, A. K.; Bleicher, S. J.; Anderson, C.; Silbert, C. K.; Foster, A. E. Alcohol hypoglycemia; IV. Current concepts of its pathogenesis. Diabetes 14:350-361, 1965.

Gimenez, E. R.; Vallejo, N. E.; Roy, E.; Lis, M.; Izurieta, E. M.; Rossi, S.; Capuccio, M. Percutaneous alcohol intoxication. Clin. Toxicol. 1:39-48, 1968.

Goldstein, D. B. Pharmacological aspects of physical dependence on ethanol. Life Sci. 18:553-562, 1976.

Graham, T.; Baulk, K. Effect of alcohol ingestion on man's thermoregulatory responses during cold water immersion. Aviat. Space Environ. Med. 51:155-159, 1980.

Greenberg, L. A. The definition of an intoxicating beverage. Q. J. Stud. Alcohol 16:316-325, 1955.

Gumpel, R. C.; Kaufman, E. H. Alcohol-induced hypoglycemia. N. Y. State J. Med. 64:1014-1017, 1964.

Haggard, H. W.; Greenberg, L. A. Studies in the absorption, distribution and elimination of ethyl alcohol. II. The excretion of alcohol in urine and expired air; and the distribution of alcohol between air and water, blood and urine. J. Pharmacol. Exp. Ther. 52:150-166, 1934a.

Haggard, H. W.; Greenberg, L. A. Studies in the absorption,

distribution and elimination of ethyl alcohol. III. Rate of oxidation of alcohol in the body. J. Pharmacol. Exp. Ther. 52:167-178, 1934b.

Hammond, K. B.; Rumack, B. H.; Rodgerson, D. O. Blood ethanol; a report of unusually high levels in a living patient. J. A. M. A. 226:63-64, 1973.

Harger, R. N.; Forney, R. B. Aliphatic alcohols. In Progress in Chemical Toxicology. Vol. 1, A. Stolman (Ed.). Academic Press, New York, 1963.

Hayes, S. L.; Pablo, G.; Radomski, T.; Palmer, R. F. Ethanol and oral diazepam absorption. N. Engl. J. Med. 296:186-189, 1977.

Himwich, H. E. The physiology of alcohol. J. A. M. A. 163:545-549, 1957.

Hunt, W. A.; Majchrowicz, E. Suppression of the ethanol withdrawal syndrome by aliphatic diols. J. Pharmacol. Exp. Ther. 213:9-12, 1980.

Jacobsen, E. The metabolism of ethyl alcohol. Pharmacol. Rev. 4:107-135, 1952.

Jetter, W. W. Studies in alcohol. I. The diagnosis of acute alcoholic intoxication by a correlation of clinical and chemical findings. Am. J. Med. Sci. 196:475-487, 1938a.

Jetter, W. W. Studies in alcohol. II. Experimental feeding of alcohol to non-alcoholic individuals. Am. J. Med. Sci. 196:487-493, 1938b.

Johnson, D. A.; Lee, N. M.; Cooke, R.; Loh, H. Adaptation to ethanol-induced fluidization of brain lipid bilayers: cross-tolerance and reversibility. Mol. Pharmacol. 17:52-55, 1980a.

Johnstone, R. E.; Reier, C. E. Acute respiratory effects of ethanol in man. Clin. Pharmacol. Ther. 14:501-508, 1973.

Johnstone, R. E.; Witt, R. L. Respiratory effects of alcohol intoxication. J. A. M. A. 222:486, 1972.

Jorgensen, H. E.; Wieth, J. O. Dialysable poisons. Lancet 1:81-84, 1963a.

Kaye, S.; Haag, H. B. Terminal blood alcohol concentrations in ninety-four fatal cases of acute alcoholism. J. A. M. A. 165:451-452, 1957.

Kaye, S.; Haag, H. B. Study of death due to combined action of alcohol and paraldehyde in man. Toxicol. Appl. Pharmacol. 6:316-320, 1964.

Kim, S. S.; Hodgkinson, R. Acute ethanol intoxication and its prolonged effect on a full term neonate. Anesth. Analg. 55:602-603, 1976.

Kisson, B.; Begleiter, H. The Biology of Alcoholism, Vol. 1, Biochemistry. Plenum Press, New York, 1971.

Koblin, D. D.; Deady, J. E.; Dong, D. E.; Eger, E. E. II. Mice tolerant to nitrous oxide are also tolerant to alcohol. J. Pharmacol. Exp. Ther. 213:309-312, 1980.

Le Blanc, A. E.; Kalant, H. Ethanol-induced cross tolerance to several homologous alcohols in the rat. Toxicol. Appl. Pharmacol. 32:123-128, 1975.

Lehmann, K. B.; Flury, F. Toxicology and Hygiene of Industrial Solvents. The Williams & Wilkins Co., Baltimore, 1938.

Levy, R.; Elo, T.; Hanenson, I. B. Intravenous fructose treatment of acute alcohol intoxication -- effects on alcohol metabolism. Arch. Intern. Med. 137:1175-1177, 1977.

Lieber, C. S.; DeCarli, L. M. Ethanol oxidation by hepatic microsomes; adaptive increase after ethanol feeding. Science 162:917-918, 1968.

Lieber, C. S.; DeCarli, L. M. The role of the hepatic microsomal ethanol oxidizing system (MEOS) for ethanol metabolism in vivo. J. Pharmacol. Exp. Ther. 181:279-287, 1972.

Loomis, T. A. A study of the rate of metabolism of ethyl alcohol with special reference to certain factors reported as influencing this rate. Q. J. Stud. Alcohol 11:527-537, 1950.

Lundquist, F. The determination of ethyl alcohol in blood and tissues. Methods Biochem. Anal. 7:217-251, 1959.

MacGregor, D. C.; Schonbaum, E.; Bigelow, W. G. Acute toxicity studies on ethanol, propanol and butanol. Can. J. Physiol. Pharmacol. 42:689-696, 1964.

Marc-Aurele, J.; Schreiner, G. E. The dialysance of ethanol and methanol: A proposed method for the treatment of massive intoxication by ethyl or methyl alcohol. J. Clin. Invest. 39:802-807, 1960.

McCreery, M. J.; Hunt, W. A. Physico-chemical correlates of alcohol intoxication. Neuropharmacology 17:451-461, 1978.

Mezey, E. Ethanol metabolism and ethanol-drug interactions. Biochem. Pharmacol. 25:869-875, 1976.

Misra, P. S.; Lefevre, A.; Ishii, H.; Rubin, E.; Lieber, C. S. Increase of ethanol, meprobamate and pentobarbital metabolism after chronic ethanol administration in man and in rats. Am. J. Med. 51:346-351, 1971.

Moss, M. H. Alcohol-induced hypoglycemia and coma caused by alcohol sponging. Pediatrics 46:445-447, 1970.

Neame, P. B.; Joubert, S. M. Postalcoholic hypoglycemia and toxic hepatitis. Lancet 2:893-897, 1961.

Newman, H. W.; Wilson, R. H. L.; Newman, E. J. Direct determination of maximal daily metabolism of alcohol. Science 116:328-329, 1952.

Poklis, A.; Pearson, M. A. An unusually high blood ethanol level in a living patient. Clin. Toxicol. 10:429-431, 1977.

Reinke, L. A.; Kauffman, F. C.; Belinsky, S. A.; Thurman, R. G. Interaction between ethanol metabolism and mixed-function oxidation in perfused rat liver: inhibition of p-nitroanisole o-demethylation. J. Pharmacol. Exp. Ther. 213:70-78, 1980.

Rubin, E.; Gang, H.; Misra, P. S.; Lieber, C. S. Inhibition of drug metabolism by acute ethanol intoxication. Am. J. Med. 49:801-806, 1970.

Rubin, E.; Lieber, C. S. Hepatic microsomal enzymes in man and rat. Induction and inhibition by ethanol. Science 162:690-691, 1968.

Rubin, E.; Lieber, C. S. Alcoholism, alcohol and drugs. Science 172:1097-1102, 1971.

Sellers, E. M.; Kalant, H. Drug therapy: alcohol intoxication and withdrawal. N. Engl. J. Med. 294:757-762, 1976.

Sellers, E. M.; Lang, M.; Koch-Weser, J.; LeBlanc, E.; Kalant, H. Interaction of chloral hydrate and ethanol in man; I. Metabolism. Clin. Pharmacol. Ther. 13:37-49, 1972.

Sharkawi, M. Inhibition of alcohol dehydrogenase by dimethyl formamide and dimethyl sulfoxide. Toxicol. Lett. 4:493-497, 1979.

Sharkawi, M.; Caille, G. Disulfiram enhances ethanol pharmacological activity and impairs its elimination. Toxicol. Lett. 4:485-491, 1979.

Steer, P.; Marwell, R.; Werk, E. E., Jr. Clinical alcohol hypoglycemia and isolated adrenocortiotrophic hormone deficiency. Ann. Intern. Med. 71:343-398, 1969.

Tobon, F.; Mezey, E. Effect of ethanol administration on hepatic ethanol and drug-metabolizing enzymes and on rates of ethanol degradation. J. Lab. Clin. Med. 77:110-121, 1971.

Tucker, H. St. G., Jr.; Porter, W. B. Hypoglycemia following alcoholic intoxication. Am. J. Med. Sci. 204:559-566, 1942.

Turai, L.; Somogyi, E.; Cserhati, E.; Kelemen, J. Uber akute Alkolholvergiftungen in Kindesalter. Acta Paediatr. Acad. Sci. Hung. 2:137-148, 1961.

Turai, L.; Somogyi, E.; Cserhati, E.; Kelemen, J. Uber akute Alkoholvergiftungen in Kindesalter. Through Toxic Episodes Childhood. Acta Paediatr. Acad. Sci. Hung 3:4, 1962.

Varma, B. K.; Cincotti, J. Mouthwash induced hypoglycemia. Am. J. Dis. Child 132:930-931, 1978.

Verron, G. Alkoholvergiftungen in Kindesalter. Monatsschr. Kinderheilkd. 117:96-99, 1969.

von Wartburg, J. P. Biochemische Aspekte des Alkoholismus. Chimia 33:79-83, 1978.

Walder, A. I.; Redding, J. S.; Faillace, L.; Steenberg, R. W. Rapid detoxification of the acute alcoholic with hemodialysis. Surgery 66:201-207, 1969.

Webster, R. W. Legal Medicine and Toxicology. W. B. Saunders Co., Philadelphia, 1930.

Zeiner, A. R.; Paredes, A.; Christensen, H. D. The role of acetaldehyde in mediating reactivity to an acute dose of ethanol among different racial groups. Alcoholism 3:11-18, 1979.

Zysset, T.; Preisig, R.; Bircher, J. Increased systemic availability of drugs during acute ethanol intoxication: studies with mephenytoin in the dog. J. Pharmacol. Exp. Ther. 213:173-178, 1980.

ETHYLENE GLYCOL

Ethylene glycol is a colorless, almost odorless liquid. In industry it finds many uses as a solvent and as a starting material in chemical syntheses. Around the home it is found in a few cosmetic preparations, but "permanent type" automobile antifreeze is the principal source of poisonings. Formulae illustrating the chemical (but not necessarily metabolic) interrelationships of some common glycols and their derivatives are shown in Figure III-4.

Toxicology of ethylene glycol: More than 50 human fatalities from the ingestion of ethylene glycol have been reported, and the mean lethal dose appears to be about 100 ml. in adults (Laug et al., 1939). Inhalation is not generally hazardous because the glycol has a low vapor pressure (Wiley et al., 1936), but chronic poisoning, evidenced by nystagmus and recurrent attacks of unconsciousness, has been reported in a group of women exposed to vapors emanating from ethylene glycol heated above 100° C. (Troisi, 1950).

Only minor skin irritation and skin penetration are described, but the FDA has ruled that preparations intended for repeated topical application should contain no more than 5% of this glycol. Acute iridocyclitis has followed accidental eye contact (Sykowski, 1951). Rats exposed continuously to vapor concentrations of 12 mg./cubic meter sometimes showed corneal damage and apparent blindness without signs of systemic intoxication (Coon et al., 1970).

In man the sequence of events following acute ingestion is well documented. Although alcoholic beverages are often consumed concomitantly, it is clear that ethylene glycol alone can produce an inebriation like that from ethanol. Sometimes the symptoms may be delayed and more persistent than after ethanol (Berman et al., 1957; Brekke, 1930; Flanagan and Libcke, 1964; Friedman et al., 1962; Kahn and Brotchner, 1950; Smith, 1951). Such patients may present a difficult diagnostic problem (Giromini et al., 1964), but the absence of an odor of alcohol in the breath should prove helpful in the differential diagnosis (Kahn and Brotchner, 1950).

In the more fulminating form of the intoxication, victims lapse into profound coma punctuated with seizures. Life-threatening complications that may occur in this period include respiratory failure secondary to central nervous depression, cardiovascular collapse (Friedman et al., 1962; Hagemann and Chiffelle, 1948), pulmonary edema (Friedman et al., 1962; Kahn and Brotchner, 1950; Milles, 1946; Pons and Custer, 1946), and severe metabolic acidosis (Flanagan and Libcke, 1964; Friedman et al., 1962; Giromini et al., 1964; Hagemann and Chiffelle, 1948; Hagstam et al., 1965; Nadeau et al., 1954; Wacker et

al., 1965). Without treatment, death may occur in 8 to 24 hours.

Those who die promptly in the phase of central depression may escape significant renal pathology (Pons and Custer, 1946), but the survivors almost invariably experience acute renal failure (Berman et al., 1957; Flanagan and Libcke, 1964; Friedman et al., 1962; Hagstam et al., 1965; Kahn and Brotchner, 1950; Levy, 1960; Reidenberg et al., 1964; Ross, 1956; Smith, 1951). Victims who die late in obvious uremia exhibit marked renal pathology, including destruction of epithelial cells, interstitial edema, focal hemorrhagic necrosis in the cortex, extensive hydropic degeneration, numerous cellular casts and birefringent oxalate crystals in the convoluted tubules (Flanagan and Libcke, 1964; Friedman et al., 1962; Levy, 1960; Schreiner and Maher, 1965; Smith, 1951).

Pathological changes, however, are not limited to the kidney. Exudative changes perhaps due to capillary damage have been observed in the brain. The leptomeninges may show hyperemia (Boemke, 1943; Hagemann and Chiffelle, 1948; Pons and Custer, 1946; Ross, 1956) or vascular oxalosis (Bove, 1966; Giromini et al., 1964; Kersting and Nielsen, 1965; Smith, 1951). Spinal fluid pressure and protein content may be elevated. Both the etiology and significance of these changes appear to be unexplained, since they sometimes precede significant renal pathology (Pons and Custer, 1946). Exudative, congestive and hemorrhagic changes also occur in the pericardium (Hagemann and Chiffelle, 1948). Patients who survive for several days before death show central hepatic lobular hydropic degeneration (Smith, 1951), but congestion may be the only liver pathology in those who die in the early phases of the poisoning (Pons and Custer, 1946).

The mortality rate in untreated cases of severe ethylene glycol poisoning is high, but a milder intoxication, presumably reflecting the ingestion of a smaller dose, is also recognized. Here the acute illness is bypassed, and the initial symptoms of alcohol inebriation may be followed by a clearing of the sensorium and an asymptomatic period of several days before the onset of renal failure (Friedman et al., 1962, Levy, 1960; Reidenberg et al., 1964; Smith, 1951). Oliguria may be persistent (50 days in one elderly woman), but improvement in renal function can be anticipated in those who survive (Collins et al., 1970).

As with other aliphatic alcohols, the metabolism of ethylene glycol is probably linked closely to the biochemical and physiological derangements it produces in mammals. Depending on the oral dose and the laboratory species, only small amounts of unchanged glycol are excreted in the urine, (Gessner et al., 1961). Perhaps the initial central nervous depression is due to the glycol *per se*. Each hydroxyl group in turn is oxidized in a series of steps. Thus, the major metabolites in order of their appearance are glycoaldehyde, glycolic acid and glyoxylic acid. Each successive metabolite is more toxic and produces greater renal damage in rats than its precursor (Bove, 1966).

Several pathways exist for the metabolism of glyoxylic acid, but no one of them appears to be quantitatively more important than the others. Oxidation to oxalic acid results in a characteristic calcium oxalate crystalluria and sometimes deposits of oxalate in liver (Zarembski and Hodgkinson, 1967), kidneys and brain (Gaultier *et al.*, 1976). Oxidation to formic acid and carbon dioxide occurs to only a slight extent. Glycine and several keto acids are also recognized minor metabolites (Clay and Murphy, 1977; Parry and Wallach, 1974).

Although the terminal events of renal failure are similar, the suggestion (Milles, 1946) that ethylene glycol poisoning should be treated like systemic OXALATE poisoning (see p. III-326) with soluble calcium salts does not appear to have been pursued extensively. One seriously poisoned patient received massive calcium therapy with recovery; however, reexamination after 2 years suggested permanent brain damage (Grant, 1952). Signs consistent with hypocalcemic tetany have been described in man (Hagstam *et al.*, 1965; Ross, 1956), but the evidence is not impressive. A mild hypocalcemia, however, is a common finding (Parry and Wallach, 1974).

Some patients have complained of dimness of vision (Friedman *et al.*, 1962), but permanent ocular injury like that produced by METHYL ALCOHOL is very rare in systemic ethylene glycol poisoning. Presumably, this difference is related to the fact that formate is only a minor metabolite in the case of ethylene glycol. Bilateral optic atrophy occurred in an elderly man who consumed a half pint in divided doses over 48 hours (Ahmed, 1971a). The metabolic acidosis induced by ethylene glycol, however, can be as severe as that produced by METHYL ALCOHOL (see p. III-275).

Unlike the acidosis produced by methanol, the acidosis due to ethylene glycol intoxication cannot be ascribed to the accumulation of formic acid. Some experimental results appear to implicate glyoxylic acid as the responsible metabolite (McChesney *et al.*, 1972), whereas others show a better correlation between the blood concentration of glycolic acid and the degree of acidosis (Chou and Richardson, 1978; Clay and Murphy, 1977). Whatever metabolite or metabolites are responsible, the administration of sodium bicarbonate to control acidosis usually produces symptomatic improvement (Flanagan and Libcke, 1964; Friedman *et al.*, 1962; Nadeau *et al.*, 1954; Pendras, 1963; Wacker *et al.*, 1965), and perhaps prevents more serious sequelae.

Recent evidence indicates that the initial steps in the oxidation of ethylene glycol are mediated by alcohol dehydrogenase, the liver enzyme also responsible for the metabolism of ethanol. This circumstance suggested that ethanol might serve as a competitive substrate and retard the metabolic transformation of the glycol to its more toxic metabolites. Similar reasoning led to the ethyl alcohol therapy of methanol poisoning (see p. III-277). Peterson and colleagues (1963) were able to double the LD_{50} of ethylene glycol in rats by antidoting them with ethanol. The urinary excretion of unchanged glycol in the first 24 hours in alcohol-treated rats was twice that of control animals, whereas in monkeys glycol excretion was increased 10-fold. As evaluated in mice, some alkyldiol compounds, such as propylene glycol or 1,3-butanediol, were almost twice as effective as ethanol in preventing death (Holman *et al.*, 1979).

Ethyl alcohol was employed clinically in two cases in which potentially lethal doses of ethylene glycol were consumed (Wacker *et al.*, 1965). Although the equivalent of 95% ethanol was administered for 4 days at an average rate of 11 ml./hr., it was still necessary to employ vigorous bicarbonate therapy to control acidosis. By comparison with untreated cases, however, both patients emerged from coma rapidly and oxaluria disappeared in 18 hours. Without ethanol, oxaluria has persisted for as long as 5 days (Flanagan and Libcke, 1964). Such therapy, however, must be initiated soon after ingestion, perhaps within 8 hours (Wacker *et al.*, 1965). Pyrazole and 4-methylpyrazole, which are potent inhibitors of alcohol dehydrogenase, afford significant protection against the toxic effects of ethylene glycol in mice, rats, dogs and monkeys, also indicating that the glycol is normally metabolized to more toxic products *via* the ethyl alcohol route (Chou and Richardson, 1978; Mundy *et al.*, 1974; Van Stee *et al.*, 1975).

Schreiner *et al.* (1959) indicate that ethylene glycol is dialyzable and that, in addition to the usual uremic indications for hemodialysis, early institution of this procedure may appreciably lower the body burden of unmetabolized glycol. Pendras (1963) also demonstrated the feasibility of this procedure by recovering ethylene glycol in the dialysate from poisoned dogs. The dialyzability of this glycol has been confirmed in several clinical episodes (e.g., Hagstam *et al.*, 1965; Michelis *et al.*, 1976; Pendras, 1963). Indeed, early and vigorous treatment with diuretics, ethanol, sodium bicarbonate and hemodialysis may prevent an impending renal shutdown (Stokes and Aueron, 1980; Underwood and Bennett, 1973).

It appears likely that one or more intermediary metabolites of ethylene glycol are specific nephrotoxins (Berman et al., 1957). Deposition of calcium or magnesium oxalate crystals within the kidneys and urinary tract is no longer regarded as sufficient to explain the observed pathological changes (see OXALATE p. III-326). Mild glomerular damage and azotemia in the absence of crystalluria have been described in monkeys (Roberts and Seibold, 1969).

In contrast, when animals are fed small quantities of ethylene glycol over a period of several months, kidney tubular atrophy is undoubtedly aggravated by oxalate production and retention as calcium oxalate stones in renal tubules, kidney, pelvis and urinary bladder (Lepkovsky et al., 1935; Morris et al., 1942). Glycolic acid or ethylene glycol chronically fed to rats results in more severe oxaluria and kidney oxalate deposition in males than in females (Richardson, 1965; Tanret et al., 1961). Liver homogenates from male rats oxidize glycolic acid to oxalate more rapidly than similar preparations from females (Richardson, 1965). Castrated animals treated with sex hormones of the opposite sex respond to ethylene glycol feeding like the opposite sex (Tanret et al., 1962). Vitamin B_6 deficiency also abolished this sex difference and makes females more susceptible to ethylene glycol-induced oxaluria (Richardson, 1965). Such studies may eventually prove to have significance in elucidating the pathogenesis of oxalosis (see p. III-327).

A hemorrhagic diathesis characterized by multiple deficiencies of clotting factors (VII, IX, X and prothrombin) occurred among male mice kept in pine shavings sterilized with ethylene oxide. Single gavage doses of ethylene glycol were subsequently found to produce a specific depression of factor X activity in some strains of male mice (Meier et al., 1962). The significance of these findings for man is not yet clear.

Toxicology of ethylene glycol derivatives: With respect to the many commercially important derivatives of ethylene glycol (see Figure III-4), by far the largest body of clinical experience and experimental data relates to diethylene glycol. In the 1930s, a therapeutic preparation of 10% sulfanilamide in about 70% diethylene glycol was marketed without adequate toxicity testing in animals and without evaluation by either the FDA or the AMA Council on Pharmacy and Chemistry. Before this product could be withdrawn from the market, it was implicated in 105 uremic deaths (Calvery and Klumpp, 1939; Geiling and Cannon, 1938; Leech, 1937). Although sulfanilamide alone sometimes produces kidney damage, the evidence was overwhelming that diethylene glycol was the sole agent responsible for this tragedy (Geiling and Cannon, 1938).

Because it served as the drug vehicle, dieth-

ylene glycol was consumed by these patients in a relatively strict regimen of divided doses for 6 to 13 days (Calvery and Klumpp, 1939). Under these conditions, victims exhibited nausea, vomiting, headache, diarrhea, abdominal pain, and additional signs and symptoms commonly associated with acute renal failure. There appear to be no clinical reports of massive single ingestion episodes in man, but the above experience indicates that 2 to 3 oz. in divided doses are enough to cause fatal renal injury (Calvery and Klumpp, 1939). Similar episodes in South Africa involved sedative mixtures intended for children (Bowie and McKenzie, 1972).

Thus, both ethylene glycol and diethylene glycol are more hazardous to man than implied by single-dose oral toxicity data in laboratory animals. Ethylene glycol in animals falls in toxicity class 2, and diethylene glycol is also rated 2 or even 1 (Smyth et al., 1941a).

Despite opinions to the contrary (Schreiner and Maher, 1965), the renal pathology in the patients who had ingested the diethylene glycol product closely resembled that in victims of ethylene glycol poisoning, except that oxalate crystals were absent (Leech, 1937). Moreover, central lobular hydropic degeneration of the liver, pulmonary edema, pericardial hemorrhage, and distention of the leptomeningeal veins are also encountered in both situations (Leech 1937; Smith, 1951).

Although clinical experience is less extensive, the major renal findings and some of the incidental changes in diethylene glycol poisoning are also seen after dioxane (Smyth et al., 1941a; see also Section II) and after the simple glycol ethers of both ethylene glycol (Rowe, 1962) and diethylene glycol (Kesten et al., 1939). Hexylene glycol (2-methyl-2,4-pentanediol) used to impregnate the mesh of burn dressings has also been implicated in the production of coma and acute renal failure (Procter, 1966).

Of several glycol derivatives given by mouth to animals, only ethylene glycol and its simple esters elevated the urinary excretion of oxalate (Wiley et al., 1938). The structure of diethylene glycol and all derivatives of ethylene glycol containing a stable ether linkage (Group B of Figure III-4) appears to preclude their metabolism to oxalate. These findings support the concept that oxaluria per se plays a minor role in the pathogenesis of acute renal failure. Although adequate metabolic studies were not encountered, it would appear equally unlikely that ether-bridged compounds can be metabolized to glycolic or glyoxylic acids. Perhaps this is the reason that the metabolic acidosis encountered with ethylene glycol is only rarely described with diethylene glycol (Bowie and McKenzie, 1972) and similar compounds (but see below).

Among the various low-molecular-weight eth-

Group A	Ethylene glycol and its mono- and diesters, e.g., ethylene glycol diformate, ethylene glycol monoacetate	$\begin{array}{cc} CH_2-CH_2 \\ | \quad\quad | \\ OH \quad OH \end{array}$	$\begin{array}{cc} CH_2-CH_2 \\ | \quad\quad | \\ OH \quad O-C-R \\ \quad\quad\quad \| \\ \quad\quad\quad O \end{array}$
Group B	Diethylene glycol and its mono- and diesters, mono- and diethers, and ether-esters	$CH_2-CH_2-O-CH_2-CH_2$ with OH on each end	
	Ethylene glycol and its mono- and diethers and ether-esters	$\begin{array}{cc} CH_2-CH_2 \\ | \quad\quad | \\ OH \quad O-R \end{array}$	
	Dioxane	$\begin{array}{c} CH_2-CH_2 \\ O \quad\quad O \\ CH_2-CH_2 \end{array}$	
Group C	Propylene glycol	$\begin{array}{cc} CH_2-CH-CH_3 \\ | \quad\quad | \\ OH \quad OH \end{array}$	
	Polyethylene glycols	$CH_2-CH_2-O-(CH_2-CH_2-O)_n-CH_2-CH_2$ with OH on each end	

Figure III-4. Typical glycols of commerce and their chemical derivatives.

ylene glycol derivatives, the presence of an ether linkage appears to predispose to more intense renal damage, *e.g.*, diethylene glycol, dipropylene glycol, dioxane, and monomethyl, ethyl and butyl ethers of diethylene glycol (Kesten *et al.*, 1939). In contrast, the toxicity of simple esters resembles that of the parent glycol, to which they are promptly hydrolyzed in the body. An important exception, however, is the high toxicity of formate esters (Smyth *et al.*, 1941a), which may reflect a hazard of the acid moiety that exceeds that of the glycol. A mixed ether-ester tends to share the acute toxicity of the ether rather than that of the relatively labile ester (Smyth, 1952).

Chronic poisonings from vapors of monoalkyl ethers of ethylene glycol, particularly methyl Cellosolve and butyl Cellosolve, have occurred in the U.S.A. Toxic encephalopathy and evidence of bone marrow depression without hemolysis were the key findings (Greenburg *et al.*, 1938; Parsons and Parsons, 1938). In rats but not dogs, hemoglobinuria was also observed. Butyl Cellosolve produced these effects at somewhat lower vapor concentrations than ethyl or methyl Cellosolve (Werner *et al.*, 1943a, c). Lung, kidney and liver changes have also been observed with most simple ethers of ethylene glycol (Werner *et al.*, 1943a; Rowe, 1962), suggesting that the acute toxic syndrome may resemble that produced by diethylene glycol.

Simple ethers of ethylene glycol are more acutely toxic than the parent alcohol; on the basis of animal data most of them fall in toxicity class 3 (Smyth *et al.*, 1941a). The ethers of diethylene glycol (Carbitols) are also more toxic than the parent glycol; they are found in toxicity class 2 (Smyth *et al.*, 1941a). As is true of the glycols, these ethers may be even more hazardous to man than to test animals. Intense exposures of man to any of these derivatives might be predicted to result in some central nervous depression, mild liver damage, perhaps pulmonary edema, and death in acute renal failure. Perhaps the nephrotoxic propensity is aggravated by intravascular hemolysis with some members of the series (Carpenter *et al.*, 1956; von Oettingen and Jirouch, 1931), but the clinical evidence is not convincing (Browning, 1965). One clinical report described an unexpectedly severe metabolic acidosis. Two adults were profoundly acidotic 18 hours after each ingested 100 ml. of the monomethyl ether of ethylene glycol (Nitter-Hauge, 1970).

Toxicology of polyglycols and propylene glycol: After ethylene and diethylene glycols, the next member in the ascending homologous series is triethylene glycol. It is the lowest molecular weight polymer (about 200) that is commonly called a "polyethylene glycol"; it corresponds approximately to PEG 200. Through PEG 600 the polymers are liquids at room temperature; above PEG 1000 they are solids (the so-called Carbowaxes). As a general rule the toxicity to laboratory animals appears to decrease the higher the degree of polymerization, but in all cases extremely large doses are required to kill (toxicity class 1). The acute oral lethal dose divided by the molecular weight is roughly a constant through nonaethylene glycol

(Smyth *et al.*, 1941a, 1950). Deaths appear to arise from renal injuries rather than from primary central nervous depression.

Some confusion exists in the literature with regard to the higher polymers of ethylene glycol, particularly as evaluated on a subacute or chronic basis. Improvements in synthetic processes since 1941 resulted in noticeably less toxic polymers (Smyth *et al.*, 1950). In more recent long-term feeding experiments in rats and dogs, there appear to be no essential distinctions among polyethylene glycols from PEG 200 through 4000, but compounds with a molecular weight of 6000 and greater are definitely less toxic (Smyth *et al.*, 1955). The intravenous LD_{50} of PEG 300 in rats is about 7 ml./kg. (Carpenter and Shaffer, 1952). PEG 400 has been given intravenously to humans in 1-gm. doses, and about 80% is recovered in the urine in 12 hours (Shaffer *et al.*, 1950). When given to monkeys for 13 weeks in daily doses of 2 to 4 ml./kg., PEG 200 induced mild oxalate crystalluria in the renal cortex, which was not associated with other clinical or pathological findings (Prentice and Majeed, 1978).

Above PEG 1000, gastrointestinal absorption is negligible in rats, but even PEG 6000 is excreted to a high degree in human urine after intravenous administration (Shaffer and Critchfield, 1947). Percutaneous toxicity and local reactions were absent in a series from PEG 300 through 9000 applied to rabbit skin (Tusing *et al.*, 1954). Compared to other derivatives discussed here, the polyethylene glycols are essentially innocuous.

Propylene glycol appears to be much less toxic than any of the other low-molecular-weight glycols. It is employed as a solvent in drugs, cosmetics and foods. Information about the experimental animal toxicity of this and many other glycols has been reviewed exhaustively (Rowe, 1962).

Symptomatology:

A. Ethylene glycol and its metabolic precursors (Group A compounds in Figure III-4).
 1. Central nervous depression characterized by transient exhilaration, drunkenness, ataxia, vertigo progressing to stupor and finally coma, with or without a transient period of convulsions. Death from respiratory arrest or perhaps cardiovascular collapse, or else a slow clearing of the sensorium.
 2. When only ethylene glycol has been consumed, there is no alcohol odor on the breath.
 3. Nausea, vomiting, abdominal pain, de-

hydration, weakness, muscle tenderness.
 4. Hyperpnea may indicate either severe metabolic acidosis or pulmonary edema.
 5. Perhaps carpopedal spasm or other signs of hypocalcemic tetany.
 6. Lumbar pain, albuminuria, hematuria, oliguria progressing to anuria.
 7. Acute renal failure with uremia, peripheral edema, ascites, pulmonary edema, drowsiness, cyanosis, coma, and death in 7 to 10 days.

B. Diethylene glycol and Group B compounds (Figure III-4).
 1. Central nervous depression, although probably less prominent than with ethylene glycol (see A1 above).
 2. No hypocalcemic tetany or metabolic acidosis (see A4 and A5 above), with the possible exception of poisonings due to ethylene glycol monomethyl ether.
 3. Nausea, vomiting, and sometimes diarrhea.
 4. Prominent headache. Later abdominal and lumbar pain and costovertebral angle tenderness.
 5. Transient polyuria and then oliguria, progressing to anuria.
 6. Acute renal failure as in A7 above.
 7. Less critical pathological lesions may appear in brain, lungs, liver, meninges and heart.
 8. Observations in animals suggest the remote possibility of pulmonary edema, intravascular hemolysis and bone marrow depression, at least with some ether derivatives of ethylene and diethylene glycols.

C. Polyethylene glycols and propylene glycol (Group C in Figure III-4). Essentially innocuous but very large doses produce renal injuries in experimental animals. Furthermore, propylene glycol can produce central nervous depression in large doses.

Treatment:

A. Ethylene glycol and Group A substances (Figure III-4).
 1. Gastric lavage with water (p. I-8). Syrup of ipecac may be a safe way to empty the stomach if given promptly after the ingestion (p. I-2).
 2. Supportive measures against central nervous depression, including the administration of oxygen and artificial respiration as needed (pp. IV-12 and 7-12).
 3. Because convulsions have been de-

scribed during the comatose state, an-aleptic drugs should probably be avoided. If convulsions become intense and persistent, the intravenous admin-istration of diazepam or a short-acting barbiturate drug may become neces-sary (p. IV-37).

4. Try to distinguish between convulsive seizures and muscle spasms due to hy-pocalcemia. If in doubt, parenteral cal-cium therapy is recommended (p. IV-74).

5. Although cerebral edema has been de-scribed, it is not likely to require spe-cific attention, but if the cerebrospinal fluid pressure is very high, decompress as suggested on pp. IV-43–46).

6. If hypotension becomes severe, vaso-constrictor drugs may be required to support the blood pressure (p. IV-16), but avoid infusing large volumes of fluid.

7. Early in the course of the intoxication, it is probably wise to attempt to estab-lish a brisk flow of dilute urine in order to promote the excretion of ethylene glycol and its metabolites. Both man-nitol (p. IV-52) and furosemide (p. IV-22) have been used, even in the early oliguric phase.

8. Be cautious and conservative about correcting mild dehydration and elec-trolyte imbalances, but severe meta-bolic acidosis necessitates vigorous treatment with sodium bicarbonate, although mild acidosis is perhaps best ignored. No data are yet available to establish whether bicarbonate therapy to alkalinize the urine serves to protect the kidneys against nephrotoxic me-tabolites of ethylene glycol.

9. Hemodialysis (or peritoneal dialysis) to reduce blood and tissue levels of ethylene glycol and its metabolites, to correct severe acidosis, and to forestall the development of uremia.

10. If facilities for hemodialysis or perito-neal dialysis are unavailable and es-pecially if central nervous depression is not profound, ethyl alcohol may be administered in an attempt to inhibit the metabolism of ethylene glycol to its more toxic metabolites. Try the whiskey or ethanol regimen suggested for methyl alcohol poisoning (p. III-277). Perhaps pyrazole or 4-methyl-pyrazole will prove eventually to be the antidote of choice.

11. Miscellaneous supportive measures for impending acute renal failure (pp. IV-51–56).

B. Diethylene glycol and Group B substances (Figure III-4).

1. Gastric lavage with water (p. I-8). Syrup of ipecac may be a safe way to empty the stomach if given promptly after the ingestion (p. I-2).

2. Supportive measures against central nervous depression, including the ad-ministration of oxygen and artificial respiration as needed (pp. IV-7–14).

3. Avoid analeptic drugs for reasons de-scribed under A3 above.

4. If hypotension becomes severe, vaso-constrictor drugs may be required to support the blood pressure (p. IV-16) but avoid infusing large volumes of fluid.

5. See comment under A5 above regard-ing cerebral edema.

6. Watch for metabolic acidosis and/or hypocalcemia tetany, particularly with some of the formate esters and mon-oalkyl ethers.

7. Diuretic therapy as outlined under A7 above deserves a trial, but no clinical experience can be cited in diethylene glycol poisoning.

8. The value of early hemodialysis to re-move diethylene glycol and related substances has not been established, but it may prove to be a worthwhile measure in severe poisonings.

9. Miscellaneous supportive measures for impending acute renal failure (pp. IV-51–56).

Laboratory:

1. Analytical methods (*e.g.*, gas chromatog-raphy) are available for several of the gly-cols and for some of their metabolites. In one massive ingestion the serum ethylene glycol concentration reached 450 mg./100 ml. (Michelis *et al.*, 1976).

2. Frequent determinations of blood electro-lytes, especially CO_2 and chloride (to detect and monitor metabolic acidosis), calcium (to detect impending hypocalcemia) and potassium (to evaluate renal failure).

3. EEG and lumbar puncture if coma per-sists.

4. Repeated urinalyses and renal function tests.

5. Liver function tests and hematological studies.

References:

Ahmed, M. M. Ocular effects of antifreeze poisoning. Br. J. Ophthalmol. *55*:854-855, 1971a.

Berman, L. B.; Schreiner, G. E.; Feys, J. The nephrotoxic lesion of ethylene glycol. Ann. Intern. Med. 46:611-619, 1957.

Boemke, F. Beitrag zur Toxikologie und Pathologie des Athylenglykols (Glysantin). Virchow Arch. Pathol. Anat. 310:106, 1943.

Bove, K. E. Ethylene glycol toxicity. Am. J. Clin. Pathol. 45:46-50, 1966.

Bowie, M. D.; McKenzie, D. Diethylene glycol poisoning in children. S. Afr. Med. J. 46:931-934, 1972.

Brekke, A. Two cases of poisoning by ethylene glycol; acute uremia cured by unilateral decapsulation of kidney. Norsk. mag. f. laegevidensk 91:381-388, 1930.

Browning, E. Toxicity and Metabolism of Industrial Solvents. Elsevier Publishing Co., Amsterdam, 2nd ed, 1965.

Calvery, H. O.; Klumpp, T. G. Toxicity for human beings of diethlene glycol with sulfanilamide. South. Med. J. 32:1105-1109, 1939.

Carpenter, C. P.; Pozzani, U. C.; Weil, C. S.; Nair, J. H., III; Keck, G. A. Smyth, H. F., Jr. The toxicity of butyl cellosolve solvent. Arch. Ind. Health 14:114-131, 1956.

Carpenter, C. P.; Shaffer, C. B. A study of the polyethylene glycols as vehicles for intramuscular and subcutaneous injection. J. Am. Pharm. Assoc., Sci. Ed., 41:27-29, 1952.

Chou, J. Y.; Richardson, K. E. The effect of pyrazole on ethylene glycol toxicity and metabolism in the rat. Toxicol. Appl. Pharmacol. 43:33-44, 1978.

Clay, K. L.; Murphy, R. C. On the metabolic acidosis of ethylene glycol intoxication. Toxicol. Appl. Pharmacol. 39:39-49, 1977.

Collins, J. M.; Hennes, D. M.; Holzgang, C. R.; Gourley, R. T.; Porter, G. A. Recovery after prolonged oliguria due to ethylene glycol. Arch. Intern. Med. 125:1059-1062, 1970.

Coon, R. A.; Jones, R. A.; Jenkins, L. J., Jr.; Siegel, J. Animal inhalation studies on ammonia, ethylene glycol, formaldehyde, dimethylamine, and ethanol. Toxicol. Appl. Pharmacol. 16:646-655, 1970.

Flanagan, P.; Libcke, J. H. Renal biopsy observations following recovery from ethylene glycol nephrosis. Am. J. Clin. Pathol. 41:171-175, 1964.

Friedman, E. A.; Greenberg, J. B.; Merrill, J. P.; Dammin, G. J. Consequences of ethylene glycol poisoning; report of four cases and review of the literature. Am. J. Med. 32:891-902, 1962.

Gaultier, M.; Conso, F.; Rudler, M.; Leclerc, J. P.; Mellerio, F. Intoxication aigue par l'ethylene glycol. Eur. J. Toxicol. Environ. Hyg. 9:373-379, 1976.

Geiling, E. M. K.; Cannon, P. R. Pathologic effects of Elixir Sulfanilamide (diethylene glycol) poisoning clinical and experimental correlations: final report. J. A. M. A. 111:919-926, 1938.

Gessner, P. K.; Parke, D. V.; Williams, R. T. The metabolism of C¹⁴-labelled ethylene glycol. Biochem. J. 79:482-489, 1961.

Giromini, M.; De Freudenreich, J.; Jenny, M.; Haenni, B. Acidose metabolique par intoxication a l'Antigel. Schweiz. Med. Wochenschr. 94:1687-1690, 1964.

Grant, A. P. Acute ethylene glycol poisoning treated with calcium salts. Lancet 2:1252-1253, 1952.

Greenberg, L.; Mayers, M. R.; Goldwater, L. J.; Burke, W. J.; Moskowitz, S. Health hazards in the manufacture of "fused collars"; I. Exposure to ethylene glycol monomethyl ether. J. Ind. Hyg. Toxicol. 20:134-147, 1938.

Hagemann, P. O.; Chiffelle, T. R. Ethylene glycol poisoning. A clinical and pathologic study of three cases. J. Lab. Clin. Med. 33:573-584, 1948.

Hagstam, K. E.; Ingvar, D. H.; Paatela, M.; Tallqvist, H. Ethylene-glycol poisoning treated by haemodialysis. Acta Med. Scand. 178:599-606, 1965.

Holman, N. W., Jr.; Mundy, R. L.; Teague, R. S. Alkyldiol antidotes to ethylene glycol toxicity in mice. Toxicol. Appl. Pharmacol. 49:385-392, 1979.

Kahn, H. S.; Brotchner, R. J. A recovery from ethylene glycol (antifreeze) intoxication; a case of survival and two fatalities from ethylene glycol including autopsy findings. Ann. Intern. Med. 32:284-294, 1950.

Kersting, E. J.; Nielsen, S. W. Experimental ethylene glycol

poisoning in the dog. Am. J. Vet. Res. 27:574-582, 1965.

Kesten, H. D.; Mulinos, N. G.; Pomerantz, L. Pathologic effects of certain glycols and related compounds. Arch. Pathol. 27:447-465, 1939.

Laug, E. P.; Calvery, H. O.; Morris, H. J.; Woodward, G. The toxicology of some glycols and derivatives. J. Ind. Hyg. Toxicol. 21:173-201, 1939.

Leech, P. N. Elixir of Sulfanilamide-Massengill. Chemical, pharmacologic, pathologic and necropsy reports; preliminary toxicity reports on diethylene glycol and sulfanilamide. J. A. M. A. 109:1531-1539, 1937.

Lepkovsky, S.; Ouer, R. A.; Evans, H. M. The nutritive value of the fatty acids of lard and some of their esters. J. Biol. Chem. 108:431-438, 1935.

Levy, R. I. Renal failure secondary to ethylene glycol intoxication. J. A. M. A. 173:1210-1213, 1960.

McChesney, E. W.; Goldberg, L.; Harris, E. S. Reappraisal of the toxicology of ethylene glycol. IV. The metabolism of labelled glycollic and glyoxylic acids in the rhesus monkey. Food Cosmet. Toxicol. 10:655-670, 1972.

Meier, H.; Allen, R. C.; Hoag, W. G. Spontaneous hemorrhagic diathesis in inbred mice due to single or multiple "prothrombin-complex" deficiencies. Blood 19:501-514, 1962.

Michelis, M. F.; Mitchell, B.; Davis, B. B. "Bicarbonate resistant" metabolic acidosis in association with ethylene glycol intoxication. Clin. Toxicol. 9:53-60, 1976.

Milles, G. Ethylene glycol poisoning with suggestions for its treatment as oxalate poisoning. Arch. Pathol. 41:631-638, 1946.

Morris, H. J.; Nelson, A. A.; Calvery, H. O. Observations on the chronic toxicities of propylene glycol, ethylene glycol, diethylene glycol, ethylene glycol mono-ethyl ether and diethylene glycol mono-ethyl ether. J. Pharmacol. Exp. Ther. 74:266-273, 1942.

Mundy, R. L.; Hall, L. M.; Teague, R. S. Pyrazole as an antidote for ethylene glycol poisoning. Toxicol. Appl. Pharmacol. 28:320-322, 1974.

Nadeau, G.; Cote, R.; Delaney, F. J. Two cases of ethylene glycol poisoning. Can. Med. Assoc. J. 70:69-70, 1954.

Nitter-Hauge, S. Poisoning with ethylene glycol monomethyl ether. Acta Med. Scand. 188:277-280, 1970.

Parry, M. F.; Wallach, R. Ethylene glycol poisoning. Am. J. Med. 57:143-150, 1974.

Parsons, C. E.; Parsons, M. E. M. Toxic encephalopathy and "granulopenic anemia" due to volatile solvents in industry; report of two cases. J. Ind. Hyg. Toxicol. 20:124-133, 1938.

Pendras, J. Ethylene glycol poisoning as an indication for hemodialysis. Clin. Res. 11:249, 1963.

Peterson, D. I.; Peterson, J. E.; Hardinge, M. G.; Wacker, W. E. C. Experimental treatment of ethylene glycol poisoning. J. A. M. A. 186:955-957, 1963.

Pons, C. A.; Custer, R. P. Acute ethylene glycol poisoning; a clinicopathologic report of eighteen fatal cases. Am. J. Med. Sci. 211:544-552, 1946.

Prentice, D. E.; Majeed, S. K. Oral toxicity of polyethylene glycol (PEG 200) in monkeys and rats. Toxicol. Lett. 2:119-122, 1978.

Procter, D. S. C. Coma in burns - the cause traced to dressings. S. Afr. Med. J. 40:1116-1120, 1966.

Reidenberg, M. M.; Powers, D. V.; Sevy, R. W.; Bello, C. T. Acute renal failure due to nephrotoxins. Am. J. Med. Sci. 247:25-29, 1964.

Richardson, K. E. Endogeneous oxalate synthesis in male and female rats. Toxicol. Appl. Pharmacol. 7:507-515, 1965.

Roberts, J. A.; Seibold, H. R. Ethylene glycol toxicity in the monkey. Toxicol. Appl. Pharmacol. 15:624-631, 1969.

Ross, I. P. Ethylene glycol poisoning with meningoencephalitis and anuria. Br. Med. J. 1:1340-1342, 1956.

Rowe, V. K. Glycols and derivatives of glycols. In Industrial Hygiene and Toxicology, Edited by F. A. Patty, Vol. II. Toxicology. 2nd ed. Edited by D. W. Fassett and D. D. Irish. Interscience Publishers, Inc., New York, 1962.

Schreiner, G. E.; Maher, J. F. Toxic nephropathy. Am. J. Med. 38:409-499, 1965.

Schreiner, G. E.; Maher, J. F.; Marc-Aurele, J.; Knowlan, K.; Alvo, M. Ethylene glycol - two indications for hemodialysis.

Trans. Am. Soc. Artif. Intern. Organs 5:81, 1959.

Shaffer, C. B.; Critchfield, F. H. The absorption and excretion of the solid polyethylene glycols ("Carbowax" compounds). J. Pharm. Sci. 36:152-157, 1947.

Shaffer, C. B.; Critchfield, F. H.; Nair, J. H., III. The absorption and excretion of a liquid polyethylene glycol. J. Pharm. Sci. 39:340-344, 1950.

Smith, D. E. Morphologic lesions due to acute and subacute poisoning with antifreeze. Arch. Pathol. 51:423-433, 1951.

Smyth, H. F., Jr. Physiological Aspects of the Glycols and Related Compounds. In Glycols, p. 300-327. Edited by G. O. Curme, Jr. and F. Johnston. Reinhold Publishing Corp., New York, 1952.

Smyth, H. F., Jr.; Carpenter, C. P.; Weil, C. S. The toxicology of the polyethylene glycols. J. Am. Pharm. Assoc., Sci. Ed., 39:349-354, 1950.

Smyth, H. F., Jr.; Carpenter, C. P.; Weil, C. S. The chronic oral toxicology of the polyethylene glycols. J. Am. Pharm. Assoc., Sci. Ed., 44:27-30, 1955.

Smyth, H. F., Jr.; Seaton, J.; Fischer, L. The single dose toxicity of some glycols and derivatives. J. Ind. Hyg. Toxicol. 23:259-268, 1941a.

Stokes, J. B.; Aueron, F. Prevention of organ damage in massive ethylene glycol ingestion. J. A. M. A. 243:2065-2066, 1980.

Sykowski, P. Ethylene glycol toxicity. Am. J. Ophthalmol. 34:1599-1600, 1951.

Tanret, P.; Thomas, J.; Cottenot, F. Evolution des depots oxaliques et lipidiques au cours de la lithiase renale experimentale par l'ethylene-glycol et l'acide oxalique. C. R. Soc. Biol. (Paris) 155:1025-1027, 1961.

Tanret, P.; Thomas, J.; Thomas, E.; Cottenot, F. Influence du sexe sur les formations de depots d'oxalate de calcium dans les reins chez le Rat intoxique par l'ethylene-glycol. C. R. Soc. Biol. (Paris) 156:1285-1287, 1962.

Troisi, F. M. Chronic intoxication by ethylene glycol vapour. Br. J. Ind. Med. 7:65-69, 1950.

Tusing, T. W.; Elsea, T. R.; Sauveue, A. B. The chronic dermal toxicity of a series of polyethylene glycols. J. Pharm. Sci. 43:489-490, 1954.

Underwood, F.; Bennett, W. M. Ethylene glycol intoxication. Prevention of renal failure by aggressive management. J. A. M. A. 226:1453-1454, 1973.

Van Stee, E. W.; Harris, A. M.; Horton, M. L.; Back, K. C. The treatment of ethylene glycol toxicosis with pyrazole. J. Pharmacol. Exp. Ther. 192:251, 1975.

von Oettingen, W. F.; Jirouch, E. H. Pharmacology of ethylene glycol and some of its derivatives in relation to their chemical constitution and physical chemical properties. J. Pharmacol. Exp. Ther. 42:355-372, 1931.

Wacker, W. E. C.; Haynes, H.; Drayan, R.; Fisher, W.; Coleman, J. E. Treatment of ethylene glycol poisoning with ethyl alcohol. J. A. M. A. 194:1231-1233, 1965.

Werner, H. W.; Mitchell, J. L.; Miller, J. W.; von Oettingen, W. F. The acute toxicity of vapors of several monoalkyl ethers of ethylene glycol. J. Ind. Hyg. Toxicol. 25:157-163, 1943a.

Werner, H. W.; Mitchell, J. L.; Miller, J. W.; von Oettingen, W. F. Effects of repeated exposure of dogs to monoalkyl ethylene glycol ether vapors. J. Ind. Hyg. Toxicol. 25:409-414, 1943c.

Wiley, F. H.; Hueper, W. C.; Bergen, D. S.; Blood, F. R. The formation of oxalic acid from ethylene glycol and related solvents. J. Ind. Hyg. Toxicol. 20:269-277, 1938.

Wiley, F. H.; Hueper, W. C.; von Oettingen, W. F. Toxicity and potential dangers of ethylene glycol. J. Ind. Hyg. Toxicol. 18:123-126, 1936.

Zarembski, P. M.; Hodgkinson, A. Plasma oxalic acid and calcium levels in oxalate poisoning. J. Clin. Pathol. 20:283-285, 1967.

FERROUS SALTS

Ferrous salts are widely used in the treatment of iron-deficiency anemias. Ferrous carbonate, chloride, fumarate (32.9% Fe by weight), gluconate (12.5% Fe), lactate (23.9% Fe), and glutamate have all been prescribed, but the sulfate is the most popular iron preparation in the United States. The official U.S.P. tablets contain 300 mg. $FeSO_4 \cdot 7H_2O$ or an equivalent amount of dried (anhydrous) ferrous sulfate containing 60 mg. computed as elemental iron. It is also available as a syrup and as elixirs. Ferric salts (e.g., the ammonium citrate and hydroxide) and even metallic iron powder ("reduced iron") have been employed in the treatment of anemia. The latter, however, is no longer a significant market product. Carbonyl iron is a reduced form of high bioavailability and apparent low toxicity (Sachs and Houchin, 1978).

Chelated forms of iron include iron choline citrate. These preparations when given by mouth are claimed to be less irritating to the gastric mucosa (Franklin et al., 1958), but no convincing evidence exists to prove that they are less hazardous than the inorganic salts when given in equivalent bioavailable doses. Small amounts of soluble copper and manganese salts are often included along with iron compounds in preparations for the treatment of iron-deficiency anemia. These additives do not contribute sig-nificantly to the toxicity of ferrous sulfate preparations (Forbes, 1947; Somers, 1947), but the evidence that they improve the therapeutic result has always been suspect.

Toxicology: Iron is potentially toxic in all of its dosage forms, and a single toxic syndrome is common to them all. As tested in several animal species, five different iron compounds proved to lie in toxicity class 3 (Somers, 1947; Hoppe et al., 1955). Elemental iron is significantly less toxic in rats than soluble salts (Boyd and Shanas, 1963a). For the purposes of the discussion below, ferrous sulfate may be taken as representative. In the body, the ferrous ion is believed to be rapidly oxidized to Fe^{3+}.

The incidence of acute accidental intoxication with ferrous sulfate appears to parallel its use in medicine. Very few authenticated case reports of iron poisoning of any type can be found in the medical literature of the decades prior to 1947, when iron was in disrepute as a therapeutic agent (Forbes, 1947). It was so universally regarded as innocuous when reinstated in the treatment of anemia that such signs as severe shock and hematemesis were often not recognized as consequences of known prior ingestions of excessive amounts of ferrous sulfate (Hertzog et al., 1943; Howard, 1949). The number of such reported cases continues to grow steadily. A 50%

mortality rate was reported in one early selected series of severe cases (Aldrich, 1958; Cann and Verhulst, 1960d), but more recent experience suggests that a considerably lower mortality can be anticipated (Barr and Fraser, 1968; Fischer *et al.*, 1971; Greengard and McEnery, 1968; James, 1970). In a review of 474 cases published in 1971, there was a mortality of about 1% (Westlin, 1971).

Most of the reported deaths from iron poisoning have occurred in infants and young children who ingested ferrous sulfate tablets because of the sweet candy or chocolate coating. In the case of infants and young children it is usually difficult to determine with any degree of certainty the number of tablets swallowed, but in fatal cases the quantities are invariably in gross excess of customary therapeutic doses. Recoveries have occurred following the ingestion of as many as 70 tablets (0.3 gm. each), perhaps because substantial but unknown portions were promptly removed by vomiting (Cann and Verhulst, 1960d); however, serious sequelae and deaths have followed as few as 15 tablets (Amerman *et al.*, 1958; Duffy and Diehl, 1952; Hoppe *et al.*, 1955).

In general the ingestion of up to 10 tablets by a child is associated with mild poisoning, whereas moderate to severe intoxication follows ingestion of 20 tablets or more (James, 1970). On a body weight basis 20 to 60 mg. (computed as elemental iron) per kg. (body weight) is a mildly to moderately toxic dose whereas 200 to 250 mg./kg. is a life-threatening dose (Robotham and Lietman, 1980; Stein *et al.*, 1976a). The latter often results in serum iron levels of 500 μg./100 ml. or higher.

Iron poisoning in adults is very rare (Eriksson *et al.*, 1974; Henriksson *et al.*, 1979; Wallack and Winkelstein, 1974), but adults appear to be as susceptible as infants and children if appropriate amounts are consumed. In one adult female 42 mg. iron/kg. produced only epigastric pain whereas in another 180 mg./kg. produced a severe poisoning (Eriksson *et al.*, 1974). Death has been reported in an adult who ingested at one time ¼ lb. of the sulfate (Foucar *et al.*, 1948). Iron poisoning poses special problems in pregnancy. In one case both fetus and mother died perhaps because of a decision to withhold chelation therapy (Strom *et al.*, 1976).

Acute iron poisoning may occur in a number of distinct phases (Aldrich, 1958). Ferrous sulfate can exert an intensely corrosive action on the gastric mucosa, particularly at the pyloric end. Epigastric pain and vomiting may begin within 10 to 60 minutes, followed over the next 6 to 8 hours by shock, coma and death (Charney, 1961; Curtiss and Kosinski, 1954; Davis and Gibbs, 1956; Duffy and Diehl, 1952; Murphy *et al.*, 1951; Smith *et al.*, 1950; Swift *et al.*, 1952;

Thomson, 1947). Vomitus may contain particles of tablets and be brown in color, but blood is also frequently found. Hematemesis may occur even in the absence of ulceration apparently because of capillary dilation and diapedesis (Jacobs *et al.*, 1965). Watery diarrhea sometimes with ribbons of bowel mucosa further contributes to cardiovascular collapse from fluid and electrolyte loss.

If the victim survives this initial phase, a quiescent period usually follows with some clinical improvement. Some victims ultimately progress to complete recovery, but others relapse within 12 hours into fatal secondary shock (Aldrich, 1958; Prain, 1949; Thomson, 1950) or pneumonitis resulting from the aspiration of vomitus (Forbes, 1947).

In relapse a profound metabolic acidosis is often observed (Reissmann and Coleman, 1955). Acidosis has been ascribed to the hydrolysis of ferric ions in blood, but increases in lactic and citric acids also occur. Respiratory changes characteristic of acidosis are frequently noted. Although the severity of symptoms shows some correlation with serum iron levels (Franklin *et al.*, 1958), acidosis is not always reversed when the serum iron concentration is lowered with a chelating agent (Felts *et al.*, 1962a). Undoubtedly acidosis contributes to cardiovascular collapse. Phenylephrine produced no blood pressure response in dogs that were hypotensive because of iron poisoning until their acidosis was controlled with THAM (Felts *et al.*, 1962a).

Other factors that are postulated to contribute to peripheral circulatory collapse include a direct effect of iron in vascular walls (Roberts *et al.*, 1975), the production or release of ferritin, which may be identical with v.d.m. or vasodepressor material (Demulder, 1958; Jacobs *et al.*, 1965; Schafir, 1961; Smith, 1952), hemoconcentration because of increased capillary leakage, decreases in the production of plasma proteins because of liver injury, and possible release of bacterial toxins from the gut (Jacobs *et al.*, 1965; Shafir, 1961).

Postmortem examination usually reveals liver damage consisting of periportal hemorrhagic necrosis (Large, 1961; Luongo and Bjornson, 1954). Among some survivors delicate fibrosis of the liver (mild cirrhosis) has been described. Derangements of liver function such as hypoglycemia, elevated blood ammonia, multiple coagulation defects due to impaired synthesis of clotting factors, etc., are common in iron poisoning (Brown and Gray, 1955; de Castro *et al.*, 1977; Henriksson *et al.*, 1979; Greenblatt *et al.*, 1976; Witzelben and Chaffey, 1962), and occasionally death has been ascribed to acute hepatic failure (Covey, 1964; Gleason *et al.*, 1979).

Late pyloric stenosis, similar to that incurred by survivors of mineral acid ingestion (p. III-8), and intestinal obstruction secondary to infarction (see below) are well known (Crosskey, 1952; Gandhi and Robarts, 1962; Ross, 1953; Warden et al., 1958; Wilmers and Heriot, 1954). Endoscopy and fluoroscopy are mandatory procedures to assess the extent of the damage once the acute phase has subsided. Changes have been reported as late as 6 years after ingestion. Gastrectomy may be necessary in cases of severe scarring and fibrosis (Gezernik et al., 1980). A single tablet of ferrous sulfate ingested by an elderly woman became lodged in the hypopharynx and produced local ulceration there (Abbarah et al., 1976).

Iron does not appear to impair renal function directly (Enerbäck and Lundin, 1965), and even renal failure secondary to shock appears to be a rare occurrence. Neurologic sequelae (abnormal EEG, hyperkinetic and destructive behavior) have been reported at least once (Barr and Fraser, 1968).

Biochemical and physiological mechanisms underlying iron poisoning are not understood. Perhaps iron can initiate circulatory or respiratory collapse directly. Methemoglobinemia is not responsible for the cyanosis (Swift et al., 1952), even though one patient unresponsive to oxygen was said to show a rapid improvement in color after methylene blue (Smith et al., 1950). Toxic doses of iron can be absorbed through the intact mucosa of both the small and large bowel of rabbits and dogs (Franklin et al., 1958; Reissmann et al., 1955), but preexisting damage to the mucosa is believed to facilitate absorption and promote toxicity (Demulder, 1958; Prain, 1949). Serum iron is strongly bound to a plasma protein known as transferrin, which is normally only 20 to 45% saturated; the binding capacity is equivalent to 3.3 mg. of iron per liter (National Academy of Science, 1979). Signs of systemic iron poisoning appear only after this reserve binding capacity is saturated.

Because many brands of ferrous sulfate tablets are enteric coated and therefore insoluble in gastric juice, gastric lavage may be ineffective in removing them. If emesis can be induced or has already occurred, an examination of the vomitus may reveal the state of the ingested material and indicate the proper course of further therapy. Whether the tablets are enteric coated or not, an X-ray of the abdomen is useful for revealing their presence and for evaluating the success of emesis, gastric lavage, catharsis or enemas (Green, 1971; Hosking, 1969; James, 1970). Positive X-ray evidence for the continued presence of tablets after failure to evacuate the stomach by conventional means led to the performance of a successful gastrotomy in one case (Peterson and Fifield, 1980). Segmental necrosis of the small intestines is common with enteric coated tablets (Smith et al., 1950; Swift et al.,

1952). Small bowel resection may be necessary to remove areas of necrosis (Walsh, 1980; Roberts et al., 1975).

Experimental treatment: Rats receiving ferrous sulfate by stomach tube have been shown to tolerate lethal doses if given promptly a soluble phosphate salt (Sisson and Bronson, 1958). This and later work (Bronson and Sisson, 1960) are the basis for the phosphate treatment which has been widely recommended in the past. Not only has its effectiveness not been proved in human victims of iron poisoning, but in at least two cases complications of hypocalcemia and hyperphosphatemia indicated that systemic phosphate poisoning was superimposed on the pre-existing iron intoxication (Bachrach et al., 1979; Geffner and Opas, 1980); see also Phosphates in Section II. Moreover, an in vitro study indicated that neither sodium bicarbonate nor phosphate (diluted Fleet Phosphosoda oral solution) was effective in precipitating iron at acidic pH values (Czajka et al., 1981).

Although research on the therapeutic role of chelating agents in iron poisoning has been extensive, no totally satisfactory drug or procedure has been developed. Dimercaprol (BAL, p. III-50) increased the mortality of experimental animals given near mean lethal doses of iron (Edge and Somers, 1948). In spite of this evidence that the BAL-iron complex is more toxic than iron alone, BAL has received a limited clinical trial. Its use has met only indifferent success (Roxburgh, 1949; Shoss, 1954), and it is best avoided in favor of less toxic and more effective agents.

Considerably more experience has accumulated with EDETATE CALCIUM DISODIUM (p. III-163) and chemically related structures, e.g., DTPA or diethylenetriaminepentaacetic acid. In dogs edetate prolonged survival time perhaps by lowering serum iron concentrations, but mortality was not decreased (Bronson and Sisson, 1960). It has been used in a number of clinical cases with ultimate survival of the victims (Barrie and Wilson, 1962; Covey, 1964; Dugdale and Powell, 1964; Piotrowska and Warnecka, 1966; Schafir, 1961; Simpson and Blunt, 1960). Some of these reports indicate decreases in serum iron concentration together with a hastening of urinary excretion. Not all investigators, however, are enthusiastic about the clinical response of the edetate-treated patient. Chelated iron may also be excreted in bile, but the importance of this route has not been defined in man (Haddock et al., 1965). Even early treatment has failed at times to prevent death (Dugdale and Powell, 1964). These polycarboxylic acid-type chelators are probably not as safe or effective as deferoxamine (below).

Deferoxamine (DFOM) is an iron chelating agent introduced for use in primary and secondary hemochromatosis and in acute iron poisoning (Moeschlin and Schnider, 1963). DFOM was derived from naturally occurring iron complexes, siderochromes, and its affinity for ferric iron is very high and quite specific. It is absorbed from the gastrointestinal tract to some extent (Whitten et al., 1966). It can be given intravenously if the rate of administration is carefully controlled, but the intramuscular route is preferred. Its antidotal capacity in acute iron poisoning is small but significant. When given by mouth 0.5 to 2 hours after an LD$_{50}$ of ferrous sulfate, all guinea pigs survived; 80% survived an LD$_{100}$ under similar circumstances (Moeschlin and Schnider, 1963). Only 3 of 9 dogs survived when enteral and parenteral DFOM was started 1 hour after an oral LD$_{100}$ of ferrous sulfate (Whitten et al., 1965).

When several chelating agents (including some not available for clinical use) were tested in equimolar doses in mice, DFOM by mouth immediately after ferrous sulfate was much more effective than edetate. Other experimental drugs were even more active than DFOM (Nigrovic and Catsch, 1965). When administration of the chelating agent was delayed for only 30 minutes, however, it was no longer effective by mouth. In contrast intraperitoneal DFOM retained highly significant antidotal activity even when its administration was delayed. Thus, early therapy with DFOM is critical for success, and both oral and parenteral administration appear to be indicated.

Because even the maximal benefits of DFOM are small and rigidly dictated by the circumstances of its employment, the clinical experience is difficult to interpret (Dugdale and Powell, 1964; Henderson et al., 1963; Jacobs et al., 1965; McEnery and Greengard, 1966; Perlmutter and Sanders, 1966; Santos and Pisciotta, 1964; Shapiro and Barbezat, 1964; Whelan et al., 1966). In all of the above reports victims survived and many experienced an abatement of clinical symptoms when DFOM was administered. In a controlled series of mild to moderate poisonings, the combination of oral and parenteral DFOM seemed to have no significant effect on serum iron levels when compared to a control group that received only supportive care or a group that received only oral DFOM. All patients receiving DFOM, however, showed an increased urinary iron excretion (Leikin et al., 1967). Whitten et al. (1965) successfully treated 13 children, mostly with a combination of oral and intravenous DFOM, but they remained unconvinced that the DFOM therapy was responsible for the recoveries. In a much larger but uncontrolled study involving 172 patients (Westlin, 1966), DFOM was judged to have produced clinical improvement in most victims, and the overall mortality was only 1.7%.

The recommended dose of deferoxamine (Desferal) mesylate in children (Westlin, 1966) is 5 to 10 gm. by gastric tube at the conclusion of lavage. If the patient is not in shock, also give 1 gm. intramuscularly, followed by 0.5 gm. i.m. every 4 hours for 2 doses and, if indicated, every 4 to 12 hours thereafter. If the patient is in shock, the intravenous route is preferable. By infusion, the rate of administration should not exceed 15 mg./kg. per hour. Overly rapid intravenous administration may produce tachycardia, hypotension, erythema and urticaria.

Exchange transfusion has produced good clinical results (Amerman et al., 1958; Tomlinson, 1964) and compares favorably (Whitten, 1963) or is superior to chelation therapy (Movassaghi et al., 1969) in animal studies. Even without exchange, transfusions of fresh whole blood may be of value (Emmanouilides, 1959) both to treat shock and to provide additional iron-binding capacity. Under ordinary circumstances hemodialysis is probably of little value because of the plasma protein binding of iron (Demulder, 1958). The possible beneficial effects of including protein in the dialysis fluid to trap dialyzed iron does not appear to have been explored. The effect of contemporaneous administration of chelating agents on the efficiency of peritoneal dialysis (Covey, 1964; Lavender and Bell, 1970) or hemodialysis (Felts et al., 1962a) has been disputed.

Symptomatology:

1. Severe gastritis or gastroenteritis with abdominal pain, retching, and prolonged vomiting, beginning 10 to 60 minutes after ingestion. Vomitus may become bloody. Diarrhea is sometimes violent; the feces are watery and later tarry. Dehydration becomes intense.
2. Shock, pallor, cyanosis and coldness. Rapid, weak or imperceptible pulse, low blood pressure, rapid and shallow respirations.
3. Sometimes breathing is deep and rapid, reflecting an accompanying metabolic acidosis.
4. Drowsiness, hyporeflexia, dilated pupils, coma. Vasomotor instability, shock or coma and a serum iron level in great excess of the total iron-binding capacity (see Laboratory below) are poor prognostic signs.
5. Liver injury, consisting of hemorrhagic necrosis which is usually reversible.
6. Death from shock, usually in 4 to 5 hours. Sometimes following apparent recovery, pneumonia with fever or secondary shock may cause death 1 to 3 days later.
7. Among survivors pyloric stenosis and mild hepatic cirrhosis may be encountered as

persistent sequelae, but recovery is usually complete.

Treatment:

1. Induce vomiting by administering promptly syrup of ipecac (p. I-2) if enteric-coated tablets are known to have been ingested. If a readily soluble form of iron was consumed, it may be better to swallow promptly activated charcoal (p. I-4). Although charcoal does not bind ferrous iron tightly, it has a moderately high binding capacity at gastric pH values (Smith *et al.*, 1967a). (Once in the alkalinity of the duodenum, dissolved iron presumably hydrolyzes promptly to form insoluble oxides.) Milk of magnesia may be an effective alternative to activated charcoal. In a recent rat study, milk of magnesia prevented or delayed the absorption of a lethal dose of ferrous sulfate (Chadwick *et al.*, 1982).

2. Gastric lavage with water or 5% sodium bicarbonate solution. We currently believe that neither the safety nor efficacy of the widely recommended phosphate lavage fluid has been adequately established (see text above).

3. An X-ray of the abdomen may show the presence of intact tablets, which can sometimes be removed by further lavage or by administering a saline cathartic.

4. Deferoxamine mesylate (5 to 10 gm.) in water may be left in the stomach. Whereas this procedure is not endorsed by the FDA, the evidence commonly cited against oral deferoxamine (Whitten *et al.*, 1965, 1966) is not so convincing in our opinion as the evidence for its efficacy and safety (see text above).

5. In a patient not in shock, give 1.0 gm. deferoxamine intramuscularly followed by 0.5 gm. every 4 to 12 hours. Do not exceed 6 gm. in 24 hours. For patients in cardiovascular collapse the drug may be given by slow intravenous infusion not to exceed 15 mg./kg. per hour. The initial intravenous dose of 1 gm. may be followed by two 0.5-gm. doses 4 hours apart.

6. Intravenous 5% glucose in saline to correct dehydration. See pp. IV-66–67. Watch for evidence of acidosis and treat vigorously if present (pp. IV-69–72).

7. Transfusion with plasma or whole blood if shock becomes severe (p. IV-18).

8. Oxygen therapy as indicated (p. IV-12).

9. Exchange transfusion or plasmapheresis may be employed particularly in the event of renal shutdown, but hemodialysis is of little or no value for removing iron.

10. For supportive treatment of liver injury see p. IV-59–63.

11. Antibiotics at the first sign of infection. See pp. IV-85–86.

12. Observe the patient carefully for signs of relapse (48 hours) or late stricture formation (several days to weeks).

Laboratory:

1. It is important to differentiate between mild and severe cases when planning therapy. Rapid methods for determining the approximate serum iron level are useful for this purpose (Cooper *et al.*, 1971; Fischer, 1967; Hosking, 1969a). If the serum iron is in excess of the total iron binding capacity or has an absolute value of greater than 400 to 500 μg./dl., the patient should be regarded as severely poisoned (Fischer *et al.*, 1971; Westlin, 1971).

2. Once deferoxamine therapy has been started, the single most useful serum index of the need for additional therapy is the iron binding capacity. Values for total serum iron may be misleading because some methods do and some do not measure that iron complexed with deferoxamine (Gevirtz and Wasserman, 1966).

3. A change in color of the urine from straw to "vin rose" or "port wine" indicates excretion of the DFOM-iron complex. Its persistence indicates the need for continued chelation therapy (Greengard, 1975).

4. Hyperglycemia and leukocytosis frequently accompany high serum iron levels (James, 1970).

5. Multiple blood coagulation defects have been reported, but massive hemorrhage is uncommon.

References:

Abbarah, T. R.; Fredell, J. E.; Ellenz, G. B. Ulceration by oral ferrous sulfate. J. A. M. A. *236*:2320, 1976.
Aldrich, R. A. Acute iron toxicity. In *Iron in Clinical Medicine*, Edited by R. O. Wallerstein and S. R. Mettier. University of Calif. Press, Berkeley, 1958.
Amerman, E. E.; Brescia, M. A.; Aftahi, F. Ferrous sulfate poisoning. J. Pediatr. *53*:476-478, 1958.
Bachrach, L.; Correa, A.; Levin, R.; Grossman, M. Iron poisoning: complications of hypertonic phosphate lavage therapy. J. Pediatr. *94*:147-149, 1979.
Barr, D. G. D.; Fraser, D. K. B. Acute iron poisoning in children. Role of chelating agents. Br. Med. J. *1*:737-741, 1968.
Barrie, H.; Wilson, B. D. R. Calcium disodium edathamil in the treatment of ferrous sulfate poisoning. J. A. M. A. *180*:244-246, 1962.
Boyd, E. M.; Shanas, M. N. The acute oral toxicity of reduced iron. Can. Med. Assoc. J. *89*:171-175, 1963a.
Bronson, W. R.; Sisson, T. R. C. Studies on acute iron poisoning. Am. J. Dis. Child. *99*:18-26, 1960.
Brown, R. J. K.; Gray, J. D. The mechanism of acute ferrous sulfate poisoning. Can. Med. Assoc. J. *73*:192-197, 1955.
Cann, H. M.; Verhulst, H. L. Accidental poisoning in young children, the hazards of iron medication. Am. J. Dis. Child. *99*:688-691, 1960d.
Chadwick, E. W.; Corby, D. G.; Decker, W. J. Is milk of

magnesia a potentially effective antidote for acute iron poisoning? Vet. Human Toxicol. 24:298, 1982.

Charney, E. A fatal case of ferrous sulfate poisoning. J. A. M. A. 178:326-327, 1961.

Cooper, H. A.; Ekblad, M. D.; Fairbanks, V. F. Emergency semiquantitative estimation of plasma iron concentration in acute iron poisoning. Am. J. Dis. Child. 122:19-21, 1971.

Covey, T. J. Ferrous sulfate poisoning. J. Pediatr. 64:218-226, 1964.

Crosskey, P. H. Pyloric stenosis after ferrous sulfate poisoning. Br. Med. J. 2:285, 1952.

Curtiss, C. D.; Kosinski, A. A. Fatal case of iron intoxication in a child. J. A. M. A. 156:1320-1328, 1954.

Czajka, P. A.; Konrad, J. D.; Duffy, J. P. Iron poisoning - an in vitro comparison of bicarbonate and phosphate lavage solutions. J. Pediatr. 98:491-494, 1981.

Davis, D. W.; Gibbs, G. E. Iron poisoning. Am. Pract. Dig. Treat. 7:1092-1094, 1956.

de Castro, F. J.; Jaeger, R.; Gleason, W. A. Liver damage and hypoglycemia in acute iron poisoning. Clin. Toxicol. 10:287-289, 1977.

Demulder, R. Iron metabolism, biochemistry, and clinical pathological physiology - review of recent literature. Arch. Intern. Med. 102:254-301, 1958.

Duffy, T. L.; Diehl, A. M. Ferrous sulfate poisoning, report of three cases. J. Pediatr. 40:1-5, 1952.

Dugdale, A. E.; Powell, L. W. Acute iron poisoning; its effects and treatment. Med. J. Aust. 2:990-992, 1964.

Edge, N. D.; Somers, G. F. The effect of dimercaprol (BAL) in acute iron poisoning. Q. J. Pharm. Pharmacol. 21:364-369, 1948.

Emmanouilides, G. C. Acute ferrous sulfate poisoning in children, report of five cases. Clin. Proc. Child. Hosp. Wash. 15:291-299, 1959.

Enerbäck, L.; Lundin, P. M. The effect of overloading with complex iron preparations on the morphology and function of the rat kidney. Toxicol. Appl. Pharmacol. 7:525-534, 1965.

Eriksson, F.; Johansson, S. V.; Hellstedt, H.; Strandberg, O.; Wester, P. O. Iron intoxication in two adult patients. Acta Med. Scand. 196:231-236, 1974.

Felts, J. H.; Barringer, M.; Meredith, J. H. Combined chelation, hemodialysis and alkalinization, a possible treatment for iron poisoning. Trans. Am. Soc. Artif. Intern. Organs. 8:229-234, 1962a.

Fischer, D. S. A method for the rapid detection of acute iron toxicity. Clin. Chem. 13:6-11, 1967.

Fischer, D. S.; Parkman, R.; Finch, S. C. Acute iron poisoning in children. The problem of appropriate therapy. J. A. M. A. 218:1179-1184, 1971.

Forbes, G. Poisoning with preparations of iron, copper and manganese. Br. Med. J. 1:367-370, 1947.

Foucar, F. H.; Gordon, B. S.; Kaye, S. Death following ingestion of ferrous sulfate. Am. J. Clin. Pathol. 18:971-973, 1948.

Franklin, M.; Rohse, W. G.; Huerga, J.; Kemp, C. R. Chelate iron therapy. J. A. M. A. 166:1685-1693, 1958.

Gandhi, R. K.; Robarts, F. H. Hourglass stricture of the stomach and pyloric stenosis due to ferrous sulfate poisoning. Br. J. Surg. 49:613-617, 1962.

Geffner, M. E.; Opas, L. M. Phosphate poisoning complicating treatment for iron ingestion. Am. J. Dis. Child. 134:509-510, 1980.

Gevirtz, N. R.; Wasserman, L. R. The measurement of iron and iron-binding capacity in plasma containing deferoxamine. J. Pediat. 68:802-804, 1966.

Gezernik, W.; Schmaman, A.; Chappell, J. S. Corrosive gastritis as a result of ferrous sulphate ingestion. S. Afr. Med. J. 57:151-154, 1980.

Gleason, W. A.; Demello, D. E.; Decastro, F. J.; Connors, J. J. Acute hepatic failure in severe iron poisoning. J. Pediatr. 95:138-140, 1979.

Green, V. A. Iron ingestions; the Childrens Mercy Hospital. Clin. Toxicol. 4:245-252, 1971.

Greenblatt, D. J.; Allen, M.; Koch-Weser, J. Accidental iron poisoning in childhood. Six cases including one fatality. Clin. Pediat. 15:835-838, 1976.

Greengard, J. Iron poisoning in children. Clin. Toxicol. 8:575-597, 1975.

Greengard, J.; McEnery, J. T. Iron poisoning in children. G. P. 37:88-93, 1968.

Haddock, E. P.; Zapolski, E. J.; Rubin, M.; Princiotto, J. V. Biliary excretion of chelated iron. Proc. Soc. Exp. Biol. Med. 120:663-668, 1965.

Henderson, F.; Vietti, T. J.; Brown, B. Desferrioxamine in the treatment of acute toxic reaction to ferrous gluconate. J. A. M. A. 186:1139-1142, 1963.

Henriksson, P.; Nilsson, L.; Nilsson, I. M.; Stenberg, P. Fatal iron intoxication with multiple coagulation defects and degradation of factor VIII and factor XIII. Scan. J. Haematol. 22:235-240, 1979.

Hertzog, A. J.; Karstrom, A. E.; Bechel, M. J. Accidental amphetamine sulfate poisoning. J. A. M. A. 121:256-257, 1943.

Hoppe, J. O.; Marcell, G. M. A.; Tainter, M. L. A review of the toxicity of iron compounds. Am. J. Med. Sci. 230:558-571, 1955.

Hosking, C. S. Radiology in the management of acute iron poisoning. Med. J. Aust. 1:576-579, 1969.

Hosking, C. S. A simple, rapid method of determining the approximate serum iron level in acute iron poisoning. Med. J. Aust. 1:981-982, 1969a.

Howard, S. J. Poisoning by ferrous sulfate. Br. Med. J. 2:1298, 1949.

Jacobs, J.; Greene, H.; Gendel, B. R. Acute iron intoxication. N. Engl. J. Med. 273:1124-1127, 1965.

James, J. A. Acute iron poisoning; assessment of severity and prognosis. J. Pediatr. 77:117-119, 1970.

Large, H. L., Jr. A case of iron intoxication caused by Roncovite with a note on striation of portal blood flow. Am. J. Clin. Pathol. 35:427-434, 1961.

Lavender, S.; Bell, J. A. Iron intoxication in an adult. Br. Med. J. 2:406-408, 1970.

Leikin, S.; Vossough, P.; Mochir-Fatemi, F. Chelation therapy in acute iron poisoning. J. Pediatr. 71:425-430, 1967.

Luongo, M. A.; Bjornson, S. S. The liver in ferrous sulfate poisoning. N. Engl. J. Med. 251:995-999, 1954.

McEnery, J. T.; Greengard, J. Treatment of acute iron ingestion with deferoxamine in 20 children. J. Pediatr. 68:773-779, 1966.

Moeschlin, S.; Schnider, U. Treatment of primary and secondary hemochromatosis and acute iron poisoning with a new, potent iron-eliminating agent (Desferrioxamine-B). N. Engl. J. Med. 269:57-66, 1963.

Movassaghi, N.; Purugganan, G. G.; Leikin, S. Comparison of exchange transfusion and deferoxamine in the treatment of acute iron poisoning. J. Pediatr. 75:604-608, 1969.

Murphy, J. W.; Neustein, C.; Hoffman, A. C.; Winters, H. V.; Gaskins, A. L. Acute iron poisoning. Report of a case and review of the literature. Arch. Pediatr. 68:303-308, 1951.

National Academy of Science. Iron. Subcommittee on Iron, Committee on Medical and Biologic Effects of Environmental Pollutants, Div. of Medical Sciences, Assembly of Life Sciences, NRC, University Park Press, Baltimore, 1979.

Nigrovic, V.; Catsch, A. Tierexperimentell Untersuchungen zur Behandlung der akuten Eisenvergiftung. Naunyn Schmiedebergs Arch. Pharmakol. 251:225-232, 1965.

Perlmutter, R.; Sanders, B. Use of desferrioxamine in treatment of acute ferrous sulfate intoxication. Calif. Med. 104:313-314, 1966.

Peterson, C. D.; Fifield, G. C. Emergency gastrotomy for acute iron poisoning. Ann. Emerg. Med. 9:262-264, 1980.

Piotrowska, E.; Warnecka, A. A case of acute iron poisoning. (Also abstracted in Drug Digests 2: No. 2, 88, 1967.). Pediatr. Pol. 41:213-215, 1966.

Prain, J. H. Fatal poisoning of an infant by antianaemic pills containing iron, manganese and copper. Br. Med. J. 2:1019-1020, 1949.

Reissmann, K. R.; Coleman, T. J. Acute intestinal iron intoxication: II. Metabolic, respiration and circulatory effects of absorbed iron salts. Blood 10:46-51, 1955.

Reissmann, K. R.; Coleman, T. J.; Budai, B. S.; Moriarity, L. R. Acute intestinal iron intoxication: I. Iron absorption, serum iron and autopsy findings. Blood 10:35-45, 1955.

Roberts, R. J.; Nayfield, S.; Soper, R.; Kent, T. H. Acute iron intoxication with intestinal infarction managed in part by small bowel resection. Clin. Toxicol. 8:3, 1975.

Robotham, J. L.; Lietman, P. S. Acute iron poisoning: a review. Am. J. Dis. Child. 139:875-879, 1980.

Ross, F. G. M. Pyloric stenosis and fibrous stricture of stomach due to ferrous sulfate poisoning. Br. Med. J. 2:1200-1202, 1953.

Roxburgh, R. C. Fersolate poisoning. Proc. R. Soc. Med. 42:85-86, 1949.

Sachs, P. V.; Houchin, D. N. Comparative bioavailablility of elemental iron powders for repair of iron deficiency anemia in rats. Studies of efficacy and toxicity of carbonyl iron. Am. J. Clin. Nutr. 31:566-573, 1978.

Santos, A. S.; Pisciotta, A. V. Acute iron intoxication. Am. J. Dis. Child. 107:424-427, 1964.

Schafir, M. The management of acute poisoning by ferrous sulfate. Pediatrics 27:83-94, 1961.

Shapiro, N.; Barbezat, G. O. A case of acute iron poisoning treated with desferrioxamine-B. S. Afr. Med. J. 58:461-463, 1964.

Shoss, J. Ferrous sulfate poisoning. A case treated with BAL. J. Pediatr. 44:77-78, 1954.

Simpson, K.; Blunt, A. Acute ferrous sulfate poisoning treated with edathamil calcium-disodium. Lancet 2:1120-1122, 1960.

Sisson, T. R. C.; Bronson, W. R. Studies in the treatment of acute iron poisoning. Am. J. Dis. Child. 96:463-465, 1958.

Smith, J. P. The pathology of ferrous sulfate poisoning. J. Pathol. 64:467-472, 1952.

Smith, R. P.; Gosselin, R. E.; Henderson, J. A.; Anderson, D. M. Comparison of the absorptive properties of activated charcoal and Alaskan montmorillonite for some common poisons. Toxicol. Appl. Pharmacol. 10:95-104, 1967a.

Smith, R. P.; Jones, C. W.; Cochran, W. E. Ferrous sulfate toxicity; report of a fatal case. N. Engl. J. Med. 243:641-645, 1950.

Somers, G. F. Relative toxicity of some therapeutic iron preparations. Br. Med. J. 2:201-203, 1947.

Stein, M.; Blayney, D.; Feet, T.; Goeigen, T. G.; Micik, S.; Nahan, W. L. Acute iron poisoning in children. West. J. Med. 125:289-297, 1976a.

Strom, R. L.; Schiller, P.; Seeds, A. E.; Bensel, R. T. Fatal iron poisoning in a pregnant female. Minn. Med. 59:483-489, 1976.

Swift, S. C.; Cefalu, V.; Rubell, E. B. Ferrous sulfate poisoning. Report of a fatal case. J. Pediatr. 40:6-10, 1952.

Thomson, J. Two cases of ferrous sulfate poisoning. Br. Med. J. 1:640-641, 1947.

Thomson, J. Ferrous sulfate poisoning; its incidence, symptomatology, treatment and prevention. Br. Med. J. 1:645-646, 1950.

Tomlinson, B. Ferrous-sulfate poisoning treated by exchange transfusion. Lancet 2:1015, 1964.

Wallack, M. K.; Winkelstein, A. Acute iron intoxication in an adult. J. A. M. A. 229:1333-1334, 1974.

Walsh, P. V. Slow-release iron tablet and gangrene of Meckel's diverticulum. Br. J. Clin. Prac. 34:258, 1980.

Warden, M. R.; Munro, G. A.; Lanier, R. R. Fibrous stricture of the stomach due to iron (Feosol) poisoning. Radiology 71:732-734, 1958.

Westlin, W. F. Deferoxamine in the treatment of acute iron poisoning. Clin. Pediatr. 5:531-535, 1966.

Westlin, W. F. Deferoxamine as a chelating agent. Clin. Toxicol. 4:597-602, 1971.

Whelan, G.; Fazio, V.; Biggs, J. C. Acute iron intoxication, a case treated by chelation. Am. J. Med. 41:626-628, 1966.

Whitten, C. F. Accidental iron poisoning in children. J. Natl. Med. Assoc. 55:503-509, 1963.

Whitten, C. F.; Gibson, G. W.; Good, M. H.; Goodwin, J. F.; Brough, A. J. Studies in acute iron poisoning; 1. Desferrioxamine in the treatment of acute iron poisoning: clinical observations, experimental studies, and theoretical considerations. Pediatrics 36:322-335, 1965.

Whitten, C. F.; Yoo-Chen, C.; Gibson, G. W. Studies in acute iron poisoning; further observations on desferrioxamine in the treatment of acute experimental iron poisoning. Pediatrics 38:102-110, 1966.

Wilmers, M. J.; Heriot, A. J. Pyloric stenosis complicating acute poisoning by ferrous sulfate. Lancet 2:68-69, 1954.

Witzleben, C. L.; Chaffey, N. J. Distribution as a determinant of iron hepatotoxicity. Nature 195:90-91, 1962.

FLUORIDE

Sodium fluoride (NaF) and sodium fluosilicate (Na_2SiF_6) were once employed widely as insecticides (ant, roach and beetle powders) and occasionally as rodenticides. Sodium fluoride has been used internally as an anthelminic in swine (*never* in man) and externally as a delousing powder on poultry and cattle. Sodium fluoride preparations for the prevention of dental caries are available in several forms, *e.g.*, tablets (chewable, acidulated phosphate, etc.), liquids, rinses, gels, dentrifices and lozenges. Fluoride concentrations and the total amount of fluoride in a single container are safely limited by law (Hennon *et al.*, 1964; Hodge, 1963); the safety of these preparations in the home has been discussed (Duxbury *et al.*, 1982).

Dentrifices containing stannous fluoride (SnF_2), sodium fluoride or the most widely used sodium monofluorophosphate constitute sources of absorbable fluoride but not ones likely to be hazardous (Desphande and Bester, 1964; Segreto *et al.*, 1961). Cryolite (Na_3AlF_6), an insoluble sodium fluoaluminate, is sometimes dusted on vegetable or fruit crops as an insecticide; thousands of tons are employed in mixtures with bauxite (Al_2O_3) in electrolysis pots to produce aluminum. Although infrequently found outside of laboratories and various industries, HF as a gas (hydrogen fluoride) and as an aqueous solution (hydrofluoric acid) warrants consideration because it is a very hazardous form of fluoride. Some commercially available rust removers contain dangerous quantities of HF in solution (see also Section VI, General Formulations).

Worker errors and malfunctioning of automatic fluoridation equipment have occasionally led to toxic concentrations of fluoride in drinking water; in the resulting mini-epidemics of acute fluoride poisoning, no deaths have occurred, but the potential exists for mass poisonings (Hoffman *et al.*, 1980; Vogt *et al.*, 1982).

Chronic endemic fluorosis due to high concentrations of natural fluoride in local water supplies is characterized by mottling of the teeth, osteosclerotic changes in the skeleton and rarely central nervous system involvement (Dean, 1936; Hodge and Smith, 1965; Kilborn *et al.*, 1950; Linsman and McMurray, 1943; Marier *et al.*, 1963; Rosenzweig and Abkewitz, 1963; Sauer-brunn *et al.*, 1965; Singh and Jolly, 1961). Oste-osclerosis may also occur in industrial fluorosis from chronic occupational exposures to fluoride dusts and vapors (Hodge and Smith, 1977). Fluorosis illustrates important toxicological properties of fluoride but not ones that are relevant to acute fluoride poisoning.

Fluoride poisoning can be induced by any soluble compound which dissociates fluoride ion (Greenwood, 1940; Larner, 1950; McClure, 1933; Smith *et al.*, 1960a; Zipkin and Likins, 1957). Fluoro-organic compounds are becoming more widely used; in general the high stability of the C-F bond contributes to their relatively low toxicities, but some are metabolized to yield fluoride ions in significant amounts (*e.g.*, methoxyfluorane). See also FLUOROACETATE, p. III-193, and specific compounds in Section II.

Toxicology of soluble fluoride salts: More than 600 fatalities in the United States between 1933 and 1965 have been ascribed to the ingestion of soluble inorganic fluorides (Hodge and Smith, 1965); because of both accidental and suicidal ingestions, the number continues to rise. From a study of these cases one concludes that a single dose of 5 to 10 gm. (70 to 140 mg./kg.) of sodium fluoride by mouth is almost certain to be lethal in an untreated adult (Hodge and Smith, 1965). Less than 1 gm. by mouth, however, has caused dangerous poisoning (Bell, 1936; Greenwood, 1940) whereas 120 gm. has been survived, probably because of prompt vomiting (Abukurah *et al.*, 1972). Six grams have been administered intravenously to a teenager without signs of systemic toxicity, but the dosage was given intermittently over a period of 9 days (Black *et al.*, 1949). The systemic toxicity of sodium fluosilicate is about equal to that of sodium fluoride (Greenwood, 1940), whereas the less soluble cryolite is much less toxic (Larner, 1950).

A remarkable mass poisoning, involving 263 victims of whom 47 died, occurred at the Oregon State Hospital when NaF roach powder mistaken for powdered milk was added to scrambled eggs (Lidbeck *et al.*, 1943). The prepared dish was rejected by some because of a salty or soapy taste and produced numbness of the mouth in others. Toxic signs and symptoms consisted of abrupt and severe nausea, vomiting and diarrhea, followed promptly by abdominal burning and cramps. In many cases blood was noted in the vomitus and feces. General collapse was evidenced by pallor, weakness, shallow pulse and respirations, weak heart sounds, wet cold skin, cyanosis, mydriasis and coma. Some victims also experienced a thick, mucoid discharge from the mouth and nose, paralysis of the muscles of deglutition, painful carpopedal spasms of the extremities and localized or generalized urticaria.

In other poisoning episodes additional signs and symptoms have been reported: headache, convulsions and muscle weakness (Roholm, 1937; Vogt *et al.*, 1982). The course of acute fluoride poisoning is generally rapid with death often in 2 to 4 hours; if a victim survives the first 24 hours, the prognosis is good (Hodge and Smith, 1965).

Besides ingestion fluoride gains access to the body by inhalation of dusts, fumes and vapors (Hodge and Smith, 1977; Kaltreider *et al.*, 1972), but significant penetration of the intact skin probably occurs only with HF (see below). When present as a soluble salt, fluoride is readily absorbed from the alimentary tract, but even 2% solutions of NaF kill mucosal cells and may result in severe corrosive gastroenteritis. In part this corrosiveness is due to a toxic action on mucosal capillaries and is seen even after parenteral administration (Sollmann, 1957). Most of the mucosal erosion, however, occurs in the stomach, where gastric acid converts ionic fluoride to hydrofluoric acid (HF). Because this HF is largely un-ionized ($pK_a = 3.8$), it rapidly penetrates mucous membranes. A common result is corrosive gastritis with gastric hemorrhages. Because sodium fluosilicate (silicofluoride) releases F^- quickly only in alkaline media, the stomach is sometimes (but not always) spared a corrosive injury in fluosilicate poisoning (*e.g.*, Yolken *et al.*, 1976). Because ingested NaF is converted to HF in the stomach, the vomitus is generally irritating and sometimes corrosive; it can injure the esophagus, mouth, lips and eyes. In one case the vomitus was shown to be capable of etching glass (Peters, 1948). Emesis and esophageal ulceration were undoubtedly responsible for the rare esophageal stricture that developed a few days after the ingestion of sodium fluoride (Abukurah *et al.*, 1972).

Fluoride is a "general protoplasmic poison," but it is not possible yet to describe in detail the mechanisms by which it produces death (Hodge and Smith, 1965). At least four major functional derangements are recognized: (1) enzyme inhibition, (2) hypocalcemia, (3) cardiovascular collapse and (4) specific organ damage. Inhibition of one or more of the enzymes controlling cellular respiration and glycolysis may result in critical biochemical defects (Hodge and Smith, 1965). For example, hyperkalemia, which has been recognized recently in poisoned humans and dogs (Baltazar *et al.*, 1980; Yolken *et al.*, 1976), is probably due to a failure of cell metabolism to provide enough ATP to sustain the normally high K^+ gradient between cells and extracellular fluids. Another example may be metabolic acidosis, which has been observed in fluoride poisoning but not adequately studied (Abukurah *et al.*, 1972; Simpson *et al.*, 1980; Whitford *et al.*, 1979; Yolken *et al.*, 1976). Inhibition of cholinesterase activity noted *in vitro*, however, probably plays no role in fluoride poisoning (Dybing and Loe, 1956).

Fluoride poisoning can lead to severe hypocalcemia in which reductions occur in the plasma levels of both total calcium and ionic calcium. Hypomagnesemia has also been recognized (Abukurah *et al.*, 1972; Simpson *et al.*, 1980; Tepperman, 1980). Whatever the mechanism of the hypocalcemia (see below), its most spectacular consequence is tetany, *i.e.*, painful, involuntary muscle contractions, initially of the distal extremities (carpopedal spasm, twitching of limb muscles, laryngospasm, cardiospasm, etc.). Tetany is never the first sign in acute fluoride poisoning; it may not appear for several hours and sometimes not at all, in spite of severe hypocalcemia (Tepperman, 1980). In hypocalcemic tetany the plasma (or serum) calcium level is usually 7 mg./dl. or less; latent tetany can often be demonstrated at somewhat higher levels. Calcium levels as low as 2.2 and 2.6 mg./dl. have been measured in sera obtained from fluoride victims *in extremis* (Tepperman, 1980; Rabinowitch, 1945).

Tetany is generally regarded as due to spontaneous discharges arising in the distal axons of motor neurones. An additional mechanism may operate in fluoride poisoning. Thus fluoride in concentrations as low as 0.5 mmol. (which have been found in many human victims of fluoride poisoning) facilitates neuromuscular transmission at vertebrate motor end plates, apparently by increasing the sensitivity of cholinergic receptors to acetylcholine; allegedly this effect is not due to hypocalcemia or to the inhibition of cholinesterase (Koketsu and Gerard, 1956). Whether or not tetany is ever a primary cause of death in fluoride poisoning is unclear. Victims of massive doses often die of cardiovascular derangments without signs of overt tetany.

Cardiovascular collapse is probably the commonest proximal cause of death in acute fluoride poisoning (Geiger, 1936; Lidbeck *et al.*, 1943; Maletz, 1935; Roholm, 1937; Sharkey and Simpson, 1933). Hypotension and circulatory shock arise from a combination of many factors: fluid and electrolyte losses due to vomiting and diarrhea, intragastric bleeding due to intense corrosive gastritis, central vasomotor depression and perhaps direct depression of vascular smooth muscle (Caruso and Hodge, 1965; Leone *et al.*, 1956). Sinus tachycardia is undoubtedly the commonest cardiac finding in fluoride poisoning, but serious cardiac arrhythmias also occur frequently. In older clinical reports (Roholm, 1937), these arrhythmias were not well characterized;

case histories often described episodes such as sudden onset of shortness of breath, loss of pulse and death (*e.g.*, Maletz, 1935). In modern times electrocardiograms have demonstrated that these episodes are periods of transient ventricular fibrillation (Abukurah *et al.*, 1972; Baltazar *et al.*, 1980; Simpson *et al.*, 1980), sometimes preceded by ventricular tachycardia (Yolken *et al.*, 1976). Ventricular fibrillation in fluoride poisoning appears to be responsive to resuscitative measures such as intravenous lidocaine and cardioversion, but multiple recurrences are the rule. Whereas some of these victims could not be saved (Baltazar *et al.*, 1980; Simpson *et al.*, 1980), remarkable recoveries have been reported (Abukurah *et al.*, 1972; Yolken *et al.*, 1976).

Many conditions are acknowledged to promote abnormal mechanisms of the heart beat; in fluoride poisoning predisposing factors include hypotension (with consequent myocardial hypoxia), acidosis, hypocalcemia, hypomagnesemia and hyperkalemia, all of which have been noted above. The relative importance of these factors has not been assessed, but it is noteworthy that among four recent fluoride victims who developed ventricular fibrillation, two did not have prefibrillatory hypotension of significance (Baltazar *et al.*, 1980; Yolken *et al.*, 1976), two had normal plasma potassium levels (Abukurah *et al.*, 1972; Simpson *et al.*, 1980), and one had only mild acidosis (Baltazar *et al.*, 1980). All four patients had demonstrated hypocalcemia or clinical signs thereof, but at least in one of them (Baltazar *et al.*, 1980), the prefibrillatory ECG showed a much more prominent hyperkalemic effect (peaked T waves) than hypocalcemic effect (prolonged QT). In dogs infused continuously for 1 hour with fluoride solutions, no ECG evidence of hypocalcemia appeared until 85% of an average lethal dose was injected; no cardiac signs of hypocalcemia were detected in those dogs who died after receiving only 70% of the average dose (Leone *et al.*, 1956). Intense, acute hypocalcemia in rats (produced by sodium polyphosphate infusions) led to prompt bradycardia, AV blockade and cardiac arrest but not ventricular fibrillation (Gosselin *et al.*, 1953). Furthermore, ventricular fibrillation has not been described in OXALATE poisoning (p. III-326), in which hypocalcemia also occurs. Thus the exact cause of ventricular arrhythmias in fluoride poisoning remains uncertain.

In addition to cardiovascular, neuromuscular and gastrointestinal derangements, acute fluoride poisoning causes major adverse effects on two other organ systems, the brain and the kidneys. The more critical dysfunctions are those of the brain. Toxic signs occasionally include headache, excessive salivation, nystagmus and dilated pupils. Transient convulsions have been described (Roholm, 1937), but lethargy, stupor and coma are far more common, and death is often ascribed to respiratory failure, presumably of central origin (*e.g.*, Rabinowitch, 1945). Whatever the causes of these brain derangements, it is noteworthy that coma and respiratory arrest may develop in the presence of a normal blood pressure (Yolken *et al.*, 1976). Apparently the central neural effects of fluoride are not solely secondary to an inadequate cerebral circulation.

The same type of inference can be made about the renal disorders. Because profound shock from any cause can damage the kidneys irreversibly, it is not surprising that some victims of fluoride poisoning are anuric at death (*e.g.*, Simpson *et al.*, 1980). Mild renal pathology (acute congestion and cloudy swelling of tubular cells) has been described in human fatalities (Carr, 1936; Geiger, 1936), as well as degenerative tubular lesions in dosed animals (Hodge and Smith, 1965). Death due to acute renal failure, however, appears to be unknown in humans or animals acutely poisoned with fluoride (Taylor *et al.*, 1961a). Chronic exposure does not result in significantly more renal injury (Pindborg, 1957; Taylor *et al.*, 1961b). Mild and completely reversible renal effects, however, appear to be common in acute fluoride poisoning, even in patients who are not hypotensive. For example, two normotensive victims of ingested fluoride were noted to have proteinuria (described as 2+) on hospital admission (Abukurah *et al.*, 1972; Yolken *et al.*, 1976). Proteinuria has also been reported in acutely dosed rats (Taylor *et al.*, 1961a). In a subacute exposure due to elevated fluoride levels in drinking water, polyuria and presumably secondary polydipsia have been reported once in humans. In rats infused with sodium fluoride, polyuria can be induced without changes in arterial blood pressure or glomerular filtration rate; because it is vasopressin-resistant, the condition resembles nephrogenic diabetes insipidus (Rush and Willis, 1982). This tubular concentrating defect may persist for a few days, but recovery is eventually complete (Whitford and Stringer, 1978).

Hypocalcemia has been suggested as the mechanism underlying many diverse signs and symptoms in fluoride poisoning, particularly if death is delayed. Some of these suggestions, however, are not tenable. For example, terminal petechial hemorrhages in the skin and internal organs have been attributed to a clotting defect resulting from depression of plasma levels of ionized calcium (Carr, 1936). As with OXALATE (p. III-174), however, it appears unlikely that plasma calcium levels can be depressed sufficiently to impair clotting without inducing fatal tetany or cardiac arrest. Depressions of plasma ionized calcium has been suggested as

the cause of cardiac disturbances, which are prominent *in extremis* (Leone *et al.*, 1956; Lu *et al.*, 1965). At least in some species, however, fluoride interferes with both the contractile power of the heart and the mechanism of beat in a way that cannot be ascribed to hypocalcemia (Sollmann, 1957); as noted above, an associated hyperkalemia may be more critical to cardiac function than the hypocalcemia of fluoride poisoning. Finally, it is unlikely that calcium binding plays a role in manifestations of central nervous system poisoning such as depression, occasional epileptiform convulsions and respiratory failure.

The usual explanation of the hypocalcemia in fluoride poisoning is that F^- precipitates calcium *in vivo* as highly insoluble CaF_2, which is thought to accumulate promptly in bone. Because magnesium fluoride also has a low water solubility (although 5 times greater than that of CaF_2), hypomagnesemia may arise by a similar mechanism (Hodge and Smith, 1965; Simpson *et al.*, 1980). To restore the plasma calcium level to normal, however, in a man who had ingested a large dose of sodium fluoride, calcium salts had to be injected in amounts far in excess of the molar amount of fluoride that disappeared from the plasma and extracellular fluid. This observation prompted Simpson *et al.* (1980) to suggest the hypothesis that the hypocalcemia of fluoride poisoning may arise from the conversion of plasma hydroxyapatite to fluorapatite and its subsequent deposition in bone. That an exchange of fluoride and hydroxyl ions occurs in bone apatite has long been known (Hodge and Smith, 1965). According to the new hypothesis, fluoride-induced hypocalcemia is due not to the precipitation of CaF_2 but to the deposition in bone crystals of newly formed fluorapatite that serves as a nucleation catalyst for further calcification. The data and hypothesis, however, do not preclude the precipitation of some calcium as CaF_2 in renal tubular fluid, urine and perhaps other sites. That homeostatic mechanisms to correct hypocalcemia are operative in fluoride poisoning (Simpson *et al.*, 1980) is evidenced by high plasma levels of parathormone (from the parathyroid glands) and of alkaline phosphatase (presumably from bone).

Whatever the mechanism, fluoride almost certainly does accumulate rapidly in bone during acute fluoride poisoning. Though temporary, its large accretion in bone serves to protect vulnerable soft tissues and organs. Most of the sequestered fluoride, however, is eventually released but only slowly. If renal function is not seriously impaired (see above), it is excreted in urine. In this way the body burden of fluoride is safely lowered but only over a long period of time, probably several days or a few weeks. The full pharmacokinetic pattern of fluoride has not been measured, but an early plasma half-life of about 1.4 hours was reported in two fluoride-poisoned patients (Berman *et al.*, 1973; Yolken *et al.*, 1976). This rapid initial clearance represented the combined processes of sequestration in bone, renal excretion and removal by hemodialysis or by peritoneal dialysis. Whereas hemodialysis was thought to have been responsible for 30% of the loss (Berman *et al.*, 1973), peritoneal dialysis (Yolken *et al.*, 1976) was judged to have been ineffective in removing fluoride. The contribution of bone to the removal of fluoride is presumably reflected in a plasma fluoride half-life of 8 to 10 hours measured in a toxic, anuric patient who was not dialyzed (Simpson *et al.*, 1980).

The renal clearance of fluoride is much higher than that of chloride or bromide. Although generally less than that of inulin or creatinine (Waterhouse *et al.*, 1980), occasional fluoride clearances appear to exceed the glomerular filtration rate (*e.g.*, Yolken *et al.*, 1976), suggesting that F^- is not only filtered at the glomerulus but that it may also be secreted into the tubular fluid. Tubular resorption, however, is almost always the dominant process. By reducing water and solute resorption, osmotic and high-ceiling diuretics can enhance the renal clearance of fluoride (Abukurah *et al.*, 1972). More impressive elevations in the urinary excretory rate, however, have been produced by intravenous infusions of sodium bicarbonate. In anesthetized rats infused continuously with sodium fluoride to death, treatment with isotonic sodium bicarbonate led to lower plasma fluoride levels and to higher renal clearances than in rats treated with isotonic saline (Whitford *et al.*, 1979). Similarly rats made alkalotic before NaF infusions excreted fluoride faster than did acidotic rats; in the former the fluoride clearance was about half that of inulin and in the latter one-quarter (or less) that of inulin (Reynolds *et al.*, 1978). In the strong pH-dependence of its excretory rate, fluoride is similar to SALICYLATE (p. III-368); both acids have similar pK_a values (3.8 and 3.5, respectively). Whether fluoride excretion in man is as pH dependent as in the rat needs to be studied.

In addition to the advantage gained by alkalinizing the urine, the deliberate induction of a systemic metabolic alkalosis may be protective to victims of fluoride poisoning in other ways. When groups of anesthetized, nephrectomized rats were infused continuously with sodium fluoride, the alkalotic group survived longer, tolerated higher fluoride doses and died with higher plasma fluoride levels than did the acidotic group (Reynolds *et al.*, 1978). When intact rats suffering from fluoride poisoning were treated with infusions of isotonic NaCl or isotonic $NaHCO_3$, the rats receiving the bicarbonate (with or without concomitant acetazolamide)

showed significantly higher tolerance to the lethal action of fluoride. In all cases the alkalotic group had higher terminal fluoride levels in the plasma and lower tissue-to-plasma fluoride concentration ratios in heart but not in brain (Reynolds *et al.*, 1978; Whitford *et al.*, 1979). These data support the hypothesis that a systemic bicarbonate alkalosis enhances the pH gradient between extracellular fluid and the more acidic intracellular fluid and that consequently it lowers the intracellular fluoride concentration at any given extracellular F^- level, in accord with the principles of non-ionic diffusion. Thus an induced alkalosis may spare fluoride-sensitive intracellular mechanisms. Whether or not a metabolic alkalosis can be produced safely in a person with acute fluoride poisoning remains to be explored, but the rodent studies serve to emphasize that any metabolic or respiratory acidosis should be vigorously corrected.

Besides the treatment of acidosis and dehydration and the use of conventional measures to counteract overt or impending shock, the major challenge to the therapist is to administer calcium salts as quickly as possible (Abukurah *et al.*, 1972; Peters, 1948). As described above, parenteral injections of calcium serve both to correct hypocalcemia and to accelerate the deposition of fluoride into bone. Because the administration of calcium chloride may lead to a chloride acidosis, calcium gluconate is far preferable. Conventional doses of calcium salts are listed in Section IV (p. IV-74), but much larger quantities may be required in acute fluoride poisoning, sometimes as much as 110 mmol. calcium in adults, which is equivalent to 500 ml. of 10% calcium gluconate infused intravenously over a period of a few hours (Abukurah *et al.*, 1972; Simpson *et al.*, 1980). Plasma calcium analyses are important to avoid under- or overtreatment, but in an emergency the prolonged QT interval of the ECG may be used as a sign that more calcium is required. Although its exact contribution to the derangements of fluoride poisoning is unknown, hypomagnesemia should also be corrected by the injection of $MgSO_4$ (see p. IV-75).

If the patient is anuric and remains anuric or oliguric after the arterial blood pressure is restored to near normal levels, hemodialysis may be useful to remove toxic amounts of fluoride (Berman *et al.*, 1973). Probably peritoneal dialysis is also effective (see p. IV-56), in spite of the negative experience of Yolken *et al.*, (1976), who may have grossly underestimated the amount of fluoride removed (see Simpson *et al.*, 1980). Because of the many reported cases of ventricular arrhythmias, all acutely ill victims of fluoride poisoning should be subjected to continuous cardiac monitoring, and all available defibrillatory equipment and antifibrillatory drug solutions (*e.g.*, lidocaine) should be mobilized for possibly emergency use.

Toxicology of hydrofluoric acid: The ingestion of an estimated 1.5 gm. of hydrofluoric acid produced sudden death without gross pathologic damage (Curry, 1962). On the other hand, the repeated ingestion of small amounts of HF (Calenoff, 1962) has resulted in moderately advanced fluoride osteosclerosis in man. Thus, HF is capable of inducing the systemic manifestations of both acute and chronic fluoride poisoning. It possesses an additional hazard, however, because of its intense corrosivity.

Respiratory exposure to high concentrations of hydrofluoric acid fumes characteristically results in ulcerative tracheobronchitis and hemorrhagic pulmonary edema in man and animals (Mayer and Guelich, 1963; Rosenholtz et al., 1963). This local reaction is equivalent to that caused by gaseous hydrogen chloride or sulfur dioxide (Machle et al., 1934). For the management of the adult respiratory distress syndrome, see pp. IV-14–16. Even though pulmonary involvement may dominate the clinical picture and pathologic findings, systemic fluoride poisoning may still be the cause of death.

Similarly, HF can be absorbed percutaneously to produce severe systemic poisoning. Such was the case in one skin burn due to 5 gm. of pure anhydrous liquid HF (chilled and under pressure until the vessel burst); about 2.5% of the body surface area was estimated to have been contaminated (Burke et al., 1973). In a remarkably similar episode, the patient experienced severe hypocalcemia and multiple attacks of ventricular fibrillation but no pulmonary edema; he died in asystole after 9.5 hours (Tepperman, 1980). Blood fluoride levels in such patients are sometimes comparable to those found in persons dying after ingestion of neutral salts (Greendyke and Hodge, 1964).

Skin contact with anhydrous HF and solutions above 30% produces immediate pain, but reactions to more dilute solutions may be delayed for many hours. The pain is said to be excruciating and unusually persistent. Healing is delayed, and necrotic changes may continue to occur beneath a layer of tough coagulated skin to produce deep penetrating ulcers (Jones, 1939; Klauder et al., 1955). Because of the severity of hydrofluoric acid burns, considerable experimental work has been directed at more effective methods of management. Sodium bicarbonate washes have been recommended as a first aid measure (Jones, 1939), but boric acid solutions are probably superior. The local infiltration of calcium gluconate to bind fluoride as a less soluble complex is said to relieve pain and promote healing (Blunt, 1964; Paley and Siefter, 1941), but in an experimental study in rats, HF dermal burns penetrated less and healed faster when 10% magnesium acetate or sulfate was substituted for 10% calcium gluconate as the infiltrating solution (Harris et al., 1981). This use of magnesium solutions deserves a clinical trial in man. Magnesium oxide pastes as recommended below are of demonstrated value, and soaking in a 0.2% solution of Hyamine 1622 in iced alcohol or water has been recommended (Reinhardt et al., 1966). Boric acid forms complexes with fluoride and may be useful in treating local lesions (Marcovitch and Stanley, 1942).

Symptomatology:

A. Ingestion of soluble fluoride salts (*e.g.*, NaF).

   1. Salty or soapy taste, salivation, nausea. Repeated small doses (as in drinking water) may produce no other symptoms, but polyuria and polydipsia have also been reported.

   2. Large doses lead promptly to burning or crampy abdominal pain, intense vomiting and diarrhea, often with hematemesis and melena. Dehydration and thirst.

   3. Muscle weakness, tremors, and rarely transient epileptiform convulsions, preceded or followed by progressive central nervous depression (lethargy, coma and respiratory arrest, even in the absence of circulatory failure).

   4. Shock characterized by pallor, weak and thready pulse (sometimes irregular), shallow unlabored respiration, weak heart sounds, wet cold skin, cyanosis, anuria, dilated pupils, followed almost invariably by death in 2 to 4 hours.

   5. Even in the absence of shock, arrhythmias may occur, especially multiple episodes of ventricular fibrillation leading eventually to cardiac arrest.

   6. If the victim survives a few hours, paralysis of the muscles of deglutition, carpopedal spasm, and painful spasms of the extremities.

   7. Occasionally localized or generalized urticaria.

   8. The above signs and symptoms are related to a variety of metabolic disorders that may occur in acute fluoride poisoning, including hypocalcemia (which may be the only invariable finding), hypomagnesemia, metabolic and/or respiratory acidosis and sometimes hyperkalemia.

B. Local actions of HF vapor or aqueous solutions.

   1. Superficial or deep burns of the skin and mucous membranes of the diges-

tive and/or respiratory tracts. Necrotic ulcers are painful and heal slowly. Percutaneous absorption may lead to systemic fluoride poisoning; see A above.

2. For symptoms (and treatment) after the inhalation of HF or F_2, see pp. IV-14–16.

Treatment:

A. Ingestion of soluble fluoride salts (*e.g.*, NaF).

1. Obtain a blood specimen for analysis (see below) and start an intravenous infusion of glucose in isotonic saline.

2. Inject intravenously 30 ml. of 10% calcium gluconate solution slowly. Repeat in 10 to 20 minutes and/or whenever latent or overt tetany appears.

3. Unless vomiting has been extensive, perform gentle gastric lavage with lime water or a 1% solution of calcium chloride or milk. Then give orally several ounces of lime water at frequent intervals if retained, or aluminum hydroxide gels. Such gels are particularly useful because they are demulcents, antacids and effective binders of fluoride ions.

4. Institute continuous cardiac monitoring and prepare for possible endotracheal intubation (p. IV-4), assisted ventilation (p. IV-7), DC cardioversion (p. IV-30), and ventricular pacing (p. IV-30).

5. Treat shock vigorously by the administration of saline, plasma, or whole blood (p. IV-17). Give oxygen as needed. Keep the patient warm.

6. Correct dehydration and institute forced alkaline diuresis by infusing sodium bicarbonate (p. IV-72), unless the patient is anuric or severely oliguric. The goal is to create a brisk flow of urine with a pH of 7 or higher (preferably 7.5). Discontinue fluids and electrolytes (except calcium) if anuria develops (p. IV-53).

7. If tetany or latent tetany appears (p. IV-74), start an intravenous infusion of 10% calcium gluconate at a rate of 1 to 3 ml./minute, until the plasma calcium level returns to normal. Prolongation of the QT interval in the ECG indicates the need for more calcium, but hypercalcemia (p. IV-73) should be avoided. Some adult victims of fluoride poisoning have required 500 ml. of 10% calcium gluconate (110 mmol. Ca^{2+}).

8. In addition to hypocalcemia, chemical analyses of plasma (see below) may demonstrate hypomagnesemia (p. IV-75), hyperkalemia (p. IV-72) or a severe metabolic acidosis (p. IV-69). Each of these derangements may have to be corrected, especially the metabolic acidosis.

9. Ventricular tachycardia-fibrillation in fluoride poisoning is frequently responsive to such therapeutic measures as DC cardioversion (p. IV-30) and intravenous lidocaine (p. IV-25), but multiple recurrences have been reported. One patient (Abukurah *et al.*, 1972) required DC countershock 63 times over 12 hours, but he survived. Therefore vigorous resuscitative efforts are appropriate.

10. In an anuric patient extracorporeal hemodialysis (p. IV-55) is an efficient way to remove fluoride. If the patient survives, renal function usually resumes spontaneously before a state of severe azotemia is reached.

B. Treatment of HF burns of skin where HF concentration was 20% or more (Iverson *et al.*, 1971; Reinhardt *et al.*, 1966; Scharnweber, 1969).

1. Wash all exposed areas copiously with cold tap water. Alkaline soap may also be helpful, especially in promoting the wettability of surfaces; a weak borax solution can also achieve the same result.

2. Irrigate exposed eyes with large volumes of water or weak boric acid solution followed by water.

3. Infiltrate exposed area with 10% calcium gluconate. Use a 30-gauge needle and small volumes that do not distend tissues (0.5 ml./cm.²). Relief of pain by infiltration is a useful index to the adequacy of treatment. If the patient cannot tolerate the pain, local anesthesia may be given prior to calcium gluconate. In some cases, topical application of a 2.5% calcium gluconate gel controls pain and makes injections unnecessary (Browne, 1974).

4. If further treatment is to be delayed, soak areas in iced magnesium sulfate solution (25%).

5. Anesthetize area, excise burn eschar and debride it. Do not hesitate to remove fingernails or toenails since HF apparently passes through these structures without visible damage.

6. Anticipate pulmonary edema (p. IV-14).

C. Treatment of HF burns of the skin where HF concentration was less than 20% (Dibbell *et al.*, 1970; Reinhardt *et al.*, 1966).

1. Spray water over affected area. Remove contaminated clothing and accessories.
2. Immerse affected skin area in an ice-cold aqueous or alcoholic (95% ethyl alcohol) solution of Hyamine 1622 or some similar high-molecular weight quaternary ammonium salt such as benzalkonium chloride (Zephiran). Use wet gauze compresses in which ice cubes are wrapped, if the lesion cannot be immersed. Keep this solution away from the eyes. Interrupt the soaking occasionally to avoid cold injury. If this soaking is continued for 1 to 4 hours, local infiltration with calcium gluconate is thought to be unnecessary and undesirable.
3. If blisters form, institute debridement as described above.
4. After soaking, apply a magnesium oxide-petrolatum ointment or a steroid ointment.

Laboratory:

1. Probably the easiest method for measuring the fluoride concentration in body fluids in victims of fluoride poisoning is use of the Orion fluoride-specific electrode. The diffusion method of Taves (*viz.*, Waterhouse *et al.*, 1980) is also useful for estimating inorganic fluoride. Blood fluoride levels in 5 fatal cases ranged from 3.5 to 15.5 mg./L. (Gettler and Ellerbrook, 1939), but at least one patient with an initial serum level of 14 mg./L. survived (Yolken *et al.*, 1976). For data about tissue concentrations, see Hodge and Smith (1965).
2. Chemical analyses of blood plasma (or serum) are essential for detecting and evaluating hypocalcemia, hypomagnesemia, hyperkalemia and metabolic acidosis. Concentration estimates both of total calcium and of ionic calcium (the later by electrometric methods) are desirable.
3. Chemical controls are also essential for the intelligent management of fluid and electrolyte therapy.

References:

Abukurah, A. R.; Moser, A. M., Jr.; Baird, C. L.; Randall, R. E., Jr.; Setter, J. G.; Blanke, R. V. Acute sodium fluoride poisoning. J. A. M. A. *222*:816-817, 1972.

Baltazar, R. F.; Mower, M. M.; Funk, M. Acute fluoride poisoning leading to fatal hyperkalemia. Chest *78*:660-663, 1980.

Bell, R. D. Poisoning by sodium fluoride. Br. Med. J. *1*:886, 1936.

Berman, L.; Taves, D.; Mitra, S.; Newmark, K. Inorganic fluoride poisoning: treatment by hemodialysis. N. Engl. J. Med. *289*:922 1973.

Black, M. M.; Kleiner, I. S.; Bolker, H. The toxicity of sodium fluoride in man. N. Y. State J. Med. *49*:1187-1188, 1949.

Blunt, C. P. Treatment of hydrofluoric acid skin burns by injection with calcium gluconate. Ind. Med. Surg. *33*:869-871, 1964.

Browne, T. D. The treatment of hydrofluoric acid burns. J. Soc. Occup. Med. *24*:80-89, 1974.

Burke, W. J.; Hoegg, V. R.; Phillips, R. E. Systemic fluoride poisoning resulting from a fluoride skin burn. J. Occup. Med. *15*:39-41, 1973.

Calenoff, L. Osteosclerosis from intentional ingestion of hydrofluoric acid. Am. J. Roentgenol. Radium Ther. Nucl. Med. *87*:1112-1115, 1962.

Carr, J. L. Acute fluorine poisoning. Calif. Med. *44*:83-87, 1936.

Caruso, F. S.; Hodge, H. C. The effect of oral doses of sodium fluoride on blood pressure in dogs. J. Dent. Res. *44*:99-101, 1965.

Curry, A. S. Twenty-one uncommon cases of poisoning. Br. Med. J. *1*:687-689, 1962.

Dean, H. T. Chronic endemic fluorosis. J. A. M. A. *107*:1269-1273, 1936.

Deshpande, S. S.; Bester, J. F. Absorption and retention of fluoride from ingested stannous fluoride dentifrice. J. Pharm. Sci. *53*:803-807, 1964.

Dibbell, D. G.; Iverson, R. E.; Jones, W.; Laub, D. R.; Madison, M. S. Hydrofluoric acid burns of the hand. J. Bone Joint Surg. 52A:931-936, 1970.

Duxbury, A. J.; Leach, F. N.; Duxbury, J. T. A review - Acute fluoride toxicity. Br. Dental J. *153*:64-66, 1982.

Dybing, O.; Loe, L. V. Fluoride poisoning and cholinesterases in rats. Acta Pharmacol. Toxicol. *12*:364-368, 1956.

Geiger, J. C. Poisoning due to the ingestion of a mixture of sodium bicarbonate and sodium fluoride. Calif. Med. *44*:81-83, 1936.

Gettler, A. O.; Ellerbrook, L. Toxicology of fluorides. Am. J. Med. Sci. *197*:625-638, 1939.

Gosselin, R. E.; Tidball, C. S.; Megirian, R.; Maynard, E. A.; Downs, W. L.; Hodge, H. C. Metabolic acidosis and hypocalcemia as toxic manifestations of polymeric phosphates. J. Pharmacol. Exp. Ther. *108*:117-127, 1953.

Greendyke, R. M.; Hodge, H. C. Accidental death due to hydrofluoric acid. J. Forensic Sci. *9*:383-390, 1964.

Greenwood, D. A. Fluoride intoxication. Physiol. Rev. *20*:582-616, 1940.

Harris, J. C.; Rumack, B. H.; Bregman, D. J. Comparative efficacy of injectable calcium and magnesium salts in the therapy of hydrofluoric acid burns. Clin. Toxicol. *18*:1027-1032, 1981.

Hennon, D. K.; Stookey, G. K.; Muhler, J. C. Fluoride retention in rats receiving various vitamin-sodium fluoride preparations. J. Pediatr. *64*:272-277, 1964.

Hodge, H. C. Fluoride tablets: Questions and answers. J. Pediatr. *63*:454-458, 1963.

Hodge, H. C.; Smith, F. A. Biological effects of inorganic fluorides. In *Fluorine Chemistry*, Vol. IV. Edited by J. H. Simons. Academic Press, Inc., New York, 1965.

Hodge, H. C.; Smith, F. A. Occupational fluoride exposure. J. Occup. Med. *19*:12-39, 1977.

Hoffman, R.; Mann, J.; Calderone, J.; Trumbull, J.; Burkhart, M. Acute fluoride poisoning in a New Mexico elementary school. Pediatrics *65*:897-900, 1980.

Iverson, R. E.; Laub, D. R.; Madison, M. S. Hydrofluoric acid burns. Plast. Reconstr. Surg. *48*:107-112, 1971.

Jones, A. T. The treatment of hydrofluoric acid burns. J. Ind. Hyg. Toxicol. *21*:205-212, 1939.

Kaltreider, N. L.; Elder, M. J.; Cralley, L. V.; Colwell, M. O. Health survey of aluminum workers with special reference to fluoride exposure. J. Occup. Med. *14*:531-541, 1972.

Kilborn, L. G.; Outerbridge, T. S.; Lei, H. Fluorosis with report of an advanced case. Can. Med. Assoc. J. *62*:135-141, 1950.

Klauder, J. V.; Shelanski, L.; Gabriel, K. Industrial uses of compounds of fluorine and oxalic acid; cutaneous reaction and calcium therapy. Arch. Ind. Health *12*:412-419, 1955.

Koketsu, K.; Gerard, R. W. Effects of sodium fluoride on nerve-muscle transmission. Am. J. Physiol. *186*:278-282, 1956.

Larner, J. Toxicological and metabolic effects of fluorine-containing compounds. Ind. Med. Surg. *19*:535-539, 1950.

Leone, N. C.; Geever, E. F.; Moran, N. C. Acute and subacute toxicity studies of sodium fluoride in animals. Pub. Health Rep. *71*:459-467, 1956.

Lidbeck, W. L.; Hill, I. B.; Beeman, J. A. Acute sodium fluoride poisoning. J. A. M. A. *121*:826-827, 1943.

Linsman, J. F.; McMurray, C. A. Fluoride osteosclerosis from drinking water. Radiology *40*:474-484, 1943.

Lu, F. C.; Grewal, R. S.; Rice, W. B.; Graham, R. C. B.; Allmark, M. G. Acute toxicity of sodium fluoride for rhesus monkeys and other laboratory animals. Acta Pharmacol. Toxicol. *22*:99-106, 1965.

Machle, W.; Thamann, F.; Kitzmiller, K.; Cholak, J. The effects of the inhalation of hydrogen fluoride. I. The response following exposure to high concentrations. J. Ind. Hyg. Toxicol. *16*:129-145, 1934.

Maletz, L. Report of a fatal case of fluoride poisoning. N. Engl. J. Med. *213*:370-372, 1935.

Marcovitch, S.; Stanley, W. W. A study of antidotes for fluorine. J. Pharmacol. Exp. Ther. *74*:235-238, 1942.

Marier, J. R.; Rose, D.; Boulet, M. Accumulation of skeletal fluoride and its implications. Arch. Environ. Health *6*:664-671, 1963.

Mayer, L.; Guelich, J. Hydrogen fluoride (HF) inhalation and burns. Arch. Environ. Health *7*:445-447, 1963.

McClure, F. J. Review of fluorine and its physiological effects. Physiol. Rev. *13*:277-300, 1933.

Paley, A.; Seifter, J. Treatment of experimental hydrofluoric acid corrosion. Proc. Soc. Exp. Biol. Med. *46*:190-192, 1941.

Peters, J. H. Therapy of acute fluoride poisoning. Am. J. Med. Sci. *216*:278-285, 1948.

Pindborg, J. J. The effect of .05 per cent dietary sodium fluoride on the rat kidney. Acta Pharmacol. Toxicol. *13*:36-45, 1957.

Rabinowitch, I. M. Acute fluoride poisoning. Can. Med. Assoc. J. *52*:345-349, 1945.

Reinhardt, C. F.; Hume, W. G.; Linch, A. L.; Wetherhold, J. M. Hydrofluoric acid burn treatment. Am. Ind. Hyg. Assoc. J. *27*:166-171, 1966.

Reynolds, K. E.; Whitford, G. M.; Pashley, D. H. Acute fluoride toxicity: the influence of acid-base status. Toxicol. Appl. Pharmacol. *45*:415-427, 1978.

Roholm, K. *Fluorine Intoxication.* H. K. Lewis, London, 1937.

Rosenholtz, M. J.; Carson, T. R.; Weeks, M. H.; Wilinski, F.; Ford, D. F. Oberst, F. W. A toxicopathologic study in animals after brief single exposures to hydrogen fluoride. Am. Ind. Hyg. Assoc. J. *24*:253-261, 1963.

Rosenzweig, K. A.; Abkewitz, I. Prevalence of endemic fluorosis in Israel at medium fluoride concentrations. Pub. Health Rep. *78*:77-80, 1963.

Rush, G. F.; Willis, L. R. Renal tubular effects of sodium fluoride. J. Pharmacol. Exp. Ther. *223*:275-279, 1982.

Sauerbrunn, B. J. L.; Ryan, C. M.; Shaw, J. F. Chronic fluoride intoxication with fluorotic radiculomyelopathy. Ann. Intern. Med. *63*:1074-1078, 1965.

Scharnweber, H. C. Treatment of hydrofluoric acid burns of the skin by immediate surgical excision. Ind. Med. Surg. *38*:31-32, 1969.

Segreto, V. A.; Yeary, R. A.; Brooks, R.; Harns, N. O. Toxicity study of stannous fluoride in Swiss strain mice. J. Dent. Res. *40*:623, 1961.

Sharkey, T. P.; Simpson, W. M. Accidental sodium fluoride poisoning, report of eight cases, with one fatality. J. A. M. A. *100*:97-100, 1933.

Simpson, E.; Rao, L. G. S.; Evans, R. M.; Wilkie, W.; Rodger, J. C.; Lakhani, A. Calcium metabolism in a fatal case of sodium fluoride poisoning. Ann. Clin. Biochem. *17*:10-14, 1980.

Singh, A.; Jolly, S. S. Endemic fluorosis. Q. J. Med. *30*:357-372, 1961.

Smith, F. A.; Downs, W. L.; Hodge, H. C.; Maynard, E. A. Screening of fluorine-containing compounds for acute toxicity. Toxicol. Appl. Pharmacol. *2*:54-58, 1960a.

Sollmann, T. *A Manual of Pharmacology.* 8th Ed., W. B. Saunders Co., Philadelphia, 1957.

Taylor, J. M.; Gardner, D. E.; Scott, J. K.; Maynard, E. A.; Downs, W. L. Smith, F. A.; Hodge, H. C. Toxic effects of fluoride on the rat kidney. II. Chronic effects. Toxicol. Appl. Pharmacol. *3*:290-314, 1961b.

Taylor, J. M.; Scott, J. K.; Maynard, E. A.; Smith, F. A.; Hodge, H. C. Toxic effects of fluoride on the rat kidney. I. Acute injury from single large doses. Toxicol. Appl. Pharmacol. *3*:278-289, 1961a.

Tepperman, P. B. Fatality due to acute systemic fluoride poisoning following a hydrofluoric acid skin burn. J. Occup. Med. *22*:691-692, 1980.

Vogt, R. L.; Witherell, L.; LaRue, D.; Klaucke, D. N. Acute fluoride poisoning associated with an on-site fluoridator in a Vermont elementary school. Am. J. Pub. Health *72*:1168-1169, 1982.

Waterhouse, C.; Taves, D.; Munzer, A. Serum inorganic fluoride: changes related to previous fluoride intake, renal function and bone resorption. Clin. Sci. *58*:145-152, 1980.

Whitford, G. M.; Stringer, G. I. Duration of the fluoride-induced urinary concentrating defect in rats. Proc. Soc. Exp. Biol. Med. *157*:44-49, 1978.

Whitford, G. M.; Reynolds, K. E.; Pashley, D. H. Acute fluoride toxicity: Influence of metabolic alkalosis. Toxicol. Appl. Pharmacol. *50*:31-39, 1979.

Yolken, R.; Kinecny, D.; McCarthy, P. Acute fluoride poisoning. Pediatrics *58*:90-93, 1976.

Zipkin, I.; Likins, R. C. Absorption of various fluorine compounds from the gastrointestinal tract of the rat. Am. J. Physiol. *191*:549-550, 1957.

FLUOROACETATE

Sodium fluoroacetate or Compound 1080 is a synthetic, water-soluble, nonvolatile salt, with a faint odor like vinegar; it is usually mixed with a black dye. As a rodenticide, it has no equal in terms of potency, stability, and acceptability in rodent baits and drinking water (Dieke and Richter, 1946b). However, because of its very high toxicity for birds and mammals, including man and domestic animals, the use of this substance has been limited by law to licensed pest control operators.

Fluoroacetate is also a constituent of some poisonous plants, notably *Acacia georginae*, a perennial shrub of Australia that has poisoned cattle and sheep (Oelrichs and McEwan, 1962). The same is true of at least two species of *Dichapetalum* in South and West Africa (Vickery and Vickery, 1972). Domestic animals such as cats and dogs may be poisoned by eating rodents and birds killed by fluoroacetate poisoned bait.

Fluoroacetamide and certain derivatives of 2-fluoroethanol are also potent rodenticides and insecticides and are toxic to mammals presumably because of metabolic oxidation to fluoroacetate. Indeed, indirect evidence indicates that a wide variety of compounds of the general formula $F(CH_2)_n Z$ may be metabolized to fluoroacetate if Z can be removed by metabolism and if n is an even number. A molecule with an ω-fluorine on an unbranched carbon chain should always be suspected as a potential metabolic source of fluoroacetate (Pattison, 1959).

Toxicology: The very high acute toxicity of sodium fluoroacetate constitutes a real hazard, and at least 16 human fatalities were reported by 1959 (Pattison, 1959). As little as 0.1 mg./kg. has proved lethal for dogs and cats (Chenoweth, 1949). Estimates of the mean lethal dose in man range from 2 to 10 mg./kg.; 5 mg./kg. is probably the best single value (Gajdusek and Luther, 1950; Harrisson *et al.*, 1952a and b).

In experimental studies the lethal dose is essentially the same by all routes of administration (Spector, 1955). Ingestion is certainly the most likely mode of poisoning, but there is one report of a near-fatal intoxication in which the inhalation of sodium fluoroacetate powder may have played a major role. The author of this communication was also the victim (Williams, 1948). The compound appears to be absorbed promptly from the alimentary tract, but initial symptoms are commonly delayed for one or several hours (Pattison, 1959). Absorption does not occur through intact skin.

Fluoroacetate is a delayed convulsant. The fluoroacetate ion is not poisonous itself but is converted to fluorocitric acid, which blocks the tricarboxylic acid cycle, an essential mechanism of energy production in mammalian cells (Clark and Riker, 1950; Farah *et al.*, 1950; Furchgott, 1950). This blockade is due to inhibition of the enzyme aconitase, so that citrate cannot be converted to isocitrate. Toxic effects do not appear immediately; time is required for the "lethal synthesis" of fluorocitrate (Liebecq and Peters, 1949; Peters *et al.*, 1953; Peters, 1957). This metabolic lesion manifests itself principally in disturbed activities of the central nervous system and of the heart. Poisoned rats show high concentrations of fluoroacetate in the heart and brain with comparatively low concentrations in the liver (Hagan *et al.*, 1950).

Dogs die of convulsions or of subsequent respiratory paralysis, but in man, monkeys, horses (Frick and Boebel, 1946) and rabbits, central nervous excitation is usually incidental, and the dangerous and fatal complication is ventricular fibrillation (Brockmann *et al.*; 1955; Chenoweth, 1949). After successful resuscitation from cardiac arrest, a poisoned child was left with severe neurologic impairment (McTaggart, 1970). Convulsions, however, may be the only significant sign of poisoning. In a nonfatally poisoned infant only mild emesis and sinus tachycardia preceded four brief episodes of seizure activity over a 12-hour period that began 20 hours after ingestion; recovery was uneventful thereafter (Reigart *et*

al., 1975). An 18-month-old girl with repeated convulsions died in coma 96 hours after ingesting an estimated 23 mg./kg. fluoroacetamide (WHO Information Circular No. 11, 1963, as cited by Hayes (1982)).

Chronic poisoning with sodium fluoroacetate is improbable, but renal changes resembling nephrosis have occurred in rats given either acutely lethal or repeated sublethal injections of fluorocitrate (Cater and Peters, 1961). In the only alleged case of chronic human poisoning, a rabbit exterminator in New Zealand was exposed repeatedly during preparation of fluoroacetate bait over a period of 10 years. He presented with severe and progressive lesions of the renal tubular epithelium and with milder hepatic, neurologic and thyroid dysfunctions (Parkin *et al.*, 1977).

Except for its conversion to fluorocitrate, the metabolism of fluoroacetate is not known. A liver defluorinating enzyme system has been described in rats; it is stimulated *in vitro* by glutathione. The observation that prior depletion of liver glutathione in rats increases their susceptibility to death by fluoroacetate suggests that defluorination is an important detoxication pathway *in vivo* (Kostyniak, 1979).

In experimental poisonings in monkeys, parenteral monoacetin (glyceryl monoacetate) has proved to be an effective antidote. It appears to serve as an acetate donor to block fluoroacetate metabolism in a competitive manner (Chenoweth *et al.*, 1951). Although perhaps less well documented experimentally, acetamide or ethyl alcohol in approximately the same doses as monoacetin may have value in fluoroacetate poisonings (Gitter, 1956; Hutchens *et al.*, 1949). In rats the LD_{50} of 2-fluoroethanol was increased 20-fold by ethanol treatment, whereas that for 2-chloroethanol was increased about 4-fold. Monkeys were also protected (Peterson *et al.*, 1968). These antidotes have had no clinical trial, as far as we know.

Some early observations suggested that other 2-halogenated acetates had pharmacological actions similar to but weaker than 2-fluoroacetate (Clark and Riker, 1950; Farah *et al.*, 1950). The intraperitoneal LD_{50} values in mice of iodo-, bromo-, and chloro-acetates are 45, 85 and 270 mg./kg., respectively. In rats the subcutaneous LD_{50} values of fluoro-, iodo-, and chloro-acetates are 5, 60, and 108 mg./kg., respectively (Hayes *et al.*, 1973). Thus, all are appreciably toxic, but even the iodo derivative is less toxic than fluoroacetate (Le Poidevin, 1965). Unlike fluoroacetate some of these compounds have inhibitory effects on glycolysis. Although their toxic mechanisms are not well understood, they are sulfhydryl acetylating agents, whereas fluoroacetate is not (Pattison, 1959).

Symptomatology:

1. Prompt epigastric distress and vomiting in one reported case. (Vomiting and defecation are frequent in poisoned dogs.)
2. Apprehension, auditory hallucinations, nystagmus, tingling sensation of nose, facial twitching, numbness of face. These and other central nervous effects appear gradually after a latency of several hours.
3. Central nervous excitation, progressing to epileptiform convulsions.
4. Severe central nervous depression between and subsequent to the convulsive episodes, but death is seldom due to respiratory failure in humans poisoned with fluoroacetate.
5. Disturbances in the mechanism of the heart beat usually appear only after the convulsive phase.
6. Pulsus alternans, long sequences of ectopic beats (often multifocal), and ventricular tachycardia may disintegrate into ventricular fibrillation and death.

Treatment:

1. Induce vomiting immediately if possible.
2. Gastric lavage with tap water unless convulsions (or imminent convulsions) make this impractical.
3. Instill into the stomach sodium or magnesium sulfate in water (15 to 30 gm.).
4. Although the clinical efficacy of monoacetin (glyceral monoacetate) is not established, it probably should be administered if available. The recommended dose is 0.5 ml./kg. of undiluted fluid intramuscularly every half hour for several hours and then at a reduced level for at least 12 hours. In the same dose monoacetin may also be given intravenously after dilution with 5 parts of sterile isotonic saline. No preparation of monoacetin is known to be available on the pharmaceutical market. The usual commercial fluid has large amounts of free glycerine (due to hydrolysis favored by heat and exposure to sunlight), and the assay is seldom better than 70%. The exigency of an overt poisoning, however, probably warrants the use of even nonsterile commercial material. Irrespective of impurities, injections may be expected to produce some sedation and vasodilatation. The site of intramuscular injection must be varied because of local pain and edema. In the event that parenteral administration is not feasible, the patient may drink a mixture of 100 ml. of monoacetin in 500 ml. of water. Repeat after 1 hour.
5. If monoacetin is not available, acetamide or ethyl alcohol may be given in the same doses.
6. A short-acting barbiturate drug or diazepam may be tried in the control of convulsions (pp. IV-35–39).
7. Oxygen therapy and artificial ventilation, as required (pp. IV-12 and 7–12).
8. It is doubtful that digitalis is ever warranted. Parenteral procainamide or quinidine may be given a therapeutic trial (p. IV-25), but in experimental poisonings these drugs have proved much less successful than monoacetin in controlling cardiac arrhythmias.
9. If possible, monitor the electrocardiogram continuously and secure chest electrodes for external electrical defibrillation if it becomes necessary. See pp. IV-26–31.

Laboratory:

1. The cardiac status should be monitored repeatedly by an electrocardiogram. Any pattern of alteration in the mechanical or electrical heart beat indicates a need for more monoacetin.
2. Hyperglycemia and glycosuria have been noted in some experimental studies.
3. The significance of black, tarry blood in poisoned animals needs explanation (*e.g.*, Frick and Boebel, 1946).
4. Data on serum calcium and citrate levels would be of interest in clinical and experimental poisonings.

References:

Brockmann, J. L.; McDowell, A. V.; Leeds, W. G. Fatal poisoning with sodium fluoroacetate. J. A. M. A. *159*:1529-1532, 1955.

Cater, D. B.; Peters, R. A. The occurrence of renal changes resembling nephrosis in rats poisoned with fluorocitrate. Br. J. Exp. Pathol. *42*:278-289, 1961.

Chenoweth, M. B. Monofluoroacetic acid and related compounds. Pharmacol. Rev. *1*:383-424, 1949.

Chenoweth, M. B.; Kandel, A.; Johnson, L. B.; Bennett, D. R. Factors influencing fluoroacetate poisoning. Practical treatment with glycerol monoacetate. J. Pharmacol. Exp. Ther. *102*:31-49, 1951.

Clark, D. A.; Riker, W. F., Jr. The effect of fluoroacetate on the sartorius muscle of the frog. J. Pharmacol. Exp. Ther. *99*:118-131, 1950.

Dieke, S. H.; Richter, C. P. Comparative assays of rodenticides on wild Norway rats. I. Toxicity. Public Health Rep. (U. S.) *61*:672-679, 1946b.

Farah, H.; West, T. C.; Angel, R. The action of sodium fluoroacetate on intestinal smooth muscle. J. Pharmacol. Exp. Ther. *98*:234-244, 1950.

Frick, E. J.; Boebel, F. W. Clinical observation of "1080" poisoning. Vet. Med. *41*:196-197, 1946.

Furchgott, R. F. The effect of sodium fluoroacetate on the contractility and metabolism of intestinal smooth muscle. J. Pharmacol. Exp. Ther. *99*:1-15, 1950.

Gajdusek, D. C.; Luther, G. Fluoroacetate poisoning. A review and report of a case. Am. J. Dis. Child. *79*:310-320, 1950.

Gitter, S. The influence of acetamide on citrate accumulation after fluoroacetate poisoning. Biochem. J. *63*:182-187, 1956.

Hagan, E. C.; Ramsey, L. L.; Woodward, G. Absorption, distribution and excretion of sodium fluoroacetate (1080) in rats. J. Pharmacol. Exp. Ther. *99*:432-434, 1950.

Harrisson, J. W. E.; Ambrus, J. L.; Ambrus, C. M. Fluoroacetate (1080) poisoning. Ind. Med. Surg. *21*:440-442, 1952b.

Harrisson, J. W. E.; Ambrus, J. L.; Ambrus, C. M.; Rees, E. W.; Peters, R. H., Jr.; Reese, L. C.; Baker, T. Acute poisoning with sodium fluoroacetate (Compound 1080). J. A. M. A. 149:1520-1522, 1952a.

Hayes, F.; Short, R.; Gibson, J. Differential toxicity of monochloroacetate, monofluoroacetate and monoiodoacetate in rats. Toxicol. Appl. Pharmacol. 26:93-102, 1973.

Hayes, W. J., Jr. Pesticides Studied In Man. Williams & Wilkins, Baltimore, 1982.

Hutchens, J. O.; Wagner, H.; Podolsky, B.; McMahon, T. M. The effect of ethanol and various metabolites on fluoroacetate poisoning. J. Pharmacol. Exp. Ther. 95:62-70, 1949.

Kostyniak, P. J. Defluorination: a possible mechanism of detoxification in rats exposed to fluoroacetate. Toxicol. Lett. 3:225-228, 1979.

Le Poidevin, N. The toxicity of some halogenated fatty acids and their derivatives. Acta Pharmacol. Toxicol. 23:98-102, 1965.

Liebecq, C.; Peters, R. A. The toxicity of fluoroacetate and the tricarboxylic acid cycle. Biochim. Biophys. Acta 3:215-230, 1949.

McTaggart, D. R. Poisoning due to fluoroacetate (1080). Med. J. Aust. 2:641-642, 1970.

Oelrichs, P. B.; McEwan, T. The toxic principle of Acacia georginae. Queensl. J. Agric. Sci. 19:1, 1962.

Parkin, P. J.; McGiven, A. R.; Bailey, R. R. Chronic sodium monofluoroacetate (Compound 1080) intoxication in a rabbiter. NZ Med. J. 85:93-99, 1977.

Pattison, F. L. M. Toxic Aliphatic Fluorine Compounds. Elsevier Press, Inc., New York, 1959.

Peters, R.; Wakelin, R.; Buffa, P. Biochemistry of fluoroacetate poisoning, the isolation and properties of the fluorotricarboxylic acid inhibitor of citrate metabolism. Proc. R. Soc. London B 140:497-507, 1953.

Peters, R. A. Mechanism of the toxicity of the active constituents of Dichapetalum cymosum and related compounds. Adv. Enzymol. 18:113, 1957.

Peterson, D. I.; Peterson, J. E.; Hardinge, M. G. Protection by ethanol against the toxic effects of monofluoroethanol and monochloroethanol. J. Pharm. Pharmacol. 20:465-468, 1968.

Reigart, J. R.; Brueggeman, J. L.; Keil, J. E. Sodium fluoroacetate poisoning. Am. J. Dis. Child. 129:1224-1226, 1975.

Spector, W. S. Handbook of Toxicology. Vol. I, W. B. Saunders Co., Philadelphia, 1955.

Vickery, B.; Vickery, M. L. Fluoride metabolism in Dichapetalum toxicarium. Phytochem. 11:1905-1909, 1972.

Williams, A. T. Sodium fluoroacetate poisoning. Hosp. Corps Q. 21:16-18, 1948.

FORMALDEHYDE

Formaldehyde gas (HCHO) in solution may be present around the home as a constituent of antiseptics, deodorizing preparations, and fumigants. It may also slowly leach out of improperly "cured" polymeric foams made from formaldehyde and urea and used as wall and ceiling insulation in homes (see below). Formaldehyde-type resins are currently being used to wrinkle-proof fabrics, and occupational exposures with toxic reactions have occurred in establishments handling women's clothes (Bourne and Seferman, 1959). Formaldehyde has a pungent odor with a suffocating effect. Formalin is an aqueous solution containing not less than 37% (by weight) of formaldehyde and small amounts of methanol, ethanol or both (0 to 15%, to prevent polymerization). Embalming fluids contain appreciable amounts of formalin (see Section VI, General Formulations).

Toxicology: The largest oral dose of formalin from which recovery has been reported is 4 oz. (Allen et al., 1970; Hale, 1922), but the more recent case necessitated total gastrectomy. The ingestion of 1 oz. has caused death within 3 hours (Kline, 1925). Probably the mean lethal dose in adults is about 1 to 2 oz. If the patient survives the first 48 hours, the prognosis is good, and a rapid recovery is the rule.

Formaldehyde probably reacts quickly with the mucosa of the alimentary and respiratory tracts. In vitro and in vivo it combines with a variety of functional groups to form addition products or to initiate polymerization reactions. Sulfhydryl reagents, such as BAL, cysteine or mercaptoethanol, antagonize the lethal effects of injected formaldehyde in rats and mice (Guerri et al., 1977).

Formaldehyde is rapidly oxidized to formic acid in various tissues, especially the liver and erythrocytes (Malorny et al., 1965). Following intravenous infusions of formaldehyde into cynomolgus monkeys, it was eliminated with a half-life of 1.5 minutes, and blood formate concentrations increased concomitantly (McMartin et al., 1979). Much of the formate, at least in laboratory rodents, is oxidized to carbon dioxide and water. Significant amounts, however, may be excreted as formate salts in the urine, and some is converted metabolically to labile methyl groups after activation by tetrahydrofolic acid (Malorny et al., 1965). See also METHYL ALCOHOL (p. III-276) for further details of formate metabolism.

The ingestion of formalin leads promptly to inflammation, ulceration and/or coagulation necrosis (fixation or tanning to a leather-like consistency) of the gastrointestinal mucosa (Gaál, 1931). Formaldehyde resembles mineral acids (see p. III-8) in that corrosive damage with late strictures occurs commonly in the stomach without extensive esophageal involvement (Bartone et al., 1968; Roy et al., 1962; Steigmann and Dolehide, 1956; Vinson and Harrington, 1929), but esophageal strictures have occurred (Allen et al., 1970). Furthermore tissue destruction may extend as far as the jejunum (Gaál, 1931). Circulatory collapse and kidney damage may also occur soon after ingestion (Böhmer, 1934; Steigmann and Dolehide, 1956).

Whether or not sufficient unreacted formaldehyde is absorbed to produce systemic effects is not established. Vertigo, fright, loss of consciousness or coma were prominent features of early reported cases (Böhmer, 1934; Kline, 1925; March, 1927; Webster, 1930). Undoubtedly metabolic acidosis (Allen et al., 1970) both from formic acid production and lactic acidemia (Malorny et al., 1965), together with a compromised circulation, contributed to these central neural manifestations.

Inhaled vapors are very irritating to the eyes, nose and upper respiratory tract; high concentrations may produce edema or spasm of the larynx. Severe obstructive tracheobronchitis may result from inhalation (Ely, 1910), but pulmonary edema is uncommon (Kline, 1925). Severe lung changes, however, may be the consequence of aspiration of ingested formalin in combination with stomach acid (Böhmer, 1934; Gonzales et al., 1954; Kline, 1925). The susceptibility of mucous membranes to the irritative actions of formaldehyde is diminished by repeated exposure. Contact with vapor or solution causes the skin to become white, rough, hard and anesthetic, due to superficial coagulation necrosis; with long exposure, dermatitis and hypersensitivity frequently result (Sollmann, 1957).

Data on the effects of long term exposure to low levels of formaldehyde are scant, but preliminary results indicate that formaldehyde vapor is carcinogenic in rats; squamous cell carcinomas of the nasal cavity are described. Occupational exposures to the gas have a propensity for inducing asthma (Hendrick and Lane, 1977), and allergic-type reactions have been reported in some individuals at concentrations below the odor threshold of about 0.8 ppm (Loomis, 1979).

Polymeric foams of phenol-formaldehyde and of urea-formaldehyde are materials commonly used for home insulation. Mice exposed to the thermal decomposition products of the latter material developed a cardiomyopathy. These products were judged to be more irritating and toxic than those produced by comparable treatment of wood (Anderson et al., 1979). Following the widespread use of these polymers in homes in the northeastern United States in the 1970s, complaints ranging from eye and throat irritation to breathing difficulties, headache, nausea, sleeplessness, skin rashes and epistaxis came to the attention of health agencies (De Murcie, 1978). It is widely held that small amounts of formaldehyde gas escaping from the foam insulation are responsible for these signs and symptoms and that only very sensitive individuals are affected (Consumer Product Safety Commission, 1979). Especially in new buildings and mobile homes, formaldehyde vapor concentrations range as high as 3.7 ppm (Dally et al., 1981). The true magnitude of this problem and its health implications are unclear at present. In 1982 urea-formaldehyde foam insulation was banned in residential and school buildings (Consumer Product Safety Commission, 1982).

In a homologous aliphatic series of aldehydes the toxicity appears to decrease with increasing molecular weight. Unsaturated aldehydes are more toxic than their saturated homologues (Salem and Cullumbine, 1960; Skog, 1950). Central depressant activity becomes more pronounced as the aliphatic chain length increases, but unsaturated aldehydes such as acrolein and crotonaldehyde resemble formaldehyde in their predilection to produce respiratory tract injury (Skog, 1950). For a discussion of the systemic actions of acetaldehyde, see DISULFIRAM, p. III-159. Whether or not intravenous infusions of formaldehyde mimic the sympathomimetic effects of acetaldehyde is in dispute (Egle and Hudgins, 1974; James and Bear, 1968). In any event, as indicated above, inhaled and ingested formaldehyde may not reach the systemic circulation in significant amounts.

When given systemically, both methanol and formaldehyde are metabolized to formic acid in many species. Presumably methanol passes through a formaldehyde stage although the latter has never been identified in poisoned patients. Formate is responsible for the retinal damage and systemic acidosis in methanol poisoning in primates (see p. III-276), but only acidosis (Allen et al., 1970) has been reported after ingestion or inhalation of formaldehyde. The distinction may be simply one of dose, but it is also possible that ingested formaldehyde is largely fixed in the gut and so does not yield as much formic acid as an equimolar dose of methanol.

Symptomatology:
  A. Inhalation.
    1. Irritation of mucous membranes, especially of eyes, nose and upper respiratory tract.
    2. With higher concentration, cough, dysphagia, bronchitis, pneumonia, edema or spasm of the larynx. Pulmonary edema is uncommon.
  B. Ingestion.
    1. Immediate intense pain in mouth, pharynx, and stomach.
    2. Nausea, vomiting, hematemesis, abdominal pain, and occasionally diarrhea (which may be bloody).
    3. Pale, clammy skin, and other signs of shock.
    4. Difficult micturition, hematuria, anuria.
    5. Vertigo, convulsions, stupor, and coma.
    6. Death due to respiratory failure.
  C. Skin contact
    1. Irritation and hardening of skin. Strong solutions produce coagulation necrosis.
    2. Dermatitis and hypersensitivity from prolonged or repeated exposure.
Treatment:
    1. Administer by mouth one or more of the following: water, milk, 0.2% ammo-

nia water (2 to 3 teaspoonfuls of household ammonia water diluted with 1 pint of water), ammonium acetate (3 teaspoonfuls in water), egg whites, activated charcoal. Ammonium salts are probably effective because they transform formaldehyde into methenamine (March, 1927).

2. Demulcents: milk, eggs, aluminum hydroxide gels.

3. Morphine for the control of pain (p. IV-32).

4. Combat shock by the intravenous administration of isotonic saline, plasma, or whole blood (pp. IV-17–20).

5. To correct acidosis, give sodium bicarbonate or M/6 sodium lactate solution intravenously (p. IV-72).

6. Assist ventilation, if indicated (pp. IV-7–12).

7. Penicillin or other antibiotic if an infection appears (pp. IV-85–86).

8. Wash affected skin with large quantities of soap and water.

Laboratory: Urinalysis may reveal red blood cells (sometimes gross hematuria) and casts. The acid-base status and electrolyte levels in blood should be monitored. Data on blood formate levels would be useful.

References:

Allen, R. E.; Thoshinsky, M. J.; Stallone, R. J.; Hunt, T. K. Corrosive injuries of the stomach. Arch. Surg. *100*:409-413, 1970.

Anderson, R. C.; Stock, M. F.; Sawin, R.; Alarie, Y. Toxicity of thermal decomposition products of urea formaldehyde and phenol formaldehyde foams. Toxicol. Appl. Pharmacol. *51*:9-17, 1979.

Bartone, N. F.; Grieco, R. V.; Henn, B. S., Jr. Corrosive gastritis due to ingestion of formaldehyde. J. A. M. A. *203*:50-51, 1968.

Bohmer, K. Formalinvergiftung. Dtsch. Z. Gesamte Gerichte, Med. *23*:7-18, 1934.

Bourne, H. G., Jr.; Seferman, S. Wrinkle-proofed clothing may liberate toxic quantities of formaldehyde. Ind. Med. Surg. *28*:232-233, 1959.

Consumer Product Safety Commission. Ban of urea-formaldehyde foam insulation. Federal Register *47*:14366-14419, April 2, 1982.

Consumer Product Safety Commission. Urea-formaldehyde foam insulation; public hearings. Federal Register *44*:69578-69581, 12/3/79.

Dally, K. A.; Hanrahan, L. P.; Woodbury, M. A.; Kanarek, M. S. Formaldehyde exposure in nonoccupational environments. Arch. Environ. Health *36*:277-284, 1981.

De Murcie, D. The formaldehyde health controversy. Mass. Physician *37*:18-21, 1978.

Egle, J. L., Jr.; Hudgins, P. M. Dose-dependent sympathomimetic and cardioinhibitory effects of acrolein and formaldehyde in the anesthetized rat. Toxicol. Appl. Pharmacol. *28*:358-366, 1974.

Ely, F. A. Formaldehyde poisoning. J. A. M. A. *54*:1140-1141, 1910.

Gaal, A. Von. Zur Kenntis der anatomischen Veranderungen bei der Formalinvergiftung. Zentralbl. Allg. Pathol. *51*:257-262, 1931.

Gonzales, T. A.; Vance, M.; Helpern, M.; Umberger, C. J. *Legal Medicine, Pathology and Toxicology*, 2nd ed. Appleton-Century-Crofts, New York, 1954.

Guerri, C.; Godfrey, W.; Grisolia, S. Protection against toxic effects of formaldehyde in vitro, and of methanol or formaldehyde in vivo, by subsequent administration of SH reagents. Physiol. Chem. Phys. *8*:543-550, 1977.

Hale, B. L. Formaldehyde poisoning. J. A. M. A. *78*:452, 1922.

Hendrick, D. J.; Lane, D. J. Occupational formalin asthma. Brit. J. Ind. Med. *34*:11-18, 1977.

James, T. N.; Bear, E. S. Cardiac effects of some simple aliphatic aldehydes. J. Pharmacol. Exp. Ther. *163*:300-308, 1968.

Kline, B. S. Formaldehyde poisoning, with report of a fatal case. Arch. Intern. Med. *36*:220-228, 1925.

Loomis, T. A. Formaldehyde toxicity. Arch. Pathol. Lab. Med. *103*:321-324, 1979.

Malorny, G.; Reitbrock, N.; Schneider, M. Die Oxydation des Formaldehyds zu Ameisensaure im Blut, ein Beitrag zum Stoffwechsel des Formaldehyds. Naunyn Schmiedebergs Arch. Pharmakol. *250*:419-436, 1965.

March, G. H. Formalin poisoning. Recovery. Br. Med. J. *2*:687, 1927.

McMartin, K. E.; Martin-Amat, G.; Noker, P. E.; Tephly, T. R. Lack of a role for formaldehyde in methanol poisoning in the monkey. Biochem. Pharmacol. *28*:645-649, 1979.

Roy, M., Jr.; Calonje, M. A.; Mouton, R. Corrosive gastritis after formaldehyde ingestion. Report of a case. N. Engl. J. Med. *266*:1248-1250, 1962.

Salem, H.; Cullumbine, H. Inhalation toxicities of some aldehydes. Toxicol. Appl. Pharmacol. *2*:183-187, 1960.

Skog, E. A toxicological investigation of lower aliphatic aldehydes. 1. Toxicity of formaldehyde, acetaldehyde, propionaldehyde and butyraldehyde, as well as of acrolein and crotonaldehyde. Acta Pharmacol. Toxicol. *6*:299-318, 1950.

Sollmann, T. *A Manual of Pharmacology.* 8th Ed., W. B. Saunders Co., Philadelphia, 1957.

Steigmann, F.; Dolehide, R. A. Corrosive (acid) gastritis, management of early and late cases. N. Engl. J. Med. *254*:981-986, 1956.

Vinson, P. P.; Harington, S. W. Cicatricial stricture of the stomach without involvement of the esophagus following the ingestion of formaldehyde. J. A. M. A. *93*:917-918, 1929.

Webster, R. W. *Legal Medicine and Toxicology.* W. B. Saunders Co., Philadelphia, 1930.

HYDROGEN SULFIDE

Hydrogen sulfide (H_2S) is a colorless gas, heavier than air, possessing the odor of rotten eggs. It is generated in several industries, and is present in sewers ("sewer gas") and cesspools and among the products of putrefaction everywhere (Mitchell and Davenport, 1924). Hydrogen sulfide may be encountered in vast amounts in association with petroleum ("sour crude") and other natural gas deposits (Burnett et al., 1977).

It is employed in ton quantities in the preparation of heavy water for use as the moderator in nuclear reactors (National Research Council, 1979). Poisonings have occurred in or near tanks for the processing and storage of liquid manure now widely used to dispose of large volumes of livestock wastes (Morse et al., 1981; Osbern and Crapo, 1981). Tanneries use sodium sulfide to remove hair from hides (Smith and Gosselin,

1979). It may be generated from decomposing protein in the holds of fishing vessels (Anon., 1978; Glass et al., 1980).

Hydrogen sulfide is released in vivo from ingested or injected soluble inorganic sulfide salts. From time to time it has been asserted that the gas is generated in large quantities in the human bowel by bacteria (Division of Industrial Hygiene, 1941; Weisiger et al., 1980), but sophisticated analyses of human flatus have failed to confirm its presence (National Research Council, 1979).

Barium and strontium sulfides have been used as depilatories. In trace amounts calcium sulfide has been tried as a food preservative. Calcium polysulfide is sometimes employed as an agricultural insecticide and fungicide. Sodium sulfide has many industrial uses.

Toxicology of sulfide: Vapor concentrations of H_2S as low as 0.005% (50 ppm) in air may cause toxic symptoms, and 0.1 to 0.2% is usually fatal within a few minutes (Ahlborg, 1951; American Petroleum Institute, 1948j; Manufacturing Chemists' Association, Inc., 1950c; Smith and Gosselin, 1964). Because the body has an inherently large capacity for detoxifying sulfide (Haggard, 1925; Weber and Lendle, 1965), the toxicity of gas mixtures is more closely related to concentration than to length of exposure (O'Donoghue, 1961; Smith and Gosselin, 1964).

Odor is not a dependable way to detect this gas because in dangerous concentrations it is said to produce a rapid paralysis of the olfactory nerve endings (American Petroleum Institute, 1948j). Susceptibility to hydrogen sulfide may vary among individuals, and it has been suggested that sensitivity may be increased by previous exposure (Ahlborg, 1951; American Petroleum Institute, 1948j) although others deny that either tolerance or sensitivity can be acquired (Poda, 1966).

It is likely that the intensity of exposure accounts for the very diverse courses of hydrogen sulfide poisoning. In extremely high vapor concentrations (e.g., 1000 ppm) a few breaths can lead to abrupt loss of consciousness. If, however, the exposure is terminated promptly, recovery is also rapid. Somewhat lower vapor concentrations allow enough time for a variety of systemic and local effects to become manifest. The latter are described first.

At low concentrations of hydrogen sulfide (e.g., 50 to 200 ppm) the toxic symptoms are due chiefly to local tissue irritation rather than to systemic actions. The most characteristic effect is on the eye, where the superficial injury to the conjunctiva and cornea is known to workers in tunnels, caissons and sewers as "gas eye." This keratoconjunctivitis is manifested after several hours or days of exposure as a scratchy, irritated sensation with tearing or burning. Recovery is

almost always complete and spontaneous unless secondary infection occurs (Grant, 1974).

Often there is also involvement of the respiratory tract with cough, dyspnea and perhaps pulmonary edema (Haggard, 1925). Evidence of severe pulmonary edema has been found at autopsy and in survivors of respiratory exposures (Adelson and Sunshine, 1966; Breysse, 1961b; Kemper, 1966; Kleinfeld et al., 1964; Simson and Simpson, 1971; Wine et al., 1968), but pulmonary involvement does not appear to be a regular feature of even intensive exposure to this gas (Ahlborg, 1951; Milby, 1962) perhaps because time is necessary for the local irritancy of the agent to express itself. Except for those cases with lung edema, the tissue pathology in victims of H_2S poisoning may be limited to petechial hemorrhages and congestion of brain and lungs, greyish-green cyanosis, and green to purple discoloration of blood, viscera and cerebral cortex (Adelson and Sunshine, 1966; Breysse, 1961b; Freireich, 1946; Simson and Simpson, 1971).

Soluble salts of sulfides are alkaline, and sodium sulfide may produce caustic burns (see also LYE, p. III-245). Sodium and other soluble sulfides are promptly and completely hydrolyzed in body fluids (Haggard, 1921) so that in terms of their systemic effects no toxicological distinctions are recognized between them and hydrogen sulfide. Several reported cases of intoxication by commercial products containing barium sulfide suggest prominent contributions of sulfide to the intoxication, although concomitant barium poisoning cannot be ruled out (Gould et al., 1973; Jobba and Rengei, 1971).

Sulfide and cyanide produce similar effects on the chemoreceptors of the carotid body and are about equipotent in producing respiratory stimulation (Anichkov and Belen'kii, 1948). In addition to increasing ventilation, small parenteral doses of sulfide in laboratory animals produce a fleeting rise followed by a profound (perhaps irreversible) fall in blood pressure. Death, however, is invariably a result of central respiratory paralysis (Haggard et al., 1922; Heymans et al., 1932; Owen and Gesell, 1931; Winder and Winder, 1933). The latter process may be accelerated in respiratory exposures because of the initial stimulation of breathing mediated through the carotid body (Yant, 1930). There are also at least two reports of myocardial involvement, one of them with persistent atrial fibrillation (cited in Simson and Simpson, 1971).

Humans exposed to high concentrations of hydrogen sulfide experience headache, nausea, dizziness, confusion and weakness of the extremities, followed by a precipitous lapse into unconsciousness. Because sulfide is so rapidly detoxified in the body, any decrease in the exposure intensity may result in a rapid and spontaneous revival. Thus, highly labile states of consciousness have characterized many poisoning episodes (Adelson and Sunshine, 1966; Ahlborg, 1951; Freireich, 1946; Kleinfeld et al., 1964; McCabe and Clayton, 1952; Milby, 1962; Poda, 1966). If the exposure is sufficiently intense and sustained, victims rapidly become apneic and exhibit anoxic convulsions, perhaps with opisthotonos and risus sardonicus (Hurwitz and Taylor, 1954; Kemper, 1966).

Survivors of acute toxic episodes sometimes show neurologic sequelae such as amnesia, intention tremor, neurasthenia, disturbance of equilibrium or more serious brain stem and cortical damage (Ahlborg, 1951; Aufdermaur and Tonz, 1970; Hurwitz and Taylor, 1954; Kemper, 1966; McCabe and Clayton, 1952; Poda, 1966; Zeyer, 1955), but complete recovery is the general rule (Kleinfeld et al., 1964). No truly cumulative effects are recognized (Manufacturing Chemists' Assoc., Inc., 1950c), but adequate precedents exist to predict that recurrent, acute but mild exposures may summate in terms of hypoxic tissue damage to produce neurologic deficits like those occurring in survivors of other severe asphyxiant poisonings (see also CARBON MONOXIDE, p. III-97 and CYANIDE, p. III-126).

The toxicity of hydrogen sulfide, its speed of action, the clinical picture of intoxications, its potentiation by other asphyxiants (Hofer, 1926), together with certain enzymatic studies (Nicholls, 1975; Smith et al., 1977), all suggest that the hydrosulfide anion, like cyanide, produces its major toxic effects through inhibition of cytochrome oxidase. Furthermore, hydrosulfide also forms stable complexes with heme-type porphyrinic structures when the iron is in the trivalent state. Thus animals can be protected against sulfide poisoning by the prior induction of methemoglobinemia (Smith and Gosselin, 1964). Injections of sodium nitrite similarly antidoted sulfide poisoning as demonstrated in mice (Scheler and Kabisch, 1963). The mechanism of these effects is attributed to a competition for free sulfide between tissue cytochrome oxidase and circulating methemoglobin, the latter binding sulfide in an inactive form called sulfmethemoglobin. The latter slowly releases sulfide to endogenous detoxication processes (Scheler and Kabisch, 1963; Smith and Gosselin, 1964).

The ferric heme groups of methemoglobin bind hydrosulfide less tenaciously than cyanide (Smith and Gosselin, 1966). In mice with a 33% methemoglobinemia, the LD_{50} of cyanide is 3.3 times greater than in normal mice, whereas the LD_{50} of sulfide is 2.4 times greater (Smith and Gosselin, 1966; Smith, 1967a). The injection of sodium nitrite has been employed successfully in the resuscitation of two human victims of severe hydrogen sulfide poisoning (Peters, 1981; Stine et al., 1976).

Although artificial respiration and oxygen therapy probably should not be neglected as therapeutic adjuncts, significant protective or antidotal effects of oxygen have not been demonstrated experimentally (Smith et al., 1976). Sulfhemoglobin (in contrast to sulfmethemoglobin) has never been encountered in those who survived hydrogen sulfide poisoning, but its postmortem formation may be responsible for the various tissue discolorations described above.

The first acid dissociation constant of hydrogen sulfide is about 10^{-7} M, so that in body fluids dissociated and undissociated hydrogen sulfide exist in about equal proportions. The undissociated acid, however, penetrates biological membranes more rapidly than the hydrosulfide (HS^-) anion (Beerman, 1924). Indeed, under appropriate circumstances hydrogen sulfide can penetrate the intact skin to produce signs of systemic intoxication (Walton and Witherspoon, 1925). Several deaths have followed the application of ammonium sulfide permanent wave solutions (Bunce et al., 1941; Laug and Draize, 1942), and systemic poisonings are said to have resulted from the cutaneous application of salves containing elemental sulfur (Basch, 1926).

Evidence has been obtained for the presence of a sulfide oxidase in mammalian liver (Baxter and Van Reen, 1958a; Sörbo, 1960), but important nonenzymatic mechanisms for sulfide detoxication are also recognized. Sulfide tends to undergo spontaneous oxidation to nontoxic products such as polysulfides, thiosulfate or sulfate, and these reactions are catalyzed by heavy metals particularly in the presence of protein (Baxter and Van Reen, 1958b; Denis and Reed, 1927). A reaction with endogenous disulfide bonds may constitute an important detoxication mechanism, and a potential antidotal approach is the administration of oxidized glutathione (Smith and Abbanat, 1966). Apparently by complex formation, cobaltous chloride also significantly protects mice against death by sulfide or cyanide (Smith, 1969). It has been suggested that excretion by the lungs may also play a significant role in decreasing hydrogen sulfide toxicity in nonrespiratory exposures (Atkinson and Fitzpatrick, 1911–12), but neither hydrogen sulfide nor the postulated metabolites methanethiol and dimethyl sulfide were found on the breath of mice given near-lethal systemic doses of sodium sulfide (Susman et al., 1978).

Symptomatology:
   A. Low to moderately high vapor concentrations
      1. *Irritant actions.*

Eyes: painful conjunctivitis, photophobia, lacrimation, and corneal opacity.

Respiratory tract: rhinitis with anosmia, tracheobronchitis with pain and cough, pulmonary edema with dyspnea, sometimes late bronchopneumonia.

Skin: direct contact (as a solution) may produce erythema and pain.

2. *Gastrointestinal effects:* profuse salivation, nausea, vomiting, diarrhea.
3. *Central nervous effects:* giddiness, headache, vertigo, amnesia, confusion, and unconsciousness.
4. *Miscellaneous:* tachypnea, palpitations, tachycardia, arrhythmia, sweating, weakness, and muscle cramps.

B. Very high vapor concentrations
1. Sudden collapse and unconsciousness, with or without a warning cry.
2. Death from prompt respiratory paralysis, usually with a terminal asphyxial convulsion.
3. After sublethal exposures coma may disappear promptly, but full recovery is usually slow; the patient may have a residual cough, cardiac dilatation, slow pulse, peripheral neuritis, albuminuria, and some degree of amnesia or of psychic disturbance. Recovery is eventually complete in most nonfatal cases.

Treatment:
1. Remove immediately to fresh air. Keep at rest and comfortably warm.
2. If respirations are depressed, artificial respiration without interruption until normal breathing is restored. See pp. IV-7–12.
3. Administer oxygen (p. IV-12) and continue even after spontaneous breathing is established. If pulmonary edema ensues, see p. IV-14.
4. In severe poisonings treat with amyl nitrite and sodium nitrite as for cyanide poisoning (p. III-127), but omit sodium thiosulfate injection (Smith *et al.*, 1976).
5. Atropine sulfate (0.6 mg. intramuscularly) may contribute some symptomatic relief.
6. Conjunctivitis may be relieved by the instillation of 1 drop of olive oil in each eye and sometimes by 3 to 4 drops of epinephrine solution (1:1000) at frequent intervals (*e.g.*, 5 minutes). Occasionally local anesthetics and hot or cold compresses are necessary to control the pain.
7. Antibiotics at the first hint of pulmonary infection. See pp. IV-85–86.

Laboratory: Urine may contain albumin, casts, and a few red blood cells. High concentrations of hydrosulfide ion have been analyzed quantitatively in the blood of fatally poisoned humans (Osbern and Crapo, 1981). The presence of H_2S in air can be detected by lead-acetate test paper.

References:

Adelson, L.; Sunshine, I. Fatal hydrogen sulfide intoxication, report of three cases occurring in a sewer. Arch. Pathol. *81*:375-380, 1966.

Ahlborg, G. G. Hydrogen sulfide poisoning in shale oil industry. Arch. Ind. Health *3*:247-266, 1951.

American Petroleum Institute. API toxicological review (Hydrogen sulfide). New York, 1948j.

Anichkov, S. V.; Belen'kii, M. L. *Pharmacology of the Carotid Body Chemoreceptors.* The Macmillan Co., New York, 1963.

Anonymous. Hydrogen-sulphide poisoning. Lancet *1*:28-29, 1978.

Atkinson, J. P.; Fitzpatrick, C. B. Further observations on the tolerance of gases by the circulatory apparatus. Proc. Soc. Exp. Biol. Med. *9*:25-26, 1911-12.

Aufdermaur, F.; Tonz, O. Kindliche Jauchegasvergiftungen bei Benutzung "rustikaler" Aborte. Schweiz. Med. Wochenschr. *100*:894-896, 1970.

Basch, F. Uber Schwefelwasserstoffvergiftung bei ausserlicher Applikation von elementarem Schwefel in Salbenform. Naunyn Schmiedebergs Arch. Pharmakol. *111*:126-132, 1926.

Baxter, C. F.; Van Reen, R. Some aspects of sulfide oxidation by rat liver preparations. Biochim. Biophys. Acta *28*:567-572, 1958a.

Baxter, C. F.; Van Reen, R. The oxidation of sulfide to thiosulfate by metalloprotein complexes and by ferritin. Biochim. Biophys. Acta *28*:573-578, 1958b.

Beerman, H. Some physiological actions of hydrogen sulfide. J. Exp. Zool. *41*:33-43, 1924.

Breysse, P. A. Hydrogen sulfide fatality in a poultry feather fertilizer plant. Am. Ind. Hyg. Assoc. J. *22*:220-222, 1961b.

Bunce, A. H.; Parker, F. P.; Lewis, G. T. Accidental death from absorption of heatless permanent wave solution. J. A. M. A. *116*:1515-1517, 1941.

Burnett, W. W.; King, E. G.; Grace, M.; Hall, W. F. Hydrogen sulfide poisoning: review of 5 years' experience. Can. Med. Assoc. J. *117*:1277-1280, 1977.

Denis, W.; Reed, L. The action of blood on sulfides. J. Biol. Chem. *72*:385-394, 1927.

Division of Industrial Hygiene, National Institutes of Health, U. S. Public Health Service. Hydrogen sulfide, its toxicity and potential dangers. Public Health Rep. (U. S.) *56*:684-692, 1941.

Freireich, A. W. Hydrogen sulfide poisoning. Report of two cases, one with fatal outcome, from associated mechanical asphyxia. Am. J. Pathol. *22*:147-155, 1946.

Glass, R. I.; Ford, R.; Allegra, D. T.; Markel, H. L. Deaths from asphyxia among fishermen. J. A. M. A. *244*:2193-2194, 1980.

Gould, D. B.; Sorrell, M. R.; Lupariello, A. D. Barium sulfide poisoning. Arch. Intern. Med. *132*:891-894, 1973.

Grant, W. M. *Toxicology of the Eye.* 2nd ed. Charles C Thomas, Springfield, Ill, 1974.

Haggard, H. W. The fate of sulfides in the blood. J. Biol. Chem. *44*:519-529, 1921.

Haggard, H. W. Toxicology of hydrogen sulfide. J. Ind. Hyg. Toxicol. *1*:113-121, 1925.

Haggard, H. W.; Henderson, Y.; Charlton, T. J. The influence of hydrogen sulfide upon respiration. Am. J. Physiol. *61*:289-297, 1922.

Heymans, C.; Bouckaert, J. J.; Von Euler, U. S.; Dautrebande, L. Sinus carotidiens et reflexes vasomoteurs. Arch. Int. Pharmacodyn. Ther. *43*:86-110, 1932.

Hofer, R. Uber die Wirkung von Gasgemischen. Naunyn Schmiedebergs Arch. Pharmakol. *111*:183-205, 1926.

Hurwitz, L. J.; Taylor, G. L. Poisoning by sewer gas with unusual sequelae. Lancet *1*:1110-1112, 1954.

Jobba, G.; Rengei, B. Uber die Neopol-Vergiftung. Arch. Toxikol. 27:106-110, 1971.

Kemper, F. D. A near-fatal case of hydrogen sulfide poisoning. Can. Med. Assoc. J. 94:1130-1131, 1966.

Kleinfeld, M.; Giel, C.; Russo, A. Acute hydrogen sulfide intoxication, an unusual source of exposure. Ind. Med. Surg. 33:656-660, 1964.

Laug, E. P.; Draize, J. H. The percutaneous absorption of ammonium hydrogen sulfide and hydrogen sulfide. J. Pharmacol. Exp. Ther. 76:179-188, 1942.

Manufacturing Chemists' Association, Inc. Chemical safety data sheet, SD-36 (Hydrogen sulfide). Washington, D. C., 1950c.

McCabe, L. C.; Clayton, G. D. Air pollution by hydrogen sulfide in Poza Rica, Mexico. An evaluation of the incident of Nov. 24, 1950. Arch. Ind. Hyg. Occup. Med. 6:199-213, 1952.

Milby, T. H. Hydrogen sulfide intoxication. Review of the literature and report of unusual accident resulting in two cases of nonfatal poisoning. J. Occup. Med. 4:431-438, 1962.

Mitchell, C. W.; Davenport, S. J. Hydrogen sulfide literature. Public Health Rep. (U. S.) 39:1-13, 1924.

Morse, D. L.; Woodbury, M. A.; Rentmeester, K.; Farmer, D. Death caused by fermenting manure. J. A. M. A. 244:63-64, 1981.

National Research Council, Committee on Medical and Biologic Effects of Environmental Pollutants, Subcommittee on Hydrogen Sulfide. Hydrogen Sulfide. University Park Press, Baltimore, 1979.

Nicholls, P. The effect of sulphide on cytochrome aa₃. Isosteric and allosteric shifts of the reduced α peak. Biochem. Biophys. Acta 396:24-35, 1975.

O'Donoghue, J. G. Hydrogen sulfide poisoning in swine. Can. J. Comp. Med. 25:217-219, 1961.

Osbern, L. N.; Crapo, R. O. Dung lung: A report of toxic exposure to liquid manure. Ann. Intern. Med. 95:312-314, 1981.

Owen, H.; Gessell, R. Peripheral and central chemical control of pulmonary ventilation. Proc. Soc. Exp. Biol. Med. 28:765-766, 1931.

Peters, J. W. Hydrogen sulfide poisoning in a hospital setting. J. A. M. A. 246:1588-1589, 1981.

Poda, G. A. Hydrogen sulfide can be handled safely. Arch. Environ. Health 12:795-800, 1966.

Scheler, W.; Kabisch, R. Uber die antagonistische Beeinflussung der akuten H₂S-Vergiftung bei der Maus durch Methamoglobinbildner. Acta Biol. Med. Ger. 11:194-199, 1963.

Simson, R. E.; Simpson, G. R. Fetal hydrogen sulfide poisoning associated with industrial waste exposure. Med. J. Aust.

1:331-334, 1971.

Smith, L.; Kruszyna, H.; Smith, R. P. The effect of methemoglobin on the inhibition of cytochrome c oxidase by cyanide, sulfide or azide. Biochem. Pharmacol. 26:2247-2250, 1977.

Smith, R. P. The oxygen and sulfide binding characteristics of hemoglobins generated from methemoglobin by two erythrocytic systems. Mol. Pharmacol. 3:378-385, 1967a.

Smith, R. P. Cobalt salts; effects on cyanide and sulphide poisoning and on methemoglobinemia. Toxicol. Appl. Pharmacol. 15:505-516, 1969.

Smith, R. P.; Abbanat, R. A. Protective effects of oxidized glutathione in acute sulfide poisoning. Toxicol. Appl. Pharmacol. 9:209-217, 1966.

Smith, R. P.; Gosselin, R. E. The influence of methemoglobinemia on the lethality of some toxic anions; II. Sulfide. Toxicol. Appl. Pharmacol. 6:584-592, 1964.

Smith, R. P.; Gosselin, R. E. On the mechanism of sulfide inactivation by methemoglobin. Toxicol. Appl. Pharmacol. 8:159-172, 1966.

Smith, R. P.; Gosselin, R. E. Hydrogen sulfide poisoning. J. Occup. Med. 21:93-97, 1979.

Smith, R. P.; Kruszyna, R.; Kruszyna, H. Management of acute sulfide poisoning. Arch. Environ. Health 31:166-169, 1976.

Sorbo, B. On the mechanism of sulfide oxidation in biological systems. Biochim. Biophys. Acta 38:349-351, 1960.

Stine, R. J.; Slosberg, B.; Beacham, B. E. Hydrogen sulfide intoxication. Ann. Intern. Med. 85:756-758, 1976.

Susman, J. L.; Hornig, J. F.; Thomae, S. C.; Smith, R. P. Pulmonary excretion of hydrogen sulfide, methanethiol, dimethyl sulfide and dimethyl disulfide in mice. Drug Chem. Toxicol. 1:327-338, 1978.

Walton, D. C.; Witherspoon, M. G. Skin absorption of certain gases. J. Pharmacol. Exp. Ther. 26:315-324, 1925.

Weber, H. D.; Lendle, L. Toxische Wirkungsbedingungen von Schwefelwasserstoff und Behandlungsmoglichkeiten der akuten Vergiftung. Arch. Toxicol. 20:290-312, 1965.

Weisiger, R. A.; Pinkus, L. M.; Jakoby, W. B. Thiol s-methyltransferase: suggested role in detoxication of intestinal hydrogen sulfide. Biochem. Pharmacol. 29:2885-2887, 1980.

Winder, C. V.; Winder, H. O. The seat of action of sulfide on pulmonary ventilation. Am. J. Physiol. 105:337-352, 1933.

Winek, C. L.; Collom, W. D.; Wecht, C. H. Death from hydrogen sulphide fumes. Lancet 1:1096, 1968.

Yant, W. P. Hydrogen sulfide in industry - occurrence, effects, and treatment. Am. J. Public Health 20:598-608, 1930.

Zeyer, H. G. Schwefelwasserstoff-Polyneuritis und -Encephalopathie. Arch. Gewerbepath. Gewerbehyg. 13:687-693, 1955.

HYPOCHLORITE

Hypochlorite salts (e.g., sodium, potassium, calcium, magnesium) serve as disinfectants, bleaches, and deodorizers. Specifically they are used to disinfect contaminated utensils, large masses of organic matter (excreta), and occasionally water for drinking. Dilute aqueous solutions (0.5 to 5%) are sometimes used medicinally as foot baths. Under a host of trade names, dilute hypochlorites are found in almost every home in the form of laundry bleach or as the active constituent of "liquid household bleach" (usually about 5% sodium hypochlorite, NaOCl).

Commercial solutions of household bleach are made by adding gaseous chlorine to 12 to 15% sodium hydroxide solutions until the alkalinity is just neutralized: the mixture is then diluted to about 5% NaOCl for the consumer market (Griffith, 1962). Because even a little too much Cl_2 means an acidic solution of hypochlorite that is unstable, manufacturers with inadequate production controls use too little chlorine and market a product with a free alkalinity that may run as high as 1% NaOH. In contrast "neutral" preparations have a pH of 9 to 10 with a very low titratable alkalinity. All hypochlorite solutions are unstable, especially if acidified; slowly decomposing on contact with air they become less toxic with age.

Occasionally so-called concentrated bleaches are marketed, apparently for home use, with sodium hypochlorite concentrations of 9 to 15 percent. Products intended for industrial use (e.g., commercial laundry bleach, dairy sanitizers, disinfectants for swimming pools, etc.) may have much higher hypochlorite concentrations (over 50%), but in these products the active ingredient is more apt to be calcium hypochlorite than sodium hypochlorite.

The concentration of a hypochlorite solution or powder is often stated in terms of "available chlorine" or "active chlorine." This is the percentage of gaseous chlorine (gm. Cl_2 per 100 ml. solution or per 100 gm. solid) which can be released by the hypochlorite if it oxidizes chloride ions that are present in excess in these preparations (often as added sodium chloride). Although in chlorinated soda the stated concentrations of sodium hypochlorite and of available chlorine are essentially equal, chlorinated lime is usually equivalent to no more than 70% of its weight in available chlorine. These values vary with the method of preparation, the age, the technique of storage, etc.

In some laundry bleaches other oxidizing agents, such as peroxides and perborates, serve as the active ingredient. At one time calcium hypochlorite (as chlorinated lime) was the principal constituent of dry bleaching powders, but some modern preparations contain other sources of active chlorine such as dichlorodimethylhydantoin and trichloroisocyanuric acid, which slowly form hypochlorite in aqueous solutions. In the textile industry reducing bleaches are sometimes used; they may contain sulfites, hydrosulfites or oxalic acid.

Toxicology: The toxicity of hypochlorite arises from its corrosive activity on skin and mucous membranes. Most of this corrosiveness stems from the oxidizing potency of the hypochlorite itself, a capacity which is measured in terms of "available chlorine" (see above). The alkalinity of some preparations (see above) may contribute substantially to the tissue injury and mucosal erosion. According to some authorities, acidic solutions would be more dangerous than alkaline ones because of the presence of free chlorine and hypochlorous acid (HOCl). Due to its low ionization and consequent lack of charge, this acid is probably able to penetrate mucous membrane more deeply than does the hypochlorite ion. Hence acidic antidotes are inadvisable and probably dangerous (Done, 1961a). Both the acid and salt appear to be rapidly inactivated (reduced) by protein (Strange et al., 1951) and other tissue constituents, and probably little, if any, reaches the circulation. All systemic symptoms, therefore, are thought to be secondary to local tissue injury and shock.

As with other strictly corrosive agents, lethality is more intimately related to concentration than to dose (i.e., conc. × vol.). The ingestion of hypochlorite solutions with "available chlorine" concentrations as low as 0.5% is rarely if ever a threat to life. Although no exact clinical data are available, solutions with 4 to 6% available chlorine are probably lethal to adults only in oral doses of many ounces, but as little as 1 oz. may be dangerous if the concentration is 15% or more. With bleaches, as well as other caustic agents, death is usually due to complications of severe local injury, such as toxemia, shock, perforation, hemorrhage, infection and obstruction.

Liquid bleach containing 4 to 6% sodium hydrochlorite (usually 5.25%) is the commonest hypochlorite in the home. Poison statistics prepared by the National Clearinghouse for Poison Control Centers indicate a high incidence of accidental bleach ingestion by children, but few if any of these cases have been described in the medical literature. One infers that hypochlorite as present in liquid household bleach is rather innocuous. It is recognized that it induces emesis promptly in children and presumably in adults, as well as in dogs. In dogs it is 5 times more potent as an emetic than syrup of ipecac (Carter and Griffith, 1961). Other reactions are uncommon. No reports of fatal poisonings were located in the medical literature, but a successful suicide investigated by the New York City Office of the Medical Examiner is said to have been due to the ingestion of sodium hypochlorite. Fabre et al. (1957) suggest that 4 to 8 oz. of Javelle water (2.5% active chlorine) may produce death, but the ingestion of 1 quart of a 5% solution has been survived (Strange et al., 1951).

Nevertheless liquid household bleach with 5% sodium hypochlorite is not always benign. Done (1961a) tells of an 18-month-old girl who swallowed a "few tablespoonsful" and immediately coughed, choked and vomited. Gastric lavage with a weak vinegar solution was performed within 10 minutes. Promptly thereafter she became lethargic and was admitted to a local hospital in a state of coma. Her temperature was 103.2°F., pulse 160, respirations 88, and blood pressure unobtainable. Rales and rhonchi were audible, and clonic convulsive movements persisted until death, which occurred, in spite of vigorous treatment, 19 hours after ingestion. Postmortem examination revealed focal necrosis, hemorrhage, and superficial erosion of the gastric mucosa, but the presumptive cause of death was an acute tracheobronchitis and obstructive atelectasis secondary to bronchial exudates. Done inferred that bleach solution was aspirated into the trachea. He speculated about the possibility of a relationship between the gastric lavage with dilute vinegar and the intense and unexpected state of hyperchloremic acidosis in this patient.

Esophageal stricture is often mentioned as a possible late complication of hypochlorite poisoning. A 47-year-old man who survived the ingestion of 1 quart of liquid household bleach was eventually readmitted for a total gastrectomy because of a cicatricial injury of the stomach, but his esophagus appeared to be healthy (Strange *et al.*, 1951). French *et al.* (1970), however, describe two cases, one in an infant and one in an adult, where each had consumed several ounces of bleach (5.25% sodium hypochlorite). Both eventually developed esophageal strictures which required interposition of the colon as a by-pass. They were the only two to develop strictures among 160 patients examined after bleach ingestion over a period of 10 years. In 393 hypochlorite cases seen at the Children's Hospital in Columbus, Ohio, in 1960 and 1961, Landau and Saunders (1964) found no esophageal stricture or perforation. Similarly, 129 cases, of which 65 were examined within 4 days of ingestion, were negative on esophagoscopy except for two instances of very mild injury (Pike *et al.*, 1963). German experience, as represented by 23 accidental ingestions of hypochlorite bleach, is similarly benign (Muhlendahl *et al.*, 1978.)

However, 21 patients in another series of 150 cases were described as having ulcerative esophagitis (Cardona and Daly, 1964), and 9 of 31 patients were said to have severe esophageal burns with two examples of narrowing of the lumen (Yarington, 1965).

Undiluted liquid bleach (Clorox) instilled into the upper esophagus of rabbits and dogs produced no permanent esophageal lesions unless the lower end of the esophagus was occluded, in which case half of the dogs died from esophageal perforation, mediastinitis and pleurisy (Landau and Saunders, 1964). The cat esophagus is said to resemble the human esophagus more closely than does the dog. Again when the esophagus has occluded, contact with commercial household bleaches for 3 minutes was sufficient to result in late strictures in some cats (Weeks and Ravitch, 1969). Even preparations containing 0.5% sodium hydroxide, which represents a high free alkalinity for a commercial household bleach preparation, led to no permanent damage to the unoccluded dog esophagus.

From these observations one concludes that procedures which are instituted in lye poisoning to prevent esophageal strictures (p. III-250) are usually unnecessary and therefore undesirable after the ingestion of liquid household bleach. With respect to solid hypochlorite bleaches, the issue is not so clear. No ingestions of calcium hypochlorite (chlorinated lime) have come to our attention, but the powder is known to be intensely irritating on mucous membranes and has caused conjunctivitis, corneal ulcers, nasal ulcers, nasal septal necrosis, laryngeal edema, etc. Presumably the organic sources of chlorine, such as trichloroisocyanuric acid, are less dangerous because they release chlorine more slowly.

Only symptomatic and supportive measures are available in the treatment of hypochlorite poisoning. A solution of sodium thiosulfate (hyposulfite) will reduce any unreacted material with which it comes in contact, but it is not generally available or required, and its efficacy as an antidote is unproved. Since even neutral or alkaline hypochlorite salts may be converted to hypochlorous acid by the acidity of gastric juice, mild alkali therapy by mouth may be beneficial, if given promptly. When indicated, surgical measures such as tracheotomy or gastrectomy may be lifesaving.

Available chlorine is frequently found in public water supplies. Occasional cases of asthma and so-called functional colitis have been attributed to this mode of contact (Sheldon and Lovell, 1949; Watson and Kibler, 1933). Other unusual modes of exposure have been described. For example, a 7-year-old girl suffered chronic gastroduodenitis apparently because of a persistent habit of sucking on her white socks that had been heavily bleached (Loeb and King, 1974).

Occasionally cases of poisoning are encountered as a result of mixing hypochlorite solutions with various other types of household preparations. The danger of mixing bleach and ammonia is discussed under AMMONIA, p. III-22. Some toilet bowl cleaners (hydrochloric acid, sodium bisulfate) or rust removers (hydrofluoric or oxalic acids) are sufficiently acidic to liberate chlorine gas from bleach. See NITROGEN OXIDES, p. III-323, for the management of victims exposed to such pulmonary irritants. Despite a report to the contrary (Faigel, 1964), in our experience vinegar is not acidic enough to produce chlorine evolution when mixed with bleach. The addition of hypochlorite bleach to solutions of phenolic disinfectants, however, may generate toxic polychlorinated phenols (Lynch *et al.*, 1975). Mixtures of bleach and lye (oven or drain cleaners) pose no special safety problems beyond those inherent in each substance alone; indeed, alkalis tend to stabilize hypochlorite (Gleason *et al.*, 1964).

Symptomatology:

1. Pain and inflammation of the mouth, pharynx, esophagus, and stomach. Erosion of mucous membranes, chiefly of the stomach.
2. Vomiting. The vomitus may be bright red or resemble coffee grounds (hemorrhage).
3. Circulatory collapse, with cold and clammy skin, cyanosis, and shallow respirations.
4. Confusion, delirium, coma.
5. Edema of pharynx, glottis and larynx, with stridor and obstruction.
6. Perforation of the esophagus or stomach, with mediastinitis or peritonitis.
7. The inhalation of hypochlorous acid fumes causes severe respiratory tract irritation and pulmonary edema.

8. Skin contact may cause vesicular eruptions and eczematoid dermatitis.

Treatment:

1. Swallow immediately milk, egg white, starch paste, milk of magnesia, aluminum hydroxide gel, or magnesium trisilicate gel. If available, a few ounces of 1% sodium thiosulfate solution may be ingested and left in the alimentary tract. Avoid sodium bicarbonate because of the release of carbon dioxide. Do not use acidic antidotes. Do not induce vomiting.

2. Milk of magnesia (1 oz.) left in the stomach is useful as a mild antacid, adsorbent, demulcent, and cathartic.

3. Demulcents, such as starch, egg white, milk, gruel as necessary.

4. Opiates for the control of pain (p. IV-32).

5. Treat shock vigorously with intravenous fluids (p. IV-17).

6. Prompt surgical intervention when indicated, *e.g.*, tracheotomy, gastrectomy. See p. IV-6. Routine esophagoscopy, however, is probably unwarranted after ingestion of the usual liquid household laundry bleach (5.25% sodium hypochlorite).

7. If spilled on skin, wash with liberal quantities of water and apply a paste of baking soda.

Laboratory: Check blood for electrolyte and acid-base disorders.

References:

Cardona, J. C.; Daly, J. F. Management of corrosive esophagitis. Analysis of treatment, methods, and results. N. Y. State J. Med. *64*:2307-2313, 1964.

Carter, R. O.; Griffith, J. F. Factors relating to accidental ingestion hazard. Soap Chemical Specialties *37*:49-52 and 57-60, 1961.

Done, A. K. Salt Lake City County General Hospital, Utah. Personal Communication (1961). An informal report about this case was written by Dr. Done for the Bull. of Supplementary Material, Clinical Toxicology of Commercial Products. (Edited by M. N. Gleason, R. E. Gosselin and H. C. Hodge.) 5(No. 7):13-14, 1961a.

Fabre, R.; Truhaut, R.; Regneir, M. T. *Traitement d'urgence des intoxications.* . G. Doin et Cie, Paris, 1957.

Faigel, H. C. Mixtures of household cleaning agents. N. Engl. J. Med. *271*:618, 1964.

French, R. J.; Tabb, H. G.; Rutledge, L. J. Esophageal stenosis produced by bleach; report of two cases. South. Med. J. *63*:1140-1144, 1970.

Gleason, M. N.; Gosselin, R. E.; Hodge, H. C. Mixing of chlorine bleach with other household cleaning agents. Bull. Supplementary Materials, Clinical Toxicology of Commercial Products 8(No. 5):8-11, 1964.

Griffith, J. F. Personal communication. Procter and Gamble Company, Feb. 1962.

Landau, G. D.; Saunders, W. H. The effect of chlorine bleach on the esophagus. Arch. Otolaryngol. *80*:174-176, 1964.

Loeb, F. X.; King, T. L. Chronic duodenitis due to laundry bleach. Am. J. Dis. Child *128*:256-257, 1974.

Lynch, R. E.; Lee, G. R.; Kushner, J. P. Porphyria cutanea tarda associated with disinfectant misuse. Arch. Intern. Med. *135*:549-552, 1975.

Muhlendahl, K. E. v.; Oberdisse, U.; Krienke, E. G. Local injuries by accidental ingestion of corrosive substances by children. Arch. Toxicol. *39*:299-324, 1978.

Pike, D. G.; Peabody, J. W., Jr.; Davis, E. W.; Lyons, W. S. A re-evaluation of the dangers of Clorox ingestion. J. Pediatr. *63*:303-305, 1963.

Sheldon, J. M.; Lovell, R. G. Asthma due to halogens. Am. Practitioner *4*:43-44, 1949.

Strange, D. C.; Finneran, J. C.; Shumacker, H. B., Jr.; Bowman, D. E. Corrosive injury of the stomach; report of a case caused by ingestion of Clorox and experimental study of injurious effects. Arch. Surg. *62*:350-357, 1951.

Watson, S. H.; Kibler, C. S. Drinking water as a cause of asthma. J. Allergy *5*:197-198, 1933.

Weeks, R. S.; Ravitch, M. M. Esophageal injury by liquid chlorine bleach; experimental study. J. Pediatr. *74*:911-916, 1969.

Yarington, C. T., Jr. Ingestion of caustic: A pediatric problem. J. Pediatr. *67*:674-677, 1965.

IMIPRAMINE

Imipramine (*e.g.*, Tofranil), the first successful "tricyclic antidepressant," is selected here as typifying this entire group of drugs, although amitryptyline (*e.g.*, Elavil) is probably the most popular example today. Tricyclic antidepressants are widely used in the management of psychiatric depression. They are also used sometimes in children for the treatment of enuresis, but because they are potent and dangerous, they probably should be reserved for intractable cases (Goel and Shanks, 1974).

The mechanisms responsible for the therapeutic efficacy of tricyclic antidepressants have not been adequately identified, but as a class these drugs have a bewildering array of pharmacologic effects: sedation, cholinergic receptor blockade (antimuscarinic), α-adrenergic receptor blockade, inhibition of catecholamine uptake mechanism at adrenergic nerve endings, blockade of H1 and H2 histamine receptors, and a quinidine-like effect on the heart (impairment of both conduction and contractility). Because tricyclics are said to prevent the centrally-mediated antihypertensive action of clonidine, it is possible that they block α_2- as well as α_1-adrenergic receptors. The inhibition of the adrenergic neuronal reuptake mechanism accounts for the potentiated responses to injected catecholamines and for the potentiation of the central and peripheral stimulant actions of amphetamines. Which, if any, of these effects is related to the therapeutic use of the tricyclics is not known, but at least some of the toxic effects described below can be accounted for by the antimuscarinic, alpha-blocking, and quinidine-like actions. Many of these actions are shared by the chemically related phenothiazine tranquilizers; see CHLORPROMAZINE, p. III-109.

Imipramine and amitriptyline are both demethylated in the liver to yield the active metabolites, desipramine and nortriptyline respectively. The latter compounds are also marketed as drugs (e.g., Norpramin, Aventyl). Protriptyline (Vivactil), trimipramine (Surmontil) and doxepin (e.g., Adapin, Sinequan) are similar drugs. Newer agents include the tricyclic antipsychotic drug loxapine (Loxitane) and its desmethyl analog, amoxapine (Asendin). Maprotiline (Ludiomil) is described as a tetracyclic antidepressant; it shares, however, many of the same adverse effects as the tricyclics.

Toxicology: Tricyclics have produced many serious and fatal intoxications in infants, children and adults, but there is an impression that their effects are not so dramatic or dangerous in adults as in children (Noble and Matthew, 1970). In either case there is considerable variation in reported lethal doses in humans. Indeed, variations among patients may be more important than any differences among the various drugs.

Imipramine always produces severe symptoms or death when the ingested dose exceeds 20 mg./kg. Adults have succumbed to 500 to 750 mg., but several have survived doses of 1 gm. or more (more than 5 gm. in one case); few children could tolerate such a dose (Brophy, 1967; Fréjaville et al., 1966; Hall, 1970; Steel et al., 1967).

Nortriptyline has produced severe intoxications in adults in doses of 600 and 950 mg. (Duke and Horton, 1969; Stinnett et al., 1968), but 2 to 3 times these doses have been survived (Rendoing et al., 1969). Doses of 1000 to 2500 mg. of desipramine have produced severe poisonings in adults (Bucher and Stucki, 1967; Heitmann and Kunst, 1968; Tchen et al., 1966; Williams, 1964). Four mg./kg. of amitriptyline produced mild signs of intoxication in a child (Fendrick, 1962); the mean lethal dose by mouth for an adult would appear to be 1000 mg. (Beighton and Hardingham, 1966; Davies and Allaye, 1963b; Lloyd et al., 1967; Mehrotra, 1965). Adult therapeutic doses of these drugs are about 60 to 100 mg. per day. They appear to be at least one order of magnitude more toxic to man than to laboratory rodents (Meyers et al., 1966).

Tricyclic overdoses lead to a wide variety of syndromes, all of which can be dangerous and difficult to manage. Two organ systems which are principally affected are the heart and the central nervous system. Cardiac and CNS disorders may coexist or they may occur singly. Death may result from functional impairment of either organ system or in some cases from aspiration pneumonitis (Bickel et al., 1967; Fréjaville et al., 1966). Aspiration, however, may not have been responsible for 2 fatal cases of pneumonitis encountered after amitriptyline overdoses (Marshall and Moore, 1973; Sunshine and Yaffe, 1963). Reported fatality rates in hospitalized victims of tricyclic poisoning vary from about 0.5 to 5%.

Cardiac arrhythmias and conduction defects occur in most severe poisonings and create major problems in management. The documented accumulation of tricyclics in high concentrations in the myocardium is presumably responsible for these disorders. The initial sinus tachycardia has been ascribed to an anticholinergic (antimuscarinic) action at cardiac vagal nerve endings. Some of the arrhythmias may be due to circulating epinephrine; the myocardium is thought to be especially responsive to endogenous catecholamines because the reuptake system at cardiac adrenergic nerve endings is blocked. Hypotension compromises coronary flow and so may predispose to disordered mechanisms of beat. Finally, direct myocardial toxic effects are also believed to play an important role (Alexander and Nino, 1969; Chahine and Castellanos, 1971).

Marked ECG changes in imipramine poisoning include prolonged QT interval, widening of QRS complexes, depression of ST segments and T wave changes, configurations often associated with myocardial infarctions (Barnes et al., 1968; Freeman et al., 1969; Davis et al., 1968; Sacks et al., 1968; Thorstrand, 1976). A QRS interval of greater than 100 msec. is said to be common in severe poisonings and suggests a high tricyclic blood level (Bailey et al., 1978; Thorstrand, 1976). As in digitalis poisoning, almost every possible rhythm and conduction defect has been described: atrial and ventricular tachycardias, flutters and fibrillations; various types of blocks and bradyarrhythmias (rarely seen except as a late phenomenon); multifocal extrasystoles; and cardiac arrest. These disturbances may be accompanied by profound hypotension presumably due to low cardiac output (Starkey and Lawson, 1980), although the shock may be partly vasogenic (Langou et al., 1980).

Severe cardiac derangements almost always begin within 6 hours after the ingestion and usually last no longer than 1 to 2 days. In some cases sudden cardiac arrest occurred, even at a time when vital signs were stable or improving (Davies and Allaye, 1963a; Masters, 1967). Indeed a risk of cardiac arrest may exist for several days, although the danger appears to be low after the first 24 hours. With perhaps one exception (Sueblinvong and Wilson, 1969), survivors suffer no permanent cardiac damage. In contrast to quinidine poisoning, children seem to be even more susceptible than adults to serious cardiac complications in tricyclic poisoning (e.g., Arneson, 1961; Giles, 1963). Tricyclics are also especially dangerous in persons with preexisting cardiovascular disease (Muller et al., 1961). Substantial numbers of overdosed adults, however, develop no cardiac effects more ominous than mild sinus tachycardia (Noble and Matthew, 1970; Sedal et al., 1972; Thorstrand, 1976).

Among the tricyclic antidepressant drugs

available on the market today, at least minor differences are recognized in terms of their cardiotoxic potential. For example, amitriptyline and doxepin are more arrhythmogenic than imipramine, at least in dogs (Brown and Leversha, 1979). The demethylated derivatives of imipramine and amitriptyline may be slightly more cardiotoxic than the parent drugs (Nicotra et al., 1981). The 2-hydroxy metabolites of imipramine and of desipramine are said to be significantly more cardiotoxic than the parent compounds. On the other hand overdoses of loxapine and amoxapine have produced severe brain dysfunction without cardiac effects other than sinus tachycardia (Kulig et al., 1982; Peterson, 1981). On occasion, however, significant ECG disorders have been observed in amoxapine poisoning (Bock et al., 1982). All of these drugs are capable of producing coma, convulsions and other forms of neurologic damage (e.g., Goldberg and Spector, 1982).

The central nervous system manifestations of tricyclic overdosage can be as complicated and as dangerous as the cardiac effects (Fréjaville et al., 1966; Fasoli and Glauser, 1981). Patients, particularly those in the pediatric age range, are apt to show fluctuating states of consciousness, ranging from drowsiness or coma to agitation, delirium, hallucinations and twitching. Grand mal convulsions may occur even in the comatose patient, as well as frequent myoclonic jerks (Arneson, 1961; Petit et al., 1977). Deep coma and respiratory depression are signs of severe poisoning (Brown et al., 1971; Sunshine and Yaffe, 1963). The fluctuating neurologic signs may include periods of hyperirritability with choreiform movements, cogwheel rigidity of the extremities, and opisthotonus (Fréjaville et al., 1966). Hypothermia and less commonly hyperpyrexia are described (Giles, 1963; Harthorne et al., 1963; Nicotra et al., 1981; Lee, 1961). Tendon reflexes may be hyperactive or depressed.

The antimuscarinic activity of tricyclic antidepressants is expressed in terms of dry mouth, urinary retention, absent bowel sounds, hot dry skin and sinus tachycardia; mydriasis, sometimes with blurred vision and pupillary paralysis, is particularly common (Bailey et al., 1978). The delirium, twitching and hyperpyrexia may all be manifestations of central anticholinergic activity, but the convulsions almost certainly represent a different central mechanism.

Coma is often brief (a few hours) but it may last for many days. Even after the patient has regained consciousness, abnormal EEG patterns, extrapyramidal signs and acute psychosis have been observed; sometimes permanent brain damage occurs (Alajem and Albagli, 1962; Sueblinvong and Wilson, 1969; Sedal et al., 1972). Although tricyclic antidepressants are not generally regarded as addictive, a withdrawal syndrome has been described in patients who had been treated over prolonged periods of time (Agbayewa, 1981).

As a group the tricyclics are rapidly and completely absorbed from the gastrointestinal tract. Plasma levels, however are never very high, and in fatal poisonings the liver concentrations of free drug and metabolites were 3- to 20-fold higher than the blood levels (Munksgaard, 1969). Imipramine is extensively metabolized. Some 20 urinary metabolites have been identified provisionally; besides desmethylimipramine, major metabolites are the 2-hydroxy derivatives of both imipramine and desipramine. In nontoxic doses only 40% of the total radioactivity of an oral dose in man is excreted in the urine over 24 hours and 75% is excreted after 3 days (Crammer et al., 1969). Very little of this excreted radioactivity is likely to have been in the form of biologically active molecules.

Therapeutic considerations: Because of the threat of tachyarrhythmias leading to cardiac arrest, continuous cardiac monitoring for at least 24 hours is important in any severely ill, tricyclic-poisoned patient, particularly if the QRS interval is greater than 100 msec. As in QUINIDINE poisoning (p. III-355), the various types of circulatory disorders encountered in tricyclic poisoning require different programs of therapy.

Although hypertension has been reported in a few cases (Giles, 1963; Peterson, 1981), hypotension is often observed; it is sometimes severe and ominous, especially that occurring in association with bradycardia in the late stages of severe poisonings (e.g., Ruddy, 1972). This bradycardia has been successfully managed with a transvenous pacemaker (Sueblinvong and Wilson, 1969). In most cases the hypotension probably reflects a low cardiac output due to impaired contractility of the myocardium (but see Langou et al., 1980, for a contrary opinion). Accordingly vasoconstrictor drugs are generally inappropriate. Metaraminol led to further deterioration of the cardiac status in at least one case (Colvard, 1968), and methoxamine had no beneficial actions in another (Garrison and Moffitt, 1962).

Drugs with positiove inotropic actions on the myocardium may have a useful role in tricyclic poisoning. Isoproterenol has been tried in severely poisoned children (Ruddy, 1972) and adults (Moccetti et al., 1971). Intravenous isoproterenol enhanced the survival rate of nortriptyline- and amitriptyline-poisoned cats (Lum et al., 1982); a selective β_1-adrenergic agonist such as dobutamine might have been superior, but all adrenergic agonists increase the risk of ventricular tachycardia. Digitalis appears to have been lifesaving in a 2.5-year-old boy who had consumed 1 gm. imipramine (Sueblinvong and Wilson, 1969), and ouabain proved to be effective in imipramine-poisoned dogs (Laddu and Somani,

1969). In spite of these demonstrations, cardiac glycosides are often regarded as dangerous in tricyclic poisoning because they too can induce conduction defects and arrhythmias. Intravenous glucagon was tested against refractory cardiac failure in one patient (Ruddy, 1972). In most cases, however, the hypotension does not require specific attention; it often disappears as the tachycardia subsides.

That vagal blockade plays a role in generating the sinus tachycardia and other supraventricular tachycardias (atrial, nodal) of tricyclic poisoning is suggested by their sensitivity to injections of pyridostigmine (Pearson *et al.*, 1969; Rasmussen, 1965; Torchiana *et al.*, 1972), neostigmine (Royds and Knight, 1970; Lloyd *et al.*, 1967) and physostigmine (Slovis *et al.*, 1971). With a reduction in the ventricular rate, the blood pressure and arterial circulation may improve. More surprisingly, intraventricular conduction defects (wide QRS, bundle branch blocks) may also improve with physostigmine therapy, as evidenced by narrowing and normalization of bizarre QRS complexes (Tobis and Das, 1976; Wright, 1976); apparently these conduction defects are rate-sensitive. It is difficult, however, to distinguish between a supraventricular tachycardia with bundle branch block and/or aberrant AV conduction on the one hand and a ventricular tachycardia on the other; published reports of tricyclic poisonings do not resolve this issue. A true ventricular tachycardia that slows with anticholinesterase therapy is presumably due to a pacemaker in the ventricular conducting system, probably the proximal portion such as the bundle of His or the main bundle branches, which in mammals are known to be innervated by the vagus. Whatever the mechanism, slowing of the rate and occasionally reversion to a sinus rhythm have been observed after intravenous physostigmine therapy (*e.g.*, Wright, 1976), but severe bradycardia and even asystole have also been induced in tricyclic poisoned adults, even when a 2 mg. dose of physostigmine was injected slowly (Pentel and Peterson, 1980).

Ventricular tachycardias arising from ectopic foci in the distal myocardium or from reentry mechanisms not involving proximal portions of the Purkinje apparatus are almost certainly refractory to cholinergic stimuli. Because such tachycardias may deteriorate into ventricular fibrillation (*e.g.*, Freeman *et al.*, 1969; Sesso *et al.*, 1973), they should be treated vigorously. In tricyclic poisonings success has been reported with many antiarrhythmic (antifibrillatory) drugs, including procainamide (Ruddy, 1972), propranolol (Roberts *et al.*, 1973; Sesso *et al.*, 1973) and phenytoin sodium (Moccetti *et al.*, 1971). In conscious, amitriptyline-poisoned rabbits, intravenous clonidine and verapamil, alone or in combination, were the most effective drugs for restoring a sinus rhythm (El-Hage *et al.*, 1982), but no clinical trials have been reported in humans. Potassium chloride by infusion has been used successfully at least once (Penny, 1968); it should be particularly valuable in treating tachycardias in the small minority of tricyclic-poisoned patients with distinct hypokalemia (Goldberg and Spector, 1982; Thorstrand, 1976). Because of its short duration, the ease of controlling the response and the relatively small risk of inducing AV blockade, intravenous lidocaine is probably the most widely used of the conventional antiarrhythmic drugs in tricyclic poisonings.

The single most effective measure, however, for ameliorating or terminating serious arrhythmias in poisoned children and dogs (but not guinea pigs) is said to be an infusion of sodium bicarbonate or of the amine buffer THAM (Brown 1976a and b). Poisoned adults also respond well to sodium bicarbonate infusions (Slovis *et al.*, 1971), but the precise nature of the sensitive tachyarrhythmias has not been adequately documented. Sodium lactate (1 M) infusions have also been recommended on the basis of extensive trials (Fréjaville *et al.*, 1966). The pretreatment acid-base status of many of these patients was not specified. Whether the beneficial effects of sodium bicarbonate and sodium lactate are due to a sodium effect, the correction of acidosis, or the production of alkalosis remains unclear. Respiratory alkalosis from hyperventilation may also have a beneficial, though transient effect. One theory is that alkalosis enhances tricyclic binding to plasma proteins. In a series of 68 poisonings, however, no relationship was found between ECG abnormalities and pre-treatment serum levels of sodium, potassium or bicarbonate (Serafimovski *et al.*, 1975).

It is doubtful that all patients whose cardiovascular status improved with sodium bicarbonate treatment were initially acidotic, because significant acidosis is not found in most victims of tricyclic overdoses (Thorstrand, 1976). Acidosis is not rare, however; those in deep coma usually have a mixed acidosis, partly respiratory and partly metabolic (Sutherland *et al.*, 1977). In a few instances, particularly in post-ictal and in hyperpyrexic patients, this acidosis was found to be intense and associated with high anion gaps (*e.g.*, Goldberg and Spector, 1982). Certainly any acidosis, metabolic or respiratory, should be treated promptly and vigorously in victims of tricyclic poisoning, whatever the cardiac status.

For the neurologic deficits, a variety of therapeutic measures is available. In the presence of respiratory depression, ventilatory assistance has the highest priority. Agitation and convulsions can be controlled with barbiturates, but these drugs are thought to potentiate markedly the respiratory depression (Fréjaville *et al.*, 1966; Stark and Bethune, 1965). For this reason, diazepam is probably the drug of choice for controlling convulsions (Young and Galloway, 1971). Sometimes intravenous phenytoin sodium is used for this purpose (Kulig *et al.*, 1982).

Besides its usefulness in overcoming some of the cardiac disturbances, intravenous physostigmine has been shown to correct rapidly and dramatically both coma and convulsions in some patients with tricyclic poisoning (Munoz, 1976; Slovis *et al.*, 1971; Tobis and Das, 1976; Wright, 1976). It is also effective against choreiform movements in man and other neurologic signs in dogs (Burks *et al.*, 1974; Torchiana *et al.*, 1972). These favorable but usually brief responses to physostigmine are presumably due to its ability to penetrate the blood-brain barrier and to antagonize cholinergic blockade in the brain. In one patient poisoned with doxepin, physostigmine produced a favorable but transient response. In attempting to repeat the phenomenon, neostigmine was given in error with no response. When the error was discovered and physostigmine was reinjected, another favorable response ensued (Janson *et al.*, 1977). A beneficial reaction to intravenous physostigmine, usually within 5 minutes, has been used as an aid in diagnosing intoxications due to tricyclic antidepressants or to other central anticholinergic poisons (Aquilonius and Hedstrand, 1978). To sustain a therapeutic action, an effective dose may have to be repeated every half hour.

Physostigmine therapy, however, can be dangerous, and its proper role in the management of tricyclic poisoning is in dispute. Not all therapists find it effective in suppressing convulsions (*e.g.*, Starkey and Lawson, 1980), and Aquilonius and Hedstrand (1978) are not persuaded that it decreases mortality in poisoned humans. There is little merit in awakening a comatose patient if he is then confused and combative. Furthermore the drug may trigger seizures and produce severe cholinergic signs (*e.g.*, bronchorrhea and bronchospasm) even in patients overdosed with tricyclics (Aquilonius and Hedstrand, 1978; Newton, 1975). Physostigmine in subtoxic doses does increase the seizure activity and lethality of several tricyclics in mice and rats (Vance *et al.*, 1977; Wiezorek and Kaestner, 1982). Probably physostigmine should be reserved for life-threatening complications after they have proven refractory to other forms of therapy.

The common approaches to hastening elimination of a drug, such as forced diuresis (Lloyd and Hart, 1965; Ward and Tin-Myint, 1965), peritoneal dialysis (Halle and Collipp, 1969a), extracorporeal hemodialysis (Harthorne *et al.*, 1963; Pall *et al.*, 1976) and even exchange trans-

fusion (Louis *et al.*, 1970; Sidiropoulos and Bickel, 1971), do not benefit dramatically victims of tricyclic overdoses. Relatively small amounts of drug can be recovered by these procedures, probably because the tricyclics have a very large volume of distribution (10 to 60 L./kg.) in the body and are extensively bound to tissues and to plasma proteins. In an *in vitro* model system, hemodialysis against soybean oil was found to be superior to aqueous dialysis; besides drug in the dialysate, the polyvinyl chloride tubing of the apparatus was found to absorb imipramine (Asbach *et al.*, 1977). A few patients have been treated with apparent success by hemoperfusion over activated charcoal or XAD-4 resin (Diaz-Buxo *et al.*, 1978; Trafford *et al.*, 1977). Even though only small amounts of tricyclics were recovered, rapid clearance of the blood may have been temporarily beneficial (Heath *et al.*, 1982). Although most therapists are skeptical about the effectiveness of any form of hemoperfusion in tricyclic poisoning, at least several reports agree that hemoperfusion over Amberlite resins is superior to that over activated charcoal (Heath *et al.*, 1980a; Pedersen *et al.*, 1978; Trafford *et al.*, 1980a).

The discovery that a sizeable amount of imipramine is secreted into the stomach and that another component undergoes extensive enterohepatic recycling has led to the suggestion that repeated doses of activated charcoal may be helpful. In one case continuous aspiration of gastric contents for 24 hours removed much more drug than did urinary excretion (Gard *et al.*, 1973). Certainly charcoal is effective in reducing absorption of these drugs from the gastrointestinal tract (Crome *et al.*, 1977a).

Symptomatology:

1. After a latent period of 1 to 12 hours (usually less than 6 hours), increasing agitation, restlessness and motor disturbances, including involuntary jerky movements and spasticity.
2. Atropinic signs and symptoms, including dryness of the mouth and eventually mydriasis (sometimes with photophobia and blurred vision), sinus tachycardia, urinary retention, absent bowel sounds, hot dry skin, fixed dilated pupils.
3. Extreme agitation, delirium, auditory and visual hallucinations.
4. Twitching, exaggerated tendon reflexes, myoclonic jerks, choreiform movements, cogwheel rigidity of the limbs. Generalized tonic-clonic convulsions or opisthotonus may occur spontaneously or be precipitated by external stimuli. Positive Babinski sign. Nystagmus.
5. Drowsiness may progress rapidly to coma,

with depression of tendon reflexes, respiratory depression, and apnea. Particularly in children, coma may be accompanied by rapidly fluctuating neurologic states, ranging from flaccidity to hyperirritability and convulsions. Abnormal EEG patterns. Coma and associated neurologic signs may persist for several days but usually subside after 24 hours.

6. Mild hypothermia is common, but dangerous hyperpyrexia does occur. Together with the convulsions, fever may lead to severe metabolic acidosis.

7. Independent of the neurological derangements and sometimes even in their absence, circulatory disorders evidenced by tachycardia, arrhythmias, hypotension (although hypertension is occasionally observed) and in severe poisonings cardiac arrest. Hypotension may lead to circulatory shock.

8. ECG abnormalities include widening of the QRS, prolonged QT interval, marked changes in ST segment and T waves. Sinus tachycardia is the commonest rate disorder, but almost every recognized abnormal mechanism of beat has been reported, including conduction defects (AV blockade, bundle branch blocks, etc.) and both atrial and ventricular tachyarrhythmias. Ventricular tachycardia may lead to brief episodes of ventricular fibrillation (which either revert or end in asystole). Bradyarrhythmias are also ominous and often presage cardiac arrest.

9. Oliguria or anuria, aspiration pneumonitis, late cardiac arrest and persisting neuropsychiatric disorders may complicate or interrupt convalescence. Among survivors recovery is usually complete in 2 to 5 days. Permanent brain damage is rare, and irreversible cardiac injury is almost unknown.

Treatment:

1. If the patient is comatose or severely obtunded, insert a cuffed endotracheal tube (p. IV-4) to protect the airway. Support ventilation (pp. IV-7-12) and administer oxygen (p. IV-12), as indicated.

2. Control extreme agitation, preconvulsive hyperreflexia and convulsions with intravenous diazepam (5 to 10 mg. in adults); see p. IV-37. Alternatively, intravenous physostigmine may be tried (see 11 below).

3. In severely ill patients, especially those with prolonged QRS complexes (greater than 100 msec.), institute continuous cardiac monitoring. Be prepared to defibrillate with DC countershocks (p. IV-30) and to administer cardiac massage (p. IV-26).

4. Perform gastric aspiration and lavage (p. I-8). Because of delayed gastric emptying, it may be worthwhile even many hours after the ingestion. Do not use ipecac, except perhaps in the presymptomatic phase shortly after the ingestion.

5. Instill into the stomach activated charcoal and sodium sulfate (p. I-12). To trap drug and active metabolites secreted into the stomach or duodenum (through bile), it may be useful to administer a slurry of activated charcoal every few hours.

6. Dehydration, acidosis and hypokalemia may require parenteral fluid therapy (p. IV-69-73), but the deficits are usually mild. Avoid excessive fluid therapy.

7. Tachycardias, tachyarrhythmias, bradycardia, bradyarrhythmias, conduction defects and hypotension are all said to respond favorably to intravenous injections or infusions of sodium bicarbonate (p. IV-72). A safe and still effective dose has not been adequately defined, but children have received 0.5 to 2 mEq./kg. (apparently as 0.5 to 2 M solutions) by slow intravenous injection (Brown, 1976a). Avoid higher doses unless required to correct a demonstrated acidosis (p. IV-69).

8. If sodium bicarbonate does not correct severe bradycardia, a transvenous pacemaker (p. IV-30) may be required.

9. Mild hypotension should be treated cautiously, if at all. Severe hypotension and shock, however, warrant serious attention. The cautious infusion of blood volume expanders (e.g., saline, plasma) and perhaps the administration of vasoconstrictor drugs have been suggested (Langou et al., 1980). On the other hand, if shock is cardiogenic in type (high central venous pressure) and the heart rate is not excessive, a slow infusion of isoproterenol, dopamine, dobutamine or glucagon may raise cardiac output and blood pressure. Alternatively, rapid digitalization with ouabain may be tried. See pp. IV-20-21.

10. Ventricular tachycardia or frequent ventricular premature beats warrants a trial with intravenous lidocaine (p. IV-25) to prevent ventricular fibrillation. Other antiarrhythmic drugs may be effective but are probably more dangerous (pp. IV-23-26).

11. Supraventricular tachycardias and probably some "high" ventricular tachycardias may slow down and even revert to a sinus rhythm after physostigmine treatment. An intravenous test dose in adults is 1 to 2 mg. physostigmine salicylate, injected no faster than 1 mg./minute, repeated in 10 to 15 minutes up to a total dose of 4

mg. If the response is favorable, 2 mg. doses may be reinjected at 20- to 60-minute intervals, as required. If the response is not favorable, give no more physostigmine. In children the usual test dose is 0.5 mg., repeated if necessary at 10-minute intervals to a total dose of 2 mg. The injections may also terminate hallucinations, convulsions and coma, but because of occasional dangerous untoward reactions (see text above), physostigmine should probably be restricted to life-threatening anticholinergic crises. Never use it in the presence of bradycardia.

12. Mild hypothermia may require no attention, but hyperpyrexia always requires vigorous therapy; see p. IV-84.

13. Severe and prolonged intoxication may warrant hemoperfusion (through Amberlite XAD-4), but forced diuresis, peritoneal dialysis and hemodialysis are not worthwhile.

14. Be alert for signs of pneumonia and treat incipient infections vigorously (see pp. IV-85–86).

Laboratory:

1. In the absence of a reliable history, a chemical analysis of the plasma for imipramine may be crucial in the diagnosis. Drug and metabolite levels in plasma have been found to correlate statistically with some of the clinical signs and ECG disorders (Nicotra *et al.*, 1981; Petit *et al.*, 1977), but the correlations are not impressive (Bailey *et al.*, 1978). Moreover, the range of plasma concentrations reported in toxic patients is so wide (less than 100 to more than 1700 ng. imipramine per ml.) that knowledge of an individual plasma level appears to have little prognostic value (Bailey *et al.*, 1978; Langou *et al.*, 1980).

2. Plasma analyses for the assessment of acidosis and the detection of hypokalemia are important guides in therapy.

References:

Agbayewa, M. O. Withdrawal sysmptoms after tricyclic antidepressants. Can. Med. Assoc. J. *125*:420–422, 1981.

Alajem, N.; Albagli, C. Severe imipramine poisoning in an infant. Am. J. Dis. Child. *103*:702-705, 1962.

Alexander, C. S.; Nino, A. Cardiovascular complications in young patients taking psychotropic drugs. Am. Heart J. *78*:757-769, 1969.

Aquilonius, S. -M.; Hedstrand, U. The use of physostigmine as an antidote in tricyclic anti-depressant intoxication. Acta Anaesthesiol. Scand. *22*:40–45, 1978.

Arneson, G. A. Near fatal case of imipramine overdosage. Am. J. Psychiatry *117*:934-936, 1961.

Asbach, H. W.; Holz, F.; Mohring, K.; Schuler, H. W. Lipid hemodialysis versus charcoal hemoperfusion in imipramine poisoning. Clin. Toxicol. *11*:211–219, 1977.

Bailey, D. N; Vandyke, C.; Langou, R. A.,; Jatlow, P. I.

Tricyclic antidepressants - plasma levels and clinical findings in overdose. Am J. Psychiatr. *135*:1325–1328, 1978.

Barnes, R. J.; Kong, S. M.; Wu, R. W. Y. Electrocardiographic changes in amitriptyline poisoning. Br. Med. J. *27*:222-223, 1968.

Beighton, P.; Hardingham, M. Amitriptyline poisoning treated by forced diuresis. Practitioner *197*:354-357, 1966.

Bickel, M. H.; Brochon, R.; Friolet, B.; Herrmann, B.; Stofer, A. R. Clinical and biochemical results of a fatal case of desipramine intoxication. Psychopharmacologia *10*:431-436, 1967.

Bock, J. L; Cummings, K. C.; Jatlow, P. I. Amoxapine overdose: a case report. Clin. Res. Rep. *139*:1619–1620, 1982.

Brophy, J. J. Suicide attempts with psychotherapeutic drugs. Arch. Gen. Psychiatry *17*:652-657, 1967.

Brown, T. C. K.; Dwyer, M. E.; Stocks, J. G. Antidepressant overdosage in children - a new menace. Med. J. Aust. *2*:848-851, 1971.

Brown, T. C. K. Sodium bicarbonate treatment for tricyclic antidepressant arrhythmias in children. Med. J. Aust. *2*:380–382, 1976a.

Brown, T. C. K. Tricyclic antidepressant overdosage: Experimental studies on the management of circulatory complications. Clin. Toxicol. *9*:255–272, 1976b.

Brown, T. C. K.; Leversha, A. Comparison of the cardiovascular toxicity of three tricyclic antidepressant drugs: imipramine, amitriptyline, and doxepin. Clin. Toxicol. *14*:253–256, 1979.

Bucher, H. W.; Stucki, P. Kardiale Komplikationen bei einer Vergiftung mit Desipramin (Pertofran). Schweiz. Med. Wochenschr. *97*:519-521, 1967.

Burks, J. S.; Walker, J. E.; Rumack, B. H.; Ott, J. E. Tricyclic antidepressant poisoning; reversal of coma, choreoathetosis, and myoclonus by physostigmine. J. A. M. A. *230*:1405-1407, 1974.

Chahine, R. A.; Castellanos, A., Jr. Myocardial toxicity produced by desipramine overdosage. Chest *59*:566-568, 1971.

Colvard, C., Jr. Overdosage of desipramine hydrochloride with marked electrocardiographic abnormalities. South. Med. J. *61*:1218-1222, 1968.

Crammer, J. L.; Scott, B.; Rolfe, B. Metabolism of ¹⁴C-imipramine. II. Urinary metabolites in man. Psychopharmacologia *15*:207-225, 1969.

Crome, P.; Dawling, S.; Braithwaite, R. A.; Masters, J.; Walkey, R. Effect of activated charcoal on absorption of nortriptyline. Lancet *2*:1203–1205, 1977a.

Davies, D. M.; Allaye, R. Amitriptyline poisoning. Lancet *2*:543, 1963a.

Davies, D. M.; Allaye, R. Amitriptyline poisoning. Lancet *2*:643, 1963b.

Davis, J. M.; Bartlett, E.; Termini, B. A. Overdosage of psychotropic drugs: A review. Dis. Nerv. Syst. *29*:157-164 and 246-256, 1968.

Diaz-Buxo, J. A.; Farmer, C. D.; Chandler, J. T. Hemoperfusion in the treatment of amitriptyline intoxication. Trans. Am. Soc. Artif. Intern. Organs *24*:699–703, 1978.

Duke, W. W.; Horton, J. P. Nortriptyline (Aventyl) overdosage. South. Med. J. *62*:1348-1349, 1969.

El-Hage, A.; Balazs, T.; West, W. L. Protective effects of clonidine and verapamil in experimental amitriptyline poisoning in rabbits. J. Toxicol. Clin. Toxicol. *19*:321–335, 1982.

Fasoli, R. A.; Glauser, F. L. Tricyclic antidepressant overdose. Clin. Toxicol. *18*:155–163, 1981.

Fendrick, G. M. Amitriptyline poisoning. N. Engl. J. Med. *267*:1031-1032, 1962.

Freeman, J. W.; Mundy, G. R.; Beattie, R. R.; Ryan, C. Cardiac abnormalities in poisoning with tricyclic antidepressants. Br. Med. J. *2*:610-611, 1969.

Fréjaville, J. P.; Nicaise, A. M.; Christoforov, B.; Sraer, J. D.; Pebay-Peyroula, F.; Gaultier, M. Etude statistique d'une seconde centaine d'intoxications aigues par les derives de l'iminodibenzyle (tofranil, pertofran, G34, surmontil) et ceux du dihydrobenzocyclohepadiene (laroxyl, elavil). Bull. Soc. Med. Hop. Paris *117*:1151-1175, 1966.

Gard, H.; Knapp, D.; Walle, T.; Gaffney, T.; Hanenson, I. Qualitative and quantitative studies on the disposition of amitriptyline and other tricyclic antidepressant drugs in man as it relates to the management of the overdosed patient. Clin. Toxicol. 6:571-584, 1973.

Garrison, H.F.; Moffitt, E. M. Imipramine hydrochloride intoxication. J. A. M. A. 179:456-458, 1962.

Giles, H. M. Imipramine poisoning in childhood. Br. Med. J. 2:844-846, 1963.

Goel, K. M.; Shanks, R. A. Amitriptyline and imipramine poisoning in children. Br. Med. J. 1:261-263, 1974.

Goldberg, M. J.; Spector, R. Amoxapine overdose - Report of 2 patients with severe neurologic damage. Ann. Intern. Med. 96:463, 1982.

Hall, R. Tricyclic antidepressant tranquilizers. Bull. Natl. Clearinghouse for Poison Control Centers, May-June, 1970.

Halle, M. A.; Collipp, P. J. Amitriptyline hydrochloride poisoning. Unsuccessful treatment by peritoneal dialysis. N. Y. State J. Med. 69:1434-1436, 1969a.

Harthorne, J. W.; Marcus, A. M.; Kaye, M. Management of massive imipramine overdosage with mannitol and artificial dialysis. N. Engl. J. Med. 268:33-36, 1963.

Heath, A.; Wickstrom, I.; Ahlmen, J. Haemoperfusion in tricyclic antidepressant poisoning. Lancet 1:155, 1980a.

Heath, A.; Wickstrom, I.; Martenson, E.; Ahlmen, J. Treatment of antidepressant poisoning with resin hemoperfusion. Human Toxicol. 1:361-371, 1982.

Heitmann, R.; Kunst, H.Todlich verlaufene Vergiftung mit Pertofran. Dtsch. Med. Wochenschr. 93:117-120, 1968.

Janson, P. A.; Watt, J. B.; Hermos, J. A. Doxepin overdose. Success with physostigmine and failure with neostigmine in reversing toxicity. J.A.M.A. 237:2632-2633, 1977.

Kulig, K.; Rumack, B. H.; Sullivan, J. B., Jr.; Brandt, H.; Spyker, D. A.; Duffy, J. P.; Shipe, J. R. Amoxapine overdose. J.A.M.A. 248:1092-1094, 1982.

Laddu, A. R.; Somani, P. Desipramine toxicity and its treatment. Toxicol. Appl. Pharmacol. 15:287-294, 1969.

Langou, R. A.; Vandyke, C.; Tahan, S. R.; Cohen, L. S. Cardiovascular manifestations of tricyclic antidepressant overdose. Am. Heart J. 100:458-464, 1980.

Lee, F. I. Imipramine overdosage - report of a fatal case. Br. Med. J. 1:338-339, 1961.

Lloyd, T. W.; Hart, D. R.; Torode, J. A. Amitriptyline poisoning. Lancet 2:716-717, 1967.

Lloyd, T. W.; Hart, D. R. Amitriptyline poisoning. Lancet 2:554, 1965.

Louis, C.; Olbing, H.; Bohlmann, H. G.; Phillippou, A.; Heimsoth, V. Zur Behandlung der Imipramin-Vergiftung beim Kind. Dtsch. Med. Wochenschr. 95:2078-2082, 1970.

Lum, B. K. B.; Follmer, C. H.; Lockwood, R. H.; Thomas, H. M. Experimental studies on the effects of physostigmine and of isoproterenol on toxicity produced by tricyclic antidepressants. J. Toxicol. Clin. Toxicol. 19:51-65, 1982.

Marshall, A.; Moore, K. Pulmonary disease after amitriptyline overdosage. Brit. Med. J. 1:716-717, 1973.

Masters, A. B. Delayed deaths in imipramine poisoning. Br. Med. J. 3:866-867, 1967.

Mehrotra, T. N. Amitriptyline poisoning. Lancet 2:544-545, 1965.

Meyers, D. B.; Small, R. M.; Anderson, R. C. Toxicology of nortriptyline hydrochloride. Toxicol. Appl. Pharmacol. 9:152-159, 1966.

Moccetti, T.; Lichtlen, P.; Albert, H.; Meier, E.; Imbach, P. Kardiotoxizitat der trizyklischen Antidepressiva. Schweiz. Med. Wochenschr. 101:1-10, 1971.

Muller, O. F.; Goodman, N.; Bellet, S. The hypotensive effect of imipramine hydrochloride in patients with cardiovascular disease. Clin. Pharmacol. Ther. 2:300-307, 1961.

Munksgaard, E. C. Concentrations of amitriptyline and its metabolites in urine, blood and tissue in fatal amitriptyline poisoning. Acta Pharmacol. Toxicol. 27:129-134, 1969.

Munoz, R. A. Treatment of tricyclic intoxication. Am. J. Psychiatry 133:1085-1087, 1976.

Newton, R. W. Physostigmine salicylate in the treatment of tricyclic antidepressant overdose. J.A.M.A. 231:941-943, 1975.

Nicotra, M. B.; Rivera, M.; Pool, J. L.; Noall, M. W. Tricyclic antidepressant overdose: Clinical and pharmacological observations. Clin. Toxicol. 18:599-613, 1981.

Noble, J.; Matthew, H. Acute poisoning by tricyclic antidepressants: Clinical features and management of 100 patients. Clin. Toxicol. 2:403-421, 1970.

Pall, H.; Kleinberger, G.; Kotzaurek, R.; Pichler, M.; Szeless, S. Schwere Leponex - Vergiftung und ihre Intensivbehandlung. Wein. Klin. Wochenschr. 88:179-181, 1976.

Pearson, J. D.; Jones, E. S.; Gabbe, D. M. Cardiac arrest and arrhythmias due to self poisoning with imipramine. Anaesthesia 24:69-71, 1969.

Pedersen, R. S.; Jorgensen, K. A.; Olesen, A. S.; Christensen, K. N. Charcoal haemoperfusion and antidepressant overdose. Lancet 1:719, 1978.

Penny, R. Imipramine hydrochloride poisoning in childhood. Am. J. Dis. Child. 116:181-186, 1968.

Pentel, P.; Peterson, C. D. Asystole complicating physostigmine treatment of tricyclic antidepressant overdose. Ann. Emerg. Med. 9:588-590, 1980.

Peterson, C. D. Seizures induced by acute loxapine overdose. Am. J. Psychiatry 138:1089-1091, 1981.

Petit, J. M.; Spiker, D. G.; Ruwitch, J. F.; Ziegler, V. E.; Weiss, A. N. Tricyclic antidepressant plasma levels and adverse effects after overdose. Clin. Pharmacol. Ther. 21:47-51, 1977.

Rasmussen, J. Amitriptyline and imipramine poisoning. Lancet 2:850-851, 1965.

Rendoing, J.; Pasalis, C. C.; Gisselmann, A. Intoxication aigue par la nortriptyline. Presse Med. 77:439-440, 1969.

Roberts, R. J.; Mueller, S.; Lauer, R. M. Propranolol in the treatment of cardiac arrhythmias associated with amitriptyline intoxication. J. Pediatr. 82:65-67, 1973.

Royds, R. B.; Knight, A. H. Tricyclic antidepressant poisoning. Practitioner 204:282-286, 1970.

Ruddy, J. M. Management of tricyclic antidepressant ingestion in children with special reference to use of glucagon. Med. J. Aust. 1:630-633, 1972.

Sacks, M. H.; Bonforte, R.J.; Lasser, R. P.; Dimich, I. Complications of imipramine intoxication. J. A. M. A. 205:588-590, 1968.

Sedal, L.; Koerman, M. G.; Williams, F. O.; Mushin, G. Overdosage of tricyclic antidepressants; report of two deaths and a prospective study of 24 patients. Med. J. Aust. 2:74-79, 1972.

Serafimovski, N.; Thorball, N.; Asmussen, I.; Lunding, M. Tricyclic antidepressive poisoning with special reference to cardiac complications. Acta Anaesthesiologica Scand. Suppl. 57:55-63, 1975.

Sesso, A. M.; Snyder, R. C.; Schott, C. E. Propranolol in imipramine poisoning. Am. J. Dis. Child. 126:847-849, 1973.

Sidiropoulos, D.; Bickel, M. H. Eine todliche Vergiftung mit Imipramin in kleiner Dosis bei einem Kleinkind. Schweiz. Med. Wochenschr. 101:851-853, 1971.

Slovis, T. L.; Ott, J. E.; Teitelbaum, D. T.; Lipscomb, W. Physostigmine therapy in acute tricyclic antidepressant poisoning. Clin. Toxicol. 4:451-459, 1971.

Stark, J. E.; Bethune, D. W. Amitriptyline poisoning. Lancet 2:390, 1965.

Starkey, I. R.; Lawson, A. A. H. Poisoning with tricyclic and related antidepressants - a ten-year review. Q. J. Med. 49:33-49, 1980.

Steel, C. M.; O'Duffy, J.; Brown, S. S. Clinical effects and treatment of imipramine and amitriptyline. Br. Med. J. 3:663-667, 1967.

Stinnett, J. L.; Valentire, J.; Abrutyn, E. Nortriptyline hydrochloride overdosage. J. A. M. A. 204:69-71, 1968.

Sueblinvong, V.; Wilson, J. F. Myocardial damage due to imipramine intoxication. J. Pediatr. 74:475-478, 1969.

Sunshine, P.; Yaffe, S. J. Amitriptyline poisoning. Am. J. Dis. Child. 106:501-506, 1963.

Sutherland, G. R.; Park, J.; Proudfoot, A. T. Ventilation and acid-base changes in deep coma due to barbiturate or tricyclic antidepressant poisoning. Clin. Toxicol. 11:403-412, 1977.

Tchen, P.; Weatherhead, A. D.; Richards, N. G. Acute intoxication with desipramine. N. Engl. J. Med. 274:1197, 1966.

Thorstrand, C. Clinical features in poisonings by tricyclic antidepressants with special reference to the ECG. Acta Med. Scand. 199:337-344, 1976.

Tobis, J.; Das, B. N. Cardiac complications in amitriptyline poisoning. J.A.M.A. *235*:1474-1476, 1976.

Torchiana, M. L.; Wenger, H. C.; Lagerquist, G.; Morgan, G. M.; Stone, C. A. Pharmacological antagonism of the toxic manifestations of amitriptyline and protriptyline in dogs. Toxicol. Appl. Pharmacol. *21*:383-389, 1972.

Trafford, J. A. P.; Jones, R. H.; Evans, R.; Sharp, P.; Sharpstone, P.; Cook, J. Haemoperfusion with R-004 Amberlite resin for treating acute poisoning. Br. Med. J. *2*:1453-1456, 1977.

Trafford, A.; Sharpstone, P.; O'Neal, H. Haemoperfusion in tricyclic antidepressant poisoning. Lancet *1*:155, 1980a.

Vance, M. A.; Ross, S. M.; Millington, W. R.; Blumberg, J. B. Potentiation of tricyclic antidepressant toxicity by physo-

stigmine in mice. Clin. Toxicol. *11*:413-421, 1977.

Ward, F. G.; Tin-Myint, B. Amitriptyline poisoning. Lancet *2*:910, 1965.

Wiezorek, W. D.; Kaestner, I. Effects of physostigmine on acute toxicity of tricyclic antidepressants and benzodiazepines in mice and rats. Arch. Toxicol. Suppl. *5*:133-135, 1982.

Williams, A. J. Desipramine overdosage. Br. Med. J. *1*:371-372, 1964.

Wright, S. P. Usefulness of physostigmine in imipramine poisoning. A dramatic response in a child resistant to other therapy. Clin. Pediatr. *15*:1123-1128, 1976.

Young, J. A.; Galloway, W. H. Treatment of severe imipramine poisoning. Arch. Dis. Child. *46*:353-355, 1971.

IODINE

Iodine, one of the oldest antiseptics in modern medicine, still maintains its popularity because it is economical and moderately effective as a skin antiseptic, bactericide, fungicide, amebicide, and counterirritant. It is used most frequently as the official USP tincture (2% iodine and 2% NaI in 50% alcohol), but it is also available as Strong Iodine Solution, also known as Lugol's solution (5% iodine and 10% KI in aqueous solution) (Gershenfeld and Witlin, 1950; Nye, 1937). The strong iodine tincture (7%) and iodine ointment (4%) have been virtually eliminated. The iodide salts make no significant contribution to the toxicity of these mixtures.

The discussion below is probably also relevant to the ingestion of liquid bromine. If only because of its higher concentration, the reaction to liquid bromine is likely to be far more severe than that following ingestion of the common iodine preparations. No cases of liquid bromine ingestion can be cited, but the gas is known to be intensely irritating (see Section II).

Toxicology: Accidental and suicidal poisonings from iodine are not uncommon, but fatalities are rare (Moore, 1938). Reported lethal doses in adults range from a few tenths of a gram to more than 20 gm. Probably the mean lethal dose lies between 2 and 4 gm. of free iodine or 1 to 2 oz. of the strong tincture (Reese, 1874; Webster, 1930). Because the symptoms after a sublethal dose may be as distressing as those after a lethal dose, it may be difficult to estimate the amount ingested or to make a realistic prognosis (Moore, 1938).

Poisoning is due largely to the highly corrosive action of iodine on the gastrointestinal tract, an action which arises at least in part from the oxidizing potential of this element. Food present in the digestive tract rapidly inactivates iodine by converting it to comparatively harmless iodide. If death intervenes, it is usually within 48 hours (Finkelstein and Jacobi, 1937).

Other routes of administration are occasionally a source of poisoning. Inhalation of iodine vapor is very irritating to mucous membranes, and both upper airway and pulmonary effects have been described in laboratory animals (Amdur, 1978). Application of iodine to the skin may rarely give rise to a hypersensitivity reaction in the form of fever and generalized skin eruption that has proved fatal (Seymour, 1937). Local inflammatory reactions (burns) were not uncommon after cutaneous application of the strong tincture. Death following application of iodine tincture to a third of the body surface is said to have occurred (Moore, 1938).

The nervous, circulatory, and renal disturbances which follow the ingestion of iodine are ascribed to corrosive gastroenteritis and attending shock (Finkelstein and Jacobi, 1937). The renal lesion, which sometimes resembles acute tubular necrosis, may be exacerbated by a hemolytic anemia (Dyck *et al.*, 1979). A metabolic acidosis of significant proportions (plasma bicarbonate 11 mmol./L.) was observed 3 hours after ingestion of Lugol's solution. At 5 hours the serum lactate was 13 mmol./L. (Dyck *et al.*, 1979), in contrast to normal values of 0.6 to 1.8.

Although free iodine may remain in the alimentary tract for several hours after ingestion, most if not all is converted to inorganic iodide or organically bound iodine before or during intestinal absorption (Moore, 1938). The blood plasma reveals principally iodide and a small amount of protein-bound iodine. The evidence is insufficient, however, to rule out the possibility that small amounts of free iodine reach the circulation and exert direct systemic effects on parenchymal organs. Traces of free iodine have been reported in saliva, sweat and urine (Webster, 1930).

In a large series of patients who were esophagoscoped because of iodine ingestion, the incidence of ulcerative esophagitis was only 5% (Cardona and Daly, 1964). However, a late fatal esophageal stenosis and a late pyloric stenosis have each been reported at least once (Finkelstein and Jacobi, 1937; Wilensky and Kaufman, 1939).

The iodide ion probably plays no significant role in the acute toxicity of iodine. Simple iodide salts are noncorrosive and relatively benign. They are principally active as expectorants and diuretics. A mild toxic syndrome called "iodism" results from chronic iodide overdoses and from the repeated administration of small amounts of iodine. Iodism is characterized by salivation, coryza, sneezing, conjunctivitis, headache, laryngitis, bronchitis, stomatitis, parotitis, enlargement of the submaxillary glands, and skin rashes. Except for discontinuing the medication, treatment is rarely required (Barker and Wood, 1940; Ehrich and Seifter, 1949; Paull, 1959). See also Iodide Salts in Section II.

Symptomatology:
1. Burning pain in the mouth and esophagus. The lips and mucous membranes are stained brown.
2. Severe corrosive gastroenteritis evidenced by vomiting, abdominal pain, and diarrhea. The vomitus is blue if starch is present in the stomach. Occasionally the feces become bloody.
3. Hypotension, tachycardia, cyanosis, and other signs of shock.
4. Headache, dizziness, delirium, collapse, and stupor.
5. Death may be due to circulatory collapse, asphyxiation from edema of the glottis, aspiration pneumonia, or pulmonary ema.
6. Occasionally hemorrhagic nephritis (with oliguria or anuria) becomes apparent within 1 to 3 days. It is probably a sequel to severe shock and/or intravascular hemolysis.
7. Late esophageal and pyloric stenosis have each been reported at least once.

Treatment:
1. Swallow *promptly* milk, starch, flour, or eggs.
2. Gastric lavage with a solution of starch (1 to 10%), of sodium thiosulfate (1%), or of protein (egg white, milk).
3. Fluid and electrolyte replacement for the correction of dehydration, shock, and acid-base imbalances (pp. IV-64, 17, 69).
4. Supportive measures for the treatment of circulatory collapse (p. IV-17).
5. Opiates for the control of pain (p. IV-32).
6. Preparations for an emergency tracheostomy in case signs of laryngeal obstruction appear (p. IV-6).
7. Antibiotic therapy if an infection appears (pp. IV. 85–86).
8. Supportive treatment in anticipation of renal failure if shock has been severe. See pp. IV-51–55.

Laboratory:
1. The urine may reveal albumin, casts, red blood cells, and leukocytes.
2. Evidence of hemolysis may be found.
3. Metabolic acidosis (lactic acidemia) has been reported.

References:

Amdur, M. O. Respiratory response to iodine vapor alone and with sodium chloride aerosol. J. Toxicol. Environ. Health 4:619-630, 1978.

Barker, W. H.; Wood, W. B., Jr. Severe febrile iodism during the treatment of hyperthyroidism. J. A. M. A. 114:1029-1038, 1940.

Cardona, J. C.; Daly, J. F. Management of corrosive esophagitis. Analysis of treatment, methods, and results. N. Y. State J. Med. 64:2307-2313, 1964.

Dyck, R. F.; Bear. R. A.; Goldstein, M. B.; Halperin, M. L. Iodine-iodide toxic reaction: case report with emphasis on the nature of the metabolic acidosis. Can. Med. Assoc. J. 120:704-706, 1979.

Ehrich, W. E.; Seifter, J. Thrombotic thrombocytopenic purpura caused by iodine. Report of a case. Arch. Pathol. 47:446-449, 1949.

Finkelstein, R.; Jacobi, M. Fatal iodine poisoning. A clinicopathologic and experimental study. Ann. Intern. Med. 10:1283-1296, 1937.

Gershenfeld, L.; Witlin, B. Iodine as an antiseptic. Ann. N. Y. Acad. Sci. 53:172-182, 1950.

Moore, M. The ingestion of iodine as a method of attempted suicide. N. Engl. J. Med. 219:383-388, 1938.

Nye, R. N. Relative in vitro activity of certain antiseptics in aqueous solution. J. A. M. A. 108:280-287, 1937.

Paull, A. M. Toxic reactions to iodine. R. I. Med. J. 42:96-99, 1959.

Reese, J. J. A Manual of Toxicology. J. B. Lippincott Co., Philadelphia, 1874.

Seymour, W. B., Jr. Poisoning from cutaneous application of iodine. A rare aspect of its toxicologic properties. Arch. Intern. Med. 59:952-966, 1937.

Webster, R. W. Legal Medicine and Toxicology. W. B. Saunders Co., Philadelphia, 1930.

Wilensky, A. O.; Kaufman, P. A. Pyloric stenosis following ingestion of tincture of iodine. Am. J. Surg. 43:779-782, 1939.

IPECAC

Other than the crude drug the commonly encountered forms of ipecac are the fluidextract, the syrup, and, in combination with opium, a powder (Dover's powder). Repeated attempts have been made to remove the fluidextract from the market, but it is used in the preparation of the popular syrup. The chief pharmacological activities of these preparations are attributable to their alkaloid content. The only alkaloid of therapeutic importance in ipecac is emetine, which is sometimes employed in an isolated form as a parenteral solution. Emetine once enjoyed considerable renown as the drug of choice in amebic hepatitis. Although it is gradually being replaced by less toxic agents, emetine still finds occasional use in refractory cases and in those where the relief of symptoms is urgent. Ipecac is often included in cough preparations as an expectorant, but it is known in toxicology principally for its emetic action.

Syrup of ipecac is widely recommended by pediatricians and poison control centers. In many localities it has been distributed and stored in home medicine cabinets in the form of

1 oz. (30 ml.) bottles for emergency use. The recommended dose of syrup of ipecac as an emetic after ingestion episodes in children is from 10 to 20 ml., repeated once if no effect occurs after 20 to 25 minutes (Reid, 1970). The adult dose is 30 ml.

In a study of 250 children who vomited following syrup of ipecac (usually a single dose of 20 ml.), it was found that an average time of 19 minutes was required to induce emesis (Robertson, 1962). Eighty-eight percent of these children vomited in 30 minutes or less, which compares favorably with the time usually required to complete an adequate gastric lavage. Furthermore, considerable experimental evidence exists to show that emesis is more effective, at least in dogs and children, in emptying the stomach than is gastric lavage (Abdallah and Tye, 1967; Boxer et al., 1969; Corby et al., 1967; Reid, 1970); see also Section I. Whether or not water is given before or after ipecac appears not to influence the outcome (Bukis et al., 1978), but milk delayed the onset of emesis by an average of 10 minutes (Varipara and Oderda, 1977).

Reports comparing the efficacy of various emetic agents continue to appear. Although Karlsson and Norén (1965) found that 0.25 gm. of copper sulfate as a 1% solution induced vomiting in a higher proportion of treated children than syrup of ipecac and with a shorter latency, most pediatricians regard copper sulfate as a dangerous drug and avoid its use.

In puppies given a barium sulfate meal, intramuscular apomorphine had a much shorter latency and produced more complete recovery of barium sulfate than did syrup of ipecac. Indeed, the effects of the latter were unpredictable, and some animals exhibited drowsiness without vomiting even in repeated doses (Corby et al., 1967). In a similar study in dogs, subcutaneous or intraocular apomorphine was judged to have a shorter latency of action, a better recovery of a barium meal and a greater margin of safety than lobeline or syrup of ipecac (Abdallah and Tye, 1967). Berry and Lambdin (1963) employed intramuscular apomorphine in 55 pediatric patients. The onset of emesis was rapid but vomiting was often protracted and some patients became very depressed. The experience of MacLean (1973) with subcutaneous apomorphine was similar. Because smaller doses are required, intravenous apomorphine has been suggested as a route which may avoid such side effects, but it has not yet received an adequate clinical trial (Gosselin and Smith, 1966).

Toxicology: The minimal lethal dose of emetine hydrochloride given orally in the form of enteric coated capsules is 15 to 20 mg./kg. for rabbits and cats (Anderson and Leake, 1930). The intraperitoneal LD_{50} in mice is 62 mg./kg. and in rats is 17 mg./kg. (Gimble et al., 1948).

Of the major alkaloids of ipecac, cephaeline is said to be twice as toxic as emetine when given subcutaneously in white rats, whereas psychotrine is apparently not fatal in animals even in doses up to 1 gm./kg. (Walters and Koch, 1917). Prior to improved analytical techniques, wide variations in toxicity were noted among various preparations of emetine and ipecac (Lake, 1918; Levy and Rowntree, 1916).

The cumulative nature of emetine poisoning was noted when cats and rabbits were found to tolerate doses of 1.5 to 4 mg./kg. for a few days even though this regimen eventually killed them (Dale, 1915). The sum of the daily doses that culminate in death approaches the acutely fatal single dose (Radomski et al., 1952; Rosen et al., 1935).

The fatal dose of emetine in man may be as low as 20 mg./kg. (Anderson and Reed, 1934; Brem and Konwaler, 1955). Ipecac fluidextract, which is 14.3 times more concentrated than the syrup, contains about 2% total alkaloids. The proportions of emetine and cephaeline vary from near equality to a fourfold preponderance of emetine. Toxic or even fatal effects might be anticipated in man with doses above 2 oz. of the fluidextract. Only 10 ml. produced death in a 4-year-old child (Bates and Grunwald, 1962).

In the few deaths ascribed to the syrup, other important factors were believed contributory. In one bizarre case an adult woman consumed 3 to 4 bottles per day after meals over a 3-month period to lose weight. She presented with paroxysmal supraventricular tachycardia, which was converted to a slower sinus tachycardia with propranolol and edrophonium. Eventually, however, she went into cardiac failure from which she could not be resuscitated. It was estimated that she had consumed a total dose of 5.7 to 7.6 gm. emetine (Adler et al., 1980). A 14-month-old child given the syrup in the recommended dose after chewing on the leaves of an "amaryllis" plant continued to vomit over the next 2 days, and eventually expired in cardiorespiratory arrest. On postmortem examination the entire stomach including the pylorus was found to have herniated into the left pleural space. A preexisting diaphragmatic defect was suspected as being contributory, although none could be demonstrated (Robertson, 1979).

When prior ingestion of a phenothiazine antiemetic drug prevented vomiting even after 90 ml. of the syrup, cardiac arrhythmias were the major manifestation of overdosage (MacLeod, 1963). In one study, however, 81% of 63 patients who had ingested drugs with alleged antiemetic effects vomited following a single dose of syrup of ipecac (Manoguerra and Krenzelok, 1978).

In contrast to emetine, which has acquired a stigmatic reputation, only a dozen human fatalities or serious intoxications have been attributed to galenical preparations of ipecac (Manno and Manno, 1977). Several poisonings resulted from confusion between the syrup and fluidextract when the latter was used in attempts to induce emesis in patients suspected of accidental poisoning (Allport, 1959; Bates and Grunwald, 1962; Miser and Robertson, 1978; Smith and Smith, 1961; Speer et al., 1963). Death resulted from the compulsive ingestion of *vinum ipecacuanhae*, a hydroalcoholic preparation used in England (Harrison, 1908). The cardinal signs in these cases were violent and persistent vomiting and later bloody diarrhea, together with cardiac irregularities.

Autopsy findings of esophagitis and congestion with mucosal erosions of the entire gastrointestinal tract are consistent with the irritant action of ipecac and its alkaloids on these mucosal surfaces. Although stimulation of the chemoreceptor trigger zone in the brain stem appears to be responsible for vomiting after conventional doses of ipecac or emetine (Bhargava et al., 1961; Eggleston and Hatcher, 1915), gastrointestinal irritation probably contributes to the protracted vomiting after large doses. In Allport's case (1959) marked inflammation with luminal constriction was discovered by esophagoscopy 1 month after ingestion of ipecac fluidextract. It is difficult to know whether such lesions are due to primary irritation by the drug or to excessive exposure of these mucosal surfaces to stomach acid during prolonged vomiting.

Besides their irritancy, ipecac and emetine are recognized as drugs possessing specific cardiotoxicity (Marino, 1961a). The effects may take the form of mild, reversible depression or inversion of T waves (Baer, 1951), progressing to bradycardia, disturbances in intraventricular conduction (Boyd and Scherf, 1941), atrial fibrillation (Sayid, 1935), myocardial infarction (Cera, 1956), or fatal myocarditis (Brem and Konwaler, 1955). In guinea pigs emetine cardiotoxicity is potentiated by forced exercise, as judged by ECG changes and coronary signs (Marino, 1961b).

Because emetine shows a predilection for accumulating in muscular organs, its cardiotoxicity has been postulated to arise from an interference with the biochemical basis of contractility (Parmer and Cottrill, 1949) or with observed disturbances in the metabolism of carbohydrate (Diamant, 1958). Characteristic lesions in the form of an interstitial edema of heart muscle with a spreading apart of individual fibers occur in poisoned animals; necrosis of some fibers is also seen (Rinehart and Anderson, 1931). Focal interstitial cell proliferation in the myocardium and epicardial hemorrhage were observed in human fatalities from ipecac (Smith and Smith, 1961; Speer et al., 1963). Some evidence (see

review by Manno and Manno, 1977) suggests, however, that emetine has blocking effects on adrenergic neurons, ganglia and myoneural junctions.

The cardiac depression noted above, in combination with fluid losses from vomiting, may precipitate peripheral circulatory collapse in the acutely poisoned patient. Because of the danger of cardiac arrest, emetine is no longer used intravenously, but local inflammatory reactions frequently follow subcutaneous injections.

Symptomatology:
A. Following oral ingestion of ipecac galenicals or alkaloids the signs and symptoms are chiefly gastrointestinal.
   1. Nausea, vomiting, diarrhea, cramping abdominal pain, bloody vomitus or feces, dehydration.
   2. Rarely cardiac disorders, as described below.
B. The subcutaneous injection of therapeutic doses or overdoses of emetine may produce any or all of the above, usually to a less severe degree, but the chief hazard is one of cardiotoxicity.
   1. Increased pulse rate, hypotension, precordial pain, dyspnea, fatigue and abnormal ECG changes which are first manifested in the T wave.
   2. Bradycardia, prolonged atrioventricular conduction times, atrial tachycardia and fibrillation, myocardial infarction or cardiac arrest.
   3. Profound shock from cardiac depression and fluid loss as the result of vomiting.

Treatment:
1. In the brief asymptomatic period after ingesting a toxic dose of any ipecac preparation, swallow a slurry of activated charcoal (p. I-4). If vomiting does not begin promptly, empty the stomach by lavage with water.
2. No specific antidotes or pharmacological antagonists are known to be effective against the cardiac damage.
3. Vomiting may possibly be controlled by parenteral administration of chlorpromazine or its congeners (see p. IV-49), but only large doses are likely to be effective.
4. General supportive measures for shock, as indicated (pp. IV-17–21).
5. If possible, monitor the electrocardiogram continuously. Insert transvenous pacemaker electrodes if the ventricular rate shows a progressive decline. See pp. IV-30–31.
6. Maintain bedrest until the ECG is normal.

Laboratory: Frequent electrocardiographic tracings may be of prognostic value. Quantitative methods for the determination of emetine are available but are not of prognostic help (Adler *et al.*, 1980; Parmer and Cottrill, 1949). Albuminuria has been reported.

References:

Abdallah, A. H.; Tye, A. A comparison of the efficacy of emetic drugs and stomach lavage. Am. J. Dis. Child. *113*:571-575, 1967.

Adler, A. G.; Walinsky, P.; Krall, R. A.; Cho, S. Y. Death resulting from ipecac syrup poisoning. J. A. M. A. *243*:1927-1928, 1980.

Allport, R. B. Ipecac is not innocuous. Am. J. Dis. Child. *98*:786-787, 1959.

Anderson, H. H.; Leake, C. D. Oral toxicity of emetine hydrochloride and certain related compounds in rabbits and cats. Am. J. Trop. Med. *10*:249-259, 1930.

Anderson, H. H.; Reed, A. C. Untoward effects of anti-amebic drugs. Am. J. Trop. Med. Hyg. *14*:269-281, 1934.

Baer, L. J. Electrocardiographic effects of emetine hydrochloride. Milit. Surgeon *109*:120-128, 1951.

Bates, T.; Grunwald, E. Ipecac poisoning, a report of two cases of ingestion of fluid extract of ipecac. Am. J. Dis. Child. *103*:169-173, 1962.

Berry, F. A.; Lambden, M. A. Apomorphine and levallorphan tartrate in acute poisonings. Am. J. Dis. Child. *105*:160-163, 1963.

Bhargava, K. P.; Gupta, P. C.; Chandra, O. Effect of ablation of the chemoreceptor trigger zone (CT zone) on the emetic response to intraventricular injection of apomorphine and emetine in the dog. J. Pharmacol. Exp. Ther. *134*:329-331, 1961.

Boxer, L.; Anderson, F. D.; Rowe, D. S. Comparison of ipecac-induced emesis with gastric lavage in treatment of acute salicylate ingestion. J. Pediatr. *74*:800-803, 1969.

Boyd, L. J.; Scherf, D. Electrocardiogram in acute emetine intoxication. J. Pharmacol. Exp. Ther. *71*:362-372, 1941.

Brem, T. H.; Konwaler, B. E. Fatal myocarditis due to emetine hydrochloride. Am. Heart J. *50*:476-481, 1955.

Bukis, D.; Kuwahara, L.; Robertson, W. O. Results of forcing fluids: Pre- versus post-ipecac. Vet. Hum. Toxicol. *20*:90-91, 1978.

Cera, L. J. Emetine toxicity with electrocardiographic abnormalities. Circulation *14*:33-37, 1956.

Corby, D. G.; Lisciandro, R. C.; Lehman, R. H.; Decker, W. J. The efficiency of methods used to evacuate the stomach after acute ingestions. Pediatrics *40*:871-874, 1967.

Dale, H. H. A preliminary note on chronic poisoning by emetine. Br. Med. J. *2*:895, 1915.

Diamant, E. J. Carbohydrate metabolism in emetine-poisoned rats. J. Pharmacol. Exp. Ther. *122*:465-473, 1958.

Eggleston, C.; Hatcher, R. A. The seat of emetic action of various drugs. J. Pharmacol. Exp. Ther. *7*:225-253, 1915.

Gimble, A. I.; Davison, C.; Smith, P. K. Studies on the toxicity, distribution and excretion of emetine. J. Pharmacol. Exp. Ther. *94*:431-438, 1948.

Gosselin, R. E.; Smith, R. P. Trends in the therapy of acute poisonings. Clin. Pharmacol. Ther. *1*:279-299, 1966.

Harrison, R. T. A case of ipecacuanha poisoning. Lancet *2*:536, 1908.

Karlsson, B.; Noren, L. Ipecacuanha and copper sulfate as emetics in intoxications in children. Acta Pediatr. Scand. *54*:331-335, 1965.

Lake, G. C. On the toxicity of emetine hydrochloride, with special reference to the comparative toxicity of various market preparations. U. S. Public Health Serv., Hyg. Lab. Bull. No. 113, 1918.

Levy, R. L.; Rowntree, L. G. On the toxicity of varous commercial preparations of emetine hydrochloride. Arch. Intern. Med. *17*:420-443, 1916.

MacLean, W. C., Jr. A comparison of ipecac syrup and apomorphine in the immediate treatment of ingestion of poisons. J. Pediatr. *82*:121-124, 1973.

MacLeod, J. Ipecac intoxication - use of cardiac pacemaker in management. N. Engl. J. Med. *268*:146-147, 1963.

Manno, B. R.; Manno, J. E. Toxicology of ipecac: a review. Clin. Toxicol. *10*:221-242, 1977.

Manoguerra, A. S.; Krenzelok, E. P. Rapid emesis from high-dose ipecac syrup in adults and children intoxicated with antiemetics or other drugs. Am. J. Hosp. Pharm. *35*:1360-1362, 1978.

Marino, A. Electrocardiographic and behavioral effects of emetine. Science *133*:385-386, 1961a.

Marino, A. Physical stress and emetine cardiotoxicity. Experientia *171*:116-117, 1961b.

Miser, J. S.; Robertson, W. O. Ipecac poisoning. West. J. Med. *128*:440-443, 1978.

Parmer, L. G.; Cottrill, C. W. Distribution of emetine in tissues. J. Lab. Clin. Med. *34*:818-821, 1949.

Radomski, J. L.; Hagan, E. C.; Fuyat, H. N.; Nelson, A. A. The pharmacology of ipecac. J. Pharmacol. Exp. Ther. *104*:421-426, 1952.

Reid, D. H. S. Treatment of the poisoned child. Arch. Dis. Child. *45*:428-433, 1970.

Rinehart, J. F.; Anderson, H. H. Effect of emetine on cardiac muscle. Arch. Pathol. *11*:546-553, 1931.

Robertson, W. O. Ipecac - a slow or fast emetic?. Am. J. Dis. Child. *103*:136-139, 1962.

Robertson, W. O. Syrup of ipecac associated fatality; a case report. Vet. Hum. Toxicol. *21*:87-89, 1979.

Rosen, E. A.; Martin, R. R.; David, N. A. Cumulative toxicity of emetine hydrochloride in guinea pigs. Proc. Soc. Exp. Biol. Med. *33*:289-291, 1935.

Sayid, I. A. Auricular fibrillation after emetine injection. Lancet *2*:556, 1935.

Smith, R. P.; Smith, D. M. Acute ipecac poisoning, report of a fatal case and review of the literature. N. Engl. J. Med. *265*:523-525, 1961.

Speer, J. D.; Robertson, W. O.; Schultz, L. R. Ipecacuanha poisoning, another fatal case. Lancet *1*:475-477, 1963.

Varipara, R. J.; Oderda, G. M. Effects of milk on ipecac-induced emesis. N. Engl. J. Med. *296*:112-113, 1977.

Walters, A. D.; Koch, E. W. Pharmacological studies of the ipecac alkaloids and some synthetic derivatives of cephaeline. I. Studies on toxicity. J. Pharmacol. Exp. Ther. *10*:73-81, 1917.

ISOPROPYL ALCOHOL

Isopropyl alcohol (2-propanol, isopropanol) is an important industrial solvent and a disinfectant, but in the home it is found principally in rubbing alcohol, skin lotions, hair tonics, aerosol products, deicing and antifreeze preparations (Macht, 1920; von Oettingen, 1943; Zakhari *et al.*, 1977).

Toxicology: According to clinical experience isopropyl alcohol is more toxic than ethyl alcohol and less toxic than methyl alcohol. Unlike methanol, it produces no retinal injury (Fuller and Hunter, 1927). Its acute potency as a central nervous depressant is about twice that of ethanol (Grant, 1923; Morris and Lightbody, 1938; Wallgren, 1960). The probable lethal dose for an adult is 8 oz. (240 ml.), but as little as 20 ml. in water can produce symptoms (Grant, 1923; Fuller and Hunter, 1927). Individuals with a tolerance for ethyl alcohol are also relatively tolerant of isopropyl alcohol (Mendelson *et al.*, 1957), and a chronic alcoholic is reported to have survived the ingestion of about 1 pint of 70% isopropyl alcohol (Chapin, 1949), whereas another died after 1.3 pints (Adelson, 1962).

Although an initial phase of exhilaration is said to be lacking (Browning, 1965), the signs and symptoms of isopropyl alcohol poisoning are similar to those of ethanol intoxication. In both cases death after an acute exposure is usually preceded by respiratory arrest in deep coma, characteristically within a few hours after the ingestion (Adelson, 1962). If gas exchange is maintained by artificial ventilation, large doses can be survived, but, as with other aliphatic alcohols (see ETHYL ALCOHOL, p. III-167), high blood alcohol levels eventually induce serious cardiac toxicity. It may manifest itself in disordered mechanisms of beat (*e.g.*, atrial arrest) or simply as severe arterial hypotension. Dehydration and hemorrhagic gastritis may be other factors contributing to the genesis of extreme hypotension.

In isopropyl alcohol poisoning hypotension is a bad prognostic sign (Adelson, 1962). If severe and persistent, shock may lead to serious (Chapin, 1949, Juncos and Taguchi, 1968) or even fatal (Adelson, 1962) renal injury after a period of several days. At least mild hepatic dysfunction has been described in man (Chapin, 1949), and in rats isopropyl alcohol like ethanol (but unlike other aliphatic alcohols) increases significantly the triglyceride content of the liver. Severe liver injuries, however, have not been observed. Human volunteers consuming isopropyl alcohol in a daily dose of 6.4 mg./kg. for 6 weeks failed to develop significant alterations in the chemical or cellular composition of the blood or urine or in the ability of the liver to excrete sulfobromophthalein (Wills *et al.*, 1969). Like ethyl alcohol, isopropanol intensifies and potentiates the toxic effects of CARBON TETRA-CHLORIDE (p. III-101) in experimental animals and probably in man (Folland *et al.*, 1976).

Besides potency there are two important toxicological distinctions between isopropyl alcohol and ethanol. Isopropyl alcohol induces a more frequent and more prominent gastritis with pain, nausea, vomiting and hemorrhage (Fuller and Hunter, 1927; Lehman and Chase, 1944). Indeed vomiting with aspiration is a serious threat and dangerous complication in clinical isopropyl alcohol poisonings, even though this substance, when diluted to 70% or less, has a low aspiration hazard in anesthetized rats (Gerarde and Ahlstrom, 1966a).

Another distinction is the longer duration of intoxication induced by isopropyl alcohol. This difference can probably be ascribed to two facts. First, isopropyl alcohol is metabolized, at least in man, more slowly than is ethanol (Fuller and Hunter, 1927; Morris and Lightbody, 1938; Williams, 1959b). The kinetics of its elimination in dogs and rats does not resemble that for either ethanol or methanol (Abshagen and Riebrock, 1969). Second, the major metabolite (Williams 1959b) is acetone, another central nervous depressant. The oxidation of isopropanol to acetone probably involves alcohol dehydrogenase, and the rate of metabolism cannot be accelerated to a useful degree by the administration of insulin or glucose (Lehman, 1946).

Because physiological mechanisms for disposing of this alcohol are inherently slow, hemodialysis should prove to be a useful procedure. Indeed it appears to have been responsible for the rapid recovery of two men, each of whom reputedly ingested a quart of rubbing alcohol, presumably consisting of 70% isopropanol (Freireich *et al.*, 1967; King *et al.*, 1970). Peritoneal dialysis was employed successfully in a mentally retarded adult who had consumed 1 pint (Dua, 1974).

Absorption through the skin does not seem to be a significant portal of entry (Boughton, 1944). However, the accidental inhalation of vapors during and following sponging with isopropyl alcohol in poorly ventilated areas has produced deep coma, a hazard that is not generally recognized. Perhaps alcohol rubs to reduce fever and to alleviate muscular aches are employed more often than is warranted (Garrison, 1953; McFadden and Haddow, 1969; Senz and Goldfarb, 1958). Isopropyl alcohol is readily absorbed from the bowel, and one schizophrenic individual attempted suicide with a self-administered enema (Corbett and Meier, 1968).

Isopropyl alcohol is occasionally encountered as an ingredient in illicit alcoholic beverages and in preparations not intended for ingestion, such as some shaving lotions. Other ingredients, notably volatile aromatics such as menthol, camphor, methyl salicylate and naphthalene, may complicate the clinical picture and produce a syndrome of frank central stimulation with motor restlessness, extreme apprehension, hallucinations and general disorientation (Gadsden *et al.*, 1958; Smith, 1959b).

Normal propyl alcohol (propanol-1) may be slightly more toxic than isopropyl alcohol (Wallgren, 1960), but it appears to induce many of the same biological effects (Browning, 1965). Although *n*-propyl alcohol is not often encountered, a human fatality has been ascribed to its ingestion (Durwald and Degen, 1956).

Symptomatology:
1. Dizziness, incoordination, headache, confusion, stupor and coma.
2. Gastroenteritis with vomiting, hematemesis, and diarrhea.
3. Hypotension, with or without bradycardia, and sometimes severe circulatory collapse.

4. Persistent coma with hypothermia.
5. Death by respiratory arrest.
6. Late manifestations: aspiration pneumonia; kidney and liver dysfunctions, which are usually mild and transient, but the renal impairment may be serious.

Treatment:

1. Gastric lavage with water. Large amounts of isopropyl alcohol have been removed even when lavage was delayed (Light and Marx, 1969).
2. Caffeine sodium benzoate, 0.5 gm. subcutaneously, may be helpful to counteract central nervous depression, but vigorous analeptic therapy is dangerous and ill-advised (see pp. IV-41–42). Oxygen and artificial ventilation as needed (see pp. IV-7–14).
3. Intravenous glucose and saline to correct dehydration, electrolyte deficiencies, possibly acidosis, and shock (pp. IV-66–67, 69–72). Blood and possibly pressor drugs may have to be infused to control severe hypotension (pp. IV-16–20).
4. Hemodialysis to reduce blood and tissue levels of isopropyl alcohol (p. IV-55).
5. Prophylactic measures in anticipation of disturbances in liver (p. IV-60) and kidney (p. IV-52) function.

Laboratory:

1. Severe acetonuria and acetonemia are encountered in isopropyl alcohol poisoning (Ashkar and Miller, 1971) but also in diabetes mellitus and the ketoacidosis of ethanol intoxication and of cyanide poisoning. The absence of starvation, glycosuria or acidosis (normal pH, normal anion gap, normal serum bicarbonate) in the presence of acetone in the breath and urine suggests isopropyl alcohol poisoning.
2. Function tests to detect and evaluate possible liver and kidney disturbances.
3. Cardiac function should be assessed with repeated electrocardiograms.
4. Isopropyl alcohol can be detected and measured in blood and gastric contents. Blood levels of 150 mg./100 ml. are associated with deep coma (McCord *et al.*, 1948). One child recovered after a blood level of 520 mg./100 ml. (Visudhiphan and Kaufman, 1971).
5. The significance of increased cerebrospinal fluid protein (Visudhiphan and Kaufman, 1971) in severe poisoning is unknown; the same is true of hemolysis and myopathy (Juncos and Taguchi, 1968).

References:

Abshagen, U.; Riebrock, N. Kinetik der Elimination von 2-Propanol und seines Metaboliten Aceton bei Hund und Ratte. Naunyn Schmiedebergs Arch. Pharmakol. *264*:110-118, 1969.

Adelson, L. Fatal intoxication with isopropyl alcohol (rubbing alcohol). Am. J. Clin. Pathol. *38*:144-151, 1962.

Ashkar, F. S.; Miller, R. Hospital ketosis in the alcoholic diabetic; a syndrome due to isopropyl alcohol intoxication. South. Med. J. *64*:1409-1410, 1971.

Boughton, L. L. Relative toxicity of ethyl and isopropyl alcohols as determined by long term rat feeding and external application. J. Am. Pharm. Sci. *33*:111-113, 1944.

Browning, E. *Toxicity and Metabolism of Industrial Solvents.* Elsevier Publishing Co., Amsterdam, 2nd ed, 1965.

Chapin, M. A. Isopropyl alcohol poisoning with acute renal insufficiency. J. Maine Med. Assoc. *40*:288-290, 1949.

Corbett, J.; Meier, G. Suicide attempted by rectal administration of drug. J. A. M. A. *206*:2320-2321, 1968.

Dua, S. L. Peritoneal dialysis for isopropyl alcohol poisoning. J. A. M. A. *230*:35, 1974.

Durwald, W.; Degen, W. Eine todliche Vergiftung mit n-Propyl Alkohol. Arch. Toxikol. *16*:85, 1956.

Folland, D. S.; Schaffner, W.; Ginn, H. E.; Crofford, O. B.; McMurray, D. R. Carbon tetrachloride toxicity potentiated by isopropyl alcohol. J. A. M. A. *236*:1853-1856, 1976.

Freireich, A. W.; Cinque, T. J.; Xanthaky, G.; Landau, D. Hemodialysis for isopropanol poisoning. N. Engl. J. Med. *277*:699-700, 1967.

Fuller, H. C.; Hunter, O. B. Isopropyl alcohol - an investigation of its physiologic properties. J. Lab. Clin. Med. *12*:326-349, 1927.

Gadsden, R. H.; Mellette, R. R.; Miller, W. C., Jr. Scrap iron intoxication. J. A. M. A. *168*:1220-1224, 1958.

Garrison, R. F. Acute poisoning from use of isopropyl alcohol in tepid sponging. J. A. M. A. *152*:317-318, 1953.

Gerarde, H. W.; Ahlstrom, D. B. The aspiration hazard and toxicity of a homologous series of alcohols. Arch. Environ. Health *13*:457-461, 1966a.

Grant, D. H. The pharmacology of isopropyl alcohol. J. Lab. Clin. Med. *8*:382-386, 1923.

Juncos, L.; Taguchi, J. T. Isopropyl alcohol intoxication. J. A. M. A. *204*:732-734, 1968.

King, L. H.; Bradley, K. P.; Shires, D. L. Hemodialysis for isopropyl alcohol poisoning. J. A. M. A. *211*:1855, 1970.

Lehman, A. J. Effect of insulin, insulin-dextrose, and water diuresis on metabolism of isopropyl alcohol. Proc. Soc. Exp. Biol. Med. *62*:232-234, 1946.

Lehman, A. J.; Chase, H. F. The acute and chronic toxicity of isopropyl alcohol. J. Lab. Clin. Med. *29*:561-567, 1944.

Light, F. B.; Marx, G. F. The value of gastric aspiration in a comatose child. Anesthesiology *31*:478-480, 1969.

Macht, D. I. A toxicological study of some alcohols with especial reference to isomers. J. Pharmacol. Exp. Ther. *16*:1-10, 1920.

McCord, W. M.; Switzer, P. K.; Brill, H. H., Jr. Isopropyl alcohol intoxication. South. Med. J. *41*:639-642, 1948.

McFadden, S. W.; Haddow, J. E. Coma produced by topical application of isopropanol. Pediatrics *43*:622-623, 1969.

Mendelson, J.; Wexler, D.; Leiderman, P. H.; Solomon, P. A study of addiction to nonethyl alcohols and other poisonous compounds. Q. J. Stud. Alcohol *18*:561-580, 1957.

Morris, H. J.; Lightbody, H. D. The toxicity of isopropanol. J. Ind. Hyg. Tox. *20*:428-434, 1938.

Senz, E. H.; Goldfarb, D. L. Coma in a child following use of isopropyl alcohol in sponging. J. Pediatr. *53*:322-323, 1958.

Smith, R. P. Poisoning with Old Spice shaving lotion. A case report. Bull. Suppl. Material, Clinical Toxicology of Commercial Products (Edited by M. N. Gleason, R. E. Gosselin and H. C. Hodge.) II (no. 11):12, 1959b.

Visudhiphan, P.; Kaufman, H. Increased cerebrospinal fluid protein following isopropyl alcohol intoxication. N. Y. State J. Med. *71*:887-888, 1971.

von Oettingen, W. F. Aliphatic alcohols: their toxicity and potential dangers in relation to their constitution and their fate in metabolism. Public Health Bull. No. 281, 1943.

Wallgren, H. Relative intoxicating effects on rats of ethyl, propyl and butyl alcohols. Acta Pharmacol. Toxicol. *16*:217-222, 1960.

Williams, R. T. *Detoxification Mechanisms*, 2nd ed. John Wiley and Sons, Inc., New York, 1959b.

Wills, J. H.; Jameson, E. M.; Coulston, F. Effects on man of daily ingestion of small doses of isopropyl alcohol. Toxicol. Appl. Pharmacol. 15:560-565, 1969.

Zakhari, S.; Leibowitz, M.; Levy, P.; Aviado, D. M. Isopropanol and Ketones in the Environment. CRC Press, Cleveland, Ohio, 1977.

KEROSENE

Kerosene (kerosine) is one of several petroleum distillates prepared by the fractionation of crude petroleum oil. In order of decreasing volatility the major fractions are: petroleum ether or benzine, gasoline, mineral spirits, kerosene, fuel oil, lubricating oils, paraffin wax, and asphalt or tar. These fractions consist chiefly of aliphatic or straight-chain hydrocarbons of the alkane series. Petroleum ether or benzine is composed largely of pentane and hexane, whereas kerosene is predominantly hydrocarbons lying between nonane and hexadecane. All fractions and particularly kerosene contain appreciable amounts of aromatic or unsaturated ring hydrocarbons (e.g., toluene and xylene) and saturated rings or cycloparaffins (sometimes called naphthenes). Petroleum products obtained by "cracking" processes also contain unsaturated straight-chain molecules (olefins and diolefins) (American Petroleum Institute, 1948i).

Kerosene and related compounds are used as illuminating fuels, heating fuels, motor fuels, vehicles for many insecticides and fungicides (Reingold and Lasky, 1947), cleaning agents and paint thinners. Kerosene and gasoline can be found around homes, garages and farms, often in containers originally designed for beverages. Since the turn of the century (Hamilton, 1897), the ingestion of these hydrocarbon mixtures has caused numerous fatalities, particularly in children and infants. The incidence of poisoning by kerosene in the South is several times that in the rest of the United States. Overall mortality is low but hospitalization may be required in a high proportion of ingestion episodes (Press, 1962).

Toxicology: It is becoming increasingly apparent that the prognosis in most cases of kerosene ingestion hinges on whether or not aspiration occurred when the material was ingested or later during eructation or vomiting (Baldachin and Melmed, 1964; Foley et al., 1954; McNally, 1956; Olstad and Lord, 1952).

The mean lethal dose cannot be stated with certainty. Provided that aspiration does not occur, 4 to 6 oz. by the oral route may be a reasonable estimate for an average adult, although twice this amount has been tolerated and less than ½ oz. has caused death. Perhaps this estimate is too low since oral LD_{50} values in rats, rabbits and guinea pigs exceed 20 ml./kg. In fatal poisonings, death may occur within 2 to 24 hours after ingestion. It has been stated that the difference between the lethal dose in cases of uncomplicated ingestion and those where as-

piration occurs may be as great as the difference between a pint and a teaspoonful (Richardson and Pratt-Thomas, 1951). Aspiration, however, is a tragically frequent occurrence in infants and children, but the pediatric patient whose chest film is normal when first seen and who is still asymptomatic after 6 hours of observation is believed to be out of danger (Anas et al., 1981).

The characteristic lesion resulting from the aspiration of liquid hydrocarbons into the tracheobronchial tree is an acute, fulminating, hemorrhagic and often fatal bronchopneumonia; it may appear within minutes or be delayed for several hours (Soule and Foley, 1957). The progress of the pulmonary disease may be followed roentgenographically by observing the extent to which the lung field becomes opacified (Gershon-Cohen et al., 1953; Lesser et al., 1943; Reynolds and Bonte, 1960). Early and widespread pulmonary changes can be seen even in the absence of clinical signs (Brünner et al., 1964), and conversely pulmonary symptoms may precede lung X-ray changes (Vaziri et al., 1980). Death may result from asphyxia secondary to intense pulmonary edema and consolidation (Heacock, 1949; Lavenstein, 1945; Scott, 1944). Children who survive hydrocarbon pneumonitis usually recover clinically within 3 to 5 days, but adults sometimes have a protracted course (Mayock et al., 1961), and secondary bacterial infections may lead to chronic respiratory disease such as bronchiectasis.

Occasionally pseudocysts or pneumatoceles develop and resolve spontaneously over several weeks or months (Bagdassarian and Weiner, 1965; Campbell, 1970; Dragsted and Rodbro, 1965). Pneumatoceles characteristically appear as late unexpected findings on chest films without evidence of pneumothorax or empyema (Bergeson et al., 1975). In one large series of cases pneumatoceles appeared to be most commonly associated with charcoal lighter fluid as opposed to other common petroleum products (Harris and Brown, 1976).

How kerosene reaches the lungs has been the subject of much speculation. Aside from aspiration, the possibility that blood-borne hydrocarbons are hazardous to the lungs has received attention. Some studies report pulmonary lesions in rats, a species that cannot vomit, after kerosene gavage (Ashkenazi and Berman, 1961; Deichmann et al., 1944). Benign pulmonary lesions in elderly patients who habitually use mineral oil for laxative purposes can be seen in X-ray (Schneider, 1949). Carefully controlled studies, however, some on large animal species including monkeys, indicate that kerosene presented as a single oral dose is not a significant hazard in terms of pneumonitis *after* it has been absorbed (Foley *et al.*, 1954; Huxtable *et al.*, 1964; Wolfsdorf *et al.*, 1972; Wolfe *et al.*, 1970).

Kerosene and related hydrocarbons are also irritating to skin and mucous membranes, and percutaneous absorption is sometimes significant. On prolonged or extensive contact, kerosene and its congeners can produce epidermal necrolysis (Barnes and Wilkinson, 1973). A 12-year-old boy who was partially immersed in a pool of gasoline for an hour presented with hypotension and a "scald" of 50% of his body surface. Transient hematuria occurred, followed by abdominal tenderness, an elevated blood level of amylase, disseminated intravascular coagulation and nonoliguric renal failure. Autopsy revealed epidermal loss of skin, cerebral edema, diffuse bilateral pneumonia, biventricular cardiac enlargement, toxic nephrosis, fatty infiltration of the liver and peripancreatic fat necrosis (Walsh *et al.*, 1974). Perhaps the percutaneous route of exposure carries a special risk for renal damage. One adult who used diesel fuel as a shampoo developed oliguria and acute renal failure requiring hemodialysis (Barrientos *et al.*, 1977). Another who cleaned his hands and arms with diesel fuel for several weeks developed acute tubular necrosis (Crisp *et al.*, 1979).

The chief systemic reaction to kerosene and related petroleum hydrocarbons is central nervous depression (Reed *et al.*, 1950; Steiner, 1947). Hydrocarbons of all types induce central nervous depression, but the aliphatic hydrocarbons (which predominate in petroleum distillates) are said to produce profound coma with an inhibition of deep tendon reflexes, whereas the coma from aromatic hydrocarbons is characterized by motor restlessness, tremors, and hyperactive reflexes (von Oettingen, 1940).

Less kerosene is required to produce anesthesia when it is inhaled as a vapor than when it is ingested as a liquid, apparently because absorption from the bowel is slow and incomplete (Bratton and Haddow, 1975; Dice *et al.*, 1982; Mann *et al.*, 1977), but because of its low volatility kerosene is seldom hazardous as a vapor (American Petroleum Institute, 1948i). Gasoline, however, may produce symptoms at a concentration of 0.1% in air (Drinker *et al.*, 1943). Inhalation of jet airplane fuel, which is said to resemble kerosene in its composition, has produced an intoxication (Davies, 1964), as also has inhalation of synthetic hydrocarbon jet lubricating oil (Montgomery *et al.*, 1977).

There appears to be a narrow margin between the anesthetic and lethal doses (von Oettingen, 1940), but in nonfatal poisonings serious aftereffects are almost never encountered (Reed *et*

al., 1950). Cigarette lighter fluid has been "sniffed" by teenagers for its euphoric effects. The syndrome closely resembles ethyl alcohol inebriation. Although some children have indulged in this practice for several years, there is rarely clear evidence of permanent sequelae (Ackerly and Gibson, 1964; Glaser, 1966). Peripheral neuropathy with symmetrical motor involvement in distal lower limbs has been reported after chronic gasoline sniffing (Gallassi *et al.*, 1980).

Although one adult who injected himself intravenously with 3 to 4 ml. of kerosene survived with minimal systemic effects (Green, 1977), another experienced pleuritic chest pain, epigastric discomfort and dyspnea within 2 hours, followed by a severe hemorrhagic pneumonitis. The appearance of chest X-ray changes lagged several hours behind the symptoms. He also developed fever and leukocytosis in the absence of a demonstrable bacterial infection. The pathology was otherwise confined to the lungs, and the lesions eventually resolved completely (Vaziri *et al.*, 1980). When injected into the tail vein of rats, kerosene caused severe lung damage, but when given into the portal vein, hepatic necrosis was the primary lesion (Bratton and Haddow, 1975).

In the aliphatic series, narcotic potency increases with the chain length at least through octane (von Oettingen, 1940), but very large molecules (hexadecane and above) are essentially innocuous, apparently because they are not absorbed from the alimentary tract. Consequently, petroleum fractions above kerosene (*e.g.*, lubricating oils and paraffin oils) are much less toxic than kerosene itself and are essentially benign if refined by the removal of unsaturated derivatives. In experimental animals, cycloparaffins (naphthenes) have a greater narcotic potency and lethality than do aliphatic hydrocarbons with the same boiling point (von Oettingen, 1940).

Besides central nervous depression and local irritation, mild and presumably reversible lesions of a degenerative and sometimes hemorrhagic nature are occasionally reported in visceral organs such as the liver, kidneys, bone marrow and spleen (Ashkenazi and Berman, 1961; Barrientos *et al.*, 1977; Narasimhan and Granla, 1967; Steiner, 1947; Walsh *et al.*, 1974). Exposure to gasoline vapors was implicated in severe fatty changes in the liver and myocardium and death secondary to systemic fat emboli, which occurred during anesthesia for repair of injuries in an aircraft accident (Tonge *et al.*, 1969). Sometimes the myocardium is so sensitized that small amounts of endogenous epinephrine precipitate ventricular fibrillation and sudden death, but aromatic solvents like benzene are probably more hazardous in this respect (see also XYLENE, p. III-397). In one child abnormalities of the ECG and vectorcardiogram persisted more than 8 months after furniture polish ingestion (James et al., 1971a), but parenchymal injuries are usually of short duration.

The relation between toxic signs and symptoms and the chemical composition of petroleum distillates has not been adequately established. Although pure samples of aliphatic hydrocarbons like hexane have been used experimentally to induce typical acute toxic reactions, unsaturated hydrocarbons, aromatic rings, and naphthenes undoubtedly contribute to the usual clinical intoxication. For example, the aromatic constituents are particularly irritating to skin and mucous membranes (see XYLENE, p. III-401). When given by gavage to rats without aspiration, significant differences in lethality were noted among three shale-derived and one petroleum-derived jet fuels. Although the responsible ingredients are not known, the greater toxicity of some of them appeared to be associated with the nitrogenous fraction (Parker et al., 1981).

Gasoline (plain or leaded) is said to be more toxic than kerosene in children (Nunn and Martin, 1934). If this distinction is valid, it may be due to differences in aliphatic chain length or to differences in nonaliphatic constituents. In any case, gasoline or other petroleum product additives such as tetraethyl lead and the cresyl phosphates do not contribute appreciably to the acute toxicity (Dooley, 1963). In view of the variation in molecular composition among different petroleum fractions and among different samples of the same fraction, it is surprising that the clinical syndrome of acute intoxication is as uniform as described.

The aspiration hazard appears to be related to the viscosity and perhaps to the surface tension of any liquid. As measured by an aspiration-hazard test in which 0.2 ml. of solvent is placed in the mouth of an anesthetized rat, Gerarde (1963) found that pulmonary lesions and death are more frequent the lower the viscosity of an aliphatic hydrocarbon or hydrocarbon mixture. Petroleum distillate fractions with viscosities above 70 to 80 SSU at body temperature (100°F.) were essentially benign in this test, and kerosene with a viscosity of 32 was safe only if blended with lubricating oils to form solutions with viscosities of about 70 and above. Gerarde (1963) emphasized that aspiration is a phenomenon which occurs within the time of one inhalation. In a conscious victim various physiological protective mechanisms act promptly to prevent further aspiration. The viscosity of a solvent determines not only the likelihood of its entry into the trachea but also the rate and extent of its penetration into the terminal bronchioles and alveoli. Thus both the frequency of aspiration and the severity of the resulting pulmonary pathology are closely related to the solvent viscosity.

Lighter fluid, gasoline, kerosene (Gerarde, 1963) and some commercial furniture polishes (Huxtable et al., 1964) have viscosities below 45 SSU and all are highly toxic by aspiration. Hydrocarbons of even lower viscosity have very low boiling points; they too are dangerous by aspiration. They tend to produce rapid exitus, not because of pulmonary edema but because of cardiac arrest, central respiratory paralysis or asphyxia by displacement of alveolar air with hydrocarbon vapor (Gerarde, 1963). Viscous materials like paints, glues, asphalt, rubber cement, etc. may contain high concentrations of hydrocarbons but represent an insignificant aspiration hazard.

Furniture polishes are a frequent source of exposure of small children to hydrocarbons. In a large series of cases pneumonia was felt to be more common after ingestion of kerosene, furniture polish and lighter fluid than after other petroleum products, the most severe cases being those due to furniture polish (Harris and Brown, 1976). There is a distinct clinical impression that furniture polishes with a mineral seal oil base (see Section II) are more hazardous than those containing kerosene (Mintz, 1966; Press, 1962). This impression was not confirmed by the aspiration test in rats, in which such a product produced pathological changes and mortality rates identical with those induced by kerosene (Ring and Nelson, 1966).

Forms of therapy: The only uncontroversial course of treatment is symptomatic and supportive. Because of the danger of aspiration, emetics should never be prescribed; on the other hand, the antiemetics are also contraindicated because of the possibility of synergistic central depression (Gerarde, 1959). The value versus the danger of gastric lavage is still a subject of controversy and investigation (Press, 1962). Lavage is not indicated if vomiting of any appreciable extent has occurred. It is probably also contraindicated if the patient is comatose. The extreme view has been taken that, if lavage is employed, its primary purpose should be to prevent regurgitation and subsequent aspiration (Blattner, 1951; Richardson and Pratt-Thomas, 1951). Perhaps a person who has swallowed and retained two or more ounces of kerosene (1 ml./kg.) is a candidate for gastric aspiration and lavage, but the more common and more acceptable indication is the ingestion of a petroleum solvent containing a highly toxic solute such as one of the pesticides.

If lavage is judged to be justified in spite of the recognized risk of inducing vomiting and aspiration, certain special precautions are recommended in addition to the procedural details outlined on p. I-10. As always, remove the gastric contents before instilling lavage fluid. Keeping the head and chest lowered and pinching off the lavage tube prior to its rapid withdrawal help to minimize the incidence of aspiration (Carithers, 1955). In a comatose patient and perhaps in a conscious patient whose respiratory tract has been anesthetized topically by a spray (Wycoff, 1959), an endotracheal tube with an inflatable balloon can protect the lungs (Foley et al., 1954). A lavage tube with a balloon that can be inflated within the esophagus has also been recommended. In a large cooperative study it was concluded that gastric lavage performed according to local practices in seven hospitals did no harm, but no conclusive evidence was generated to indicate that it was beneficial (Press, 1962). The same was true of an experimental study in rats (Ring and Nelson, 1966). In another large series at a single hospital, however, it was concluded that complications were more common with lavage than without it (Cachia and Fenech, 1964).

Other measures that may reduce the toxicity of ingested kerosene include the administration of activated charcoal. In rats given kerosene by gastric intubation, the prompt administration of a slurry of activated charcoal (in an amount of about 0.5 gm. for each gram of hydrocarbon) resulted in kerosene blood levels that were significantly lower than in control animals over a 12-hour period (Chin et al., 1969). Whether this trapping of kerosene by adsorption is genuinely beneficial needs to be tested in clinical patients.

Another technique recommended by some British authorities is the ingestion of several ounces of mineral oil (medicinal-grade liquid petrolatum). If the attempt does not induce vomiting, several possible benefits can be cited. First, mineral oil is a demulcent that may reduce gastric irritation and so minimize eructation and vomiting. Second, kerosene and mineral oil are fully miscible, and the mixture has a higher viscosity than kerosene alone, so that aspiration may be less likely when and if vomiting does occur (Gerarde, 1963). Third, mineral oil is a mild cathartic; it may accelerate the fecal excretion of kerosene by reducing its transit time to the rectum and perhaps by inhibiting its intestinal absorption. When given to rats under conditions in which there was no possibility of aspiration, mineral oil, in a volume equal to or half that of a previously administered volume of either pure hendecane (C_{11}) or kerosene, reduced hendecane absorption and prevented mortality due to hendecane and kerosene. After four years of clinical experience, these physicians concluded that this mineral oil treatment resulted in shorter hospitalization in some cases and no hospitalization in others (Ashkenazi and Berman, 1961). Beamon et al. (1976), however, concluded that, when given to patients who had ingested hydrocarbons, both mineral oil and olive oil resulted in a higher incidence of pneumonia. Additional studies of this practice appear to be warranted.

In kerosene poisoning with pulmonic involvement, several reports (Mayock et al., 1961; Jamison and Wallace, 1964) describe clinical improvement coincidental with steroid therapy, even when instituted as long as 2 weeks after the beginning of respiratory symptoms. In a cooperative, double-blind study involving 71 children, however, methylprednisolone resulted in no objective evidence of significant improvement in mild to moderately severe hydrocarbon pneumonitis (Marks et al., 1972). In guinea pigs dexamethasone even in combination with antibiotics increased significantly the number of positive lung cultures after kerosene gavage (Brown et al., 1974). No evidence of a significant beneficial effect was obtained in studies with dogs (Steele et al., 1972) or with baboons (Wolfsdorf and Kündig, 1974).

Symptomatology (see also XYLENE, p. III-397):

A. Inhalation.
   1. An odor of kerosene on the breath.
   2. Transient euphoria ("naphtha jag"), resembling alcoholic intoxication.
   3. Burning sensation in the chest.
   4. Headache, tinnitus, nausea.
   5. Weakness, restlessness and incoordination.
   6. Confusion and disorientation, leading to drowsiness and eventually coma, sometimes with convulsions.
   7. Vasomotor disturbances causing, for example, cyanosis of the extremities.
   8. Rarely sudden death, presumably due to ventricular fibrillation.
   9. Death usually due to respiratory arrest.
B. Ingestion.
   1. Local irritation with burning sensation in mouth, esophagus, and stomach. Odor of kerosene on breath, clothing or vomitus.
   2. Vomiting, eructation and diarrhea with blood-tinged feces.
   3. Drowsiness and any of the other signs and symptoms described above may be observed after ingestion, but the usual clinical course is quite benign unless liquid hydrocarbon is aspirated into the respiratory tract.
   4. The sudden development of rapid breathing, cyanosis, tachycardia and low-grade fever are the usual signs of pulmonary involvement, generally secondary to unrecognized aspiration. Bas-

ilar rales rapidly progress to massive pulmonary edema or to pneumonic hemorrhage, infiltration and secondary infection. Death may result from asphyxia within a few hours.

5. Severe or untreated cases may develop confluent pneumonia, cardiac dilatation, hepatosplenomegaly, urinary changes consisting of albuminuria with cells and casts, and atrial fibrillation-flutter associated with cardiac failure.

6. Complete recovery of pulmonary function is the general rule in surviving children. If only the lungs are affected, such children are apt to be clinically well within 3 to 5 days, but a secondary bacterial pneumonia may interrupt convalescence, especially in adults.

Treatment:

1. Emetics are definitely contraindicated, and activated charcoal has not been established as effective in clinical studies (see Section I).

2. A controversial method of trapping ingested kerosene is to swallow several ounces of mineral oil (white petrolatum); see discussion above.

3. In general the potential benefits of gastric lavage do not justify the risk in cases of kerosene ingestion. Exceptions are indicated in the test above. If and when warranted by special circumstances, the procedure should be performed with at least some of the precautions described above. Copious amounts of water or 3% sodium bicarbonate may be used. It may or may not be useful to instill 30 to 60 ml. of mineral oil in the stomach at the conclusion of lavage and to follow this with a saline cathartic in water (*e.g.*, sodium sulfate). See also Section I (pp. I-8–12).

4. If coma develops, be prepared to protect the airway with a cuffed endotracheal tube, to relieve respiratory obstruction (p. IV-2) and to provide ventilatory assistance (pp. IV-7–12).

5. If frequent ventricular premature beats or other arrhythmias occur, institute cardiac monitoring.

6. Parenteral antibiotic therapy, if indicated, for bacterial invasion of the lungs. See pp. IV-85–86.

7. Supportive treatment of pulmonary edema by the use of positive-pressure oxygen therapy (pp. IV-14–16).

8. Avoid epinephrine because of possible adverse effects on the sensitized myocardium. Avoid alcohol which may promote absorption from the bowel. A cleansing enema with or without activated charcoal may help remove unabsorbed kerosene.

Laboratory:

1. A double gastric fluid level may be noted in an upright frontal chest film, particularly if a glassful of water is first consumed to provide an aqueous layer. As little as 5 ml. of kerosene in the stomach may be detectable (Daffner and Jimenez, 1973). X-rays are also of value in the diagnosis of pulmonary lesions. In adults serial determination of vital capacity may be helpful.

2. Repeated electrocardiograms are desirable to detect myocardial damage and conduction defects.

3. An unexpected and unexplained hemoglobinemia has been reported occasionally in man and experimental animals. When possible, an attempt should be made to detect it. It occurred after gasoline ingestion in a child with apparently normal red cells. Exposure of red cells to gasoline vapor *in vitro* resulted in rapid and extensive hemolysis (Stockman, 1977).

4. With the exception of leukocytosis, blood disorders are rarely seen in acute poisonings; in chronic exposures they are presumably due to the small content of benzene which is present in all but highly purified samples (Hiebel *et al.*, 1963; Johnson, 1955).

5. Albumin, sugar and acetone have been reported in the urine even in the absence of renal failure. Hypoglycemia has been reported in some animals (Narasimhan and Ganla, 1967).

6. Chemical methods are available for the determination of kerosene in blood on the basis of aromatic content (Gerarde and Skiba, 1960; Guertin and Gerarde, 1959). Hydrocarbons have been recovered from lung tissue and identified by gas chromatography and infrared spectroscopy (Johnston *et al.*, 1965).

References:

Ackerly, W. C.; Gibson, G. Lighter fluid "sniffing." Am. J. Psychiatr. *120*:1056-1061, 1964.

American Petroleum Institute. API toxicological review (Kerosene). New York, 1948i.

Anas, N.; Namasonthi, V.; Ginsburg, C. M. Criteria for hospitalizing children who have ingested products containing hydrocarbons. J.A.M.A. *246*:840-847, 1981.

Ashkenazi, A. E.; Berman, S. E. Experimental kerosene poisoning in rats, use of C¹⁴-labelled hendecane as an indicator of absorption. Pediatrics *28*:642-649, 1961.

Bagdassarian, O. M.; Weiner, S. Pneumatocele formation complicating hydrocarbon pneumonitis. Am. J. Roentgen. *95*:104-111, 1964.

Baldachin, J.; Melmed, R. N. Clinical and therapeutic aspects of kerosene poisoning. A series of 200 cases. Br. Med. J. *2*:28-30, 1964.

Barnes, R. L.; Wilkinson, D. S. Epidermal necrolysis from clothing impregnated with paraffin. Br. Med. J. *4*:466-467, 1973.

Barrientos, A.; Ortuno, M. T.; Morales, J. M.; Tello, F. M.;

Rodicio, J. L. Acute renal failure after use of diesel fuel as shampoo. Arch. Intern. Med. 137:1217, 1977.

Beamon, R. F.; Siegel, C. J.; Landers, G.; Green, V. Hydrocarbon ingestion in children: a six-year retrospective study. J. Am. Coll. Emerg. Phys. 5:771-775, 1976.

Bergeson, P. S.; Hales, S. W.; Lastgarten, M. D.; Lipow H. W. Pneumatoceles following hydrocarbon ingestion. Report of three cases and review of the literature. Am. J. Dis. Child. 129:49-54, 1975.

Blattner, R. J. Comments on current literature. Kerosene poisoning. J. Pediatr. 39:391-392, 1951.

Bratton, L.; Haddow, J. E. Ingestion of charcoal lighter fluid. J. Pediat. 87:633-636, 1975.

Brown, J.; Burke, B.; Dajani, A. S. Experimental kerosene pneumonia: Evaluation of some therapeutic regimens. J. Pediatr. 84:396-401, 1974.

Brunner, S.; Rovosing, H.; Wulf, H. Roentgenographic changes in the lungs of children with kerosene poisoning. Am. Rev. Resp. Dis. 89:250-254, 1964.

Cachia, E. A.; Fenech, F. F. Kerosene poisoning in children. Arch. Dis. Child. 39:502-504, 1964.

Campbell, J. G. Pneumatocele formation following hydrocarbon ingestion. Am. Rev. Resp. Dis. 101:414-418, 1970.

Carithers, H. A. Accident prevention in childhood - the kerosene hazard. J. A. M. A. 159:109-111, 1955.

Chin, L.; Picchioni, A. L.; Duplisse, B. R. Comparative antidotal effectiveness of activated charcoal, Arizona montmorillonite, and evaporated milk. J. Pharm. Sci. 58:1353-1356, 1969.

Crisp, A. J.; Bhalla, A. K.; Hoffbrand, B. I. Acute tubular necrosis after exposure to diesel oil. Br. Med. J. 2:177-178, 1979.

Daffner, R. H.; Jimenez, J. P. The double gastric fluid level in kerosene poisoning. Radiology 106:383-384, 1973.

Davies, N. E. Jet fuel intoxication. Aerosp. Med. 35:481-482, 1964.

Deichmann, W. B.; Kitzmiller, K. V.; Withrup, S.; Johansmann, R. Kerosene intoxication. Ann. Intern. Med. 21:803-823, 1944.

Dice, W. H.; Ward, G.; Kelley, J.; Kilpatrick, W. R. Pulmonary toxicity following gastrointestinal ingestion of kerosene. Ann. Emerg. Med. 11:138-142, 1982.

Dooley, A. E. Toxicity of petroleum product additives. Arch. Environ. Health 6:324-328, 1963.

Dragsted, P. J.; Rodbro, P. Pseudocysts of the lungs in kerosene poisoning. Chest 48:87-90, 1965.

Drinker, P.; Yaglou, C. P.; Warren, M. F. The threshold toxicity of gasoline vapor. J. Ind. Hyg. Toxicol. 25:225-232, 1943.

Foley, J. C.; Dreyer, N. B.; Soule, A. B.; Woll, E. Kerosene poisoning in young children. Radiology 62:817-829, 1954.

Gallassi, R.; Montagna, P.; Pazzaglia, P.; Cirignotta, F.; Lugaresi, E. Peripheral neuropathy due to gasoline sniffing. A case report. Eur. Neurol. 19:419-421, 1980.

Gerarde, H. W. Toxicological studies on hydrocarbons. V. Kerosene. Toxicol. Appl. Pharmacol. 1:462-474, 1959.

Gerarde, H. W. Toxicological studies on hydrocarbons. IX. The aspiration hazard and toxicity of hydrocarbons and hydrocarbon mixtures. Arch. Environ. Health 6:329-341, 1963.

Gerarde, H. W.; Skiba, P. Toxicological studies on hydrocarbons; VI. A colorimetric method for the determination of kerosine in blood. Clin. Chem. 6:327-331, 1960.

Gershon-Cohen, J.; Bringhurst, L. S.; Byrne, R. N. Roentgenography of kerosene poisoning (chemical pneumonitis). Am. J. Roentgenol. Radium Ther. Nucl. Med. 69:557-562, 1953.

Glaser, F. B. Inhalation psychosis and related states. Arch. Gen. Psychiatry 14:315-322, 1966.

Green, D. O. Intravenous energine - a case report. Clin. Toxicol. 10:283-286, 1977.

Guertin, D. L.; Gerarde, H. W. Toxicological studies on hydrocarbons. IV. An ultraviolet spectrophotometric method for the quantitative determination of benzene and alkylbenzenes in blood. Arch. Ind. Health 20:262-265, 1959.

Hamilton, W. C. Death from drinking coal oil. Med. News 71:214-215, 1897.

Harris, V. J.; Brown, R. Pneumatoceles as a complication of chemical pneumonia after hydrocarbon ingestion. Am. J. Roentgenol. Rad. Ther. Nucl. Med. 125:531-537, 1976.

Heacock, C. H. Pneumonia in children following the ingestion of petroleum products. Radiology 53:793-797, 1949.

Hiebel, J.; Gant, H. L.; Schwartz, S. O.; Friedman, I. A. Bone marrow depression following exposure to kerosene. A report of 3 cases. Am. J. Med. Sci. 246:185-191, 1963.

Huxtable, K. A.; Bolande, R. D.; Klaus, M. Experimental furniture polish pneumonia in rats. Pediatrics 34:228-235, 1964.

James, F. W.; Kaplan, S.; Benzing, G. Cardiac complications following hydrocarbon ingestion. Am. J. Dis. Child. 121:431-433, 1971a.

Jamison, K. E.; Wallace, E. R. Kerosene pneumonitis treated with adrenal steroids. Calif. Med. 100:43-44, 1964.

Johnson, D. E. Hypoplastic anemia following chronic exposure to kerosene. J. Am. Med. Wom. Assoc. 10:421-424, 1955.

Johnston, G. W.; Hoch, W. S.; Butz, W. C. Recovery of hydrocarbons from lung tissue in fatal ingestion of furniture polish, characterization by gas chromatography and infrared spectroscopy. Am. J. Clin. Path. 43:570-574, 1965.

Lavenstein, A. F. Ingestion of kerosene complicated by pneumonia, pneumothorax, pneumopericardium and subcutaneous emphysema. J. Pediatr. 26:395-400, 1945.

Lesser, L. I.; Weens, H. S.; McKay, J. D. Pulmonary manifestations following ingestion of kerosene. J. Pediatr. 23:352-364, 1943.

Mann, M. D.; Pirie, D. J.; Wolfsdorf, J. Kerosene absorption in primates. J. Pediatr. 91:495-498, 1977.

Marks, M. I.; Chicme, L.; Legere, G.; Hillman, E. Adrenocorticosteroid treatment of hydrocarbon pneumonia in children, a cooperative study. J. Pediatr. 81:366-369, 1972.

Mayock, R. L.; Borzorgnia, N.; Zinsser, H. F. Kerosene pneumonitis treated with adrenal steroids. Ann. Intern. Med. 54:559-566, 1961.

McNally, W. D. Kerosene poisoning in children. J. Pediatr. 48:296-299, 1956.

Mintz, A. A. Furniture polish intoxication. South. Med. J. 59:1010-1014, 1966.

Montgomery, M. R.; Wier, G. T.; Zieve, F. J.; Anders, M. W. Human intoxication following inhalation exposure to synthetic jet lubricating oil. Clin. Toxicol. 11:423-426, 1977.

Narasimhan, M. J., Jr.; Ganla, V. G. Experimental studies on kerosene poisoning. Acta Pharmacol. Toxicol. 25:214-224, 1967.

Nunn, J. A.; Martin, F. M. Gasoline and kerosene poisoning in children. J. A. M. A. 103:472-474, 1934.

Olstad, R. B.; Lord, R. M., Jr. Kerosene intoxication. Am. J. Dis. Child. 83:446-453, 1952.

Parker, G. A.; Bogo, V.; Young, R. W. Acute toxicity of conventional versus shale-derived JP5 jet fuel: light microscopic, hematologic, and serum chemistry studies. Toxicol. Appl. Pharmacol. 57:302-317, 1981.

Press, E. Cooperative kerosene poisoning study. Evaluation of gastric lavage and other factors in the treatment of accidental ingestion of petroleum distillate products. Pediatrics 29:648-674, 1962.

Reed, E. S.; Leikin, S.; Kerman, H. D. Kerosene intoxication. Am. J. Dis. Child. 79:623-632, 1950.

Reingold, I. M.; Lasky, I. I. Acute fatal poisoning following ingestion of a solution of DDT. Ann. Intern. Med. 26:945-947, 1947.

Reynolds, J.; Bonte, F. J. Kerosene pneumonitis. Tex. State J. Med. 56:34-38, 1960.

Richardson, J. A.; Pratt-Thomas, H. R. Toxic effects of varying doses of kerosene administered by different routes. Am. J. Med. Sci. 221:531-536, 1951.

Ring, R.; Nelson, J. D. Hydrocarbon pneumonitis in rats, comparison of mineral seal oil furniture polish and kerosene toxicities with an evaluation of gastric lavage. Arch. Environ. Health 13:749-752, 1966.

Schneider, L. Pulmonary hazard of the ingestion of mineral oil in the apparently healthy adult. N. Engl. J. Med. 240:284-291, 1949.

Scott, E. P. Pneumonia, pneumothorax and emphysema following ingestion of kerosene. J. Pediatr. 25:31-34, 1944.

Soule, A. B., Jr.; Foley, J. C. Poisoning from petroleum distillates, the hazards of kerosene and furniture polish. J. Maine Med. Assoc. 48:103-110, 1957.

Steele, R. W.; Conklin, R. H.; Mark, H. M. Corticosteroids and antibiotics for the treatment of fulminant hydrocarbon aspiration. J. A. M. A. 219:1434-1437, 1972.

Steiner, M. M. Syndromes of kerosene poisoning in children. Am. J. Dis. Child. 74:32-44, 1947.

Stockman, J. A. More on hydrocarbon-induced hemolysis. J. Pediatr. 90:848, 1977.

Tonge, J. I.; Hurley, R. N.; Ferguson, J. Systemic fat embolism associated with the toxic effects of aviation-fuel inhalation and general anesthesia. Lancet 1:1059-1063, 1969.

Vaziri, N. D.; Smith, P. J.; Wilson, A. Toxicity with intravenous injection of naphtha in man. Clin. Toxicol. 16:335-343, 1980.

von Oettingen, W. F. Toxicity and potential dangers of aliphatic and aromatic hydrocarbons. Public Health Bull. No. 255, 1940.

Walsh, W. A.; Scarpa, F. J.; Brown, R. S.; Ashcraft, K. W.; Green, V. A.; Holder, T. M.; Amoury, R. A. Gasoline immersion burn. N. Engl. J. Med. 291:830, 1974.

Wolfe, B. M.; Brodeur, A. E.; Shields, J. B. The role of gastrointestinal absorption of kerosene in producing pneumonitis in dogs. J. Pediatr. 76:867-873, 1970.

Wolfsdorf, J.; Kundig, H. Dexamethasone in the management of kerosene pneumonia. Pediatrics 53:86-90, 1974.

Wolfsdorf, J.; Paed, D.; Kungdig, H. Kerosene poisoning in primate. S. Afr. Med. J. 46:619-621, 1972.

Wycoff, C. C. Aspiration during induction of anesthesia, its prevention. Anesth. Analg. 38:5-13, 1959.

LEAD

Lead and its salts are used in a wide variety of processes in and out of industry. For example, the metal is used in printer's type, storage battery plates, solder, electric cable covering, bearing alloys, pipes, and gun shot. The carbonate, chromate, and various oxides are found in paints and pottery glaze; "white lead" is the carbonate (Klein et al., 1970; Leonard and Lynch, 1958). Salts like the arsenate have been used in agriculture as insecticidal sprays (Nelson et al., 1973). Occasionally solutions of the subacetate serve in medicine as external astringents. Cases of lead poisoning have been traced to illicit alcoholic beverages such as "moonshine" (Asokan et al., 1974; Whitfield et al., 1972). The inks on colored pages of popular magazines contain startlingly high concentrations of lead (Hankin et al., 1973). The burning of magazines (Perkins and Oski, 1976) and battery casings (Dolcourt et al., 1981) for home heating has resulted in poisonings.

Some of the more unusual sources of lead poisoning include inadequately ventilated indoor firing ranges (Landrigan et al., 1975; Fischbein et al., 1979), surma, which is a mascara-like pigment which is applied to the conjunctival surfaces for cosmetic purposes in some Asian societies (Ali et al., 1978), Asian herbal remedies (Lightfoote et al., 1977) and aphrodisiacs (Brearly and Forsythe, 1978), lead transported into homes on the contaminated clothing of exposed workers (Baker et al., 1977), lead pigments in tapestries (Fischbein et al., 1982) and the deliberate ingestion of lead carbonate by an artist in the hope of inducing hallucinations that would lead to more creative imagery (Chiba et al., 1980).

Pica (perverted appetite) is a frequent exposure factor in chronic plumbism, particularly among children in lower socioeconomic classes (Greenberg et al., 1958; Millican et al., 1956). Since pica is recognized to be a manifestation of an iron-deficiency anemia in some children (Lanzkowsky, 1959), it is tempting to speculate that correction of the anemia is a way to prevent pica and lead poisoning in these cases. However, other complex environmental factors such as low calcium diets (Snowdon and Sanderson, 1974) and an inherited deficiency in red cell glucose-6-phosphate dehydrogenase activity (McIntire and Angle, 1972) or sickle-cell anemia (Anku and Harris, 1974) may play important, if poorly understood, roles in the epidemiology of lead poisoning. Symptomatic lead poisoning occurs throughout the year but displays a seasonal incidence with a peak in the spring and summer months. The interested reader is referred to the following epidemiological studies: Blanksma et al. (1969), Chisolm and Harrison (1956), Ingalls et al. (1961), Lin-Fu (1973), and Rapaport and Rubin (1941).

Epidemic lead poisoning has been associated with ancient societies; some historians believe that it contributed to the fall of the Roman Empire. Studies of lead in 1600-year-old Peruvian skeletons, however, revealed concentrations three orders of magnitude below those of modern Englishmen and Americans (Ericson et al., 1979). Blood levels in remote Himalayan populations are substantially below those in members of industrialized societies (Piomelli et al., 1980). Childhood plumbism in U.S. slums has been referred to as "the silent epidemic." It has been suggested that the results of many laboratory and field studies on lead exposure have been confounded by the fact that the reagents, nutrients and control populations were contaminated far in excess of "natural" levels (Settle and Patterson, 1980).

Toxicology: Lead is poisonous in all forms (Fairhall and Sayers, 1940). It is one of the most hazardous of the toxic metals because the poison is cumulative and the toxic effects are many and severe. The intestinal and respiratory channels are the usual routes by which lead enters the body. Thus systemic lead poisoning can result from the inhalation of airborne lead particulate matter or fumes (Hammond et al., 1981; Zimmer, 1961) or from the ingestion of lead in water, food, etc.

At least in rats intestinal lead absorption resembles calcium transport in that it is bidirectional (Aungst and Fung, 1981) and rate-limited, so that that the blood lead level is not a linear function of the oral dose (Aungst et al., 1981). In rats intestinal absorption is greater in suckling animals than in dams, so that the young acquire higher brain concentrations (Mykkanen et al., 1979). In healthy humans the kinetics of lead metabolism fit a three-compartment model. The first compartment, in which lead has a half-life of about 35 days, includes the blood; it receives lead absorbed from the gut, delivers some of it to the urine and communicates with the other two pools. The second compartment, in which lead has about the same half-life, encompasses soft tissues, contains only about half as much lead as the blood and loses some of it to hair, nails, sweat, saliva, bile and other digestive secretions. The third compartment, the skeleton, contains the vast bulk of the total body burden; here lead has a very long half-life, although bones may differ in their rates of lead turnover (Rabinowitz et al., 1976). The lead content of dense human bone increases steadily with age whereas in spongy bone lead reaches a plateau or even decreases (Gross et al., 1975). In exposed workers the apparent blood lead half-life was positively correlated with the duration of exposure and with the blood lead concentration at the time of termination of exposure (O'Flaherty et al., 1982).

Intoxication from a single exposure is unusual, but it has resulted from both accidental and intentional ingestion of solutions of soluble lead salts (Karlog and Möller, 1958; Karpatkin, 1961). After the immediate gastrointestinal reaction subsides, a threat remains that severe and even fatal attacks may reappear within days or weeks. These delayed and persistent reactions are usually indistinguishable from the signs and symptoms of typical chronic plumbism (saturnism), where intoxication arises from the cumulative retention of lead from repeated small exposures (see below). Like the latter, the delayed reaction may develop insidiously or with dramatic suddenness. The ingestion of metallic lead may lead to an acute attack after a long (45 days in one case) asymptomatic period (Biehusen and Pulaski, 1956). Thus the acute and chronic syndromes may merge, and both are discussed below.

Following ingestion of a large amount of any soluble lead salt (especially the acetate, carbonate or chromate), the initial signs and symptoms are due largely to local irritation of the alimentary tract. If absorption is sufficient, pain, leg cramps, muscle weakness, paresthesias, depression, coma, and death may follow within 1 or 2 days. Fatal poisonings of this acute type have been described after the ingestion of lead acetate and carbonate in doses which usually exceed 30

gm. (Karpatkin, 1961; Webster, 1930). Rarely a hemolytic crisis may occur in acute or subacute plumbism (Miwa et al., 1981; Nortier et al., 1980; Valentine et al., 1976).

If sufficient lead is retained after a single exposure, a syndrome identical with chronic intoxication may develop within weeks or months. Many acute poisonings, however, subside without sequelae, since the absorption of lead from the bowel is inherently slow and incomplete (Cantarow and Trumper, 1944; Kehoe et al., 1933a-c, 1935). Presumably this outcome is also favored by vigorous treatment. As long as the body, however, contains excessive amounts of lead fixed in the tissues (notably bone, see Voight and Larsson, 1959), symptomatic recurrences are an ever-present threat. Whether insidious or sudden in onset, a recurrence may occur without an exciting incident or may be precipitated by any stressful situation such as fever, acidosis, alkalosis (Byers and Maloof, 1954), or deleading therapy (Smith, 1959a). In all cases these episodes are regularly associated with a definite and characteristic rise in the lead concentration of the body fluids and excreta.

Cases of lead poisoning due to retained bullets are reported only rarely but represent potentially life-threatening reactions (Linden et al., 1982). Victims of lead shot who experience toxic symptoms almost immediately have been described in the European literature, but almost all cases in the United States have involved the dissolution of a single bullet over several months to more than 20 years (Dillman et al., 1979). The diagnosis of lead poisoning may not be made until the time of postmortem examination (DiMalo and Garriott, 1980). Bullets in joint spaces are said to be more likely to cause toxic complications than are bullets lodged in soft tissues (Linden et al., 1982). An accelerated mobilization and sudden onset of signs and symptoms may be triggered by such stresses as thyrotoxicosis (Cagin et al., 1978) or other endocrinopathy, infection, and alcoholism (Linden et al., 1982). To prevent a clinical exacerbation due to the stresses of surgery, it is probably prudent to employ chelation therapy (see below) before any operative intervention (Linden et al., 1982).

Intoxication from multiple exposures is the usual pattern; it represents a response to the accumulative retention of lead from repeated small intakes. Chronic plumbism expresses itself in many diverse ways, but three major clinical syndromes are recognized. The *alimentary type* is characterized by anorexia, a metallic taste, constipation, and severe abdominal cramps (lead colic) due to intestinal spasm and sometimes associated with rigidity of the abdominal wall, leading to misdiagnoses and even surgical intervention (Berger and Lundberg, 1951). Lead-induced abdominal pain is a sensitive index of intoxication and may occur before significant elevation of blood lead levels (Dahlgren, 1978). Extreme colonic dilation (megacolon) with a remarkable return to normal after successful chelation therapy has been reported (Richardson and Buisseret, 1981).

The *neuromuscular type* is characteristic of adult plumbism but has occasionally been reported in children (Feldman *et al.*, 1977; Seto and Freeman, 1964); it consists of peripheral neuritis which is usually painless and limited to the extensor muscles. A wrist drop is the most characteristic lesion of lead palsy. Weakness or paralysis may occasionally be accompanied by muscular wasting, arthralgia and myalgia, but sensation is otherwise unaffected (Boothby *et al.*, 1974). As produced in laboratory animals, a decrease in motor nerve conduction velocity is associated with segmental demyelination (Fullerton, 1966; Myers *et al.*, 1980a). In humans slowing of motor and sensory nerve conduction velocities, especially in the arm nerves, showed a close correlation with increasing blood lead levels (Seppalainen *et al.*, 1979).

The *cerebral type* of lead poisoning has been called lead encephalopathy. Although rare in adults (Crutcher, 1963; Cirksena *et al.*, 1962; Morris *et al.*, 1964; Whitfield *et al.*, 1972), it is the most common type in children. Sometimes a child who is fully conscious and alert on admission lapses into a terminal coma within a few hours (Alexander and Delves, 1972), but more characteristically children present in convulsions (Harris, 1976) or preconvulsive stages as described under "Symptomatology" below. Encephalopathy is a complication in about 50% of pediatric lead poisonings, and before the introduction of combined chelation therapy (see below) in 1964, the mortality rate among children developing cerebral involvement was about 25%. In those with encephalopathy, such long-term sequelae as neurologic defects, retarded mental development and chronic hyperactivity are more likely than in those with intense exposure but no encephalopathy (Rummo *et al.*, 1979; Sachs *et al.*, 1979). Of those who survived, one-third had permanent neurologic sequelae (Popoff *et al.*, 1963; Smith *et al.*, 1963b; Sanford, 1955), but the incidence of permanent injury appears to be lower today.

In lead encephalopathy of childhood the brain is characteristically swollen and may appear hyperemic or pale. Exudates containing plasma proteins are present. Lesions are found throughout the brain but in greatest abundance in the hemispheres and cerebellum (Blackman, 1937). In at least one adult, however, there was a remarkable focal abnormality which led to the incorrect diagnosis of a cerebral glioma (Powers *et al.*, 1977). An unusual form of calcification of the cerebrum was noted in surveys and routine autopsies in Queensland, Australia; it correlated

positively with the lead content of bones (Tonge *et al.*, 1977). After surviving for 40 years in a state of severe mental deterioration that followed an episode of lead encephalopathy at the age of 2 years, an individual was found to have in his brain neurofibrillary tangles characteristic of Alzheimer's presenile dementia (Niklowitz and Mandybur, 1975). Lead inclusion bodies have been found in the anterior horn cells and the neurons of the substantia nigra in rhesus monkeys given lead chronically (Osheroff *et al.*, 1982).

Edema and hemorrhage presumably due to capillary dysfunction occurred in the cerebellum of nursing rat pups although tissue lead levels were no higher there than in other regions, suggesting a special sensitivity of cerebellar capillaries (Goldstein *et al.*, 1974). The mitochondria of capillary endothelial cells from the cortex of rats accumulated electron-dense deposits when the cells were suspended in culture medium containing lead. Since the lead accumulation was in mitochondrial areas known to contain high concentrations of calcium, lead may have been interfering with calcium function in these regions (Silbergeld *et al.*, 1980). In guinea pigs given a tracer dose of ^{210}Pb, the choroid plexus accumulated lead to concentrations 70 times higher than that in CSF or brain substance, suggesting the existence of an active transport process (O'Tuama *et al.*, 1976).

Lead inhibits γ-glutamyl transpeptidase more intensively in young rat pups than in older ones (Scheri *et al.*, 1981). Adenyl cyclase activity in many rat tissues including brain is inhibited by low concentrations of lead and by several other heavy metals; only lead, however, also stimulated phosphodiesterase activity (Nathanson and Bloom, 1976). In children exposed to lead, elevations in urinary catecholamine metabolites have been noted (Silbergeld and Chisolm, 1976). Various influences of lead on cholinergic (Modak *et al.*, 1975), dopaminergic (Silbergeld and Alder, 1978), and noradrenergic (Golter and Michaelson, 1975; Taylor *et al.*, 1978) functions in brain have been described, but no unified hypothesis has appeared to explain these effects.

Several studies (Grandjean *et al.*, 1979; Needleman *et al.*, 1979; Valciukas *et al.*, 1978) in children and adults with mild degrees of lead retention have revealed subtle psychological dysfunctions at blood lead levels above 40 μg./dl.; these disorders included impairments of long-term memory, psychomotor performance, verbal and visiospatial abstraction, auditory and speech processing, nonadaptive behavior in the classroom and general intelligence scales.

In any type of chronic plumbism, the patient may show facial pallor, a gingival lead line, mild jaundice, anemia, basophilic stippling of the red blood cells, albuminuria, cylindruria, porphyrinuria, and excessive urinary and blood concentrations of lead (Byers, 1959; Cohen and Ahrens, 1959; Jenkins and Mellins, 1957). Half of one series of cases exhibited metaphyseal dysplasia (Pease and Newton, 1962), but the diagnostic reliability of "lead lines" in long bone x-rays has been challenged (Sartain et al., 1964).

Although temporary disturbances in renal function are well known, lead is not generally recognized as a dangerous nephrotoxin. In man, at least two types of renal dysfunction are recognized. The first is a temporary disorder of the proximal tubules. The reabsorption of amino acids, glucose and some electrolytes is impaired. In rats an increased excretion of sodium and, to a lesser extent, potassium resulted in hyponatremia (Suketa et al., 1979). Renal sodium- and potassium-dependent ATPase activity was markedly decreased after lead administration to rats, as well as potassium-dependent phosphatase activity (Suketa et al., 1979, 1981). Complete recovery of renal function is the rule at least in short-term plumbism of childhood (Tepper, 1963). In rats, however, lead exposure during infancy caused permanent but subtle renal dysfunction (Mailman et al., 1978).

In adults with prolonged and intensive exposures to lead, a chronic and progressive nephrotic syndrome is recognized (Emmerson, 1963; Lilis et al., 1968, 1979; Morgan et al., 1966; Wedeen et al., 1975, 1979). In many of these patients, the functional disorder is associated with tubular atrophy and interstitial nephritis (Wedeen et al. 1979). Unlike the tubular lesion above, this nephropathy is only sometimes improved by chelation therapy (Wedeen et al., 1979). Because glomerular and tubular immunoglobulin deposition was found in many biopsy specimens examined by techniques of immunofluorescence, it has been suggested that an autoimmune reaction contributes to the interstitial nephritis (Wedeen et al., 1979).

So-called saturnine gout (Ball and Sorenson, 1969; Batuman et al., 1981) has been ascribed in years past to a renal lesion and consequent hyperuricemia. Giant tophi have been observed in humans (Orfanos and Kunzig, 1975), but many clinical differences between saturnine gout and the inherited form of gout are recognized. Indeed, studies in pigs have suggested that the two conditions differ even at the molecular level. Lead injections in pigs greatly increased the urinary excretion of guanine and resulted in guanine concretions in and around joints, not concretions of sodium urate. Perhaps lead inhibition of guanine aminohydrolase (guanase) is responsible for saturnine gout rather than a renal lesion (Farkas et al., 1978), but hyperuricacidemia accompanies the disease in most (if not all) human patients (e.g., Orfanos and Kunzig, 1975). Pathognomonic intranuclear inclusions can often be seen in the epithelium of the proximal tubule, but their significance is unknown (Choie and Richter, 1972).

The nephrotic syndrome is often accompanied by arterial hypertension (Lilis et al., 1968). In the past the pallor of lead poisoning has been ascribed in part to direct spasmogenic effects of lead on blood vessels. In dogs acute intravenous lead in small doses increased plasma renin activity (Mouw et al., 1978) whereas in chronically exposed rats lead appeared to inhibit renin synthesis and release, as well as to reduce the plasma concentration of angiotensin II (Victery et al., 1982).

As with lead-induced kidney dysfunction, the anemia and other hematologic disorders of lead poisoning (Griggs, 1964) sometimes complicate the illness (Berk et al., 1970; Moosa and Harris, 1969), but they are rarely the primary cause of death. In contrast to the rare hemolytic crisis in acute plumbism, the usual anemia of chronic poisoning is of the hypochromic, normocytic type and has little clinical significance except in advanced cases (Hutchinson and Stark, 1961; Wolman, 1956). Large dilated red cells, some shaped like four-leaf clovers, have been found in peripheral blood (Canberk et al., 1978). An apparently inducible, lead-binding protein of low molecular weight has been isolated from the red cells of exposed individuals (Raghavan and Gonick, 1977). Calcium and lead compete for binding sites on the red cell membrane (Ong and Lee, 1980a), but a considerable fraction of blood lead penetrates into red cells and binds to hemoglobin (Ong and Lee, 1980b).

Lead has complex, multiple and still incompletely understood effects on heme synthesis (Fujii, 1979). It is a potent and specific inhibitor of the activity of δ-aminolevulinic acid dehydratase, a component enzyme in the biosynthesis of hemoproteins and cytochromes. The discovery that lead forms a specific complex with the substrate δ-aminolevulinic acid points to this interaction as the inhibitory mechanism (Baxter et al., 1979). A fluorescent porphyrin in the red cells of lead-poisoned patients and in iron deficiency anemia has been identified as zinc protoporphyrin (Lamola and Yamane, 1974). This pigment (ZPP) may accumulate to even higher levels than in patients with erythropoietic protoporphyria, but the characteristic photosensitivity does not occur in plumbism because the pigment does not diffuse out of the erythrocyte (Piomelli et al., 1975). The ZPP is apparently bound to the heme sites on hemoglobin (Lamola et al., 1975), and its detection by fluorescence constitutes the basis for a portable field device (hematofluorometer) useful in screening for lead poisoning (Fischbein et al., 1978).

Hepatitis and hepatic failure, together with more common manifestations of lead poisoning, were prominent in a series of cases (Beattie *et al.*, 1975, 1979) involving lead and opium pills, which were crushed, suspended in water and self-injected intravenously. Although hepatotoxicity in these cases was ascribed to the bizarre route of exposure, liver damage also occurred (Nortier *et al.*, 1980) following a single massive ingestion of red lead (lead tetroxide). In isolated rat hepatocytes lead induces changes in intracellular calcium homeostasis and in calcium-mediated hepatocyte functions (Pounds *et al.*, 1982a and b). Evidence for lead-induced disturbances in glucose homeostasis has also been obtained in rats (Stevenson *et al.*, 1976). Despite these uncommon reports of hepatotoxic actions of lead and its well known effects on the heme biosynthetic pathway, lead had only minimal effects on cytochrome P450-dependent drug metabolizing activity in workmen with biochemical signs of lead poisoning (Fischbein *et al.*, 1977). Diffuse degenerative changes in the myocardium have been described in rats given lead in their drinking water for 6 weeks (Asokan, 1974).

Lead is clearly teratogenic in laboratory animals (EPA, Air Quality Criteria Document for Lead, in revision). It is not known with certainty whether or not it is teratogenic in humans. In the guinea pig lead crosses the placenta into the fetal circulation faster than mercury but slower than methylmercury or cadmium (Kelman and Walter, 1980). A survey of almost 12,000 samples of human umbilical cord blood taken in the United States between 1979 and 1981 showed that mean values of lead decreased by about 11% per year; the levels were higher in infants born in the summer than in the winter (Rabinowitz and Needleman, 1982). An apparent association between minimally elevated blood levels of lead and microcephaly among rural children (mean age 7 years) was ascribed to probable prenatal exposure (Routh *et al.*, 1979). Mild transplacental lead poisoning and evidence for abnormally high levels of lead without symptoms have been described in human newborns (Singh *et al.*, 1978; Timpo *et al.*, 1979).

In spite of the multiplicity of symptoms, acute crises in chronic plumbism are treated in essentially the same way as acute lead poisoning, according to the outline below. These measures are designed to reduce the concentration of free lead in blood and body fluids by preventing the absorption or resorption of lead from the alimentary tract and by promoting the urinary and biliary excretion of lead without damage to the excretory organs.

Treatment of inorganic lead poisoning: In symptomatic episodes the most effective single therapeutic agent that has received FDA approval is the calcium disodium salt of ethylenediaminetetraacetic acid (EDTA) known as edetate calcium disodium (CaNa$_2$EDTA), (Bess-

man *et al.*, 1954; Chisolm and Harrison, 1957; Cotter, 1954; Crutcher, 1963; Haritos, 1961; Leckie and Tompsett, 1958; Sidbury, 1955; Tanis, 1955). This compound forms a stable, soluble, nontoxic, virtually nonionic complex with lead ions. The result of administration is usually a considerable rise in the urinary excretion of lead and at least a transient suppression of toxic signs and symptoms, sometimes including even the manifestations of lead encephalopathy (Bessman *et al.*, 1954; Radwan *et al.*, 1982). For a detailed discussion of the uses and hazards of this compound, see EDETATE CALCIUM DISODIUM, p. III-163.

Calcium trisodium penetate (DTPA), a chelating agent closely related to CaNa$_2$EDTA, is not generally available in the United States. Its efficacy in lead mobilization is about equivalent to that of CaNa$_2$EDTA (Albahary and Guillaume, 1966; Brugsch *et al.*, 1965; Hammond, 1971). Because the lead-EDTA complex is dialyzable, hemodialysis has been attempted after loading the patient with the chelating agent. Although the clinical benefits were adjudged insignificant in one case (Smith *et al.*, 1965), lead excretion may be significantly increased in patients with renal insufficiency (Mehbod, 1967). In the experience of Pedersen (1978), who managed a patient after a single massive ingestion of 40 gm. of lead oxide, the blood lead half-life was 96 hours when given CaNa$_2$EDTA alone but only 9 hours when infusions of the chelator were combined with extracorporeal hemodialysis. Experience with combined hemodialysis and chelation therapy against some forms of mercury (see p. III-270) has also been encouraging.

Dimercaprol (BAL) also forms a complex with lead, but for reasons that are not fully understood, BAL alone has seldom proved useful in the treatment of clinical lead poisoning (Bradley and Baumgartner, 1958; Germuth and Eagle, 1948; Ryder and Kehoe, 1947; Weatherall, 1948). The lead mobilizing patterns of BAL and CaNa$_2$EDTA differ and complement each other. BAL appeared to be less effective in removing lead from the brain and other soft tissues, whereas it seemed to be superior in animals at sequestering lead from bony structures (Aronson and Hammond, 1964). More recent evidence suggests that therapy with CaNa$_2$EDTA (and perhaps all chelating agents) results primarily in removal of lead from bone. This is followed by a redistribution of lead from soft tissues to the skeleton (Hammond *et al.*, 1967). This hypothesis is difficult to reconcile with observations on an adult with lead encephalopathy, polyneuropathy and anemia; during CaNa$_2$EDTA therapy the encephalopathy and anemia improved but the polyneuritis intensified (Dubi *et al.*, 1979).

Penicillamine has also been used with apparent success as a systemic antidote in lead poisoning (Boulding and Baker, 1957; Harris, 1958). The isomer of penicillamine used in these and other early trials was not specified. Probably the racemic mixture (D,L form) was prescribed, but since the early to mid-1960s D-penicillamine has been used almost exclusively. In terms of efficacy, no distinctions are recognized between D- and D,L-penicillamine (cf. Westerman et al., 1965, with Hammond, 1973). In contrast, N-acetyl-D-penicillamine proved inactive in promoting the urinary excretion of lead in two patients whose output responded favorably to D-penicillamine (Cramer, 1974). Albahary and Guillaume (1966), Hammond (1973) and Westerman et al. (1965), however, found D- and D,L-penicillamines, whether given by mouth or intravenously, to be inferior to DTPA and to CaNa$_2$EDTA in accelerating lead excretion. Results with combined DTPA and penicillamine were equivocal. Because it can be given by mouth, penicillamine has found particular utility in mild and uncomplicated plumbism (Goldberg et al., 1963; Marcus, 1982; Ohlsson, 1962; Selander et al., 1966; Wyllie et al., 1963), and in prolonged or supplementary therapy (Vitale et al., 1973). In one large program of ambulatory treatment, however, there were several adverse reactions to penicillamine but none to CaNa$_2$EDTA (Sachs et al., 1970). In spite of the large amount of favorable experience, D-penicillamine is not yet officially sanctioned by the FDA for use in lead poisoning.

Newer agents not yet generally available or approved in the United States include 2,3-dimercaptosuccinic acid (DMSA) and sodium 2,3-dimercaptopropane-1-sulfonate (DMPS). In terms of their efficacy in promoting the urinary excretion of lead in acutely poisoned rats, Hofmann and Segewitz (1975) found DTPA to be superior to DMPS, which was in turn superior to D-penicillamine. In minimally lead-poisoned rats, DMSA was as effective as BAL, and both were superior to CaNa$_2$EDTA or D-penicillamine, when the chelating agents were administered intraperitoneally; however, DMSA was almost as effective by mouth as by the intraperitoneal route and significantly more effective than oral D-penicillamine (Graziano et al., 1978). In five lead-poisoned smelter workers, DMSA appeared to be effective and well tolerated (Friedheim et al., 1978). Ascorbic acid given orally to lead-exposed rats was said to be as effective as equimolar amounts of parenteral CaNa$_2$EDTA, and the combination was more than twice as effective as either given alone (Goyer and Cherian, 1979). In calves thiamine given together with lead prevented signs of toxicity and death and resulted in lower tissue levels of lead (Bratton et al., 1981).

Repeated warnings have been made against the oral prophylactic use of CaNa$_2$EDTA or other chelating agents to prevent lead toxicity in exposed workers (e.g., Lilis and Fischbein, 1976). Sodium citrate, D-penicillamine, CaNa$_2$EDTA and BAL, all given by mouth, increased lead absorption from the gastrointestinal tract of rats, and all except CaNa$_2$EDTA increased the amount of lead retained in the body (Jugo et al., 1975).

In the management of acute encephalopathy the best combination of agents is CaNa$_2$EDTA and BAL. In one series of cases therapy was judged successful in 21 of 22 children (Coffin et al., 1966). In another series no deaths occurred with the combination, whereas a 25% mortality would be expected with CaNa$_2$EDTA alone (Chisolm, 1968). Flap craniectomy to reduce the high intracranial pressure of acute encephalopathy is unsatisfactory (Greengard et al., 1962), and the results of a trial with parenteral steroids and mild hypothermia were inconclusive (Greengard et al., 1965). Osmotic decompression of the brain has apparently been successful (Greengard, 1961; Katz, 1960). Even if death is prevented, however, 25% of children with lead encephalopathy or recurrent but less severe bouts of plumbism sustain permanent brain injury. Thus, many authorities recommend vigorous prophylactic deleading therapy as in the case of asymptomatic children with blood lead in the range of 50 to 80 µg./100 ml. (Chisolm, 1973; Sachs et al., 1970). In general, lead poisoning is treated more vigorously in children than in adults, whether there are symptoms or not.

Toxicology of alkyl lead: Tetraethyl and tetramethyl lead are lipid-soluble liquids of high volatility that have been employed as gasoline additives. Ordinarily, their presence in gasoline does not contribute significantly to the acute oral toxicity of the hydrocarbon mixture (see KEROSENE, p. III-222). Prolonged compulsive "sniffing" of gasoline, however, has resulted in severe encephalopathy and death (Boeckx et al., 1977; Hansen and Sharp, 1978; Law and Nelson, 1968; Robinson, 1978; Valpey et al., 1978). Some cases had features in common with chronic inorganic lead poisoning, suggesting that some of the retained alkyl lead was degraded to inorganic lead (Robinson, 1978). Large numbers of children residing in isolated communities may be exposed to lead by this practice (Boeckx et al., 1977; Kaufman and Wiese, 1978; Seshia et al., 1978).

In contrast to lead salts, these alkyl derivatives are capable of rapidly penetrating the intact skin (Laug and Kunze, 1948). Although their record of safety under ordinary use conditions was regarded in the past as good, the mean blood lead level in one survey of filling station operators and garage workers was more than twice that in a control population of clerks and students (Moore et al., 1976). Besides occasional skin contact with liquid gasoline, such workers are also exposed to the lead of automobile exhaust gas, which consists of inorganic fumes and particulates arising from the thermal decomposition of alkyl lead.

The acute oral LD_{50} of tetraethyl lead in rats is 14 mg./kg. (Schroeder et al., 1972). Schepero (1964) found oral lethal doses in rats to be about 17 mg./kg for tetraethyl lead and 108 mg./kg. for tetramethyl lead. Despite its faster clearance, tetraethyl lead is more toxic than tetramethyl lead in rhesus monkeys, too (Heywood et al., 1978). In a massive human skin exposure to tetramethyl lead, the individual remained asymptomatic even though his urinary lead excretion was higher than that reported in victims severely poisoned by tetraethyl lead (Gething, 1975). Studies of the pulmonary uptake, distribution and elimination of these two alkyl leads in humans failed to reveal differences which could explain the distinctions in toxicity (Heard et al., 1979).

As with alkyl mercury (p. III-267) and alkyl tin compounds (see Section II), the chief derangement occurs within the central nervous system and manifests itself as insomnia, fatigue, nightmares, restlessness, irritability, weakness, ataxia, tremors, tinnitus, delusions, suicidal tendencies, psychosis, mania, and convulsions (Beattie et al., 1972; Cassells and Dodds, 1946; Machle, 1935; Sanders, 1964). There is a clinical impression, however, that this type of intoxication has a better prognosis than the closely related acute encephalopathy of chronic plumbism in children. If the acute phase is survived, recovery without sequelae is the rule.

Chronic sniffing of leaded gasoline, however, can induce very disabling neurological deficits. Among children and adolescents who engage in this practice, a common syndrome consisted of tremors, exaggerated tendon reflexes, incoordination and cerebellar signs (including myoclonus) in varying combinations (Seshia et al., 1978). Abnormal electroencephalograms were observed in more than half the patients, but only two instances of peripheral neuropathy were detected. The prognosis for neurologic recovery is surprisingly good if the patient can be persuaded in time to discontinue the sniffing habit. If not, the disease tends to be progressive in spite of intermittent therapeutic efforts, and the victim is likely to die during an acute toxic episode (Boeckx et al., 1977). In one case he became chronically demented before his demise (Valpey et al., 1978).

The onset of symptoms after alkyl leads is more rapid than after lead salts, but rats may not show signs of poisoning for several days after dosing (in some cases more than a week). Pathologic processes are found in the brain and other organs (Valpey et al., 1978), but they have not as yet suggested a mechanism for the intoxica-

tion (Schepero, 1964). Single injections of triethyl lead in mice failed to produce cerebral edema, but the total number of glial cells fell initially and then returned to normal although the distribution among the various types was altered (Sturrock, 1979). In one human case of massive ingestion of pure tetraethyl lead the patient survived 36 hours. The initial signs and symptoms were referable to a greatly increased intracranial pressure, but the terminal event was pulmonary edema (Stasik et al., 1969). In single exposures toxic signs and symptoms sometimes do not reach peak intensity for 1 to 2 weeks (Beattie et al., 1972). Many cases have occurred under conditions where it was difficult to ascertain whether the skin or the lungs was the primary portal of entry (Bini and Bollea, 1947; Cassells and Dodds, 1946; Stasik et al., 1969).

Like tetraalkyl tin compounds, the toxicity of tetraalkyl leads appears to depend on their conversion in vivo to the trialkyl forms (Aldridge et al., 1962; Cremer and Callaway, 1961). In rats 24 hours after an intravenous dose of tetraethyl lead, half the total lead in soft tissues was in the triethyl form and inorganic lead made up the remainder (Bolanowska, 1968). Eventually the distribution in the body resembles that after the administration of inorganic lead salts.

The management of acute poisoning by tetraethyl lead is unsatisfactory. Penicillamine and edetate calcium disodium increased the urinary excretion of lead without dramatic clinical improvement (Beattie et al., 1972; Kitzmiller et al., 1954; Law and Nelson, 1968). At least these treatments did not exacerbate the course of the poisoning. The combination of BAL and edetate calcium disodium appears to have been useful in treating a case of encephalopathy due to sniffing leaded gasoline (Hansen and Sharp, 1978), but the efficacy of the therapeutic regime (below) for lead encephalopathy has not been adequately established for alkyl lead intoxication. In most acute cases signs and symptoms subside promptly as the lead is excreted in urine, and chelation therapy is thus unnecessary. The chronic neurologic syndrome resulting from repeated inhalation of leaded gasoline appears to respond to the same forms of chelation therapy (see below) as does chronic plumbism due to inorganic lead exposures (Seshia et al., 1978).

Symptomatology:

A. *Acute poisoning by ingestion only.*

 1. An astringent and metallic taste in the mouth, dry throat, thirst.
 2. Burning abdominal pain, nausea, and vomiting. The vomitus may appear milky due to the presence of lead chloride. The abdominal pain may become colicky and severe.
 3. Sometimes diarrhea, less often consti-

pation. The stools may be bloody, or black due to the presence of lead sulfide.

4. Peripheral circulatory collapse (shock).

5. Neuromuscular symptoms include muscular weakness, pain, and cramps, especially in the legs.

6. Central nervous system manifestations include headache, insomnia, paresthesias, depression, coma, and death.

7. Though usually of secondary concern, kidney damage may result in oliguria, albuminuria, and cylindruria. The renal lesion may be due to the mildly nephrotoxic action of lead, to disturbances in kidney circulation, or to the products of intravascular hemolysis (Beaver, 1961; Danilooić, 1958; Radašević et al., 1961). Renal lesions may assume increased importance if edetate calcium disodium therapy is instituted; see p. III-163.

8. An acute hemolytic crisis sometimes develops and results in anemia and hemoglobinuria.

9. Death may occur within 1 or 2 days, but recovery is the rule. Convalescence is slow and may be interrupted by episodes like those seen in typical chronic poisoning (see text above).

B. *Lead encephalopathy* in chronic lead poisoning (as manifested in children).

1. Headache and insomnia.

2. Persistent vomiting, which is sometimes projectile. A typical lead colic may or may not be present.

3. Visual disturbances, choked optic disks.

4. Irritability, restlessness, delirium, hallucinations.

5. Convulsions and coma.

6. The intracranial pressure is characteristically high. The cerebrospinal fluid is generally unremarkable except for an elevation of total protein.

7. Death from exhaustion and respiratory failure. The mortality rate is high; recovery is slow and frequently incomplete.

C. *Chronic plumbism without encephalopathy.* See text above.

Treatment:

A. *Acute poisoning by ingestion.*

1. Unless vomiting is extensive, lavage the stomach with tap water or a 1% solution of sodium or magnesium sulfate. Leave 15 to 30 gm. of magnesium sulfate in 6 to 8 ounces of water in the stomach, both as an antidote and as a cathartic.

2. Egg white and milk are useful demulcents.

3. For abdominal pain atropine sulfate and other antispasmodics should be given a trial, but morphine may become necessary.

4. Intravenous calcium chloride or calcium gluconate (see p. IV-74) may cause a temporary suppression of lead colic and other untoward symptoms (Johnstone, 1957a; Wilenty, 1949).

5. Dehydration, shock, and electrolyte disturbances should be treated by the parenteral administration of isotonic saline (pp. IV-64–67).

6. Give edetate calcium disodium (CaNa$_2$EDTA) by slow intravenous drip or by intramuscular injection; see p. III-165 for doses and techniques. If the intestinal contents are suspected to hold significant amounts of lead, the administration of a saline cathartic and/or a cleansing enema is recommended before instituting chelation therapy. These measures, however, should not be allowed to delay EDTA administration appreciably.

7. In severe poisonings and particularly in encephalopathy, also give BAL in divided doses up to 24 mg./kg. per 24 hours (Chisolm, 1968); see p. III-165 for details.

B. *Additional measures for lead encephalopathy.* The treatment measures outlined above are generally appropriate, with emphasis on both BAL and CaNa$_2$EDTA. In addition, large doses of diazepam or barbiturate drugs may be necessary to control extreme degrees of central nervous excitation, but Chisolm (1968) prefers paraldehyde because of the lead-induced disturbance in prophyrin metabolism. Occasionally intracranial decompression may become advisable. Intravenous infusions of hypertonic urea have been successfully employed in controlling cerebral edema and in reducing intracranial pressure (Greengard, 1961; Katz, 1960); see pp. IV-43–46.

C. *Chronic plumbism without encephalopathy.*

1. During asymptomatic periods in chronic plumbism, chelation therapy may or may not be indicated. The younger the patient and the higher the blood level of lead (or other evidence of a high body burden), the more appropriate are therapeutic efforts to promote lead excretion. The following recommendations are based on those of Chisolm (1968), as interpreted and expanded by Green et al. (1976) and Seshia et al. (1978), with minor modifications.

(a) In children with blood Pb > 100 μg./dl., give a full course of BAL and CaNa$_2$EDTA as in lead encephalopathy; see p. III-165 for details. Speed is imperative because such children are prone to encephalopathy, the onset of which can be unpredictable and fulminating. After the course of BAL-EDTA, give oral D-penicillamine 10 mg./kg. three or four times daily (0.5 to 1 hour before meals); some therapists prefer 20 mg./kg. twice daily. Continue the course of D-penicillamine for 1 to 6 months or until the blood concentration of lead falls below 50 μg./dl. in two consecutive specimens and the 24-hour urine contains less than 0.1 mg. Pb.

(b) In asymptomatic children with blood Pb levels between 50 and 100 μg./dl., give intramuscular CaNa$_2$EDTA (12.5 mg./kg. per dose) 4 times daily; see p. III-165 for details. These injections are repeated for 3 to 5 days, during which time urinary and blood levels of lead should be monitored. A subsequent course of oral D-penicillamine may or may not be indicated.

(c) In asymptomatic adults with blood levels of lead above 100 μg./dl., intramuscular CaNa$_2$EDTA, as under (b) above for 3 to 5 days. A subsequent course of oral D-penicillamine (250 mg. three times daily) may or may not be indicated.

(d) In asymptomatic adults with blood levels of lead between 80 and 100 μg./dl., a 1- to 3-month course of oral D-penicillamine (250 mg. 3 or 4 times daily) may be useful; it should be taken when the stomach is empty (*e.g.*, 0.5 to 1 hour before meals).

(e) In asymptomatic adults with blood levels of lead between 50 and 80 μg./dl., chelation therapy may be unnecessary. The EDTA lead mobilization test (p. III-165) may be helpful in reaching a decision.

2. Symptomatic episodes in chronic plumbism are treated, with respect to chelation therapy, exactly like acute poisonings (see A), except when encephalopathy is the dominant feature (then see B).

3. Chronic chelation therapy with CaNa$_2$EDTA or D-penicillamine promotes urinary losses of essential metals, such as zinc, copper, iron and others. During "rest periods" between courses of chelators, dietary supplements of zinc and perhaps of the other elements are advisable.

Laboratory:

1. The many laboratory aids for the diagnosis of chronic lead poisoning are beyond the scope of this discussion. This subject has been reviewed by the American Academy of Pediatrics (1969). In general a 24-hour specimen of urine is preferable to a single sample (even when corrected by conventional means) for a chemical determination of lead (Byers *et al.*, 1954; Molyneux, 1964). A blood analysis for lead is helpful if the blood sample is taken and stored in specially cleaned glassware (Bessman and Layne, 1955). Findings of more than 40 to 50 μg. of lead per 100 ml. of whole blood or 0.1 mg. per liter of urine (24-hour specimen) are considered pathognomonic of lead poisoning. In alkyl lead poisoning, the urinary output of lead is a much more sensitive indicator of exposure than is the blood level (Gething, 1975).

2. Various lead mobilization tests involving a trial dose of CaNa$_2$EDTA or D-penicillamine have been described (Ohlsson, 1963; Whitaker *et al.*, 1962). A specific procedure utilizing CaNa$_2$EDTA is described on p. III-165. The degree to which lead excretion is enhanced by such a provocative test may aid in reaching or rejecting a diagnosis of lead poisoning. It may also indicate whether or not chelation therapy is appropriate in an asymptomatic person with only a borderline elevation in the blood lead level (Saenger *et al.*, 1982).

3. Modern alternative diagnostic tests include urinary δ-aminolevulinic acid (Davis and Andelman, 1967), red cell δ-aminolevulinic acid dehydratase activity (Weissberg *et al.*, 1971) and lead levels in hair (Kopito *et al.*, 1969).

4. Fluorescence of free erythrocyte protoporphyrin constitutes the basis for a rapid and simple diagnostic technique (Whitaker and Vietti, 1959).

5. An early but nonspecific sign may be an increase in the urinary excretion of coproporphyrins (Harrold *et al.*, 1952; Maloof, 1950; Pinto *et al.*, 1952).

6. Glucosuria (Roxburgh and Haas, 1959) and occasionally aminoaciduria are described (Chisolm and Leahy, 1962; Wilson *et al.*, 1953). In lead encephalopathy, the protein content of the CSF is slightly elevated.

7. A low ^{131}I uptake in the presence of otherwise normal thyroid function has been described (Sandstead *et al.*, 1969).

References:

Albahary, C.; Guillaume, J. Saturnisme et penicillamine. Presse Med. *74*:2193-2196, 1966.

Aldridge, W. N.; Cremer, J. E.; Threlfall, C. J. Trialkylleads and oxidative phosphorylation: A study of the action of trialkylleads upon rat liver mitochondria and rat brain cortex slices. Biochem. Pharmacol. 11:835-846, 1962.

Alexander, F. W.; Delves, H. T. Death from acute lead poisoning. Arch. Dis. Child. 47:446-448, 1972.

Ali, A. R.; Smales, O. R. C.; Aslam, M. Surma and lead poisoning. Br. Med. J. 2:915-916, 1978.

American Academy of Pediatrics. Subcommittee on Accidental Poisoning. Prevention, diagnosis and treatment of lead poisoning in childhood. Pediatrics 44:291-298, 1969.

Anku, V. D.; Harris, J. W. Peripheral neuropathy and lead poisoning in a child with sickle-cell anemia - Case report & review of literature. J. Pediatrics 85:337-340, 1974.

Aronson, A. L.; Hammond, P. B. Effect of two chelating agents on the distribution and excretion of lead. J. Pharmacol. Exp. Ther. 146:241-251, 1964.

Asokan, S. K.; Vansant, J.; Bassett, W. B., Jr.; Nardone, D. Delayed recognition of lead encephalopathy in two "moonshine" drinkers. S. Med. J. 67:1440-1442, 1974.

Asokan, S. K. Experimental lead cardiomyopathy: myocardial structural changes in rats given small amounts of lead. J. Clin. Med. 84:20-25, 1974.

Aungst, B. J.; Fung, H. L. Kinetic characterization of in vitro lead transport across the rat small intestine. Mechanism of intestinal lead transport. Toxicol. Appl. Pharmacol. 61:39-47, 1981.

Aungst, B. J.; Dolce, J. A.; Fung, H. L. The effect of dose on the disposition of lead in rats after intravenous and oral administration. Toxicol. Appl. Pharmacol. 61:48-57, 1981.

Baker, E. L.; Jr.; Folland, D. S.; Taylor, T. A.; Frank, M.; Peterson, W.; Lovejoy, G.; Cox, D.; Houseworth, J.; Landrigan, P. J. Lead poisoning in children of lead workers. Home contamination with industrial dust. N. Engl. J. Med. 296:260-261, 1977.

Ball, G. V.; Sorenson, L. B. Pathogenesis of hyperuricemia in saturnine gout. N. Engl. J. Med. 280:1199-1202, 1969.

Batuman, V.; Maesaka, J. K.; Haddad, B.; Tepper, E.; Landy, E.; Wedeen, R. P. The role of lead in gout nephropathy. N. Engl. J. Med. 304:520-524, 1981.

Baxter, C. S.; Wey, H. E.; Cardin, A. D. Evidence for specific lead-δ-aminolevulinate complex formation by carbon-13 nuclear magnetic resonance spectroscopy. Toxicol. Appl. Pharmacol. 47:477-482, 1979.

Beattie, A. D.; Briggs, J. D.; Canavan, J. S. F.; Doyle, D.; Mullin, P. J.; Watson, A. A. Acute lead poisoning. Five cases resulting from self-injection of lead and opium. Q. J. Med. 44:275-284, 1975.

Beattie, A. D.; Moore, M. R.; Goldberg, A. Tetraethyl-lead poisoning. Lancet 2:12-15, 1972.

Beattie, A. D.; Mullin, P. J.; Baxter, R. H.; Moore, M. R. Acute lead poisoning: an unusal cause of hepatitis. Scott. Med. J. 24:318-321, 1979.

Beaver, D. L. The ultrastructure of the kidney in lead intoxication with particular reference to intranuclear inclusions. Am. J. Pathol. 39:195-208, 1961.

Berger, K. E.; Lundberg, E. A. Intestinal volvus precipitated by lead poisoning. J. A. M. A. 147:13-16, 1951.

Berk, P. D.; Tschudy, D. P.; Shephey, L. A.; Waggoner, J. G.; Berlin, N. I. Hematologic and biochemical studies in a case of lead poisoning. Am. J. Med. 48:137-144, 1970.

Bessman, S. P.; Layne, E. C., Jr. A rapid procedure for the determination of lead in blood or urine in the presence of organic chelating agents. J. Lab. Clin. Med. 45:159-166, 1955.

Bessman, S. P.; Rubin, M.; Leiken, S. The treatment of lead encephalopathy - a method for the removal of lead during the acute stage. Pediatrics 14:201-208, 1954.

Biehusen, F. C.; Pulaski, E. J. Lead poisoning after ingestion of a foreign body retained in the stomach. N. Engl. J. Med. 254:1179-1181, 1956.

Bini, L.; Bollea, G. Fatal poisoning by lead-benzine. J. Neuropathol. Exp. Neurol. 6:271-278, 1947.

Blackman, S. S., Jr. The lesions of lead encephalitis in children. Bull. Johns Hopkins Hosp. 61:1-61, 1937.

Blanksma, L. A.; Sachs, H. K.; Murray, E. F.; O'Connell, M. J. Incidence of high blood lead levels in Chicago. Pediatrics 44:661-667, 1969.

Boeckx, R. L.; Postl, B.; Coodin. F. J. Gasoline sniffing and tetraethyl lead poisoning in children. Pediatrics 60:140-145, 1977.

Bolanowska, W. The distribution and excretion of triethyl lead in rats. Br. J. Ind. Med. 25:203-208, 1968.

Boothby, J. A.; de Jesus, P. V.; Rowland, L. P. Reversible forms of motor neuron disease: lead neuritis. Arch. Neurol. 31:18-23, 1974.

Boulding, J. E.; Baker, R. A. The treatment of metal poisoning with penicillamine. Lancet 2:985, 1957.

Bradley, J. E.; Baumgartner, R. J. Subsequent mental development of children with lead encephalopathy as related to type of treatment. J. Pediatr. 53:311-315, 1958.

Bratton, G. R.; Zmudzki, J.; Belland, M. C.; Warnock, L. G. Thiamin (vitamin B_1) effects on lead intoxication and deposition of lead in tissues: Therapeutic potential. Toxicol. Appl. Pharmacol. 59:164-172, 1981.

Brearley, R. L.; Forsythe, A. M. Lead poisoning from aphrodisiacs: potential hazard in immigrants. Br. Med. J. 2:1748-1749, 1978.

Brugsch, H. G.; Colombo, N. J.; Pagnotto, L. D. Chelation by calcium trisodium penetate in workers exposed to lead. N. Engl. J. Med. 272:993-996, 1965.

Byers, R. K. Lead poisoning: review of the literature and report on 45 cases. Pediatrics 23:585-603, 1959.

Byers, R. K.; Maloof, C. A. Edathamil calcium-disodium (Versenate) in treatment of lead poisoning in children. Am. J. Dis. Child. 87:559-569, 1954.

Byers, R. K.; Maloof, C. A.; Cushman, M. Urinary excretion of lead in children. Diagnostic application. Am. J. Dis. Child. 87:548-558, 1954.

Cagin, C. R.; Ditsy-Puray, M.; Westerman, M. P. Bullets, lead poisoning, and thyrotoxicosis. Ann. Intern. Med. 89:509-511, 1978.

Canberk, A.; Sehirli, I.; Canberk, Y.; Kogancuoglu, H. Urine δ-aminolevulinic acid and erythropoietic activity in human lead intoxication. Toxicol. Appl. Pharmacol. 44:257-261, 1978.

Cantarow, A.; Trumper, M. Lead Poisoning. The Williams & Wilkins Co., Baltimore, 1944.

Cassells, D. A. K.; Dodds, E. C. Tetraethyl lead poisoning. Br. Med. J. 2:681-685, 1946.

Chiba, M.; Toyoda, T.; Inaba, Y.; Ogihara, K.; Kikuchi, M. Acute lead poisoning in an adult from ingestion of paint. N. Engl. J. Med. 303:459, 1980.

Chisolm, J. J., Jr. The use of chelating agents in the treatment of acute and chronic lead intoxication in childhood. J. Pediatr. 73:1-38, 1968.

Chisolm, J. J., Jr. Management of increased lead absorption and lead poisoning in children. N. Engl. J. Med. 289:1016-1018, 1973.

Chisolm, J. J., Jr.; Harrison, H. E. The exposure of children to lead. Pediatrics 18:943-958, 1956.

Chisolm, J. J., Jr.; Harrison, H. E. The treatment of acute lead encephalopathy in children. Pediatrics 19:2-20, 1957.

Chisolm, J. J., Jr.; Leahy, N. B. Aminoaciduria as a manifestation of renal tubular injury in lead intoxication and a comparison with patterns of aminoaciduria seen in other diseases. J. Pediatr. 60:1-17, 1962.

Choie, D. D.; Richter, G. W. Lead poisoning; rapid formation of intranuclear inclusions. Science 177:1194-1195, 1972.

Cirksena, W. J.; Deller, J. J.; Marcarelli, J. L. Adult chronic lead intoxication. Report of an unusual source. Arch. Environ. Health 4:183-190, 1962.

Coffin, R.; Phillips, J. L.; Staples, W. I.; Spector, S. Treatment of lead encephalopathy in children. J. Pediatr. 69:198-206, 1966.

Cohen, G. J.; Ahrens, W. E. Chronic lead poisoning. J. Pediatr. 54:271-284, 1959.

Cotter, L. H. Treatment of lead poisoning by chelation. J. A. M. A. 155:906-908, 1954.

Cramer, K. D-Penicillamine and N-acetyl-D-penicillamine in lead poisoning. Postgrad. Med. J. 50:14-16, 1974.

Cremer, J. E.; Callaway, S. Further studies on the toxicity of some tetra- and trialkyl lead compounds. Br. J. Ind. Med. 18:277-282, 1961.

Crutcher, J. C. Clinical manifestations and therapy of acute lead intoxication due to the ingestion of illicitly distilled alcohol. Ann. Intern. Med. 59:707-715, 1963.

Dahlgren, J. Abdominal pain in lead workers. Arch. Environ. Health 33:156-159, 1978.

Danilooic, V. Chronic nephritis due to ingestion of lead-contaminated flour. Br. Med. J. 1:27-28, 1958.

Davis, J. R.; Andelman, S. L. The detection of early lead poisoning using the Davis test for urinary ALA. Arch. Environ. Health 15:53-59, 1967.

Dillman, R. O.; Crumb, C. K.; Lidsky, M. J. Lead poisoning from a gunshot wound - report of a case and review of the literature. Am. J. Med. 66:509-514, 1979.

DiMalo, V.; Garriott, J. A fatal case of lead poisoning due to a retained bullet. Vet. Human Toxicol. 22:390-391, 1980.

Dolcourt, J. L.; Finch, C.; Coleman, G. D.; Klimas, A. J.; Milar, C. R. Hazard of lead exposure in the home from recycled automobile storage batteries. Pediatrics 68:225-230, 1981.

Dubi, J.; Schneider, P.; Regli, F. L'intoxication saturnine. Schwiez. Med. Wschr. 109:123-127, 1979.

Emmerson, B. T. Chronic lead nephropathy. The diagnostic use of calcium EDTA and the association with gout. Aust. N. Z. J. Med. 12:310-324, 1963.

EPA. Air Quality Criteria Document for Lead, in revision.

Ericson, J. E.; Shirahata, H.; Patterson, C. C. Skeletal concentrations of lead in ancient Peruvians. N. Engl. J. Med., 300:946-951, 1979.

Fairhall, L. T.; Sayers, R. R. The relative toxicity of lead and some of its common compounds. Public Health Bull. No. 253, 1940.

Farkas, W. R.; Starrawitz, T.; Schneider, M. Saturnine gout: lead-induced formation of guanine crystals. Science 199:786-787, 1978.

Feldman, R. G.; Hayes, M. K.; Yeanes, R.; Aldrich, F. D. Lead neuropathy in adults and children. Arch. Neurol. 34:481-488, 1977.

Fischbein, A.; Alvares, A. P.; Anderson, K. E.; Sassa, S.; Kappas, A. Lead intoxication among demolition workers: the effect of lead on the hepatic cytochrome P-450 system in humans. J. Toxicol. Environ. Health 3:431-437, 1977.

Fischbein, A.; Daum, S. M.; Davidow, B.; Slavin, G.; Alvares, A. P.; Sassa, S.; Anderson, K. E.; Kappas, A.; Eisinger, J.; Blumberg, W. E.; Winicow, E. H.; Selikoff, I. J. Lead hazard among iron workers; dismantling lead-painted elevated subway line in New York City. N.Y. State J. Med. 78:1250-1259, 1978.

Fischbein, A.; Rice, C.; Sarkozi, L.; Kon, S. H.; Petrocci, M.; Selikoff, I. J. Exposure to lead in firing ranges. J.A.M.A. 241:1141-1144, 1979.

Fischbein, A.; Wallace, J.; Anderson, K. E.; Sassa, S.; Kon, S.; Rohl, A. N.; Kappas, A. Lead poisoning in an art conservator. J.A.M.A. 247:2007-2009, 1982.

Friedheim, E.; Graziano, J. H.; Popovac, D.; Dragovic, D.; Kaul, B. Treatment of lead poisoning by 2,3-dimercaptosuccinic acid. Lancet 2:1234-1235, 1978.

Fujii, H. Role of red cell pyrimidine 5'-nucleotidase in experimental lead poisoning. Arch. Toxicol. 43:59-64, 1979.

Fullerton, P. M. Chronic peripheral neuropathy produced by lead poisoning in guinea pigs. J. Neuropathol. Exp. Neurol. 25:214-236, 1966.

Germuth, F. G., Jr.; Eagle, H. The efficacy of BAL (2, 3-dimercaptopropanol) in the treatment of experimental lead poisoning in rabbits. J. Pharmacol. Exp. Ther. 92:397-410, 1948.

Gething, J. Tetramethyl lead absorption: a report of human exposure to a high level of tetramethyl lead. Br. J. Indust. Med. 32:329-333, 1975.

Goldberg, A.; Smith, J. A.; Lockhead, A. C. Treatment of lead poisoning with oral penicillamine. Br. Med. J. 1:1270-1275, 1963.

Goldstein, G. W.; Asbury, A. K.; Diamond, I. Pathogenesis of lead encephalopathy. Uptake of lead and reaction of brain capillaries. Arch. Neurol. 31:382-389, 1974.

Golter, M.; Michaelson, I. A. Growth, behavior, and brain

catecholamines in lead-exposed neonatal rats: A reappraisal. Science 187:359-361, 1975.

Goyer, R. A.; Cherian, M. G. Ascorbic acid and EDTA treatment of lead toxicity in rats. Life Sci. 24:433-438, 1979.

Grandjean, P.; Arnvig, E.; Beckmann, J. Psychological dysfunctions in males occupationally exposed to inorganic lead. Manage. Control Heavy Met. Environ. Int. Conf., pp. 85-88, 1979.

Graziano, J. H.; Leong, J. K.; Friedheim, E. 2,3-Dimercaptosuccinic acid: A new agent for the treatment of lead poisoning. J. Pharmacol. Exp. Ther. 206:696-700, 1978.

Green, V. A.; Wise, G. W.; Callenbach, J. Lead poisoning. Clin. Toxicol. 9:33-51, 1976.

Greenberg, M.; Jacobziner, H.; McLaughlin, M. C.; Fuerst, H. T.; Pellitteri, O. Proceedings - A study of pica in relation to lead poisoning. Pediatrics 22:756-760, 1958.

Greengard, J. Lead encephalopathy in children. Intravenous use of urea in its management. N. Engl. J. Med. 264:1027-1030, 1961.

Greengard, J.; Adams, B.; Berman, E. Acute lead encephalopathy in young children. Evaluation of therapy with a corticosteroid and moderate hypothermia. J. Pediatr. 66:707-711, 1965.

Greengard, J.; Voris, D. C.; Hayden, R. The surgical therapy of acute lead encephalopathy. J. A. M. A. 180:660-664, 1962.

Griggs, R. C. Lead poisoning: Hematologic aspects. In Progress in Hematology, Vol. IV. (C. V. Moore and E. B. Brown, Ed.) Grune and Stratton, New York, 1964.

Gross, S. B.; Pfitzer, E. A.; Yeager, D. W.; Kehoe, R. A. Lead in human tissues. Toxicol. Appl. Pharmacol. 32:638-651, 1975.

Hammond, P. B. The effects of chelating agents on the tissue distribution and excretion of lead. Toxicol. Appl. Pharmacol. 18:296-310, 1971.

Hammond, P. B. The effects of D-penicillamine on the tissue distribution and excretion of lead. Toxicol. Appl. Pharmacol. 26:241-246, 1973.

Hammond, P. B.; Aronson, A. L.; Olson, W. C. The mechanism of mobilization of lead by ethylenediaminetetraacetate. J. Pharmacol. Exp. Ther. 157:196-206, 1967.

Hammond, P. B.; O'Flaherty, E. J.; Garside, P. S. The impact of air-lead on blood-lead in man. A critique of the recent literature. Food Cosmet. Toxicol. 19:631-638, 1981.

Hankin, L.; Heichel, G. H.; Botsford, R. A. Lead poisoning from colored printing inks. Clin. Pediatr. 12:654-655, 1973.

Hansen, K. S.; Sharp, F. R. Gasoline sniffing, lead poisoning, and myoclonus. J.A.M.A. 240:1375-1376, 1978.

Haritos, N. P. Chronic lead intoxication; a report of 24 treated cases at Children's Hospital. Clin. Proc. Child. Hosp., Wash. 17:110-115, 1961.

Harris, C. E. C. A comparison of intravenous calcium disodium versenate and penicillamine in lead poisoning. Can. Med. Assoc. J. 79:664-666, 1958.

Harris, I. Lead encephalopathy: Case reports. S. Afr. Med. J. 50:1371-1373, 1976.

Harrold, G. C.; Meek, S. F.; Padden, D. A. A coproporphyrin III test as a measure of lead damage. II. Considering lead dusts of relatively large particle size. Arch. Ind. Hyg. Occup. Med. 6:24-31, 1952.

Heard, M. J.; Wells, A. C.; Newton, D.; Chamberlain, A. C. Human uptake and metabolism of tetraethyl- and tetramethyllead vapor labelled with lead-203. Manage. Control Heavy Met. Environ. Int. Conf., pp. 103-108, 1979.

Heywood, R.; James, R. W.; Sortwell, R. J.; Prentice, D. E.; Barry, P. S. I. The intravenous toxcity of tetra-alkyl lead compounds in rhesus monkeys. Toxicol. Lett. 2:187-197, 1978.

Hofmann, V., Segewitz, G. Influence of chelation therapy on acute lead intoxication in rats. Arch. Toxicol. 34:213-225, 1975.

Hutchison, H. E.; Stark, J. M. The anaemia of lead poisoning. J. Clin. Pathol. 14:548-549, 1961.

Ingalls, T. H.; Tiboni, E. A.; Werrin, M. Lead poisoning in Philadelphia, 1955-1960. Arch. Environ. Health 3:575-579, 1961.

Jenkins, C. D.; Mellins, R. B. Lead poisoning in children; a study of forty six cases. Arch. Neurol. 77:70-78, 1957.

Johnstone, R. T. A re-examination of the picture of plumbism. Ind. Med. Surg. 26:323-326, 1957a.

Jugo, S.; Maljkovic, T.; Kostial, K. Influence of chelating agents on the gastrointestinal absorption of lead. Toxicol. Appl. Pharmacol. 34:259-263, 1975.

Karlog, O.; Moller, K. O. Three cases of acute lead poisoning; analyses of organs for lead and observations on polarographic lead determinations. Acta Pharmacol. Toxicol. 15:8-15, 1958.

Karpatkin, S. Lead poisoning after taking Pb acetate with suicidal intent; report of a case with a discussion of the mechanism of anemia. Arch. Environ. Health 2:679-684, 1961.

Katz, R. A. Intravenous urea in the therapy of increased intracranial pressure with lead encephalopathy. N. Engl. J. Med. 262:870-872, 1960.

Kaufman, A.; Wiese, W. Gasoline sniffing leading to increased lead absorption in children. Clin. Pediatrics 17:475-477, 1978.

Kehoe, R. A.; Thamann, F.; Cholak, J. On normal absorption and excretion of lead. Lead absorption and lead excretion in modern American life. J. Ind. Hyg. Toxicol. 15:273-288, 1933a.

Kehoe, R. A.; Thamann, F.; Cholak, J. Sources of normal lead absorption. J. Ind. Hyg. Toxicol. 15:290-300, 1933b.

Kehoe, R. A.; Thamann, F.; Cholak, J. Lead absorption and excretion in infants and children. J. Ind. Hyg. Toxicol. 15:301-305, 1933c.

Kehoe, R. A.; Thamann, F.; Cholak, J. Normal absorption and excretion of lead. J. A. M. A. 104:90-92, 1935.

Kelman, B. J.; Walter, B. K. Transplacental movements of inorganic lead from mother to fetus. Proc. Soc. Exp. Biol. Med. 163:278-282, 1980.

Kitzmiller, K. V.; Cholak, J.; Kehoe, R. A. Treatment of organic lead (tetraethyl) intoxication with edathamil calcium disodium. Arch. Ind. Hyg. Occup. Med. 10:312-318, 1954.

Klein, M.; Namer, R.; Harpur, E.; Corbin, R. Earthenware containers as a source of fatal lead poisoning. N. Engl. J. Med. 283:669-672, 1970.

Kopito, L.; Briley, A. M.; Shwachman, H. Chronic plumbism in children, diagnosis by hair analysis. J. A. M. A. 209:243-248, 1969.

Lamola, A. A.; Yamane, T. Zinc protoporphyrin in the erythrocytes of patients with lead intoxication and iron deficiency anemia. Science 186:936-938, 1974.

Lamola, A. A.; Piomelli, S.; Pohfitzpatrick, M. B.; Yamane, T.; Harber, L. C. Erythropoietic protoporphyria and lead intoxication - molecular basis for difference in cutaneous photosensitivity 2. Different binding of erythrocyte protoporphyrin to hemoglobin. J. Clin. Invest. 56:1528-1535, 1975.

Landrigan, P. J.; McKinney, A. S.; Hopkins, L. C.; Rhodes, W. W., Jr.; Price, W. A.; Cox, D. H. Chronic lead absorption. J.A.M.A. 234:394-397, 1975.

Lanzkowsky, P. Investigation into the aetiology and treatment of pica. Arch. Dis. Child. 34:140-148, 1959.

Laug, E. P.; Kunze, F. M. The penetration of lead through the skin. J. Ind. Hyg. Toxicol. 30:256-259, 1948.

Law, W. R.; Nelson, E. R. Gasoline sniffing by an adult. J. A. M. A. 204:144-146, 1968.

Leckie, W. J. H.; Tompsett, S. L. The diagnostic and therapeutic use of edathamil calcium disodium (EDTA, Versene) in excessive inorganic lead absorption. Q. J. Med. 27:65-82, 1958.

Leonard, A. R.; Lynch, G. Dishware as a possible source of lead poisoning. Calif. Med. 89:414-416, 1958.

Lightfoote, J.; Blair, H. I.; Cohen, J. R. Lead intoxication in an adult caused by Chinese herbal medication. J.A.M.A. 238:1539, 1977.

Lilis, R.; Gavrilescu, N.; Nestorescu, B.; Dumitriu, C.; Roventa, A. Nephropathy in chronic lead poisoning. Br. J. Ind. Med. 25:196-202, 1968.

Lilis, R.; Fischbein, A. Chelation therapy in workers exposed to lead: a critical review. J.A.M.A. 235:2823-2824, 1976.

Lilis, R.; Valciukas, J.; Fischbein, A.; Andrews, G.; Selikoff, I.

J.; Blumberg, W. Renal function impairment in secondary lead smelter workers: correlations with zinc protoporphyrin and blood lead levels. J. Environ. Pathol. Toxicol. 2:1447-1474, 1979.

Lin-Fu, J. S. Lead exposure and toxicity in children. N. Engl. J. Med. 289:1229-1233 and 1289-1293, 1973.

Linden, M. A.; Manton, W. I.; Stewart, R. M.; Thal, E. R.; Feit, H. Lead poisoning from retained bullets. Pathogenesis, diagnosis and management. Ann. Surgery 195:305-313, 1982.

Machle, W. F. Tetra-ethyl lead intoxication and poisoning by related compounds of lead. J. A. M. A. 105:578-585, 1935.

Mailman, R. B.; Krigman, M. R.; Mueller, R. A.; Mushak, P.; Breese, G. R. Lead exposure during infancy permanently increases lithium-induced polydipsia. Science 201:637-639, 1978.

Maloof, C. C. Role of porphyrins in occupational diseases. I. Significance of coproporphyrinuria in lead workers. Arch. Ind. Hyg. Occup. Med. 1:298-307, 1950.

Marcus, S. M. Experience with D-penicillamine in treating lead poisoning. Vet. Human Toxicol. 24:18-20, 1982.

McIntire, M. S.; Angle, C. R. Air lead: relation to lead in blood of black school children deficient in glucose-6-phosphate dehydrogenase. Science 177:520-522, 1972.

Mehbod, H. Treatment of lead intoxication, combined use of peritoneal dialysis and edetate calcium disodium. J. A. M. A. 201:972-974, 1967.

Millican, F. K.; Lourie, R. S.; Layman, E. M. Emotional factors in the etiology and treatment of lead poisoning; a study of pica in children. Am. J. Dis. Child. 91:144-152, 1956.

Miwa, S.; Ishida, Y.; Takegawa, S.; Urata, G.; Toyoda, T. A case of lead intoxication: clinical and biochemical studies. Am. J. Hematol. 11:99-105, 1981.

Modak, A. T.; Weintraub, S. T.; Stavinoha, W. B. Effect of chronic ingestion of lead on the central cholinergic system in rat brain regions. Toxicol. Appl. Pharmacol. 34:340-347, 1975.

Molyneux, M. K. B. Use of single urine samples for the assessment of lead absorption. Br. J. Ind. Med. 21:203-209, 1964.

Moore, P. J.; Pridmore, S. A.; Gill, G. F. Total blood lead levels in petrol venders. Med. J. Aust. 1:438-440, 1976.

Moosa, A.; Harris, F. Erythrocyte hypoplasia due to lead poisoning; a devastating, yet curable disease. Clin. Pediatr. 8:400-402, 1969.

Morgan, J. M.; Hartley, M. W.; Miller, R. E. Nephropathy in chronic lead poisoning. Arch. Intern. Med. 118:17-29, 1966.

Morris, C. E.; Heyman, A.; Pozefsky, T. Lead encephalopathy caused by ingestion of illicitly distilled whiskey. Neurology 14:493-499, 1964.

Mouw, D. R.; Vander, A. J.; Cox, J.; Fleischer, N. Acute effects of lead on renal electrolyte excretion and plasma renin activity. Toxicol. Appl. Pharmacol. 46:435-447, 1978.

Myers, R. R.; Powel, H. C.; Shapiro, H. M.; Costello, M. L.; Lampert, P. W. Changes in endoneurial fluid pressure, permeability, and peripheral nerve ultrastructure in experimental lead neuropathy. Ann. Neurology 8:392-401, 1980a.

Mykkanen, H. M.; Dickerson, J. W. T.; Lancaster, M. C. Effect of age on the tissue distribution of lead in the rat. Toxicol. Appl. Pharmacol. 51:447-454, 1979.

Nathanson, J. A.; Bloom, F. E. Heavy metals and adenosine cyclic 3',5'-monophosphate metabolism: possible relevance to heavy metal toxicity. Mol. Pharmacol. 12:390-398, 1976.

Needleman, H. L.; Gunnol, C.; Leviton, A.; Reed, R.; Peresie, H.; Maher, C.; Barrett, P. Deficits in psychologic and classroom performance of children with elevated dentine lead levels. N. Engl. J. Med. 300:689-695, 1979.

Nelson, W. C.; Lykins, M. H.; Mackey, J.; Newill, V. A.; Finklea, J. F.; Hammer, D. I. Mortality among orchard workers exposed to lead arsenate spray; a cohort study. J. Chronic Dis. 26:105-118, 1973.

Niklowitz, W. J.; Mandybur, T. I. Neurofibrillary changes following childhood lead encephalopathy. J. Neuropathol. Exp. Neurol. 34:445-455, 1975.

Nortier, J. W. R.; Sangster, B.; van Kestern, R. G. Acute lead poisoning with hemolysis and liver toxicity after ingestion of red lead. Vet. Human Toxicol. 22:145-147, 1980.

O'Flaherty, E. J.; Hammond, P. B.; Lerner, S. I. Dependence of apparent blood lead half-life on the length of previous lead exposure in humans. Fund. Appl. Toxicol. 2:44-54, 1982.

Ohlsson, W. T. L. Penicillamine as lead-chelating substance in man. Br. Med. J. 1:1454-1456, 1962.

Ohlsson, W. T. L. Detection of exposure to lead by a mobilization test with peroral penicillamine. Occup. Health Rev. 15:14-18, 1963.

Ong, C. N.; Lee, W. R. Interaction of calcium and lead in human erythrocytes. Br. J. Ind. Med. 37:70-77, 1980a.

Ong, C. N.; Lee W. R. Distribution of lead-203 in human peripheral blood in vitro. Br. J. Ind. Med. 37:78-84, 1980b.

Orfanos, C. E.; Kunzig, M. Chronic lead intoxication - lead gout with giant tophi on skin, nephropathia and porphyria. Der. Hautarzt 26:581-584, 1975.

Osheroff, M. R.; Uno, H.; Bowman, R. E. Lead inclusion bodies on the anterior horn cells and neurons of the substantia nigra in the adult rhesus monkey. Toxicol. Appl. Pharmacol. 64:570-576, 1982.

O'Tuama, L. A.; Kim, C. S.; Gatzy, J. T.; Krigman, M. R.; Mushak, P. The distribution of inorganic lead in guinea pig brain and neural barrier tissues in control and lead-poisoned animals. Toxicol. Appl. Pharmacol. 36:1-9, 1976.

Pease, C. N.; Newton, G. G. Metaphyseal dysplasia due to lead poisoning in children. Radiology 79:233-240, 1962.

Pedersen, R. S. Lead poisoning treated with haemodialysis. Scand. J. Urol. Nephrol. 12:189-190, 1978.

Perkins, K. C.; Oske, F. A. Elevated blood lead in a 6-month-old breast fed infant. Role of newsprint logs. Pediatrics 57:426-476, 1976.

Pinto, S. S.; Einert, C.; Roberts, W. J.; Winn, G. S.; Nelson, K. W. Coproporphyrinuria; study of its usefulness in evaluating lead exposure. Arch. Ind. Hyg. Occup. Med. 6:496-507, 1952.

Piomelli, S.; Lamola, A. A.; Pohfitzpatrick, M. B.; Seaman, C.; Harber, L. C. Erythopoietic protoporphyria and lead intoxication - molecular basis for difference in cutaneous photosensitivity 1. Different rates of disappearance of protoporphyrin from erythrocytes, both in vivo and in vitro. J. Clin. Invest. 56:1519-1527, 1975.

Piomelli, S.; Cerash, L.; Cerash, M. B.; Seaman, C.; Mushak, P.; Glover, B.; Padgett, R. Blood lead concentrations in a remote Himalayan population. Science 210:1135-1137, 1980.

Popoff, N.; Weinberg, S.; Feigin, I. Pathologic observations in lead encephalopathy. Neurology 13:101-112, 1963.

Pounds, J. G.; Wright, R.; Morrison, D.; Casciano, D. A. Effect of lead on calcium homeostasis in the isolated rat hepatocyte. Toxicol. Appl. Pharmacol. 63:389-401, 1982a.

Pounds, J. G.; Morrison, D.; Wright, R.; Casciano, D. A.; Shaddock, J. G. Effect of lead on calcium-mediated cell function in the isolated rat hepatocyte. Toxicol. Appl. Pharmacol. 63:402-408, 1982b.

Powers, J. M.; Rowe, S. E.; Earlywine, G. R. Lead encephalopathy simulating a cerebral neoplasm in an adult. J. Neurosurg. 46:816-819, 1977.

Rabinowitz, M. B.; Wetherill, G. W.; Kopple, J. D. Kinetic analysis of lead metabolism in healthy humans. J. Clin. Invest. 58:260-270, 1976.

Rabinowitz, M. B.; Needleman, H. L. Temporal trends in the lead concentrations of umbilical cord bloods. Science 216:1429-1431, 1982.

Radasevic, Z.; Saric, M.; Beritic, T.; Knezevic, J. The kidney in lead poisoning. Br. J. Ind. Med. 18:222-230, 1961.

Radwan, H.; Braun, H.; Bar-Sela, S.; Kott, E. Lead encephalopathy treated by versenate (Ca-EDTA). Eur. Neurol. 21:157-160, 1982.

Raghavan, S. R. V.; Gonick, H. C. Isolation of low-molecular weight lead-binding protein from human erythrocytes. Proc. Soc. Exp. Biol. Med. 155:164-167, 1977.

Rapaport, M.; Rubin, M. I. Lead poisoning. A clinical and experimental study of the factors influencing the seasonal incidence in children. Am. J. Dis. Child. 61:245-255, 1941.

Richardson, J. H.; Buisseret, P. D. Richardson, J. H.; Buisseret, P. D. Acquired megacolon associated with acute lead poisoning. Br. Med. J. 283:104-105, 1981.

Robinson, R. O. Tetraethyl lead poisoning from gasoline sniffing. J.A.M.A. 240:1373-1374, 1978.

Routh, D. K.; Mushak, P.; Boone, L. A new syndrome of elevated blood lead and microcephaly. J. Ped. Psychol. 4:67-76, 1979.

Roxburgh, R. C.; Haas, L. The diagnostic importance of glycosuria in lead poisoning in childhood. Arch. Dis. Child. 34:70-73, 1959.

Rummo, J. H.; Routh, D. K.; Rummo, N. J.; Brown, J. F. Behavioral and neurological effects of symptomatic and asymptomatic lead exposure in children. Arch. Environ. Health 34:120-124, 1979.

Ryder, H. W.; Kehoe, R. A. The effect of dithiopropanol (BAL) on human lead intoxication. J. Lab. Clin. Med. 32:1423, 1947.

Sachs, H. K.; Blanksma, L. A.; Murray, E. F.; O'Connell, M. J. Ambulatory treatment of lead poisoning: Report of 1, 555 cases. Pediatrics 46:389-396, 1970.

Sachs, H. K.; McCaughran, D. A.; Krall, V.; Rozenfeld, I. H.; Yongsmith, N. Lead poisoning without encephalopathy - effect of early diagnosis on neurologic and psychologic salvage. Am. J. Dis. Child. 133:786-790, 1979.

Saenger, P.; Rosen, J. F.; Markowitz, M. Diagnostic significance of edetate disodium calcium testing in children with increased lead absorption. Am. J. Dis. Child. 136:312-315, 1982.

Sanders, L. W. Tetraethyl lead intoxication. Arch. Environ. Health 8:270-277, 1964.

Sanford, H. N. Lead poisoning in young children. Postgrad. Med. 17:162-169, 1955.

Sanstead, H. H.; Stant, E. G.; Brill, A. B.; Arias, L. I.; Terry, R. T. Lead intoxication and the thyroid. Arch. Intern. Med. 123:632-635, 1969.

Sartain, P.; Whitaker, J. A.; Martin, J. The absence of lead lines in bones of children with early lead poisoning. Am. J. Roentgenol. 91:597-601, 1964.

Schepero, G. W. H. Tetraethyl lead and tetramethyl lead, comparative experimental pathology; I. Lead absorption and pathology. Arch. Environ. Health 8:277-295, 1964.

Scheri, R.; Beuthin, F. C.; Louis-Ferdinand, R. T. Effect of lead acetate on the kinetics of γ-glutamyl transpeptidase activity from neonatal rat pup brain. Drug Chem. Toxicol. 4:363-371, 1981.

Schroeder, T.; Avery, D. D.; Cross, H. A. The LD_{50} value of tetraethyl lead. Experientia 28:425-426, 1972.

Selander, S.; Cramer, K.; Hallberg, L. Studies in lead poisoning. Oral therapy with penicillamine; relationship between lead in blood and other laboratory tests. Br. J. Ind. Med. 23:282-291, 1966.

Seppalainen, A. M.; Hernberg, S.; Kock, B. Relationship between blood lead levels and nerve conduction velocities. Neurotoxicology 1:313-332, 1979.

Seshia, S. S.; Rajani, K. R.; Boeckx, R. L.; Chow, P. N. The neurological manifestations of chronic inhalation of leaded gasoline. Develop. Med. Child. Neurol. 20:323-334, 1978.

Seto, D. S. Y.; Freeman, J. M. Lead neuropathy in childhood. Am. J. Dis. Child. 107:337-342, 1964.

Settle, D. M.; Patterson, C. C. Lead in albacore. Guide to lead pollution in Americans. Science 207:1167-1176, 1980.

Sidbury, J. B., Jr. Lead poisoning. Treatment with disodium calcium ethylenediaminetetraacetate. Am. J. Med. 18:932-946, 1955.

Silbergeld, E. K.; Chisolm J. J., Jr. Lead poisoning: Altered urinary catecholamine metabolites as indicators of intoxication in mice and children. Science 192:153-155, 1976.

Silbergeld, E. K.; Adler, H. S. Subcellular mechanisms of lead neurotoxicity. Brain Res. 148:451-467, 1978.

Silbergeld, E. K.; Wolinsky, J. S.; Goldstein, G. W. Electron probe microanalysis of isolated brain capillaries poisoned with lead. Brain Res. 189:369-376, 1980.

Singh, N.; Donovan, C. M.; Hanshaw, J. B. Neonatal lead intoxication in a prenatally exposed infant. J. Pediatr. 93:1019-1021, 1978.

Smith, H. D. Lead poisoning in children and its therapy with EDTA. Ind. Med. Surg. 28:148-151, 1959a.

Smith, H. D.; Boehner, R. L.; Carney, T.; Majors, W. J. The sequelae of pica with and without lead poisoning. Am. J. Dis. Child. 105:609-616, 1963b.

Smith, H. D.; King, L. R.; Margolin, E. G. Treatment of lead encephalopathy. Am. J. Dis. Child. *109*:322-324, 1965.

Snowdon, C. T.; Sanderson, B. A. Lead pica in rats. Science *183*:92-94, 1974.

Stasik, M.; Byczkowska, Z.; Szendzikowski, S.; Fiedorczuk, Z. Acute tetraethyl lead poisoning. Arch. Toxikol. *24*:283-291, 1969.

Stevenson, A.; Merali, Z.; Kacew, S.; Singhal, R. L. Effects of subacute and chronic lead treatment on glucose homeostasis and renal cyclic AMP metabolism in rats. Toxicology *6*:265-275, 1976.

Sturrock, R. R. A quantitative histological study of the efects of acute triethyl lead poisoning on the adult mouse brain. Neuropathol. Appl. Neurobiol. *5*:419-431, 1979.

Suketa, Y.; Hasegawa, S.; Yamamoto, T. Changes in sodium and potassium in urine and serum of lead-intoxicated rats. Toxicol. Appl. Pharmacol. *47*:203-207, 1979.

Suketa, Y.; Ujiie, M.; Okada, S. A possible mechanism for changes in renal K$^+$-dependent phosphatase activity in lead-treated rats. Toxicol. Appl. Pharmacol. *59*:230-237, 1981.

Tanis, A. L. Lead poisoning in children, including nine cases treated with edathamil calcium-disodium. Am. J. Dis. Child. *89*:325-331, 1955.

Taylor, D.; Nathanson, J.; Hoffer, B.; Olson, L.; Seiger, A. Lead blockade of norepinephrine-induced inhibition of cerebellar purkinje neurons. J. Pharmacol. Exp. Ther. *206*:371-381, 1978.

Tepper, L. B. Renal function subsequent to childhood plumbism. Arch. Environ. Health *7*:76-85, 1963.

Timpo, A. E.; Amin, J. S.; Casalino, M. B.; Yuceoglu, A. M. Congenital lead intoxication. J. Pediatr. *94*:765-767, 1979.

Tonge, J. I.; Burry, A. F.; Saal, J. R. Cerebellar calcification: a possible marker of lead poisoning. Pathology *9*:289-300, 1977.

Valciukas, J. A.; Lilis, R.; Fischbein, A.; Selikoff, I. J.; Eisinger, J.; Blumberg, W. E. Central nervous system dysfunction due to lead exposure. Science *201*:465-467, 1978.

Valentine, W. N.; Paglia, D. E.; Fink, K.; Madokoro, G. Lead poisoning - association with hemolytic anemia, basophilic stippling, erythrocyte pyrimidine 5'-nucleotidase deficiency, and intraerythrocytic accumulation of pyrimidine. J. Clin. Invest. *58*:926-932, 1976.

Valpey, R.; Sumi, S. M.; Copars, M. K.; Gobe, G. J. Acute and chronic progressive encephalopathy due to gasoline sniffing. Neurology *28*:507-510, 1978.

Victery, W.; Vander, A. J.; Markel, H.; Katzman, L.; Shulak, J. M.; Germain, C. Lead exposure begun *in utero* decreases renin and angiotensin II in adult rats. Proc. Soc. Exp. Biol. Med. *170*:63-67, 1982.

Vitale, L. F.; Rosalinasbailon, A.; Folland, D.; Brennan, J. F.; McCormick, B. Oral penicillamine therapy for chronic lead poisoning in children. J. Pediatr. *83*:1041-1045, 1973.

Voight, G. E.; Larsson, L. E. Distribution of lead and mercury in femur of acutely poisoned rats. Acta Pathol. Microbiol. Scand. *47*:256-258, 1959.

Weatherall, M. Effects of BAL and BAL glucoside in acute lead acetate poisoning. Br. J. Pharmacol. *3*:137-145, 1948.

Webster, R. W. *Legal Medicine and Toxicology.* W. B. Saunders Co., Philadelphia, 1930.

Wedeen, R. P.; Maesaka, J. K.; Weiner, B.; Lipat, G. A.; Lyons, M. M.; Vitale, L. F.; Joselow, M. M. Occupational lead nephropathy. Am. J. Med. *59*:630-641, 1975.

Wedeen, R. P.; Mallik, D. K.; Batuman, V. Detection and treatment of occupational lead nephropathy. Arch. Intern. Med. *139*:53-57, 1979.

Weissberg, J. B.; Lipschutz, F.; Oski, F. A. δ-Aminolevulinic acid dehydratase activity in circulating blood cells. N. Engl. J. Med. *284*:565-569, 1971.

Westerman, M. P.; Pfitzer, E.; Ellis, L. D.; Jensen, W. N. Concentrations of lead in bone in plumbism. N. Engl. J. Med. *273*:1246-1250, 1965.

Whitaker, J. A.; Austin, W.; Nelson, J. D. Edathamil calcium disodium (Versenate) diagnostic test for lead poisoning. Pediatrics *29*:384-388, 1962.

Whitaker, J. A.; Vietti, T. J. Fluorescence of the erythrocytes in lead poisoning in children; an aid to rapid diagnosis. Pediatrics *24*:734-738, 1959.

Whitfield, C. L.; Chien, L. T.; Whitehead, J. D. Lead encephalopathy in adults. Am. J. Med. *52*:289-298, 1972.

Wilenty, W. C. Treatment of lead intoxication. J. A. M. A. *139*:823-825, 1949.

Wilson, V. K.; Thomas, M. L.; Dent, C. E. Amino-aciduria in lead poisoning; a case in childhood. Lancet *2*:66-68, 1953.

Wolman, I. J. Hematology of lead poisoning in childhood. Am. J. Med. Sci. *232*:688-693, 1956.

Wyllie, J.; Petermann, H.; Petermann, E. Effect of penicillamine in promoting lead excretion. Can. Med. Assoc. J. *88*:1155-1159, 1963.

Zimmer, F. E. Lead poisoning in scrap-metal workers. J. A. M. A. *175*:238-240, 1961.

LINDANE

Benzene hexachloride or BHC (more properly called hexachlorocyclohexane) in its various forms was formerly a widely used insecticide, especially in the control of cotton insects. Technical BHC is a mixture with the following approximate isomeric composition: α 65 to 70%, β 6 to 8%, γ 12 to 15%, δ 2 to 5 %, and others 5 to 10%. These isomers differ qualitatively and quantitatively in biological activity. The α and γ isomers are central nervous stimulants; the β and δ are depressants. In a mixture of these isomers it is possible that one component may antidote another (Council on Pharmacy and Chemistry, 1951).

When it was discovered that almost all the insecticidal activity of BHC resided with the γ isomer, the latter rapidly supplanted BHC and became the insecticide known as lindane. Technical lindane is at least 99% γ-BHC. BHC as such is no longer produced in the United States. The future of lindane is also in doubt, since it is currently on the Rebuttable Presumption Against Registration list of the EPA. The registration of some lindane products for certain uses has already been cancelled, including its use in continuous vaporizers, on some agricultural crops and dairy cattle and in dairy barns and milk rooms.

Toxicology: The mean lethal dose of technical BHC may be about 400 mg./kg. when ingested by man. The γ isomer (lindane) has the highest acute toxicity; its lethal dose is perhaps 125 mg./kg. (Hayes, 1982). Rather few human fatalities have been ascribed to either BHC or lindane, but many nonfatal poisonings have been reported (reviewed by Hayes, 1982). In the United States many of these poisonings occurred in children who swallowed lindane pellets intended for use in vaporizers (Joslin *et al.*, 1960; Starr and Clifford, 1972). For example, within 30 minutes after ingesting an estimated 1.5 gm. lindane, a 2½-year-old girl exhibited irritability and grand mal convulsions. With supportive care she recovered within 24 hours. Serum levels of lindane were high initially but fell rapidly. Considerable amounts were recovered in the first stool samples (Starr and Clifford, 1972).

At least two group poisonings have resulted from the ingestion of food contaminated with lindane. In Australia, four out of five members of a family who ate a homemade dessert containing lindane experienced vomiting and convulsions after a latent period that averaged 5 hours (Wilson, 1959). Each of 11 adults who drank Nescafé in which lindane was inadvertently substituted for sugar received a dose of about 86 mg./kg. (Bambov et al., 1966, as summarized by Hayes, 1982). The interval from ingestion to the onset of malaise varied from 20 minutes to 4 hours and averaged about 1 hour. All survived but only after periods of severe convulsions.

A 36-year-old man who ingested lindane-contaminated food had grand mal seizures for 2 hours. Also present were severe acidemia, muscle weakness and pain, headache, episodic hypertension, myoglobinuria and eventually acute renal failure and anemia. Pancreatitis developed on the 13th day. A muscle biopsy on the 15th day showed widespread necrosis and regeneration of muscle fibers (Munk and Nantel, 1977).

BHC is absorbed through all portals including the intact skin. Severe and even fatal vapor exposures have resulted from using electric vaporizers in the home (Council on Pharmacy and Chemistry, 1952a, 1954). In these chronic vapor exposures, aplastic anemia and other hematological disorders (e.g., agranulocytosis) are described (Friberg and Martensson, 1953; Loge, 1965; West, 1967; see also pp. IV-101–105). The registrations for continuous type vaporizers have been cancelled, but "one-shot" vaporizers are still registered. Lindane has been associated with aplastic anemia under other conditions of exposure as well (Gewin, 1959; Stiegliz et al., 1967).

More recently 1% lindane as a cream, lotion or shampoo has been introduced as a medical treatment for scabies and lice (Kwell, Gamene). Of six cases of alleged neurotoxicity associated with the use of this type of product, at least five were judged to be due to accidental ingestion or inappropriate application (Kramer et al., 1980). Some children exhibited seizures after total body applications or after applications that were left on longer than the recommended 24 hours (Lee and Groth, 1977). Percutaneous absorption with measurable blood levels of lindane has been documented in infants and children treated with 1% lotion although the correlation between blood concentration and amount of lindane applied was poor (Ginsburg et al., 1977). Convulsions and death can be produced in weanling rabbits by topical doses used on human infants, but young adult rabbits given the same dose

showed only anorexia and mild excitement (Hanig et al., 1976). An inappropriately large droplet size in emulsified cattle dip was held responsible for the absorption of toxic and even fatal amounts from a normally safe concentration (Ray et al., 1975).

The rapidity with which symptoms develop after ingesting BHC varies with the isomer: the γ is fastest (within 1 hour, e.g.., Nicholls, 1958), the α slowest (within 24 hours), and the technical or commercial mixture is intermediate (usually within 2 hours but sometimes as late as 12 hours, e.g., Danopoulos et al., 1953). Death from the pure γ isomer is usually prompt (24 hours), whereas from the others it may be delayed several days. The pathology resembles that caused by DDT; liver damage and hyaline changes in the renal tubules are described most often (Joslin et al., 1960).

In rats given BHC by mouth the material was 80% absorbed when given as a solution in olive oil but only 6% absorbed when given as an aqueous suspension. The highest concentrations were found in adipose tissue and the lowest in blood and muscle. Peak values were reached in 2 to 5 days. By 2 weeks after intraperitoneal administration, 34% of the dose was recovered in the feces mostly unchanged and only 5% in the urine (Koss and Koransky, 1975).

Although symptoms and treatment are similar, lindane is more acutely toxic than DDT. Moreover, it may modify brain function for days and even weeks after a single exposure. Following a single dose of lindane the threshold for pentylenetetrazole-induced seizures first decreases and then increases after 2 days to above normal. At a time when the convulsive threshold is increased, the brain content of γ-aminobutyric acid is also elevated (Hulth et al., 1978).

Rats made cachectic by feeding a low protein diet were twice as susceptible to the acute toxic effects of lindane as were animals fed a normal diet (Boyd and Chen, 1968). Like all other members of the halogenated hydrocarbon class of insecticides, lindane exposure leads to increases in liver and kidney weight and the induction of hepatic microsomal drug-metabolizing enzymes in rats (Kolmodin-Hedman et al., 1971; Pelissier and Albrecht, 1976).

Symptomatology (from technical BHC or the γ isomer):

1. After ingestion a latent period varying from about ½ hour to several hours.
2. Hyperirritability and central nervous excitation: notably vomiting, faintness, tremor, restlessness, muscle spasms, ataxia, and clonic and tonic convulsions.
3. Infants and children may experience hyperpyrexia presumably as a consequence of the convulsions.

4. Postictal coma of variable duration, leading eventually (within 24 hours) to respiratory failure and death.

5. A second bout of convulsions may occur after consciousness is regained. Retrograde amnesia is described.

6. Pulmonary edema (with cyanosis and dyspnea) was observed in two fatally poisoned children.

7. From exposure to lindane vapors (and its thermal decomposition products), headache, nausea, vomiting, irritation of eyes, nose, and throat. Repeated exposure may lead to agranulocytosis or even fatal aplastic anemia.

8. Dermatitis and urticaria occasionally.

Treatment:

1. Perform gastric lavage or administer activated charcoal (see Section I), followed by saline cathartics but not mineral oil or digestible oils because they may promote absorption (Morgan *et al.*, 1977).

2. Sedatives and anticonvulsants. Diazepam, pentobarbital or phenobarbital in amounts adequate to control convulsions (p. IV-37).

3. Calcium gluconate intravenously may be used in conjunction with anticonvulsants in the control of convulsions. See p. IV-74.

4. Rest and quiet.

5. Do *not* use epinephrine because ventricular fibrillation may result.

Laboratory: Increases in SGPT, prothrombin time and coagulation time have been observed in animals (Kashiyap *et al.*, 1976).

References:

Boyd, E. M.; Chen, C. P. Lindane toxicity and protein-deficient diet. Arch. Environ. Health *17*:156-163, 1968.

Council on Pharmacy and Chemistry, A. M. A. Toxic effects of technical benzene hexachloride and its principal isomers. J. A. M. A. *147*:571-574, 1951.

Council on Pharmacy and Chemistry, A. M. A. Health hazards of electric vaporizing devices for insecticides. J. A. M. A. *149*:367-369, 1952a.

Council on Pharmacy and Chemistry, A. M. A. Abuse of insecticide fumigating devices. J. A. M. A. *156*:607, 1954.

Danopoulos, E.; Melissinos, K.; Katsas, G. Serious poisoning by hexachlorocyclohexane. Clinical and laboratory observations on five cases. Arch. Ind. Hyg. Occup. Med. *8*:582-587, 1953.

Friberg, L.; Martensson, J. Case of panmyelophthisis after exposure to chlorphenothane and benzene hexachloride. Arch. Ind. Hyg. Occup. Med. *8*:166-169, 1953.

Gewin, H. M. Benzene hydrochloride and aplastic anemia. J. A. M. A. *171*:1624-1625, 1959.

Ginsburg, C. M.; Lowry, W.; Reisch, J. S. Absorption of lindane (gamma-benzene hexachloride) in infants and children. J. Pediatr. *91*:998-1000, 1977.

Hanig, J. P.; Yoder, P. D.; Krop, S. Convulsions in weanling rabbits after a single topical application of 1% lindane. Toxicol. Appl. Pharmacol. *38*:463-469, 1976.

Hayes, W. J., Jr. *Pesticides Studied In Man*. Williams & Wilkins, Baltimore, 1982.

Hulth, L.; Hoglund, L.; Bergman, A.; Moller, L. Convulsive properties of lindane, lindane metabolites and the lindane isomer α-hexachlorocyclohexane: effects on the convulsive threshold for pentylenetetrazole and the brain content of γ-aminobutyric acid (GABA) in the mouse. Toxicol. Appl. Pharmacol. *46*:101-108, 1978.

Joslin, E. F.; Forney, R. L.; Huntington, R. W.; Hayes, W. J., Jr. A fatal case of lindane poisoning. Proc. of 1958 Seminar of National Association of Coroners, published privately, 1960.

Kashiyap, S. K.; Gupta, S. K.; Bhatt, H. V.; Shah, M. P. Acute oral toxicity of hexachlorocyclohexane (BHC) in albino rats. Ind. J. Med. Res. *64*:768-772, 1976.

Kolmodin-Hedman, B.; Alexanderson, B.; Sjoqvist, F. Effect of exposure to lindane on drug metabolism: decreased hexobarbital sleeping-times and increased antipyrene disappearance rate in rats. Toxicol. Appl. Pharmacol. *20*:299-307, 1971.

Koss, G.; Koransky, W. Studies on toxicology of hexachlorobenzene l. Pharmacokinetics. Arch. Toxicol. *34*:203-212, 1975.

Kramer, M. S.; Hutchinson, T. A.; Rudnick, S. A.; Leventhal, J. M.; Feinstein, A. R. Operational criteria for adverse drug reactions in evaluating suspected toxicity of a popular scabicide. Clin. Pharmacol. Ther. *27*:149-155, 1980.

Lee, B.; Groth, P. Scabies: transcutaneous poisoning during treatment (letter). Pediatrics *59*:643, 1977.

Loge, J. P. Aplastic anemia following exposure to benzene hexachloride (Lindane). J. A. M. A. *193*:110-114, 1965.

Morgan, D. P.; Dotson, J. B.; Lin, L. I. Effectiveness of activated charcoal, mineral oil, and castor oil in limiting gastrointestinal absorption of a chlorinated hydrocarbon pesticide. Clin. Toxicol. *11*:61-70, 1977.

Munk, Z. M.; Nantel, A. Acute lindane poisoning with development of muscle necrosis. Can. Med. Assoc. J. *117*:1050-1054, 1977.

Nicholls, R. W. A case of acute poisoning by benzene hexachloride. Med. J. Aust. *1*:42-43, 1958.

Pelissier, M. A.; Albrecht, R. Teneur minimale du regime en lindane induisant les monoxygenases microsomales chez le rat. Food Cosmet. Toxicol. *14*:297-301, 1976.

Ray, A. C.; Norris, J. D., Jr.; Reagor, R. D. Benzene hexachloride poisoning in cattle. J. Am. Vet. Assoc. *166*:1180-1182, 1975.

Starr, H. G., Jr.; Clifford, N. J. Acute lindane intoxication. Arch. Environ. Health *25*:374-375, 1972.

Stieglitz, R.; Stobbs, H.; Schuettman, W. Knochenmarkschaden nach beruflicher Einwirkung des Insektizids Gamma-hexachlorcyclohexan (Lindan). Acta Haematol. *38*:337-350, 1967.

West, I. Lindane and hematological reactions. Arch. Environ. Health *15*:97-101, 1967.

Wilson, J. S. Lindane poisoning in a family. Med. J. Aust. *2*:684, 1959.

LITHIUM

Lithium is the lightest metal known, but in nature it exists only as lithium ions or salts. Lithium bromide was once used as a hypnotic and sedative. Lithium chloride was employed formerly as a table salt substitute and more recently in the management of manic depressive psychosis and less frequently of unipolar depression (Gershon, 1970). Lithium carbonate, however, is now more widely used for these medicinal purposes. With some lithium salts, the anion probably determines the major toxicity, *e.g.*, lithium chromate and dichromate, lithium fluoride, lithium oxalate, lithium selenate and selenite.

Toxicology: The acute toxicity of lithium salts is difficult to assess. Most poisonings have occurred over weeks to months of chronic intake, not from single ingestion episodes; only 12 of the 100 cases reviewed by Hansen and Amdisen (1978) were due to acute overdoses. Moreover, the toxicity of lithium is almost certainly determined in important measure by the concomitant sodium intake. Little systematic work has been done to assess lithium toxicity at various controlled levels of sodium intake, but high sodium intake protects rat kidneys against injury by lithium (Shou, 1958a).

The acute oral LD_{50} of lithium carbonate in rats is about 710 mg./kg. (Smyth *et al.*, 1969b), placing it near the borderline between toxicity classes 3 and 4. That is not inconsistent with the few reports of single massive ingestions by humans. In one such episode a 58-year-old woman consumed 22.5 gm. of lithium carbonate together with 1.25 gm. of thioridazine. Within an hour she experienced vomiting and profuse diarrhea, but, when the gastrointestinal symptoms subsided within a few hours, she was found to be normal in a physical examination that included a complete neurologic workup. Her serum lithium reached 8.2 mEq./L. at 2.5 hours after ingestion and was 1.7 mEq./L. even at 48 hours (see below). The authors of this report believe that the thioridazine also ingested could not have prevented the usual effects of lithium (Horowitz and Fisher, 1969). The remarkable absence of symptoms in this case may have been due to the known slow rate of penetration of lithium into the brain (Shou, 1958b).

A relatively benign course was also followed by an adult male who ingested 36 gm. while on regular maintenance therapy. His serum lithium peaked at 3 mEq./L. at about 5 hours and was 2.2 mEq./L. 3 hours later following lavage, activated charcoal, aminophylline and fluid therapy. An ensuing bradycardia and idioventricular rhythm were ascribed to hypokalemia. It responded to intravenous potassium chloride, and the patient recovered fully in a few days (Habibzadeh and Zeller, 1977).

Several more recent reports of massive overdoses point to a remarkable delay between ingestion and the onset of toxicity. One adult female was seen 1 to 2 hours after ingesting 60 gm. of lithium carbonate in combination with 15 gm. chlorpromazine and 0.9 gm. flurazepam. She had vomited twice and was lavaged with the recovery of some particulate matter. A slurry of 100 gm. of activated charcoal was left in the stomach. Her serum lithium rose progressively from 3.7 mEq./L. on admission to a peak of 14 mEq./L. at about 48 hours with few overt signs of toxicity. At 45 hours she was slightly drowsy, but 4 hours later she was in a profound coma. Both peritoneal dialysis and hemodialysis were instituted, and the serum lithium fell rapidly to less than 2 mEq./L. without any change in the level of consciousness. Respiratory and cardiac complications eventually led to her demise (Achong *et al.*, 1975).

Except for her eventual recovery, a similar course was followed by another patient who ingested 12 gm. in combination with 375 mg. flurazepam and 1.5 gm. doxepin. She was seen 3 hours after ingestion and lavaged. Peritoneal dialysis was instituted when the serum lithium level reached 5.9 mEq./L. Despite continued dialysis the serum level continued to rise to 9.6 mEq./L. at 48 hours. Dialysis was discontinued after 1 week because an infection developed in the peritoneal cavity. After 11 days in coma recovery was nearly complete by the 18th day (Marshall and Kesson, 1981). An adult male who also ingested 12 gm. was discharged after lavage, only to be readmitted 9 hours later complaining of thirst and blurred vision. He was treated conservatively with fluids, electrolytes and mannitol and made a complete recovery (Shneerson, 1978).

Even when a sudden rise in serum lithium was noted during the course of chronic therapy (to 6.8 mEq./L.), the clinical status did not become alarming until the 3rd day. Again despite effective treatment which reduced the level to 1.9 mEq./L., the patient was comatose for 18 days and finally died (Amdisen *et al.*, 1975). These cases suggest that a slow and/or erratic absorption of lithium from the gastrointestinal tract must contribute to the delayed and insidious appearance of toxicity, and that lithium transport between blood and brain is inherently slow.

When used therapeutically in affective disorders, lithium is taken in multiple doses every day over long periods of time; the total daily dose ranges from 0.9 to 2.4 gm. as Li_2CO_3. The optimal therapeutic plasma level is believed to lie between 0.6 and 1.5 mEq./L. Toxic effects are usually severe at steady plasma levels of 2 mEq./L. or greater (Gershon, 1970), and sustained levels of 4 mEq./L. are often fatal (Herrero, 1973).

In the peripheral sympathetic nervous system lithium increases the ability of adrenergic nerve terminals to sequester norepinephrine. Thus, the effects of injected or endogenously released norepinephrine are attenuated (Gershon, 1970). Perhaps this mechanism operating in the central nervous system is responsible for the therapeutic actions of lithium in the manic phases of affective disorders, but it does not appear to be related to the toxic effects of the drug. An interference with cyclic-AMP-mediated processes that are regulated by polypeptide hormones has also been postulated as a mechanism for some effects of lithium (*e.g.*., Singer and Rotenberg, 1973). In toxic concentrations lithium inhibits monoamine oxidase as well (Beaty *et al.*, 1981).

When lithium is taken daily, a prodromal syndrome is recognized; it precedes full-blown intoxication by several days to a week. The signs of vomiting, diarrhea, drowsiness, coarse tremor, muscle twitching, and slurred speech can in part be confused with the spontaneous advent of a depressive phase of a manic disorder. Except for this possible confusion, lithium intoxication in psychiatric patients takes the same form as in individuals without affective disorders (Corcoran *et al.*, 1949; Greenfield *et al.*, 1950; Hanlon *et al.*, 1949; Shou *et al.*, 1968b; Stern, 1949). The central nervous system and muscles are primarily affected, with tremor, muscular and reflex hyperirritability, confusion, coma, EEG abnormalities, mental lapses, attacks of hyperextension of the arms and legs, neurologic asymmetries and cutaneous hyperesthesia and hyperalgesia. An acute generalized sensorimotor peripheral neuropathy developed over several weeks in one patient but cleared completely (Brust *et al.*, 1979). These and other signs below cannot as yet be ascribed to any single pathologic mechanism.

Although prominent on intravenous administration to animals, toxic reactions of the heart and circulation are not usually life-threatening in man. Electrocardiographic changes such as flattening and sometimes inversion of T-waves can be demonstrated even at relatively low doses. One manic-depressive patient, however, developed marked arrhythmias and bundle branch block during therapy. The former, but not the latter, disappeared on withdrawing lithium. When lithium was resumed, the patient died, and interstitial myocarditis was found at autopsy (Tseng, 1971). Perimyocarditis was found at autopsy of another case (Amdisen *et al.*, 1975).

Reports of toxic changes in bone marrow have been disputed (Shou, 1957). A significant but reversible leukocytosis with a trend toward neutrophilia and lymphocytopenia occurs during periods of lithium ingestion. This effect, however, does not appear to be dose-related or dependent on the concentration of lithium in peripheral blood (Shopsin *et al.*, 1971).

Lithium has poorly understood effects on the thyroid. In rats triiodothyronine pretreatment increased the acute toxicity of lithium but blocked its hypothermic effect (Sanghvi *et al.*, 1971). A significant decrease in serum protein-bound iodine and clinical hypothyroidism have occured (Rogers and Whybrow, 1971). A high incidence of goiter was noted in another series of patients although all affected remained clinically euthyroid (Shou *et al.*, 1968a). Myxedema has been reported at least once (Luby *et al.*, 1971).

Concomitant dehydration (Pi and Surawicz, 1978), administration of diuretic drugs (König *et*

al., 1978), and restricted sodium intake are generally acknowledged to enhance the toxicity of lithium (Coppen and Shaw, 1967). In an otherwise stabilized individual, weight loss due to dieting or disease can lead to lithium intoxication (Tonks, 1977). A potentially lethal interaction between lithium and physostigmine, which can be prevented by atropine, has been described in rats (Davis and Hatoum, 1980). Concurrent use of methyldopa (Byrd, 1977), tetracycline, indomethacin, haloperidol, thioridazine, carbamazepine or phenytoin may increase the risk of lithium toxicity (Medical Letter, 1980; Speirs and Hirsch, 1978). Various diuretics may interfere with the renal excretion of lithium and so induce lithium poisoning.

Acute renal failure is sometimes the cause of death in animals (Shou, 1957), and in rats a sixfold increase in plasma renin suggested that both direct toxicity to the renal tubule and circulatory disturbances contributed to the acute renal failure (Thomsen and Olesen, 1978). In humans renal insufficiency often predisposes to lithium poisoning (Amdisen and Skjoldborg, 1969; Gautier *et al.*, 1972; Lee *et al.*, 1971; Shou *et al.*, 1968b). The converse is also true. Lithium is now known to produce nephrogenic diabetes insipidus, distal renal tubular acidosis and impairment of renal concentrating ability, all by unknown mechanisms (Chan *et al.*, 1981). Perhaps these contribute to the risk of lithium toxicity in a vicious cycle. Proximal tubular damage as assessed by renal biopsy, with recovery of normal renal function after withdrawal of lithium, has been documented (Lavender *et al.*, 1973), and ultrastructural changes have been noted in the distal convoluted tubules and collecting ducts (Davies and Kincaid-Smith, 1979; Myers *et al.*, 1980).

Lithium penetrates the placental barrier, and poisoning characterized by cyanosis, lethargy and flaccid muscle tone has been recognized in the newborn. As judged by plasma lithium levels, infants do not appear to be unusually susceptible to its toxic effects (Wilbanks *et al.*, 1970; Woody *et al.*, 1971). In contrast, the elderly are said to be more sensitive although this may represent poor hydration (Van der Velde, 1971). Lithium poisoning in one infant was thought to be prolonged by breast feeding when the mother continued on the drug (Tunnejen and Herz, 1972). Lithium is teratogenic in rats, and malformed infants have been born of mothers using the drug (Aoki and Ruedy, 1971; Vacaflor *et al.*, 1970).

Aside from developmental anomalies, complete recovery is the general rule among survivors of lithium intoxication. However, two adults exposed to toxic levels for prolonged periods of time exhibited permanent damage to the basal ganglia and cerebellar connections (Von Hartitzsch *et al.*, 1972). Two of 23 cases became permanently demented; one of the two was also ataxic (Hansen and Amdisen, 1978). Some patients with renal insufficiency failed to regain normal renal function (Hansen and Amdisen, 1978; Myers *et al.*, 1980).

Extracorporeal hemodialysis is effective in reducing serum lithium levels although a rebound phenomenon has been observed (Amdisen and Skjoldborg, 1969). Peritoneal dialysis would appear to be worthwhile if an artificial kidney is not available (Lavender *et al.*, 1973; Wilson *et al.*, 1971). In one case dramatic improvement followed within minutes after intravenous infusion of 1 liter of ⅙ M sodium lactate, but the patient's pretreatment acid-base status was not clearly defined (Gaind and Saran, 1970). Bicarbonate, lactate, acetazolamide, urea and aminophylline are said to hasten the renal excretion of lithium (Thomsen, 1969). Raising the sodium intake did not increase lithium clearance (Thomsen, 1969). In the absence of intense vomiting or diarrhea, the victim of lithium poisoning is apt to have an elevated body water content (Coppen and Shaw, 1967).

Symptomatology:
1. In patients not previously exposed to the drug or those in whom a single massive ingestion is superimposed on chronic therapy, only vomiting and diarrhea may be provoked initially. Such patients, however, should be hospitalized because the toxic syndrome may be delayed for hours to days after ingestion (see text above).
2. In patients taking the drug daily, prodromal signs may include apathy, sluggishness, drowsiness, slurred speech, blurred vision, nystagmus, weakness, ataxia, lethargy, tinnitus, tremor and muscle twitching.
3. Profuse and varied central nervous system and muscle signs include: hyperreflexia, muscle fasciculations, choreiform movements, spasticity, parkinsonism, delirium, anxiety, stupor, coma and epileptiform seizures. Because lithium is slowly cleared from the cerebrospinal fluid, toxic effects can be expected to persist several days after the drug has been discontinued and even after plasma concentrations have been lowered by effective treatment.
4. In patients in prolonged coma, late pulmonary complications such as atelectasis, bronchopneumonia and pulmonary edema.
5. Renal concentrating defects and nephrogenic diabetes insipidus with polydipsia and polyuria are common findings with therapeutic doses; they tend to disappear when therapy is stopped.
6. Renal failure with albuminuria may indicate permanent tubular damage.
7. Rarely myocarditis with arrhythmias, conduction defects and hypotension. T-wave depression in the ECG is a common, benign and reversible effect.

Treatment:
1. In single ingestion episodes, give syrup of ipecac and/or perform gastric lavage (see Section I), if productive vomiting has not already occurred. Although we can cite no data, it seems unlikely that activated charcoal binds lithium to a useful degree; therefore it is best avoided in lithium poisonings.
2. Fluid and electrolyte replacement for the correction of dehydration and acid-base imbalances (pp. IV-64–72). Overhydration may precipitate pulmonary edema.
3. Infusion of urea or mannitol (p. IV-52), alkalinization of the urine (p. IV-72) and aminophylline increase lithium excretion in patients with good renal function.
4. Extracorporeal or peritoneal hemodialysis (pp. IV-55–57) to decrease lithium levels and control uremia in severe intoxications. If a massive overdose is known with certainty to have been ingested, it may be prudent to institute these measures even in the absence of positive clinical findings because of severe delayed toxicity (see text above).
5. Diazepam for the suppression of abnormal motor activity. See pp. IV-35–39.
6. Supportive treatment for central nervous depression. See pp. IV-39–43.

Laboratory: Blood plasma lithium levels may help in diagnosis and prognosis. Toxicity is common at sustained plasma levels at 2 mEq./L. and above; steady levels above 4 mEq./L. are often fatal. Frequent electrocardiograms to assess cardiac status.

References:

Achong, M. R.; Fernandez, P. G.; McLeod, P. J. Fatal self-poisoning with lithium carbonate. Can. Med. Assoc. J. *112*:868-870, 1975.

Amdisen, A.; Gottfries, C. G.; Jacobsson, L.; Winblad, B. Grave lithium intoxication with fatal outcome. Acta Psychiatrica Scand., Suppl. No. *255*:25-33, 1975.

Amdisen, A.; Skjoldborg, H. Haemodialysis for lithium poisoning. Lancet *2*:213, 1969.

Aoki, F. Y.; Ruedy, J. Severe lithium intoxication; management without dialysis and report of a possible teratogenic effect of lithium. Can. Med. Assoc. J. *105*:847-848, 1971.

Beaty, O., III.; Collis, M. G.; Shepherd, J. T. Action of lithium on the adrenergic nerve ending. J. Pharmacol. Exp. Ther. *218*:309-317, 1981.

Brust, J. C. M.; Hammer, J. S.; Challenor, Y.; Healton, E. B.; Lesser, R. P. Acute generalized polyneuropathy accompanying lithium poisoning. Ann. Neurol. *6*:360-362, 1979.

Byrd, G. J. Lithium carbonate and methyldopa: apparent interaction in man. Clin. Toxicol. *11*:1-4, 1977.

Chan, W. Y.; Mosca, P.; Rennert, O. W. Lithium nephrotoxicity: A review. Ann. Clin. Lab. Sci. *11*:343-349, 1981.

Coppen, A.; Shaw, D. M. The distribution of electrolytes and water in patients after taking lithium carbonate. Lancet *2*:805-806, 1967.

Corcoran, A. C.; Taylor, R. D.; Page, I. H. Lithium poisoning from the use of salt substitutes. J. A. M. A. *139*:685-688, 1949.

Davies, B.; Kincaid-Smith, P. Renal biopsy studies of lithium and prelithium patients and comparison with cadaver transplant kidneys. Neuropharmacology *18*:1001-1002, 1979.

Davis, W. M.; Hatoum, N. S. Synergism of the toxicity of physostigmine and neostigmine by lithium or by a reserpine-like agent (Ro4-1284). Toxicology *17*:1-7, 1980.

Gaind, R.; Saran, B. M. Acute lithium poisoning. Postgrad. Med. J. *46*:629-631, 1970.

Gautier, J.; Breteau, M.; Lamisse, F.; Bienvenu, P.; Ginies, G. L'intoxication aigue par le carbonate de lithium. Sem. Hop. Paris *48*:125-131, 1972.

Gershon, S. Lithium in mania. Clin. Pharmacol. Ther. *11*:168-187, 1970.

Greenfield, I.; Zuger, M.; Bleak, R. M.; Bakal, S. F. Lithium chloride intoxication. N. Y. State J. Med. *50*:459-460, 1950.

Habibzadeh, M. A.; Zeller, N. H. Cardiac arrhythmia and hypopotassemia in association with lithium carbonate overdose. South. Med. J. *70*:628-630, 1977.

Hanlon, L. W.; Romaine, M., III; Gilroy, F. J.; Deitrick, J. E. Lithium chloride as a substitute for sodium chloride in the diet, observations on its toxicity. J. A. M. A. *139*:688-692, 1949.

Hansen, H. E.; Amdisen, A. Lithium intoxication. Q. J. Med. *47*:123-144, 1978.

Herrero, F. A. Lithium carbonate toxicity. J. A. M. A. *226*:1109-1110, 1973.

Horowitz, L. C.; Fisher, G. U. Acute lithium toxicity. N. Engl. J. Med. *281*:1369, 1969.

Konig, P.; Kufferle, B.; Lenz, G. Ein Fall von Lithiumintoxikation bei therapeutischen Lithiumdosen infolge zusatzlicher Gabe eines Diuretikums. Wien. Klin. Wochenschr. *90*:380-382, 1978.

Lavender, S.; Brown, J. N.; Berrill, W. T. Acute renal failure and lithium intoxication. Postgrad. Med. J. *49*:277-279, 1973.

Lee, R. V.; Jempol, L. M.; Brown, W. V. Nephrogenic diabetes insipidus and lithium intoxication. N. Engl. J. Med. *284*:93-94, 1971.

Luby, R. D.; Schwartz, D.; Rosenbaum, H. Lithium carbonate-induced myxedema. J. A. M. A. *218*:1298-1299, 1971.

Marshall, A. M.; Kesson, C. M. Severe lithium poisoning. Drug Intell. Clin. Pharm. *15*:598-599, 1981.

Medical Letter. Another look at lithium. Medical Letter, Inc., New Rochelle, N. Y. *22*:17-19, February 22, 1980.

Myers, J. B.; Morgan, T. O.; Carney, S. L.; Ray, C. Effects of lithium on the kidney. Kidney Intern. *18*:601-608, 1980.

Pi, H. T.; Surawicz, F. G. Severe neurotoxicity and lithium therapy. Clin. Toxicol. *13*:479-486, 1978.

Rogers, M. P.; Whybrow, P. C. Clinical hypothyroidism occurring during lithium treatment; two case histories and a review of thyroid function in 19 patients. Am. J. Psychiatry *128*:158-160, 1971.

Sanghvi, I.; Shopsin, B.; Gershon, S. The effects of sub-acute administration of triiodothyronine (T$_3$) on the acute toxicity of lithium in the rat. Life Sci. (I) *10*:1217-1223, 1971.

Shneerson, J. M. Acute lithium intoxication. Br. J. Clin. Pract. *32*:232-237, 1978.

Shopsin, B.; Friedmann, R.; Gershon, S. Lithium and leukocytosis. Clin. Pharmacol. Ther. *12*:923-928, 1971.

Shou, M. Biology and pharmacology of the lithium ion. Pharmacol. Rev. *9*:17-58, 1957.

Shou, M. Lithium studies; 1. Toxicity. Acta Pharmacol. Toxicol. *15*:70-84, 1958a.

Shou, M. Lithium studies; 3. Distribution between serum and tissue. Acta Pharmacol. Toxicol. *15*:115-124, 1958b.

Shou, M.; Amdisen, A.; Jensen, S. E.; Olsen, T. Occurrence of goitre during lithium treatment. Br. Med. J. *3*:710-713, 1968a.

Shou, M.; Amdisen, A.; Trap-Jensen, S. Lithium poisoning. Am. J. Psychiatry *125*:520-527, 1968b.

Singer, I.; Rotenberg, D. Mechanisms of lithium action. N. Engl. J. Med. *289*:254-260, 1973.

Smyth, H. F., Jr.; Carpenter, C. P.; Weil, C. S.; Pozzani, U. Z.; Striegel, J. A.; Nycum, J. S. Range finding toxicity data: List VII. Am. Ind. Hyg. Assoc. J. *30*:470-476, 1969b.

Speirs, J.; Hirsch, S. R. Severe lithium toxicity with "normal" serum concentrations. Br. Med. J. *1*:815-817, 1978.

Stern, R. L. Severe lithium chloride poisoning with complete recovery; report of case. J. A. M. A. *139*:710-711, 1949.

Thomsen, K. Renal lithium elimination in man and active treatment of lithium poisoning. Acta Psychiatr. Scand., Suppl. No. *207*:83-84, 1969.

Thomsen, K.; Olesen, O. V. Lithium-induced acute renal failure in the rat. Toxicol. Appl. Pharmacol. *45*:155-161, 1978.

Tonks, C. M. Lithium intoxication induced by dieting and saunas. Br. Med. J. *2*:1396-1397, 1977.

Tseng, H. L. Interstitial myocarditis probably related to lithium carbonate intoxication. Arch. Pathol. *92*:444-448, 1971.

Tunnejen, W. W.; Herz, C. G. Toxic effects of lithium in newborn infants; a commentary. J. Pediatr. *81*:804-807, 1972.

Vacaflor, L.; Lehmann, H. E.; Ban, T. A. Side effects and teratogenicity of lithium carbonate treatment. J. Clin. Pharmacol. *10*:387-389, 1970.

Van Der Velde, C. D. Toxicity of lithium carbonate in elderly patients. Am. J. Psychiatry *127*:1075-1077, 1971.

Von Hartitzsch, B.; Hoenich, N. A.; Leigh, R. J.; Wilkinson, R.; Frost, T. H. Weddel, A.; Posen, G. A. Permanent neurological sequelae despite hemodialysis for lithium intoxication. Br. Med. J. *4*:757-759, 1972.

Wilbanks, G. D.; Bressler, B.; Peete, C. H., Jr.; Cherny, W. B.; London, W. L. Toxic effects of lithium carbonate in a mother and newborn infants. J. A. M. A. *213*:865-867, 1970.

Wilson, J. H. P.; Donker, A. J. M.; Van Der Hem, G. K.; Wientjes, J. Peritoneal dialysis for lithium poisoning. Br. Med. J. *2*:749-750, 1971.

Woody, J. N.; London, W. L.; Wilbanks, G. D., Jr. Lithium toxicity in a newborn. Pediatrics *47*:94-96, 1971.

LYE

The strong corrosive alkalis known as "lye" include caustic soda, caustic potash, sodium and potassium hydroxides, carbonates, oxides and peroxides. Some highly alkaline phosphates, *e.g.*, trisodium phosphate, produce injuries similar to that of lye (Palmer, 1958). Lithium hydride (see also Section II) and related compounds react vigorously on contact with moisture to generate lithium hydroxide and hydrogen gas, which may ignite spontaneously. The resulting tissue damage may be more intense than that from lye.

Lyes are commonly used as cleaning agents and are present in many washing powders, some denture cleaners, some non-phosphate "ecology" detergents, drain-pipe cleaners and paint removers. Most of the reported cases of poisoning have resulted from the careless practice of leaving lye solutions in beverage containers within the reach of a thirsty child. The incidence of fatal poisonings by lye in the South is several times that in the rest of the United States. (Arena, 1955; Brown and Kiser, 1942). Lye burns of the mouth continue to be common in children, but deep esophageal and gastric injuries are more common among suicidal adults (Hawkins *et al.*, 1980).

Urine sugar reagent tablets, *e.g.*, Clinitest, contain anhydrous sodium hydroxide together with small amounts of copper sulfate, sodium bicarbonate and citric acid. They represent a potential hazard in the homes of many diabetics. Despite opinions to the contrary (Rabinowitz and Tchang, 1961), the nature of the lesion in most cases of Clinitest tablet ingestion resembles that following any corrosive alkali; the other ingredients make no contribution to the ingestion syndrome. A single tablet is a dangerous dose (Bloomer and Kirchner, 1955; Burton and Zawadzki, 1962; Canby, 1957; Danzig and Loebel, 1965; Lasky and Picard, 1956; Owens, 1954; Tomsovic and Jaird, 1958: Zimmerman, 1959). AMMONIA ingestion involves some special problems because of its volatility; see p. III-21.

Toxicology: The strong alkalis are markedly corrosive and penetrating. This property is due to their solubilizing reactions with protein and collagen, saponifying effect on lipids, and dehydrating action on tissue cells (Houck *et al.*, 1962). The corroded areas are soft, gelatinous and friable, and often exhibit a brownish discoloration. The term "liquefaction necrosis" is often associated with lye injury, as distinct from "coagulation necrosis," which is the tissue response to mineral ACIDS (p. III-8) and which often leaves supporting structures intact. Although initial responses of the dermis may be similar (Houck *et al.*, 1962), ultimate tissue destruction with lye is more intense than with acids. The latter, however, produce the more fulminating illness.

Sometimes the first mouthful of lye solution makes further swallowing impossible because of intense pain and spasm. Systemic reactions are due solely to local tissue injury, but their intensity cannot be dependably predicted from the size of the dose. As with most caustic solutions, concentration is more critical than volume. In the rabbit esophagus a 10-second exposure to a 1 N solution of sodium hydroxide (4%) produced necrosis of the mucosa and submucosa with some involvement of the inner longitudinal layers. With a 3 N solution necrotic damage extended to the circular muscle. A 5 N solution damaged the outer longitudinal muscle, and with 7 N sodium hydroxide necrosis extended through the esophageal wall and into the periesophageal tissues (Krey, 1952). In terms of total dose caustic alkalis have killed adult humans who ingested less than 10 gm.

Based on old experimental data summarized by Muhlendahl *et al.* (1978), corrosive injuries of the esophagus and presumably of other mucous membranes are unlikely with concentrations of sodium hydroxide below 1%. Even with 1% solutions (pH 13.4), the damage was slight and did not penetrate into the muscularis. By contrast, sodium metasilicate solutions of pH 13 are highly corrosive (Schneider, 1970). The difference is the buffer capacity of sodium metasilicate solutions, which means that the high pH is well sustained in the presence of tissue components that quickly neutralize dilute sodium hydroxide.

At equimolar concentrations, sodium, lithium and potassium hydroxide solutions have equal pH values. Thus a 1% solution of NaOH (pH 13.4) is equivalent to 0.6% LiOH and 1.3% KOH. If these three solutions are also equally injurious, then each is likely to cause nonpenetrating mucosal burns in the mouth and esophagus that heal readily. Some evidence, however, suggests that KOH may be more damaging than NaOH (Ashcraft and Padula, 1974). Intact skin is not so sensitive as mucous membranes, and lye concentrations of a few percent can generally be tolerated on the skin briefly. Even the eye is not usually injured permanently by small volumes of 1% sodium hydroxide if the solution is removed promptly by washing the conjunctival sac with large amounts of water (Grant, 1974; Griffith *et al.*, 1980).

Traditional drain cleaners consist of granular lye in very high concentrations, some approaching 100%. In the 1960s several liquid drain cleaners were introduced in the American market. Ranging from 25 to 36.5% sodium or potassium hydroxide in water, they are less concentrated than the granular products, but it is generally agreed that they are more hazardous (Hawkins *et al.*, 1980; Leape *et al.*, 1971; Martel, 1972; Ritter *et al.*, 1971). In experiments with cats, exposure for 1 second to 1 ml. was sufficient to cause full-thickness esophageal necrosis (Leape *et al.*, 1971). Even products that were less than 10% lye produced severe damage after 30 seconds (Ashcraft and Padula, 1974). Solid granular caustics tend to adhere to the mucosa of the tongue, palate, glossopharynx and upper esophagus, where they induce deep, irregularly arranged burns, whereas liquid lye products more often cause diffuse damage throughout the esophagus, not infrequently the stomach and sometimes even the duodenum and lower tract (Cello *et al.*, 1980; Ritter *et al.*, 1968).

In an experimental study Testa (1938) administered caustic soda in a barium meal to dogs and observed the gastrointestinal progress of this fluid mass by fluoroscopy. It followed the magenstrasse to the antrum, where it induced pylorospasm, trapping the corrosive at that site. Autopsy confirmed that this was the locus of the greatest necrotic damage. Subsequent investigations have confirmed that lye administration to an erect dog produces a hemorrhagic gastritis (Bosher *et al.*, 1951).

In humans, however, because of anatomical differences, the neutralizing effect of stomach acid and perhaps other factors, it is usually true that lye powders and granules elicit an esophageal injury rather than a gastric one. In a series of 116 cases of corrosive esophageal stricture (more than 100 due to lye), the incidence of concomitant pyloric obstruction was less than 20% (Heindl, 1926). Occasional occurrences of both injuries from lye are described in the English language medical literature (Bolstad, 1948; Clearfield et al., 1969; Davis et al., 1972; Vinson and Hartman, 1925), as well as a few examples of pyloric obstruction without esophageal involvement (Asch and Herter, 1971; Boikan and Singer, 1930; Messersmith et al., 1970). With liquid lye products, the stomach as well as the esophagus tends to be injured, as noted above. In one case massive necrosis and multiple perforations of the small and large intestines to the level of the sigmoid colon resulted in death (Sperling and Wheeler, 1974). Lye, therefore, differs from corrosive acids both in some fundamental aspects of the tissue injury and in the gross anatomical site of greatest damage.

The presence of lye burns in the mouth is not a reliable indication of esophageal involvement, and the absence of oral lesions is no guarantee that an injury of the lower tract has not occurred. Thus, severe esophageal stenosis has been reported in patients without detectable burns of the oral cavity (Alford and Harris, 1959; Cody, 1954; Hardin, 1956: Viscomi et al., 1961), particularly with liquid lye products (Cello et al., 1980; Muhlendahl et al., 1978). The existence of esophageal and gastric burns cannot be reliably inferred from the presence or location of symptoms (Cello et al., 1980), but among children, severe esophageal burns were always accompanied by one or more of the following signs and symptoms: visible burns in the oral cavity, hypersalivation, retching, vomiting, retrosternal or epigastric pain, cardiovascular collapse, airway obstruction (Muhlendahl et al., 1978). Presumably children with an uncertain history of ingestion and without any of these signs or symptoms do not require treatment. Otherwise there appears to be no alternative to an early diagnostic esophagoscopy, unless one elects to treat all cases on presumptive evidence (Cannon and Chandler, 1963; Cardona and Daly, 1971; Cleveland et al., 1963; Cody, 1954; Kaplan et al., 1961; Middelkamp et al., 1961; Viscomi et al., 1961; Waggoner, 1958; Yurich, 1959).

In a large series of patients esophagoscoped because of a history of lye ingestion, 40 to 60% exhibited esophageal lesions (Alford and Harris, 1959; Cardona and Daly, 1971; Cleveland et al., 1963; Kaplan et al., 1961). Perhaps only half of such patients eventually develop a stricture that requires treatment (Alford and Harris, 1959). No portion of the esophagus appears particularly susceptible or resistant to stricture formation. When lesions were classified according to location (cricopharyngeus, middle third, cardia and multiple sites), the incidence of strictures was roughly equal in all categories (Alford and Harris, 1959; Owens, 1954). Sometimes severe and poorly understood motility disturbances precede frank stricture (Moody and Garrett, 1969).

Death after lye ingestion may result from any one of several complications: circulatory shock, asphyxia due to glottic or laryngeal edema, perforation of the esophagus with mediastinitis, intercurrent infection or inanition due to late stricture formation. Pulmonary complications are frequently overlooked (Stothers, 1952) and may result from aspiration secondary to regurgitation or overflow or from lye-induced fistulas between the esophagus and the trachea (Ray et al., 1974). In an extreme example complete pulmonary necrosis occurred (Danrigal et al., 1962). Aspiration pneumonitis is always a potential hazard during esophagoscopy or bougienage (Alford and Harris, 1959; Fatti et al., 1956). Laryngeal or tracheal stenosis may occur late in the illness. Carcinoma may appear at the site of a chronic stricture (Lansing et al., 1969).

Forms of therapy: The extent and severity of a lye injury and its clinical course are probably influenced importantly by any first aid measures that may be applied within the first minute (or perhaps half minute) after the initial exposure. Although strong alkalies in general do not injure tissues as rapidly as strong acids, the need for prompt intervention is recognized by all therapists. The traditional forms of first aid involve attempts first to dilute the lye by swallowing water if possible and by washing contaminated body surfaces (skin, eyes, mouth), and second to neutralize the lye by the subsequent (or concurrent) use of any available, mildly acidic solution, such as citrus fruit juice or diluted household vinegar.

In 1977, the safety of acidic diluents was challenged (Rumack and Burrington, 1977) on the assumption that excessively high temperatures would be generated in vivo by the rapid release of the heat of neutralization (13.4 kcal./mol. OH^- neutralized), which is unavoidable when H^+ and OH^- ions combine. The demonstration that high temperatures can be attained in test tube neutralization is not adequate evidence that in vivo neutralization is dangerous. For example, the ingestion of several ounces of a dilute aqueous solution assures that the heat generated is moved convectively and distributed over a large mucosal surface area. High mucosal blood flows can rapidly dissipate large amounts of heat generated in the esophagus and stomach and so prevent local tissue temperatures from reaching the same peak values as the luminal contents.

Whether it is more harmful to use acidic diluents than not to use them can be established only by clinical experience or animal experiments. Animal studies can be cited that purport to demonstrate a favorable (Leape, 1974) and an unfavorable (Weiss et al., 1978b) response to neutralization, but neither demonstration is particularly convincing. The latter study has been published only in abstract form, and a later (1979) analysis of the microscopic pathology failed to detect significant differences among the various treatment regimens.

The assertion that attempts to neutralize ingested lye are dangerous and ill-advised has been widely disseminated in the medical and lay press. Apparently it has been embraced by many persons. We consider it an interesting hypothesis, but until definitive animal or human data can be produced to prove or disprove it, we believe that the traditional use of dilute acid should not be abandoned as a first aid measure in lye poisoning.

Of course, neutral buffers can be substituted for dilute acids, but they too generate heat when they neutralize and their speed of neutralization is not significantly different from that of unbuffered acid. Fresh milk is a nearly neutral buffer readily available in most American homes. In terms of its ability to reduce the pH of sodium hydroxide solutions to a noninjurious level (e.g., pH 9.5), fresh milk has the same neutralizing capacity as an equal volume of a solution consisting of 1 part of white vinegar in 34 parts of water (unpublished titration curves from our laboratory). More specifically, 6 to 7 oz. of fresh milk "neutralizes" 1 teaspoonful of 1 N NaOH. Because of inevitable delays in preparing diluted vinegar (probably a 1:3 dilution would be serviceable), fresh milk may be the antidote of choice in most home situations, but laboratories and workshops should have stronger buffers or acids ready for lye accidents. In any case the goal in our opinion is not to neutralize all of the ingested lye but only that part which may be retained temporarily within the esophagus. With liquid lye preparations, the amount so retained is likely to be a very small fraction of the ingested dose (assuming no retention due to preexisting esophageal disease).

In 1920 Salzer introduced a regimen for the management of lye ingestion injuries; it included recommendations for early prophylactic dilatation of the esophagus beginning within a few days of the ingestion episode. Despite initial skepticism these recommendations were eventually widely accepted in this country and used through the early 1950s (Crowe, 1944; Finnerty, 1954; Gellis and Holt, 1942; Hanckel, 1951; Holinger et al., 1954; Kernodle et al., 1948; Waggoner, 1958; Webb and Woolsey, 1949). Perforation and aspiration accidents occurred on occasion, but the mortality record was surprisingly low. Certainly the wry comment that "sooner or later all cases of esophageal stricture die of the bougie" was undeserved. The evidence is overwhelming that early dilation reduces the incidence of late esophageal stenosis, but there is something to be said for the criticism that many ingestion episodes would not have resulted in stricture even without treatment (Cody, 1954; Kaplan et al., 1961).

Once stricture formation has occurred, most authorities agree that efforts at dilatation should be continued until it is apparent that esophageal function cannot be restored without surgery. Surgical approaches to esophageal stenosis are varied and inventive. Yudin and his successor, Petrov, in Moscow together performed an incredible 634 reconstructions (Betts et al., 1955). The reader is referred to surgical texts and the following reports: Burford et al., 1953; Finnerty, 1954; Holinger et al., 1954; Leegaard, 1945; Nardi, 1957; Ogura et al., 1961; Thomas and Dedo, 1977; Yudin, 1944. Unhappily, further stricture formation sometimes occurs at the site of anastomosis (Cody, 1954).

In the early 1950s an alternative regimen to the Salzer technique was proposed, namely the prophylactic administration of cortisone or related steroids. Presumably by inhibiting fibroplasia, cortisone may decrease granulation and scar tissue contracture. This hypothesis was supported by experimental work in a number of animal species (Krey, 1952; Rosenberg et al., 1951; Weisskopf, 1952), and soon all investigators agreed that cortisone significantly decreased the incidence of stricture formation in laboratory animals (Haller and Bachman, 1964; Johnson, 1963). In the absence of cortisone, intercurrent thoracic infection was recognized to play an important but perhaps not decisive role in survival (Bosher et al., 1951). With cortisone, however, bacterial invasion became a major problem, and the mortality rose (Haller and Bachman, 1964; Rosenberg et al., 1951). The addition of intensive broad-spectrum antibiotic therapy to cortisone treatment radically decreased the mortality, while the incidence of stricture remained low (Haller and Bachman, 1964; Johnson, 1963; Rosenberg et al., 1953; Weisskopf, 1952). In a large-scale study in dogs, bougienage in combination with steroids led to a lower incidence of stricture formation than either alone (Knox et al., 1967).

This excellent experimental work was quickly followed by clinical application. In early trials cortisone failed to prevent strictures in two patients who were not treated until the 4th and 10th day after lye ingestion (Ray and Morgan, 1956; Smith et al., 1953c). When steroid therapy is started within 24 to 48 hours of caustic ingestion, clinical results bear out the experimental work, and this regimen has received enthusiastic support (Borja et al., 1969; Cannon and Chandler, 1963; Cardona and Daly, 1971; Cleveland et al., 1963; Middelkamp et al., 1961; Ray and Morgan, 1956; Viscomi et al., 1961). It appears to be particularly useful in moderate burns but not in severe injuries due to liquid lye (Hawkins et al., 1980), where prompt surgical intervention may be required (see below).

Not all therapists, however, are persuaded that steroid therapy after lye ingestion is safe and effective (DiCostanzo et al., 1980; Kirsh et al., 1978). Even proponents admit that steroids do not entirely prevent stricture formation, particularly in the case of severe burns (Bikhazi et al., 1969), but those that do occur appear to be less dense, more pliable and yield to dilatation more readily than in cases not so treated (Cardona and Daly, 1971). The use of intraluminal stents is discussed under "Treatment" below. Because it is necessary to start steroid therapy early to be maximally effective, it is axiomatic that an early diagnostic esophagoscopy be performed. Indeed, to spare the patient without esophageal burns unnecessary expense and treatment, there appears to be no alternative. In experienced hands the procedure is said to be safe if the esophagoscope is not passed beyond the first burned area (Cardona and Daly, 1971). The procedure is said to be significantly more hazardous in pediatric patients where an esophagogram may be the best alternative (Borja et al., 1969), but with modern flexible fiberoptic instruments, many earlier restrictions on endoscopy have been removed (Cello et al., 1980).

Esophagoscopy, X-rays and/or laparotomy may reveal the presence of burns or eschars in danger of perforation. Immediate and aggressive surgical intervention may be dictated by such findings (Allen et al., 1970; Ashbaugh et al., 1971; Ray et al., 1974; Shaw et al., 1969). For example, if endoscopy or laparotomy reveals blackening of the gastric mucosal and serosal surfaces, indicating deep (full thickness) necrosis of the stomach wall, an immediate gastrectomy is imperative (Davis et al., 1972; Kirsh et al., 1978; Mills et al., 1979; Ray et al., 1974). Because the esophagus is almost always severely burned in such cases, an exploratory right thoracotomy is conducted. If the esophagus is necrotic, total esophagostomy is also performed, with later reconstruction by colon interposition (Kirsh et al., 1978; Ray et al., 1974).

In a provocative experimental study in dogs, established strictures were treated with bougienage and either prednisolone or the lathyrogenic agent, β-aminopropionitrile. The latter inhibits the formation of intramolecular covalent bonds in newly synthesized collagen, and it appeared to restore normal deglutition and to increase esophageal diameter better than the steroid treatment (Butler et al., 1977; Madden et al., 1973). Penicillamine-induced lathyrism was also effective in preventing lye-induced esophageal strictures in rats (Gehanno and Guedon, 1981).

Symptomatology:

1. The ingestion of lye causes swallowing to become painful and difficult almost immediately (dysphagia). A burning pain extends down the esophagus to the stomach (retrosternal and epigastric pain). Contaminated areas of the lips, chin, tongue, and pharynx become edematous and covered with exudate. Profuse salivation. Because of pharyngeal and esophageal edema, it may become impossible after a few hours to swallow even saliva. Mucous membranes are at first white but later brown, edematous, gelatinous, and necrotic.

2. The vomitus is thick and slimy due to mucus; later it may contain blood and shreds of mucous membrane.

3. The pulse is often rapid and feeble; respirations are fast and shallow; the skin is cold and clammy; collapse ensues.

4. Death due to shock, asphyxia from glottic edema or intercurrent infection (pneumonia) commonly occurs on the second or even the third day. Aspiration pneumonitis has been described.

5. Convalescence may be interrupted during the first week by esophageal perforation or perhaps even gastric perforation. Mediastinitis may present as severe substernal pain with fever.

6. If complications do not appear, liquids and soft food can be swallowed with comparative ease within 5 to 7 days. It should be recognized, however, that in most cases this absence of distress merely marks a latent period and that esophageal strictures will develop within weeks or months unless effective treatment is instituted.

Treatment:

1. Dilute ingested alkali by drinking immediately large volumes of water or milk, if possible. Acid diluents may also be useful. For information about their antidotal role, see the text above. Wash contaminated skin and accessible areas of mucous membrane extensively with running tap water. See below for treatment of eye injuries.

2. Gastric lavage and emetics are contraindicated because of the danger of gastric or esophageal perforation.

3. Vegetable oil in small quantities (e.g., 1 teaspoonful) given frequently by mouth and applied to all denuded areas. If swallowing is possible, other demulcent drinks may be helpful (e.g., milk, egg white, aluminum gels).

4. Analgesics should be given liberally to relieve pain (p. IV-31). Parenteral atropine may help to suppress hypersalivation.

5. Treat shock by the intravenous administration of electrolyte solutions, plasma, and whole blood (p. IV-17). Keep the patient warm.

6. As soon as pain and shock are controlled, attempts to establish the presence or ab-

sence of esophageal and/or gastric injury are recommended. A barium swallow under fluoroscopic observation may demonstrate esophageal dysfunction, but negative findings on the first day or two are not adequate to rule out significant mucosal damage. A more definitive diagnostic procedure is esophagoscopy under local or general anesthesia. It is relatively safe if done early in the illness (*e.g.*, first day), particularly with flexible fiberoptic endoscopy, and if the tube is not inserted beyond areas with submucosal lesions. Even in the absence of visible burns patients should be reexamined periodically for at least a year. Frequent barium esophagograms may reveal the presence of developing strictures.

7. Prompt and aggressive surgical intervention, when indicated, as with severe laryngeal edema or with mucosal lesions judged likely to lead to esophageal or gastric perforation. Massive and diffuse necrosis may necessitate an emergency esophagogastrectomy (see text above). If asphyxia appears, a tracheostomy may be required (p. IV-6).

8. In the presence of penetrating mucosal burns of the esophagus that are considered unlikely to perforate, prompt and vigorous corticosteroid therapy is recommended. Therapy should start as soon as possible and preferably no later than 48 hours. Even young children should receive the equivalent of about 60 mg. of prednisone per day in divided doses. This dose should be maintained for several days and then gradually reduced by no more than 5 mg. per day over a period of 2 to 3 weeks. If practical, the oral route of administration is employed. Potassium supplementation may be desirable while large doses of steroids are being employed.

9. During the period of intense steroid therapy a broad-spectrum antibiotic, such as one of the tetracyclines (see pp. IV-89–90), should be administered prophylactically. Otherwise antibiotic therapy is withheld unless signs of secondary infection appear.

10. During steroid-antibiotic therapy, some therapists (*e.g.*, Balasegaram, 1975) pass and keep in the esophagus a Levin or similar tube to maintain patency of the esophageal lumen, as an aid to later bougienage if it becomes necessary. Elaborate intraluminal stents have been recommended (Mills *et al.*, 1978). Other physicians (*e.g.*, DiCostanzo *et al.*, 1980) believe that any indwelling tube delays and compromises esophageal healing and increases the risk of perforation and infection.

11. As an alternative to steroid-antibiotic therapy, a clinical trial of penicillamine as a lathyrogenic agent in preventing strictures appears to be warranted. For the results of trials in rats, see Gehanno and Guedon (1981).

12. Some therapists insist on early total parenteral alimentation to promote esophageal healing (DiCostanzo *et al.*, 1980). Others give liquids and soft foods as tolerated, but in most instances the parenteral administration of fluids and carbohydrates is necessary for the first week. For dietary management, see pp. IV-75–78. In severe cases gastrostomy or jejunostomy may be useful to maintain the patient's nutritional status while resting the esophagus.

13. If esophageal strictures cannot be prevented, they may be corrected by bougienage. Otherwise reconstructive surgery may become imperative.

14. In case of surface burns on skin or eyes, wash with large amounts of cold running water. Probably hydrocortisone should be instilled in the conjunctival sac of an injured eye, but, if possible, consult an ophthalmologist or a more specialized treatise (*e.g.*, Grant, 1974).

Laboratory:

1. Blood analyses to detect dehydration, acidosis or other electrolyte imbalances.

References:

Alford, B. R.; Harris, H. H. Chemical burns of the mouth, pharynx and esophagus. Ann. Otol. Rhinol. Laryngol. *68*:122-128, 1959.

Allen, R. E.; Thoshinsky, M. J.; Stallone, R. J.; Hunt, T. K. Corrosive injuries of the stomach. Arch. Surg. *100*:409-413, 1970.

Arena, J. M. The problem of accidental poisoning in children as it exists today. J. A. M. A. *159*:1537-1539, 1955.

Asch, M. J.; Herter, F. F. Lye ingestion causing pyloric stenosis without esophageal injury. N. Y. State J. Med. *71*:455-457, 1971.

Ashbaugh, D. G.; Jenkins, D. W.; Gainey, M. D. Gastroscopy in corrosive burn of the stomach. J. A. M. A. *216*:1638-1639, 1971.

Ashcraft, K. W.; Padula, R. T. The effect of dilute corrosives on the esophagus. Pediatrics *53*:226-232, 1974.

Balasegaram, M. Early management of corrosive burns of the oesophagus. Br. J. Surg. *62*:444-447, 1975.

Betts, R. H.; Thomas, T.; Gopinath, N. Cervical esophagojejunostomy for extensive stricture of the esophagus. Surgery *38*:553-565, 1955.

Bikhazi, H. B.; Thompson, E. R.; Shumrick, D. A. Caustic ingestion; current status. Arch. Otolaryngol. *89*:770-773, 1969.

Bloomer, W. E.; Kirchner, J. A. Esophageal stricture. Conn. Med. J. *19*:91-92, 1955.

Boikan, W. S.; Singer, H. A. Gastric sequelae of corrosive poisoning. Arch. Intern. Med. *46*:342-357, 1930.

Bolstad, D. S. Pyloric obstruction and stricture of esophagus following ingestion of lye (sodium hydroxide mixed with sodium bicarbonate). Arch. Otolaryngol. *47*:180-184, 1948.

Borja, A. R.; Ransdell, H. T., Jr.; Thomas, T. V.; Johnson, W.

Lye injuries of the esophagus; analysis of ninety cases of lye ingestion. J. Thorac. Cardiovasc. Surg. 57:533-538, 1969.

Bosher, L. H., Jr.; Burford, T. H.; Ackerman, L. The pathology of experimentally produced lye burns and strictures of the esophagus. J. Thorac. Cardiovasc. Surg. 21:483-489, 1951.

Brown, H. W.; Kiser, G. Epidemiology of lye poisoning in the United States. Am. J. Public Health 32:822-830, 1942.

Buford, T. H.; Webb, W. R.; Ackerman, L. Caustic burns and their surgical management, a clinico-experimental correlation. Ann. Surg. 138:453-460, 1953.

Burton, J. F.; Zawadzki, E. S. Death from Clinitest tablets. J. Forensic Sci. 7:357-362, 1962.

Butler, C.; Madden, J. W.; Davis, W. M.; Peacock, E. E. Morphologic aspects of experimental esophageal lye strictures. II Effect of steroid hormones, bougienage, and induced lathyrism on acute lye burns. Surgery 81:431-435, 1977.

Canby, J. P. Clinitest produced esophageal stricture: Report of two cases. J. Pediatr. 50:68-70, 1957.

Cannon, S.; Chandler, J. R. Corrosive burns of the esophagus: Analysis of one hundred patients. Eye Ear Nose Throat Mon. 42:35-44, 1963.

Cardona, J. C.; Daly, J. F. Current management of corrosive esophagitis; an evaluation of results in 239 cases. Ann. Otol. Rhinol. Laryngol. 80:521-527, 1971.

Cello, J. P.; Fogel, R. P.; Boland, R. Liquid caustic ingestion-spectrum of injury. Arch. Intern. Med. 140:501-504, 1980.

Clearfield, H. R.; Shin, Y. H.; Schreibman, B. K. Emphysematous gastritis secondary to lye ingestion. Am. J. Dig. Dis. 14:195-199, 1969.

Cleveland, W. W.; Chandler, J. R.; Lawson, R. B. Treatment of caustic burns of the esophagus. J. A. M. A. 186:262-264, 1963.

Cody, C. C., III. Recent trends in management of esophageal strictures. Ann. Otol. Rhinol. Laryngol. 63:1120-1139, 1954.

Crowe, J. T. Poisoning due to lye. Value of Bokay prophylactic dilation in prevention of early strictures of the esophagus. Am. J. Dis. Child. 68:9-12, 1944.

Danrigal, A.; Dumont, G.; Derobert, L. Necrose totale du poumon par caustique. Med. Leg. Domm. Corpor. 42:68-69, 1962.

Danzig, L. S.; Loebel, A. S. Clinitest tablet ingestion and stricture of the esophagus. J. A. M. A. 192:1092, 1965.

Davis, L. L.; Raffersperger, J.; Novak, G. M. Necrosis of the stomach secondary to ingestion of corrosive agents. Chest 62:48-51, 1972.

Di Costanzo, J.; Noirclerc, M.; Jouglard, J.; Escoffier, J. M.; Cano, N.; Martin, J.; Gauthier, A. New therapeutic approach to corrosive burns of the upper gastrointestinal tract. Gut 21:370-375, 1980.

Fatti, L.; Marchand, P.; Crawshaw, G. R. The treatment of caustic strictures of the esophagus. Surg. Gynecol. Obstet. 102:195-206, 1956.

Finnerty, J. J. The late treatment of caustic strictures of the esophagus. Surg. Clin. North Am. 34:353-361, 1954.

Gehanno, P.; Guedon, C. Inhibition of experimental esophageal lye strictures by penicillamine. Arch. Otolaryngol. 107:145-147, 1981.

Gellis, S. S.; Holt, L. E., Jr. Treatment of lye ingestion by Salzer method. Ann. Otol. Rhinol. Laryngol. 51:1086-1088, 1942.

Grant, W. M. Toxicology of the Eye. 2nd ed. Charles C Thomas, Springfield, Ill, 1974.

Griffith, J. F.; Nixon, G. A.; Bruce, R. D.; Reer, P. J.; Bannan, E. A. Dose-response with chemical irritants in the albino rabbit eye as a basis for selecting optimum testing conditions for predicting hazard to the human eye. Toxicol. Appl. Pharmacol. 55:501-513, 1980.

Haller, J. A., Jr.; Bachman, K. The comparative effect of current therapy on experimental caustic burns of the esophagus. Pediatrics 34:236-245, 1964.

Hanckel, R. W. Lye burns of the esophagus. Ann. Otol. Rhinol. Laryngol. 60:22-38, 1951.

Hardin, J. C., Jr. Caustic burns of esophagus; 10-year analysis. Am. J. Surg. 91:742-748, 1956.

Hawkins, D. B.; Demeter, M. J.; Barnett, T. E. Caustic inges-

tion-controversies in management - review of 214 cases. Laryngoscope 90:98-109, 1980.

Heindl, A., Jr. Klinische Beobachtungen an 137 gutartigen Oesophagusstenosen der I. chir. Universitatsklinik, Wein, 1901-1925. Dtsch. Z. Chir. 199:252-269, 1926.

Holinger, P. H.; Johnston, K. C.; Potts, W. J.; DaCunha, F. The conservative and surgical management of benign strictures of the esophagus. J. Thorac. Cardiovasc. Surg. 28:345-366, 1954.

Houck, J. C.; DeAngelo, L.; Jacob, R. A. The dermal chemical response to alkali injury. Surgery 51:503-507, 1962.

Johnson, E. E. A study of corrosive esophagitis. Laryngoscope 73:1651-1696, 1963.

Kaplan, J.; Gandhi, K.; Elsen, J., Jr.; Oppenheimer, P. Early esophagoscopy for diagnosis of esophageal burns. Arch. Otolaryngol. 73:52-53, 1961.

Kernodle, G. W.; Taylor, G.; Davison, W. C. Lye poisoning in children. Am. J. Dis. Child. 75:135-142, 1948.

Kirsh, M. M.; Peterson, A.; Brown, J. W.; Orringer, M. B.; Ritter, F.; Sloan, H. Treatment of caustic injuries of the esophagus. A 10 year experience. Ann. Surg. 188:675-678, 1978.

Knox, W. G.; Scott, J. R.; Zintel, H. A.; Guthrie, R.; McCabe, R. E. Bougienage and steroids used singly or in combination in experimental corrosive esophagitis. Ann. Surg. 166:930-940, 1967.

Krey, H. On treatment of corrosive lesions in esophagus: Experimental study. Acta Otolaryngol. Suppl. 102:1-49, 1952.

Lansing, P. B.; Ferrante, W. A.; Ochsner, J. L. Carcinoma of the esophagus at the site of lye stricture. Am. J. Surg. 118:108-111, 1969.

Lasky, M. I.; Picard, H. N. Stricture of esophagus due to accidental ingestion of urine testing tablets (Clinitest). Ill. Med. J. 109:30-31, 1956.

Leape, L. L. New liquid lye drain cleaners. Clin. Toxicol. 7:109-114, 1974.

Leape, L. L.; Ashcraft, K. W.; Scarpelli, D. G.; Holder, T. M. Hazard to health - liquid lye. N. Engl. J. Med. 284:578-581, 1971.

Leegaard, T. Corrosive injuries of the oesophagus, with particular reference to the treatment of acute corrosive oesophagitis. J. Laryngol. Otol. 60:389-414, 1945.

Madden, J. W.; Davis, W. M.; Butler, C., II; Peacock, E. E., Jr. Experimental esophageal lye burn. II. Correcting established strictures with beta-aminopropionitrile and bougienage. Ann. Surg. 178:277-284, 1973.

Martel, W. Radiological features of esophagogastritis secondary to extremely caustic agents. Radiology 103:31-36, 1972.

Messersmith, J. K.; Oglesby, J. E.; Mahoney, W. D.; Baugh, J. H. Gastric erosions from alkali ingestion. Am. J. Surg. 119:740-742, 1970.

Middelkamp, J. N.; Cone, A. J.; Ogura, J. H.; Higgins, C. R., Jr.; Lowe, G. A. Endoscopic diagnosis and steroid and antibiotic therapy of acute lye burns of the esophagus. Laryngoscope 21:1354-1362, 1961.

Mills, L. J.; Estrera, A. S.; Platt, M. R. Avoidance of esophageal stricture following severe caustic burns by the use of an intraluminal stent. Ann. Thorac. Surg. 28:60-65, 1979.

Moody, F. G.; Garrett, J. M. Esophageal achalasia following lye ingestion. Ann. Surg. 170:775-784, 1969.

Muhlendahl, K. E. v.; Oberdisse, U.; Krienke, E. G. Local injuries by accidental ingestion of corrosive substances by children. Arch. Toxicol. 39:299-324, 1978.

Nardi, G. L. Surgical treatment of lye strictures of the esophagus by mediastinal colon transplant without resection. N. Engl. J. Med. 256:777-780, 1957.

Ogura, J. H.; Roper, C. L.; Burford, T. H. Functional restoration of the food passages in extensive stenosing caustic burns of the pharynx and esophagus. Laryngoscope 71:885-902, 1961.

Owens, H. Chemical burns of the esophagus. The importance of various chemicals as etiologic agents in stricture formation. Arch. Otolaryngol. 60:482-486, 1954.

Palmer, E. D. Esophageal corrosion by attempted suicide in the army. U. S. Armed Forces Med. J. 9:728-735, 1958.

Rabinowitz, J. G.; Tchang, S. Esophageal stricture following ingestion of Clinitest tablets. Am. J. Roentgenol. Radium Ther. Nucl. Med. 86:579-581, 1961.

Ray, E. S.; Morgan, D. L. Cortisone therapy of lye burns of the esophagus. J. Pediatr. 49:394-397, 1956.

Ray, J. F., III; Myers, W. O.; Lawton, B. R.; Lee, F. Y.; Wenzel, F. J.; Sautter, R. D. The natural history of liquid lye ingestion: rationale for aggressive surgical approach. Arch. Surg. 109:436-439, 1974.

Ritter, F. N.; Gago, O.; Kirsh, M. M.; Komurn, R. M.; Orvald, T. O. The rationale of emergency esophagogastrectomy in the treatment of liquid caustic burns of the esophagus and stomach. Ann. Otol. Rhinol. Laryngol. 80:513-520, 1971.

Ritter, F. N.; Newman, M. H.; Newman, D. E. A clinical and experimental study of corrosive burns of the stomach. Ann. Otol. Rhinol. Laryngol. 77:830-842, 1968.

Rosenberg, N.; Kunderman, P. J.; Vroman, L.; Moolten, S. E. Prevention of experimental lye strictures of the esophagus by cortisone. Arch. Surg. 63:147-151, 1951.

Rosenberg, N.; Kunderman, P. J.; Vroman, L.; Moolten, S. E. Prevention of experimental esophageal stricture by cortisone. II. Control of suppurative complications by penicillin. Arch. Surg. 66:593-598, 1953.

Rumack, B. H.; Burrington, J. D. Caustic ingestions: a rational look at diluents. Clin. Toxicol. 11:27–34, 1977.

Salzer, H. Frubehandlung der Speiserohrenveratzung. Wein Klin. Wochenschr. 33:307, 1920.

Schneider, C. J., Jr. The ingestion hazard of dishwasher detergents and liquid waxes and polishes. Cornell Aeronautical Laboratory, Inc. Report No. VZ2926-D-7 prepared for the National Commission on Product Safety, 1970.

Shaw, A.; Garvey, J.; Miller, B. Lye burn requiring total gastrectomy and colon substitution for esophagus and stomach in a two-year-old boy. Surgery 65:837-844, 1969.

Smith, V. M.; Compton, J. R.; Palmer, E. D. Cortisone and acute lye corrosion of the esophagus. Arch. Otolaryngol. 58:235-244, 1953c.

Sperling, H. V.; Wheeler, M. J. An unusual complication of lye ingestion. J. A. M. A. 228:871, 1974.

Stothers, H. H. Chemical burns and strictures of the esophagus. Arch. Otolaryngol. 56:262-276, 1952.

Testa, G. F. Contributo radiologico e sperimentale allo studio delle lesiono esofagee e gastriche nelle causticazioni du alcali. Radiol. Med. (Torino) 25:17-51, 1938.

Thomas, A. N.; Dedo, H. H. Pharyngogastrostomy for treatment of severe caustic stricture of the pharynx and esophagus. J. Thorac. Cardiovasc. Surg. 73:817-822, 1977.

Tomsovic, E. J.; Jarid, H. Cicatricial stenosis of esophagus following ingestion of single urine-sugar reagent tablet. J. Pediatr. 53:608-614, 1958.

Vinson, P. P.; Hartman, S. W. Pyloric obstruction due to swallowing a solution of concentrated lye. Med. Clin. North Am. 8:1037-1040, 1925.

Viscomi, G. J.; Beekhuis, G. J.; Whitten, C. F. An evaluation of early esophagoscopy and corticosteroid therapy in the management of corrosive injury of the esophagus. J. Pediatr. 59:356-360, 1961.

Waggoner, L. G. Diagnosis and management of chemical burns of the esophagus. Laryngoscope 68:1790-1813, 1958.

Webb, B.; Woolsey, D. S. Lye burns of the esophagus. J. A. M. A. 141:384-386, 1949.

Weisskopf, A. Effects of cortisone on experimental lye burn of the esophagus. Ann. Otol. Rhinol. Laryngol. 61:681-691, 1952.

Weiss, L. R.; Seabaugh, V. M.; McLaughlin, J., Jr.; Orzel, R. A.; Krop, S. Effectiveness of first-aid treatment for lesions induced by alkali. Fed. Proc. 37:505, 1978b.

Yudin, S. S. The surgical reconstruction of 80 cases of artificial esophagus. Surg. Gynecol. Obstet. 78:561-583, 1944.

Yurich, E. L. Early diagnosis and treatment of corrosive burns of the esophagus. Laryngoscope 69:131-140, 1959.

Zimmerman, C. Esophageal stricture from accidental ingestion of Clinitest tablets. Am. J. Dis. Child. 97:101-103, 1959.

MARIHUANA

The name marihuana (or marijuana) generally refers to a mixture of cut, dried and ground flowers, leaves and stems of *Cannabis sativa* (also inappropriately called *Cannabis indica*), an annual weed commonly known as hemp or Indian hemp. It is frequently ingested or smoked to induce states of intoxication. Some users become intensely habituated to this practice. Marihuana is known by many slang names: pot, grass, Mary Jane, tea, weed, etc. In India dried mature leaves are called bhang. In all cases the active constituents are a series of tetrahydrocannabinols, which are most prevalent in the resin produced by the flowering tops of the plant (Farnsworth, 1969). The powdered resin is called hashish or simply "hash"; in the form of a hard brown cake it is known in India as charas. In the United States marihuana is commonly smoked in pipes or cigarettes ("joints" or "reefers"), sometimes in a mixture with tobacco.

Tetrahydrocannabinols represent one group of more than 30 "cannabinoids" found in the plant; they possess in common three 6-membered rings, a single phenolic hydroxyl group, and an amyl side chain. Some of these compounds are essentially devoid of biological activity. The principal psychoactive components are the *trans* isomers of l-Δ^9-tetrahydrocannabinol (Δ^9-THC) and in considerably smaller amounts

l-Δ^8-tetrahydrocannabinol (dibenzopyran nomenclature). By a different numbering system (monoterpene) these components are known as the Δ^1 and $\Delta^{1(6)}$ isomers, respectively. Both are hallucinogenic and have similar activities and potencies in man (Hollister and Gillespie, 1973). When isolated, they are unstable viscous oils (Waller, 1971). When marihuana is smoked, small additional quantities of Δ^9-THC may be produced by the pyrolysis of cannabinolic acids (freshly harvested plants contain considerable quantities of Δ^9-THC acid precursors according to Doorenbos *et al.*, 1971), but the psychopotency of cannabis preparations is generally found to parallel the content of Δ^9-THC (Nahas, 1973). This content varies markedly among strains of cannabis found in different parts of the world; it also varies with conditions of growth (climate, soil, humidity, etc.). In some domestic strains levels of Δ^9-THC are less than 0.2%, but 1 to 1.5% is probably typical of Mexican-grown marihuana, whereas Asian strains (Thailand) may produce 4 to 6% yields and Columbian plants 3 to 3.5% (Doorenbos *et al.*, 1971; Institute of Medicine, 1982; Nahas, 1973). A product with 1% Δ^9-THC is considered to be of good quality on the illicit market. Hashish tends to be 5 to 10 times more potent.

Toxicology: With perhaps one exception, in

which a potent preparation of hashish was smoked (Heyndrickx et al., 1969), human fatalities from cannabis have not been described. However, one individual, in whom the diagnosis of cannabis intoxication was confirmed by radioimmunoassay, was found in grade III coma with flexed arms, extended legs and some features of decorticate rigidity. He recovered fully over 4 days (Garrett et al., 1977).

Acute toxicity data are difficult to interpret because botanical preparations vary markedly in composition and potency (Waller, 1971; Nahas, 1973). Although a standardized reference-grade marihuana is now available from the National Institute of Mental Health, most modern toxicity studies have been restricted to Δ^9-trans-THC. Whereas this compound is undoubtedly the principal psychotropic constituent of marihuana (see above), it is not established that it is exclusively responsible for the acute lethality or the subacute or chronic toxicities of the botanical mixture (Nahas, 1973).

Toxicity studies on Δ^9-trans-THC are complicated by its extreme insolubility in water. It is commonly dissolved in sesame oil or distributed in an emulsion of isotonic saline and polysorbate 80 with or without sesame oil. The emulsion is more toxic than the oil solution (Mantilla-Plata and Harbison, 1974; Rosenkrantz et al., 1974). Rhesus monkeys survived doses as high as 9000 mg. Δ^9-THC in oil per kilogram of body weight, given at one time by stomach tube (Thompson et al., 1974). With such massive doses considerable quantities, which presumably were not absorbed, were found in the feces. Perhaps part of the dose was lost in vomitus. In rats, which cannot vomit, mean lethal doses are 666 or 800 mg./kg. when administered by stomach tube as an emulsion and 1270 mg./kg. when presented as an oil solution (Phillips et al., 1971; Rosenkrantz et al., 1974). Suspended in a solution of albumin, to which THC tightly binds, 2000 mg./kg. failed to kill (Harris, 1971). One infers that it is almost impossible to ingest enough marihuana to contain a lethal dose of Δ^9-THC.

By parenteral routes, however, this material is not so benign. The intravenous mean lethal dose of Δ^9-THC in an emulsion is about 30 to 40 mg./kg. in mouse and rat (Phillips et al., 1971; Rosenkrantz et al., 1974) and about 100 mg./kg. in the rhesus monkey (Thompson et al., 1974). At least in rats the mean lethal dose by inhalation (when calculated on the basis of the amount retained) is believed to be essentially the same as the intravenous lethal dose (Rosenkrantz et al., 1974).

Few marihuana users have access to such large quantities of active material. The usual marihuana cigarette weighs 0.3 to 1 gm. and seldom contains more than 20 mg. Δ^9-THC, which is the amount in standardized cigarettes developed at the National Institute of Mental

Health for experimental purposes (Waller, 1971). Perhaps a typical illicit cigarette weighs 1 gm. and contains about 10 mg. Δ^9-THC. When such reefers are "smoked" by a machine designed to mimic a human smoker, about half of the contained quantity of THC is destroyed by heat (pyrolysis), about one-quarter is left in the butt and about one-quarter is delivered in the smoke (Truitt, 1971). When the cigarette was fully consumed (Manno et al., 1970; Rosenkrantz et al., 1974), as much as half of the Δ^9-THC was recovered in smoke. Of course the quantity inhaled is not the same as the quantity absorbed; the latter is sometimes assumed to be half the former (Galanter et al., 1972). Studies in which pure Δ^9-THC was injected into experienced volunteers indicate that about 2 mg. is a threshold dose and 3 to 5 mg. a desirable dose for psychic effects; these quantities are equivalent to smoking two joints of good quality. Inhaled doses of more than 15 mg. are avoided by most experienced users because undesirable distortions of mood and perception may be induced (e.g., Pearl et al., 1973). Similarly oral doses exceeding 35 mg. are regarded as undesirable (Perez-Reyes et al., 1973).

Somatic responses to these low doses are mild in human subjects. The resting heart rate is commonly elevated in a dose-dependent fashion (Johnson and Domino, 1971; Roth et al., 1973). Except for sinus tachycardia, ECG abnormalities are few and trivial. Ventricular premature contractions have been reported (Johnson and Domino, 1971), but they are infrequent and probably do not account for the occasional syncopal episodes during "highs." Vagovagal reflexes with severe bradycardia are responsible for some of these fainting attacks (Roth et al., 1973). Postural hypotension may also be responsible, perhaps because reflex venoconstriction is impaired (Perez-Reyes et al., 1973). At rest the blood pressure may be slightly elevated or depressed; an elevation is more common. The exercise tolerance of persons who are subject to angina pectoris is decreased. The increase in workload of the heart, although transient, may be dangerous to those with hypertension, cerebrovascular disease and coronary atherosclerosis (Institute of Medicine, 1982).

Other somatic signs and symptoms include conjunctival irritation (even when THC is administered by injection), increased body sway, an occasional dry mouth and an increased appetite with a preference for sweet foods. Headache, nausea and vomiting are sometimes experienced (Weil, 1970). With the usual doses there are no constant effects on pupil size, respirations or body temperature.

Higher doses in man may induce tremor, rigidity, incoordination and hyperreflexia, as well as the psychic effects described below. On six occasions oral consumption of marihuana cigarette butts resulted in urinary retention, which necessitated catheterization, in a 55-year-old man who did not experience this reaction after smoking the drug (Burton, 1979).

In the massive doses administered to laboratory animals, many additional somatic effects have been described. Shortly after the intravenous injection of lethal doses, rats and mice were ataxic and hyperresponsive to sound and touch. They then became progressively depressed although still responsive to external stimuli. Loss of righting reflex, dyspnea and bradypnea preceded coma, apnea and death (Phillips *et al.*, 1971; Rosenkrantz *et al.*, 1974). In addition, tremors, diarrhea and lacrimation were noted after intravenous and oral doses (Phillips *et al.*, 1971). Hypothermia and hypotension are frequently described (*e.g.*, Rosenkrantz *et al.*, 1974) Experiments have failed to establish the mechanisms of THC-induced hypotension in dogs (Harris, 1971; Hardman *et al.*, 1971).

In subacute studies in monkeys receiving daily doses of Δ^9-THC, anorexia, constipation, hypothermia, bradycardia, bradypnea, lethargy and drowsiness were noted (Thompson *et al.*, 1974). Moribund monkeys were sacrificed. Autopsy findings included pancreatic and testicular atrophy, ulcerative colitis, vacuolar nephrosis and liver enlargement. Laboratory findings included leukocytosis, elevated BUN and increased prothrombin time, but the two latter effects were also present in a mild form in controls treated only with the sesame oil vehicle. The oil may also have contributed to the hemorrhagic pneumonitis and severe emphysema seen in monkeys treated by the intravenous route (Thompson *et al.*, 1974). Lung edema and hemorrhage have also been reported in intravenously dosed dogs (Harris, 1971) and rats (Phillips *et al.*, 1971), even when oil was not used as the vehicle.

The recreational use of marihuana is based of course on its psychologic effects. A mild degree of inebriation ("social high") is usually sought by inhaling smoke containing 3 to 10 mg. Δ^9-THC or by ingesting somewhat higher doses. The psychological and behavioral reactions of humans to these low doses have been catalogued and discussed in great detail by many observers (*e.g.*, Bromberg, 1934; Weil and Zinberg, 1969; Tart, 1970). The quality, intensity and duration of the "high" are influenced by many factors, including the potency of the preparation, the route and speed of administration, the social setting and the experience and mood of the user. When a small amount of marihuana is smoked, psychic effects appear within minutes and may last only 2 to 3 hours (Weil *et al.*, 1968). For an equivalent peak effect an oral dose must be 2 to 4 times higher (Lieberman and Lieberman, 1971). After ingestion the latency is usually 30 to 60 minutes, and the duration is usually 3 to 5 hours but sometimes as long as 12 hours. Studies with Δ^9-THC by mouth demonstrate that the latency and duration are highly dependent on the vehicle (Perez-Reyes *et al.*, 1973).

The first psychic response to the inhalation of marihuana smoke is apt to be a feeling of uneasiness or jitteriness, usually followed promptly by a sense of relaxation and well being. Time seems to slow down, colors appear to be more vivid, and ideas are perceived as unusually profound. Speech is apt to be disconnected, perhaps because of difficulties with immediate recall (Weil and Zinberg, 1969). The mood may vary from one of jocularity to one of meditation in a dreamlike state. Eventually drowsiness is usually experienced, followed by sleep from which the subject awakens with no physiological aftereffects and no memory loss (Bromberg, 1934). Irrelevant to this treatise are the many recent investigations designed to evaluate objectively the cognitive behavior and motor performance of human and animal subjects in this state of mild inebriation (but see National Commission on Marihuana and Drug Abuse, 1972).

Dysphoria, however, may occur instead of euphoria. Novice users in particular may experience panic reactions in which they become apprehensive and tearful but not disoriented. Simple reassurance is usually the only treatment required (Weil, 1970). Given an adequate dose, however, even experienced users sometimes have unpleasant "trips." These episodes usually involve visual and sometimes auditory hallucinations, often preceded by distortions of visual perception and by brief impressions of vividly colored flashing lights (Bromberg, 1934; Wikler, 1970). The hallucinations are not unlike those described after LSD and other hallucinogens. Factors that predispose to cannabis hallucinations are unknown, but dose is believed to be one important determinant (Isbell and Jasinski, 1969). Whereas some subjects appear to enjoy their hallucinations, others become terrified but not necessarily disoriented (Keeler, 1968). The hallucinatory phase is usually brief, and sequelae are uncommon. A rare and bizarre phenomenon is one or more spontaneous recurrences of hallucinations ("flashbacks") days or weeks after the original experience (Weil, 1970).

A more serious adverse reaction pattern to cannabis is usually referred to as an acute toxic psychosis (Bromberg, 1934; Talbott and Teague, 1969). Unlike the responses described above, this uncommon syndrome may last several days (up to 2 weeks) after a single acute exposure. In addition to hallucinations and other clinical features described above, the victim experiences depersonalization, emotional depression, delusions, paranoid ideation, restlessness, disorientation, and delirium. In this confusional state he may seriously injure himself or others. The treatment is usually the same as for acute schizophrenia (Talbott and Teague, 1969). Indeed some of these patients may have been compensated schizophrenics whose defenses were temporarily destroyed by marihuana, but cannabis psychoses have also occurred in individuals without known prior personality disorders (Talbott and Teague, 1969).

The chronic use of cannabis involves additional risks. For example, the development of tolerance may encourage the use of increasing doses. Acquired tolerance to the behavioral and even the lethal effects of THC is well established in laboratory animals (Harris, 1971; Hardman *et al.*, 1971; Kosersky *et al.*, 1974), and in man too tolerance develops to many effects of the drug (Williams *et al.*, 1946; Institute of Medicine, 1982; Nahas, 1973). Physical dependence as evidenced by a mild withdrawal syndrome can also appear rapidly in man (Williams *et al.*, 1946), but physical dependence is likely to be significant only in heavy and continuous consumers ("potheads"). Withdrawal symptoms commonly include restlessness, irritability, jitteriness and insomnia, with disturbances in EEG sleep patterns. Addiction in the sense of compulsive behavior to acquire the drug is not, however, a feature of marihuana use (Institute of Medicine, 1982).

Heavy smokers of marihuana and hashish experience varying degrees of respiratory tract irritation, leading to bronchitis, pharyngitis, sinusitus and uvula edema (Tennant *et al.*, 1971). The acute response to inhaled smoke is bronchodilation even in asthmatics, but chronic use leads inevitably to various degrees of bronchoconstriction. Although definitive data are lacking, it seems likely that marihuana smoking may be a cause of lung cancer as is cigarette smoking (Institute of Medicine, 1982).

Other medical problems have been described in chronic users of cannabis. Reversible, suppressive effects upon testicular function (low sperm counts, abnormal sperm morphology) have been observed in human users and in exposed laboratory rodents. In mice and rats ovarian function can also be suppressed by crude marihuana extracts and by Δ^9-tetrahydrocannabinol. The reproductive consequences of these effects, however, have not been established (Institute of Medicine, 1982). In mice and rats marihuana and Δ^9-THC are embryotoxic but not teratogenic (Rosenkrantz, 1979), except at very high doses (Institute of Medicine, 1982). An earlier inference that cannabis may induce liver disease in heavy users (Kew *et al.*, 1969) has not been substantiated. Rarely neurologic disorders are encountered, but the long-term physical and psychological consequences of chronic cannabis consumption have not yet been settled and are still under study.

The mechanisms responsible for the various central nervous system effects of cannabis are unknown. In laboratory animals THC has been shown to have anticonvulsant and analgesic activities (Harris, 1971); it prolongs hexobarbital sleeping time but intensifies the excitatory effects of amphetamines (Forney, 1971). Spontaneous motor activity is reduced, but treated animals are hypersensitive to noise and touch. This spectrum of activity with its admixture of excitatory and inhibitory components is unlike that of any other psychotropic agent. A genetically unique colony of rabbits has been identified; its members respond with non-fatal seizures to only the psychoactive cannabinoids (Martin and Consroe, 1976).

Although cannabis hallucinations are not notably different from those induced by other hallucinogens, no cross-tolerance with LSD, psilocybin or mescaline can be demonstrated (Isbell and Jasinski, 1969). Presumably different brain mechanisms are involved. As compared with LSD, THC and other cannabis preparations induce more prolonged euphoria, more prominent sedation, less sympathetic activity (*i.e.*, no pupillary dilatation as with LSD), less frequent tremors and hyperreflexia, and fewer and less severe "flashbacks" (Hollister *et al.*, 1968). A clinical diagnosis, however, is often impossible, in part because street marihuana is sometimes "cut" with other psychoactive substances, such as amphetamine, heroin, cocaine and even camphor (Taylor *et al.*, 1970).

Intravenous marihuana: A severe and potentially fatal reaction is provoked by the intravenous injection of crude aqueous extracts of marihuana. Because such preparations contain large amounts of insoluble material, at least some of which may be biologically inert, it is likely that the particles may act as microemboli and induce a nonspecific "foreign body reaction." Such signs and symptoms as hyperventilation, pulmonary edema or effusions (Vaziri *et al.*, 1981), acute pulmonary hypertension and infarction, transient thrombocytopenia and leukocytosis (Henderson and Pugsley, 1968), chills, fever, myalgia, arthralgia, rhabdomyolysis and mild disturbances in liver function (Farber and Huertas, 1976; Mims and Lee, 1977; Payne and Brand, 1975) might be explicable on this nonspecific basis.

A growing number of case reports, however, strongly suggests that a unique syndrome of marihuana intoxication is superimposed on the non-specific reactions. This syndrome is heralded by a fulminant gastroenteritis, evidenced by vomiting, diarrhea, crampy abdominal pain and delayed gastrointestinal bleeding (King and Cowen, 1969; Vaziri *et al.*, 1981). Both intense peripheral vasoconstriction (Henderson and Pugsley, 1968) and vasodilatation (Vaziri *et al.*,

1981) have been described, but hypotension, sinus tachycardia and hypovolemic shock with transitory renal failure are common. All cases reported to date have recovered fully over days to weeks with only supportive care.

Metabolism: Metabolic studies in laboratory rodents show that radiolabeled Δ^9-THC enters brain but does not accumulate there preferentially. Highest concentrations are found in lung tissue after inhalation and intravenous administration (references cited by Nahas, 1973). Radioactivity derived from labeled Δ^9-THC is excreted in urine and bile. In man more is eventually eliminated in feces than in urine, even after parenteral administration (Lemberger et al., 1971). Large quantities of radioactive label, however, are retained in the body for surprisingly long periods; only half to three-quarters of a dose is recovered in human excreta in 72 hours (Lemberger et al., 1972a); a week or more is required for complete elimination of a single dose.

Metabolites of Δ^9-THC account for the radioactivity retained in plasma and tissues. Based on the low concentrations of unmodified Δ^9-THC detectable in plasma after the first hour (Lemberger et al., 1971), its biotransformation is thought to be rapid. Oxidative enzymes in liver microsomes play a major role in the metabolic inactivation of Δ^9-THC (Wall, 1971). The first metabolite in the sequence is 11-hydroxy-Δ^9-THC, and the second is the 8,11-dihydroxy derivative (Nahas, 1973). Probably side chain oxidation also occurs. Many unidentified polar metabolites are found in tissues and excreta (e.g., Lemberger et al., 1972a; Perez-Reyes et al., 1973). The 11-hydroxy metabolite of Δ^9-THC is now recognized to be psychoactive; it is as effective and perhaps even more potent than unmodified Δ^9-THC (Lemberger et al., 1972b; Kosersky et al., 1974). Cross-tolerance between these two compounds has been demonstrated (Kosersky et al., 1974). Several investigators have proposed that the psychic effects of cannabis are due not to Δ^9-THC but to its 11-hydroxy metabolite, but this view is not widely held at the present time. In mice death after Δ^9-THC appears to be due to unmetabolized compound, since mortality was enhanced by pretreatments that blocked the enzymatic conversion of THC to hydroxy metabolites (Mantilla-Plata and Harbison, 1974).

Therapeutic considerations: Acute marihuana intoxication is generally not a major challenge to the therapist. Only conservative measures are warranted because the prognosis for complete recovery is usually excellent. Novice marihuana users who become panicky usually respond well to simple reassurance or mild sedation (Weil, 1970). In using sedatives, however, caution is required because of the known additive effects between cannabis and other central nervous system depressants such as barbiturates and alcohol (Dalton et al., 1975; Forney, 1971). Patients who are confused and hallucinating may need to be restrained to prevent injuries, but aggressive behavior is rare, and most individuals can be successfully "talked down" (see "Treatment" below) (Taylor et al., 1970).

No drug antagonist or antidote to cannabis is known. Even if available, it would seldom be required. Patients who are comatose from overdoses of cannabis may require intensive supportive care, as with other central nervous depressants. Analeptics, however, should be avoided because at least in animals the toxicity of tetrahydrocannabinols is enhanced by amphetamine and other stimulants such as cocaine and caffeine (Hardman et al., 1971). Even pressor agents should be used only with caution, because in dogs Δ^9-THC is known to potentiate cardiovascular effects of epinephrine and norepinephrine (Harris, 1971). In man amphetamine and marihuana have additive effects on heart rate and blood pressure (Evans et al., 1976). Propranolol particularly in combination with atropine blocks the cardiovascular responses to acute marihuana intoxication and to intravenous Δ^9-THC (Benowitz et al., 1979; Sulkowski et al., 1977).

In general, however, drug therapy is best avoided, except for the use of chlorpromazine or other phenothiazine tranquilizers in those individuals with frightening hallucinations, paranoid ideation or other psychotic manifestations (Garrett et al., 1977; Taylor et al., 1970). For this purpose some physicians prefer a minor tranquilizer such as chlordiazepoxide. The same principles apply to the clinical management of poisonings with other hallucinogens (Consroe, 1973), although phenothiazines are regarded as hazardous (Gershon et al., 1965) and thus are avoided in treating the delirium of atropine overdosage (Taylor et al., 1970).

For purposes of illicit transport, balloons or condoms are sometimes filled with marihuana or other drugs, tied shut and swallowed. These may be recovered later by self-induced vomiting or passed with feces. Large numbers have been swallowed resulting in intestinal obstruction. They may or may not be apparent on abdominal X-ray. In one case rupture of such a balloon resulted in only mild signs of intoxication; thus, conservative management is indicated. However, if such balloons contain more potent drugs, e.g., COCAINE (p. III-114), surgical intervention for their removal may be justified (Dassel and Punjabi, 1979; Vowels and Harvey, 1980).

Symptomatology (acute intoxication by ingestion or by inhalation of marihuana smoke):
    1. An initial transient period of uneasiness

or even apprehension and panic, followed by relaxation and usually euphoria.

2. Sinus tachycardia. Occasional ventricular premature beats. Orthostatic (postural) hypotension with rare syncopal attacks.
3. Conjunctival injection. Normal pupil size.
4. Sometimes a dry mouth, increased appetite for sweet foods. Less often headache, nausea and vomiting.
5. Various and changing psychic moods ranging from jocularity to dreamlike meditation, usually followed by sleep.
6. With higher doses distortions of visual perception and sometimes sensations of flashing colored lights, at first only with the eyes closed, culminating in complex visual and auditory hallucinations.
7. Ataxia, tremor and hyperreflexia.
8. Increasing confusion, restlessness, disorientation and delirium.
9. Sometimes elaborate paranoid delusions and severe emotional depression, which may persist for days after the acute phase of intoxication.
10. As inferred from animal studies, central nervous depression with deepening coma, medullary depression, bradypnea, bradycardia, and hypotension.
11. Death from respiratory arrest or perhaps cardiovascular collapse.

Treatment:

1. If poisoning is due to recent ingestion (*e.g.*, within 2 hours), empty the stomach and perform gastric lavage. Use caution if the patient is drowsy (see Section I). The safety and efficacy of emetics are not established in cannabis poisoning.
2. Even several hours after the ingestion of marihuana, the oral administration of a saline cathartic (by installation through a stomach tube if necessary) is probably worthwhile. Give 15 to 30 gm. of sodium sulfate.
3. Try to keep the patient in a supine or sitting position to avoid syncopy due to orthostatic hypotension.
4. If the victim is frightened but well oriented, simple reassurance may be adequate.
5. If the victim is confused, disoriented and frightened by hallucinations, a prolonged "talkdown" is required. Keep the patient in a quiet room with a therapist present at all times. Remove extraneous stimuli such as bright lights and unnecessary noise. Try to establish verbal contact. Talk slowly and simply. Try to give the victim a sense of reality ("This is a book. Feel it"). Simple repetitive concrete statements by the therapist may help the patient to verbalize his experience and to

become reoriented. Alternating periods of confusion and of mental clarity can be anticipated. See also pp. IV-33–35.
6. If the hallucinations are particularly terrifying or if paranoid delusions become prominent, administer intramuscular chlorpromazine (25 mg.). Other phenothiazine tranquilizers may be preferable: fluphenazine hydrochloride 1.2 mg.; prochlorperazine 10 to 20 mg.; trifluoperazine hydrochloride 1 to 2 mg. The latter is said to have the fewest autonomic side effects. However, if the history or examination suggests that atropine, scopolamine or any other anticholinergic drug has also been consumed, avoid all phenothiazines. Try chlordiazepoxide or diazepam instead.
7. If disorientation is accompanied by extreme restlessness and hyperactivity, gentle restraint may be required to prevent the victim from injuring himself and others. See p. IV-35.
8. If he is comatose, maintain a patent airway and administer artificial respiration as required (see pp. IV-2–12).
9. Propranolol has been shown to block most of the cardiovascular effects of marihuana smoke. Thus it may be useful in managing the intoxicated patient with poor cardiac reserve or cardiac arrhythmia.
10. Avoid all analeptic drugs.

Laboratory:

1. Monitor the ECG at intervals if the pulse becomes irregular.
2. Analyse blood sugar. Current evidence indicates that hyper- and hypoglycemia are rare.
3. Radioimmunoassays can be used to detect and quantify THC in the urine. The most sensitive but elaborate method for analyzing cannabinoids is a combination of gas-liquid chromatography and mass spectrometry.

References:

Benowitz, N. L.; Rosenberg, J.; Rogers, W.; Bachman, J.; Jones, R. T. Cardiovascular effects of intravenous delta-9-tetrahydrocannabinol: Autonomic nervous mechanisms. Clin. Pharmacol. Ther., *25*:440-446, 1979.

Bromberg, W. Marihuana intoxication; a clinical study of *Cannabis sativa* intoxication. Am. J. Psychol. *91*:303-330, 1934.

Burton, T. A. Urinary retention following cannabis ingestion. J. A. M. A. *242*:351, 1979.

Consroe, P. Treatment of acute hallucinogenic drug toxicity; specific pharmacological intervention. Am. J. Hosp. Pharm. *30*:85-86, 1973.

Dalton, W. S.; Martz, R.; Lemberger, L.; Rodda, B. E.; Forney, R. B. Effects of marihuana combined with secobarbital. Clin. Pharmacol. Ther. *18*:298-304, 1975.

Dassel, P. M.; Punjabi, E. Ingested marihuana-filled balloons. Gastroenterol. *76*:166-169, 1979.

Doorenbos, N. J.; Fetterman, P. S.; Quimby, M. W.; Turner,

C. E. Cultivation, extraction and analysis of *Cannabis sativa* L. Ann. N. Y. Acad. Sci. *191*:3-12, 1971.

Evans, M. A.; Martz, R.; Rodda, B. E.; Lemberger, L.; Forney, R. B. Effect of marijuana-dextroamphetamine combination. Clin. Pharmacol. Ther. *20*:350-358, 1976.

Farber, S. J.; Huertas, V. E. Intravenously injected marihuana syndrome. Arch. Intern. Med. *136*:337-339, 1976.

Farnsworth, N. R. Pharmacognosy and chemistry of 'Cannabis sativa'. J. Am. Pharm. Assoc. *9*:410-415, 1969.

Forney, R. B. Toxicology of marihuana. Pharmacol. Rev. *23*:279-291, 1971.

Galanter, M.; Wyatt, R.; Lemberger, L.; Weingartner, H.; Vaughan, T.; Roth, W. Effects on humans of delta-9-tetrahydrocannabinol administered by smoking. Science *176*:934-936, 1972.

Garrett, C. P. O.; Braithwaite, R. A.; Teale, J. D. Unusual case of tetrahydrocannabinol intoxication confirmed by radioimmunoassay. Br. Med. J. *2*:166, 1977.

Gershon, S.; Neubauer, H.; Sundland, D. Interaction between some anticholinergic agents and phenothiazines. Clin. Pharmacol. Ther. *6*:749-756, 1965.

Hardman, H.; Domino, E.; Seevers, M. General pharmacological actions of some synthetic tetrahydrocannabinol derivatives. Pharmacol. Rev. *23*:295-315, 1971.

Harris, L. General and behavioral pharmacology. Pharmacol. Rev. *23*:285-294, 1971.

Henderson, A.; Pugsley, D. Collapse after intravenous injection of hashish. Br. Med. J. *3*:229-230, 1968.

Heyndrickx, A.; Scheiris, C.; Schepens, P. Toxicological study of a fatal intoxication by man due to Cannabis smoking. J. Pharm. Belg. *24*:371-375, 1969.

Hollister, L.; Gillespie, H. Delta-8- and delta-9-tetrahydrocannabinol. Clin. Pharmacol. Ther. *14*:353-357, 1973.

Hollister, L.; Richards, R.; Gillespie, H. Comparison of tetrahydrocannabinol and synhexyl in man. Clin. Pharmacol. Ther. *9*:783-791, 1968.

Institute of Medicine. *Marijuana and Health*. National Academy Press, Washington, D. C., 1982.

Isbell, H.; Jasinski, D. A comparison of LSD-25 with (-)delta-9-*trans*-tetrahydrocannabinol (THC) and attempted crosstolerance between LSD and THC. Psychopharmacologia *14*:115-123, 1969.

Johnson, S.; Domino, E. Some cardiovascular effects of marihuana smoking in normal volunteers. Clin. Pharmacol. Ther. *12*:762-768, 1971.

Keeler, M. Marihuana induced hallucination. Dis. Nerv. Syst. *29*:314-315, 1968.

Kew, M.; Bersohn, I.; Siew, S. Possible hepatotoxicity of Cannabis. Lancet *1*:578-579, 1969.

King, A.; Cowen, D. Effect of intravenous injection of marihuana. J. A. M. A. *210*:724-725, 1969.

Kosersky, D. S.; McMillan, D.; Harris, L. Delta-9-tetrahydrocannabinol and 11-hydroxy-delta-9-tetrahydrocannabinol; behavior effects and tolerance development. J. Pharmacol. Exp. Ther. *189*:61-65, 1974.

Lemberger, L.; Axelrod, J.; Kopin, I. Metabolism and disposition of Δ^9-tetrahydrocannabinol in man. Pharmacol. Rev. *23*:371-380, 1971.

Lemberger, L.; Crabtree, R.; Rowe, H. 11-Hydroxy-delta-9-tetrahydrocannabinol; pharmacology, disposition, and metabolism of a major metabolite of marihuana in man. Science *177*:62-64, 1972b.

Lemberger, L.; Weiss, J.; Watanabe, A.; Galanter, I.; Wyatt, R.; Cardon, P. Delta-9-tetrahydrocannabinol. N. Engl. J. Med. *286*:685-688, 1972a.

Lieberman, C.; Lieberman, B. Marihuana—a medical review. N. Engl. J. Med. *284*:88-91, 1971.

Manno, J.; Kiplinger, G.; Haine, S.; Bennett, I.; Forney, R. Comparative effects of smoking marihuana or placebo on human motor and mental performance. Clin. Pharmacol. Ther. *11*:808-815, 1970.

Mantilla-Plata, B.; Harbison, R. Effects of phenobarbital and SKF 525A pretreatment, sex, liver injury, and vehicle on delta-9-tetrahydrocannabinol toxicity. Toxicol. Appl. Pharmacol. *27*:123-130, 1974.

Martin, P.; Consroe, P. Cannabinoid induced behavioral convulsions in rabbits. Science *194*:965-967, 1976.

Mims, R. B.; Lee, J. H. Adverse effects of intravenous cannabis tea. J. Nat. Med. Assoc., *69*:491-495, 1977.

Nahas, G. *Marihuana- Deceptive Weed*. Raven Press, New York, 1973.

National Commission Marihuana and Drug Abuse. *Marihuana: A Signal of Misunderstanding*. Appendix, Vol. 1, Washington, D. C., U. S. Government Printing Office, March 1972.

Payne, R. J.; Brand, S. N. The toxicity of intravenously used marihuana. J. A. M. A. *233*:351-354, 1975.

Pearl, J.; Domino, E.; Rennick, P. Short-term effects of marijuana smoking on cognitive behavior in experienced male users. Psychopharmacologia *31*:13-24, 1973.

Perez-Reyes, M.; Lipton, M.; Wall, M.; Brine, D.; Davis, K.; Timmons, M. The clinical pharmacology of orally administered delta-9-tetrahydrocannabinol. Clin. Pharmacol. Ther. *14*:48-55, 1973.

Phillips, R.; Turk, R.; Forney, R. Acute toxicity of delta-9-tetrahydrocannabinol in rats and mice. Proc. Soc. Exp. Biol. Med. *136*:260-263, 1971.

Rosenkrantz, H. Effects of cannabis on fetal development of rodents. In *Marijuana: Biological Effects*, G. G. Nahas and W. D. M. Paton, editors. Pergamon Press, N. Y., 1979.

Rosenkrantz, H.; Heyman, I.; Braude, M. Inhalation, parenteral and oral LD50 values of delta-9-tetrahydrocannabinol in Fischer rats. Toxicol. Appl. Pharmacol. *28*:18-27, 1974.

Roth, W.; Tinklenberg, J.; Kopell, B.; Hollister, L. Continuous electrocardiographic monitoring during marihuana intoxication. Clin. Pharmacol. Ther. *14*:533-540, 1973.

Sulkowski, A.; Vachon, L.; Rich, E. S., Jr. Propranolol effects on acute marihuana intoxication in man. Psychopharmacol. *52*:47-53, 1977.

Talbott, J.; Teague, J. Marihuana psychosis. J. A. M. A. *210*:299-302, 1969.

Tart, C. Marijuana intoxication; common experiences. Nature *226*:701-704, 1970.

Taylor, R. L.; Maurer, J. I.; Tinklenberg, J. R. Management of "bad trips" in an evolving drug scene. J. A. M. A. *213*:422-425, 1970.

Tennant, F.; Preble, M.; Prendergast, T.; Ventry, P. Medical manifestations associated with hashish. J. A. M. A. *216*:1965-1969, 1971.

Thompson, G.; Fleischman, R.; Rosenkrantz, H.; Braude, M. Oral and intravenous toxicity of delta-9-tetrahydrocannabinol in rhesus monkeys. Toxicol. Appl. Pharmacol. *27*:648-665, 1974.

Truitt, E. G. Biological disposition of tetrahydrocannabinols. Pharmacol. Rev. *23*:273-278, 1971.

Vaziri, N. D.; Thomas, R.; Sterling, M.; Seiff, K.; Pahl, M. V.; Davila, J.; Wilson, A. Toxicty with intravenous injection of crude marijuana extract. Clin. Toxicol. *18*:353-366, 1981.

Vowels, M.; Harvey, P. M. Ingestion of hashish oil-filled condoms. Med. J. Aust. *2*:509-510, 1980.

Wall, M. E. The in vitro and in vivo metabolism of tetrahydrocannabinol (THC). Ann. N. Y. Acad. Sci. *191*:23-37, 1971.

Waller, C. W. Chemistry of marihuana. Pharmacol. Rev. *23*:265-272, 1971.

Weil, A. T. Adverse reactions to marihuana. N. Engl. J. Med. *282*:997-1000, 1970.

Weil, A. T.; Zinberg, N. Acute effects of marihuana on speech. Nature *222*:434-437, 1969.

Weil, A. T.; Zinberg, N. E.; Nelson, J. M. Clinical and psychological effects of marihuana in man. Science *162*:1234-1242, 1968.

Wikler, A. Clinical and social aspects of marihuana intoxication. Arch. Gen. Psychiatry *23*:320-325, 1970.

Williams, E. G.; Himmelsbach, C. K.; Wikler, A. Studies on marihuana and pyrahexyl compound. Public Health Rep. *61*:1059-1083, 1946.

MEPROBAMATE

Meprobamate is a drug widely known under the brand names Equanil and Miltown. The compound was synthesized originally for possible use as a muscle relaxant; it was found subsequently to be a potent anticonvulsant and to exhibit a marked taming effect when administered to monkeys. The behavior observed in these animals suggested a loss of fear, hostility, and aggressiveness without marked impairment of appetite or loss of interest in the surroundings. When first introduced, meprobamate appeared to represent a new type of drug—one which was active centrally but which lacked those prominent effects on the autonomic nervous system seen after other tranquilizers such as reserpine and chlorpromazine. More precisely, meprobamate is said to exert a selective action on the thalamus and also to inhibit multineuronal spinal reflexes (Berger, 1954, 1956).

Meprobamate was widely acclaimed on its introduction to clinical medicine in about 1954. Its popularity led to its use in a multitude of psychopathological states both alone and in combination with many other types of drugs, particularly those used in chronic and debilitating diseases. It is apparent that meprobamate's wide availability to depressed and mentally disturbed patients invited its frequent use as an instrument of attempted suicide (McKown et al., 1963).

A drug that is closely allied chemically and used in much the same manner as meprobamate is phenaglycodol (Ultran); presumably much of the following discussion is pertinent also to this compound. Also related and apparently capable of producing similar toxic syndromes are mephenesín, carisoprol and emylcamate. The common benzodiazepine drugs, which are rapidly replacing meprobamate in clinical medicine, are discussed under DIAZEPAM, p. III-138.

Toxicology: Acute toxicity studies (Table III-6) on laboratory animals have demonstrated that meprobamate is four to five times less toxic than most barbiturates, in accordance with reports of its early clinical trials (Borrus, 1955, 1957; Selling, 1955).

Table III-6.
Experimental Acute Toxicity Studies with Meprobamate

Species	Route	LD_{50} (mg./kg.)
Mice	Intraperitoneal	800[a]
Mice	Oral	1100[b]
Rats	Oral	1600[b]

[a] Berger (1956).

[b] Wyeth Laboratories (1958a).

Shortly after its introduction, reports of attempted suicide by the ingestion of massive doses began to appear in the clinical literature. These reports establish that meprobamate in large doses (10 to 40 gm.) is unexpectedly hazardous in man in that it may induce profound and persistent hypotension (Algeri et al., 1959; Allen et al., 1977; Belaval and Widen, 1958; Blumberg et al., 1959; Briggs, 1959; Deisher, 1956; Ferguson et al., 1960; Scott et al., 1956; Shane and Hirsh, 1956; Woodward, 1957). Because it has been observed even in the absence of muscular flaccidity, this hypotension has been ascribed to a direct action of the drug on the vasomotor center (Ferguson et al., 1960).

It is important not to confuse the syndrome with acute barbiturate intoxication because after meprobamate a precipitous fall in blood pressure may occur in what appears to be a lightly comatose patient. The importance of frequent measurements of vital signs is emphasized. Both blood volume expanders and levarterenol (Blumberg et al., 1959) or ephedrine sulfate (Briggs, 1959) have been used in attempts to maintain the arterial blood pressure. There is, however, the ever present danger that overhydration will lead to severe pulmonary edema, particularly when the right atrial or pulmonary wedge pressure is elevated. Some evidence suggests that the hypotension may be secondary to acute cardiac failure, and at least one patient responded very well to infusions of isoproterenol (Lhoste et al., 1977).

If hypotension is averted, the prognosis is generally good. In one massive ingestion episode, however, a favorable response to fluid therapy as indicated by a complete return to consciousness was followed by sudden death. Because the stomach was found to contain large amounts of meprobamate, it was presumed that the improved circulatory status facilitated the further absorption of a lethal dose (Jenis et al., 1969).

Undoubtedly coma is the most frequently described sign in meprobamate intoxication. It is usually characterized by areflexia and a lack of response to sensory stimuli (Algeri et al., 1959; Charet et al., 1956; McKown et al., 1963; Shane and Hirsh, 1956; Woodward, 1957), although both signs may be absent (Ferguson et al., 1960).

Respiratory depression has been noted and attributed to respiratory center inhibition (Woodward, 1957), but it is rarely severe enough to compromise survival. Excess oronasal secretions or relaxation of the pharyngeal wall (Algeri et al., 1959) may present a problem in terms of airway obstruction. Most patients do not require respiratory assistance and neither do poisoned animals (Berger, 1954; Ferguson et al., 1960;

Scott *et al.*, 1956). Both dilated and constricted pupils have been observed, and muscular relaxation is more often present than not (Hiestand, 1956; Lockhart, 1956; Shane and Hirsh, 1956). Exceptional occurrences include such paradoxical reactions as extreme excitement with therapeutic doses (Friedman and Marmelzat, 1956) or motor hyperexcitability in the form of repeated myoclonic seizures of an epileptiform nature following the ingestion of 20 gm. (Troy *et al.*, 1958).

In two fatalities in women, doses of 12 gm. (240 mg./kg.) and 20 gm. (350 mg./kg.) were ingested (Powell *et al.*, 1958). Since both women were found dead, it was no more than an assumption that they succumbed to cardiovascular collapse. Others given adequate medical care have survived doses of nearly 40 gm. (Hiestand, 1956; Woodward, 1957). Eight grams has been estimated as an adult dose that produces dangerous symptoms, but is not usually fatal (Brophy, 1967). In a review of 720 poisoning episodes (Davis *et al.*, 1968), there were only 16 fatalities among 129 patients who consumed the drug in the 12- to 40-gm. dose range.

Profound meprobamate intoxication is associated with plasma levels of 20 mg./100 ml. Most patients appear to be comatose at levels above 10 mg./100 ml., whereas consciousness returns at levels below 5 mg./100 ml. (Maddock and Bloomer, 1967). Therapeutic plasma levels are about 1 mg./100 ml. Meprobamate is rapidly metabolized. It has been predicted that in an otherwise healthy adult a plasma level of 25 mg./100 ml. would decline in 24 hours to levels associated with restoration of consciousness.

Hemodialysis may cut this time period in half, and mannitol diuresis may reduce it by one-third (Maddock and Bloomer, 1967). In an actual case mannitol was successfully employed with results consonant with the above prediction (Powers and Lubin, 1966). In another patient with an initial serum level of 12 mg./100 ml., peritoneal dialysis resulted in an average clearance of only 3.5 ml./min. (Dymeut *et al.*, 1965). In dogs a saline-furosemide diuresis resulted in a significant increase in meprobamate clearance (Gibson *et al.*, 1974).

Both resin (Hoy *et al.*, 1980) and charcoal (Crome *et al.*, 1977) hemoperfusions have been performed successfully in severely poisoned patients. The resin hemoperfusion cartridge extracted considerable drug at rates approaching the plasma flow through it (about 200 ml./minute), but total recovery was only a small fraction of the ingested dose (Hoy *et al.*, 1980). Nevertheless, both patients showed rapid clinical improvement. The major benefit of the procedure may have been to improve the blood pressure and so to restore normal renal and hepatic function. In another massive ingestion (36 gm.) a gastrotomy performed more than 40 hours later

recovered a tarry mass of activated charcoal from which almost 25 gm. of meprobamate was recovered (Schwartz, 1976). These procedures for promoting the removal of meprobamate should be reserved for severely intoxicated patients.

Sensitivity reactions to doses as low as 1 tablet in patients without a previous history of allergy or prior exposure to the drug have also been reported. The effects include stomatitis and proctitis (Brachfeld and Bell, 1959), pruritic eruptions (Charkes, 1958; Corley and Brundage, 1957), purpura (Carmel and Dannenberg, 1956), pronounced anaphylactoid reaction (Nevins, 1960), fatal allergic collapse (Adlin *et al.*, 1958), and a fatal case of aplastic anemia (Meyer *et al.*, 1957). Meprobamate appears to exert a potentiating effect on certain central depressants. In fatal human poisonings, blood and tissue levels of meprobamate were significantly lower in those cases where alcohol and/or barbiturates were also consumed (Felby, 1970).

Addiction with apparent withdrawal symptoms has been produced in mice (Swinyard *et al.*, 1957) and dogs (Essig, 1958) following clinical experiences in which convulsive seizures were noted in a few patients after the abrupt withdrawal of the drug (Barsa and Kline, 1956; Johnson, 1962; Lemere, 1956; Tucker and Wilensky, 1957). In at least one case in which the patient consumed 10 gm. per day, withdrawal resulted in death (Swanson and Okada, 1963). The addicting and intoxicating properties are said to resemble those of the barbiturates (Essig, 1964). In some cases of physical dependence on meprobamate, the patient has had a previous history of addiction to alcohol, to barbiturates or to narcotics (Mohr and Mead, 1958; Ewing and Fullilove, 1957; Essig and Ainslie, 1957). It is apparent that addiction is not predicated solely on the prolonged administration of clinically effective doses; the personality of the subject, previous drug history, and the size of the dose are important deciding factors (Boyd *et al.*, 1958).

Symptomatology:

1. The course of the intoxication is characterized by a notable lack of autonomic involvement.
2. Drowsiness, relaxation, stupor, sleep, coma, areflexia, muscular flaccidity, hypothermia, lack of response to sensory stimuli, pupils fixed and unresponsive to light.
3. Slow pulse and moderate depression of the blood pressure.
4. Severe and persistent hypotension which may appear at any time during the intoxication probably constitutes the chief hazard.

5. Respiration may or may not be depressed. Occasional atelectasis or pulmonary edema.

6. Less frequently observed are paradoxical reactions ranging from extreme excitement to epileptiform seizures.

7. Anxiety, restlessness, confusion and convulsions during recovery suggest physical dependence due to heavy drug consumption over a long period of time.

Treatment:

1. If the patient is awake and neither loss of consciousness nor convulsions are imminent, give by mouth syrup of ipecac (p. I-2) or a slurry of activated charcoal (p. I-4).

2. Gastric lavage with warm water or saline as soon as practical, if productive vomiting is not produced by syrup of ipecac or if ipecac cannot be used. Precautions against aspiration are essential (p. I-10), especially in the comatose patient. Gastric lavage (or the induction of emesis) may be useful many hours after the original ingestion to remove unabsorbed drug.

3. After lavage leave in the stomach 15 to 30 gm. of sodium sulfate in water as an osmotic cathartic.

4. Symptomatic and supportive treatment with frequent monitoring of vital signs.

5. Correct airway obstruction (p. IV-2), give oxygen (p. IV-12) or administer artificial respiration (p. IV-7), as warranted.

6. If hypotension appears, prompt and persistent therapeutic measures including expansion of the blood volume (p. IV-18) and/or the administration of pressor agents such as metaraminol or levarterenol (p. IV-17). A cautious infusion of isoproterenol, dobutamine or dopamine may also be useful to enhance cardiac output (p. IV-21).

7. Avoid barbiturates or use sparingly even in the presence of epileptiform convulsions because these drugs may lead to intense central nervous depression if meprobamate is still present in the body. Convulsions after symptomatic recovery usually indicate a withdrawal reaction (see above). In this case barbiturates are both useful and generally safe, although diazepam may be better.

8. Hemodialysis (pp. IV-56–57) or mannitol diuresis (p. IV-52) or perhaps saline-furosemide diuresis, in the severely intoxicated patient. Because of the uncertain cardiovascular status, however, fluids should be infused with caution, and urinary output should be monitored carefully.

9. Hemoperfusion with Amberlite XAD-4 resin may be necessary after massive overdoses (Hoy *et al.*, 1980). See p. IV-57.

Laboratory: Numerous methods are available for the determination of meprobamate in biological fluids (Sunshine, 1966).

References:

Adlin, E. V.; Sher, P. B.; Berk, N. G. Fatal reaction following the ingestion of meprobamate. Arch. Intern. Med. *102*:484-489, 1958.

Algeri, E. J.; Katsas, G. G.; McBay, A. J. Toxicology of some new drugs. Glutethimide, meprobamate, and chlorpromazine. J. Forensic Sci. *4*:111-134, 1959.

Allen, M. D.; Greenblatt, D. J.; Noel, B. J. Meprobamate overdosage: a continuing problem. Clin. Toxicol. *11*: 501-515, 1977.

Barsa, J. A.; Kline, N. S. Use of meprobamate in the treatment of psychotic patients. Am. J. Psychiatry *112*:1023, 1956.

Belaval, G. S.; Widen, A. L. Meprobamate toxicity. U. S. Armed Forces Med. J. *9*:1691-1702, 1958.

Berger, F. M. The pharmacological properties of 2-methyl-2-*n*-propyl-1,3-propanediol dicarbamate (Miltown), a new interneuronal blocking agent. J. Pharmacol. Exp. Ther. *112*:413-423, 1954.

Berger, F. M. Meprobamate, its pharmacologic properties and clinical uses. Int. Rec. Med. *169*:184-196, 1956.

Blumberg, A. G.; Rosett, H. L.; Dobrow, A. Severe hypotensive reactions following meprobamate overdosage. Ann. Intern. Med. *51*:607-612, 1959.

Borrus, J. C. Study of effect of Miltown (2-methyl-2-*n*-propyl-1,3-propanediol dicarbamate) on psychiatric states. J. A. M. A. *157*:1596-1598, 1955.

Borrus, J. C. Meprobamate in psychiatric disorders. Med. Clin. North Am. *41*:327-337, 1957.

Boyd, L. J.; Cammer, L.; Mulinos, M. G.; Huppert, V. F.; Hammer, H. Meprobamate addiction. J. A. M. A. *168*:1839-1843, 1958.

Brachfeld, J.; Bell, E. C. Stomatitis and proctitis as manifestations of meprobamate idiosyncrasy. J. A. M. A. *169*:1321-1322, 1959.

Briggs, G. W. Meprobamate toxicity. Med. Bull. U. S. Army Europe *16*:137-139, 1959.

Brophy, J. J. Suicide attempts with psychotherapeutic drugs. Arch. Gen. Psychiatry *17*:652-657, 1967.

Carmel, W. J.; Dannenberg, T. Nonthrombocytopenic purpura due to Miltown (2-methyl-2-*n*-propyl-1,3-propanediol dicarbamate). N. Engl. J. Med. *255*:770-771, 1956.

Charet, R.; Brill, B.; Elloso, C. Coma after Miltown overdose. Ann. Intern. Med. *45*:1211-1213, 1956.

Charkes, N. D. Meprobamate idiosyncrasy; report of a case and review of the literature. Arch. Intern. Med. *102*:584-593, 1958.

Corley, B. L.; Brundage, F. Reaction following ingestion of 400 mg. of meprobamate. Calif. Med. *86*:183, 1957.

Crome, P.; Higgenbottom, T.; Elliott, J. A. Severe meprobamate poisoning -- successful treatment with haemoperfusion. Postgrad. Med. J. *53*:698-699, 1977.

Davis, J. M.; Bartlett, E.; Termini, B. A. Overdosage of psychotropic drugs: A review. Dis. Nerv. Syst. *29*:157-164 and 246-256, 1968.

Deisher, J. B. Ingestion of 12 grams of meprobamate with recovery. Northwest Med. *55*:1083-1085, 1956.

Dymeut, P. G.; Curtis, D. D.; Gourrich, G. E. Meprobamate poisoning treated by peritoneal dialysis. J. Pediatr. *67*:124-126, 1965.

Essig, C. F. Withdrawal convulsions in dogs following chronic meprobamate intoxication. Arch. Neurol. *80*:414-417, 1958.

Essig, C. F. Addiction to nonbarbiturate sedative and tranquilizing drugs. Clin. Pharmacol. Ther. *5*:334-343, 1964.

Essig, C. F.; Ainslie, J. D. Addiction to meprobamate (Equanil, Miltown). J. A. M. A. *164*:1382, 1957.

Ewing, J. A.; Fullilove, R. E. Addiction to meprobamate. N.

Engl. J. Med. *257*:76-77, 1957.

Felby, S. Concentrations of meprobamate in the blood and liver following fatal meprobamate poisoning. Acta Pharmacol. Toxicol. *28*:334-337, 1970.

Ferguson, M. J.; Germanos, S.; Grace, W. J. Meprobamate overdosage. A report on the management of five cases. Arch. Intern. Med. *106*:237-239, 1960.

Friedman, H. T.; Marmelzat, W. L. Adverse reactions to meprobamate. J. A. M. A. *162*:628-630, 1956.

Gibson, T. P.; Ketter, K. A.; Delle, M.; DiBona, G. F. Enhanced renal tubular secretion of meprobamate; role of saline-furosemide diuresis. Clin. Toxicol. *7*:29-35, 1974.

Hiestand, E. C. Overdosage with meprobamate - presentation of a case. Ohio State Med. J. *52*:1306-1307, 1956.

Hoy, W. E.; Rivero, A.; Marin, M. G.; Rieders, F. Resin hemoperfusion for treatment of a massive meprobamate overdose. Ann. Intern. Med. *93*:455-456, 1980.

Jenis, E. H.; Payne, R. J.; Goldbaum, L. R. Acute meprobamate poisoning. J. A. M. A. *207*:361-362, 1969.

Johnson, A. M. Chronic meprobamate intoxication. N. Engl. J. Med. *267*:145, 1962.

Lemere, F. Habit-forming properties of meprobamate. Arch. Neurol. *76*:205-206, 1956.

Lhoste, F.; Lemaire, F.; Rapin, M. Treatment of hypotension in meprobamate poisoning (letter). N. Engl. J. Med. *296*:1004, 1977.

Lockhart, W. E. Suicidal Miltown, hazard of overhydration in treatment. Southwest. Med. *37*:428, 1956.

Maddock, R. K., Jr.; Bloomer, H. A. Meprobamate overdosage, evaluation of its severity and methods of treatment. J. A. M. A. *201*:999-1003, 1967.

McKown, C. H.; Verhulst, H. L.; Crotty, J. J. Overdosage effects and danger from tranquilizing drugs. J. A. M. A. *185*:425-430, 1963.

Meyer, L. M.; Heever, W. L.; Bertscher, R. W. Aplastic anemia after meprobamate (2-methyl-2-n-propyl-1,3-propanediol dicarbamate) therapy. N. Engl. J. Med. *256*:1232-1233, 1957.

Mohr, R. C.; Mead, B. T. Meprobamate addiction. N. Engl. J. Med. *259*:865-868, 1958.

Nevins, D. M. Anaphylactoid reaction following administration of one meprobamate tablet. Ann. Intern. Med. *53*:192-193, 1960.

Powell, L. W.; Mann, G. T.; Kaye, S. Acute meprobamate poisoning. N. Engl. J. Med. *259*:716-718, 1958.

Powers, D. V.; Lubin, J. D. Use of mannitol in acute meprobamate intoxication. Anesth. Analg. *45*:422-424, 1966.

Schwartz, H. S. Acute meprobamate poisoning with gastrotomy and removal of a drug-containing mass. N. Engl. J. Med. *295*:1177-1178, 1976.

Scott, P. A. L.; Grimshaw, L.; Molony, H. M. P. Hypotensive episodes following treatment with meprobamate. Lancet *2*:1158-1159, 1956.

Selling, L. S. Clinical study of a new tranquilizing drug. Use of Miltown (2-methyl-2-n-propyl-1,3-propanediol dicarbamate). J. A. M. A. *157*:1594-1596, 1955.

Shane, A. M.; Hirsh, S. Three cases of meprobamate poisoning. Can. Med. Assoc. J. *74*:908-909, 1956.

Sunshine, I. *Handbook of Analytical Toxicology.* Chemical Rubber Co., Cleveland, 1966.

Swanson, L. A.; Okada, T. Death after withdrawal of meprobamate. J. A. M. A. *184*:780-781, 1963.

Swinyard, E. A.; Chin, L.; Fingl, E. Withdrawal hyperexcitability following chronic administration of meprobamate to mice. Science *125*:739-741, 1957.

Troy, C. A.; Gershon, S.; Morgan, P. J. A case of meprobamate coma with convulsions. Med. J. Aust. *2*:667-668, 1958.

Tucker, K.; Wilensky, H. A clinical evaluation of meprobamate therapy in a chronic schizophrenic population. Am. J. Psychiatry *113*:698-703, 1957.

Woodward, M. G. Attempted suicide with meprobamate. Northwest. Med. *56*:321-322, 1957.

Wyeth Laboratories. Brochure (Meprobamate). Wyeth Laboratories, Philadelphia, 1958a.

MERCURY

A host of mercury compounds has served in clinical medicine as antiseptics, antisyphilitics, cathartics, and diuretics. The occupational uses and hazards of mercury are legion; some unusual or important examples are fingerprint photographers (Agate and Buckell, 1949), dentists (McCord, 1961), hatters (Neal and Jones, 1938), medical laboratory personnel (Noe, 1959) and painters. Allergic dermatitis is a frequent complication arising from sensitization to mercuric sulfide (cinnabar), the red pigment usually employed in tattoos (Davis, 1960; Goldberg, 1959). Modern agriculture also employs many organic and inorganic derivatives of mercury in the form of dusts, wettable powders, solutions and fumigant vapors; these preparations serve as fungicides and as seed and cereal protectants. Many forms of paper contain mercury, and one person is known to have become intoxicated as a result of paper pica, perhaps secondary to an iron deficiency anemia (Olynyk and Sharpe, 1982). A polyvinyl alcohol preservative used in the collection of fecal specimens for examination of parasitic infestations contains 4.5% mercuric chloride (Seidel, 1980). Hair bleaches have also been a cause of poisonings (Wustner *et al.*, 1975).

As indicated below, all forms of mercury are poisonous if absorbed. Each has given rise to typical mercury intoxication under appropriate circumstances; this includes the free metal, calomel, mercurial antiseptic dyes, mercury-containing pesticides and mercurial diuretic drugs. The poisonous actions of mercury are usually associated with the mercuric ion, which these inorganic and organic materials furnish rapidly or slowly. Alkyl and some other organic mercurials, however, may have toxic effects due to the parent compound. Acute poisoning is perhaps the major threat in the home and on the farm, but, because mercury is a cumulative poison, subacute and chronic intoxications are recognized, particularly in industry.

Toxicology of inorganic mercury salts: One of the commonest and most toxic salts of mercury is mercuric chloride ($HgCl_2$), commonly known as bichloride of mercury or corrosive sublimate. The oral LD_{50} is 10 mg./kg. in mice and 37 mg./kg. in rats. Human fatalities have resulted from as little as 0.5 gm. by mouth, although the mean lethal dose in adults probably lies between 1 and 4 gm. The alimentary effects of many mercury compounds (notably mercuric chloride) are so rapid that the course and prognosis are determined largely by events within the first 10 to 15 minutes, particularly by the intervention of vomiting or a therapeutic lavage.

Acute systemic mercurialism may end fatally within a few minutes, but death (in uremia) is usually delayed 5 to 12 days.

Ionizable mercuric salts like mercuric chloride are corrosive. When ingested, necrosis begins immediately in the mouth, throat, esophagus, and stomach. Within a few minutes violent pain, profuse vomiting and severe purging are experienced, and the patient may die within a few hours from peripheral vascular collapse secondary to fluid and electrolyte losses (Augustine, 1956; Lowe, 1959). If the patient survives this phase, the primary gastroenteritis usually subsides spontaneously within a few days, but severe hemorrhagic colitis has occurred as late as 9 days following ingestion (Sanchez-Sicillia et al., 1963).

A second phase, developing within 1 to 3 days after the exposure, is characterized by stomatitis, membranous colitis, and tubular nephritis (nephrosis). This second phase, which is seen even with noncorrosive preparations of mercury and is independent of the portal of entry, is associated with a slow and prolonged excretion of mercury by the salivary glands, the gastrointestinal mucosa, and the kidneys. Death in this phase is usually the result of complete renal failure (Troen et al., 1951).

Mental and nervous symptoms are uncommon in acute mercurialism, in contrast to chronic mercury poisoning (Breiger and Rieders, 1959), but central nervous system involvement is common with some organic mercury compounds (see below). Ultrastructural changes have been described in rat hepatocytes (Desnoyers and Chang, 1975), but mercury is not usually a significant hepatotoxin. Sometimes a nephrotic syndrome is the major or sole indication of mercury intoxication, particularly after chronic exposure (e.g., Cook and Yates, 1969). In some instances it has been ascribed to an allergic response (Becker et al., 1962; Kazantzis et al., 1962), but direct nephrotoxic actions are well known.

The primary renal lesion in acute mercurialism appears to be a generalized increase in the permeability of the tubular epithelium. Transient polyuria and then anuria are regarded as consequences of the permeability change. It has been suggested that the anuria is due to complete resorption of tubular fluid because of the colloid oncotic pressure of peritubular fluid, not because of tubular blockade (Bank et al., 1967; Gottlieb and Coye, 1962; Rodin and Crowson, 1962). In dogs, however, the proximal convoluted tubules may become so filled with the cytoplasmic debris of sloughed epithelial cells that the back pressure can lead to a cessation of filtration (Baehler et al., 1977).

Some metabolic changes in rat kidney after acute renal failure induced by mercuric chloride suggest that the metal may have a direct effect on mitochondrial electron transport (Trifillis et al., 1981). Kidney uptake of mercury is markedly enhanced by excess cysteine, and the uptake of mercuric cysteine is slowed by an excess of histidine or lysine, suggesting that the metal complex is actively transported (Richardson et al., 1975a). Rats were shown to acquire resistance to mercuric chloride nephrotoxicity, but cross-resistance to other nephrotoxic agents (potassium chromate, biphenyl, hexachloro-1,3-butadiene) did not occur (Kluwe, 1982). Conversely, pretreatment with sodium chromate, p-aminophenol, sodium maleate or uranyl acetate in doses sufficient to cause renal damage offered protection against mercury renal damage. These effects were not related to the renal contents of metallothionein or mercury (Tandon et al., 1980).

In pregnant women absorbed ionic mercury is also a hazard to the fetus, but most reported fetal poisonings have been traced to mercury vapor (see elemental mercury below) or to organic mercurials, especially methyl mercury (Koos and Longo, 1976). In animal tests all forms of mercury have proven to be teratogenic. Many mercury compounds (including mercuric chloride in concentrations of 1 to 5%) are irritating to the skin and may produce dermatitis with or without vesication. Contact with the eyes causes ulceration of the conjunctiva and cornea.

Absorbed ionic mercury is excreted primarily in urine and feces (Friberg and Vostal, 1972). Although not a major mechanism for its metabolism or excretion, reductive pathways in animals and presumably in man are capable of converting Hg^{2+} to the free metal, which can be excreted in the expired breath. A dose-dependent increase in this conversion was observed after ethanol in mice, as evidenced by a 10-fold increase in the expired mercury vapor (Dunn et al., 1981). The converse reaction is also well established, and at least part of an absorbed dose of elemental mercury vapor is oxidized to the mercuric ion (see below).

Toxicology of elemental mercury: Metallic mercury (quicksilver) constitutes a special case among mercury compounds because dangerous symptoms are commonly encountered only after inhalation of the vapor. Liquid mercury is absorbed through the intact skin of man and animals, but no quantitative estimates of the rate of penetration appear to be available (Friberg and Vostal, 1972). In most cases of poisonings allegedly due to percutaneous exposure, inhalation cannot be ruled out as the major route of mercury entry. Only small amounts of mercury are absorbed after the oral administration of the liquid metal to rats (Bornmann et al., 1970). The accidental release of large quantities of metallic mercury into the gastrointestinal tract during surgical manipulations produced no more serious reaction than nonpersistent fistulous tracts (Cantor, 1951). In an exceptional case, however, a preexisting small bowel fistula apparently allowed mercury to accumulate in retroperitoneal tissues, where conditions may have been more favorable for oxidation of Hg^0 to Hg^{2+}. The patient died with signs like those seen in systemic poisonings by mercuric salts (Bredfeldt and Moeller, 1978). In most cases broken glass is the chief hazard associated with the accidental biting of mercury thermometers.

In a case of intravenous self-administration of liquid mercury, pulmonary embolization terminated life before there were signs of systemic intoxication (Conrad et al., 1957). In several other cases, however, one involving intravenous injection of as much as 20 ml., the systemic signs and symptoms of malaise, pleuritic chest pain and shortness of breath resolved quickly, and hypoxemia and respiratory alkalosis were no longer apparent at the end of a week (Celli and Khan, 1976). Embolization is also a potential hazard of accidents during some cardiac catheterization procedures (Buxton et al., 1965). Mercury depots are clearly and bizarrely visible on X-ray (Schulz and Beskind, 1960; Teitelbaum and Ott, 1969; Vas et al., 1980) over periods of years without signs of systemic intoxication (Ambre et al., 1977; Chitakara et al., 1978). It has been suggested, however, that such deposits in the lung fields may also arise from aspiration of ingested liquid mercury (Stanojevich and Kostitch, 1968). Rupture of a mercury filled bag on the end of an intestinal tube resulted in aspiration and mercury deposits that were visible on X-ray for 22 years (Dzau et al., 1977).

Respiratory exposure to mercury vapor results in high initial concentrations in the lungs (Kudsk, 1965; Teisinger and Fiserova-Bergerova, 1965). Most of this lung burden is absorbed rapidly, but a small depot is absorbed slowly (Berlin et al., 1969a; Gage, 1961; Hayes and Rothstein, 1962). High concentrations exist transiently in brain and probably explain the preponderance of central nervous system signs, as opposed to renal damage, seen after this route of exposure (Berlin and Johansson, 1964; Magos, 1968a). Indeed, some evidence suggests that mercury penetrates into the nervous system primarily as the elemental form (Berlin et al., 1969b; Magos, 1967, 1968a). The kidneys, however, eventually accumulate the greatest share of the total body burden (Hayes and Rothstein, 1962), presumably because atomically dispersed mercury is oxidized to ionic mercury rather promptly. A large share (98%) of mercury vapor in blood is concentrated in the red cells, where it may be gradually oxidized to Hg^{2+} and then released into the plasma, so that the red cell-to-plasma ratio falls to about 2 within 20 hours (Cherian et al., 1978). (Many organomercurials follow a similar pattern of distribution and redistribution in blood.) It has been alleged that

after a respiratory exposure to mercury vapor appreciable amounts of mercury are excreted in sweat (Sunderman, 1978).

A unique reaction occurs on massive vapor exposures as in confined spaces or on heating the liquid, namely acute pulmonary edema (Burke and Quagliana, 1963; Campbell, 1948; Matthes et al., 1958; Milne et al., 1970; Natelson et al., 1971; Snodgrass et al., 1981a; Tennant et al., 1961). In fatal cases diffuse interstitial pneumonitis with profuse fibrinous exudation was observed at autopsy. If the exposure is not fatal, recovery from the acute illness usually occurs over several days to weeks with only mild exertional dyspnea and a dry cough persisting for longer periods (Hallee, 1969; Moutinho et al., 1981; Seaton and Bishop, 1978). Perhaps this acute lung reaction is auto-protective since renal sequelae and central nervous system involvement were absent in survivors. See also NITROGEN OXIDES (p. III-323 and pp. IV-14–16) for management of pulmonary complications.

Most human exposures to mercury vapor, however, are mild but prolonged. In these cases pulmonary symptoms are rare, and significant pulmonary lesions do not occur. The hazard here is the accumulation of enough mercury in various organs and tissues to produce chronic mercury poisoning.

Chronic mercury poisoning: Long-term, low-level exposure to mercury vapor is a common hazard in varous industries and among dentists. The inhalation of dusts of inorganic mercuric salts is also an occupational hazard in some industrial plants. Whether the exposure is to elemental or ionic mercury, or even to organomercurials that breakdown in vivo to release the mercuric ion (see aryl and alkoxyalkyl mercury below), chronic mercurialism is believed to express itself in the same diverse ways; only alkyl mercury poisoning is clinically distinctive (see below). Even the portal of entry does not influence significantly the nature of the symptom complex, unless the daily dose is large enough to provoke an acute reaction. If enough mercury is retained in the body after a large single dose, the signs and symptoms of chronic mercury poisoning may appear gradually as the victim recovers from his acute injuries, but this sequence is uncommon today.

The predominant manifestations are neurologic. The violent gastrointestinal reactions elicited in acute poisonings are absent, but excessive salivation (ptyalism), anorexia, digestive disturbances, vague abdominal distress and mild diarrhea are common. Renal involvement is usually absent or mild, although a few, possibly hypertensive individuals develop nephrosis, i.e., intense proteinuria without azotemia (Becker et al., 1962). Peripheral neuropathies are described (e.g., Hryhorczuk et al., 1982; Levine et al., 1982); in one patient it was the only sign of mercurialism (Iyer *et al.*, 1976). Both motor and sensory nerves may be affected, with numbness and weakness but rarely complete paralysis or muscle atrophy. Sometimes muscle fasciculations and pain with or without tenderness have been described. The central nervous system, however, is the principal target of damage.

Tremors are frequently encountered; they typically involve the hands and fingers, less often eyelids, lips, cheeks, tongue and legs, and they are usually fine (but later coarse and irregular), bilateral and exaggerated by intention (Neal and Jones, 1938). Tendon reflexes may be hypo- or hyperactive. Various forms of motor control may become impaired (slurred or scanning speech, ataxic gait). Ptosis and visual disturbances are reported occasionally, but only rarely (*e.g.*, Hryhorczuk *et al.*, 1982) has constriction of the visual fields been ascribed to any form of mercurialism except that induced by alkyl mercury (see below). Deafness and other sensory losses are sometimes reported (Wustner *et al.*, 1975).

At least as common as tremors in chronic mercury poisoning is a syndrome known as erethism. It has long been recognized and associated with occupational exposures to mercury (Neal and Jones, 1938; Smith, 1978). Erethism consists of subtle or dramatic changes in behavior and personality: depression, despondency, fearfulness, restlessness, irritability, irascibility, timidity, indecision, and easy embarrassment. These psychic and behavioral characteristics are often accompanied by insomnia, drowsiness, headache and fatigue. In advanced cases, memory loss, hallucinations and mental deterioration may occur. It is alleged that Sir Isaac Newton went mad for a period of 1 year while engaged heavily in alchemy. Recent analyses of samples of his hair showed high concentrations of mercury (Broad, 1981).

In addition to ptyalism, a metallic taste is a common complaint. Gingivitis of various grades has often been described; in advanced cases it led to "pyorrhea" and the loosening of teeth. Other occasional manifestations of mucosal inflammation include stomatitis, pharyngitis, conjunctivitis and otitis. A dark, bluish line may appear along the gingival margins (Neal and Jones, 1938). It is less common and less impressive than a characteristic discoloration of the anterior lens surface, known as mercurialentis, which is a diagnostically useful sign of chronic mercury exposure (Atkinson, 1943; Parameshvara, 1967). Skin signs include abnormal blushing, dermatographia, excessive sweating and irregular erythematous or macular rashes. Because of anorexia, painful mouth and digestive disorders, victims of advanced mercurialism may be pale and cachectic, according to descriptions in the older literature.

Acrodynia: Subacute or chronic mercurialism occasionally manifests itself by an uncommon syndrome known as acrodynia (Warkany and Hubbard, 1948; 1953). Infantile acrodynia was first described in 1828, but many adult cases have been reported since. It is also called "pink disease" because of the color of the extremities. The manifestations include apathy, anorexia, flush, fever, a nephrotic syndrome with albuminuria and generalized edema, diaphoresis, photophobia, insomnia and most characteristically a pruritic and sometimes painful scaling or peeling of the skin of the hands and feet with bullous lesions. Atypical cases of unknown etiology but apparently not due to mercury are also recognized. The term, acrodynia, is also used for the condition in rats caused by pyridoxine (vitamin B_6) deficiency, which has some features in common with the acrodynia of mercurialism.

Most early cases were associated with the use of insoluble mercurous chloride (calomel) as a laxative or diuretic (Bivings and Lewis, 1948; Cheek, 1960; Clements, 1960; Warkany and Hubbard, 1948). However, the syndrome has also been induced by exposure to metallic mercury (Alexander and Rosario, 1971; Johnson *et al.*, 1978), ammoniated mercury (Snaiman and Flagler, 1971), mercurial antiseptics such as merbromin and thiomersal (Matheson *et al.*, 1980; Yeh *et al.*, 1978), alkoxyalkyl mercury fungicides (Prediger, 1976) and a phenylmercury fungicide in paint (Hirschman *et al.*, 1963).

Urinary mercury levels are characteristically low in acrodynia, suggesting a hypersensitivity reaction. Increased excretion of catecholamines and other signs of sympathetic nervous system dysfunction often accompany the disease (Hirschman *et al.*, 1963). In the case reported by Johnson *et al.* (1978), the disease was thought to have an autoimmune basis; it was accompanied by a profound neutropenia and terminated fatally. In describing a congenitally agammaglobulinemic adult who had received γ-globulin injections for 15 years, Matheson *et al.* (1980) pointed out that most available globulin preparations contain thiomersal as a bacteriostatic agent. In a case reported by Yeh *et al.* (1978) a neonate had been treated with local applications of merbromin for only 5 days.

Although some favorable responses have been reported, the value of BAL is not established in acrodynia (Bivings and Lewis, 1948; Warkany and Hubbard, 1953). Two cases appeared to respond favorably to *N*-acetyl-D,L-penicillamine (Aronow and Fleischmann, 1976; Hirschman *et al.*, 1963), with transient improvement in another (Johnson *et al.*, 1978). Fortunately, in most cases recovery follows spontaneously when the exposure is terminated. Furthermore, acrodynia has become exceedingly uncommon since mercurial ointments and other medicinal forms of mercury are no longer used in pediatrics.

Toxicology of aryl and alkoxyalkyl mercury: These two classes of organomercurials are rather similar in terms of toxicity, instability *in vivo*, tissue distribution, retention and excretion; they differ markedly from alkyl mercury compounds discussed below (Swensson and Ulfvarson, 1963). In the aryl mercurials, mercury is joined by a Hg-to-carbon bond to an aromatic ring such as benzene, toluene, phenol, cresol, nitrophenol, etc. The commonest examples are phenylmercuric salts of inorganic acids (*e.g.*, hydrochloric, nitric, boric, etc.) or of organic acids (*e.g.*, acetate, salicylate, oleate, benzoate, etc.). Phenylmercuric salts are widely employed in agriculture. For example, seeds treated with them to prevent fungal growth and then fed to hens led to the production of mercury-contaminated eggs (Englander *et al.*, 1980). Various alkoxyalkyl mercurials such as methoxyethylmercuric chloride and acetate are also used as agricultural fungicides. Several alkoxyalkyl compounds of mercury long served in medicine as mercurial diuretics; they have, however, been discarded for this purpose.

In terms of acute LD_{50} values in rats and mice, most organic mercury derivatives tested are somewhat less lethal than mercuric chloride (summarized by Friberg and Vostal, 1972). For example, the oral LD_{50} of phenylmercuric acetate is reported to be 22 mg.(of Hg)/kg. in rats and 26 in mice. On the other hand, the oral LD_{50} of methoxyethyl mercury acetate is only 10 to 16 mg. (of Hg)/kg. in rats, which is less than the reported LD_{50} of mercuric chloride. Phenylmercuric acetate is known to be well absorbed through all portals, including intact skin.

Signs and symptoms in acutely poisoned men and test animals have not been adequately described. Local irritant effects are well established, such as dermatitis and burns from skin exposures to phenylmercuric salts (Goldwater *et al.*, 1964; Ladd *et al.*, 1964). Blistering has occurred when methoxyethyl mercury acetate was applied to the skin in high concentrations, and pulmonary symptoms have arisen when methoxyethyl mercury oxalate or silicate was inhaled (Friberg and Vostal, 1972). In terms of systemic effects the only well documented acute reaction is sudden death during intravenous mercurial diuretic therapy (Barker *et al.*, 1942; DeGraff and Nadler, 1942). Most of these deaths were ascribed to cardiac arrest or ventricular fibrillation, but rarely respiratory failure was observed without cardiac manifestations. Hypersensitivity reactions have also been reported (Ladd *et al.*, 1964).

No unequivocal central neural effects have been recognized in acute exposures. Even an attempted suicide with phenyl mercury is said to have elicited no significant neurological signs (Ishida, 1970, as cited by Hayes, 1982). The same was true of a suicidal ingestion of 5.7 gm. of methoxyethyl mercury chloride, which elicited

vomiting and chemical burns of the mouth and throat but little else (Köppel *et al.*, 1982). Most intoxications by aryl and alkoxyalkyl mercury, however, have not been detected until after repeated or continuous exposures of long duration. Even then, the number of reported poisonings, aside from skin rashes, is remarkably low (Ladd *et al.*, 1964).

In subacute and chronic poisonings and probably sometimes in the late stages of acute poisonings, these organomercurials appear to produce intoxication syndromes that are in practice indistinguishable from those induced by inorganic mercury. For example, renal damage has been reported in rats and mice given repeated parenteral doses of phenylmercuric salts and of alkoxyalkyl mercurials. Death in renal failure, as well as the production of a nephrotic syndrome, has been ascribed to mercurial diuretics (Freeman *et al.*, 1962; Robillard *et al.*, 1976; Scott, 1964; Wallner and Herman, 1950). Nephrosis also appeared in a 60-year-old man who for 5 years had handled grain treated with methoxyethyl mercury silicate (Strunge, 1970). A 5-year-old boy exposed to a methoxyethyl mercury seed disinfectant developed acrodynia (Prediger, 1976). As in chronic inorganic mercury poisoning, neurological signs (tremor, motor and sensory nerve disorders) have been detected in a few individuals chronically exposed to these forms of organic mercury (Friberg and Vostal, 1972; Hayes, 1982). A 39-year-old farmer who had used no precautions in dusting oat seeds with phenylmercuric acetate over a period of 5 to 6 years and who excreted large amounts of mercury in the urine died of an apparently progressive neurologic disease resembling amyotrophic lateral sclerosis (Brown, 1954). Five other farmers similarly exposed were said to have various motor disabilities.

That the syndromes of chronic intoxication induced by inorganic mercury and by many organic mercurials are very similar is probably explained by the rapid metabolic breakdown of these mercurials to the mercuric ion. For example, studies on the fate and excretion of phenylmercuric acetate in rats, dogs and chicks indicate that phenyl mercury is absorbed intact from many portals, transported largely in red blood cells, metabolized in the liver and perhaps elsewhere to release inorganic mercury, which in the rat is excreted mostly in feces (Daniel and Gage, 1971; Miller *et al.*, 1960). Within 2 to 4 days, essentially all of the phenyl mercury was broken down. Hydroxylation of the phenyl ring was thought to precede rupture of the carbon-to-mercury bond; hydroxyphenyl mercury compounds decompose spontaneously in the presence of acid and cysteine or BAL (Canty and Kishimoto, 1975; Daniel and Gage, 1971). Methoxyethyl mercury salts and at least some of the mercurial diuretics may be even more labile. In rats subcutaneously injected methoxyethyl mercury chloride decomposed (either spontaneously or enzymatically) with a half-time of about 1 day to release inorganic mercury that largely migrated to the kidneys and was eventually excreted (Daniel et al., 1971).

Perhaps because these various forms of organic mercury are so rapidly converted to inorganic mercury, they do not appear to cross the blood-brain barrier appreciably. Thus, shortly after single exposures the brains of laboratory mammals contain much less mercury than do other organs and tissues; kidneys and liver accumulate the major burden (Berlin and Ullberg, 1963a–c; Gage, 1964; Swensson and Ulfvarson, 1967; Takeda et al., 1968). With time the retained mercury is redistributed, so that the blood/brain concentration ratio falls toward 1.0 (Friberg and Vostal, 1972). As with inorganic salts of mercury, repeated exposure to these organomercurials causes slow but progressive increases in brain levels of mercury.

Toxicology of alkyl mercury: Methyl, ethyl, n-propyl and perhaps n-butyl mercury derivatives (Takeda et al., 1968) are virulent neurotoxins on either acute or chronic exposure (e.g., Okinaka et al., 1964). They are especially hazardous because of their volatility, their ability to penetrate epithelial and blood-brain barriers and their persistence in vivo. Methyl mercury was absorbed 15 to 35 times more rapidly from ligated segments of the rat gastrointestinal tract than was mercuric chloride (Sasser et al., 1978). The mean half-life in man is 65 days, but the range was 40 to 105 days (Bakir et al., 1973). By contrast, mercury in the form of phenylmercuric salts (above) is much safer because phenylmercurials are less volatile, much less able to enter the brain, much more readily metabolized and so more rapidly excreted.

Toxic encephalopathy of epidemic proportions with high mortality occurred as a result of the ingestion of sea foods obtained from Minamata Bay in Japan (Minamata disease) (Tsubaki and Irukayama, 1977). The waters were highly polluted with industrial wastes containing mercury compounds (Matsumoto et al., 1965). Ionic mercury is readily methylated by microorganisms in detritus and sediments under bodies of water. After methylation the mercury enters into and is concentrated in natural food chains. Minamata disease is characterized by progressive muscular weakness, loss of vision, paralysis, coma and death. More than 100 persons died or suffered severe neurologic damage and 17 babies were born in the area with infantile cerebral palsy. A milder outbreak occurred among fish-eating Indians and Inuits in Ontario (Wheatley et al., 1979).

In Iraq consumption of seed grain treated with methyl mercury fungicides resulted in more than 6,500 hospital admissions and 500 deaths (Clarkson et al., 1976). Patients exhibited paresthesias of hands and feet and around the mouth, dysarthria, ataxia, concentric constriction of visual fields (tunnel vision) and hearing loss (Bakir et al., 1973). Three members of a family in Almagordo, New Mexico, were similarly afflicted after consumption of pork from swine that had been fed methyl mercury treated grain (Pierce et al., 1972). Thus methyl mercury is seen to pass through food chains unchanged (Snyder and Seelinger, 1976).

Not only does methyl mercury readily cross the placenta (Koos and Longo, 1976), but suckling infants may acquire high levels via breast milk (Amin-Zaki et al., 1976). In a group of 32 infants exposed prenatally, there were 9 cases of cerebral palsy. Although the mothers usually improved, damage to the fetal nervous system may be permanent. After 5 years developmental retardation, exaggerated tendon reflexes and pathologic extensor plantar reflexes (minimal brain damage syndrome) were still apparent (Amin-Zaki et al., 1979). In children poisoned after birth the degree of recovery was related to the severity of the intoxication. Children with mild to moderate poisoning slowly but steadily improved. All had residual general hyperreflexia. Ataxia and motor weakness disappeared in some but visual changes improved less completely. Of 17 children who were blind, only 5 recovered partial sight. Almost half of a severely poisoned group were left physically and mentally incapacitated (Amin-Zaki et al., 1978). In a few cases the neuromuscular disorder was said to respond well to neostigmine (Rustam et al., 1975).

In man the effects of methyl mercury are critically dependent on the dose, i.e., the dose-response curve appears to be very steep. Paresthesias are associated with an estimated total body burden of 40 mg., whereas death occurred at an estimated 200 mg. (Bakir et al., 1973). Given by mouth as single doses to animals, however, mercuric chloride is more toxic than methyl mercury, although both fall into toxicity class 5 (Clarkson, 1972).

Given by mouth to healthy volunteers the radiolabel of methyl mercury (^{203}Hg) accumulated in the liver (half the total dose) and in the head (10% of the dose). It was excreted primarily in the feces, but urinary excretion increased with time up to 30 days (Aberg et al., 1969). In the blood it is largely bound to red cells or hemoglobin (Lundgren et al., 1967). In the victims of Minamata disease mercury was widely distributed. Residual deposits were readily detected in the kidneys, liver and reticuloendothelial system, with lesser but detectable amounts in the thyroid, adrenal glands, spermatocytes of testis, pancreas and skin. It tended to accumulate more slowly in nervous tissue and to remain there for longer periods of time (Okabe and Takeuchi, 1980). A correlation was noted between the concentration of mercury in maternal hair and the severity of intoxication both in mothers and in the children delivered from them (Amin-Zaki *et al.*, 1979; Marsh *et al.*, 1981). In two fatal cases involving ethyl mercury in Iraq, 8 to 10 ppm were found in the kidney, 6 to 7 ppm in liver, 3 to 5 ppm in cerebellum and 15 ppm in blood (Hilmy *et al.*, 1976).

Remarkable species differences are recognized in methyl mercury poisoning; sheep and hens, for example, do not respond with neurologic signs (Hilmy *et al.*, 1978). Age is a significant factor in toxicity in humans; transplacental intoxication may be the worst and younger children are more susceptible than older ones (Snyder and Seelinger, 1976). Young rats are more susceptible than those 18 days of age, and the increased toxicity is associated with a decreased whole body clearance (Thomas *et al.*, 1982). The long half-life in neonatal rats appears to be due to an impaired ability to secrete mercury (perhaps in the form of a glutathione complex) into bile, which is a major route of elimination in adults (Ballatori and Clarkson, 1982). When rat tissues were depleted of glutathione by pretreatment with diethyl maleate, mercury deposition in kidney, red cells and to a lesser extent brain was also decreased (Richardson and Murphy, 1975). In mice, however, older animals were said to be more susceptible, and males were more susceptible than females. Toxicity was also greater at low ambient temperatures (Nomiyama *et al.*, 1980) and when alcohol was consumed concurrently in the drinking water (Takahashi *et al.*, 1978).

Methyl mercury has effects on brain neurotransmitters (Taylor and DiStefano, 1976) and on the enzymes which synthesize them (Tsuzuki, 1981). Protein synthesis is inhibited in both brain and liver (Omata *et al.*, 1978; 1980). As studied in human fetal neurons and astrocytes in tissue culture, damage to plasma membranes and neurotubular injury are early features of methyl mercury toxicity. These changes occur more readily in neurons than in astrocytes, but eventually irreversible degeneration occurs in both cell types (Choi *et al.*, 1981). These degenerative changes presumably underlie the clinical syndrome of amyotrophic lateral sclerosis, which has been documented in 11 individuals in Iraq who consumed bread prepared from wheat treated with the seed disinfectant Granosan M (Kantarjian, 1961).

Forms of treatment: Extensive clinical experience with dimercaprol (BAL) has established it as the antidote of choice in acute poisonings due to inorganic mercury salts, where the critical target organ is usually the kidneys (Longcope and Leutscher, 1946; Swensson and Ulfvarson, 1967). When introduced in 1945–1946, it made obsolete an earlier antidote that had enjoyed some success, namely sodium formaldehyde sulfoxylate (Rosenthal, 1935; Wolpaw and Alpers, 1942).

BAL is maximally effective when given early in the course of an acute episode and is often lifesaving under those circumstances. In general, it enhances the renal excretion of mercury, and it usually (but not always) decreases the amount of metal retained in the kidney (Gabard, 1976b; Swensson and Ulfvarson, 1967). In some cases it also promotes the fecal excretion of mercury (Longcope and Leutscher, 1946; Swensson and Ulfvarson, 1967), presumably because of the biliary secretion of the BAL-mercury complex. Probably the complex can be resorbed in the bowel (enterohepatic cycling), which could explain why BAL does not always increase the mercury content of feces (Gabard, 1976b). When injected in rats shortly after an injection of mercuric chloride, BAL caused a small increase in the brain content of mercury (Magos, 1968b), but when begun a few hours later, a 5-day course of BAL therapy led to lower mercury levels in the brains of treated animals than of untreated controls (Gabard, 1976b). Caution is indicated with BAL therapy in cases of acute renal insufficiency, where it may aggravate the renal damage or manifest its own toxicity (see p. III-50) (Doolan *et al.*, 1953). Because of the biliary excretory route, however, renal failure is not an absolute contraindication to BAL therapy.

BAL is much less effective in acrodynia and in chronic mercurialism, where the brain is the critically diseased organ. Although it often provokes an increase in urinary mercury, the rise is usually small in terms of the estimated body burden, and the clinical improvement, if any, is typically marginal (Battigelli, 1960). The same is often true of other chelating agents, such as D-penicillamine and its *N*-acetyl isomers (see below). A trial course of therapy with one or another chelator is probably warranted, however, because some patients have experienced considerable improvement. Often a 10-day or 2-week course with D-penicillamine is followed by a rest period of 1 to 2 weeks and then a 7- to 10-day trial of BAL (or vice versa). With BAL (*e.g.*, Sunderman, 1978), D-penicillamine (Iyer *et al.*, 1976; Markowitz and Schaumburg, 1980), and *N*-acetyl-D,L-penicillamine (Aronow and Fleischmann, 1976; Smith and Miller, 1961), favorable clinical and biochemical responses have been charted. Even when cases of alkyl mercury poisoning are excluded, however, failures of chelation therapy probably outnumber successes in chronic mercurialism, although the contrary opinion has been expressed with respect to *N*-acetyl-D,L-penicillamine (Kark *et al.*, 1971).

Although BAL has also been used in treating acute pneumonitis due to the inhalation of mercury vapor in high concentrations (Tennant *et al.*, 1961), its efficacy for this purpose is not established. Because of the tendency for absorbed mercury vapor to enter the brain (Berlin and Johansson, 1964; Berlin *et al.*, 1969b) and for BAL therapy to increase mercury levels in the brain (Berlin and Lewander, 1965), the penicillamines (see below) are probably preferable to BAL as antidotes in acute vapor exposures (Snodgrass *et al.*, 1981). For the same two reasons (Berlin and Rylander, 1964), it is possible that BAL should be withheld in any acute poisoning due to a phenylmercuric salt. On the other hand BAL proved to be highly effective in protecting rats against the lethal actions of phenyl mercury hydroxide injected subcutaneously (Swensson and Ulfvarson, 1967). In the same study BAL accelerated the demise of rats given subcutaneous methoxyethyl mercury hydroxide. As noted above, clinical experience with these forms of organic mercury is too limited to settle the issue. Certainly BAL is not useful in methyl mercury poisoning (see below).

In contrast to BAL, D-penicillamine and *N*-acetyl-D,L-penicillamine are effective chelating agents when taken by mouth. In test animals and human patients they are useful in both acute (Aposhian and Aposhian, 1959; Swensson and Ulfvarson, 1967) and chronic mercurialism (*e.g.*, Hirschman *et al.*, 1963; Kark *et al.*, 1971; Smith and Miller, 1961). In view of the long history and widespread use of the penicillamines, it is disconcerting to learn that they have not received FDA approval as therapeutic agents in mercury poisoning and that *N*-acetyl-D,L-penicillamine is not even available in the United States as a pharmaceutical. There should be no hesitancy, however, about using these "orphan drugs" when indicated, and the acetyl derivative is available from the Aldrich Chemical Co. of Milwaukee, Wisconsin. These two penicillamines are usually used in the same dose (250 mg. every 6 hours, *i.e.*, 4 times daily); in this dose they are usually well tolerated. Perhaps the *N*-acetyl form is less toxic, but until more experience accumulates, one should assume that it can elicit all the toxic reactions reported after D-penicillamine (see latter in Section II).

As noted above, the penicillamines appear to be superior to BAL in treating acute poisoning by mercury vapor and chronic mercurialism of almost any form. Not yet established, however, is their antidotal effectiveness in acute poisonings by phenyl mercury or alkoxyalkyl mercury, and their value in alkyl mercury intoxication is equivocal. In acute poisonings due to the ingestion of inorganic salts of mercury, intramuscular BAL is far preferable to oral penicillamine for three reasons: vomiting may prevent retention of penicillamine; penicillamine may enhance the gastrointestinal absorption of mercury; and once absorbed, penicillamine is less successful than

BAL in preventing death, at least in rats given Hg^{2+} by parenteral routes (*e.g.*, Swensson and Ulfvarson, 1967). Furthermore, the penicillamines are probably contraindicated in the presence of a severe renal injury because they promote mercury excretion only by that route; unlike BAL, they do not enhance the biliary (fecal) excretion of the metal (Yonaga and Morita, 1981).

In some countries varous other sulfhydryl chelating agents have been tested and approved. D-Penicillamine, *N*-acetyl-D-penicillamine and 2,3-dimercaptosuccinic acid (DMSA), when given in equimolar doses to rats at 48 and 54 hours after mercuric chloride, were all able to reduce the mercury content of the kidneys, but DMSA was by far the most effective. Only DMSA significantly increased the urinary excretion of mercury (Tandon and Magos, 1980). Gabard (1976b) tested 15 chelating agents (not including DMSA) in rats and found that the most favorable effects on urinary excretion and organ content of mercury were obtained with sodium 2,3-dimercaptopropane-1-sulfonate (DMPS). Neither DMSA nor DMPS is presently an approved drug in the United States.

In spite of a few apparent clinical successes, edetate calcium disodium (p. III-163) is probably contraindicated in all forms of mercurialism (Glömme and Gustavson, 1959). Hemodialysis and peritoneal dialysis may be helpful in renal insufficiency, but they have little or no value for removing mercury, presumably because it is bound tightly to plasma and tissue proteins (Doolan *et al.*, 1953; Fishman *et al.*, 1948; Kahn *et al.*, 1977; Leumann and Brandenberg, 1977; Sanchez-Sicillia *et al.*, 1963). As noted below, however, dialysis techniques may be useful in conjunction with chelation therapy to remove some of the low molecular weight chelates of mercury.

Methyl and other alkyl derivatives of mercury pose more formidable problems in therapy than other mercurials because they are rapidly absorbed and penetrate quickly into the brain (Thomas and Smith, 1982). When given one day after three daily doses of methyl mercury in dogs or several days after methyl mercury in rats, BAL was less effective than D-penicillamine in preventing the occurrence of toxic signs (Zimmer and Carter, 1978; 1979). Other experimental evidence and clinical impressions (Engleson and Herner, 1952; Glömme and Gustavson, 1959; Lundgren and Swensson, 1960) suggest that BAL has only limited usefulness in alkyl mercury poisonings and may even exacerbate the nervous symptoms. In mice and pregnant rats given single doses of methyl mercury, *N*-acetyl-D,L-penicillamine was judged to be superior to D-penicillamine and several other sulfhydryl chelators in mobilizing mercury from various tissues (Aaseth, 1976; Aaseth *et al.*, 1976). BAL was not used in the Iraq epidemic but D-penicillamine was. The results were quite variable: dramatic falls in blood mercury levels occurred in some patients but not in others (Bakir *et al.*, 1973).

Both DMSA and DMPS appeared to be superior to other agents when tested under comparable conditions in methyl mercury poisoned animals (Aaseth and Friedheim, 1978; Gabard, 1976c; Planas-Bohne, 1981). DMSA was judged to be better than DMPS in removing mercury from the brains of poisoned mice (Aaseth and Friedheim, 1978), whereas DMPS was superior to DMSA in removing mercury from the kidneys (Gabard, 1976a; Planas-Bohne, 1981). In rats DMSA was effective in reversing toxic signs when given even as late as 5 days after methyl mercury (Magos *et al.*, 1978). In patients in the Iraq epidemic the mean half-life of methyl mercury was about 65 days. It decreased to 10 days in patients receiving DMPS whereas it was 17 to 26 days in patients treated with D-penicillamine or *N*-acetyl-D,L-penicillamine (Clarkson *et al.*, 1981).

A synthetic thiolated resin was also used in Iraqi victims to thwart the enterohepatic recycling of methyl mercury (Clarkson *et al.*, 1973). It decreased the plasma half-life in eight of these patients to 20 days. Other polymeric resins are in the developmental stages (Harbison *et al.*, 1977; Takahashi *et al.*, 1975).

In contrast to the experience with lead chelates, promising results have been obtained using a combination of chelation and extracorporeal hemodialysis. Perhaps the effort was successful because the chelator was infused into arterial blood just before it entered the dialyzer. Both the complex and the chelating agents (D-penicillamine, *N*-acetyl-D,L-penicillamine, cysteine and acetylcysteine) were found to be highly dialyzable, so that very little of the free chelator was returned to the systemic circulation (Kostyniak *et al.*, 1975). Rates of removal of methyl mercury from dogs were increased by a factor of 100 (Kostyniak *et al.*, 1977). This technique has been tried in at least two patients, one of whom was said to have shown considerable improvement (Al-Abbasi *et al.*, 1978). Although most of the experience has been accrued with cysteine, in dogs DMSA was superior to cysteine by a factor of about two (Kostyniak, 1982). Conventional hemodialysis after intramuscular injections of BAL was of little use in a victim of acute mercuric cyanide poisoning (Leumann and Brandenberger, 1977).

Symptomatology: (For information about respiratory exposures, chronic exposures and organomercurials, see text above.)

　A. *First phase after ingestion of inorganic mercury salts*

1. Burning pain, sense of constriction, and ashen discoloration of the mucous membrane in mouth and pharynx, occurring immediately after the ingestion of corrosive mercury salts.
2. Within a few minutes intense epigastric pain, followed by diffuse abdominal pain and associated with almost continuous vomiting of mucoid material, which frequently contains blood and shreds of mucous membrane.
3. Severe purging, with liquid, bloody feces and considerable tenesmus.
4. Metallic taste, excessive salivation and thirst.
5. A rapid, weak pulse; shallow breathing; pallor; prostration; collapse, and death.
6. Signs and symptoms listed above are not encountered with mercury compounds of low irritancy or with portals of entry other than the mouth. In these cases the first clinical evidence of poisoning may be phase 2 (see B).

　B. *Second phase.* If death does not intervene, phase 2 begins in 1 to 3 days in untreated cases (unless vomiting so effectively removed the poison that absorption was negligible).

1. The gastroenteritis described above tends to subside in about 36 hours under the influence of local treatment.
2. Mercurial stomatitis may (or may not) appear within 24 to 36 hours. It is characterized by a glossitis and ulcerative gingivitis. Salivation is marked (ptyalism). In chronic neglected cases severe infections, loosening of teeth, and necrosis of the jaw are major complications.
3. Necrosis of the renal tubules is evident within 2 to 3 days. In sequence the results are transient polyuria, albuminuria, cylindruria, hematuria, anuria, and eventual death associated with azotemia and renal acidosis, or recovery within 10 to 14 days.
4. Especially in untreated cases, a membranous colitis may first appear many days after the original exposure. It is evidenced by dysentery, tenesmus, ulceration of the colonic mucosa, and hemorrhage. Liver necrosis sometimes develops. In neglected cases collapse and death may occur weeks after the start of the illness.
5. Rarely neurologic signs and symptoms (*e.g.*, tremors, peripheral neuropathies) may appear late in the course of a slow convalescence after an acute exposure. In these atypical cases the syndrome of acute mercurialism is succeeded by that of chronic mercurialism (see text above).

Treatment: (Speed is imperative.)

1. As soon as possible, drink milk (with or without raw egg whites stirred into it) or a slurry of activated charcoal (see p. 1-4) to help precipitate mercury in the stomach.

2. Gastric lavage with tap water, milk, or 2 to 5% solution of sodium bicarbonate, unless spontaneous vomiting is intense and productive.

3. Administer through the lavage tube 0.5 to 1 oz. of sodium or magnesium sulfate in 6 to 8 oz. of water (unless spontaneous purging has already begun) and a slurry of activated charcoal.

4. Administer BAL (dimercaprol) intramuscularly as a 10% solution in oil. If given within 3 hours after ingestion, severe renal damage may be prevented. Dosage schedules are suggested in Table III-2 (p. III-52). See p. III-51 also for information about the clinical toxicity of BAL and for a discussion about the basis of the doses recommended. Collect urine before and after BAL therapy for mercury analyses.

5. Demulcents (*e.g.*, milk of magnesia, starch, bismuth subcarbonate) and analgetic drugs may be useful and necessary.

6. Because the BAL-mercury complex excreted in bile may be partly resorbed in the bowel, it is probably useful to administer activated charcoal every few hours, starting as soon as vomiting subsides.

7. Treat shock (peripheral vascular collapse) by correcting dehydration and electrolyte imbalances (see pp. IV-17 and 64–67).

8. If renal insufficiency develops, see p. IV-53 for the management of acute renal failure.

9. The maintenance of an adequate nutritional status (see p. IV-75) may be troublesome if stomatitis or colitis become severe or persistent.

10. If toxic signs or symptoms recur after an apparent recovery, another course of chelation therapy is warranted. BAL is still appropriate, but a trial with D-penicillamine or with N-acetyl-D,L-penicillamine may be preferable (see text above). Either penicillamine is given by mouth, usually with an empty stomach, in a dose of 250 mg. 4 times daily in adults or 10 mg./kg. 3 times daily in children, for 5 to 10 days. After the ingestion of inorganic mercury, BAL should always be used first. If chosen for a second course of chelation therapy, penicillamine should be withheld until ingested mercury is cleared out of the bowel.

11. Watch for late cicatricial gastric stenosis in those who survive the ingestion of corrosive mercuric salts (Gonzales *et al.*, 1962).

Laboratory:

1. Various methods are available for the quantitative analysis of mercury in blood, urine, feces and hair, but no reliable analytical procedure is simple. The degree of exposure and severity of symptoms are not highly correlated with mercury levels in tissues or excreta (Goldwater and Nicolau, 1966). Considerable overlap exists in the ranges of mercury found in the general population, in exposed asymptomatic individuals and in overtly ill patients. In the general population, excluding those with known exposures, mercury concentrations are said to range from <0.005 to 0.07 ppm in whole blood and from <0.001 to 0.22 ppm (but only rarely above 0.05) in urine (Hayes, 1982). Thus, an analytic value of more than 0.1 ppm (10 μg./dl.) in either blood or urine suggests an unusual exposure. Mercury accumulates in hair as the hair grows at its root; concentrations in newly formed hair average about 250 times greater than concurrent blood levels. Mean (or median) values of mercury in the hair of the general population range from 2 to 9 ppm. Although the intestinal tract is an important excretory route for mercury, apparently too few specimens of feces have been analyzed to establish normal limits.

2. Determination of β_2-microglobulins has been recommended as a useful test for evaluating renal tubular function (Pesce *et al.*, 1977).

3. Electroencephalographic changes may be correlated closely with the clinical state, particularly in methyl mercury intoxication (Brenner and Snyder, 1980).

References:

Aaseth, J. Mobilization of methyl mercury *in vivo* and *in vitro* using N-acetyl-DL-penicillamine and other complexing agents. Acta Pharmacol. Toxicol. *39*:289–301, 1976.

Aaseth, J.; Wannag, A.; Norseth, T. The effect of N-acetylated DL-penicillamine and DL-homocysteine Thiotactone on the mercury distribution in adult rats, rat foetuses and Macaca monkeys after exposure to methyl mercuric chloride. Acta Pharmacol. Toxicol. *39*:302–311, 1976.

Aaseth, J.; Friedheim, E. A. N. Treatment of methyl mercury poisoning in mice with 2,3-dimercaptosuccinic acid and other complexing thiols. Acta Pharmacol. Toxicol. *42*:248–252, 1978.

Aberg, B.; Ekman, L.; Falk, R.; Persson, G.; Snihs, J. O. Metabolism of methyl mercury (^{203}Hg) compounds in man. Arch. Environ. Health *19*:478-484, 1969.

Agate, J. N.; Buckell, M. Mercury poisoning from fingerprint photography; occupational hazard of policemen. Lancet *2*:451-453, 1949.

Al-Abbasi, A. H.; Kostyniak, P. J.; Clarkson, T. W. An extracorporeal complexing hemodialysis system for the treatment of methyl mercury poisoning. III. Clinical applications. J. Pharmacol. Exp. Ther. *207*:249–254, 1978.

Alexander, J. F.; Rosario, R. A case of mercury poisoning acrodynia in a child of 8. Can. Med. Assoc. J. *104*:929–930, 1971.

Ambre, J. J.; Welsh, M. J.; Svare, C. W. Intravenous elemental mercury injection: blood levels and excretion of mercury. Ann. Intern. Med. 87:451–453, 1977.

Amin-Zaki, L.; Elhassani, S.; Majeed, M. A.; Clarkson, T. W.; Doherty, R. A.; Greenwood, M. R.; Giovanoli-Jakubczak, T. Perinatal methylmercury poisoning in Iraq. Am. J. Dis. Child. 130:1070–1076, 1976.

Amin-Zaki, L.; Majeed, M. A.; Clarkson, T. W.; Greenwood, M. R. Methylmercury poisoning in Iraqi children: clinical observations over two years. Br. Med. J. 1:613–616, 1978.

Amin-Zaki, L.; Majeed, M. A.; Elhassani, S. B.; Clarkson, T. W.; Greenwood, M. R.; Doherty, R. A. Prenatal methyl-mercury poisoning—clinical observations over 5 years. Am. J. Dis. Child. 133:172–177, 1979.

Aposhian, H. V.; Aposhian, M. M. N-Acetyl-DL-penicillamine, a new oral protective agent against the lethal effects of mercuric chloride. J. Pharmacol. Exp. Ther. 126:131-135, 1959.

Aronow, R.; Fleischmann, L. E. Mercury poisoning in children. The value of N-acetyl-DL-penicillamine in a combined therapeutic approach. Clin. Pediatr. 15:936–945, 1976.

Atkinson, W. S. A colored reflex from the anterior capsule of the lens which occurs in mercurialism. Am. J. Ophthal. 26:685–688, 1943.

Augustine, J. R. Mercury bichloride (corrosive sublimate) poisoning. Can. Med. Assoc. J. 74:371-372, 1956.

Baehler, R. W.; Kotchen, T. A.; Burke, J. A.; Galla, J. H.; Bhathenia, D. Considerations on the pathophysiology of mercuric chloride-induced acute renal failure. J. Lab. Clin. Med. 90:330–340, 1977.

Bakir, F.; Damluji, S. F.; Amin-Zaki, L.; et al. . Methyl mercury poisoning in Iraq. Science 181:230-241, 1973.

Ballatou, N.; Clarkson, T. W. Developmental changes in the biliary excretion of methylmercury and glutathione. Science 216:61–63, 1982.

Bank, N.; Mutz, B. F.; Aynedjian, H. S. The role of "leakage" of tubular fluid in anuria due to mercury poisoning. J. Clin. Invest. 46:695-704, 1967.

Barker, M. H.; Lundberg, H. A.; Thomas, M. E. Sudden death and mercurial diuretics. J. A. M. A. 119:1001-1004, 1942.

Battigelli, M.C. Mercury toxicity from industrial exposures. A critical review of the literature, Part II. J. Occup. Med. 2:394–399, 1960.

Becker, C. G.; Becker, E. L.; Mahler, J. F.; Schreiner, G. E. Nephrotic syndrome after contact with mercury; a report of five cases, three after the use of ammoniated mercury ointment. Arch. Intern. Med. 110:178-186, 1962.

Berlin, M.; Fazackerley, J.; Nordberg, G. The uptake of mercury in the brains of mammals exposed to mercury vapor and to mercuric salts. Arch. Environ. Health 18:719-729, 1969b.

Berlin, M.; Johansson, L. G. Mercury in mouse brain after inhalation of mercury vapor and after intravenous injection of mercury salt. Nature 204:85-86, 1964.

Berlin, M.; Lewander, T. Increased brain uptake of mercury caused by 2,3-dimercaptopropanol (BAL) in mice given mercuric chloride. Acta Pharmacol. Toxicol. 22:1–7, 1965.

Berlin, M.; Nordberg, G. F.; Serenius, F. On the site and mechanism of mercury vapor resorption in the lung. Arch. Environ. Health 18:42-50, 1969a.

Berlin, M.; Rylander, R. Increased brain uptake of mercury induced by 2, 3-dimercaptopropanol (BAL) in mice exposed to phenylmercuric acetate. J. Pharmacol. Exp. Ther. 146:236-240, 1964.

Berlin, M.; Ullberg, S. Accumulation and retention of mercury in the mouse. I. An autoradiographic study after a single intravenous injection of mercuric chloride. Arch. Environ. Health 6:589-601, 1963a.

Berlin, M.; Ullberg, S. Accumulation and retention of mercury in the mouse. II. An autoradiographic comparison of phen-ylmercuric acetate with inorganic mercury. Arch. Environ. Health 6:602-609, 1963b.

Berlin, M.; Ullberg, S. Accumulation and retention of mercury in the mouse. III. An autoradiographic comparison of meth-ylmercuric dicyandiamide with inorganic mercury. Arch. Environ. Health 6:610-616, 1963c.

Bivings, L.; Lewis, G. Acrodynia: A new treatment with BAL.

J. Pediatr. 32:63-65, 1948.

Bornmann, G.; Henke, G.; Alfes, H.; Mollmann, H. Uber die enterale Resorption von metallischen. Quecksilber. Arch. Toxikol. 26:203-209, 1970.

Bredfeldt, J. E.; Moeller, D. D. Systemic mercury intoxication following rupture of a Miller-Abbott tube. Am. J. Gastroen-terol. 69:478–480, 1978.

Breiger, H.; Rieders, F. Contemporary views on ancient oc-cupational diseases, chronic lead and mercury poisoning. J. Chronic Dis. 9:177-184, 1959.

Brenner, R. P.; Snyder, R. D. Late EEG findings and clinical status after organic mercury poisoning. Arch. Neurol. 37:282–284, 1980.

Broad, W. J. Sir Isaac Newton: Mad as a hatter. Science 213:1341-1344, 1981.

Brown, I. A. Chronic mercurialism, a cause of the clinical syndrome of amyotrophic lateral sclerosis. Arch. Neurol. Psych. 72:674-681, 1954.

Burke, W. J.; Quagliana, J. M. Acute inhalation mercury intoxication. J. Occup. Med. 5:157-160, 1963.

Buxton, J. T., Jr.; Hewitt, C; Gadsden, R. H.; Bradham, G. B. Metallic mercury embolism. J. A. M. A. 193:573-575, 1965.

Campbell, J. S. Acute mercurial poisoning by inhalation of metallic vapor in an infant. Can. Med. Assoc. J. 58:72-75, 1948.

Cantor, M. O. Mercury lost in the gastrointestinal tract. Re-port of an unusual case. J. A. M. A. 146:560-561, 1951.

Canty, A. J.; Kishimoto, R. British anti-Lewisite and organo-mercury poisoning. Nature 253:123-125, 1975.

Celli, B.; Khan, M. A. Mercury embolization of the lung. N. Engl. J. Med. 295:883-885, 1976.

Cheek, D. B. On the nature of pink disease. Med. J. Aust. 1:153-155, 1960.

Cherian, M. G.; Hursh, J. B.; Clarkson, T. W.; Allen, J. Radioactive mercury distribution in biological fluids and excretion in human subjects after inhalation of mercury vapor. Arch. Environ. Health 33:109–114, 1978.

Chitkara, R.; Seriff, N. S.; Kinas, H. Y. Intravenous self-administration of metallic mercury in attempted suicide – report of a case with serial roentgenographic and physio-logic studies over an 18-month period. Chest 73:234–236, 1978.

Choi, B. H.; Cho, K. H.; Lapham, L. W. Effects of methylmer-cury on human fetal neurons and astrocytes in vitro: a time-lapse cinematographic and electron microscopic study. En-viron. Res. 24:61–74, 1981.

Clarkson, T. W. Recent advances in the toxicology of mercury with emphasis on the alkyl mercurials. C. R. C. Critical Rev. Toxicol. 1:203-234, 1972.

Clarkson, T. W.; Small, H.; Norseth, T. Excretion and absorp-tion of methyl mercury after polythiol resin treatment. Arch. Environ. Health 26:173-176, 1973.

Clarkson, T. W.; Amin-Zaki, L.; Al-Tikriti, S. K. An outbreak of methylmercury poisoning due to consumption of contam-inated grain. Fed. Proc. 35:2395–2399, 1976.

Clarkson, T. W.; Magos, L.; Cox, C.; Greenwood, M. R.; Amin-Zaki, L.; Majeed, M. A.; Al-Damleeji, S. F. Tests of efficacy of antidotes for removal of methylmercury in human poi-soning during the Iraq outbreak. J. Pharmacol. Exp. Ther. 218:74–83, 1981.

Clements, F. W. The rise and decline of pink disease. Med. J. Aust. 1:922-925, 1960.

Conrad, M. E., Jr.; Sanford, J. P.; Preston, J. A. Metallic mercury embolization - clinical and experimental. Arch. Intern. Med. 100:59-65, 1957.

Cook, T. A.; Yates, P. O. Fatal mercury intoxication in a dental surgery assistant. Br. Dent. J. 127:553-555, 1969.

Daniel, J. W.; Gage, J. C. The metabolism by rats of phenyl-mercury acetate. Biochem. J. 122:24P, 1971.

Daniel, J. W.; Gage, J. C.; Lefevre, P. A. The metabolism of methoxyethylmercury salts. Biochem. J. 121:411–415, 1971.

Davis, R. G. Hazards of tattooing. Report of two cases of dermatitis caused by sensitization to mercury (cinnabar). U. S. Armed Forces Med. J. 11:261-280, 1960.

DeGraff, A. C.; Nadler, J. E. A review of the toxic manifesta-tions of mercurial diuretics in man. J. A. M. A. 119:1006-1011, 1942.

Desnoyers, P. A.; Chang, L. W. Ultrastructural changes in rat hepatocytes following acute mercury intoxication. Environ. Res. *9*:224–239, 1975.

Doolan, P. D.; Hess, W. C.; Kyle, L. H. Acute renal insufficiency due to bichloride of mercury. Observations on gastrointestinal hemorrhage and BAL therapy. N. Engl. J. Med. *249*:273-276, 1953.

Dunn, J. D.; Clarkson, T. W.; Magos, L. Interaction of ethanol and inorganic mercury: Generation of mercury vapor *in vivo*. J. Pharmacol. Exp. Ther. *216*:19–23, 1981.

Dzau, V. J.; Szabo, S.; Chang, Y. C. Aspiration of metallic mercury. A 22-year follow-up. J.A.M.A. *238*:1531–1532, 1977.

Englender, S. J.; Landrigan, P. J.; Greenwood, M. R.; Atwood, R. G.; Clarkson, T. W.; Smith, J. C. Organic mercury exposure from fungicide-contaminated eggs. Arch. Environ. Health *35*:224–228, 1980.

Engleson, G.; Herner, T. Alkyl mercury poisoning. Acta Paediatr. Scand. *41*:289–294, 1952.

Fishman, A. P.; Kroop, I. G.; Leiter, E.; Hyman, A. The management of anuria in acute mercurial intoxication. N. Y. State J. Med. *48*:2393-2396, 1948.

Freeman, R. B.; Maher, J. F.; Schreiner, G. E.; Mostofi, F. K. Nephrotoxicity of mercurial diuretics. Ann. Intern. Med. *57*:34-43, 1962.

Friberg, L.; Vostal, J. *Mercury in the Environment.* . C. R. C. Press, Chemical Rubber Company, Cleveland, Ohio, 1972.

Gabard, B. Treatment of methylmercury poisoning in the rat with sodium 2,3-dimercaptopropane-1-sulfonate. Influence of dose and mode of administration. Toxicol. Appl. Pharmacol. *38*:415–424, 1976a.

Gabard, B. Excretion and distribution of inorganic mercury in rat as influenced by several chelating agents. Arch. Toxicol. *35*:15–24, 1976b.

Gabard, B. Improvement of oral chelation treatment of methylmercury poisoning in rats. Acta Pharmacol. Toxicol. *39*:250–255, 1976c.

Gage, J. C. The distribution and excretion of inhaled mercury vapor. Br. J. Ind. Med. *18*:287-294, 1961.

Gage, J. C. Distribution and excretion of methyl and phenylmercury salts. Br. J. Ind. Med. *21*:197-202, 1964.

Glomme, J.; Gustavson, K. H. Treatment of experimental acute mercury poisoning by chelating agents BAL and EDTA. Acta Med. Scand. *164*:175-182, 1959.

Goldberg, H. I. Mercurial reaction in a tattoo. Can. Med. Assoc. J. *80*:203-204, 1959.

Goldwater, L. J.; Ladd, A. C.; Berkhout, D. G.; Jacobs, M. J. Acute exposure to phenylmercuric acetate. J. Occup. Med. *6*:227–228, 1964.

Goldwater, L. J.; Nicolau, A. Absorption and excretion of mercury in man. IX. Persistence of mercury in blood and urine following cessation of exposure. Arch. Environ. Health *12*:196-198, 1966.

Gonzalez, L. L.; Zinniger, M. M.; Altemeier, W. A. Cicatrical gastric stenosis caused by ingestion of corrosive substances. Ann. Surg. *156*:84-89, 1962.

Gottlieb, L. I.; Coye, R. D. Effect of mercuric chloride on serum protein catabolism and protein content of rabbit kidney. Am. J. Physiol. *202*:1121-1124, 1962.

Hallee, T. J. Diffuse lung disease caused by inhalation of mercury vapor. Am. Rev. Respir. Dis. *99*:430–436, 1969.

Harbison, R. D.; Jones, M. M.; MacDonald, J. S.; Pratt, J. T.; Coates, R. L. Synthesis and pharmacological study of a polymer which selectively binds mercury. Toxicol. Appl. Pharmacol. *42*:445-454, 1977.

Hayes, A. D.; Rothstein, A. The metabolism of inhaled mercury vapor in the rat studied by isotope techniques. J. Pharmacol. Exp. Ther. *138*:1-40, 1962.

Hayes, W. J., Jr. *Pesticides Studied in Man.* Williams & Wilkins, Baltimore, Md. 1982.

Hilmy, M. I; Rahim, S. A.; Abbas, A. H. Normal and lethal mercury levels in human beings. Toxicology *6*:155–159, 1976.

Hilmy, M. I.; Rahim, S. A.; Abbas, A. H.; Taka, R. Y. Toxicity of organic mercury in sheep and hens. Clin. Toxicol. *12*:445–456, 1978.

Hirschman, S. Z.; Feingold, M.; Boylen, G. Mercury in house paint as a cause of acrodynia. Effect of therapy with N-acetyl-D,L-penicillamine. N. Engl. J. Med. *269*:889-893, 1963.

Hryhorczuk, D. O.; Meyers, L., Jr.; Chen, G. Treatment of mercury intoxication in a dentist with N-acetyl-D,L-penicillamine. Clin. Toxicol. *19*:401-408, 1982.

Iyer, K.; Goodgold, J.; Eberstein, A.; Berg, P. Mercury poisoning in a dentist. Arch. Neurol. *33*:788–790, 1976.

Johnson, K. G.; Evanger, A.; Van Meter, W. Elemental mercury poisoning manifest by acrodynia and neutropenia. Vet. Human Toxicol. *20*:404–409, 1978.

Kahn, A.; Denis, R.; Blum, D. Accidental ingestion of mercuric sulphate in a 4-year old child. Management with BAL and peritoneal dialysis. Clin. Pediatr. *16*:956–958, 1977.

Kantarjian, A. D. A syndrome clinically resembling amyotrophic lateral sclerosis following chronic mercurialism. Neurology *11*:639-644, 1961.

Kark, R. A. P.; Poskanzer, D. C.; Bullock, J. D.; Boylen, G. Mercury poisoning and its treatment with N-acetyl-D,L-penicillamine. N. Engl. J. Med. *285*:10-16, 1971.

Kazantzis, G.; Schiller, K. F. R.; Asscher, A. W.; Drew, R. G. Albuminuria and the nephrotic syndrome following exposure to mercury and its compounds. Q. J. Med. *31*:403-418, 1962.

Kluwe, W. M. Developed resistance to mercuric chloride nephrotoxicity—failure to protect against other nephrotoxicants. Toxicol. Letters *12*:19–25, 1982.

Koos, B. J.; Longo, L. D. Mercury toxicity in the pregnant woman, fetus and newborn infant—Review. Am. J. Obstet. Gynecol. *126*:390–409, 1976.

Koppel, C.; Baudisch, H.; Keller, F. Methoxyethylmercury chloride poisoning: clinical findings and in vitro experiments. Clin. Toxicol. *19*:391–400, 1982.

Kostyniak, P. J.; Clarkson, T. W.; Cestero, R. V.; Freeman, R. B.; Abbasi, A. H. An extracorporeal complexing hemodialysis system for the treatment of methylmercury poisoning. I. *In vitro* studies of the effects of 4 complexing agents on the distribution and dialyzability of methylmercury in human blood. J. Pharmacol. Exp. Ther. *192*:260–269, 1975.

Kostyniak, P. J.; Clarkson, T. W.; Abbasi, A. H. An extracorporeal complexing hemodialysis system for the treatment of methylmercury poisoning. II. In vivo application in the dog. J. Pharmacol. Exp. Ther. *203*:253–263, 1977.

Kostyniak, P. J. Mobilization and removal of methylmercury in the dog during extracorporeal complexing hemodialysis with 2,3-dimercaptosuccinic acid (DMSA). J. Pharmacol. Exp.Ther. *221*:63–68, 1982.

Kudsk, F. N. Absorption of mercury vapor from the respiratory tract in man. Acta Pharmacol. Toxicol. *23*:250-262, 1965.

Ladd, A. C.; Goldwater, L. J.; Jacobs, M. B. Absorption and excretion of mercury in man. V. Toxicity of phenylmercurials. Arch. Environ. Health *9*:43-52, 1964.

Leumann, E. P.; Brandenberger, H. Hemodialysis in a patient with acute mercuric cyanide intoxication. Concentrations of mercury in blood, dialysate, urine, vomitus and feces. Clin. Toxicol. *11*:301–308, 1977.

Levine, S. P.; Cavender, G. D.; Langolf, G. D.; Albers, J. W. Elemental mercury exposure – peripheral neurotoxicity. Br. J. Ind. Med. *39*:136–139, 1982.

Longcope, W. T.; Leutscher, L. A., Jr. The treatment of acute mercury poisoning by BAL. J. Clin. Invest. *25*:557-567, 1946.

Lowe, B. Acute mercury poisoning. N. Engl. J. Med. *261*:409-410, 1959.

Lundgren, K. -D.; Swensson, A. A survey of results of investigations on some organic mercury compounds used as fungicides. Am. Ind. Hyg. Assoc. J. *21*:308-311, 1960.

Lundgren, K. -D.; Swensson, A.; Ulfvarson, U. Studies in humans on the distribution of mercury in the blood and the excretion in urine after exposure to different mercury compounds. Scand. J. Clin. Lab. Invest. *20*:164-166, 1967.

Magos, L. Mercury-blood interaction and mercury uptake by the brain after vapor exposure. Environ. Res. *1*:323-337, 1967.

Magos, L. Uptake of mercury by the brain. Br. J. Ind. Med. *25*:315-318, 1968a.

Magos, L. Effect of 2,3-dimercaptopropanol (BAL) on urinary

excretion and brain content of mercury. Br. J. Ind. Med. 25:152–154, 1968b.

Magos, L.; Peristianis, G. C.; Snowden, R. T. Post exposure preventive treatment of methylmercury intoxication in rats with dimercaptosuccinic acid. Toxicol. Appl. Pharmacol. 45:463–475, 1978.

Markowitz, L.; Schaumburg, H. H. Successful treatment of inorganic mercury neurotoxicity with N-acetyl-penicillamine despite an adverse reaction. Neurology 30:1000–1001, 1980.

Marsh, D. O.; Myers, G. J.; Clarkson, T. W.; Amin-Zaki, L.; Tikriti, S.; Majeed, M. A.; Dabbagh, A. R. Dose-response relationship for human fetal exposure to methylmercury. Clin. Toxicol. 81:1311–1318, 1981.

Matheson, D. S.; Clarkson, T. W.; Gelfand, E. W. Mercury toxicity (acrodynia) induced by long-term injection of gammaglobulin. J. Pediatr. 97:153–155, 1980.

Matsumoto, H.; Koya, G.; Takeuchi, T. Fatal Minamata disease. A neuropathological study of two cases of intrauterine intoxication by a methyl mercury compound. J. Neuropathol. Exp. Neurol. 24:563–574, 1965.

Matthes, F. T.; Kirschner, R.; Yow, M. D.; Brennan, J. C. Acute poisoning associated with inhalation of mercury vapor. Pediatrics 22:675–687, 1958.

McCord, C. P. Mercury poisoning in dentists. Ind. Med. Surg. 30:554, 1961.

Miller, V. L.; Klavano, P. A.; Csonka, E. Absorption, distribution and excretion of phenylmercuric acetate. Toxicol. Appl. Pharmacol. 2:344–352, 1960.

Milne, J.; Christophers, A.; DeSilva, P. Acute mercurial pneumonitis. Br. J. Ind. Med. 27:334–338, 1970.

Moutinho, M. E.; Tompkins, A. L.; Rowland, T. W.; Banson, B. B.; Jackson, A. H. Acute mercury vapor poisoning – fatality in an infant. Am. J. Dis. Child. 135:42–44, 1981.

Natelson, E. A.; Blumenthal, B. J.; Fred, H. L. Acute mercury vapor poisoning in the home. Chest 59:677–678, 1971.

Neal, P. A.; Jones, R. R. Chronic mercurialism in the hatter's fur cutting industry. J. A. M. A. 110:337–343, 1938.

Noe, F. S. Mercury as a potential hazard in medical laboratories. N. Engl. J. Med. 261:1002–1006, 1959.

Nomiyama, K.; Matsui, K.; Nomiyama, H. Effects of temperature and other factors on the toxicity of methyl mercury in mice. Toxicol. Appl. Pharmacol. 56:392–398, 1980.

Okabe, M.; Takeuchi, T. Distribution and fate of mercury in tissues of human organs in minamata disease. Neurotoxicology 1:607–624, 1980.

Okinaka, S.; Yoshikawa, M.; Mozia, T.; et al. . Encephalopathy due to an organic mercury compound. Neurology 14:69–73, 1964.

Olynyk, F.; Sharpe, D. H. Mercury poisoning in paper pica. N. Engl. J. Med. 306:1056, 1982.

Omata, S.; Sakimura, K.; Tsubaki, H.; Sugano, H. In vivo effect of methyl mercury on protein synthesis in the brain and liver of the rat. Toxicol. Appl. Pharmacol. 44:367–378, 1978.

Omata, S.; Horigome, T.; Momose,Y.; Kambayashi, M.; Mochizuki, M.; Sugano, H. Effect of methylmercury chloride on the in vivo rate of protein synthesis in the brain of the rat: Examination with the injection of a large quantity of 14C-valine. Toxicol. Appl. Pharmacol. 56:207–215, 1980.

Parameshvara, V. Mercury poisoning and its treatment with N-acetyl-D,L-penicillamine. Br. J. Ind. Med. 24:73–76, 1967.

Pesce, A. J.; Hanenson, I.; Sethi, K. β_2-Microglobulinuria in a patient with nephrotoxicity secondary to mercuric chloride ingestion. Clin. Toxicol. 11:309–315, 1977.

Pierce, P. E.; Thompson, G. F.; Likosky, W. H.; Nickey, L. N.; Barthel, W. F.; Hinman, A. R. Alkyl mercury poisoning in humans. J. A. M. A. 220:1439–1442, 1972.

Planas-Bohne, F. The influence of chelating agents on the distribution and biotransformation of methyl mercuric chloride in rats. J. Pharmacol. Exp. Ther. 217:500–504, 1981.

Prediger, V. Ausloesung einer Akrodynie durch Aufnahme von Saatbeizmitteln. Monatsschr. Kinderheilkd. 124:36–37, 1976.

Richardson, R. J.; Wilder, A. C.; Murphy, S. D. Uptake of mercury and mercury-amino acid complexes by rat renal cortex slices. Proc. Soc. Exp. Biol. Med. 150:303–307, 1975a.

Richardson, R. J.; Murphy, S. D. Effect of glutathione depletion on tissue deposition of methylmercury in rats. Toxicol. Appl. Pharmacol. 31:505–519, 1975.

Robillard, J. E.; Rames, L. K.; Jensen, R. L.; Roberts, R. J. Peritoneal dialysis in mercurial diuretic intoxication. J. Pediatr. 88:79–81, 1976.

Rodin, A. E.; Crowson, C. N. Mercury nephrotoxicity in the rat. 2. Investigation of the intracellular site of mercury nephrotoxicity by correlated serial time histologic and histoenzymatic studies. Am. J. Path. 41:485–499, 1962.

Rosenthal, S. M. Use of sodium formaldehyde sulfoxylate in mercury poisoning. J. Pharmacol. Exp. Ther. 54:34–41, 1935.

Rustam, H.; Von Burg, R.; Amin-Zaki, L.; Hassani, E. S. E. Evidence for a neuromuscular disorder in methylmercury poisoning. Clinical and electrophysiological findings in moderate to severe cases. Arch. Environ. Health 30:190–195, 1975.

Sanchez-Sicillia, L.; Seto, D. S.; Nakamoto, S.; Kolff, W. J. Acute mercurial intoxication treated by hemodialysis. Ann. Intern. Med. 59:692–706, 1963.

Sasser, L. B.; Jarboe, G.E.; Walter, B. K.; Kelman, B. J. Absorption of mercury from ligated segments of the rat gastrointestinal tract. Proc. Soc. Exp. Biol. Med. 157:57–60, 1978.

Schulz, E.; Beskind, H. Systemic deposition of metallic mercury. J. Pediatr. 57:733–737, 1960.

Scott, E. P. The medical bag: Another source of accidental poisoning. A case of near fatal apparent mercury poisoning. Clin. Pediatr. 3:706–708, 1964.

Seaton, A.; Bishop, C. M. Acute mercury pneumonitis. Br. J. Ind. Med. 35:258–261, 1978.

Seidel, J. Acute mercury poisoning after polyvinyl alcohol preservative ingestion. Pediatrics 66:132–134, 1980.

Smith, A. D. M.; Miller, J. W. Treatment of inorganic mercury poisoning with N-acetyl-DL-penicillamine. Lancet 1:640–642, 1961.

Smith, D. L., Jr. Mental effects of mercury poisoning. South. Med. J. 71:904–905, 1978.

Snaiman, K. F.; Flagler, D. G. Mercury poisoning with central and peripheral nervous system involvement treated with penicillamine. Pediatrics 48:639–642, 1971.

Snodgrass, W.; Sullivan, J. B.; Rumack, B. H.; Hashimoto, C. Mercury poisoning from home gold ore processing. Use of penicillamine and dimercaprol. J. A. M. A. 246:1929–1931, 1981a.

Snyder, R. D.; Seelinger, D. F. Methyl mercury poisoning. Clinical follow-up and sensory nerve conduction studies. J. Neurol. Neurosurg. Psychiat. 39:701–704, 1976.

Stanojevich, M.; Kostitch, H. A case of mercury fixation in the lungs. Poumon Coeur 24:693–698, 1968.

Strunge, P. Nephrotic syndrome caused by a seed disinfectant. J. Occup. Med. 12:178–179, 1970.

Sunderman, F. W.; Sr. Clinical response to therapeutic agents in poisoning from mercury vapor. Ann. Clin. Lab. Sci. 8:259–269, 1978.

Swensson, A.; Ulfvarson, U. Toxicology of mercury compounds used as fungicides. Occup. Health Rev. 15:5–11, 1963.

Swensson, A.; Ulfvarson, U. Experiments with different antidotes in acute poisoning by different mercury compounds. Effect on survival and on distribution and excretion of mercury. Int. Arch. Gewerbepath. Gewerbhyg. 24:12–50, 1967.

Takahashi, H.; Hirayama, K.; Ikegami, Y. Resin for methyl mercury elimination in rats. Kumamoto Med. J. 28:60, 1975.

Takahashi, H.; Shibue, Y.; Fukushima, Y. Factors affecting the toxicity of methyl mercury. Chudokuken Ho 11:14–16, 1978.

Takeda, Y.; Kunugi, T.; Hoshino, O.; Urita, T. Distribution of inorganic, aryl, and alkyl mercury compounds in rats. Toxicol. Appl. Pharmacol. 13:156–164, 1968.

Tandon, S. K.; Magos, L.; Cabral, J. R. P. Protection against mercuric chloride by nephrotoxic agents which do not induce thionein. Toxicol. Appl. Pharmacol. 52:227–236, 1980.

Tandon, S. K.; Magos, L. Effect of kidney damage on the mobilisation of mercury by thiol-complexing agents. Br. J. Ind. Med. 37:128–132, 1980.

Taylor, L. L.; DiStefano, V. Effects of methyl mercury on brain biogenic amines in the developing rat pup. Toxicol. Appl. Pharmacol. *38*:489-497, 1976.

Teisinger, J.; Fiserova-Bergerova, V. Pulmonary retention and excretion of mercury vapors in man. Ind. Med. Surg. *34*:580-584, 1965.

Teitelbaum, D. T.; Ott, J. E. Elemental mercury self-poisoning. Clin. Toxicol. *2*:243-248, 1969.

Tennant, R.; Johnston, H. J.; Wells, J. B. Bilateral pneumonitis from inhalation of mercury vapor. Conn. Med. *25*:106-109, 1961.

Thomas, D. J.; Smith, J. C. Effects of coadministered low molecular weight thiol compounds on short term distribution of methyl mercury in the rat. Toxicol. Appl. Pharmacol. *62*:104-110, 1982.

Thomas, D. J.; Fisher, H. L.; Hall, L. L.; Mashak, P. Effects of age and sex on retention of mercury by methyl mercury-treated rats. Toxicol. Appl. Pharmacol. *62*:445-454, 1982.

Trifillis, A. L.; Kahng, M. W.; Trump, B. F. Metabolic studies of HgCl$_2$-induced acute renal failure in the rat. Exp. Mol. Pathol. *35*:14-24, 1981.

Troen, P.; Kaufman, S. A.; Katz, K. H. Mercuric bichloride poisoning. N. Engl. J. Med. *244*:459-463, 1951.

Tsubaki, T.; Irukayama, K. *Minamata Disease: Methyl Mercury Poisoning in Minamata and Nugata, Japan*. Kodansha Ltd., Japan & Elsevier Scientific Publishing Co., New York, 1977.

Tsuzuki, Y. Effect of chronic methyl mercury exposure on activities of neurotransmitter enzymes in rat cerebellum. Toxicol. Appl. Pharmacol. *60*:379-381, 1981.

Vas, W.; Tuttle, R. J.; Zylak, C. J. Intravenous self-administration of metallic mercury. Radiology *137*:313-315, 1980.

Wallner, A.; Herman, L. Mercurial diuretics. Some hazards of mercuhydrin. Report of two cases with one death. Ann.

Intern. Med. *32*:1190-1197, 1950.

Warkany, J.; Hubbard, D. M. Mercury in the urine of children with acrodynia. Lancet *1*:829-830, 1948.

Warkany, J.; Hubbard, D. M. Adverse mercurial reactions in the form of acrodynia and related conditions. Am. J. Dis. Child. *81*:335-373, 1951.

Warkany, J.; Hubbard, D. M. Acrodynia and mercury. J. Pediat. *42*:365-386, 1953.

Wheately, B.; Barbeau, A.; Clarkson, T. W.; Lapham, L. W. Methyl mercury poisoning in Canadian Indians - the elusive diagnosis. Can. J. Neurol. Sci. *6*:417-422, 1979.

Wolpaw, R.; Alpers, N. The treatment of acute mercury poisoning with sodium formaldehyde sulfoxylate with a review of twenty cases. J. Lab. Clin. Med. *27*:1387-1395, 1942.

Wustner, H.; Orfanos, C. E.; Steinbach, H.; Kaferstein, H.; Herpers, H. Nail changes and loss of hair: cardinal signs of mercury poisoning from hair bleaches. Dtsch. Med. Wochenschr. *100*:1694-1697, 1975.

Yeh, T. F.; Pildes, R. S.; Firor, H. V. Mercury poisoning from mercurochrome therapy of an infected omphalocele. Clin. Toxicol. *13*:463-467, 1978.

Yonaga, R.; Morita, K. Comparison of the effect of N(2,3-dimercaptopropyl) phthalamidic acid DL-penicillamine, and dimercaprol on the excretion of tissue retention of mercury in mice. Toxicol. Appl. Pharmacol. *57*:197-207, 1981.

Zimmer, L. J.; Carter, D. E. Efficacy of 2, 3-dimercaptopropanol and D-penicillamine on methyl mercury induced neurological signs and weight loss. Life Sci. *23*:1025-1034, 1978.

Zimmer, L.; Carter, D. E. Effects of complexing treatment administered with the onset of methyl mercury neurotoxic signs. Toxicol. Appl. Pharmacol. *51*:29-38, 1979.

METHYL ALCOHOL

Methyl alcohol (methanol, wood alcohol) is a widely used solvent in paint removers and windshield washer fluids. It is used in gasoline antifreeze fluids and with ethanol and soap as a solid canned fuel. Small amounts of methanol are found in expired breath of normal subjects (Ericksen and Kularni, 1963), and a possible metabolic source for endogenous methanol is recognized (Axelrod and Daly, 1965). The purpose or significance of endogenous methanol and its accumulation in alcoholic subjects during prolonged periods of drinking (Majchrowicz and Mendelson, 1971) are not yet understood.

Toxicology: Methyl alcohol is readily absorbed from the gastrointestinal and respiratory tracts. In a case allegedly involving percutaneous absorption, a dominant component of vapor inhalation could not be ruled out (Kahn and Blum, 1979). As little as 2 teaspoonfuls is considered toxic if ingested. The fatal dose in man lies between 2 and 8 oz.; this range implies a high variation in individual susceptibility (Sollmann, 1957). Death may be prompt, but it is usually delayed for several days, and the mortality rate is high. The prognosis improves if treatment is instituted before visual disturbances appear (Bennett *et al.*, 1953; Benton and Calhoun, 1953).

When methanol consumption is not accompanied by the intake of ethyl alcohol, inebriation and subsequent drowsiness are said to be mild and transient. This phase may be followed by an entirely asymptomatic interval. The characteristic signs and symptoms develop in rapid succession after a latency of 6 to 30 hours (usually 12 to 18) following the initial intake (Jacobson *et al.*, 1945; Kaplan and Levreault, 1945; Röe, 1955b). Because these late effects are produced by pure samples, impurities are thought to play no important role in the toxicity of methyl alcohol (Sollmann, 1957).

The latent period is believed to represent the time required for the metabolic transformation of methanol to the form responsible for the delayed toxic effects. Individual differences in the rates of these reactions may account for the wide variations in individual susceptibility. Since these reactions occur primarily in the liver, pre-existing liver damage, such as cirrhosis, may delay metabolism, making that individual appear more resistant. A very limited experience with infants suggests that the clinical picture is like that in adults in all important respects (Kahn and Blum, 1979).

The symptoms that appear after the initial inebriation result from a combination of factors, of which a characteristic metabolic acidosis appears to be the trigger (Röe, 1946). The severity of essentially all late symptoms in methanol poisoning is said to be proportional to the intensity of this delayed acidosis (Bennett *et al.*, 1953; Cooper *et al.*, 1952; Dethlefs and Naraqi, 1978).

Central nervous depression is due partly to acidosis and partly to cerebral edema (Kenney and Mellinkoff, 1951; Sollmann, 1957), but monkeys adequately treated with bicarbonate still die from central nervous depression (Potts, 1955). Acidosis is the result of methanol oxidation to formic acid (Bastrup, 1947; Lund, 1948), which accumulates and reduces severely the body's alkali reserve. For unknown reasons other organic acids including lactic acid are said to accumulate also (Harrop and Benedict, 1920). Coincident with the onset of acidosis, vision often becomes severely impaired.

In contrast to human exposures, a long latent period, relatively high toxicity, acidosis, and ocular injury are *not* features of methyl alcohol intoxication in nonprimate laboratory animals (Gilger and Potts, 1955; Röe, 1955a). These prominent species differences are responsible for much confusion in the scientific literature. It is now known that several species of monkeys can serve as experimental models for the human syndrome (Clay *et al.*, 1975). Administration of doses of 3 gm. methanol per kg. body weight to rhesus and pigtail monkeys results in a mild central nervous depression, a latent period and then severe metabolic acidosis, coma and death. In these animals the onset of the acidosis coincided with an accumulation of formic acid in blood and a decrease in the bicarbonate content of plasma (McMartin *et al.*, 1976). Formate may account for all (Clay *et al.*, 1975) or for about half of the anion gap during the acidosis (McMartin *et al.*, 1976). Sixty and 100% of the anion gap was formate in two human patients (McMartin *et al.*, 1980).

The administration of pyrazole or 4-methylpyrazole, which are potent inhibitors of alcohol dehydrogenase, blocks formate accumulation and the occurrence of acidosis by greatly decreasing the rate of oxidation of methanol to formate. These biochemical effects are accompanied by an amelioration of the clinical signs of intoxication (McMartin *et al.*, 1976).

Based on the now well-established concept that formic acid is responsible for the delayed effects in methanol poisoning, one infers that measures which accelerate formate oxidation or utilization should also be useful in therapy. It appears that formate metabolism proceeds via a folic acid-dependent pathway (Makar and Tephly, 1977; McMartin *et al.*, 1977). The evidence is that folic acid deficient monkeys and rats were more sensitive to methanol than control animals and that folate preloading of nondeficient monkeys increased the rate of formate oxidation to carbon dioxide. Data from an *in vitro* system suggest that methionine deficiency may also retard the oxidation of formate (Billings and Tephly, 1979). Like folic acid, calcium 5-formyl tetrafolate (citrovorum factor, Leucovorin) also stimulated the oxidation of formate

to CO_2 and inhibited the accumulation of formic acid in the blood of methanol-poisoned monkeys (Noker *et al.*, 1980). In contrast to folic acid, Leucovorin was effective in reversing the course of methanol poisoning in monkeys even when given after the alcohol (Noker *et al.*, 1980).

The monkey model of human methyl alcohol poisoning extends to the ocular toxicity as well. Formate accumulation in blood parallels the occurrence of eye damage. Formate infusions in monkeys produce ocular damage even when they are buffered to prevent systemic acidosis (Martin-Amat *et al.*, 1978). Morphologic studies on monkey eyes after methanol poisoning have suggested that the retinal damage may be due to disruption in neural axoplasmic flow.

Visual disturbances, which are a distinctive aspect of methanol poisoning in man, may become evident soon after acidosis begins. Dilated, unreactive pupils and dimness of vision are characteristic. The ocular lesion, which involves chiefly the ganglion cells of the retina, is a destructive inflammation followed by atrophy. In the acute phase the retina is congested and edematous, and the edges of the optic disk may be blurred. The result is bilateral blindness, which is usually permanent unless treatment is prompt and energetic. Even if complete blindness is avoided, residual scotomata are common (Benton and Calhoun, 1953; Röe, 1948). The electroretinogram is said to have diagnostic and prognostic significance in methyl alcohol poisoning (Ruedemann, 1962).

Except for optic atrophy, permanent neurologic sequelae are exceedingly rare, but difficulties in speech have been noted on at least one occasion (Naraqi *et al.*, 1979). Motor dysfunction with rigidity, spasticity and hypokinesis of unknown etiology has also been reported. Levodopa provided some functional relief (Guggenheim *et al.*, 1971).

At one time it was widely accepted that formaldehyde generated metabolically from methyl alcohol was responsible for the ocular toxicity (Potts and Johnson, 1952; Praglin *et al.*, 1955). Considerable doubt now exists about the role of formaldehyde in methanol poisoning. Formaldehyde has yet to be identified in blood or tissues from methanol-poisoned primates or human victims, and formaldehyde is known to have a half-life of only 1.5 minutes when infused into monkeys (McMartin *et al.*, 1979). Ocular damage has never been reported after human cases of formaldehyde ingestion. Finally, the characteristic eye injury can be produced in monkeys by formate infusions, as noted above. Thus it is unlikely that formaldehyde is the cause of retinal injury in methanol poisoning.

Outside of acid-base disturbances, elevation of serum amylase has been the most striking laboratory abnormality observed with any degree of regularity in man (Naraqi *et al.*, 1979), and pancreatic necrosis has been demonstrated at autopsy (Bennett *et al.*, 1952). These findings have suggested that pancreatitis may be the cause of the severe abdominal pain that frequently accompanies methanol intoxication (Kaplan, 1962; Yant and Shrenk, 1937).

Therapeutic considerations: Ethyl alcohol, when consumed at the same time as methyl alcohol, prolongs the latent period before toxic symptoms appear. It has also been observed that some of the severe symptoms of methanol poisoning are alleviated by the ingestion of ethanol, and for this reason the recommended treatment includes the administration of ethanol by mouth, by stomach tube and/or by intravenous infusion. A blood ethyl alcohol level of about 0.1% is regarded as optimal (Röe, 1946). In extreme cases the ethanol may be given intravenously as a dilute solution in bicarbonate or saline (Agner *et al.*, 1949).

The mechanism of this protection lies in the ability of ethyl alcohol to inhibit the metabolic oxidation of methanol, even though this rate is inherently slow (Gilger *et al.*, 1956, 1959; Zatman, 1946). Like ethanol, the metabolism of methanol proceeds at a rate that is constant and independent of concentration within wide limits. In some species, *e.g.*, man and monkey, both substances are acted upon by the same enzyme, alcohol dehydrogenase (Kini and Cooper, 1961; Makar *et al.*, 1968), whereas in rats methanol oxidation requires liver catalase, which is inhibited by ethanol (Smith, 1961a; Tephly *et al.*, 1964; Van Harken *et al.*, 1965). This explanation of the antidotal effectiveness of ethanol has been proved in rats by experiments using radioactively labeled alcohols (Bartlett, 1950a and b).

Pyrazole, a potent inhibitor of alcohol dehydrogenase, has also been suggested on theoretical grounds as a methanol antidote (Lester and Benson, 1970). Because formate is probably detoxified by one carbon pathways, the administration of large doses of folic acid may also be helpful (Herken *et al.*, 1969). Significant antidotal effects of BAL, cysteine and mercaptoethanol have been demonstrated in rats and mice, but the basis for these effects and any possible role in human poisoning remain to be elucidated (Guerri *et al.*, 1977).

Extracorporeal hemodialysis has been employed successfully in numerous instances of methyl alcohol poisoning, some of which presented with grave prognostic signs (Austin *et al.*, 1961; Cowen, 1964; Felts *et al.*, 1962b; Jørgensen and Wieth, 1963a; McCoy *et al.*, 1979; Pfister *et al.*, 1966; Shinaberger, 1961). In other cases, however, hemodialysis failed to prevent permanent ocular defects or death, probably because it was instituted too late in the course of the intoxication (Gonda *et al.*, 1978). Prompt hemodialysis is recommended when the blood methanol concentration exceeds 50 mg./100 ml.

(Cowen, 1964), when an ounce or more of methanol has been ingested, when acidosis becomes evident, or when a visual abnormality is recognized (Gonda *et al.*, 1978). Both methanol and formate are dialyzable substances (Marc-Aurele and Schreiner, 1960). Even during hemodialysis it is considered vital to administer bicarbonate and especially ethanol (Gonda *et al.*, 1978); they should be given by mouth or vein despite some inevitable losses to the dialysis fluid. McCoy *et al.* (1979) estimated the dialysance of methanol as 98 ml./minute and that of ethanol as 100 to 120 ml./minute. Another indication for dialysis is the oliguria that sometimes occurs in severe methanol intoxications (Closs and Solberg, 1970).

Peritoneal dialysis has also been employed successfully on occasion (Stinebaugh, 1960; Wenzl *et al.*, 1968), but it is clearly less efficient than a modern artificial kidney (Keyvan-Larijarni and Tannenberg, 1974). Forced fluid diuresis is even less efficient. In one series of patients the clearance of methanol by peritoneal dialysis was 5 to 10 times the clearance by forced fluid diuresis (Kane *et al.*, 1968).

Symptomatology:

1. A latency usually of 12 to 18 hours, during which time the only clinical signs are those of a generally mild and transient state of inebriation as after ethanol.
2. Headache, anorexia, weakness, fatigue, leg cramps, vertigo, restlessness.
3. Nausea, occasionally vomiting and diarrhea. Violent abdominal pain, back pain, leg pain.
4. Apathy or delirium progressing sometimes rapidly to coma. Rarely excitement, mania and convulsions.
5. Dimness of vision with dilated pupils, reacting poorly, if at all, to light, followed often by bilateral blindness (transient or permanent). Eyes are often sensitive to pressure, and eye movements are painful.
6. Breathing is rapid and shallow, not usually deep and labored (Kussmaul type) as seen in other types of metabolic acidosis.
7. Mild tachycardia is common, but the blood pressure is usually well maintained.
8. Death in coma is due to respiratory failure or rarely to circulatory collapse.
9. Protracted convalescence with asthenia. Blindness is usually permanent.

Treatment:

1. Gastric lavage with 3 to 5% sodium bicarbonate, leaving some solution in the stomach after the lavage.
2. Ethanol treatment is designed to produce and sustain an ethanol blood level of about 100 mg./dl. A loading dose of 0.6 gm./kg. (expressed as pure ethanol) can be achieved by sipping diluted 100-proof

whiskey in an amount of 1.5 ml./kg. over a period of 15 to 30 minutes. The maintenance dose varies; for 100-proof whiskey it amounts to about 0.2 to 0.3 ml./kg. every hour by mouth or by stomach tube. McCoy *et al.* (1979) recommend that after the oral loading dose (see above) diluted ethanol be infused intravenously at a rate of 66 mg./kg. (expressed as pure ethanol) per hour in nondrinkers and 154 mg./kg. per hour in chronic tolerant drinkers. If hemodialysis is initiated, the infusion should be increased by 103 mg./kg. per hour.

3. Give 4 gm. sodium bicarbonate by mouth (or by stomach tube if necessary) every 15 minutes until the arterial blood pH is normal. Repeat the course of alkali treatment as indicated. Even when fully corrected, the acidosis may recur at any time during the first several days. Avoid sodium lactate as an alkalinizing agent since lactate metabolism may be impaired in these patients. Check blood pH or plasma CO_2 content or combining power, preferably every hour. Also see pp. IV-69–72.

4. Oxygen and artificial ventilation if respirations become weak and insufficient (pp. IV-7–14).

5. Protect patient's eyes from light.

6. Morphine for abdominal pain (unless respiration is depressed).

7. Dextrose, saline and sodium bicarbonate may be administered intravenously.

8. Hemodialysis in severe cases where the response to alkali treatment may be delayed or incomplete. See pp. IV-55–56.

9. Check cerebrospinal fluid pressure. If elevated, treat brain edema as outlined on pp. IV-43–46.

10. Based on studies in monkeys, repetitive doses of Leucovorin calcium injection 2 mg./kg. i.m. at 0, 4, 8, 12 and 18 hours after methanol might be expected to help reverse the course of the poisoning (Noker *et al.*, 1980).

Laboratory:

1. Check blood alcohol level and arterial blood pH or plasma CO_2 combining power (or urine acidity) at repeated intervals (preferably every hour, since relapses are common).

2. Measure serum amylase (see text).

3. Hypokalemia of severe proportions has been reported (Tonning *et al.*, 1956).

4. Blood methanol concentrations in 6 fatal cases ranged from 110 to 240 mg./100 ml. (Harger *et al.*, 1938). A few patients with blood concentrations above 500 mg./100 ml. have survived with vigorous treatment. The methanol half-life is about 8 hours. Caution is indicated in interpreting published blood concentrations of methanol because many methods in common use do not distinguish between methanol and ethanol. Poisoned patients are apt to have ingested both alcohols or to have been given ethanol therapeutically.

5. Specific methods are available for measuring formate in body fluids (Makar *et al.*, 1975).

References:

Agner, K.; Hook, O.; Von Porat, B. The treatment of methanol poisoning with ethanol, with report of two cases. Q. J. Stud. Alcohol 9:515-522, 1949.

Austin, W. H.; Lope, C. P.; Burnham, H. N. Treatment of methanol intoxication by hemodialysis. N. Engl. J. Med. 265:334, 1961.

Axelrod, J.; Daly, J. Pituitary gland: Enzymic formation of methanol from S-adenosylmethionine. Science 150:892-893, 1965.

Bartlett, G. R. Combustion of C^{14}-labelled methanol in intact rat and its isolated tissues. Am. J. Physiol. 163:614-618, 1950a.

Bartlett, G. R. Inhibition of methanol oxidation by ethanol in the rat. Am. J. Physiol. 163:619-621, 1950b.

Bastrup, J. Th. On the excretion of formic acid in experimental poisoning with methyl alcohol. Acta Pharmacol. Toxicol. 3:312-322, 1947.

Bennett, I. L., Jr.; Cary, F. H.; Mitchell, G. L.; Cooper, M. N. Acute methyl alcohol poisoning; a review based on experiences in an outbreak of 323 cases. Medicine 32:431-463, 1953.

Bennett, I. L., Jr.; Nation, T. C.; Olley, J. F. Pancreatitis in methyl alcohol poisoning. J. Lab. Clin. Med. 40:405-409, 1952.

Benton, C. D.; Calhoun, F. D., Jr. The ocular effects of methyl alcohol poisoning; report of a catastrophe involving 320 persons. Am. J. Ophthalmol. 36:1677-1685, 1953.

Billings, R. E.; Tephly, T. R. Studies on methanol toxicity and formate metabolism in isolated hepatocytes. The role of methionine in folate-dependent reactions. Biochem. Pharmacol. 28:2985-2991, 1979.

Clay, K. L.; Murphy, K. C.; Watkins, W. D. Experimental methanol toxicity in the primate. Analysis of metabolic acidosis. Toxicol. Appl. Pharmacol. 34:49-61, 1975.

Closs, K.; Solberg, C. O. Methanol poisoning. J. A. M. A. 211:497-499, 1970.

Cooper, M. N.; Mitchell, G. L.; Bennett, I. L.; Cary, F. H. Methyl alcohol poisoning. An account of the 1951 Atlanta epidemic. J. Med. Assoc. Ga. 61:48-51, 1952.

Cowen, D. L. Extracorporeal dialysis in methanol poisoning. Ann. Intern. Med. 61:134-135, 1964.

Dethlefs, R.; Naraqi, S. Ocular manifestations and complications of acute methyl alcohol intoxication. Med. J. Aust. 2:483-485, 1978.

Eriksen, S. P.; Kulkarni, A. B. Methanol in normal human breath. Science 141:639-640, 1963.

Felts, J. H.; Templeton, T. B.; Wolff, W. A.; Meredith, J. H.; Hines, J. Methanol poisoning treated by hemodialysis. South. Med. J. 55:46-47, 1962b.

Gilger, A. P.; Farkas, I. S.; Potts, A. M. Studies on the visual toxicity of methanol. X. Further observations on the ethanol therapy of acute methanol poisoning in monkeys. Am. J. Ophthalmol. (Part II of July) 48:153-161, 1959.

Gilger, A. P.; Potts, A. M. Studies on the visual toxicity of methanol. V. The role of acidosis in experimental methanol poisoning. . Am. J. Ophthalmol. (Part II of Feb.) 39:63-86, 1955.

Gilger, A. P.; Potts, A. M.; Farkas, I. S. Studies on the visual toxicity of methanol. IX. The effect of ethanol on methanol poisoning in the rhesus monkey. Am. J. Ophthalmol. (Part II of Oct.) 42:244-252, 1956.

Gonda, A.; Gault, H.; Churchill, D.; Hollomby, D. Hemodialysis for methanol intoxication. Am. J. Med. 64:749-758, 1978.

Guerri, C.; Godfrey, W.; Grisolia, S. Protection against toxic effects of formaldehyde in vitro, and of methanol or formaldehyde in vivo, by subsequent administration of SH reagents. Physiol. Chem. Phys. 8:543-550, 1977.

Guggenheim, M. A.; Couch, J. R.; Weinberg, W. Motor dysfunction as a permanent complication of methanol ingestion. Arch. Neurol. 24:550-554, 1971.

Harger, R. N.; Johnson, S. L.; Bridwell, E. G. Detection and estimation of methanol with results in human cases of methanol poisoning. J. Biol. Chem. 123:1, 1938.

Harrop, G. A., Jr.; Benedict, E. M. Acute methyl alcohol poisoning associated with acidosis. Report of a case. J. A. M. A. 74:25-27, 1920.

Herken, W.; Rietbruck, N.; Henschler, D. Zum Mechanismus der Methanolvergiftung. Arch. Toxikol. 24:214-228, 1969.

Jacobson, B. M.; Russell, H. K.; Grimm, I.; Fox, E. C. Acute methyl alcohol poisoning. Report of eighteen cases. Naval Med. Bull. 44:1099-1106, 1945.

Jorgensen, H. E.; Wieth, J. O. Dialysable poisons. Lancet 1:81-84, 1963a.

Kahn, A.; Blum, D. Methyl alcohol poisoning in an 8-month-old boy -- An unusual route of intoxication. J. Pediatr. 94:841-843, 1979.

Kane, R. L.; Talbert, W.; Harlan, J.; Sizemore, G.; Cataland, S. A methanol poisoning outbreak in Kentucky. Arch. Environ. Health 17:119-129, 1968.

Kaplan, A.; Levreault, G. U. Methyl alcohol poisoning, report of forty-two cases. Naval Med. Bull. 44:1107-1111, 1945.

Kaplan, K. Methyl alcohol poisoning. Am. J. Med. Sci. 244:170-174, 1962.

Kenney, A. H.; Mellinkoff, S. M. Methyl alcohol poisoning. Ann. Intern. Med. 34:331-338, 1951.

Keyvan-Larijarni, H.; Tannenberg, A. Methanol intoxication. Arch. Intern. Med. 134:293-296, 1974.

Kini, M. M.; Cooper, J. R. The biochemistry of methanol poisoning. III. The enzymic pathway for the conversion of methanol to formaldehyde. Biochem. Pharmacol. 8:207-215, 1961.

Lester, D.; Benson, G. O. Alcohol oxidation in rats inhibited by pyrazole, oximes and amides. Science 169:282-283, 1970.

Lund, A. Excretion of methanol and formic acid in man after methanol consumption. Acta Pharmacol. Toxicol. 4:205-212, 1948.

Majchrowicz, E.; Mendelson, J. H. Blood methanol concentrations during experimentally induced ethanol intoxication in alcoholics. J. Pharmacol. Exp. Ther. 179:293-300, 1971.

Makar, A. B. Tephly, T. R. Methanol poisoning. VI: role of folic acid in the production of methanol poisoning in the rat. J. Toxicol. Environ. Health 2:1201-1209, 1977.

Makar, A. B.; McMartin, K. E.; Palese, M.; Tephly, T. R. Formate assay in body fluids. Application to methanol poisoning. Biochem. Med. 13:117-126, 1975.

Makar, A. B.; Tephly, T. R.; Mannering, G. J. Methanol metabolism in the monkey. Mol. Pharmacol. 4:471-483, 1968.

Marc-Aurele, J.; Schreiner, G. E. The dialysance of ethanol and methanol: A proposed method for the treatment of massive intoxication by ethyl or methyl alcohol. J. Clin. Invest. 39:802-807, 1960.

Martin-Amat, G.; McMartin, K. E.; Hayreh, S. S.; Hayreh, M. D.; Tephly, T. R. Methanol poisoning: ocular toxicity produced by formate. Toxicol. Appl. Pharmacol. 45:201-208, 1978.

McCoy, H. G.; Cipolle, R. J.; Ehlers, S. M.; Sawchuck, R. J.; Zaske, D. E. Severe methanol poisoning. Application of a pharmacokinetic model for ethanol therapy and hemodialysis. Am. J. Med. 67:804-807, 1979.

McMartin, K. E.; Ambre, J. J.; Tephly, T. R. Methanol poisoning in human subjects. Role for formic acid accumulation in the metabolic acidosis. Am. J. Med. 68:414-418, 1980.

McMartin, K. E.; Makar, A. B.; Martina, G.; Palese, M.; Tephly, T. R. Methanol poisoning. I. The role of formic acid in the development of metabolic acidosis in the monkey and the reversal by 4-methylpyrazole. Biochem. Med. 13:319-333, 1976.

McMartin, K. E.; Martin-Amat, G.; Makar, A. B.; Tephly, T. R. Methanol poisoning. V. Role of formate metabolism in the monkey. J. Pharmacol. Exp. Ther. 201:564-572, 1977.

McMartin, K. E.; Martin-Amat, G.; Noker, P. E.; Tephly, T. R. Lack of a role for formaldehyde in methanol poisoning in the monkey. Biochem. Pharmacol. 28:645-649, 1979.

Naraqi, S.; Dethlefs, R. F.; Slobodniuk, R. A.; Sairere, J. S. An outbreak of acute methyl alcohol intoxication. Aust. N. Z. J. Med. 9:65-68, 1979.

Noker, P. E.; Eells, J. T.; Tephly, T. R. Methanol toxicity: treatment with folic acid and 5-formyl tetrahydrofolic acid. Alcohol. Clin. Exp. Res. 4; 378-383, 1980.

Pfister, A. K.; McKenzie, J. V.; Dinsmore, H. P.; Edman, C. D. Extracorporeal dialysis for methanol intoxication. J. A. M. A. 197:1041-1043, 1966.

Potts, A. M. The visual toxicity of methanol. VI. The clinical aspects of experimental methanol poisoning treated with base. Am. J. Ophthalmol. (Part II of Feb.) 39:86-92, 1955.

Potts, A. M.; Johnson, L. V. Studies on the visual toxicity of methanol. I. The effect of methanol and its degradation products on retinal metabolism. Am. J. Ophthalmol. (Part II of May) 35:107-133, 1952.

Praglin, J.; Spurney, R.; Potts, A. M. An experimental study of electroretinography. I. The electroretinogram in experimental animals under the influence of methanol and its oxidation products. Am. J. Ophthalmol. (Part II of Feb.) 39:52-62, 1955.

Roe, O. Methanol poisoning. Its clinical course, pathogenesis and treatment. Acta Med. Scand. Suppl. No. 182:1-253, 1946.

Roe, O. The ganglion cells of the retina in case of methanol poisoning in human beings and experimental animals. Acta Ophthalmol. 26:169-182, 1948.

Roe, O. Uber den Wert der tierexperimentellen Untersuchungen fur das Studium der Toxizitat des Methanols. Schweiz. Med. Wochenschr. 85:813-820, 1955a.

Roe, O. Metabolism and toxicity of methanol. Pharmacol. Rev. 7:399-412, 1955b.

Ruedemann, A. D., Jr. The electroretinogram in chronic methyl alcohol poisoning in human beings. Am. J. Ophthalmol. 54:34-53, 1962.

Shinaberger, J. H. Treatment of methanol poisoning by extracorporeal dialysis. Arch. Intern. Med. 108:937-939, 1961.

Smith, M. E. Interrelations in ethanol and methanol metabolism. J. Pharmacol. Exp. Ther. 134:233-237, 1961a.

Sollmann, T. A Manual of Pharmacology. 8th Ed., W. B. Saunders Co., Philadelphia, 1957.

Stinebaugh, B. J. The use of peritoneal dialysis in methyl alcohol poisoning. Arch. Intern. Med. 105:613-617, 1960.

Tephly, T. R.; Parks, R. E., Jr.; Mannering, G. J. Methanol metabolism in the rat. J. Pharmacol. Exp. Ther. 143:292-300, 1964.

Tonning, D. J.; Brooks, D. W.; Harlow, C. M. Acute methyl alcohol poisonings in 49 naval ratings. Can. Med. Assoc. J. 74:20-27, 1956.

Van Harken, D. R.; Tephly, T. R.; Mannering, G. J. Methanol metabolism in the isolated perfused rat liver. J. Pharmacol. Exp. Ther. 149:36-42, 1965.

Wenzl, J. E.; Mills, S. D.; McCall, J. T. Methanol poisoning in an infant. Am. J. Dis. Child. 116:445-447, 1968.

Yant, W. P.; Shrenk, H. H. Distribution of methanol in dogs after inhalation and administration by stomach tube and subcutaneously. J. Ind. Hyg. Toxicol. 19:337-345, 1937.

Zatman, L. J. The effect of ethanol on the metabolism of methanol in man. Biochem. J. 40:lxvii-lxviii, 1946.

METHYL BROMIDE

Methyl bromide and methyl chloride are gases at ordinary temperatures whereas methyl iodide is a volatile liquid. The iodide is encountered infrequently, but it is an intermediate in methylation reactions. Both the chloride and the bromide have been used as refrigerants. Methyl bromide is also found in some fire extinguishers and is used as an insecticidal fumigant. When used as a fumigant for various foodstuffs in years past, methyl bromide caused more fatalities among California workmen than any other agricultural chemical (Hine, 1969). At low vapor concentrations (which may produce poisonings over a long period of time), methyl bromide and methyl chloride are not detectable by taste or odor.

Toxicology: Each of these halogenated methanes has produced death in man. The major signs and symptoms of the intoxication are referable to the central nervous system (*e.g.*, Kegel *et al.*, 1929; Prain and Smith, 1952; Garland and Camps, 1945). Based on animal experimentation the toxicity of this series increases in the order: methyl chloride, methyl bromide (Sayers *et al.*, 1929), methyl iodide (von Oettingen, 1964), but all produce similar toxic syndromes in man. Ethyl chloride and bromide appear to resemble their corresponding methyl homologues but are less toxic (Irish *et al.*, 1941; Sayers *et al.*, 1929). Monohalomethanes are not importantly renotoxic or hepatotoxic. Those halogenated hydrocarbon solvents whose potential for producing death in renal or hepatic failure predominates over actions on the nervous system are discussed under CARBON TETRACHLORIDE, p. III-101.

Coma or convulsions are often the immediate cause of death from methyl bromide (Clarke *et al.*, 1945; Longley and Jones, 1965; Prain and Smith, 1952; Viner, 1945), unless massive exposure to the respiratory tract precipitates pulmonary edema (Miller, 1943; Prain and Smith, 1952; Wyers, 1945). This clinical impression is clearly supported by animal experimentation, wherein subacutely exposed rabbits exhibited a delayed nervous system reaction, but more intensively exposed animals developed pulmonary edema (Irish *et al.*, 1940, 1941). In some cases thermal decomposition of methyl bromide to more irritant products has been inferred (Miller *et al.*, 1961; von Oettingen, 1946a).

Both central and peripheral neurologic deficits may persist; organic brain syndrome has occurred (Goulon *et al.*, 1975; Greenberg, 1971). Profound psychological depression because of prolonged convalescence is troublesome (Hine, 1969). Low-level subacute exposures to the vapor have produced a syndrome of polyneuropathy without overt central manifestations (Kan-

tarjian and Shaheen, 1963). Whether the injury is central or peripheral, a slow but eventually complete recovery is the rule (Carter, 1945; DeJong, 1944; Drawneek *et al.*, 1964; Ingram, 1951; Johnstone, 1945).

Sufficient percutaneous absorption of methyl bromide can occur to produce death in man (Jordi, 1953), and if evaporation is delayed in any way such as by gloves, boots or other clothing, it is an intense vesicant on human skin. The blisters produced by methyl bromide are enormous but rarely deep enough to destroy the entire skin layer (Butler *et al.*, 1945; Rathus and Landy, 1961; Thomson, 1945; Watrous, 1942; Wyers, 1945). Like other vesicants, including lewisite, methyl bromide inhibits skin glycolysis at the hexokinase level (Dixon and Needham, 1946). Methyl iodide is also a vesicant, but methyl chloride is not.

Methyl chloride sometimes produces death in pulmonary edema (Kegel *et al.*, 1929; McNally, 1946), but in exposed animals its occurrence is not a regular or predictable phenomenon (Dunn and Smith, 1947; Smith and von Oettingen, 1947a–c). Instead, neurologic involvement as with methyl bromide is characteristic. Early signs may be confused with influenza whereas more severe poisonings can be confused with viral encephalitis or meningitis except that there is usually no fever (Scharnweber *et al.*, 1974). Convulsive episodes occur frequently and are often described as Jacksonian in character (Baker, 1927; Gorham, 1934; Hansen *et al.*, 1953; Jones, 1942a; MacDonald, 1964). Unlike the more highly chlorinated methanes, methyl chloride appears to cause only mild narcosis in animals (von Oettingen, 1949), and extremely labile levels of consciousness are sometimes seen in man (Muscat-Baron, 1963). Thus, the neurologic symptoms of methyl chloride and methyl bromide are similar.

In one fatal case of methyl iodide intoxication, the victim died in profound coma, but oliguria and "bronchopneumonia" were also reported (Garland and Camps, 1945). In the case reported by Appel *et al.* (1975), coma, oliguric renal failure and pulmonary congestion were also noted, as well as seizures and prominent cerebellar and parkinsonian signs. At 5 months his neurologic examination was normal but mild psychiatric disturbances persisted. Disturbances in brain lipid metabolism and increased serum lipids were noted in rabbits injected with methyl iodide (Hasegawa *et al.*, 1971).

Renal failure due to tubular necrosis may be a late sequelae after any one of these three monohalomethanes, but these lesions are uncommon and usually of mild proportions (Benat and Courtney, 1948; Hasegawa *et al.*, 1971; Prain and Smith, 1952; Repko and Lasley, 1979; Spevak et al., 1976; Viner, 1945). Similarly, there have been occasional reports of jaundice, elevations of liver enzyme activity in serum and abnormal liver function tests suggestive of mild hepatotoxicity after exposure to methyl bromide and methyl chloride (Repko and Lasley, 1979; Spevak et al., 1976; Verberk et al., 1979; Wood, 1951). In a 6-year-old boy, signs of liver involvement in conjunction with encephalopathy after exposure to vapors of methyl bromide were at first mistaken for Reye's syndrome (Shield et al., 1977). Intravascular hemolysis was noted at least once after inhalation of methyl chloride (Mackie, 1961).

It seems unlikely that dehalogenation or hydrolysis to methyl alcohol and free halide plays a significant role in the toxicity of methyl iodide or methyl bromide. In a fatal case of methyl iodide poisoning neither methyl alcohol nor unusually large concentrations of iodide were found in the urine or cerebrospinal fluid (Garland and Camps, 1945). Although exceptions can be cited (Longley and Jones, 1965; Viner, 1945), blood inorganic bromide levels in methyl bromide poisoning are not so high as those associated with intoxication by bromide salts (Benatt and Courtney, 1948; Collins, 1965; Drawneek et al., 1964), but the blood bromide level does show some correlation with the severity of the clinical symptoms. It has been demonstrated clearly that rabbits tolerate blood levels after sodium bromide administration many times higher than bromide levels associated with death after methyl bromide exposure; they are also much more tolerant to the vapors of methyl alcohol than the vapors of methyl bromide (Irish et al., 1941). Although water is essential for its activity, methyl bromide is a much more effective disinfectant of anthrax spores than hydrogen bromide or methanol vapor (Kolb et al., 1952). To explain these differences it was once postulated that bromide distribution after methyl bromide differs from that after inorganic bromide (Miller and Haggard, 1943), but most observations would appear to be better accounted for by postulating direct toxic actions of all three monohalomethanes.

In contrast to methyl bromide, early reports of methyl chloride intoxications describe an increase in urinary formate excretion which paralleled the severity of the clinical syndrome (Baker, 1927; Kegel et al., 1929). Later experience (Jones, 1942a) and critical animal studies (Smith and von Oettingen, 1947a-c) failed to confirm this observation. Formaldehyde and methyl alcohol, however, are said to be detectable in mice after inhalation or intraperitoneal administration of methyl chloride (Subjbert, 1967), but a clear-cut demonstration of significant concentrations of these metabolites in man

is lacking. Several symptoms of methyl chloride poisoning in man are similar to those elicited by methyl alcohol, notably the characteristic latent period (Smith and von Oettingen, 1947a-c), acidosis (Hartman et al., 1955; Weinstein, 1937), visual disturbances (Baker, 1930; Gorham, 1934; Hansen et al., 1953; Mackie, 1961), persistent vomiting (Birch, 1935; Sharp, 1930), abdominal pain (Weinstein, 1937) and mental confusion like alcoholic inebriation (Hansen et al., 1953; Jones, 1942a).

Unlike the blindness from methanol, however, visual disturbances after methyl chloride exposure are mild and fully reversible. It has been suggested that they may result from a temporary paralysis of the ciliary muscle (Baker, 1927). The acid-base status in patients acutely poisoned by either methyl chloride or bromide deserves more attention to ascertain whether reports of acidosis can be ascribed to protracted vomiting or to specific metabolic effects (see also METHYL ALCOHOL, p. III-275). Probably some conversion to methanol occurs, but the major nervous system effects of methyl chloride like methyl bromide are best ascribed to the chemical per se or to its reaction products with tissue ligands.

Both methyl iodide (Buckell, 1949) and methyl bromide (Lewis, 1948) have an ability to inhibit irreversibly certain enzyme systems in vitro. This effect appears to involve sulfhydryl groups and probably requires a methylation reaction. Methyl chloride has been shown to S-methylate cysteine residues of serum albumin and reduced glutathione in human red blood cells and in ground brain, liver and kidneys of rats and guinea pigs (Redford-Ellis and Gowenlock, 1971a and b). In intact exposed rats, methyl chloride lowered nonprotein sulfhydryl levels (largely reduced glutathione) in liver, kidneys and lungs (but not blood), apparently by combining enzymatically with —SH groups (Dodd et al., 1982). Dimercaprol (BAL) has been shown to protect mice poisoned with methyl iodide (Buckell, 1949). Although BAL was apparently ineffective in reversing the course of 7 clinical cases of methyl bromide intoxication (Rathus and Landy, 1961), it may be of benefit if started in the latent period preceding toxic symptoms. At least one patient was treated with N-acetylcysteine (see ACETAMINOPHEN, p. III-5). It appeared to do no harm and it may have been of benefit (Zatuchni and Hong, 1981).

Probably all three of these halogenated methanes function as alkylating agents. With methyl chloride, a major target molecule appears to be tissue reduced glutathione (Dodd et al., 1982), leading to the formation of N-acetyl-S-methylcysteine, but probably the bromide and iodide are also metabolized to methyl mercapturic acid (Chasseaud, 1976). Both methyl chloride and methyl iodide are mutagenic in vitro even without metabolic activation, and the latter is carcinogenic in mice (Fishbein, 1980).

Symptomatology (3 to 12 hours after inhalation of vapor):

1. Dizziness and headache.
2. Anorexia, nausea, vomiting, and abdominal pain.
3. Lassitude, profound weakness, slurring of speech, and staggering gait.
4. Transient blurring of vision, diplopia, sometimes strabismus, and even temporary blindness.
5. Mental confusion, mania, tremors, and epileptiform convulsions, perhaps with a Jacksonian-type of progression.
6. Rapid respirations, associated with signs of severe pulmonary edema, cyanosis, pallor and collapse. Pulmonary edema, convulsions and mental confusion may occur independently of one another.
7. Coma, areflexia and death from respiratory or circulatory collapse.
8. Low-level subacute vapor exposures have produced a syndrome of persistent numbness in the hands and legs, impaired superficial sensation, muscle weakness, unsteadiness of gait and absent or hypoactive distal tendon reflexes.
9. Late sequelae include bronchopneumonia after severe pulmonary lesions, renal failure with anuria due to tubular degeneration, and severe weakness with or without evidence of paralysis. These difficulties, however, tend to subside within a few weeks or months, and complete recovery is the rule. Hepatic failure does not occur, but jaundice and other evidence of mild hepatic injury are noted occasionally.

Treatment:

1. Remove promptly from a contaminated atmosphere.
2. If the patient is first seen in the asymptomatic (latent) period, a therapeutic trial with *N*-acetylcysteine or dimercaprol (BAL) should be considered. Use the dosage schedules on pp. III-6 and 52 respectively.
3. Quickly remove any contaminated clothing. Methyl bromide can penetrate ordinary rubber gloves. All contaminated clothing should be carefully aerated before being reworn. Wash contaminated skin carefully with water. Blistered areas are best covered with a sterile Vaseline dressing, which should be changed as indicated.
4. Restrain the confused or maniacal patient (p. IV-35). Treat convulsions by the parenteral administration of anticonvulsive drugs. See p. IV-37 for the technique of administering barbiturates or diazepam.
5. Severe metabolic acidosis has not been described, but any marked acidosis must be corrected by the cautious administration of alkali. The problem is complicated by the threat of pulmonary edema and perhaps of renal shutdown; except for these complications, acidosis should be treated vigorously. See p. IV-71.
6. Administer positive pressure oxygen for impending pulmonary edema. See p. IV-14 for supportive treatment in this syndrome, which is sometimes the proximal cause of death.
7. Because of central nervous depression with coma and respiratory paralysis, artificial ventilation may become necessary (pp. IV-7–12).
8. Even if asymptomatic, the patient should be kept under observation for at least 48 hours.
9. Treat rare cases of late renal failure according to the principles on pp. IV-52–55.

Laboratory:

1. Frequent chemical determinations of the blood electrolytes, particularly the plasma CO_2 and chloride levels, to detect and measure a metabolic acidosis. The urine, if any, may contain albumin, cells, and casts.
2. No simple chemical tests are available for the diagnosis of methyl bromide poisoning, but low concentrations of bromide ion appear in the blood and perhaps in the cerebrospinal fluid of persons exposed to methyl bromide (Clarke *et al.*, 1945). Its detection may be of diagnostic value.

References:

Appel, G. B.; Galen, R.; O'Brien, J.; Schoenfeldt, R. Methyl iodide intoxication. A case report. Ann. Intern. Med. *82*:534-536, 1975.

Baker, H. M. Intoxication with commercial methyl chloride. J. A. M. A. *88*:1137-1138, 1927.

Baker, H. M. Industrial methyl chloride poisoning. Am. J. Public Health *20*:291-295, 1930.

Benatt, A. J.; Courtney, T. R. B. Uraemia in methyl bromide poisoning. A case report. Br. J. Ind. Med. *5*:21-25, 1948.

Birch, C. A. Toxic effects of methyl chloride gas. Lancet *1*:259-260, 1935.

Buckell, M. 2, 3-Dimercapto-1-propanol (BAL) and methyl iodide intoxication. Nature *163*:330, 1949.

Butler, E. C. B.; Perry, K. M. A.; Williams, J. R. F. Methyl bromide burns. Br. J. Ind. Med. *2*:30-31, 1945.

Carter, A. B. Methyl bromide poisoning, effects on the nervous system. Br. Med. J. *1*:43-45, 1945.

Chausseaud, L. F. Conjugation with glutathione and mercapturic acid excretion. In *Glutathione: Metabolism and Function.* (Arias, I. M. and W. B. Jakoby, eds.). New York, Raven Press, pp. 77-114, 1976.

Clarke, C. A.; Roworth, C. G.; Holling, H. E. Methyl bromide poisoning, an account of four recent cases met with in one of H. M. ships. Br. J. Ind. Med. *2*:17-23, 1945.

Collins, R. P. Methyl bromide poisoning, a bizarre neurological disorder. Calif. Med. 103:112-116, 1965.

DeJong, R. N. Methyl bromide poisoning with special reference to nervous system manifestations. J. A. M. A. 125:702-703, 1944.

Dixon, M.; Needham, D. M. Biochemical research on chemical warfare agents. Nature 158:432-438, 1946.

Dodd, D. E.; Bus, J. S.; Barrow, C. S. Nonprotein sulfhydryl alterations in F-344 rats following acute methyl chloride inhalation. Toxicol. Appl. Pharmacol. 62:228-236, 1982.

Drawneek, W.; O'Brien, M. J.; Goldsmith, H. J.; Bourdillon, R. E. Industrial methyl bromide poisoning in fumigators. Lancet 2:855-856, 1964.

Dunn, R. C.; Smith, W. W. Acute and chronic toxicity of methyl chloride. IV. Histopathologic observations. Arch. Pathol. 43:296;300, 1947.

Fishbein, L. Potential carcinogenic and mutagenic industrial chemicals. I. Alkylating agents. J. Toxicol. Environ. Health 6:1133-1177, 1980.

Garland, A.; Camps, F. E. Methyl iodide poisoning. Br. J. Ind. Med. 2:209-211, 1945.

Gorham, A. B. Medical aspects of methyl chloride. Br. Med. J. 1:529-530, 1934.

Goulon, M.; Nouailhat, F.; Escourolle, R.; Zarranz-Imirizaldu, J. J. Grosbuis, S.; Levy-Alcover, M. A. Intoxication par le bromure de methyle. Trois observations, dont une mortelle. Etude neuropathologique d'un cas de stupeur avec myoclonies suivi pendant cinq ans. Rev. Neurologique 131:445-468, 1975.

Greenberg, J. O. The neurological effects of methyl bromide poisoning. Ind. Med. Surg. 40:27-29, 1971.

Hansen, H.; Weaver, N. K.; Venable, F. S. Methyl chloride intoxication, report of fifteen cases. Arch. Ind. Health 8:328-334, 1953.

Hartman, T. L.; Wacker, W.; Roll, R. M. Methyl chloride intoxication: report of two cases, one complicating pregnancy. N. Engl. J. Med. 253:552-554, 1955.

Hasegawa, H.; Sato, M.; Suzuki, H. Experimental study of methyl iodide poisoning. Ind. Health 9:36-45, 1971.

Hine, C. H. Methyl bromide poisoning, a review of ten cases. J. Occup. Med. 11:1-10, 1969.

Ingram, F. R. Methyl bromide fumigation and control in the date packing industry. Arch. Ind. Health 4:193-198, 1951.

Irish, D. D.; Adams, E. M.; Spencer, H. C.; Rowe, V. K. Response attending exposure of laboratory animals to vapors of methyl bromide. J. Ind. Hyg. Toxicol. 22:218-230, 1940.

Irish, D. D.; Adams, E. M.; Spencer, H. C.; Rowe, V. K. Chemical changes of methyl bromide in relation to its physiological effects. J. Ind. Hyg. Toxicol. 23:408-411, 1941.

Johnstone, R. T. Methyl bromide intoxication of a large group of workers. Ind. Med. Surg. 14:495-497, 1945.

Jones, A. M. Methyl chloride poisoning. Q. J. Med. 11:29-43, 1942a.

Jordi, A. U. Methyl bromide through the intact skin: A report of one fatal and two non-fatal cases. J. Aviation Med. 24:536-539, 1953.

Kantarjian, A. D.; Shaheen, A. S. Methyl bromide poisoning with nervous system manifestations resemblng polyneuropathy. Neurology 13:1054-1058, 1963.

Kegel, A. H.; McNally, W. D.; Pope, A. S. Methyl chloride poisoning from domestic refrigerators. J. A. M. A. 93:353-358, 1929.

Kolb, R. W.; Schneiter, R.; Floyd, E. P.; Byers, D. H. Disinfective action of methyl bromide, methanol and hydrogen bromide on anthrax spores. Arch. Ind. Health 5:354-364, 1952.

Lewis, S. E. Inhibition of SH enzymes by methyl bromide. Nature 161:692-693, 1948.

Longley, E. O.; Jones, A. T. Methyl bromide poisoning in man. Ind. Med. Surg. 34:499-502, 1965.

MacDonald, J. D. C. Methyl chloride intoxication: Report of 8 cases. J. Occup. Med. 6:81-84, 1964.

Mackie, I. J. Methyl chloride intoxication. Med. J. Aust. 1:203-205, 1961.

McNally, W. D. Eight cases of methyl chloride poisoning with three deaths. J. Ind. Hyg. Toxicol. 28:94-97, 1946.

Miller, B. H.; Navone, R.; Ota, M. Irritation from residual bromides after methyl bromide fumigation. Public Health Rep. (U. S.) 76:216-218, 1961.

Miller, D. P.; Haggard, H. W. Intracellular penetration of bromide as a feature in toxicity of alkyl bromides. J. Ind. Hyg. Toxicol. 25:423-433, 1943.

Miller, J. W. Fatal methyl bromide poisoning. Arch. Pathol. 36:505-507, 1943.

Muscat-Baron, J. M. A case of methyl chloride poisoning. Br. Med. J. 2:365-366, 1963.

Prain, J. H.; Smith, G. H. Methyl bromide; clinicopathologic report of 8 cases of poisoning. Br. J. Ind. Med. 9:44-49, 1952.

Rathus, E. M.; Landy, P. J. Methyl bromide poisoning. Br. J. Ind. Med. 18:53-57, 1961.

Redford-Ellis, M.; Gowenlock, A. H. Studies on the reaction of chloromethane with human blood. Acta Pharmacol. Toxicol. 30:36-48, 1971a.

Redford-Ellis, M.; Gowenlock, A. H. Studies on the reaction of chloromethane with preparations of liver, brain and kidney. Acta Pharmacol. Toxicol. 30:49-58, 1971b.

Repko, J. D.; Lasley, S. M. Behavioral, neurological, and toxic effects of methyl chloride: a review of the literature. CRC Crit. Rev. Toxicol. 6:283-302, 1979.

Sayers, R. R.; Yant, W. P.; Thomas, B. G. H.; Berger, L. B. Physiological response attending exposure to vapors of methyl bromide, methyl chloride, ethyl bromide and ethyl chloride. Public Health Bull. No. 185, 1929.

Scharnweber, H. C.; Spears, G. N.; Cowles, S. R. Chronic methyl chloride intoxication in six industrial workers. J. Occup. Med. 16:112-113, 1974.

Sharp, B. B. Toxic effects of methyl chloride gas. Br. Med. J. 1:336, 1930.

Shield, L. K.; Coleman, T. L.; Markesbery, W. R. Methyl bromide intoxication: neurologic features, including simulation of Reye syndrome. Neurology 27:959-962, 1977.

Smith, W. W.; Von Oettingen, W. F. The acute and chronic toxicity of methyl chloride. I. Mortality resulting from exposures to methyl chloride in concentrations of 4000 to 300 parts per million. J. Ind. Hyg. Toxicol. 29:47-52, 1947a.

Smith, W. W.; Von Oettingen, W. F. The acute and chronic toxicity of methyl chloride. II. Symptomatology of animals poisoned by methyl chloride. J. Ind. Hyg. Toxicol. 29:123-128, 1947b.

Smith, W. W.; Von Oettingen, W. F. The acute and chronic toxicity of methyl chloride. III. Hematology and biochemical studies. J. Ind. Hyg. Toxicol. 29:185-189, 1947c.

Spevak, L.; Nadj, V.; Felle, D. Methyl chloride poisoning in four members of a family. Br. J. Ind. Med. 33:272-274, 1976.

Subjbert, L. Untersuchungen uber den Abbau des Methylchlorids bei Mausen. Arch. Toxikol. 22:233-235, 1967.

Thomson, G. R. A case of burning and slight poisoning by methyl bromide. Br. J. Surg. 33:91-92, 1945.

Verberk, M. M.; Rooyakkers-Beemster, T.; De Vlieger, M.; Van Vliet, A. G. M. Bromine in blood, EEG and transaminases in methyl bromide workers. Br. J. Ind. Med. 36:59-62, 1979.

Viner, M. Methyl bromide poisoning: A new industrial hazard. Can. Med. Assoc. J. 53:43-45, 1945.

von Oettingen, W. F. The toxicity and potential dangers of methyl bromide with special reference to its use in the chemical industry in fire extinguishers and in fumigation. Natl. Insts. Health Bull. No. 185, 1946a.

von Oettingen, W. F. The Halogenated Hydrocarbons of Industrial and Toxicological Importance. Elsevier Publishing Co., New York, 1964.

von Oettingen, W. F.; Powell, C. C.; Sharpless, N. E.; Alford, W. C.; Pecora, L. J. Relation between the toxic action of chlorinated methanes and their chemical and physiochemical properties. Natl. Insts. Health Bull. No. 191, 1949.

Watrous, R. M. Methyl bromide, local and mild systemic toxic effects. Ind. Med. Surg. 11:575-579, 1942.

Weinstein, A. Methyl chloride (refrigerator) gas poisoning, an industrial hazard. J. A. M. A. 108:1603-1605, 1937.

Wood, M. W. Cirrhosis of the liver in a refrigeration engineer attributed to methyl chloride. Lancet 1:508-509, 1951.

Wyers, H. Methyl bromide intoxication. Br. J. Ind. Med. 2:24-

29, 1945.

Zatuchni, J.; Hong, K. Methyl bromide poisoning seen initially as psychosis. Arch. Neurol. 38:529-530, 1981.

MORPHINE

Morphine and other natural alkaloids of opium serve many uses in clinical medicine. Powdered opium, tincture of opium (laudanum), camphorated tincture of opium (paregoric) and Pantopon have been largely supplanted by various salts of morphine. Codeine, oxycodone, dihydromorphinone (Dilaudid), and methyldihydromorphinone (metopon) are available derivatives of morphine currently used in therapy. Heroin, a derivative of morphine that is illegal in the United States, is important because it is the favorite opiate of narcotic addicts, but the management of chronic addiction and of the withdrawal syndrome is beyond the scope of this manual. The problem has been well discussed elsewhere (Fraser and Grider, 1953; Lewis and Zinberg, 1964; Wikler, 1952; Zinberg and Lewis, 1964). In recent years clonidine has shown some promise as an adjunct to the management of the abstinence syndrome (Masini et al., 1981), and naloxone (see below) has been used to evaluate the severity of the state of narcotic dependence (Wang et al., 1974). Although its structure is unlike that of the morphine alkaloids, the synthetic drug methadone produces a similar toxic syndrome. Specific comments concerning many of these and related drugs can be found in Section II.

Toxicology: Acute morphine poisoning may arise from a suicidal act, from an error in an addict's estimation of his own tolerance, or from accidental overdosage in therapy. Homicidal poisoning is rare (Webster, 1930). Iatrogenic intoxication has been reported often in victims of traumatic shock, who may appear to require large or repeated doses only because the drug is poorly absorbed from parenteral sites until an adequate circulation is reestablished.

In a non-addicted adult who is not in pain, 60 mg. of morphine by mouth is generally a toxic dose; 100 mg. is almost always toxic and the probable lethal dose lies between 120 and 250 mg. (2 to 4 grains) (Eddy, 1941; Webster, 1930). By parenteral routes, doses much in excess of 30 mg. are likely to be dangerous (Jaffe and Martin, 1980). These estimates, however, are not well established. In the extensive literature compilation of Eddy (1941), survivors outnumbered non-survivors in all reported dose ranges (including doses as high as 20 to 120 grains). Such surveys, however, are apt to be grossly biased by the inclusion of unrecognized or unreported addicts with marked degrees of acquired tolerance. On the other hand, it is inconceivable that the more than 1100 preoperative surgical patients who tolerated 0.5 to 3.0 mg./kg. morphine injected intravenously at the Massachusetts General Hospital were all addicts (Lowenstein et al., 1969). In a subset of these patients, 7 subjects (24 to 71 years old) without apparent heart or lung disease were compared with 8 subjects (37 to 66 years old) with aortic stenosis. All were given intravenously 1.0 mg./kg. morphine at a rate of 10 mg./minute, and all were monitored carefully for 1 hour, at which time surgical anesthesia was induced with one of the inhalation agents. During the one-hour test period, all subjects were encouraged to breath deeply, and none even required ventilatory assistance (!). It is difficult to reconcile this experience of Lowenstein et al. (1969) with the conventional toxic dose estimates above.

Infants and young children are thought to be more susceptible on a body weight basis, but this time-honored impression has been denied by at least one competent investigator (Eddy, 1941). Elderly persons and patients with myxedema are comparatively intolerant of morphine and other opiates, whereas patients with hyperthyroidism and those in severe pain have a high tolerance (Jaffe and Martin, 1980). The highest levels of tolerance, however, are encountered in narcotic addicts, some of whom take more than 1000 mg. of morphine daily, with few objective signs other than miosis and constipation (Isbell and White, 1953; Wikler, 1952). In nonaddicts, therapeutic doses of morphine may be dangerously potentiated by alcohol or barbiturates (Eerola, 1961; Moeller, 1952).

Morphine is absorbed through all mucous membranes, including the buccal, nasal and respiratory mucosae. The nature of the toxic syndrome is not determined by the portal of entry. Before the turn of this century ingestion was the commonest mode of poisoning (Bartlett, 1897), but parenteral self-administration is now a far more common cause of death among addicts (Helpern and Rho, 1966). Signs and symptoms begin within 20 to 40 minutes after ingestion (Webster, 1930).

Once established, morphine poisoning presents most of the classical features of central nervous depression. Although not diagnostic, the triad of coma, pinpoint pupils and profoundly depressed respiration strongly suggests morphine poisoning. In acute morphinism death occurs typically within 6 to 12 hours (Webster, 1930). The patient who survives the first 24 hours has a favorable prognosis. Death, even in the addict, is nearly always due to respiratory failure (Helpern and Rho, 1966).

If not the cause of death, circulatory insufficiency is at least often contributory. When present, cardiovascular collapse is usually a consequence of severe anoxia from inadequate lung ventilation. Complete right bundle branch block occurred in a severe case of methadone poisoning in a toddler (Ratcliffe, 1963). Paroxysmal atrial fibrillation was a feature in six cases of heroin intoxication (Labi, 1969). Addicts who lose consciousness with one limb under their body may present with the crush syndrome and its attendant renal impairment (Schrieber et al., 1971). However, myoglobinuria and other signs of the crush syndrome occurred in an adult male several days after inhaling ("snorting") a mixture of heroin, cocaine and powdered sugar without loss of consciousness (D'Agostino and Arnett, 1979).

Next to respiratory failure the most common lethal complication of acute morphinism is pulmonary edema (Duberstein and Kaufman, 1971; Helpern and Rho, 1966; Morrison et al., 1970; Steinberg and Karliner, 1968). Perhaps some cases are due to aspiration of gastric contents (Warnock et al., 1972), but they appear to be the exception rather than the rule. Some evidence for seasonal variation has been cited in support of an allergic etiology (Morrison et al., 1970). The intravenous route does not appear to be obligatory for the induction of narcotic pulmonary edema. For example, ingestions of methadone, heroin, propoxyphene, levorphanol and barbiturates have provoked the reaction (Frand et al., 1972a; Raskin, 1976; Turner, 1977). Although acute left ventricular failure might conceivably underlie narcotic-induced lung edema, morphine in doses up to 3 mg./kg. has been given safely to nonaddict patients with minimal circulatory reserve (Lowenstein et al., 1969). The common adulterants of street heroin have come under suspicion, but none has been established as the causative agent. Milk is widely reputed among addicts to be an antagonist to heroin overdose. Its intravenous administration resulted in pulmonary edema in what must be an exceptional case (Drenick, 1970). Some addicts prefer the intranasal route ("snorting"). Conceivably, particulate narcotic might find its way into the lung under such circumstances and precipitate the reaction (Hirsch and Adelson, 1972).

The protein content of pulmonary edema fluid from five heroin-poisoned patients was equal to that of their plasma, whereas the edema fluid from five patients with acute left ventricular failure contained less than half the protein of plasma (Katz et al., 1972). This finding, however, may reflect differences in the severity of the two reactions rather than any fundamental difference in etiology. Others insist that the effects of heroin pulmonary edema on lung function are similar to those of pulmonary edema due to other causes (Frand et al., 1972b). Aside from an unproven direct effect of narcotics on the lung, the most likely explanation for the edema is an increase in the permeability of the alveolar wall or capillaries because of the severe hypoxia (Duberstein and Kaufman, 1971; Garriott and Sturner, 1973). Addicts also have many infectious pulmonary complications because of the use of non-sterile injection techniques (Stern et al., 1968).

Opium, laudanum, paregoric, and Pantopon owe their toxicity to their contents of morphine. Alkaloids related to morphine have qualitatively similar actions, but many of them are weaker depressants and stronger stimulants. For example, thebaine is a weak narcotic and a potent convulsant, and toxic doses of codeine and meperidine (see Section II) produce restlessness and excitement rather than coma (Eddy, 1939; Rumler and Weigel, 1963; Steinhaus and Tatum, 1950). Barbiturates antagonize these signs of central stimulation, but over-titration compounds the risk of respiratory failure (Winter and Flataker, 1956). When a series of eight narcotic drugs was evaluated in dogs, an inverse correlation was noted between narcotic potency and both the convulsive potency and degree of cardiovascular depression (de Castro et al., 1979).

Morphine is metabolized in man by conjugation of one or both hydroxyl groups, primarily with glucuronic acid and to a minor extent with sulfate. Eventually 60 to 80% of a dose is excreted in the urine, but perhaps as much as one-third of the dose is passed into the bile with enterohepatic recycling. As much as 10% may be recovered in the feces, and 5% appears as expired carbon dioxide. This pattern is not altered much with chronic dosing (Caldwell and Sever, 1974). Because newborn rats and human infants have a limited capacity for carrying out conjugation reactions (Yeh and Krebs, 1980), they may have a greater sensitivity to morphine and other narcotics.

Heroin is hydrolyzed by human serum cholinesterase to 6-acetylmorphine. This pathway is sufficiently important that heroin potency in man may be influenced by plasma cholinesterase activity or genotype (Lockridge et al., 1980). Except for the detection of small amounts of heroin and 6-acetylmorphine in the urine, the pattern indicated above for morphine in general holds for heroin as well (Yeh et al., 1976).

Codeine and oxycodone have higher oral-to-parenteral potency ratios than morphine because of less intensive first-pass metabolism in the liver. About 10% of the total dose of codeine is demethylated to morphine. Codeine is found in the urine as such, as morphine, as norcodeine and as various conjugates (Nomof et al., 1977).

Therapeutic considerations: A vigorous program of symptomatic and supportive treatment has saved many victims of morphine poisoning. The single most important element in therapy is the correction of anoxia by all available means: the maintenance of a patent airway, the administration of oxygen, the use of artificial ventilation, and the injection of specific narcotic antagonists.

Given parenterally, specific antagonists such as naloxone promptly reverse the respiratory depression, coma and hypotension from overdoses of morphine, codeine, all semisynthetics and almost all synthetic narcotics (Chase et al., 1952; Domino et al., 1953; Eckenhoff et al., 1952; Fraser et al., 1952; Marx and Love, 1953; Strober, 1954). Under appropriate conditions most of the other recognized actions of morphine are reduced or abolished (Hart and McCawley, 1944; Lasagna, 1954; Unna, 1943). The beneficial effects of these drugs in the treatment of morphinism have been ascribed to a competition between antagonist and narcotic for morphine receptor sites in critical tissues.

Despite the established efficacy of nalorphine and levallorphan (see Section II), naloxone has clearly emerged as the antagonist of choice. It is 6 times more potent than levallorphan and 30 times more potent than nalorphine in antagonizing the respiratory depression induced by meperidine (Foldes et al., 1963; Sadove et al., 1963). Its major advantage, however, is its almost complete lack of agonistic (morphine-like) activity particularly with respect to respiratory depression (Foldes et al., 1969). Thus, it not only reverses rapidly the respiratory depression due to narcotic agonists, but it does not compound the respiratory depression in patients whose coma is due to a non-narcotic central nervous depressant. For example, the drug is not dangerous when given to patients poisoned by barbiturates, but both nalorphine and levallorphan are hazardous in such circumstances (Buchner et al., 1972; Evans et al., 1973). Indeed, in rats naloxone delayed the development and duration of barbiturate coma and decreased lethality (Furst et al., 1977). Finally, naloxone antagonizes the toxic effects of pentazocine, whereas nalorphine does not.

A potentially dangerous interaction between morphine and propranolol has been documented in the laboratory. To a lesser extent the same is true for the combination of morphine and practolol, as well and the combination of propranolol and other narcotics. The increased narcotic lethality is prevented by naloxone, suggesting that it is unrelated to β-adrenergic receptor blockade (Davis and Hatoum, 1979; Winter, 1974). A similar pattern of increased lethality that is antagonized by naloxone has been reported for morphine with choline (Ho et al., 1979) and with the catechol-O-methyl transferase inhibitors, tropolone and 3,5-dihydroxy-4-methoxybenzoic acid (Davis et al., 1979). Perhaps all these interactions have their basis in an interference with morphine metabolic detoxication. The dangers of the combination of pentazocine and tripelennamine are discussed under ANTIHISTAMINICS (p. III-38).

Narcotic poisoning in neonates: Heroin-addicted mothers or those on methadone maintenance programs deliver infants that often show signs of withdrawal within hours of birth (Sussman, 1963a). Low birth weights, hyperactivity, irritability, tremors, regurgitation and diarrhea are common, but respiratory depression is not usually prominent (Kahn et al., 1969; Blatman, 1974; Reddy et al., 1971). An ineffectual sucking reflex is said to be common, and it may interfere seriously with postpartum feeding (Kron et al., 1976). Seizures are encountered occasionally, and there are a few reports of still-births (Cravey and Reed, 1981). Methadone withdrawal in the newborn is not associated with a high mortality or prolonged morbidity (Harper et al., 1974), but the severity of the reaction correlates closely with the maternal methadone dose schedule (Harper et al., 1977; Ostrea et al., 1976). Methadone doses should be lowered as soon as possible in late pregnancy to prevent the withdrawal reaction in the neonate. Even after the withdrawal syndrome is controlled, however, continued vigilance is warranted; at least one infant has died under circumstance suggesting methadone transmission via breast milk (Smialek et al., 1977). In the absence of respiratory impairment, neonates with narcotic dependencies have been managed with phenobarbital, chlorpromazine, paregoric or diazepam (Nathenson et al., 1971). The latter was judged more effective in restoring the sucking reflex (Kron et al., 1976). Naloxone should not be used in neonates with suspected physical dependence.

Even in nonaddicted mothers a neonatal syndrome much like a withdrawal reaction has been reported when codeine-containing medications were used prior to delivery (Mangurten and Benawra, 1980). Respiratory depression, however, is more common in neonates when morphine or meperidine is given during labor (Evans et al., 1976a). Naloxone, even in repeated doses, has been used safely in infants under one year of age who were accidentally poisoned acutely with morphine or methadone (Gober et al., 1979; Sesso and Rodzvilla, 1975; Simons, 1973). One 2½-year-old child who had ingested propoxyphene was unresponsive to the usual therapeutic dose, but did finally respond to 2 mg. naloxone, which is 20 times the recommended dose (Moore et al., 1980). Before injecting naloxone, it may be wise to remove endotracheal tubes. The response is so rapid that one child gagged and aspirated because the tube was left in place (Curnock, 1978).

Symptomatology:

1. Supralethal doses of morphine produce prompt coma, but sublethal doses usually

lead to a transient period of euphoria and exhilaration, characterized by a sensation of warmth and comfort, appearing within half an hour after ingestion.

2. Gradual drowsiness, dizziness, heaviness of the head, weariness, diminution of sensibility, loss of pain and other modalities of sensation.

3. Vomiting with little or no nausea.

4. A transient excitement state, characterized by extreme restlessness, delirium, and rarely epileptiform convulsions, is sometimes seen in children and rarely in adult women.

5. Bilateral miosis, progressing to pinpoint pupils, which do not react to light or accommodation. The pupils may dilate during terminal asphyxia.

6. Itching of the skin and nose, sometimes with skin rashes and urticaria.

7. Coma, with muscular relaxation and depressed or absent superficial and deep reflexes. A Babinski toe sign may appear.

8. Marked slowing of the respiratory rate with inadequate pulmonary ventilation and consequent cyanosis. Breathing becomes stertorous and irregular (Cheyne-Stokes or Biot).

9. The pulse is slow and the blood pressure gradually falls to shock levels. Urine formation ceases or is reduced to a very low rate.

10. The skin is cold and pale and shows a mottled cyanosis. The body temperature falls.

11. Death within 6 to 12 hours is usually due to respiratory arrest and consequent asphyxia.

12. Sometimes shock, severe but rapidly clearing pulmonary edema, hypostatic pneumonia or aspiration pneumonia contribute significantly to the fatal outcome.

13. During the recovery phase, itching, headache, nausea, vomiting, confusion, and obstipation may require attention. A symptomatic relapse may signal developing bronchopneumonia.

Treatment:

1. Even several hours after the ingestion of morphine, gastric lavage may be beneficial, because the drug often induces pylorospasm. A potassium permanganate solution (1:5000) or 1 ml. of tincture of iodine in a liter (quart) of water makes a satisfactory lavage fluid, but it is not established that these solutions are superior to tap water. Precautions against aspiration are essential. Emetics are rarely successful and are potentially dangerous. Save gastric contents for analysis.

2. Leave in the stomach 15 to 30 gm. of sodium sulfate in water as a saline cathartic and a slurry of activated charcoal (see Section I).

3. In morphine overdosage due to subcutaneous or intramuscular injection, a tourniquet or ice bag may be used to delay absorption.

4. Try to keep the patient awake by mild continuous stimulation that arouses but does not exhaust him. Moderately intense stimuli constitute an effective antidote against an impending morphine coma.

5. Correct airway obstruction. The insertion of an oropharyngeal airway or endotracheal tube is usually advisable in a comatose patient who has no gag reflex. See p. IV-3.

6. Continuous or intermittent oxygen therapy is usually indicated, but there is no justification for the use of O_2-CO_2 mixtures. See pp. IV-12–14.

7. Sometimes the inhalation of oxygen causes an arrest of spontaneous breathing. Artificial ventilation is then essential. Do not wait for respiratory arrest, but give mechanical assistance whenever the rate or depth of breathing is clearly inadequate (pp. IV-7–12).

8. The usual adult dose of naloxone is 0.4 to 2.0 mg. intravenously, intramuscularly or subcutaneously. The intravenous route is recommended for emergency situations. Repeat 2 to 5 times at 2- to 3-minute intervals if necessary to achieve the desired degree of narcotic antagonism (as evidenced, for example, by an improvement in pulmonary ventilation) up to a total dose of 10 mg. The dose in children and neonates is 0.01 mg./kg., which can be increased to 0.1 mg./kg. It may be wise to remove an endotracheal tube prior to injecting naloxone to prevent gagging and aspiration when the narcosis lightens. To sustain a beneficial effect, it may be necessary to readminister naloxone at intervals. Keep the patient under continuous surveillance. Failure to obtain significant improvement with naloxone suggests that the condition may be due to concurrent disease or non-narcotic drugs.

9. Maintain hydration and electrolyte balance by the slow administration of modest amounts of fluid and salts, but avoid overhydration. Diuretic drugs are without beneficial effects.

10. Hypotension is treated indirectly by the administration of oxygen. Sometimes a plasma transfusion is useful.

11. Good nursing is essential. The body temperature should be maintained if possible. Perhaps antibiotic therapy is advisable as prophylaxis against pneumonia (see pp. IV-85–86). By repeatedly changing the pa-

tient's posture, hypostatic pneumonia and decubitus ulcers are avoided. See p. IV-83.

Laboratory:

1. None of the routine laboratory tests has diagnostic or prognostic significance in acute morphinism. A variety of chemical tests and at least one bioassay procedure are practical ways of detecting morphine and related alkaloids in biological fluids and excreta (Elliot *et al.*, 1964). Modern analytical and immunologic techniques are sensitive to nano- and picogram levels (Alder *et al.*, 1972; Nakamura, 1978). Even in fatal cases, however, a wide range of blood morphine concentrations has been reported (Richards *et al.*, 1976).

2. Liver damage has been reported in mice with associated changes in serum hepatic enzyme activity (Needham *et al.*, 1981).

References:

Adler, F. L.; Liu, C. T.; Catlin, D. H. Immunological studies on heroin addiction. I. Methodology and application of a hemagglutination inhibition test for detection of morphine. Clin. Immunol. Immunopathol. *1*:53-68, 1972.

Bartlett, E. J. An examination of forty-three published cases of opium or morphine poisoning. Boston Med. Surg. J. *137*:674-675, 1897.

Blatman, S. Narcotic poisoning of children (1) through accidental ingestion of methadone and (2) in utero. Pediatrics *54*:329-332, 1974.

Buchner, L. H.; Cimino, J. A.; Raybin, H. W.; Stewart, B. Naloxone reversal of methadone poisoning. N. Y. State J. Med. *72*:2305-2309, 1972.

Caldwell, J.; Sever, P. S. The biochemical pharmacology of abused drugs. III. Cannabis, opiates and synthetic narcotics. Clin. Pharmacol. Ther. *16*:989-1013, 1974.

Chase, H. F.; Boyd, R. S.; Andrews, P. M. N-Allylnormorphine in treatment of dihydromorphinone and methorphinan overdosage. J. A. M. A. *150*:1103-1104, 1952.

Cravey, R. H.; Reed, D. Placental transfer of narcotic analgesic in man. Clin. Toxicol. *18*:911-914, 1981.

Curnock, D. A. Respiratory depression due to unsuspected narcotic ingestion treated with naloxone. Arch. Dis. Child. *53*:508-509, 1978.

D'Agostino, R. S.; Arnett, E. N. Acute myoglobinuria and heroin snorting. J. A. M. A. *241*:277, 1979.

Davis, W. M.; Hatoum, N. S.; Khalsa, J. H. Toxic interaction between narcotic analgesics and inhibitors of catechol-*O*-methyltransferase. Toxicology *14*:217-227, 1979.

Davis, W. N.; Hatoum, N. S. Lethal synergism between morphine or other narcotic analgesics and propranolol. Toxicology *14*:141-151, 1979.

de Castro, J.; Van de Water, A.; Wouters, L.; Xhonneux, R.; Reneman, R.; Kay, B. Comparative study of cardiovascular neurological and metabolic side-effects of light narcotics in dogs. Acta Anesthesiol. Belg. *30*:5-99, 1979.

Domino, E. F.; Pelikan, E. W.; Traut, E. F. Nalorphine (Nalline) antagonism to racemorphan (Dromoran) intoxication. J. A. M. A. *153*:26-27, 1953.

Drenick, E. J. Heroin overdose complicated by intravenous injection of milk. J. A. M. A. *213*:1687, 1970.

Duberstein, J. L.; Kaufman, D. Y. Clinical study of epidemic of heroin intoxication and heroin-induced pulmonary edema. Am. J. Med. *51*:704-714, 1971.

Eckenhoff, J. E.; Elder, J. D., Jr.; King, B. D. N-Allylnormorphine in the treatment of morphine or Demerol narcosis. Am. J. Med. Sci. *223*:191-197, 1952.

Eddy, N. B. Studies of morphine, codeine and their derivatives. XIV. The variation with age in the toxic effects of morphine, codeine and some of their derivatives. J. Pharmacol. Exp. Ther. *66*:182-201, 1939.

Eddy, N. B. Toxicity. In: *The Pharmacology of the Opium Alkaloids*, edited by H. Krueger, N. B. Eddy, and M. Sumwalt. U. S. Public Health Report, Suppl. No. 165, 1941.

Eerola, R. The effect of ethanol on the toxicity of hexobarbital, thiopental, morphine, atropine and scopolamine, an experimental study in mice. Ann. Med. Exp. Biol. Fenn. 39: Suppl. No. 3, 1961.

Elliot, H. W.; Nomof, N.; Parker, K.; Dewey, M. L.; Way, E. L. Comparison of the nalorphine test and urinary analysis in the detection of narcotic use. Clin. Pharmacol. Ther. *5*:405-413, 1964.

Evans, J. M.; Hogg, M. I. J.; Rosen, M. Reversal of narcotic depression in the neonate by naloxone. Br. Med. J. *2*:1098-1100, 1976a.

Evans, L. E. J.; Roscoe, P.; Swanson, C. P.; Prescott, L. F. Treatment of drug overdosage with naloxone, a specific narcotic antagonist. Lancet *1*:452-455, 1973.

Foldes, F. F.; Duncalf, D.; Kuwabara, S. The respiratory, circulatory and narcotic antagonistic effects of nalorphine, levallorphan and naloxone in anaesthetized subjects. Can. Anaesth. Soc. J. *16*:151-161, 1969.

Foldes, F. F.; Lunn, J. N.; Moore, J.; Brown, I. M. N-Allylnoroxymorphone: A new potent narcotic antagonist. Am. J. Med. Sci. *245*:23-30, 1963.

Frand, U. I.; Shim, C. S.; Williams, M. H. Methadone-induced pulmonary edema. Ann. Intern. Med. *76*:975-979, 1972a.

Frand, U. I.; Shim, C. S.; Williams, M. H. Heroin-induced pulmonary edema, sequential studies of pulmonary function. Ann. Intern. Med. *77*:29-35, 1972b.

Fraser, H. F.; Grider, J. A. Treatment of drug addiction. Am. J. Med. *14*:571-577, 1953.

Fraser, H. F.; Wikler, A.; Eisenman, A. J.; Isbell, H. Use of *N*-Allylnormorphine in treatment of methadone poisoning in man. Report of two cases. J. A. M. A. *148*:1205, 1952.

Furst, Z.; Foldes, F. F.; Knoll, J. Influence of naloxone on barbiturate anesthesia and toxicity in rat. Life Sciences *20*:921-926, 1977.

Garriott, J. C.; Sturner, W. Q. Concentrations and survival periods in acute heroin fatalities. N. Engl. J. Med. *289*:1276-1278, 1973.

Gober, A. E.; Kearns, G. L; Yokel, R. A.; Danziger, L. Repeated naloxone administration for morphine overdose in a 1-month-old infant. Pediatrics *63*:606-608, 1979.

Harper, R. G.; Solish, G.; Feingold, E.; Gerstenwoolf, N. B.; Sokal, M. M. Maternal ingested methadone, body fluid methadone and the neonatal withdrawal syndrome. Am. J. Obstet. Gynecol. *129*:417-424, 1977.

Harper, R. G.; Solish, G. I.; Purow, H. M.; Sang, E.; Panepinto, W. C. The effect of a methadone treatment program upon pregnant heroin addicts and their newborn infants. Pediatrics *54*:300-305, 1974.

Hart, E. R.; McCawley, E. L. The pharmacology of N-allylnormorphine as compared with morphine. J. Pharmacol. Exp. Ther. *82*:339-348, 1944.

Helpern, M.; Rho, Y. -M. Deaths from narcotism in New York City, incidence, circumstances and postmortem findings. N. Y. State J. Med. *66*:2391-2407, 1966.

Hirsch, C. S.; Adelson, L. Acute fatal intranasal narcotism. Hum. Pathol. *3*:71-73, 1972.

Ho, I. K.; Loh, H. H.; Way, E. L. Toxic interactions between choline and morphine. Toxicol. Appl. Pharmacol. *51*:203-208, 1979.

Isbell, H.; White, W. M. Clinical characteristics of addictions. Am. J. Med. *14*:558-565, 1953.

Jaffe, J. H.; Martin, W. R. Opioid analgesics and antagonists. In *The Pharmacological Basis of Therapeutics*. (Gilman, A. G.; Goodman, L. S.; Gilman, A., editors). Macmillan Publishing Co. Inc., pp. 494-534, 1980.

Kahn, E. J.; Neumann, L. L.; Polk, G. A. The course of the heroin withdrawal syndrome in newborn infants treated with phenobarbital or chlorpromazine. J. Pediatr. *75*:495-500, 1969.

Katz, S.; Aberman, A.; Frand, U. I.; Stein, I. M.; Fulop, M. Heroin pulmonary edema, evidence for increased pulmonary capillary permeability. Am. Rev. Resp. Dis. 106:472-474, 1972.

Kron, R. E.; Litt, M.; Phoenix, M. D.; Finnegan, L. P. Neonatal narcotic abstinence - effects of pharmacotherapeutic agents and maternal drug usage on nutritive sucking behavior. J. Pediatr. 38:637-641, 1976.

Labi, M. Paroxysmal atrial fibrillation in heroin intoxication. Ann. Intern. Med. 71:951-959, 1969.

Lasagna, L. Nalorphine (N-allylnormorphine). Practical and theoretical considerations. Arch. Intern. Med. 94:532-558, 1954.

Lewis, D. C.; Zinberg, N. E. Narcotic usage. II. A historical perspective on a difficult medical problem. N. Engl. J. Med. 270:1045-1050, 1964.

Lockridge, O.; Mottershaw-Jackson, N.; Eckerson, H. W.; La Da, B. N. Hydrolysis of diacetylmorphine (heroin) by human serum cholinesterase. J. Pharmacol. Exp. Ther. 215:1-3, 1980.

Lowenstein, E.; Hallowell, P.; Levine, F. H.; Daggett, W. M.; Austen, W. G. Cardiovascular response to large doses of intravenous morphine in man. N. Engl. J. Med. 281:1389-1393, 1969.

Mangurten, H. H.; Benawra, R. Neonatal codeine withdrawal in infants of nonaddicted mothers. Pediatrics 65:159-160, 1980.

Marx, F. J.; Love, J. Effectiveness of N-allylnormorphine in the management of acute morphine poisoning. Ann. Intern. Med. 39:635-640, 1953.

Masini, E.; Blandina, D.; Mannaioni, P. F.; Luciani, G. Clonidine and naloxone for rapid opiate detoxication: Comparison between treatments. Clin. Toxicol. 18:1021-1026, 1981.

Moeller, K. O. Death due to therapeutic doses of morphine or morphine-scopolamine in patients under influence of alcohol or barbituric acid. Ugeskr. Laeger 114:1785-1793, 1952.

Moore, R. A.; Rumack, B. H.; Conner, C. S.; Peterson, R. G. Naloxone, underdosage after narcotic poisoning. Am. J. Dis. Child. 134:156-158, 1980.

Morrison, W. J.; Wetherill, S.; Zyroff, J. The acute pulmonary edema of heroin intoxication. Radiology 97:347-351, 1970.

Nakamura, G. R. Toxicologic assessments in acute heroin fatalities. Clin. Toxicol. 13:75-87, 1978.

Nathenson, G. G.; Golden, S.; Litt, I. F. Diazepam in the management of the neonatal narcotic withdrawal syndrome. Pediatrics 48:523-527, 1971.

Needham, W. P.; Shuster, L.; Kanel, G. C.; Thompson, M. L. Liver damage from narcotics in mice. Toxicol. Appl. Pharmacol. 58:157-170, 1981.

Nomof, N.; Elliott, H. W.; Parker, K. D. Actions and metabolism of codeine (methylmorphine) administration by continuous intravenous infusion to humans. Clin. Toxicol. 11:517-529, 1977.

Ostrea, E. M.; Chavez, C. J.; Strauss, M. E. Study of factors that influence severity of neonatal narcotic withdrawal. J. Pediatr. 88:642-645, 1976.

Raskin, M. M. N. Pulmonary edema of acute overdose reaction and near-drowning: some radiographic and physiologic comparisons. South Med. J. 69:1063-1065, 1976.

Ratcliffe, S. G. Methadone poisoning in a child. Br. Med. J. 1:1069-1070, 1963.

Reddy, A. M.; Harper, R. G.; Stern, G. Observations on heroin and methadone withdrawal in the newborn. Pediatrics 48:353-358, 1971.

Richards, R. G.; Reed, D.; Cravey, R. H. Death from intravenously administered narcotics: a study of 114 cases. J.

Forensic Sci. 21:467-482, 1976.

Rumler, W.; Weigel, W. Uber die Codeinvergiftung im Kindesalter. Ein Problem der Pharmakologie und Toxikologie des wachsenden Organismus. Monatsschr. Kinderheillkd. 111:241-246, 1963.

Sadove, M. S.; Balagot, R. C.; Hatano, S.; Jobgen, E. A. Study of a narcotic antagonist, N-allylnoroxymorphone. J. A. M. A. 183:666-668, 1963.

Schreiber, S. N.; Liebowitz, M. R.; Berenstein, L. H.; Srinivasan, K. Limb compression and renal impairment (crush syndrome) complicating narcotic overdose. N. Engl. J. Med. 284:368-369, 1971.

Sesso, A. M.; Rodzvilla, J. P. Naloxone therapy in a seven-month-old with methadone poisoning. Clin. Pediatr. 14:388-389, 1975.

Simons, P. S. The treatment of methadone poisoning with nalaxone (Narcan). J. Pediatr. 83:846-847, 1973.

Smialek, J. E.; Monforte, J. R.; Aronow, R.; Spitz, W. U. Methadone deaths in children. J. A. M. A. 238:2516-2517, 1977.

Steinberg, A. D.; Karliner, J. S. The clinical spectrum of heroin pulmonary edema. Arch. Intern. Med. 122:122-127, 1968.

Steinhaus, J. E.; Tatum, A. L. An experimental study of cocaine intoxication and its treatment. J. Pharmacol. Exp. Ther. 100:351-361, 1950.

Stern, W. Z.; Spear, P. W.; Jacobson, H. G. The roentgen findings in acute heroin intoxication. Am. J. Roentgenol. Radium Ther. Nucl. Med. 103:522-532, 1968.

Strober, M. Treatment of acute heroin intoxication with nalorphine (Nalline) hydrochloride. J. A. M. A. 154:327-328, 1954.

Sussman, S. Narcotic and methamphetamine use during pregnancy, effect on newborn infants. Am. J. Dis. Child. 106:325-330, 1963a.

Turner, J. E.; Richards, R. G. A fatal case involving levorphanol. J. Analyt. Toxicol. 1:103-104, 1977.

Unna, K. Antagonistic effect of N-allylnormorphine upon morphine. J. Pharmacol. Exp. Ther. 79:27-31, 1943.

Wang, R. I. H.; Wiesen, R. L.; Lamid, S.; Roh, B. L. Rating the presence and severity of opiate dependence. Clin. Pharmacol. Therap. 16:653-658, 1974.

Warnock, M. L.; Ghanremani, G. G.; Rattenborg, C.; Ginsberg, M.; Valenzuela, J. Pulmonary complication of heroin intoxication. J. A. M. A. 219:1051-1053, 1972.

Webster, R. W. Legal Medicine and Toxicology. W. B. Saunders Co., Philadelphia, 1930.

Wikler, A. Opiate Addiction. Psychological and Neurophysiological Aspects in Relation to Clinical Problems. Charles C Thomas, Springfield, Ill, 1952.

Winter, C. A.; Flataker, L. Effect of N-allylnormorphine upon massive doses of narcotic drugs. Proc. Soc. Exp. Biol. Med. 93:158-160, 1956.

Winter, J. C. Propranolol and morphine: a lethal interaction. Arch. Intern. Pharm. Ther. 212:195-198, 1974.

Yeh, S. Y.; Gorodetzky, C. W.; McQuinn, R. L. Urinary excretion of heroin and its metabolites in man. J. Pharmacol. Exp. Ther. 196:249-256, 1976.

Yeh, S. Y.; Krebs, H. A. Development of narcotic drug metabolizing enzymes in the newborn rat. J. Pharmacol. Exp. Ther. 213:28-32, 1980.

Zinberg, N. E.; Lewis, D. C. Narcotic usage. I. A spectrum of a difficult medical problem. N. Engl. J. Med. 270:989-993, 1964.

MUSHROOM TOXINS

Poisoning from toxic mushrooms (toadstools) is called mycetismus. Poisonous species are common in North America and are difficult for the inexperienced to distinguish from edible varieties. Homespun methods of differentiation are invariably fallacious and therefore dangerous; for example, taste is no adequate criterion since the deadly *Amanita phalloides* is said to have a delicious flavor. In spite of a rich folklore, silver coins have no proper role in the safety evaluation of wild mushrooms. In the United States Amanitas are responsible for most diagnosed cases of mushroom fatalities, but more than 70 species representing many genera are capable of inducing toxic reactions in man.

There are no accurate statistics on the incidence of mushroom poisoning or even on the number of fatal cases. Mushroom ingestions are said to have been responsible for about 1% of the 35,000 cases of accidental poisoning recorded annually by the National Clearinghouse for Poison Control Centers in Washington, D.C., but the true incidence is undoubtedly higher (Lincoff and Mitchel, 1977). Block *et al.* (1955) estimated that about 50 persons die in the United States each year from ingesting toxic mushrooms, but others regard this figure as too high, perhaps by a factor of 2 (R.W. Buck, personal communication, 1967), perhaps by a factor of 10 (K.F. Lampe, personal communication, 1982). On a worldwide basis, estimates range from 50 to 300 mushroom-related deaths per year (Lincoff and Mitchel, 1977). Most of these deaths are due to cyclopeptide poisoning (Group I toxins), but gyromitrin-containing mushrooms (Group II toxins) are sometimes responsible especially in eastern Europe. The other varieties of mushroom toxins are rarely lethal.

A history of eating noncultivated mushrooms is usually the first clue that a physician elicits in diagnosing mycetismus. A specific diagnosis, however, requires botanical identification of the mushroom and/or chemical identification of its toxin(s) in the patient's blood or excreta. Many elegant books are available to help the amateur mushroom collector (*e.g.*, Miller, 1972), but for a reliable species identification the services of an expert are usually required. The following discussion does not address the subject of how to recognize or identify a toxic mushroom; the presumption is that an identification has already been made.

Toxicology: The ingestion of toxic mushrooms may induce any of many diverse sets of signs and symptoms. At least three distinctive clinical syndromes have long been recognized and named mycetismus choleriformis, mycetismus nervosa and mycetismus cerebralis (Alder 1961; Ford, 1923). The modern practice, however, is to classify poisonings due to the ingestion of fleshy fungi according to the toxic principles believed to be responsible. This convention leads to some difficulties because not all mushroom toxins have been identified, not even all of the lethal ones (see Group VIII below). Some fungi possess more than one type of toxin and so sometimes lead to "mixed" intoxications. In spite of these and some other difficulties, the following discussion is organized according to a classification proposed by Lincoff and Mitchel (1977), involving 7 separate groups of mushroom toxins, with the addition here of an eighth group to include the unidentified renal toxin found in

some species of *Cortinarius*. The numerical designation of each group is arbitrary and differs in different treatises.

Whereas this classification encompasses the mushroom toxins that are known to be involved most often in clinical poisonings, it is important to recognize that the toxic potential of many mushrooms has not yet been explored. Isolated clinical reports indicate toxic signs and symptoms that cannot be ascribed to known toxins (Lampe, 1979). Future studies will certainly reveal new toxic principles.

Group I. Cyclopeptides

A frequently lethal illness preceded by a long latency arises from the ingestion of a series of cyclic polypeptides found in several species of *Amanita*, notably the "death cap," *A. phalloides* (Wieland and Wieland, 1959) and several related species (Block *et al.*, 1955) known as the "destroying angels" (*A. verna, A. virosa, A. bisporigera*). Some of the same cyclopeptides are also found in three species of *Galerina* (*G. autumnalis, G. marginata, G. venenata*), which have also produced clinical poisonings (Grossman and Malbin, 1954). Smaller but still dangerous amounts have been reported in *A. brunnescens* and *A. tenuifolia* (Tyler, 1963). Very small and almost certainly safe amounts have been detected in a bewildering array of unrelated mushrooms including several edible ones, notably *Boletus edulis* and *Cantharellus cibarius* (Faulstich and Cochet-Meilhac, 1976).

Ingestion is followed by an asymptomatic latent period of 6 to 15 or even 20 hours, although this characteristic feature may be obscured by a concurrent illness due to the ingestion of some other food poison. The cyclopeptide intoxication begins as a severe gastroenteritis (Lampe, 1978; Lewes, 1948), sometimes with associated cardiovascular collapse, prostration, delirium and coma. Death may occur at this stage ("cerebral death"), but after a day or two the patient often seems to improve, at least for a short time. The most characteristic manifestations do not occur until the 3rd or 4th day after the ingestion, when liver swelling, tenderness and other signs of hepatic cell necrosis appear. Severe damage may also arise in the renal tubular epithelium, myocardium and brain. Death may occur within 5 to 10 days; it is due to liver failure (Van der Veer and Farley, 1935; Harrison *et al.*, 1965), to renal failure (Myler *et al.*, 1964), to cerebral damage with attending coma (Abul-Haj *et al.*, 1963) or to cardiac arrest. Liver failure is probably the commonest cause of death. No satisfactory treatment for poisoning by *A. phalloides* is recognized.

Studies beginning in 1937 led to the chemical identification of the toxic principles in *A. phalloides* (Wieland and Wieland, 1959; Wieland,

1968). Aside from a hemolytic basic protein (phallolysin), which has been known for a long time and which is apparently inactive by mouth, all of the toxins of *A. phalloides* are cyclic polypeptides with molecular weights varying from about 800 to 1100, but they may exist in mushroom cells as parts of large molecular complexes.

Two groups of polypeptides are recognized. The phallotoxins (which includes phalloidin) possess in common a cyclic heptapeptide skeleton with some unusual amino acids (Wieland, 1968). At least in the case of phalloidin, which probably is not active systemically when given by mouth (Wieland, 1968), the cytotoxicity of the injected polypeptide is associated with a thioether linkage between cysteine and tryptophan in the toxin molecule (Wieland and Wieland, 1959). Phalloidin (and presumably the other phallotoxins) bind to and promptly damage cytoplasmic membranes of the liver cell, including the plasma membrane, lysosome membranes and especially the endoplasmic reticulum (Fiume and Laschi, 1965; Wieland, 1968). Their mode of action has been reviewed (Chilton, 1978; Lampe, 1978), but it is unlikely that they contribute to the ingestion toxicity of *A. phalloides* either because of their limited absorption from the alimentary tract or for other unexplained reasons.

The long delayed hepatotoxic response seen in human poisonings is due to the other group of cyclic polypeptides, the amatoxins, consisting of at least 6 molecular species, including α-, β-, and γ-amanitin and especially the α component (Wieland and Wieland, 1959). These amatoxins possess in common a cyclic octapeptide skeleton (Wieland, 1968). They are more toxic than the phallotoxins, and, unlike the latter, they damage the nucleolus and later the nucleus of liver cells (Fiume and Laschi, 1965). In laboratory rodents the mean lethal dose of α-amanitin is only 0.1 mg./kg. (Wieland, 1965). Man is said to be even more susceptible. A single specimen of *A. phalloides* or as little as 20 to 30 gm. may contain enough of this constituent (perhaps 7 mg.) to kill a man, but the amounts of amatoxins appear to be highly variable. For example, some specimens in the Pacific Northwest are said to be rich in β-amanitin but almost devoid of α-amanitin (Tyler *et al.*, 1966). *A. verna* and *A. virosa* sometimes lack both (Yocum and Simons, 1977).

Biochemical mechanisms involved in the cytotoxicity of these polypeptides have been investigated in several laboratories. Mice (but not rats) are particularly sensitive to the nephrotoxicity of these toxins (Fiume *et al.*, 1969), but liver injury is usually the major lesion in man (*e.g.*, Menu and Faure, 1967). There appears to be a prompt decrease or cessation of bile flow, a reduction in liver glycogen, hypoglycemia with or without an initial phase of hyperglycemia, a fall in the RNA content of liver nuclei, and a failure of liver cell protein synthesis (Wieland, 1965; Fiume and Stirpe, 1966; Wieland and Wieland, 1959), but whether or not any of these effects is the primary lesion has not been established. The ability of α-amanitin to inhibit RNA polymerase II (Lindell *et al.*, 1970) has been useful in biochemical research. The failure of transcription is probably the molecular defect responsible for hepatic necrosis (Faulstich, 1979; Lampe, 1978).

A bewildering variety of pharmacological agents has been reported to protect mice against lethal doses of phallotoxins and in some cases against amatoxins (Floersheim, 1972a–c). The list includes high doses of penicillin, chloramphenicol, phenylbutazone, cytochrome *c*, vitamin C and many others. Floersheim (1972a–c) has suggested that they may be effective by displacing Amanita toxins from binding sites on plasma proteins and so accelerating their excretion in the urine before they are able to induce liver and renal injury, but at least α-amanitin does not bind to serum albumin (Fiume *et al.*, 1977).

The list of experimental antidotes continues to grow (reviewed by Lampe, 1978, and by Floersheim, 1978) and includes rifampicin, cysteamine, and silymarin (obtained from the Mediterranean milk thistle). *A. phalloides* even contains a nontoxic cyclodecapeptide (antamanide) that protects against phalloidin (reviewed by Chilton, 1978). To be effective, however, most of these agents must be administered before or within a few minutes after a lethal dose of the toxic cyclopeptides. Aside from a limited study in dogs, the only animals in which they have been tested are laboratory mice and rats. Except for large doses of penicillin G and thioctic acid (see below) and rarely of cytochrome *c*, none of these antidotes has received a clinical trial, and so none can be recommended unequivocally. In a person with no penicillin allergy, however, large doses of penicillin G can do no harm, and the recommended dose of 250 mg./kg. given daily by continuous intravenous infusion appears to be beneficial in human victims (Moroni *et al.*, 1976), as in dogs (Floersheim *et al.*, 1978). Penicillin is believed to act by inhibiting amatoxin uptake by hepatocytes (Faulstich, 1979). If so, its utility is probably limited to the first 24 or perhaps 48 hours after ingestion.

Since 1963 the European literature has referred to the successful use of thioctic acid in clinical Amanita poisonings. Although this substance is ineffective prophylactically and therapeutically in poisoned mice (Floersheim, 1972c), Kubicka and Alder (1968) report survival in 39 out of 40 treated human cases. Many favorable clinical reports were published in Poland, Italy and France, and some apparent successes have been noted in the United States (*e.g.*, Bartter *et al.*, 1980; Finestone *et al.*, 1972; Teutsch and Brennan, 1978). Thioctic acid, usually called α-lipoic acid in the current biochemical literature, is sometimes regarded as one of the B vitamins. An experimental treatment regimen involving intravenous α-lipoic acid is outlined below (see "Treatment"). More experience is required to establish its role in Amanita poisoning, but early enthusiasm has certainly waned, and most experts today appear to be skeptical if not negative. Certainly the value of thioctic acid has not been demonstrated in experimental animals or in a controlled clinical study.

Approved therapy of Amanita poisoning in man is strictly symptomatic and supportive, with emphasis on measures to limit absorption of the amatoxins and to promote their elimination. A horse serum antitoxin prepared at the Pasteur Institute in Paris has been recommended at various times (Block *et al.*, 1955), but its effectiveness has been denied (Menu and Faure, 1967; Wieland, 1968), and it is no longer available. With the development of a radioimmunoassay with an amatoxin sensitivity of about 0.5 ng./ml. (Faulstich, 1979), it has been established that appreciable amounts of toxin are found in human blood plasma for at least 24 hours after the ingestion of *A. phalloides* (Busi *et al.*, 1977), that these toxins are excreted in urine (Costantino *et al.*, 1977) and bile (Busi *et al.*, 1979), that some of the toxin filtered in the kidney may be resorbed into or through the renal tubules (Faulstich, 1979) and that toxin eliminated in bile is partly resorbed in the gut. Forced diuresis may be useful in promoting the renal excretion of these polypeptides, but whether an osmotic diuresis is superior to a water diuresis is not clearly established (Langer *et al.*, 1980). Because activated charcoal binds them very tightly, its oral administration has been recommended to interrupt the enterohepatic circulation, although in the presence of nausea an indwelling duodenal tube with continuous suctioning may be more practical.

Whereas hemodialysis (Elliott *et al.*, 1961) and peritoneal dialysis (Myler *et al.*, 1964) have long been used in anuric mushroom victims and in those with hepatic failure, Tholen *et al.* (1966) may have been the first to emphasize that hemodialysis should be instituted early in the course of the poisoning to remove the toxin. With molecular weights of about 900, the amatoxins have been shown to be readily dialyzable from plasma protein solutions (Seeger and Bartels, 1976). In various series of human *A. phalloides* poisonings, attempts have been made to compare amatoxin removal by peritoneal dialysis with that by plasmapheresis, exchange transfusion and forced diuresis (Costantino and Damia, 1977; Langer *et al.*, 1980). All of these modes of therapy appeared to be useful if instituted within the first 36 hours after the ingestion. Extracorporeal hemodialysis is in general more efficient than peritoneal dialysis, but hemoperfusion through activated charcoal has been extolled as superior to all of the other measures in promoting amatoxin elimination (Faulstich, 1979; Wauters *et al.*, 1978). More data are needed, but it appears that hemoperfusion may be worthwhile during the first 48 hours after the ingestion (Faulstich, 1979). Both extracorporeal hemodialysis and hemoperfusion require heparinization of the patient. Heparin is probably safe during the first 48 hours because amatoxin-induced coagulation defects are not usually prominent that early in the intoxication.

In clinical poisonings by *A. phalloides*, the fatality rate is about 50% according to Alder (1961) or about 30% according to Grzymala (1965). In the United States, where true *A. phalloides* has a more limited distribution than in Europe (Litten, 1975), experience with cyclopeptide poisoning does not appear to be quite so grim, but accurate statistics are unavailable. Hepatic coma is a bad prognostic sign, but complete recoveries have occurred (*e.g.*, Teutsch and Brennan, 1978). Perhaps improvements in supportive care are responsible for the apparent reduction in fatality rates in Europe. For example, Moroni *et al.* (1976) reported no deaths in 33 persons with *A. phalloides* poisoning treated with penicillin G, thioctic acid and other agents listed below.

Symptomatology (Group I):
1. Asymptomatic period of 6 to 15 hours after ingestion (sometimes not manifested if other toxic fungi with short latent periods were ingested at the same time).
2. Sudden onset of abdominal pain, usually colicky.
3. Nausea, violent vomiting and severe bloody or blood-streaked diarrhea.
4. Rapidly developing weakness, restlessness and eventual apathy.
5. Dehydration, with extreme thirst.
6. Muscle cramps and twitching.
7. Cyanosis, cold clammy skin, and other signs of shock. Hypotension and tachycardia may persist for many days.
8. Somnolence leading to coma and sometimes death as early as the 2nd day in young children ("cerebral death").
9. A phase of distinct clinical improvement is often described after 1 to 2 days, especially if dehydration, electrolyte imbalances and shock have been corrected by therapy.
10. Tender enlargement of the liver, with jaundice apparent within 3 to 5 days, due

to hepatic cell degeneration, which may progress to massive acute yellow atrophy.

11. Oliguria or anuria, secondary to renal tubular damage, occurs in only a small fraction of cases if circulatory shock is avoided.

12. Delirium, hallucinations, sometimes convulsions, and eventually coma.

13. Cardiac arrhythmias and hypotension.

14. Because of severe blood coagulation defects, massive internal hemorrhages may occur.

15. Death in 5 to 8 days may be due to cellular damage in the central nervous system, liver, kidneys, or heart. In various series the fatality rate has ranged from 0 to 100%; 30% is a widely quoted value. Death may occur as late as 7 to 8 days after the ingestion.

Treatment (Group I):

1. If spontaneous vomiting has not already been extensive and productive, induce emesis with syrup of ipecac (p. I-2), and/or perform gastric lavage with water or potassium permanganate solution (1:5000). Save the gastric contents.

2. Activated charcoal, several tablespoonfuls in water by mouth. If vomiting does not prevent its retention, this dose of activated charcoal should be given every few hours to interrupt the early enterohepatic cycling of the amatoxins. Alternatively, a tube can be introduced into the duodenum with continuous aspiration.

3. Saline catharsis with sodium sulfate (15 to 30 gm. in water) by mouth. High colonic enemas may also help to stimulate prompt evacuation. A clinical impression persists that the sooner and the more vigorous the purging, whether spontaneous or induced by treatment, the less severe is the late injury to vital organs.

4. Meperidine (Demerol) for the control of pain. Morphine is best avoided because it may delay purging.

5. Correct dehydration and shock by the intravenous administration of replacement fluids (pp. IV-66 and 17).

6. Intravenous infusions of glucose when and if hypoglycemia appears.

7. To promote amatoxin excretion and to limit renal involvement, try to maintain a brisk urine flow during the first 2 days, if necessary by using mannitol (p. IV-52).

8. Early extracorporeal hemodialysis or better hemoperfusion over activated charcoal (p. IV-57) is also judged worthwhile during the first 3 days to eliminate the toxin.

9. Intravenous corticosteroids have been recommended, e.g., 20 to 40 mg. dexamethasone daily, in the hope of inhibiting toxin fixation in the liver. As with items 10 and 11 below, the value of this form of therapy has not been demonstrated objectively.

10. Another experimental regimen that is alleged to protect the liver (see text above) is the intravenous infusion of large doses of penicillin G (250 mg./kg. daily) during the first 2 days.

11. A trial with intravenous thioctic acid (α-lipoic acid) may or may not be useful (see text above). It has been administered in glucose solution by slow intravenous infusion (300 mg. over 24 hours daily for several days). For details about procuring and using this agent, see thioctic acid in Section II.

12. Digitalis may be given a trial if hypotension persists after rehydration is completed.

13. Institute supportive treatment for impending renal and hepatic insufficiencies (pp. IV-52 and 60).

Laboratory (Group I):

1. Because prognosis and treatment vary drastically with the type of mushroom, a species identification is always desirable. If a large enough piece of the fungus is available, an expert can recognize it from various botanical characteristics. A simple spot test for detecting amatoxins was described by Meixner (see Beutler and Vergeer, 1980); it should be a useful screening procedure, especially with A. virosa, specimens of which may or may not contain amatoxins. A rapid and comparatively simple chromatographic isolation of phalloides toxins has been proposed as a practical method of identification (Block et al., 1955). The procedure is said to require only 0.1 gm. of fresh A. phalloides; it should prove distinctly useful, although radioimmunoassays (see below) are now more widely used. Phalloidin and β-amatoxin were successfully isolated from the liver of a boy who died of mushroom poisoning (Abul-Haj et al., 1963).

2. A kit for a simple radioimmunoassay with an amatoxin sensitivity of about 0.5 ng./ml. is now available (Faulstich, 1979). It has been used successfully to quantify the toxins in serum, urine and duodenal juice (see text above).

3. Repeated biochemical tests of liver function and kidney function are important. Serum transaminase levels (SGOT, SGPT, LDH) are particularly sensitive indices of liver injury, as are blood levels of coagulation factors synthesized in the liver.

4. Blood electrolyte levels should be monitored to evaluate the progress of replace-

ment therapy with water and salt (pp. IV-64–67, 69–72).

5. Blood glucose determinations to detect severe hypoglycemia.

Group II. Gyromitrins and MMH

Many (but perhaps not all) species of the genus *Gyromitra* contain a group of chemically related toxins, known as gyromitrins, that decompose to release monomethylhydrazine (MMH). These so-called false morels or brain fungi (also known in Europe as lorels or lorchels) are popular springtime mushrooms, and *G. esculenta* in particular is often collected as food in eastern Europe, sometimes in France and Italy and rarely in the United States, except perhaps in the Pacific northwest. Various other ascomycetes, notably members of the genus *Helvella*, are suspected to contain the same or related poisons (Lincoff and Mitchel, 1977).

In the fungi MMH is bound as the *N*-methyl-*N*-formylhydrazines of several low molecular weight aliphatic aldehydes. The first to be isolated was the hydrazone of acetaldehyde, originally named gyromitrin (List and Luft, 1968), now sometimes called ethylidene gyromitrin. Subsequently the corresponding hydrazones of 3-methylbutanal, pentanal and hexanal were detected (Pyysalo, 1975). One kilogram of fresh *G. esculenta* from central Europe contained 1.2 to 1.6 gm. (0.12 to 0.16%) of potassium iodate-reducing materials, calculated as ethylidene gyromitrin (List and Luft, 1968). The oral LD_{50} values of these hydrazones in rabbits range from about 50 to 300 mg./kg., the ethylidene analogue being the most toxic (Pyysalo, 1975). Rats appear to be more tolerant, the oral LD_{50} being 320 mg./kg. From data on food poisoning outbreaks, the lethal dose of ethylidene gyromitrin is estimated to be 20 to 50 mg./kg. in adult humans and 10 to 50 mg./kg. in children (cited by Niskanen *et al.*, 1976).

The gyromitrins are moderately volatile, but in boiling water (Pyysalo, 1976) and in stomach acid they are hydrolyzed to *N*-methyl-*N*-formylhydrazine (MFH) and then to the highly volatile MMH. That the breakdown is extensive and the MMH is absorbed have been demonstrated in mice given gyromitrin by mouth (von Wright *et al.*, 1978). The toxicity of gyromitrins is usually ascribed to this MMH produced *in vivo*. However, respiratory exposure of monkeys to MMH vapor (reviewed by Back and Thomas, 1970) produces among other effects methemoglobinemia, intravascular hemolysis, hematuria, early hypoglycemia and convulsions, none of which is a common feature of human gyromitrin poisonings, although each has been observed in isolated cases (Franke *et al.*, 1967; Hendricks, 1940). Possibly other mushroom constituents

suppress some of these effects or possibly the dose of MMH in mushroom poisonings is too small to elicit them. Almost certainly the hydrophilic MMH and the more lipophilic gyromitrins have different patterns of distribution *in vivo*. The concept that the toxicity of gyromitrins is due entirely to the release of MMH is still a hypothesis and one not entirely consonant with experimental data (*cf.* Braun *et al.*, 1979).

The chief clinical feature in common between MMH poisoning and gyromitrin poisoning is late liver necrosis with coma. When due to the ingestion of mushrooms of the genus *Gyromitra*, this liver injury is preceded by a period of severe gastroenteritis (Franke *et al.*, 1967). Possibly a metabolite of MMH, like the acetylhydrazine metabolite of the drug isoniazid, acts as an alkylating agent to induce liver cell necrosis (Lampe, 1978). If this theory proves to be correct, *N*-acetylcysteine may be useful to protect the liver, as in acetaminophen poisoning (p. III-5). Thioctic acid is not recommended in gyromitrin intoxication.

Hydrazine and its methyl derivatives act as vitamin B_6 antagonists. They are said to combine with and inactivate pyridoxal-5-phosphate and to inhibit its biosynthesis. The loss of pyridoxal phosphate reduces the activity of several enzymes that require it as a coenzyme, including those involved in the metabolism of GABA (γ-aminobutyric acid). Convulsions in hydrazine poisoning have been ascribed to abnormally low levels of GABA in the brain. Part of the evidence in support of these interactions is the demonstration that pyridoxine, the vitamin precursor of pyridoxal phosphate, is effective as an antidote in suppressing the convulsions of 1,1-dimethylhydrazine poisoning in animals (Back and Thomas, 1970). It also appears capable of correcting both the hyperexcitability (Frierson, 1965) and coma (Kirklin *et al.*, 1976) observed in men acutely poisoned by hydrazine. In animals the convulsions of MMH are more difficult to control and higher doses are required (Back and Thomas, 1970). Parenteral doses as high as 25 mg./kg. have been recommended for humans poisoned by MMH, but smaller amounts in combination with diazepam may be more effective in suppressing these convulsions (George *et al.*, 1982).

In gyromitrin poisoning, however, convulsions and other neurological disorders are rare until the stage of hepatic coma. Whereas pyridoxine is able to suppress some of the visceral actions of gyromitrin (Braun *et al.*, 1979), we know of no evidence that it protects the liver cell against gyromitrins or prevents hepatic injury by MMH. Nevertheless, it is usually recommended in poisonings due to these mushrooms (Lampe, 1978); almost certainly it can due no harm.

Poisonings from ingesting mushrooms of the

genus *Gyromitra* are peculiarly unpredictable. Many persons have and continue to eat these wild fungi, notably *G. esculenta*, apparently with impunity. This mushroom is especially popular in Poland and eastern Europe, where most of the reported poisonings have occurred. Indeed, wild *G. esculenta* was once a mushroom of commerce in Poland and Germany, amounting to 350,000 kg. per year in 1930 (Chilton, 1978). Like the illness itself, the fatality rate is highly variable: 14.7% (74 out of 513) in the series reported from Central Europe by Franke *et al.* (1967), 1 of 11 Swiss cases according to Alder (1961), 6 of 138 cases in Poland according to Grzymala (1965c). Lincoff and Mitchel (1977) state that "only about 20 *Gyromitra* poisonings have been reported in North America since 1900, but half of these were fatal."

The failure of *G. esculenta* to produce intoxications consistently is explicable in part by the ways it is prepared for eating. The usual mode of cooking, which has long been known to reduce the risk of poisoning, is to parboil the mushroom and to discard the water. Boiling them for 10 minutes in large volumes of water or drying them thoroughly has been shown to remove or destroy over 99% of the hydrazine content (Pyysalo, 1976). These techniques, however, are not always sufficient, and highly variable clinical responses, ranging from no symptoms to death, have been described among individuals who ate from the same batch of cooked *G. esculenta* (Hendricks, 1940). Susceptibility and resistance to gyromitrin poisoning cannot be reliably predicted.

Symptomatology (Group II):

1. Symptoms commonly begin abruptly 6 to 8 hours after ingestion (as early as 2 hours and as late as 20 hours).
2. Prominent headache, fatigue, dizziness, sensation of abdominal bloating.
3. Nausea and vomiting that may persist intermittently for several hours.
4. Watery diarrhea (rarely bloody) occurs but is not invariable (it is always seen in Group I poisonings).
5. Abdominal pain, muscle cramps, perhaps loss of motor control or transient paralysis.
6. Usually a complete recovery in 2 to 4 days, but occasionally jaundice appears after about 36 to 40 hours. Hepatomegaly and splenomegaly occur. The liver becomes painful. Hepatic necrosis leads to liver failure, coma and death.
7. Intravascular hemolysis has been reported at least once, with secondary renal failure, but clear-cut evidence of hemolysis is rarely encountered in human poisonings (Hendricks, 1940).

Treatment (Group II):

1. The early induction of emesis and/or gastric lavage is likely to be useful. The efficacy of activated charcoal has not been demonstrated but it can do no harm (see Section I).
2. Control distressing vomiting with antiemetic drugs (p. IV-49).
3. Meperidine for abdominal and muscle pain (p. IV-32).
4. Correct dehydration and electrolyte imbalances by intravenous infusions (pp. IV-64–73).
5. Test for and, if necessary, correct hypoglycemia, which is commonly encountered in early MMH poisoning in monkeys but not often observed in gyromitrin poisonings in man until the stage of liver failure.
6. Pyridoxine hydrochloride (in adults 5 gm. as 50 ml. of a 10% solution, injected intravenously over a period of 3 to 5 minutes), repeated every few hours or perhaps more often if neurologic signs are encountered (see text above). This is a much larger dose of pyridoxine than has been used or recommended previously in mushroom poisoning, but it has been given successfully and apparently safely in isoniazid poisoning (see Section II). An unpublished study, however, is said to have revealed sensory nerve damage in individuals who compulsively ingested 2 to 6 gm. daily over long periods.
7. Whether early peritoneal dialysis, hemodialysis or hemoperfusion are useful in removing the toxin or its precursors is not established, but these measures are beneficial in hepatic coma (p. IV-55).
8. General supportive measures for overt liver failure (pp. IV-61–63).
9. If intravascular hemolysis is detected, protect the kidneys by maintaining a diuresis with injected mannitol (p. IV-52) and perhaps by alkalinizing the urine with injected sodium bicarbonate (p. IV-72).

Group III. Coprine and Cyclopropanone

Coprine is a water-soluble thermostable compound present in the wild mushroom *Coprinus atramentarius* and in a few other less common species of the same genus (Lincoff and Mitchel, 1977). This mushroom is commonly known as the "inky cap," but the name is sometimes applied to other species of the same genus because in aging all of them tend to deliquesce to form ink-like droplets containing microscopic black spores. With the aid of a bioassay, coprine was isolated from *C. atramentarius* and its structure was determined in 1975 (Hatfield and Schaumberg, 1975; Lindberg *et al.*, 1975). It can be described as the γ-glutamyl conjugate of 1-aminocyclopropanol. A kilogram of fresh *C. atramentarius* is said to contain about 160 mg. coprine. At this level neither coprine nor its metabolites have any intrinsic toxicity that is recognized clinically, and the mushroom is commonly classified as edible (Miller, 1972).

Coprine is hydrolyzed *in vivo* to glutamic acid and 1-aminocyclopropanol. The latter is slowly hydrolyzed (half-time 30 minutes at 27°C. and pH 7.4) to cyclopropanone hydrate (Wiseman and Abeles, 1979). Cyclopropanone (but not coprine and probably not 1-aminocyclopropanol) is a potent inhibitor of liver low-K_m acetaldehyde dehydrogenase *in vivo* and *in vitro* (Tottmar and Lindberg, 1977; Wiseman and Abeles, 1979). When ethyl alcohol is administered during this state of inhibition, its metabolite acetaldehyde accumulates in the blood. In rats pretreated with coprine by stomach tube at doses of 7, 27 and 81 mg./kg., the blood acetaldehyde levels during ethanol metabolism were 10, 20 and 40 times higher than those in control rats given ethanol alone (Tottmar and Lindberg, 1977). The defect in acetaldehyde metabolism does not appear immediately; in mice given by stomach tube a lyophilized powder of *C. atramentarius*, a latency of 3 to 6 hours preceded the state of inhibition (Genest *et al.*, 1968). Once established, the enzyme defect persists for several days. For example, abnormal accumulations of acetaldehyde after an ethanol challenge were still detectable in rats 6 days after they received 81 mg./kg. coprine (Tottmar and Lindberg, 1977).

The coprinus-alcohol reaction in man is similar to that in laboratory mammals, and the same biochemical mechanisms are believed to be responsible. The mushroom produces no illness unless alcohol is consumed. After the inhibition of acetaldehyde dehydrogenase is established, which may not occur until an hour or more after the mushroom is eaten (the latent period in man is not known with certainty), the ingestion of even small amounts of ethanol leads promptly to an illness consisting of sensations of warmth, flushing, fullness and throbbing in the neck veins, tingling in the fingers, severe headache, nausea, vomiting, chest pain, tachycardia, hypertension and confusion (Reynolds and Lowe, 1965; Lampe, 1978). These signs and symptoms, which are ascribed to acetaldehydemia, usually last for only 2 to 4 hours, but the state of abnormal sensitivity to alcohol may persist for several days. No deaths have been reported, but one victim experienced esophageal rupture from violent retching (Mayer *et al.*, 1971).

The studies summarized above establish that the condition of abnormal sensitivity to alcohol induced by coprine and *C. atramentarius* is equivalent biochemically and clinically to the state induced by the drug disulfiram. For more information about the symptomatology and treatment of the coprinus-alcohol reaction, see DISULFIRAM (p. III-161).

Group IV. Muscarine

This alkaloid was first isolated in 1869 from the mushroom *Amanita muscaria*, of which it is a very minor constituent (Waser, 1961). At measured concentrations of less than 0.0003% in fresh specimens of *A. muscaria* and *A. pantherina*, muscarine is almost never responsible for symptoms in poisonings by these two mushrooms; their principal toxins are in Group V (see below). Only occasional specimens of *A. muscaria* have been reported to cause mild muscarinic effects such as sweating and salivation (Lampe, 1978; Waser, 1967). In contrast, many (perhaps 30) species of *Inocybe* and at least 6 species of *Clitocybe* have been found to contain 0.1 to 0.5% muscarine (dry weight) according to chromatographic assays (Chilton, 1978; Tyler, 1963). The ingestion of any of these mushrooms is likely to produce muscarine poisoning.

Although first isolated in 1869, the structural formula of muscarine was not established until the 1950s (Chilton, 1978; Waser, 1961). It is a small, heat-stable, quaternary ammonium compound with a tetrahydrofuran ring (molecular weight 174). Four stereoisomers exist, and all have been detected in *Inocybe* spp. (Catalfomo and Eugster, 1970). Muscarine itself is designated L-(+)-muscarine and is the principal form of the alkaloid in most mushrooms. Where found, *epi-* and *allo-* and *epi-allo-* muscarines usually occur in descending amounts. L-(+)-Muscarine is also several hundred times more potent in biological test systems than the next most active diasteriomer, *epi*-muscarine (Chilton, 1978). Therefore one would expect lower estimates of muscarine in mushrooms from bioassays calibrated against pure (+)-muscarine than from chemical assays which before 1970 did not distinguish among the isomers. The converse, however, is widely reported. For example, *I. napipes* with 0.73% (dry weight) muscarine by chromatography was found to contain over 3% muscarine in a rat bioassay (Malone *et al.*, 1962). A similar disparity has been reported in many other species of *Inocybe*. The substance or substances responsible for much of the muscarine-like activity have not been identified, but candidates include choline and acetylcholine, both of which are present in many fungi.

Pure muscarine and muscarine-containing mushrooms produce similar effects *in vivo*. All of these effects are ascribed to the stimulation by muscarine of a group of receptors on various smooth muscles, exocrine glands and cardiac pacemaker cells. Many (but not all) of these receptors are innervated by parasympathetic postganglionic neurones, which employ acetylcholine as their neurotransmitter. Thus, acetylcholine is the physiological agonist for these muscarine-sensitive receptors. Probably because it is not destroyed by the enzyme cholinesterase, muscarine is a somewhat more potent agonist than acetylcholine. Over the past century muscarine has been a valuable research tool for locating and studying these muscarinic-cholinergic receptors, but it is not used and never has been widely used as a therapeutic agent. Probably because of its cationic charge, it does not appear to cross the blood-brain barrier, and so only peripheral receptors are believed to be involved in its toxic actions. Atropine is regarded as a complete pharmacologic antagonist of muscarine because it blocks the same subset of cholinergic receptors that muscarine excites. In adequate doses atropine can suppress all of the known signs and symptoms of muscarine poisoning, but even without treatment most victims recover within a few hours.

The most sensitive and definitive sign of muscarine poisoning is excessive sweating (Jelliffe, 1937; Lampe, 1978). Also common are nausea, vomiting and abdominal colic. Less commonly reported signs include salivation, rhinorrhea, blurred vision (presumably due to ciliospasm) and watery diarrhea (Lampe, 1978). Other effects listed below are rather infrequent, but they do occur in severe poisoning. Poisonings are probably more common than one might infer from the small number of published reports, but deaths are rare. In Switzerland between 1919 and 1958, Alder (1961) collected 38 cases of muscarine poisoning due to the ingestion of *Inocybe patouillardii* or *Clitocybe dealbata* (*sudorifica*); 3 deaths were recorded. Over a 10-year period in Poznan, Poland, 17 cases of *I. patouillardii* were reported with no deaths (Grzymala, 1965c). The oral lethal dose of muscarine in laboratory animals is not known. We know of no basis for the suggestion that 0.3 to 0.5 gm. is a lethal dose in man (Lincoff and Mitchel, 1977).

Symptomatology (Group IV):
1. Sweating is usually the first, most sensitive and most definitive sign. It commonly appears within 15 to 30 minutes after ingestion, rarely beyond 1 hour. The victim's skin and clothing may be drenched.
2. Salivation, nausea, vomiting, colic and watery diarrhea.
3. Miosis (but not always), blurring of vision, lacrimation.
4. Dyspnea, wheezing, rales.
5. Slow and irregular pulse, hypotension.
6. Restlessness, weakness, but usually no confusion.
7. Rarely death within a few hours due to cardiac arrest, cardiovascular collapse, or conceivably respiratory tract obstruction.

Treatment (Group IV):
1. Atropine sulfate, 2 mg., intramuscularly, repeated in 10 to 15 minutes, if necessary, to suppress sweating. Sweating is the best single indicator of the need for additional atropine. Doses adequate for this purpose will control almost all of the other visceral effects of muscarine. Salivation and bradycardia, however, are other useful and important indicators.
2. Unless spontaneous vomiting is judged to have been adequate to empty the stomach, syrup of ipecac or gastric lavage may be considered, but atropine alone should be sufficient to control signs and symptoms if the only toxin is muscarine.
3. If signs of respiratory tract obstruction are not corrected by atropinization, suctioning and/or the administration of a bronchodilator drug (*e.g.*, epinephrine) may be indicated. See pp. IV- 4 and 15.
4. The arterial circulation is rarely inadequate if cardiac arrest, bradycardia, bradyarrhythmias and respiratory tract obstruction are controlled by atropine. However, dehydration, if any, should be corrected by the parenteral administration of fluids.

Group V. Ibotenic Acid and Muscimol

Ibotenic acid is a water-soluble amino acid with an isoxazole ring. It can be extracted from *Amanita muscaria* (popularly known as the "fly agaric"), *A. pantherina* (the "panther agaric"), *A. cothurnata* (which may be a subspecies or variant of the panther mushroom), *A. strobiliformis* (in Japan), and some possibly hybrid specimens of *A. gemmata*, but it does not occur in any other genus of mushroom or in any other species of Amanita tested (Benedict *et al.*, 1966; Chilton and Ott, 1976). A single clinical report of a poisoning, however, suggests that it may also be a constituent of *A. crenulata* (Buck, 1965).

Ibotenic acid is unstable, and especially in acid it decarboxylates spontaneously to yield muscimol (also known as pantherine). Thus mushroom extracts contain both compounds, even though muscimol may not be a normal constituent of fresh specimens. The combined concentration is about 0.18% (dry weight basis) in *A. muscaria* and as much as 0.46% in *A. pantherina* (Benedict *et al.*, 1966). Trace amounts of muscazone, which can be produced by photoisomerization of ibotenic acid, have also been reported (Chilton, 1978). Other potentially toxic compounds (*e.g.*, stizolobic and stizolobinic acids) have been identified especially in *A. pantherina* (Chilton and Ott, 1976). Muscarine is also present (see Group IV above), but the amounts are generally too small to contribute to the clinical toxicity of these mushrooms.

Independent work in three laboratories in Japan, England and Switzerland during the 1960s served to establish the presence and identities of ibotenic acid and muscimol (reviewed by Chilton, 1978). These compounds were promptly recognized as the constituents responsible for the fly-killing property of these mushrooms. Indeed, the long-known "flyicidal" activity of *A. muscaria* (from which it presumably derives its name) served as an invaluable assay during the isolation and purification of ibotenic acid. More recently toxicologists have come to believe that these two compounds are the elusive intoxicants responsible for the psychomotor reactions experienced after ingesting these mushrooms. An earlier hypothesis that the toxic ingredient is a tropine alkaloid ("pilzatropine") has been rejected.

The hallucinogenic property of *A. muscaria* has been known since the early eighteenth century when the first of many travelers told of remote Siberian tribesmen who prized this mushroom and consumed it mostly in religious rites (Lincoff and Mitchel, 1977; Wasson, 1967). Largely on linguistic grounds, Wasson (1968) has suggested that the fly agaric was the "soma" consumed by Vedic priests of ancient India to attain ecstacy and immortality. The popularization of this and related ethnopharmacologic theories led to the deliberate ingestion of *A. muscaria* and *A. pantherina* by many persons dedicated to exploring altered states of consciousness. The testimony of these mycophagists is mixed (Ott, 1978). The intoxication is regarded as pleasant by some and exceedingly disagreeable by others, but in contrast to the psilocybin experience (see Group VI below), hallucinations are neither common nor particularly inspiring. Nevertheless, in the Pacific northwest *A. pantherina* is now collected and eaten (raw or cooked) for recreational purposes (Lincoff and Mitchel, 1977; Ott, 1978). Specimens, however, vary widely in potency; darkly pigmented ones appear to be the most active and contain the largest amounts of ibotenic acid and muscimol (Benedict *et al.*, 1966). Techniques of preparation for eating also vary; boiling in large amounts of water extracts at least some of the ibotenic acid and muscimol; peeling and discarding the skin appears to reduce potency. Because of intrinsic variations and diverse methods of culinary preparation, a "safe" dose of *A. pantherina* cannot be stated, and some alarming intoxications have been reported in the United States, Europe and South Africa, especially in children (reviewed by Lampe, 1978; Lincoff and Mitchel, 1977). Deaths, however, are rare.

Certainly the panther agaric is more toxic, more psychoactive and richer in ibotenic acid

than is *A. muscaria* (Benedict *et al.*, 1966). In contrast to *A. pantherina* no prominent variations in the contents of ibotenic acid or muscimol were found among western specimens of the fly agaric, even among the several color variants of this mushroom. Nevertheless, *A. muscaria* of northeastern United States is commonly regarded by mycophagists as lacking in any significant psychoactivity, especially the yellow-orange variety. At least all of this deliberate and in some cases accidental experimentation has served to establish that *Amanita muscaria* is not the deadly mushroom that it was once held to be.

Both ibotenic acid and muscimol are now available in good purity, and both have been tested singly in laboratory animals (mice, rats, kittens, etc.) and in human volunteers. The LD_{50} of muscimol in rats is 45 mg./kg. by mouth and about 4.5 mg./kg. by intravenous injection; corresponding values for ibotenic acid are 129 and 42 mg./kg. (Theobald *et al.*, 1968). Because the decarboxylation product muscimol is also 5 to 10 times more active than ibotenic acid in man, it is presumed that muscimol is the chief psychoactive agent *in vivo*, perhaps only because it crosses the blood-brain barrier more readily. Threshold oral doses in adult humans are about 7.5 to 10 mg. muscimol and 20 to 90 mg. ibotenic acid (Theobald *et al.*, 1968; Waser, 1967). Symptoms usually begin within an hour and last 3 to 4 hours (although more persistent effects have been observed in some test animals).

Both the time course and the signs and symptoms (as described below under "symptomatology") are similar to those encountered in poisonings due to ibotenic acid-containing mushrooms (*e.g.*, Buck, 1963; Lincoff and Mitchel, 1977; Ott, 1978; Wasson, 1968). Some clinical intoxications by these mushrooms last longer than 4 hours, especially those produced by *A. pantherina*, but the difference may be simply one of effective dose. Nausea and vomiting are more common after ingestion of mushrooms than of ibotenic acid or muscimol. Indeed, muscimol has an antiemetic action against apomorphine-induced vomiting in dogs (Theobald *et al.*, 1968). Aside from nausea, however, gastrointestinal symptoms are not usually prominent in poisonings by these mushrooms. When gut reactions are encountered, they are usually ascribed to unknown irritants in the mushrooms, not to ibotenic acid or muscimol and not to muscarine, which is seldom present in clinically significant amounts (but see Lampe, 1978; Waser, 1967).

The mechanisms by which ibotenic acid and muscimol alter central neural activity have received attention (reviewed by Chilton, 1978). Ibotenic acid is described as a conformationally restricted derivative of glutamic acid and muscimol of γ-aminobutyric acid (GABA). Both GABA and glutamic acid are putative central neurotransmitters. In contrast to the mushroom toxins, neither glutamic acid nor GABA cross the mammalian blood-brain barrier appreciably. When administered intrathecally, glutamic acid activates spinal interneurones and Renshaw cells, as does ibotenic acid. In contrast, intrathecal GABA and muscimol inhibit firing of some central neurones. When administered systemically, however, ibotenic acid and muscimol produce in laboratory animals rather similar effects, consisting chiefly of a central inhibition of motor activity with essentially no change in peripheral autonomic activity (Theobald *et al.*, 1968). In cats, rabbits and rats, both compounds induce similar EEG alterations, consisting of synchronization at low doses and high-voltage spikes at high doses (Scotti de Carolis *et al.*, 1969; Theobald *et al.*, 1968). Thus, within the central nervous system both ibotenic acid and muscimol appear to behave as false neurotransmitters.

No pharmacologic antagonists for these central actions are known. Physostigmine is ineffective, and atropine is said to intensify the delirium (Lincoff and Mitchel, 1977). A potentially dangerous drug interaction has been demonstrated in rabbits; after a high dose of muscimol, they reacted to a small intravenous dose of diazepam or phenobarbital with flaccid paralysis and an almost complete disappearance of cortical electrical activity for periods of about one hour (Scotti de Carolis *et al.*, 1969).

Symptomatology (Group V):

1. After a latent period of 0.5 to 1.5 hours, drowsiness and fatigue, followed by a period of sleep (with "visions") and nothing else if the dose is small.
2. Inconstant but generally mild signs of gastrointestinal irritation (nausea, sometimes vomiting).
3. Signs similar to those in an alcohol intoxication: dizziness, ataxia, slurred speech, restlessness, erratic and sometimes maniacal behavior, sometimes interrupted by periods of somnolence.
4. Various emotional responses are described, ranging from excitement and elation to fear and withdrawal.
5. At the subjective level, hallucinations have been reported, but they are neither common nor spectacular. As in most delirious patients, illusions are based on misinterpretations of sensory information (*e.g.*, distortions of time and space, misidentification of persons, etc.).
6. Twitching of the limbs and tremors may occur. Except in periods of excessive motor activity the vital signs are usually normal.
7. Signs and symptoms gradually subside over

a period of 3 to 4 hours, although they may persist for 8 hours after ingesting *A. pantherina*. Some residual feelings (*e.g.*, headache) may continue for several more hours.

8. Death is rare but has been reported in a few children. As with some other classes of toxic mushrooms, children may react in bizarre and unpredictable ways. In addition to the delirium described above, various neurologic syndromes have been observed in children who ate *A. pantherina*: they include loss of consciousness, violent tonic-clonic convulsions, loss of tendon reflexes, unreactive pupils, etc.

Treatment (Group V):

1. If the patient has not vomited spontaneously and if he is not already delirious, empty the stomach with syrup of ipecac (p. I-2) or with gastric lavage (p. I-8).
2. Do not use atropine because it has intensified the delirium of some individuals who ingested *A. muscaria* and *A. pantherina*. Do not use physostigmine; it is without benefit in this intoxication.
3. Because small doses of diazepam and barbiturates have induced paralysis in muscimol-pretreated animals, it may be unsafe to treat this form of delirium with these tranquilizers. If grand-mal convulsions occur, however, the cautious use of diazepam is recommended. See pp. IV-35–39.
4. Presumably the hallucinations and the maniacal behavior that they sometimes inspire are responsive to the phenothiazine tranquilizers and to haloperidol. Because of uncertain interactions, however, it is probably safer to avoid drug intervention and to manage the delirium with "talk-down" techniques and restraint as described under MARIHUANA (p. III-257).

Group VI. Psilocybin and Psilocin

Several 4- and 5-hydroxylated tryptamine derivatives have been detected in a variety of wild mushrooms (Hofmann *et al.*, 1958; Tyler, 1958, 1963; Wieland *et al.*, 1953). The 5-hydroxy compounds (serotonin, bufotenine) are of minor toxicologic interest because the quantities ingested in fungi are almost never enough to produce their characteristic actions on peripheral tissues and because the blood-brain barrier largely excludes them from critical sites within the brain (see Section II). In contrast, the 4-hydroxytryptamine derivatives (psilocybin, psilocin) and/or their metabolites appear to pass readily from blood to brain, where they are strongly psychotropic and in large doses hallucinogenic.

The eventual discovery of psilocybin as an hallucinogen began in the 1950s with investigations by R. Gordon Wasson, Roger Heim, Rolf Singer and others into the use of so-called "magic mushrooms" in religious rituals by Indian tribes of southern Mexico (Lincoff and Mitchel, 1977; Singer, 1978). The practice, which proved to be widespread throughout Meso-America, probably dates back thousands of years. It was vividly described in the 16th century by various Spanish observers. The Aztec name for the sacred mushrooms was teonanacatl, but tribes in different locales were found to designate different species of psychoactive mushrooms as their teonanacatl. Heim later identified most of them as members of the genus *Psilocybe*, but specimens of *Stropharia*, *Conocybe* and *Panaeolus* were also included. From one of the hallucinogenic species *Psilocybe mexicana*, Hofmann et al. (1958) isolated, identified and later synthesized psilocybin.

In the 1960s and 1970s popular accounts of these investigations generated widespread interest and the formation of cults devoted to finding and consuming psilocybin-containing mushrooms for mystical and recreational purposes. Dedicated thrill-seekers soon discovered that it is unnecessary to travel to Mexico; species of *Psilocybe* are distributed worldwide. They are, however, generally rather insignificant looking little brown mushrooms ("LBM's"), often growing on cow dung in meadows. They are not likely to be mistaken for edible mushrooms or to be consumed accidentally as food, but some of them can be confused with lethal *Galerina* (see Group I above). The favorite species along the Gulf coast is *P. cubensis* ("blue legs"), whereas in the Pacific northwest *P. semilanceata* ("liberty bells") and the very potent *P. baeocystis* are commonly harvested (Lincoff and Mitchel, 1977).

The possession of psilocybin and psilocin and of mushrooms containing them is illegal in the United States (Schedule I controlled substances), but kits for growing *P. cubensis* from authentic spores (which contain no psilocybin) have been sold by mail order. Black market mushrooms represented as *Psilocybe* have often proved to be common grocery store *Agaricus bisporus* spiked with LSD, DOM or PCP (see Section II). The same is true of powders sold illicitly and misrepresented as pure psilocybin (Cheek and Newell, 1970).

Psilocybin is *O*-phosphoryl-4-hydroxy-*N*,*N*-dimethyltryptamine and psilocin is its dephosphorylated metabolite. Psilocin is probably the pharmacologically active form, but both compounds behave alike *in vivo*, presumably because phosphatases rapidly convert psilocybin to psilocin (Chilton, 1978). Mushrooms contain far more psilocybin, which is the more stable compound and which can be extracted by boiling water. Unlike psilocybin, psilocin readily autooxidizes to a blue pigment of uncertain composition. The development of a blue or blue-green stain on the freshly exposed tissue of the cap or stem is used by amateur collectors to identify psilocybin-containing mushrooms, but various species of *Boletus*, which contain no hallucinogens, also have a bluing reaction when bruised or cut.

Assays by the Federal Bureau of Narcotic and Dangerous Drugs have revealed a range of 0.2 to 0.49% (w/w) psilocybin in dried specimens of *Psilocybe* spp. (Chilton, 1978). The true range of variation, however, is probably considerably larger because mushrooms of some species (so-called "psilocybin-latent" species) are reported to differ markedly in psilocybin-psilocin content at different seasons and in different parts of the world (Lincoff and Mitchel, 1977). Furthermore, it is not certain that these two indoles are the only hallucinogens present in these fungi. Unlike other species of *Psilocybe, P. baeocystis* also contains the monomethyl and nonmethylated analogues of psilocybin, named baeocystin and nor-baeocystin respectively. Their pharmacological activities, however, have not yet been described (Lampe, 1978). Specimens of *Gymnopilus (Pholiota) spectabilis* which were said to contain an unidentified indole but no psilocybin appeared to cause a typical psilocybin-like illness in three adults who ate small quantities of them (Buck, 1967). In Japan *G. spectabilis* has been called the "big laughing mushroom" (Lincoff and Mitchel, 1977). The identity of its hallucinogenic principle is unknown but it is probably related to psilocybin and psilocin.

In general, the clinical signs and symptoms reported in those who ingest psilocybin-containing mushrooms (Hyde et al., 1978; Lampe, 1978; Lincoff and Mitchel, 1977; Verrill, 1914) closely parallel those produced by pure samples of psilocybin and psilocin (Hollister, 1961d; Hollister and Hartman, 1962; Jacobsen, 1963). In a nontolerant adult the effective oral dose of psilocybin is usually 3.5 to 12 mg. (Usdin and Efron, 1972), which is contained in 1 to 4 gm. of dried *P. mexicana*. This is equivalent to about 15 to 20 mushrooms, depending upon their size, but much larger numbers (more than 50) have been consumed. With more potent species such as *P. baeocystis*, a satisfactory dose may consist of 5 or fewer specimens. The mushrooms may be eaten fresh and raw, dried and raw, or cooked.

Signs and symptoms commonly begin in 15 to 30 minutes. Intense and persistent yawning is common. The psychic effects may be judged pleasant and even ecstatic or disagreeable and sometimes terrifying, depending upon the dose, the personality and expectations of the user, and the social setting in which the experience occurs. In a "good trip" the subject remains well oriented. Visual distortions are commonly reported, including characteristically a wavy or undulating distortion of viewed flat surfaces.

True hallucinations tend to occur only with excessive doses. The psychic and sensory effects usually subside in 2 to 4 hours after swallowing pure psilocybin (Hollister, 1961d), but after ingesting mushrooms they occasionally persist for periods as long as 6 to 8 hours. If the episode lasts longer than 6 to 8 hours, one should seek another causative agent, such as PCP, LSD or one of the phenylethylamine hallucinogens.

Most intoxications are so brief and mild that no medical treatment is required, but sometimes a disoriented or panicky subject may require diazepam or one of the antipsychotic tranquilizers. Intravenous physostigmine (4 mg.) is said to have suppressed hallucinations and other signs of intoxication in a 21-year-old man who had ingested 30 specimens of *P. semilanceata*, but his recovery may have been entirely coincidental (Van Poorten *et al.*, 1982).

The lethal dose of psilocybin in man is not known. No deaths have been reported in adults from eating psilocybin or psilocybin-containing mushrooms, although one dedicated experimentalist is reported to have consumed deliberately 40 mg. psilocybin. Lincoff and Mitchel (1977) suggest that "the ingestion of 100 or even 50 psilocybes may be life-threatening."

In young children the record is not so benign. In addition to hallucinations, convulsions and loss of consciousness were described in a young girl (11 years old?) who had eaten a small piece of *Copelandia* (also called *Panaeolus*) *cyanescens* (Heim *et al.*, 1966). A 4-year-old boy became comatose for a short time after eating *Panaeolus foenisecii* (Miller, 1972). Admittedly the toxicological assessment of the genus *Panaeolus* is far from complete, and toxins other than psilocybin may contribute, but at least in Heim's case (1966) an adult who consumed mushrooms from the same collection experienced a typical psilocybin intoxication. In another episode two children, ages 4 and 9, became dizzy, weak, disoriented and incoherent. Atropine-like effects were prominent (dry mouth, dry and flushed skin, hyperpyrexia), and intermittent tonic-clonic convulsions occurred. The child with the higher fever (106°F.) died on the third hospital day. This tragedy was attributed to the ingestion of *Psilocybe baeocystis*, but the mushroom fragment may have been misidentified (McCawley *et al.*, 1966, as summarized by Lampe, 1978).

Tolerance to psilocybin and cross-tolerance with LSD, DMT and mescaline are described (see Section II). According to one hypothesis all of these hallucinogens act by suppressing input to serotonergic neurones whose cell bodies are located in the raphe nuclei of the midbrain and whose axons terminate in the forebrain. Impulses in this system normally serve to prevent one from being alerted or distracted by repetitive or irrelevant sensory stimuli. The result of suppressing this inhibitory system is heightened sensory awareness, sensory distortions, confusion and hallucinations. Hallucinogenic amphetamines are thought to cause the same disinhibition by a more indirect action on the raphe nuclei. The psychic experience induced by psilocybin is accompanied by mild signs of excess sympathetic tone (slight tachycardia, mydriasis, etc.), but some of these somatic effects may be due to direct stimulation of peripheral serotonin receptors. In general they are much less prominent than with LSD.

Symptomatology (Group VI):
1. Within 10 to 30 minutes after ingesting pure psilocybin (or perhaps a little longer after eating a psilocybin-containing mushroom), anxiety and tension appear.
2. Giddiness or dizziness, fatigue, drowsiness and often intense yawning.
3. Weakness, twitching, shivering, hot or cold sensations, paresthesias of the extremities, numbness of the lips.
4. Nausea but no vomiting (usually).
5. Within 30 to 60 minutes, visual distortions (altered shapes, intensified colors, blurred or sharpened outlines and kaleidoscopic color patterns, usually only with the eyes closed), increased auditory acuity, distortions of time sense.
6. Euphoria or other mood changes (*e.g.*, sadness), feelings of unreality and of depersonalization, difficulty in concentrating and in expressing thoughts.
7. Sweating, yawning, tearing, facial flush, dilated pupils, tachycardia.
8. Within 1 to 2 hours, an intensification of the visual effects (see above) and particularly a wavy, undulating distortion of viewed flat surfaces.
9. Dream-like meditation.
10. Usually within 2 to 4 hours but sometimes only after 6 to 8 hours, all of these effects disappear with no residue except perhaps headache and a sense of fatigue.
11. Rarely a schizophrenic-like state may be induced. In one case (Hyde *et al.*, 1978) it lasted 4 days and probably represented the activation of latent paranoid schizophrenia.
12. In young children additional toxic reactions have been reported, including fixed dilated pupils, hyperpyrexia, coma and intermittent tonic-clonic convulsions.

Treatment (Group VI):
1. Administer syrup of ipecac or perform gastric lavage, if possible within 30 minutes of the ingestion.
2. In most cases the intoxication is so mild and brief that no specific medical treat-

ment is needed, but children should be observed carefully for possible fever, coma and convulsions.

3. A frightened victim may require only reassurance. A confused or disoriented person may sometimes be managed by simple "talkdown" techniques, as in marihuana poisoning (p. III-257).

4. Diazepam and particularly the antipsychotic tranquilizers (*e.g.*, chlorpromazine and haloperidol) are said to suppress all of the psychic effects of psilocybin and psilocin. See pp. IV-33–35.

Group VII. Gastrointestinal Irritants

When eaten either cooked or raw, mushrooms of many species and genera are known to produce transient but often severe gastroenteritis with little or no evidence of other systemic reactions. Although not everyone is affected, these mushrooms cause vomiting and diarrhea with such high frequency that allergies are not likely to be responsible. With few exceptions, relevant toxins have not been extracted or identified. In the few instances where a toxic substance has been isolated, its role in clinical poisonings remains unsettled.

The most troublesome fungi in Group VII are those large enough and common enough to tempt the unwary mycophagist and those most easily confused with safe and edible species (Lincoff and Mitchel, 1977). Especially hazardous are the species in which these characteristics happen to coincide with a toxin of high potency. According to Lampe (1978), the mushrooms most commonly encountered in severe Group VII intoxications are the following five: *Chlorophyllum molybdites* (also called *Lepiota morganii*), *Entoloma lividum* (*Rhodophyllus lividum* or *R. sinuatus*), *Tricholoma pardinum*, *Omphalotus olearius* (*Clitocybe illudens*, *Pleurotus olearius*) and *Paxillus involutus*.

Perhaps *C. molybdites* is the one most often involved in gastroenteritis leading to hospitalization in North America (Lampe, 1978). A typically severe case was described by Picchioni (1965). Paradoxically, a few individuals claim to eat this mushroom with impunity and to enjoy it (Lincoff and Mitchel, 1977). The same is true of *Paxillus involutus*, but here the distinction is geographic in that specimens growing in parts of western North America may be safe but certainly not those growing in eastern United States or in Europe (Bschor and Mallach, 1963; Lincoff and Mitchel, 1977). A 10-year study in Poznan, Poland, revealed 109 reported cases of *Paxillus involutus* poisoning leading to 93 hospitalizations and 1 death (Grzymala, 1965c).

Much anecdotal literature supports the concept that a single species of mushroom may produce specimens of high toxicity in one locale and of low toxicity in another. This variability appears to be especially true of the gastrointestinal toxins of Group VII. Because many poisonings have been reported, almost all mycologists advise against eating boletes with red pores or with flesh that stains blue when bruised, but some persons have found them harmless and palatable. Varying methods of culinary preparation may account for some of these inconsistencies but not for most of them.

Any comprehensive list of mushroom species that may induce a simple (but often violent) gastroenteritis is long and imposing; it encompasses essentially all established genera, including *Agaricus, Boletus, Chlorophyllum, Entoloma, Gomphus, Hebeloma, Lactarius, Lycoperdon, Morchella, Naematoloma, Paxillus, Pholiota, Polyphorus, Ramaria, Russula, Scleroderma, Tricholoma* and *Verpa*. For information about individual species that have been implicated, see more detailed treatises (*e.g.*, Lincoff and Mitchell, 1977; Miller, 1972).

Characteristically the illness from Group VII toxins begins ½ to 4 hours after the ingestion. According to reviews by Tyler (1963) and by Lincoff and Mitchel (1977), unusually long latencies of 8 to 14 hours have been observed in a few individuals after eating any of 3 species of *Gomphus* (especially *G. floccosus*, also called *Cantharellus floccosus*). Signs and symptoms from Group VII fungi consist largely of nausea, vomiting, diarrhea and severe crampy abdominal pain. Significant differences exist; for example, both *Chlorophyllum molybdites* and *Omphalotus olearius* produce violent emesis, but only the former tends to cause intense diarrhea, which sometimes becomes bloody. In severe poisonings dehydration may lead to circulatory collapse (*e.g.*, Picchioni, 1965).

A characteristic feature of poisonings by Group VII toxins is the absence of intense sweating (Group IV), delirium (Group V), hallucinations (Group VI) and hepatorenal damage (Groups I and II). In terms of these criteria questions have been raised about some of the mushrooms listed above. For example, *O. olearius* in southern Europe is said to contain muscarine or a muscarine-like substance and to produce "increased perspiration" and "increased salivation" (Maretic, 1967; Maretic *et al.*, 1975). These quotations do not sound like the intense sweating and sialorrhea of true muscarine poisoning (see Group IV above). Several North American reports of poisonings by *O. olearius* (commonly called the jack-o'-lantern mushroom) note explicitly the absence of sweating, salivation and tearing (summarized by Lincoff and Mitchel, 1977). In a Vermont poisoning involving 5 adults seen by one of us (R.E.G.), sweating was no greater than that often provoked by anxiety, and salivation was no greater than that which often accompanies nausea. In neither of the two patients given a large parenteral dose of atropine was vomiting suppressed. There are similarly unconvincing inferences of muscarine in some of the boletes with red pores.

In a few mushroom treatises, liver and/or kidney damage have been ascribed to ingestions of *Paxillus involutus*, *Naematoloma fasciculare* (the "sulfur cap") and *Entoloma lividum*, but profound circulatory shock secondary to gastroenteritis may have been responsible for these uncommon visceral injuries (Bschor and Mallach, 1963; Herbich *et al.*, 1966).

No definitive therapy is available. Vomiting usually prevents the retention of adsorbents and demulcents, and one hesitates to administer parenteral antiemetics, antispasmodics or antidiarrhea drugs during the acute phase in fear of slowing elimination of the poison. If dehydration and electrolyte imbalances are prevented by parenteral fluid therapy, recovery almost always occurs spontaneously within a few hours (although vomiting and diarrhea occasionally persist for a couple of days after eating *Chlorophyllum molybdites*). Some victims have required hospitalization for several days. Death is rare and limited to the very young and the very old (whose lack of tolerance to dehydration and electrolyte disorders is well documented) and to those with preexisting, debilitating diseases.

Symptomatology (Group VII):
1. Asymptomatic period of ½ to 4 hours after the ingestion (but as long as 8 to 14 hours after eating *Gomphus floccosus*).
2. Nausea and violent vomiting for a period of several hours. Sometimes vomiting is the only significant effect.
3. Intense diarrhea may or may not occur. Feces are occasionally blood-streaked. Severe crampy abdominal pain.
4. Minimal or absent are such muscarinic signs as sweating, salivation and tearing.
5. Headache, fatigue, bitter taste, perioral paresthesias.
6. Dehydration leading to hypotension and shock in severe poisonings.
7. Faintness, pallor, chills, tingling, leg cramps.
8. Restlessness, confusion and coma.
9. Death (due to circulatory collapse) is rare. Recovery without sequelae is usually complete in 1 to 3 days.

Treatment (Group VII):
1. If spontaneous vomiting has not already begun, induce emesis with syrup of ipecac and/or perform gastric aspiration and lavage with tap water. Save the gastric contents and vomitus.
2. Meperidine by injection for the control of severe pain. Morphine is best avoided because it may delay purging and fecal elimination of the toxin.
3. After the stomach has been emptied by extensive vomiting or lavage, retching may be partly suppressed by parenteral antiemetic medication; see p. IV-49.
4. Avoid atropine unless muscarinic signs are prominent (*e.g.*, intense sweating, profuse salivation).
5. Prevent or correct dehydration and electrolyte imbalances by fluid therapy (pp. IV-64–73).
6. Treat circulatory shock vigorously; see pp. IV-17–20.

Laboratory (Group VII):
1. Try to find an expert to identify the offending mushroom on the basis of its morphology (or that of its microscopic spores), using gastric contents or vomitus if a fresh specimen is unavailable.
2. Blood electrolyte levels should be monitored to evaluate parenteral replacement therapy.

Group VIII. Cortinarius Nephrotoxin

As demonstrated by many clinical poisonings and by several toxicity tests in laboratory animals, at least 3 species of the genus *Cortinarius* contain one or more potent nephrotoxins. The renal injury is remarkable in that it appears only after a latent period of 3 to 14 days. Grzymala (1962, 1965a) was the first to recognize the relationship between renal damage and the antecedent ingestion of *Cortinarius orellanus*, when he investigated an epidemic of more than one hundred poisonings in the Konin district of Poland in 1952. *C. orellanus* is found not only in Poland but throughout central Europe (Germany, Austria, Italy, Switzerland, France). It must have claimed many unrecognized victims because it was considered to be an edible species before Grzymala's study.

At least two other species of *Cortinarius*, namely *C. gentilis* and *C. speciosissimus*, produce similar poisonings and presumably contain the same nephrotoxin(s) (Mottonen *et al.*, 1975). These two species occur in Finland and probably throughout Scandinavia. The first recognized human poisonings by *C. speciosissimus* were reported in Finland in 1974 (Hulmi *et al.*, 1974); at least 3 cases have occurred in Scotland (Short *et al.*, 1980). A report that this species was found on the west coast of the United States has not been confirmed. *C. gentilis* but not *C. orellanus* is known to occur in North America (Lampe, 1978). No renal injuries, however, have been ascribed to eating any *Cortinarius* on this continent. The genus, however, is a very large one, with hundreds of known species, many of uncertain edibility.

The structure of the nephrotoxin is still in doubt. Grzymala (1962) isolated from *C. orellanus* a pale-yellow to colorless, crystalline substance which he named orellanine. Its concentration in the dried mushroom is 1 to 1.5% (Antkowiak and Gessner, 1979), so that a specimen of average size is likely to contain 15 to 20 mg. (Lincoff and Mitchel, 1977). The oral LD_{50} in cats, mice and guinea pigs ranged from 4.9 to 8.3 mg./kg. It acted slowly over several days to cause damage mainly to the kidneys and liver (Grzymala, 1962). Orellanine is soluble in alkali but not in neutral or acidic aqueous solutions; according to Antkowiak and Gessner (1979) it is a polyphenol, probably the bis-*N*-oxide of 3,3′,4,4′-tetrahydroxy-2,2′-bipyridyl. Others, however, consider orellanine to be a mixture. Using somewhat different extraction and separation procedures, Kurnsteiner and Moser (1981) isolated a toxin of high water solubility that is readily destroyed by UV light. It too proved to be a slow-acting poison. Mice died as late as 10 days after an intraperitoneal dose; even after a massive dose ($10\times LD_{100}$), death did not occur before 48 hours. The LD_{50} was not determined, but the intraperitoneal LD_{100} in mice was about 10 mg./kg. Kurnsteiner and Moser (1981) suggest that their toxin may be a peptide combined with the polyphenol of Antkowiak and Gessner. No attempt to characterize the structure of the nephrotoxin(s) of *C. speciosissimus* has been reported, but as present in the mushroom, it too is resistant to drying, freezing and normal cooking procedures.

The first signs and symptoms of the intoxication are usually thirst, nausea, vomiting, abdominal pain and diarrhea (or sometimes constipation). Characteristically this symptom complex does not begin until 2 to 4 days after the ingestion (Grzymala, 1965a; Marichal *et al.*, 1977; Short *et al.*, 1980), but this long latent period cannot be recognized if various Group VII mushrooms are eaten at the same time (*e.g.*, Favre *et al.*, 1976). A toxic component distinct from the nephrotoxin may be responsible for this early gastrointestinal phase of the intoxication; at least a rapidly acting toxin, as assayed in mice, has been separated from the slow acting one by Sephadex fractionation of a methanol extract of *C. orellanus* (Kurnsteiner and Moser, 1981). Similarly, the transient and usually mild liver injury that follows ingestion of *C. orellanus* (Grzymala, 1965a; Favre *et al.*, 1976) may be due to a component other than the nephrotoxic one, because *C. speciosissimus* does not produce liver damage in man (Hulmi *et al.*, 1974; Short *et al.*, 1980) or in rats (Mottonen *et al.*, 1975). The renal injury, which is heralded by such signs and symptoms as muscle pains, lumbar pain, head-

ache, anorexia, chills and night sweats, is often not evident clinically until a week or more after the ingestion.

There is general agreement that the renal lesion is primarily an interstitial nephritis, with interstitial edema, infiltration of lymphocytes, plasma cells and eventually polymorphonuclear leukocytes, together with tubular necrosis, and later fibrosis, tubular dilation and epithelial atrophy (Favre *et al.*, 1976; Marichal *et al.*, 1977; Mottonen *et al.*, 1975; Nieminen *et al.*, 1975; Short *et al.*, 1980). The glomeruli are generally normal, although a mild mesangial reaction has been described (Short *et al.*, 1980). Perhaps the interstitial inflammation and tubular necrosis are due to different toxins because pretreatment of rats with phenobarbital intensified the tubular damage in the cortex but had no effect on the inflammation in the outer medullary zone produced by the gastric administration of a dried homogenate of *C. speciosissimus* (Nieminen, 1976).

In rats as well as man, the inflammatory reaction and subsequent scarring are apt to be patchy, with some nephrons appearing to be spared (Favre *et al.*, 1976; Nieminen *et al.*, 1975; Short *et al.*, 1980). The damage, however, can be so intense and widespread that irreversible renal failure results, necessitating chronic intermittent hemodialysis or kidney transplantation (Marichal *et al.*, 1977; Short *et al.*, 1980). There is an impression that individuals may differ markedly in sensitivity to this nephrotoxin; about 25% of dosed rats appear to be resistant to the toxin(s) of *C. speciosissimus*, even after large doses (Nieminen and Pyy, 1976). Hypersensitivity, however, has not been implicated, and immunofluorescence studies on human renal biopsies are generally negative (Favre *et al.*, 1976; Short *et al.*, 1980).

A fatality rate of 15% was cited by Grzymala (1965a) in the 1952 series of Polish cases. With modern techniques of managing chronic renal failure, however, these deaths should be largely preventable. No specific forms of therapy are known for *Cortinarius* poisoning. An assertion that resin hemoperfusion can protect those who have eaten toxic Cortinarii even 5 days after the ingestion requires confirmation (Heath *et al.*, 1980). At least in rats the nephritis can be detected microscopically as early as 2 days after the intragastric instillation of *C. speciosissimus* (Nieminen *et al.*, 1975).

Symptomatology (Group VIII):

1. If toxic Cortinarii but no other toxic mushrooms are ingested, there is characteristically an asymptomatic latent period of 2 to 4 days. With very small doses it is

possible that the first clinical signs are those of renal dysfunction, in which case the latent period may be as long as 14 days.

2. Nausea, vomiting, diarrhea (rarely constipation) and abdominal pain of varying intensity. The vomiting may subside, but the other gastrointestinal symptoms usually persist for many days.

3. Severe anorexia, intense thirst, headache, chilly sensations (without fever), muscle pains, night sweats.

4. *C. orellanus* but not *C. speciosissmus* may cause transient liver damage, as evidenced by right upper quadrant pain, hepatomegaly, jaundice, elevations of serum enzymes (SGOT), etc. Hepatic failure is not complete, and liver function recovers spontaneously, sometimes even before renal impairment is recognized.

5. The kidney injury becomes first evident clinically 3 to 14 days after the ingestion (typically about 1 week). Signs and symptoms include bilateral lumbar pain, oliguria, hematuria, anuria, twitching, and increasing somnolence.

6. Death in renal failure or recovery after 1 week or more. Spontaneous recovery may be signaled by a period of intense diuresis.

7. Severe anorexia, intermittent nausea, night sweats and weakness may persist for weeks and months, even after normal renal function has been restored.

Treatment (Group VIII):

1. If the mushroom is identified as a toxic *Cortinarius* shortly after the ingestion, empty the stomach with syrup of ipecac or gastric lavage. The toxin or toxins, however, are thought to be absorbed promptly; certainly the long latent period is not due to delayed absorption from the alimentary tract. Save gastric contents for possible identification of mushroom fragments or spores.

2. The value of early hemodialysis and hemoperfusion is not yet established. However, if many specimens of toxic Cortinarii were eaten, particularly if the ingestion was repeated on two or more consecutive days, the prognosis is ominous enough to warrant heroic measures, of which hemoperfusion holds the most promise (Heath 1980). See pp. IV-57–58.

3. No specific forms of therapy are known. Because of the uncertain functional status of the liver and kidneys, caution should be used in prescribing any drug for symptomatic relief.

4. Supportive measures for impending renal failure (pp. IV-52–53) and for the management of overt renal failure (pp. IV-53–55).

Laboratory (Group VIII):

1. Because no chemical method is established for the identification of these nephrotoxins, diagnosis must be based on identification of the mushrooms. The services of a mycologist are almost essential.

2. Liver and renal function tests are useful for prognosis and the evaluation of therapy.

3. The clinical chemistry laboratory plays an essential role in the management of acute and chronic renal failure (pp. IV-52–55).

References (all groups):

Abul-Haj, S. K.; Ewald, R. A.; Kazyak, L. Fatal mushroom poisoning. N. Engl. J. Med. *269*:223-227, 1963.

Alder, A. E. Erkennung und Behandlung der Pilzvergiftungen. Dtsch. Med. Wochenschr. *86*:1121-1127, 1961.

Antkowiak, W. Z.; Gessner, W. P. The structures of orellanine and orelline. Tetrahedron Letters *21*:1931–1934, 1979.

Back, K. C.; Thomas, A. A. Aerospace problems in pharmacology and toxicology. Ann. Rev. Pharmacol. *10*:399, 1970.

Bartter, F. C.; Berkson, B.; Gallelli, J.; Hiranaka, P. Thioctic acid in the treatment of poisoning with alpha-amanitin. In *Amanita Toxins and Poisoning*. H. Faulstich, B. Kommerell and T. Wieland (editors). Verlag Gerhard Witzstrock, New York, pp. 197-202, 1980.

Benedict, R. G.; Tyler, V. E., Jr.; Brady, L. R. Chemotaxonomic significance of isoxazole derivatives in *Amanita* species. Lloydia *29*:333-342, 1966.

Beutler, J. A.; Vergeer, P. P. Amatoxins in American mushrooms: evaluation of the meixner test. Mycologia *72*:1142–1149, 1980.

Block, S. S.; Stevens, R. L.; Barreto, A.; Murrill, W. A. Chemical identification of the Amanita toxin in mushrooms. Science *121*:505-506, 1955.

Braun, R.; Kremer, J.; Rau, H. Renal functional response to the mushroom poison gyromitrin. Toxicology *13*:187-196, 1979.

Bschor, F.; Mallach, H. J. Vergiftungen durch den Kahlen Krempling (Paxillus involutus), eine geniessbare Pilzart. Arch. Toxikol *20*:82-95, 1963.

Buck, R. W. Toxicity of Amanita muscaria. J. A. M. A. *185*:663, 1963.

Buck, R. W. Poisoning by *Amanita crenulata*. N. Engl. J. Med. *272*:475-476, 1965.

Buck, R. W. Psychedelic effect of *Pholiota spectabilis*. N. Engl. J. Med. *276*:391–392, 1967.

Busi, C.; Fiume, L.; Costantino, D.; Borroni, M.; Ambrosino, G.; Olivotto, A.; Bernardini, D. The determination of amanitines in the serum of patients poisoned by amanita phalloides. La Nouvelle Presse Medicale *6*:2855-2857, 1977.

Busi, C.; Fiume, L.; Costantino, D.; Langer, M.; Vesconi, F. Amanita toxins in gastroduodenal fluid of patients poisoned by the mushroom Amanita phalloides. N. Engl. J. Med. *300*:800, 1979.

Catalfomo, P.; Eugster, C. Muscarine and muscarine isomers in selected *Inocybe* species. Helv. Chim. Acta *53*:848-851, 1970.

Cheek, F. E.; Newell, S. Deceptions in the illicit drug market. Science *167*:1276, 1970.

Chilton, W. S. Chemistry and mode of action of mushroom toxins. In *Mushroom Poisoning: Diagnosis and Treatment.*, B. H. Rumack and E. Salzman (editors). CRC Press, Inc, 1978.

Chilton, W. S.; Ott, J. Toxic metabolites of *Amanita pantherina*, *A. cothurnata*, *A. muscaria* and other *Amanita* species. Lloydia *39*:150-157, 1976.

Costantino, D.; Brega, A.; Langer, M.; Fiume, L.; Gavazzini, V.; Vesconi, S. Busi, C.; Iapichino, G.; Rivolta, E. Contributo allo studio dilla Cinetica della Amanitina nell'uomo. Anest. e. Rianim. *18*:267-274, 1977.

Costantino, D.; Damia, G. L'Intoxication phalloidienne. Resultats de diverses therapeutiques chez 47 malades. Nouvelle Presse Medicale 6:2315-2317, 1977.

Elliott, W.; Hall, M.; Kerr, D. N. S.; Rolland, C. F.; Smart, G. A.; Swinney, J. Mushroom poisoning. Lancet 2:630-633, 1961.

Faulstich, H. New aspects of amanita poisoning. Klin. Wochenschr. 57:1143-1152, 1979.

Faulstich, J.; Cochet-Meilhac, M. Amatoxins in edible mushrooms. FEBS Lett. 64:73-75, 1976.

Favre, H.; Leski, M.; Christeler, P.; Vollenweider, E.; Chatelanat, F. Cortinarius orellanus, a toxic mushroom provoking delayed acute renal failure. Schweiz. Med. Wochenschr. 106:1097-1102, 1976.

Finestone, A.; Berman, R.; Widmer, B.; Markowitz, J. Thioctic acid treatment of acute mushroom poisoning. Pa. Med. 75:49-51, 1972.

Fiume, L.; Laschi, R. Lesioni ultrastrutturali prodotte nelle cellule parenchimali epatiche dalla falloidina e dalla α-amanitina. Sperimentale 115:288-297, 1965.

Fiume, L.; Marinozzi, V.; Nardi, F. The effects of amanitin poisoning on mouse kidney. Br. J. Exp. Pathol. 50:270-276, 1969.

Fiume, L.; Sperti, S.; Montanaro, L.; Busi, C.; Costantino, D. Amanitins do not bind to serum albumin. Lancet 1:1111, 1977.

Fiume, L.; Stirpe, F. Decreased RNA content in mouse liver nuclei after intoxication with α-amanitin. Biochim. Biophys. Acta 123:634-645, 1966.

Floersheim, G. L. Curative potencies against α-amanitin poisoning by cytochrome c. Science 177:808-809, 1972a.

Floersheim, G. L. Antidotes to experimental α-amanitin poisoning. Nature 236:115-117, 1972b.

Floersheim, G. L. Neue Gesichtspunkte zur Therapie von Vergiftungen durch den grunen Knollenblatterpilz (Amanita phalloides). Schweiz. Med. Wochenschr. 102:901-909, 1972c.

Floersheim, G. L. Experimental basis for the treatment of deathcap (Amanita phalloides) poisoning. Schweiz. Med. Wochenschr. 108:185-197, 1978.

Floersheim, G. L.; Eberhard, M.; Tschumi, P.; Duckert, F. Effects of penicillin and silymarin on liver enzymes and blood clotting factors in dogs given a boiled preparation of Amanita phalloides. Toxicol. Appl. Pharmacol. 46:455-462, 1978.

Ford, W. W. A new classification of mycetismus (mushroom poisoning). Trans. Assoc. Am. Physicians 38:225-229, 1923.

Franke, S.; Freimuth, U.; List, P. H. Uber die Giftigkeit der Fruhjahrslorchel Gyromitra (Helvella) esculenta Fr. Arch. Toxikol. 22:293-332, 1967.

Frierson, W. B. Use of pyridoxine HCl in acute hydrazine and UDMH intoxication. Indus. Med. Surg. 34:650-651, 1965.

Genest, K.; Coldwell, B. B.; Hughes, D. W. Potentiation of ethanol by Coprinus atramentarius in mice. J. Pharm. Pharmacol. 20:102-106, 1968.

George, M. E.; Pinkerton, M. K.; Back, K. C. Therapeutics of monomethylhydrazine intoxication. Toxicol. Appl. Pharmacol. 63:201-208, 1982.

Grossman, C. H.; Malbin, B. Mushroom poisoning: a review of the literature and report of 2 cases. Ann. Intern. Med. 40:249-259, 1954.

Grzymala, S. L'isolement de l'orellanine, poison de Cortinarius orellanus Fries et l'etude de ses effets anatomo-pathologiques. Bull Soc. Mycol. France 78:394-404, 1962.

Grzymala, S. Etude clinique des intoxications par les champignons du genre Cortinarius orellanus Fr. Bull. Med. Leg. Toxicol. Med. 8:60-70, 1965a.

Grzymala, S. Les Recherches sur la frequence des intoxications par les champignons. Bull. Med. Legale 8:200-210, 1965c.

Harrison, D. C.; Coggins, C. H.; Welland, F. H.; Nelson, S. Mushroom poisoning in five patients. Am. J. Med. 38:787-792, 1965.

Hatfield, G. M.; Schaumberg, J. P. Isolation and structural studies of coprine, the disulfiram-like constituent of Coprinus atramentarius. Lloydia 38:489-496, 1975.

Heath, A.; Delin, K.; Eden, E.; Martensson, E.; Selander, D.; Wickstrom, I.; Ahlmen, J. Haemoperfusion with amberlite resin in the treatment of self-poisoning. Acta Med. Scand. 207:455-460, 1980.

Heim, R.; Hofmann, A.; Tscherter, H. Sur une intoxication collective a syndrome psilocybien causee en France par un Copelandia. C.R. Acad. Sci., Ser. D. 262:519-523, 1966.

Herbich, J.; Lohwag, K.; Rotter, R. Todliche Vergiftung mit dem grunblattrigen Schwefelkopf. Archiv. Toxikol. 21:310-320, 1966.

Hofmann, A.; Heim, R.; Brack, A.; Kobel, H. Psilocybin, ein psychotroper Wirkstoff aus dem mexikanischen Rauschpilz Psilocybe mexicana Heim. Experientia 14:107-109, 1958.

Hollister, L. E. Clinical, biochemical and psychologic effects of psilocybin. Arch. Intern. Pharmacodyn. Ther. 130:42-52, 1961d.

Hendricks, H. V. Poisoning by false morel (Gyromitra esculenta). Report of a fatal case. J. A. M. A. 114:1625, 1940.

Hollister, L. E.; Hartman, A. M. Mescaline, lysergic acid diethylamide and psilocybin: comparison of clinical syndromes, effects on color perception and biochemical measures. Comp. Psychiatr. 3:235, 1962.

Hulmi, S.; Sipponen, P.; Forsstrom, J.; Vilska, J. Mushroom poisoning caused by Cortinarius speciosissimus. Duodecim, 90:1044-1050, 1974.

Hyde, C.; Glancy, G.; Omerod, P.; Hall, D.; Taylor, G. S. Abuse of indigenous psilocybin, mushrooms: A new fashion and some psychiatric complications. Brit. J. Psychiat. 132:602-604, 1978.

Jacobsen, E. The clinical pharmacology of the hallucinogens. Clin. Pharmacol. Ther. 4:480-503, 1963.

Jelliffe, S. E. Some notes on poisoning by Clitocybe dealbata (Sow.) var. sudorifica (Peck). N. Y. State J. Med. 37:1357-1361, 1937.

Kirklin, J. K.; Watson, M.; Bondoc, C. C.; Burke, J. F. Treatment of hydrazine-induced coma with pyridoxine. N. Engl. J. Med. 294:938-939, 1976.

Kubicka, J.; Alder, A. E. Ueber eine neuere Behandlungsmethode der Vergiftung durch den Knollenblatterpilz. Praxis 57:1304-1306, 1968.

Kurnsteiner, H.; Moser, M. Isolation of a lethal toxin from Cortinarius orellanus Fr. Mycopathologia 74:65-72, 1981.

Lampe, K. F. Pharmacology and therapy of mushroom intoxications. In Mushroom Poisoning: Diagnosis and Treatment. B. H. Rumack and E. Salzman (editors). CRC Press, Inc, 1978.

Lampe, K. F. Toxic fungi. Ann. Rev. Pharmacol. Toxicol. 19:85-104, 1979.

Langer, M.; Vesconi, S.; Sapichino, G.; Costantino, D.; Radrizzani, D. The early removal of amatoxins in the treatment of Amanita Phalloides poisoning. Klin. Wochenschr. 58:117-123, 1980.

Lewes, D. "Mushroom" poisoning due to Amanita phalloides. Br. Med. J. 2:383-385, 1948.

Lincoff, G.; Mitchel, D. H. Toxic and Hallucinogenic Mushroom Poisoning. Van Nostrand Reinhold Co, 1977.

Lindberg, P.; Bergman, R.; Wickberg, B. Isolation and structure of coprine, a novel physiologically active cyclopropanone derivative from Coprinus atramentarius and its synthesis via 1-aminocyclopropanol. J. Chem. Soc. Chem. Commun. 23:946-947, 1975.

Lindell, T. J.; Weinberg, F.; Morris, P. W.; Roeder, R. G.; Rutter, W. J. α-Amanitin: specific inhibitor of nuclear RNA polymerase II. Science 170:447-449, 1970.

List, P. H.; Luft, P. Gyromitrin, das Gift der Fruhjahrslorchel. Arch. Pharm. (Wein-heim) 301:295-305, 1968.

Litten, W. The most poisonous mushrooms. Sci. Am. 231:90-101, 1975.

Malone, M. H.; Robichaud, R. C.; Tyler, V. E., Jr.; Brady, L. R. Relative muscarinic potency of thirty Inocybe species. Lloydia 25:231-237, 1962.

Maretic, Z. Poisoning by the mushroom, Clitocybe olearia Marie. Toxicon 4:263-267, 1967.

Maretic, Z.; Russell, F. E.; Golobic, V. Twenty-five cases of poisoning by the mushroom Pleurotus olearius. Toxicon 13:379-381, 1975.

Marichal, J. F.; Triby, F.; Wiederkehr, J. L.; Carbiener, R. Insuffisance renale chronique apres intoxication par champignons de type *Cortinarius orellanus* Fries. Nouv. Presse Med. *6*:2973-2975, 1977.

Mayer, J. H.; Herlocker, J. E.; Parisian, J. Esophageal rupture after mushroom-alcohol ingestion. N. Engl. J. Med. *285*:1323, 1971.

Menu, J. P.; Faure, J. L'Intoxication Par Les Champignons. Masson & Cie, editeurs, Paris, 1967.

Miller, O. *Mushrooms of North America*. E. P. Dutton, New York, 1972.

Moroni, F.; Fantozzi, R.; Masini, E.; Mannaioni, P. F. Trend in therapy of Amanita phalloides poisoning. Arch. Toxicol. *36*:111-115, 1976.

Mottonen, M.; Nieminen, L.; Heikkila, H. Damage caused by two Finnish mushrooms, *Cortinarius speciosissimus* and *Cortinarius gentilis* on the rat kidney. Zeitschr. f. Naturforsch. *30C*:668-671, 1975.

Myler, R. K.; Lee, J. C.; Hopper, J., Jr. Renal tubular necrosis caused by mushroom poisoning. Arch. Intern. Med. *114*:196-204, 1964.

Nieminen, L. Effect of drugs on mushroom poisoning induced in the rat by *Cortinarius speciosissimus*. Arch. Toxicol. *35*:235-238, 1976.

Nieminen, L.; Pyy, K. Individual variation in mushroom poisoning induced in the male rat by *Cortinarius speciosissimus*. Med. Biol. *54*:156-158, 1976.

Nieminen, L.; Mottonen, M.; Terri, R.; Ikonen, S. Nephrotoxicity of *Cortinarius speciosissimus*: a histological and enzyme histochemical study. Exp. Path. *11*:239-246, 1975.

Niskanen, A.; Pyysalo, H.; Rimaila-Parnanen, E.; Hartikka, P. Short-term peroral toxicity of ethylidene gyromitrin in rabbits and chickens. Fd. Cosmet. Toxicol. *14*:409-415, 1976.

Ott, J. Recreational use of hallucinogenic mushrooms in the United States. In *Mushroom Poisoning: Diagnosis and Treatment* (Rumack, B.H.; Salzman, E., editors), CRC Press, 1978.

Picchioni, A. L. Mushroom poisoning. Am J. Hosp. Pharm. *22*:634, 1965.

Pyysalo, H. Some new toxic compounds in false morels, *Gyromitra esculenta*. Nataswissenshoften *8*:395, 1975.

Pyysalo, H. Tests for gyromitrin, a poisonous compound in false morel gyromitra esculenta. Z. Lebensmitt-Untersuch. Forschung. *160*:325-330, 1976.

Reynolds, W. A.; Lowe, F. H. Mushrooms and a toxic reaction to alcohol. N. Engl. J. Med. *272*:630-631, 1965.

Scotti de Carolis, A.; Lipparini, F.; Longo, V. G. Neuropharmacological investigations on muscimol, a psychotropic drug extracted from *Amanita muscaria*. Psychopharmacologia (Berl.) *15*:186-195, 1969.

Seeger, R.; Bartels, O. Elimination of toxic peptides from *Amanita phalloides* by charcoal perfusion *in vitro*. Dtsch. Med. Wochenschr. *101*:1456-1458, 1976.

Short, A. I. K.; Watling, R.; MacDonald, M. K.; Robson, J. Poisoning by *Cortinarius speciosissimus*. Lancet *2*:942-944, 1980.

Singer, R. Hallucinogenic mushrooms. In *Mushroom poisoning: Diagnosis and Treatment*. (B.H. Rumack and E. Salzman, Eds.). CRC Press, pp. 201-214, 1978.

Teutsch, C.; Brennan, R. W. Amanita mushroom poisoning with recovery from coma: a case report. Ann. Neurol. *3*:177-179, 1978.

Theobald, W.; Buch, O.; Kunz, H. A.; Krupp, P.; Stenger, E. G.; Heimann, H. Pharmakologische und experimentalpsy-

chologische Untersuchungen mit 2 Inhaltsstoffen des Fliegenpilzes (*Amanita Muscaria*). Arzneim. Forsch. *18*:311-315, 1968.

Tholen, H.; Frohlich, T.; Huber, F.; Massini, M. A. Early haemodialysis in poisoning by Amanita phalloides. Ger. Med. Mon. *11*:89-91, 1966.

Tottmar, O.; Lindberg, P. Effects on rat liver acetaldehyde dehydrogenases *in vitro* and *in vivo* by coprine, the disulfiram-like constituent of *Coprinus atramentarius*. Acta Pharmacol. Toxicol. *40*:476-481, 1977.

Tyler, V. E., Jr. Occurrence of serotonin in hallucinogenic mushroom. Science *128*:718, 1958.

Tyler, V. E., Jr. Poisonous mushrooms. Prog. Chem. Toxicol. *1*:339-389, 1963.

Tyler, V. E., Jr.; Benedict, R. G.; Brady, L. R.; Robbers, J. E. Occurrence of Amanita toxins in American collections of deadly Amanita. J. Pharm. Sci. *55*:590-593, 1966.

Usdin, E.; Efron, D.H. Psychotropic Drugs and Related Compounds. 2nd ed., DHEW Publ. no. 72-9074, U.S. Gov. Printing Office, Washington, 1972.

Van der Veer, J. B.; Farley, D. L. Mushroom poisoning (mycetismus). Report of four cases. Arch. Intern. Med. *55*:773-791, 1935.

VanPoorten, J. F.; Stienstra, R.; Dworacek, B.; Moleman, P.; Rupreht, J. Physostigmine reversal of psilocybin intoxication. Anesthesiology *56*:313, 1982.

Verrill, A. E. A recent case of mushroom intoxication. Science *40*:408-410, 1914.

von Wright, A.; Pyysalo, H.; Niskanen, A. Quantitative evaluation of metabolic formation of methylhydrazine from acetaldehyde-*N*-methyl-*N*-formyl-hydrazone, the main poisonous compound of *Gyromitra esculenta*. Toxicol. Lett. *2*:261-265, 1978.

Waser, P. G. Chemistry and pharmacology of muscarine, muscarone and some related compounds. Pharmacol. Rev. *13*:465-515, 1961.

Waser, P. G. The pharmacology of Amanita muscaria. In: Ethnopharmacologic Search for Psychoactive Drugs, edited by D. Efron, B. Holmstedt and N. Kline. Proceedings of symposium held in San Francisco, 1967, pp. 419-439, 1967.

Wasson, R. G. Fly agaric and man. In: Ethnopharmacologic Search for Psychoactive Drugs, edited by D. Efron, B. Holmstedt and N. Kline. Proceedings of symposium held in San Francisco, 1967, pp. 405-414, 1967.

Wasson, R. G. *Soma: Divine Mushrooms of Immortality*. Harcourt Brace Janonovich Inc., New York, 1968.

Wauters, J. P.; Rossel, C.; Farquet, J. J. Amanita phalloides poisoning treated by early charcoal haemoperfusion. Br. Med. J. *2*:1465, 1978.

Wieland, O. Changes in liver metabolism induced by the poisons of Amanita phalloides. Clin. Chem. *11*:323-338, 1965.

Wieland, T. Poisonous principles of mushrooms of the genus Amanita. Science *159*:946-952, 1968.

Wieland, T.; Motzel, W.; Merz, H. Uber das Vorkommen von Bufotenine im gelben Knollenblatterpilz. Ann. Chem. *581*:10-16, 1953.

Wieland, T.; Wieland, O. Chemistry and toxicology of Amanita phalloides. Pharmacol. Rev. *11*:87-107, 1959.

Wiseman, J. S.; Abeles, R. A. Mechanism of inhibition of aldehyde dehydrogenase by cyclopropanone hydrate and the mushroom toxin coprine. Biochemistry *18*:427-435, 1979.

Yocum, R. R.; Simons, D. M. Amatoxins and phallotoxins in Amanita species of the Northeastern United States. Lloydia *40*:178-190, 1977.

NAPHTHALENE

Naphthalene (naphthalin or tar camphor) is a white crystalline solid of very low solubility in water. It is an ingredient of some moth repellents and toilet bowl deodorants and was once used as an intestinal vermifuge and wood preservative.

Toxicology: Although it may be delayed for several days, a hemolytic crisis constitutes the most spectacular reaction in naphthalene poisoning (*e.g.*, Athreya *et al.*, 1961; Chusid and Fried, 1955; Dawson *et al.*, 1958; Mackell *et al.*, 1951; Schafer, 1951; Zinckham and Childs, 1958).

It is seen most commonly in individuals of dark skinned races, notably American and some African Negroes, Arabs and other Semites, Mediterranean peoples, Caucasians of Latin extraction and various Asians (Dacie, 1967).

Particularly susceptible individuals are believed to possess a genetically determined metabolic defect which is sex-linked and finds its full expression in males. This defect results in a deficiency in glucose-6-phosphate dehydrogenase activity of red blood cells. Another consequence of the defect is that the erythrocyte is impaired in its ability to maintain a balance between its stores of oxidized and reduced glutathione. Thus, hemolysis and the appearance of Heinz bodies in red cells incubated with challenge chemicals (see below), abnormally low levels of glucose-6-phosphate dehydrogenase activity, decreased concentrations of reduced glutathione and an inability of the red cell to respond to methylene blue by an increase in methemoglobin reductase activity (see also ANILINE, p. III-33) all constitute useful diagnostic criteria in screening potential reactors (Dacie, 1967; Brewer et al., 1962).

Naphthalene is only one example of a wide variety of chemical compounds known to trigger the hemolytic crisis in sensitive individuals (Beutler, 1959; Gross et al., 1958). A spectrum of activity is recognized from aspirin, which produces only a mild reaction in sensitive Negroes, to the much more potent phenylhydrazine, acetylphenylhydrazine and acetanilid. Naphthalene and most other chemicals that can precipitate the reaction lie somewhere between these two extremes (Kellermeyer et al., 1962). These substances include: 8-aminoquinoline antimalarials, particularly primaquine; some sulfonamides such as sulfamethoxypyridazine and sulfisoxazole; several nitrofurans; compounds of vegetable origin such as the active ingredient in fava beans; and a large group of additional and diverse compounds (Dacie, 1967).

The intensity of the reaction presumably depends upon the extent of the red cell defect, at least in some cases on the size of the dose, and on the nature of the trigger compound. Sometimes other extra-erythrocytic factors also play important roles (Kellermeyer et al., 1962). In the absence of a challenging chemical, however, there are no overt manifestations of the defect.

As seen after naphthalene the classic features of this blood dyscrasia include fragmentation of red cells with anisocytosis and poikilocytosis, icterus, severe anemia with nucleated red cells, leukocytosis, and dramatic decreases in hemoglobin, hematocrit and red cell count (Anziulewicz et al., 1959). More severe reactions also include Heinz body formation (Hanssler, 1964; Irle, 1964; Valaes et al., 1963; Zuelzer and Apt, 1949), hemoglobinuria (Abelson and Henderson, 1951; Gidron and Leurer, 1956; Valaes et al., 1963) and mild methemoglobinemia (Grigor et al., 1966; Haggerty, 1956; Hanssler, 1964; Valaes et al., 1963). The hemolytic episode tends to be self-limiting because damage occurs most intensively in older cells, i.e., those approaching the normal life span of 100 to 120 days (Dacie, 1967). The chief threat to life in young infants is kernicterus, which carries a high mortality (Naiman and Kosoy, 1964; Valaes et al., 1963). In older children and adults the hemolytic crisis may be followed by renal tubular blockade and acute renal failure (Gidron and Leurer, 1956; MacGregor, 1954).

Naphthalene is also toxic in normal individuals without recognized blood cell defects. It is difficult, however, to estimate the lethal dose in nonsensitive individuals because the red cell abnormality has not been excluded convincingly in most reported cases of poisoning. In the total population a wide range of individual susceptibility exists, and among sensitive individuals minute doses have induced dangerous reactions (Naiman and Kosoy, 1964; Valaes et al., 1963).

The mean lethal dose in nonsensitive adults may lie between 5 and 15 gm., but no convincing evidence can be cited in support of this estimate. Six grams have been survived (Gidron and Leurer, 1956), but 2 gm. over a 2-day period killed a 6-year-old child (Sollmann, 1957). The nature of the syndrome appears to be essentially the same in sensitive and nonsensitive victims; the threshold dose constitutes the probable distinction. Indeed, hemolytic episodes have been reported in infants with normal red cell glucose-6-phosphate dehydrogenase activity (Valaes et al., 1963) and normal glutathione stability (Jacobziner and Raybin, 1964).

Heinz body formation does not always occur (Anziulewicz et al., 1959) or may be of mild proportions (Bregman, 1954; Cock, 1957), and a dark urine (with negative benzidine reaction) may reflect the presence of naphthalene metabolites instead of hemoglobinuria (Bregman, 1954). Positive spectroscopic evidence for methemoglobinemia is not always obtained (Mackell et al., 1951) or may be seen only transiently (Grigor et al., 1966). At least one investigator (Haggerty, 1956) noted that the serum of a poisoned patient was brown, suggesting that hemolysis may be a prerequisite to methemoglobin formation, as it is chlorate poisoning (see BROMATE, p. III-74). In plasma, ferric heme groups of methemoglobin tend to exchange with albumin to form methemalbumin, which retains some of the spectroscopic properties of methemoglobin (Fairley, 1941a and b).

In addition to ingestion naphthalene is toxic by vapor inhalation after spontaneous sublimitation or in electric vaporizing devices (Hanssler, 1964; Irle, 1964; Naiman and Kosoy, 1964; Valaes *et al.*, 1963). Systemic reactions have occurred after dressing infants in clothing stored with naphthalene mothballs, suggesting that percutaneous absorption may occur (Cock, 1957; Grigor *et al.*, 1966). This process may be facilitated by applications of baby oil (Dawson *et al.*, 1958; Schafer, 1951). Transplacental naphthalene poisoning has also occurred (Anziulewicz *et al.*, 1959; Zinckham and Childs, 1958).

With the exception of dermatitis due to hypersensitivity with positive patch tests, reports of naphthalene poisoning in industry are rare (Fanburg, 1940; Gerarde, 1960). Corneal ulceration and cataracts following exposure to vapor and dust can be demonstrated experimentally and occur occasionally in man (Adams, 1930; Ghetti and Mariani, 1956; Meyer, 1955). The OSHA TWA (time-weighted average) for an 8-hour day is 10 ppm in air.

In mice nonciliated bronchiolar epithelial (Clara) cells are selectively damaged by intraperitoneal naphthalene. Following exfoliation of Clara cells the remaining ciliated cells show morphological abnormalities. Regeneration of Clara cells was followed by a return to normal morphology of ciliated cells (Mahvi *et al.*, 1977). A similar phenomenon has not been described in man.

Transfusions of whole blood are clearly indicated in the treatment of severe hemolytic reactions (Beutler, 1959), but no specific therapeutic measures are recognized. Because naphthalene *per se* is nonhemolytic (even in shed blood from sensitive patients), a metabolite is indicated as the active compound (Zuelzer and Apt, 1949).

Naphthalene is metabolized to yield a variety of hydroxy- and methylthio- derivatives in rats (Bock *et al.*, 1976; Stillwell *et al.*, 1978). In these two groups of metabolites α-naphthol and 1-methylthionaphthalene are the most prominent urinary constituents. The initial metabolite is apparently a 1,2-epoxide produced in the liver by mixed function oxidase. This reactive compound is subsequently converted to naphthalene dihydrodiol and to α-naphthol. Both compounds are excreted as such and as glucuronide conjugates. Mercapturic acid conjugates are also quantitatively important in the rat (Chen and Dorough, 1979). Naphthalene dihydrodiol may be further converted in the eye to yield 1,2-naphthoquinone, a known cataractogenic agent.

The hemolytic potential of naphthalene derivatives decreases in the order: α-naphthol, β-naphthol, α-naphthoquinone, β-naphthoquinone (Mackell *et al.*, 1951). As noted above, some metabolites of naphthalene are excreted as glucuronides (Williams, 1959b). The inadequacy of this and other detoxication mechanisms in the newborn (Brown, 1957) may explain their susceptibility to naphthalene poisoning.

In contrast to naphthalene, the only reported effects of methylated naphthalene in man are skin irritation and skin photosensitization (Gerarde, 1960). Chlorinated derivatives of naphthalene frequently produce an acneiform eruption of the skin and various degrees of liver necrosis. See Polychlorinated naphthalenes in Section II.

Symptomatology:
  A. *Surface contact.*
    1. Naphthalene cataracts and ocular irritation have been produced experimentally in rabbits and have been described in man.
    2. Skin irritation and, in the case of a sensitized person, severe dermatitis. Lesions clear spontaneously as soon as the exposure is terminated.
    3. Percutaneous absorption is apparently inadequate to produce acute systemic reactions except in newborns (see below).
  B. *Inhalation of vapor.*
    1. Headache, confusion, and excitement.
    2. Nausea and sometimes vomiting, and extensive sweating.
    3. Dysuria, hematuria, and the acute hemolytic reaction described below.
    4. Rarely optic neuritis is encountered.
  C. *Ingestion.*
    1. Abdominal cramps with nausea, vomiting and diarrhea.
    2. Headache, profuse perspiration, listlessness, confusion.
    3. In severe poisoning, coma with or without convulsions.
    4. Irritation of the urinary bladder, presumably due to excretory products of naphthalene metabolism. Signs and symptoms include urgency, dysuria, and the passage of a brown or black urine with or without albumin and casts; usually these effects disappear within a few days, and they should be distinguished from a hemolytic reaction.
    5. Acute intravascular hemolysis is the most characteristic sign, particularly in persons with red cell glucose-6-phosphate dehydrogenase deficiency. It often begins on the third day and is accompanied by anemia, leukocytosis, fever, hemoglobinuria, jaundice, renal insufficiency, and sometimes disturbances in liver function.
    6. In the absence of adequate supportive treatment, death may result from acute renal failure in adults or kernicterus in young infants.

Treatment:

1. Induce emesis and/or perform gastric lavage with large amounts of warm water (see Section I), whenever poisoning by mouth is suspected.
2. Instill a saline cathartic such as magnesium or sodium sulfate in water (15 to 30 gm.).
3. Demulcents such as milk, egg white, gelatin, or other protein solutions may be useful after the stomach is emptied, but oils should be avoided because they may promote absorption.
4. Contaminated eyes or skin should be flushed with warm water, followed by the application of a bland ointment.
5. A severe anemia due to hemolysis may require small repeated blood transfusions preferably with red cells from a non-sensitive individual. Cortisone therapy (p. IV-100) appears to have been beneficial in a few cases of naphthalene hemolysis.
6. In the event of intravascular hemolysis with hemoglobinuria, protect the kidneys by promoting a brisk flow of dilute urine; an osmotic diuretic such as mannitol is often used for this purpose (p. IV-52). It may also be helpful to alkalinize the urine by giving small amounts of sodium bicarbonate, but many investigators doubt the efficacy of this measure in preventing blockage of renal tubules.
7. In the event of kernicterus, hemodialysis and exchange transfusions may be required.
8. Supportive measures in the case of acute renal failure (see p. IV-53).

Laboratory:

1. Laboratory findings are often indicative of a severe hemolytic anemia. Red cell fragmentation with anisocytosis, poikilocytosis, Heinz body formation and methemoglobinemia are accompanying phenomena. Efforts should be made to ascertain whether methemoglobin formation occurs in red cells or in plasma.
2. α-Naphthol is present in the urine, and its detection may be necessary for a definitive diagnosis.
3. Patients should be screened for red cell glucose-6-phosphate dehydrogenase deficiency, but not until several weeks after the ingestion episode.

References:

Abelson, S. M.; Henderson, A. T. Moth ball poisoning. U. S. Armed Forces Med. J. 2:491-493, 1951.

Adams, D. R. A study of the correlation between the biochemical and intra-ocular changes induced in rabbits by the administration of naphthalene. Br. J. Ophthalmol. 14:545-576, 1930.

Anziulewicz, J. A.; Dick, H. J.; Chiarulli, E. E. Transplacental naphthalene poisoning. Am. J. Obstet. Gynecol. 78:519-521, 1959.

Athreya, B. H.; Swain, A. K.; Dickstein, B. Acute hemolytic anemia due to the ingestion of naphthalene. Indian J. Child. Health 10:305-308, 1961.

Beutler, E. The hemolytic effect of primaquine and related compounds, A review. Blood 14:103-139, 1959.

Bock, K. W.; Van Ackeren, G.; Lorch, F.; Birke, F. W. Metabolism of naphthalene to naphthalene dihydrodiol glucuronide in isolated hepatocytes and in liver microsomes. Biochem. Pharmacol. 25:2351-2356, 1976.

Bregman, R. Moth ball poisoning, a case presentation. Clin. Proc. Child. Hosp. D. C. 10:1-3, 1954.

Brewer, G. J.; Tarlov, A. R.; Alving, A. S. The methemoglobin reduction test for primaquine-type sensitivity of erythrocytes. J. A. M. A. 180:386-388, 1962.

Brown, A. K. Studies on the neonatal development of the glucuronide conjugating system. Am. J. Dis. Child. 94:510, 1957.

Chen, K. C.; Dorough, H. W. Glutathione and mercapturic acid conjugations in the metabolism of naphthalene and 1-naphthyl N-methylcarbamate (carbaryl). Drug Chem. Toxicol. 2:331-354, 1979.

Chusid, E.; Fried, C. T. Acute hemolytic anemia due to naphthalene ingestion. Am. J. Dis. Child. 89:612-614, 1955.

Cock, T. C. Acute hemolytic anemia in the neonatal period. Am. J. Dis. Child. 94:77-79, 1957.

Dacie, J. V. The Haemolytic Anaemias, Congenital and Acquired. Part IV. Drug-Induced Haemolytic Anaemias, Paroxysmal Nocturnal Haemoglobinuria, Haemolytic Disease of the Newborn, 2nd ed. Grune and Stratton, Inc., New York, 1967.

Dawson, J. P.; Thayer, W. W.; Desforges, J. F. Acute hemolytic anemia in the newborn infant due to naphthalene poisoning; report of two cases with investigations into the mechanism of the disease. Blood 13:1113-1125, 1958.

Fairley, N. H. Methaemalbumin. Part I. Clinical aspects. Q. J. Med. 10:95-114, 1941a.

Fairley, N. H. Methaemalbumin. Part II. Its synthesis, chemical behavior, and experimental production in man and monkeys. Q. J. Med. 10:115-138, 1941b.

Fanburg, S. J. Exfoliative dermatitis due to naphthalene. Arch. Dermatol. 42:53-58, 1940.

Gerarde, H. W. Toxicology and Biochemistry of Aromatic Hydrocarbons. Elsevier, Amsterdam, 1960.

Ghetti, G.; Mariani, L. Alterazioni oculari du naftalina; ricerche cliniche e sperimentali. Med. Lav. 47:533-538, 1956.

Gidron, E.; Leurer, J. Naphthalene poisoning. Lancet 1:228-230, 1956.

Grigor, W. G.; Robin, H.; Harley, J. D. An Australian varient on "full-moon disease." Med. J. Aust. 2:1229-1230, 1966.

Gross, R. T.; Hurwitz, R. E.; Marks, P. A. An hereditary enzymatic defect in erythrocyte metabolism: Glucose-6-phosphate dehydrogenase deficiency. J. Clin. Invest. 37:1176-1184, 1958.

Haggerty, R. J. Naphthalene poisoning. N. Engl. J. Med. 255:919-920, 1956.

Hanssler, H. Lebensbedrohliche Naphthalinvergiftung bei einem Saugling durch Vaporindampfe. Dtsch. Med. Wochenschr. 89:1794-1797, 1964.

Irle, U. Akute hamolytisch Anamie durch Naphthalin-Inhalation bei zwei Fruhgeborenen und einem Neugeborenen. Dtsch. Med. Wochenschr. 89:1798-1800, 1964.

Jacobziner, H.; Raybin, H. W. Naphthalene poisoning. N. Y. State J. Med. 64:1762-1763, 1964.

Kellermeyer, R. W.; Tarlov, A. R.; Brewer, G. J.; Carson, P. E.; Alving, A. S. Hemolytic effect of therapeutic drugs, clinical considerations of the primaquine-type hemolysis. J. A. M. A. 180:388-394, 1962.

MacGregor, R. R. Naphthalene poisoning from the ingestion of moth balls. Can. Med. Assoc. J. 70:313-314, 1954.

Mackell, J. V.; Rieders, F.; Brieger, W.; Bauer, E. L. Acute hemolytic anemia due to ingestion of naphthalene moth balls. Pediatrics 7:722-728, 1951.

Mahvi, D.; Bank, H.; Harley, R. Morphology of a naphthalene-induced bronchiolar lesion. Am. J. Pathol. 86:559-572, 1977.

Meyer, R. T. The medical significance of lenticular opacities (cataract) before the age of fifty. N. Engl. J. Med. 252:622-

628, 1955.

Naiman, T. L.; Kosoy, M. H. Red cell glucose-6-phosphate dehydrogenase deficiency - a newly recognized cause of neonatal jaundice and kernicterus in Canada. Can. Med. Assoc. J. 91:1243-1249, 1964.

Schafer, W. B. Acute hemolytic anemia related to naphthalene. Report of a case in a newborn infant. Pediatrics 7:172-174, 1951.

Sollmann, T. A Manual of Pharmacology. 8th Ed., W. B. Saunders Co., Philadelphia, 1957.

Stillwell, W. G.; Bouwsma, O. J.; Thenot, J. P.; Horning, M. G.; Griffin, G. W.; Ishikawa, K. Takaku, M. Methylthio metabolites of naphthalene excreted by the rat. Res. Commun. Chem. Pathol. Pharmacol. 20:509-530, 1978.

Valaes, T.; Doxiadis, S. A.; Fessas, P. Acute hemolysis due to naphthalene inhalation. J. Pediatr. 63:904-915, 1963.

Williams, R. T. Detoxification Mechanisms, 2nd ed. John Wiley and Sons, Inc., New York, 1959b.

Zinkham, W. H.; Childs, B. A defect of glutathione metabolism in erythrocytes from patients with a naphthalene-induced hemolytic anemia. Pediatrics 22:461-471, 1958.

Zuelzer, W. W.; Apt, L. Acute hemolytic anemia due to naphthalene poisoning. J. A. M. A. 141:185-190, 1949.

NICOTINE

Nicotine (1-methyl-2-(3-pyridyl)pyrrolidine) is a colorless, volatile, and strongly alkaline liquid, which on exposure to air acquires a brown color and a tobacco-like odor. It is readily soluble in water and forms salts with acids. The alkaloid is obtained from the dried leaves and stems of *Nicotiana tobacum* and *Nicotiana rustica* (Tso, 1972), where it occurs in concentrations of 0.5 to 8% with citric and malic acids (usually 1 to 3%). Nicotine is encountered most frequently in tobacco products and now rarely in insecticide preparations. For use as an insecticide it was usually marketed as a 40% solution of the sulfate, but free nicotine has also been used (Stevenson, 1933). Occasionally nicotine is used in animal "tranquilizing" darts (Feurt et al., 1958).

Tobacco is employed not only for smoking, chewing and snuffing, but it has been used in enemas and poultices. Cigarette tobacco varies in its nicotine content, but common blends contain 15 to 25 mg. per cigarette, with a current trend toward lower levels (Tso, 1972). However, when a cigarette is smoked by machine to mimic an average smoker's technique, the smoke contains less than 3 mg. per cigarette. Periodical analyses by the FTC and others indicate that the smoke of most American brands contains 0.3 to 2.6 mg. nicotine and 8 to 43 mg. tar (Anon., 1972; Moore et al., 1967). The total dose of nicotine retained from smoking a small cigar is about 1 to 4.5 mg. (Armitage et al., 1978). As shown in recent times, manufacturers can produce cigarettes of almost any tar and nicotine yield. Animal studies suggest, however, that components other than nicotine in the particulate phase of cigarette smoke contribute significantly to the acute lethal effects (Bernfeld, 1975).

Reactions from chronic exposure to tobacco and nicotine (e.g., Kepp, 1938; Maffei and Miami, 1962; Thienes, 1960) are not considered in this manual, but they have been reviewed authoritatively (Larson and Silvette, 1971; National Clearinghouse for Smoking and Health, 1971). In view of the ubiquitous distribution of tobacco, nicotine poisoning is reported with surprising infrequency today, but when nicotine insecticides were popular in the 1920s and 1930s, fatal poisonings were common (reviewed by Larson et al., 1961).

Toxicology: Nicotine is one of the most toxic of all poisons and acts with great rapidity. It is absorbed from the alimentary canal, respiratory tract and intact skin (Faulkner, 1933; Lockhart, 1933). Percutaneous absorption is many times faster with the free alkaloid than with its acid salts (Faulkner, 1933). A self-limited illness known as "green-tobacco sickness" has been described in young men handling uncured tobacco leaves in the field; it consists of pallor, vomiting and prostration and is probably due to the percutaneous absorption of nicotine from wet leaves (Gehlbach et al., 1974).

The major effects of nicotine, aside from local caustic actions, are a transient stimulation and subsequent depression or paralysis of the central nervous system, all peripheral autonomic ganglia, and motor end-plates in skeletal muscles. In addition smooth muscle cells are excited, perhaps directly, by the alkaloid, an action that may be partly responsible for the observed vasoconstriction and intestinal movements. These phasic neural and neuromuscular actions of nicotine lead to complex and variegated clinical syndromes.

Lethal doses of nicotine and its salts have been established in many animal species (reviewed by Larson et al., 1961). The oral LD_{50} of nicotine in the dog is about 10 mg./kg. For an adult human the mean lethal dose has been estimated to be 30 to 60 mg. (0.5 to 1.0 mg./kg.), but a few milligrams may produce a serious illness and even death (Larson et al., 1961). An adult male game warden (who was a habitual smoker) accidentally shot himself in the thigh with an animal "tranquilizing" dart containing nicotine. The dose of 3.6 mg./kg. produced a desperate but nonfatal poisoning (Brady et al., 1979).

Marked tolerance to the alkaloid is acquired by confirmed smokers. The ingestion of an insecticide solution with as much as 2 gm. of nicotine has been survived (Ahn, 1952). In lethal poisonings postmortem examination often reveals congestion and hyperemia of the brain, meninges and many visceral organs, especially the kidneys (Beeman and Hunter, 1937). Sometimes hemorrhages are described in the gastrointestinal tract and lung (Adebahr and Voight, 1963).

Tobacco is much less toxic than expected from its nicotine content. Apparently intestinal absorption of nicotine as present in tobacco is so slow that metabolic inactivation sometimes keeps pace with absorption. Spontaneous vomiting may also remove much unabsorbed alkaloid. On the other hand, serious poisonings and death have occurred from contamination of an infant's formula with tobacco (Reynolds, 1914), the use of aqueous infusions of tobacco as enemas (Garcia-Estrada and Fischman, 1977; Oberst and McIntyre, 1953; Willis, 1937), swallowing tobacco quids, ingesting residues from pipes and many other bizarre circumstances (Polson and Tattersall, 1959). Probably all toddlers who ingest tobacco or tobacco products should be treated prophylactically with activated charcoal and/or gastric lavage (see below).

In fatal cases of nicotine poisoning, death is usually rapid; it occurs nearly always within 1 hour and occasionally within 5 minutes (McNally, 1920, 1922; Moore, 1962). According to the traditional view, death is due to paralysis of the respiratory muscles. Paralysis of medullary centers controlling respiration requires a larger dose (Gold and Brown, 1935). Artificial respiration is uniformly successful in preventing death in dogs given lethal doses of nicotine if started before the circulation fails and continued until muscle paralysis disappears. Circulatory failure is not necessarily permanent. If heart action can be initiated by external cardiac massage or intracardiac epinephrine while respirations are maintained, death may be prevented (Franke and Thomas, 1936). If the patient survives 4 hours, the prognosis is good.

Nicotine first stimulates and later depresses the central nervous system to produce tremors, then clonic convulsions, followed by tonic-extensor convulsions and death. Thus, despite assertions to the contrary, it appears that there are important central components in the lethal actions of nicotine. These central actions can be blocked in varying degrees by a variety of agents including antiparkinsonian drugs, antihistaminics, anticonvulsants, anesthetics, adrenergic blocking drugs and phenothiazines (Bovet and Longo, 1951; Cahen and Lynes, 1951; Laurence and Stacey, 1953; Yamamoto et al., 1966).

Caramiphen (Parpanit) hydrochloride and diethazine (Diparcol) hydrochloride, two drugs with complex actions on the central and autonomic nervous systems, have been extolled in the control of experimental nicotine poisoning (Heymans and DeVleeschhouwer, 1948; Heymans and Estable, 1949). Given intravenously in large doses, diethazine has protected dogs against 100 to 200 lethal doses of nicotine. Although this degree of effectiveness cannot be anticipated in man for many reasons, caramiphen and diethazine deserve clinical trials in acute nicotine poisoning. Unhappily, neither drug is made in the United States or available to physicians here.

Following intravenous administration to dogs and monkeys, nicotine was rapidly distributed to many tissues. At 5 minutes the adrenal medulla and the cerebral cortex contained the highest concentrations (Tsujimoto et al., 1975). The major pathway for nicotine metabolism in the rabbit and rat appears to be hydroxylation on the alpha position of the pyrrolidine ring, followed by further oxidation to cotinine (Adir et al., 1980; Hucker et al., 1960). This pathway is induced by chronic ethanol treatment of rats, which also increases both the total plasma clearance and the apparent volume of distribution of nicotine (Adir et al., 1980).

The elimination of nicotine is complete within 16 hours; about 80 to 90% is detoxified and the remainder is excreted unchanged in the urine (Ganz et al., 1951; Larson and Haag, 1942). The maintenance of an acid urine is said to accelerate excretion, but it is doubtful that this observation has clinical significance (Haag and Larson, 1942).

Many naturally occurring and synthetic derivatives of nicotine have been tested as potential insecticides. By intraperitoneal injection d-nornicotine is 3 to 4 times more acutely toxic to rats and guinea pigs than nicotine. l-Nornicotine, d-nicotine and l-nicotine are all equitoxic (Hicks and Sinclair, 1947). Besides nornicotine only anabasine, dihydronicotyrine and 5'-methylnornicotine have toxicities similar to that of nicotine (Mattila and Vartiainen, 1963; Yamamoto et al., 1962).

Thirteen nicotine-related alkaloids present or reputedly present in cigarette smoke were compared separately with nicotine in 9 mammalian test systems (Clark et al., 1965). In contrast to their lethality (above), none was as potent as nicotine in these test systems. Only nornicotine and anabasine have potencies of the same order of magnitude as nicotine. Since nicotine is by far the most prevalent alkaloid in tobacco smoke, it is believed to be solely responsible for the nicotine-like effects in man and experimental animals (Clark et al., 1965).

N'-Nitrosonornicotine, a potential carcinogen, has been positively identified in unburned tobacco; its concentration of 2 to 89 ppm is among the highest reported for any environmental nitrosamine (Hoffmann et al., 1974). Lobeline, an alkaloid from Lobelia inflata, has actions similar to those of nicotine, but it is much less potent.

It is found in commercial anti-smoking tablets and lozenges.

Symptomatology:

1. Burning sensation in mouth and throat, salivation, nausea, abdominal pain, vomiting and diarrhea. Gastrointestinal reactions are less severe but do occur after cutaneous and respiratory exposures.
2. Systemic effects include agitation, headache, sweating, dizziness, auditory and visual disturbances, confusion, weakness, and incoordination. The victim may collapse suddenly and with little prodromata only a short time after ingesting a nicotine solution.
3. At first respirations are deep and rapid, the blood pressure is high, and the pulse is slow. Intense vagal stimulation may cause transient cardiac standstill or paroxysmal atrial fibrillation (Ahn, 1952, 1953). The pupils are generally constricted.
4. Central nervous excitation is also evidenced by tremors and sometimes by clonic-tonic convulsions.
5. As depression develops, the pupils dilate, the blood pressure falls, and the pulse becomes rapid and often irregular. Faintness, prostration, cyanosis and dyspnea progress to collapse.
6. Death from paralysis of respiratory muscles, usually only a few minutes after collapse.

Treatment (speed is *imperative*):

1. For ingested poison, administer 6 to 8 heaping teaspoonfuls of activated charcoal (p. I-4) as a slurry in water.
2. Because nicotine induces vomiting by stimulating the chemoreceptor trigger zone of the brainstem, it seems inadvisable to administer syrup of ipecac, which acts by the same mechanism.
3. Unless spontaneous emesis is vigorous and productive, gastric lavage with 0.5% solution of tannic acid or a 1:5000 solution of potassium permanganate. Use water if these solutions are not immediately available.
4. If nicotine is spilled on the skin, wash thoroughly and *immediately* with diluted vinegar and/or cold running water.
5. Artificial ventilation (p. IV-7) and oxygen therapy (p. IV-12) until spontaneous breathing is adequate or until the heart ceases to beat. Central respiratory stimulants are rarely if ever indicated. Keep the airway clear (p. IV-2). Profuse salivation may require continuous oral suction.
6. If severe or persistent, convulsions may be controlled with small intravenous doses of barbiturates or diazepam (p. IV-37).

7. Most of the visceral manifestations can be controlled by various combinations of autonomic blocking drugs, such as atropine and phenoxybenzamine (Dibenzyline). Caramiphen (Parpanit) hydrochloride and diethazine (Diparcol) hydrochloride, which have been extolled in the control of experimental nicotine poisoning (see above), are not available in the United States.

Laboratory:

1. Secretion of the adrenal medulla may cause an elevation of blood sugar, but laboratory data are rarely of diagnostic or prognostic help in acute nicotine poisoning.
2. Nicotine blood levels in habitual smokers are said to average less than 0.03 mg./100 ml., whereas concentrations of 1 mg./100 ml. or more have been reported in fatal nicotine poisonings (McBay, 1966). Some data on postmortem tissue concentrations in human deaths are also available (McNally, 1922; Tiess and Nagel, 1966).

References:

Adebahr, G.; Voight, G. E. Morphologische Veranderungen bei der akuten todlichen Nicotin vergiftung. Dtsch. Z. Ges. Gerichtl. Med. 54:304-315, 1963.

Adir, J.; Wildfeuer, W.; Miller, R. P. Effect of ethanol pretreatment on the pharmacokinetics of nicotine in rats. J. Pharmacol. Exp. Ther. 212:274-279, 1980.

Ahn, Von B. Paroxysmal auricular fibrillation in acute nicotine poisoning. Cardiologia 21:765-772, 1952.

Ahn, Von B. A further case of paroxysmal auricular fibrillation in acute nicotine poisoning. Acta Med. Scand. 145:28-33, 1953.

Anon. FTC compromises on cigarette ads. Consumer Rep. 37:470-471, 1972.

Armitage, A.; Dollery, C.; Houseman, T.; Kohner, E.; Lewis, P. J.; Turner, D. Absorption of nicotine from small cigars. Clin. Pharmacol. Ther. 23:143-151, 1978.

Beeman, J. A.; Hunter, W. C. Fatal nicotine poisoning. A report of twenty-four cases. Arch. Pathol. 24:481-485, 1937.

Bernfeld, P. Acute toxicity of smoke from different brands of cigarettes measured in mice. Toxicol. Appl. Pharmacol. 31:413-420, 1975.

Bovet, D.; Longo, G. The action in nicotine-induced tremors of substances effective in parkinsonism. J. Pharmacol. Exp. Ther. 102:22-30, 1951.

Brady, M. E.; Ritschel, W. A.; Saelinger, D. A.; Cacini, W.; Patterson, J. Animal model and pharmacokinetic interpretation of nicotine poisoning in man. Int. J. Clin. Pharmacol. Biopharm. 17:12-17, 1979.

Cahen, R. L.; Lynes, T. E. Nicotinolytic drugs. I. Drugs inhibiting nicotine-induced tremors. J. Pharmacol. Exp. Ther. 103:44-53, 1951.

Clark, M. S. G.; Rand, M. J.; Vanov, S. Comparison of pharmacological activity of nicotine and related alkaloids occurring in cigarette smoke. Arch. Int. Pharmacodyn. Ther. 156:363-379, 1965.

Faulkner, J. M. Nicotine poisoning by absorption through the skin. J. A. M. A. 100:1664-1665, 1933.

Feurt, S. D.; Jenkins, J. H.; Hayes, F. A.; Crockford, H. A. Pharmacology and toxicology of nicotine with special reference to species variation. Science 126:1054-1055, 1958.

Franke, F. E.; Thomas, J. E. The treatment of acute nicotine poisoning. J. A. M. A. 106:507-512, 1936.

Ganz, A.; Kelsey, F. E.; Geiling, E. M. K. Excretion and tissue distribution studies on radioactive nicotine. J. Pharmacol. Exp. Ther. 103:209-214, 1951.

Garcia-Estrada, H.; Fischman, C. M. An unusual case of nicotine poisoning. Clin. Toxicol. *10*:391-393, 1977.

Gehlbach, S. H.; Williams, W. A.; Perry, L. D.; Woodall, J. S. Green-tobacco sickness; An illness of tobacco harvesters. J. A. M. A. *229*:1880-1883, 1974.

Gold, H.; Brown, F. A contribution to the pharmacology of nicotine. J. Pharmacol. Exp. Ther. *54*:143-144, 1935.

Hagg, H. B.; Larson, P. S. Studies on the fate of nicotine in the body. I. The effect of pH on the urinary excretion of nicotine by tobacco smokers. J. Pharmacol. Exp. Ther. *76*:235-239, 1942.

Heymans, C.; De Vleeschhouwer, G. R. Actions pharmacologiques de l'ester diethylaminoethylique de l'acide. Arch. Int. Pharmacodyn. Ther. *75*:307-324, 1948.

Heymans, C.; Estable, J. J. On new nicotinolytic compounds. Science *109*:122, 1949.

Hicks, C. S.; Sinclair, D. A. Toxicities of optical isomers of nicotine and nornicotine. Aust. J. Exp. Biol. Med. Sci. *25*:83-86, 1947.

Hoffmann, D.; Hecht, S. S.; Ornaf, R. M.; Wynder, E. L. N'-Nitrosonornicotine in tobacco. Science *186*:265-267, 1974.

Hucker, H. B.; Gillette, J. R.; Brodie, B. B. Enzymatic pathway for the formation of cotinine, a major metabolite of nicotine in rabbit liver. J. Pharmacol. Exp. Ther. *129*:94-100, 1960.

Kepp, F. R. V. Nikotin-Polyneuritis. Arch. Toxikol. *9*:115-116, 1938.

Larson, P. S.; Haag, H. B. Studies on the fate of nicotine in the body. II. On the fate of nicotine in the dog. J. Pharmacol. Exp. Ther. *76*:240-244, 1942.

Larson, P. S.; Haag, H. B.; Silvette, H. *Tobacco. Experimental and Clinical Studies.* Williams and Wilkins Co., Baltimore, Md, 1961.

Larson, P. S.; Silvette, H. *Tobacco. Experimental and Clinical Studies.* Supplement I and Supplement II. Williams & Wilkins Co., Baltimore, 1968 and 1971.

Laurence, D. R.; Stacey, R. S. Mechanism of the prevention of nicotine convulsions by hexamethonium and by adrenaline blocking agents. Br. J. Pharmacol. *8*:62-65, 1953.

Lockhart, L. P. Nicotine poisoning. Br. Med. J. *1*:246-247, 1933.

Maffei, G.; Miami, P. Experimental tobacco poisoning. Arch. Otolaryngol. *75*:386-396, 1962.

Mattila, M.; Vartiainen, A. The lethal dose, pressor effect and intestinal activity of some pyrrolidine N-substituted nornicotine derivatives. Acta Pharmacol. Toxicol. *19*:330-336,

1963.

McBay, A. J. Law-medicine notes, chemical findings in poisonings. N. Engl. J. Med. *274*:1257-1258, 1966.

McNally, W. D. A report of five cases of poisoning by nicotine. J. Lab. Clin. Med. *5*:213-217, 1920.

McNally, W. D. A report of five cases of nicotine poisoning. J. Lab. Clin. Med. *8*:83-85, 1922.

Moore, G. E.; Bross, I.; Shamberger, R.; Bock, F. G. Tar and nicotine retrieval from fifty-six brands of cigarettes. Cancer *20*:323-332, 1967.

Moore, H. W. Acute nicotine poisoning, poison case report of month. J. S. C. Med. Assoc. *58*:445, 1962.

National Clearinghouse for Smoking and Health. *The Health Consequences of Smoking.* A report of the Surgeon General. USDHEW, PHS Publication No. (HSM) 71-7513, U. S. Government Printing Office, Washington, D. C, 1971.

Oberst, B. B.; McIntyre, R. A. Acute nicotine poisoning. Pediatrics *11*:338-340, 1953.

Polson, C. J.; Tattersall, R. N. *Clinical Toxicology.* J. B. Lippincott Co., Philadelphia, 1959.

Reynolds, H. S. A case of acute poisoning of peculiar origin. J. A. M. A. *62*:1723, 1914.

Stevenson, H. M. Acute nicotine poisoning as noted in the manufacture and use of nicotine insecticides. Calif. Med. *38*:92-95, 1933.

Thienes, C. H. Chronic nicotine poisoning. Ann. N. Y. Acad. Sci. 90: Article 1, 239-248, 1960.

Tiess, D.; Nagel, K. H. Akute todliche Vergiftung mit "Nikotin 95/98%". Beitrag zur Analytik des Giftes am frischen, gelagerten und formalinfixierten Organmaterial. Arch. Toxikol. *22*:68-70, 1966.

Tso, T. C. Physiology and Biochemistry of Tobacco Plants. Dowden, Hutchinson and Ross, Inc., Stroudsburg, Pa, 1972.

Tsujimoto, A.; Nakashima, T.; Tanino, S.; Dohi, T.; Kurogochi, Y. Tissue distribution of [³H]nicotine in dogs and rhesus monkeys. Toxicol. Appl. Pharmacol., *32*:21-31, 1975.

Willis, H. W. Acute nicotine poisoning. Report of a case in a child. J. Pediatr. *10*:65-68, 1937.

Yamamoto, I.; Kamimura, H.; Yamamoto, R.; Sakai, S.; Goda, M. Studies on nicotinoids as an insecticide. Agric. Biol. Chem. *26*:709-716, 1962.

Yamamoto, I.; Otori, K.; Inoki, R. Pharmacological studies on antagonists against nicotine-induced convulsions and death. Jap. J. Pharmacol. *16*:402-415, 1966.

NITRITE

Inorganic nitrite salts and organic nitrites and nitrates are available in many homes as medicinal agents, *e.g.*, amyl nitrite, nitroglycerin, sodium nitrite and sweet spirits of niter. Epidemics and isolated episodes of intoxications have occurred when sodium nitrite was mistaken for sodium chloride in the preparation of food or when nitrite salts were used overzealously in the treatment of meat products (Aquanno *et al.*, 1981, Bakshi *et al.*, 1967; Buch, 1952; Greenberg *et al.*, 1945; McQuiston, 1936; Padberg and Martin, 1939; Singley, 1962; Tepperman *et al.*, 1951; Thwailes, 1956). The use of nitrates and nitrites in cured meats has its roots in antiquity (Binkerd and Kolari, 1975). Most reports of human nitrate poisoning, however, concern infants fed well water contaminated with nitrites (see below). Nitrite is of some environmental concern because of its propensity to react with some amines to generate carcinogenic nitrosamines (Wolff and Wasserman, 1972).

Toxicology of inorganic nitrite salts: The two basic actions of sodium nitrite *in vivo* are the relaxation of smooth muscle, especially of small blood vessels, and in toxic doses the conversion of hemoglobin to methemoglobin. The same dual toxicity is shared by many inorganic and organic nitrates and nitrites, but the high molecular weight aliphatic compounds such as nitroglycerin (see below) are generally much more potent in producing vascular collapse than in generating methemoglobin. By contrast, some aromatic nitro (and amino) compounds are powerful methemoglobin formers but not directly acting vasodilators (see ANILINE, p. III-31). Other aromatic nitro compounds appear to have neither action (*e.g.*, dinitrophenol, p. III-156).

In most cases (but see below) sodium nitrite must be swallowed (or injected) to produce poisoning. Its fate in the body is not well known, but it disappears rapidly, and in some species its effects outlast the detectable presence of nitrite in the blood (Sinclair and Jones, 1967). In rats it crosses the placental barrier to generate methemoglobin in the fetus (Gruener et al., 1973). Although tolerance to the vascular effects of nitrites is well known, little tolerance develops to methemoglobin formation (Diven et al., 1964). Cumulative toxic effects are not well characterized (Druckrey et al., 1963; Musil, 1966). In contrast to some methemoglobin formers, small doses of sodium nitrite in man fail to accelerate erythrocyte destruction (Beutler and Mikus, 1961).

Several fatal cases of acute sodium nitrite poisoning can be cited (Barton, 1954; Greenburg et al., 1945; Manley, 1945; McQuiston, 1936; Naidue and Rao, 1936; Padberg and Martin, 1939; Palmer, 1933; Singley, 1962). A 17-month-old child died after 450 mg. (32 mg./kg.) of sodium nitrite given intravenously in the mistaken impression of acute cyanide poisoning (Berlin, 1970). Most cases, however, have occurred under circumstances that make estimation of the dose difficult if not impossible. The ingestion of 130 mg. produced a severe poisoning in a 2-month-old infant (Oppé, 1951), but the oral mean lethal dose for adults is probably about 1 gm., if administered at one time.

In an unusual industrial accident three workmen were sprayed with a molten mixture of sodium and potassium nitrates, producing extensive burns over 30 to 70% of their body surfaces. One man died with 65% methemoglobin whereas the other two, with 56 and 42% methemoglobin, respectively, were treated successfully with methylene blue and exchange transfusions (Harris et al., 1979). Although this methemoglobinemia was ascribed to absorption of nitrate, its fulminating character suggests that it was due to nitrite, which can be generated from nitrates by extremely high temperatures.

Signs and symptoms of nitrite poisoning include intense cyanosis, nausea, vertigo, vomiting, collapse, spasms of abdominal pain, tachycardia, tachypnea, coma, convulsions and death (Bakshi et al., 1967; Barton, 1954; Greenberg et al., 1945; McQuiston, 1936; Oppé, 1951). Injection and inflammation of gastric and intestinal mucosa are described at autopsy (Barton, 1954; McQuiston, 1936).

Although the reaction of nitrite ion with hemoglobin has been studied for many years (e.g., Kiese, 1966; Smith and Olson, 1973), no clear picture of the precise mechanism involved has yet emerged. The red cells of patients with malignant disease and pregnant women are said to be especially sensitive to nitrite (Metcalf, 1961). Human red cells deficient in glucose-6-phosphate dehydrogenase are also more sensitive to the methemoglobin-generating activities of nitrite than normal red cells (Calabrese et al., 1980), but nitrite does not trigger a Heinz body

hemolytic anemia in such cells as do many other drugs and chemicals (e.g., naphthalene, p. III-307).

As evaluated in laboratory rodents, a nitrite-generated methemoglobinemia differs in several respects from that produced by other chemicals. The onset of the methemoglobinemia is delayed, and circulating levels are uniquely sustained (Smith et al., 1967). Nitrite may inhibit methemoglobin reductase activity in mouse red cells (Kruszyna et al., 1982). Free nitrite ion can form a weak complex with ferric heme groups (Smith, 1967b). Thus a reaction mixture of nitrite and hemoglobin may contain oxyhemoglobin, methemoglobin and the nitrite-methemoglobin complex. Nitrite also appears to inhibit transiently the hepatic microsomal mixed function oxidase system (Friedman and Sawyer, 1974), although the physiological significance of the effect for oxidative drug metabolism is questionable (Kohl et al., 1978).

Given appropriate therapy, victims of nitrite poisoning have survived even though 75 to 78% of the circulating blood pigment was in the form of methemoglobin (Tepperman et al., 1951). Probably the least effective approach to the management of an overwhelming methemoglobinemia is the administration of ascorbic acid (Bolyai et al., 1972; Carnick et al., 1946; Gibson, 1943). Exchange transfusion has been used successfully, at least once in nitrite-methemoglobinemia (Kirby, 1955), but methylene blue has been widely employed with almost universal success. It acts promptly to accelerate methemoglobin reduction, and in appropriate doses a clearing of cyanosis and clinical improvement should occur in 1 to 2 hours.

This rapid therapeutic response to methylene blue suggests that the methemoglobinemia induced by sodium nitrite is responsible for the major signs and symptoms of intoxication. For a more complete discussion of the use of methylene blue in methemoglobinemia, see ANILINE, p. III-33. Oxygen at 4 atmospheres significantly decreased mortality and methemoglobin levels in rats after nitrite (Goldstein and Doull, 1971). Methylene blue and hyperbaric oxygen had additive effects in protecting mice against death by nitrite (Sheehy and Way, 1974).

Whatever the source of nitrite, the syncope or shock induced by large doses is due initially to the pooling of blood in dilated postarteriolar vessels, notably venules and even large veins (Wilkins et al., 1937). Doses that produce no symptoms or only slight circulatory changes in man when in the supine position can induce syncope when the victim is upright (Weiss et al., 1937). This vasodilation is not blocked by atropine or by any recognized drug. Epinephrine, whose principal vascular action is the constriction of arterioles, is ineffective and perhaps dangerous here (Wilkins et al., 1938), as is pitressin, whose chief effects are exerted on the coronary bed (Stead et al., 1939). Probably epinephrine and related compounds should be strictly prohibited; they intensify the arteriolar constriction that is generated by spontaneous reflexes in the nitrite-poisoned patient, with the result that tissue blood flow is further compromised.

Reflex tachycardia is the rule, but a vagovagal reflex may induce transient bradycardia just before complete collapse (Wilkins et al., 1937). Eventually this shocklike state is complicated by oxygen lack which arises from circulatory inadequacy (stagnant anoxia) and from a reduction in the oxygen-carrying capacity of the blood due to methemoglobin formation, of which the latter is more important (Asbury and Rhoad, 1964).

Nitrite is secreted in saliva in normal subjects and into gastric juice, particularly in achlorhydric subjects. Bacteria capable of reducing nitrate to nitrite and of catalyzing nitrosamine formation especially in the presence of thiocyanate can survive in neutral gastric juice (Ruddell et al., 1976; Walters et al., 1979). Most intestinal and urinary nitrate is believed to have a dietary origin, but mammals, including the germ-free rat, produce some metabolic nitrate, presumably from organic nitrogenous substrates (Witter et al., 1981).

Reduction of nitrate salts to nitrite: Nitrite intoxication is encountered most frequently among neonates who consume water contaminated with nitrates. Nitrate as such does not produce methemoglobinemia. Indeed sodium and potassium nitrates are for the most part rapidly absorbed and excreted unchanged, causing few reactions other than diuresis and perhaps catharsis (Melville, 1965). Under some circumstances, however, appreciable amounts of nitrate are converted to nitrite.

In 1940, Schwartz and Rector reported a case of severe (57%) methemoglobinemia in a 2-week-old infant. The etiology of this disorder was unrecognized at the time, but in 1945 Comly reported two similar cases and made reference to many unpublished incidents. The syndrome initially suggested congenital heart disease, but spectroscopic tests revealed profound methemoglobinemia. A common history in these cases was residence in a rural area where the home water supply was a well. Comly (1945) found these waters to be heavily contaminated with nitrates and coliform bacteria. Similar cases (Ferrant, 1946; Faucett and Miller, 1946) emphasized that the reaction is peculiar to the neonate, i.e., other members of the family were not affected. Cornblath and Hartmann (1948) found that sensitive neonates had gastric pH values above 4. Thus ingested bacteria may escape destruction in the stomach and proliferate in the upper gastrointestinal tract. Many strains of bacteria are known that avidly reduce nitrate to nitrite.

Municipal water supplies which contained nitrate in sufficient concentrations to induce the reaction were never implicated (Anon., 1950), presumably because they were free of gross bacterial contamination. Additional reports confirmed that this syndrome was limited to the first 3 months of life. Furthermore, the observed delay in the appearance of the reaction supports the concept that an appropriate intestinal flora has to be established to convert dietary nitrate to nitrite (Bucklin and Myint, 1960; Carlisle, 1950; Downs, 1950; Fawns and Aldridge, 1954; Goluboff and Wheaton, 1961; Lecks, 1950; Miller, 1971; Rosenfield and Huston, 1950; Walliker and Baxter, 1949; Wood, 1949).

The relative importance of additional factors that may also predispose the neonate to nitrate methemoglobinemia remains to be established. A high incidence of dyspepsia in susceptible infants has been noted and may be linked to alterations in gastrointestinal flora (Lachhein et al., 1960). High circulating levels of fetal hemoglobin may contribute to the severity of the reaction (Busing, 1961). Infants may consume larger amount of nitrate relative to total hemoglobin than do adults (Thal et al., 1961). Knotek and Schmidt (1964) traced many of their cases to *Bacillus subtilis* spores which contaminated dried milk formulas rather than well water, and Simon et al. (1964) noted that infants fed acidified (lactic and citric acid) dried milk preparations failed to develop the syndrome. The neonate has an immature methemoglobin reductase system (Busing, 1961). Detailed biochemical and pathologic studies, however, have failed to reveal any important distinctions between methemoglobinemia from well water and that from nitrite intoxication (Werner et al., 1965; Wuttke, 1965).

Perhaps the above discussion also has relevance to the occasional reports of severe and even fatal methemoglobinemia following the use of bismuth subnitrate as an antidiarrheal agent (Miller, 1945; Roe, 1933; Wallace 1947) and silver nitrate treatment of burns (Ternberg and Luce, 1968). In the latter case the burn surface is probably the source of bacterial contamination and the injured area permits systemic absorption of nitrite. Nitrates are found in high concentrations in many foods (Fassett, 1966a), but only nitrate-rich, unprocessed spinach has been involved in frank poisonings. Spinach possesses enzyme systems for nitrate reduction (Hölscher and Natzschka, 1964; Phillips, 1971).

Toxicology of organic nitrites and nitrates: Simple aliphatic nitrites such as ethyl nitrite, butyl nitrite, isobutyl nitrite and amyl nitrite are volatile liquids that are readily absorbed from the lungs. They appear to be weak methemoglobin-generating agents when inhaled, but at least ethyl nitrite and butyl nitrite cause profound methemoglobinemia when ingested (see also Section II). Nitroglycerin is absorbed when placed on the skin (Schwartz, 1946) or swallowed, but a prompt and potent vasodilator action is best obtained by absorption through the oral or buccal mucosa.

High molecular weight aliphatic organic nitrites (octyl nitrite) and nitrates (glyceryl trinitrate, pentaerythritol tetranitrate, triethanolamine trinitrate) are used as coronary vasodilators, and intoxications are characterized by cardiovascular and central nervous reactions. In general these compounds are not methemoglobin formers in man (Matsumoto et al., 1961; von Oettingen, 1946b). The metabolism of nitroglycerin (glyceryl trinitrate) is poorly understood, but the molecule can be partially denitrated enzymatically in the liver (Needleman et al., 1969). Its biological effects appear to outlast its detectable presence in blood (Crandell et al., 1929). Tolerance and cross tolerance among this group of compounds are well known (Crandell et al., 1931), and wide variations in sensitivity are recognized among individuals not previously exposed to these agents (Leuth and Hanks, 1938). The lethal dose of nitroglycerin has been estimated as 200 mg. but 1200 mg. have been tolerated with only slight effects (Rabinowitch, 1944) and a dose of 24 mg. has produced a severe intoxication (see below).

Nervous signs and symptoms are common in poisoning due to organic nitrates. To what extent these effects are due to elevated intracranial pressure and to cerebral anoxia rising from circulatory collapse is not established, but noncirculatory causes have not been ruled out.

An unusual intoxication was seen by one of us (R.E.G.) in consultation (unpublished observations). In a suicidal gesture an obese 47-year-old woman ingested 24 mg. nitroglycerin (60 therapeutic doses) without vomiting. When seen at the hospital emergency room 15 minutes later, she was convulsing and semicomatose without cyanosis. The systolic blood pressure was moderately elevated (150/80), and the pulse was fast (104). The respiratory rate of 24 increased gradually over several hours to a level of 120 per minute. Breathing finally became Cheyne-Stokes in character. Convulsions subsided promptly, perhaps because of the intramuscular administration of amobarbital (only 40 mg.), and consciousness was regained in 3 to 4 hours. At this time, however, she became apneic and was placed in a respirator. With the restoration of spontaneous breathing hyperventilation re-

turned. About 7 hours after the ingestion the more common symptoms of numbness, tingling, excitement, headache and flushing were noted. Recovery was eventually complete.

Symptomatology:
1. A prompt fall in blood pressure.
2. A roaring sound in the ears, a headache which is persistent and throbbing, with associated vertigo, a generalized tingling sensation, palpitations, and visual disturbances.
3. The skin is flushed and perspiring, later cold and cyanotic.
4. Nausea and vomiting. The ingestion of nitrites may also cause colic and diarrhea.
5. Syncope, especially when attempting to stand upright.
6. Methemoglobinemia, with attendant cyanosis and anoxia.
7. Hyperpnea; later dyspnea and slow breathing.
8. The pulse may be slow, dicrotic, and intermittent.
9. Increased intraocular tension and intracranial pressure.
10. Collapse and coma, followed by clonic convulsions.
11. Death due to circulatory collapse.

Treatment:
1. Keep patient recumbent in a shock position and comfortably warm. Passive movements of the extremities may aid venous return.
2. Gastric lavage with tap water or perhaps with a 1:5000 solution of potassium permanganate (if the nitrite was taken orally).
3. Administer oxygen (p. IV-12) and artificial ventilation if necessary (p. IV-7). Hyperbaric oxygen decreases both mortality and methemoglobin levels in animals given sodium nitrite. Its efficacy is not established in poisonings due to organic nitrates and nitrites.
4. Methylene blue (1% solution) in a dose of 1 to 2 mg./kg. intravenously, or 5 mg./kg. orally in less severe cases of methemoglobinemia.
5. Transfusion with whole blood or plasma expanders (p. IV-17). Avoid epinephrine and other vasoconstrictor drugs.

Laboratory: Simple spectrophotometric methods for the determination of methemoglobin and oxyhemoglobin even in the presence of methylene blue are available and can be used to monitor levels well below that at which cyanosis is clinically evident (Smith, 1971). By customary tests in a clinical laboratory (e.g., the formation of acid hematin or cyanomethemoglobin), the blood "hemoglobin" level is typically normal, whereas the blood oxygen-carrying capacity is measurably low (in the absence of effective treatment). The difference is a sensitive and practical index of methemoglobinemia in nitrite poisoning.

References:

Anon. (Editorial) Nitrates in well water and methemoglobin-emia in infants. Am. J. Public Health 40:866-867, 1950.

Aquanno, J. J.; Chan, K. M.; Dietzler, D. N. Accidental poisoning of two laboratory technologists with sodium nitrite. Clin. Chem. 27:1145-1146, 1981.

Asbury, A. C.; Rhode, E. A. Nitrite intoxication in cattle: The effects of lethal doses of nitrite on blood pressure. Am. J. Vet. Res. 25:1010-1013, 1964.

Bakshi, S. P.; Fahey, J. L.; Pierce, L. E. Sausage cyanosis - acquired methemoglobinemic nitrite poisoning. N. Engl. J. Med. 277:1072, 1967.

Barton, G. M. G. A fatal case of sodium nitrite poisoning. Lancet 1:190-191, 1954.

Berlin, C. M., Jr. The treatment of cyanide poisoning in children. Pediatrics 46:793-796, 1970.

Beutler, E.; Mikus, B. J. The effect of sodium nitrite and para-aminopropiophenone administration on blood methemoglo-bin levels and red blood cell survival. Blood 18:455-467, 1961.

Binkerd, E. F.; Kolari, O. E. The history and use of nitrate and nitrite in the curing of meat. Fd. Cosmet. Toxicol. 13:655-661, 1975.

Bolyai, J. Z.; Smith, R. P.; Gray, C. T. Ascorbic acid and chemically induced methemoglobinemia. Toxicol. Appl. Pharmacol. 21:176-185, 1972.

Buch, O. Massenvergiftung durch Natriumnitrit. Arch. Toxi-kol. 14:53-55, 1952.

Bucklin, R.; Myint, M. K. Fatal methemoglobinemia due to well water nitrates. Ann. Intern. Med. 52:703-705, 1960.

Busing, K. -H. Trinkwasserbedingte Sauglings Methamoglo-binamie. Med. Klin. 56:177-181, 1961.

Calabrese, E. J.; Moore, G. S.; Ho, S. C. Low erythrocyte glucose-6-phosphate dehydrogenase (G-6-PD) activity and susceptibility to nitrite-induced methemoglobin formation. Bull. Environ. Contam. Toxicol. 25:837-840, 1980.

Carlisle, M. C. Well water methemoglobinemia; report of 2 cases. Tex. Med. 46:703-707, 1950.

Carnick, M.; Polis, B. D.; Klein, T. Methemoglobinemia. Treatment with ascorbic acid. Arch. Intern. Med. 78:296-302, 1946.

Comly, H. H. Cyanosis in infants caused by nitrates in well water. J. A. M. A. 129:112-116, 1945.

Cornblath, M.; Hartmann, A. F. Methemoglobinemia in young infants. J. Pediatr. 33:421-425, 1948.

Crandell, L. A.; Leake, C. D.; Lovenhart, A. S.; Muehlberger, C. W. The rate of elimination of glyceryl trinitrate from the blood stream after intravenous administration in dogs. J. Pharmacol. Exp. Ther. 37:283-296, 1929.

Crandell, L. A.; Leake, C. D.; Lovenhart, A. S.; Muehlberger, C. W. Acquired tolerance to and cross tolerance between the nitrous and nitric acid esters and sodium nitrite in man. J. Pharmacol. Exp. Ther. 41:103-119, 1931.

Diven, R. H.; Reed, R. E.; Pistor, W. J. The physiology of nitrite poisoning in sheep. Ann. N. Y. Acad. Sci. 111:Art 2, 638-643, 1964.

Downs, E. F. Cyanosis of infants caused by high nitrate concentrations in rural water supplies. Bull. WHO 3:165-169, 1950.

Druckrey, H.; Steinhoff, D.; Beuthner, H.; Schneider, H.; Klarner, P. Prufung von Nitrit auf chronisch toxische Wir-kung an Ratten. Arzneim. Forsch. 13:230-232, 1963.

Fassett, D. W. Nitrates and nitrites. In Intoxicants Occurring Naturally in Foods. NAS-NRC Publ. No. 1354 Wash., D. C., 1966a.

Faucett, R. L.; Miller, H. C. Methemoglobinemia occurring in infants fed milk diluted with well water of high nitrate content. J. Pediatr. 29:593-596, 1946.

Fawns, H. T.; Aldridge, A. G. V. Methaemoglobinaemia due to nitrates and nitrites in drinking water. Br. Med. J. 2:575-576, 1954.

Ferrant, M. Methemoglobinemia. Two cases in newborn in-fants caused by nitrates in well water. J. Pediatr. 29:583-592, 1946.

Friedman, M. A.; Sawyer, D. R. Inhibition of mouse-liver microsomal enzyme functions after oral administration of sodium nitrite. Food Cosmet. Toxicol. 12:195-200, 1974.

Gibson, Q. H. The reduction of methemoglobin by ascorbic acid. Biochem. J. 37:615-618, 1943.

Goldstein, G. M.; Doull, J. Treatment of nitrite-induced met-hemoglobinemia with hyperbaric oxygen. Proc. Soc. Exp. Biol. Med. 138:137-139, 1971.

Goluboff, N.; Wheaton, R. Methylene blue induced cyanosis and acute hemolytic anemia complicating the treatment of methemoglobinemia. J. Pediatr. 58:86-89, 1961.

Greenberg, M.; Birnkrant, W. B.; Schifter, J. J. Outbreak of sodium nitrite poisoning. Am. J. Public Health 35:1217-1220, 1945.

Gruener, N.; Shuval, H. I.; Behroozi, K.; Cohen, S.; Shechter, H. Methemoglobinemia induced by transplacental passage of nitrites in rats. Bull. Environ. Contam. Toxicol. 9:44-48, 1973.

Harris, J. C.; Rumack, B. H.; Peterson, R. G.; McGuire, B. M. Methemoglobinemia resulting from absorption of nitrates. J. A. M. A. 242:2869-2871, 1979.

Holscher, P.; Natzschka, J. Methemoglobin in young infants due to nitrite in spinach. Ger. Med. Mon. 9:325-327, 1964.

Kiese, M. The biochemical production of ferrihemoglobin-forming derivatives from aromatic amines, and mechanisms of ferrihemoglobin formation. Pharmacol. Rev. 18:1091-1161, 1966.

Kirby, N. G. Sodium nitrite poisoning treated by exchange transfusion. Lancet 1:594-595, 1955.

Knotek, Z.; Schmidt, P. Pathogenesis, incidence and possibil-ities of preventing alimentary nitrate methemoglobinemia in infants. Pediatrics 34:78-83, 1964.

Kohl, R.; Wulff, U.; Netter, K. J. Effect of nitrite on micro-somal cytochrome-P-450. Xenobiotica 8:359-364, 1978.

Kruszyna, R.; Kruszyna, H.; Smith, R. P. Comparison of hydroxylamine, 4-dimethylaminophenol and nitrite protec-tion against cyanide poisoning in mice. Arch. Toxicol. 49:191-202, 1982.

Lachhein, L.; Thal, W.; Harnack, O. Methamoglobinamien durch Brunnenwasser bei Sauglingen. Dtsch. Gesun-dheitsw. 15:2339-2343, 1960.

Lecks, H. J. Methemoglobinemia in infancy. Am. J. Dis. Child. 79:117-123, 1950.

Lueth, H. C.; Hanks, T. G. Unusual reaction of patients with hypertension to glyceryl trinitrate. Arch. Intern. Med. 62:97-108, 1938.

Manley, C. H. A fatal case of sodium nitrite poisoning. Analyst 70:50, 1945.

Matsumoto, H.; Hylin, J. W.; Miyahara, A. Methemoglobine-mia in rats injected with 3-nitropropanoic acid, nitrite, and nitroethane. Toxicol. Appl. Pharmacol. 3:493-499, 1961.

McQuiston, T. A. C. Fatal poisoning by sodium nitrite. Lancet 2:1153-1154, 1936.

Melville, K. I. Coronary vasodilators: The nitrites and other agents. In Drill's Pharmacology in Medicine, 3rd ed. (J. R. DiPalma, Ed.). McGraw Hill Book Co., New York, 1965.

Metcalf, W. K. A biochemical change in the blood in preg-nancy and malignant disease. Phys. Med. Biol. 5:259-269, 1961.

Miller, G. E. Bismuth subnitrate poisoning with methemoglo-binemia. Gastroenterology 4:430-434, 1945.

Miller, L. W. Methemoglobinemia associated with well water. J. A. M. A. 216:1642-1643, 1971.

Musil, J. Der Einfluss einer chronischen Natriumnitrit Intox-ikation auf Ratten. Acta Biol. Med. Ger. 16:388-394, 1966.

Naidue, S. R.; Rao, P. V. Case of nitrite poisoning. Br. Med. J. 1:1300, 1936.

Needleman, P.; Blehm, D. J.; Rotskoff, K. S. Relationship between glutathione-dependent denitration and the vasodilator effectiveness of organic nitrate. J. Pharmacol. Exp. Ther. 165:286-288, 1969.

Oppe, T. E. Methaemoglobinemia due to sodium nitrite. Lancet 1:1051, 1951.

Padberg, L. R.; Martin, T. Three fatal cases of nitrite poisoning. J. A. M. A. 113:1733, 1939.

Palmer, A. A. Fatal poisoning by sodium nitrite. Med. J. Aust. 2:113-114, 1933.

Phillips, W. E. J. Naturally occurring nitrite in foods in relation to infant methemoglobinemia. Food Cosmet. Toxicol. 9:219-223, 1971.

Rabinowitch, I. M. Acute nitroglycerine poisoning. Can. Med. Assoc. J. 50:199-202, 1944.

Roe, H. E. Methemoglobinemia following the administration of bismuth subnitrate. Report of a fatal case. J. A. M. A. 101:352-354, 1933.

Rosenfield, A. B.; Huston, R. Infant methemoglobinemia in Minnesota due to nitrates in well water. Minn. Med. 33:787-796, 1950.

Ruddell, W. S. J.; Bone, E. S.; Hill, M. J.; Blendis, L. M.; Walters, C. L. Gastric-juice nitrite. Lancet 2:1037-1040, 1976.

Schwartz, A. M. The cause, relief and prevention of headaches arising from contact with dynamite. N. Engl. J. Med. 235:541-544, 1946.

Schwartz, A. S.; Rector, E. J. Methemoglobinemia of unknown origin in a two week old infant. Am. J. Dis. Child. 60:652-659, 1940.

Sheehy, M. H.; Way, J. L. Nitrite intoxication: protection with methylene blue and oxygen. Toxicol. Appl. Pharmacol. 30:221-226, 1974.

Simon, C.; Manzke, H.; Kay, H.; Mrowetz, G. Uber Vorkommen, Pathogense und Moglichkeiten zur Prophylaxe der durch Nitrit verursachten Methamoglobinamie. Z. Kinderheilkd. 91:124-138, 1964.

Sinclair, K. B.; Jones, D. I. H. Nitrite toxicity in sheep. Res. Vet. Sci. 8:65-70, 1967.

Singley, T. L. III. Secondary methemoglobinemia due to the adulteration of fish with sodium nitrite. Ann. Intern. Med. 57:800-803, 1962.

Smith, R. P. The nitrite methemoglobin complex - its significance in methemoglobin analyses and its possible role in methemoglobinemia. Biochem. Pharmacol. 16:1655-1664, 1967b.

Smith, R. P. Spectrophotometric determination of methemoglobin and oxyhemoglobin in the presence of methylene blue. Clin. Toxicol. 4:273-285, 1971.

Smith, R. P.; Alkaitis, A. A.; Shafer, P. R. Chemically induced methemoglobinemias in the mouse. Biochem. Pharmacol. 16:317-328, 1967.

Smith, R. P.; Olson, M. V. Drug-induced methemoglobinemia. Semin. Hematol. 10:253-268, 1973.

Stead, E. A., Jr.; Kunkel, P.; Weiss, S. Effect of pitressin in circulatory collapse induced by sodium nitrite. J. Clin. Invest. 18:673-678, 1939.

Tepperman, J.; Marquardt, R.; Reifenstein, G. H.; Lozner, E. L. Methemoglobinemic cyanosis, report of an epidemic due to corning extract substituted for maple syrup. J. A. M. A. 146:923-925, 1951.

Ternberg, J. L.; Luce, E. Methemoglobinemia: A complication of the silver nitrate treatment of burns. Surgery 63:328-330, 1968.

Thal, W.; Lachhein, L.; Martinek, M. Welche Hamoglobinkonzentrationen sind bei Brunnenwasser-Methamoglobinamie noch mit den Leben vereinbar?. Arch. Toxikol. 19:25-33, 1961.

Thwailes, C. A case of methemoglobinemia due to sodium nitrite poisoning. Med. J. Aust. 2:185-186, 1956.

von Oettingen, W. F. Effects of aliphatic nitrous and nitric acid esters on the physiological functions with special reference to their chemical constitution. Natl. Insts. Health Bull. No. 186, 1946b.

Wallace, W. M. Methemoglobinemia in an infant as a result of the administration of bismuth subnitrite. J. A. M. A. 133:1280-1281, 1947.

Walliker, G. W.; Baxter, E. H. Methemoglobinemia. A cause of cyanosis in infants and children. Arch. Pediatr. 66:143-156, 1949.

Walters, C. L.; Carr, F. P. A.; Dyke, C. S.; Saxby, M. J.; Smith, P. L. R.; Walker, R. Nitrite sources and nitrosamine formation in vitro and in vivo. Fd. Cosmet. Toxicol. 17:473-479, 1979.

Weiss, S.; Wilkins, R. W.; Haynes, F. W. Nature of circulatory collapse induced by sodium nitrite. J. Clin. Invest. 16:73-84, 1937.

Werner, U.; Thal, W.; Wuttke, W. -D. Schwerste und letal verlaufene Methamoglobinamien durch nitrathaltigs Brunnenwasser bei jungen Sauglingen. Dtsch. Med. Wochenschr. 90:124-127, 1965.

Wilkins, R. W.; Haynes, F. W.; Weiss, S. Role of venous system in circulatory collapse induced by sodium nitrite. J. Clin. Invest. 16:85-91, 1937.

Wilkins, R. W.; Weiss, S.; Haynes, F. W. Effect of epinephrine in circulatory collapse induced by sodium nitrite. J. Clin. Invest. 17:41-51, 1938.

Witter, J. P.; Gatley, S. J.; Balish, E. Evaluation of nitrate synthesis by intestinal microrganisms in vivo. Science 213:449-450, 1981.

Wolff, I. A.; Wasserman, A. E. Nitrates, nitrites and nitrosamines. Science 177:15-19, 1972.

Wood, K. I. Well water methemoglobinemia. N. Y. State J. Med. 49:2576, 1949.

Wuttke, W. -D. Zur Morphologie der Brunnenwassermethamoglobinamie bei Sauglingen. Frankfurt Z. Pathol. 74:363-370, 1965.

NITROGEN OXIDES

Gaseous mixtures of the oxides of nitrogen, commonly called nitrous fumes, contain varying proportions of the following five oxides: nitrous oxide (N_2O), nitric oxide (NO), nitrogen trioxide (N_2O_3), nitrogen dioxide (NO_2, with its dimer N_2O_4), and nitrogen pentoxide (N_2O_5). Of these constituents, NO and NO_2 are the principal hazards. Nitric oxide, which is the principal oxide of nitrogen in smog, is a colorless gas that is slowly oxidized to nitrogen dioxide by oxygen in air under appropriate photochemical conditions (Sancier et al., 1962). Except for high concentrations of NO in the gases from electric arc welding

(Elkins, 1946), nitrogen dioxide is the chief constituent of nitrous fumes; it is a reddish-brown gas, which exists at low temperatures as the colorless tetroxide. The conversion of NO_2 to N_2O_4 is a rapid and reversible reaction, and the equilibrium depends only upon the temperature; at 35°C. the mixture consists of about 70% N_2O_4 and 30% NO_2 (McNally, 1942).

Numerous industrial and nonindustrial sources of nitrous fumes are recognized (von Oettingen, 1941a). The oxides are released in the reaction between nitric acid and any organic material; in the exhaust from metal cleaning processes; in the gases from electric arc welding; in electroplating, engraving, and photogravure operations; in dynamite blasting (Derrick and Johnson, 1943; Muller, 1969); in diesel engine exhaust; in the burning of some fabrics and of nitrocellulose, *e.g.*, nonsafety photographic and X-ray film (Terrill *et al.*, 1978); and in the combustion of some shoe polishes (LaFleche *et al.*, 1961). Perhaps the most important source, however, is the internal combustion engine (Guidotti, 1978).

In years past, isolated cases of severe symptoms and death of unknown etiology have been reported in farmers who were working in or near silos (LeRossignol, 1932; Schroeppel, 1953). It was recognized in 1956 that this syndrome ("silo-fillers' disease") resulted from an acute exposure to oxides of nitrogen (Lowery and Shuman, 1956). The mechanisms by which the toxic oxides are produced in silos and the similarity to industrial exposures have been established (Delaney *et al.*, 1956; Grayson, 1956). Assayed samples of silo gas contained 0 to 140 ppm NO, 8 to 360 ppm NO_2 and 0.2 to 9% CO_2 (Giddens *et al.*, 1970). In contrast to silo-fillers' disease, "farmers' lung" appears to be a nonspecific interstitial pulmonary reaction to dusts laden with fungi or their products (Studdert, 1953). The differential diagnosis between these two states is not difficult once either is suspected (Bringhurst *et al.*, 1959; Dickie and Rankin, 1958).

Nitrogen oxides are emphasized in this compilation chiefly because they typify a large number of irritant gases which produce acute pulmonary reactions when inhaled: *viz.*, chlorine (Cl_2), fluorine (F_2), bromine (Br_2), sulfur dioxide (SO_2), hydrogen chloride (HCl), hydrogen fluoride (HF), hydrogen sulfide (H_2S), ozone (O_3), phosgene ($COCl_2$), chloropicrin (CCl_2-NO_2), 1-chloro-1-nitroethane and -nitropropane, dichloronitroethane (Ethide), perfluoro-isobutylene, and ethylene oxide. Smoke inhalation may also have features in common with the inhalation of respiratory tract irritants (Webster *et al.*, 1967). These and many other gaseous irritants have been studied as potential chemical warfare agents. Some are important propellant fuels in rockets. Several are used currently as agricultural fumigants. Many are prominent constituents of air pollution (Amdur, 1962).

Toxicology: Of the five principal oxides of nitrogen, nitrous oxide (N_2O) is a mild anesthetic used in medicine and dentistry and is comparatively harmless. The principal target organ for the other oxides of nitrogen is the lung. With respect to the characteristic pulmonary lesion, nitric oxide is less dangerous than nitrogen dioxide. Little is known about the toxicology of nitrogen trioxide and of nitrogen pentoxide. Nitrogen dioxide, with its dimer N_2O_4, is the largest component of most fumes and causes most of the damage.

Only very high vapor concentrations induce prompt or immediate distress. Usually there are no symptoms at the time of exposure, except perhaps for a slight and transient cough, mild fatigue, and brief nausea. The acute danger period arises 5 to 72 hours later, when a slowly evolving but progressive inflammation of the lungs causes profuse exudation into the alveolar spaces (Tse and Bockman, 1970; von Oettingen, 1941a). Fluid loss from the blood produces massive pulmonary edema and severe hemoconcentration. Because of impaired gas exchange in the lungs, breathing becomes rapid and cyanosis becomes intense. Death is usually due to asphyxia within a few hours after respiratory symptoms begin (Lindquist, 1944; Nichols, 1930; Rignér and Swenson, 1961; Schiötz, 1945).

If the victim does not die during the initial phase of pulmonary edema and inflammation, signs and symptoms of pulmonary insufficiency may persist and even progress over periods of weeks and months; such persons may die within a few weeks from ventilatory insufficiency (Lowery and Schuman, 1956) or become permanently disabled because of their exertional dyspnea (Becklake *et al.*, 1957). This pattern, however, is not the common one. Most survivors appear to recover fully within a few days or a few weeks after the acute exposure (*e.g.*, Camiel and Berkhan, 1944). However, even if X-rays of the lungs indicate complete clearing (Milne, 1969; Tse and Bockman, 1970), only a cautious prognosis is warranted. Thus many patients have experienced a second acute pulmonary reaction 2 to 6 weeks after the first (Milne, 1969; Nichols, 1930; Tse and Bockman, 1970).

This relapse may arise abruptly and progress rapidly; associated signs and symptoms are cough, tachypnea, dyspnea, fever, tachycardia and cyanosis (Nichols, 1930; Tse and Bockman, 1970). The patient may be even more intensely ill during this relapse than during the initial reaction (McAdams and Krop, 1955; Milne, 1969), and deaths have occurred. Chest films during this period almost always show fine nodular infiltrates throughout all lung fields (Lowery and Schuman, 1956; Milne, 1969; Tse and Bockman, 1970), an appearance that has provoked a misdiagnosis of miliary tuberculosis. At postmortem examination the pathologic diagnosis is bronchiolitis obliterans (Lowery and Schuman, 1956; McAdams, 1955). Survivors recover slowly over periods of many months; they may or may not be left with chronic pulmonary dysfunction or with abnormal lung fields by X-ray (Milne, 1969; Tse and Bockman, 1970).

The relation between vapor concentration and duration of lethal exposure has been defined in laboratory animals (Gray et al., 1952, 1954a and b; LaTowsky et al., 1941; Tollman et al., 1941), but these data are seldom useful to the physician who has no convenient way of estimating the intensity of exposure except in terms of the clinical response. The typical reaction to nitrous fumes is delayed and insidious because nitrogen oxides are largely absorbed by and react with pulmonary alveolar structures and terminal respiratory bronchi. The upper respiratory tract is largely spared (Nichols, 1930), perhaps because these gases have a low solubility in aqueous media and because they are only slowly hydrolyzed.

This is not true of many irritant gases. For example, ammonia, formaldehyde, hydrochloric, sulfuric (Amdur et al., 1952a and b; Goldman and Hill, 1953), acetic (Amdur, 1961), and hydrofluoric acids are said to act mainly on the upper portions of the respiratory tract. Chlorine, fluorine, bromine, chloropicrin, dichloronitroethane, hydrogen sulfide, sulfur dioxide (Greenwald, 1954; Murray, 1946), acrolein, and ethylene oxide act on all portions. Nitrous fumes, phosgene, ozone, phosphorus trioxide, and phosphorus chlorides act chiefly on the alveolar walls (Sollmann, 1957). The deep response to toxic gases depends on whether the primary reaction is on the alveolar membrane or the pulmonary capillaries. Only capillary damage results in pulmonary edema (Gross et al., 1967).

Unlike nitrogen oxides, those irritant vapors that attack the mucosa of the upper respiratory tract (see above) usually give prompt and adequate warning. Irritation of mucous membranes results in conjunctivitis, rhinitis, pharyngitis, and bronchitis. High vapor concentrations cause immediate pain and choking, temporary reflex arrest of breathing (in expiration), spasmodic closure of the glottis, bronchoconstriction, reflex slowing of the heart, and prompt asphyxial syncope. Excessive spasm or edema of the glottis may be directly fatal. Asthmatic breathing and violent coughing may lead to disruptive emphysema, with the appearance of subcutaneous blebs of air in the neck.

Although some of the deep pulmonary irritants produce metabolic acidosis, as well as CO_2 retention (Gailitis et al., 1958), the alkali reserve of blood and tissues is not seriously depleted. In nonfatal cases convalescence is usually slow and often complicated by general asthenia, various respiratory infections, weak and irregular cardiac action, cardiac dilatation, recurrent asthmatic attacks, chronic bronchitis and bronchiolitis fibrosa obliterans, chronic pulmonary insufficiency, and rarely diffuse pulmonary fibrosis and emphysema (Becklake et al., 1957; Grayson, 1957; von Oettingen, 1941a; Leib et al., 1958; McAdams and Krop, 1955; Tse and Bockman,

1970). Persistent lung malfunction, however, is sufficiently uncommon to suggest that in some reported cases it was due to pre-existing chronic bronchitis (Ramirez and Dowell, 1971).

American astronauts on the Apollo-Soyuz mission were briefly exposed by accident to NO_2 during reentry into the Earth's atmosphere. In addition to clinical and X-ray findings indicative of diffuse pneumonitis, they had elevated urinary levels of hydroxylysine glycosides, suggestive of collagen breakdown in the pulmonary parenchyma (Hatten et al., 1977).

Forms of therapy: The treatment of pulmonary edema outlined below is appropriate after an exposure to any fume or vapor which is a primary lung irritant. Prednisone allegedly produced dramatic benefits in severe cases of silo-fillers' disease (Gailitis et al., 1958; Lowery and Shuman, 1956). Gailitis et al. (1958) emphasized that prolonged therapy may be required. A common therapeutic emergency similar in many respects to irritant gas inhalation is the aspiration of stomach contents into the lungs, an occasional complication of obstetric anesthesia (Mendelson, 1946). The intravenous administration of high doses of hydrocortisone has been successfully employed in such cases (Berris and Kasler, 1965; Dines et al., 1961; Hausmann and Lunt, 1955); similarly, intramuscular prednisone and other corticosteroids have been regarded as lifesaving (Lowery and Schuman, 1956; Tse and Bockman, 1970). However, similar claims about the benefits of steroid therapy in kerosene pneumonitis are no longer generally accepted (see p. III-223).

Absorption spectra characteristic of diene conjugation and typical of peroxidized polyenoic fatty acids can be found in rat lung lipids after animals are exposed to nitrogen dioxide. These peroxidative changes fit the time course of lung damage and can be partially blocked by pretreatment of the animals with large doses of α-tocopherol (Thomas et al., 1968). α-Tocopherol (vitamin E) deficiency intensified the suppression of glutathione peroxidase activity in the lungs and blood of mice exposed to NO_2, and vitamin E supplementation at least partially prevented that effect (Ayaz and Csallany, 1978). In combination with NO_2 exposure, vitamin E deficiency resulted in greater weight loss and decreased survival of mice (Csallany and Ayaz, 1978).

The simultaneous inhalation of compounds that furnish free sulfhydryl groups or compounds with disulfide bonds protects against the lethal effects of nitrogen dioxide and ozone (Fairchild et al., 1959). Perhaps in the early stages after exposure, a therapeutic trial with N-acetylcysteine (Mucomyst) by aerosolization or direct instillation is justified. The safety of this material is well established (see ACETAMIN-OPHEN, p. III-2).

Pretreatment with thiourea derivatives also affords protection but probably by a different mechanism since an interrelationship appears to exist between these gases and thyroid activity. Increased thyroid activity but not hypermetabolism *per se* increases the susceptibility of rodents to ozone and nitrogen dioxide (Fairchild and Graham, 1963). Many irritant gases produce an apparently nonspecific elevation of hepatic alkaline phosphatase activity (Murphy et al., 1964b). Changes in the oxygen consumption, lactic dehydrogenase and aldolase activities of various tissues have also been recognized (Buckley and Balchum, 1965).

Even with exposure levels below those associated with histologic damage, alterations in respiratory patterns are detectable. Nitrogen dioxide produces an increase in respiratory frequency (Freeman et al., 1966; Murphy et al., 1964a), and sulfur dioxide exposures result in increased pulmonary air flow resistance. The latter is ascribed to reflex bronchoconstriction (Frank, 1964); it can be prevented by atropine or complete cold block of the cervical vagosympathetic nerve (Nadel et al., 1965).

Systemic effects of absorbed nitrogen oxides: There can be little doubt that at least some oxides of nitrogen are absorbed to produce systemic effects. About 50 to 60% of an inhaled dose of NO_2 was retained by rhesus monkeys during quiet respiration. The gas was distributed throughout the lung and retained there for long periods after exposure, but part of the retained material was found in systemic blood (Goldstein et al., 1977). When young human adults were exposed to 1 or 2 ppm for 3 hours daily for 3 days, the following changes were noted in blood chemistry: a decrease in red cell membrane acetylcholine esterase activity, an increase in red cell peroxidized lipids, a decrease in red cell glucose-6-phosphate dehydrogenase, and decreases in total hemoglobin and hematocrit (Posin et al., 1978). Pretreatment with well-known microsomal enzyme inducing agents significantly prolonged the survival time of rats exposed to NO_2, but it was not clear whether this represented a hepatic or a pulmonary effect of the inducers (Sagai, 1978). Mice gavaged with solutions of morpholine and then exposed to NO_2 (0.2 to 50 ppm for 4 hours) showed time- and dose-dependent increases (up to 1,000-fold) in total body content of *N*-nitrosomorpholine (Iqbal et al., 1980).

It has long been known that nitric oxide (NO) reacts with hemoglobin in solution to form nitric oxide hemoglobin (NO-Hb, nitrosylhemoglobin). The NO binds to the same ferrous heme sites as oxygen and carbon monoxide (CO), but the af-finity of NO for these sites is 1,400 times greater than that of CO, which in turn is bound 250 times more tightly than oxygen. Moreover, NO affects the oxygen dissociation curve in the same manner as CO (see CARBON MONOXIDE, p. III-95), resulting in a greater compromise in oxygen transport than would be predicted on the basis of the loss in oxygen capacity alone (Kon et al., 1977). Because early reports (Sancier et al., 1962) failed to show any NO-Hb in the blood of animals exposed to NO, these *in vitro* binding studies were regarded as laboratory curiosities. With the demonstration that normal human blood contains 20 nanomoles of NO per ml., however, interest in NO-Hb has been renewed. The NO in blood was not related to smoking, and comparable levels were found in monkeys. Rats had lower levels as did one apparently unique human subject. Whether the NO is of environmental or endogenous origin is not yet known (Freemen et al., 1978).

More recent studies have shown that when mice were exposed to about 10 ppm NO for one hour, NO-Hb could be detected in blood by electron spin resonance. It reached a maximum concentration of 0.13% of the total hemoglobin within 20 minutes and remained at this steady state level. With termination of exposure NO-Hb disappeared from blood, with a half-life of several minutes. A dose-response relationship was shown between blood NO-Hb and ambient NO between 2 and 10 ppm. Rabbit blood behaved differently in that the NO-Hb spectrum was seen only after the addition of dithionite (Oda et al., 1975). When mice were exposed to mixtures of NO and CO, the same blood concentrations of NO-Hb and CO-Hb were generated as in exposures to the same partial pressures of each gas alone, indicating the absence of any interactions in binding (Oda et al., 1976). The blood levels of NO-Hb are far below predictions based on the *in vitro* binding affinity, by which an ambient concentration of only 0.4 ppm should have produced 50% saturation. Either NO is rapidly metabolized or it fails to reach hemoglobin *in vivo* or NO-Hb itself is rapidly metabolized (Oda et al., 1976).

Subsequent experiments with mice exposed to 40 ppm NO showed a peak NO-Hb level of 0.7%, but a 5% methemoglobinemia with a similar time course was also noted. The conversion of NO-Hb to methemoglobin has been studied *in vitro*: it requires the presence of molecular oxygen (Case et al., 1979). Exposure of mice to 40 ppm NO_2 generated 0.2% NO-Hb but no methemoglobin (Oda et al., 1980). Others, however, have reported methemoglobinemia in animals exposed to either NO or NO_2 (Case et al., 1979). A linear relationship exists between NO-Hb in blood and ambient concentrations of either NO or NO_2, but NO always generated higher levels than equivalent concentrations of NO_2 between 20 and 80 ppm. With 80 ppm NO (but not NO_2), methemoglobin levels in mice exceeded 15 percent (Oda *et al.*, 1980).

Mice exposed to 40 ppm NO_2 also had elevated concentrations of blood nitrite and even higher concentrations of nitrate (Oda *et al.*, 1981). Nitrite and nitrate are also postulated as products of the decomposition reaction of NO-Hb as generated by NO (Yoshida *et al.*, 1980).

The pathophysiological significance of low levels of NO-Hb is not yet known, but the consequences of severe methemoglobinemia are generally appreciated (see ANILINE and NITRITE, pp. III-31 and 314). Several reports have indicated that NO_2 can cause a significant methemoglobinemia (Cutlip, 1966; MacQuiddy *et al.*, 1941; Toothill, 1967). Three adults who died almost immediately after entering a silo presumably as a result of exposure to oxides of nitrogen had postmortem methemoglobin levels of 38 to 44% (Fleetham *et al.*, 1978).

Symptomatology:

1. Usually no symptoms occur at the time of exposure, with the exception of a slight cough and perhaps fatigue and nausea. Exposure to low concentrations may result in impaired pulmonary defense mechanisms (macrophages, cilia) with complications as in no. 10 below.
2. Only very concentrated nitrous fumes produce prompt coughing, choking, headache, nausea, abdominal pain, and dyspnea (tightness and burning pain in the chest).
3. A symptom-free period follows exposure and lasts for 5 to 72 hours.
4. Fatigue, uneasiness, restlessness, cough, hyperpnea, and dyspnea appear insidiously, as the adult respiratory distress syndrome gradually develops.
5. Increasingly rapid and shallow respirations, cyanosis, mild or violent coughing with frothy expectoration, and physical signs of pulmonary edema (*e.g.*, rales and rhonchi). The vital capacity is rapidly reduced. A serous exudate may develop in the pleural cavity, but its volume is usually small.
6. Anxiety, mental confusion, lethargy, and finally loss of consciousness.
7. A weak, rapid pulse, dilated heart, venous congestion, intense cyanosis, and severe hemoconcentration. Circulatory collapse is secondary to anoxia and hemoconcentration.
8. An asphyxial death due to blockade of gas exchange in the lungs. Death commonly occurs within a few hours after the first evidence of pulmonary edema.
9. Sometimes a second acute phase follows the initial pulmonary reaction after a quiescent period of several weeks. Cough, tachypnea, dyspnea, fever, tachycardia and cyanosis at this stage are usually due to bronchiolitis obliterans. The relapse may be abrupt and fulminating, leading either to death or a slow convalescence.
10. In nonfatal cases, convalescence may be complicated by infectious bronchitis, bronchiolitis obliterans, pneumonia and general asthenia. Rarely diffuse pulmonary fibrosis may develop.

Treatment:

1. Terminate the exposure immediately. If encountered shortly after exposure, instruct the patient to breathe deeply.
2. Enforce *complete* rest (bed or chair) for 24 to 48 hours, whether toxic signs and symptoms are recognized or not. Keep the victim comfortably warm.
3. During the presymptomatic period the inhalation of a sodium bicarbonate-sodium chloride aerosol has been suggested as a prophylactic measure (Grayson, 1957). Its effectivenss has not been demonstrated. Clinical trials with antioxidants appear to be warranted. Vitamin E in the form of α- or mixed tocopherols can be given by mouth in doses of several hundred milligrams. *N*-Acetylcysteine (Mucomyst) by aerosolization or direct instillation in accord with the manufacturer's recommendations may be worthwhile.
4. As soon as the victim begins to cough, has difficulty breathing, or feels slightly fatigued, start oxygen therapy (Fleming, 1943). Pure oxygen should be administered by any method which ensures high inspiratory concentrations. Nasal prongs are usually tried first. If oxygenation is inadequate, use oxygen with continuous distending airway pressure (pp. IV-12–15). Hyperbaric oxygen (1.8 atmospheres) increased the incidence of pulmonary edema when given together with NO_2 to dogs (Shechter *et al.*, 1975).
5. The removal of frothy exudate from the respiratory tract is a major therapeutic problem. Suctioning, postural drainage, and other measures are discussed on pp. IV-15–16.
6. Bronchospasm is corrected by the inhalation of aerosols of albuterol, isoetharine, metaproterenol, or terbutaline (p. IV-15).
7. Most drugs are ineffective and possibly harmful; in this category are atropine, epinephrine, expectorants, emetics, sedative

drugs (except for small doses of morphine), and usually cardiac glycosides. In a few instances rapid digitalization with a drug like ouabain may be advisable.

8. Cardiovascular collapse is strictly secondary to anoxia and to hemoconcentration. Venesection and replacement of blood by isotonic saline are regarded as useful measures in some clinics and as dangerous procedures in others. Venesection should certainly be avoided once circulatory collapse has become established. The use of rotating tourniquets (as described on p. IV-23) may be beneficial during the stage of intense venous congestion.

9. An emergency tracheostomy under local anesthesia (p. IV-6) may make it possible to remove foam more efficiently by a suctioning catheter, but usually complicates the administration of oxygen.

10. Artificial ventilation may become necessary, but unless airway obstruction can be corrected, it is seldom effective. Ventilatory assistance by intermittent positive pressure is described on pp. IV-7–12.

11. In the presence of a severe, confirmed methemoglobinemia a cautious trial with methylene blue (p. III-34) may be justified. The safety and efficacy of this procedure have not been established in man or animals poisoned with nitrogen oxides.

12. Give penicillin and/or other antibiotics in large doses as soon as evidence of a respiratory infection appears. See pp. IV-85–86.

13. Steroid therapy has been recommended to minimize the inflammatory reaction and to prevent pulmonary and bronchiolar fibrosis, but many disagree. Prednisone has been given to exposed adults in amounts of 30 to 80 mg. daily in divided doses. How long to continue steroid therapy is a difficult question.

14. Patients should be closely observed for at least 6 weeks. Relapses are described.

Laboratory:

1. Methemoglobinemia may be detected by comparing the oxygen-carrying capacity of blood with the concentration of hemoglobin measured by the color of acid hematin. Methemoglobinemia sometimes results from inhalation of nitrogen oxides, but few quantitative estimations have been reported in clinical poisonings. More data are highly desirable.

2. In addition to CO_2 retention, a mild metabolic acidosis may be detectable. It seldom warrants specific treatment.

3. Various methods have been devised for sampling and analyzing air samples for nitrogen oxides, but they are seldom available to the nonindustrial physician.

References:

Amdur, M. O. The respiratory response of guinea pigs to the inhalation of acetic acid vapor. Am. Ind. Hyg. Assoc. J. 22:1-5, 1961.

Amdur, M. O. Air pollution and human health - acute biologic effects. N. Engl. J. Med. 266:348-349, 1962.

Amdur, M. O.; Schulze, R. Z.; Drinker, P. Toxicity of sulfuric acid mist to guinea pigs. Arch. Ind. Hyg. Occup. Med. 5:318-329, 1952a.

Amdur, M. O.; Silverman, L.; Drinker, P. Inhalation of sulfuric acid mist by human subjects. Arch. Ind. Hyg. Occup. Med. 6:305-313, 1952b.

Ayaz, K. L.; Csallany, A. S. Long-term NO_2 exposure of mice in the presence and absence of Vitamin E. II. Effect on glutathione peroxidase. Arch. Environ. Health 33:285-296, 1978.

Becklake, M. R.; Goldman, H. I.; Bosman, A. R.; Freed, C. C. The long-term effects of exposure to nitrous fumes. Am. Rev. Resp. Dis. 76:398-409, 1957.

Berris, B.; Kasler, D. Pulmonary aspiration of gastric acid - Mendelson's syndrome. Can. Med. Assoc. J. 92:905-907, 1965.

Bringhurst, L. S.; Byrne, R. N.; Gershon-Cohen, J. Respiratory disease of mushroom workers, farmers' lung. J. A. M. A. 171:15-18, 1959.

Buckley, R. D.; Balchum, O. J. Acute and chronic exposures to nitrogen dioxide. Arch. Environ. Health 10:220-223, 1965.

Camiel, N. R.; Berkhan, H. S. Inhalation pneumonia from nitric fumes. Radiology 42:175-182, 1944.

Case, G. D.; Dixon, J. S.; Schooley, J. C. Interactions of blood metalloproteins with nitrogen oxides and oxidant air pollutants. Environ. Res. 20:43-65, 1979.

Csallany, A. S.; Ayaz, K. L. Long-term NO_2 exposure of mice in the presence and absence of vitamin E. I. Effect on body weights and lipofuscin pigments. Arch. Environ. Health 33:285-291, 1978.

Cutlip, R. C. Experimental nitrogen dioxide poisoning in cattle. Pathol. Vet. 3:474-485, 1966.

Delaney, L. T., Jr.; Schmidt, H. W.; Stroebel, C. F. Silo-fillers' disease. Mayo Clin. Proc. 31:189-198, 1956.

Derrick, E. H.; Johnson, D. W. Three cases of poisoning by irrespirable gases. Med. J. Aust. 2:355-358, 1943.

Dickie, H. A.; Rankin, J. Farmers' lung, an acute granulomatous interstitial pneumonitis occurring in agricultural workers. J. A. M. A. 167:1069-1076, 1958.

Dines, D. E.; Baker, N. G.; Scantland, W. A. Aspiration pneumonitis - Mendelson's syndrome. J. A. M. A. 176:229-231, 1961.

Elkins, H. B. Nitrogen dioxide - rate of oxidation of nitric oxide and its bearing on the nitrogen dioxide content of electric arch fumes. J. Ind. Hyg. Toxicol. 28:37-41, 1946.

Fairchild, E. J., II; Graham, S. L. Thyroid influence on the toxicity of respiratory irritant gases, ozone and nitrogen dioxide. J. Pharmacol. Exp. Ther. 139:177-184, 1963.

Fairchild, E. J., II; Murphy, S. D.; Stokinger, H. E. Protection by sulfur compounds against the air pollutants ozone and nitrogen dioxide. Science 130:861-862, 1959.

Fleetham, J. A.; Tunnicliffe, B. W.; Munt, P. W. Methemoglobinemia and the oxides of nitrogen. N. Engl. J. Med. 298:1150, 1978.

Fleming, A. J. A method for handling cases gassed with nitrous fumes. Ind. Med. Surg. 12:127-131, 1943.

Frank, N. R. Studies on the effects of acute exposure to sulfur dioxide in human subjects. Proc. R. Soc. Med. 57:1029-1033, 1964.

Freeman, G.; Dyer, R. L.; Juhos, L. T.; St. John, G. A.; Anbar, M. Identification of nitric oxide (NO) in human blood. Arch. Environ. Health 33:19-23, 1978.

Freeman, G.; Furiosi, N. J.; Haydon, G. B. Effects of continuous exposure of 0. 8 ppm NO_2 on respiration of rats. Arch.

Environ. Health 13:454-456, 1966.

Gailitis, J.; Burns, L. E.; Nally, J. B. Silo-fillers' disease. Report of a case. N. Engl. J. Med. 258:543-544, 1958.

Giddens, W. E., Jr.; Whitehair, C. K.; Sleight, S. D. Nitrogen dioxide (silogas) poisoning in pigs. Am. J. Vet. Res. 31:1779-1786, 1970.

Goldman, A.; Hill, W. T. Chronic bronchopulmonary disease due to inhalation of sulfuric acid fumes. Arch. Ind. Hyg. Occup. Med. 8:205-211, 1953.

Goldstein, E.; Peek, N. F.; Parks, N. J.; Hines, H. H.; Steffey, E. P.; Tarkington, B. Fate and distribution of inhaled nitrogen dioxide in rhesus monkeys. Am. Rev. Respir. Dis. 115:403-412, 1977.

Gray, E. L.; Goldberg, S. B.; Patton, F. M. Toxicity of the oxides of nitrogen. III. Effect of chronic exposure to low concentrations of vapors from red fuming nitric acid. Arch. Ind. Hyg. Occup. Med. 10:423-425, 1954b.

Gray, E. L.; MacNamee, J. K.; Goldberg, S. B. Toxicity of NO_2 vapors at very low levels. Arch. Ind. Hyg. Occup. Med. 6:20-21, 1952.

Gray, E. L.; Patton, F. M.; Goldberg, S. B.; Kaplan, E. Toxicity of the oxides of nitrogen. II. Acute inhalation toxicity of nitrogen dioxide, red fuming nitric acid, and white fuming nitric acid. Arch. Ind. Hyg. Occup. Med. 10:418-422, 1954a.

Grayson, R. R. Silage gas poisoning. Nitrogen dioxide pneumonia, a new disease in agricultural workers. Ann. Intern. Med. 45:393-408, 1956.

Grayson, R. R. Nitrogen dioxide pneumonia. A recently discovered malady in silo-fillers. GP 16:90-99, 1957.

Greenwald, I. Effects of inhalation of low concentrations of sulfur dioxide upon man and other mammals. Arch. Ind. Hyg. Occup. Med. 10:455-475, 1954.

Gross, P.; Rinehart, W. E.; DeTreville, R. T. P. The pulmonary reactions to toxic gases. Am. Ind. Hyg. Assoc. J. 28:315-321, 1967.

Guidotti, T. L. The higher oxides of nitrogen: inhalation toxicology. Environ. Res. 15:443-472, 1978.

Hatten, D. V.; Leach, C. S.; Nicogossian, A. E.; Di Ferrante, H. Collagen breakdown and nitrogen dioxide inhalation. Arch. Environ. Health 32:33-36, 1977.

Hausmann, W.; Lunt, R. L. The problem of the treatment of peptic aspiration pneumonia following obstetric anaesthesia (Mendelson's syndrome). J. Obstet. Gynaecol. Br. Commonw. 62:509-512, 1955.

Iqbal, Z. M.; Dahl, K.; Epstein, S. S. Role of nitrogen dioxide in the biosynthesis of nitrosamines in mice. Science 207:1475-1477, 1980.

Kon, K.; Maeda, N.; Shiga, T. Effect of nitric oxide on the oxygen transport of human erythrocytes. J. Toxicol. Environ. Health 2:1109, 1977.

LaFleche, L. R.; Boiven, C.; Leonard, C. Nitrogen dioxide - a respiratory irritant. Can. Med. Assoc. J. 84:1438-1443, 1961.

LaTowsky, L. W.; MacQuiddy, E. L.; Tollman, J. P. Toxicology of oxides of nitrogen. I. Toxic concentrations. J. Ind. Hyg. Toxicol. 23:129-133, 1941.

Leib, G. M. P.; Davis, W. N.; Brown, T.; McQuiggan, M. Chronic pulmonary insufficiency secondary to silo-fillers' disease. Am. J. Med. 24:471-474, 1958.

LeRossignol, W. J. Irritants and gases affecting workers in silo. J. A. M. A. 98:2307, 1932.

Lindquist, T. Nitrous gas poisoning among welders using acetylene flame. Study of 16 cases including 4 deaths. Acta Med. Scand. 118:210-243, 1944.

Lowery, T.; Shuman, L. M. "Silo-fillers' disease" - a syndrome caused by nitrogen dioxide. J. A. M. A. 162:153-160, 1956.

MacQuiddy, E. L.; LaTowsky, L. W.; Tollman, J. P.; Finlayson, A. I. Toxicology of oxides of nitrogen. II. Physiological effects and symptomatology. J. Ind. Hyg. Toxicol. 23:134-139, 1941.

McAdams, A. J., Jr. Bronchiolitis obliterans. Am. J. Med. 19:314-322, 1955.

McAdams, A. J.; Krop, S. Injury and death from red fuming nitric acid. J. A. M. A. 158:1022-1024, 1955.

McNally, W. D. Nitric oxide fumes. Ind. Med. Surg. 11:207-210, 1942.

Mendelson, C. L. The aspiration of stomach contents into the lungs during obstetric anesthesia. Am. J. Obstet. Gynecol. 52:191-205, 1946.

Milne, J. E. H. Nitrogen dioxide inhalation and bronchiolitis obliterans. A review of the literature and report of a case. J. Occup. Med. 11:538-547, 1969.

Muller, B. L. Nitrogen dioxide intoxication after a mining accident. Respiration 26:249-261, 1969.

Murphy, S. D.; Davis, H. V.; Zaratzian, V. L. Biochemical effects in rats from irritating air contaminants. Toxicol. Appl. Pharmacol. 6:520-528, 1964b.

Murphy, S. D.; Ulrich, C. E.; Frankowitz, S. H.; Xintaras, C. Altered function in animals inhaling low concentrations of ozone and nitrogen dioxide. Am. Ind. Hyg. Assoc. J. 25:246-253, 1964a.

Murray, W. A. Bronchiostenosis and atelectasis from sulfur dioxide. Can. Med. Assoc. J. 54:599-600, 1946.

Nadel, J. A.; Salem, H.; Tamplin, B.; Tokiwa, Y. Mechanism of bronchoconstriction during inhalation of sulfur dioxide. J. Appl. Physiol. 20:164-167, 1965.

Nichols, B. H. The clinical effects of the inhalation of nitrogen dioxide. Am. J. Roentgenol. Radium Ther. Nucl. Med. 23:516-520, 1930.

Oda, H.; Kusumoto, S.; Nakajima, T. Nitrosyl-hemoglobin formation in the blood of animals exposed to nitric oxide. Arch. Environ. Health 30:453-456, 1975.

Oda, H.; Nogami, H.; Kusumoto, S.; Nakajima, T. Nitrosylhemoglobin and carboxyhemoglobin in blood of mice simultaneously exposed to nitric oxide and carbon monoxide. Bull. Environ. Contam. Toxicol. 16:582-587, 1976.

Oda, H.; Nogami, H.; Nakajima, T. Reaction of hemoglobin with nitric oxide and nitrogen dioxide in mice. J. Toxicol. Environ. Health 6:673-678, 1980.

Oda, H.; Tsubone, H.; Suzuki, A.; Ichinose, T. Alterations of nitrite and nitrate concentrations in the blood of mice exposed to nitrogen dioxide. Environ. Res. 25:294-301, 1981.

Posin, C.; Clark, K.; Jones, M. P.; Patterson, J. V.; Buckley, R. T.; Hackney, J. D. Nitrogen dioxide inhalation and human blood biochemistry. Arch. Environ. Health 33:318-324, 1978.

Ramirez, J.; Dowell, A. R. Silo-filler disease; nitrogen dioxide-induced lung injury. Ann. Intern. Med. 74:569-576, 1971.

Rigner, K.; Swenson, A. The late prognosis of nitrous fume poisoning, a follow-up study. Acta Med. Scand. 170:291-299, 1961.

Sagai, M. The effect of enzyme-inducing agents in the survival times of rats exposed to lethal levels of nitrogen dioxide. Toxicol. Appl. Pharmacol. 43:169-174, 1978.

Sancier, K. M.; Freeman, G.; Mills, J. S. Electron spin resonance of nitric oxide-hemoglobin complexes in solution. Science 137:752-754, 1962.

Schiotz, E. H. Welding regarded from the medical point of view. Acta Med. Scand. 121:537-552, 1945.

Schroeppel, J. E. Death in a silo. J. A. M. A. 153:893, 1953.

Shechter, Y.; Pelled, B.; Alroy, G.; Lightig, C.; Tirosh, M. Deleterious effects of hyperbaric oxygen treatment on mortality and pathological changes in nitrogen dioxide-poisoned dogs. Respiration 32:210-216, 1975.

Sollmann, T. A Manual of Pharmacology. 8th Ed., W. B. Saunders Co., Philadelphia, 1957.

Studdert, T. C. Farmers' lung. Br. Med. J. 1:1305-1309, 1953.

Terrill, J. B.; Montgomery, R. R.; Reinhardt, C. F. Toxic gases from fires. Science 200:1343-1347, 1978.

Thomas, H. V.; Mueller, P. K.; Lyman, R. L. Lipoperoxidation of lung lipids in rats exposed to nitrogen dioxide. Science 159:532-534, 1968.

Tollman, J. P.; LaTowsky, L. W.; MacQuiddy, E. L.; Schonberger, S. Toxicology of the oxides of nitrogen. III. Gross and histological pathology. J. Ind. Hyg. Toxicol. 23:141-147, 1941.

Toothill, C. The chemistry of the in vivo reaction between haemoglobin and various oxides of nitrogen. Br. J. Anaesth. 39:405-412, 1967.

Tse, R. L.; Bockman, A. A. Nitrogen dioxide toxicity; report of four cases in firemen. J. A. M. A. 212:1341-1344, 1970.

von Oettingen, W. F. Toxicity and potential dangers of nitrous fumes. U. S. Public Health Serv. Public Health Bull. No. 272, 1941a.

Webster, J. R.; McCabe, M. M.; Karp, M. Recognition and management of smoke inhalation. J. A. M. A. *201*:287-290, 1967.

Yoshida, K.; Kasama, K.; Kitabatake, M.; Okuda, M.; Smai, M. Metabolic fate of nitric oxide. Int. Arch. Occup. Environ. Health *46*:71-77, 1980.

OXALATE

Oxalic acid and its salts are commonly used as bleaches, rust and ink eradicators, and metal cleaners. Their presence around the home has led to occasional accidental poisoning, particularly because of the resemblance between oxalic acid and Epsom salts (magnesium sulfate), and between potassium hydrogen oxalate and cream of tartar (potassium acid tartrate). In the nineteenth century, oxalic acid was a common instrument of suicide in England and Wales (Witthaus, 1911). Many plants contain oxalate, notably rhubarb leaves, *Dieffenbachia* or "dumbcane," beets, spinach, mangold, halogeton, sorrel, purslane, dock, greasewood and Russian thistle (Drach and Maloney, 1963; Fassett, 1966b; Kingsbury, 1964; Steinberg and Brown, 1939); however, claims that oxalate was responsible for poisoning by at least some of these sources have been disputed. Potential metabolic sources of oxalate include ethylene glycol, glyoxylic acid, glycolic acid and glyoxal. See also ETHYLENE GLYCOL, p. III-172.

Toxicology: When ingested in large doses, oxalic acid and its soluble salts act as severe corrosive agents on the alimentary tract mucosa. Although this corrosive action may be slightly more marked with the free acid than with its soluble salts, acidity itself is not responsible, and the administration of dilute alkali is unwarranted and unwise. Symptoms appear almost immediately, and death may occur within a few minutes apparently as a result of severe gastroenteritis and secondary shock (Webster, 1930). In spite of intense corrosion, gastric perforation is said to be rare (Brown and Gettler, 1922). Purging may continue for more than 1 week, with death from exhaustion in neglected cases (Witthaus, 1911). Early gangrene has been reported from prolonged immersion of the hands in oxalate solutions (Grolnick, 1929; Klauder *et al.*, 1955).

If the victim does not die quickly from the local gastrointestinal injury, absorption and consequent systemic intoxication may become manifest. With dilute oxalate solutions, it is possible that gastrointestinal symptoms may be entirely absent; symptoms are then delayed, and the first evidence of poisoning may be muscle twitching, cramps or central nervous depression. The neuromuscular effects can be explained largely by the calcium-complexing action of oxalate, which depresses the level of ionized calcium in body fluids.

This form of hypocalcemia is said to produce severe disturbances in the functions of the heart and of the brain (Polson and Tattersall, 1959), but it is not clear that these organs are primary targets in oxalate poisoning. In contrast to FLUORIDE poisoning (p. III-185), in which both hypocalcemia and severe ventricular arrhythmias occur, the weak and "thready" pulse often described in oxalate poisoning (Witthaus, 1911) is probably secondary to poor coronary perfusion because of severe hypotension. A primary cardiac action, however, cannot be ruled out; indeed, it is inevitable if the plasma level of ionic calcium becomes very low (Dvorackova, 1966). Similarly, the disturbances in brain function may or may not be secondary to circulatory collapse; their relationship to hypocalcemia is far from clear. In fatally poisoned sheep, the cerebrospinal fluid calcium did not reflect the systemic hypocalcemia, nor did fetal plasma levels in pregnant ewes (Littledike *et al.*, 1976).

Total plasma calcium is also depressed presumably due to the deposition of calcium oxalate in soft tissues of the kidney, liver and other organs (Zarembski and Hodgkinson, 1967). Renal injury is usually demonstrable in oxalate poisoning (Brown and Gettler, 1922); kidney lesions assume increasing importance if death is delayed beyond 2 days (Polson and Tattersall, 1959). The origin of the kidney damage is not clearly understood. Dunn *et al.* (1924) did not believe that the deposition of calcium oxalate in the renal tubules played an important role. They maintained that the lesions are in effect an ischemic necrosis caused by vascular stasis. Although perhaps less important, mechanical injury may result from crystals of calcium and magnesium oxalate which precipitate within the kidneys and urinary tract.

The mean lethal dose for an adult probably lies between 15 and 30 gm., and death usually occurs within a few hours (Webster, 1930). Convalescence is characteristically slow, especially if there is much damage to the gastrointestinal tract. Esophageal strictures, although reported (Brown and Gettler, 1922), are apparently an uncommon complication. A teen-ager experienced cardiac arrest within 30 minutes after the accidental intravenous administration of 1.2 gm. of sodium oxalate. Heart action was revived after 5 minutes by cardiac massage, but the patient never regained consciousness and died on the fourth day (Dvorackova, 1966).

By virtue of their avidity for calcium, oxalic acid and oxalate salts are sometimes used as anticoagulants in blood specimens drawn for chemical analysis. Despite suggestions to the contrary (Howard, 1932; Robb, 1919), bleeding tendencies or coagulation defects are not a feature of oxalate poisoning or oxalosis (see below). It is generally recognized that the plasma level of ionized calcium cannot be reduced by 50% without inducing severe hypocalcemic tetany. The larger reductions that are necessary to delay significantly the normal clotting mechanisms are incompatible with life (Bard, 1961). The observations of Steinberg and Brown (1939) that extracts from oxalate-containing plants (sorrel, beets, citrus fruits, rhubarb) accelerated clotting time prompted the occasional use of oxalic acid as a hemostatic to control bleeding as a result of surgery (Blain and Campbell, 1942) and even in hemophilia (Page *et al.*, 1940). This paradoxical effect could not be duplicated by Foster (1940) and apparently remains unexplained.

Severe and even fatal cases of rhubarb ingestion are recognized among livestock (Kingsbury, 1964) and perhaps man in the United States (Robb, 1919). The reported signs and symptoms resemble those induced systemically by oxalate. It has been suggested that damage to the rumen may be a key lesion and that livestock may therefore be more sensitive to oxalate by mouth than is man (James *et al.*, 1971b; Littledike *et al.*, 1976). The leaves of rhubarb are said to contain higher concentrations of oxalate than the stalks (Kingsbury, 1964). Perhaps this is the reason that the stalks can be consumed with impunity in prepared dishes. Oxalic acid, however, begins to sublime at the temperature of boiling water (Howard, 1932), so that cooking may further lower the oxalate content of the stalks. In the poison case described by Robb (1919) the rhubarb was cooked, but both stalks and leaves were consumed.

European reports frequently involve raw rhubarb ingestion (Kalliala and Kauste, 1964; Streicher, 1964; Tallqvist and Vaananen, 1960), and many of the toxic signs and symptoms described differ from those of oxalate poisoning. Initial symptoms of nausea and vomiting are delayed for several hours, and ketosis and evidence of liver involvement are reported. The terminal events, however, are quite clearly associated with acute renal failure. Whether these differences relate to cooked vs. raw rhubarb or European vs. domestic varieties is not clear. Further investigation on these points is indicated (Fassett, 1966b).

Primary hyperoxaluria is a rare idiopathic disease which may have hereditary origins. The characteristics of hyperoxaluria, oxalate crystals in the urinary tract and widespread oxalate deposits throughout the body (oxalosis) suggest an inborn error of metabolism (Hodgkinson and Zarembski, 1968). A state of oxalosis has been produced in experimental animals by the chronic feeding of ETHYLENE GLYCOL (see p. III-174). Primary hyperoxaluria does not resemble acute oxalate poisoning and seems to have little in common with the rarely described chronic oxalate poisoning (Howard, 1932). Exogenous, oxalate administration produces no greater rise in urinary oxalate excretion in patients with primary hyperoxaluria than in normal subjects, but feeding ascorbate, glycine or glycolic acid increases oxaluria. Primary hyperoxaluria probably represents an overproduction of oxalate, possibly due to a defect in glycolic acid metabolism. All regimens of therapy attempted in this disorder have been unsuccessful, and renal failure is the inevitable cause of death (Frederick *et al.*, 1963; Marshall and Horwith, 1959; Stauffer, 1960). The relationship between oxalosis and systemic oxalate poisoning may afford a fruitful area for investigation.

Symptomatology:

1. Burning pain in throat, esophagus, and stomach. Exposed areas of mucous membrane turn almost immediately an opaque white, but unlike the mineral acids there are no corrosive actions on the lips and face.
2. Vomiting (often bloody or with a coffee-ground appearance), intense burning pain, severe purging.
3. The pulse becomes weak, irregular, and sometimes imperceptible. Hypotension and the usual signs of cardiovascular collapse appear.
4. If death is delayed for a few hours, nervous or neuromuscular symptoms develop: headache, muscle cramps (particularly of the jaw and extremities), tetany, sometimes convulsions, stupor, coma, and death.
5. Renal damage, as evidenced by oliguria, albuminuria, and hematuria may persist for weeks.

Treatment (must be prompt):

1. Give immediately by mouth a dilute solution of any soluble calcium salt: calcium lactate, lime water, finely pulverized chalk or plaster (suspended in a large volume of water), or even milk. Large amounts of calcium are required to inactivate oxalate by precipitating it as the insoluble calcium salt. Do not give an emetic drug.
2. Perform gastric lavage carefully or not at all if severe mucosal injury is already evident. Dilute lime water (calcium hydroxide) makes a good lavage fluid if used in large quantities.
3. Administer by slow intravenous injection 10 to 20 ml of calcium gluconate (10% solution) or of calcium chloride (5% solution). This injection may have to be repeated frequently to prevent hypocalcemic tetany. Calcium gluconate (10 ml.) may also be

given intramuscularly every few hours. Calcium compounds are never given subcutaneously; even the intramuscular route is hazardous in infants because of the incidence of sloughing. See also p. IV-74.

4. In severe cases parathyroid extract (100 USP units) given intramuscularly.

5. Morphine may be necessary for the control of pain.

6. Treat shock by the cautious intravenous injection of isotonic saline solution. Check for metabolic acidosis and infuse sodium bicarbonate if necessary (p. IV-72).

7. Watch for edema of the glottis and the late formation of esophageal strictures.

8. Useful demulcents by mouth include milk of magnesia, bismuth subcarbonate, and mineral oil.

9. Prophylactic and therapeutic measures in anticipation of renal damage. See pp. IV-52–55.

Laboratory: Hematuria and albuminuria may be prominent. Oxalate crystals are probably always present in the urine of a poisoned patient, but they cannot be considered diagnostic. The ECG may show prolonged Q-T intervals, even when rate corrected. Increases in plasma phosphate and magnesium, as well as marked hyperglycemia in the face of an inappropriately low plasma insulin level, were observed in poisoned sheep (Littledike *et al.*, 1976).

References:

Bard, P. *Medical Physiology*, 11th ed. C. V. Mosby Co., St. Louis, 1961.

Blain, A. W.; Campbell, K. N. Hemostatic effect of oxalic acid. Arch. Surg. 44:1117-1125, 1942.

Brown, S. A.; Gettler, A. O. A study of oxalic acid poisoning. Proc. Soc. Exp. Biol. Med. 19:204-208, 1922.

Drach, G.; Maloney, W. H. Toxicity of the common houseplant *Dieffenbachia*; report of a case. J. A. M. A. 184:1047-1048, 1963.

Dunn, J. S.; Haworth, A.; Jones, N. A. The pathology of oxalate nephritis. J. Pathol. 27:299-318, 1924.

Dvorackova, I. Todliche Vergiftung nach intravenoser Verabreichung von Natriumoxalat. Arch. Toxikol. 22:63-67, 1966.

Fassett, D. W. Oxalates. In *Toxicants Occurring Naturally in Foods.* . N. A. S. -N. R. C. Publication No. 1354, Washington, D. C., 1966b.

Foster, R. H. K. On the role of oxalic acid in blood clotting. Proc. Soc. Exp. Biol. Med. 44:136-139, 1940.

Frederick, E. W.; Rabkin, M. T.; Ritchie, R. H., Jr.; Smith, L. H., Jr. Studies on primary hyperoxaluria. I. *In vivo* demonstration of a defect in glyoxylate metabolism. N. Engl. J. Med. 269:821-829, 1963.

Grolnick, M. Case of early gangrene due to oxalic acid immersion. N. Y. State J. Med. 29:1461, 1929.

Hodgkinson, A.; Zarembski, P. M. Oxalic acid metabolism in man; a review. Calcif. Tissue Res. 2:115-132, 1968.

Howard, C. D. Chronic poisoning by oxalic acid, with report of case and results of study concerning volatilization of oxalic acid from aqueous solutions. J. Ind. Hyg. Toxicol. 14:283-290, 1932.

James, M. P.; Seawright, A. A.; Steele, D. P. Experimental acute ammonium oxalate poisoning of sheep. Aust. Vet. J. 47:9-17, 1971b.

Kalliala, H.; Kauste, O. Ingestion of rhubarb leaves as cause of oxalic acid poisoning. Ann. Paediatr. Fenn. 10:228-231, 1964.

Kingsbury, J. M. *Poisonous Plants of the United States and Canada.* Prentice-Hall, Inc., Englewood Cliffs, N. J., 1964.

Klauder, J. V.; Shelanski, L.; Gabriel, K. Industrial uses of compounds of fluorine and oxalic acid; cutaneous reaction and calcium therapy. Arch. Ind. Health 12:412-419, 1955.

Littledike, E. T.; James, L.; Cook, H. Oxalate (halogeton) poisoning of sheep: certain physiopathologic changes. Am. J. Vet. Res. 37:661-666, 1976.

Marshall, V. F.; Horwith, M. Oxalosis. J. Urol. 82:278-284, 1959.

Page, R. C.; Russell, H. K.; Rosenthal, R. L. Effect on oxalic acid intravenously on blood coagulation time in three hemophiliacs. Ann. Intern. Med. 14:78-86, 1940.

Polson, C. J.; Tattersall, R. N. *Clinical Toxicology.* J. B. Lippincott Co., Philadelphia, 1959.

Robb, H. F. Death from rhubarb leaves due to oxalic acid poisoning. J. A. M. A. 73:627-628, 1919.

Stauffer, M. Oxalosis. Report of a case with a review of the literature and discussion of the pathogenesis. N. Engl. J. Med. 263:386-390, 1960.

Steinberg, A.; Brown, W. R. A new concept regarding mechanism of clotting and the control of hemorrhage. Am. J. Physiol. 126:638, 1939.

Streicher, E. Akutes Nierenversagen und Ikterus nach einer Vergiftung Rhubarberblattern. Dtsch. Med. Wochenschr. 89:2379-2381, 1964.

Tallqvist, H.; Vaananen, I. Death from oxalic acid in rhubarb leaves. Ann. Paediatr. Fenn. 6:144, 1960.

Webster, R. W. *Legal Medicine and Toxicology.* W. B. Saunders Co., Philadelphia, 1930.

Witthaus, R. A. *Manual of Toxicology.* Wm. Wood & Co., New York, 1911.

Zarembski, P. M.; Hodgkinson, A. Plasma oxalic acid and calcium levels in oxalate poisoning. J. Clin. Pathol. 20:283-285, 1967.

PARAQUAT

Paraquat is the best known of a group of bipyridilium herbicides, which also includes diquat, morfamquat, chlormequat and difenzoquat. These valuable herbicide/desiccants destroy green plant tissue on contact with minimal systemic translocation. They are almost instantaneously inactivated on contact with soils, particularly clay, to which they bind tenaciously. Their unique value is that spraying on one day can be followed by reseeding on the next, even without ploughing. As implied by the suffix to their generic names, all are quaternary ammonium compounds. Paraquat, diquat, and morfamquat each contain two pyridine rings with quaternized nitrogens. In paraquat the pyridine rings of the bipyridyl nucleus are joined in the para-positions, and both nitrogens are substituted with methyl groups.

The herbicidal activity of paraquat is dependent on active photosynthesis, during which it competes with NADP for electrons furnished by a transfer system in the chloroplast. A single electron addition to paraquat produces methyl viologen, a free radical resonating structure with a blue color. It has been used as a redox indicator in laboratories for many years. Methyl viologen can react with molecular oxygen to regenerate paraquat ion and to yield such toxic and reactive products as hydrogen peroxide, superoxide anion and peroxide anion. All of these are potentially toxic to plant cell membranes. In animal and human cells the initial electron transfer cannot be initiated by photosynthesis, but there appear to be similarities between the herbicidal effects and the toxic effects in man (see below).

Paraquat is available as the dichloride, dibromide and dimethanosulfate salts, all of which appear to be equitoxic when the lethal doses are expressed in terms of the paraquat ion content. The more popular commercial formulations of paraquat include: Grammoxone, a 20% aqueous concentrate; Preeglene Extra, a mixture of 9% paraquat and 9% diquat; and Weedol, a 2.5% granular formulation. Presumably because of its greater safety, only the latter is sold to the general public; however, determined individuals and toddlers have consumed enough of the granular product to produce severe poisonings and death (Beebeejaum *et al.*, 1971; Cooke *et al.*, 1973; McDonagh and Martin, 1970). Most serious poisonings and deaths have involved the liquid concentrates.

During the mid-1970s, public controversy surrounded a program of aerial spraying of illicit marihuana crops in Mexico with paraquat, and the practice was suspended in 1978. During this period, paraquat-contaminated marihuana is known to have entered the United States. No known cases of paraquat poisoning or any other long-term effects were reported as being associated with this source of exposure.

Toxicology: Although paraquat is an excellent herbicide, it has a less than enviable record of safety. Since its registration in 1965, it has been responsible for hundreds of human deaths. The clinical syndrome induced by ingestion of paraquat-diquat mixtures (Gardner, 1972; Toner *et al.*, 1970) and products containing only diquat as the active ingredient (Schonborn *et al.*, 1971; Vanholder *et al.*, 1981) suggest that there are no important toxicological distinctions between diquat and paraquat. Human poisonings by other bipyridilium herbicides have not yet come to our attention.

Considerable variability appears to exist in the lethal dose by mouth both because substantial amounts may be removed by prompt vomiting and because of erratic and incomplete absorption from the gastrointestinal tract (Haley, 1979; Vandijk *et al.*, 1975). In many cases of accidental ingestion, death occurred eventually, even though the victim thought that he had promptly spit out all of the solution which had entered his mouth (Smith and Heath, 1976). On the other hand, the ingestion of an ounce of the 20% concentrate has been survived with vigorous

treatment (Thomas *et al.*, 1977). As noted in Section II, there are also considerable species differences in susceptibility to paraquat, but man may be among the most sensitive. The prudent view is that any amount can be dangerous.

Deaths or serious poisonings have followed the inhalation of sprays (George and Hedworth-Whitty, 1980), accidental or deliberate skin application for topical parasites (Hodgkinson, 1982; Wohlfahrt, 1981), and hypodermic injections (Almog and Tal, 1967; Harley *et al.*, 1977). Except for severe blistering and excoriation resulting from repeated dermal application and local ulcers of the mouth, esophagus and stomach from ingestion, the toxic syndrome is independent of the route of administration. As evaluated by repeated daily doses for 90 days in rats, paraquat has only a modest propensity for producing chronic or cumulative toxicity; the chronicity factor was 5.2 (Kimbrough and Gaines, 1970).

The survival time in fatally poisoned humans is also highly variable; death may occur at any time from a few hours to a month after ingestion (Parkinson, 1980). A "typical" intoxication has three stages, beginning with local corrosive burns, vomiting (sometimes blood-stained) and diarrhea (sometimes strongly positive for occult blood). Within a few days usually transient but extensive clinical signs and laboratory evidence signal toxic damage to the liver, kidneys and heart. Within a week, dyspnea, cyanosis, oxygen dependence and X-ray opacities in the lungs herald the onset of a relentless pulmonary fibrosis, often with hemorrhagic pulmonary edema (Grabensee *et al.*, 1971). In severe poisonings this sequence of events may be greatly accelerated. As noted below, paraquat poisoning involves multiple organ systems, and numerous possible causes of death are recognized aside from the lung lesions.

The most regular early sign of paraquat poisoning, irrespective of the route of administration, is vomiting. After ingestion, vomiting is usually followed by substernal and epigastric pain. Diarrhea is less common. Within 24 hours victims may complain of sore throat and difficulty in swallowing due to ulceration in the esophagus. Excoriated lips and ulcers on the tongue, buccal mucosa and pharynx are often visible (Bullivant, 1966; Campbell, 1968; Fennelly *et al.*, 1968; Harrison *et al.*, 1972; Pasi and Hine, 1971). In one case a child expelled the entire lining of his esophagus (Malone *et al.*, 1971). If concentrates are splashed in the eyes, the resulting lesions may resemble those produced by strong alkali (Cant and Lewis, 1968).

Acute renal failure may complicate attempts to remove paraquat by forced diuresis, which is a potentially dangerous form of therapy because victims are already prone to develop pulmonary edema (Howard, 1979). A proximal tubular dysfunction is suggested by findings of proteinuria, glucosuria, aminoaciduria, and increased excretion of phosphorus, sodium and urate (Vaziri et al., 1979). Histological damage to the loops of Henle (Hargreave et al., 1969) and tubular necrosis (Parkinson, 1980) have both been observed in fatal poisonings. In many cases, patients survived the episode of acute renal failure with a documented improvement in the glomerular filtration rate only to succumb eventually to the lung lesions (Copland et al., 1974; McKean, 1968; Vaziri et al., 1979). In other cases, however, the renal failure was of sufficient severity to have been judged contributory to demise; in these cases, death occurred in 5 days or less (Parkinson, 1980; Vanholder et al., 1981). In contrast to paraquat, the kidney is the primary if not the exclusive target organ for morfamquat in all animal species studied (Smith and Heath, 1976).

Jaundice and increased serum transaminase activity were noted in one patient who survived only 2 days, although the liver was normal by histological examination (Hargreave et al., 1969). Indeed, the hepatic involvement is often more transient and of milder proportions than the renal injury, but occasionally in massive ingestions, extensive centrilobular necrosis and acute hepatic failure are believed to have contributed to early demise (Parkinson, 1980; von der Hardt and Cardesa, 1971; Matsumoto et al., 1980). Bile duct lesions have been described as well, and in some patients who survived more than a week, intrahepatic cholestasis developed (Matsumoto et al., 1980).

Toxic myocarditis, congestive failure, cardiac arrest and circulatory collapse (perhaps secondary to cardiac damage) may also contribute to early death (Oreopoulos et al., 1968; Hargreave et al., 1969; Nagi, 1970; Parkinson, 1980; von der Hardt and Cardesa, 1971). Focal myocardial necrosis has been found postmortem (Masterson and Roche, 1970). Cerebral hemorrhages have occurred in several victims (Grant et al., 1980; Mukada et al., 1978; Vanholder et al., 1981). The distribution of the hemorrhages was unusual, and they were said to resemble those in thiamine deficiency. Perhaps paraquat damages selectively the cerebral blood vessels (Grant et al., 1980).

In five cases a rapidly progressive normochromic anemia appeared within a few days after ingestion. Examination of the marrow suggested a selective aplasia of the erythroid cell line. In one survivor the peripheral red cell counts and marrow morphology returned to normal by 6 months (Lautenschlager et al., 1974). In one victim with intense cyanosis, appreciable levels of methemoglobin together with a few Heinz bodies were detected. Methylene blue was effective in reversing the methemoglobinemia,

but the patient then experienced a late hemolytic episode. His red cells were not deficient in glucose-6-phosphate dehydrogenase (Ng et al., 1982). Methemoglobin formation by paraquat has been confirmed in vitro in human blood (Watanabe and Ogata, 1982). Adrenal cortical necrosis involving the zonae fasciculata and reticularis has been described at least once (Nagi, 1970). In all cases of damage to other organs, however, the lungs were invariably involved to a greater or lesser extent.

In patients who survive for more than a week, the ultimate determinant of continued survival is usually the severity of the lung involvement. The pulmonary pathology has been divided into two phases, an initial transient and destructive phase, which is rarely seen in humans postmortem, and a late proliferative phase (Smith and Heath, 1976). From animal studies it has been inferred that the destructive phase may involve damage to the alveolar epithelium. Although paraquat has no direct effects on pulmonary surfactant in vitro, surfactant is reduced or absent in poisoned animals due both to decreased synthesis and to increased degradation (Etherton and Gresham, 1979; Manklelow, 1967; Meerbach and Grabner, 1978). Whether or not surfactant loss is a critical event in the destructive phase is not known, but the alveolar damage is held responsible for occasional cases of early pulmonary edema (Smith and Heath, 1976).

The proliferative phase presents clinically as a restriction of lung volume, a decrease in arterial oxygen tension, an increasing alveolar-to-arterial oxygen tension gradient and a late intrapulmonary shunt (Cooke et al., 1973). The pulmonary pathology in both animals and man has been extensively reviewed (Smith and Heath, 1976). Briefly, the critical events appear to be a widespread and intensive proliferation of fibroblastic tissue in the alveolar spaces, which eventually obliterates the deep lung architecture. Death is the result of respiratory failure secondary to anoxic hypoxia (Adachi et al., 1978; Cooke et al., 1973; Dearden et al., 1978; Matthew et al., 1968). In desperate cases, lung transplants have been attempted, but no patient has survived such an operation to date (Cooke et al., 1973; Matthew et al., 1968). In nonfatal cases, complete recovery appears to be the general rule.

Absorption and disposition: Animal studies (rats, guinea pigs, monkeys) suggest that paraquat and diquat are poorly absorbed from the gastrointestinal tract and from subcutaneous sites (Daniel and Gage, 1966; Murray and Gibson, 1974). In rats, more than half the oral dose was still present in the gastrointestinal tract 32 hours after dosing, and 17 and 14% of the total dose were eventually excreted in feces and urine, respectively. Disagreement exists over whether or not small amounts of metabolites are found in rat urine after oral administration. Although it has been suggested that paraquat may be extensively metabolized by gut microflora, biotransformation is not an important protective mechanism against this poison (Daniel and Gage, 1966; Murray and Gibson, 1974). In both humans and animals, irrespective of the route of administration, peak serum concentrations are reached very early and decline rapidly thereafter. Peak concentrations in rats are achieved within an hour; in humans, little is found in serum after the first day (Fairshter et al., 1979; Murray and Gibson, 1974). As evaluated in 79 patients, individuals with plasma concentrations of less than 2.0, 0.3 or 0.1 mg./L. at 4, 10 or 24 hours after ingestion, respectively, are apt to survive (Proudfoot et al., 1979). A urinary excretion of more than 1 mg./hr. beyond 8 hours of ingestion is said to be associated with a high mortality (Wright et al., 1978). Paraquat, however, is eliminated in a complex pharmacokinetic pattern, which in dogs involves at least a triexponential function (Hawksworth et al., 1981).

In many cases the appearance of lung damage is delayed for periods of up to a week after the decline in plasma concentration even to undetectable levels. This delayed onset originally led to the concept of paraquat as a "hit-and-run poison." This concept was abandoned with the discovery that paraquat is actively concentrated in the lungs, kidneys and perhaps other organs and tissues. Because it is slowly released from these sites, detectable amounts may be present in the urine and feces for weeks after exposure (Murray and Gibson, 1974; Tompsett, 1970).

As shown by studies with metabolic inhibitors, with hypoxia and with other organic bases that interact competitively, paraquat is actively accumulated in mouse renal cortical slices (Ecker et al., 1975a). In intact dogs, rats and mice, paraquat is both freely filtered in glomeruli and actively secreted into renal tubular fluid at least at low doses; the same is probably true of diquat (Ecker et al., 1975b; Hawksworth et al., 1981; Lock, 1979). At higher doses or at 24 hours after a single toxic dose, both impairment in renal function and decreased paraquat clearance are evident. Thus, early renal failure induced by paraquat results in impairment of its own clearance and substantially increases its uptake into "slow" compartments, notably the lungs (Hawksworth et al., 1981). Even with normal renal function any organic base that is also actively secreted has the potential for decreasing paraquat clearance, as also does any drug or intervention that decreases effective renal blood flow, e.g., β_2-adrenergic agonists such as isoproterenol (Maling et al., 1978).

Paraquat is also actively and selectively sequestered by the lungs probably over many days (Rose et al., 1980). The active uptake process is inhibited competitively by a number of amines (Ross and Krieger, 1981). This process is oxygen-dependent, but it exhibits an unusual resistance to hypoxia (Montgomery et al., 1980). Paraquat concentrations in lung and kidney tissue correlate with lethality in rats, and the lungs eventually reach concentrations in excess of those in any other organ or tissue (Sharp et al., 1972). There is, however, no preferential subcellular localization in lungs or other tissues, with paraquat being found in all cell fractions (Ilett et al., 1974).

Mechanism: Research on the mechanism of paraquat toxicity has proceeded along two broad lines. The first has attempted to relate the mechanism of its herbicidal activity (see above) to its effects in mammalian cells (Smith and Heath, 1976). The second has been to draw analogies between paraquat and other compounds known to be metabolized to highly reactive intermediates or free radicals, e.g., acetaminophen and carbon tetrachloride. Neither approach has been entirely satisfactory to date, and almost all relevant observations have been disputed.

In support of the concept that paraquat is converted in vivo to a free radical which, in turn, reacts with molecular oxygen to form such toxic intermediates as superoxide anion, the following evidence has been offered. The target organ, the lungs, is the best oxygenated of any in the body. The lung lesions have many features in common with acute oxygen poisoning (Smith and Heath, 1976). High ambient oxygen tensions increase paraquat lethality in rats and intensify the lung injury (Fisher, 1973). Exposure of rats to high oxygen tensions while treating them with bacterial endotoxins results in an increase in antioxidant enzyme activity in the lung, including superoxide dismutase. Such treated rats exhibit a prolonged survival time after dosing with paraquat relative to control groups (Frank, 1981). Similarly, survival times are prolonged in rats made tolerant to high oxygen tensions by oxygen exposure alone (Bus et al., 1976). Deficiency in the antioxidant, vitamin E (Block, 1979), or in selenium, which is normally incorporated into such antioxidant enzymes as glutathione peroxidase (Cross et al., 1977), enhanced paraquat toxicity to rats, but vitamin E administration failed to affect mortality or lung pathology in poisoned rats (Redetzki et al., 1980).

Reports that the administration of superoxide dismutase to paraquat poisoned rats both prolongs and increases their survival (Autor, 1974; Wasserman and Blick, 1978) have been disputed (Patterson and Rhodes, 1982). There was no correlation between the ability of three bipyridilium herbicides to form free radicals in tissue homogenates and the extent of the damage which they produce in vivo in lung, kidney and liver (Baldwin et al., 1975).

As indicated above, evidence for paraquat metabolism to any form is scant, and it does not appear to be covalently bound to tissue proteins or nucleotides (Ilett *et al.*, 1974). There is evidence both for (Bus *et al.*, 1976) and against (Keeling and Smith, 1982) paraquat-induced depletion of reduced glutathione in various target organs. Evidence exists both for and against the hypothesis that paraquat initiates lipid peroxidation in target organs (Bus *et al.*, 1975; Kornbrust and Mavis, 1980; Shu *et al.*, 1979).

Miscellaneous observations which may be relevant but have yet to be fully exploited in elucidating the mechanism of paraquat toxicity include the failure to find significant organ pathology in lethally poisoned rabbits (Butler and Kleinerman, 1971). An inhibition of DNA synthesis has been reported in cell culture systems (Carmines *et al.*, 1981) and in several target organs in intact rats (Van Osten and Gibson, 1975). In isolated perfused rat lungs an early effect of paraquat is a reversible decrease in the endothelial cell uptake of serotonin (Block and Schoen, 1982).

Forms of treatment: If the victim is seen within hours of ingestion, vigorous attempts to limit the gastrointestinal absorption of paraquat may be the single most important therapeutic intervention (Howard, 1979). Numerous adsorbents bind paraquat tenaciously, including Amberlite CG-120, magnesium trisilicate, activated charcoal (Staiff *et al.*, 1973), bentonite and Fuller's earth (Clark, 1971; Okonek *et al.*, 1982). There is little basis for selecting any one of these over the others, but activated charcoal may be the most readily available. It should be administered repeatedly in combination with a saline cathartic to hasten transit time through the bowel (Fairshter *et al.*, 1976; Smith *et al.*, 1974a). Whole-gut irrigation via a nasogastric tube has been tried at least twice, apparently with success (Greig and Streat, 1978; Okonek *et al.*, 1976).

Since paraquat is both filtered and actively secreted by the kidney, forced diuresis in the early stages of poisoning may be worthwhile. The fact that forced diuresis can be initiated rapidly must be weighed against the risks of an impending decrease in renal function and the imminent development of pulmonary edema. Even among the patients who achieved a brisk diuresis, not all survived (Greig and Streat, 1978; Grundies *et al.*, 1971; Mickleson and Fulton, 1971; Fisher *et al.*, 1971). Of the other possible modalities for removing absorbed paraquat, peritoneal dialysis is said to be less efficacious than forced diuresis (Fisher *et al.*, 1971).

In *in vitro* experimental models, paraquat is well dialyzed by artificial kidneys (Grundies *et al.*, 1971). The efficiency of the procedure depends on the plasma concentration of paraquat. At 1 to 2 ppm, toxicologically significant amounts probably cannot be removed, but at 20 ppm the clearance was 70 ml./min. at a blood flow of 100 ml./min. (Okonek *et al.*, 1976). Because plasma concentrations peak early and fall rapidly, the process is discouragingly inefficient. In one case, hemodialysis instituted 17 hours after ingestion and continued for 8 hours removed only 2% of the calculated absorbed dose (Spector *et al.*, 1978), but the survival of two patients was ascribed to immediate, intensive and prolonged dialysis (Eliahou *et al.*, 1973).

In *in vitro* trials, hemoperfusion over coated activated charcoal was 5 to 7 times more efficient than hemodialysis (Okonek *et al.*, 1976). The results of both *in vitro* studies and *in vivo* hemoperfusions in poisoned dogs indicated that a cation exchange resin (Zerolit 225 SRC 21) was superior to uncoated activated charcoal as an adsorbent (Maini and Winchester, 1975). Two teenagers were both successfully treated by unprecedented "continuous" hemoperfusions for 8 hr./day over 2 to 3 weeks (Okonek *et al.*, 1979). An exchange blood transfusion of over twice the calculated blood volume failed to save a severely poisoned infant (Mickleson and Fulton, 1971).

The compelling evidence that high oxygen tensions exacerbate paraquat-induced lung damage poses an agonizing dilemma for the therapist when signs of hypoxia are apparent in the patient. Hypoxic environments (finally 10% oxygen after stepwise decreases from 14%) protected mice against death. In hypoxic and paraquat-poisoned guinea pigs, even a brief exposure to room air led to pulmonary edema and death (Rhodes *et al.*, 1976). To reduce the pO_2 to which the lungs were exposed, the inspired oxygen content was lowered to 15% while arterial blood was circulated through a membrane oxygenator, but the patient died of brain damage; at autopsy, the pulmonary lesions were found to be extensive (Klaff *et al.*, 1977). Probably oxygen therapy is best avoided until its need becomes critical.

In rats the expectorants ammonium chloride and potassium iodide prevented the paraquat-induced decrease in lung surfactant activity, the increase in pulmonary resistance and the decrease in lung compliance; it is not clear, however, that they would have prevented death (Cambar and Aviado, 1970). Daily niacin therapy prolonged survival and modestly decreased mortality in paraquat-poisoned rats (Brown *et al.*, 1981). The anti-inflammatory and anti-edemogenic drug, eriodictyol, prevented the signs of acute pulmonary insufficiency and the decreases in lung compliance and respiratory minute volume provoked by paraquat in rats (Aviado *et al.*, 1974). An early report about the successful use of immunosuppressant therapy has since been refuted (Malcomson and Beesley, 1975).

Symptomatology:
  A. Ingestion, usually of liquid concentrates. Except for local lesions (below), signs and

symptoms of systemic intoxication are independent of the route of exposure and formulation (*i.e.*, liquid or granular).

1. Burning discomfort or pain in mouth, pharynx, esophagus and abdomen (substernal or epigastric); prompt and repeated vomiting with hematemesis; diarrhea with bloody stools; headache.
2. Death may occur in 24 hours or less due to fulminating pulmonary or cerebral hemorrhage or to renal, hepatic or cardiac failure.
3. When smaller amounts or dilute solutions are consumed, sore throat and dysphagia within 24 hours; excoriated lips; ulcers of the tongue, buccal mucosa and pharynx.
4. Within 1 to 6 days, signs of acute renal failure, including oliguria, increases in plasma BUN and creatinine, proteinuria, glucosuria and aminoaciduria.
5. Signs of hepatotoxicity, such as pain in right upper quadrant due to an enlarged and tender liver, jaundice and elevations in serum transaminase activity.
6. Signs of toxic myocarditis or signs of pulmonary congestion and early pulmonary edema that may or may not reflect acute cardiac failure.
7. Cyanosis may be due to anoxic hypoxia or methemoglobinemia; the latter has been reported at least once.
8. Signs of adrenal cortical necrosis, such as fever, abdominal pain, lethargy, somnolence, hypovolemic vascular shock.
9. Any or all of the above may be followed by a period of improvement lasting as long as 2 weeks.
10. Generalized rales and progressively decreasing pulmonary function: reduced arterial oxygen saturation, cyanosis, restriction in lung volume, increasing alveolar-to-arterial oxygen tension gradient, intrapulmonary shunt, granular changes in X-rays of the lung fields.
11. Respiratory failure secondary to anoxemia.
12. In survivors the general rule is that recovery is eventually complete, although pulmonary function tests may be abnormal for months.
13. Occasionally persistent anemia due to selective suppression of erythropoiesis in bone marrow.

B. Spills on the skin.
1. Severe skin irritation, blistering and excoriation, especially with repeated applications.

2. Loss of fingernails or toenails, followed by normal regeneration.
3. Systemic signs of intoxication as above but usually milder.

C. Inhalation of sprays.
1. Nose bleeds, headache, coughing, sore throat.
2. Systemic signs of intoxication as above but usually milder.

D. Splashes in the eye.
1. Severe inflammation reaching maximal intensity in 12 to 24 hours.
2. Loss of conjunctival epithelium and superficial layers of the cornea.
3. Perhaps penetrating lesions as in lye injuries, but with proper care recovery is usually complete.
4. Systemic signs have not been reported from this route of exposure.

Treatment: Potentially the most desperate and challenging type of intoxication in modern clinical toxicology.

A. Ingestion.
1. If liquid concentrates (20% or more) have been consumed, swallow promptly large quantities of milk, egg whites or gelatin solutions. If these or other protein solutions are not available, give 200 to 500 ml. of a 30% suspension of activated charcoal, bentonite or Fuller's earth. A slurry of granular household laundry detergent or a hand dishwashing liquid well diluted with water may be swallowed, in a dose of about 0.1–0.2 gm./kg. to precipitate paraquat, if protein solutions are unavailable. Because of possible mucosal injury and because intense vomiting is likely to occur spontaneously, emetic drugs are probably best avoided. Cautious gastric lavage using more dilute suspensions of protein solutions or adsorbents.
2. If dilute solutions (2% or less) or granular formulations were swallowed, administer syrup of ipecac (p. I-2) and/ or perform gastric lavage using the lavage fluids listed above.
3. Leave in the stomach 200 to 500 ml. of a 30% suspension of activated charcoal or bentonite, together with 30 gm. magnesium sulfate. Readminister the adsorbent as often as practical, *i.e.*, every 2 to 4 hours, for several days, with magnesium sulfate as required to sustain diarrhea.
4. Begin forced diuresis (p. IV-52), but check repeatedly for impending pulmonary edema.
5. Hypoxic atmospheres (10 to 15% O_2) protect animals and have been tried in

several clinical cases, although not successfully. If this form of therapy is
attempted, maintain the arterial oxygen tension at > 40 mm Hg at all times.

6. Methemoglobinemia responds to
methylene blue (p. III-34), but this
drug may precipitate a late hemolytic
crisis.

7. Steroids for adrenal cortical failure (p.
IV-100).

8. In the event of renal failure, start extracorporeal hemodialysis (p. IV-55)
or, better, hemoperfusion (p. IV-57).
Unusually prolonged periods of either
operation may be required, but their
effectiveness in removing paraquat
falls precipitiously with time after
ingestion.

9. Daily chest films, arterial oxygen tension measurements, pulmonary function studies and chest auscultations.

10. Monitor for signs of renal, hepatic or
cardiac failure and institute appropriate therapies (pp. IV-52, IV-60 and IV-
22).

11. Oxygen therapy is best withheld until
the arterial tension falls to critical
levels. Oxygen requirements may be
reduced by sedation.

B. Spills on the skin.

1. Thorough washing with soap and water; treat local injury with bland preparations that may contain local anesthetics, steroids and/or antibiotics.

2. If dermal exposure to liquid concentrates was extensive, any or all measures above beginning with no. 4 can be
instituted, as indicated.

C. Inhalation of sprays.

1. If exposure has been severe, any or all
measures above beginning with no. 4
can be instituted, as indicated.

D. Splashes in the eye.

1. Irrigate with water for 10 to 15 minutes.

2. Antibiotics to control infection.

3. Consult with ophthalmologist.

Laboratory:

1. Methods are available for determining
paraquat in blood, urine and tissues (Fisher
et al., 1971). Such determinations, however,
are primarily useful only in confirming the
diagnosis. The Chevron Chemical Company has offered to perform urine and dialysate analyses at no cost; call (415)-233-
3737.

2. Monitor carefully fluid and electrolyte balance during forced diuresis and forced diarrhea.

3. Tests for renal and hepatic function at least
during the first week.

4. Monitor ECG continuously.

5. Repeated chest films, chest auscultations
and arterial oxygen tension determinations.

6. Evidence in human serum has been obtained for lipid peroxidation (Yasaka *et al.*,
1981).

References:

Adachi, H.; Yokota, T.; Fiyihara, S.; Nakamura, H.; Uchino,
F. Two autopsy cases of paraquat poisoning. Tokohu J.
Exp. Med. *125*:331–339, 1978.

Almog, C.; Tal, E. Death from paraquat after subcutaneous
injection. Br. Med. J. *3*:721, 1967.

Autor, A.P. Reduction of paraquat toxicity by superoxide
dismutase. Life Sciences *14*:1309–1319, 1974.

Aviado, D.M.; Bacalzo, L.V., Jr.; Belej, M.A. Prevention of
acute pulmonary insufficiency by eriodictyol. J. Pharmacol.
Exp. Ther. *189*:157–166, 1974.

Baldwin, R.C.; Pasi, A.; MacGregor, J.T.; Hine, C.H. The rates
of radical formation from the dipyridylium herbicides paraquat, diquat and morfamquat in homogenates of rat lung,
kidney and liver: An inhibitory effect of carbon monoxide.
Toxicol. Appl. Pharmacol. *32*:298–304, 1975.

Beebeejaum, A.R.; Beevers, G.; Rogers, W.N. Paraquat poisoning—prolonged excretion. Clin. Toxicol. *4*:397–407, 1971.

Block, E.R. Potentiation of acute paraquat toxicity by vitamin
E deficiency. Lung *156*:195–203, 1979.

Block, E.R.; Schoen, F.J. Depression of serotonin uptake by
rat lungs exposed to paraquat. J. Pharmacol. Exp. Ther.
221:254–260, 1982.

Brown, O.R.; Heitkamp, M.; Sing, C.S. Niacin reduces paraquat toxicity in rats. Science *212*:1510–1512, 1981.

Bullivant, C.M. Accidental poisoning by paraquat: Report of
two cases in man. Br. Med. J. *21*:1272–1273, 1966.

Bus, J.S.; Aust, S.D.; Gibson, J.E. Lipid peroxidation: A possible mechanism for paraquat toxicity. Res. Commun.
Chem. Pathol. Pharmacol. *11*:31–38, 1975.

Bus, J.S.; Cagen, S.Z.; Olgaard, M.; Gibson, J.E. A mechanism
of paraquat toxicity in mice and rats. Toxicol. Appl. Pharmacol. *35*:501–513, 1976.

Butler, C.; Kleinerman, J. Paraquat in the rabbit. Br. J. Ind.
Med. *28*:67–71, 1971.

Cambar, P.J.; Aviado, D.M. Bronchopulmonary effects of
paraquat and expectorants. Arch. Environ. Health *20*:488–
494, 1970.

Campbell, S. Death from paraquat in a child. Lancet *1*:144,
1968.

Cant, J.S.; Lewis, D.R.H. Ocular damage due to paraquat and
diquat. Br. Med. J. *3*:59, 1968.

Carmines, E.L.; Carchman, R.A.; Borzelleca, J.F. Investigations into the mechanism of paraquat toxicity utilizing a
cell culture system. Toxicol. Appl. Pharmacol. *58*:353–362,
1981.

Clark, D.G. Inhibition of the absorption of paraquat from the
gastrointestinal tract by absorbents. Br. J. Ind. Med.
28:186–188, 1971.

Cooke, N.J.; Flenley, D.C.; Matthew, H. Paraquat poisoning.
Serial studies of lung function. Q. J. Med. *42*:683–692, 1973.

Copland, G.M.; Kolin, A.; Shulman, H.S. Fatal pulmonary
intra-alveolar fibrosis after paraquat ingestion. N. Engl. J.
Med. *291*:290–292, 1974.

Cross, C.E.; Reddy, K.A.; Hasegawa, G.K.; Chiu, M.M.; Tyler,
W.S.; Omaye, S.T. Paraquat toxicity; effects of selenium
deficiency and anti-inflammatory drug pretreatments. Biochem. Mech. Paraquat Toxic. *1*:201–211, 1977.

Daniel, J.W.; Gage, J.C. Absorption and excretion of diquat
and paraquat in rats. Br. J. Indust. Med. *23*:133–136, 1966.

Dearden, L.C.; Fairshter, R.D.; McRae, D.M.; Smith, W.R.;
Glauser, F.L.; Wilson, A.F. Pulmonary ultrastructure of the
late aspects of human paraquat poisoning. Am. J. Pathol.
93:667–680, 1978.

Ecker, J.L.; Gibson, J.E.; Hook, J.B. *In vitro* analysis of the
renal handling of paraquat. Toxicol. Appl. Pharmacol.

34:170-177, 1975a.

Ecker, J.L.; Hook, J.B.; Gibson, J.E. Nephrotoxicity of paraquat in mice. Toxicol. Appl. Pharmacol. 34:178-186, 1975b.

Eliahou, H.E.; Almog, C.; Gura, V.; Iaina, A. Treatment of paraquat poisoning by hemodialysis. Isr. J. Med. Sci. 9:459-462, 1973.

Etherton, J.E.; Gresham, G.A. Early bronchiolar damage following paraquat poisoning in mice. J. Pathol. 128:21-27, 1979.

Fairshter, R.D.; Rosen, S.M.; Smith, W.R.; Glauser, F.L.; McRae, D.M.; Wilson, A.F. Paraquat poisoning: new aspects of therapy. Q. J. Med. 45:551-565, 1976.

Fairshter, R.D.; Dabivaziri, N.; Smith, W.R.; Glauser, F.L.; Wilson, A.F. Paraquat poisoning—analytical toxicologic study of 3 cases. Toxicology 12:259-266, 1979.

Fennelly, J.J.; Gallagher, R.T.; Carroll, R.J. Paraquat poisoning in a pregnant woman. Br. Med. J. 21:722-723, 1968.

Fisher, H.K.; Humphries, M.; Bails, R. Paraquat poisoning. Ann. Int. Med. 75:731-736, 1971.

Fisher, H.K. Enhancement of oxygen toxicity by the herbicide paraquat. Am. Rev. Resp. Dis. 107:246-252, 1973.

Frank, L. Prolonged survival after paraquat. Role of the lung antioxidant enzyme systems. Biochem. Pharmacol. 30:2319-2324, 1981.

Gardner, A.J.S. Pulmonary oedema in paraquat poisoning. Thorax 27:132-135, 1972.

George, M.; Hedworth-Whitty, R.B. Non-fatal lung disease due to inhalation of nebulised paraquat. Br. Med. J. 280:902, 1980.

Grabensee, B.; Keltmann, G.; Murtz, R.; Borchard, F. Paraquat poisoning, Deut. Med. Woch. 96:498-506, 1971.

Grant, H.C.; Lantos, P.L.; Parkinson, C. Cerebral damage in paraquat poisoning. Histopathology 4:185-195, 1980.

Greis, D.; Streat, S.J. Intentional paraquat poisoning: case report. N.Z. Med. J. 88:12-13, 1978.

Grundies, H.; Kolmar, D.; Bernhold, I. Paraquat intoxication. Deut. Med. Woch. 96:588, 1971.

Haley, T.J. Review of the toxicology of paraquat. Clin. Toxicol. 14:1-46, 1979.

Hargreave, T.B.; Gresham, G.A.; Karayannopoulos, S. Paraquat poisoning, Postgr. Med. J. 45:633-635, 1969.

Harley, J.B.; Grinspan, S.; Root, R.K. Paraquat suicide in a young woman: results of therapy directed against the superoxide radical. Yale J. Biol. Med. 50:481-488, 1977.

Harrison, L.C.; Dortimer, A.C.; Murphy, K.J. Fatalities due to the weedkiller paraquat. Med. J. Austr. 2:774-777, 1972.

Hawksworth, G.M.; Bennett, P.N.; Davies, D.S. Kinetics of paraquat elimination in the dog. Toxicol. Appl. Pharmacol. 57:139-145, 1981.

Hodgkinson, R. Fatal paraquat poisoning. Med. J. Australia, 2:120, 1982.

Howard, J.K. Recent experience with paraquat poisoning in Great Britain: A review of 68 cases. Vet. Hum. Toxicol. 21 Suppl.:213-216, 1979.

Ilett, K.F.; Stripp, B.; Menard, R.H.; Reid, W.D.; Gillette, J.R. Studies on the mechanism of the lung toxicity of paraquat: comparison of tissue distribution and some biochemical parameters in rat and rabbits. Toxicol. Appl. Pharmacol. 28:216-226, 1974.

Keeling, P.L.; Smith, L.L. Relevance of NADPH depletion and mixed disulphide formation in rat lung to the mechanism of cell damage following paraquat administration. Biochem. Pharmacol. 31:3243-3249, 1982.

Kimbrough, R.D.; Gaines, T.B. Toxicity of paraquat to rats and its effect on rat lungs. Toxicol. Appl. Pharmacol. 17:679-690, 1970.

Klaff, L.J.; Levin, P.J.; Potgieter, P.D.; Losman, J.G.; Nochomovitz, L.E.; Ferguson, A.D. Treatment of paraquat poisoning with the membrane oxygenator: a case report. S. Afr. Med. J. 51:203-205, 1977.

Kornbrust, D.J.; Mavis, R.D. The effect of paraquat on microsomal lipid peroxidation in vitro and in vivo Toxicol. Appl. Pharmacol. 53:323-332, 1980.

Lautenschlager, J.; Grabensee, R.; Pottgen, W. Paraquat intoxication and isolated aplastic anaemia. Deut. Med. Woch. 99:2348-2351, 1974.

Lock, E.A. The effect of paraquat and diquat on renal function in the rat. Toxicol. Appl. Pharmacol. 48:327-336, 1979.

Maini, R.; Winchester, J.F. Removal of paraquat from blood by haemoperfusion over sorbent materials. Br. Med. J. 3:281-282, 1975.

Malcolmson, E.J.; Beesley, J.B. Unsuccessful immunosuppressant therapy of paraquat poisoning. Br. Med. J. 3:650-651, 1975.

Maling, H.M.; Saul, W.; Williams, M.A.; Brown, E.A.B.; Gillette, J.R. Reduced body clearance as the major mechanism of the potentiation by β_2-adrenergic agonists of paraquat lethality in rats. Toxicol. Appl. Pharmacol. 43:57-72, 1978.

Malone, J.D.G.; Carmody, M.; Keogh, B.; O'Dwyer, W.F. Paraquat poisoning: a review of nineteen cases. J. Irish Med. Assoc. 64:59, 1971.

Manklelow, B.W. The loss of pulmonary surfactant in paraquat poisoning: a model for the study of the respiratory distress syndrome. Br. J. Exp. Pathol. 48:366-369, 1967.

Masterson, J.G.; Roche, W. Another paraquat fatality. Br. Med. J. 2:482, 1970.

Matsumoto, T.; Matsumori, H.; Kuwabara, N.; Fukuda, Y.; Ariva, R. A histopathological study of the liver in paraquat poisoning—An analysis of fourteen autopsy cases with emphasis on bile duct injury. Acta Pathol. Jpn. 30:859-870, 1980.

Matthew, H.; Logan, A.; Woodruff, M.F.A.; Heard, B. Paraquat poisoning—lung transplantation. Br. Med. J. 3:759-763, 1968.

McDonagh, B.J.; Martin, J. Paraquat poisoning in children. Arch. Dis. Child. 45:425-427, 1970.

McKean, W.I. Recovery from paraquat poisoning. Br. Med. J. 3:292, 1968.

Meerbach, W.; Grabner, R. Lung alterations after paraquat poisoning. Exp. Pathol. 16:168-179, 1978.

Mickleson, K.N.; Fulton, D.B. Paraquat poisoning treated by a replacement blood transfusion: case report. N.Z. Med. J. 74:26-27, 1971.

Montgomery, M.R.; Wyatt, I.; Smith, L.L. Oxygen effects on metabolism and paraquat uptake in rat lung slices. Exp. Lung Res. 1:239-250, 1980.

Mukada, T.; Sasano, N.; Sato, K. Autopsy findings in a case of acute paraquat poisoning with extensive cerebral purpura. Tohoku J. Exp. Med. 125:253-263, 1978.

Murray, R.; Gibson, J. Paraquat disposition in rats, guinea pigs and monkeys. Toxicol. Appl. Pharmacol. 27:283-291, 1974.

Nagi, A.H. Paraquat and adrenal cortical necrosis. Br. Med. J. 2:669, 1970.

Ng, L.L.; Naik, R.B.; Polak, A. Paraquat ingestion with methaemoglobinaemia treated with methylene blue. Br. Med. J. 284:1445-1446, 1982.

Okonek, S.; Hofmann, A.; Henningsen, B. Efficacy of gut lavage, hemodialysis, and hemoperfusion in the therapy of paraquat or diquat intoxication. Arch. Toxicol. 36:43-51, 1976.

Okonek, S.; Baldamus, C.A.; Hofmann, A.; Schuster, C.J.; Bechstein, P.B.; Zoller, B. Two survivors of severe paraquat intoxication by "continuous hemoperfusion". Klin. Wochenschr. 57:957-959, 1979.

Okonek, S.; Setyadharma, H.; Borchet, A.; Krienke, E.G. Activated charcoal is as effective as Fuller's earth or bentonite in paraquat poisoning. Klin. Wochenschr. 60:207-210, 1982.

Oreopoulos, D.G.; Soyannwo, M.A.O.; Sinniah, R.; Fenton, S.S.A.; McGeown, M.G.; Bruce, J.H. Acute renal failure in a case of paraquat poisoning. Br. Med. J. 23:749-750, 1968.

Parkinson, C. The changing pattern of paraquat poisoning in man. Histopathology 4:171-183, 1980.

Pasi, A.; Hine, C.H. Paraquat poisoning. Proc. West. Pharmacol. Soc. 14:169-172, 1971.

Patterson, C.E.; Rhodes, M.L. The effect of superoxide dismutase on paraquat mortality in mice and rats. Toxicol. Appl. Pharmacol. 62:65-72, 1982.

Proudfoot, A.T.; Stewart, M.S.; Levitt, T. Widdop, B. Paraquat poisoning: significance of plasma-paraquat concentrations. Lancet 2:330-332, 1979.

Redetzki, H.M.; Wood, C.D.; Grafton, W.D. Vitamin E and paraquat poisoning. Vet. Human Toxicol. 22:395–397, 1980.

Rhodes, M.L.; Zavala, D.C.; Brown, D. Hypoxic protection in paraquat poisoning. Lab. Invest. 35:496–500, 1976.

Rose, M.S.; Smith, L.L.; Wyatt, I. Toxicology of herbicides with special reference to the bipyridiliums. Ann. Occup. Hyg. 23:91–94, 1980.

Ross, J.H.; Krieger, R.I. Structure-activity correlation of amines inhibiting active uptake of paraquat (methyl viologen) into rat lung slices. Toxicol. Appl. Pharmacol. 59:238–249, 1981.

Schonborn, H.; Schuster, H.P.; Kossling, K. Klinik und Morphologie der akuten peroralen Diquatintoxikation (Reglone). Arch. Toxikol. 27:204–216, 1971.

Sharp, C.W.; Ottolenghi, A.; Posner, H.S. Correlation of paraquat toxicity with tissue concentrations and weight loss of the rat. Toxicol. Appl. Pharmacol. 22:241–251, 1972.

Shu, H.; Talcott, R.E.; Rice, S.A.; Wei, E.T. Lipid peroxidation and paraquat toxicity. Biochem. Pharmacol. 28:327–331, 1979.

Smith, L.L.; Wright, A.; Wyatt, I.; Rose, M.S. Effective treatment for paraquat poisoning in rats and its relevance to treatment of paraquat poisoning in man. Br. Med. J. 4:561–569, 1974a.

Smith, P.H.; Heath, D. Paraquat. CRC Crit. Rev. Toxicol. 4:411–445, 1976.

Spector, D.; Whorton, D.; Zachary, J.; Slavin, R. Fatal paraquat poisoning: tissue concentrations and implications for treatment. Johns Hopkins Med. J. 142:110–113, 1978.

Staiff, D.C.; Irle, G.K.; Felsenstein, W.C. Screening of various adsorbents for protection against paraquat poisoning. Bull. Environ. Contam. Toxicol. 10:193, 1973.

Thomas, P.D.; Thomas, D.; Chan, Y.L.; Clarkson, A.R. Paraquat poisoning is not necessarily fatal. Med. J. Aust. 2:564–

565, 1977.

Tompsett, S.L. Paraquat poisoning. Acta Pharmacol. Toxicol. 28:346–358, 1970.

Toner, P.G.; Vetters, J.M.; Spilg, W.G.S.; Harland, W.A. Fine structure of the lung lesion in a case of paraquat poisoning. J. Pathol. 102:182–185, 1970.

Vandijk, A.; Maes, R.A.A.; Prost, R.H.; Daize, J.M.C.; Vanheyst, A.N.P. Paraquat poisoning in man. Arch. Toxicol. 34:129–136, 1975.

Vanholder, R.; Colardyn, R.; Dereuck, J.; Praet, M.; Lameire, N.; Ringoir, S. Diquat intoxication—report of 2 cases and review of the literature. Am. J. Med. 70:1267–1271, 1981.

Van Osten, G.K.; Gibson, J.E. Effect of paraquat on the biosynthesis of deoxyribonucleic acid, ribonucleic acid and protein in the rat. Fd. Cosmet. Toxicol. 13:47–54, 1975.

Vaziri, N.D.; Ness, R.L.; Fairshter, R.D.; Smith, W.R.; Rosen, S.M. Nephrotoxicity of paraquat in man. Arch. Intern. Med. 139:172–174, 1979.

von der Hardt, H.; Cardesa, A. Die histopathologischen Fruhveranderungen nach paraquat–intoxikation. Klin. Wschr. 49:544–550, 1971.

Wasserman, B.; Block, E.R. Prevention of acute paraquat toxicity in rats by superoxide dismutase. Aviation Space Environ. Med. 49:805–809, 1978.

Watanabe, S.; Ogata, M. Methemoglobin formation by paraquat. Acta Medica Okayama 36:495–499, 1982.

Wohlfahrt, D.J. Paraquat poisoning in Papua New Guinea. Papua New Guinea Med. J. 24:164–167, 1981.

Wright, N.; Yeoman, W.B.; Hale, K.A. Assessment of severity of paraquat poisoning. Br. Med. J. 2:396, 1978.

Yasaka, T.; Ohya, I.; Matsumoto, J.; Shiramizu, T.; Sasagun, Y. Acceleration of lipid peroxidation in human paraquat poisoning. Arch. Intern. Med. 141:1169–1171, 1981.

PARATHION

Parathion (*O,O*-diethyl-*O*-*p*-nitrophenyl thiophosphate) is one of several related organic phosphorus insecticides which possess great potency and a wide range of usefulness in modern agriculture (Casida, 1964; Heath, 1961; O'Brien, 1960). See Section II for information about many of these related insecticides. Parathion is a yellow to dark brown liquid of low vapor pressure, insoluble in water and kerosene, stable in the presence of moisture but hydrolyzed rapidly by alkali. Technical parathion is available commercially as the active ingredient of various dusts, wettable powders, emulsifiable concentrates, and aerosols, all of which act on the insect as contact and stomach poisons. The chemical is retained on the surface of plants and fruit, clothing and mechanical equipment, all of which may remain toxic for days (Anderson *et al.*, 1965; Ganelin *et al.*, 1964; Kanagaratnam *et al.*, 1960; Quinby and Lemmon, 1958; Warren *et al.*, 1963). Decontamination is difficult; articles known to have been in contact with parathion are best destroyed if economically feasible. Because of its high toxicity parathion is not used in the home or barn.

Toxicology: Organophosphorus insecticides are among the most poisonous materials commonly used for pest control. In terms of toxic actions to man, they are related to one another and also to a group of chemical warfare agents

known as the nerve gases (Grob, 1956). Among these compounds parathion has an intermediate toxicity (DuBois and Coon, 1952; Hayes, 1963). Absorption to a dangerous degree can occur through any portal including the intact skin (Grob, 1956). Although many human fatalities have been traced unequivocally to parathion, the probable lethal dose in man is best inferred from animal experimentation. On this basis 10 to 20 mg. is an estimate of the *minimal* oral dose which is acutely lethal to an adult, whereas the mean lethal dose is probably 300 mg. (4 mg./kg.). On the other hand, 120 mg. has killed an adult, and children have died after only 2 mg. of parathion, a dose of about 0.1 mg./kg. (Hayes, 1963). Young animals are more susceptible than adults of the same species (DuBois, 1971) and the same may be true of human children (Klugman, 1959).

Most occupational accidents involving parathion and its chemical relatives are ascribed to dermal exposure, and at least a few cases are known in which the possibility of concurrent oral intake was precluded (Introna, 1959; Petty, 1957; Reichert, 1978). In man parathion is at least 10 times less toxic by skin application than by inhalation and about 3 times less toxic by ingestion than by inhalation (Hartwell *et al.*, 1964). Ingestion, however, is a genuine hazard. An epidemic involving 79 persons killed 17 of them in Jamaica in 1976; they had all consumed wheat flour that had been contaminated with parathion in international commerce (Diggory *et al.*, 1977).

As assessed by the urinary excretion of metabolites, the rate of absorption of parathion from human skin varies directly with the ambient temperature (Funckes *et al.*, 1963). As little as one drop of concentrated material represents a very real danger to life if splashed in the eye (de Ong, 1956). Obviously great caution is necessary in handling parathion and related compounds, and the therapist should certainly protect himself, at least by wearing natural rubber gloves and apron, if the patient's skin or clothing appears to be contaminated with active material.

Parathion and its relatives are known to inhibit the enzyme cholinesterase in all parts of the body by phosphorylating the active site (Holmstedt, 1959). Toxic signs and symptoms are regarded as indirect consequences of this enzyme inactivation. According to this interpretation a poisoned tissue is unable to prevent local accumulation of acetylcholine, which acts as an excitatory substance in low concentration and a paralytic substance in high concentration (DuBois, *et al.*, 1949).

Although this explanation is a useful one, it is well to recognize that it is little more than a good working hypothesis. During both poisoning and convalescence, experimental animals and man exhibit poor correlations between the severity of toxic signs and symptoms on the one hand and tissue levels of enzyme activity or of acetylcholine on the other hand, even in such target organs as the brain. For example, cholinesterase inhibition appears before and lasts much longer than clinically detectable evidences of poisoning (Hamblin and Golz, 1955; Davies *et al.*, 1967; Payne and Robinson, 1962; Holmstedt, 1959). In rats the time courses of such neurologic effects as changes in visually evoked potentials and maximal electroshock seizure patterns differ from the time course of acetylcholinesterase inhibition (Woolley, 1976). Acetylcholine levels remain elevated as long as cholinesterase inhibition persists. In spite of this persistence experimental animals exhibit clinical recovery, suggesting that tolerance to acetylcholine develops at the receptor level (Brodeur and DuBois, 1964).

Although the inhibition of cholinesterase appears to be partially reversible for several hours after an acute exposure, there is a progressive and irreversible inactivation of enzyme following repeated exposures or prolonged contact (Hobbinger, 1956). It is probable that this cumulative biochemical lesion is repaired chiefly through the regeneration of new enzyme. In one poisoned infant the rate of restoration of plasma cholin-

esterase occurred at a rate consonant with liver protein synthesis, but the regeneration of red cell cholinesterase occurred faster than would be predicted from erythropoietic rates (Mackey, 1966). Under these circumstances a clinical intoxication is possible from small repeated subclinical exposures. The situation is particularly hazardous because of the narrow margin between the dose which is just sufficient to produce symptoms and that which is adequate to kill.

Based on the above hypothesis toxic signs and symptoms can be classified with respect to the tissue site of enzyme inhibition; thus the pharmacologist refers to the muscarinic, nicotinic, and central nervous effects of organophosphorus insecticides (Grob and Harvey, 1953; Grob, 1956; Holmstedt, 1959; Koelle and Gilman, 1949). Such a classification is not particularly useful to the clinical toxicologist, whose principal concerns are the sequence and intensity of signs and symptoms.

Both sequence and latency of symptoms depend to some extent on the portal of entry. For example, respiratory tract symptoms appear first during an inhalation exposure to parathion, whereas gastrointestinal effects are more prominent when the poison is swallowed. A skin exposure may reveal itself before systemic manifestations by the appearance of local sweating and local twitching or fasciculations (but no erythema or skin irritation). An ocular exposure with liquid parathion is always manifested by prompt miosis and other ocular disturbances, which may or may not be present after exposures by other routes (Milby *et al.*, 1964). The onset of symptoms is probably quickest after inhalation (a few minutes) and slowest after a primary cutaneous exposure (insidious onset after a latency of one or more hours) (Andersen and Jersild, 1949; Annis and Williams, 1953; Batchelor and Walker, 1954; Dixon, 1957; Gilsenan, 1957; Grob *et al.*, 1949; Johnston, 1953; Wishahi *et al.*, 1958).

Whatever the portal of entry, severe respiratory distress eventually appears in major intoxications. Although mucus secretion, bronchospasm, and pulmonary edema may be disabling and confuse the diagnosis (Bernstein and Gould, 1968; Bledsoe and Seymour, 1972; Velhanayagam, 1962), fatalities in man are usually due to respiratory failure on the basis of central nervous paralysis. Even coma, areflexia and apnea do not preclude a favorable outcome if immediate and energetic treatment is instituted. Respiratory acidosis should be anticipated, but a metabolic component may also be present (Annis and Williams, 1953; Boelcke *et al.*, 1970; Prinz, 1969).

In contrast to parathion, poisonings by TEPP, paraoxon, and nerve gases always develop at a rapid rate. In part this difference may arise from the fact that pure parathion and several related insecticides (*e.g.*, malathion, guthion) are not true cholinesterase poisons until they are converted *in vivo* to active products (Holmstedt, 1959; Murphy *et al.*, 1968). Such cholinesterase inhibitors arising by "lethal synthesis" require more sustained therapy than those which are toxic *per se* (Namba and Hiraki, 1958; Teitelman *et al.*, 1975). The active metabolite of parathion is paraoxon, a conversion mediated by microsomal enzymes in the liver. Parathion is not converted to paraoxon by enzymes in human skin; the local reactions at sites of skin absorption (see above) are probably due to active contaminants in commercial grades of parathion. Although paraoxon is slowly hydrolyzed by skin enzymes (Fredriksson *et al.*, 1961), it is many times more hazardous than parathion by this route of administration (Nabb *et al.*, 1966).

At least part of the wide spectrum of activity exhibited by organophosphorus insecticides relates to differences in their relative rates of metabolism to toxic forms and their rates of detoxication (Becker *et al.*, 1964; Dahm *et al.*, 1962; Gaines *et al.*, 1966). Similarly, interspecies differences in toxicity can be ascribed at least in part to metabolic differences (Murphy, 1971; Potter and O'Brien, 1964; Taylor *et al.*, 1965), which also sometimes lead to unexpected interactions when two pesticides are administered simultaneously (Black *et al.*, 1975; DuBois, 1958; Keplinger and Deichmann, 1967; Triolo and Coon, 1966). Tissue distribution may also explain some differences in the activity of various agents. For example, phosphoramides penetrate the central nerve system poorly (DuBois, 1971).

Whereas chronic exposure to parathion and related pesticides may cause persistent symptoms, survivors of acute, single-dose exposures usually recover rapidly. Indeed toxic signs and symptoms tend to disappear long before measured levels of cholinesterase have returned to normal. Long-term sequelae are rare but are described; they tend to be neuropsychiatric disorders, peripheral neuropathies, or myopathies.

Reversible but persistent neuropsychiatric sequelae have been ascribed to chronic exposure to parathion and similar compounds (Dille and Smith, 1964; Gershon and Shaw, 1961) or to unusually severe acute poisoning episodes. Disorientation, depersonalization, hallucinations, abnormal EEG patterns and subjective symptoms like those experienced during temporal lobe epileptic auras may persist many weeks (Brown, 1971; Leuzinger *et al.*, 1971). Increased levels of anxiety associated with lowered levels of plasma cholinesterase have been reported in exposed sprayers when compared to nonexposed farmers (Levin *et al.*, 1976). In one patient scopolamine had beneficial effects (Sidell, 1974).

Certain organophosphorus compounds, *e.g.*, isopestox, mipafox, *S,S,S*-tributyl phosphorotri-

thioate and diisopropylfluorophosphate, produce demyelination of the spinal cord and peripheral nerves in chickens in a manner similar to TRI-*ORTHO*-CRESYL PHOSPHATE (p. III-388). Long axons are primarily affected. The result may be a chronic syndrome in man (Namba *et al.*, 1971). The lesions are apparently unrelated to cholinesterase inhibition (Aldridge and Johnson, 1971) but are due to inhibition of a different protein, the so-called neurotoxic esterase. The latter is inappropriately named since neurotoxicity results from inhibition of this enzyme. Parathion and malathion are generally believed not to produce these lesions, but a polyneuritis has been reported at least once following an attempted suicide with parathion (Voiculescu *et al.*, 1971). In rats paraoxon produced a grouped skeletal muscle fiber necrosis (Wecker *et al.*, 1978). Perhaps Voiculescu's case above was a myopathy instead of a neuropathy.

Davignon *et al.* (1965) found a significantly higher incidence of leukopenia and neurologic signs (miosis, loss of reflexes, tremor, ataxia) among apple growers exposed to organophosphates than in a control population. Hyporeflexia, as measured by the isometric force generated by the achilles tendon reflex, was found in one group of chronically exposed workers (Rayner *et al.*, 1972). Durham *et al.* (1965), however, were unable to demonstrate significant impairment of mental alertness in an exposed population.

Treatment of parathion poisoning: Three major principles of therapy are artificial respiration when needed, the administration of atropine in large doses to control the visceral actions of the poison, including the cardiovascular effects and probably some of the central nervous actions (but not skeletal muscle paralysis), and the injection of pralidoxime chloride (2-PAM) or a related systemic anticholinesterase antidote (Durham and Hayes, 1962; Wilson and Ginsberg, 1955; Wilson, 1958). Most of the clinical experience has involved 2-PAM (Erdmann, 1960; Funckes, 1960; Grob and Johns, 1958a-d; Jacobziner and Raybin, 1961e; Namba and Hiraki, 1958; Quinby and Clappison, 1961; Quinby *et al.*, 1963; Read and Combes, 1961; Rosen, 1960).

2-PAM is effective when given with atropine against most organophosphorus anticholinesterase compounds of all types. Exceptions in which 2-PAM appeared to be ineffective or only marginally effective in animal screening tests include poisonings by dimefox, dimethoate, OMPA, phorate and tabun (Davies and Green, 1959; Done, 1961b). 2-PAM has been of benefit in human cases of phosdrin poisoning although the effects were said to be less dramatic than against parathion (Quinby, 1964). Clinical experience in malathion and tetraethylpyrophosphate poisonings shows considerable promise (Arnan, 1962;

Gitelson *et al.*, 1966; Quinby, 1964). It has also been employed with apparent success in human intoxications from Azodrin, demeton, diazinon, dichlorvos, disulfoton, EPN, guthion, isofluro-phate, methyl demeton, phosphamidon and others (*e.g.*, Davies *et al.*, 1967; Namba *et al.*, 1971).

Since the combination of 2-PAM and atropine is more effective than either drug alone, 2-PAM is never used without atropine, although the converse is sometimes true. Therapy with 2-PAM and other oxime enzyme reactivators (e.g., DAM) is relatively ineffective if delayed (Erdmann, 1960; Gough and Shellenberger, 1977–78). Neither 2-PAM nor 1,1'-trimethylenebis(4-formyl pyridinium bromide) dioxime (TMB-4) penetrates the central nervous system very well (Fleischer *et al.*, 1960), suggesting that their major antidotal activity is exerted peripherally. The issue, however, is not settled. Some animal tests indicate limited reactivation of brain cholinesterase by systemically administered 2-PAM (reviewed by Namba *et al.*, 1971). Furthermore, 2-PAM has produced prompt recovery from coma and convulsions in a few parathion-poisoned patients in whom the improvement could not be attributed to beneficial effects on respiration or blood pressure (Funckes, 1960; Namba *et al.*, 1971).

Clearly much remains to be learned about brain cholinesterase and the course and severity of the intoxication. For example, a *d*-hydropyridinium derivative of 2-PAM, pro-2-PAM, has been synthesized; it readily crosses the blood-brain barrier to reactivate brain acetylcholinesterase inhibited by organophosphates (Bodor *et al.*, 1975). Moreover, pro-2-PAM is much less acutely toxic to mice than 2-PAM. The two oximes are equally effective in reactivating blood cholinesterases, but surprisingly pro-2-PAM was less effective in protecting mice against death, suggesting that there is no correlation between brain acetylcholinesterase reactivation and survival (Boskovic *et al.*, 1980).

In the United States only 2-PAM is available as an approved drug, but in European countries considerable experience has accrued with toxogonin (obidoxim), a reactivator that is very closely related to TMB-4 (Knolle, 1970). A late disturbance in liver function has been ascribed to toxogonin (Barckow and Neuhaus, 1969; Boelcke and Kamphenkel, 1970; Teitelman *et al.*, 1975). Against *p*-nitrophenyl-di-*n*-butyl-phosphinate, a soman-like agent, TMB-4 was much more effective than 2-PAM (Harris *et al.*, 1979a).

Common errors in therapy include insufficient doses of atropine (Freeman and Epstein, 1955; Gordon and Frye, 1955; Grob and Harvey, 1953; Grob, 1956), failure to establish a patent airway, ineffective artificial respiration, and neglect of the patient after signs and symptoms have been

temporarily controlled. Any severely poisoned patient is in danger for at least 24 hours. One severely poisoned patient received 3.9 gm. of atropine over 16 days and 92 gm. of 2-PAM over 23 days before recovering fully (Warriner *et al.*, 1977). Although the antimuscarinic effects of atropine and atropine-like drugs are well known to be crucial in treating organophosphorus poisoning, it has been suggested that the anticonvulsant properties of these drugs become important in the management of very severe poisonings (Green *et al.*, 1977).

Exchange transfusion has been successfully performed in at least one critically ill patient (Boelcke *et al.*, 1970). Six of 11 patients who had consumed more than a lethal dose (5 to 45 gm.) of methyl parathion survived following extracorporeal hemodialysis, even though the largest amount removed from a single patient was only 390 mg. Clinical recovery was said to parallel the decreasing serum level of parathion (Gal *et al.*, 1970). Experimental studies in which the pesticides were added to blood *in vitro* indicated that nitrostigmine could not be dialyzed, but that demeton-*S*-methylsulfoxide and dimethoate were cleared at rates of 53 and 59 ml./minute, respectively. Hemoperfusion over coated charcoal was more efficient, with respective clearances of 84 and 88 ml./minute, and in this case nitrostigmine was also cleared at a rate of 59 ml./minute. The results with nitrostigmine were confirmed in a single poisoned patient (Okonek, 1976). In a patient who had consumed 100 to 150 gm. of parathion, the clearance by XAD-4 resin at a blood flow of 100 ml./minute was 83 ml./minute; this clearance was 40% higher than that with activated charcoal. Even so, the patient did not survive (Pentz and Brunn, 1979).

Both in Europe and in the United States phenothiazine tranquilizers have been employed for their antiemetic and calming effects in organophosphate poisonings. In at least one case that appeared near recovery, the administration of promazine on postexposure days 9 through 12 led to a recurrence of some signs of the original intoxication and eventual death in respiratory failure (Arterberry *et al.*, 1962). In laboratory animals chlorpromazine and promazine in single or repeated doses after parathion led to a 2-fold increase in mortality, but they did not alter the toxicity of phosdrin (Gaines, 1962). Several phenothiazine and nonphenothiazine antihistaminics are reversible and competitive inhibitors of pseudo-cholinesterase but not of rat brain acetylcholinesterase (Fernandez *et al.*, 1975).

In addition to phenothiazines, barbiturates, chlordiazepoxide, meprobamate and reserpine (but not alcohol) potentiated parathion toxicity in rats (Weiss and Orzel, 1967). This potentiation occurs only with organophosphates that have prominent actions in the central nervous system and may be related to central cholinergic processes (Proctor *et al.*, 1964). In treating human victims of parathion poisoning, these drugs are usually avoided.

In rhesus monkeys poisoned by soman, intravenous diazepam suppressed both the EEG manifestations of seizure activity and the overt convulsions. Atropine failed to control either, but the combination doubled the lethal dose of soman. All the animals were comatose for varying periods, but those that recovered were alert with some residual muscular weakness on the following day (Lipp, 1972). In conscious rabbits, however, diazepam compounded the respiratory depression produced by soman. Atropine alone prevented respiratory depression, but less effectively so when given with diazepam (Johnson and Wilcox, 1975). In fluostigmine poisoned rats, phenytoin, when given with atropine and an oxime reactivator, increased the LD_{50} significantly over that in animals given the latter two drugs only. Pentobarbital, diazepam, trimethadione and phensuximide prolonged life but did not prevent death (Grudzinska *et al.*, 1979).

Symptomatology:
1. Nausea is often the first symptom, followed by vomiting, abdominal cramps, diarrhea, and excessive salivation (sialorrhea). Hypothermia has been reported in animals and at least once in man as an early sign (Cupp *et al.*, 1975).
2. Headache, giddiness, vertigo, and weakness.
3. Rhinorrhea and a sensation of tightness in the chest are common in inhalation exposures.
4. Blurring or dimness of vision, miosis (with fixed pinpoint pupils), tearing, ciliary muscle spasm, loss of accommodation, and ocular pain. None of these eye effects is diagnostically dependable except in primary ocular exposures. Indeed, mydriasis is sometimes seen (Eitzman and Wolfson, 1967; Davies *et al.*, 1967), probably due to sympatho-adrenal discharge.
5. Bradycardia or tachycardia. Varying degrees of AV heart block are described, as well as atrial arrhythmias.
6. Loss of muscle coordination, slurring of speech, fasciculations and twitching of muscles (particularly of the tongue and eyelids), and generalized profound weakness.
7. Mental confusion, disorientation, and drowsiness.
8. Difficulty in breathing, excessive secretion of saliva and of respiratory tract mucus, oronasal frothing, cyanosis, pulmonary rales and rhonchi, and hypertension (presumably due to asphyxia).
9. Random jerky movements, incontinence, convulsions, and coma.
10. Death primarily due to respiratory arrest arising from failure of the respiratory center, paralysis of respiratory muscles, intense bronchoconstriction, or all three.

Treatment:
1. Atropinize the patient immediately. In an adult the usual dose is 1 to 4 mg. of the sulfate (or other salt) given intramuscularly or better intravenously (if there is no cyanosis). The maintenance of full atropinization may require 2-mg. doses at intervals of 10 to 60 minutes for many hours. Because of their high tolerance, poisoned patients commonly receive too little atropine, rarely too much. The need for more atropine can be recognized by the continuation or recurrence of those toxic symptoms described above; excessive salivation is a particularly useful criterion (but not eye signs). It is said that atropine is dangerous in the presence of anoxia and that cyanosis should be corrected before atropinization (Hayes, 1965; Holmstedt, 1959), but this is not always possible.
2. Relieve upper airway obstruction (see p. IV-2). Mucus and other respiratory tract secretions may have to be aspirated constantly (p. IV-4). Endotracheal intubation or tracheotomy may become necessary (see p. IV-4).
3. In the presence of established symptoms administer 2-PAM (2-pyridine aldoxime methochloride, pralidoxime chloride, Protopam chloride). The initial adult dose is 1 to 2 gm., preferably as an intravenous infusion in 100 ml. saline over a period of 15 to 30 minutes. For a more rapid effect it can be injected i.v. as a 5% solution in water over a period of not less than 5 minutes. In children the initial dose should be 20 to 40 mg./kg. By reactivating parathion-poisoned cholinesterase, these oximes may cause a prompt restoration of skeletal muscle strength. If weakness persists, maintenance doses may be given periodically by intramuscular or subcutaneous routes or continuously by intravenous infusion (Done, 1961b). For example, a second dose of 1 to 2 gm. may be administered after 1 hour, as indicated. Oximes and atropine have entirely different modes of action and do not interfere with each other's antidotal activity. Therefore both should be used, or atropine alone may suffice in milder poisonings. See Section II (pralidoxime chloride) for information about the clinical toxicity of 2-PAM (see also Jager and Stagg, 1958), but with careful administration this drug is usually well tolerated (Quinby, 1964).

4. Give oxygen and artificial ventilation as needed (see p. IV-7). In addition to upper tract obstruction, pulmonary edema may occur (Quinby and Clappison, 1961) and may require treatment (p. IV-14).
5. Gastric lavage with 5% sodium bicarbonate solution may be warranted after the ingestion of parathion, if spontaneous vomiting is not prompt and profuse.
6. Wash any contaminated areas of skin with soap and water or still better with 95% ethyl alcohol (Fredricksson, 1961). Irrigate the eyes with water or saline solution.
7. Administer cautiously by the intravenous route isotonic saline to correct dehydration and electrolyte imbalances. Give sodium bicarbonate for metabolic acidosis. See pp. IV-64–67, 69–73.
8. Never give theophylline, or theophylline-ethylenediamine (aminophylline). Avoid central depressant drugs such as morphine, barbiturates, reserpine, phenothiazines and other tranquilizers of all sorts. Rarely diazepam may be justified in the management of the convulsive phase, but the latter can generally be prevented or treated by adequate atropinization and the correction of asphyxia.
9. Keep the patient under constant observation for a period of 24 to 36 hours. Symptoms may persist for a month (Kunst et al., 1970).
10. Hemoperfusion may be worthwhile after massive exposures, but more experience is required before its role can be properly evaluated.

Laboratory:

1. Repeated blood analyses for cholinesterase activity are valuable in establishing the diagnosis, particularly if the pre-exposure level is known. The test can now be done in the laboratories of most general hospitals. Atropine does not interfere with this test. The measurement of the urinary excretion of p-nitrophenol (a metabolite common to parathion, chlorthion and EPN), however, may be a more sensitive index of exposure intensity than plasma or red cell cholinesterase levels (Arterberry et al., 1961; Roan et al., 1969). Tissue levels of organophosphorus pesticides have also been measured in fatal cases (Fazekas and Rengei, 1967; Lores et al., 1978).
2. ECG records are useful, although cardiac blocks rarely occur in clinical poisonings in the absence of asphyxia.
3. Severe hypoglycemia occurred in a fatally poisoned child. Both parathion and methacholine produce decreases in blood glucose levels in mice, apparently due to hyperinsulinemia from direct stimulation of islet secretion (Hruban et al., 1963). Malathion intoxication, however, produced hyperglycemia in a mother and son (Meller et al., 1981).

References:

Aldridge, W. N.; Johnson, M. K. Side effects of organophosphorus compounds: Delayed neurotoxicity. Bull. W. H. O. 44:259-263, 1971.

Andersen, A. H.; Jersild, T. Poisoning by diethylparanitrophenylthiophosphate. Acta Pharmacol. Toxicol. 5:129-134, 1949.

Anderson, L. S.; Warner, D. L.; Parker, J. E.; Bluman, N.; Page, B. D. Parathion poisoning from flannelette sheets. Can. Med. Assoc. J. 92:809-813, 1965.

Annis, J. W.; Williams, J. W. Change in electrolytes in a case of parathion poisoning. J. A. M. A. 152:594-596, 1953.

Arnan, A. Accidental poisoning from agricultural pesticides. Bull. W. H. O. 26:109-120, 1962.

Arterberry, J. D.; Bonifaci, R. W.; Nash, E. W.; Quinby, G. E. Potentiation of phosphorus insecticides by phenothiazine derivatives. J. A. M. A. 182:848-850, 1962.

Arterberry, J. D.; Durham, W. F.; Elliott, J. W.; Wolfe, H. R. Exposure to parathion. Arch. Environ. Health 3:476-485, 1961.

Barckow, D.; Neuhaus, G. Zur Behandlung der schweren Parathion-(E605)-Vergiftung mit dem Cholinesterase-reaktivator Obidoxim (Toxogonin). Arch. Toxikol. 24:133-146, 1969.

Batchelor, G. S.; Walker, K. C. Health hazards involved in use of parathion in fruit orchards of north central Washington. Arch. Ind. Hyg. Occup. Med. 10:522-529, 1954.

Becker, E. L.; Punte, C. L.; Barbaro, J. F. Acute toxicity of alkyl and phenylalkylphosphonates in the guinea pig and rabbit in relation to their anticholinesterase activity and their enzymatic inactivation. Biochem. Pharmacol. 13:1229-1237, 1964.

Bernstein, S.; Gould, J. H. Parathion poisoning in children. J. Med. Soc. N. J. 65:199-203, 1968.

Black, W. D.; Talbot, R. B.; Wade, A. E. A study of the effect of ovex on parathion and paraoxon toxicity in rats. Toxicol. Appl. Pharmacol. 33:393-400, 1975.

Bledsoe, F. H.; Seymour, E. Q. Acute pulmonary edema associated with parathion poisoning. Radiology 103:53-56, 1972.

Bodor, N.; Shek, E.; Higuchi, T. Delivery of a quaternary pyridinium salt across the blood-brain barrier by its dihydropyridine derivative. Science 190:155-156, 1975.

Boelcke, G.; Butigan, N.; Davar, H.; Erdmann, W. D.; Gaaz, J. W.; Nenner, M. Neue Erfahrungen bei der toxikologisch kontrollierten Therapie einer ungewohnlich schweren Vergiftung mit Nitrostigmin (E 605 forte). Dtsch. Med. Wochenschr. 95:2516-2521, 1970.

Boelcke, G.; Kamphenkel, L. Der Einfluss der Nitrostigmin-Vergiftung und der spezifischen Antidot-Therapie mit Obidoxim auf die Bilirubin-Clearance und den Gallefluss der Ratte. Arch. Toxicol. 26:210-219, 1970.

Boskovic, B.; Tadic, V.; Kasic, R. Reactivating and protective effects of pro-2-PAM in mice poisoned with paraoxon. Toxicol. Appl. Pharmacol. 55:32-36, 1980.

Brodeur, J.; DuBois, K. D. Studies on the mechanism of acquired tolerance by rats to O,O-diethyl S-2-(ethylthio)ethyl phosphorodithioate (Di-Syston). Arch. Int. Pharmacodyn. Ther. 149:560-570, 1964.

Brown, H. W. Electroencephalographic changes and disturbance of brain function following human organophosphate exposure. Northwest. Med. 70:845-846, 1971.

Casida, J. E. Esterase inhibitors as pesticides. Science 146:1011-1017, 1964.

Cupp, C. M.; Kleiber, G.; Reigart, R.; Sandifer, S. H. Hypothermia in organophosphate poisoning and response to PAM. J. S. C. Med. Assoc. 71:166-168, 1975.

Dahm, P. A.; Kopecky, B. E.; Walker, C. B. Activation of organophosphorus insecticides by rat liver microsomes. Toxicol. Appl. Pharmacol. 4:683-696, 1962.

Davies, D. R.; Green, A. L. The chemotherapy of poisoning by organophosphate anticholinesterases. Br. J. Ind. Med. 16:128, 1959.

Davies, J. E.; Davis, J. H.; Frazier, D. E.; Mann, J. B.; Reich, G. A.; Tocci, P. M. Disturbances of metabolism in organophosphate poisoning. Ind. Med. Surg. 36:58-62, 1967.

Davignon, L. F.; St. -Pierre, J.; Charest, G.; Tourangeau, F. J. A study of the chronic effects of insecticides in man. Can. Med. Assoc. J. 92:597-602, 1965.

De Ong, E. R. Chemistry and Uses of Pesticides, 2nd ed. Reinhold Publishing Corp., New York, 1956.

Diggory, H. J. P.; Landrigan, P. J.; Latimer, K. P.; Ellington, A. C.; Kimbrough, R. D.; Liddle, J. A.; Cline, R. E.; Smrek, A. L. Fatal parathion poisoning caused by contamination of flour in international commerce. Am J. Epidemiol. 106:145-153, 1977.

Dille, J. R.; Smith, P. W. Central nervous system effects of chronic exposure to organophosphate insecticides. Aerosp. Med. 35:474-478, 1964.

Dixon, E. M. Dilatation of the pupils in parathion poisoning. J. A. M. A. 163:444-445, 1957.

Done, A. K. Clinical pharmacology of systemic antidotes. Clin. Pharmacol. Ther. 2:750-793, 1961b.

DuBois, K. P. Potentiation of the toxicity of insecticidal organic phosphates. Arch. Ind. Health 18:488-496, 1958.

DuBois, K. P. The toxicity of organophosphorus compounds to mammals. Bull. W. H. O. 44:233-240, 1971.

DuBois, K. P.; Coon, J. M. Toxicology of organic phosphorus-containing insecticides to mammals. Arch. Ind. Hyg. Occup. Med. 6:9-13, 1952.

DuBois, K. P.; Doull, J.; Salerno, P. R.; Coon, J. M. Studies on the toxicity and mechanism of action of p-nitrophenyldiethyl-thiophosphate (parathion). J. Pharmacol. Exp. Ther. 95:79-92, 1949.

Durham, W. F.; Hayes, W. J., Jr. Organic phosphorus poisoning and its therapy. Arch. Environ. Health 5:21-47, 1962.

Durham, W. F.; Wolfe, H. R.; Quinby, G. E. Organophosphorus insecticides and mental alertness. Arch. Environ. Health 10:55-66, 1965.

Eitzman, D. V.; Wolfson, S. L. Acute parathion poisoning in children. Am. J. Dis. Child. 114:397-400, 1967.

Erdmann, W. D. Parathion (E605) poisoning treated with the antidote PAM (pyridine-2-aldoxime methiodide). Ger. Med. Mon. 5:304-311, 1960.

Fazekas, I. G.; Rengei, B. Methylparathion-gehalt menschlicher Organe nach todlichen "Wofatox" Vergiftungen. Arch. Toxikol. 22:381-386, 1967.

Fernandez, G.; Diaz Gomez, M. I.; Castro, J. A. Cholinesterase inhibition by phenothiazine and nonphenothiazine antihistaminics: Analysis of its postulated role in synergizing organophosphate toxicity. Toxicol. Appl. Pharmacol. 31:179-190, 1975.

Fleisher, J. H.; Hansa, J.; Killos, P. J.; Harrison, C. S. Effects of 1,1-trimethylenebis(4-formylpyridinium bromide) dioxime (TMB-4) on cholinesterase activity and neuromuscular block following poisoning wiith sarin and DFP. J. Pharmacol. Exp. Ther. 130:461-468, 1960.

Fredricksson, T. Percutaneous absorption of parathion and paraoxon. Arch. Environ. Health 3:185-188, 1961.

Fredricksson, T.; Farrior, W. L., Jr.; Witter, R. F. Studies on the percutaneous absorption of parathion and paraoxon. Acta Derm. Venereol. 41:335-343, 1961.

Freeman, G. F.; Epstein, M. A. Therapeutic factors in survival after lethal cholinesterase inhibition by phosphorus insecticides. N. Engl. J. Med. 253:266-270, 1955.

Funckes, A. J. Treatment of severe poisoning with 2-pyridine aldoxime methiodide (2-PAM). Arch. Environ. Health 1:404-406, 1960.

Funckes, A. J.; Hayes, G. R.; Hartwell, W. V. Urinary excretion of paranitrophenol by volunteers following dermal exposure to parathion at different ambient temperatures. J. Agric. Food Chem. 11:455-457, 1963.

Gaines, T. B. Poisoning by organic phosphorus pesticides potentiated by phenothiazine derivatives. Science 138:1260-1261, 1962.

Gaines, T. B.; Hayes, W. J., Jr.; Linder, R. E. Liver metabolism

of anticholinesterase compounds in live rats: Relation to toxicity. Nature 209:88-89, 1966.

Gal, G.; Simon, L.; Rengei, B.; Mindszentry, L.; Ember, M. Hemodialysis in the treatment of poisoning by methyl parathion. Res. Commun. Chem. Pathol. Pharmacol. 1:553-560, 1970.

Ganelin, R. S.; Mail, G. A.; Cueto, C., Jr. Hazards of equipment contaminated with parathion. Arch. Environ. Health 8:826-828, 1964.

Gershon, S.; Shaw, F. H. Psychiatric sequelae of chronic exposure to organophosphorus insecticides. Lancet 1:1371-1374, 1961.

Gilsenan, L. A fatal case of parathion poisoning. Med. J. Aust. 2:251, 1957.

Gitelson, S.; Aladjemoff, L.; Ben-Hador, S.; Katznelson, R. Poisoning by a malathion-xylene mixture. J. A. M. A. 197:819-821, 1966.

Gordon, A. S.; Frye, C. W. Large doses of atropine, low toxicity and effectiveness in anticholinesterase intoxication. J. A. M. A. 159:1181-1184, 1955.

Gough, B. J.; Shellenberger, T. E. In vivo inhibition of rabbit whole blood cholinesterase with organophosphate inhibitors and reactivation with oximes. Drug Chem. Toxicol. 1:25-43, 1977-78.

Green, D. M.; Muir, A. W.; Stratton, J. A.; Inch, T. D. Dual mechanism of the antidotal action of atropine-like drugs in poisoning by organophosphorous anti-cholinesterases. J. Pharm. Pharmacol. 29:62-64, 1977.

Grob, D. Manifestations and treatment of poisoning due to nerve gas and other organic phosphate anticholinesterase compounds. Arch. Intern. Med. 98:221-239, 1956.

Grob, D.; Garlick, W. L.; Merrill, G. C.; Fremuth, H. C. Death due to parathion, an anticholinesterase insecticide. Ann. Intern. Med. 31:899-904, 1949.

Grob, D.; Harvey, A. M. The effects and treatment of nerve gas poisoning. Am. J. Med. 14:52-63, 1953.

Grob, D.; Johns, R. J. Treatment of anticholinesterase intoxication with oximes, use in normal subjects and in patients with myasthenia gravis. J. A. M. A. 166:1855-1858, 1958a.

Grob, D.; Johns, R. J. Use of oximes in the treatment of intoxication by anticholinesterase compounds in normal subjects. Am. J. Med. 24:497-511, 1958b.

Grob, D.; Johns, R. J. Use of oximes in the treatment of intoxication by anticholinesterase compounds in patients with myasthenia gravis. Am. J. Med. 24:512-518, 1958c.

Grob, D.; Johns, R. J. Treatment of anticholinesterase intoxication with oximes. Neurology 8:897-902, 1958d.

Grudzinska, E.; Gidynska, T.; Rump, S. Therapeutic value of anticonvulsant drugs in poisoning with an organophosphate. Arch. Int. Pharmacodyn. Ther. 238:344-350, 1979.

Hamblin, D. O.; Golz, H. H. Parathion poisoning - a brief review. Ind. Med. Surg. 24:65-72, 1955.

Harris, L. W.; Stitcher, D. L.; Heyl, W. C.; Lieske, C. N.; Lowe, J. R.; Clark, J. H.; Broomfield, C. A. The effects of atropine-oxime therapy in cholinesterase activity and survival of animals intoxicated with p-nitrophenyl di-n-butylphosphinate. Toxicol. Appl. Pharmacol. 49:23-29, 1979a.

Hartwell, W. V.; Hayes, G. R., Jr.; Funckes, A. J. Respiratory exposure of volunteers to parathion. Arch. Environ. Health 8:820-825, 1964.

Hayes, W. J., Jr. Clinical Handbook on Economic Poisons. USPHS Publication No. 476. U. S. Government Printing Office, Washington, D. C., 1963.

Hayes, W. J., Jr. Parathion poisoning and its treatment. J. A. M. A. 192:49-50, 1965.

Heath, D. F. Organophosphorus Poisons, Anticholinesterases and Related Compounds. Pergamon Press, New York, 1961.

Hobbinger, F. Chemical reactivation of phosphorylated human and bovine true cholinesterases. Br. J. Pharmacol. 11:295-303, 1956.

Holmstedt, B. Pharmacology of organophosphorus cholinesterase inhibitors. Pharmacol. Rev. 11:567-688, 1959.

Hruban, Z.; Schulman, S.; Warner, N. E.; DuBois, K. P.; Bunnag, S.; Bunnag, S. C. Hypoglycemia resulting from insecticide poisoning. J. A. M. A. 184:590-593, 1963.

Introna, F. Acute poisoning by percutaneous absorption of

E605. Riv. Infort. Mal. Prof. *46*:1222–1231, 1959.

Jacobziner, H.; Raybin, H. W. Parathion poisoning successfully treated with 2-PAM (pralidoxime chloride). N. Engl. J. Med. *265*:436–437, 1961e.

Jager, B. V.; Stagg, G. N. Toxicity of diacetyl monoxime and of pyridine-2-aldoxime methiodide in man. Bull. Johns Hopkins Hosp. *102*:203, 1958.

Johnson, D. D.; Wilcox, W. C. Studies on the mechanism of the protective and antidotal actions of diazepam in organophosphate poisoning. Europ. J. Pharmacol. *34*:127–132, 1975.

Johnston, J. M. Parathion poisoning in children. J. Pediatr. *42*:286–291, 1953.

Kanagaratnam, K.; Boon, W. H.; Hoh, T. K. Parathion poisoning from contaminated barley. Lancet *1*:538–542, 1960.

Keplinger, M. L.; Deichmann, W. B. Acute toxicity of combinations of pesticides. Toxicol. Appl. Pharmacol. *10*:586–595, 1967.

Klugman, H. B. Parathion poisoning. S. Afr. Med. J. *33*:899–901, 1959.

Knolle, J. Die klinische Bedeutung der Cholinesterasenbestimmung im Blut bei akuten Intoxikationen mit phosphororganischen Insecticiden. Klin. Wochenschr. *48*:1157–1168, 1970.

Koelle, G. B.; Gilman, A. Anticholinesterase drugs. J. Pharmacol. Exp. Ther. *95*:166–216, 1949.

Kunst, H.; Collard, W.; Heitmann, R.; Mobius, W.; Ritter, U. Uber die Behandlung von Alkylphosphatvergiftung. Dtsch. Med. Wochenschr. *95*:2513–2516, 1970.

Leuzinger, S.; Pasi, A.; Dolder, R. Synoptische Auswertung von 536 Alkylphosphatvergiftungen. Schweiz. Med. Wochenschr. *101*:563–570, 1971.

Levin, H. S.; Rodnitzky, R. L.; Mick, D. L. Anxiety associated with exposure to organophosphate compounds. Arch. Gen. Psychiat. *33*:225–228, 1976.

Lipp, J. A. Effect of diazepam upon soman-induced seizure activity and convulsions. Electroenceph. Clin. Neurophysiol. *32*:557–560, 1972.

Lores, E. M.; Bradway, D. E.; Moseman, R. F. Organophosphorous pesticide poisonings in humans: determination of residues and metabolites in tissues and urine. Arch. Environ. Health *33*:270–276, 1978.

Mackey, R. W. Parathion poisoning in a young infant. Am. J. Dis. Child. *3*:321–323, 1966.

Meller, D.; Fraser, I.; Kryger, M. Hyperglycemia in anticholinesterase poisoning. Can. Med. Assoc. J. *124*:745–747, 1981.

Milby, T. H.; Ottoboni, F.; Mitchell, H. W. Parathion residue poisoning among orchard workers. J. A. M. A. *189*:351–356, 1964.

Murphy, S. D. Mechanisms of pesticide interactions in vertebrates. Residue Rev. *25*:201–221, 1971.

Murphy, S. D.; Lauwerys, R. R.; Cheever, K. L. Comparative anticholinesterase action of organophosphorus insecticides in vertebrates. Toxicol. Appl. Pharmacol. *12*:22–35, 1968.

Nabb, D. P.; Stein, W. J.; Hayes, W. J., Jr. Rate of skin absorption of parathion and paraoxon. Arch. Environ. Health *12*:501–505, 1966.

Namba, T.; Hiraki, K. PAM (pyridine-2-aldoxime methiodide) therapy for alkylphosphate poisoning. J. A. M. A. *166*:1834–1839, 1958.

Namba, T.; Nolte, C. T.; Jackrel, J.; Grob, D. Poisoning due to organophosphate insecticides, acute and chronic manifestations. Am. J. Med. *50*:475–492, 1971.

O'Brien, R. D. *Toxic Phosphorus Esters.* Academic Press, Inc., New York, 1960.

Okonek, S. Probable progress in therapy of organophosphate poisoning—extracorporeal hemodialysis and hemoperfusion. Arch. Toxicol. *35*:221–227, 1976.

Payne, J. R.; Robinson, B. R. Pyridine-2-aldoxime methiodide, a valuable agent for phosphate poisoning. Calif. Med. *96*:330–334, 1962.

Pentz, R.; Brunn, J. Hemoperfusion with XAD-4 resin in the treatment of a severe parathion intoxication. Arch. Toxicol. *42*:311–315, 1979.

Petty, C. S. Organic phosphate insecticide poisoning: An agricultural occupational hazard. J. La. St. Med. Soc. *109*:158–164, 1957.

Potter, J. L.; O'Brien, R. D. Parathion activation by livers of aquatic and terrestial vertebrates. Science *144*:55–56, 1964.

Prinz, H. J. Eine schwere percutane Vergiftung mit Parathion (E605). Arch. Toxikol. *25*:318–328, 1969.

Proctor, C. D.; Ridlon, S. A.; Fudema, J. J.; Prabhu, V. G. Extension of tranquilizer action by anticholinesterases. Toxicol. Appl. Pharmacol. *6*:1–8, 1964.

Quinby, G. E. Further therapeutic experience with pralidoximes in organic phosphorus poisoning. J. A. M. A. *187*:202–206, 1964.

Quinby, G. E.; Clappison, G. B. Parathion poisoning, a near-fatal pediatric case treated with pyridine aldoxime methiodide (2-PAM). Arch. Environ. Health *3*:538–543, 1961.

Quinby, G. E.; Lemmon, A. B. Parathion residues as a cause of poisoning in crop workers. J. A. M. A. *166*:740–746, 1958.

Quinby, G. E.; Loomis, T. A.; Brown, H. W. Oral occupational parathion poisoning treated with 2-PAM iodide (2-pyridine aldoxime methiodide). N. Engl. J. Med. *268*:639–643, 1963.

Rayner, M. D.; Popper, J. S.; Carvalho, E. W.; Hurov, R. Hyporeflexia in workers chronically exposed to organophosphate insecticides. Res. Commun. Chem. Pathol. Pharmacol. *4*:595–606, 1972.

Read, W. T.; Combes, M. A. A new specific antidote for organic phosphate ester poisoning. Pediatrics *28*:950–955, 1961.

Reichert, E. R.; Klemmer, H. W.; Haley, T. J. A note on dermal poisoning from Mevinphos and parathion. Clin. Toxicol. *12*:33–35, 1978.

Roan, C. C.; Morgan, D. P.; Cook, N.; Paschal, E. H. Blood cholinesterases, serum parathion concentrations and urine p-nitrophenol concentrations in exposed individuals. Bull. Environ. Contam. Toxicol. *4*:362–369, 1969.

Rosen, F. S. Toxic hazards, parathion. N. Engl. J. Med. *262*:1243–1244, 1960.

Sidell, F. R. Soman and sarin; clinical manifestations and treatment of accidental poisoning by organophosphates. Clin. Toxicol. *7*:1–17, 1974.

Taylor, W. J. R.; Kalow, W.; Sellers, E. A. Poisoning with organophosphorus insecticides. Can. Med. Assoc. J. *93*:966–970, 1965.

Teitelman, U.; Adler, M.; Levy, I.; Dikstein, S. Treatment of massive poisoning by the organophosphate pesticide methidathion. Clin. Toxicol. *8*:277–282, 1975.

Triolo, A. J.; Coon, J. M. The protective effect of aldrin against the toxicity of organophosphate anticholinesterases. J. Pharmacol. Exp. Ther. *154*:613–623, 1966.

Velhanayagam, A. V. A. "Folidel" (parathion) poisoning. Br. Med. J. *2*:986–987, 1962.

Voiculescu, V.; Gheorghiu, M.; Cioran, C.; Dumitrescu, C.; Plaiasu, D. Polyneuritis due to organophosphate insecticide (parathion and dipterex) poisoning. Neurol. Psychiatr. Neurochir. *16*:535–539, 1971.

Warren, M. C.; Conrad, J. P., Jr.; Bocian, J. J.; Hayes, M. Clothing-borne epidemic. Organic phosphate poisoning in children. J. A. M. A. *184*:266–268, 1963.

Warriner, R. A.; Nies, A. S.; Hayes, W. J. Severe organophosphate poisoning complicated by alcohol and turpentine ingestion. Arch. Environ. Health *32*:203–205,1977.

Wecker, L.; Kiauta, T.; Dettbarn, W. D. Relationship between acetylcholinesterase inhibition and the development of a myopthy. J. Pharmacol. Exp. Ther. *206*:97–104, 1978.

Weiss, L. R.; Orzel, R. A. Enhancement of toxicity of anticholinesterases by central depressant drugs in rats. Toxicol. Appl. Pharmacol. *10*:334–339, 1967.

Wilson, I. B. A specific antidote for nerve gas and insecticide (alkylphosphate) intoxication. Neurology *8* (Suppl. No. 1):41–43, 1958.

Wilson, I. B.; Ginsberg, S. A powerful reactivator of alkylphosphate-inhibited acetylcholinesterase. Biochim. Biophys. Acta *18*:168–174, 1955.

Wishahi, A.; Aboul-Dahab, Y. W.; Sherif, Y.; El-Darawg, Z. Parathion poisoning (phosphorus compound). A report on 22 children in an outbreak. Arch. Pediatr. *75*:387–396, 1958.

Woolley, D. E. Some aspects of the neurophysiological basis of insecticide action. Fed. Proc. *35*:2610–2617, 1976.

PHENOL

Phenol (carbolic acid) and cresols are marketed in many forms and sold widely for their antiseptic activity. They are often used in homes and on farms as disinfectants, barn deodorants, sanitizers, etc. (see also Section VI, General Formulations). Phenol is available as pure crystals or as a liquefied preparation (88% C_6H_5OH with about 10% water). Dilute phenol solutions (1 to 2%) are used medicinally as antipruritic preparations for the skin. Their repeated use over large skin areas or on particularly moist areas (axillary region, groin, feet) should be avoided (Calvery, 1942; Cronin and Brauer, 1949). Camphor and other substances with similar physicochemical properties interact with phenol both to reduce its corrosive properties and to impede percutaneous absorption. However, severe local necrotic damage (Calvery, 1942; Hubler, 1943) and fatal systemic poisoning (Miller, 1942) have followed the use of this combination, which was once endorsed for "athlete's foot."

Lord Lister in 1865 selected phenol for trial in the prevention and therapy of sepsis. Phenolic preparations were used to cleanse skin areas prior to surgery, which was often conducted in rooms disinfected by carbolic acid sprays. Phenol compresses were employed as wound dressings. Whereas this use of phenol demonstrated the feasibility of asepsis, the literature of this era is rich with allusions to both acute and chronic phenol poisonings resulting from these practices. Phenol is now recognized as a general protoplasmic poison which is toxic to all cells.

An early antiseptic preparation of phenol known as "lysol" was obtained by boiling a mixture of heavy tar oils with vegetable oils in the presence of a strong alkali such as potassium or sodium hydroxide. Although the phenol concentration of "lysol" was 8- to 10-fold less than pure or liquefied phenol, ingestion episodes still resulted in typical signs of phenol poisoning. The clinical picture, however, was often complicated by the more intense corrosive activity of the added alkali (see also LYE, p. III-245). During the 1930s "lysol" was a frequent choice in attempted suicides. This mixture, of course, must not be confused in its composition or toxicity with the brand name product described in Section V.

Toxicology: Although many sources indicate that phenolic preparations were responsible for an astonishing number of poisonings in years past (Hodge and Scharfe, 1937; Webster, 1930; Witthaus, 1911), little of this potential wealth of information seems to have found its way into the English language medical literature. Perhaps in part because so few modern reports of phenol poisoning exist, the mechanisms by which phenol exerts its characteristic effects are only poorly understood. The case reports selected for discussion below span more than a half-century of medical literature. They illustrate features that older authorities (*e.g.*, Reese, 1874; von Oettingen, 1949; Webster, 1930; Witthaus, 1911) recognized as pathognomonic of phenol poisoning, as well as aspects that were unusual and even bizarre.

Phenol and the three isomeric cresols produce identical symptoms in poisoned animals and all exhibit toxicity of about the same magnitude (Deichmann and Keplinger, 1962). The oral mean lethal dose (LD_{50}) in rats is 530 mg./kg.; similar values have been reported in the dog, rabbit, and monkey. No reliable estimates of the mean lethal dose in man can be offered. Certainly 1 gm. by mouth is a dangerous dose, even though more than one hundred times this amount has been survived (Webster, 1930; Witthaus, 1911). Much evidence exists to suggest that in man phenol may be considerably less toxic by mouth than by absorption from wounds, body cavities or even intact unbroken skin. The safest viewpoint is to regard any amount of phenol as dangerous.

After ingestion, white or brownish stains and areas of necrosis may be noted about the face, mouth and esophagus. As with most caustic solutions, concentration appears to be more critical than volume with respect to the local response. Ten percent solutions of phenol regularly produce corrosion, and occasionally skin necrosis is seen with solutions as dilute as 1% (Deichmann and Keplinger, 1962). The corrosive damage following phenol or even "lysol" ingestion, however, is much milder than that following strong alkali or mineral acids. Moreover, the local effects can be strongly mitigated by the presence of any vehicle with an affinity for phenol. In 177 cases of "lysol" ingestion only 11 exhibited ulcerative esophagitis (Cardona and Daly, 1964). Hodge and Scharfe (1937) have commented on the rarity of late esophageal strictures, and Turner (as cited by Schulenburg, 1941) may have reported the only existing example of pyloric stenosis without esophageal involvement. Laryngeal edema and pulmonary edema as a result of aspiration have also been recognized (Bethune and Court, 1954).

Sometimes there is only mild pain or discomfort because phenol demyelinates or otherwise destroys many types of nerve fibers (Berry and Olszewski, 1963). Solutions of phenol (6%) in glycerine are sometimes employed in medical practice to produce nerve blocks. The spread of phenol beyond the intended site (stellate ganglion) resulted in infarction of the cervical cord with extensive paralysis in one patient and neurolysis of the cervical posterior roots with respiratory arrest in another (Superville-Sovak et al., 1975).

As judged by animal studies (Deichmann and Keplinger, 1962), absorption from the bowel begins promptly, but appreciable amounts may remain in the stomach for some hours. If this pattern is also true of man, gastric lavage would appear to be generally worthwhile and relatively safe because of the low incidence of corrosive damage. In 27 cases of phenol poisoning by mouth, a 10% ethanol solution was judged to offer no advantage over water as a lavage fluid. Indeed, the symptoms appeared to be more severe when phenol and alcohol were ingested concomitantly (Clarke and Brown, 1906).

Irrespective of the route of exposure there can be no doubt that the major hazard of phenol poisoning stems from its systemic effects. Severe and fatal phenol poisonings have occurred after such superficial exposure as to suggest hypersensitivity or idiosyncrasy. Lucas and Lane (1895) treated hundreds of patients with 5% carbolic acid compresses before noting collapse in two young patients. Brown (1895) reported a case of unconsciousness within 5 minutes of rubbing a child's head with carbolic acid. In many cases profound coma occurred in less than 30 minutes, demonstrating the remarkable speed with which phenol can be absorbed through human skin (Bethune and Court, 1954; Evans, 1952; McCord and Munster, 1924; Miller, 1942; Smith, 1922; Turtle and Dolan, 1922). Again, in many of these cases the exposure to phenol would appear to have been negligible by the standards of medical practice of that day.

Either as a solution or as a vapor, phenol penetrates intact skin rapidly. Phenol vapors are also well absorbed by the lungs (Piotrowski, 1971). Although the onset of phenol poisoning can be surprisingly abrupt, the dangerous phase of the intoxication is usually complete in 24 hours.

An initial phase of central nervous stimulation, seen regularly in poisoned animals (Deichmann and Keplinger, 1962; Witthaus, 1911) and sometimes in children (Webster, 1930), may be only fleeting or altogether absent in human adults. In mice, for example, phenol was the only monosubstituted benzene in a large series of compounds to produce convulsions regularly. Of the dihydroxybenzenes, resorcinol (meta) and quinol (hydroquinone) (para) were similar to phenol in convulsant activity whereas catechol (ortho) was more potent by a factor of about 2.5 (Angel and Rogers, 1972).

A profound fulminating central nervous depression with coma, hypothermia, loss of vasoconstrictor tone, cardiac depression and respiratory arrest are the more common manifestations of systemic phenol poisoning in man. However, stertorous breathing, mucous rales, froth at the mouth and nose and frank pulmonary edema are mentioned so frequently that one hesitates to attribute these pulmonary complications entirely to aspiration pneumonitis (Bennett et al., 1950; Bethune and Court, 1954; Clarke and Brown, 1906; Hartigan, 1900; Lucas and Lane, 1895; Miller, 1942; Reese, 1874; Semple, 1925; Smith, 1922; Stajduhar-Caric, 1968; Turtle and Dolan, 1922). Indeed, in many of the above cases the original contact with phenol was cutaneous rather than by mouth. If phenol has a propensity to produce pulmonary edema, this phenomenon does not seem to be generally recognized, and its mechanism is not at all clear.

In addition to respiratory deaths of both central and pulmonary origin and cardiac deaths from hypovolemic shock or myocardial depression (Anderson, 1869), renal complications are seen frequently and sometimes may progress to acute failure (Brown, 1895; Turtle and Dolan, 1922; Vance, 1945). Ventricular arrhythmias appear to be a rare complication (Haddad et al., 1979). A slight elevation of serum bilirubin has been reported once (Evans, 1952), but hepatic damage does not appear to be a feature of acute phenol poisoning. Hyperbilirubinemia in newborns has been associated with exposure to mixtures of phenols used as disinfectants and detergents (Needham et al., 1980; Wysowski et al., 1978). That the bilirubin may have been due to accelerated red cell destruction rather than hepatic damage is suggested by the fact that several phenolic compounds have been implicated as causes of methemoglobinemia or Heinz body hemolytic anemia or both (Fertman and Fertman, 1955; Kurechi et al., 1980; Lebowitz, 1980; Smith and Olson, 1973).

Very little is known about the metabolic effects of phenol. It does not appear to share the ability of many of its derivatives, such as DINITROPHENOL (p. III-156) or pentachlorophenol, to uncouple oxidative phosphorylation. At least, hypermetabolism has not been recognized, and hypothermia rather than hyperpyrexia is usually described, although the latter is not unknown (Witthaus, 1911). Sodium bicarbonate by mouth or vein has been recommended as therapy (Gibbs, 1931), and on at least two occasions it effected rather dramatic relief, particularly of the respiratory symptoms (Bennett et al., 1950; Smith, 1922). The results of meager acid-base studies (Bennett et al., 1950) are not consistent, however, with an acidosis of severe enough proportions to account for the moribund status of some patients. Perhaps confusion stems from the latency of the metabolic derangements. In one woman who ingested 1 oz. of 89% phenol, only a mild acidosis was present after 4 hours, but at 18 hours her arterial pH was down to 7.25. During the first 24 hours she appeared to have a mixed acid-base disturbance (respiratory alkalosis and metabolic acidosis) reminiscent of SALICYLATE (p. III-368) poisoning (Haddad et al., 1979).

Almost all case reports of phenol poisoning describe acute or single-dose exposures. An epidemic of mild and perhaps "chronic" phenol poisoning, however, occurred when wells in southern Wisconsin became contaminated by spilled phenol. The illness was characterized by diarrhea, dark urine, and sores and burning in the mouth (Baker et al., 1978).

Animal studies indicate that the extent of percutaneous absorption of phenol depends more upon the magnitude of the skin area exposed than on the concentration of the applied solution. Although the injury caused by local contact with phenol tends in general to retard percutaneous absorption (Deichmann and Keplinger, 1962; Conning and Hayes, 1970), immediate steps are always indicated to remove unabsorbed material from the skin. The most effective procedure for skin decontamination, however, remains a subject of active and vigorous controversy. Contrary recommendations, often supported by experimental evidence, abound in the literature. Alcohol (Keating and Travell, 1943), mineral oil (Gibbs, 1931), vegetable oils such as castor, olive or cottonseed (Deichmann and Keplinger, 1962; Goodman and Geiger, 1935; Harkness, 1931), glycerin (Conning and Hayes, 1970) and polyethylene glycols with or without methyl alcohol (Brown et al., 1975; Pullin et al., 1978), all have their supporters and detractors. In the absence of any unanimity, plain water would appear to be the procedure of choice. Before washing a contaminated area of skin, however, liquefied or solid phenol should be removed by blotting with any absorbent material.

Renal excretion is the principal route of elimination. Peritoneal dialysis was judged ineffective in removing cresol ingested in the form of British Lysol (Thomas, 1969). In man 90% of a nontoxic oral dose (0.01 mg./kg.) of ^{14}C-labeled phenol was excreted in 24 hours, principally as the sulfate (77% of the excreted label) and as the glucuronide (16%), with small amounts of sulfate and glucuronide conjugates of a metabolite, hydroquinone (Capel et al., 1972). With larger doses free (unmetabolized) phenol can presumably be found in the urine. At least it has been reported in rabbit urine (Deichmann and Keplinger, 1962). Rabbits also oxidize appreciable amounts of phenol to carbon dioxide and water (Deichmann and Keplinger, 1962). Considerable species differences are recognized in phenol metabolism (Capel et al., 1972; Kao et al., 1979). Experiments in cats suggest that hydroquinone formation is an obligatory step for phenol poisoning (Miller et al., 1976b). Studies

in rats indicate that the major site of phenol conjugation to the sulfate or glucuronide is the intestines rather than the liver (Powell et al., 1974).

Symptomatology:

1. Burning pain in mouth and throat. White necrotic lesions in mouth, esophagus and stomach. Abdominal pain, vomiting (less common than with other corrosives), and bloody diarrhea.
2. Pallor, sweating, weakness, headache, dizziness, tinnitus.
3. Shock: weak irregular pulse, hypotension, shallow respirations, cyanosis, pallor, and a profound fall in body temperature.
4. Possibly fleeting excitement and confusion, followed by unconsciousness. Convulsions are rarely seen except in children (and most animals).
5. Stertorous breathing, mucous rales, rhonchi, frothing at nose and mouth and other signs of pulmonary edema are sometimes seen. Characteristic odor of phenol on the breath.
6. Scanty, dark-colored or "smoky" urine. If death does not occur promptly, moderately severe renal insufficiency may appear.
7. Methemoglobinemia, Heinz body hemolytic anemia and hyperbilirubinemia have been reported occasionally.
8. Death from respiratory, circulatory or cardiac failure.
9. If spilled on skin, pain is followed promptly by numbness. The skin becomes blanched, and a dry opaque eschar forms over the burn. When the eschar sloughs off, a brown stain remains.

Treatment:

1. If the patient is alert and able to swallow, have him drink a slurry of activated charcoal in water (p. I-4). Do not offer an emetic drug.
2. Careful gastric lavage with water if there are no deep burns in the mouth or pharynx. Older recommendations to lavage with olive oil or with other vegetable oils (salad, castor, cottonseed) do not appear to be supported by convincing data. In any case avoid mineral oil (a poor solvent for phenol) and alcohol (which facilitates the gastric absorption of phenol).
3. Remove contaminated clothing instantly. Carefully blot up any free liquid on the skin with care to avoid spreading it. Use any absorbent material, such as cotton wool swabs. The therapist should wear gloves or otherwise protect his skin from

contamination. Finally (and promptly) wash external exposed areas with copious amounts of running water.

4. Demulcents: egg white, milk, gruel p.o. if phenol has been mouthed or swallowed.

5. External heat in moderation to maintain the body temperature.

6. Morphine or meperidine for pain, if necessary.

7. Sodium bicarbonate may provide relief of symptoms even though the patient is not severely acidotic (p. IV-72). The rationale is not understood.

8. Oxygen therapy and artificial respiration as needed (pp. IV-12 and 7). Watch for signs of pulmonary edema, which may develop rapidly. (p. IV-14).

9. Hypotension may reflect vasogenic (p. IV-16) or cardiogenic (p. IV-20) shock (or both). Monitor ECG. Correct dehydration and oligemia with parenteral fluids, but infuse cautiously because of the uncertain pulmonary, cardiac and renal status. Digitalis is seldom effective.

10. Supportive measures for impending renal insufficiency (p. IV-52).

11. Watch for esophageal stricture, even though it occurs only rarely after phenol poisoning.

Laboratory:

1. Phenol can be detected in urine, where it is excreted unchanged or as a glucuronide or ethereal sulfate. A small fraction is oxidized to hydroquinone, pyrocatechol, and unknown substances, which impart a green to black color to the urine.

2. Frequent urinalyses to reveal albumin, red blood cells, and casts.

3. Acid-base balance should be investigated vigorously. See pp. IV-69–72.

4. Serum bilirubin may be slightly elevated. Liver function tests may be indicated, but hemolysis is the likely cause of the hyperbilirubinemia.

References:

Anderson, W. Fatal misadventure with carbolic acid. Lancet 1:179, 1869.

Angel, A.; Rogers, K. J. An analysis of the convulsant activity of substituted benzenes in the mouse. Toxicol. Appl. Pharmacol., 21:214-229, 1972.

Baker, E. L.; Landrigan, P. J.; Bertozzi, P. E.; Field, P. H.; Basteyns, B. J.; Skinner, H. G. Phenol poisoning due to contaminated drinking water. Arch. Environ. Health 33:89-94, 1978.

Bennett, I. L.; James, D. F.; Golden, A. Severe acidosis due to phenol poisoning. Report of two cases. Ann. Intern. Med. 32:324-327, 1950.

Berry, R.; Olszewski, J. Pathology of intrathecal phenol injection in man. Neurology 13:152-154, 1963.

Bethune, M.; Court, D. Vaporizing fluids containing phenols in the treatment of whooping cough. Br. Med. J. 1:1494-1495, 1954.

Brown, V. K. H.; Box, V. L.; Simpson, B. J. Decontamination procedures for skin exposed to phenolic substances. Arch. Environ. Health 30:1-6, 1975.

Brown, W. H. A curious case of carbolic acid poisoning. Lancet 1:543, 1895.

Calvery, H. O. Warning on the use of phenol-camphor in cases of "athlete's foot." J. A. M. A. 119:366, 1942.

Capel, I. D.; French, M. R.; Millburn, M.; Smith, R. L.; Williams, R. T. The fate of ¹⁴C phenol in various species. Xenobiotica 2:25-34, 1972.

Cardona, J. C.; Daly, J. F. Management of corrosive esophagitis. Analysis of treatment, methods, and results. N. Y. State J. Med. 64:2307-2313, 1964.

Clarke, T. W.; Brown, E. D. The value of alcohol in carbolic acid poisoning. A clinical and experimental study. J. A. M. A. 46:782-790, 1906.

Conning, D. M.; Hayes, M. J. The dermal toxicity of phenol: an investigation of the most effective first-aid measures. Br. J. Ind. Med. 27:155-159, 1970.

Cronin, T. D.; Brauer, R. O. Death due to phenol contained in Foille. J. A. M. A. 139:777-779, 1949.

Deichmann, W. B.; Keplinger, M. L. Phenols and Phenolic Compounds. In *Industrial Hygiene and Toxicology*, edited by F. A. Patty, *Vol. II. Toxicology,* 2nd ed., pp. 1363-1408. Edited by D. W. Fassett and D. D. Irish. Interscience Publishers, Inc., New York, 1962.

Evans, S. J. Acute phenol poisoning. Br. J. Ind. Med. 9:227-229, 1952.

Fertman, M. H.; Fertman, M. B. Toxic anemias and Heinz bodies. Medicine 34:131-192, 1955.

Gibbs, O. S. Treatment of carbolic acid poisoning. Br. Med. J. 1:581-582, 1931.

Goodman, L.; Geiger, A. J. Therapy in carbolic acid poisoning. Am. J. Med. Sci. 190:206-219, 1935.

Haddad, L. M.; Dimond, K. A.; Schweistris, J. E. Phenol poisoning. Case report. JACEP 8:267-269, 1979.

Harkness, A. H. Primary treatment of carbolic acid poisoning. Br. Med. J. 1:686-687, 1931.

Hartigan, W. Poisoning by lysol. Br. Med. J. 2:1498, 1900.

Hodge, G. E.; Scharfe, E. E. Stricture of the esophagus. Can. Med. Assoc. J. 37:541-547, 1937.

Hubler, W. R. Ulceration of the feet following single application of camphor-phenol mixture. J. A. M. A. 123:990, 1943.

Kao, J.; Bridges, J. W.; Faulkner, J. K. Metabolism of C-14phenol by sheep, pig, and rat. Xenobiotica 9:141-147, 1979.

Keating, J. O.; Travell, J. Comparison of antidotes for phenol burns of the skin. Fed. Proc. 2:83, 1943.

Kurechi, T.; Kikugawa, K; Nishizawa, A. Transformation of hemoglobin A into methemoglobin by sesamol. Life Sci. 26:1675-1681, 1980.

Lebowitz, R. L. Intravesical chemical cauterization and methemoglobinemia. Pediatrics 65:630, 1980.

Lucas, R. C.; Lane, W. A. Two cases of carbolic acid coma induced by application of carbolic acid compresses to the skin. Lancet 1:1362-1364, 1895.

McCord, C. P.; Munster, D. K. Phenol poisoning from ink. J. A. M. A. 83:843, 1924.

Miller, F. G. Poisoning by phenol. Can. Med. Assoc. J. 46:615-616, 1942.

Miller, J. J.; Powell, G. M.; Olavesen, A. H.; Curtis, C. G. The toxicity of dimethoxyphenol and related compounds in the cat. Toxicol. Appl. Pharmacol. 38:47-57, 1976b.

Needham, L. L.; Hill, R. H.; Paschal, D. C.; Sirmans, S. L. Determination of three germicidal phenols in serum of infants with hyperbilirubinemia. Clin. Chim. Acta 107:261-266, 1980.

Piotrowski, J. K. Evaluation of exposure to phenol: absorption of phenol vapour in the lungs and through the skin and excretion of phenol in urine. Br. J. Ind. Med. 28:172-178, 1971.

Powell, G. M.; Miller, J. J.; Olavesen, A. H.; Curtis, C. G. Liver as major organ of phenol detoxication. Nature 252:234-235,

1974.

Pullin, T. G.; Pinkerton, M. N.; Johnston, R. V.; Kilian, D. J. Decontamination of the skin of swine following phenol exposure: a comparison of the relative efficacy of water versus polyethylene glycol/industrial methylated spirits. Toxicol. Appl. Pharmacol. 43:199-206, 1978.

Reese, J. J. A Manual of Toxicology. J. B. Lippincott Co., Philadelphia, 1874.

Schulenburg, C. A. R. Corrosive stricture of the stomach without involvement of esophagus. Lancet 2:367-368, 1941.

Semple, H. F. Lysol poisoning. Br. Med. J. 2:774, 1925.

Smith, H. E. Absorption of carbolic acid through the skin. Lancet 2:1359, 1922.

Smith, R. P.; Olson, M. V. Drug-induced methemoglobinemia. Semin. Hematol. 10:253-268, 1973.

Stajduhar-Caric, Z. Acute phenol poisoning. Singular findings in a lethal case. J. Forensic Med., 15:41-42, 1968.

Superville-Sovak, B.; Rasminsky, M.; Finlayson, M. H. Complications of phenol neurolysis. Arch. Neurol, 32:226-228,

1975.

Thomas, B. B. Peritoneal dialysis and lysol poisoning. Br. Med. J. 3:720, 1969.

Turtle, W. R. M.; Dolan, T. A case of rapid and fatal absorption of carbolic acid through the skin. Lancet 2:1273-1274, 1922.

Vance, B. M. Intrauterine injection of "Lysol" as an abortifacient. Arch. Pathol. 40:395-398, 1945.

von Oettingen, W. F. Phenol and its derivatives: the relation between their chemical constitution and their effect on the organism. Natl. Insts. Health Bull. No. 190, 1949.

Webster, R. W. Legal Medicine and Toxicology. W. B. Saunders Co., Philadelphia, 1930.

Witthaus, R. A. Manual of Toxicology. Wm. Wood & Co., New York, 1911.

Wysowski, D. K.; Flynt, J. W., Jr.; Goldfield, M.; Altman, R.; Davis, A. T. Epidemic neonatal hyperbilirubinemia and use of a phenolic disinfectant detergent. Pediatrics 61:165-170, 1978.

PHOSPHORUS

Acute phosphorus poisoning early in this century was caused by the ingestion of match tips, fireworks and quack nostrums (Dwyer and Helwig, 1925; Humphreys and Halpert, 1931; LaDue et al., 1944; Stacey, 1921; Webster, 1930). There is no scientific basis for the medicinal use of phosphorus, and legislation together with international trade agreements has largely eliminated it from the above sources (Ward, 1928).

Modern matches that can be struck on any rough surface contain either red phosphorus (see below) or phosphorus sesquisulfide, together with potassium chlorate and glue. Safety matches which must be ignited on a prepared surface have tips containing potassium chlorate and antimony sulfide, whereas the striking surface consists of red phosphorus (or the sesquisulfide), sand and glue (Witthaus, 1911; see also Section VI). The principal toxic hazard of either type of match relates to its content of chlorate rather than phosphorus; see also BROMATE, p. III-74.

Acute phosphorus poisoning, however, is still encountered with surprising regularity after the ingestion of rat poisons or roach powders where yellow (also called white) phosphorus may be present in concentrations up to 5% (Caley and Kellock, 1955; Cushman and Alexander, 1966; Diaz-Rivera et al., 1950; Fletcher and Galambos, 1962; Greenberger et al., 1964; Rubitsky and Myerson, 1949). Because of the emergence of warfarin-resistant strains of rats, phosphorus rodenticides may be used increasingly (Simon and Pickering, 1976).

Toxicology: Elemental phosphorus occurs in two common forms. "Red" phosphorus is non-volatile, insoluble, unabsorbable, and thus nontoxic in single oral doses, unless it is contaminated with traces of yellow phosphorus (Witthaus, 1911). Repeated doses of red phosphorus, however, may induce systemic phosphorus poisoning. "Black phosphorus" is another inert, nontoxic allotropic form of the element.

Elemental yellow (or white) phosphorus is a translucent solid, which has a distinct odor resembling garlic. It is practically insoluble in water but readily soluble in most oils. Although stable under water, the element is converted by boiling alkali to the hypophosphorus ion ($H_2PO_2^-$) and phosphine. On exposure to air, phosphorus fumes and may flame spontaneously as it oxidizes to the sesquioxide (P_2O_3). Inhalation of phosphorus fumes can produce symptoms of acute phosphorus poisoning (Heimann, 1946).

Skin contact produces painful second and third degree burns as a result of both chemical and thermal damage (Jones, 1942b). This property has long been exploited as a weapon in warfare. During the Vietnam conflict sporadic reports appeared of sudden unexpected deaths of patients who had suffered relatively minor white phosphorus burns. Experiments with rabbits indicated that phosphorus is absorbed through areas of burned skin to produce a sudden and marked reversal of the serum calcium/phosphorus ratio and ECG changes (see below) like those encountered after phosphorus ingestion (Bowen et al., 1971).

Phosphorus is a general protoplasmic poison whose toxicity is enhanced when it is dissolved in solvents such as alcohol or digestible fats and oils like castor oil (Atkinson, 1921; Dwyer and Helwig, 1925). Although liquid petrolatum is said to retard absorption and decrease phosphorus toxicity, phosphorus is still rapidly absorbed when given to rats by mouth in mineral oil. It accumulates primarily in the liver, where peak levels are reached 2 to 3 hours after toxic oral doses (Ghoshal et al., 1971). Finely divided particles and emulsions are more toxic than coarse grained preparations, and bile salts are said to be important for phosphorus absorption (Witthaus, 1911).

Perhaps because of the water content and the low oxygen tension, particles of elemental phosphorus are stable for relatively long periods of time in the alimentary tract. One wonders if aerophagia might not promote ignition of phosphorus within the gut and so explain the occasional report of gastrointestinal necrosis, ulceration and perforation (Wechsler and Wechsler, 1951). Pieces inserted under the skin and into the peritoneum and liver of animals were found encapsulated at autopsy (Witthaus, 1911). The free element, however, is thought to be the toxic form in tissues, and it has been recovered from blood, liver, brain and fetuses *in utero* (Webster, 1930; Witthaus, 1911). Some phosphorus is thought to be slowly oxidized to harmless acids, which are gradually excreted by the kidneys (Sollmann, 1957; Witthaus, 1911).

The acute fatal dose of yellow phosphorus for an adult is between 50 and 100 mg. (Sollmann, 1957; Webster, 1930), or about 1 mg./kg. Recovery, however, has occurred after 0.8 and 1.5 gm. (Diaz-Rivera *et al.*, 1950; Newburger *et al.*, 1948), whereas only 3 mg. proved lethal to a 2-year-old child (Webster, 1930). The prognosis is generally poor, and the fatality rate is about 50% (Diaz-Rivera *et al.*, 1950; LaDue *et al.*, 1944; Rubitsky and Myerson, 1949). In examining the records of 802 poisonings Witthaus (1911) concluded the average survival time to be 5 to 6 days. Deaths in the first 2 days are due to peripheral vascular collapse, although signs of acute renal failure are seen as early as 24 to 48 hours. Later in the course of poisoning, death is due to cardiac, hepatic or renal failure or rarely to postconvulsive central nervous depression (Diaz-Rivera *et al.*, 1950).

Although contrary opinions have been expressed (Diaz-Rivera *et al.*, 1950), the classical picture of acute phosphorus poisoning develops in three stages (LaDue *et al.*, 1944; Rubitsky and Myerson, 1949; Witthaus, 1911). Gastrointestinal symptoms occurring shortly after ingestion arise from local irritation, but unlike the response to a truly corrosive poison the effects may not be immediately evident and sometimes are so mild as to escape recognition (Witthaus, 1911). Vomiting is almost always present; early hematemesis may reflect gastric erosion, whereas late hematemesis usually indicates a depression of plasma prothrombin secondary to hepatic damage (Diaz-Rivera *et al.*, 1950). "Expulsion of smoke from the mouth" probably describes phosphorus fumes (Fletcher and Galambos, 1962), and vomitus and feces may be luminescent or fuming (Chretien, 1945; Cushman and Alexander, 1966; Witthaus, 1911). Other symptoms in this period are secondary to the gastroenteritis or impending peripheral vascular collapse.

In many cases stage 2 is a relatively symptom-free period of several days. Patients have been discharged prematurely during this period (Wechsler and Wechsler, 1951). In the experience of Diaz-Rivera *et al.* (1950), however, pa-

tients were rarely free of symptoms. An intensification of the toxic syndrome after 48 hours is described.

In the third stage of systemic intoxication, the liver undergoes acute degeneration and fatty infiltration with accompanying metabolic disturbances. Indeed, nonspecific signs of injury may be seen in hepatic cells as early as one hour after the ingestion of phosphorus. Gastrointestinal symptoms again become severe. Hemorrhages may occur at many sites (Hann and Veale, 1910) because of depletion of clotting factors. Vitamin K may improve coagulation times (Fletcher and Galambos, 1962), but transfusions of fresh whole blood may be required in patients with severe hepatic damage. Phosphorus may also act directly to inhibit protein synthesis in the liver (Barker *et al.*, 1963; Pani *et al.*, 1972).

Prominent biochemical differences are recognized between the hepatotoxic effects of phosphorus and of other agents, *e.g.*, carbon tetrachloride (Pani *et al.*, 1972). Hypoglycemia is often observed (Althausen and Thoenes, 1932; McIntosh, 1927; McLean *et al.*, 1929); its early appearance (stage 1) is a grave prognostic sign, as is early azotemia, hepatomegaly or toxic delirium (Diaz-Rivera *et al.*, 1950). Early liver pathology includes fatty changes in Kupffer cells (Lawrence and Huffman, 1929a), focal necrosis, fatty metamorphosis and parenchymatous degeneration with acute inflammation of the portal canals. The late phase, which may be persistent, resembles early portal cirrhosis (Greenberger *et al.*, 1964; LaDue *et al.*, 1944; Mallory, 1933).

Death in acute renal failure is not common, but fatal cases with cortical necrosis have been described (Perry, 1953). Renal function studies of a nonlethal poisoning suggested a disturbance in proximal tubular function (Cushman and Alexander, 1966). Hypocalcemia and hypophosphatemia are described in some patients (Cushman and Alexander, 1966), but hyperphosphatemia with normal serum calcium levels are reported in others (Diaz-Rivera *et al.*, 1950).

Electrocardiographic changes may reflect a direct toxic action of phosphorus on the myocardium or may be secondary to metabolic disturbances; they include moderate T wave and S-T segment alterations (Dathe and Nathan, 1946; Diaz-Rivera *et al.*, 1961; Newburger *et al.*, 1948), sino-atrial tachycardia (Chretien, 1945), prolongation of Q-T interval, abnormalities in rhythm and low voltage of the QRS complex (Diaz-Rivera *et al.*, 1961). The ECG changes can be prolonged, lasting as long as 3 months in one case (Matsumoto *et al.*, 1972). They can mimic those of acute myocardial infarction, and death has occurred in cardiac standstill in the early phase of the intoxication (Pietras *et al.*, 1968; Talley *et al.*, 1972) or from myocardial damage more than 2 days after ingestion (Schellmann *et al.*, 1979).

Acidosis has been described (Webster, 1930); presumably it is of mild proportions except *in extremis*. Monocytosis occurs in poisoned animals (Lawrence and Huffman, 1929b) but is uncommon in man. Instead, lymphocytosis and polycythemia even with adequate hydration occur regularly (Diaz-Rivera *et al.*, 1950).

No satisfactory therapy for phosphorus poisoning has been devised. The commonest form of systemic intoxication involves hepatic necrosis, often with hepatoencephalopathy. Indeed acute phosphorus poisoning is often used as an animal model for testing measures of supportive therapy in hepatic insufficiency (Burnell *et al.*, 1976; Horak *et al.*, 1979). In this stage, exchange transfusions may be marginally helpful (Marin *et al.*, 1971), and poisoned dogs appear to benefit from cross-circulation with healthy dogs (Burnell *et al.*, 1976). Therapeutic interventions, however, have not been demonstrably successful in preventing liver cell damage after known exposures to phosphorus, but free radical scavengers, such as acetylcysteine or α-tocopherol, do not appear to have been tested. In spite of earlier claims of success, corticosteroid therapy is not effective in preventing phosphorus-induced liver injury, in delaying the onset of coma or in reducing mortality (Marin *et al.*, 1971).

In contrast to acute poisoning, chronic phosphorus intoxication, once common in some industries because of inhalation of phosphorus fumes, is virtually unknown in modern times. It was characterized by cachexia, anemia, bronchitis and necrosis of the mandible, the so-called "phossy" or "Lucifer's" jaw (Heimann, 1946; Ward, 1928). Other bones may be involved as demonstrated by chronic systemic administration to animals (Adams and Sarnat, 1940; Fleming *et al.*, 1942). Even in acute phosphorus poisoning dense growth lines in all extremities proximal to the epiphyseal lines ("phosphorschicht") have been described (Blumenthal and Lesser, 1938). These lesions, however, are unimportant in the acute syndrome of phosphorus poisoning described above.

Symptomatology:

A. Acute poisoning—typically in 3 stages.

1. *First stage*—symptoms due to local irritation, occurring within a few minutes or few hours after exposure and lasting from 8 hours to 3 days. Except for thermal burns on the body surface, effects are not immediate.

    a. Skin contact produces painful penetrating second and third degree burns, which heal slowly. These lesions represent both chemical and thermal damage.

    b. Ingestion produces a sensation of warmth or a burning pain in the throat and abdomen, with intense thirst.

    c. Nausea, vomiting, diarrhea, severe abdominal pain. A garlic odor from breath and excreta is highly suggestive of phosphorus poisoning (garlic, Lewisite, and arsenic must be ruled out). Luminescent vomitus and feces are essentially diagnostic of phosphorus.

    d. Shock may be severe enough to cause death in 24 to 48 hours.

2. *Second stage*—an almost symptom-free period of several days (8 hours to several weeks), during which the patient seems to be recovering.

3. *Third stage*—symptoms of systemic toxicity from absorbed poison.

    a. Nausea, protracted vomiting, diarrhea; massive hematemesis may occur.

    b. Liver tenderness and enlargement, jaundice, pruritus.

    c. Hemorrhages into skin, mucous membranes, and viscera, due to injury of blood vessels and inhibition of blood clotting (low plasma levels of prothrombin and fibrinogen).

    d. Renal damage is evidenced by oliguria, hematuria, casts, albuminuria, and sometimes anuria.

    e. Cardiovascular collapse, due to a direct, toxic action of phosphorus on heart muscle and blood vessels, usually late in the course of the poisoning.

    f. Central nervous involvement resulting in convulsions, confusion, and coma. If the patient survives, cerebral symptoms of hepatic encephalopathy may persist for a long time.

    g. Death occurs usually in 4 to 8 days, but it may be delayed 3 weeks. Irreversible shock, hepatic failure, central nervous system damage, massive hematemesis, or renal insufficiency may be the proximal cause of death.

B. Chronic poisoning (from ingestion or inhalation). Cachexia, anemia, bronchitis, general debility, necrosis of mandible—all associated with lowered resistance to infection and defective tissue repair.

Treatment:

1. Care should be taken to protect both patient and attendant from vomitus, gastric washings, and feces, since the phosphorus in them can cause burns of skin and eyes. Probably emetic drugs should not be given, unless a long delay is anticipated before lavage can be initiated.

2. Even many hours after an ingestion, perform gastric lavage, using copious quantities of one of the following solutions:

   a. Potassium permanganate (1:5000) is probably preferable; it may convert phosphorus to various oxides (acids), which are comparatively harmless.

   b. Cupric sulfate solution (0.2%) acts as an emetic and as an antidote by coating the phosphorus particles with insoluble copper phosphide. Unless the lavage fluid is promptly removed, there is a risk of copper poisoning.

   c. Tap water if the solutions described above are not immediately available.

3. Liquid petrolatum (100 to 200 ml.) should be introduced into the stomach following lavage and left there. Avoid digestible fats and oils.

4. Isotonic solutions of sodium chloride and of sodium lactate parenterally to combat shock, dehydration, and acidosis (pp. IV-64–67, 69–72). Glucose infusions may be required to correct hypoglycemia. Calcium gluconate may be required if hypocalcemia appears (p. IV-74).

5. Morphine and other opiates to control pain.

6. Vitamin K_1 in large doses (e.g., 65 mg. slowly by intravenous drip) may in part combat hypoprothrombinemia, but transfusions with *fresh* whole blood may be necessary to correct the coagulation defect and anemia.

7. Supportive treatment for delirium and convulsions (pp. IV-33 and 35).

8. General supportive measures for hepatic insufficiency (p. IV-61) and more rarely renal failure (p. IV-52).

9. Corticoid therapy has been recommended for severe shock. See text above.

10. Treat skin burns by washing with warm water or with 1 percent cupric sulfate solution, and then apply bland ointments. As long as unoxidized phosphorus remains embedded in the skin, the contaminated area should be kept submerged in water or copper sulfate solution. Visible pieces of phosphorus should be removed surgically.

Laboratory:

1. Phosphorus can be demonstrated chemically in vomitus and feces, which may "smoke" or fume.

2. Urine may contain albumin, bile pigments, casts, blood and amino acids. Measure and record the output of urine.

3. Blood chemistry: low blood sugar, high nonprotein nitrogen, high bilirubin, low fibrinogen, low prothrombin. Both hypo- and hyperphosphatemia have been described. Hypocalcemia may or may not occur.

4. Hematological data are variable: leukopenia or leukocytosis, anemia or polycythemia, lymphocytosis.

5. Frequent electrocardiographic recordings may reveal cardiac damage.

References:

Adams, C. O.; Sarnat, R. G. Effects of yellow phosphorus and arsenic trioxide on growing bones and growing teeth. Arch. Pathol. 20:1192-1202, 1940.

Althausen, T. L.; Thoenes, E. Influence on carbohydrate metabolism of experimentally induced hepatic changes. II. Phosphorus poisoning. Arch. Intern. Med. 50:58-75, 1932.

Atkinson, H. V. The treatment of acute phosphorus poisoning. J. Lab. Clin. Med. 1:148-150, 1921.

Barker, E. A.; Smuckler, E. A.; Benditt, E. P. Effects of thioacetamide and yellow phosphorus poisoning on protein synthesis in vivo. Lab. Invest. 12: 955-960, 1963.

Blumenthal, S.; Lesser, A. Acute phosphorus poisoning. Am. J. Dis. Child. 55:1280-1287, 1938.

Bowen, T. E.; Whelan, T. J., Jr.; Nelson, T. G. Sudden death after phosphorus burns. Ann. Surg. 174:779-784, 1971.

Burnell, J. M.; Dennis, M. B., Jr.; Clayson, K. J.; Smuckler, E. A.; Cleft, R. A. Evaluation in dogs of cross-circulation in the treatment of acute hepatic necrosis induced by yellow phosphorus. Gastroenterology 71:827-831, 1976.

Caley, J.; Kellock, I. Acute yellow phosphorus poisoning. Lancet 1:539, 1955.

Chretien, T. E. Acute phosphorus poisoning. Report of a case with recovery. N. Engl. J. Med. 232:247-249, 1945.

Cushman, P., Jr.; Alexander, B. H. Renal phosphate and calcium excretory defects in a case of acute phosphorus poisoning. Nephron 3:123-128, 1966.

Dathe, R. A.; Nathan, D. A. Electrocardiographic changes resulting from phosphorus poisoning. Report of a case. Am. Heart J. 31:98-102, 1946.

Diaz-Rivera, R. S.; Collazo, P. J.; Pons, E. R.; Tirregrosa, M. Y. Acute phosphorus poisoning in man; a study of 56 cases. Medicine 29:269-298, 1950.

Diaz-Rivera, R. S.; Ramos-Morales, F.; Garcia-Palmieri, M. R.; Ramirez, E. A. The electrocardiographic changes in acute phosphorus poisoning in man. Am. J. Med. Sci. 241:758-765, 1961.

Dwyer, H. L.; Helwig, F. C. Phosphorus poisoning in a child from the ingestion of fireworks. J. A. M. A. 84:1254-1256, 1925.

Fleming, R. B. L.; Miller, J. W.; Swayne, V. R., Jr. Some recent observations on phosphorus toxicology. J. Ind. Hyg. Toxicol. 24:154-158, 1942.

Fletcher, G. F.; Galambos, J. T. Phosphorus poisoning in humans. Arch. Intern. Med. 112:846-852, 1962.

Ghoshal, A. K.; Porta, E. A.; Hartroft, W. S. Isotopic studies on the absorption and tissue distribution of white phosphorus in rats. Exp. Mol. Pathol. 14:212-219, 1971.

Greenberger, N. J.; Robinson, W. L.; Isselbacher, K. J. Toxic hepatitis after the ingestion of phosphorus with subsequent recovery. Gastroenterology 47:179-183, 1964.

Hann, R. G.; Veale, R. A. A fatal case of poisoning by phosphorus with unusual subcutaneous haemorrhages. Lancet 1:163-164, 1910.

Heimann, H. Chronic phosphorus poisoning. J. Ind. Hyg. Toxicol. 28:142-150, 1946.

Horak, W.; Polterauer, P.; Renner, F.; Silberbauer, K.; Rauhs, R.; Muhlbacher; Funovics, J. Plasmaperfusion uber Aktivkohle und Amberlite XAD-7 bei der phosphor-induzierten Lebernekrose des Hundes. Gastroenterology 17:90-98, 1979.

Humphreys, E. M.; Halpert, B. Acute phosphorus poisoning: Report of case due to ingestion of fireworks. Am. J. Dis. Child. 41:354-359, 1931.

Jones, A. T. Treatment of phosphorus burns. Br. Med. J. 2:244-245, 1942b.

LaDue, J. S.; Schenken, J. R.; Kuker, L. H. Phosphorus poisoning. A report of 16 cases with repeated liver biopsies in a recovered case. Am. J. Med. Sci. 208:223-233, 1944.

Lawrence, J. S.; Huffman, M. M. Fatty changes in the Kupffer cells in the liver of the guinea pig in phosphorus poisoning. Arch. Pathol. 7:809-812, 1929a.

Lawrence, J. S.; Huffman, M. M. An increase in the number of monocytes in the blood following subcutaneous administration of yellow phosphorus in oil. Arch. Pathol. 7:813-819, 1929b.

Mallory, F. B. Phosphorus and alcoholic cirrhosis. Am. J. Pathol. 9:557-567, 1933.

Marin, G. A.; Montoya, C. A.; Sierra, J. L.; Senior, J. R. Evaluation of corticosteroid and exchange-transfusion treatment of acute yellow-phosphorus intoxication. N. Engl. J. Med. 284:125-128, 1971.

Matsumoto, S.; Kohri, Y.; Tanaka, K.; Tsuchiya, G. A case of acute phosphorus poisoning with various electrocardiographic changes. Jap. Circ. J. 36:963-970, 1972.

McIntosh, R. M. Acute phosphorus poisoning. Report of a case with recovery. Am. J. Dis. Child. 34:595-602, 1927.

McLean, S.; MacDonald, A.; Sullivan, R. C. Acute phosphorus poisoning from ingestion of roach paste: Report of a fatal case in a child. J. A. M. A. 93:1789-1793, 1929.

Newburger, R. A.; Beaser, S. B.; Schwachman, H. Phosphorus poisoning with recovery accompanied by electrocardiographic changes. Am. J. Med. 4:927-930, 1948.

Pani, P.; Gravela, E.; Mazzarino, C.; Burdino, E. On the mechanism of fatty liver in white phosphorus poisoned rats.

Exp. Mol. Pathol. 16:201-209, 1972.

Perry, J. W. Phosphorus poisoning with cortical necrosis of kidney: Report of 2 fatal cases. Aust. N. Z. J. Med. 2:94-98, 1953.

Pietras, R. J.; Stavrakos, C.; Gunnar, R. M.; Tobin, J. R., Jr. Phosphorus poisoning simulating acute myocardial infarction. Arch. Intern. Med. 122:430-434, 1968.

Rubitsky, H. J.; Myerson, R. M. Acute phosphorus poisoning. Arch. Intern. Med. 83:164-178, 1949.

Schellmann, B.; Zober, A.; Zink, P. Suizidale Phosphorvergiftung. Arch. Toxicol. 42:303-309, 1979.

Simon, F. A.; Pickering, L. K. Acute yellow phosphorus poisoning. J. A. M. A. 235:1343-1344, 1976.

Sollmann, T. A Manual of Pharmacology. 8th Ed., W. B. Saunders Co., Philadelphia, 1957.

Stacy, W. C. Dangers of phosphorus in fireworks. J. A. M. A. 77:1514, 1921.

Talley, R. C.; Linhart, J. W.; Trevino, A. J.; Moore, L.; Beller, B. M. Acute elemental phosphorus poisoning in man. Am. Heart J. 84:139-140, 1972.

Ward, E. F. Phosphorus necrosis in the manufacture of fireworks. J. Ind. Hyg. Toxicol. 10:314-330, 1928.

Webster, R. W. Legal Medicine and Toxicology. W. B. Saunders Co., Philadelphia, 1930.

Wechsler, L.; Wechsler, R. L. Phosphorus poisoning: The latent period and unusual gastrointestinal lesions. Gastroenterology 17:279-283, 1951.

Witthaus, R. A. Manual of Toxicology. Wm. Wood & Co., New York, 1911.

PYRETHRUM

Pyrethrum has been known and used as an insecticide for many years. Even with the advent of many new agents, pyrethrum is still considered so effective that it is included in most household sprays today. The source of this material is the flowers of the pyrethrum plant, *Chrysanthemum cinerariaefolium* (Shepard, 1939). The insecticide can be prepared by drying and grinding the flowers to a powder, which contains 1 to 3% active material. A more efficient method is the extraction of active ingredients with a solvent such as alcohol, kerosene or naphtha. The activity and toxicity of pyrethrum reside in at least six esters of complex alcohols and acids, called pyrethrin I and II, cinerin I and II, and jasmolin I and II, known collectively as pyrethrins. When isolated, these esters are viscous liquids, insoluble in water, and quickly decomposed by mild acid and alkali. They are also unstable in the environment because of exposure to light and air. Available are purified extracts containing 20 to 35% pyrethrins and a refined grade (termed "pale") containing 60% active ingredients.

Pyrethrum is sometimes used as a dust, and the term "insect powder" on the label is legally proper only if the product contains pyrethrum powder. A more common formulation is the extract in a suitable solvent or vehicle for use as a household, garden or livestock spray. Pyrethrum preparations frequently contain a synergist which is added to increase their stability and insecticidal effectiveness; these include sesamex, piperonyl butoxide, piperonyl cyclonene, *n*-octyl

sulfoxide of isosafrole, *n*-propyl isome, and *N*-isobutylundecylenamide.

Several semisynthetic derivatives of chrysanthemumic and related acids have been developed for use as insecticides. These compounds, known as pyrethroids, are generally more effective insecticides than the native pyrethrins and less toxic toward mammals. Compounds now in use include allethrin (Ambrose and Robbins, 1951; Carpenter *et al.*, 1950; Starr *et al.*, 1950a and b), cyclethrin (Carpenter *et al.*, 1954), barthrin (Ambrose, 1963; Masri *et al.*, 1964a and b), dimethrin (Ambrose, 1964; Masri *et al.*, 1964a and b), bioallethrin (Verschoyle and Barnes, 1972), bioresmethrin (Abernathy and Casida, 1973), and phenolthrin (Fujimoto *et al.*, 1973).

Toxicology: Natural pyrethrins are only moderately toxic to warm-blooded animals by oral administration but highly toxic by parenteral routes (Ambrose and Robbins, 1951; Shimkin and Anderson, 1936). When dissolved in dimethyl sulfoxide, the oral LD_{50} in rats is 260 to 420 mg./kg. for pyrethrin I and more than 600 mg./kg. for pyrethrin II (Casida *et al.*, 1971). In contrast, the intravenous lethal doses are 5 and 1 mg./kg., respectively (Verschoyle and Barnes, 1972). These differences between oral and parenteral toxicities are presumably a consequence of rapid metabolic detoxication. Thus rats can ingest over a 24-hour period a dose which is lethal if taken at one time, and can maintain this intake every day of their lives without apparent injury (Carpenter *et al.*, 1950).

In man the fatal oral dose of the naturally

occurring mixture of pyrethrins is 1 to 2 gm./kg., as inferred from data on rats and guinea pigs. Since the pyrethrin concentration of pyrethrum powder is about 1 to 3% and of insecticide sprays is usually 1 to 2%, serious poisonings are highly improbable, but the death of a 2-year-old child has been attributed to the ingestion of ½ oz. (15 gm.) of a pyrethrum concentrate (Hayes, 1963). Kerosene and naphtha, the common solvents in pyrethrum sprays, are generally more hazardous than the "active ingredients." See also KERO-SENE, p. III-220.

In general synthetic analogues of pyrethrins (sometimes called pyrethroid insecticides) are much less acutely toxic to rats and presumably to man than are the natural pyrethrins. The synthetic pyrethroids (and presumably the natural ones as well) are rapidly absorbed and distributed through body tissues, including the brain. Symptoms of intoxication in rats are observed between ½ and 1½ hours after ingestion when brain concentrations are maximal (Miyamoto et al., 1971).

The toxic mechanism of pyrethrum and pyrethroids in mammals is not well characterized. These substances are central nervous stimulants and can induce convulsions. In gerbils, large toxic doses cause hyperglycemia, reduced glucose tolerance, and a reduction in total serum proteins (Karel and Saxena, 1975). Increased liver and kidney weights were noted in animals chronically fed either synthetic or natural pyrethrins (Ambrose, 1963, 1964), together with the reversible appearance of unusual cytoplasmic inclusion bodies in hepatic cells (Masri et al., 1964b; Kimbrough et al., 1968). The functional significance of the hepatic lesion has not been defined.

There is conflicting evidence about the metabolism of the pyrethrins in mammals. Pyrethrins I and II are said to be detoxified rapidly by hydrolysis of the ester linkage to chrysanthemumic acid and an alcohol. The latter in most cases is oxidized to the aldehyde and acid, which is excreted as such or conjugated with glucuronide (Ambrose, 1963; Masri et al., 1964a). More recent evidence, however, indicates that in rats the cyclopropane carboxylic ester bond of chrysanthemumic acid is relatively stable as present in pyrethrin I, pyrethrin II and the semisynthetic allethrin (Casida et al., 1971). The principal metabolites in rat urine are oxidation products, involving side chain oxidation in both the acid and alcohol moieties (Casida et al., 1971).

On the other hand, ester hydrolysis is the principal metabolic fate of at least some semisynthetic pyrethrins, such as resmethrin, permethrin, and phenothrin (Abernathy and Casida, 1973; Elliot et al., 1976; Miyamoto et al., 1974). For these compounds, ester hydrolysis of the trans-isomer (termed bioresmethrin, bio-

permethrin, biophenothrin) occurs rapidly in liver microsomes, but the cis-isomers are hydrolyzed more slowly by an oxidative process requiring NADPH (Veda et al., 1975; Miyamoto et al., 1971). Perhaps because of rapid hydrolysis, the trans-isomer of resmethrin is significantly less toxic than the cis-isomer in mammals. The products, which are slowly excreted in bile and urine, can be demonstrated in body tissues up to 3 weeks after ingestion (Miyamoto et al., 1971).

The synergists commonly found in pyrethrum formulations (as listed above) possess even lower acute toxicities in laboratory mammals than do pyrethrins. Although these additives enhance insecticidal potency, there is no evidence that they increase the mammalian toxicity of fresh pyrethrum (Starr et al., 1950a and b). The issue, however, deserves more study, particularly since the demonstration that side-chain oxidation is a prominent feature of the metabolic inactivation of pyrethrin I and II in rats (Casida et al., 1971). The mixed-function oxidase system of mammalian liver microsomes is known to be responsible for such enzymatic oxidations. By substrate competition, insecticidal synergists, particularly those of the methylenedioxybenzene type, are capable of inhibiting this system of liver enzymes (Casida et al., 1966; Anders, 1968). The inference is that the synergists might inhibit the enzymatic detoxication of at least some pyrethrins and consequently enhance their toxicity not only to insects (Casida et al., 1966) but perhaps also to man.

Neither the natural nor the synthetic pyrethrins are believed to be significantly absorbed through intact skin. No toxic effects were observed in rats or rabbits after large dermal applications (1.5 gm./kg.) of pyrethrin (Malone and Brown, 1968). In spite of the low primary toxicity of pyrethrins, skin contact and inhalation may cause allergic attacks in sensitive people; severe dermatitis, asthma, vasomotor rhinitis and anaphylactoid reactions have been reported. Persons sensitive to ragweed pollen are particularly prone to react to pyrethrins (Feinberg, 1934; Garratt and Bigger, 1923; McCord et al., 1921; Ramirez, 1930; Sulzberger and Weinberg, 1930). Barthrin and dimethrin, however, produced no primary irritation, sensitization or allergic reactions when tested on human volunteers (Ambrose 1963, 1964).

As tested on the isolated cockroach giant axon, allethrin in minute concentrations produces a repetitive discharge, an increase in the negative afterpotential and finally a conduction block (Narahashi, 1962a and b, 1971; Narahashi and Anderson, 1967). The repetitive discharges in arthropod nerves are apparently due to a prolongation of the enhanced sodium conductance occurring during the action potential. This effect is similar to that of DDT (p. III-135), and like DDT, pyrethroids are more toxic at low temperatures than at high ones (Casida, 1980).

Symptomatology (largely inferred from animal studies):
1. Numbness of lips and tongue, sneezing, nausea, vomiting, and diarrhea.
2. Headache, restlessness, tinnitus, incoordination, clonic convulsions, stupor, and prostration.
3. Death due to respiratory paralysis.
4. Skin contact may cause dermatitis, sometimes with an associated eosinophilia.
5. Hydrocarbon solvents such as kerosene may produce pulmonary edema (p. III-220).

Treatment:
1. Generally no treatment is required after ingestion of the usual dilute pyrethrum powder (see text above). The chief hazard of most commercial solutions resides in the solvent; see 7 below.
2. The decision to empty the stomach or not is largely predicated on information about other constituents in the ingested product. With liquid preparations containing kerosene or a related petroleum distillate, do not induce emesis (see p. III-220). Otherwise syrup of ipecac (p. I-2) or a slurry of activated charcoal (p. I-4) may be administered.
3. If the amount ingested is estimated to contain a lethal or near-lethal dose of pyrethrum (see text above) or of any other ingredient in the mixture, cautious gastric lavage may be performed, even though the product is composed largely of kerosene or a related petroleum distillate. See p. I-10 and pp. III-222–223 for special precautions. Furthermore, it may be advisable to premedicate the patient with diazepam or a barbiturate drug.
4. Administer a saline cathartic, e.g., 15 to 30 gm. sodium sulfate in water and perhaps a slurry of activated charcoal (p. I-12). Avoid all oils and fats, which promote the intestinal absorption of pyrethrum.
5. Symptomatic and supportive treatment with oxygen (p. IV-12), artificial ventilation (p. IV-7), diazepam for convulsions (p. IV-37), and parenteral fluids.
6. Wash skin promptly with generous quantities of water.
7. See treatment of kerosene and naphtha poisoning (p. III-224), if signs or symptoms are due to the vehicle.
8. Symptomatic and supportive measure for allergic manifestations such as asthma, rhinitis, anaphylaxis and dermatitis.

Laboratory: No common laboratory tests have diagnostic or prognostic value.

References:

Abernathy, C. O.; Casida, J. E. Pyrethroid insecticides; esterase cleavage in relation to selective toxicity. Science 179:1235-1236, 1973.

Ambrose, A.; Robbins, D. J. Comparative toxicity of pyrethrins and allethrin. Fed. Proc. 10:276-277, 1951.

Ambrose, A. M. Toxicologic studies on pyrethrin-type esters of chrysanthemumic acid. I. Chrysanthemumic acid, 6-chloropiperonyl ester (Barthrin). Toxicol. Appl. Pharmacol. 5:414-426, 1963.

Ambrose, A. M. Toxicologic studies on pyrethrin-type esters of chrysanthemumic acid. II. Chrysanthemumic acid, 2, 4-dimethyl benzyl ester. Toxicol. Appl. Pharmacol. 6:112-120, 1964.

Anders, M. W. Inhibition of microsomal drug metabolism by methylenedioxybenzenes. Biochem. Pharmacol. 17:2367-2370, 1968.

Carpenter, C. P.; Weil, C. S.; Pozzani, U. C.; Smyth, H. F., Jr. Comparative acute and subacute toxicities of allethrin and pyrethrins. Arch. Ind. Hyg. Occup. Med. 2:420-432, 1950.

Carpenter, C. P.; Weil, C. S.; Pozzani, U. C.; Smyth, H. F., Jr. Acute and subacute toxicity of cyclethrin. Arch. Ind. Hyg. Occup. Med. 10:162-168, 1954.

Casida, J. E. Pyrethrum flowers and pyrethroid insecticides. Environ. Health Perspect. 34:189-202, 1980.

Casida, J. E.; Engle, J. L.; Essac, E. G.; Kamienski, F. X.; Kuwatsuka, S. Methylene-C14-dioxyphenyl compounds: Metabolism in relation to their synergistic action. Science 153:1130-1133, 1966.

Casida, J. E.; Kimmel, E. C.; Elliott, M.; Janes, N. F. Oxidative metabolism of pyrethrins in mammals. Nature 230:326-327, 1971.

Chikamoto, T. The toxicity of chrysanthemyl-, allethronyl-, and piperonyl piperonylates and the higher homologues. Agric. Biol. Chem. 28:633-638, 1964.

Elliot, M.; Janes, N. F.; Pulman, D. A.; Gaughan, L. G.; Unai, T.; Casida, J. E. Radiosynthesis and metabolism in rats of the 1R isomers of the insecticide permethrin. J. Agric. Food Chem. 24:270-276, 1976.

Feinberg, G. M. Pyrethrum sensitization; its importance and relation to pollen allergy. J. A. M. A. 102:1557-1558, 1934.

Fujimoto, K.; Itaya, N.; Okuno, Y.; Kadota, T.; Yamaguchi, T. A new insecticidal pyrethroid ester. Agric. Biol. Chem. 37:2681-2682, 1973.

Garratt, J. R.; Bigger, J. W. Asthma due to insect powder. Br. Med. J. 2:764, 1923.

Hayes, W. J., Jr. Clinical Handbook on Economic Poisons. USPHS Publication No. 476. U. S. Government Printing Office, Washington, D. C., 1963.

Karel, A. K.; Saxena, S. C. Investigation on the acute toxic effect of pyrethrum on the blood glucose and of glucose administration on the acute pyrethrum toxicity in Meriones hurrianae Jerdon (Rodentia). Arch. Int. Physiol. Biochim. 83:19-25, 1975.

Kimbrough, R. D.; Gaines, T. B.; Hayes, W. J., Jr. Combined effect of DDT, pyrethrum, and piperonyl butoxide on rat liver. Arch. Environ. Health 16:333-341, 1968.

Malone, J. C.; Brown, N. C. Toxicity of various grades of pyrethrum to laboratory animals. Pyrethrum Post 9:3-8, 1968.

Masri, M. S.; Hendrickson, A. P.; Cox, A. J., Jr.; DeEds, F. Subacute toxicity of two chrysanthemumic acid esters: Barthrin and dimethrin. Toxicol. Appl. Pharmacol. 6:716-725, 1964b.

Masri, M. S.; Jones, F. T.; Lundin, R. E.; Bailey, G. F.; DeEds, F. Metabolic fate of two chrysanthemumic acid esters: Barthrin and dimethrin. Toxicol. Appl. Pharmacol. 6:711-715, 1964a.

McCord, C. P.; Kilker, C. H.; Minister, D. K. Pyrethrum dermatitis. A record of the occurrence of occupational dermatoses among workers in the pyrethrum industry. J. A. M. A. 77:448-449, 1921.

Miyamoto, J.; Nishida, T.; Veda, K. Metabolic fate of resmethrin, 5-benzyl-3-furylmethyl-dl-trans- chrysanthemate in the rat. Pest. Biochem. Physiol. 1:293-306, 1971.

Miyamoto, J.; Nishida, T.; Veda, K. Metabolic fate of resmethrin, 5-benzyl-3-furylmethyl-dl-trans- chrysanthemate in the rat. Pest. Biochem. Physiol. 1:293-306, 1971.

Miyamoto, J.; Suzuki, T.; Nakae, C. Metabolism of phenothrin or 3-phenoxybenzyl d-trans-chrysanthemumate in mammals. Pesticide Biochem. Physiol. 4:438-450, 1974.

Narahashi, T. Nature of the negative after-potential increased by the insecticide allethrin in cockroach giant axons. J. Cell. Physiol. 59:67-76, 1962b.

Narahashi, T. Mode of action of pyrethroids. Bull. WHO 44:337-345, 1971.

Narahashi, T.; Anderson, N. C. Mechanism of the excitation block by the insecticide allethrin applied externally and internally to squid giant axons. Toxicol. Appl. Pharmacol. 10:529-547, 1967.

Ramirez, M. A. Pyrethrum; an etiologic factor in vasomotor rhinitis and asthma. J. Allergy 1:149-155, 1930.

Shepard, H. H. *The Chemistry and Toxicology of Insecticides.* Burgess Publishing Co., Minneapolis, 1939.

Shimkin, M. B.; Anderson, H. H. Acute toxicities of rotenone and mixed pyrethrins in mammals. Proc. Soc. Exp. Biol. Med. 34:135-138, 1936.

Starr, D. F.; Ferguson, P.; Salmon, T. N. Toxicity of allethrin to rats. Soap Sanit. Chemicals 26:108-109, 1950a.

Starr, D. F.; Ferguson, P.; Salmon, T. N. Toxicity of a synthetic pyrethrin. Soap Sanit. Chemicals 26:139-143, 1950b.

Sulberger, M. B.; Weinberg, C. B. Dermatitis due to insect powder. J. A. M. A. 95:111-112, 1930.

Veda, K.; Gaughan, L. C.; Casida, J. E. Metabolism of four resmethrin isomers by liver microsomes. Pest. Biochem. Physiol. 5:280-294, 1975.

Verschoyle, R. D.; Barnes, J. M. Toxicity of natural and synthetic pyrethrins in rats. Pest. Biochem. Physiol. 2:308-311, 1972.

QUINIDINE

Quinine and quinidine are a stereoisomeric pair of cinchona alkaloids useful in treating malaria. Chloroquine and hydroxychloroquine are synthetic antimalarials that also possess the quinoline nucleus. Some of these compounds have proved effective not only against malaria but against other protozoan infections as well and are widely used in areas where these diseases are endemic. Certain other therapeutic applications, such as the use of quinidine in cardiac arrhythmias and chloroquine in rheumatoid arthritis, have led to renewed interest in the pharmacology and toxicology of these drugs. Quinidine is available as the following medicinal salts: sulfate, gluconate, and polygalacturonate. All are marketed in tablets for oral use, including a 300 mg. extended-release tablet of quinidine sulfate. The sulfate and gluconate are also available in ampuls for i.v. or i.m. injection.

Toxicology: Data on the animal toxicity of quinine and quinidine are complex because the lethal dose is critically dependent on the rate of administration. During intravenous infusion in cats, the fatal dose of quinine was found to be 100 mg./kg. at an injection rate of 5 mg./kg. per minute, but it rose to 140 mg./kg. if the rate of infusion was slowed to 2 mg./kg. per minute (Weiss and Hatcher, 1927a). Similar observations have been made with quinidine in cats (Weiss and Hatcher, 1927b) and other species (Gordon et al., 1925). Given intravenously to rabbits, chloroquine appears to be somewhat more toxic. Doses of 15 to 40 mg./kg. produced severe cardiotoxicity (Kubásta et al., 1967). Based on single lethal oral doses in rats and mice, all of these drugs lie in toxicity classes 3 and 4. Although clinical data indicate that persons with heart disease are much more sensitive than laboratory rodents to the lethal effects of quinidine sulfate, both children and adults with healthy hearts have survived after ingesting more than 300 mg./kg. (Reimold et al., 1973a; Woie and Oyri, 1974).

The toxic actions of quinidine (and quinine) can be classified into four categories: allergic (and idiosyncratic), gastrointestinal, central neural and cardiovascular. True allergic reactions, representing sensitization from prior exposures, are not uncommon but are rarely life-threatening. The more frequent are various skin eruptions and drug fevers. In 6 reported cases, the fever was associated with a reversible hepatitis, involving granulomatous and/or necrotic lesions in the liver (Koch et al., 1976). The more serious reactions are thrombocytopenic purpura and hemolytic anemia (Bishop et al., 1959; Lyon and DeGraff, 1965). Thus, neither malaria nor a red cell enzyme defect is a prerequisite for severe intravascular hemolysis during quinine or quinidine therapy (Lang and Jones, 1964).

Idiosyncratic reactions of a non-allergic nature are also recognized. For example, even small doses induce nausea, vomiting and diarrhea in some susceptible individuals. The intolerance of others is manifested by a toxic syndrome known as cinchonism, occurring at dose levels well tolerated by most persons (see below). A progressive (but reversible) dementia in a 72-year-old woman on chronic quinidine therapy appears to represent an unusual idiosyncratic reaction (Gilbert, 1977). A more common and more dangerous form of idiosyncracy consists of transient but recurrent paroxysms of ventricular fibrillation after even small therapeutic doses (Kaplinsky et al., 1972; Selzer and Wray, 1964). Individuals in whom quinidine promptly and markedly lengthens the Q-T interval appear to be particularly prone to ventricular flutter and fibrillation, as probably are persons with spontaneously long Q-T's (Koster and Wellens, 1976). To reduce the incidence and severity of these various allergic and idiosyncratic reactions, physicians often administer a "test-dose" before beginning a regular course of therapy; for quinidine sulfate the usual test dose is 0.2 gm. (Lyon and DeGraff, 1965).

Central neural reactions are encountered in normal individuals, too, if the dose of quinidine is large enough. The nausea and vomiting are largely if not exclusively of central origin. Acutely poisoned individuals have also experienced lethargy, irritability, drowsiness, confusion, ataxia, twitching, delirium, coma and convulsions (Kerr et al., 1971; Reimold et al., 1973a; Shub et al., 1978; Woie and Oyri, 1974). In subacute and chronic exposures the central effects commonly present as the syndrome known as cinchonism. This state, which can be induced by all cinchona alkaloids and by cinchophen, is characterized by tinnitus, headache, vertigo, nausea and disturbed vision. The term quinidine amblyopia arose because of the frequency of blurred vision, photophobia, diplopia, nyctalopia, defective color perception and constricted fields of vision (Lincoff, 1955); see also below.

Sudden syncope and convulsions may or may not represent a direct action of quinidine on the central nervous system. When followed by focal neurologic deficits, they suggest acute cerebral ischemia due to an arterial embolus (usually arising from a mural thrombus in a diseased left atrium). Quinidine-induced cardiac standstill may be responsible, but it is rare in the absence of complete atrioventricular block (Thomson, 1956). Transient and recurrent paroxysms of ventricular tachycardia or fibrillation are probably the commonest cause of quinidine syncope (Selzer and Wray, 1964; Ranier-Pope et al., 1962). In some cases, however, convulsions occur without evidence of acute cerebral ischemia, respiratory acidosis (Kerr et al., 1971), or cardiac arrhythmia; in these cases convulsions are believed to represent a direct effect of the alkaloid on the brain.

Another central neural effect is respiratory arrest, which has long been recognized as the immediate cause of death in many laboratory animals acutely poisoned with quinidine (Weiss and Hatcher, 1927b). In these test animals the heart is observed to continue to beat for several minutes after breathing has ceased (Gordon et al., 1925). This phenomenon, however, is infrequently described in the clinical literature (Reimold et al., 1973a). In the acutely poisoned man death is usually due to cardiac arrest, e.g., asystole or ventricular fibrillation (Acierno and Gruber, 1951).

While less important than the cardiac effects, the vascular actions of quinidine and quinine contribute importantly to the toxic syndrome by inducing a state of blood vessel paralysis (Luchi et al., 1963; Lyon and DeGraff, 1965). The result is a low peripheral vascular resistance and hypotension that is relatively refractory to sympathetic nerve stimulation and to adrenergic vasoconstrictor drugs (Luchi et al., 1963; Reimold et al., 1973a; Kerr et al., 1971). With therapeutic doses of quinidine, the hypotension is entirely of vascular origin. With toxic doses, however, it is in part a consequence of a severe depression in the contractile strength of the heart (Luchi et al., 1963).

Quinidine and quinine are properly described as general cardiac depressants, but the cardiac actions of quinidine are more intense than those of quinine. Besides their negative inotropic actions, they inhibit spontaneous diastolic depolarization at all myocardial pacemaker sites, slow rates of depolarization and of conduction, lengthen the effective refractory period, and raise the electrical threshold. In some cases the result is a failure of impulse formation and propagation in the heart, with consequent cardiac standstill. However, because not all regions of the heart muscle are equally affected, abnormal stimulus reentry mechanisms may develop in the non-uniform myocardium, with consequent tachyarrhythmias. Disorders of conduction are most apparent within the specialized conducting apparatus of the ventricle (Purkinje fibers). The result is varying degrees of intraventricular block (long QRS and Q-T). Prolongation of the QRS duration by 50% (e.g., from 80 to 120 msec.) is taken empirically as evidence of excessive quinidine effect. Effects on atrioventricular conduction are variable, but mild degrees of AV block are common. Together with prominent U waves these ECG changes occur after both therapeutic and toxic doses of quinidine, the intensity paralleling the dose. Indeed most of the toxic effects on the heart are extensions of the therapeutically useful actions.

Except for quinidine's vagal-blocking effect, which may be important in some clinical uses of the drug but which is probably irrelevant in quinidine poisoning, the cardiac actions of quinidine are remarkably similar to those of another antiarrhythmic drug, procainamide. The same is true of quinine. For example, an adult woman died in cardiac arrest 4 hours after ingesting 20 gm. of quinine sulfate (Winek et al., 1974). As an adulterant in heroin, quinine has produced AV conduction defects in addicts (Lupovich et al., 1970).

Biochemical mechanisms responsible for the myocardial actions of quinidine and quinine are not known. Experimental studies, largely on isolated perfused hearts, indicate that quinidine reduces the permeability of heart muscle to several electrolytes (briefly reviewed by Brandfonbrener et al., 1966). Even with little or no change in the resting transmembrane potential, the sodium influx and the potassium outflow are lowered during excitation and recovery, respectively (Choi et al., 1972a). At the same time the K^+ influx may be enhanced (Choi et al., 1972b). In several experimental preparations, these permeability changes have led to significant increases in the myocardial content of potassium (Choi et al., 1972a; Conn and Wood, 1960), although this is not a universal finding (*e.g.*, Brown *et al.*, 1961). Presumably other organs and tissues also extract K⁺ from the extracellular fluid under the influence of quinidine. At least mild hypokalemia has been reported in several persons with quinidine poisoning (Kerr *et al.*, 1971; Reimold *et al.*, 1973a). In some cases it cannot be accounted for in terms of potassium losses in vomitus and feces. In one 24-year-old woman hypokalemia and nodal extrasystoles were observed for several months after an acute poisoning by 12.5 gm. of quinine hydrochloride (Reimold *et al.*, 1970). Sometimes the plasma sodium level is also low.

Acidosis that is only partly respiratory in origin is a regular feature of quinidine intoxication in dogs (Bellet *et al.*, 1959a; Luchi *et al.*, 1963). Although often mentioned in the clinical literature, acidosis has not been well characterized or documented in human quinidine poisonings (*e.g.*, Kerr *et al.*, 1971), but an unequivocal metabolic acidosis was demonstrated in the patient of Shub *et al.* (1978).

Other quinoline drugs: Among drugs possessing the quinoline ring (see above), chloroquine has been responsible for a larger number of recently reported fatalities than any of the others (Bäumler and Lüdin, 1963; Cann and Verhulst, 1961; Carson *et al.*, 1967; Kiel, 1964; Larkworthy, 1971; Markowitz and McGinley, 1964; Mason *et al.*, 1964; McCann *et al.*, 1975; Robinson *et al.*, 1970; Wilkey, 1973). Doses of about 1 gm. have regularly produced death in children (Cann and Verhulst, 1961; Markowitz and McGinley, 1964, Mason *et al.*, 1964, McCann *et al.*, 1975), and 3 gm. was fatal to two adults (Don Micheal and Aiwazzadeh, 1970; Kiel, 1964). The onset of symptoms is extremely rapid, and many victims die within 2 hours. Visual disturbances sometimes precede the abrupt onset of circulatory shock terminating in cardiac arrest. Pressor amines, if effective at all, produce only temporary improvement in the circulatory status. Hyperexcitability or convulsions herald demise. Autopsy findings are limited to congestion and edema of the lungs and brain.

These reports on chloroquine fatalities support a speculative characterization of intoxication by the chloroquine-quinidine-quinine group of drugs (Cann and Verhulst, 1961) and perhaps others containing the quinoline nucleus. The cases involving chloroquine had many features in common with cases of quinine intoxication (Hillman and Harpur, 1961). Poisoning due to an overdose of hydroxychloroquine (Plaquenil) showed some similarities (Graham, 1960), and several therapeutic misadventures with quinidine (Wasserman *et al.*, 1958; Bailey, 1960) contributed details to what may be a syndrome common to the quinoline nucleus.

In acute poisonings due to any of these sub-stances cardiac arrest may occur as early as 30 minutes after the onset of toxic symptoms. In chloroquine intoxication cardiac arrest is due to direct myocardial action, anoxia, or both. Given intravenously to rabbits, chloroquine produces rapid cardiotoxicity: complete AV block, ventricular standstill, extrasystoles, tachycardia and fibrillation, with respiratory arrest secondary to anoxia (Kubăsta *et al.*, 1967). As with quinidine, neural and idiosyncratic reactions have also been ascribed to chloroquine. For example, at least four persons experienced convulsions after therapeutic doses of chloroquine (Torrey, 1968).

With acute overdoses many if not all of these drugs also produce temporary visual disturbances. Quinine overdoses in particular sometimes produce total blindness without any other prominent signs or symptoms (*e.g.*, Robertson and Raman, 1979; Sabto *et al.*, 1981). This blindness is usually ascribed to retinal vasoconstriction; it appears to respond to stellate ganglion blockade (Robertson and Raman, 1979), although a complete recovery of vision also occurs in almost all untreated cases.

Even with recommended dosage regimens, ocular abnormalities are recognized (Henkind and Rothfield, 1963). They are particularly well established for chloroquine and are associated with long term therapy (Ellsworth and Zeller, 1961; Hobbs *et al.*, 1961; Ormrod, 1962; Reed and Campbell, 1962; Sataline and Farmer, 1962). Severe visual field defects and permanent retinal damage have occurred (Frisius and Beyer, 1969). Of possible relevance is the observation that the eyes of pigmented but not albino rats accumulate extremely high concentrations of chloroquine, hydroxychloroquine and desethylchloroquine during chronic feeding trials (McChesney *et al.*, 1965, 1967). Less frequent side effects include peripheral neuropathy (Loftus, 1963) and brief episodes of toxic psychosis (Frisius and Beyer, 1969; Sapp, 1964).

Treatment of quinidine poisoning: Most courses of therapy recommended in quinidine and quinine poisoning have proved ineffectual. Certainly no single regimen is widely accepted at the present time. Presumably the primary goal of treatment should be to sustain the cardiac mechanism until the drug is eliminated. Fortunately quinidine and its hydroxy metabolites are rapidly excreted in the urine, especially in an acid urine (Gerhardt *et al.*, 1969), so that the critical period is probably only a few hours in most poisonings.

No antidote is known to counter all phases of the cardiotoxicity of quinidine or quinine. Many different drugs have been explored in experimental poisonings with variable but largely indifferent success. The list includes lanatoside C (Brandfonbrener *et al.*, 1968), dihydroouabain (Brown *et al.*, 1961), isoproterenol (Gottsegen and Östör, 1963), angiotensin with and without calcium (Luchi *et al.*, 1963) and THAM (Sierra *et al.*, 1962). Of these drugs the cardiotonic glycosides are almost certainly useless. Sodium lactate, however, has attracted more attention than any other single agent.

In dogs (Bellet *et al.*, 1959a) and perhaps in man, some of the cardiotoxic effects of quinidine may disappear promptly during or after the intravenous infusion of a 1 M sodium lactate solution. Such ECG disorders as widening of the QRS complex, prolongation of the P-R interval, and changes in the T waves and S-T segments (but not AV dissociation seen in severe poisoning) were reduced or completely suppressed by these infusions. In dogs molar sodium lactate abolished similar electrocardiographic disturbances in procainamide poisoning (Bellet *et al.*, 1959b) and in hyperkalemia due to the infusion of potassium chloride (Bellet and Wasserman, 1957). In quinidine poisoning, where the arterial pressure is apt to be very low, rises toward normotensive levels have been observed. The early clinical experience with molar sodium lactate was encouraging (Bailey, 1960; Wasserman *et al.*, 1958), but even in controlled experimental poisonings its usefulness was not established to everyone's satisfaction (Lee, 1960; Luchi *et al.*, 1963; Sierra *et al.*, 1962). Apparently it is used only rarely at the present time, as judged by the scarcity of clinical publications.

Rational treatment probably requires the therapist to recognize that the cardiotoxicity of quinidine can assume two distinct forms. The first pattern (Type I) involves a failure of cardiac stimulus formation or propagation, terminating in ventricular standstill. The second pattern (Type II) is one of abnormal stimulus formation, leading to ventricular tachyarrhythmias and terminating in ventricular fibrillation. The terminology used here is original, but the distinction is believed to be important because the two situations demand entirely different programs of therapy.

Stimulus failure (Type I) can be regarded as a progressive state involving a weakening of impulse formation (pacemaker failure) and a gradual impairment of conduction, particularly through the specialized conducting system of the AV junction and ventricle. Failure of adequate perfusion accompanied by a lengthening of the QRS interval by 50% or more (120 to 140 msec. or longer) is sometimes regarded as a sign that vigorous measures may be required to sustain the cardiac beat (Bellet, 1963). Perhaps an infusion of 1 molar sodium lactate is useful under these circumstances (Wasserman *et al.*, 1958), but it is not always effective (Ranier-Pope *et al.*, 1962), and probably one of the catecholamine drugs is preferable. Epinephrine, norepinephrine (levarterenol) and isoproterenol are all capable

of stimulating atrial pacemakers and of narrowing a wide QRS or of accelerating a slow idioventricular pacemaker in the presence of complete heart block. They also increase the stroke volume and cardiac output by stimulating the quinidine-depressed myocardium (Luchi *et al.*, 1963). At least in experimental animals the lethality of quinidine is distinctly reduced (Gottsegen and Östör, 1963).

It has been asserted but not established that isoproterenol accomplishes these changes with a smaller risk than epinephrine of inducing ventricular tachycardia or fibrillation (Nickel and Thibaudeau, 1961). Because isoproterenol is a vasodilator and levarterenol a vasoconstrictor, the latter would appear to be preferable in the hypotensive patient. In quinidine-poisoned dogs, however, levarterenol did not increase peripheral vascular resistance (Luchi *et al.*, 1963); the elevation in blood pressure was due entirely to cardiac stimulation. In a severely poisoned 16-year-old girl who had ingested 8 gm. of quinidine sulfate (117 mg./kg.), neither hypotension nor oliguria were responsive to infusions of dopamine, isoproterenol, norepinephrine (levarterenol) or mixtures thereof (Shub *et al.*, 1978).

If an infusion of isoproterenol or levarterenol fails to sustain an adequate heart rate and stroke volume in Type I poisoning, electrical pacing of the ventricles may be indicated, but the attempt is apt to be unsuccessful because of the high threshold of the quinidine-poisoned heart (Kerr *et al.*, 1971). Certainly all antifibrillatory drugs should be avoided in Type I poisonings. Except in cases of severe hypokalemia (see above), even potassium should be withheld. Thus quinidine and potassium induce similar aberrations of the ECG, and mild hypokalemia protects dogs against quinidine-induced intraventricular conduction failure and raises the lethal dose of quinidine (Brandfonbrener *et al.*, 1966). Survival of a 42-year-old woman who ingested 100 coated (long-acting) tablets of quinidine sulfate (total dose 20 gm.) was ascribed (perhaps wrongly) to hypokalemia produced by hemodialysis (Woie and Oyri, 1974).

In contrast, the abnormal mechanism of ventricular activation in Type II poisoning usually involves a rapid heart rate. The therapist's aim is to moderate and control the ventricular tachycardia and to prevent its deterioration into ventricular fibrillation. Under these circumstances potassium may be a useful agent, and it has been infused in victims of quinidine poisoning (Kerr *et al.*, 1971; Reimold *et al.*, 1973a). Except when used to correct preexisting hypokalemia, however, potassium should probably be discarded in favor of an antifibrillatory drug that is less apt to compromise AV conduction. Both propranolol (Seaton, 1966) and lidocaine (Shub *et al.*, 1978; Kaplinsky *et al.*, 1972) have been used successfully to terminate ventricular rhythms in quinidine poisoning and to restore a supraventricular mechanism. Phenytoin (diphenylhydantoin) sodium would probably be superior to propranolol and perhaps to lidocaine under these circumstances. Ventricular fibrillation may necessitate defibrillation by DC electroshocks (Ranier-Pope et al., 1962), but ventricular contractions may resume spontaneously after brief, recurring periods of fibrillation (Selzer and Wray, 1964).

To employ these therapeutic regimens correctly, it is necessary of course to recognize both types of poisoning and to distinguish between them. In practice it is sometimes difficult to differentiate between ventricular tachycardia (Type II) and a supraventricular mechanism with bundle branch block or other conduction defect (Type I) (Rivers and Boyd, 1973). Furthermore clinical signs of both patterns can sometimes be found in a single person. For example, Type I patients occasionally exhibit ventricular premature beats (Kerr et al., 1971; Reimold et al., 1973a), and Type II patients often show widening of the QRS before a ventricular mechanism becomes established (Selzer and Wray, 1964). To predict the ultimate or definitive pattern, one notes that persons with chronic heart disease, especially in congestive failure, usually exhibit a Type II reaction to quinidine overdoses (Selzer and Wray, 1964; Thomson, 1956). In persons with structurally sound hearts, Type I is thought to be the more common pattern (Kerr et al., 1971; Woie and Oyri, 1974). Even when quinidine appeared to induce ventricular tachycardia in otherwise healthy hearts, the disorder was well tolerated and fibrillation did not occur (Reimold et al., 1973a; Rivers and Boyd, 1973; Shub et al., 1978).

Whatever the mechanism of the heart beat, anoxia and respiratory acidosis should be corrected by administering oxygen and mechanically supporting breathing, as necessary. To sustain the cerebral and coronary circulations, severe hypotension requires attention. As noted above, adrenergic vasoconstrictor drugs such as levarterenol and methoxamine tend to be ineffective in raising the peripheral vascular resistance in quinidine poisoning (Luchi et al., 1963). However, β-adrenergic agonists such as levarterenol, epinephrine and presumably isoproterenol raise the blood pressure by increasing the cardiac output through mechanisms described above (Luchi et al., 1963; Lyon and DeGraff, 1965). These drugs are unquestionably useful in Type I poisonings (see above). Although one hesitates to recommend them in Type II poisonings because they might provoke or potentiate multifocal ventricular tachycardia and fibrillation, intravenous isoproterenol is said to have been lifesaving in a cardiac patient with ventric-

ular flutter-fibrillation due to quinidine (Nickel and Thibaudeau, 1961). Angiotensin is one pressor agent to which blood vessels appear to remain sensitive in quinidine poisoning. Especially when infused with edetate calcium disodium, angiotensin raised the peripheral vascular resistance, cardiac output and blood pressure in quinidine-intoxicated dogs (Luchi et al., 1963). This regimen, however, does not appear to have been tested in clinical poisonings.

Although quinidine reduces the contractile strength of the myocardium, poisoned children and adults with structurally sound hearts tolerate intravenous fluids well (Kerr et al., 1971; Reimold et al., 1973a; Woie and Oyri, 1974). Presumably these infusions of saline and of glucose in water are helpful in raising the blood pressure and promoting urine flow.

Elimination of quinidine and quinine: The pharmacokinetics of quinidine in patients with arrhythmias were studied after single therapeutic doses (2 to 6 mg./kg. of the gluconate i.v., and 2 to 10 mg./kg. of the sulfate p.o.). With intravenous administration the apparent volume of distribution averaged 3.0 liters/kg. The mean half-life of elimination from the plasma was 7.8 hours. Total body clearance was 4.8 ml./minute per kg., of which the renal clearance was only 1.0 ml./minute per kg. Thus only about 20% of administered quinidine was excreted in the urine. Most was metabolized in the liver to various ring hydroxy derivatives, which were promptly excreted by the kidneys. As predicted, elimination was abnormally slow in a patient with cirrhosis and hepatic insufficiency (Conrad et al., 1977). On the basis of this kinetic pattern, one would also predict that massive overdoses of quinidine would yield much longer half-lives of elimination and smaller clearance values than those above, but the only relevant datum located was a single plasma half-life of 18.8 hours during forced diuresis in a 3-year-old girl with a retained dose of 1600 mg. quinidine sulfate (Reimold et al., 1973a).

After filtration at the glomerulus, unmetabolized quinidine and quinine are apparently resorbed by passive back-diffusion in the distal renal tubule. This resorption was only slightly inhibited by a mannitol-induced osmotic diuresis, as judged by a disappointingly small rise in the rate of quinine excretion (Donadio et al., 1968). The resorption can be largely prevented, however, if the tubular fluid is made acidic enough to promote the ionization of these weak organic bases. In an experimetal study in man, lowering the urine pH from above 7.5 to less than 6.0 resulted in an almost 10-fold increase in urinary quinidine excretion (Gerhardt et al., 1969). Acidification also promotes the excretion of the other quinoline drugs (Jailer et al., 1947). In the presence of an acid urine, the excretory rate of quinidine did not appear to be particularly sensitive to the rate of urine flow, as influenced by furosemide (Reimold *et al.*, 1973a), but only high flow rates were tested. In treating the acidosis of quinidine poisoning, one should presumably avoid alkalinizing the urine.

Various other techniques have been tested for accelerating the elimination of quinidine and quinine. An exchange transfusion was employed successfully in severe quinine poisoning (Burrows *et al.*, 1972). In mild quinine poisoning, peritoneal dialysis removed only 11 percent of the ingested dose over a period of 16 hours (Markham *et al.*, 1967). The experience of Donadio *et al.* (1968) was even less encouraging. Although about 10% (145 mg.) of the retained dose of quinidine sulfate was recovered from a 3-year-old child during 8 hours of hemodialysis, the kidneys maintained a somewhat higher rate of elimination (Reimold *et al.*, 1973a). Hemodialysis in an adult removed even less quinidine (Woie and Oyri, 1974). The poor dialyzability of quinidine and quinine has been ascribed to their extensive binding to plasma proteins. A much more rapid extraction was accomplished by hemoperfusion through a canister of uncoated charcoal, but the procedure had to be aborted after one hour because of clotting (Shub *et al.*, 1978). It is unlikely that hemodialysis or hemoperfusion is worthwhile in quinidine poisoning except after massive overdoses in persons with preexisting liver or kidney disease or in those whose hypotension and consequent oliguria are refractory to attempts at cardiovascular resuscitation.

Symptomatology:
1. Lethargy, drowsiness, irritability.
2. Tinnitus, headache, vertigo, nausea, disturbed vision (which together are called "cinchonism").
3. Vomiting, diarrhea, abdominal pain, hot flushed skin, sweating.
4. Severe hypotension due to cardiovascular collapse, with cold sweating, pallor, cyanosis and dyspnea.
5. Apprehension, restlessness, confusion, twitching.
6. Coma punctuated with brief periods of generalized convulsions.
7. Sudden syncope in the absence of most other signs and symptoms suggests ventricular fibrillation (sometimes transient) or rarely arterial embolism.
8. Respiratory depression with periods of apnea.
9. Cardiac arrests and death due to quiescent or fibrillating ventricles.
10. Allergic responses include skin rashes, drug fever, thrombocytopenia purpura and hemolytic anemia.

Treatment:
1. If extensive vomiting has not occurred, empty the stomach by administering syrup of ipecac or performing gastric lavage. Leave a slurry of activated charcoal in the stomach.
2. Monitor the electrocardiogram, continuously if possible. Also measure at frequent intervals the arterial blood pressure and other vital signs.
3. Begin a slow intravenous infusion of glucose in water or isotonic saline, to sustain the blood pressure and promote urine flow and as a vehicle for drugs as required. Use caution in patients with preexisting heart disease and check the venous pressure often.
4. Be prepared to administer oxygen and artificial respiration as required.
5. Drugs against delirium or coma are neither safe nor necessary in most cases of quinidine poisoning. If the cerebral circulation and pulmonary ventilation are well maintained, signs of brain dysfunction are minimized but not necessarily prevented. Small doses of diazepam may be required to suppress convulsions (p. IV-37).
6. If the ECG indicates a Type I poisoning (slow pulse with long QRS; see text above):
   a. Infuse levarterenol or isoproterenol intravenously if the QRS widens to 0.14 sec. or more (see p. IV-24).
   b. Insert a transvenous pacemaker catheter into the right ventricle and prepare to pace the ventricles if the rate is not maintained by drugs (p. IV-30).
   c. Avoid antifibrillatory drugs and digitalis.
   d. Infuse potassium only to correct severe hypokalemia (p. IV-73). A mild degree of hypokalemia may be protective.
7. If the ECG indicates a Type II poisoning (ventricular tachyarrhythmia; see text above):
   a. Correct any significant degree of hypokalemia by slowly infusing potassium chloride (p. IV-73).
   b. In the presence of multifocal ventricular tachycardia, with or without periods of ventricular fibrillation, inject phenytoin sodium or lidocaine intravenously (p. IV-25).
   c. Infuse levarterenol (p. IV-17) only if hypotension is severe.
   d. Electric countershock to terminate ventricular fibrillation (p. IV-30).
8. External cardiac massage in the event of cardiac standstill or refractory ventricular fibrillation. Such extreme measures as cardiopulmonary bypass may be war-

ranted to salvage patients with structurally sound hearts.

9. Correct any severe metabolic acidosis, but try to avoid alkalinizing the urine. Diuresis may or may not be helpful in promoting quinidine secretion, but oliguria should be corrected. Peritoneal dialysis is not worthwhile, and hemodialysis and hemoperfusion are warranted only in those few patients in whom diuretic and cardiovascular drugs fail to correct oliguria and in patients with preexisting liver disease that might impair the metabolic detoxification of quinidine.

Laboratory: Electrocardiograms will indicate a characteristic widening of the QRS complex ("intraventricular block") and sometimes of the P-R interval, as well as the appearance of cardiac arrhythmias. Blood chemical determinations may indicate a metabolic acidosis and either hypo- or hyperkalemia. Blood electrolyte and pH determinations are required for the proper evaluation of treatment. Methods that are available for the determination of quinine and quinidine in human plasma are also applicable to other members of this group (Brodie and Udenfriend, 1943). Therapeutic plasma levels are 2.3 to 5.0 μg./ml. Whereas serum quinidine concentrations of 8 to 10 μg./ml. are usually considered toxic levels, the ECG is probably a better measure of clinical toxicity (Bellet, 1963).

References:

Acierno, L. J.; Gruber, R. Utility and limitations of intravenous quinidine in arrhythmias. Am. Heart J. *41*:733-741, 1951.

Bailey, D. J. Cardiotoxic effects of quinidine and their treatment. Arch. Intern. Med. *105*:13-22, 1960.

Baumler, J.; Ludin, M. Todliche suicidale Vergiftung mit chloroquine. Arch. Toxikol. *20*:96-101, 1963.

Bellet, S. *Clinical Disorders of the Heart Beat*. Lea and Febiger, Philadelphia, 1963.

Bellet, S.; Hamdan, G.; Somlyo, A.; Lara, R. The reversal of cardiotoxic effects of quinidine by molar sodium lactate. An experimental study. Am. J. Med. Sci. *237*:165-176, 1959a.

Bellet, S.; Hamdan, G.; Somlyo, A.; Lara, R. A reversal of the cardiotoxic effects of procaine amide by molar sodium lactate. Am. J. Med. Sci. *237*:177-189, 1959b.

Bellet, S.; Wasserman, F. The effects of molar sodium lactate in reversing the cardiotoxic effect of hyperpotassemia. Arch. Intern. Med. *100*:565-575, 1957.

Bishop, R. C.; Spencer, H. H.; Bethel, F. H. Quinidine purpura. Report of six cases. Ann. Intern. Med. *50*:1227-1240, 1959.

Brandfonbrener, M.; Kjobech, C.; Cooper, E. The effect of digitalization on quinidine toxicity. Am. Heart J. *76*:249-251, 1968.

Brandfonbrener, M.; Kronholm, J.; Jones, H. R. The effect of serum potassium concentration on quinidine toxicity. J. Pharmacol. Exp. Ther. *154*:250-254, 1966.

Brodie, B. B.; Udenfriend, S. The estimation of quinine in human plasma with a note on the estimation of quinidine. J. Pharmacol. Exp. Ther. *78*:154-158, 1943.

Brown, T. E.; Grupp, G.; Acheson, G. H. The effect of quinidine on the potassium balance of the dog heart. J. Pharmacol. Exp. Ther. *133*:84-89, 1961.

Burrows, A. W.; Hambleton, G.; Hardman, M. J.; Wilson, B. D. R. Quinine intoxication in a child treated by exchange transfusion. Arch. Dis. Child. *47*:304-305, 1972.

Cann, H. M.; Verhulst, H. L. Fatal acute chloroquine poisoning in young children. Pediatrics *27*:95-102, 1961.

Carson, J. W., Jr.; Barringer, M. L.; Jones, R. E. Fatal chloroquine ingestion: An increasing hazard. Pediatrics *40*:449-450, 1967.

Choi, S. J.; Roberts, J.; Kelliher, G. J. The effect of propranolol and quinidine on ^{22}Na- and ^{42}K-exchange in the cat papillary muscle. Europ. J. Pharmacol. *20*:10-21, 1972a.

Choi, S. J.; Roberts, J.; Kelliher, G. J.; Modification of the action of propranolol and quinidine on ^{22}Na- and ^{42}K-exchange by reserpine. Europ. J. Pharmacol. *20*:22-33, 1972b.

Conn, H. L.; Wood, J. C. Acute effects of quinidine on K exchange and distribution in the dog ventricle. Am J. Physiol. *199*:151-156, 1960.

Conrad, K. A.; Molk, B. L.; Chidsey, C. A. Pharmacokinetic studies of quinidine in patients with arrhythmias. Circulation *55*:1-7, 1977.

Don Micheal, T. A.; Aiwazzadeh, S. The effects of acute chloroquine poisoning with special reference to the heart. Am. Heart J. *79*:831-842, 1970.

Donadio, T. V., Jr.; Whelton, A.; Gilliland, P. F.; Cirksena, W. J. Peritoneal dialysis in quinine intoxication. J. A. M. A. *204*:274, 1968.

Ellsworth, R. J.; Zeller, R. W. Chloroquine (Aralen)-induced retinal damage. Arch. Ophthalmol. *66*:269-272, 1961.

Frisius, H.; Beyer, K. H. Klinik, Toxicologie und Therapie einer schweren Chininvergiftung. Arch. Toxikol. *24*:201-213, 1969.

Gerhardt, R. E.; Knooss, R. F.; Thyrum, P. T.; Luchi, R. J.; Morris, J. J., Jr. Quinidine excretion in aciduria and alkaluria. Ann. Intern. Med. *71*:927-933, 1969.

Gilbert, G. J. Quinidine dementia. J.A.M.A. *237*:2093-2094, 1977.

Gordon, B.; Matton, M.; Levine, S. A. The mechanism of death from quinidine and a method of resuscitation. An experimental study. J. Clin. Invest. *1*:497-517, 1925.

Gottsegen, G.; Ostor, E. Prevention of the cardiotoxic effect of quinidine by isoproterenol. Am. Heart J. *65*:102-109, 1963.

Graham, J. D. P. An overdose of Plaquenil. Br. Med. J. *1*:1256, 1960.

Henkind, P.; Rothfield, N. F. Ocular abnormalities in patients treated with synthetic antimalarial drugs. N. Engl. J. Med. *269*:433-439, 1963.

Hillman, E.; Harpur, E. R. Quinine poisoning. N. Engl. J. Med. *264*:138-139, 1961.

Hobbs, H. E.; Eadie, S. P.; Sommerville, F. Ocular lesions after treatment with chloroquine. Br. J. Ophthalmol. *45*:284-297, 1961.

Jailer, J. W.; Rosenfeld, M.; Shannon, J. A. The influence of orally administered alkali and acid on the renal excretion of quinacrine, chloroquine and Santoquine. J. Clin. Invest. *26*:1168-1172, 1947.

Kaplinsky, E.; Yahini, J. H.; Barzilai, J.; Neufeld, H. N. Quinidine syncope; report of a case successfully treated with lidocaine. Chest *62*:764-766, 1972.

Kerr, F.; Kenoyer, G.; Bilitch, M. Quinidine overdose, neurological and cardiovascular toxicity in a normal person. Br. Heart J. *33*:629-631, 1971.

Kiel, F. W. Chloroquine suicide. J. A. M. A. *190*:398-400, 1964.

Koch, M. J.; Seeff, L. B.; Crumley, C. E.; Rabin, L.; Burns, W. A. Quinidine hepatotoxicity. A report of a case and review of the literature. Gastroenterol. *70*:1136-1140, 1976.

Koster, R. W.; Wellens, H. J. J. Quinidine-induced ventricular flutter and fibrillation without digitalis therapy. Am J. Cardiol. *38*:519-523, 1976.

Kubasta, M.; Vykydal, M.; Zmestal, A.; Gikalovova, I. Cardiotoxicity of chloroquine in rabbits. Arch. Toxikol. *22*:373-380, 1967.

Lang, P. A.; Jones, C. C. Acute renal failure precipitated by quinine sulfate in early pregnancy. J. A. M. A. *188*:464-466, 1964.

Larkworthy, W. Acute chloroquine poisoning. Practitioner *207*:212-214, 1971.

Lee, Y. Quinidine intoxication. An experimental study of the effect of molar sodium lactate and potassium chloride. Am. Heart J. *60*:785-798, 1960.

Lincoff, M. H. Quinine amblyopia. Arch. Ophthalmol. *53*:382-384, 1955.

Loftus, L. R. Peripheral neuropathy following chloroquine therapy. Can. Med. Assoc. J. *89*:917-920, 1963.

Luchi, R. J.; Helwig, J., Jr.; Conn, H. L., Jr. Quinidine toxicity and its treatment. Am. Heart J. *65*:340-348, 1963.

Lupovich, P.; Piewski, R.; Sapira, J. D.; Juselius, R. Cardiotoxicity of quinine as an adulterant. J. A. M. A. *212*:1216, 1970.

Lyon, A. F.; DeGraff, A. C. Antiarrhythmic drugs. III. Quinidine toxicity. Am. Heart J. *70*:139-141, 1965.

Markham, T. N.; Dodson, V. N.; Eckberg, D. L. Peritoneal dialysis in quinine sulfate intoxication. J. A. M. A. *202*:1102-1103, 1967.

Markowitz, H. A.; McGinley, J. M. Chloroquine poisoning in a child. J. A. M. A. *189*:950-951, 1964.

Mason, J. R.; Khan, K.; Frewing, H. L. Fatal chloroquine poisoning: Two more cases. J. A. M. A. *188*:187, 1964.

McCann, W. P.; Permisohn, R.; Palmisana, P. A. Fatal chloroquine poisoning in a child: Experience with peritoneal dialysis. Pediatrics *55*:536-538, 1975.

McChesney, E. W.; Banks, W. F., Jr.; Fabian, R. J. Tissue distribution of chloroquine, hydroxychloroquine and desethylchloroquine in the rat. Toxicol. Appl. Pharmacol. *10*:501-513, 1967.

McChesney, E. W.; Banks, W. F., Jr.; Sullivan, D. J. Metabolism of chloroquine and hydroxychloroquine in albino and pigmented rats. Toxicol. Appl. Pharamcol. *7*:627-636, 1965.

Nickel, S. N.; Thibaudeau, Y. Quinidine intoxication treated by isoproterenol (Isuprel). Can. Med. Assoc. J. *85*:81-83, 1961.

Ormrod, J. N. Two cases of chloroquine-induced retinal damage. Br. Med. J. *1*:918-919, 1962.

Rainier-Pope, C. R.; Schrire, V.; Beck, W.; Barnard, C. N. The treatment of quinidine-induced ventricular fibrillation by closed-chest resuscitation and external defibrillation. Am. Heart J. *63*:582-590, 1962.

Reed, H.; Campbell, A. A. Central scotomata following chloroquine therapy. Can. Med. Assoc. J. *86*:176-178, 1962.

Reimold, E. W.; Reynolds, W. J.; Fixler, D. E.; McElroy, L. Use of hemodialysis in the treatment of quinidine poisoning. Pediatrics *52*:95-99, 1973a.

Reimold, W. V.; Larbig, D.; Kochsiek, K. Hypokaliamie und Herzrhythmusstorungen infolge Chininvergiftung. Dtsch. Med. Wochenschr. *95*:517-521, 1970.

Rivers, R. P. A.; Boyd, R. D. H. Quinidine toxicity in a normal heart. Acta Paediatr. Scand. *62*:391-395, 1973.

Robertson, D. H.; Raman, K. R. Quinine poisoning—An unusual indication for stellate ganglion blockade. Anaesthesia *34*:1041-1042, 1979.

Robinson, A. E.; Copper, A. I.; Camps, F. E. The distribution of chloroquine in man after fatal poisoning. J. Pharm. Pharmacol. *22*:700-703, 1970.

Sabto, J.; Pierce, R. M.; West, R. H.; Gurr, F. W. Hemodialysis, peritoneal dialysis, plasmapheresis and forced diuresis for the treatment of quinine overdose. Clin. Nephrol. *16*:264-268, 1981.

Sapp, O. L., III. Toxic psychosis due to quinacrine and chloroquine. J. A. M. A. *187*:373-375, 1964.

Sataline, L. R.; Farmer, H. Impaired vision after prolonged chloroquine therapy. N. Engl. J. Med. *266*:326-347, 1962.

Seaton, A. Quinidine-induced paroxysmal ventricular fibrillation treated with propranolol. Br. Med. J. *1*:1522-1523, 1966.

Selzer, A.; Wray, H. W. Quinidine syncope; paroxysmal ventricular fibrillation occurring during treatment of chronic atrial arrhythmias. Circulation *30*:17-26, 1964.

Shub, C.; Gau, G. T.; Sidell, P. M.; Brennan, L. A. The management of acute quinidine intoxication. Chest *73*:173-178, 1978.

Sierra, M. A.; Keyes, M. H.; Williams, R. M.; Becker, D. J.; Silverblatt, C. W.; Gardner, W. R.; Wasserman, F. The effect of 2-amino-2-hydroxymethyl-1, 3-propanediol (THAM) in experimental quinidine intoxication. Am. J. Cardiol. *10*:562-569, 1962.

Thomson, G. M. Quinidine as a cause of sudden death. Circulation *14*:757-765, 1956.

Torrey, E. F. Chloroquine seizures. J. A. M. A. *204*:867-870, 1968.

Wasserman, F.; Brodsky, L.; Dick, M. M.; Kathe, J. H.; Rodensky, P. L. Successful treatment of quinidine and procaine amide intoxication. Report of three cases. N. Engl. J. Med. *259*:797-802, 1958.

Weiss, S.; Hatcher, R. II. Studies on quinine. J. Pharmacol. Exp. Ther. *30*:327-333, 1927a.

Weiss, S.; Hatcher, R. III. Studies on quinidine. J. Pharmacol. Exp. Ther. *30*:335-345, 1927b.

Wilkey, I. S. Chloroquine suicide. Med. J. Aust. *1*:396-397, 1973.

Winek, C. L.; Davis, E. R.; Collom, W. D.; Shanor, S. P. Quinine fatality; case report. Clin. Toxicol. *7*:129-132, 1974.

Woie, L.; Oyri, A. Quinidine intoxication treated with hemodialysis. Acta Med. Scand. *195*:237-239, 1974.

RESERPINE

Reserpine is a pure crystalline alkaloid derived from the roots of *Rauwolfia serpentina*, a small shrub growing wild in certain regions of India and other tropical countries. The powdered whole root and extracts thereof have been used for centuries in Indian folk medicine for a variety of purposes, and these preparations, together with the purified alkaloids, are now employed by physicians throughout the world for the control of hypertension and for the production of tranquilization. Its popularity, however, is waning as more effective antihypertensives and tranquilizers are becoming available. Deserpidine (11-desmethoxyreserpine) is derived from a related species of the genus *Rauwolfia*. Ajmaline, a Rauwolfia alkaloid used to manage cardiac arrhythmias in Europe, has caused several severe poisonings; see in Section II.

Toxicology: Reserpine alkaloids exert significant effects both on the central nervous system and on many peripheral tissues. Central actions would appear to arise from effects within the hypothalamus and the limbic system. In terms of the hypothalamus, the response appears to be a sustained increase in the amount of spontaneous neural activity in the centers that control the parasympathetic nervous system (Brodie *et al.*, 1959). This enhanced activity is reflected peripherally in such signs and symptoms as miosis, bradycardia, nasal stuffiness, increased hunger (and eventually weight gain), enhanced gastric acid secretion, nausea, diarrhea and excessive salivation (Hollister, 1961b). At the same time central sympathetic tone may or may not be inhibited.

In any case it is definitely established that there is a significant reduction in the responses to sympathetic nerve activity because of a highly characteristic type of nerve blockade that appears to be restricted to the peripheral terminals of sympathetic adrenergic nerves. This blockade is associated with marked reductions in the levels of endogenous norepinephrine not only in adrenergic nerves but also in such critical organs as the heart, blood vessels, chromaffin tissue, and even the adrenal medulla. At some of these sites the effective tissue concentration of catecholamines falls by more than 90%. This depletion is due to the failure of the mechanisms responsible for the storage of norepinephrine (and some other amines) within intracellular granular vesicles. As a result stored catecholamines are freed within cells and then subjected to metabolic inactivation by intracellular monoamine oxidase. Since norepinephrine serves as the transmitter substance in adrenergic nerves, the affected nerves are not able to carry regulatory impulses to peripheral effector organs. A consistent fall in blood pressure reflects widespread vasodilatation secondary to loss of vasoconstrictor tone, but a reduction in the force of cardiac contraction may be contributory.

Central neural actions of reserpine are also revealed in terms of various psychic, emotional and motor responses. These reactions have been ascribed to a fall in the brain concentrations of norepinephrine (Holzbauer and Vogt, 1956) and of serotonin (Brodie et al., 1961), but a concomitant depletion of brain dopamine is more recently held to be responsible (Carlsson, 1974). In this category are included responses that may be desired therapeutically, such as sedation and reduction in emotional tension, as well as unwanted side effects that are commonly encountered in therapy, such as excessive drowsiness, fatigue, apathy, headache, confusion, dizziness, hallucinations, nightmares, anxiety and agitation (Parker and Murphy, 1961). Emotional depression is both a common consequence of reserpine therapy and at times an alarming one, because at least in older patients suicide is believed to be a real danger.

Other central manifestations of reserpine may be related to the spontaneous electrical seizures which are described in the amygdala and other portions of the limbic cortex of reserpine-poisoned animals (Killam and Killam, 1957). Although clinical convulsions have not been described in patients who received large overdoses of reserpine, even conventional doses appear to increase sensitivity to such convulsive stimuli as electroshock, insulin hypoglycemia, and convulsant drugs (Bracha and Hess, 1956; Foster and Gayle, 1956). Motor difficulties of central origin are often encountered with conventional doses and particularly with large doses. These disturbances include muscle spasm, tremor, masklike face with bowed shoulders, and various types of dystonia, all of which usually return to normal following cessation of therapy (Stead and Wing, 1955). These states are said to respond favorably to the same drugs that are used in parkinsonism, but l-dopa should be avoided. For more information about the tardive dyskinesias induced by many neuroleptic drugs including reserpine, see CHLORPROMAZINE, p. III-111.

The magnitude of the lethal dose is not well established. Animal studies suggest that reserpine and its congeners lie near the borderline between toxicity classes 3 and 4 in terms of the single oral mean lethal dose (Harrisson et al., 1955; Parker and Murphy, 1961). Although the drug is readily absorbed from the gastrointestinal tract, it is in part metabolized by the intestinal mucosa, perhaps accounting for its higher toxicity by parenteral routes (Stitzel, 1976). For example, the intravenous LD_{50} for the rabbit and rat is approximately 10 mg./kg. (Ciba, 1955), and as little as 1 mg./kg. injected subcutaneously in the cat produces severe circulatory failure within 24 hours (Zaimis, 1961).

When first introduced into clinical medicine in the United States., some patients received daily doses as large as 20 mg. by mouth, but because of the high incidence of side effects, the currently recommended dose varies between 0.1 and 1.0 mg. per day in the adult human. A 20-month-old male child ingested 260 mg. of reserpine (Serpasil); he slept most of the next 3 days but could be aroused at any time, and recovery was eventually complete (Hubbard, 1955). In three children ranging in age from 2 to 4 years (two of whom ingested less than 25 mg.), coma, bradycardia and hypothermia were the cardinal signs. Hypertension (170/110 mm. Hg) and sinus tachycardia developed in the youngest child. Contrary to expectation there was an increase in the urinary excretion of free catecholamines in the two younger children on the first postingestion day, with no striking changes in the excretory pattern of catecholamine metabolites (Loggie et al., 1967). In a review of 151 cases of Rauwolfia alkaloid ingestion as reported to the National Clearinghouse, about a third exhibited flush and some form of central depression. Only one case of coma and two cases of hypotension were reported (McKown et al., 1963). A mild congenital intoxication in the newborn has been described (Platou, 1961). In all the above cases complete recovery ensued, which is fortunate since no effective antidote is known.

On the other hand the opinion has been expressed that young children may be more resistant than adults to toxic doses of reserpine. Although no acute poisonings in man have ended fatally to our knowledge, there are many reasons for caution in making optimistic prognoses. The effective oral dose and by inference the toxic dose vary considerably from individual to individual. A long latent period before the appearance of toxic signs and symptoms is character-

III-364 SECTION III. THERAPEUTICS INDEX

istic and is noted even after the parenteral administration of reserpine. Once established, the toxic syndrome may last for many days, perhaps more than 1 week.

Although considerable variation is found in the amounts of unchanged drug and metabolites eliminated in the feces, some material is always present even after parenteral administration. This observation points to an enterohepatic shunt for reserpine, which may be sizeable in some patients (Stitzel, 1976). After oral administration of labeled reserpine to humans, radioactivity could be detected in plasma, urine and feces for 11 to 12 days. Only 8% of the dose was eliminated in the urine in 4 days, chiefly as methyl reserpate, trimethyoxybenzoic acid. and its sulfate and glucuronide conjugates. The drug is acted upon by serum esterases and hydrolytic and microsomal enzymes in the liver (Pfeifer *et al.*, 1976). Although initial concentrations in plasma exceed those in red cells, reserpine is bound much more tenaciously to the latter (Maas *et al.*, 1969).

The toxic syndrome due to a massive overdose appears to consist of an exaggeration and intensification of all of those effects and side effects that arise from therapeutic doses. Various degrees of central nervous depression, with or without catatonia, have been described, but relevant reports are few (Plummer *et al.*, 1954; Jacobziner and Raybin, 1961f; Hubbard, 1955). Coma is usually of long duration, but it may be of rather mild intensity in that the patient can sometimes be aroused by intense or even by gentle stimuli. Peripheral vasodilatation with conjunctival injection and a generalized blush (particularly of the face) is prominent and persistent; it undoubtedly contributes to the fall in body temperature that is usually noted. A hyperchlorhydria which is unaffected by atropine, methantheline or epinephrine is regularly induced in man by therapeutic doses (Schneider and Clark, 1956). In individuals with a predisposition to peptic ulcer, massive gastrointestinal hemorrhage or perforation may occur (Duncan and Fleeson, 1959).

Severe cardiovascular collapse is potentially the most dangerous complication (Pfeifer *et al.*, 1976). At least mild hypotension is a consistent finding, except in young children (see above). Presumably vasodilatation is largely responsible for this hypotension, but an impairment in the contractile force of the heart may contribute to an important degree. At least in cats severe circulatory failure 24 hours after 1 mg./kg. of reserpine (subcutaneously) has been ascribed to weakened cardiac contractions. The hearts were enlarged and flabby and exhibited severe degenerative microscopic changes of the myocardium (Zaimis, 1961). Electron miscroscopic studies of hearts from reserpine-treated mice and dogs re-

vealed mitochondrial damage (Sun *et al.*, 1968), presumably responsible for an uncoupling of oxidative phosphorylation (Schwartz and Lee, 1960). Ouabain improved considerably the contractile force of the heart and raised the level of the arterial blood pressure in reserpine-poisoned cats (Zaimis, 1961). Clinical experience, however, suggests that combined therapy with reserpine and digitalis may lead to a high incidence of cardiac arrhythmias (Dick *et al.*, 1962).

In general drug therapy must be approached with great caution in the reserpinized patient. For example, these alkaloids potentiate the actions of many sedative, hypnotic, and anesthetic drugs, so that anesthesia and surgery are apt to be poorly tolerated (Ziegler and Lovette, 1961; Smessaert and Hicks, 1961; Pfeifer *et al.*, 1976). Similarly epinephrine and norepinephrine (levarterenol) may give rise to exaggerated vascular and cardiac reactions in reserpine-poisoned individuals. In contrast some drugs are less active after reserpine. Although it has been recommended for the control of various side effects in reserpine therapy (Feinblatt *et al.*, 1956), ephedrine and related amines are usually less active and sometimes almost inactive in reserpinized animals. In general supportive measures that do not involve extensive drug therapy are probably safest and are expected to suffice in most cases.

Symptomatology (after a latency of one or more hours):

1. Sedation, reduction in emotional tension, and sleep.
2. Drowsiness, apathy, fatigue, anxiety, headache, dizziness, confusion, restlessness and hallucinations.
3. An agitated depression may lead to a suicide attempt.
4. Signs and symptoms of increased parasympathetic nervous activity, such as nasal stuffiness, miosis, excessive salivation, intense gastric acid secretion, sensations of hunger (leading to frequent feedings and eventual weight gain), nausea with anorexia, and sometimes both vomiting and diarrhea.
5. Excessive secretory and motor activity of the stomach may lead eventually to the formation of a peptic ulcer with pain, hemorrhage, and perforation.
6. Evidence of blockade of peripheral adrenergic nerves, such as peripheral vasodilatation, bradycardia, occasional failure of the ejaculatory reflex, etc.
7. Motor disturbances, apparently of the extrapyramidal system, characterized by stiffness with aching pain in the legs, tremors, and various types of dystonia and catatonia.
8. In chronic therapy hormonal disturbances

have been described, notably mild feminization of adult males (gynecomastia and lactation).

9. After a single massive dose most of the effects noted above are not encountered. Instead the patient becomes sleepy and eventually comatose; he may or may not be arousable. Coma or sleep may last for several days.

10. Associated with the coma there is commonly widespread blushing, conjunctival injection, hypotension with bradycardia, and hypothermia. The hypotension, which often persists for several days, may be mild or severe. In one 2-year-old an initial phase of hypertension has been reported (Loggie *et al.*, 1967).

11. Recovery is the rule, but cardiovascular collapse may become a threat to life.

Treatment:

1. In the acutely poisoned patient who is not in coma, emesis should be induced or gastric lavage performed (see Section I), even several hours after ingestion of the alkaloid. Leave in the stomach a saline cathartic and activated charcoal (p. I-12) to prevent enterohepatic recycling.

2. Annoying parasympathomimetic side effects during reserpine therapy can often be controlled with atropine or other anticholinergic drugs in small doses.

3. Although often inactive in reserpinized animals, small doses of ephedrine and related amines have been recommended for the suppression of these same side effects.

4. Epigastric pain and other signs of a peptic ulcer may require local antacid therapy (aluminum hydroxide, aluminum trisilicate, etc.).

5. Stiffness, tremors, and other evidence of motor dysfunction can often be controlled by drugs useful in the management of parkinsonism, but the safer course is to discontinue reserpine therapy and wait for spontaneous recovery.

6. The characteristic coma with hypotension generally responds to conservative supportive therapy. Analeptic drugs are probably more dangerous than beneficial, because their convulsant potential seems to be exaggerated by reserpine.

7. Use blankets and the external application of mild heat to maintain the body temperature at a normothermic level.

8. Unless the blood pressure becomes very low, avoid vasopressor drugs, which may prove to be inactive (*e.g.*, ephedrine) or which may lead to an exaggerated cardiovascular response (*e.g.*, epinephrine, levarterenol).

9. Because of the uncertain cardiac status in reserpine poisoning, avoid rapid intravenous infusions for the purpose of raising the arterial blood pressure.

10. Although not described in clinical poisonings, rapid digitalization with ouabain or acetylstrophanthidin may aid in the maintenance of an adequate circulation (IV-21), although there may be a high risk of cardiac arrhythmias.

Laboratory: Frequent electrocardiograms may aid in the detection of myocardial damage, although injury currents have not been reported in reserpine-poisoned humans.

References:

Bracha, S.; Hess, J. P. Death occurring during combined reserpine-electroshock treatment. Am. J. Psychiatr. *113*:257, 1956.

Brodie, B. B.; Spector, S.; Shore, P. A. Interaction of drugs with norepinephrine in the brain. Pharmacol. Rev. 11: Part 2, 548-564, 1959.

Brodie, B. B.; Sulser, F.; Costa, E. Psychotherapeutic drugs. Ann. Rev. Med. *12*:349-368, 1961.

Carlsson, A. Antipsychotic drugs and catecholamine synapses. J. Psychiat. Res. *11*:57-64, 1974.

Ciba Pharmaceutical Products, Inc. Serpasil in Psychiatry. Brochure. Summit, N. J, 1955.

Dick, H. L. H.; McCawley, E. L.; Fisher, W. A. Reserpine-digitalis toxicity. Case reports of cardiac arrhythmias occurring during reserpine-digitalis therapy and a review of the literature with supporting animal experiments. Arch. Intern. Med. *109*:503-506, 1962.

Duncan, D. A.; Fleeson, W. Reserpine-induced gastrointestinal hemorrhage. J. A. M. A. *170*:1661, 1959.

Feinblatt, T. M.; Feinblatt, H. M.; Ferguson, E. A., Jr. Rauwolfia-ephedrine as a hypotensive-tranquilizer. J. A. M. A. *161*:424-426, 1956.

Foster, M. W., Jr.; Gayle, R. F., III. Chlorpromazine and reserpine as adjuncts in electroshock treatment. South. Med. J. *49*:731-735, 1956.

Harrisson, J. W. E.; Packman, E. W.; Smith, E.; Hosansky, N.; Salkin, R. Toxicity and chemistry of 11-desmethoxyreserpine (Raunormine) (3, 4, 5-trimethoxybenzoic acid ester of methyl 11-desmethoxyreserpate), an alkaloid from *Rauwolfia canescens*. . J. Pharm. Sci. *44*:688-693, 1955.

Hollister, L. E. Current concepts in therapy, complications from psychotherapeutic drugs. N. Engl. J. Med. *264*:345-347, 1961b.

Holzbauer, M.; Vogt, M. Depression by reserpine of the noradrenaline concentration in the hypothalamus of the cat. J. Neurochem. *1*:8-11, 1956.

Hubbard, B. A., Jr. Reserpine. J. A. M. A. *157*:468, 1955.

Jacobziner, H.; Raybin, H. W. Briefs on accidental chemical poisoning in New York City. N. Y. State J. Med. *61*:3153-3156, 1961f.

Killam, E. K.; Killam. K. F. The influence of drugs on central afferent pathways. In *Brain Mechanisms and Drug Actions, A Symposium,* p. 71-98. Edited by W. S. Field. Charles C Thomas, Springfield, Ill, 1957.

Loggie, J. M. H.; Saito, H.; Kahn, I.; Fenner, A.; Gaffney, T. E. Accidental reserpine poisoning: clinical and metabolic effects. Clin. Pharmacol. Ther. *8*:692-695, 1967.

Maas, A. R.; Jenkins, B.; Shen, Y.; Tannenbaum, P. Studies on absorption, excretion, and metabolism of ^{3}H-reserpine in man. Clin. Pharmacol. Ther. *10*:366-371, 1969.

McKown, C. H.; Verhulst, H. L.; Crotty, J. J. Overdosage effects and danger from tranquilizing drugs. J. A. M. A. *185*:425-430, 1963.

Parker, J. M.; Murphy, C. W. Reserpine - a comparison of chronic toxicity in animals with clinical toxicity. Can. Med. Assoc. J. *84*:1177-1180, 1961.

Pfeifer, H. J.; Greenblatt, D. J.; Koch-Wesen, J. Clinical toxicity of reserpine in hospitalized patients: a report from the Boston collaborative drug surveillance program. Am. J. Med. Sci. 271:269-276, 1976.

Platou, R. V. Poisonings in children. Lancet 81:548-551, 1961.

Plummer, A. J.; Earl, A.; Schneider, J. A.; Trapold, J.; Barnes, W. Pharmacology of Rauwolfia alkaloids including reserpine. Ann. N. Y. Acad. Sci. 59: Art. 1, 8-21, 1954.

Schneider, E. M.; Clark, M. L. Hyperchlorhydria induced by intravenous reserpine. Response to various therapeutic agents. Am. J. Dig. Dis. 1:22-30, 1956.

Schwartz, A.; Lee, K. S. Effect of reserpine on heart mitochondria. Nature 188:948-949, 1960.

Smessaert, A. A.; Hicks, R. G. Problems caused by Rauwolfia drugs during anesthesia and surgery. N. Y. State J. Med.

61:2399-2403, 1961.

Stead, J. S.; Wing, J. K. Parkinsonism during treatment with reserpine. Lancet 1:823-824, 1955.

Stitzel, R. E. The biological fate of reserpine. Pharmacol. Rev. 28:179-205, 1976.

Sun, S.; Sohal, R. S.; Colcolough, H. L.; Burch, G. E. Histochemical and electron microscopic studies on the effects of reserpine on the heart muscle of mice. J. Pharmacol. Exp. Ther. 161:210-221, 1968.

Zaimis, E. Reserpine-induced circulatory failure. Nature 192:521-523, 1961.

Ziegler, C. H.; Lovette, J. B. Operative complications after therapy with reserpine and reserpine compounds. J. A. M. A. 176:916-919, 1961.

ROTENONE

Rotenone is a widely used insecticide, combining the qualities of effectiveness against insects and relatively low toxicity for plants and mammals. It is used in dusts and sprays, alone and in combination with pyrethrins and sometimes other insecticides and with fungicides. It has also been employed clinically for the external treatment of chiggers (2% lotion) and scabies (10% emulsion).

Many plant sources of rotenone are known, particularly Derris grown in Malaya and the East Indies, and Lonchocarpus (familiarly known as cubé) grown in Central and South America (Haag and Taliaferro, 1940). The latter is now the principal source of commercial rotenone in the United States. These plants have been known for many centuries and used for poisoning arrow heads, for poisoning fish, and even for suicide (Shepard, 1939). In addition to fish, rotenone is highly toxic to birds (Cutkomp, 1943). Apparently the fresh derris root has a much higher toxicity than the dried powdered root from which rotenone is extracted. Only in recent years, however, have the active principles been isolated and widely utilized. The roots are dried, ground, and extracted with solvents such as chloroform and benzene.

The so-called fish poison plants contain other active ingredients besides rotenone, namely deguelin, toxicarol, tephrosin, and sumatrol—all chemically related to rotenone but less effective as insecticidal agents. Besides these natural rotenoids, several derivatives of rotenone have been chemically prepared—dihydrorotenone isorotenone, dehydrorotenone, etc., each of which is more active against certain insects than is the parent compound, but none of which is in common use at the present time. Most of these substances are less toxic to mammals than is rotenone (Ambrose and Haag, 1937).

Toxicology: Rotenone is relatively free of hazards in normal use, because of 1) the low percentage (1 to 5%) commonly used in formulations; 2) the unstable nature of rotenone (it decomposes rapidly in light and air); 3) its irritant actions when ingested, causing prompt vomiting (Ambrose and Haag, 1936; Haag, 1931); and 4) its low solubility in water (Santi and Toth, 1965). No human fatalities have been reported.

Rotenone, however, is more toxic to mammals than pyrethrins and approaches the toxicity of DDT. Although the mean lethal dose by mouth varies widely among common species of laboratory mammals, a reasonable estimate for man is 0.3 to 0.5 gm./kg. Since in animals rotenone is hundreds of times more toxic intravenously than orally, gastrointestinal absorption is presumably slow and incomplete (Buckingham, 1930; Santi and Toth, 1965; Shepard, 1939; Shimkin and Anderson, 1936). Because of poor absorption, coarse particles of solid rotenone are much less toxic than fine powders. Fats and oils promote absorption and so enhance toxicity (Haag and Taliaferro, 1940). Prolonged feeding experiments in animals have failed to demonstrate pathologic effects other than growth depression (Brooks and Price, 1961; Hansen et al., 1965).

Rotenone is a central nervous poison. Given intravenously to test animals, it produces vomiting, incoordination, muscle tremors, clonic convulsions and respiratory failure (Shepard, 1939; Shimkin and Anderson, 1936). No clinical reports of systemic poisoning in man were located. Although not a primary irritant, derris root and other rotenone preparations have caused dermatitis in humans (Dorne and Friedman, 1940).

Rotenone metabolism in laboratory mammals is mediated by NADP-linked hepatic microsomal enzymes. A half-dozen polar metabolites have been tentatively identified; the toxicity of some of these rotenoids to mice is of the same order of magnitude as the parent compound (Fukami et al., 1967). Öberg (1961) and Horgan et al. (1968) observed that rotenone inhibits mitochondrial oxidations involving NAD in a manner similar to amobarbital. Ernster et al. (1963), however, concluded that rotenone blocks NAD-flavin linked electron transport in a more specific manner than barbiturates. This blockade was not antagonized by 2,4-dinitrophenol or NAD and cytochrome c, but was overcome by vitamin K_3 (menadione sodium bisulfite), which apparently activates a bypass of the rotenone sensitive site (Ernster *et al.*, 1963). The respiratory depression and fall in arterial blood pressure in rabbits produced by intravenous rotenone can also be blocked by contemporaneous administration of menadione (Santi and Toth, 1965).

Various compounds known as insecticidal synergists, such as piperonyl butoxide and sesamex, are often added to commercial formulations of rotenone to enhance its insecticidal effectiveness. Apparently they act by inhibiting the enzymatic detoxication of rotenone in target pests. In large doses, however, these synergists are capable of inhibiting the NADP-linked microsomal enzyme system of mammalian liver (see PYRETHRUM, pp. III-354–355, for references). Therefore they may prolong the biological life and enhance the toxicity of rotenone in mammals. No definitive data were located, but this possibility should be explored in experimental animals.

When tested on the isolated guinea pig ileum or rabbit bowel, rotenone is 100 times more potent as a spasmolytic than papaverine, and its effects are more persistent after washing (Santi *et al.*, 1963). The vasodilator effects after arterial injection in dogs also mimic those of papaverine but are more profound, suggesting that papaverine may also influence mitochondrial energy metabolism. Although effects on the isolated heart can be demonstrated, cardiac action persists in the rotenone-poisoned animal even after respiratory arrest (Santi and Toth, 1965).

Symptomatology (largely inferred from animals studies):

1. Numbness of oral mucous membranes, nausea, vomiting and gastric pain.
2. Muscle tremors, incoordination, clonic convulsions and stupor. At least in rabbits and dogs, some of these effects are due to severe hypoglycemia.
3. Respiratory stimulation, followed by depression. The immediate cause of death is asphyxia from respiratory arrest.
4. Skin irritation from local application.
5. Severe pulmonary irritation from inhalation of dust.
6. With liquid preparations, aspiration of the solvent or vehicle, which is often kerosene or a related petroleum hydrocarbon, may produce pulmonary edema and pneumonitis (p. III-220).

Treatment:

1. The decision to empty the stomach or not is largely predicated on information about other constituents in the ingested product. With liquid preparations containing kerosene or a related petroleum distillate, do not induce emesis (see p. III-220). Otherwise syrup of ipecac (p. I-2) or a slurry of activated charcoal (p. I-4) may be administered.
2. If the amount ingested is estimated to contain a lethal or near-lethal dose of rotenone (see text above) or of any other ingredient in the mixture, cautious gastric lavage may be performed, even though the product is composed largely of kerosene or a related petroleum distillate. See p. I-10 and p. III-222 for special precautions. Furthermore, it may be advisable to premedicate the patient with diazepam or a barbiturate drug.
3. Administer a saline cathartic, *e.g.*, 15 to 30 gm. sodium sulfate in water and perhaps a slurry of activated charcoal (p. I-12). Avoid all oils and fats, which promote the intestinal absorption of rotenone.
4. Symptomatic and supportive treatment with oxygen (p. IV-12), artificial ventilation (p. IV-7), barbiturates (p. IV-37), and parenteral fluids.
5. Based on the experimental studies in laboratory animals described above, a trial with large parenteral doses of menadione (vitamin K_3) appears to be warranted. Use the water-soluble menadione sodium bisulfite (10 or more mg. i.v. or i.m.) or menadiol sodium diphosphate (75 mg. i.v.).
6. Administer glucose intravenously to correct hypoglycemia.
7. Wash skin with liberal quantities of water.
8. Treat pulmonary complications in the same way as those arising from the aspiration of kerosene (p. III-224) or the inhalation of nitrogen oxides (p. III-323).

Laboratory: Because severe hypoglycemia has been reported in some animals, a blood sugar test is desirable.

References:

Ambrose, A. M.; Haag, H. B. Toxicological study of derris. Ind. Eng. Chem. *28*:815-821, 1936.

Ambrose, A. M.; Haag, H. B. Toxicological studies of derris - comparative toxicity and elimination of some constituents of derris. Ind. Eng. Chem. *29*:429-431, 1937.

Brooks, I. C.; Price, R. W. Studies on the chronic toxicity of Pro-Noxfish, a proprietary synergized rotenone fish toxicant. Toxicol. Appl. Pharmacol. *3*:49-56, 1961.

Buckingham, D. E. Action of rotenone upon mammals when taken by mouth, preliminary report. Ind. Eng. Chem. *22*:1133-1134, 1930.

Cutkomp, L. K. Toxicity of rotenone and derris extract administered orally to birds. J. Pharmacol. Exp. Ther. *77*:238-246, 1943.

Dorne, M.; Friedman, T. B. Derris root dermatitis. J. A. M. A. *115*:1268-1270, 1940.

Ernster, L.; Dallner, G.; Azzone, G. F. Differential effects of rotenone and Amytal on mitochondrial electron and energy transfer. J. Biol. Chem. *238*:1124-1131, 1963.

Fukami, J.; Yamamoto, I.; Casida, J. E. Metabolism of rotenone *in vitro* by tissue homogenates from mammals and insects. Science 155:713-716, 1967.

Haag, H. B. Toxicological studies of Derris elliptica and its constituents. I. Rotenone. J. Pharmacol. Exp. Ther. 43:193-208, 1931.

Haag, H. B.; Taliaferro, I. Toxicological studies on cube. J. Pharmacol. Exp. Ther. 69:13-20, 1940.

Hansen, W. H.; Davis, K. J.; Fitzhugh, O. G. Chronic toxicity of cube. Toxicol. Appl. Pharmacol. 7:535-542, 1965.

Horgan, D. J.; Singer, T. P.; Casida, J. E. Studies on respiratory chain-linked reduced nicotinamide adenine dinucleotide-dehydrogenase. XIII. Binding sites of rotenone, piericidin A and amytal in the respiratory chain. J. Biol. Chem. 243:839-843, 1968.

Oberg, K. E. The site of the action of rotenone in the respiratory chain. Exp. Cell Res. 24:163-164, 1961.

Santi, R.; Ferrari, M.; Toth, C. E. Papaverine-like pharmacological properties of rotenone. J. Pharm. Pharmacol. 15:697-698, 1963.

Santi, R.; Toth, C. E. Toxicology of rotenone. Il Farmaco 20:270-279, 1965.

Shepard, H. H. The Chemistry and Toxicology of Insecticides. Burgess Publishing Co., Minneapolis, 1939.

Shimkin, M. B.; Anderson, H. H. Acute toxicities of rotenone and mixed pyrethrins in mammals. Proc. Soc. Exp. Biol. Med. 34:135-138, 1936.

SALICYLATE

Salicylic acid (*ortho*-hydroxybenzoic acid) and its derivatives (*e.g.*, aspirin) are an important class of compounds widely used in clinical medicine as analgetics, antipyretics, fungistatics, keratolytics, rubefacients, and antirheumatics (Smith and Smith, 1966). The annual consumption exceeds that of any other group of drugs. The same is true of the morbidity and mortality due to overdosage. Salicylate poisoning is encountered frequently; in children it is usually due to willful ingestion and in adults to suicidal or therapeutic administration (Meyer, 1961). The incidence of severe poisoning in children, however, has decreased substantially in recent years due to the introduction of safety packaging, a decrease in the number of tablets of flavored children's aspirin per package and the rising popularity of other analgetic-antipyretic drugs such as ACETAMINOPHEN (p. III-2).

Toxicology: The common derivatives of salicylic acid produce substantially the same toxic syndrome ("salicylism"). Phenyl salicylate (salol) poisoning is unique in that the chief effects are due to phenol, which is liberated by hydrolysis in the intestinal tract and probably in other tissues too. In toxic doses, salicylamide (which is not metabolized to salicylic acid) produces more central nervous depression and a syndrome that is less lethal than true salicylism (Done, 1959). Except for severe local irritation, methyl salicylate (oil of wintergreen) is not notably different in its toxic actions from the therapeutically useful salicylates (Davison *et al.*, 1961).

The mean lethal dose of sodium salicylate or acetylsalicylic acid (ASA, aspirin) by mouth probably lies between 20 and 30 gm. in adults, although less than 1 gm. of aspirin has killed and 130 gm. have been survived (Gilman *et al.*, 1980). Toxic effects usually appear whenever 10 gm. or more is ingested in single or divided doses over a period of 12 to 24 hours (Dubow and Soloman, 1948). On a molar basis methyl salicylate is no more toxic than sodium salicylate in experimental animals (Davison *et al.*, 1961). The deplorable clinical record of poisonings by the methyl

ester (Stevenson, 1937) is probably related to the fact that it is a liquid and so can be ingested more easily in large doses. In an infant, 4 ml. have proved lethal and, in an adult, 6 ml. Children (especially under the age of 3 years) are disproportionately more susceptible than adults to the toxic actions of all salicylates (Erganian *et al.*, 1947). Fay (1969) recommends hospitalization for any young child who ingests more than 1.9 gm. aspirin (*e.g.*, 25 baby aspirin tablets or 6 adult tablets). Symptoms are often delayed several hours (Crichton and Elliot, 1960).

Although many rheumatic patients have been poisoned by the intravenous administration of salicylates, most cases of salicylism are due to ingestion. Methyl and phenyl salicylates sometimes produce systemic poisoning by penetrating intact skin (von Weiss and Lever, 1964), but the percutaneous absorption of salicylic acid and its other derivatives reaches toxic levels only when large skin areas are covered with the drug in a suitable base (*e.g.*, lanolin) and/or when the skin has been damaged by preexisting disease, *e.g.*, psoriasis, ichthyosis, or when the stratum corneum has been deliberately removed (Birmingham *et al.*, 1979; Cawley *et al.*, 1953; Davies *et al.*, 1979; Taylor and Halprin, 1975; Wüthrich *et al.*, 1970).

The major toxic signs and symptoms arise from stimulation and terminal depression of the central nervous system. Central excitation reveals itself in many ways: emesis, hyperpnea, headache, tinnitus, confusion, bizarre behavior (Greer *et al.*, 1965) or mania and generalized convulsions. Asterixis is an unusual sign of salicylate toxicity in adults on chronic therapy (Anderson, 1981). Death is usually due to respiratory failure or cardiovascular collapse while in a state of coma (Riley and Worley, 1956). Occasionally paradoxical hyperthermia with or without convulsions is a prominent and even lethal complication (Dodd *et al.*, 1937; Segar and Holliday, 1958). Severe sensory disturbances, such as tinnitus, deafness and dimness of vision, are common during the acute phase (Kapur, 1965; Meyers *et al.*, 1965), but permanent neurological deficits are rare among survivors. An EEG abnormality that persisted for 5 weeks was found in one adult who had consumed 20 to 30 aspirin tablets daily (Bronn and Wilson, 1971).

In a few cases the cerebral manifestations of salicylate toxicity appear to have been exacerbated by cerebral edema of uncertain etiology. In two children judged to be only moderately intoxicated, coma occurred 24 to 48 hours after ingestion, at a time when the serum salicylate was rapidly declining. They responded to the administration of mannitol (Dove and Jones, 1982). Two other infants exhibited oliguria and fluid retention in the face of adequate hydration, a syndrome resembling that of inappropriate antidiuretic hormone secretion. Mannitol was only transiently effective, but strict fluid restriction resulted in a prompt and satisfactory diuresis (Temple et al., 1976). Cerebral edema was thought to play a role in a slowly developing stupor in an adult receiving both aspirin and dichlorphenamide, a carbonic anhydrase inhibitor (Hurwitz et al., 1980).

Less common features of acute salicylism include sweating, skin eruptions, gastrointestinal and other hemorrhages (Fishler, 1964; Graham and Parker, 1948; Kossover and Kaplan, 1961), pulmonary edema especially in older patients on chronic therapy (Granville and Sergeant, 1960; Heffner and Sahn, 1981; Greenstein, 1963), renal disturbances including renal failure (Robin et al., 1959; Snodgrass et al., 1981), and pancreatitis (Sussman, 1963b). A bleeding tendency may be manifest by hematemesis, melena or petachiae in the skin and mucous membranes. Salicylate-induced hypoprothrombinemia is usually responsible, but aspirin and to a lesser extent other salicylates also inhibit platelet aggregation. In addition to hypoprothrombinemia, an aspirin-induced hepatitis is recognized; it is rare and usually associated with chronic therapy and appears over days to weeks. This form of hepatitis is said to be more common in children with active rheumatic fever or collagen diseases, who are receiving high doses (Travers and Hughes, 1978; Zimmerman, 1981; Zucker et al., 1975). Salicylates are notorious gastric irritants (St. John, 1975), and a fatal peritonitis resulted from gastric perforation after an overdose of enteric coated tablets (Farrand et al., 1975).

In addition to these and other dose-dependent reactions, signs of drug idiosyncrasy or hypersensitivity are common (Feinberg, 1952; Samter and Beers, 1968). For example, hemolytic anemia is sometimes induced in individuals with a genetic deficiency of glucose-6-phosphate dehydrogenase (Shahidi and Westring, 1970). Some experimental evidence suggests that aspirin and sodium salicylate may aggravate hemolysis in pyruvate kinase deficiency as well (Glader, 1976; Monti and Bucar, 1976).

Many of the toxic effects outlined above are due to or aggravated by a severe disturbance in acid-base balance (Eichenholz et al., 1961; Farber et al., 1949; Guest et al., 1945; Singer, 1954; Winters et al., 1959). Many factors contribute to this imbalance, but the chief cause is prolonged hyperventilation from central stimulation, resulting in varying degrees of respiratory alkalosis. This disorder may be aggravated by a metabolic alkalosis which results from vomiting. In the poisoned adult, alkalosis commonly persists until the stage of terminal respiratory failure.

Young children with salicylate overdosage react differently from adults in one important respect, namely the prompt development of ketosis (Barnett et al., 1942), which converts an initial alkalosis into an uncompensated acidosis. Metabolic acidosis is usually well established in the salicylate-poisoned child before he is seen by the physician, whereas the adult patient is more commonly in a state of respiratory alkalosis under the same circumstances (Anderson et al., 1976; Berg, 1977; Brown et al., 1967a). If, however, other drugs such as central nervous system depressants were ingested at the same time, they may shift the balance in a poisoned adult to a respiratory acidosis (Gabow et al., 1978). Acidosis in poisoned adults is associated with impaired consciousness and is a grave prognostic finding (Proudfoot and Brown, 1969). Perhaps renal tubular dysfunction plays a role in these acid-base disturbances (Campbell and Mac-Laurin, 1958). Urinary excretion of ketone acids, Krebs cycle acids, uric acid, glucose and protein may all be elevated (Andrews et al., 1961; Ben-Ishay, 1964; Berry and Guest, 1963; Schwartz and Landy, 1965).

Ketosis in salicylate-poisoned children has not been adequately explained, but there is an impression that it may be secondary to a primary disorder in carbohydrate metabolism. Salicylate causes an early and significant rise in oxygen consumption (Tenney and Miller, 1955). In the dog this increase (which may be twofold) is due to the uncoupling of oxidative phosphorylation in skeletal muscle and perhaps other tissues. Perhaps because of this stimulation, a small decrease in tissue oxygen tension develops, in spite of hyperpnea and accelerated blood flow (increased cardiac output). This tissue anoxia has been ascribed to a salicylate-induced decrease in red cell 2,3-diphosphoglycerate. This decrease results in an increase in the oxygen affinity of hemoglobin (Kravath et al., 1972) and a consequent reduction in the amount released in tissue capillaries.

Hyperglycemia has been reported in salicylate-poisoned adults (Schadt and Purnell, 1958), but an overwhelming and refractory hypoglycemia appears to be more common in children (Cotton and Fahlberg, 1964; Limbeck et al., 1965;

Mortimer and Lepow, 1962; Pickering, 1964). Hypoglycemia can occur in patients whose subsequent glucose tolerance patterns are normal and not modified by therapeutic doses of salicylate. Salicylate-induced hypoglycemia does not appear to involve high blood insulin levels. In acutely poisoned mice the brain glucose was only 33% of control despite normal plasma glucose levels. When glucose was given with salicylate, survival was significantly increased (Thurston et al., 1970).

It is often said that the toxic effects of salicylates are manifested at plasma levels in excess of 30 mg./100 ml. (Brown et al., 1967a; Coombs et al., 1945). However, a poor correlation between blood salicylate levels and the clinical severity of the intoxication is sometimes found (Done, 1960; Surapathana et al., 1970). At least two factors are held responsible for this poor correlation: protein binding and blood pH. Because of intensive protein binding, the serum concentration of unbound or free salicylate is a more relevant index of potential toxicity than the total concentration (Buchanan et al., 1975; Reed and Palmisano, 1975). However, techniques for making such measurements are rarely available in clinical laboratories. Because the pH of CSF is well maintained at or near normal values even during systemic acidosis (Leusen, 1972), a low blood pH tends to force salicylates into the CSF in accord with the principles of nonionic diffusion. In 10 infants the intensity of the intoxication, as judged by the degree of acidosis, correlated more closely with salicylate levels in cerebrospinal fluid than with salicylate levels in serum (Buchanan and Rabinowitz, 1974).

Despite a wide variation in blood levels at death, rats given salicylate under various conditions had a very narrow range of brain salicylate concentrations (Hill, 1973). The latter finding suggests that death in these animals was due to a primary central nervous system effect. Rats made alkalotic by bicarbonate infusions had lower brain, muscle and liver salicylate concentrations and excreted more drug in the urine than rats made acidotic by carbon dioxide inhalation or the administration of acetazolamide (Hill, 1971, 1973). Thus, the increased frequency of acidosis in children appears to account for the greater severity of their intoxication syndrome. Conversely, the respiratory alkalosis of adults may be an autoprotective mechanism.

Intrauterine salicylate intoxication is recognized when mothers take the drug late in pregnancy (Lynd et al., 1976). Salicylates are excreted in breast milk and nursing infants have been poisoned by that route (Clark and Wilson, 1981). Although salicylates are not teratogenic, their regular ingestion during pregnancy has been associated with lower birth weights, increased perinatal mortality, ante- and postpartum hemorrhage, prolonged gestation and complicated deliveries (Collins and Turner, 1975; Turner and Collins, 1975).

Hastening salicylate elimination: Therapy for salicylism is symptomatic and supportive, with major emphasis on correction of the acid-base imbalance and acceleration of salicylate excretion. In the final analysis recovery depends upon urinary excretion, since 70 to 80% of a given dose can eventually be retrieved in the urine in the form of salicylate and its metabolites. In order to improve renal function, prompt attempts should be made to correct dehydration and shock.

Excretion, however, is inherently slow; about 50% of a given dose is eliminated in 24 hours in poisoned patients. Thus in previously healthy persons with untreated salicylate poisoning, the average plasma (or serum) half-life of salicylate is said to be 20 to 22 hours (Cummings et al., 1964; Done, 1960). Although considerable variation exists, the plasma half-life of salicylate in therapeutic doses is only 5 hours (Levy and Hollister, 1964). Generalizations about half-life, however, are dangerous when the complex elimination patterns are known to be both dose- and time-dependent (Bedford et al., 1965; Levy et al., 1972). For example, aspirin is almost completely hydrolyzed to salicylic acid, which is eliminated by renal excretion, by conjugations with glycine and glucuronic acid and by conversion to gentisic acid. The products of the conjugation are rapidly excreted, but the two conjugation reactions are easily saturable, resulting in a decreased systemic clearance of salicylate with increasing dose (Levy, 1981).

Elimination is distinctly faster if the urine is alkaline (pH above 7.0) than if it is acid (Gutman et al., 1955; MacPherson et al., 1955). The administration of sufficient sodium bicarbonate to alkalinize the urine is always a useful procedure if the urine is acidic (Kaplan and Del Carmen, 1958; Oliver and Dyer, 1960; Whitten et al., 1961). The poisoned adult may have an alkaline urine because of his respiratory alkalosis. Under these circumstances the therapeutic administration of alkali is unwarranted and dangerous.

By inducing a diuresis with parenteral fluids and bicarbonate, Cumming et al. (1964) reduced the mean plasma salicylate half-life to 7.5 hours in poisoned patients. An alternative measure, which presumably corrects systemic acidosis and also hastens excretion by inducing an osmotic diuresis, is the intravenous use of an amine buffer of low toxicity, namely tris(hydroxymethyl)aminomethane (Strauss and Nahas, 1960). Considerably more experience has been accumulated with another osmotic diuretic, mannitol, and with "loop diuretics" such as furosemide (Berg, 1977). Even without bicarbonate treatment, mannitol reduced the mean plasma salicylate half-life to 12 hours in three patients (Ghose and Joekes, 1964). In combination with adequate bicarbonate therapy, its efficiency is much improved (Lawson et al., 1969; Prowse et al., 1970; Savage et al., 1969). This regimen has disadvantages in that it leads invariably to hypokalemia (Lawson et al., 1969) and sometimes to pulmonary edema secondary to mannitol retention (Morgan et al., 1968). In one study alkaline glucose diuresis was not significantly different from alkaline mannitol in terms of promoting salicylate excretion (Prowse et al., 1970). As noted above, glucose administration may have other advantages, too.

Experiments in dogs have shown that the administration of acetazolamide (Diamox) is followed by an increase in the renal excretion of salicylate. However, this effect is achieved only at the expense of aggravating any systemic acidosis, which increased the mortality of salicylate-poisoned animals (Kaplan and Del Carmen, 1958). Drugs like acetazolamide produce a respiratory acidosis because of inhibition of red blood cell carbonic anhydrase (Liddell and Maren, 1975). In spite of this adverse experimental evidence, acetazolamide has been employed clinically (Feuerstein et al., 1960; Schwartz et al., 1959). In order to avoid acetazolamide-induced acidosis, Morgan and Polak (1969) also gave their patients bicarbonate. This combination was superior to bicarbonate alone in salicylate-poisoned puppies, but the authors hesitate to recommend its use in acidotic children (Reimold et al., 1973b). The advantage of the procedure is that large amounts of fluids are not required. In terms of the renal clearance of salicylate, however, acetazolamide in combination with bicarbonate was not significantly different from mannitol in combination with sodium lactate (Morgan and Polak, 1971). Benzolamide, another carbonic anhydrase inhibitor, produces maximal alkalinization of the urine in mice in doses that do not result in systemic acidosis (Liddell and Maren, 1975).

The lack of specific systemic antidotes for salicylate poisoning and the frequency and severity of intoxications have inspired the use of drastic therapeutic regimens. Among them considerable clinical experience has been accumulated with the use of exchange transfusion (Adams et al., 1957; Diamond and DeYoung, 1958; Earle, 1961; Done and Otterness, 1956; Leiken and Emmanouilides, 1960; Millar and Bowman, 1961; Rentsch et al., 1959; Yampolsky and Perry, 1960). The procedure is usually restricted to infants and young children.

Despite a high degree of plasma protein binding by salicylate (Smith et al., 1946), hemodialysis is apparently effective in removing circulating drug as well as compensating for renal failure (Doolan et al., 1951; Jørgensen and Wieth, 1963b; Levy, 1967; Magness and Murray, 1961; Thomsen and Dalgard, 1958). The plasma half-life of salicylate in dogs or human patients can be reduced with a modern apparatus to 4 to 6 hours (James et al., 1962; Jørgensen and Wieth, 1963b). Indications for hemodialysis include coma, impending circulatory collapse, rising plasma salicylate levels in the range of 70 to 100 mg./100 ml., oliguria, and failure of the urine to become alkaline in response to a standard dose of bicarbonate (Beveridge et al., 1964; Schlegel et al., 1966). With special adaptations in the apparatus the procedure has been performed safely and effectively in a 7-month-old infant (Fine et al., 1968). Although extracorporeal hemodialysis is recognized as an efficient means of ridding the body of salicylate, delays frequently encountered in preparation for this procedure tend to offset its advantage over alkaline diuresis (Dukes et al., 1963).

Peritoneal dialysis has been employed for the same indications as hemodialysis also with success (Elliott and Crichton, 1960; Halle and Collipp, 1969b; Etteldorf et al., 1961; Rhamy and Segar, 1961). Although the inclusion of 5% albumin in the dialysis fluid to trap salicylate and prevent back diffusion improves the efficiency of peritoneal dialysis (Schlegel et al., 1966; Summitt and Etteldorf, 1964), at best this procedure is about as effective as alkaline diuresis in terms of the salicylate clearance (James et al., 1962).

A more rapid method for removing salicylate is hemoperfusion through a coated-charcoal column. The technique has been used infrequently in salicylate-poisoned patients (e.g., Winchester et al., 1981). As evaluated experimentally in dogs, hemoperfusion over encapsulated charcoal was as effective as extracorporeal hemodialysis with no important adverse effects (Brookings and Ramsey, 1975). Hemodialysis, however, has an advantage over hemoperfusion in that it also tends to correct acid-base and electrolyte disturbances (Winchester et al., 1981). Most patients with acute salicylism require neither procedure.

Symptomatology:
1. A large oral dose of salicylate, particularly of the acid or the methyl ester, causes mild burning pain in the throat and stomach and usually prompt vomiting. An asymptomatic interval of several hours may follow these initial symptoms.
2. Deep and rapid breathing (hyperpnea), apathy, and lassitude are important early signs of systemic poisoning.
3. Anorexia, nausea, vomiting, thirst, and occasionally diarrhea, probably all of central nervous origin.
4. Headache, fullness in the head, dizziness,

tinnitus, difficulty in hearing and dimness of vision.

5. Irritability, restlessness, confusion, disorientation.
6. Delirium, mania, generalized convulsions.
7. Deep coma and death due to respiratory failure and/or cardiovascular collapse.
8. Miscellaneous reactions which are occasionally encountered:
   a. High fever, especially in children, with associated thirst and profuse perspiration.
   b. Hemorrhagic phenomena, commonly evidenced by petechiae in the skin and mucous membranes, hematemesis, or melena.
   c. Various skin eruptions are described, usually only after chronic medication. Some of these lesions may represent drug allergies.
9. Instead of typical salicylism as described above, an occasional patient exhibits a true idiosyncrasy or acquired hypersensitivity. The following allergic responses to salicylate have been described: angioneurotic edema, hives, laryngeal edema and consequent asphyxia, and especially asthma.

Treatment:

1. Pending gastric lavage, use emetics such as syrup of ipecac or delay gastric emptying and absorption by swallowing a slurry of activated charcoal (see p. I-4). Do not give ipecac after charcoal.
2. Gastric lavage with water or perhaps sodium bicarbonate solution (3 to 5%). Methyl salicylate is said to delay gastric emptying time; lavage may be used effectively up to 6 hours after ingestion. As much as 20 gm. of salicylate has been recovered in washings 9 hours after ingestion (Matthew *et al.*, 1966). Mild alkali delays salicylate absorption from the stomach and perhaps slightly from the duodenum.
3. Saline catharsis with sodium or magnesium sulfate (15 to 30 gm. in water).
4. Take an immediate blood sample for an appraisal of the patient's acid-base status. A pH determination on an anaerobic sample of arterial blood is best. An analysis of the plasma salicylate concentration should be made at the same time. Laboratory controls are almost essential for the proper management of severe salicylism.
5. In the presence of an established acidosis, alkali therapy is essential, but at least in the adult, alkali should be withheld until its need is demonstrated by chemical analysis. The intensity of treatment depends upon the intensity of acidosis (see p. IV-

69). In the presence of vomiting, intravenous sodium bicarbonate is the most satisfactory form of alkali therapy (p. IV-72).

6. Correct dehydration and hypoglycemia (if present) by the intravenous administration of glucose in water or in isotonic saline. The administration of glucose may also serve to remedy the ketosis which is often seen in poisoned children.
7. Even in patients without hypoglycemia, infusions of glucose adequate to produce distinct hyperglycemia are recommended to prevent glucose depletion in the brain. This recommendation is based on impressive experimental data in animals; see text.
8. Renal function should be supported by correcting dehydration and incipient shock. Overhydration is not justified. An alkaline urine should be maintained by the administration of alkali if necessary, with care to prevent a severe systemic alkalosis (p. IV-69). As long as the urine remains alkaline (pH preferably above 7.5), the administration of an osmotic diuretic such as mannitol or perhaps THAM (see p. IV-52) is useful, but one must be careful to avoid hypokalemia. Supplements of potassium chloride should be included in parenteral fluids (see 5-7 above).
9. Small doses of barbiturates, diazepam, paraldehyde, or perhaps other sedative drugs (but probably not morphine) may be required to suppress extreme restlessness and convulsions (see p. IV-35).
10. For hyperpyrexia, use sponge baths (see p. IV-84).
11. The presence of petechiae or other signs of a hemorrhagic tendency calls for large doses of vitamin K and perhaps ascorbic acid. See p. III-396 for a discussion of the treatment of hypoprothrombinemia. Small transfusions may be necessary, since bleeding in salicylism is not always due to a prothrombin deficit.
12. Hemodialysis and hemoperfusion have proved useful in salicylate poisoning, as have peritoneal dialysis and exchange transfusions, but alkaline diuretic therapy (see 8 above) is probably sufficient in all except fulminating cases.

Laboratory:

1. In toxic patients the blood plasma salicylate concentration usually exceeds 30 mg./100 ml., but remarkable exceptions have been reported.
2. The patient's acid-base status must be appraised by the best methods available, and determinations should be repeated at frequent intervals. Because salicylate poi-

soning is a mixed metabolic and respiratory disturbance (Proudfoot and Brown, 1969), the best method for measuring an uncompensated acidosis or alkalosis is a pH determination on an anaerobic sample of arterial blood.

3. Blood analyses may also reveal any or all of the following:
   a. Ketosis.
   b. Hypoglycemia or hyperglycemia.
   c. Hypoprothrombinemia.
   d. Prolonged blood coagulation time (rare).
   e. Elevation of glutamic oxalacetic and pyruvic transaminase activities (Manso *et al.*, 1956).
   f. Hypocalcemia has been reported in rats (Kato *et al.*, 1982).

4. Urinalysis may reveal albumin, casts, red blood cells and white blood cells, acetone and diacetic acid. Amino-aciduria with a preponderance of S-containing amino acids similar to patterns reported in hepatic injury has been observed.

References:

Adams, J. T.; Bigler, J. A.; Green, O. C. A case of methyl salicylate intoxication treated by exchange transfusion. J. A. M. A. 165:1563-1565, 1957.

Anderson, R. J. Asterixis as a manifestation of salicylate toxicity. Ann. Intern. Med. 95:188-189, 1981.

Anderson, R. J.; Potts, D. E.; Gabow, P. A.; Rumack, B. H.; Schrier, R. W. Unrecognized adult salicylate intoxication. Ann. Intern. Med. 85:745-748, 1976.

Andrews, B. F.; Bruton, O. C.; Knoblock, E. C. Amino-aciduria in salicylate intoxication. Am. J. Med. Sci. 240:411-414, 1961.

Barnett, H. L.; Powers, J. R.; Benward, J. H.; Hartmann, A. F. Salicylate intoxication in infants and children. J. Pediatr. 21:214-223, 1942.

Bedford, C.; Cummings, A. J.; Martin, B. K. A kinetic study of the elimination of salicylate in man. Br. J. Pharmacol. 24:418-431, 1965.

Ben-Ishay, D. Aminoaciduria induced by salicylates. J. Lab. Clin. Med. 63:924-932, 1964.

Berg, K. J. Acute acetylsalicylic acid poisoning: treatment with forced alkaline diuresis and diuretics. Eur. J. Clin. Pharmacol. 12:111-116, 1977.

Berry, H. K.; Guest, G. M. The effects of salicylate intoxication on amino acid excretions in rats. Metabolism 12:760-770, 1963.

Beveridge, G. W.; Forshall, W.; Munro, J. F.; Owen, J. A.; Weston, I. A. G. Acute salicylate poisoning in adults. Lancet 1:1406-1409, 1964.

Birmingham, B. K.; Greene, D. S.; Rhodes, C. T. Systemic absorption of topical salicylic acid. Int. J. Dermatol. 18:228-231, 1979.

Bronn, G. L.; Wilson, W. P. Salicylate intoxication and the CNS. Dis. Nerv. Syst. 32:135-140, 1971.

Brookings, C. H.; Ramsey, J. D. Salicylate removal by charcoal haemoperfusion on experimental intoxication in dogs - assessment of efficacy and safety. Arch. Toxicol. 34:243-252, 1975.

Brown, S. S.; Cameron, J. C.; Matthew, H. Plasma salicylate levels in acute poisoning in adults. Br. Med. J. 2:738-739, 1967a.

Buchanan, N.; Kundig, H.; Eyberg, C. Experimental salicylate intoxication in young baboons. J. Pediatrics 86:225, 1975.

Buchanan, N.; Rabinowitz, L. Infantile salicylism - a reappraisal. J. Pediatr. 84:391-395, 1974.

Campbell, E. J. M.; MacLaurin, R. E. Acute renal failure in salicylate poisoning. Br. Med. J. 1:503-505, 1958.

Cawley, E. P.; Peterson, N. T.; Wheeler, C. E. Salicylic acid poisoning in dermatological therapy. J. A. M. A. 151:372-374, 1953.

Clark, J. H.; Wilson, W. G. Breast-fed infant with metabolic acidosis caused by salicylate. Clin. Pediatr. 20:53-54, 1981.

Collins, E.; Turner, G. Maternal effects of regular salicylate ingestion in pregnancy. Lancet 2:335-337, 1975.

Coombs, F. S.; Warren, H. A.; Higley, C. S. Toxicity of salicylates. J. Lab. Clin. Med. 30:378-379, 1945.

Cotton, E. K.; Fahlberg, V. I. Hypoglycemia with salicylate poisoning. Am. J. Dis. Child. 108:171-173, 1964.

Crichton, J. U.; Elliot, G. B. Salicylate - a dangerous drug in infancy and childhood. A survey of 58 cases of salicylate poisoning. Can. Med. Assoc. J. 83:1144-1147, 1960.

Cumming, G.; Dukes, D. C.; Widdowson, G. Alkaline diuresis in treatment of aspirin poisoning. Br. Med. J. 2:1033-1036, 1964.

Davies, M. G.; Briffa, D. V.; Greaves, M. W. Systemic toxicity from topically applied salicylic acid. Br. Med. J. 1:661, 1979.

Davison, C.; Zimmerman, E. F.; Smith, P. K. On the metabolism and toxicity of methyl salicylate. J. Pharmacol. Exp. Ther. 132:207-211, 1961.

Diamond, E. F.; DeYoung, V. R. Acute poisoning with oil of wintergreen treated by exchange transfusion. Am. J. Dis. Child. 95:309-310, 1958.

Dodd, K.; Minot, A. S.; Arena, J. M. Salicylate poisoning: an explanation of more serious manifestations. Am. J. Dis. Child. 53:1435-1446, 1937.

Done, A. K. Uses and abuses of antipyretic therapy. Pediatrics 23:774-780, 1959.

Done, A. K. Salicylate intoxication, significance of measurements of salicylate in blood in cases of acute ingestion. Pediatrics 26:800-807, 1960.

Done, A. K.; Otterness, L. J. Exchange transfusion in the treatment of oil of wintergreen (methyl salicylate) poisoning. Pediatrics 18:80-85, 1956.

Doolan, P. D.; Walsh, W. P.; Kyle, L. H.; Wishinsky, H. Acetylsalicylic acid intoxication. A proposed method of treatment. J. A. M. A. 146:105-106, 1951.

Dove, D. J.; Jones, T. Delayed coma associated with salicylate intoxication. J. Pediatrics 100:493-496, 1982.

Dubow, E.; Soloman, N. H. Salicylate tolerance and toxicity in children. Pediatrics 1:495-504, 1948.

Dukes, D. C.; Blainey, J. D.; Cumming, G.; Widdowson, G. The treatment of severe aspirin poisoning. Lancet 2:329-331, 1963.

Earle, R., Jr. Congenital salicylate intoxication - report of a case. N. Engl. J. Med. 265:1003-1004, 1961.

Eichenholz, A.; Mulhausen, R.; Redleaf, P. The nature of the acid-base disturbance in salicylate intoxication. J. Lab. Clin. Med. 58:816-823, 1961.

Elliott, G. B.; Crichton, J. U. Peritoneal dialysis in salicylate intoxication. Lancet 2:840-842, 1960.

Erganian, J. A.; Forbes, J. B.; Case, D. M. Salicylate intoxication in the infant and young child. J. Pediatr. 30:129-145, 1947.

Etteldorf, J. N.; Dobbins, W. T.; Summitt, R. L.; Rainwater, W. T.; Fischer, R. L. Intermittent peritoneal dialysis using 5 per cent albumin in the treatment of salicylate intoxication in children. J. Pediatr. 58:226-236, 1961.

Farber, H. R.; Yiengst, M. J.; Shock, N. W. The effect of therapeutic doses of aspirin on the acid-base balance of the blood in normal adults. Am. J. Med. Sci. 217:256-262, 1949.

Farrand, R. J.; Green, J. H.; Howorth, C. Enteric-coated aspirin overdose and gastric perforation. Br. Med. J. 4:85-86, 1975.

Fay, R. Salicylate poisoning in children. N. Y. State J. Med. 69:3155-3156, 1969.

Feinberg, S. M. Drug allergy - some clinical and immunological aspects. Ann. Allergy 10:260-269, 1952.

Feuerstein, R. C.; Finberg, L.; Fleishman, E. Acetazolamide for aspirin poisoning. Pediatrics 25:215-227, 1960.

Fine, R. N.; Stiles, Q.; DePalma, J. R.; Donnell, G. N. Hemodialysis in infants under 1 year of age for acute poisoning. Am. J. Dis. Child. 116:657-661, 1968.

Fishler, J. J. Effects of aspirin, acetaminophen and salicylamide on gastric mucosa of dogs. Am. J. Dig. Dis. 9:465-470, 1964.

Gabow, P. A.; Anderson, R. J.; Potts, D. E.; Schrier, R. W. Acid-base disturbances in salicylate-intoxicated adult. Arch. Intern. Med. 138:1481-1484, 1978.

Ghose, R. R.; Joekes, A. M. Treatment of severe aspirin poisoning without dialysis. Lancet 1:1409-1412, 1964.

Gilman, A. G.; Goodman, L. S.; Gilman, A. Goodman and Gilman's Pharmacological Basis of Therapeutics, 6th ed. The MacMillan Publishing Co., Inc., New York, 1980.

Glader, B. E. Salicylate induced injury of pyruvate-kinase-deficient erythrocytes. N. Engl. J. Med. 294:916-918, 1976.

Graham, J. D. P.; Parker, W. A. The toxic manifestations of sodium salicylate therapy. Q. J. Med. 17:153-163, 1948.

Granville, K. L.; Sergeant, H. G. S. Pulmonary edema due to salicylate intoxication. Lancet 1:575-577, 1960.

Greenstein, S. M. Pulmonary edema due to salicylate intoxication. Dis. Chest 44:552-553, 1963.

Greer, H. D., III; Ward, H. P.; Corbin, K. B. Chronic salicylate intoxication in adults. J. A. M. A. 193:555-558, 1965.

Guest, G. M.; Rapoport, S.; Roscoe, C. The effect of salicylates on the electrolyte structure of the blood plasma. II. The action of therapeutic doses of sodium salicylate and acetylsalicylic acid in man. J. Clin. Invest. 24:707-774, 1945.

Gutman, A. B.; Yu, T. F.; Sirota, J. H. A study by simultaneous clearance techniques of salicylate excretion in man. J. Clin. Invest. 34:711-721, 1955.

Halle, M. A.; Collipp, P. J. Treatment of methyl salicylate poisoning by peritoneal dialysis. N. Y. State J. Med. 69:1788-1789, 1969b.

Heffner, J. E.; Sahn, S. A. Salicylate-induced pulmonary edema - clinical features and prognosis. Ann. Intern. Med. 95:405-409, 1981.

Hill, J. B. Experimental salicylate poisoning: Observations on the effects of altering blood pH on tissue and plasma salicylate concentrations. Pediatrics 47:658-665, 1971.

Hill, J. B. Salicylate intoxication. N. Engl. J. Med. 288:1110-1113, 1973.

Hurwitz, G. A.; Wingfield, W.; Cowart, T. D.; Jollow, D. J. Toxic interaction between salicylates and a carbonic anhydrase inhibitor: the role of cerebral edema. Vet. Human Toxicol., 22 Suppl. 2:42-44, 1980.

James, J. A.; Kimbell, L.; Read, W. T. Experimental salicylate intoxication. I. Comparison of exchange transfusion, intermittent peritoneal lavage and hemodialysis as a means of removing salicylate. Pediatrics 29:442-447, 1962.

Jorgensen, H. E.; Wieth, J. O. Dialysable poisons. Lancet 1:81-84, 1963b.

Kaplan, S. A.; Del Carmen, F. T. Experimental salicylate poisoning. Observations on the effects of carbonic anhydrase inhibitor and bicarbonate. Pediatrics 21:762-770, 1958.

Kapur, Y. P. Ototoxicity of acetylsalicylic acid. Arch. Otolaryngol. 81:134-138, 1965.

Kato, Y.; Senzaki, H.; Ogara, H. Aspirin-induced hypocalcemia in the rat. Toxicol. Appl. Pharmacol. 64:64-71, 1982.

Kossover, M. F.; Kaplan, M. H. The role of salicylates in massive gastrointestinal hemorrhage. Am. J. Gastroenterol. 35:445-455, 1961.

Kravath, R. E.; Abel, G.; Colli, A.; McNamara, H.; Cohen, M. I. Salicylate poisoning - effect on 2, 3-diphosphoglycerate levels in the rat. Biochem. Pharmacol. 21:2656-2658, 1972.

Lawson, A. A. H.; Proudfoot, A. T.; Brown, J. S.; MacDonald, R. H.; Fraser, A. G.; Cameron, J. C.; Matthew, H. Forced diuresis in the treatment of acute salicylate poisoning in adults. Q. J. Med. 38:31-48, 1969.

Leiken, S. L.; Emmanouilides, G. C. The use of exchange transfusion in salicylate intoxication. Report of 7 cases. J. Pediatr. 57:715-720, 1960.

Leusen, I. Regulation of cerebrospinal fluid composition with reference to breathing. Physiol. Rev. 52:1-56, 1972.

Levy, G. Comparative pharmacokinetics of aspirin and acetaminophen. Arch. Intern. Med. 141:279-281, 1981.

Levy, G.; Hollister, L. E. Variation in rate of salicylate elimination by humans. Br. Med. J. 2:286-288, 1964.

Levy, G.; Tsuchiya, T.; Amsel, L. P. Limited capacity for salicyl phenolic glucuronide formation and its effect on the kinetics of salicylate elimination in man. Clin. Pharmacol. Ther. 13:258-268, 1972.

Levy, R. I. Overwhelming salicylate intoxication in an adult, acid-base changes during recovery with hemodialysis. Arch. Intern. Med. 119:399-402, 1967.

Liddell, N. E.; Maren, T. H. CO$_2$ retention as a basis for increased toxicity of salicylate with acetazolamide - avoidance of increased toxicity with benzolamide. J. Pharmacol. Exp. Ther. 195:1-7, 1975.

Limbeck, G. A.; Ruvalcaba, R. H. A.; Samols, E.; Kelly, V. C. Salicylates and hypoglycemia. Am. J. Dis. Child. 109:165-167, 1965.

Lynd, P. A.; Andreasen, A. C.; Wyatt, R. J. Intrauterine salicylate intoxication in a newborn. A case report. Clin. Pediatr. 15:912-913, 1976.

MacPherson, C. R.; Milne, M. D.; Evans, B. M. The excretion of salicylate. Br. J. Pharmacol. 10:484-489, 1955.

Magness, J. L.; Murray, J. B. Treatment of salicylate intoxication using extracorporeal hemodialysis. J. Lancet 81:253-254, 1961.

Manso, C.; Taranta, A.; Nydick, I. Effect of aspirin administration on serum glutamic oxaloacetic and glutamic pyruvic transaminases in children. Proc. Soc. Exp. Biol. Med. 93:84-88, 1956.

Matthew, H.; Mackintosh, T. F.; Tompsett, S. L.; Cameron, J. C. Gastric aspiration and lavage in acute poisoning. Br. Med. J. 1:1333-1337, 1966.

Meyer, R. J. Acetylsalicylic acid (aspirin) poisoning, epidemiology. Am. J. Dis. Child. 102:17-24, 1961.

Meyers, E. N.; Bernstein, J. M.; Fostiropolous, G. Salicylate ototoxicity. N. Engl. J. Med. 273:587-590, 1965.

Millar, R. J.; Bowman, J. Oil of wintergreen (methyl salicylate) poisoning treated by exchange transfusion. Can. Med. Assoc. J. 84:956-957, 1961.

Monti, M.; Bucar, I. Red cell organic phosphates during administration of salicylates. Scand. J. Haematol. 16:295-299, 1976.

Morgan, A. G.; Bennett, J. M.; Polak, A. Mannitol retention during diuretic treatment of barbiturate and salicylate overdosage. Q. J. Med. 37:589-606, 1968.

Morgan, A. G.; Polak, A. Acetazolamide and sodium bicarbonate in treatment of salicylate poisoning in adults. Br. Med. J. 1:16-19, 1969.

Morgan, A. G.; Polak, A. The excretion of salicylate in salicylate poisoning. Clin. Sci. 41:475-484, 1971.

Mortimer, E. A.; Lepow, M. L. Varicella with hypoglycemia possibly due to salicylates. Am. J. Dis. Child. 103:583-590, 1962.

Oliver, T. K.; Dyer, M. E. The prompt treatment of salicylism with sodium bicarbonate. Am. J. Dis. Child. 99:553-565, 1960.

Pickering, D. Salicylate poisoning: The diagnosis when its possibility is denied by the parents. Acta Paediatr. Scand. 53:501-504, 1964.

Proudfoot, A. T.; Brown, S. S. Acidaemia and salicylate poisoning in adults. Br. Med. J. 2:547-550, 1969.

Prowse, K.; Pain, M.; Marston, A. D.; Cumming, G. The treatment of salicylate poisoning using mannitol and forced alkaline diuresis. Clin. Sci. 38:327-337, 1970.

Reed, J. R.; Palmisano, P. A. Central nervous system salicylate. Clin. Toxicol. 8:623-631, 1975.

Reimold, E. W.; Worthen, H. G.; Reilly, T. D., Jr. Salicylate poisoning, comparison of acetazolamide administration and alkaline diuresis in the treatment of experimental salicylate intoxication in puppies. Am. J. Dis. Child. 125:668-674, 1973b.

Rentsch, J. B.; Bradley, A.; Marsh, S. B. Two cases of salicylate intoxication successfully treated by exchange transfusion. Am. J. Dis. Child. 98:778-785, 1959.

Rhamy, R. K.; Segar, W. E. Treatment of renal suppression

associated with acute salicylate poisoning. J. Urol. *86*:205-210, 1961.

Riley, H. D., Jr.; Worley, L. Salicylate intoxication. Pediatrics *18*:578-594, 1956.

Robin, E. D.; Davis, R. P.; Rees, A. B. Salicylate intoxication with reference to the development of hypokalemia. Am. J. Med. *26*:869-882, 1959.

Samter, M.; Beers, R. F. Intolerance to aspirin. Ann. Intern. Med. *68*:975-983, 1968.

Savage, T. M.; Ward, J. D.; Simpson, B. R.; Cohen, R. D. Treatment of severe salicylate poisoning by forced alkaline diuresis. Br. Med. J. *1*:35-36, 1969.

Schadt, D. C.; Purnell, D. C. Salicylate intoxication in an adult. Arch. Intern. Med. *102*:213-216, 1958.

Schlegel, R. J.; Altstatt, L. B.; Canales, L.; Goiser, J. L.; Alexander, J. L.; Gardner, L. I. Peritoneal dialysis for severe salicylism: an evaluation of indications and results. J. Pediatr. *69*:553-562, 1966.

Schwartz, R.; Fellers, F. X.; Knapp, J.; Yaffe, S. The renal response to administration of acetazoleamide (Diamox) during salicylate intoxication. Pediatrics *23*:1103-1114, 1959.

Schwartz, R.; Landy, G. Organic acid excretion in salicylate intoxication. J. Pediatr. *66*:658-666, 1965.

Segar, W. E.; Holliday, M. A. Physiological abnormalities of salicylate intoxication. N. Engl. J. Med. *259*:1191-1198, 1958.

Shahidi, N. T.; Westring, D. W. Acetylsalicylic acid induced hemolysis and its mechanism. J. Clin. Invest. *49*:1334-1340, 1970.

Singer, R. B. The acid base disturbance in salicylate intoxication. Medicine *33*:1-13, 1954.

Smith, M. J. H.; Smith, P. K. *The Salicylates.* Interscience Publishers, New York, 1966.

Smith, P. K.; Gleason, H. L.; Stoll, C. G.; Ogorzalek, S. Studies on the pharmacology of salicylates. J. Pharmacol. Exp. Ther. *87*:237-255, 1946.

Snodgrass, W.; Rumack, B. H.; Peterson, R. G.; Holbrook, M. L. Salicylate toxicity following therapeutic doses in young children. Clin. Toxicol. *18*:247-259, 1981.

St. John, J. B. Gastric mucosal damage by aspirin. CRC Crit. Rev. Toxicol. *3*:317-344, 1975.

Stevenson, C. S. Oil of wintergreen (methyl salicylate) poisoning, report of three cases, one with autopsy, and a review of the literature. Am. J. Med. Sci. *193*:772-788, 1937.

Strauss, J.; Nahas, G. G. Use of amine buffer (THAM) in treatment of acute salicylate intoxication. Proc. Soc. Exp. Biol. Med. *105*:348-351, 1960.

Summitt, R. L.; Etteldorf, J. N. Salicylate intoxication in children - experience with peritoneal dialysis and alkalini-zation of the urine. J. Pediatr. *64*:803-814, 1964.

Surapathana, L.; Futrakul, P.; Campbell, R. A. Salicylism revisited, unusual problems in diagnosis and management. Clin. Pediatr. *9*:658-661, 1970.

Sussman, S. Severe salicylism and acute pancreatitis. Calif. Med. *99*:29-32, 1963b.

Taylor, J. R.; Halprin, K. M. Percutaneous absorption of salicylic acid. Arch. Dermatol. *111*:740-743, 1975.

Temple, A. R.; George, D. J.; Done, A. K.; Thompson, J. A. Salicylate poisoning complicated by fluid retention. Clin. Toxicol. *9*:61-68, 1976.

Tenney, S. M.; Miller, R. M. The respiratory and circulatory actions of salicylate. Am. J. Med. *19*:498-508, 1955.

Thomsen, A. C.; Dalgard, O. Z. Haemodialysis in acute acetylsalicylic acid poisoning. Am. J. Med. *25*:484-486, 1958.

Thurston, J. H.; Pollock, P. G.; Warren, S. K.; Jones, E. M. Reduced brain glucose with normal plasma glucose in salicylate poisoning. J. Clin. Invest. *49*:2139-2145, 1970.

Travers, R. L.; Hughes, G. R. V. Salicylate hepatotoxicity in systemic lupus erythematosus: a common occurrence? Br. Med. J. *2*:1532-1533, 1978.

Turner, G.; Collins, E. Fetal effects of regular salicylate ingestion in pregnancy. Lancet *1*:338, 1975.

von Weiss, J. F.; Lever, W. F. Percutaneous salicylic acid intoxication in psoriasis. Arch. Dermatol. *90*:614-619, 1964.

Whitten, C. F.; Kesaree, N. M.; Goodwin, J. F. Managing salicylate poisoning in children, an evaluation of sodium bicarbonate therapy. Am. J. Dis. Child. *101*:178-194, 1961.

Winchester, J. F.; Gelfand, M. C.; Helliwell, M.; Vale, J. A.; Goulding, R.; Shreiner, G. E. Extracorporeal treatment of salicylate or acetaminophen poisoning - is there a role? Arch. Int. Med. *141*:370-374, 1981.

Winters, R. W. Salicylate intoxication in infants and children. Pediatrics *23*:255-257, 1959.

Winters, R. W.; White, J. S.; Hughes, M. C.; Ordway, N. K. Disturbances of acid-base equilibrium in salicylate intoxication. Pediatrics *23*:260-285, 1959.

Wuthrich, B.; Zabrodsky, S.; Storck, H. Percutaneous vergiftung durch Resorcin. Salicylsaure and weisse Pracipitatsalbe. Pharm. Acta Helv. *45*:453-460, 1970.

Yampolsky, J.; Perry, S. W. The treatment of poisoning in children by exchange transfusion. A review of the literature and report of a case. South. Med. J. *53*:1169-1172, 1960.

Zimmerman, H. J. Effects of aspirin and acetaminophen on the liver. Arch. Intern. Med. *141*:333-342, 1981.

Zucker, P.; Daum, F.; Cohen, M. I. Aspirin hepatitis. Am. J. Dis. Child. *129*:1433-1434, 1975.

STRYCHNINE

Strychnine is prepared from dried ripe seeds of *Strychnos nux-vomica*, which contain 1.1 to 1.4% (rarely 2%) strychnine and about an equal amount of a closely related alkaloid, brucine. In clinical medicine strychnine was used traditionally as a stomachic and unjustifiably as a stimulant and tonic, in the form of alkaloidal salts (nitrate, sulfate, phosphate), various elixirs and syrups (Haslam, 1965), nux vomica tincture (0.12% strychnine), nux vomica fluid extract (1.0 to 1.2% strychnine), and the dried powdered extract of *S. nux-vomica* (7 to 7.7% strychnine). Cathartic and tonic tablets, containing irrational mixtures of cathartics, belladonna and strychnine, are still obtainable; attracted by their sugar coating many children have poisoned themselves with these tablets (Clement and Holloway, 1964; Murray, 1926; Ross and Brown, 1935; Stannard, 1969).

Strychnine is a long-established rodenticide, commonly used at bait concentrations of about 0.5%. Although such bait is usually refused by rats, the material is useful in the control of mice, gophers, squirrels, prairie dogs, porcupines, rabbits, moles, and other predatory animals and birds. The ingestion of strychnine bait has caused human poisoning. Strychnine was formerly an important source of suicidal and homicidal poisonings (Aikman, 1930), but recognized cases are now comparatively infrequent.

Toxicology: Strychnine is a potent convulsant. When taken by mouth, the mean lethal dose in man probably lies between 100 and 120 mg. (1.5-2 mg./kg.). A dose as small as 16 mg. has killed an adult, and 30 mg. is usually a threat to life; in contrast, recovery has followed the ingestion of more than 2000 mg. (Witthaus, 1911). When administered by the subcutaneous route, the lethal dose is less by one-half to two-thirds. On a body weight basis, children may be slightly more refractory to strychnine than are adults (Sollmann, 1957).

The lethality of nux vomica is believed to parallel its content of strychnine. Brucine is not a major toxicological problem; although it may act as a local anesthetic agent and perhaps as a paralytic substance, it produces convulsions only in relatively large doses (40 times the effective dose of strychnine, according to Webster, 1930).

After the ingestion of strychnine or nux vomica, untoward symptoms commonly begin within 10 to 30 minutes (occasionally after a delay of 1 hour). Often without warning of any kind, the patient falls in a violent convulsion, but usually there are prodromal signs and symptoms. Soon any mild sensory stimulus triggers a violent generalized convulsion. A transient clonic phase is quickly followed by spasm of all skeletal muscles; the stronger muscles dominate and produce a posture characteristic of spinal convulsions (see "Symptomatology"). Tetanic contractions of the diaphragm, thoracic and abdominal muscles stop respiration, so that anoxia and cyanosis develop quickly.

After the convulsion, the victim is relaxed, depressed, and exhausted. Because sensation is unaffected, the convulsions are painful and engender overwhelming fear. As many as 10 convulsions, separated by intervals of 10 to 15 minutes, may be experienced, but death commonly occurs between the second and fifth paroxysm. In an isolated case involving a massive overdose (estimated at 3.4 gm.), the patient expired within 15 minutes with little or no evidence of the classical symptoms (Lloyd and Pedley, 1953). The exact mechanism of strychnine's action on the cerebrospinal axis is not clearly established, but the drug apparently acts similarly on all portions of the central and peripheral nervous systems to increase excitability.

Included in the differential diagnosis of strychnine convulsions are the following clinical entities: tetanus, hydrophobia, spinal meningitis, epilepsy, and hysteria. Infectious tetanus and hydrophobia (rabies) produce prodromal malaise and a less fulminating course than strychnine poisoning. Pharyngeal and glottic spasm are more marked in rabies than in strychnine intoxication. The high fever of spinal meningitis is distinctive. In convulsive attacks of epilepsy, consciousness is always lost. Some cases of hysteria are very difficult to distinguish from strychnine poisoning (Sollmann, 1957).

Death is commonly due to asphyxia from respiratory arrest during or between convulsions. Respiratory failure may arise from anoxic damage cumulating during each convulsive episode or from exhaustion of medullary nerve centers because of over-stimulation. Both types of injury

can be prevented if convulsions are aborted early in the course of poisoning.

Strychnine effects on other organ systems are usually of secondary interest (Dusser de Barenne, 1933). At doses above the convulsive threshold this alkaloid increases discharges in sympathetic nerves and produces tachycardia and hypertension, even when convulsions are prevented (in dogs) by anesthesia and muscle paralyzants (Sofola and Odusote, 1976). By reducing central sympathetic outflow, diazepam may protect the heart from excessive stimulation.

To prevent or abort convulsions, rapidly acting intravenous barbiturate drugs are satisfactory central nervous depressants (Dawson and Taft, 1931; Fenten, 1933; Kempf et al., 1933; Priest, 1938; Rose, 1935; Swanson, 1933; Wheelock, 1932). More recently diazepam has been successfully employed to control convulsions. It is effective at levels producing less central nervous system depression than the barbiturates (Harden and Griggs, 1971; Heidrich et al., 1969; Herishanu and Landau, 1972; Jackson et al., 1971; Maron et al., 1971). Other options are described in Section IV (pp. IV-35–39).

Thiopental in a water-miscible mineral oil suspension has been used rectally in infants (Symons and Boyle, 1963), but the degree of sedation is more difficult to control. Intravenous mephenesin has been used to good advantage to control muscular rigidity (Jacoby and Boyle, 1956; Swissman and Jacoby, 1964); perhaps other centrally acting muscle relaxants such as methocarbamol should also be tried in strychnine poisoning. Curariform drugs and succinylcholine (Hawkins, 1962; Sgaragli and Mannaioni, 1973; Statham, 1956) are said to be useful, but they obligate the therapist to intubation and artificial respiration (p. IV-9). A barbiturate is also indicated in conjunction with these peripherally acting muscle relaxants to control anxiety and restlessness and to mitigate the influence of sensory stimuli.

Much less satisfactory or ineffective in the convulsing patient are atropine (Statham, 1956; Wescoe and Green, 1948), morphine (Aikman, 1930), chloroform (Gettler and St. George, 1935; Lovegrove, 1963), apomorphine (Gold and Gold, 1933; Haggard and Greenberg, 1932), intramuscular paraldehyde (Hawkins, 1962), tribromoethanol (Stalberg and Davidson, 1933) and intramuscular phenobarbital (Swissman and Jacoby, 1964). Hypothermia has been employed in severe poisonings (Cotton and Lane, 1966), presumably to decrease oxygen demand, but its efficacy is not established.

Strychnine is largely detoxified in the liver (Priestly et al., 1931), and its rate of metabolism can be increased in animals by pretreatment with phenobarbital or other inducers of microsomal enzyme activity (Howes and Hunter, 1966; Tsukamoto *et al.*, 1964). At least four metabolites appear after incubation of strychnine with rabbit liver slices. One of these, 2-hydroxystrychnine, is about 100-fold less toxic than the parent compound (Tsukamoto *et al.*, 1964). Deacetylation also results in a loss of biological activity (Dey, 1965). Approximately 20% of a sublethal dose escapes in the urine unchanged, but the percent excreted decreases with increasing dose (Weiss and Hatcher, 1922). The suggestion has been made that forced diuresis and peritoneal lavage may hasten strychnine elimination (Hatcher and Smith, 1917; Teitelbaum and Ott, 1970). In a massive ingestion episode where mannitol diuresis was used, however, only 1% of the dose was recovered in the urine in 24 hours (Sgaragli and Mannaioni, 1973).

Significant cumulative toxicity is not recognized (Hatcher and Eggleston, 1918). Since both detoxication and excretion are comparatively fast, the prognosis in strychnine poisoning is good if the patient can be kept alive for the first 5 to 6 hours (Witthaus, 1911).

Symptomatology (beginning 15 to 30 minutes after ingestion):

1. Without warning the patient may fall into a violent convulsion, but often prodromal symptoms are described, such as restlessness, apprehension, heightened acuity of perception (hearing, vision, feeling, etc.), abrupt movements, hyperreflexia, and especially muscular stiffness of the face and legs. Rarely vomiting occurs.

2. A minor sensory stimulus may suddenly trigger a violent generalized convulsion which lasts from 0.5 to 2 minutes. At first the movements are intermittent (clonic), but a spinal tetanic phase quickly intervenes. The body typically arches in hyperextension (opisthotonos), so that in a supine position the body is supported by the heels and head. The legs are adducted and extended, the arms are flexed over the chest or rigidly extended, and the fists are tightly clenched. The jaw is rigidly clamped (trismus), the face is fixed in a grin (risus sardonicus), and the eyes protrude in a fixed stare. Because the muscles of respiration are involved in a sustained spasm, breathing ceases and deep cyanosis appears. Consciousness is retained during the convulsion, which is painful, and the patient remains apprehensive and fearful throughout the illness.

3. Between convulsions, muscular relaxation is typically complete. Breathing resumes and the cyanosis lessens. Cold perspiration covers the skin. Dilated pupils may contract. The patient sometimes falls asleep from exhaustion. Reflex irritability usually remains low for a period of 10 to 15 minutes, when hyperexcitability quickly returns, and sudden stimuli such as a noise or even a draft of air may precipitate another paroxysm.

4. One to ten such attacks occur before recovery or death from respiratory arrest. In the absence of effective treatment, most victims do not tolerate more than 5 convulsions, and death commonly occurs within 1 to 3 hours after the ingestion of a fatal dose. As the poisoning progresses, the convulsions may become more violent and the intermissions shorter.

5. Repeated convulsions may lead to lactic acidemia, hyperkalemia, hyperthermia and dehydration.

6. If the patient survives the first 5 to 6 hours, the prognosis is good. There are few serious sequelae among survivors. Rarely rhabdomyolysis, myoglobinuria and consequent renal damage may result from violent, uncontrolled convulsions.

Treatment:

1. Treatment is designed primarily to prevent convulsions and thus to protect medullary centers from excessive stimulation and from anoxia.

2. If it can be done before the development of reflex hyperexcitability, the induction of emesis is desirable, but a safer procedure is the ingestion of a slurry of 6 to 8 heaping teaspoonful of activated charcoal (p. I-4) in a few ounces of water (Chin *et al.*, 1969). Gastric lavage is postponed until the patient is fully premedicated.

3. Protect patient from harming himself during convulsions, and reduce all sensory stimulation to a minimum by keeping him in a comfortably warm, quiet and darkened room. Avoid all unessential procedures, and exclude all visitors. Each succeeding convulsion reduces the patient's chances of survival. See pp. IV-35–39.

4. Inject intravenously sufficient amounts of diazepam (0.1–0.2 mg./kg.) to prevent further convulsive paroxysms. It may be repeated if necessary at 10 to 15-minute intervals up to a maximal dose of 30 mg. (in adults). If necessary, this regimen may be repeated cautiously in 2 to 4 hours. A short acting barbiturate drug such as amobarbital sodium (Amytal) or pentobarbital sodium (Nembutal) is also useful. An adequate dose usually produces loss of consciousness, and more than 0.5 gm. by slow intravenous injection may be necessary (p. IV-37).

5. If neither diazepam nor a satisfactory bar-

biturate is immediately available, convulsions can often be controlled temporarily by the inhalation of ether. See p. IV-39.

6. Neuromuscular blocking agents (*e.g.*, curare) may have adjunctive value in the management of strychnine convulsions. At least limited experience with curariform drugs has been encouraging. The therapist who has experience with muscle relaxants having central sites of action (*e.g.*, mephenesin) may find them useful adjuvants (see p. IV-39).

7. If postconvulsive depression or an overdose of anticonvulsant drug causes apnea, artificial respiration becomes essential. Keep the airway clear and administer oxygen (p. IV-2 and 12). See also p. IV-7.

8. The patient must be kept under constant observation for many hours. Wakefulness, hyperreflexia, and muscular twitching signal a need for additional doses of barbiturate or diazepam.

9. After convulsions and reflex irritability have been suppressed, gastric lavage can be safely performed. A dilute potassium permanganate solution (1:5000) is probably best. The iodide in tincture of iodine (1 teaspoonful in a glass of water) forms an insoluble strychnine salt, which may temporarily delay absorption, but a slurry of activated charcoal is probably more effective.

10. Metabolic acidosis from lactic acidemia (p. IV-69), hyperkalemia (p. IV-72), hyperthermia (p. IV-84) and dehydration (p. IV-64) may all require attention. In general, however, measures to correct these metabolic derangements can and should be postponed until the convulsions are suppressed

11. During recovery, maintain a brisk urine flow if there is clinical or laboratory evidence of rhabdomyolysis and myoglobinuria.

Laboratory: Blood analyses to detect acidosis, hyperkalemia and other metabolic disorders. A high serum level of creatine phosphokinase may indicate rhabdomyolysis. A leukocytosis is commonly observed; it is presumably associated with the release of epinephrine from the adrenal medulla. Methods are available for the isolation and identification of strychnine in stomach contents and other organs.

References:

Aikman, J. Strychnine poisoning in children. J. A. M. A. *95*:1661-1665, 1930.

Chin, L.; Picchioni, A. L.; Duplisse, B. R. Comparative antidotal effectiveness of activated charcoal, Arizona montmorillonite, and evaporated milk. J. Pharm. Sci. *58*:1353-1356, 1969.

Clement, J. A.; Holloway, A. M. Suicidal strychnine poisoning. Lancet *1*:983, 1964.

Cotton, M. S.; Lane, D. H. Massive strychnine poisoning; a successful treatment. J. Miss. State Med. Assoc. *7*:466-468, 1966.

Dawson, W. T.; Taft, C. H., Jr. Suppression of strychnine convulsions by barbiturates. Proc. Soc. Exp. Biol. Med. *28*:917-918, 1931.

Dey, P. K. Protective action of lemon juice and ascorbic acid against lethality and convulsive property of strychnine. Naturwissenschaften *1*:164, 1965.

Dusser de Barenne, J. G. The mode and site of action of strychnine on the nervous system. Physiol. Rev. *13*:325-335, 1933.

Fenton, B. C. Use of sodium amytal in strychnine poisoning. J. A. M. A. *101*:1333, 1933.

Gettler, A. O.; St. George, A. V. Toxicology in children. Am. J. Clin. Pathol. *5*:466-488, 1935.

Gold, D.; Gold, H. Apomorphine as an antidote to strychnine poisoning. J. A. M. A. *100*:1589-1590, 1933.

Haggard, H. W.; Greenberg, L. A. Antidotes for strychnine poisoning. J. A. M. A. *98*:1133-1136, 1932.

Harden, J. A.; Griggs, R. C. Diazepam treatment in a case of strychnine poisoning. Lancet *2*:372-373, 1971.

Haslam, M. T. Accidental strychnine poisoning. Br. Med. J. *1*:1191, 1965.

Hatcher, R. A.; Eggleston, C. The fate of strychnine in the body. J. Pharmacol. Exp. Ther. *10*:281-319, 1918.

Hatcher, R. A.; Smith, M. I. The elimination of strychnine by the kidneys. J. Pharmacol. Exp. Ther. *9*:27-41, 1917.

Hawkins, G. F. Two cases of strychnine poisoning in children. Br. Med. J. *2*:26, 1962.

Heidrich, H.; Ibe, K.; Klinge, D. Akute Vergiftung mit Strychnin-N-oxydhydrochlorid (Movellan-Tabletten) und ihre Behandlung mit Diazepam. Arch. Toxikol. *24*:188-200, 1969.

Herishanu, Y.; Landau, H. Diazepam in the treatment of strychnine poisoning. Br. J. Anaesth. *44*:747-748, 1972.

Howes, J. F.; Hunter, W. H. The stimulation of strychnine metabolism in rats by some anticonvulsant compounds. J. Pharm. Pharmacol. *18*:52s-57s, 1966.

Jackson, G.; Ng, S. H.; Diggle, G. E.; Bourke, I. G. Strychnine poisoning treated successfully with diazepam. Br. Med. J. *3*:519-520, 1971.

Jacoby, J.; Boyle, J. The treatment of strychnine poisoning with mephenesin. J. Lab. Clin. Med. *48*:270-273, 1956.

Kempf, G. F.; McCallum, J. T. C.; Zerfas, L. G. A successful treatment for strychnine poisoning. Report of eleven cases. J. A. M. A. *100*:548-551, 1933.

Lloyd, J. T. A.; Pedley, E. Acute strychnine poisoning after a massive dose. Br. Med. J. *2*:429-430, 1953.

Lovegrove, F. T. B. Three cases of strychnine poisoning. Med. J. Aust. *1*:783, 1963.

Maron, B. J.; Krupp, J. R.; Tune, B. Strychnine poisoning successfully treated with diazepam. J. Pediatr. *78*:697-699, 1971.

Murray, L. M. An analysis of sixty cases of drug poisoning. Arch. Pediatr. *43*:193-196, 1926.

Priest, R. E. Strychnine poisoning successfully treated with sodium amytal. Report of two cases. J. A. M. A. *110*:1440, 1938.

Priestly, J. T.; Markowitz, J.; Mann, F. C. Studies on the physiology of the liver. XX. Detoxicating function of the liver with special reference to strychnine. Am. J. Physiol. *96*:696-708, 1931.

Rose, T. Strychnine poisoning with recovery. Med. J. Aust. *1*:213, 1935.

Ross, J. R.; Brown, A. Strychnine poisoning in children. Can. Med. Assoc. J. *32*:282, 1935.

Sgaragli, G. P.; Mannaioni, P. F. Pharmacokinetic observations on a case of massive strychnine poisoning. Clin. Toxicol. *6*:533-540, 1973.

Sofola, O. A.; Odusote, K. A. Sympathetic cardiovascular effects of experimental strychnine poisoning in dogs. J. Pharmacol. Exp. Ther. *196*:29-34, 1976.

Sollmann, T. *A Manual of Pharmacology*. 8th Ed., W. B. Saunders Co., Philadelphia, 1957.

Stalberg, S.; Davidson, H. S. The newer treatment of strychnine poisoning. Report of an unusual case. J. A. M. A. 101:102-105, 1933.

Stannard, M. W. Child death due to Easton's tablets. Practitioner 203:668-669, 1969.

Statham, C. Case of strychnine poisoning. Br. Med. J. 2:1101-1102, 1956.

Swanson, E. E. The antidotal effect of sodium amytal in strychnine poisoning. J. Lab. Clin. Med. 18:933-934, 1933.

Swissman, N.; Jacoby, J. Strychnine poisoning and its treatment. Clin. Pharmacol. Ther. 5:136-140, 1964.

Symons, A. J. C.; Boyle, A. K. Accidental strychnine poisoning. A case report. Br. J. Anaesth. 35:54-55, 1963.

Teitelbaum, D. T.; Ott, J. E. Acute strychnine intoxication. Clin. Toxicol. 3:267-273, 1970.

Tsukamoto, H.; Oguri, K.; Watabe, T.; Yoshimura, H. Metabolism of drugs. XLI. The metabolic fate of strychnine in rabbit liver. J. Biochem. 55:394-400, 1964.

Webster, R. W. Legal Medicine and Toxicology. W. B. Saunders Co., Philadelphia, 1930.

Weiss, S.; Hatcher, R. A. Studies on strychnine. J. Pharmacol. Exp. Ther. 19:419-482, 1922.

Wescoe, W. C.; Green, R. E. On the mechanism of the convulsant action of strychnine, the lack of atropine antagonism. J. Pharmacol. Exp. Ther. 94:78-84, 1948.

Wheelock, M. C. Strychnine poisoning. J. A. M. A. 99:1862, 1932.

Witthaus, R. A. Manual of Toxicology. Wm. Wood & Co., New York, 1911.

THALLIUM

Salts of thallium serve as active ingredients in pesticides used to control rats, mice, ground squirrels, prairie dogs, moles and such insects as ants and cockroaches. Thallous (monovalent) sulfate is the only form used in pesticidal formulations; it is 80% thallium metal (Council on Drugs, 1957). Despite their high toxicity thallium salts were once used internally as a temporary depilatory in cases of favus and ringworm of the scalp and externally as a cream depilatory in cases of hypertrichosis. These uses have been practically abandoned. The record of thallium poisoning in man has become so notorious that many countries including the United States ban or strictly regulate its sale. In Europe thallium is claimed to be more prevalent than arsenic as a homicidal agent (Klöppel and Weiler, 1978). Intoxication has occurred after exposure to organic compounds of thallium (Richeson, 1958).

Toxicology: As evidenced by its trivalent compounds, the element thallium belongs in the aluminum family, but monovalent thallium salts are more closely related, chemically and toxicologically, to divalent lead, although the acute toxicity of thallium compounds is much higher (Moeschlin, 1965). There is, however, no relationship between lead and thallium in terms of exposure as judged by blood levels in urban children (Singh et al., 1975).

The ingestion of any thallous salt is followed, after a latent period of 12 to 24 hours, by a severe hemorrhagic gastroenteritis and consequent circulatory collapse (shock). Probably this enteritis is due to vascular actions of absorbed thallium. In children early signs of rhinorrhea and conjunctivitis may be confused with upper respiratory infections (Grossman, 1955; Grulee and Clark, 1951).

Delirium, convulsions, and coma may appear rapidly, but more often the acute reaction subsides, only to be replaced by the gradual development of the following (in any combination): mild gastrointestinal disturbances, polyneuritis, encephalopathy, skin eruptions (Schwartzman and Kirschbaum, 1962), and hepatorenal injury (Fischl, 1966). Subarachnoid hemorrhage, bone marrow depression and increased radiopacity of the liver have been reported (Grunfeld and Hinostroza, 1964). Degenerative changes in mitochondria and other subcellular structures have been observed (Herman and Bensch, 1967). A distal axonal degeneration in motor and sensory nerves may account for a peripheral neuropathy of varying severity (Cavanagh et al., 1974; Kennedy and Cavanagh, 1976). The most characteristic sign is alopecia, but it appears only in cases where death is delayed for at least 20 days (Prick et al., 1955). These delayed effects are usually persistent and may prove fatal. Convalescence is slow (Munch et al., 1933; Prick et al., 1955).

As with lead, this subacute syndrome may develop without a recognized acute illness, especially if small quantities of thallium salts are ingested daily. Subacute and chronic intoxications are associated with the cumulative tissue retention of thallium, presumably in the form of sparingly soluble thallous chloride. Any sudden release of thallium from these tissue stores may precipitate acute toxic symptoms as in lead poisoning (Council on Drugs, 1957). Over a period of 1 month about 70% of an administered dose is excreted, largely in urine and partly in bile (Lund, 1956).

Thallium and potassium show interrelationships in some tissues, e.g., the red blood cell (Gehring and Hammond, 1964). Thallous ion has a 10-fold greater affinity for sodium-potassium activated ATPase than potassium, and thallium is apparently transported into cells by the potassium pump mechanism (Inturrisi, 1969). It is not clear whether such an interrelationship is responsible for the electrocardiographic changes observed in experimental thallium poisoning (Grunfeld et al., 1963). Arterial hypertension, sinus tachycardia and increased urinary excretion of catecholamines have been described in several patients (Bank et al., 1972; Merguet et al., 1969). Hypotension observed in rats may be due to direct vascular smooth muscle relaxation and a negative chronotropic effect;

the latter has been demonstrated in isolated guinea pig atria (Lameijer and Van Zwieten, 1976).

The mean lethal dose in an adult is probably about 1 gm. of thallium sulfate. Two patients survived 1.3 gm. but another died after 3.2 gm. (Grunfeld and Hinostroza, 1964). Single doses of 4 mg. per kg. of body weight have caused toxic reactions in children (Munch, 1928). The difference between a depilatory and a toxic dose is small and allows no margin for idiosyncrasy.

Forms of therapy: Thallium poisoning appears to be refractory to most antidotal procedures that have been attempted. Dimercaprol (BAL) appears to have no influence on the excretion or the toxicity of thallium in rats (Lund, 1956). Although high doses are said to produce occasional improvement in human thallotoxicosis (Grunfeld and Hinostroza, 1964), most reports indicate that, if BAL is beneficial at all, its effects are not dramatic (Arnan, 1962; Fischl, 1966; Mazzei and Schaposnik, 1949; Reed et al., 1963; Stein and Perlstein, 1959; Welty and Berrey, 1950).

Edetate calcium disodium proved disappointing in acute thallium intoxications in rats (Lund, 1956), dogs (Skelley and Gabriel, 1964), and humans (Chamberlain et al., 1958; Reed et al., 1963; Smith and Doherty, 1964). Penicillamine failed to relieve symptoms or increase urinary thallium excretion in a single case (Smith and Doherty, 1964). Thiouracil has been used in therapy, but its role is poorly understood (Bedville and Spragg, 1956). Various sulfur containing amino acids have been tried experimentally and largely abandoned (Gross et al., 1948; Heyndrickx, 1957; Lund, 1956; Taber, 1964).

Diphenylthiocarbazone (dithizon), an organic reagent used for the estimation of some heavy metals, has been investigated as a potential thallium antidote. Dithizon is said to afford good protection to rats (Lund, 1956) apparently by primarily increasing the fecal excretion of thallium (Schwetz et al., 1967). Opinions differ with respect to its effects on acute thallium poisoning in the dog (Doak et al., 1965; Mathew and Low, 1960; Skelley and Gabriel, 1964), and limited clinical experience has resulted in no clear-cut consensus (Arena et al., 1965; Mathews and Anzarut, 1968; Reed et al., 1963; Smith and Doherty, 1964). Although the findings have been disputed, dithizon is said to have diabetogenic and goitrogenic actions (Lund, 1956; Stavinoha et al., 1959). In dogs loss of zinc from the tapetum lucidum, necrosis, secondary retinal detachment and blindness occurred with dithizon, but no damage occurred in monkeys, which are devoid of a tapetal layer in the eye (Budinger, 1961). Pathologic changes in the prostate glands of dogs have been similarly ascribed to zinc mobilization (Lo et al., 1960).

Diethyldithiocarbamate (dithiocarb, the monomer of disulfiram) appears to be about as potent as dithizon in accelerating total thallium excretion in poisoned rats, but it hastens both urinary and fecal elimination (Schwetz et al., 1967). However, dithiocarb had only minimal antidotal effects in guinea pigs (Righetti and Moeschlin, 1971). Data in rats indicate that dithiocarb effects a redistribution of thallium into brain (Rauws et al., 1969). Dithiocarb is well tolerated by rats and dogs (Sunderman et al., 1967). Again, limited clinical experience was encouraging in some cases (Bass, 1963; Reiders and Cordova, 1965; Sunderman, 1967), but signs of intoxication were thought to be intensified in others (Keller et al., 1971; Kamerbeek et al., 1971a).

Daily intravenous injections of 0.3 to 1.0 gm. of sodium iodide have been employed in an attempt to precipitate insoluble thallium iodide in the tissues (Fairweather et al., 1955). An equivalent amount of sodium thiosulfate is given later by cautious intravenous injection (10 to 20 ml. of 3% solution) to mobilize the thallium in small quantities for excretion; if acute symptoms are reactivated by this procedure, thiosulfate treatment is stopped and iodide substituted. Again proof of the usefulness of this technique is incomplete (Reed et al., 1963), and it is doubtful that there is any method of inactivating the metal once it has been absorbed.

The rate of removal of thallium from rats and dogs was increased by elevations of dietary potassium, and rats fed a high-potassium diet were more resistant to the acute lethal effects of thallium (Gehring and Hammond, 1967). Nevertheless potassium did not appear to have antidotal effects in acute thallium poisoning in guinea pigs (Righetti and Moeschlin, 1971). In patients potassium supplementation led to a 2- to 3-fold increase in thalliuresis, but at least transiently signs of poisoning were aggravated (Bank et al., 1972; Gartel et al., 1978; Papp et al., 1969).

Ferric ferrocyanide (Prussian blue) and similar coordination complexes with cobalt and nickel can bond thallium tenaciously and prevent its absorption from the gastrointestinal tract (Manninen et al., 1976; Van der Stock and de Schepper, 1978). It appears to be superior to activated charcoal in this respect (Dvorak, 1969; Heydlauf, 1969). In thallium-poisoned humans doses of about 10 gm. twice daily by duodenal tube for 10 to 14 days appeared to increase the fecal excretion of thallium and to produce a favorable clinical response (Kamerbeek et al., 1971b; Van der Merwe, 1972). A problem with this approach is that chronic thallium intoxication commonly results in intestinal hypomotility or paralytic ileus, which is often resistant to laxatives. Perhaps this accounts for the more favorable response when the drug is given in the acute phase of the illness as opposed to the chronic phase (Stevens *et al.*, 1974).

Finally, opinions are also divided as to the efficacy of hemodialysis (Paulsen *et al.*, 1972; Piazolo *et al.*, 1971). Hemodialysis has been used in combination with forced diuresis (Drasch and Hauck, 1977); the former is said to be three times more effective than the latter, but hemoperfusion was the most efficient procedure of all (Moeschlin, 1980).

Symptomatology:

1. Symptoms usually appear within 12 to 24 hours after a single toxic dose or after several weeks of small daily doses.
2. In acute poisonings gastrointestinal effects are dominant: severe paroxysmal abdominal pain (colic), vomiting and diarrhea.. The vomitus and stools are often bloody. In severe cases, tremors, delirium, convulsions, paralysis, coma and death, sometimes within 1 to 2 days.
3. In subacute poisonings, signs and symptoms referable to the alimentary tract include intermittent intestinal colic, nausea, vomiting, diarrhea, achlorhydria, stomatitis, excessive salivation and gingival discoloration (comparable to the lead line).
4. Neuromuscular symptoms include tremors, leg pains, paresthesias of the hands and feet, and a frank peripheral polyneuritis, principally in the legs.
5. Ocular and facial palsies and retrobulbar neuritis lead to severe and sometimes permanent disability.
6. A toxic psychosis, delirium, convulsions and other signs of encephalopathy.
7. Tachycardia, hypertension and arrhythmias indicate autonomic sympathetic dysfunction.
8. Skin eruptions, including keratinization, petechiae and ecchymoses.
9. Central lobular necrosis of the liver and damage to the renal tubular epithelium. The hepatorenal lesions *per se* are rarely lethal.
10. The loss of hair (alopecia) is usually reversible unless repeated exposures are allowed. The lesion is apparently due to a metabolic disturbance in the hair follicle, perhaps of circulatory or neurotropic origin.

Treatment:

1. Immediate measures include administration of an emetic, or gastric lavage with water or perhaps better with a 1% solution of sodium or potassium iodide (in order to form insoluble thallium iodide). The instillation of a slurry of activated charcoal may reduce intestinal absorption and so promote fecal excretion (Lund, 1956).
2. Unless diarrhea is already established, produce catharsis with sodium or magnesium sulfate (15 to 30 gm.) in water or with castor oil (1 oz.)
3. Administer demulcents orally such as milk, starch paste, aluminum oxide gels, bismuth subcarbonate, etc.
4. Peripheral vascular collapse (shock) should be treated with parenteral fluids and electrolytes (pp. IV-17-20).
5. The efficacy of any of the elaborate therapeutic measures and antidotes mentioned in the text above remains to be established in clinical poisonings when absorption has already occurred.
6. Symptomatic and supportive treatment for the various signs and symptoms of central nervous origin. Trihexyphenidyl (Artane) has been found effective in relieving tremor.
7. To protect the heart against tachyarrhythmias, propranolol is useful.
8. Because of possible disturbances in calcium metabolism, the daily ingestion of several grams of calcium gluconate, lactate or chloride is recommended. Ample quantities of milk may be substituted.
9. If achlorhydria develops, nutrition may be improved by the administration of diluted hydrochloric acid before each meal. One regimen is to sip through a straw (to minimize exposure of the teeth) 4 to 8 oz. of water containing 5 to 10 ml. of 10% hydrochloric acid.

Laboratory:

1. Urinalysis may reveal aminoaciduria (Fischl, 1966), albuminuria and an increase in cells and casts.
2. In spite of obvious central neural involvement, the cerebrospinal fluid and its pressure are usually unremarkable (Prick *et al.*, 1955).
3. A definitive diagnosis may require chemical or spectrographic analysis of body fluids or excreta for thallium (Wilson and Hausman, 1964). Concentrations in saliva may be 15-fold higher than those in urine (Richelmi *et al.*, 1980).
4. Repeated electrocardiograms are desirable. Increased urinary excretion of catecholamine metabolites has been described.

References:

Arena, J. M.; Watson, G. A.; Sakhadeo, S. S. Fatal thallium poisoning. Clin. Pediatr. *4*:267-270, 1965.

Arnan, A. Accidental poisoning from agricultural pesticides. Bull. W. H. O. *26*:109-120, 1962.

Bank, W. J.; Pleasure, D. E.; Suzuki, K.; Nigro, M.; Katz, R. Thallium poisoning. Arch. Neurol. *26*:456-464, 1972.

Bass, M. Thallium poisoning; a preliminary report. J. Am. Osteopath. Assoc. 63:229-235, 1963.

Bedville, B. L.; Spragg, G. S. Report of a case of thallium poisoning treated with thiouracil. Med. J. Aust. 2:222-223, 1956.

Budinger, J. Diphenylthiocarbazone blindness in dogs. Arch. Pathol. 71:304-310, 1961.

Cavanagh, J. B.; Fuller, N. H.; Johnson, H. R. M.; Ruge, P. The effects of thallium salts, with particular reference to the nervous system changes. Q. J. Med. 43:293-319, 1974.

Chamberlain, P. H.; Stavinoha, W. B.; Davis, H.; Knicker, W. T.; Panos, T. C. Thallium poisoning. Pediatrics 22:1170-1182, 1958.

Council on Drugs, A. M. A. Thallotoxicosis - a recurring problem. J. A. M. A. 165:1567-1568, 1957.

Doak, R. L.; Schmidtke, R. P.; Wallach, J. D.; Davis, L. E.; Niemeyer, K. H. Thallium intoxication: A specific antidote, supportive therapy and clinical evaluation. Vet. Med. 60:1227-1231, 1965.

Drasch, G.; Hauck, G. Verlaufskontrolle der Intensivtherapie von Thalliumintoxikationen. Arch. Toxicol. 38:209-215, 1977.

Dvorak, P. Kolloidale Hexacyanoferrate (II) als Antidote bei der Thallium-Intoxikation. Z. Gesamte Exp. Med. 151:89-92, 1969.

Fairweather, M. J.; Stovell, V.; Santiago, P.; Adams, K. P.; Davis, J.; Campbell, W. Thallium poisoning in children. Tex. Med. 51:466-468, 1955.

Fischl, J. Aminoaciduria in thallium poisoning. Am. J. Med. Sci. 251:40-42, 1966.

Gartel, B.; Innis, R.; Moses, H., III. Clinical conferences at the Johns Hopkins Hospital. Thallium poisoning. The Johns Hopkins Med. J. 142:27-31, 1978.

Gehring, P. J.; Hammond, P. B. The uptake of thallium by rabbit erythrocytes. J. Pharmacol. Exp. Ther. 145:215-221, 1964.

Gehring, P. J.; Hammond, P. B. The interrelationship between thallium and potassium in animals. J. Pharmacol. Exp. Ther. 155:187-201, 1967.

Gross, P.; Ranne, E.; Wilson, J. W. Studies on the effect of thallium poisoning of the rat; the influence of cystine and methionine on alopecia and survival periods. J. Invest. Dermatol. 10:119-134, 1948.

Grossman, H. Thallotoxicosis. Report of a case and a review. Pediatrics 16:868-872, 1955.

Grulee, C. G., Jr.; Clark, E. H. Thallotoxicosis in a preschool nursery. Am. J. Dis. Child. 81:47-51, 1951.

Grunfeld, O.; Batilana, G.; Aldana, L.; Hinostroza, G.; Larrea, P. Electrocardiographic changes in experimental thallium poisoning. Am. J. Vet. Res. 24:1291-1296, 1963.

Grunfeld, O.; Hinostroza, G. Thallium poisoning. Arch. Intern. Med. 114:132-138, 1964.

Herman, M. M.; Bensch, K. G. Light and electron microscopic studies of acute and chronic thallium intoxication in rats. Toxicol. Appl. Pharmacol. 10:199-222, 1967.

Heydlauf, H. Ferric-cyanoferrate (II): an effective antidote in thallium poisoning. Eur. J. Pharmacol. 6:340-344, 1969.

Heyndrickx, A. Treatment of thallium poisoning in mice. Toxicological analysis by radioactivation. Acta Pharmacol. Toxicol. 14:20-26, 1957.

Inturrisi, C. E. Thallium-induced dephosphorylation of a phosphorylated intermediate of the (sodium and thallium-activated) ATPase. Biochem. Biophys. Acta 178:630-633, 1969.

Kamerbeek, H. H.; Rauws, A. G.; Ten Ham, M.; Van Heijst, A. N. P. Dangerous redistribution of thallium by treatment with sodium diethyldithiocarbamate. Acta Med. Scand. 189:149-154, 1971a.

Kamerbeek, H. H.; Rauws, A. G.; Ten Ham, M.; Van Heijst, A. N. P. Prussian blue in therapy of thallotoxicosis. Acta Med. Scand. 189:321-324, 1971b.

Keller, R.; Thimme, W.; Dissman, W.; Buschmann, H. J.; Dross, K.; Daugs, J. Thallium vergiftung mit Verbrauchskoagulopathie. Schweiz. Med. Wochenschr. 101:511-515, 1971.

Kennedy, P; Cavanagh, J. B. Spinal changes in the neuropathy of thallium poisoning--a case with neuropathological studies. J. Neurol. Sci. 29:295-301, 1976.

Kloppel, A.; Wiler, G. Beitrag Zur Schwermetallvergiftung insbesondere durch Thallium. Dtsch. Med. Wochenschr. 103:75-76, 1978.

Lameijer, W.; Van Zwieten, P. A. Acute cardiovascular toxicity of thallium (1) ions. Arch. Toxicol. 35:49-61, 1976.

Lo, M.; Hall, T.; Wjitmire, W. Some effects of dithizone on the canine prostate. Cancer 13:401-411, 1960.

Lund, A. The effect of various substances on the excretion and the toxicity of thallium in the rat. Acta Pharmacol. Toxicol. 12:260-268, 1956.

Manninen, V.; Malkonen, M.; Skulskii, I. A. Elimination of thallium in rats as influenced by prussian blue and sodium chloride. Acta Pharmacol. Toxicol. 39:256-261, 1976.

Mathew, G. W.; Low, D. G. Thallium intoxication in dogs. J. Am. Vet. Med. Assoc. 137:544-549, 1960.

Mathews, J.; Anzarut, A. Thallium poisoning. Can. Med. Assoc. J. 99:72-75, 1968.

Mazzei, E. S.; Schaposnik, F. Subacute poisoning by thallium treated with BAL. Br. Med. J. 2:791-792, 1949.

Merguet, P.; Schumann, H. J.; Murata, T.; Rausch-Stroomann, J. G.; Schroder, E.; Paar, D.; Bock, K. D. Untersuchungen zur Pathogenese von Hypertonie und Sinustachykardie bei der Thalliumvergiftung des Menschen. Arch. Klin. Med. 216:1-20, 1969.

Moeschlin, S. Poisoning, Diagnosis and Treatment. 1st Amer. Ed., Grune and Stratton, New York, 1965.

Moeschlin, S. Thallium poisoning. Clin. Toxicol. 17:133-146, 1980.

Munch, J. C. The toxicity of thallium sulfate. J. Pharm. Sci. 17:1086-1093, 1928.

Munch, J. C.; Ginsburg, H. M.; Nixon, C. E. The 1932 thallotoxicosis outbreak in California. J. A. M. A. 100:1315-1319, 1933.

Papp, J. P.; Gay, P. C.; Dodson, V. N.; Pollard, H. M. Potassium chloride treatment in thallotoxicosis. Ann. Intern. Med. 71:119-123, 1969.

Paulson, G.; Vergara, G.; Young, J.; Bird, M. Thallium intoxication treated with dithizone and hemodialysis. Arch. Intern. Med. 129:100-103, 1972.

Piazolo, P.; Franz, H. E.; Brech, W.; Walb, D.; Wilk, G. Behandlung der Thalliumvergiftung mit der Hamodialyse. Dtsch. Med. Wochenschr. 96:1217-1222, 1971.

Prick, J. J. G.; Smitt, W. G. S.; Muller, L. Thallium Poisoning. Elsevier Press, Inc., New York, 1955.

Rauws, A. G.; Ten Ham, M.; Kamerbeek, H. H. Influence of the antidote dithiocarb on distribution and toxicity of thallium in the rat. Arch. Int. Pharmacodyn. Ther. 182:425-426, 1969.

Reed, D.; Crawley, J.; Faro, S. N.; Pieper, S. J.; Kurland, L. T. Thallotoxicosis. J. A. M. A. 183:516-522, 1963.

Reiders, F.; Cordova, V. F. Effect of sodium diethyldithiocarbamate on urinary thallium excretion in man. Pharmacologist 7:162, 1965.

Richelmi, P.; Bono, F.; Guardia, L.; Ferrini, B.; Manzo, L. Salivary levels of thallium in acute human poisoning. Arch Toxicol. 43:321-325, 1980.

Richeson, E. M. Industrial thallium intoxication. Ind. Med. Surg. 27:607-619, 1958.

Righetti, P.; Moeschlin, S. The therapeutic effect of dithiocarb (DTC) and potassium chloride on experimental thallium poisoning in guinea pigs. Clin. Toxicol. 4:165-171, 1971.

Schwartzman, R. M.; Kirschbaum, J. O. The cutaneous histopathology of thallium poisoning. J. Invest. Dermatol. 39:169-173, 1962.

Schwetz, B. A.; O'Neil, P. V.; Voelker, F. A.; Jacobs, D. W. Effects of diphenylthiocarbazone and diethyldithiocarbamate on the excretion of thallium by rats. Toxicol. Appl. Pharmacol. 10:79-88, 1967.

Singh, N. P.; Bogden, J. D.; Joselew, M. M. Distribution of thallium and lead in children's blood. Arch. Environ. Health 30:557-558, 1975.

Skelley, J. F.; Gabriel, K. L. Thallium intoxication in the dog. Ann. N. Y. Acad. Sci. 111:612-617, 1964.

Smith, D. H.; Doherty, R. A. Thallitoxicosis. Report of three cases in Massachusetts. Pediatrics 34:480-490, 1964.

Stavinoha, W. B.; Emerson, G. A.; Nash, J. B. The effect of some sulfur compounds on thallotoxicosis in mice. Toxicol.

Appl. Pharmacol. *1*:638-646, 1959.

Stein, M. D.; Perlstein, M. A. Thallium poisoning. Report of two cases. Am. J. Dis. Child. *98*:80-85, 1959.

Stevens, W.; Van Peteghem, C.; Heyndrickx, A.; Barbier, F. Eleven cases of thallium intoxication treated with Prussian blue. Int. J. Clin. Pharmacol. Ther. Toxicol. *10*:1-22, 1974.

Sunderman, F. W., Jr. Diethyldithiocarbamate therapy of thallotoxicosis. Am. J. Med. Sci. *253*:209-220, 1967.

Sunderman, F. W.; Poynter, O. E.; George, R. B. The effects of the protracted administration of the chelating agent, sodium diethyldithiocarbamate (dithiocarb). Am. J. Med. Sci. *254*:24-33, 1967.

Taber, P. Chronic thallium poisoning: Rapid diagnosis and

treatment. J. Pediatr. *65*:461-463, 1964.

Van der Merwe, C. F. The treatment of thallium poisoning; a report of two cases. S. Afr. Med. J. *46*:960-961, 1972.

Van der Stock, J.; de Schepper, J. The effect of Prussian blue and sodium-ethylenediaminetetraacetic acid on the faecal and urinary elimination of thallium by the dog. Res. Vet. Sci. *25*:337-342, 1978.

Welty, J. A.; Berrey, B. H. Acute thallotoxicosis. Report of two cases treated with BAL. J. Pediatr. *37*:756-758, 1950.

Wilson, W. J., Jr.; Hausman, R. The determination of thallium in organs and body fluids by a flame spectrophotometric method. J. Lab. Clin. Med. *64*:154-159, 1964.

THIRAM

Thiram (tetramethylthiuram disulfide) is the methyl analog of disulfiram or Antabuse; it is a white powder which is almost insoluble in water. Thiram is an important agricultural fungicide and is used in industry as a rubber accelerator. Together with related compounds, it has served successfully as an insecticide and as a repellent against the Japanese beetle. It is also used as a fungicide and a bacteriostat in medicated soaps.

Toxicology: No systemic poisonings in man have been reported to our knowledge, but a fatality due to the zinc salt of a thiram metabolite (ziram) has been reported (Buklan, 1974). Animal tests suggest two toxic syndromes: that due to the inherent toxicity of thiram and that induced by ethyl alcohol in those who have ingested otherwise insignificant amounts of thiram (Barnes and Fox, 1955; Hald et al., 1952). A few instances of the latter syndrome have been reported in man after topical exposures (e.g., Reinl, 1966). The thiram-alcohol reaction, which is equivalent to the disulfiram (Antabuse)-alcohol reaction, is not described here; for its symptomatology and treatment, see the discussion of DISULFIRAM on p. III-159. Perhaps because of inadequate exposure, thiram and its congeners rarely induce this sensitization to alcohol in man, although it has occurred.

Thiram is a moderately severe irritant of mucous membranes and a mild irritant of intact skin (Council on Pharmacy and Chemistry, 1955), as well as a potent skin sensitizer (Shelley, 1964). On the basis of single oral doses (aqueous suspensions) in laboratory animals, the mean lethal dose lies near 0.5 gm./kg. (higher in rats, lower in rabbits) (Barnes and Fox, 1955; Gaines, 1969; Weiss and Orzel, 1967). The toxicity is known to be greater in the presence of fats, oils, and fat solvents which promote absorption.

The ethyl analogue (tetraethylthiuram disulfide or disulfiram) is about 10 times less toxic than thiram and is a much weaker irritant (Hanzlik and Irvine, 1921). Both compounds, however, produce similar toxic effects, and many of the following observations are abstracted from reports about disulfiram, which has been more extensively studied.

Animals killed by single oral doses of disulfi-

ram or thiram show hyperemia and focal ulceration of the gastrointestinal tract, focal necrosis of liver and renal tubules, and patchy demyelinization seen first in the cerebellum and medulla (Child and Cramp, 1952). As judged by clinical signs and symptoms (see below), the human brain is also affected. Furthermore, severe but reversible peripheral neuropathies have been encountered during disulfiram therapy (Bradley and Hewer, 1966; Hayman and Wilkins, 1956; Mokri et al., 1981; Supprian, 1969); they commonly involve both motor and sensory functions. In one patient receiving 0.5 gm. disulfiram daily for 5 months, degeneration of microtubules and neurofilaments in axons progressed to axonal degeneration with demyelinization; unmyelinated axons were spared (Moddel et al., 1978). Hepatotoxicity, possibly of idiosyncratic origin, has also been reported in patients on disulfiram therapy (Ranek and Andreasen, 1977). For a summary of autopsy findings in a single human fatality due to a metabolite of thiram, see Ziram in Section II.

Single oral doses of 6 gm. disulfiram (Antabuse) and even 8 gm. (Audier et al., 1961) have been well tolerated, but the recommended clinical dose (0.25 to 1.0 gm. daily) has occasionally produced fatigue, sleepiness, headache, dizziness, mild gastrointestinal disorders, unpleasant taste, lowered blood pressure, reduced potency, minor confusional states and severe dermatitis (Martensen-Larsen, 1953; Barefoot, 1951; Rathod, 1958; Bennett et al., 1951). Doses of 1.5 gm. daily are said to produce definite behavioral changes. Lethargy, impaired memory span, bizarre behavior, emotional lability (acute organic brain syndrome) in a group of nonpsychotic subjects and intensified psychotic symptoms in schizophrenics have been described (Heath et al., 1965; Knee and Razani, 1974; Liddon and Satran, 1967; Weddington et al., 1980). It is difficult to evaluate the primary clinical toxicity of disulfiram because some of the reported poisonings were probably induced by ethyl alcohol and not by an overdose of the drug (e.g., Kellner, 1953). As noted before (p. III-159), the alcohol-disulfiram reaction may be very severe, and it is almost impossible to prove that alcohol was not consumed by an uncooperative disulfiram-treated patient.

A young woman who consumed at one time 18 gm. of disulfiram reportedly without alcohol (Waris, 1954) was sick for 4 days with headache, vomiting, gastric pain and diarrhea. Another girl (15 years old) took 19 tablets (presumably 9.5 gm.) and was found to be somnolent but not comatose; later she became agitated, confused and incoherent (Audier et al., 1961). Tendon reflexes were absent in all extremities for a period of 1 week, but recovery was eventually complete. In another unsuccessful suicide a woman of 40 years swallowed 16 tablets and exhibited only a mild tachycardia and depressed tendon reflexes. A 4-year-old boy was sleepy and eventually comatose after 20 tablets. Persistent EEG abnormalities suggested permanent brain damage; however, the child also had severe pneumonitis, presumably secondary to aspiration of vomitus (Schmoigl, 1970). A 2-year-old boy who ingested an estimated 2.5 gm. disulfiram was asymptomatic for about 12 hours, when vomiting and drowsiness occurred. He recovered after 4 days, but only after experiencing severe ataxia, hallucinations, uncontrollable arm movements, irritability and speech difficulty (Manoguerra and Kearney, 1982).

At least three biochemical mechanisms can be proposed as a basis for the central nervous system toxicity of disulfiram. Certain key sulfhydryl enzymes (e.g., hexokinase, amino acid oxidases) are inhibited by sulfide-disulfide exchange with disulfiram, thiram and ferbam (Neims et al., 1966; Strömme, 1963, 1965; Owens and Rubinstein, 1964). In several species (Casier and Merlevede, 1962; Melson and Weigelt, 1967) at least small amounts of disulfiram and thiram are converted in vivo to carbon disulfide. One team of investigators (Merlevede and Casier, 1961) has reported an extraordinary 50% conversion in man. The reaction involves the rapid reduction of disulfiram and presumably thiram by reticulocytes and perhaps other cells to yield diethyl and dimethyl dithiocarbamic acid respectively (Cobby et al., 1977; Strömme, 1963); both of the latter dissociate into carbon disulfide and dialkylamine. CARBON DISULFIDE (p. III-90) is a well known neurotoxin. (For additional information about the metabolism of disulfiram, see p. III-160.) Finally, disulfiram in vivo has been established as a potent inhibitor of dopamine-β-hydroxylase. It, therefore, interferes with norepinephrine biosynthesis and ultimately leads to tissue norepinephrine depletion and dopamine accumulation (Goldstein and Nakajima, 1966; Hashimoto et al., 1965b; Musacchio et al., 1966).

Chronic administration of disulfiram has produced behavioral and neurological effects in man, perhaps due to carbon disulfide generated by metabolic breakdown of the drug (Rainey, 1977). As noted above, the behavioral abnormalities include drowsiness, confusion, headache, nausea, loss of libido and rarely psychoses. The neurological disorders include ataxia, slurred speech, weakness (including ptosis), Parkinsonian tremor, and peripheral neuritis. Chronic exposure to thiram in industry also appears to be responsible for neuropsychiatric effects (Cherpak et al., 1971). Thiram is teratogenic in hamsters and mice but perhaps not in rats (summarized by Fishbein, 1976). Perhaps disulfiram is teratogenic in humans (Nora et al., 1977). The carcinogenic potential of thiram and its congeners is not well established.

Symptomatology (the primary toxic reaction, *not* that induced by alcohol, as inferred in part from clinical reports of disulfiram overdoses):

1. Nausea, vomiting, diarrhea, anorexia, weight loss. Nausea and emesis may be persistent and the diarrhea copious.
2. Headache, lethargy, dizziness, ataxia, confusion, drowsiness, emotional lability and coma.
3. Delirium, tremor, catatonia and hallucinations have occurred with large repeated doses of disulfiram, apparently in the absence of ethanol intake.
4. Reduction in blood pressure, not usually severe unless fluid and electrolyte deficits are extensive.
5. Suppression of tendon reflexes.
6. Hypotonia and, within a few hours or a few days, flaccid paralysis. In animals this disorder appears first in the hind limbs and is a type of ascending paralysis (Landry's syndrome). The muscles retain responsiveness to mechanical and electrical stimulation. If death does not occur, recovery of acutely poisoned animals tends to be complete within 1 or 2 weeks.
7. Respiratory paralysis and death.
8. Severe dermatitis and hepatitis probably represent hypersensitivity reactions.
9. Peripheral neuropathies in patients on chronic disulfiram therapy tend to disappear spontaneously over periods of a few months after the therapy is discontinued.

Treatment:

1. If the victim is alert and has not yet vomited, give syrup of ipecac (p. I-2) and/or perform gastric lavage with tap water. Disulfiram tablets have been found in the stomach even 4 hours after ingestion.
2. Leave in the stomach 15 to 30 gm. of sodium sulfate in water and perhaps a slurry of activated charcoal (p. I-12). Avoid fats, oils and lipid solvents, which enhance intestinal absorption.

3. Rigorously prohibit ethyl alcohol in all forms for at least 10 days.

4. Correct water and electrolyte deficits by infusing isotonic saline or balanced salt solutions (pp. IV-64–73). These infusions are also useful to sustain the blood pressure.

5. Because of the reported inhibition of hexokinase (Strömme, 1965), it might be worthwhile to induce mild hyperglycemia with an infusion of glucose.

6. Artificial respiration (p. IV-7) and oxygen therapy (p. IV-12), as needed. Oxygen administration, however, should probably be restricted to short periods because disulfiram and one of its major metabolites (diethyldithiocarbamate) enhance the pulmonary toxicity of oxygen, at least in rats (Forman et al., 1980).

7. Symptomatic and supportive treatment for various gastrointestinal symptoms (p. IV-49) and neurological complications.

8. In managing thiram or disulfiram poisonings characterized by delirium and/or psychotic behavior, centrally active drugs should be used cautiously, if at all, because of the many adverse interactions with disulfiram that have been described (e.g., with phenytoin, morphine, chlorpromazine). Small doses of diazepam may be helpful, but antipsychotic drugs such as chlorpromazine sometimes make the situation worse (Knee and Razani, 1974).

Laboratory: Tests to detect and evaluate possible disturbances of liver and kidney function should be conducted repeatedly. Hypercholesterolemia may be detected; it occurs frequently in the course of disulfiram therapy and can be corrected by taking 50 mg. pyridoxine daily (Major and Goyer, 1978).

References:

Audier, M.; Serradimigni, A.; Bille, J.; Francois, G. A propos de deux cas de tentative de suicide par disulfiram. Presse Med. 69:2074, 1961.

Barefoot, S. W. Acneform eruption produced by use of tetraethylthiuram disulfide. J. A. M. A. 147:1653, 1951.

Barnes, B. A.; Fox, L. E. Screening some thiuram disulfides and related compounds for acute toxicity and Antabuse-like activity. J. Pharm. Sci. 44:756-759, 1955.

Bennett, A. E.; McKeever, L. G.; Turk, R. E. Psychotic reaction during tetraethylthiuram disulfide (Antabuse) therapy. J. A. M. A. 145:483-484, 1951.

Bradley, W. G.; Hewer, R. L. Peripheral neuropathy due to disulfiram. Br. Med. J. 2:449-450, 1966.

Buklan, A. I. Acute poisoning with ziram. (as cited in Chem. Abstracts 82:133715b) Sud. -Med. Ekopert. 17:51, 1974.

Casier, H.; Merlevede, E. On the mechanism of the disulfiram-ethanol intoxication symptoms. Arch. Int. Pharmacodyn. Ther. 139:165-176, 1962.

Cherpak, V. V.; Bezuglyi, V. P.; Kaskevich, L. M. Sanitary-hygienic characteristics of working conditions and health of persons working with tetramethylthiuram disulfide. (as cited in Chem. Abstracts 76:54976) Vrach. Delo 10:136-139, 1971.

Child, G. P.; Cramp, M. The toxicity of tetraethylthiuram disulfide (Antabuse) to mouse, rat, rabbit and dog. Acta Pharmacol. Toxicol. 8:305-314, 1952.

Cobby, J.; Mayersohn, M.; Selliah, S. The rapid reduction of disulfiram in blood and plasma. J. Pharmacol. Exp. Ther. 202:724-731, 1977.

Council on Pharmacy and Chemistry, A. M. A. Outlines of information on pesticides. Part 1, Agricultural fungicides. J. A. M. A. 157:237-241, 1955.

Fishbein, L. Environmental health aspects of fungicides. I. Dithiocarbamates. J. Toxicol. Environ. Health 1:713-735, 1976.

Forman, H. J.; York, J. L.; Fisher, A. B. Mechanism for the potentiation of oxygen toxicity by disulfiram. J. Pharmacol. Exp. Ther. 212:452-455, 1980.

Gaines, T. B. Acute toxicity of pesticides. Toxicol. Appl. Pharmacol. 14:515-534, 1969.

Goldstein, M.; Nakajima, K. The effects of disulfiram on the repletion of brain catecholamine stores. Life Sci. 5:1133-1138, 1966.

Hald, J.; Jacobsen, E.; Larsen, V. The Antabuse effect of some compounds related to Antabuse and cyanamide. Acta Pharmacol. Toxicol. 8:329-337, 1952.

Hanzlik, P. J.; Irvine, A. The toxicity of some thioureas and thiuram disulfides. J. Pharmacol. Exp. Ther. 17:349-355, 1921.

Hashimoto, Y.; Ohi, Y.; Imaizumi, R. Inhibition of brain dopamine-β-oxidase in vivo by disulfiram. Jap. J. Pharmacol. 15:445-446, 1965b.

Hayman, M.; Wilkins, P. A. Polyneuropathy as a complication of disulfiram therapy of alcoholism. Q. J. Stud. Alcohol 17:601-607, 1956.

Heath, R. G.; Nesselhof, W.; Bishop, M. P.; Byers, L. W. Behavioral and metabolic changes associated with administration of tetraethylthiuram disulfide (Antabuse). Dis. Nerv. Syst. 26:99-104, 1965.

Kellner, K. Ein Fall von Antabus-Vergiftung. Med. Klin. 48:1034-1036, 1953.

Knee, S. T.; Razani, J. Acute organic brain syndrome: a complication of disulfiram therapy. Am. J. Psychiatry 131:1281-1282, 1974.

Liddon, S. C.; Satran, R. Disulfiram (Antabuse) psychosis. Am. J. Psychiatry 123:1284-1289, 1967.

Major, L. F.; Goyer, P. F. Effects of disulfiram and pyridoxine on serum cholesterol. Ann. Intern. Med. 88:53-56, 1978.

Manoguerra, A. S.; Kearney, T. E. Acute disulfiram toxicity. Vet. Hum. Toxicol. 24:282, 1982.

Martensen-Larsen, O. Five years experience with disulfiram in the treatment of alcoholics. Q. J. Stud. Alcohol 14:406-408, 1953.

Melson, F.; Weigelt, H. The influence of tetramethyl thiuram and carbon disulfide on the enzymes monoaminoxidase and alcoholdehydrogenase. In Toxicology of Carbon Disulphide, edited by H. Brieger and J. Teisinger. Excerpta Medica Foundation, Amsterdam, pp. 100-103, 1967.

Merlevede, E.; Casier, H. Teneur en sulfure de carbone de l'air expire chez des personnes normales ou sous l'influence de l'alcool ethylique au cours du traitement par l'antabuse (disulfiram) et le diethyldithiocarbamate de soude. Arch. Int. Pharmacodyn. Ther. 132:427-453, 1961.

Moddel, G.; Bilbao, J. M.; Payne, D.; Ashby, P. Disulfiram neuropathy. Arch. Neurol. 35:658-660, 1978.

Mokri, B.; Ohnishi, A.; Dyck, P. J. Disulfiram neuropathy. Neurology 31:730-735, 1981.

Musacchio, J. M.; Goldstein, M.; Anagnoste, B.; Poch, G.; Kopin, L. J. Inhibition of dopamine-β-hydroxylase by disulfiram in vivo. J. Pharmacol. Exp. Ther. 152:56-61, 1966.

Neims, A. H.; Coffey, D. S.; Hellerman, L. Interaction between tetraethylthiuram disulfide and the sulfhydryl groups of D-amino acid oxidase and of hemoglobin. J. Biol. Chem. 241:5941-5948, 1966.

Nora, A. H.; Nora, J. J.; Blu, J. Limb-reduction anomalies in infants born to disulfiram-treated alcoholic mothers. Lancet 2:664, 1977.

Owens, R. G.; Rubinstein, J. H. Chemistry of the fungicidal action of tetramethylthiuram disulfide (thiram) and ferbam.

Contrib. Boyce Thompson Inst. *22*:241-258, 1964.

Rainey, J. M. Disulfiram toxicity and carbon disulfide poisoning. Am. J. Psychiatr. *134*:371-378, 1977.

Ranek, L.; Andreasen, P. B. Disulfiram hepatotoxicity. Br. Med. J. *2*:94-96, 1977.

Rathod, N. H. Toxic effects of disulfiram therapy, with two case reports. Q. J. Stud. Alcohol *19*:418-427, 1958.

Reinl, W. Alkoholuberempfindlichkeit nach Umgang mit dem Fungicid Tetramethylthiuramdisulfid (TMTD). Arch. Toxikol. *22*:12-15, 1966.

Schmoigl, S. Akute Disulfiram-Vergiftung bei einer Kleinkind. Nervenarzt *41*:89-92, 1970.

Shelley, W. B. Golf-course dermatitis due to thiram fungicide. J. A. M. A. *188*:415-417, 1964.

Stromme, J. H. Effects of diethyldithiocarbamate and disulfiram on glucose metabolism and glutathione content of human erythrocytes. Biochem. Pharmacol. *12*:705-715,

1963.

Stromme, J. H. Metabolism of disulfiram and diethyldithiocarbamate in rats with demonstration of an *in vivo* ethanol-induced inhibition of the glucuronic acid conjugation of the thiol. Biochem. Pharmacol. *14*:393-410, 1965.

Supprian, U. Uber einen Fall von Antabusintoxikation. Nervenarzt *40*:276-277, 1969.

Waris, E. Antabusforgiftning utan alkohol (Antabuse poisoning without alcohol). Nord. Med. *51*:455, 1954. As abstracted in Q. J. Stud. Alcohol 16:361, 1955.

Weddington, W. W.; Marks, R. C.; Verghese, J. P. Disulfiram encephalopathy as a cause of the catatonia syndrome. Am. J. Psychiatry *137*:1217-1219, 1980.

Weiss, L. R.; Orzel, R. A. Enhancement of toxicity of anticholinesterases by central depressant drugs in rats. Toxicol. Appl. Pharmacol. *10*:334-339, 1967.

TOXAPHENE

Toxaphene is a complex mixture of chlorinated derivatives of camphene, principally octachlorocamphene, but some commercial products consist of at least 175 polychlorinated 10-carbon compounds (Casida *et al.*, 1974). The technical or insecticidal grade is an amber-colored waxy solid with a mild pine odor. It is prepared commercially as dusts, sprays and wettable powders. It is a relatively slow-acting residual insecticide, which has been used extensively against cotton insects and grasshoppers. It has also been used for the control of insects resistant to DDT, but it is not considered safe for household application (Council on Pharmacy and Chemistry, 1952b).

Toxaphene is the last remaining representative of the "hard type" halogenated hydrocarbon insecticides to be used almost without restrictions in the United States. At the time of this writing, however, its future status is in doubt since it is on the Rebuttable Presumption Against Registration list of the EPA.

Toxicology: The compound is absorbed through the intact skin, respiratory tract and gastrointestinal tract (Council on Pharmacy and Chemistry, 1952b). The mean lethal dose (LD_{50}) by mouth is 80 to 90 mg./kg. in rats (Boyd and Taylor, 1971; Gaines, 1969), but many other values have been reported, perhaps reflecting the variable intestinal absorption of toxaphene. Acute toxicity in rats is potentiated at least 3-fold by protein deficiency (Boyd and Taylor, 1971). Intestinal absorption is increased by the presence of digestible oils, and liquid preparations (oil solvents) penetrate the skin far more readily than do dusts or powders (Johnston and Eden, 1952; Lackey, 1949a and b).

At least eight human fatalities have occurred (Haun and Cueto, 1967; McGee *et al.*, 1952; Pollack, 1953). Although not definitely ascertained, the lethal oral dose for an adult is estimated to be 2 to 7 gm., representing a toxicity about 4 times that of DDT (Council on Pharmacy and Chemistry, 1952b; Hayes, 1963.) As might be expected in such a complex mixture, the hazards of toxaphene may be due in large measure to relatively minor but highly toxic subfractions (Nelson and Matsumura, 1975; Pollock and Kilgore, 1980; Saleh *et al.*, 1977).

Toxic symptoms in acute poisoning usually appear within 1 hour, and death occurs within 4 to 8 hours. The onset of symptoms is characteristically abrupt (von Oettingen, 1955). Generalized convulsions constitute the only definitive manifestation of the intoxication, but cyanosis has appeared before convulsions at least once (Pollack, 1953). Measures which are used to combat camphor poisoning (see p. III-85) may be useful in toxaphene poisoning too (Lehman, 1948), but therapy has not been fully evaluated in human intoxications. The control of convulsions is always desirable, but may not be decisive. In one case signs of improvement in a quiescent patient were followed by a fever spike and death in respiratory collapse (Hayes, 1963).

Two agricultural workers with histories of heavy exposure to chlorinated camphene sprays (aqueous emulsions) experienced sudden exertional dyspnea, tachycardia, weakness and low blood pressure. The symptoms were considered mild relative to the extensive radiological findings of miliary shadows in both lungs. One victim also presented with hilar adenopathy, but in neither case did a diagnosis of tuberculosis appear to fit the clinical picture. Both patients recovered promptly on cortisone, streptomycin and isoniazid (Warraki, 1963).

Rats metabolically dechlorinate toxaphene (Casida *et al.*, 1974). In several organisms and environmental systems, this reaction is a reductive dechlorination, sometimes a dehydrochlorination (Saleh *et al.*, 1977). In part toxaphene is also metabolized by NADPH-dependent mixed function oxidase in rat hepatic microsomal enzyme preparations, but the relative importance of this oxidative pathway in relation to reductive dechlorination remains unknown (Chandurkar and Matsumura, 1979). Like other chlorinated hydrocarbon insecticides, toxaphene induces hepatic microsomal enzyme activity (Welch et al., 1971).

Lesions arise in the liver and renal tubules of chronically exposed animals (Lackey, 1949b; Lackey and Weed, 1951). At doses that result in overt maternal toxicity, toxaphene is teratogenic in mice and rats (Chernoff and Carver, 1976). Even without prior activation by exposure to liver homogenates, toxaphene is mutagenic in the *Salmonella* test (Hooper et al., 1979). Finally, toxaphene is highly carcinogenic in mice and rats (Reuber, 1979).

Toxaphene is less readily stored in body fat than is DDT (von Oettingen, 1955). Its accumulation in adipose tissue of broiler chickens has been documented (Bush et al., 1978). Like DDT, it probably is concentrated in natural food chains.

Symptomatology:

1. Reflex hyperexcitability, evidenced by tremor, salivation, and vomiting. When present, emesis is apparently always secondary to reflex excitation and not to local gastrointestinal irritation.
2. Generalized epileptiform convulsions of variable duration. Symptoms are precipitated or aggravated by external stimuli.
3. Death due to exhaustion and respiratory failure.
4. Mild irritation of skin after dermal exposures but little if any sensitization.

Treatment:

1. A slurry of activated charcoal followed by gastric lavage with tap water.
2. Saline cathartics, *e.g.,* sodium or magnesium sulfate (15 to 30 gm.) in water.
3. Demulcents, but avoid oils.
4. Barbiturates to control convulsions (thiopental, phenobarbital, or pentobarbital). Convulsions are best managed if treatment is begun before their appearance; if convulsions have already developed, use a short-acting drug like thiopental sodium, and give a full anesthetic dose. Perhaps diazepam is even better. See pp. IV-35–39.
5. Wash off any poison which may have contacted the skin. Use liberal amounts of soap and running water.
6. Avoid epinephrine, as a precaution against possible ventricular fibrillation.
7. Protect patient from strong external stimuli, which may precipitate convulsions.
8. As soon as the convulsions are controlled, treat any associated metabolic disorders, such as dehydration (p. IV-64) and acidosis (p. IV-69).

Laboratory: Repeated tests are desirable to detect and evaluate possible disturbances in liver and kidney function. See pp. IV-52 and 59.

References:

Boyd, E. M.; Taylor, F. I. Toxaphene toxicity in protein-deficient rats. Toxicol. Appl. Pharmacol. *18*:158-167, 1971.

Bush, P. B.; Tanner, J. T.; Kiker, J. T.; Page, R. K.; Booth, N. H.; Fletcher, O. J. Tissue residue studies on toxaphene in broiler chickens. J. Agric. Food Chem. *26*:126-130, 1978.

Casida, J. E.; Holmstead, R. L.; Khalifa, S.; Knox, J. R.; Ohsawa, T.; Palmer, K. J.; Wong, R. Y. Toxaphene insecticide; a complex biodegradable mixture. Science *183*:520-521, 1974.

Chandurkar, P. S.; Matsumura, F. Metabolism of a toxicant B and toxican C of toxaphene in rats. Bull. Environ. Contam. Toxicol. *21*:539-547, 1979.

Chernoff, N.; Carver, B. D. Fetal toxicity of toxaphene in rats and mice. Bull. Environ. Contam. Toxicol. *15*:660-664, 1976.

Council on Pharmacy and Chemistry, A. M. A. Pharmacological properties of toxaphene, a chlorinated hydrocarbon insecticide. J. A. M. A. *149*:1135-1137, 1952b.

Gaines, T. B. Acute toxicity of pesticides. Toxicol. Appl. Pharmacol. *14*:515-534, 1969.

Haun, E. C.; Cueto, C., Jr. Fatal toxaphene poisoning in a 9-month-old infant. Am. J. Dis. Child. *113*:616-618, 1967.

Hayes, W. J., Jr. Clinical Handbook on Economic Poisons. USPHS Publication No. 476. U. S. Government Printing Office, Washington, D. C., 1963.

Hooper, N. K.; Ames, B. N.; Saleh, M. A.; Casida, J. E. Toxaphene, a complex mixture of polychloroterpenes and a major insecticide, is mutagenic. Science *205*:591-593, 1979.

Johnston, B. L.; Eden, W. G. The toxicity of aldrin, dieldrin, and toxaphene to rabbits by skin absorption. J. Econ. Entomol. *46*:702-703, 1952.

Lackey, R. W. Observations on the acute and chronic toxicity of toxaphene in the dog. J. Ind. Hyg. Toxicol. *31*:117-154, 1949a.

Lackey, R. W. Observations on the precutaneous absorption of toxaphene in the rabbit and dog. J. Ind. Hyg. Toxicol. *31*:155-157, 1949b.

Lackey, R. W.; Weed, O. Treatment of acute toxaphene poisoning in the dog. South. Med. J. *44*:165-166, 1951.

Lehman, A. J. The toxicology of the newer agricultural chemicals. Q. Bull. Assoc. Food Drug Officials *12*:82-89, 1948.

McGee, L. C.; Reed, H. L.; Fleming, J. P. Accidental poisoning by toxaphene; review of toxicology and case reports. J. A. M. A. *149*:1124-1126, 1952.

Nelson, J. O.; Matsumura, F. Simplified approach to studies of toxic toxaphene components. Bull. Environ. Contam. Toxicol. *13*:464-470, 1975.

Pollock, G. A.; Kilgore, W. W. Toxicities and description of some toxaphene fractions: isolation and identification of a highly toxic component. J. Toxicol. Environ. Health *6*:115-125, 1980.

Pollock, R. W. Toxaphene poisoning - report of a fatal case. Northwest Med. *52*:293-294, 1953.

Reuber, M. D. Carcinogenicity of toxaphene: a review. J. Toxicol. Environ. Health *5*:729-748, 1979.

Saleh, M. A.; Turner, W. V.; Casida, J. E. Polychlorobornane components of toxaphene: structure-toxicity relations and metabolic reductive dechlorination. Science *198*:1256-1258, 1977.

von Oettingen, W. F. The Halogenated Hydrocarbons, Toxicity and Potential Dangers. Public Health Service Publication No. 414, U. S. Government Printing Office, Washington, D. C., 1955.

Warraki, S. Respiratory hazards of chlorinated camphene. Arch. Environ. Health *7*:253-256, 1963.

Welch, R. M.; Levin, W.; Kuntzman, R.; Jacobson, M.; Conney, A. H. Effect of halogenated hydrocarbon insecticides on the metabolism and uterotropic action of estrogens in rats and mice. Toxicol. Appl. Pharmacol. *19*:234-246, 1971.

TRI-*ORTHO*-CRESYL PHOSPHATE

Tri-*o*-cresyl phosphate (TOCP), also known as tri-*o*-tolyl phosphate, occurs as a contaminant in industrial-grade tricresyl phosphate, which contains predominately the *meta*- and *para*-isomers. Modern mixtures contain less than 1% of the *ortho*-isomer although in years past as much as 20% might have been found (personal communication Dr. Gerard Egan, Exxon Corp., April, 1978). Tricresyl phosphate has been used in a variety of industrial processes and materials, including commerical plasticizers, nitrocellulose solvents, lubricants, gasoline additives, flame retardants and a cooling fluid in machine guns.

Since the demonstration that TOCP is capable of causing a neurotoxic paralysis (Smith *et al.*, 1930), a few other organophosphorus compounds have been shown to produce similar effects. Table III-7 lists some of them (Watanabe

and Sharma, 1973). That this toxic response involves neuronal degeneration in the central and peripheral nervous systems has been well documented in man and susceptible animal species (Davies, 1963). More recently, chemically unrelated compounds such as hexane, methyl-*n*-butyl ketone and acrylamide have been recognized as producing a similar syndrome (see also Section II).

Toxicology: Human neuropathies of epidemic proportion due to TOCP have been reviewed by Davies (1963). In established cases of human exposure, the neurotoxic effects have generally been nonlethal. In a well documented outbreak occurring in the southern United States in early 1930, approximately 20,000 people were poisoned (Smith and Elvove, 1930). The paralysis proved to be due to the presence

Table III-7.
Characteristics of Some Neurotoxic Compounds[a]

Neurotoxic Compounds	Chemical Name	Delay Between Exposure and Paralysis (Days)	Duration of Paralysis (Days)	Reference
TOTP (TOCP)	Tri-*o*-tolyl phosphate	8–14	No complete recovery	Barnes and Denz, 1953
DFP	Diisopropylphosphorofluoridate	11–12	No complete recovery	Witter and Gaines, 1963
Mipafox (Isopestox)	Bis-(monoisopropylamino)-fluoro-phosphate	12–24	No complete recovery	Majno and Karnovsky, 1961
DEF	*S,S,S,*-Tributyl phosphorotrithioate	14–28	>30	Gaines, 1969
Merphos	Tributyl phosphorotrithioite	3–21	>90	Gaines, 1969
Dursban (Dowco 179)	*O,O*-Diethyl *O*-(3,5,6-trichloro-2-pyridyl)-phosphorothioate	3–18	10–20	Gaines, 1969
EPN	*O*-Ethyl *O-p*-nitrophenyl phenylphosphonothioate	—[b]	>330	Gaines, 1969
Carbophenothion (Trithion)	*S-*(*p*-Chlorophenylthio)methyl *O,O*-diethylphosphorodithioate	—[b]	35–53	Gaines, 1969
Abate (Bithion)	*O,O*-Dimethyl phosphorothioate *O,O*-diester with 4,4' thiodiphenol	—[b]	6–31	Gaines, 1969
Ruelene (Dowco 132)	4-*tert*-Butyl-2-chlorophenyl methyl methylphosphoramidate	—[b]	4–64	Gaines, 1969
Ethion (Embathion, Nialate)	*O,O,O',O',*-Tetraethyl *S,S'*-methylenebisphosphorodithioate	—[b]	7–71	Gaines, 1969
Acrylamide		Days to weeks	Months	See Section II
Hexane		Weeks to months	Months	See Section II
Methyl-*n*-butyl ketone		Weeks to months	Months	See Section II

[a] Species tested in all cases (except the last three compounds) were chickens, all birds atropinized except for those treated with TOTP.

[b] No significant delay in onset of paralysis.

of TOCP in a contaminated ginger extract used for beverage production ("ginger paralysis"). This demonstration shed light on earlier reports of neuropathies due to triaryl phosphates in tuberculosis patients being treated with phosphocreosote. A large-scale intoxication by TOCP occurred in Morocco in 1959 in which approximately 10,000 people were affected (Albertini *et al.*, 1968). This tragedy resulted from cooking with a mixture of olive oil and lubricating oil, the latter containing TOCP. Tri-o-cresyl phosphate polyneuritis linked to contaminated flour sacking material has also been reported (Sorokin, 1969). Several cases have been associated with the footwear industry. In 1951 two industrial workers were paralyzed by the pesticide mipafox (Bidstrup and Bonnell, 1954).

Clinical features of the human neuropathy included pain in the calves and paresthesias of hands and feet. The first objective sign was slapping of the feet on the floor while walking, followed by increasing unsteadiness. As the condition progressed, wasting of the intrinsic muscles of the hands became apparent. Transient high stepping was accompanied by an inability to stand still (Burley, 1932; Sorokin, 1969). The appearance of spasticity 1 year after the ingestion of TOCP and after apparent recovery from flaccid paralysis has been described (Godfrey, 1961).

Species differences in response to TOCP are recognized. The chicken and cat have been widely utilized to investigate the syndrome because their responses are similar to those of man. Rabbit, guinea pig, monkey and dog react inconsistently. Rats and mice have been reported to be relatively resistant to the severe paralysis in spite of nervous tissue damage (Majno and Karnovsky, 1961). The clinical signs of paralysis cannot be produced in young chickens or rats (Barnes and Denz, 1953; Taylor, 1967).

Degeneration of nerves induced by TOCP has been demonstrated at various sites in the central and peripheral nervous systems. The onset of paralysis occurs approximately 8 to 14 days after exposure (Davies, 1963). It is generally accepted that the principal degeneration occurs in the medulla, spinal cord and sciatic nerve (Barnes and Denz, 1953; Cavanagh, 1954; Fenton, 1955). Pathological features described in the hen suggested an anterior horn disease like poliomyelitis associated with peripheral axonal degeneration (Cavanagh and McDermot, 1961). In the peripheral nervous system, the sciatic nerve was most affected, and distal portions of the nerves degenerated first (Cavanagh, 1954). In the cat, the peripheral nerves of largest diameter and greatest length were more prone to be affected (Cavanagh, 1964). In the cat central nervous system, fiber length rather than fiber diameter appeared to be the important factor (Cavanagh and Patangia, 1965). Degeneration in the human spinal

anterolateral columns (Chaudhuri, 1965) and muscle lesions have been reported (Smith and Lillie, 1931; Vora *et al.*, 1962). Follow-up studies of human poisonings and postmortem inspections demonstrated participation of the long spinal pathways in the process (Zeligs, 1938; Aring, 1942).

The description of TOCP intoxication as a specific demyelinating disease (Smith and Lillie, 1931) has proven to be misleading. Bischoff (1967, 1970) has shown that the initial alterations in the sciatic nerve and spinal cord occurred in the axoplasm and included proliferation of smooth endoplasmic reticulum and degeneration of neurofilaments. Mitochondrial clustering and altered spatial relationships between the axon and Schwann cell membranes were demonstrated. It is now believed that TOCP acts primarily on the axon, particularly myelinated fibers, and that myelin disintegration is secondary to axonal destruction (Prineas, 1969). Studies on spinal cord synaptic morphology in TOCP-treated chickens and cats demonstrated clumping of vesicles, mitochondrial swelling and obliteration of the synaptic cleft (Illis *et al.*, 1966; Ahmed, 1971b).

The physiologic disposition of TOCP has been studied in several species. Gross and Grosse (1932) reported accumulations of TOCP in the rabbit gastrointestinal wall, liver and spleen after an intravenous dose. Dermal exposure of a dog resulted in the presence of TOCP in all examined tissues in the following sequence of descending concentration: liver > kidney > lung > nervous tissue > bone (Hodge and Sterner, 1943). Myers *et al.* (1955) found active esterase inhibitors in the urine of rats and rabbits after intraperitoneal injections of TOCP. In the rabbit, enterohepatic circulation of TOCP or its metabolites was demonstrated. In the chicken, an oral dose of TOCP was shown to accumulate over a two-week period only in nervous tissue; other tissues showed an initial increase followed by a decline (Watanabe and Sharma, 1973). The major metabolite of TOCP, CBDP (2-o-(cresyl)-4H-1:3:2 benzodioxaphosphoran-2-one), a cyclic saligenin phosphate, has been shown to accumulate in chicken liver for a long period after an oral dose of TOCP (Sharma and Watanabe, 1974).

The excretion of TOCP has been regarded as very slow. Smith and Stohlman (1943) detected the substance in cat urine and feces 6 days after an intravenous dose. After dermal absorption in two human subjects, 0.1 and 0.4% of the administered dose were excreted in urine within 3 days (Hodge and Sterner, 1943). In the chicken, 26.5% of an orally administered dose was excreted over a 72-hour period; unmetabolized TOCP accounted for nearly 99% of the excreted material (Sharma and Watanabe, 1974).

Highly purified samples of TOCP do not affect

the serum enzyme, cholinesterase. The metabolism of TOCP, however, has been shown to produce potent esterase inhibitors (Aldridge, 1954; Myers *et al.*, 1955; Davison, 1955; Casida, 1961). Eto *et al.* (1962) reported that the primary antiesterase metabolite in rats and chickens is CBDP; two additional metabolites corresponding to hydroxylated TOCP and hydroxylated CBDP were detected. The initial hydroxylation of TOCP occurs in the liver, and the cyclization reaction yielding CBDP is catalyzed by an albumin fraction in the plasma (Eto *et al.*, 1967). The CBDP metabolite has been observed to be more potent than TOCP both in the inhibition of cholinesterase and in the production of axonal damage (Casida *et al.*, 1961; Bleiberg and Johnson, 1965).

The neuropathy produced by TOCP is not associated with typical signs or symptoms of cholinesterase inhibition, but because many neurotoxic agents are antiesterases, the cholinesterase enzymes have been studied extensively. Inhibition of butyrylcholinesterase was postulated as a basis of the neuropathy (Earl and Thompson, 1952), but not all butyrylcholinesterase inhibitors are neurotoxic (Davison, 1953). Pseudocholinesterase inhibition has long been regarded by most investigators as incidental to the genesis of neurotoxicity (Aldridge, 1954; Hine *et al.*, 1956; Cavanagh and Holland, 1961; Witter and Gaines, 1963). Johnson (1969, 1970, 1975) believes that a "neurotoxic esterase" was inhibited selectively *in vivo* by diisopropylfluorophosphate and mipafox. Because carbamylation or sulfonylation of this enzyme was shown not to produce axonal damage, it was concluded that the nature of the group transferred to the active site determined the neurotoxic response.

Several studies have focused on lipid metabolism because of the similarity of TOCP intoxication to Wallerian degeneration, in which extensive alteration of lipids is known to occur (Berry *et al.*, 1965a). Based on lipid analyses, one cannot differentiate between primary and secondary effects, including those of starvation (Majno and Karnovsky, 1961; Joel *et al.*, 1967; Morazain and Rosenberg, 1970). The incorporation of phospholipid precursors was shown not to be affected by TOCP administration (Webster, 1954; Taylor, 1965; Sheltawy and Dawson, 1969). Cholesterol levels in TOCP-treated chickens have been observed to be high (Johnson and Weiss, 1965; Berry and Cevallos, 1966; Morazain and Rosenberg, 1970).

The antiesterase hypotheses and superficial similarities between TOCP intoxication and vitamin deficiencies have stimulated numerous studies of therapeutic regimes based on atropine, oximes and vitamins. Atropine and oximes were found to be completely ineffective in treating the delayed neuropathy of TOCP (Bleiberg and

Johnson, 1965; Davies, 1972). The conversion of TOCP to CBDP is reputedly inhibited *in vitro* by SKF 525-A (2-ethylaminoethyl-2,2-diphenylvalerate), but SKF 525-A was found to be ineffective in preventing TOCP intoxication (Bleiberg and Johnson, 1965; Morazain and Rosenberg, 1970). Varying levels of thiamine, *O*-acetyl thiamine, oxythiamine, tocopherol and *O*-acetyl tocopherol, in addition to complete mixtures of vitamins, proved to be ineffective in alleviating TOCP, CBDP or DFP neurotoxic paralysis (Casida *et al.*, 1961; Baron and Casida, 1962). Chambers and Casida (1967) demonstrated beneficial effects in TOCP-dosed chickens from pretreatment with high levels of nicotinic acid analogs. The onset of paralysis was delayed for several days, but complete prevention of the neurotoxic signs was not achieved.

Glees (1960) reported that cortisone administered three days prior to TOCP and every third day thereafter protected chickens from the TOCP neuropathy. In other animal studies cortisone acetate administered simultaneously with TOCP provided a limited improvement in the TOCP-induced ataxic condition (Baron and Casida, 1962). O'Brien (1967) suggested that TOCP neurotoxicity might involve an autoimmune component, but studies in the chicken have failed to support this hypothesis (Watanabe and Sharma, 1976).

Interactions of TOCP with other substances have been studied. The simultaneous intraperitoneal administration of TOCP or CBDP and pentobarbital was observed to prolong the sleeping time (Buttar *et al.*, 1968). Oral administration of TOCP 24 hours prior to an intraperitoneal injection of hexobarbital caused a reduction in sleeping time (Lynch and Coon, 1972). TOCP potentiated the effects of sarin, soman, physostigmine (McKay *et al.*, 1971) and malathion in rats and mice (Murphy *et al.*, 1959; Casida, 1961; Cohen and Murphy, 1971). Reduction in the toxicity of parathion and EPN were produced in mice by TOCP pretreatment (Lynch and Coon, 1972).

To date no satisfactory correlation has been established between neurotoxic potential and chemical structure among organophosphorus compounds (Aldridge and Barnes, 1961, 1966; Johnson, 1975), and no proposed mechanism explains adequately TOCP-induced delayed neuropathy. Furthermore, no specific treatment and no adequate palliative therapy (except physiotherapy) have been proven effective.

Symptomatology (according to Albertine *et al.*, 1968):

1. Sudden diarrhea and nausea or vomiting during or shortly after ingestion. Gastrointestinal upset is seldom prolonged more than 48 hours, and abatement is also ab-

rupt. These signs may reflect cholinesterase inhibition.

2. The above is followed by an asymptomatic latent period of 8 to 35 days.

3. Feverish feeling in spite of a normal body temperature, brief episodes of diarrhea, conjunctivitis, rhinitis, pharyngitis and laryngitis accompanied by dysphagia, lasting several days to a week.

4. Sensory disturbances including paresthesias or causalgias in distal parts of extremities, particularly the toes, feet and lower parts of the legs. Cramping pains in calves.

5. At 10 to 40 days after the beginning of the prodromal stage, there is a surprisingly abrupt onset of flaccid paralysis (within hours) with rapid progression over several days. First seen in toe muscles, it spreads proximally from the periphery. Paralysis of fingers and hand muscles may lag 4 to 5 days behind signs in the lower extremities.

6. Severity of the intoxication can be assessed only after the complete picture of paralysis is established over 8 to 10 days. All gradations are recognized from mild to total paresis. In severe poisonings the most serious stage is reached in the second or third month, followed by no change or slow recovery.

7. Hyperhiderosis with cold, moist, cyanotic hands and feet.

8. Flaccid paralysis may be followed by spasticity of the lower extremities ranging from hyperreflexia to clonus, hypertonus and a markedly spastic gait characterized by high steps and foot drop, ("Jake walk"). These signs of extrapyramidal involvement are more severe in children and are more slowly and less completely reversed than are peripheral nerve lesions.

9. Except in the elderly, those with preexisting heart disease or intercurrent infections, the prognosis is favorable and mortality is low. About three fourths of all cases recover to the point of not requiring further treatment after 1 to 2 years. Only 5% remain totally incapacitated.

Treatment:

1. In the absence of spontaneous vomiting, administer a slurry of activated charcoal (p. I-4), followed by gastric lavage (p. I-8).

2. Saline cathartics, *e.g.*, sodium or magnesium sulfate (15 to 30 gm.) in water.

3. Daily doses of vitamin B_1 (300 mg.), together with 1000 μg. vitamin B_{12} by intramuscular injection, over 45 days may have a protective effect on the nervous system, if begun early, but no effect on regeneration of peripheral motor neurons in controlled trials.

4. Corticosteroids with dosage adjusted and tapered in accord with individual tolerances over a 30-day period may hasten regeneration. See p. IV-100.

5. Pilocarpine (10 to 20 mg. daily in divided doses by subcutaneous injection) resulted in a surprising but temporary improvement in motor activity in some patients. The rationale for this treatment is unknown.

6. Aspirin or phenylbutazone for muscle pains.

7. Physiotherapy, occupational therapy, sports and orthopedic programs.

Laboratory: Not generally relevant. True and pseudocholinesterase may be markedly inhibited for 2 to 3 days but not during the later period of the progressive neuropathy.

References:

Ahmed, M. M. Synaptic morphology in the spinal cord of normal and tricresylphosphate (TCP) poisoned hen. Acta Neuropathol. *17*:302-309, 1971b.

Albertini, A. V.; Gross, D.; Zinn, W. M. *Triaryl-phosphate Poisoning in Morocco 1959.* Georg Thieme Verlag, Stuttgart, 1968.

Aldridge, W. N. Tricresyl phosphates and cholinesterase. Biochem. J. *56*:185-189, 1954.

Aldridge, W. N.; Barnes, J. M. Neurotoxic and biochemical properties of some triaryl phosphates. Biochem. Pharmacol. *6*:177-188, 1961.

Aldridge, W. N.; Barnes, J. M. Further observations on the neurotoxicity of organophosphorous compounds. Biochem. Pharmacol. *15*:541-548, 1966.

Aring, C. D. The systemic nervous affinity of triorthocresyl phosphate (Jamaica ginger palsy). Brain *65*:34-47, 1942.

Barnes, J. M.; Denz, F. A. Experimental demyelination with organo-phosphorus compounds. J. Pathol. Bacteriol. *65*:597-605, 1953.

Baron, R. L.; Casida, J. E. Enzymatic and antidotal studies on the neurotoxic effect of certain organophosphates. Biochem. Pharmacol. *11*:1129-1136, 1962.

Berry, J. F.; Cevallos, W. H. Lipid class and fatty acid composition of peripheral nerves from normal and organophosphorus-poisoned chickens. J. Neurochem. *13*:117-124, 1966.

Berry, J. F.; Cevallos, W. H.; Wade, R. R. Lipid class and fatty acid composition of an intact peripheral nerve and during Wallerian degeneration. J. Am. Oil Chem. Soc. *42*:492-500, 1965a.

Bidstrup, P. A.; Bonnell, J. A. Anticholinesterase - paralysis in man following poisoning by cholinesterase inhibitors. Chem. Ind. (London) *24*:674-676, 1954.

Bischoff, A. The ultrastructure of tri-ortho-cresyl phosphate poisoning 1. Studies on myelin and axonal alterations in the sciatic nerve. Acta Neuropathol. *9*:158-174, 1967.

Bischoff, A. The ultrastructure of tri-ortho-cresyl phosphate poisoning 2. Studies on the spinal cord. Acta Neuropathol. *15*:142-155, 1970.

Bleiberg, M. J.; Johnson, H. Effects of certain metabolically active drugs and oximes on tri-o-cresyl phosphate toxicity. Toxicol. Appl. Pharmacol. 7:227-235, 1965.

Burley, B. T. Polyneuritis from tricresyl phosphate. J. A. M. A. *98*:298-304, 1932.

Buttar, H. S.; Tyrrell, D. L.; Taylor, J. D. Effect of tri-o-cresyl phosphate, tri-o-cresyl thiophosphate and 2-(o-cresyl)-4*H*:1:3:2-benzodioxaphosphoran-2-one on pentobarbital induced sleeping time in mice. Arch. Int. Pharmacodyn. Ther. *172*:373-379, 1968.

Casida, J. E. Specificity of substituted phenyl phosphorus compounds for esterase inhibition in mice. Biochem. Pharmacol. *5*:332-342, 1961.

Casida, J. E.; Eto, M.; Baron, R. L. Biological activity of a tri-o-cresyl phosphate metabolite. Nature 191:1396-1397, 1961.

Cavanagh, J. B. The toxic effects of tri-ortho-cresyl phosphate on the nervous system: experimental study in hens. J. Neurol. Neurosurg. Psychiat. 17:163-172, 1954.

Cavanagh, J. B. Peripheral nerve changes in ortho-cresyl phosphate poisoning in the cat. J. Path. Bact. 87:365-383, 1964.

Cavanagh, J. B.; Holland, P. Localization of cholinesterases in the chicken nervous system and the problem of selective neurotoxicity of organophosphorous compounds. Br. J. Pharmacol. 16:218-230, 1961.

Cavanagh, J. B.; McDermot, V. Sensory terminal degeneration in ortho-cresyl phosphate poisoning. Lancet 2:583-584, 1961.

Cavanagh, J. B.; Patangia, G. N. Changes in the central nervous system in the cat as the result of tri-o-cresyl phosphate poisoning. Brain 38:165-180, 1965.

Chambers, H. W.; Casida, J. E. Protective activity of nicotinic acid derivatives and their 1-alkyl-2- and 1-alkyl-6-pyridones against selected neurotoxic agents. Toxicol. Appl. Pharmacol. 10:105-118, 1967.

Chaudhuri, R. N. Paralytic disease caused by consumption of flour contaminated with tricresyl phosphate. Tran. Roy. Soc. Trop. Med. Hyg. 59:98, 1965.

Cohen, S. D.; Murphy, S. D. Malathion potentiation and inhibition of hydrolysis of various carboxylic esters by TOTP in mice. Biochem. Pharmacol. 20:575-587, 1971.

Davies, D. R. Neurotoxicity of organophosphorous compounds. In Handbuch der Experimentellen Pharmakologie, edited by G. Koelle, Vol. XV, p. 860-882. Springer-Verlag, New York, 1963.

Davies, D. R. Effect of oximes and atropine on delayed neurotoxic effects of DFP and sarin on chicken. Biochem. Pharmacol. 21:3145-3151, 1972.

Davison, A. N. Some observations on the cholinesterases of the central nervous system after the administration of organophosphorous compounds. Br. J. Pharmacol. 8:212-216, 1953.

Davison, A. N. The conversion of schradan (OMPA) and parathion into inhibitors of cholinesterase by mammalian liver. Biochem. J. 61:203-209, 1955.

Earl, C. J.; Thompson, R. H. S. The inhibitory action of tri-ortho-cresyl phosphate on cholinesterases. Br. J. Pharmacol. 7:261-269, 1952.

Eto, M.; Casida, J. E.; Eto, T. Hydroxylation and cyclization reactions involved in the metabolism of tri-o-cresyl phosphate. Biochem. Pharmacol. 11:337-352, 1962.

Eto, M.; Oshima, Y.; Casida, J. E. Plasma albumin as a catalyst in cyclization of diaryl o-(α-hydroxy)-tolyl phosphates. Biochem. Pharmacol. 16:295-308, 1967.

Fenton, J. C. B. The nature of the paralysis in chickens following organophosphorous poisoning. J. Path. Bact. 69:181-189, 1955.

Gaines, T. B. Acute toxicity of pesticides. Toxicol. Appl. Pharmacol. 14:515-534, 1969.

Glees, P. Effect of cortisone on degenerating nerve fibers in birds. Nature 187:327, 1960.

Godfrey, C. M. An epidemic of triorthocresyl phosphate poisoning. Can. Med. Assoc. J. 85:689-691, 1961.

Gross, E.; Grosse, A. Ein Beitrag zur Toxikologie des Ortho-trikresylphosphates. Arch. Exp. Pathol. Pharmacol. 168:473-514, 1932.

Hine, C. H.; Dunlap, M. K.; Rice, E. G.; Coursey, M. M.; Gross, R. M.; Anderson, H. H. Neurotoxicity and anticholinesterase activities of some substituted phenyl phosphates. J. Pharmacol. Exp. Ther. 116:227-234, 1956.

Hodge, H. C.; Sterner, J. H. The skin absorption of triorthocresyl phosphate as shown by radioactive phosphorous. J. Pharmacol. Exp. Ther. 79:225-235, 1943.

Illis, L.; Patangia, G. N.; Cavanagh, J. B. Boutons terminaux and tri-ortho-cresyl phosphate neurotoxicity. Exp. Neurol. 14:160-174, 1966.

Joel, C. D.; Moser, H. W.; Majno, G.; Karnovsky, M. L. Effects of bis-(monoisopropylamino)-fluoro phosphine oxide (mipafox) and of starvation of the lipids in the nervous system of the hen. J. Neurochem. 14:479-488, 1967.

Johnson, H.; Weiss, L. R. Histochemical differentiation between concentration of free cholesterol and cholesterol ester for the assessment of pesticide-induced demyelination. Toxicol. Appl. Pharmacol. 7:486, 1965.

Johnson, M. K. A phosphorylation site in brain and the delayed neurotoxic effect of some organophosphorous compounds. Biochem. J. 111:487-495, 1969.

Johnson, M. K. Organophosphorous and other inhibitors of brain "neurotoxic esterase" and the development of delayed neurotoxicity in hens. Biochem. J. 120:523-531, 1970.

Johnson, M. K. The delayed neuropathy caused by some organophosphorous esters: Mechanism and challenge. C. R. C. Crit. Rev. Toxicol. 3:289-316, 1975.

Lynch, W. T.; Coon, J. M. Effects of TOTP pretreatment on the toxicity and metabolism of parathion and paraoxon in mice. Toxicol. Appl. Pharmacol. 21:153-165, 1972.

Majno, G.; Karnovsky, M. L. A biochemical and morphological study of myelination and demyelination-III. Effect of an organophosphorous compound (mipafox) on the biosynthesis of lipid by nervous tissue of rats and hens. J. Neurochem. 8:1-16, 1961.

McKay, D. H.; Jardine, R. V.; Adie, P. The synergistic action of 2-(o-cresyl)-4H-1,3,2-benzodioxaphosphorin-2-oxide with soman and physostigmine. Toxicol. Appl. Pharmacol. 20:474-479, 1971.

Morazain, R.; Rosenberg, P. Lipid changes in tri-o-cresyl phosphate induced neuropathy. Toxicol. Appl. Pharmacol. 16:461-474, 1970.

Murphy, S. D.; Anderson, R. L.; DuBois, K. P. Potentiation of toxicity of malathion by tri-ortho-tolyl phosphate. Proc. Soc. Exp. Biol. Med. 100:483-487, 1959.

Myers, D. K.; Rebel, J. B. J.; Veeger, C.; Kemp, A.; Simons, E. G. L. Metabolism of triarylphosphates in rodents. Nature 176:259-260, 1955.

O'Brien, R. D. Insecticides - Action and Metabolism. Academic Press, New York, 1967.

Prineas, J. Triorthocresyl phosphate myopathy. Arch. Neurol. 21:150-156, 1969.

Sharma, R. P.; Watanabe, P. G. Time related disposition of tri-o-tolylphosphate (TOTP) and metabolites in chicken. Pharm. Res. Comm. 6:475-484, 1974.

Sheltawy, A.; Dawson, R. M. C. The metabolism of polyphosphoinositides in hen brain and sciatic nerve. Biochem. J. 111:157-165, 1969.

Smith, M. I.; Elvove, E. Pharmacological and chemical studies of the course of so-called ginger paralysis. Public Health Repts. No. 45:1703-1716, 1930.

Smith, M. I.; Elvove, E.; Frazier, W. H. The pharmacological actions of certain phenol esters with specific reference to the etiology of so called ginger paralysis. Publ. Health Rep. (Wash.) 45:2509-2524, 1930.

Smith, M. I.; Lillie, R. D. The histopathology of tri-ortho-cresyl phosphate poisoning. Arch. Neurol. Psychiat. 26:976-992, 1931.

Smith, M. I.; Stohlman, E. F. A comparative study of three phosphoric esters of orthocresol. J. Pharmacol. Exp. Ther. 51:217-236, 1934.

Sorokin, M. Ortho cresyl phosphate neuropathy: Report of an outbreak in Fiji. Med. J. Aust. 1:506-508, 1969.

Taylor, J. D. The effect of tri-ortho-cresyl phosphate intoxication on phospholipid synthesis in cat spinal cord. Can. J. Physiol. Pharmacol. 43:715-721, 1965.

Taylor, J. D. A neurotoxic syndrome produced in cats by a cyclic phosphate metabolite of tri-o-cresyl phosphate. Toxicol. Appl. Pharmacol. 11:538-545, 1967.

Vora, D. D.; Dastur, D. K.; Braganca, B. Z.; Parihar, L. M.; Iyer, C. G. S.; Fondekar, R. B.; Prabhakaran, K. Toxic polyneuritis in Bombay due to orthocresyl phosphate poisoning. J. Neurol. Neurosurg. Psychiat. 25:234-242, 1962.

Watanabe, P. G.; Sharma, R. P. Persistence of tri-o-tolyl-phosphate (TOTP) and metabolites in chicken tissues as related to neurotoxicity. In Pesticides and the Environment, p. 503-512. Intercontinental Medical Book Corp., New York, 1973.

Watanabe, P. G.; Sharma, R. P. Lymphatic tissue response in chickens treated with tri-o-tolyl phosphate. J. Toxicol. Environ. Health *1*:777-786, 1976.

Webster, G. R. The distribution and metabolism of phosphorous in normal and demyelinating nervous tissue of the chicken. Biochem. J. *57*:153-158, 1954.

Witter, R. F.; Gaines, T. B. Relationship between depression of brain or plasma cholinesterase and paralysis in chickens caused by certain organic phosphorous compounds. Biochem. Pharmacol. *12*:1377-1386, 1963.

Zeligs, M. A. Upper motor neuron sequelae in "Jake" paralysis; a clinical followup study. J. Nerv. Mental Dis. *87*:464-470, 1938.

TURPENTINE

Turpentine, gum turpentine, oil of turpentine, and spirits of turpentine are essentially synonymous names. Turpentine is a common solvent found in many homes, workshops and barns, not infrequently in a container that was originally designed for a beverage. The ingredients of turpentines are the same regardless of source or method of preparation but wide variations in proportions are recognized. All consist principally of terpenes, the chief ones being α-pinene, β-pinene and Δ^3-carene (Mirov *et al.*, 1962; Smith, 1964b; Williams and Bannister, 1962). Turpentine is used in mixing oil-base paints and in removing paint stains. Medicinally it has been used externally as a "stupe," internally for "worms," and in various forms as an expectorant and abortifacient. It is a solvent for waxes and is found in various kinds of polish.

Toxicology: Turpentine is readily absorbed from the gastrointestinal tract, skin and respiratory tract (Chapman, 1941). Many accidental poisonings through ingestion have been reported and include several fatalities (Craig, 1953). As little as 15 ml. (½ oz.) has proved fatal to a child (Harbeson, 1936), but a few children have survived 2 and even 3 oz. (Jacobziner and Raybin, 1961g). The mean lethal dose in adults probably lies between 4 and 6 oz. (Grapel, 1901; Maitland, 1931; Stanwell, 1901). It has been claimed that oxidation products of turpentine produced by prolonged exposure to air are more toxic and more irritating (Pirilä *et al.*, 1964; Rundberg, 1937). The acute toxicity of turpentine is less than that of most volatile oils such as eucalyptus, sassafras, camphor and wintergreen (Craig, 1953).

Turpentine is a local irritant (Nelson *et al.*, 1943) and a central neural depressant. In addition to the usual signs and symptoms of gastroenteritis, coughing and choking often occur after ingestion (Jacobziner and Raybin, 1961g). Such distress does not establish conclusively that the solvent was aspirated into the tracheobronchial tree because it is probable that the respiratory tract can be irritated by the vapors of volatile constituents that are excreted by the lungs. Significant aspiration, however, can definitely occur, as shown by the aspiration-hazard test of Gerarde (see p. III-222). In patients aspiration may lead to pulmonary edema and pneumonitis with dyspnea, cyanosis and fever, but pulmonary pathology is not so common or severe as in kerosene poisoning (Beamon *et al.*, 1976; see also p. III-220).

One third of a series of 255 patients admitted with a history of "hydrocarbon" ingestion had consumed turpentine. In this series turpentine constituted the largest group, followed by furniture polish and then kerosene. About half of the patients were lavaged and about half were given ipecac. The ensuing pulmonary complications were more severe in the group that was lavaged (Ng *et al.*, 1974), but no evidence was presented to indicate whether the difference was significant in the turpentine subgroup.

Occasional findings of dysuria, hematuria (Monnet and Thomé, 1961), albuminuria and glycosuria may reflect the ability of turpentine to irritate the urinary bladder and kidneys, but these lesions appear to be transient and completely reversible; death is rarely if ever due to renal failure (but see Chapman, 1941). Although often encountered in the older literature (*e.g.*, Witthaus, 1911; Browning, 1965), a toxic nephritis is seldom seen today; in Jacobziner's series of 450 ingestion cases (1961), renal damage was not reported once. It has, however, occurred not only after ingestion but also after chronic skin contact with the liquid and prolonged respiratory exposure to high concentrations of the vapor (Chapman, 1941).

The usual vapor exposure during painting with oil-base paint containing turpentine appears to have no toxicological significance. There was no evidence of pulmonary lesions in rats and mice exposed to lethal concentrations of turpentine vapor. Instead, following an increase in respiratory rate with a decrease in tidal volume, animals convulsed and went into sudden apnea. The brain and spleen contained the highest concentrations of volatile constituents (Sperling *et al.*, 1967).

Keplinger (1962) reported that the composition of domestic turpentine changed considerably after the Naval Stores Act of 1923. Turpentine manufactured in the United States today is alleged to be more "pure," notably because of the removal of a constituent that was largely responsible for its former activity as a skin rubifacient and eczematogenic agent (Pirilä *et al.*, 1964; Thrysin, 1937). The latter is said to be a hydroperoxide of Δ^3-carene. Perhaps these modifications are also related to the apparent rarity of renal lesions in current poisonings. If so, foreign turpentine may not be so benign. The practice of mixing turpentine with methyl alcohol, benzene, formaldehyde, phenols, etc., is apparently obsolete (McCord, 1926a).

Chemical peritonitis has occurred on at least three occasions when turpentine was instilled into the uterus to effect abortion (Bingham and Cutler, 1936; Martini, 1957; Quander and Moseley, 1964). Pain was excruciating in all cases. Inflammatory and necrotic changes in pelvic organs were noted in one case (Bingham and Cutler, 1936), and passage of a 4 cm. fetus preceded the development of acute pulmonary edema in another (Quander and Moseley, 1964).

A useful review of the toxicology of turpentine in laboratory animals has been published by Sperling (1969). It includes data on blood and tissue levels and histological changes after vapor exposures, together with evidence that non-lethal exposures induce hepatic microsomal enzymes.

Symptomatology:

1. Burning pain in mouth and throat, abdominal pain, nausea, vomiting and occasionally diarrhea.
2. Mild respiratory tract symptoms are often noted: they include coughing, choking, dyspnea and even cyanosis. Aspiration and perhaps even systemic absorption of turpentine may lead to pulmonary edema and pneumonitis.
3. Transient excitement, ataxia, confusion and finally stupor, which is the commonest severe symptom. Convulsions occur occasionally, usually not until several hours after ingestion, when they may interrupt a deep coma.
4. Occasionally painful urination, albuminuria, hematuria. The urine may have an odor resembling that of violets (also in eucalyptol poisoning). The renal lesion is usually transient.
5. Odor of turpentine on breath and in vomitus.
6. Fever and tachycardia are common.
7. Death is usually due to respiratory failure.

Treatment:

1. Syrup of ipecac to induce vomiting if the patient is alert and if the ingested dose exceeded 1 ounce.
2. If the patient is drowsy or stuporous, cautious gastric lavage with tap water or weak sodium bicarbonate solution. If vomiting has not occurred, it is always worthwhile to empty the stomach because appreciable amounts of turpentine can be recovered many hours after ingestion. Use precautions such as a cuffed tube to prevent aspiration (p. III-222). It may be useful to give a few ounces of mineral oil at the conclusion of the lavage.
3. Saline catharsis with sodium or magnesium sulfate (15 to 30 gm.) in water.
4. If coma occurs, protect the airway with a cuffed endotracheal tube to relieve obstruction (p. IV-4) and to facilitate ventilatory assistance (p. IV-9).
5. Parenteral fluids to promote a mild diuresis.
6. Codeine for pain. Avoid morphine because of possible respiratory depression.
7. Stimulants (*e.g.*, doxapram) may be useful (see pp. IV-41–42).
8. Oxygen therapy, and other measures against pulmonary edema and pneumonitis (pp. IV-14–16), as indicated.

Laboratory: Glycosuria, hematuria and albuminuria may be demonstrated, but they rarely occur in modern poisonings.

References:

Beamon, R. F.; Siegel, C. J.; Landers, G.; Green, V. Hydrocarbon ingestion in children: a six-year retrospective study. J. Am. Coll. Emerg. Phys. *5*:771-775, 1976.

Bingham, E. M.; Cutler, O. I. Chemical peritonitis following intrauterine injection. Calif. Med. *44*:45-46, 1936.

Browning, E. *Toxicity and Metabolism of Industrial Solvents.* Elsevier Publishing Co., Amsterdam, 2nd ed, 1965.

Chapman, E. M. Observations of the effect of paint on the kidneys with particular reference to the role of turpentine. J. Ind. Hyg. Toxicol. *23*:277-289, 1941.

Craig, J. O. Poisoning by the volatile oils in childhood. Arch. Dis. Child. *28*:475-483, 1953.

Grapel, F. G. Turpentine poisoning. Br. Med. J. *1*:340, 1901.

Harbeson, A. E. A case of turpentine poisoning. Can. Med. Assoc. J. *35*:549-550, 1936.

Jacobziner, H.; Raybin, H. W. Turpentine poisoning. Arch. Pediatr. *78*:357-364, 1961g.

Keplinger, M. L. Personal communication. Hercules Powder Company, Wilmington, Del, April, 1962.

Maitland, F. B. Toxicity and fatal dose of turpentine. Br. Med. J. *2*:77, 1931.

Martini, A. P. Peritonitis following intrauterine injection of turpentine. Obstet. Gynecol. *9*:523, 1957.

McCord, C. P. Occupational dermatitis from wood turpentine. J. A. M. A. *86*:1979, 1926a.

Mirov, N. T.; Zavarin, E.; Bicho, J. G. Composition of gum turpentine of pines, *Pinus nelsonii* and *Pinus occidentalis.* J. Pharm. Sci. *51*:1131-1135, 1962.

Monnet, P.; Thome, J. Intoxication aigue par l'essence de terebenthine chez un enfant de 23 mois. Pediatrie *16*:270-273, 1961.

Nelson, K. W.; Ege, J. F., Jr.; Ross, M.; Woodman, L. E.; Silverman, L. Sensory response to certain industrial solvent vapors. J. Ind. Hyg. Toxicol. *25*:282-285, 1943.

Ng, R. C.; Darwish, H.; Stewart, D. A. Emergency treatment of petroleum distillate and turpentine ingestion. CMA J. *111*:537-538, 1974.

Pirila, V.; Siltanen, E.; Pirila, L. On the chemical nature of the eczematogenic agent in oil of turpentine. Dermatologica *128*:16-21, 1964.

Quander, M. F.; Moseley, J. E. Abortion, chemical peritonitis and pulmonary edema following intrauterine injection of turpentine. Obstet. Gynecol. *24*:572-574, 1964.

Rundberg, G. Turpentine eczema in Swedish painters. An occupational hygiene investigation. Hygiea *99*:209-249, 1937.

Smith, R. H. Variation in the monoterpenes of *Pinus ponderosa* Laws. Science *143*:1337-1338, 1964b.

Sperling, F. In vivo and in vitro toxicology of turpentine. Clin. Toxicol. *2*:21-35, 1969.

Sperling, F.; Marcus, W. L.; Collins, C. Acute effects of turpentine vapor on rats and mice. Toxicol. Appl. Pharmacol. *10*:8-20, 1967.

Stanwell, F. S. Turpentine poisoning. Br. Med. J. *1*:640-641, 1901.

Thrysin, E. Turpentine eczema in Swedish painters. Hygiea *99*:268-287, 1937.

Williams, A. L.; Bannister, M. H. Composition of gum turpentines from twenty-two species of pines grown in New Zealand. J. Pharm. Sci. *51*:970-975, 1962.

Witthaus, R. A. *Manual of Toxicology*. Wm. Wood & Co., New York, 1911.

WARFARIN

Warfarin, 3-(α-acetonylbenzyl)-4-hydroxycoumarin, is an effective rodenticide available commercially as a powdered concentrate with 0.5% active material. Finished baits commonly contain 0.025% active material (Hayes, 1963). Warfarin was developed at the University of Wisconsin as an outgrowth of studies on hydroxycoumarin derivatives in relation to hemorrhagic disease in cattle (Krieger, 1952).

Warfarin is practically insoluble in water but it dissolves freely in alkaline solutions because it forms a sodium salt. Warfarin sodium USP (*e.g.*, Coumadin) is widely used in clinical medicine as a therapeutic anticoagulant.

Several other hydroxycoumarin derivatives are also marketed as rodenticides. Various acyl and aryl indandiones also kill rodents (and other mammals) by similar mechanisms. Collectively these two classes of compounds are sometimes called anticoagulant rodenticides. Bentley (1972) summarized information about the worldwide uses of these materials in pest control. Additional comments about several of the individual compounds can be found in Section II.

Toxicology: Warfarin is completely absorbed from the alimentary tract (O'Reilly *et al.*, 1963), and apparently also through the skin. At least severe intoxications have resulted from repeated skin contact (Green, 1955; Fristedt and Sterner, 1965). Warfarin is extensively metabolized in both man and animals, but unique and perhaps active metabolites occur in man (Lewis and Trager, 1970).

Warfarin acts upon the liver specifically to inhibit prothrombin formation. In toxic doses it is also injurious to blood vessels, as evidenced by widespread dilatation and engorgement and by an increase in capillary fragility. Both hypoprothrombinemia and vascular injury predispose to fatal internal hemorrhage, which is the basis of its effectiveness as a rodenticide and of its potential toxicity to man (Hayes and Gaines, 1950; Hayes, 1963; Heisey *et al.*, 1956). The stress induced by mild to moderate warfarin poisoning has been suggested as one of the possible causes of Reye's syndrome (Mogilner *et al.*, 1974).

The inhibition of prothrombin formation does not become apparent until the body's prothrombin reserves are consumed. Multiple doses are usually required to maintain the inhibition of synthesis until these reservoirs are depleted. If sufficiently large, a single dose may prove effective after a latency of several days (Wisconsin Alumni Research Foundation, 1951; Back *et al.*, 1978), but in 29 single ingestion episodes reported to the Boston Poison Center no signs of hemorrhage or even depression of plasma prothrombin occurred (Brewer and Haggerty, 1957). The same was true of 100 cases followed by the Poisons Service of Guy's Hospital in London (Goulding, 1968).

The acute oral single-dose LD_{50} of warfarin sodium in male rats is 100 mg./kg. and in female rats 9 mg./kg., with the highest mortality rates between the 4th and 10th post-treatment days (Back *et al.*, 1978). This 10-fold sex difference in sensitivity is not observed in humans. An increased sensitivity in protein-deficient rats, however, may extend to man (Colvin and Wang, 1974).

For an intake of 100 mg./kg., the average adult man would have to eat 3 lb. of a warfarin concentrate (0.5%) or about 60 lb. of a strong rat bait (0.025%). In contrast, the daily ingestion for 6 days of as little as 1 to 2 mg./kg. (corresponding to about 1 lb. of 0.025% bait per day) has produced a near fatal illness in an adult person (Holmes and Love, 1952). A Korean family of 14 persons lived for a period of 15 days on a diet of warfarinized cornmeal with an estimated individual intake of warfarin which varied between 1 and 2 mg./kg. each day; all of these persons became severely ill with hemorrhages and 2 died (Lange and Terveer, 1954).

Other instances of repeated challenge in humans (including some examples of criminal poisonings) led to a similar syndrome (Ikkala *et al.*, 1964; Nilsson, 1957; Pribilla, 1966). Warfarin and the closely related bishydroxycoumarin have produced virtually identical effects whether after iatrogenic overdoses or after self administration by malingerers (Cosgriff, 1953; O'Reilly *et al.*, 1962; Rosenbloom and Crane, 1946; Schlevin and Lederer, 1944; Stafne and Moe, 1951). Perhaps some of these instances of factitious hemorrhagic disease were the result of psychotic illnesses (Eldore *et al.*, 1979; Gelfand and Mitani, 1979). The intentional poisoning of two siblings by their mother using various drugs, including warfarin, was felt to be a bizarre form of child abuse (Hvizdala and Gellady, 1978).

In its effect on the blood coagulation mechanism, warfarin is among the more potent of the hydroxycoumarin derivatives (Ingram, 1961). Vascular lesions may also be more prominent with warfarin than with its congeners. A single large dose produces no untoward signs or symptoms until clinical evidence of hemorrhage, which is usually apparent on the second, third, or fourth day, but a significant change in the blood prothrombin level can be detected within 24 hours. After a single intravenous injection of the sodium salt (about 1 mg./kg.), the maximal response in man is usually reached in 48 hours, and recovery is essentially complete by the fifth day. The fairly long plasma half-life (7 days in one would-be suicide) is due at least in part to intensive enterohepatic recycling (Jähnchen and Meinertz, 1977).

Except for potency, warfarin does not differ markedly from other inhibitors of prothrombin such as bishydroxycoumarin (Dicumarol), ethylbiscoumacetate (Tromexan), acenocoumarol (Sintrom), coumachlor, cyclocoumarol, phenprocoumon, and nicoumalone. All of these suppress the hepatic formation of prothrombin and of factors VII, IX and X to produce the clotting defect. Vitamin K specifically antagonizes these deficiencies; large and repeated doses are necessary for effective treatment (Ingram, 1961). The same is true in poisonings by indandiones (see below), but these compounds possess additional pharmacological actions.

Indandiones: In contrast to the hydroxycoumarins, experiments have not so clearly established the mechanism of death after various 2-acyl-1,3-indandiones, which are also used as rodenticides and sometimes as insecticides. Phenindione, diphenadione and anisindione are examples of therapeutically useful drugs of this type. Multiple-dose toxicity in animals clearly involves the same hemorrhagic phenomena as with the hydroxycoumarins (Saunders et al., 1955).

Massive single oral doses, however, killed rats and rabbits within 2 to 12 hours (Kabat et al., 1944). In these acute exposures hemorrhages were not usually found on postmortem examination, and prothrombin levels were not invariably depressed. Animals receiving these single lethal doses of substituted indandiones (100 to 200 mg./kg.) exhibited labored breathing, progressive muscular weakness, hyperexcitability, pulmonary congestion, venous engorgement, and cardiac standstill in systole (Kabat et al., 1944). It is not established that vitamin K protects against this syndrome. Again in contrast to hydroxycoumarins, clinical side effects of indandiones include agranulocytosis, pyrexia, diarrhea, hepatitis, renal tubular necrosis, exfoliative dermatitis and paralysis of accommodation (Ingram, 1961).

A rare and occasionally lethal complication of therapeutic doses of hydroxycoumarin and indandione congeners involves multiple skin lesions characterized by petechia, ecchymoses and hemorrhagic infarcts with necrosis. The mechanism of this reaction is not well understood (Adams and Pass, 1960; Nalbandian et al., 1965). Another complication arises because warfarin (and perhaps other anticoagulants of this group)

is strongly bound to plasma proteins but can be displaced by phenylbutazone or oxyphenbutazone administered concomitantly, to produce a hemorrhagic diathesis during normal warfarin maintenance therapy (Aggeler et al., 1967).

Symptomatology (onset after a few days or few weeks of repeated ingestion):
1. Epistaxis and bleeding gums.
2. Pallor and sometimes petechial rash.
3. Massive ecchymoses and/or hematomata, especially of the elbows, knees and buttocks.
4. Blood in urine and feces.
5. Occasionally paralysis due to cerebral hemorrhage.
6. Hemorrhagic shock and death.

Treatment:
1. Empty the stomach with syrup of ipecac (p. I-2) and/or perform gastric lavage with tap water (p. I-4), if possible within a few hours after ingestion of a single large dose.
2. Vitamin K is a specific antidote. Vitamin K_1 emulsion is the preferred form. The initial subcutaneous or intramuscular dose in adults is 5 to 10 mg. (up to 25 mg.), repeated once if necessary. Only in victims who are bleeding severely or otherwise in serious distress should the drug be given intravenously and then at a rate no faster than 1 mg./min. If necessary on subsequent days, vitamin K_1 should be continued at a reduced level until the prothrombin time returns to normal. Vitamin K_1 is preferable to K_1 oxide (dose 0.5 to 2.5 mg.) and certainly preferable to menadione or menadione sodium bisulfite. Caution: large doses of vitamin K in the premature or neonatal infant have produced hemolytic anemia, Heinz body formation, jaundice and kernicterus. These reactions have followed doses in excess of 15 mg./kg. (Nyhan, 1961).
3. Small transfusions of carefully matched whole blood may be necessary as a temporary source of prothrombin and of red blood cells. Fresh blood is preferable to stored blood to supply accessory coagulation factors.
4. Cholestyramine 4 gm. three times daily for 10 days can decrease plasma half-life by preventing enterohepatic recycling (Jähnchen and Meinertz, 1977; Meinertz et al., 1977).
5. Vitamin C is no substitute for Vitamin K, but ascorbic acid may be a useful adjunct to K therapy, as judged by animal studies. At least a dose of 100 mg. of ascorbic acid several times a day can do no harm.
6. After the control of hemorrhage and repair of the coagulation defect, replacement iron therapy is desirable to correct any second-

ary anemia. Ferrous sulfate at a dose of 0.3 gm. t.i.d. is recommended.

7. In some cases accessible hematomas should be aspirated after the clotting power of the blood is restored to normal.

Laboratory:

1. The principal diagnostic test is a demonstration of markedly reduced prothrombin activity in blood plasma, as measured by the method of Quick or one of its modifications. The test should be repeated at least twice daily until a normal prothrombin time is established.

2. The blood clotting time and the bleeding time may be prolonged, but these values are not necessarily abnormal.

3. Blood is often demonstrable in urine and feces.

4. Secondary anemia (hypochromic, microcytic) may be marked.

References:

Adams, C. W.; Pass, B. J. Extensive dermatitis due to warfarin sodium (Coumadin). Circulation 22:947-948, 1960.

Aggeler, P. M.; O'Reilly, R. A.; Leong, L.; Kowitz, P. E. Potentiation of anticoagulant effect of warfarin by phenylbutazone. N. Engl. J. Med. 276:496-501, 1967.

Back, N.; Steger, R.; Glassman, J. M. Comparative acute oral toxicity of sodium warfarin and microcrystalline warfarin in the Sprague-Dawley rat. Pharmacol. Res. Commun. 10:445-452, 1978.

Bentley, E. W. A review of anticoagulant rodenticides in current use. Bull. W. H. O. 47:275-280, 1972.

Brewer, E.; Haggerty, R. J. Rat poisons. I. Warfarin. N. Engl. J. Med. 267:145-146, 1957.

Colvin, H. W.; Wang, W. L. Toxic effects of warfarin in rats fed different diets. Toxicol. Appl. Pharmacol. 28:337-348, 1974.

Cosgriff, S. W. Hemorrhage due to self-medication with bishydroxycoumarin. J. A. M. A. 153:547-548, 1953.

Eldore, A.; Zylber-Katz, E.; De-Nour, A. K. Single case study. Anticoagulant abuse: a psychotic syndrome? J. Nerv. Ment. Dis. 167:442-446, 1979.

Fristedt, B.; Sterner, N. Warfarin intoxication from percutaneous absorption. Arch. Environ. Health 11:205-208, 1965.

Gelfand, R.; Mitani, G. Single case study. Surreptitious use of warfarin. J. Nerv. Ment. Dis. 167:447-449, 1979.

Goulding, R. Toxicological case records. Practitioner 200:319-320, 1968.

Green, P. Haemorrhagic diathesis attributed to warfarin poisoning. Can. Med. Assoc. J. 72:769-770, 1955.

Hayes, W. J., Jr. Clinical Handbook on Economic Poisons. USPHS Publication No. 476. U. S. Government Printing Office, Washington, D. C., 1963.

Hayes, W. J., Jr.; Gaines, T. B. Control of Norway rats with residual rodenticide warfarin. Public Health Rep. 65:1537-1555, 1950.

Heisey, S. R.; Saunders, J. P.; Olson, K. C. Some anticoagulant properties of 2-acyl-1, 3-indandiones and warfarin in rabbits. J. Agric. Food Chem. 4:144-147, 1956.

Holmes, R. W.; Love, J. Suicide attempt with warfarin, a bishydroxycoumarin-like rodenticide. J. A. M. A. 148:935-937, 1952.

Hvizdala, E. V.; Gellady, A. M. Intentional poisoning of two siblings by prescription drugs. Clin. Pediatr. 17:480-482, 1978.

Ikkala, E.; Myllyla, G.; Nevanlinna, H. R.; Pelkonen, R.; Pyorala, K. Haemorrhagic diathesis due to criminal poisoning with warfarin. Acta Med. Scand. 176:201-203, 1964.

Ingram, G. I. C. Anticoagulant therapy. Pharmacol. Rev. 13:279-328, 1961.

Jahnchen, E.; Meinertz, T. Pharmakokinetische Aspekte der Uberdosierung und Intoxikation mit oralen Antikoagulantien. Arzneimittel-Forschung 27:1849-1856, 1977.

Kabat, H.; Stohlman, E. F.; Smith, M. I. Hypoprothrombinemia induced by administration of indandione derivatives. J. Pharmacol. Exp. Ther. 80:160-170, 1944.

Krieger, C. H. From arsenic to warfarin - the story of rodenticides. J. Agric. Food Chem. 7:46-50, 1952.

Lange, P. F.; Terveer, J. Warfarin poisoning. Report of fourteen cases. U. S. Armed Forces Med. J. 5:872-877, 1954.

Lewis, R. J.; Trager, W. F. Warfarin metabolism in man; identification of metabolites in urine. J. Clin. Invest. 49:907-913, 1970.

Meinertz, T.; Gilfrich, H. J.; Bork, R.; Jahnchen, E. Treatment of phenprocoumon intoxication with cholestyramine. Brit. Med. J. 2:439-440, 1977.

Mogilner, B. M.; Freeman, J. S.; Blashar, Y.; Pincus, F. E. Reye's syndrome in three Israeli children. Possible relationship to warfarin toxicity. Isr. J. Med. Sci. 10:1117-1125, 1974.

Nalbandian, R. M.; Mader, I. J.; Barrett, J. L.; Pearce, J. F.; Rupp, E. C. Petechia, ecchymoses and necrosis of skin induced by coumarin congeners. J. A. M. A. 192:603-608, 1965.

Nilsson, I. M. Recurrent hypothrombinaemia due to poisoning with a dicumarol-containing rat-killer. Acta Haematol. 17:176-182, 1957.

Nyhan, W. L. Toxicity of drugs in the neonatal period. J. Pediatr. 59:1-20, 1961.

O'Reilly, R. A.; Aggeler, P. M.; Gibbs, J. O. Hemorrhagic state due to surreptitious ingestion of bishydroxycoumarin. N. Engl. J. Med. 267:19-24, 1962.

O'Reilly, R. A.; Aggeler, P. M.; Leong, L. S. Studies on the coumarin anticoagulant drugs: The pharmacodynamics of warfarin in man. J. Clin. Invest. 42:1542-1551, 1963.

Pribilla, O. Mord durch Warfarin. Arch. Toxikol. 21:235-249, 1966.

Rosenbloom, D.; Crane, J. J. Massive hematuria due to dicumarol overdosage. J. A. M. A. 132:924-925, 1946.

Saunders, J. P.; Heisey, S. R.; Goldstone, A. D.; Bay, E. C. Comparative toxicities of warfarin and some 2-acyl-1, 3-indandiones in rats. J. Agric. Food Chem. 3:762-765, 1955.

Schlevin, E. L.; Lederer, M. Uncontrollable hemorrhage after dicumarol therapy with autopsy findings. Ann. Intern. Med. 21:332-342, 1944.

Stafne, W. A.; Moe, A. E. Hypoprothrombinemia due to dicumarol in a malingerer; a case report. Ann. Intern. Med. 35:910-911, 1951.

Wisconsin Alumni Research Foundation. Warfarin - re Toxicity. Brochure. Madison, Wisc, Nov., 1951.

XYLENE

Xylene (in three isomeric forms) is taken here as prototypical of aromatic hydrocarbon solvents such as toluene, ethyl benzene, cumene, mesitylene and other simple alkyl-substituted benzenes. In the following discussion, comments are made about many of the individual agents and about benzene, but see also Section II. In commerce the alkyl benzenes are often found as contaminants of one another, but since the late 1950s commercial toluene and xylene have been virtually benzene-free (Browning, 1965). For example, a product known as "mixed xylenes"

(Carpenter *et al.*, 1975) contains 65% *m*-xylene, 19% ethylbenzene, 8% each of *o*- and *p*-xylene, 0.1% toluene but no benzene. Because of its unique toxic potential (see below), benzene has been banned as an ingredient in products intended for use in the home. It is, however, present in gasoline in concentrations up to 2% in the United States and up to 16% in some European countries (McDermott and Vos, 1979; Young *et al.*, 1978).

Xylenes, toluene and the other alkyl benzenes, as well as benzene itself, are widely used in industry. Except for benzene, they are found around the home as vehicles in paints, in paint removers, in degreasing cleaners, lacquers, glues and cements and as solvent/vehicles for insecticides and other pesticides. For many years the principal commercial source of aromatic hydrocarbons was the destructive distillation of bituminous coal, but for the past several decades petroleum has been a major source (Gerarde, 1960).

Toxicology: Benzene, toluene and the various xylenes are toxic by all portals of entry, but percutaneous absorption is generally too slow to produce signs of acute systemic poisoning (Wolf *et al.*, 1956). Instead, skin contact often results in a characteristic dermatitis attributed to removal of the protective fat of the skin (von Oettingen, 1940; Wolf *et al.*, 1956). As judged primarily in laboratory animals, essentially the same train of signs follows the acute administration of any one of these compounds, as well as other simple alkyl-substituted benzenes (see also Section II). Moreover, the acute toxic syndrome is essentially the same whether the compounds are given by injection, by gavage or by inhalation. However, exposure to vapors carries with it prominent laryngeal and bronchial irritation, and severe pulmonary edema is a common but not invariant finding in fatally poisoned humans (Carter, 1928; Gerarde, 1960; Morley *et al.*, 1970; Winek *et al.*, 1967).

When given by mouth to adult rats, xylene (mixed isomers but more than 50% *meta-*) was the most toxic, followed by benzene and then toluene. The respective LD$_{50}$ values were 4.9, 6.0 and 7.7 ml./kg. (the specific gravity for each was about 0.87). Thus, these materials appear to lie near the borderline between toxicity classes 2 and 3 (Kimura *et al.*, 1971; Wolf *et al.*, 1956).

There is a widespread impression in the clinical literature, however, that humans are much more susceptible than are rodents to the acute toxicity of aromatic hydrocarbons by mouth. Adult lethal doses in the range of 15 ml. are frequently mentioned. Sollmann (1957) refers to two nineteenth century cases in which the ingestion of 9 to 12 ml. benzene is said to have caused serious collapse. Gerarde (1960) notes, however, that capsules containing up to 4 or 5 gm. of benzene have been administered daily, together with olive oil, to victims of chronic myelogenous leukemia; the only effects ascribed to this treatment were headache, vertigo, gastrointestinal distress, impotence and renal dysfunction. If xylene and toluene are as acutely toxic as benzene in man, 15 to 30 ml. is a reasonable estimate of the human lethal dose by mouth (toxicity class 4).

The ingestion of any of these solvents, however, must be a rare event. Aside from episodes involving highly toxic solutes, no well documented human cases have come to our attention. Gerarde (1960) mentioned a single episode in which the ingestion of 1 tablespoonful of benzene (12 to 15 ml.) caused collapse, bronchitis and pneumonia. An acute hemorrhagic pneumonitis is highly likely if any of these aromatic solvents is aspirated into the lungs (Gerarde, 1960). As in kerosene poisoning (p. III-220), it is possible that aspiration poses a greater threat to life than does gastrointestinal absorption, but resolution of this issue required more data. Almost all serious and fatal poisonings in man to date have been the result of respiratory exposures to high vapor concentrations (Hamilton, 1931; Longley *et al.*, 1967; Morley *et al.*, 1970).

In acute exposures all of these aromatic hydrocarbons produce basically similar toxic reactions, consisting primarily of local irritation and central nervous excitation and depression. The signs and symptoms resemble those of ethyl alcohol inebriation with euphoria and all stages of central nervous depression up to anesthesia and respiratory arrest (Longley *et al.*, 1967). Vapor concentrations of toluene of 10,000 to 30,000 ppm may produce anesthesia in less than one minute. If such levels are achieved gradually, the victim may be unaware of the danger.

The usual signs of central nervous depression, such as emotional lability, impaired motor coordination, slurred speech, ataxia, nystagmus, stupor and coma, may be punctuated by episodes of neuroirritability, for which the physiologic basis is not well understood. Unlike the aliphatic petroleum hydrocarbons, where deep coma is associated with depressed reflexes (see KEROSENE, p. III-221), aromatic hydrocarbons induce states of unconsciousness which are accompanied by tremors, motor restlessness, hypertonus, jactitations and generally hyperactive reflexes (Carpenter *et al.*, 1975; Cohen *et al.*, 1978; von Oettingen, 1940). In animals areflexia does not occur until near-fatal doses are reached. Perhaps benzene is a more prominent neuroirritant than xylene or toluene.

Death is usually due to respiratory arrest and consequent asphyxia (Svirbely *et al.*, 1943; von Oettingen, 1940). Occasionally, however, sudden death has been reported in vapor exposures under circumstances which impute the heart as the critical organ. Animal experiments show that benzene sensitizes the myocardium to epinephrine, so that even the endogenous hormone may precipitate sudden and fatal ventricular fibrillation (Nahum and Hoff, 1934).

Coma has lasted as long as 15 hours after a 19-hour exposure to toluene vapor (Morley et al., 1970), and muscular weakness has persisted for more than a week after benzene intoxication. In animal tests a xylene coma has the longest duration and a benzene coma the shortest. If death does not supervene, however, complete recovery is the general rule. Only mild and temporary impairments have been noted in liver and kidney function (Hamilton, 1931; Longley et al., 1967; Morley et al., 1970).

Despite rather minor differences in acute single-dose toxicity, major distinctions exist among the members of this group with respect to the effects of chronic or repeated exposures. At least in part these differences appear to have their basis in the metabolic pathways by which these solvents are handled in vivo.

Xylene: Human volunteers exposed repeatedly to m-xylene vapor retained about 60% of the inhaled material in the lung. The estimated daily uptake was recovered almost quantitatively as m-methylhippuric acid in the urine (Riihimaki et al., 1979). Similarly, humans excrete p-methylhippuric acid after exposure to p-xylene (Ogata et al., 1970). In rats, however, p-xylene is partly converted to p-tolualdehyde in the liver. The latter is in turn transported to the lung where it inactivates pulmonary microsomal enzymes (Patel et al., 1978).

In the blood m-xylene is largely bound to plasma proteins. Unchanged xylene is excreted chiefly via the lungs, but it amounts to less than 5% of the absorbed dose. Elimination in expired air and in urine (as methylhippuric acid) follows a two-phase pattern in man, with an initial half-life of about 1 hour and a slow phase with a half-life of about one day. The data suggest accumulation of xylene in adipose tissue with repeated exposures (Riihimaki et al., 1979). Exercise promotes redistribution into subcutaneous fat (Engstroem and Riihimaki, 1979).

Exposure of human subjects to 90 ppm m-xylene produces acute effects on reaction time, manual coordination, body balance and the EEG. Although tolerance to these effects developed over one work week, it was largely lost over the weekend (Savolainen et al., 1980). Concomitant ingestion of ethyl alcohol potentiated the deleterious behavioral effects of xylene in animals (Savolainen et al., 1978). Alcohol also potentiated the weak hepatic microsomal enzyme-inducing effects of xylene, and the combination produced liver damage at doses of xylene which were not effective alone (Elovaara et al., 1980). None of the three isomers of xylene appears to be teratogenic (Ungvary et al., 1980).

Toluene: Side-chain oxidation to carboxylic acids is the preferred route for metabolism of mono-n-alkyl derivatives of benzene, but the introduction of phenolic hydroxyl groups is an alternative route (Gerarde and Ahlstrom, 1966b). The extent of ring hydroxylation increases with increasing dose and with increasing length of the alkyl side-chain. The phenolic hydroxyls tend to be conjugated with sulfate, whereas the carboxylic acids tend to be conjugated with glycine. Thus toluene in man is metabolized via benzyl alcohol to benzoic acid and is excreted largely as hippuric acid. The latter can be used as an index of toluene exposure (Pagnotto and Lieberman, 1967; Wilczok and Bieniek, 1978; von Oettingen et al., 1942). However, hippurate is a normal constituent of human urine whereas o-cresol, a minor metabolite of toluene, is not. The urinary output of o-cresol has been shown to be linearly related to toluene exposure (Angerer, 1979; Pfaffli et al., 1979). As with xylene, toluene tends to concentrate in fat and to be eliminated from such depots slowly (Pyykko et al., 1977).

The industrial experience with toluene has been generally good. Hepatomegaly, lymphocytosis and minor deviations in red cell volume and corpuscular hemoglobin concentration have been associated with exposure (Greenburg et al., 1942) but not chromosome aberrations (Maki-Paakkanen et al., 1980).

The euphoric and central depressant effects of toluene and other aromatics are sought out habitually by some individuals (Grabski, 1961; Satran and Dodson, 1963) and apparently are responsible for the widespread practice of inhaling glues, paint thinners, fingernail polish removers, cleaning fluids, etc. among antisocial children, teenagers and adults (Glaser, 1966; Press and Done, 1967). Similar habituations are recognized to aliphatic hydrocarbon mixtures (see also KEROSENE, p. III-221). It is common practice to empty tubes of "airplane cement" or even pure solvents into large plastic bags that can be placed over the head of the "sniffer." Circumstances surrounding several deaths suggested that narcosis was followed by asphyxiation in the plastic bag (Collom and Winek, 1970; Winek and Collom, 1971). Cardiac deaths, however, cannot be ruled out. The known propensity of aromatic hydrocarbons to sensitize the myocardium to circulating epinephrine (see above) may potentiate the effects of the "diving reflex" in which irritant vapors trigger apnea, bradycardia, vasomotor changes and perhaps cardiac arrhythmias (Allison, 1978).

Since the prohibition of benzene as a solvent in household glues, one potential serious adverse reaction (see below) has been circumvented. In glues where hexane is present, with or without toluene, a polyneuropathy may occur in habitual sniffers (see Hexane in Section II). Otherwise, gross pathophysiologic changes in solvent abusers are surprisingly rare (Hayden et al., 1976;

Massengale *et al.*, 1963). Occasionally "sniffers" are reported to have an abnormal incidence of vague neurologic signs, hepatomegaly, mild impairment of renal function, hemorrhagic diathesis, eosinophilia and acute elevations of intracranial pressure (O'Brien *et al.*, 1971; Press and Done, 1967). Some sniffers complain of gastrointestinal disorders, including nausea, vomiting, abdominal pain and hematemesis (Streicher *et al.*, 1981). After many years of solvent abuse a few individuals have developed persistent and even permanent cerebellar dysfunctions. Peripheral nerves are largely spared, and the encephalopathy can be induced by pure toluene as well as glues and other mixtures (Boor and Hurtig, 1977; Knox and Nelson, 1966; Malm and Lying-Tunell, 1980).

A potentially more serious and life-threatening reaction to repeated toluene abuse is hypokalemic muscle paralysis, presumably secondary to renal tubular acidosis (Bennett and Forman, 1980; Kroeger *et al.*, 1980; Taher *et al.*, 1974). It appears likely that toluene or a toxic metabolite produces a type I renal distal tubular defect which may be accompanied by systemic acidosis and an inappropriately high urine pH (Taher *et al.*, 1974). Another cause of systemic acidosis is the metabolism of toluene and other alkyl benzenes to organic acids, as evidenced by a so-called "anion gap" in blood plasma. In toluene abusers, the anion gap, which may be as high as 39 mEq./L., has been ascribed to the accumulation of benzoate and/or hippurate (Fischman and Oster, 1979). Both organic acid acidosis and renal tubular acidosis contribute to potassium wasting. In the acute situation, where only 3 to 5 days of toluene abuse occurred, the renal tubular defect was probably more critical in generating potassium loss (Taher *et al.*, 1974). Some of these patients presented with obviously impaired renal function, but others without azotemia had a high anion gap metabolic acidosis, hypophosphatemia and hypokalemia. Rarely the tubular injury leads to severe azotemia and hyperkalemia (Russ *et al.*, 1981). Perhaps the renal lesion impairs the tubular acid secretory mechanism, which would ordinarily clear these metabolites of toluene at very rapid rates. Whether or not recurrent calculi are an associated problem (Kroeger *et al.*, 1980) is not clear.

Benzene: Among the aromatic solvents benzene is unique because its oxidative metabolism involves obligatory ring hydroxylation. This fact is thought to play a critical role in the bone marrow injury that follows exposure to benzene. It is now believed that older reports ascribing myelotoxic effects to toluene, xylene and even aliphatic hydrocarbon solvents are best ascribed to benzene contamination of those materials (Hough *et al.*, 1944).

The first step in benzene metabolism is probably oxidation to an arene oxide by hepatic microsomal enzyme systems (cytochrome P450, mixed function oxidase). Benzene oxide may undergo nonenzymatic isomerization to form a phenol, or it may be hydrated by epoxide hydrase to a catechol. Arene oxide glutathione transferase may lead to conjugation, or the oxide may escape this detoxication by reacting with essential cellular nucleophiles to produce damage or death of the cell (Jerina and Daly, 1974). Covalent binding of unidentified metabolite(s) has been demonstrated in liver, kidney and bone marrow after single and repeated doses in mice (Longacre *et al.*, 1981). Benzene, however, produces only minimal liver and kidney toxicity (Wirtschafter and Cronyn, 1964), in contrast to the intense damage from CARBON TETRACHLORIDE (p. III-101) or ACETAMINOPHEN (p. III-2).

A large fraction of the phenol is converted in rats to phenyl sulfate or phenyl glucuronide (Gerarde and Ahlstrom, 1966b; Snyder *et al.*, 1967a), but as the dose of benzene was increased, more free phenol was excreted in the urine. The activity of the sulfating enzyme systems was high in adult male rats relative to that in young female rats. These sex and age differences correlate with the leukopenic action of benzene and suggest that sulfation is a detoxication reaction (Ikeda *et al.*, 1961; Ikeda, 1964).

It has been stated that measures which inhibit benzene metabolism protect animals against the bone marrow toxicity (Kocsis and Snyder, 1975), but conflicting observations have appeared in the literature. For example, partial hepatectomy reduced both benzene metabolism and the ability of benzene to block iron uptake into red blood cells (Sammett *et al.*, 1979). At least two groups, however, have reported that phenobarbital induction of hepatic microsomal enzymes increased benzene metabolism but protected against leukopenia (Gill *et al.*, 1979; Ikeda and Ohtsuji, 1971). Experimentally induced alterations in benzene metabolism do not influence the acute toxicity of the solvent (Drew and Fouts, 1974).

There is also disagreement about whether or not benzene stimulates its own metabolism by enzyme induction (Saito *et al.*, 1973). Perhaps the basis for this confusion and apparently contradictory observations lies in the hypothesis that benzene metabolism leads to the generation of reactive intermediates, which can bind to cytochrome P450, resulting in an inhibition of benzene metabolism (Gonasun *et al.*, 1973). Some evidence suggests that this metabolite is not the epoxide (see above) but something that lies beyond the phenol stage of metabolism (Tunek *et al.*, 1978).

Further confusion is generated by the uncertainty about whether the putative toxic metabolite is generated in the liver and transported to the bone marrow or whether it is generated *in situ*. Phenol and an unidentified metabolite are produced from benzene by rabbit bone marrow (Andrews *et al.*, 1979). In rat bone marrow, catechol and hydroquinone persisted longer than phenol or benzene after systemic dosing with the latter (Rickert *et al.*, 1979). In human lymphocytes in culture, catechol and to a lesser extent hydroquinone were more potent than phenol or benzene in effecting sister chromatid exchanges and in delaying cell division (Morimoto and Wolff, 1980). Ingested ethanol enhances the hematotoxicity of inhaled benzene in mice (Snyder *et al.*, 1981).

Chronic benzene exposure eventually leads to pancytopenia where the initial leukopenia is followed by thrombocytopenia and anemia. Anemia may be responsible for such signs and symptoms as weight loss, weakness, fatigue, headache, lethargy, etc. Thrombocytopenia leads to hemorrhagic tendencies, including petechiae, easy bruising, epistaxses, bleeding from the gums and menorrhagia. A neutropenia or even agranulocytosis may be responsible for sudden overwhelming infections (Cohen *et al.*, 1978; Haley, 1977). At one time or another, however, almost every known type of blood dyscrasia has been ascribed to benzene exposure, including paradoxical increases in the numbers of formed elements in peripheral blood and hyperplasia of the marrow in the presence of pancytopenia (Hunter, 1939; Mallory *et al.*, 1939). Serious abnormalities in the peripheral blood have been found in exposed workers in the complete absence of physical signs or symptoms and vice versa. There are enormous and unexplained differences in individual sensitivity (Greenburg *et al.*, 1939).

Whatever metabolite is responsible for the bone marrow toxicity, it is manifested as a severe disturbance in DNA and RNA synthesis (Moeschlin and Speck, 1967; Kissling and Speck, 1972). The cytotoxicity, however, is expressed both as disturbances in precursor cell differentiation and in phases of the cell cycle (Irons *et al.*, 1979; Kocsis and Snyder, 1975). Increased chromosomal aberrations have been found in peripheral lymphocytes many years after exposure (Forni *et al.*, 1971; Picciano, 1979; Tough and Brown, 1965).

For decades benzene occupied an anomalous position in that most authorities agreed that it was the one chemical where a reasonable cause-and-effect relationship had been established for acute myelogenous leukemia in humans (Cronkite, 1961) but not for carcinogenesis in laboratory animals. A carcinogenic potential has now been demonstrated in rats after daily oral gavage for one year (Maltoni and Scarnato, 1979). Cases are now appearing in the clinical literature in which exposures producing acute myelotoxicity were followed many years later by leukemia (Aksoy *et al.*, 1974; DeGowen, 1963; Vigliani and Saita, 1964; Vigliani and Forni, 1976). Benzene is also embryotoxic and teratogenic in rats (Kuna and Kapp, 1981).

Pharmacokinetic studies reveal no gross differences between benzene and xylene. In male rats exposed to 500 ppm benzene, the steady state concentrations in various tissues were: 12 μg./gm. blood, 37 μg./gm. bone marrow and 164 μg./gm. fat (Rickert *et al.*, 1979). Benzene was eliminated more slowly in rats of either sex which had more body fat. Its slower elimination in female rats than in male rats was also ascribed to differences in body fat content (Sato *et al.*, 1975). Perhaps this difference is the basis for the clinical impression that human females are more susceptible to benzene toxicity than males. In human subjects the proportion of inhaled benzene that was retained and eventually excreted as phenol in the urine was greater in heavier subjects. Only a small fraction of the retained benzene was eliminated unchanged in exhaled air (Hunter and Blair, 1972).

Symptomatology:

A. *Acute ingestion or inhalation:*
1. Ingestion causes a burning sensation in the mouth and stomach, also nausea, vomiting and salivation. Hematemesis may occur.
2. Substernal pain, cough and hoarseness are described.
3. Aspiration into the tracheobronchial tree, either during ingestion or subsequent to vomiting or eructations, is likely to produce a severe hemorrhagic pneumonitis.
4. In vapor exposures a transient euphoria is sometimes observed.
5. Headache, giddiness, vertigo, ataxia and tinnitus.
6. Confusion, stupefaction and coma.
7. Often associated with this coma are tremors, motor restlessness, hypertonus and hyperactive reflexes, but frank convulsions rarely occur except in association with terminal asphyxia.
8. Death from respiratory failure or from sudden ventricular fibrillation.
9. Skin contact with liquid may cause erythema and even blisters if the contact is prolonged. Hemorrhagic inflammatory lesions develop on mucous membranes in contact with liquid.

B. *Chronic or repeated inhalation (solvent sniffers):* Because most solvent abusers use many solvents and solvent mixtures, including aromatic hydrocarbons (mostly toluene), aliphatic hydrocarbons (especially gasoline), volatile esters and ketones, and halogenated hydrocarbon solvents, it is not usually possible to designate which agent is responsible for each toxic sign and symptom. Toluene alone, however, is believed to be capable of generating the three syndromes described below (Streicher *et al.*, 1981).

1. Severe muscle weakness leading to limb paralysis, associated with hypokalemia due to renal tubular acidosis (see text above). Cardiac arrhythmias often accompany the hypokalemia. Sensory function and tendon reflexes are not impaired.
2. Gastrointestinal complaints, including abdominal pain, nausea, vomiting and hematemesis but no significant abdominal tenderness or palpable abdominal masses.
3. Neuropsychiatric complaints, including (a) lethargy, hallucinations, coma or (b) headache, dizziness, syncope or (c) paresthesias and peripheral neuropathy or (d) cerebellar ataxia and other cerebellar signs.

Treatment:

1. Because of the aspiration hazard, avoid emetic drugs, whenever practical. However, if the ingested xylene (or other aromatic hydrocarbon solvent) contains a dangerous amount of a toxic solute (*e.g.*, pesticide) and if gastric lavage cannot be initiated promptly, it may be advisable to proceed with the induction of emesis (p. I-2-4).
2. Cautious gastric lavage with warm water. Observe all precautions described on pp. I-10 and 11 and p. III-222. One or two ounces of mineral oil may be instilled and left in the stomach at the completion of lavage.
3. Sodium or magnesium sulfate (15 to 30 gm. dissolved in water) as a saline cathartic.
4. General supportive measures, including oxygen administration (p. IV-12), artificial ventilation (p. IV-7) and parenteral fluids, as indicated.
5. Avoid epinephrine because of its possible adverse effect on the sensitized myocardium. Avoid all digestible fats, oils and alcohol, which might promote intestinal absorption.
6. If eyes or skin are affected, wash thoroughly and apply a bland analgetic ointment.
7. If pulmonary edema or consolidation occurs, treat as in kerosene poisoning (p. III-224). See also pp. IV-14–16.
8. Because of the possibility of ventricular fibrillation, monitor the ECG continuously and be prepared to administer external cardiac massage (p. IV-26). Secure and keep available an electrical defibrillator (p. IV-30).
9. In chronic solvent abusers, correct dehydration (p. IV-64), acidosis (p. IV-71), hypokalemia (p. IV-73) and hypophosphatemia. Usually toxic signs and symptoms (except those due to neuropathies and to cerebellar lesions) disappear within a few days after fluid and electrolyte abnormalities are corrected.

Laboratory:

1. Methods are available for the quantitative estimation of aromatic hydrocarbons in blood (Guertin and Gerarde, 1959).
2. Urinary excretion of *o*-, *m*- and/or *p*-methylhippuric acids after exposure to the respective xylene isomers (see above), *o*-cresol or hippuric acid after toluene (Pagnotto and Lieberman, 1967; Svirbely *et al.*, 1944), and phenol after benzene exposure (Hough *et al.*, 1944; Rainsford and Davies, 1965) may serve as indices of exposure.
3. Severe hypokalemia and hypophosphatemia may occur after chronic exposure to toluene (and presumably xylene), as well as hyperchloremic or anion-gap acidosis.
4. High serum creatine phosphokinase levels, without infarction in heart or brain, suggest rhabdomyolysis, as does myoglobinuria. These findings are common in chronic toluene abusers (Streicher *et al.*, 1981).
5. Chronic solvent abusers also show hematuria and albuminuria frequently but rarely renal failure.
6. Complete hematological and bone marrow studies are always appropriate.

References:

Aksoy, M.; Erdem, S.; DinCol, G. Leukemia in shoe-workers exposed chronically to benzene. Blood 44:837-841, 1974.

Allison, D. J. Reflexes from the nose. N. Engl. J. Med. 299:1468, 1978.

Andrews. L. S.; Sasame, H. A.; Gillette, J. R. H-3-Benzene metabolism in rabbit bone marrow. Life Sci. 25:567-572, 1979.

Angerer, J. Occupational chronic exposure to organic solvents. VII. Metabolism of toluene in man. Int. Arch. Occup. Environ. Health 43:63-67, 1979.

Bennett, R. H.; Forman, H. R. Hypokalemic periodic paralysis in chronic toluene exposure. Arch. Neurol. 37:673, 1980.

Boor, J. W.; Hurtig, H. I. Persistent cerebellar ataxia after exposure to toluene. Ann. Neurol. 2:440-442, 1977.

Browning, E. *Toxicity and Metabolism of Industrial Solvents.* Elsevier Publishing Co., Amsterdam, 2nd ed, 1965.

Carpenter, C. P.; Kinkead, E. R.; Geary, D. L., Jr.; Sullivan, L. J.; King, J. M. Petroleum hydrocarbon toxicity studies. V. Animal and human response to vapors of mixed xylenes. Toxicol. Appl. Pharmacol. 33:543-558, 1975.

Carter, G. Fatal case of accidental poisoning by benzol vapour. Br. Med. J. 2:794-795, 1928.

Cohen, H. S.; Freedman, M. L.; Goldstein, B. D. The problem of benzene in our environment: clinical and molecular considerations. Am. J. Med. Sci. 275:124-136, 1978.

Collom, W. D.; Winek, C. L. Detection of glue constituents in fatalities due to "glue sniffing". Clin. Toxicol. 3:125-130, 1970.

Cronkite, E. P. Evidence for radiation and chemicals as leukemogenic agents. Arch. Environ. Health 3:297-303, 1961.

DeGowen, R. L. Benzene exposure and aplastic anemia followed by leukemia 15 years later. J. A. M. A. 185:748-751, 1963.

Drew, T.; Fouts, R. The lack of effects of pretreatment with phenobarbital and chlorpromazine on the acute toxicity of benzene in rats. Toxicol. Appl. Pharmacol. 27:183-193, 1974.

Elovaara, E.; Collan, Y.; Pfaffli, P.; Vainio, H. The combined toxicity of technical grade xylene and ethanol in the rat. Xenobiotica 10:435-445, 1980.

Engstroem, J.; Riihimaki, V. Distribution of m-xylene to subcutaneous adipose tissue in short-term experimental human exposure. Scand. J. Work Environ. Health 5:126-134, 1979.

Fischman, C. M.; Oster, J. R. Toxic effects of toluene. J. A. M. A. 241:1713-1715, 1979.

Forni, A. M.; Cappelini, A.; Pacifico, E.; Vigliani, E. C. Chromosome changes and their evolution in subjects with past exposure to benzene. Arch. Environ. Health 23:385-391, 1971.

Gerarde, H. W. Toxicology and Biochemistry of Aromatic Hydrocarbons. Elsevier, Amsterdam, 1960.

Gerarde, H. W.; Ahlstrom, D. B. Toxicologic studies on hydrocarbons. XI. Influence of dose on the metabolism of mono-n-alkyl derivatives of benzene. Toxicol. Appl. Pharmacol. 9:185-190, 1966b.

Gill, D. P.; Kempen, R. R.; Nash, J. B.; Ellis, S. Modifications of benzene myelotoxicity and metabolism by phenobarbital SKF-525A and 3-methylcholanthrene. Life Sci. 25:1633-1640, 1979.

Glaser, F. B. Inhalation psychosis and related states. Arch. Gen. Psychiatry 14:315-322, 1966.

Gonasun, L. M.; Witmer, C.; Kocsis, J. J.; Snyder, R. Benzene metabolism in mouse liver microsomes. Toxicol. Appl. Pharmacol. 26:398-406, 1973.

Grabski, D. A. Toluene sniffing producing cerebellar degeneration. Am. J. Psychiatry 118:461-462, 1961.

Greenburg, L.; Mayers, M. R.; Goldwater, L.; Smith, A. R. Benzene (benzol) poisoning in the rotogravure printing industry in New York City. J. Indust. Hyg. Toxicol. 21:395-420, 1939.

Greenburg, L.; Mayers, M. R.; Heimann, R.; Moskowitz, S. The effects of exposure to toluene in industry. J. A. M. A. 118:573-578, 1942.

Guertin, D. L.; Gerarde, H. W. Toxicological studies on hydrocarbons. IV. An ultraviolet spectrophotometric method for the quantitative determination of benzene and alkylbenzenes in blood. Arch. Ind. Health 20:262-265, 1959.

Haley, T. J. Evaluation of the health effects of benzene inhalation. Clin. Toxicol. 11:531-548, 1977.

Hamilton, A. Benzene (benzol) poisoning. Arch. Pathol. 11:434-454, 601-637, 1931.

Hayden, J. W.; Comstock, E. G.; Comstock, B. S. The clinical toxicology of solvent abuse. Clin. Toxicol. 9:169-184, 1976.

Hough, V. H.; Gunn, F. D.; Freeman, S. Studies on toxicity of commercial benzene and of mixtures of benzene, toluene and xylene. J. Ind. Hyg. Toxicol. 26:296-306, 1944.

Hunter, C. G.; Blair, D. Benzene: pharmacokinetic studies in man. Ann. Occup. Hyg. 15:193-199, 1972.

Hunter, F. T. Chronic exposure to benzene (benzol) II. The clinical effects. J. Indust. Hyg. Toxicol. 21:331-354, 1939.

Ikeda, M. Enzymatic studies on benzene intoxication. J. Biochem. 55:231-243, 1964.

Ikeda, M.; Murakami, H.; Nishio, M. The correlation between detoxicating enzyme activity and benzol susceptibility. Arch. Biochem. Biophys. 93:670-671, 1961.

Ikeda, M.; Ohtsuji, H. Phenobarbital-induced protection against toxicity of toluene and benzene in the rat. Toxicol. Appl. Pharmacol. 20:30-43, 1971.

Irons, R. D.; Heck, H.; Moore, B. J.; Muirhead, K. A. Effects of short-term benzene administration on bone marrow cell cycle kinetics in the rat. Toxicol. Appl. Pharmacol. 51:399-409, 1979.

Jerina, D. M.; Daly, J. W. Arene oxides: A new aspect of drug metabolism. Science 185:573-582, 1974.

Kimura, E. T.; Ebert, D. M.; Dodge, P. W. Acute toxicity and limits of solvent residue for sixteen organic solvents. Toxicol. Appl. Pharmacol. 19:699-704, 1971.

Kissling, M.; Speck, B. Further studies on experimental benzene induced aplastic anemia. Blut 25; 97-103, 1972.

Knox, J. W.; Nelson, J. R. Permanent encephalopathy from toluene inhalation. N. Engl. J. Med. 275:1494-1496, 1966.

Kocsis, J. J.; Snyder, R. Current concepts of benzene toxicity. CRC Crit. Rev. Toxicol. 3:265-288, 1975.

Kroeger, R. M.; Moore, R. J.; Lehman, T. H.; Giesy, J. D.; Skeeters, C. E. Recurrent urinary calculi associated with toluene sniffing. J. Urol. 123:89-91, 1980.

Kuna, R. A.; Kapp, R. W., Jr. The embryotoxic/teratogenic potential of benzene vapor in rats. Toxicol. Appl. Pharmacol. 57:1-7, 1981.

Longacre, S. L.; Kocsis, J. J.; Snyder, R. Influence of strain differences in mice in the metabolism and toxicity of benzene. Toxicol. Appl. Pharmacol. 60:398-409, 1981.

Longley, E. O.; Jones, A. T.; Welch, R.; Lomaesv, O. Two acute toluene episodes in merchant ships. Arch. Environ. Health 14:481-487, 1967.

Maki-Paakkanen, J.; Husgafvel-Pursiainen, K.; Kalliomaki, P. L.; Tuominen, J.; Sorsa, M. Toluene-exposed workers and chromosome aberrations. J. Toxicol. Environ. Health 6:775-781, 1980.

Mallory, T. B.; Gall, E. A.; Brinkley, W. J. Chronic exposure to benzene (benzol). III. The pathologic results. J. Indust. Hyg. Toxicol. 21:355-393, 1939.

Malm, G.; Lying-Tunell, U. Cerebellar dysfunction related to toluene sniffing. Acta Neurol. Scand. 62:188-190, 1980.

Maltoni, C.; Scarnato, C. First experimental demonstration of the carcinogenic effects of benzene. Long-term bioassays on Sprague-Dawley rats by oral administration. Med. Lav. 70:352-357, 1979.

Massengale, O. N.; Glaser, H. H.; LeLievre, R. E.; Dodds, J. B.; Klock, M. E. Physical and psychological factors in glue sniffing. N. Engl. J. Med. 269:1340-1344, 1963.

McDermott, H. J.; Vos, G. A. Service station attendants' exposure to benzene and gasoline vapors. Am. Indust. Hyg. Assoc. J. 40:315-321, 1979.

Moeschlin, S.; Speck, B. Experimental studies on the mechanism of action of benzene on the bone marrow (radioautographic studies using ³H-thymidine). Acta Haematol. 38:104-111, 1967.

Morimoto, K.; Wolff, S. Increase of sister chromatid exchanges and perturbations of cell division kinetics in human lymphocytes by benzene metabolites. Cancer Res. 40:1189-1193, 1980.

Morley, R. D.; Eccteston, W.; Douglas, C. P.; Greville, W. E. J.; Scott, D. J.; Anderson, J. Xylene poisoning; a report on one fatal case and two cases of recovery after prolonged unconsciousness. Br. Med. J. 3:442-443, 1970.

Nahum, L. H.; Hoff, H. E. The mechanism of sudden death in acute benzene poisoning. J. Pharmacol. Exp. Ther. 50:336-345, 1934.

O'Brien, E. T.; Yeoman, W. B.; Hobby, J. A. E. Hepatorenal damage from toluene in a "glue sniffer." Br. Med. J. 2:29-30, 1971.

Ogata, M.; Tomokuni, K.; Takatsuka, Y. Urinary excretions of hippuric acid and m- or p-methylhippuric acid in the urine of persons exposed to vapors of toluene and m- or p-xylene as a test of exposure. Br. J. Indust. Med. 27:43-50, 1970.

Pagnotto, L. D.; Lieberman, L. M. Urinary hippuric acid excretion as an index of toluene exposure. Am. Ind. Hyg. Assoc. J. 28:129-134, 1967.

Patel, J. M.; Harper, C.; Drew, R. J. The biotransformation of p-xylene to a toxic aldehyde. Drug Metab. Dispos. 6:368-374, 1978.

Pfaffli, P. Savolainen, H.; Kalliomaki, P. L.; Kalliokoski, P. Urinary o-cresol in toluene exposure. Scand. J. Work Environ. Health 5:286-289, 1979.

Picciano, D. Cytogenetic study of workers exposed to benzene. Environ. Res. 19:33-38, 1979.

Press, E.; Done, A. K. Solvent sniffing, physiologic effects and community control measures for intoxication from the intentional inhalation of organic solvents. I and II. Pediatrics *39*:451-461 and 611-622, 1967.

Pyykko, K.; Tahti, H.; Vapaatalo, H. Toluene concentrations in various tissues of rats after inhalation and oral administration. Arch. Toxicol. *38*:169-176, 1977.

Rainsford, S. G.; Davies, T. A. L. Urinary excretion of phenol by men exposed to vapor of benzene: A screening test. Br. J. Ind. Med. *22*:21-26, 1965.

Rickert, D. E.; Baker, T. S.; Bus, J. S.; Barrow, C. S.; Irons, R. D. Benzene disposition in the rat after exposure by inhalation. Toxicol. Appl. Pharmacol. *49*:417-423, 1979.

Riihimaki, V.; Pfaffli, P.; Savolainen, K.; Pekari, K. Kinetics of *m*-xylene in man. General features of absorption, distribution, biotransformation and excretion in repetitive inhalation exposure. Scand. J. Work Environ. Health *5*:217-231, 1979.

Russ, G.; Clarkson, A. R.; Woodroffe, A. R.; Seymour, A. E.; Cheng, I. K. P. Renal failure from "glue sniffing". Med. J. Aust. *2*:121-122, 1981.

Saito, F. U.; Kocsis, J. J.; Snyder, R. Effect of benzene on hepatic drug metabolism and ultrastructure. Toxicol. Appl. Pharmacol. *26*:209-217, 1973.

Sammett, D.; Lee, E. W.; Kocsis, J. J.; Snyder, R. Partial hepatectomy reduces both metabolism and toxicity of benzene. J. Toxicol. Environ. Health *5*:785-792, 1979.

Sato, A.; Nakajima, T.; Fujiwara, Y.; Murayama, N. Kinetic studies on sex difference in susceptibility to chronic benzene intoxication with special reference to body fat content. Br. J. Indust. Med. *32*:321-328, 1975.

Satran, R.; Dodson, V. N. Toluene habituation. N. Engl. J. Med. *268*:719-721, 1963.

Savolainen, H.; Vainio, H.; Helojoki, M.; Elovaara, E. Biochemical and toxicological effects of short-term, intermittent xylene inhalation exposure and combined ethanol intake. Arch. Toxicol. *41*:195-205, 1978.

Savolainen, K.; Riihimaki, V.; Seppalainen, A. M.; Linnoila, M. Effects fo short-term meta-xylene exposure and physical exercise on the central nervous system. Int. Arch. Occup. Environ. Health *45*:105-121, 1980.

Snyder, C. A.; Erlichman, M. N.; Laskin, S.; Goldstein, B. D.; Albert, R. E. The pharmacokinetics of repetitive benzene exposure at 300 and 100 ppm in AKR mice and Sprague-Dawley rats. Toxicol. Appl. Pharmacol. *57*:164-171, 1981.

Snyder, R.; Uzuki, F.; Gonasum, L.; Bromfield, E.; Wells, A. The metabolism of benzene *in vitro*. Toxicol. Appl. Pharmacol. *11*:346-360, 1967a.

Sollmann, T. *A Manual of Pharmacology.* 8th Ed., W. B. Saunders Co., Philadelphia, 1957.

Streicher, H. Z.; Gabow, P. A.; Moss, A. H.; Kono, D.; Kaehny, W. D. Syndromes of toluene sniffing in adults. Ann. Intern. Med. *94*:758-762, 1981.

Svirbely, J. L.; Dunn, R. C.; von Oettingen, W. F. The acute toxicity of vapors of certain solvents containing appreciable amounts of benzene and toluene. J. Ind. Hyg. Toxicol. *25*:366-373, 1943.

Svirbely, J. L.; Dunn, R. C.; von Oettingen, W. F. The chronic toxicity of moderate concentrations of benzene and of mixtures of benzene and its homologues for rats and dogs. J. Ind. Hyg. Toxicol. *26*:37-46, 1944.

Taher, S. M.; Anderson, R. J.; McCartney, R.; Popovtzer, M.; Schrier, R. W. Renal tubular acidosis associated with toluene "sniffing". N. Engl. J. Med. *290*:765-768, 1974.

Tough, I. M.; Brown, W. M. C. Chromosome aberrations and exposure to ambient benzene. Lancet *1*:684, 1965.

Tunek, A.; Platt, K. L.; Bentley, P.; Oerch, F. Microsomal metabolism of benzene to species irreversibly binding to microsomal protein and effects of modifications of this metabolism. Mol. Pharmacol. *14*:920-929, 1978.

Ungvary, G.; Tatrai, E.; Hudak, A.; Barcza, G.; Lorincz, M. Studies on the embryotoxic effects of *ortho-*, *meta-* and *para*-xylene. Toxicology *18*:61-74, 1980.

Vigliani, E. C.; Forni, A. Benzene and leukemia. Environ. Res. *11*:122-127, 1976.

Vigliani, E. C.; Saita, G. Benzene and leukemia. N. Engl. J. Med. *271*:872-876, 1964.

von Oettingen, W.; Neal, P. A.; Donahue, D. D. The toxicity and potential dangers of toluene. J. A. M. A. *118*:579-584, 1942.

von Oettingen, W. F. Toxicity and potential dangers of aliphatic and aromatic hydrocarbons. Public Health Bull. No. 255, 1940.

Wilczok, T.; Bieniek, G. Urinary hippuric acid concentration after occupational exposure to toluene. Br. J. Ind. Med. *35*:330-334, 1978.

Winek, C. L.; Collom, W. D. Benzene and toluene fatalities. J. Occup. Med. *13*:259-261, 1971.

Winek, C. L.; Collom, W. D.; Wecht, C. H. Fatal benzene exposure by glue sniffing. Lancet *1*:683, 1967.

Wirtschafter, Z. T.; Cronyn, M. W. Relative hepatotoxicity, pentane, trichloroethylene, benzene, carbon tetrachloride. Arch. Environ. Health *9*:180-185, 1964.

Wolf, M. A.; Rowe, V. K.; McCollister, D. D.; Hollingsworth, R. L.; Ogen, F. Toxicological studies of certain alkylated benzenes and benzene. Arch. Ind. Health *14*:387-398, 1956.

Young, R. J.; Rinsky, R. A.; Infante, P. F. Benzene in consumer products. Science *199*:248, 1978.

SECTION IV

Supportive Treatment in Acute Chemical Poisoning

Contents

INTRODUCTION

In clinical toxicology, good patient management involves much more than terminating the toxic exposure and administering a chemical antidote or pharmacological antagonist. The alert physician is attentive to every symptom that arises during the entire course of an illness, symptoms that contribute to the patient's suffering whether they have serious prognostic import or not. In the course of offering symptomatic relief, the therapist inevitably gives support to those organ systems that are working to preserve physical and chemical homeostasis. The maintenance of homeostasis, which operates spontaneously and automatically in health, often becomes so inadequate in a poison victim that the physician must attempt to regulate many physiological parameters at the same time. It is this attempt that is called supportive treatment. In most poisonings good supportive therapy is more important than the "correct" antidote.

First aid, emergency treatment and general supportive therapy are phases of a continuum with no well-defined boundaries between them. The principles and techniques of removing poison from a victim's skin, eye and stomach are outlined in Section I. With respect to ingested poisons, this decontamination involves emptying the stomach by inducing emesis or by gastric lavage, trapping the poison by adsorbents such as activated charcoal, and speeding the transit of the toxin through the intestinal tract by the administration of an appropriate cathartic. Other first aid measures, including such high priority items as the correction of respiratory tract obstruction, the administration of artificial ventilation and cardiac resuscitation, are discussed here in Section IV.

The physician-toxicologist often has no direct involvement in these early phases of this therapeutic continuum. In the United States today, the initial care of the patient is often in the hands of those who serve in rescue squads and on ambulance teams, most of whom are now accredited emergency medical technicians. Thus, some parts of Section IV are addressed primarily to these and related paramedics.

Section IV describes those measures of supportive treatment that are believed to be most appropriate in cases of acute chemical poisoning. The material is presented as a series of topics under the relevant organ system (see "Contents"). Although functional pathology is briefly outlined, the emphasis in this section is on therapy and the techniques of therapy. Specific poisons are mentioned only to illustrate special clinical problems. Unless indicated to the contrary, all recommended doses are designed for an adult person of average size. In children, doses are usually reduced in proportion to the body weight or body surface area.

The details of treatment must be conditioned always by the facilities, the training and experience of the therapist, and by those many features that are unique to each patient's intoxication. Every clinical situation is influenced by so many indeterminate and intangible factors that there is no place for dogmatism in therapeutics. In this spirit the following remarks are offered as suggestions, not as rigorous prescriptions and prohibitions.

RESPIRATION

Respiratory Obstruction

It is always imperative to assure a free and patent airway. As long as spontaneous breathing continues, signs of airway obstruction include inspiratory retraction at the neck or intercostal spaces, dissociation of diaphragmatic from intercostal movements ("rocking boat respiration" or "paradoxical respiration"), audible wheezes or rhonchi, snoring, laryngeal stridor, and large quantities of secretions in the oropharynx. A variety of signs and symptoms arises from the attending anoxia; they include cyanosis, restlessness, depression, confusion, and lethargy. Restlessness is a particularly common early symptom; cyanosis is an unreliable sign until late in the course of asphyxia.

The following measures in sequence are employed to relieve obstruction in various parts of the respiratory tract:

1. Remove dentures and any debris from the mouth.
2. Position the patient in a lateral Trendelenburg or supine with the head extended (tilted back) and the jaw jutting forward.
3. Establish an oropharyngeal or nasopharyngeal airway.
4. Suction the pharynx, larynx, and trachea, as necessary, through the mouth or nose.
5. Pass an endotracheal tube or esophageal obturator airway if the above measures are insufficient or if the trachea needs to be protected against the threat of vomiting and aspiration.
6. If endotracheal intubation is impractical, perform a cricothyrotomy, or a standard tracheotomy, preceded in either case by a percutaneous needle cricothyrostomy if the patient's condition is critical.
7. Remove mucus by suctioning through the tracheostomy tube either blindly or under direct observation with a bronchoscope.
8. Relieve patchy atelectasis by chest physiotherapy and by rolling the patient periodically.

These procedures are discussed in detail below. For a more complete discussion, consult Section I, pp. 1–28, *Atlas of Emergency Medicine*, Ed. 2, by P. Rosen and G. Sternbach, published by Williams & Wilkins, Baltimore, 1983. Also see

"Standards for cardiopulmonary resuscitation (CPR) and emergency care," *JAMA* 227:836–868, 1974.

During attempts to correct respiratory tract obstruction, the victim is likely to benefit from intermittent or continuous oxygen therapy (p. IV-12). If he is completely apneic, artificial ventilation (pp. IV-7–12) takes precedence over all efforts to correct partial obstruction. From time to time, however, artificial respiration can and should be interrupted as necessary to permit procedures for improving airway patency.

Obstruction of the oropharynx. Such obstruction is often due to muscle relaxation that allows the mandible to drop backward and to press the root of the tongue against the relaxed posterior pharyngeal wall (Fig. IV-1A). This problem can usually be avoided by keeping the victim on his side with his head low. This lateral head-down position is also valuable in minimizing the aspiration of vomitus.

If the tongue has already slipped into the pharynx, as is often true of the unconscious patient in the supine position, it must be lifted forward. This is accomplished by a maneuver known as the head-tilt chin-lift, two variants of which are illustrated in Fig. IV-1. The rescuer places one hand on the victim's forehead, the other under the neck at the base of the skull,

with the fingertips behind the angle of the mandible. The head is then tilted backward by applying pressure on the victim's forehead while lifting the neck with the other hand (Fig. IV-1B). Alternatively, the fingers of one hand are placed under the chin against the bony mandible, *not* against the soft tissues in the floor of the mouth. An upward and forward motion of this hand at the same time that pressure is applied to the forehead by the other hand serves to tilt the head backward and to carry the tongue forward (Fig. IV-1C). If these procedures are not successful in relieving the obstruction, the jaw thrust maneuver (p. IV-7) should be tried. In all cases the position of head extension must be maintained or the tongue will slip back into the hypopharynx.

In the absence of a gag reflex, the tongue is best held in place by the insertion of a hard rubber or plastic oropharyngeal airway. This device is merely slid along the roof of the mouth until its ventral curvature hooks the root of the tongue and carries it forward. Some therapists prefer to slide it along the buccal surface (*i.e.*, the cheek) and then rotate it downward 90° to hook the base of the tongue. Alternatively, it is inserted with its convexity against the surface of the tongue and then rotated 180°. A no. 5 airway is suitable for adults, a no. 3 for children, and a

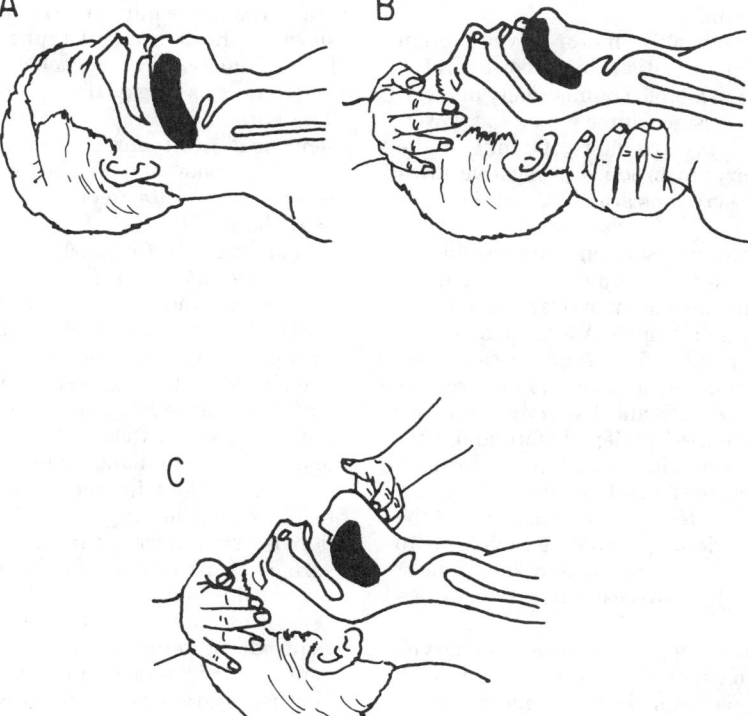

Figure IV-1. Obstruction of the oropharynx by the base of the tongue (*shaded*) due to relaxation and retraction of the mandible (*A*) and two versions (*B* and *C*) of the head-tilt chin-lift maneuver that relieves this obstruction.

no. 1 for infants. Only unconscious or obtunded patients tolerate oropharyngeal airways.

If trismus prevents instrumentation through the mouth or if the gag reflex is active, a nasopharyngeal airway is used instead. First shrink the nasal mucous membranes by topical application of a decongestant such as 0.5% phenylephrine solution. Choose the side with the wider air passage. If desired, a local anesthetic solution can be instilled. Place a water-soluble gel in the nostril as a lubricant. Commercial nasopharyngeal airways have a small curvature. Insert the device so that its concave surface faces the convexity of the floor of the nasal cavity. Some degree of nasal bleeding is not uncommon at the time of insertion. Because the end of the tube lies in the hypopharynx, it may provoke gagging and vomiting, especially in children. In general, however, it is better tolerated than is an oropharyngeal airway.

Suctioning the airway. Suctioning the airway is necessary to remove mucus and other secretions from the hypopharynx and tracheobronchial tree. Sometimes the oropharynx can be wiped out with a finger covered with a gauze pad, but for the lower tract a small flexible catheter is required. Clean or, if practical, aseptic technique should be employed; sterile, disposible plastic catheters are often used. Catheters of various sizes are available; a 6 Fr. is usually appropriate for the newborn whereas 12 to 14 Fr. are used in adults.

A catheter attached to a motor-driven suction pump is best, but a satisfactory foot-operated suction pump is available commercially and can serve where there is no source of electric power. Of course a large syringe (50 to 100 ml.) can be used, if necessary, to produce a negative pressure, but thick secretions are difficult to remove with a syringe.

Electrically powered suction units installed in treatment centers should provide air flows up to 30 liters/min. and a vacuum of over 300 mm. Hg when the tube is clamped. With such a high suction capacity, both fluids and gases are removed from the upper airways. Therefore it is desirable to oxygenate and hyperventilate any severely compromised patient before and after using these suction units. Furthermore, the suction should not be turned on until after the catheter is inserted to the desired depth, and the duration of a suctioning should be limited to 10 to 15 seconds. Keep the suction on at least intermittently while the catheter is being extracted.

If the patient is deeply narcotized, the larynx and trachea can usually be entered blindly with the suctioning catheter. If the coma is not intense, this maneuver may induce reflex (vagal) bradycardia, reflex spasm of the laryngeal muscles and adduction of the cords. Laryngospasm is usually transient, but if it persists and completely occludes the airway, the physician must proceed to endotracheal intubation. If a solid foreign body is suspected in the larynx, it should be visualized through a laryngoscope and removed before intubating the trachea.

Endotracheal intubation. If the conservative measures outlined above fail to establish a good airway, endotracheal intubation or some form of tracheostomy becomes advisable. To prevent if not cure respiratory obstruction, one or the other of these measures is almost invariably instituted when the apneic patient reaches a modern treatment center. Either procedure circumvents obstruction due to excessive oropharyngeal secretions or to inflammatory edema of the pharynx and larynx. Intubation is the safer procedure and is almost always tried first; it is usually all that is required. Unlike a pharyngeal airway, an indwelling tube in the trachea prevents respiratory obstruction due to spasm or edema of the vocal cords; it also allows the trachea and even the major bronchi to be suctioned with considerable efficiency by a small catheter passed periodically through the endotracheal tube.

Endotracheal intubation, however, is not free of problems. Unless the larynx is first cleared of foreign bodies, a tube may push them down into the trachea or bronchi. When obstruction is due to an inflammatory reaction of the larynx and upper tract, this inflammation may subside only slowly in the presence of a tube (or other foreign body). Finally, an endotracheal tube can be tolerated only as long as the cough reflex is absent. The patient in coma or under anesthesia presents no difficulty in this regard, but even simple sedation makes it possible for most conscious persons to tolerate an endotracheal tube once it is in place.

Endotracheal tubes are available commercially in various sizes; size 7.5 or 8.5 is appropriate for most adults. As an airway for assisted ventilation, for preventing aspiration and for preventing or correcting upper tract obstruction, one chooses a tube bearing an inflatable rubber cuff near the beveled end, in order to ensure a tight seal within the trachea. Models with soft and highly compliant balloon cuffs are much safer than older stiff models. A metal stylet may be placed inside the endotracheal tube to make it more rigid during the act of insertion. The surface of the tube should be lubricated with a water-soluble gel.

Before any attempt to insert the tube, a patient who is breathing inadequately should be ventilated vigorously; for this purpose a mask-and-bag system is widely used in emergency treatment centers. The conscious patient may need a sedative and almost always a local anesthetic such as cocaine applied on the hypopharynx. If muscle tone is high, a muscle-paralyzing drug such as intravenous succinylcholine may be required. By paralyzing striated muscle, one also prevents or terminates laryngospasm, in the presence of which intubation is almost always possible but only at the cost of some trauma to the cords. After the paralyzing agent has produced good relaxation, discontinue ventilatory assistance and remove any oropharyngeal or nasopharyngeal airway. The patient is now ready for intubation.

With the aid of a laryngoscope, the pharynx and larynx are checked to establish that no foreign bodies are present. Under direct observation through the laryngoscope, the endotracheal tube is then passed into the mouth and through the glottis. It is advanced until the entire inflatable cuff lies just below the larynx, *i.e.*, beyond the vocal cords; if passed too far, the end may become impacted in the right main bronchus. When the tube is in proper position, the stylet is removed, and the balloon is inflated with air until an air leak can no longer be heard around the cuff when the patient breathes or is respired. With a properly selected tube, this seal should be achieved with a cuff pressure of less than 30 mm. Hg. With young children (less than 8 years old), the cuff is generally *not* inflated. An oral airway or bite block is then reinserted to prevent the patient from biting the endotracheal tube when muscle strength returns. The free end of the tube is taped to the cheek.

Because of the danger of inducing trauma, this procedure is best reserved for the physician with special training, but this injunction, like some of the pretreatments described above, may have to be ignored in critical emergencies. Oral endotracheal intubation, however, is impractical if an injury or disease prevents the head from being extended or if the patient cannot lie in the supine position (*e.g.*, during the distress of an asthmatic attack or of pulmonary edema). Under these circumstances passage of an endotracheal tube may be attempted blindly through the nose. Nasotracheal intubation, however, is difficult, and the possibilities for inducing trauma are considerable, but once in place, a nasotracheal tube can often be tolerated and maintained safely for long periods (*e.g.*, 3 to 4 weeks). As noted below, a temporary but useful alternative to endotracheal intubation is passage of an esophageal obturator airway.

A properly positioned endotracheal tube offers no certain guarantee against respiratory obstruction. The tube may kink, or it may become occluded by mucous plugs; either complication may arise insidiously or with alarming rapidity. It may be necessary to pass a suction catheter down the tube every few minutes or only infrequently, but a trained person should be in constant attendance as long as intubation is contin-

ued. To prevent necrotizing tracheobronchitis, air or oxygen delivered to an endotracheal tube should be preheated and prehumidified.

Intubation is usually continued as long as the patient tolerates it. The tube is removed when the victim begins to cough or "buck on the airway." By this time his cough reflex is usually sufficient to ensure the expulsion of secretions. In any case it is undesirable to leave an endotracheal tube in place any longer than necessary. Modern endotracheal tubes with low-pressure high-volume cuffs have been maintained *in situ* successfully for continuous periods up to 3 to 4 weeks, but the usual duration of intubation is less than 1 week. Complications such as mucosal ulceration, tracheal wall necrosis and late stenosis are rare as long as the intracuff air pressure is held below 30 mm. Hg. (usually 20 to 25 mm.). An external pilot balloon on most commercial tubes is a very useful pressure-regulating device. When a tube is finally removed, the patient should be kept under careful observation because obstruction may occur immediately from laryngeal spasm or after a few hours from laryngeal edema; both complications are rare.

Esophageal obturator airway. In general, emergency medical technicians (EMTs) and other rescue personnel are not certified to pass endotracheal tubes. A safer and easier procedure, which has become popular in the field, is insertion of an esophageal obturator airway (EOA). Like the endotracheal tube, it protects the comatose patient against oropharyngeal obstruction and against aspiration of vomitus, and it provides a channel both for assisted ventilation (p. IV-9) and for the delivery of oxygen (p. IV-13). It is, however, used only as an emergency airway.

The esophageal obturator looks like a blind endotracheal tube with an inflatable cuff near the sealed tip. It is passed blindly through the mouth into the esophagus until the cuff lies somewhere in the middle third of the esophagus. Once the cuff is inflated, vomiting is impossible, and the gastric contents cannot be regurgitated or aspirated. The portion of the tube that lies in the pharynx has multiple perforations. Air or oxygen pumped or blown into the obturator airway flows out of these holes and through the glottis into the lungs, if it cannot escape through the mouth or nose. To seal the facial orifices, a special plastic oronasal mask with an inflated cuff is firmly pressed to the face; it has a port through which the obturator tube exits.

As soon as the unconscious victim reaches a medical treatment center, the esophageal obturator airway is removed. Because this act may induce gastric regurgitation, it is standard practice to pass a cuffed endotracheal tube *before* deflating and removing the esophageal obturator cuff. Unlike the obturator, a properly seated endotracheal tube prevents obstruction due to laryngeal spasm or edema. Because of this and other advantages, the endotracheal tube is the preferred airway.

Tracheostomy. Surgical relief of upper airway obstruction is necessary if more conservative measures are unsuccessful. Tracheostomy is performed instead of endotracheal intubation when the latter cannot be accomplished or cannot be tolerated. It is also indicated if the upper tract is severely inflamed, as, for example, after the ingestion of corrosive poisons. Tracheostomy, however, appears to lead to many more long-term complications, such as tracheal stenosis, than does endotracheal intubation.

Provided that the incision can be made promptly enough, tracheostomy can be and should be an orderly surgical procedure, involving sterile technique and local anesthesia. However, in near-terminal asphyxia due to or complicated by upper airway obstruction, the physician may have no choice except to perform an emergency tracheostomy without anesthesia and without sterile equipment. In most cases, however, it is safer and quicker to pass an endotracheal tube or even to insert a large gauge needle (15 G or larger) through the midline of the cricothyroid membrane, thereby gaining enough time to prepare for a regular tracheostomy. In the so-called needle cricothyrostomy, it is useful to insert a second needle, one for the continuous flow of oxygen and the other to allow for exhalation.

Two different operative procedures are in vogue to accomplish a definitive tracheostomy. The new technique is called a cricothyrostomy or a cricothyroidotomy. It is simpler, faster and easier than the standard operation. It has been performed often by nonsurgical medical personnel, and the incidence of complications is low, even when used for prolonged periods. Because of the small size of the cricothyroid membrane, however, it is impractical in patients younger than about 3 years.

To perform a cricothyrostomy, extend the neck if possible. Locate by palpation the cricothyroid membrane, which lies between the inferior prominence of the thyroid cartilage and the cricoid cartilage just inferior to it. Because these two cartilages are so close to the skin surface, the thickness of soft tissues to be penetrated and therefore the amount of bleeding are small. Prep the skin, and infiltrate the area with a local anesthetic solution. Make a vertical skin incision about 4 cm. long, usually at or just off the midline. Divide the platysma to expose the cricothyroid membrane, which is then opened with a short transverse incision. No cartilage is cut. The elasticity of the cricothyroid membrane allows the opening to be dilated enough to accommodate standard cuffed tracheostomy tubes. For most adults a 5- to 6-mm. tube is appropriate, which is slightly smaller than used for lower tracheotomies. Before it is introduced, withdraw any endotracheal tube that may be present, and remove any blood from the trachea by suctioning through the incision. After the tracheostomy tube is inserted, its lateral flanges can be sutured to the skin. After suctioning the trachea through the tube, inflate the cuff.

A "standard" tracheostomy formerly called for an incision through the skin and subcutaneous tissues from the laryngeal prominence (Adam's apple) to the suprasternal notch. A more conservative technique employs a 6-cm. long midline skin incision from the first to the fourth tracheal rings. The dissection is carried down to the anterior cervical fascia, through which the thyroid isthmus may be seen if hemostasis has been maintained by clamping or tying bleeders. The thyroid isthmus can often be avoided by pushing it upward and incising below this area. Otherwise the isthmus must be sectioned. A rectangular window about 2 by 4 mm. is cut in the anterior wall of the trachea by excising the anterior portion of one tracheal ring. The third ring is a recommended site, but others have been used. After bleeding is controlled and debris is removed from the tracheal mucosa through the stoma, a cuffed tracheostomy tube is inserted caudally and fixed in place.

With any type of tracheostomy or cricothyrostomy, it is essential to deliver only preheated and prehumidified air (or oxygen) to the tracheostomy tube or stoma. Stomal infections are not uncommon, in spite of aseptic surgical technique. The inflated cuffs on tracheostomy tubes present the same problems and concerns as those described above for cuffed endotracheal tubes (p. IV-5). Like patients with endotracheal tubes, patients with tracheostomies require suctioning of the trachea to remove secretions. Sterile suctioning catheters and gloves should be used. The suction pump should not be on while the catheter is being inserted through the tracheostomy tube, but intermittent suction should be employed during withdrawal of the catheter.

Bronchoscopy. Even in a tracheostomized patient, however, bronchoscopy with suctioning under direct observation sometimes proves to be the only satisfactory way of cleaning the major bronchi of obstructive plugs. In spite of bronchoscopy, secretions, edema and foreign bodies may remain in the smaller air passages to produce scattered regions of obstruction and consequent atelectasis. These regions may be identified by x-rays or by the absence of breath sounds over corresponding areas of the chest wall. Pounding these areas energetically with cupped palms helps to dislodge mucous plugs. Forceful hyperventilation by rebreathing may help. Drainage of the lower air passages is also promoted by rolling the patient from one side to the other periodically and by elevating the foot of the bed. For other techniques, see p. IV-15. Pneumonia is an almost inevitable complication of lower airway obstruction, but perhaps it is best to wait for frank signs of infection before instituting antibiotic therapy (p. IV-85).

Artificial Ventilation

If breathing movements are inadequate or absent, ventilatory assistance is imperative; it becomes possible only after major airway obstruction has been corrected. Because direct insufflation methods of artificial respiration are always available, they are generally employed first. Once the victim reaches a modern emergency treatment center, however, some kind of mechanical ventilatory device is likely to be used, especially a mask-and-bag system (p. IV-10). Manual methods of artificial respiration, such as the back-pressure arm-lift method of Holger-Nielson, are no longer recommended.

If the initiation of assisted ventilation does not cause cyanosis to disappear or subside markedly within a minute, an explanation should be sought promptly. If the circulation remains adequate by clinical criteria (*e.g.*, palpable pulses in carotid and radial areas), persistent cyanosis suggests unrecognized respiratory obstruction. Sometimes the fault is the technique of the therapist. If unexplained difficulties continue, other approved methods of artificial respiration should be tried.

Once the therapist has assured himself that his procedure of artificial ventilation is the best available, it must be continued until the patient responds or until cardiac action has ceased beyond any reasonable doubt. (For the management of cardiac arrest, see pp. IV-26–31). Below are summarized clinically useful methods of artificial respiration.

Mouth-to-mouth and mouth-to-nose insufflation. These methods (sometimes called direct insufflation methods) are ancient techniques of artificial respiration. Because of hygienic and esthetic objections, they did not become popular until their superiority was established conclusively. These procedures are more effective than any manual methods of ventilatory resuscitation, especially if there is partial airway obstruction, as is usually the case. Direct insufflation methods are always available, but, except for obstetricians, physicians largely ignored them until the 1950s. In November 1958 an *ad hoc* committee appointed by the National Academy of Sciences and the National Research Council reviewed data on artificial respiration obtained through research projects supported by the U.S. Department of Defense, the American Red Cross, and others. There was unanimous agreement that the mouth-to-mouth (or mouth-to-nose) technique of artificial respiration is the most practical one for ventilating an apneic victim of any age in the absence of special equipment or help from a second person, regardless of the cause of respiratory arrest.

Mouth-to-mouth and mouth-to-nose techniques have the advantage of providing both volume and pressure needed to inflate the victim's lungs immediately. These maneuvers also afford to the rescuer more information than is provided by any other method about the volume, pressure, and timing needed to ventilate the victim. This is an important advantage because the unconscious flaccid patient who is not breathing or who is underbreathing often has an upper air passage that is partially obstructed. As noted before (Fig. IV-1*A*), this obstruction is usually due to the base of the tongue sagging into the posterior wall of the pharynx when the mandible relaxes. Until the chin and tongue are properly positioned (p. IV-3), no method of artificial respiration can be performed successfully.

With upper tract obstruction promptly detected and corrected, mouth-to-mouth insufflation becomes a practical way of providing ventilatory assistance even to a person much larger than the therapist, without excessive fatigue. Furthermore, the operator is able to sense quickly any weak spontaneous respiratory movements and to synchronize his efforts with those of the patient. Although the therapist must hyperventilate moderately when resuscitating an adult victim, dizziness and other signs of hypocapnea are not usually a serious problem if the respiratory rate is slow, even when the procedure is continued for a long time.

The proper technique of mouth-to-mouth and mouth-to-nose resuscitation, as recommended by the American Red Cross, is illustrated in Fig. IV-2*A–D* and described in a series of explicit instructions below.

1. Roll the patient on his back so that the face is up (supine position). If foreign matter is visible in the mouth, wipe it out quickly with your fingers or a cloth wrapped around your fingers.

2. To prevent or relieve obstruction of the oropharynx due to sagging of the tongue, perform the head-tilt chin-lift maneuver (Fig. IV-1 on p. IV-3), and then keep the hands in place to sustain this position (Fig. IV-2*A*). Alternatively, a jaw thrust maneuver can be performed as follows: with the fingers of each hand behind the angles of the mandible, lift the jaw upward forcefully while tilting the head backward. The jaw thrust is best accomplished from a location at the top of the victim's head.

3. With the airway open, the rescuer should

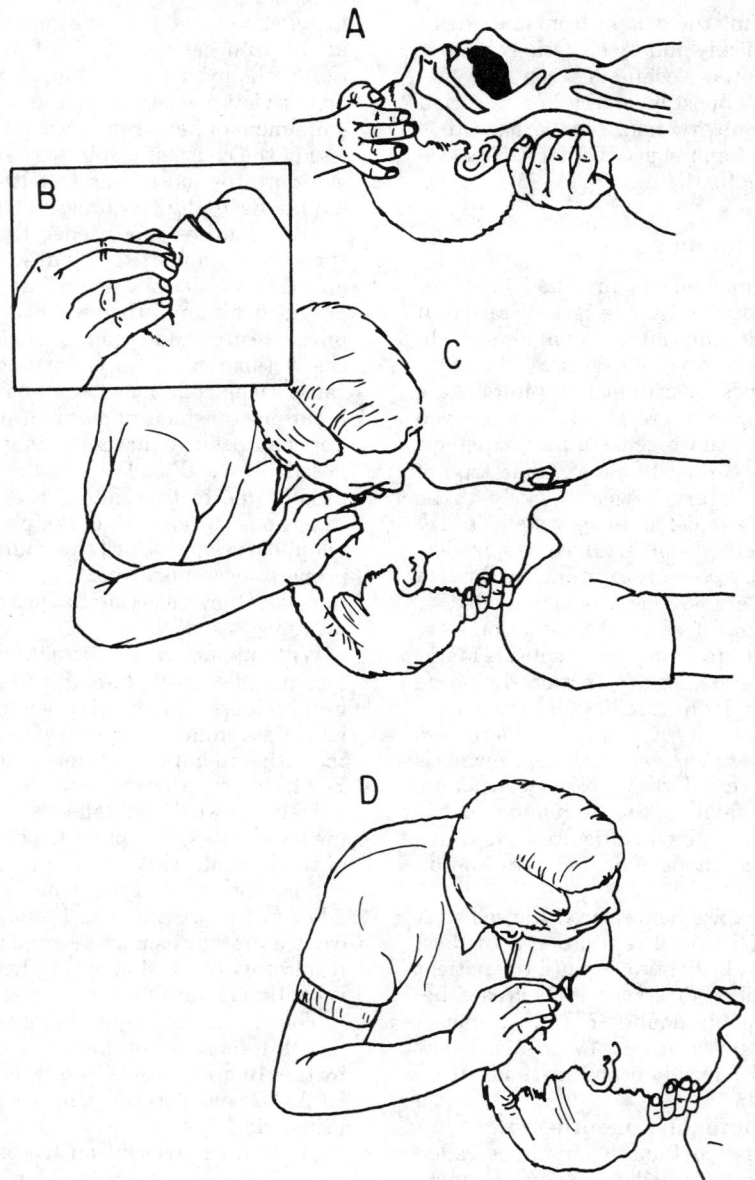

Figure IV-2. Mouth-to-mouth resuscitation, consisting of (*A*) the head-tilt chin-lift maneuver, (*B*) pinching to occlude the nostrils, (*C*) exhaling forcefully into the victim's mouth, (*D*) listening and watching the victim exhale.

be able to determine whether or not the victim is breathing. Listen by placing the ear next to the victim's mouth and nose, watch for movements of the chest and abdomen, and try to feel any exhaled air.

4. If no spontaneous breathing can be detected or if the respiratory movements are clearly inadequate, inflate the victim's lungs as described below (no. 5). The usual recommendation is to begin with 4 or 5 quick full breaths without allowing the

victim's lungs to deflate fully in-between breaths. Then stop for 5 to 10 seconds to check the carotid arterial pulse. If no heart action can be detected in this way, the diagnosis is cardiac arrest, and cardiopulmonary resuscitation must be instituted (see p. IV-26). Otherwise proceed with no. 5.

5. Take a moderately deep breath, and at the same time occlude the victim's nose by pinching the nostrils shut (Fig. IV-2*B*).

Instead of pinching, it is sometimes possible to block the nostrils with your cheek. Keep your mouth open and place it over the victim's mouth as firmly as you can in order to prevent air leakage (Fig. IV-2*C*). Exhale forcefully, blowing air into the patient's mouth while watching the chest rise. Usually air can be blown through the victim's teeth even though they may be clenched, but, in case of difficulty, try the following instruction (no. 6).

6. As an alternative to instruction no. 5, close the victim's mouth by pinching his lips with your fingers and place your mouth over his nose in order to deliver air. This is known as the mouth-to-nose method.

7. As soon as you see the chest rise, you have probably delivered an adequate breath. Remove your mouth, turn your head to the side, and listen for the return rush of air caused by the passive elastic recoil of the victim's chest (Fig. IV-2*D*). With the adult patient, repeat the operation every 5 seconds (12 breaths per minute) until he breathes spontaneously at an adequate rate and depth.

8. When the victim is an infant or young child, proceed as above, but in this case place your mouth over both his mouth *and* nose to make a relatively leak-proof seal, and breathe out only a shallow puff of air. The rate should be maintained at about 20 per minute.

9. If air exchange is inadequate, recheck the position of the head and jaw. If obstruction persists, quickly turn the victim on his side and deliver several sharp blows between the shoulder blades in the hope of dislodging foreign matter or perform an abdominal thrust. To accomplish the latter, straddle a supine victim and place the heel of one of your hands over the epigastrium (not over the xiphoid process), with the other hand on top of it. Compress the victim's abdomen with a rapid upward thrust of your hands and repeat several times if necessary. Because this procedure is apt to induce vomiting, the victim's head should be positioned to the side in the hope of avoiding aspiration. Again sweep your finger through his mouth to remove obstructing material.

10. As with any method of positive-pressure lung inflation, mouth-to-mouth insufflation may force air into the stomach and lead to gastric distension. The latter is apt to compromise pulmonary ventilation and the systemic circulation and may lead to vomiting and consequent aspiration. When and if a tympanic bulge appears in the epigastrium, prompt decompression is advisable. A manual technique is always available. Place the victim on his side (preferably his left side), and turn his head slightly downward, but avoid any severe angulation that might impede the ejection of vomitus from the mouth. Exert moderate pressure in the epigastrium so that gas and gastric fluid are expelled through the mouth. Then clean the mouth (see no. 1 above) and continue the resuscitation.

Mouth-to-tube and mouth-to-mask methods. These methods of artificial respiration are simply variants on the mouth-to-mouth technique. In all cases the therapist's expired air is used to inflate the patient's lungs, which then deflate passively when the operator removes his mouth. Various pieces of simple equipment can be used to make the process of insufflation easier, but since these devices are not necessary, no time should be wasted locating them. As with mouth-to-mouth resuscitation, one seeks to deliver a larger-than-normal tidal volume of about 1 liter (10 to 15 ml./kg.) to an adult victim, at a somewhat slower-than-normal frequency of 10 to 12 breaths per minute.

A properly positioned endotracheal tube provides a nearly ideal airway, and the therapist can readily inflate the victim's lungs by blowing into the tube. In order that this air does not escape back around the tube before the lungs are inflated, it is desirable and in most cases essential to use an endotracheal tube with an inflatable rubber cuff to form an air seal in the trachea (p. IV-4). The esophageal obturator airway can be used like the endotracheal tube for mouth-to-tube ventilation, provided that the special oronasal mask is available to seal the nose and mouth (p. IV-5). With more elaborate devices the therapist's hands can be freed for other duties. For example, by mounting a specially designed twin-valve assembly on the end of an endotracheal tube and then connecting it to the operator's mouth by a flexible rubber hose, artificial respiration can be continued while external cardiac massage is performed (p. IV-27), but this apparatus is not generally available.

If a tracheostomy has been performed (p. IV-6), the tracheostomy tube can be used in the same way as an endotracheal tube for mouth-to-tube resuscitation. In a person who has had a laryngectomy, there may be no tube in the tracheal stoma. By pressing his mouth around the stoma, the therapist can usually perform effective mouth-to-stoma resuscitation. In an occasional "laryngectomee," however, the larynx has not been removed, and the trachea still communicates with the pharynx and mouth. To perform mouth-to-stoma insufflation under these circumstances, the operator's hands must be used to seal the victim's nose and mouth.

Unlike mouth-to-tube resuscitation, mouth-to-mask techniques require the operator to take precautions against pharyngeal obstruction due to a retracted tongue (p. IV-3). Mouth-to-mask resuscitation is not widely practiced because its principal advantage over mouth-to-mouth or mouth-to-nose insufflation is simply an esthetic one. Because of occasional difficulties in achieving a good seal between the face and mask, some operators regard mouth-to-mask resuscitation as more difficult and less reliable than the mouth-to-mouth procedure.

The converse opinion, however, is also held, especially with the availability of a small oronasal mask called a "pocket mask" (Laerdal Medical Corp., Armonk, N.Y. 10504). This clear plastic device has an inflated cuff to provide an airtight seal to the face and a small inlet tube through which a continuous flow of oxygen can be introduced, if a supply is available. The mask is held in place by a strap around the victim's head, but when the operator blows into an open port in the mask, he uses both hands to clamp the mask tightly to the victim's face so that the air does not escape but is forced into the lungs. As before, the patient exhales passively when the operator removes his mouth. To prevent the tongue from obstructing the pharynx, the neck should be extended (head tilted backward) and the mandible should be supported in a forward position (p. IV-3). With the pocket mask, many therapists consider mouth-to-mask resuscitation to be easier than the established mouth-to-mouth technique, and tidal volumes in excess of 1 liter can usually be achieved.

Masks of other designs have been recommended. Perhaps the most widely available is the oronasal mask used for clinical anesthesia. By removing the bag, a large port (22 mm. diameter) becomes available on the mask; the operator periodically blows air through it, as described above. In a related procedure he both exhales and inhales through a flexible rubber tube (preferably equipped with a mouthpiece) connected to the mask. Here the mask must be modified by drilling into it an air vent which can be alternately opened and blocked by the operator's thumb. In this unusual technique the therapist necessarily rebreathes to some extent, and so hypocapnia and respiratory alkalosis are avoided.

Still more elaborate equipment has been tested. Valves on a specially designed mask enable the operator to inhale fresh air (with some rebreathing) while the victim exhales through a different port. Another interesting variant is illustrated in Figure IV-3. Here a therapist with a gas mask and canister is safely ventilating an apneic subject while both of them are in a toxic atmosphere. Although this apparatus is not marketed and is therefore unavailable even to first

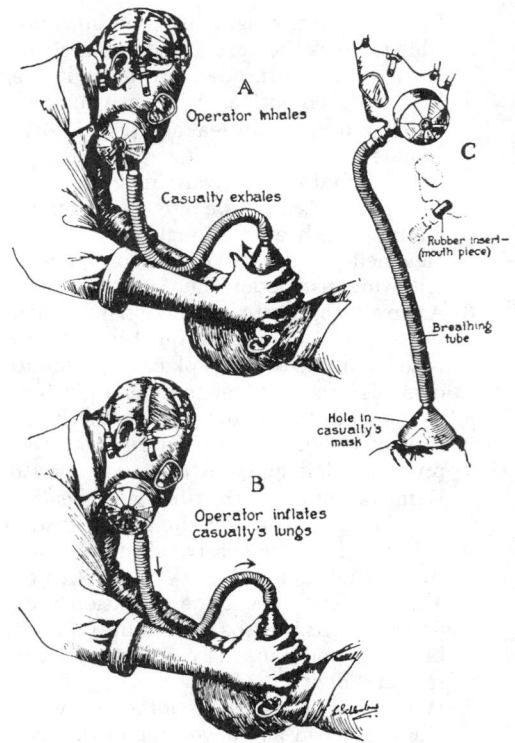

Figure IV-3. Special equipment for ventilating an apneic patient in a toxic atmosphere. (Courtesy of Directorate of Medical Research, Chemical Warfare Laboratories, Army Chemical Center.)

aid squads, its utility is obvious when the victim cannot be evacuated, as in gas warfare or large-scale industrial accidents. Further research and development in the technology of resuscitation needs to be encouraged.

Mechanical devices for ventilatory resuscitation. Artificial respiration by mechanical devices is easier and less tiring than by direct insufflation. For the patient, however, the principal advantage of mechanical ventilators is that they allow oxygen-rich gas to be administered. Anyone who requires ventilatory assistance can profit by supplemental oxygen. Of course a patent airway must be established first in all instances (pp. IV-2–7).

For short-term resuscitation, especially in the field, manually operated devices are popular. Widely used are several completely portable hand-operated bag-and-mask resuscitators. Between the bag and mask there is a small chamber in which one-way valves are mounted to eliminate rebreathing. These devices employ environmental air or medicinal oxygen and can deliver an adequate volume to the victim with each manual squeeze of the bag. The operator senses the degree of inspiratory resistance by the pressure required to squeeze the bag, and he ascertains the degree of inflation by watching the chest wall rise. The rubber bag is so constructed that it promptly self-inflates when the operator relaxes his hand. When oxygen is used, it flows continuously through the valve assembly between the mask and the bag, and so high flow rates are required (15 to 20 liters/min.). By removing the mask, the bag can be connected through the valve assembly directly to an endotracheal tube.

A similar, simple resuscitative apparatus that can be found in the emergency room of most hospitals consists of an anesthesia face mask connected to a reservoir bag by means of a right-angle elbow with a nipple for the oxygen supply. With the mask held firmly on the face and oxygen running to fill the bag, active inflation of the lungs can be obtained by manual compression of the bag. In this case the bag is not self-inflating, and a continuous flow of oxygen is required to keep the bag full.

Bag-and-mask resuscitation, however, requires considerable practice. The self-inflating apparatus described above is rather bulky, and inexperienced operators find it awkward to hold the mask tightly on the victim's face with one hand while squeezing the bag with the other. Tests have shown that many operators generate tidal volumes of no more than 500 or 600 ml., in contrast to the 1-liter volumes that can often be achieved with mouth-to-mouth or mouth-to-mask resuscitation. For these reasons, other kinds of portable ventilators are preferred by many rescuers.

One popular device is a hand-operated demand-valve assembly available in several designs, particularly the Robert Shaw design, which is made by several companies. It connects the hose from the pressure regulator of a medicinal oxygen tank to an oronasal mask or endotracheal tube. When the operator's thumb activates the valve, oxygen quickly inflates the victim's lungs. By watching the chest wall, the therapist quickly senses how long to keep his thumb on the demand valve, but as a safety feature, the apparatus has a blow-off valve set to open at a pressure of 50 or 60 cm. water. Again exhalation is passive through an expiratory port that prevents rebreathing. As noted below, gastric distension can be generated by any method of assisted ventilation based on positive inspiratory pressures; it may be particularly common with demand-valve devices because they deliver brief but rather high-pressure pulses. Because the oxygen is not pre-humidified, this and related techniques of resuscitation are intended to be used for short periods only.

In addition to these manually operated devices, many automatic or semiautomatic portable resuscitators have been marketed. All machines involve a positive-pressure inspiratory phase and a passive expiratory one. Most operate on the principle that pressure from a cylinder of oxygen, properly reduced, forcefully inflates the lungs. Inflation is controlled by a release valve which is actuated at a predetermined pressure and interrupts the flow of oxygen. If resistance to the flow of oxygen is encountered, the pressure releases too early to effect lung inflation, and the device starts to recycle at a high frequency, in some cases with a chattering sound. Portable resuscitators of this general design were formerly carried in the vehicles of many municipal fire departments, FAST squads and ambulances, but they have been largely replaced with simpler and more reliable devices, notably masks with hand-operated oxygen demand valves (above).

For more prolonged ventilatory assistance, particularly of patients with endotracheal or tracheostomy tubes, still more elaborate machines are available. Manufacturers include Bear, Bird, Emerson, Monaghan, Ohio, and Puritan-Bennett. These machines provide humidified oxygen at various concentrations and temperatures (which are often adjustable), and they serve to control and to monitor various respiratory parameters. Of course they are less portable than the devices described above, or not portable at all, but because of wheels they are mobile. When properly adjusted, these machines are both safe and reliable. Although a full-face or oronasal mask can be used, a cuffed endotracheal tube is the usual mechanism for connecting the patient to this kind of apparatus.

In general these hospital-type ventilators are electrically or pneumatically powered and serve to inflate the lungs by generating intermittently a positive pressure in the upper airway. Expiration is passive, but it may be retarded by adding a resistance or exit pressure that slows exhalation. Cycling is automatic and controlled by a preset pressure (as described above), a preset volume, or a preset time. Some ventilators can be operated in more than one of these modes. Furthermore, some machines can be set to function as either a controller or an assistor of ventilation. In the former mode the device cycles automatically and does not follow the patient's spontaneous respiratory movements. In the latter it generates a positive pressure to augment each tidal volume that is initiated by negative airway pressure produced by the patient's spontaneous inspiratory efforts. Mixed modes of operation are possible and commonly used as, for example, intermittent mandatory ventilation.

Several studies have demonstrated that machines that deliver a specified tidal volume (volume-preset or volume-limited ventilators) are preferable to pressure-set variable-volume devices. At least they are more effective in ventilating patients with reduced pulmonary compliance from such states as atelectasis, pneumonia, pulmonary edema and adult respiratory distress syndrome (p. IV-14). High airway pressures may be required, and these ventilators permit high (and variable) pressures, but an upper limit is set to prevent barotrauma of the lungs. Among the desirable features of volume-preset machines are built-in alarm systems, the precise control of oxygen concentrations and the option to introduce positive end-expiratory pressure (see below). These features are difficult and in some cases impossible to achieve in pressure-preset apparatuses.

In resuscitating an adult victim, a volume-preset ventilator is usually set initially to deliver each minute 10 to 12 tidal volumes, each of about 10 to 15 ml./kg. (body weight). Arterial blood gases are then measured to ascertain the adequacy of the ventilation, and appropriate adjustments are then made in the machine controls. Even with this somewhat larger-than-normal minute volume, the arterial Po_2 may be unacceptably low because of such pulmonary lesions as interstitial edema and/or atelectasis.

Alveolar collapse is believed to occur during expiration when there is a deficiency of pulmonary surfactant, as is probably true in most victims of the adult respiratory distress syndrome (ARDS). To overcome this collapse as well as the abnormally high alveolar-to-arterial oxygen gradient and consequent hypoxemia, a ventilator may be set to operate in the PEEP mode ("positive end-expiratory pressure"). In effect, exhalation occurs against a machine-generated pressure that is set between 5 and 30 cm. water. To fill the lungs, the ventilator generates even higher pressures during the inspiratory phases (30 to 60 cm. water); thus the airway pressure is above barometric pressure throughout the respiratory cycle. With PEEP an oronasal mask is often unsatisfactory, and a cuffed endotracheal tube is far preferable.

Because expiration is still passive (i.e., does not involve contraction of the expiratory muscles), the end-expiratory lung volume (functional residual capacity) is elevated by PEEP, and thus alveoli are stabilized above their collapsing volumes. The selection of an appropriate positive end-expiratory pressure can be difficult. Pressures that are excessive may induce pneumothorax, and they tend to reduce cardiac output by impeding venous return into the thorax. In spite of these problems, PEEP is an important feature of ventilatory assistance for victims of ARDS (p. IV-14).

Besides the ventilators described above, there are Drinker or tank-type respirators ("iron-lungs"), as well as the cuirass and breathing jacket. They are used chiefly for patients with weakness of the respiratory muscles in whom respiratory tract obstruction is judged to be only a remote possibility (e.g., post-poliomyelitis victims). The ventilatory reserve power of these machines is generally inadequate whenever the airway resistance is high or the lung-thorax compliance is low. For this and other reasons, they are almost never used in clinical toxicology. Based on an entirely different principle, electrophrenic stimulators, when available, may be effective in the management of apnea of central nervous origin, but success with this method apparently required much practice, and the device is not used in current practice. High frequency ventilation is a new but still experimental technique beyond the scope of this manual.

Except for the electrophrenic respirator, all of the resuscitation devices listed above employ positive-presssure inspiration, i.e., pressure within the mask or airway exceeds that outside the chest. One possible consequence, if the patient is not intubated with a cuffed endotracheal tube, is that air or oxygen is forced down the esophagus into the stomach, particularly if flow resistance is encountered at or below the glottis. By elevating the diaphragm, gastric distension is apt to compromise pulmonary ventilation and the systemic circulation, and it may also lead to vomiting and consequent aspiration. The therapist must check for this complication by examining the epigastrium frequently; when distended, it must be decompressed immediately. Manual methods are available (p. IV-9). Occasionally decompression can be accomplished by passing a Levine tube, but a stiffer gastric tube is preferable. Sometimes a long nasotracheal tube is introduced intentionally into the esophagus, and a Levine tube is then easily threaded through it. With modern methods of resuscitation, gastric dilatation is regarded as a major problem since any procedure effective in ventilating the lungs in the presence of abnormal airway resistance is necessarily capable of inflating the stomach.

Oxygen Therapy

Probably all patients who must be assisted in their respiratory efforts could profit from the simultaneous administration of oxygen at higher concentrations than in air. Such oxygen, however, is not usually essential, and artificial respiration should never be delayed in order to find a source of it.

There are at least six clinical situations, however, in which oxygen therapy is unquestionably beneficial. They occur under the following circumstances: when traumatic injury interferes with full respiratory excursions, whether spontaneous or induced by a resuscitator; when respiratory tract obstruction cannot be entirely eliminated; when there exists an impediment to the diffusion of oxygen across alveolar walls, as in pulmonary edema; when the oxygen transport mechanism of the blood is inadequate, as in severe anemia or carbon monoxide poisoning; when the cardiac output is abnormally low, as in cardiopulmonary resuscitation with external cardiac compression; and when oxygen utilization by tissues is defective, as in cyanide or sulfide poisoning.

In all of these situations it is worthwhile to maintain in the inspired air an oxygen concentration of 40% or higher, i.e., at least twice that in normal air. The lower value can be achieved by feeding pure oxygen continuously from a tank of compressed gas at a rate of 6 liters/min. through a nasal cannula which terminates just behind the soft palate. A more convenient and more comfortable way to deliver oxygen is through a set of nasal prongs, which are soft plastic funnel-shaped tubes inserted just inside each nostril and held in place by a strap behind the ears. Oxygen flow rates of 1 to 4 liters/min. usually result in inspiratory concentrations of 24 to 36% O_2, whereas flow rates of 4 to 6 liters/min. yield 30 to 45%, but actual values vary with the patient's breathing pattern. Similar low-to-moderate O_2 concentrations can be achieved by delivering oxygen to the entry port of a simple oronasal mask, i.e., one without valves and without a reservoir bag.

With nasal or oronasal administration, the oxygen should be humidified by bubbling it through sterile water before it enters the catheter or mask. This precaution is even more crucial when oxygen is deliverd by endotracheal or tracheostomy tube. Some devices use aerosolizers to ensure high humidity.

Except for a mouthpiece and noseclip or an endotracheal tube, only oronasal masks of special design ("non-rebreathers") allow oxygen concentrations as high as 90 to 95% to be attained regularly in inspired air. Many designs are available; they are constructed of rubber, rigid plastic, malleable plastic, or combinations of these materials. In these high-flow systems, pure oxygen is fed in continuously at a rate fast enough to prevent deflation of the reservoir bag during inspiration (usually more than 10 liters/min). One-way valves prevent rebreathing and so avoid dilution of incoming oxygen by expired air. Other models possess demand valves so that oxygen flows only during inspiration and so the supply is conserved.

Some masks are so constructed that inspired O_2 concentrations can be regulated at specified values by controlling the rate at which pure O_2 flows into the device (HAFOE or venturi masks); levels of 24 to 48% can be attained with com-

mercially available models. Some designs allow positive pressures to be created within the mask, especially during expiration; see "Adult Respiratory Distress Syndrome" below for a discussion of positive-pressure oxygen therapy, i.e., oxygen therapy with positive airway pressure.

Masks are uncomfortable and tend to be used only for short-term therapy. Most delirious patients tolerate hoods and tents better than face masks. The same is true of infants and young children, for whom the hood (sometimes called a face tent) is especially useful. Even when properly used, however, hoods and tents (and especially tents) seldom allow inspiratory oxygen concentrations above 40 to 50% and then only at high flow rates (above 10 liters/min.)

In almost all patients the administration of pure oxygen is safe for at least several hours. Without good indications, inspiratory oxygen concentrations should not be held at 90 to 100% for more than 12 hours, because inflammation may develop within the respiratory tract (cough, sputum, substernal pain). If oxygen therapy is expected to be prolonged, a concentration of 60% is generally preferable to 100%, or the two levels can be used alternately. The lower concentration is entirely satisfactory in most cases, but sometimes pure oxygen is essential (e.g., traumatic chest injuries, pulmonary edema, CO poisoning) although in some of these cases (e.g., ARDS), the use of PEEP (p. IV-12) or of CPAP (p. IV-15) allows one to use lower oxygen concentrations. Even during short periods some patients with chronic pulmonary disease (e.g., emphysema) tolerate pure oxygen poorly for several reasons (e.g., respiratory acidosis, marginal atelectasis, loss of hypoxic drive).

Inspiratory oxygen tensions higher than 1 atmosphere can be obtained by placing the patient in a compression chamber and raising the ambient pressure until the partial pressure of oxygen exceeds 1 atmosphere (hyperbaric oxygen). Oxygen tensions of 2 to 2.5 atmospheres have been recommended for treating severe carbon monoxide poisoning. At least two problems are encountered. First, so few compression chambers are available in the United States that this form of therapy is rarely feasible. Second, signs and symptoms due to adverse effects of oxygen on the lungs are commonly encountered after 6 to 8 hours at a Po_2 of 2 atmospheres. The effects may include pulmonary edema, hemorrhage, pneumonia, hyalin membrane formation, and alveolar cell dysfunction. At higher pressures the latency is even shorter. Above 2.5 atmospheres the first manifestations of oxygen toxicity are usually neural rather than respiratory.

In principle, hyperbaric oxygen should be helpful in treating patients with severe pulmonary edema and other acute diffuse pulmonary diseases that induce hypoxia. In practice, however, much of this hypoxemia is due to ventilation-perfusion imbalance, and here oxygen at 1 atmosphere with positive airway pressure is likely to be superior to hyperbaric oxygen without extra airway pressure (p. IV-15).

Victims of poisoning do not require the respiratory stimulus of exogenous carbon dioxide. The practice of administering CO_2-O_2 mixtures to correct underbreathing is ill-advised for at least two reasons: in states of intoxication the respiratory center may be relatively insensitive to even dangerously high concentrations of CO_2, and an abnormally high level of arterial CO_2 inevitably exists in any patient who underventilates. Even though the addition of CO_2 to inspired air leads to marked hyperpnea, the procedure produces or intensifies, but never corrects, a respiratory acidosis. Underbreathing requires ventilatory assistance, not CO_2.

The continuous administration of CO_2 (usually 2 to 5% in O_2) was once claimed to be beneficial in carbon monoxide poisoning. Carbon dioxide here serves both as a respiratory stimulant and a promoter of carboxyhemoglobin dissociation. Even in this case, however, the administration of CO_2 is no longer recommended because of the dangers of respiratory acidosis. Indeed, exogenous CO_2 has no legitimate therapeutic uses.

Adult Respiratory Distress Syndrome

Acute diffuse infiltrative lesions of the lungs may arise from the inhalation of a variety of poisonous gases and vapors. The X-ray findings reflect an abnormal accumulation of fluid in the alveolar walls or alveolar spaces, together with variable numbers of inflammatory and alveolar cells. The fluid is derived from the blood plasma. In contrast to cardiogenic pulmonary edema, hydrostatic pressure in pulmonary capillaries is not elevated (pulmonary capillary wedge pressure less than 20 mm. Hg), but the edema fluid tends to be much richer in protein than that of the cardiac patient. Two interrelated functional deficits are responsible for the patient's distress: hypoxemia because of poor gas exchange in some lung regions with consequent ventilation-perfusion imbalance and a decrease in lung compliance because of interstitial edema with a consequent rise in the effort and work of breathing. Airway resistance may also rise due to mucosal edema, mucus accumulation and smooth muscle contraction. The illness is called the adult respiratory distress syndrome (ARDS).

Sometimes a latency of many hours separates the toxic exposure from the first appearance of signs and symptoms. An increase in the respiratory rate may be the first sign of impending ARDS. Gradually (or in some cases abruptly) other signs and symptoms emerge, including restlessness, anxiety, cough, expectoration, chest tightness, substernal pain, dyspnea, cyanosis, rales and rhonchi. Hypoxemia and occasionally CO_2 retention develop. After exposure to the pyrolysis products of some plastics (e.g., Teflon) or the fumes of some metals (e.g., cadmium), fever may be a prominent feature of the illness.

After a known exposure, physical exercise must be avoided. Even in an asymptomatic individual, complete rest should be prescribed for at least 24 hours. At the first evidence of impending ARDS, oxygen administration should be commenced by the quickest and most expeditious means available. Soft nasal prongs are widely used, and oxygen is first delivered to them at very slow flow rates (0.5 to 1 liter/min.). Adjustments in the flow rate are made as dictated by measurements of arterial blood Po_2, Pco_2 and pH. If inspiratory O_2 concentrations above 40% are required to sustain the arterial Po_2 above 60 mm. Hg, a high-flow oronasal mask with valves is usually substituted for the nasal prongs, as described above. In mild cases, positive airway pressure breathing is not usually necessary (for more severe poisonings, see below).

Because of their recognized anti-inflammatory actions, glucocorticoids have been recommended often in the therapy of ARDS, especially when due to an exogenous poison, such as kerosene or one of the irritant gases. Current opinion, however, holds that these hormones are ineffective in this and related pulmonary disorders, except for those with a primary allergic origin. This unfavorable opinion is supported by controlled studies of kerosene poisoning in dogs and baboons. Because adrenocorticosteroid therapy leads often to troublesome adverse effects, a trial course in ARDS is unwarranted.

Bacterial pneumonia is a common late complication of ARDS, and at least in adult patients, this condition may represent one of the few defensible indications for prophylactic antibiotic therapy (pp. IV-85–97). The frightened or anxious patient deserves mild sedation; a small dose of diazepam or one of its congeners is likely to be beneficial, but full doses of any sedative should be avoided. Unless the pulmonary disorder is of cardiac origin, morphine is used only with extreme caution, if at all, but sometimes an intravenous dose of 2 to 6 mg. is helpful.

If pulmonary edema and respiratory distress intensify, the patient should sit upright, and a high concentration of oxygen should be delivered with positive airway pressure. This form of treatment is sometimes referred to informally as positive-pressure oxygen therapy. A more correct and less ambiguous phrase is "continuous distending airway pressure," of which two forms are recognized. PEEP or "positive end-expiratory pressure" is the name used when the procedure includes active ventilatory assistance (see p. IV-12). If the patient is not underbreathing, one uses a technique called CPAP or "continuous positive airway pressure." In either case, the therapy serves to correct or reduce atelectasis by producing a larger-than-normal end-expiratory lung volume (p. IV-12). In this way ventilation-perfusion imbalance is lessened, alveolar-arterial oxygen gradients are reduced, and the arterial Po_2 rises.

Several other events contribute to the improvement. Although the absolute gas pressure within the lungs is elevated only slightly, the increase also favors the diffusion of oxygen across edematous alveolar walls. Perhaps positive pressure within the lungs also promotes the resorption of fluid in the alveoli, but it is more likely that the effect is on the rate of edema formation. Thus the elevated thoracic pressure tends to retard venous return, with the result that the pulmonary capillary hydrostatic pressure and filtration rate are lowered. In any case the improvement in the arterial Po_2 means that the inspiratory O_2 concentration can be gradually lowered from peak levels of 90 to 95% to less than 50%, where oxygen toxicity is unlikely (p. IV-13).

CPAP is usually accomplished by connecting the patient to the same hospital-type multipurpose respiratory machine used for PEEP (p. IV-12), which is then operated in the CPAP mode. In this mode the machine generates in the airway an almost steady positive pressure that can be set within the range of 0 to 20 cm. water (sometimes even higher). With an adult patient, the usual connection is through an indwelling endotracheal tube with an inflated cuff (p. IV-4). In a young child, the cuff is generally left uninflated. In neonates, CPAP can be generated through nasal prongs.

Although less satisfactory and less comfortable, CPAP can also be produced by using a special high-flow oronasal mask equipped with elaborate exhalation valves that are interchangeable. Depending upon the valve rating and upon how tightly the mask fits the patient's face, oxygen (or air) flowing into the mask at recommended flow rates generates within the mask a positive pressure of 5, 7.5, 10, 12, 15, or 20 cm. water (the fit is not always good enough to achieve the highest pressure levels). Whenever the patient takes a breath, the mask pressure tends to drop momentarily by about 20%, but the pressure is almost constant throughout the respiratory cycle. Of course this positive pressure facilitates inspiration, but expiration requires some degree of active effort by the patient. High mask pressures lead to elevated pulmonary and intrathoracic pressures that may impede venous return and reduce cardiac output. They may also force air down the esophagus into the stomach and produce dangerous degrees of gastric dilatation (p. IV-9).

In some cases of ARDS flow resistance in the small pulmonary air passages contributes significantly to the victim's dyspnea. Narrowing of the lumen may be due to one or more of the following disorders: the accumulation of mucous or serous secretions, mucosal edema, submucosal hyperemia and bronchospasm. Secretions are presumably responsible for the coarse rhonchi that can be heard through the chest wall, but bronchospasm is the usual cause of prolonged expiratory wheezes. A patient with such a wheeze cannot be expected to tolerate CPAP, at least not until his bronchospasm is suppressed.

Bronchospasm can often be corrected by oral inhalation of a β-adrenergic agonist. To avoid excessive cardiac stimulation, one of the selective $β_2$ agonists is usually chosen. Four such drugs are not marketed in the United States: albuterol, isoetharine, metaproterenol and terbutaline; they are available as solutions for aerosolization ("nebulization") and/or dose-metered pressurized inhalers. Epinephrine is similarly packaged for inhalation; although its excitatory effects on the heart may be undesirable, the mucosal vasoconstriction that results from its α-adrenergic activity may be helpful in reducing air flow resistance. If one or more of these adrenergic agonists fails to produce prompt relief, intravenous aminophylline is often tried. The recommended loading dose of 6 mg./kg. is infused over a period of about 30 minutes. If the therapeutic response is judged inadequate and no signs of toxicity appear (p. III-17), an additional 3 mg./kg. of aminophylline can be infused slowly. To administer aminophylline concurrently with a $β_2$-adrenergic agonist is said to be safe and effective.

Respiratory tract secretions are an inevitable feature of ARDS. They may be thick and mucoid or thin and frothy. Upper tract secretions can usually be coughed up and expectorated, but thick fluids in the smaller air passages cannot be raised so easily. After bronchospasm is corrected, various forms of chest physiotherapy are employed to help dislodge mucus plugs within bronchioles and terminal airways. For example, therapists use cupped hands to percuss the chest and chest wall vibrators with large contact pads to vibrate the thorax and lung parenchyma. These procedures are accompanied by a maneuver known as postural drainage, consisting of laying the patient on his side and then tilting the body headdown to such an angle that the contralateral mainstem bronchus assumes an almost vertical orientation. Accumulated secretions then flow downward into the trachea within a few seconds or few minutes. The intended result is a paroxysm of coughing with the production of sputum. If the patient begins to choke instead of expectorate, he should be promptly suctioned (p. IV-4).

Inspissated secretions indicate the need to increase the humidity of the inspired air, to check the patient's state of water balance and to correct any dehydration (p. IV-64). To facilitate the removal of especially viscous secretions, acetylcysteine (Mucomyst) may be administered as an aerosol through a face mask, mouthpiece or tracheal stoma, but many therapists believe that the drug is effective only if its solution is instilled into a bronchus when thick material is encountered during bronchoscopy. Acetylcysteine serves to reduce the viscosity of respiratory tract mucus by opening disulfide cross-linkages. This mucolytic, liquifying action may increase the volume of tracheobronchial secretions and intensify coughing. In case of choking, a suction machine should be readily available (p. IV-4).

Large quantities of frothy or foamy exudate within the respiratory tract presents a different problem. Presumably such proteinaceous fluid is derived by excessive filtration through damaged alveolar capillaries and venules. Suctioning may be imperative (p. IV-4), but the use of ethyl alcohol as an antifoaming agent is no longer recommended. A possible therapeutic role for other surface-active agents does not appear to have been explored. Currently accepted forms of therapy are directed toward lowering hydrostatic pressures in the pulmonary microvasculature with the hope of reducing rates of filtration and thus controlling the volume of the exudate. As noted above, positive airway pressure (PEEP and CPAP) tends to lower pulmonary blood pressure by slowing venous return. If possible, pulmonary vascular pressures should be monitored with a Swan-Ganz catheter to assess the efficacy of this and other treatments. Besides oxygen therapy with CPAP, other measures that may be useful to reduce edema formation in the lungs are the same as those employed against cardiogenic pulmonary edema (p. IV-22), namely rapid dehydration by administration of "loop diuretics" (p. IV-22), the use of nitroprusside or nitroglycerin to decrease preload (p. IV-22), phlebotomy and possibly rotating venous tourniquets (p. IV-23).

CIRCULATION

Two major categories of circulatory disorders follow exposures to toxic chemicals: those due to faulty vasomotor tone or abnormal capillary permeability, and those due to inadequacy of the heart as a pump.

Blood Vessels

Angiitis, thrombosis, internal bleeding, excessive capillary transudation, and all degrees of vasodilation and vasoconstriction have resulted from exogenous poisons. The most common complication is profound and persistent hypotension, leading to the familiar syndrome of peripheral vascular collapse or shock. Two major types must be distinguished, to be designated in this report as vasogenic shock and oligemic shock. In both instances there is believed to be a disparity between the circulating blood volume and the volume capacity of the vascular circuit. In vasogenic shock the vascular volume is too large, and in oligemic shock the blood volume is too small. In both cases the return of venous blood is insufficient to enable the heart to maintain an adequate cardiac output.

Vasogenic shock. This condition might better be described as shock due to vasomotor paralysis or paralytic vasodilatation. In some cases it is due to a defect in the responsiveness of vascular smooth muscle to neural and hormonal stimuli, as in quinidine and quinine posioning. In other cases the primary disorder appears to be depressed activity in the vasomotor centers of the brainstem, with the result that blood vessels are deprived of normal tonic vasoconstrictor stimuli. In either case there is hypotension due to widespread vasodilatation without primary loss of circulating fluid. Paralytic hypotension cannot be distinguished reliably from oligemic shock by physical signs, although the former is not so consistently accompanied by thirst or profound hemoconcentration and the skin is not always cold and clammy.

Inactivity of the brainstem vasomotor centers has long been held responsible for hypotension in poisonings by hypnotic and depressant drugs. At least with respect to barbiturates this explanation is no longer tenable. M. H. Weil and H. Shubin (Diagnosis and Treatment of Shock, Williams and Wilkins, Baltimore, 1967) have demonstrated that normal or even high peripheral vascular resistance accompanies the hypotension of barbiturate intoxication, indicating that the vasomotor centers, sympathetic vasoconstrictor nerves and arteriolar smooth muscles are functionally intact. Circulatory failure in barbiturate poisoning appears to be due to a complex mixture of oligemic and cardiogenic shock (p. III-55), not primarily as failure of vasomotion. On the other hand, the hypotension in chlorpromazine, reserpine and clonidine poisonings is probably due to a failure to maintain sympathetic vasoconstrictor tone.

It should be noted, however, that arterioles and related resistance vessels are not the only parts of the vascular circuit that are normally subjected to important vasoconstrictor influences. The compliance of small and large veins depends upon venomotor tone that is sustained under normal circumstances by both humoral and neural stimuli. Thus, vasogenic shock may represent a failure of vasoconstriction in precapillary resistance vessels or in postcapillary capacitance vessels or both. For example, nitrite shock is recognized to be due almost exclusively to dilatation of venules and veins (p. III-315). The fact that resistance vessels appear to function normally in most victims of barbiturate poisoning does not exclude the possibility of paralytic venodilatation as a significant element in the genesis of the characteristic circulatory failure.

Two types of pharmacological agents are available in the control of vasogenic shock: peripherally acting vasoconstrictor drugs and centrally acting analeptic drugs. The latter are employed to raise the level of spontaneous or reflex activity in vasomotor centers of the central nervous system. In subconvulsive doses they are effective only when the central nervous system is depressed or inhibited. Even here they are useless if the poison has rendered the vascular smooth muscle insensitive to the adrenergic nerve transmitter substance. The actions of analeptic drugs are complex and variable; their effects on the blood pressure are usually transient and frequently undependable. In fact they are probably less effective as pressor agents than as respiratory stimulants. For information about the use of analeptic drugs, see Table IV-3 (p. IV-42).

More precise and more dependable control of paralytic hypotension can usually be secured by administering peripherally acting vasoconstrictor drugs. Even in situations where the vascular smooth muscle is relatively insensitive to constrictor stimuli, as in quinidine poisoning, an effective dose can sometimes be found. To what extent the resulting pressor response is due to cardiac stimulation rather than vasoconstriction is usually difficult to surmise. Furthermore, the relative importance of arteriolar and venous constriction in the drug management of vasogenic shock has not been adequately assessed. Most of the clinically useful drugs are of the adrenergic type; they mimic or substitute for the sympathetic neurotransmitter. For example, phenylephrine (Neo-Synephrine) hydrochloride in doses of 2 to 10 mg. or methoxamine (Vasoxyl) hydrochloride in doses of 15 mg. can be injected intramuscularly; in much smaller doses both can also be given by slow intravenous injection.

Probably the drug of choice, however, is levarterenol (l-norepinephrine). It lacks the vasodilator properties of epinephrine. Given intravenously its effects are immediate but transient. Excellent control of the arterial blood pressure can be obtained by the slow infusion of levarterenol (e.g., Levophed, 4 ml. or 4 mg. in 1 liter of saline or glucose solution, given intravenously at an approximate rate of 1 ml. per minute). It is apparent that this procedure demands frequent observations of the blood pressure, preferably at 3- to 10-minute intervals or continuously if possible. Cardiac arrhythmias are seldom encountered but are a potential source of danger. Severe local lesions due to ischemia occur if the solution is allowed to extravasate. If such extravasation is recognized promptly and stopped, local necrosis can often be prevented by infiltrating the subcutaneous area with a solution of phentolamine (Regitine) or of piperoxan (Benodaine), each in a dose of about 5 mg. dissolved in 10 or 20 ml. of isotonic saline.

Because no cumulative effects are recognized at the recommended rates of administration, these infusions may be continued almost indefinitely. The procedure, however, cannot be recommended without reservation because neither cardiac nor renal responses of a chronic nature have been thoroughly explored. If the infusion is continued for many hours or days, it becomes advisable on terminating therapy to decrease gradually the rate of administration, because abrupt withdrawal often leads to a precipitous fall in blood pressure.

Oligemic shock. Oligemic shock is a consequence of absolute hypovolemia i.e., a critically small circulating blood volume. Depending upon its genesis, it is variously known as surgical shock, hemorrhagic shock, and traumatic shock. In chemical intoxications, abnormal permeability of blood vessels may cause the leakage of prodigious amounts of plasma, with or without red blood cells, into tissues, serous cavities, and particularly the lumen of the gastrointestinal tract. The extent of concealed hemorrhage and of plasma depletion by leakage is frequently underestimated. The same is true of severe losses of body water and salt (p. IV-66), which may also lead to oligemic shock.

The usual progression of signs and symptoms includes restlessness, thirst, hemoconcentration, hypotension, oliguria, grayish pallor, and a cold, moist skin. The mental state may vary from excitement to stupor. Peripheral pulses are usually weak and rapid. These classical signs and symptoms, however, may not appear until the venous return and cardiac output become severely reduced. One of the earliest manifestations of shock is a sustained decline in blood pressure when the subject changes from the recumbent to the sitting position (this sign is more significant in a young patient than an elderly one). In contrast, the arterial pressure is generally well maintained while the patient stays recumbent, until the blood volume is reduced by more than 20%.

Therapy is principally an endeavor to repair and to maintain an adequate circulation by restoring the circulating volume, whether the deficit is due to loss of blood or to exudation of plasma. Vasoconstrictor drugs are rarely effective or necessary because compensatory reflexes generate and usually maintain maximal vasoconstriction in this syndrome. Indeed, there is evidence that this reflex constriction may itself be harmful by compromising the blood flow in critical organs. This evidence has led to the suggestion that adrenergic blocking drugs such as phenoxybenzamine (Dibenzyline) may be useful in treating oligemic shock that proves refractory to liberal intravenous replacement therapy. Late in the course of shock, however, vasodilatation may occur spontaneously. Unless this complication occurs, vasoconstrictor drugs should be avoided.

The ideal replacement fluid in the treatment of oligemic shock is blood plasma or whole blood. They alone provide important blood coagulation factors which other replacement fluids may deplete by dilution. Until the specific need of each patient can be determined, transfusions with whole blood are preferable. If a rise in the venous hematocrit is subsequently demonstrable, plasma or a plasma expander should be substituted for blood. Isotonic saline (0.9% NaCl) is less valuable than plasma; although it may correct hemoconcentration and restore the circulating volume, these actions are usually transient. Isotonic saline, however, has an invaluable role in the emergency control of shock while preparations are made for transfusions with blood, plasma, or plasma substitute. Moreover, in the patient whose circulatory collapse is due exclusively to losses of body water and salt (e.g., by extensive vomiting, diarrhea, etc.), the administration of isotonic saline or a balanced salt solution (Ringer's) may be the only treatment required (p. IV-66). In fully established oligemic shock, the average patient probably requires about 20 ml. of whole blood or plasma expander per kg. of body weight; in some cases 10 ml. per kg. is sufficient.

Besides transfusion reactions due to immunologic incompatibilities (mismatching), whole blood transfusions present a small but distinct danger of inducing the viral disease known as homologous serum hepatitis. The same risk exists with the use of single-donor human plasma, whether frozen or fresh. A convenient test for the presence of hepatitis B antigen makes it possible to identify and discard specimens containing the B virus. At present, most post-transfusion hepatitis is said to be of the non-A, non-B variety, for which no screening test exists. The incidence of serum hepatitis, however, is only 2 to 3 cases per 10,000 transfusions in many parts of the United States (e.g., New Hampshire and Vermont).

On the other hand commercial pooled human plasma carries such a high risk of hepatitis B virus that it is not used as such in current clinical practice. Gentle heat treatment (e.g., 60°C. for 10 hours) is said to inactivate the virus, but the resulting product, sold as a 5% solution labeled "plasma protein fraction (human)," has fallen into disfavor because its rapid infusion has caused unexplained hypotension. Most pooled human plasma is used to prepare specialized protein fractions useful for passive immunization and for treating blood coagulation defects. Another important product of the fractionation process is serum albumin, which is freed of hepatitis virus by gentle heat sterilization. Human serum albumin (5% sterile solution) is an excellent though expensive substitute for plasma in treating hypovolemic shock.

Except for the expense of serum albumin and the danger of hepatitis with blood plasma, these proteins are thought to be preferable to all other plasma expanders. Stroma-free hemoglobin is the subject of vigorous current investigation as a plasma substitute. Globin, the protein derived from hemoglobin, has been tested and found inferior; many lots proved to be nephrotoxic. By acid hydrolysis, bone gelatin can be reduced to molecular sizes which are appropriate for intravenous use. When so processed, gelatin is a safe, stable, and cheap plasma expander, which is well retained in the circulation but is eventually metabolized completely to amino acids of nutritional value. Because of gelation at room temperature, the infusion equipment must be kept warm during the administration of this material. At present, none of these proteins is used clinically as a plasma expander in the United States.

Polyvinylpyrrolidone (PVP) is an inert synthetic polymer and probably the cheapest of all plasma expanders. It is said to have been used extensively by German troops in World War II. It is an effective and apparently safe therapeutic agent in the control of shock. Although no specific tissue injury has yet been ascribed to PVP, a potential hazard must be acknowledged because this polymer is not metabolized and yet is excreted only slowly by the kidneys. Consequently large amounts are stored chiefly in the reticuloendothelial system for periods of many years, and chronic disease arising from this tissue retention has not been thoroughly excluded.

PVP has many commercial uses (see Section II), but it is rarely, if ever, used as a plasma volume expander in the United States.

Dextran, a mixture of large, branched polymers of glucose, is a cheap, stable and generally safe plasma expander. Partial hydrolysis and fractionation have led to the availability of two forms of dextran; one has an average molecular weight of 70,000 or 75,000, the other of 40,000. Both are available in sterile, pyrogen-free isotonic saline or 5% dextrose; the concentrations are 6% (Dextran 70) and 10% (Dextran 40). Both solutions have been used extensively and found to be effective plasma expanders when infused intravenously. About half of an infused dose is excreted by the kidneys over a period of 24 hours; the rest is slowly oxidized over a period of several weeks. There appears to be no long-term storage in tissues. Dextran, however, is antigenic, and untoward reactions (e.g., itching, urticaria, joint pain, etc.) occur in about 10% of individuals who receive it. In massive doses, however, antibody production does not usually occur, and the incidence of anaphylaxis is very low. Dextrans have been stockpiled for national defense. Hetastarch (also known as hydroxyethyl starch) resembles dextran and is also available clinically as a plasma volume expander. Only further clinical experience, however, can clarify the proper roles of dextrans and hetastarch in the management of shock.

Any available peripheral vein is adequate for the administration of replacement fluid in shock. Intra-arterial transfusions have no compelling advantages over intravenous ones. Subcutaneous routes of fluid administration are distinctly undependable in peripheral vascular collapse. When transfusions are administered intermittently through a needle, a superficial vein at one of the following sites is usually chosen: back of hands, forearms, antecubital fossa, or ankle. Only a large needle should be used (15 to 18 gauge), and it should be taped to the skin. It is usually advisable to restrain the limb as well. If a satisfactory superficial vein cannot be seen or palpated, even after application of a tourniquet, a surgical cut-down is necessary. After surgical exposure, the vein should be cannulated, preferably with a polyethylene tube rather than a metal needle because the latter is likely to produce local phlebitis and thrombosis if kept in situ for long periods. A polyethylene catheter is useful, therefore, in two situations: when one is unable to insert and maintain within a vein a needle of proper size, and when one anticipates a need for frequent or continuous intravenous therapy over a period of one or more days.

Superficial veins at many sites have been catheterized successfully, particularly veins in the forearm, the cephalic vein at the shoulder, the external jugular vein, and, in infants, various scalp veins. For large-bore catheters the internal jugular vein has become a popular channel. The preferred vessel for a cut-down, however, is usually the saphenous vein, which is often palpable on the anteromedial aspect of the lower leg or on the dorsum of the foot, and which in the adult can be located specifically 1 cm. anterior to and 1 cm. superior to the medial malleolus. At this site the saphenous vein is found superficial to the fascia by dissecting through the skin and subcutaneous tissues. The vein is tied, and a small incision is made in the vessel wall proximal to this tie. A polyethylene tube is chosen with a diameter as large as can be accommodated easily by the exposed vein. To ensure sterility, catheters are best stored in 0.1% aqueous solution of benzalkonium chloride (e.g., Zephiran). The appropriate catheter is inserted into the vein through the incision and threaded for a distance of several inches toward the heart. The tube should be held in place by a tight ligature encircling the cannulated portion of the vein. A second tie anchors the catheter to the body surface where it passes through the skin incision. Between infusions, the cannula is left in situ filled with a dilute heparin solution and sealed with a short stylus in the free end.

The rate of administration of intravenous replacement fluid depends upon the severity of the deficit. In routine blood transfusions, a slow rate is always employed, especially for the first 50 ml. which are best injected no faster than 2 ml./min. In oligemic shock, however, fast rates of administration are frequently required. Provided that whole blood has been properly cross-matched, it may be given to the patient in severe shock as rapidly as the cardiac action allows. With conventional equipment the gravity method may prove too slow, even when a large needle is used and when the container of blood is elevated as high as possible. The rate of flow can be hastened by stripping the tube from above downward with a lubricated thumb and forefinger. Sometimes a three-way metal stopcock and syringe can be used to pump blood into a peripheral vein. Also available are special transfusion sets that sustain very high flow rates. In most cases, however, the conventional gravity method of transfusion is satisfactory because an injection rate of 1 liter/hour usually serves to maintain an adequate circulation.

The transfusion is stopped when signs of shock disappear and when urine flow is resumed at a rate of at least 40 ml./hour. The transfusion should also be terminated if rapid or labored breathing, flushed facies, venous distention, a gallop rhythm, or pulmonary rales develop.

Another procedure commonly employed in the treatment of shock is to elevate the foot of the bed or the patient's feet so that his head is several inches lower than his legs. This measure promotes the return of blood from the large venous reservoirs of the legs and abdomen. The patient is covered with one or more blankets, but all attempts to restore a normal skin temperature by the local application of heat should be strictly prohibited. Oxygen inhalation (p. IV-12) is frequently employed; not all authorities agree that it is a useful measure, but with proper technique it certainly can do no harm. Drugs should be used only cautiously and sparingly in these patients, and the only dependable route of administration in the presence of severe circulatory collapse is the intravenous channel.

Heart

Heart failure. Chemical agents may impair the circulation by the production of many types of cardiac lesions. The mechanisms that initiate and control the beat may become deranged (see discussion of cardiac arrhythmias, p. IV-23), or the heart muscle itself may lose some of its contractile strength. A myocardial injury may be direct or indirect, diffuse or focal, reversible or irreversible. Regardless of the nature of the cardiac disorder, heart failure appears whenever the pumping action does not keep pace with the circulatory requirements of the body.

Cardiac failure manifests itself in many ways. Any one of at least three clinical syndromes may result from a cardiac injury of toxic origin. The three syndromes are a hypotensive shocklike state, congestive heart failure, and acute pulmonary edema. Although the distinctions are somewhat artificial, this classification serves to emphasize that three different programs of therapy are available. The clinical management of each syndrome is outlined below.

Hypotension of cardiac origin (cardiogenic shock) must be distinguished from vasomotor paralysis and from oligemic shock, because treatments differ even though these conditions present many clinical features in common. In the shocklike state of diffuse myocarditis or focal myocardial infarction, various signs and symptoms usually direct attention to the heart. For example, pain, anxiety, and a sensation of oppression in the chest are common. The arterial blood pressure is low; the peripheral veins may or may not be collapsed. The arterial pulse is soft, small, and readily compressible. The heart rate is usually fast and often irregular. Electrocardiograms may reveal conduction defects, arrhythmias, and injury currents indicative of myocardial ischemia or necrosis. The heart sounds have a poor quality, and a gallop rhythm is usually present.

Perhaps the most specific finding, however, is cardiac dilatation; it may be evidenced by a diffuse and feeble apical thrust which is displaced to the left or is lost entirely. Dilatation of the left ventricle sometimes causes relative insufficiency of the mitral valve and a consequent systolic murmur. Elevation of venous pressure is another cardinal finding. Any shocklike syndrome accompanied by venous hypertension is almost certainly of cardiac origin. With the exception of venous congestion and perhaps cardiac dilatation, the disorders outlined above may be either causes or consequences of peripheral vascular collapse, but whenever they appear early in the course of circulatory insufficiency, it is reasonable to assume that the primary defect is within the heart.

The first and principal aim of treatment is a reduction of all circulatory stresses so as to ensure maximal rest for the heart. Oxygen consumption and tissue metabolism are minimized by the maintenance of complete bed rest. If recumbency causes labored breathing or other distress, rest in a chair is prescribed. A patient's evaluation of his own comfort is probably the best index to the proper resting posture. Even the mildest exercise (e.g., self-feeding) is usually prohibited. Ideally, continuous cardiac monitoring should be instituted.

Among other attempts to decrease the circulatory load, the therapist prevents or corrects any abnormal elevations in the circulating blood volume. In contrast to the hypotension of peripheral vascular collapse, vasoconstrictor drugs and intravenous fluids are strictly prohibited in the usual conservative regimen. Sodium chloride in any form is withheld, and even the intake of water is sometimes restricted. Occasionally, however, hypovolemia occurs in cardiogenic shock, and it may become necessary to correct volume deficits by the slow and cautious infusion of saline, plasma or albumin solutions while monitoring the central venous pressure.

Elevations of body temperature are corrected by antipyretic drugs and by other appropriate measures, because a fever raises the circulatory requirements of all tissues. For the same reason infections are suppressed by intensive antibiotic therapy (p. IV-86). Whenever possible, all types of mental excitement are avoided and anxieties are minimized. Mental and physical repose and adequate sleep can usually be ensured by the regular administration of simple sedatives or tranquilizers such as chlordiazepoxide, diazepam and hydroxyzine. Pain is vigorously suppressed with analgetic drugs.

Occasionally pain of cardiac origin justifies a trial with a coronary vasodilator such as sublingual or intravenous nitroglycerin. For intravenous therapy, ampuls containing 50 mg. nitroglycerin in 10 ml. of an alcohol-glycol solvent are marketed under the name Tridil. The contents must be diluted with 500 ml. 5% dextrose or 0.9% sodium chloride before injection. The infusion rate must be precisely controlled with a pump that has an exact but adjustable delivery. The recommended dose rate is 5 μg./min. at the onset, to be increased every 3 to 5 minutes until an effect is encountered. The optimal dose differs widely among individuals.

Cyanosis calls for prompt oxygen therapy (p. IV-12), which may also suppress pain and dyspnea. Severe arrhythmias and tachycardias require one of the antifibrillary drugs (see p. IV-25). Any systemic metabolic disorder that might contribute to myocardial weakness must be corrected, including such disturbances as hypoglycemia, hypokalemia, hypocalcemia, and severe acidosis. In cases of diffuse myocarditis or myocardial infarction, digitalis and other cardiac glycosides are often ineffective and sometimes even dangerous, at least in conventional doses. If used cautiously, however, they have limited value in both preventing and treating heart failure associated with myocarditis or infarction.

If, in spite of the therapeutic efforts enumerated above, the patient fails to rally, the problem may be that the blood pressure is too low to sustain an adequate coronary circulation. Under these circumstances the therapeutic stratagem may have to be altered radically. Peripheral vasoconstrictors are seldom effective, but drugs that temporarily enhance the contractile strength of the heart may raise the arterial blood pressure, improve tissue perfusion, and initiate progressive clinical improvement. Agonists of the β_1-adrenergic receptor have been used for this purpose.

Although a potent β-agonist, isoproterenol has two major undesirable and potentially dangerous effects; it tends to produce considerable tachycardia and widespread peripheral vasodilatation, so that the mean arterial blood pressure may fall instead of rise. Dopamine and dobutamine cause much less tachycardia and little or no change in peripheral vascular resistance in doses that exert positive inotropic actions on the heart and raise the cardiac output. These drugs are ineffective by mouth and both are rapidly metabolized. For a sustained action, a continuous intravenous infusion is required. Besides cardiogenic shock, intractable congestive heart failure refractory to full doses of digitalis is sometimes responsive to these infusions. They are not administered, however, to patients with tachyarrhythmias or with oligemia until these disorders are corrected.

Dopamine hydrochloride (Intropin) is marketed in ampuls, to be dissolved and diluted in isotonic saline or dextrose solution to a concentration of 400 to 800 μg./ml. The recommended rate of the initial infusion is 2 to 5 μg./kg. per minute, to be increased gradually to 20 to 50 μg./kg. per minute as required. Dobutamine hydrochloride (Dobutrex) should also be diluted to concentrations of 250 to 1000 μg./ml. before in-travenous infusion at recommended rates that range from 2.5 to 15 μg./kg. per minute. During infusions with either drug, patients should be monitored carefully and continuously. If possible, the following measurements should be performed: arterial blood pressure, ECG, pulmonary wedge pressure, central venous pressure and cardiac output.

Congestive heart failure is a similar syndrome arising from subacute or chronic inadequacy of the heart as a pump, usually due to valvular disease, to weakness of the myocardium, or to an excessive frequency of cardiac contraction. Associated with a low cardiac output and insufficient tissue blood flow, the renal excretion of water and electrolytes becomes defective. Over a period of several days or several weeks, salt and water accumulate in the body in excessive amounts. These events lead to edema, congestion, cough, dyspnea, orthopnea, anorexia, nausea, venous distention, anxiety, and profound weakness, among many other signs and symptoms.

Whatever the original cause of congestive failure, the chief corrective measure, aside from removing the cause whenever feasible, is the administration of digitalis or a related cardiotonic glycoside. When properly used, these drugs are safe and usually effective; in the presence of congestive heart failure, the only contraindication to their use is digitalis poisoning itself. Standardized preparations of whole-leaf digitalis (from *Digitalis purpurea*) used to be given orally, but the isolated and purified glycosides such as digoxin and digitoxin are preferred in current practice and are essential for parenteral administration.

With digitalis and its congeners, the proper dose must be individualized. For optimal effect this dose must often approach the toxic range, but no rational excuse exists for maintaining a patient in severe digitalis poisoning (for its recognition and treatment, see p. III-146). For each of the common purified cardiac glycosides and popular mixtures thereof, an average "digitalizing dose" and a maintenance dose have been suggested in Section II. In most cases the initial digitalizing dose should be divided and given as aliquots over a period of a few hours or a few days. If a prompt response is essential, a full dose can usually be administered at one time with a reasonable degree of impunity. For example, the "digitalizing dose" of digitoxin for an average adult is 1.0 to 1.5 mg. orally or intravenously. It produces maximal cardiac effects within 4 to 12 hours. The action is persistent (2 to 3 weeks) and cumulative, and its maintenance usually requires only 0.1 mg. daily.

A more prompt response can be obtained with intravenous digoxin, but in very urgent cases intravenous ouabain (G-strophanthin) should be substituted. An average "digitalizing dose" of ouabain (0.3 to 0.5 mg. in adults) produces cardiac actions which begin within 5 minutes, are maximal in 0.5 to 2 hours, and are over in about 24 hours. No single dose schedule is adequate for all patients, but because these drugs are often lifesaving, they should never be withheld from a patient in congestive heart failure.

Ancillary treatment includes all of the measures specified under "hypotension of cardiac origin" (p. IV-20). Specifically, rest, oxygen therapy, sedation, and restrictions on the intake of salt (and rarely of water) are proper and useful procedures.

To further reduce cardiac work, especially in the patient whose congestive heart failure is associated with cardiac pain, vasodilator therapy has been explored. Both sodium nitroprusside and nitroglycerin have been given intravenously to lessen preload and afterload, i.e., to lower an elevated diastolic filling pressure by promoting venodilatation and to lower the arterial pressure by causing arteriolar dilatation. Nitroprusside is capable of accomplishing both of these goals, with the result that pulmonary vascular congestion is relieved and cardiac output is enhanced, at least in some cases. Nitroglycerin is apt to relieve pulmonary congestion without any prominent effect on cardiac output, presumably because its dilator action is stronger on capacitance vessels (veins) than on resistance vessels (arterioles). To utilize either of these agents safely and effectively, it is important, if not essential, to monitor the ECG, arterial blood pressure, intracardiac pressures, pulmonary wedge (capillary) pressure and cardiac output. For this purpose right heart catheterization is performed, and a thermister-tipped pulmonary floating catheter (Swan-Ganz catheter) is introduced. The way nitroglycerin is administered intravenously is described on p. IV-20.

As noted above, an entirely different stratagem is sometimes adopted in cases of intractable congestive heart failure refractory to full doses of digitalis. Thus, instead of reducing cardiac work to allow the heart more time for repair, an attempt is made to enhance cardiac output and coronary blood flow by infusing inotropic drugs such as dopamine or dobutamine (p. IV-21). Because of the risks of inducing tachycardia, arrhythmias and angina, these drugs have a very limited role.

In most cases of congestive heart failure, diuretic drugs are appropriate, even though the improved renal blood flow that results from digitalis itself may stimulate the excretion of extra salt and water. Oral doses of urea, theophylline, theobromine, acidifying salt such as ammonium chloride, acetazolamide (Diamox) and other carbonic anhydrase inhibitors, all are capable of promoting a clinically useful diuresis, but the most sustained and most dependable diuresis is that induced by one of the thiazide drugs (chlorothiazide and hydrochlorothiazide), by ethacrynic acid or by furosemide.

Ethacrynic acid (Edecrin) and furosemide (Lasix) have entirely replaced mercurial diuretics in current practice. Both of these agents are capable of inducing intense diuresis whatever the acid-base status of the patient. In some patients these so-called "loop diuretics" have been effective when other diuretics have failed. Both are active by mouth, and both exhibit a rapid onset of action (usually within half an hour) and a comparatively short duration of action (6 to 8 hours). For an even more rapid effect a lyophilized preparation of sodium ethacrynate is available in vials; when reconstituted by adding 50 ml. of isotonic glucose or saline, it can be slowly injected intravenously (0.5 to 1.0 mg./kg.). This solution is too irritating for administration by other parenteral routes. Furosemide is also available in ampuls for slow intravenous injection (adult dose 20 to 40 mg. in 2 to 4 ml.); this preparation can also be given intramuscularly. If a prompt diuresus results, the dose of furosemide can be repeated 2 hours later. If not, the dose can be increased in increments of about 20 mg. to a daily maximum of 200 to 400 mg.

Because of rapid and massive depletion of body water and electrolytes, both ethacrynic acid and furosemide may induce such adverse reactions as weakness, dizziness, lethargy, leg cramps, anorexia, thirst, vomiting, diarrhea, and mental confusion. Some electrolyte replacement therapy, especially supplements of potassium, may be required (see pp. IV-72–73).

Even with a good diuretic response, massive pleural effusion and ascites generally warrant thoracentesis and abdominal paracentesis, respectively. Net losses of body water and salt can also be accomplished by intermittent peritoneal lavage (p. IV-56) with any commercially available balanced salt solution that has been rendered hyperosmotic by the addition of glucose in a concentration of 4 to 7%. In this way 1 liter or more of body water can be removed within an hour or two.

Cardiogenic pulmonary edema may develop as one aspect of congestive heart failure, but it often occurs acutely in persons who show no signs of systemic visceral congestion or peripheral edema. The etiology of this condition is not simple and much remains to be explained, but according to one reasonable hypothesis, pulmonary congestion and eventual edema develop because the injured or diseased left ventricle pumps less blood than the right. If this explanation is sound, the condition is properly called acute left ventricular failure.

Probably pulmonary edema of cardiac origin

is always preceded by a period of hypertension and vascular congestion in the pulmonary circuit. Sometimes pathological reflexes arising from congested lungs cause bronchoconstriction and wheezing ("cardiac asthma"). With or without recognized prodromata, pulmonary edema may appear with dramatic suddenness and alarming intensity. Once established, signs and symptoms of cardiogenic pulmonary edema are essentially indistinguishable from those of the adult respiratory distress syndrome (p. IV-14).

Good supportive treatment involves all of the measures outlined for the adult respiratory distress syndrome (ARDS) due to irritant gases (pp. IV-14–16). These measures include complete rest, oxygen therapy with CPAP (p. IV-15) or some other form of positive airway pressure such as PEEP (p. IV-12), bronchodilator therapy when indicated (p. IV-15), postural drainage (p. IV-15) and airway suctioning as tolerated. In addition, a small intravenous dose of morphine sulfate (2 to 6 mg. in an adult) may slow the respiratory rate, reduce dyspnea and improve oxygenation. Rapid "digitalization," preferably with intravenous ouabain (p. IV-21), is desirable if the patient has received no form of digitalis previously, but these glycosides are not so effective in acute pulmonary edema as in the more chronic syndrome of congestive heart failure.

If the patient's condition worsens and hypoxemia intensifies, more drastic measures are required. The appearance of large amounts of frothy exudate in the respiratory tract suggests an excessively high filtration pressure in the alveolar capillaries. Unless the plasma protein levels are low, a high filtration pressure implies pulmonary hypertension. This inference can and should be verified by the introduction of a Swan-Ganz catheter (p. IV-22). Therapy is then directed toward reducing pulmonary hypertension and so decreasing the rate of lung edema formation. One stratagem is to decrease venous return by inducing intense venodilatation or by blood trapping with rotating venous tourniquets. Another stratagem is to reduce the blood volume by phlebotomy of 1 or 2 pints or by producing systemic dehydration.

The rapid induction of a body water deficit can be accomplished by peritoneal lavage or hemodialysis with a hypertonic fluid (see above), but unless there are other indications for dialysis, it is easier and safer to use one of the rapidly acting, high-ceiling diuretic drugs, such as intravenous ethacrynic acid or furosemide. As noted above, serum electrolyte levels must be carefully monitored during the resulting diuresis because hypokalemia may become severe enough to require K^+ administration.

Drugs that produce systemic venodilatation lower the diastolic filling pressure and stroke volume of the right ventricle, so that the pulmonary capillary pressure (wedge pressure) almost invariably falls. As noted on p. IV-22, both sodium nitroprusside and nitroglycerin relieve pulmonary hypertension when infused intravenously, and so they reduce the likelihood of cardiogenic pulmonary edema. Furthermore, they probably reduce pulmonary capillary filtration rates and so serve to moderate an existing pulmonary edema whatever its etiology. It is important, however, to monitor responses to these drugs carefully (p. IV-22). For information about the technique of infusing nitroglycerin, see p. IV-20.

An entirely different procedure that has a similar therapeutic goal is the use of rotating venous tourniquets to trap blood. One starts with blood pressure cuffs on one arm and both thighs. The cuff pressures are held at about the diastolic arterial level. Every 20 minutes one of the cuffs in sequence is removed and reinflated on the unoccupied limb. The procedure is an old one, but no data on its efficacy were located.

Attempts have been made to control pulmonary edema by the intravenous administration of a hypertonic solution of glucose or sucrose (e.g., 50 to 100 ml. of a 50% solution). These injections may have transiently beneficial effects, but they are rarely worthwhile and are sometimes dangerous. Hypertonic human serum albumin has been recommended. In principle, a protein solution should be more effective than solutions of highly permeant solutes like glucose, but it too should be avoided whenever the pulmonary edema is likely to be due to abnormally high capillary permeability, as in many cases of the adult respiratory distress syndrome (p. IV-14).

Cardiac arrhythmias. Many abnormalities of rate and rhythm are encountered in victims of poison. These disturbances may be due to diffuse or focal myocarditis, with or without necrosis, but often there is no intrinsic cardiac lesion. In these instances the primary derangement lies within those portions of the autonomic nervous system that control the cardiac mechanisms. An electrocardiogram is required for a definitive diagnosis of most abnormal rhythms, but a competent bedside examination is often adequate to rule out the more dangerous abnormalities. In any case, an ECG tells nothing about the etiology of the disorder; it does not distinguish between those of toxic and those of nontoxic origin.

An abnormal mechanism of beat is comparatively benign if the ventricles are driven at a tolerable rate by an atrial pacemaker (or by the atrioventricular node). In this category are most cases of atrial tachycardia, atrial premature beats, atrial fibrillation, and all types of sinus rhythm. Most patients with these disorders require no treatment directed specifically toward the heart. The offending chemical agent, if any, should be removed, and rest and sedation are generally indicated. Sometimes digitalization is advisable to protect the ventricles from an excessive rate of stimulation by overactive atria.

In three types of situations, specific treatment is necessary for disordered mechanisms of beat. The first category includes any patient with an extremely fast ventricular rate, whether regular or not. Whatever its cause, extreme tachycardia may lead to severe circulatory embarrassment and eventually to cardiac failure. Treatment of the latter is outlined above. Exhaustion and failure of the heart, however, can often be prevented by measures which moderate or terminate the tachycardia.

In most cases dangerously high heart rates originate in supraventricular foci (*e.g.*, atrial tachycardia, flutter, and fibrillation). In each of these disturbances a normal sinus rhythm may be restored by one of the so-called "antifibrillatory" drugs (see below), with or without the prior administration of a rapidly acting cardiac glycoside. However, in many patients and especially those with paroxysmal atrial tachycardia and paroxysmal fibrillation, a normal sinus rhythm can be restored more quickly and more safely by inducing reflex vagal discharge or by injecting a drug that mimics vagal actions on the heart. Such drugs are neostigmine (i.m.) and methacholine (s.c.).

Rarely supraventricular tachycardias and arrhythmias are refractory to all of these measures. Some of the more desperate of these refractory cases can be treated by electric countershock delivered, as in ventricular fibrillation (p. IV-30), through electrodes applied to the chest wall where the skin has been prepared with liberal amounts of electrode paste. For such a potentially painful procedure, the patient must first be anesthetized (*e.g.*, i.v. thiopental sodium) or at least intensively sedated; for this purpose intravenous diazepam (Valium) has proved useful in a dose of 5 to 10 mg. injected over a period of 1 to 2 minutes. The therapist must be prepared to insert an artificial pacemaker if the physiological pacemaker in the sinoatrial node fails to become active when the abnormal beats are terminated. Another hazard of countershock is the distinct possibility of inducing ventricular fibrillation. The threat is said to be less with an instrument that delivers direct current (DC) rather than AC pulses, especially if the timing of the stimulus can be controlled by the patient's own ventricular electrical complex so as to avoid the "vulnerable period," which occurs during the T-wave of the ECG. Various machines that generate these so-called "synchronized" pulses can be procured (p. IV-30). In any case, the physician who elects this form of treatment must be ready to defibrillate the ventricles if necessary.

The second type of disordered cardiac mechanism requiring active therapy is extreme bradycardia. This is equivalent to transient cardiac standstill, which leads to repeated episodes of syncope and sometimes convulsions (Adams-Stokes syndrome). It can be prevented by any drug that enhances the rate. For example, the sinus bradycardia encountered occasionally in anticholinesterase poisoning (*e.g.*, parathion) responds to large doses of atropine. When the ventricular rate is slow because of complete atrioventricular heart block (AV block), a trial dose of atropine sulfate (*e.g.*, 1 to 2 mg. intravenously or intramuscularly) may be advisable; it serves to restore a supraventricular rhythm whenever the block is due to abnormal vagal activity or its equivalent.

Even if the block cannot be removed by this or other measures, an unacceptably slow ectopic pacemaker in the ventricle can often be accelerated by the cautious administration of epinephrine (0.1 to 0.4 ml. of 1:1000 epinephrine hydrochloride, i.m.) or other sympathomimetic drugs (*e.g.*, ephedrine sulfate 30 mg. p.o.). In states of intoxication, however, epinephrine and pressor drugs like it are best avoided because many toxic agents (*e.g.*, halogenated hydrocarbons) sensitize the heart even to conventional doses of epinephrine, so that fatal ventricular fibrillation is occasionally induced.

Perhaps a safer and even more effective drug than epinephrine is isoproterenol hydrochloride (*e.g.*, Isuprel), administered sublingually in doses of 10 to 20 mg. every 2 to 4 hours to maintain an adequate ventricular rate. The daily dose should not exceed 60 mg. A faster and perhaps more dependable response can be obtained by the subcutaneous, intramuscular or intravenous injection of isoproterenol. To establish an intravenous infusion, 10 ml. of a 1:5000 solution (2 mg.) is diluted in 50 ml. of 5% dextrose solution and administered initially at a rate of 5 μg./min. (1.25 ml. of the diluted mixture per min.) or about half this rate in children. The infusion rate, however, should be readjusted promptly according to the patient's responses. Continuous cardiac monitoring is almost essential, and the blood pressure should be checked at frequent intervals. Obviously such an infusion is no more than a temporary measure. In chronic cases of complete heart block, chlorothiazide and prednisone are said to be useful adjuncts.

If an adequately rapid ventricular rate is not maintained by these several drugs, it becomes essential to provide the heart with an artificial pacemaker. The technique of using externally generated electrical pulses delivered through transvenous pacemaker electrodes is discussed below under the management of cardiac arrest (p. IV-30).

The third and final group of disorders in the cardiac mechanism that require specific treatment consists of those rhythms which tend to deteriorate spontaneously into ventricular fibrillation and consequent death. Frequent premature beats of ventricular origin and ventricular tachycardia are recognized to be dangerous in this respect, and generally these conditions should be treated promptly with one of the antifibrillatory drugs. Procainamide hydrochloride or one of several salts of quinidine (*e.g.*, sulfate, hydrochloride, gluconate) is a common choice when oral medication can be tolerated.

One satisfactory dosage schedule for quinidine sulfate in the adult consists of an oral test dose of 0.2 gm. for the detection of hypersensitivity; in the absence of an untoward reaction it is followed by 300 to 400 mg. every 2 to 3 hours for about 5 doses but almost certainly not for more than 9 doses (cumulative amount less than 3.6 gm.). This regimen is interrupted if the disordered rhythm reverts to normal or if significant toxicity develops (see p. III-355).

Instead of quinidine, procainamide hydrochloride (Pronestyl) may be given a trial by the oral, intramuscular, or occasionally the intravenous route. The oral dose for an average adult is 1 gm., followed by a maintenance dose of 250 to 500 mg. every 2 to 4 hours. By the intramuscular route, 200 to 400 mg. is repeated every 20 minutes until 1 gm. is given; the effect can be maintained thereafter by 500 to 1000 mg. every 6 hours.

In a small minority of patients with atrial fibrillation from any cause, treatment with quinidine or procainamide induces an abrupt and potentially dangerous rise in the ventricular rate before a sinus rhythm is restored. To protect the heart in the event of such a "paradoxical" ventricular response, patients with atrial fibrillation are often pretreated with digoxin or other digitalis preparations before quinidine or procainamide is administered.

In severe emergencies, procainamide can be administered intravenously, either by continuous infusion or by intermittent injection. In the latter technique, 100 mg. is given by direct i.v. injection over a period of 2 minutes. The injection is repeated at 5-minute intervals until the arrhythmia is suppressed or the cumulative dose reaches 1000 mg. or severe toxicity is encountered. The ECG and arterial blood pressure should be monitored before each injection. To sustain a therapeutic response, a continuous infusion at a rate of 2 to 6 mg./min. replaces the intermittent injections.

Lidocaine hydrochloride (*e.g.*, Xylocaine) has been used successfully in the same way as procainamide. Because its latency and duration of action are so brief, at least when given by the intravenous route, its actions are rather easy to control, and it is usually preferred over procainamide in emergencies. An initial dose of 50 to 100 mg. (1 to 2 mg./kg.) can be injected intravenously over a period of 2 to 4 minutes. If the tachyarrhythmia is not corrected, a second usually smaller dose can be administered after 5 to 15 minutes. To sustain a beneficial effect, a continuous infusion may be established after a successful bolus dose. The infusion rate is usually 1 to 4 mg. lidocaine per minute, but the total dose should not exceed 200 or 300 mg. in an hour. Because of its very short duration of action, an overdose of lidocaine is believed to be less dangerous than an overdose of procainamide.

Procainamide and quinidine are similar in their actions on the heart, and there is little basis for choosing between them. Of course quinidine is more expensive, and parenteral preparations are not readily available. Hypersensitivity reactions to both drugs are recognized. With chronic procainamide therapy this reaction may take the form of a lupus-like syndrome, which resembles disseminated lupus erythematosus but which disappears when procainamide therapy is discontinued. In addition to drug allergy, both compounds may precipitate severe functional disturbances in the cardiac action, especially when they are administered parenterally. For example, a fall in systolic blood pressure of as much as 20 mm. of mercury is an indication that injections should be discontinued at least temporarily. These drugs have successfully arrested primary ventricular rhythms only to result in fatal cardiac standstill because of an unrecognized but coexistent conduction block between the normal atrial pacemaker and the ventricles. The same castastrophe is possible with any antifibrillatory drug, but lidocaine and particularly phenytoin are safer in this respect because they themselves do not impair junctional transmission in the usual doses.

Phenytoin sodium (Dilantin sodium) has emerged as the antifibrillatory drug of choice in suppressing the ventricular and supraventricular tachyarrhythmias of digitalis poisoning (p. III-151). Certainly procainamide has proved to be dangerous in this condition, in part because it can compromise the already defective mechanism of impulse transmission through the AV node. By contrast, phenytoin sometimes improves impaired junctional transmission. In mild digitalis poisoning it may be given by mouth in doses of 100 to 200 mg. three to four times daily.

In severe poisoning parenteral administration of phenytoin sodium is necessary; the intravenous route is preferred because of uncertainties in rates of absorption from intramuscular depots. Each ampul of the parenteral preparation contains 100 mg. drug in 2 ml. of a glycol-alcohol-water mixture at pH 12. The drug precipitates if this solution is diluted with conventional infusion fluids. Therefore the commercial solution is administered without dilution by the intermittent injection method, as described for procainamide (see above). Thus, 100 mg. phenytoin sodium is injected over a period of 2 minutes or more, so that the injection rate does not exceed 50 mg./min. The arterial blood pressure and ECG are monitored just before each injection. The injection is repeated at 5-minute intervals until the arrhythmia is suppressed or serious toxicity is encountered (*e.g.*, cardiovascular collapse or CNS depression) or the cumulative dose reaches 1000 mg. In most cases with a successful outcome, only 500 to 600 mg. was required.

Patients with severe derangements in the mechanism of heart beat may require at any time externally applied electrical pulses to defibrillate the ventricles and/or endocardially applied pulses to stimulate the ventricles regularly in order to maintain an effective cardiac action. Such severely ill patients should probably be put to bed and kept under continual observation. One effective and efficient way of doing this is to connect the patient to any one of several commercial machines which monitors continuously the electrocardiogram and sounds an alarm whenever the frequency of the ventricular complex rises above or falls below pre-set limits that are chosen by the therapist.

Cardiac arrest. This phrase is used commonly to mean the cessation of any ventricular action that is adequate to pump blood. Generally this means that the ventricles are either quiescent or fibrillating. Severe myocardial anoxia and profound vagal inhibition are the two factors most often responsible for the sudden termination of effective contractions in a structurally sound heart. These factors often arise in chemical poisonings and occasionally produce cardiac arrest. Given prompt and vigorous resuscitation, many of these victims can be saved.

A presumptive diagnosis of cardiac arrest is proper when peripheral pulses suddenly disappear, the blood pressure becomes undetectable, or auscultation fails to reveal audible heart sounds. Any one of three cardiac states may exist: feeble but coordinated beating, ventricular fibrillation, or total standstill. The true situation becomes evident when an electrocardiogram is recorded or when the heart is exposed to view. Differentiation is important for choosing the proper definitive treatment but is unnecessary for initiating emergency resuscitation.

Since cardiac arrest must be resolved within 2 to 4 minutes, if the patient is to recover without residual brain damage, a predetermined plan of action is essential. The details of the plan depend upon how many therapists are available.

With a silent precordium and absent arterial pulsations, one first searches for evidence that the central nervous system is still viable. The search should occupy no more than 5 to 10 seconds. If the pupils are not dilated maximally and if they still respond to light, thumping the precordium may serve to initiate cardiac action, but cardiac compression (sometimes called cardiac massage) is the resuscitative measure having the highest priority until the arrival of equipment for electrical defibrillation and/or artificial pacing. When a cardiac accident occurs on the surgical operating table, an emergency thoracotomy may be called for; it allows the heart to be emptied by manual squeezing. In most cases, however, thoracotomy is unwarranted, and external rather than internal cardiac massage is indicated. Elderly patients with stiff rib cages undoubtedly constitute an exception to this generalization.

External cardiac compression is accomplished by applying pressure over the lower sternum to depress it. With lateral displacement of the heart restricted by the pericardium and mediastinum, this maneuver serves to compress the heart between the sternum and the vertebral bodies. With rhythmically applied pressure, blood in the ventricles is squeezed into the arteries. In this way the therapist attempts to induce in a patient with either cardiac arrest or ventricular fibrillation a level of cardiac output adequate to prevent irreversible brain damage but not adequate to induce consciousness. The latter is highly unlikely since the induced cardiac output is only about one-quarter to one-third of normal, even when compression is properly performed. The procedure usually produces palpable pulses in the femoral and carotid arteries but not in the radial artery. Sometimes a blood pressure cuff over the brachial artery reveals a systolic pressure of 80 to 100 mm. of mercury. Recommended techniques of external cardiac massage are described in an explicit series of instructions below.

Of course cardiac compression is only part of the resuscitation process. It does not move appreciable amounts of air into and out of the lungs. Without pulmonary ventilation even brisk cerebral blood flow has no survival value. The combined procedure of artificial ventilation and external cardiac compression is known as cardiopulmonary resuscitation (CPR).

If no one else is present or immediately available, it is possible for one person to perform CPR by interrupting the cardiac compression every 15 seconds in order to inflate the patient's lungs with fresh air twice in rapid succession. If a ventilating machine, such as a manually triggered pneumatically powered device, is present, it should be used. Otherwise mouth-to-mouth resuscitation is indicated (p. IV-7).

With an adequate number of trained personnel, other procedures become practical. Pulsations of the carotid and femoral arteries can be sought as indices that cardiac massage is effective. The pupil size and pupillary light reflex can also be checked at frequent intervals. The victim's legs can be elevated (8 to 10 inches) to aid venous return to the heart. A surgical cutdown on a peripheral vein (p. IV-19) makes it possible to begin an infusion of isotonic saline. An indwelling venous cannula provides a convenient channel for administering any drugs that may be prescribed. Except for epinephrine, however, drugs should probably be avoided until a specific diagnosis is established. For this purpose an ECG should be located. With an electrocardiogram to distinguish between ventricular fibrillation and asystole, attempts at more definitive treatment become practical (see below).

Sometimes spontaneous heart sounds are faintly audible over the precordium even in the absence of any detectable arterial pulsations. Such a patient obviously requires cardiopulmonary resuscitation. With the arrival of a second therapist, a trial injection of epinephrine becomes practical. A 1:1000 aqueous solution of epinephrine should be diluted 10-fold with isotonic saline, and 0.5 to 2.0 ml. of the diluted solution should be injected intravenously. The closer to the heart the more effective is this injection. The right jugular vein is usually a satisfactory site, but if the chest is open, the needle is inserted directly into the right atrium.

Since this injection occasionally precipitates ventricular fibrillation, the therapist must be prepared to deal with this complication. Epinephrine is ineffective against fibrillation, although it may be useful in preparing the heart for electrical defibrillation.

Until the cardiac mechanism recovers spontaneously (which rarely occurs) or until an electrical defibrillator or an artificial external pacemaker is obtained, the circulation is maintained by continuous cardiac massage. Obviously successful resuscitation requires the cooperative efforts of many people. Cardiac compression is a fatiguing maneuver, and even a physically fit therapist will probably be exhausted after 15 to 20 minutes. With a team of two or more rescuers, assignments should probably be exchanged every 5 or 10 minutes.

Cardiopulmonary resuscitation (CPR) is illustrated in Figures IV-4 through IV-7, and the correct technique, together with associated procedures, is described in the following series of instructions.

Step 1—Preliminary diagnosis. Successful resuscitation is impossible unless cardiac arrest is recognized promptly. Check for heart sounds and examine the pupils. In the unconscious, apneic, and pulseless patient, pupils that are not maximally dilated and that do react to light constitute the most useful evidence of central nervous system viability. If an electrical defibrillator and artificial pacemaker are available, proceed directly to Steps 6 and 7 (but see 5).

Step 2—Prepare patient. Place the victim in a supine position on a firm surface, such as the

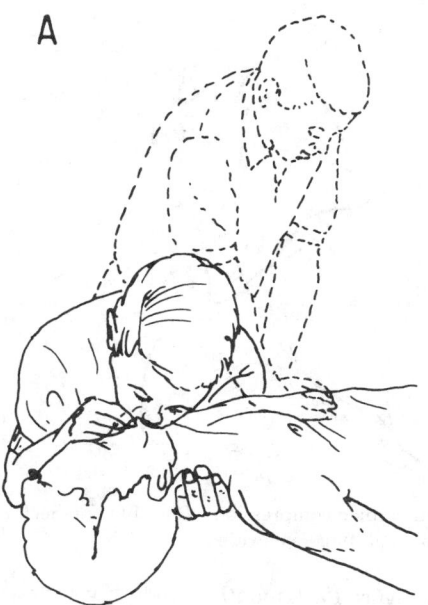
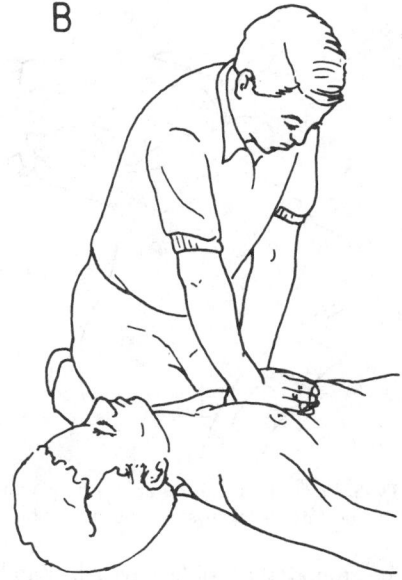

Figure IV-4. Cardiopulmonary resuscitation (CPR) by one rescuer, starting with (*A*) two quick full lung inflations, followed by (*B*) 15 chest compressions.

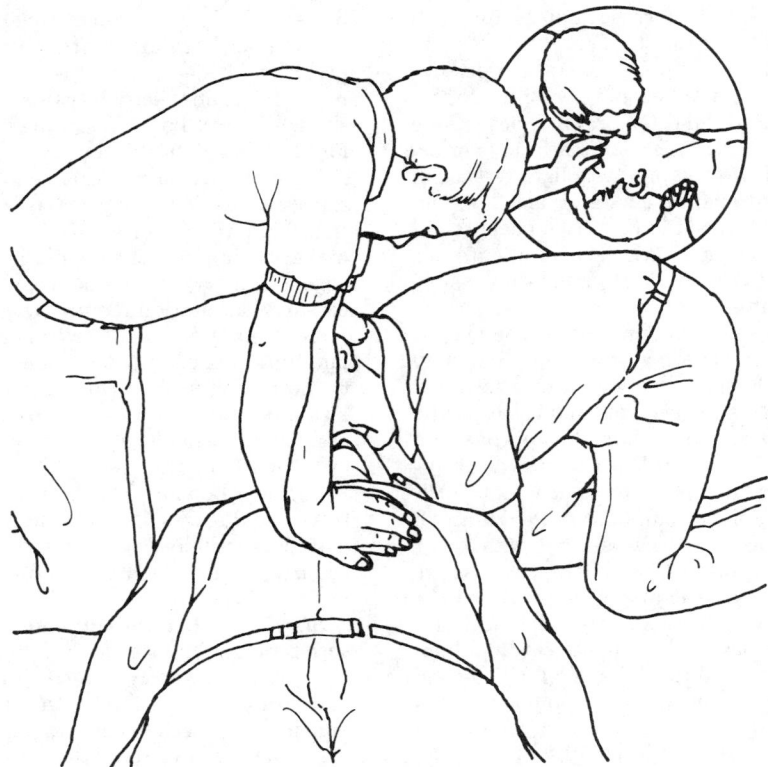

Figure IV-5. Two-rescuer cardiopulmonary resuscitation (CPR). The operator on the left is just releasing chest compression, while the operator on the right quickly inflates the victim's lungs once (at the end of every 5 compressions). Compression rate of 60 per minute continues without interruption.

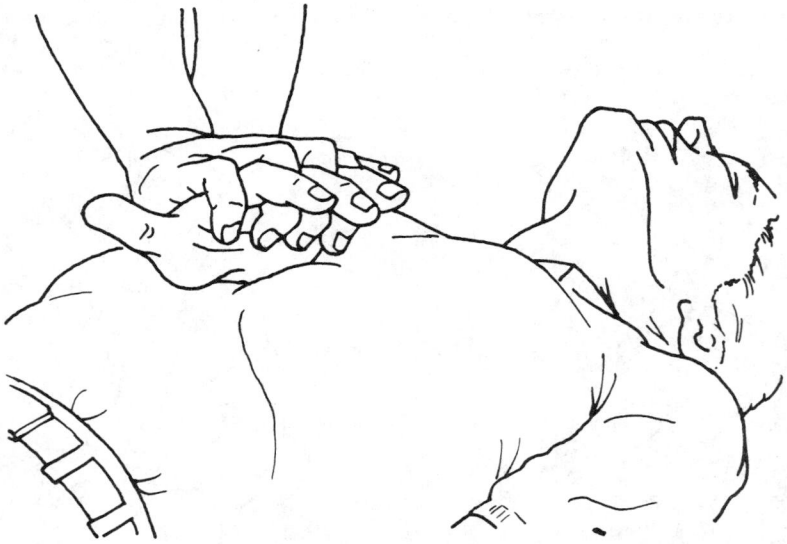

Figure IV-6. Position of the therapist's hands during external cardiac compression. Note that the heel of one hand is on the victim's lower sternum (not xiphoid process), with all fingers elevated.

floor or the ground. If possible, have a bystander summon an ambulance and locate others who can help with the resuscitation.

Step 3—Begin artificial respiration. As noted in Figure IV-4, mouth-to-mouth ventilation can be accomplished intermittently by the same operator who performs cardiac compression, but it is obviously preferable to divide these responsi-

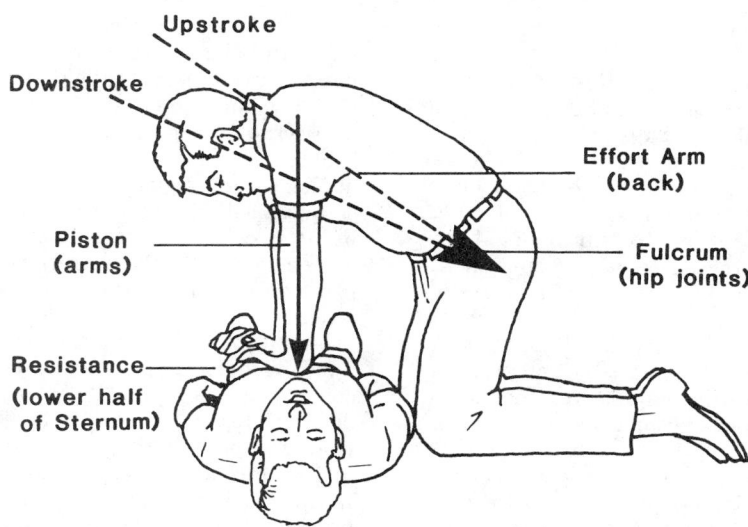

Figure IV-7. The mechanics of external cardiac compression, in which each downstroke depresses the victim's sternum 1.5 to 2 inches (adult victim).

bilities between two therapists working together. For the proper techniques of mouth-to-mouth resuscitation or alternative procedures, see pp. IV-7-10.

With a single rescuer, the CPR cycle begins with two quick full lung inflations (Fig. IV-4A). As illustrated in Figure IV-4B, the therapist then raises himself on his knees and proceeds to initiate repetitive chest compression (as described in Step 4 below). After 15 chest compressions at a rate of about 80 per minute, the operator returns to the victim's head and again fully inflates the victim's lungs twice in rapid succession. By providing the second breath before the victim's lungs can empty completely, the ventilatory phase of CPR can be reduced to 4 to 5 seconds. The cycle of chest compressions and inflations is continued, so that about 60 cardiac compressions are accomplished each minute.

With a team of two rescuers, the members position themselves on opposite sides of the victim. One operator provides uninterrupted chest compression at a frequency of 60 per minute. The other therapist interposes between compressions one full lung inflation after every 5 compressions. Figure IV-5 illustrates a moment when the operator on the left is releasing chest pressure as the operator on the right delivers a quick breath into the victim's mouth.

Step 4—Institute compression. Pressure is delivered through the heel of one hand, which is placed over the lower sternum (not the xiphoid process or the costochondral junctions). As seen in Figure IV-6, a second hand rests on top of the first. The fingers may or may not be intermeshed, but they should not rest on the victim's chest or bear any of the pressure.

With the arms stiff, pressure is applied vertically downward, so that the sternum of the adult victim moves 1.5 to 2 inches toward the vertebral column (Fig. IV-7). At the end of each stroke, the operator lifts his trunk by rotating at the hips and so releases completely pressure on the sternum, thereby allowing elastic recovery of the chest wall and spontaneous cardiac filling from the venous reservoirs. Whenever possible, the hands should remain in contact with the chest wall to avoid the need to reposition them. The compression and release phases are of equal duration, and the cycle is repeated about once a second (60 per minute). The rhythmic motion should be smooth, without jabs or jerkiness.

Obviously less depression of the sternum is required in infants and children. Because the rib cage is more flexible, children up to 10 years old require no more than the force that can be delivered through the heel of one hand and a compression depth of 1 to 1.5 inches. In newborn infants the pressure of two fingers is often sufficient to produce the desired compression depth of 0.5 inch. Because the cardiac ventricles of the infant lie high in the chest, the midsternum (between the nipples) is the proper location for the pressure. A rate as high as 100 to 120 per minute should probably be maintained in infants.

Every minute or two, CPR can be interrupted for 4 or 5 seconds to check for spontaneous arterial pulses. If cardiac activity does not resume after a few minutes, massage may be interrupted long enough (4 to 5 seconds) to inject epinephrine. A solution made by diluting 0.2 ml. of 1:1000 aqueous epinephrine can be injected either intravenously as described above or directly into the heart by plunging the needle through the chest wall to the left of the xiphoid process. Even if the drug fails to elicit spontaneous heart beats, the prognosis is far from hopeless and cardiac compression should be continued.

Step 5—Electrocardiographic diagnosis. If possible an ECG tracing should be secured. For this purpose cardiac massage can be interrupted for a few moments. Whatever the atrial action, the ECG will presumably demonstrate either that the ventricles are quiescent (no electrical activity) or else that they are fibrillating. In the latter instance proceed to Step 6, but in the former instance one can omit Step 6 and proceed directly to Step 7. If an ECG machine is unavailable but an electric defibrillator happens to be at hand, it is probably reasonable and proper to use it as described in Step 6, even though the problem may be one of ventricular standstill and not fibrillation.

Step 6—Defibrillation. If an adequate electrical defibrillator is at hand, proceed to use it without delay. If it is not immediately available, maintain cardiac massage until it can be obtained. In the presence of adequate cardiac massage, procainamide (Pronestyl) hydrochloride in a dose of about 200 mg. administered intravenously or directly into the atrium is sometimes successful in terminating ventricular fibrillation, but electrical defibrillation (countershock) is much more dependable.

Clinically useful machines are marketed by many companies: Becton-Dickinson, Burdick, Birtcher, Hewlett Packard, Litton, General Electric and others. Some machines are line-powered and other battery-powered. Early models, which may still be found in some smaller hospitals, provide 60-cycle AC pulses with intensities as high as 750 volts and durations of between 0.15 and 0.5 second. With electrodes on the chest surface (see below), a pulse of 450 volts AC for 0.25 second is an effective countershock in most adults. Presumably a child requires considerably less.

All modern defibrillators, however, deliver DC pulses, specifically modified condensor discharges with intensities up to 400 watt-seconds (also called joules) and pulse durations of about 2 milliseconds. Furthermore, if the victim's heart is generating any electrical activity that can be recognized as a ventricular complex, the modern machine automatically delivers its discharge a few milliseconds after the QRS. This so-called "synchronization" tends to minimize the chance that the countershock is delivered during the "vulnerable" period of the ventricle, which is normally contemporaneous with the descending limb of the T-wave. By avoiding the vulnerable period, it is believed that synchronized DC shocks are less likely than AC shocks to induce ventricular fibrillation.

For external defibrillation, electrodes of large surface area are usually employed. They must be pressed firmly against the chest and held in place with insulated handles, preferably with hand guards to protect the therapist. To reduce skin resistance the electrode sites are first prepared by applying and massaging the areas with conventional electrode paste. One electrode is applied to the region of the manubrium or the suprasternal notch and the other to the region of the apical thrust. Because of the high voltage and current (several amperes), no one should be in direct contact with the patient when the shock is delivered. To prevent damage, the electrocardiograph should be disconnected momentarily.

When the current is turned on, a brief tonic convulsion is observed. If the first countershock does not terminate ventricular fibrillation and restore a normal rhythm, a second shock of higher intensity can be tried after a few seconds. In treating ventricular fibrillation with synchronized DC pulses, some therapists prefer to start with a maximal countershock of 400 watt-seconds. Others try up to two shocks of 200 to 300 watt-seconds each before using the maximal level. With infants and young children, the shock intensity is 2 watt-seconds per kg. (body weight). Sometimes an injection of epinephrine as described above serves to "strengthen" the fibrillation and make it more susceptible to interruption by countershock. If ventricular fibrillation ceases but no other cardiac mechanism intervenes, external cardiac compression should be resumed until an artificial pacemaker can be provided.

Step 7—Artificial pacemakers. Instruments are available to generate electrical pulses that may excite the electrically silent and quiescent ventricles so as to produce effective mechanical systole. The electrodes are either applied to the chest wall (external pacemaker) or are buried within the chest (internal or transthoracic pacemaker). In practice external electrodes are no longer used except as an emergency standby technique until direct pacing can be initiated. With an electrode assembly mounted inside a special needle, it is possible to penetrate the chest and to insert the electrodes into the right ventricular wall. Whereas this device has obvious utility in extreme emergencies, electrodes implanted in the myocardium have generally proved to be unsatisfactory over extended periods of time.

At present endocardial pacing with a "transvenous pacemaker" is the preferred method, whether the need is expected to be temporary or permanent. This device consists of bipolar electrodes that are sealed into the tip of a special flexible catheter. The catheter is inserted into the external jugular or cephalic vein, and with the aid of an obturator the tip is advanced and wedged in the apex of the right ventricle, so that the electrodes are applied to the endocardial surface. Wires within the catheter can be connected to an external pulse generator and power source, or a miniature generator and battery can be implanted under the skin in the right axilla or pectoral area. Except as a temporary measure in an emergency, external pacemaker circuits are no longer used. A variety of stimulus parameters can be selected. Some of the available circuits sense any spontaneous activity within the ventricle and generate pulses only when the natural frequency falls below some predetermined level ("demand" system). Because of the small power requirements of these devices, the lithium power supply needs to be replaced in most patients only every 6 years.

Step 8—Late supportive treatment. As more personnel and facilities are mobilized, supportive treatment can be extended in scope and intensity. Respiratory tract secretions may require suctioning (p. IV-4), and an endotracheal tube may be inserted (p. IV-4). Even after spontaneous respirations are restored, most of these patients can probably profit from oxygen therapy (p. IV-12). The slow intravenous infusion of epinephrine, isoproterenol, calcium salts, or perhaps ouabain may improve the cardiac action and raise the arterial blood pressure. Acidosis is frequently observed and requires prompt attention (p. IV-71). The same is true of several complications that arise occasionally because of overly vigorous chest massage, *i.e.*, fractures of the sternum and ribs, separated costochondral junctions, pneumothorax, subcutaneous emphysema, and lacerations of the liver. If neurological damage is evidenced by hyperpyrexia, persisting coma, dilated pupils, continuing apnea, or convulsions, the extent of the hypoxic brain injury can perhaps be minimized by the induction of hypothermia. At the same time an intravenous infusion of urea (p. IV-45) has been recommended to reduce cerebral edema and to lower the cerebrospinal fluid pressure, even if one chooses not to subject such a critically ill patient to the diagnostic tests that might be required to demonstrate a high intracranial pressure.

However successful the resuscitation, one must seek and remove the causes of cardiac arrest before one can be confident that recovery is assured. If practical, the electrocardiogram of these patients should be monitored continuously for several hours and perhaps for several days, so that any recurrence of cardiac arrest can be recognized and corrected promptly.

CENTRAL NERVOUS SYSTEM

Pain

The suppression of pain is one of the first and most important elements in supportive treatment. Universally endorsed standards of professional conduct attest to its high priority. Pain, especially persistent pain, generates fear, anxiety, irritability, and exhaustion. Besides preventing psychic disturbances, the control of pain may forestall the disorganization of many somatic functions, since through reflex and hormonal mechanisms intense pain exerts noxious influences on many organ systems. Sometimes these undesirable reactions to pain serve to perpetuate the offending stimulus, creating so-called "vicious cycles." A simple if somewhat mundane example is the pain of muscle spasm which generates more spasm, and so more pain. Certain types of visceral pain (*e.g.*, from myocardial ischemia) may potentiate and perhaps cause severe vasomotor collapse. Of course pain is not always detrimental, and a physician should hesitate to suppress it completely, until its diagnostic and prognostic values have been fully exploited.

The systemic administration of analgesic drugs is not always necessary to control pain. Thus, many types of visceral pain are erased effectively by spasmolytic drugs. For example, atropine sulfate eradicates the pain of colic by inhibiting the intestinal spasm which generates it. Similarly nitrites and other antispasmodics are sometimes effective against biliary and renal colic. Isolated neuritic pain can usually be controlled by infiltration with a local anesthetic solution, such as procaine hydrochloride. Topical anesthetic drugs in the form of ointments and solutions may effectively inhibit pain arising from localized cutaneous and mucosal lesions. Pain from integumentary structures often responds to the local application of heat, especially moist heat. Sometimes cold applications are preferable, notably when an inflamed or itching skin is the source of distress.

In most cases, however, pain requires the administration of a true analgesic drug, *i.e.*, one whose effects are mediated at least in part by actions within the central nervous system. Among the safest and most effective compounds of this type are the salicylates, notably acetylsalicylic acid or aspirin. Oral doses of 0.3 to 0.6 gm. every 2 to 4 hours are often adequate to control superficial pain and particularly pain of a neuralgic, myalgic, or arthralgic character. When pain is not effectively controlled by aspirin, it is often supplemented by small amounts of codeine phosphate (*e.g.*, 8 to 32 mg.).

Several factors, however, limit the usefulness

of aspirin and other salicylates. For example, bleeding time is prolonged by even therapeutic doses. Furthermore, the oral route is the only appropriate channel for administering them. Absorption from the rectum is slow and undependable, and although the intravenous route is available for solutions of sodium salicylate, these infusions are somewhat hazardous and distinctly inconvenient. In many chemical poisonings, gastrointestinal damage precludes oral medication. Since salicylates are often irritating to even the normal gastric mucosa and sometimes produce ulceration, salicylate therapy is of limited value in clinical toxicology.

Sharing the analgesic, antipyretic and antiinflammatory activities of the salicylates are a group of synthetic drugs which, like the salicylates, act by inhibiting prostaglandin synthesis *in vivo*. The list includes ibuprofen, naproxen and fenoprofen. They are used chiefly for the control of symptoms in rheumatoid arthritis. Only oral preparations are marketed, and like aspirin, they sometimes irritate the gastric mucosa. For these reasons they too are rarely useful in clinical toxicology. Acetaminophen is a popular non-narcotic analgesic drug. In therapeutic doses it tends to be well tolerated and does not prolong bleeding time and does not cause gastric erosion. It also can be administered only by the oral route.

Propoxyphene (dextropropoxyphene, Darvon) hydrochloride is a synthetic analgesic drug that binds to and activates opioid receptors in the brain. It is effective against mild and moderate pain when given by mouth alone or together with salicylates or acetaminophen. Unlike the latter it has no antipyretic activity. In dose and duration of action, it resembles codeine, but its potency is less. Its addiction liability may be even less than that of codeine. Because of its low toxicity in conventional doses (32 to 65 mg.), it is sometimes employed where other non-narcotic analgesics fail, but because it can be given safely only by the oral route, its use in clinical toxicology is limited.

Pentazocine is a more potent and effective synthetic opioid than propoxyphene. As an analgesic agent it can be given orally as the hydrochloride in a dose of 50 mg. or parenterally as a solution of the lactate salt in a dose of 30 to 50 mg. At least when given by the oral route, it seems to induce less physical dependence than morphine, but peculiar patterns of abuse by parenteral routes have been described (see Section II). As an analgesic, it is less effective than morphine and many of morphine's congeners. Furthermore, because it possesses weak antagonistic activity at opioid receptors, as well as agonistic actions, it can induce dysphoria and signs of withdrawal reactions in narcotic addicts.

Morphine and other naturally occurring and semisynthetic narcotic alkaloids furnish dependable and intense analgesia by many routes of administration. Their use should be restricted to patients in whom non-narcotic analgesic drugs are inadequate. Adequate control, however, is a matter of judgment, and physicians and patients often have different opinions on this subject. An impression persists that some physicians and particularly young ones are so reluctant to prescribe morphine or its congeners that their patients are deprived of the levels of relief from pain and anxiety that they deserve. Except in individuals with a history of drug abuse, the risk of iatrogenic addiction has probably been overemphasized. Most chemical injuries are of short duration, and the need for pain relief is correspondingly short-lived.

Admittedly morphine therapy may be complicated by such problems as addiction, physical dependence, tolerance, medullary depression (especially of the respiratory center), spasm of smooth muscle, reflex vomiting, constipation, urinary retention, idiosyncrasies, pruritus, and urticaria. With respect to physical dependence, addiction, and tolerance, all of the narcotic alkaloids share the liabilities of morphine. Codeine is probably the drug of choice in most cases where the non-narcotic analgesics are insufficient.

At first small oral doses (8 to 32 mg.) of codeine sulfate or phosphate are tried in conjunction with salicylates or acetaminophen. An alternative semisynthetic narcotic is oxycodone; in the United States it is available only in products which contain aspirin (Percodan) or acetaminophen (Percocet). If these are inadequate, codeine salts can be given in parenteral doses as high as 60 mg. (i.m. or s.c.) and repeated every 3 to 4 hours as required.

If a more powerful analgesic is necessary, one of the following is tried: meperidine (Demerol) hydrochloride 80 to 100 mg., p.o. or i.m., every 2 to 4 hours as necessary; methadone hydrochloride, 5 to 10 mg., p.o., i.m., or s.c., at intervals of 3 to 5 hours as required; hydromorphone (dihydromorphinone, Dilaudid) hydrochloride, 1 to 2 mg., p.o. or s.c., every 3 or 4 hours as necessary; levorphanol tartrate, 2 or 3 mg., s.c. or p.o., every 6 to 8 hours as necessary. Because of its slightly greater tendency to produce stupefaction, euphoria, and addiction, morphine is best reserved for cases where a euphoric tranquility is desired, as well as relief from pain. The average adult dose of morphine sulfate is 5 to 15 mg., s.c. or 8 to 20 mg., p.o., but in the presence of severe pain larger amounts may be necessary.

All of the narcotic analgesics are detoxified principally in the liver. They should be prescribed sparingly if at all in cases of liver disease, myxedema, adrenal insufficiency, and other states of reduced metabolism. If poisoning results from overdosages of morphine or its congeners, institute treatment as outlined on p. III-287). Narcotics should never be administered according to a fixed schedule but should be given only at times of actual need. As soon as the severe phase of a painful illness ceases, all narcotics should be withheld. In some patients an iatrogenic addiction can arise after only a few days of repeated medication, and so the physician should be alert for withdrawal symptoms as soon as the administration of any narcotic drug is discontinued.

Frequently pain is experienced in the absence of peripheral stimulation from significant pathophysiological or pathoanatomical disturbances. Clinically this type of pain is seen as a hysterical conversion symptom or else as one manifestation of depression. In these instances analgesic drugs are unpredictable and usually ineffective. At times, sedation may be more appropriate, particularly when there is accompanying anxiety. In contrast, when pain arises from recognized pathological foci, sedative drugs alone are inappropriate because in the presence of such unrelieved pain, they may induce restlessness and even delirium.

Delirium

The word delirium is as confusing as the state it is intended to denote. The problem is not that the word lacks a definition but that it has been defined in several contradictory ways by different experts. For example, G. L. Engel, J. Romano and Z. J. Lipowski have used the word to encompass most, if not all, states of confusion, i.e., situations in which a person has an inability to think with his usual speed and clarity. In all cases the basis of the victim's confusion is presumed to be one or more derangements in the chemistry of the brain. These derangements can be produced by one or a combination of etiological factors, such as intoxication with drugs and other chemicals, infection, fever, circulatory disturbance, trauma, tumor, and toxemia based on some systemic metabolic or endocrine disturbance. Previous editions of this manual have adopted this global view of delirium as a form of cerebral insufficiency.

In general, however, clinical toxicologists use the term delirium in a more restricted sense. Thus, R. D. Adams and others exclude confusional states that are chronic, progressive and essentially irreversible, such as the confusion of dementia. Also excluded are acute confusional states that are associated with impaired arousal and decreased psychomotor activity, as, for example, the transient confusion and even agitation that may occur in an early stage of progressive central nervous system depression (pp. IV-39–43).

What remains in the restricted nosology of delirium are those confusional states that are reversible, have a generally abrupt onset and are not accompanied by stupor or other reduced states of arousal. The patients are characteristically alert, excited, and sometimes agitated; they commonly experience sensory distortions (illusions) and hallucinations. Indeed the victim's confusion appears to result from a heightened alertness that causes him to become so distracted by repetitive or irrelevant sensory stimuli that he cannot sustain any line of thought. As a result he is preoccupied with his own illusory and hallucinatory experiences and is relatively inattentive to the therapist and others. In some cases the confusion and the excitement may culminate in generalized convulsions.

The clinical toxicologist commonly encounters delirium in patients experiencing withdrawal reactions (abstinence syndrome) after chronic intoxications with alcohol (delirium tremens), barbiturates and other sedative drugs. In addition, grand mal convulsions from any cause may lead to a brief postconvulsive period of delirium. Acute intoxications with various drugs and chemicals are also a common cause of delirium; the list includes aminophylline, amphetamines, atropine, caffeine, camphor, cocaine, some ergot alkaloids (e.g., LSD), imipramine and other tricyclic antidepressants, marihuana, mescaline, psilocybin, salicylates, and strychnine. Somewhat atypical forms of delirium are occasionally reported in poisonings due to the convulsant insecticides (DDT, chlordane, lindane) and also in poisonings due to lithium, quinine (and quinidine), thallium, and lead. Various systemic infections may produce delirium, such as typhoid fever, pneumonia, septicemia, etc. The same is true of some vascular, neoplastic and infectious diseases of the central nervous system, although in these cases there are often associated focal or lateralizing neurological signs.

Although specific tests are necessary in the clinical examination to demonstrate milder forms of delirium, the full-blown syndrome is readily apparent. Here, due to a failure of cognitive functions, the patient's mental responses become disorganzed, his orientation to time and place becomes faulty, and his memory and ability to concentrate become impaired. There is particular difficulty in comprehending and remembering recent stimuli. Restlessness, tremulousness, anxiety, frightening dreams or insomnia, tremors and hyperactive tendon reflexes are often present. With still further progression, gross confusion and disorientation become apparent. A patient's previous attempts to overcome the defect through heightened effort can no longer conceal the disturbance. There may be a concurrent impairment of motor skills, first seen in feeding, toilet care, speech, and writing; in extreme cases incontinence and gross untidiness occur. Final stages are characterized by incoherence, convulsions, stupor, and finally coma.

No brief description can include the wide range of psychological and behavioral aberrations seen in delirium. As the vulnerable psychological functions of control, integration, and inhibition are affected, there emerge highly individual manifestations determined by the patient's lifelong personal experiences and cultural background. There may be gross amounts of anxiety, at times progressing to panic; in other patients, marked depression and withdrawal are sometimes observed. Some experienced drug abusers have learned how to control their fears and to enjoy their state of self-induced delirium (for example, see Group VI Mushroom Toxins in Section III). Blatant misidentification may occur in the form of visual and auditory illusions. Where hallucinations are present, their specific content reflects the patient's distinctly personal preoccupations and conflicts.

The diagnosis of delirium requires the demonstration of a defect in formal intellectual functions, in order to distinguish it from other psychological disorders. The simplest test is to ask the patient to provide factual data about the date, his present location, and recent events. Another useful procedure to test attention, concentration, and retention is the serial subtraction of numbers, e.g., 3 from 100, from 97, etc. The results of these or similar simple tests, coupled with general clinical observations, are usually sufficient to establish the diagnosis. Although a psychiatrist may be invaluable in establishing the diagnosis and in suggesting treatment, delirium should be regarded as a medical problem, not a psychological one.

The first objectives in the management of delirium are the detection and removal of its causes. In acute poisonings this entails the use of any detoxifying or antidotal measures that are available. General supportive treatment should be directed at the maintenance of oxygenation, circulation, and electrolyte balance, since disruption of these vital processes will lead to further impairment of brain metabolism. If cerebral edema or other causes of elevated intracranial pressure are suspected, the possibility of decompressing the cranial cavity should be explored (p. IV-43). Of course any drug that might be responsible for the delirium should be avoided.

Another important objective is the prevention or suppression of any uncontrolled behavior that might lead to injury, exhaustion, or death. Overexertion, excitement, panic, aggressive outbursts, attempts to escape, wandering off in a confused manner, and suicidal behavior all occur unpredictably in severe forms of delirium. Preventive measures should be based upon an understanding of the psychological phenomena in delirium. Frequent observations are extremely important. Besides the necessity for vigilance on the part of the staff, the mere presence of another person is a source of considerable comfort and reassurance to some delirious patients. If feasible, the same person, either a doctor or nurse, should be available as much of the time as possible; the presence of several individuals or frequent changes in personnel only contribute to the confusion. As a familiar and recognizable person, a member of the family may serve well as an attendant.

Because of the cognitive defect, efforts should be made to help the patient with his orientation by reminding him frequently where he is and why. To minimize the risk of misinterpretation all procedures should be explained to him in simple terms with emphasis on their helpful or therapeutic qualities rather than their physiological mechanisms. Instructions and requests when necessary should be brief, simple and repeated more than once because of the difficulty in grasping and retaining information.

The delirious patient is managed best in a relatively bare, well lighted room. Distracting objects such as wall paper with elaborate designs may be misinterpreted as frightening illusory figures. Because darkness and semidarkness contribute to sensory deprivation, the room should remain illuminated at night. If the patient cannot be observed at all times, it is better to keep the mattress on the floor than to risk a fall from bed. Similarly, serious injury or death may be averted by having windows securely locked. In addition, the general principles of good nursing care should be employed, such as attention to nutrition and cleanliness, in spite of what may be viewed as the patient's lack of cooperation. Vital signs should be observed and recorded regularly.

Except in the delirium of a withdrawal reaction (see below), chemical sedation should be avoided whenever possible. Delirium is usually a reversible disorder, and the above measures will generally ensure the patient's safety and provide for his care until the disorder subsides. Drugs should not be used as a substitute for vigilant care. Random overactivity, confused speech, and restlessness are not indications for sedative drugs, but if convulsions are judged to be imminent, anticonvulsant therapy may be instituted (p. IV-36). The danger of administering sedative drugs is that of adding to the cerebral metabolic disturbance and so prolonging and intensifying the state of delirium. Only when a patient's extreme overactivity threatens him with exhaustion, when he is unresponsive to the general measures outlined above, or when it is impossible to implement these measures, the cautious use of sedatives or tranquilizers may be justified.

The phenothiazine and butyrophenone tranquilizers are generally superior to conventional hypnotic-sedative drugs in suppressing excessive psychomotor activity whenever a hallucinogenic chemical is responsible (*e.g.*, cocaine, amphetamines, psilocybin, marihuana, phencyclidine, etc., but *not* atropine). Chlorpromazine in adult doses of 50 to 100 mg., administered orally or intramuscularly, repeated in several hours if necessary, is effective, but side effects of chlorpromazine (see Section III) and its congeners limit their usefulness. Of particular relevance is the hypotensive reaction that occurs not infrequently a short time after the first parenteral dose. Fainting and injury can be avoided by keeping the patient recumbent for the first hour. Haloperidol in oral or intramuscular doses as high as 2 to 5 mg. is also highly effective and may be somewhat safer than the phenothiazines.

In summary, when excitatory, hallucinogenic and psychotomimetic chemicals are responsible for delirium, drugs that are central nervous system depressants should be used sparingly if at all and then only to reduce extreme degrees of agitation so that the patient can rest intermittently. On the other hand, when delirium occurs during a withdrawal reaction from alcohol or from any of the sedative-hypnotic drugs (such as the barbiturates, meprobamate, etc.), drug therapy tends to be more aggressive, probably because uncontrolled delirium often leads to status epilepticus in the individual with a high degree of physical dependence.

In managing delirium in withdrawal reactions of the alcohol-sedative type (it occurs only rarely in the narcotic abstinence syndrome), antipsychotic drugs such as chlorpromazine, haloperidol and their congeners are not useful and may even be hazardous by increasing the risk of seizures. The drugs of choice here are the shorter acting hypnotics and tranquilizers. Bromides and barbiturates, particularly the long acting ones, should be avoided. Paraldehyde can be administered orally in doses of 8 to 15 ml. mixed with cold fruit juice to make it more palatable. If necessary it can be administered by rectum, but this procedure itself may frighten and further agitate a delirious patient. Chloral hydrate in oral doses of 0.5 to 1.5 gm. has also been used but is probably less effective. Diazepam and its congeners are widely used. Sometimes a short-acting barbiturate drug (*e.g.*, pentobarbital) is preferred (see also p. IV-37).

In general, high doses are required, whichever drug is selected, because these patients have high degrees of tolerance and cross-tolerance to sedative-hypnotic drugs. The aim of drug therapy is to suppress or prevent signs and symptoms of full-blown delirium. Tremulousness, irritability and insomnia usually indicate a need for more medication, but beneficial responses may be delayed for several hours even with effective doses. Once the patient is comfortable (which may require a mild degree of intoxication) and his status has become stable, drug doses can be gradually reduced over a period of days to weeks, as the state of physical dependence is slowly dissipated.

Episodes of wild excitement with serious assaultive or self-destructive behavior are seen occasionally in delirious patients. For such cases many general hospitals have available a bare security room with locked screened windows. Rarely the patient has to be forcibly restrained to protect himself or others. Once the decision is reached, it should be implemented quickly and unwaveringly by experienced personnel present in large enough numbers to accomplish the task with the least chance of injury to the patient and staff. To avoid peripheral nerve injuries, the patient should be positioned so as to minimize the chances of bruising vulnerable spots (*e.g.*, elbow, lateral aspect of knee, etc.). Mechanical devices such as wrist, ankle, or full-sheet restraints should be used only as a last resort and then only long enough to make provisions for more definitive care.

Convulsions

The present discussion is restricted to the acute convulsive episodes seen in chemical poisonings. Omitted are the many problems of managing chronic convulsive disorders such as idiopathic or traumatic epilepsy. One must acknowledge, however, that a poison victim may also suffer from epilepsy and that any toxic convulsion may represent the chemical activation of latent epilepsy. Many metabolic disturbances can be induced by chemical agents, and such disorders as hypocapnia from hyperventilation, cerebral anoxia, cortisone overdosage, water intoxication, and hypoglycemia are more apt to precipitate convulsions in an epileptic than in a nonepileptic.

Even in persons with no stigma of epilepsy, the following compounds regularly induce convulsions if ingested in sufficient amounts: strychnine, picrotoxin, pentylenetetrazol (Metrazol), amphetamine, camphor, DDT and many other chlorinated insecticides, and parathion and its congeners. Often toxic doses of cocaine, tetracaine, various antihistaminic drugs, salicylates, and fluoroacetate salts cause generalized convulsions. Occasionally a general anesthetic is responsible. If one includes atypical cases, almost all drugs and common chemicals have been reported as the cause of seizures, but in many fatal poisonings terminal convulsions are simply anoxic or asphyxial in origin.

Although there are many different ways in which chemicals induce hyperexcitability and consequent convulsions, a single program of supportive treatment is applicable to all cases, if supplemented by appropriate specific therapy. In every case the first consideration is to prevent the patient from injuring himself during those periods when a seizure renders him helpless. For example, he should be laid on the floor or at least prevented from rolling off the bed. His collar is loosened, and artificial dentures and detachable dental bridges are removed between convulsive paroxysms. If the patient has no gag reflex, an oropharyngeal airway is best used to hold the tongue forward; this prevents it from occluding the oropharynx and also from being chewed; the removal of saliva and other secretions is made easier by the use of this device. For the correct technique of insertion, see p. IV-3. To minimize the aspiration of vomitus the patient is kept on his side, if possible with his head facing downward.

All diagnostic and therapeutic procedures are held to a minimum; for example, gastric lavage is postponed until adequate premedication suppresses all convulsive activity. Since paroxysms are precipitated in some victims by very mild stimuli, sensory stimulation should be reduced by keeping the patient in a comfortably warm, quiet, and darkened room. Even visits by professional assistants should be as infrequent as practical.

Anoxia and an oxygen debt can be corrected rapidly by administering pure oxygen between convulsions if this can be accomplished without triggering another paroxysm. If natural breathing is not resumed as soon as the skeletal muscles relax at the end of a seizure, artificial respiration (p. IV-7) must be initiated immediately. If convulsions recur at frequent intervals over a long period, the parenteral administration of water, salt, and glucose becomes advisable (pp. IV-65–67).

Severe metabolic acidosis due to intense lactic acidemia can also arise during acute episodes of recurring convulsions. Although this acidosis may subside rapidly when the convulsions are suppressed, sodium bicarbonate therapy is often indicated (p. IV-71). Similarly, convulsions generate heat, and the resulting hyperthermia may warrant attention (p. IV-84). Intense and sustained contractions of skeletal muscles sometimes lead to rhabdomyolysis, as evidenced by high serum levels of creatine phosphokinase. On rare occasions the resulting myoglobinemia damages renal tubules. The maintenance of a mild diuresis, however, usually protects the kidneys.

In most cases these supportive measures must be accompanied by appropriate specific treatment. Examples of definitive treatment include atropine in poisoning by parathion and other anticholinesterase substances, glucose in hypoglycemic attacks, oxygen in anoxic convulsions, osmotic decompression in cases of cerebral edema (p. IV-45), and vigorous measures to reduce the body temperature in febrile convulsions (p. IV-84). Many patients, however, also require anticonvulsant drugs, *i.e.*, agents which depress the central nervous system generally or the motor apparatus specifically, without regard to the cause of the original hyperexcitability, as noted below.

Any illness that consists of continuous or frequent seizures of the grand mal type is called status epilepticus, whatever its etiology. If status epilepticus is allowed to persist, an asphyxial death from respiratory arrest becomes almost inevitable because convulsions cause progressive damage to the respiratory center in two ways: from exhaustion which attends violent overstimulation and from anoxia which develops each time tetanic contractions of the respiratory muscles stop breathing movements. Other causes of death from status epilepticus include circulatory failure and bronchopneumonia (mainly from aspiration). By preventing or aborting convulsions early in the course of poisoning, these various complications can be avoided, and time is gained during which specific treatment can be instituted or natural mechanisms of detoxication can be mobilized.

Drugs useful in preventing or reducing the frequency of seizures in chronic epilepsy are seldom effective in treating an actual convulsion or aborting an imminent one, whatever its cause. For example, even when injected intravenously, phenobarbital and mephobarbital act too slowly to be drugs of choice in a convulsing patient (see below). Although trimethadione (Tridione) protects animals against experimental seizures of many types and has been recommended in the clinical management of tetanus and status epilepticus, it is now generally regarded as ineffective in the treatment of status epilepticus. Mesantoin and phenacemide (Phenurone) are known to prevent or modify drug-induced convulsions in experimental animals, but their value as treatment agents does not appear to match their effectiveness as prophylactic drugs. In the presence of an actual or an impending convulsion, the best treatment in most cases is the immediate parenteral administration of diazepam or any barbiturate drug with a short latency and short duration of action.

Parenteral diazepam (Valium) is now widely

accepted as the drug of choice in treating status epilepticus. It is effective in suppressing convulsions from many causes, including chemical poisoning, drug withdrawal reactions, epilepsy, head trauma, brain tumors, etc. It is particularly recommended against the convulsions sometimes encountered in patients with considerable degrees of central nervous depression, as in imipramine and chlorpromazine poisonings, where barbiturates are dangerous because they are more apt to induce apnea. As an anticonvulsant, diazepam is usually administered intravenously in a dose of 0.1 to 0.2 mg./kg. (see Table IV-1). The intramuscular route is inferior but permissible if convulsions prevent an intravenous injection. When only the intravenous route is used and the injection is made slowly (*e.g.*, over a period of at least 1 to 2 minutes), the response

Table IV-1
Parenteral Therapy for the Suppression of Convulsions

Drug	Form	Route[a]	Dose (Adult)[b]	Technique
Diazepam (*e.g.*, Valium)	Sterile soln.: 0.5% (5 mg./ml.) containing water, propylene glycol, alcohol and preservatives	i.v. or i.m.	5–10 mg. (1–2 ml.), up to a total dose of about 30 mg.	Initial adult dose is 1–2 ml. (i.v.), repeated as necessary at 10–15-min. intervals to a total dose of about 6 ml. The sequence can be repeated after 2–4 hours, *if necessary*
Lorazepam (*e.g.*, Ativar)	Sterile soln.: 0.2 and 0.4%, containing water, PEG-400, propylene glycol and preservatives	i.v. or i.m.	8 mg.	For i.v., dilute with equal vol. sterile water or saline. Inject 4 mg. not faster than 2 mg./min. Repeat after 15 min. *if necessary*
Pentobarbital sodium (*e.g.*, Nembutal sodium)	Sterile soln.: 5%, containing water, propylene glycol, and alcohol, or a freshly prepared aqueous solution	i.v. or i.m.	0.2–0.5 gm. (4–10 ml.) or 3–7 mg./kg.	In an adult the initial dose is 2–3 ml. (100–150 mg.) injected i.v. over a period of at least 2 min. Then wait 2–5 min. and repeat *as necessary*
Amobarbital sodium (*e.g.*, Amytal sodium)	Sterile soln.: 5%. Only freshly prepared aqueous solutions are suitable. Sterile ampul contains 0.25 or 0.5 gm. of dry powder	i.m. or i.v.	0.3–0.6 gm. (6–12 ml.)	For i.v. injection, use approximately the same volumes and timing as for pentobarbital. For i.m. injections, 10% solutions are preferable (but not required)
Phenobarbital sodium	Aqueous solutions must be freshly prepared, but stable, sterile propylene glycol-water solutions are available (60 or 130 mg./ml.)	i.m. or i.v.	0.26–0.78 gm.	Start with 0.26 gm (i.m.) (2 × 130 mg.). Repeat in 30 min. *as necessary*. Can also be given i.v. but long latency invites overdosage
Thiopental sodium (*e.g.*, Pentothal sodium)	Sterile soln.: 2.5%. Only freshly prepared aqueous solutions are suitable	i.v. *only* (avoid extravasation)	0.1–0.2 gm. (4–8 ml.)	In an average adult, 3–5 ml. can be injected i.v. without delay. Then wait 1 min. and repeat injection *if necessary*. Supplemental doses of 1–3 ml. are given as required (*e.g.*, every 5 min.), but the total cumulative dose should be kept below 1.0 gm. (40 ml.).

[a] In general, the i.v. route is preferred if convulsions are imminent or have already begun.
[b] Except for thiopental sodium, these doses are not anesthetic in convulsing patients. Much larger doses of barbiturates in the anesthetic range are sometimes required to control convulsions.

is so prompt that the dose can often be adjusted accordingly. Mixing or diluting diazepam with infusion fluids is not recommended; the commercial solution (5 mg./ml.) is usually injected directly by syringe.

Adverse reactions to intravenous diazepam include local irritation (phlebitis) with venous thrombosis. In elderly, debilitated or chemically depressed individuals, diazepam-induced apnea, hypotension and cardiac arrest have been described. None of these reactions, however, is common, and a slow injection rate reduces the risk of any of these complications. The principal disadvantage of intravenous diazepam is not its toxicity but its short duration of action. Convulsions may be suppressed for only 10 to 15 minutes, although an hour is probably more typical. Whereas additional doses can be given, tolerance has been reported to develop rapidly, and diazepam is not regarded as an appropriate drug for maintenance control of recurrent convulsive disorders.

Because of their longer durations of action, two related benzodiazepines have been recommended in place of diazepam: clonazepam (Clonopin) and lorazepam (Ativan). The latter in particular may displace diazepam as the drug of choice in status epilepticus; see Table IV-1 for recommended doses and injection techniques.

Phenytoin (Dilantin) sodium has long been a mainstay in the treatment of status epilepticus. It has a much longer duration of action than diazepam, and it causes less central nervous depression than the barbiturates (see below). Intravenous phenytoin sodium has been widely used in the management of status epilepticus, particularly in idiopathic epilepsy and in postoperative convulsions in neurosurgical patients. A sterile solution containing 50 mg./ml. is available; the recommended adult dose is 150 to 250 mg. injected no faster than 50 mg./min., followed 30 minutes later by 100 to 150 mg. if necessary. Fröscher (*Treatment of Status Epilepticus*, University Park Press, Baltimore, 1979) recommends much larger doses, namely 1000 mg. on the first day, partly i.v. and partly p.o. Even when given i.v., however, the drug has a long latency (5 to 20 minutes), and it may induce severe hypotension if injected too rapidly.

Of more concern is the question of whether phenytoin sodium is effective against convulsions induced by convulsant poisons, such as strychnine. Although Fröscher (*ibid.*) insists that it is an important drug in the management of status epilepticus from any cause, there are very few clinical reports that describe its successful use in poisonings by analeptic drugs or convulsants. In animals it is generally ineffective not only in treating but also in preventing convulsions induced by analeptic drugs and by electroshock. Therefore, we cannot recommend phenytoin sodium as a reliable anticonvulsant in clinical toxicology.

Barbiturate drugs have long been used successfully in the management of convulsions in chemical poisonings and in drug withdrawal reactions. With barbiturates the intramuscular route is often satisfactory and always safer than the intravenous channel. Because solutions of the sodium salts are locally irritating due to their alkalinity, no more than 5 ml. should be injected at any one intramuscular site. A violent and persistent convulsion, however, usually warrants intravenous therapy. Solutions of the sodium salts of thiopental, pentobarbital, and amobarbital are usually employed; phenobarbital sodium is hazardous by the intravenous route chiefly because the delay in its onset of action may mislead the therapist into giving too much.

The effective duration of action is the principal distinction among these barbiturates (see p. III-53). In the dose ranges recommended in Table IV-1, phenobarbital is the most persistent and thiopental is the most transient. If thiopental sodium is used to counteract a convulsant poison for more than 15 to 30 minutes, more drug is usually required than is recommended in Table IV-1. The larger the cumulative dose of thiopental the slower is the recovery from its effects; if enough is given to saturate body storage depots (chiefly adipose tissue), thiopental's actions are as persistent as those of pentobarbital.

Appropriate doses and proper techniques for injecting barbiturates into convulsing patients are outlined in Table IV-1. Smaller amounts are sometimes adequate, and for this reason all doses are administered fractionally. No more than a just adequate dose is ever used, because the barbiturate effect should not be allowed to extend into the phase of central nervous depression, which most convulsant poisons induce eventually. Except for phenobarbital, the barbiturate doses in Table IV-1 are sufficient to induce deep hypnosis if not anesthesia in normal adults—but not all victims of stimulant poisons. On the other hand, anesthesia is often unnecessary to control convulsions. For treating infants and children, the proper adult dose is reduced in proportion to the body weight or to the body surface area., Elderly persons and those with parenchymal liver disease require much less than recommended in Table IV-1. Overdosage with barbiturates requires treatment as outlined on p. III-58. After convulsions have been controlled, wakefulness, twitching, and hyperreflexia signal a need for more anticonvulsant drug.

Because of its ultrashort duration of action, thiopental (Pentothal sodium) is sometimes preferred when the convulsive phase is expected to be transient (*i.e.*, up to 30 minutes). This barbiturate, however, produces more untoward reactions than its congeners; among the occasional alarming effects observed during intravenous administration are a profound fall in arterial blood pressure, severe respiratory depression with cyanosis, varying degrees of laryngospasm, bronchospasm, hiccupping, sneezing, and coughing. The anesthesiologist who administers this drug in preparation for surgery minimizes the incidence of these reactions by premedication with intramuscular atropine and a conventional barbiturate, like pentobarbital, but premedication is obviously impractical in the emergency treatment of convulsions.

Clearly one should hesitate to use thiopental unless equipment is available for the administration of oxygen and artificial ventilation. Shock and a history of asthma are also important contraindications. Thiopental-induced laryngospasm and bronchospasm are usually self-limiting, but whenever these reactions are encountered, thiopental injections are best replaced by the inhalation of ether. Usually endotracheal intubation is practical in the presence of laryngospasm, but in general the procedure should be reserved for a trained anesthetist. (p. IV-4). If the longer duration of action is not expected to be critical, pentobarbital sodium is probably preferable to thiopental sodium in the hands of everyone except the expert.

Other drugs that have been recommended for suppressing convulsions in status epilepticus include lidocaine, chloral hydrate, paraldehyde and the inhalation anesthetics. In spite of the paradox that an overdose of lidocaine can induce convulsions (see p. III-118), intravenous lidocaine has been used successfully in status epilepticus in Europe (Fröscher, *op. cit.*). This use is neither approved nor widely recognized in the United States. Similarly, chloral hydrate seems to have few proponents today, except for those who manage alcohol and drug withdrawal reactions; the ratio of its anticonvulsant to sedative activity is rather low.

Paraldehyde has uses that are similar to those of chloral hydrate. Its anticonvulsant activity is undeniable, and it was once a major drug in the control of status epilepticus. It is still sometimes recommended for this purpose. Plastic syringes and needles cannot be used because paraldehyde is a solvent for many plastics. The intravenous route produces prompt effects but is considered dangerous. Deep intramuscular injection is painful, and absorption is slow and erratic. When oral administration is impractical, as in status epilepticus, paraldehyde can be administered rectally after dilution with 2 parts of vegetable oil (or mineral oil). A mixture of equal parts of

diethyl ether and oil has been used in the same way. Both of these solutions are given as retention enemas in a dose of 0.5 to 1 ml. of the mixture per kg. of body weight. Because the level of anesthesia cannot be effectively controlled when the rectum is used as the route of administration, supplemental doses of barbiturates are best avoided.

If other available measures fail to suppress status epilepticus, general anesthesia can be induced with one of the inhalation agents, usually ether or nitrous oxide. Under these circumstances, however, it is difficult to know how long to sustain the anesthetic state or how to judge the patient's need for more conventional anticonvulsant therapy.

Substances which relax skeletal muscles are recommended occasionally as adjuvants to the anticonvulsive drugs. Two categories of muscle relaxants are recognized: those which act on central nervous synapses, such as meprobamate and diazepam, and those which act peripherally to produce a neuromuscular blockade, such as curare (*d*-tubocurarine), gallamine (Flaxedil), decamethonium (C-10, Syncurine), and succinylcholine (Anectine). Each of these drugs has received clinical trials in cases of electroshock therapy, tetanus, or status epilepticus. As noted above, diazepam is now used as a primary agent in the control of convulsions rather than as an adjuvant.

With the possible exceptions of meprobamate, diazepam and their congeners, these muscle relaxants have no effect on the neurologic basis of convulsions. They act only to modify convulsions by weakening or paralyzing skeletal muscles and so prevent the fractures, luxations, and pain of violent seizures. Because the intensity of the drug response cannot be accurately predicted or controlled, a complete flaccid paralysis sometimes results. This is not necessarily a tragic complication, since artificial ventilation is practicable when apnea is due to flaccid paralysis and not when due to convulsive spasm. However, all equipment necessary for rapid resuscitation, such as endotracheal intubation, controlled artificial ventilation, oxygen administration, and suction, should be on hand. The therapist without special apparatus and special training is ill advised to use any of these skeletal muscle relaxants in the control of convulsions.

Central Nervous Depression

As used here, the phrase "central nervous depression" is equivalent to the toxicologists' "narcosis" and is not related to the syndrome of psychic depression or melancholia. Central nervous depression follows overdoses of many drugs and toxic chemicals, all of which presumably interfere with brain metabolism. In its severest form, this syndrome culminates in respiratory arrest as a result of general reflex paralysis. In its milder forms it may mimic any stage of clinical anesthesia: headache, inattention, vertigo, confusion, agitation, drowsiness, stupor, and coma—often with a terminal convulsion which is probably due to anoxia or asphyxia.

Coma is a state of unconsciousness from which the victim cannot be aroused. In coma the vital signs are generally reduced, and reflexes are frequently depressed or absent. Various regulatory centers in the medulla oblongata are commonly inhibited, notably the vasomotor center with consequent vasodilatation and hypotension, and the respiratory center with consequent underbreathing and cyanosis. Circulatory insufficiency may be aggravated by the hypoxia which stems from inadequate pulmonary ventilation.

To characterize the intensity of coma in clinical terms, various classification schemes have been proposed. Table IV-2 summarizes one classification that recognizes four progressive stages of deepening coma. Although the original proposal was intended to describe barbiturate poisoning only, the classification has been widely used (sometimes with considerable strain) to characterize comas due to all kinds of non-narcotic drugs and chemicals.

In any single patient, clinical signs may change rapidly as the intensity of coma fluctuates. Good care requires that the the patient's status be monitored continuously as long as coma persists.

Table IV-2
An Intensity Classification of Coma[a]

Stage I:	Patient is comatose but withdraws from painful stimuli, such as pinching or venipuncture. Deep tendon reflexes are intact. No depression of respirations or blood pressure
Stage II:	No withdrawal from painful stimuli, such as pinching or venipuncture. Most reflexes are intact. No depression of respirations or blood pressure
Stage III:	No withdrawal from painful stimuli. Most reflexes are depressed, but respirations and blood pressure are only slightly depressed, if at all
Stage IV:	No withdrawal from painful stimuli. Most reflexes are depressed or absent. Respiratory rate is less than 8 per minute and/or systolic blood pressure is less than 85 mm. Hg

[a] Slightly modified from Arieff and Friedman (*Am. J. Med. Sci.*, 266:405–426, 1973), which in turn was inspired by a classification of Reed, Driggs and Foote (*Ann. Intern. Med.*, 37:290–303, 1952).

This is a difficult objective to achieve unless the patient is kept in an intensive care unit of a modern hospital. With most depressant drugs, the prognosis for eventual recovery is good if the coma does not reach stage IV.

In deeply comatose states (usually stage IV), early deaths are most often due to respiratory arrest or to cardiovascular collapse, but delayed fatalities may arise from anyone or any aggregate of the following complications: cerebral edema, pulmonary edema, hypostatic pneumonia, lung abscess, hyperpyrexia without infection, and irreversible renal failure. An occasional patient who survives severe and prolonged hypoxia during the acute phase may suffer residual neurological lesions.

Of course coma may arise from many causes; the differential diagnosis is extensive. When poison is responsible, the etiology is usually established through a history provided by the victim's family or friends. If no reliable history is immediately available, diagnostic clues are sought in terms of the physical examination, especially the neurological examination. The existence of lateralizing neurological signs suggests a focal lesion in the central nervous system, such as a tumor, infection or hemorrhage. A lumbar puncture that produces bloody or xanthochromic spinal fluid supports a diagnosis of a cerebrovascular accident. Many focal lesions in the cranium can be detected and localized by computerized tomography (CT). CT is now an invaluable tool in diagnosing the cause of coma.

If the CT scan and spinal fluid are normal and the neurological signs are bilaterally symmetrical and cardiopulmonary function is grossly intact, the presumptive diagnosis is an intoxication due to some exogenous or endogenous chemical. Sometimes the issue can be clarified quickly by a chemical screening procedure performed on blood or urine; for examples, see Section III under Laboratory for each congener. Sometimes a careful physical examination reveals clinical signs that are more apt to be generated by one coma-producing chemical than by another; for example, see Section III under Symptomatology for each congener. In general, however, even the most elaborate clinical examination is not adequate to establish convincingly the chemical basis of a patient's comatose state.

When the cause of coma cannot be established promptly and unequivocally by the measures outlined above, it is a routine practice in many treatment centers to administrate in sequence an i.v. bolus of glucose, an i.v. injection of naloxone (Narcan) and an i.v. (or i.m.) injection of thiamine. The first two injections are potentially both diagnostic and therapeutic because prompt arousal after the first establishes a presumptive diagnosis of hypoglycemic coma and arousal after the second indicates a narcotic overdose.

The thiamine is included on the premise that the coma may represent an alcoholic encephalopathy of the Wernicke-Korsakoff variety. Large doses of these agents are used. In adult patients 50 to 100 ml. of 50% glucose is injected; in children the dose is usually 1 gm./kg. (up to 50 gm.). With naloxone (Narcan) hydrochloride a single dose as large as 2 mg. is often administered to comatose adults (for children, see p. III-287). The adult dose of thiamine hydrochloride is 100 mg. under these circumstances. Even if these injections do not relieve the coma, it is believed that they do no significant harm.

Almost every patient in deep coma requires prompt, intensive, sustained, and multifaceted treatment. Unless glucose or naloxone prove to be curative, the whole armamentarium of the therapist may be needed. The highest priority usually goes to the correction of anoxia. Any one or group of the following measures may be necessary: the removal of airway obstruction (p. IV-2), oxygen administration (p. IV-12), artificial ventilation (p. IV-7), and perhaps analeptic therapy (see below). If anoxia can be minimized, cardiovascular collapse is often avoided.

Mild degrees of hypotension are properly ignored, but severe circulatory failure deserves treatment as outlined under vasogenic shock (p. IV-16). Dehydration and electrolyte disturbances must be corrected (pp. IV-64–75), and if coma persists, a program of parenteral alimentation is instituted (p. IV-76). The periodic intake of even small amounts of glucose or other carbohydrate is usually sufficient to prevent the ketosis and acidosis of starvation.

The parenteral administration of a wide-spectrum antibiotic is no longer considered an advisable prophylactic measure, but overt infection must be treated promptly and vigorously (p. IV-85). The patient should be examined repeatedly for signs of urinary retention, and if the bladder is distended, it should be emptied by catheterization if other measures fail (p. IV-51). To prevent hardening of the colonic contents and fecal impactions, an occasional oil retention enema is desirable. Defects in temperature regulation have to be compensated artificially (p. IV-84); hypothermia due to abnormally rapid heat loss and minimal heat production is the usual problem requiring attention, but toxic fevers also occur. Repositioning the patient in his bed at frequent intervals minimizes the occurrence of such complications as hypostatic pneumonia, decubitus ulcers, and venous thrombosis (p. IV-83).

The proper role of stimulant or analeptic drugs, once a topic of serious controversy, is now generally neglected or ignored. With the exception of specific narcotic antagonists in the treatment of opiate overdoses, analeptics are regarded at the present time by most therapists as unnecessary and even hazardous because they distract attention from the essential elements of supportive treatment. In the past 30 to 35 years a large number of reports describing the successful treatment of barbiturate poisoning without stimulants emphasizes by indirection that analeptics had often been used unnecessarily. The comatose patient who moves in response to a painful stimulus, whose respirations and blood pressure are not depressed severely and whose swallowing and cough reflexes are intact has no need for an arousal drug, and none should be given. In more deeply comatose patients the vital signs may require active support, but measures other than analeptic drugs are available in any modern hospital with an intensive care unit. In many such institutions, analeptics have been effectively banished.

The opprobrium which these drugs are now accorded may not be entirely appropriate because not all victims of poison have access to the resources of modern intensive care units and the physician teams that operate them. The value of analeptic therapy has been proved repeatedly in experimental poisonings in laboratory animals. It seems likely that, properly employed, they could become useful adjuvants in managing deeply comatose patients, particularly when no resources are available for monitoring continuously the vital signs. Even when there seems to be a clear and compelling need, however, analeptic therapy is never a substitute for the supportive measures described above; it is properly regarded as only one and probably a minor phase of general supportive treatment.

Whereas camphor and strychnine have long been acknowledged to be obsolete as medicinal agents, the status of many other central nervous stimulants is ambiguous. Within modern times many analeptics have been recommended; the list includes various amphetamines, bemegride, caffeine and related methyl xanthines, doxapram, ephedrine, ethamivan, methylphenidate, nikethamide, pentylenetetrazol, and picrotoxin.

Appropriately or not, most of these agents are no longer marketed in the United States. Among the available ones, only a few can be purchased in forms suitable for parenteral administration. In any case physicians experienced in the use of analeptic drugs are believed to be few in number. Of course these considerations do not apply to the narcotic antagonists, such as nalorphine, naloxone or levallorphan, which are not general excitatory drugs. Their effectiveness in treating states of coma due to morphine and its congeners is well established and widely recognized (p. III-286).

Table IV-3 lists doses and methods of administering general analeptics currently available for parenteral use. Regardless of the cause of central nervous depresssion, these drugs are

Table IV-3
Analeptic Therapy in Central Nervous Depression

Drug	Form	Route	Adult Dose[a]	Comment
Doxapram (Dopram)	Sterile soln. of hydrochloride: 20 mg./ml. (in 20 ml. multiple dose vials)	i.v.	1. Priming dose: 1.0 mg./kg. in mild depression, 2.0 mg./kg. in moderate depression 2. Maintenance: repeat once after 5–10 min. and then hourly or i.v. infusion at hourly rate not to exceed 3 mg./kg.	Recommended maximal dose is 3 gm. in 24 hours. Maintenance doses given only to patients who show beneficial responses to priming dose
Nikethamide (Coramine)	Sterile soln.: 25%	i.v., i.m., s.c., (p.o.)	1–5 ml. by any route	Probably safer but certainly less effective than the above in most situations
Caffeine	Mixed salt with sodium benzoate. Sterile soln.: 0.50 gm./2 ml., equivalent to 250 mg. caffeine	i.v., i.m., (p.o.), (rectal)	0.5–1.0 gm. every 1–3 hours as necessary, usually by the intramuscular route. Do not exceed 6 gm. in 24 hours	Generally safe, but a single dose may remain effective for several hours. With repeated doses, cumulative toxicity may occur if the primary poison is detoxified first

[a] These doses are regarded as appropriate in severe grades of depression; they should be adjusted for the depth of coma and the response to treatment.

given, if at all, only with the intent of raising and maintaining the general level of reflex excitability and of restoring protective reflexes, until sufficient time passes to allow detoxication and excretion of the original poison. A beneficial response consists of an increase in rate or depth of breathing and rise in the blood pressure toward normotensive levels. In the apneic patient spontaneous respirations may be induced. Thus the major therapeutic value of these medicinals is their analeptic actions on the medullary centers of respiration and vasomotion. At the same time there may be improvement in muscle tone and the appearance of spontaneous movements. To be effective, large and repeated doses may be required, but these agents should not be used to restore consciousness because the attempt may precipitate convulsions. Any convulsive seizure induced by an analeptic drug is followed by a phase of depression which may dangerously aggravate the primary intoxication.

Of the three drugs listed in Table IV-3, doxapram seems to be the only one that continues to attract medical attention. It can stimulate breathing in doses that cause little generalized excitation. This respiratory stimulation arises from excitation of carotid chemoreceptors at low doses and from excitation of medullary respiratory neurons at higher doses. Nikethamide appears to lack the first of these two actions. With the recommended i.v. dose of doxapram (Table IV-3), the tidal volume tends to increase, and there is an associated small rise in the breathing frequency. These respiratory effects usually occur in 20 to 40 seconds, peak at 1 to 2 minutes and disappear after 5 to 12 minutes. These actions, however, cannot be induced regularly in deeply comatose patients without using excessive doses.

The blood pressure may also rise moderately after an injection of doxapram, allegedly because of cardiac stimulation and not peripheral vasoconstriction. Perhaps catecholamine release is involved in this cardiac action. Caffeine can also stimulate the heart, but the rise in blood pressure after caffeine is due at least in part to excitation of the medullary vasomotor center with consequent peripheral vasoconstriction.

Any of the clinically useful analeptics may produce a convulsive seizure if given in immoderate amounts. An impending convulsion may be signaled by hyperreflexia, spontaneous movement, muscle twitching, and the sudden restoration of responsiveness to painful stimuli. In the presence of these signs, analeptic therapy should be terminated or at least interrupted. Diazepam should be available for immediate intravenous injection if a convulsion occurs. Other unwanted subconvulsive reactions to stimulant drugs are straining, coughing, sneezing, laryngospasm, cardiac arrhythmias, retching, and vomiting. These effects may be difficult to control.

Various considerations of a miscellaneous nature are sometimes of paramount importance in treating central nervous system depression. In any victim of poison, increased intracranial pressure warrants investigation and treatment according to the principles discussed below. Many chemicals that induce severe grades of central nervous depression circulate in the blood as dialyzable substances. The excretion of barbiturates, glutethimide, alcohols, and many other depressants can be promoted by hemoperfusion, hemodialysis or intermittent peritoneal dialysis (pp. IV-55–58). Hydration or even overhydration, when accompanied by the administration of an osmotic diuretic, may accelerate the renal excretion of an intoxicant (pp. III-55 and IV-52), providing that the kidneys and circulatory system have not been damaged. By speeding recovery and particularly by shortening the phase of coma, these techniques may forestall the development of fatal complications.

Elevated Intracranial Pressure

Exogenous chemicals may produce a variety of diffuse and even localized lesions within the cranium that lead to significant elevations in the cerebrospinal fluid pressure. As measured in the ventricles of the human brain, the mean CSF pressure is normally 65 to 195 mm. CSF (or water), which is equivalent to about 5 to 15 mm. Hg. Any abnormal space-occupying mass of sufficient size within the cranium leads to intracranial hypertension. The mass may be localized and discrete (e.g., tumor, abscess, hematoma, aneurysm, etc.), wide-spread but discrete (e.g., dilatation of intracranial arteries or veins, petechial hemorrhages, etc.) or diffuse (e.g., brain edema). In clinical toxicology brain edema (often misnamed cerebral edema) is probably the commonest cause of intracranial hypertension.

In some poisonings, however, the primary intracranial pathology appears to be a vasculitis with congestion, thrombosis, and hemorrhage. Arsenic poisoning, particularly with organic arsenicals, may lead to a hemorrhagic encephalitis with multiple symmetrical foci of hemorrhagic necrosis and sometimes gross cerebral hemorrhage. In contrast, edematous swelling without hemorrhage is the rule in lead encephalopathy. Of course hemorrhage in the brain as elsewhere may occur in any bleeding diathesis, notably in poisonings due to warfarin and other agents that induce hypoprothrombinemia.

Three types of brain edema are recognized by R. A. Fishman (*Cerebrospinal Fluid in Diseases of the Nervous System*, W. B. Saunders, Philadelphia, 1980); they are called vasogenic edema, cellular (cytotoxic) edema and interstitial edema. The latter is also known as hydrocephalic edema because it is best characterized in obstructive hydrocephalus. The genesis of this form of brain edema is an obstruction to the flow of CSF within the ventricles or a blockade of CSF absorption in the subarachnoid space. The ventricles (at least those rostal to the obstruction) are dilated, and the periventricular white matter is grossly edematous from CSF that has crossed the ependymal membrane. Interstitial brain edema of this type is not likely to arise from exposure to exogenous poisons.

On the other hand both vasogenic edema and cytotoxic edema of the brain have been ascribed to chemical insults. Vasogenic edema is a consequence of an abnormal rise in the permeability of brain capillaries. The endothelium of these capillaries is normally characterized by unusually tight cellular junctions, so that large hydrophilic molecules like proteins cannot diffuse from blood to brain or do so very slowly. This state of exclusion has long been called the "blood-brain barrier." If the functional integrity of this barrier is compromised, protein and water leak into the substance of the brain, which then becomes swollen. The white matter is more vulnerable than the gray matter to the resulting distortions of brain architecture. The protein content of the CSF rises, and the volume of the ventricles decreases as the brain tissue swells. Brain edema and swelling in lead encephalopathy (p. III-228) have been ascribed to this type of capillary injury. Enhanced capillary permeability is also thought to account for the edema of purulent meningitis and the localized edema around such focal brain lesions as a tumor, abscess, trauma, infarction and hemorrhage.

In cellular (cytotoxic) edema of the brain the primary injury is to the neurons and glial cells. The breakdown of metabolic products within damaged cells leads to osmotic transfer of water from the extracellular space to the intracellular space. The swelling of cells raises the intracranial pressure and reduces the volume of the ventricles. The commonest cause of cellular edema is hypoxia or asphyxia, as, for example, during cardiac arrest. Perhaps the histotoxic anoxia of cyanide and hydrogen sulfide poisonings also initiates the process of neuronal and glial swelling. A less common cause of cellular edema of the brain is acute plasma hypo-osmolality because of dilutional hyponatremia, inappropriate ADH secretion or acute sodium depletion (p. IV-68). Still another form of osmotic disequilibrium that may result in cellular edema of the brain occurs when the plasma solute concentration of a patient with chronic plasma hyperosmolality is suddenly reduced to normal by medical treatment. This situation sometimes arises in the therapy of diabetic ketoacidosis and during hemodialysis of uremic patients.

The three types of brain edema described above may coexist, and distinctions are not always practical. For example, cardiac arrest promptly produces cellular edema of neurons and glia, but vasogenic edema may intervene later, perhaps because capillary endothelial cells are slower to express an anoxic injury. Indeed, whatever the cause, brain edema that is acute, intense and diffuse eventually raises the intracranial pressure enough to compress the microvasculature. Thus, ischemia and tissue anoxia are both causes and consequences of brain edema.

In many states of intoxication the neuropathology has been ascribed to brain anoxia. In addition to diffuse edema, a few petechial hemorrhages are not uncommon, and if the victim survives for 2 or 3 days, cloudy swelling and diffuse cellular necrosis can be recognized in microscopic sections of his brain. These anoxic lesions have been described in acute fatalities due to ether, chloroform, morphine, barbiturates, and probably many other central nervous system depressants. Similar lesions in carbon monoxide poisoning have also been ascribed to brain anoxia. Perhaps the same is true of the increased intracranial pressure described in patients acutely intoxicated with ethyl, methyl, and isopropyl alcohols.

Sometimes exogenous poisons create chronic elevations of intracranial pressure that last for months or years. One example is a syndrome known as pseudotumor cerebri or benign intracranial hypertension (although it is not always benign). Besides a high intracranial pressure (frequently 300 to 600 mm. CSF), the absence of localizing neurological signs is a requirement of the diagnosis. It is also necessary to rule out mass lesions, obstructive hydrocephalus, hypertensive encephalopathy and some other established causes of intracranial hypertension. The only symptoms may be headache and blurring or dimness of vision, which is usually associated with papilledema. The syndrome has been ascribed to many etiological agents and states (reviewed by Fishman, *op. cit.*), but the pathogenesis is not well understood. Brain edema seems to be the only consistent pathological finding. Among the exogenous chemicals held responsible for clinical cases of pseudotumor cerebri are vitamin A and tetracycline in excessive doses. Cases have also been ascribed to Kepone after industrial exposures. Probably some of the other chlorinated hydrocarbon insecticides are also capable of inducing this illness.

Of course an elevation in the intracranial pressure may be due to a disease process that is concurrent with but independent of a chemical insult, or the relationship may be very indirect. For example, trauma, tumor, infection (abscess, meningitis, encephalitis), and postinfectious states of allergy (postinfectious encephalitis) are all recognized causes of abnormally high cerebrospinal fluid pressure. The same is true of renal and hepatic failure in some instances.

Significant elevations of the intracranial pressure are not always easy to recognize. Papilledema (choked disc) is an important sign that occurs reasonably early in many cases but not in all. Various deviations in the vital signs, such as arterial hypertension, bradycardia and respiratory slowing (the Cushing triad), are apt to be late manifestations unless the pathology induces an early compression or displacement of the brain stem. Similarly, cardiac arrhythmias, pulmonary edema and upper gastrointestinal hemorrhage are late and uncommon responses to elevated intracranial pressure. Headache and altered states of consciousness are common in clinical toxicology but they are not diagnostic of brain edema because there are so many other causes.

A lumbar puncture can provide definitive evidence of an elevation in the cerebrospinal pressure. Except when portions of the brain have already herniated below the tentorium or into the foramen magnum, a high lumbar spinal fluid pressure is always indicative of an elevation in the intracranial pressure. A lumbar puncture is a generally safe procedure except when there is a localized space-occupying mass in the brain (tumor, abscess, or hemorrhage). If one uses precautions to prevent the escape of spinal fluid, the hazard of herniation is reduced but not eliminated. The danger is so real that in modern medical centers lumbar puncture is postponed in any suspected cases until computerized tomography (CT) rules out an intracranial mass lesion or an obstruction or displacement of the ventricular system. In the absence of CT, similar information can sometimes be obtained by various echo devices or by arteriography.

Certainly it is easier to diagnose an increase in the intracranial pressure than it is to evaluate its contribution to the morbidity of any victim of poison. Perhaps because lumbar puncture is not a routine procedure in clinical toxicology, there is only meager evidence about the role of elevated intracranial pressure in the morbidity and mortality of poison victims. Now that there are available reasonably safe and moderately effective ways of reducing such pressure, the question deserves much more attention than it has received in the past. Lowering the cerebrospinal fluid pressure is certainly a more rational form of therapy than an analeptic drug whenever medullary depression is due to high intracranial pressure.

The treatment of intracranial hypertension also presents problems. Although it has been done often, especially in pseudotumor cerebri, one cannot safely reduce pressure in the cranium by draining cerebrospinal fluid from the subarachnoid space anywhere around the spinal cord. In the presence of high intracranial pressure, any attempt to do so may cause the brain to herniate downward at one of two common sites: either the uncus may slip below the tentorial notch or the cerebellum may herniate through the foramen magnum and compress the medulla. Both complications are more common when the cranium contains an abnormal space-occupying mass such as a tumor, abscess, or hematoma. If any one of these lesions is suspected, it should be located with the aid of CT, as noted above.

Many neurosurgical techniques have been used to remove aliquots of CSF directly from the cranial cavity, both from the subarachnoid space and from the brain ventricles. Although the resulting drop in intracranial pressure tends to be disappointingly transient, these procedures are sometimes tried, especially in Reye's syndrome. Patients with pseudotumor cerebri are even provided occasionally with surgical shunts to remove CSF. In most patients with brain edema, however, removing CSF from the ventricles seems to hasten obliteration of the ventricular space by promoting further brain swelling. Interest has recently revived in a radical and highly controversial surgical procedure known as hemicraniectomy. It may be an effective method of decompression when brain edema is regional but not when it is general. In any case it is limited to life-threatening and intractable disease and then only if it can be demonstrated that brain stem function is still intact.

In the medical treatment of acute brain edema, the head is elevated, and any angulation of the neck that might impede venous drainage from the cranial cavity is avoided. Some of these patients need ventilatory support (pp. IV-7–12). Indeed, artificially induced hyperventilation (respiratory alkalosis) lowers acutely the intracranial pressure by producing cerebral vasoconstriction. The effect, however, lasts only as long as the arterial plasma CO_2 tension is maintained at subnormal levels (usually 28 to 32 mm. Hg). Even when respiratory alkalosis is not contraindicated, this method of lowering intracranial pressure is useful for only short periods, as, for example, during a neurosurgical operation.

The systemic administration of glucocorticoids, particularly dexamethasone, has proven effective against the vasogenic edema associated with brain tumor (primary and metastatic), brain abscess and head trauma. In one dosage regimen 10 mg. dexamethasone is injected intravenously, followed by 4 mg. every 6 hours by intramuscular or intravenous injection, but a priming dose as high as 200 mg. in the first 6 hours has also been employed. The use of dexamethasone in brain infarction and in Reye's syndrome is still controversial. In the opinion of R. A. Fishman (*op. cit.*), the effectiveness of steroid therapy against cellular (cytotoxic) brain edema (see above) has not been demonstrated convincingly.

In most cases of brain edema, however, decompression can be accomplished at least temporarily by the intravenous infusion of an osmotically active solute that penetrates into the brain more slowly than water can migrate out of it. In the past, hypertonic solutions of sodium chloride, albumin, sucrose, dextrose and urea have all been employed, but mannitol and glycerol are now believed to be superior to the other substances. These "dehydrating" agents are most effective in cases of diffuse cerebral swelling, but they have also been used with apparent benefit in cases of tumor, presumably because peritumoral edema was reduced. A subdural hematoma is regarded as a contraindication to osmotic decompression of the cranium because decompression may increase the potential subdural space and so favor further hemorrhage. Perhaps a similar hazard exists in the presence of localized intracerebral hemorrhage, but diffuse petechial hemorrhages do not rule out this therapeutic measure.

Mannitol is available for intravenous injection in concentrations ranging from 5 to 25%; 20 and 25% solutions are usually used for osmotic decompression of the brain. Recommended doses range from 0.5 to 2.5 gm./kg. Any simple statement of dosage, however, tends to be misleading because the efficacy of the procedure depends upon producing and sustaining (for an undefined period) an elevation in the plasma osmotic pressure of at least 10 milliosmoles per liter; a 20 to 30 milliosmolal rise is usually sought. For this objective the rate of infusion may be just as important as the total dose. In most clinics these mannitol infusions have been completed in 5 to 20 minutes. If repeated hyperosmolal therapy is expected to be necessary, it is probably wiser to choose the smaller dose and the shorter infusion time.

Because mannitol and to a lesser extent glycerol in the recommended doses are diuretic, an indwelling bladder catheter is desirable in the comatose patient to avoid overdistension of the bladder. The body dehydration and salt losses produced by this treatment must eventually be corrected (p. IV-66), but rehydration should be conducted slowly and cautiously. Osmotic therapy is not appropriate in the presence of renal or cardiac insufficiency.

A glycerol (*i.e.*, glycerin) solution suitable for intravenous infusion is available commercially in England but not the United States. To avoid hemolysis the concentration of glycerol (in isotonic saline) should not exceed 10%; for the same reason the infusion rate should not exceed 4.5 ml./min. Glycerol, however, is usually administered by mouth or in comatose patients by nasogastric tube. The dose by this route is usually 1 to 1.5 gm./kg. as a 50 to 75% solution. In some cases a maintenance dose of 0.5 to 1.0 gm./kg. has been given every 3 to 4 hours. Unlike mannitol, glycerol is metabolized and therefore adds to the caloric load. Clinical experience with mannitol is more extensive than with glycerol.

To assess the efficacy and progress of osmotic decompression of the brain, it is desirable to monitor intermittently or continuously both the plasma osmolality and the intracranial pressure. For the latter purpose a variety of extradural and subdural devices can be inserted through the skull. In very few case reports, however, has either of these measurements been described. Although the data are incomplete and highly variable, it appears that both mannitol and glycerol in the recommended doses are capable of lowering the intracranial pressure by 50% or even more within 1 to 2 hours. The pressure then gradually returns to pretreatment levels over a period of 2 to 8 hours, unless the underlying defect has been repaired.

In hyperosmolal therapy the reduction in the volume of the brain and the lowering of the intracranial pressure are due to shifts of water from brain into the CSF and into the blood. This migration of water occurs only while the osmolality of the plasma exceeds that of the CSF and brain. In brain regions where capillary walls may be damaged, the solute concentration gradient from blood to brain is poorly sustained. Thus osmotic decompression is likely to be less successful with vasogenic edema than with other types of edema (see above).

Even with a normal blood-brain barrier, significant amounts of injected mannitol and glycerol eventually diffuse across the capillary wall and accumulate in the brain itself. With a falling solute concentration in the plasma due to urinary excretion, the osmotic gradient between blood and brain may then become reversed, so that water moves back into the brain substance. In some cases the intracranial pressure rises to a level that exceeds the pretreatment level. Such "rebound" rises are infrequent, but they are alarming and dangerous. To avoid rebound phenomena, the therapist should use the smallest dose of mannitol or glycerol that proves to be effective.

The need for another course of hyperosmolal therapy or at least for another diagnostic lumbar puncture can be recognized by increasing somnolence or deepening coma, by dilated or unequal pupils, and by changing vital signs, such as irregular or periodic breathing, bradycardia, and mounting hypertension. If necessary, hypertonic solutions of mannitol or glycerol may be infused many times over a period of a few days, but numerous precautions must be taken. With repeated therapy it becomes essential to monitor the plasma osmolality and electrolyte levels, to measure the intake and output of fluids and to take appropriate corrective measures if dehydration or overhydration are detected. The progressive accumulation of osmoles in blood (and by inference in tissues) must be avoided because excessive osmolality can itself induce coma, which has been reported as a complication of glycerol therapy. Osmotic decompression of the brain is not a practical form of chronic treatment.

Induced hypothermia is another modality of treatment for dangerous elevations of intracranial pressure due to diffuse brain edema. It can be used alone or in combination with hyperosmolal therapy. Many reasons might be cited in support of the premise that this form of treatment should be ideal for protecting the edematous brain against permanent damage. In practice, however, the benefits have not been clearly demonstrated. Deep hypothermia is not easy to induce or sustain safely; apparently it has been used in rather few medical centers for this purpose.

Barbiturate anesthesia has recently attracted attention as an experimental mode of treatment for brain edema. By continuous titration with intravenous thiopental sodium, patients have been kept under controlled anesthesia for periods of one or more weeks. The procedure does lower the intracranial pressure, but the mechanisms responsible and the ultimate results in terms of morbidity and mortality are still topics of controversy.

Suicide

As judged by admissions to municipal hospitals, a large proportion of acute chemical poisonings in adults arises from acts of suicidal intent. Many varieties of drugs and toxic chemicals are ingested. For many decades, barbiturate drugs were the most popular poisons, but they are much less available in the home now than formerly because they are less frequently prescribed and because of greater legal restrictions on their movement in commerce. Recent trends in suicides have not been well defined, but during the past decade many depressed persons have consumed large quantities of antidepressant medication (tricyclic antidepressants, lithium, etc), along with ethyl alcohol, as agents in attempted suicide. Deliberate overdoses of aspirin and of diazepam are often described, and carbon monoxide has long been a favorite instrument of suicide.

As soon as medical treatment removes any threat to the patient's survival, the attending physician should evaluate carefully the meaning of the suicide attempt. Since almost everyone who attempts suicide is a potential repeater, no patient should be dismissed until there is an adequate opportunity to judge the seriousness of his suicidal intent, risk of another trial, and the possible need for such preventive measures as hospitalization and psychiatric care. Intelligent appraisal of the patient requires an elementary understanding of suicidal behavior in our culture, some knowledge of the psychiatric disorders in which it occurs, and close attention to the patient's mental status. The following remarks are intended as a guide for the general practitioner who is confronted with an emergency situation. Beyond the necessary immediate decisions, consultation with a psychiatrist is essential for details about the specific psychiatric diagnosis and treatment.

The act of suicide, reflecting in most cases severe psychological disturbances, may occur in a variety of psychiatric disorders. A useful way of categorizing suicide attempts, without evoking considerations of diagnosis, was offered by J. M. Weiss (*Psychiatry*, *20:* 17, 1957), who described three broad types. The first is the suicide gesture in which the patient is fairly confident that the outcome will not be fatal. The second is a more genuine attempt in which the person thinks that he may die but is not certain, *i.e.*, "a gamble with death." The last type is represented by the suicide act that is based on a deep and unambiguous intent to end life, and in most of these cases death would have resulted if the act had not been aborted through intervention.

These three types of suicidal behavior may be viewed on a spectrum of increasingly probable lethality. Although they do not fit into existing diagnostic categories in any highly specific fashion, the first and third types can be illustrated by and understood in terms of two groups of psychiatric disorders. The second type, in which the intent is uncertain, is generally the most difficult to appraise and may occur in any kind of emotional illness.

The first type, the suicide gesture, is the one encountered most frequently in the hospital emergency room. This form of behavior occurs in persons with personality trait disturbances, usually hysterical in nature. The gesture of suicide, typically melodramatic and impulsive, occurs in the midst of conflict with another person. Elements of revenge, retaliation, and coercion toward the other person are evident. Simultaneously the act may be prompted by less obvious determinants, such as the need to satisfy some more or less obscure psychological goal. Some degree of emotional depression is frequently present. Commonly there is a history of previous threats or actual gestures. Although the patient does not want to die, poor judgment may lead to serious injury or death. The risk of miscalculation is substantially greater if he is under the influence of alcohol or some other psychotropic drug when he makes his decision. On the other hand the attempt may be so blatantly inadequate as an act of self-destruction that the true intent seems obvious. Nevertheless the circumstances should be evaluated with care. The corroborative account of a relative or other informant will enable the physician to be more secure in his judgment.

Once the effects of the self-administered poison are controlled and convalescence begins, these patients often appear remorseful. Rarely is there any *immediate* threat of another attempt, particularly when the act served its "purpose" of successfully coercing the environment or of bringing about the desired reunion with another person. The danger of repetition is lessened further if there is a feeling of relief and gratitude or if some associated depression has been relieved through the dramatic episode. Whatever danger exists is mitigated by the physician who manages during his ministrations to control or avoid anxieties of his own and who is careful not to be provoked by the patient into anger or criticism. For these patients hospitalization may be unnecessary, but a psychiatric evaluation is important before the patient is released.

The third type of act, that based on serious intent, is usually related to major emotional depression. Here the physician should be familiar with the signs and symptoms of the depressive state, whether the diagnosis be psychoneurotic depression, psychotic depression, manic-depressive psychosis, or involutional melancholia. Although less often true of neurotic depression than of other types, an intense depression is commonly expressed by a characteristic group of clinical features. They consist of loss of interest, feelings of guilt (expressed as worthlessness or self-deprecation in severe cases), hopelessness, pessimism, and persistent thoughts of suicide. Either agitation or else retardation of thinking and movement may be seen. In agitated depressions the victim experiences exaggerated worry over real or imaginary situations and displays overt signs of discrete or diffuse anxiety. In contrast, the withdrawn patient is inactive, undemonstrative, and uncommunicative.

The vegetative signs of serious depression include persistent anorexia with weight loss, constipation, absence of sexual desire or potency, cessation or diminution of menstruation, and sleep disturbances with a typical pattern of awakening early. Patients frequently experience the greatest discomfort in the early morning upon awakening, with gradual improvement as the day progresses.

In the manic-depressive psychosis, mania or

hypomania may precede or follow the depressed phase. It is a somewhat ephemeral state characterized by optimism, well-being, and overactivity, in which the patient attempts to deny or ward off the depressive feeling from conscious awareness. The manic attack may terminate in suicide with little warning.

In states of depression suicide is said to occur more frequently at the onset and during early recovery than during the phase of deepest melancholy. In-patient psychiatric treatment is always indicated following an unsuccessful suicide attempt by a severely depressed patient.

The hysterical personality disorder and the psychotic depressive reaction are used here as examples of clinical categories in which are often seen the least serious and most serious acts of suicide, respectively. However, clinical studies reveal that suicide is attempted in a large number of psychiatric illnesses including affective psychoses (manic-depressive psychosis, involutional melancholia, psychotic depression), personality disorders, chronic alcoholism, delirium, dementia, and schizophrenia. Other less traditional categories include panic states (*e.g.*, sexual panics), pathological grief, reaction to despair and frustration, physical disfigurement, and learning of incurable disease. In these so-called reactive depressions, where the patient's distress is a response to a real external situation that is unfortunate and sometimes genuinely tragic, suicide is a distinct possibility whenever the emotional reaction is exaggerated out of proportion to the precipitating stimulus. Finally, severe states of emotional depression may occur at specific stages of various organic diseases. For example, the prolonged convalescence from acute or chronic arsenic poisoning is sometimes associated with severe melancholia; luetic paresis and pernicious anemia are said to be other examples.

The delirious or demented patient may present the least predictable risk of suicide. His confusion, disorientation, and tendency to misinterpret what he hears and sees may lead to panic and uncontrolled behavior. For example, he may leap from a window, misidentifying it as a door, in an attempt to escape from an imaginary situation which frightens him. Although the resulting death should not be classified as suicide because it was unintentional, the victim of delirium should be protected against himself in the same way as the person who seeks his own destruction. The clinical management of the delirious patient is described on p. IV-34.

As noted before, the most severe and most persistent of the suicidal urges occur in psychotically depressed patients. In schizophrenia suicidal impulses may arise in response to hallucinations or to paranoid delusions. Thus self-mutilation and death may represent the patient's

obedience to instructions he has heard in his hallucinations. On the other hand, when a paranoid person tries suicide, it represents an attempt to escape the painful persecutions which he mistakenly ascribes to a real or imaginary individual or group. The perseverance of suicidal behavior in the psychotic patient is sometimes extraordinary. At any time he may engage in such violent acts of self-destruction as throwing himself from a window, hanging himself with bed clothes, multilating himself with a knife, or raiding the hospital pharmacy for poisons. It is the duty of the physician to restrain this type of patient and in every other way to curtail his opportunities for violence.

Regardless of the clinical diagnosis, a physician may be aided in his appraisal of any patient as a suicide risk by a knowledge of some of the social and interpersonal factors that are often related to the act. For example, most grave acts of suicidal intent are performed by males, by elderly people, by those who are single, divorced or widowed, and by retired individuals, especially those recently retired. The attempt may occur in the wake of a recent death in the family or in situations where the patient feels that he is unwanted and a burden. Less earnest and less dangerous threats and gestures of suicide are likely to occur among females, young people, and married persons. In this group, problems that are commonly associated with suicide include the break-up of a marriage or engagement, a frustrated love relationship, and marital incompatibility.

A person belonging to this less dangerous group is more likely to announce to people around him, sometimes in a threatening or dramatic way, his intention to commit suicide. He is also more apt to make the gesture or attempt under circumstances where help will be forthcoming. On the other hand, in the earnest and serious trial, a declaration of intent may have been made only in a very disguised fashion or perhaps not at all. Certainly most persons make some kind of effort, consciously or subconsciously, to reveal their preoccupation with thoughts of suicide in what has been called the "cry for help." The assertion that the risk of suicide is low among those who talk about it is invalid even as a generalization.

In summary, the physician's judgment of the risk that remains after an unsuccessful suicide should be based upon a number of factors. First, he should attempt to obtain a detailed history of the events surrounding the act. If not incapacitated by his self-imposed illness, the patient is a primary source of these data. During the interview, the physician should make observations about the patient's personality structure (whether immature, histrionic, and provocative, as in the hysterical personality) and mood (whether depressed as manifested by tears, withdrawal, melancholic facial expressions, retardation). It is appropriate and sometimes helpful to question the patient directly about his feelings on the subject of suicide. The physician should search for signs and symptoms of a psychotic disorder. Where possible, a relative or other witness to the act should also be interviewed. If there is a farewell note, it should be evaluated carefully as another important source of clues about the meaning of the act. The nature and severity of the self-inflicted injury are major pieces of evidence. From all of these data the physician reaches an opinion about the patient's original intent, i.e., whether the act was largely a gesture, a more borderline "gamble with death," or a serious venture in self-destruction.

In evaluating further risk, the physician must consider the patient's current mental status and the various social and interpersonal factors that so often influence social behavior. These considerations may serve as more important predictors of further risk than a diagnosis of the underlying psychiatric disorder. For example, an elderly, retired, recently widowed male living alone who attempts suicide without prior communication is probably a poor risk even if there are no specific signs and symptoms upon which to base a diagnosis of depression, dementia, etc. Certainly the psychological seriousness of an act is not always correlated with its medical severity. A provocative suicide gesture by a person with a mildly hysterical character may lead to a drug-induced coma of dangerous intensity because of miscalculation or ignorance. Conversely, the individual who is profoundly dedicated to killing himself may err by taking too small a dose. In general, however, attempts at shooting, stabbing, hanging, and jumping from a height tend to reflect a more serious intent than the ingestion of drugs.

Finally, a psychiatrist should be consulted about any patient who tries suicide. Appropriate management usually consists of hospitalization on a general medical ward with careful observation until such consultation is obtained. Above all, before the patient is discharged, the physician should acquire a reasonable understanding of any suicide attempt in its psychological, social, and medical framework.

GASTROINTESTINAL TRACT

Mouth Care

After emergency decontamination (Section I), the local treatment of chemical burns in the mouth involves scrupulous oral hygiene. The practice of oral hygiene is also beneficial to many other types of patients, notably those who are comatose or in whom intubation is being maintained. Dryness of the mouth is best avoided by ensuring systemic hydration (p. IV-65). Dried secretions within the mouth are removed by swabbing with cotton pledgets moistened with a mild alkaline mouthwash. Cracking of the lips is prevented by the use of cold cream. Stomatitis can sometimes be controlled locally by mouth washes of 0.02% potassium permanganate, but infectious stomatitis also deserves systemic antibiotic therapy (p. IV-86). Even in patients with chemical burns of the mouth and throat, however, antibiotic therapy is no longer regarded as an advisable prophylactic measure; instead it should be reserved for cases with frank infection.

Nausea and Vomiting

The treatment of severe gastritis, which frequently accompanies chemical poisonings, depends upon the nature of the toxic agent (see Section II). Associated with gastritis, there is often severe nausea and vomiting. If the patient is semiconscious or unconscious, the aspiration of vomitus into the trachea is a major hazard; it can be minimized by keeping the victim on his side with his head slightly lower than his trunk. Better protection of the airway against the dangers of aspirated vomitus is obtained by the insertion of a cuffed endotracheal tube (p. IV-4).

However distressing to a conscious patient, no attempt (except perhaps gastric lavage—techniques and precautions of which are described in Section I) should be made to stop repeated emesis until it is reasonably certain that the vomitus no longer contains appreciable amounts of the ingested poison. The decision usually depends upon the duration of emesis and the volume of vomitus. In any case, the control of nausea and vomiting may be very difficult or even impossible in these cases.

Mild nausea associated with gastric irritation sometimes responds to sips of warm water, mild tea, or bland antacid preparations like alumina gels or milk of magnesia. Atropine sulfate given subcutaneously in doses of 0.3 to 1.2 mg., is often helpful. In some cases relief follows parenteral sedation (e.g., i.m. sodium phenobarbital or secobarbital), but morphine and other opium derivatives should be withheld. Many of the antihistaminic drugs have a mildly antiemetic action. Chlorpromazine (Thorazine) and some of the other phenothiazine tranquilizers (e.g., prochlorperazine) are effective in the control of nausea and vomiting from a variety of causes; prochlorperazine (Compazine) edisylate may be given intramuscularly in a dose of 5 to 10 mg. three or four times a day, but it is best avoided after exposure to hepatic toxins. In the presence of abdominal distension, nausea and vomiting may prove intractable to all measures except abdominal decompression (see below).

Losses of essential electrolytes through intensive vomiting can and *must* be addressed promptly by replacement therapy. Among the individual deficits which may arise are dehydration (p. IV-64), salt depletion (p. IV-66), hypochloremic alkalosis (p. IV-69), rarely metabolic acidosis (p. IV-69), and hypopotassemia (p. IV-72). Especially in young children, these deficiencies may reach alarming proportions within a short time. After water and electrolyte balances are restored, the administration of simple nutrients is usually desirable. As long as gastritis and vomiting persist, parenteral alimentation must be provided (p. IV-76).

In general, sips of warm water or tea may be offered within 12 to 24 hours after the nausea of acute gastritis subsides. Milk or strained gruel is sometimes preferred. At first the intake should be limited to 1 or 2 teaspoonfuls every half hour. If tolerated, a few salted crackers or dry toast may be added. Eventually small servings of a regular diet are given a trial. Although vomiting may be precipitated if oral feedings are inaugurated too soon or too zealously, eating should be resumed as soon as tolerated because parenteral alimentation is expensive and carries some risk of complications. For more detailed suggestions about the resumption of oral feedings, see p. IV-77.

Abdominal Distension

In acute chemical poisoning abdominal distension is usually paralytic in origin, and may indicate rupture of the stomach or bowel with generalized peritonitis. In any case prompt recognition is imperative. If the problem is one of simple paralytic ileus, gastric decompression is a useful prophylactic and therapeutic measure. If begun promptly, no other treatment is required.

Continuous gastric decompression is accomplished by nasogastric intubation. A no. 18 F Salem sump tube is appropriate for adults; plastic tubes are better tolerated than those made of rubber. To ensure proper gastric emptying of both air and fluid, the proper position of the tube tip in the gastric antrum should be confirmed by abdominal X-ray. A constant negative pressure is maintained by Wangensteen bottles or by a suction machine. The Salem sump tube is usually preferable to the double-lumen Miller-Abbott tube in the treatment of paralytic ileus because the inflated balloon of the Miller-Abbott tube is not carried into the small intestine when there is no effective peristalsis. The tube must be flushed periodically to prevent blockage.

With a nasogastric tube, abdominal decompression is usually effected within 12 to 18 hours, if at all, but suction may have to be continued prophylactically for several days. As long as it is maintained, the physician must correct repeatedly an inevitable hypochloremic alkalosis by administering parenterally isotonic saline or balanced salt solution (p. IV-71). Losses of potassium by gastric suction may be considerable. To maintain proper electrolyte balance these losses should be compensated by the inclusion of potassium salts in the parenteral infusions (p. IV-73).

In addition to gastric intubation, deflation of the colon may become important; it may be promoted by a rectal tube, usually a no. 38 F catheter. The procedures described above are usually more effective and safer than the administration of cholinergic drugs (see management of urinary retention below).

Diarrhea

As in the case of emesis, the physician should hesitate to suppress any diarrhea that might be beneficial in removing ingested poison. It is difficult to evaluate the importance of this excretory route in toxicology, but reasonably prompt evacuation would seem to be desirable in most cases.

Part of the poison eliminated in feces may represent material absorbed from and then re-excreted into the gastrointestinal tract. Thus appreciable quantities of many alkaloids, and perhaps of most, can be found in bile irrespective of the route of administration. To some extent this biliary excretion is nullified by the intestinal resorption of active poison. To minimize this enterohepatic recycling, a brisk passage of intestinal contents is thought to be desirable. As described in Section I, saline cathartics can be used to accomplish this purpose (*e.g.*, sodium or magnesium sulfate in doses of 30 gm. in water). High colonic irrigation is seldom warranted.

On the other hand, violent purging undoubtedly does more harm than good. At least mild attempts should be made to suppress any diarrhea which becomes persistent and copious. If it is reflex in origin, subcutaneous atropine sulfate (dose 0.3 to 1.2 mg.) is helpful. Good relief of pain and intestinal spasm is often provided by intramuscular meperidine (Demerol) hydrochloride (50 to 100 mg.) or codeine sulfate (30 to 60 mg.) every 3 hours. Hot or cold compresses on the abdomen may be of some value. If oral medication is not contraindicated, a mild antidiarrheal action can be obtained from kaolin (10 gm. with 1 ounce of water), activated charcoal (one or more tablespoonfuls), bismuth subcarbonate (1.0 gm.), or aluminum oxide gels. These agents also serve as adsorbents and may delay passage of toxic chemicals across the intestinal mucosa. Paregoric (camphorated tincture of opium) and other morphine preparations should be withheld or used only sparingly to control the pain of severe cramps. The paramount consideration, however, is the correction of dehydration and electrolyte imbalances that often result from persistent diarrhea (pp. IV-64–67, 69–73).

URINARY SYSTEM

Urinary Retention

Toxic agents may cause acute urinary retention by producing either bladder atony or vesicle neck spasm. In either instance a full bladder demands prompt drainage. This can be accomplished most readily by urethral catheterization. It is now generally recognized that such catheterization, particularly the use of an indwelling catheter, predisposes to urinary tract infection. Consequently this procedure should be undertaken only when absolutely necessary. The use of drugs, as discussed below, may be tried first to relieve urinary retention if there are no contraindications to their administration. An indwelling catheter (e.g., Foley catheter with a 5-ml. bag) should be utilized only when clearly required and never solely for the convenience of physicians and nurses. Finally, it should be removed as soon as practicable.

Inability to catheterize a patient usually means errors in technique, a poor choice of catheter or the presence of a urethral stricture or large prostate. The male urethra has the form of an S curve. If the penis is held under slight tension at right angles to the legs and abdomen, one curve of the S is thereby eliminated. Lubricate the catheter well. Avoid catheters which are too large for the urethral lumen and also those which are so small that they buckle within the urethra. Nos. 18, 20, and 22 F appear to be most easily introduced in most adult patients by most physicians. The use of a stylet by an inexperienced operator is inadvisable, as it may result in urethral tears or perforations. If the bladder is suspected to contain more than 500 ml. of urine, decompression should be accomplished slowly over a period of 10 to 20 minutes.

With continuous drainage maintained through an indwelling catheter, it was a common practice to irrigate the catheter and bladder periodically in the hope of suppressing bacterial growth within the organ. Many clinicians, however, now feel that the closed drainage system should not be interrupted for bladder irrigation, especially with patients in whom a catheter is expected to remain for only a short time, i.e., less than a week. Prophylactic antibiotics do not effectively prevent infection but merely predispose to the emergence of antibiotic-resistant organisms within the urinary tract. Similarly, chemotherapy of urinary infections is usually unsuccessful when a catheter is in place and frequently leads only to a change in the type of infective organism.

Although urethral catheterization is usually more effective, urinary retention from bladder atony or vesicle neck spasm can sometimes be controlled by drugs. The two most widely used are bethanechol chloride (Urecholine) and neostigmine methylsulfate. Urecholine is employed in doses of 10 to 30 mg. orally (and perhaps as high as 50 mg.) or 2.5 to 5 mg. subcutaneously; neostigmine is given subcutaneously in doses of 0.5 to 1.0 mg. Although these drugs may be given several times daily, their actions are uncertain and frequently include unpleasant cholinergic side effects such as sweating, lacrimation, salivation, and intestinal cramps. In some patients these unwanted actions may be controlled by the simultaneous administration of atropine (0.3 to 0.6 mg.) without materially reducing the drug's effectiveness.

With bethanechol and other parasympathomimetic drugs, there is always the remote possibility of a catastrophic untoward reaction such as cardiac arrest, especially when the subcutaneous route is used. In any case these agents should never be tried in patients who are known or suspected to have asthma, heart disease, or any mechanical obstruction within the bowel or urinary tract such as a urethral stricture or prostate enlargement whether benign or malignant. Before using these drugs, a careful history should be taken to determine if the patient had any voiding difficulties prior to the onset of urinary retention that might indicate the presence of an obstructive lesion.

However obtained, urine specimens should be saved because they may prove invaluable to the physician treating a victim of poison. For example, a urine sample provides material for toxicological examination, as well as a means of appraising the patient's state of renal function, hydration, acid-base balance, etc.

Pathogenesis of Renal Injury

Renal damage occurs often in chemical poisonings. The kidneys, however, are not always the primary site of injury in chemically induced renal failure. Azotemia and other signs of impaired renal function may be due to prerenal or postrenal causes. Postrenal failure arises from acute obstructive lesions in the outflow tract. Sometimes obstruction is due to the precipitation of exogenous chemicals within the kidney tubules, particularly the collecting ducts, but usually the renal pelves and ureters are also involved. Among the poorly soluble substances that form such precipitates are uric acid, cystine, methotrexate and some of the sulfonamide drugs. Retrograde pyeloureterograms may be required to establish the diagnosis of obstructive uropathy.

Prerenal failure reflects an impairment of blood flow to the kidneys resulting in low rates of glomerular filtration. The usual causes are dehydration, sepsis, hypotension and cardiac failure. In some clinics measurements of the fractional excretion of sodium (i.e., U/P concentration ratio) are thought to be helpful in distinguishing prerenal azotemia (low ratio) from acute tubular necrosis (high ratio). Simple, practical methods of ruling out dehydration and hypotension as causes of oliguria are described on p. IV-53.

True nephrotoxins attack the kidneys directly. Although glomerular injuries are recognized, the tubular epithelium appears to be the more vulnerable site. Based on the work of J. Oliver, two types of tubular lesions are now recognized. Specific damage of the tubular cells, results from the local action of various nephrotoxic agents. The proximal tubules are most often involved, although some nephrotoxins initially attack the loop of Henle. In either case the injury often progresses to segmental necrosis. Typically its appearance is delayed 2 to 4 days after exposure. Once established the disorder involves all of the nephrons of both kidneys, but the process tends to be completely reversible as the damaged tubular epithelium regenerates.

In contrast to this symmetrical involvement of all nephrons, patchy lesions have also been described. The latter appear to result from prolonged renal ischemia, usually secondary to shock or severe reduction of the circulating blood volume but probably sometimes due to intense renal vasoconstriction. The disorder is characterized by necrosis of tubular cells and frequently dissolution of the tubular basement membrane. The latter process is believed to result in permanent destruction of the particular nephron involved, as evidenced by the eventual formation of a fibrous scar. Because this type of lesion is most frequently observed following massive tissue injury associated with prolonged vascular collapse, acute renal failure complicating such an event has a much poorer prognosis than the renal damage due to a specific nephrotoxic substance. Insofar as shock is preventable, the ischemic, disruptive type of lesion may be avoidable. Both varieties of renal tubular damage may coexist in a victim of poison.

Suspected Renal Injury

Opinions vary concerning the proper management of the asymptomatic person who has re-

ceived a potentially toxic dose of a recognized kidney poison. Of course if dimercaprol (BAL), edetate calcium disodium (Ca-Na$_2$-EDTA), or some other acceptable chelating agent is available and appropriate, it should be used without delay. Although there is no convincing evidence that a simple water diuresis speeds the excretion of any toxic substance, increased urine flow induced by an osmotic diuretic may promote the excretion of any solute, toxic or otherwise, that is normally resorbed by the renal tubular epithelium. Furthermore, there are at least theoretical advantages in maintaining a dilute tubular fluid during the excretion of a primary nephrotoxic chemical. A brisk flow within the renal tubules may also be useful in preventing blockage due to denatured protein or other cellular debris.

Therefore, in the absence of edema or other evidence of overhydration, an attempt to induce an osmotic diuresis with mannitol is advisable in most instances. The contents of a single 50-ml. ampul of 25% mannitol can be injected intravenously in a few minutes. If this measure leads to a urine flow of 2 to 3 ml. per minute or greater within the next half hour, a sustained mannitol diuresis should then be attempted. It can be achieved either by repeated intravenous injections of 50-ml. aliquots of 25% mannitol or by the continuous infusion of 5 or 10% mannitol at 5 to 10 ml. per minute. The effectiveness of mannitol or any other osmotic diuretic drug depends upon its prompt renal excretion. If it is not excreted, the result may be fluid retention, expansion of the extracellular fluid volume, hyponatremia, hyperosmolality, edema and dangerous circulatory congestion. In the presence of edema or other evidence of fluid overload, mannitol and other osmotic diuretics should be avoided. In such cases, intravenous furosemide (p. IV-22) may serve to establish a diuresis.

In order to prevent either over- or under-hydration during the course of diuretic treament, an hourly flow sheet recording intake, output, and fluid balance should be kept. Frequent weighing of the patient is another simple and useful guide. Frequent measurements of serum electrolyte levels are almost essential for monitoring massive diuretic therapy (so-called "forced diuresis").

Alkalinization of the urine by cautiously administering sodium bicarbonate (p. IV-72) may also have some protective action on the kidneys in the preoliguric phase, especially in poisonings by various organic acids (e.g., sulfonamide drugs) and by some heavy metals (e.g., uranium salts). Of course, treatment must be cautious enough to ensure that overhydration and a systemic alkalosis are avoided.

Mild Renal Injury

Although a transient phase of spontaneous polyuria is sometimes noted, the first objective evidence of renal injury is expected to be oliguria. Early in the clinical course, however, it may be difficult to distinguish between oliguria due to dehydration or other hemodynamic abnormality (prerenal failure) and oliguria due to injury of the renal tubules. If there are clinical signs of dehydration, 1 liter of 5% dextrose in water (or in saline if there is evidence of a salt deficit) should be given intravenously over a 2-hour period. If dehydration is the sole cause of oliguria, an increase in urine flow promptly ensues. Similarly, if oliguria is due to a reduction in the glomerular filtration rate caused by hypotension, then the intravenous administration of a vasopressor agent or other shock therapy (p. IV-17) can be expected to accelerate the flow of urine without delay.

In the absence of evident dehydration or shock, a single intravenous injection of mannitol, as described above, may be a useful way to assess an acute state of oliguria. If the response is one of diuresis, one concludes that the renal tubules are not obstructed or at least not severely obstructed. Under these circumstances it is usually advisable to continue mannitol administration in order to maintain a mild diuresis.

If urinary flow is not restored to normal levels by these measures, a presumptive diagnosis of acute tubular necrosis is warranted, and further management should proceed as outlined below. Under no circumstances should one attempt to "force" a diuresis by the continued administration of diuretic drugs or of parenteral fluids once gross deficits in body water and electrolytes have been corrected. As noted above, hyponatremia, hyperosmolality and circulatory overloading with consequent congestive heart failure and pulmonary edema have resulted from such misguided therapy. The restitution of urine flow following initial therapy provides no assurance against kidney damage, because the renal effects of nephrotoxic substances may not appear for several days after exposure. Consequently close observation and attention to body fluid and electrolyte balances are indicated until it becomes apparent that the kidneys have been spared.

After a chemical injury to the kidneys, conventional tests of renal function are not worthwhile during the oliguric phase. The 24-hour urine volume, daily body weight and serum potassium level are the information of greatest value. Even after the resumption of normal urine flow, tubular function may be restored so slowly that no final appraisal of residual damage is possible for weeks or even months. Eventually studies of urinary protein excretion, the blood urea nitrogen level, serum creatinine concentration, and the 24-hour creatinine clearance are useful in demonstrating complete recovery.

Acute Renal Failure

The pathogenesis of this disorder is described above (p. IV-51). Whether kidney damage is mild or severe, the principles of diagnosis and treatment are the same. Acute intrinsic renal failure means tubular necrosis. In this state complete anuria is rare; daily urine volumes usually range between 100 and 300 ml. In this phase of oliguria the basic problem is the nearly total absence of renal adjustments to the water and electrolyte balance of the body. The therapist must try to compensate for this lack of homeostatic control. The major problems requiring attention during the oliguric phase are the maintenance of water balance and the prevention of hyperkalemia. As noted below, the acidosis that accompanies acute renal failure does not usually warrant treatment.

The state of water balance can be judged best by daily observations of the body weight. A daily weight loss of 300 gm. (or about ½ lb.) is usually desired because the catabolism of body fat and protein generates this amount of water each day. Thus if the intake of fluid were sufficient to hold the body weight constant, overhydration would result. All other expenditures of body water, however, are replaced. The daily water requirement approximates measurable losses from the kidneys and from the gastrointestinal tract, plus insensible water loss from skin and lungs (approximately 900 ml. per day in the afebrile patient), minus the water of oxidation from the catabolism of body fat and proteins (about 300 ml. per day). Thus the daily water allowance usually amounts to about 600 ml. plus all sensible water loss in excretions, but in the presence of fever or a high environmental temperature insensible water losses are much higher (p. IV-64). The simplest and perhaps most useful rule is to restrict the fluid intake to an amount that will sustain a body weight loss of about 300 gm. each day or perhaps slightly more if the intake of food is very poor. This fluid restriction may or may not generate excessive thirst.

Similarly, the intake of sodium chloride should not exceed demonstrable losses. Unless diarrhea is present, such losses are usually very small. Urinary excretion of salt in the oliguric patient is generally so scant that it can be ignored.

The most serious electrolyte abnormality during the oliguric phase is elevation of the serum potassium concentration. Its determination every day is highly desirable in order that therapy may be instituted when and if toxic levels are approached. Some physicians consider the electrocardiogram to be a more reliable index of clinically significant hyperkalemia (p. IV-72).

Several methods are available for combating hyperkalemia. First among these is the diet, which should be high in calories, carbohydrate and fat, but free of protein and potassium. Since body cells are rich in potassium, protein catabolism must be kept to a minimum, and this is accomplished by the daily intake of at least 100 gm. of carbohydrate. If nausea does not preclude the ingestion of food and fluids, the patient can be encouraged to sip a solution prepared by dissolving in his daily allowance of water 100 gm. of lactose (which is not so sweet and therefore is less nauseating than glucose or sucrose). For variety and to raise the daily intake to 1000 to 1800 calories if practical, one may also provide sour balls and other hard sugar candy, butter balls (consisting of equal parts of powered sugar and salt-free sweet butter), and/or an equal mixture of ginger ale and Karo syrup. If nausea or severe anorexia prevents intake by mouth, the minimal requirement of 100 gm. of carbohydrate can be approached by the slow intravenous infusion of 10% glucose in water (p. IV-76), subject to the previously defined restriction on the daily fluid intake. The use of the anabolic steroid norethandrolone (Nilevar) in a dose of 10 mg. twice daily may help to retard protein catabolism.

A second method for preventing or treating hyperkalemia is the use of the cation exchange resin Kayexalate in the sodium form. A dose of 15 gm. (about 5 teaspoonfuls) administered orally three or four times daily serves to decrease the serum potassium level rapidly, especially when it is given with sorbitol to prevent obstipation. The latter drug is prescribed as a 70% solution; 5 ml. should be given with each dose of Kayexalate. If a more rapid reduction of the serum potassium level must be accomplished, 5 ml. of 70% sorbitol should be given orally every 2 hours until diarrhea is established, and 5 ml. about twice daily thereafter to maintain loose stools. If oral medication is not tolerated, Kayexalate and sorbitol may be administered by retention enema (200 ml. of 25% sorbitol and 40 gm. of resin every 6 hours). For the prevention rather than correction of hyperkalemia, 5 gm. of Kayexalate by mouth four times daily usually suffices.

Despite a strict dietary regimen and the use of Kayexalate and sorbitol, life-endangering hyperkalemia may intervene. In that event, a mixture of glucose and insulin can be used to foster the migration of potassium into tissue cells. For this purpose crystalline insulin is dissolved in 10% glucose in water (1 unit for each 2 to 3 gm. of glucose) and infused intravenously. It serves as a stop-gap measure until some form of hemodialysis can be instituted. The introduction of effective methods for intermittent peritoneal dialysis has greatly reduced the use of the artificial kidney, and has made it possible to carry out dialysis in virtually every general hospital.

The principles and uses of dialysis are described on pp. IV-55–56.

On the regimen described above, patients invariably develop some degree of metabolic acidosis before the restoration of renal tubular function. This acidosis is usually not severe, and no attempt is made to correct it unless it becomes intense enough to lead to distressing symptoms. Even in a patient who is markedly hyperpneic, the acidosis should be only partially corrected, if at all. One practice is to administer small repeated doses of sodium citrate by mouth or sodium lactate by vein until the severe symptoms subside. More vigorous efforts to treat the acidosis of renal failure may cause such dangerous complications as hypocalcemic tetany and/or convulsions.

In addition to metabolic acidosis, hyponatremia and to a lesser degree hypochloremia develop frequently during the oliguric state. These deviations from normal, however, are not marked if overhydration has been avoided by the recommended restriction of fluid. This hyponatremia, like the acidosis, is usually well tolerated, whereas attempts to correct it by increasing the salt intake are apt to precipitate cardiac failure and pulmonary edema. Intractable pulmonary edema may occur with or without peripheral edema and hypertension. When it appears in a patient with acute renal failure, rapid digitalization is indicated, even though the cardiac glycosides are frequently ineffective in this cardiovascular crisis. The emergency treatment of pulmonary edema is outlined on pp. IV-14 and 23.

Oliguria may persist for periods ranging from a few hours to 3 weeks (average 10 to 12 days), but as the renal tubules begin to regenerate, oliguria is gradually replaced by a phase of normal or supranormal urine flow. Although the onset of diuresis signals probable recovery, the polyuric phase is also associated with a high mortality and demands scrupulous vigilance for a period of at least 1 week. Normal renal function is not regained for some time, as evidenced by the fact that the blood urea level often continues to rise for another 5 days.

Urine volumes during the stage of polyuria may reach as high as 3 to 5 liters daily, especially if the prescribed loss of body weight was not attained during the oliguric phase. Even if overhydration was avoided, some degree of polyuria may occur, and under these circumstances the daily losses of water and of electrolytes (now including both sodium and potassium) must be replaced to avoid serious states of depletion. The need for such replacement is best gauged by measuring not only the daily volume of urine but also the amounts of sodium and potassium contained in it, in order that equal quantities can be administered during the subsequent 24-hour period. However, if the prescribed loss of body weight was not achieved during the oliguric phase, a genuine excess of body water can be assumed to exist at the beginning of polyuria. Under these circumstances complete replacement of the fluid loss is undesirable because it serves to perpetuate an obligatory diuresis. As soon as possible, parenteral replacement therapy should cease. With a falling level of blood urea and a declining hyperkalemia, the patient should be placed on an unrestricted diet as tolerated.

Miscellaneous clinical problems that may arise during acute renal failure include the following gastrointestinal disturbances: anorexia, nausea, vomiting, diarrhea, and abdominal distension. The diarrhea, which usually occurs late in the oliguric stage, may be profuse and persistent. These intestinal losses of water and electrolytes (except for potassium during the phase of oliguria) must be replaced in like measure through parenteral routes (pp. IV-64–67). The symptomatic control of these disorders is outlined on pp. IV-49–51.

The most common mental symptom in acute renal failure is somnolence, but confusion, coma, tremor and asterixis are also encountered. Attempts to correct these disorders with drugs are generally unwise. Indeed, any drug therapy must be conducted with caution, since renal excretion is normally a major mechanism for disposing of medicinal agents. In the presence of renal damage, therefore, drugs should be either avoided or used only sparingly. Recommended doses of antibiotics, when required by patients with renal failure, have been published (C. Kunin, *Annals of Internal Medicine, 67:* 151, 1967).

A rapidly developing anemia, which is usually normochromic and normocytic, is a constant feature of renal insufficiency. It arises because of deficient erythropoiesis. Apparently it is self-limiting and usually well tolerated, in contrast to the blood transfusions which are sometimes used to correct or ameliorate it. A bleeding tendency is also sometimes observed in uremia. Thrombocytopenia is occasionally the cause, but probably more often a platelet deficiency in one or more of the clotting factors is responsible. In the presence of acute renal failure, however, blood transfusions are hazardous because of the ease with which congestive heart failure can be precipitated in these patients.

If tubular regeneration is delayed or is so grossly incomplete that renal failure persists in spite of the supportive measures outlined above, other complications may arise. Even with intense hemodialysis, deaths occur in this group of patients. The proximal cause of death is apt to be infection or malnutrition or rarely gastrointestinal hemorrhage from stress ulcers. In such severely ill patients kidney transplantation may be considered a justifiable procedure. If so, blood transfusions are usually required to prepare the patient for surgery, in spite of the evident danger of such transfusions. Washed red blood cells may be preferable to whole blood in order to reduce the antigenic load.

Hemodialysis

This name refers to the therapeutic procedure whereby unwanted solutes in the blood plasma are allowed to diffuse across a dialysis membrane into a solution provided by the therapist. This solution, the dialysate, is replaced continuously or intermittently with fresh solution of carefully defined composition, so that diffusional transport is allowed to continue. In preparing solutions suitable for hemodialysis, all diffusible solutes should in theory be present in concentrations approximating those in an ultrafiltrate of normal blood plasma. In practice many variations in composition have been used satisfactorily. Obviously any unwanted substance or substances in the patient's blood should be omitted in preparing dialysis fluid.

Hemodialysis is useful in at least two kinds of cases, both of which are encountered in clinical toxicology. The first is the patient in acute renal failure, whether due to a nephrotoxic poison or not. Hemodialysis here serves to reduce the level of azotemia and especially to lower the plasma level of potassium (p. IV-53). For this potentially lifesaving maneuver, the dialysate solution is prepared without potassium. With appropriately hypertonic solutions, hemodialysis can also be used to achieve a negative fluid balance, as, for example, in the overhydrated oliguric patient.

The second type of patient in whom hemodialysis is distinctly beneficial may or may not have defective renal function, but his blood plasma contains a high concentration of a dialyzable poison that is being excreted or metabolized so slowly as to jeopardize his survival. Under these circumstances hemodialysis speeds recovery by removing some of the circulating poison.

Table IV-4 lists some of the substances that are known to be dialyzable. It is improper to infer, however, that hemodialysis is necessarily a worthwhile procedure against all of these poisons. For some agents, removal by dialysis is so slow, relative to rates of metabolic inactivation and renal excretion, that hemodialysis is almost worthless. In this category are poisonings due to phenothiazine tranquilizers, chloroquine, copper, iron, etc. For many other poisons the issue is unclear because of insufficient clinical experience.

On the other hand, hemodialysis has almost certainly proved useful in poisonings due to salicylates, barbiturates, glutethimide, methaqualone, bromide, chlorate, lithium and potassium. In each case the benefit was ascribed to significant reductions in the blood level of the poison. Success has also been claimed in cases of intoxication by ethyl, methyl and isopropyl alcohols, ethylene glycol, boric acid, meprobamate, ethchlorvynol, chloral hydrate, phenacetin, acetaminophen and thiocyanate. With further experience recommendations may be extended to other substances (*e.g.*, bromate, fluoride), but other techniques such as hemoperfusion (see p. IV-57) may eventually supersede hemodialysis.

Table IV-4
Dialyzable Poisons[a]

Barbiturates[b]	Antidepressants	Metals	Miscellaneous Substances
Amobarbital	Amphetamine	Calcium	Aniline
Barbital	Isocarboxazid	Lithium[b]	Boric acid
Butabarbital	Methamphetamine	Magnesium	Camphor
Butalbital	Pargyline	Potassium	Carbon tetrachloride
Cyclobarbital	Phenelzine	Sodium	Chlorate
Pentobarbital	Tranylcypromine	Strontium	Chloroquine
Phenobarbital			Chlorpropamide
Secobarbital	Alcohols	Halides	Colchicine
	Ethanol[b]	Bromide	Cyclophosphamide
Depressants, Sedatives,	Ethylene glycol	Chloride	Dinitro-*ortho*-cresol
and Tranquilizers	Isopropyl alcohol	Iodide	Diquat
Chloral hydrate	Methanol[b]	Fluoride[b]	Ergotamine
Chlordiazepoxide			Eucalyptus oil
Diazepam	Analgesics	Endogenous Toxins	5-Fluorouracil
Diphenhydramine	Acetaminophen	Ammonia	Mannitol
Ethchlorvynol	Acetophenetidin	Bilirubin	Methotrexate
Ethinamate	Acetylsalicylic acid[b]	Cystine	Paraquat
Glutethimide[b]	Dextropropoxyphene	Endotoxin	Procainamide
Meprobamate	Methylsalicylate[b]	Lactic acid	Sodium citrate
Methaqualone		Urea	Thiocyanate[b]
Methyprylon	Anticonvulsants	Uric Acid[b]	Toluene
Paraldehyde	Methsuximide		Trichloroethylene
Phenytoin	Phenytoin		
Primidone	Primidone		

[a] Slightly modified and reproduced with permission from J. F. Winchester, M. C. Gelfand, J. H. Knepshield and G. E. Schreiner, *Transactions of the American Society for Artificial Internal Organs*, 23:762–842, 1977.
[b] Kinetics of dialysis thoroughly studied and/or clinical experience extensive.

When faced with a severe intoxication due to any drug product not listed above, the physician is well advised to telephone the manufacturer in order to ascertain the dialyzability of the active ingredients.

Extracorporeal hemodialysis is an effective but rather elaborate procedure. Several kinds of artificial kidneys are marketed. In all designs, coils of cellulose dialysis tubing are bathed on the outside by a large volume of a wash solution that is oxygenated, warmed, and stirred continuously. Blood is removed continuously from one of the patient's peripheral arteries (usually the brachial); it is pumped through the dialysis tubing and back into a peripheral vein. To prevent coagulation, heparin is added, and to ensure against emboli, the blood is filtered before it is returned to the patient. Because the artificial kidney generally requires more blood than can be safely furnished by the patient, the machine is primed with donor blood before it is connected to the patient. Obviously considerable equipment and experience are required for successful extracorporeal hemodialysis, and so its use should be limited to large and adequately staffed medical centers.

Peritoneal Dialysis

The same limitations do not apply to *in vivo* techniques of hemodialysis, the most popular and successful of which is peritoneal dialysis. In this procedure the peritoneum and especially the mesentery serve as dialysis membranes. The available surface area is said to be equivalent to the filtering surface of all the renal glomeruli. Dialysis fluid is injected into the peritoneal cavity and removed periodically, after which fresh fluid is instilled. The mesothelial lining of the peritoneal cavity is usually regarded as an inert semipermeable membrane through which only macromolecules like the plasma proteins fail to pass.

Unlike the cellulose tubing of the artificial kidney, however, the permeability of mesentery and peritoneum can be modified reversibly by drugs in various ways that may prove eventually to be clinically useful (H. G. Hare, H. Valtin and R. E. Gosselin, *Journal of Pharmacology and Experimental Therapeutics*, 145: 122, 1964). Solute transport rates into and out of the peritoneal cavity can be enhanced by numerous drugs added to the peritoneal fluid, including streptokinase, isoproterenol, dipyridamole, nitroprusside, dopamine, gastrointestinal hormones and prostaglandins (reviewed by J. F. Maher, *Kidney International 18* (suppl. 10): S-117, 1980). The feasibility of using these drugs during dialysis of poison victims has not yet been adequately demonstrated.

These efforts serve to emphasize a notable disadvantage of peritoneal dialysis, namely the relatively slow rates at which it clears the blood of unwanted solutes (R. E. Gosselin and R. P. Smith, *Clinical Pharmacology and Therapeutics*, 7: 279, 1966). For example, barbiturates are removed only 10 to 50% as fast as with a modern extracorporeal hemodialyzer. The same disparity exists for several other dialyzable poisons.

Whatever the numerical value of the peritoneal dialysance, removal by dialysis can be made faster if it is possible to trap the diffusing solute within the peritoneal cavity and so minimize back-diffusion. For example, the inclusion of 5% serum albumin in dialysis fluid has been shown to improve the efficiency of peritoneal dialysis in clearing the blood of salicylates and barbiturates. Probably cheaper and more effective trapping agents could be developed.

The principle of nonionic diffusion has also been exploited to speed the dialytic clearance. Thus, the peritoneum and mesentery, like other biological membranes, appear to be more permeable to uncharged molecules than to those bearing an electrical charge. If buffers are used to maintain the pH of dialysis fluid sufficiently different from that of the blood, an unwanted substance that enters the peritoneal cavity in its undissociated form may become ionized to such an extent that its escape is inhibited. In accordance with these expectations, barbiturates accumulate in the peritoneal cavity faster when the dialysis fluid is buffered at pH 10 than when it is unbuffered. There have been only a few attempts to exploit these principles in toxicology, and the safety of using dialysis fluids at unphysiological pH levels has not been thoroughly demonstrated. In any case the procedure appears to have only limited utility. On theoretical grounds it is possible to predict that the only poisons that might be trapped at an appreciable

rate by this mechanism are weak acids and weak bases with pK values between 5 and 8 (Gosselin and Smith, *loc. cit.*).

For intermittent peritoneal dialysis, a nonirritating plastic catheter with many small holes is used. It is inserted with a trochar through the smallest possible midline incision, about one-third of the way from the umbilicus to the pubic symphysis. A sterile pyrogen-free solution is then introduced into the peritoneal cavity by gravity feed; later it is removed by gravity drainage, sometimes aided by gentle pressure on the abdomen toward the end of the flow. The process is then repeated, and all volumes introduced and removed are carefully recorded. Samples of the dialysate are kept for chemical analysis. The larger the volume of fluid injected into the peritoneal cavity and the more frequently it is replaced, the faster is the process of removing undesirable substances from the blood. When the plasma potassium level must be lowered quickly, an exchange rate of 2 liters every hour is recommended in adults. Exchanging 2 liters every 2 hours, however, is sufficient in most cases. Neither pain nor infection has proved to be a frequent complication.

Disposable sets for intermittent peritoneal dialysis are available commercially; they contain all the necessary equipment and solutions, as well as detailed instructions for carrying out the relatively simple procedures. The advantages of this method over the artificial kidney are many: it does not require a team of physicians; it does not entail arterial and venous cut-downs or donor blood; it is relatively inexpensive; it can be used in newborn infants. In the rare instance that peritoneal lavage is contraindicated because of recent abdominal surgery or peritonitis, the patient may have to be transferred to a medical center for treatment by an artificial kidney or by hemoperfusion.

Hemoperfusion

In the past dozen years considerable interest has developed in a process called hemoperfusion. By various techniques the patient's blood is allowed to flow through a column or canister packed with a finely divided solid adsorbent such as activated charcoal or one of the synthetic resins, usually nonionic but occasionally an ion-exchange resin. The blood may or may not require filtration to remove particles of adsorbent before it is returned to the patient. The charcoal or resin removes circulating poisons as well as some dissolved physiologic substances, but except for rare cases of hypocalcemia and of hypoglycemia, the extraction of normal blood chemicals appears to present no difficulties in hemoperfusions of short duration. A more common and more serious problem is platelet removal by the device. At least modest reductions in platelet count are commonly reported but not bleeding tendencies. In 1980 an entire issue of *Clinical Toxicology* (volume 17(4)) was devoted to reports describing the techniques, advantages, and shortcomings of hemoperfusion in clinical poisonings; some of these reports are cited below.

In many ways hemoperfusion is simpler than hemodialysis, and it is said to be more easily mastered (Rosenbaum *et al.*, pp. 493–500, *loc. cit.*). The principal advantage of hemoperfusion, however, is its greater efficiency in removing most poisons, as evidenced by higher measured values of the plasma or blood clearance. For lipid-soluble drugs and poisons, the highest clearance rates have been achieved with adsorptive columns containing the uncoated, uncharged resin, Amberlite XAD-4. In general, uncoated activated charcoal or charcoal coated with various protective semipermeable layers (*e.g.*, cellulose nitrate with albumin, acrylic hydrogel, etc.) do not permit such rapid rates of removal (Rosenbaum *et al.*, pp. 493–500; also Gelfand and Winchester, pp. 583–602, *loc. cit.*).

With the Amberlite XAD-4, plasma clearance values of some drugs (*e.g.*, ethchlorvynol, glutethimide, and some of the barbiturates) commonly approach the rate of plasma flow through the adsorbent column. In one study the plasma clearance of digoxin in dogs actually exceeded the plasma flow rate, demonstrating that the column also removed digoxin bound to blood cells. With each successive hour of continuous hemoperfusion (sessions often last 2 to 10 hours), the extraction ratio and therefore the computed plasma clearance are apt to decrease, indicating a tendency for the column to approach its adsorption capacity. With commercial canisters containing 200 to 600 gm. of charcoal or resin, however, the hourly decrements are generally small in the case of those poisons which the adsorbent binds with high affinities.

In order to exploit this efficient removal, it is necessary to sustain high rates of blood flow through these canisters. In adults, even when toxic and hypotensive, it is often possible to achieve blood flow rates of 200 to 300 ml./min. by inserting inlet and outlet cannulas percutaneously into the vena cava via the femoral vein

and by using a roller pump to move the blood through the circuit. Unlike extracorporeal hemodialysis devices, hemoperfusion canisters can be primed with physiological saline solution; extra blood is not required. The patient, however, must be adequately heparinized before venous cannulas are introduced. Because of this heparin and the expected loss of blood platelets, patients with a potential bleeding problem (*e.g.*, those with liver insufficiency) are not appropriate candidates for this procedure.

Whereas clearance values are useful for comparing hemoperfusion with hemodialysis and for evaluating various kinds of hemoperfusion canisters, a high value for the plasma or blood clearance does not guarantee that the procedure is useful in treating patients who may be overdosed with that substance. As has been pointed out several times (*e.g.*, Gibson, pp. 501–513; also Garella and Lorch, pp. 515–527, *loc. cit.*) with drugs that have large volumes of distribution due to extensive binding to tissue cells or due to large solubilites in fat, high clearances do not yield large recoveries, at least not large in terms of the ingested dose. For this reason the tricyclic antidepressants, for example, are not good candidates for hemoperfusion in spite of their high clearance values; the same is probably true of the cardiac glycosides in most cases. As with hemodialysis, in order to qualify as a rational mode of therapy, hemoperfusion should also remove a target substance at a rate that is high relative to its combined rates of renal excretion and metabolic detoxication.

Further experience is necessary before any concensus is achieved with respect to which kinds of intoxications are appropriately treated by hemoperfusion. As with most other active interventions, the procedure is probably best reserved for seriously ill patients with high blood levels. Limited experience to date suggests that the following poisons can be removed at clinically significant rates by hemoperfusion canisters that are commercially available today: many barbiturates (perhaps all except the ultrashort-acting ones), ethchlorvynol, glutethimide, meprobamate, methaqualone, methyprylon, theophylline and salicylates (Chang, pp. 529–542; also Rosenbaum *et al.*, pp. 493–500; also Gelfand and Winchester, pp. 583–602, *loc. cit.*).

LIVER

Prompt recognition and effective management of chemically induced liver damage require an understanding of the basic mechanisms by which chemicals may affect hepatic structure and function. In addition one must recognize that there exists a high degree of intrinsic individual variation in susceptibility to hepatotoxic agents. Only part of this variability can be ac-

counted for by such factors as age, nutritional status, and preexisting liver disease.

Pathogenesis of Liver Injury

Acutely hepatotoxic agents attack hepatocytes, in some cases specific organelles of the hepatocyte initially. The result is the intracellular accumulation of fat or cell necrosis or both. Examples of such hepatotoxic chemicals are listed in Table IV-5. The excessive accumulation of fat (triglycerides predominantly) does not necessarily lead to death of the hepatocyte or a major loss of liver function. Hepatocyte necrosis, however, leads to hepatic failure whenever large numbers of parenchymal cells are killed. Typical lesions involve all hepatocytes throughout the entire liver and progress ultimately to cell lysis. Initially the hepatocyte damage may be "zonal" within the liver lobule. Thus some chemicals in Table IV-5 characteristically affect the centrolobular region first whereas others attack midzonal or periportal areas. The necrosis induced acutely by all of these agents is not accompanied by prominent local inflammatory reactions.

All of the agents in Table IV-5 tend to induce

Table IV-5
Examples of Acutely Hepatotoxic Chemicals[a]

Chemical	Produces Necrosis	Produces Fatty Liver
Carbon tetrachloride	×	×
Chloroform	×	×
Trichloroethylene	×	×
Tetrachloroethane	×	×
Bromobenzene	×	
Dimethylnitrosamine	×	×
Dimethylaminoazobenzene	×	×
Thioacetamide	×	
Pyrrolizidine alkaloids	×	×
Aflatoxin	×	×
Penicillum islandicum	×	×
Amanita phalloides	×	
Tannic acid	×	
Phosphorus	×	×
Ethionine		×
Azaserine	×	×
Cycloheximide		×
Tetracycline		×
Cerium		×
Beryllium	×	
Allyl alcohol	×	
Allyl formate		×
Ethanol		×
Methotrexate		×
Mithramycin	×	
Mitomycin C		×
Puromycin		×
Urethane	×	
Galactosamine	×	×
Acetaminophen	×	
Phenacetin	×	
Furosemide	×	
Emetine		×

[a] Reproduced (with slight modifications) from Chapter 10 by G. L. Plaa in Cassarett and Doull's *Toxicology*, Ed. 2, Macmillan Publishing Co., New York, 1980. See original for literature references.

liver cell damage in a predictable pattern and to an extent roughly proportional to the intensity and duration of the toxic exposure. Evidence of liver dysfunction usually appears after a brief latent period (1 to 7 days), and parenchymal cell destruction is often extensive.

Another group of hepatotoxic chemicals also characteristically provokes hepatocyte necrosis but with intense local inflammatory reactions. This disease tends to be progressive like viral hepatitis. All well-established examples are drugs, some of which are listed in Table IV-6 under "viral-like hepatitis." This type of toxic response occurs in very low incidence among exposed individuals, and susceptible persons cannot be identified beforehand. Furthermore no relationship is recognized between dose and the intensity of the damage. An allergic basis is suspected.

Another class of chemicals produces hepatic dysfunction apparently without attacking hepatocytes directly. The lesion here is bile stasis with dilation of the canaliculi. This type of intrahepatic biliary obstruction leads to early jaundice and ultimately to mild focal hepatocyte necrosis, usually with ultimate recovery. Many diverse drugs are capable of inducing this type of liver lesion; some prominent examples are listed in Table IV-6 under "intrahepatic cholestasis." These drugs produce hepatic dysfunction in an unpredictably small fraction of exposed individuals without relation to dosage. These episodes, which may represent hypersensitivity reactions, commonly follow latent periods of 3 to 5 weeks and rarely lead to significant liver cell destruction.

Finally, overt liver disease may follow an accidental or iatrogenic toxic exposure and yet be unrelated to it. For example, many authorities now attribute the liver damage associated with the administration of cinchophen to intercurrent viral hepatitis.

Recognition of Toxic Liver Injury

The impressive functional reserve and regenerative capacity of the liver may effectively mask mild drug-induced liver damage unless it is sought assiduously by the proper clinical, chemical, and biopsy means. After appropriate latent periods, anorexia, nausea, vomiting, and right upper quadrant distress may indicate acute liver damage. In the "allergic" hepatic dysfunction produced by the phenothiazine tranquilizers like chlorpromazine, gastrointestinal symptoms are less intense, and itching, transient fever, and dark urine are usually the earliest evidences of liver injury. On physical examination, tender liver enlargement is the chief sign of all forms of hepatic inflammation and necrosis.

In searching for early laboratory evidence of liver disease, which may precede any clinical

Table IV-6
Examples of Drug-Associated Liver Injury[a]

Intrahepatic Cholestasis

Chlorpromazine	Ectylurea
Prochlorperazine	p-Aminosalicylic acid
Promazine	Chlorthiazide
Trifluoperazine	Thiouracil
Thioridazine	Methimazole
Mepazine	Carbimazole
Carbamazepine	Propylthiouracil
Amitriptyline	Metahexamide
Imipramine	Carbutamide
Iprindole	Acetohexamide
Chlordiazepoxide	Tolbutamide
Diazepam	Tolazamide
Methyltestosterone	Chlorpropamide
Norethandrolone	Sulfanilamide
Methandrolone	Sulfadiazine
Fluoxymestrone	Erythromycin estolate
Mestranol	Troleandomycin
Norethynodrel	Sodium oxacillin
Estradiol	Nitrofurantoin
Arsphenamine	Oxyphenisatin
Carbarsone	Phenindione

Viral-like Hepatitis

Iproniazid	Isoniazid
Phenylisopropylhydrazine	Pyrizinamide
Nialamide	Halothane
Phenelzine	Methoxyflurane
Tranylcypromine	p-Aminosalicylic acid
Imipramine	Ethionamide
Cinchophen	Zoxazolamine
6-Mercaptopurine	Acetohexamide
α-Methyldopa	Indomethacin
Carbamazepine	Trimethobenzamide
Ethacrynic acid	Phenindione
Phenylbutazone	Sulfamethoxazole
Colchicine	Sulfisoxazole
Oxyphenisatin	Papaverine
Dantrolene	Ibufenac

[a] Reproduced (with slight modifications) from Chapter 10 by G. L. Plaa in Cassarett and Doull's *Toxicology*, Ed. 2, Macmillan Publishing Co., New York, 1980. See original for literature references.

symptoms, no single liver function test is invariably satisfactory. In each instance the most sensitive test for diagnostic and prognostic purposes is determined by the pattern of cell damage. Thus, a battery of tests that assess different parameters of liver function should be performed at appropriate intervals after the toxic exposure. In general, however, the plasma prothrombin time is a good indicator of the severity of liver damage, the serum level of glutamic-pyruvic transaminase reflects in part the rate and extent of hepatocellular destruction, and the serum level of alkaline phosphatase is a sensitive indicator of an obstructive hepatic reaction (cholestasis) as induced by drugs listed in Table IV-6. Before the clinical appearance of jaundice, bilirubinuria, which is a common and rather nonspecific sign of liver damage of all types, may be detected with the simple Ictotest.

When the true nature or extent of liver injury following a toxic exposure is unclear, percutaneous needle biopsy of the liver can often provide information of both diagnostic and prognostic importance. In experienced hands it is a safe procedure if the patient is cooperative and if there is no bleeding diathesis.

Mild or Suspected Liver Damage

Many chemicals employed in industry, in the home, and in medical practice produce symptoms *suggestive* of liver damage (*i.e.*, gastrointestinal disturbances) and induce transient hepatic dysfunction of uncertain significance. In such cases the aims of the therapist are to prevent further injury, to detect signs of advancing damage, and to alleviate symptoms. The most important measures are those taken to prevent further exposure to the presumed offending agent and to avoid exposure to any other potentially hepatotoxic substance.

The patient is usually most comfortable at home on bed-and-chair activity during observation and recovery. Although there is no justification for strict bedrest, premature and excessive exertion may accentuate signs and symptoms of acute liver dysfunction. There is no clinical proof that special diets or vigorous vitamin supplementation hastens recovery or prevents progressive liver damage. One should, however, provide a well balanced diet of a moderate to high caloric content, as tolerated (p. IV-79). At the same time one of the commercially available multiple vitamin preparations (p. IV-80) is perhaps worthwhile.

If anorexia or vomiting prevents an adequate intake of food or fluid, intravenous infusions of glucose solutions (5 or 10% in water), by supplying at least 100 gm. of carbohydrate daily, will minimize protein catabolism (p. IV-76) and combat dehydration. In most cases of suspected or mild liver dysfunction no specific drugs are required to control symptoms. If restlessness, anorexia and nausea are troublesome, however, careful administration of diazepam (Valium), 2 to 10 mg. by mouth 2 to 4 times daily, or prochlorperazine (Compazine), 5 mg. orally twice daily, may be helpful. Of course the latter drug is rigorously avoided if any phenothiazine derivative is suspected to have been the offending agent.

Persistent vomiting, fever, increasing weakness and marked right upper quadrant tenderness should alert the attending physician to the possibility of serious hepatocellular damage (see below) or intercurrent intra-abdominal disease. On the other hand, when the physical examination and laboratory tests of liver function indicate recovery, the patient should be encouraged to increase his activities progressively for several days. Then a final set of appropriate liver function tests should be performed to confirm his ability to tolerate normal or near-normal activity.

Overt Hepatocellular Damage

Profound anorexia and nausea with persistent vomiting, dark urine and deepening jaundice, increasing hepatic discomfort and tenderness, and signs of altered consciousness are indicative of rapidly progressive, potentially fatal liver cell damage. Patients with such ominous signs and symptoms should be hospitalized, the exact nature and extent of the liver damage investigated, and vigorous supportive therapy initiated. Basic supportive care in such cases includes: (1) strict bed rest, because asthenia and confusion often make ambulation both difficult and hazardous; (2) careful regulation of the daily caloric intake, body weight, and fluid balance, because anorexia and vomiting contribute to further debility and liver damage and because renal dysfunction may accompany advancing liver failure; (3) avoidance of all unnecessary medication; (4) frequent determinations of serum bilirubin and transaminase as indices of liver cell damage; (5) analyses to reveal plasma concentrations of electrolytes, urea, prothrombin, and albumin as guides for further therapy. Prothrombin time may be the best single indicator of the severity of the liver injury, and it should be measured frequently.

An adequate caloric intake must be ensured in order to maintain hepatic glycogen stores (which may protect against further toxic damage), to minimize ketosis and tissue wasting, and to avoid the rare complication of severe hypoglycemia. Without proper attention intake is often erratic and limited by severe anorexia. Frequent small and palatable feedings of carbohydrate-rich solids and liquids should be encouraged but not to the extent that vomiting is induced. Feedings with a high fat content are often poorly tolerated but are not harmful, whereas protein-rich food should be given only with extreme caution (see discussion of "Hepatic Coma" below).

Daily multiple vitamin supplements may be administered by oral or parenteral routes (p. IV-80). Vitamin K has special significance in liver insufficiency, as noted below. If less than 1500 calories are ingested in any 24-hour period, a glucose solution (5 or 10% in water) should be given by slow intravenous infusion. Glucose by any route promotes glycogenesis; fructose and invert sugar are said to be even more efficient precursors of liver glycogen, but if given slowly, glucose is just as satisfactory as fructose.

Patients in all stages of hepatic cell insufficiency have a reduced tolerance of water and salt. Whereas edema and ascites are often major complications and sometimes preterminal states in subacute and chronic liver disease, especially in the presence of fibrosis, they are not common in acute toxic hepatitis. Progressive fluid retention may be a problem, however, as evidenced by a rapid gain in weight, a falling urine output despite adequate hydration, and ultimately the formation of dependent edema or ascites. Under these circumstances the intake of fluid should be restricted to simple replacement of sensible and insensible water losses (p. IV-64). At the same time it is important to restrict the sodium intake, sometimes to levels as low as 0.5 gm. of sodium chloride (200 mg. sodium) per day. Usually the control of salt and water intake does not need to be as strict as in acute renal insufficiency. If renal function is well maintained in the presence of liver disease, the judicious use of combinations of spironolactone (Aldactone) and furosemide (p. IV-22) may help to minimize fluid retention, but great caution must be exercised in the use of agents like chlorothiazide for this purpose (see discussion of "Hepatic Coma," p. IV-63).

In contrast to the hyperkalemia of renal failure, necrosis of the liver may lead to hypokalemia and a clinically significant depletion of body potassium. Many factors can contribute to potassium loss, notably vomiting, diarrhea, and the intensive use of diuretic drugs, but the principal cause is usually an excessive renal excretion of potassium under the influence of high levels of endogenous aldosterone. Any severe deficit should be corrected by the cautious administration of potassium salts (p. IV-73).

Potassium losses can also be reduced by suppressing vomiting with an effective antiemetic agent such as prochlorperazine (Compazine) in very small doses. Similarly sedative or tranquilizing drugs are sometimes used in controlling diarrhea, abdominal discomfort, and restlessness, which may accompany acute liver damage, but adverse drug reactions are frequent. Occasionally diphenhydramine hydrochloride (e.g., Benadryl) is a useful mild antiemetic with some sedative actions; it appears to be safer than most of the other available agents. In general, however, one attempts to avoid drugs in the presence of liver damage or else uses them with extreme caution, as noted under the management of hepatic coma (p. IV-64).

Spontaneous bleeding, as manifested by nosebleeds, ecchymoses at sites of venipuncture, or occult gastrointestinal hemorrhage, is a grave sign that usually signifies extensive hepatocellular dysfunction. The intravenous or intramuscular administration of vitamin K is indicated (p. III-396); it may serve on occasion to reduce the hazard of extensive bleeding. Fresh whole blood can also be administered; it is of some value in the management of hypoprothrombinemia when and if the latter becomes refractory to vitamin K therapy. Transfusions of whole blood and plasma are used also to control anemia and hypoproteinemia. Furthermore, such transfusions may be effective in restoring urine flow when and if oliguria intervenes during the course of liver failure, as is sometimes true even when there is no other evidence of hypovolemic shock. For this purpose human serum albumin, especially a salt-poor preparation, is usually well tolerated (p. IV-18).

Many substances have been extolled for their ability to prevent the deposition or to accelerate the removal of fat from the liver; these lipotropic agents include choline, methionine, cysteine, inositol, lipocaic, liver extract, and vitamin B_{12}. In spite of impressive demonstrations in the laboratory, clinicians have seldom found anything favorable to say about these substances, and currently none of them is recommended in the treatment of acute hepatic failure. Similarly there is no satisfactory clinical or experimental evidence that justifies the use of adrenocortical steroids or corticotropin in the therapy of acute toxic injuries of the liver. The administration of hormones complicates the management of these critically ill patients without offering any demonstrable benefits.

In summary, no therapy is recognized to be effective in reversing the metabolic impact of a hepatotoxic injury. The physician's opportunity is to provide optimal supportive care that permits survival of the patient until liver necrosis ceases and regeneration occurs. During the reparative phase the diet continues to be of concern. Although there is no evidence that excess protein speeds liver regeneration, a high-protein, high-carbohydrate, high-caloric diet is usually recommended. Unless nausea and vomiting intervene, the nutrition of an uncooperative or anorectic patient can sometimes be maintained by tube feeding; a high-protein formula for tube feeding is described in Table IV-11 (p. IV-82). As recovery progresses, a needle biopsy may be undertaken to exclude the possibility of residual liver injury. Whereas an occasional patient develops post-necrotic cirrhosis, good supportive treatment usually ensures complete recovery or perhaps merely focal hepatic scarring that has little functional significance.

Hepatic Coma

Any intense and generalized failure of hepatic cell function, either because of liver cell destruction or because portal blood has been shunted away from the liver (portal-caval shunts), leads to a characteristic syndrome of grave import known as hepatic coma. The physician must be alert to the earliest manifestations of this complication, seek out all factors known to contribute to its genesis, and undertake a careful and methodical program to prevent its progression and fatal termination. Obviously all of the problems considered in the discussion of "Overt Hepatocellular Damage" (p. IV-61) are relevant here, but additional considerations of diagnosis and treatment arise when liver failure progresses to the stage of impending hepatic coma.

This clinical syndrome has three major components: disturbances of mental function, abnormal neurological findings, and abnormalities of the electroencephalogram. The mental status ranges from early and inconstant confusion with somnolence and untidiness to complete disorientation, excitement, and finally deepening coma, sometimes with terminal seizures. Neurological examination reveals variable weakness, hyper- or hyporeflexia, rigidity of the limbs, Babinski sign, and a peculiar "flapping tremor" of the outstretched hands, arms, and tongue. These flapping motions, known as asterixis, are not a true tremor but rather a nonrhythmic lapse of position alternating with corrective movements. Asterixis is an important clue to impending hepatic coma, but it is not absolutely pathognomonic since it occurs in other conditions, such as long-term heart failure, chronic obstructive pulmonary disease and even some drug overdoses.

The typical electroencephalogram shows bilaterally symmetrical slow-wave activity (2 to 3 per second) that is almost unique to hepatocerebral intoxication. During the acute phase of liver cell injury the appearance of mild confusion, undue restlessness or sleepiness, or an inconstant "flapping" of the extended hands should prompt the physician to confirm the diagnosis of impending hepatic coma with an electroencephalogram.

All aspects of supportive therapy recommended for patients with overt hepatocellular damage (p. IV-61) are relevant and appropriate in the presence of hepatic coma after an acute toxic insult. Other measures are also available; they are designed to remove various specific factors which are known to precipitate or potentiate hepatic coma. When vigorously pursued, these measures may lead to dramatic clinical improvement.

First and foremost are a series of procedures designed to reduce blood and brain levels of ammonia, because endogenous ammonia intoxication is at least in part a cause of coma in advanced liver disease. These abnormally high concentrations of ammonia arise because the injured liver fails to detoxify this physiological substance, which is formed largely within the gut and kidneys by the deamination of amino acids.

At least four measures are regarded as clinically useful for lowering the rate of ammonia production. They are: (1) reducing protein intake temporarily to 20 to 30 gm. daily or even to zero if hepatic coma is observed to progress rapidly; (2) preventing obstipation and ensuring frequent bowel movements with gentle enemas and mild laxative agents if necessary (e.g., lactulose, milk of magnesia or sodium sulfate); (3) reducing the number of ammonia-forming bacteria in the bowel by administering poorly absorbed antibiotics such as neomycin sulfate, 3 gm. daily in divided doses by mouth (by nasogastric tube if necessary); and (4) the strict interdiction of agents known to increase blood ammonia levels, such as chlorothiazide and acetazolamide. Of these measures, the third is

the most controversial because of the potential systemic toxicity of antibiotics. Lactulose appears to be a useful agent because it induces a controlled diarrhea and also because it is metabolized to acidic molecules by bacteria in the colon. Acidification of the colonic contents tends to trap ammonia as the ammonium ion, which is excreted in feces. The usual dose of lactulose syrup is 2 to 3 tablespoonfuls (30 to 45 ml., containing 20 to 30 gm. of lactulose) three or four times daily.

In addition to these prophylactic measures, attempts to reduce actively the blood ammonia concentration have been employed when the level is high and when coma is profound. In addition to lactulose already mentioned, recommendations here include the slow intravenous infusion of glutamic acid, or arginine, or of a commercially available conjugate of these two amino acids, but these agents have not been proven in clinical trials to be efficacious. An alternative possibility is intermittent peritoneal dialysis (p. IV-56). Its potential usefulness in the management of hepatic coma does not seem to have been explored, but it might prove to be an effective way of removing endogenous ammonia and at the same time correcting some of the other electrolyte and fluid disorders that are commonly found in these patients. In any case any measure that lowers the concentration of ammonia in the brain can be expected to lessen the intensity of hepatic coma.

In addition to ammonia intoxication other electrolyte imbalances, though not serious in themselves, may potentiate significantly the central nervous system manifestations of liver disease. This is particularly true of hypokalemic alkalosis, which often arises in advanced liver disease because of losses of body potassium through vomiting and diarrhea, vigorous diuretic therapy, and the endogenous secretion of aldosterone. At the same time patients in hepatic coma often hyperventilate, so that respiratory and metabolic alkalosis coexist, but only the latter requires attention. The only therapy needed is the administration of potassium chloride, usually by parenteral routes (p. IV-73), in order to correct the body deficit. As noted previously (p. IV-61), patients with advanced liver disease tend to accumulate fluid, especially if the intakes of water and salt are not carefully regulated. The result of inadequate fluid restriction is almost invariably a dilutional hyponatremia (p. IV-68). Unless hyponatremia is very severe, it is unnecessary and unwise to attempt to restore the level of plasma sodium by administering sodium chloride.

Intercurrent infections are recognized as common "potentiating" factors in patients who are critically ill with liver disease. An unrecognized pneumonia or urinary tract infection may intensify the signs and symptoms of hepatic coma. Of course all infections should be detected promptly and treated vigorously with any appropriate chemotherapeutic agent (p. IV-85). As noted below, however, unusually small doses may prove to be effective. Furthermore conventional doses of drugs such as streptomycin may lead to serious intoxication because of defective drug metabolism and because of frequently associated renal failure. Blood levels of antibiotics should be monitored often when appropriate analytic techniques are available.

Sometimes the onset of hepatic coma can be traced to the unwise administration of a sedative hypnotic drug. The metabolism and detoxication of foreign substances may be severely impaired in patients with extensive liver parenchymal disease. Consequently, drug intolerances are often encountered, particularly with sedatives. Fortunately, most of the distressing symptoms in liver disease can be controlled without medication. Except for occasional restlessness and vomiting, there is usually no pressing need for sedative, hypnotic, or analgesic drugs. (Even pruritis is uncommon in toxic hepatitis). The magnitude of drug intolerance in liver disease has not been adequately delineated, but there is no reason to believe that it is restricted to central nervous system depressants. Caution is imperative, therefore, in the administration of all drugs; doses should be kept small and prescriptions should be limited to strict necessity. Certainly in the presence of impending hepatic coma, all narcotics, sedatives, and tranquilizing drugs should be prohibited.

Unless complicated by the unwise administration of a sedative or hypnotic drug, central nervous system depression in hepatic coma does not progress to the stage of respiratory arrest or cardiovascular collapse. Death when it occurs can usually be ascribed to a severe intercurrent infection, such as aspiration pneumonitis, or to some other complication of stasis (p. IV-83). More rarely there are other proximal causes of death: terminal convulsions, hemorrhage and shock (pp. IV-35 and 17), and acute renal failure (p. IV-53). Nevertheless, with vigorous supportive treatment many patients in hepatic coma can be saved. Victims with acute toxic injury of the liver have an especially good prognosis. If life can be sustained, most of them will recover without residual liver damage.

ELECTROLYTES AND WATER BALANCE

In a variety of clinical situations, the intake of water and minerals becomes insufficient to meet normal or exaggerated metabolic needs or to correct excessive losses. Imbalances of water and salt create such states as dehydration, edema, acidosis, alkalosis, shock, muscle cramps, oliguria, and fever. Each of these conditions is encountered frequently in acute chemical poisonings. Many of these disorders are interdependent. The several processes which work to maintain constancy in the chemical composition of tissues and body fluids are so closely allied that no one component can be disturbed without inducing shifts in others. Thus, metabolic acidosis and dehydration, for example, are often found to accompany one another.

For simplicity in presentation, however, disorders in the metabolism of water and specific electrolytes are discussed separately. Because deficiency states are the ones most commonly encountered in clinical toxicology, they are given the most attention. In the following discussion, the emphasis is placed on diagnosis and treatment, but at least a rudimentary appreciation of mechanism is essential for the rational management of patients with disturbances in salt and water metabolism.

Dehydration

Even when no fluid is admitted, the body continues to excrete water. It also continues to produce water by the oxidation of tissue solids. For excretory needs, water is extracted from the blood, interstitial liquid, and intracellular fluid. Water produced metabolically by the oxidation of food or tissue fuels amounts to about 300 ml. daily in an average adult. The daily obligatory water expenditure of a healthy person includes 500 to 700 ml. for urinary excretion, 500 to 600 ml. as insensible evaporation from the skin, 400 to 500 ml. as vapor exhaled in expired air, and perhaps 100 ml. in feces. Thus, with no water intake a body water deficit accumulates at the rate of more than 1 liter a day.

These values of loss represent minimal estimates for an inactive afebrile, adult patient resting in bed in a temperate environment. Physical activity, elevation of air temperature, or exposure to a source of radiant energy such as the sun immediately raises the basal water loss through the skin. An air temperature of 80°F. induces active sweating even in a resting person. Water losses in sweat have been known to exceed 14 liters a day under conditions of extreme work and heat (E. F. Adolph *et al., Physiology of Man in the Desert*, Interscience Publishers, New York, 1947).

Many pathological states create unavoidable losses of fluid. Two to five liters of water may be eliminated daily in any one of the following ways: vomiting, diarrhea, febrile sweating, and drainage of an intestinal fistula or of a suctioning catheter in the stomach or bowel. Tubular lesions may so impair the concentrating power of the kidney that the irreducible volume of urine exceeds 2 liters daily. Draining fistulas in the abdominal and thoracic cavities are sometimes major sources of fluid loss, and the weeping of exudate into dressings over burned or otherwise injured areas of skin may contribute substantially to the total output of water.

In infants and children both physiological and pathological losses of fluid are greater in proportion to the body weight than in adults. A major reason is that the skeletomuscular system, which in adults contains a large proportion of the body water (and electrolytes), is underdeveloped in the young, whereas the visceral organs, which are chiefly responsible for the losses, are relatively large. The differential is also due to the higher metabolic rate of the child, to his proportionately larger surface area through which water vaporizes, to his extra metabolic demands for growth, and in the very young to the reduced capacity of the immature kidney to produce a concentrated urine. If water expenditure is compared with body metabolism instead of body weight, minimal losses are about the same in infants and adults and amount to 80 to 170 ml. (depending upon the urine specific gravity) per 100 calories of metabolic heat. This means that the average, healthy, 10-kg. baby eliminates 3 to 4 times as much fluid per kg. of body weight as the adult of average size.

An exclusive depletion of body water is uncommon. It arises in an otherwise healthy person only when he is physically deprived of potable water, as when lost in the desert or at sea. In contrast, the sick or poisoned patient may suffer a simple water deficit because of lesions which prevent him from ingesting fluid. Disorders such as pharyngitis, esophagitis, cardiospasm, stricture, and generalized weakness may make it impossible to drink, whereas apathy, drowsiness, stupor, and coma may erase any desire for needed water. In contrast to combined salt and water deficits described subsequently, simple water depletion is due almost always to inadequate intake, not to excessive loss.

There are a few exceptions to the last generalization, *i.e.*, conditions in which primary water deficits arise because of excessive losses of body water. The first example is intensive sweating. Because sweat is a hypotonic secretion (*i.e.*, it is less salty than blood plasma), it robs the body of more water than electrolytes. Even healthy men with an adequate source of drinking water rarely maintain hydration while working in the heat, and the resulting water deficit is repaid surprisingly slowly. Other examples are diabetes insipidus and impairments in the renal concentrating mechanism that accompany some disorders of calcium and potassium metabolism. In each of these situations there is an abnormal renal ex-

cretion of water without a proportional excretion of salt.

The above circumstances give rise to primary deficits in body water only if the victim is unable to drink in response to his usual sensations of intense thirst. For example, the person with diabetes insipidus who becomes comatose for any reason is in danger of severe dehydration within a short period of time. In a somewhat similar way, any comatose patient who is fed a high protein intake by gavage experiences a diuresis due to the excretion of urea ("solute diuresis"). Unless the intake of fluid is correspondingly large, the result is a primary depletion of body water, a condition that may not be recognized promptly because of the large volume of urine.

The signs and symptoms of dehydration depend upon any associated deficits of electrolyte. Simple water depletion generates thirst and often little else. Salivary secretions become thick and scanty, and the mucous membranes of the mouth and throat become dry. Subcutaneous tissues lose much of their turgor and elasticity. Progressive weakness arises, and in severe grades of dehydration mental confusion and hallucination may occur. Until dehydration is advanced, the blood volume is well maintained at the expense of intracellular fluid, and hemoconcentration is not as marked as would otherwise be true. Hypernatremia is always present in primary water depletion, but because the kidneys do not usually respond by excreting extra salt, water and only water is required to restore health. A water deficit which equals 2% of the body weight constitutes a clinically mild dehydration, 4% a moderate dehydration, and 6% a severe dehydration. Water starvation which reaches about 15% of the body weight, or 20 to 22% of the body water, is believed to be fatal in most cases (Adolph *et al.*, 1947, *op. cit.*).

The treatment of dehydration is simply the administration of water in amounts sufficient to correct the deficit. The oral route is preferred, but all channels of administration are appropriate. For parenteral use, water must be rendered isotonic or at least isosmotic; when there is no deficit of body salt, this is usually accomplished by the addition of 5% glucose. The route of administration is a less important decision than the quantity of fluid.

Unfortunately the extent of a water deficit can seldom be established with accuracy at the bedside or even in the laboratory. The patient's body weight is the most useful simple index, but it cannot be interpreted unless his normal or hydrated weight is known. In most cases this information becomes available only after a cure. With healthy kidneys subjected to a normal solute load, a daily urine volume in excess of 1 liter or a rate of urine flow above 0.6 ml. per hour per kg. (2 ml. per hour per kg. in infants) is inconsistent with a significant depletion of body water. In the absence of cardiac or renal disease, it is proper to continue the administration of water until a stage of mild diuresis is reached.

Dehydration should be prevented as well as corrected. In most severe poisonings, it is desirable to delineate fluid requirements carefully by maintaining a chart of daily expenditures through all channels. Continuous losses of water from the skin, respiratory tract, and urine cannot be prevented or even depressed beyond a fixed level. For the average afebrile adult resting in bed on a low caloric diet, this irreducible minimum lies between 1500 and 2000 ml. each day. Even in such a patient, the intake should exceed this minimal loss to provide a margin of safety. Occasionally the parenteral administration of grossly excessive amounts of water induces in severely ill patients overhydration and water intoxication (p. IV-68), but usually an excess of intake over obligatory loss is excreted harmlessly as extra urine.

Salt Depletion

Body deficits of sodium chloride arise almost invariably from extraordinary losses of salt, not from primary restrictions of intake. Salt is never eliminated without water, but unlike water the obligatory losses of sodium chloride are very small in a healthy person. For example, if salt is removed from the diet, normal kidneys conserve this electrolyte by excreting a salt-free urine. The normal salt content of feces is small, and water lost by vaporization in a temperate environment is essentially salt-free.

The secretion of sweat, however, normally robs the body of sodium chloride, which is present in sweat in concentrations of 0.1 to 0.4%. Under conditions of extreme heat, more than 20 gm. of salt can be lost in a day by this avenue. Furthermore, substantial amounts of sodium chloride are present in most pathological excretions, including vomitus, diarrheal stools, the drainage from various fistulas, the chyme from an ileostomy opening, the transudate from burned and eroded areas of skin, the returns from a suctioning catheter in the stomach or bowel, and the urine from any kidney which cannot conserve salt. Daily losses of NaCl in these fluids may total more than 30 gm. In most of these cases, coexisting deficits of water and salt are both significant and are often accompanied by profound disorders of acid-base balance (p. IV-69).

In a few situations, however, the body deficit of salt is proportionately greater than the deficit of water, so that the clinical problem is largely one of salt depletion. A common example is the person who compensates for severe water loss by drinking but does nothing about contemporaneous losses of sodium chloride. Thus men working in the heat may suffer primary salt depletion if they replace the water lost in sweat but not the salt. A similar problem arises when the physician attempts to treat a mixed deficit by infusing isotonic glucose solution instead of isotonic saline. A rarer example is provided by the patient who washes salt out of his body by drinking water while his stomach is being emptied continuously by a suctioning catheter.

In these patients, in whom there are no shortages of body water, the only signs of salt depletion may be muscle weakness and painful muscle spasms. These so-called "heat cramps" often occur in the calf muscles, abdominal muscles, and intrinsic muscles of the hand, particularly during periods of physical activity.

Usually body deficits of salt and of water coexist. Sometimes the losses of salt are proportionately greater than those of water, as for example in renal salt-wasting disease, the cerebral salt-wasting syndrome, and adrenocortical insufficiency. Unlike the healthy person, these patients continue to excrete salt even when their intakes of salt and of water are severely curtailed. Their body fluids tend to become hypotonic, but this tendency stimulates a water diuresis so that an equivalent amount of water is removed with the salt. The result is an "isotonic contraction" of the extracellular fluid volume. Eventually this fluid compartment is so reduced in volume that the pituitary secretes antidiuretic hormone which terminates the water diuresis. Renal salt loss continues, however, and the result is hyponatremia. Because the osmotic pressure of the extracellular fluid is lowered, water migrates into the tissue cells to equalize the osmotic pressures. This shift further reduces the volumes of extracellular fluid and of circulating blood. Although the plasma concentration of sodium remains low, hemoconcentration is revealed by elevations in the plasma protein concentration and in the hematocrit.

In clinical toxicology probably the commonest deficits arise from equivalent losses of salt and of water. Such losses are almost entirely at the expense of the extracellular fluid volume, in contrast to primary water depletion in which cellular dehydration also occurs. In the former instance thirst is mild or absent, and the mucous membranes are not characteristically desiccated. Anorexia and nausea are common, and vomiting often prevents repletion by the oral route. Headache, giddiness, tendency to orthostatic fainting, and a profound sense of exhaustion are often described. A reduction in the blood pressure and in the volume of the pulse may progress to a typical state of oligemic shock (p. IV-17). Factors which incline to circulatory collapse include not only the reduction in blood volume but also the marked rise in blood viscosity because of hemoconcentration. Reflex vasoconstriction induced by the hypotension reduces renal blood flow, and kidney function becomes impaired. Thus, in clinically significant salt deficiency, the blood urea concentration is elevated.

In principle, sodium chloride is all that is necessary to correct a simple salt deficit. Since large doses of salt are poorly tolerated by mouth, especially when nausea is present, saline solutions by parenteral channels are preferred. Although hypertonic solutions (e.g., 3% NaCl) have been used successfully, overdoses produce such adverse effects on the circulation (e.g., hypertension) that these solutions are not recommended. In any case, normal physiological saline (0.85 to 0.9% NaCl) is adequate since the body retains the salt that it needs and quickly excretes the excess fluid as urine. To avoid overloading the heart, the intravenous infusion of isotonic saline should probably be restricted to a rate of about 500 ml. per hour in an average adult except in cases of frank shock. In contrast, physiological saline is a poor replacement fluid in primary *water* deprivation, and it may even aggravate the symptoms; in these cases only water and electrolyte-poor solutions are appropriate for reparation.

In the usual mixed deficit, the proper replacement fluid depends on the nature of the shortage. When losses arise from vomiting, physiological saline is usually sufficient; when due to extensive sweating, hypotonic saline is required. The latter can be obtained by mixing isotonic saline and 5% glucose in water in an appropriate ratio, or the two solutions can be administered alternately. Within broad limits, the proper proportions are not critical. Of more concern, if oligemic shock is imminent (p. IV-17), is the speed with which a saline solution can be infused.

As outlined above, the clinical history and physical examination aid in evaluating the nature and intensity of mixed deficits. Laboratory determinations are also helpful. A small urine volume of high specific gravity is characteristic of patients whose principal defect is a lack of body water. Except in Addison's disease, some types of renal disease, and a few other rare metabolic disorders, a salt deficiency is denoted by the absence or near absence of NaCl in urine. Plasma levels of sodium and chloride may be moderately low, but a salt deficit is accommodated chiefly by reductions in the volume of blood and extracellular fluid and not by reductions in electrolyte concentrations. Hemoconcentration, as evidenced by high plasma levels of protein, is usually more striking in states of salt depletion than in water deficits of compa-rable intensity. The blood urea concentration is also higher because of reduced renal blood flow and impaired kidney function.

Methods for determining the plasma and extracellular fluid volumes are too complicated for extensive or routine application. No test and no series of tests define precisely the extent of any deficit. The response of the patient to treatment and the clinical experience of the therapist are the best guides. The patient who excretes 1500 ml. of urine daily with a chloride content in excess of 100 mEq. per liter has presumably recovered from any shortages of either water or salt.

Excesses of Salt and Water

A body surplus of only sodium chloride arises solely through excessive intake. The deliberate ingestion of salt to induce vomiting was a medically recommended procedure many years ago but not now. It produced several fatalities in children. Although prompt vomiting usually protects against an acute overdose of sodium chloride, some individuals retained enough to cause severe hypernatremia. Salt poisoning has also resulted from accidental ingestions, from errors in formulating infant diets and from the inappropriate use of hypertonic saline solutions in gastric lavage.

Signs and symptoms of salt poisoning include intense thirst, vomiting, diarrhea, fever, prostration, muscle twitching and rigidity, convulsions, coma and death. Vomiting and diarrhea are due at least in part to a violent inflammatory reaction of the gastrointestinal mucosa produced by hypertonic salt solutions. As a result the victim cannot correct the hypernatremia by drinking water. The high osmolality of extracellular fluids extracts water from all tissue cells, but the brain is probably the most critically injured organ, at least in fatal cases. A plasma sodium concentration of 274 mEq./L. has been reported in a neonate who survived, but levels of about 180 are more typical.

Healthy adult human kidneys respond to hypernatremia by excreting urine with a high sodium concentration; the maximal concentration is about 270 to 290 mEq./L. Such concentrations, however, are associated with low urine volumes, and consequently sodium excretion is slow, particularly when water losses from vomiting and diarrhea compromise renal blood flow and glomerular filtration. Indeed, many salt-poisoned patients are described as anuric or oliguric. In infants and young children the renal concentrating mechanism is underdeveloped, which accounts for their higher vulnerability in salt poisoning. In any case, whenever the hypernatremia exceeds the capacity of the kidneys to correct it, therapeutic intervention is essential.

In this case, as with any marked deviation from normal in the osmolality of body fluids, therapy should be paced so as to correct the abnormality slowly (*i.e.*, over many hours or perhaps even a few days for a full correction).

Whereas intravenous infusions of isotonic glucose in water are appropriate therapy to correct the hypernatremia of dehydration by diluting the extracellular compartment, this procedure can be dangerous when hypernatremia is due to an excessive body load of sodium. In the latter instance infusions of glucose in water lead to abnormal volume expansion of the blood and extracellular fluid compartments. The arterial blood pressure may then climb to hypertensive levels, which can quickly compromise the ability of the heart to sustain an adequate output. Cardiogenic pulmonary edema (p. IV-22), peripheral edema and other signs of congestive heart failure (p. IV-21) may develop rapidly. If the sodium overload is not too great, however, the slow administration of water (usually in the form of an infusion of 5% glucose in water, *never* saline in any dilution) may be sufficient treatment for the patient whose kidney function is well preserved.

The optimal therapy of hypernatremia due to an excessive body burden of sodium is not well established. One regimen is the intravenous administration of one of the "high-ceiling" or "loop" diuretics, sodium ethacrynate or furosemide (p. IV-22). These drugs lead to the excretion of large volumes of urine with the same osmolality and the same sodium concentration as the plasma. As soon as the drug is administered, a continuous infusion of 5% glucose in water is required to compensate for the fluid losses during the massive diuresis. Potassium replacement therapy is likely to be required too. Some therapists have used peritoneal dialysis successfully to remove sodium rapidly from the body. Sodium-free dialysis fluid has been formulated with 7 to 8% glucose to prevent its absorption from the peritoneal cavity. Volumes of 15 to 50 ml./kg. have been instilled and removed after 2 hours. See Section II under "Sodium Chloride" for references to published reports. Obviously plasma electrolyte levels must be carefully monitored throughout these procedures.

A surplus of body water can be achieved by drinking faster than the kidneys are able to make urine. In otherwise normal adults a rate in excess of 10 to 14 ml./min. is required. Compulsive water drinking of this magnitude is sometimes observed in emotionally disturbed individuals. Polydipsia has also been ascribed to the use of thioridazine and perhaps of other phenothiazine tranquilizers. The result is a syndrome known as water intoxication. The same derangement can arise in treating mixed water-salt deficits by infusing too much water (with glucose) and too little sodium chloride.

A surplus of body water without a surplus of salt can also result from the persistent renal excretion of too much sodium and too little water. This dichotomy arises in the syndrome of inappropriate (*i.e.*, excessive) secretion of the antidiuretic hormone (ADH). Inappropriate ADH secretion occurs in a variety of diseases (*e.g.*, various malignancies, chronic lung disease, CNS disorders); occasional cases have been ascribed to the use of tricyclic antidepressants, to narcotics and to chlorpropamide. Whenever water is the only body constituent in excess, the disorder leads to an expansion in the volumes of the extracellular and intracellular fluid compartments, with consequent hyponatremia and hypoproteinemia. Plasma sodium levels well below 120 mEq./L. have been observed. Because of this hemodilution, other blood solutes may also be present in abnormally low concentrations (*e.g.*, BUN). The serum osmolality is generally below 270 milliosmoles per kg. water.

Water intoxication usually presents with complaints of weight gain, weakness and lethargy. Mental confusion may be apparent, but the victim is typically apathetic rather than excited (p. IV-33). Neither hypertension nor pitting edema is usually present. Convulsions have been described. Death occurs in coma.

In addition to identifying and treating whatever disease state may be responsible for the water intoxication, the therapist should limit the patient's fluid intake to about 900 ml. daily (adult). In mild to moderate states of intoxication, no other therapy may be required. Thus fluid restriction induces a steady decrease in body water and body weight and a progressive increase in the plasma sodium concentration. A more vigorous course of therapy is required if the victim is stuporous, comatose or convulsing. Hypertonic saline solution (usually 5% NaCl) is then infused intravenously, usually in amounts of 200 to 300 ml. (adult). Whereas this procedure will raise the plasma sodium level much faster than simply restricting fluid intake, it may induce congestive heart failure, particularly if the saline solution is infused too rapidly. To reduce the risk, it is probably advisable to administer intravenous sodium ethacrynate or furosemide (p. IV-22) at the beginning of the hypertonic saline infusion. Thus these high-ceiling diuretics are useful adjuvants in the management both of hyponatremia and of hypernatremia.

Body excesses limited either to salt or to water are uncommon, but coexisting surpluses of both substances are encountered frequently. The plasma sodium concentration may be high, low or normal, depending on which component is present in greater excess. Among the many diseases in which excessive quantities of both salt and water tend to accumulate *in vivo*, congestive heart failure, liver failure and kidney failure are probably the examples most often encountered by the clinical toxicologist. The management of water and electrolyte balance in these three states is discussed on pp. IV-21, 61 and 53, respectively.

Acidosis and Alkalosis

States of acidosis and alkalosis are frequently superimposed upon deficits or excesses of both water and salt. Although acid-base imbalances are associated with alterations in the concentration of many ions, only variations in the hydrogen ion concentration (pH) are essential in generating those untoward signs or symptoms that are characteristic of acidosis and alkalosis. Much of the confusion in the medical literature about the mechanics of acid-base disorders arises from the circuity of the chemical methods commonly used for detecting and evaluating these disturbances. Misunderstanding would diminish if present methods were largely replaced with reliable determinations of pH on anaerobic samples of arterial blood. Unless "arterialized," venous blood is unsatisfactory because specimens from different sites vary in hydrogen ion concentration and so reflect local tissue conditions that may obscure the systemic reaction. In contrast, systemic arterial blood has the same composition in all parts of the body.

If properly measured in arterial blood or plasma, a hydrogen ion concentration below 3.5×10^{-8} M (pH above 7.45) is diagnostic of alkalosis, whereas a hydrogen ion concentration above 4.5×10^{-8} M (pH below 7.35) is pathognomonic of acidosis. As stated here the limits are arbitrary, but the generalization is valid irrespective of the etiology of the disorder. Although the physician cannot distinguish by this test between a respiratory and a metabolic acidosis, at least he cannot confuse acidosis with alkalosis.

Because of practical difficulties in measuring arterial pH and because the arterial pH may be *almost* normal in states of acidosis and alkalosis that are described as "compensated," plasma concentrations of other ions are sometimes analyzed instead, with the implicit intent of using these data to infer the existence of deviations in hydrogen ion concentration. In this respect, the ions of major interest are sodium (Na^+), chloride (Cl^-), and particularly bicarbonate (HCO_3^-). Together with a clinical history and physical examination, these chemical determinations are adequate guides in most clinical situations. In cases of respiratory acidosis or alkalosis, however, the plasma bicarbonate concentration may be misleading if not dangerously deceptive. For example, some salicylate-poisoned patients have been treated incorrectly because such laboratory evidence was misinterpreted.

Whenever abnormal plasma electrolyte levels imply a severe disorder of acid-base balance that is not fully consistent with the clinical evidence, a measurement of the arterial pH is required. For this purpose blood must be obtained anaerobically in a special vacuum tube or in a well oiled syringe containing heparin (or some other anticoagulant). With modern instrumentation (*e.g.*, glass electrode and accessories), the determination is simple and relatively reliable. Even the discomfort of an arterial puncture can be avoided by sampling venous blood that has been arterialized by inducing rapid blood flow through intense local vasodilatation (*e.g.*, immersing the arm in warm water). Even capillary blood has been employed. Thus a specimen that is approximately anaerobic can be obtained by inserting the tip of a capillary tube deep into a droplet of blood as the blood wells up from a stab wound at the finger tip.

If no facilities are available for the chemical analysis of blood, a crude but useful substitute is litmus paper to determine the reaction of freshly voided urine. Usually the urine is acid in the presence of a systemic acidosis and alkaline in alkalosis. Unfortunately there are many exceptions to this generalization (*e.g.*, renal disease, urinary tract infection, etc.), and so the reaction of urine is often an unreliable guide to therapy in disorders of acid-base balance.

Table IV-7 is a conventional classification of acid-base disorders. Examples of each type can be found in the realm of clinical toxicology. From this table it is apparent, for example, that a metabolic acidosis may arise in three ways: (*a*) the retention of nonvolatile acids or acid-forming salts as a result of immoderate intake or defective excretion; (*b*) the excessive metabolic production of physiological acids, such as lactic acid, or of abnormal metabolites such as formic acid; and (*c*) the depletion of sodium bicarbonate stores by the elimination of alkaline body fluids, as in certain cases of profuse diarrhea. Similarly, a metabolic alkalosis might arise in three ways (*a*) excessive intakes of alkali or alkalinizing salts; (*b*) the elimination of chloride ion as hydrochloric acid and the consequent retention of sodium as $NaHCO_3$, as during the extensive vomiting of gastric acid; and (*c*) severe potassium depletion, as may occur during diuretic therapy, particularly in the presence of primary or secondary hyperaldosteronism (see p. IV-72).

Respiratory acidosis and alkalosis are due to underbreathing and overbreathing, respectively, and are associated with changes in the plasma concentration of carbonic acid. These changes, however, are not reflected in any predictable way by alterations in the plasma levels of Na^+,

Table IV-7
Classification of Acid-Base Disturbances[a]

ACIDOSIS

I. Respiratory acidosis: increased plasma carbonic acid
  A. Conditions in which there is interference with the excretion of CO_2
    1. Pulmonary and cardiac disease
    2. Central nervous system depression
    3. Anesthesia
    4. Asphyxial states
  B. Breathing in an atmosphere containing excessive quantities of CO_2
II. Metabolic acidosis: depletion of plasma sodium bicarbonate
  A. Accumulation of nonvolatile acids
    Medication with HCl, NH_4Cl, ammonium mandelate, etc.
    Ingestion or inhalation of acids or acid anhydrides
    Increased production of metabolic acids
    1. Diabetes mellitus
    2. Starvation
    3. Cyclic vomiting of children
    4. Methyl alcohol poisoning (also ethylene glycol, etc.)
    Decreased excretion of metabolic acids
    1. Toxic nephritis
    2. Renal insufficiency from any cause
  B. Excessive loss of sodium bicarbonate
    1. Diarrhea
    2. Losses through intestinal fistulas or catheters
    3. Renal tubular acidosis

ALKALOSIS

I. Respiratory alkalosis: depletion of plasma carbonic acid
  A. Overbreathing
    1. Hysteria
    2. Encephalitis (sometimes)
    3. Anoxic anoxemia
    4. Poisoning with salicylate, etc.
II. Metabolic alkalosis: increased plasma sodium bicarbonate
  A. Immoderate intake of alkalies
  B. Excessive loss of hydrochloric acid
    1. Vomiting
    2. Continuous gastric lavage
  C. Potassium depletion (if severe)

[a] Reproduced with slight modifications from James A. Dauphinee, Chapter 12, p. 354, *Clinical Nutrition*, edited by N. Jolliffe, F. F. Tisdall, and P. R. Cannon, 1950, with permission of the publisher, Paul B. Hoeber, Inc., New York.

Cl^-, or HCO_3^-; any ionic shifts that are observed are usually efforts at renal compensation for the primary disorder. Respiratory alkalosis is a response to toxic doses of many central nervous stimulants, notably salicylates and various analeptics. Respiratory acidosis probably occurs as a terminal event in every fatal poisoning when breathing ceases or becomes grossly inadequate. Anoxia, however, is then much more important than the acidosis which accompanies it.

If the laboratory diagnosis of acid-base disorders is difficult, recognition by physical diagnosis is thoroughly impractical. On the other hand, once the nature of the disturbance has been established by combining the evidence from the laboratory, from the bedside, and from the history, then changing signs and symptoms are often helpful in evaluating the progress of therapy. Except in respiratory acidosis, where symptoms of anoxia are usually dominant, the acidotic patient commonly complains of generalized malaise, weakness, dull headache, abdominal pain, nausea, and vomiting. Signs of dehydration, circulatory insufficiency, and various grades of stupor or coma are often present. Hyperpnea is a common sign; respirations are usually rapid but sometimes slow and deep (Kussmaul).

An established alkalosis is characterized clinically by abnormal irritability, restlessness, and neuromuscular hyperexcitability which is indistinguishable from that of hypocalcemic tetany (see p. IV-74). Forceful vomiting is common, and a considerable degree of dehydration may accompany the disturbance. Respirations are either enhanced, as in respiratory alkalosis, or moderately depressed as in many cases of metabolic alkalosis. Note that a patient who is hyperventilating may be suffering from respiratory alkalosis or from severe metabolic acidosis. It is apparent that water and salt depletions usually coexist with and contribute to the symptomatology of acid-base disorders.

Prompt and effective treatment is often lifesaving in cases where the acidity or alkalinity of the body is severely deranged. When respiratory acidosis arises from acute respiratory depression, asphyxia, or pulmonary edema, acidosis is generally incidental to hypoxia, and treatment is directed chiefly at the relief of this associated oxygen lack (p. IV-12). Tetany due to hyperventilation (respiratory alkalosis) is usually best controlled by rebreathing into a paper bag. Parenteral calcium therapy (p. IV-74) may become necessary. Hyperpnea can often be suppressed by sedation and in the case of hysteria by reassurance or more sophisticated forms of psychotherapy.

In metabolic alkalosis, as seen after persistent vomiting, physiological saline with or without glucose is always an excellent replacement fluid because bicarbonate excess is accompanied by hypochloremia and usually by a sodium deficit. When salt is administered, the chloride deficit is corrected by the retention of Cl^-, and the bicarbonate surplus is eliminated as urinary $NaHCO_3$. Indeed, sodium and chloride are essential for the renal compensation of metabolic alkalosis. With a sodium deficit or volume depletion, the kidneys conserve sodium and fail to excrete sodium bicarbonate, in spite of an intense systemic alkalosis.

Thus, the therapy of metabolic alkalosis is essentially the same as that for salt and water depletion (see p. IV-66). The principal difference is that more attention should be paid to potassium balance when treating metabolic alkalosis. Hypokalemia is usually present. To the extent that it is due to the sequestration of extracellular potassium within tissue cells under the influence of alkalemia, the hypokalemia may correct itself when the kidneys are provided with enough NaCl solution to rectify the alkalosis. If the alkalosis, however, arose because of extensive vomiting or diarrhea, the loss of potassium may have created a significant body deficit. Potassium replacement therapy is then warranted (p. IV-73).

In a few patients, sodium chloride infusions alone are insufficient to permit the kidneys to repair a metabolic alkalosis by excreting sodium bicarbonate and retaining chloride. In these individuals the kidneys cannot conserve chloride effectively despite the severe hypochloremia that always accompanies metabolic alkalosis. The condition has been called a chloride-wasting nephropathy. It arises in several disorders of adrenocortical function, including primary (and probably secondary) aldosteronism, Cushing's syndrome, and licorice poisoning (see Section II), and in severe potassium depletion from any cause. Thus, K^+ in renal tubular cells is required for the renal conservation of chloride. In the chloride-wasting nephropathy, potassium (usually as the chloride) has to be administered before the kidneys can process sodium chloride by excreting $NaHCO_3$ and retaining Cl^-. Apparently the potassium deficit does not have to be fully corrected to restore renal tubular function. This failure of renal conservation of chloride also explains why severe body deficits of potassium are sometimes the cause of metabolic alkalosis (see Table IV-7).

Acidifying agents, such as ammonium chloride or hydrochloride acid, are much less useful than sodium and potassium chlorides because they fail to rectify the sodium and potassium deficits which almost invariably accompany metabolic alkalosis. Only dangerous levels of alkalosis require the ingestion of diluted hydrochloric acid or acid salts. Occasionally sodium chloride with or without KCl fails to correct the alkalosis because of severe renal disease and consequent failure to excrete sodium bicarbonate. Acid salts such as arginine or lysine hydrochlorides may be useful in this situation.

Metabolic acidosis too is usually accompanied by dehydration and salt depletion, and often it disappears as soon as these two associated deficits are corrected by the conservative therapeutic measures already described (pp. IV-66 and 67). Indeed infusions of saline or of balanced salt solutions are the mainstay of the clinical management of metabolic acidosis. If the acidosis is severe, however, alkali therapy is usually warranted (see below). In addition, because potassium depletion often arises during the course of metabolic acidosis, it may also require replacement therapy (p. IV-73) in order to avoid the severe hypokalemia that may otherwise appear as soon as the acidosis and dehydration are corrected. To a lesser extent, the same tends to be true of calcium. When the production of ketone bodies (organic acids and ketones derived from fat metabolism) becomes excessive because of depletion of tissue glycogen reservoirs, the administration of glucose is also beneficial. Of course the diabetic also requires large doses of insulin.

In severe acidemia, when the plasma pH falls below 7.2, saline infusions may not be adequate, and more aggressive treatment is indicated, notably alkali therapy. The two common alkalinizing salts are sodium bicarbonate and sodium lactate, the latter being metabolized to sodium bicarbonate in the body. Sodium bicarbonate is obviously preferable whenever lactate metabolism is impaired, as is presumably true in any situations with spontaneous lactic acidemia and probably in many cases with large anion gaps that are only partially explained (*e.g.*, poisonings by salicylate, ethanol, methanol, formaldehyde, fluoride, fluoroacetate, toluene, strychnine and other convulsants, etc.). Indeed, as an agent for the treatment of acidosis, sodium lactate is regarded as obsolete at many medical centers, at least in adult patients.

If there is no vomiting or pathology of the upper alimentary tract, sodium bicarbonate and sodium lactate are given best by mouth. The inclusion of glucose and water promotes the intestinal absorption of electrolytes in cholera and perhaps in other diarrheal diseases. For intravenous infusions, sodium lactate is marketed as a ⅙ molar solution (M/6 or 1.75%). Sterile solutions of sodium bicarbonate (available in ampuls containing 44 mEq. in 50 ml., 7.5%) are commonly injected in concentrations up to 5% (usually 1.2% or M/7), either alone or mixed with isotonic saline. The intravenous route is usually chosen in preference to the subcutaneous path.

In whatever way one classifies the severity of acidosis, the more extreme the disorder the more alkali therapy is required. No criteria, however, are available for predicting with a useful degree of accuracy the alkali needs of acidotic patients. The intensity and duration of therapy must be controlled by the progression of signs and symptoms, by repeated analyses of plasma sodium, chloride, and bicarbonate, and/or by measurements of the alkalinity of the urine. As a general rule, whenever the plasma bicarbonate level is below 15 mEq. per liter (33 vol. %), a reasonable initial dose of M/6 sodium lactate or M/6 NaHCO$_3$ is 25 ml. per kg. of body weight (or 6.0 ml. per kg. with 5% NaHCO$_3$). Given by slow intravenous drip, these doses may have to be repeated several times, but as the bicarbonate concentration of plasma reaches 20 mEq. per liter, parenteral and probably even oral alkali therapy should be discontinued to avoid over-alkalinization. Infusions of physiological saline, however, are properly continued until the associated deficits of salt and water are entirely erased (p. IV-67).

Disorders of Potassium Balance

Both hypo- and hyperkalemia are encountered in victims of poison. Dangerously high levels of potassium are rarely found except in patients with defective renal function. Because of rapid excretion, simple potassium salts have a low oral toxicity in a normal person. However, extensive tissue injury, acute rhabdomyolysis and acute acidosis may cause K$^+$ to be released from tissue cells faster than even normal kidneys can excrete it. In severe grades of renal injury and particularly in states of anuria, dietary potassium accumulates in the body. Even when no potassium is ingested, catabolism gradually releases intracellular potassium and causes a progressive rise in the extracellular concentration.

When the level in blood plasma reaches about twice normal or 7 to 8 mEq. per liter, the patient frequently exhibits muscle weakness, hyporeflexia, paresthesias, anxiety, restlessness, and disturbances of cardiac rhythm. Because these signs are variable and often occur too late for effective therapy, the early detection and proper management of potassium intoxication demand frequent chemical analyses of plasma or serum. If reliable laboratory measurements are unavailable, repeated electrocardiograms may help to detect hyperkalemia, but they furnish no information from which a quantitative value of the extracellular K$^+$ concentration can be estimated. The first electrocardiographic sign of potassium intoxication is usually an increase in the amplitude of the T wave; eventually various cardiac arrhythmias, including episodes of asystole, presage complete cardiac arrest (p. IV-26). The clinical management of hyperkalemia is described on pp. IV-53–54.

Hypokalemia is evidenced by plasma or serum potassium concentrations below the normal range of 3.5 to 5.0 mEq. per liter (or 14 to 20 mg./100 ml.). Probably a profound intracellular deficit of potassium always accompanies hypokalemia (except in a few rare instances, such as respiratory alkalosis, barium poisoning, and familial periodic paralysis). Because this cation is plentiful in all ordinary foods, deficiency states commonly arise only when losses are excessive.

Partial depletion of cellular potassium and its incomplete replacement by the cellular penetration of extracellular sodium have been described in many pathological states, including diarrhea, hemorrhage, shock, trauma, diabetic coma, metabolic acidosis, hypochloremic alkalosis, and severe dehydration. In respiratory alkalosis, the hypokalemia is due entirely to the migration of extracellular K$^+$ into tissue cells; the same phenomenon at least partially accounts for the hypokalemia of metabolic alkalosis. In the patient with diabetic acidosis, hypokalemia may appear only after the initiation of therapy, particularly the administration of insulin and alkaline salts. Especially in infants and children, the alkalosis and dehydration of profuse vomiting and the acidosis and dehydration of severe diarrhea are both accompanied by substantial losses of potassium. The hypokalemia reported in chronic toluene abusers is said to be due to excessive urinary losses because of renal tubular acidosis (p. III-400). Adrenocortical overactivity (*e.g.*, Cushing's syndrome) and licorice poisoning also lead to large urinary losses of potassium. The intense hypokalemia of barium poisoning (p. III-61) has not been fully explained.

The clinical manifestations of potassium depletion include weakness, lethargy, and abdominal distention. The most distinctive sign, however, is muscle atony progressing to flaccid paralysis. Cardiac disturbances include tachycardia, arrhythmias, and ventricular dilatation. Subacute and chronic potassium deficiencies lead to a recently recognized but well established nephropathy. These effects are not sufficiently definitive to suggest the correct diagnosis unless the physician is alert to the possibility of this complication. In any conditions that promote excessive losses of potassium, the blood plasma level should be analyzed repeatedly. If no adequate laboratory facilities are available, a suspicion of hypokalemia is stongly supported by electrocardiographic findings of prolonged QT interval, flattening of the T wave, appearance of a prominent U wave, and depression of the ST segment.

The correction of a potassium deficit requires considerable caution, particularly if the renal status is uncertain. The oral route is the safest way to administer potassium salts but is clearly impractical in the presence of vomiting or severe diarrhea. A common oral dose of a potassium salt (usually the chloride but sometimes the nitrate or acetate) is 1 to 2 gm. in solution (often dissolved in milk) 3 to 6 times in a 24-hour period.

By intravenous or other parenteral channels, potassium must be infused very slowly to avoid even transient periods of hyperkalemia, which might produce heart block and cardiac arrest. Except in cases of profound paralysis induced by hypokalemia, potassium salts should not be given by any route at a rate exceeding 15 to 20 mEq. per hour (1 to 1.5 gm. KCl), and the total dose does not usually need to be greater than 150 mEq. (11 gm. KCl); often 15 to 45 mEq. (1 to 3 gm.) is sufficient. For parenteral administration potassium chloride is generally chosen; it is available in sterile ampuls containing 20 mEq. (10 ml.) or 40 mEq. (20 ml.). Before infusion this solution is diluted with isotonic saline or glucose in water, so that the K^+ concentration does not exceed 40 to 60 mEq. per liter. Darrow's solution, which contains NaCl, sodium lactate, and KCl (2.7 gm. per liter), has proved particularly effective in infants by intravenous infusion or more rarely by hypodermoclysis; the recommended maximal dose is 80 ml. per kg., and it should be spaced over a period of 4 to 8 hours.

Disorders of Blood Calcium

Calcium retention and depletion are dependent on many complex factors, including the dietary levels of calcium and vitamin D, endoge-nous vitamin D, parathyroid activity, acid-base balance, bone growth and mineralization, bone resorption and disease, renal function, lactation, and many other circumstances. Within broad limits the dietary calcium level is comparatively unimportant, but mild deficiency states during active growth, pregnancy, and lactation have been ascribed to inadequate calcium intake. Indeed calcium and iron are the only minerals in which American diets are sometimes regarded as deficient. Milk is the best source of calcium; 1 quart contains about 1.3 gm., which equals the daily requirement of the average child. Milk-free diets, unless carefully designed, tend to be deficient in absorbable calcium. For example, due to the oxalic acid of spinach and the phytic acid of cereals, most calcium in these foods cannot be assimilated.

Probably vitamin D is more often a critical dietary component than is calcium. Inadequate intake of vitamin D is responsible for infantile and juvenile rickets, and sometimes osteomalacia in adults. Persistent overdoses of vitamin D, when accompanied by high calcium diets, may led to hypercalcemia and metastatic calcification of soft tissues. In states of calcium deficiency, however, vitamin D sometimes produces hypocalcemia by promoting the mineralization of bone (*e.g.*, in the rachitic child given vitamin D but not extra calcium). In general, however, profound alterations of calcium balance are less often due to dietary factors than to disease states such as parathyroid disease and other metabolic disorders of bone, renal insufficiency, malabsorption syndrome, etc.

Chronic defects in calcium metabolism are less often of concern to the toxicologist than are acute disturbances. These conditions are not often recognized unless accompanied by abnormally high or low levels of ionic calcium in blood and extracellular fluid. Of the total calcium in blood plasma (10 mg./100 ml. or 2.5 mM), only about half is present as the simple ion Ca^{2+}. According to one estimate (Neuman and Neuman, *The Chemical Dynamics of Bone Mineral*, University of Chicago Press, 1958), the calcium in normal blood plasma is partitioned as follows: ionic 53%, protein-bound 33% (7% attached to globulins and 26% to albumin), 6% as a bicarbonate complex, 3% as a citrate complex, and 3% as a soluble phosphate complex. Since only the protein-bound element is nondiffusible, 66% of the total calcium can be found in ultrafiltrates. Whereas variations in this normal pattern over long periods of time may have many metabolic consequences, acute physiological disturbances are due solely to alterations in the ionic calcium level.

The chief effects of transient hypercalcemia are those on the heart, muscles and nerves. If the plasma concentration of ionic calcium rises to 1.5 times its normal value (concentrations of total and ionic calcium tend to parallel each other in this range), muscle weakness, constipation, and such mental states as disorientation and confusion may occur. As the calcium reaches levels 2 to 5 times normal, vagal bradycardia, sinus arrhythmia, shifting pacemaker, varying degrees of heart block, ventricular premature beats, ventricular tachycardia, and finally ventricular fibrillation may develop. This syndrome can be produced by the parenteral administration of soluble, ionizable calcium salts; it also occurs in acute parathyroid crises (hyperparathyroidism) and in the hypercalcemia of malignancy. Because of limited intestinal absorption, dangerous hypercalcemia cannot be induced by the ingestion of calcium compounds, even when massive doses are swallowed.

Any considerable reduction in the ionic calcium activity produces tetany. When the total blood calcium is low, as well as the level of Ca^{2+}, the condition is called hypocalcemic tetany. When the concentration of chemically bound calcium rises in proportion to the fall in the ionic fraction (e.g., during infusions of sodium edetate), the condition is called normocalcemic tetany. The distinction is important only because most clinical chemistry laboratories report only values of total calcium or the total exclusive of that bound to a tight chelating agent such as EDTA. Electrometric methods are available, however, for estimating the concentration of ionic calcium.

An impending or latent tetany may be detected with the aid of several diagnostic procedures. The Chvostek sign, Trousseau phenomenon, and peroneal sign are useful ways of exposing neuromuscular hyperexcitability. Electrical stimulation of a motor nerve (the Erb test) is used occasionally. Both the rheobase and chronaxie of peripheral nerve are decreased when the extracellular level of ionic calcium is low. Frank or manifest tetany reveals itself as carpal and pedal spasm, laryngospasm, tremors and twitching, pain (probably due to muscle spasm), convulsive seizures of all types, gastrointestinal disorders such as cardiospasm and vomiting, and occasionally many other signs and symptoms. In the neonatal period, laryngospasm (leading to cyanosis) and irritability are sometimes the only manifestations. Tetany may have a sudden onset and alarming intensity, or the disturbance may be mild and persistent.

Hypocalcemic tetany is due to dietary inadequacies of calcium and vitamin D as in rickets and some forms of osteomalacia, to certain types of gastrointestinal tract disease (malabsorption syndrome), to excessive utilization as in pregnancy, to excessive loss as in lactation, to hypoparathyroidism, and to idiopathic states such as neonatal tetany. Normocalcemic tetany occurs in metabolic and respiratory alkalosis (see p. IV-70), because a rise in pH allows the plasma proteins to bind more calcium and so reduce the Ca^{2+} concentration. Toxic doses of soluble fluorides and oxalates may also cause normocalcemic tetany (pp. III-187 and 326). Under some poorly defined circumstances, infusions of sodium phosphate and of sodium citrate produce tetany.

The prompt administration of ionic calcium is sufficient to control both hypocalcemic and normocalcemic tetany. Given by mouth, calcium salts act too slowly to employ in manifest tetany, but the oral route is preferred in states of latent tetany. Calcium chloride, gluconate, and lactate are the common medicinal salts; calcium gluceptate is also available. The recommended oral dose in an adult is 1 to 2 gm. of $CaCl_2 \cdot 2H_2O$, 2 to 4 gm. of calcium lactate, and 1 to 3 gm. of calcium gluconate, repeated every few hours as necessary. Of these preparations, probably the chloride produces gastric irritation most often; to avoid vomiting, it should be given only in a highly diluted formula.

Calcium salts should never be injected subcutaneously, and the intramuscular route is sometimes dangerous, particularly in infants. For example, even calcium gluconate, which is the least irritating preparation, occasionally produces sloughing when injected intramuscularly as a 10% solution. For this reason the only acceptable route for parenteral administration is the intravenous channel. The usual adult dose of calcium gluconate is 10 to 30 ml. of a 10% sterile solution (0.45 mEq. Ca^{2+}/ml.), injected slowly to avoid severe tachycardia and flushing. Some adult victims of acute fluoride poisoning, however, have required as much as 220 mEq. calcium, which is equivalent to 500 ml. of 10% calcium gluconate infused intravenously over a few hours. Such massive infusions require careful monitoring of the plasma calcium concentration and of the ECG.

Calcium chloride is sometimes infused in concentrations of 5 to 10%; for example, 5 to 20 ml. of a 5% solution can be administered if the rate is kept below 2 ml. per minute. Unlike the lactate or gluconate which are metabolized, repeated doses of calcium chloride may produce a systemic acidosis. In an acidotic patient (e.g., one with renal insufficiency), the gluconate is always preferred to the chloride.

Other measures are also useful in the control of tetany. For example, rebreathing, as into a paper bag, may suppress the alkalotic tetany of hyperventilation. A single injection of parathyroid extract (Parathyroid Injection, U.S.P.) is sometimes sufficient, after a latency of a few hours, to control mild hypocalcemia for a period of several days, but this treatment is not recommended unless the tetany is due to parathyroid insufficiency. In contradistinction to manifest tetany, latent tetany can often be controlled, whatever its origin, by the oral administration of vitamin D (25,000 to 50,000 units per day) or of dihydrotachysterol (2.5 mg. per day), together with a calcium-rich diet.

Disorders of Magnesium Balance

The normal concentration of magnesium in human blood plasma is 1.6 to 2.2 mEq./L., about one-third of which is bound to plasma proteins. Toxic responses may be seen at serum concentrations as low as 3 to 4 mEq./L., but threshold effects are hard to recognize because of the frequent coexistence of other abnormal states such as renal insufficiency, hypocalcemia, acidosis, hyperkalemia and digitalis therapy. At magnesium concentrations of 10 to 15 mEq./L., such lethal complications as cardiac arrest or respiratory paralysis may occur.

Magnesium poisoning secondary to the oral intake of magnesium-containing antacids or laxatives occurs rarely if ever in healthy adults consuming recommended doses. Even soluble magnesium salts are so slowly absorbed that their ingestion generally causes nothing more than purging. However, massive overdoses, conventional doses in elderly and/or uremic patients, incorrectly formulated hemodialysis fluids and overzealous use of magnesium-containing enemas have all led to dangerous and even fatal intoxications. In chronic renal insufficiency hypermagnesemia may occur even without an abnormally high intake, but plasma levels then rarely exceed 5 mEq./L.

The intoxication syndrome can be insidious in onset and erroneously ascribed to the failure of multiple organ systems in elderly uremic patients. With single large overdoses, however, death often occurs in less than 24 hours. Early signs and symptoms include nausea, vomiting, malaise and confusion. Deep tendon reflexes are decreased. Central nervous system depression may progress through coma to medullary paralysis. However, magnesium also causes a loss of muscle power by decreasing the neuronal release of acetylcholine at myoneural junctions. Thus central respiratory depression may be compounded by depressed function of the respiratory musculature.

Hypotension may be due to peripheral vasodilation or to decreased cardiac output secondary to conduction defects. Bradycardia is common, with such ECG changes as a prolonged PR and widened QRS, leading eventually to arrest in diastole.

All magnesium-containing medications should be withdrawn. It is said that the respiratory effects can be antagonized to some extent by the intravenous administration of calcium salts, but in at least one case vigorous therapy with calcium did not prevent a fatal outcome (*Anesthesiology 32*: 378, 1970). Peritoneal or extracorporeal hemodialysis against fluids devoid of magnesium does not appear to have been explored as a form of treatment.

In the context of clinical toxicology hypomagnesemia has been reported in acute fluoride poisoning (see p. III-187), in chronic alcoholism (especially with hepatic cirrhosis), and in patients on long-term diuretic therapy for heart failure (*British Medical Journal, 3*: 620, 1972). In the latter study five patients with mild hypomagnesemia were also found to have significantly depressed magnesium levels in skeletal muscle. Serum magnesium levels as low as 0.48 mEq./L. have been reported in acute fluoride poisoning (*Annals of Clinical Biochemistry, 17*: 10, 1980). Clinical features said to be associated with magnesium deficiency include muscle cramps, paresthesias, exaggerated tendon reflexes and neuromuscular disorders similar to those seen in hypocalcemia. Indeed both hypocalcemia and hypokalemia are often associated with hypomagnesemia.

Severe magnesium deficiency warrants parenteral replacement therapy. For this purpose magnesium sulfate is usually infused intravenously. The official U.S.P. salt is $MgSO_4 \cdot 7H_2O$, one gram of which is equivalent to 4.06 millimoles. It is available as a sterile 50% solution which is diluted for slow intravenous infusion. Doses of 2 to 4 gm. (17 to 34 mEq.) have been given daily in divided doses. During such infusions, the therapist should check the deep-tendon reflexes repeatedly; as long as they are active, respiratory paralysis from hypermagnesemia is unlikely. Monitoring the ECG is also desirable. Perhaps an injectable calcium salt should be on hand to counteract a magnesium sulfate overdose, but a useful Ca^{2+}-Mg^{2+} antagonism has not been clearly demonstrated. If hypomagnesemia and hypocalcemia coexist, both deficits should be corrected at the same time (see p. IV-74).

NUTRITION

The subject of nutrition has multifold significance for the clinical toxicologist. Good nutrition is protective against many poisons, notably hepatotoxic substances. Whatever the causative agent, an acute injury is often accompanied by large losses of nutrients, while at the same time tissue damage creates extraordinary metabolic demands for many dietary factors. Damage to the gastrointestinal mucosa sometimes impairs digestion and absorption severely. Liver damage leads to poor utilization of those nutrients which are absorbed. Protein and vitamin deficiencies lead to anorexia, which intensely complicates healing and repair. Finally, poor nutrition is almost always instrumental in prolonging convalescence far beyond that of the well nourished patient.

Physiological and psychological stresses alter body metabolism. One type of reaction is a nonspecific response described by H. Selye and called the "general adaptation syndrome." The pituitary-adrenal system is known to be involved in all reactions to stress and specifically in the acquisition and maintenance of the general adaptation syndrome. Whereas the nutritional status of experimental animals affects the course of the adaptation syndrome, the converse is also true.

In chemical poisonings, however, the major metabolic alterations are not stereotyped, but arise from specific pathological effects of the particular toxin causing the stress. In the laboratory, diets protective against one type of poison are found to enhance the harmful effects of another. For example, diets rich in fat increase the toxicity of 2,4,6-trinitrotoluene (TNT) but diminish the toxicity of cyanide. The acute toxicity of rotenone is augmented by a fatty diet, but the chronic toxicity is decreased. In selenium and arsphenamine poisonings, liver glycogen appears to be spared better by dietary protein than by carbohydrate, whereas in carbon tetrachloride poisoning a high carbohydrate diet with a moderate amount of protein is judged to be best. Although it would be inexcusably naive to translate these laboratory demonstrations directly into clinical practice, eventually special diets may become available to the physician for protection against and supportive treatment of specific chemical insults. It is certain that no one diet will prove optimally effective in managing all forms of poisoning.

Parenteral Feeding

In many severe poisonings, mucosal lesions of the alimentary tract prevent the patient from retaining, digesting, or assimilating ingested food or fluid. Only parenteral channels are then available for the administration of nutrient substances. Modern regimens of parenteral alimentation appear to be nutritionally adequate, but oral feedings should be resumed as soon as possible because parenteral alimentation is generally expensive, inconvenient, annoying to the patient, and potentially dangerous because of numerous untoward reactions.

In the adult the intravenous route is the only parenteral channel suitable for the efficient administration of nourishment. Particularly with hypertonic solutions, hypodermoclyses are uncomfortable and unsatisfactory because both water and solute are absorbed slowly from sub-

cutaneous depots. In infants and young children, however, this route is sometimes preferred; especially when the area is infiltrated with hyaluronidase, the mobilization of fluid and solute is comparatively fast. The water and electrolyte requirements of adult and pediatric patients are outlined on pp. IV-64–73. Besides water and salts, intravenous feedings are limited largely to the administration of glucose or other monosaccharides, vitamins, amino acid mixtures, alcohol, and serum proteins. To meet high caloric requirements, fat emulsions have been administered successfully by the intravenous route, but toxicity is often associated with their use over prolonged periods, as described below. Their ultimate usefulness remains to be determined.

Unlike the young child or infant, the well-nourished adult person is well endowed to tolerate short periods of fasting. Of the 1600 to 2000 calories needed daily by the average adult resting in bed, glucose from tissue glycogen is the major metabolic fuel during the initial hours of fasting. After glycogen is depleted, tissue stores of fat and protein are consumed. The result is at least a mild ketosis, a negative nitrogen balance, and a gradual wasting of all tissues. Although the daily administration of 100 gm. of glucose furnishes only a quarter to a fifth of the caloric requirement, this amount of carbohydrate is sufficient to prevent ketosis and to reduce the catabolism of tissue proteins to a minimal level. For 100 gm. of glucose (d-glucose or dextrose), 1 liter of a 10% aqueous solution can be administered intravenously. To prevent sugar from spilling into the urine, about 2 hours is required for this infusion in a person of average size, because the maximal rate of glucose utilization lies between 0.5 and 0.7 gm. per kg. per hour. Invert sugar and levulose are said to be utilized faster than d-glucose and may be substituted for it.

In addition to carbohydrate, a parenteral preparation of the water-soluble vitamins (B-complex and ascorbic acid) is desirable in amounts which match the standard maintenance recommendations of the National Research Council (p. IV-81). Of course daily losses of water and electrolytes must be replaced, but in other respects a modest amount of glucose with vitamin supplements is an acceptable parenteral feeding for an illness of short duration.

A practical solution for the problem of maintaining a patient's nutrition over a period of many days solely by parenteral alimentation has presented formidable obstacles (but see below). Raising the carbohydrate intake to match the caloric needs is a difficult task and one of limited value (except in the patient with parenchymal liver disease). To avoid overhydration, hypertonic solutions are required. The repeated injection of glucose in concentrations above 10% often induces phlebitis, although under special circumstances concentrations up to 50% (usually 20 to 25%) have been administered without complications through a small plastic cannula threaded into one of the larger veins (*e.g.*, jugular, superior or inferior vena cava). In assimilating carbohydrate, intracellular stores of potassium are replenished at the expense of the extracellular fluid; to prevent hypokalemia during high carbohydrate feedings, potassium in the form of a balanced salt solution (*e.g.*, Ringer's) is serviceable. For its food value ethyl alcohol has been given intravenously in concentrations of 5 to 6%, but its intoxicating potential is a hazard, and it is never safe in an unconscious patient.

Although infusions of human plasma proteins are sometimes valuable in supporting the circulatory and immunologic systems, they are not effective nutrients. Mixtures of amino acids and small polypeptides are the only useful sources of nitrogen when only parenteral routes of administration are available. Acid and enzymatic hydrolysates of casein and of other proteins (*e.g.*, lactalbumin, bovine blood, yeast, beef) have been employed intravenously and subcutaneously, usually in concentrations of 5% in water (which is slightly hypertonic). In general these commercial mixtures furnish about 15 amino acids, including the 8 that are essential for man (tryptophan is destroyed by acid hydrolysis and so must be added). If injected too rapidly, these sterile mixtures sometimes induce untoward reactions such as nausea, vomiting, abdominal pain, flushing, hypotension, chills, and fever, as well as occasional localized phlebitis. Such reactions appear to be particularly common when single amino acids are infused in large doses (*e.g.*, Floyd *et al.*, *Journal of Clinical Investigation, 45:* 1487, 1966), and if only for this reason, single amino acids should not be used for parenteral alimentation. Two to three hours should be allowed for the intravenous injection of 1 liter of a 5% amino acid solution. Of course amino acid infusions are contraindicated in patients with hepatic coma, anuria or metabolic diseases that impair nitrogen utilization.

The parenteral administration of protein hydrolysates tends to spare the breakdown of tissue protein, provided that tissue glycogen and fat can be mobilized to provide enough carbohydrate and fatty acids to meet the caloric requirements of the fasting patient. This condition, however, rarely lasts for more than a few days. Thereafter, infused amino acids are largely deaminated and oxidized, as long as the caloric needs are not met by exogenous carbohydrate and lipid. The result may be a considerable rise in blood urea nitrogen, especially in patients with impaired renal or hepatic function. Under these circumstances a negative nitrogen balance occurs even when liberal quantities of amino acids are infused.

To achieve a long-term positive nitrogen balance by parenteral alimentation, amino acid infusions are not sufficient; one must also provide carbohydrate and/or lipid in amounts sufficient to meet most if not all the caloric needs. As noted above, it is difficult to administer parenterally enough carbohydrate for this purpose, but a commercial fat emulsion is now available for intravenous infusion. Intralipid 10% (Cutter Laboratories, Inc.) is a 10% emulsion largely of soybean oil, which consists of triglycerides of predominantly unsaturated fatty acids. It is a useful source of calories and of essential fatty acids for patients requiring complete parenteral alimentation for extended periods (usually more than 5 days). Although Intralipid 10% is generally well tolerated in recommended doses (for adults the initial dose is 500 ml. infused into a central vein over a 4-hour period), both early and delayed adverse reactions are described. The former include dyspnea, flushing, cyanosis, allergic reactions, hyperlipemia and hypercoagulability; the latter include hepatomegaly and splenomegaly, jaundice (due to centrolobular cholestasis), thrombocytopenia and leukopenia. In general, intravenous fat emulsions are contraindicated in those with severe liver damage, pulmonary disease, anemia or a disorder of blood coagulation. Electrolyte or other nutrient solutions should not be mixed with Intralipid 10%, but glucose and amino acid mixtures can and should be administered concurrently with intravenous fat emulsions, so that the latter supplies no more than 60% of the patient's total caloric intake.

Thus, because of technical advances in solution preparation, total nutritional maintenance by the intravenous route (hyperalimentation) is now feasible but difficult. Solutions containing amino acids, dextrose, vitamins and minerals have been used alone and with intravenous fat emulsions to maintain body weight even in severe burn patients for long periods of time. Others with gastrointestinal disorders have been adequately fed in this way for weeks or months. To prevent damage to vessel walls, these hypertonic solutions should be infused only into large central veins. Another aspect to the very considerable hazards of hyperalimentation is the necessity for a 24-hour intravenous drip. Strict attention to aseptic techniques during solution preparation, storage and administration is necessary to avoid an overwhelming and potentially fatal bacterial or fungal invasion. In toxicology hyperalimentation finds particular utility in the management of patients who have ingested corrosive agents, where healing is helped by placing the gut at rest.

Resumption of Oral Feeding

Because of the somewhat unsatisfactory status of parenteral alimentation, oral feedings should be reinstituted as soon as possible. The best treatment for acute gastritis, however, is absolute rest for the stomach for several days. The only reliable criterion for determining when to start feeding is the patient's response to a test meal. To prepare the stomach for food, lavage with warm water containing a small amount of sodium bicarbonate has been recommended but is usually regarded as unnecessary. Unless severe mucosal lesions of the alimentary tract are suspected, a trial feeding is usually safe after a period of 12 to 24 hours without nausea or pain.

The initial feeding is limited to a few sips (about 1 teaspoonful) of warm water, dilute tea, or milk. If well tolerated, 1 teaspoonful of milk or strained gruel is offered every ½ hour. The size and frequency of feedings are gradually increased as the patient's tolerance to food rises. A few salted crackers or dry toast are added to the diet. Eventually small servings of cooked cereal, soft boiled eggs, mashed potatoes, and other bland foods are offered. As described subsequently (p. IV-80), vitamin requirements are best met by daily supplementation.

The conviction that "bland" foods like those listed above induce less gastric acid production than conventional meals is an old one, but recent studies have led some nutritionists to challenge this belief. Nevertheless, foods that are traditionally regarded as strong stimulators of acid secretion are commonly avoided, including acid foods, coarse foods, alcoholic beverages, condiments and spices, meat extracts, and meat soups. All fried and greasy foods are withheld, as are items which tend to produce flatulence. The patient's own appetite is one excellent guide in determining how fast to restore a normal menu, but a regular diet, perhaps in small amounts, can usually be resumed as soon as it is clear that the test feedings described above are well tolerated.

To maintain the nutrition of a severely poisoned patient, treatment must be individualized. The physician should check frequently the patient's reactions to feeding and should determine whether the food prescribed is actually served and eaten. Too early or too zealous resumption of oral feeding after a long abstinence may precipitate nausea, vomiting, pain, intestinal distention, and diarrhea. For the management of nausea and vomiting, see p. IV-49. For diarrhea induced by diet, canned applesauce or commercial pectin, fed alone or with meals, is generally effective, but diarrhea caused by indiscreet feeding must be distinguished from that due to poison (IV-50), to undernutrition, or to infection.

Even when no complications are encountered, it is advisable at the resumption of oral feedings for someone to sit beside the patient at meals to help and encourage him. Because food acquires profound emotional significance during periods of stress, feeding problems, which so often complicate convalescence, can often be prevented by the therapist who spends a few minutes with the patient at meal times.

General Diets

A mild intoxication of short duration only rarely disturbs the nutrition of an otherwise healthy person to an extent that is clinically significant. In these cases, a diet which meets normal requirements is generally sufficient. If any nutritional inadequacy is suspected, a high protein supplement and one or two maintenance multivitamin tablets (p. IV-80) may be added to the regular diet each day. General hospital diets are designed to meet the Recommended Dietary Allowances of the National Research Council; these recommendations are judged to be appropriate for the average normal adult person. A general hospital diet contains approximately 2200 calories, 75 gm. of protein, 100 gm. of fat, and 250 gm. of carbohydrate. Vitamins and minerals are present in the recommended amounts.

No diet is adequate if it is not consumed. Although everyone agrees that hospital patients rarely eat all foods served, data on actual intake are scanty. G. G. Duncan (*Journal of the American Dietetic Association, 25:* 330, 1949) analyzed 6 successive meals of 78 patients on a medical ward. The average daily consumption was 1870 calories out of the 2430 calories which were served. Of the 105 gm. of protein which were presented daily, only 81 gm. were ingested. Of 49 patients who received supplementary feedings, only 14 ingested 100 gm. or more of protein. Of the 29 patients not receiving supplementary feedings, only 1 patient consumed more than 100 gm. of protein. Studies of patients on surgical and obstetrical wards showed still lower intakes of food and protein. Duncan believes that food consumption was best in those patients whose illness directed the therapist's attention to the patient's diet.

Probably the food intake of any patient can be improved by heeding his individual needs. The management of anorexia is discussed below under the topic of high caloric diets. These general considerations are not usually applicable to the infant. Although nutrition is often a crucial factor in the survival of a poisoned baby, the topic of infant feeding during periods of illness cannot be reduced to simple generalizations—except for the rule that sudden and frequent changes of formula and alternate periods of fasting and gorging must be avoided. If a baby or young child has persistent diarrhea, tolerates food poorly, or does not gain weight, a pediatric specialist should be consulted.

Perhaps the most important consideration in the nutrition of an accidentally poisoned child is the prevention of undesirable attitudes toward food. Many cases of chronic anorexia stem from an illness during which the child was forced to eat so that he could be "built up." Coaxing and cajoling are not likely to have beneficial effects. Some parents need to be reassured that a child's lack of appetite is temporary and that given a choice of good foods the child will eat enough to maintain good nutrition. They should be told, too, that no one food need be forced upon a reluctant child. The parents should try to serve vegetables which the child likes and to find substitutes for those which he resists. If fruits are consumed in quantity, a temporary diet with no vegetables is probably more desirable than a life-long aversion to these dietary staples. Milk is practically essential for an adequate supply of calcium. By the use of dry skim milk, some of the daily milk requirement can be incorporated into solid food such as custards, mashed potatoes, and cereals. Milk shakes served with straws are often accepted when plain milk is not.

Every child should be encouraged and given an opportunity to feed himself at meals. Interest in eating is often stimulated by letting him plan his own menu on special occasions. For the small child, large portions of food and large glasses of milk are overwhelming to the psyche if not to the stomach. Modest servings at frequent intervals are preferable.

High Caloric Diets

A daily intake of 1600 to 2000 calories is sufficient for the average afebrile inactive adult patient with a minor injury or illness, but 2500 to 4000 calories may be required after severe trauma or disease. A large number of calories is necessary not only to meet energy demands but also to ensure efficient utilization of dietary protein. Of the dozens of established therapeutic diets, none is more useful to the clinical toxicologist than a high caloric, high protein diet. In one form or another this dietary regimen is used widely for the nutritional rehabilitation of patients convalescing from serious disease, surgery, trauma, and similar stressful conditions that cause the destruction of body protein and the depletion of vitamin stores. Probably a high protein intake should be started even during the catabolic stage of injury since the end of the catabolic stage and the beginning of the anabolic phase cannot be determined accurately by clinical criteria. Although assimilation is poor in the early stages of convalescence, the overall benefit to the patient easily justifies the effort and expense of establishing a protein-rich diet.

The Recommended Dietary Allowance for a normal 70-kg. man is 56 gm. of protein daily (0.8 gm. per kg). For tissue synthesis in injury and disease, however, 2 to 4 gm. per kg. is recommended. The poisoned child needs protein for growth as well as repair. The Recommended Dietary Allowance for the normal child is 2 gm. per kg. per day in early childhood to 1.2 gm. per kg. in late childhood and adolescence. Little reliable information is available about the long-range effects of acute injury upon growth. In practice an injured child may be given as much protein food as he can tolerate. Four cups of milk, 2 ounces of meat, 1 egg, 2 slices of bread, and 2 servings of vegetables contains approximately 60 gm. of protein, which more than meets the Recommended Dietary Allowance for the 8-year-old child weighing 27 kg. (59 lb.). It can be seen that high intakes of protein require careful planning and that considerable ingenuity may become necessary to stimulate appetite.

Table IV-8 outlines an adult diet which is rich in protein and carbohydrate and moderately plentiful in fat. A representative menu is found in Table IV-9. This diet supplies 3000 calories daily, of which approximately a third is derived from fat. Higher levels of fat are undesirable because they delay absorption, depress appetite, and sometimes cause gastrointestinal disturbances, particularly in patients with liver disease. In liver disease this intolerance may require the elimination of fatty foods. To keep down the fat content, skim milk can be substituted for some or all of the whole milk. Gravies and salad dressings are usually eliminated in these high-caloric diets; vinegar or lemon juice and sugar may be used on salads. The amount and proportion of carbohydrate can be raised easily by the addition of more jelly, sugar, or hard candy. In liver disease carbohydrate levels between 350 and 500 gm. daily are sought.

Table IV-9 shows that a protein intake over 130 gm. daily is difficult to achieve. If the patient fails to eat the prescribed amount of meat or other bulky protein foods, or if a still higher protein intake is desired, the incorporation of dry skim milk is an acceptable and comparatively inexpensive way of fortifying liquid milk, fruit drinks, cereal, and desserts. Despite the enthusiasm of some physicians for oral mixtures of amino acids, they are generally unpalatable and expensive, and offer no nutritional advantages over food protein except in patients who lack proteolytic enzymes. Even in these patients amino acids are properly considered short-range therapy and are best presented as medicine, not as food. In any case avoid large doses of any single amino acid because even their oral administration may lead to the same toxic reactions as those encountered during intravenous infusions (see p. IV-77).

A high caloric intake requires correspondingly large amounts of dietary supplements, notably the water-soluble vitamins. In severe injury the same catabolic reaction which raises the caloric

Table IV-8
High-Protein, High-Carbohydrate, Moderate-Fat Diet—Daily Allowance for Adults[a]

Food	Servings	Grams	Calories	Approximate Composition		
				Protein (gm.)	Carbohydrate (gm.)	Fat (gm.)
Milk	6 cups	1440	990	51	72	54
Meat or fish	2 (large)	180	575	46	—	43
Eggs	2	100	160	13	—	12
Fruit	2	200	140	1	30	—
Vegetables	2	200	50	3	10	—
Potato	1	150	125	3	30	—
Bread, cereal	5	—	400	13	75	—
Butter	1 tbs.	15	105	—	—	11
Jam, jelly, sugar, or honey	5 tbs.	—	275	—	70	—
Dessert	—	—	175	3	30	5
Total			3000	133	317	125

[a] Figures from "Food Composition Table for Short Method of Dietary Analysis," by J. M. Leichaenring and E. D. Wilson, Journal of the American Dietetic Association, 27: 386, 1951.

Table IV-9
High-Protein, High-Carbohydrate, Moderate-Fat Diet for Adults

Suggested Meal Pattern	Sample Menu
Breakfast	*Breakfast*
Citrus fruit	Orange juice
Cereal	Oatmeal, brown sugar
Two eggs	Soft-cooked eggs
Toast, butter, jelly	Toast, butter, jelly
Milk	Milk
Beverage, if desired	Coffee, sugar
10 A.M. Milk	Glass of milk
Lunch	*Lunch*
Meat	Pot roast
Potato	Mashed potato
Vegetable	Green beans
Bread, butter, jelly	Bread, butter, jelly
Dessert	Rice pudding
Milk	Milk
Beverage, if desired	
3 P.M. Milk	Vanilla malted milk
Dinner	*Dinner*
Soup	Beef broth with rice
Meat or meat substitute	Baked hash
	Carrot and celery sticks
Vegetable	Bread, butter, jelly
Bread, butter, jelly	Applesauce
Fruit	Milk
Milk	Tea
Beverage, if desired	
Bedtime	*Bedtime*
Milk	Milk
Sandwich	Liverwurst sandwich

and protein requirements also depletes tissue vitamin stores. Table IV-10 lists the recommended daily vitamin allowances in health (usually contained in a general hospital diet). The recommendations for a severely ill patient are about five times the allowances for normal maintenance. In any abnormal state with an intense catabolic reaction, 1 or 2 *therapeutic* tablets or capsules are administered daily for the first 2 or 3 days; then 1 tablet a day is given until convalescence is well established, when 1 or 2 of the standard *maintenance* tablets becomes adequate and is continued until the patient is well. Brewers' yeast is an inexpensive source of B vitamins and is also rich in protein. It is best dispensed as a medicine; 1 or 2 ounces mixed with water can be consumed with a "chaser" of fruit or vegetable juice. If oral feeding is impractical in the acute phase of an illness, these vitamin allowances can usually be satisfied by parenteral preparations.

Very little reliable information is available about the specific vitamin requirements of a poisoned person. In acute intoxications of short duration, supplementary vitamin A is probably unnecessary, except in hepatic disease where storage or availability may be subnormal. Even in liver disease a daily supplement of more than 5000 units of vitamin A is unnecessary, and very large doses are toxic (see Section II). As described on p. III-395, vitamin K is essential in correcting hypoprothrombinemia induced by certain therapeutic and toxic substances (*e.g.*, dicoumarol, warfarin). Ascorbic acid (cevitamic acid), however, is the vitamin which has attracted the most attention in clinical toxicology. Subclinical deficiency states of vitamin C have been blamed for poor resistance to infection, defective immunological responses, and impaired detoxication reactions. Although these

Table IV-10
Recommended Daily Dietary Allowances for Vitamins[a]

Vitamin		Men (23–50 yr.)	Women (23–50 yr.)	Children (1–3 yr.)
Vitamin A	μg. retinol (or equivalent)	1000	800	400
Vitamin D	μg. cholecalciferol (or equivalent)	5	5	10
Vitamin E	mg. d-α-tocopherol (or equivalent)	10	8	5
Vitamin C	mg.	60	60	45
Thiamin	mg.	1.4	1.0	0.7
Niacin	mg.	18	13	9
Riboflavin	mg.	1.6	1.2	0.8
Vitamin B_6	mg.	2.2	2.0	0.9
Folacin	μg.	400	400	100
Vitamin B_{12}	μg.	3.0	3.0	2.0

[a] Recommended by the Food and Nutrition Board, National Research Council (1980), and intended to provide for individual variations among most "normal" persons. For other age ranges, see ninth revised edition of *Recommended Dietary Allowances*, published by National Academy of Sciences, Washington, D.C.

claims are not well substantiated, a chemically demonstrable depletion of plasma and tissue vitamin C is adequate justification for daily supplementation. Single doses as high as 1 gm. have been recommended. In general, however, massive doses of vitamins are unnecessary, and this practice diverts attention from the importance of an adequate diet and the need of educating the patient in good eating habits.

In prescribing a high caloric diet the chief problem is usually the difficulty which the patient has in consuming it. Although high caloric supplementary feedings are generally recommended (and necessary) in a high-protein, high-carbohydrate diet, they are clearly undesirable if they depress the appetite severely. Whenever appetite becomes a serious limitation, concentrated sugar and fruits should not be served between meals. A small meal at bedtime is probably best; milk with a sandwich or cereal adds appreciably to the daily intake, especially if the milk is fortified by the addition of dried skim milk or an emulsified fat preparation. Sometimes a patient with anorexia responds to a regimen of two meals a day. If practical, these meals should be served at 8:00 A.M. and 4:30 P.M. to coincide with possible periods of maximal hunger contractions. No between-meal feedings are then served. At meal time the patient is told to eat all the food offered. When he does so, the quantity served is gradually increased. When the patient shows that he is willing and able to eat a third meal, it can then be introduced at noon. Later, as a normal appetite is regained, meal times can be altered to fit the hospital or family routine.

Tube Feeding (Enteric Alimentation)

Aside from intravenous hyperalimentation (p. IV-76), tube feeding (gavage) is the only satis- factory way of providing adequate nourishment for some patients, notably those with obstacles to eating, such as severe anorexia, corrosive lesions of the mouth and perhaps of the esophagus, paralysis of the swallowing muscles, and varying grades of stupor or coma. For the clinical toxicologist the most frequent indication for tube feeding is probably intractable anorexia, such as that sometimes encountered during the prolonged convalescence from various debilitating poisons like arsenic. To counteract severe anorexia, conservative methods, which include specially prepared appetizing dishes, good nursing care, persuasion, and fortified liquid drinks, are often inadequate. Under these circumstances, tube feeding is a practical and effective way of insuring an appropriate diet as long as the alimentary tract is able to digest and assimilate food.

The usual technique involves intubation of the stomach with a nasogastric tube. Gavage is generally impractical, however, in the presence of severe gastric lesions, and as a substitute in some clinics duodenal feeding has been accomplished by the use of an Einhorn tube threaded into the duodenum. Nutrient enemas are rarely worthwhile and never satisfy metabolic needs. Water and salt are undoubtedly absorbed from the large intestine, and probably also alcohol and glucose in very small amounts, but no other nutritional factors are believed to pass through the colonic mucosa.

The success of tube feedings depends greatly on the attitude and cooperation of the patient. If possible the procedure is explained carefully to the patient, and his consent is obtained. Several sources of difficulty may be encountered. A major danger is the regurgitation and aspiration of a feeding into the trachea; with proper technique this should not occur, except rarely in patients with no swallowing reflex (when tube feeding is inevitably hazardous). During continuous tube feeding, care is taken to prevent the accumulation of food in the stomach with consequent gastric dilatation and upper abdominal fullness. When the liquid formula is administered intermittently, any gastric residue can be aspirated before a fresh feeding is added. The diarrhea frequently induced by high caloric formulas can usually be controlled by reducing the quantity fed or by adding applesauce or commercial pectin. Liquid diets grossly contaminated with putrefactive bacteria sometimes cause violent untoward gastrointestinal reactions. Although formerly a source of difficulty, gastric tubes seldom become clogged with modern liquid formulas. In spite of the best professional care, some patients cannot or will not tolerate continual intubation. In these exceptional patients the anxiety, hostility, or restlessness induced by a gastric tube probably makes its use unwise.

A small (2 to 3 mm. external diameter) nasogastric tube is preferred. Plastic tubes cause less irritation than soft rubber tubes. A polyvinyl catheter, which is softer and more flexible than one of polyethylene, is said to be preferable; to insert this tube its rigidity may have to be increased temporarily by chilling it. In most patients the tube can be left in place almost indefinitely, or it may be passed for each feeding and then withdrawn. Continuous or intermittent feeding is permissible. For example, liquid formulas may be administered at a rate of 100 ml. per hour, for a total of 2400 ml. in 24 hours, providing that the epigastrium is observed frequently for signs of gastric distension. For interval feeding, the total daily quantity is divided into 4 to 8 equal aliquots, each of which is injected into the tube from a 50-ml. syringe through a no. 15 gauge needle fitted tightly into the lumen of the tube. If limited to 300 ml., an individual feeding need take only a few minutes in an adult. All formulas should be warmed to body temperature before administration. Concentrated mixtures should not be fed abruptly or in great quantity to patients who have been fasting. For the first few days of feeding, a diluted formula is used, and only one-third to one-half of the total daily allowance is administered. Tube feeding is discontinued as soon as a patient recovers an adequate appetite.

Many satisfactory liquid formulas have been described for administration by gastric tube. One representative example is outlined in Table IV-11. Although more costly, a powdered concentrate which can be suspended in water is more convenient, and mixtures of this type are available on the commercial market. One product (Sustagen, by Mead Johnson & Company) contains in a recommended daily ration (400 gm. suspended in 800 ml. of water) 94 gm. of milk protein, 266 gm. of carbohydrate, and 14 gm. of fat, totaling 1560 calories, along with adequate minerals and vitamins. Because of its high osmolality, the patient generally needs more water than that supplied by the formula; supplemental water is also useful to flush the tube. Unless the water intake is adequate, a high protein intake leads occasionally to severe azotemia and hypernatremia. These complications are not uncommon in comatose patients who fail to receive extra fluids (p. IV-65). For patients who are sensitive to milk, a lower osmolality, lower calorie, lactose-free formula based on soybean protein is available (Isocal, Mead Johnson).

Table IV-11
Tube Feeding—High-Protein, Moderate-Carbohydrate, Low-Fat Formula—Daily Allowance for Adults[a]

Ingredient	Quantity		Calories	Approximate Composition		
				Protein (gm.)	Carbohydrate (gm.)	Fat (gm.)
Skim milk	2 qt.	2000 gm.	720	70	102	2
Skim milk powder (dried)	6 oz.	180 gm.	652	64	94	2
Brewers' yeast powder	1 oz.	30 gm.	82	11	11	1
Whites of 2 eggs	—	—	30	7	—	—
Corn syrup (e.g., Karo)	4 oz.	120 gm.	343	—	89	—
Ascorbic acid (ground tablet)	—	100 mg.				
Fish liver oil concentrate						
Vitamin A		5000 I.U.				
Vitamin D		1000 I.U.				
Total			1827	152	296	5

Directions: Beat up whites of eggs and add corn syrup. Make a paste by adding a small amount of skim milk to dried skim milk powder and brewers' yeast powder. The beaten egg whites and paste can then be stirred into the remaining amount of skim milk.

[a] F. J. Ingelfinger and C. L. Holt: *Medical Clinics of North America*, 30: 1024, 1946. Reproduced (with modifications) by permission of the publishers, W. B. Saunders Co., Philadelphia.

MISCELLANEOUS

Problems of Stasis

The word "stasis" is used here to include all physiological disturbances arising from immobilization in bed. Among the more common problems of prolonged and complete bed rest are hypostatic pneumonia, venous thrombosis, decubitus ulcers, constipation, cystitis, muscle atrophy and contractures, and demineralization of bone with associated nephrolithiasis. Directly or indirectly, most of these complications are due to a sluggish microcirculation.

The major emphasis is prevention. Bed rest should not be enforced when unnecessary or any longer than essential—particularly in elderly patients, since they are more susceptible to disorders of stasis than are the young. Even in the acute phase of an intoxication or illness, most patients can be properly allowed to sit upright for bowel movements and even to get out of bed briefly. In most cases a patient with adequate strength can and should be encouraged to spend several hours each day sitting in a chair and to take mild and graded exercise. In cases of paralysis and of coma, the hazards of stasis can be minimized by repositioning the victim in bed at frequent intervals (perhaps every hour) and by passive exercise of the limbs, together with vigorous massage.

In some situations more specific prophylactic measures are available. The danger of infection can be minimized by careful nursing technique. With particularly susceptible patients, the use of gowns and masks by nurses and physicians may be desirable. For those who are comatose, whose cough reflex is depressed, or who have been exposed to an irritant vapor, brief periods of hyperventilation have been artificially induced by rebreathing into a paper bag or using a Dali-Schwartz tube. Such hyperventilation is believed to promote the circulation and lymphatic drainage of the lungs and to expel mucous plugs which create regions of atelectasis. Both rebreathing and the administration of 5% carbon dioxide in oxygen, however, are hazardous in acidotic patients. A far more effective way to prevent or correct atelectasis is the use of constant positive airway pressure (CPAP) (p. IV-14).

To forestall venous thrombosis, which occurs most often in the vessels of the limbs and pelvis, one avoids tight dressings and constrictive clothing (e.g., garters), and prevents gaseous distension of the bowel, fecal impaction, urinary retention, dehydration, shock, bruising and other forms of blunt trauma, and septicemia. Any person on prolonged bed rest should move his legs often; if this is impossible, passive exercise and massage become essential.

To prevent rashes and bed sores, cleanliness is ensured by washing frequently with a hard soap of good quality. To avoid maceration, the skin is kept dry, if necessary by applying rubbing alcohol and then talcum powder or a bland ointment, especially in intertriginous areas and regions subject to pressure. Bed sheets are kept clean, dry, and free of wrinkles and crumbs. By changing the patient's position repeatedly and by giving him support on inflated rings, a constantly shifting air mattress or lambs wool, one protects areas over bony prominences which are particularly vulnerable to pressure necrosis, such as the buttocks, back, elbows, knees, and heels.

The use of antibiotics for the prevention of infection in the bedridden patient is now generally condemned. There is little evidence that their administration will forestall infection, and when infection occurs during prophylactic antibiotic therapy, it is usually due to an organism that is quite resistant to the commonly used antibacterial agents. Staphylococcal and Gram-negative infections are a particularly serious threat to the severely ill or debilitated hospital patient.

In spite of customary care, disorders of stasis cannot always be prevented. The appropriate treatment varies with the specific complication, but all relevant curative measures should be pursued vigorously. Bronchopneumonia arising in an area of hypostatic congestion requires intensive antibiotic therapy (p. IV-86). With any evidence of phlebothrombosis or thrombophlebitis (e.g., pain or tenderness in an extremity, a measured increase in calf diameter, unexplained fever, tachycardia), an immediate surgical consultation is desirable.

Superficial phlebitis is usually limited to the superficial saphenous vein and responds adequately to such conservative measures as immobilization of the leg (for at least the first 3 to 4 days), elevation of the extremities, local application of heat, and drugs for the control of pain. Perhaps the use of anticoagulant drugs is worthwhile to limit the extension of the thrombus or thrombi. Thrombosis in the deep venous system of the leg or pelvis is a far more serious problem and if neglected may result in pulmonary emboli.

Whether the diagnosis is phlebothrombosis or thrombophlebitis (these may well represent different stages of the same pathological process), the measures listed above are judged to be appropriate. Some kind of surgical intervention is commonly elected. The simplest of the useful surgical operations is proximal vein ligation, especially if it can be accomplished high in the thigh. Anticoagulant therapy may or may not be used after this operation, or it may be preferred to surgery. Heparin is usually selected; its inhibitory actions on the clotting mechanism are multiple, profound, and almost immediate. In contrast, dicoumarol and related anticoagulant drugs are not effective until 24 to 48 hours after administration. Some physicians prefer to continue with heparin for as long as 7 to 10 days before switching to dicoumarol. Although a phlebitis with thrombosis is obviously an inflammatory process, infection is rarely involved. Only when bacteremia betrays the rare case with septic thrombi or emboli is antibiotic therapy warranted.

Decubitus ulcers should be treated promptly and vigorously. Proper débridement by surgical techniques or by soaking the affected areas with solutions containing hydrolytic enzymes is indicated. Systemic antibiotic therapy should be instituted if a spreading infection or bacteremia is evident. After filling the ulcer with Gelfoam powder, the application of a gauze dressing under slight pressure may promote healing. In a few cases where the ulcer is clean, skin grafts are used to accelerate epithelialization and healing. If regeneration continues to be abnormally slow, the diet should be investigated, and if necessary nutritional supplements should be prescribed (pp. IV-75–82).

Disturbances of Body Temperature

The control of hyperpyrexia and of hyperthermia has occasionally been lifesaving. In each case, proper therapy depends upon the mechanism of the derangement in body temperature. Fevers may arise from many causes, including infections, parenterally introduced foreign proteins (e.g., milk, peptone), bacterial pyrogens, intravascular hemolysis and other types of rapid tissue breakdown, some central nervous lesions (e.g., basilar hemorrhages), severe dehydration, and the application of intense heat (e.g., sun, hot air, diathermy).

Febrile states are also induced by toxic doses of many drugs, including the convulsants, cocaine, atropine, dinitrophenol and derivatives, thyroid hormone, epinephrine and ephedrine, and some samples of methylene blue. Rarely antipsychotic drugs of the phenothiazine and butyrophenone series induce an illness characterized by high fever, hypertonus and rhabdomyolysis; for more information about this "malignant neuroleptic syndrome," see "Chlorpromazine" in Section III. This syndrome resembles closely that produced in genetically predisposed individuals by inhalation anesthetics such as halothane and perhaps by succinylcholine; this rare reaction is known as malignant hyperpyrexia.

Whenever the air is cooler than the body, a fall in deep body temperature to hypothermic levels may result from severe exposure (e.g., cold air, ice water), destruction of vasoconstrictor tone (e.g., spinal cord section), drugs which depress heat production (e.g., anesthetics and central depressants), and peripherally acting vasodilator drugs (e.g., nitrites, magnesium salts, anesthetic agents). In contrast, specific antipyretic drugs such as salicylates, acetaminophen, quinine, antipyrine, etc., do not produce hypothermia in therapeutic doses because they lower an elevated body temperature only to normothermic levels.

Aside from its diagnostic and prognostic value, fever has little clinical significance. Only rarely does it threaten a patient's life or even contribute appreciably to his malaise. In general, only when a fever exceeds 105 or 106°F. are direct and energetic attempts to reduce the temperature justified. Valid exceptions to this conservative rule are recognized, notably in poisonings due to such metabolic stimulants as dinitrophenol and its many derivatives used in modern agriculture. Hot weather and a mild elevation of body temperature appear to enhance the toxicity of these agents, and vigorous efforts to hold the temperature at a normal or even subnormal level are warranted.

The hypothermic patient also does not usually require treatment designed specifically to raise his body temperature. For example, the person who has spent a winter night outdoors in an alcoholic coma is often seriously ill, but in most cases reduction in body temperature is not a crucial factor in his survival. Provided that the circulation is maintained, bed rest in a conventionally warm room is sufficient to produce a gradual restoration of a normal body temperature. In profound hypothermia (rectal temperature below 80°F.), however, specific attempts at artificial rewarming are probably advisable. The safest and most efficacious procedure for heating the hypothermic person has not yet been defined. Peritoneal dialysis with fluids preheated to 96.6°F. was effective in one case of severe barbiturate poisoning with attendant hypothermia (see "Barbiturates" in Section III).

Until recent times many ritualistic forms of hydrotherapy were performed on patients with abnormally high and low body temperatures. Today the procedures are simpler, and the therapeutic claims for them are more modest. For example, in extreme fever (hyperpyrexia), various cooling applications are used; these include sponging the skin with tepid water or with alcohol, the application of cold compresses on the forehead and neck, sprinkling water on the skin while it is being fanned, and immersion in baths of cool water or use of mechanically operated "ice blankets." Water temperatures below 78°F. are rarely used, not only because they are sometimes painful but also because they generate reflex vasoconstriction which impairs their effectiveness. To reduce the deep body temperature, a brisk cutaneous circulation must be promoted and maintained, usually by vigorous massage. Ice packs, ice water baths, and ice water enemas are unnecessarily violent and dangerous.

In many cases of extreme hyperpyrexia (*e.g.*, cerebral hemorrhage), antipyretic drugs are ineffective and in some cases are potentially dangerous (*e.g.*, atropine poisoning), but if other measures fail, they should be tried. When oral medication is not retained or cannot be tolerated, sodium salicylate can be administered rectally as a 2% solution (usually containing a little starch or acacia as an emollient), but absorption is not dependable by this route.

Dantrolene sodium (Dantrium) has been used successfully in the "malignant neuroleptic syndrome" (see above). It appears to act by interfering with calcium release from the sarcoplasmic reticulum of skeletal muscles. As a result, muscle spasm, rhabdomyolysis, hypermetabolism and hyperpyrexia are all suppressed. In the closely related syndrome known as malignant hyperpyrexia, it is recommended that dantrolene sodium be given by continuous rapid intravenous push, beginning with a minimal dose of 1 mg./kg. and continuing until symptoms subside or the cumulative dose reaches 10 mg./kg. This regimen may be repeated if signs and symptoms reappear later. In some cases oral dantrolene sodium is given for 1 to 3 days in doses of 1 to 2 mg./kg. 4 times daily. Whether these doses are optimal for the malignant neuroleptic syndrome is not yet established. Dantrolene sodium is potentially hepatotoxic, but the commonest adverse effects (at least with chronic oral medication) are drowsiness, weakness, fatigue and diarrhea.

Infections

In probably no area of supportive treatment does the physician have at his disposal so many effective and safe drugs as in the control of bacterial and mycotic infections. The modern revolution in the chemotherapy of infectious disease has brought spectacular opportunities and responsibilities. As evidenced by the continuing high consumption of antibiotics and other antibacterial agents, there is no lack of awareness of these drugs or of their therapeutic potential. It is appropriate here only to emphasize that the control of infection is an important aspect of clinical toxicology and to mention some of the problems that arise in the therapeutic use of current antibacterial drugs.

Victims of poison are abnormally susceptible to intercurrent infections for many reasons: damage to mucous membranes and other physical barriers to infection, inadequate drainage of the tracheobronchial tree and other duct systems (*e.g.*, urinary bladder), impaired circulation to critical tissues, defective nutrition, leukopenia or agranulocytosis, etc. Catheterization and other manipulations by the physician may also break down normal barriers and further enhance the risk of bacterial invasion. Infection enhances appreciably the morbidity and probably also the mortality rate in chemical intoxications.

Within the past two decades there has occurred a major revision in the attitudes of medical scientists and practitioners concerning the use of drugs for preventing bacterial infections. The prophylactic administration of antibiotics is no longer generally accepted as a sound medical practice, except in a few specific instances such as the prevention of streptococcal infections in patients with rheumatic heart disease.

Even though the clinical toxicologist recognizes that his patient is very apt to develop an intercurrent infection, it is usually inadvisable to try to protect him with drugs. The attempt to do so tends to suppress the normal bacterial flora and to produce a selective environment in which resistant organisms thrive. Instead of preventing infection, one merely increases the chance that infection, if and when it occurs, is due to yeast or bacteria that are difficult or even impossible to eradicate with available chemotherapeutic agents. This unfortunate consequence of misguided therapy is more likely to occur in hospitalized patients because a large variety of drug-resistant pathogens can now be found in almost all hospital environments.

Obviously the hazard of prophylactic chemotherapy is greater if one employs a drug with a relatively broad spectrum of antibacterial effectiveness and if one uses large doses over a long period of time. Although such practices generally deserve to be condemned, there may be occasions when short-term prophylactic drug therapy offers an acceptable degree of protection to the acutely toxic patient during the first few critical days of his illness, without exposing him to an excessive risk. It is now understood that such occasions are much rarer than was formerly recognized.

With the growing recognition that prophylactic chemotherapy may be dangerous, emphasis has shifted to other preventive measures. The risk of infection can be minimized by careful nursing techniques. It may be advisable to isolate particularly susceptible patients and to require the professional staff to use gowns and masks in ministering to them. For those who are comatose, whose cough reflex is depressed, or who have been exposed to an irritant vapor, periods of induced hyperventilation have been used to promote the circulation and lymphatic drainage of the lungs and to expel mucous plugs, which may create regions of atelectasis and infection. It is now recognized that these complications can be prevented more successfully by the use of CPAP (p. IV-15). Early bronchoscopy at the first signs of atelectasis may also help to forestall pneumonia. Although one attempts to insure good drainage from the tracheobronchial tree, the urinary bladder, and other body cavities, catheterization should be avoided if possible. If it becomes necessary, clean or sterile technique should be employed. Other measures that are useful in preventing infections are discussed under "Problems of Stasis" (p. IV-83).

Without the false security of prophylactic antibiotic therapy, physicians are probably more alert to the early signs and symptoms of clinical infection. Of course one watches for fever and other physical signs of an overt infectious process. In addition the severely poisoned patient probably deserves frequent white blood cell counts and chest films. With even minimal evidence of infection, appropriate specimens should be obtained for culture. Sometimes cultures of sputum, urine, and other excretions and secretions are obtained even before a clinical infection is suspected, in order that the therapist may be forearmed with knowledge about the predominant bacterial flora. Of course a report from the bacteriology laboratory is of little help if an inadequate specimen was obtained or if it was mishandled before it reached the laboratory. In any case the demonstrated presence of a pathogen is not synonymous with clinical infection; it is the patient and never the culture which warrants treatment.

As soon as there are unequivocal signs and symptoms of infection and adequate material has been obtained for culture, the question of chemotherapy arises. With a severely ill patient it is not always possible to postpone a decision until a report from the bacteriology laboratory is available. Even if such a delay is permissible, an antibiotic or other chemotherapeutic agent must usually be selected before studies on the drug sensitivity of the pathogen can be completed. Without information about the culture, various clues may help the therapist choose an effective antibiotic from the large list that is currently available.

The first clue is the location of the infectious process. Tissue sites favored by various common pathogens are summarized in Table IV-12. Another readily available clue is provided by a Gram stain on material from the site of infection. Although not a substitute for a culture, a stained smear is helpful because some antibacterial agents are recognized to be effective only against Gram-positive bacteria, whereas other agents are active only against Gram-negative pathogens. This distinction is illustrated by the generalizations in Table IV-13, but some drugs are effective against many pathogens of both categories and their placement in Table IV-13 is arbitrary. Finally one's initial selection of a chemotherapeutic agent may be based on reports of earlier cultures obtained "prophylactically." Unless a history of hypersensitivity can be elicited, one of the penicillins is usually tried first in Gram-positive infections and perhaps one of the tetracyclines in Gram-negative infections.

Of course the ultimate choice of an antibiotic or antibiotic combination is dictated by the culture findings and, with a persistent infection, by studies on the drug sensitivity of the responsible organisms. Table IV-13 (pp. IV-87–91) lists the more useful antibiotics and some of the pathogens against which they are particularly effective. In each case are summarized available dosage forms and a dosage regimen that is usually adequate for an adult patient.

The only other considerations of practical significance that are apt to arise in selecting a chemotherapeutic agent are its cost and its toxicity. Some of the untoward reactions that have been ascribed to each of the currently popular antimicrobial agents are listed in Table IV-14
(continued on p. IV-97)

Table IV-12
Common Pathogens at Various Sites of Infection

Site	Pathogens
Respiratory tract	Pneumococcus (*Streptococcus pneumoniae*), Mycoplasma, Staphylococcus, Streptococcus, Klebsiella-Enterobacter, *Escherichia coli*, *Haemophilus influenzae*
Genitourinary tract	*E. coli*, Klebsiella-Enterobacter, Pseudomonas, Proteus, Enterococci, Staphylococcus, Streptococcus
Gastrointestinal tract	Salmonella, Shigella, Staphylococcus, *E. coli* (especially in infants), Campylobacter, Yersinia, Clostridia
Blood	Staphylococcus, Streptococcus, Pneumococcus, *E. coli*, Klebsiella-Enterobacter, Enterococci
Skin	Staphylococcus, Streptococcus, Enterobacteriaceae, *H. influenzae*
Central nervous system	Pneumococcus, *H. influenzae* (in young children), *Neisseria meningitides*, Mycobacteria, Streptococcus
Wounds	Staphylococcus (*Staphylococcus aureus*), Streptococcus (group A), Clostridia, Gram-negative bacilli, Enterococcus, *Bacteroides fragilis*

Table IV-13
Antibiotics Useful Against Common Pathogens

Name and Common Trade Names	Dosage Forms	Dosage Regimens (Adult)	Uses and Other Comments
A. *Chiefly for infections caused by Gram-positive pathogenic bacteria*			
Cephalosporins[a] Many trade names Cephalexin Keflex Cephalothin Keflin	Oral cap. Sterile soln.	250–500 mg., q.6h. i.m. 0.5–2.0 gm., q.4–6h. i.v. about the same dose by slow infusion	Active against most Gram-positive cocci including penicillinase-producing staphylococci and many strains of Gram-negative bacilli. Used as alternatives to penicillin in allergic patients but sometimes cross-allergies occur. Generally not recommended for treatment of meningitis because of poor penetration into CSF.
Clindamycin[a] Cleocin	Oral cap. Sterile soln.	p.o. 150–450 mg., q.6h. i.m. or i.v. 300–600 mg., q.6h.	A derivative of lincomycin with a similar antibacterial spectrum. Should be reserved for anaerobic infections outside the central nervous system and as an alternative for treatment of some staphylococcal infections in patients allergic to penicillin.
Erythromycin (and various esters) Erythrocin Ilotycin	Oral cap. and tab. Sterile drug Topical ointment	p.o. 250–500 mg., q.6h. i.v. 250–1000 mg., q.6h.	Drug of choice against *Mycoplasma pneumoniae* and *Legionella pneumophila* and for treating respiratory infections in patients allergic to penicillin. Not recommended for treatment of severe staphylococcal infections because of rapid development of resistance.
Lincomycin[a] (as hydrochloride) Lincocin	Oral capsules, drops and syrup Sterile drug	p.o. 500 mg., q.6–8h. in adults, 10–15 mg./kg. in children, q.6–8h. i.m. 600 mg., q.8h., 10 mg./kg., q.8h. in children i.v. about the same doses as i.m.	Similar to clindamycin in activity and adverse effects but less effective. Not drug of first choice for any infection.
Penicillins Many trade names			All varieties of penicillin are effective against Group A streptococci, pneumococci, neisseria, clostridia, and some staphylococci. Penicillin is also available as inhalation powders, troches, nasal solutions, topical powders, and suppositories.
	Potassium penicillin G buffered tab. and sterile powder	p.o. 400,000 to 800,000 u., q.6h. i.v. or i.m. 5,000,000 u., q.d. (or higher)	Parenteral crystalline penicillin G is first choice for severe infections.
	Potassium penicillin V tab. Penicillin V cap. or tab.	p.o. 400,000 to 800,000 u., q.6h. Same as above	Preferred for oral treatment of non-penicillinase-producing staphylococci and other Gram-positive cocci.

[a] May be useful against penicillin-resistant staphylococci.

Table IV-13—*Continued*

Name and Common Trade Names	Dosage Forms	Dosage Regimens (Adult)	Uses and Other Comments
A. Chiefly for infections caused by Gram-positive pathogenic bacteria—Continued			
Penicillins—*continued*	Procaine penicillin G (aq. suspension)	i.m. 300,000–600,000 u., q.12–24h.	Long-acting for less severe Group A streptococci, pneumococci, gonococci, *Treponema pallidum*.
	Benzathine penicillin G (aq. suspension)	i.m. 600,000–1,200,000 u., once (repeated monthly for rheumatic fever)	For treatment of rheumatic fever, Group A streptococcal pharyngitis, and syphilis.
	Cloxacillin,[a] oral cap.	p.o. 0.5–1.0 gm., q.6h.	Particularly useful in oral therapy of infections caused by penicillinase-producing staphylococci.
	Dicloxacillin[a] oral cap.	p.o. 0.5–1.0 gm., q.6h.	See above.
	Sodium oxacillin,[a] sterile (also oral cap.)	i.m. or i.v. 250–2000 mg., q.4–6h.	Particularly useful in the systemic therapy of severe infections caused by penicillinase-producing staphylococci.
	Nafcillin,[a] sterile (also cap.)	i.v. 500–1500 mg., q.4h.	For severe infections. See above.
	Sodium methicillin[a] powder	i.m. or i.v., 25–50 mg./kg., q.8h. in neonates	Rarely used in adults because of risk of interstitial nephritis. Commonly used in neonates.
Vancomycin[a] Vancocin	Sterile drug (as hydrochloride)	Only i.v., 0.125–0.5 gm., q.6–12h.	An effective alternative to the penicillins for endocarditis caused by *Streptococcus viridans* or *Enterococcus*, for severe staphylococcal infections, and for penicillin-resistant pneumococcal infections. Oral treatment can be life-saving in patients with antibiotic-associated colitis due to *Clostridium difficile*.
B. Chiefly for infections caused by Gram-negative pathogenic bacteria			
Amikacin Amikin	Sterile soln.	i.m. 5–7.5 mg./kg., q.8–12h. (for patients with normal renal function)	Aminoglycoside derived from kanamycin often useful against Gram-negative bacterial strains resistant to kanamycin, gentamicin and tobramycin and its use should be reserved for this purpose.
Amoxicillin Amoxil Larotid Polymox	Oral capsules, drops and powder for oral suspension.	p.o. 250–500 mg., q.8h.	At least as effective as oral ampicillin for most infections except shigellosis. Contraindicated in patients allergic to penicillins.
Ampicillin Omnipen Penbritin Polycillin	Oral cap. and suspensions. Sterile drug, sodium salt	p.o. 0.5–1.0 gm., q.6h. i.m. or i.v. 0.5–3.0 gm., q.6h.	A semisynthetic penicillin. One of the drugs of choice against *Shigella* and *Haemophilus influenzae* (but some strains are now resistant), also effective against many other Gram-negative and -positive bacteria. Not used in infections due to penicillinase-producing organisms or in patients sensitive to penicillin. Useful against urinary tract infections. Systemic infections may require addition of gentamicin or tobramycin.

[a] May be useful against penicillin-resistant staphylococci.

Table IV-13—*Continued*

Name and Common Trade Names	Dosage Forms	Dosage Regimens (Adult)	Uses and Other Comments
B. Chiefly for infections caused by Gram-negative pathogenic bacteria—Continued			
Carbenicillin Geocillin Geopen Pyopen	Oral tab. (indenyl sodium salt) Disodium salt, sterile	p.o. 382–764 mg., q.6h. i.v. or i.m. 1–5 gm., q.4–6h.	A semisynthetic penicillin useful against *Pseudomonas*, ampicillin-resistant *Proteus* and some other Gram-negative bacilli, especially *Enterobacter* and *Serratia. Klebsiella* are generally resistant. Often used in combination with gentamicin, amikacin or tobramycin. Even susceptible organisms may become resistant during treatment.
Chloramphenicol (and various ester salts) Chloromycetin	Oral tab. Sterile drug Otic drops	p.o. 7.5–12.5 mg./kg., q.6h. i.v. 7.5–25 mg./kg., q.6h.	Useful against typhoid (salmonellosis) and *H. influenzae* meningitis. Effective against many other Gram-negative and -positive organisms, but use is restricted by its toxicity. Also available as eye drops, ointments, topical creams. Should be used *only* when less hazardous drugs are ineffective.
Demeclocycline Declomycin	Oral cap., tab., drops, and syrup	p.o. 100–300 mg., q.6–12h.	Like other tetracyclines, effective against a wide variety of Gram-negative and -positive pathogens including some rickettsiae.
Doxycycline Vibramycin	Cap.	p.o. 100 mg. q.12h. for first day, 50 mg. q.12h. thereafter	Less gastrointestinal disturbance than other tetracyclines.
Gentamicin Garamycin	Sterile soln.	i.m. or i.v. 1–2 mg./kg., q.8h.	The drug of choice for hospital-acquired Gram-negative sepsis. Severely ill patients may require addition of a second drug such as a cephalosporin. Also used with penicillin G or ampicillin for treatment of endocarditis caused by *Enterococcus*. Ineffective against anaerobic bacteria.
Kanamycin[a] (as the sulfate) Kantrex Klebcil	Cap. Aerosol Sterile drug	p.o. 1.0 gm., q.6h. (larger doses in hepatic coma) 250 mg., q.12h. by inhalation i.m. 5–7.5 mg./kg., q.8–12h. i.v. rarely	An aminoglycoside active against some Gram-negative bacilli but often not hospital-acquired pathogens. Poorly absorbed in gut; used p.o. as an alternative to chloramphenicol and ampicillin only to treat enteric infections and like neomycin to reduce normal intestinal flora in hepatic coma. Largely replaced by gentamicin or tobramycin. Useful for short term therapy only in systemic infections due to most Gram-negative bacteria and to otherwise resistant staphylococci.
Neomycin sulfate Mycifradin	Oral tablet	p.o. 500 mg., q.4h. More in hepatic coma	Same antibacterial spectrum as kanamycin. Parenteral formulations have no rational use because of their toxicity.

[a] May be useful against penicillin-resistant staphylococci.

Table IV-13—*Continued*

Name and Common Trade Names	Dosage Forms	Dosage Regimens (Adult)	Uses and Other Comments
B. Chiefly for infections caused by Gram-negative pathogenic bacteria—Continued			
Oxytetracycline Terramycin	Cap., tab. and syrup	p.o. 250–500 mg., q.6h.	Wide variety of Gram-negative and -positive organisms, including some rickettsiae, and *Mycoplasma pneumoniae.*
	Sterile drug	i.v. 200–500 mg., q.6–12h. i.m. 100 mg., q.8h. or 150 mg., q.12h.	Only if oral medication is impractical. For severe infections only. Also available in ophthalmic solutions, ointments, powders, troches, etc.
Piperacillin Pipracil	Sterile powder	i.m. 3–4 gm., q.4–6h.	A piperazine derivative similar to carbenicillin but with a wider spectrum particularly against Pseudomonas, *Klebsiella* pneumoniae and *Bacteroides fragilis.* For serious infections use in combination with an aminoglycoside.
Polymyxin B (as the sulfate) Aerosporin	Sterile powder	i.m. or i.v. but rarely so used.	Not absorbed when given orally. Generally should not be used parenterally.
	Ointments, lotions, etc., mixed with other antibiotics		Used topically in combination with other antibiotics for the treatment of infected wounds, for irrigation of the catheterized bladder to prevent or suppress bacteriuria, and for treatment of otitis externa.
Polymyxin E Colistin sulfate Coly-Mycin E	Oral suspension	2–5 mg./kg., q.8h.	Similar to polymyxin B in antibacterial activity. Used p.o. in infants and children for diarrhea from enteric pathogens.
Sodium colistimethate	Sterile drug	i.m. or i.v. 0.8–1.6 mg./ kg., q.8h.	For severe systemic and urinary tract infections due to sensitive organisms, esp. *Pseudomonas aeruginosa.*
Spectinomycin Trobicin	Sterile powder	i.m. 2 gm. once	A single-dose alternative treatment for urogenital or anal gonorrhea. Not effective against syphilis.
Streptomycin as its salts (also dihydro-streptomycin)	Sterile drug	i.m. 0.5–1.0 gm., q.12h; also i.v. rarely	Rarely used p.o. at present. Still drug of choice against *Francisella tularensis.* Poorly absorbed in gut. Effective against some Gram-negative organisms but usually used with other drugs. Dihydrostreptomycin is not given i.v. or intrathecally. Also available as topical ointments, solutions, aerosols.
Tetracycline (and its salts) Achromycin Panmycin Polycycline Tetracyn Sumycin	Cap., syrup	p.o. 250–500 mg., q.6h.	Same antibacterial spectrum as oxytetracycline and demethylchlortetracycline.
	Sterile drug (as the hydrochloride)	i.v. 200–500 mg., q.6–12h.	Only if oral medication is impractical. For severe infections only. Also available as aerosols, ointments, ophthalmic powder, troches, etc.

Table IV-13—*Continued*

Name and Common Trade Names	Dosage Forms	Dosage Regimens (Adult)	Uses and Other Comments
		B. Chiefly for infections caused by Gram-negative pathogenic bacteria—Continued	
Tobramycin Nebcin	Sterile powder	i.m. or i.v. 1.0–2.0 mg./kg., q.8h. (for patients with normal renal function)	Aminoglycoside with action similar to that of gentamicin. More effective against *P. aeruginosa* and less effective against *Serratia*. Addition of a cephalosporin may be necessary for severely ill patients.
		C. For mycotic infections	
Amphotericin B Fungizone	Sterile drug	Only i.v. 0.25 mg./kg. over 2–6 h. each day, increasing to 0.5–1.0 mg./kg. daily	For hosptial treatment of deep (systemic) mycotic diseases. Rarely given intrathecally (in coccidioidal meningitis). Because serious adverse effects are frequent, used only for severe infections when less hazardous drugs are ineffective.
	Cream, ointment, lotion		Treatment of monilia infections of skin and mucous membranes.
Flucytosine Ancobon	Capsules: 250 and 500 mg.	Only p.o. 12.5 to 38 mg./kg., q.6h.	Used with amphotericin B in treatment of cryptococcal infection (pulmonary, meningitis) and systemic candidiasis. Avoid in renal insufficiency.
Griseofulvin Grifulvin Fulvicin	Tab. Suspension	Only p.o. 500 mg., q.24h.	Effective in the systemic treatment of superficial fungus infections (dermatomycoses). Should be used only if topical clotrimazole or miconazole is ineffective.
Ketoconazole Nizoral	Tab.	p.o. single-dose: 200 mg./day for superficial mycoses; 1000 mg./day for systemic mycoses	Therapeutic activity in paracoccidioidomycosis, blastomycosis, coccidioidomycosis, histoplasmosis, chronic mucocutaneous candidiasis and resistant dermatophyte infections.
Miconazole Monistat	Sterile soln. Also skin cream	An initial test dose of 200 mg. i.v.; i.v. 300–800 mg., q.8h. over period of 30 to 60 min.	Synthetic imidazole derivative active against yeasts and filamentous fungal infections. May be of some value for patients with disseminated coccidioidomycosis and paracoccidioidomycosis.
Nystatin Mycostatin	Oral tab.	p.o. 500,000 to 1,000,000 u., q.8h.	Poorly absorbed from gut but effective in suppressing *Candida albicans* in the alimentary tract.
	Oral suspension.		Treatment of candidiasis in oral cavity.
	Creams, ointments, powders	Topical 100,000 u./ml.	Also effective topically against moniliasis of mouth, vagina, skin.

Table IV-14
Adverse Effects of Antimicrobial Drugs[a]

* **ACEDAPSONE** (*Hansolar*)—Probably same as dapsone

AMANTADINE (*Symmetrel*)
  Frequent: Livedo reticularis and ankle edema; insomnia; dizziness; lethargy
  Occasional: Depression; psychosis; confusion; slurred speech; congestive heart failure; orthostatic hypotension; urinary retention; GI disturbance; rash; visual disturbance; sudden loss of vision; increased seizures in epilepsy
  Rare: Convulsions; leukopenia; neutropenia; eczematoid dermatitis; oculogyric episodes
  (INTERACTION: Hallucinations, confusion, nightmares with anticholinergics)

AMIKACIN (*Amikin*)
  Occasional: Vestibular damage; renal damage; fever; rash
  Rare: Auditory damage; CNS reactions; blurred vision; nausea; vomiting; neuromuscular blockage and apnea, may be reversible with calcium salts; paresthesias; hypotension
  (INTERACTIONS: Increased nephrotoxicity with cephalosporins, polymyxins; ototoxicity with ethacrynic acid; neuromuscular blockade with curariform drugs)

AMINOSALICYLIC ACID—See Para-aminosalicylic acid

AMOXICILLIN—See Penicillins

AMPHOTERICIN B (*Fungizone*)
  Frequent: Renal damage; hypokalemia; thrombophlebitis at site of injection; nausea, chills, fever, vomiting during infusions
  Occasional: Hypomagnesemia; normocytic, normochromic anemia
  Rare: Hemorrhagic gastroenteritis; blood dyscrasias; rash; blurred vision; peripheral neuropathy; convulsions; anaphylaxis; arrhythmias; acute liver failure; reversible nephrogenic diabetes insipidus; hearing loss; acute pulmonary edema; spinal cord damage with intrathecal use
  (INTERACTIONS: Concurrent use may increase toxicity of other nephrotoxic agents, curariform drugs, and digitalis glycosides; decreased anticandidal effect with miconazole; acute pulmonary reactions, sometimes fatal, with leukocyte transfusions in patients with granulocytopenia)

AMPICILLIN—See Penicillins

AMPICILLIN-PROBENECID (*Polycillin-PRB*; *Probampacin*; *Trojacillin-Plus*)
  Probably same as for ampicillin, except rashes could be caused by either component and may be more frequent.

* **BACAMPICILLIN**—See Penicillins

BACITRACIN
  Frequent: Renal damage; local pain with i.m. use; GI disturbance

  Occasional: Blood dyscrasias; rash
  (INTERACTION: Concurrent use may increase toxicity of other nephrotoxic agents)

CAPREOMYCIN (*Capastat*)
  Occasional: Renal damage; eighth-nerve damage; hypokalemia
  Rare: Allergic reactions; neuromuscular blockade and apnea with large i.v. doses, reversed by neostigmine or calcium gluconate
  (INTERACTIONS: Increased toxicity with other ototoxic or nephrotoxic agents)

CARBENICILLIN—See Penicillins

CEFOXITIN—See Cephalosporins

CEPHALOSPORINS (*cefaclor—Ceclor*; *cefadroxil—Duricef, Ultracef*; *cefamandole—Mandol*; cefazolin—*Ancef, Kefzol*; *cefotaxime—Claforan*; *cefoxitin—Mefoxin*; cephalexin—*Keflex*, and others; cephaloglycin—*Kafocin*; cephalothin—*Keflin*; cephapirin—*Cefadyl*; cephradine—*Anspor, Velosef*; *moxalactam—Moxam*)
  Frequent: Thrombophlebitis with i.v. use; serumsickness-like reaction with prolonged parenteral administration
  Occasional: Allergic reactions, rarely anaphylactic; GI disturbance; hypoprothrombinemia, hemorrhage with cefamandole and moxalactam; rash and arthritis with cefaclor
  Rare: Hemolytic anemia; hepatic dysfunction; blood dyscrasias; renal damage; pseudomembranous colitis; convulsions; *Antabuse*-like reaction after alcohol ingestion with cefamandole and moxalactam
  (INTERACTIONS: Toxic renal damage may be potentiated by concurrent use of aminoglycosides, probenecid, or rapid-acting diuretics such as furosemide or ethacrynic acid)

CHLORAMPHENICOL (*Chloromycetin*; and others)
  Occasional: Blood dyscrasias; gray syndrome in infants; GI disturbance
  Rare: Aplastic anemia, even with eye drops or ointment, possibly leukemia; allergic and febrile reactions; peripheral neuropathy; optic neuritis and other CNS injury; pseudomembranous colitis
  (INTERACTIONS: *Antabuse*-like symptoms with alcohol; increased anticoagulant effect with dicumarol; increased hypoglycemia with sulfonylureas; increased phenytoin toxicity; increased effects of barbiturates)

* **CINOXACIN** (*Cinobac*)—Probably same as nalidixic acid

CLINDAMYCIN (*Cleocin*)
  Frequent: Diarrhea; allergic reactions
  Occasional: Pseudomembranous colitis, sometimes severe, can occur even with topical use
  Rare: Blood dyscrasias; esophageal ulceration
  (INTERACTIONS: Neuromuscular blockade with

---

* Relatively new drug; the possibility that other adverse effects will appear is greater than with older drugs.

[a] Reproduced with modifications and with permission from *Handbook of Antimicrobial Therapy*, The Medical Letter, New Rochelle, New York, 1982.

Table IV-14—*Continued*

curariform drugs; increased diarrhea, colitis with diphenoxylate-atropine (*Lomotil*) and similar agents)

* CLOFAZIMINE (*Lamprene*)
Frequent: Pigmentation of skin, cornea, retina and urine discoloration with prolonged high dosage
Occasional: Epigastric distress; diarrhea; headache; splenic infarction with high doses

CLOXACILLIN—See Penicillins

COLISTIMETHATE—See Polymyxins

* CYCLACILLIN—See Penicillins

CYCLOSERINE (*Seromycin*)
Frequent: Coma; anxiety; depression; confusion; disorientation; hallucinations; paranoia
Occasional: Peripheral neuropathy; liver damage; malabsorption syndrome; folate deficiency
Rare: Seizures
(INTERACTION: Increased convulsions with chronic alcohol abuse)

DAPSONE (*Avlosulfon*; and others)
Frequent: Rash; transient headache; GI irritation; anorexia
Occasional: Cyanosis due to methemoglobinemia and sulfhemoglobinemia; other blood dyscrasias including hemolytic anemia; nephrotic syndrome; liver damage; peripheral neuropathy; hypersensitivity reactions; increased risk of lepra reactions; insomnia; irritability; uncoordinated speech; agitation; acute psychosis
Rare: Renal papillary necrosis; severe hypoalbuminemia; epidermal necrolysis; optic atrophy; agranulocytosis

DEMECLOCYCLINE—See Tetracyclines

DICLOXACILLIN—See Penicillins

DOXYCYCLINE—See Tetracyclines

ERYTHROMYCINS (*Erythrocin*; and others)
Occasional: Stomatitis; GI disturbance; cholestatic hepatitis with erythromycin estolate in adults
Rare: Allergic reactions, including severe respiratory distress; pseudomembranous colitis; hemolytic anemia; hepatotoxicity with other erythromycins; transient hearing loss with high doses, prolonged use, or in patients with renal insufficiency
(INTERACTION: Increased effect of theophylline)

ETHAMBUTOL (*Myambutol*)
Occasional: Optic neuritis; allergic reactions; GI disturbance; mental confusion; precipitation of acute gout
Rare: Peripheral neuritis; possibly renal damage

ETHIONAMIDE (*Trecator-SC*)
Frequent: GI disturbance
Occasional: Liver damage; CNS disturbance including peripheral neuropathy; allergic reactions; gynecomastia
Rare: Hypothyroidism; optic neuritis; acute gouty arthritis
(INTERACTION: May increase hypoglycemia with sulfonylureas)

FLUCYTOSINE (*Ancobon*)
Frequent: GI disturbance, including severe diarrhea and ulcerative colitis; rash; hepatic dysfunction; blood dyscrasias, including pancytopenia and fatal agranulocytosis
Occasional: Confusion; hallucinations

FURAZOLIDONE (*Furoxone*)
Frequent: Nausea; vomiting
Occasional: Allergic reactions, including pulmonary infiltration; headache; orthostatic hypotension; hypoglycemia; polyneuritis
Rare: Hemolytic anemia in G-6-PD deficiency and infants less than one month old
(INTERACTIONS: *Antabuse*-like reaction with alcohol; possible hypertensive crisis with other monoamine oxidase inhibitors, tyramine-containing foods or beverages, sympathomimetic amines such as phenylephrine, ephedrine, and amphetamines, and with levodopa; hyperpyrexia and convulsions with tricyclic antidepressants; hyperpyrexia, hypertension, or hypotension and coma with meperidine)

GENTAMICIN (*Garamycin*; and others)
Occasional: Vestibular damage; renal damage; rash
Rare: Auditory damage; neuromuscular blockade and apnea, reversible with calcium or neostigmine; disturbed mental function; polyneuropathy; anaphylaxis
(INTERACTIONS: Increased nephrotoxicity with cephalosporins, polymyxins and possibly methicillin, and furosemide; ototoxicity with ethacrynic acid; neuromuscular blockade with curariform drugs)

GRISEOFULVIN (*Fulvicin-U/F*; and others)
Occasional: GI disturbance; allergic and photosensitivity reactions
Rare: Proteinuria; blood dyscrasias; mental confusion; paresthesias; exacerbation of lupus erythematosus; fixed-drug eruption; reversible liver damage; lymphadenopathy
(INTERACTION: Decreased effects of oral anticoagulants)

HETACILLIN—See Penicillins

* HYDROXYSTILBAMIDINE
(*Hydroxystilbamidine Isethionate*)
Frequent: Hypotension; vomiting; renal damage
Occasional: Liver damage; neuropathies

ISONIAZID
Occasional: Peripheral neuropathy; liver damage, potentially fatal, particularly in patients more than 35 years old; glossitis and GI disturbance; allergic reactions; fever
Rare: Blood dyscrasias; depression, agitation, auditory and visual hallucinations, paranoia; optic neuritis; hyperglycemia; folate and vitamin B_6 deficiency; pellagra-like rash; keratitis; lupus erythematosus-like syndrome; chronic liver injury; cirrhosis; Stevens-Johnson syndrome
(INTERACTIONS: Psychotic episodes, ataxia with disulfiram (*Antabuse*); enhanced toxicity of pheny-

---

* Relatively new drug; the possibility that other adverse effects will appear is greater than with older drugs.

Table IV-14—Continued

toin; increased incidence of hepatitis with alcohol or rifampin; diminished isoniazid effect with aluminum antacids, and in some patients with chronic alcohol abuse; hypertensive crisis with food rich in mono-amines)

KANAMYCIN (*Kantrex*; *Klebcil*)
Occasional: Eighth-nerve damage affecting mainly hearing that may be irreversible and may not be detected until after therapy has been stopped (most likely with renal impairment); renal damage
Rare: Rash; fever; peripheral neuritis; parenteral or intraperitoneal administration may produce neuro-muscular blockade and apnea, not reversed by neo-stigmine or calcium gluconate
(INTERACTIONS: Increased nephrotoxicity with cephalosporins, polymyxins; ototoxicity with other ototoxic drugs, ethacrynic acid; neuromuscular blockade with curariform drugs)

* **KETOCONAZOLE** (*Nizoral*)
Frequent: Nausea and vomiting
Occasional: Gynecomastia; abdominal pain; rash; itching; dizziness; constipation; diarrhea; fever and chills; photophobia; headache
Rare: Hepatitis; transient elevated transaminase; severe epigastric burning and pain

LINCOMYCIN (*Lincocin*)
Frequent: Diarrhea, sometimes progressing to se-vere pseudomembranous colitis
Occasional: Allergic reactions, rarely anaphylactic
Rare: Blood dyscrasias; hypotension with rapid i.v. injection
(INTERACTIONS: Neuromuscular blockade with curariform drugs; decreased lincomycin effect with kaolin-pectin (*Kaopectate*); increased diarrhea, col-itis with diphenoxylate-atropine (*Lomotil*) and sim-ilar agents)

METHACYCLINE—See Tetracyclines
METHENAMINE MANDELATE (*Mandelamine*; and others) and
METHENAMINE HIPPURATE (*Hiprex*; *Urex*)
Occasional: GI disturbance; dysuria; allergic reac-tions

METHICILLIN—See Penicillins
METHISAZONE (*Marboran*)
Frequent: Severe vomiting; nausea; anorexia
Occasional: Diarrhea; transient fluid retention; al-lergic reactions
Rare: Hyperbilirubinemia
(INTERACTION: Increased toxicity with alcohol)
METRONIDAZOLE (*Flagyl*; and others)
Frequent: Nausea; headache; dry mouth; metallic taste
Occasional: Vomiting; diarrhea; insomnia; weak-ness; stomatitis; vertigo; paresthesias; rash; urethral burning; phlebitis at injection site
Rare: Encephalopathy; pseudomembranous colitis; ataxia; reversible neutropenia
(INTERACTION: Increased anticoagulant effect; mild *Antabuse*-like reaction with alcohol)

* **MEZLOCILLIN**—See Penicillins
* **MICONAZOLE** (*Monistat i.v.*)
Occasional: Phlebitis; thrombocytosis; chills; pru-ritis; rash; vomiting; hyperlipidemia; dizziness; blurred vision
Rare: Anemia; thrombocytopenia; hyponatremia; renal insufficiency; anaphylaxis; cardiac and respi-ratory arrest
(INTERACTIONS: Increased effect of oral antico-agulants; decreased anticandidal effect with ampho-tericin B)
MINOCYCLINE—See Tetracylines
* **MOXALACTAM**—See Cephalosporins
NAFCILLIN—See Penicillins
NALIDIXIC ACID (*NegGram*)
Frequent: GI disturbance; rash; visual disturbance
Occasional: CNS disturbance; acute intracranial hypertension in young children; photosensitivity re-actions, sometimes persistent; convulsions; hyper-glycemia
Rare: Cholestatic jaundice; blood dyscrasias; ar-thralgia or arthritis; lupus-like syndrome; confusion, depression, excitement, visual hallucinations
(INTERACTION: Increased effect of oral antico-agulants)
* **NATAMYCIN** (*Natacyn*)
Rare: Conjunctival chemosis, hyperemia
NEOMYCIN (*Mycifradin*; and others)
Occasional: Eighth-nerve and renal damage, same as with kanamycin but hearing loss may be more frequent and severe and may occur with oral, intra-articular, irrigant, or topical use; GI disturbance; malabsorption with oral use; contact dermatitis with topical use
Rare: Neuromuscular blockade and apnea that may be reversed by intravenous neostigmine or calcium gluconate; pseudomembranous colitis
(INTERACTIONS: Increased nephrotoxicity with other nephrotoxic drugs; increased ototoxicity with ethacrynic acid and other ototoxic drugs; neuromus-cular blockade with curariform drugs; possible de-creased digoxin effect)
NITROFURANTOIN (*Furadantin*; and others)
Frequent: GI disturbance; allergic reactions, in-cluding pulmonary infiltration
Occasional: Lupus-like syndrome; blood dyscra-sias; hemolytic anemia; peripheral neuropathy, sometimes severe; pulmonary fibrosis
Rare: Cholestatic jaundice; chronic active hepatitis, sometimes fatal; trigeminal neuralgia; crystalluria; increased intracranial pressure; lactic acidosis; se-vere hemolytic anemia in G-6-PD deficiency
NOVOBIOCIN (*Albamycin*)
Frequent: Cholestatic jaundice; allergic reactions; GI disturbance; neonatal hyperbilirubinemia
Occasional: Severe blood dyscrasias
NYSTATIN (*Mycostatin*; and others)
Occasional: Allergic reactions; GI disturbance
OXACILLIN—See Penicillins

* Relatively new drug; the possibility that other adverse effects will appear is greater than with older drugs.

Table IV-14—*Continued*

OXOLINIC ACID (*Utibid*)
Frequent: CNS disturbance; nausea
Occasional: GI disturbance; anorexia; pruritis
Rare: Allergic reactions; blood dyscrasias; photophobia
(INTERACTION: May increase effect of oral anticoagulants)

OXYTETRACYCLINE—See Tetracyclines

***PARA*-AMINOSALICYLIC ACID (PAS)**
Frequent: GI disturbance
Occasional: Allergic reactions; liver damage; renal irritation; blood dyscrasias; thyroid enlargement; malabsorption syndrome
Rare: Acidosis; hypokalemia; encephalopathy; vasculitis; hypoglycemia in diabetics
(INTERACTION: Increased toxicity with probenecid)

PAROMYCIN (*Humatin*)
Frequent: GI disturbance; renal damage
Occasional: Eighth-nerve damage (mainly auditory)

PENICILLINS (amoxicillin—*Amoxil*, and others; ampicillin—*Polycillin*, and others; *bacampicillin—*Spectrobid*; carbenicillin—*Geocillin, Geopen, Pyopen*; cloxacillin—*Tegopen*, and others; *cyclacillin—*Cyclapen-W*; dicloxacillin—*Dycill, Dynapen, Pathocil*; hetacillin—*Versapen*; methicillin—*Azapen, Celbenin, Staphcillin*; *mezlocillin—*Mezlin*; nafcillin—*Nafcil, Unipen*; oxacillin—*Prostaphlin*, and others; penicillin G; penicillin V; *piperacillin—*Pipracil*; ticarcillin—*Ticar*)
Frequent: Allergic reactions, rarely anaphylactic; rash (more common with ampicillin and amoxicillin than with other penicillins); diarrhea (most common with ampicillin)
Occasional: Hemolytic anemia
Rare: Hepatic damage with semisynthetic penicillins; granulocytopenia or agranulocytosis with semisynthetic penicillins; renal damage with semisynthetic penicillins and penicillin G; muscle irritability and seizures, usually after high doses in patients with impaired renal function; hyperkalemia and arrhythmias with i.v. potassium penicillin G given rapidly; bleeding diathesis; thrombocytopenia with methicillin and mezlocillin; pseudomembranous colitis with ampicillin, amoxicillin, carbenicillin, or penicillin; terror, hallucinations, disorientation, agitation, bizarre behavior and neurological reactions with high doses of procaine penicillin G, oxacillin, and ticarcillin; hypokalemic alkalosis and/or sodium overload with high doses of carbenicillin, ticarcillin, or nafcillin; platelet dysfunction with high doses of carbenicillin, ticarcillin or methicillin; hemorrhagic cystitis with methicillin or carbenicillin; gastrointestinal bleeding with dicloxacillin; tissue damage with extravasation of nafcillin
(INTERACTIONS: Increased nephrotoxicity with aminoglycosides; decreased effect of oral contraceptives with ampicillin)

PENTAMIDINE ISETHIONATE (*Lomidine*)
Frequent: Hypotension; hypoglycemia; vomiting; blood dyscrasias; renal damage; pain at injection site
Occasional: May aggravate diabetes; shock; liver damage
Rare: Herxheimer-type reaction; acute pancreatitis

POLYMYXINS (colistimethate—*Coly-Mycin*; polymyxin B—*Aerosporin*; and others)
Occasional: Renal damage; peripheral neuropathy; thrombophlebitis at i.v. injection site with polymyxin B
Rare: Allergic reactions; neuromuscular blockade and apnea with parenteral administration, not reversed by neostigmine but may be by i.v. calcium chloride
(INTERACTIONS: Increased nephrotoxicity with aminoglycosides; neuromuscular blockade with curariform drugs)

PROBAMPACIN (ampicillin-probenecid—*Polycillin-PRB*; and others)
Probably same as for ampicillin, except that either component can cause rashes, which therefore are likely to be more frequent

PYRAZINAMIDE (*Aldinamide*)
Occasional: Liver damage; hyperuricemia; GI disturbance; arthralgia
Rare: Photosensitivity reactions

RIFAMPIN (*Rifadin*; *Rimactane*)
Occasional: Liver damage; GI disturbance; allergic reactions
Rare: Flu-like syndrome, sometimes with thrombocytopenia, hemolytic anemia, shock, and renal failure, particularly with intermittent therapy; acute organic brain syndrome; may color skin, urine, tears and soft contact lenses orange; renal damage; severe proximal myopathy
(INTERACTIONS: Decreased effect of oral anticoagulants, barbiturates, digitoxin, oral hypoglycemics, quinidine, oral contraceptives, corticosteroids; increased hepatotoxicity with isoniazid; may cause methadone withdrawal symptoms in patients on methadone)

RIFAMPIN-ISONIAZID (*Rifamate*; *Rimactane/INH*)—See individual drugs

SPECTINOMYCIN (*Trobicin*)
Occasional: Urticaria; dizziness; nausea; chills and fever

STREPTOMYCIN
Frequent: Eighth-nerve damage (mainly vestibular), sometimes permanent; paresthesias; rash; fever
Occasional: Pruritis; anaphylaxis; renal damage
Rare: Blood dyscrasias; neuromuscular blockade and apnea with parenteral administration, usually reversed by neostigmine; optic neuritis; hepatic necrosis; myocarditis; hemolytic anemia and renal failure; pseudomembranous colitis; toxic erythema
(INTERACTIONS: Increased nephrotoxicity with cephalosporins, polymyxins; ototoxicity with etha-

* Relatively new drug; the possibility that other adverse effects will appear is greater than with older drugs.

Table IV-14—*Continued*

crynic acid; neuromuscular blockade with curari-form drugs)

SULFAMETHOXAZOLE-TRIMETHOPRIM

(*Bactrim*; *Septra*)—See Trimethoprim-Sulfame-thoxazole

SULFONAMIDES

Frequent: Allergic reactions (rash, photosensitivity and drug fever)

Occasional: Kernicterus in newborn; renal damage; liver damage; Stevens-Johnson syndrome (particularly with long-acting sulfonamides); hemolytic anemia; other blood dyscrasias; vasculitis

Rare: Transient acute myopia; pseudomembranous colitis

(INTERACTIONS: Long-acting sulfonamides: increased effect of oral anticoagulants; increased hypoglycemia with sulfonylureas; increased thiopental effects with sulfisoxazole)

TETRACYCLINES (demeclocycline—*Declomycin*; doxycycline—*Vibramycin*, and others; methacycline—*Rondomycin*; minocycline—*Minocin*; oxytetracycline—*Terramycin*, and others; tetracycline hydrochloride— *Achromycin*; and others)

Frequent: GI disturbance; bone lesions and staining and deformity of teeth in children up to 8 years old, and in the newborn when given to pregnant women after the fourth month of pregnancy.

Occasional: Malabsorption; enterocolitis; photosensitivity reactions (most frequent with demeclocycline); vestibular toxicity with minocycline; increased azotemia with renal insufficiency (except doxycycline) but exacerbation of renal failure with doxycycline has been reported; renal insufficiency with demeclocycline in cirrhotic patients; parenteral doses may cause serious liver damage, especially in pregnant women and patients with renal disease receiving 1 gm. or more daily; esophageal ulcerations; phototoxicity with demeclocycline and sometimes with other tetracyclines; hyperpigmentation with minocycline

Rare: Allergic reactions, including anaphylaxis; pseudomembranous colitis; blood dyscrasias; increased intracranial pressure; fixed-drug eruptions; diabetes insipidus with demeclocycline; transient acute myopia; blurred vision, diplopia, papilledema; photo-onycholysis and onycholysis; acute interstitial nephritis with minocycline; altered thyroid function with minocycline; aggravation of myasthenic symptoms with i.v. injection, reversed with calcium

(INTERACTIONS: Nephrotoxicity with methoxyflurane; decreased tetracycline effects with oral antacids, bismuth subsalicylate, zinc sulfate, iron; decreased doxycycline effects with barbiturates, carbamazepine, phenytoin; decreased efficacy of oral contraceptives)

TICARCILLIN—See Penicillins

TOBRAMYCIN (*Nebcin*)—Probably same as with gentamicin

* TRIFLURIDINE (*Viroptic*)

Occasional: Burning or stinging; palpebral edema

Rare: Epithelial keratopathy; hypersensitivity reactions

* TRIMETHOPRIM (*Proloprim*; *Trimpex*)

Frequent: Nausea, vomiting with high doses

Occasional: Megaloblastic anemia, thrombocytopenia, neutropenia; rash

Rare: Pancytopenia

TRIMETHOPRIM-SULFAMETHOXAZOLE

(*Bactrim*; *Septra*)

Frequent: Rash; nausea and vomiting

Occasional: Hemolysis in G-6-PD deficiency; acute megaloblastic anemia; granulocytopenia; thrombocytopenia; pseudomembranous colitis; kernicterus in newborn

Rare: Agranulocytosis; aplastic anemia; hepatotoxicity; Stevens-Johnson syndrome; fever; confusion; depression; hallucinations; deterioration in renal disease; intrahepatic cholestasis

(INTERACTIONS: Prolonged prothrombin time with warfarin (*Coumadin*; others); neutropenia, thrombocytopenia with azathioprine (*Imuran*) in renal allograft recipients)

TROLEANDOMYCIN (*TAO*)

Occasional: Stomatitis; GI disturbance; cholestatic jaundice

Rare: Allergic reactions

(INTERACTIONS: Increased effect of theophylline, carbamazepine; jaundice with oral contraceptives)

VANCOMYCIN (*Vancocin*)

Frequent: Thrombophlebitis; chills, fever

Occasional: Eighth-nerve damage (mainly hearing) especially with large or continued doses (more than 10 days), in presence of renal damage, and in the elderly

Rare: Renal damage; peripheral neuropathy; urticaria; neutropenia; hypotension with rapid i.v. administration

(INTERACTIONS: Increased toxicity with other ototoxic or nephrotoxic agents)

VIOMYCIN (*Viocin*)

Frequent: Eighth-nerve damage (vestibular and hearing) with large or continued doses (more than 10 days) or in presence of renal damage

Occasional: Rash; renal damage; electrolyte disturbances

(INTERACTIONS: Increased toxicity with other ototoxic and nephrotoxic agents; neuromuscular blockade with curariform drugs)

VIDARABINE (*Vira-A*)

Occasional: GI disturbance; nausea, vomiting; weakness; thrombophlebitis; fluid overload

Rare: Confusion; blood dyscrasias; CNS symptoms; neurological deterioration; coma and death in renal failure

---

* Relatively new drug; the possibility that other adverse effects will appear is greater than with older drugs.

(pp. IV-92–96). As noted on pp. IV-98–99 it is difficult if not impossible to estimate the true incidence of these drug reactions or to distinguish between those of allergic and those of nonallergic origin.

Of course many useful chemotherapeutic agents are not antibiotics. For example, methenamine mandelate (Mandelamine) is an adequate drug in many urinary tract infections, as long as the urine has been acidified (pH about 5), and various nitrofuran derivatives are effective in diverse infectious processes. A host of synthetic compounds is employed in curing or controlling infections due to mycobacteria, malaria parasites, amoeba, and many other pathogens. However, of all types of synthetic antimicrobial agents, sulfonamides ("sulfas") are still the most generally useful.

An unnecessarily large number of sulfonamide drugs is marketed. For systemic infections due to susceptible bacteria, oral doses of sulfisoxazole, sulfamethoxazole or sulfadiazine are sometimes used, but antibiotics (see Table IV-13) tend to be preferred. Sulfamethizole, sulfacytine and sulfonamide mixtures (e.g., trisulfapyrimidines) are also effective but are commonly reserved for urinary tract infections. For enteric infections poorly absorbed drugs are sometimes employed to ensure high local concentrations within the intestinal tract; the common enteric "sulfa" is phthalylsulfathiazole (Sulfathalidine). Sulfasalazine is widely used in ulcerative colitis and regional enteritis.

The dose varies with the preparation and with the nature and location of the infection, but a typical adult dose of a systemically active sulfonamide drug is 3 to 6 gm. initially, followed by 1 gm. every 4 to 6 hours. Children are sometimes given relatively larger doses, namely 0.06 to 0.12 gm. per pound of body weight for the first 24 hours, half as an initial dose and half as six equal maintenance doses. With drugs like sulfameter and sulfadimethoxine, which are excreted only slowly, adequate blood levels can be maintained by a single dose each day (0.5 gm. for adults). For more detailed information about dosage, see Section II.

If oral medication cannot be tolerated, sodium salts of several systemically effective sulfonamides (the diethanolamine salt in the case of sulfisoxazole) are available as sterile solutions for intravenous administration. This use is rare today.

All clinically useful sulfonamides are remarkably innocuous to common laboratory animals, but untoward reactions of the hypersensitivity type are not uncommon in clinical patients. Such reactions as headache, dizziness, mild confusion, and nausea do not necessarily warrant withdrawal of the drug. On the other hand the offending compound should be discontinued and perhaps another sulfonamide derivative substituted cautiously if any of the following disturbances appear: vomiting, diarrhea, fever, dermatitis, leukopenia, and microscopic hematuria. Immediate, complete, and unqualified cessation of all sulfonamide therapy is imperative if any of the following severe reactions are encountered: gross hematuria, renal colic, anuria, hepatitis, peripheral neuritis, agranulocytosis, hemolytic anemia, and aplastic anemia. For further information about these and other untoward reactions, see "Sulfonamides" in Section II or consult Section II for listings of specific sulfonamide drugs.

Drug Reactions

The words "drug hypersensitivity" and "drug idiosyncrasy" are used to denote adverse drug reactions which are unrelated to the recognized pharmacological actions of the drug, which are not markedly dose-dependent, and which cannot be produced regularly in all persons. The term hypersensitivity is used in reference to allergic states, where it is established or suspected that the adverse effects of a drug depend upon the development of an immunological reaction.

The term idiosyncrasy is best limited to those untoward reactions mediated by nonimmunological means. One form of idiosyncrasy is called hyper-reactivity, and it is manifested as an exaggerated response to therapeutic doses of the drug or to even smaller doses. For example, the tinnitus from quinine is a predictable toxic response. When it occurs at an abnormally low dose, it may be called an idiosyncrasy, or the patient may be referred to as a hyper-responder. Other idiosyncratic reactions, however, are atypical in qualitative terms and not extensions of known pharmacological effects. In general, the mechanisms responsible for idiosyncratic reactions are unknown, but at least some of them have a genetic predisposition.

The field of pharmacogenetics encompasses drug reactions which have a hereditary basis. For example, the hemolytic anemia following exposure to a wide variety of drugs and chemicals has as its basis an inherited deficiency in the red blood cell enzyme, glucose-6-phosphate dehydrogenase. One may also inherit a resistance to a drug effect, such as that to the anticoagulant effects of warfarin. Although the phrase "drug reaction" is often used in the following discussion, all generalizations are equally applicable to nonmedicinal compounds.

Nature and scope. The emphasis in Sections II and III of this manual rests on syndromes of frank overdosage, consisting of those psychic and somatic reactions which are strictly dose-dependent and so are largely predictable. In the case of drugs, many of these toxic syndromes reflect undesirable extensions or exaggerations of effects which in proper intensity are therapeutically useful. Omitted from the summaries in Section II and III are most untoward reactions after customary doses; these infrequent and erratic effects generally belong to the category of idiosyncrasy or hypersensitivity. With many substances and particularly nonmedicinal chemicals, the distinction between toxic responses and idiosyncratic or hypersensitivity reactions is obscure. Because the techniques of clinical and laboratory diagnosis furnish no *certain* clues, differentiation has often rested ultimately upon statistical analyses of actual "poisonings" in both laboratory animals and clinical patients.

If only to determine the appropriate supportive treatment, it is important to try to distinguish between those reactions which are inherent in the toxicity of the offending chemical and those responses which are characteristic of or peculiar to the "poisoned" individual. With only an isolated case, a proper evaluation is often impossible. Many kinds of obstacles block an unequivocal conclusion. First, toxic reactions and idiosyncratic or hypersensitivity reactions may coexist after a massive exposure. The intensity of the clinical response is not a relevant criterion. Many of the common indicators of allergy may be absent, even when the drug reaction is definitely on an immunological basis. A negative skin test has no diagnostic significance, since with most reactions to drugs, the patient's skin exhibits no prompt response to an intradermal injection of the offending chemical. Passive transfer tests are also diagnostically undependable. Eosinophilia is encountered only occasionally.

At the statistical level the most useful data to the clinical toxicologist are the true incidence of each untoward reaction to each dosage level of each drug or chemical. Although the available information about any single compound is inadequate, the following general impressions are commonly accepted. High doses of any substance regularly produce a toxic syndrome which is similar, at least in a qualitative sense, from one person to the next, and is generally related to the pharmacological actions of the drug. Lower doses, in the so-called pharmacological range, produce a group of effects that develop uniformly in almost everyone and that include therapeutically useful responses plus normal "side effects."

Hypersensitivity or idiosyncratic reactions may develop after even smaller doses; they occur in *low* incidence and often bear the imprint of allergy. This group of phenomena is more stereotyped in its clinical manifestations than are the pharmacological and toxicological responses. The character of the lesion is more distinctively a property of the patient than a specific attribute of the agent. Thus a given patient may react in

the same way to various unrelated chemicals, whereas a single substance may induce radically different syndromes in different individuals. At least for some compounds, however, both the frequency of these adverse reactions and to a lesser degree the patterns of response are predictable in a statistical sense.

The clinical manifestations of drug allergy are highly diverse (E.-S.K. Assem, Drug Allergy. In *Textbook of Adverse Drug Reactions*, D.M. Davies, Ed., Oxford University Press, 1977). Fortunately serious reactions are rare although minor reactions are frequently encountered. Single or multiple organ systems may be involved, *e.g.*, skin, formed elements of the blood, liver, blood vessels, bronchi, kidneys and heart. In any single individual, the intensity and route of exposure appear to be important determinants of the reaction pattern. In spite of other areas of disagreement, most authorities apparently agree that chemicals differ significantly in their capacities to induce sensitization and that these differences are revealed by the frequency of untoward reactions and to a limited extent also by the nature of the lesions and the target organs of damage.

Although genuine differences surely exist, it is not definitely established that certain current drugs deserve a good reputation any more than that some others warrant a bad reputation with respect to untoward reactions. There is widespread concern about the erroneous impressions that arise because of current methods of reporting drug toxicity. When reported in the literature, a single case of a rare but severe illness such as aplastic anemia arising during and allegedly due to the administration of a drug has been known to prejudice many physicians against the drug, especially if it is a new one. This prejudice often stimulates the publication of other isolated case reports and also promotes the indiscriminate damning of the drug for a host of poorly documented reactions. Collecting such case histories into review articles tends to compound the suspicions of the uncritical reader. Thus the original case report may act as the trigger for a chain reaction that reflects discredit on a drug and implies at the same time that alternative drugs are relatively free of risk.

In most instances, however, the original case, like isolated cases generally, is almost impossible to evaluate without statistical data that are rarely available. For example, to interpret intelligently the allegedly causal role of a drug in the production of aplastic anemia, one must usually know the incidence of this dyscrasia in both the presence and absence of the drug, as encountered in the general population, in patients with diseases commonly treated by the drug, and in patients with and without histories of other allergies. Even if the drug's guilt can be established by statistically valid correlations, the magnitude of the risk must be measured against the hazard and effectiveness of alternative drugs or of no drugs at all. The complaint has been raised that therapeutic nihilists are counterattacking under the banner of drug allergy.

The following criteria are listed by E.-S.K. Assem (*op. cit.*) as useful in the diagnosis of drug hypersensitivity: (*a*) no correlation with known pharmacological properties of the drug, (*b*) no linear relationship to dosage, (*c*) recognition of a reaction that conforms to patterns of known allergic responses (see below), (*d*) an induction period required on primary exposure but not on readministration, (*e*) disappearance on cessation of exposure and reappearance on readministration of a small dose (sometimes a dangerous diagnostic test), (*f*) occurrence in a minority of exposed persons, and (*g*) the possibility of desensitization. Obviously most of these criteria are nonspecific. Other experts would include a history of allergy or evidence of other allergic diseases. The latter evidence includes the similarity between reactions to drugs and reactions to conventional allergens, the occasional demonstration of a positive skin test, the marked sensitivity and specificity of the patient's acquired capacity to react to a drug, and finally the success of antiallergy therapy and sometimes of desensitization procedures.

On the basis of these and related criteria, E.-S.K. Assem concludes that drug reactions consisting of rash, angioneurotic edema, serum sickness syndrome, anaphylaxis, and asthma are usually allergic in origin. Jaundice, acute yellow atrophy, and optic neuritis are probably nonallergic. Granulocytopenia, thrombocytopenia, anemia, and polyneuritis may belong in one or the other category. However, because of the periportal eosinophilia that characterizes the hepatitis of some patients taking such phenothiazine tranquilizers as chlorpromizine, most authorities believe that this hepatitis is allergic in origin. In all cases a reaction is more likely allergic when a priming or a sensitizing dose has preceded the toxic episode and is more likely nonallergic when long continued administration or the use of large doses appears to have played an etiological role.

The reaction pattern is sufficiently stereotyped in most cases of drug hypersensitivity to be an aid in diagnosis. Skin eruptions are the commonest clinical manifestation, particularly contact-type dermatitis, urticaria, and various exanthemal rashes. Less frequent skin expressions of drug hypersensitivity are exfoliative dermatitis, erythema multiforme-like rashes, acneform eruptions, bullous lesions, purpura simplex, photosensitizations, simple pruritus, and fixed eruptions. Systemic syndromes are comparatively rare; they are usually represented by one or more of the following reactions: bronchial asthma, fever, serum-sickness type of illness, shock of the anaphylactic variety, hepatitis, all kinds of blood dyscrasias, polyneuritis, and periarteritis nodosum. With each of these lesions, a constellation of medicinal agents is commonly associated.

The particular drugs which are held to be frequently responsible for each type of reaction are listed by Assem (*op. cit.*), by E. W. Martin (*Hazards of Medication*, 2nd ed., J.B. Lippincott, 1978), by M. N. Dukes (*Side Effects of Drugs*, No. 7, Elsevier, 1983) and by others. Such lists are never exhaustive and, for reasons noted before, some examples probably represent erroneous associations, but these compilations are useful guides in alerting the physician to the areas of greatest risk. For example, the drugs responsible for the largest variety of hypersensitivity reactions, as judged by published reports, are sulfonamides, mercurials, penicillins, iodides, arsenicals, gold salts, streptomycin, barbiturates, and quinine. A more modern list might omit the mercurials, iodides, and arsenicals, which are less often used today; it would emphasize the penicillins and other antibiotics and would add the phenothiazine tranquilizers. As an example, see Table IV-15 (pp. IV-102–104), which is limited to hematological reactions. Extensive tables of drugs implicated in various types of hypersensitivity reactions can be found in Martin (*ibid.*).

Antiallergic therapy. Having arrived at a presumptive diagnosis of chemical or drug hypersensitivity and having recognized that its mechanism is probably allergic, the physician is ready to institute antiallergic supportive treatment. In all severe and most mild reactions, the first practical measure is the rigorous exclusion of the presumptive allergen or allergens. Insofar as practical, no drug with a high allergenic liability is used in treating these reactions. This precaution helps avoid the superimposition of one allergy on another, with the confusion that inevitably attends this complication. In addition, skin and mucous membranes in the process of reacting to one allergen appear to be more susceptible to sensitization by others, perhaps only because normal physical barriers are temporarily impaired during many allergic crises.

In most cases, discomfort subsides and repair begins soon after the exclusion of the offending drug or chemical. In these cases no other treatment is warranted. The universal temptation to treat skin lesions with topical applications of various medicaments should particularly be suppressed. Only if considerable distress persists after removal of the allergen does the potential benefit from local treatment justify the risk. Only drugs known to have a low capacity to sensitize by topical application should be considered—such as glycerin, mineral oil, lanolin, zinc oxide, some cold creams, ichthyol, and talc.

Some hypersensitivity crises warrant systemic drug therapy. Allergic bronchial asthma, urticaria, giant hives, and anaphylactoid shock often respond most quickly to an intramuscular injection of epinephrine. Unnecessarily large doses of this drug are frequently used. Except for the occasional person who is slightly refractory because of repeated use, any amount in excess of 0.5 ml. of 1:1000 aqueous epinephrine contributes little or nothing except unpleasant side effects; often 0.2 ml. is a therapeutically effective single dose in the adult. Sometimes a slow intravenous injection of aminophylline is beneficial, particularly in the severely distressed or epinephrine-resistant asthmatic. For longer durations of action, intramuscular injections of epinephrine in oil (usual adult dose 1 ml. of 1:1000 solution) are occasionally useful.

Antihistaminic drugs (H_1 blockers) have also been used to combat the effects of histamine released during allergic reactions to drugs. They are particularly useful in acute urticarial reactions, where it is reasonable to give 10 mg. chlorpheniramine maleate intramuscularly or perhaps intravenously, if epinephrine alone does not control the symptoms. In morbilliform eruptions, where there is probably little histamine release, only the anesthetic, antipruritic actions of the drug may be operative. Antihistaminic drugs have relatively persistent effects. Except for bronchial asthma, the same allergic reactions responsive to epinephrine can be controlled occasionally by antihistaminic drugs; the latter are also useful in the serum-sickness syndrome and particularly in allergic rhinitis and conjunctivitis. Many hypersensitivity disorders that do not respond appreciably to antihistamine therapy can be successfully prevented by administering the drug before exposure to the allergen.

Antihistaminics, however, are not innocuous, and many cases of skin sensitization have been ascribed to both their local and systemic administration. Probably because it is more extensively used, tripelennamine (Pyribenzamine) has been blamed for more untoward reactions than have its competitors, but none is free of risk. Some clinicians and particularly dermatologists believe that the adverse effects of antihistaminic drugs outweight the beneficial results.

Among antiallergic drugs the greatest popularity currently rests with the various adrenal glucocorticoids. The principal adrenocortical steroid is cortisol (also known as hydrocortisone); it can be administered by all routes (oral, i.m., i.v., inhalation, topically). Many naturally occurring and semisynthetic derivatives of cortisol are also available and widely used. Although these drugs act too slowly to be useful for the immediate treatment of anaphylaxis, almost every type of allergic lesion has been reported to respond to them with dramatic improvement. Not every case benefits, however.

The mechanisms by which these hormones accomplish their beneficial actions are not understood, but presumably they suppress tissue reactivity only, without disturbing the underlying allergic state. For example, they are said to reduce the inflammatory reaction to many injurious agents, both chemical and physical. The steroid hormones have been shown to inhibit the release of arachidonic acid from cell membranes and so to slow the synthesis of prostaglandins. Because of the multiple roles of prostaglandins in inflammation, this inhibition of synthesis accounts for part of the anti-inflammatory response to steroid hormones. The suppression of inflammatory processes persists only as long as hormone treatment is continued, unless the underlying allergic mechanism subsides spontaneously in the interim.

The need of some patients for prolonged and intensive therapy enhances the risk of metabolic side effects. These distressing and in some cases dangerous side effects include hypokalemia, edema, moon face, congestive heart failure, hyperglycemia, glucosuria, increased susceptibility to infections, peptic ulcer, hirsutism, acne, girdle obesity, osteoporosis, disorders of mood and behavior (see also Section II under Corticosteroids). Fortunately these adverse effects are rarely encountered if the course of therapy is limited to 2 to 3 days, even when high doses are used.

In acute adrenal cortical insufficiency, which is a rare event in clinical toxicology but has been reported in paraquat poisoning (p. III-330), replacement therapy is essential to survival. It consists of infusions of glucose and sodium chloride solutions, together with hydrocortisone sodium succinate. A common stat intravenous dose of this steroid in adults is 100 mg., followed by a slow infusion of about 100 mg. every 8 hours, but the proper dose varies widely among individuals. The administration of a mineralocorticoid may also be required, such as 0.1 to 0.2 mg. fludrocortisone acetate by mouth.

In severe allergic reactions, however, mineralocorticoids are ineffective and undesirable because they induce sodium retention and potassium excretion (see above). In the management of allergic disorders, prednisone has widely replaced cortisol for oral use because of a little less difficulty with electrolyte control during therapy; it has about 4 times the anti-inflammatory potency of cortisol. A common daily dose of oral prednisone is 1 mg./kg. in children and 40 to 60 mg. in adults, in both cases in divided amounts. In life-threatening situations when parenteral steroid therapy is warranted, the intravenous infusion of dexamethasone sodium phosphate in daily doses of 8 to 12 mg. is appropriate. Like some other steroids fluorinated in the 9α position, dexamethasone has an anti-inflammatory (antiallergic) potency about 25 times greater than cortisol, with almost no capacity to induce sodium retention. Whatever the steroid, if it is administered systemically over a period of several days or weeks, especially in high doses, it is likely to suppress the activity of the patient's own adrenal glands. Abrupt cessation of corticosteroid therapy is then risky; instead, the dose must be gradually reduced over periods of 1 or more weeks.

In some types of cutaneous, conjunctival, and mucosal sensitization, the topical application of adrenocorticoids in the form of ointments and solutions is sufficient. For example, hydrocortisone, prednisolone, fludrocortisone acetate, fluorometholone, and other derivatives are marketed in bland ointments. Because of high effectiveness, broad spectrum of action, and relative freedom from severe toxicity, this group of drugs represents a major advance in the pharmacological control of allergic disease.

Blood dyscrasias. Essentially every known variety of blood dyscrasia has been reported as an expression of drug reaction. On the other hand, only moderate numbers of drugs and chemicals have been implicated. Table IV-15 is a compilation produced by Dr. Eric Martin and his associates. As in the case of an earlier compilation sponsored by the American Medical Association, the table does not indicate the frequency of occurrence or the intensity of the reactions. More blood dyscrasias are reported in association with exposures to chloramphenicol than to any other single substance. The next largest number of cases is associated with tetracyclines and penicillins. Aspirin and phenobarbital are reported moderately often, but these associations may also have been spurious, reflecting only the high frequency with which these drugs are employed.

Probably many drugs not listed in Table IV-15 can also have significant adverse effects on the blood. A more complete list would include hydralazine, dapsone (Avlosulfon), diphenhydramine (Benadryl), and heparin; the latter is a common cause of thrombocytopenia. Blood dyscrasias have also been ascribed to DDT, chlordane and lindane (see Section III) and to several other environmental chemicals such as benzene (p. III-308) and probably other petroleum hydrocarbons. Whether lists such as Table IV-15 are ever complete enough to be genuinely useful is debatable.

Major adverse hematological responses to drugs and chemicals include the following: leukopenia, agranulocytosis, thrombocytopenia, hemolytic and other anemias, and pancytopenia (aplastic anemia). Various mechanisms operating singly or jointly appear to be responsible for these disturbances in the cellular composition of blood. Three classes of pathological events are recognized: inhibition of blood cell production in bone marrow; acceleration of blood cell destruc-

tion at intravascular and extravascular sites (*e.g.*, spleen, liver); and effects on the morphology and function of blood elements but not on their numbers. An example of the latter category is the well known actions of aspirin on platelets. Bone marrow suppression by exogenous chemicals may reflect either damage to stem cells or inhibition of some aspect of the maturation process. Accelerated peripheral removal includes the processes of thrombolysis, intra- and extra-vascular hemolysis, perhaps autoagglutination and sequestration, and secondary hypersplenism. Probably marrow suppression is more common than enhanced peripheral destruction, but neither the site nor mechanism of action is known for most of the chemicals listed in Table IV-15.

In a few cases, however, mechanisms have been identified. For example, thrombocytopenias induced by quinine, quinidine, and probably heparin are due to thrombolysis, not to impaired production. High blood levels of ethanol also destroy platelets, but the resulting thrombocytopenia only occasionally leads to bleeding episodes. In the case of quinine and quinidine (but probably not heparin or ethanol), an immunologic mechanism is often involved; these drugs function as haptens, and the resulting immune complex deposition on cells can result in either thrombolysis or extravascular hemolysis (mostly in the spleen). A similar mechanism is responsible for rare cases of hemolytic anemia due to cephalosporins and for the agranulocytosis produced by aminopyrine. Blood dyscrasias that develop occasionally during the lupus-like syndrome caused by hydralazine and by procainamide also involve immunologic mechanisms. A nonimmunologic mechanism is definitely established as responsible for the hemolytic crisis produced by many chemicals in those individuals who have red cells deficient in glucose-6-phosphate dehydrogenase activity (see p. III-308). Some examples of drug-induced marrow suppression have been traced to inhibition of heme synthesis, to disorders of folic acid metabolism and to disturbances in DNA and RNA synthesis (see p. III-401).

Although the incidence of blood dyscrasias is low relative to the exposure rate to most of the drugs listed in Table IV-15, many of these hematological disorders are a severe threat to life. Examples include platelet counts below 20,000/μl. and leukocyte counts below 1000/μl. Several unique problems of diagnosis and treatment arise in the clinical management of these patients. Although the clinical history (including the occupational history) often serves to direct attention to the offending chemical, it is difficult and often impossible in an isolated case to establish the chemical's mechanism of action. Aside from an examination of the bone marrow, any attempt to determine mechanism is usually un-

Table IV-15
Drugs which Can Induce Blood Dyscrasias[a]

Drug	Agranulocytosis (Leukopenia)	Aplastic Anemia	Hemolytic Anemia	Megaloblastic Anemia	Pancytopenia	Thrombocytopenia
Acetanilid			✕			
Acetazolamide (Diamox)		✕			✕	✕
Acetophenetidin		✕	✕		✕	✕
Acetylphenylhydrazine			✕			
Acetylsalicylic acid (Aspirin)	✕	✕	✕		✕	✕
Allyl-isopropyl-acetylcarbamide (Sedormid)						✕
Aminopyrine (Pyramidon)	✕	✕	✕			
Amodiaquine (Camoquin)		✕				
Antihistamines		✕				
Antineoplastics		✕				
Antipyrine (Phenazone)			✕			
Arabinoside				✕		
Arsenicals (Organic)		✕				
Arsenobenzenes						✕
Azathioprine (Imuran)	✕			✕		✕
Barbiturates		✕		✕	✕	✕
Busulfan (Myleran)					✕	✕
Butazolidin	✕	✕			✕	✕
Carbamazepine (Tegretol)	✕	✕				✕
Carbimazole		✕				
Carbutamide		✕				
Cephalothin Sodium (Keflin)			✕	✕		✕
Chloramphenicol (Chloromycetin)	✕	✕	✕		✕	✕
Chlordiazepoxide (Librium)	✕	✕				
Chlorothiazide (Diuril)	✕	✕			✕	✕
Chlorpromazine (Thorazine)	✕		✕			
Chlorpropamide (Diabinese)		✕			✕	✕
Cinchophen	✕					
Clofibrate (Atromid-S)	✕	✕				
Colchicine	✕	✕				✕
Cyclophosphamide (Cytoxan)	✕	✕				✕
Cytarabine (Cytosar)	✕			✕		✕
Cytosine arabinoside	✕			✕		✕
Diaminophenylsulfone			✕			
Digitalis glycosides	✕	✕			✕	✕
Dimercaprol (BAL)			✕			
Dipyrone	✕	✕				✕
Ethchlorvynol (Placidyl)			✕			✕
Ethosuximide (Zarontin)	✕	✕				
5-Fluorouracil				✕		
Furaltadone			✕			
Furazolidone (Furoxone)			✕			
Gold compounds		✕			✕	✕
Hydantoins		✕				✕
Hydrochlorothiazide (Hydrodiuril)						✕
Hydroxyurea (Hydrea, Hydroxycarbamide)	✕			✕		✕
Hydroflumethiazide (Diucardin, Saluron)	✕	✕				✕

[a] Modified and reproduced with permission from *Hazards of Medication*, by E. W. Martin, 2nd ed., pp. 314–316, J. B. Lippincott Co., Philadelphia, 1978.

Table IV-15—*Continued*

Drug	Agranulo-cytosis (Leukopenia)	Aplastic Anemia	Hemolytic Anemia	Megalo-blastic Anemia	Pancyto-penia	Thrombo-cytopenia
Imipramine (Tofranil)	×					
Indomethacin (Indocin)	×	×	×			×
Iothiouracil (Itrumil)	×					
Isoniazid			×			
Melphalan (Alkeran)		×				×
Mepazine (Pacatal)	×	×			×	
Mephenytoin (Mesantoin)	×	×	×	×	×	×
Meprobamate (Equanil, Miltown)	×	×			×	×
6-Mercaptopurine (Purinethol)	×			×		×
Mesoridazine (Serentil)	×	?[b]	?[b]		?[b]	?[b]
Methicillin (Staphcillin)	×		×			×
Methimazole (Tapazole)	×	×			×	×
Methophenobarbital				×		
Methyldopa (Aldomet)	×	×	×		×	×
Methylene blue			×			
Methylthiouracil		×				
Nitrofurantoin (Furandantin)			×			
Nitrofurazone (Furacin)			×			
Novobiocin						×
Oxyphenbutazone (Tandearil)	×	×				
Pamaquine			×			
Para-aminosalicylic acid			×			
Paradione	×	×			×	×
Penicillin	×	×	×		×	×
Pentaquine			×			
Pentazocine (Talwin)	×					
Phenacemide (Phenurone)		×				
Phenindione	×					
Phenothiazines	×	×	×	×	×	×
Phenylbutazone (Butazolidin)	×	×			×	×
Phenylhydrazine			×			
Phenytoin sodium				×		
Plasmoquine			×			
Potassium perchlorate		×				
Primaquine			×			
Primidone (Mysoline)		×		×		
Probenecid (Benemid)			×			
Procainamide (Pronestyl)	×	×				
Procarbazine (Matulane)	×	×				×
Prochlorperazine (Compazine)	×					
Promazine (Sparine)	×					
Propylthiouracil	×					×
Pyrimethamine (Daraprim)	×			×	×	×
Quinacrine (Atabrine)		×	×			×
Quinidine	×	×	×		×	×
Quinine			×			×
Rifampin (Rifadin, etc.)	×		×			×
Streptomycin	×	×	×		×	×
Stibophen (Fuadin)			×			×
Sulfonamides:	×	×	×		×	×
Sulfasalazine (Azulfidine)			×			

Table IV-15—*Continued*

Drug	Agranulo-cytosis (Leukopenia)	Aplastic Anemia	Hemolytic Anemia	Megalo-blastic Anemia	Pancyto-penia	Thrombo-cytopenia
Sulfacytine (Renoquid)	?[b]	?[b]	?[b]		?[b]	?[b]
Sulfadiazine	X		X			
Sulfamethizole	X	X			X	
Sulfamethoxazole (Gantanol)	X	X	X			X
Sulfisoxazole (Gantrisin)		X	X		X	X
Sulfoxone			X			
Tetracycline	X		X		X	X
Thiacetazone (Seroden, etc.)		X	X			
Thiazolsulfone (Promizole)			X			
Thiocyanates		X				
Thioguanine	X			X		X
Thioridazine (Mellaril)	X					
Thiouracil	X					X
Tolbutamide (Orinase)	X	X			X	X
Triamterene (Dyrenium)			X	X		
Trimethadione (Tridione)	X	X			X	X
Tripelennamine (Pyribenz-amine)	X					
Vincristine	X	X				
Vitamin K water-soluble ana-logues			X			

[b] A question mark (?) indicates an early indication or a definite possibility of occurrence with a drug that was relatively new when the data collection was suspended. Several drugs in this table are no longer marketed.

necessary in current practice for reasons noted below.

To identify, however, and then to remove the chemical substance that triggered the dyscrasia is always a worthwhile and even essential procedure. Although this measure does not guarantee a prompt or spontaneous recovery, many hematological disorders subside within a few days after the exposure is terminated. The problem of identifying the exogenous cause, however, can be formidable. Except for the occasional demonstration of specific antibodies, the only conclusive proof is the administration of a small test dose after the patient has fully recovered. The procedure is distinctly risky and is obviously unavailable when the information is most needed. Ordinary skin tests are essentially worthless.

The principles of supportive treatment in cases of blood dyscrasia are the exclusion of the causative agent, replacement therapy, protection against infection, stimulation of hematopoiesis, and suppression of the metabolic or immunologic processes responsible for the abnormality.

Replacement therapy entails transfusions usually of separated blood components such as packed red cells, platelets or rarely white cells. In this way the specific needs of each patient can be met with less chance of a transfusion reaction. Only with some hemorrhagic diatheses is whole blood preferred, and then the blood should be freshly obtained from a single donor. With all of these preparations, at least mild reactions (fever, hives, etc.) are common, particularly in patients who receive multiple transfusions. In some medical centers these individuals are pretreated before each tranfusion with an antihistaminic drug (H₁ blocker), an antipyretic (usually acetaminophen) and, if necessary, 100 mg. i.v. hydrocortisone.

Large amounts of platelet-rich plasma with platelet hematocrits of about 70% are generated by modern cell separators from the blood of single or multiple donors. At present these platelet suspensions can be stored up to 72 hours before they become unstable. Each processed pint of donor blood yields enough platelets to raise the platelet count in an adult recipient by 10,000 to 15,000/μl.; it is not uncommon to infuse six such units of separated platelets in a single transfusion. How long donor platelets survive and function in the recipient cannot be predicted; survival time is known to be quite variable. Repeated platelet tranfusions, however, have proved to be highly effective in preventing and controlling severe hemorrhagic crises in thrombocytopenic patients.

To protect the leukopenic person against infection is always a major concern because even simple infections tend to explode into alarming septicemias when the blood possesses few or no granulocytes. The practice of keeping these patients under a heavy blanket of antibiotics, however, is no longer acceptable. The long continued administration of broad-spectrum antibacterial drugs or mixtures of various narrow-spectrum agents leads inevitably to profound changes in the microbial flora of the skin and mucous membranes. Drug-resistant organisms and particularly fungi emerge as the dominant forms. An uncontrollable systemic infection from the invasion of these pathogens then becomes probable. The alternative procedure is to withhold prophylactic chemotherapy. Even the agranulocytic patient often keeps free of clinically significant infection for long periods if he practices simple measures of personal hygiene and if he is kept in a protective environment. Of course intensive antibiotic therapy is prescribed at the earliest sign of infection, preferably with massive doses of several drugs at the same time.

Almost all attempts to stimulate hemopoietic activity in a depressed bone marrow or to accelerate directly the output of an active marrow are unsuccessful. A small percentage of patients with marrow failure, however, appear to respond to androgen therapy. In the occasional patient in whom marrow failure is due to immune phenomena (*e.g.*, antibodies or suppressor T-cells), immunosuppressive therapy may restore hemopoiesis. Marrow transplantation is reserved for the most severe and persistent cases of marrow failure, when and if a suitable donor is available.

In those dyscrasias due to accelerated blood cell destruction, immunosuppressive therapy, notably in the form of corticosteroids, has a distinctly higher success rate than in marrow failure. This is particularly true in the idiopathic forms of thrombocytopenia purpura and acquired hemolytic anemias of the Coombs-positive type, both of which are often examples of autoimmune disorders. Some cases of drug-induced thrombocytopenia and hemolytic anemia are also responsive to glucocorticoid therapy. Presumably these patients have an underlying drug allergy. Some specific drugs known to have been responsible for such allergies are mentioned above. How often an immunologic mechanism is responsible for drug-induced thrombocytopenia or hemolytic anemia is not established, but a therapeutic trial with glucocorticoids is not recommended by most hematologists as a routine procedure.

One of the important arguments against steroid therapy in patients with drug-induced dyscrasias is that it is often unnecessary. Thus, most of these patients improve rapidly after they are isolated from the offending chemical, and during their period of high vulnerability they can usually be sustained by the other supportive measures described above, notably by replacement therapy. Furthermore, it is probable that most cases of drug-induced blood dyscrasias do not have an immunologic basis and so are refractory to steroid therapy. Indeed, except with thrombocytopenia and hemolytic anemia, the success rate is likely to be very low.

Clearly these arguments are not compelling, and the physician who chooses a therapeutic trial with glucocorticoids cannot be fairly criticized if his patient has a life-threating blood dyscrasia other than agranulocytosis. (In the latter case the chances of success hardly justify the added risk of infection associated with steroid therapy). In the case of a hemolytic anemia, one would clearly want to rule out an inherited deficiency in red cell glucose-6-phosphate dehydrogenase activity before starting a trial with steroids. The usual regimen is 1 mg./kg. of prednisone daily for a period of at least one week, followed by a gradual tapering of the dose (p. IV-100). Splenectomy, however, is almost never justified in the treatment of drug-induced blood dyscrasias. Splenectomy is most effective against congenital hemolytic anemia and autoimmune thrombocytopenia, although it is sometimes used in autoimmune hemolytic anemias, too.

Nursing Care

In a severely poisoned patient, no adequate program of supportive treatment can be managed without the active cooperation of a well trained nurse. In current practice, the busy physician makes many crucial decisions but often leaves their implementation to others. This is proper and appropriate whenever trained nurses are available. On the other hand, every medical practitioner should be reasonably familiar with nursing procedures, if only because he may be required to instruct members of the patient's family in the techniques of patient care in the home. It is not possible or appropriate to describe here the art and science of nursing, but it is proper to outline some of the nursing services that have proved to be so beneficial both to severely ill and convalescing patients. The most effective way for the physician to review this topic is to spend a few days as a patient in a hospital bed.

A capable and diligent nurse exerts many beneficial influences on the patient and on the course of his illness. First a nurse performs all services specified by the physician with respect to medications, activity, diet, fluids, etc. He or she observes and records periodically the patient's vital signs and any other relevant clinical data. These general and specific observations supplement and often complement the physician's own examinations. In such areas as the patient's response to food, consumption of fluids, urine output, number of bowel movements, duration of sleep, vital signs during sleep, etc., the nurse's report is often the only source of reliable information.

Particularly for the seriously ill person, a nurse performs many services. He or she protects his skin by keeping him clean and dry. The nurse makes him comfortable and relaxed by massaging his back and limbs, by repositioning him frequently in bed, by rearranging his pillow, and by passive exercises when appropriate. The nurse furnishes blankets and hot packs when he is chilled, and alcohol sponging, ice packs and fanning when he is hot. The nurse spares his strength by giving physical support whenever he must be moved, furnishes encouragement, and if necessary assistance when he eats, drinks, voids, etc. The nurse keeps indwelling catheters clean and patent and ensures the proper functioning of venoclysis sets and other equipment.

A good nurse is not only the ally of the physician but often the chief confidante of the patient. In the role as a sympathetic helper, the nurse often becomes one of the principal supports of the patient's morale. A good nurse almost invariably acts as an intermediary between patient, family physician, and hospital. Finally, the trained nurse is qualified to perform in an emergency most of the lifesaving procedures of resuscitation available to physicians.

SECTION V

Trade Name Index

Jean Braddock, Editor
Patricia Greeno, Applications Programmer
Winston Lee, Pharm.D., Toxicologist[1]
Grant Lum, Pharm.D., Toxicologist[2]
Lawrence Fleckenstein, Pharm.D., Toxicologist[3]

INTRODUCTION

In this section are listed alphabetically by trade name over 15,000 non-food products that might be ingested accidentally or suicidally. Lists of ingredients in these products were contributed and edited by the companies that manufacture and/or market the products.

Directions for Use

1. As a general rule the products are listed by their registered trade names, which are printed in capital letters. Unless obvious from the name of the product, the category of use is indicated under the trade name, *e.g.*, rodenticide, silver polish, dishwasher detergent. The intended use category of a product is added as a further guide to its identification, but no definitive or complete statement of how the product is to be used is included. The manufacturer's name is added in abbreviated form; the complete name and address can be found in Section VII, Manufacturers' Index.

With few exceptions the ingredients of the products are listed, many with percentages or amounts, and asterisks are placed after the ingredients expected to be responsible for major toxic effects if the product is ingested in harmful amounts or otherwise misused. The asterisk directs the reader to consult Section II for toxicity information about that ingredient. A dagger placed after an asterisk indicates that the substances cannot be located in Section II under the identical name but is listed under a synonym or is represented by a closely related substance,

the name of which is stated under the product information.

Example: BIG CAT
General cleaner concentrate
(Calgon Corp., Commercial Div.)

Dodecylbenzene sulfonate*†
Fatty amide
Water

† See Alkyl aryl sodium sulfonates

An ingredient name unlisted in Section II is daggered to indicate the appropriate Section II entry if and only if it bears an asterisk. It should also be noted that ingredient names are sometimes preceded by a modifying word, *e.g.*, Technical Piperonyl butoxide. The internal capital (in this example "P") indicates that the modifier should be disregarded when the reader looks up the ingredient in Section II.

2. In arranging alphabetically the trade names in Section V, spacing between words, punctuation, numbers, and non-letter symbols have been ignored. The order of each entry progresses through each letter of the trade name in turn. For example, in ACME CHLORDANE 45% SPRAY, the "45%" is disregarded.

Trade names beginning with the abbreviation "DR." or "MR." are therefore alphabetized with product names beginning with the letters DR or MR, and will not be found under "DOCTOR" or "MISTER."

Numbers that are an integral part of the trade name (*i.e.*, replacing words) are listed as though spelled out.

Example: 6–12 = SIX-TWELVE
20/20 = TWENTY/TWENTY

---

[1] Director, Drug Information Service, Alta Bates Hospital, Berkeley, California.
[2] Veterans Administration Hospital, San Diego, California.
[3] Walter Reed Army Medical Center, Washington, D.C. 20012.

In cases of ambiguity the product descriptions have been repeated in full in two alphabetical locations. For example, A-1 is listed at the beginning of the A's and also as if spelled out as A-ONE.

Letter groups or words ending in a number precede the next alphabetical sequence.

Example: BR-5512
              BRACEOIL

3. Products whose trade names include all toxicologically significant ingredients and percentages have been omitted from this edition, e.g., HOPKINS 5% SEVIN DUST.

However, if the product contains toxic ingredients in addition to the substance stated in the ingredient name, the formula is presented.

Example: HOPKINS MALATHION 57%
              EMULSIFIABLE LIQUID
              Insecticide
              (Hopkins Agric.)

              Malathion* 57.00%
              Xylene-range aromatic
                 solvent* 29.36%

4. When only a generic term appears in the trade name, the manufacturer's name is prefixed in capitals.

Example: DAP GENERAL PURPOSE
                    CEMENT

5. Some manufacturers prefer that the name of the company precede the trade name of their product. In this case the product is usually cross-indexed. For example, VICKS VAPORUB is also indexed under VAPORUB, with the notation: See VICKS VAPORUB. We suggest that the users of the book look for a product under the manufacturer's name if they cannot locate it under the trade name alone. Cross-indexing is extensive but not complete.

6. For some commonly used products or product lines, ingredient information was not available for this edition. In a number of cases, the manufacturer has supplied directions for obtaining emergency assistance.

Example: PAPER MATE PENS & RE-
                    FILLS
              (Gillette Co., Paper Mate
              Div.)

              The Gillette Co., Paper Mate
              Div., Boston, Mass. 02199, will
              receive collect phone calls
              from poison control centers or
              physicians asking for emer-
              gency toxicological informa-
              tion about the company's
              products.

Phone: 617-421-7000

Comprehensive listings of the formulations of some cosmetics and paint manufacturers are included in the Trade Name Index. To avoid excessive duplication, the entries for most manufacturers in these two categories consist only of the company name, address, and telephone number, with a reference to Section VI, General Formulations, where toxicity estimates of similar products are given, together with lists of ingredients and percentages frequently found in such products.

7. The designation "'76 Ed." in the lower right hand corner of a product entry indicates that no revised information about its composition has been received from the manufacturer since the compilation of the 1976 (fourth) edition. Because these manufacturers have had several opportunities to edit their listings during the preparation of the present edition, it is reasonable to assume that in many cases there have been no changes in composition.

8. With a possible choice of innumerable products on the market that are eligible for inclusion in this section, the limitations of time and space made selectivity a necessity. The products chosen for this edition are, for the most part, items with large sales volumes. It is recommended that owners of the first four editions keep them as companion volumes. Many products described in the previous editions are currently off the market, but many can still be found on shelves in homes, garages, and barns. Reference to these earlier descriptions may prove useful in emergencies.

9. For information about any product whose trade name cannot be located in this section, a telephone call to the manufacturer may be indicated (see Section VII). In the interim, Section VI (General Formulations) may provide valuable guidance about the composition of commercial mixtures which are marketed for the same or similar purposes.

All of the material in Section V is also part of the CTCP data base, which is one of the computerized components of the NIH-EPA Chemical Information System (CIS). The data in the "product module" of this component are structured for the rapid search and retrieval of information keyed to the following subjects: (1) trade names, (2) manufacturers' names, (3) ingredients, and (4) product use categories. Searches can be made on any of these elements, singly or in combination. Toxicity information can also be accessed through the Section II part of the data base (known as the "toxicity module") and through other components of CIS.

The CTCP component in CIS also includes many products for which there was no room in this book, plus discontinued and obsolete formulas. The computerized data base is updated periodically.

The information in Section V was compiled from product data supplied by the manufacturers. The ingredients listed in this section are those which were present at the time the data were furnished by the manufacturers. Ingredient changes are not uncommon. Neither the authors nor the manufacturers accept any responsibility for differences which may exist between the product composition as listed in this section and as subsequently found in the marketplace.

How to Use the Asterisks in This Index

For every commercial product described, an asterisk has been assigned to those ingredients (or classes of ingredients) which in our opinion might be responsible for toxic signs and symptoms if the product were ingested rapidly in harmful amounts. In all cases this situation implies unequivocal misuse of the product; no attempt has been made to evaluate the toxic hazard, if any, arising from proper or recommended methods of use. However innocuous a commercial mixture, there exists almost invariably an amount sufficient to provide a toxic dose of each ingredient. **In principle the asterisk should designate only that single ingredient (or class of ingredients) whose lethal dose is contained in the least quantity of the mixture.** Obviously uncertainties arose in assigning some asterisks, and in many mixtures several constituents were starred because the concentration of each was believed to be significant relative to its intrinsic toxicity. On the other hand, all components of some products were judged to be so benign that no attempt was made to assign an asterisk to any of them. In many instances the manufacturer listed the ingredients of his product without stating the percentage composition. In these instances asterisks were assigned from a knowledge of what similar products contain wherever a particular ingredient was suspected to be present in a concentration that might contribute significantly to the toxicity of the commercial mixture. Obviously no absolute toxicity is implied by any asterisk since no fixed limits were established for issuing them.

For specific toxicity information, Section II should be consulted under the name of each ingredient that possesses an asterisk in Section V. For each toxic ingredient and by inference for every product in which this ingredient is starred, Section II outlines a possible and, as closely as we can predict, the probable toxic syndrome and, by suitable reference to Section III, directs attention to an appropriate program of treatment. Section II also provides a categorical estimate of the lethality of each separate ingredient in terms of a numerical "toxicity rating" (see Introduction to Section II). Given the percentage composition of a commercial formula (Section V) and the intrinsic toxicities of its starred ingredients (Section II), the physician has adequate information to reach provisional answers to such questions as: how much of this product can be ingested without endangering life?—or, how much will probably kill? Unfortunately, these questions can seldom if ever be answered with the desired degree of precision or reliability, but even approximate and tentative answers are useful in formulating a realistic prognosis whenever the physician knows how much of a potential intoxicant has been ingested.

To reach a useful estimate of the toxicity of a product (in the absence of direct data), its chemical composition (Section V) must be evaluated in terms of the established toxicities of its separate ingredients (Section II), notably those ingredients which bear an asterisk in the listings of Section V. One of the best ways to organize one's efforts is to try to assign a toxicity rating to each product (in contradistinction to the ratings of Section II, which describe only isolated ingredients). To do this, basic assumptions are required. In the Introduction to Section VI, the subsection entitled "How to Assign Toxicity Ratings to Products" outlines various rules and conventions that we have evolved in selecting toxicity ratings for the sample formulas of Section VI. In our contacts with medical practitioners, we have become convinced that these ratings are a practical way of answering the physicians' question: how toxic is it? That the assignment of toxicity ratings is a feasible procedure is attested by the examples in Section VI, General Formulations.

ACKNOWLEDGMENTS

This revision of Section V should be dedicated to its contributing manufacturers. With few exceptions the descriptions of the thousands of products listed here were provided by them. Editing and re-editing were done by these companies, who deleted old products, informed us of changes of formulas, and added new products to our lists. The composition of these new products provided a basis for selecting many new items for inclusion in Section II (Ingredients Index). Some of the toxicity data about these substances were contributed by company research laboratories and their consultants, as is indicated in the list of source-references appended to Section II. The addresses listed in Section VII were taken from the letterheads of the thousands of manufacturers with whom we have corresponded. Without the collaboration of these manufacturers, there would have been no *Clinical Toxicology of Commercial Products*. Physicians who turn to this reference book for information can join with the authors in this expression of gratitude to the many companies and their members who have made this revised edition possible.

We also gratefully recognize our continuing indebtedness to Marion Gleason, retired, whose insight and imagination sparked the creation of CTCP. Mrs. Gleason was responsible for compiling and editing the product information in the first four editions of CTCP. We have benefited from her dedication, experience, and training in carrying on her work in this fifth edition.

We particularly wish to acknowledge the help of the many specialists and staff workers who have made the present publication of this section possible. Drs. Fleckenstein, Lum, and Lee have spent many hours assessing the toxicity of product formulas and assigning asterisks to those ingredients with the potential for causing toxic effects. We are deeply grateful for their expert assistance.

Patricia Greeno was responsible for maintaining the computer data base from which this section was printed and for the associated programming. She also trained the CTCP staff members in the use of the project programs. Her efficiency and hard work made the recording and updating of product data in our computer files a smoothly running operation.

We would also like to thank the editorial assistants who worked on this edition: David Span, Richard Patterson, Marli Weiner, Karen Thireos, and Judy Bristow. Katherine Foster volunteered her long secretarial experience in helping us meet the publisher's deadline. Last of all, we are deeply indebted to Sharon Zyga, who for the past year has donated her time and energy to this project. She assisted the editor in proof-reading all of the galleys for Section V, kept our data base up-to-date, and cheerfully turned her hand to any task that needed doing.

To the publishers and printers of CTCP we give a special note of appreciation for their continuing help with the preparation of the Trade Name Index. We particularly wish to thank Ray Reter, Book Production Sponsor, and Frederick Boone, Data Processing Manager.

A

A-1

Hand rubbing compound
(McAleer)

Kerosene
Sodium stearate
Paraffin oil
Tripoli (semidecomposed silica)
'76 Ed.

A A FLY SPRAY, FOREMOST 4840

See FOREMOST 4840 A A FLY SPRAY

A.A.I.

Animal area insecticide
(Puritan Chem. Co.)

Active ingredients: 100%
  Petroleum distillate *
  2,2-Dichlorovinyl dimethyl phosphate and related compounds (DDVP) *
  N-Octyl bicycloheptene dicarboximide
  Technical Piperonyl butoxide
  Pyrethrins

AAPRI COSMETICS

Aapri Cosmetics
P.O. Box 1090
Placentia, Calif. 92670

24-hour emergency phone
number: 617-421-7000

AATCC STANDARD DETERGENT #124

Institutional and industrial cleaning product

Procter & Gamble Co.
Ivorydale Technical Center
Cincinnati, Ohio 45217

Phone: 513-562-1100

AATREX 4L

Herbicide
(Ciba-Geigy Ag. Div.)

Atrazine * 40.8%
Related compounds 2.2%

AATREX NINE-O

Herbicide
(Ciba-Geigy Ag. Div.)

Atrazine * 85.5%
Related compounds 4.5%

AATREX 80W

Herbicide
(Ciba-Geigy Ag. Div.)

Atrazine * 76%
Related compounds 4%

A-B-A TABLETS
(Cramer Products)

Phenacetin	162.000 mg.
Atropine sulfate	0.050 mg.
Dicalcium phosphate	40.000 mg.
FD & C 28-A Pea-pod Green	0.171 mg.
Aspirin (10% gran.) *	226.800 mg.
Cornstarch	5.000 mg.
Zinc stearate	4.000 mg.
Sterotex	4.000 mg.
Caffeine (anhydrous)	32.400 mg.

ABATE MANUFACTURING CONCENTRATE

Mosquito larvicide and insecticide
(Amer. Cyanamid, Agric. Div.)

O,O,O',O'-Tetramethyl O,O'-
thiodi-p-phenylene
phosphorothioate * 90.0%/w

A.B.C. - ALUMINUM BODY CLEANER (Liquid)

See GUNK A.B.C. - ALUMINUM BODY CLEANER (Liquid)

ABC ALUMINUM WELDING FLUX NO. 8
(Anti-Borax)

Potassium chloride 1-10%
Sodium chloride * 30-47%
Lithium chloride * 30-47%

ABCO AC-60

Concentrated chemical cleaner; municipal and industrial use
(ABCO, Inc.)

Muriatic acid *

ABCO D-300

Germicide and detergent sanitizer for institutional and industrial use
(ABCO, Inc.)

Nonylphenoxypoly (ethyleneoxy)
ethanol iodine complex (providing 0.8% available iodine) 9.40%
Phosphoric acid (85%) * 3.50%

ABCO GF-250

Disinfectant, sanitizer, deodorizer; for hospital use
(ABCO, Inc.)

n-Alkyl (60% C14, 30% C10, 5% C12, 5% C18) dimethyl benzyl
ammonium chlorides * 2.565%
n-Alkyl (50% C12, 30% C14, 17% C16, 3% C18) dimethyl ethylbenzyl ammonium chlorides * 2.565%

ABCO GSS-66 GRANULAR SOIL STERILANT

Municipal & industrial use
(ABCO, Inc.)

2-Methoxy-4,6-
bis(isopropylamino)-s-triazine .. 5.0%
Sodium chlorate * 40.0%
Sodium metaborate 50.0%

ABCO IMPROVED W.K-245

Herbicide
(ABCO, Inc.)

Isooctyl ester of 2,4,5-trichloro-
phenoxyacetic acid * 64.2%

ABCO ODC 150-1

Germicidal detergent-deodorizer concentrate
(ABCO, Inc.)

n-Alkyl (60% C14, 30% C16, 5% C12, 5% C18) dimethyl benzyl
ammonium chlorides * 1.758%
n-Alkyl (68% C12, 32% C14) dimethyl ethylbenzyl ammonium
chlorides * 1.758%
Sodium metasilicate * 2.216%
Sodium hydroxide * 1.050%
Ethylene diamine tetraacetic acid
tetrasodium salt 0.573%
Essential oils 0.228%

ABCO ODC-150-P

General purpose hospital germicidal cleaner concentrate
(ABCO, Inc.)

Ortho-benzyl-para-chlorophenol .. 3.1%
Soap 15.1%
Isopropyl alcohol 2.91%

ABCO PR-126

Paint stripper
(ABCO, Inc.)

Methanol *

ABCO PS-23

Coating and paint stripper
(ABCO, Inc.)

Methyl alcohol *

ABCO T.F.-75 TURF FUNGICIDE

Professional use only
(ABCO, Inc.)

Thiram (Tetramethylthiuram disulfide) * 75%

ABCO WKC-5

Aquatic weed control
(ABCO, Inc.)

Diquat dibromide (6,7-Dihydrodi-
pyrido(1,2-a:2:1'-c)pyrazidinium
dibromide) * 2.383%

Starred ingredients (*) may be responsible for major toxic effects; consult Section II.

ABCO WK 24-D
Herbicide - broadleaf weed control
(ABCO, Inc.)

Dimethylamine salt of 2,4-dichlo-
rophenoxyacetic acid * 49.0%

ABCO W.K.-DT 133
Herbicide; non-crop areas
(ABCO, Inc.)

Isooctyl ester of 2,4-dichlorophen-
oxyacetic acid * 34.0%
Isooctyl ester of 2,4,5-trichloro-
phenoxyacetic acid * 32.5%

ABCO WKNS-8
Herbicide
(ABCO, Inc.)

Aliphatic petroleum distillates *   83.27%
Xylene * 9.65%
Prometon   (2,4-Bis(isopropyl-
amino)-6-methoxy-s-triazine) .   0.86%

ABCO WKS-65 BRUSH KILLER
Herbicide; non-crop areas
(ABCO, Inc.)

Isooctyl ester of 2,4-dichlorophen-
oxyacetic acid * 46.0%
Isooctyl ester of 2,4,5-trichloro-
phenoxyacetic acid 10.5%
Isooctyl ester of silvex (2-(2,4,5-
Trichlorophenoxy)propionic
acid) 10.6%

ABCO WKS-74M SELECTIVE WEED KILLER
Herbicide
(ABCO, Inc.)

Potassium salt of 2-(2-methyl-4-
chlorophenoxy)propionic   acid
(MCPP) * 25.9%

ABCO WKS-74 SELECTIVE WEED KILLER
*Control of turf and lawn broadleaf
weeds*
(ABCO, Inc.)

Dimethylamine salt of 2-(2-methyl-
4-chlorophenoxy)propionic
acid * 16.2%
Dimethylamine salt of 2,4-dichlo-
rophenoxyacetic acid * 16.1%

ABDEC DROPS
*Multivitamin supplement for infants
and children*
(Parke-Davis)

Each 1.0 ml.:
Vitamin A .... 1500 IU
Vitamin D .... 400 IU
Plus multivitamins

ABDEC DROPS WITH FLUO-RIDE
Multivitamin supplement for infants
(Parke-Davis)

Each 1.0 ml.:
Vitamin A .... 1500 IU
Vitamin D .... 400 IU
Fluoride .... 0.25 mg.
Plus multivitamins

ABDEC MULTIPLE VITAMIN CAPSULES
(Parke-Davis)

Each capsule:
Vitamin A ...... (3 mg.) 10,000 units
Vitamin D ...... (10 mcg.) 400 units
Plus multivitamins

ABDOL WITH MINERALS
Vitamin-mineral deficiency states
(Parke-Davis)

Each capsule:
Vitamin A ...... (1.5 mg.) 5000 units
Vitamin D ...... (10 mcg.) 400 units
Plus multivitamins and minerals

ABFEX
Insecticide - household insect control
(ABCO, Inc.)

Petroleum distillates * 99.112%
Technical Piperonyl butoxide .. 0.740%
Pyrethrins 0.148%

ABFEX AEROSOL SPRAY
Insecticide - household insect control
(ABCO, Inc.)

Petroleum distillates * 18.8%
Technical Piperonyl butoxide 1.0%
Pyrethrins 0.2%

ABFICIDE
Household insect control
(ABCO, Inc.)

Petroleum distillates * 99.52%
Pyrethrins 0.48%

ABFICIDE AEROSOL SPRAY
Household insect control
(ABCO, Inc.)

Pyrethrins 0.5%
Technical Piperonyl butoxide 4.0%
Petroleum distillates * 15.5%

ABSORBINE ARTHRITIC PAIN LOTION
*Temporary relief from minor pains of
arthritis, rheumatism*
(Young, W.F.)

Methyl salicylate *
Methyl nicotinate
Menthol *
Isopropyl alcohol 3%
Cetyl alcohol 1%

ABSORBINE ATHLETE'S FOOT POWDER
(Young, W.F.)

Benzethonium chloride *
Zinc stearate
Parachlorometaxylenol
Aluminum chlorhydroxy allantoinate
Menthol *
Inert ingred.: 86.4%
Corn starch
Magnesium carbonate

ABSORBINE JR.
Rubefacient, counterirritant solution
(Young, W.F.)

Wormwood
Thymol *
Chloroxylenol *
Menthol *
Acetone *
Essential oils *
Tinctures

A.B.T./(AFTER BURN RELIEF)
(Bullard)

8-Hydroxyquinoline .... <1%
Liquid petrolatum USP .... >10%
Rosemary oil USP * .... >10%
Oil of linseed 1-10%

ACARABEN 4E
Miticide
(Ciba-Geigy Ag. Div.)

Chlorobenzilate 45.5%
Xylene * 43.5%

ACCELERASE-PB
Treatment of nervous indigestion
(Organon)

Each capsule:
Lipase .... 4,000 N.F. Units
Amylase .... 15,000 N.F. Units
Protease .... 15,000 N.F. Units
Mixed conjugated
Bile salts .... 65 mg.
Cellulase .... 2 mg.
Calcium carbonate .... 20 mg.
Belladonna alkaloids (levo)
(87.5% hyoscyamine and 12.5%
atropine as sulfates) .... 0.2 mg.
Phenobarbital * .... 16 mg.

ACCELERATE
Herbicide
(Pennwalt)

Endothall (as monomethyl-
cocoamine salt)(liquid
concentrate) * .... 0.52 lb./gal.

ACCELERATOR 45C
Various industrial uses
(Parker Div.)

Solution containing:
Hydrofluoric acid * 20%

ACCLEAN, FORMULA HC-500

See KLENZADE ACCLEAN, FORMULA HC-500

AC COMPOUNDS
Acidic cleaning & oxide removal solution for use on metals
(Whitfield Chem.)

Phosphoric acid * .... >10%

ACEDOVAL
Analgesic, antipyretic
(Vale)

Each tablet:
Dover's powder (represents
  1.5 mg. opium) .... 15.0 mg.
Phenacetin * .... 162.0 mg.
Caffeine (anhydrous) ...... 8.1 mg.
Camphor .... 16.2 mg.

ACEDYNE
(Vale)

Each tablet:
Phenacetin * .... 32.4 mg.
Aspirin * .... 32.4 mg.
Caffeine anhydrous ...... 3.2 mg.
Atropine sulfate ...... 0.032 mg.
Magnesium trisilicate ...... 64.8 mg.

ACEITE VEGETAL LIQUID CLEANSER
(Kolmar Labs.)

Emulsifier .... >50%
Emollient 10-25%
Water 5-10%

ACETEST
Urine ketone test reagent tablet
(Ames)

Each tablet:
Sodium borate * .... 73.0 mg.
Sodium nitroferricyanide (Sodium nitroprusside) * ..... 1.0 mg.
Aminoacetic acid (Glycine) ... 9.0 mg.
Disodium phosphate .... 94.0 mg.
Lactose .... 20.0 mg.
Corn starch .... 2.5 mg.
Magnesium stearate .... 0.5 mg.

ACETO AGRICULTURAL CHEMICALS

Aceto Agricultural Chemicals Corp.
126-02 Northern Blvd.
Flushing, N.Y. 11368

Phone: 212-898-2300

ACETOJEN
Analgesic
(Jenkins Labs.)

Each tablet:
Aspirin * .... 3 1/2 gr.
Phenacetin (acetanilid
  deriv.) * .... 2 1/2 gr.
Caffeine .... 1/4 gr.
Tinc. Gelsemium * .... 3 min.

ACETOJEN, JR.
Analgesic
(Jenkins Labs.)

Each tablet:
Acetylsalicylic acid * ...... 1 1/2 gr.
Phenacetin * .... 1 gr.
Hyoscyamus extract (total alkaloids 0.0002 gr.) .... 0.0125 gr.
Gelsemium extract ...... 0.0125 gr.

ACETYCOL TABLETS
For rheumatism and arthritis
(OJF)

Each tablet:
Colchicine .... 0.5 mg.
Sodium salicylate * .... 500 mg.

ACID-GRO

See RA-PID-GRO ACID-GRO

ACIDINE
Antacid
(Consolid. Royal)

Magnesium trisilicate
Dried Aluminum hydroxide gel
Calcium carbonate
Sodium bicarbonate
Oil peppermint
Small amounts of Malt diatase, Bismuth
  subcarbonate, Papain

'76 Ed.

ACID MANTLE (CREME & LOTION)
Dermatological, protectant, emollient
(Dorsey Labs.)

Aluminum acetate
Emollient vehicle

ACIDULIN
For hydrochloric acid deficiency
(Lilly, Eli)

Each Pulvule:
Glutamic acid hydrochloride . 340 mg.

ACI-JEL
Therapeutic vaginal jelly
(Ortho)

Acetic acid 0.92%
Oxyquinoline sulfate 0.025%
Ricinoleic acid 0.7%
Boric acid * 3%
Glycerin 5%

ACITABS
Antacid
(Chex)

Each tablet:
Sugar .... 19.0 gr.
Aluminum hydroxide gel ..... 4.5 gr.
Pepsin .... 1.0 gr.
Corn syrup
Oil of peppermint
Essential oils

'76 Ed.

ACL-59
Chlorinating swimming pool water
(Pool Equipment, Inc.)

Potassium dichloroisocyanurate
(available chlorine 59%) * 100%

'76 Ed.

ACME ALL ROUND DUST
Insecticide, fungicide
(PBI/Gordon)

Methoxychlor, technical 5.00%
Zineb 5.20%
Rotenone 0.75%
Other cube resins 1.20%

ACME BAGWORM SPRAY
Insecticide
(PBI/Gordon)

Toxaphene * 20.00%
Kelthane 3.60%
Xylene * 68.50%

ACME BORDEAUX MIXTURE
Fungicide
(PBI/Gordon)

Copper sulfate (12.75% metallic
  copper) * 50%
Lime 50%

ACME CHLORDANE 45% SPRAY
Insecticide
(PBI/Gordon)

Technical Chlordane * 45.0%
Petroleum distillates * 50.00%

ACME CHLORDANE 72% SPRAY
Insecticide
(PBI/Gordon)

Technical Chlordane * 72.0%
Petroleum distillates * 23.0%

ACME CRABGRASS KILLER
(PBI/Gordon)

Monosodium acid
  methanearsonate * 16.6%

ACME DOG & CAT REPELLENT (Aerosol)
(PBI/Gordon)

Methyl nonyl ketone 1.90%

ACME DORMANT OIL SPRAY
(PBI/Gordon)

Paraffinic petroleum oil *† 96.0%

†*See* Kerosene

ACME EMO-NIK
Insecticide
(PBI/Gordon)

Selected Petroleum oil * 80%/w
Nicotine alkaloid * 1.50%/w

ACME FRUIT TREE SPRAY
Insecticide, fungicide
(PBI/Gordon)

Captan 12%
Methoxychlor technical * 12%
Malathion * 6%

ACME GARDEN GUARD
Insecticide
(PBI/Gordon)

Rotenone 1.00%
Other cube resins 1.60%

ACME GARDEN WEED PREVENTER
(PBI/Gordon)

Dimethyl tetrachloroterephthalate
(Dacthal) 2.5%

ACME GARDEN WEED PREVENTER SPRAY
Herbicide
(PBI/Gordon)

Dimethyl
tetrachloroterephthalate * 75.00%

ACME INDOOR PLANT SPRAY (Aerosol)
Insecticide
(PBI/Gordon)

Pyrethrins 0.02%
Rotenone 0.13%
Other cube resins 0.13%
Technical Piperonyl butoxide 0.25%
Petroleum distillates 0.18%

ACME LIME SULFUR SPRAY
Dip for control of sarcoptic mange of hogs; lice & psoroptic scabies of sheep & cattle
(PBI/Gordon)

Calcium polysulfides * 29%

Total combined sulfur not less than 23%

ACME 50% MALATHION SPRAY
Insecticide
(PBI/Gordon)

Tech. Malathion * 50%
Aromatic petroleum distillate * 42%

ACME PESTROY 25% METHOXYCHLOR
Insecticide
(PBI/Gordon)

Methoxychlor * 25.00%
Xylene *

ACME PRUNING SEALER
Seals moisture out on rose canes, shrub & tree wounds
(PBI/Gordon)

Gilsonite 22.0%
Mineral spirits * 23.0%
Inert ingredients:
  Propellents 55.0%

ACME RED RIVER VEGETABLE SPRAY
Insecticide-fungicide
(PBI/Gordon)

Sevin * 25.00%
Zineb 38.00%

ACME RED SPIDER & MITE SPRAY
Miticide
(PBI/Gordon)

Kelthane * 18.50%

ACME ROSE DUST
Insecticide & fungicide
(PBI/Gordon)

Captan 7.000%
Malathion 4.000%
Methoxychlor 5.000%
Dinocap (Dinitro-(1-methylhep-
  tyl)phenyl crotonate) 0.675%
Other nitrophenols & derivatives,
  chiefly dinitro (1-methylheptyl)
  phenol 0.075%

ACME ROSE & FLOWER SPRAY (Aerosol)
Insecticide
(PBI/Gordon)

Pyrethrins 0.020%
N-Octyl bicycloheptene
  dicarboximide 0.300%
Rotenone 0.100%
Other cube resins 0.200%
Methoxyclor 0.300%
Dichlone 0.120%
Karathane 0.113%
Other related nitrp phenols,
  chiefly dinitro methyl heptyl
  phenol 0.012%
Petroleum distillate 0.115%

ACME SLUG & SNAIL BAIT
(PBI/Gordon)

Metaldehyde * 2.75%

ACME SUPER BRUSH KILLER
Herbicide
(PBI/Gordon)

Dimethylamine salt of 2,4-dichlo-
  rophenoxyacetic acid * 27.59%
Dimethylamine salt of 2-(2-
  methyl-4-chlorophenoxy) propionic acid * 13.86%
Dimethylamine salt of dicamba
  (3,6-Dichloro-o-anisic acid) ... 2.76%

ACME SUPER CHICKWEED KILLER
(PBI/Gordon)

2-(2-Methyl-4-
  chlorophenoxy)propionic acid, diethanolamine salt * 13.7%
2,4-Dichlorophenoxyacetic acid, diethanolamine salt * 13.6%
Dicamba, diethanolamine salt (3,6-
  Dichloro-o-anisic acid) 1.3%

ACME TOMATO FRUIT SET SPRAY (Aerosol)
Growth regulator
(PBI/Gordon)

Beta-naphthoxy acetic acid 0.004%

ACME TOMATO, VEGETABLE DUST
(PBI/Gordon)

Sevin * 3.0%
Zineb 5.2%
Sulphur 20.0%

ACME VEGETATION KILLER
(PBI/Gordon)

2-Methoxy-4,6-bis (isopropylamino)-s-triazine (Prometone) 3.6%
2,4-Dichloro phenoxyacetic acid
  (2,4-D) 1.0%
Aromatic petroleum distillates * . 88.6%

ACME WASP & HORNET JET SPRAY
(PBI/Gordon)

Resmethrin 0.150%
Related compounds 0.020%
Aromatic petroleum
  hydrocarbons 0.199%
Petroleum distillate * 26.375%

ACME WEED-N-GRASS KILLER
(PBI/Gordon)

Sodium cacodylate 5.2%
Dimethylarsinic acid 0.9%

Starred ingredients (*) may be responsible for major toxic effects; consult Section II.

ACME WEED-NO-MORE SPOT WEEDER
(PBI/Gordon)

2,4-Dichlorophenoxyacetic acid, dimethylamine salt	0.620%
2-(2-Methyl-4-chlorophenoxy)propionic acid, dimethylamine salt	0.281%
Dicamba, dimethylamine salt (3,6-Dichloro-o-anisic acid)	0.064%

ACME YARD AND PATIO FOGGER
Kills & repels mosquitoes, flies, gnats and wasps
(PBI/Gordon)

Resmethrin	0.250% w/w
Related compounds	0.034%
2-Hydroxyethyl-n-octyl sulfide	0.950%
Related compounds	0.050%
Aromatic petroleum solvent	0.332%

ACNAVEEN BAR
For acne & oily skin
(CooperCare)

Aveeno colloidal oatmeal	50%
Sulfur	2%
Salicylic acid *	2%

ACNE-AID CREAM
For acne
(Stiefel Labs.)

Sulfur	2.5%
Resorcinol *	1.25%
Para-chloro-meta-xylenol	0.375%
Microporous cellulose	

ACNE-AID DETERGENT SOAP
For acne
(Stiefel Labs.)

Sulfated surfactants and Hydrocarbon hydrotropes	6.3%

ACNE AID LOTION (Clear & Tinted)
(Stiefel Labs.)

Sulfur	10%
Alcohol	10%

ACNEDERM LOTION
For use in the treatment of acne and allied skin conditions
(Lannett)

Dispersible Sulfur	5%
Zinc oxide	10%
Zinc sulfate	1%
Alcohol	21%/vol.

ACNEDERM MEDICATED SOAP
For the treatment of acne and allied skin conditions
(Lannett)

Zinc oxide	2%
Zinc sulfate	1%
Colloidal Sulfur	5%
Penetrating non-soap base	

ACNE-DOME CREME & LOTION
Acne treatment
(Dome)

Colloidal Sulfur	4%
Resorcinol monoacetate (equiv. to 2% resorcinol) *	3%
Acid pH vehicle: Oil in water, emulsion-type creme containing a buffered solution of Aluminum acetate	

ACNE-DOME MEDICATED CLEANSER
Soapless cleanser for control of acne & seborrhea
(Dome)

Colloidal Sulfur	2%
Salicylic acid *	2%
Acid pH vehicle	

ACNESARB LOTION
Acne therapy
(C & M Pharmacal)

Salicylic acid *	3%
Boric acid *	2%
Hyamine 10X (quaternary germicide) *	
Isopropyl alcohol *	63%
Purified water	

ACNO ASTRINGENT
(Baker-Cummins)

Isopropanol *	
Water	
Polyoxyethylene lauryl ethers	

ACNO LOTION
Acne treatment
(Baker-Cummins)

Sulfur	3%
Salicylic acid *	2%

ACNOMEL ACNE CAKE
(MenJ Labs.)

Resorcinol	1%
Sulfur	8%

ACNOMEL ACNE CREAM
(MenJ Labs.)

Resorcinol *	2%
Sulfur	8%
Alcohol	11% w/w

ACNOPHILL (PLAIN)
For acne
(Torch)

Sulfur precipitated	5%
Potassium and zinc sulfides & polysulfides *†	5%
Zinc oxide	10%
Hydrophilic vehicle ad.	100%

'76 Ed.

†*See* Sulfide salts

ACNOTEX LOTION
For acne therapy
(C & M Pharmacal)

Sulfur	8%
Salicylic acid *	2.25%
Hyamine 10X *	
Propylene glycol	
Powder base	
Acetone *	
Isopropyl alcohol *	22%
Color	
Perfume	
Purified water	

ACNYCIN CREAM
Antiseptic-antibiotic
(Columbia Med.)

Hexachlorophene	0.5%
Sulfur	5%
Resorcinol *	2%
Zinc oxide	

ACNYL CREAM
For acne
(Pharmex)

Resorcinol *	2%
Sulfur	8%
Hexachlorophene	0.25%

ACORN RAT & MOUSE KILLER
(Lowman Co.)

Warfarin	0.025%

ACOTIN
Analgesic
(Watkins Products, Inc.)

Each tablet:
Aspirin *	5 gr.
Caffeine	

ACOTUS COUGH SYRUP
(Whorton)

Each teaspoonful:
Phenylephrine hydrochloride *	5 mg.
Guaiacol glyceryl ether	100 mg.
Menthol	1 mg.
Dextromethorphan hydrobromide *	5 mg.
Alcohol (by volume)	10%

'76 Ed.

Starred ingredients (*) may be responsible for major toxic effects; consult Section II.

ACOUSTI-BOND ADHESIVE
No. 57
(Bogert, A.Z.)

Resinous binder (derived from
  rosin and/or modified rosin) .. 40-46%
Petroleum naphtha 8%
Clay 43-49%
Isopropanol 3%

ACOUSTI-gum
Adhesive
(Templar)

Clays
Rosin derivatives
Synthetic resins
Dissolved in Petroleum solvent *

ACP

See ALSOL ACP

ACRA-SEAL
*Automotive, electrical, industrial,
  household use; waterproofs and rust-
  proofs*
(Radiator)

Aromatic solvents *
Chlorinated solvents *

'76 Ed.

ACTAMIN
Analgesic
(Buffington)

Each tablet:
  Acetaminophen * .... 325 mg.

ACTI-CIL
Herbicide
(National Chemsearch)

Heavy Aromatic naphtha * 50.00%
Petroleum base oil 46.51%
Bromacil 0.60%
Pentachlorophenol 0.80%
Other Chlorophenols 0.09%

ACTICORT LOTION 25
Anti-inflammatory, antipruritic
(Baker-Cummins)

Hydrocortisone 0.25%

ACTICORT LOTION 100
Anti-inflammatory, antipruritic
(Baker-Cummins)

Hydrocortisone 1%

ACTIDIL SYRUP
Antihistaminic
(Burroughs Wellcome)

Each 5 cc:
  Triprolidine HCl * .... 1.25 mg.

ACTIDIL TABLETS
Antihistaminic
(Burroughs Wellcome)

Each tablet:
  Actidil (Triprolidine
    hydrochloride) * .... 2.5 mg.

ACTIFED-C
Expectorant
(Burroughs Wellcome)

Each 5 cc:
  Codeine phosphate * .... 10 mg.
  Actidil (Triprolidine HCl) * .. 2 mg.
  Sudafed (Pseudoephedrine
    HCl) * .... 30 mg.
  Glyceryl guaiacolate
    (Guaifenesin) .... 100 mg.
Preservatives:
  Methylparaben 0.1%
  Sodium benzoate 0.1%

ACTIFED SYRUP
Antihistaminic, decongestant
(Burroughs Wellcome)

Each 5 cc.:
  Actidil (Triprolidine
    hydrochloride) * .... 1.25 mg.
  Sudafed (Pseudoephedrine
    hydrochloride) * .... 30 mg.
Preservatives:
  Sodium benzoate 0.1%
  Methylparaben 0.1%

ACTIFED TABLETS
Antihistaminic, decongestant
(Burroughs Wellcome)

Each tablet:
  Actidil (Triprolidine
    hydrochloride) * .... 2.5 mg.
  Sudafed (Pseudoephedrine
    hydrochloride) * .... 60 mg.

ACTION ALGI-CURE
Aquarium algicide
(General Developments Corp.)

Monuron (3-(p-Chorophenyl)-1,1-
    dimethylurea) 0.75%
Simazine (2-Chloro-4,6-bis(ethyl-
    amino)-s-triazine) 0.55%
Atrazine (2-Chloro-4-ethylamino-6-
    isopropylamino-s-triazine) .. 0.2%
Dichlone (2,3-Dichloro-1,4-
    naphthoquinone) 0.1%

'76 Ed.

ACTION BLEACH PACKETS
(Colgate-Palmolive)

Alkaline mixture of inorganic salts:
  Sulfate
  Phosphate *
  Carbonate *†
Synthetic detergent 2%
Organic bleaching agent
  which yields Sodium hy-
  pochlorite in alkaline
  solution .... approx. 20%

'76 Ed

†*See* Sodium carbonate

ACTION GERMICIDAL CLEANER

See PIONEER ACTION GERMICI-
DAL CLEANER

ACTOL EXPECTORANT SYRUP
(Beecham Labs.)

Each 5 ml.:
  Noscapine* .... 30 mg.
  Guaifenesin .... 200 mg.
  Alcohol* 12.5%
  Flavoring .... q.s.

ACTOL EXPECTORANT TABLETS
(Beecham Labs.)

Each tablet:
  Noscapine* .... 30 mg.
  Guaifenesin .... 200 mg.

ACTUSOL
Oil & grease emulsifier
(DuBois Chem.)

Potassium vegetable oil soaps
Kerosene fraction of petroleum *
Straight chain glycol

AD
(Colgate-Palmolive)

Combined amount: .... approx. 15%
  Alkyl aryl sulfonate *
  Nonionic detergent (alkyl phenol ethox-
    ymer)
Combined amount: .... approx. 75%
  Phosphates *
  Sodium sulfate
  Sodium silicate *

'76 Ed.

ADAPETTES
*Contact lens solution; in purse/pocket
  size*
(Burton, Parsons & Co.)

Thimerosal 0.004%

ADAPIN CAPSULES
Antianxiety, antidepressant
(Pennwalt, Pharm. Div.)

Each capsule:
  Doxepin HCl * 10, 25, 50, 75
                          or 100 mg.

ADAPT
*Cushioning solution for hard contact
  lenses*
(Burton, Parsons & Co.)

Thimerosal 0.004%
EDTA 0.1%

Starred ingredients (*) may be responsible for major toxic effects; consult Section II.

ADDIT
Carpet cleaner
(Sanitek)

Nonionic surfactants	10%
Isopropanol	10%
Dipropylene glycol monomethyl ether (Cellosolve)	5%
Perfume, Dye, Anionic surfactant, Potassium hydroxide	trace
Water	balance

ADEFLOR CHEWABLE TABLETS
Prevention of dental caries
(Upjohn)

Each 0.5 or 1 mg. tablet:
Fluoride (as sodium fluoride)	0.5 mg.; 1 mg.
Vitamin A	4000 I.U.
Vitamin D	400 I.U.
Plus multivitamins and minerals	

ADEFLOR DROPS
Prevention of dental caries
(Upjohn)

Each 0.6 ml.:
Fluoride (as sodium fluoride)	0.5 mg.
Vitamin A	2000 I.U.
Vitamin D	400 I.U.
Ascorbic acid	50.0 mg.
Pyridoxine hydrochloride	1.0 mg.

ADEFLOR M TABLETS
Dietary supplement
(Upjohn)

Each tablet:
Vitamin A	6000 I.U.
Vitamin D	400 I.U.
Fluoride (as sodium fluoride)	1 mg.
Iron (from 91.27 mg. ferrous fumarate) *	30 mg.
Plus multivitamins and minerals	

ADHESIVE PRIMERS NO. 1642

See KNIGHT ADHESIVE PRIMERS NO. 1642

ADIOS, DEL

See DEL ADIOS

ADIPEX-P CAPSULES
Anorectic
(Lemmon Co.)

Phentermine hydrochloride (equiv. to 24 mg. of Phentermine base) *	30 mg.

ADIPEX-P TABLETS
Anorectic
(Lemmon Co.)

Each tablet:
Phentermine hydrochloride (equiv. to 30 mg. of Phentermine base) *	37.5 mg.

ADMIRABLE RUG SHAMPOO
(Uncle Sam)

Blend of Synthetic detergents & surfactants *
Optical brightener
Formaldehyde *
Dye
Water

ADOCAINE OINTMENT
Topical anesthetic
(Wesley Pharm.)

Cod liver oil	
Vitamin A	850 U/gm.
Vitamin D	85 U/gm.
Benzalkonium chloride	
Allantoin	0.25%
Zinc oxide	5%
Diperodon hydrochloride	0.25%
Lanolin-petrolatum base	

ADORN HAIR SPRAYS
(Gillette Co., Personal Care Div.)

The Gillette Co., Personal Care Div., Boston, Mass. 02199 will receive collect phone calls from poison control centers or physicians asking for emergency toxicological information about the company's products.

Phone: 617-421-7000

ADRENOSEM SALICYLATE SYRUP
(Beecham Labs.)

Each 5 ml.:
Adrenochrome semicarbazone (present as 65 mg. carbazochrome salicylate) *	2.5 mg.

ADRENOSEM SALICYLATE TABLETS
(Beecham Labs.)

Each tablet:
Adrenochrome semicarbazone (present as 65 mg. carbazochrome salicylate) *	2.5 mg.

ADSORBOCARPINE
For treatment of glaucoma
(Burton, Parsons & Co.)

Pilocarpine HCl *	1%; 2% or 4%

ADSORBONAC (2% and 5%)
Aid in reducing corneal edema
(Burton, Parsons & Co.)

Sodium chloride	2% or 5%
Polyvinylpyrrolidone	1.67%
Thimerosal (as preservative)	0.002%
EDTA (as preservative)	0.05%

ADVANCED COATING & CHEMICALS PRODUCTS
Specialty coatings

Advanced Coating & Chemicals
4343 Temple City Blvd.
Temple City, Calif. 91780

Phone: 213-579-6270

ADVANCE LIQUID
(C-Z Chemical)

n-Alkyl (55% C16, 20% C14, 20% C12, 5% C18) dimethyl benzyl ammonium chloride *	6.4%
Non-ionic wetting agent	4.5%
Soda ash *	3.0%
Tetrasodium pyrophosphate *	84.1%

'76 Ed.

AERO ACRYLIC AND WAX REMOVER (No Phosphate)
(Boyle-Midway)

Water	
Combined amount:	1-10%
Sequestrant	
Carbonate *†	
Sulfonate	
Nonionic surfactant	
Ammonia	<1%

†*See* Sodium carbonate

AEROCAINE
Topical anesthetic, antiseptic
(Aeroceuticals)

Benzyl alcohol (N.F.) *	22.7%
Benzocaine (N.F.)	13.6%
Hexachlorophene (USP)	0.5%
Benzethonium chloride (USP)	0.5%

'76 Ed.

AEROCEUTICALS AEROSOL MERTHIOLATE
First aid antiseptic spray
(Aeroceuticals)

Merthiolate	0.033%
Thimerosal (after application the conc. approx. 1:1000)	
Alcohol	22%

'76 Ed.

AEROLATE
For emphysema, asthma
(Fleming)

III (each capsule):	
Theophylline *	1 gr.
JR. (each capsule):	
Theophylline *	2 gr.
SR. (each capsule):	
Theophylline *	4 gr.

Starred ingredients (*) may be responsible for major toxic effects; consult Section II.

AEROLATE LIQUID
Bronchodilator
(Fleming)

Each 15 ml.:
Theophylline * .... 160 mg.
Tangerine flavored base

AERO-MASTER FOGGING AND CONTACT SPRAY
(Aero-Master)

Tetramethrin 0.48%
3-Phenoxybenzyl d-cis and trans 2,
2-dimethyl-2-(2-methyl-
propenyl)
cyclopropanecarboxylate 0.15%
Other isomers 0.01%
Aromatic petroleum distillate 1.60%
Petroleum distillate * 97.69%

AERO-MASTER FOGGING INSECTICIDE
(Aero-Master)

Resmethrin 0.250%
Related compounds 0.034%
Aromatic petroleum
hydrocarbons 0.331%
Petroleum distillate * 99.375%

AERO-MASTER FOGGING INSECTICIDE MILL FOGGING FORMULA
(Aero-Master)

Petroleum oils * 98.866%
Technical Piperonyl butoxide .. 0.810%
Pyrethrins 0.324%

AERO-MASTER SPRAYING AND FOGGING INSECTICIDE
(Aero-Master)

Pyrethrins 0.50%
Piperonyl butoxide (technical) .. 1.00%
N-Octyl bicycloheptene
dicarboximide 1.67%
Petroleum distillate * 96.83%

AERO-MASTER SUPER FOGGING INSECTICIDE
(Aero-Master)

Resmethrin 0.500%
Related compounds 0.068%
Aromatic petroleum
hydrocarbons 0.662%
Petroleum distillate * 98.750%

AERO-MASTER SYNALTRANS-D INSECTICIDE
(Aero-Master)

d-trans Allethrin (allyl homolog
of Cinerin I) 0.250%
Piperonyl butoxide, technical .. 0.500%
N-Octyl bicycloheptene
dicarboximide 0.825%
Petroleum distillate * 98.425%

AER-O-MATIC CLOSET FRESHNER
Clothes moth killer
(Allied Block)

Active ingred.:
Paradichlorobenzene * 99%
Inert ingred.:
Essential oils 1%

AER-O-MATIC MOTH KILLER
(Allied Block)

Naphthalene * 99%
Essential oil 1%

AER-O-MATIC MOTH KILLER CRYSTALS
(Allied Block)

Paradichlorobenzene * 100%

AER-O-MATIC REFILL MOTH KILLER
(Allied Block)

Paradichlorobenzene * 99%
Essential oils 1%

AEROPURE
*Concentrated air sanitizer and deodor-
izer*
(Aeroceuticals)

Isopropanol 7.80%
Triethylene glycol 3.90%
Essential oils * 3.00%
Methyldodecyl benzyl trimethyl
ammonium chloride 0.12%
Methyldodecylxylylene bis (trime-
thyl ammonium chloride) 0.03%
'76 Ed.

AEROSEB-DEX (Aerosol)
For dermatoses
(Herbert Labs.)

Dexamethasone 0.01%
Alcohol 68.5%
Isopropyl myristate
Propellant (Butane)

AEROSEB-HC
Topical aerosol spray
(Herbert Labs.)

Hydrocortisone 0.5%
Alcohol 68%
Isopropyl myristate
Propellant (Butane)

AEROSPORIN STERILE POWDER
Antibiotic
(Burroughs Wellcome)

Each 20 cc:
Polymyxin B sulfate .... 500,000 units

AEROTHERM
First aid spray for burns
(Aeroceuticals)

Benzyl alcohol (N.F.) * 22.7%
Benzocaine (N.F.) 13.6%
Hexachlorophene (USP) 0.5%
'76 Ed.

AEROWAX
(Boyle-Midway)

Solids: 15%
Synthetic waxes
Emulsifiers (anionic and nonionic)
Plasticizers
Resins
Acrylic polymer
Ammonia .... <1%
Water

AFCO CSD
Cleaner - sanitizer - deodorant
(Fergusson, Alex. C., Co.)

Sodium carbonate * 22.21%
Alkyl dimethyl benzyl ammonium
chlorides 5.56%

AFCO SUPER-CHLOR
Germicide, disinfectant
(Fergusson, Alex. C., Co.)

Dichloro-s-triazinetrione * 23.5%

A-FIL CREAM
Prevents sunburn and suntan
(CooperCare)

Titanium dioxide 5%
Menthyl anthranilate 5%

AFRIN (NASAL SOLUTION and NASAL SPRAY)
Nasal decongestant
(Schering)

Each cc:
Oxymetazoline hydrochloride   0.5 mg.
Glycine   3.8 mg.
Sorbitol solution (equiv. to 40
mg. sorbitol) .... 57.1 mg.
Phenylmercuric acetate ..... 0.02 mg.
Benzalkonium chloride ...... 0.2 mg.
Sodium hydroxide (to adjust pH to a
weak acid sol. (5.5-6.5))
Purified water, q.s. .... 1 cc

AFRIN PEDIATRIC NOSE DROPS
(Schering)

Oxymetazoline hydrochloride ... 0.025%

Starred ingredients (*) may be responsible for major toxic effects; consult Section II.

AFTA AFTER SHAVE SKIN CONDITIONER
(Mennen)

Water
SD Alcohol 40 *
PEG-8 distearate
Fragrance
Triethanolamine
Carbomer-934
PEG-2 stearate
D&C Green #5
FD&C Yellow #5

AFTER TAN
(Aloe Creme)

Aloe vera plant gel

AGFA RODINAL BLACK AND WHITE FILM DEVELOPER
(Braun North America)

Potassium hydroxide * 4.7%
p-Aminophenol

AGILE
Liquid laundry builder
(Diversey Wyandotte)

Sodium hydroxide*

AGORAL
Cathartic
(Warner-Lambert)

Each 15 ml.:
  Mineral oil .... 4.2 gm.
  Phenolphthalein .... 0.2 gm.

AGRO-CHEM BRAND CAPTAN 15 + 30% SULFUR
Fungicide
(Arizona)

Captan 15.00%
Sulfur * 30.00%

AGRO-CHEM BRAND CRYOLITE 50 DUST
Insecticide
(Arizona)

Sodium fluoaluminate (Fluorine expressed as elemental 27.1%) . 50.00%

AGRO-CHEM BRAND DIAZINON 14G
Insecticide
(Arizona)

Diazinon * 14%

AGRO-CHEM BRAND DIBROM 8EC
Insecticide
(Arizona)

Naled * 58%
Xylene * 20%

AGRO-CHEM BRAND DINITRO WEED KILLER
(Arizona)

Dinoseb (2-sec-Butyl-4,6-dinitrophenol) * 55%

AGRO-CHEM BRAND DI-SYSTON 6.5 + TERRACLOR 6.5
Insecticide and fungicide
(Arizona)

O,O-Diethyl   S-2-(ethylthio)ethyl phosphorodithioate * 6.50%
Pentachloronitrobenzene 6.50%

AGRO-CHEM BRAND ENDRIN 1.6E
Insecticide
(Arizona)

Endrin * 19.7%
Aromatic petroleum solvent 72.8%

AGRO-CHEM BRAND GWK
Herbicide
(Arizona)

Dinoseb * 30.25%

AGRO-CHEM BRAND MALATHION 5-E
Insecticide
(Arizona)

Malathion * 57%
Xylene range aromatic solvent * ... 32%

AGRO-CHEM BRAND MALATHION EC-57
Insecticide
(Arizona)

Malathion * 57%
Aromatic petroleum solvent * 32%

AGRO-CHEM BRAND METHYL PARATHION 4-E
Insecticide
(Arizona)

Methyl parathion * 45.52%
Xylene range aromatic solvent .. 48.20%

AGRO-CHEM BRAND PAIR EM6-3
Insecticide
(Arizona)

Parathion * 57.8%
Methyl parathion 27.5%
Related compounds 1.45%
Xylene 6.44%

AGRO-CHEM BRAND PARATHION 2
Insecticide
(Arizona)

Parathion * 2.00%

AGRO-CHEM BRAND PARATHION 4E
Insecticide
(Arizona)

Parathion * 46.69%
Aromatic petroleum solvent 47.60%

AGRO-CHEM BRAND PERTHANE EC-48
Insecticide
(Arizona)

Perthane 42.2%
Related reaction products 5.8%
Aromatic petroleum solvent * 47.5%

AGRO-CHEM BRAND PHOSDRIN 4E
Insecticide
(Arizona)

Phosdrin * 30%
Related compounds 20%

AGRO-CHEM BRAND PHOSPHAMIDON 8 SPRAY
Insecticide
(Arizona)

Phosphamidon * 74.5%
Related compounds 3.5%

AGRO-CHEM BRAND SEVIN 10 DUST
Insecticide
(Arizona)

Carbaryl * 10.00%

AGRO-CHEM BRAND SEVIN 10 WITH 50% SULFUR
Insecticide and fungicide
(Arizona)

Carbaryl * 10.00%
Sulfur * 50.00%

AGRO-CHEM BRAND THIMET 6.5 + TERRACLOR 6.5
Insecticide and fungicide
(Arizona)

Phorate * 6.50%
Pentachloronitrobenzene 6.50%

AGRO-CHEM BRAND THIODAN 2E
Insecticide
(Arizona)

Endosulfan * 24.00%
Aromatic petroleum solvent * ... 69.5%

Starred ingredients (*) may be responsible for major toxic effects; consult Section II.

AGRO-CHEM BRAND TORBIDAN 28
Insecticide
(Arizona)

Toxaphene	66.6%
Methyl parathion *	16.8%
Aromatic petroleum solvent	11.6%

AGRO-CHEM BRAND TOXAPHENE 6E
Insecticide
(Arizona)

Toxaphene *	60.0%
Aromatic petroleum solvent *	35.5%

AGRO-CHEM BRAND TOXAPHENE 6-E METHYL PARATHION 3-E
Insecticide
(Arizona)

Toxaphene	52.5%
Methyl parathion *	26.3%
Xylene	15.2%

AGRO-CHEM BRAND ZM 8% FUNGICIDE DUST
(Arizona)

Manganese	1.6%
Zinc	0.2%
Ethylene bisdithiocarbamate ion	6.2%

AGROX FLOWABLE
Seed treatment
(Chipman Inc.)

Maneb *	25.0%

AGROX N-M
Seed treatment
(Chipman Inc.)

Maneb *	50.0%

AGROX 2-WAY
Seed treatment
(Chipman Inc.)

Captan	35.46%
Related derivatives	2.04%
Diazinon *	25.00%

AGROX 3-WAY
Seed treatment
(Chipman Inc.)

Captan	31.68%
Related derivatives	1.82%
Diazinon *	11.00%
Lindane *	16.60%

AGSCO DB-GREEN
Insecticide-fungicide seed treatment
(Agsco)

Maneb	50.00%
Lindane *	18.75%

AGSCO TOXAPHENE
Insecticide
(Agsco)

Toxaphene *	60%
Xylene type solvent *	36%
Emulsifiers	4%

AGWAY ABATE 4E
Insecticide, larvicide
(Agway)

O,O,O',O'-Tetramethyl O,O'-thiodi-p-phenylene phosphorothioate	43.0%
Aromatic petroleum solvent *	39.0%

AGWAY ALFALFA SPRAY 22E
Insecticide
(Agway)

Methoxychlor (technical) *	23.787%
Malathion *	23.807%
Xylene *	43.510%

AGWAY AMMATE WEED & BRUSH KILLER
(Agway)

Ammonium sulfamate *	46.5%

AGWAY ANT AND ROACH SPRAY
Insecticide
(Agway)

Pyrethrins	0.045%/wt.
Tech. Piperonyl butoxide	0.090%/wt.
N-Octyl bicycloheptene dicarboximide	0.150%/wt.
Ronnel	1.000%/wt.
Tech. Chlordane	1.500%/wt.
Petroleum distillates *	93.265%/wt.

AGWAY BOOSTER PLUS E
(Agway)

Paraffin base petroleum oil *†	83%
Surfactant blend	16%

†*See* Petroleum distillate

AGWAY CHARGER-E
Spray adjuvant and wetting agent
(Agway)

Octylphenoxy polyethoxyethanol *†

†*See* Alkyl phenoxy polyethoxy ethanols

AGWAY CHLORDANE 8E
Insecticide
(Agway)

Active ingred. (by wt.):

Technical Chlordane *	72.0%
Petroleum distillate *	18.0%

AGWAY CIODRIN CONCENTRATE
Insecticide
(Agway)

Active ingred. (by wt.):

Dimethyl phosphate of alpha-methylbenzyl 3-hydroxy-cis-crotonate *	25.0%
Xylene	63.7%

AGWAY CRANBERRY HERBICIDE 13.1G
(Agway)

Sodium N-1-naphthylphthalamate	8.1%
Isopropyl N-(3-chlorophenyl) carbamate	5.0%

AGWAY CROP SPRAY
Insecticide
(Agway)

Technical Piperonyl butoxide	60.0%
Pyrethrins	6.0%

AGWAY CYGON 2-E
Insecticide
(Agway)

Dimethoate *	23.40%

AGWAY DAIRY DUST
Insecticide; veterinary
(Agway)

Dimethyl phosphate of alpha-methylbenzyl 3-hydroxy-cis-crotonate *	3.0%

AGWAY DIAZINON AG500
Insecticide
(Agway)

O,O-Diethyl O-(2-isopropyl-6-methyl-4-pyrimidinyl) phosphorothioate *	48%
Xylene *	36%

AGWAY DUAL GARDEN ORCHARD SPRAY
Insecticide, fungicide
(Agway)

Active ingred. (by wt.):

Captan	15.0%
Malathion *	7.5%
Methoxychlor (technical)	15.0%

AGWAY DUAL STOCK SPRAY
Insecticide
(Agway)

Dimethyl phosphate of alpha-methylbenzyl 3-hydroxy-cis-crotonate	1.00%
2,2-Dichlorovinyl dimethyl phosphate	0.24%
Related compounds	0.01%
Petroleum hydrocarbons *	98.75%

Starred ingredients (*) may be responsible for major toxic effects; consult Section II.

AGWAY DUAL STOCK SPRAY CONCENTRATE
Insecticide
(Agway)

Dimethyl phosphate of alpha-methylbenzyl 3-hydroxy-cis-
crotonate * 10.0%
2,2-Dichlorovinyl dimethyl phosphate 2.3%
Related compounds 0.2%
Petroleum hydrocarbons 77.0%

AGWAY DUOCIDE CONCENTRATE
Rodenticide
(Agway)

2-Pivalyl-1,3-indandione ..... 0.50%/wt.

AGWAY DUOCIDE RAT BAIT STATION
(Agway)

2-Pivalyl-1,3-indandione 0.025%/w

AGWAY DURSBAN 2EC
Insecticide
(Agway)

Chlorpyrifos (O,O-Diethyl O-(3,5,6-
trichloro-2-pyridyl)
phosphorothioate) * 22.4%
Aromatic petroleum derivative
solvent * 44.1%

AGWAY DURSBAN 2EC LAWN INSECTICIDE
(Agway)

Chlorpyrifos (O,O-Diethyl O-(3,5,6-
trichloro-2-pyridyl)
phosphorothioate) * 22.4%
Xylene * 44.1%

AGWAY ENDRIN 1.6E
Insecticide
(Agway)

Endrin * 19.40%
Xylene range aromatic hydrocarbon solvent 74.60%

AGWAY FENTEX 4E
Insecticide
(Agway)

Fenthion * 46.50%
Xylene * 44.89%

AGWAY FOAMING ACID CLEANSER
(Agway)

Mineral acid *

AGWAY GARDEN VEGETABLE DUST
Insecticide
(Agway)

Malathion * 5.6%
Methoxychlor (technical) 5.0%
Captan 7.0%

AGWAY GLYODEX 50-16W
Fungicide
(Agway)

Glyodin (2-Heptadecyl glyoxalidine acetate) * 50.00%
Dodine (n-Dodecylguanidine
acetate) * 16.00%

AGWAY HOOF ROT TREAT
For cattle and sheep
(Agway)

Methylrosaniline chloride *
Coal tar hydrocarbons * 35%
Santophen 1 (o-Benzyl-p-
chlorophenol) 0.0075%
Soap
Coal oil
Vegetable oils

AGWAY HORNET AND WASP SPRAY
(Agway)

Pyrethrins 0.10%
Piperonyl butoxide (technical) .. 0.20%
N-Octyl bicycloheptene
dicarboximide 0.33%
o-Isopropoxyphenyl
methylcarbamate 0.50%
Petroleum distillate * 83.87%

AGWAY INHIBITOR 3 E
Growth inhibitor
(Agway)

Diethanolamine salt of 6-hydroxy-3-
(2H)-pyridazione *† 58%

†*See* Maleic hydrazide

AGWAY IODINE 7%
Antiseptic; veterinary
(Agway)

Iodine (U.S.P.) * .... 7% w/v
Potassium iodide (U.S.P.) .... 5% w/v
Alcohol .... 85.0% v/v

AGWAY IODINE TEAT DIP
For use on dairy cows
(Agway)

Nonyl phenoxypolyethoxy
ethanol-iodine complex (providing 1.0% titratable iodine) 11.35%

AGWAY KELTHANE 1.5EC
Miticide
(Agway)

1,1-Bis(p-chlorophenyl)-2,2,2-
trichloroethanol 18.5%
Xylene * 73.0%

AGWAY LINDANE 20EC
Insecticide
(Agway)

Gamma isomer of benzene hexachloride from lindane * 20.00%
Xylene * 54.00%

AGWAY LIQUID BACTERICIDE AND TEAT DIP
(Agway)

Sodium hypochlorite * 8.4%

AGWAY LIQUID PIPELINE CLEANSER
(Agway)

Potassium hydroxide * .... >10%

AGWAY LIVESTOCK SPRAY
Insecticide
(Agway)

Petroleum distillate * ..... 99.565%/wt.
2,2-Dichlorovinyl dimethyl
phosphate .... 0.186%/wt.
Related compounds .... 0.014%/wt.
Piperonyl butoxide,
technical .... 0.210%/wt.
Pyrethrins .... 0.025%/wt.

AGWAY LOUSE POWDER
Veterinary insecticide
(Agway)

O,O-Diethyl O-(3-chloro-4-methyl-2-
oxo-(2H)-1-benzopyran-7-yl)
phosphorothioate * 1%

AGWAY MALATHION 5E
Insecticide
(Agway)

Active ingred. (by wt.):
Malathion * 55.00%
Xylene * 36.20%

AGWAY MALATHION GRAIN SPRAY
Insecticide
(Agway)

Malathion * 55.0%
Xylene * 36.2%

AGWAY MALATHION INSECT SPRAY
(Agway)

Malathion * .... 55.00%/wt.
Petroleum distillate .... 35.00%/wt.

AGWAY METHOXYCHLOR 2-E
Insecticide
(Agway)

Methoxychlor (technical) 24.0%
Xylene * 69.0%

Starred ingredients (*) may be responsible for major toxic effects; consult Section II.

AGWAY METHOXYCHLOR 5G
For control of mosquito larvae
(Agway)

Methoxychlor (technical)	5%
Heavy aromatic naphtha *	24%

AGWAY METHOXYCHLOR M-2E
Insecticide
(Agway)

Methoxychlor (technical)	23.7%
Heavy aromatic naphtha *	71.3%

AGWAY ORCHARD MOUSE BAIT - COATED
Rodenticide; wax coated cracked corn
(Agway)

Zinc phosphide *	2%

AGWAY ORCHARD MOUSE BAIT - COATED OATS
(Agway)

Zinc phosphide *	2%

AGWAY PARATHION 8 EC
Insecticide
(Agway)

Parathion *	81.7%
Xylene	6.2%

AGWAY PHOSPHAMIDON 8 E
Insecticide
(Agway)

Phosphamidon *	74.5%
Related compounds	3.5%

AGWAY POTATO STORAGE AREAS & EQUIPMENT DISINFECTANT
(Agway)

Hyamine 2389 * Methyldodecylbenzyl trimethyl ammonium chloride *	8.00%
Methyldodecylxylylene bis(trimethyl ammonium chloride) *	2.00%

AGWAY POULTRY DUST
Insecticide
(Agway)

Carbaryl (1-Naphthyl N-methylcarbamate) *	5.0%/wt.

AGWAY PREEMERGENT GARDEN WEED KILLER
(Agway)

Dacthal	5%/w

AGWAY PREMERGE
Herbicide
(Agway)

2-sec-Butyl-4,6-dinitrophenol, as the alkanolamine salts (of the ethanol and isopropanol series) *	51.0%

AGWAY PROTECTOR-3L SEED TREATMENT
Fungicide
(Agway)

2-(Thiocyanomethylthio) benzothiazole*	30.0%

AGWAY RESIDUAL FLY SPRAY 2E
(Agway)

Fenthion *	25.2%
Aromatic petroleum distillate *	69.8%

AGWAY ROACH-ANT KILLER
Pressurized spray
(Agway)

O,O-Diethyl O-(2-isopropyl-4-methyl-6-pyrimidinyl) phosphorothioate	0.500%
Pyrethrins	0.052%
Technical Piperonyl butoxide	0.261%
Petroleum distillate *	69.187%

AGWAY ROSE & FLORAL SPRAY
Insecticide, fungicide, miticide
(Agway)

Active ingred. (by wt.):

Pyrethrins	0.025%
Technical Piperonyl butoxide	0.256%
Rotenone	0.128%
Other cube extractives	0.256%
Folpet	0.700%
Carbaryl	1.000%
Petroleum distillate	0.060%

AGWAY ROTENONE 4W
Insecticide
(Agway)

Rotenone *	4.00%
Other cube resins	8.00%

AGWAY SERAFUME
Fumigant
(Agway)

Carbon tetrachloride *	76.5%
Carbon bisulfide	10.0%
Ethylene dichloride	10.0%
Ethylene dibromide	3.5%

AGWAY SPACE SPRAY
Insecticide
(Agway)

Technical Piperonyl butoxide	2.50%
Pyrethrins	0.30%
Petroleum distillate *	96.87%

AGWAY SYSTEMIC TREE & SHRUB SPRAY
Insecticide
(Agway)

S-(2-(Ethylsulfinyl)ethyl)O,O-di-methyl phosphorothioate	6.0%
Methoxychlor (technical)	5.0%
1,1-Bis(p-chlorophenyl)-2,2,2-trichloroethanol	0.9%
Xylene *	49.6%

AGWAY TEPP 40E
Insecticide
(Agway)

Tetraethyl pyrophosphate *	40.00%
Other ethyl phosphates *	60.00%

AGWAY THIODAN 2E
Insecticide
(Agway)

Endosulfan *	23.70%
Aromatic petroleum distillate *	69.00%

AGWAY THIODAN 3E
Insecticide
(Agway)

Endosulfan *	33.7%
Xylene base aromatic petroleum solvent *	59.7%

AGWAY TOTAL WEED KILLER
(Agway)

2-Methoxy-4,6-bis(isopropylamino)-s-triazine	1.6%/wt.
Petroleum hydrocarbons *	90.6%/wt.

AGWAY TOXAPHENE 6E
Insecticide
(Agway)

Active ingred. (by wt.):

Toxaphene *	60.0%
Xylene *	35.0%

AGWAY VIRMIST CONCENTRATED AEROSOL INSECT KILLER
(Agway)

Pyrethrins	1.07%
Technical Piperonyl butoxide	2.14%
N-Octyl bicycloheptene dicarboximide	2.14%
Petroleum hydrocarbons *	11.60%

AGWAY WEED KILLER "66"
(Agway)

2,4-D Amine (Triethanolamine salt of 2,4-dichlorophenoxy-acetic acid)(equiv. to 2,4-dichlorophenoxyacetic acid 38.6%)) *	64.7%/wt.

Starred ingredients (*) may be responsible for major toxic effects; consult Section II.

AHOY LIQUID DETERGENTS (Green, Pink & Lemon)
(Great Atlantic & Pacific)

Sodium linear alkyl benzene sulfo-
nate (52% active) * 27.0%
Ammonium ethoxylated primary
alcohol sulfate 5.0%
Sodium xylene sulfonate (50%
active) 2.5%
Urea 0.5%
Formaldehyde (37%) 0.3%
Dye, perfume .... trace
Opacifier (not in Green
formulation) .... trace

pH 6.5-7.5

A-H TABLETS
Antihistaminic; veterinary
(Jensen-Salsbery Labs.)

Each tablet:
Doxylamine
succinate * .... 25 mg.; 100 mg.

AIM FLUORIDE DENTIFRICE
(Lever Bros.)

Sodium monofluorophosphate .. <1%
Hydrogenated Starch
hydrolyzate 40-50%
Water 25-30%
Hydrated Silica 10-20%
Polyethylene glycol 1-5%
Sodium alkyl sulfate 1-3%
Ethyl alcohol 1-3%
Flavor .... <2%
Cellulose gum .... <1%
Sodium saccharin .... <1%
Sodium benzoate .... trace
Colorants .... trace

AIM, FORMULA PL-400

See KLENZADE AIM, FORMULA PL-
400

AIM (MINT) FLUORIDE DENTIFRICE
(Lever Bros.)

Sodium monofluorophosphate .. <1%
Hydrogenated Starch
hydrolyzate 40-50%
Water 25-30%
Hydrated Silica 10-20%
Polyethylene glycol 1-5%
Sodium alkyl sulfate 1-3%
Ethyl alcohol 1-3%
Flavor .... <2%
Cellulose gum .... <1%
Sodium saccharin .... <1%
Sodium benzoate .... trace
Colorants .... trace

AIR-DIS

See C-Z AIR-DIS

AIRE-CON
*Air deodorizer, moth proofer and mil-
dew preventative*
(Hysan Corp.)

Combined amount: 100%
Paradichlorobenzene *
Perfume

AIR-GLY
Air sanitizer, conditioner, deodorizer
(Hysan Corp.)

Isopropyl alcohol *
Triethylene glycol
Propylene glycol
Methyldodecylbenzyl trimethylammo-
nium chloride *
Inert ingredients: 80.73%
Dichlorodifluoromethane
Trichloromonofluoromethane
Petroleum distillate *
Perfume

AIROMA HEART
(Carson Chem. Corp.)

Paradichlorobenzene * 99%
Essential oil 1%

'76 Ed.

AIR SWEET DEODORIZING BLOCKS
(Uncle Sam)

Paradichlorobenzene *
Essential oils

AIR SWEET PERFUME SPRAY
(Uncle Sam)

Essential oils *
Emulsifiers
Water

AIR-TOX
Insecticide
(Bonide)

Pyrethrins 0.25%
Technical Piperonyl butoxide ... 2.00%
Petroleum distillate * 12.75%

AIR TREET
Air conditioner, sanitizer, deodorizer
(Hysan Corp.)

Isopropyl alcohol *
Triethylene glycol
Propylene glycol
Methyldodecylbenzyl trimethyl-
ammonium chloride *
Inert ingredients: 80.73%
Dichlorodifluoromethane
Trichloromonofluoromethane
Petroleum distillate *
Perfume

AIRWICK PROFESSIONAL PRODUCTS A-500
*Disinfectant-detergent, odor counter-
actant*
(Airwick)

Active ingred.: 15.36%
Quaternary ammonium compounds *
Inert ingred.: 84.64%
Inorganic builders
Nonionic detergent
Essential oils and aromatics
Urea
Dye

AIRWICK PROFESSIONAL PRODUCTS A.B.C.
Heavy duty bowl cleaner
(Airwick)

Hydrochloric acid * 23.00%
n-Alkyl dimethyl benzyl ammonium chlorides 0.05%
Bis(tri-n-butyltin)oxide 0.01%

pH less than 1.0

AIRWICK PROFESSIONAL PRODUCTS A-33 DRY
*Disinfectant detergent, odor counter-
actant*
(Airwick)

Quaternary ammonium chlorides * 11.6%
Tetrasodium ethylenediamine
tetraacetate 1.0%
Essential oils and aromatics 1.0%
Nonionic detergent .... <15%
Inorganic alkaline builders .... <60%
Urea .... <20%
Dye .... <1%

pH 9.6-10.0 (at use dilution)

AIRWICK PROFESSIONAL PRODUCTS A-125 DRY
Powdered hard surface cleaner
(Airwick)

Alkaline builders *† 76%
Detergent (nonionic and anionic) . <20%
Essential oils and aromatics * .... <5%
Dye .... <1%

pH 10.5-11.5 (at use dilution)

†*See* Builders (detergents)

AIRWICK PROFESSIONAL PRODUCTS A-3 LIQUID
*Disinfectant, detergent, odor counter-
actant*
(Airwick)

Water .... approx. 90%
Nonionic detergent 5.0%
Quaternary ammonium
compounds * 2.5%
Essential oils and aromatics ...... <1.0%
Sodium carbonate
(anhydrous) .... <1.0%
Tetrasodium ethylenediamine
tetraacetate .... <1.0%

pH 9.6-10.2

Starred ingredients (*) may be responsible for major toxic effects; consult Section II.

AIRWICK PROFESSIONAL PRODUCTS A-33 LIQUID
Detergent, disinfectant, odor counteractant
(Airwick)

Water	approx. 85%
Nonionic detergent	<5%
Phosphate	<5%
Quaternary ammonium chloride *	3%
Dye	<1%
Essential oils and aromatics	<1%
Tetrasodium ethylenediamine tetraacetate	<1%

pH 10.0-11.5 (at use dilution)

AIRWICK PROFESSIONAL PRODUCTS A-125 LIQUID
Heavy duty detergent, odor counteractant
(Airwick)

Water	90%
Nonionic detergents	6.5%
Alkaline builders	<5%
Borax	<5%
Essential oils and aromatics	<1%
Color	<1%

pH 8.3-9.3

AIRWICK PROFESSIONAL PRODUCTS AQUINOC
Insecticide deodorant for trash
(Airwick)

Active ingred.:	
Synthetic pyrethroids	0.250%
Related compounds	0.034%
Inert ingred.:	99.716%
Nonionic surfactant	
Dye	
Essential oils and aromatics	
Water	

pH 6.2-7.8

AIRWICK PROFESSIONAL PRODUCTS ARREST BUFFABLE DETERGENT RESISTANT FLOOR FINISH
(Airwick)

Water	approx. 80%
Acrylic copolymer	approx. 12%
Polyethylene wax	approx. 5%
Plasticizing agents	approx. 1%
Coalescing agents	<5%
Surfactant	<1%
Preservative	<1%

pH 8.9-9.1

AIRWICK PROFESSIONAL PRODUCTS ASEPTICARE
Disinfectant/air sanitizer/odor counteractant
(Airwick)

Quaternary ammonium compounds	0.30%
Ethanol	62.74%
Isopropanol	0.42%
Essential oils	0.30%
Water	<15.00%
Hydrocarbon propellant	<21.00%
Corrosion inhibitor	<1.00%
Glycol	<1.00%

AIRWICK PROFESSIONAL PRODUCTS BAC-TEX
Bacteriostatic rug shampoo
(Airwick)

Water	approx. 65%
Anionic detergents	<20%
Sodium lauryl sulfate	9.0%
Isopropanol	5.0%
Optical brighteners	<1%
Phenols	0.7%
Essential oils and aromatics	0.4%
Tetrasodium ethylenediamine tetraacetate	0.2%

pH 8.0-9.0 (at use dilution)

AIRWICK PROFESSIONAL PRODUCTS BRAWN
Lime remover and descaler
(Airwick)

Water	approx. 55%
Phosphoric acid *	<20%
Glycolic acid	<15%
Nonionic detergent	<5%
Antifoam agent	<1%
Dye	<1%
Corrosion inhibitor	<1%

AIRWICK PROFESSIONAL PRODUCTS CBC BOWL CLEANER
(Airwick)

Phosphoric acid *	18%
Nonionic detergent	<1%
Corrosion inhibitors	<1%
Essential oils and aromatics	<1%
Water	approx. 80%

pH <1.0

AIRWICK PROFESSIONAL PRODUCTS CBC PLUS
Toilet bowl cleaner
(Airwick)

Phosphoric acid *	18%
Nonionic detergent	<1%
Corrosion inhibitors	<1%
Thickener	<1%
Dye	<1%
Water	approx. 75%

pH <2

AIRWICK PROFESSIONAL PRODUCTS CONFIDENCE
Floor polish
(Airwick)

Water	approx. 84.0%
Copolymer emulsion	<12.0%
Polyethylene wax emulsion	<3.0%
Plasticizing agent	>5.0%
Resin	>1.5%
Preservative	<1.0%

pH 8.7-9.0

AIRWICK PROFESSIONAL PRODUCTS DEFIANCE DETERGENT RESISTANT FLOOR FINISH
(Airwick)

Water	approx. 80%
Copolymer emulsion	10.0%
Polyethylene wax emulsion	5.5%
Plasticizing agent	approx. 1%
Ammonium hydroxide	<1%
Resin	1.5%
Coalescing agents	<5%
Preservative	1%

pH 8.9-9.1

AIRWICK PROFESSIONAL PRODUCTS ENTACIDE
Insecticide aerosol
(Airwick)

Active ingred.:	
Pyrethrins	0.30%
Piperonyl butoxide (technical)	0.60%
N-Octyl bicycloheptene dicarboximide	1.00%
Petroleum distillate	1.35%
Inert ingred.:	
Essential oils and aromatics	0.30%
Combined amount:	96.45%
Water	
Hydrocarbon propellant	

AIRWICK PROFESSIONAL PRODUCTS ENTACIDE R
Residual insecticide aerosol
(Airwick)

Active ingred.:	
Diazinon	0.500%
Pyrethrins	0.045%
Piperonyl butoxide (technical)	0.090%
N-Octyl bicycloheptene dicarboximide	0.151%
Petroleum distillates *	89.710%
Inert ingred.:	9.504%
Essential oils and aromatics *	
Hydrocarbon propellant	

Starred ingredients (*) may be responsible for major toxic effects; consult Section II.

AIRWICK PROFESSIONAL PRODUCTS ESCAPE STRIPPER
Ammoniated synthetic detergent
(Airwick)

Water	approx. 85%
Nonionic detergent	<5%
Monoethanolamine	5%
Ammonium hydroxide *	<5%
Phosphate	<5%
Dye	<1%
Chelating agent	<1%
Cellosolve	<5%

pH 12.0-12.5

AIRWICK PROFESSIONAL PRODUCTS F/H
Detergent/disinfectant
(Airwick)

Water	91.6%
Quaternary ammonium compounds *	5.12%
Nonionic detergent	5.00%
Sodium carbonate	2.20%
EDTA	1.08%

pH 11.5-11.9

AIRWICK PROFESSIONAL PRODUCTS FOAM-TEX
Dry foam rug shampoo
(Airwick)

Isopropanol	<10%
Essential oils and aromatics	<1%
Optical brighteners	<1%
Chelating agent	<1%
Water	approx. 80%
Anionic detergents	<10%
Preservative	<1%

pH 6.5-7.2 at use dilution of 1:8

AIRWICK PROFESSIONAL PRODUCTS GOLD LABEL LIQUID, GREEN LABEL LIQUID, RED LABEL LIQUID
Odor counteractant
(Airwick)

Water	approx. 95%
Nonionic emulsifiers	<5%
Anionic emulsifiers	<5%
Essential oils and aromatics *	<5%
Dye	<1%
Preservative	<1%

pH 6.0-7.0

AIRWICK PROFESSIONAL PRODUCTS GOLD LABEL MIST
Odor counteractant spray
(Airwick)

Water	approx. 70%
Isobutane (propellant)	<25%
Essential oils and aromatics	<1%
Corrosion inhibitors	<1%
Emulsifiers	<2%

AIRWICK PROFESSIONAL PRODUCTS OMEGA
Detergent, disinfectant, odor counteractant
(Airwick)

Active ingred.:	
Quaternary ammonium compounds *	12.00%
EDTA	3.12%
Sodium carbonate	0.50%
Essential oils and aromatics	0.50%
Inert ingred.:	83.88%
Water	
Nonionic detergent	
Amphoteric detergent	
Dye	

pH 10.5-11.5

AIRWICK PROFESSIONAL PRODUCTS OMNIPAK
Powdered detergent/stripper
(Airwick)

Alkaline builders *†	65%
Anionic and nonionic detergents	<20%
EDTA salt	3%
Sodium metasilicate pentahydrate *	<13%
Essential oils and aromatics	<1%
Dye	<1%
Silicone emulsion	<1%

pH 10.5-11.5 (at use dilution)

†*See* Builders (detergents)

AIRWICK PROFESSIONAL PRODUCTS PADLOCK SEALER
(Airwick)

Water	approx. 80%
Acrylic polymer	approx. 15%
Glycol	approx. 3%
Plasticizing agents	<1%
Ammonium hydroxide	<1%
Surfactant	<1%
Preservative	<1%

pH 9.3-9.7

AIRWICK PROFESSIONAL PRODUCTS PRO-TEX
Rug shampoo
(Airwick)

Water	approx. 60%
Anionic detergent *	approx. 25%
Ethylene glycol monoethyl ether	10%
Essential oils and aromatics	<1%
Optical brighteners	<1%
Chelating agent	<1%
Preservative	<1%

pH 8.5-9.8 at use dilution of 1:40

AIRWICK PROFESSIONAL PRODUCTS SENTRY LIQUID
Toilet bowl cleaner/deodorant
(Airwick)

Synthetic detergents solution	approx. 70%
Essential oils and aromatics *	<15%
Dye solution	<10%
Chelating agent	<5%
Monoethanolamine	<5%
Preservative	<5%
Silicone	<1%

pH 9.1-9.9

AIRWICK PROFESSIONAL PRODUCTS SENTRY SOLID
Toilet bowl cleaner/deodorant
(Airwick)

Inorganic builders	<70%
Water	<15%
Essential oils and aromatics *	<5%
Dye	<1%
Silicone	<1%
Synthetic detergents	<10%

AIRWICK PROFESSIONAL PRODUCTS SOLIDAIRE
Green Label, Red Label, Blue Label, Gold Label, Silver Label, Citrus, Spearmint
Solid gel odor counteractants
(Airwick)

Water	approx. 95%
Gelling agents	<5%
Essential oils and aromatics *	<5%
Coloring agent	<1%
Emulsifier	<1%
Preservative	<1%

pH 7

AIRWICK PROFESSIONAL PRODUCTS SOLIDAIRE PLUS
Copper, Orange, Purple
Odor counteractants
(Airwick)

Water	<85%
Gelling agents	<5%
Essential oils and aromatics *	<10%
Pigment	<1%
Emulsifier	<5%
Preservative	<1%
Glycol	5%

AIRWICK PROFESSIONAL PRODUCTS SPRITZ
Liquid solvent detergent cleaner
(Airwick)

Water	<90%
Butyl Cellosolve *	<10%
Detergent	5%
Sodium metasilicate pentahydrate	1%
Dye	<1%
Essential oils and aromatics	<0.1%

pH 12.0-13.0

AJAX ALL-PURPOSE CLEANER
(Colgate-Palmolive)

Ammonium	approx. 1%
Tetrapotassium pyrophosphate	approx. 10%
Sodium carbonate	approx. 3%
Synthetic detergents	approx. 6%

'76 Ed.

AJAX CLEANSER (With Bleach and Disinfectant)
(Colgate-Palmolive)

Trichloro-s-triazinetrione	0.50%
Sodium dodecyl benzene sulfonate	3.65%
Trisodium phosphate	3.95%
Sodium bromide	0.70%
Silica	90%

'76 Ed.

AJAX LAUNDRY DETERGENT
(Colgate-Palmolive)

Combined amount:	14%
Alkyl benzene sulfonate *	
Soap	
Nonionic surfactant	
Inorganic builders:	74.6%
Phosphate *	
Silicate *	
Sodium sulfate	
Color, perfume, and minor ingredients	1.8%
Moisture	9.5%

'76 Ed.

AJAX LIQUID DETERGENT
(Colgate-Palmolive)

Alkyl aryl sulfonate *	approx. 15%
Ethoxylated alcohol sulfate	approx. 20%
Alcohol	approx. 6%
Organic builders and stabilizers	approx. 6%

'76 Ed.

AJAX TOILET BOWL CLEANER
(Colgate-Palmolive)

Water	72%
Hydrochloric acid *	26%
Opacifier	1%
Ethoxylated alkyl phenol	
Dehydroabietylamine ethoxylate	
Isopropanol	

AJAX WINDOW CLEANER WITH HEXAMMONIA
(Colgate-Palmolive)

Water	>90%
Combined amount:	3%
Ethylene glycol monoethyl ether	
Propylene glycol monomethyl ether	
Isopropyl alcohol	4%
Combined amount:	<1%
Sodium nitrite	
Sodium phosphate	
Anionic detergent	
Ammonium hydroxide	

'76 Ed.

AKRO-FLINT
Two component epoxy used as high gloss enamel; interior-exterior
(Akron Paint & Varnish Co.)

Lead free
Ketone solvents *

AKROS ALUMINUM PAINT
(Akron Paint & Varnish Co.)

Aluminum pigment
Mineral spirits *

AKROS BLACK ENAMEL
(Akron Paint & Varnish Co.)

Carbon black
Mineral spirits *

AKROS EGGSHELL ENAMEL
(Akron Paint & Varnish Co.)

Titanium pigment
Mineral spirits *

AKROS FLOOR & TRIM ENAMEL
(Akron Paint & Varnish Co.)

Titanium pigment
Mineral spirits *

AKROS PAINT PRODUCTS
Paints, varnishes & industrial finishes

Akron Paint & Varnish Co.
Firestone Park Sta.
Box 2765
Akron, Ohio 44301

Phone: 216-773-8911

See PAINTS, Section VI, General Formulations

AKROS PLIOLITE FLOOR ENAMEL
(Akron Paint & Varnish Co.)

Titanium pigment
Aromatic solvent *

AKROS SHINGLE STAINS
(Akron Paint & Varnish Co.)

Titanium pigment
Mineral spirits *

AKROS TRAFFIC & CURB PAINT
(Akron Paint & Varnish Co.)

Yellow:
Lead chromate *
Mineral spirits *

White:
Lead	trace
Titanium pigment	
Mineral spirits *	

AKROS VINYL LATEX
(Akron Paint & Varnish Co.)

Titanium pigment
Latex

AKROS WHITE ENAMEL
(Akron Paint & Varnish Co.)

Titanium pigment
Mineral spirits *

AKTROL
Neutralizes excessive pool alkalinity
(Modern Pool Products)

Sulphuric acid *

ALANAP
Herbicide
(Uniroyal Chem.)

Sodium N-1-naphthylphthalamate	23.7%

ALANAP LIQUID
Herbicide
(Uniroyal Chem.)

Sodium N-1-naphthylphthalamate	23%

ALAR-85
Plant growth regulant
(Uniroyal Chem.)

Succinic acid 2,2-dimethyl hydrazide	85.0%

ALASKA DEODORIZED FISH FERTILIZER
(Alaska)

Organic nitrogen	4%
Ammoniacal nitrogen	1%
Total Nitrogen	5%
Available Phosphoric acid	1%
Water-soluble Potash	1%

Starred ingredients (*) may be responsible for major toxic effects; consult Section II.

AL-AY (C.T. GREEN)
Nasal decongestant
(Bowman Pharm.)

Each tablet:
Phenylephrine HCl		5 mg.
Chlorpheniramine maleate		2 mg.
Aspirin *		162 mg.
Caffeine		15 mg.
Aminoacetic acid		162 mg.

AL-AY (S.C.T. DARK GREEN)
Nasal decongestant
(Bowman Pharm.)

Each tablet:
Phenylephrine HCl		5 mg.
Chlorpheniramine maleate		2 mg.
Acetaminophen *		160 mg.
Caffeine		15 mg.

ALBALON-A LIQUIFILM STERILE OPHTHALMIC SOLUTION
(Allergan Pharm.)

Naphazoline HCl	0.05%
Antazoline phosphate	0.50%
Polyvinyl alcohol	1.40%

ALBALON LIQUIFILM
Ophthalmic solution
(Allergan Pharm.)

Naphazoline HCl	0.1%
Polyvinyl alcohol	1.4%

ALBERTO-CULVER CO. COSMETIC PRODUCTS
Cosmetics and toiletries

Alberto-Culver Co.
2525 Armitage Ave.
Melrose Park, Ill. 60160

Phone: 312-450-3175

See COSMETICS, Section VI, General Formulations

ALBERTO VO5 CONDITIONING HAIRDRESSING, REGULAR
(Alberto-Culver)

Mineral oil light
Petrolatum
Lanolin
PEG-8 dilaurate
Paraffin
Isopropyl myristate
Fragrance
BHA

ALBERTO VO5 EXTRA BODY SHAMPOO
(Alberto-Culver)

Water
Sodium laureth sulfate
Lauramide DEA
Sodium chloride
Fragrance
Phosphoric acid
Methylparaben
Formaldehyde
FD & C Yellow #5
FD & C Red #40
FD & C Blue #1

ALBERTO VO5 HAIRSETTING GEL
(Alberto-Culver)

Water
SD Alcohol 40
PVP
Glycerine
Carbomer-940
Oleth-20
Diisopropanolamine
Fragrance
Methylparaben
Formaldehyde
Hydrolyzed animal protein
EDTA
FD & C Yellow #6
D & C Red #19

ALBERTO VO5 HAIRSETTING LOTION (Extra Hold)
(Alberto-Culver)

Water
SD Alcohol 40
PVP K30
Formaldehyde
Oleth-20
Fragrance
FD & C Yellow #5
FD & C Red #40

ALBERTO VO5 HAIRSETTING LOTION (Natural Hold)
(Alberto-Culver)

Water
SD Alcohol 40
PVP K30
Formaldehyde
Oleth-20
Fragrance
FD & C Red #40

ALBERTO VO5 HAIR SPRAY
(Alberto-Culver)

SD Alcohol 40
Isobutane/propane
Methylene chloride
Ethyl ester of PVM/MA copolymer
Fragrance
Aminomethyl propanol
Other ingredients

ALBERTO VO5 HOT OIL TREATMENT
(Alberto-Culver)

Water
Cocotrimonium chloride
PEI-1500
PEI-1500 hydrochloride
Acetamide MEA
Hydroxyethylcellulose
Oleth-20
Fragrance
Methylparaben
Polyquaternium 10
FD & C Yellow #6

ALBERTO VO5 HOT PROTEIN PAC
(Alberto-Culver)

Water
Polawax
Ethylene glycol stearate
Arlacel 165
Avitex ML
Acetylated Lanolin
Albumen (Lanalbine CG)
Quaternium 33
Stearalkonium chloride
Isopropyl myristate
Mineral oil
Lanolin alcohol
Quaternium 31
PPG-2 lanolin ether
Lauryl alcohol
Formaldehyde
Fragrance
Preservatives
FD & C Yellow #6
FD & C Yellow #5

ALBERTO VO5 NON-AEROSOL HAIR SPRAY
Pump bottle
(Alberto-Culver)

SD Alcohol 40
Ethyl ester of PVM/MA copolymer
Aminomethyl propanol
Fragrance

ALBERTO VO5 SHAMPOO FOR DRY HAIR
(Alberto-Culver)

Water
Sodium laureth sulfate
Lauramide DEA
Sodium chloride
Fragrance
Phosphoric acid
Methylparaben
Formaldehyde
FD & C Yellow #5
FD & C Blue #1

Starred ingredients (*) may be responsible for major toxic effects; consult Section II.

ALBERTO VO5 SHAMPOO FOR NORMAL HAIR
(Alberto-Culver)

Water
Sodium laureth sulfate
Lauramide DEA
Sodium chloride
Fragrance
Phosphoric acid
Methylparaben
Formaldehyde
FD & C Yellow No. 6

ALBERTO VO5 SHAMPOO FOR OILY HAIR
(Alberto-Culver)

Water
Sodium laureth sulfate
Lauramide DEA
Sodium chloride
Fragrance
Phosphoric acid
Methylparaben
Formaldehyde
Sodium sulfite
FD & C Blue

ALBERTO VO5 SHAMPOO W/ESSENCE OF JOJOBA
(Alberto-Culver)

Water
Sodium laureth sulfate
Lauramide DEA
Sodium chloride
Fragrance
Phosphoric acid
Methylparaben
Formaldehyde
Jojoba oil
Caramel
FD & C Red #4
FD & C Red #33

ALBERTO VO5 SHAMPOO W/ESSENCE OF NEUTRAL HENNA
(Alberto-Culver)

Water
Sodium laureth sulfate
Lauramide DEA
Sodium chloride
Fragrance
Phosphoric acid
Methylparaben
Formaldehyde
Henna extract
Caramel

ALBORADA MOISTURIZING CREAM
(Jeffrey Martin, Inc.)

Purified water
Isopropyl palmitate
Mineral oil
Stearic acid
Cetyl alcohol
Lanolin
Sorbitol
Glyceryl stearate
Petrolatum
Dimethicone
Tocopheryl acetate
Retinyl palmitate
Ergocalciferol
Allantoin
Pyridoxine-HCl
Panthenol
PEG-100-stearate
Vegetable oil
Carbomer-940
Triethanolamine
Methylparaben
Butylparaben
Imidazolidinyl urea
Quaternium-15
Fragrance

AL-BRITE
Concentrated aluminum cleaner & brightener
(ABCO, Inc.)

Hydrofluoric acid *

ALBUSTIX
Urine protein test reagent strip
(Ames)

Tetrabromphenol blue
FD & C Yellow
Citrate buffer
Bibulous strip of cellulose

ALCOJET
Cleaner for hospital, laboratory & industrial glassware by machine methods
(Alconox)

Complex phosphate *
Silicates
Wetting agents (Polyoxyethylene ester of mixed fatty & rosin acids)

AL-CON, MUNICHEM
See MUNICHEM AL-CON

ALCONEFRIN (12, 25 & 50)
Decongestant nose drops
(Alcon)

Phenylephrine HCl
    Alconefrin 12: 0.16%
    Alconefrin 25: 0.25%
    Alconefrin 50: 0.50%

Preservatives:
    Benzalkonium chloride
    Sodium bisulfite

ALCONOX
Laboratory detergent
(Alconox)

Hydrocarbon sulfonates (derived from linear alkylates, biodegradable) *†
Complex phosphates *

†*See* Alkyl aryl sodium sulfonates

ALCO-REX
Rubefacient
(Rexall)

Absolute Alcohol * 70%

'76 Ed.

ALCOTABS
Detergent tablets
(Alconox)

Hydrocarbon sulfonates (derived from linear alkylates, biodegradable) *†

†*See* Alkyl aryl sodium sulfonates

ALERMINE
Antihistamine
(Direct Div.)

Each tablet:
    Chlorpheniramine maleate * .... 4 mg.

ALERTACAPS
See DEWITT'S ALERTACAPS

ALERT-PEP CAPSULES
Induces alert clear thought, heightens muscular & mental capacities
(Approved Pharm.)

Each capsule, time disintegration (6-8 hours):
    Caffeine * .... 200 mg.

'76 Ed.

ALEVAIRE
Detergent aerosol for inhalation
(Breon Labs.)

Superinone (brand of tyloxapol) . 0.125%
Sodium bicarbonate 2%
Glycerin 5%

ALEXANDRA DE MARKOFF COSMETICS

Alexandra De Markoff
Sub. of Charles of the Ritz Group, Ltd.
40 W. 57th St.
New York, N.Y. 10019

Phone: 212-621-7300

See COSMETICS, Section VI, General Formulations

Starred ingredients (*) may be responsible for major toxic effects; consult Section II.

ALFA-TOX
Insecticide
(Ciba-Geigy Ag. Div.)

Methoxychlor (technical) 20%
Diazinon 10%
Aromatic petroleum derivative
solvent * 63%

ALGAECIDE B BRIQUETTES
(Lester Labs.)

Sodium pentachlorophenate *
Related compounds

'76 Ed.

ALGAE KIL
To control algae growth in swimming pools
(Haviland Products Co.)

n-Alkyl dimethyl benzyl ammonium
chloride * 10%

'76 Ed.

ALGATROL
For control of algae in swimming pools
(Kem Mfg. Co.)

n-Alkyl (C14-50%, C12-40%, C16-
10%)dimethyl benzyl ammo-
nium chlorides * 10.00%

ALGEM
Swimming pool algaecide
(Modern Pool Products)

Alkenyl dimethyl ethyl ammonium
bromide * 10%

ALGEM CONCENTRATE
Algaecide for swimming pools
(Modern Pool Products)

Alkenyl (C18 90%, C16 10%) dimethyl
ethyl ammonium bromide * 75%

ALGEPON XR CONCENTRATE
Cationic fulling & scouring auxiliary to minimize dye migration
(Arkansas Co.)

Combination of:
Quaternary nitrogen
compound *† .... approx. 10%
Pyrrolidone derivative ... approx. 35%

'76 Ed.

†*See* Cationic surfactants

ALGEX
Liquid algae & slime control
(Lester Labs.)

Quaternary ammonium chlorides *
Organic tin *†
Isopropyl alcohol *

'76 Ed.

†*See* Organotin compounds

ALGEX CONCENTRATE RUB
Analgesic
(Approved Pharm.)

Menthol *
Camphor *
Methyl salicylate *
Eucalyptus *

'76 Ed.

ALGICIDE 28X

See BIO-GUARD ALGICIDE 28X

ALGI-CURE

See ACTION ALGI-CURE

ALGIMYCIN GLB-X
For algae control in ornamental ponds and pools
(Great Lakes Biochemical)

Monuron (3-(p-Chlorophenyl)-1,1-
dimethylurea) 1.50%
Simazine (2-Chloro-4,6-
bis(ethylamino)-s-triazine) 1.10%
Atrazine (2-Chloro-4-ethylamino-6-
isopropylamino-s-triazine) 0.4%

ALGIMYCIN PLL-C
For algae control in ponds, lakes, lagoons
(Great Lakes Biochemical)

Copper as metallic in the form of: Chelate of copper citrate *, Chelate of
copper gluconate * 5%

ALISED
Antacid, antispasmodic
(Elder)

Each tablet:
Phenobarbital * .... 8.0 mg.
Atropine sulfate * .... 0.13 mg.
Calcium carbonate .... 226.0 mg.
Magnesium carbonate ..... 162.0 mg.

ALKAD
Additive for control of pH and bacteria in water coolant systems
(Whitfield Chem.)

Potassium tetraborate * .... >10%
Dithiocarbamates 5-10%

ALKAGEL TABLETS
Antacid
(Towne, Paulsen)

Each tablet:
Co-precipitate gel: .... 400 mg.
Aluminum hydroxide
Magnesium carbonate
Glycine .... 50 mg.

ALKALOL
Antiseptic alkaline solution
(Alkalol)

Alcohol 0.05%
Thymol *
Eucalyptol *
Menthol *
Camphor *
Benzoin
Potassium alum
Potassium chlorate *
Sodium bicarbonate
Sodium chloride
Oils of:
Sweet birch, Spearmint, Pine, Cassia

ALKA-SELTZER EFFERVESCENT ANTACID
(Miles Labs., Inc.)

Each tablet:
Sodium bicarbonate * ...... 1008 mg.
Citric acid .... 800 mg.
Potassium bicarbonate * ... 300 mg.

In water the product contains the following
ions:
Sodium .... 276 mg.
Potassium .... 117 mg.
Citrates .... 788 mg.
Bicarbonate .... 123 mg.

ALKA-SELTZER EFFERVESCENT PAIN RELIEVER AND ANTACID
(Miles Labs., Inc.)

Each tablet:
Aspirin * .... 324 mg.
Sodium bicarbonate .... 1904 mg.
Citric acid .... 1000 mg.

In water the product contains the following
ions:
Acetylsalicylate .... 322 mg.
Sodium .... 521 mg.
Citrates .... 985 mg.
Bicarbonate .... 337 mg.

ALKA-SELTZER PLUS COLD MEDICINE
(Miles Labs., Inc.)

Each tablet:
Phenylpropanolamine
bitartrate * .... 24.08 mg.
Chlorpheniramine maleate   2.00 mg.
Acetylsalicylic acid
(Aspirin) * .... 324.00 mg.

Starred ingredients (*) may be responsible for major toxic effects; consult Section II.

ALKASOL
Liquid paint stripper cleaner
(Whitfield Chem.)

Combined amount:	>10%
Sodium hydroxide *	
and/or	
Potassium hydroxide *	
Glycols	>10%

ALKASTRIP
Paint stripper, cleaner
(Whitfield Chem.)

Caustic soda *	>10%
Sodium or potassium phenolates *	>10%

ALKA-2 CHEWABLE ANTACID
(Miles Labs., Inc.)

Each tablet:
Calcium carbonate	500 mg.

ALKETS TABLETS
Antacid
(Upjohn)

Each tablet:
Calcium carbonate	
(precipitated)	780 mg.
Magnesium carbonate	130 mg.
Magnesium oxide	65 mg.

Sucrose, Starch, Calcium stearate, Mineral oil, Artificial flavor, and Color

ALKYD SANI-FLAT (WHITE 204-01)
Interior paint
(Benjamin Moore)

Pigment:	61.6%
Titanium dioxide (type II)	23.6%
Calcium carbonate	15.7%
Silicates	60.7%
Vehicle:	38.4%
Alkyd varnish:	55.8%
Soya alkyd resin	35.8%
Mineral spirits *	64.2%
Mineral spirits *	41.4%
Naphthas	2.4%
Driers	0.4%

ALLANO HAND AND BODY LOTION

See AMWAY ALLANO HAND AND BODY LOTION

ALLBEE C-800 PLUS IRON
Vitamin supplement with iron
(Robins)

Each tablet:
Iron	27 mg.
Plus multivitamins	

ALL-BRANDS WAX REMOVER
(Lehn & Fink)

Ammonium hydroxide	minor
Sodium metasilicate	minor
Ethylene glycol monobutyl ether	minor
Monoethanolamine	minor

ALLCLEAR, WARDLEY'S

See WARDLEY'S ALLCLEAR

"all", CONCENTRATED (Low Phosphate)

See CONCENTRATED "all" (Low Phosphate)

"all", CONCENTRATED (Nonphosphate)

See CONCENTRATED "all" (Nonphosphate)

ALLERDEC CAPSULES
Hay fever & pollen allergy relief
(Towne, Paulsen)

Each capsule:
Phenylpropanolamine HCl *	25 mg.
Chlorpheniramine maleate *	1 mg.
Methapyrilene HCl *	5 mg.
Pyrilamine maleate *	5 mg.

ALLEREST CHILDREN'S CHEWABLE TABLETS
Decongestant, antihistaminic
(Pharmacraft)

Each chewable tablet:
Phenylpropanolamine *	9.4 mg.
Chlorpheniramine	1.0 mg.

ALLEREST EYE DROPS
(Pharmacraft)

Methyl cellulose	
Naphazoline HCl	0.012%
Disodium edetate	0.100%
Benzalkonium chloride	0.010%
Boric acid	
Sodium borate	

ALLEREST NASAL SPRAY
(Pharmacraft)

Phenylephrine	0.5%

ALLEREST TABLETS
Decongestant, antihistaminic
(Pharmacraft)

Each tablet:
Phenylpropanolamine *	18.75 mg.
Chlorpheniramine	2.00 mg.

ALLEREST TIME CAPSULES
Decongestant, antihistaminic
(Pharmacraft)

Each capsule:
Chlorpheniramine maleate	4 mg.
Phenylpropanolamine HCl *	50 mg.

ALLERGAN ATROPINE SULFATE
Ophthalmic solutions
(Allergan Pharm.)

Atropine sulfate *	1%; 2%; and 4%
Chlorobutanol (chloral derivative as a preservative)	0.5%
Boric acid	
Sodium citrate	
Purified water	

ALLERGESIC TABLETS
Anti-allergy tablet
(Vitarine)

Each tablet:
Phenylpropanolamine hydrochloride *	18.7 mg.
Chlorpheniramine maleate *	2.0 mg.

ALLERGEX AEROSOL
House dust inhibitor
(Hollister-Stier Labs.)

Dow 500M or Carbowax 1500
Roccal *
GE 60 Silicone Antifoam
Triton X-45
Triton X-100
Sodium nitrate *
Morpholine *
Methyl hydroxybenzoate
Water
Isobutane (propellant)

ALLERGICAPS
Symptomatic relief of hayfever, colds & allergies
(Approved Pharm.)

Each capsule:
Phenylpropanolamine HCl *	25 mg.
Chlorpheniramine maleate *	1 mg.
Methapyrilene fumarate	5 mg.

'76 Ed.

ALLERSTAT
Decongestant-antihistaminic
(Lemmon Co.)

Each capsule:
Phenylpropanolamine hydrochloride *	25 mg.
Phenylephrine hydrochloride *	2.5 mg.
Pheniramine maleate *	12.5 mg.
Pyrilamine maleate *	12.5 mg.

Starred ingredients (*) may be responsible for major toxic effects; consult Section II.

ALLEVIATE FOOD PLANT FOGGING SPRAY (OIL BASE)
Insecticide (indoor)
(Fairfield American)

Allethrin	1.25%
Related compounds	0.14%
Piperonyl butoxide	5.00%
Petroleum distillate *	93.61%

"all", FLUFFY (Low Phosphate)

See FLUFFY "all" (Low Phosphate)

"all", LIQUID (Low Phosphate)

See LIQUID "all" (Low Phosphate)

"all", LIQUID (Nonphosphate)

See LIQUID "all" (Nonphosphate)

ALLRAT
Rodenticide
(B&G Co.)

3-(alpha-Acetonylfurfuryl)-4-hydroxycoumarin	0.025%

ALL SEASON WINDSHIELD WASHER
(Texaco Canada Ltd.)

Methyl alcohol *
Surfactant *
Dye

ALL SEASON 10W-30 MOTOR OIL
(Marathon Oil Co.)

Additives, containing Zinc alkyl dithiophosphate, Olefin copolymer	20%
Mineral oil	balance

ALLWITE LIQUID, GRIFFIN

See GRIFFIN ALLWITE LIQUID

ALLYLGESIC
Sedative, analgesic
(Elder)

Each tablet:
Acetaminophen *	100 mg.
Aluminum aspirin *	100 mg.
Aspirin *	150 mg.
Diallyl barbituric acid *	15 mg.

ALLYLGESIC W/ ERGOTAMINE
Migraine headaches
(Elder)

Each capsule:
Ergotamine tartrate *	1 mg.
Acetaminophen *	100 mg.
Aluminum aspirin *	100 mg.
Aspirin *	150 mg.
Allobarbital *	15 mg.

ALMAY CHIP RESISTANT TOP COAT
(Almay)

Butyl acetate *
Petroleum distillate naphtha
Nitrocellulose
Isopropanol
Ethyl acetate
Dibutyl phthalate
Polyester resin
Camphor

ALMAY CLEAN AND GENTLE DAILY SHAMPOO
(Almay)

Water
Sodium laureth sulfate
TEA lauryl sulfate
Sodium chloride
Lauramide DEA
Citric acid
Disodium EDTA
Methylparaben
Propylparaben
Imidazolidinyl urea
Benzophenone-4
FD & C Yellow No. 5
FD & C Blue No. 1
D & C Red No. 33

ALMAY CLEAN AND GENTLE OIL-FREE CONDITIONER
(Almay)

Water
Propylene glycol
Stearalkonium chloride
Hydroxyethylcellulose
Emulsifying wax NF
Magnesium aluminum silicate
Methylparaben
Propylparaben
Imidazolidinyl urea
Benzophenone-4
Citric acid
FD & C Yellow No. 5
D & C Green No. 5

ALMAY CUTICLE TREATMENT OIL
(Almay)

Castor oil
PEG-40 sorbitan peroleate
Propylene glycol isostearate
Mineral oil
Propylparaben
BHA
D & C Red No. 17

ALMAY DEEP CLEANSING COLD CREAM
(Almay)

Mineral oil
Water
Beeswax
Synthetic Spermaceti
Sodium borate
Glyceryl stearate
Methylparaben
Propylparaben

ALMAY DEEP MIST GENTLE GEL MASK
(Almay)

Water
SD Alcohol 40
PVP
Carbomer 940
Triethanolamine
Methylparaben
Choleth 24
Propylparaben
FD & C Blue No. 1
D & C Yellow No. 10

ALMAY DEEP MIST PURIFYING FRESHENER
(Almay)

Water
SD Alcohol 40
Sorbitol
Polysorbate 80
Methylparaben
Propylparaben
Tetrasodium EDTA
FD & C Yellow No. 6
D & C Red No. 33
D & C Yellow No. 10

ALMAY DEEP MIST PURIFYING TONER
(Almay)

Water
SD Alcohol 40
Sorbitol
Polysorbate-80
Trisodium EDTA
D & C Red No. 33
FD & C Blue No. 1

ALMAY DEEP PORE CLEANSING MASK
(Almay)

Water
Kaolin
SD Alcohol 40
Bentonite
Fuller's earth
Propylene glycol
Glyceryl stearate SE
Methylparaben
Propylparaben
Sodium polymethacrylate
May contain: Iron oxides, Ultramarine blue, Titanium dioxide

ALMAY ENAMEL QUICK DRY
(Almay)

Cyclomethicone
Safflower oil
Oleic acid
Propylparaben
BHA
Methylparaben

ALMAY EXTRA LIGHT FORMULA FACIAL CLEANSER
(Almay)

Water
Stearic acid
Propylene glycol
Oleic acid
Potassium hydroxide
Methylparaben
Propylparaben
Imidazolidinyl urea

ALMAY FRESH FINISH BALANCED MAKEUP
(Almay)

Water
Talc
Titanium dioxide
Mineral oil
Propylene glycol
Stearic acid
Imidazolidinyl urea
Triethanolamine
Magnesium aluminum silicate
Glyceryl stearate
Cetyl alcohol
Cellulose gum
Methylparaben
Propylparaben
Sodium polymethacrylate
May contain: Iron oxides, Ultramarine blue

ALMAY FRESH GLOW MOISTURIZING MAKEUP
(Almay)

Water
Mineral oil
Octyl hydroxystearate
Squalene
Propylene glycol
Stearic acid
Glyceryl stearate SE
Triethanolamine
Magnesium aluminum silicate
Propylparaben
Methylparaben
Imidazolidinyl urea
Cellulose gum
May contain: Talc, Titanium dioxide, Iron oxides, Ultramarine blue

ALMAY FRESH LOOK OIL-FREE MAKEUP
(Almay)

Water
Glycerin
Talc
PEG-4
Magnesium aluminum silicate
Sodium polymethacrylate
Imidazolidinyl urea
PVP
Methylparaben
Cellulose gum
Titanium dioxide
Propylparaben
Iron oxides

ALMAY GENTLE ACTION ENAMEL REMOVER
(Almay)

Butyl acetate *
Ethyl acetate
n-Butyl alcohol
Propylene glycol dicaprylate/dicaprate

ALMAY HIGH GLOSS NAIL GUARD
(Almay)

Butyl acetate *
Toluene
Nitrocellulose
Ethyl acetate
Polyester resin
Isopropyl alcohol
Dibutyl phthalate
Camphor
Acrylates copolymer
UV absorber-1

ALMAY LONGER LASTING LASHES WATERPROOF MASCARA
(Almay)

Petroleum distillate or C11-12 Isoparaffin or C10-13 Isoparaffin or C11-13 Isoparaffin
Talc
Hydrogenated Castor oil
Beeswax
Alkylated PVP
Quaternium-18 hectorite
Microcrystalline wax
Propylene carbonate
Castor oil
Polybutene
Mineral oil
Lanolin oil
Propylparaben
Methylparaben
Imidazolidinyl urea
Propylene glycol
BHA
Propyl gallate
Citric acid
May contain: Titanium dioxide, Iron oxides, Chromium hydroxide green, Ultramarine blue

ALMAY MOISTURE RICH LIPSTICK (FROSTED AND CREME)
(Almay)

Castor oil
Lanolin oil
Myristyl myristate
Isopropyl lanolate
Microcrystalline wax
Octyl dodecanol
TriLaurin
Cetyl alcohol
Ozokerite
Candelilla wax
Carnauba
Propylparaben
Propylene glycol
BHA
Propyl gallate
Citric acid
May contain: Safflower glyceride, Titanium dioxide, Iron oxides, D & C Red No. 3 aluminum lake, D & C Red No. 6 barium lake, D & C Red No. 7 calcium/strontium lake, D & C Red No. 9 barium lake, D & C Red No. 19 aluminum lake, D & C Red No. 30 lake, D & C Yellow No. 5 aluminum lake, D & C Orange No. 17 lake, D & C Yellow No. 6 aluminum lake, D & C Red No. 36 lake, Mica, Bismuth oxychloride, Carmine

ALMAY MOISTURIZING EYE MAKEUP REMOVER PADS
(Almay)

Soft cotton flannel pads saturated with:
Light mineral oil
Propylene glycol dicaprylate/dicaprate
Propylparaben
Methylparaben

ALMAY NON-OILY EYE MAKEUP REMOVER
(Almay)

Water
Poloxamer 184
Amphoteric-6
Imidazolidinyl urea
Methylparaben
Propylparaben

ALMAY OIL CONTROL FACIAL CLEANSER
(Almay)

Water
Ammonium lauryl sulfate
SD Alcohol 40
Oleyl alcohol
Methylparaben
Propylparaben
D & C Green No. 5
FD & C Yellow No. 6
FD & C Red No. 33
D & C Yellow No. 10

ALMAY OIL CONTROL PURIFYING PORE LOTION
(Almay)

Water
SD Alcohol 40
Polysorbate-80
Tetrasodium EDTA
FD & C Blue No. 1
FD & C Yellow No. 5

ALMAY PROFESSIONAL FORMULA EYEBROW AND LINER PENCILS
(Almay)

TriLaurin
Polyethylene
Talc
Japan wax
Octyl dodecanol
Carnauba
Methylparaben
Propylparaben
Butylparaben
BHA
BHT
Citric acid
May contain: Titanium dioxide, Mica, Ultramarine blue, Ferric ammonium ferrocyanide, Iron oxides, Chromium oxide greens, Chromium hydroxide green

ALMAY PROTECTIVE BASE COAT
(Almay)

Butyl acetate *
Isopropanol
Toluol
Ethyl acetate
Polyvinyl butyral
Nitrocellulose
Dibutyl phthalate
Polyester resin
Ferric ferrocyanide

ALMAY PROTEIN CONDITIONING HAIRSPRAY (NON-AEROSOL)
(Almay)

SD Alcohol 40
Butyl ester of PVM/MA copolymer
Water
Animal protein derivative
Aminomethyl propanol
Dimethicone copolyol
Trisodium EDTA

ALMAY PURE AND GENTLE EVERYDAY CONDITIONING SHAMPOO
(Almay)

Water
Sodium laureth sulfate
TEA-lauryl sulfate
Propylene glycol
Hydrolyzed Animal protein
Glycol stearate and other ingredients
Lauramide DEA
Sodium chloride
Hydropropyl methylcellulose
Methylparaben
Imidazolidinyl urea
Disodium EDTA-copper
Citric acid
Propylparaben

ALMAY REGULAR AND EXTRA HOLD PROTEIN CONDITIONING HAIRSPRAY (AEROSOL)
(Almay)

SD Alcohol 40
Isobutane
Butyl ester of PVM/MA copolymer
Butane
Propane
Dimethicone copolyol
Animal protein derivative
Aminomethyl propanol

ALMAY RIDGE FILLING PRE-COAT
(Almay)

Butyl acetate *
Ethyl acetate
Talc
Nitrocellulose
Polyester resin
Dibutyl phthalate
Isopropyl alcohol
Butyl alcohol
Camphor
Polyvinyl butyral
Stearalkonium hectorite
Titanium dioxide
May contain: Iron oxides

ALMAY SHEER FINISH TRANSLUCENT PRESSED POWDER
(Almay)

Talc
Magnesium stearate
Mineral oil
Zinc oxide
Imidazolidinyl urea
Methylparaben
Propylparaben
May contain: Ultramarine blue, Iron oxides, Titanium dioxide

ALMAY SHINE FREE BLOTTING POWDER
(Almay)

Talc
Hydrated Silica
Kaolin
Water
Mineral oil
Titanium dioxide
Imidazolidinyl urea
Methylparaben
Propylparaben
May contain: Iron oxides, Titanium dioxide

ALMAY TRANSLUCENT FINISH FACE POWDER
(Almay)

Talc
Magnesium stearate
Isopropyl palmitate
Kaolin
Methylparaben
Propylparaben
Imidazolidinyl urea
May contain: Iron oxides, Titanium dioxide, Ultramarine blue

ALNYTE
Insomnia relief
(Mayer Labs.)

Each tablet:
  Methapyrilene HCl * .... 25 mg.
  Scopolamine aminoxide HBr . 0.2 mg.
  Salicylamide * .... 250 mg.

          '76 Ed.

ALO-BODY
(Aloe Creme)

Aloe vera plant gel

ALO-FACE MOISTURE PLUS
(Aloe Creme)

Aloe vera plant gel

ALO-HANDS
(Aloe Creme)

Aloe vera plant gel

ALO-LEGS
(Aloe Creme)

Aloe vera plant gel

ALO-LIPSTICK (MOISTURE PLUS)
(Aloe Creme)

Aloe vera plant gel

ALO-MOISTURE PLUS BEAUTY MATTE
(Aloe Creme)

Aloe vera plant gel

Starred ingredients (*) may be responsible for major toxic effects; consult Section II.

ALO-MOISTURE PLUS NIGHT CREME
(Aloe Creme)

Aloe vera plant gel

ALO-OINTMENT
(Aloe Creme)

Aloe vera plant gel

ALOPHEN PILLS
Cathartic
(Parke-Davis)

Each pill:
   Phenolphthalein .... 60 mg.

ALO-SUNBURN RELIEF LOTION
(Aloe Creme)

Aloe vera plant gel

ALO-TONE THE SKIN TONER
(Aloe Creme)

Aloe vera plant gel

ALO-VITALIZING SKIN CLEANSER
(Aloe Creme)

Aloe vera plant gel

ALO-V LUSTERIZING SHAMPOO
(Aloe Creme)

Aloe vera plant gel

ALPHA CHALKBOARD CHALK
(Weber Costello)

Calcium carbonate 95%
Vegetable binder 5%

ALPHACOLOR BRILLIANTS, CHALK PASTELS, AND DRY TEMPERA
Art material
(Weber Costello)

Earth oxides or nontoxic organic pigments

ALPHACOLOR LIQUID TEMPERA
Water-base paint
(Weber Costello)

Nontoxic earth oxides or organic pigments
Nontoxic organic binders

ALPHA-KERI (BATH OIL & SPRAY)
Water-dispersible, antipruritic oil
(Westwood Pharm.)

Kerohydric brand of dewaxed, oil-soluble keratin-moisturizing fraction of lanolin
Mineral oil
Nonionic emulsifiers

'76 Ed.

ALPHAMUL
Laxative
(Lannett)

Castor oil emulsion 60%

ALPHASITE CHALKBOARD CHALK
(Weber Costello)

Calcium carbonate 95%
Vegetable binder 5%

ALPHOSYL (Lotion-Lubricating Cream)
For psoriasis
(Reed & Carnrick)

Allantoin 2%
Special Coal tar extract * 5%

ALSOL ACP
Carburetor purge
(Alsol)

Isopropyl alcohol
Aromatic solvent *

'76 Ed.

ALSOL ALUMINUM BRIGHTENER & CLEANER
Automotive
(Alsol)

Acids *
Halides *†
Butyl Cellosolve

'76 Ed.

†*See* Fluoride

ALSOL AUTO WASH, POWDER
(Alsol)

Synthetic detergents *
Alkaline salts *

'76 Ed.

ALSOL BLACK RUBBER DRESSING
Automotive
(Alsol)

Petroleum solvents *

'76 Ed.

ALSOL CREME WAX
Automotive
(Alsol)

Petroleum distillates *

'76 Ed.

ALSOLDER 500
Solder
(Harris, J.W.)

Cadmium * 83%
Zinc 17%

ALSOL FLOOR CLEANER, POWDER
(Alsol)

Synthetic detergents *
Alkaline salts *

'76 Ed.

ALSOL HAND RUBBING COMPOUND
Automotive
(Alsol)

Petroleum distillates *

'76 Ed.

ALSOL HAND SOAP
(Alsol)

Lanolin
Alkaline salts *

'76 Ed.

ALSOL HEAVY DUTY GENERAL PURPOSE CLEANER
(Alsol)

Synthetic detergents *
Alkaline salts *

'76 Ed.

ALSOL LABEL REMOVER
(Alsol)

Glycol ethers *

'76 Ed.

ALSOL LIQUID SOLVENT CAR WAX
(Alsol)

Petroleum solvents *

'76 Ed.

Starred ingredients (*) may be responsible for major toxic effects; consult Section II.

ALSOL METAL PARTS CLEANER
Automotive
(Alsol)

Cresols *
Chlorinated solvents *
Petroleum distillates *

'76 Ed.

ALSOL MOTOR WASH REGULAR
(Alsol)

Petroleum solvents *

'76 Ed.

ALSOL MOTOR WASH SPECIAL
(Alsol)

Petroleum solvents *
Glycols *†

'76 Ed.

†*See* Ethylene glycol

ALSOL ODORLESS MOTOR WASH
(Alsol)

Petroleum solvents *
Glycols *†

'76 Ed.

†*See* Ethylene glycol

ALSOL PARTSITE
(Alsol)

Petroleum solvents *

'76 Ed.

ALSOL PINE OIL DISINFECTANT
(Alsol)

Pine oil * 60%
Soap 20%

'76 Ed.

ALSOL RUBBER LUBRICANT
Automotive
(Alsol)

Butyl Cellosolve *

'76 Ed.

ALSOL RUB-R-KLEEN
(Alsol)

Synthetic detergents *
Alkaline salts *

'76 Ed.

ALSOL 61 CLEANER
(Alsol)

Petroleum solvents *

'76 Ed.

ALSOL SPOT REMOVER, PERFUMED
(Alsol)

Petroleum solvents *
Chlorinated solvents *

'76 Ed.

ALSOL STEAM JENNY CLEANER, LIQUID
(Alsol)

Synthetic detergents *
Alkaline salts *

'76 Ed.

ALSOL SYNTHETIC RUBBING & POLISHING COMPOUND
Automotive
(Alsol)

Petroleum distillates *
Abrasive

'76 Ed.

ALSOL TAR REMOVER LACQUER CLEANER
(Alsol)

Petroleum solvent *
Chlorinated hydrocarbons *

'76 Ed.

ALSOL TOP LUBE AND VALVE LUBRICANT
Automotive
(Alsol)

Petroleum base oils *

'76 Ed.

ALSOL TRANSFLUSH
Purges transmission system of gums, carbons, etc.
(Alsol)

Methanol *

'76 Ed.

ALSOL TRU-GLO
Cleaner & polisher
(Alsol)

Petroleum distillate *
Terpene solvent *

'76 Ed.

ALSOL 2 PHASE CARBURETOR CLEANER
Automotive
(Alsol)

Cresols *
Chlorinated hydrocarbons *

'76 Ed.

ALSOL UPHOLSTERY SHAMPOO
Automotive
(Alsol)

Synthetic detergent *
Isopropanol *

'76 Ed.

ALUCAINE
Skin ointment
(Jenkins Labs.)

Benzocaine 5%
Carbolic acid * 1.39%
Ichthammol 1.39%
Balsam Peru 0.46%
Exsiccated Alum 3.7%
Oil cade *
Oil eucalyptus *

ALUDROX SUSPENSION AND TABLETS
Antacid
(Wyeth Labs.)

Suspension (each 5 ml.):
  Aluminum hydroxide gel . . . . . 307 mg.
  Magnesium hydroxide . . . . 103 mg.

Tablets (each):
  Dried Aluminum hydroxide gel 233 mg.
  Magnesium hydroxide . . . . 83 mg.

ALUMADRINE
For respiratory infections
(Fleming)

Each tablet:
  Acetaminophen * . . . . 500 mg.
  Phenylpropanolamine * . . . . . 25 mg.
  Chlorpheniramine maleate . . . 4 mg.

ALUMIN-NU POWER ALUMINUM SIDING, AWNING, AND MOBILE HOME CLEANER
(Alumin-Nu)

Hydrofluoric acid * . . . . <1.1%

ALUMIN-NU POWER EXTERIOR VINYL SIDING, AWNING, MOBILE HOME, DOOR & WINDOW CLEANER
(Alumin-Nu)

Hydrofluoric acid * . . . . <1.1%

Starred ingredients (*) may be responsible for major toxic effects; consult Section II.

ALUMINUM BLACK TOUCH-UP
(Birchwood Casey)

Phosphoric acid *
Selenium dioxide *
Fluoboric acid *
Nickel sulfate *
Copper sulfate *
Methanol

ALUMIZOL
Dressing for superficial wounds and abrasions
(King Pharmaceutical)

Aluminum (very fine powder)
Zinc oxide
Mineral oil
White petrolatum
Starch

ALUPRIN
Buffered analgesic
(Lemmon Co.)

Each tablet:
　Aspirin * .... 300 mg.
　Buffered with Dried Aluminum hydroxide gel, Magnesium hydroxide

ALURATE ELIXIR (Red)
Sedative, hypnotic
(Roche)

Each 5 ml.:
　Alurate (Aprobarbital) * ...... 40 mg.
　Alcohol 20%

ALUWETS
Wet dressing
(Stiefel Labs.)

Aluminum chloride hexahydrate

AMACO MODELING CLAY
(American Art Clay Co.)

This product bears the AP Seal issued by the Crayon, Water Color and Craft Institute, Inc. This seal certifies that the product contains no materials in sufficient quantities to be toxic or injurious to the human body even if ingested.

AMAZING SPRAY
All purpose cleaner and degreaser
(Snee, W.G., Co.)

Active ingred.: 25%
　Butyl Cellosolve *
　Sodium metasilicate *
　Tripolyphosphate *
　Ninex 24 Detergent

AMBER GRANULES
Institutional and industrial cleaning product

Procter & Gamble Co.
Ivorydale Technical Center
Cincinnati, Ohio 45217

Phone: 513-562-1100

AMBODRYL HYDROCHLORIDE
Antihistamine
(Parke-Davis)

Each Kapseal:
　Bromodiphenhydramine
　　hydrochloride * .... 25 mg.

AMBRITE COLORED MOLDED CHALK
(American Crayon Co.)

This product bears the CP Seal issued by the Crayon, Water Color and Craft Institute, Inc. This seal certifies that the product contains no materials in sufficient quantities to be toxic or injurious to the human body even if ingested.

AMBRITE T

See CHAPMAN AMBRITE T

AMBROCIDE
Wood preservative
(Chapman Chem.)

Benzene hexachloride, gamma
　isomer * 8.28%
Benzene hexachloride, other
　isomers 14.72%
Petroleum distillate * 69.5%
　　　　　　　　　　　　　'76 Ed.

AMBROID LIQUID CEMENT
Adhesive
(Ambroid)

Nitrocellulose type of cement:
　Alcohol * 50%
　Ketones * 50%
　Allyl isothiocyanate (Synthetic oil
　　of mustard) .... trace

AMBROID PLASTIC CEMENT
Adhesive
(Ambroid)

Styrene plastic 28%
Hydrocarbons *† 72%
Allyl isothiocyanate (Oil of
　mustard) .... trace

†See Adhesives, Section VI, General Formulations

AMBROSIA COSMETIC PRODUCTS

Ambrosia Cosmetics, Inc.
1950 S. Ocean Dr.
Hallendale, Fla. 33009

Phone: 305-454-5323

See COSMETICS, Section VI, General Formulations

AMBUSH BATH OIL
Sizes - 1/2 oz., & 1 oz.
(Dana Perfumes)

Essential oils * .... >1%
Aromatic chemicals
Isopropyl myristate

AMBUSH DRY PERFUME
Sachet - 1 oz.
(Dana Perfumes)

Essential oils * .... >1%
Aromatic chemicals
Talc
Magnesium silicate
Iron oxide

AMBUSH DUSTING POWDER (4 oz.), SHAKER BATH POWDER (2 oz.), DELUXE DUSTING POWDER (8 oz.)
(Dana Perfumes)

Essential oils * .... >1%
Aromatic chemicals
Talc
Zinc stearate
Magnesium carbonate

AMBUSH EAU DE COLOGNE
Sizes - 2 oz., 4 oz., 8 oz., & 16 oz.
(Dana Perfumes)

Essential oils * .... >1%
Aromatic chemicals
Specially denatured Alcohol (39-C) *
Deionized water
FD & C Yellow #6
FD & C Yellow #5

AMBUSH, FOREMOST 4812-ES

See FOREMOST 4812-ES AMBUSH

AMBUSH INSECTICIDE
For control of insects on cotton
(ICI Americas)

Permethrin * 25.6%

AMBUSH MIST CONCENTRATE (Glass Bottle)
Sizes - 1/2, 1 oz.
(Dana Perfumes)

Essential oils * .... >1%
Aromatic chemicals
Specially denatured Alcohol (39-C) *
Dichlorotetrafluoroethane
beta-Carotene in saturated solution

AMBUSH PERFUME
Sizes - 1/8, 1/4, 1/2, & 1 oz.
(Dana Perfumes)

Essential oils * .... >1%
Aromatic chemicals
Specially denatured Alcohol (39-C) *

Starred ingredients (*) may be responsible for major toxic effects; consult Section II.

AMBUSH PERFUME MIST
(Glass Bottle)
Aerosol - 1/4 oz.
(Dana Perfumes)

Essential oils * .... >1%
Aromatic chemicals
Specially denatured Alcohol (39-C) *
Carotene
D & C Red #17
Dichlorotetrafluoroethane

AMBUSH SKIN PERFUME OIL
Size - 1/4 oz.
(Dana Perfumes)

Essential oils * .... >1%
Aromatic chemicals
Isopropyl myristate

AMBUSH SOAP
Size - 3.5 oz.
(Dana Perfumes)

Essential oils .... >1%
Aromatic chemicals
Coconut oil
Glycerin
Tallow
Lanolin
Water

AMBUSH SOLID COLOGNE
Size - 2 oz.
(Dana Perfumes)

Essential oils * .... >1%
Aromatic chemicals
Specially denatured Alcohol (39-C) *
Deionized water
Sodium stearate
Propylene glycol
Cetyl alcohol

AMBUSH SPRAY COLOGNE
Aerosol - 3 oz.
(Dana Perfumes)

Essential oils * .... >1%
Aromatic chemicals
Specially denatured Alcohol (39-C) *
Dichlorodifluoromethane
Dichlorotetrafluoroethane

AMBUSH SPRAY COLOGNE (COLORED)
Aerosol - 2 oz.
(Dana Perfumes)

Essential oils * .... >1%
Aromatic chemicals
Specially denatured Alcohol (39-C) *
Dichlorotetrafluoroethane
beta-Carotene

AM CAPS
(Cramer Products)

Ammonia * 15-22%
Ethyl alcohol 35-40%

AMCHEM AMINE 2,4,5-T FOR RICE
Herbicide
(Amchem)

Triethylamine salt of 2,4,5-trichlo-
rophenoxyacetic acid * 56.8%

AMCHEM NAA-800
For control of pre-harvest drop of apples
(Amchem)

Potassium salt of naphthalene
acetic acid * 24.3%

AMCHEM WEED KILLER 650
(Amchem)

2,4-Dichlorophenoxyacetic acid,
isopropyl ester * 45.1%

AMCO
Adhesive
(Ambroid)

Nitrocellulose type of cement
  Alcohols * 20%
  Hydrocarbons *† 60%
  Ketones * 20%
Allyl isothiocyanate (synthetic oil
  of mustard) .... trace
†See Adhesives, Section VI, General Formulations

AMEN
Progestin
(Carnrick Labs.)

Each tablet:
  Medroxyprogesterone acetate . 10 mg.

AMERCOAT 67 ANTI-FOULING
Coating
(Ameron)

Metallic copper 10-20%
Rosin 20-25%
Coal tar 5-10%
Pine oil 0-5%
Inert ingredients: 25-35%
  Pigments *†
Xylol * 15-20%
Mineral spirits 0-5%

†See Dyes and Pigments, Section VI, General Formulations

AMERCOAT 70 ANTI-FOULING
Coating
(Ameron)

Metallic copper 20-25%
Rosin 20-25%
Coal tar 5-10%
Pine oil 0-5%
Inert ingredients: 20-30%
  Pigments *†
Xylol * 10-15%
Mineral spirits 5-10%

†See Dyes and Pigments, Section VI, General Formulations

AMERCOAT 2035 ANTI-FOULING
Coating
(Ameron)

Tributyltin fluoride * 10-15%
Vinyl acetate resin 5-10%
Rosin 5-10%
Inert ingredients 30-35%
Mixed Hydrocarbons 15-20%
Ketone 20-25%

AMERICAINE AEROSOL
Surface pain & itching
(American Critical Care)

Benzocaine 20%
In a base of Polyethylene glycol-200
Hydrocarbons as propellants

AMERICAINE FIRST AID BURN OINTMENT
(American Critical Care)

Benzocaine 20%
Benzethonium chloride 0.1%
Polyethylene glycols-300 & 4000

AMERICAINE FIRST AID SPRAY TOPICAL ANESTHETIC
(American Critical Care)

Benzocaine 10.0%
Benzethonium chloride 0.1%
Alcohol (USP) .... 25% v/v
Polyethylene glycol-300
Propylene glycol

AMERICAINE HEMORRHOIDAL OINTMENT
(American Critical Care)

Benzocaine 20%
Benzethonium chloride 0.1%
Polyethylene glycols-300 & 4000

AMERICAINE-OTIC
Topical anesthetic ear drops
(American Critical Care)

Benzocaine 20%
Benzethonium chloride 0.1%
Glycerin 1%
Polyethylene glycol-300

Starred ingredients (*) may be responsible for major toxic effects; consult Section II.

AMERICAN CRAYON WAX CRAYONS
(American Crayon Co.)

This product bears the CP Seal issued by the Crayon, Water Color and Craft Institute, Inc. This seal certifies that the product contains no materials in sufficient quantities to be toxic or injurious to the human body even if ingested.

AMERICAN CYANAMID PESTICIDE PRODUCTS

American Cyanamid Company
Agricultural Division
Berdan Ave.
Wayne, N.J. 07470

Office phone: 201-831-2000

Emergency (24 hr.): 201-835-3100

AMERICAN DRIPLESS OIL
Lubricant
(American Grease Stick)

Naphtha (Aliphatic petroleum) *	79%
Combined amount:	15%
Mineral oil	
Aluminum stearate	
Sorbitan mono-oleate	6%

AMERICAN FAST DRY PENETRATING SEAL-A25
Penetrating sealer for wood & linoleum floors
(American-Lincoln)

Nonvolatile:	30%
Tung oil	
Ester gum	
Modified Phenolic resin	
Volatile:	70%
Mineral spirits *	

AMERICAN GYM FINISH A-60
Surface finish for wood floors
(American-Lincoln)

Nonvolatile:	42%
Tung oil	
Ester gum	
Modified Phenolic resin	
Volatile:	58%
Mineral spirits *	

AMERICAN HOECHST CORP., ANIMAL HEALTH PRODUCTS
Veterinary pharmaceuticals

American Hoechst Corp.
Animal Health Div.
Route 202-206 North
Somerville, N.J. 08876

Phone: 201-685-2696

AMERICAN INKS AND COATINGS PRODUCTS
Paints and printing inks

American Inks and Coatings Corp.
P.O. Box 803
Valley Forge, Pa. 19482

Phone: 215-272-8866

AMERICAN LAFRANCE MULTI-PURPOSE DRY CHEMICAL EXTINGUISHER
(American LaFrance)

Mono-ammonium phosphate

AMERICAN LAFRANCE PURPLE K DRY CHEMICAL EXTINGUISHER
(American LaFrance)

Potassium bicarbonate

AMERICAN LAFRANCE REGULAR DRY CHEMICAL EXTINGUISHER
(American LaFrance)

Sodium bicarbonate

AMERICAN PENTRA-SEAL
Penetrating sealer for wood & linoleum floors
(American-Lincoln)

Nonvolatile:	36%/v
Tung oil	
Ester gum	
Modified Phenolic resin	
Volatile:	64%/v
Mineral spirits *	

AMERICAN SUPER LUSTRE FINISH
Non-wax wax finish for resilient floors
(American-Lincoln)

Nonvolatile:	14%
Synthetic wax	
Modified resins	
Oleic acid	

AMERTAN
Antiseptic ointment for burns
(Lilly, Eli)

Tannic acid	5%
Merthiolate	1:5000

AMESEC (ENSEALS & PULVULES)
Nocturnal asthma and allergic manifestations
(Lilly, Eli)

Each Enseal or Pulvule:
Amobarbital *	25 mg.
Ephedrine hydrochloride *	25 mg.
Aminophylline *	130 mg.

AMFEX INHALER
For colds & hay fever
(Approved Pharm.)

Each inhaler:
l-Desoxyephedrine base *
2 Amino-heptane
Phenylephrine HCl *
Menthol *
Aromatics

'76 Ed.

AMIBEN
Preemergence herbicide
(Amchem)

Ammonium salt of Amiben (3-Amino-2,5-dichlorobenzoic acid) *	23.4%

AMIBEN GRANULAR
Preemergence herbicide
(Amchem)

Ammonium salt of Amiben (3-Amino-2,5-dichlorobenzoic acid) *	10.8%

AMINE 4D
Herbicide
(Diamond Shamrock Corp.)

Dimethylamine salt of 2,4-dichlorophenoxyacetic acid *	47.4%

AMINE 6D
Herbicide
(Diamond Shamrock Corp.)

Dimethylamine salt of 2,4-dichlorophenoxyacetic acid *	65.6%

AMINE-FOUR HERBICIDE
(Dow)

Active inged.:
2,4-Dichlorophenoxyacetic acid, alkanolamine salts *	57.1%
Inert ingred.:	
Water plus sequestering agents	42.9%

AMINO-CERV CERVICAL CREME
(Milex)

Urea	8.34%
Sodium propionate	0.50%
Methionine	0.83%
Cystine	0.35%
Inositol	0.83%
Benzalkonium chloride	0.000004%

Starred ingredients (*) may be responsible for major toxic effects; consult Section II.

AMINODUR DURA-TABS
Bronchodilator
(Berlex Labs.)

Each tablet:
Aminophylline * .... 300 mg.

AMINODYNE COMPOUND
Analgesic
(Bowman Pharm.)

Each tablet:
Acetaminophen * .... 162.0 mg.
Aspirin .... 226.8 mg.
Caffeine .... 32.4 mg.

AMINO TRIAZOLE WEEDKILLER 90
Herbicide
(Amer. Cyanamid, Agric. Div.)

3-Amino-1,2,4-triazole 90.0%/w

AMITONE TABLETS
Antacid
(Norcliff Thayer)

Each tablet:
Calcium carbonate .... 350 mg.
Sugar/Starch .... 500 mg.
Peppermint flavor 1%

AMITROL-T
Herbicide
(Amchem)

3-Amino-1,2,4-triazole 21.1%

AMIZINE
Herbicide
(Amchem)

3-Amino-1,2,4-triazole 15.0%
2-Chloro-4,6-bis (ethylamino)-s-
triazine * 45.0%

AMLAB ANTI-ITCH CREAM
Antibiotic, antihistaminic, anesthetic
(Amlab)

Benzocaine 3%
Pyrilamine maleate * 1%
Methylparaben 0.1%
Cetyldimethylbenzyl ammonium
chloride 0.1%
In a base containing:
Glycerine 5%
Lanolin 1%

AMLAB ANTI-ITCH LOTION
Medicated; for the temporary relief of itching skin
(Amlab)

Diphenhydramine hydrochloride * 1%
Pramoxine hydrochloride 0.5%
Titanium dioxide 1%
Zinc oxide 4%
Glycerine 5%
In a soothing emollient base

AMLAB BUQUETS
Stimulant diuretic
(Amlab)

Each tablet:
Theobromine sodio salicylate * 55 mg.
Oleoresin Capsicum
Extract Buchu
Extract Uva ursi
Extract Juniper berries

AMLAB DRAWING SALVE
For skin irritations
(Amlab)

Ammonium ichthiosulfonate
Methyl salicylate *
Pine tar *
Rosin

"AMMATE" WEED AND BRUSH KILLER SOLUTION
(Du Pont)

Ammonium sulfamate * 48.4%

"AMMATE" X-NI WEED AND BRUSH KILLER
(Du Pont)

Ammonium sulfamate * 95%

"AMMATE" X WEED AND BRUSH KILLER
(Du Pont)

Ammonium sulfamate * 95%

AM + MEDIC

See AMWAY AM + MEDIC

AMMENS MEDICATED POWDER
(Bristol-Myers)

Zinc oxide
Boric acid *
Corn starch
Talc
Aromatic oils

AMMORID DIAPER RINSE
(Kinney)

Methylbenzethonium chloride * 5%
Buffering agents 95%

AMMORID OINTMENT
For diaper rash, etc.
(Kinney)

Benzethonium chloride *
Zinc oxide
Lanolin base

AMOBAM
Fungicide
(Fike Chemicals)

Diammonium ethylene bisdithiocarbamate *

AMOCAL
Expectorant
(Jenkins Labs.)

Each tablet:
Pyrilamine maleate * .... 5 mg.
Phenylephrine hydrochloride 2 mg.
Ammonium chloride .... 1 gr.
Calcium (iodized) .... 1/2 gr.
Powdered Ipecac .... 1/16 gr.
Tartar emetic .... 1/136 gr.
Benzoic acid .... 1/68 gr.
Extract Licorice .... 1 gr.

AMOCAL JR.
Expectorant
(Jenkins Labs.)

Each tablet:
Pyrilamine maleate * .... 3 mg.
Phenylephrine hydrochloride 1 mg.
Ammonium chloride .... 1/2 gr.
Calcium (iodized) .... 1/16 gr.
Powdered Ipecac .... 1/16 gr.
Tartar emetic .... 1/136 gr.
Benzoic acid .... 1/68 gr.
Extract Licorice .... 1 gr.

AMOCO ALFALFA INSECTICIDE
(Amoco)

Active ingredients by weight:
Methoxychlor, technical 23.8%
Malathion (O,O-Dimethyl di-
thiophosphate of diethyl
mercaptosuccinate) 23.84%
Xylene * 46.10%

AMOCO BRUSH KILLER - M
(Amoco)

Active ingredients by weight:
Propylene glycol butyl ether esters of 2,4-dichlorophenoxy-
acetic acid * 36.0%
Propylene glycol butyl ether esters of 2,4,5-trichlorophenoxy-
acetic acid 34.1%

AMOCO 2,4-D LV ESTER - M
Herbicide
(Amoco)

Active ingredients by weight:
Propylene glycol butyl ether esters of 2,4-dichlorophenoxy-
acetic acid (equivalent to 44.9%
of 2,4-dichlorophenoxyacetic
acid) * 72.8%

Starred ingredients (*) may be responsible for major toxic effects; consult Section II.

AMOCO 2,4-D WEED KILLER NO. 2 - M
Herbicide
(Amoco)

Active ingredients by weight:
Dimethylamine salt of 2,4-dich-lorophenoxyacetic acid (equiv-alent to 40.9% 2,4-dichloro-phenoxyacetic acid) * 49.3%

AMOCO 2,4-D WEED KILLER NO. 5 - M
(Amoco)

Active ingredients by weight:
Butyl esters of 2,4-dichlorophen-oxyacetic acid (equivalent to 46.76% 2,4-dichlorophenoxy-acetic acid) * 58.6%

AMOCO MALATHION SPRAY
Insecticide
(Amoco)

Active ingredients by weight:
Malathion * 57.0%
Xylene * 37.0%

AMOCO MCPA WEED KILLER - M
(Amoco)

Active ingredients by weight:
Dimethylamine salt of 2-methyl-4-chlorophenoxyacetic acid (MCPA) (2-methyl-4-chloro-phenoxyacetic acid equivalent 42.5%) * 52.1%

AMOCO METHOXYCHLOR SPRAY
Insecticide
(Amoco)

Active ingredients by weight:
Methoxychlor, technical 25.1%
Xylene * 70.1%
Petroleum hydrocarbons 2.8%

AMOCO MOSQUITO SPRAY CONCENTRATE
(Amoco)

Active ingredients by weight:
Fenthion (O,O-Dimethyl O-4-(methylthio)-m-tolyl phosphorothioate) * 24.18%
Aromatic petroleum distillate * 71.00%

AMOCO THIMET 15-G
Insecticide
(Amoco)

Active ingredients by weight:
Phorate (O,O-Diethyl S-(ethyl-thio)-methyl phosphorodithioate) * 15.0%

AMOCO 2,4,5-T LV ESTER - M
Herbicide
(Amoco)

Active ingredients by weight:
Propylene glycol butyl ether es-ters of 2,4,5-trichlorophenoxy-acetic acid (equivalent to 45.0% of 2,4,5-trichlorophenoxyacetic acid) * 69.2%

AMOCO TOXAPHENE SPRAY
Insecticide
(Amoco)

Active ingredients by weight:
Toxaphene (technical chlori-nated camphene, chlorine content 67 to 69%) * 59.58%
Aromatic petroleum derivative solvent 6.62%
Petroleum oil 26.10%

AMODRINE
Bronchial antispasmodic with sedative
(Searle, G.D., & Co.)

Each tablet:
Aminophylline * .... 100 mg.
Racephedrine hydrochloride * 25 mg.
Phenobarbital .... 8 mg.

AMONIDRIN TABLETS
Expectorant
(OJF)

Each tablet:
Ammonium chloride .... 200 mg.
Guaifenesin .... 100 mg.

AMOXIL CAPSULES
Antibiotic therapy
(Beecham Labs.)

Each capsule:
Amoxicillin .... 250 mg.; 500 mg.

AMOXIL FOR ORAL SUSPENSION
Antibiotic therapy
(Beecham Labs.)

Each 5 ml.:
Amoxicillin .... 125 mg.; 250 mg.

AMOXIL PEDIATRIC DROPS FOR ORAL SUSPENSION
Antibiotic therapy
(Beecham Labs.)

Each ml.:
Amoxicillin .... 50 mg.

AMPHOJEL SUSPENSION AND TABLETS
Antacid
(Wyeth Labs.)

Suspension (available with or without fla-vor) each 5 ml.:
Aluminum hydroxide gel .... 320 mg.

Tablets (each):
Dried Aluminum hy-droxide gel .... 0.3 gm.; 0.6 gm.

AMPHYL DISINFECTANT-DEODORANT-DETERGENT
(Nat'l Labs. Div.)

Soap, anhydrous 44.0%
o-Phenylphenol * 15.0%
p-tert-Amylphenol 6.3%
Alcohol 4.7%

AMPHYL SPRAY DISINFECTANT-DEODORANT
(Nat'l Labs. Div.)

o-Phenylphenol 0.136%
3,4',5-Tribromosalicylanilide ... 0.019%
3,5-Dibromosalicylanilide 0.005%
Alcohol * 78.500%

AM SOL
Weed Killer
(FMC Corp., Agricultural Chem. Div.)

Dimethylamine salt of 2,4-dichlo-rophenoxy acetic acid * 49.5%

AMWAY ALLANO HAND AND BODY LOTION
Aerosol foam hand lotion
(Amway Corp.)

	approx. %
Water	80%
PPG-5-ceteth-20	5%
Isobutane	4%
Stearic acid	2%
Isopropyl palmitate	2%
Polawax A-31	2%
Acetylated Lanolin alcohol	2%
Triethanolamine	1%
PEG-40 sorbitan peroleate	1%
Carbomer 941	<1%
Methylparaben	<1%
Allantoin	<1%
Imidazolidinyl urea	<1%
Phenyl dimethicone	<1%
Propylparaben	<1%
Glyceryl stearate	<1%
Stearamidoethyl diethylamine	<1%
Perfume	<1%

AMWAY AM + MEDIC
First aid spray
(Amway Corp.)

Isobutane (propellant) ..... approx. 80%
SD Alcohol 40 .... approx. 10%
Isopropyl palmitate .... approx. 8%
Benzocaine .... <1%
Menthol .... <1%
Triclosan .... <1%

Starred ingredients (*) may be responsible for major toxic effects; consult Section II.

AMWAY ANTI-TARNISH SILVER POLISH
(Amway Corp.)

	approx. %
Water	70%
Aluminum silicate	10%
Dithio bis-(stearyl propionate)	5%
Calcium carbonate	5%
Coconut diethanolamide or Diethanolamide of lauric acid	5%
Ammonium carbonate	5%
Soap	1%
Carboxyvinyl polymer	<1%
Ammonium hydroxide	<1%
Perfume	<1%
Dye	<1%

AMWAY ARTISTRY II CREAMY CLEANSING LOTION
(Amway Corp.)

Water
Mineral oil
Propylene glycol
Isopropyl palmitate
PEG-20 stearate
Sodium myreth sulfate
Cetyl alcohol
Triethanolamine
Methylparaben
Carbomer-941
Fragrance
Allantoin
Potassium sorbate
Propylparaben
Benzoic acid

AMWAY ARTISTRY II SKIN FRESHENER
(Amway Corp.)

Water
SD Alcohol 40 (Ethanol) *
Propylene glycol
Polysorbate 80
Allantoin
Fragrance
D & C Red No. 33
FD & C Yellow No. 5

AMWAY AUTOMATIC DISHWASHER COMPOUND - LIMITED PHOSPHATE FORMULA
(Amway Corp.)

	approx. %
Sodium tripolyphosphate hexahydrate	45%
Sodium metasilicate pentahydrate *	20%
Sodium carbonate *	20%
Sodium sulfate	15%
Sodium dichloroisocyanurate dihydrate	2%
Nonionic surfactant	2%

AMWAY AUTOMATIC DISHWASHER COMPOUND - STANDARD FORMULA
(Amway Corp.)

	approx. %
Sodium tripolyphosphate hexahydrate *	75%
Sodium metasilicate pentahydrate *	20%
Sodium dichloroisocyanurate dihydrate	1%
Nonionic surfactant	1%

AMWAY BLUE POWER
Automatic toilet bowl cleaner
(Amway Corp.)

	approx. %
Urea	40%
Nonionic surfactant	20%
Sodium sulfate	15%
Water	10%
Linear sodium alkyl aryl sulfonate	7%
Blue dye	5%
Sodium tallowate	1%
Pine oil	1%
Tetrasodium EDTA	<1%
Sodium o-phenylphenate	<1%
Silicone emulsion	<1%

AMWAY BORONIA CONCENTRATED AIR FRESHENER (Aerosol)
(Amway Corp.)

	approx. %
Methylene chloride *	70%
SD Alcohol 40 (Ethanol)	10%
Isobutane (propellant)	10%
Propane (propellant)	5%
Perfume	3%
Meelium	1%

AMWAY BOWL CLEANER II
(Amway Corp.)

	approx. %
Sodium bisulfate *	85%
Sodium carbonate	13%
Citric acid	1%
Silica	<1%
Nonionic surfactant	<1%
Pine oil	<1%
Dye	<1%

AMWAY BUFF-UP FURNITURE POLISH
(Amway Corp.)

	approx. %
Water	45%
Odorless Petroleum distillates *	25%
Silicone emulsion blend	10%
Isobutane (propellant)	10%
Propane (propellant)	5%
Polyglycerol oleate	2%
Carnauba wax	1%
Synthetic crystalline Wax	<1%
Microcrystalline Wax	<1%
Organic amine	<1%
Tall oil fatty acid or Oleic acid	<1%
Perfume	<1%

AMWAY BUG SPRAY
Aerosol insecticide
(Amway Corp.)

	approx. %
Water	70%
Isobutane (propellant)	30%
Propane (propellant)	3%
SBP-1382/Bioallethrin concentrate 10-6.25	2%

AMWAY CHROME AND GLASS CLEANER
Abrasive cleaner
(Amway Corp.)

	approx. %
Silicon dioxide	70%
Water	25%
Stearic acid	3%
Diethylene glycol monoethyl ether	2%
Calcium oxide	2%
Barium sulfate	1%
Primary alkyl polyoxyethylene alcohol	<1%
Sodium borate decahydrate	<1%
Perfume	<1%

AMWAY CONCRETE FLOOR CLEANER
(Amway Corp.)

	approx. %
Sodium metasilicate pentahydrate *	60%
Sodium carbonate *	40%
Nonionic surfactant	3%
Pine oil	<1%

AMWAY CORPORATION

Amway Corporation
7575 East Fulton Road
Ada, Michigan 49355
Amway employees on twenty-four hour call are authorized to give information to physicians and Poison Control Centers.

Phone: 616-676-6307

AMWAY DAYBREAK CONCENTRATED AIR FRESHENER
(Amway Corp.)

	approx. %
Isobutane (propellant)	50%
Isopropyl alcohol*	40%
Water	5%
Perfume	3%
Meelium	3%
Ethanolamine	<1%

Starred ingredients (*) may be responsible for major toxic effects; consult Section II.

AMWAY DETER DOUBLE ACTIVE ANTI-PERSPIRANT SPRAY
(Amway Corp.)

	approx. %
Isobutane (propellant)	60%
Cyclomethicone	20%
Propane (propellant)	10%
Aluminum chlorohydrate	10%
Propylene glycol dicaprylate/dicaprate	2%
Quaternium-18 bentonite	<1%
SD Alcohol 40 (Ethanol)	<1%
Silicon dioxide	<1%
Perfume	<1%

AMWAY DETER DOUBLE ACTIVE FOOT DEODORANT SPRAY
(Amway Corp.)

	approx. %
Isobutane (propellant)	70%
Propane (propellant)	15%
Cyclomethicone	15%
Talc	4%
Silicon dioxide	<1%
Perfume	<1%
Triclosan	<1%
Quaternium-18 bentonite	<1%
SD Alcohol 40 (Ethanol)	<1%
Menthol	<1%

AMWAY DETER DOUBLE ACTIVE ROLL-ON ANTI-PERSPIRANT
(Amway Corp.)

	approx. %
Water	60%
Aluminum chlorohydrate *	20%
Glyceryl stearate and PEG-100 stearate	4%
Mineral oil	4%
Propylene glycol	4%
Aluminum chloride	3%
Magnesium aluminum silicate	1%
Octyl dodecanol	1%
Cetearyl alcohol and Ceteareth-20	1%
Glycine	<1%
Allantoin	<1%
Perfume	<1%
Benzethonium chloride	<1%

AMWAY DETERGENT RESISTANT FLOOR POLISH
(Amway Corp.)

	approx. %
Water	80%
Acrylic copolymer	10%
Diethylene glycol monoethyl ether	3%
Emulsified Polyethylene	2%
Alkali soluble resin	2%
Tributoxyethyl phosphate	1%
Ammonium hydroxide	<1%
Formaldehyde	<1%
Fluorochemical surfactant	<1%

AMWAY d-15 INSECT REPELLENT
(Amway Corp.)

	approx. %
1,1,1-Trichloroethane *	45%
SD Alcohol 40 (Ethanol)	15%
N,N-Diethyl-m-toluamide (DEET) *	15%
Isobutane (propellant)	7%
Perfume	<1%

AMWAY d-15 INSECT REPELLENT TOWELETTE
(Amway Corp.)

	approx. %
SD Alcohol 40	50%
Towelette	40%
DEET (N,N-Diethyl-m-toluamide)	11.26%
Fragrance	<1%

AMWAY DISH DROPS
Liquid detergent
(Amway Corp.)

	approx. %
Water	60%
Sodium alkyl aryl sulfonate *	25%
Ammonium lauryl polyether sulfate	5%
Coconut diethanolamide	5%
Sodium xylene sulfonate	2%
Magnesium sulfate	<1%
Citric acid	<1%
Formaldehyde	<1%
Perfume	<1%

AMWAY DRAIN MATE LIQUID DRAIN CLEANER
(Amway Corp.)

	approx. %
1,1,1-Trichloroethane *	85%
Odorless Mineral spirits *	10%
Pine oil	5%
Dye	<1%

AMWAY DRIFAB WATER REPELLENT SPRAY
(Amway Corp.)

	approx. %
1,1,1-Trichloroethane *	90%
Odorless Mineral spirits	4%
Carbon dioxide (propellant)	4%
Hydrocarbon resin	<1%
Refined wax	<1%
Aluminum chelate	<1%

AMWAY DRY CHLORINE BLEACH
Powdered laundry bleach
(Amway Corp.)

	approx. %
Sodium sulfate	80%
Sodium dichloroisocyanurate *	15%
Sodium carbonate *	10%
Mineral oil	<1%

AMWAY ENGINE DEGREASER
Aerosol solvent cleaner
(Amway Corp.)

	approx. %
Petroleum distillates *	80%
Pine oil	10%
Ethoxylated linear alcohol	10%
Carbon dioxide (propellant)	3%

AMWAY ENGINE DEGREASER CONCENTRATE
Solvent cleaner
(Amway Corp.)

	approx. %
Petroleum distillates *	80%
Pine oil	10%
Ethoxylated linear alcohol	10%

AMWAY FLOOR WAX
(Amway Corp.)

	approx. %
Water	60%
Polymer-polyethylene blend	35%
Diethylene glycol monoethyl ether	2%
Alkali soluble resin	2%
Tributoxyethyl phosphate	1%
Ethylene glycol	<1%
Ammonium hydroxide	<1%
Formaldehyde	<1%
Fluorochemical surfactant	<1%

AMWAY GERMICIDAL CONCENTRATE
Liquid disinfectant
(Amway Corp.)

	approx. %
Water	80%
n-Alkyl dimethyl benzyl ammonium chloride *	15%
SD Alcohol 40 (Ethanol)	2%

AMWAY GREEN MEADOWS CONCENTRATED AIR FRESHENER
(Amway Corp.)

	approx. %
Isobutane (propellant)	50%
Isopropyl alcohol *	40%
Water	5%
Perfume	3%
Meelium	3%
Ethanolamine	<1%

AMWAY INDUSTROCLEAN
(Amway Corp.)

	approx. %
Water	90%
2-Butoxyethanol *	5%
Sodium carbonate	3%
Sodium alkyl aryl sulfonate	2%
Sodium metasilicate pentahydrate *	2%
Sodium EDTA	<1%
Coconut alkanolamide	<1%

Starred ingredients (*) may be responsible for major toxic effects; consult Section II.

AMWAY KOOL WASH
Liquid detergent
(Amway Corp.)

	approx. %
Water	65%
Sodium alkyl aryl sulfonate *	20%
Sodium lauryl ether sulfate	5%
Coconut diethanolamide	5%
SD Alcohol 40 (Ethanol)	2%
Fluorescent whitening agents	<1%
Polyvinylpyrrolidone	<1%
Formaldehyde	<1%
Citric acid	<1%
Perfume	<1%

AMWAY L.O.C. HIGH SUDS
Liquid detergent
(Amway Corp.)

	approx. %
Water	90%
Ammonium lauryl polyether sulfate	5%
Sodium alkyl aryl sulfonate	3%
Coconut diethanolamide	3%
Sodium chloride	1%
Sodium EDTA	<1%
Citric acid	<1%
Formaldehyde	<1%
Perfume	<1%

AMWAY L.O.C. REGULAR
Liquid detergent
(Amway Corp.)

	approx. %
Water	80%
Primary alcohol ethoxylate	10%
Coconut diethanolamide	10%
Tetrasodium EDTA	<1%
Dye	<1%
Citric acid	<1%
Perfume	<1%

AMWAY METAL CLEANER PASTE
(Amway Corp.)

	approx. %
Water	50%
Silicon dioxide	30%
Diatomaceous earth	10%
Calcium chloride	5%
Citric acid	5%
Sodium lauryl sulfate	1%
Xanthan gum	<1%

AMWAY MOTH CRYSTALS
Insect repellent
(Amway Corp.)

Paradichlorobenzene *	approx. 100%
Perfume	<1%

AMWAY MOUTH REFRESHER
Mouthwash
(Amway Corp.)

	approx. %
Water	85%
Sorbitol	10%
SD Alcohol 38B (Ethanol)	5%
Polysorbate-80	<1%
Dipropylene glycol methyl ether	<1%
Sodium saccharin	<1%
Citric acid	<1%
Zinc chloride	<1%
Flavor	<1%

AMWAY NEUTRALODOR AIR FRESHENER
(Amway Corp.)

	approx. %
Water	65%
Isobutane (propellant)	15%
Isoparaffinic hydrocarbon	10%
Propane (propellant)	3%
Isopropyl alcohol	2%
Polyglycerol oleate	<1%
Perfume	<1%
Meelium	<1%

AMWAY OVEN CLEANER
(Amway Corp.)

	approx. %
Water	85%
Sodium hydroxide *	9%
Sulfonated carboxylated starch	4%
Soap	1%
Magnesium sulfate	<1%
Nonionic ether surfactant	<1%

AMWAY OVEN 'N' GRILL
Aerosol oven protectorant
(Amway Corp.)

	approx. %
1,1,1-Trichloroethane *	90%
Carbon dioxide (propellant)	5%
Dimethylpolysiloxane	3%

AMWAY POINTS NORTH AFTER SHAVE
(Amway Corp.)

	approx. %
SD Alcohol 40 *	65%
Water	30%
Perfume *	2%
Diisopropyl adipate	1%
Citric acid	<1%
Uvinul D-50	<1%
Emcol E-607	<1%
Dye	<1%

AMWAY REDU
Rust stain remover
(Amway Corp.)

	approx. %
Sodium hydrosulfite *	70%
Sodium carbonate	25%
Sodium tripolyphosphate	5%

AMWAY REMOVE FABRIC SPOT CLEANER
(Amway Corp.)

	approx. %
1,1,1-Trichloroethane *	50%
Isobutane (propellant)	25%
Silica	10%
Isopropyl alcohol	5%
Naphtha	5%
Propane (propellant)	5%

AMWAY RINSE AID FOR DISHWASHERS
(Amway Corp.)

	approx. %
Nonionic surfactant *	80%
SD Alcohol 40 (Ethanol)	5%
Propylene glycol	5%
Water	5%
Sodium benzoate	<1%

AMWAY RUG & UPHOLSTERY SHAMPOO
(Amway Corp.)

	approx. %
Water	90%
Sodium lauryl sulfate	5%
Disodium lauric monoethanolamide - sulfosuccinate half ester	2%
Lauryl alcohol	<1%
Sodium sulfate	<1%
Formaldehyde	<1%

AMWAY S-A-8 LIMITED PHOSPHATE (JAPAN)
Laundry detergent
(Amway Corp.)

Sodium carbonate *	<45%
Sodium tripolyphosphate	<25%
Sodium metasilicate *	<15%
Nonionic surfactant	<15%
Minor constituents	<5%

AMWAY S-A-8 LIQUID LAUNDRY DETERGENT
(Amway Corp.)

	approx. %
Water	50%
Nonionic surfactant *	35%
Sodium alkyl aryl sulfonate	10%
Diethanolamine	5%
SD Alcohol 40 (Ethanol)	2%
Sodium stearate	<1%
Fluorescent whitening agents	<1%
Dye	<1%
Perfume	<1%

AMWAY S-A-8 NO PHOSPHATE
Laundry detergent
(Amway Corp.)

Sodium carbonate *	<65%
Sodium metasilicate pentahydrate *	<25%
Nonionic surfactant	<20%
Minor constituents (brighteners, fragrance)	<4%

Starred ingredients (*) may be responsible for major toxic effects; consult Section II.

AMWAY S-A-8 PLUS - MODIFIED
Laundry detergent
(Amway Corp.)

	approx. %
Sodium tripolyphosphate *	65%
Liquid Sodium silicate	15%
Nonionic surfactant	10%
Water	5%
Sodium carbonate	3%
Sodium carboxymethyl cellulose	2%
Sodium hydroxide	<1%
Fluorescent whitening agent	<1%
Perfume	<1%

AMWAY SATINIQUE HAIR SPRAY WITH PROTEIN
(Amway Corp.)

	approx. %
SD Alcohol 40 (Ethanol)	60%
Isobutane (propellant)	30%
Propane (propellant)	6%
Octylacrylamide/Acrylates/ Butylaminoethyl meth- acrylate polymer	2%
Protein derivative	<1%
Aminomethyl propanol	<1%
PPG-26 oleate	<1%
Perfume	<1%

AMWAY SEE SPRAY WINDOW CLEANER
(Amway Corp.)

	approx. %
Water	80%
Isopropyl alcohol	10%
Isobutane (propellant)	4%
2-Butoxyethanol	3%
Ammonium hydroxide	2%
Propane (propellant)	<1%
Ammonium lauryl ether sulfate	<1%
Silicone emulsion	<1%

AMWAY SEPTIC TANK AIDS
Septic tank treatment tablets
(Amway Corp.)

	approx. %
Bacterial enzymes	50%
Corn sugar binder	25%
Calcium sulfate	5%
Sodium thiosulfate	5%
Active dry Yeast	5%
Aerobic and anaerobic bacteria culture	5%
Sodium sulfate	2%
Nonionic surfactant	1%
Octo sucrose acetate	<1%
Dye	<1%
Perfume	<1%

AMWAY SHOE SPRAY
(Amway Corp.)

	approx. %
Methylene chloride * or	60%
Combined amount:	60%
Methylene chloride *	30%
1,1,1-Trichloroethane *	30%
Isobutane (propellant)	15%
Ethylene glycol ethyl ether acetate	5%
SD Alcohol 40 (Ethanol) or Isopropanol	5%
Propane (propellant)	5%
Ethyl cellulose	1%
Dibutyl phthalate	<1%
2-Butoxyethanol	<1%
Lanolin	<1%
Dimethyl silicone	<1%

AMWAY SILICONE GLAZE DETERGENT RESISTANT CAR POLISH
(Amway Corp.)

	approx. %
Water	45%
Odorless Mineral spirits *	35%
Aluminum silicate	5%
Silicone resin	5%
Calcined Diatomaceous earth	5%
Oleic acid	2%
Oxidized microcrystalline Wax	2%
Dimethyl silicone	1%
Morpholine	<1%
Ammonium hydroxide	<1%
Carboxyvinyl polymer	<1%
Dye	<1%

AMWAY SMASHING WHITE LAUNDRY BOOSTER
(Amway Corp.)

	approx. %
Water	75%
Sodium hexametaphosphate	20%
Tetrapotassium pyrophosphate	5%
Formaldehyde	<1%
Dye	<1%
Perfume	<1%

AMWAY TONGA AFTER SHAVE
(Amway Corp.)

	approx. %
SD Alcohol 40 *	60%
Water	35%
Perfume	2%
Diisopropyl adipate	1%
Citric acid	<1%
Uvinul D-50	<1%
Emcol E-607	<1%
Dye	<1%

AMWAY TONGA COLOGNE
(Amway Corp.)

	approx. %
SD Alcohol 40 *	65%
Water	30%
Perfume	4%
Citric acid	<1%
Uvinul D-50	<1%
Emcol E-607	<1%
Dye	<1%

AMWAY TONGA SPRAY DEODORANT
(Amway Corp.)

	approx. %
SD Alcohol (Ethanol)	45%
Trichloroethane	20%
Isobutane (propellant)	20%
Methylene chloride	10%
Propane (propellant)	2%
Isopropyl palmitate	2%
Zinc phenolsulfonate	<1%
Perfume	<1%
Triclosan	<1%

AMWAY TOOTHPASTE
(Amway Corp.)

	approx. %
Dicalcium phosphate	45%
Water	20%
Sorbitol	20%
Glycerine	10%
Sodium carboxymethylcellulose	<1%
Magnesium aluminum silicate	<1%
Sodium benzoate	<1%
Methylparaben	<1%
Propylparaben	<1%
Sodium saccharin	<1%
Sodium lauryl sulfate	<1%
Flavor	<1%

AMWAY TRIZYME
Enzyme pre-soak for laundry
(Amway Corp.)

	approx. %
Sodium sulfate	60%
Sodium tripolyphosphate *	35%
Nonionic surfactant	5%
Enzymes	2%
Fluorescent whitening agents	<1%
Perfume	<1%

AMWAY VINYL AND LEATHER CLEANER
(Amway Corp.)

	approx. %
Water	80%
Odorless Mineral spirits	10%
Diethylene glycol monoethyl ether	3%
Fatty acid	2%
Dimethyl polysiloxane fluid	2%
Nonionic surfactant	2%
Triethanolamine	<1%
Perfume	<1%

AMWAY VINYL TOP DRESSING
(Amway Corp.)

	approx. %
Water	85%
Silicone emulsion	8%
Amino-functional Silicone emulsion	8%
Formalin	<1%
Perfume	<1%

Starred ingredients (*) may be responsible for major toxic effects; consult Section II.

AMWAY WATER SOFTENING COMPOUND, LIMITED PHOSPHATE
(Amway Corp.)

	approx. %
Sodium sesquicarbonate *	55%
Sodium tripolyphosphate hexahydrate *	45%

AMWAY WAX REMOVER
(Amway Corp.)

	approx. %
Water	70%
Tall oil fatty acid or Oleic acid	7%
Mixed Fatty acid diethanolamide	5%
Isopropanol	5%
Ammonium hydroxide *	4%
Primary alkyl polyoxyethylene alcohol	3%
Pine oil	2%
Tetrasodium EDTA	<1%

AMWAY WONDER MIST
Aerosol lubricant
(Amway Corp.)

	approx. %
Trichloroethane *	65%
Isobutane (propellant)	15%
White mineral oil	10%
Propane (propellant)	5%
Silicone wax	2%
Soap	2%

AMWAY ZOOM SPRAY CLEANER CONCENTRATE
(Amway Corp.)

	approx. %
Water	80%
2-Butoxyethanol *	5%
Sodium carbonate	5%
Sodium alkyl aryl sulfonate	3%
Methoxy propanol	2%
Coconut alkanolamide	1%
Sodium EDTA	<1%
Dye	<1%

AMYTAL ELIXIR
Sedative
(Lilly, Eli)

ELIXIR (Each fluid ounce):

Amobarbital *	4 gr.
Alcohol	34%

AMYTAL SODIUM PULVULES, USP CAPSULES
Sedative
(Lilly, Eli)

Each capsule:
Amobarbital sodium * .... 1 gr.; 3 gr.

ANACAINE OINTMENT
Topical anesthetic
(Gordon Labs.)

Benzocaine	10%
Boric acid *	5%
Cream base	

ANACIN ANALGESIC TABLETS
(Whitehall Labs.)

Each tablet:
Aspirin *
Caffeine

ANADONE
For control of convulsions in dogs
(Bio-Ceutic)

Each tablet:
Primidone * .... 250 mg.

ANADROL-50 TABLETS
Treatment of aplastic anemia
(Syntex Labs.)

Each tablet:
Oxymetholone .... 50 mg.

ANAHIST, SUPER, NASAL SPRAY

See SUPER ANAHIST NASAL SPRAY

ANALBALM
Counter-irritant, local analgesic
(Central Pharmacal Co.)

Methyl salicylate *
Camphor *
Menthol *

ANALGESINE, LIQUID
External analgesic
(Elder)

Methyl salicylate, synthetic *	4.8%
Camphor, synthetic *	1.7%
Menthol (racemic) *	1.2%

ANALGETS
Analgesic
(Vale)

Each wafer:

Aspirin *	64.8 mg.
Magnesium trisilicate	64.8 mg.

ANAPAC (SUPER) COLD TABLETS AC (ANTI-COUGH)

See SUPER ANAPAC COLD TABLETS AC (ANTI-COUGH)

ANAPAC TABLETS, SUPER

See SUPER ANAPAC TABLETS

ANAPLEX
Anthelmintic for dogs and cats
(Bio-Ceutic)

Each capsule (for 25 lb. animal):

Dichlorophene	2.5 gm.
Toluene *	3.0 gm.

ANAPRIME OPHTHAKOTE OPHTHALMIC SOLUTION VETERINARY
Anti-inflammatory, antibacterial agent
(Syntex Agribusiness)

Flumethasone	0.01%
Neomycin sulfate (equivalent to 0.35% neomycin base)	0.5%
Polymixin B sulfate	10,000 units/cc

In a Hydroxypropyl methylcellulose vehicle containing:
Polyethylene glycol 4000
Propylene glycol
Methylparaben
Propylparaben
Citric acid
Sodium hydroxide and/or sulfuric acid to adjust pH

ANAPRIME OPHTHALMIC SOLUTION VETERINARY
Anti-inflammatory, antibacterial agent
(Syntex Agribusiness)

Flumethasone	0.01%
Neomycin sulfate (equiv. to 0.35% neomycin base)	0.5%
Polymixin B sulfate	10,000 units/cc

In a solution of:
Propylene glycol
Polyethylene glycol 4000
Citric acid
Sodium hydroxide to adjust pH

ANAPRIME SUSPENSION VETERINARY
Anti-inflammatory agent
(Syntex Agribusiness)

Flumethasone	0.2%

Solution:
Propylene glycol
Benzyl alcohol
Sodium chloride
Polysorbate 80
Citric acid and sodium hydroxide to adjust pH
Purified water

ANASPAZ
Antispasmodic-antisecretory
(Ascher, B.F.)

Each tablet:
l-Hyoscyamine sulfate * ... 0.125 mg.

ANASPAZ PB
Antispasmodic-antisecretory
(Ascher, B.F.)

Each tablet:

l-Hyoscyamine sulfate *	0.125 mg.
Phenobarbital *	15 mg.

Starred ingredients (*) may be responsible for major toxic effects; consult Section II.

ANATHESIA MOP

See DURHAM'S ANATHESIA MOP

ANAVERM-1

Anthelmintic; veterinary
(Direct Div.)

Each capsule:
Toluene * .... 120 mg.
Dichlorophene .... 100 mg.

ANAVERM-2.5

Anthelmintic; veterinary
(Direct Div.)

Each capsule:
Toluene * .... 300 mg.
Dichlorophene .... 250 mg.

ANAVERM-5

Anthelmintic; veterinary
(Direct Div.)

Each capsule:
Toluene * .... 600 mg.
Dichlorophene .... 500 mg.

ANAVERM-10

Anthelmintic; veterinary
(Direct Div.)

Each capsule:
Toluene * .... 1.2 gm.
Dichlorophene .... 1.0 gm.

ANAVERM-25

Anthelmintic; veterinary
(Direct Div.)

Each capsule:
Toluene * .... 3.0 gm.
Dichlorophene .... 2.5 gm.

ANAVERM-40

Anthelmintic; veterinary
(Direct Div.)

Each capsule:
Toluene * .... 4.8 gm.
Dichlorophene .... 4.0 gm.

ANBESOL

Antiseptic, anesthetic
(Whitehall Labs.)

Benzocaine
Phenol *
Iodine *
Alcohol

ANCHO-DINE

See ANCHOR ANCHO-DINE

ANCHOR ANCHO-DINE

Iodine supplement and expectorant;
veterinary
(Anchor Labs)

Active ingred.:
Ethylenediamine dihydriodide
(equiv. 20 gr./oz.) 4.600%
Guaranteed analysis:
Iodine (not less than 3.695%)
Salt (NaCl) (not less than 91.000%, not
more than 95.400%) *

ANCHOR ANCOSUL

Veterinary; antibacterial
(Anchor Labs)

Each bolus:
Sulfadimethoxine * .... 15 gm.

ANCHOR BLOOD STOPPER

Antihemorrhagic; veterinary
(Anchor Labs)

Ferrous sulfate (exsiccated) * 84%
Potassium alum (crystalline powder) 6%
Talc 10%

ANCHOR CALDEX

For milk fever in cattle; veterinary
(Anchor Labs)

Calcium gluconate (as calcium
borogluconate) .... 23% w/v
Dextrose monohydrate .... 10% w/v
Distilled water .... 71% w/v

ANCHOR CALDEX, M.P.

For cattle & sheep milk fever; veteri-
nary
(Anchor Labs)

Each 100 cc:
Calcium gluconate (as the
borogluconate) .... 23.0% w/v
Dextrose .... 25.0% w/v
Magnesium chloride .... 4.5% w/v
Phosphorus (as sodium
hypophosphite) .... 1.0% w/v

ANCHOR CALF SCOUR BOLUS

Treatment of bacterial calf diarrhea
(Anchor Labs)

Each bolus:
Neomycin sulfate equiv. to
neomycin .... 300 mg.
Activated Attapulgite
Pectin

ANCHOR CALF SCOUR FORMULA

(Anchor Labs)

Each fl. oz.:
Neomycin base (as sulfate) ... 175 mg.
Activated Attapulgite
Pectin
Homatropine methylbromide
Inert ingred.:
Sodium benzoate
Methylparaben
Propylparaben
Benzoic acid

ANCHOR CANINE WORMER No. 25

For large dogs
(Anchor Labs)

Each capsule:
2,2'-Methylenebis(4-chloro-
phenol) (Dichlorophene) ... 2.5 gm.
Methylbenzene (Toluene) * .. 3.0 gm.

ANCHOR DEHORN PASTE

Veterinary
(Anchor Labs)

Sodium hydroxide * 32%
Calcium hydroxide & water 68%

ANCHOR DERMA-SECT

Insecticidal shampoo; veterinary
(Anchor Labs)

Gamma isomer of benzene hexachloride from lindane 0.097%

ANCHOR DOG VITAMINS

(Anchor Labs)

Each tablet:
Vitamin A .... 1000 IU
Vitamin D2 .... 100 IU
Iron .... 1.2 mg.
Plus vitamins and minerals

ANCHOR FEN-ARSENATE DRENCH

Wormer; veterinary
(Anchor Labs)

Phenothiazine (12.50 gm./fl.
oz.) .... 42.46% w/v
Lead arsenate (0.50 gm./fl.
oz.) * .... 1.69% w/v

ANCHOR FERRO-TREET

Veterinary
(Anchor Labs)

Oral Iron *†

†*See* Iron salts

Starred ingredients (*) may be responsible for major toxic effects; consult Section II.

ANCHOR FLEA, LICE AND TICK SPRAY
For dogs and cats
(Anchor Labs)

Carbaryl *	1.00%
Pyrethrins	0.06%
Piperonyl butoxide (technical)	0.60%
Butoxypolypropylene glycol	5.00%
Petroleum distillate *	20.00%

ANCHOR GENERAL DISINFECTANT
(Anchor Labs)

Nonylphenoxypoly (ethyleneoxy) ethanol-iodine complex	13.76%
Phosphoric acid	5.95%

ANCHOR GENTLE IODINE SPRAY
Veterinary; topical antiseptic
(Anchor Labs)

Nonylphenoxypoly (ethyleneoxy) ethanol-iodine complex (equiv. to 2.50% titratable iodine)	12.50% w/w
Isopropyl alcohol *	65.00% w/w

ANCHOR HYDRO-LITE
Veterinary; for preventing dehydration
(Anchor Labs)

Vitamin A	400,000 units/lb.
Ethylenediamine dihydriodide	
Calcium gluconate	
Calcium hypophosphite	
Cobalt sulfate monohydrate *	
Copper sulfate pentahydrate *	
Ferrous (Iron) sulfate *	
Magnesium sulfate	
Manganese sulfate monohydrate	
Potassium chloride	
Sodium chloride	
Zinc sulfate	
Sodium bicarbonate	

ANCHOR ISOLITE
Drinking water antibacterial; veterinary
(Anchor Labs)

Each oz.:	
Sodium sulfathiazole *	0.67 oz.
Nutritional ingred.:	
Vitamin A	12,500 IU/oz.
Vitamin D3	1,800 IU/oz.
Ethylenediamine dihydriodide	
Potassium chloride	
Calcium gluconate	
Sodium bicarbonate	
Ferrous (iron) sulfate	
Zinc sulfate	
Cobalt sulfate monohydrate	
Manganese sulfate monohydrate	
Copper sulfate pentahydrate	
Calcium hypophosphite	
Magnesium sulfate	
Sodium chloride	

ANCHOR LITTER-MATE
For baby pig scours & pneumo-enteritis
(Anchor Labs)

Each 3 cc.:	
Neomycin base (as sulfate)	4.4 mg.
Activated Attapulgite (colloidal)	
Pectin	
Inert ingred.:	
Sodium benzoate	0.12% w/v
Methylparaben	0.18% w/v
Benzoic acid	0.10% w/v
Propylparaben	0.02% w/v

ANCHOR MANGE LOTION
(Anchor Labs)

Gamma isomer of benzene hexachloride from lindane	0.10%
Rotenone	0.12%
2,2'-Methylenebis(4-chlorophenol) (Dichlorophene)	0.50%
Benzyl benzoate *	30.00%
Isopropyl alcohol *	68.38%

ANCHOR NEOMYCIN SOLUTION
Veterinary; antibiotic
(Anchor Labs)

Each ml.:	
Neomycin sulfate (equiv. to 140 mg. neomycin base)	200 mg.

ANCHOR PIPERAZINE
Water wormer; veterinary
(Anchor Labs)

Active ingred.:	
Piperazine base (from piperazine monohydrochloride)	17.10% w/v
Inert ingred.:	
Sodium benzoate (as preservative)	0.10% w/v

ANCHOR PIPRA-POWDER "53"
Wormer - veterinary
(Anchor Labs)

Piperazine base	53%

ANCHOR PURGOLAX RUMEN BOLUS
Antacid-laxative for cattle
(Anchor Labs)

Active ingred./bolus:	
Nux vomica (as powdered extract, equiv. to 0.115 gr. strychnine)	10 gr.
Tartar emetic *	10 gr.
Ginger	3 gr.
Capsicum	3 gr.
Magnesium oxide	276 mg.
Cobalt sulfate monohydrate	100 mg.
Inert ingred.:	
Excipients with artificial color and flavor	q.s.

ANCHOR RONNEL SCREW WORM & EAR TICK SPRAY
Veterinary
(Anchor Labs)

Ethyl alcohol	45.65%
Propylene glycol	15.00%
FD & C Blue #1	0.05%
Xylene *	15.50%
Korlan 8	3.80%
A-70	20.00%

ANCHOR STRONG IODINE TINCTURE
Veterinary
(Anchor Labs)

Iodine *	7.0% w/v
Potassium iodide	5.0% w/v
Isopropyl alcohol (99%)	86.67% v/v

ANCHOR SULFA-UREA BOLUSES
Veterinary
(Anchor Labs)

Each bolus:	
Urea	207 gr.
Sulfanilamide	33 gr.
Sulfathiazole	5 gr.

ANCHOR SUL-LITE
Antibacterial; veterinary
(Anchor Labs)

Each fluid oz.:	
Sodium sulfamethazine *	12.5% w/v
Inert ingred.:	88.10%
Orthophenylphenol	
Ethylenediamine dihydriodide	
Potassium chloride	
Calcium gluconate	
Sodium bicarbonate	
Sodium phosphate dibasic heptahydrate	
Magnesium sulfate trihydrate	
Manganese sulfate monohydrate	
Ferric ammonium citrate	
Cobalt sulfate monohydrate	
Zinc sulfate	
Copper sulfate pentahydrate	
Sodium citrate	

ANCHOR TRIPLE SULFA BOLUS
Veterinary; antibacterial
(Anchor Labs)

Sulfathiazole *	90 gr.
Sulfanilamide *	90 gr.
Sulfamethazine *	60 gr.

ANCO GAS LINE ANTIFREEZE
Dryer and freeze protection for gasoline
(The Anderson Co.)

Methyl alcohol *	>98%

Starred ingredients (*) may be responsible for major toxic effects; consult Section II.

ANCOSUL

See ANCHOR ANCOSUL

ANCO WINDSHIELD WASHER ANTI-FREEZE
Preparation for washer reservoirs in wintertime
(The Anderson Co.)

Methyl alcohol *	>95%
Polyether alcohol surfactant	1%

ANCO WINDSHIELD WASHER SOLVENT
Preparation for washer reservoirs
(The Anderson Co.)

Polyether alcohol surfactant	1%
Sodium sulfosuccinate surfactant	1%

ANC TABLETS
Relief of minor aches and pains
(Friendly Labs.)

Each tablet:
Aspirin *	3 1/2 gr.
N-Acetyl-p-aminophenol	1/2 gr.
Caffeine	1 gr.
Salicylamide	2 gr.

ANDREA RAAB COSMETICS

Andrea Raab Corp.
4702 Glenwood Rd.
Brooklyn, N.Y. 11234

Phone: 212-252-8800

See COSMETICS, Section VI, General Formulations

ANDREW JERGENS TOILETRIES & COSMETICS

Andrew Jergens Co.
2535 Spring Grove Ave.
Cincinnati, Ohio 45214

Phone: 513-421-1400

See COSMETICS, Section VI, General Formulations

AN-DU-SEPTIC WHITE CHALK

See CRAYOLA AN-DU-SEPTIC WHITE CHALK

ANDYLATE-FORTE
Antipyretic, analgesic, circulatory stimulant
(Vita Elixir Co.)

Each tablet:
Aceto-p-aminophenol (Acetaminophen) *	3 gr.
Salicylamide *	3 gr.
Caffeine	1/4 gr.

ANDYLATE RUB
Temporary relief to minor aches and pain
(Vita Elixir Co.)

Methyl nicotinate
Methyl salicylate *
Camphor *
Dipropylene glycol salicylate
Oil of cassia
Oleoresin of Capsicum
Oleoresin of Ginger

ANDYLATE TABLETS
Antipyretic, analgesic
(Vita Elixir Co.)

Each tablet:
Sodium salicylate *	10 gr.

ANECAL CREAM
Skin irritations
(Lannett)

Benzocaine	3%
Calamine	5%
Zinc oxide	5%

ANEXSIA-D
Analgesic, antitussive
(Beecham Labs.)

Each tablet:
Hydrocodone bitartrate *	7 mg.
Phenacetin *	150 mg.
Aspirin *	230 mg.
Caffeine	30 mg.

ANEXSIA WITH CODEINE
Analgesic, antitussive
(Beecham Labs.)

Each tablet:
Codeine phosphate *	30 mg.
Phenacetin *	160 mg.
Aspirin *	225 mg.
Caffeine	32 mg.

ANGIJEN
Hypertension
(Jenkins Labs.)

Each tablet:
Pentaerythritol tetranitrate *	10 mg.

ANGIJEN NO. 1
Hypertension
(Jenkins Labs.)

Each tablet:
Pentaerythritol tetranitrate *	20 mg.
Phenobarbital *	15 mg.

ANIMA-SPRA
Insecticide for dogs, cats
(Goshen Labs.)

Pyrethrins	0.025%
Rotenone	0.128%
Other cube extractives	0.236%
Piperonyl butoxide	0.256%
Petroleum distillates	0.102%

ANITA OF DENMARK COSMETICS

Anita of Denmark Inc.
P.O. Box 2246
Palm Springs, Calif. 92263

Phone: 714-320-7481

See COSMETICS, Section VI, General Formulations

ANO BRUSH CLEANER
(Reliable Paste)

Mineral spirits *	>70%
Isopropanol	about 10%
Detergent	balance

ANODYNOS
Analgesic
(Buffington)

Each tablet:
Aspirin *
Salicylamide
Acetaminophen *
Caffeine

ANODYNOS DHC TABLETS
Analgesic & antipyretic
(Berlex Labs.)

Each tablet:
Dihydrocodeinone bitartrate	5 mg.
Aspirin *	227 mg.
Caffeine	32.4 mg.
Acetaminophen *	150 mg.

ANODYNOS FORTE
Cold relief tablets; antihistaminic-decongestant
(Buffington)

Each capsule shaped tablet:
Chlorpheniramine maleate	2 mg.
Phenylephrine hydrochloride *	10 mg.
Salicylamide	
Acetaminophen *	
Caffeine	

ANSAR 529 H.C.
Herbicide
(Diamond Shamrock Corp.)

Monosodium acid methanearsonate *	48.35%

ANSEMCO (NO. 2 & NO. 8)
Analgesic
(Elder)

Each No. 2 tablet:
Aspirin *	259.2 mg.
Phenacetin *	129.6 mg.
Caffeine	16.2 mg.

Each No. 8 tablet:
Aspirin *	226.8 mg.
Phenacetin *	162.0 mg.
Caffeine	16.2 mg.
Phenobarbital	16.2 mg.

Starred ingredients (*) may be responsible for major toxic effects; consult Section II.

ANTAGONATE TABLETS
Antihistaminic
(Dome)

Chlorpheniramine maleate * ..... 4 mg.

ANTAPRIN
Analgesic
(Cameron Medical Corp.)

Each tablet:
Aspirin * .... 5 gr.
Aluminum hydroxide glycine
Calcium carbonate

ANTCHEK ANT TRAP
(Linck)

Baygon * 0.250%

ANTEPAR SYRUP & TABLETS
Anthelmintic
(Burroughs Wellcome)

SYRUP:
Piperazine citrate anhy-
drous (equiv. to 500 mg.
of piperazine hexa-
hydrate) .... 550 mg/cc

TABLETS:
Piperazine citrate anhy-
drous (equiv. to 500 mg.
of piperazine hexa-
hydrate) .... 550 mg./tab.

ANT-GO

See SWEENEY'S ANT-GO

ANTHON HORSE WORMER
(Cutter (Brand) Bayvet Div. Cutter Labs.)

Active ingred.: 90%
Trichlorfon *
Inert ingred.: 10%
Colloidal Silica
Dextrose

ANTHRA-DERM OINTMENT
Psoriasis
(Dermik)

Anthralin *† 0.1%; 0.25%;
0.5%; or 1.0%
White petrolatum
Unsaturated fatty acid ester

†*See* Anthracene oil

ANTI-BAC B
Chlorinated sanitizer
(Diversey Wyandotte)

Sodium dichloroisocyanurate * 27.0%

ANTI-BORAX BRAZING FLUX NO. 2
(Anti-Borax)

Borax 1-20%
Boracic acid * 20-80%

ANTI-BORAX SILVER SOLDER PASTE FLUX NO. 16
(Anti-Borax)

Potassium carbonate *†
Potassium fluoborate *
Boracic acid *

Alkaline pH

†*See* Lye

ANTI-DUST WHITE CHALK

See CRAYOLA ANTI-DUST WHITE CHALK

ANTILIRIUM TABLETS
Cholinesterase
(OJF)

Each tablet:
Physostigine salicylate * .... 1 mg.

ANTI-SPOR CLIPPER OIL
Disinfectant and lubricant for clipper blades used in barber and beauty salons
(Nu-Vita Products Div.)

p-tertiary Amyl phenol 1%
Inert ingredients: 99%
Petroleum distillate (kerosene) *

ANTISTONE

See UNIVERSAL ANTISTONE

ANTI-TERGE HAND CREAM
Protective cream
(Comfort)

Silicones
Lanolin

ANTIVERT TABLETS, ANTIVERT/25 TABLETS, & ANTIVERT/25 CHEWABLE TABLETS
Antihistamine
(Roerig)

Each tablet:
Meclizine HCl * 12.5 mg.; and 25 mg.

ANT-JEX REDWOOD ANT STAKES
Insecticide
(General Pest Service)

Arsenic trioxide * 0.25%
Inert ingred.: 99.75%
Sugar, Honey, Water, Pectin, Citric acid

'76 Ed.

ANT-KIL POWDER

See DURHAM'S ANT-KIL POWDER

ANTNO
Ant killer
(Twin City Exterminating Co.)

Antimony potassium tartrate * 2%

'76 Ed.

ANTOR, EMULSIFIABLE CONCENTRATE
Herbicide
(Hercules Incorporated)

N-Chloroacetyl-N-(2,6-diethyl-
phenyl)glycine ethyl ester * 48%

ANTRENYL BROMIDE
Peptic ulcer, as adjunctive therapy
(CIBA Pharmaceutical)

Each tablet:
Oxyphenonium bromide *† .... 5 mg.

†*See* Atropine

ANTRIN
Analgesic
(Vale)

Each tablet:
Aspirin * .... 320 mg.
Valbase: .... 130 mg.
Dihydroxyaluminum aminoacetate

ANTRIN JUNIOR
Analgesic
(Vale)

Each tablet:
Aspirin * .... 81.0 mg.
Valbase: .... 64.8 mg.
Dihydroxyaluminum aminoacetate

ANTROCOL
Antisecretory-sedative
(Poythress, Wm. P.)

Each tablet or capsule:
Atropine sulfate * .... 0.195 mg.
Phenobarbital * .... 16 mg.

ANTROL ANT KILLER
(Boyle-Midway)

Sodium arsenite * 0.61%

ANTROL ANT KILLER SPRAY
(Boyle-Midway)

DDVP	0.20%
Baygon *	0.50%
Petroleum distillate *	83.03%
Propellant	

ANTROL ANT POWDER
(Boyle-Midway)

Baygon *	2.00%

ANTROL ANT TRAPS
(Boyle-Midway)

Baygon *	2.00%

ANTURANE TABLETS & CAPSULES
Chronic or intermittent gouty arthritis
(CIBA Pharmaceutical)

Sulfinpyrazone *	Tablets - 100 mg.
	Capsules - 200 mg.

ANTUSSAL SYRUP
(Vale)

Each fl. oz.:

Alcohol	1.5%
Phenylpropanolamine hydrochloride *	30.0 mg.
Pyrilamine maleate *	80.0 mg.
Ammonium chloride	518.4 mg.
Tolu syrup	q.s.

ANULAN SUPPOSITORIES
Rectal suppositories
(Lannett)

Bismuth resorcin compound *†
Bismuth subgallate
Zinc oxide
Boric acid *
Balsam Peru

†*See* Resorcinol

ANUPHEN SUPPOSITORIES
Analgesic, antipyretic
(Comatic)

Each suppository:
Acetaminophen *　120 mg.; 650 mg.

ANVITA
Medicated vaginal suppositories
(Schmidt)

Boric acid *	34%
Alum	0.5%
Thymol	1:13,000
Monochlorthymol	1:40,000
Phenylmercuric borate	1:2,000
Aromatics	<0.1%
Cocoa butter	q.s.

A.O.K.
Starting fluid
(Pyroil)

Combined amount:	<1%
High molecular weight esters	
Mixture of oxygenated unsaponifiable hydrocarbons	
Ethyl ether *	>90%

'76 Ed.

A-1
Hand rubbing compound
(McAleer)

Kerosene *
Sodium stearate
Paraffin oil
Tripoli (semidecomposed silica)

'76 Ed.

AORACILLIN-B
(Vita Elixir Co.)

Each tablet:	
Penicillin G (crystalline)	500,000 & 200,000 units

APACHE
Alkaline laundry compound
(Diversey Wyandotte)

Sodium hydroxide *
Alkaline salts

A&P ANTISEPTIC MOUTHWASH & GARGLE
(Great Atlantic & Pacific)

Ethyl alcohol	25.7%
Boric acid	0.5%
Eucalyptol	trace
Menthol	trace
Benzoic acid	trace
Methyl salicylate	trace
Color	trace
Water	balance

A&P ANT & ROACH KILLER
Household aerosol insecticide
(Great Atlantic & Pacific)

Pyrethrins	0.05%
Piperonyl butoxide	0.10%
N-Octyl bicycloheptene dicarboximide	0.17%
O-Isopropoxyphenyl methylcarbamate	0.50%
Isopropanol	7.50%
Methylene chloride	14.00%
Hydrocarbon propellant	20.00%
Petroleum distillate *	57.70%

A&P ASTRINGENT MOUTHWASH & GARGLE
(Great Atlantic & Pacific)

Ethyl alcohol	5.0%
Zinc chloride	0.2%
Flavors, color	trace
Water	balance

A&P AUTOMATIC DISHWASHER DETERGENT
(Great Atlantic & Pacific)

Sodium tripolyphosphate	30.0%
Sodium silicate *	16.0%
Nonionic surfactant	1.5%
Potassium dichloroisocyanurate	1.5%
Perfume	trace
Sodium sulfate	balance

pH (1% solution) - 10.5

A&P BUG KILLER II
Household aerosol insecticide
(Great Atlantic & Pacific)

Petroleum distillate	9.25%
Multicide Intermediate 2084	2.00%
Hydrocarbon propellant	30.00%
Water	balance

APCABUFF
(Approved Pharm.)

Each tablet:	
Aspirin *	3 1/4 gr.
Phenacetin *	2 1/2 gr.
Caffeine	1/2 gr.
Co-buffered with:	
Aluminum & magnesium hydroxide complex	

'76 Ed.

A.P.C. COMPLETE WATER TREATMENT FOR SWIMMING POOLS
(Modern Pool Products)

Calcium hypochlorite (available chlorine 70%) *

A.P.C. ICHTHYAMER OINTMENT 20%
For minor burns, bruises, boils
(Am. Pharmaceutical)

Brand of Ichthammol ointment

APCO 360
Solvent
(Oklahoma Refining)

Paraffins *	48%
Naphthenes *	40%
Aromatics *	11%
Olefins *	1%

APCO 467
Solvent
(Oklahoma Refining)

Paraffins *	42%
Naphthenes *	45%
Aromatics *	11%
Olefins *	2%

APCO 125, DEPOLARIZED

See DEPOLARIZED APCO 125

Starred ingredients (*) may be responsible for major toxic effects; consult Section II.

APCO 140, DEPOLARIZED

See DEPOLARIZED APCO 140

APCO 467, DEPOLARIZED

See DEPOLARIZED APCO 467

APCOTHINNER
Paint thinner
(Oklahoma Refining)

Paraffins *	53%
Naphthenes *	36%
Aromatics *	10%
Olefins	1%

A.P.C. WITH DEMEROL
Analgesic, spasmolytic, sedative, anti-pyretic
(Winthrop Labs.)

Each tablet:
Aspirin *	200 mg.
Phenacetin *	150 mg.
Caffeine *	30 mg.
Demerol hydrochloride *	30 mg.

APEX MOTH CAKES, CRYSTALS AND NUGGETS
(Clean Home)

Paradichlorobenzene *

'76 Ed.

A&P FLYING INSECT KILLER (Aerosol)
(Great Atlantic & Pacific)

Water	61.0%
Hydrocarbon propellant	30.0%
Petroleum distillate	6.4%
Synthetic Pyrethroid	2.5%
Perfume	trace

A&P FRESHENER(S)
Floral, Evergreen, Lilac, Spice, Lemon; aerosol air freshener
(Great Atlantic & Pacific)

Ethylene oxide condensate of a fatty acid	<1.25%
Diethyl phthalate	<1.00%
Ethyl alcohol	<1.00%
Perfume oil	<0.75%
Diglycol laurate (neutral)	<0.50%
Hydrocarbon propellant (Isobutane 85% - Propane 15%)	<35.00%
Water	balance

APHCO HEMORRHOIDAL OINTMENT & SUPPOSITORIES
(Am. Pharmaceutical)

Bismuth subcarbonate
Bismuth subgallate
Bismuth subiodide
Peruvian balsam
Resorcinol *
Benzocaine
Zinc oxide
Boric acid *

A&P LEMON FURNITURE POLISH (Aerosol)
(Great Atlantic & Pacific)

Silicone emulsion	<10%
Hydrocarbon propellant (Isobutane 85% - Propane 15%)	<5%
Isoparaffinic hydrocarbon	<0.75%
Wax	<0.50%
Morpholine	trace
Oleic acid	trace
Water	balance

A&P ORAL HYGIENIC MOUTHWASH & GARGLE
(Great Atlantic & Pacific)

Ethyl alcohol	18.5%
Glycerin	10.0%
Flavors, colors, other ingredients	trace
Water	balance

APO SUN CREAM WITH PABA
Sun screen
(Reynes Products, Inc.)

Purified water
TEA stearate
Mineral oil
Ethyl dihydroxypropyl PABA
Propylene glycol
Glycerin
Acetylated lanolin
Glyceryl stearate
Cetyl alcohol
Methylparaben
Propylparaben

A-POXIDE CAPSULES
Minor tranquilizer
(Abbott)

Each capsule:
Chlordiazepoxide hydrochloride (USP) *	5 mg.; 10 mg.; 25 mg.

APPEDRINE TABLETS
Appetite control
(Thompson Med.)

Each tablet:
Phenylpropanolamine HCl *	25 mg.
Caffeine *	100 mg.

Each three (3) tablets:
Vitamin A	5000 IU
Vitamin D	400 IU

Sodium carboxymethyl cellulose
Plus Multivitamins and minerals

APPET-IRON
(Columbia Med.)

Each tsp.:
Vitamin B1	10 mg.
Vitamin B12	25 mcg.
Ferric pyrophosphate	250 mg.

APPROVE
Soap for industrial and office use
(Calgon Corp., Commercial Div.)

Triclosan
Soap
Fatty amide
Emollients
Water

APPROVED PHARMACEUTICAL COLD SORE LOTION
(Approved Pharm.)

Benzoin *
Storax *
Tolu *
Camphor *
Isopropyl alcohol *

'76 Ed.

APPROVED PHARMACEUTICAL CORN REMOVER LOTION
(Approved Pharm.)

Isopropyl alcohol *
Salicylic acid *
Flexible Collodion *

'76 Ed.

APPROVED PHARMACEUTICAL DIURETIC PILLS
(Approved Pharm.)

Each pill:
Methylene blue	1/2 gr.
Ext. Uva ursi	1/4 gr.
Ext. Buchu	1/8 gr.
Couch grass	1/2 gr.
Corn silk	1/2 gr.
Oil juniper	1/20 gr.

'76 Ed.

APPROVED PHARMACEUTICAL NAIL BITING & THUMB SUCKING LIQUID
(Approved Pharm.)

Capsicum *
Aloes *
Tolu *
Alcohol

'76 Ed.

Starred ingredients (*) may be responsible for major toxic effects; consult Section II.

APPROVED PHARMACEUTICAL PYRIDENE TABLETS
Urinary tract analgesic
(Approved Pharm.)

Phenylazo-diaminopyridene
HCl * .... 100 mg.

'76 Ed.

APPROVED PHARMACEUTICAL SUPER STRENGTH PAIN RELIEVER
(Approved Pharm.)

Each tablet:
N-Acetyl-p-aminophenol * .. 1 1/2 gr.
Caffeine .... 1 gr.
Aspirin * .... 3 1/2 gr.
Salicylamide .... 2 gr.

'76 Ed.

APPROVED PHARMACEUTICAL TEETHING LOTION
(Approved Pharm.)

Benzocaine
Iodine *
Alcohol

'76 Ed.

APPROVED PHARMACEUTICAL TOOTHACHE LIQUID
(Approved Pharm.)

Oil of cloves *
Oil of cassia *
Benzocaine
Iodine *
Alcohol

'76 Ed.

APRO HEMORRHOIDAL OINTMENT
(Approved Pharm.)

Hyoscyamine sulfate *
Chloroform
Alcohol
Diperodon
Chloral hydrate *
Menthol *
Camphor *
Zinc oxide

'76 Ed.

APRO HEMORRHOIDAL SUPPOSITORIES
(Approved Pharm.)

Bismuth subgallate
Bismuth oxyiodide
Resorcin *
Diperodon
Peru balsam *
Boric acid *
Zinc oxide
Cocoa butter

'76 Ed.

A&P SHAVE CREAM (Regular, Lemon-Lime and Menthol)
(Great Atlantic & Pacific)

Stearic acid 6.4%
Glycerine 6.0%
Triethanolamine 5.0%
Hydrocarbon propellant 4.0%
Sodium lauryl sulfate 1.5%
Coconut fatty acid 1.5%
Stearyl alcohol 0.5%
Menthol (in Menthol product) .. 0.5%
Perfume (in Regular and Lemon-
Lime product) 0.5%

A&P SPRAY STARCH
(Great Atlantic & Pacific)

Starch 5.00%
Sulfonated Castor oil 0.50%
Sodium borate 0.25%
Silicone emulsion 0.10%
Minor components .... trace
Isobutane/propane propellant .. 7.00%
Water .... balance

APTREX
Non-selective weed killer
(Certified Labs.)

Monuron trichloroacetate (3-(p-
Chlorophenyl)-1,1-dimethylurea
trichloroacetate) 3.20%
Isooctyl ester of 2,4-dichlorophen-
oxyacetic acid 0.50%

A&P WINDOW CLEANER WITH AMMONIA
(Great Atlantic & Pacific)

Isopropanol 8.0%
Ethylene glycol monoisobutyl
ether 2.5%
Nonyl alkyl phenol polyglycol
ether .... trace
Triethanolamine lauryl sulfate . trace
Dye .... trace
Ammonia .... trace
Water .... balance

pH - 9.5-10.5

A&P WINDOW SPRAY WITH AMMONIA
(Great Atlantic & Pacific)

Isopropanol 7.5%
Ethylene glycol monoisobutyl
ether 2.5%
Nonyl alkyl phenol polyglycol
ether .... trace
Triethanolamine lauryl sulfate . trace
Ammonia .... trace
Hydrocarbon propellant 4.5%
Water .... balance

pH - 9.5-10.5

A-200 PYRINATE LIQUID
Pediculicide
(Norcliff Thayer)

Pyrethrins 0.165%
Piperonyl butoxide (tech.) 2.000%
Deodorized Kerosene 5.000%

AQUA-BAN TABLETS
Diuretic
(Thompson Med.)

Each tablet:
Ammonium chloride
Caffeine *

AQUACARE CREAM
Dry skin cream
(Herbert Labs.)

Urea .... 2 %
Benzyl alcohol *
Emollient base

AQUACARE/HP CREAM
(Herbert Labs.)

Purified water
Urea 10%
Oleth-3 phosphate
Cetyl stearyl glycol
Petrolatum
Triethanolamine
Synthetic Spermaceti
Carbomer 934
Glycerin
Mineral oil
Lanolin alcohol
Lanolin oil
Benzyl alcohol
Perfume

AQUACARE/HP LOTION
(Herbert Labs.)

Purified water
Urea 10%
Oleth-3 phosphate
Petrolatum
Synthetic Spermaceti
Glycerin
Triethanolamine
Mineral oil
Lanolin alcohol
Cetyl stearyl glycol
Lanolin oil
Carbomer 934
Benzyl alcohol
Perfume

Starred ingredients (*) may be responsible for major toxic effects; consult Section II.

AQUACARE LOTION
Dry skin lotion
(Herbert Labs.)

Urea .... 2 %
Benzyl alcohol *
Emollient base

AQUA CHECK
*Test strip for swimming pool water free
    chlorine and pH reagent*
(Ames)

Bromthymol blue
Vanillin azine
Syringealdazine

AQUACHLORAL
SUPPRETTES
Rectal sedative
(Webcon)

Each suppository:
Chloral hydrate * .... 5 gr.; 10 gr.;
                            or 15 gr.

AQUACIDE
*Insecticide; institutional and industrial
    use*
(Schneid)

Pyrethrins 0.10%
Piperonyl butoxide (technical) 0.20%
Essential oils 0.30%
N-Octyl bicycloheptene
    dicarboximide 0.33%
Petroleum distillate 0.48%

'76 Ed.

AQUA-CIDE
(CONCENTRATE)
Control of algae in swimming pools
(Hysan Corp.)

N-Alkyl (60% C14, 30% C16, 5% C12,
    5% C18) dimethyl benzyl ammo-
    nium chlorides * 5.00%
N-Alkyl (50% C12, 30% C14, 17%
    C16, 3% C18) dimethyl ethylben-
    zyl ammonium chlorides * 5.00%

AQUADENE
*Potable water treatment (sequestering
    agent)*
(Stiles-Kem)

Complex Polyphosphates * 50%

AQUADERM MOISTURE
LOTION
(C & M Pharmacal)

Purified water
Glycerine 20%
Propylene glycol 10%
Salicylic acid 0.25%
Octoxynol-9 (nonionic
    penetrant) 0.03%
FD & C Red No. 40 .... 0.0001%
Fragrance

AQUA-DUCE TABLETS
Diuretic
(Columbia Med.)

Each tablet:
Po. ext. Buchu .... 32.4 mg.
Po. ext. Uva Ursi .... 32.4 mg.
Po. ex. Corn silk .... 32.4 mg.
Po. ext. Juniper .... 16.2 mg.
Caffeine * .... 16.2 mg.

AQUA ETHION 8
INSECTICIDE

See NIAGARA AQUA ETHION 8 IN-
    SECTICIDE

AQUA-FLOW
Hard lens rewetting solution
(CooperVision Pharm.)

Polyvinyl alcohol
Hydroxyethylcellulose
Sodium bicarbonate
Sodium chloride
Potassium chloride
Benzalkonium chloride
Trisodium edetate

AQUA-FRESH
Toothpaste
(Beecham Products)

Sodium monofluorophosphate

AQUAGENE-1 SPRAY
ADJUVANT

See UNICO AQUAGENE-1 SPRAY
    ADJUVANT

AQUA KEM
*Deodorant for use in portable toilet
    holding tanks*
(Thetford Corp.)

Formaldehyde * 34%
Methanol * 11%
Nonionic surfactant .... <3%
Perfume oil .... <2%
Cellulose derivative .... <1%
Acid Blue #9 .... <1%
Water .... balance

AQUA KEM TOSS INS
*Deodorizer for use in portable toilet
    holding tanks*
(Thetford Corp.)

Paraformaldehyde * 80%
Sodium silico aluminate 10%
Inorganic phosphate .... <5%
Perfume oil .... <5%
Acid Blue #9 .... <5%

AQUA KILL, MUNICHEM

See MUNICHEM AQUA KILL

AQUA-KLEEN 20
Herbicide
(Amchem)

2,4-Dichlorophenoxyacetic acid, bu-
    toxy ethanol ester * 29.0%

AQUA LACTEN LOTION
For rough or chapped skin
(Herald Pharm.)

Cetyl alcohol
Propylene glycol monostearate, pure
Light Liquid petrolatum
Petrolatum Snow White
Urea 10%
Lactic acid 2%
Sodium lauryl sulfate
Propylparaben
Methylparaben

AQUALAND ALGAECIDE
Algae control in swimming pools
(Aqualand)

n-Alkyl (50% C12, 30% C14, 17% C16,
    3% C18) dimethyl ethylbenzyl am-
    monium chlorides * 5%
n-Alkyl (60% C14, 30% C12,
    5% C18) dimethyl benzyl ammo-
    nium chlorides * 5%

AQUALAND CHLORINE
CONCENTRATE
Swimming pool treatment
(Aqualand)

Potassium dichloro-s-
    triazinetrione * 97%

AQUALAND DRY
CHLORINATING
CHEMICAL
*For algae and bacteria control in swim-
    ming pools*
(Aqualand)

Sodium   dichloro-s-triazinetrione
    dihydrate   (available   chlorine
    56%) * 100%

AQUALAND STABILIZED
CHLORINATING TABLETS
*For algae and bacteria control in swim-
    ming pools*
(Aqualand)

Trichloro-s-triazinetrione (available
    chlorine 85%) * 99.5%

AQUALENE SOLUBLE OIL
(Crescent Oil)

Mineral oil
Petroleum sulfonate *

Starred ingredients (*) may be responsible for major toxic effects; consult Section II.

AQUAMED LOTION
For dry, itchy or chapped skin
(Herald Pharm.)

Cetyl alcohol
Propylene glycol monostearate, pure
Light liquid petrolatum
Petrolatum, Snow White, USP
Sorbitan monostearate
Sodium lauryl sulfate *
Propylparaben
Methylparaben

AQUAMINT COSMETIC PRODUCTS
Cosmetics and toiletries

Aquamint Laboratories, Inc.
P.O. Box 7
St. Charles, Ill. 60174

Phone: 312-584-1251

See COSMETICS, Section VI, General Formulations

AQUA PHOS KIL 6

See NIAGARA AQUA PHOS KIL 6

AQUA PURER, WARDLEY'S

See WARDLEY'S AQUA PURER

AQUA-SHED WATERPROOF FLOOR WAX
(Uncle Sam)

Polyethylene
Waxes
Resins (modified phenolic & styrene maleic anhydride)
Ammonia *
Morpholine *
Oleic acid
Potassium hydroxide *

AQUASONIC 100 ULTRASOUND TRANSMISSION GEL
(Parker Labs.)

Polymer
Humectant
Deionized/ultraviolet Water
Food color (FDA approved)
Perfume
Methylparaben
Propylparaben

pH 6.50 to 6.95

AQUATAG
Diuretic
(Direct Div.)

Each tablet:
  Benzthiazide * .... 25 mg.; 50 mg.

AQUATHOL
Herbicide
(Pennwalt)

Endothall (as disodium salt)
(liquid concentrate) * .. 1.46 lbs./gal.

AQUATHOL GRANULAR
Herbicide
(Pennwalt)

Endothall (as dipotassium salt) * .. 7.2%

AQUATHOL K
Herbicide
(Pennwalt)

Endothall (as dipotassium salt) * .... 3 lbs./gal.

AQUATHOL PLUS
Herbicide
(Pennwalt)

Endothall * .... 1.7 lbs./gal.
Silvex as potassium salts ... 2.4 lbs./gal.

AQUATHOL PLUS GRANULAR
Herbicide
(Pennwalt)

Endothall * 3.6%
Silvex as potassium salts 5.0%

AQUA TONIC, WARDLEY'S

See WARDLEY'S AQUA TONIC

AQUA VELVA AFTER SHAVING LOTION
(Williams, J.B.)

Alcohol (denatured with colocynth) *
Glycerin

AQUA VELVA SILICONE LATHER
(Williams, J.B.)

Triethanolamine soap
Lanolin oil
Silicone
Propellants

AQUAZINE
Algicide
(Ciba-Geigy Ag. Div.)

Simazine * 80%

AQUET
Detergent
(Manostat)

Alkyl aryl polyethylene glycol *
Trace amount of water

AQUINOC

See AIRWICK PROFESSIONAL PRODUCTS AQUINOC

AQWADRIL-50
Diuretic
(Wesley Pharm.)

Each tablet:
  Hydrochlorothiazide * .... 50 mg.

AQWESIDE
Diuretic-antihypertensive
(Wesley Pharm.)

Each tablet:
  Trichlormethiazide * .... 4 mg.

AQWESINE-25 & -50
Antihypertensive
(Wesley Pharm.)

Each tablet:
  Hydrochlorothiazide * .... 25 or 50 mg.
  Reserpine .... 0.125 mg.

ARAB BUG-DETH
(Federal Chem.)

Baygon 0.500%
2,2-Dichlorovinyl dimethyl phosphate (DDVP) 0.093%
Related compounds 0.007%
Petroleum distillate * 39.390%
Inerts: Chlorinated solvent and CO_2 * 60.010%

ARAB CRACK & CREVICE ROACH CONTROL (Aerosol)
(Federal Chem.)

Chlorpyrifos 0.500%

ARAB FLEA & TICK SPRAY MIST (Aerosol)
(Federal Chem.)

Carbaryl 0.500%
Rotenone 0.100%
Rotenoids and other Cube extractives 0.200%
Pyrethrins I and II 0.050%
Technical Piperonyl butoxide ... 0.250%
Butoxypolypropylene glycol 2.500%

ARAB FLY & MOSQUITO SPRAY (Aerosol)
(Federal Chem.)

Resmethrin 0.200%
Related compounds 0.028%
d-trans Allethrin (allyl homolog of Cinerin I) 0.400%
Related compounds 0.030%
Aromatic petroleum hydrocarbons 0.272%
Petroleum distillate 6.500%

Starred ingredients (*) may be responsible for major toxic effects; consult Section II.

ARAB FOGERATOR (Aerosol)
Insecticide
(Federal Chem.)

2,2-Dichlorovinyl dimethyl phosphate (DDVP)	0.46%
Related compounds	0.04%
Pyrethrins	0.50%
Technical Piperonyl butoxide	2.50%
Petroleum distillates *	16.45%

ARAB 45 TERMITE CONTROL CONCENTRATE
(Federal Chem.)

Technical Chlordane *	45%
Petroleum distillate *	50%
Inerts: Emulsifier	5%

ARAB LAWN AND GARDEN

See ARAB LAWN-GARD

ARAB LAWN-GARD
Insecticide
(Federal Chem.)

Diazinon *	25.0%
Aromatic petroleum derivative solvent *	55.7%

ARAB PATIO & GARDEN INSECT SPRAY (Water-based Aerosol)
(Federal Chem.)

Resmethrin	0.200%
Related compounds	0.028%
d-trans Allethrin (allyl homolog of Cinerin I)	0.150%
Related compounds	0.012%
Aromatic petroleum hydrocarbons	0.272%
Petroleum distillate	6.500%

ARAB POWER PAK INSECT FOGGER (Aerosol)
Insecticide
(Federal Chem.)

Pyrethrins	0.500%
Technical Piperonyl butoxide	1.000%
N-Octyl bicycloheptene dicarboximide	1.000%
Refined Petroleum oil	8.000%

ARAB ROACH AND ANT SPRAY
Insecticide
(Federal Chem.)

Diazinon	0.500%
Pyrethrins	0.105%
Technical Piperonyl butoxide	0.525%
Petroleum distillates *	98.870%

ARAB U-DO-IT TERMITE CONTROL CONCENTRATE
Insecticide
(Federal Chem.)

Technical Chlordane *	72.00%
Petroleum distillate *	23.00%
Inerts (Emulsifier)	5.0%

ARAB WASP & HORNET SPRAY
(Federal Chem.)

Baygon	0.500%
2,2-Dichlorovinyl dimethyl phosphate (DDVP)	0.325%
Related compounds	0.025%
Petroleum distillate *	39.140%
Inerts: Chlorinated solvents and CO_2 *	60.010%

ARACAIN RECTAL OINTMENT
(Commerce Drug)

Benzocaine
Carbolic acid *
Menthol *
Thymol *
Zinc oxide
Boric acid *
Tannic acid *
Sulfur
Oils of Eucalyptus *, Tar, Juniper tar

ARALEN PHOSPHATE TABLETS
For malaria, extraintestinal amebiasis
(Winthrop Labs.)

Each tablet:	
Chloroquine phosphate *	500 mg.

ARALEN PHOSPHATE WITH PRIMAQUINE PHOSPHATE, USP
For malaria prophylaxis only
(Winthrop Labs.)

Each tablet:	
Aralen phosphate (brand of chloroquine phosphate, USP)(equiv. to 300 mg. base) *	500 mg.
Primaquine phosphate (equiv. to 45 mg. base) *	79 mg.

"ARASAN" 50 RED-ND SEED PROTECTANT
(Du Pont)

Thiram *	50%

"ARASAN" 50 RED SEED PROTECTANT
(Du Pont)

Thiram *	50%

"ARASAN" 70-S SEED PROTECTANT
(Du Pont)

Thiram *	70%
Methoxychlor	2%

ARBOR FOOT SALVE
(Washington Hom.)

Thuya occidentalis HPUS *†

†*See* Essential oils

ARCO AQUATIC WEEDKILLER
Herbicide
(Atlantic Richfield Co.)

Petroleum oil *	99.8%

'76 Ed.

ARCO HOUSEHOLD OIL
(Atlantic Richfield Co.)

Petroleum distillates *	98.3%

'76 Ed.

ARCO LIGHTER FLUID
(Atlantic Richfield Co.)

Petroleum distillates *	100%

'76 Ed.

ARCO MOTOR OIL
(Atlantic Richfield Co.)

Oil-soluble Zinc-phosphorus type compound *†
Oil-soluble Barium or calcium sulfonate *
Refined Mineral oil *

'76 Ed.

†*See* Zinc salts

ARCONOMY POWDER
(Armour-Dial, Inc.)

Sodium soap	75-100%
Moisture	1-5%
Minor ingredients (total)	1-5%

ARCO SELECTIVE WEEDKILLER NO. 1 AND WEEDKILLER "A"
Herbicides
(Atlantic Richfield Co.)

Petroleum hydrocarbon *	100%

'76 Ed.

Starred ingredients (*) may be responsible for major toxic effects; consult Section II.

ARDELL HAIR CARE PRODUCTS

Ardell, Inc.
30601 Carter Rd.
Solon, Ohio 44139

Phone: 216-248-3700

See COSMETICS, Section VI, General Formulations

A-REST
Growth regulator
(Elanco Prod.)

Ancymidol 0.0264%

AR-EX COSMETICS

Ar-Ex Products Co.
1036 W. Van Buren
Chicago. Ill. 60607

Phone: 312-226-5241

See COSMETICS, Section VI, General Formulations

ARGESIC TABLETS
Analgesic
(Econo Med)

Each tablet:
Phenyltoloxamine citrate * .. 30 mg.
Magnesium salicylate .... 600 mg.

ARGYROL S.S. 10%
Anti-infective
(CooperVision Pharm.)

Each fl. oz.:
Mild Silver
  protein *† ...... 100 mg. silver/ml.
Calcium disodium
  edetate .... 11 mg./ml.

†*See* Silver salts

ARGYROL S.S. 20% DROPPERETTE
Anti-infective
(CooperVision Pharm.)

Each fl. oz.:
Mild Silver
  protein *† ...... 200 mg. silver/ml.
Calcium disodium
  edetate .... 11 mg./ml.

†*See* Silver salts

ARIEL
Granular laundry detergent
(Procter & Gamble)

Complex sodium phosphate * . 50-74%
Sodium sulfate 10-24%
Sodium alkyl benzene sulfonate . 5-9%
Water 5-9%
Sodium alkyl ethoxylate sulfate . 1-4%
Alkyl ethoxylate 1-4%
Sodium silicate 1-4%
Enzymes 1-4%
Soap 1-4%
Minor ingredients, each .... trace

pH of 1% solution 10.0

ARKOLENE GN
Biodegradable plus humectant anionic wetting agent
(Arkansas Co.)

Linear   alkyl   ammonium
  sulfonate * .... approx. 30%

'76 Ed.

ARKO SCOUR AA
Scouring agent
(Arkansas Co.)

Ethoxylated alcohol ...... approx. 40%
Solvent (Xylol type) *† ... approx. 45%

'76 Ed.

†*See* Xylene

ARLAC
Alkaline laundry compound
(Diversey Wyandotte)
Sodium hydroxide *
Alkaline salts

ARMADEX
Appetite control
(Arman Drug Co.)

Each three capsules:
Sodium
  carboxymethylcellulose .....300 mg.
Benzocaine .... 9.0 mg.
Vitamin A (Palmitate) .4000 USP units
Vitamin D (Calciferol)400 USP units
Vitamin C (Ascorbic acid) .....30 mg.
Iron (as fumarate) ....10 mg.
Plus multivitamins & minerals

ARMAN'S EAR DROPS
For softening of ear wax
(Arman Drug Co.)

Benzalkonium chloride 1:1000
Chlorobutanol (anhydrous) 1%
Benzocaine
Urea
Base:
  Propylene glycol
  Glycerine

ARM & HAMMER CARPET DEODORIZER (SCENTED & UNSCENTED)
(Church & Dwight)

Sodium bicarbonate *
Perfume (Scented only) 0.35%

ARM & HAMMER CAT LITTER DEODORIZER
(Church & Dwight)

Sodium bicarbonate *

ARM & HAMMER LAUNDRY DETERGENT
(Church & Dwight)

Anionic surfactant *
Nonionic surfactant
Sodium carbonates *
Sodium silicate *

ARM & HAMMER OVEN CLEANER
(Church & Dwight)

Potassium glycolate *†
Potassium acetate *†
Calcium carbonate

†*See* Potassium salts

ARM & HAMMER WASHING SODA
(Church & Dwight)

Sodium carbonate (hydrated) * .. 100%

ARMITE ANTI-SEIZE NO. 609
Sealant and anti-seize compound for threaded fittings and gaskets
(Balkamp, Inc.; Mfr., Armite Labs.)

Pure metallic Lead powder * 72%
Petroleum oil * 20%
Petroleum grease (Barium soap 15%) . 8%

ARMITE MIRACLE FORMULA 12/34 AEROSOL/BULK
Penetrant, lubricant, corrosion inhibitor
(Balkamp, Inc.; Mfr., Armite Labs.)

Mineral spirits * 70%
Mineral oil * 21%
Petrolatum 6%
Emulsifiers 3%
Carbon dioxide (Aerosol)

Starred ingredients (*) may be responsible for major toxic effects; consult Section II.

ARMOHEX LIQUID HEXACHLOROPHENE SOAP CONCENTRATE (Institutional)
(Armour-Dial, Inc.)

Moisture and volatile	50-75%
Potash soap *	25-50%
Glycerin	1-5%
PEG-75 lanolin	1-5%
Hexachlorophene	0.75%
Minor ingredients (total)	0.1-1%

ARMOHEX LIQUID HEXACHLOROPHENE SOAP - READY TO USE; Red and Natural (Institutional)
(Armour-Dial, Inc.)

Moisture and volatile	75-100%
Potash soap *	10-25%
Hexachlorophene	0.25%
Minor ingredients (total)	1-5%

ARMOR ALL CLEANER
General purpose cleaner
(Armor All Products)

Water solution/Glycol ether *	90%
Coconut superamide	
Antimicrobial agent	1%

ARMOR ALL PROTECTANT
Protective treatment for most polymer materials
(Armor All Products)

Polydimethyl siloxane (water solution/emulsion)	>90%
Antimicrobial agent	<1%

ARMOR ALL ULTRA-PLATE
Hard surface protective treatment and polish
(Armor All Products)

Odorless Mineral spirits *	>20%
Amino functional Polydimethyl siloxane	<10%
Diatomaceous earth and fillers	<10%
Water	>50%

ARMORCOTE PRODUCTS

See COOK'S ARMORCOTE PRODUCTS

ARMOR-TILE REDUCER

See COOK'S ARMOR-TILE REDUCER

A.R.M. TABLETS (ALLERGY RELIEF MEDICINE)
(MenJ Labs.)

Each tablet:
Chlorpheniramine maleate *	4.0 mg.
Phenylpropanolamine HCl *	37.5 mg.

ARNUCLANS
Hematinic
(Wesley Pharm.)

Each tablet:
Strychnine sulfate *	1/150 gr.
Iron arsenate	1/67 gr.
Thiamine hydrochloride	1 mg.

AROTEX 8302

See INTEX 8302 AROTEX

ARREST BUFFABLE DETERGENT RESISTANT FLOOR FINISH

See AIRWICK PROFESSIONAL PRODUCTS ARREST BUFFABLE DETERGENT RESISTANT FLOOR FINISH

ARRID CREAM
Antiperspirant deodorant
(Carter Products)

Aluminum chlorohydrate *	<25%
Aluminum chloride	<5%
Water	
Waxes and emollient oils	
Nonionic emulsifiers	
Glycerine	
Dimethicone	
Hydroxypropyl methylcellulose	
Fragrance	
Preservative	

ARRID EXTRA DRY LIGHT POWDER
Deodorant/antiperspirant
(Carter Products)

Aluminum chlorohydrate	<13%
Oils	
Talc	
Mineral dispersant	
Hydrocarbons	
Perfume (Scented, Unscented, Baby Fresh)	

ARRID EXTRA DRY NON-AEROSOL SPRAY
Antiperspirant deodorant
(Carter Products)

Aluminum sesquichlorohydrate	<20%
Alcohol	
Water	
Emollient oils	
Nonionic emulsifiers	
Fragrance	

ARRID EXTRA DRY POWDER ROLL-ON
Antiperspirant deodorant
(Carter Products)

Aluminum chlorohydrate *	<50%
Aluminum chloride	<5%
Talc and Silica	
Nonionic emulsifiers, esters and ethers	
Fragrance (Regular, Baby Fresh)	

ARRID EXTRA DRY SPRAY
Deodorant/antiperspirant
(Carter Products)

Aluminum chlorohydrate	<13%
Oils	
Mineral dispersant	
Hydrocarbons	
Perfume (Scented and Unscented)	

ARRID ROLL-ON
Antiperspirant deodorant
(Carter Products)

Aluminum zirconium complex	<25%
Water	
Nonionic emulsifiers	
Magnesium aluminum silicate	
Cyclomethicone	
Fragrance	

ARRID SPRAY DEODORANT
(Carter Products)

Anhydrous Alcohol
Zinc phenolsulfonate *
Propylene glycol
Perfume
Hydrocarbons

ARRID XX ROLL-ON
Antiperspirant deodorant
(Carter Products)

Aluminum chlorohydrate *	<25%
Water	
Nonionic emulsifiers	
Magnesium aluminum silicate	
Fragrance	
Color	

ARRID XX SPRAY
Deodorant/antiperspirant
(Carter Products)

Aluminum chlorohydrate	<13%
Oils	
Mineral dispersant	
Hydrocarbons	
Perfume (Scented and Unscented)	

ARRIVE
Detergent-germicide
(Puritan Chem. Co.)

Active ingred.:	15.2%
n-Alkyl (60% C14, 30% C16, 5% C12, 5% C18) dimethyl benzyl ammonium chloride *	
n-Alkyl (68% C12, 32% C14) dimethyl ethylbenzyl ammonium chloride *	
Tetrasodium ethylene diamine tetraacetate	
Sodium carbonate	
Essential oils	
Inert ingred.:	84.8%
Water	
Perfume	
Dye	

Starred ingredients (*) may be responsible for major toxic effects; consult Section II.

ARROW
Acid detergent and lime solvent; industrial use
(National-Purity Soap)

Organic acids *
Nonionic wetting agents

pH of 1% solution 2.5

ARROW CHROME PROTECTOR
(Arrow Labs.)

Mineral oil, light
Oleic acid
Triethanolamine
Non-ionic detergent *

'76 Ed.

ARROW CHROME RUST REMOVER
(Arrow Labs.)

Oxalic acid *
Hydrochloric acid *

'76 Ed.

ARROW HEAVY DUTY STEAM CLEANING COMPOUND
(Arrow Labs.)

Caustic soda *

'76 Ed.

ARROW LEATHER MAGIC
(Arrow Labs.)

Sodium metasilicate
Isopropanol
Sodium alkyl sulfate *
Triethanolamine lauryl sulfate *
Fatty amide-condensate
Sulfonated ketones
Hydrophilic wax-cyclohexanone-amine
  wax (Vegamin wax)
Anhydrous fatty acid-amine condensate

'76 Ed.

ARROW MAGIC REMOVER
(Arrow Labs.)

Mineral spirits *
Orthodichlorobenzene *
Xylol *

'76 Ed.

ARROW PURPLE MAGIC
(Arrow Labs.)

Sodium alkyl sulfate *
Triethanolamine lauryl sulfate *
Fatty amide-condensate
Anhydrous fatty acid-amine condensate
Sulfonated ketones
Hydrophilic wax-cyclohexanone-amine
  wax (Vegamin wax)

'76 Ed.

ARROW STEAM CLEANER CONCENTRATE NO. 351
(Arrow Labs.)

Caustic soda *

'76 Ed.

ARROW WHITE TIRE MAGIC
(Arrow Labs.)

Alcohol *
Alkali *

'76 Ed.

ARRYL
Antiseptic oral wash
(Rogers Park)

Carbamide (Synthetic urea)
Sodium alkyl aryl sulfonate *

ARSEPHENO CATTLE DRENCH

See MARTIN'S ARSEPHENO CATTLE DRENCH

ARSEPHENO SHEEP & GOAT DRENCH

See MARTIN'S ARSEPHENO SHEEP & GOAT DRENCH

ARSONATE LIQUID
Post-emergence weed control of cotton
(Diamond Shamrock Corp.)

Monosodium acid
  methanearsonate * 51.0%

AR-SULFA SOLUBLE POWDER
Veterinary bactericide
(Salsbury)

Sodium sulfathiazole
  sesquihydrate * 100%

ARTEX LIP TINT
Embalming supply
(Royal Bond)

Isopropanol *
Acetone *

ARTEX PAINT SOLVENT & CLEANER
(Artex)

Aromatic hydrocarbons * 98.9%
Non-aromatic hydrocarbons 1.1%

ARTEX ROLL-ON DECORATOR PAINT
Regular line, Brite & Wild, Gemtex
(Artex)

Mineral spirits * .... approx. 40%
Modified Urethane oil resin approx. 40%
Organic pigments (no toxic
  heavy metals) .... approx. 20%

ARTEX ROLL-ON DECORATOR PAINT MAGIC GLO
(Artex)

Acrylic ester .... approx. 50%
Toluene * .... approx. 30%
Organic pigments (no toxic
  heavy metals) .... approx. 20%

ARTEX ROLL-ON DECORATOR PAINT XTRA GLO
(Artex)

Acrylic copolymer .... approx. 35%
Cellosolve * .... approx. 33%
Organic pigments (no toxic
  heavy metals) .... approx. 18%
Acetone * .... approx. 12%
N-Propyl acetate .... <2%

ARTEX TIP CLEANER
Solvent cleaner
(Artex)

Mineral spirits * 100%

ARTHOL
(Towne-Paulsen)

Each tablet:
  Acetaminophen * .... 250 mg.
  Salicylamide .... 250 mg.
  Vitamin C .... 50 mg.

ARTHRALGEN TABLETS
Analgesic, antipyretic
(Robins)

Each tablet:
  Salicylamide .... 250 mg.
  Acetaminophen * .... 250 mg.
  Ascorbic acid .... 25 mg.

ARTHRITIS STRENGTH BUFFERIN
Analgesic
(Bristol-Myers)

Each tablet:
  Aspirin * .... 7 1/2 gr.
  Di-Alminate:
    Aluminum glycinate
    Magnesium carbonate

ARTISTRY II CREAMY CLEANSING LOTION

See AMWAY ARTISTRY II CREAMY CLEANSING LOTION

Starred ingredients (*) may be responsible for major toxic effects; consult Section II.

ARTISTRY II SKIN FRESHENER

See AMWAY ARTISTRY II SKIN FRESHENER

ARTRA SKIN TONE CREAM
Skin bleaching agent
(Plough)

Cetyl alcohol
Starfol wax (Glyceryl stearate)
Methylparaben
Hydroquinone * .... 2.0% w/w
Perfume
Sodium sulfite

A.S.A. COMPOUND
Antipyretic, analgesic, antirheumatic
(Lilly, Eli)

Each Pulvule:
  Acetophenetidin * .... 0.16 gm.
  Acetylsalicylic acid * ...... 0.227 gm.
  Caffeine .... 0.0325 gm.

ASAFEN TABLETS
Analgesic
(Rawleigh)

Each tablet:
  Aspirin * .... 3 gr.
  Phenacetin * .... 3 gr.
  Caffeine .... 1/3 gr.

'76 Ed.

ASALCO NO. 1
Analgesic
(Jenkins Labs.)

Each tablet:
  Acetylsalicylic acid * .... 3 1/2 gr.
  Acetophenetidin * .... 2 1/2 gr.
  Caffeine .... 1/2 gr.

ASALCO NO. 2
Anodyne, analgesic with sedative effects
(Jenkins Labs.)

Each tablet:
  Dover's powder (powdered opium, 1/40 gr.) * .... 1/4 gr.
  Acetylsalicylic acid * .... 3 1/2 gr.
  Acetophenetidin * .... 2 1/2 gr.
  Caffeine .... 1/2 gr.
  Tincture Gelsemium .... 2 mg.

ASBRON G INLAY-TABS & ELIXIR
Bronchodilator, expectorant
(Dorsey Labs.)

Each tablet or 15 ml.:
  Theophylline sodium glycinate * .... 300 mg.
  Guaifenesin (Glyceryl guaiacolate) .... 100 mg.
  Alcohol (Elixir only) 15%

ASCAP COMPOUND
Cold remedy
(Maxim Chem.)

Salicylamide * .... 5 gr.
Acetophenetidin * .... 2 1/2 gr.
Caffeine .... 1/2 gr.

'76 Ed.

ASCAP "P" COMPOUND
Cold remedy
(Maxim Chem.)

Salicylamide * .... 5 gr.
Acetophenetidin * .... 2 1/2 gr.
Caffeine .... 1/2 gr.
Phenobarbital * .... 1/4 gr.

'76 Ed.

ASCORBICAP
Treatment of vitamin C deficiency
(ICN Pharm.)

Each timed-release capsule:
  Ascorbic acid .... 500 mg.

ASCRIPTIN A/D
Buffered analgesic & antipyretic for arthritis therapy
(Rorer, W.H., Inc.)

Each tablet:
  Aspirin * .... 325 mg.
  Maalox (Magnesium-aluminum hydroxide) .... 300 mg.

ASCRIPTIN TABLETS
Analgesic, antipyretic, anti-inflammatory
(Rorer, W.H., Inc.)

Each tablet:
  Aspirin * .... 325 mg.
  Maalox (Magnesium-aluminum hydroxide) .... 150 mg.

ASCRIPTIN WITH CODEINE
Analgesic, antipyretic, anti-inflammatory
(Rorer, W.H., Inc.)

Each tablet:
  Aspirin * ....325 mg.
  Maalox (Magnesium-aluminum hydroxide) ....150 mg.
  Codeine phosphate * 15 mg. or 30 mg.

ASEPTICARE

See AIRWICK PROFESSIONAL PRODUCTS ASEPTICARE

ASEPTIC-CLEAN
Hard surface cleaner, sanitizer, odor counteractant
(National-Purity Soap)

Alkyl (60% C14, 30% C16, 10% C12) dimethylbenzyl ammonium chloride * 9.0%
Tetrasodium ethylenediamine tetraacetate 1.9%
Trisodium phosphate 1.0%
Nonionic detergent (100% active) .. 7.0%

ASID-O-PHY
Liquid acid cleaner
(Diversey Wyandotte)

Phosphoric acid*

ASMACOL
Bronchospasm due to asthma
(Vale)

Each tablet:
  Butabarbital * .... 15 mg.
  Aminophylline * .... 180 mg.
  Phenylpropanolamine hydrochloride * .... 25 mg.
  Chlorpheniramine maleate * .. 2 mg.
Buffered with:
  Dihydroxyaluminum aminoacetate .... 120 mg.

ASMA-KETS A.H. TABLETS WITH ANTIHISTAMINE
For relief of bronchial asthma
(Rexall)

Each tablet:
Theophylline (anhydrous) * .... 2 gr.
Ephedrine sulfate * .... 3/8 gr.
Chlorpheniramine maleate ...... 2 mg.

'76 Ed.

ASMA-LIEF PEDIATRIC SUSPENSION
For the relief of bronchial asthma and hay fever
(Columbia Med.)

Each 5 ml.:
  Theophylline * .... 65 mg.
  Ephedrine HCl * .... 12 mg.
  Phenobarbital .... 4 mg.

ASMA-LIEF TABLETS
For bronchial asthma & hay fever
(Columbia Med.)

Each tablet:
  Theophylline * .... 2 gr.
  Ephedrine HCl * .... 3/8 gr.
  Phenobarbital .... 1/8 gr.

ASMASET CAPSULES
For bronchial asthma
(Premo)

Each capsule:
  Aminophylline * .... 130 mg.
  Ephedrine HCl * .... 25 mg.
  Amobarbital * .... 25 mg.

'76 Ed.

Starred ingredients (*) may be responsible for major toxic effects; consult Section II.

ASMAVERT
For bronchial asthma or hay fever
(Nephron)

Each tablet:
  Chlorpheniramine maleate .... 2 mg.
  Ephedrine sulfate * .... 3/8 gr.
  Theophylline * .... 2 gr.

ASMINOREL IMPROVED
Antiasthmatic
(Direct Div.)

Each tablet:
  Ephedrine sulfate * .... 25 mg.
  Theophylline * .... 130 mg.
  Hydroxyzine HCl .... 10 mg.

ASMINYL
For paroxysms of bronchial asthma
(OJF)

Each tablet:
  Phenobarbital sodium .... 8 mg.
  Ephedrine sulfate * .... 26 mg.
  Theophylline hydrous * ..... 130 mg.

A-SPA-SPRA
Insecticide; veterinary
(Goshen Labs.)

Pyrethrins 0.5%
Piperonyl butoxide 4.0%
Petroleum distillates * 10.5%

ASPERGUM
Analgesic chewing gum tablets
(Plough)

Each tablet:
  Aspirin * .... 3 1/2 gr.

ASPHAC-G TABLETS
Analgesic
(Central Pharmacal Co.)

Each tablet:
  Aspirin * .... 250 mg.
  Phenacetin * .... 120 mg.
  Caffeine (anhydrous) ...... 15 mg.

ASPIRBAR TABLETS
Sedative-analgesic
(Lannett)

Each tablet:
  Phenobarbital .... 1/4 gr.
  Aspirin * .... 10 gr.

ASPIRSED
Analgesic and sedative
(Bio-Factor Labs.)

Each tablet:
  Aspirin * .... 5 gr.
  Phenobarbital .... 1/2 gr.
                                '76 Ed.

ASPON
Insecticide
(Stauffer)

Aspon (O,O,O,O-Tetrapropyl dithiopyrophosphate) *

ASTHMABAN TABLETS
*For temporary relief of bronchial
  asthma*
(Jeffrey Martin, Inc.)

Each tablet:
  Ephedrine hydrochloride * ... 25 mg.

ASTHMACON
Antiasthmatic
(CMC Research Div.)

Each capsule:
  Aminophylline * .... 130 mg.
  Ephedrine HCl * .... 25 mg.
  Amobarbital * .... 25 mg.

ASTHMAID
(Pharmex)

Phenobarbital .... 1/8 gr.
Theophylline * .... 2 gr.
Ephedrine sulfate .... 3/8 gr.

ASTRING-O-SOL
Mouthwash concentrate
(Winthrop Labs.)

Alcohol 70%
Zinc chloride, USP 0.42%
Fluid extract of Myrrh 0.56%
Methyl salicylate, USP * 4.62%

ASTYPTODYNE
Household antiseptic
(Astyptodyne)

Oil of southern pine *
                                '76 Ed.

ASULOX
Herbicide
(Rhone-Poulenc)

Sodium salt of asulam (methyl
  sulfanilylcarbamate) 37.2%

ATABRINE
HYDROCHLORIDE
For malaria, giardiasis, and tapeworm
(Winthrop Labs.)

Each tablet:
  Quinacrine hydrochloride * .. 100 mg.

ATARAX
Tranquilizer, antihistamine
(Roerig)

Tablets (each):
  Hydroxyzine HCl * .. 10 mg.; 25 mg.;
                        50 mg.; 100 mg.

Syrup (each 5 ml.):
  Hydroxyzine HCl .... 10 mg.

ATARAXOID
Steroid therapy
(Pfizer)

Each tablet:
  Prednisolone .... 2.5 mg.; 5.0 mg.
  Hydroxyzine HCl .... 10 mg.

AT EASE
Paste abrasive scouring cleaner
(Shaklee)

Nonionic surfactant
Silica flour
Perfume & Colorant .... small amounts

A-10 WOOD PRESERVING CONCENTRATE

See CRE-O-TOX A-10 WOOD PRE-
  SERVING CONCENTRATE

ATIVAN
Management of anxiety disorders
(Wyeth Labs.)

Each tablet:
  Lorazepam* .... 0.5 mg.; 1.0 mg.;
                        or 2.0 mg.

ATLACIDE
Herbicide
(Chipman Inc.)

Sodium chlorate * 59.2%

ATLAS DOOR-EASE
(Atlas Supply Co.)

See DOOR-EASE

ATLAS LOCK-EASE
(Atlas Supply Co.)

See LOCK-EASE

ATOMIC BALM
(Cramer Products)

Paraffin 3.75%
Lanolin (USP)(anhydrous) 5.00%
Petrolatum (NF)(amber) 75.00%
Oleoresin capsicum 0.50%
Turpentine 0.50%
Methyl salicylate (USP) * 12.50%
Menthol, technical 2.75%

ATOMIC RUB-DOWN LINIMENT
(Cramer Products)

Mineral oil (NF) 42.50%
Petrolatum (NF)(amber) 30.00%
Camphor (USP) 0.15%
Turpentine-gum spirits 16.07%
Methyl salicylate (USP) * 10.00%
Oleoresin capsicum 0.39%
Turpentine 0.39%
Bay oil (Myrcia oil) 0.50%

ATOX 1%
(Chipman Inc.)

Rotenone 1%

ATRATOL 8P
Pelleted herbicide
(Ciba-Geigy Ag. Div.)

Atrazine	7.6%
Atrazine related compounds	0.4%
Sodium chlorate *	40.0%
Sodium metaborate	47.0%

ATRATOL 80W
Herbicide
(Ciba-Geigy Ag. Div.)

Atrazine *	71.3%
Related compounds	3.7%
Prometon	5.0%

ATROBARB
Sedative, antispasmodic, antiemetic
(Jenkins Labs.)

Each No. 1 tablet:
Phenobarbital sodium (bar-bituric acid derivative) * .	1/8 gr.
Atropine sulphate	1/1000 gr.

Each No. 2 tablet:
Phenobarbital sodium (bar-bituric acid derivative) * .	1/4 gr.
Atropine sulphate	1/500 gr.

Each No. 3 tablet:
Phenobarbital sodium (bar-bituric acid derivative) * .	1/4 gr.
Atropine sulphate	1/250 gr.

ATROPHATE
Ophthalmic ointment for dogs
(Burns-Biotec)

Atropine sulfate *	1%
Lanolin (anhydrous)	
White petrolatum	
Mineral oil	
Water (Purified)	

ATROPINE SULFATE S.O.P.
Sterile ophthalmic ointments
(Allergan Pharm.)

Atropine sulfate *	0.5%; 1.0%
Chlorobutanol (chloral derivative as a preservative)	0.5%
White petrolatum	
Mineral oil	
Nonionic lanolin derivatives	
Purified water	

ATROPISOL OPHTHALMIC SOLUTION
Mydriatic
(CooperVision Pharm.)

Each 5 ml.:
Atropine sulfate *	0.5%, 1.0%, 2.0%
Isotonic, buffered aqueous solution of:	
Boric acid	
Sodium carbonate	
Potassium chloride	
Benzalkonium chloride	0.01%
Disodium edetate	0.01%

A-200 PYRINATE LIQUID
Pediculicide
(Norcliff Thayer)

Pyrethrins	0.165%
Piperonyl butoxide (tech.)	2.000%
Deodorized kerosene	5.000%

AURA
Automatic dishwasher detergent
(Calgon Corp., Commercial Div.)

Chlorinated trisodium phosphate *
Complex Phosphates *

AURAGREEN
Colorant
(Mallinckrodt, Inc.)

Malachite green *
Auramine
Crystal violet (Gentian violet) *

AURALCORT EAR DROPS
(Wesley Pharm.)

Each 7 ml. dropper:
Neomycin sulfate	3.5 mg.
Polymixin B sulfate	2000 Units
Hydrocortisone	0.1%
Antipyrine	5%
Dibucaine hydrochloride	0.25%

AURALGESIC DROPS
Ear drops
(Wesley Pharm.)

Glycerine
Antipyrine
Benzocaine

AURAPHENE-B EAR DROPS
Wax softening and removal
(Reese Chem.)

Chloroxylenol
Benzalkonium chloride
Acetic acid
Glycerin

AURIMITE
Antibacterial, antipruritic; veterinary
(Burns-Biotec)

Active ingred. (by wt.):
Dioctyl sodium sulfosuccinate .	1.952%
Benzocaine	1.952%
Tyrothricin	0.039%
Technical Piperonyl butoxide .	0.49%
Petroleum distillate	0.18%
Pyrethrins	0.04%
Hydrocortisone	0.032%
Inert ingred.:	
Isopropyl alcohol	4.882%
Propylene glycol	
Color	

AUROCAINE
Otic analgesic
(Vita Elixir Co.)

Benzocaine	0.15 gm.
Antipyrine *	0.70 gm.
Glycerol	q.s.

AURO EAR DROPS
For softening wax
(Commerce Drug)

Propylene glycol
Phenacetin *
8-Hydroxyquinoline
Urea peroxide
Carbopol 941

AUSTIN'S A-1 BLEACH
(Austin, J.)

Sodium hypochlorite * . . . . . . | 5.25%/wt.

AUSTIN'S CARPET & UPHOLSTERY CLEANER
(Austin, J.)

Ammonia 26° . . . . | 3%

AUSTIN'S LIQUID WIPE AWAY
Cleaner
(Austin, J.)

Ammonia 26° . . . . | 3%

AUSTIN'S WINDOW CLEANER
(Austin, J.)

Ammonia 26° . . . . | 4%

AUTO-KLEEN BLO-DRI
Car wash detergent
(National-Purity Soap)

Nonionic combination surfactant *
Cationic emulsion polish

AUTOMATE 1, FORMULA 2062

See KLENZADE AUTOMATE 1, FORMULA 2062

AUTOMATE 2, FORMULA 2124

See KLENZADE AUTOMATE 2, FORMULA 2124

AUTOMATE 3, FORMULA 2125

See KLENZADE AUTOMATE 3, FORMULA 2125

AUTOMATIC VANISH SOLID
Solid in-tank bowl cleaner
(Drackett)

Urea	
Nonionic detergent	<15%
Water	
Perfume	
Preservative	<1.0%
Dye	

Starred ingredients (*) may be responsible for major toxic effects; consult Section II.

AUTOMATIC VANISH TOILET BOWL CLEANER (LIQUID)
Liquid, in-tank, toilet bowl cleaner
(Drackett)

Anionic and non-ionic
detergents . . . . <10%/wt.
Perfume
Dye
Water

AVADEX
Herbicide
(Monsanto)

Diallate (S-(2,3-Dichloroallyl)-
diisopropylthiocarbamate) * . . . 45.7%

AVADEX BW
Herbicide
(Monsanto)

Triallate (S-(2,2,3-Trichloroallyl)-
diisopropylthiocarbamate) * . . . 46.3%

AVALON NU-CHALK COLORED MOLDED CHALK
(Avalon Industries)

This product bears the AP Seal issued by the Crayon, Water Color and Craft Institute, Inc. This seal certifies that the product contains no materials in sufficient quantities to be toxic or injurious to the human body even if ingested.

AVALON NU-CHALK WHITE MOLDED CHALK
(Avalon Industries)

This product bears the AP Seal issued by the Crayon, Water Color and Craft Institute, Inc. This seal certifies that the product contains no materials in sufficient quantities to be toxic or injurious to the human body even if ingested.

AVASOL
Vitamin supplement
(Wesley Pharm.)

Each capsule:
Vitamin A palmitate
(solubilized) . . . . 10,000 I.U.

AVC CREAM
For relief of symptoms of vulvo vaginitis
(Merrell Dow)

Each tube:
Sulfanilamide * 15.0%
Aminacrine hydrochloride 0.2%
Allantoin 2.0%

AVC/DIENESTROL CREAM
In atrophic vaginitis complicated by infection
(Merrell Dow)

Each 4 oz. tube:
Dienestrol 0.01%
Sulfanilamide 15.0%
Aminacrine hydrochloride 0.2%
Allantoin 2.0%
Water-miscible base:
Lactose
Propylene glycol
Stearic acid
Diglycol stearate
Trolamine
Buffered with lactic acid to approx.
pH 4.5

AVC/DIENESTROL SUPPOSITORIES
In atrophic vaginitis complicated by infection
(Merrell Dow)

Each suppository:
Dienestrol . . . . 0.70 mg.
Sulfanilamide* . . . . 1.05 gm.
Aminacrine hydrochloride . . 0.014 gm.
Allantoin . . . . 0.14 gm.
Lactose
Polyethylene glycol 400
Polysorbate 80
Polyethylene glycol 4000
Glycerin
Buffered with lactic acid to approx. pH 4.5

AVC SUPPOSITORIES
For relief of symptoms of vulvo vaginitis
(Merrell Dow)

Each suppository:
Sulfanilamide * . . . . 1.05 gm.
Aminacrine hydrochloride . . 0.014 gm.
Allantoin . . . . 0.14 gm.
Lactose

AVEENO-BAR
For sensitive skin
(CooperCare)

Aveeno colloidal oatmeal 50%
Lanolin derivative

AVEENO COLLOIDAL OATMEAL
For bath/soothe irritated skin
(CooperCare)

Specially milled flour of Oatmeal . . 100%

AVEENO LOTION
For minor skin irritations
(CooperCare)

Colloidal Oatmeal
Aqueous lotion base

AVEENO OILATED
For dry skin conditions
(CooperCare)

Aveeno colloidal oatmeal
Liquid petrolatum
Hypoallergenic Lanolin fraction

AVENTYL HCl (Pulvules & Liquid)
Mental depression, and anxiety-tension states
(Lilly, Eli)

PULVULES (each):
Nortriptyline
hydrochloride * . . . 10 mg. or 25 mg.

LIQUID (each 5 ml.):
Nortriptyline
hydrochloride * . . . . 10 mg.
Alcohol

AVI-TAB
Tonic; veterinary, avian
(Salsbury)

Copper sulfate (copper metallic
5.3%) * 21%
Ext. Nux vomica (strychnine 1.2 gr./
oz.) 4%
Areca nut 10%
Kamala
Mustard
Oleoresin capsicum
Anise oil
Potassium iodide 1.4%
Sulfates of cobalt, iron, manganese, zinc

AVITROL CONCENTRATE
For the control of gulls
(Avitrol Corp.)

4-Aminopyridine * 25%

AVITROL CORN CHOPS
For the control of sparrows, blackbirds, and cowbirds
(Avitrol Corp.)

Active ingred.:
4-Aminopyridine * 0.50%
Inert ingred.:
Corn chops 99.31%
Hydrogen chloride 0.19%

AVITROL CORN CHOPS - PEANUT BUTTER
For the control of starlings
(Avitrol Corp.)

Active ingred.:
4-Aminopyridine * 0.80%
Inert ingred.:
Corn chops 79.1%
Peanut butter 19.8%
Hydrogen chloride 0.3%

AVITROL DOUBLE STRENGTH CORN CHOPS
For the control of blackbirds, cowbirds, and starlings
(Avitrol Corp.)

Active ingred.:
4-Aminopyridine * 1.00%
Inert ingred.:
Corn 98.62%
Hydrogen chloride 0.38%

Starred ingredients (*) may be responsible for major toxic effects; consult Section II.

AVITROL DOUBLE STRENGTH WHOLE CORN
For the control of crows
(Avitrol Corp.)

Active ingred.:
4-Aminopyridine * 1.00%
Inert ingred.:
Corn 98.62%
Hydrogen chloride 0.38%

AVITROL MIXED GRAINS
For the control of sparrows, blackbirds, and cowbirds
(Avitrol Corp.)

Active ingred.:
4-Aminopyridine * 0.50%
Inert ingred.:
Mixed grains 99.31%
Hydrogen chloride 0.19%

AVITROL PELLETIZED FEED
For the control of starlings
(Avitrol Corp.)

Active ingred.:
4-Aminopyridine * 1.00%
Inert ingred.:
Pelletized feed 98.62%
Hydrogen chloride 0.38%

AVITROL POWDER MIX
For the control of starlings
(Avitrol Corp.)

4-Aminopyridine * 50%

AVITROL SORGHUM
For the control of sparrows, blackbirds, and cowbirds
(Avitrol Corp.)

Active ingred.:
4-Aminopyridine * 0.50%
Inert ingred.:
Sorghum 99.31%
Hydrogen chloride 0.19%

AVITROL WHEAT
For the control of sparrows, blackbirds, and cowbirds
(Avitrol Corp.)

Active ingred.:
4-Aminopyridine * 0.50%
Inert ingred.:
Wheat 99.31%
Hydrogen chloride 0.19%

AVITROL WHOLE CORN
For the control of pigeons
(Avitrol Corp.)

Active ingred.:
4-Aminopyridine * 0.50%
Inert ingred.:
Corn 99.31%
Hydrogen chloride 0.19%

AVON ACCOLADE, CUCUMBER, DELICATE BEAUTY, MOISTURE SECRET, ENVIRA, SKINPLICITY, TRACY - ALL SIZES
(Avon)

Water
Alcohol
Astringent
Emollients
Nutrients
Emulsifiers
pH adjusters
Surfactants
Skin conditioners
Fragrance
Chelating agents
Certified colors
Preservatives
U.V. absorbers

AVON ACTIVE AID ANTISEPTIC SPRAY - 3 oz.
(Avon)

Propellant
Alcohol
Emollients
Topical anesthetic
Preservatives
Fragrance

AVON ACTIVE AID FIRST AID CREAM - 1.5 oz.
(Avon)

Water
Emollients
Emulsifiers
Topical anesthetic
Film-former
pH adjusters
Preservatives
Fragrance

AVON ACTIVE AID PROTECTIVE SHIELD - 1.5 oz.
(Avon)

Emollients
Thickeners
Sunscreen agent
Fillers
Preservatives
Fragrance

AVON ACTIVE AID SKIN COMFORT LOTION - 8 oz.
(Avon)

Water
Emollients
Emulsifiers
Preservatives
Fragrance
pH adjuster
Thickeners
Certified colors

AVON AEROSOL ANTI-PERSPIRANT DEODORANT, DRI-N-DELICATE - 4 oz.
(Avon)

Propellant
Anti-perspirant
Emollients
Suspending agents
Fragrance

AVON AEROSOL ANTI-PERSPIRANT DEODORANT, MEN'S
ON DUTY 24, ULTRA-DRY (Regular or Unscented) - 4.7 oz.
(Avon)

Propellant
Anti-perspirant
Emollients
Film former
Fragrance

AVON AEROSOL DEODORANT - FAMILY, PERFUMED - 4, 7 oz.
(Avon)

Alcohol
Propellant
Deodorant
Emollients
Fragrance

AVON AEROSOL MISTS AND SPRAYS - ALL FRAGRANCES - ALL SIZES
(Avon)

Alcohol
Propellant
Fragrance
U.V. absorber
Certified colors

AVON AFTER SHOWER SMOOTHER, SKIN-SO-SOFT - 4 oz.
(Avon)

Water
Alcohol
Propellant
Emulsifiers
Emollients
Lubricants
Thickeners
Fragrance
Neutralizers
Certified colors

AVON AMERICAN SPORTSTER SHAMPOO/ SHOWER SOAP FOR MEN - 5 oz.
(Avon)

Water
Anionic detergent
Nonionic detergent
Emollients
pH adjusters
Fragrance
Preservatives
Sequestering agent
Certified colors

AVON BLUE TRANQUILITY FRESHENER - 8 oz.
(Avon)

Water
Alcohol
Emollients
Anionic detergents
Fragrance
Solar salt
Thickeners
Certified colors
U.V. absorber
pH adjuster

AVON BUBBLE BATH AND FOAMING BATH OIL, ALL TYPES, ALL FRAGRANCES, ALL SIZES
(Avon)

Water
Detergents
Fragrance *
Preservatives
Foam stabilizers
Emulsifiers
pH adjusters
Solar salt
Anti-oxidant
U.V. absorber
Emollients
Alcohol
Certified colors
Sequestering agent

AVON BUBBLE BATH, CHILDREN'S - ALL SIZES
(Avon)

Water
Detergents
Foam stabilizers
Fragrance *
pH adjusters

AVON BUBBLE BATH GEL - ALL FRAGRANCES - 4, 6 oz.
(Avon)

Water
Detergents
Fragrance
Preservatives
Foam stabilizers
Thickeners
pH adjuster
Certified colors
Sequestering agent
U.V. absorber

AVON CLEAN AND LIVELY - 7 oz.
Shampoo
(Avon)

Water
Detergents
Stabilizers
Emulsifiers
Preservatives
Fragrance
pH adjusters
Astringents
Bath salts
Sequestering agent
Certified colors
U.V. absorber

AVON CLEAR SKIN CONCENTRATE
COLOR-TREATED HAIR, SUPER HI-LIGHT GEL, SUPER HI-LIGHT LIQUID - 3, 5, 8 oz.
Shampoo
(Avon)

Water
Detergents
Fragrance
Preservatives
Certified colors
U.V. absorber
Emollients
pH adjusters
Thickeners
Sequestering agent

AVON CLEAR SKIN MEDICATED ASTRINGENT - 12 oz.
(Avon)

Alcohol
Water
Emulsifiers
Astringent
Keratolytic agent
Emollients
Fragrance
Certified colors
U.V. absorbers

AVON CLEAR SKIN MEDICATED LOTION - 4 oz.
(Avon)

Water
Alcohol
Colloidal Sulfur
Thickeners
Calamine compound
Fragrance

AVON COLOGNE, BOYS' AND GIRLS' - ALL FRAGRANCES - ALL SIZES
(Avon)

Water
Alcohol
Surfactants
Fragrance
Certified colors
U.V. absorber
Sequestering agent

AVON COLOGNE ICE, COLOGNE STICK - ALL FRAGRANCES - ALL SIZES
(Avon)

Alcohol
Water
Emulsifiers
Fragrance
Thickeners
Anti-oxidant
Sequestering agent
Certified colors

AVON CONCENTRE, GLACE - ALL FRAGRANCES - 1 oz.
(Avon)

Emollients
Fragrance
Film-former
Anti-oxidant

AVON CREAM ANTI-PERSPIRANT DEODORANT, DRI-N-DELICATE, HABIT - 1.5, 2 oz.
(Avon)

Water
Anti-perspirant
Emulsifiers
Buffering agent
Fragrance
Preservatives
Certified colors

AVON CREAM PERFUME OR CREAM SACHET - ALL FRAGRANCES - ALL SIZES
(Avon)

Water
Emulsifiers
Emollients
Fragrance
Surfactants
Preservatives
Sequestering agent
Alcohol
Certified colors
U.V. absorber

AVON CREME COLOGNE, RENEWABLE-TOCCARA - 1.0 oz.
(Avon)

Water
Emollients
Fragrance
Emulsifiers
Film-formers
pH adjusters
Thickeners
Preservatives
Suspending agents

Starred ingredients (*) may be responsible for major toxic effects; consult Section II.

AVON CRYSTALS - MINERAL SPRING - 12 oz.
(Avon)

Inorganic salts
Emollients
Filler
Fragrance *
Anionic detergents
Certified colors

AVON CUTICLE REMOVER - 1 oz.
(Avon)

Water
Emollients
Emulsifiers
pH adjusters
Thickeners
Fragrance

AVON DANDRUFF SHAMPOO - GEL AND LIQUID; GENTLE LOTION, HI-LIGHT-DRY, NORMAL, OILY - ALL SIZES
(Avon)

Water
Detergents
Emulsifiers
Thickeners
pH adjusters
Fragrance
Preservatives
Certified colors
U.V. absorber
Emollients

AVON DEMISTICK AND SOLID PERFUME COMPACT - ALL FRAGRANCES - ALL SIZES
(Avon)

Emollients
Waxes
Fragrance
Preservatives
Certified colors
Thickeners

AVON DEODORANT BODY POWDER - FEELIN' FRESH AND SPORTIF, 8 oz.
(Avon)

Talc
Bath salts
Emulsifiers
Fragrance

AVON ELEGANCE SKIN TONIC - 6 oz.
(Avon)

Demineralized water
Alcohol
Astringent
Surfactants
Emollients
pH adjusters
Certified colors
Fragrance

AVON EMOLLIENT MIST - ALL FRAGRANCES - ALL SIZES
(Avon)

Alcohol
Propellant
Emollients
Water
Fragrance
Emulsifiers

AVON EMOLLIENT SHOWER GEL - SKIN-SO-SOFT - 6 oz.
(Avon)

Emollients
Water
Thickeners
pH adjuster
Fragrance
Certified colors

AVON ENAMELS - 0.5 oz.
(Avon)

Solvents
Film-former
Plasticizers
Alcohol
Certified colors
Resins
Pearling agents
Thickeners
U.V. absorber

AVON ESSENCE OF BALSAM: HI-LIGHT DANDRUFF; PROTEIN DANDRUFF; PROTEM DANDRUFF - ALL SIZES
(Avon)

Water
Detergents
pH adjusters
Fragrance
Preservatives
Certified colors
Emulsifiers
Protein additive
Emollients
Thickeners
U.V. absorber

AVON FACE LOTIONS - AFTER-SHAVE AND CONDITIONER FOR DRY OR SENSITIVE SKIN - ALL TYPES, ALL SIZES
(Avon)

Water
Alcohol
Emollients
Emulsifiers
Fragrance
pH adjusters
Healing agent
Thickeners
Certified colors
U.V. absorber

AVON FACE LOTIONS - AFTER-SHAVE, BRACING AND PRE-SHAVE - ALL TYPES, ALL FRAGRANCES, ALL SIZES
(Avon)

Alcohol
Water
Fragrance
Emollients
Emulsifiers
Astringent
Anti-oxidant
Certified colors
pH adjusters
Sequestering agent
U.V. absorber

AVON FANCY FEET AEROSOL FOOT SPRAY - 4 oz.
(Avon)

Alcohol
Propellant
Deodorants
Emollients
Emulsifiers
Astringent
Fragrance

AVON FANCY FEET FOOT CARE CREAM - 3 oz.
(Avon)

Water
Emollients
Emulsifiers
Thickeners
Abrasives
pH adjusters
Barrier agent
Preservatives
Fragrance

AVON FLUFF - BIRD OF PARADISE - 3 oz.
Cologne
(Avon)

Water
Emollients
Propellant
Emulsifiers
Fragrance
Thickeners
Preservatives
Certified colors
Anti-oxidant

Starred ingredients (*) may be responsible for major toxic effects; consult Section II.

AVON FRESHENERS - ALL
TYPES - ALL
FRAGRANCES - 6, 8, 10, 12
oz.
(Avon)

Alcohol
Water
Fragrance
Certified colors
Preservatives
Emollients
Emulsifiers
Thickeners
U.V. absorber
Pearling agent
Sequestering agent

AVON GELEE - ALL
FRAGRANCES - ALL SIZES
(Avon)

Alcohol
Water
Fragrance
Thickeners
pH adjusters
Emulsifiers
Sequestering agent
Certified colors
U.V. absorber

AVON HELLO SUNSHINE
FUNSHINE NAIL TINTS -
0.5 oz.
(Avon)

Alcohol
Resins
Water
Certified colors

AVON HENNA RICH LIQUID
- 8 oz.
Shampoo
(Avon)

Water
Surfactants
Stabilizers
Conditioners
Emulsifiers
Preservatives
Fragrance
Suspending agents
Certified colors

AVON JEWELRY CLEANER -
8 oz.
(Avon)

Water
Detergents
pH adjusters
Fragrance
Preservatives

AVON KEEP CLEAR ANTI-
DANDRUFF - 7 oz.
Shampoo
(Avon)

Water
Detergents
pH adjusters
Stabilizers
Antimicrobials
Thickeners
Fragrance
pH adjusters
Emollients
Alcohol
Certified colors

AVON KWICKETTES - ALL
FRAGRANCES
(Avon)

Alcohol
Water
Fragrance
Emollients
Emulsifiers
Sequestering agent
Anti-oxidant

AVON LEMON VELVET,
RAINING VIOLETS,
MOISTURIZED FRICTION
LOTION - ALL SIZES
(Avon)

Alcohol
Water
Emollients
Fragrance
Anti-oxidant
U.V. absorber

AVON LIGHT PERFUME
AND FRAGRANCE DEMOS
- ALL FRAGRANCES - 1
DRAM
(Avon)

Alcohol
Fragrance
Certified colors
U.V. absorber

AVON LIQUID ANTI-
PERSPIRANT, ON DUTY 24
- 2 oz.
(Avon)

Alcohol
Anti-perspirant
Emollients
Water
Emulsifiers
Buffering agent
Fragrance

AVON LIQUID
DEODORANT, PERFUMED
- 2 oz.
(Avon)

Alcohol
Water
Deodorant
Fragrance
Emollients

AVON LOTION SHAMPOO -
ZANY COLOGNE - 10 oz.
(Avon)

Water
Detergents
Conditioners
Film-formers
Foam stabilizers
Thickeners
Fragrance
Preservatives
pH adjuster
Suspending agents
Emollients
Colors

AVON MEN'S AND
WOMEN'S - ALL
FRAGRANCES - ALL SIZES
(Avon)

Alcohol
Water
Fragrance
Emollients
Certified colors
U.V. absorbers
Anti-oxidant
Sequestering agent

AVON MEN'S REGULAR
LIQUID - 2, 4 oz.
Hair dressing
(Avon)

Alcohol
Water
Emollients
Film-formers
Fragrance
Certified colors

AVON MINERAL SPRING
MOISTURIZING BODY
RUB - 8 oz.
(Avon)

Water
Alcohol
Emulsifiers
Emollients
Thickeners
Fragrance
Certified colors

AVON NAIL MENDER - 0.5
oz.
(Avon)

Solvents
Alcohol
Resins

Starred ingredients (*) may be responsible for major toxic effects; consult Section II.

AVON NATURAL COLOGNE SPRAY - ALL FRAGRANCES - ALL SIZES
(Avon)

Alcohol
Fragrance
U.V. absorber
Certified colors

AVON NATURALLY GENTLE GEL AND LIQUID - ALL SIZES
Shampoo
(Avon)

Water
Detergents
Emulsifiers
Preservatives
Fragrance
U.V. absorber
Certified colors
Foam stabilizers
Bath salts
pH adjusters

AVON NEW VITALITY CONDITIONING - 8 oz.
Shampoo
(Avon)

Detergents
Water
Stabilizers
Conditioners
Thickeners
Emulsifiers
Anti-oxidant
Emollients
Fragrance
Preservatives
Certified colors

AVON NEW VITALITY HOT CONDITIONING TREATMENT - 0.75 oz.
(Avon)

Water
Emollients
Emulsifiers
Detergents
Resins
Thickeners
Preservatives
Fragrance
Certified colors

AVON OILY LIQUID - ALL TYPES - ALL SIZES
Nail polish remover
(Avon)

Solvents
Water
Fragrance
Certified colors
Spreading agent
Alcohol
Emollients
Emulsifiers

AVON PAD SAMPLES - ALL FRAGRANCES
Cologne
(Avon)

Alcohol
Fragrance
Water
Emollients
U.V. absorber
Anti-oxidant
Certified colors

AVON PERFECT BALANCE TONING ASTRINGENT - 6 oz.
(Avon)

Water
Alcohol
Astringent
Emulsifiers
Fragrance

AVON PERFECT BALANCE TONING FRESHENER - 6 oz.
(Avon)

Water
Astringent
Alcohol
Fragrance
Emulsifiers
U.V. absorbers
Anti-oxidant
Certified colors

AVON PERFUME - ALL FRAGRANCES - ALL SIZES
(Avon)

Alcohol
Fragrance
Water
Emollients
Certified colors
U.V. absorber

AVON PERFUME LUSTRE, RENEWABLE-TOCCARA - 0.4 oz.
(Avon)

Water
Emollients
Fragrance
Opacifiers
Emulsifiers
Film-formers
pH adjusters

AVON PERFUME PENCIL
(Avon)

Emollients
Thickeners
Fragrance
Preservatives

AVON PERFUME, SOLID - HELLO SUNSHINE - 0.25 oz.
(Avon)

Emollients
Fragrance
Anti-caking agent
Preservatives

AVON POWDER ANTI-PERSPIRANT DEODORANT - ULTRA-DRY - 7 oz.
(Avon)

Propellant
Anti-perspirant
Emollients
Barrier agent
Suspending agent
Talc
Fragrance

AVON POWDERED BUBBLE BATH CONCENTRATE - ALL FRAGRANCES - 2 oz.
(Avon)

Surfactants
Anticaking agents
Water
Fragrance
Nonfat dry milk solids
Certified colors

AVON PRODUCTS

Avon Products, Inc.
Suffern, N.Y. 10901

All calls for emergency medical information should be directed to the following special telephone number: 914-357-2012 (Collect). Information will always be available at the above number at any time of the day or night.

AVON PROTEIN CONDITIONING FOR MEN - 3 oz.
Shampoo
(Avon)

Water
Detergents
Emulsifiers
Protein additive
Fragrance
Preservatives
pH adjusters
Certified colors
Sequestering agent

Starred ingredients (*) may be responsible for major toxic effects; consult Section II.

AVON PROTEIN CREME DANDRUFF - 3 oz.
Shampoo
(Avon)

Water
Detergents
Foam stabilizers
Emulsifiers
Anti-dandruff agent
pH adjusters
Fragrance
Protein additive
Certified colors
Preservatives

AVON PROTEM CREME WITH PROTEIN - 6 oz.
Shampoo
(Avon)

Water
Detergents
Soap
Thickeners
Emollients
Fragrance
Anti-oxidant
Preservatives
Protein additive
Certified colors

AVON RESILIENT LOTION FOR ADDED BODY - 8 oz.
Shampoo
(Avon)

Water
Detergents
Conditioners
Film-formers
Thickeners
Emulsifiers
Preservatives
Fragrance
Sequestering agent
Thickeners
Certified colors

AVON ROLLETTE - ALL FRAGRANCES - 0.33 oz.
(Avon)

Alcohol
Water
Fragrance
Emollients
Emulsifiers
Thickeners
U.V. absorber
Anti-oxidant
Sequestering agent
pH adjusters
Certified colors

AVON ROLL-ON ANTI-PERSPIRANT DEODORANT - ALL FRAGRANCES - 2, 4 oz.
(Avon)

Water
Anti-perspirant
Emulsifiers
Emollients
Fragrance
Thickeners
Sequestering agent
Preservatives
Certified colors

AVON ROOM AND WARDROBE FRESHENER - ALL FRAGRANCES - 6, 7 oz.
(Avon)

Propellant
Alcohol
Fragrance
Solvent

AVON ROOM AND WARDROBE FRESHENER - WATER-BASED - ALL FRAGRANCES - 6, 7 oz.
(Avon)

Water
Propellant
Defoaming agent
Surfactant
Fragrance
Preservatives
Corrosion inhibitor

AVON SALON SYSTEM - BALANCED, FRESHENING, MOISTURE RICH - 7 oz.
Shampoo
(Avon)

Water
Surfactants
Foam stabilizers
Fragrance
Preservatives
Certified colors
U.V. absorbers
Emollients
Conditioners
Bath salts
pH adjusters
Astringent
Suspending agents

AVON SHAMPOO, NON-TEAR, SWEET PICKLES - 12 oz.
(Avon)

Water
Emulsifiers
Amphoteric detergents
Emollients
pH adjusters
Fragrance
Preservatives

AVON SKIN BRACER, ROOKIE BOY'S, SURE WINNER - 2.75 oz.
(Avon)

Water
Alcohol
Detergents
Fragrance
Chelating agents
Preservatives

AVON SPRAY - ALL FRAGRANCES - 6 oz.
(Avon)

Propellant
Alcohol
Fragrance

AVON SPRAY ANTI-PERSPIRANT DEODORANT, ON DUTY 24 - 4 oz.
(Avon)

Alcohol
Anti-perspirant
Emollients
Water
Emulsifiers
Buffering agent
Fragrance

AVON SPRAY COLOGNE, RENEWABLE-TOCARRA - 1.25 oz.
(Avon)

Water
Alcohol
Fragrance
Film-former
Detergents
Preservative
pH adjuster
Suspending agents

AVON SPRAY ESSENCE - ALL FRAGRANCES - 0.25 oz., 1.25 oz.
(Avon)

Alcohol
Propellant
Fragrance
Certified colors

AVON SPUNSILK SPUNCOLOR NAIL ENAMELS - 0.5 oz.
(Avon)

Solvents
Coloring agents
Pearling agents
U.V. absorber

Starred ingredients (*) may be responsible for major toxic effects; consult Section II.

AVON STEPPING OUT COMFORT SPRAY - 5 oz.
(Avon)

Propellant
Alcohol
Water
Astringent and Bacteriostat
Fragrance
Preservatives

AVON STICK ANTI-PERSPIRANT, ON DUTY 24 - 2.5 oz.
(Avon)

Emollients
Anti-perspirant
Alcohol
Talc
Fragrance
Emulsifiers

AVON STICK DEODORANT FOR MEN - 2.25 oz.
(Avon)

Alcohol
Water
Emulsifiers
Emollients
Fragrance
Certified colors
Sequestering agent

AVON STRENGTHENER WITH NYLON AND PROTEIN - 0.5 oz.
Nail care
(Avon)

Solvents
Plasticizers
Resins
Alcohol
Protein additive
Certified colors

AVON SUNNY MORN SHAMPOO - ALL FRAGRANCES - 8 oz.
(Avon)

Water
Detergents
Foam stabilizers
Emollients
Emulsifiers
Fragrance
Preservatives
Thickeners
Anti-oxidant
Sequestering agent
Certified colors
U.V. absorber

AVON SUPER BASE COAT - 0.5 oz.
(Avon)

Solvents
Resins

AVON SUPER NAIL DRY - 0.5 oz.
(Avon)

Emollients
Drying agents
Preservatives

AVON SUPER TOP COAT - 0.5 oz.
(Avon)

Solvents
Resins
Alcohol

AVON SWIVEL UP ANTI-PERSPIRANT DEODORANT, DRI-N-DELICATE - 1.5, 2 oz.
(Avon)

Water
Anti-perspirant
Emulsifiers
Buffering agent
Fragrance
Preservatives
Certified colors

AVON TIMELESS FRAGRANCE DEMO - 1 DRAM
(Avon)

Alcohol
Emollients
Fragrance

AVON TIME-RELEASE ANTI-PERSPIRANT DEODORANT PROTECTION ON DUTY 24 - 7 oz.
(Avon)

Propellant
Anti-perspirant
Emollients
Encapsulated fragrance
Thickeners

AVON ULTRA AND ULTRALIGHT CREME PERFUME - ALL FRAGRANCES - 0.66 oz.
(Avon)

Water
Emulsifiers
Fragrance
Preservatives
Surfactants
Thickeners
pH adjusters
U.V. absorber
Certified colors
Anti-oxidant

AVON ULTRA COLOGNE MIST - ALL FRAGRANCES - ALL SIZES
(Avon)

Propellant
Alcohol
Emollients
Fragrance

AVON ULTRA COLOGNE, ULTRA COLOGNE SPRAY - ALL FRAGRANCES - ALL SIZES
(Avon)

Alcohol
Fragrance
Emollients
Water
Certified colors
U.V. absorber
Anti-oxidant

AVON ULTRA PERFUME ROLLETTE - TIMELESS, UNSPOKEN - 0.33 oz.
(Avon)

Alcohol
Emollients
Fragrance
Thickeners
Certified colors
U.V. absorber

AVON ULTRA PURSE CONCENTRE - ALL FRAGRANCES - 0.33 oz.
(Avon)

Alcohol
Emollients
Fragrance
Water
Thickeners
Certified colors
U.V. absorber

AVON ULTRA WEAR NAIL ENAMEL - ALL COLORS - 0.5 oz.
(Avon)

Solvents
Resins
Pigments

A.V.P.-NATAL-FA
Prenatal supplement
(A.V.P. Pharmaceuticals)

Vitamin A (acetate)	8000 IU
Vitamin D (ergocalciferol)	400 IU
Iodine (potassium iodide)	150 mcg.
Iron (ferrous fumerate)	60 mg.
Plus multivitamins and minerals	

A-10 WOOD PRESERVING CONCENTRATE

See CRE-O-TOX A-10 WOOD PRE-SERVING CONCENTRATE

AXION

Granular laundry pre-soak preparation
(Colgate-Palmolive)

Linear Alkyl benzene
  sulfonate * .... approx. 12%
Inorganic salts: .... approx. 75%
  Sodium phosphate *
  Sulfate
  Silicate
Moisture .... approx. 10%
Alcalase (proteolytic enzyme
  product of industrial
  fermentation) 0.75%

'76 Ed.

AXOTAL TABLETS

Analgesic, antipyretic, sedative
(Adria)

Each tablet:
  Butalbital (USP) * .... 50 mg.
  Acetaminophen (USP) ...... 325 mg.
  Caffeine (USP) .... 40 mg.

AYDS AM/PM CAPSULES

Appetite suppressant
(Campana)

Each Yellow capsule:
  Phenylpropanolamine HCl * . 50 mg.
  Caffeine .... 200 mg.

Each Blue capsule:
  Phenylpropanolamine HCl * . 25 mg.

  Contains color additives including FD
  & C Yellow No. 5 (Tartrazine)

AYDS APPETITE SUPPRESSANT DROPLETS

(Campana)

Each 0.6 ml.:
  Phenylpropanolamine HCl * .. 25 mg.

AYDS EXTRA STRENGTH CAPSULES

Appetite suppressant
(Campana)

Each capsule:
  Phenylpropanolamine HCl * . 75 mg.
  Caffeine .... 200 mg.

  Contains color additives including FD
  & C Yellow No. 5 (Tartrazine)

AYERST LABORATORIES PRODUCTS

Ayerst Laboratories
685 Third Ave.
New York, N.Y. 10017

Phone: 212-878-5996
Outside of business hours: 212-986-1000

AYRCAP S.R.

Bronchodilator
(Ascher, B.F.)

Each capsule:
  Theophylline * .... 260 mg.
  Pseudoephedrine
    hydrochloride * .... 50 mg.
  Butabarbital * .... 15 mg.

AYR LIQUID

Bronchodilator
(Ascher, B.F.)

Each 15 ml.:
  Theophylline * .... 130 mg.
  Pseudoephedrine
    hydrochloride * .... 25 mg.
  Butabarbital * .... 8 mg.
  Alcohol 20%

AYRTAB

Bronchodilator
(Ascher, B.F.)

Each tablet:
  Theophylline * .... 100 mg.
  Guaifenesin .... 100 mg.

AZIUM TABLETS AND ORAL SOLUTION

Anti-inflammatory; veterinary
(Burns-Biotec)

Each tablet:
  Crystalline
    Dexamethasone .... 0.25 mg.

Oral Solution (each ml.):
  Dexamethasone .... 1 mg.; 2 mg.
  Polyethylene glycol 400 ...... 500 mg.
  Benzyl alcohol .... 9 mg.
  Methylparaben .... 1.8 mg.
  Propylparaben .... 0.2 mg.
  Alcohol (2 mg. solution) 4.75%

AZIZA FROSTED SHADOW TRIO (ALL SHADES)

(Chesebrough-Pond's)

Talc .... >50%
Mica .... >10-25%
Iron oxides .... >5-10%
Titanium dioxide .... >5-10%
Zinc stearate .... >5-10%
Mineral oil .... >5-10%
Colors .... >1-5%

AZIZA SHINE-ON LIPGLOSS (ALL SHADES)

(Chesebrough-Pond's)

Lanolin oil .... >25-50%
Cyclomethicone .... >10-25%
Polyterpene resin .... >10-25%
Isopropyl palmitate .... >5-10%
PVP/eicosene copolymer ..... >5-10%
Ethylene/acrylate copolymer .. >5-10%
Stearalkonium hectorite ...... >1-5%
Propylene carbonate .... >1-5%
Titanium dioxide .... >0.1-1%
Colors .... >0.1-1%
Iron oxides .... >0.1-1%
Fragrance .... >0.1-1%
Methylparaben .... >0.1-1%
BHA .... >0.1-1%
Propylparaben .... >0.1-1%

AZIZA SOFT TOUCH CREME SHADOW (ALL SHADES)

(Chesebrough-Pond's)

Isodecyl oleate .... >25-50%
Polyglyceryl-3 diisostearate .... >10-25%
Kaolin .... >5-10%
Titanium dioxide .... >5-10%
Hydrogenated Castor oil ...... >5-10%
Acetylated Lanolin .... >1-5%
Colors .... >1-5%
Ceresin .... >1-5%
Stearic acid .... >1-5%
Iron oxides .... >1-5%
Silica .... >0.1-1%
Methylparaben .... >0.1-1%
BHA .... >0.1-1%

AZIZA WATERPROOF MASCARA (ALL SHADES)

(Chesebrough-Pond's)

Petroleum distillate .... >25-50%
Water .... >25-50%
Iron oxides .... >10-25%
Pentaerythritol rosinate ...... >1-5%
Zinc stearate .... >1-5%
Beeswax .... >1-5%
Carnauba .... >1-5%
Talc .... >1-5%
Ceresin .... >1-5%
Paraffin .... >1-5%
Sodium magnesium silicate .... >1-5%
Aluminum stearate .... >1-5%
DMDM hydantoin .... >0.1-1%
Methylparaben .... >0.1-1%
Propylparaben .... >0.1-1%

AZMA-ESE TABLETS

Treatment of asthma symptoms
(DePree)

Theophylline (anhydrous) *
Glyceryl guaiacolate
Ephedrine HCl *

AZMAR TABLETS

For bronchial asthma & hay fever
(Approved Pharm.)

Each tablet:
  Theophylline * .... 100 mg.
  Ephedrine hydrochloride * .. 25 mg.
  Methapyrilene
    hydrochloride * .... 16.6 mg.

'76 Ed.

AZO GANTANOL

Antibacterial-analgesic for urinary tract infections
(Roche)

Each tablet:
  Sulfamethoxazole .... 500 mg.
  Phenazopyridine HCl * ...... 100 mg.

AZO GANTRISIN

Antibacterial-analgesic for urinary tract infections
(Roche)

Each tablet:
  Sulfisoxazole .... 500 mg.
  Phenazopyridine HCl * ...... 50 mg.

Starred ingredients (*) may be responsible for major toxic effects; consult Section II.

AZOLATE TABLETS
Treatment of lower urinary tract infections
(Amfre-Grant)

Each tablet:
Phenazopyridine HCl * ...... 25 mg.
Methenamine mandelate * ... 250 mg.

AZO-SOXAZOLE TABLETS
(Columbia Med.)

Each tablet:
Sulfisoxazole * .... 500 mg.
Phenylazo-diaminopyridine
HCl .... 50 mg.

AZO-STANDARD TABLETS
Urinary analgesic
(Webcon)

Each tablet:
Phenazopyridine
hydrochloride * .... 1 1/2 gr.

AZOSTIX
Test for blood urea nitrogen
(Ames)

Urease
Bromthymol blue
Citric acid
Bovine albumin
Gelatin USP PFS flakes
Polyethylene glycol
Tris (hydroxymethyl) aminomethane
Ethyl cellulose
Benzene
Acetamide

AZTEC CLEAR
(Dow)

Ethyl alcohol 79.4%
Homomenthyl salicylate 7.0%

AZTEC CREAMY
(Dow)

Water 80.7%
Emollients 10.0%
Homomenthyl salicylate 7.0%

AZTEC SUNSCREEN
(Dow)

Ethyl alcohol 71.4%
Homomenthyl salicylate 6.0%
Amyl-p-dimethylaminobenzoate .. 2.0%

B

BAB-O CLEANSER
Household cleanser
(Purex Corp.)

Siliceous abrasive .... >90%
Alkaline builder 1-5%
Anionic surfactant 1-2%
Organic chlorine bleaching agent . <2%
Coloring agent .... <1%
Perfume .... <1%

BABYLON PERFUME, COLOGNE, TOILET WATER
(Parfums Duvelle)

Alcohol (denatured with diethyl phthalate) *

BABY MAGIC BABY OIL
(Mennen)

Mineral oil
Lanolin
Fragrance

BABY MAGIC BATH
(Mennen)

Water
Sodium laureth sulfate
Cocamido propyl betaine
PEG-78 glyceryl monococoate
PEG-30 glyceryl monococoate
Fragrance
Methylparaben
Propylparaben
Citric acid
Propylene glycol
FD & C Yellow #5
FD & C Red #4

BABY MAGIC LOTION
(Mennen)

Water
Glycerin
Glyceryl stearate
Mineral oil
Cetyl alcohol
PEG-100 stearate
Lanolin alcohol
Fragrance
Lanolin
Benzalkonium chloride
D & C Red #19
FD & C Yellow #5

BABY MAGIC POWDER
(Mennen)

Talc
Fragrance
Methylbenzethonium chloride *

BABY MAGIC SHAMPOO
(Mennen)

Water
Polysorbate-20
Amphoteric-20
Sodium laureth sulfate
PEG-150 distearate
Citric acid
Fragrance
Quaternium-15
FD & C Yellow #5
FD & C Red #4

BACARATE
Appetite suppressant
(Direct Div.)

Each tablet:
Phendimetrazine tartrate * ... 35 mg.

BACCO-RESIST
Anti smoking lozenge
(Vita Elixir Co.)

Lobeline sulfate .... 1/64 gr.

BACIMYCIN OINTMENT
For superficial skin infections
(Merrell Dow)

Each gm.:
Bacitracin (supplied as zinc
bacitracin) .... 500 units
Neomycin base (supplied as
neomycin sulfate) .... 3.5 mg.
Petrolatum base

BACKES' TOY PISTOL CAPS
(Backes', M., Sons)

Antimony sulfide * 47.5%
Potassium chlorate 47.5%
Red amorphous phosphorus * 4.0%
Carbonate of magnesium .... trace

'76 Ed.

BACK-UP ALGICIDE INHIBITOR

See BIO-GUARD BACK-UP ALGICIDE-INHIBITOR

BAC-OFF, DEL

See DEL BAC-OFF

BACON'S C-K TEA
Cathartic
(Brown Mfg.)

Senna leaves 34 1/2%
Mandrake root * 22%
Aromatic herbs 43 1/2%

'76 Ed.

BAC-STOP
Liquid iodophor sanitizer cleaner
(Diversey Wyandotte)

Butoxy monoether of polyoxypropylene - polyoxyethylene glycol
- iodine complex (providing
1.75% titratable iodine)* 12.675%
Phosphoric acid * 3.750%
Citric acid 2.000%

BACTA-LIFE

See BLUE SEAL BACTA-LIFE

BAC-TEX

See AIRWICK PROFESSIONAL PRODUCTS BAC-TEX

Starred ingredients (*) may be responsible for major toxic effects; consult Section II.

BACTILIN
Detergent-germicide
(Puritan Chem. Co.)

Sodium carbonate 3.0%
n-Alkyl (60% tetradecyl, 30% hexadecyl, 5% dodecyl, 5% octadecyl)
  dimethyl benzyl ammonium
  chlorides * 1.6%
n-Alkyl (50% dodecyl, 30% tetradecyl, 17% hexadecyl, 3% octadecyl)
  dimethyl benzyl ammonium
  chlorides * 1.6%
Anhydrous Sodium metasilicate ... 1.0%

BACTINE ANTISEPTIC/ ANESTHETIC FIRST-AID SPRAY AEROSOL
(Miles Labs., Inc.)

Benzalkonium chloride ...... 0.13% w/w
Lidocaine hydrochloride .... 2.50% w/w

BACTINE ANTISEPTIC FIRST-AID SPRAY LIQUID
(Miles Labs., Inc.)

Alcohol .... 3.17% w/w
Benzalkonium chloride ...... 0.13% w/w
Lidocaine hydrochloride .... 2.50% w/w

BACTINE HYDROCORTISONE SKIN CARE CREAM
(Miles Labs., Inc.)

Hydrocortisone 0.5%

BACTOCILL
Antibiotic therapy
(Beecham Labs.)

Each capsule:
  Oxacillin sodium .... 250 mg.; 500 mg.

BACTOX PINE ODOR DISINFECTANT
(Lester Labs.)

Soap
Pine oil *
Sodium orthobenzyl-parachlorophenate
Isopropanol *

'76 Ed.

BADGER MULTI-PURPOSE DRY CHEMICAL EXTINGUISHER
(Badger-Powhatan)

Mono-ammonium phosphate

BADGER PURPLE K DRY CHEMICAL EXTINGUISHER
(Badger-Powhatan)

Potassium bicarbonate

BADGER REGULAR DRY CHEMICAL EXTINGUISHER
(Badger-Powhatan)

Sodium bicarbonate

BAFIX
Germicidal spray & wipe cleaner and surface deodorant; institutional & commercial use
(Hysan Corp.)

N-Alkyl (60% C14, 30% C16, 5%
  C12, 5% C18) dimethyl benzyl
  ammonium chloride 0.076%
N-Alkyl (50% C12, 30% C14, 17%
  C16, 3% C18) dimethyl ethyl-
  benzyl ammonium chloride .. 0.076%
Sodium metasilicate 0.24%
Essential oils 0.20%
Inert ingredients: 99.408%
  Detergents *
  Cleaners
  Builder *
  Propellant

BAG BALM
Ointment; veterinary
(Dairy Assoc.)

Petrolatum 88%
Lanolin 7%
8-Oxyquinolin sulfate 0.3%
Sanitas 1.8%
Water 2.9%

B & A HYGIENIC POWDER
Vaginal douche
(Eastern Research Labs.)

Sodium bicarbonate
Potassium alum
Borax *
Oil of eucalyptus *
Menthol *
Synthetic Methyl salicylate (synthetic oil
  of wintergreen) *

'76 Ed.

BAIN DE SOLEIL PRODUCTS

Bain de Soleil
40 W. 57th St.
New York, N.Y. 10019

Phone: 212-621-7327

See COSMETICS, Section VI, General
Formulations

BAINICIDE
Insect spray
(Lester Labs.)

Petroleum distillates *
Piperonyl butoxide
Pyrethrins
Essential oils *

'76 Ed.

BAKER'S CLEANER & SHAMPOO
(Baker, C.P.)

Alcohol 1-10%
Alcohol sulfate 1-10%

'76 Ed.

BAKERSEAL
Thread sealing and lubricating compound
(Radiator)

Petroleum distillates *

'76 Ed.

BAKER'S FURNITURE POLISH
(Baker, C.P.)

Sulfonated vegetable oil 1-10%
Neutral petroleum oil *† .... >10%

'76 Ed.

†*See* Petroleum distillate

BAKER'S INSTANTANEOUS SILVER POLISH
(Baker, C.P.)

Infusorial earth
Soap
Glycerin

'76 Ed

BAKER'S METAL POLISH
(Baker, C.P.)

Oleic acid 1-10%
Alcohol 1-10%
Ammonia 1-10%
Silica

'76 Ed

BALAN (GRANULAR)
Selective herbicide
(Elanco Prod.)

N-Butyl-N-ethyl-a,a,a-trifluoro-2,6-
  dinitro-p-toluidine (Balan) 2.5%

BALAN L.C.
Selective herbicide
(Elanco Prod.)

N-Butyl-N-ethyl-a,a,a-trifluoro-2,6-
  dinitro-p-toluidine * 19.4%

BALKAMP ALUMINUM JELLY
(Balkamp, Inc.; Mfr., Woodhill Chemi
  cal)

Phosphoric acid * 15%

BALKAMP ANTI-SEIZE BRUSH TOP
(Balkamp, Inc.; Mfr., Loctite Corp.)

Mineral oil *	60%
Fillers	40%

BALKAMP ANTI-SEIZE SPRAY
(Balkamp, Inc.; Mfr., Loctite Corp.)

Mineral oil *	21%
Dichloromethane *	65%
Fillers	10%
Carbon dioxide	3%

BALKAMP BATTERY CLEANER
(Balkamp, Inc.; Mfr., Aerosol Systems, Inc.)

Water	89%
Sodium bicarbonate	5%

BALKAMP BATTERY TERMINAL PROTECTOR
(Balkamp, Inc.; Mfr., Aerosol Systems, Inc.)

Xylene *	30%
Chlorinated solvent	25%

BALKAMP BELT DRESSING (#4-249, #4-255, #4-257)
(Balkamp, Inc.; Mfr., Cling Surface Co.)

Petroleum distillates *	30%/wt.
Combined amount:	70%/wt.
Solid Petroleum fraction of an asphaltic nature	
Heavy bodied Mineral oil fraction of crude, and unrefined wool grease	

BALKAMP BELT DRESSING #4-4770 (Aerosol)
(Balkamp, Inc.; Mfr., Cling Surface Co.)

Base product	75%
Petroleum distillates *	
Solid petroleum fraction of an asphaltic nature, heavy bodied mineral oil fraction of crude, and unrefined wool grease	
Methylene chloride *	
Propane	25%

BALKAMP BOLT SEALER
(Balkamp, Inc.; Mfr., Woodhill Chemical)

Methyl ethyl ketone
Toluol *

BALKAMP BOOT CEMENT
Tire repair
(Balkamp, Inc.; Mfr., H.B. Egan Mfg. Co.)

Combined amount:	approx. 80%
Rubber solvent *	
1,1,1-Trichloroethane (Chlorinated solvent) *	

BALKAMP CHOKE CLEANER
(Balkamp, Inc.; Mfr., Aerosol Systems, Inc.)

Methylene chloride	15%
Xylene *	37%
2-Butoxyethanol	5%
Orthodichlorobenzene	10%

BALKAMP CONTACT CEMENT
(Balkamp, Inc.; Mfr., Woodhill Chemical)

Combined amount:	80%
Toluol *	
Acetone *	
Naphtha *	

BALKAMP dgf-123
Lubricant (dry film type) applied via aerosol spray
(Balkamp, Inc.; Mfr., Miracle Power)

Graphite
Chlorinated solvents *
Isopropanol *
Aliphatic hydrocarbon propellant

BALKAMP DOOR-EASE
(Balkamp, Inc.)

See DOOR-EASE

BALKAMP DRIPLESS OIL
Lubricant
(Balkamp, Inc.; Mfr., American Grease Stick)

Naphtha (Aliphatic petroleum) *	79%
Mineral oil + Aluminum stearate	15%
Sorbitan mono-oleate	6%

BALKAMP ENGINE DEGREASER
(Balkamp, Inc.; Mfr., Aerosol Systems, Inc.)

Aromatic naphtha *	92%
Alkyl aryl polyethyl alcohol (detergent)	8%

BALKAMP E-POX-E CEMENT
(Balkamp, Inc.; Mfr., Woodhill Chemical)

Epoxy resin
Amine hardener

BALKAMP E-POX-E GLUE
(Balkamp, Inc.; Mfr., Woodhill Chemical)

Epoxy resin
Amine hardener

BALKAMP E-POX-E STEEL
(Balkamp, Inc.; Mfr., Woodhill Chemical)

Epoxy resin
Amine hardener

BALKAMP FAST CURE M/C
(Balkamp, Inc.; Mfr., Loctite Corp.)

Epoxy resin
Hardener

BALKAMP FIBERGLASS REPAIR KIT
(Balkamp, Inc.; Mfr., Woodhill Chemical)

Resin portion:	
Epoxy resin	100%
Hardener portion:	
Amine resin	100%

BALKAMP FIRE GUM EXHAUST SEALER
(Balkamp, Inc.; Mfr., Holt-Lloyd)

Alkaline product *†

pH=12.1

†*See* Alkaline salts

BALKAMP FORMULA V
(Balkamp, Inc.; Mfr., Woodhill Chemical)

Tetrahydrofuran *	24%
Acetone	50%

BALKAMP GASKET CEMENT
Automotive
(Balkamp, Inc.; Mfr., H.B. Egan Mfg. Co.)

Combined amount:	90%
Rubber solvent *	
1,1,1-Trichloroethane (Chlorinated solvent) *	

BALKAMP GASKET COMPOUND
(Balkamp, Inc.; Mfr., Loctite Corp.)

Polyester resins

BALKAMP GLASS ADHESIVE
(Balkamp, Inc.; Mfr., Loctite Corp.)

Mixed Polyurethane and polyester resins

BALKAMP GUN GUM MUFFLER BANDAGE KIT
(Balkamp, Inc.; Mfr., Holt-Lloyd)

Alkaline product *†

pH 11.5

†*See* Alkaline salts

Starred ingredients (*) may be responsible for major toxic effects; consult Section II.

BALKAMP GUN GUM MUFFLER SEAL
(Balkamp, Inc.; Mfr., Holt-Lloyd)

Alkaline product *†

pH 12.2

†See Alkaline salts

BALKAMP HOUSEHOLD OIL
(Balkamp, Inc.; Mfr., Panef Mfg. Co.)

Lubricating oil - petroleum distillate *

BALKAMP IGNITION & BATTERY SEALER
(Balkamp, Inc.; Mfr., Aerosol Systems, Inc.)

Xylene *	30%
Chlorinated solvent	25%

BALKAMP JACK OIL
Automotive
(Balkamp, Inc.; Mfr., Southwest Petro-Chem)

Mineral oil *	>99%
Rust proofing and antioxidation agents, antiscuffing additives	<1%

BALKAMP KLEAN AND PRIME
(Balkamp, Inc.; Mfr., Loctite Corp.)

Methyl chloroform *	approx. 90%
Isopropanol *	approx. 10%

BALKAMP LIQUID BUFFER
Inner tube repair
(Balkamp, Inc.; Mfr., H.B. Egan Mfg. Co.)

Combined amount:	100%
Rubber solvent *	
1,1,1-Trichloroethane (Chlorinated solvent) *	

BALKAMP LIQUID HARDENER
(Balkamp, Inc.; Mfr., Dynatron/Bondo)

Methyl ethyl ketone peroxides *

BALKAMP LIQUID SOLDER
(Balkamp, Inc.; Mfr., Woodhill Chemical)
Toluol *
Methyl ethyl ketone

BALKAMP LIQUID STEEL
(Balkamp, Inc.; Mfr., Woodhill Chemical)

Methyl ethyl ketone
Toluol *

BALKAMP LITH-EASE
(Balkamp, Inc.)

See LITH-EASE

BALKAMP LOCK DEFROSTER
(Balkamp, Inc.; Mfr., Panef Mfg. Co.)

Propylene glycol	58.28%
Rust inhibitor (Sodium 2-mercaptobenzothiazole)	0.03%
De-ionized water	41.69%

BALKAMP LOCK-EASE
(Balkamp, Inc.)

See LOCK-EASE

BALKAMP LOCK N SEAL
(Balkamp, Inc.; Mfr., Loctite Corp.)

Polyester resins

BALKAMP LUB-A-CABLE
(Balkamp, Inc.; Mfr., Panef Mfg. Co.)

Mineral spirits (Aliphatic hydrocarbon) *	96%
Colloidal Graphite	4%

BALKAMP LUB-A-GRAPH
(Balkamp, Inc.; Mfr., Panef Mfg. Co.)

Mineral spirits (Aliphatic hydrocarbon) *	96%
Colloidal Graphite	4%

BALKAMP NAVAL JELLY
(Balkamp, Inc.; Mfr., Woodhill Chemical)

Phosphoric acid *

BALKAMP PART-EASE
(Balkamp, Inc.)

See PART-EASE

BALKAMP PENETRANT
(Balkamp, Inc.; Mfr., American Grease Stick)

Petroleum distillate *	91%
2-Butyl alcohol	5%
Glycerol mono-oleate	4%

BALKAMP PENETRATING OIL
(Balkamp, Inc.; Mfr., Panef Mfg. Co.)

Petroleum distillate *	74%
Mineral spirits (Aliphatic hydrocarbon) *	26%

BALKAMP PIPE SEALANT WITH TEFLON
(Balkamp, Inc.; Mfr., Loctite Corp.)

Polyester resins	41%
Octanol	12%
Fillers	36%
Polyester plasticizer	11%

BALKAMP PLASTIC ALUMINUM
(Balkamp, Inc.; Mfr., Woodhill Chemical)

Toluol *
Methyl ethyl ketone
Aluminum (atomized)

BALKAMP PLASTIC RUBBER
(Balkamp, Inc.; Mfr., Woodhill Chemical)

Toluol *

BALKAMP PLASTIC-RUBBER CEMENT
(Balkamp, Inc.; Mfr., H.B. Egan Mfg. Co.)

Methyl ethyl ketone *	48%
Toluol *	48%

BALKAMP QUICK SET
(Balkamp, Inc.; Mfr., Loctite Corp.)

Methyl cyanoacrylate monomer*†

†See Methyl-2-cyanoacrylate

BALKAMP RuGLYDE
Rubber lubricant
(Balkamp, Inc.; Mfr., American Grease Stick)

Potassium vegetable oil soap	7.0%
Ethylene glycol	1.3%
Corrosion inhibitors	<1.0%
Sequestering agent	<1.0%
Water	91.7%

BALKAMP SIL-GLYDE
(Balkamp, Inc.)

See SIL-GLYDE

BALKAMP SLEEVE RETAINER
(Balkamp, Inc.; Mfr., Loctite Corp.)

Mixed Polyurethane and polyester resins

BALKAMP SPRAY BELT DRESSING #4-256
(Balkamp, Inc.; Mfr., Cling Surface Co.)

Petroleum distillate *	17%
Chlorinated solvent as Methylene chloride	25 1/2%
Petroleum derived resins	42 1/2%
Propane	15%

Starred ingredients (*) may be responsible for major toxic effects; consult Section II.

BALKAMP STARTING FLUID
(Balkamp, Inc.; Mfr., United States Aviex Co.)

Unrefined Ethyl ether * 80-90%

BALKAMP STUD N BEARING MOUNT
(Balkamp, Inc.; Mfr., Loctite Corp.)

Polyester resins

BALKAMP SUPER GLUE 3
(Balkamp, Inc.; Mfr., Woodhill Chemical)

Cyanoacrylate ester * 95%

BALKAMP TINS-TYTER PERFECT BOND TINNING FLUID
(Balkamp, Inc.; Mfr., Remont, Inc.)

Zinc chloride *

BALKAMP TIRE SEALANT
(Balkamp, Inc.; Mfr., Bernzomatic Corp.)

Urethane
Toluol *
Isopropyl alcohol (anhydrous)
Isopropyl acetate
Tergitol
Dichlorodifluoromethane

BALKAMP TRIM CEMENT
(Balkamp, Inc.; Mfr., Woodhill Chemical)

Aliphatic naphtha *

BALKAMP TUBE CEMENT
Automotive
(Balkamp, Inc.; Mfr., H.B. Egan Mfg. Co.)

Combined amount: 100%
  Rubber solvent *
  1,1,1-Trichloroethane (Chlorinated solvent) *

BALKAMP UNDERCOATER
(Balkamp, Inc.; Mfr., Aerosol Systems, Inc.)

Asphalt 33%
Petroleum distillate * 22%

BALKAMP WHITE GREASE
(Balkamp, Inc.; Mfr., Panef Mfg. Co.)

White lithium grease 100%

BALKAMP WHITE PLASTIC RUBBER
(Balkamp, Inc.; Mfr., Woodhill Chemical)

Toluol * 50%

BALKAMP WICK N' LOCK
(Balkamp, Inc.; Mfr., Loctite Corp.)

Polyester resin

BALKAMP WINDOW SEALER
(Balkamp, Inc.; Mfr., Woodhill Chemical)

Toluol *
Methyl ethyl ketone

BALL O' PERFUME
Air deodorant
(Curran)

Paradichlorobenzene *

'76 Ed.

BALMEX BABY POWDER
(Macsil, Inc.)

Balsan (specially purified balsam Peru)
Zinc oxide
Talc
Starch
Calcium carbonate

BALMEX EMOLLIENT LOTION
Infant's skin conditioner
(Macsil, Inc.)

Lanolin oil
Balsan (specially purified balsam Peru) *
Silicone

BALMEX OINTMENT
Emollient, protective, anti-inflammatory, healing ointment
(Macsil, Inc.)

Balsan (specially purified balsam Peru)
Vitamin A
Vitamin D
Zinc oxide
Bismuth subnitrate
Silicone base

BALNETAR
Water dispersible emollient-tar
(Westwood Pharm.)

Westwood tar (equiv. to crude coal tar USP) * 2.5%
Alpha-Keri (dewaxed, oil-soluble, keratin-moisturizing fraction of lanolin)
Mineral oil
Nonionic emulsifier

'76 Ed.

BALTIMORE PAINT & CHEMICAL PRODUCTS

Baltimore Paint & Chemical Co.
1370 Ontario St.
Cleveland, Ohio 44113
Phone: 216-566-2000

See PAINTS, Section VI, General Formulations

BAM
Odor controlled insecticide; industrial and institutional use
(Scientific International)

Pyrethrins 0.250%
Technical Piperonyl butoxide ... 0.500%
N-Octyl bicycloheptene
  dicarboximide 0.500%
Petroleum distillate 1.000%
Inert ingred.: 97.750%
  Volatile solvents
  Propellants

BAMBU WAX
(Zecol)

Silicone
Aromatic solvent *
Petroleum wax
Aliphatic solvent
Silica
Amine oleate

'76 Ed.

BAN-A-BUG
Residual spray
(Wipp Pest Control)

Tech. Chlordane 2%

BAN ACHE
Penetrating heat lotion
(Reese Chem.)

Methyl salicylate *
Oil of eucalyptus
Menthol
Camphor

BANACID
Antacid tablets
(Buffington)

Each tablet:
  Aluminum hydroxide
  Magnesium hydroxide
  Magnesium trisilicate

BANALG LINIMENT
Rubefacient, counterirritant
(OJF)

Menthol *
Camphor *
Methyl salicylate *
Eucalyptus oil *

BAN AMINE WEED KILLER

See UNICO BAN AMINE WEED KILLER

Starred ingredients (*) may be responsible for major toxic effects; consult Section II.

BAN ANTI-PERSPIRANT
Cream deodorant
(Bristol-Myers)

Aluminum sesquichlorohydrate
Water
Glyceryl stearate
Propylene glycol
Stearyl alcohol
Glycine
Isopropyl palmitate
Ceteareth-20
Isopropyl myristate
Titanium dioxide
Fragrance
Isopropyl stearate
D & C Yellow No. 10
D & C Red No. 19

BAN BASIC (Regular & Neutral Scent)
Non-aerosol anti-perspirant spray
(Bristol-Myers)

Aluminum chlorohydrate
Aluminum chloride
SD Alcohol 40 * 80%/v
Water
PPG-11 stearyl ether
Laureth-4
Glycine
Fragrance
Laureth-23

BANCAP CAPSULES
Analgesic
(OJF)

Each capsule:
  Salicylamide .... 200 mg.
  Acetaminophen * .... 300 mg.

BANCAP WITH CODEINE CAPSULES
Analgesic
(OJF)

Each capsule:
  Codeine phosphate .... 1 mg.
  Salicylamide .... 200 mg.
  Acetaminophen * .... 300 mg.

BANNER DISINFECTANT SPRAY (HOSPITAL GRADE)
(Banner Mfg. Co.)

Orthophenylphenol 0.176%
4-Chloro-2-cyclopentylphenol .. 0.028%
Essential oils 0.300%
Alcohol 49.950%
Sodium nitrite *

'76 Ed.

BANNER TOILET BOWL CLEANER
(Banner Mfg. Co.)

Hydrogen chloride * 24.57%
n-Alkyl dimethyl benzyl ammonium chlorides 0.30%
n-Alkyl dimethyl ethylbenzyl ammonium chlorides 0.30%

'76 Ed.

BANODOR
Odor counteractant; institutional and commercial use
(National-Purity Soap)

Quaternary ammonium compounds *
Essential oils

BAN QUICK DRY ROLL-ON ANTI-PERSPIRANT DEODORANT
(Bristol-Myers)

Aluminum chlorohydrate *

BAN ROLL-ON ANTI-PERSPIRANT DEODORANT
(Bristol-Myers)

Aluminum chlorohydrate *

BANSECT FLEA & TICK COLLAR FOR CATS
(Miller-Morton)

Naled * 10%

BANSECT FLEA & TICK COLLAR FOR DOGS
(Miller-Morton)

Naled * 15%

BAN-SMOKE CHEWING GUM
To combat tobacco habit
(Thompson Med.)

Benzocaine
Dextrose
Oil of anise
Oil of peppermint
Oil of wintergreen
Oil of cinnamon
Oil of clove

BAN SUPER SOLID ANTI-PERSPIRANT DEODORANT (Neutral, Fresh or Spice Scent)
(Bristol-Myers)

Active ingred.:
  Aluminum chlorohydrate *
Other ingred.:
  Octyl palmitate
  Stearyl alcohol
  Paraffin
  PEG-25 propylene glycol stearate
  Fragrance *
  Titanium dioxide
  BHT

BANTRON
Smoking deterrent
(Campana)

Each tablet:
  Lobeline sulfate *
  Slow and fast acting antacids

BANVEL HERBICIDE
(Velsicol)

Dimethylamine salt of Dicamba *   48.2%
Dimethylamine salt of related
  acids 12.0%

BARBASOL BRUSHLESS
Shaving cream
(Leeming Div.)

Glyceryl stearate
Lanolin
Liquid petrolatum
Boric acid .... approx. 1.5-2.0%

BARBATOSE #2 BLUE
Sedative
(Vale)

Each tablet:
  Barbital * .... 64.8 mg.
  Hyoscyamus .... 8.1 mg.
  Passiflora extract .... 16.2 mg.
  Valerian extract .... 16.2 mg.

BARBATRO NO. 2
Sedative, anticholinergic
(Elder)

Each tablet:
  Phenobarbital * .... 1/4 gr.
  Atropine sulfate .... 1/250 gr.

BARBELOID
Antispasmodic
(Vale)

Each tablet:
  Phenobarbital * .... 16.2000 mg.
  Hyoscyamine sulfate * ... 0.1037 mg.
  Atropine sulfate .... 0.0194 mg.
  Scopolamine
    hydrobromide .... 0.0065 mg.

BARBER SHOP SHAVING SOAP
(Williams, J.B.)

Sodium and potassium soaps

BARC GREASELESS CREAM
For lice, nits, crablice
(Commerce Drug)

Isobornyl thiocyanoacetate *
Other related terpenes
Dioctyl sodium sulfosuccinate *

BARCO-DYNE
Detergent, sanitizer, disinfectant
(Barco)

Nonphenylether of polyethylene
  glycol-iodine complex (providing
  0.8% available iodine) 17.0%
Phosphoric acid * 5.5%

'76 Ed.

Starred ingredients (*) may be responsible for major toxic effects; consult Section II.

BARCO-SOL
Liquid bowl cleaner
(Barco)

Hydrochloric acid *

'76 Ed.

BARDAHL ADDITIVES & LUBRICANTS

Bardahl Manufacturing Corp.
P.O. Box 70607
1400 N.W. 52nd St.
Seattle, Wash. 98107

In the event of a medical emergency, call the following phone number for 24-hour-a-day service: 206-634-5252

BARDAHL CARBURETOR CLEANER
(Bardahl Mfg. Corp.)

Aromatic solvents *
Polyglycols

BARDAHL ENGINE TUNE UP
(Bardahl Mfg. Corp.)

Aromatic solvents characterized by Xylene *
Aliphatic solvent
Ethylene glycol-n-butyl ether

BARDAHL FUEL SYSTEM TREATMENT
Gasoline additive
(Bardahl Mfg. Corp.)

Aromatic solvents characterized by Xylene *
Amine type dispersant

BARDAHL GAS LINE ANTI-FREEZE
(Bardahl Mfg. Corp.)

Methyl alcohol * 20%

BARDAHL MOTORCYCLE INJECTION OIL
2 Stroke lubricant
(Bardahl Mfg. Corp.)

Petroleum solvents *
Mineral oil *
Calcium sulfonate
Amine dispersant
Green Automate dye

BARDAHL OUTBOARD MOTOR OIL
2 Stroke lubricant
(Bardahl Mfg. Corp.)

Petroleum solvents *
Mineral oil *
Calcium sulfonate
Amine dispersant
Green Automate dye

BARDAHL SNOWMOBILE OIL
2 Stroke lubricant
(Bardahl Mfg. Corp.)

Petroleum solvents *
Mineral oil *
Calcium sulfonate
Amine dispersant
Green Automate dye

BARDAHL TOP OIL
Gasoline additive
(Bardahl Mfg. Corp.)

Aromatic solvents characterized by Xylene *
Light mineral oil
Amine type dispersant

BARDAHL VBA MOTORCYCLE 2 STROKE
2 Stroke lubricant
(Bardahl Mfg. Corp.)

Petroleum solvents *
Mineral oil *
Calcium sulfonate
Amine dispersant
Green Automate dye

BAR-D-K, CABOT'S

See CABOT'S BAR-D-K

BARE ELEGANCE MOISTURIZING BODY SHAMPOO, FRESH JASMINE
(Gillette Co., Personal Care Div.)

TEA-lauryl sulfate	Glycol stearate
Lauramide DEA	Methylparaben
Cocoamidopropyl	Propylparaben
betaine	Tetrasodium
Propylene glycol	EDTA
Glycerin	Fragrance
Boric acid	
Sodium chloride	
Quaternium-19	

BARE ELEGANCE MOISTURIZING BODY SHAMPOO, FRESH SPRING
(Gillette Co., Personal Care Div.)

TEA-lauryl sulfate	Glycol stearate
Lauramide DEA	Methylparaben
Cocoamidopropyl	Propylparaben
betaine	Tetrasodium
Propylene glycol	EDTA
Glycerin	Fragrance
Boric acid	
Sodium chloride	
Quaternium-19	

BARE ELEGANCE MOISTURIZING BODY SHAMPOO, UNSCENTED
(Gillette Co., Personal Care Div.)

TEA-lauryl sulfate	Glycol stearate
Lauramide DEA	Methylparaben
Cocoamidopropyl	Propylparaben
betaine	Tetrasodium
Propylene glycol	EDTA
Glycerin	
Boric acid	
Sodium chloride	
Quaternium-19	

BARICIDE

See CHEMFORM BARICIDE

BAR KEEPERS FRIEND
Cleanser & polish
(SerVaas Labs.)

by weight
Oxalic acid (as the dihydrate) * 10%
Silica (amorphous) 87%
Sodium carbonate 2%
Nonionic surfactant .... <1%
Perfume .... trace

BAR KEEPERS FRIEND LIQUID CLEANSER
(SerVaas Labs.)

Water 50-55%
Feldspar † 30-35%
Citric acid 5-10%
Cab-O-Sil 1-5%
Nonionic soap 1-5%
Perfume .... <1%

†*See* Aluminum silicate

BAR KEEPERS FRIEND SHINY SINKS
(SerVaas Labs.)

Water 50-55%
Feldspar † 30-35%
Citric acid 5-10%
Cab-O-Sil 1-5%
Nonionic soap 1-5%
Perfume .... <1%

†*See* Aluminum silicate

BAR KEEPERS FRIEND SOFT CLEANSER
(SerVaas Labs.)

Water 50-55%
Feldspar † 30-35%
Citric acid 5-10%
Cab-O-Sil 1-5%
Nonionic soap 1-5%
Perfume .... <1%

†*See* Aluminum silicate

Starred ingredients (*) may be responsible for major toxic effects; consult Section II.

BARRAGE INDUSTRIAL STRENGTH BOWL CLEANSE
(Nat'l Labs. Div.)

n-Alkyl (C12 40%, C14 50%, C16 10%) dimethyl benzyl ammonium chlorides	0.05%
Hydrogen chloride *	19.00%

BARSEB HC
For seborrheic dermatitis of the scalp
(Barnes-Hind)

Hydrocortisone	1%
Salicylic acid	0.5%
Isopropyl alcohol *	45%
Propylene glycol	
Isopropyl myristate	
Ascorbic acid	
Citric acid	

BARSEB THERA-SPRAY
For seborrheic dermatitis of the scalp
(Barnes-Hind)

Each bottle (84 gm.):
Hydrocortisone	360 mg.
Salicylic acid *	288 mg.
Benzalkonium chloride	14 mg.
Alcohol	46 gm.
Propylene glycol	
Isopropyl myristate	
Butane (propellant)	

BARTLETT'S FIXED COPPER (W.P.)
Fungicide
(Bartlett, N.M.)

Fixed Copper *	53%

BARTLETT'S MALATHION
Insecticide
(Bartlett, N.M.)

Malathion *	25%; 50%

BARTLETT'S PARATHION W.P.
Insecticide
(Bartlett, N.M.)

Parathion *	15%

BARTLETT'S PHOSDRIN
Miticide
(Bartlett, N.M.)

Phosdrin (Alpha isomer of mevinphos) *	60%

BARTON'S SPOT REMOVER
(Dyanshine)

Petroleum naphtha *
1,1,1-Trichlorethane *

BASALJEL CAPSULES AND SWALLOW TABLETS
Antacid
(Wyeth Labs.)

Each capsule or swallow tablet:
Dried basic Aluminum carbonate gel (equiv. to 608 mg. dried aluminum hydroxide gel or 500 mg. aluminum hydroxide)

BASALJEL SUSPENSION & EXTRA STRENGTH SUSPENSION
Antacid
(Wyeth Labs.)

Suspension (each 5 ml.):
Basic Aluminum carbonate gel (equiv. to 400 mg. aluminum hydroxide)

Extra strength suspension (each 5 ml.):
Basic Aluminum carbonate gel (equiv. to 1000 mg. aluminum hydroxide)

BASIC-G
Liquid germicidal concentrate
(Shaklee)

Quaternary germicides	12.500%
Tetrasodium EDTA	3.420%
Nonionic surfactants	
Ethyl alcohol	
Sodium sesquicarbonate	
Color & Perfume	small amounts

BASKET O'FLOWERS AIR FRESHENER
(Curran)

Paradichlorobenzene *

'76 Ed.

BATHING JEWELS
Bath oil capsules (small & large)
(Delagar)

Each capsule:
Mineral oil	30 min. or 80 min.
Perfume oil *	2.5%
Nonionic surfactant	1.25%
Isostearic acid in Yellow (Exotic perfume), Red (Rose perfume), Green (Pine perfume), Lilac (Lilac perfume)	2.00%

'76 Ed.

BATH-O-VEL
For bathing the dermatologically ill patient
(Torch)

Sulfated oil
Water softeners
Emulsifying agents
Distilled water

'76 Ed.

BAXIMIN OINTMENT
(Columbia Med.)

Each gram:
Polymyxin B sulfate	5000 units
Bacitracin	400 units
Neomycin sulfate	5 mg.

BAXINETS
Antibacterial-anesthetic for throat irritations
(Columbia Med.)

Each troche:
Cetylpyridinium chloride	2.5 mg.
Benzocaine	10 mg.

BAYER ADULT ASPIRIN
Analgesic
(Glenbrook Labs.)

Acetylsalicylic acid *	5.0 gr.

BAYER CHILDREN'S ASPIRIN
Analgesic, pediatric
(Glenbrook Labs.)

Acetylsalicylic acid *	1.25 gr.

BAYER CHILDREN'S COLD TABLETS
Analgesic-decongestant
(Glenbrook Labs.)

Phenylpropanolamine HCl *	3.125 mg.
Aspirin *	81 mg.

BAYER CHILDREN'S COUGH SYRUP
Decongestant - antitussive
(Glenbrook Labs.)

Each 5 ml.:
Phenylpropanolamine HCl *	9 mg.
Dextromethorphan hydrobromide	7.5 mg.
Alcohol	5%

BAYER DECONGESTANT COLD TABLETS
Analgesic-decongestant-antihistaminic
(Glenbrook Labs.)

Aspirin *	325 mg.
Phenylpropanolamine HCl	12.5 mg.
Chlorpheniramine maleate	2 mg.

BAYER TIMED-RELEASE ASPIRIN
Sustained-release analgesic
(Glenbrook Labs.)

Acetylsalicylic acid *	10.0 gr.

BAYGON
Insecticide
(Mobay Chemical Corp.)

Propoxur (2-(1-Methylethoxy)phenol methylcarbamate) *

Starred ingredients (*) may be responsible for major toxic effects; consult Section II.

BAYMIX CRUMBLES
Cattle feed supplement (medicated) for control of roundworms
(Cutter (Brand) Bayvet Div. Cutter Labs.)

Coumaphos 0.32%

BAYPAX
Insecticide
(Biocerta)

Baygon tech. * 1.0%
Petroleum distillate * 83.75%

'76 Ed.

BAYTEX
Insecticide
(Mobay Chemical Corp.)

Fenthion (O,O-Dimethyl O-(3-methyl-4-(methylthio)phenyl) phosphorothioate) *

BC (POWDER & TABLETS) ORIGINAL FORMULA
(Block Drug)

Powder:
Aspirin * .... 650 mg.
Salicylamide .... 195 mg.
Caffeine * .... 32 mg.

Each tablet:
Aspirin * .... 325 mg.
Salicylamide .... 95 mg.
Caffeine * .... 16 mg.

BDC CHLORINATED CLEANER
Pipeline and tank cleaner for dairies
(Birchmore Dairy Supply)

Sodium tripolyphosphate .... >35%
Soda ash * .... >40%
Sodium metasilicate * .... <15%
Sodium dichloroisocyanurate ..... <3%

BEACON SELF-POLISHING FLOOR WAX
(Lehn & Fink)

Ammonium hydroxide .... minor
Ethylene glycol .... minor
Formaldehyde .... minor
Dipropylene glycol monomethyl ether .... minor

BEARFAST
Adhesive
(Ambroid)

Nitrocellulose type of cement
Alcohols * 20%
Hydrocarbons *† 60%
Ketones * 20%
Allyl isothiocyanate (synthetic oil of mustard) .... trace

†*See* Adhesives, Section VI, General Formulations

BEARIN' SEAL
To prevent leaks in engine oil seals
(Radiator)

Petroleum distillates *

'76 Ed.

BEAR LAMP BLACK
(Monsanto)

Fine pure Carbon powder

BEAR-OX 22
Granular weed killer
(Stewart Sanitary Supply)

Bromacil 2%
Diuron 2%

BEAR-OX 150
Nonselective weed and grass killer
(Stewart Sanitary Supply)

Sodium metaborate tetrahydrate (Boron trioxide equivalent 22.6%) 66.5%
Sodium chlorate * 30.0%
Bromacil 1.5%

BEAR-OX 486
Nonselective weed and grass killer
(Stewart Sanitary Supply)

Sodium chlorate * 30%
Sodium metaborate tetrahydrate (Boron trioxide equivalent 23.3%) 68%

BEAT IT DOG REPELLENT
(Senoret)

Bone oil 7%
Allyl isothiocyanate * 1%

BEATSALL CRYSTALS

See MEYER'S BEATSALL CRYSTALS

BEATSALL FOG SPRAY

See MEYER'S BEATSALL FOG SPRAY

BEAUCOUP
Germicidal detergent
(Huntington Labs.)

Active ingred.: 22.24%
Sodium lauryl sulfate 5.24%
Sodium o-phenylphenate 4.95%
Sodium o-benzyl-p-chlorophenate 4.20%
Sodium p-tert amyl phenate * 2.10%
Tetrasodium ethylene diamine tetraacetate 2.00%
Sodium carbonate 1.90%
Isopropyl alcohol 1.65%
Essential oils 0.20%
Inert ingred.: 77.76%
Water
2-Methyl-2,4-pentanediol
Urea
Sodium tripolyphosphate *
Sodium sulfite *

BEAU KREML HAIR DRESSING
(Williams, J.B.)

Alcohol (denatured with colocynth) *
Polyalkalene glycols

BEAUTI-BOWL
Toilet bowl deodorant
(Curran)

Paradichlorobenzene *

'76 Ed.

BEAUTY BATH
Bath oil capsules (small & large)
(Delagar)

Each capsule:
Mineral oil .... 30 min. or 80 min.
Perfume oil * 2.5%
Nonionic surfactant 1.25%
Isostearic acid in Yellow (Exotic perfume), Red (Rose perfume), Green (Pine perfume), Lilac (Lilac perfume) 2.00%

'76 Ed.

BEAUTY COAT
(Park Chem.)

Water
Polyester resin
Silicone
Isopropanol *
Wetting agent *

BECKSPAR GAY VELVET
Paint for interior plaster walls
(Akron Paint & Varnish Co.)

Titanium pigment
Latex

BEECHAM COSMETICS

Beecham Cosmetics
875 N. Michigan Ave.
Chicago, Ill. 60611

Phone: 312-951-7000

See COSMETICS, Section VI, General
  Formulations

BEECHAM LABORATORIES BABY OINTMENT
*For skin irritations such as prickly
  heat, diaper rash, sunburn and wind-
  burn*
(Beecham Labs.)

Aluminum hydroxide
Zinc oxide
Boric acid *
Benzoin
Tolu balsam *
Storax
0.2% Phenol
Lanolin-petrolatum base

BEE CHEMICAL CO. PRODUCTS
Liquid colorants & coatings for plastics

Bee Chemical Co.
2700 E. 170th
Lansing, Ill. 60438

Phone: 312-474-7000

BEELITH
Vitamin B6, magnesium supplement
(Beach Pharm.)

Each tablet:
  Magnesium oxide * .... 600 mg.
  Vitamin B6 (Pyridoxine HCl) . 25 mg.

BEE-NIP
Insecticide
(NIP-CO)

Pyrethrins 0.10%
Piperonyl butoxide (technical) . 0.20%
N-Octyl bicycloheptene
  dicarboximide 0.33%
o-Isopropoxyphenyl
  methylcarbamate * 0.50%
Isoparaffinic hydrocarbons * 83.87%

BEETLE KIL
Insecticide
(Sonford Products)

Benzene hexachloride, gamma
  isomer * 11.4%
Benzene hexachloride, other
  isomers * 13.0%
DDT * 11.4%
Petroleum distillate 60.2%

BEETLE LOG TOX
Wood preservative & insecticide
(Sonford Products)

Benzene hexachloride, gamma
  isomer 7.16%
Benzene hexachloride, other
  isomers 8.24%
Pentachlorophenol * 29.40%
Solvents 55.20%

BEE-WASP

See VIRCHEM BEE-WASP

BE-FREE
Anti-smoking aid
(Coronet Medical)

Benzocaine .... 1/20 gr.
Colloidal Kaolin
Powdered Licorice
Calcium carbonate
Soluble Saccharine
Oil of peppermint
Oil of cinnamon
Oil of anise

                                    '76 Ed.

BEHOLD
Aerosol furniture polish
(Drackett)

Wax
Silicone oil
Paraffin hydrocarbon solvent ... 30-40%
Emulsifiers
Water 40-50%
Perfume
Hydrocarbon propellant
Preservative

BEHOLD PUMP SPRAY FURNITURE POLISH
Non-aerosol furniture polish
(Drackett)

Wax
Silicone oil
Petroleum distillate .... <10%
Emulsifiers
Water .... >75%
Hydrocarbon propellant
Trace amounts of Morpholine, Preserva-
  tive, Perfume, Lanolin

BELAC POWDER
Antacid
(Moffet Inc.)

Each oz.:
  Magnesium carbonate .... 63 gr.
  Calcium carbonate .... 370 gr.

BELAP
Anticholinergic-sedative
(Lemmon Co.)

Each tablet:
  Phenobarbital * .... 16.2 mg.
  Belladonna extract * .... 10.8 mg.

BELFER
Dietary supplement
(OJF)

Each tablet:
  Ascorbic acid .... 50 mg
  Iron (as ferrous fumarate, fer-
    rous sulfate, ferrous
    gluconate) .... 17 mg
  Plus vitamins B12, B6, B1, B2

BELLADENAL TABLETS & BELLADENAL-S (SPACETABS)
Antispasmodic and anticholinergic
(Sandoz)

Each tablet & Spacetab:
  Bellafoline (levorotatory alka-
    loids of belladonna, as
    malates) .... 0.25 mg
  Phenobarbital * .... 50 mg

BELLADOL (ELIXIR & TABLETS)
Sedative, antispasmodic
(Premo)

Each tablet & 5 cc:
  Phenobarbital (1/4 gr.) * ... 16.2 mg
  Hyoscyamine sulfate * ...... 0.1037 mg
  Atropine sulfate .... 0.0194 mg
  Hyoscine hydrobromide ... 0.0065 mg
  Alcohol (elixir) 23%/

                                    '76 Ed

BELLAFEDROL A-H TABLETS
Antihistamine with antispasmodic
(Lannett)

Each tablet:
  Pyrilamine maleate * .... 12.5 mg
  Chlorpheniramine maleate ... 1 mg
  Phenylephrine HCl .... 2.5 mg
  Ext. Belladonna .... 6 mg

BELLAFOLINE TABLETS
Antispasmodic and anticholinergic
(Sandoz)

Each tablet:
  Bellafoline (levorotatory alka-
    loids of belladonna) ...... 0.25 mg

BELLALPHEN
Antispasmodic-sedative
(CMC Research Div.)

Each tablet:
  Phenobarbital * .... 1/4 g
  Atropine sulfate .... 0.0194 mg
  Hyoscyamine sulfate * ...... 0.1037 mg
  Hyoscine hydrobromide ... 0.0065 mg

BELL-ANS
Antacid, digestant
(Bell & Co.)

Each tablet:
  Sodium bicarbonate 78.91
  Ginger 2.45
  Wintergreen *† 1.81

†*See* Wintergreen oil

Starred ingredients (*) may be responsible for major toxic effects; consult Section II.

B.E.L.L. DROPS
For adult horses and cattle
(Daniels, Dr. A.C.)

Each ml.:
Aconite FE * . . . . 0.10 ml.
Belladonna root FE * . . . . . . 0.25 ml.
Digitalis FE * . . . . 0.25 ml.
Nux vomica FE * . . . . 0.375 ml.

BELLERGAL-S AND BELLERGAL TABLETS
Autonomic stabilizer
(Dorsey Labs.)

BELLERGAL TABLETS (each):
Ergotamine tartrate . . . . 0.3 mg.
Bellafoline (levorotatory alka-
loids of belladonna, as
malates) . . . . 0.1 mg.
Phenobarbital * . . . . 20.0 mg.

BELLERGAL-S TABLETS (each):
Ergotamine tartrate . . . . 0.6 mg.
Bellafoline (levorotatory alka-
loids of belladonna, as
malates) . . . . 0.2 mg.
Phenobarbital * . . . . 40.0 mg.

BELL LABS. RODENT CAKE
(Bell Labs., Inc.)

Diphacinone 0.005%
Blend of food grade cereals 99.995%

BELT-EASE
Belt dressing
(American Grease Stick)
(Marketed by: Chrysler Corp., Parts
Div.)

Combined amount: 80%
Polybutene (Butylene
polymer) 35.7%
Naphtha (aliphatic) * 35.7%
1,1,1-Trichloroethane * 28.6%
Carbon dioxide 2%

BENACHLOR
Antihistamine, expectorant
(Jenkins Labs.)

Each 5 cc:
Diphenhydramine
hydrochloride * . . . . 12.5 mg.
Ammonium chloride . . . . 130 mg.
Sodium citrate . . . . 55 mg.
Menthol . . . . 1.11 mg.
Alcohol 5%

BENADRYL (CAPSULES & ELIXIR)
Antihistaminic
(Parke-Davis)

ELIXIR (each 5 ml.):
Diphenhydramine
hydrochloride * . . . . . 12 1/2 mg.

CAPSULES (each):
Diphenhydramine
hydrochloride * . . . . . 50 mg.; 25 mg.

BENDECTIN
For nausea and vomiting of pregnancy
(Merrell Dow)

Each tablet:
Decapryn (Doxylamine
succinate) * . . . . 10 mg.
Pyridoxine hydrochloride . . . . . 10 mg.

BENDIX HIGH TEMPERATURE BRAKE FLUID
(Bendix)

Polyoxyalkyleneglycolether type brake
fluid *†

'76 Ed.

†*See* Brake fluids, Section VI, General Formulations

BENDIX PARTS CLEANER (METACLENE)
(Bendix)

Cresol *
Petroleum hydrocarbons
Ethylene dichloride
Aqueous potassium soap saponified from
refined tall oil
Sodium bichromate *

'76 Ed.

BENDIX PARTS CLEANER (SPEEDCLENE)
(Bendix)

Cresol *
Petroleum hydrocarbons
Aqueous potassium soap saponified from
refined tall oil
Sodium bichromate *

'76 Ed.

BENDIX STARTING FLUID
(Bendix)

Diethyl ether (major ingred.) *
Petroleum hydrocarbons *
Lubrizol 917 . . . . trace
Carbon dioxide propellant

'76 Ed.

BENDIX SUPER HEAVY DUTY BRAKE FLUID
(Bendix)

Ethyl ether of diethylene glycol *
Ethyl ether of ethylene glycol *
Propylene glycol
Polyalkylene glycols

'76 Ed.

BENDYLATE
Antihistamine
(Direct Div.)

CAPSULES (each):
Diphenhydramine
HCl * . . . . 25 mg.; 50 mg.

ELIXIR (each 5 ml.):
Diphenhydramine
HCl * . . . . 12.5 mg.
Alcohol 14%

BENDYNE COSMETIC PRODUCTS

Bendyne, Ltd.
150 Fifth Ave.
New York, N.Y. 10011

Phone: 212-691-0040

See COSMETICS, Section VI, General
Formulations

BENEMID TABLETS
To increase excretion of uric acid
(MSD)

Each tablet:
Probenecid * . . . . 0.5 gm.

BENESAN
Insecticide
(Chipman Inc.)

Gamma isomer of benzene hexachlor-
ide (from lindane) * 50%

BEN-GAY
Rubefacient, counterirritant
(Leeming Div.)

Menthol *
Lanolin
Methyl salicylate *

BENISONE CREAM
Topical steroid/anti-inflammatory
(CooperCare)

Betamethasone benzoate 0.025%
Water-washable emollient cream base

BENISONE GEL
Topical steroid/anti-inflammatory
(CooperCare)

Betamethasone benzoate 0.025%
Alcohol
Water
Disodium edetate
Propylene glycol
Carboxyvinyl polymer
Diisopropanolamine

BENJAMIN MOORE PAINT PRODUCTS

See MOORE, BENJAMIN, PAINT
PRODUCTS

Starred ingredients (*) may be responsible for major toxic effects; consult Section II.

"BENLATE" DF FUNGICIDE
(Du Pont)

Benomyl 75%

"BENLATE" FUNGICIDE
(Du Pont)

Benomyl 50%

BENNETT'S PAINT PRODUCTS

Bennett's Glass & Colorizer Paint
65 W. First S.
Salt Lake City, Utah 84101

Phone: 801-486-2211

See PAINTS, Section VI, General Formulations

"BENOMYL" 50W FUNGICIDE
(Du Pont)

Benomyl 50%

BENOQUIN CREAM
Depigmenting agent
(Elder)

Monobenzyl ether of
  hydroquinone * 20%

BENOXYL (5 & 10) LOTION
Antibacterial, mild keratolytic medication
(Stiefel Labs.)

Benzoyl peroxide .... 5% or 10%

BENSULFOID LOTION
Acne treatment
(Poythress, Wm. P.)

Bensulfoid (33% sulfur on
  bentonite) 6%
Resorcinol * 2%
Thymol 0.5%
Hexachlorophene (preservative
  only) 0.1%
Zinc oxide 6%
Alcohol (by volume) 12%
Perfume
Cosmetic colors
Emulsifiers
Absorbents

BENTEC
Powdered laundry bleach
(Diversey Wyandotte)

Trichloroisocyanurate acid*

BENVICIDE
Gaseous sterilizing agent for use in commercial gas sterilizers
(Ben Venue Labs.)

Ethylene oxide * 11%/w
Inert ingredients:
  Trichloromonofluoromethane
    (G-11) 78.2%/w
  Dichlorodifluoromethane (G-
    12) 10.8%/w

BENVICIDE 12
For use in commercial gas sterilizer
(Ben Venue Labs.)

Ethylene oxide * 12%/w
Dichlorofluoromethane (G-12) 88%

BENWOOD INTERIOR STAIN (WALNUT 237-60)
(Benjamin Moore)

Pigment: 47.4%
  Calcium carbonate 93.6%
  Silicates 2.2%
  Tinting colors 4.2%
Vehicle: 52.6%
  Alkyd varnish: 41.1%
    Soya alkyd resin 59.4%
    Mineral spirits 40.6%
  Mineral spirits * 58.3%
  Driers 0.6%

BENWOOD SATIN FINISH VARNISH
For interior use
(Benjamin Moore)

Pigment: 4.8%
  Silicates 100%
Vehicle: 95.2%
  Alkyd varnish: 80.0%
    Soya alkyd resin 43.7%
    Mineral spirits * 56.3%
  Mineral spirits * 19.4%
  Driers 0.6%

BENWOOD URETHANE FINISH - LOW LUSTRE (435-00)
For interior use
(Benjamin Moore)

Pigment: 5.7%
  Silicates 100.0%
Vehicle: 94.3%
  Varnish: 89.5%
    Polyurethane resin,
      Class 1 .... 49.2%
    Mineral spirits * 50.8%
  Mineral spirits * 10.4%
  Driers 0.1%

BENYLIN COUGH SYRUP
(Parke-Davis)

Each 5 ml.:
  Benadryl * .... 12.5 mg.
  Alcohol 5%

BENZAC
Acne gel
(Owen Labs.)

Benzoyl peroxide * 5%; 10%
Polyoxyethylene lauryl ethers ... 6%
Alcohol 30%

BENZAGEL
For treatment of acne
(Dermik)

Active ingred.:
  Benzoyl peroxide .... 5 or 10%
Inactive ingred.:
  Carbomer 940
  Sodium hydroxide
  Dioctyl sodium sulfosuccinate
  Alkyl polyglycol ether
  Fragrance
  Alcohol 14%

BENZALOIDS
(Jenkins Labs.)

Each lozenge:
  Benzocaine .... 5.0 mg.
  Calcium iodized .... 12.0 mg.
  Eucalyptol .... 0.35 mg.
  Methenamine .... 6.5 mg.
  Menthol .... 0.2 mg.

BENZEDREX INHALER
Nasal decongestant
(MenJ Labs.)

Propylhexedrine * .... 250 mg.
Menthol
Aromatics

BENZEDRINE (TABLETS & SPANSULE CAPSULES)
Indicated for narcolepsy and exogenous obesity
(SK&F)

TABLETS (each):
  Amphetamine sulfate * . 5 mg.; 10 mg.

SPANSULES (each sustained release capsule):
  Amphetamine sulfate * .... 15 mg.

BENZODENT
Denture analgesic
(Vicks Toiletry Products Div).

Petrolatum
Sodium carboxymethyl cellulose
Benzocaine .... 20% (w/w)
8-Hydroxyquinoline sulfate .. 0.1%
Eugenol 0.4%

BENZO-MENTH LOZENGES
(Vale)

Benzocaine .... 2.2 mg
Benzoic acid
Menthol *
Oils of eucalyptus *
Wintergreen *
Peppermint

Starred ingredients (*) may be responsible for major toxic effects; consult Section II.

BERKEM 90
Swimming pool floor and walls cleaner
(Modern Pool Products)

Sodium hydroxide *

BERKITE-4
Anti-algae specific
(Modern Pool Products)

Dichlone (2,3-Dichloro-1,4-
naphthoquinone) 1.5%

BERKITE-13
Anti-algae specific
(Modern Pool Products)

Dichlone (2,3-Dichloro-1,4-
naphthoquinone) 4.9%

BERRY-SET

See SCIENCE BERRY-SET

BESCO CRAYONS
(Binney & Smith)

Wax blend
Non-toxic pigments

BESCO INSECT SPRAY
(Besco Corp.)

Active ingred.: 100%
Petroleum distillate *
Technical Piperonyl butoxide
Pyrethrins *

BESCO MINT-
DISINFECTANT
(Besco Corp.)

Active ingred.: 2.5%
Methyldodecylbenzyltrimethyl ammonium chloride *
Methyldodecylxylene bis(trimethyl ammonium chloride) *†

†*See* Cationic surfactants

BESCO ODORLESS
DISINFECTANT
(Besco Corp.)

Active ingred.: 2.5%
Methyldodecylbenzyltrimethyl ammonium chloride *
Methyldodecylxylene bis(trimethyl ammonium chloride) *†

†*See* Cationic surfactants

BEST-ALL CLEANER
(Hillyard Chem.)

Alkali *
Synthetic detergent *

'76 Ed.

BESTINE SOLVENT AND
THINNER
(Union Rubber)

Hexane *

BESTOL
Mouthwash, gargle
(Etna Chem.)

Alcohol 69%/v
Tincture of Myrrh
Benzoin
Formaldehyde *
Thymol *
Eucalyptol *

'76 Ed.

BEST-TEST ONE COAT
CEMENT
Pressure sensitive adhesive
(Union Rubber)

Natural rubber 12.0%
Hexane * 82.0%
Terpene phenolic resin 6.0%
Fragrance 0.1%
Processing aid 0.1%

BEST-TEST PAPER
CEMENT
(Union Rubber)

Hexane * 91.5%
Natural rubber 8.3%

BETACIDE
Algicide, germicide, disinfectant
(Weil Chem.)

n-Alkyl (60% C14, 30% C16, 5% C12, 5%
C18) dimethyl benzyl ammonium chlorides *
n-Alkyl (50% C12, 30% C14, 17% C16, 3%
C18) dimethyl ethylbenzyl ammonium
chlorides *

BETALAX
Laxative
(Vernon Labs.)

Magnesium hydroxide
Magnesium carbonate
Salol *
Beta naphthol benzoate
Malt diastase
Papain
Oil of peppermint
Anise

BETAMIX
Herbicide
(NOR-AM)

Phenmedipham * 8.0%/w
Desmedipham * 8.0%/w

BETANAL
Herbicide
(NOR-AM)

Phenmedipham * .... 15.9%/w.

BETANEX
Herbicide
(NOR-AM)

Desmedipham 16.0%/w

BETASAN
Herbicide
(Stauffer)

Betasan (S-(O,O-Diisopropyl phosphorodithioate) of N-(2-mercapoethyl) benzenesulfonamide) *

BETA-SECT
For control of flies and mosquitos
(Certified Labs.)

Xylene * 81.0%
Beta-butoxy-beta-thiocyano-di-
ethyl ether 5.3%
Petroleum distillates 4.7%
Naled 4.6%

BETZ C-5P (Pellets)
*Microorganism control agent; indus-
trial use*
(Betz Labs.)

Active ingred.: 48%
1,3-Dichloro-5,5-dimethylhydantoin *
Inert ingred.: 52%
Includes solubilizing and dispersing
agents

BETZ ENTEC 369
Fungicide and bactericide; industrial
(Betz Entec)

Sodium dimethyldithiocarbamate .. 15%
Nabam * 15%

BETZ ENTEC 340 (Liquid)
Slime control agent; industrial use
(Betz Entec)

Active ingred.:
N-Alkyl (C12-5%, C14-60%, C16-
30%, C18-5%) dimethyl benzyl
ammonium chloride * 24.0%
Bis(tributyltin)oxide 4.75%
Inert ingred.: 71.25%
Includes solubilizing and dispersing
agents

BETZ ENTEC 343 (Pellets)
*Microorganism control agent; indus-
trial use*
(Betz Entec)

Active ingred.: 91%
1,3-Dichloro-5,5-dimethylhydantoin
(provides 60.0% available chlorine) *
Inert ingred.: 9%
Includes solubilizing and dispersing
agents

BETZ ENTEC 345A
Industrial water treatment
(Betz Entec)

2,2-Dibromo-3-
nitrilopropionamide * 5%

Starred ingredients (*) may be responsible for major toxic effects; consult Section II.

BETZ ENTEC 346 (Powder)
Slime control agent; industrial use
(Betz Entec)

Active ingred.: 54%
  Sodium dichloro-s-triazinetrione dihydrate *
Inert ingred.: 46%
  Includes solubilizing and dispersing agents

BETZ ER-10
Industrial water treatment
(Betz Labs.)

2,2-Dibromo-3-
nitrilopropionamide * 20%

BETZ ER-11
Bactericide and fungicide; industrial
(Betz Labs.)

Sodium pentachlorophenate * 79%
Sodium salts of other chlorophenols 11%

BETZ SLIME-TROL DP-508
Slime control agent; industrial
(Betz Labs.)

2,2-Dibromo-3-
nitrilopropionamide * 20%

BETZ SLIME-TROL RX-17 (Liquid)
Slime control agent; industrial use
(Betz Labs.)

Sodium pentachlorophenate * 24.7%
Sodium 2,4,5-trichlorophenate 9.1%
Sodium salts of other
  chlorophenates 2.9%
Sodium dimethyl dithiocarbamate 4.0%
N-Alkyl (C12 40%, C14 50%, C16 10%) dimethyl benzyl ammonium
chloride 5.0%

BETZ SLIME-TROL RX-28 (Liquid)
Slime control agent; industrial use
(Betz Labs.)

3,5-Dimethyl tetrahydro-2H-1,3,5-
thiadiazine-2-thione * 21.0%

BETZ SLIME-TROL RX-34 (Liquid)
Slime control agent; industrial use
(Betz Labs.)

Sodium dimethyl
  dithiocarbamate * 15.0%
Nabam (Disodium ethylene
  bisdithiocarbamate) * 15.0%

BETZ SLIMICIDE C-57
Slime control agent; industrial
(Betz Labs.)

Sodium dimethyldithiocarbamate .. 15%
Nabam * 15%

BETZ SLIMICIDE J-12 (Liquid)
Slime control agent; industrial use
(Betz Labs.)

N-Alkyl (C12 5%, C14 60%, C16 30%,
C18 5%) dimethyl benzyl ammonium chloride * 24.0%
Bis (tributyltin) oxide 5.0%

BETZ SLIMICIDE 242 (Liquid)
Slime control agent; industrial use
(Betz Labs.)

Active ingred.:
  Dodine (Dodecylguanidine
  acetate) * 10.0%
  Isopropanol * 30.0%
Inert ingred.: 60.0%
  Includes solubilizing and dispersing agents

BETZ SLIMICIDE 508 (Liquid)
Slime control agent; industrial
(Betz Labs.)

Active ingred.: 20.0%
  2,2-Dibromo-3-nitrilopropionamide *
Inert ingred.: 80.0%
  Includes solubilizing and dispersing agents

BEVILL'S
For removal of corns & calluses
(Bevill)

Alcohol *
Ether *
Salicylic acid *
Oil of wintergreen *
Tincture Ferric chloride *

BEVILL'S LOTION
For symptomatic relief of skin fungus infections
(Bevill)

Salicylic acid *
Methyl salicylate *
Ether 8%
Ethyl alcohol 68%

BEVRO KLENE

See KLENZADE BEVRO KLENE

BEWON ELIXIR
Dietary supplement
(Wyeth Labs.)

Each 5 ml.:
  Thiamine hydrochloride ..... 0.25 mg.
  Alcohol 16%

BEXTON 4L HERBICIDE
(Dow)

Active ingred.: 41.75%
  Propachlor *
Inert ingred.: 58.25%
  Water
  Clay
  Wetting agents

B.F.I.
Antiseptic dusting powder
(Beecham Products)

Bismuth-formic-iodide *†
Zinc phenolsulfonate *
Bismuth subgallate
Amol (Mono-n-amyl hydroquinone ether)
Potassium alum
Boric acid *
Menthol *
Eucalyptol *
Thymol *
Inert diluents

†*See* Iodine

BGO
An antiseptic, antifungal, soothing ointment
(Calotabs)

Iodoform *
Salicylic acid *
Sulphur (precipitated)
Zinc oxide
1% Phenol (liquefied)
Calamine
Menthol *
Petrolatum
Lanolin
Mineral oil
1% Undecylenic acid

B-75 GOLDEN (ALL SOLUBLE BORAX BASE INDUSTRIAL SKIN CLEANSER)
(Sugar Beet)

Soap 25%
Borax * 75%

'76 Ed.

BGS 116 GOPHER BAIT
Rodenticide
(B&G Co.)

Strychnine alkaloid * .... 0.35%/wt.

BICEP
Herbicide
(Ciba-Geigy Ag. Div.)

Atrazine * 20.8%
Atrazine related compounds 1.1%
Metolachlor 27.5%

BICHOLAX
Laxative
(Elder)

Each tablet:
  Phenolphthalein .... 32.4 mg
  Cascara extract 1-3
  Sodium glycocholate
  Aloin

BiCOZENE CREME
Anti-itch medication
(Creighton Products)

Benzocaine 6%
Resorcinol * 1.66%
In a cream base

Starred ingredients (*) may be responsible for major toxic effects; consult Section II.

BIDETTE DISPOSABLE DOUCHE
(Youngs Drug Products)

Water
Sodium lactate *
Nonoxynol-9
Polysorbate-20
Lactic acid *
Fragrance
Benzalkonium chloride
Methylparaben
Propylparaben

BIDETTE MIST (Aerosol)
Feminine deodorant
(Youngs Drug Products)

Isobutane
SD Alcohol 40
Isopropyl myristate
Fragrance

BIDETTE POWDER (Aerosol)
Feminine deodorant
(Youngs Drug Products)

Isobutane
SD Alcohol 40
Talc
Isopropyl myristate
Fragrance

BIDRIN MISCIBLE
Insecticide
(FMC Corp., Agricultural Chem. Div.)

Dimethyl phosphate of 3-hydroxy N,N-dimethyl-cis-crotonamide * . 75%

BIG BLOW SUPER FOGGING INSECT KILLER
Institutional and commercial use
(Hysan Corp.)

Pyrethrins 0.30%
Piperonyl butoxide technical 0.60%
N-Octyl bicycloheptene
  dicarboximide 1.00%
Petroleum distillates 8.10%

BIG CAT
General cleaner concentrate
(Calgon Corp., Commercial Div.)

Dodecylbenzene sulfonate *†
Fatty amide
Water

†See Alkyl aryl sodium sulfonates

BIG C-D CATTLE SPRAY
Insecticide
(Techne Corp.)

Petroleum hydrocarbons * 98.57%
Dimethyl phosphate of alpha
  methylbenzyl 3-hydroxy-cis-
  crotonate * 1.00%
2,2-Dichlorovinyl dimethyl
  phosphate 0.24%
Related compounds 0.01%

'76 Ed.

BIG CHIEF BLEACH
(Patterson Labs.)

Sodium hypochlorite * 5.25%

BIG-HED LINIMENT
(Humco)

Chlorothymol *
Gum camphor *
Oils origanum artificial *
Camphor sassafrassy *
Sassafras artificial *
Pine oil *
Spirits turpentine *
Mineral spirits *

BIG SIG II
Fine line writing pen
(Sanford Corp.)

Dyes
Glycols
Water
Phenol (as preservative) .... <1%

BIG 6 MALATHION DUST
Insecticide
(Hess & Clark)

Malathion * 6%

BIG STICK PANEL & FOAM ADHESIVE 6018

See WELDWOOD BIG STICK PANEL
  & FOAM ADHESIVE 6018

BIKE AID
Lubricant, penetrant, inhibitor; dry film lubricant
(Dri-Slide)

Molybdenum disulfide *
Light petroleum hydrocarbons and derivatives *

BIKINI FLOOR WAX
(Uncle Sam)

Polyethylene
Resins (modified phenolic)
Waxes
Ammonia *
Oleic acid
Morpholine *
Plasticizer
Styrene plastic emulsified
Acrylic plastic emulsified (metal cross-linked)

BILAMIDE TABLETS
Antispasmodic with cholagogue
(Norgine Labs.)

Each tablet:
  Phenobarbital * .... 8 mg.
  Homatropine methylbromide . 1.4 mg.
  Dried Ox bile .... 200 mg.

BILAX
Laxative
(Leo Products)

Extr. Rhubarb
Aloe *
Buckthorn
Olibanum galbanum
Myrrh praep.

BILEX TABLETS
Antispasmodic
(Moffet Inc.)

Each tablet:
  Atropine sulfate .... 1/500 gr.
  Magnesium sulfate * .... 5 gr.
  Oxgall (granular) .... 1 gr.

BILEZYME PLUS
Bile acids, digestive enzymes
(Geriatric Pharm.)

Each tablet:
  Phenobarbital * .... 8 mg.
  Homatropine methylbromide . 2.5 mg.
  Gerilase .... 30 mg.
  Geriprotase .... 6 mg.
  Dehydrocholic acid .... 200 mg.
  Desoxycholic acid .... 50 mg.

BILI-LABSTIX
Urine pH, protein, glucose, ketones, bilirubin and blood test reagent strip
(Ames)

pH PAD:
  Methyl red
  Bromthymol blue
  Sodium citrate
  Tween 21
  Plasdone K29-32
  Polyethylene glycol
  Viscarin
PROTEIN PAD: .... See ALBUSTIX
GLUCOSE PAD: .... See CLINISTIX
KETONE PAD: .... See KETOSTIX
BILIRUBIN PAD: ... See ICTOSTIX
OCCULT BLOOD
  PAD: .... See HEMASTIX

BILOCOMP TABLETS
(Lannett)

Each tablet:
  Bile salts .... 1 1/2 gr.
  Extract Cascara .... 1/2 gr.
  Phenolphthalein .... 1/2 gr.
  Oleoresin capsicum .... 1/20 m.

BIN-FUME GRAIN FUMIGANT
(Industrial Fumigant)

Carbon tetrachloride * 82.3%
Carbon bisulfide 16.3%
Pentane 0.4%
Sulfur dioxide 1.0%

BINGMAN'S HORSE WORM GRANULES
(Bingman Labs.)

Piperazine dihydrochloride (equiv. to
  17% piperazine base) 34%

Starred ingredients (*) may be responsible for major toxic effects; consult Section II.

BINGMAN'S MEDICATED OINTMENT
Veterinary
(Bingman Labs.)

Dichlorophene *
Isopropyl alcohol *
Propylene glycol
Oil of camphor *
Oil of red thyme
Oil of eucalyptus *
Iodine *
Lanolin
Petrolatum

BINGMAN'S PIPERAZINE SOLUBLE POWDER DRINKING WATER WORMER
Veterinary
(Bingman Labs.)

Each 100 cc:
Piperazine .... 34.0 gm.

BINGO DRAIN PIPE OPENER
(Huntington Labs.)

Potassium hydroxide *

BINNEY & SMITH PROJECTION CHALK
For use with light colored chalkboard
(Binney & Smith)

Major constituents:
Calcium sulfate
Non-toxic pigment
Minor constituent:
Non-toxic coating

B-I-N PRIMER - SEALER
(Zinsser, Wm., & Co.)

Pigment: 32.75%
Titanium dioxide 58%
Silicates 42%
Vehicle-Pure white shellac cut 3
lbs./gal. in: 67.25%
Glycol ether *
Special Industrial Solvent No. 4 (approx. percentage composition by volume):
Ethyl alcohol 80%
Methyl alcohol 4%
Isopropyl alcohol * 15%
Methyl isobutyl ketone 1%

BIO-88
Spreader-activator (non-ionic) for agricultural sprays
(Kalo)

Alkyl polyethoxy ethanol *
Free fatty acids
Isopropanol *

BIO-CAD
Turf fungicide
(Scientific International)

Cadmium chloride (total cadmium (Cd) 12.3%) * 20.1%

BIO-CEUTIC MANGE LOTION
Veterinary
(Bio-Ceutic)

Rotenone 0.12%
Gamma isomer of benzene hexachloride from lindane 0.10%
Dichlorophene (2,2'-Methylene-bis(4-chlorophenol)) 0.50%
Benzyl benzoate * 30.00%
Isopropyl alcohol * 68.38%
Inert ingred. including artificial color and odor 0.90%

BIO-CEUTIC PAD SEAL
Foot care for dogs and horses
(Bio-Ceutic)

Dichlorophene 10.0%
p-Chloro-m-cresol 0.5%
Inert ingred.:
Isopropyl alcohol (99%) (equiv. to 78.75% by vol.) * 59.5%
Propellants 30.0%

BIO-CEUTIC STRONGER TINCTURE OF IODINE
Topical antiseptic; veterinary
(Bio-Ceutic)

Iodine * 7%
Potassium iodide 5%
Isopropyl alcohol 86.67%
Distilled water .... q.s.

BIO-CEUTIC WOUND SPRA (Aerosol)
Veterinary
(Bio-Ceutic)

Methyl violet 0.06%
Furfuryl alcohol 0.60%
Tetrahydro furfuryl alcohol 0.03%
Urea 0.60%
Isopropanol * 18.00%
Propylene glycol 20.71%
Inert ingred.:
Trichlorofluoromethane 30.00%
Dichlorodifluoromethane 30.00%

BIO-CHECKS
Weed killer for lawns and golf courses
(Scientific International)

Disodium methanearsonate anhydrous (equivalent to 15% disodium methanearsonate hexahydrate) * 9.45%

BIO-CUSTOM BLEND
Liquid turf fertilizer
(Scientific International)

Total nitrogen 16%
Available Phosphoric acid 4%
Soluble Potash 8%
Sources:
Ammonia *
Ammonium nitrate *
Phosphoric acid *
Muriate of potash *

BIO-DAYSED
Daytime sedative
(Bio-Factor Labs.)

Each tablet:
Butabarbital sodium * . 1/4 gr.; 1/2 gr.

'76 Ed.

BIODIN
Iodine therapy for livestock and poultry
(Whitmoyer)

Ethylenediamine dihydriodide * .. 9.2%

BIO-DONNAL (ELIXIR & TABLETS)
(Bio-Factor Labs.)

Each 5 cc & tablet:
Atropine sulfate .... 0.0194 mg.
Hyoscyamine sulfate * .... 0.1037 mg.
Hyoscine hydrobromide ... 0.0065 mg.
Phenobarbital (1/4 gr.) * .. 16 mg.
Alcohol (elixir) 20%

'76 Ed.

BIO-ESTYL
Estrogen therapy
(Bio-Factor Labs.)

Each tablet:
Ethinyl estradiol .. 0.02 mg.; 0.05 mg.

'76 Ed.

BIO-FILM
Spreader-sticker for agricultural sprays
(Kalo)

Alkylarylpolyethoxy ethanol
Free and combined fatty acids
Glycol ethers
Di-alkyl benzenedicarboxylate
Isopropanol *

BIO-GUARD ALGICIDE-INHIBITOR
(Bio-Lab)

Alkyl (C14, 90%; C12, 5%; C16, 5%) dimethyl dichlorobenzyl ammonium chloride * 35%
Alkyl (C14, 90%; C12, 5%; C16, 5%) dimethyl ethyl ammonium bromide 5%
Inert ingred.: 60%
Water
Ethylenediaminetetraacetic acid, tetrasodium salt
Color

BIO-GUARD ALGICIDE 28X
For swimming pools
(Bio-Lab)

Alkyl (58%, C14; 28%, C16; 14%, C12) dimethyl benzyl ammonium chloride * 10%

BIO-GUARD BACK-UP ALGICIDE-INHIBITOR
For swimming pools
(Bio-Lab)

Active ingred.:
Alkyl (C14, 90%; C12, 5%; C16, 5%) dimethyl dichlorobenzyl ammonium chloride * 35%
Alkyl (C14, 90%; C12, 5%; C16, 5%) dimethyl ethyl ammonium bromide 5%

Inert ingred.:
Water, Ethylenediaminetetraacetic acid, Tetrasodium salt, Color .. 60%

BIO-GUARD BALANCE PAK 200
pH increaser in swimming pools
(Bio-Lab)

Alkaline salts *

BIO-GUARD BREAK-POINT FR-65
Rids pool of organic waste
(Bio-Lab)

Calcium hypochlorite * 65%

BIO-GUARD BURN OUT
Rids pool of organic waste
(Bio-Lab)

Calcium hypochlorite * 65%

BIO-GUARD BURN OUT 35
Rids pool of organic waste
(Bio-Lab)

Lithium hypochlorite (contains 35% available chlorine) * 29%

BIO-GUARD CLC CALCIUM HYPOCHLORITE
Algicide for swimming pools
(Bio-Lab)

Calcium hypochlorite * 65%

BIO-GUARD KLEEN-IT FILTER DESCALER & CLEANER
For swimming pools
(Bio-Lab)

Contains acids *

BIO-GUARD KUSTOM KLOR II FORMULATED CHLORINATING GRANULES WITH WATER CONDITIONERS
For white plaster pools
(Bio-Lab)

Trichloro-s-triazinetrione * 55.6%

BIO-GUARD LAUNDRI-STAT T-521F
Chemical bacteriostat, fungistat for fabric treatment
(Bio-Lab)

Alkyl (C14, 90%; C12, 5%; C16, 5%) dimethyl dichlorobenzyl ammonium chloride * 33.5%
Tributyltin neodecanoate 7.9%

BIO-GUARD LOK-UP WINTER ANTIFREEZE
Recirculating system antifreeze in swimming pools
(Bio-Lab)

Propylene glycol

BIO-GUARD LOK-UP WINTERIZER ALGAECIDE
(Bio-Lab)

Alkyl (C14, 90%; C12, 5%; C16, 5%) dimethyl dichlorobenzyl ammonium chloride * 35%
Alkyl (C14, 90%; C12, 5%; C16, 5%) dimethyl ethyl ammonium bromide 5%

BIO-GUARD LOK-UP WINTER SHOCK
Chlorinating treatment for swimming pools
(Bio-Lab)

Sodium dichloro-s-triazinetrione * 99.5%

BIO-GUARD LOK-UP WINTERTROL
Algae preventative in swimming pools
(Bio-Lab)

Alkyl (C14, 58%; C16, 28%; C12, 14%) dimethyl benzyl ammonium chloride * 10%

BIO-GUARD LO 'N SLO pH DECREASER
For swimming pools
(Bio-Lab)

Sodium bisulfate * 88%

BIO-GUARD MSA ALGICIDE
(Bio-Lab)

Copper (as elemental) * 7.1%
Alkyl (C14, 90%; C12, 5%; C16, 5%) dimethyl dichlorobenzyl ammonium chloride 2.5%

BIO-GUARD NO. 90 ORGANIC CHLORINE CONCENTRATE
For white plaster pools
(Bio-Lab)

Trichloro-s-triazinetrione (available chlorine 90.2%) * 100%

BIO-GUARD SHOK 'N LOK CHLORINATED STABILIZER
For swimming pools
(Bio-Lab)

Sodium dichloro-s-triazinetrione * . 34%

BIO-GUARD SPOT KILL SUPER ALGAE DESTROYER
For white plaster pools only
(Bio-Lab)

Trichloro-s-triazinetrione * 99%

BIO-GUARD STATUS QUO CHLORINE CARTRIDGES
Pool water disinfecting agent
(Bio-Lab)

Trichloro-s-triazinetrione (available chlorine - 89%) * 99.0%

BIO-GUARD STINGY STICK
Chlorine cartridges for swimming pools
(Bio-Lab)

Trichloro-s-triazinetrione (available chlorine 89%) * 100%

BIO-GUARD SUPER 90 CHLORINE CONC.
(Bio-Lab)

Trichloro-s-triazinetrione (available chlorine 90.2%) * 100%

BIO-GUARD SUPER SOLUBLE ORGANIC CHLORINE CONCENTRATE
For swimming pools
(Bio-Lab)

Sodium dichloro-s-triazinetrione (available chlorine 62%) * 100%

BIO-GUARD SURFACE CLEANER
For all types of pool surfaces
(Bio-Lab)

Phosphoric acid *
Muriatic acid *
Synthetic detergent

BIO-GUARD SWIMMING POOL ALGICIDE 28-10
(Bio-Lab)

Alkyl (58% C14, 28% C16, 14% C12) dimethyl benzyl ammonium chloride * 10%

Starred ingredients (*) may be responsible for major toxic effects; consult Section II.

BIO-GUARD SWIMMING POOL ALGICIDE 28-40
(Bio-Lab)

Alkyl (58% C14, 28% C16, 14% C12) dimethyl benzyl ammonium chloride * 40%

BIO-GUARD TABGARD CHLORINATING TABLETS
For swiming pools
(Bio-Lab)

Trichloro-s-triazinetrione (available chlorine 90%) * 100%

BIO-LENE
Disinfectant
(Bio-Lab)

Cresylic acid * 50%
Anhydrous soaps 32%

BIO-LUTONE
Progestogen therapy
(Bio-Factor Labs.)

Each tablet:
  Ethisterone (Anhydrohydroxy-progesterone) .... 10 mg.

'76 Ed.

BIO-SEC 153
Insecticide
(Bio-Lab)

Piperonyl butoxide technical 0.481%
Pyrethrins 0.048%
Petroleum distillate * 99.471%

BIO-SEC 170
Insecticide
(Bio-Lab)

Piperonyl butoxide technical 0.64%
Pyrethrins 0.06%
Petroleum oil * 99.30%

BIO-SEC 240
Insecticide
(Bio-Lab)

Piperonyl butoxide technical 1.27%
Pyrethrins 0.13%
Petroleum oil * 98.60%

BIO-SELECT
Weed killer for golf courses
(Scientific International)

Potassium salt of 2-(2-methyl-4-chlorophenoxy) propionic acid (MCPP) * 25.9%

BIO-STIK
Lip balm
(Commerce Drug)

Benzocaine
Camphor *
Menthol *
Allantoin

BIOTHESIN
Gastrointestinal sedative
(Vale)

Each tablet:
  Benzocaine .... 16.2 mg.
  Cerium oxalate *† .... 129.6 mg.
  Bismuth subnitrate .... 129.6 mg.

†*See* Oxalate salts

BIOTOLENE
Acute otitis media, softening and removing cerumen
(King Pharmaceutical)

Benzocaine 1.5%
Cetalkonium chloride 0.25%
Chlorobutanol 0.25%
Propylene glycol base with 8-hydroxyquinoline

BIOTRES
Topical antibiotic ointment; antibacterial
(Central Pharmacal Co.)

Each gm.:
  Zinc bacitracin (U.S.P.) .. 500 units
  Polymyxin B sulfate (U.S.P.) .... 10,000 units

BIO-TYTRA
Antibacterial, anesthetic for sore throat
(Approved Pharm.)

Each troche:
  Cetylpyridinium chloride ..... 2.5 mg.
  Benzocaine .... 10 mg.

'76 Ed.

BIPECTOL
Treatment of diarrhea
(Vale)

Each wafer:
  Opium (equiv. to 5 m. paregoric) * .... 1.2 mg.
  Bismuth hydroxide .... 32.4 mg.
  Kaolin colloidal .... 162.0 mg.
  Pectin NF .... 32.4 mg.

BIPHETAMINE (7 1/2, 12 1/2, 20)
Anorexiant, as cation exchange resin complex of sulfonated polystyrene
(Pennwalt, Pharm. Div.)

Each capsule:
  d-Amphetamine * .. 3.75 mg.; 6.25 mg.; or 10 mg.
  dl-Amphetamine * .. 3.75 mg.; 6.25 mg.; or 10 mg.

BIRCHCLEEN ACID CLEANER
Dairy use
(Birchmore Dairy Supply)

Phosphoric acid * .... >30%
Hydroxyacetic acid .... <15%

BIRCHCLEEN BULK TANK CLEANER
Dairy use
(Birchmore Dairy Supply)

Sodium tripolyphosphate .... >35%
Soda ash * .... >35%
Sodium metasilicate * .... <20%
Sodium dichloroisocyanurate ..... >2%
Alkyl aryl sulfonate .... <4%

BIRCHCLEEN CHLORINATED PIPELINE CLEANER
Dairy use
(Birchmore Dairy Supply)

Sodium tripolyphosphate .... >35%
Soda ash * .... >40%
Sodium metasilicate * .... <15%
Sodium dichloroisocyanurate ..... <3%

BIRCHCLEEN IODINE UDDER WASH
Cleaner sanitizer
(Birchmore Dairy Supply)

Nonylphenoxypoly (ethyleneoxy) ethanol-iodine complex (providing 1.75% titratable iodine) 14.25%
Phosphoric acid * 12.50%

BIRD "NEPOLON" COATINGS
(Bird & Son)

Neoprene 1-20%
Chlorosulphonated polyethylene .. >10%
Xylene (or other high B.P. aromatic solvent) * .... >10%
Water insoluble lead base curing agent 1-10%
Phenolic & phenolic resinous compounds 1-10%
Glycol ether .... <10%
Non-lead inorganic coloring pigments & fillers 1-20%

BIRD ROOF COATINGS AND CEMENT
(Bird & Son)

Asphalt .... >10%
Petroleum solvents (substantially aliphatic) * .... >10%
Fillers: 1-10%
  Rock dust
  Talc
  Soapstone
  Asbestos

BIRD TANGLEFOOT
Bird repellent
(Tanglefoot)

Polybutenes *
Hydrogenated Castor oil

Starred ingredients (*) may be responsible for major toxic effects; consult Section II.

BISILAD
Intestinal protective adsorbent
(Central Pharmacal Co.)

Each 15 ml.:
Bismuth subgallate .... 0.15 g.
Kaolin, colloidal .... 5.5 g.
Benzoic acid (preservative) 0.075%
Lugol's solution (preservative) 0.1%
Aromatized suspension:
  Thymol
  Menthol
  Eucalyptus oil
  Methyl salicylate

BISMA REX GEL
Antacid - absorbent
(Rexall)

Each 5 cc:
Aluminum hydroxide 1-5%
Magnesium hydroxide 1-5%
Oil of peppermint .... <1%

'76 Ed.

BISODOL POWDER
Antacid
(Whitehall Labs.)

Sodium bicarbonate
Magnesium carbonate
Oil of peppermint

BISODOL TABS
Antacid
(Whitehall Labs.)

Calcium carbonate
Magnesium hydroxide

BISONITE CONCRETE FLOOR ENAMEL
(Bisonite Co.)

Pigment: 22.5%
  Titanium dioxide 100.0%
Vehicle: 77.5%
  Butadiene-styrene resin 25.6%
  Plasticizer 3.9%
  Chlorinated paraffin
  Tung oil
  High flash Naphtha * 38.5%
  Mineral spirits * 32.0%

BISONITE PAINT PRODUCTS

Bisonite Co. Inc.
2250 Military Rd.
Tonawanda, N.Y. 14150

Phone: 716-693-6130

BISONITE RUBBER BASE MASONRY PAINT
(Bisonite Co.)

Pigment: 49.3%
  Titanium dioxide 33.4%
  Zinc oxide 11.1%
  Magnesium silicate 41.1%
  Diatomaceous silica 14.4%
Vehicle: 50.7%
  Butadiene-styrene resin 13.9%
  Chlorinated paraffin 13.9%
  High flash Naphtha * 40.0%
  Mineral spirits * 32.2%

BISSELL COMMERCIAL RUG SHAMPOO
(Bissell)

Anionic synthetic detergents
Synthetic antisoil resin
Chelate .... trace
Ammonium hydroxide .... trace

BISSELL FOAM RUG CLEANER (Aerosol)
(Bissell)

Anionic synthetic detergents
Synthetic clay thickener

BISSELL MINI SHAMPOO (Aerosol)
Small area carpet cleaning
(Bissell)

Anionic synthetic detergents
Synthetic clay thickener

BISSELL NOT ON THE CARPET (Aerosol)
To clean pet accidents
(Bissell)

Anionic synthetic detergents
Synthetic clay thickener

BISSELL ONE STEP CARPET CLEANER (Aerosol)
(Bissell)

Anionic synthetic detergents
Synthetic clay thickener

BISSELL ONE STEP FIBERGLASS & BATHROOM CLEANER
(Aerosol)
(Bissell)

Chelate
Ethylene glycol, Butyl ether*
Anionic synthetic detergent
Naphtha*
Dowicide A*

BISSELL ONE STEP OVEN CLEANER (Aerosol)
(Bissell)

Sodium hydroxide *
Thickeners
Detergent

BISSELL ONE STEP SPOT LIFTER (Aerosol)
(Bissell)

Silica absorbent
1,1,1,-Trichloroethane *
Hydrocarbon propellant

BISSELL UPHOLSTERY SHAMPOO (Aerosol)
(Bissell)

Anionic synthetic detergents
Synthetic clay thickener

BISSELL WALL TO WALL RUG SHAMPOO
(Bissell)

Anionic synthetic detergents
Synthetic antisoil resin
Chelate .... trace
Ammonium hydroxide .... trace

BITE-X
Stops nailbiting
(Bite-X Corp.)

Sucrose octa-acetate

BITEX ACID & ALKALI RESISTANT PAINT
(Knight, M. A.)

Coal tar base *
Industrial Aromatic solvents *
Petroleum naphtha solvents *

BI-ZETS
For sore throat
(Reese Chem.)

Each lozenge:
Benzocaine .... 10 mg.
Cetyl pyridinium chloride ..... 2 mg.

BIZ (Lower Phosphate Formula)
Laundry pre-soak
(Procter & Gamble)

Sodium tripolyphosphate 25-49%
Sodium bicarbonate 25-49%
Sodium perborate * 25-49%
Alkyl ethoxylate 1-4%
Enzymes .... <1%
Minor ingredients, each .... <1%

pH (1% solution) - 9.3

BIZ (Non-Phosphate Formula)
Laundry pre-soak
(Procter & Gamble)

Sodium bicarbonate	25-49%
Sodium perborate *	25-49%
Sodium sulfate	10-24%
Sodium silicate (not meta)	5-9%
Sodium carbonate	5-9%
Alkyl ethoxylates	1-4%
Sodium alkyl benzene sulfonate	1-4%
Enzymes	<1%
Minor ingredients, each	<1%

pH (1% solution) - 9.3

BIZ (Phosphate Formula)
Laundry pre-soak
(Procter & Gamble)

Sodium tripolyphosphate *	50-74%
Sodium perborate	25-49%
Alkyl ethoxylate	1-4%
Enzymes	<1%
Minor ingredients, each	<1%

pH (1% solution) - 9.3

BIZOLIN-100 & BIZOLIN-200
Anti-inflammatory for dogs
(Bio-Ceutic)

Each tablet:
Phenylbutazone * ....100 mg.; 200 mg.

BK-BK
Cleaner
(Pennwalt)

Sodium hydroxide *

B-K-C.C.A.
Alkaline detergent
(Pennwalt)

Sodium carbonate *
Sodium orthosilicate
Alkali phosphate

B-K CHLORINE-BEARING POWDER
Bactericide, disinfectant, deodorant
(Pennwalt)

Calcium hypochlorite *	50%

B-KLEER
Alkaline detergent
(Pennwalt)

Sodium hydroxide *
Alkaline phosphate

B-K LIQUID
Bactericide
(Pennwalt)

Sodium hypochlorite *	5.25%

B-K-Z TABLETS
For diarrhea
(Sutliff & Case)

Each chewable tablet:
Kaolin	370 mg.
Bismuth subgallate	60 mg.
Zinc phenosulfonate *	16 mg.
Opium, powdered *	5 mg.

'76 Ed.

BLACK AND WHITE BLEACHING CREAM
(Plough)

Cetyl alcohol	
Starfol wax (Glyceryl stearate)	
Methylparaben	
Hydroquinone *	2.0% w/w
Perfume	
Sodium sulfite	

BLACK BAND FLOOR WAX
Industrial grade
(McAleer)

Morpholine oleate *
Vegetable waxes
Terpene phenolic resins *†
Shellac
Borax *
Ammonia *
Colloidal silica

'76 Ed.

†*See* Terpenes and Phenol

BLACK DRAUGHT
Laxative
(Chattem)

Casanthranol *
Other vegetable products

BLACK EAGLE MEDICINE BALL
Laxative
(C.T.S. Labs)

Methyl salicylate *
Senna *
Buckthorn
Mandrake
Uva ursi
Elecampane

BLACK FLAG ADULT FLEA KILLER
(Boyle-Midway)

Tetramethrin	0.200%
d-(cis, trans) Phenothrin	0.382%
Other isomers	0.018%
Petroleum distillate	14.400%
Methylene chloride	40.000%
1,1,1-Trichloroethane *	17.000%
Hydrocarbon propellant	28.000%

BLACK FLAG ANT & ROACH KILLER
(Boyle-Midway)

Baygon *	0.50%
DDVP	0.20%
Petroleum distillate *	83.03%
Propellant	

BLACK FLAG ANT TRAPS
(Boyle-Midway)

Baygon *	2.00%

BLACK FLAG AUTOMATIC ROOM FOGGER FORMULA S
(Boyle-Midway)

Tetramethrin	0.200%
d-(cis,trans) Phenothrin	0.382%
Other isomers	0.018%
Petroleum distillate	14.000%
1,1,1-Trichloroethane	17.000%
Methylene chloride *	40.000%
Hydrocarbon propellant	

BLACK FLAG DEAD AIM ANT & ROACH KILLER
(Boyle-Midway)

DDVP	0.20%
Baygon *	1.00%
Petroleum distillate *	79.12%
Propellant	

BLACK FLAG FLEA AND TICK KILLER RUG AND ROOM SPRAY
(Boyle-Midway)

Tetramethrin	0.400%
d-(cis,trans) Phenothrin	0.287%
Other Isomers	0.013%
Water	
Hydrocarbon propellant	

BLACK FLAG FLYING INSECT KILLER
(Boyle-Midway)

Resmethrin	0.080%
Related compounds	0.011%
d-trans Allethrin	0.160%
Related compounds	0.012%
Piperonyl butoxide (technical)	0.800%
Aromatic petroleum solvent *	1.191%
1,1,1-Trichloroethane *	<2%
Hydrocarbon propellant and water	

BLACK FLAG FLYPORT
Insect trap
(Boyle-Midway)

Insect attractant
Adhesive

BLACK FLAG GYPSY MOTH AND CATERPILLAR INSECT KILLER
(Boyle-Midway)

d-trans Allethrin	0.3%
Piperonyl butoxide (technical)	1.5%
Petroleum distillates	3.0%
Surface active agents, fragrance, and corrosion inhibitors	5.0%
Water and hydrocarbon propellant	approx. 90.0%

BLACK FLAG HOUSE & GARDEN INSECT KILLER IMPROVED SUPER SPRAY
(Boyle-Midway)

Resmethrin	0.100%
Related compounds	0.014%
d-trans Allethrin	0.200%
Related compounds	0.015%
Piperonyl butoxide (technical)	0.800%
Aromatic petroleum solvent *	1.133%
1,1,1-Trichloroethane*	<2%
Hydrocarbon propellant and water	

BLACK FLAG INSECT SPRAY
(Boyle-Midway)

Methoxychlor (tech.)	0.75%
Lethane 384	1.00%
Essential oil	0.20%
Petroleum distillates *	98.05%

BLACK FLAG LARGE AREA AUTOMATIC ROOM FOGGER FORMULA S
(Boyle-Midway)

Tetramethrin	0.200%
d-(cis,trans)Phenothrin	0.382%
Other isomers	0.018%
Petroleum distillate	14.400%
1,1,1-Trichloroethane	17.000%
Methylene chloride *	40.000%
Hydrocarbon propellant	

BLACK FLAG LIQUID ANT & ROACH KILLER
(Boyle-Midway)

Baygon *	0.50%
DDVP	0.20%
Petroleum distillates *	86.13%

BLACK FLAG LIQUID PROFESSIONAL POWER ANT & ROACH KILLER
(Boyle-Midway)

Baygon *	0.950%
DDVP and related compounds	0.200%
Petroleum distillates *	82.120%
Combined amount:	<20%
Methylene chloride	
Glycol ether solvent	
Mineral oil	

BLACK FLAG OUTDOOR FOGGER
(Boyle-Midway)

Resmethrin	0.200%
Related compounds	0.028%
MGK Repellant 874	0.475%
Related compounds	0.025%
Petroleum distillates	0.272%
Propellant	

BLACK FLAG PRE-ADULT FLEA KILLER
(Boyle-Midway)

Methoprene	0.15%
Methylene chloride	55.00%
1,1,1-Trichloroethane *	<20.00%
Other solvents	<1.00%
Propellant	approx. 25.00%

BLACK FLAG PROFESSIONAL POWER ANT & ROACH KILLER (Aerosol)
(Boyle-Midway)

DDVP	0.20%
Baygon *	1.00%
Petroleum distillate *	79.12%
Propellant	

BLACK FLAG PROFESSIONAL POWER FLYING INSECT KILLER
(Boyle-Midway)

d-trans Allethrin	0.50%
Piperonyl butoxide (technical)	1.40%
Propellant	

BLACK FLAG PROFESSIONAL POWER HOUSE & GARDEN INSECT KILLER
(Boyle-Midway)

Pyrethrins	0.50%
Piperonyl butoxide (technical)	1.50%
Petroleum distillate	5.00%
Propellant	

BLACK FLAG ROACH KILLER SPECIAL CITY FORMULA
(Boyle-Midway)

DDVP	0.20%
Baygon *	1.00%
Petroleum distillate *	79.12%
Propellant	

BLACK FLAG ROACH MOTEL
(Boyle-Midway)

Insect attractant
Adhesive

BLACK FLAG ROACH POWDER
(Boyle-Midway)

Pyrethrins	0.1%
Piperonyl butoxide (technical)	1.0%
Petroleum distillate *	58.9%
Silica gel	40.0%

BLACK FLAG ROACH TRAPS
Insecticide
(Boyle-Midway)

Baygon *	2%

BLACK FLAG SOLID INSECT KILLER
Vaporizing insect strip
(Boyle-Midway)

DDVP *	20.0%

BLACK FLAG SUPER SPRAY DO-IT-YOURSELF PROFESSIONAL STRENGTH BUG KILLER
(Boyle-Midway)

Chlorpyrifos *	0.50%
Xylene range aromatic solvent	0.33%
Water and emulsifiers	99.17%

BLACK FLAG TRIPLE ACTIVE BUG KILLER
(Boyle-Midway)

d-trans Allethrin	0.30%
Piperonyl butoxide (technical)	1.50%
Petroleum distillates	3.00%
Hydrocarbon propellant and water	

BLACK FLAG WASP, BEE AND HORNET KILLER
(Boyle-Midway)

Baygon *	0.50%
DDVP	0.20%
Petroleum distillates *	61.02%
Propellant	

BLACK JACK ROOF CEMENT
(Gibson-Homans)

Asphalt	>10%
Petroleum spirits *	>10%
Asbestos fiber	1-10%
Whiting	>10%

BLACK MAGIC
Adhesive
(Miracle Adhesives)

Rubber
Resin
Pigments
Aliphatic petroleum hydrocarbon *

Starred ingredients (*) may be responsible for major toxic effects; consult Section II.

BLACK STRAND & BROWN STRAND HAIR COLORING
(Strand)

Capsules:
Para-phenylenediamine
Resorcinol *
Duponal C

Bottle:
Hydrogen peroxide, 10-volume
strength *

BLACK TITE

See DAP BLACK TITE

BLAISDELL CLINICAL GLASS MARKER (569T Red only)
(Berol/Blaisdell)

Waxes
Dry pigment
Acid azo pigment
Barium salt *
Kaolin clays
Titanium dioxide

BLAISDELL HI-TEMP MARKER (1371T Green only)
For marking permanency at high temperatures
(Berol/Blaisdell)

Waxes
Chromium oxide pigments
Black iron oxide pigment *
Bentonite clay

BLAISDELL HYDRO-MARKER
Water soluble markers
(Berol/Blaisdell)

Water soluble waxes
Dry pigments *†
Titanium dioxide

†*See* Industrial Crayons, Section VI, General Formulations

BLAK-RAY FLUORESCENT READMISSION INKS
(Ultra-Violet)

Alcohols *	>70%
Coumarin derivative dyes	<1%
Urea formaldehyde resins	0-10%
Esters	0-10%

BLAK-RAY INVISIBLE FLUORESCENT OFFSET PRINTING INK A 716-A
(Ultra-Violet)

Linseed oil varnishes	>7%
Calcium carbonate	<10%
Colloidal Silica	<10%
Fluorescent pigments *†	<10%

†*See* Pigments, Section VI, General Formulations

BLAK-RAY PERMANENT FLUORESCENT MARKING INKS
(Ultra-Violet)

Esters	0-25%
Alcohols *	50-90%
Butyl Cellosolve *	0-40%
Cellulose acetate butyrate	0-10%
Styrene copolymer resin	0-5%
Coumarin derivative dyes	<5%

BLAK-RAY REMOVABLE FLUORESCENT MARKING INKS
(Ultra-Violet)

Alcohols *	0-50%
Glycols *	<10%
Triethyl phosphate	0-10%
Vinyl resins	0-15%
Zn-Cd sulfide	0-10%
Coumarin derivative dyes	<1%

BLAST
Alkaline cleaning compound
(DuBois Chem.)

Caustic soda *
Complex sodium salts of silicates, carbonates and phosphates
Soap
Nonionic surfactant

BLAZE FURNACE CEMENT
(Gibson-Homans)

Sodium silicate *	>10%
Asbestos fiber	1-10%
Whiting	>10%
Water	>10%

BL BUSAN 30
Fungicide
(Buckman Labs.)

2-(Thiocyanomethylthio) benzothiazole *	30%

BL BUSAN 40
Slimicide, fungicide
(Buckman Labs.)

Potassium N-hydroxymethyl-N-methyldithiocarbamate *	40%

BL BUSAN 52
Slimicide, fungicide
(Buckman Labs.)

Potassium N-hydroxymethyl-N-methyldithiocarbamate *	32%
Sodium 2-mercaptobenzothiazole *	8%

BL BUSAN 72
Fungicide
(Buckman Labs.)

2-(Thiocyanomethylthio) benzothiazide *	60%

BL BUSAN 83
Water treatment
(Buckman Labs.)

Potassium dimethyldithiocarbamate *	20%
Tetrasodium ethylenediaminetetraacetate	1%

BL BUSAN 85
Slimicide
(Buckman Labs.)

Potassium dimethyldithiocarbamate *	50%

BL BUSAN 11-M1
Preservative
(Buckman Labs.)

Barium metaborate (calculated as BaB204-H20)	90%

BL DIMET
Slimicide
(Buckman Labs.)

Potassium dimethyldithiocarbamate *	50%

BL DISA
Water treatment
(Buckman Labs.)

Potassium dimethyldithiocarbamate *	20%
Tetrasodium ethylenediaminetetraacetate	1%

BLEN
(Reily Chem.)

Liquid detergent *†

†*See* Detergents, Section VI, General Formulations

BLENDOR
Embalming supply; fluid dye & internal cosmetic
(Royal Bond)

Carbitol *
Isopropanol *

BLEPHAMIDE LIQUIFILM
Ophthalmic suspension
(Allergan Pharm.)

Sulfacetamide sodium	10%
Prednisolone acetate	0.2%
Phenylephrine HCl	0.12%
Polyvinyl alcohol	1.4%

BLEPHAMIDE S.O.P.
Ophthalmic ointment
(Allergan Pharm.)

Sulfacetamide sodium	10.0%
Prednisolone acetate	0.2%
Phenylmercuric acetate	0.0008%

Mineral oil
White petrolatum
Nonionic lanolin derivatives

Starred ingredients (*) may be responsible for major toxic effects; consult Section II.

BLEPH-10 LIQUIFILM
Ophthalmic solution
(Allergan Pharm.)

Sulfacetamide sodium	10%
Polyvinyl alcohol	1.4%

BLINK-N-CLEAN
Hard contact lens solution
(Allergan Pharm.)

Polyoxyl 40 stearate	
Polyethylene glycol 300	
Chlorobutanol (chloral derivative as a preservative)	0.5%

BLINX
Ophthalmic irrigating solution
(Barnes-Hind)

Alkaline borate buffer:
Boric acid	
Sodium borate	
Phenylmercuric acetate	0.004%

BLISTAID COLD SORE LOTION
(Columbia Med.)

Isopropyl alcohol *
Gum benzoin
Camphor *
Menthol *

BLIST-AWAY
For cold sores, sore lips, fever blisters
(Amlab)

Benzocaine Hexatyn (Oxyquinoline sulfate)
Tripelennamine HCl *
Zirconium oxide
Polyvinylpyrrolidone
Lanolin
Allantoin
Camphor *
Menthol *
Flesh-tinted cream base

BLISTEX LIP OINTMENT
(Blistex)

Phenol	0.405%
Camphor	1.000%
Base:	balance
Mineral oil	
Beeswax	
Petrolatum	
Paraffin	
Lanolin	
Polyglyceryl-3	
Diisostearate	
Spirits of ammonia	

BLISTIK LIP BALM
(Blistex)

Octyl dimethyl PABA	1.5%
Allantoin	1.0%
Base:	balance
Mineral oil	
Paraffin	
Petrolatum	
Beeswax	
Bituminus hydrocarbons	

BLIS-TO-SOL AEROSOL
Athletes foot
(Chattem)

Salicylic acid *
Benzoic acid *
Thymol *

BLIS-TO-SOL LIQUID
Athletes foot
(Chattem)

Undecylenic acid *	
Salicylic acid *	
Thymol *	
Acetone *	18% w/w

BLIS-TO-SOL POWDER
Athletes foot
(Chattem)

Salicylic acid *
Benzoic acid *
Thymol *

BLISTR-KLEAR
Lip medication
(Miller-Morton)

Camphor	<1%
Lanolin	
Alcohol	40%

BLITZ RAT BAIT
(Blitz Products)

Warfarin (3-(alpha-Acetonylbenzyl)-4-hydroxycoumarin)	0.025%
N'-(2-Quinoxalinyl) sulfanilamide	0.025%
Inert ingred.:	99.950%
Cereal base	

'76 Ed.

BLOSSOM-SET

See SCIENCE BLOSSOM-SET

BLOXODOR CRYSTALS, LILAC
Deodorant
(Hillyard Chem.)

Para-dichlorobenzene *

'76 Ed.

BL TCMTB
Fungicide
(Buckman Labs.)

2-(Thiocyanomethylthio) benzothiazole *	80%

BLUBORO POWDER ASTRINGENT SOAKING SOLUTION
(Herbert Labs.)

Aluminum sulfate
Calcium acetate

BLU-BOY
Automatic toilet bowl cleaner
(Northwest Sanitation)

Water	>30%
Ethoxylated alkylphenols *	25%
Carbamide	>43%
Neptune blue	>2%

BLUE BARREL LAUNDRY SOAP BAR
(Purex Corp.)

Sodium tallow-coconut oil soap	>40%
Silicon dioxide	10-15%
Sodium silicate (not meta) *	10-15%
Sodium chloride	<1%
Glycerine	<1%
Perfume	<1%
Water	balance

BLUE CROSS COSMETIC PRODUCTS

Blue Cross Beauty Products, Inc.
1341 W. First St.
Los Angeles, Calif. 90026

Phone: 213-626-8101

See COSMETICS, Section VI, General Formulations

BLUE DEATH RAT AND MOUSE BAIT HIDE-A-PACK

See MASTER MIX BLUE DEATH RAT AND MOUSE BAIT HIDE-A-PACK

BLUE DEATH RAT BAIT

See MASTER MIX BLUE DEATH RAT BAIT

BLUE-DEATH SUGAR BAIT FLY-KILLER
Insecticide
(Texas Phenothiazine Co.)

Dimethyl(2,2,2-trichloro-1-hydroxyethyl)phosphonate (Dipterex)	1%

'76 Ed.

BLUE DRAGON GARDEN DUST
Insecticide
(Dragon)

Carbaryl *	2%

BLUE FOAM
(Park Chem.)

Water
Non-ionic surfactants
Dye

Starred ingredients (*) may be responsible for major toxic effects; consult Section II.

BLUE FYTE LOCK-ON
Room deodorant; institutional and commercial use
(Hysan Corp.)

Paradichlorobenzene
N-Alkyl (50% C12, 30% C14, 17% C16, 3% C18) dimethyl benzyl ammonium chlorides *
Lauryl methacrylate
Paraformaldehyde *
Inert ingredients: 2.10%
　Essential oils
　Nonyl phenoxy polyoxyethylene ethanol
　Calcium silicate
　Water

BLUE GROTTO
Hospital disinfectant
(Hysan Corp.)

Active ingred.: 43.89%
　Isopropyl alcohol *
　Potassium laurate
　Alpha and beta terpineols *
　4- and 6-Chloro-2-phenyl phenol *
　o-Benzyl-p-chlorophenol *
　Essential oils
　Sodium salt of ethylene diamine tetra-
　　acetic acid
　Orthophenylphenol *
　2,4,5-Trichlorophenol *
　p-tert-Amylphenol *
Inert ingred.: 56.11%
　Water

BLUE LUSTRE HOME CARE PRODUCTS

Earl Grissmer Co., Inc.
7950 Castleway Dr.
Indianapolis, Ind. 46250

Phone: 317-842-0820

BLUE POWER

See AMWAY BLUE POWER

BLUE RIBBON BLEACH
(Patterson Labs.)

Sodium hypochlorite * 5.25%

BLUE RIBBON RINSE
Fabric softener
(Patterson Labs.)

Patterson Labs., Inc.
11930 Pleasant Ave.
Detroit, Mich. 48217

Phone: 313-843-4500

BLUE RIBBON SUDSY-DETERGENT AMMONIA
(Patterson Labs.)

Ammonia * 5.2%

BLUE SEAL BACTA-LIFE
Septic tank activator
(Cloroben Chem. Corp.)

Yeast (nutmeg) 98%
Dehydrated enzymes 2%

'76 Ed.

BLUE SEAL BOILER CLEANER
(Cloroben Chem. Corp.)

Trisodium phosphate * 66 1/2%
Sodium sulfate anhydrous 33%
Sodium dichromate 1/2%

'76 Ed.

BLUE SEAL BOILER STOP-LEAK COMPOUND
(Cloroben Chem. Corp.)

Rust inhibitors *†

'76 Ed.

†*See* Rust control, Section VI, General Formulations

BLUE SEAL CESSPOOL CLEANER
(Cloroben Chem. Corp.)

Sodium hydroxide * 100%

'76 Ed.

BLUE SEAL CLOSET BOWL CLEANER
(Cloroben Chem. Corp.)

Sodium bisulfate * 100%

'76 Ed.

BLUE SEAL CUTTING OIL
(Cloroben Chem. Corp.)

Mineral oils
Sulfur
Chlorine *

'76 Ed.

BLUE SEAL DRAIN PIPE SOLVENT
(Cloroben Chem. Corp.)

Sodium hydroxide * 85%
Sodium nitrate 7 1/2%
Aluminum dross 7%

'76 Ed.

BLUE SEAL ENAMEL CLEANER
(Cloroben Chem. Corp.)

Abrasive 88%
Sodium tripolyphosphate (fines) ... 5%
Alkyl aryl sulfonate 5%
Trisodium phosphate (fines) 2%

'76 Ed.

BLUE SEAL PIPE JOINT CEMENT
(Cloroben Chem. Corp.)

Silicates
Carbonates
Oxides and sulfates of calcium, magnesium and barium
Mineral and vegetable oils

'76 Ed.

BLUE SEAL ROOT RAIDER
(Cloroben Chem. Corp.)

Sodium hydroxide * 96 1/2%
Aluminum dross 3 1/2%

'76 Ed.

BLUE STAR OIL BASE INSECTICIDE
(Huntington Labs.)

Petroleum distillate * 96.85%
Technical Piperonyl butoxide ... 3.00%
Pyrethrins 0.15%

BLUE STAR OINTMENT
For skin irritations
(Bourland)

Salicylic acid *
Benzoic acid
Synthetic Oil of wintergreen *
Anhydrous wool fat
Yellow petrolatum
Camphor *

BLUE STAX
Hairdressing & conditioner
(King Research)

Petrolatum
Mineral oil
Lanolin
Paraffin
Isopropyl myristate
PEG-8 dilaurate
Oleyl alcohol
Fragrance
D & C Violet 2
D & C Green 6
Captan

BLUE STREAK ANT BAIT
Control of the western harvester ant
(Texas Phenothiazine Co.)

Heptachlor (Heptachlorotetrahydro-4,7-methanoindene) 1.22%
Related compounds 0.78%

'76 Ed.

BLUE STREAK PAINT REMOVER
(Klean-Strip)

Chlorinated hydrocarbons * ..... >70%
Alcohol (<4% methanol) .... >20%
Thickeners & Inhibitors .... <5%

Starred ingredients (*) may be responsible for major toxic effects; consult Section II.

BLUE STUFF
Rug shampoo
(Paul Koss)

Water
Isopropyl alcohol * 8-12%
Sodium lauryl sulfate 3-5%
Lauroyl diethanolamide 2-4%
Tetrasodium EDTA .... <1%
Dye .... trace
Brightener .... trace
Formalin .... trace

BLUE TAG CYTHION-5E
Insecticide for use on stored grains
(Terminal Grain)

Malathion * 57%
Xylene * 30%

'76 Ed.

BLU-KOTE, DR. NAYLOR'S
(Dauber Bottle or Spray Bomb)

See DR. NAYLOR'S BLU-KOTE
(Dauber Bottle or Spray Bomb)

BLU-MAGIK
Detergent
(National Chemicals, Inc.)

Nonylphenol polyglycol ether (Nonyl-
phenoxypoly (ethyleneoxy) ethanol) *
Hydroxyacetic acid *
Isopropanol *

BLU-WHITE
Laundry additive
(Purex Corp.)

Anionic surfactant 5-10%
Nonionic surfactant 1-5%
Sodium tetraborate (anhydrous) 1-3%
Fluorescent whitening agent .... <1%
Pigment dyes .... <1%
Perfume .... <1%
Sodium sulfate .... balance

B-NINE-SP
Plant growth regulant
(Uniroyal Chem.)

Succinic acid 2,2-dimethyl
hydrazide 85.0%

BOB'S GYPSY RUB
LINIMENT NO. 2
(Smith, C.G., Products Co.)

Menthol *
Methyl salicylate *
Oil of eucalyptus *
Camphorated oil *
Isopropyl alcohol * 28 1/3%

'76 Ed.

BOBWHITE AUTOBODY
FILLER WITH CREAM
HARDENER
(Bondo Corp.)

Polyester resin
Metallic naphthenate &
aniline derivative as
promoters .... very small amt.
Benzoyl peroxide as catalyst * 50%
Filler:
Talc

'76 Ed.

BODYMAN FLEXIBLE
BONDO AUTOBODY
FILLER WITH CREAM
HARDENER
(Bondo Corp.)

Polyester resin (flexible type)
Metallic naphthenates & ani-
line derivative as pro-
moters .... small amt.
Benzoyl peroxide cream as
catalyst * 50%
Filler:
Talc

'76 Ed.

BODY ON TAP (Dry Hair)
Beer enriched shampoo
(Bristol-Myers)

Water
Beer
Sodium laureth sulfate
Lauramide DEA
Glycerin
Hexylene glycol
Hydrolyzed animal protein
PEG-150 distearate
Quaternium-6
Sodium lauryl sulfate
Fragrance
Laneth-10 acetate
Hydroxypropyl methylcellulose
Methylparaben
Citric acid
Sodium cetyl sulfate
Laureth-3
Formaldehyde
Disodium EDTA
Propylparaben
D & C Yellow No. 10
FD & C Red No. 4
D & C Green No. 5

BODY ON TAP (Normal Hair)
Beer enriched shampoo
(Bristol-Myers)

Water
Beer
Sodium laureth sulfate
Lauramide DEA
Sodium lauryl sulfate
Hexylene glycol
Hydrolyzed animal protein
PEG-150 distearate
Quaternium-6
Fragrance
Sodium cetyl sulfate
Laureth-3
Methylparaben
Hydroxypropyl methylcellulose
Citric acid
Formaldehyde
Disodium EDTA
Propylparaben
D & C Yellow No. 10
FD & C Red No. 4
D & C Green No. 5

BODY ON TAP (Oily Hair)
Beer enriched shampoo
(Bristol-Myers)

Water
Beer
Sodium laureth sulfate
Lauramide DEA
Sodium lauryl sulfate
Hexylene glycol
Hydrolyzed animal protein
PEG-150 distearate
Fragrance
Quaternium-6
Sodium cetyl sulfate
Laureth-3
Methylparaben
Citric acid
Formaldehyde
Disodium EDTA
Propylparaben
D & C Yellow No. 10
FD & C Red No. 4
D & C Green No. 5

BOIL EASE
Anesthetic drawing salve
(Commerce Drug)

Benzocaine
Resin cerate
Ichthammol
Carbolic acid *
Thymol *
Camphor *
Juniper tar

BOILER BRITE
Boiler scale remover
(Lester Labs.)

Sulfamic acid *
Chelates
Corrosion inhibitors *†

'76 Ed.

†*See* Rust control, Section VI, General
Formulations

BOILERENE
(Lester Labs.)

Phosphates *
Chelates
Alkali *

'76 Ed.

BOILER-LAX
Boiler cleaner
(Radiator)

Aminosulfonic acid *

'76 Ed.

BOILnSOAK
For soft contact lens care
(Burton, Parsons & Co.)

Sodium chloride	0.7%
Thimerosal (as preservative)	0.001%
Disodium edetate (as preservative)	0.1%

BOLARIS
Bowl cleaner
(Rawleigh)

N-Alkyl (60% C14, 30% C16, 5% C12, 5% C18) dimethyl benzyl ammonium chloride	0.05%
Bis (tributyltin) oxide	0.01%
Hydrogen chloride *	23.00%

'76 Ed.

BOLD 3 (Formula 1)
Granular laundry detergent
(Procter & Gamble)

Sodium sulfate	25-49%
Complex sodium phosphates	10-24%
Sodium alkyl benzene sulfonate	10-24%
Sodium sulfate	10-24%
Water	5-9%
Sodium aluminosilicates	5-9%
Ditallow dimethyl ammonium chloride	1-4%
Alkyl ethoxylate	1-4%
Alkyl alcohol	1-4%
Minor ingredients, each	trace

pH (1% solution) - 10.4

BOLD 3 (Formula 2)
Granular laundry detergent
(Procter & Gamble)

Sodium aluminosilicates	25-49%
Sodium sulfate	25-49%
Sodium alkyl benzene sulfonate	10-24%
Sodium silicate	5-9%
Water	5-9%
Sodium carbonate	5-9%
Ditallow dimethyl ammonium chloride	1-4%
Sodium tetraborate	1-4%
Alkyl alcohol	1-4%
Minor ingredients, each	trace

pH (1% solution) - 10.4

BOLD 3 (Formula 3)
Granular laundry detergent
(Procter & Gamble)

Sodium aluminosilicates	25-49%
Sodium sulfate	10-24%
Sodium alkyl benzene sulfonate	10-24%
Sodium carbonate	10-24%
Water	5-9%
Ditallow dimethyl ammonium chloride	1-4%
Sodium silicate	1-4%
Polyacrylamide	1-4%
Alkyl alcohol	1-4%
Sodium tetraborate	1-4%
Sodium toluene sulfonate	1-4%
Minor ingredients, each	trace

pH (1% solution) - 10.9 max.

BOLD 3 (Formula 4)
Granular laundry detergent
(Procter & Gamble)

Sodium aluminosilicates	25-49%
Sodium alkyl benzene sulfonate	10-24%
Sodium sulfate	10-24%
Sodium silicate	10-24%
Water	5-9%
Sodium carbonate	5-9%
Ditallow dimethyl ammonium chloride	1-4%
Alkyl ethoxylate	1-4%
Sodium tetraborate	1-4%
Sodium toluene sulfonate	1-4%
Alkyl alcohol	1-4%
Minor ingredients, each	trace

pH (1% solution) - 10.9 max.

BOLO
Chemical lawn trimmer
(Puritan Chem. Co.)

Sodium cacodylate	4.5%
Dimethylarsinic acid (Cacodylic acid)	0.78%

Total Arsenic (as elemental)(all in water soluble form 2.53%)

BOMBANE JET STREAM
Screw worm, ear tick control; veterinary
(Martin, C. J.)

Gamma isomer of benzene hexachloride *	3.15%
Pine oil *	20.00%

BOMBARD INSECT SPRAY
Insecticide
(Uncle Sam)

Pyrethrum
Synergists
Petroleum distillate *

BONAIR
Deodorant
(Lester Labs.)

Paradichlorobenzene *

'76 Ed.

BON AMI PRODUCTS

Faultless Starch/Bon Ami Co.
1025 W. 8th St.
Kansas City, Missouri 64101

Phone: 816-421-7075

BONAT CONTROLLED pH CONTROLLED SYSTEM CONDITIONING SHAMPOO
(Bonat)

Water	50-65%
Amphoteric-2	20-30%
Lauramide DEA	5-10%
Glycol stearate and other ingredients	<5%
Laureth-23	<2%
Stearamine oxide	<2%
Citric acid	<2%
Quaternium-19	<2%
Fragrance	<1%
Quaternium-15	<1%
Tetrasodium EDTA	<1%
Wheat germ oil	<1%

BONAT CONTROLLED pH CONTROLLED SYSTEM SHAMPOO
(Bonat)

	percentage range
Sodium lauryl sulfate *	25.0-38.0%
Sodium laureth sulfate *	25.0-35.0%
Water	25.0-35.0%
Cocamide DEA	5.0-10.0%
Citric acid	<2.0%
Fragrance	<1.0%
Methylparaben	<1.0%

BONAT CONTROLLED pH SALON PERM SYSTEM LOTION
Permanent wave lotion
(Bonat)

	percentage range
Water	85.0-97.0%
Ammonium thioglycolate *	5.0-12.0%
Ammonium hydroxide *	<2.0%
Styrene/acrylamide copolymer	<1.0%
Laureth-23	<1.0%
Fragrance	<1.0%

May contain: PEG-60 lanolin (<1%), Oleyl alcohol (<1%), D & C Yellow #11 (trace)

BONAT COSMETIC PRODUCTS
Hair sprays, waving lotions, shampoos

Bonat, Inc.
250 Lackawanna Ave.
West Paterson, N.J. 07424

Phone: 201-256-3400

See COSMETICS, Section VI, General Formulations

BONATE
(Suppositoria Labs.)

Each suppository:
 Bismuth subgallate
 Bismuth resorcin comp.
 Balsam Peru *
 Benzocaine
 Zinc oxide
 Boric acid *

BONAT FRAGRANT PERM LOTION
Permanent wave lotion
(Bonat)

	percentage range
Water	80.0-95.0%
Ammonium thioglycolate	3.0-9.0%
Ethanolamine *	<5.0%
Styrene/acrylamide copolymer	<1.0%
Laureth-23	<1.0%
Fragrance	<1.0%

BONAT HAIR STRENGTH 10
Hair conditioner
(Bonat)

Water	75-85%
Laneth-40	5-12%
Butylene glycol	5-10%
Bis-2-hydroxyethyl tallow ammonium chloride	<6%
Hydrolyzed animal protein	<6%
Fragrance	<1%
Imidazolidinyl urea	<1%
Methylparaben	<1%
Propylparaben	<1%

BONAT THIN WHITE NEUTRALIZER
Permanent wave
(Bonat)

	percentage range
Water	85.0-98.0%
Hydrogen peroxide *	<5.0%
Styrene/acrylamide copolymer	<1.0%
Fragrance	<1.0%
Boric acid	<1.0%
Phosphoric acid	<1.0%

BONDEX SILICONE WATERPROOFING
For exterior masonry
(Bondex)

Silicones	3.15%
Mineral spirits *	87.7%

BONDO
Extra flexible white plastic filler
(Bondo Corp.)

Polyester resin
Promoters: .... very small amount
 Metallic Naphthenate
 Aniline derivative
Benzoyl peroxide (as catalyst) * 50%
Filler:
 Talc

'76 Ed.

BOND-O-LOK
Zinc phosphating agent
(Whitfield Chem.)

Phosphoric acid *	>10%
Acid Zinc salts *	>10%

BONIDE AMMATE X WEED & BRUSH KILLER
Herbicide
(Bonide)

Ammonium sulfamate * 95%

BONIDE ANT DUST
Insecticide
(Bonide)

Diazinon * 1.0%

BONIDE ASPON 2E
Organophosphorus soil insecticide
(Bonide)

O,O,O,O-Tetrapropyl dithiopyrophosphate 25.67%
Xylene range aromatic hydrocarbon solvent * 66.30%

BONIDE BLUE DEATH .75% ROTENONE GARDEN DUST
Insecticide
(Bonide)

Rotenone	0.75%
Other Cube resins *	1.50%

BONIDE BORER-MINER KILLER
(Bonide)

Gamma isomer of benzene hexachloride from lindane * 20.00%

BONIDE BORER-MINER KILLER-5
(Bonide)

Gamma isomers of benzene hexachloride from Lindane * 5%

BONIDE BRUSHKIL
Herbicide
(Bonide)

Dimethylamine salt of 2,4-Dichlorophenoxyacetic acid * 13.0%
Dimethylamine salt of Dicamba (3,6-Dichloro-o-anisic acid) 1.5%
Dimethylamine salt of related acids 0.3%

BONIDE BUG FOG
Fog or spray insecticide
(Bonide)

Petroleum distillate * 81.1%
Aromatic petroleum derivative solvent * 12.2%
Methoxychlor (technical) 5.0%
Beta-butoxy beta-thiocyano diethyl ether 1.7%

BONIDE BULB DUST
Controls thrips and disease
(Bonide)

Methoxychlor, technical	5.0%
Thiram *	10.0%

BONIDE CHICKWEED, CLOVER AND BENT GRASS KILLER
(Bonide)

Polypropoxypropyl ester of Silvex * 13.5%

BONIDE CHICKWEED & CLOVER KILLER
(Bonide)

Dimethylamine salt of Dicamba (3,6-Dichloro-o-anisic acid) * .. 13.0%
Dimethylamine salt of related acids 2.1%

BONIDE CHLORDANE 74% E
Termite control
(Bonide)

Technical Chlordane *	74%
Petroleum distillate *	20%

BONIDE COMPLETE FRUIT TREE SPRAY
Insecticide, fungicide, aphicide, miticide, scalicide
(Bonide)

Captan	12.0%
Malathion	6.0%
Methoxychlor, technical	12.0%
Carbaryl	0.3%
Aromatic petroleum solvent *	36.5%

BONIDE COMPLETE FRUIT TREE SPRAY (Powder)
(Bonide)

Captan	15.0%
Methoxychlor, technical *	15.0%
Malathion	7.5%

BONIDE COPPER SPRAY OR DUST
Fungicide
(Bonide)

Copper ((in basic copper sulphate) expressed as metallic) * 7%

BONIDE CRABGRASS & BROADLEAF WEED KILLER
(Bonide)

Dodecylammonium methanearsonate *	8.00%
Octylammonium methanearsonate *	8.00%
Octyl ammonium salt of 2,4-dichlorophenoxyacetic acid *	8.16%

BONIDE CRABGRASS PREVENTER AND WEED KILLER
(Bonide)

Tupersan	2.75%

BONIDE CUKE AND MELON DUST
Insecticide/fungicide
(Bonide)

Rotenone *	1%
Other Cube extractives *	2%
Copper ((in basic copper sulphate) expressed as metallic) *	7%

BONIDE DANDELION KILLER
(Bonide)

Sodium salt of 2,4-Dichlorophenoxyacetic acid	1.77%

BONIDE DURSBAN 2E INSECTICIDE
(Bonide)

Chlorpyrifos (O,O-Diethyl O-(3,5,6-trichloro-2-pyridyl) phosphorothioate) *	24.5%
Xylene *	68.9%

BONIDE EVERGREEN-FLOWER INSECT SPRAY
(Bonide)

Malathion	15.0%
Methoxychlor, technical	5.0%
Carbaryl	2.5%
1,1-Bis (p-chlorophenyl)-2,2,2-trichloroethanol	1.0%
Aromatic petroleum derivative solvents *	23.5%

BONIDE FLOWER-VEGETABLE 4-IN-1 SPRAY
Aphicide, miticide, insecticide, fungicide
(Bonide)

Malathion	9.4%
Technical Methoxychlor	9.5%
2,4-Dinitro-6-octyl phenyl crotonate	1.4%
2,6-Dinitro-4-octyl phenol crotonate Nitrooctyl phenols (principally dinitro)	0.1%
Aromatic petroleum solvents *	13.5%

BONIDE FLYING & CRAWLING INSECT KILLER
(Bonide)

Pyrethrins	0.25%
Technical Piperonyl butoxide	2.00%
Petroleum distillate *	12.75%

BONIDE FOAMING JET ACTION WEED KILLER
(Bonide)

Triethanolamine salt of 2,4-Dichlorophenoxyacetic acid	1.25%
Triethanolamine salt of Silvex (2-(2,4,5-Trichlorophenoxy) propionic acid)	1.16%

BONIDE FRUIT, SHADE, ORNAMENTAL TREE & WOODY EVERGREEN INSECTICIDE
(Bonide)

N-(Mercaptomethyl)-phthalimide S-(O,O-dimethylphosphorodithioate) *	12.5%

BONIDE GARDEN DUST FOR VEGETABLES-FLOWERS
Insecticide, fungicide
(Bonide)

Pyrethrins	0.03%
Technical Piperonyl butoxide	0.30%
Rotenone *	0.50%
Other cube resins	1.00%
Sulfur (4-5 microns)	25.00%
Copper (in basic copper sulfate)(expressed as metallic) *	5.00%

BONIDE GRASS-N-WEED KILLER
(Bonide)

Cacodyllic acid *	

BONIDE GRASS-N-WEED KILLER JET SPRAY
(Bonide)

Ammonium sulfamate	9.5%

BONIDE GRUB CHINCH BUG & SOD WEBWORM KILLER
(Bonide)

O,O-Diethyl O-(2-isopropyl-4-methyl-6-pyrimidinyl) phosphorothioate *	10%

BONIDE HORNET WASP & BEE BOMB
(Bonide)

Pyrethrins	0.10%
b-Butoxy-b-thiocyanodiethyl ether *	1.85%
Petroleum distillate *	76.00%

BONIDE HOUSEHOLD FLEA KILLER SPRAY INSECTICIDE
(Bonide)

Beta-butoxy beta'-thiocyano diethyl ether (Lethane) *	3.1%/wt.
Petroleum distillates *	71.9%/wt.

BONIDE HOUSE PLANT SHINE SPRAY
(Bonide)

Petroleum oil *	98%

BONIDE HOUSE PLANT, WHITEFLY, APHID AND SPOTTED MITE SPRAY
(Bonide)

Tetramethrin	0.250%
Related compounds	0.034%
Resmethrin	0.106%
Related compounds	0.014%
Petroleum distillate	9.000%

BONIDE KELTHANE EC
Agricultural miticide
(Bonide)

Kelthane	18.5%
Xylene *	73.0%

BONIDE KILBRUSH
Herbicide
(Bonide)

Butyl 2,4,5-trichlorophenoxyacetate	9.8%
Butyl 2,4-dichlorophenoxyacetate *	20.0%

BONIDE LAWN AND GARDEN INSECT CONTROL W/DIAZINON 12 1/2% E
(Bonide)

O,O-Diethyl O-(2-isopropyl-4-methyl-6-pyrimidinyl) phosphorothioate *	12.5%
Aromatic petroleum derivative solvent *	67.7%

Starred ingredients (*) may be responsible for major toxic effects; consult Section II.

BONIDE LAWN AND GARDEN INSECT CONTROL W/DIAZINON 25% E
(Bonide)

O,O-Diethyl O-(2-isopropyl-4-methyl-6-pyrimidinyl) phosphorothioate *	25.0%
Aromatic petroleum derivative solvent *	55.2%

BONIDE LAWN AND ORNAMENTAL INSECTICIDE
(Bonide)

Chlorpyrifos *	24.5%
Xylene *	68.9%

BONIDE LAWN AND TURF FUNGICIDE
(Bonide)

4,6-Dichloro-N-(2-chlorophenyl)-1,-3,5-triazin-2-amine *	50%

BONIDE LAWN CHINCH BUG & SOD WEBWORM CONTROL
(Bonide)

Chlorpyrifos *	2.3%
Aromatic petroleum derivative solvent	4.0%

BONIDE LAWN DISEASE CONTROL
(Bonide)

Thiram *	10%

BONIDE LAWN FUNGICIDE
(Bonide)

Zineb *	50.0%
Cadmium chloride *	7.5%
Thiram *	6.4%

BONIDE LAWN WEED KILLER (GRANULES)
Herbicide
(Bonide)

Triethanolamine salt of 2,4-dichlorophenoxyacetic acid *	8.35%

BONIDE LIQUID COPPER FUNGICIDE 4E
(Bonide)

Copper salts of fatty and rosin acids (copper as metallic, 4%) *	48%

BONIDE MALATHION 50% E INSECTICIDE
(Bonide)

Malathion *	50%
Xylene *	39%

BONIDE METHOXYCHLOR 25% E INSECTICIDE
(Bonide)

Methoxychlor, technical	25%
Xylene *	63%
Heavy aromatic Naphtha	7%

BONIDE MOLETOX II POISON BAIT MOLE & GOPHER KILLER
(Bonide)

Zinc phosphide *	2%

BONIDE MOLETOX POISON PEANUTS MOLE & GOPHER KILLER
(Bonide)

Arsenic trioxide *	1.5%

BONIDE MOSQUITO FOG OIL OR SPRAY
(Bonide)

Methoxychlor, technical	25.00%
Beta-butoxy beta'-thiocyano diethyl ether	1.85%
Aromatic petroleum derivative solvent *	70.65%

BONIDE OIL & LIME SULPHUR SPRAY
Insecticide for dormant shrubs, roses, trees and fruit trees
(Bonide)

Calcium polysulfides *	5.0%
Petroleum oils *	80.0%

BONIDE "ONE-SHOT" RAT KILLER
Rodenticide
(Bonide)

Red squill powder *	10%

BONIDE ORCHARD MOUSE BAIT
(Bonide)

Zinc phosphide *	2%

BONIDE ORGANIC GREENHOUSE, HOUSEPLANT & VEGETABLE SPRAY CONCENTRATE
Insecticide
(Bonide)

Pyrethrins	1%
Piperonyl butoxide, technical	10%
Petroleum distillate *	79%

BONIDE PENTIDE
Wood preservative - termite repellent
(Bonide)

Pentachlorophenol *	4.4%
Other chlorophenols	0.6%
Petroleum hydrocarbons *	91.63%

BONIDE PRUNING-WOUND BOMB
(Bonide)

Asphalt solids	21%
Petroleum distillate *	22%
Pine oil	1%

BONIDE RABBIT-DEER REPELLENT & BULB SAVER
(Bonide)

Thiram *	11.0%
Acrylic polymer resins	11.0%

BONIDE ROACH & ANT KILLER SPRAY
(Bonide)

b-Butoxy-b-thiocyanodiethyl ether *	3.1%/wt.
Petroleum distillates *	71.9%/wt.

BONIDE ROACH, ANT & SPIDER KILLER
(Bonide)

Chlorpyrifos (O,O-Diethyl O-(3,5,6-trichloro-2-pyridyl) phosphorothioate) *	0.5%
Pyrethrins	0.1%
Technical Piperonyl butoxide	0.2%
N-Octyl bicycloheptene dicarboximide	0.3%
Aromatic petroleum derivative solvent *	1.0%

BONIDE ROSE AND FLOWER SPRAY OR DUST
Insecticide/fungicide
(Bonide)

Folpet	6.5%
Carbaryl *	4.0%
Methyl naphthalenes	1.9%
Aromatic petroleum derivative solvents *	1.1%
1,1-Bis(p-chlorophenyl)-2,2,2-trichloroethanol	1.0%
Malathion	1.0%

BONIDE ROSE & FLORAL SPRAY BOMB
Insecticide/fungicide
(Bonide)

Carbaryl	0.750%
Folpet	0.500%
Malathion	0.500%
1,1-Bis(p-chlorophenyl)-2,2,2-trichloroethanol	0.075%

Starred ingredients (*) may be responsible for major toxic effects; consult Section II.

BONIDE ROSE SPRAY INSTANT ALL LIQUID
Insecticide/fungicide
(Bonide)

Carbaryl *	10.00%
Captan	10.00%
2,4-Dinitro-6-octyl phenyl crotonate and 2,6-Dinitro-4-octyl phenyl crotonate	0.90%
Nitrooctyl phenols (principally dinitro)	0.10%
1,1-Bis(p-chlorophenyl)-2,2,2-trichloroethanol	0.50%
Malathion	0.96%

BONIDE ROTENONE-COPPER DUST FOR POTATO-TOMATO-VEGETABLE GARDENS
Insecticide, fungicide
(Bonide)

Copper (in basic copper sulfate)(expressed as metallic) *	7.00%
Rotenone	0.35%
Other cube resins	0.65%
Methyl naphthalenes	1.30%

BONIDE ROTENONE 5 ORGANIC INSECTICIDE
(Bonide)

Rotenone *	5.0%
Other Cube resins *	10.0%

BONIDE ROTOSYN INSECT DUST
(Bonide)

Rotenone	0.35%
Other Cube resins	0.65%
Methyl naphthalenes	1.30%

BONIDE SEVIN 2 FLOWABLE INSECTICIDE
(Bonide)

Carbaryl *	22.5%

BONIDE SLUG & SNAIL KILLER W/ZECTRAN
Meal bait
(Bonide)

Mexacarbate (4-(Dimethylamino)-3,5-xylyl methylcarbamate) *	2.0%

BONIDE SOIL FUMIGANT
(Bonide)

Vapam *	32.7%

BONIDE STUMP OUT
Stump remover
(Bonide)

Sodium bisulfite
Sulfur *

BONIDE SWEET CORN & FRUIT SPRAY-DUST
(Bonide)

Powdered stem of Ryania speciosa *	40%

BONIDE SYSTEMIC GRANULES
Insecticide
(Bonide)

O,O-Diethyl S-(2,-(ethylthio)ethyl) phosphorodithioate *	2%

BONIDE SYSTEMIC INSECTICIDE
(Bonide)

Dimethoate *	23.4%

BONIDE TETRAMETHRIN SPRAY BOMB
Insecticide
(Bonide)

Tetramethrin	0.200%
Resmethrin	0.191%
Other isomers	0.009%
Petroleum distillate	9.250%

BONIDE TOMATO-POTATO DUST
Insecticide - fungicide
(Bonide)

Carbaryl *	3.0%
Maneb	4.8%

BONIDE TOMATO-POTATO VEGETABLE
Insecticide/fungicide
(Bonide)

Maneb	5.6%
Endosulfan *	3.0%

BONIDE TOM CAT
Rodenticide
(Bonide)

Warfarin	0.025%

BONIDE TREE-TOX
Fruit tree dust or spray
(Bonide)

Methoxychlor, technical	6.0%
Captan	6.0%
Malathion	3.0%
Carbaryl	0.5%

BONIDE TRIP-L-KIL
Insecticide
(Bonide)

Malathion *	3.00%
Methoxychlor, technical	3.00%
b-Butoxy-b-thiocyanodiethyl ether *	0.53%
Xylene *	6.66%
Petroleum distillate *	86.65%

BONIDE TURFCIDE 10 G FUNGICIDE
(Bonide)

Pentachloronitrobenzene *	10%

BONIDE TURF & ORNAMENTAL HERBICIDE 75% W.P.
(Bonide)

Dimethyl tetrachloroterephthalate	75%

BONIDE VEGETABLE-FLORAL DUST OR SPRAY
Insecticide and fungicide
(Bonide)

Carbaryl	1.25%
Rotenone	0.50%
Other cube resins	1.00%
Copper (in basic copper sulphate) expressed as metallic *†	7.00%
Methyl naphthalenes	0.85%

†*See* Cupric sulfate

BONIDE VEGETABLES & FRUIT TREES SPRAY
Insecticide
(Bonide)

Carbaryl *	13.5%
Malathion *	13.5%

BONIDE V-1
Fog, mist or spray insecticide
(Bonide)

Mineral oil *	99.50%
2,2-Dichlorovinyl dimethyl phosphate	0.46%
Related compounds	0.04%

BONIDE WEED KILLER
(Bonide)

Dimethylamine salt of 2,4-Dichlorophenoxyacetic acid *	13.0%
Dimethylamine salt of Dicamba (3,6-Dichloro-o-anisic acid)	1.5%
Dimethylamine salt of related acids	0.3%

BONIDE WEED SEEDLING KILLER (GRANULES)
Herbicide
(Bonide)

S-Ethyl dipropylthiocarbamate (Eptam)	2.3%

BONIDE ZECTRAN 1E INSECTICIDE
(Bonide)

Mexacarbate *	11%
Aromatic petroleum derivative solvent *	58%

Starred ingredients (*) may be responsible for major toxic effects; consult Section II.

BONIDE ZECTRAN 2E INSECTICIDE (LIQUID)
(Bonide)

4-(Dimethylamino)-3,5-xylyl
  methylcarbamate * 22%
Aromatic petroleum derivative
  solvent * 31%

BONINE CHEWABLE TABLETS
Motion sickness
(Pfipharmecs)

Each tablet:
  Meclizine hydrochloride* ...... 25 mg.

BONNE BELL COSMETIC PRODUCTS

Bonne Bell, Inc.
Georgetown Row
18519 Detroit Ave.
Lakewood, Ohio 44107

Phone: 216-221-0800

See COSMETICS, Section VI, General
  Formulations

BONTRIL PDM
Anoretic
(Carnrick Labs.)

Each tablet:
  Phendimetrazine tartrate * ... 35 mg.

BONUS D
Herbicide
(Scott, O.M.)

Neburon 2.00%
Carrier base: Fertilizer 35-0-0

B.O.P. - BRUSH-ON-PARTS CLEANER

See GUNK B.O.P. - BRUSH-ON-
  PARTS CLEANER

BO-PEEP AMMONIA
(Purex Corp.)

Ammonia * 1-5%
Nonionic surfactant .... <2%
Colorant .... <1%
Perfume .... <1%
Water .... balance

May contain an opacifier at trace level

BORA FAB
Laundry bleach and detergent booster
(National-Purity Soap)

Energized Borax *
Active Oxygen .... 10.0% min.

pH of 1%-5% solutions 10.0-10.4

BORAPAX SUPREME
Industrial skin cleanser
(Calgon Corp., Commercial Div.)

Soap
Borax *
Emollients
Urea

BORATEEM
Laundry aid
(U.S. Borax)

Borax * 98.4%
Sodium alkylbenzene sulfonate ... 0.4%
Carboxymethylcellulose and
  brighteners 1.0%

BORATE-48, FERTILIZER

See FERTILIZER BORATE-48

BORATE-68, FERTILIZER

See FERTILIZER BORATE-68

BORAXO
Powdered hand soap
(U.S. Borax)

Toilet soap 25.0%
Borax * 75.0%
Perfume *

BORAXO DISINFECTANT TILE AND PORCELAIN CLEANER
(U.S. Borax)

Tetrasodiumethylene-
  diaminetetraacetate 9.13%
Isopropanol * 5.00%
5-Chloro-2-
  (2, 4-dichlorophenoxy) phenol .. 0.07%

BORAXO LIQUID LOTION SOAP
(U.S. Borax)

Anhydrous Soap
Lanolin
Fillers
Water

BORAXO WATERLESS HAND CLEANER
(U.S. Borax)

Mineral oil
Water
Nonoxynol-6, Propylene glycol
TEA-oleate
Pigment
Perfume *
Lanolin

BORDERLAND BLACK REPELLENT
Blackbird repellent
(Borderland Prod.)

3,5-Dimethyl-4-
  (methylthio)phenol methylcarbamate (Methiocarb) * 18.75%

BORERKIL
Insecticide
(Lethelin)

Lindane (Gamma isomer of benzene
  hexachloride) * 2.0%

BORER-SOL

See DEXOL BORER-SOL

BO-RID 10H-15K SOIL STERILANT
Herbicide
(Bogle)

Bromacil (5-Bromo-3-sec-butyl-6-
  methyluracil) 4%
Diuron   (3-(3,4-Dichlorophenyl)-1,1-
  dimethylurea) 6%
                              '76 Ed.

BO-RID 10H SOIL STERILANT
Herbicide
(Bogle)

Bromacil (5-Bromo-3-sec-butyl-6-
  methyluracil) 4%
                              '76 Ed.

BO-RID 15H SOIL STERILANT
Herbicide
(Bogle)

Bromacil (5-Bromo-3-sec-butyl-6-
  methyluracil) 6%
                              '76 Ed.

BO-RID 20H SOIL STERILANT
Herbicide
(Bogle)

Bromacil (5-Bromo-3-sec-butyl-6-
  methyluracil) 8%
                              '76 Ed.

BO-RID 10K SOIL STERILANT
Herbicide
(Bogle)

Diuron   (3-(3,4-Dichlorophenyl)-1,1-
  dimethylurea) 4%
                              '76 Ed.

BO-RID 15K SOIL STERILANT
Herbicide
(Bogle)

Diuron   (3-(3,4-Dichlorophenyl)-1,1-
  dimethylurea) 6%

'76 Ed.

BO-RID 20K SOIL STERILANT
Herbicide
(Bogle)

Diuron   (3-(3,4-Dichlorophenyl)-1,1-
  dimethylurea) 8%

'76 Ed.

BO-RID 25K SOIL STERILANT
Herbicide
(Bogle)

Diuron   (3-(3,4-Dichlorophenyl)-1,1-
  dimethylurea) * 10%

'76 Ed.

BO-RID 40K SOIL STERILANT
Herbicide
(Bogle)

Diuron   (3-(3,4-Dichlorophenyl)-1,1-
  dimethylurea) * 16%

'76 Ed.

BO-RID PARABO CRYSTALS
Insecticide
(Bogle)

Paradichlorobenzene * 100%

'76 Ed.

BO-RID TCA-CHLORATE WEED KILLER, SPECIAL-A
Herbicide
(Bogle)

Sodium chlorate * 18.76%
Sodium trichloroacetate 6.25%
Calcium chloride 11.25%

'76 Ed.

BO-RID TCA-CHLORATE WEED KILLER, SPECIAL-C
Herbicide
(Bogle)

Sodium chlorate * 19.62%
Sodium trichloroacetate 9.81%
Calcium chloride 11.77%

'76 Ed.

BO-RID TCA-CHLORATE WEED KILLER, SPECIAL-D
Herbicide
(Bogle)

Sodium chlorate * 28.49%
Sodium trichloroacetate 14.24%
Calcium chloride 17.09%

'76 Ed.

BOROFAX OINTMENT
Emollient
(Burroughs Wellcome)

Boric acid * 5%
Lanolin

BOROLEUM
*For relief of discomforts due to head
  colds, sinus, hayfever, minor nasal
  and skin irritations*
(Sinclair Pharm.)

Menthol *
Camphor *
Eucalyptol *
Methyl salicylate *
Boracic acid . . . . <1/4 of 1%
Petrolatum

BOROLID
Antiseptic solution
(Whorton)

Benzoic acid
Acetanilid *
Thymol *
Oil cassia
Methyl salicylate *
Oil peppermint
Oil eucalyptus *
Boric acid *
Zinc chloride *

'76 Ed.

BORONIA CONCENTRATED AIR FRESHENER (Aerosol)

See AMWAY BORONIA CONCEN-
  TRATED AIR FRESHENER (Aerosol)

BOROSORB
Emollient
(Torch)

Boric acid * 10%
Hydrophilic vehicle . . . . ad. 100%

'76 Ed.

BOSS GRANULES
Laundry soap
(National-Purity Soap)

Anhydrous Soap chips 92%
Silicates
Wetting agent - nonionic *
Phosphate (P2O5) 5.8%

pH of 1% solution 11.0

BOSTON POLISH

See BUTCHER'S BOSTON POLISH

B & O SUPPRETTES
Analgesic, antispasmodic, sedative
(Webcon)

NO. 15A (each suppository):
  Powdered Opium * . . . . 30 mg.
  Belladonna extract . . . . 1/4 gr.

NO. 16A (each suppository):
  Powdered Opium * . . . . 60 mg.
  Belladonna extract . . . . 1/4 gr.

BOTTOMKOTE PAINT
(International Paint)

Copper *
Mineral spirits *
Aromatics *†
Pigments - no lead

†*See* Aromatic hydrocarbon solvent

BOUNCE
Dryer-added fabric softener
(Procter & Gamble)

Rayon fabric sheet coated with the follow-
ing:
  Polyhydric ester 70-95%
  Dialkyldimethylammonium
    salt 10-25%
  Perfume 1-4%
  Minor ingredients, each . . . . . .   <1%

BOUNTY FLOOR FINISH

See BUTCHER'S BOUNTY FLOOR
  FINISH

BOVINOL CIOVAP
(Amoco)

Active ingredients by weight:
  Dimethyl phosphate of alpha-
    methylbenzyl-3-hydroxy-cis-
    crotonate * 1.00%
  2,2-Dichlorovinyl dimethyl
    phosphate 0.23%
  Related compounds 0.02%

BOVINOL INSECTICIDE
Insecticide
(Amoco)

Active ingredients by weight:
  Ronnel (O,O-Dimethyl O-(2,4,5-
    trichlorophenyl)phosphorothi-
    oate) 1.00%
  Mineral oil * 98.48%

BOVINOL STOCK SPRAY WITH VAPONA
Insecticide
(Amoco)

Active ingredients by weight:
  2,2-Dichlorovinyl dimethyl
    phosphate 0.93%
  Related compound 0.07%
  Petroleum distillate * 99.00%

Starred ingredients (*) may be responsible for major toxic effects; consult Section II.

BOVINOL SUPER STOCK SPRAY
Insecticide
(Amoco)

Active ingredients by weight:
Pyrethrins 0.10%
Piperonyl butoxide, technical . 0.20%
N-Octyl bicycloheptene
dicarboximide 0.33%
Di-n-propyl isocinchomeronate 0.20%
Petroleum distillate * 99.17%

BOWES B-133 SELF-VULCANIZING CEMENT
(Bowes)

Toluol * .... >90%

BOWES DISC & DRUM DOT 3 MOTOR VEHICLE BRAKE FLUID
(Bowes)

Polyalkylene oxide ethers *†

†*See* Brake fluids, Section VI, General Formulations

BOWES LEAK FINDER
(Bowes)

Synthetic detergents *

BOWES LIQUID CAR WASH
(Bowes)

Synthetic detergent *

BOWES LIQUID STOP LEAK
(Bowes)

Isopropanol 9%
Sulfonate base

BOWES LIQUID WHITE SIDEWALL CLEANER
(Bowes)

Caustic (pH approx. 13) *

BOWES POWER AID
(Bowes)

Methanol * 98.5%

BOWES RUST ROUT
(Bowes)

Water-soluble oil

BOWES SOLVENT & CLEANER
(Bowes)

Rubber solvent * .... >90%

BOWES SUPER RADIATOR FLUSH
(Bowes)

Sodium chromate * 16%

BOWES TRANSMISSION SEALER-CONDITIONER
(Bowes)

Triaryl phosphate *

BOWES TUBELESS TIRE BONDING COMPOUND
(Bowes)

Toluol * .... >80%

BOWES WINDSHIELD WASHER ANTIFREEZE
(Bowes)

Methanol * .... >80%

BOWL CLEAN (HEAVY DUTY & SUPER EMULSION)
Liquid toilet bowl cleaners
(Hillyard Chem.)

Hydrochloric acid *

'76 Ed.

BOWL CLEAN, REGULAR & SUPER
(Hillyard Chem.)

Hydrochloric acid *

'76 Ed.

BOWL CREME
Cleans, disinfects, deodorizes toilets & urinals
(Varley, James)

Hydrogen chloride * 27.64%
Para-diisobutyl phenoxy ethoxy
ethyl dimethyl benzyl ammonium chloride 0.20%
o-Benzyl p-chlorophenol 0.15%

BOWLENE
Toilet bowl cleaner
(Climaco)

Sodium bisulfate *

BOWL KLEAN

See SCHNEID'S BOWL KLEAN

BOWL POWER
Toilet bowl cleaner
(Lehn & Fink)

Granular Calcium hypochlorite * .. 65%

BOWL QUICK
Institutional and industrial cleaning product

Procter & Gamble Co.
Ivorydale Technical Center
Cincinnati, Ohio 45217

Phone: 513-562-1100

BOWMAN COLD TABLET (C.T. YELLOW OBLONG)
(Bowman Pharm.)

Each tablet:
Acetaminophen * .... 324.0 mg.
Phenylpropanolamine HCl . 24.3 mg.
Caffeine .... 16.2 mg.

BOWMAN COUGH SYRUP
(Bowman Pharm.)

Each 5 cc.:
Guaifenesin .... 100.0 mg.
Phenylpropanolamine HCl * 12.5 mg.
Dextromethorphan HBr ... 10.0 mg.
Alcohol 15%

BOWTUSSIN D.M. (GREEN)
(Bowman Pharm.)

Each 5 cc.:
Guaifenesin .... 100 mg.
Dextromethorphan HBr * ... 15 mg.
Alcohol 15%

BOW-WOW FLEA KILLER
(Sweeney, W. R.)

Pyrethrins 0.5%

BOYLEX
Drawing salve
(Approved Pharm.)

Diperodon
Hexachlorophene
Rosin cerate
Ichthammol
Carbolic acid *
Juniper tar
Thymol *
Camphor *

'76 Ed.

BOYSEN PAINT PRODUCTS

Boysen Paint Co.
P.O. Box 23543
Oakland, Calif. 94623

Phone: 415-653-9211

See PAINTS, Section VI, General Formulations

Starred ingredients (*) may be responsible for major toxic effects; consult Section II.

B-P ASEPTO DISINFECTANT DEODORANT
Aerosol disinfectant, air sanitizer and deodorant
(Bard-Parker)

Orthophenylphenol	0.176%
p-tert.-Amylphenol	0.044%
Essential oils	0.300%
Alcohol	53.460%

B-P CHLOROPHENYL
For surgical and dental instruments
(Bard-Parker)

Sodium salt of 2,2'-methylenebis(3,4,6-trichloro-phenol) (Hexachlorophene)	1.00%
Isopropanol	8.75%

B-P GERMICIDE
For surgical & dental instruments
(Bard-Parker)

Isopropanol *	65.26%
Methanol	2.75%
Formaldehyde *	8.00%
Sodium salt of 2,2'-methylenebis(3,4,6-trichloro-phenol) (Hexachlorophene)	0.50%

BP LO-VOL 4D
Herbicide
(Diamond Shamrock Corp.)

2,4-Dichlorophenoxyacetic acid, bu-toxy propyl esters *	72.8%

BPN OINTMENT
Antibiotic agent
(Norwich-Eaton)

Bacitracin	500 units/gm.
Polymyxin B (as sulfate)	5000 units/gm.
Neomycin (as sulfate)	3.5 mg./gm.
Petrolatum base	

B.P.P.-LEMMON
Antidiarrheal
(Lemmon Co.)

Each tablet:
Powdered Opium (equiv. to 0.3 ml. paregoric) *	1.2 mg.
Bismuth subgallate	120 mg.
Pectin	15 mg.
Kaolin	120 mg.
Zinc phenolsulfonate *	15 mg.

B.P.P. WAFERS
Antidiarrheal
(Wesley Pharm.)

Each wafer:
Opium *	1.2 mg.
Bismuth hydroxide	1/2 gr.
Kaolin colloidal	2 1/2 gr.
Pectin N.F.	1/2 gr.
Flavored base	q.s.

BPS GLOSS REMOVER
(BPS Paint Co.)

Xylol *
Ethanol

BPS PAINT THINNER
(BPS Paint Co.)

Petroleum distillate *

BPS PAINT & VARNISH REMOVER (Non-Flammable)
(BPS Paint Co.)

Methylene chloride *
Methanol *

BPS WATER REPELLENT CLEAR COATING
For exterior masonry surfaces
(BPS Paint Co.)

Silicone resin	5.0%
Petroleum distillates *	95.0%

BQ COLD TABLETS
Analgesic, decongestant, antihistamine
(Bristol-Myers)

Each tablet:
Acetaminophen	325 mg.
Phenylpropanolamine HCl *	12.5 mg.
Chlorpheniramine maleate	2 mg.

B.Q.R.
For colds
(Calotabs)

Alcohol	8 1/2%
Fluid extract Cascara sagrada aromatic	
Sodium salicylate *	
Syrup of Ipecac *	
Menthol *	
Balsam Peru	
Elixir lactated Pepsin	

BR-5512
Heavy duty cleaner
(DuBois Chem.)

Caustic soda *
Sodium salts of phosphates and silicates
Nonionic surfactant

BRACEOIL
Veterinary - external analgesic
(Thoroughbred)

Menthol	0.250%
Camphor *	1.023%
Thymol	0.100%
Capsicum	0.200%
Methyl salicylate *	2.300%
Oil of distilled pine	
Oil of juniper	
Salicylic acid	0.660%
Cyncal 14 (Alkyl di-methyl-ben-zyl ammonium chlorides)	50 ppm
Gov't. Alcohol (S.D.A.) *	75%/vol.

BRADLEY, MILTON, TOYS AND SCHOOL SUPPLIES

Milton Bradley Co.
P.O. Box 2209
Springfield, Mass. 01101

Phone: 413-525-6411

BRAGGI TOILETRIES
(Revlon)

Revlon, Inc.
767 Fifth Ave.
New York, N.Y. 10153

Phone: 212-572-5000

Revlon Research Center, Inc.
945 Zerega Ave.
Bronx, N.Y. 10473

Phone: 212-824-9000

See COSMETICS, Section VI, General Formulations

BRAND-EM-OL

See FRANKLIN BRAND-EM-OL

BRANDY HARVEST COLOGNES

Brandy Harvest Colognes
53-06 39th Ave.
Woodside, N.Y. 11377

Phone: 212-899-1279

See COSMETICS, Section VI, General Formulations

BRASIVOL
Acne scrub cleaner, three grades (fine, medium, rough)
(Stiefel Labs.)

Synthetic Aluminum oxide particles
Surfactant cleansing base
Polyoxyethylene lauryl ether

BRASS BLACK TOUCH-UP
(Birchwood Casey)

Selenium dioxide *
Methanol

BRASSO
Brass polish
(French, R. T.)

Kerosene *	60-70%
Fatty acids	8%
Anhydrous Ammonia	0-1%
Chalk	25-30%
Perfume	0-0.13%

BRAUN SHAVER CLEANING FLUID
(Braun North America)

n-Propanol *	90.0%
Tetrachloroethylene	9.5%
Petroleum distillates	0.5%

Starred ingredients (*) may be responsible for major toxic effects; consult Section II.

BRAVE NO PHOSPHATE LAUNDRY DETERGENT
(Wakefern; supplier, Witco Chem.)

Sodium carbonate *
Sodium sulfate
Anionic surfactant (Sodium tridecyl benzene sulfonate)
Sodium silicate (1:2.4 ratio)(not meta)
Sodium chloride
Moisture
Sodium carboxymethylcellulose
Anti-caking agents
Fluorescent whiteners
Perfume
Blue coloring (if applicable)

BRAVO 500
Fungicide
(Diamond Shamrock Corp.)

Chlorothalonil ... 40.4%

BRAVO 6F
Fungicide
(Diamond Shamrock Corp.)

Chlorothalonil
(Tetrachloroisophthalonitrile) ... 54%

BRAVO W-75
Fungicide
(Diamond Shamrock Corp.)

Chlorothalonil
(Tetrachloroisophthalonitrile) ... 75%

BRAWN

See AIRWICK PROFESSIONAL PRODUCTS BRAWN

BRAWNY
Degreaser
(Holcomb)

Kerosene * ... >10%

'76 Ed.

BRAWNY FLOOR WAX

See BUTCHER'S BRAWNY FLOOR WAX

BREACOL DECONGESTANT COUGH MEDICATION, REGULAR AND MENTHOLATED
Antitussive-decongestant-antihistaminic
(Glenbrook Labs.)

Each 5 ml.:
Synephenol-D (brand of Phenylpropanolamine HCl) * ... 37.5 mg.
Dextromethorphan hydrobromide ... 10 mg.
Chlorpheniramine maleate ... 4 mg.
Alcohol ... 10%

BREAK-POINT FR-65

See BIO-GUARD BREAK-POINT FR-65

BREASE ANTITUSSIVE
(King Pharmaceutical)

Each 5 cc:
Potassium iodide * ... 324 mg.
Glycerylguaiacolate ... 100 mg.
Chlorpheniramine maleate ... 2 mg.
Ephedrine sulfate * ... 4 mg.

BREATH O' PINE
All purpose cleaner
(Brondow, Inc.)

Pine oil * ... 40%
Neutral soap ... 15%
Isopropyl alcohol ... 5%

BREEZEE MIST FOOT POWDER
Anti-perspirant, fungicide and deodorant
(Pedinol)

Aluminum chlorohydroxide *
Undecylenic acid *
Zinc undecylenate *
Menthol *

BREEZE (Low Phosphate)
Powder laundry detergent
(Lever Bros.)

Sodium sulfate * ... 20-45%
Sodium polyphosphate * ... 20-30%
Anionic detergent ... 10-20%
Sodium silicate ... 5-10%
Water ... 5-10%
Sodium carbonate ... 0-5%
Cellulosic ... <1%
Perfume ... <1%
Optical dye ... trace

BREEZE (Nonphosphate)
Powder laundry detergent
(Lever Bros.)

Sodium carbonate * ... 30-40%
Sodium sulfate * ... 10-30%
Anionic detergent ... 10-20%
Sodium silicate ... 10-20%
Water ... 1-5%
Cellulosic ... <1%
Perfume ... <1%
Optical dye ... trace

BRETOL
Germicide
(Fine Organics, Inc.)

Cetyl dimethyl ethyl ammonium bromide * ... 100%

'76 Ed.

BREVICON 21- AND 28-DAY TABLETS
Oral contraceptive agent
(Syntex F.P.)

Each active tablet (21/package):
Norethindrone ... 0.5 mg.
Ethinyl estradiol ... 0.035 mg.

28-Day package also contains 7 inert tablets

BREWER INSTITUTIONAL DESCALER
Dishmachine scale remover
(Brewer Chem.)

Phosphoric acid * ... 90-100%
Glycolic acid ... <5%

BREWER SUPER RINSE AID
Liquid dishmachine rinse detergent
(Brewer Chem.)

Modified terminated Alkyl aryl ether ... approx. 40%
Isopropyl alcohol ... <5%

BREWER SUPER SOUR
Laundry neutralizer
(Brewer Chem.)

Citric acid (anhydrous)* ... 50-60%

BREXIN CAPSULES
Decongestant
(Savage Labs.)

Each capsule:
Pseudoephedrine hydrochloride (USP) * ... 60 mg.
Pyrilamine maleate (USP) ... 30 mg.
Guaifenesin (USP) ... 100 mg.

BREXIN L.A. CAPSULES
Temporary relief of cold symptoms, allergic rhinitis, sinusitis
(Savage Labs.)

Each capsule:
Chlorpheniramine maleate (USP) * ... 8 mg.
Pseudoephedrine hydrochloride (USP) * ... 120 mg.

BREXIN LIQUID
Temporary relief of cough, cold symptoms
(Savage Labs.)

Each 5 ml.:
Pseudoephedrine hydrochloride (USP) * ... 30 mg.
Pyrilamine maleate (USP) ... 15 mg.
Guaifenesin (USP) ... 100 mg.

BRICKLEEN-DC
For cleaning dark colored brick work
(Haviland Products Co.)

Phosphoric acid *
Hydrochloric acid *
Non-ionic surfactant

'76 Ed.

BRICKLEEN LC
For cleaning light colored brick work
(Haviland Products Co.)

Sulfuric acid *
Hydrochloric acid *
Non-ionic surfactant

'76 Ed.

BRICON BACKRUBBER INSECTICIDE

See FRANKLIN BRICON BACKRUB-
BER INSECTICIDE

BRIDAL BOUQUET BATH OIL
(Dana Perfumes)

Essential oils * .... >1%
Mineral oil
Isopropyl myristate
Lanolin oil
Tegester (Spreading agent)

BRIDAL BOUQUET DUSTING POWDER
(Dana Perfumes)

Essential oils * .... >1%
Aromatic chemicals
Talc
Zinc stearate
Magnesium carbonate

BRIDAL BOUQUET EAU DE COLOGNE
Size - 4 oz.
(Dana Perfumes)

Essential oils * .... >1%
Aromatic chemicals
Specially denatured Alcohol (39-C) *
Deionized water

BRIDAL BOUQUET PERFUME
Sizes - 1/8, 1/4, 1/2, & 1 oz.
(Dana Perfumes)

Essential oils * .... >1%
Aromatic chemicals
Specially denatured Alcohol (39-C) *

BRIDAL BOUQUET PRESSED BATH POWDER CAKE
Size - 4 oz.
(Dana Perfumes)

Essential oils * .... >1%
Aromatic chemicals
Talcs
Stearates
Salts

BRIDAL BOUQUET SPRAY COLOGNE
Aerosol - 3 oz.
(Dana Perfumes)

Essential oils * .... >1%
Aromatic chemicals
Specially denatured Alcohol (SD39C) *
Dichlorodifluoromethane
Dichlorotetrafluoroethane

BRIGADE (Test Market)
Automatic toilet bowl cleaner; Bleach Cake: Off-White Bar
(Procter & Gamble)

Hypochlorite salts (mostly
  calcium) * 25-49%
Sodium chloride 25-49%
Sodium metasilicate 5-9%
Misc. salts (mostly calcium and
  sodium) 5-9%
(Total available chlorine, 40%)

pH (1% solution) - 11.4

BRIGHTENIZE
Aluminum cleaner
(Holcomb)

Ammonium bifluoride 1-10%
Phosphoric acid * .... >10%

'76 Ed.

BRIGHT SHINE
Automotive finishes
(McAleer)

Mineral spirits *
Waxes
Silicone oils
Diatomaceous earth
Amyl acetate *

'76 Ed.

BRIGHT WATER LAUNDRY DETERGENT
Dry laundry detergent
(Great Atlantic & Pacific, mfr.; Compass Foods, dist.)

Sodium linear alkyl benzene
  sulfonate .... <17%
Sodium carbonate * .... <30%
Sodium silicate .... <10%
Sodium carboxymethylcellulose <2%
Optical brighteners .... <1%
Sodium chloride .... <10%
Dye .... trace
Sodium sulfate and moisture ... balance

BRILCO
Insecticide
(Brilco Labs.)

Pyrethrins 0.50%
Piperonyl butoxide (technical) .. 1.00%
N-Octyl bicycloheptene
  dicarboximide 1.50%
Chlorpyrifos (O,O-Diethyl O-(3,-
  5,6-trichloro-2-
  pyridyl)phosphorothioate) * .. 2.53%
Aromatic petroleum distillate * . 1.42%
Petroleum distillate * 87.88%

BRILIATE
For relief of nervous tension
(Approved Pharm.)

Each capsule:
  Phenyltoloxamine citrate * .. 88 mg.
  Salicylamide * .... 130 mg.

'76 Ed.

BRILLO CLEANSER
Household cleanser
(Purex Corp.)

Siliceous abrasive .... >85%
Alkaline builder 1-10%
Anionic surfactant 1-3%
Organic chlorine bleaching agent . <2%
Coloring agent .... <1%
Perfume .... <1%

BRILLO HOUSEHOLD CLEANER
Aqueous all purpose cleaner
(Purex Corp.)

Anionic surfactant 5-10%
Nonionic surfactant .... <5%
Alkaline builder 5-10%
Alkanolamide .... <5%
Sequestering agents .... <1%
Ammonia .... <1%
Opacifier .... <1%
Perfume .... <1%
Water .... balance

BRILLO KOSHER SOAP
(Purex Corp.)

Sodium coconut oil soap ...... >45%
Potassium coconut oil soap .... >15%
Glycerine 5-10%
Coloring agent .... <1%
Perfume .... <1%
Water .... balance

BRILLO RED KOSHER SOAP
(Purex Corp.)

Sodium coconut oil soap ...... >90%
Coloring agent .... <1%
Perfume .... <1%
Water .... balance

BRILLO SOAP PADS
Pot and pan scrubber
(Purex Corp.)

Sodium tallow-coconut oil soap ... >45%
Steel wool .... >43%
Nonionic surfactant 1-3%
Antioxidant 1-2%
Paraffin wax 1-2%
Coloring agent .... <1%
Perfume .... <1%

BRINKS
Invisible permanent ink
(Sanford Corp.)

Aromatic solvent:
  Xylene *
  Toluene *
Dyes
Resins

Starred ingredients (*) may be responsible for major toxic effects; consult Section II.

BRIOSCHI
Antacid
(Brioschi, Inc.)

Tartaric acid
Sodium bicarbonate

BRISK CAPSULES
For fatigue & hangover
(Pharmex)

Each timed disintegration capsule:
  Caffeine * . . . . 250 mg.

BRITE EYES LIQUID BLEACH
(National Allied Products)

Sodium hypochlorite * 5.25%
Water & salt 94.75%

BRITE KLEEN
Liquid detergent
(Kay Chem. Co.)

Anionic detergent * 20-35%
Chelating agent 2-4%

BRITE-KLENZ (FORMULA HC-19, FORMULA HC-20)

See KLENZADE BRITE-KLENZ (FORMULA HC-19, FORMULA HC-20)

BRITE MAGIC
Adhesive
(Miracle Adhesives)

Rubber
Resin
Pigments
Aliphatic petroleum hydrocarbon *

BRITEN-ZIT
Cleaner
(Hillyard Chem.)

Liquid soap

'76 Ed.

BRITE SPECIAL
Aluminum brightener
(Calgon Corp., Commercial Div.)

Hydrofluoric acid *
Ethylene oxide adduct
Sulfuric acid *

BRITEWAY CLEANER DISINFECTANT DEODORANT
(Dolge)

Soap 13.3%
Isopropanol 7.5%
o-Benzyl-p-chlorophenol 5.0%

BROADCIDE
Non-selective broad leaf weed killer
(Malter International)

Dimethylamine salt of 2,4-dichlo-
  rophenoxyacetic acid 4.94%
Potassium salt of 2-(2-methyl-4-
  chlorophenoxy)propionic acid
  (MCPP) * 12.95%

BROCADE DEODORANT TOILET BAR
(Safeway Stores)

Sodium soap 84%
Salt, Glycerine, Titanium dioxide,
  Perfume 3%
Deodorant (Trichlorocarbanilide) . . 1%
Moisture 12%

BROCADE LIQUID DETERGENT
(Safeway Stores)

Linear Alkyl aryl sulfonate
  (Na) * 18%
Linear Alcohol ethoxy sulfate
  (NH4) 10%
Lauric diethanolamide 4%
Sodium xylene sulfonate 8%
Combined amount: 0.5%
  Perfume
  Dye
  Polystyrene polymer
Water . . . . balance

BROCADE TOILET BAR
(Safeway Stores)

Sodium soap 85%
Salt, Glycerine, Titanium dioxide,
  Perfume 3%
Moisture 12%

BROMAT
Germicide
(Fine Organics, Inc.)

Cetyl trimethyl ammonium
  bromide * 100%

'76 Ed.

BROMEPAPH ELIXIR
(Columbia Med.)

Each 5 ml.:
  Brompheniramine maleate * . . . 4 mg.
  Phenylephrine HCl * . . . . 5 mg.
  Phenylpropanolamine HCl * . . . 5 mg.
  Alcohol 2.3%

BROMEPAPH EXTENDED-ACTION TABLETS
(Columbia Med.)

Each tablet:
  Brompheniramine maleate * . . 12 mg.
  Phenylephrine HCl * . . . . 15 mg.
  Phenylpropanolamine HCl * . . 15 mg.

BROMFED CAPSULES
Antihistamine - decongestant
(Muro Pharm.)

Each timed release capsule:
  Brompheniramine maleate . . . 12 mg.
  Pseudoephedrine HCl * . . . . . 120 mg.
  Nu-Pareil (Sucrose & starch) . 50%
  Hydrogenated Castor oil . . . . . <5%
  Pharmaceutical glaze . . . . <10%

BROMFED-PD CAPSULE
Antihistamine - decongestant
(Muro Pharm.)

Each timed release capsule:
  Brompheniramine maleate . . . . 6 mg.
  Pseudoephedrine HCl * . . . . . . 60 mg.
  Nu-Pareil . . . . >50%
  Hydrogenated Castor oil . . . . . <5%
  Pharmaceutical glaze . . . . <10%

BROMIDROSIS POWDER, DR. SCHOLL'S

See DR. SCHOLL'S BROMIDROSIS POWDER

BROMI-LOTION
Antiperspirant
(Gordon Labs.)

Aluminum hydroxychloride *†

†*See* Aluminum chlorohydroxide

BROMINAL
Postemergence weed killer
(Amchem)

Octanoic acid ester of Bromoxynil
  (3,5-Dibromo-4-
  hydroxybenzonitrile) * 33.4%

BROMINAL PLUS
Postemergence weed killer
(Amchem)

Octanoic acid ester of Bromoxynil
  (3,5-Dibromo-4-
  hydroxybenzonitrile) * 30.7%
Butoxyethanol ester of 2-Methyl-4-
  chlorophenoxy acetic acid 33.4%

BROMI-TALC
Deodorant foot powder
(Gordon Labs.)

Potassium alum
Bentonite
Talc

BROM-O-GAS
Fumigant
(Great Lakes Chem. Corp.)

Methyl bromide * 98%
Chloropicrin * 2%

BROMO-SECT W.E.
Control of flies and mosquitoes
(National Chemsearch)

Xylene * 81.0%
Beta-butoxy-beta-thiocyano-di-
ethyl ether 5.3%
Petroleum distillates 4.7%
Naled 4.6%

BROMO SELTZER
Analgesic antacid
(Warner-Lambert)

Each 80 gr.:
Acetaminophen * .... 325 mg.
Sodium bicarbonate ...... 2.781 gm.
Citric acid (when dissolved
forms sodium citrate - 2.848
gm.) .... 2.224 gm.

BRONATE
Herbicide
(Rhone-Poulenc)

Octanoic acid ester of
bromoxynil * 31.7%
Isooctyl ester of 2-methyl-4-chloro-
phenoxyacetic acid 34.0%

BRONCAJEN
(Jenkins Labs.)

Each tablet:
Pyrilamine maleate * .... 10 mg.
Phenylephrine HCl .... 2 mg.
Potassium guaiacol sulfonate .. 2 gr.
Ammonium chloride .... 2 gr.
Ipecac .... 1/8 gr.

BRONCHOBID
Bronchodilator
(Glaxo Inc.)

Each Duracap capsule:
Theophylline (anhydrous) * .. 260 mg.
Ephedrine hydrochloride * ... 35 mg.

BRONITIN
Asthmatic antispasmodic
(Whitehall Labs.)

Theophylline *
Ephedrine *
Methapyrilene HCl *
Glyceryl guaiacolate

BRONITIN MIST
Asthmatic bronchodilator
(Whitehall Labs.)

Epinephrine bitartrate *

BRONKAID MIST
Bronchodilator aerosol
(Winthrop Labs.)

Epinephrine 0.5%
Alcohol 33.0%
Ascorbic acid, USP 0.19%
Propellants:
Dichlorodifluoromethane
Dichlorotetrafluoromethane

BRONKAID TABLETS
Bronchodilator/expectorant
(Winthrop Labs.)

Each tablet:
Epinephrine sulfate, USP .... 24 mg.
Theophylline anhydrous,
USP * .... 100 mg.
Guaifenesin .... 100 mg.

BRONKODYL (CAPSULES & ELIXIR)
Bronchodilator
(Breon Labs.)

Each capsule:
Theophylline * ..... 100 mg.; 200 mg.

Elixir (each 15 ml.):
Theophylline * .... 80 mg.
Alcohol .... 20% v/v

BRONKOLIXIR
Bronchodilator, decongestant
(Breon Labs.)

Each 5 ml.:
Ephedrine sulfate * .... 12 mg.
Guaifenesin .... 50 mg.
Theophylline .... 15 mg.
Phenobarbital .... 4 mg.
Alcohol .... 19% v/v

BRONKOMETER
Bronchodilator
(Breon Labs.)

Each nebulizer contains:
Isoetharine mesylate ...... 0.61% w/w
Alcohol .... 30% w/w
Saccharin
Menthol
Ascorbic acid (preservative) 0.1% w/w
Fluorochlorohydrocarbons (propellants)

BRONKOSOL
Bronchodilator
(Breon Labs.)

Each ml.:
Isoetharine HCl 1%
Aqueous-glycerin solution containing:
Sodium chloride
Citric acid
Sodium hydroxide
Methylparaben
Propylparaben
Acetone sodium bisulfite

BRONKOSOL UNIT DOSE contains only
0.25% isoetharine HCl per ml.

BRONKOTABS
Bronchodilator, decongestant
(Breon Labs.)

Each tablet:
Ephedrine sulfate * .... 24 mg.
Theophylline * .... 100 mg.
Phenobarbital .... 8 mg.
Guaifenesin .... 100 mg.

BRO-NO-MOR
For infectious coryza in poultry; veter-inary
(Hilltop)

Sodium sulfathiazole ... 12.5 gm./100 cc.

'76 Ed.

BROWN'S N&B LINIMENT
For man or beast
(Brown Medicine Co.)

Alcohol *† 63 1/2%
Pine tar oil *
Carbolic acid *
Thyme oil *
Barbadoes tar
Turpentine *

†*See* Isopropyl alcohol

BROZONE

See DOW BROZONE

BRUCE ACRYLIC FOR WOOD
(Armour-Dial, Inc.)

Rule 66 Mineral spirits * 75-100%
Neocryl B-705 .... 5-10%
Piccotex 120 .... 1-5%
Minor ingredients (total) 0.1-1%

BRUCE CLEAN AND WAX FOR WOOD
(Armour-Dial, Inc.)

Rule 66 Mineral spirits * 75-100%
Paraffins and waxes 5-10%
Minor ingredients (total) 1-5%

BRUCE CLEANING WAX FOR WOOD (Industrial)
(Armour-Dial, Inc.)

Rule 66 Mineral spirits * 75-100%
Paraffins and waxes 5-10%
Minor ingredients (total) 1-5%

BRUCE DARK TONE WAX
(Armour-Dial, Inc.)

Rule 66 Mineral spirits * 75-100%
Waxes 10-25%
Minor ingredients (total) 1-5%

BRUCE DEEP CLEANER FOR WOOD
(Armour-Dial, Inc.)

Rule 66 Mineral spirits * 75-100%
Paraffin wax 1-5%
Minor ingredients (total) 1-5%

Starred ingredients (*) may be responsible for major toxic effects; consult Section II.

BRUCE 5-MINUTE WAX AND ACRYLIC REMOVER
(Armour-Dial, Inc.)

Water	75-100%
Tripropylene glycol methyl ether	1-5%
Ammonia	0.1-1%
Minor ingredients (total)	1-5%

BRUCE FLOOR CLEANER
(Industrial)
(Armour-Dial, Inc.)

Rule 66 Mineral spirits *	75-100%
Paraffin wax	1-5%
Minor ingredients (total)	1-5%

BRUCE LIQUID PASTE WAX FOR WOOD
(Armour-Dial, Inc.)

Rule 66 Mineral spirits *	75-100%
Waxes	10-25%
Minor ingredients (total)	0.1-1%

BRUCE 1-STEP FOR WOOD
(Armour-Dial, Inc.)

Rule 66 Mineral spirits *	75-100%
Neocryl B-705	5-10%
Piccotex 120	1-5%
Minor ingredients (total)	0.1-1%

BRUCE PASTE WAX
(Armour-Dial, Inc.)

Rule 66 Mineral spirits *	75-100%
Shellwax	10-25%
Other waxes	5-10%
Minor ingredients (total)	1-5%

BRUDER PAINT PRODUCTS

M. A. Bruder & Sons, Inc.
600 Reed Rd.
Broomall, Pa. 19008

Phone: 215-353-5100

See PAINTS, Section VI, General Formulations

BRULIN'S 2,4-D LIQUID WEED KILLER - 20%
(Brulin)

Dimethylamine salt of 2,4-D dichlorophenoxyacetic acid *	24.7%

BRULIN'S EM-50
Insecticide
(Brulin)

Malathion *	50%
Xylene *	35%

BRULIN'S FORMULA #350 INSECTICIDE
(Brulin)

Piperonyl butoxide technical	1.75%
Pyrethrins	0.35%
Petroleum distillate *	97.90%

BRULIN'S NON-SELECTIVE WEED KILLER
Herbicide
(Brulin)

Sodium arsenite *	45.5%

BRULIN'S 7-X CONCENTRATE
Insecticide
(Brulin)

Beta-butoxy beta'-thiocyano diethyl ether *	10.5%
Malathion (O,O-Dimethyl dithiophosphate of diethyl mercaptosuccinate) *	18.0%
Petroleum hydrocarbons *	71.5%

BRUNING PAINT PRODUCTS

Bruning Paint (Maryland)
601 S. Haven St.
Baltimore, Md. 21224

Phone: 301-342-3636

See PAINTS, Section VI, General Formulations

BRUSHKILLER 170
Herbicide
(Amchem)

2,4-Dichlorophenoxypropionic acid, butoxyethanol ester *†	31.1%
2,4-Dichlorophenoxyacetic acid, butoxyethanol ester *	31.8%

†*See* 2-(2,4-Dichlorophenoxy)propionic acid

BRUSHKILLER 171
Herbicide
(Amchem)

2,4-Dichlorophenoxypropionic acid, butoxyethanol ester *†	21.7%
2,4-Dichlorophenoxyacetic acid, butoxyethanol ester *	17.7%

†*See* 2-(2,4-Dichlorophenoxy)propionic acid

BRUSH-RHAP AMINE A-2D-2T
Herbicide
(Vertac)

Dimethylamine salt of 2,4-dichlorophenoxyacetic acid (equiv. to 20.5% of 2,4-dichlorophenoxyacetic acid) *	24.7%
Triethylamine salt of 2,4,5-trichlorophenoxyacetic acid (equiv. to 20.5% of 2,4,5-trichlorophenoxyacetic acid) *	28.6%

BRUSH-RHAP A-4T
Herbicide
(Vertac)

Triethylamine salt of 2,4,5-trichlorophenoxyacetic acid (equiv. to 40.8% of 2,4,5-T acid) *	57.0%

BRUSH-RHAP LV 2D-2T
Herbicide
(Vertac)

2-Ethylhexyl ester of 2,4-dichlorophenoxyacetic acid (equiv. to 23% of 2,4-dichlorophenoxyacetic acid) *	34.7%
2-Ethylhexyl ester of 2,4,5-trichlorophenoxyacetic acid (equiv. to 23% of 2,4,5-trichlorophenoxyacetic acid) *	33.1%

BRUSH-RHAP LV-4T
Herbicide
(Vertac)

2-Ethylhexyl ester of 2,4,5-trichlorophenoxyacetic acid (equiv. to 45.4% of 2,4,5-trichlorophenoxyacetic acid) *	65.3%

BRUSH-RHAP LV-6T
Herbicide
(Vertac)

2-Ethylhexyl ester of 2,4,5-trichlorophenoxyacetic acid (equiv. to 60.4% of 2,4,5-trichlorophenoxyacetic acid) *	87.0%

BRUSH-RHAP OXY-4T
Herbicide
(Vertac)

Butoxy-ethanol ester of 2,4,5-trichlorophenoxyacetic acid (equiv. to 44.9% of 2,4,5-trichlorophenoxyacetic acid) *	62.5%

BRYKO
(Pennwalt)

Non-ionic detergent

Starred ingredients (*) may be responsible for major toxic effects; consult Section II.

BRYLCREEM
Hair dressing
(Beecham Products)

Mineral oil
Beeswax
Calcium hydroxide
Stearic acid

BTC-2125
Disinfectant
(Onyx)

Alkyl dimethyl ethylbenzyl ammonium chloride *
Alkyl dimethyl benzyl ammonium chloride *

BTC 50% USP
Germicide
(Onyx)

Alkyl dimethyl benzyl ammonium chloride USP *

BUBBLE CLUB LIQUID
Bubble bath
(Purex Corp.)

Anionic surfactant	7-15%
Alkanolamide	1-5%
Solubilizer	1-5%
Ethyl alcohol	<1%
Coloring agent	<1%
Perfume	<1%
Water	balance

BUBBLE JEWELS
Bath oil capsules
(Delagar)

Each capsule:
Mineral oil	
Perfume oil *	2.5%
Nonionic surfactant	1.25%
Isostearic acid (in yellow (Exotic perfume), red (Rose perfume), green (Pine perfume), and lilac (Lilac perfume))	2.00%

'76 Ed.

BUBBLE-LITES
(Noma-World Wide)

Each vial:
Methylene chloride *	3 1/2 cc

BUCACET IMPROVED THROAT LOZENGE
(Lemmon Co.)

Each lozenge:
Cetylpyridinium chloride	2.5 mg.
Terpin hydrate	10 mg.
Benzocaine	15 mg.
Sodium citrate	32.4 mg.
Mannitol	
Sorbitol	

BUCHU, JUNIPER AND POTASSIUM ACETATE N.F.

See LILLY BUCHU, JUNIPER AND POTASSIUM ACETATE N.F.

BUCKLEY'S MIXTURE
Cough and cold remedy
(Buckley)

Ammonium carbonate	3.06%
Potassium bicarbonate	5.34%
Menthol	0.44%
Camphor	0.044%
Canada balsam	0.43%
Oil of Pine needles	0.076%
Tincture of Capsicum	0.05%
Glycerin	6.01%

BUCKLEY'S WHITE RUB
For muscular aches and pains
(Buckley)

Menthol *	3.588%
Camphor *	2.829%
Turpentine	1.346%
Methyl salicylate *	1.204%
Thymol	0.703%
Oil of cedar leaf	0.541%
Oleoresin of Capsicum	0.007%

BUCODERM CAPSULES
Control of pruritis and dermatoses in dogs
(Burns-Biotec)

Each capsule:
Prednisolone	5 mg.
Chlorpheniramine maleate *	1 mg.
Pyrilamine maleate *	1 mg.
Fatty acids	100 mg.
Vitamin A palmitate	5,000 IU
Inositol	8.5 mg.
Vitamin D2	150 IU
Vitamin E (as d-alpha Tocopheryl acid succinate)	5 IU

BUCTRIL
Herbicide
(Rhone-Poulenc)

Octanoic acid ester of bromoxynil *	33.8%

BUDENE
Synthetic rubber products and tires
(Goodyear)

Polybutadiene

BUELL CLEANER LQ-M NO. 555
(Polychem Corp.)

Water
Polyoxypropylene-polyoxyethylene block copolymer
Sodium xylene sulfonate
Anionic phosphate ester, potassium salt
Tetrasodium EDTA
Quaternium-15
Citric acid
FD & C Yellow #5

BUELL CLEANER-LQ NO. 444
(Polychem Corp.)

Sodium dodecyl benzene sulfonate
Water
Propylene glycol
Linear Alcohol ethoxylate
Oleic diethanolamide
Tetrasodium EDTA
Sodium xylene sulfonate

BUELL CLEANER-M NO. 333
(Polychem Corp.)

Sodium tripolyphosphate
Sodium metasilicate
Sodium carbonate
Urea
Terminated linear Alcohol ethoxylate
Tetrasodium EDTA

BUELL CLEANER NO. 222
(Polychem Corp.)

Sodium tripolyphosphate
Sodium carbonate
Sodium sulfate
Sodium bicarbonate
Sodium dodecyl benzene sulfonate
Sodium sesquicarbonate
Urea
Tetrasodium EDTA
Polyoxyethylene octyl phenyl ether
Sodium carboxymethyl cellulose

BUELL INSTRUMENT LUBRICANT NO. 999
(Polychem Corp.)

Water
Polybutene
Propylene glycol
Oleth-2
Oleth-20
Triethanolamine oleate
Sulfated Castor oil
DMDM hydantoin
Methylparaben
Propylparaben

BUENO
Herbicide
(Diamond Shamrock Corp.)

Monosodium acid methanearsonate *	35.19%

BUENO-6
Herbicide
(Diamond Shamrock Corp.)

Monosodium acid methanearsonate *	48.35%

BUFACET
For headache, neuralgia & common colds
(Jenkins Labs.)

Each tablet:
Acetylsalicylic acid *	3 1/2 gr.
Acetophenetidin *	2 1/2 gr.
Caffeine alkaloid	1/2 gr.
Aromatics	q.s.

Starred ingredients (*) may be responsible for major toxic effects; consult Section II.

BUFFABLE FLINT
Liquid floor polish
(Sanitek)

Acrylic polymer emulsion	10.4%
Diethylene glycol monoethyl ether (Cellosolve)	4.0%
Polyethylene emulsion	3.3%
Rosin maleate resin	1.5%
Tributoxyethyl phosphate	0.9%
Nonionic surfactant	0.3%
Formalin, Ammonia, Fluoro-chemical surfactant	trace
Water	balance

BUFFADYNE LEMMON
Buffered analgesic & antipyretic
(Lemmon Co.)

Each tablet:
Aspirin *	230 mg.
Phenacetin *	150 mg.
Caffeine	30 mg.

Buffered with Aluminum hydroxide gel (Dried), Magnesium hydroxide

BUFFALO DRY CHEMICAL RECHARGE
For fire extinguishers
(Norris Industries)

Sodium bicarbonate
Diatomaceous earth
Polysiloxane coating

'76 Ed.

BUFFAPRIN
Analgesic
(Buffington)

Each tablet:
Aspirin *
Buffered with Magnesium oxide

BUFFERIN
Analgesic
(Bristol-Myers)

Each tablet:
Aspirin *	5 gr.

Di-Alminate:
Aluminum glycinate
Magnesium carbonate

BUFFER-X
Spreader-activator-buffer for agricultural sprays
(Kalo)

Alkylarylpolyethoxy ethanol
Free and combined fatty and phosphatic acids
Isopropanol *

BUFFETS (SCORED)
Analgesic
(Bowman Pharm.)

Each tablet:
Aspirin *	226 mg.
Phenacetin	160 mg.
Caffeine	32 mg.

Buffered with Aluminum hydroxide gel

BUFFINOL
Analgesic
(Clapp, Otis)

Each tablet:
Aspirin *
Buffered with Magnesium oxide

BUFF-N-GLO
(Uncle Sam)

Acrylic & styrene polymers (metal cross-linked)
Resins (modified phenolic)
Wax
Ammonia *
Morpholine *
Plasticizers
Surfactants
Oleic acid
Potassium hydroxide *
Water

BUFF STUFF
Spray buff material
(Paul Koss)

Water	<95%
Modified Acrylic emulsion	
Morpholine *	<2%

pH 9.4-9.6

BUFF-UP FURNITURE POLISH

See AMWAY BUFF-UP FURNITURE POLISH

BUG BUSTER, GOOD-LIFE

See GOOD-LIFE BUG BUSTER

BUG-DETH

See ARAB BUG-DETH

BUG DEVIL
Fumigant
(Lester Labs.)

Ethylene dichloride *
Carbon tetrachloride *

'76 Ed.

BUG-E-VICT DUST, EXCELCIDE

See EXCELCIDE BUG-E-VICT DUST

BUG-GETA SNAIL & SLUG PELLETS
(Chevron)

Metaldehyde *	3.25%/w

Chevron emergency phone number: 415-233-3737

BUG-NIP
Insecticide for house & garden
(NIP-CO)

Pyrethrins	0.250%
n-Octyl sulfoxide of isosafrole	1.100%
Related compounds	0.150%
Petroleum distillate	1.000%

BUG-OFF
Insect repellent; industrial and institutional use
(Scientific International)

N,N-Diethyl-meta-toluamide	3.78%
Other isomers	0.42%
N-Octyl bicycloheptene dicarboximide (MGK 264)	1.20%
2,3:4,5-Bis(2-butylene)tetrahydro-2-furaldehyde	0.30%
Di-n-propyl isocinchomeronate	0.30%

BUGSBEGONE
Roach spray
(Carpenter, W.D.)

o-Isopropoxyphenyl methylcarbamate	1%
2-Butoxyethanol *	9%
Petroleum distillate *	90%

BULB-SAVER
Fungicide
(Nott)

Thiram *	10.0%

BULK LYSOL BRAND DISINFECTANT
(Nat'l Labs. Div.)

Soap	16.50%
o-Phenylphenol	2.80%
o-Benzyl-p-chlorophenol	2.70%
Alcohol	1.80%
Xylenols *	1.50%
Isopropyl alcohol	0.90%
Tetrasodium ethylenediaminetetraacetate	0.76%

BULLARD'S A.B.T./(AFTER BURN RELIEF)

See A.B.T./(AFTER BURN RELIEF)

BULLARD'S MEDICATED OINTMENT-R
All-purpose first-aid cream
(Bullard)

Ichthammol	1%
Camphor	<1%
Menthol	<1%
Zinc oxide	1-10%
Isopropyl alcohol *	
8-Hydroxyquinoline benzoate	<1%
Vanishing cream base	>10%

Starred ingredients (*) may be responsible for major toxic effects; consult Section II.

BULLDOG LINOLEUM PASTE
Adhesive
(Templar)

Clays
Water solution of:
  Wood sugars
  Calcium lignosulfonates

BULL-DOG WART REMOVER
(Commerce Drug)

Flexible Collodion
Salicylic acid *

BULLS-EYE
*Flexible body filler with cream harde-
ner*
(Bondo Corp.)

Polyester resin
Promoters: . . . . very small amount
  Metallic Naphthenate
  Aniline derivative
Benzoyl peroxide (as
  catalyst) * 50%
Filler:
  Talc

'76 Ed.

BULLS EYE SHELLAC (3 lb. cut)
(Zinsser, Wm., & Co.)

Pure Shellac 30.7%
Special Industrial Solvent No.
  4 (approx. percentage com-
  position by volume): 69.3%
  Ethyl alcohol 80%
  Methyl alcohol 4%
  Isopropyl alcohol * 15%
  Methyl isobutyl ketone 1%

BULLS EYE SPRAY SHELLAC
(Zinsser, Wm., & Co.)

Non-volatile:
  Shellac resin 11.8%
Volatile:
  Ketones * 28.4%
  Alcohols * 39.5%
Propellant:
  Aliphatic hydrocarbons (Pro-
  pane-Isobutane) 20.3%

BUMINTEST
Urine protein reagent tablet
(Ames)

Each tablet:
  Boric acid * . . . . 56 mg.
  Sulfosalicylic acid * . . . . 400 mg.
  Sodium bicarbonate

BUQUETS
See AMLAB BUQUETS

BURDEO
Non-irritating deodorant gel
(Hill Dermaceuticals)

Aluminum acetate basic
Boric acid *
Hexachlorophene

BUREN IMPROVED TABLETS
Urinary analgesic
(Ascher, B.F.)

Each tablet:
  Phenazopyridine
    hydrochloride * . . . . 150 mg.
  Butabarbital * . . . . 15 mg.
  l-Hyoscyamine sulfate . . . . . 0.125 mg.

BURNISHINE
Silver polishing cream
(Burnishine)

Soap
Silica
Soda ash
Camphor *
Sassafras

BURNISHINE ALUMINUM BRIGHTENER
(Burnishine)

Acids *
Emulsifiers
Surface active agents
Organic solvents

BURNISHINE CHROME AND METAL POLISH
(Burnishine)

Petroleum solvents *
Abrasives
Emulsifiers
Residual agents

BURNISHINE MOW-POWER
Conditioner for lawn mower engines
(Burnishine)

Isopropanol *
o-Dichlorbenzene *
Range oil *
Rust inhibitors

BURN OUT
See BIO-GUARD BURN OUT

BURN OUT 35
See BIO-GUARD BURN OUT 35

BURNTAME
Burn and sunburn aerosol spray
(Cross)

Benzocaine 20%

BUROTOR
Astringent
(Torch)

Emulsion Aluminum acetate 5%

'76 Ed.

BURST LAUNDRY DETERGENT
(Colgate Palmolive)

Combined amount: 14%
  Alkyl benzene sulfonate *
  Soap
  Nonionic surfactant
Inorganic builders: 74.6%
  Phosphate *
  Silicate *
  Sodium sulfate
Color, perfume and minor
  ingredients 1.8%
Moisture 9.5%

'76 Ed.

BUTALAN ELIXIR
Sedative
(Lannett)

Each 30 cc.:
  Sodium butabarbital * . . . . 0.2 gm.

BUTALIX
Sedative
(Vale)

Each fl. oz.:
  Alcohol 10%
  Sodium butabarbital * . . . . . . 200 mg.

BUTATRAX SOLU-CAPS
Tranquilizer
(Sutliff & Case)

Each Solu-Cap:
  Amobarbital * . . . . 20 mg.
  Butabarbital * . . . . 30 mg.

'76 Ed.

BUTAZOLIDIN ALKA CAPSULES
Antiarthritic, anti-inflammatory agent
(Geigy Pharmaceuticals)

Each capsule:
  Phenylbutazone * . . . . 100 mg.
  Dried Aluminum hydroxide gel 100 mg.
  Magnesium trisilicate . . . . 150 mg.

BUTAZOLIDIN TABLETS
Antiarthritic - anti-inflammatory agent
(Geigy Pharmaceuticals)

Each tablet:
  Phenylbutazone * . . . . 100 mg.

Starred ingredients (*) may be responsible for major toxic effects; consult Section II.

BUTCHER'S AEROSOL SPRAY CLEANING POLISH
(Butcher Polish)

	approx. % by wt.
Silicone emulsion	7%
Isobutane/propane 90/10	4%
Wax	<1%
Perfume	trace
Water	balance

BUTCHER'S BOSTON POLISH
Solvent-based paste wax
(Butcher Polish)

Waxes	
Mineral spirits *	65%
Turpentine *	14%
Oil soluble dye	

BUTCHER'S BOUNTY FLOOR FINISH
(Butcher Polish)

	approx. % by wt.
Metal crosslinked all Acrylic polymer	29.5%
Nonionic polyethylene emulsion	7.0%
Diethylene glycol monomethyl ether	2.5%
Polyester type resin	<1.0%
Tributoxyethyl phosphate	<1.0%
Dibutyl phthalate	<1.0%
Dipropylene glycol monomethyl ether	<1.0%
Amphoteric fluorosurfactant	<1.0%
Silicone antifoam emulsion	<1.0%
Water	balance

BUTCHER'S BRAWNY FLOOR WAX
(Butcher Polish)

	approx. % by wt.
Blend of emulsifiable copolymers, Resins, Polyethylenes, Waxes (including carnauba wax)	15%
Tall oil fatty acid	1%
Morpholine	1%
Potassium hydroxide	<1%
Tributoxyethyl phosphate	<1%
Anionic fluorosurfactant	<1%
Preservative	<1%
Water	balance

BUTCHER'S BRIGHT WASHROOM CLEANER
(Butcher Polish)

	approx. % by wt.
Ethylene glycol monobutyl ether *	5%
Polyalkoxylated primary alcohol	2%
Tetrapotassium pyrophosphate	1%
Ammonia 26°	1%
Sodium metasilicate	<1%
Alkyl dimethylbenzyl ammonium chloride	<1%
Tetrasodium ethylenediamine tetraacetate	<1%
Corrosion inhibitor	<1%
Isobutane/Propane (90/10)	5%
Water and Perfume	balance

BUTCHER'S CAPTAIN QUICK STRIPPER
(Butcher Polish)

	approx. % by wt.
Monoethanolamine	4%
Ethylene glycol monobutyl ether *	3%
Sodium metasilicate	2%
Sodium hydroxide	<1%
Ethylene diamine tetraacetic acid	<1%
Amphoteric surfactant	<1%
Alkyl polyoxyalkalene ether	<1%
Sodium dioctyl sulfosuccinate	<1%
Lauryl dimethylamine oxide	<1%
Phosphate ester	<1%
Dye	trace
Water	balance

BUTCHER'S CHARGE BOWL CLEANER
(Butcher Polish)

	approx. % by wt.
Hydrochloric acid (20°) *	27%
Polyalkoxylated primary alcohol	3%
Alkyl dimethyl benzyl ammonium chloride	2.5%
Polyethylene based opacifier	2%
Ethylene thiourea	<1%
Perfume	<1%
Water	balance

BUTCHER'S COLONEL CUTTER SUPER STRIPPER
(Butcher Polish)

	approx. % by wt.
Monoethanolamine	6.0%
Ethylene glycol monobutyl ether *	6.5%
Sodium metasilicate	4%
Ammonia 26°	1%
Amphoteric surfactant	1%
Sodium hydroxide and EDTA acid	<1%
Phosphate ester surfactant	<1%
Sodium dioctyl sulfosuccinate	<1%
Lauryl dimethyl amine oxide	<1%
Dye and water	balance

BUTCHER'S FLOOR CLEANER & WAX REMOVER
(Butcher Polish)

	approx. % by wt.
Monoethanolamine	4%
Ethylene glycol monobutyl ether *	3%
Sodium metasilicate	2%
Ethylene diamine tetraacetic acid	<1%
Alkyl polyoxyalkalene ether	<1%
Sodium dioctyl sulfosuccinate	<1%
Sodium hydroxide	<1%
Lauryl dimethylamine oxide	<1%
Phosphate ester	<1%
Amphoteric surfactant	<1%
Dye	trace
Water	balance

BUTCHER'S FLO PASTE WAX
(Butcher Polish)

Waxes	
Mineral spirits *	88%
Perfume	

BUTCHER'S FOOTLIGHTS CARPET SHAMPOO
(Butcher Polish)

	approx. % by wt.
Modified Fatty alcohol sulfate	33%
Diethylene glycol monoethyl ether	1%
Primary amyl acetate	<1%
Optical brightener	<1%
Water	balance

BUTCHER'S GREEN STRIPE FLOOR WAX
(Butcher Polish)

	approx. % by wt.
Waxes	12%
Polyester resin	3%
Tall oil fatty acid	1%
Morpholine	1%
Potassium hydroxide	<1%
Tributoxyethyl phosphate	<1%
Fluorosurfactant	<1%
Preservative	<1%
Water	balance

BUTCHER'S LIQUID STOVE POLISH
(Butcher Polish)

	approx. % by wt.
Tall oil fatty acid	8%
Lampblack	5%
Carbon black	3%
Potassium hydroxide	<2%
Boiled Linseed oil	<2%
Graphite	1%
Lignosulfonate	<1%
Water	balance

BUTCHER'S PASTE STOVE POLISH
(Butcher Polish)

	approx. % by wt.
Graphite	15%
Tall oil fatty acid	13%
Carbon black	6%
Potassium hydroxide	2%
Colloidal Magnesium aluminum silicate	2%
Lampblack	1%
Water	balance

BUTCHER'S QUEST GERMICIDE CLEANER
(Butcher Polish)

Alkyl polyoxyalkalene ether	4%
Combined amount:	3%
n-Alkyl dimethyl benzyl ammonium chlorides *	
n-Alkyl dimethyl ethylbenzyl ammonium chlorides *	
Sodium carbonate	3%
Tetrasodium ethylene diamine tetraacetate	3%
Ethyl alcohol	<1%
Dye	trace
Perfume	trace
Water	balance

BUTCHER'S RED ROCKET DEGREASER
(Butcher Polish)

	approx. % by wt.
Ethylene glycol monobutyl ether *	4%
Diethylene glycol monoethyl ether *	4%
Sodium carbonate	3%
Anionic surfactant	2%
Sodium hydroxide	1%
Sodium metasilicate	1%
Sodium dioctyl sulfosuccinate	<1%
Amphoteric surfactant	<1%
Tetrasodium ethylenediamine tetraacetate	<1%
Balance:	
Water	
Red dye	
Silicone antifoam emulsion	

BUTCHER'S TILE WAX
(Butcher Polish)

Waxes
Sodium stearate
Butyl p-hydroxybenzoate
Tall oil fatty acid

BUTCHER'S WHITE DIAMOND BOWLING ALLEY WAX
(Butcher Polish)

Waxes	
Mineral spirits *	65%
Turpentine *	14%

BUTESIN PICRATE OINTMENT
For minor burns
(Abbott)

Butamben picrate	1%

BUTIBEL (ELIXIR AND TABLETS)
Antispasmodic-sedative
(McNeil Pharm.)

Each tablet/5 cc:
Sodium butabarbital *	15 mg.
Belladonna extract	15 mg.

BUTIBEL-ZYME TABLETS
Digestive aid
(McNeil Pharm.)

Each tablet:
Sodium butabarbital *	15 mg.
Belladonna extract	15 mg.
Proteolytic enzyme standardized	10 mg.
Amylolytic enzyme standardized	20 mg.
Cellulolytic enzyme standardized	5 mg.
Lipolytic enzyme standardized	100 mg.
Iron ox bile (45% cholic acid)	30 mg.

BUTICAPS
Daytime sedative
(McNeil Pharm.)

Each capsule:
Sodium butabarbital *	15 mg.; 30 mg.; 50 mg.; 100 mg.

BUTISOL SODIUM ELIXIR/ TABLETS
Daytime sedative
(McNeil Pharm.)

Sodium butabarbital *
Elixir (per 5 cc):	30 mg.
Tablets:	15 mg.; 30 mg.; 50 mg.; or 100 mg.
Alcohol (Elixir)	7%

BUTORINAL TABLETS
Analgesic, relaxant
(Pharmex)

Each tablet:
Isobutyl allylbarbituric acid *	3/4 gr.
Aspirin *	3 gr.
Phenacetin *	2 gr.
Caffeine	2/3 gr.

BUTOXONE
Herbicide
(Rhone-Poulenc)

Dimethylamine salt of 4-(2,4-dichlorophenoxy)butyric acid *	23.0%

BUTOXONE AMINE
Herbicide
(Rhone-Poulenc)

Dimethylamine salt of 4-(2,4-dichlorophenoxy)butyric acid *	26.2%

BUTOXONE ESTER
Herbicide
(Rhone-Poulenc)

Isooctyl ester of 4-(2,4-dichlorophenoxy)butyric acid *	38.6%

BUTOXONE SB
Herbicide
(Rhone-Poulenc)

Dimethylamine salt of 4-(2,4-dichlorophenoxy)butyric acid *	23.0%

BUTTERFLY TABLETS
(Cramer Products)

Calcium carbonate	500 mg.

BUTYL CAL-SEAL
Caulking compound
(Calbar)

Soybean oil
Polybutene
Soya lecithin
Butyl rubber
Mineral spirits *
Magnesium silicate
Calcium carbonate
Titanium dioxide

BUTYL 4D
Herbicide
(Diamond Shamrock Corp.)

Butyl ester of 2,4-dichlorophenoxyacetic acid *	53.6%

BUTYL 6D
Herbicide
(Diamond Shamrock Corp.)

Butyl ester of 2,4-dichlorophenoxyacetic acid *	73.5%

BUTYL-FLEX

See DAP BUTYL-FLEX

BUTYN DENTAL OINTMENT
(Abbott)

Butacaine	4%
Special ointment base	q.s.

BUTYRAC 118
Herbicide
(Amchem)

4-(2,4-Dichlorophenoxy) butyric acid, dimethylamine salt *	25.0%

BUTYRAC 175
Postemergence herbicide
(Amchem)

4-(2,4-Dichlorophenoxy) butyric acid, dimethylamine salt *	23.0%

BUTYRAC ESTER
Herbicide
(Amchem)

4-(2,4-Dichlorophenoxy) butyric acid, butoxy ethanol ester *	33.5%

BUX TEN GRANULAR
Insecticide
(Chevron)

m-(1-Methylbutyl)phenyl methylcarbamate *	7.5%
m-(1-Ethylpropyl)phenyl methylcarbamate *	2.5%

Chevron emergency phone number: 415-233-3737

BUZZ OFF
Insecticide: equine spray and rub-on
(Bio-Ceutic)

Pyrethrin	0.05%
Methoxychlor	0.50%
Butoxypolypropylene glycol	10.00%
Piperonyl butoxide	0.50%

BVMO-G FLAVORTABS
Geriatric supplement for dogs and cats
(Burns-Biotec)

Each tablet:
Diethylstilbestrol	0.05 mg.
Methyltestosterone	1 mg.
Thyroid	16.2 mg.
Plus multivitamins and minerals	

BY-SAW
Temporary relief of constipation
(Friendly Labs.)

Extract of Bile NF
Phenolphthalein yellow
Ext. Cascara sagrada *
Aloin *
Podophyllin *

BZQ 50
Used in the manufacture of plastic automotive patching compounds
(U.S. Peroxygen)

Benzoyl peroxide in phthalate-type ester plasticizer *

'76 Ed.

C

CABOT, SAMUEL, PAINT PRODUCTS
Paints, stains and wood preservatives

Samuel Cabot, Inc.
One Union St.
Boston, Mass. 02108

Phone: 617-723-7740

See PAINTS, Section VI, General Formulations

CABOT'S BAR-D-K
Wood preservative
(Cabot, Samuel)

Pentachlorophenol (technical) * 5%

CABOT'S PENTA-WOOD-SEAL
Wood preservative
(Cabot, Samuel)

Pentachlorophenol (technical) * 5%

CACHET MOISTURE CREME SOAP
(Chesebrough-Pond's)

Water	>50%
Sodium C14-16 olefin sulfonate	>10-25%
Cocamidopropyl betaine	>5-10%
Lauramide DEA	>1-5%
Linoleamide DEA	>1-5%
Glycol stearate	>0.1-1%
Fragrance	>0.1-1%
Disodium EDTA	>0.1-1%
DMDM hydantoin	>0.1-1%
Phosphoric acid	>0.1-1%
Methylparaben	>0.1-1%
Propylparaben	0.1% or less

CACHET MOISTURIZING BODY LOTION
(Chesebrough-Pond's)

Water	>50%
Glycerin	>1-5%
Mineral oil	>1-5%
Stearic acid	>1-5%
Glycol stearate and other ingred.	>1-5%
Acetylated Lanolin alcohol	>0.1-1%
Triethanolamine	>0.1-1%
Glyceryl stearate	>0.1-1%
Fragrance	>0.1-1%
Cetyl alcohol	>0.1-1%
Dimethicone	>0.1-1%
Magnesium aluminum silicate	>0.1-1%
Methylparaben	>0.1-1%
Propylparaben	0.1% or less
Carbomer-934	0.1% or less
Disodium EDTA	0.1% or less

C-A-D
Fungicide for turf
(National Chemsearch)

Cadmium chloride (equiv. to 12.2% as metallic cadmium) * 20.1%

CADDY
Turf fungicide
(Cleary)

Cadmium chloride * 20.1%

'76 Ed.

CADMINATE
Turf fungicide
(Mallinckrodt, Inc.)

Cadmium succinate * 60%

CADOPHILL
Eczema, seborrhea
(Torch)

Oil of cade (Juniper tar) *	5%
Sulfur precipitated	5%
Salicylic acid *	3%
Hydrophilic vehicle ad.	100%

'76 Ed.

CAFACETIN (C.T. GREEN)
(Bowman Pharm.)

Each tablet:
Phenacetin	162.0 mg.
Aspirin *	259.2 mg.
Gelsemium extract	4.9 mg.
Caffeine	16.2 mg.

CAFECON (Timed Disintegration Capsules)
Stimulant
(CMC Research Div.)

Each capsule:
Caffeine (1,3,7-Trimethylxanthine) * ..... 100 mg.

CAFERGOT (TABLETS & SUPPOSITORIES)
For migraine & other vascular headaches
(Sandoz)

Tablets (each):
Ergotamine tartrate USP *	1 mg.
Caffeine USP *	100 mg.

Suppositories (each):
Ergotamine tartrate USP *	2 mg.
Caffeine USP *	100 mg.

CAFERGOT P-B (TABLETS & SUPPOSITORIES)
For vascular headaches
(Sandoz)

Tablets (each):
Ergotamine tartrate USP *	1 mg.
Caffeine USP *	100 mg.
Bellafoline (levorotatory alkaloids of belladonna, as malates)	0.125 mg.
Pentobarbital sodium USP *	30 mg.

Suppositories (each):
Ergotamine tartrate USP *	2 mg.
Caffeine USP *	100 mg.
Bellafoline (levorotatory alkaloids of belladonna, as malates)	0.25 mg.
Pentobarbital sodium USP *	60 mg.

CAFOTAN TABLETS
Muscular aches & pains
(Premo)

Each tablet:
Aspirin *
Caffeine alkaloid *

'76 Ed.

CAF-TROL BOLUSES
For treatment of calf scours
(Hilltop)

Neomycin base (as sulfate)	125 mg.
Kaolin	3,750 mg.
Potassium chloride	100 mg.
Calcium gluconate	160 mg.
Magnesium carbonate	18 mg.
Sodium chloride	680 mg.
Sodium bicarbonate	448 mg.

'76 Ed.

Starred ingredients (*) may be responsible for major toxic effects; consult Section II.

CALADRYL (CREAM & LOTION)
For skin irritations
(Parke-Davis)

Benadryl hydrochloride * 1%
Calamine base

CAL-A-GRIN LOTION
Skin astringent
(Rogers Park)

Prepared neo-calamine
Magma of Bentonite
Carbolic acid liquefied *
Grindelia robusta fl. ext.
Sulfur precipitated
Benzocaine

CALA-HIST CALAMINE PLUS SPRAY
For itching of skin irritations
(Approved Pharm.)

Zirconium oxide 1%
Benzocaine 1%
Camphor 0.1%
Menthol 0.1%
Calamine 1%
'76 Ed.

CALCIDRINE SYRUP
Sedative, expectorant
(Abbott)

Each 5 ml.:
  Calcium iodide (anhydrous) .. 152 mg.
  Codeine * .... 8.4 mg.
  Alcohol 6%

CALDECORT
Antifungal, antipruritic, antiinflammatory
(Pennwalt, Pharm. Div.)

Hydrocortisone as the acetate 0.5%

CALDESENE OINTMENT
Promotes healing of diaper rash
(Pharmacraft)

Zinc oxide
Cod liver oil .... 15% w/w
Lanolin
Petrolatum
Talc

CALDESENE POWDER
Antibacterial, antifungal
(Pharmacraft)

Calcium undecylenate 10%

CALDEX
See ANCHOR CALDEX

CALDEX, M.P.
See ANCHOR CALDEX, M.P.

CALEATE OINTMENT
Relief of itching, pain & discomfort of skin poisoning
(Elder)

Pyrilamine maleate 0.125%
Zinc oxide 4.35%
Neo-calamine 4.35%

CALGON
Water conditioner & softener
(Beecham Products)

Vitreous sodium phosphate (Sodium hexametaphosphate)

CALGON BATH OIL BEADS
Bath water & skin conditioner
(Beecham Products)

Vitreous sodium phosphate (Sodium hexametaphosphate)
Fatty acid esters

CALGON BOUQUET
Bath water conditioner
(Beecham Products)

Vitreous sodium phosphate (Sodium hexametaphosphate)

CALGON BUBBLE BATH
Water conditioner and bubble bath
(Beecham Products)

Vitreous sodium phosphate (Sodium hexametaphosphate)
Anionic surfactant *

CALGON HAND CLEANSING LOTION
For industrial and office use
(Calgon Corp., Commercial Div.)

Glycols and glycol ethers *
Aliphatic hydrocarbons *
Emulsifying agents
Water

CALGONITE
Household dishwashing machine detergent
(Beecham Products)

Sodium tripolyphosphate *
Sodium silicate
Trisodium phosphate *
Sodium hypochlorite .... small amount
Nonionic surfactants .... small amount

CALGON SILICONE LOTION
For industrial use
(Calgon Corp., Commercial Div.)

Dimethyl polysiloxane 10%
Emulsifying agents
Water

CALICARB NO.1
Antacid
(Jenkins Labs.)

Each tablet:
  Calcium carbonate .... 4 gr.
  Magnesium carbonate ...... 2 1/2 gr.
  Bismuth subnitrate .... 1 gr.
  Powdered Ipecac .... 1/250 gr.
  Aromatics .... q.s

CAL-ICE
Antiseptic skin cream
(Commerce Drug)

Benzocaine
Calamine
Menthol *
Camphor *

CALICYLIC CREME
For removal of heavy callus
(Gordon Labs.)

Salicylic acid * 10%
Cream base

CALIFORNIA PAINT PRODUCTS

California Products Corp.
169 Waverly
Cambridge, Mass. 02139

Phone: 617-547-5300

See PAINTS, Section VI, General Formulations

CAL JET ALGAECIDE LIQUID
For swim pools
(Coastal Industries)

Alkyl dimethyl benzyl ammonium chloride (QUAT) * 7.5%
Sodium carbonate 2.5%
Water

CAL JET ALGAECIDE TABLETS
For swim and splasher pools
(Coastal Industries)

Dodecylbenzyl trimethyl ammonium chloride * 7.5%
Sodium carbonate * 92.5%

CALLAHAN'S SOLDERING FLUID
(Callahan)

Zinc ammonium chloride *
'76 Ed.

Starred ingredients (*) may be responsible for major toxic effects; consult Section II.

CALMOL 4 HEMORRHOIDAL SUPPOSITORIES
(Leeming Div.)

Norwegian cod liver oil
Lanolin
Zinc oxide
Bismuth subgallate
Balsam Peru
Cocoa butter base

CALOCIDE
Skin astringent
(Consolid. Royal)

Ammonium alum
Zinc sulfate *
Tannic acid

'76 Ed.

CALO-CLOR
Fungicide
(Mallinckrodt, Inc.)

Mercurous chloride * 60%
Mercuric chloride * 30%

CALODEX CREAM
(Wesley Pharm.)

Calamine
Pyrilamine *
Diperodon hydrochloride

CALO-GRAN
Turf fungicide for snow mold control
(Mallinckrodt, Inc.)

Mercurous chloride * 1.8%
Mercuric chloride * 0.9%

CALOTABS
Laxative
(Calotabs)

Each tablet:
Dioctyl sodium
    sulfosuccinate * .... 100 mg.
Casanthranol * .... 30 mg.

CALSA IMPROVED
Analgesic
(Amlab)

Each tablet:
Acetaminophen * .... 250 mg.
Salicylamide .... 250 mg.

CALSUL DORMANT SPRAY

See DEXOL CALSUL DORMANT SPRAY

CALSUXAPHEN CAPSULES
Sedative
(Lannett)

Each capsule:
Calcium succinate .... 2 1/2 gr.
Salicylamide * .... 4 gr.
Phenobarbital * .... 1/8 gr.
Ascorbic acid .... 30 mg.

CALVIN KLEIN COSMETICS

Calvin Klein Cosmetics Corp.
9 W. 57th St.
New York, N.Y. 10019

Phone: 212-759-8888

See COSMETICS, Section VI, General Formulations

CAMA
Buffered analgesic
(Dorsey Labs.)

Each tablet:
Aspirin (USP) * ..... (10 gr.) 600 mg.
Magnesium hydroxide
    (USP) .... 150 mg.
Aluminum hydroxide
    (dried gel) (USP) ... 150 mg.

CAMADINE
Analgesic
(Wesley Pharm.)

Each tablet:
Salicylamide .... 1 gr.
Acetophenetidin * .... 1/4 gr.
Caffeine citrate .... 1/10 gr.
Atropine sulfate .... 1/2000 gr.

CAMALOX (SUSPENSION & TABLETS)
Antacid
(Rorer, W.H., Inc.)

Each 5 ml. or tablet:
Magnesium hydroxide ...... 200 mg.
Aluminum hydroxide .... 225 mg.
Calcium carbonate .... 250 mg.

CAMAY
Soap bar
(Procter & Gamble)

Soap from animal and vegetable
    fats 75-100%
Water 10-24%
Fatty acid 5-10%
Perfume 1-4%
Sodium chloride 1-4%
Minor ingredients, each .... <1%

pH (1% solution) - 10.0

CAMEO ALUMINUM & STAINLESS STEEL CLEANER
(Purex Corp.)

Siliceous abrasive .... >80%
Corn starch 5-10%
Sulfamic acid 4-7%
Anionic surfactant 1-5%
Sodium silicofluoride * .... <3%
Perfume .... <1%

CAMEO COPPER CLEANER
(Purex Corp.)

Siliceous abrasive .... >80%
Sulfamic acid .... <6%
Perfume .... <1%
Anionic surfactant .... <4%
Nonionic surfactant .... <1%

CAMEO COSMETIC PRODUCTS

Cameo, Inc.
322 Ryder Rd.
Toledo, Ohio 43615

Phone: 419-531-5381

See COSMETICS, Section VI, General Formulations

CAMFO CREME

See FALK'S CAMFO CREME

CAMICIDE
Insect spray
(Campbell Chemicals, Inc.)

Refined Petroleum oil * 99.05%
N-Octyl bicycloheptene
    dicarboximide 0.50%
Technical Piperonyl butoxide ... 0.30%
Pyrethrins 0.15%

'76 Ed.

CAMPA CHEM
Deodorant for use in portable toilet holding tanks
(Thetford Corp.)

Formaldehyde * 20%
Methanol 6%
Nonionic surfactant .... <3%
Perfume oil .... <1%
Acid Blue #9 .... <1%
Water .... balance

CAMPA CHEM POWDER DEODORANT
Deodorizer for use in portable toilet holding tanks
(Thetford Corp.)

Paraformaldehyde * 80%
Sodium silico aluminate 10%
Inorganic phosphate .... <5%
Perfume oil .... <5%
Acid Blue #9 .... <5%

Starred ingredients (*) may be responsible for major toxic effects; consult Section II.

CAMPHO-PHENIQUE LIQUID
Topical anesthetic/antimicrobial
(Winthrop Labs.)

Phenol, USP	4.66%
Camphor, USP *	10.85%
Light mineral oil	84.08%
Aromatics	

CAMPHO-PHENIQUE POWDER
Topical anesthetic/antimicrobial
(Winthrop Labs.)

Camphor, USP *	4.375%
Phenol, USP *	2.000%
Talc	

CAMPTEX
(Texaco Canada Ltd.)

Petroleum distillate *

CAMTROPIN
Common cold and hay fever
(Jenkins Labs.)

Each tablet:
Caffeine alkaloid	1/12 gr.
Camphor	1/5 gr.
Atropine sulphate	1/600 gr.

CANDEX CREME & LOTION
Treatment of infections caused by Candida species (Monilia)
(Dome)

Each gram or ml.:
Nystatin (USP)	100,000 units
Carboxy vinyl polymer	
Sodium lauryl sulfate	
Hexadecyl alcohol	
Cetyl alcohol	
Dowicil 200	
Sodium hydroxide	
Citric acid	
Sodium citrate	
Purified water	

CANDLE-LITE'S CITRONELLA CANDLES
Mosquito and gnat repellent aid
(Candle-lite)

Active ingred.:	
Citronella oil	2%
Inert ingred.:	
Paraffin wax	98%

CANDO SILVER POLISH
(Wright, J.A.)

Water	
Diatomaceous earth	
Soap	
Sodium sesquicarbonate	<2%
or	
Sodium carbonate	<3%
Essential oil	
Dye	

CANEX
Acaricide - veterinary
(Pitman-Moore)

Rotenone	0.12%
Other ether extractions of cube	0.20%

CANINE CAPS

See MARTIN'S CANINE CAPS

CANOE AFTER SHAVE LOTION
Size - 3 11/16 oz.
(Dana Perfumes)

Essential oils *	>1%
Aromatic chemicals	
Alcohol 96	
Deionized water	
Menthol *	
Cremophor RH40 (PEG hydrogenated castor oil)	
Propylene glycol	
Aluminum chlorhydroxy allantoinate	

CANOE ANTI-PERSPIRANT SPRAY
Size - 5 oz.
(Dana Perfumes)

Essential oils *	>1%
Aromatic chemicals	
Cabosil M-5	
ArPacel 85	
PPG 14 butyl ether	
Aluminum chlorhydrate	
Chlorofluorocarbons	

CANOE DEODORANT STICK
Size - 2 3/4 oz.
(Dana Perfumes)

Essential oils *	>1%
Aromatic chemicals	
Propylene glycol	
Specially denatured Alcohol (SD40)	
Deionized water	
Sodium stearate	

CANOE DUSTING POWDER (TALC)
Size - 4 oz.
(Dana Perfumes)

Essential oils	>1%
Aromatic chemicals	
Talc	
Magnesium carbonate	
Iron oxide	

CANOE EAU DE COLOGNE
Sizes - 3 11/16 oz., 8 7/16 oz., 15 7/8 oz., & 32 7/16 oz.
(Dana Perfumes)

Essential oils *	>1%
Aromatic chemicals	
Specially denatured Alcohol (SD39-C) *	
Deionized water	

CANOE ROYALE COLOGNE
(Dana Perfumes)

Essential oils *	>1%
Aromatic chemicals	
Alcohol *	
Deionized water	

CANOE SOAP ON-A-ROPE
(Dana Perfumes)

Essential oils	>1%
Aromatic chemicals	
Tallow	
Glycerol	
Coconut oil	
Lanolin	
Water	

CANOE SOAP TOTE
(Dana Perfumes)

Tallow	
Essential oils	>1%
Aromatic chemicals	
Coconut oil	
Glycerine	
Lanolin	
Water	

CANOE SPRAY BODY TALC
Size - 8 oz.
(Dana Perfumes)

Essential oils	1%
Aromatic chemicals	
Talc	
Hydrocarbons (Isopar 687)	
Isopropyl myristate	
Trichlorofluoromethane	
Dichlorodifluoromethane	

CANTHARONE CANTHARIDIN COLLODION
Topical wart remover
(Seres Labs.)

Cantharidin *	0.7%
Acetone	
Flexible Collodion	
Ethocel	
Ether	35.0%
Alcohol	11.0%

CAN-TROL
Herbicide
(Rhone-Poulenc)

Sodium salt of 4-(2-methyl-4-chlorophenoxy)butyric acid *	23.5%

CAPAROL + MSMA WITH SURFACTANT
Herbicide
(Ciba-Geigy Ag. Div.)

Prometryn	8.4%
Monosodium acid methanearsonate *	33.6%

Starred ingredients (*) may be responsible for major toxic effects; consult Section II.

CAPAROL 80W
Herbicide
(Ciba-Geigy Ag. Div.)

Prometryn * 80%

CAPITAL WITH CODEINE
Analgesic
(Carnrick Labs.)

Each tablet:
Acetaminophen * .... 325 mg.
Codeine phosphate .... 30 mg.

CAPITAL WITH CODEINE SUSPENSION
Analgesic
(Carnrick Labs.)

Each 5 ml.:
Acetaminophen * .... 120 mg.
Codeine phosphate * .... 12 mg.

CAPRI CONCENTRATED FABRIC SOFTENER
(Industrial Equities)

Quaternary ammonium
compound * 5-10%
Fluorescent whitening agent ... <1%
Preservative .... <1%
Colorant .... <1%
Perfume .... <1%
Water .... balance

CAPRI LIQUID DISHWASHING DETERGENT
(Industrial Equities)

Anionic surfactant 6-12%
Hydrotrope 1-3%
Alkanolamide .... <1%
Ethyl alcohol .... <1%
Opacifier .... <1%
Colorant .... <1%
Perfume .... <1%
Water .... balance

CAPRON PAIN RELIEF CAPSULES
Analgesic
(Vitarine)

Each capsule:
Acetaminophen * .... 65 mg.
Aspirin * .... 227 mg.
Phenacetin * .... 162 mg.
Caffeine (anhydrous) .... 32.4 mg.

CAPTAIN KELLY FIRE EXTINGUISHER (5B:C)
(Gillette Appliance Div.)

Bicarbonated salt
Propellant

CAPTAIN QUICK STRIPPER

See BUTCHER'S CAPTAIN QUICK STRIPPER

CAPTAN MOLYSLICK
Insecticide
(MFA Oil Co.)

Captan 25%

CARBAX EMOLLIENT
For skin irritations
(Moss, Belle)

Propylene glycol
Polyethylene glycols

CARB-LIFE

See SILOO CARB-LIFE

CARB MEDIC
Carburetor cleaner
(Radiator)

Diacetone alcohol *
Aromatic solvents *

'76 Ed.

CARBO-CHLOR
Metal cleaner, spot remover, grease and tar remover
(Sunnyside)

1,1,1-Trichloroethane *

CARBOFF
Carbon remover
(Holcomb)

Cresol * .... >10%
Methylene chloride .... >10%
Trichlorethylene 1-10%

'76 Ed.

CARBOLINEUM WOOD PRESERVATIVE & INSECTICIDE
(Carbolineum)

Carbolineum Wood Preserving Co.
6683 N. 40th St.
Milwaukee, Wis. 53223

Phone: 414-353-5040

CARBOLIN OIL

See MARTIN'S CARBOLIN OIL

CARBONA CLEANING FLUID
(Carbona)

Combined amount: 25%
Trichloroethane * 75%
Perchloroethylene * 25%
Petroleum solvent * 75%

CARBONA NO. 10 SPECIAL SPOT REMOVER
(Carbona)

Combined amount: 25%
Perchloroethylene * 25%
1,1,1-Trichloroethane * 75%
Petroleum solvent * 75%

CARBONA PIN-POINT OILER
(Carbona)

Lightweight mineral lubricating oil   100%

CARBONA RUG & UPHOLSTERY SHAMPOO
(Carbona)

Combined amount: 19%
Sodium lauryl sulfate 90%
Dimethylene oxide 10%
Ethylene glycol monobutyl ether . 2.8%
Aqueous solution 78.2%
Preservative and optical
brightener .... <1.0%

CARBONA SHAMPOOZER FOR RUGS & UPHOLSTERY
(Carbona)

Sodium lauryl sulfate .... <1.0%
Sodium lauroyl sarcosinate ...... <1.0%
Ethylene glycol monobutyl ether . <1.0%
Preservative .... <1.0%
Optical brightener .... <1.0%
Aqueous solution 98.0%

CARBONA SPRAY FOAM RUG SHAMPOO
(Carbona)

Maleic anhydride-styrene
copolymer 2.3%
Ethylene glycol monomethyl ether 2.4%
Aqueous solution 84.1%
Lauric acid amide .... <1.0%
Sodium hydroxide .... <1.0%
Stearic acid .... <1.0%
Silica .... <1.0%
Ammonia .... <1.0%
Optical brightener .... <1.0%
Isobutane propellent 8.0%

CARBONA SPRAY SPOT REMOVER
(Carbona)

Perchloroethylene * 16%
1,1,1-Trichloroethane * 25%
Methylene chloride * 15%
Silica 4%
Propellant:
Freon 12 .... 32%
Isobutane 8%

CARBONA TILE & JOINT CLEANER
(Carbona)

Dow Corning Emulsion 921	4.00%
Versene	3.00%
Neutronyx 656 (Onyx Chem. Co.)	3.37%
Ethylene glycol monoethyl ether	3.37%
Wall-Wipe:	86.60%
Versene	2.37%
Neutronyx 656	3.54%
Ethylene glycol monoethyl ether	3.54%
Aqueous solution	90.45%

CARBONA WALL-WIPE
(Carbona)

Versene	2.37%
Neutronyx 656 (Onyx Chem. Co.)	3.54%
Ethylene glycol monoethyl ether	3.54%
Aqueous solution	90.45%

CARBON-MET - C.M. (Liquid; Ready to Use)

See GUNK C.M. - CARBON-MET (Liquid; Ready to Use)

CARB-O-SEP
Turkey blackhead preventive
(Whitmoyer)

p-Ureidobenzenearsonic acid (equiv. to 62.39 grains arsenic trioxide per oz. of Carb-O-Sep) *†	37.5%

†*See* Arsenic trioxide

CARBOTABS
Digestant, antacid
(Jenkins Labs.)

Each tablet:
Papain	1/32 gr.
Magnesium carbonate	1 gr.
Sodium bicarbonate	3 1/3 gr.
Pancreatin	1/32 gr.
Calcium carbonate	3/4 gr.

CARBRITAL KAPSEALS
Sedative hypnotic combination
(Parke-Davis)

Each Kapseal:
Pentobarbital sodium *	1 1/2 gr.
Carbromal *	4 gr.

CARCO CATTLE SPRAY
(Carpenter, W.D.)

Pyrethrins	0.05%
Technical Piperonyl butoxide	0.10%
N-Octyl bicycloheptene dicarboximide	0.16%
Di-n-propyl isocinchomeronate	0.20%
Petroleum distillate *	99.49%

CARCO FARM DISINFECTANT
(Carpenter, W.D.)

Sodium orthophenylphenate *	98%

CARDI-KOFF TABLETS
Cardiac weakness; veterinary
(Hart-Delta, Inc.)

Each tablet:
Digitalis *	484 mcg.
Strophanthin	13 mcg.
Sparteine sulfate	1.62 mcg.
Nitroglycerin *	approx. 130 mcg.
In a base of cactus powders	

'76 Ed.

CARDILATE-P TABLETS
Coronary vasodilator, sedative
(Burroughs Wellcome)

Each tablet:
Erythrityl tetranitrate *	10 mg.
Phenobarbital *	15 mg.

CARDILATE TABLETS
Coronary vasodilator
(Burroughs Wellcome)

Each tablet:
Erythrityl tetranitrate *	5 mg.; 10 mg.

CARDOXIN
Cardiotonic glycoside
(Vita Elixir Co.)

Each tablet:
Digoxin USP *	0.25 mg.

CARDUI
Tonic, antispasmodic
(Chattem)

Blessed thistle	
Alcohol	19%/v
Golden seal	

CARESS BEAUTY BAR
(Lever Bros.)

Acyl isethionate	45-55%
Fatty acids	15-25%
Sodium soap	10-15%
Water	5-10%
Sodium isethionate	1-5%
Anionic detergent	1-5%
Perfume	1-5%
Mineral oil	1-5%
Sodium chloride	<2%
Titanium dioxide	<1%
Colorants	trace

CAR-FRESHNER DEODORIZERS
(Car-Freshner)

Absorbent carrier containing:
Essential oils *
Animal aromatic extracts *†
Artificial aromatic products *†

†*See* Essential oils

CARGILL I-D/25-10
For treatment of seeds; soil insect & disease control
(Cargill)

Captan	10.0%
Heptachlor *	25.0%
Related compounds	9.7%
99% Gamma chlordane	
1% Nonachlor	

CARIN
Insecticide
(Techne Corp.)

Carbaryl (1-Naphthyl N-methyl-carbamate) *	24.4%

'76 Ed.

CARMEL FORMULA F-2
Insecticide
(Carmel Chem. Corp.)

Pyrethrins	0.20%
Piperonyl butoxide, technical	0.25%
Petroleum distillate *	99.55%

CARMEL FORMULA F-3
Insecticide
(Carmel Chem. Corp.)

Petroleum distillate *	97.75%
N-Octyl bicycloheptene dicarboximide	2.00%
Pyrethrins	0.25%

CARMEL FORMULA F-5
Insecticide
(Carmel Chem. Corp.)

Pyrethrins	0.5%
Technical Piperonyl butoxide	1.0%
N-Octyl bicycloheptene dicarboximide	1.0%
Petroleum distillate *	97.5%

CARMEL FORMULA F-500
Insecticide
(Carmel Chem. Corp.)

Resmethrin	0.500%
Related compounds	0.068%
Aromatic petroleum hydrocarbons	0.662%
Petroleum hydrocarbons *	98.750%

Starred ingredients (*) may be responsible for major toxic effects; consult Section II.

CARMEL FORMULA GH-18
Insecticide
(Carmel Chem. Corp.)

Naled *	10%
Aromatic petroleum distillate *	45%
Petroleum distillate	45%

CARMEL FORMULA GH-19
Insecticide
(Carmel Chem. Corp.)

Petroleum distillate *	90.0%
2,2-Dichlorovinyl dimethyl phosphate *	9.3%
Related compounds	0.7%

CARMEL FORMULA GH-20
Insecticide
(Carmel Chem. Corp.)

Petroleum distillate	95.0%
Dithione or Sulfotepp (Tetraethyl dithionopyrophosphate) *	4.5%
Related phosphates	0.5%

CARMEL FORMULA GH-21
Insecticide
(Carmel Chem. Corp.)

Kelthane	10.00%
Vapona (and related compounds) *	8.00%
Lethane *	2.50%
Petroleum distillate *	79.50%

CARMEL FORMULA GH-27
Insecticide
(Carmel Chem. Corp.)

Petroleum distillate	45%
Aromatic petroleum distillate *	45%
Diazinon	10%

CARMEL FORMULA GH-31
Insecticide
(Carmel Chem. Corp.)

Petroleum distillate *	88%
Kelthane *	12%

CARMEL FORMULA GH-33
Insecticide
(Carmel Chem. Corp.)

Aromatic petroleum distillate *	45%
Petroleum distillate	45%
Decachlorobis (2,4-cyclopentadiene-1-yl) *	10%

CARMEL FORMULA GH-40
Fungicide
(Carmel Chem. Corp.)

Dinitro (1-methylheptyl) phenyl crotonate	0.78%
Dinitro (1-methylheptyl) phenol and related compounds	0.22%
Cupric 8-quinolinolate	2.00%

CARMEL FORMULA GH-44
Insecticide
(Carmel Chem. Corp.)

Beta-butoxy-beta′-thiocyano diethyl ether	2.50%
Malathion	14.00%
Xylene *	15.00%
Petroleum distillate	67.75%

CARMEL FORMULA GH-60
Insecticide
(Carmel Chem. Corp.)

Resmethrin	0.500%
Related compounds	0.068%
Aromatic petroleum hydrocarbons	0.662%
Petroleum hydrocarbons *	98.750%

CARMEL FORMULA MU-8
Insecticide
(Carmel Chem. Corp.)

Petroleum distillate *	90.0%
Vapona *	10.0%

CARMEL FORMULA MU-9
Insecticide
(Carmel Chem. Corp.)

Petroleum distillate *	90.0%
Vapona	10.0%

CARMEL FORMULA MU-12
Insecticide
(Carmel Chem. Corp.)

Malathion *	44.7%
Beta-butoxy-beta′-thiocyanodiethyl ether *	19.8%
Petroleum distillate	35.5%

CARMEL FORMULA MU-13
Insecticide
(Carmel Chem. Corp.)

Malathion *	3.00%
Beta-butoxy-beta′-thiocyanodiethyl ether	1.76%
Petroleum distillate *	95.24%

CARMEL FORMULA MU-14
Insecticide
(Carmel Chem. Corp.)

Petroleum distillate *	99.00%
2,2-Dichlorovinyl dimethyl phosphate	0.93%
Related compounds	0.07%

CARMEL FORMULA MU-15
Insecticide
(Carmel Chem. Corp.)

Petroleum distillate *	80.00%
2,2-Dichlorovinyl dimethyl phosphate *	18.60%
Related compounds	1.40%

CARMEL FORMULA MU-16
Insecticide
(Carmel Chem. Corp.)

Petroleum distillate *	99%
Naled (1,2-Dibromo-2,2-dichloroethyl dimethylphosphate)	1%

CARMEL FORMULA MU-17
Insecticide
(Carmel Chem. Corp.)

Petroleum distillate	80%
Naled *	20%

CARMEL FORMULA MU-39
Insecticide
(Carmel Chem. Corp.)

Malathion	23.75%
Ethylene dichloride	10.00%
Xylene *	15.00%
Petroleum oils	50.00%

CARMEX
Cold sores, chapped lips
(Carma)

Menthol *	approx. 1.0%
Camphor *	2.0%
Phenol	0.5%
Salicylic acid *	approx. 1.0%
Base:	
Lanolin	
Petrolatum	

CARMILAX BOLETS
Antacid and mild laxative for cattle
(Norden Labs.)

Each Bolet:

Magnesium hydroxide	27.0 gm.
Nux vomica powdered extract (equiv. to strychnine 7 mg.) *	100.0 mg.
Ginger	200.0 mg.
Capsicum	70.0 mg.

CARMILAX POWDER
Rumen stimulant, mild laxative, carminative; veterinary
(Norden Labs.)

Each lb.:

Magnesium hydroxide	361.0 gm.
Extract of Nux vomica (strychnine alkaloid 0.045 gm.)	0.62 gm.
Capsicum	1.3 gm.
Ginger	1.3 gm.

CAROID LAXATIVE TABLETS
(Winthrop Labs.)

Each tablet:

Cascara sagrada ext.	50 mg.
Phenolphthalein white	32.4 mg.

CAROLATE
Therapeutant
(Bartlett, F.A.)

Salicylic acid *	26.77%
Urea	9.21%
Copper sulfate (crystalline) *	1.78%

CARON COSMETIC PRODUCTS
Carone perfume

Caron Corp.
40 W. 57th St.
New York, N.Y. 10019

Phone: 212-582-1144

See COSMETICS, Section VI, General Formulations

CAROSEL CONCENTRATE
Tree disease
(Bartlett, F.A.)

Helione orange	10%
8-Hydroxyquinoline sulfate	2%
Malachite green *	5%

CARPENTER'S FACE FLY TREATMENT
Veterinary
(Carpenter, W.D.)

Pyrethrins	0.060%
Technical Piperonyl butoxide	0.120%
N-Octyl bicycloheptene dicarboximide	0.200%
Di-n-propyl isocinchomeronate	0.400%
Petroleum distillates *	99.220%

CARPET LUSTER
(Klean-Strip)

Sodium lauryl sulfate *	>90%
Disinfectants, Dyes, & Wetting agents	<10%

CARPETSHEEN
Carpet cleaner
(Hillyard Chem.)

Petroleum distillates *

'76 Ed.

CARSON CHEM. CORP. BOWL DEODORANT
(Carson Chem. Corp.)

Paradichlorobenzene *	99%
Essential oil	1%

'76 Ed.

CARSON CHEM. CORP. CEDAR MOTH BLOCK
(Carson Chem. Corp.)

Paradichlorobenzene *	99%
Essential oil	1%

'76 Ed.

CARSON CHEM. CORP. CLOSET FRESHNER
(Carson Chem. Corp.)

Paradichlorobenzene *	99%
Essential oil	1%

'76 Ed.

CARSON CHEM. CORP. GARBAGE CAN FRESHNER
(Carson Chem. Corp.)

Paradichlorobenzene *	99%
Essential oil	1%

'76 Ed.

CARSON CHEM. CORP. LAVENDER SACHET
(Carson Chem. Corp.)

Paradichlorobenzene *	99%
Essential oil	1%

'76 Ed.

CARSON CHEM. CORP. MOTH BALLS
(Carson Chem. Corp.)

Naphthalene *	100%

'76 Ed.

CARSON CHEM. CORP. MOTH CAKE
(Carson Chem. Corp.)

Paradichlorobenzene *	99%
Essential oil	1%

'76 Ed.

CARSON CHEM. CORP. MOTH FLAKES
(Carson Chem. Corp.)

Naphthalene *	100%

'76 Ed.

CARSON CHEM. CORP. VAPORIZER & VAPORIZER REFILL
(Carson Chem. Corp.)

Paradichlorobenzene *	100%

'76 Ed.

CARSON CHEW-CHECK
Stops licking & chewing of bandages, furniture, rugs, etc.; veterinary
(Carson Chemicals, Inc.)

Neutral oils
Flavoring oils

CARSON F. T. SEVIN DIP
Veterinary - insecticide and antimicrobial agent
(Carson Chemicals, Inc.)

Carbaryl	8%
Lindane	3.9%
Aromatic solvent *	68%

CARSON GROOM
Veterinary - therapeutic shampoo
(Carson Chemicals, Inc.)

Lanolized base	
Pyrethrins	0.05%
Technical Piperonyl butoxide	0.5%

CARSON KITTY FLEA & TICK POWDER
(Carson Chemicals, Inc.)

Carbaryl *	5.0%

CARSON PESTICIDAL SHAMPOO
Insecticide; veterinary
(Carson Chemicals, Inc.)

Technical Piperonyl butoxide	0.50%
Pyrethrins	0.05%

CARSON PRODUCTS CO.
Cosmetics and toiletries

Carson Products Co.
P.O. Box 22309
Savannah, Ga. 31403

Phone: 912-232-8114

See COSMETICS, Section VI, General Formulations

CARSON SCARLET WOUND SPRAY
Veterinary
(Carson Chemicals, Inc.)

Menthol *
Oil of camphor *
Eucalyptus oil *
Pine oil
Thyme oil *
Peru balsam
Biebrich scarlet red & vegetable oil

CARSON SCREW WORM BOMB
Veterinary
(Carson Chemicals, Inc.)

Lindane	3%
Xylol *	12%
Mineral oil	15%

Starred ingredients (*) may be responsible for major toxic effects; consult Section II.

CARTER'S BALL TIP TUBE MARKER
(Carter's Ink)

Ketones *
Vinyl lacquer
Pigment

'76 Ed.

CARTER'S CHECK PROTECTOR INK
(Carter's Ink)

Dyes or pigments
Non-drying natural oils

'76 Ed.

CARTER'S CLOTH MARKING INK - BLACK
Stamping indelible
(Carter's Ink)

Carbitol (butyl) *
Propylene glycol
Dyes
Resin

'76 Ed.

CARTER'S CLOTH MARKING INK - WHITE
Stamping indelible
(Carter's Ink)

Turpentine *
Varnish
Pigments
Cobalt dryer *

'76 Ed.

CARTER'S CONTACT GLU
(Carter's Ink)

Rubber
Ketones *
Toluol *

'76 Ed.

CARTER'S, DR., K & B TEA

See DR. CARTER'S K & B TEA

CARTER'S EPOXY CEMENT
(Carter's Ink)

Part A:
    Epoxy resin
Part B:
    Amine hardener

'76 Ed.

CARTER'S GLOW COLOR MARKERS
(Carter's Ink)

Pigment *
Resin
Xylene *

'76 Ed.

CARTER'S GOLD INK
(Carter's Ink)

Gold bronze powder *
Alcohol
Dextrine
Phenol *
Wetting agent

'76 Ed.

CARTER'S HOUSEHOLD CEMENT
(Carter's Ink)

Nitrocellulose resin
Ketones *
Alcohol *
Aromatics *

'76 Ed.

CARTER'S INK ERADICATORS
(Carter's Ink)

Sodium hypochlorite
Sodium bicarbonate
Sodium phosphate

'76 Ed.

CARTER'S LAUNDRY INK
(Carter's Ink)

Cresylic acid *
Turpentine
Dyes
Phenol *
Resin

'76 Ed.

CARTER'S LITTLE PILLS
Laxative
(Carter Products)

Podophyllum * . . . .   <5 mg.
Aloes . . . .   <16 mg.

CARTER'S MUCILAGE
(Carter's Ink)

Dextrin
Borax *
Urea
Peroxide
Formaldehyde *

'76 Ed.

CARTER'S NUMBERING MACHINE INK
(Carter's Ink)

Non-drying oils
Dyes or pigments

'76 Ed.

CARTER'S OPAQUE STAMP PAD INKS
(Carter's Ink)

Glycol ether *
Alcohol *
Resin
Dyes or pigments
Tannic acid

'76 Ed.

CARTER'S POWER MODEL CEMENT
Household cement
(Carter's Ink)

Cellulose acetate resin
Ketones *
Alcohols
Lacquer
Toluene *
Butyl acetate *

'76 Ed.

CARTER'S PRICE MARKER CLEANER
(Carter's Ink)

Butanol *
Diacetone alcohol *

'76 Ed.

CARTER'S PROJECTOR MARKER
(Carter's Ink)

Urea
Sodium benzoate
Dyes
Glycol
Resin
Alcohol

'76 Ed.

CARTER'S RIGID PLASTIC MODEL CEMENT
(Carter's Ink)

Polystyrene
Toluene *

'76 Ed.

CARTER'S RUBBER CEMENT
(Carter's Ink)

Rubber
Petroleum solvent *
Resin

'76 Ed.

CARTER'S RUBBER CEMENT THINNER
(Carter's Ink)

Petroleum solvent *

'76 Ed.

CARTER'S SCHOOL PASTE
(Carter's Ink)

Dextrine
Borax *
Phenol *
Dioxin
Trisodium phosphate

'76 Ed.

CARTER'S SILVER INK
(Carter's Ink)

Aluminum powder
Dextrine
Dioxin
Bichromate of soda *†

'76 Ed.

†See Dichromate salts (soluble)

CARTER'S STAMP PAD INKS
(Carter's Ink)

Glycerine
Glycol *
Dyes
Phenol *
Glycol ether *

'76 Ed.

CARTER'S STYLE WRITER
(Carter's Ink)

Dyes
Humectant
Surfactant *
Sodium benzoate *
Glycol *†

'76 Ed.

†See Ethylene glycol

CARTER'S TEMPERA COLORS
(Carter's Ink)

Alcohol
Gum solution
Pigments *
Phenol *

'76 Ed.

CARTER'S TYPE CLEANER
(Carter's Ink)

Trichloroethane *

'76 Ed.

CARTER'S VINYL PLASTIC CEMENT
(Carter's Ink)

Vinyl chloride-vinyl acetate copolymer
Plasticizer
Ketones *
Toluol *

'76 Ed.

CARTER'S WHITE INK
(Carter's Ink)

Pigments
Gum solution
Preservative

'76 Ed.

CARTER'S WHITE MARKER
(Carter's Ink)

Pigment
Resin
Xylene *

'76 Ed.

CARTER'S WRITING INKS
(Carter's Ink)

Gum solution
Cellosolve
Phenol *
Formaldehyde
Sulfuric acid
Dyes

'76 Ed.

CARTRAX-10 & CARTRAX-20 TABLETS
Vasodilator, antianxiety agent
(Roerig)

Each Cartrax-10 tablet (yellow):
  Pentaerythritol tetranitrate * . 10 mg.
  Hydroxyzine hydrochloride ... 10 mg.

Each Cartrax-20 tablet (white):
  Pentaerythritol tetranitrate * . 20 mg.
  Hydroxyzine hydrochloride ... 10 mg.

CARVEN COSMETIC PRODUCTS

Carven Parfums
630 Fifth Ave.
New York, N.Y. 10020

Phone: 212-489-2445

See COSMETICS, Section VI, General Formulations

CARZOL SP
Miticide, insecticide
(NOR-AM)

Formetanate hydrochloride * ... 92%/w

CASCADE (Formula 1)
Automatic dishwasher detergent
(Procter & Gamble)

Complex sodium phosphates 25-49%
Water 25-49%
Sodium silicates 10-24%
Chlorinated trisodium phosphate 10-24%
Propylene/ethylene oxide
  condensate................. 1-4%
Minor ingredients, each .... trace

pH (1% solution) - 10.4

CASCADE (Formula 2)
Automatic dishwasher detergent
(Procter & Gamble)

Complex sodium phosphates 25-49%
Water 25-49%
Sodium silicates 10-24%
Chlorinated trisodium phosphate 10-24%
Alkyl ethoxylate 1-4%
Minor ingredients, each .... trace

pH (1% solution) - 10.6

CASCADE (Formula 3)
Automatic dishwasher detergent
(Procter & Gamble)

Complex sodium phosphates 25-49%
Sodium sulfate 10-24%
Water 10-24%
Sodium silicate 10-24%
Chlorinated trisodium phosphate 10-24%
Propylene/ethylene oxide
  condensate................. 5-9%
Minor ingredients, each .... trace

pH (1% solution) - 10.8

CASCADE (Formula 4)
Automatic dishwasher detergent
(Procter & Gamble)

Complex sodium phosphates 25-49%
Sodium sulfate 10-24%
Sodium silicate 10-24%
Water 10-24%
Sodium carbonate 10-24%
Sodium chloride 5-9%
Alkyl ethoxylate 1-4%
Sodium dichlorocyanurate 1-4%
Minor ingredients, each .... trace

pH (1% solution) - 10.9

Starred ingredients (*) may be responsible for major toxic effects; consult Section II.

CASCANYL
Cathartic
(Wesley Pharm.)

Each tablet:
Belladonna P.E. .... 1/8 gr.
Podophyllin * .... 3/20 gr.
Aloin .... 1/4 gr.
Oleoresin ginger .... 1/16 gr.
Ext. Cascara sagrada .... 1/4 gr.

CASCO
Institutional and industrial cleaning product

Procter & Gamble Co.
Ivorydale Technical Center
Cincinnati, Ohio 45217

Phone: 513-562-1100

CASECT
Pour-on cattle insecticide
(Bio-Ceutic)

Trichlorfon * 8%

CAS-EVAC
Cathartic
(Parke-Davis)

Cascara sagrada *
Alcohol 18%

CASITE LEAK STOP & RUST STOP
Radiator additive
(Hastings Mfg. Co.)

Hydrocarbon, Amide, Carboxylate, Hydroxy, and Potassium radicals

CASITE MOTOR HONEY
Lubricant additive
(Hastings Mfg. Co.)

Hydrocarbon, Hydrocarbon polymer, and Carboxylate radicals

CASITE OIL FORTIFIER
Lubricant additive
(Hastings Mfg. Co.)

Hydrocarbon, Amide, Carboxylate, Dithiophosphate, Sulfurized olefin, Sulfonate, Calcium, Sodium, and Zinc radicals

CASITE SMOOTH SEAL
Transmission fluid additive
(Hastings Mfg. Co.)

Hydrocarbon, Amide, Carboxylate, Dithiophosphate, Sulfonate, Barium, and Zinc radicals

CASITE SPRAY-LUBE
Lubricant
(Hastings Mfg. Co.)

Hydrocarbon, Carboxylate, and Hydroxy radicals
Propane propellant

CASITE TUNE-UP
Fuel additive
(Hastings Mfg. Co.)

Hydrocarbon, Amide, and Carboxylate radicals

CASTADERM
Dermatological lotion
(Lannett)

Boric acid *
Resorcin *
Acetone
Solution Carbol fuchsin

CASTORIA, FLETCHER'S
See FLETCHER'S CASTORIA

CASWELL-MASSEY COSMETIC PRODUCTS
Colognes & men's toiletries

Caswell-Massey Co., Ltd.
575 Lexington Ave.
New York, N.Y. 10022

Phone: 212-355-5775

See COSMETICS, Section VI, General Formulations

CASYLLIUM
Laxative
(Upjohn)

Each 6 gm.:
Fluidextract Cascara
(debittered) .... 3 ml.
Psyllium husk powder .... 4.1 gm.
Prune powder .... 1.2 gm.

CATRON
Screw worm and ear tick spray
(Bio-Ceutic)

Ronnel 2.5%
Xylene 0.5%

CAULK-O-SEAL
Caulking compound
(Calbar)

Soybean oil
Polybutene
Soya lecithin
Mineral spirits *
Magnesium silicate
Calcium carbonate
Titanium dioxide

CAVALIER SHOE POLISHES
(Kiwi Polish)

The Kiwi Polish Co. PTY, Ltd.
Route 662
Douglassville, Pa. 19518

Phone: 215-326-5800

CAVOS
Embalming fluid
(Embalmers')

Formaldehyde *

CAVREX
Embalming fluid
(Embalmers')

Formaldehyde *

CBC BOWL CLEANER
See AIRWICK PROFESSIONAL PRODUCTS CBC BOWL CLEANER

CBC PLUS
See AIRWICK PROFESSIONAL PRODUCTS CBC PLUS

C. & C. DROPS COUGH SYRUP
For farm animals
(Daniels, Dr. A.C.)

Each fl. oz.:
F.E. Belladonna leaf * .... 15 min.
F.E. Lobelia * .... 5 min.
Potassium guaiacolsulphonate 15 gr.
Potassium chlorate * .... 15 gr.
Ammonium chloride .... 30 gr.
Licorice-syrup base .... q.s.

CCS-318
Emulsion cleaner
(Calgon Corp., Commercial Div.)

Petroleum distillates *
Synthetic emulsifiers *

C.D. - CORROSION DIGESTER (Powder)
See GUNK C.D. - CORROSION DIGESTER (Powder)

C-D DUST
See DR. ROGERS' C-D DUST

Starred ingredients (*) may be responsible for major toxic effects; consult Section II.

C.D.M. EXPECTORANT
Antihistaminic antitussive cough expectorant
(Lannett)

Each 5 ml.:
Dextromethorphan
  hydrobromide .... 10 mg.
Chlorpheniramine maleate .... 1 mg.
Phenylephrine HCl .... 5 mg.
Sodium citrate .... 15 mg.
Glyceryl guaiacolate .... 25 mg.

CDQ
Disinfectant, deodorizer, cleaner
(Brulin)

n-Alkyl (60% C14, 30% C16, 5% C12,
  5% C18) dimethyl benzyl ammonium chlorides * 1.6%
n-Alkyl (68% C12, 32% C14) dimethyl
  ethyl benzyl ammonium
  chlorides * 1.6%
Essential oils 0.6%
Monoethanolamine 3.5%

CDQ AEROSOL
Disinfectant, deodorizer, cleaner
(Brulin)

n-Alkyl (60% C14, 30% C16, 5%
  C12, 5% C18) dimethyl benzyl
  ammonium chlorides 0.076%
n-Alkyl (50% C12, 30% C14, 17%
  C16, 3% C18) dimethyl ethyl
  benzyl ammonium chlorides .. 0.076%
Essential oils 0.20%
Sodium metasilicate 0.24%

CEBETINIC TABLETS
Dietary supplement
(Upjohn)

Each tablet:
Iron (from 324 mg. ferrous
  gluconate) * .... 37.5 mg.
Plus multivitamins

"CEDAR CLOSET" MOTH CAKE
(Curran)

Paradichlorobenzene *

'76 Ed.

CEDAR PARA LOG
(Curran)

Paradichlorobenzene *

'76 Ed.

CEDAR VALLEY HOG OIL
External treatment
(Cedar Valley Dist.)

Menthyl salicylate * ..... 0.5-5%/vol.
Mineral oil * .... 95-99.5%/vol.

CEDILANID TABLETS
Cardiac glycoside
(Sandoz)

Each tablet:
Lanatoside C, N.F. * .... 0.5 mg.

CED R WOOD CAKE
(Carson Chem. Corp.)

Paradichlorobenzene * 99%
Essential oil 1%

'76 Ed.

CEETOLAN CONCENTRATE
Mouth wash concentrate
(Lannett)

Cetyldimethylbenzylammonium chloride

Two-fl.-oz. bottle diluted with
one gallon water makes anti-septic mouth
wash 1:5500 of active ingredient

CELCURE
Wood preservative
(American Celcure)

Copper sulphate (anhydrous) * .. 3.84%
Sodium dichromate (anhydrous) * 5.01%
Chromic acid (anhydrous) 0.20%

'76 Ed.

CELESTONE CREAM
Anti-inflammatory, antiallergic, antipruritic
(Schering)

Each gram:
Betamethasone .... 2 mg.
Base:
Stearic acid
Propylene glycol monostearate
Isopropyl myristate
Propylene glycol
Polyoxyethylene sorbitan monopalmitate
Sorbitol
Purified water
Methylparaben .... 1 mg.
Butyl p-hydroxybenzoate ...... 4 mg.

CELESTONE SYRUP AND TABLETS
Anti-inflammatory corticosteroid
(Schering)

Each 5 cc and tablet:
Betamethasone .... 0.6 mg.
Alcohol (syrup only) .... <1%

CELLO-SEAL
Tissue sealer
(Royal Bond)

Acetone *
Dimethylphthalate

CELOPON
Biodegradable anionic detergent
(Arkansas Co.)

Sodium methyl oleyl taurate *

'76 Ed.

CEL-TON-SA BRAND HERB TEA
Cathartic
(C.T.S. Labs.)

Senna leaves *

CEL-TON-SA MENTHOLATED ANALGESIC OINTMENT
(C.T.S. Labs.)

Menthol *
Camphor *
Eucalyptus oil *
Thymol *
Oil of mustard
Oil of nutmeg
Oil of peppermint
Oil of cajeput

CEL-TON-SA SNOW WHITE LINIMENT
Rubefacient
(C.T.S. Labs.)

Methyl salicylate *
Gum of camphor *
Stronger Ammonia water
Oleic acid
Triethanolamine
Stearic acid

CEL-TON-SA SUPERIOR IRON TABLETS
(C.T.S. Labs.)

Iron (Ferrous sulphate) *

CEM-REM
Cement & concrete sealer, coating
(Speco)

Styrene-butadiene
Aliphatic solvent *†

'76 Ed.

†*See* Petroleum naphtha

CEM-SEAL
Floor seal
(Hillyard Chem.)

Aromatic solvent naphtha *

'76 Ed.

Starred ingredients (*) may be responsible for major toxic effects; consult Section II.

CENALENE (ELIXIR AND TABLETS)
Mental energizer
(Central Pharmacal Co.)

ELIXIR (each 5 ml.):
Pentylenetetrazol *	100 mg.
Thiamine hydrochloride	1.67 mg.
Niacinamide	7.5 mg.
Cyanocobalamin	2.5 mcg.
Alcohol	15%

TABLETS (each):
Pentylenetetrazol *	100 mg.
Thiamine mononitrate	1.67 mg.
Niacinamide	7.5 mg.
Cyanocobalamin	2.5 mcg.

CENOL ANT AND ROACH KILLER
Insecticide
(Cenol)

Pyrethrins	0.050%
Piperonyl butoxide, technical	0.100%
N-Octyl bicycloheptene dicarboximide	0.166%
o-Isopropoxyphenyl methylcarbamate	0.500%
Petroleum distillate *	84.700%

CENOL DAIRY CATTLE SPRAY
Insecticide
(Cenol)

Pyrethrins	0.04%
Technical Piperonyl butoxide	0.08%
N-Octyl bicycloheptene dicarboximide	0.13%
2,3,4,5-Bis(delta-2-butylene)-tetrahydrofurfural	0.20%
Petroleum distillate *	99.55%

CENOL FLOWER & VEGETABLE DUST
Insecticide, fungicide
(Cenol)

Pyrethrins	0.030%
Piperonyl butoxide technical	0.300%
Rotenone	0.500%
Other cube resins	1.000%
Sulfur	25.000%
Copper (basic copper sulfate expressed as metallic) *	5.000%

CENOL GARDEN DUST
Insecticide
(Cenol)

Rotenone	1%
Other cube resins	2%

CENOL HOUSE & GARDEN INSECTICIDE
(Cenol)

Pyrethrins	0.25%
Technical Piperonyl butoxide	0.80%
Petroleum distillate	1.00%

CENOL KILL QUICK FOGGING SPRAY SBP-1382
Insecticide
(Cenol)

(5-Benzyl-3-furyl)methyl-2,2-dimethyl-3-(2-methylpropenyl) cyclopropanecarboxylate	0.200% w/w
Related compounds	0.027%
Aromatic petroleum hydrocarbons	0.265%
Petroleum distillate *	99.500%

CENOL ROACH & HOUSEHOLD INSECT SPRAY
(Cenol)

Pyrethrins	0.05%
Piperonyl butoxide (technical)	0.26%
O,O-Diethyl O-(2-isopropyl-6-methyl-4-pyrimidinyl) phosphorothioate	0.50%
Petroleum distillates *	99.12%

CENOL TOMATO DUST
Insecticide, fungicide
(Cenol)

Pyrethrins	0.030%
Piperonyl butoxide technical	0.300%
Rotenone	0.500%
Other cube resins	1.000%
Sulfur	25.000%
Copper (basic copper sulfate expressed as metallic) *	5.000%

CEN-O-PHEN
Germicidal detergent
(Central Chem.)

Isopropyl alcohol	10%
Ortho-benzyl-para-chlorophenol	5.4%
Para-tertiary amyl phenol *	5.3%
Ortho-phenolphenate	4.3%

'76 Ed.

CEN-PE-CO DIESEL-KLENZ
(Central Petroleum)

Oxidized hydrocarbons

CEN-PE-CO FACE FLY TREATMENT
Insecticide; veterinary
(Central Petroleum)

Pyrethrins	0.06%
Piperonyl butoxide, technical	0.12%
N-Octyl bicycloheptene dicarboximide	0.20%
Di-n-propyl isocinchomeronate	0.40%
White mineral oil (National Formulary Grade)	99.22%

CEN-PE-CO MOTOR-KLENZ
(Central Petroleum)

Oxidized hydrocarbons

CEN-PE-CO NEVER-LITE STOCK SPRAY
Insecticide
(Central Petroleum)

Pyrethrins	0.075%
Piperonyl butoxide, technical	0.150%
N-Octyl bicycloheptene dicarboximide	0.250%
Di-n-propyl isocinchomeronate	0.200%
Petroleum distillate *	99.325%

CEN-PE-CO NEW CATTLE OIL
Insecticide
(Central Petroleum)

Malathion	2.00%
Di-n-propyl isocinchomeronate	0.20%
N-Octyl bicycloheptene dicarboximide	0.20%
Mineral oil *	97.60%

CEN-PE-CO OILS
(Central Petroleum)

Mineral oil	
Phosphorus	trace
Zinc	trace
Barium	trace
May also contain Calcium	

CEN-PE-CO SUPER DAIRY & BEEF CATTLE SPRAY
Insecticide
(Central Petroleum)

Ciodrin	1.00%
2,2-Dichlorovinyl dimethyl phosphate	0.23%
Related compounds	0.02%
Petroleum hydrocarbons *	98.57%

CEN-PE-CO SUPER 100 BARN & STOCK SPRAY
Insecticide
(Central Petroleum)

Pyrethrins	0.10%
Piperonyl butoxide, technical	0.20%
N-Octyl bicycloheptene dicarboximide	0.33%
Di-n-propyl isocinchomeronate	0.40%
Petroleum distillate*	98.97%

CENTENNIAL 25
Liquid floor polish
(Sanitek)

Acrylic polymer emulsion	18.2%
Diethylene glycol monoethyl ether (Cellosolve)	5.8%
Polyethylene emulsion	2.7%
Rosin maleate alkali soluble resin	2.2%
Tributoxyethyl phosphate	1.5%
Nonionic surfactant	0.4%
Formalin, Ammonia, Defoamer, Fluorochemical surfactant	trace

Starred ingredients (*) may be responsible for major toxic effects; consult Section II.

CENTEX
Herbicide
(National Chemsearch)

Sodium chlorate *	18.00%
Sodium metaborate	9.00%

CENTOX SPRAY
Insecticide
(Central Chem.)

Chlordane	<3%
Technical Piperonyl butoxide	<2%
Pyrethrins	<2%
Petroleum oil *	balance

'76 Ed.

CENTRAL'S DISHWASHING COMPOUNDS, 44-A, 44-P AND NUFOME
(Central Chem.)

Central Chemical Company, Inc.
3130 Brinkerhoff Rd.
Kansas City, Kan. 66115

Phone: 913-621-6542

CENTRAL'S RESIDUAL SPRAY
Insecticide
(Central Chem.)

Diazinon	0.50%
Piperonyl butoxide technical	0.375%
Pyrethrins	0.075%
Deodorized Petroleum oil *	99.05%

'76 Ed.

CENTRAX CAPSULES
Management of anxiety disorders
(Parke-Davis)

Each capsule:
Prazepam* ......5 mg.; 10 mg.; 20 mg.

CENTRAX TABLETS
Management of anxiety disorders
(Parke-Davis)

Each tablet:
Prazepam* .... 10 mg.

CEO-TWO
Evacuant suppository
(Beutlich, Inc.)

Each suppository:
Sodium bicarbonate
Potassium bitartrate
Polyethylene glycol water soluble base

CEPACOL
Antibacterial mouthwash/gargle
(Merrell Dow)

Alcohol	14%
Cetylpyridinium chloride	1:2000
Phosphate buffers	
Aromatics	

CEPACOL ANESTHETIC TROCHES
(Merrell Dow)

Each tablet:
Ceepryn (Cetylpyridinium chloride)	1:1500
Benzocaine	
Aromatics	
Green citrus-flavored hard candy base	

CEPACOL THROAT LOZENGES
(Merrell Dow)

Cetylpyridinium chloride	1:1500
Benzyl alcohol	0.3%
Aromatics	

CEPASTAT LIQUID
Antiseptic anesthetic mouthwash/gargle
(Merrell Dow)

Phenol *	1.4%
Eugenol	
Menthol	
Glycerin	

CEPASTAT SORE THROAT LOZENGES
Antiseptic anesthetic
(Merrell Dow)

Each lozenge:
Phenol *	1.45%
Menthol	0.12%
Eucalyptol oil	0.04%

Base:
Sorbitol

CEPHULAC SYRUP
Treatment of portal systemic encephalopathy
(Merrell Dow)

Each 15 ml.:
Lactulose	10 gm.

Syrup:
Lactose
Galactose
Other sugars

CERABON TABLETS
Oral antibiotic; dogs and cats
(Elanco Prod.)

Each tablet:
Dihydrostreptomycin sulfate (equiv. to 50 mg. dihydrostreptomycin base)	
Carob flour	0.5 gm.

CEREFOLIUS, FLUID

See FLUID CEREFOLIUS

CERFEX SPACKLING COMPOUND
(United Gilsonite)

Gypsum
Animal glue
Zinc sulfate *

CERISSA TOILETRIES

Revlon, Inc.
767 Fifth Ave.
New York, N.Y. 10153

Phone: 212-572-5000

Revlon Research Center, Inc.
945 Zerega Ave.
Bronx, N.Y. 10473

Phone: 212-824-9000

See COSMETICS, Section VI, General Formulations

CEROSE COMPOUND CAPSULES
Bronchial, nasal decongestant; antitussive
(Ives Labs.)

Each capsule:
Chlorpheniramine maleate	2.0 mg.
Phenylephrine hydrochloride *	7.5 mg.
Dextromethorphan hydrobromide *	10.0 mg.
Terpin hydrate *	64.8 mg.
APAP (Acetaminophen) *	194.0 mg.
Ascorbic acid	25.0 mg.

CEROSE-DM
Antihistaminic-sedative expectorant
(Ives Labs.)

Each 5 cc:
Dextromethorphan hydrobromide *	10 mg.
Phenindamine tartrate *	5 mg.
Phenylephrine hydrochloride *	5 mg.
Fluid extract of Ipecac	0.17 m.
Glycerin	40 m.
Potassium guaiacolsulfonate	86 mg.
Sodium citrate	3 gr.
Citric acid	1 gr.
Alcohol	2 1/2%

CERTICIDE
Insecticide
(Certified Labs.)

Petroleum distillates *	99.429%
Technical Piperonyl butoxide	0.476%
Pyrethrins	0.095%

CERTIFIED ALGAECIDE
Depresses algae growth
(Certified Labs.)

Methyldodecylbenzyl trimethyl ammonium chloride *	8%
Methyldodecylxylylene bis (trimethyl ammonium chloride)	2%

CERTIFIED AS-655 WEED KILLER
(Certified Labs.)

Sodium arsenite * 40.00%

CERTIFIED C-400 CRAB GRASS KILLER
(Certified Labs.)

Dodecyl ammonium
methylarsonate * 8.0%
Octyl ammonium methylarsonate * 8.0%

CERTIFIED C-300 SELECTIVE WEED KILLER
Kills woody plants
(Certified Labs.)

Isooctyl ester of 2,4-dichlorophen-
oxyacetic acid * 24.5%
Isooctyl ester of 2,4,5-trichloro-
phenoxyacetic acid * 11.7%

CERTIFIED C-100 WEED KILLER
(Certified Labs.)

Sodium chlorate * 18.00%
Sodium metaborate (anhydrous) 6.00%

CERTIFIED C-795 WEED KILLER
(Certified Labs.)

Sodium chlorate * 18.00%
Sodium metaborate (anhydrous) 5.96%

CERTIFIED HC-200 CONCENTRATE
Insecticide
(Certified Labs.)

Active ingredients: 100%
Refined Mineral oil
Technical Piperonyl butoxide
N-Octyl bicycloheptene
dicarboximide *
Pyrethrins *

CERTIFIED HOME PRODUCTS DIAPER PAIL DEODORIZER, NON-TOXIC
(Certified Home Prod.)

Gypsum 40%
Sand 40%
Essential oil 1.0%

CERTI-FOG CONCENTRATE
Insecticide for use in food plants, schools, storage buildings, etc.
(Certified Labs.)

Combined amount: 100%
Petroleum distillates *
N-Octyl bicycloheptene dicarboximide
Technical Piperonyl butoxide
Pyrethrins

CERTOX INSECT KILLER
Insecticide
(York Chem.)

Diazinon 0.5%
Pyrethrum
Piperonyl butoxide

CERTREX 50-C
(Mobil Oil)

Aromatic petroleum oil *

CERUSOL
For constipation, bloat, otitis; veterinary
(Burns-Biotec)

Dioctyl sodium sulfosuccinate (in
a solvent base) .... 5% w/w
Certified color
Methylparaben
Propylparaben

CETABUFF
Analgesic
(Wesley Pharm.)

Each tablet:
Aspirin * .... 3 1/2 gr.
Phenacetin * .... 2 1/2 gr.
Caffeine .... 1/2 gr.
Co-buffered with an Aluminum magnesium hydroxide complex

CETACAINE
Topical anesthetic
(Cetylite)

Benzocaine 14.0%
Butyl aminobenzoate 2.0%
Tetracaine hydrochloride 2.0%
Benzalkonium chloride 0.5%
Cetyl dimethyl ethyl ammonium
bromide 0.005%

CETACET
Analgesic, antipyretic
(Wesley Pharm.)

Each capsule:
Dover's powder .... 24.3 mg.
Phenacetin * .... 2 gr.
Aspirin * .... 3 gr.
Caffeine .... 1/2 gr.

CETAMIDE
Ophthalmic ointment
(Alcon)

Active ingred. (each gm.):
Sodium sulfacetamide 10%
Preservatives:
Methylparaben 0.05%
Propylparaben 0.01%
Inactive ingred.:
White petrolatum
Anhydrous liquid Lanolin
Mineral oil

CETAPRED
Ophthalmic ointment
(Alcon)

Active ingred. (each gm.):
Sulfacetamide sodium 10%
Prednisolone acetate 0.25%
Preservatives:
Methylparaben 0.05%
Propylparaben 0.01%
Inactive ingred.:
White petrolatum
Anhydrous liquid Lanolin
Mineral oil

CETASED
Analgesic
(Wesley Pharm.)

Each tablet:
Aspirin * .... 3 1/2 gr.
Phenacetin * .... 2 1/2 gr.
Caffeine .... 1/2 gr.
Phenobarbital .... 1/4 gr.

CETATS
Germicide
(Fine Organics, Inc.)

Cetyl trimethyl ammonium
tosylate * 100%

'76 Ed.

CETOL
Germicide
(Fine Organics, Inc.)

Cetyl dimethyl benzyl ammonium
chloride * 100%

'76 Ed.

CETRO-CIROSE
Sedative, antitussive
(Ives Labs.)

Each fl. oz.:
Codeine phosphate * .... 1/2 gr.
Fl. extr. of Ipecac .... 1 m.
Glycerin .... 240 m.
Potassium guaiacolsulfonate .. 8 gr.
Sodium citrate .... 18 gr.
Citric acid .... 6 gr.
Alcohol 1 1/2%

CETYLCIDE
Disinfectant
(Cetylite)

Cetyl dimethyl ethyl ammonium
bromide * 6.5%
Benzalkonium chloride (Alkyl (50%
C12, 30% C14, 17% C6, 3% C18)
dimethyl benzyl ammonium
chloride) * 6.5%
Isopropyl alcohol * 13.0%
Sodium nitrite

Starred ingredients (*) may be responsible for major toxic effects; consult Section II.

CEVIM-T
Vitamins
(Russ Pharm.)

Each tablet:
Vitamin A (palmitate) .... 10,000 I.U.
Vitamin D (Ergocalciferol) 400 I.U.
Iodine (Potassium iodide) 0.15 mg.
Iron (Ferrous sulfate) ..... 12.00 mg.
Plus multivitamins and minerals

C-4 SOLUBLE CRESYLIC DISINFECTANT
(Coopers Creek Chem.)

Active ingreds.: 75%
Cresylic acids *
Soap

C-4 TREE WOUND & PRUNING DRESSING
(Coopers Creek Chem.)

Aliphatic hydrocarbons * 35%
Petroleum distillate * 19%
Copper naphthenate (equiv. to metallic copper 1%) 6%

CHACON ANT, SPIDER AND ROACH SPRAY (Aerosol)
(Chacon Chem. Corp.)

Pyrethrins 0.050%
Technical Piperonyl butoxide ... 0.100%
N-Octyl bicycloheptene dicarboximide 0.166%
O-Isopropoxyphenyl methylcarbamate * 0.500%
Petroleum distillates * 69.184%

CHACON BERMUDA GRASS CONTROL
(Chacon Chem. Corp.)

Copper sulfate (anhydrous) * .. 12.780%
Zinc sulfate (anhydrous) 4.495%

CHACON BORDOIL COPPER-OIL FUNGICIDE
(Chacon Chem. Corp.)

Copper sulfate (anhydrous) * 6.4%
Petroleum oil * 30.0%

CHACON BROAD-LEAF WEED KILLER
(Chacon Chem. Corp.)

2,4-Dichlorophenoxyacetic acid, propylene glycol butyl ether esters *† 20.0%

†See 2,4-D esters

CHACON 50% CHLORDANE SPRAY
(Chacon Chem. Corp.)

Technical Chlordane * 50.0%
Aromatic petroleum derivative solvent * 46.5%

CHACON CRABGRASS CONTROL
(Chacon Chem. Corp.)

Disodium methanearsonate * 12.6%

CHACON CUTWORM & SOWBUG CONTROL
(Chacon Chem. Corp.)

Carbaryl * 5%

CHACON DOG & CAT REPELLENT (Aerosol)
(Chacon Chem. Corp.)

Methyl nonyl ketone 1.9%
Related compound 0.1%

CHACON DU-O-CIDE MULTI-PURPOSE GARDEN SPRAY
(Chacon Chem. Corp.)

Copper oleate *† 15.00%
Pyrethrins 0.40%
Rotenone 1.25%
Other cube extractives 1.25%
Light medium Petroleum oils ... 15.00%

†See Copper

CHACON EARWIG CONTROL
(Chacon Chem. Corp.)

Carbaryl * 5%

CHACON FRUIT AND VEGETABLE DUST
(Chacon Chem. Corp.)

Malathion * 5%
Carbaryl * 5%
Sulfur * 30%

CHACON FRUIT AND VEGETABLE SPRAY
(Chacon Chem. Corp.)

Malathion * 6.50%
Carbaryl * 6.50%

CHACON HOUSE AND GARDEN INSECT SPRAY (Aerosol)
(Chacon Chem. Corp.)

d-trans Allethrin (allyl homolog of Cinerin I) 0.25%
Piperonyl butoxide (technical) 0.80%
N-Octyl bicycloheptene dicarboximide 0.40%
Petroleum distillate 8.05%

CHACON HOUSE PLANT INSECT SPRAY (Aerosol)
(Chacon Chem. Corp.)

Pyrethrins 0.056%
Petroleum distillate 0.224%

CHACON LAWN & GARDEN FUNGICIDE
(Chacon Chem. Corp.)

Tetrachloroisophthalonitrile 9.0%
Copperoxychloride sulfate (copper expressed as elemental by wt. 1.2%) * 2.0%

CHACON 50% MALATHION
(Chacon Chem. Corp.)

Malathion * 50.00%
Aromatic petroleum derivative solvent * 40.37%

CHACON ROSE AND FLOWER SPRAY (Aerosol)
(Chacon Chem. Corp.)

Pyrethrins 0.020%
Rotenone 0.100%
Other cube resins 0.200%
Dichlone 0.120%
Methoxychlor (technical) 0.300%
N-Octyl bicycloheptene dicarboximide 0.300%
2,4-Dinitro-6-octyl phenyl crotonate
2,6-Dinitro-4-octyl phenyl crotonate 0.091%
Nitrooctyl phenols (principally dinitro) 0.005%

CHACON ROSE & FLOWER DUST
(Chacon Chem. Corp.)

Malathion * 5%
Carbaryl * 5%
Sulfur * 30%

CHACON SCALE AND SPIDER MITE CONTROL
(Chacon Chem. Corp.)

Malathion * 6.50%
Light medium Petroleum oil * .. 81.50%

CHACON SEVIN LIQUID GARDEN SPRAY
(Chacon Chem. Corp.)

Carbaryl * 5%

CHACON SPURGE & OXALIS CONTROL
(Chacon Chem. Corp.)

Sodium thiocyanate * 25.0%

Starred ingredients (*) may be responsible for major toxic effects; consult Section II.

CHACON SYSTEMIC INSECT CONTROL FOR POTTED PLANTS
(Chacon Chem. Corp.)

S-(2-(Ethylsulfinyl)ethyl) O,O-dimethyl phosphorothioate * 6.7%

CHACON SYSTEMIC SPRAY WITH FUNGICIDE
(Chacon Chem. Corp.)

Carbaryl*	5.00%
S-(2-(Ethylsulfinyl)ethyl) O,O-dimethyl phosphorothioate*	5.00%
2,4-Dinitro-6-octyl phenyl crotonate	1.46%
2,6-Dinitro-4-octyl phenyl crotonate	
Nitrooctyl phenols (principally dinitro)	0.10%
Aromatic petroleum derivative solvent*	29.37%

CHACON TOMATO BLOSSOM SPRAY (Aerosol)
(Chacon Chem. Corp.)

p-Chlorophenoxyacetic acid 0.0042%

CHACON VEGETABLE & TOMATO INSECT SPRAY (Aerosol)
(Chacon Chem. Corp.)

Pyrethrins	0.056%
Rotenone	0.125%
Other cube resins	0.250%
Petroleum distillate	0.225%

CHACON WEED-O-KIL COMPLETE WEED KILLER
(Chacon Chem. Corp.)

2,4-bis(Isopropylamino)-6-methoxy-s-triazine	2.50%
Pentachlorophenol *	1.00%
Other Chlorophenols and related compounds	0.12%

CHAIR-LOC
Wood sweller
(Chair Loc)

Rosin soap (reaction product of rosin and triethanolamine)	18.4%
Propylene glycol (industrial)	15.6%
Denatured alcohol	11.1%
Ammonia (28%)	1.5%
Dextrin	7.6%
Milk casein	3.6%
Remainder (water)	42.2%

CHANEL NO. 5 BODY LOTION
(Chanel, Inc.)

Water	>50%
Alcohol	<20%
Emollient esters	7-10%
Nonionic surfactant	<3%
Film former	<1%
Polyol-humectant	<5%
Preservatives	<0.1%
Sequesterant	<0.1%
Color	trace

CHANEL NO. 5 EAU DE COLOGNE
(Chanel, Inc.)

Alcohol *	>50%
Water	10-20%
Fragrance *†	1-5%
Color	trace

†*See* Essential oils

CHANEL NO. 5 EAU DE TOILETTE
(Chanel, Inc.)

Alcohol *	>50%
Water	5-15%
Fragrance *†	1-5%
Color	trace

†*See* Essential oils

CHANEL NO. 5 OIL FOR THE BATH
(Chanel, Inc.)

Emollient ester	45-55%
Emollient alcohol	10-15%
Mineral oil	<25%
Lanolin derivative	<5%
Nonionic surfactant	<5%
Fragrance *†	<5%

†*See* Essential oils

CHANEL NO. 5 PERFUME
(Chanel, Inc.)

Alcohol	>50%
Fragrance *†	15-30%

†*See* Essential oils

CHANEL NO. 5 SPRAY COLOGNE
(Chanel, Inc.)

Alcohol *	>50%
Water	10-20%
Fragrance *†	<5%

†*See* Essential oils

CHANEL NO. 5 SPRAY PERFUME
(Chanel, Inc.)

Alcohol *	>50%
Fragrance *†	<15%

†*See* Essential oils

CHANEL NO. 19 EAU DE COLOGNE
(Chanel, Inc.)

Alcohol *	>50%
Water	<20%
Fragrance *†	1-5%
Color	trace

†*See* Essential oils

CHANEL NO. 19 EAU DE TOILETTE
(Chanel, Inc.)

Alcohol *	>50%
Water	<20%
Fragrance *†	1-5%
Color	trace

†*See* Essential oils

CHANEL NO. 19 PERFUME
(Chanel, Inc.)

Alcohol *	>50%
Fragrance *†	<25%

†*See* Essential oils

CHANEL NO. 22 BATH OIL
(Chanel, Inc.)

Emollient ester	45-55%
Emollient alcohol	10-15%
Mineral oil	<25%
Lanolin derivative	<5%
Nonionic surfactant	<5%
Fragrance *†	<5%

†*See* Essential oils

CHANEL NO. 22 EAU DE COLOGNE
(Chanel, Inc.)

Alcohol *	>50%
Water	<20%
Fragrance *†	1-5%
Color	trace

†*See* Essential oils

CHANEL NO. 22 PERFUME
(Chanel, Inc.)

Alcohol	>50%
Fragrance *†	20-40%

†*See* Essential oils

CHANEL NO. 22 SPRAY PERFUME
(Chanel, Inc.)

Alcohol *	>50%
Fragrance *†	10-30%

†*See* Essential oils

CHAPERONE DEODORANT SPRAY
For household, dogs and cats
(Sudbury Lab.)

G-11 (glycol)	0.2%
G-4 (glycol)	0.1%
Delta extra	5.0%
Menthols racemic, USP *	2.0%
Propellent	

'76 Ed.

CHAPERONE FLEA & TICK AEROSOL SPRAY FOR DOGS & CATS
(Sudbury Lab.)

Pyrethrins	0.025%
Piperonyl butoxide, tech.	0.256%
Rotenone	0.128%
Other cube extractives	0.236%
Petroleum distillates	0.102%

'76 Ed.

CHAPERONE FOAM SHAMPOO
For dogs, cats
(Sudbury Lab.)

Piperonyl butoxide, tech.	0.880%
Pyrethrins	0.088%
Petroleum oil	0.352%

'76 Ed.

CHAPERONE, LIQUID
Dog repellent
(Sudbury Lab.)

Oil of lemongrass *	11.0%
Synthetic Oil of mustard	0.2%

'76 Ed.

CHAPERONE NEW AEROSOL LIQUID DOG OR CAT REPELLENT (INDOOR)
(Sudbury Lab.)

Oil of lemongrass	2.0%
Synthetic Oil of mustard	0.1%
Propellant and inert ingredients	93.0%

'76 Ed.

CHAPERONE NEW AEROSOL LIQUID DOG OR CAT REPELLENT (OUTDOOR)
(Sudbury Lab.)

Oil of lemongrass	6.9%
Propellant and other inert ingredients	98%

'76 Ed.

CHAPERONE REPEL-O ROPE
Animal repellent
(Sudbury Lab.)

Oil of lemongrass *	11.0%
Synthetic Oil of mustard	0.2%

'76 Ed.

CHAPERONE SQUIRREL REPELLENT
(Sudbury Lab.)

Paradichlorobenzene *	98%
Oil of lemongrass	0.5%

'76 Ed.

CHAP-ET LIP BALM
Flavors: Cherry, Grape, Lemon, Orange, Regular, Bubble Gum
(Stanback)

Active ingred.:	
Octyl dimethyl PABA	1.50%
Other ingred.:	
Petrolatum, Wax, Mineral oil	>80%
Isopropyl myristate	>10%
Flavors	<3%
Camphor (Regular only)	0.5%
Colors:	trace
FD & C Red #3	
FD & C Blue #1	
FD & C Yellow #5	
FD & C Yellow #6	

CHAPMAN AMBRITE T
Insecticidal wood preservative
(Chapman Chem.)

Benzene hexachloride, gamma isomer *	6.63%
Benzene hexachloride, other isomers	8.27%
Pentachlorophenol *	17.20%
Other chlorinated phenols	2.00%
Xylene *	31.10%

'76 Ed.

CHAPMAN BHC-1 EMULSIFIABLE CONCENTRATE
Insecticide
(Chapman Chem.)

Benzene hexachloride, gamma isomer *	11.3%
Benzene hexachloride, other isomers	17.0%
Methylated naphthalene *	56.7%

'76 Ed.

CHAPMAN BUCHANAN SPECIAL BLEND STAIN CONTROL
For control of blue stain and mold in softwoods and hardwoods
(Chapman Chem.)

Sodium pentachlorophenate *	55.3%
Sodium salts of other chlorophenols	7.7%
Borax (Sodium tetraborate decahydrate)	30.0%

'76 Ed.

CHAPMAN PENTA GENERAL WEED KILLER
(Chapman Chem.)

Pentachlorophenol	6.88%
Other chlorophenols	0.80%
Aromatic petroleum derivative solvent *	89.00%

'76 Ed.

CHAPMAN PENTA PLUS 40
Wood preservative, soil poison
(Chapman Chem.)

Pentachlorophenol *	35.3%
Other chlorinated phenols	4.1%
Aromatic petroleum derivative solvent *	41.0%

'76 Ed.

CHAPMAN PENTA PRESERVATIVE CONCENTRATE 1 TO 10
Wood preservative
(Chapman Chem.)

Pentachlorophenol *	34.1%
Other chlorinated phenols	4.9%
Aromatic petroleum solvents *	30.0%
Inert ingred.:	
Special Solvents	29.0%
Other	2.0%

'76 Ed.

CHAPMAN PENTA-WR CONCENTRATE 1 TO 3
Wood preservative
(Chapman Chem.)

Pentachlorophenol *	14.90%
Other chlorophenols	2.16%
Petroleum distillate *	55.33%
Inert ingred.:	
Water repellents	26.71%

'76 Ed.

CHAPMAN PENTA-WR CONCENTRATE 1 TO 5
Wood preservative
(Chapman Chem.)

Pentachlorophenol *	21.00%
Other chlorophenols	3.04%
Petroleum distillate *	37.20%
Inert ingred.:	
Water repellents	37.50%

'76 Ed.

CHAPMAN PENTA-WR WATER REPELLENT WOOD PRESERVATIVE READY-TO-USE
(Chapman Chem.)

Pentachlorophenol *	4.37%
Other chlorinated phenols	0.63%
Petroleum hydrocarbons *	81.80%
Inert ingred.:	
From chlorinated phenols	0.20%
Other	13.00%

'76 Ed.

CHAPMAN PERMATOX 155
Fungicide - wood preservative
(Chapman Chem.)

Potassium 2,3,4,6-tetrachloro-phenate *	31.43%
Potassium 2,4,5-trichlorophenate	7.34%
Potassium salts of other chlorophenols	8.50%

'76 Ed.

CHAPMAN PERMATOX 10-S
Wood preservative
(Chapman Chem.)

Borax *	57.0%
Sodium pentachlorophenate *	31.6%
Sodium salts of other chlorophenols	4.4%

'76 Ed.

CHAPMAN POL-NU
Wood preservative
(Chapman Chem.)

Pentachlorophenol	9.05%
Other chlorinated phenols	1.05%
Aromatic petroleum derivative solvent *	80.48%

'76 Ed.

CHAPMAN POL-NU 15-15
Wood preservative
(Chapman Chem.)

Pentachlorophenol *	12.97%
Other chlorinated phenols	1.51%
(Equiv. to 15.1% pentachlorophenol, technical)	
Creosote *	15.46%
Aromatic petroleum derivative solvent *	60.47%

'76 Ed.

CHAPMAN POL-NU PAK
Wood preservative
(Chapman Chem.)

Pentachlorophenol *	9.14%
Other chlorinated phenols	1.07%
(Equiv. to 10.66% pentachlorophenol, technical)	
Aromatic petroleum derivative solvent *	81.17%

'76 Ed.

CHAPMAN PQ-8
Fungicide concentrate - wood preservative
(Chapman Chem.)

Copper 8-quinolinolate	5.40%

'76 Ed.

CHAPMAN PQ-10
Fungicide - wood preservative
(Chapman Chem.)

Copper 8-quinolinolate	5.00%
Pentachlorophenol *	17.60%
Tetrachlorophenol	2.40%

'76 Ed.

CHAPMAN Q-SAN CONCENTRATE 1 TO 3
Water repellent wood preservative
(Chapman Chem.)

Copper 8-quinolinolate	0.96%

Note: May be mixed by user by adding one part of concentrate to 3 parts of any of the following:
Mineral spirits *
VM and P Naphtha *
Stoddard solvent *
Xylol *

'76 Ed.

CHAPMAN TIMPREG
Wood preservative
(Chapman Chem.)

Pentachlorophenol *	9.21%
Other chlorinated phenols	1.07%
(Equiv. to 10.7% technical pentachloro-phenol)	
Creosote	15.00%
Sodium fluoride *	15.00%
Aromatic petroleum derivative solvent *	51.30%

'76 Ed.

CHAPMAN TIMPREG B
Wood preservative
(Chapman Chem.)

Pentachlorophenol *	8.95%
Other chlorinated phenols	1.04%
(Equiv. to 10.69% technical pentachlo-rophenol)	
Sodium tetraborate, anhydrous	15.50%
Aromatic petroleum derivative solvent *	67.74%

'76 Ed.

CHAPMAN TIMPREG B (SPECIAL)
Wood preservative
(Chapman Chem.)

Pentachlorophenol *	9.41%
Other chlorinated phenols	1.09%
(Equiv. to 10.88% technical pentachlo-rophenol)	
Creosote	15.46%
Sodium tetraborate, anhydrous	15.50%
Aromatic petroleum derivative solvent *	51.91%

'76 Ed.

CHAPMAN TIMPREG PAK
For control of decay and as an aid in protection against termites
(Chapman Chem.)

Pentachlorophenol *	9.21%
Other chlorinated phenols	1.07%
(Equiv. to 10.7% pentachlorophenol, technical)	
Creosote	15.00%
Sodium fluoride *	15.00%
Aromatic petroleum derivative solvent *	51.30%

'76 Ed.

CHAPMAN WEED-FREE G
Granular herbicide
(Chapman Chem.)

Bromacil (5-Bromo-3-sec-butyl-6-methyluracil)	1.84%
Diuron (3-(3,4-Dichlorophenyl)1,1-dimethylurea)	0.92%
Sodium trichloroacetate (trichloro-acetic acid equiv. 5.13%)	5.81%
Dimethylamine salt of 2,3,6-trich-lorobenzoic acid	0.39%
Dimethylamine salt of other chlor-inated benzoic acids	0.26%

'76 Ed.

CHAP-OFF CREAM
For cold sores, fever & sun blisters
(Approved Pharm.)

Menthol *
Camphor *
Benzoin
Quaternary ammonium compound *

'76 Ed.

Starred ingredients (*) may be responsible for major toxic effects; consult Section II.

CHAP STICK FLAVORS
(Cherry, Grape, Mint, Strawberry, Orange, Lemon-Lime)
Lip emollient
(Miller-Morton)

Petrolatums	44%
Padimate O	1.5%
Lanolin (USP)	1.0%
Flavor	
Waxes	
Mineral oil	

CHAP STICK REGULAR
Lip emollient
(Miller-Morton)

Petrolatums	44%
Padimate O	1.5%
Lanolin (USP)	1.0%
Camphor (USP)	0.8%
Waxes	
Mineral oil	

CHAP STICK SPF-15
(Miller-Morton)

Petrolatums	44%
Padimate O	7%
Oxybenzone	3%
Lanolin	0.5%
Camphor (USP)	0.8%
Waxes	
Mineral oil	

CHARDONNA TABLETS
Antispasmodic-sedative
(Rorer, W.H., Inc.)

Each tablet:
Phenobarbital *	15 mg.
Extract Belladonna (belladonna alkaloids, 0.18 mg.) *	15 mg.

CHARGE BOWL CLEANER

See BUTCHER'S CHARGE BOWL CLEANER

CHARGER-E

See AGWAY CHARGER-E

CHARGERS
Stimulant
(DePree)

Caffeine *

CHARGO
Carbon remover and oven cleaner for industrial and institutional use
(Scientific International)

Caustic potash *

CHARLES OF THE RITZ COSMETICS

Charles of the Ritz Group Ltd.
40 W. 57th St.
New York, N.Y. 10019

Phone: 212-621-7327

See COSMETICS, Section VI, General Formulations

CHARLIE COSMETICS & TOILETRIES

Revlon, Inc.
767 Fifth Ave.
New York, N.Y. 10153

Phone: 212-572-5000

Revlon Research Center, Inc.
945 Zerega Ave.
Bronx, N.Y. 10473

Phone: 212-824-9000

See COSMETICS, Section VI, General Formulations

CHARO SCATTER-PAKS
Odor adsorber
(Requa)

Activated Charcoal

CHARSYLL
Aid in relief of constipation; adsorbent, antacid
(Friendly Labs.)

Psyllium seed husks
Activated charcoal
Dextrose

CHASE-MM ANT AND ROACH
Insecticide
(Chase Prod.)

Pyrethrins	0.050%
Technical Piperonyl butoxide	0.100%
N-Octyl bicycloheptene dicarboximide	0.166%
O,O-Diethyl O-(2-isopropyl-6-methyl-4-pyrimidinyl)phosphorothioate	0.500%
Petroleum distillate *	74.184%

'76 Ed.

CHASE-MM ANT KILLER
Insecticide
(Chase Prod.)

Sodium arsenate *	0.95%

'76 Ed.

Total arsenic (as metallic) all in water soluble form 0.39%

CHASE-MM FLYING INSECT KILLER
(Chase Prod.)

Pyrethrins	0.25%
Technical Piperonyl butoxide	0.50%
N-Octyl bicycloheptene dicarboximide	0.50%
Petroleum distillate	9.15%

'76 Ed.

CHASE-MM HOUSE AND GARDEN INSECT KILLER
(Chase Prod.)

Pyrethrins	0.25%
Technical Piperonyl butoxide	0.50%
N-Octyl bicycloheptene dicarboximide	0.50%
Petroleum distillate	9.15%

'76 Ed.

CHASE-MM INSECT REPELLENT
(Chase Prod.)

N,N-Diethyl-meta-toluamide	3.78%
Other isomers	0.42%
N-Octyl bicycloheptene dicarboximide	1.20%
2,3:4,5-Bis(2-butylene)tetrahydro-2-furaldehyde	0.30%
Di-n-propyl isocinchomeronate	0.30%

'76 Ed.

CHASE-MM LONG RANGE JET WASP SPRAY
(Chase Prod.)

Pyrethrins	0.15%
Technical Piperonyl butoxide	0.30%
N-Octyl bicycloheptene dicarboximide	0.53%
Technical Chlordane	2.00%
Petroleum distillate *	62.02%

'76 Ed.

CHASE-MM PATIO PATROL
(Chase Prod.)

Pyrethrins	0.20%
Technical Piperonyl butoxide	1.00%
Technical Methoxychlor	1.00%
2-Hydroxyethyl-n-octyl sulfide	0.95%
Related compounds	0.05%
Petroleum distillate	0.92%

'76 Ed.

CHATEAU CONCENTRATED FABRIC SOFTENER
(Industrial Equities)

Quaternary ammonium compound *	5-10%
Fluorescent whitening agent	<1%
Preservative	<1%
Colorant	<1%
Perfume	<1%
Water	balance

CHATEAU LIQUID DISHWASHING DETERGENT
(Industrial Equities)

Anionic surfactant	6-12%
Hydrotrope	1-3%
Alkanolamide	<1%
Ethyl alcohol	<1%
Opacifier	<1%
Colorant	<1%
Perfume	<1%
Water	balance

CHECK-FLY AND WORM CONTROL

See PURINA CHECK-FLY AND WORM CONTROL

CHECKMATE I
Steam system treatment
(Stiles-Kem)

Cyclohexamine *
Water
Sodium sulfite *

CHECKMATE II
Steam boiler treatment
(Stiles-Kem)

Aquadene *
Cyclohexamine *
Water

CHEER (Formula 1)
Granular laundry detergent
(Procter & Gamble)

Complex sodium phosphates	25-49%
Sodium carbonate	10-24%
Sodium sulfate	10-24%
Sodium alkyl ethoxylate sulfate	10-24%
Water	5-9%
Sodium silicate	5-9%
Sodium alkyl benzene sulfonate	1-4%
Sodium toluene sulfonate	1-4%
Minor ingredients, each	trace

pH (1% solution) - 10.9 max.

CHEER (Formula 2)
Granular laundry detergent
(Procter & Gamble)

Sodium sulfate	25-49%
Complex sodium phosphates	25-49%
Sodium alkyl benzene sulfonate	10-24%
Water	5-9%
Sodium silicate	1-4%
Sodium toluene sulfonate	1-4%
Minor ingredients, each	trace

pH (1% solution) - 10.9 max.

CHEER (Formula 3)
Granular laundry detergent
(Procter & Gamble)

Sodium sulfate	25-49%
Complex sodium phosphates	10-24%
Sodium alkyl benzene sulfonate	10-24%
Sodium carbonate	10-24%
Sodium aluminosilicate	5-9%
Water	5-9%
Sodium silicate	1-4%
Sodium toluene sulfonate	1-4%
Minor ingredients, each	trace

pH (1% solution) - 10.9 max.

CHEER (Formula 4)
Granular laundry detergent
(Procter & Gamble)

Complex sodium phosphates	25-49%
Sodium sulfate	25-49%
Sodium alkyl benzene sulfonate	10-24%
Water	5-9%
Sodium silicate	5-9%
Sodium toluene sulfonate	1-4%
Minor ingredients, each	trace

pH (1% solution) - 10.9 max.

CHEER (Formula 5)
Granular laundry detergent
(Procter & Gamble)

Sodium sulfate	25-49%
Sodium carbonate	10-24%
Sodium silicate	10-24%
Sodium alkyl benzene sulfonate	10-24%
Sodium alkyl ethoxylate sulfate	5-9%
Water	1-4%
Polyethylene glycol	1-4%
Minor ingredients, each	trace

pH (1% solution) - 10.9 max.

CHEK LEMON-LIME & CHEK MINT
Glycol air sanitizers; aerosol
(Kem Mfg. Co.)

Triethylene glycol	4.5%
Propylene glycol	3.0%
n-Alkyl (50% C14, 40% C12, 10% C16)dimethyl benzyl ammonium chloride	0.1%

CHEK-R-FURAN, PURINA

See PURINA CHEK-R-FURAN

CHEK-R-MYCIN

See PURINA CHEK-R-MYCIN

CHEL-IRON LIQUID
For iron-deficiency anemia
(Kinney)

Each tsp. (5 cc):
Ferrocholinate (equiv. to elemental iron, 50 mg.) * ... 0.417 gm.
In nonalcoholic Sorbitol vehicle

CHEL-IRON PEDIATRIC DROPS
For prevention, treatment of iron-deficiency anemia
(Kinney)

Each cc:
Ferrocholinate (equiv. to elemental iron, 25 mg.) * ... 0.208 gm.
In nonalcoholic, Sorbitol vehicle

CHEL-IRON TABLETS
For iron-deficiency anemia
(Kinney)

Each tablet:
Ferrocholinate (equiv. to elemental iron, 40 mg.) * ... 0.33 gm.

CHEMFORM BARICIDE
Concentrated insecticide spray
(Chemical Formulators)

Malathion *	16.0%
Methoxychlor (technical)	16.0%
Petroleum distillates *	63.0%

'76 Ed.

CHEMFORM BRAND SEVIN
Insecticide
(Chemical Formulators)

SPRAY POWDER:	
Sevin *	50%
GARDEN DUST:	
Sevin *	5%

'76 Ed.

CHEMFORM BUTOXY BRUSH KILLER
Herbicide
(Chemical Formulators)

2,4-Dichlorophenoxyacetic acid, butoxy ethoxy propanol esters *	28.0%
2,4,5-Trichlorophenoxyacetic acid, butoxy ethoxy propanol esters	13.3%
Inert ingred.:	58.7%
Emulsifier	
Solvents	

'76 Ed.

CHEMFORM 72% CHLORDANE
Insecticide, spray concentrate
(Chemical Formulators)

Chlordane (technical) *	72.0%
Petroleum distillate	23.2%

'76 Ed.

Starred ingredients (*) may be responsible for major toxic effects; consult Section II.

CHEMFORM DIOXY WEED KILLER
Herbicide, home & farm
(Chemical Formulators)

Dimethylamine salt of 2,4-dichlo-
rophenoxyacetic acid * 49.4%

'76 Ed.

CHEMFORM EVERGREEN SPRAY CONCENTRATE
Insecticide
(Chemical Formulators)

Malathion * 30%
Toxaphene (Chlorinated
camphene) * 20%
Xylols * 45%

'76 Ed.

CHEMFORM HOME TERMITE CONCENTRATE
Insecticide
(Chemical Formulators)

Chlordane (technical) * 47.00%
Inert ingred.:
Alkyl aryl sulfonate emulsifier   4.00%
Petroleum solvent * 44.00%

'76 Ed.

CHEMFORM METHOXYCHLOR 2 EC
Insecticide
(Chemical Formulators)

Active ingred.:
Methoxychlor (technical) * 25.0%
Petroleum distillate (xylene
bottoms) * 70.0%
Inert ingred.:
Alkyl aryl sulfonate (wetting
agent) 5.0%

'76 Ed.

CHEMFORM ROSE AND FLORAL DUST
Insecticide-fungicide
(Chemical Formulators)

Sevin (1-Naphthyl N-methylcarbamate) * 2.0%
Lindane (Gamma isomer of benzene
hexachloride) 1.0%
Tedion (2,4,5,4'-Tetrachlorodi-
phenyl sulphone) 0.5%
Maneb (manganese as metallic
0.99%) (Manganese ethylenebisdithiocarbamate) 6.4%
Sulfur - 325 fine ground 20.0%

'76 Ed.

CHEMFORM TOMATO DUST
Insecticide-fungicide
(Chemical Formulators)

Maneb (metallic manganese 0.99%)
(Manganese
ethylenebisdithiocarbamate) 4.8%
Sevin (Carbaryl) * 2.0%

'76 Ed.

CHEM HOE 2EC
Herbicide
(PPG Industries, Chem. Div.)

Isopropyl carbanilate 26%
Emulsifier 6%
Isophorone 34%
Xylene * 34%

CHEM HOE FL4
Herbicide
(PPG Industries, Chem. Div.)

Isopropyl carbanilate * 43%
Water 44%
Potassium chloride 10%
Emulsifier 3%

CHEM HOE 15G
Herbicide
(PPG Industries, Chem. Div.)

Isopropyl carbanilate * 15%
Sand and surfactant 85%

CHEMICAL MACE
*Aerosol non-lethal weapon for use by
police as an alternative to billy club
or firearm*
(Smith & Wesson/General Ordnance)

2-Chloroacetophenone (Phenylchloromethyl ketone) * .. 0.9% w/w
Inert carriers

CHEMIGUM
Oil resistant rubber products
(Goodyear)

Synthetic rubber copolymer of:
Butadiene
Acrylonitrile *

CHEM-REM CHEMICAL RESISTANT PAINT
(Speco)

Metallic pigments of Chrome *, Iron, Alu-
minum, Copper *, Titanium
Lampblack with various hydrocarbon ve-
hicles
Resins
Plasticizers
Coal tar solvents *

'76 Ed.

CHEMTROL NO. 1-5
*Antimicrobial compound used in indus-
trial water treatment*
(Zimmite Corp.)

Active ingred.:
Methylene bis(thiocyanate) * .. 5.0%
Inert ingred.:
Dimethylformamide 95.0%

CHEMTROL NO. 2A
*Antimicrobial compound used in indus-
trial water treatment*
(Zimmite Corp.)

n-Alkyl (C18 90%, C16 10%)
trimethyl ammonium chloride* .. 45%

CHEMTROL NO. 12
*Antimicrobial compound used in
industrial water treatment*
(Zimmite Corp.)

n-Alkyl (C18 90%, C16 10%)
trimethyl ammonium chloride * 35%
Bis(tributyltin)oxide* 8%

CHEMTROL NO. 19
*Antimicrobial compound used in indus-
trial water treatment*
(Zimmite Corp.)

Poly (oxyethylene (dimethyliminio)
ethylene (dimethyliminio)-ethyl-
ene dichloride) * 30%

CHEMTROL NO. 20
*Antimicrobial compound used in indus-
trial water treatment*
(Zimmite Corp.)

2,2-Dibromo-3-nitrilopropionamide * 5%

CHEMTROL 21
*Antimicrobial compound used in indus-
trial water treatment*
(Zimmite Corp.)

2,2-Dibromo-3-
nitrilopropionamide * 20%

CHEMTROL NO. 24
*Antimicrobial compound used in indus-
trial water treatment*
(Zimmite Corp.)

Sodium dimethyldithiocarbamate .. 15%
Nabam * 15%

CHEMTROL 28
*Antimicrobial compound used in indus-
trial water treatment*
(Zimmite Corp.)

Methylenebis(thiocyanate) * 10%

Starred ingredients (*) may be responsible for major toxic effects; consult Section II.

CHEMTROL NO. 840
Antimicrobial compound used in industrial water treatment
(Zimmite Corp.)

Sodium hypochlorite * 12.5%

CHEMWEED-265 SELECTIVE WEED KILLER
Herbicide
(National Chemsearch)

Potassium salt of 2-(2-methyl-4-chlorophenoxy) propionic acid *

CHEQ ANTIPERSPIRANT/ DEODORANT SPRAY (NON-AEROSOL)
(Almay)

Aluminum chlorohydrex
SD Alcohol 40
Isopropyl palmitate
Isopropyl myristate
Stearic acid
Trisodium EDTA

CHEQ EXTRA DRY ANTIPERSPIRANT/ DEODORANT SPRAY (AEROSOL)
(Almay)

Aluminum chlorohydrate
Isobutane
Cyclomethicone
Isopropyl myristate
Butane
Propane
Isopropyl isostearate
Silica
Sorbitan trioleate

CHEQ ROLL-ON ANTIPERSPIRANT/ DEODORANT
(Almay)

Aluminum chlorohydrate
Water
Glyceryl stearate
PEG-75 lanolin oil
Propylene glycol
Lauryl lactate
Mineral oil
PEG-8 laurate
Magnesium aluminum silicate
Laneth-10 acetate
PEG-4 oleate
Lanolin alcohol
Methylparaben
Propylparaben

CHEQ SOFT POWDER EXTRA DRY ANTIPERSPIRANT/ DEODORANT SPRAY (AEROSOL)
(Almay)

Aluminum chlorohydrate
Isobutane
Cyclomethicone
Talc
Butane
Propane
Silica
Sorbitan trioleate

CHERACOL COUGH SYRUP
(Upjohn)

Each 5 ml.:
    Codeine phosphate * .... 10 mg.
    Guaifenesin .... 100 mg.
    Alcohol 3%

CHERACOL D FAMILY COUGH SYRUP
(Upjohn)

Each 5 ml.:
    Dextromethorphan
      hydrobromide .... 10 mg.
    Guaifenesin .... 100 mg.
    Alcohol 3%

CHERALIN SYRUP
Cough expectorant and sedative
(Lannett)

Each fl. oz.:
    Chloroform .... 2 mins.
    Potassium guaiacol sulfonate . 8 gr.
    Ammonium chloride .... 8 gr.
    Antimony and Potassium
      tartrate .... 1/12 gr.

CHERALIN WITH CODEINE
Cough expectorant and sedative
(Lannett)

Each fl. oz.:
    Chloroform .... 2 mins.
    Potassium guaiacol sulfonate . 8 gr.
    Ammonium chloride .... 8 gr.
    Antimony and Potassium
      tartrate .... 1/12 gr.
    Codeine phosphate * .... 1 gr.

CHERATHOR COUGH SYRUP
(Towne, Paulsen)

Each fl. oz.:
    Dextromethorphan HBr ..... 45 mg.
    Pyrilamine maleate * .... 40 mg.
    Methapyrilene HCl * .... 20 mg.
    Ammonium chloride .... 520 mg.
    Potassium guaiacol sulfonate . 520 mg.
    Antimony potassium tartrate . 5 mg.
    Chloroform .... 2 m.
    Alcohol 5%

CHERO-TRISULFA-V
Multiple sulfonamide therapy
(Vita Elixir Co.)

Each 5 cc:
    Sulfadiazine * .... 0.166 gm.
    Sulfacetamide * .... 0.166 gm.
    Sulfamerazine * .... 0.166 gm.
    Sodium citrate .... 0.500 gm.

CHERROSOTE COUGH SYRUP
(Rexall)

Alcohol 2%
Chloroform .... <1%
Calcium creosote sulfonate ..... <1%
Calcium guaiacol sulfonate ..... <1%
Wild cherry bark 1-10%
White pine bark 1-10%
Spikenard root .... <1%
Balm of Gilead buds .... <1%
Blood root .... <1%
Sassafras bark .... <1%
Ammonium chloride 1-5%
Tartar emetic * .... <1%

'76 Ed.

CHERRY CHLORASEPTIC LOZENGES
Topical anesthetic-antiseptic
(Norwich-Eaton)

Each lozenge:
    Phenol * .... 34 mg.
    Sodium hydroxide .... 1.3 mg.
    Flavor
    Dye
    Sugar solids
    Syrup solids
    Water

CHERRY CHLORASEPTIC MOUTHWASH AND GARGLE
Topical anesthetic-antiseptic
(Norwich-Eaton)

Phenol * 1.4%
Sodium hydroxide 0.05%
Glycerin 1.2%

CHERRY CHLORASEPTIC SPRAY
Topical anesthetic-antiseptic
(Norwich-Eaton)

Phenol * 1.5%
Sodium hydroxide 0.05%
Glycerin 1.2%
Flavor

CHERRY KLOP INSECT KILLER
(Hysan Corp.)

Pyrethrins 0.30%
Piperonyl butoxide technical 0.60%
N-Octyl bicycloheptene
    dicarboximide 1.00%
Petroleum distillates 8.10%

Starred ingredients (*) may be responsible for major toxic effects; consult Section II.

CHEVRON PRODUCTS

Standard Oil Co. of California
Environmental Health Center
P.O. Box 1272
Richmond, CA 94802

Emergency medical consultation
concerning Chevron or Ortho products
may be obtained on a 24-hour basis from
Chevron's Poison Information Center.

Emergency phone number: 415-233-3737

CHEVRON WEED KILLER CONCENTRATE "D"
(Chevron)

Diquat dibromide * 35.3%/w

Chevron emergency phone number: 415-233-3737

CHEW-CHECK

See CARSON CHEW-CHECK

CHEW-NOT
Repellent for rabbits, deer & meadow mice
(Nott)

Thiram * 20.0%

CHEX
Breath deodorant
(Chex)

Each tablet:
Chlorophyll .... 2 mg.
Essential oils * .... 7 mg.
Sugar
Corn syrup
Menthol *
Methyl salicylate *

'76 Ed.

CHEXIT
Decongestant, antihistaminic, antitussive, expectorant, analgesic
(Dorsey Labs.)

Each tablet:
Phenylpropanolamine
hydrochloride * .... 25 mg.
Pheniramine maleate * .... 12.5 mg.
Pyrilamine maleate * .... 12.5 mg.
Dextromethorphan
hydrobromide .... 30 mg.
Terpin hydrate .... 180 mg.
Acetaminophen * .... 325 mg.

CHICK-CHICK
Easter egg dyes
(Doxsee Food Corp.)

Salt
US certified colors for yellow, orange & red 3%
US certified colors for green, blue & lavender 1 1/2%

CHIGGEREX
Relief from insect bites
(Scherer Labs.)

Benzocaine
Camphor *
Menthol *
Clove oil *
Olive oil
Peppermint oil
Water and Pegosperse base

CHIGGERTOX
Relief from insect bites
(Scherer Labs.)

Benzocaine
Benzyl benzoate
Soft soap
Isopropanol base

CHILDREN'S CO-TYLENOL LIQUID COLD FORMULA
Decongestant-analgesic
(McNeil Consumer Products Co.)

Each 5 ml.:
Acetaminophen * .... 160 mg.
Chlorpheniramine maleate ... 1 mg.
Pseudoephedrine
hydrochloride * .... 15 mg.

CHILDREN'S HOLD
4 hour cough suppressant & decongestant
(Beecham Products)

Each lozenge:
Dextromethorphan
Phenylpropanolamine *

CHILDREN'S TYLENOL CHEWABLE TABLETS
Analgesic-antipyretic
(McNeil Consumer Products Co.)

Each tablet:
Acetaminophen * .... 80 mg.

CHILDREN'S TYLENOL ELIXIR
Analgesic-antipyretic
(McNeil Consumer Products Co.)

Each 5 ml.:
Acetaminophen * .... 120 mg.

CHILL-IT
Canned refrigerant
(Speco)

Cellulose derivatives
Glycol blends
Water-soluble dye
Rust inhibitors (Nuodex 545)

'76 Ed.

CHIMERE CLEANSING GEL
(Chesebrough-Pond's)

Water .... >50%
Sodium C14-16 olefin
sulfonate .... >10-25%
Cocamidopropyl betaine ...>5-10%
Lauramide DEA .... >1-5%
Linoleamide DEA .... >1-5%
Fragrance .... >0.1-1%
Disodium EDTA .... >0.1-1%
DMDM hydantoin .... >0.1-1%
Phosphoric acid .... >0.1-1%
Methylparaben .... >0.1-1%
Propylparaben .... 0.1% or less
Propylene glycol .... 0.1% or less
Color .... 0.1% or less

CHIMERE CONDITIONING BATH & BODY OIL
(Chesebrough-Pond's)

Mineral oil .... >25-50%
Isopropyl palmitate .... >25-50%
Fragrance * .... >1-5%
Nonoxynol-4 .... >0.1-1%

CHIMERE LIQUID SOAP
(Chesebrough-Pond's)

Water .... >50%
Sodium C-14-16 olefin
sulfonate 10-20%
Cocamidopropyl betaine ... 5-10%
Lauramide DEA 1-5%
Linoleamide DEA 1-5%
Glycol stearate 1-5%
Propylene glycol .... <0.1%
Colors .... <0.1%
Methylparaben 0.1-1%
Propylparaben 0.1-1%
Fragrance 0.1-1%
Disodium EDTA 0.1-1%
DMDM hydantoin 0.1-1%
Phosphoric acid 0.1-1%

CHIMERE PERFUMED POWDER MITT
(Chesebrough-Pond's)

Talc .... >50%
Fragrance 1-5%

CHIMERE PERFUMED SHAKER TALC
(Chesebrough-Pond's)

Talc .... >50%
Fragrance 1-5%

CHIMERE SKIN REFRESHER SPRAY
(Chesebrough-Pond's)

SD Alcohol 40 .... >50%
Water .... >10-25%
Propylene glycol .... >1-5%
Fragrance .... >1-5%
Colors .... 0.1% or less

Starred ingredients (*) may be responsible for major toxic effects; consult Section II.

CHINOSOL
Antiseptic
(Vernon Labs.)

Each tablet:
Oxyquinoline sulfate * .... 3/5 gr.

CHIPCO RONSTAR G
Herbicide
(Rhone-Poulenc)

Oxadiazon 2.0%

CHIPCO TURF HERBICIDE "D"
(Rhone-Poulenc)

Dimethylamine salt of 2,4-dichlo-
rophenoxyacetic acid * 47.29%

CHIPCO TURF HERBICIDE MCPP
Herbicide
(Rhone-Poulenc)

2-(2-Methyl-4-
chlorophenoxy)propionic acid, diethanolamine salt * 32.8%

CHIPCO TURF KLEEN
Herbicide
(Rhone-Poulenc)

Diethanolamine salt of 2-(2-
methyl-4-chlorophenoxy)
propionic acid * 16.20%
Diethanolamine salt of 2,4-dichlo-
rophenoxyacetic acid * 15.48%

CHIPMAN ANT AND GRUB KILLER
Insecticide
(Chipman Inc.)

Chlordane 5.0%

CHIPMAN B-3 DUAL PURPOSE SEED TREATMENT
(Chipman Inc.)

Technical Diazinon * 11.0%
Gamma BHC (from lindane) * ... 16.6%
Captan 33.5%

CHIPMAN BRUSH KILLER 76
Herbicide
(Chipman Inc.)

Iso-octyl ester 2,4-dichlorophenoxy
acid (2,4-D acid equiv. 38.4 oz./Imperial
gal.) *
Iso-octyl ester 2,4,5-trichlorophenoxy-
acetic acid (2,4,5-T acid equiv. 38.4 oz./
Imperial gal.) *

CHIPMAN BRUSH KILLER 128
Herbicide
(Chipman Inc.)

Each gal.:
2,4-D acid equiv. * .... 64 oz.
2,4,5-T acid equiv. * .... 64 oz.

CHIPMAN CUCURBIT DUST
Fungicide, insecticide
(Chipman Inc.)

Methoxychlor, tech. 3.0%
Zineb (Zinc ethylene
bisdithiocarbamate) 3.9%

CHIPMAN D-L PLUS SEED TREATMENT
Insecticide, fungicide
(Chipman Inc.)

Diazinon * 15.0%
Gamma BHC (from lindane) * 25.0%
Captan 15.0%

CHIPMAN FERBAM WETTABLE POWDER
Fungicide
(Chipman Inc.)

Ferbam (Ferric
dimethyldithiocarbamate) * 76%

CHIPMAN GARDEN DUST
Insecticide, fungicide
(Chipman Inc.)

Folpet (Phaltan) 5%
Malathion * 4%
Carbaryl * 5%

CHIPMAN GARDEN FUNGICIDE
Wettable powder fungicide
(Chipman Inc.)

Technical Captan 50%

CHIPMAN GRAIN PROTECTANT
Seed treatment
(Chipman Inc.)

Malathion 0.5%

CHIPMAN LIMAX SLUG KILLER PELLETS
Insecticide
(Chipman Inc.)

Metaldehyde * 2.75%

CHIPMAN LIVESTOCK SPRAY
Insecticide
(Chipman Inc.)

Crotoxyphos * 1%
Dichlorvos 0.25%

CHIPMAN LOUSE POWDER
Insecticide
(Chipman Inc.)

Rotenone 0.5%

CHIPMAN PREMIUM LAWN WEEDKILLER
Herbicide
(Chipman Inc.)

2,4-D equiv. * ..... 20 oz./Imperial gal.
Mecoprop (d-isomer) 20 oz./Imperial gal.

CHIPMAN ROSE DUST OR SPRAY
Insecticide, fungicide
(Chipman Inc.)

Folpet 5%
Malathion * 4%
Carbaryl * 5%

CHIPMAN TCA
Herbicide
(Chipman Inc.)

TCA equiv. (sodium salt 95%) * ... 84%

CHIPMAN TRI-COP WP
(Chipman Inc.)

Basic Copper sulfate * 53.0%

CHIPTOX
Herbicide
(Rhone-Poulenc)

Sodium salt of 2-methyl-4-chloro-
phenoxyacetic acid * 23.7%

CHLORACET CAPSULES
Relief in colds, allergies & influenza
(Jenkins Labs.)

Each capsule:
Chlorpheniramine maleate .. 4 mg.
Salicylamide .... 3 gr.
Phenacetin * .... 2 gr.
Caffeine .... 1/2 gr.
Ascorbic acid .... 50 mg.
Methamphetamine HCl ..... 1.25 mg.

CHLORAGESIC
Analgesic rub
(La Crosse)

Each oz.:
Chloral hydrate * .... 10 gr.
Methyl salicylate *
Menthol *

CHLORAMATE UNICELLES
Relief of allergies
(Reid-Provident)

Each timed-release capsule:
Chlorpheniramine maleate * .. 12 mg.

Starred ingredients (*) may be responsible for major toxic effects; consult Section II.

CHLORASEPTIC CHILDREN'S LOZENGES
Control of minor sore throat pain
(Norwich-Eaton)

Benzocaine .... 5 mg.
Grape flavorings

CHLORASEPTIC-DM LOZENGES
Topical anesthetic-antiseptic; antitussive
(Norwich-Eaton)

Each lozenge:
Phenol * .... 34 mg.
Sodium hydroxide .... 1.3 mg.
Dextromethorphan
   hydrobromide * .... 10 mg.
Flavor
Glycerin
Agar
Caramel
Sugar solids
Syrup solids
Water

CHLORASEPTIC GEL
Relief of discomfort from minor mouth and gum irritations
(Norwich-Eaton)

Phenol * 1.4%

CHLORASEPTIC LOZENGES
Topical anesthetic-antiseptic
(Norwich-Eaton)

Each lozenge:
Phenol * .... 34 mg.
Sodium hydroxide .... 1.3 mg.
Flavor
Dye
Sugar solids
Syrup solids
Water

CHLORASEPTIC MOUTHWASH AND GARGLE
Topical anesthetic-antiseptic
(Norwich-Eaton)

Phenol * 1.4%
Sodium hydroxide 0.05%
Glycerin 1.2%

CHLORASEPTIC SPRAY
Topical anesthetic-antiseptic
(Norwich-Eaton)

Phenol * 1.5%
Sodium hydroxide 0.05%
Glycerin 1.2%

CHLOR-A-TYL
(Jenkins Labs.)

Each tablet:
Acetyl-p-aminophenol * .... 160 mg.
Chlorpheniramine maleate .. 1 mg.
Phenylephrine HCl * .... 7 1/2 mg.
Ascorbic acid .... 15 mg.

CHLORBIOTIC
Ophthalmic ointment for dogs and cats
(Burns-Biotec)

Each gram:
Chloramphenicol (in a light mineral oil) .... 10 mg.
White petrolatum
Polyoxyethylene sorbitan monostearate
   base

CHLORCAIN
Anesthetic throat lozenges
(Jenkins Labs.)

Each tablet:
Cetylpyridinium chloride ..... 4 mg.
Sodium propionate .... 10 mg.
Benzocaine .... 6 mg.

CHLOR-DIS PINK, FOREMOST 1651

See FOREMOST 1651 CHLOR-DIS PINK

CHLOREA GRANULAR
Herbicide
(Rhone-Poulenc)

Sodium chlorate * 40.0%
Sodium metaborate 51.0%
Diuron 2.4%

CHLOR-F-RIN TABLETS
Antihistamine
(Moffet Inc.)

Each tablet:
Chlorpheniramine maleate, USP 4 mg.
Phenylephrine HCl, USP * .... 5 mg.

CHLOR-HISTINE ELIXIR
(Columbia Med.)

Each 5 ml.:
Phenylephrine HCl * .... 5.0 mg.
Chlorpheniramine maleate .. 1.0 mg.
Chloroform * .... 13.5 mg.
Menthol * .... 1.0 mg.
Sodium bisulfite 0.1%
Alcohol 5.0%

CHLORINATED KLEER-MOR FORMULA HC-10

See KLENZADE CHLORINATED KLEER-MOR FORMULA HC-10

CHLOR-KIL HOME & GARDEN INSECTICIDE
(Durham's)

Technical Chlordane 5%

'76 Ed.

CHLOR-MAL 96, MUNICHEM

See MUNICHEM CHLOR-MAL 96

CHLOROPTIC
Ophthalmic solution
(Allergan Pharm.)

Chloramphenicol 0.5%

CHLOROPTIC-P S.O.P.
Sterile ophthalmic ointment
(Allergan Pharm.)

Chloramphenicol 1.0%
Prednisolone alcohol 0.5%
Chlorobutanol (chloral derivative as
   a preservative) 0.5%
White petrolatum
Mineral oil
Polyoxyl 40 stearate
Polyethylene glycol 300
Nonionic lanolin derivatives

CHLOROPTIC S.O.P.
Sterile ophthalmic ointment
(Allergan Pharm.)

Chloramphenicol 1.0%
Chlorobutanol (chloral derivative as
   a preservative) 0.5%
White petrolatum
Mineral oil
Polyoxyl 40 stearate
Polyethylene glycol 300
Nonionic lanolin derivatives

CHLOR-O-SAN

See UNIVERSAL CHLOR-O-SAN

CHLOROTHANE
Liquid analgesic
(Eastern Research Labs.)

Each fl. oz.:
Chloroform * .... 90 m.
Chloral hydrate * .... 8 gr.
Alcohol 26%/v
Isopropyl alcohol * 11%/v
Methyl salicylate *
Menthol *
Camphor *
Acetone

'76 Ed.

CHLORPAX
Insecticide
(Biocerta)

Chlordane technical 2%
Aliphatic petroleum distillates * .. 98%

'76 Ed.

CHLORPAX EMULSION CONCENTRATE
(Biocerta)

Chlordane, tech. * 73.0%
Petroleum distillates * 22.0%

'76 Ed.

Starred ingredients (*) may be responsible for major toxic effects; consult Section II.

CHLORTERP
(Jenkins Labs.)

Each tablet:
Terpin hydrate *	2 gr.
Potassium iodide	1/8 gr.
Creosote	1/10 min.
Eucalyptol	1/10 min.

CHLOR-TRIMETON EXPECTORANT
Antihistamine-decongestant-expectorant
(Schering)

Each 5 cc:
Chlorpheniramine maleate	2 mg.
Phenylephrine hydrochloride	10 mg.
Ammonium chloride	100 mg.
Sodium citrate	50 mg.
Glyceryl guaiacolate	50 mg.
Alcohol	<1%

CHLOR-TRIMETON EXPECTORANT WITH CODEINE
Antihistaminic-decongestant-expectorant-antitussive-analgesic
(Schering)

Each 5 cc:
Chlorpheniramine maleate	2 mg.
Phenylephrine hydrochloride	10 mg.
Ammonium chloride	100 mg.
Sodium citrate	50 mg.
Glyceryl guaiacolate	50 mg.
Codeine phosphate *	10 mg.
Alcohol	approx. 5.25%

CHLOR-TRIMETON REPETABS
Relief of allergic manifestations
(Schering)

Each Repetab:
Chlorpheniramine maleate *	8 mg.; 12 mg.

CHLOR-TRIMETON SYRUP
Relief of certain allergic manifestations
(Schering)

Each 5 cc:
Chlorpheniramine maleate	2 mg.

CHLOR-TRIMETON TABLETS
For relief of allergies
(Schering)

Each tablet:
Chlorpheniramine maleate *	4 mg.

CHLORTRON
Antihistamines
(Pharmex)

Each capsule (timed disintegration):
Chlor-prophenpyridamine maleate *	8 mg.; 12 mg.

Each tablet:
Chlor-prophenpyridamine maleate *	4 mg.

CHLORULAN TABLETS
Diuretic
(Lannett)

Each tablet:
Chlorothiazide *	250 mg.; or 500 mg.

CHLORZIDE
Diuretic
(Foy Labs.)

Each tablet:
Hydrochlorothiazide *	50 mg.

CHOCOLAX
Laxative
(Elder)

Each tablet:
Phenolphthalein	32.4 mg.

CHOKE-EASE (Aerosol)
Automatic choke & carburetor cleaner
(American Grease Stick)

Combined amount:	97.1%
Xylene (mixture of ortho, meta + para) *	64.7%
Diacetone alcohol	32.4%
Carbon dioxide	2.9%

CHOLAN DH
Hydrocholeretic
(Pennwalt, Pharm. Div.)

Each tablet:
Dehydrocholic acid	250.0 mg.

CHOLAN HMB
Hydrocholeretic, anti-spasmodic, mild sedative
(Pennwalt, Pharm. Div.)

Each tablet:
Phenobarbital *	8.0 mg.
Dehydrocholic acid	250.0 mg.
Homatropine methylbromide	2.5 mg.

CHOLDUN'S CHROME PROTECTOR
(Choldun)

Mineral oil, light
Oleic acid
Triethanolamine
Non-ionic detergent *

'76 Ed.

CHOLDUN'S CHROME RUST REMOVER
(Choldun)

Oxalic acid *
Hydrochloric acid *

'76 Ed.

CHOLDUN'S HEAVY DUTY STEAM CLEANING COMPOUND
(Choldun)

Caustic soda *

'76 Ed.

CHOLDUN'S LEATHER MAGIC
(Choldun)

Sodium metasilicate
Isopropanol
Sodium alkyl sulfate *
Triethanolamine lauryl sulfate *
Fatty amide-condensate
Anhydrous fatty acid-amine condensate
Sulfonated ketones
Hydrophilic wax-cyclohexanone-amine wax (Vegamin wax)

'76 Ed.

CHOLDUN'S MAGIC REMOVER
(Choldun)

Mineral spirits *
Orthodichlorobenzene *
Xylol *

'76 Ed.

CHOLDUN'S PURPLE MAGIC
(Choldun)

Sodium alkyl sulfate *
Triethanolamine lauryl sulfate *
Fatty amide-condensate
Anhydrous fatty acid-amine condensate
Sulfonated Ketones
Hydrophilic wax-cyclohexanone-amine wax (Vegamin wax)

'76 Ed.

CHOLDUN'S WHITE TIRE MAGIC
(Choldun)

Alcohol *
Alkali *

'76 Ed.

Starred ingredients (*) may be responsible for major toxic effects; consult Section II.

CHOLOXIN
Hypocholesterolemic
(Flint Labs.)

Each tablet:
Dextrothyroxine sodium,
USP * .... 1 mg.; 2 mg.;
4 mg.; 6 mg.
Lactose, USP
Sugar, powdered, USP (contains corn starch)
Acacia, USP
Povidone, USP
Polysorbate 80, USP
Magnesium stearate, USP
Talc, USP
Gelatin, USP

CHOOZ (Medicated Gum)
Antacid, digestant
(Plough)

Magnesium trisilicate
Calcium carbonate
Peppermint oil

CHORE-BOY ACID CLEANER
Dairy use
(Chore-Boy)

Phosphoric acid * .... >30%
Hydroxyacetic acid .... <15%

CHORE-BOY BULK TANK CLEANER
Dairy use
(Chore-Boy)

Sodium tripolyphosphate .... >35%
Soda ash * .... >35%
Sodium metasilicate * .... <20%
Sodium dichloroisocyanurate ..... >2%
Alkyl aryl sulfonate .... <4%

CHORE-BOY CHLORINE SANITIZER
Dairy use
(Chore-Boy)

Sodium dichloro-s-triazinetrione
(Sodium
dichloroisocyanurate) * 20.84%

CHORE-BOY GENERAL CLEANER
For dairy farm utensils
(Chore-Boy)

Sodium metasilicate * .... >10%
Nonyl phenol ethylene oxide
condensate .... >5%
Sodium tripolyphosphate .... >40%
Soda ash * .... >40%

CHORE-BOY IODINE UDDER WASH
Cleaner sanitizer
(Chore-Boy)

Nonylphenoxypoly (ethyleneoxy) ethanol-iodine complex (providing 1.75% titratable iodine) 14.25%
Phosphoric acid * 12.50%

CHORE-BOY LIQUID PIPELINE CLEANER
Institutional and industrial use
(Chore-Boy)

Caustic potash (Potassium
hydroxide) * .... >17%
Polyphosphates .... >16%
Sodium hypochlorite .... <2%

CHORE-BOY PIPELINE CLEANER
Dairy use
(Chore-Boy)

Sodium tripolyphosphate .... >35%
Soda ash * .... >35%
Sodium metasilicate * .... <15%
Sodium dichloroisocyanurate ..... <3%

CHRISTIAN DIOR COSMETIC PRODUCTS

Christian Dior Perfumes, Inc.
9 W. 57th St.
New York, N.Y. 10019

Phone: 212-759-1840

See COSMETICS, Section VI, General Formulations

CHRISTODYNE-DHC
Analgesic, antipyretic and antitussive
(Paddock Labs.)

Each tablet:
Acetyl-p-aminophenol * ..... 2 1/2 gr.
Acetylsalicylic acid * .... 3 1/2 gr.
Caffeine .... 1/2 gr.
Dihydrocodeinone bitartrate . 1/12 gr.

CHROMAGEN
Hematinic
(Savage Labs.)

Each capsule:
Ferrous fumarate USP * ..... 200 mg.
Ascorbic acid USP .... 250 mg.
Cyanocobalamin USP ...... 10 mcg.
Desiccated stomach substance 100 mg.

CHROME-GLO
Polish
(Speco)

Abrasives
Ammonia *

'76 Ed.

CHROMELIN
Complexion blender
(Summers Labs.)

Dihydroxyacetone 5%

CHROME OINTMENT
Skin irritation & burns
(Wambaugh)

Balm Gilead .... Trace amount
Lanolin base

'76 Ed.

CHROMERGE
Chromic acid solution
(Manostat)

Chromic acid *

CHRONULAC SYRUP
Laxative
(Merrell Dow)

Each 15 ml.:
Lactulose .... 10 gm.
Syrup:
Lactose
Galactose
Other sugars

CHRYSLER PARTS BELT-EASE
(Chrysler Corp., Parts Div.)

See BELT-EASE

CHRYSLER PARTS DOOR-EASE
(Chrysler Corp., Parts Div.)

See DOOR-EASE

CHRYSLER PARTS LOCK-EASE
(Chrysler Corp., Parts Div.)

See LOCK-EASE

CHRYSLER PARTS SIL-GLYDE
(Chrysler Corp., Parts Div.)

See SIL-GLYDE

CHURN-KLENE
See KLENZADE CHURN-KLENE

Starred ingredients (*) may be responsible for major toxic effects; consult Section II.

CIARA TOILETRIES

Revlon, Inc.
767 Fifth Ave.
New York, N.Y. 10153

Phone: 212-572-5000

Revlon Research Center, Inc.
945 Zerega Ave.
Bronx, N.Y. 10473

Phone: 212-824-9000

See COSMETICS, Section VI, General
Formulations

CICO LIQUID PASTE
(Carter's Ink)

Corn syrup
Tapioca flour
Phenol *
Formaldehyde *
Phosphoric acid

'76 Ed.

CIDEX ACTIVATED DIALDEHYDE
Sterilizing and disinfecting solution
(Arbrook)

Glutaraldehyde 2.0%

CIDEX FORMULA 7
*Long-life activated dialdehyde steriliz-
ing and disinfecting solution*
(Arbrook)

Glutaraldehyde 2%

CIK ROACH 'N ANT KILLER
(Hysan Corp.)

O,O-Diethyl O-(2-isopropyl-4-
methyl-6-pyrimidinyl)
phosphorothioate 0.500%
Pyrethrins 0.050%
Technical Piperonyl butoxide .. 0.262%
Petroleum distillate * 95.238%

CINCH
Dishwashing liquid
(Procter & Gamble)

Water 50-74%
Sodium alkyl ethoxylate sulfate . 10-24%
Sodium alkyl sulfate 10-24%
Ethanol 5-9%
Siliceous particles (diatomite, hy-
drated aluminum silicate) 5-9%
Alkyl amine oxide 1-4%
Sodium dicarboxylated alkyl
sulfonate 1-4%
Minor ingredients, each .... trace

pH (as is) - 8.5

CINCH FLY SPRAY FOR HORSES
(Franklin Labs.)

Pyrethrins 0.5%
Piperonyl butoxide (technical) 5.0%
Butoxypolypropylene glycol * 12.5%
Petroleum distillate 2.0%

CINCH WIPE-ON FLY REPELLENT FOR HORSES
(Franklin Labs.)

Pyrethrins 0.06%
Piperonyl butoxide (technical) .. 0.12%
N-Octyl bicycloheptene
dicarboximide 0.20%
Di-n-propyl isocinchomeronate .. 0.40%
2,3:4,5-Bis(2-butylene)tetrahydro-
2-furaldehyde 0.20%
Oil of citronella 0.05%
Refined White oil 98.97%

CINDY CONCENTRATED FABRIC SOFTENER
(Industrial Equities)

Quaternary ammonium
compound * 5-10%
Fluorescent whitening agent ... <1%
Preservative .... <1%
Colorant .... <1%
Perfume .... <1%
Water .... balance

CINDY DRYER CYCLE FABRIC SOFTENER SHEETS
(Industrial Equities)

Cationic softener * 50-60%
Nonwoven rayon substrate 37-42%
Perfume .... <1%

CINDY FABRIC SOFTENER
(Industrial Equities)

Quaternary ammonium
compound * 2-5%
Preservative .... <1%
Colorant .... <1%
Perfume .... <1%
Water .... balance

CINDY LIQUID BLEACH
(Industrial Equities)

Sodium hypochlorite * 5 1/4%
Sodium chloride .... <5%
Water .... balance

CINDY LIQUID DISHWASHING DETERGENT
(Industrial Equities)

Anionic surfactant 6-12%
Hydrotrope 1-3%
Alkanolamide .... <1%
Ethyl alcohol .... <1%
Opacifier .... <1%
Colorant .... <1%
Perfume .... <1%
Water .... balance

CIN-QUIN CAPSULES
Cardiac depressant
(Rowell)

Quinidine sulfate * .... 200 mg.; 300 mg.

CIN-QUIN TABLETS
Cardiac depressant
(Rowell)

Quinidine sulfate * .... 100 mg.; 200 mg.;
300 mg.

CIRCART
Embalming fluid
(Embalmers')

Formaldehyde *

"CIRCLE" PERFUMED ROOM DEODORANT
Floral scented
(Curran)

Paradichlorobenzene *

'76 Ed.

CIRCLETTE COLD WAVE GOLDEN LOTION
(Willat)

Mono-thioglycerol 1-10%

CIRCOL
Embalming fluid
(Embalmers')

Formaldehyde *

CIRTAN
Embalming fluid
(Embalmers')

Formaldehyde *

CITCOP 4E
Liquid copper fungicide
(Cities Service Co.)

Copper salts of fatty and rosin
acids *† 48%

†*See* Copper

Starred ingredients (*) may be responsible for major toxic effects; consult Section II.

CITRA CAPSULES
Antihistamine, decongestant, analgesic
(Boyle & Co.)

Each capsule:
Phenylephrine HCl *	10.00 mg.
Ascorbic acid	50.00 mg.
Pheniramine maleate	6.25 mg.
Chlorpheniramine maleate	1.00 mg.
Pyrilamine maleate	8.33 mg.
Salicylamide	227.00 mg.
Phenacetin	120.00 mg.
Caffeine alkaloid	30.00 mg.

CITRA FORTE CAPSULES
Antitussive, antihistaminic, analgesic
(Boyle & Co.)

Each capsule:
Hydrocodone bitartrate *	5.00 mg.
Ascorbic acid	50.00 mg.
Pheniramine maleate	6.25 mg.
Potassium citrate	150.00 mg.
Pyrilamine maleate	8.33 mg.
Chlorpheniramine maleate	1.00 mg.
Phenylephrine HCl	10.00 mg.
Salicylamide	227.00 mg.
Caffeine alkaloid	30.00 mg.
Phenacetin	120.00 mg.

CITRA FORTE SYRUP
Antitussive, antihistaminic, analgesic
(Boyle & Co.)

Each 5 cc.:
Hydrocodone bitartrate *	5.00 mg.
Ascorbic acid	30.00 mg.
Pheniramine maleate	2.50 mg.
Potassium citrate	150.00 mg.
Pyrilamine maleate	3.33 mg.
Chlorpheniramine maleate	1.00 mg.
Phenylephrine HCl	10.00 mg.
Salicylamide	227.00 mg.
Caffeine alkaloid	30.00 mg.
Phenacetin	120.00 mg.
Alcohol	2%

CITRITAN LOTION
Suntan preparation
(D'Lanerg)

Mineral oil Kaydol
Stearic acid
Cocoa butter
Coconut oil
Glyceryl monostearate SE
Sunaromes WMO (2-Ethylhexyl salicylate)
Propylparaben USP
Water
FD & C Yellow #5
Methylparaben
Triethanolamine
Perfume Lemon F1-3769-1
Perfume Lime Pon 2276

CITRITAN OIL
Suntan preparation
(D'Lanerg)

Mineral oil Kaydol
Mineral oil Blandol
Cocoa butter
Coconut oil
Sunaromes WMO (2-Ethylhexyl salicylate)
Color - Leeben suntan shade
Perfume cocoa butter

CITRITAN TAN RETAINER
Suntan preparation
(D'Lanerg)

Mineral oil Kaydol
Stearic acid
Glyceryl monostearate SE
Cocoa butter
Coconut oil
Vitamin E
Propylparaben USP
Water

CITROCARBONATE
To increase alkali reserve
(Upjohn)

Each 3.9 gm. (when dissolved):
Sodium bicarbonate	approx. 0.78 gm.
Sodium citrate (anhydrous)	approx. 1.82 gm.

CITROPYRINE ELIXIR
(International Chem.)

Each oz.:
Aspirin *	20 gr.
Sodium salicylate *	20 gr.
Sodium citrate	40 gr.

'76 Ed.

CITROVAL
Analgesic
(Vale)

Each tablet:
Phenacetin *	64.8 mg.
Aspirin *	129.6 mg.
Caffeine anhydrous	6.5 mg.
Sodium citrate	129.6 mg.

CITROX
Skin ointment
(Citrox)

Lanolin
Glycerin
Stearic acid
Sodium benzoate
Oil of lemon *
Allantoin

CJ'S COATED RAT AND MOUSE BAIT
Rodenticide
(Martin, C.J.)

Coated Warfarin

CLAIRE ROOM DEODORIZERS
Spice Aire, Lemon Aire, Mint Aire, Bel Aire, Spring Aire
(Claire)

Triethylene glycol	7.5%

CLAIROL HAIR CARE PRODUCTS

Clairol, Inc.
345 Park Ave.
New York, N.Y. 10154

Phone: 212-546-5000

See COSMETICS, Section VI, General Formulations

CL10 ALUMINUM PAINT
For interior and exterior wood, metal and masonry surfaces
(United Gilsonite)

Pigment:	13%
Aluminum paste - standard lining	100%
Vehicle:	87%
Processed Linseed oil	40%
Mineral spirits *	60%

CL25 ALUMINUM PAINT
For interior and exterior wood, metal and masonry surfaces
(United Gilsonite)

Pigment:	16.4%
Aluminum paste - standard lining	100%
Vehicle:	83.6%
Processed Linseed oil	45%
Mineral spirits *	55%

CLARIX
Industrial laundry detergent
(Diversey Wyandotte)

Sodium hydroxide*
Alkaline salts

C-20 LAUNDRY POWDER

See MT. HOOD C-20 LAUNDRY POWDER

CLAYCRETE
Powdered sculpting and modeling media
(American Art Clay Co.)

This product bears the CP Seal issued by the Crayon, Water Color and Craft Institute, Inc. This seal certifies that the product contains no materials in sufficient quantities to be toxic or injurious to the human body even if ingested.

CLAYOLA MODELING CLAY
(Binney & Smith)

Grease-type binder
Preservative
Odorant
Non-toxic pigments

CLAYTON LIGHT DUTY TANK CLEANER
For spray cleaning in aluminum tank trucks
(Clayton Mfg.)

Sodium silicate	>40%
Sodium carbonate *	>10%
Sodium phosphate	>10%
Nonionic synthetic detergent	1-10%

CLAYTON VAT COMPOUND NO. 2
(Clayton Mfg.)

Sodium silicate	>10%
Sodium hydroxide *	10-20%
Sodium phosphate	>10%
Sodium carbonate *	>10%
Soap	>10%

CLAYTON VAT COMPOUND NO. 3
(Clayton Mfg.)

Sodium carbonate	>10%
Sodium hydroxide *	>50%
Soap	>10%

CLAYTON VAT COMPOUND NO. 4
(Clayton Mfg.)

Sodium carbonate	>10%
Sodium hydroxide *	>50%
Nonionic synthetic detergent	1-10%

CLAYTON WATER CONDITIONING COMPOUNDS
Boiler feedwater conditioning compounds
(Clayton Mfg.)

COMPOUND 1A:
Sodium hydroxide *	20%
Sodium sulfite anhydrous	65%
Trisodium phosphate, anhydrous	15%
Cobalt sulfate	0.01%

COMPOUND 2A:
Sodium hydroxide *	30%
Sodium sulfite anhydrous	35%
Trisodium phosphate, anhydrous	35%
Cobalt sulfate	0.01%

COMPOUND 3A:
Sodium hydroxide *	35%
Sodium sulfite anhydrous	25%
Trisodium phosphate, anhydrous	40%
Cobalt sulfate	0.01%

CLEAN-ALL

See SOLVIT CLEAN-ALL

CLEAN AND ETCH
Concrete cleaner
(Paul Koss)

Water	<45%
Phosphoric acid (85%) *	<40%
Isopropyl alcohol	<25%
Dioctyl ester of sodium sulfosuccinic acid	
Methyl ethyl ketone	
Ethylene dichloride	
Triethanolamine	
Dye	trace

pH 2.3-2.5

CLEAN HATCH
Sanitizer, disinfectant
(Whitmoyer)

Active ingred.:
Methyldodecyl trimethyl ammonium chloride *	10.00%
Methyldodecylxylylene bis (trimethyl ammonium chloride)	2.50%
Tetrasodium ethylenediamine tetraacetate	0.38%
Sodium carbonate *	0.50%
Inert ingred.:	86.62%
Contains Sodium nitrite *	

CLEAN-N-GLEAM
(Uncle Sam)

Acrylic polymers (metal cross-linked)
Vegetable oils & Potassium hydroxide *
Synthetic detergents *
Polyethylene
Morpholine *
Water softeners
Water

CLEAN-N-SOAK
Hard contact lens cleaning and soaking solution
(Allergan Pharm.)

Cleaning agent
Phenylmercuric nitrate 1:25,000

CLEAN-O-LITE
Cleaner-sanitizer
(Hillyard Chem.)

Quaternary synthetic detergent *†

'76 Ed.

†*See* Cationic surfactants

CLEAN-OUT DRAIN OPENER
Industrial/institutional use
(Puro Chem. Co.)

Caustic soda (Sodium hydroxide) *
Caustic potash (Potassium hydroxide) *

CLEAN QUICK (Phosphate Formula or 0-Phosphate Formula)
Institutional and industrial cleaning product

Procter & Gamble Co.
Ivorydale Technical Center
Cincinnati, Ohio 45217

Phone: 513-562-1100

CLEAN START NON-AMMONIATED WAX STRIPPER
(Nat'l Labs. Div.)

Sodium metasilicate pentahydrate	minor
Ethylene glycol monobutyl ether (Butyl Cellosolve)	minor
Monoethanolamine	minor

CLEAN WALLPAPER CLEANER
(Clean Prod.)

Clean Products Co.
7275 Neville St.
Columbus, Ohio 44102

Phone: 614-252-1104

CLEAR AND DRY
Analgesic-decongestant
(Whitehall Labs.)

Phenylephrine *
Belladonna alkaloids *
Phenindamine tartrate *
Caffeine
Aspirin *
Aluminum hydroxide-magnesium carbonate co-dried gel

CLEARASIL ACNE TREATMENT STICK
(Vicks Toiletry Products Div.)

Polyoxyethylene lauryl ether	
PEG-20 sorbitan beeswax	
Titanium dioxide	
Sulfur	8.0%
Bentonite	4.0%
Resorcinol	1.0%
Iron oxides	

CLEARASIL ANTIBACTERIAL ACNE LOTION
(Vicks Toiletry Products Div.)

Benzoyl peroxide	5.0%
Water	
Propylene glycol	10.0%
Glyceryl stearate SE	
Bentonite	
Cellulose gum	
Isopropyl myristate	
Sodium citrate	
Dimethicone	
Methylparaben	
Propylparaben	

Starred ingredients (*) may be responsible for major toxic effects; consult Section II.

CLEARASIL ANTIBACTERIAL SOAP
Acne treatment/deodorant soap
(Vicks Toiletry Products Div.)

Soap from animal and vegetable fats
Triclosan 0.75%

CLEARASIL BP ACNE TREATMENT CREAM
(Vicks Toiletry Products Div.)

Benzoyl peroxide *	10.0%
Water	
Propylene glycol	10.0%
Bentonite	
Glyceryl stearate SE	
Isopropyl myristate	
Cellulose gum	
Dimethicone	
Methylparaben	
Titanium dioxide	
Iron oxide	
Propylparaben	

CLEARASIL PORE DEEP CLEANSER
(Vicks Toiletry Products Div.)

Salicylic acid	0.5%
Alcohol (Ethanol)	43.0%
Water	
Acetone	
Ceteareth-27	
Propylene glycol	
Tartaric acid	
Fragrance	
Menthol	

CLEAR DAY WINDOW CLEANER
(Industrial Equities)

Isopropyl alcohol	5-10%
Butyl Cellosolve *	2-5%
Dioctyl sodium sulfosuccinate	<1%
Polyoxyethylene sorbitan monolaurate	<1%
Colorant	<1%
Perfume	<1%
Water	balance

CLEAR EYES
Decongestant eye drops
(Abbott)

Naphazoline hydrochloride	0.012%
Boric acid	<2%
Sodium borate	
Methylcellulose (4000 CPS)	
Disodium edetate	0.1%
Benzalkonium chloride	0.01%

CLEAR-ICH MARINE, MIRACLE

See MIRACLE CLEAR-ICH MARINE

CLEAR-NOSE
Relief of nasal congestion
(Friendly Labs.)

Phenylephrine HCl USP *	1/4% sol.
Methylparaben	0.02%
Propylparaben	0.01%
Sodium bisulphite *	0.2%

CLEAR SPRAY LIQUID NET
Hair spray
(Bonat)

	percentage range
SD Alcohol 40 *	70.0-85.0%
Water	8.0-15.0%
Vinyl acetate/Crotonic acid/ Vinyl neodecanoate copolymer	3.0-6.0%
Vinyl acetate/Crotonic acid copolymer	<2.0%
Aminomethyl propanol	<1.0%
Dimethicone copolyol	<1.0%
Fragrance	<1.0%
Sodium bisulfite	<1.0%
Benzophenone-4	<1.0%

CLEARTUF PET RESINS
Synthetic resin used in bottles, textiles and films
(Goodyear)

Polyethylene terephthalate

CLEEN-BRITE
Glass cleaner
(Help)

Isopropyl alcohol *

'76 Ed.

CLEEN-WITE
Shoe polish
(Help)

Titanium dioxide
Gum tragacanth
Bentonite
Perfume

'76 Ed.

CLENS
Cleaning & disinfecting solution for hard contact lenses
(Burton, Parsons & Co.)

Benzalkonium chloride	0.02%
EDTA	0.1%

CLENZOIL
For cleaning & maintenance of fire-arms
(Clenzoil Co.)

Trichloroethylene *
Turpentine

CLERZ
Contact lens comfort drop
(CooperVision Pharm.)

Neutral hypertonic balanced Salt solution
Poloxamer 407

Sorbic acid	0.1%
Disodium edetate	0.1%
Sodium borate	0.2%

CLIMALENE
Cleaner
(Climaco)

Sodium carbonate *
Sodium perborate *

CLIMAX
Wallpaper cleaner
(Cleveland Cleaner)

Wheat flour	42.0000%
Ammonium alum	0.0060%
Water and salt solution	55.0000%
Aniline, color not certified	0.0002%
Kerosene oil	2.0000%

'76 Ed.

CLING 'N STRIP
Paint stripper
(Holcomb)

Methylene chloride *	>10%
Methanol	1-10%

'76 Ed.

CLING-SURFACE BAR & CHAIN OIL w/MOLY
(Cling-Surface)

Mineral oil 98%

CLING-SURFACE BELT DRESSING (Aerosol)
(Cling-Surface)

Mineral spirits *	17%
Methylene chloride *	30%
Propane/Isobutane	25%

CLING-SURFACE BLUE LAYOUT FLUID (Aerosol)
(Cling-Surface)

Acetone *	50%
Acetates	20%
Toluene *	10%
Propane/Isobutane	15%

CLING SURFACE ELECTRIC MOTOR CLEANER (Aerosol)
(Cling-Surface)

1,1,1-Trichloroethane * 96%

Starred ingredients (*) may be responsible for major toxic effects; consult Section II.

CLING SURFACE FAN & BELT DRESSING AND CS 50 (Non Aerosol)
(Cling-Surface)

Stoddard solvent * 30%

CLING-SURFACE GASKET REMOVER (Aerosol)
(Cling-Surface)

Methylene chloride * 70%
Propane/Isobutane 30%

CLING-SURFACE HEAVY DUTY ANTI RUST (Aerosol)
(Cling-Surface)

Lacolene 10%
Methylene chloride 10%
Propane/Isobutane 30%

CLING-SURFACE SILICONE "SUPER SLIP" (Aerosol)
(Cling-Surface)

Hexane * 30%
Heptane * 30%
Propane/Isobutane * 30%

CLINISTIX
Urine glucose reagent strip
(Ames)

Glucose oxidase
Peroxidase
FD & C Red
Ortho-tolidine dihydrochloride
Citrate buffer

CLINITEST
Urine sugar reagent tablet
(Ames)

Each tablet:
Copper sulfate .... 20.0 mg.
Citric acid .... 300.0 mg.
Sodium hydroxide * ...... 232.5 mg.
Sodium carbonate .... 80.0 mg.

CLINOMINT TOOTHPASTE

See DEWITTS'S CLINOMINT TOOTH-
PASTE

CLIPPERCIDE SPRAY FOR HAIR CLIPPERS
Germicide, fungicide; aerosol
(King Research)

o-Phenylphenol 0.25%
Isopropyl alcohol * 11.00%

CLISTIN (ELIXIR/TABLETS)
Antihistaminic
(McNeil Pharm.)

Each tablet/5 cc:
Carbinoxamine maleate *† ..... 4 mg.

†*See* Antihistaminics

CLISTIN-D TABLETS
Decongestant-analgesic
(McNeil Pharm.)

Each tablet:
Carbinoxamine maleate ...... 2 mg.
Acetaminophen * .... 300 mg.
Phenylephrine hydrochloride . 10 mg.

CLISTIN EXPECTORANT SYRUP
(McNeil Pharm.)

Each 5 cc:
Carbinoxamine maleate ... 2 mg.
Ammonium chloride ...... 120 mg.
Sodium citrate hydrous .... 120 mg.
Potassium guaiacolsulfonate 60 mg.
Benzyl alcohol .... 0.3%(v/v)

CLISTIN R-A TABLETS
Antihistamine
(McNeil Pharm.)

Each tablet:
Carbinoxamine
maleate *† .... 8 mg. or 12 mg.

†*See* Antihistaminics

CLIX SOLVENT DEGREASER & CLEANER
(National Chemsearch)

Aliphatic hydrocarbons *
Nonionic wetting agents
Anionic emulsifiers

CLOCREAM
Topical vitamin therapy
(Upjohn)

Each oz.:
Vitamins A and D (equiv. to cod
liver oil) .... 1 oz.
In a vanishing cream base

CLODERM CREAM
Topical antiinflammatory
(Ortho-Dermatology)

Clocortolone pivalate 0.1%

CLONOPIN
Anticonvulsant
(Roche)

Each tablet
Clonazepam * .... 0.5 mg.; 1 mg.;
2 mg.

CLOR-ADE
Automatic dishwasher detergent
(Calgon Corp., Commercial Div.)

Sodium silicates
Complex phosphates *
Chlorinated trisodium phosphate *
Soda ash *

CLOROPOOL
Concentrated chlorine solution for swimming pools
(Modern Pool Products)

Sodium hypochlorite * 5.25%

CLOROX LIQUID BLEACH
(Clorox)

Water .... >75%
Sodium hypochlorite * 5-10%
Sodium chloride 0.5-5%
Sodium carbonate 0.5-2%
Sodium hydroxide .... <0.5%

CLOROX 2 - ALL FABRIC DRY BLEACH
(Clorox)

Sodium carbonate * .... >75%
Sodium perborate tetrahydrate . 11-25%
Protease (from Bacillus
licheniformis) 0.5-2%
Fluorescent whitening agent .... <0.5%
Primary linear alcohol ethoxylates
(Surfactant) .... <0.5%
Ultramarine blue .... <0.5%
Fragrance .... <0.5%

CLOROZONE
Germicide, antiseptic, disinfectant, deodorant
(Consolidated Chem., Inc.)

Sodium hypochlorite * 5.0%

CLOSE-UP (MINT, GREEN) DENTIFRICE
(Lever Bros.)

Hydrogenated Starch
hydrolyzate 40-50%
Water 20-30%
Hydrated Silica 10-20%
Polyethylene glycol 1-5%
Sodium alkyl sulfate 1-3%
Ethyl alcohol 1-3%
Flavor .... <1%
Cellulose gum .... <1%
Sodium saccharin .... <1%
Sodium benzoate .... trace
Colorants .... trace

CLOSE-UP (MINT, GREEN) FLUORIDE DENTIFRICE
(Lever Bros.)

Sodium monofluorophosphate	<1%
Hydrogenated Starch	
hydrolyzate	40-50%
Water	20-30%
Hydrated Silica	10-20%
Polyethylene glycol	1-5%
Sodium alkyl sulfate	1-3%
Ethyl alcohol	1-3%
Flavor	<1%
Cellulose gum	<1%
Sodium saccharin	<1%
Sodium benzoate	trace
Colorants	trace

CLOSE-UP (RED) DENTIFRICE
(Lever Bros.)

Hydrogenated Starch	
hydrolyzate	40-50%
Water	20-30%
Hydrated Silica	10-20%
Polyethylene glycol	1-5%
Sodium alkyl sulfate	1-3%
Flavor	1-2%
Ethyl alcohol	1-2%
Cellulose gum	<1%
Sodium saccharin	<1%
Sodium benzoate	trace
Menthol	trace
Colorants	trace

CLOSE-UP (RED) FLUORIDE DENTIFRICE
(Lever Bros.)

Sodium monofluorophosphate	<1%
Hydrogenated Starch	
hydrolyzate	40-50%
Water	20-30%
Hydrated Silica	10-20%
Polyethylene glycol	1-5%
Sodium alkyl sulfate	1-3%
Flavor	1-2%
Ethyl alcohol	1-2%
Cellulose gum	<1%
Sodium saccharin	<1%
Sodium benzoate	trace
Menthol	trace
Colorants	trace

CLOUD SOFT
Cold wave lotion
(Willat)

Ammonium thioglycolate	1-10%

CLOVERINE SALVE
For minor skin irritations and burns
(Lambda Inc.)

White petrolatum
Rectified Turpentine oil
White wax
Perfume

CLOVER PHENOTHIAZINE DRENCH POWDER
Anthelmintic; veterinary
(Clover Chem.)

Phenothiazine NF *	99%
	'76 Ed.

CLOVER PHENOTHIAZINE N.F. POWDER
Anthelmintic; veterinary
(Clover Chem.)

Phenothiazine NF *	99%
	'76 Ed.

CLOVOCAIN
Dental medicine, surface anesthesia
(Vita Elixir Co.)

Benzocaine
Oil of cloves

CLOXAPEN CAPSULES
Antibiotic therapy
(Beecham Labs.)

Each capsule:
Cloxacillin sodium .. 250 mg.; 500 mg.

CL10 ALUMINUM PAINT
For interior and exterior wood, metal and masonry surfaces
(United Gilsonite)

Pigment:	13%
Aluminum paste - standard	
lining	100%
Vehicle:	87%
Processed Linseed oil	40%
Mineral spirits *	60%

CL25 ALUMINUM PAINT
For interior and exterior wood, metal and masonry surfaces
(United Gilsonite)

Pigment:	16.4%
Aluminum paste - standard	
lining	100%
Vehicle:	83.6%
Processed Linseed oil	45%
Mineral spirits *	55%

CLYO SPRAY COLOGNE (LOUISE PHILIPPE)
(Chesebrough-Pond's)

SD Alcohol 40	>50%
Water	>5-10%
Fragrance	>1-5%
Propylene glycol	0.1% or less
Colors	0.1% or less

C & M BENTONITE PASTE FOR EEG TESTS
For professional use
(C & M Pharmacal)

Calcium chloride
Bentonite
Guar gum extract
Glycerine
Purified water

C.M. - CARBON-MET (Liquid; Ready to Use)

See GUNK C.M. - CARBON-MET (Liquid; Ready to Use)

CMC CLEANER
For dairy farm utensils
(Yale Chem. Co.)

Sodium metasilicate *	>10%
Nonyl phenol ethylene oxide	
condensate	>5%
Sodium tripolyphosphate	>40%
Soda ash *	>40%

C.M.P. CARBURETOR CLEANER
(Consolidated Chem., Inc.)

Cresylic acid *
Mineral spirits *
Cocoanut dialkanolamide
Orthodichlorobenzene *
Caustic potash *

C.M.S. ANTACID POWDER
(Vernon Labs.)

Calcium carbonate
Sodium bicarbonate
Colloidal Kaolin
Papain
Magnesium carbonate
Bismuth subcarbonate
Diastase
Oil of peppermint

CM WITH PAREGORIC
(Beecham Labs.)

Each 5 ml.:
Paregoric	0.6 ml.
Zinc sulfocarbolate	10.0 mg.
Phenyl salicylate	22.0 mg.
Bismuth subsalicylate	85.0 mg.
Pepsin	45.0 mg.
Alcohol	2%
Sodium content (0.39 mEq/tablespoon)	

COA CROP OIL

See NORTHLAND COA CROP OIL

Starred ingredients (*) may be responsible for major toxic effects; consult Section II.

COAST
Deodorant soap bar
(Procter & Gamble)

Soap from animal and vegetable fats	75-100%
Water	10-24%
Fatty acid	5-9%
Sodium chloride	1-4%
Perfume	1-4%
3,4,4'-Trichlorocarbanilide	<1%
Minor ingredients, each	<1%

pH (1% solution) - 10.5

COASTAL CHLORINE STABILIZING POWDER
For swimming pools
(Coastal Industries)

2,4,6-Trihydroxy triazine (Cyanuric acid)	100%

COASTAL CONCENTRATE 50 LIQUID
Algaecide for swim pools
(Coastal Industries)

Alkyl dimethyl benzyl ammonium chloride *	50%
Water	

COASTAL FILTER POWDER
For swim pools
(Coastal Industries)

Diatomaceous earth (20 micron average diameter)

COASTAL PHENOL RED SOLUTION
For testing pH content of swim pool water
(Coastal Industries)

Water solution of Phenol red (Phenolsulfonphthalein)

COASTAL POOL WATER CLARIFIER
(Coastal Industries)

Acrylamide solution *
In water

COASTAL VINYL POOL CLEANER LIQUID
(Coastal Industries)

Ethylene glycol monobutyl ether *
Propylene glycol
Sodium bicarbonate *
Trisodium phosphate *
Water

COASTAL WINTER AID
Winterizes pool water
(Coastal Industries)

Alkyl dimethyl benzyl ammonium chloride (QUAT) *	7.5%
Complexed Copper	0.1%
Trisodium phosphate	2.4%
Water	

C-O-C-S COPODUST

See NIAGARA C-O-C-S COPODUST

CODACOL COUGH SYRUP
Antihistamine, antitussive expectorant
(Towne, Paulsen)

Each fl. oz.:

Codeine phosphate *	58 mg.
Chlorpheniramine maleate	4 mg.
Glyceryl guaiacolate	100 mg.
Chloroform	2 min.
Alcohol	2%
Glycerin	

CODALAN NO. 1
Analgesic, antitussive, antipyretic
(Lannett)

Each tablet:

Codeine phosphate *	8 mg.
Acetaminophen *	150 mg.
Salicylamide *	230 mg.
Caffeine	30 mg.

CODALAN NO. 2
Analgesic, antitussive, antipyretic
(Lannett)

Each tablet:

Codeine phosphate *	15 mg.
Acetaminophen *	150 mg.
Salicylamide *	230 mg.
Caffeine	30 mg.

CODALAN NO. 3
Analgesic, antitussive, antipyretic
(Lannett)

Each tablet:

Codeine phosphate *	30 mg.
Acetaminophen *	150 mg.
Salicylamide *	230 mg.
Caffeine	30 mg.

CODAP
Analgesic
(Direct Div.)

Each tablet:

Codeine phosphate *	25 mg.
Acetaminophen *	325 mg.

CODASA TABLETS
Analgesic
(Stayner)

Each tablet:

Codeine phosphate *	1/2 gr.
Aspirin *	5 gr.

CODEL SYRUP
Cough syrup
(Elder)

Each 5 cc:

Codeine phosphate *	5.0 mg.
Ephedrine hydrochloride *	5.5 mg.
Methapyrilene fumarate *	14.6 mg.
Ammonium chloride	110.0 mg.
Alcohol	5%/vol.

CODIMAL CAPSULES
Antihistamine, decongestant, analgesic
(Central Pharmacal Co.)

Each capsule:

Chlorpheniramine maleate	2 mg.
Pseudoephedrine hydrochloride *	30 mg.
Salicylamide	150 mg.
Acetaminophen *	150 mg.

CODIMAL DH SYRUP
Expectorant, decongestant, antihistaminic, antitussive
(Central Pharmacal Co.)

Each 5 ml.:

Hydrocodone bitartrate	1.66 mg.
Phenylephrine hydrochloride	5.0 mg.
Pyrilamine maleate *	8.33 mg.
Potassium guaiacolsulfonate	83.3 mg.

CODIMAL DM SYRUP
Expectorant, decongestant, antihistaminic, antitussive
(Central Pharmacal Co.)

Each tsp. (5 ml.):

Dextromethorphan hydrobromide *	10 mg.
Phenylephrine hydrochloride *	5 mg.
Pyrilamine maleate *	8.33 mg.
Potassium guaiacolsulfonate	83.3 mg.
Alcohol	4%

CODIMAL EXPECTORANT
Expectorant, decongestant, antitussive
(Central Pharmacal Co.)

Each 5 ml.:

Phenylpropanolamine hydrochloride *	25 mg.
Potassium guaiacolsulfonate	100 mg.

CODIMAL-L.A. CENULES
Antihistamine, decongestant
(Central Pharmacal Co.)

Each Cenule (timed-release capsule):

Chlorpheniramine maleate	8 mg.
Pseudoephedrine hydrochloride *	120 mg.

CODIMAL PH SYRUP
Expectorant, decongestant, antihistaminic, antitussive
(Central Pharmacal Co.)

Each tsp. (5 ml.):

Codeine phosphate *	10 mg.
Phenylephrine hydrochloride *	5 mg.
Pyrilamine maleate *	8.33 mg.
Potassium guaiacolsulfonate	83.3 mg.

Starred ingredients (*) may be responsible for major toxic effects; consult Section II.

CODIMAL TABLETS
Analgesic, decongestant, antihistamine
(Central Pharmacal Co.)

Each tablet:
Chlorpheniramine maleate	...	2 mg.
Pseudoephedrine hydrochloride *		30 mg.
Salicylamide		150 mg.
Acetaminophen *		150 mg.

CODINETS
Antitussive
(Wesley Pharm.)

Each tablet:
Dextromethorphan hydrobromide		1/67 gr.
P.E. Extract of Ipecac		1/67 gr.
Camphor monobromated	....	1/16 gr.
Terpin hydrate		1/4 gr.
Eucalyptol		
Menthol		

CODITRATE
Expectorant, antitussive
(Central Pharmacal Co.)

Syrup (each 15 ml.):
Hydrocodone bitartrate *	....	5 mg.
Potassium guaiacolsulfonate	..	250 mg.

Tablets (each):
Hydrocodone bitartrate *	....	2.4 mg.
Potassium guaiacolsulfonate	..	120 mg.

CODIVAL OINTMENT
(Vale)

Cod liver oil		50%
Benzocaine benzoate		1%
Zinc oxide		q.s.

CODONE
Antitussive
(Lemmon Co.)

Each tablet:
Hydrocodone bitartrate *		5 mg.

COFF-O-DYNE
Antitussive; children
(VB)

Squill *
Ipecac
Ammonium chloride
Sodium citrate
Potassium guaiacolsulfonate

COGENTIN COMPRESSED TABLETS
Parkinsonism
(MSD)

Each tablet:
Benztropine mesylate *†		0.5 mg.; 1 mg.; or 2 mg.

†*See* Atropine

COIN VEND CHEER (Phosphate Formula or 0-Phosphate Formula)
Institutional and industrial cleaning product

Procter & Gamble Co.
Ivorydale Technical Center
Cincinnati, Ohio 45217

Phone: 513-562-1100

COIN VEND TIDE (Phosphate Formula or 0-Phosphate Formula)
Institutional and industrial cleaning product

Procter & Gamble Co.
Ivorydale Technical Center
Cincinnati, Ohio 45217

Phone: 513-562-1100

COLACE
Stool softener
(Mead Johnson)

Capsules:
Docusate sodium *	...	50 mg.; 100 mg.

Syrup:
Docusate sodium *		20 mg./tsp.

Liquid (1% solution):
Docusate sodium		10 mg./ml.

COLA-KAPEC
Diarrhea, nausea, upset stomach relief
(Approved Pharm.)

Each fl. oz.:
Aluminum hydroxide gel		15 gr.
Zinc sulfocarbolate		1 gr.
Pectin		3 gr.
Kaolin		90 gr.
Coca-Cola syrup		

'76 Ed.

ColBENEMID
Chronic gout and gouty arthritis
(MSD)

Each tablet:
Probenecid *		0.5 gm.
Colchicine *		0.5 mg.

COLCH-OLATE
Arthritic pain
(Walker Pharm.)

Each oz.:
Colchicine *		1/60 gr.

'76 Ed.

COLDATE
Relief of cold symptoms
(Elder)

Each tablet:
Aspirin *		2 gr.
Phenacetin *		1 1/2 gr.
Camphor monobromated	....	1/2 gr.
Dover's Powder (Opium content, 1/40 gr.)		1/4 gr.
Caffeine		1/8 gr.

COLD-DIP
Metal cleaner, stripper, degreaser; for industrial and institutional use
(Scientific International)

Cresol *
Methylene chloride *

COLD POWER DETERGENT POWDER
(Colgate-Palmolive)

Combined amount:		75%
Sodium phosphate *		
Sodium sulfate		
Sodium silicate *		
Combined amount:		14%
Linear alkyl benzene sulfonate *		
Nonionic detergent		
Soap		
Perfume, brightener, suspending and preservative agents		2%
Moisture		9%

'76 Ed.

COLGATE INSTANT SHAVE
(Colgate-Palmolive)

Super-fatted soap
Fatty-acid diethanolamine condensate
Propylene glycol
Perfume
Propellant gas

'76 Ed.

COLGATE LOW-FOAM DETERGENT
(Colgate-Palmolive)

Alkaline mixture of:
Combined amount:		<50%
Sodium sulfate		
Pentasodium tripolyphosphate *		
Sodium carbonate *		
Sodium silicate *		
Combined amount:		<15%
Nonionic surfactants (Polyethoxylated C14-C18 even numbered alcohols)		
Alkyl aryl sulfonate wetting agent		

'76 Ed.

COLGATE TOOTHPASTE WITH MFP
(Colgate-Palmolive)

Insoluble Sodium metaphosphate
Glycerine
Sorbitol
CMC (Carboxymethyl cellulose)
Sodium lauryl sulfate
Flavor and preservative
Sodium monofluorophosphate

'76 Ed.

COLGATE WINTERFRESH GEL
Dentifrice
(Colgate-Palmolive)

Sorbitol	30%
Glycerine	25%
Silicon dioxide	<25%
Water	15%
PEG-12	<5%
Sodium lauryl sulfate	1%

Sodium monofluorophosphate
Flavor
Sodium benzoate
Cellulose gum
Sodium saccharin
Titanium dioxide
FD & C Blue No. 1

COLITUSSIN
Antihistaminic, expectorant, antitussive
(Dalin)

Each fl. oz.:
Glyceryl guaiacolate	180 mg.
Methapyrilene fumarate *	75 mg.
Ephedrine hydrochloride *	65 mg.
Ammonium chloride	600 mg.
Sodium citrate	500 mg.
Citric acid	200 mg.

'76 Ed.

COLITUSSIN PEDIATRIC
For the relief of coughs, throat and bronchial inflammations
(Dalin)

Each fl. oz.:
Glyceryl guaiacolate	120 mg.
Ammonium chloride	400 mg.
Sodium citrate	350 mg.
Fl. ext. Cocillana	0.2 cc.
Syrup tolu	2.0 cc.
Citric acid	150 mg.

'76 Ed.

COLLADERM
Moisture lotion
(C & M Pharmacal)

Purified water
Glycerine
Collagen
Allantoin
Hydroxyethylcellulose
Sorbic
Octoxynol-9

COLLA-MAC CEMENT
(Lamac)

Neoprene type rubber
Synthetic adhesive resins
Non-lead curing agents
Aromatic and ketone type solvents *

COLLA-MAC THINNER
Cement thinner
(Lamac)

Aromatic and ketone type solvents *

COLLYRIUM
Eye lotion; 6 fl. oz.
(Wyeth Labs.)

Antipyrine	0.4%
Boric acid	
Borax	
Thimerosal (mercury derivative)	not more than 0.002%

COLLYRIUM WITH EPHEDRINE
Eye drops; 1/2 fl. oz.
(Wyeth Labs.)

Boric acid
Borax
Antipyrine	0.4%
Ephedrine	0.1%
Thimerosal (mercury derivative)	not more than 0.002%

COLMA-DUR, REGULAR & GEL
(Sika Chem.)

A unit:
  Epoxy resins

B unit:
  Alkaline amines *†

†*See* Coatings, Section VI, General Formulations

COLMA JOINT SEALER NS AND SL
(Sika Chem.)

A unit:
  Polysulfide polymers *

B unit:
  Lead dioxide *

COLMA SOL
All colors except green
(Sika Chem.)

A Unit:
  Epoxy resins
  Ethylene glycol monoethyl ether *
B Unit:
  Polyamide resin
  Isopropyl alcohol
  Toluene *
  Ethylene glycol monoethyl ether *
  Aromatic alkaline amine *†

†*See* Coatings, Section VI, General Formulations

COLMA SOL GREEN
(Sika Chem.)

A Unit:
  Epoxy resins
  Ethylene glycol monoethyl ether *
B Unit:
  Polyamide resin
  Isopropyl alcohol
  Toluene *
  Ethylene glycol monoethyl ether *
  Aromatic alkaline amine *†
  Chromium oxide

†*See* Coatings, Section VI, General Formulations

COLMA SURFACE-KOTE
(Sika Chem.)

A unit:
  Epoxy resins

B unit:
  Alkaline amines *†

†*See* Coatings, Section VI, General Formulations

COL-O-CAPS
Analgesic, antipyretic
(VB)

Acetophenetidin *
Bromocamphor *
Acetylsalicylic acid *
Caffeine citrate
Salicylates *

COLOCTYL CAPSULES
Stool softener for relief of constipation
(Vitarine)

Each capsule:
  Dioctyl sodium
    sulfosuccinate * .... 100 mg.

COLOGEL
Laxative
(Lilly, Eli)

Each 100 cc:
Alcohol	5%
Methyl cellulose	9 gm.

COLONEL CUTTER SUPER STRIPPER
See BUTCHER'S COLONEL CUTTER SUPER STRIPPER

COLONIA COSMETICS
Colonia Inc.
Largo Park
Stamford, Conn. 06907

Phone: 203-348-4711

See COSMETICS, Section VI, General Formulations

Starred ingredients (*) may be responsible for major toxic effects; consult Section II.

COLONIAL-32
Rodenticide
(Colonial Prod.)

Pivalyl (2-Pivalyl-1,3-indandione) 0.025%

COLONIAL-42
Rodenticide
(Colonial Prod.)

3-(a-Acetonylbenzyl)-4-hydroxy-coumarin (Warfarin)	0.025%
Sulfaquinoxaline (N'-(2-quinoxali-nyl) sulfanilamide)	0.025%

COLONIAL DAMES COLOGNES
(Colonial Dames)

Denatured alcohol *	75%
Diethyl phthalate	1%
Perfume oil	<1%

COLONIAL DAMES COSMETIC PRODUCTS
Cosmetics and perfumes

Colonial Dames Co., Ltd.
P.O. Box 22022
Los Angeles, Calif. 90022

Phone: 213-773-6441

See COSMETICS, Section VI, General Formulations

COLONIAL DAMES DUSTING POWDER
(Colonial Dames)

Talcum	>10%
Zinc stearate	<10%
Perfume oil	<1%
Magnesium carbonate	1-10%

COLONIAL DAMES FACE CREAMS
(Colonial Dames)

Lanolin	1-10%
Lanolin derivatives	<1%
Lecithin	<1%
Cetyl alcohol	<1%
White mineral oil (USP)	>10%
Beeswax	1-10%
Petrolatum	1-10%
Stearic acid	1-10%
Gycerol monostearate	1-10%
Borax	<1%
Triethanolamine	<1%
Perfume oil	<1%
Parahydroxybenzoic acid esters	1/10-1/5%
Vitamin E (dl-alpha-Tocoph-erol acetate)	25%

COLONIAL DAMES FACE POWDER
(Colonial Dames)

Titanium dioxide	1-10%
Talcum	>10%
Zinc stearate	1-10%
Iron oxide	1-10%
Perfume oil	<1%

COLONIAL DAMES FORMULA 1886 CLEANSER
(Colonial Dames)

Isopropyl alcohol *	50%
Sorbitol	2%
Glycerin	2%
Perfume	1/5%
Allantoin	1/10%
Resorcinol	1/20%

COLONIAL DAMES LOTIONS
(Colonial Dames)

Lanolin	1-10%
Lanolin derivatives	<1%
Lecithin	<1%
Cetyl alcohol	<1%
White mineral oil (USP)	>10%
Beeswax	1-10%
Petrolatum	1-10%
Stearic acid	1-10%
Glycerol monostearate	1-10%
Borax	<1%
Triethanolamine	<1%
Perfume oil	<1%
Parahydroxybenzoic acid esters	1/10-1/5%
Vitamin E (dl-alpha-Tocoph-erol acetate)	1/10-25%

COLONIAL DAMES SKIN FRESHENER
(Colonial Dames)

Ammonium alum	2%
Magnesium sulfate	2%
Fragrance	1/10%
Denatured alcohol 40	approx. 15%
Brucine sulfate	
Tertiary Butyl alcohol *	

COLONIAL DAMES VITAMIN E MAKE-UP
(Colonial Dames)

White mineral oil (NF)	>10%
Lanolin	<1%
Stearic acid	1-10%
Beeswax	<1%
Glycerol monostearate	1-10%
Tween No. 21	<1%
Triethanolamine	<1%
Glycerin	1-10%
Sorbitol	1-10%
Perfume oil	<1%
Vitamin E (dl-alpha-Tocopherol acetate)	7%
Esters of parahydroxybenzoic acid	<1%
Purified Titanium dioxide	1-10%
Calcium carbonate	1-10%
Talcum	1-10%
Iron oxide	1-10%

COLONIAL PES-TA-REST
Insecticide
(Colonial Prod.)

(5-Benzyl-3-furyl)methyl 2,2-dimethyl-3-(2-methylpropenyl)cycloprop-anecarboxylate	0.200% w/w
Related compounds	0.028% w/w
d-trans Allethrin (allyl hom-olog of Cinerin I)	0.150% w/w
Related compounds	0.012% w/w
Aromatic petroleum hydrocarbons	0.272% w/w

COLONIAL RCS
Insecticide
(Colonial Prod.)

Diazinon	0.50%
Technical Piperonyl butoxide	0.20%
Pyrethrins	0.04%
Petroleum distillate *	74.26%
Inert ingred.:	
Propellant (Dichlorodifluoromethane)	25.00%

COLONIAL ROACH TABLETS
Insecticide
(Colonial Prod.)

Boric acid * ... 40%

COLORART COLORED MOLDED CHALK
(American Crayon Co.)

This product bears the AP Seal issued by the Crayon, Water Color and Craft Institute, Inc. This seal certifies that the product contains no materials in sufficient quantities to be toxic or injurious to the human body even if ingested.

COLORART LIQUID TEMPERA
(American Crayon Co.)

This product bears the AP Seal issued by the Crayon, Water Color and Craft Institute, Inc. This seal certifies that the product contains no materials in sufficient quantities to be toxic or injurious to the human body even if ingested.

COLORART POWDER TEMPERA
(American Crayon Co.)

This product bears the AP Seal issued by the Crayon, Water Color and Craft Institute, Inc. This seal certifies that the product contains no materials in sufficient quantities to be toxic or injurious to the human body even if ingested.

Starred ingredients (*) may be responsible for major toxic effects; consult Section II.

COLORART SEMI-MOIST WATER COLORS
(American Crayon Co.)

This product bears the AP Seal issued by the Crayon, Water Color and Craft Institute, Inc. This seal certifies that the product contains no materials in sufficient quantities to be toxic or injurious to the human body even if ingested.

COLORART WAX CRAYONS
(American Crayon Co.)

This product bears the CP Seal issued by the Crayon, Water Color and Craft Institute, Inc. This seal certifies that the product contains no materials in sufficient quantities to be toxic or injurious to the human body even if ingested.

COLORART WHITE MOLDED CHALK
(American Crayon Co.)

This product bears the AP Seal issued by the Crayon, Water Color and Craft Institute, Inc. This seal certifies that the product contains no materials in sufficient quantities to be toxic or injurious to the human body even if ingested.

COLOR CLASSICS PRESSED CRAYONS
(American Crayon Co.)

This product bears the CP Seal issued by the Crayon, Water Color and Craft Institute, Inc. This seal certifies that the product contains no materials in sufficient quantities to be toxic or injurious to the human body even if ingested.

COLOR CRAFT FINGER PAINT
(Avalon Industries)

This product bears the CP Seal issued by the Crayon, Water Color and Craft Institute, Inc. This seal certifies that the product contains no materials in sufficient quantities to be toxic or injurious to the human body even if ingested.

COLOR CRAFT LIQUID TEMPERA
(Avalon Industries)

This product bears the CP Seal issued by the Crayon, Water Color and Craft Institute, Inc. This seal certifies that the product contains no materials in sufficient quantities to be toxic or injurious to the human body even if ingested.

COLOR CRAFT MODELING CLAY
(Avalon Industries)

This product bears the CP Seal issued by the Crayon, Water Color and Craft Institute, Inc. This seal certifies that the product contains no materials in sufficient quantities to be toxic or injurious to the human body even if ingested.

COLOR CRAFT POWDER TEMPERA
(Avalon Industries)

This product bears the CP Seal issued by the Crayon, Water Color and Craft Institute, Inc. This seal certifies that the product contains no materials in sufficient quantities to be toxic or injurious to the human body even if ingested.

COLOR CRAFT SEMI-MOIST WATER COLORS
(Avalon Industries)

This product bears the CP Seal issued by the Crayon, Water Color and Craft Institute, Inc. This seal certifies that the product contains no materials in sufficient quantities to be toxic or injurious to the human body even if ingested.

COLOR CRAFT WAX CRAYONS
(Avalon Industries)

This product bears the CP Seal issued by the Crayon, Water Color and Craft Institute, Inc. This seal certifies that the product contains no materials in sufficient quantities to be toxic or injurious to the human body even if ingested.

COLORTINT, NESTLE

See NESTLE COLORTINT

COLOTONE LAXATIVE WAFERS
(Miller, C. J.)

Each wafer:
Powdered Senna leaves TV ... 10 gr.
Powdered extract Belladonna
  leaves * .... 1/8 gr.
Powdered extract Licorice and
  oil of anise .... q.s.

COLREX
Analgesic, antihistaminic, nasal decongestant
(Rowell)

Each capsule:
Chlorpheniramine maleate ... 2 mg.
Phenylephrine hydrochloride . 5 mg.
Acetaminophen * .... 325 mg.

COLREX COMPOUND CAPSULES
Comprehensive 'cold' therapeutic
(Rowell)

Each capsule:
Codeine phosphate * .... 16 mg.
Acetaminophen * .... 325 mg.
Phenylephrine hydrochloride . 10 mg.
Chlorpheniramine maleate ... 2 mg.

COLREX COMPOUND ELIXIR
Comprehensive 'cold' therapeutic
(Rowell)

Each 5 ml.:
Codeine phosphate * .... 8 mg.
Acetaminophen * .... 120 mg.
Phenylephrine hydrochloride . 5 mg.
Chlorpheniramine maleate ... 1 mg.

COLREX DECONGESTANT
Antihistaminic-decongestant
(Rowell)

Each tablet:
Chlorpheniramine maleate .... 4 mg.
Tripelennamine
  hydrochloride * .... 50 mg.
Phenylpropanolamine
  hydrochloride * .... 25 mg.
Phenylephrine hydrochloride .. 10 mg.

COLREX EXPECTORANT
(Rowell)

Each 5 cc:
Guaifenesin .... 100 mg.
Sugar free

COLREX SYRUP
Cough syrup
(Rowell)

Each 5 cc.:
Dextromethorphan
  hydrobromide * .... 10 mg.
Phenylephrine hydrochloride * 5 mg.
Chlorpheniramine maleate * .. 2 mg.
Sugar free

COLREX TROCHES
Relief of sore throat due to the common cold
(Rowell)

Each troche:
Benzocaine .... 10 mg.
Cetylpyridinium chloride ..... 2.5 mg.

COLUMA
Antacid, adsorbent
(Premo)

Aluminum hydroxide gel

'76 Ed.

COLUMBIA ANTISEPTIC POWDER
To soothe externally caused skin irritations
(Sturtevant)

Boric acid *
Carbolic acid *
Zinc oxide
Talc

Starred ingredients (*) may be responsible for major toxic effects; consult Section II.

COLUMBIA BLUE-GRAY HEMORRHOIDAL SUPPOSITORIES
(Columbia Med.)

Each suppository:
Bismuth subgallate
Bismuth resorcin comp. *†
Zinc oxide
Balsam Peru
Boric acid *
Benzocaine

†*See* Resorcinol

COLUMBIA BROMPHENIRAMINE EXPECTORANT
(Columbia Med.)

Each 5 ml.:
Brompheniramine maleate	2 mg.
Glyceryl guaiacolate	100 mg.
Phenylephrine HCl *	5 mg.
Phenylpropanolamine HCl *	5 mg.
Alcohol	3.5%

COLUMBIA EAR DROPS
(Columbia Med.)

Carbamide
Propylene glycol
Glycerine
Chlorobutanol

COLUMBIA EAR DROPS (Rx)
To relieve pain, inflammation of simple ear ache
(Columbia Med.)

Antipyrine *	0.81 gm.
Benzocaine	0.21 gm.
Glycerine USP	to make 1/2 fl. oz.

COLUMBIA PAINT PRODUCTS

Columbia Paint Co.
1517 Dodge Ave.
Helena, Mont. 59601

Phone: 406-442-7650

See PAINTS, Section VI, General Formulations

COLUMBIA PROMETHAZINE EXPECTORANT
(Columbia Med.)

Each 5 ml.:
Promethazine HCl	5 mg.
Fluid extract Ipecac	0.17 min.
Potassium guaiacol sulfonate	44 mg.
Chloroform	0.25 min.
Citric acid	60 mg.
Sodium citrate	197 mg.
Alcohol	7%

COLUMBIA PROMETHAZINE VC EXPECTORANT
(Columbia Med.)

Each 5 ml.:
Promethazine HCl	5 mg.
Phenylephrine HCl *	5 mg.
Fluid extract Ipecac	0.17 min.
Potassium guaiacol sulfonate	44 mg.
Chloroform	0.25 min.
Citric acid	60 mg.
Sodium citrate	197 mg.
Alcohol	7%

COLUMBIA THEOPHYLLINE ELIXIR
(Columbia Med.)

Each 15 ml.:
Theophylline	80 mg.
Alcohol	20%

COMAIR COSMETICS

Comair Corp.
386 N.E. 191st St.
North Miami Beach, Fla. 33179

Phone: 305-652-0331

See COSMETICS, Section VI, General Formulations

COMATIC APAP WITH CODEINE ELIXIR
Analgesic, antipyretic, antitussive
(Comatic)

Each 5 ml.:
Acetaminophen *	120 mg.
Codeine phosphate	12 mg.

COMATIC BISACODYL SUPPOSITORIES
Laxative
(Comatic)

Each suppository:
Bisacodyl	10 mg.

COMATIC DIBUCAINE OINTMENT
Topical local anesthetic
(Comatic)

Dibucaine	1%

COMATIC PHENOBARBITAL ELIXIR
Sedative/hypnotic, anticonvulsant
(Comatic)

Each 5 ml.:
Phenobarbital *	20 mg.

COMATIC PSEUDOEPHEDRINE SYRUP
Decongestant
(Comatic)

Each 5 ml.:
Pseudoephedrine HCl *	30 mg.

COMBINE
Cleaner, disinfectant
(Schneid)

Active ingredients:	17.07%
Vegetable oil soap	
Sodium o-benzyl p-chlorophenate *	
Triethanolamine dodecyl benzene sulfonate *	
Sodium dodecyl benzene sulfonate *	
Hydroxyethylethylenediamine triacetic acid trisodium salt	
Inert ingredients:	82.93%
Water	
Tetrapotassium pyrophosphate *	
Propylene glycol	

'76 Ed.

COMBISTIX
Urine protein-glucose-pH multiple reagent strip
(Ames)

Protein test area: see ALBUSTIX
Glucose test area: see CLINISTIX
pH test area: see BILI-LABSTIX

COMBOT LIQUID
Equine anthelmintic
(Haver-Lockhart (Brand) Bayvet Div. Cutter Labs.)

Trichlorfon *	12.3%

COMBOT PASTE
Equine anthelmintic and boticide
(Haver-Lockhart (Brand) Bayvet Div. Cutter Labs.)

Trichlorfon *	40%

COMET CLEANSER WITH CHLORINOL
(Procter & Gamble)

Silica	50-74%
Chlorinated trisodium phosphate *	10-24%
Sodium tripolyphosphate	5-9%
Sodium alkyl benzene sulfonate	1-4%
Sodium sulfate	1-4%
Minor ingredients, each	<1%

pH (5% solution) - 11.5

COMET CLEANSER WITH CLORINAL G (Non-Phosphate Formula)
(Procter & Gamble)

Silica	70-90%
Sodium carbonate	10-24%
Sodium acetate	1-4%
Sodium sulfate	1-4%
Sodium alkyl benzene sulfonate	1-4%
Sodium dichloro-s-triazinetrione	1-4%
Minor ingredients, each	<1%

pH (5% solution) - 11.5

COMET LIQUID DISINFECTANT CLEANSER
(Procter & Gamble)

Water	75-95%
Amorphous silicate abrasive	5-10%
Sodium or Potassium carbonate	5-10%
Clay	1-4%
Sodium alkyl sulfonate	1-4%
Sodium hypochlorite	0.5%-1.0%
Minor ingredients, each	<1%

pH - 11.4

COMET PAINT & VARNISH REMOVER
(Reliable Paste)

Toluol *	approx. 10%
Acetone *	approx. 60%
Methanol *	approx. 30%

COMFOLAX
Fecal softener
(Searle, G.D., & Co.)

Each capsule:
Dioctyl sodium sulfosuccinate (USP) * .... 100 mg.

COMFOLAX-PLUS
Fecal softener and laxative
(Searle, G.D., & Co.)

Each capsule:
Dioctyl sodium sulfosuccinate (USP) * .... 100 mg.
Casanthranol * .... 30 mg.

COMFORT COSMETIC PRODUCTS
Cosmetics and toiletries

Comfort Manufacturing Co.
1056 W. Van Buren St.
Chicago, Ill. 60607

Phone: 312-421-8145

See COSMETICS, Section VI, General Formulations

COMFORTINE
For skin irritations
(Dermik)

Vitamin A
Vitamin D
Zinc oxide
Lanolin

COM-KILL WEED KILLER
(Certified Labs.)

Sodium arsenite *	40.00%
Inert ingredients:	
Water	59.50%
Sodium dodecyl benzene sulfonate	0.50%

COMMAND HAIR SPRAY
(Alberto-Culver)

SD Alcohol 40
Isobutane
Methylene chloride
Butyl ester of PVM/MA copolymer
Aminomethyl propanol
Dimethyl phthalate
Fragrance
Other ingredients

COMMANDO INSECT REPELLENT
(MFA Oil Co.)

N,N-Diethyl-m-toluamide *	41.5%
Other isomers & related compounds	8.5%
Inert ingred.:	
Isopropyl alcohol *	50.0%

COMMANDO INSECT REPELLENT AEROSOL
(MFA Oil Co.)

N,N-Diethyl-m-toluamide *	20.75%
Other isomers & related compounds	4.25%

COMMAND SAFETY SOLVENT
(Uncle Sam)

Dichloromethane *
Tetrachloroethylene *
Stoddard solvent *

COMMERCE DRUG STYE OPHTHALMIC OINTMENT
(Commerce Drug)

Cod liver oil	
Zinc sulfate	0.25%
Yellow Mercuric oxide *	1.0%
Boric acid	5.0%

COMPAZINE CONCENTRATE
Antiemetic, tranquilizer
(SK&F)

Each ml.:
Prochlorperazine * .... 10 mg.

COMPAZINE SPANSULE CAPSULES
Antiemetic-tranquilizer
(SK&F)

Each sustained release capsule:
Prochlorperazine ..... 10 mg.; 15 mg.; 30 mg.; 75 mg.

COMPAZINE SUPPOSITORIES
Antiemetic-tranquilizer
(SK&F)

Each suppository:
Prochlorperazine .... 2 1/2 mg.; 5 mg.; 25 mg.

Glycerin
Glyceryl monopalmitate
Glyceryl monostearate
Hydrogenated coconut oil fatty acids
Hydrogenated palm kernel oil fatty acids

COMPAZINE SYRUP
Antiemetic-tranquilizer
(SK&F)

Each 5 ml.:
Prochlorperazine .... 5 mg.

COMPAZINE TABLETS
Antiemetic-tranquilizer
(SK&F)

Each tablet:
Prochlorperazine .... 5 mg.; 10 mg.; 25 mg.

COMP CLEANSER-SANITIZER-DISINFECTANT DEODORANT
(Fuld-Stalfort)

Soap	10.0%
Isopropanol	3.0%
Ortho-benzyl para-chlorophenol	2.0%

'76 Ed.

COMPEX
Compatibility agent for liquid fertilizer-pesticide mixtures
(Kalo)

Alcohol sulfates *

COM-PLEET
Herbicide
(Green Light)

Prometon	3.73%
Petroleum distillate *	80.91%

COMPLETE
Denture cleanser and toothpaste
(Vicks Toiletry Products Div.)

Calcium carbonate
Water
Glycerin
Sorbitol
Silica
Sodium lauryl sulfate
Flavor
Sodium carboxymethyl cellulose
Cellulose gum
Sodium saccharin
Methylparaben
Propylparaben

COMPO ARTERIAL, MEDIUM & HARD
Embalming fluid
(Embalmers')

Formaldehyde *

COMPO CAVITY
Embalming fluid
(Embalmers')

Formaldehyde *

COMPOUND 1080
Rodenticide
(Tull Chem.)

Sodium monofluoroacetate *

COMPOUND W
Wart remover
(Whitehall Labs.)

Ether
Alcohol
Glacial acetic acid *
Salicylic acid *
Menthol *
Camphor *
Castor oil

COMPOZ TABLETS
Nighttime sleep-aid for relief of occasional sleeplessness
(Jeffrey Martin, Inc.)

Each tablet:
Pyrilamine maleate * .... 25 mg.

COMTREX CAPSULES & TABLETS
Multi-symptom cold reliever
(Bristol-Myers)

Each capsule or tablet:
Acetaminophen * .... 325 mg.
Phenylpropanolamine HCl   12 1/2 mg.
Chlorpheniramine maleate   1 mg.
Dextromethorphan HBr ...   10 mg.

COMTREX LIQUID
Multi-symptom cold reliever
(Bristol-Myers)

Each 30 ml.:
Acetaminophen * .... 650 mg.
Phenylpropanolamine HCl .... 25 mg.
Dextromethorphan HBr .... 20 mg.
Chlorpheniramine maleate ... 2 mg.
Alcohol 20%/v

CONACETOL TABLETS
Analgesic
(CMC Research Div.)

Each tablet:
N-Acetyl-p-aminophenol * ...... 5 gr.

CONAR-A SUSPENSION
Symptomatic treatment of the common cold
(Beecham Labs.)

Each 5 ml.:
Noscapine .... 7.5 mg.
Phenylephrine hydrochloride . 5 mg.
Acetaminophen * .... 150 mg.
Guaifenesin .... 50 mg.

CONAR-A TABLETS
Symptomatic treatment of the common cold
(Beecham Labs.)

Each tablet:
Noscapine .... 15 mg.
Phenylephrine hydrochloride . 10 mg.
Acetaminophen * .... 300 mg.
Guaifenesin .... 100 mg.

CONAR EXPECTORANT
For coughs
(Beecham Labs.)

Each 5 ml.:
Noscapine * .... 15 mg.
Phenylephrine
hydrochloride * .... 10 mg.
Guaifenesin .... 100 mg.
Flavoring .... q.s.

CONAR (Sugarless)
Antitussive, nasal decongestant
(Beecham Labs.)

Each 5 ml.:
Noscapine * .... 15 mg.
Phenylephrine hydrochloride * 10 mg.
Flavoring .... q.s.

CONCECOL
Sedative, anticholinergic
(King Pharmaceutical)

Each 0.3 cc:
Sodium butabarbital * ..... 16 mg.
Hyoscyamine sulfate * ..... 0.1 mg.
Homatropine methylbromide   0.02 mg.
Hyoscine hydrobromide .... 0.007 mg.

CONCENTRATED "all" (Low Phosphate)
Powder laundry detergent
(Lever Bros.)

Sodium sulfate * 35-50%
Sodium polyphosphate * 25-35%
Water 5-10%
Nonionic detergent 5-10%
Sodium silicates 1-10%
Sodium carbonate 0-5%
Sodium soap .... <1%
Perfume .... <1%
Cellulosic .... trace
Optical dye .... trace
Colorants .... trace

CONCENTRATED "all" (Nonphosphate)
Powder laundry detergent
(Lever Bros.)

Sodium sulfate * 35-45%
Sodium carbonate * 30-40%
Sodium silicate 5-15%
Nonionic detergent 5-10%
Sodium potassium aluminum
   silicate 1-5%
Water 1-5%
Sodium soap .... <1%
Perfume .... <1%
Cellulosic .... trace
Optical dye .... trace
Colorants .... trace

CONCEN-TROL, SPRAY-TROL BRAND
See SPRAY-TROL BRAND CONCEN-TROL

CONCEPT
Hospital disinfectant, deodorant
(Hysan Corp.)

Orthophenylphenol 0.176%
Paratertiaryamylphenol 0.044%
Essential oils 0.300%
Alcohol 53.460%

CONCEPTROL
Birth control cream
(Ortho)

Nonoxynol 9 .... 5.00%

CONCLUDE (Phosphate Formula or 0-Phosphate Formula)
Institutional and industrial cleaning product

Procter & Gamble Co.
Ivorydale Technical Center
Cincinnati, Ohio 45217

Phone: 513-562-1100

C-1 IDEAL BLACK STENCIL INK
(Ideal Stencil)

Fuel oil *
Black carbon
Gloss oil (T-Glo-8Y-210) *†
Soya lecithin

†*See* Mineral spirits

CONEX
Nasal decongestant
(OJF)

Each tablet:
Chlorpheniramine maleate .. 1.0 mg.
Pyrilamine maleate * .... 12.5 mg.
Phenylpropanolamine HCl * 25.0 mg.
Phenylephrine HCl .... 2.5 mg.

CONEX D.A.
Antihistamine and decongestant
(OJF)

Each tablet:
Phenylpropanolamine HCl * .. 50 mg.
Phenyltoloxamine citrate ..... 50 mg.
In a delayed action base

CONEX LOZENGES
Anesthetic & antiseptic lozenge for throat irritations
(OJF)

Each lozenge:
Benzocaine .... 5 mg.
Methylparaben .... 2 mg.
Propylparaben .... 0.5 mg.
Cetylpyridinium chloride ..... 0.5 mg.

CONEX WITH CODEINE SYRUP
Antitussive
(OJF)

Each 5 ml.:
Chlorpheniramine maleate .... 2 mg.
Guaifenesin .... 50 mg.
Phenylpropanolamine HCl * .. 25 mg.
Codeine phosphate * .... 10 mg.

CONFIDENCE

See AIRWICK PROFESSIONAL PRODUCTS CONFIDENCE

CONGESPIRIN COLD TABLETS
Analgesic/nasal decongestant for children
(Bristol-Myers)

Each tablet:
Aspirin * .... 81 mg.
Phenylephrine hydrochloride 1 1/4 mg.

CONGESPIRIN COUGH SYRUP
For children
(Bristol-Myers)

Each 5 ml.:
Dextromethorphan
hydrobromide .... 5 mg.

CONGESS TD CAPSULES
Expectorant/bronchodilator
(Fleming)

JR (each capsule):
Guaifenesin .... 125 mg.
Pseudoephedrine HCl * ...... 60 mg.

SR (each capsule):
Guaifenesin .... 250 mg.
Pseudoephedrine HCl * ..... 120 mg.

CON-O-SYL DISINFECTANT-DEODORANT
(Nat'l Labs. Div.)

o-Phenylphenol * 11.75%
o-Benzyl-p-chlorophenol 7.82%
Tetrasodium
ethylenediaminetetraacetate .. 2.96%
Sodium dodecyl benzene
sulfonate 3.17%
Isopropyl alcohol 2.60%
Essential oils 0.30%

CONPACT PREMEASURED CLEANER
(Nat'l Labs. Div.)

Tetrasodium pyrophosphate
Sodium sulfate

CONQUER LIQUID VEGETATION KILLER
(Ciba-Geigy Ag. Div.)

Prometon 2.50%
Pentachlorophenol 1.00%
Other chlorophenols and related
compounds 0.12%

CONQUEROR SYSTEM CLEANER
Liquid caustic cleaner
(Kay Chem. Co.)

Water 20-40%
Potassium hydroxide * 60-80%

CONQUEST II
Cleaner, disinfectant, deodorant
(Federal International)

n-Alkyl (myristyl 60%, palmityl
30%, lauryl 5%, stearyl
5%)dimethyl benzyl ammonium
chlorides * 2.25%
n-Alkyl (lauryl 68%, myristyl
32%)dimethyl ethylbenzyl ammonium chlorides * 2.25%
Sodium carbonate 3.00%
Tetrasodium ethylenediamine
tetraacetate 1.00%

CONQUEST 256
Cleaner, disinfectant, deodorant
(Federal International)

n-Alkyl (myristyl 60%, palmityl
30%, lauryl 5%, stearyl
5%)dimethyl benzyl ammonium
chlorides * 6.25%
n-Alkyl (lauryl 68%, myristyl
32%)dimethyl ethylbenzyl ammonium chlorides * 6.25%
Tetrasodium ethylenediamine
tetraacetate 3.60%

CONSOLIDATED PROTECTIVE COATINGS PRODUCTS
Paints & waterproofing compounds

Consolidated Protective Coatings Corp.
1801 E. 9th St.
Cleveland, Ohio 44114

Phone: 216-771-3258

See PAINTS, Section VI, General Formulations

CONSTIBAN CAPSULES
Laxative
(Columbia Med.)

Each capsule:
Casanthranol * .... 30 mg.
Dioctyl sodium
sulfosuccinate * .... 100 mg.

CONSTOLEIN TABLETS
Laxative
(Bio-Factor Labs.)

Each tablet:
Dioctyl sodium
sulfosuccinate * .... 100 mg.
Phenolphthalein (yellow) .... 65 mg.

'76 Ed.

CONSTONATE 60 CAPSULES
Fecal softener
(Bio-Factor Labs.)

Each capsule:
Dioctyl sodium sulfosuccinate * 60 mg.

'76 Ed.

CONSTOTABS
Fecal softener
(Bio-Factor Labs.)

Each tablet:
Dioctyl sodium
sulfosuccinate * .... 100 mg.

'76 Ed.

CONTAC
Continuous action decongestant capsules
(MenJ Labs.)

Each capsule:
Chlorpheniramine maleate * .. 8 mg.
Phenylpropanolamine HCl * .. 75 mg.

Starred ingredients (*) may be responsible for major toxic effects; consult Section II.

CONTAC JR.
Cold and cough medicine for children
(MenJ Labs.)

Each 5 cc. (average teaspoon):
Phenylpropanolamine HCl *	9.375 mg.
Acetaminophen *	162.5 mg.
Dextromethorphan hydrobromide	5.0 mg.
Alcohol (by volume)	10%

CONTACTICIDE 1
Insecticide
(Research Products Co.)

Pyrethrins	0.106%
Piperonyl butoxide technical	1.000%
Petroleum hydrocarbons *	98.894%

CONTACTICIDE 2
Insecticide
(Research Products Co.)

Pyrethrins	0.20%
Piperonyl butoxide	0.40%
N-Octyl bicycloheptene dicarboximide	0.66%
Petroleum distillates *	98.74%

CONTACTICIDE 3
Insecticide
(Research Products Co.)

Pyrethrins	0.3%
Technical Piperonyl butoxide	2.5%
Petroleum distillate *	97.2%

CONTACTICIDE 5
Insecticide
(Research Products Co.)

Pyrethrins	0.50%
Technical Piperonyl butoxide	1.00%
N-Octyl bicycloheptene dicarboximide	1.67%
Petroleum distillate *	96.83%

CONTACTICIDE 30
Insecticide
(Research Products Co.)

Pyrethrins	0.3%
Piperonyl butoxide	1.0%
Petroleum distillates *	97.7%

CONTACTISOL SOLUTION
Antiseptic wetting & lubricating of hard contact lenses
(CooperVision Pharm.)

Hydroxypropyl methylcellulose	
Benzalkonium chloride	0.01%
Disodium edetate	0.01%

CONTAC-TROL, SPRAY-TROL BRAND

See SPRAY-TROL BRAND CONTAC-TROL

CONTAX WEED & GRASS KILLER
(Chevron)

Active ingred. (by wt.):
Sodium dimethylarsinate *	10.40%
Dimethylarsinic acid	1.77%

Chevron emergency phone number: 415-233-3737

CONTI CASTILE SHAMPOO WITH OLIVE OIL
(Williams, J.B.)

Potassium soap
Olive oil
Coconut oil
Linoleic acid
Isopropyl cresols

CONTI CASTILE SOAP
(Williams, J.B.)

Sodium soap
Conti USP Castile Soap
Olive oil

CONTI LANOLIN SHAMPOO
(Williams, J.B.)

Mild detergent-type Lanolin derivatives

CONTIQUE CLEANING + SOAKING SOLUTION
For contact lenses
(Alcon)

Dual Detergent system
Preservatives:
Benzalkonium chloride	0.02%
Edetate disodium	0.1%

CONTIQUE CLEANING SOLUTION
For contact lenses
(Alcon)

Dual Detergent system
Purified Water
Benzalkonium chloride	0.02%

CONTIQUE SOAKING SOLUTION
For contact lenses
(Alcon)

Benzalkonium chloride	0.01%
Edetate disodium	0.01%

CONTIQUE WETTING SOLUTION
For contact lenses
(Alcon)

Polyvinyl alcohol
Hydroxypropyl methylcellulose
Preservatives:
Benzalkonium chloride	0.004%
Edetate disodium	0.025%

CONTI SOAPLETS WITH OLIVE OIL (BEAUTY SHOPPE)
(Williams, J.B.)

Sodium soap
Olive oil
Vegetable fatty acid
Coconut oil
Castor oil

CONTREET CEMENT HARDENER
(Rooto)

Sodium silicate *

CONTROFLEX, GREEN; PHOSPHORATED SYRUP
Relief of upset stomach and nausea
(Bowman Pharm.)

Sucrose	73.0%
Orthophosphoric acid	0.3%
Peppermint flavor	

CONTROL ALL PURPOSE SPRAY

See LILLY/MILLER CONTROL ALL PURPOSE SPRAY

CONTROL CAVITY FLUID
Embalming supply
(Royal Bond)

Formaldehyde *	20%
Methanol *	
Ethanol	

CONTROL-35 GERMICIDAL CLEANER

See PIONEER CONTROL-35 GERMICIDAL CLEANER

CONTROL III DISINFECTANT
For hospital only
(Consan Pacific)

n-Alkyl (60% C14, 30% C16, 5% C18, 5% C12) dimethyl benzyl ammonium chloride *	10%
n-Alkyl (68% C12, 32% C14) dimethyl ethylbenzyl ammonium chloride *	10%

CONTROL III LABORATORY GERMICIDE
For hospital only; ready to use solution, with 1560 ppm active ingredients
(Consan Pacific)

n-Alkyl (60% C14, 30% C16, 5% C18, 5% C12) dimethyl benzyl ammonium chloride	0.0781%
n-Alkyl (68% C12, 32% C14) dimethyl ethylbenzyl ammonium chloride	0.0781%

Starred ingredients (*) may be responsible for major toxic effects; consult Section II.

COOK & DUNN PAINT PRODUCTS

Cook & Dunn Paint Corp.
167 Kossuth St.
Newark, N.J. 07101

Phone: 201-589-5580

See PAINTS, Section VI, General Formulations

COOK'S ARMORCOTE GLOSS ENAMEL (FIESTA YELLOW)
(Cook Paint & Varnish Co.)

Pigment:		20.5%
Titanium dioxide pigment	83.0%	
Hansa yellow	11.0%	
Ferrite yellow	6.0%	
Vehicle:		79.5%
Soya alkyd resin	46.0%	
Petroleum distillates *	52.4%	
Drier & anti-skinning agent *	1.6%	

COOK'S ARMORCOTE GLOSS ENAMEL (LEMON BUTTER)
(Cook Paint & Varnish Co.)

Pigment:		21.6%
Titanium dioxide pigment	93.3%	
Yellow organic nickel complex	4.0%	
Isoindolinone yellow	2.6%	
Vehicle:		78.4%
Soya alkyd resin	45.0%	
Petroleum distillates *	53.6%	
Driers & anti-skinning agent *	1.4%	

COOK'S ARMORCOTE GLOSS ENAMEL (SUNSET ORANGE)
(Cook Paint & Varnish Co.)

Pigment:		18.0%
Titanium dioxide pigment	20.0%	
Dinitroaniline orange	9.3%	
Hansa yellow	17.5%	
Ferrite yellow	19.2%	
Calcium carbonate	34.0%	
Vehicle:		82.0%
Soya alkyd resin	46.0%	
Petroleum distillates *	52.6%	
Drier & anti-skinning agent *	1.4%	

COOK'S ARMORCOTE GLOSS ENAMEL (VERDAS GREEN)
(Cook Paint & Varnish Co.)

Pigment:		13.7%
Titanium dioxide pigment	38.8%	
Phthalocyanine blue	15.8%	
Ferrite yellow	14.7%	
Calcium carbonate	30.7%	
Vehicle:		86.3%
Soya alkyd resin	47.7%	
Petroleum distillate *	50.9%	
Drier & anti-skinning agent *	1.4%	

COOK'S ARMORCOTE METAL PRIMER (RED OXIDE)
(Cook Paint & Varnish Co.)

Pigment:		42.0%
Red iron oxide *	55.0%	
Calcium borosilicate	22.0%	
Magnesium silicate	12.0%	
Zinc oxide	11.0%	
Vehicle:		58.0%
Soya alkyd resin	42.4%	
Petroleum distillate *	56.2%	
Drier	1.4%	

COOK'S ARMOR-TILE REDUCER
(Cook Paint & Varnish Co.)

Hydrogenated naphtha *†	60%
Cellosolve acetate *	40%

†*See* Naphtha

COOK'S DECCA BARN PAINT
(Cook Paint & Varnish Co.)

Pigment:		49.2%
Red iron oxide	19.8%	
Calcium carbonate	29.2%	
Aluminum & magnesium silicates	48.3%	
Cuprous oxide	2.7%	
Vehicle:		50.8%
Raw Linseed oil	24.8%	
Soya alkyd resin solids	32.9%	
Aliphatic hydrocarbons *	41.3%	
Driers	1.0%	

COOK'S 63 LACQUER THINNER
(Cook Paint & Varnish Co.)

Petroleum distillate	30%
Esters	32%
Butyl alcohol	10%
Isopropyl alcohol	13%
Xylene *	15%

COOK'S 89 LACQUER THINNER
(Cook Paint & Varnish Co.)

Petroleum distillates	30%
Ketones	18%
Isopropanol	23%
Toluene *	29%

COOK'S OIL BASE OUTSIDE WHITE
(Cook Paint & Varnish Co.)

Pigment:		61.6%
Titanium dioxide pigment	29.3%	
Zinc oxide *	26.3%	
Calcium carbonate	23.4%	
Magnesium silicate	21.0%	
Vehicle:		38.4%
Raw Linseed oil	41.2%	
Bodied Linseed oil	31.8%	
Aliphatic petroleum solvent *	26.1%	
Driers & anti-skinning agent	0.9%	

COOK'S PAINT PRODUCTS
Paints

Cook Paint & Varnish Co.
P.O. Box 389
Kansas City, Mo. 64141

Phone: 816-391-6000

See PAINTS, Section VI, General Formulations

COOK'S SHADOTONE FLAT ENAMEL
(Cook Paint & Varnish Co.)

Pigment:		55.5%
Titanium dioxide pigment	31.5%	
Silica	8.0%	
Calcium carbonate	60.5%	
Vehicle:		44.5%
Soya alkyd resin	27.0%	
Aliphatic petroleum solvent *	72.0%	
Anti-skinning agent & drier	1.0%	

COOK'S SHADOTONE PRIMER UNDERCOAT
(Cook Paint & Varnish Co.)

Pigment:		58.0%
Titanium dioxide pigment	41.0%	
Calcium carbonate	59.0%	
Vehicle:		42.0%
Soya alkyd resin	32.0%	
Aliphatic petroleum solvent *	67.0%	
Driers & anti-skinning agent	1.0%	

COOK'S SHADOTONE SATIN ENAMEL (EBONY BLACK)
(Cook Paint & Varnish Co.)

Pigment:		50.0%
Carbon black	20.0%	
Calcium carbonate	76.0%	
Iron blue	4.0%	
Vehicle:		50.0%
Soya alkyd resin	47.0%	
Aliphatic petroleum solvent *	51.0%	
Anti-skinning agent & drier	2.0%	

COOK'S SHADOTONE SATIN ENAMEL (HILITE WHITE)
(Cook Paint & Varnish Co.)

Pigment:		48.4%
Titanium dioxide pigment	50.0%	
Calcium carbonate	50.0%	
Vehicle:		51.6%
Soya alkyd resin	43.4%	
Petroleum distillates *	55.7%	
Driers & anti-skinning agents	0.9%	

COOK'S SHADOTONE SATIN ENAMEL (MEDIUM BASE)
(Cook Paint & Varnish Co.)

Pigment:		47.1%
Titanium dioxide pigment	27.0%	
Calcium carbonate	73.0%	
Vehicle:		52.9%
Soya alkyd resin	43.0%	
Low odor Mineral spirits *	56.0%	
Driers & anti-skinning agents	1.0%	

Starred ingredients (*) may be responsible for major toxic effects; consult Section II.

COOK'S SHAKE & SHINGLE HOUSE PAINT (LIGHT BASE)
(Cook Paint & Varnish Co.)

Pigment: 46.5%
  Titanium dioxide pigment ... 32.0%
  Silica & silicates 68.0%
Vehicle: 53.5%
  Soya alkyd resin 30.4%
  Raw Linseed oil 10.8%
  Petroleum distillates * 57.7%
  Driers, anti-skinning agents,
    mildewcides 1.1%

COOK'S SHAKE & SHINGLE HOUSE PAINT (MEDIUM BASE)
(Cook Paint & Varnish Co.)

Pigment: 44.1%
  Titanium dioxide pigment ... 20.6%
  Silica & silicates 79.4%
Vehicle: 55.9%
  Soya alkyd resin 29.5%
  Raw Linseed oil 10.8%
  Petroleum distillates * 58.7%
  Driers, mildewcides, anti-skin-
    ning agent 1.0%

COOK'S SHAKE & SHINGLE HOUSE PAINT (WHITE)
(Cook Paint & Varnish Co.)

Pigment: 45.2%
  Titanium dioxide pigment ... 43.7%
  Silica & silicates 56.3%
Vehicle: 54.8%
  Soya alkyd resin 29.5%
  Raw Linseed oil 10.8%
  Petroleum distillates * 58.7%
  Driers, mildewcides, anti-skin-
    ning agent 1.0%

COOK'S 357 SPRAY THINNER
(Cook Paint & Varnish Co.)

Xylol * 100%

COOK'S TIMBRETONE EPOXY GLOSS VARNISH
(Cook Paint & Varnish Co.)

Vehicle: 100.0%
  Epoxy ester resin solids 41.0%
  Petroleum distillates * 54.3%
  Driers & anti-skinning
    agents * 4.7%

COOK'S TIMBRETONE WIPING STAIN FRUITWOOD
(Cook Paint & Varnish Co.)

Pigment: 20.1%
  Burnt umber 12.5%
  Raw sienna 10.5%
  Titanium dioxide pigment ... 15.5%
  Magnesium dioxide 61.5%
Vehicle: 79.9%
  Soya alkyd resin 21.0%
  Petroleum distillate * 78.3%
  Driers 0.7%

COOK'S TIMBRETONE WIPING STAIN MAHOGANY
(Cook Paint & Varnish Co.)

Pigment: 19.3%
  Burnt umber 33.0%
  Organic red toner 3.0%
  Magnesium silicate 64.0%
Vehicle: 80.7%
  Soya alkyd resin 21.0%
  Petroleum distillate * 78.3%
  Driers 0.7%

COOK'S TIMBRETONE WIPING STAIN WALNUT
(Cook Paint & Varnish Co.)

Pigment: 20.1%
  Burnt umber 37.0%
  Magnesium silicate 63.0%
Vehicle: 79.9%
  Soya alkyd resin 21.0%
  Petroleum distillate * 78.3%
  Driers 0.7%

COOK'S UTILITY THINNING SPIRITS
(Cook Paint & Varnish Co.)

Petroleum distillate *

COOK'S WOOD WASH
(Cook Paint & Varnish Co.)

Xylene * 50%
Isopropyl alcohol 30%
Ethyl acetate 20%

COOLIES (Green)
Facial cleansing pads
(Campana)

Essential oils *
Glycerin
Alcohol
Boric acid *
Methylparaben

COOL-SAVER
Inhibits bacteria and fungus growth in coolant solutions
(Certified Labs.)

Active ingred.:
  Hexahydro-1,3,5-tris (2-hydrox-
    yethyl)-s-triazine 7.85%
Inert ingred.:
  Water 92.15%

COOPERS CREEK DIP & DISINFECTANT
(Coopers Creek Chem.)

Active ingred.: 90%
  Coal tar neutral oils *
  Soap
  Cresylic acids *

COOPERVISION GLUCOSE OPHTHALMIC OINTMENT
Topical/to reduce corneal edema
(CooperVision Pharm.)

Glucose liquid (USP) 40%
White petrolatum
Anhydrous Lanolin
Methyl and propyl parabens

COOPERVISION HOMATROPINE HYDROBROMIDE
Mydriatic
(CooperVision Pharm.)

Each 5 ml. bottle or 1 ml. dropperette
applicator:
  Homatropine hydrobromide *   2%; 5%
  Buffered aqueous solution
  Boric acid
  Potassium chloride
  Sodium carbonate
  Disodium edetate
  Benzalkonium chloride

COPAC TABLETS
Analgesic
(Towne, Paulsen)

Each tablet:
  Codeine phosphate * .... 2 mg.
  Salicylamide * .... 5 gr.
  Caffeine * .... 1/2 gr.

COPE
Analgesic
(Glenbrook Labs.)

Aspirin * .... 421 mg.
Caffeine .... 32 mg.
Dried Aluminum hydroxide gel . 25 mg.
Magnesium hydroxide .... 50 mg.

COPPER-BRITE PRODUCTS

Copper-Brite, Inc.
5147 W. Jefferson Blvd.
Los Angeles, Calif. 90016

Phone: 213-933-9331

COPPER-CURE
Preservative and water repellant
(Apperson Chemicals)

Copper naphthenate * 20%
Petroleum solvent * 80%

COPPER DRAGON DUST
Insecticide & fungicide
(Dragon)

Carbaryl * 2%
Copper * 7%

Starred ingredients (*) may be responsible for major toxic effects; consult Section II.

COPPERIN A
Food supplement
(Vernon Labs.)

Each capsule:
Iron *† .... 32.0 mg.
Copper .... 1.0 mg.

†*See* Iron salts

COPPERIN B FOR CHILDREN
Food supplement
(Vernon Labs.)

Each capsule:
Iron *† .... 32.0 mg.
Copper .... 0.25 mg.

†*See* Iron salts

COPPER-LUX PAINT
(International Paint)

Copper *
Bis(tri-n-butyltin)oxide *
Color codes #80, #81, #82

COPPER-NU
(Kester)

Hydroxyethanoic acid *

COPPERSOTE
Wood preservative
(Georgia-Carolina Oil Co.)

Copper naphthenate (copper metallic
1%) 10%
Petroleum distillate * 90%

COPPERTONE LIPKOTE
(Coppertone)

White petrolatum
White wax
Paraffin wax
Lanolin anhydrous
Butylparaben
Allantoin
Homosalate *
Camphor *
Menthol *
Perfume

COPPERTONE LOTION (Tube and Bottle)
Suntan lotion
(Coppertone)

Lanolin
Cocoa butter
Methylparaben
Homosalate *
Triethanolamine
Perfume

COPPERTONE NOSKOTE (Jar and Tube)
(Coppertone)

Cocoa butter
Yellow beeswax
Paraffin wax (Jar only)
Lanolin anhydrous
Homosalate *
Amber petrolatum
Perfume

COPPERTONE OIL (Aerosol)
Suntan oil
(Coppertone)

Combined amount: 20%
  Lanolin
  Cocoa butter
  Homosalate *
  Perfume
Freon 11 and 12 .... 80%

COPPERTONE OIL (Tube and Bottle)
Suntan oil
(Coppertone)

Lanolin
Cocoa butter
Homosalate *
Mineral oil
Propylparaben
Perfume

COPPERTONE SHADE LOTION (Tube and Bottle)
Suntan lotion
(Coppertone)

Lanolin
Cocoa butter
Methyl parasept
Homosalate *
Triethanolamine
Perfume
Escalol 506 (Padimate A)

COPPO 2
Wood preservative
(Klean-Strip)

Aliphatic hydrocarbons * 80%
Copper naphthenate * 20%

COPPO PRESERVATIVE
Wood preservative
(Klean-Strip)

Petroleum distillate * 90%
Copper naphthenate 10%

COPYCAT SEMI-MOIST WATER COLORS
(American Crayon Co.)

This product bears the AP Seal issued
by the Crayon, Water Color and Craft Institute, Inc. This seal certifies that the
product contains no materials in sufficient
quantities to be toxic or injurious to the
human body even if ingested.

CORAL CONCENTRATED FABRIC SOFTENER
(Industrial Equities)

Quaternary ammonium
  compound * 5-10%
Fluorescent whitening agent ...   <1%
Preservative ....   <1%
Colorant ....   <1%
Perfume ....   <1%
Water .... balance

CO-RAL EMULSIFIABLE LIVESTOCK INSECTICIDE
(Cutter (Brand) Bayvet Div. Cutter Labs..)

Coumaphos * 11.6%
Aromatic petroleum distillate * .. 83.4%

CORAL FABRIC SOFTENER
(Industrial Equities)

Quaternary ammonium
  compound * 2-5%
Preservative ....   <1%
Colorant ....   <1%
Perfume ....   <1%
Water .... balance

CORAL LIQUID BLEACH
(Industrial Equities)

Sodium hypochlorite * 5 1/4%
Sodium chloride ....   <5%
Water .... balance

CORAL LIQUID DISHWASHING DETERGENT
(Industrial Equities)

Anionic surfactant 6-12%
Hydrotrope 1-3%
Alkanolamide ....   <1%
Ethyl alcohol ....   <1%
Opacifier ....   <1%
Colorant ....   <1%
Perfume ....   <1%
Water .... balance

CO-RAL POUR-ON
Insecticide for cattle
(Cutter (Brand) Bayvet Div. Cutter Labs.)

Coumaphos * 4%

CO-RAL SPRAY FOAM WOUND TREATMENT
For control of screw worms, maggots, ear ticks on livestock
(Cutter (Brand) Bayvet Div. Cutter Labs.)

Coumaphos * 3.0%

CORAVAL, IMPROVED
Cold tablets
(Vale)

Each tablet:
Phenylephrine
hydrochloride * .... 2.5 mg.
Belladonna extract .... 3.2 mg.
Ammonium chloride .... 32.4 mg.
Camphor * .... 32.4 mg.

CO-RAX CONCENTRATE
Rodenticide - bait
(Prentiss)

Warfarin 0.5%

CO-RAX PELLETED BAIT
Rodenticide
(Prentiss)

Warfarin 0.025%

CORDO SPECIAL THINNER P-371
(Cordo)

Ketones *
Aromatic hydrocarbons * .... <10%

CORDO SPECIAL THINNER 200T
(Cordo)

Ketones *
Aromatic hydrocarbons * .... <10%

CORDO THINNER NO. 2027
(Cordo)

Ketones
Aromatic hydrocarbons * .... >10%

CORDROL
Treatment of inflammatory conditions
(Vita Elixir Co.)

Each tablet:
Prednisolone .... 5 mg.; 20 mg.

COREGA DENTURE ADHESIVE POWDER
(Block Drug)

Karaya gum
Ethylene oxide homopolymer
Flavors

CORICIDIN COUGH FORMULA
(Schering)

Each 5 ml.:
Chlorpheniramine maleate * ... 2 mg.
Phenylphrine HCl * .... 12.5 mg.
Guaifenesin .... 50 mg.
Ammonium HCl .... 100 mg.

CORICIDIN 'D'
Decongestant tablets
(Schering)

Each tablet:
Phenylpropanolamine HCl * ... 12.5 mg.
Aspirin * .... 325 mg.
Chlorpheniramine maleate .. 2 mg.

CORICIDIN DEMILETS
Antihistaminic with analgesic
(Schering)

Each tablet:
Aspirin * .... 80 mg.
Chlorpheniramine maleate ... 0.5 mg.
Phenylephrine HCl .... 2.5 mg.

CORICIDIN MEDILETS
Cold and hay fever tablets for children
(Schering)

Each Medilet:
Chlorpheniramine maleate ... 0.5 mg.
Aspirin * .... 80 mg.

CORICIDIN NASAL MIST
Decongestant
(Schering)

Phenylephrine hydrochloride 0.5%

CORICIDIN TABLETS
Antihistaminic with analgesic
(Schering)

Each tablet:
Chlorpheniramine maleate ... 2 mg.
Aspirin * .... 325 mg.

CORIFORTE CAPSULES
Antihistaminic, analgesic, antipyretic
(Schering)

Each capsule:
Chlorpheniramine maleate * 4 mg.
Salicylamide * .... 0.19 gm.
Phenacetin * .... 0.13 gm.
Caffeine .... 0.03 gm.
Ascorbic acid .... 0.05 gm.

CORILIN INFANT LIQUID
Antihistaminic-analgesic-antipyretic compound; pediatric
(Schering)

Each cc:
Chlorpheniramine maleate .. 0.75 mg.
Sodium salicylate * .... 80 mg.
Alcohol .... <1%
Glycine .... 25 mg.

CORN FIX
Corn remover
(Alvin Last)

Phenol liquid (88%) * 2.26%
Turpentine oil 2.40%

CORN HUSKERS LOTION
(Warner-Lambert)

Glycerin
Alcohol 5 3/4%

CORN KING CATTLE SPRAY
Insecticide
(Corn King)

Dimethyl phosphate of alpha-
methylbenzyl 3-hydroxy-cis-
crotonate (Ciodrin) * 1.00%
2,2-Dichlorovinyl dimethyl
phosphate 0.23%
Related compounds 0.02%
Petroleum hydrocarbons * ... 98.50%

CORN KING DEAD-WHITE
Insecticidal, germicidal & fungicidal paint
(Corn King)

Ronnel (O,O-Dimethyl O-(2,4,5-
trichlorophenyl)
phosphorothioate) 0.5%

CORN KING DRY INSECTICIDE
For use on livestock and poultry
(Corn King)

Malathion 4.00%

CORN KING PREMIUM STOCK SPRAY
Insecticide
(Corn King)

Toxaphene (technical chlorinated
camphene, chlorine content 67-
69%) * 45.00%
Lindane (Gamma isomer of benzene hexachloride) 2.00%
Heavy aromatic naphtha * 38.00%
Xylene 5.00%

CORN KING RABON CATTLE DUST BAG
Insecticide
(Corn King)

Rabon * 4.04%
Pyrophyllite powder .... approx. 27%
Dicalite 476 .... approx. 69%

CORN KING SULPHURIZED OIL
For sarcoptic and psoroptic mange on livestock
(Corn King)

Sulphur 0.20%
Mineral oil * 99.80%

CORONA OINTMENT
Antiseptic dressing for animals
(Corona Products)

p-Chloromercuriphenol 0.067%
Lanolin .... approx. 40%
Petrolatum .... approx. 30%

Starred ingredients (*) may be responsible for major toxic effects; consult Section II.

COROVAS TYMCAPS
Treatment of angina pectoris
(Amfre-Grant)

Each Tymcap:
Pentaerythritol tetranitrate * . . 30 mg.
Secobarbituric acid *† . . . . 50 mg.

†*See* Secobarbital sodium

CORPAREX META-KAPS
Obesity
(Sutliff & Case)

Each Meta-Kap:
Dextroamphetamine sulfate . . . 15 mg.
Amobarbital * . . . . 60 mg.

'76 Ed.

CORRECTOL LAXATIVE PILLS
(Plough)

Each tablet:
Yellow phenolphthalein . . . . . 64.8 mg.
Dioctyl sodium sulfosuccinate
(DSS) * . . . . 100 mg.

CORRY'S SLUG & SNAIL DEATH
(Matson, E.M., Jr. Co.)

Metaldehyde 2%

COR-SECT
Municipal insecticide
(ABCO, Inc.)

Petroleum hydrocarbon base oil   78.905%
Xylene * 11.50%
2,2-Dichlorovinyl dimethyl
phosphate 4.70%
Related compounds 0.35%
Methoxychlor, technical 4.09%

COR-TAR-QUIN (CREME & LOTION)
*For atopic dermatitis, anogenital prur-
itis, dermatitis venenata, allergic
eczemas*
(Dome)

Liquor carbonis
detergens * 2%
Diiodohydroxyquinoline 1%
Micronized Hydrocorti-
sone alcohol 1/4%; 1/2%; 1%
Acid pH vehicle

CORT-DOME CREME & LOTION
*Prompt relief from itching; steadily re-
duces edema, erythema, scaling*
(Dome)

Microdispersed Hy-
drocortisone
alcohol . . . . 1/8, 1/4, 1/2, or 1%
Acid pH vehicle

CORT-DOME SUPPOSITORIES
(Dome)

HIGH POTENCY (each suppository):
Hydrocortisone acetate * . . . . 25 mg.
Mixed monoglyceride base

REGULAR (each suppository):
Hydrocortisone acetate * . . . . 15 mg.
Mixed monoglyceride base

CORTEF ACETATE TOPICAL OINTMENT
Anti-inflammatory corticosteroid
(Upjohn)

Each gram:
Hydrocortisone acetate . 10 mg. (1%);
25 mg. (2.5%)
Anhydrous Lanolin
White petrolatum
Mineral oil

CORTEF FLUID ORAL SUSPENSION
Anti-inflammatory corticosteroid
(Upjohn)

Each 5 ml.:
Hydrocortisone (as 13.4 mg. hydrocortisone cypionate) . . . . 10 mg.

CORTEF TABLETS
Anti-inflammatory corticosteroid
(Upjohn)

Each tablet:
Hydrocortisone . . . . . 5 mg.; 10 mg.;
20 mg.

CORTENEMA
Hydrocortisone retention enema
(Rowell)

Each disposable unit (60 cc):
Hydrocortisone . . . . 100 mg.
Aqueous solution with:
Carboxypolymethylene
Polysorbate 80
Methylparaben 0.18%

CORTIFOAM
For ulcerative proctitis
(Reed & Carnrick)

Hydrocortisone acetate 10%
Propylene glycol
Ethoxylated stearyl alcohol
Polyoxyethylene-10-stearyl ether
Cetyl alcohol
Methyl and propyl parabens
Triethanolamine
Water
Inert propellants:
Dichlorodifluoromethane
Dichlorotetrafluoroethane

CORTIN 1/2% or 1% CREAM
For eczemas
(C & M Pharmacal)

Hydrocortisone 1/2%; 1%
Iodochlorhydroxyquin 3%
Washable base

CORTISPORIN CREAM
*Topical anti-infective & anti-inflam-
matory*
(Burroughs Wellcome)

Each gram:
Polymyxin B sulfate . . . . 10,000 units
Neomycin sulfate (equiv.
to 3.5 mg. neomycin
base) . . . . 5 mg.
Gramicidin . . . . 0.25 mg.
Hydrocortisone acetate . . . . 5 mg.
Methylparaben
(preservative) 0.25%
Base:
Liquid petrolatum
White petrolatum
Emulsifying wax
Propylene glycol
Polyoxyethylene polyoxypropylene
compound
Purified water

CORTISPORIN OINTMENT (TOPICAL)
Anti-inflammatory & antibacterial
(Burroughs Wellcome)

Each gram:
Polymyxin B sulfate . . . . 5,000 units
Bacitracin zinc . . . . 400 units
Neomycin sulfate (equiv. to
3.5 mg. neomycin base) . . . . 5 mg.
Hydrocortisone . . . . 10 mg.
Special white petrolatum . . . . q.s.

CORTISPORIN OPHTHALMIC OINTMENT
Anti-infective/steroid
(Burroughs Wellcome)

Each gram:
Aerosporin
(Polymyxin B sulfate) . . . 10,000 units
Bacitracin zinc . . . . 400 units
Neomycin sulfate (equiv. to
3.5 mg. neomycin base) . . . . 5 mg.
Hydrocortisone . . . . 10 mg.
White petrolatum . . . . q.s.

CORTISPORIN OPHTHALMIC SUSPENSION
Anti-infective/steroid
(Burroughs Wellcome)

Each cc:
Polymyxin B sulfate . . . . 10,000 units
Neomycin sulfate (equiv.
to 3.5 mg. neomycin
base) . . . . 5 mg.
Hydrocortisone . . . . 10 mg.
Thimerosal 0.001%
Cetyl alcohol
Glyceryl monostearate
Liquid petrolatum
Mineral oil
Polyoxyl 40 stearate
Propylene glycol
Water for injection

Starred ingredients (*) may be responsible for major toxic effects; consult Section II.

CORTISPORIN OTIC SOLUTION
For external ear infections
(Burroughs Wellcome)

Each cc.:
Aerosporin (Polymyxin B sulfate)	10,000 Units
Neomycin sulfate (equiv. to 3.5 mg. neomycin base)	5 mg.
Hydrocortisone	10 mg. (1%)
Cupric sulfate	
Glycerin	
Hydrochloric acid	
Propylene glycol	
Water for injection	
Potassium metabisulfite (preservative)	0.1%

CORTISPORIN OTIC SUSPENSION
Ear infections
(Burroughs Wellcome)

Each cc:
Polymyxin B sulfate	10,000 units
Neomycin sulfate (equiv. to 3.5 mg. neomycin base)	5 mg.
Hydrocortisone	10 mg.
Thimerosal	0.01%
Cetyl alcohol	
Propylene glycol	
Polysorbate 80	
Water for injection	

CORT-QUIN CREME
For infectious dermatoses, stubborn eczemas
(Dome)

Microdispersed Hydrocortisone alcohol	1/2%; 1/4%
Diiodohydroxyquin	1%
Acid pH vehicle	

CORTRIL TOPICAL OINTMENT
(Pfipharmecs)

Hydrocortisone	1.0%

CORYBAN-D COLD CAPSULES
Decongestant cold capsules
(Pfipharmecs)

Each capsule:
Caffeine	30 mg.
Chlorpheniramine maleate	2 mg.
Phenylpropanolamine HCl *	25 mg.

CORY-EZE
For relief of colds; analgesic, antipyretic, antihistaminic
(Bio-Factor Labs.)

Each tablet:
Chlorphenist (Chlorpheniramine maleate, USP)	2 mg.
Salicylamide	3 gr.
Acetophenetidin *	2 gr.
Caffeine	1/4 gr.
Camphor monobromated	1/4 gr.
Methamphetamine	0.5 mg.
Atropine sulfate	1/500 gr.

'76 Ed.

CORYZAID
Decongestant
(Elder)

Each tablet:
Salicylamide *	150 mg.
Caffeine	15 mg.
Phenylephrine hydrochloride *	10 mg.
Chlorpheniramine maleate	2 mg.

CORYZTIME SR CAPSULES
Decongestant
(Elder)

Each capsule:
Phenylpropanolamine hydrochloride *	50 mg.
Chlorpheniramine maleate	8 mg.
Atropine sulfate *	0.36 mg.

COSMAFLO
Medium firming arterial fluid
(Royal Bond)

Formaldehyde index *	22%
Methanol *	

COSMATONE
Tinting liquid
(Royal Bond)

Isopropanol *

COSMERICA COSMETICS

Cosmerica
4241 Redwood Ave.
Los Angeles, Calif. 90066

Phone: 213-823-0015

See COSMETICS, Section VI, General Formulations

COTORAN + MSMA WITH SURFACTANT
Herbicide
(Ciba-Geigy Ag. Div.)

Fluometuron *	13.2%
Monosodium acid methanearsonate	27.6%

COTORAN 80WP
Herbicide
(Ciba-Geigy Ag. Div.)

Fluometuron *	80%

COTROL-D TABLETS
Nasal decongestant & bronchodilator
(Beecham Labs.)

Each tablet:
Pseudoephedrine hydrochloride *	60 mg.
Chlorpheniramine maleate	4 mg.

COTTON STATES CHLORDANE 45% EMULSIFIABLE
Insecticide
(Cotton States Chem.)

Tech. Chlordane *	45.0%
Petroleum distillate *	45.0%

COTTON STATES 72% CHLORDANE EMULSIFIABLE
Insecticide
(Cotton States Chem.)

Tech. Chlordane *	72.0%
Petroleum distillate *	16.0%

COTTON STATES MALATHION EMULSIFIABLE 57
Insecticide
(Cotton States Chem.)

Malathion, tech. *	57%
Aromatic petroleum distillates *	35%

COTTON STATES 4 LB. METHYL PARATHION
Insecticide
(Cotton States Chem.)

Methyl parathion *	44%
Aromatic petroleum distillates *	50%

COTTON STATES SEVIN SUPER TOMATO DUST
Insecticide, fungicide
(Cotton States Chem.)

Zineb	6.0%
1-Naphthyl N-methylcarbamate (Sevin) *	10.00%

C-O-TWO DRY CHEMICAL RECHARGE
For fire extinguishers
(Norris Industries)

Sodium bicarbonate
Diatomaceous earth
Polysiloxane coating

'76 Ed.

Starred ingredients (*) may be responsible for major toxic effects; consult Section II.

C-O-TWO KARBALOY LOADED STREAM RECHARGE
For fire extinguishers
(Norris Industries)

Potassium carbonate
Sodium dichromate *
Ethylene glycol

'76 Ed.

C-O-TWO MULTI-PURPOSE DRY CHEMICAL RECHARGE
For fire extinguishers
(Norris Industries)

Monoammonium phosphate
Diatomaceous earth
Tricalcium phosphate
Polysiloxane coating

'76 Ed.

C-O-TWO PURPLE K DRY CHEMICAL RECHARGE
For fire extinguishers
(Norris Industries)

Potassium bicarbonate
Diatomaceous earth
Tricalcium phosphate
Polysiloxane coating

'76 Ed.

C-O-TWO SUPER-KEM DRY CHEMICAL RECHARGE
For fire extinguishers
(Norris Industries)

Potassium chloride
Diatomaceous earth
Tricalcium phosphate
Polysiloxane coating

'76 Ed.

COTY COSMETICS AND TOILETRIES

Coty, Div. of Pfizer, Inc.
235 E. 42nd St.
New York, N.Y. 10017

Phone: 212-573-3500

See COSMETICS, Section VI, General Formulations

CO-TYLENOL COLD FORMULA LIQUID
Decongestant-analgesic
(McNeil Consumer Products Co.)

Each 30 ml.:
Acetaminophen * .... 650 mg.
Chlorpheniramine maleate ... 4 mg.
Pseudoephedrine
hydrochloride * .... 60 mg.
Dextromethorphan
hydrobromide * .... 20 mg.

CO-TYLENOL COLD FORMULA TABLETS/CAPSULES
Decongestant-analgesic
(McNeil Consumer Products Co.)

Each tablet:
Acetaminophen * .... 325 mg.
Chlorpheniramine maleate ... 2 mg.
Pseudoephedrine
hydrochloride * .... 30 mg.
Dextromethorphan
hydrobromide .... 10 mg.

COUMADIN TABLETS
Anticoagulant
(Endo Labs.)

Crystalline Sodium warfarin USP *
Lavender tablet: .... 2 mg.
Orange tablet: .... 2 1/2 mg.
Peach tablet: .... 5 mg.
Yellow tablet: .... 7 1/2 mg.
White tablet: .... 10 mg.

COUNTERPAIN RUB
Analgesic balm
(Squibb)

Methyl salicylate *
Eugenol *
Menthol *

COUNTESS MARITZA COSMETIC PRODUCTS
Perfumes, colognes, & men's toiletries

Countess Maritza Cosmetic Co., Inc.
14 Aquarium Dr.
Secaucus, N.J. 07094

Phone: 201-866-8780

See COSMETICS, Section VI, General Formulations

COVER GIRL PRODUCTS

Noxell Corporation
P.O. Box 1799
Baltimore, Md. 21203

Phone: 301-628-7300

COVICONE CREAM
Protective skin cream
(Abbott)

Silicone (Dimethylpolysiloxane)
Nitrocellulose
Castor oil
Suspended in a greaseless vanishing cream base

COWLEY'S RAT & MOUSE POISON
(Cowley, S.L.)

Arsenic trioxide * 1.5%

COW MAT CEMENT
Specialized cement for dairy farmers
(Goodyear)

Natural rubber and synthetic rub-
ber copolymer: 10-15%
Styrene
Butadiene
Toluene * 5-10%
Rubber solvent naphtha * 80-90%

CO-XAN SYRUP
Expectorant, decongestant, antitussive, bronchodilator
(Central Pharmacal Co.)

Each 15 ml.:
Theophylline sodium glycinate
(equiv. to 165 mg.
theophylline) * .... 330 mg.
Codeine phosphate * .... 15 mg.
Ephedrine hydrochloride * ... 25 mg.
Glyceryl guaiacolate .... 100 mg.
Alcohol 10%

COX FLIGHT POWER
Model fuel
(Cox, L.M.)

Methanol * 65%
Nitromethane * 15%
Castor oil 18%
Dow #1180.6 Lub. Fluid 2%

COX GLOW POWER
Model fuel
(Cox, L.M.)

Methanol * 70%
Nitromethane 10%
Castor oil 18%
Dow #1180.6 Lub. Fluid 2%

COX RACE POWER
Model fuel
(Cox, L.M.)

Methanol * 50%
Nitromethane * 30%
Castor oil 18%
Dow #1180.6 Lub. Fluid 2%

CPC
Germicide
(Fine Organics, Inc.)

Cetyl pyridinium chloride * 100%

'76 Ed.

CPC CHLORINATED DONUT TABLETS, CONCENTRATED
Swimming pool use
(Kiefer-McNeil)

Trichloro-s-triazinetrione * 100%

C.P.C. CLEAR PROTECTIVE COATING
(Paul Koss)

Water .... >90%
Silicone emulsion (40%)

pH 7.0

CPC CONCENTRATED CHLORINATED 1-INCH TABLETS
Swimming pool use
(Kiefer-McNeil)

Trichloro-s-triazinetrione * 100%

CPC CONCENTRATED CHLORINATING GRANULES
Swimming pool use
(Kiefer-McNeil)

Sodium dichloro-s-triazinetrione * 100%

CPC END-O-ALGE 2
Algicide for use in swimming pools, reservoirs, etc.
(Kiefer-McNeil)

Copper (as elemental) derived from
Copper triethanolamine
complex * 7%

CPC HALF POUNDER CHLORINATED TABLETS
Swimming pool use
(Kiefer-McNeil)

Trichloro-s-triazinetrione * 99.5%

CPC pH DRY ACID
Swimming pool use
(Kiefer-McNeil)

Sodium bisulfate * 92.1%

CPC pH SODA ASH
Swimming pool use
(Kiefer-McNeil)

Sodium carbonate * 99.58%

CPC RED PLUG CARTRIDGE WITH CONCENTRATED CHLORINATED TABLETS
Swimming pool use
(Kiefer-McNeil)

Trichloro-s-triazinetrione * 100%

CPC SUPER CONCENTRATED END-O-ALGE
Swimming pool use
(Kiefer-McNeil)

n-Alkyl (60% C14, 30% C16, 5% C12,
5% C18) dimethyl benzyl ammonium chlorides * 42%
n-Dialkyl (60% C14, 30% C16, 5% C12,
5% C18) methyl benzyl ammonium
chlorides 8%

CP SWEET KILL
Dry fly bait
(Colonial Prod.)

2,2-Dichlorovinyl dimethyl
phosphate 0.46%/w
Related compounds 0.04%/w

CR-55
Metal surface conditioning solution
(Whitfield Chem.)

Chromic acid * .... >10%
Phosphoric acid * .... >10%

CRABGRAX DSMA
Herbicide
(Dolge)

Disodium methanearsonate
anhydrous * 15.7%

CRAB-NO CRABGRASS KILLER, GOOD-LIFE

See GOOD-LIFE CRAB-NO
CRABGRASS KILLER

CRACKLETONE GLAZES

See DUNCAN CERAMICS CRACKLETONE GLAZES (CR 800 Series)

CRAFTINT ACRYLIC POLYMER COLORS
(Craftint)

Acrylic emulsion
Organic pigments *
Inorganic pigments *

CRAFTINT OIL COLORS
(Craftint)

Vegetable oils
Paint grade organic and inorganic pigments *

CRAIG-MARTIN MILK OF MAGNESIA TOOTHPASTE
(Comfort)

Glycerin CP
Corn starch
Gum tragacanth
Saccharin
Soap
Calcium carbonate
Magma

CRAMERGESIC
(Cramer Products)

Paraffin 7.435%
Lanolin (USP)(anhydrous) 5.000%
Petrolatum (NF)(amber) 70.000%
Oleoresin capsicum 0.065%
Camphor (USP) 2.000%
Methyl salicylate (USP) * 12.000%
Menthol (technical) 3.500%

CRAMER'S COLD SPRAY
(Cramer Products)

Propellent 11/12 .... 100%

CRAMER'S FLEXIBLE REUSABLE COLD PACKS
(Cramer Products)

Soft water 78.000%
Cellosize QP-100M 2.000%
Sodium chloride 20.000%
Pylaklor S-400 Turquoise Blue . 0.001%

CRAMER'S FOOT POWDER
(Cramer Products)

Talc 80.00%
Corn starch 19.00%
Benzoic acid (USP) 0.75%
8-Hydroxyquinoline sulfate 0.15%
Thymol crystals 0.10%

CRAMER'S HAND CLEANER CREAM
(Cramer Products)

Soft water 50.90%
Glycerine (USP) 1.50%
Carbopol 934 .... 0.50%
Sodium hydroxide 0.10%
Ethomeen C/25 .... 0.50%
Energetic S 5.00%
Deodorized Kerosene * 40.00%
Mineral oil (NF) 1.25%
Neutralizer (Mala #33 or Lemon
40R 4787) 0.25%

CRAMER'S INSTANT DELUXE COLD PACKS
(Cramer Products)

Ammonium nitrate .... 5 oz.
Water .... 6 oz.

CRAMER'S MASSAGE LOTION
(Cramer Products)

Water
Stearic acid
Mineral oil
Cetyl alcohol
Triethanolamine
Fragrance
Quaternium-15
Magnesium stearate
Propylparaben
Lanolin
Olive oil
Propylene glycol
Menthol

Starred ingredients (*) may be responsible for major toxic effects; consult Section II.

CRAMER'S MOUTHWASH
(Cramer Products)

Soft water	75.1200%
Sorbitol solution (USP)	24.4500%
Citric acid (USP)	0.0720%
Sodium saccharin (NF)	0.0080%
Tween 60	0.2500%
Peppermint flavor	0.1000%
D & C Green #5	0.0001%

CRAMER'S ROSIN BAGS
(Cramer Products)

Florex AA/RVM 100/up (Fullers earth)	44.45%
Bentonite powder	22.22%
F.F. Wood rosin	33.33%

CRAMER'S SALT TABLETS
(Cramer Products)

Salt *	95%
Paraffin	5%

CRAMER'S TAPE REMOVER
(Cramer Products)

Methylene chloride	25%
Petroleum distillate *	75%

CRAMER'S VITAMIN & MINERAL TABLETS
(Cramer Products)

Vitamin A (acetate)	5000 USP units
Vitamin D (ergocalciferol)	400 USP units
Iron (from 50 mg. ferrous sulfate)	10 mg.
Iodine (as potassium iodine)	0.15 mg.
Plus multivitamins and minerals	

CRATER 2X FLUID
(Texaco, Inc.)

Petroleum lubricating oil
Trichloroethane *
Pine tar *

CRATER 5X FLUID
(Texaco Inc.)

Petroleum lubricating oil
Trichloroethane *
Pine tar *

CRAYOGRAPH PRESSED CRAYONS
(American Crayon Co.)

This product bears the CP Seal issued by the Crayon, Water Color and Craft Institute, Inc. This seal certifies that the product contains no materials in sufficient quantities to be toxic or injurious to the human body even if ingested.

CRAYOLA AN-DU-SEPTIC WHITE CHALK
(Binney & Smith)

Whiting base
Starch binder

CRAYOLA ANTI-DUST WHITE CHALK
(Binney & Smith)

Whiting base
Starch binder

CRAYOLA ART & CRAFT GLUE
(Binney & Smith)

Acetate resin emulsion

CRAYOLA COLORED ART CHALK
(Binney & Smith)

Non-toxic extender pigment base
Starch binder
Non-toxic color pigments

CRAYOLA COLORED DRAWING CHALK
(Binney & Smith)

Calcium sulfate
Non-toxic colors

CRAYOLA COLORED POSTER CHALK
(Binney & Smith)

Calcium sulfate
Non-toxic colors

CRAYOLA CRAYONS
(Binney & Smith)

Wax blend
Non-toxic pigments

CRAYOLA EASY-OFF CRAYONS
(Binney & Smith)

Wax blend
Detergent
Non-toxic pigments

CRAYOLA E-Z-SYTE POLYCHROMATIC CHALK
(Binney & Smith)

Non-toxic extender pigment base
Starch binder
Non-toxic colored pigment

CRAYOLA FINGER PAINT
(Binney & Smith)

Soluble Starches
Preservative
Odorant
Non-toxic pigments

CRAYOLA FINGER PAINT POWDER
(Binney & Smith)

Soluble Starches
Preservative
Non-toxic pigments

CRAYOLA KLEERWAE COLORED CHALK
(Binney & Smith)

Non-toxic extender pigment base
Starch binder
Non-toxic color pigments

CRAYOLA POWDER PAINT
(Binney & Smith)

Soluble starches
Preservative
Non-toxic pigments

CRAYOLA TEMPERA PAINT
(Binney & Smith)

Soluble starches
Glycerine
Preservative
Odorant
Non-toxic pigments

CRAYOLA WATER COLORS
(Binney & Smith)

Water-soluble base
Organic plasticizer
Non-toxic pigments

CRAYOLA WHITE CHALK
(Binney & Smith)

Calcium sulfate

CRAYOLA WHITE PASTE
(Binney & Smith)

Starch
Corn syrup
Preservative
Water

CRAYOLET CRAYONS
(Binney & Smith)

Wax blend
Non-toxic pigments

Starred ingredients (*) may be responsible for major toxic effects; consult Section II.

CRAZY FOAM
Children's foam soap
(American Aerosol Corp.)

Sodium soap
Fatty free acids
Protein stabilizers
Wetting agents - Surfactant
Perfume
Propellant

CREAMALIN (LIQUID & TABLETS)
Antacid
(Winthrop Labs.)

Each 5 ml. or tablet:
  Short polymer Aluminum hy-
    droxide gel .... 320 mg.
  Magnesium hydroxide .... 75 mg.

CREAM SUDS (Phosphate Formula or 0-Phosphate Formula)
Institutional and industrial cleaning product

Procter & Gamble Co.
Ivorydale Technical Center
Cincinnati, Ohio 45217

Phone: 513-562-1100

CREAMY LIME BATH BUBBLES
(House of Lowell, Inc.)

TEA-lauryl sulfate *
Lauramide DEA
Modified Polystyrene latex
Perfume *
Formaldehyde
D & C color

CREMESONE
Treatment of allergic dermatitis and skin diseases
(Dalin)

Each gram:
  Hydrocortisone alcohol
    (micronized) .... 5 mg.
Dalicreme base adjusted to pH 4.6:
  Stearic acid
  Propylene glycol
  Dibasic potassium phosphate
  Glyceryl monostearate S.E.
  Monobasic potassium phosphate
  Polyoxyethylene sorbitan monostearate
  Sorbitan monostearate
  Acetylated lanolin-alcohol extract
  Methyl paraben and propyl paraben
  Deionized water
  Essential oils

'76 Ed.

CREOFECTANT (Canada Only)

See FRANKLIN CREOFECTANT
(Canada Only)

CREOMULSION
Antitussive
(Creomulsion)

Beechwood creosote *
Cascara
Ipecac
Menthol *
White pine
Wild cherry
Alcohol 1%

CREOMULSION FOR CHILDREN
Antitussive
(Creomulsion)

Beechwood creosote *
Cascara
Ipecac
Menthol *
White pine
Wild cherry
Alcohol 0.7%

CRE-O-TOX A-10 WOOD PRESERVING CONCENTRATE
(Cre-O-Tox)

Pentachlorophenol, technical * 40%
Petroleum distillate 33%

CRE-O-TOX EMULSIFIABLE CHLORDANE CONCENTRATE 8
Termite soil poisoning agent
(Cre-O-Tox)

Technical Chlordane * 72%
Petroleum distillate * 21%

CRESEPTOL
Disinfectant & deodorant
(Royal Bond)

Phenol *
Caustic soda *

CREST FLUORIDE GEL
Toothpaste
(Procter & Gamble, Health & Personal Care Div.)

Sodium fluoride 0.243%
Hydrated Silica 15-30%
Sorbitol 35-60%
Glycerin 15-25%
Sodium alkyl sulfate 1-6%
Trisodium phosphate 1-4%
Minor ingredients .... <1%
Water .... balance

CREST FLUORIDE TOOTHPASTE (Regular and Mint Flavor)
(Procter & Gamble, Health & Personal Care Div.)

Sodium fluoride 0.243%
Hydrated Silica 15-30%
Sorbitol 35-60%
Glycerin 15-25%
Sodium alkyl sulfate 1-6%
Trisodium phosphate 1-4%
Minor ingredients .... <1%
Water .... balance

CRESYLATE
For the treatment of external otitis
(Recsei Labs.)

m-Cresyl acetate (v/v) * 25%
Isopropanol (v/v) 25%
Chlorobutanol 1%
Benzyl alcohol 1%
Castor oil (in Propylene glycol) 5%

pH adjusted to 4.5

CRETEX
Concrete cleaner
(Lester Labs.)

Mild Acids *
Detergents *

'76 Ed.

CRISTALLE FRAGRANCE
(Chanel, Inc.)

Alcohol * .... >50%
Water .... <20%
Fragrance *† 2-5%

†*See* Essential oils

CRISTALLE SPRAY FRAGRANCE
(Chanel, Inc.)

Alcohol * .... >50%
Water .... <20%
Fragrance *† 2-5%

†*See* Essential oils

CRISTAL SEAL
Concrete sealer
(Sanitek)

Blend of: 75.0%
  Toluene *
  Xylene *
Polystyrene resin 23.1%
Chlorinated paraffin resin 1.9%

CROAKS
Residual insecticide concentrate; professional use
(Puritan Chem. Co.)

Aromatic petroleum distillate * .. 88.0%
o-Isopropoxyphenyl
  methylcarbamate * 4.0%

Starred ingredients (*) may be responsible for major toxic effects; consult Section II.

C-RON
Iron deficiency anemia
(Rowell)

Each tablet:
  Ferrous fumarate (iron, 66
    mg.) * .... 200 mg.
  Ascorbic acid .... 100 mg.

C-RON FA
Iron deficiency anemia
(Rowell)

Each tablet:
  Ferrous fumarate (iron, 66
    mg.) * .... 200 mg.
  Ascorbic acid .... 600 mg.
  Folic acid .... 0.5 mg.

C-RON FORTE
Iron deficiency anemia
(Rowell)

Each tablet:
  Ferrous fumarate (iron, 66
    mg.) * .... 200 mg.
  Ascorbic acid .... 600 mg.

C-RON FRECKLES
Iron deficiency anemia
(Rowell)

Each chewable tablet:
  Ferrous fumarate (iron, 33
    mg.) * .... 100 mg.
  Ascorbic acid .... 50 mg.

CROP RIDER 20% AQUA GRANULAR
Herbicide
(Diamond Shamrock Corp.)

Isooctyl ester of 2,4-dichlorophen-
  oxyacetic acid * 27.6%

CROW-CHEX
Dry bird repellent
(Borderland Prod.)

Copper oxalate * 4.00%

Inert ingred.:
  Ferric oxide 33.92%
  Silicon dioxide 2.94%
  Aluminum oxide 1.03%
  Acid insolubles 0.55%
  Inert materials 57.56%

CRUEX MEDICATED CREAM
Antifungal, antibacterial
(Pharmacraft)

Zinc undecylenate * 20.0%
PCMX 3.0%

CRUEX MEDICATED SQUEEZE POWDER
Antifungal
(Pharmacraft)

Calcium undecylenate 10.0%

CRUEX (SPRAY-ON POWDER)
Medicated powder
(Pharmacraft)

Calcium undecylenate 10.0%
Talc base

CRUSADER
Industrial skin cleanser
(Calgon Corp., Commercial Div.)

Vegetable scrubbers
Soap
Emollients
Detergent salts *†

†*See* Detergents (synthetic)

CRUST BUSTER
Lime and scale remover
(Conklin Co.)

Hydrochloric acid *

CRYOLITE
Insecticide
(FMC Corp., Agricultural Chem. Div.)

Sodium fluoaluminate ...... 90.00%/wt.

CRYSTAL ALGAECIDE
Swimming pool algaecide
(Malter International)

Methyldodecylbenzyl trimethyl
  ammonium chloride * 4.0%
Methyldodecylxylylene bis (trimethyl ammonium chloride) 1.0%
Water 95.0%

CRYSTAL CLEAR GLASS CLEANER
(Paul Koss)

Water .... >70%
Isopropyl alcohol * .... <30%
Sodium lauryl sulfate .... trace
Dye .... trace

pH 6.3-6.7

CRYSTALITE
(Texaco Inc.; Texaco Canada Ltd.)

Water-white Kerosine *

CRYSTALLITE
Anti-bacterial glass cleaner
(Puritan Chem. Co.)

Active ingredients: 23.05%
  Isopropanol *
  4′,5-Dibromosalicylanilide *
  3,4′,5-Tribromosalicylanilide *
Inert ingredients: 76.95%
  Synthetic organic detergents
  Cleaning solvents *†
  Corrosion inhibitors

†*See* Aromatic hydrocarbon solvent

CRYSTALTONE GLAZES
See DUNCAN CERAMICS CRYS-
TALTONE GLAZES (20000 Series)

CRYSTAL WHITE LIQUID
(Colgate-Palmolive)

Alkyl aryl sulfonate * ..... approx. 10%
Organic foam builders
Sodium sulfate
Ethyl alcohol .... <3%
Ethoxylated alcohol sulfate approx. 10%

                                '76 Ed.

CRYSTODIGIN
Congestive heart failure
(Lilly, Eli)

Each tablet:
  Digitoxin * .... 0.05 mg.; 0.15 mg.;
           0.1 mg.; or 0.2 mg.

C S P CLEANER
(Hillyard Chem.)

Phosphoric acid *

                                '76 Ed.

C & S POWDER
See PURINA C & S POWDER

CTC
See MFA CTC

C3 COLD COUGH CAPSULES
(MenJ Labs.)

Each capsule:
  Chlorpheniramine maleate .. 4.0 mg.
  Phenylpropanolamine HCl * 50.0 mg.
  Dextromethorphan
    hydrobromide .... 30.0 mg.

C-20 LAUNDRY POWDER
See MT. HOOD C-20 LAUNDRY
POWDER

CULLIGAN STANDARD SOAP SOLUTION
(Culligan)

Isopropyl alcohol * 57.0%
Potassium oleate 20.0%
Potassium hydroxide * 2.0%
Methyl salicylate .... <0.1%
Water 21.0%

CUNIPHEN
Industrial bactericide
(Ventron)

Solubilized Dihydroxydichlorodiphenylmethane (Dichlorophene or
  G-4) * 20%

Starred ingredients (*) may be responsible for major toxic effects; consult Section II.

CUPRACIDE
Water repellent preservative
(Honolulu Wood Treating Co.)

Copper-8-quinolinolate 0.35%
Petroleum hydrocarbons * 89.40%

CUPREX
Pediculicide
(Beecham Products)

Tetralin *
Copper oleate *
Combined amount: 69%
　Liquid paraffin
　Acetone *

CUPRINOL CLEAR WOOD PRESERVATIVE NO. 20
(Darworth)

Zinc naphthenate (equiv. to metallic
　zinc 2%) 24%
Mineral spirits * 70%

'76 Ed.

CUPRINOL GREEN WOOD PRESERVATIVE NO. 10
(Darworth)

Copper naphthenate (equiv. to metallic
　copper 2%) 24%
Mineral spirits * 59%

'76 Ed.

CUPRINOL STAIN & WOOD PRESERVATIVES (Nos. 25, 30, 35, 45, 50, 55, 65, 75, 80, and 90)
(Darworth)

Bis(tri-n-butyltin) oxide 0.3%
Mineral spirits * 55-70%

'76 Ed.

CURE-IT 6-18 CREME HARDENER, FILLERITE

See FILLERITE CURE-IT 6-18 CREME HARDENER

CURE-IT 4-20 POWDER HARDENER, FILLERITE

See FILLERITE CURE-IT 4-20 POWDER HARDENER

CURL FREE HAIR PRODUCTS
(Gillette Co., Personal Care Div.)

The Gillette Co., Personal Care Div., Boston, Mass. 02199 will receive collect phone calls from poison control centers or physicians asking for emergency toxicological information about the company's products.

Phone: 617-421-7000

CURRAN PERFUMED MOTH CRYSTALS
(Curran)

Paradichlorobenzene *

'76 Ed.

CURRAN TOILET BOWL DEODORANT
(Curran)

Paradichlorobenzene *

'76 Ed.

CUSHION
Plastic adhesive for dentures
(Lambda Inc.)

Vinyl acetate resin (AYAT)
Vinyl acetate resin (AYAF)
Alcohol
Triethyl citrate
Parachlorometaxylenol

CUSHION GRIP (Thermoplastic)
Denture adhesive
(Plough)

Polyvinyl acetate .... approx. 75%
Denatured alcohol (SD38B) approx. 25%

CUTAR
Bath oil emulsion
(Summers Labs.)

Coal tar solution * 7 1/2%

CUTICURA ACNE CREAM
(Cuticura)

Ucon 50 HB-400
Allantoin
Albagel premium
Diisopropyl adipate
Adol 158
Silicone fluid
Polyoxy 40 stearate (USP)
Titanium dioxide
Iron oxides
2-Phenoxyethanol
Benzoyl peroxide
Alcohol
Perfume

CUTICURA OINTMENT
(Cuticura)

Liquid petrolatum, Protol
Yellow petrolatum, NF
Paraffin wax
Yellow beeswax, synthetic
Isopropyl palmitate
Precipitated Sulphur USP
Oxyquinoline *
Pine oil
Phenol USP *
Rose geranium

CUTICURA SHAMPOO
(Cuticura)

Duponol WA paste
Sodium stearate
Methyl paraben (USP)
Alrosol B
Lanogel 41
Silicone
Salicylic acid (USP) *
Perfume *
Sulfur
Protein
Sodium ethylene diamine tetraacetate

CUTRINE-PLUS
Algaecide for lakes and trout ponds
(Applied Biochemists)

Copper as elemental (from mixed
　copper ethanolamine complexes) * 9.0%

CYALUME LIGHTSTICK
Lightstick - emergency light/marker
(American Cyanamid)

Colored liquid in polyethylene tube (7.5 ml.):
　Dibutyl phthalate .... about 91%
　Aromatic oxalic ester ..... about 8%
　Aromatic hydrocarbon .... about 0.1%
Colorless liquid in glass capsule (2.5 ml.):
　Dimethyl phthalate .... about 82%
　t-Butyl alcohol .... about 14%
　Hydrogen peroxide .... about 4%

CYANIDE SORE OINTMENT
(Wambaugh)

Picric acid * .... <1%
Lanolin base

'76 Ed.

CY-AN-IN
Plating solution
(Indium Corp. of Amer.)

Potassium cyanide *
Potassium hydroxide

CY-BAN
Insecticide
(Farnam Co.)

Dimethyl phosphate of alpha-methylbenzyl-3-hydroxy-cis-
　crotonate * 14.40%
Petroleum hydrocarbons 72.85%

'76 Ed.

CYDONOL MASSAGE LOTION
(Gordon Labs.)

Isopropyl alcohol * 60%/v
Methyl salicylate *
Benzalkonium chloride *

Starred ingredients (*) may be responsible for major toxic effects; consult Section II.

CYGON 2-E SYSTEMIC INSECTICIDE
(Amer. Cyanamid, Agric. Div.)

O,O-Dimethyl-S-(N-methylcar-
bamoylmethyl)
phosphorodithioate * 23.4%/w

CYGON SC-9 SYSTEMIC INSECTICIDE
(Amer. Cyanamid, Agric. Div.)

O,O-Dimethyl-S-(N-
methylcarbamoylmethyl)-
phosphorodithioate * 95.0%/w

CYGON SYSTEMIC 25
(Amer. Cyanamid, Agric. Div.)

O,O-Dimethyl-S-(N-
methylcarbamoylmethyl)-
phosphorodithioate * 25.0%/w

CYGON 400 SYSTEMIC INSECTICIDE
(Amer. Cyanamid, Agric. Div.)

O,O-Dimethyl-S-(N-
methylcarbamoylmethyl)-
phosphorodithioate * 43.5%/w

CYLERT TABLETS
*CNS stimulant for childhood hyperki-
nesis*
(Abbott)

Pemoline *
Tablets .... 18.75 mg., 37.5 mg.
                              and 75 mg.
Chewable tablets .... 37.5 mg.

CYPREX 65-W FRUIT FUNGICIDE
(Amer. Cyanamid, Agric. Div.)

n-Dodecylguanidine acetate * . 65.0%/w

CYSTEX TABLETS
*Analgesic for kidney and bladder irri-
tations*
(CooperVision Pharm.)

Methenamine .... 162 mg.
Sodium salicylate * .... 97 mg.
Salicylamide .... 65 mg.
Benzoic acid .... 32 mg.

CYSTISED, IMPROVED
(Jenkins Labs.)

Each tablet:
Methenamine * .... 40.8 mg.
Salol * .... 18.1 mg.
Methylene blue .... 5.4 mg.
Benzoic acid .... 4.5 mg.
Hyoscyamine .... 0.03 mg.
Atropine sulfate .... 0.03 mg.
Gelsemium * .... 6.1 mg.

CYSTISED, REGULAR
(Jenkins Labs)

Each tablet:
Methenamine * .... 2 gr.
Salol * .... 1/2 gr.
Methylene blue .... 1/10 gr.
Benzoic acid .... 1/8 gr.
Hyoscyamine alkaloid ..... 1/2000 gr.
Atropine sulfate .... 1/1000 gr.

CYSTOLITHIA
Urinary antiseptic, demulcent
(Whorton)

Each fl. oz.: .... 40 gr.
Methenamine *
Eupatorium
Stigmata Maydis
Triticum
Saw Palmetto aa.
Alcohol 12%/v

'76 Ed.

CYTHION "THE PREMIUM GRADE MALATHION"
Insecticide
(Amer. Cyanamid, Agric. Div.)

O,O-Dimethyl phosphorodithioate of diethyl mercapto-
succinate * 91.0%/w

CYTOBIN
*Treatment of hypothyroid activity in
dogs*
(Norden Labs.)

Each tablet:
L-Triiodothyronine (as
the sodium salt) * ... 60 or 120 mcg.

CYTROL AMITROLE-T LIQUID WEED KILLER
Herbicide
(Amer. Cyanamid, Agric. Div.)

3-Amino-1,2,4-triazole 21.1%/w
Ammonium thiocyanate * 19.1%/w
Hydrochloric acid (HCl) * 9.8%/w

C-Z AIR-DIS
Deodorant, sanitizer
(C-Z Chemical)

Isopropyl alcohol * 12%
Triethylene glycol
Propylene glycol 12%
Para di-isobutyl phenoxy ethoxy ethyl di-
methyl benzyl ammonium chloride *
Dichlorodifluoromethane (Freon 12)
Trichloromonofluoromethane (Freon 11)
Petroleum distillate *

'76 Ed.

C-Z ASPHALT TILE WAX
(C-Z Chemical)

Carnauba wax

'76 Ed.

C-Z BOILER COMPOUND
(C-Z Chemical)

Sodium hydroxide * 60%

'76 Ed.

C-Z 25 CONCENTRATED GERMICIDE
(C-Z Chemical)

Alkyl dimethyl benzyl ammonium
chlorides * 10%

'76 Ed.

C-Z DEODORANT BLOCS & CRYSTALS
(C-Z Chemical)

Paradichlorobenzene * 90%

'76 Ed.

C-Z DRAIN PIPE OPENER
(C-Z Chemical)

Sodium hydroxide * 75%

'76 Ed.

C-Z EKONO CLEANER
(C-Z Chemical)

Vegetable oils

'76 Ed.

C-Z KLENKLOR
Bactericide, germicide
(C-Z Chemical)

Sodium hypochlorite * . 3.25%
Sodium phosphate * ... approx. 92.25%

'76 Ed.

C-Z LIGHT SPIRIT WAX
(C-Z Chemical)

Carnauba wax

'76 Ed.

C-Z LINDANE
Insecticide
(C-Z Chemical)

Gamma isomer of benzene hexachloride (from lindane) * 99%
Other isomers of benzene hexachloride 1%

'76 Ed.

C-Z MARVEL-BAC CONCENTRATED GERMICIDE
(C-Z Chemical)

Methyl dodecyl benzyl trimethyl ammonium chloride * 11%

'76 Ed.

Starred ingredients (*) may be responsible for major toxic effects; consult Section II.

C-Z NO GERM DISINFECTANT
(C-Z Chemical)

Soap
Isopropyl alcohol 10%
Chloro-o-phenyl phenol * 30.475%

'76 Ed.

C-Z NU-GLO
Scrub soap
(C-Z Chemical)

Coconut and vegetable oil soaps

'76 Ed.

CZO LOTION
Astringent, emollient, antipruritic
(Elder)

Each fl. oz.:
Calamine .... 30 gr.
Zinc oxide .... 30 gr.

C-Z PENA GYM SEALER HEAVY DUTY
(C-Z Chemical)

Tung oil
Bakelite resins

'76 Ed.

C-Z PENASEAL
(C-Z Chemical)

Tung oil
Bakelite resins

'76 Ed.

C-Z PINALENE DISINFECTANT
(C-Z Chemical)

Pine oil * 73%
Soap
Isopropyl alcohol 7%

'76 Ed.

C-Z RAT & MOUSE KILLER
(C-Z Chemical)

Warfarin (3-(a-Acetonylbenzyl)-4-
hydroxycoumarin) 0.025%

'76 Ed.

C-Z SEALA-FLOR
Concrete floor sealer
(C-Z Chemical)

Tung oil
Bakelite resin

'76 Ed.

C-Z SELF POLISHING FLOOR WAX
(C-Z Chemical)

Carnauba wax 7%

'76 Ed.

C-Z SEPTIC CAUSTIC CRYSTALS
Toilet treatment
(C-Z Chemical)

Sodium hydroxide * 75%

'76 Ed.

C-Z SUPER WAX HEAVY DUTY
(C-Z Chemical)

Carnauba wax

'76 Ed.

C-Z TOILET BOWL CLEANER
(C-Z Chemical)

Bisulfate of soda * 80%

'76 Ed.

C-Z VELVEEN
Liquid toilet soap
(C-Z Chemical)

Cochine coconut oil
Vegetable oils

'76 Ed.

C-Z WATERLESS HAND CLEANER
(C-Z Chemical)

Hexachlorophene
Lanolin

'76 Ed.

C-Z WHIFF WITH CHLOROPHYLL & X-ON
Toilet bowl cleaner
(C-Z Chemical)

Hydrogen chloride * 13.96%
Formaldehyde 1.00%

'76 Ed.

C-Z 3X SERVICE CLEANER
Toilet cleaner
(C-Z Chemical)

Hydrochloric acid * 85%

'76 Ed.

C-Z ZIP MECHANIC'S BORATED HAND SOAP
(C-Z Chemical)

Lanolin
Borax 7.5%

'76 Ed.

D

DACAMINE
Herbicide
(Diamond Shamrock Corp.)

N-Oleyl-1,3-propylenediamine salt
of 2,4-Dichlorophenoxyacetic
acid * 21.9%
2,4-Dichlorophenoxyacetic acid * . 11.1%

DACAMINE 4D
Herbicide
(Diamond Shamrock Corp.)

N-Oleyl-1,3-propylenediamine salt
of 2,4-Dichlorophenoxyacetic
acid * 31.6%
2,4-Dichlorophenoxyacetic acid * . 25.4%

DACID ACID CLEANER
Dairy use
(Yale Chem. Co.)

Phosphoric acid * .... >30%
Hydroxyacetic acid .... <15%

DACONATE 6 TURF HERBICIDE
(Diamond Shamrock Corp.)

Monosodium acid methanearsonate * 48.35%

DACONIL 2787
Fungicide; wettable powder
(Diamond Shamrock Corp.)

Chlorothalonil
(Tetrachloroisophthalonitrile) ... 75%

DACONIL 2787 FLOWABLE (6F)
Fungicide
(Diamond Shamrock Corp.)

Chlorothalonil 54%

DACONIL 2787 FLOWABLE FUNGICIDE TURF CARE (500F)
(Diamond Shamrock Corp.)

Chlorothalonil
(Tetrachloroisophthalonitrile) .. 40.4%

DACRIOSE
Ophthalmic irrigating solution
(CooperVision Pharm.)

Boric acid *
Potassium chloride
Sodium carbonate
Benzalkonium chloride 0.01%
Disodium edetate 0.01%

DACTHAL FLOWABLE TURF HERBICIDE
Preemergence herbicide
(Diamond Shamrock Corp.)

Dimethyl
tetrachloroterephthalate * 54.7%

DACTHAL G-2.5
Preemergence herbicide
(Diamond Shamrock Corp.)

Dimethyl tetrachloroterephthalate   2.5%

DACTHAL G-5
Herbicide
(Diamond Shamrock Corp.)

Dimethyl tetrachloroterephthalate .. 5%

DACTHAL W-75 & DACTHAL W-75 FOR TURF
Herbicides
(Diamond Shamrock Corp.)

Dimethyl tetrachloroterephthalate * 75%

DAIRY-DU SPRAY
Insecticide
(An-Fo)

Pyrethrins 0.06%
Piperonyl butoxide (technical) .. 0.12%
N-Octyl bicycloheptene dicar-
boximide 0.20%
Di-n-propyl isocinchomeronate .. 0.40%
Petroleum distillate * 99.22%

DALAPON 85
Herbicide
(Diamond Shamrock Corp.)

2,2-Dichloropropionic acid, sodium
salt of Dalapon * 85%

DAL-E-RAD 120
Herbicide
(Vineland Chem.)

Monosodium acid methanearsonate * 51.19%

DALEX SYRUP
Antitussive, expectorant, decongestant, antihistaminic
(Dalin)

Each fl. oz.:
  Dextromethorphan
    hydrobromide * .... 45 mg.
  Phenylephrine
    hydrochloride * .... 15 mg.
  Chlorpheniramine maleate ...   6 mg.
  Glyceryl guaiacolate .... 180 mg.
  Ammonium chloride .... 600 mg.
  Buffered with Sodium citrate, Citric acid
                                      '76 Ed.

D-ALGAE
Depresses algae growth in swimming pools
(National Chemsearch)

Alkyl (60% C14, 25% C12, 15% C16)
  dimethyl   benzyl   ammonium
  chlorides * 5.0%

DALICOTE
Antipruritic, antiseptic for relief of non-specific dermatoses
(Dalin)

Hexachlorophene
Pyrilamine maleate *
Tetracaine hydrochloride
Tyrothricin
Dimethyl polysiloxane
Zinc oxide
Camphor
                                      '76 Ed.

DALICOTE VETERINARY
Antipruritic, antiseptic for relief of non-specific dermatoses
(Dalin)

Hexachlorophene
Pyrilamine maleate *
Tetracaine hydrochloride
Tyrothricin
Dimethyl polysiloxane
Zinc oxide
Camphor
                                      '76 Ed.

DALICREME
Medicated, healing skin cream
(Dalin)

Vitamin A (fish liver
  oil) .... 700 USP units/gm.
Vitamin D (irradiated
  ergosterol) .... 70 USP units/gm.
Benzocaine 0.1%
Di-isobutyl cresoxy ethoxy ethyl dimethyl
  benzyl ammonium chloride *
                                      '76 Ed.

DALIDERM
For relief from superficial fungus infections of the skin
(Dalin)

Di-isobutyl cresoxy ethoxy ethyl dimethyl
  benzyl ammonium chloride *
Carbolic acid *
Benzoic acid *
Salicylic acid *
Resorcin *
Camphor *
Tannic acid *
Solution of Coal tar *, Chlorthymol *
Ethyl alcohol 66%
                                      '76 Ed.

DALIDERM POWDER
For relief of itching, burning feet and athlete's foot
(Dalin)

Zinc undecylenate *
Sodium propionate
Di-isobutyl cresoxy ethoxy ethyl dimethyl
  benzyl ammonium chloride *
Salicylic acid *
Boric acid *
Aluminum acetate
Exsiccated Alum
Aromatized oils
                                      '76 Ed.

DALIDERM, VETERINARY
For treatment of nonspecific dermatoses in small and large animals
(Dalin)

Ethyl alcohol 66%
Quaternary ammonium compound *
Tannic acid *
Salicylic acid *
Resorcin *
Camphor *
Chlorothymol *
                                      '76 Ed.

DALIDOME POWDER PACKETS
For wet-dressings
(Dome)

Zinc sulfate *
Copper sulfate *
Camphor *

DALIDYNE
For treatment of herpes simplex, cancrum, stomatitis
(Dalin)

Ethyl alcohol 61%
Benzyl alcohol *
Quaternary ammonium compound *
Benzocaine
Tannic acid *
Analgesics *†
                                      '76 Ed.

†*See* Salicylic acid

DALIFORT TABLETS
Vitamin deficiency treatment
(Dalin)

Each tablet:
Vitamin A .... 25,000 USP units
Vitamin D .... 1,000 USP units
Iron (as ferrous gluconate) ... 15 mg.
Polyvitamins & minerals

'76 Ed.

DALIGESIC
Analgesic balm
(Dalin)

Camphor *
Eucalyptol *
Menthol USP *
Methyl salicylate *
Oleoresin capsicum
Glyceryl mono oleate
Diglycol laurate S
Diglycol stearate

'76 Ed.

DALIHIST AQUEOUS NASAL SPRAY
Decongestant, antihistaminic, antibiotic
(Dalin)

Phenylephrine HCl * 0.5%
Pyrilamine maleate * 0.15%
Tyrothricin 0.02%
Cetyl benzyl dimethyl ammonium
  chloride 0.04%
In aqueous isotonic solution

'76 Ed.

DALIHIST PEDIATRIC
Decongestant, antihistaminic, antibiotic
(Dalin)

Phenylephrine HCl * 0.25%
Pyrilamine maleate 0.075%
Tyrothricin 0.01%
Cetyl benzyl dimethyl ammonium
  chloride 0.02%
In aqueous isotonic solution

'76 Ed.

DALISEPT
For relief of burns, sunburn, diaper rash
(Dalin)

Vitamin A (fish liver oil)
Vitamin D (irradiated ergosterol)
Tyrothricin 0.02%
Diperodon HCl 5%

'76 Ed.

DALMANE
For relief of insomnia
(Roche)

Each capsule:
Flurazepam
  hydrochloride * .. 15 mg.; or 30 mg.

DAM-TITE
Maintenance material
(Speco)

Silicone compound
In Aromatic solvent *

'76 Ed.

DANA COSMETIC PRODUCTS
Perfumes, cosmetics and toiletries

Dana Perfumes Corp.
609 Fifth Ave.
New York, N.Y. 10017

Phone: 212-751-3700

See COSMETICS, Section VI, General Formulations

DANDRICIDE RINSE
(King Research)

Water
Isopropyl alcohol *
Benzalkonium chloride
Lauryl isoquinolinium bromide *
Polysorbate 20
Fragrance
Sorbitol
Certified colors

DANDRICIDE SHAMPOO
(King Research)

Water
Cocamide DEA
TEA lauryl sulfate
Lauramide DEA
Hexylene glycol
Sodium laureth sulfate
Sodium chloride
Hydrolysed animal protein
Disodium monoundecylenamido MEA-
  sulfosuccinate
Citric acid
Imidazolidinyl urea
Methylparaben
FD & C Yellow No. 5
D & C Red No. 19
Fragrance

DANEX SHAMPOO
(Herbert Labs.)

Zinc pyrithione 1%

DANIELS, DR., PRODUCTS
See DR. DANIELS

DANILAX
See DR. DANIELS' DANILAX

DANIVOM TABLETS
See DR. DANIELS' DANIVOM TABLETS

DANTAFUR
Systemic antibacterial agent; veterinary
(Norden Labs.)

Nitrofurantoin * .... 15 mg./ml.
Alcohol 10%
Special suspending medium

DAP ACRYLIC LATEX CAULK
(DAP)

Calcium carbonate
Titanium dioxide
Plasticized Acrylic polymer emulsion
Sodium benzoate 0.02%
Benzoic acid ester
Ethylene glycol 1%

DAP ACRYLIC LATEX CAULK WITH SILICONE
(DAP)

Calcium carbonate
Titanium dioxide
Water
Ethylene glycol 1%
Acrylic latex emulsion
Benzoic acid ester
Organosilane ester

DAP ALUMINUM REPAIR
(DAP)

Ketone * .... <15%
Toluene * .... <10%
Phthalate ester
Vinyl resin
Iron oxide
Silica
Aluminum
Titanium dioxide

DAP ARCHITECTURAL GRADE CAULK (Gun Grade)
(DAP)

Calcium carbonate
Magnesium silicate
Titanium dioxide
Polymerized Vegetable oil
Polybutene
Mineral spirits .... <5%
Cobalt drier (0.005% as metal)

DAP BLACK TITE
(DAP)

Calcium carbonate
Magnesium silicate
Special blown Asphalt
Mineral spirits * .... <20%

DAP BUTYL-FLEX
(DAP)

Calcium carbonate
Magnesium silicate
Titanium dioxide
Butyl rubber solution polymer in
  Mineral spirits * .... <40%

Starred ingredients (*) may be responsible for major toxic effects; consult Section II.

DAP BUTYL GUTTER & LAP SEALER
(DAP)

Calcium carbonate
Magnesium silicate
Titanium dioxide
Butyl rubber solution polymer in
   Mineral spirits * .... <30%

DAP CONTACT CEMENT
(DAP)

Toluene * .... <10%
Methyl ethyl ketone * .... <25%
Petroleum distillate * .... <50%
Chlorinated hydrocarbon polymer
Magnesium oxide
Zinc oxide
Phenolic resin

DAP DRIVEWAY CRACK SEALANT
(DAP)

Calcium carbonate
Magnesium silicate
Mineral spirits * .... <20.0%
Asphalt
Ethylene glycol .... <0.2%

DAP EXTERIOR SPACKLING COMPOUND
(DAP)

Calcium carbonate
Plasticized Polyvinyl acetate emulsion
Water
Mineral spirits .... <2%
Fatty acid amine soap

DAP FAST-SET EPOXY GLUE
(DAP)

Part A:
  Polyamide resin
  Surfactant
Part B:
  Epoxy resin
  Silica

DAP FLEXISEAL SEALANT
(DAP)

Dioctylphthalate .... <3%
Paraffinic oil 5%
Silica
Toluene * .... <35%
Synthetic rubber
Hydrocarbon resin

DAP FOAMBOARD & PANEL ADHESIVE
(DAP)

Hydrocarbon resin
Synthetic rubber
Magnesium silicate
Aliphatic hydrocarbon solvent * ... 40%
Rosin ester resin
Carbon black

DAP FURNITURE REFINISHER
(DAP)

Acetone .... <40%
Toluene * .... <20%
Isopropanol .... <40%
VM&P Naphtha .... <6%

DAP GENERAL PURPOSE CEMENT
(DAP)

Phthalate esters
Butyl acetate .... <10%
Ketone * .... <25%
Isopropyl alcohol .... <10%
Nitrocellulose
Castor oil .... <10%

DAP HEAVY DUTY WALL COVERING ADHESIVE
(DAP)

Water
Acrylic resin
Polyvinyl acetate emulsion
Hydrous Aluminum silicates
Sodium hydroxide * .... <0.25%
Alkyl aryl polyether alcohol .... <0.35%

DAP KWIK-SEAL
(DAP)

Calcium carbonate
Titanium dioxide
Plasticized Polyvinyl acetate emulsion
Ethylene glycol .... <2%
Butyl acetate .... <1%

DAP LATEX CONCRETE SEALANT
(DAP)

Calcium carbonate
Ethylene glycol .... <2%
Benzoic acid ester
Polyvinyl acetate polymer emulsion

DAP LATEX CONSTRUCTION AND SUBFLOOR ADHESIVE
(DAP)

Calcium carbonate
Vinyl acetate emulsion
Phthalate ester

DAP LATEX GLAZING COMPOUND
(DAP)

Acrylic emulsion
Calcium carbonate
Benzoic acid ester
Fatty acid amine soap
Nonyl phenoxy ethanol .... <1%
Aluminum silicate
Ethylene glycol 2%

DAP LATEX PANEL AND DRYWALL ADHESIVE
(DAP)

Vinyl acetate emulsion
Calcium carbonate
Dipropylene glycol dibenzoate
Glycol ether .... <2%
Ethylene glycol .... <1%

DAP PACER LATEX CAULK
(DAP)

Vinyl acetate-acrylic emulsion
Polybutene
Water
Ethylene glycol .... <1%
Mineral spirits .... <3%
Calcium carbonate
Benzoic acid ester

DAP PACER PANEL AND DRYWALL ADHESIVE
(DAP)

Hydrocarbon resin
Rosin ester resin
Synthetic rubber
Hexane * 40%
Magnesium silicate
Carbon black

DAP PAINTER'S CAULK
(DAP)

Calcium carbonate
Magnesium silicate
Titanium dioxide
Bodied Vegetable oils
Calcium resinate solution
Mineral spirits .... <6%

DAP PAINTERS LATEX CAULK
(DAP)

Calcium carbonate
Ethylene glycol .... <0.5%
Mineral spirits .... <3.0%
Water
Vinyl acetate-acrylic emulsion
Polybutene
Benzoic acid ester

DAP PAINTER'S PUTTY
(DAP)

Calcium carbonate
Titanium dioxide
Pure Linseed oil

DAP PANEL & DRY WALL ADHESIVE
(DAP)

Magnesium silicate
Synthetic rubber
Hydrocarbon resin
Aliphatic hydrocarbon solvent * ... 40%
Rosin ester resin
Carbon black

Starred ingredients (*) may be responsible for major toxic effects; consult Section II.

DAP PANEL NU (AEROSOL)
(DAP)

Water
Propane-isobutane 15%
Mineral oil * .... <40%
Linseed oil
Perfume

DAP PORCELAIN TOUCH-UP
(DAP)

Titanium dioxide
Polyacrylate
Cellosolve acetate * .... <15%
N-Butyl alcohol * .... <1%
Toluene * 30%

DAP PURE LINSEED OIL PUTTY
(DAP)

Calcium carbonate
Pure Linseed oil

DAP RELY-ON
(DAP)

Calcium carbonate
Magnesium silicate
Titanium dioxide
Bodied Vegetable oils
Calcium resinate solution
Mineral spirits .... <6%

DAP RELY-ON LATEX CAULK
(DAP)

Calcium carbonate
Water
Polyvinyl acetate emulsion
Vinyl acrylic emulsion
Mineral oil 3%
Ethylene glycol .... <1%
Texanol ester alcohol
Benzoic acid ester

DAP RUBBER REPAIR (BLACK)
(DAP)

Lactol spirits * .... <25%
Toluene * .... <15%
Xylene * .... <5%
Acetone * .... <5%
Resin
Rubber
Pigment
Carbon black

DAP SPACKLING COMPOUND (INTERIOR)
(DAP)

Calcium carbonate
Plasticized Polyvinyl
Acetate resin emulsion in water

DAP STEEL REPAIR
(DAP)

Ketone * .... <15%
Toluene * .... <10%
Phthalate ester
Vinyl polymer
Silica
Aluminum
Iron oxide

DAP SURFACE DEGLOSSER
(DAP)

Mineral spirits * .... <65%
Butyl Cellosolve * .... <2%
Isopropyl alcohol * .... <10%
Toluene * .... <15%
Acetone * .... <15%
N-Butyl acetate * 1%

DAP TABLETS
*Symptoms of congestive heart failure;
veterinary*
(Hart-Delta, Inc.)

Each tablet:
  Digitoxin * .... 0.5 mg.
  Aminophylline * .... 100.0 mg.
  Potassium chloride .... 25.0 mg.
                                  '76 Ed.

DAP "1012" GLAZING COMPOUND
(DAP)

Calcium carbonate
Carbon black
Magnesium silicate
Vegetable oil
Mineral spirits .... <5%

DAP "33" GLAZING COMPOUND
(DAP)

Calcium carbonate
Magnesium silicate
Titanium dioxide
Mineral oil
Linseed oil
Soybean oil
Mineral spirits .... <1%

DAP TOPS ROOF COATING
(DAP)

Mineral spirits * 35%
Asphalt
Magnesium silicate
Aluminum
Silica gel
Vegetable oil alkyd resin
Phospholipid
Cellulosic fiber

DAP TUNG OIL VARNISH
(DAP)

Modified Tung-oil resin
Mineral spirits * .... <70%

DAP WATERLESS HAND CLEANER
(DAP)

Deodorized Kerosene blend * .... >20%
Mixed Amine oleate soaps
Water
Perfume
Lanolin
Pure food colors
Preservative 0.1%

DAP WATER WASHABLE BRUSH CLEANER
(DAP)

Methylene chloride * .... <15%
Isopropyl alcohol * .... <30%
Toluene * .... <20%
Acetone * .... <30%
VM&P Naphtha .... <10%
Surfactant

DAP WEATHERSTRIP CAULK
(DAP)

Calcium carbonate
Magnesium silicate
Hydrated Aluminum silicate
Polyisobutylene

DARA BATH LUXURIANT
Foaming bath additive
(Owen Labs.)

Cocoamide DEA
Fragrance
Purified water

DARAGEN
Hair repair shampoo
(Owen Labs.)

Collagen polypeptides
Amphoteric base

DARA SOAPLESS SHAMPOO
(Owen Labs.)

Mixture of Fatty acid amides of protein
  hydrolysates

DARBAZINE CAPSULES
*Anticholinergic, tranquilizer, anti-
  emetic - dogs and cats*
(Norden Labs.)

NO. 1 (each capsule):
  Prochlorperazine (as the mal-
    eate) (sustained release
    form) * .... 3.33 mg.
  Isopropamide (as the io-
    dide) * .... 1.67 mg.

NO. 3 (each capsule):
  Prochlorperazine (as the mal-
    eate) (sustained release
    form) * .... 10 mg.
  Isopropamide (as the io-
    dide) * .... 5 mg.

DARI-BEEF CATTLE DUST

See DR. ROGERS' DARI-BEEF CAT-TLE DUST

DARI DIP

See WASCO DARI DIP

DARK & LOVELY HAIR RELAXER - RELAXER CREAM - 420B
(Carson Products)

Water
Mineral oil
Ceteth-20
Propylene glycol
PEG-75 lanolin oil
Cetyl alcohol
DEA lauryl sulfate, Sodium laurylamino-propionate, DEA laurylaminopropion-ate
Methylparaben
Propylparaben
Calcium hydroxide

DARK & LOVELY PERMANENT HAIR COLOR
Jet Black, Black, Dark Brown, Auburn, Bright Auburn
(Carson Products)

Oxidation type dyes (example: Paraphen-ylenediamine)
Base:
Oleic acid
Ammonia

6% Peroxide developer

DARK & LOVELY PROTEIN CONDITIONER #402
(Carson Products)

Water
Glyceryl stearate
Steartrimonium hydrolyzed animal pro-tein
Cetyl lactate
Quaternium 26
Quaternium 22
Myristyl myristate
Minkamidopropyl dimethylamine
Hydroxyethylcellulose
Cetyl alcohol
Olive oil
Castor oil
Lactic acid
Quaternium 15
Corn oil, Propylene glycol, Glyceryl oleate, BHA, BHT, Propyl gallate, Citric acid
Fragrance

DARK & LOVELY PROTEIN HAIR DRESS/CONDITIONER #403
(Carson Products)

Petrolatum
Mineral oil
Lanolin
Isopropyl myristate
Trihydroxystearin
Isostearic hydrolysed animal protein
Castor oil
Olive oil
Propylene glycol
Dimethicone
Imidazolidinyl urea
Methylparaben
Propylparaben
Corn oil, Glyceryl oleate, BHA, BHT, Pro-pyl gallate, Citric acid
Fragrance

DARK & LOVELY PROTEIN SETTING LOTION #404
(Carson Products)

Water
PEG-75 lanolin oil
Quaternium-26
Hydrolyzed animal protein
Quaternium-19
Imidazolidinyl urea
Methylparaben
Propylparaben
Nonoxynol-10
Fragrance

DARK & LOVELY PROTEIN SHAMPOO #401
(Carson Products)

Water
Ammonium lauryl sulfate
Hydrolyzed animal protein
Disodium monostearamido mea-sulfosuc-cinate
Cocamidopropylamine oxide
Quaternium-23
PEG-75 lanolin
Citric acid
Quaternium-15
Ammonium chloride
Fragrance

DARPAC
Systemic analgesic
(Approved Pharm.)

Each capsule:
Acetaminophen . . . . 65 mg.
Aspirin * . . . . 227 mg.
Phenacetin * . . . . 162 mg.
Caffeine (anhydrous) . . . . 32.4 mg.

'76 Ed.

DARVOCET-N
Analgesic
(Lilly, Eli)

Each tablet:
Acetaminophen * . . . . 325 mg.
Propoxyphene napsylate * . . . 50 mg.

DARVON
Analgesic
(Lilly, Eli)

Each Pulvule:
Propoxyphene
hydrochloride * . . . . . 32 mg.; 65 mg.

DARVON COMPOUND-65
Analgesic
(Lilly, Eli)

Each Pulvule:
Propoxyphene
hydrochloride * . . . . 65 mg.
Acetylsalicylic acid * . . . . 227 mg.
Acetophenetidin * . . . . 162 mg.
Caffeine . . . . 32.4 mg.

DARVON-N (Tablets and Suspension)
Analgesic
(Lilly, Eli)

Tablets (each):
Propoxyphene napsylate * . . . 100 mg.

Suspension (each 5 ml.):
Propoxyphene napsylate * . . . 50 mg.

DARVON-N WITH A.S.A.
Analgesic
(Lilly, Eli)

Each tablet:
Aspirin * . . . . 325 mg.
Propoxyphene napsylate * . . . 100 mg.

DARVON WITH A.S.A.
Analgesic
(Lilly, Eli)

Each Pulvule:
Aspirin * . . . . 325 mg.
Propoxyphene hydrochloride * 65 mg.

DASH (Formula 1)
Granular laundry detergent
(Procter & Gamble)

Sodium sulfate 25-49%
Complex sodium phosphates 25-49%
Sodium silicate 5-9%
Water 5-9%
Sodium alkyl benzene sulfonate . 5-9%
Sodium alkyl sulfate 1-4%
Alkyl ethoxylate 1-4%
Sodium soap 1-4%
Minor ingredients, each . . . . trace
pH (1% solution) - 10.1

Starred ingredients (*) may be responsible for major toxic effects; consult Section II.

DASH (Formula 2)
Granular laundry detergent
(Procter & Gamble)

Sodium sulfate	50-74%
Sodium carbonate	10-24%
Sodium silicate	10-24%
Sodium alkyl benzene sulfonate	5-9%
Sodium alkyl ethoxylate sulfate	1-4%
Sodium soap	1-4%
Sodium alkyl sulfate	1-4%
Water	1-4%
Minor ingredients, each	trace

pH (1% solution) - 10.9 max.

DASIKON
Cold remedy
(Beecham Labs.)

Each capsule:
Chlorpheniramine maleate	2 mg.
Caffeine	32 mg.
Aspirin *	195 mg.
Phenacetin *	130 mg.
Atropine sulfate	0.065 mg.

DASIN
For relief of common cold symptoms
(Beecham Labs.)

Each capsule:
Atropine sulfate	0.13 mg.
Aspirin *	130 mg.
Phenacetin *	100 mg.
Caffeine	8 mg.
Ipecac	3 mg.
Camphor	15 mg.

DATRIL
Non-aspirin pain reliever
(Bristol-Myers)

Each tablet:
Acetaminophen *	325 mg.

DATRIL 500
Extra-strength non-aspirin pain reliever
(Bristol-Myers)

Each tablet:
Acetaminophen *	500 mg.

DAVEYITE
Tree wound dressing
(Davey)

Fibrated Asphalt
Petroleum distillates (as solvent) *

DAVOSIL PROPHYLAXIS PASTE
Cleans and polishes the teeth
(Hoyt Labs.)

Silicon dioxide
In a glycerin-water base

DAWN (Formula 2)
Dishwashing liquid
(Procter & Gamble)

Water	50-74%
Magnesium alkyl ethoxylate sulfate *	10-24%
Ethanol	5-9%
Magnesium alkyl sulfate	5-9%
Ammonium chloride	1-4%
Ammonium alkyl ethoxylate sulfate	1-4%
Ammonium xylene sulfonate	1-4%
Alkylamine oxide	1-4%
Minor ingredients, each	trace

pH (as is) - 7.0

DAWN (Formula 3)
Dishwashing liquid
(Procter & Gamble)

Water	50-74%
Magnesium alkyl ethoxylate sulfate *	10-24%
Ammonium alkyl ethoxylate sulfate	5-9%
Magnesium alkyl sulfate	5-9%
Ethanol	5-9%
Ammonium chloride	1-4%
Ammonium xylene sulfonate	1-4%
Alkylamine oxide	1-4%
Minor ingredients, each	trace

pH (as is) - 7.0

DAWSON 37 SPACE FUMIGANT
(Ferguson Fumigants)

Ethylene dibromide *	30.0%
Methyl bromide *	70.0%

DAWSON 73 SPOT FUMIGANT
(Ferguson Fumigants)

Ethylene dibromide *	70.0%
Methyl bromide *	30.0%

DAXOLIN C
Schizophrenia
(Dome)

Each ml.:
Loxapine hydrochloride *	25 mg.

DAXOLIN CAPSULES
For treatment of manifestations of schizophrenia
(Dome)

Loxapine succinate *   10 mg.; 25 mg.; 50 mg.

DAYALETS PLUS IRON FILMTAB
Multiple vitamin supplement with iron
(Abbott)

Each tablet:
Iron *	18 mg.
Multivitamins	

DAYBREAK CONCENTRATED AIR FRESHENER

See AMWAY DAYBREAK CONCENTRATED AIR FRESHENER

DAYCARE DAYTIME COLDS MEDICINE, CAPSULES

See VICKS DAYCARE DAYTIME COLDS MEDICINE, CAPSULES

DAYCARE DAYTIME COLDS MEDICINE, LIQUID

See VICKS DAYCARE DAYTIME COLDS MEDICINE, LIQUID

DAY-GLO PRODUCTS
Fluorescent paints

Day-Glo Color Corp.
4732 St. Clair
Cleveland, Ohio 44103

Phone: 216-391-7070

See PAINTS, Section VI, General Formulations

DAY, JAMES B., PAINT PRODUCTS
Paint and varnish removers

James B. Day & Co.
Day Lane
Carpentersville, Ill. 60110

Phone: 312-428-2651

See PAINTS, Section VI, General Formulations

DAYS EASE AIR FRESHENERS
(Gillette Co., Toiletries Div.)

The Gillette Co., Toiletries Div., Boston, Mass. 02199 will receive collect phone calls from poison control centers or physicians asking for emergency toxicological information about the company's products.

Phone: 617-421-7000

DAYS EASE PLUMBER SAVER DRAIN OPENER
(Gillette Co., Toiletries Div.)

Caustic soda (Lye) *

Starred ingredients (*) may be responsible for major toxic effects; consult Section II.

DAYS EASE TANK BOWL CLEANER
Solid crystalline cake
(Gillette Co., Toiletries Div.)

Urea	
Tergitol S-55	
Water	
Acid Blue 9	50%
Tetrasodium EDTA	40%
SAG 47 Silicone	

DAY'S LIQUID PINE CLEANER
(Pine, Morton S.)

Pine oil *	
Vegetable oil soap	
Lanolin	
	'76 Ed.

D-B DUST
Insecticide - veterinary
(Pro-Brand Products Co.)

Technical Methoxychlor	5.00%
Malathion	4.00%
Technical Piperonyl butoxide	1.00%
Pyrethrins	0.10%
	'76 Ed.

d-CON ANT-PRUFE
Non-aerosol liquid insecticide
(d-Con)

(5-Benzyl-3-furyl)methyl-2,2 dimethyl-3-(2-methylpropenyl) cyclopropane carboxylate	0.500%
Related compounds	0.068%
Aromatic petroleum hydrocarbons	0.912%
Petroleum distillate	0.500%

d-CON CONCENTRATE
Rodenticide
(d-Con)

Warfarin	0.3%

d-CON DOUBLE-POWER ROACH & ANT KILLS AND REPELS
(d-Con)

Pyrethrins	0.075%
Technical Piperonyl butoxide	0.150%
N-Octyl bicycloheptene dicarboximide	0.250%
2-Hydroxyethyl-n-octyl sulfide	0.950%
Other related compounds	0.050%
Petroleum distillate *	95.525%

d-CON FLYING INSECT KILLER
Water-based aerosol insecticide
(d-Con)

d-trans Allethrin (allyl homolog of Cinerin I)	0.20%
Technical Piperonyl butoxide	0.90%
N-Octyl bicycloheptene dicarboximide	0.50%

d-CON FOUR/GONE AUTOMATIC ROOM FOGGER
Insecticide
(d-Con)

Petroleum distillate *	11.83%
N-Octyl bicycloheptene dicarboximide	1.67%
Technical Piperonyl butoxide	1.00%
Pyrethrins	0.50%

d-CON HOUSE & GARDEN BUG KILLER
Water-based aerosol insecticide
(d-Con)

d-trans Allethrin (allyl homolog of Cinerin I)	0.25%
Technical Piperonyl butoxide	0.80%
N-Octyl bicycloheptene dicarboximide	0.40%
Petroleum distillate	8.05%

d-CON JET STREAM ANT & ROACH KILLER (Formula V)
Solvent based aerosol insecticide
(d-Con)

o-Isopropoxyphenyl methylcarbamate *	0.500%
2,2-Dichlorovinyl dimethyl phosphate	0.186%
Related compounds	0.014%
Aromatic solvent 140 *	83.030%

d-CON JET STREAM WASP & HORNET KILLER WITH SBP-1382
Oil based aerosol insecticide
(d-Con)

(5-Benzyl-3-furyl)methyl-2,2-dimethyl-3-(2-methylpropenyl) cyclopropanecarboxylate	0.250%
Other related compounds	0.034%
Aromatic petroleum hydrocarbons	0.332%
Petroleum distillate *	98.884%

d-CON MOUSE-PRUFE
Rodenticide
(d-Con)

Warfarin	0.054%

d-CON PELLETS
Rodenticide
(d-Con)

Warfarin	0.025%

d-CON PROFESSIONAL FORMULA ANT & ROACH KILLER
(d-Con)

Pyrethrins	0.30%
Technical Piperonyl butoxide	0.60%
N-Octyl bicycloheptene dicarboximide	1.00%
Petroleum distillate *	95.10%

d-CON PROFESSIONAL FORMULA FLYING INSECT KILLER
(d-Con)

Pyrethrins	0.50%
Technical Piperonyl butoxide	1.00%
N-Octyl bicycloheptene dicarboximide	1.00%
Petroleum distillate	2%

d-CON READY-MIXED
Rodenticide
(d-Con)

Warfarin	0.025%

d-CON RID-X SEPTIC TANK ADDITIVE
To promote waste decay in septic tanks and cesspools
(d-Con)

Sodium chloride	20%
Biological culture	40%
Inert biological carrier	40%

d-CON ROACH-PRUFE
Non-aerosol liquid insecticide
(d-Con)

(5-Benzyl-3-furyl)methyl-2,2 dimethyl-3-(2-methylpropenyl) cyclopropane carboxylate	0.500%
Related compounds	0.068%
Aromatic petroleum hydrocarbons	0.912%
Petroleum distillate	0.500%

d-CON STAY/AWAY OUTDOOR FOGGER
Water-based aerosol insecticide
(d-Con)

d-trans Allethrin (allyl homolog of Cinerin I)	0.10%
Technical Piperonyl butoxide	0.50%
Technical Methoxychlor	2.00%
2-Hydroxyethyl n-octyl sulfide	1.42%
Related compounds	0.08%
Petroleum distillate	6.00%

DC&R SPRAY FUMIGANT CONCENTRATE
Disinfectant
(Hess & Clark)

Tris(hydroxymethyl)nitromethane *	19.20%
Formaldehyde	2.02%
Trisodium phosphate	0.29%
Alkyl dimethyl benzyl ammonium chloride	0.29%

DDB
Disinfectant, deodorant, bactericide
(Modern Pool Products)

Calcium hypochlorite *	72.5%

Starred ingredients (*) may be responsible for major toxic effects; consult Section II.

DDC CONCENTRATE
Detergent, disinfectant, deodorant
(Consolidated Chem., Inc.)

Hydrogen chloride *
Dimethyl benzyl ammonium chloride *†

†*See* Cationic surfactants

D-D DISINFECTANT
(United Chemical Co., Inc.)

Sodium hypochlorite (equiv. to 5%
    available chlorine) * 5 1/4%

'76 Ed.

D-D SOIL FUMIGANT
(Morgro)

Active ingredients: 100.0%
    1,3-Dichloropropene *
    1,2-Dichloropropane
    3,3-Dichloropropene
    2,3-Dichloropropene
    Related C3 chlorinated hydrocarbons

DEAD END
Residual insect spray
(Lester Labs.)

Petroleum distillates
o-Isopropoxyphenyl methylcarbamate *

'76 Ed.

DEAD LINE BUG KILLER, MUNICHEM

See MUNICHEM DEAD LINE BUG
    KILLER

DEAD SURE
*Rodenticide for municipal, professional
and industrial use*
(MuniChem Corp.)

Warfarin (3-(a-Acetonylbenzyl)-4-
    hydroxycoumarin) 0.025%

'76 Ed.

DEANER
Learning and behavior problems; hyperkinesis
(Riker Labs.)

Each tablet:
    Deanol (as the para-
      acetaminobenzoic
      acid salt) (2-
      Dimethylamino-
      ethanol) * .... 25 mg.; 100 mg.

'76 Ed.

DEATH JET
Insecticide - wasps, bees, hornets, yellow jackets
(Southwest Research Products Co.)

Methylene chloride *	11.00%
Tetrachloroethylene *	32.00%
Trichloromonofluoromethane	20.00%
Pyrethrins I & II	0.05%
Hydrogenated Rotenone & other related cube resins	0.40%
Dichlorodifluoromethane	20.00%
Petroleum distillate *	13.75%
Pine oil	2.80%

'76 Ed.

DEBBIE CONCENTRATED FABRIC SOFTENER
(Industrial Equities)

Quaternary ammonium compound *	5-10%
Fluorescent whitening agent	<1%
Preservative	<1%
Colorant	<1%
Perfume	<1%
Water	balance

DEBBIE DRYER CYCLE FABRIC SOFTENER SHEETS
(Industrial Equities)

Cationic softener *	50-60%
Nonwoven rayon substrate	37-42%
Perfume	<1%

DEBBIE FABRIC SOFTENER
(Industrial Equities)

Quaternary ammonium compound *	2-5%
Preservative	<1%
Colorant	<1%
Perfume	<1%
Water	balance

DEBBIE HEAVY DUTY LAUNDRY DETERGENT (DRY)
(Industrial Equities)

Sodium chloride *	45-50%
Sodium carbonate *	30-35%
Nonionic surfactant	5-10%
Sodium silicate (not meta)	5-10%
Cellulosic	<2%
Fluorescent whitening agent	<1%
Perfume	<1%

DEBBIE HEAVY DUTY LAUNDRY DETERGENT (LIQUID)
(Industrial Equities)

Nonionic surfactant	20-30%
Anionic surfactant	5-10%
Diethanolamine	1-3%
Fluorescent whitening agent	<1%
Colorant	<1%
Perfume	<1%
Water	balance

DEBBIE LIQUID BLEACH
(Industrial Equities)

Sodium hypochlorite *	5 1/4%
Sodium chloride	<5%
Water	balance

DEBBIE LIQUID DISHWASHING DETERGENT
(Industrial Equities)

Anionic surfactant	6-12%
Hydrotrope	1-3%
Alkanolamide	<1%
Ethyl alcohol	<1%
Opacifier	<1%
Colorant	<1%
Perfume	<1%
Water	balance

DEBROX DROPS
For earwax control
(Marion Labs.)

Carbamide peroxide	6.5%
Anhydrous Glycerol	q.s.

DECADRON
Anti-inflammatory agent
(MSD)

Each tablet:
    Dexamethasone ..... 0.25 mg.; 0.5 mg.;
          0.75 mg.; 1.5 mg.;
          or 4 mg.

DECADRON ELIXIR
Steroid therapy
(MSD)

Each 5 cc:
    Dexamethasone .... 0.5 mg.
    Alcohol 5%
    Benzoic acid 0.1%

DECAMETH
Adrenocortical steroid therapy
(Foy Labs.)

Each tablet:
    Dexamethasone .... 0.75 mg.

DECAPRYN
Antihistaminic
(Merrell Dow)

Each tablet:
    Doxylamine succinate *
      Yellow: .... 12.5 mg.
      Orange: .... 25 mg.

DECASPRAY TOPICAL AEROSOL
Dermatological conditions
(MSD)

Each 25 gm.:
    Dexamethasone .... 10 mg.
    Inactive ingred.:
      Isopropyl myristate
      Isobutane

Starred ingredients (*) may be responsible for major toxic effects; consult Section II.

DECCA BARN PAINT

See COOK'S DECCA BARN PAINT

DECHOLIN TABLETS
Hydrocholeretic
(Dome)

Each tablet:
Dehydrocholic acid .... 250 mg.

DECLARE
Commercial dishwashing detergent
(Diversey Wyandotte)

Sodium hydroxide *
Sodium hypochlorite releasing agent

DECOBEL LANACAPS
Decongestant
(Lannett)

Each capsule:
Belladonna alkaloids .... 0.128 mg.
Phenylpropanolamine HCl * ... 50 mg.
Chlorpheniramine maleate ... 1 mg.
Pheniramine maleate * .... 12.5 mg.

DECO-DISC LOZENGES
Throat lozenges
(Wesley Pharm.)

Each lozenge:
Cetalkonium chloride .... 2.5 mg.
Benzocaine .... 10 mg.
Terpin hydrate

DECODULT
Cold remedy
(Wesley Pharm.)

Each tablet:
Panitone (Wesley brand of
    Acetaminophen) * .... 300 mg.
Chlorpheniramine maleate ... 2 mg.
Phenylephrine
    hydrochloride * .... 5 mg.

DECOGEST
Cold remedy
(Wesley Pharm.)

Each tablet:
Aspirin * .... 2.5 gr.
Chlorpheniramine maleate .. 1.25 mg.
Phenylephrine
    hydrochloride * .... 2.5 mg.
Co-buffered with an Aluminum and
    Magnesium hydroxide complex

DECOHIST
Decongestant
(Towne, Paulsen)

Each capsule:
Chlorpheniramine maleate .. 1 mg.
Phenylpropanolamine * ..... 12.5 mg.
Salicylamide .... 180 mg.
Vitamin C .... 50 mg.
Caffeine .... 15 mg.

DECOJEN
Nasal decongestant
(Jenkins Labs.)

Each tablet:
Aspirin * .... 2.5 gr.
Chlorpheniramine maleate .. 1.25 mg.
Phenylephrine HCl .... 2.5 mg.
Co-buffered with:
    Aluminum hydroxide
    Magnesium hydroxide

DECOLATE
Cold remedy
(Wesley Pharm.)

Each tablet:
Glyceryl guaiacolate .... 100 mg.
Chlorpheniramine maleate * 4 mg.
Phenylephrine
    hydrochloride * .... 5 mg.

DECOMINIC
Cold remedy
(Wesley Pharm.)

Each tablet:
Chlorpheniramine maleate .. 1 mg.
Pyrilamine maleate * .... 12.5 mg.
Phenylpropanolamine
    hydrochloride * .... 25 mg.
Phenylephrine
    hydrochloride * .... 2.5 mg.

DECOMIST
Nasal decongestant
(Wesley Pharm.)

20 cc. Squeeze bottle:
Pyrilamine maleate
Phenylephrine hydrochloride
Cetalkonium chloride
Buffered isotonic solution

DECONAMINE CAPSULES SR
Antihistaminic, decongestant
(Berlex Labs.)

Each sustained-release capsule:
Chlorpheniramine maleate * 8 mg.
d-Pseudoephedrine HCl * .... 120 mg.

DECONAMINE ELIXIR
Antihistaminic, decongestant
(Berlex Labs.)

Each 5 ml.:
Chlorpheniramine maleate * 2 mg.
d-Pseudoephedrine HCl * .... 30 mg.
Alcohol 15%

DECONAMINE SYRUP
Antihistaminic, decongestant
(Berlex Labs.)

Each 5 ml.:
Chlorpheniramine maleate * 2 mg.
d-Pseudoephedrine HCl * .... 30 mg.

DECONAMINE TABLETS
Antihistaminic, decongestant
(Berlex Labs.)

Each tablet:
Chlorpheniramine maleate * .. 4 mg.
d-Pseudoephedrine HCl * .... 60 mg.

DE-CONGESTO
For nasal congestion; aerosol
(Kem Mfg. Co.)

Oil of peppermint 0.60%
Menthol 0.30%
Oil eucalyptus 0.65%
Triethylene glycol 7.00%
Alcohol 16.05%

DECOSPAN CAPSULES
Antihistaminic, decongestant
(Wesley Pharm.)

Each capsule:
Chlorpheniramine maleate * . 8 mg.
Phenylpropanolamine
    hydrochloride * .... 50 mg.
Isopropamide (as iodide) * ... 2.5 mg.

DECO-S.P.C.
Antihistaminic-decongestant
(Wesley Pharm.)

Each tablet:
Salicylamide .... 200 mg.
Phenacetin * .... 100 mg.
Caffeine .... 15 mg.
Phenylephrine
    hydrochloride * .... 5 mg.
Chlorpheniramine maleate ... 2 mg.

DECOTUSSIN
Antitussive
(Wesley Pharm.)

Each tablet:
Dextromethorphan
    hydrobromide .... 7.5 mg.
Aspirin * .... 2.5 gr.
Chlorpheniramine maleate .. 1.25 mg.
Phenylephrine
    hydrochloride * .... 2.5 mg.
Co-buffered with an Aluminum and
    Magnesium hydroxide complex

DECOTUSSIN FORTE
Antitussive
(Wesley Pharm.)

Each tablet:
Phenylephrine hydrochloride * 5 mg.
Chlorpheniramine maleate * .. 2 mg.
Ascorbic acid .... 30 mg.
Dextromethorphan
    hydrobromide .... 10 mg.

DECO-WRITE TUBES (PAINT)
(Craftint)

Alkyd resin
Petroleum hydrocarbon solvents *
Non-toxic Pigments

Starred ingredients (*) may be responsible for major toxic effects; consult Section II.

DEC TABS
Anthelmintic for dogs and cats
(Bio-Ceutic)

Each tablet:
  Diethylcarbamazine citrate * 200 mg.

DE-CUT
Plant growth control
(Fairmount Chem. Co.)

Diethanolamine salt of 1,2-dihydro-
3,6-pyridazinedione (Maleic hydrazide) * 58%

DEEP KILL WEED KILLER
Herbicide
(National Chemsearch)

Sodium arsenite *

DEEP MAGIC CREAM & LOTION
(Gillette Co., Personal Care Div.)

The Gillette Co., Personal Care Div.,
Boston, Mass. 02199 will receive collect
phone calls from poison control centers or
physicians asking for emergency toxicological information about the company's
products.

Phone: 617-421-7000

DEEP STRENGTH MUSTEROLE
Analgesic rub
(Plough)

Methyl salicylate * 30%
Menthol 3%
Mineral oil
Water .... q.s.

DEEP TREAT 1-10 WOOD PRESERVATIVE
(Klean-Strip)

Pentachlorophenol * 40%
Petroleum solvents 60%

DEEP TREAT RTU
Wood preservative
(Klean-Strip)

Pentachlorophenol * 5.20%
Petroleum solvents * 94.8%

DEF
Defoliant
(Mobay Chemical Corp.)

S,S,S-Tributyl phosphorotrithioate *

DEFIANCE DETERGENT RESISTANT FLOOR FINISH

See AIRWICK PROFESSIONAL
PRODUCTS DEFIANCE DETER-
GENT RESISTANT FLOOR FIN-
ISH

DEFT PAINT PRODUCTS
Wood finishes

Deft, Inc.
17451 Von Karman Ave.
Irvine, Calif. 92714

Phone: 714-549-8911

See PAINTS, Section VI, General Formulations

DEFY
Agricultural broadleaf weed killer
(Kalo)

2,4-D (Dimethyl ammonium 2,4-dichloro-
phenoxy acetate) *

DEGEST 2
Ocular decongestant
(Barnes-Hind)

Naphazoline HCl 0.012%
Antipyrine 0.1%
Hydroxyethylcellulose
Povidone
Aqueous isotonic citrate buffered vehicle
Benzalkonium chloride 0.0067%
Edetate disodium 0.02%

DEGREEZER (Aerosol)
(Cling-Surface)

Toluol * 3%
1,1,1-Trichloroethane * 90%

DE-HESIVE AEROSOL
(Cramer Products)

Isopropyl alcohol 99% * 58.80%
Glycerine (USP) 0.90%
Neutralizer (Mala #33) 0.15%
Arbutus perfume 0.15%
Propane 16.00%
Isobutane 24.00%

DEHIST CAPSULES
Antihistamine and decongestant
(OJF)

Each tablet:
  Phenylephrine HCl * .... 15 mg.
  Chlorpheniramine maleate * .. 8 mg.
  Phenylpropanolamine HCl * .. 30 mg.
  Timed disintegration

DEKALB DIAZINON
Seed treatment
(DEKALB AgResearch)

O,O-Diethyl O-(2-isopropyl-6-
methyl-4-pyrimidinyl)phos-
phorothioate * 33.34%

DEKGRIP PAINT
Heavy duty marine paint
(International Paint)

Mineral spirits (or turpentine substitute) *
Pigments - no lead

DEKKO ROACH-ETTES
Insecticide
(General Pest Service)

Decachlorooctahydro-1,3,4-meth-
eno-2H-
cyclobuta(c.d.)pentalen-2-one
(Kepone) 0.125%

'76 Ed.

DEKKO SILVERFISH PAKS
Insecticide
(General Pest Service)

Decachlorooctahydro-1,3,4-meth-
eno-2H-
cyclobuta(c.d.)pentalen-2-one
(Kepone) 0.125%

'76 Ed.

DEL-A-CIDE
*Insecticide for municipal, professional
and industrial use*
(Del Chemical Corp.)

Technical Chlordane (equiv. to
7.2% octachloro-4,7-methanote-
trahydroindane and 4.8% related
compounds) * 12.00%
Mixed Aliphatic hydrocarbons * 80.84%

'76 Ed.

DEL ADIOS
*Absorbent, deodorant, bacteriostatic
for municipal, professional and industrial use*
(Del Chemical Corp.)

Isopropanol 0.27%
Alkyl (C16 10%, C18 90%) trimethyl
ammonium chloride 0.38%
Methyl salicylate 0.75%
Pine oil 3.0%

'76 Ed.

DELAGAR BATH PEARLS
(Delagar)

Each capsule:
  Mineral oil .... 80 min.
  Perfume oil * 2.5%
  Nonionic surfactant 1.25%
  Isostearic acid in yellow (Exotic
    perfume), red (Rose per-
    fume), green (Pine perfume),
    and lilac (Lilac perfume) ... 2.00%

'76 Ed.

DELAGAR BUBBLE PEARLS
Bath oil capsules
(Delagar)

Each capsule:
  Mineral oil
  Perfume oil * 2.5%
  Nonionic surfactant 1.25%
  Isostearic acid (in yellow (Exotic
    perfume), red (Rose perfume),
    green (Pine perfume), and lilac
    (Lilac perfume)) 2.00%

'76 Ed.

Starred ingredients (*) may be responsible for major toxic effects; consult Section II.

DELAGAR PEARLETTES
Bath oil capsules
(Delagar)

Each capsule:
Mineral oil .... 30 min.
Perfume oil * 2.5%
Nonionic surfactant 1.25%
Isostearic acid in yellow (Exotic
perfume), red (Rose per-
fume), green (Pine perfume),
and lilac (Lilac perfume) ... 2.00%

'76 Ed.

DEL ALGAE-KILL
*Municipal, professional and industrial
use*
(Del Chemical Corp.)

N-Alkyl (50% C14, 40% C12, 10%
C16) dimethyl benzyl ammonium chlorides * 10.00%

'76 Ed.

DEL AQUATIC WEED
KILLER
Herbicide
(Del Chemical Corp.)

Diquat dibromide * 4.35%

'76 Ed.

DEL BAC-OFF
*Germicidal sanitizer-deodorizer for
municipal, professional and industrial use*
(Del Chemical Corp.)

N-Alkyl (C14, C12, C16) dimethyl
benzylchloride 0.40%
Triethylene glycol 6.00%
Essential oil - chemical de-
odorizer 0.70%
Isopropyl alcohol * 52.70%

'76 Ed.

DELCID
Antacid
(Merrell Dow)

Each 5 cc:
Aluminum hydroxide .... 600 mg.
Magnesium hydroxide .... 665 mg.

DEL 92 CONCENTRATED
WEED KILLER
*Municipal, professional and industrial
use*
(Del Chemical Corp.)

Sodium arsenite * 44.0%

'76 Ed.

DEL DEODORANT BLOCKS
*Bacteriostatic deodorant for municipal,
institutional use*
(Del Chemical Corp.)

Paradichlorobenzene * 97.15%
Paradiisobutylcresoxyethoxyethyl
dimethyl benzyl ammonium
chloride 0.25%
Lauryl methacrylate 0.25%
Paraformaldehyde 0.25%
Essential oils 1.00%
Inert ingredients: 1.10%
Nonyl phenoxy polyoxyethylene ethanol
Synthetic calcium silicate
Water

'76 Ed.

DEL DUO FOG
Contact insecticide for municipal use
(Del Chemical Corp.)

Beta-butoxy beta'-thiocyano di-
ethyl ether * 23.6%
Malathion 18.8%
Combined amount: 57.6%
Aliphatic hydrocarbons *
Aromatic hydrocarbons *

'76 Ed.

DEL ELIMINATE
Insect repellent
(Del Chemical Corp.)

N,N-Diethyl-meta-toluamide,
tech. 4.200%
N-Octyl bicycloheptene dicarboximide 1.200%
2,3:4,5-Bis(2-butylene)tetrahydro-
2-furaldehyde 0.300%
Di-n-propyl isocinchomeronate .. 0.300%

'76 Ed.

DEL-ETE
Rodenticide
(Del Chemical Corp.)

Warfarin (3(a-Acetonylbenzyl)-4-
hydroxycoumarin) 0.025%

'76 Ed.

DELFEN CONTRACEPTIVE
CREAM
(Ortho)

Nonoxynol 9 .... 5.00%

DELFEN CONTRACEPTIVE
FOAM
(Ortho)

Nonoxynol 9 .... 12.50%

DELFETAMINE 10 MG.
For obesity
(Eastern Research Labs.)

Each tablet:
Delfetamine (dl-N-Methylamphetamine hydrochloride) * . 10 mg.

'76 Ed.

DELFETA-SED TABLETS
(Eastern Research Labs.)

Each tablet:
Sedafax (special micronized
grade of amobarbital) * .... 40 mg.
Delfetamine (dl-N-Methylamphetamine hydrochloride) ... 10 mg.

'76 Ed.

DEL FILTER FLY CONTROL
*Concentrated insecticide for use in sew-
age plants*
(Del Chemical Corp.)

Mixed Aliphatic hydrocarbons * ... 73%
Malathion 3%

'76 Ed.

DEL HEAVY DUTY WEED
AND BRUSH KILLER
SOLUTION
*Municipal, professional and industrial
use*
(Del Chemical Corp.)

Ammonium sulfamate * 48.4%

'76 Ed.

DELICATE 18
Arterial fluid; embalming supply
(Royal Bond)

Formaldehyde * 18%
Methanol *

DELICATE 25
Arterial fluid; embalming supply
(Royal Bond)

Formaldehyde * 25%
Methanol *

DEL INSECTICIDAL
SHAMPOO
Insecticide
(Chem. Spec. Co., Inc.)

Isobornyl thiocyanoacetate 4.75%
Other related terpenes 1.04%
Tech. Piperonyl butoxide 1.18%
Petroleum oil 0.93%
Pyrethrins 0.12%

'76 Ed.

DEL-KILL INSECTICIDE,
FOREMOST 4820

See FOREMOST 4820 DEL-KILL IN-
SECTICIDE

Starred ingredients (*) may be responsible for major toxic effects; consult Section II.

DEL-KILL WEED KILLER 400 LIQUID
Municipal, professional and industrial use
(Del Chemical Corp.)

Mixed Aliphatic hydrocarbons *	94.97%
2,4-Dichlorophenoxyacetic acid, isooctyl ester	1.09%
Bromacil (5-Bromo-3-sec-butyl-6-methyluracil)	0.98%
Pentachlorophenol	0.80%
Other chlorophenols	0.09%

'76 Ed.

DELLA-BRITE ACID CLEANER
(Bonewitz)

Phosphoric acid *	<40%
FD & C Red No. 2 dye	<1%
Water	qs

DELLA-CARE TEAT DIP
(Bonewitz)

Butoxypolypropoxypolyethoxy ethanol iodine complex	<10%
Polyoxyethylene polyoxypropylene propylene glycol	<10%
Sodium acetate	<2%
Acetic acid	<1%
Water	qs

DELLA-CLEAN UDDER WASH
(Bonewitz)

Nonylphenoxypolyethyleneoxy ethanol	<10%
Phosphoric acid *	<20%
a-(p-Nonylphenyl) omega hydroxy-polyoxyethylene iodine complex	<10%
Water	qs

DELLA-FLEX RUBBER CLEANER
(Bonewitz)

Sodium hydroxide *	<75%
Sodium tripolyphosphate	<5%
Sodium carbonate	<10%
Nonylphenoxypolyethyleneoxy ethanol	<1%
Linear dodecylbenzenesulfonate salt	<1%
Sodium sulfate	<15%

DELLA-REGULAR CIP CLEANER
(Bonewitz)

Sodium metasilicate *	<30%
Sodium alkyl naphthalene sulfonate	<1%
Complex phosphates	<35%
Sodium dichloroisocyanurate	<5%
Sodium carbonate *	<25%
Sodium hydroxide *	<10%

DELLA-SAN LIQUID CHLORINE SANITIZER
(Bonewitz)

Sodium hypochlorite *	<7%
Sodium hydroxide *	<2%

DELLA-SUPER LIQUID CIP SYSTEMS CLEANER
(Bonewitz)

Complex phosphates *	
Potassium silicate	<10%
Potassium hypochlorite *	<5%
Potassium hydroxide *	<20%
Water	qs

DELLA-SUPER POWDER CIP CLEANER
(Bonewitz)

Sodium metasilicate *	<20%
Sodium tripolyphosphate	<40%
Sodium hydroxide *	<15%
Sodium carbonate *	<35%
Sodium alkyl naphthalene sulfonate	<1%
Sodium dichloroisocyanurate	<5%

DELLA-WASH POWDER MANUAL CLEANER
(Bonewitz)

Sodium carbonate *	<35%
Sodium linear dodecylbenzene sulfonate	<5%
Complex phosphates	<35%
Sodium linear alkylpolyethoxy phosphate ester	<5%
Sodium metasilicate *	<20%
Sodium dichloroisocyanurate	<5%

DEL LEMON "GLYCOLIZED" ROOM DEODORANT
Air sanitizer
(Del Chemical Corp.)

Alcohol	32.33%
Triethylene glycol	7.5%

'76 Ed.

DEL LINEMAN'S WASP SPRAY
Insecticide
(Del Chemical Corp.)

Pyrethrins	0.050%
Technical Chlordane	2.000%
Pine oil	2.800%
Petroleum distillate *	11.950%
Inert ingredients:	
Methylene chloride *	16.00%
Tetrachloroethylene *	32.00%
Dichlorodifluoromethane	17.60%
Trichlorofluoromethane	17.60%

'76 Ed.

DELMO-Z SPRAY
Zinc deficiency corrective for use in dormant and foliage sprays
(Chevron)

Zinc (expressed as elemental) *†	50%

Chevron emergency phone number: 415-233-3737

†See Zinc salts

DEL MUNICIDE
Concentrated residual insecticide for municipal, professional and industrial use
(Del Chemical Corp.)

Technical Chlordane *	12.00%
Malathion	3.16%
Mixed Aliphatic hydrocarbons *	80.84%

'76 Ed.

DELNAV
Insecticide
(Hercules Incorporated)

2,3-p-Dioxanedithiol-S,S-bis-(O,O-diethyl phosphorodithioate) *	68%
Related materials	32%

DE-LOUSE-MOR
Insecticide
(Hilltop)

Refined Petroleum oil *	
Gamma isomer of benzene hexachloride *	
Other isomers of benzene hexachloride	

'76 Ed.

DEL PORCELAIN CLEANER CONCENTRATE
Municipal, professional and industrial use
(Del Chemical Corp.)

Hydrogen chloride *	7.50%
Alkyl (C14 50%, C12 40%, C16 10%) dimethyl benzyl ammonium chloride	0.05%
Inert ingredients:	92.45%
Water	
Octyl phenoxy polyethoxy ethanol	
Nonyl phenoxy polyethoxy ethanol	

'76 Ed.

DEL QUATRA-D
Disinfectant, defilmer, deodorant, detergent for municipal, industrial and professional use
(Del Chemical Corp.)

Sodium carbonate	3.0%
Tetrasodium salt of ethylene diamine, tetraacetic acid	2.2%
n-Alkyl (60% C14, 30% C16, 5% C12, 5% C18) dimethyl benzyl ammonium chlorides	1.5%
n-Alkyl (50% C12, 30% C14, 17% C16, 3% C18) dimethyl ethylbenzyl ammonium chlorides	1.5%

'76 Ed.

Starred ingredients (*) may be responsible for major toxic effects; consult Section II.

DEL RAPID-KILL
Liquid weed killer for municipal, professional, and industrial use
(Del Chemical Corp.)

Mixed Aliphatic hydrocarbons *	96.10%
Bromacil (5-Bromo-3-sec-butyl-6-methyluracil)	0.97%
Pentachlorophenol	0.79%
Other chlorophenols	0.09%

'76 Ed.

DEL SAN-O-MINT
Deodorant spray for municipal, professional, and industrial use
(Del Chemical Corp.)

Isopropanol *	32.0%
Triethylene glycol	6.0%
Propylene glycol	2.5%
Diisobutylphenoxyethoxyethyl dimethyl benzyl ammonium chloride	2.0%

'76 Ed.

DEL SELECT
Weed and brush killer solution for municipal, professional, and industrial use
(Del Chemical Corp.)

Dimethylamine salt of 2,4-dichlorophenoxyacetic acid *	49.6%

'76 Ed.

DEL SK 40 HEAVY DUTY WEED KILLER
Municipal, professional, industrial use
(Del Chemical Corp.)

Alkanolamine salts (of the ethanol and isopropanol series) of 2,4-dichlorophenoxyacetic acid *	32.5%

'76 Ed.

DEL STAPH 600
Surface disinfectant and deodorizer for use in hospitals
(Del Chemical Corp.)

Tributyltin isopropyl succinate	0.024%
Tributyltin benzoate	0.036%
Tributyltin linoleate	0.012%
Sodium ethylmercurithiosalicylate	0.002%
N-Alkyl (60% C14, 30% C16, 5% C12, 5% C18) dimethyl benzyl ammonium chloride	0.486%
Isopropanol *	39.025%

'76 Ed.

DEL SUR-KLEEN
Disinfectant, cleaner and deodorizer for municipal, professional, and industrial use
(Del Chemical Corp.)

N-Alkyl (C12 40%, C14 50%, C16 10%) dimethyl benzyl ammonium chloride	0.384%
Essential oil	0.480%
Ethylene diamine tetraacetic acid	0.960%
Trisodium phosphate	1.920%
Isopropyl alcohol	5.760%
Inert ingredients:	90.496%
Detergents	
Cleaners	
Builders	
Propellent	

'76 Ed.

DEL SWAT
Insecticide
(Del Chemical Corp.)

Pyrethrins	0.3%
Technical Piperonyl butoxide	0.6%
N-Octyl bicycloheptene dicarboximide	1.0%
Petroleum distillate *	13.1%
Inert ingredients:	
Dichlorodifluoromethane	42.5%/wt.
Trichloromonofluoromethane	42.5%/wt.

'76 Ed.

DELTA-CORTEF TABLETS
Rheumatoid arthritis and intractable bronchial asthma
(Upjohn)

Each tablet:
Prednisolone (anhydrous) ...... 5 mg.

DELTADINE DISINFECTANT
Detergent - sanitizer for hospital, dairy, and industrial use
(Delta Labs.)

Phosphoric acid *	0.60%
Nonylphenoxypoly (ethyleneoxy)-ethanol iodine complex (providing 1.75% titratable iodine)	8.75%

'76 Ed.

DELTA PET DUST
Kills ticks, fleas and lice
(Delta Labs.)

Carbaryl (1-Naphthyl-N-methylcarbamate) *	
2,2-Methylenebis(4-chlorophenol) (Dichlorophene)	
Aluminum chlorohydroxy allantoinate	
Inert ingred.:	
Pyrophyllite	94.3%

'76 Ed.

DELTA PINE OIL
Disinfectant-cleanser-deodorant
(Reily Chem.)

Active ingredients:	90.0%
Pine oil *	
Soap	
Isopropyl alcohol *	
Inert ingredient:	10.0%
Water	

DELTASONE TABLETS
Rheumatoid arthritis and intractable bronchial asthma
(Upjohn)

Each tablet:
Prednisone ...... 2.5 mg.; 5 mg.; 10 mg.; 20 mg.; 50 mg.

DELUXOL HAIR CARE PRODUCTS
Deluxol Laboratories Inc.
3733 University Blvd. W.
Jacksonville, Fla. 32217

Phone: 904-733-5386

See COSMETICS, Section VI, General Formulations

DELVAK
Alkaline cleaning compound
(Diversey Wyandotte)

Sodium hydroxide *
Alkaline salts

DEL WASP JET SPRAY
Municipal, professional and industrial use
(Del Chemical Corp.)

Pyrethrins	0.15%
Tech. Piperonyl butoxide	0.30%
N-Octyl bicycloheptene dicarboximide	0.53%
Tech. Chlordane	2.00%
Petroleum distillate *	62.02%

'76 Ed.

DEL X-IT
Insecticide
(Del Chemical Corp.)

Petroleum distillate *	99.525%
N-Octyl bicycloheptene dicarboximide	0.250%
Piperonyl butoxide (technical)	0.150%
Pyrethrins	0.075%

'76 Ed.

DEL ZON-KIL
Bug killer
(Del Chemical Corp.)

Pyrethrins	0.050%
Technical Piperonyl butoxide	0.100%
N-Octyl bicycloheptene dicarboximide	0.166%
O,O-Diethyl O-(2-isopropyl-6-methyl-4-pyrimidinyl) phosphorothioate	0.500%
Petroleum distillate *	74.184%
Inert ingredients:	25.000%
Dichlorodifluoromethane	

'76 Ed.

DEMAZIN
Decongestant-antihistamine compound
(Schering)

Each 5 ml.:
Phenylephrine HCl	2.5 mg.
Chlorpheniramine maleate *	1 mg.
Alcohol	7.5%

DEMAZIN REPETABS
For relief of nasal congestion
(Schering)

Outer and inner layer each:
Chlorpheniramine maleate *	2 mg.
Phenylephrine *	10 mg.

Total per each tablet:
Chlorpheniramine maleate *	4 mg.
Phenylephrine *	20 mg.

DEMEROL APAP TABLETS
Analgesic, antipyretic
(Breon Labs.)

Each tablet:
Demerol (Meperidine HCl) *	50 mg.
Acetaminophen (APAP) *	300 mg.

DEMEROL HYDROCHLORIDE
Analgesic, spasmolytic, sedative
(Winthrop Labs.)

TABLETS:
Meperidine hydrochloride *	50 mg.; or 100 mg.

ELIXIR (each 5 ml.):
Meperidine hydrochloride *	50 mg.

DEMERT & DOUGHERTY PRODUCTS
Automotive chemicals and household cleaners

DeMert & Dougherty, Inc.
5000 W. 41st St.
Chicago, Ill. 60650

Phone: 312-523-5600

DEMETHOCAINE
Cough & sore throat
(Elder)

Each capsule:
Dextromethorphan hydrobromide *	15.0 mg.
Benzocaine	3.0 mg.

DEMISE
Turf broadleaf weed killer
(Kalo)

2,4-D *

DEMODEK
Parasiticide - veterinary
(Fort Dodge)

Benzyl benzoate *	30%

DEMSARDEX
For control of mange in dogs
(Burns-Biotec)

Active ingred. (by wt.):
Benzyl benzoate *	36.72%
Lindane	0.54%

Inert ingred.:
Isopropyl alcohol *	62.74%

DEMULEN
Progestogen-estrogen combination
(Searle, G.D., & Co.)

Each tablet:
Ethynodiol diacetate	1 mg.
Ethinyl estradiol	50 mcg.

DEMURE DEODORANT DOUCHE (Concentrate)
Vaginal douche
(Vicks Toiletry Products Div.)

Benzethonium chloride *
In packets	3.84%
In bottles	1.92%

Fragrance (Peppermint Oil)
Lactic acid
FD & C Blue #1
FD & C Yellow #5
Methylparaben

DENALAN
Denture cleanser
(Whitehall Labs.)

Sodium peroxide *
Peppermint powder

DENOREX
For treatment of psoriasis, seborrhea, dandruff
(Whitehall Labs.)

Coal tar solution *	9.0%

Menthol *
TEA-Lauryl sulfate
Water
Hydroxypropyl methylcellulose
p-Chloro-m-xylenol

DENQUEL
Toothpaste
(Vicks Toiletry Products Div.)

Water
Calcium carbonate
Glycerin
Sorbitol
Sodium lauryl sulfate
Potassium nitrate	5%

Flavor
Silica
Cellulose gum
Xanthan gum
Sodium saccharin
Methylparaben
Propylparaben

DENTOCAIN (Adult & Mild)
Analgesic for toothache, sore gums, teething
(Dentocain)

Adult:
Ethyl alcohol	56.2%
Benzocaine	15%
Peppermint oil	0.7%

Mild:
Ethyl alcohol	56.2%
Benzocaine	10%
Peppermint oil	0.7%

DENTROL LIQUID DENTURE ADHESIVE
(Block Drug)

Sodium carboxymethylcellulose
Ethylene oxide homopolymer
Polyethylene
Mineral oil
Preservative
Flavors

DENT'S DENTAL POULTICE
(Dent, C.S.)

Each pad:
Benzocaine	36.2%
Oxyquinoline	4.0%
Thymol *	2.0%
Oleoresin capsicum	0.5%

DENT'S DOUBLE-ACTION TOOTHACHE RELIEF KIT
(Dent, C.S.)

See DENT'S TOOTHACHE DROPS TREATMENT and MARANOX

DENT'S EAR WAX DROPS
(Dent, C.S.)

Each fl. oz.:
Glycerin	95.8%
Mineral oil	3.0%
Polyoxyethlylene (5) sorbitan mono-oleate	1.2%

Starred ingredients (*) may be responsible for major toxic effects; consult Section II.

DENT'S LOTION-JEL
For toothache, teething, minor denture irritations
(Dent, C.S.)

Benzocaine	5%
Methyl and propyl parasept	<1%

DENT'S TOOTHACHE DROPS TREATMENT
(Dent, C.S.)

Alcohol	60.0%
Chlorobutanol	0.09%
Eugenol *	7.5%

DENT'S TOOTHACHE GUM
Medicated wax for cavity toothache
(Dent, C.S.)

Benzocaine	5.0%
Eugenol *	5.0%

DENTU-CREME
(Block Drug)

Dicalcium phosphate dihydrate
Calcium carbonate
Glycerine
Sodium saccharin
Micronized Silica
Sodium lauryl sulfate
Magnesium aluminum silicate
Propylene glycol
Hydroxyethylcellulose
Preservative
Flavors

DEO-MINT
Disinfectant, deodorizer
(Barco)

Isopropyl alcohol *	37.44%
Ortho-benzyl para chlorophenol	5.00%
Potassium salt of oleic & linoleic acids	1.90%
Alkyl aryl sulfonate	0.43%
Perfume & counter odorants	0.29%
Hexalene glycol	0.23%
Chelating agent	0.19%

'76 Ed.

DEOMIST
Glycol air sanitizer
(Kem Mfg. Co.)

Triethylene glycol	4.5%
Propylene glycol	3.0%
n-Alkyl (50% C14, 40% C12, 10% C16)dimethyl benzyl ammonium chloride	0.1%

DEPEND-O AUTOMATIC TOILET CLEANER AND DEODORIZER (Liquid)
(Boyle-Midway)

Nonionic surfactant	<5%
Fragrance	trace
Colorant	trace
Water	balance

DEPLETITE-25
Anorexiant
(Direct Div.)

Each tablet:
Diethylpropion HCl *	25 mg.

DEPOLARIZED APCO 125
Solvent
(Oklahoma Refining)

Paraffins *	49%
Naphthenes *	44%
Aromatics *	6%
Olefins	1%

DEPOLARIZED APCO 140
Solvent
(Oklahoma Refining)

Paraffins *	48%
Naphthenes *	46%
Aromatics *	5%
Olefins	1%

DEPOLARIZED APCO 467
Solvent
(Oklahoma Refining)

Paraffins *	46%
Naphthenes *	48%
Aromatics *	5%
Olefins	1%

DEP PRODUCTS
Hair care products

Dep Corporation
12821 W. Jefferson Blvd.
Los Angeles, Calif. 90066

Phone: 213-827-9800

See COSMETICS, Section VI, General Formulations

DE PREE ALLERGY II TABLETS
Decongestant, antihistamine
(DePree)

Chlorpheniramine maleate *
Phenylpropanolamine HCl *

DE PREE ANTI-B MIST NASAL SPRAY
Decongestant, antihistamine
(DePree)

Pyrilamine maleate
Phenylephrine HCl *
Cetalkonium chloride

DE PREE ANTI-B THROAT TROCHES
Local anesthetic, antitussive
(DePree)

Cetyl pyridinium chloride
Benzocaine
d-Methorphan

DE PREE BRONCHIAL SYRUP
Expectorant
(DePree)

Potassium guaiacolate

DE PREE BRONCHIAL SYRUP DM
Expectorant, antitussive
(DePree)

Glyceryl guaiacolate
Dextromethorphan HBr *

DE PREE CHILDREN'S COUGH SYRUP
Expectorant, decongestant, antitussive
(DePree)

Glyceryl guaiacolate
Pseudoephedrine HCl *
Dextromethorphan HBr *

DE PREE DRAWING SALVE
(DePree)

Resorcinol *
Salicylic acid *
Phenol (0.25% on a 100% basis)

DE PREE SINUS HEADACHE TABLETS
Analgesic, decongestant
(DePree)

Acetaminophen *
Phenylpropanolamine HCl *

DE PREE SLEEPING TABLETS
(DePree)

Pyrilamine maleate *

DE PREE TOOTHACHE DROPS
Local anesthetic
(DePree)

Benzocaine
Camphor *
Oil of cloves *

DE PREE TRIPLE ANTI-B OINTMENT
Topical, antibacterial
(DePree)

Bacitracin
Neomycin sulfate
Polymixin B sulfate
Petrolatum base

Starred ingredients (*) may be responsible for major toxic effects; consult Section II.

DEPROL
For depression
(Wallace Labs.)

Each tablet:
Meprobamate * . . . . 400 mg.
Benactyzine hydrochloride . . . 1 mg.

'76 Ed.

DEPUTY
Aerosol tear gas spray; personal protection
(Penguin Industries)

CN (Chloracetophenone) * 2.0%

DERAYCO TEMPERA
(Craftint)

Water soluble, non-toxic Resins
Non-toxic Pigments

DERBAC TAR MEDICATED SHAMPOO
Ectoparasiticide
(Cereal)

Pine tar *
Coconut oil

DERBY LIGHTER FLUID
(Derby Refining)

Light Petroleum distillate *

'76 Ed.

DERBY PERMANENT TYPE ANTI-FREEZE AND COOLANT
(Derby Refining)

Ethylene glycol *

'76 Ed.

DERFULE
Analgesic
(OJF)

Each capsule:
Salicylamide . . . . 130 mg.
Phenacetin * . . . . 100 mg.
Atropine sulfate . . . . 0.130 mg.
Powdered Opium . . . . 2 mg.

DERGOLENE CS
Biodegradable anionic detergent
(Arkansas Co.)

Ethoxylated fatty alcohol sulfate *†

'76 Ed.

†*See* Sodium lauryl trioxyethylene sulfate

DERGON #65
Nonionic detergent
(Arkansas Co.)

Ethoxylated alkylphenol *

'76 Ed.

DERGON BD
Biodegradable nonionic detergent
(Arkansas Co.)

Ethoxylated fatty alcohol *

'76 Ed.

DERGON MF
Nonionic detergent
(Arkansas Co.)

Polyoxyethylene fatty acid ester *

'76 Ed.

DERGON OM
Biodegradable nonionic detergent
(Arkansas Co.)

Alkanolamide

'76 Ed.

DERGON SW
Biodegradable nonionic detergent
(Arkansas Co.)

Alkanolamide . . . . approx. 75%
Linear alkyl sulfonate * . . . approx. 15%

'76 Ed.

DERGON T
Biodegradable anionic detergent
(Arkansas Co.)

Fatty acid ester sulfate *†
Alkaline builders

'76 Ed.

†*See* Anionic synthetic detergents

DERGOPEN RD
Nonionic wetting and rewetting agent
(Arkansas Co.)

Polyoxyethylene ether alcohol *†
Tridecyl alcohol

'76 Ed.

†*See* Nonionic synthetic detergents

DERGOPEN RN
Nonionic wetting and rewetting agent
(Arkansas Co.)

Polyoxyethylene ether alcohol *†

'76 Ed.

†*See* Nonionic synthetic detergents

DERIFIL TABLETS
For the control of odors originating in the digestive tract
(Rystan)

Water-soluble Chlorophyll . . . . . 100 mg.

DERMA CALM
For mange; veterinary
(Goshen Labs.)

Rotenone 1%
Isopropyl alcohol * 46%
Acetone *
Chloroform *

DERMACARE
Antiseptic skin lotion
(Jenkins Labs.)

Hexachlorophene *
Camphor *
Menthol *
Lanolin

DERMACORT CREAM & LOTION
For inflammatory skin disorders
(Rowell)

Cream:
Hydrocortisone 1%

Lotion:
Hydrocortisone 0.5%; 1%

DERM-AID CREME & LOTION
For dry skin
(Gordon Labs.)

Cetyl alcohol
Lubricating oils
Perfume

DERMALAB BATH OIL
(Derma Labs.)

Mineral oil
PEG-4 dilaurate
Sunflower seed oil
Wheat germ oil
Vitamin A
Vitamin D
Fragrance
Propylparaben
BHT

Starred ingredients (*) may be responsible for major toxic effects; consult Section II.

DERMALAB CREAM
(Unscented)
(Derma Labs.)

Water
Mineral oil
Ceteareth-5
Glycerin
Stearyl alcohol
Collagen
Lanolin alcohol
Gelatin
Carbomer-941
Triethanolamine
Methylparaben
Propylparaben
Stearic hydrazide
Imidazolidinyl urea

DERMALAB LOTION
(Unscented)
(Derma Labs.)

Water
Mineral oil
Lanolin alcohol
Ceteareth-5
Isopropyl palmitate
Sesame oil
Propylparaben
Methylparaben
Stearic hydrazide
Carbomer-940
Triethanolamine
Imidazolidinyl urea

DERMALAB SHAMPOO
(Derma Labs.)

Water
TEA lauryl sulfate
Lauramide DEA
TEA coco-hydrolyzed animal protein and
    Sorbitol
Oleyl betaine
Linoleamide DEA
Quaternium 20
NaCl
Hydroxypropyl-methyl-cellulose
Fragrance
Methylparaben
Propylparaben
FD & C Yellow #5
D & C Red #19
DMDM-hydantoin

DERMALAB SKIN
CLEANSER
(Derma Labs.)

SD Alcohol #40
Water
PPG-3-methyl-ether
Polysorbate 20
Fragrance
D & A Red #19
FD & C Blue #1

DERMALAB SOAP
(Derma Labs.)

Refined Tallow
Coconut oil
Sunflower seed oil
Glycerin
Mineral oil
Lecithin

DERMALAB X-5 SHAMPOO
(Derma Labs.)

Active ingred.:
    Salicylic acid *

Other ingred.:
    Water
    Sodium laureth sulfate
    Propylene glycol
    Cocamide DEA
    Cocamidopropyl betaine
    Ammonium lauryl sulfate
    Laureth 23
    Tetrasodium EDTA
    Methylparaben
    Propylparaben
    Fragrance

DERMALAB X-5T SHAMPOO
(Derma Labs.)

Active ingred.:
    Liquid Carbonis detergens (17% solu-
        tion)
    Salicylic acid *

Other ingred.:
    Water
    Sodium laureth sulfate
    Propylene glycol
    Cocamide DEA
    Cocamidopropyl betaine
    Ammonium lauryl sulfate
    Laureth 23
    Tetrasodium EDTA
    Methylparaben
    Propylparaben
    Fragrance

DERMA MEDICONE-HC
OINTMENT
For inflammation & swelling of der-
matoses
(Medicone)

Each gram:
    Hydrocortisone acetate .... 10.0 mg.
    Benzocaine .... 20.0 mg.
    Oxyquinoline sulfate .... 10.5 mg.
    Ephedrine hydrochloride ... 1.1 mg.
    Menthol .... 4.8 mg.
    Ichthammol .... 10.0 mg.
    Zinc oxide .... 137.0 mg.
    Petrolatum
    Lanolin
    Perfume

DERMA MEDICONE
OINTMENT
For simple pruritic and minor skin af-
fections
(Medicone)

Each gram:
    Benzocaine .... 20.0 mg.
    Oxyquinoline sulfate .... 10.5 mg.
    Menthol .... 4.8 mg.
    Ichthammol .... 10.0 mg.
    Zinc oxide .... 137.3 mg.
    Petrolatum
    Lanolin
    Perfume
    Color

DERMA-PAX
Itch-relieving lotion
(Recsei Labs.)

Pyrilamine maleate 0.22%
Pheniramine maleate 0.22%
Chlorpheniramine maleate 0.06%
Benzyl alcohol 1.0%
In Isopropanol 35% v/v with Chlorobu-
tanol, Cetylpyridinium chloride

DERMAPHILL
For skin irritations
(Torch)

Aluminum acetate basic 1.0%
Phenol (Carbolic acid) 1.0%
Menthol 0.5%
Camphor * 3.0%
Hydrophilic vehicle .... ad. 100.0%

'76 Ed.

DERMA-SECT

See ANCHOR DERMA-SECT

DERMA-SMOOTHE OIL
For dry skin
(Hill Dermaceuticals)

Refined Peanut oil-mineral oil blend

DERMA-SMOOTHE/FS OIL
For relief of the inflammatory manifes-
tations of corticosteroid-responsive
dermatoses
(Hill Dermaceuticals)

Fluocinolone acetonide 0.01%
Pramoxine HCl 0.05%
In a blend of oils with Isopropyl alcohol*
and a nonionic detergent

DERMA-SOFT CREME
Corn and callus medication
(Creighton Products)

Salicylic acid * 2.5%
In a cream base

DERMA-SONE 1% CREAM
For relief of the inflammatory manifes-
tations of corticocosteroid-responsive
dermatoses
(Hill Dermaceuticals)

Hydrocortisone alcohol 1%
Pramoxine HCl 1%
In a vanishing cream base
Also contains: Cetyl alcohol, Glyceryl mon-
    ostearate, Isopropyl myristate, Polyoxy-
    ethylene sorbitan monostearate, Sorbi-
    tan monostearate, Potassium sorbate,
    Furcelleran, and Water

Starred ingredients (*) may be responsible for major toxic effects; consult Section II.

DERMASSAGE LOTION
(Colgate-Palmolive)

Mineral oil
Stearic acid
Carbitol
Triethanolamine
Lanolin
Urea
Oxyquinoline sulfate *
Menthol .... >0.8%
Perfume
Water

'76 Ed.

DERMAVAL CREAM
(Vale)

Calamine
Zinc oxide
Camphor-phenol
Menthol
Pyrilamine maleate * 2%

DERMEZE OINTMENT
Antihistaminic, anesthetic
(Premo)

Thenylpyramine hydrochloride *
Benzocaine
Tyrothrycin

'76 Ed.

DERMIDOL
Dry skin lubricant and moisturizer
(C & M Pharmacal)

Purified water
Mineral oil
Propylene glycol
PEG 6-32 stearate
Cellulose gum
Fragrance

DERMITITE LOTION
Germicidal, bactericidal and fungicidal lotion for small animals
(Daniels, Dr. A.C.)

Lanolin .... trace
Olive oil 5%
Trace amounts of:
  Menthol
  Coon oil
  Hexamethylenebis(p-chlorophenyldiguanide)diacetate
  Alcohol
  Hexachlorophene
  Methylbenzethonium chloride
  Emollient cream base

DERMOCAINE
For skin irritations
(Walker Pharm.)

Bismuth subnitrate
Salicylic acid *
Zinc oxide
Benzocaine
Thuja
Petrolatum

'76 Ed.

DERM-O-CREME
For skin irritations
(VB)

Balsam of Peru *
Phenol *
Bismuth subnitrate
Sulfur
Castor oil
Resorcin *

DERMO-PEDIC ELBOW LOTION
(CMC Research Div.)

Allantoin 0.3%
Ethoxylated lanolin
Water

DERMO-PEDIC FOOT LOTION
(CMC Research Div.)

Allantoin 0.3%
Ethoxylated lanolin
Water

DERONIL TABLETS
Anti-inflammatory corticosteroid therapy
(Schering)

Each tablet:
  Dexamethasone .... 0.75 mg.

DE-SCALE - D.S. (Liquid)

See GUNK D.S. - DE-SCALE (Liquid)

DESENEX AEROSOL
Antifungal
(Pharmacraft)

Undecylenic acid 2.0%
Zinc undecylenate * 20.0%
Propellant: Isobutane

DESENEX DRI FOOT
Anti-perspirant foot deodorant
(Pharmacraft)

Aluminum chlorhydrate complex *
Menthol *
Alcohol 29.8%

DESENEX OINTMENT
Antifungal
(Pharmacraft)

Undecylenic acid 5%
Zinc undecylenate * 20%

DESENEX POWDER
Antifungal
(Pharmacraft)

Undecylenic acid 2.0%
Zinc undecylenate * 20%

DESENEX SOAP
Antifungal
(Pharmacraft)

Undecylenic acid 2.0%

DESENEX SOLUTION
Antifungal
(Pharmacraft)

Undecylenic acid .... 10% w/w
Isopropyl alcohol * .... 40% w/w

DES-I-CATE
Herbicide
(Pennwalt)

Endothall as monomethylcocoamine salt * .... 0.52 lb./gal.

DESITIN BABY POWDER
(Leeming Div.)

Talc

DESITIN DABAWAYS
Premoistened disposable washcloths
(Leeming Div.)

Regular:
  Disodium edetate
  Benzalkonium chloride (<0.04% in the expressed liquid)

With lotion:
  Disodium edetate
  Mineral oil
  Glycerin
  Benzalkonium chloride (<0.04% in the expressed liquid)

DESITIN OINTMENT
(Leeming Div.)

Norwegian Cod liver oil
Zinc oxide
Lanolin
Petrolatum
Talcum

DESITIN SKIN CARE LOTIONS
Hand and body lotion
(Leeming Div.)

Dimethicone
Petrolatum
Glycerin
Propylene glycol diperlargonate
Glyceryl stearate
Lanolin
Cetyl alcohol
Diethylaminoethyl stearamide phosphate
Benzalkonium chloride .... <0.05%

DESO-CREME
For athlete's foot, ringworm & fungus infections
(Columbia Med.)

Zinc undecylenate * 20%
Caprylic acid 5%
Sodium propionate 2%

Starred ingredients (*) may be responsible for major toxic effects; consult Section II.

DE-SOIL CONCENTRATED ALL PURPOSE DETERGENT
(Uncle Sam)

Diethanolamide of fatty acid
Soda ash *
Borax
Ethylenediaminetetraacetate
Wetting agents
Dye
Water

DESOXYN (TABLETS & GRADUMET TABLETS)
CNS stimulant, appetite depressant
(Abbott)

TABLETS (each):
  Methamphetamine
    hydrochloride * ... 2.5 mg; or 5 mg.

GRADUMET TABLETS (each):
  Methamphetamine
    hydrochloride * ... 5 mg.; 10 mg.;
        or 15 mg.

DE-SPROUT
Prevents onion and potato sprouting
(Fairmount Chem. Co.)

Diethanolamine salt of 1,2-dihydro-
3,6-pyridazinedione (Maleic
hydrazide) * 58%

DETER DOUBLE ACTIVE ANTI-PERSPIRANT SPRAY

See AMWAY DETER DOUBLE AC-
TIVE ANTI-PERSPIRANT SPRAY

DETER DOUBLE ACTIVE FOOT DEODORANT SPRAY

See AMWAY DETER DOUBLE AC-
TIVE FOOT DEODORANT SPRAY

DETER DOUBLE ACTIVE ROLL-ON ANTI-PERSPIRANT

See AMWAY DETER DOUBLE AC-
TIVE ROLL-ON ANTI-PERSPI-
RANT

DETERGEX CLEANSER
(Pharmaseal)

Alkaline detergent containing:
  Sodium phosphates * ... approx. 80%
  Sodium carbonate * ... approx. 20%
  Anionic wetting agent

Conc. of 1 oz/gal has pH of approx. 11

DETER-SAN
Disinfectant, deodorant, sanitizer
(United Chemical Co., Inc.)

n-Alkyl (60% C14, 30% C16, 5% C12,
  5% C18) dimethyl benzyl ammonium chloride * 2.5%
n-Alkyl (50% C12, 30% C14, 17% C16,
  3% C18) dimethyl ethyl benzyl ammonium chloride * 2.5%

                    '76 Ed.

DETIA GAS EX-B
Fumigant
(Research Products Co.)

Aluminum phosphide * 57%

DETIA PELLETS
Fumigant
(Research Products Co.)

Aluminum phosphide * 57%

DETIA TABLETS
Fumigant
(Research Products Co.)

Aluminum phosphide * 57%

DET-O-JET
Detergent and degreaser; industrial
(Alconox)

Potassium hydroxide *
Silicate of soda
Chlorine

DETOXIL POWDER
Laxative
(Fibertone)

Mucilaginous portion of Psyllium seed
  (Plantago ovata)
Dextrose
Whey

DETTOL GERMICIDE & ANTISEPTIC
(French, R. T.)

Castor oil soap
Terpineol *
p-Chloro-m-xylenol .... >5%
Water 68%
Isopropyl alcohol 16.4%

DEVASTATE 1 NON-SELECTIVE WEED KILLER, PL

See PL DEVASTATE 1 NON-SE-
LECTIVE WEED KILLER

DeVILBISS INHALANT
Steam vaporizer inhalant
(DeVilbiss)

Propylene glycol .... approx. 95%
Methyl salicylate * .... approx. 2%
Eucalyptus oil * .... approx. 2%
Menthol approx.1%

DeVILBISS VAP-O-CLEAN
Steam vaporizer cleaner
(DeVilbiss)

Citric acid (1/2 gm.) .... approx. 49%
Dextrose-corn syrup solids . approx. 49%
Hydrogenated vegetable oil   approx. 2%

DEVOID
Total weed killer; industrial use
(Puritan Chem. Co.)

Petroleum distillate * 90.11%
Bromacil (5-Bromo-3-sec-butyl-6-
  methyluracil) 1.50%
Pentachlorophenol 0.80%
Other chlorophenols 0.09%

DEVRINOL (2-E, 50 WP)
Herbicide
(Stauffer)

Devrinol (N,N-Diethyl-2-(1-naphthaleny-
loxy)propionamide)

DE-WAX-ER
(Uncle Sam)

Synthetic detergent *
Sodium metasilicate
Potassium hydroxide *
Water

DEWITT'S ABSORBENT RUB
(DeWitt International)

Green soap (NF) 11.64%
Camphor 1.63%
Menthol * 1.63%
Pine tar soap (2.78%) 0.87%
Methyl salicylate 0.71%
Oil of wormwood 0.60%
Oil of sassafras synthetic 0.54%
Orthophenylphenol 0.54%
Benzocaine 0.48%
Oleoresin capsicum 0.03%
Isopropanol alcohol ...... 75.00% v/v

DEWITT'S ALERTACAPS
(DeWitt International)

Each capsule:
  Caffeine * .... 250 mg.

Starred ingredients (*) may be responsible for major toxic effects; consult Section II.

DEWITT'S ANTACID POWDER
(DeWitt International)

Each 4 gm.:
Magnesium trisilicate	1.24 gm.
Sodium bicarbonate (275 mg. sodium per teaspoonful)	1.00 gm.
Aluminum hydroxide (dried gel)	0.60 gm.
Magnesium carbonate (heavy)	0.40 gm.

DEWITT'S BABY COUGH SYRUP
(DeWitt International)

Each teaspoonful:
Glycerin	599.11 mg.
Ammonium chloride	22.17 mg.
Glycyrrhiza extract	2.17 mg.

DEWITT'S CALAMINE LOTION
(DeWitt International)

Calamine	7.12%
Zinc oxide	7.12%

DEWITT'S CAMPHOR SPIRITS
(DeWitt International)

Camphor *	10%
Alcohol	84% v/v

DEWITT'S CLINOMINT TOOTHPASTE
(DeWitt International)

Sodium monofluorophosphate *	0.76%

DEWITT'S COLD CAPSULES
(DeWitt International)

Each capsule:
Belladonna alkaloid salts	0.160 mg.
Atropine sulfate	0.024 mg.
Scopolamine hydrobromide	0.014 mg.
Hyoscyamine sulfate	0.122 mg.
Chlorpheniramine maleate	1.000 mg.
Pheniramine maleate	12.500 mg.
Phenylpropanolamine hydrochloride *	50.000 mg.

DEWITT'S COLD SORE LOTION
(DeWitt International)

Alcohol	90.00% v/v
Camphor *	3.65%
Benzoin	1.17%
Phenol	0.29%
Menthol	0.29%

DEWITT'S DAILY MULTI VITAMINS
(DeWitt International)

Each tablet:
Vitamin A	5000 units
Vitamin D	400 units
Plus multivitamins	

DEWITT'S FLOWAWAY TABLETS
(DeWitt International)

Each tablet:
Potassium nitrate *	170.0 mg.
Uva Ursi (1-3) gran. ext.	97.5 mg.
Buchu leaves (1-4) gran. ext.	24.4 mg.
Caffeine	19.5 mg.

DEWITT'S GUMZOR
(DeWitt International)

Alcohol	22% v/v
Benzocaine	5.6%
Benzyl alcohol	2.3%
Myrrh powder	1.2%

DEWITT'S HTO MANZAN REGULAR
(DeWitt International)

Tannic acid	1.5%
Benzocaine	1.0%
Allantoin	0.5%
Phenol	0.5%
Ephedrine HCl	0.2%
Menthol	0.2%

DEWITT'S HTO MANZAN STAINLESS
(DeWitt International)

Zinc oxide *	10.00%
Benzocaine	1.00%
Phenol	0.50%
Allantoin	0.50%
Ephedrine HCl	0.19%

DEWITT'S JOGGERS LOTION
(DeWitt International)

Green soap (N.F.)	11.64%
Camphor	1.63%
Menthol *	1.63%
Pine tar soap (2.78%)	0.87%
Methyl salicylate	0.71%
Oil of wormwood	0.60%
Oil of sassafras synthetic	0.54%
Orthophenylphenol	0.54%
Benzocaine	0.48%
Oleoresin capsicum	0.03%
Isopropanol alcohol	75% v/v

DEWITT'S KOFF BALLS
(DeWitt International)

Each capsule:
Dextromethorphan hydrobromide *	15 mg.
Benzocaine	3 mg.

DEWITT'S MULTI VITAMIN WITH IRON
(DeWitt International)

Each tablet:
Vitamin A	5000 units
Vitamin D	400 units
Iron (Ferrous fumarate)	18.0 mg.
Plus multivitamins	

DEWITT'S OIL FOR EAR USE
(DeWitt International)

Each 10 drops:
Camphor *	1.5 mg.
Menthol	0.8 mg.
Cajeput oil	4.6 mg.
Thyme oil	4.6 mg.

DEWITT'S PENGUIN FEET TREAT CREAM
(DeWitt International)

Water	85.64%
Allantoin	0.18%
Vee Gum H-V	0.36%
Triethanolamine	1.66%
Stearic acid flakes	3.71%
Isopropyl myristate	2.97%
Lanolin	2.14%
Chloroxylenol	0.37%
Propylene glycol	2.23%
Menthol	0.37%
Lavender oil 35-38%	0.18%
Green color 1%	0.19%

DEWITT'S PILLS
(DeWitt International)

Each tablet:
Salicylamide *	108.2 mg.
Potassium nitrate	56.4 mg.
Uva Ursi	32.4 mg.
Buchu leaves	7.8 mg.
Caffeine	6.5 mg.

DEWITT'S PYRINYL
(DeWitt International)

Pyrethrins	0.2%
Piperonyl butoxide (technical)	20.0%
Deodorized Kerosene	0.8%

DEWITT'S TEETHING LOTION
(DeWitt International)

Alcohol	22.0% v/v
Benzocaine	5.6%
Benzyl alcohol	2.3%
Myrrh powder	1.2%

DEWITT'S TERPIN HYDRATE WITH DM
(DeWitt International)

Each 5 ml.:
Dextromethorphan hydrobromide *	10 mg.
Terpin hydrate	85 mg.
Alcohol	42% v/v

Starred ingredients (*) may be responsible for major toxic effects; consult Section II.

DEWITT'S THERA-M VITAMIN
(DeWitt International)

Each tablet:
Vitamin A (acetate) ...... 10,000 IU
Vitamin D (Ergocalciferol) . 400 IU
Iodine, elemental (as potassium iodide) .... 0.15 mg.
Iron (as ferrous sulfate) .... 12.00 mg.
Plus multivitamins and minerals

DEWITT'S THROAT LOZENGES
(DeWitt International)

Each lozenge:
Dextromethorphan
hydrobromide * .... 5.0 mg.
Phenylephrine hydrochloride 2.5 mg.
Glyceryl guaiacolate .... 12.5 mg.
Benzocaine .... 10.0 mg.
Chlorpheniramine maleate 1.0 mg.
Cetyl pyridinium chloride ... 2.0 mg.

DEWITT'S TOOTHACHE DROPS
(DeWitt International)

Oil of cloves 9.98%
Benzocaine 5.01%
Beechwood Creosote 4.83%

DEWITT'S WITCH HAZEL SALVE
(DeWitt International)

Ichthammol 10.00%
Phenol 0.50%
Benzocaine 0.25%
Witch hazel leaves 2.19%

DEXA-KLOR DUST

See DEXOL DEXA-KLOR DUST

DEXA-KLOR GRANULES

See DEXOL DEXA-KLOR GRANULES

DEXA-KLOR SOIL INSECT SPRAY

See DEXOL DEXA-KLOR SOIL INSECT SPRAY

DEXAMPEX CAPSULES 15 mg.
Central stimulant; narcolepsy treatment
(Lemmon Co.)

Each capsule:
Dextroamphetamine sulfate * . 15 mg.

DEXAMPEX (5 mg. & 10 mg.)
Central stimulant; narcolepsy treatment
(Lemmon Co.)

Each tablet:
Dextroamphetamine
sulfate * .... 5 mg.; 10 mg.

DEXATRIM CAPSULES
Appetite control
(Thompson Med.)

Each capsule:
Phenylpropanolamine HCl * . 50 mg.
Caffeine * .... 200 mg.

DEXEDRINE
Indicated for narcolepsy and exogenous obesity
(SK&F)

SPANSULES (each sustained release capsule):
Dextroamphetamine
sulfate * .... 5 mg.; 10 mg.;
or 15 mg.

TABLETS (each):
Dextroamphetamine sulfate * . 5 mg.

ELIXIR (each 5 ml.):
Dextroamphetamine sulfate * . 5 mg.
Alcohol 10%

DEXOL ACTI-DIONE PM ROSE FUNGICIDE
(Dexol)

Cycloheximide .... 0.027% w/w

DEXOL BENOMYL PLANT FUNGICIDE
(Dexol)

Benomyl 50%

DEXOL BORDEAUX MIXTURE
(Dexol)

Copper (expressed as metallic
copper) * 12.75%

DEXOL BORER-SOL
Insecticide; liquid
(Dexol)

Ethylene dichloride * 50%

DEXOL CALSUL DORMANT SPRAY
Dormant oil spray for use on shrubbery, roses, small plants, shade and fruit trees
(Dexol)

Mineral oil * 67.9%
Calcium polysulphide 1.0%

DEXOL CHLORDANE 45% TERMITE SPRAY
(Dexol)

Technical Chlordane * 45%
Deodorized Petroleum distillate * .. 50%

DEXOL CHLORDANE 73% TERMITE SPRAY
(Dexol)

Technical Chlordane * 73%
Deodorized Petroleum distillate * .. 22%

DEXOL COMPOST MAKER
(Dexol)

Available Phosphoric acid (from
phosphoric acid) * 18.5%
Calcium sulfate (derived from
gypsum) 11.4%
Sulfur (from elemental sulfur) 14.5%

DEXOL CONTACT WEED KILLER
Non selective herbicide - liquid
(Dexol)

Aromatic petroleum
hydrocarbons * 80.0%
Paraffinic & naphthenic
hydrocarbons 5.0%

DEXOL CYGON SYSTEMIC INSECTICIDE
(Dexol)

Dimethoate * 23.4%

DEXOL DEXA-KLOR DUST
(Dexol)

Bendiocarb * 1%

DEXOL DEXA-KLOR GRANULES
(Dexol)

Chlorpyrifos 0.5%

DEXOL DEXA-KLOR SOIL INSECT SPRAY
(Dexol)

Chlorpyrifos * 6.7%
Petroleum distillates * 76.8%

DEXOL DIAZINON INSECT SPRAY
(Dexol)

Diazinon * 25.0%
Aromatic petroleum derivative
solvent * 55.7%

DEXOL ENIDE LIQUID WEED CONTROL
(Dexol)

Diphenamid * .... 15.4% w/w

DEXOL ENIDE WEED CONTROL
(Dexol)

Diphenamid * .... 50% w/w

DEXOL EPTAM WEED CONTROL
(Dexol)

S-Ethyl dipropylthiocarbamate 2.3%

DEXOL FISHSOL FISH EMULSION
(Dexol)

Total Nitrogen: 5%
  Nitrate nitrogen 0.00%
  Ammoniacal Nitrogen 0.50%
  Other water soluble Nitrogen . 3.75%
  Water insoluble Nitrogen 0.75%

Available Phosphoric
  acid * 2%
Soluble Potash 2%
Chlorine .... not more than 6%

DEXOL GOPHER GASSER
(Dexol)

Toxic gas produced when burning:
  Sulfur dioxide *
  Nitrogen oxide *
  Carbon monoxide *

DEXOL IRONTONE
Soil nutrient
(Dexol)

Ferrous sulfate (Fe2O3) * 93%
  Iron expressed as metallic ... 18.6%

DEXOL KOPPERSOL MILDEW & FUNGUS SPRAY
(Dexol)

Copper oleate (copper as metallic,
  1.0%) * 11.0%
Ethylene dichloride 3.0%

DEXOL LAWN WEED KILLER
Herbicide
(Dexol)

Dimethylamine salt of 2-(2-methyl-
  4-chlorophenoxy) propionic acid 3.66%
Dimethylamine salt of 2,4-dichlo-
  rophenoxyacetic acid * 8.07%
Dimethylamine salt of Dicamba
  (3,6-Dichloro-o-anisic acid) 0.84%
Dimethylamine salts of related
  compounds 0.11%

DEXOL MALATHION (Liquid)
Insecticide
(Dexol)

Malathion * 50%
Xylene * 42%

DEXOL MANEB GARDEN FUNGICIDE
(Dexol)

Maneb * 80.0%

DEXOL MULTI PURPOSE SPRAY
Insecticide, fungicide
(Dexol)

Meta-Systox * 11.74%
Karathane 1.197%
Karathane + nitrooctyl + a mixture of 1-methylheptyl, 1-ethyl-
  hexyl and 1-propylpentyl
  isomers 0.083%

DEXOL RED SPIDER & MITE SPRAY
(Dexol)

Kelthane 0.046%

DEXOL ROOTSOL
For root-blocked sewers
(Dexol)

Copper sulfate * 96.5%

DEXOL ROOT STIMULATOR WITH VITAMIN B-1
(Dexol)

a-Naphthaleneacetic acid 0.1%

DEXOL ROSE & FLOWER DUST
Insecticide, fungicide and miticide
(Dexol)

Sevin * 5.00%
Kelthane 3.00%
Karathane 0.90%

DEXOL SOW-BUG and CUT WORM BAIT
Insecticide
(Dexol)

Carbaryl (1-Naphthyl N-
  methylcarbamate) * 5%

DEXOL SPIDER-sMITE
Insecticide; liquid
(Dexol)

Kelthane * 18.5%

DEXOL SPREADER STICKER
(Dexol)

Alkyl aryl polyoxy glycols *† 80%

†See Alkyl phenoxy polyethoxy ethanols

DEXOL STUMP REMOVER
(Dexol)

Potassium nitrate *

DEXOL SYSTEMIC GRANULES
Insecticide
(Dexol)

O,O-Diethyl S-(2-(ethylthio)ethyl)
  phosphorodithioate (Di-Syston) * 2%

DEXOL SYSTEMIC HOUSE PLANT INSECTICIDE
(Dexol)

Di-Syston * 2%

DEXOL TENDER LEAF HOUSE PLANT FOOD
(Dexol)

Total Nitrogen *† 10.00%
  Nitric nitrogen 1.5%
  Ammoniac nitrogen 8.5%
Available Phosphate (derived
  from aqua ammonium
  phosphate) * 10.00%
Potash (derived from potassium
  nitrate) * 5.00%
Chelated Iron (derived from sodium ferric diethylenetriamine
  pentaacetate) 0.10%
Chelated Zinc (derived from disodium zinc ethylenediamine
  tetraacetate dihydrate) 0.05%
Chelated Manganese (derived
  from disodium manganous ethylenediamine tetraacetate
  dihydrate) 0.05%
Sarsaponin 0.01%

†See Fertilizers, Section VI, General Formulations

DEXOL TENDER-LEAF PLANT SPRAY
Insecticide
(Dexol)

READY-TO-USE:
  Petroleum hydrocarbons 0.65%
  Nicotine, as alkaloid * 0.07%
  Triethanolamine 0.043%

CONCENTRATE:
  Petroleum hydrocarbons 42%
  Nicotine, as alkaloid * 5%
  Triethanolamine 2.1%

DEXOL TENDER LEAF PLANT STARTER
Plant stimulator with Vitamin B1
(Dexol)

a-Naphthalene acetic acid 10%

DEXOL TENDER LEAF WHITEFLY & MEALYBUG SPRAY
(Dexol)

Methoprene	0.100%
Decachlorobis	0.075%
Resmethrin	0.050%
Related compounds	0.007%

DEXOL THIRAM PLUS LAWN FUNGICIDE
(Dexol)

Cycloheximide	0.75% w/w
Thiram *	75.00% w/w

DEXOL TOMATO LIFE
Fruit set chemical; ready-to-use spray
(Dexol)

beta-Naphthoxyacetic acid ... 0.00325%

DEXOL TOMATO & VEGETABLE DUST
Insecticide-fungicide
(Dexol)

Sevin *	5.0%
Zineb	4.5%

DEXOL VAPAM SOIL AID
(Dexol)

Sodium methyldithiocarbamate
  (anhydrous) * 32.7%

DEXOL VEGETABLE GARDEN INSECT SPRAY
(Dexol)

Pyrethrins	0.02%
Piperonyl butoxide, technical	0.20%
Petroleum distillate	0.08%

DEXOL ZINEB GARDEN FUNGICIDE
(Dexol)

Zineb * 75%

DEXONE TABLETS
Adrenocortical steroid therapy
(Rowell)

Dexamethasone (USP)   0.5 mg.; 0.75 mg.;
                        1.5 mg.; 4 mg.

DEX-SALT TABLETS
(Columbia Med.)

Each tablet:
Sodium chloride *	7 gr.
Dextrose	3 gr.
Vitamin B1	1 mg.

DEXTRON-II AUTOMATIC TRANSMISSION FLUID
(Marathon Oil Co.)

Additive, containing Polymer, Dye, Boron, Sulfur, Phosphorus compounds	9%
Mineral oil	balance

DEXTROSTIX
Blood-glucose reagent strip
(Ames)

Glucose oxidase
Peroxidase
Tris (hydroxymethyl) aminomethane
Malonic acid
Malonic acid disodium salt
Diaminofluorene dihydrochloride
Ortho-tolidine dihydrochloride
Benzidene dihydrochloride

DEXTROTABS - LIME
(Cramer Products)

Dextrose	97.984%
Magnesium stearate	1.500%
Artificial citrus punch flavor 7438-SD	0.500%
FD & C Blue #1 - 38% Lake	0.008%
FD & C Yellow #5 - 38% Lake	0.008%

D-FEDA GYROCAPS & SYRUP
Oral decongestant
(Dooner Labs.)

Gyrocaps (each timed release capsule):
  Pseudoephedrine
    hydrochloride * .... 60 mg.

Syrup (each 5 ml.):
  Pseudoephedrine
    hydrochloride * .... 30 mg.

d-15 INSECT REPELLENT

See AMWAY d-15 INSECT REPELLENT

d-15 INSECT REPELLENT TOWELETTE

See AMWAY d-15 INSECT REPELLENT TOWELETTE

D-FILM
Soap film remover; industrial and institutional use
(Scientific International)

Ethylene diamine tetraacetic acid

d-FILM
Hard contact lens gel cleaner
(CooperVision Pharm.)

Poloxamer 407
Benzalkonium chloride	0.025%
Trisodium edetate	0.25%

D-5 TABLETS
Symptoms of congestive heart failure; veterinary
(Hart-Delta, Inc.)

Each tablet:
  Digitoxin * .... 0.5 mg.

'76 Ed.

D-F-T SPRAY
Flea and tick killer; deodorant spray for dogs and cats
(Carson Chemicals, Inc.)

Active ingred.:
Carbaryl *	2.50%
Pyrethrins	0.06%
Technical Piperonyl butoxide	0.60%
Butoxypolypropylene glycol	5.00%
Inert ingred. *†	91.84%

†*See* Isopropyl alcohol

DG-14
Concrete seal
(Lester Labs.)

Petroleum distillates *
Resins

'76 Ed.

DIABISMUL SUSPENSION
Antidiarrheal
(OJF)

Each 15 ml.:
Kaolin	2500 mg.
Pectin	80 mg.
Opium *	7 mg.

DIAFEN
Antihistaminic
(Riker Labs.)

Each tablet:
  Diphenylpyraline
    hydrochloride *† .... 2 mg.

'76 Ed.

†*See* Antihistaminics

DIAL DEODORANT SOAP
(Bar soap) - Gold, White, Almond and Sky blue
(Armour-Dial, Inc.)

Sodium soap	75-100%
Moisture (water)	10-25%
Glycerin	1-5%
Antimicrobial active	1-5%
Perfume	0.1-1%
Minor ingredients (total)	1-5%

Starred ingredients (*) may be responsible for major toxic effects; consult Section II.

DIAL LONG LASTING AEROSOL ANTIPERSPIRANT -
Unscented, Scented, Fresh
(Armour-Dial, Inc.)

Propellant A-46	50-75%
Aluminum chlorohydrate	10-25%
Isopropyl myristate/palmitate/ stearate	5-10%
Cyclomethicone	5-10%
Minor ingredients (total)	1-5%

DIALOG
Analgesic and antipyretic
(CIBA Pharmaceutical)

Each tablet:
Allobarbital *	15 mg.
Acetaminophen *	300 mg.

DIAL ROLL-ON ANTIPERSPIRANT -
Unscented and Scented
(Armour-Dial, Inc.)

Water	50-75%
Aluminum zirconium tetrachlorohydrex glycine active	10-25%
Minor ingredients (total)	10-25%

DIAL SHAMPOO - Gold, Balsam
(Armour-Dial, Inc.)

Moisture and volatile	75-100%
Sodium lauryl sulfate	10-25%
Lauramide DEA	1-5%
Minor ingredients (total)	1-5%

DIAMOND ANTISEPTICS
(Lilly, Eli)

Each tablet:
Mercury bichloride *	475 mg.

DIAMOND FINISH
Floor finish
(Hillyard Chem.)

Mineral spirits *

'76 Ed.

DIAMOND H CREOSOTE PRESERVATIVE
(Huggins)

Free carbon	1%
Coal tar distillates *	97%

DIAMOND H PINE OIL DISINFECTANT
(Huggins)

Anhydrous Soap	10%
Pine oil *	80%

DIAMOND SEAL
Floor seal
(Hillyard Chem.)

Mineral spirits *

'76 Ed.

DIAMOND SPAR
(Touraine Paints, Inc.)

Thinner*† and Drier*	48.2%
Non-volatile Polyhydric alcohol partially esterified with linolenic, oleic, linoleic, palmitic, and stearic acids (modified with tolylene diisocyanate)	41.4%
Non-volatile Soya alkyd resin	10.4%

'76 Ed.

†See Thinners, Section VI, General Formulations

DIAMULSIN IMPROVED
Antidiarrheal
(Vale)

Each fl. oz.:
Alcohol	5%
Opium (equiv. 60 min. opium camphorated) *	14.8 mg.
Bismuth subsalicylate	129.6 mg.
Zinc sulfocarbolate	64.8 mg.
Salol	16.2 mg.
Potassium citrate	259.2 mg.

Base:
Pectin
Kaolin

DIANABOL
Adjunctive therapy in osteoporosis
(CIBA Pharmaceutical)

Each tablet:
Methandrostenolone	2.5 mg.; 5 mg.

DIANE VON FURSTENBERG COSMETICS

Diane Von Furstenberg Inc.
Cosmetics & Fragrances Div.
745 Fifth Ave.
New York, N.Y. 10022

Phone: 212-753-1111

See COSMETICS, Section VI, General Formulations

DIANTROLE ANTISEPTIC CLEANER
(Multi-Clean Products)

Isopropyl alcohol	11.52%/wt.
Potassium salt of ortho-benzyl-para-chlorophenol	4.84%/wt.
Tetrasodium ethylene diamine tetraacetate	1.44%/wt.
Potassium oleate	1.03%/wt.
Chloro-ortho-phenylphenol	0.20%/wt.
Tetrapotassium pyrophosphate	3.09%/wt.

Triethanolamine dodecylbenzenesulfonate
Disodium-4-dodecylated oxydibenzenesulfonate
Green dye (Napthol Green B, National Aniline Co.)
Perfume
Water

'76 Ed.

DIAPAKARE POWDER
Diaper rash, prickly heat
(Paddock Labs.)

Hyamine (Diisobutyl cresoxy ethyl dimethyl benzyl ammonium chloride)	0.1%
Sodium bicarbonate	5.5%
Corn starch	qs ad

Perfume

DIAPARENE CRADOL EMULS
Seborrhea capitis
(Glenbrook Labs.)

Methylbenzethonium chloride *
Petroleum and lanolin base

DIAPARENE OINTMENT
Surface-active disinfectant
(Glenbrook Labs.)

Methylbenzethonium chloride	1:1000

DIAPARENE PERI-ANAL CREME
(Glenbrook Labs.)

Methylbenzethonium chloride	1:1000

Zinc oxide
Starch
Cod liver oil
Casein

DIAPARENE POWDER
Surface-active disinfectant
(Glenbrook Labs.)

Methylbenzethonium chloride	1:1000

DIAPER PURE
Diaper soak
(Boyle-Midway)

N-Alkyl dimethyl benzyl ammonium chloride	<1%

Cleaners (Borate*/Carbonate*) †

†*See* Borate salts and Sodium carbonate

Starred ingredients (*) may be responsible for major toxic effects; consult Section II.

DIAPER-SWEET
Diaper wash
(Staley)

A. E. Staley Mfg. Co.
2200 E. Eldorado St.
Decatur, Ill. 62525

Phone: 217-423-4411

DIAPREX OINTMENT
For skin irritation
(Moss, Belle)

Boric acid * 4.6%
Zinc oxide
Zinc stearate .... <6%
Balsam Peru
In a nonabsorbent base

DI-AP-TROL
Anorexiant
(Foy Labs.)

Each tablet:
    Phendimetrazine tartrate * .... 35 mg.

DIA-QUEL
Antidiarrheal
(Marion Labs.)

Each 5 ml.:
    Tincture of opium (equiv. to
        0.75 ml. of paregoric) * .... 0.03 ml.
    Homatropine methylbromide   0.15 mg.
    Pectin .... 24 mg.
    Alcohol .... 10%/vol.

DIARIN-5
Insecticide
(Industrial Fumigant)

Diazinon 0.5%
Piperonyl butoxide 0.261%
Pyrethrins 0.052%
Petroleum distillate * 99.187%

DIA-SOL (SPRAY)
*Foot rot and ringworm treatment in
    cattle and sheep, and thrush in horses*
(Bio-Ceutic)

Dichlorophene 10.0%
p-Chloro-m-cresol 0.5%

DIASTAY
Antidiarrheal
(Elder)

Each tablet:
    Bismuth subgallate .... 120.0 mg.
    Kaolin .... 120.0 mg.
    Pectin .... 15.0 mg.
    Zinc phenolsulfonate * ..... 15.0 mg.
    Powdered Opium * .... 1.2 mg.

DIASTIX
Urine glucose reagent strip
(Ames)

Glucose oxidase
Peroxidase
Potassium iodide
FD & C Blue
Citrate buffer

DIATROL TABLETS
Antidiarrheal
(Clapp, Otis)

Pectin
Calcium carbonate

DIAZI-TROL, SPRAY-TROL BRAND

See SPRAY-TROL BRAND DIAZI-TROL

DIBAC
*Concentrated liquid sanitizer and deo-
    dorizer*
(Diversey Wyandotte)

Sodium hypochlorite * 8.5%

DIBACTOL
Germicide
(Fine Organics, Inc.)

Myristyl dimethyl benzyl ammo-
    nium chloride * 100%

'76 Ed.

DI-BROCIDE-50
*Highly concentrated fogging insecti-
    cide; municipal and industrial use*
(Puritan Chem. Co.)

Active ingredients: 100%
    Aromatic petroleum distillate *
    Malathion *
    Naled (1,2-Dibromo-2,2-dichloroethyl
        dimethyl phosphate) *
    2,2-Dichlorovinyl dimethyl phosphate
        (DDVP) *

DIBROME SPOT FUMIGANT
Fumigant
(Industrial Fumigant)

Ethylene dibromide * 70%
Methyl bromide * 30%

DICAL-D WITH IRON, CAPSULES
Calcium, iron & vitamin therapy
(Abbott)

Each capsule:
    Dibasic Calcium phosphate ... 0.5 gm.
    Ergocalciferol (Vitamin D) ... 133 u.
    Iron pyrophosphate *† .... 87 mg.

†*See* Iron salts

DICARBOSIL
Antacid
(Norcliff Thayer)

Each tablet:
    Precipitated Calcium
        carbonate .... 500 mg.
    Sugar/Starch .... 714 mg.
    Peppermint flavoring .... <1%

DICHLOFENTHION, TECHNICAL
Insecticide, nematocide
(Mobil Chemical Co.)

Dichlofenthion (O-2,4-Dichloro-
    phenyl O,O-
    diethylphosphorothioate) * 95%

DICHLORON
Insecticide
(National Chemsearch)

Chlorpyrifos (O,O-Diethyl O-(3,-
    5,6-trichloro-2-
    pyridyl)phosphorothioate) 3.00%
2,2-Dichlorovinyl dimethyl
    phosphate 2.60%
Related compounds 0.20%
Aromatic petroleum derivative
    solvent * 90.00%

DICKEY'S OLD RELIABLE EYE WASH
(Dickey)

Dickey Drug Co.
1009 West State St.
Bristol, Va. 24201

Phone: 703-669-1116

DICKINSON'S WITCH HAZEL
(Dickinson, E.E.)

Alcohol 14%

DICODID BITARTRATE TABLETS
Narcotic analgesic
(Knoll Pharm.)

Each tablet:
    Hydrocodone bitartrate * ...... 5 mg.

DICOHIST
Antitussive, antihistaminic
(Wesley Pharm.)

Each fl. oz.:
    Dextromethorphan .... 30 mg.
    Pyrilamine maleate * .... 75 mg.
    Ammonium chloride .... 8 gr.
    Sodium citrate .... 24 gr.
    Glycerin and Sugar .... q.s.

DICUMAROL TABLETS
Anticoagulant
(Abbott)

Each tablet:
Bishydroxycoumarin *   25 mg.; 50 mg.;
       or 100 mg.

DIDEE SCENT
Diaper pail deodorant; perfumed block
(Curran)

Paradichlorobenzene *

'76 Ed.

DIDREX
Appetite depressant
(Upjohn)

Each tablet:
Benzphetamine
hydrochloride * .. 25 mg.; or 50 mg.

DIE-FLY, SUPER, SUGAR-BASE FLY-KILLER

See SUPER DIE-FLY SUGAR-BASE
     FLY-KILLER

DIESEL CHIEF
Diesel engine fuel
(Texaco Inc.; Texaco Canada Ltd.)

Kerosine-type petroleum hydrocarbons *

DIESEL MEDIC
Automotive smoke suppressant
(Radiator)

Petroleum distillates *

'76 Ed.

DIETAC ONCE-A-DAY MAXIMUM STRENGTH DIET-AID CAPSULES
(MenJ Labs.)

Each capsule:
Phenylpropanolamine HCl * .. 75 mg.

DIETAC PRE-MEAL DIET-AID DROPS
(MenJ Labs.)

Each 0.2 ml.:
Phenylpropanolamine HCl * .. 25 mg.

DIETAC 12-HOUR DIET-AID CAPSULES
(MenJ Labs.)

Each capsule:
Phenylpropanolamine HCl * . 50 mg.
Caffeine .... 200 mg.

DIETAC TWICE-A-DAY MAXIMUM STRENGTH DIET-AID CAPSULES
(MenJ Labs.)

Each tablet:
Phenylpropanolamine HCl *   37.5 mg.

DIET-TRIM TABLETS
(Pharmex)

Each tablet:
Carboxymethylcellulose ..... 7 1/2 gr.
Phenylpropanolamine * ..... 25 mg.
Benzocaine

DIET-TUSS
Cough syrup
(Approved Pharm.)

Each fl. oz.:
D-Methorphan * .... 30 mg.
Combined amount: .... 80 mg.
    Thenylpyramine HCl *
    Pyrilamine maleate *
Sodium salicylate * .... 200 mg.
Sodium citrate .... 600 mg.
Ammonium chloride .... 100 mg.
Terpin hydrate
Menthol
Aromatics

'76 Ed.

DIFFICULT STAINS
Cleaning fluid
(Albatross Chem.)

1,1,1-Trichloroethane *
Sovasol No. 4 .... <10%

DIFFUSOR SPRAY CONCENTRATE
Insecticide; institutional and industrial use
(Puritan Chem. Co.)

Petroleum distillate * 98.1%
N-Octyl bicycloheptene
    dicarboximide 1.0%
Technical Piperonyl butoxide 0.6%
Pyrethrins 0.3%

DIFUSO (Liquid)
Insecticide
(Tanglefoot)

Pyrethrins
Piperonyl butoxide tech.
Petroleum distillates *

DIF WALLPAPER STRIPPER
(Zinsser, Wm., & Co.)

Dipropylene glycol monomethyl
    ether * 13.6%
Biodegradable Detergent 13.6%
a-Amylase 1.0%
Water 71.8%

DI-GAS
Stops mildew and musty odors
(Chester Chem.)

Paraformaldehyde * 95%

'76 Ed.

DIGIFORTIS KAPSEALS
Cardiac stimulant
(Parke-Davis)

Each Kapseal:
Digitalis (U.S.P.) * .... 0.1 gm.

DIGITOXIN TABLETS
Cardiac stimulant
(Abbott)

Each tablet:
Digitoxin * .... 0.1 mg.

DIGRESS
Commercial laundry bleach
(Diversey Wyandotte)

Trichloroisocyanuric acid *

DIHYCON
Anticonvulsant, slow release
(CMC Research Div.)

ADULT (each capsule):
Diphenylhydantoin * .... 250 mg.

PEDIATRIC (each capsule):
Diphenylhydantoin * .... 125 mg.

DI-ISOPACIN
Antituberculosis combination
(CMC Research Div.)

Each tablet:
Buffered Para-aminosalicylic
    acid * .... 0.75 gm.
Isoniazid .... 25 mg.

DIJA CLEAN
Liquid detergent
(Kay Chem. Co.)

Anionic detergent * 10-25%
Propylene glycol 1-10%
Opacifier .... trace

DIKE
Radiator stop leak
(Conklin Co.)

Methyl alcohol *

DI-KILL, PL

See PL DI-KILL

DILAC
Liquid acid cleaner
(Diversey Wyandotte)

Phosphoric acid *

DILANTIN INFATABS
Anticonvulsant
(Parke-Davis)

Each tablet:
    Phenytoin * .... 50 mg.

DILANTIN SUSPENSION
Anticonvulsant
(Parke-Davis)

Each 5 cc:
    Phenytoin * .... 30 mg. & 125 mg.

DILANTIN W/ PHENOBARBITAL
Anticonvulsant with sedative
(Parke-Davis)

Each Kapseal:
    Dilantin (Phenytoin
      sodium) .... 100 mg.
    Phenobarbital * ..... 16 mg.; 32 mg.

DILAUDID HYDROCHLORIDE COUGH SYRUP
(Knoll Pharm.)

Each 5 ml.:
    Hydromorphone HCl * ...... 1 mg.
    Guaifenesin .... 100 mg.
    Alcohol 5%

DILAUDID HYDROCHLORIDE RECTAL SUPPOSITORIES
Narcotic analgesic
(Knoll Pharm.)

Each suppository:
    Hydromorphone HCl * .... 3 mg.
    Colloidal Silica 1%
    Cocoa butter base

DILAUDID HYDROCHLORIDE TABLETS
Narcotic analgesic
(Knoll Pharm.)

Each tablet:
    Hydromorphone
      HCl * .... 1 mg., 2 mg.,
                  3 mg., and 4 mg.

DILOR ELIXIR
For relief of acute bronchial asthma
(Savage Labs.)

Each 15 ml.:
    Dyphylline * .... 160 mg.

DILOR-G TABLETS AND LIQUID
Bronchodilator-expectorant
(Savage Labs.)

Each tablet:
    Dyphylline * .... 200 mg.
    Guaifenesin (USP) .... 200 mg.

Each tsp. (5 ml.):
    Dyphylline * .... 100 mg.
    Guaifenesin (USP) .... 100 mg.

DILOR TABLETS
For relief of acute bronchial asthma
(Savage Labs.)

Each tablet:
    Dyphylline * .... 200 mg.; 400 mg.

DIMACID
Antacid
(Clapp, Otis)

Magnesium carbonate
Calcium carbonate

DIMACOL
Decongestant, expectorant, cough suppressant
(Robins)

Each capsule or 5 ml.:
    Pseudoephedrine hydrochlo-
      ride, NF * .... 30 mg.
    Dextromethorphan hydrobro-
      mide, NF * .... 15 mg.
    Guaifenesin, NF .... 100 mg.
    Alcohol (liquid) 4.75%

DIMENSION SHAMPOO, CONCENTRATED GEL
(Lever Bros.)

Water 40-55%
Triethanolamine lauryl sulfate * 15-25%
Ethyl alcohol 5-15%
Corn syrup 5-15%
Cocoamide monoethanolamine .. 3-7%
Triethanolamine 1-5%
Polydimethyl siloxane .... <2%
Hydroxypropyl methylcellulose . <2%
Acrylic carboxy resin .... <2%
Lactic acid .... <1%
Cationic cellulose .... <1%
Perfume .... <1%
Sodium hydroxymethane
    sulfonate .... <1%
Colorants .... trace

DIMENSION SHAMPOO, LIQUID
(Lever Bros.)

Water 40-55%
Triethanolamine lauryl sulfate * 15-25%
Corn syrup 15-25%
Ethyl alcohol 5-15%
Cocoamide monoethanolamine .. 1-5%
Triethanolamine 1-5%
Polydimethyl siloxane .... <2%
Acrylic carboxy resin .... <1%
Cationic cellulose .... <1%
Perfume .... <1%
Lactic acid .... <1%
Hydroxypropyl methylcellulose . <1%
Sodium hydroxymethane
    sulfonate .... <1%
Colorants .... trace

DIMETANE (TABLETS, EXTENTABS, ELIXIR)
Antihistamine
(Robins)

Tablets (each):
    Brompheniramine maleate,
      USP * .... 4 mg.

Extentabs (each):
    Brompheniramine ma-
      leate, USP * .... 8 mg.; 12 mg.

Elixir (each 5 ml.):
    Brompheniramine maleate,
      USP .... 2 mg.
    Alcohol 3%

DIMETANE EXPECTORANT
Antihistaminic, decongestant, antitussive
(Robins)

Each 5 ml.:
    Brompheniramine maleate,
      USP .... 2 mg.
    Guaifenesin, USP .... 100 mg.
    Phenylephrine hydrochloride,
      USP .... 5 mg.
    Phenylpropanolamine hydro-
      chloride, USP * .... 5 mg.
    Alcohol 3.5%

DIMETANE EXPECTORANT-DC
Antihistaminic, decongestant, antitussive
(Robins)

Each 5 ml.:
    Brompheniramine maleate,
      USP .... 2 mg.
    Guaifenesin, USP .... 100 mg.
    Phenylephrine hydrochloride,
      USP .... 5 mg.
    Phenylpropanolamine hydro-
      chloride, USP * .... 5 mg.
    Codeine phosphate, USP * ... 10 mg.
    Alcohol 3.5%

DIMETAPP EXTENTABS
Antihistamine, nasal decongestant
(Robins)

Each tablet:
Brompheniramine maleate,
USP * .... 12 mg.
Phenylephrine hydrochloride,
USP * .... 15 mg.
Phenylpropanolamine hydro-
chloride, USP * .... 15 mg.

DI-MOLD POWDER
Removes and retards mildew
(Chester Chem.)

Sodium pentachlorophenate * 3.4%
Sodium salts of other chlorophenols 0.6%

'76 Ed.

DINOXOL
Herbicide
(Amchem)

2,4-Dichlorophenoxyacetic acid, butoxy ethanol ester * 31.6%
2,4,5-Trichlorophenoxyacetic acid,
butoxy ethanol ester * 30.3%

DINOXOL 64
Herbicide
(Amchem)

2,4-Dichlorophenoxyacetic acid, butoxy ethanol ester * 42.2%
2,4,5-Trichlorophenoxyacetic acid,
butoxy ethanol ester * 20.1%

DI-O-CIDE
Residual insecticide
(Midland Labs.)

Active ingredients: 100%
Refined Mineral oil
Aromatic petroleum derivative
solvent *
Methoxychlor, technical
O,O-Diethyl O-(2-isopropyl-4-methyl-6-
pyrimidinyl) phosphorothioate (Dia-
zinon) *

DI-O-GEST
Antacid powder and tablets
(Am. Pharmaceutical)

Magnesium carbonate
Calcium carbonate
Colloidal Kaolin
Tricalcium phosphate
Sodium bicarbonate
Bismuth subcarbonate
Papain
Diastase

DIO-HIST SYRUP
Antihistamine compound syrup
(Approved Pharm.)

Each fl. oz.:
D-Methorphan * .... 30 mg.
Thenylpyramine
hydrochloride * .... 80 mg.
Phenylephrine HCl * .... 20 mg.
Sodium citrate
Ammonium chloride
Antimony
Potassium tartrate .... 1/24 gr.
Menthol
Aromatics
Alcohol 1%

'76 Ed.

DIOMEDICONE
Stool softener
(Medicone)

Each tablet:
Dioctyl sodium sulfosuccinate
USP * .... 50 mg.

DIOSATE CAPSULES
Stool softener
(Towne, Paulsen)

Each capsule:
Dioctyl sodium sulfo-
succinate N.F. * .. 100 mg.; 250 mg.

DIOSTATE D TABLETS
Dietary supplement
(Upjohn)

3 tablets contain:
Vitamin D .... 400 I.U.
Calcium .... 343 mg.
Phosphorus .... 265 mg.

DIOSUX
Laxative; stool softener
(Jenkins Labs.)

Each tablet:
Dioctyl sodium sulfosuccinate * 60 mg.

DIOTHANE OINTMENT
Anesthetic, emollient
(Merrell Dow)

Diperodon 1%
8-Quinolinol benzoate salt
(preservative) 0.1%
Base:
Petrolatum
Propylene glycol
Sorbitan sesquioleate

DIOXY WEED KILLER

See CHEMFORM DIOXY WEED
KILLER

DIPEPSITOL
Digestant antacid
(VB)

Bismuth subcarbonate
Pepsin
Sodium bicarbonate
Cascara

DIPHENADRIL COUGH SYRUP
(Vitarine)

Each 30 cc:
Diphenhydramine
hydrochloride * .... 75 mg.
Ammonium chloride .... 750 mg.
Sodium citrate .... 300 mg.
Menthol .... 6 mg.
Alcohol (by vol.) 5%

DIPHEN-EX
Expectorant
(Columbia Med.)

Each fl. oz.:
Diphenhydramine HCl * ..... 80 mg.
Chloroform .... 2 gr.
Alcohol 5%

DI-PHOS-E
Insecticide
(Hub States)

Ronnel (O,O-Dimethyl O-(2,4,5
trichlorophenyl)phosphoro-
thioate) 9.81%
2,2-Dichlorovinyl dimethyl
phosphate 9.81%
Chlorinated terphenyl (58.5%
chlorine) 21.00%
Xylene * 54.66%

'76 Ed.

DIP IT
Coffee stain remover
(Economics)

Sodium phosphate *
Sodium silicate
Sodium perborate *
Synthetic wetting agent

DIP-n-DRI
Cold water soap
(Alconox)

Ester of Sodium isothionate

DIP-N-STRIP
Tank degreaser
(Holcomb)

Caustic soda * .... >10%

'76 Ed.

DIPPIT
Solution used to harden a transparency positive
(Polaroid Corp.)

Isopropanol 50% *
Stannic chloride (heavy
  metal with a pH of 1) *   small amount

DIPPITY-DO SETTING GEL & LOTION
(Gillette Co., Personal Care Div.)

The Gillette Co., Personal Care Div., Boston, Mass. 02199 will receive collect phone calls from poison control centers or physicians asking for emergency toxicological information about the company's products.

Phone: 617-421-7000

DIRENE, DR. NAYLOR'S
See DR. NAYLOR'S DIRENE

DIRGE
Residual insecticide
(Puritan Chem. Co.)

Petroleum distillate *	99.184%
O,O-Diethyl O-(2-isopropyl-6-methyl-4-pyrimidinyl)phosphorothioate	0.500%
N-Octyl bicycloheptene dicarboximide	0.166%
Technical Piperonyl butoxide	0.100%
Pyrethrins	0.050%

DIRIDONE TABLETS
Urinary anesthetic and antiseptic
(Premo)

Each tablet:
  Phenazopyridine HCl * ...... 100 mg.

'76 Ed.

DIRTEX ALL PURPOSE CLEANER, LIQUID (CONCENTRATE)
See LIQUID DIRTEX ALL PURPOSE CLEANER (CONCENTRATE)

DIRTEX CLEANER, SPRAY (AEROSOL PACK)
See SPRAY DIRTEX CLEANER (AEROSOL PACK)

DIRTEX CLEANER FOR WALLS & FLOORS (POWDER)
(Savogran)

Pyrophosphates	<20%
Sesquicarbonate of soda *	<90%

DIRYL POWDER
Insecticide - veterinary
(Pitman-Moore)

Carbaryl *	5.0%
Pyrethrins	0.1%
Technical Piperonyl butoxide	1.0%

DISANTHROL CAPSULES
Laxative
(Lannett)

Each capsule:
Dioctyl sodium sulfosuccinate *	100 mg.
Casanthranol *	30 mg.

DI-SECT
Insecticide
(National Chemsearch)

Deodorized Kerosene	30.00%
Aromatic petroleum solvents *	50.00%
2-(1-Methylethoxy)phenol methylcarbamate *	4.00%
2,2-Dichlorovinyl dimethyl phosphate	0.93%
Related compounds	0.07%

DISH DROPS
See AMWAY DISH DROPS

DISH MAGIC
Liquid dishwashing detergent
(Consolidated Chem., Inc.)

Alkyl aryl sulfonate *
Other detergents

DISHMATE
Automatic dishwasher detergent
(Calgon Corp., Commercial Div.)

Caustic soda *
Complex phosphates *
Dichloroisocyanurate *
Soda ash *

DISHWASHER "all"
Powder automatic dishwashing detergent
(Lever Bros.)

Sodium polyphosphates *	40-50%
Chlorinated orthophosphates	20-30%
Water	15-20%
Sodium silicates	10-20%
Nonionic detergent	1-5%
Sodium sulfate	0-5%
Monostearyl acid phosphate	trace
Perfume	trace
Colorants	trace

DISHWASHER "all" (Low Phosphate)
Powder automatic dishwashing detergent
(Lever Bros.)

Sodium polyphosphates *	20-30%
Chlorinated orthophosphates *	20-30%
Sodium sulfate	15-25%
Sodium silicates	10-20%
Water	10-15%
Nonionic detergent	1-5%
Monostearyl acid phosphate	trace
Perfume	trace
Colorants	trace

DISINALL
Disinfectant, sanitizer, deodorizer concentrate; industrial and institutional use
(Scientific International)

n-Alkyl (50% C12, 30% C14, 17% C16, 3% C18) dimethyl ethyl benzyl ammonium chloride *	5.0%
n-Alkyl (60% C14, 30% C16, 5% C12, 5% C18) dimethyl benzyl ammonium chloride *	5.0%

DISINALL CLEANER
Germicidal cleaner; institutional use
(Scientific International)

N-Alkyl (60% C14, 30% C16, 5% C12, 5% C18) dimethyl benzyl ammonium chlorides *	1.5%
Anhydrous Sodium metasilicate *	3.5%
Ethylenediaminetetraacetic acid	1.0%
Inert ingredients:	94.0%
Non-ionic detergents *	
Phosphate builders	
Wetting and chelating agents	
Perfume	
Dye	
Water	

DISIPAL
For symptomatic relief in Parkinson's disease
(Riker Labs.)

Each tablet:
Orphenadrine HCl (2-Dimethylaminoethyl 2-methylbenzhydryl ether hydrochloride) *	50 mg.

'76 Ed.

DISOLAN CAPSULES
Treatment of constipation
(Lannett)

Each capsule:
Dioctyl sodium sulfosuccinate *	100 mg.
Phenolphthalein	65 mg.

DISOLAN FORTE CAPSULES
Treatment of constipation
(Lannett)

Each capsule:
Casanthranol *	30 mg.
Sodium carboxymethylcellulose	400 mg.
Dioctyl sodium sulfosuccinate *	100 mg.

Starred ingredients (*) may be responsible for major toxic effects; consult Section II.

DISONATE
Stool softener
(Lannett)

Capsules:
Dioctyl sodium
　sulfosuccinate * .... 60 mg.; 100 mg.;
　　　　　　　　　　　or 240 mg.

Liquid (each 5 ml.):
　Dioctyl sodium sulfosuccinate　　10 mg.

Syrup (each 5 ml.):
　Dioctyl sodium sulfosuccinate　　20 mg.

DISOPHROL CHRONOTAB TABLETS
For nasal congestion
(Schering)

Each tablet:
Disomer (Dexbromphenira-
　mine maleate) ....　6 mg.
d-Isoephedrine sulfate * ..... 120 mg.

DISOPLEX CAPSULES
Treatment of constipation
(Lannett)

Each capsule:
Dioctyl sodium
　sulfosuccinate * .... 100 mg.
Sodium
　carboxymethylcellulose .... 400 mg.

DISPEL
Insecticide - control of household insects
(ABCO, Inc.)

Technical Piperonyl butoxide ..　0.261%
Pyrethrins ....　0.052%
Petroleum distillate * ....　99.687%

DIS-SAN
Detergent-disinfectant-deodorant-sanitizer
(ABCO, Inc.)

n-Alkyl (60% C14, 30% C16, 5%
　C12, 5% C18) dimethyl benzyl
　ammonium chlorides * ......　2.56%
n-Alkyl (68% C12, 32% C14) di-
　methyl ethylbenzyl ammonium
　chlorides * ....　2.56%
Sodium metasilicate
　(anhydrous) * ....　2.40%
Tetrasodium　ethylenediamine
　tetraacetate ....　1.00%
Phosphoric acid ....　0.2495%
Essential oils ....　0.2495%

DI-SYSTON
Insecticide
(Mobay Chemical Corp.)

Disulfoton (O,O-Diethyl S-(2-
　(ethylthio)ethyl) phosphorodithioate) *

DITHANE A-40
Fungicide
(Rohm and Haas)

Nabam (Disodium ethylene
　bisdithiocarbamate) * ....　93%
Inerts ....　7%

DITHANE D-14
Fungicide
(Rohm and Haas)

Nabam (Disodium ethylene
　bisdithiocarbamate) * ....　22%
Inerts ....　78%

DITHANE M-22
Fungicide
(Rohm and Haas)

Maneb (Manganese ethylene
　bisdithiocarbamate) * ...　80%
Inerts ....　20%

DITHANE M-22 SPECIAL
Fungicide
(Rohm and Haas)

Maneb (Manganese ethylene bisdi-
　thiocarbamate with ZnSO4) * ...　80%
Inerts ....　20%

DITHANE M-45
Fungicide
(Rohm and Haas)

Coordination product of Zinc ion &
　manganese ethylene
　bisdithiocarbamate *† ....　80%
Inerts ....　20%

†*See* Maneb and Zineb

DITOX 25
Highly concentrated fogging insecticide; municipal and industrial use
(Puritan Chem. Co.)

Active ingredients: ....　100%
　Aromatic petroleum distillate *
　Malathion *
　Naled　(1,2-Dibromo-2,2-dichloroethyl
　　dimethyl phosphate) *
　2,2-Dichlorovinyl dimethyl phosphate
　　(DDVP) *

DI-TOX E
Insecticide
(Hub States)

O,O-Diethyl　O-(3,4,6-trichloro-2-
　pyridyl)phosphorothioate .....　12.31%
2,2-Dichlorovinyl dimethyl
　phosphate * ....　11.45%
Related compounds ....　0.86%
Xylene * ....　70.38%

'76 Ed.

DIUPRES-250 COMPRESSED TABLETS
Antihypertensive agent
(MSD)

Each tablet:
Chlorothiazide * ....　250 mg.
Reserpine ....　0.125 mg.

DIUPRES-500 COMPRESSED TABLETS
Antihypertensive agent
(MSD)

Each tablet:
Chlorothiazide * ....　500 mg.
Reserpine ....　0.125 mg.

DIURIL
Diuretic/antihypertensive
(MSD)

Each tablet:
Chlorothiazide * .. 250 mg. or 500 mg.

DIVERSEY WYANDOTTE OVEN CLEANER AND DEGREASER
(Diversey Wyandotte)

Potassium hydroxide *
Synthetic detergents

DIVERSOL CX WITH ARODYNE
Sanitizer-cleaner
(Diversey Wyandotte)

Sodium hypochlorite * ....　3.25%
Sodium phosphate (expressed as
　Na3PO412H2O) * ....　91.71%
Potassium permanganate ....　0.01%
Sodium lauryl sulfate ....　0.04%

DIZAN POWDER
Anthelmintic for dogs
(Elanco Prod.)

Each teaspoonful (8.3 gm.):
Dithiazanine iodide * ....　200 mg.

DIZAN TABLETS
Anthelmintic for dogs
(Elanco Prod.)

Each tablet:
Dithiazanine iodide *　10 mg.; 50 mg.;
　　　　　　　　　　　100 mg.; 200 mg.

DIZMISS (C.T. PINK; CHEWABLE, FLAVORED)
Antinauseant
(Bowman Pharm.)

Each tablet:
Meclizine hydrochloride * .... 25 mg.

D-K
Diuretic
(Friendly Labs.)

Buchu
Sodium nitrate *
Ext. Buchu
Aloes *
Capsicum *
Ext. Juniper
Ext. Uva ursi
Ext. Stone root
Oleoresin
Potassium nitrate *

D-K-NO-MOR CARBOLINEUM POULTRY MITE KILLER
(Hilltop)

Anthracene oil (Carbolineum) * .. 100%

'76 Ed.

DK-80 WEED KILLER
Herbicide
(National Chemsearch)

Sodium arsenite *

DL HAND CLEANERS (CREAM)
(DL Skin Care Products)

Saponified alkanolamide and alkali oleates
Polyoxyethylene alcoholic biodegradable detergents
Mineral spirits (narrow
cut) * .... approx. 40%
Skin moisturizers - glycol type and lubricants - organic
Mineral oil

DOAK PHARMACAL SKIN CARE PRODUCTS

Doak Pharmacal Co., Inc.
700 Shames Dr.
Westbury, N.Y. 11590

Phone: 516-333-7222

See COSMETICS, Section VI, General
Formulations

DOCTATE 300
Stool softener
(Glaxo Inc.)

Each tablet:
Docusate sodium * .... 300 mg.

DOCTATE-P
Stool softener - stimulant laxative
(Glaxo Inc.)

Each capsule:
Docusate sodium * .... 60 mg.
Danthron .... 40 mg.

DOCTIENT HC SUPPOSITORIES
(Suppositoria Labs.)

Each suppository:
Hydrocortisone acetate .... 10 mg.
Cod liver oil
Lanolin
Zinc oxide
Bismuth subgallate
Benzocaine
Resorcin *

DOCTIENT SUPPOSITORIES
(Suppositoria Labs.)

Cod liver oil
Lanolin
Zinc oxide
Bismuth subgallate
Balsam Peru *
Benzocaine
Resorcin *

DOC-TYL-ATE
Stool softener
(Cameron Medical Corp.)

Each capsule:
Dioctyl sodium
sulfosuccinate * .... 100 mg.

DOCTYLAX TABLETS
Laxative
(Approved Pharm.)

Each tablet:
Dioctyl sodium
sulfosuccinate * .... 100 mg.
Acetophenolisatin .... 2 mg.
Prune conc. .... 3/4 gr.

'76 Ed.

DOG CHECK
Dog repellent
(Nott)

Pyridine 3.90%
Citral 0.09%
Oil of mustard 0.01%

DOG SHIELD
Dog repellent
(Medical Supply Co.)

Capsaicin (derived from oleoresin of
capsicum) 0.35%

'76 Ed.

DOGZOFF (Aerosol)
Dog repellent
(Bohlender Plant Chem.)

Allyl isothiocyanate 1.54%
Creosote * 7.7%
Petroleum *†
Rosin oil

'76 Ed.

†*See* Petroleum distillate

DOGZOFF (Liquid)
Dog repellent
(Bohlender Plant Chem.)

Allyl isothiocyanate 2.00%
Creosote * 10.00%
Petroleum *†
Rosin oil

'76 Ed.

†*See* Petroleum distillate

DOLANEX ELIXIR
Analgesic
(Lannett)

Each 5 ml.:
Acetaminophen * .... 325 mg.
Alcohol 23%

DOLAN'S NON-GRAIN RAISING STAIN
(Dolan, V.J.)

Methanol * .... >5%

'76 Ed.

DOLCIN TABLETS
Antirheumatic
(Dolcin)

Aspirin (Acetylsalicylic acid) *
Calcium succinate

DOLCOMIST
Insecticide
(Dolge)

Combined amount: 90-99%
Aliphatic petroleum hydrocarbons *
Aromatic petroleum hydrocarbons *
Piperonyl butoxide 0.5-0.9%
Pyrethrins 0.2-0.4%
Essential oils .... trace

DOLCOMIST-XL
Insecticide
(Dolge)

Combined amount: 90-97%
Aliphatic petroleum hydrocarbons *
Aromatic petroleum hydrocarbons *
Piperonyl butoxide 3-4%
Pyrethrins 0.2-0.6%
Essential oils .... trace

DOLCO PINE
Disinfectant
(Dolge)

Pine oil * 75-80%
Soap .... approx. 10%

DOLEX CREAM
Analgesic
(International Chem.)

Menthol 5%
Methyl salicylate * 10%
Lanolin 25%
Petrolatum 60%

'76 Ed.

DOLEX LIQUID
Analgesic
(International Chem.)

Menthol	5%
Methyl salicylate *	15%
Isopropyl alcohol	50%
Aqua q.s.	30%

'76 Ed.

DOLEX TABLETS
Analgesic
(International Chem.)

Each tablet:
N-Acetyl-p-aminophenol * ...... 5 gr.

'76 Ed.

DOLGE E.W.T. AMINE TYPE 2,4-D WEED KILLER
(Dolge)

Diethanolamine 2,4-
dichlorophenoxyacetate * 49.6%

DOLGE FOGGING INSECTICIDE MALATHION
(Dolge)

Mineral seal oil *	70-80%
Malathion	3-4%
Beta-butoxy-beta'-thiocyano-di-ethyl ether	1-2%
Petroleum distillate *	15-20%

DOLOR PLUS
Analgesic
(Geriatric Pharm.)

Each tablet:
Aspirin *	230 mg.
Acetaminophen *	230 mg.
Caffeine	30 mg.
Butabarbital sodium	8 mg.

DOLTHANE SEALER & FINISH
Floor varnish
(Dolge)

Mineral spirits *

DOMEBORO POWDER PACKETS AND TABLETS
Externally; inflammatory skin conditions
(Dome)

Aluminum sulfate
Calcium acetate

1 or 2 packets of 2.2 gm. or 1 or 2 tablets dissolved in a pint of water makes a Burow's solution

DOMEFORM-HC CREME (1/2%)
(Dome)

Microdispersed Hydrocortisone alcohol	0.5%
Iodochlorhydroxyquin	3.0%

Acid pH vehicle:
Oil-in-water, emulsion-type creme containing a buffered solution of Aluminum acetate

DOME-PASTE BANDAGE
For leg ulcers
(Dome)

Glycerine
Zinc oxide
Gelatine paste
Calamine

DOMERINE
Medicated shampoo
(Dome)

Salicylic acid *	2%
Allantoin	0.2%

Surface-active wetting agents

DOMOL
Bath and shower oil
(Dome)

Isopropyl sebacate
Isopropyl myristate
Mineral oil

DOMOSO
Topical solution to reduce acute swelling due to trauma in dogs and horses; veterinary
(Syntex Agribusiness)

Dimethyl sulfoxide	90%

In water

DOMOSO GEL
Topical gel to reduce acute swelling due to trauma in horses; veterinary
(Syntex Agribusiness)

Dimethyl sulfoxide	90%

Base:
Carbopol 934
Disodium edetate
Sodium hydroxide and/or Hydrochloric acid to adjust pH

DONABARB
Sedative and antispasmodic
(Elder)

Each tablet:
Phenobarbital *	1/4 gr.
Powdered extract Belladonna leaves *	1/6 gr.

DONDRIL
Cough tablets
(Whitehall Labs.)

d-Methorphan HBr *
Phenylephrine HCl *
Chlorpheniramine maleate *
Glyceryl guaiacolate

DONNABARB
Controlling pyloric spasm and vomiting in colic
(Jenkins Labs.)

Each tablet:
Phenobarbital *	1/4 gr.
Extract of Belladonna (total alkaloids 0.00156 gr.) *	1/8 gr.

DONNACIN ELIXIR & TABLETS
Anticholinergic, relaxant
(Pharmex)

Phenobarbital *	16.20 mg.
Hyoscyamine sulfate	0.0104 mg.
Atropine sulfate	0.0104 mg.
Hyoscine hydrobromide	0.00065 mg.
Alcohol	23%

DONNAFED, JR.
Coryza, rhinitis, asthmatic conditions
(Jenkins Labs.)

Each tablet:
Ephedrine hydrochloride	1/16 gr.
Extract Belladonna (total alkaloids, 0.0006 gr.)	1/20 gr.
Salicylamide	1 1/4 gr.

DONNAGEL
Antidiarrheal
(Robins)

Each 30 ml.:
Kaolin (USP)	6.0000 gm.
Pectin (USP)	142.8000 mg.
Hyoscyamine sulfate (USP)	0.1037 mg.
Atropine sulfate (USP)	0.0194 mg.
Scopolamine hydrobromide (USP)	0.0065 mg.
Sodium benzoate, NF (preservative)	60.0000 mg.
Alcohol	3.8%

DONNAGEL-PG
Antidiarrheal
(Robins)

Each 30 ml.:
Kaolin (USP)	6.0000 gm.
Pectin (USP)	142.8000 mg.
Hyoscyamine sulfate (USP)	0.1037 mg.
Atropine sulfate (USP)	0.0194 mg.
Scopolamine hydrobromide (USP)	0.0065 mg.
Sodium benzoate, NF (preservative)	60.0000 mg.
Powdered Opium, USP (equiv. to paregoric 6 ml.)	24.0000 mg.
Alcohol	5%

Starred ingredients (*) may be responsible for major toxic effects; consult Section II.

DONNA-PHENAL ELIXIR
(Columbia Med.)

Each tsp.:
Atropine sulfate	0.0194 mg.
Hyoscyamine sulfate	0.1037 mg.
Hyoscyine HBr	0.0065 mg.
Phenobarbital	16.2 mg.

DONNATAL (CAPSULES, ELIXIR, TABLETS)
Sedative, antispasmodic
(Robins)

Each capsule, tablet or 5 ml.:
Hyoscyamine sulfate	0.1037 mg.
Atropine sulfate	0.0194 mg.
Hyoscine hydrobromide	0.0065 mg.
Phenobarbital *	16.2 mg.
Alcohol (Elixir)	23%

DONNATAL EXTENTABS
Antispasmodic & sedative
(Robins)

Each tablet:
Phenobarbital (USP) *	48.6000 mg.
Hyoscyamine sulfate (USP) *	0.3111 mg.
Atropine sulfate (USP)	0.0582 mg.
Scopolamine hydrobromide (USP)	0.0195 mg.

DONNATAL No. 2
Antispasmodic & sedative
(Robins)

Each tablet:
Phenobarbital (USP) *	32.4000 mg.
Hyoscyamine sulfate (USP) *	0.1037 mg.
Atropine sulfate (USP)	0.0194 mg.
Scopolamine hydrobromide (USP)	0.0065 mg.

DONPHEN
Anticholinergic-sedative
(Lemmon Co.)

Each tablet:
Phenobarbital *	15 mg.
Hyoscyamine sulfate	0.1 mg.
Atropine sulfate	0.02 mg.
Scopolamine hydrobromide	6 mcg.

DON'T
Discourages thumb sucking & nail biting
(Commerce Drug)

Sucrate octa acetate
Isopropyl alcohol *

DOOR-EASE
Stainless stick lubricant
(American Grease Stick)
(Marketed by: Atlas Supply Co.; Balkamp, Inc.; Chrysler Corp., MoPar Div.; Chrysler Corp., Parts Div.)

Paraffin wax	24.75%
Microcrystalline wax	15.00%
Carnauba wax	2.25%
Mineral oil	36.00%
Tallow, buffing grade	5.00%
Zinc naphthenate	1.00%
Anti-chek wax (petro)	16.00%

DOOR-EASE DRIPLESS OIL
Lubricant
(American Grease Stick)

Naphtha (Aliphatic petroleum) *	80%
Combined amount:	15%
Mineral oil	
Aluminum stearate	
Sorbitan mono-oleate	5%

DORBANE TABLETS
Laxative
(Riker Labs.)

Each tablet:
Danthron (1,8-Dihydroxyanthraquinone)	75 mg.

'76 Ed.

DORBANTYL
For constipation
(Riker Labs.)

Each capsule:
Danthron (1,8-Dihydroxyanthraquinone)	25 mg.
Dioctyl sodium sulfosuccinate *	50 mg.

'76 Ed.

DORBANTYL FORTE
For constipation
(Riker Labs.)

Each capsule:
Danthron (1,8-Dihydroxyanthraquinone)	50 mg.
Dioctyl sodium sulfosuccinate *	100 mg.

'76 Ed.

DORCOL PEDIATRIC COUGH SYRUP
Decongestant, expectorant, antitussive
(Dorsey Labs.)

Each 5 ml.:
Dextromethorphan hydrobromide *	5.00 mg.
Phenylpropanolamine hydrochloride *	6.25 mg.
Guaifenesin	50.00 mg.
Alcohol	5%

DOREX COFFEE POT CLEANER
(Dorex, Inc.)

Sodium perborate tetrahydrate *	50%
Sodium sulfate	49%
Triton DF-12	1%

DOREX ICE MACHINE CLEANER
(Dorex, Inc.)

Sulfamic acid *	98.000%
O'B-Hibit	2.000%
Dye	0.001%

DOREX MINERAL SOLVENT
(Dorex, Inc.)

Hydroxyacetic acid	18.8%
Tergitol 15-S-9	0.5%
Water	80.7%

DOREX TAP & LINE CLEANER
(Dorex, Inc.)

Sodium silicate	4.5%
Potassium hydroxide *	31.1%
Water	64.4%

DORIDEN
Sedative
(USV)

Each tablet:
Glutethimide NF *	0.125 gm.; 0.25 gm. or 0.5 gm.

DORMA-REST SLEEP CAPSULES
(Pharmex)

Each capsule:
Methapyrilene HCl *	25 mg.
Scopolamine aminoxide HBr	0.2 mg.

DORME'
Antihistamine
(A.V.P. Pharmaceuticals)

Each capsule:
Promethazine hydrochloride *	12.5 mg., 25 mg., or 50 mg.

DORMUTOL CAPSULES
Sleep capsule
(Approved Pharm.)

Each capsule:
Methapyrilene HCl *	25 mg.
Scopolamine aminoxide hydrobromide *	0.20 mg.

'76 Ed.

DOROTHY GRAY BETTER-OFF FACIAL HAIR BLEACH
(Gray, D.)

Water
Hydrogen peroxide
Stearyl alcohol
Steareth-20
Mineral oil
Stearic acid
Phosphoric acid

DOROTHY GRAY COSMETICS

Dorothy Gray, Ltd.
Div. Lehn & Fink Products Group
225 Summit Ave.
Montvale, N.J. 07645

Phone: 201-573-5700

See COSMETICS, Section VI, General Formulations

DOUBLE DANDERINE
Anti-dandruff medication
(Lambda Inc.)

Benzalkonium chloride	0.2%
Perfume	
Alcohol	9.0%

DOUBLE FEATURE, COMMERCIAL

See INTEX COMMERCIAL DOUBLE FEATURE

DOUBLE-SAL
Analgesic, antipyretic
(Vale)

Each tablet:
Sodium salicylate *	648 mg.

DOUBLE-X VARNISH REMOVER
(Schalk)

Trisodium phosphate *
Sodium perborate *

'76 Ed.

DOUGH-BOY PROPHYLACTIC
(Reese Chem.)

Calomel (a mercury derivative) *	30%
Oxyquinoline benzoate	

DOUGLAS HYDRO FLOW DEFOAMER
To decrease foam in extractor cleaning machines' recovery tanks
(Scot Labs.; dist., Douglas Products)

Silicone emulsion	5–6%
Preservative	trace
Water	balance

DOUGLAS HYDRO FLOW TRAFFIC SPOTTER
Spot pretreatment for use before extraction shampooing
(Scot Labs.; dist., Douglas Products)

Gylcol ether	4–7%
Amphoteric surfactant	9–11%
Water	balance

DOVACET
Analgesic
(Vale)

Each capsule:
Dover's powder (represents 2.43 mg. opium)	24.3 mg.
Phenacetin *	129.6 mg.
Aspirin *	194.4 mg.
Caffeine	32.4 mg.

DOVALGIN TABLETS
Analgesic
(Moffet Inc.)

Each tablet:
Dover's powder	16 mg.
Salicylamide *	0.15 gm.
Phenacetin *	0.1 gm.
Caffeine	8 mg.

DOVAMIDE CAPSULES
Cold remedy
(Philips Roxane Labs.)

Each capsule:
Dover's powder (1/2 gr.) (powdered opium 3.24 mg.) *	32.4 mg.
Phenacetin *	97 mg.
Salicylamide *	194 mg.
Atropine sulfate	0.13 mg.
Caffeine	8.1 mg.
Camphor monobromated	16.2 mg.

DOVAMINE CAPSULES
(Premo)

Each capsule:
Dover's powder (1/20 gr. opium)	1/2 gr.
Methapyrilene HCl *	25 mg.
Salicylamide	3 gr.
Atropine sulfate	1/500 gr.
Caffeine	1/2 gr.
Camphor	1/4 gr.

'76 Ed.

DOVAPHEN
For relief of colds & influenza
(Jenkins Labs.)

Each tablet:
Dover's powder (opium 1.62 mg.)	16.2 mg.
Acetylsalicylic acid *	2 1/2 gr.
Acetophenetidin *	1 1/2 gr.
Caffeine alkaloid	1/8 gr.
Camphor monobromated	1/4 gr.
Atropine sulfate	1/1000 gr.

DOVAPHEN CAPSULES
Analgesic, antipyretic
(Jenkins Labs.)

Each capsule:
Dover's powder	16.2 mg.
Opium	1.62 mg.
Ipecac	1.62 mg.
Aspirin *	2 1/2 gr.
Phenacetin *	1 1/2 gr.
Caffeine	1/8 gr.
Atropine sulfate	1/1000 gr.

DOVAPHEN JR.
For discomforts of the common cold
(Jenkins Labs.)

Each tablet:
Dover's powder (opium 0.81 mg.) *	8.1 mg.
Acetophenetidin *	1/2 gr.
Atropine sulfate	1/4000 gr.
Salicylamide *	1/2 gr.
Caffeine	1/10 gr.

DOVE BEAUTY BAR
(Lever Bros.)

Acyl isethionate	45-55%
Fatty acids	15-25%
Sodium soap	10-15%
Water	5-10%
Sodium isethionate	1-5%
Anionic detergent	1-5%
Perfume	<2%
Sodium chloride	<2%
Titanium dioxide	<1%
Colorants	trace

DOVE LIQUID
Liquid dishwashing detergent
(Lever Bros.)

Water	50-60%
Anionic detergents	30-40%
Fatty alkanolamides	1-5%
Opacifier	0.5-5%
Perfume	<1%
Ethanol	<1%

DOVERCLIFF WHITE DUSTLESS CHALK
(American Crayon Co.)

This product bears the AP Seal issued by the Crayon, Water Color and Craft Institute, Inc. This seal certifies that the product contains no materials in sufficient quantities to be toxic or injurious to the human body even if ingested.

DOVERIN CAPSULES
Analgesic, antipyretic
(Lannett)

Each capsule:
Dover's powder	1/4 gr.
Phenacetin *	1 1/2 gr.
Aspirin *	2 gr.
Camphor monobromate	1/8 gr.
Caffeine	1/8 gr.
Atropine sulfate	1/500 gr.

Starred ingredients (*) may be responsible for major toxic effects; consult Section II.

DOVETS
Analgesic-antipyretic
(Wesley Pharm.)

Each tablet:
Dover's powder	15 mg.
Acetophenetidin *	2 1/2 gr.
Caffeine	1/8 gr.
Camphor	1/4 gr.

DOVOSAL (C.T. TAN, EMBOSSED)
Analgesic
(Bowman Pharm.)

Each tablet:
Dovers powder (opium content 1.62 mg.)	16.2 mg.
Aspirin	129.6 mg.
Camphor monobromated	16.2 mg.
Caffeine	8.1 mg.
Phenacetin	97.2 mg.

DOW BATHROOM CLEANER (Aerosol)
(Dow)

Sodium salt of o-phenylphenol	0.21%
Tetrasodium salt of ethylenediamine tetraacetic acid	2.78%
Detergents	0.38%
Glycol ethers	6.00%
Water	90.0%

DOW BROZONE
Soil fumigant
(Dow)

Methyl bromide *	68.6%
Chloropicrin *	1.4%

Inert ingred.:
Petroleum solvent	30%

DOW BRUSH KILLER 50-50
Herbicide
(Dow)

Active ingred.:
2,4-Dichlorophenoxyacetic acid, butyl esters *	28.7%
2,4,5-Trichlorophenoxyacetic acid, butyl esters *	27.9%
Inert ingred.:	43.4%
Emulsifiers	
Petroleum solvent *	

DOW BRUSH KILLER LV-4T
Herbicide
(Dow)

Active ingred.: 65.0%
2,4,5-Trichlorophenoxyacetic acid, isooctyl esters *	
Inert ingred.:	35.0%
Emulsifiers	
Petroleum solvent *	

DOW BRUSH KILLER LV2-2
Herbicide
(Dow)

Active ingred.:
2,4-Dichlorophenoxyacetic acid, isooctyl esters *	34.7%
2,4,5-Trichlorophenoxyacetic acid, isooctyl esters *	33.1%
Inert ingred.:	32.2%
Emulsifiers	
Petroleum solvent *	

DOW BRUSH KILLER T
Herbicide
(Dow)

Active ingred.: 56.4%
2,4,5-Trichlorophenoxyacetic acid, butyl esters *	
Inert ingred.:	43.6%
Emulsifiers	
Petroleum solvent *	

DOW BRUSH KILLER TX
Herbicide
(Dow)

Active ingred.: 69.2%
2,4,5-Trichlorophenoxyacetic acid, butoxy propyl esters *	
Inert ingred.:	31.8%
Emulsifiers	
Petroleum solvent *	

DOW BRUSH KILLER X
Herbicide
(Dow)

Active ingred.:
2,4-Dichlorophenoxyacetic acid, butoxy propyl esters *	36.0%
2,4,5-Trichlorophenoxyacetic acid, butoxy propyl esters *	34.1%
Inert ingred.:	29.9%
Emulsifiers	
Petroleum solvent *	

DOW BUTYL 400
Herbicide
(Dow)

2,4-Dichlorophenoxyacetic acid, butyl esters *	58.6%
Inerts:	41.4%
Principally Petroleum solvent *	

DOW CHEMICAL PRODUCTS

Dow Chemical U.S.A.
Midland, Michigan 48640

24-Hour Emergency Phone No.:
517-636-4400

DOW CORNING AQUARIUM SEALER
(Dow Corning Corp.)

Methyl polysiloxane	84.5%
Acetoxy functional siloxane (emits acetic acid upon exposure to moist air or water)	5.5%
Inert filler and pigment	10.0%

DOW CORNING BATHTUB CAULK
(Dow Corning Corp.)

Methyl polysiloxane	84.5%
Acetoxy functional siloxane (emits acetic acid upon exposure to moist air or water)	5.5%
Inert filler and pigment	10.0%

DOW CORNING SILICONE RUBBER SEALER
(Dow Corning Corp.)

Methyl polysiloxane	84.5%
Acetoxy functional siloxane (emits acetic acid upon exposure to moist air or water)	5.5%
Inert filler and pigment	10.0%

DOW CORNING TILE CLEANER AND PROTECTOR
(Dow Corning Corp.)

Acetate salt of amine functional polysiloxane	1.5%
Detergent *	7.5%
Ethylene glycol butyl ether	3.0%
Organic acid *	3.25%
Isopropyl alcohol	1.5%
Water	82.65%
Perfume, colorant and mineral acid	0.6%

DOW DMA-4
Herbicide
(Dow)

2,4-Dichlorophenoxyacetic acid, dimethylamine salt (2,4-dichlorophenoxyacetic acid equivalent 40.9%) *	49.3%

DOW DMA-6 WEED KILLER
Herbicide
(Dow)

Active ingred.: 69.5%
2,4-Dichlorophenoxyacetic acid, dimethylamine salt *	
Inert ingred.:	30.5%
Sequestering agent	
Water	

DOWFAX 3B2
Detergent
(Dow)

Solution of active ingredient in water	approx. 46%
Anionic surfactant *	

DOWFUME 75
Grain fumigant
(Dow)

Ethylene dichloride	70%
Carbon tetrachloride *	30%

DOWFUME C
Fumigant
(Dow)

Carbon tetrachloride *	81.3%
Carbon bisulfide	12.1%
Ethylene dibromide	6.6%

DOWFUME MC-2
Fumigant
(Dow)

Methyl bromide *	98%/wt.
Chloropicrin *	2%/wt.

DOWFUME MC-33
Fumigant
(Dow)

Methyl bromide *	67%/wt.
Chloropicrin *	33%/wt.

DOW GENERAL WEED KILLER
(Dow)

2-sec-Butyl-4,6-dinitrophenol *	55%
Inert ingred.:	45%
Primarily Toluene	

DOW-HEX SOLUTION
Post-harvest fungicide
(American Machinery Corp.)

Active ingred.:	23.98%
Sodium ortho-phenylphenate (anhydrous) (sodium ortho-phenylphenate tetrahydrate 34%) *	
Inert ingred.:	76.02%
Hexamethylenetetramine *	
Sodium hydroxide *	
Water	

DOW MCP AMINE WEEDKILLER
(Dow)

2-Methyl-4-chlorophenoxyacetic acid, dimethylamine salt (equiv. to 42.5% 2-methyl-4-chlorophenoxyacetic acid) *	52.1%

DOW MOSQUITO FOGGING CONCENTRATE
(Dow)

Active ingred.:	
Chlorpyrifos (O,O-Diethyl O-(3,-5,6-trichloro-2-pyridyl)phosphorothioate) *	61.5%
Aromatic petroleum derivative solvent *	34.5%
Inert ingred.:	
Related compounds in chlorpyrifos	4.0%

DOWNDUS MOP TREATMENT MATERIAL
(Uncle Sam)

Mineral seal oil *

DOWN & OUT
Insecticide
(Dyna Systems)

Pyrethrins	0.15%
Petroleum distillates *	63.04%
2-(1-Methylethoxy)phenol methylcarbamate *	1.00%
Technical Piperonyl butoxide	0.37%
N-Octyl bicycloheptene dicarboximide	0.37%
Petroleum distillate propellant	35.07%

DOWNY
Liquid fabric softener
(Procter & Gamble)

Water	75-100%
Ditallowdimethylammonium chloride	5-9%
Isopropanol	1-4%
Nonionic surfactant	1-4%
Minor ingredients, each	<1%

pH (undiluted) - 5.0-6.6

DOW OVEN CLEANER
(Aerosol)
(Dow)

Sodium hydroxide *	approx. 4%
Polyglycol ethers	10%
Alkanolamine	5%

DOWPER
(Dow)

Tetrachloroethylene (Perchlor) *	100.0%

DOWPER GOLDEN CS SOLVENT
(Dow)

Perchloroethylene *	98.35%
Petroleum surfactant	1.5%
Polyglycol	0.15%

DOWPON C IMPROVED GRASS KILLER
Herbicide
(Dow)

Active ingred.:	
2,2-Dichloropropionic acid, sodium salt *	46.7%
2,2-Dichloropropionic acid, magnesium salt	7.8%
Trichloroacetic acid, sodium salt *	30.6%
Inert ingred.:	
Related compounds in active ingredients	14.9%

DOWPON GRASS KILLER
(Dow)

Sodium 2,2-dichloropropionate *	85%

DOWPON M HERBICIDE
(Dow)

2,2-Dichloropropionic acid, sodium salt *	72.5%
2,2-Dichloropropionic acid, magnesium salt	12.0%
Inert ingred.:	15.5%
Related compounds	

DOW POTATO TOP KILLER
(Dow)

Active ingred.:	30.2%
2-sec-Butyl-4,6-dinitrophenol *	
Inert ingred.:	69.8%
Emulsifiers	
Petroleum solvents	

DOW PROFESSIONAL TURF INSECTICIDE
(Dow)

Active ingred.:	
Chlorpyrifos (O,O-Diethyl O-(3,5,6-trichloro-2-pyridyl)phosphorothioate) *	41.2%
Aromatic petroleum derivative solvent *	29.5%
Inert ingred.:	29.3%
Emulsifiers	
Chlorinated solvent *	

DOW SELECTIVE WEED KILLER
(Dow)

2-sec-Butyl-4,6-dinitrophenol, ammonium salt *	13.7%
Inert ingred.:	86.3%
Isopropanol	70.9%

DOW SODIUM TCA INHIBITED
Grass killer
(Dow)

Sodium trichloroacetate *	90%

DOWTHERM 209
Coolant for engines
(Dow)

Alkyl glycol alkyl ether *†	96.0%

†*See* Carbitol

DOWTHERM COOLING SYSTEM CONDITIONER
(Dow)

Water	approx. 80%
Inorganic salts *	approx. 20%
Organic salts	approx. 0.5%
Dye	approx. 0.1%

Starred ingredients (*) may be responsible for major toxic effects; consult Section II.

DOW WEED KILLER 4D
(Dow)

Active ingred.: 70.0%
  2,4-Dichlorophenoxyacetic acid, isooctyl
    esters *
Inert ingred.: 30.0%
  Emulsifiers
  Petroleum solvent *

DOWZENE
Veterinary anthelmintic
(Dow)

Piperazine 98%

DOWZENE 34
Insecticide
(Dow)

Piperazine monohydrochloride ... 44.1%

DOWZENE DHC (White)
Anthelmintic; veterinary
(Dow)

Piperazine dihydrochloride (piperazine equivalent 53.0%) 97.9%

DOXAN
Laxative
(Hoechst-Roussel)

Each tablet:
  Danthron .... 50 mg.
  Dioctyl sodium sulfosuccinate * 60 mg.

DOX BRUSH CLEANER
Paint brush cleaner
(Reliable Paste)

Approx. equal amounts of:
  Toluol *
  Acetone
  Methanol

DOXINATE
Fecal softener
(Hoechst-Roussel)

CAPSULES (each):
  Dioctyl sodium
    sulfosuccinate * .... 60 mg.; 240 mg.

PEDIATRIC DROPS SOLUTION:
  Dioctyl sodium sulfosuccinate * .. 5%

DOXYCHEL FOR ORAL SUSPENSION
Broad and medium spectrum antibiotic
(Rachelle Labs.)

Each bottle:
  Doxycycline monohydrate * . 300 mg.

DOXYCHEL HYCLATE
Broad and medium spectrum antibiotic
(Rachelle Labs.)

Each capsule:
  Doxycycline hyclate * 50 mg.; 100 mg.

D'PART INSECTICIDAL SPRAYS
(Fuld-Stalfort)

Piperonyl butoxide
Pyrethrum
Petroleum hydrocarbon *

                  '76 Ed.

D.P.O. DRAIN CLEANER
(Woodward-Wanger)

Sodium hydroxide *

                  '76 Ed.

D.P.S. DRAIN PIPE SOLVENT
(Navy Brand)

Potassium hydroxide * 45%

DRAFTITE CALK
(Gibson-Homans)

Linseed, soya oils .... >10%
Petroleum thinner 1-10%
Whiting .... >65%
Talc 1-10%

DRAGON 72% CHLORDANE SPRAY
Insecticide
(Dragon)

Chlordane 72%
Xylene * 21.9%

DRAGON FRUIT TREE SPRAY
Insecticide-fungicide
(Dragon)

Captan 7%
Malathion 5%
Methoxychlor 10%

DRAGON GARDEN WEED & GRASS PREVENTER
(Dragon)

Dacthal 5%

DRAGON LIQUID SEVIN SPRAY
Insecticide
(Dragon)

Carbaryl * 21.5%

DRAGON 50% MALATHION SPRAY
Insecticide
(Dragon)

Malathion * 50%
Xylene * 39.5%

DRAGON TOMATO DUST
Fungicide
(Dragon)

Zineb 5.0%

DRAGON TOMATO-VEGETABLE DUST
Fungicide-insecticide
(Dragon)

Carbaryl * 5%
Zineb 5%

DRAGON WEED BLASTER
(Dragon)

Sodium chlorate * 18.5%
Sodium metaborate 10.1%

DRAIN A-GO-GO
Liquid drain opener; industrial and institutional use
(Puro Co.)

Sulfuric acid *

DRAIN-AWAY LIQUID DRAIN OPENER
Industrial/institutional use
(Puro Co.)

Sulfuric acid *

DRAIN CLEAN
(Woodward-Wanger)

Sodium hydroxide *

                  '76 Ed.

DRAIN-E-ZE (Liquid)
Drain line opener
(Jancyn)

Caustic liquid * 25%

DRAIN-LAX
Drain cleaner
(Radiator)

Sulfuric acid *

                  '76 Ed.

DRAIN MATE LIQUID DRAIN CLEANER

See AMWAY DRAIN MATE LIQUID
DRAIN CLEANER

DRAIN-PEP, LIQUID

See LIQUID DRAIN-PEP

DRAINZ MARK II (Liquid)
Septic/cesspool cleaner and line opener
(Jancyn)

Caustic liquid * 45%

Starred ingredients (*) may be responsible for major toxic effects; consult Section II.

DRAMAMINE (LIQUID & TABLETS)
Antinauseant, antiemetic
(Searle, G.D., & Co.)

Liquid (each 4 ml.):
Dimenhydrinate * .... 12.5 mg.

Tablets (each):
Dimenhydrinate * .... 50 mg.

DRAMAMINE SUPPOSICONES
Antinauseant, antiemetic
(Searle, G.D., & Co.)

Each Supposicone:
Dimenhydrinate * .... 100 mg.
Esterified hydrogenated vegetable fatty
acid base

DRANO (GRANULAR)
Drain cleaner
(Drackett)

Sodium hydroxide * ... approx. 50%/wt.
Sodium nitrate .... approx. 35%/wt.
Sodium chloride
Aluminum particles

DRANO INSTANT PLUNGER
Drain cleaner, aerosol
(Drackett)

Dichlorodifluoromethane .... >80%
Dichlorotetrafluoroethane .... <10%
Hydrocarbon propellant .... <10%
Hexylene glycol .... <1%
Perfume

DRANO, KITCHEN (LIQUID)
See KITCHEN DRANO (LIQUID)

DRANO, LIQUID
See LIQUID DRANO

DRANO II (GRANULAR)
Drain cleaner
(Drackett)

Sodium hydroxide * ... approx. 50%/wt.
Sodium nitrate .... approx. 35%/wt.
Sodium chloride
Aluminum particles

DRAWS-A-LOT
(Carter's Ink)

Dyes
Humectant
Sodium benzoate
Glycol *†

'76 Ed.

†*See* Ethylene glycol

DR. CALDWELL'S SENNA LAXATIVE
(Glenbrook Labs.)

Alcohol 4.5%
Senna 7.0%
Peppermint oil
Syrup pepsin

DR. CARTER'S K & B TEA
Cathartic
(Brown Mfg.)

Senna leaves * 70 3/4%
Mandrake root * 2 3/4%
Aromatic herbs 26 1/2%

'76 Ed.

DR. DANIELS' ABSORBENT BLISTER
For horses and cattle
(Daniels, Dr. A.C.)

Red iodide mercury * 10%

DR. DANIELS' COLIC DROPS
For horses, colts, mules, cows
(Daniels, Dr. A.C.)

Nux vomica * 1-10%
Colocynth * 1-10%

DR. DANIELS' DANILAX
Liquid cathartic; veterinary
(Daniels, Dr. A.C.)

Phenolphthalein
Petrolatum

DR. DANIELS' DANIVOM TABLETS
For gastric irritation; veterinary
(Daniels, Dr. A.C.)

Cerium oxalate *
Bismuth subnitrate
Phenol *
Menthol *
Benzocaine

DR. DANIELS' EQUINE HEAVE POWDER
For temporary relief of certain respiratory conditions of horses
(Daniels, Dr. A.C.)

Powdered Nux vomica (Strychnine 0.06%) 5.0%
Arsenic trioxide * 1.0%
Powdered Lobelia * 2.0%
Powdered Strammonium 5.0%
Sodium thiosulfate tech. 14.25%
Sodium chloride 15.5%
Sodium bicarbonate 26.0%
Sodium sulfate tech. 6.25%
Camphor 1.5%
Licorice root 13.5%
Ammonium chloride 10.0%

DR. DANIELS' GALL SALVE
For harness galls, speed cracks and scratches
(Daniels, Dr. A.C.)

Ammoniated mercury * 0.5%
Carbolic acid .... <0.5%
Mutton tallow .... <0.5%
Salicylic acid .... <0.5%
Petrolatum

DR. DANIELS' GOLDEN LINIMENT
(Daniels, Dr. A.C.)

Capsicum
Oil turpentine *
Oil camphor *
Sassafras
Gum camphor *
Methyl salicylate *
Kerosene *

DR. DANIELS' HOOF DRESSING
(Daniels, Dr. A.C.)

Pine tar * .... <5%
Oil turpentine .... <5%
Coon oils

DR. DANIELS' HOOF OINTMENT AND SOFTENER
(Daniels, Dr. A.C.)

Ammoniated mercury * .... <0.5%
Carbolic acid .... <0.5%
Salicylic acid .... <0.5%
Rosin
Mutton tallow
Petrolatum

DR. DANIELS' HOPPLE CHAFE LOTION FOR HORSES
For chafing, minor cuts, galls, abrasions
(Daniels, Dr. A.C.)

Olive oil
Ether
Goulard's extract *

DR. DANIELS' LINIMENT POWDER
For horses and ponies
(Daniels, Dr. A.C.)

Borax *
Bicarbonate of soda
Castile soap
Oil camphor * 3%
Belladonna .... trace

DR. DANIELS' NEW WORM EXPELLER
Expels large roundworms (ascarids)
(Daniels, Dr. A.C.)

Each capsule:
Piperazine adipate
For cats .... 125 mg.
For puppies .... 250 mg.
For dogs .... 500 mg.

DR. DANIELS' SKIN OINTMENT
For skin irritations; veterinary
(Daniels, Dr. A.C.)

Benzocaine
Acid Salicylate *
Oil of wintergreen *
Carbolic acid *
Sulfur
Amber Petrolatum

DR. DANIELS' TAPEWORM TABLETS
Veterinary
(Daniels, Dr. A.C.)

Each tablet:
Arecoline hydrobromide * .... 1/8 gr.

DR. DANIELS' V-M CAPSULES
Veterinary
(Daniels, Dr. A.C.)

Brewers' yeast
Brewers' yeast extract
Dehydrated Lemon juice
Tricalcium phosphate

DR. DANIELS' WONDER LOTION
For skin injuries
(Daniels, Dr. A.C.)

Extract Oak bark
Alcohol .... 15%/v.

DREFT (Formula 1)
Granular laundry detergent
(Procter & Gamble)

Sodium sulfate 25-49%
Sodium carbonate 10-24%
Sodium silicate 10-24%
Sodium alkyl benzene sulfonate . 10-24%
Water 5-9%
Sodium perborate 1-4%
Sodium alkyl sulfate 1-4%
Minor ingredients, each .... trace

pH (1% solution) - 10.9 max.

DREFT (Formula 2)
Granular laundry detergent
(Procter & Gamble)

Complex sodium phosphates 25-49%
Sodium sulfate 25-49%
Sodium alkyl benzene sulfonate . 10-24%
Water 10-24%
Sodium silicate 5-9%
Sodium perborate 1-4%
Sodium soap 1-4%
Minor ingredients, each .... trace

pH (1% solution) - 10.9 max.

DRESSUP
Furniture polish aerosol
(Dolge)

Petroleum distillate * ..... approx. 50%
1,1,1-Trichloroethane * 30-35%
Isobutane/propane (50/50)
(propellant) 20%
Essential oils .... trace
White wax .... trace
Silicone .... trace

DREST (LIPID FREE HAIR DRESSING GEL)
Scalp treatment of dandruff, seborrhea & acne
(Dermik)

Benzalkonium chloride ..... 0.125% w/w
Alkyl isoquinolinium
bromides .... 0.15% w/w
S.D. Alcohol .... 14.1% w/w
In clear gel vehicle with Polyvinylpyrrolidone to control hair

DR. FENNER'S ANTISEPTIC OINTMENT
For skin burns and irritations
(Brown Mfg.)

Benzocaine
Origanum
Venice turpentine *† 3 9/10%
Oil of nutmeg
Sassafras 1%
Balsam of fir
Special base

†*See* Essential oils

'76 Ed.

DR. FENNER'S GOLDEN RELIEF
Carminative and rubefacient
(Brown Mfg.)

Each fl. oz.:
Alcohol 65%
Chloroform .... 5 m.
Turpentine * 17%
Gum myrrh
Aromatic oils
Ether .... 22 m.
Capsicum
Ammonia 4%
Gum guaiac

'76 Ed.

DR. FRED PALMER SKIN WHITENER #202
(Carson Products)

Petrolatum
Stearic acid
Propylene glycol
Cetyl alcohol
Polysorbate 61
Microcrystalline wax
Paraffin
Hydroquinone
Water
Citric acid
Sodium meta bisulfite
Methylparaben
Propylparaben
Fragrance

DR. FRED PALMER ULTRA BLEACH & TONE CREAM #203
(Carson Products)

Water
Glyceryl stearate
Glyceryl stearate & Isopropyl myristate, & Stearyl stearate
Propylene glycol
Petrolatum
Isopropyl myristate
Lanolin
Paraffin
Hydroquinone
Stearyl stearate
Fragrance
Citric acid
Sodium m-bisulfite
Sodium sulfite
Methylparaben
Propylparaben
FD & C Yellow #5

DR. HUBBARD'S SURFACE GERMICIDE & AIR DEODORIZER
(Hubbard, J.)

Alcohol * 69.30%
Mixture of: Thymol *, Oil lavender, Oil rosemary *, Oil pine, Terpinyl acetate, Oil eucalyptus *, 3,4,6-Trichlorophenol ... 1.58%

DRIAD POWDER PAINT
(Binney & Smith)

Soluble starches
Preservative
Non-toxic pigments

DRIFAB WATER REPELLENT SPRAY

See AMWAY DRIFAB WATER REPELLENT SPRAY

DRI-IT
Rinsing agent for machine dishwashing
(DuBois Chem.)

Nonionic surfactants
Isopropyl alcohol .... approx. 4%
Ethylenediaminetetraacetic acid type sequestrant

DRI KEM
Deodorizer for use in portable toilet holding tanks
(Thetford Corp.)

Paraformaldehyde *	80%
Sodium silico aluminate	10%
Inorganic phosphate	<5%
Perfume oil	<5%
Acid Blue #9	<5%

DRINOPHEN CAPSULES
Analgesic
(Lannett)

Each capsule:
Phenylpropanolamine HCl *	15 mg.
Acetylsalicylic acid *	230 mg.
Acetaminophen *	200 mg.

DRI ODO ROLL-ON ANTIPERSPIRANT
(Rawleigh)

Each 100 cc:
Chlorhydrol (Aluminum chlorhydroxide complex) *	18 gm.

'76 Ed.

DRIONE INSECTICIDE (DUST)
Indoors; dogs and cats
(Fairfield American)

Pyrethrins	1.0%
Piperonyl butoxide	10.0%
Amorphous Silica gel	40.0%
Petroleum distillate *	49.0%

DRIONE INSECTICIDE SPRAY (AEROSOL)
Indoor use
(Fairfield American)

Pyrethrins	0.1%
Piperonyl butoxide	1.0%
Silica gel	4.0%
Petroleum distillate *	4.9%
Propellant A-70	25.0%
Solvents *	65.0%

DRI-OUT
Moisture proofing agent; industrial maintenance
(Scientific International)

Petroleum distillate *

DRI-PHED EXPECTORANT WITH CODEINE
(Stayner)

Each 5 ml.:
Codeine phosphate *	10 mg.
Triprolidine HCl *	2 mg.
Pseudoephedrine HCl *	30 mg.
Guaifenesin	100 mg.
Sodium benzoate	0.1%
Methylparaben	0.1%

DRI-PHED SYRUP
(Stayner)

Each 5 ml.:
Triprolidine HCl *	1.25 mg.
Pseudoephedrine HCl *	30.00 mg.
Sodium benzoate	0.1%
Methylparaben	0.1%

DRI-PHED TABLETS
(Stayner)

Each tablet:
Triprolidine HCl *	2.5 mg.
Pseudoephedrine HCl *	60.0 mg.

DRISDOL
Antirachitic
(Winthrop Labs.)

Each drop:
Ergocalciferol (Vitamin D2)	250 units
Propylene glycol	

DRISDOL CAPSULES
For hypoparathyroidism and refractory rickets
(Winthrop Labs.)

Each capsule:
Vitamin D, USP (Ergocalciferol, USP)	50,000 units

DRI-SLIDE
Lubricant, penetrant, inhibitor, dry film lubricant
(Dri-Slide)

Molybdenum disulfide *
Light petroleum hydrocarbons and derivatives *

DRISTAN CAPSULES
Decongestant
(Whitehall Labs.)

Phenylephrine *
Chlorpheniramine *

DRISTAN COUGH FORMULA
Decongestant cough syrup
(Whitehall Labs.)

d-Methorphan HBr *
Chlorpheniramine maleate *
Phenylephrine HCl *
Sodium citrate
Glyceryl guaiacolate
Alcohol

DRISTAN INHALER
Nasal decongestant
(Whitehall Labs.)

Propylhexedrine *

DRISTAN NASAL MIST
Nasal decongestant
(Whitehall Labs.)

Phenylephrine HCl *
Pheniramine maleate *
Cetyl dimethyl benzyl ammonium chloride
Thimerosal

DRISTAN ROOM VAPORIZER
Nasal decongestant
(Whitehall Labs.)

Camphor *
Thymol *
Menthol *
Eucalyptol *
Dipropylene glycol
Triethylene glycol
Alcohol
Propellents

DRISTAN TABLETS
Analgesic-decongestant
(Whitehall Labs.)

Phenylephrine HCl *
Phenindamine tartrate *
Aspirin *
Caffeine

DRITEK
Carpet shampoo
(Sanitek)

Anionic surfactants (30% active) *	32.0%
Isopropanol	8.7%
Dipropylene glycol monomethyl ether (Cellosolve)	2.3%
Nonionic surfactant	0.9%
Tetrasodium pyrophosphate	trace
Water	balance

DRITZ TAILOR'S CHALK
(Scovill)

Clay (pure)
Vegetable dye coloring

DRIVE (Low Phosphate)
Powder laundry detergent
(Lever Bros.)

Sodium sulfate	15-45%
Sodium polyphosphates	20-30%
Anionic detergent	10-20%
Sodium silicate	5-15%
Water	5-10%
Sodium carbonate	0-5%
Cellulosic	<1%
Perfume	<1%
Optical dye	trace

DRIVE (Nonphosphate)
Powder laundry detergent
(Lever Bros.)

Sodium carbonate *	30-50%
Sodium sulfate	20-30%
Anionic detergent	15-25%
Sodium silicate	10-20%
Water	1-5%
Cellulosic	<1%
Perfume	<1%
Optical dye	<1%

DRIVE STAIN ERASER
Laundry pretreat stick
(Lever Bros.)

Sodium soap	30-50%
Fatty acids	30-40%
Sodium sulfate	20-40%
Water	5-10%
Nonionic detergent	5-10%
Sodium silicate	1-5%
Sodium chloride	<1%
Glycerol	<1%
Perfume	<1%
Caustic soda	<1%
EDTA	<1%
Colorant	<1%

DRIXORAL SUSTAINED-ACTION TABLETS
Nasal congestion
(Schering)

Each tablet:

Dexbrompheniramine maleate	6 mg.
d-Isoephedrine sulfate *	120 mg.

DRIZE M
Nasal decongestant
(Ascher, B.F.)

Each capsule:

Chlorpheniramine maleate	8 mg.
Phenylephrine hydrochloride *	20 mg.
Methscopolamine nitrate *	2.5 mg.

DRI-ZIT OIL & GREASE ABSORBENT
(Waverly Mineral Products Co.)

Aluminum-magnesium silicate	
Iron oxide	small amounts

DR. KILMER'S SWAMP ROOT
Laxative
(Lambda Inc.)

Extractives of:
Buchu leaves
Peppermint herb
Rhubarb root
Mandrake root *
Cape aloes *†
Scullcap leaves
Columbo root
Valerian root
Cinnamon
Oil of juniper *
Oil of birch *‡
Balsam copaiba
Balsam tolu
Venice turpentine

Alcohol	10 1/2%

†*See* Aloe
‡*See* Oil of sweet birch

DR. LYON'S TOOTH POWDER (REGULAR)
(Glenbrook Labs.)

Calcium carbonate

DR. MAKER'S MOUTH KOMFORT
Cold sores, fever blisters and chapped lips
(Oral Prophylactic Ass'n., Inc.)

Each fl. oz.:

Pectin	745.2 mg.
Bismuth sodium tartrate	486.0 mg.
	'76 Ed.

DR. MAYFIELD ARSONIC POWDER
For growth, scours; veterinary
(Dr. Mayfield Labs.)

Sodium arsanilate *	40%

DR. MAYFIELD PREMIX #3 POWDER
For growth, scours; veterinary
(Dr. Mayfield Labs.)

Sodium arsanilate *	10%

DR. NAYLOR'S ANTISEPTIC DUSTING POWDER
Veterinary
(Naylor)

Boric acid *	>10%
Talc	>10%
Thymol iodide	<1%
Tannic acid	<1%
Chlorothymol crystals	<1%
Oil camphor	<1%

DR. NAYLOR'S BLU-KOTE (Dauber Bottle or Spray Bomb)
Antiseptic for wounds; veterinary
(Naylor)

Acriflavine	<1%
Gentian violet	<1%
Urea	<10%
Glycerin	<10%
Isopropyl alcohol *	>10%
Sodium propionate	<10%
Sequestrene	<1%

DR. NAYLOR'S DEHORNING PASTE
Veterinary
(Naylor)

Glycerine	>10%
Iron oxide	<1%
Caustic soda (50%) *	>10%
Calcium hydroxide	>10%

DR. NAYLOR'S DIRENE
Intestinal antiseptic, antacid; veterinary
(Naylor)

Sulfaguanidine	<10%
Pectin	<10%
Aluminum hydroxide	<10%
Bismuth subnitrate	<10%
Catechu	<10%
Quebracho wood *	>10%
Carob flour	>10%
Kaolin	>10%

DR. NAYLOR'S LINITE
Veterinary
(Naylor)

Linseed oil	>10%
Turpentine *	>10%
Copper sulfate	<1%
Camphor, powd.	<1%
Phenol, 85% *	<10%
Kerosene *	>10%
Sulfuric acid, 66° *	<10%
Chloro-o-phenylphenol *	<10%
Dichlorophene tech.	<10%
Acetone	<10%

DR. NAYLOR'S MEDICATED TEAT DILATORS
Veterinary
(Naylor)

DILATOR MEDICATION:

Camphor *	>10%
Menthol	<10%
Eucalyptol *	>10%
Oils of Thyme, Clove, Thuja, Pine, Cedar leaf *	>10%
Sulfathiazole	<10%
Gentian violet	<1%
Ammonia (28%)	<1%
Castor oil	<10%
Methanol	>10%

ANTISEPTIC OINTMENT:

Petrolatum	>10%
Wax	>10%
Lanolin	>10%
Essential oils *	>10%
Color	trace

Starred ingredients (*) may be responsible for major toxic effects; consult Section II.

DR. NAYLOR'S MEDIGEN
For the appetite; veterinary
(Naylor)

Soda	>10%
Sodium sulphate	>10%
Salt *	>10%
Tricalcium phosphate	<10%
Potassium sulphate	<10%
Gentian	>10%
Colombo root	>10%
Cinchona root *	<10%
Ginger root	<10%
Cobalt	<1%
Nux vomica (Strychnine 1/2 gr. per oz. Medigen) *	5.75%

DR. NAYLOR'S RED-KOTE
(Dauber Bottle or Spray Bomb)
Antiseptic for wounds; veterinary
(Naylor)

Castor oil	>10%
Rosin	>10%
Linseed oil	>10%
Essential oils *	<10%
Hydroxyquinoline	<1%
Phenol crystals *	<10%
Biebrich scarlet red	<1%
Isopropyl alcohol	<10%

DR. NAYLOR'S STOP-A-LEAK
For cow's teats that leak milk; veterinary
(Naylor)

Ethyl acetate	>10%
Tannic acid	<10%
Iodine (7%) *	>10%
Ethyl cellulose	<10%

DR. NAYLOR'S UDDER BALM
Antiseptic ointment; veterinary
(Naylor)

Petrolatum	>10%
Lanolin	>10%
Wax	<10%
Essential oils *	<10%
Hydroxyquinoline	<1%
Color	trace

DR. NAYLOR'S UDDER LINIMENT
Veterinary
(Naylor)

Rice oil	>10%
Light mineral oil	>10%
Beta pine oil	<10%
Essential oils *	<10%
Thymol crystals	<1%
Titanium dioxide	<1%
Volclay bentonite	<10%
Color	trace

DRO BRUSHON PASTE
Insecticide
(Dro)

Malathion	2.5%
Chlordane, tech.	1.5%

'76 Ed.

DRO EMULSION KILLS ANTS
(Dro)

Tech. Chlordane	2%
Inert ingredients *	98%

'76 Ed.

DRO KILLS ROACHES
(Dro)

Petroleum distillates *
Malathion *
Chlordane, tech. *
Isobornyl thiocyanoacetate *
Other related terpenes

'76 Ed.

DRO'S NO. 49
Insecticide
(Dro)

Petroleum distillate *
Beta-butoxy-beta-thiocyano-diethyl ether *
Malathion *
Dieldrin *

'76 Ed.

DRO'S NO. 49 BOMB
Insecticide
(Dro)

O,O-Diethyl-O-(2-isopropyl-6-methyl-4-pyrimidinyl) thiophosphate	0.500%
Pyrethrins	0.100%
Piperonyl butoxide, tech.	0.250%
Petroleum distillate *	74.150%

'76 Ed.

DRO SPRAY COATING
Insecticide
(Dro)

Petroleum distillates *	70.913%
Malathion	2.500%
Chlordane, tech.	1.500%
Pyrethrins	0.025%
Piperonyl butoxide, tech.	0.062%

'76 Ed.

DR. PETER'S GOMOZO
Stimulant laxative
(Fahrney)

Each 30 ml.:
Senna fluid extract *	2 ml.
Water	
Alcohol	16%
Sucrose	
Caramel	

DR. PETTIT'S AMERICAN EYE SALVE
(Lambda Inc.)

Boric acid *	5%
White petrolatum	
Mineral oil	

DR. PIERCE'S A-NURIC TABLETS
Diuretic
(Lambda Inc.)

Powdered Buchu (as extract)	65 mg.
Powdered Couch grass (as extract)	65 mg.
Powdered Corn silk (as extract)	32.5 mg.
Powdered Hydrangea (as extract) *	32.5 mg.

DR. PIERCE'S GOLDEN MEDICAL DISCOVERY
Tonic, gastric stimulant
(Lambda Inc.)

Gentian
Berberis
Sanguinaria
Wild cherry bark
Stone root
Cascara
Stillingia

DR. PIERCE'S PLEASANT PELLETS
Laxative
(Lambda Inc.)

Stramonium (alkaloid 1/6000 gr.)
Podophyllin *
Resin jalap
Aloin *

DR. ROGERS' C-D DUST
Control of early and late blight, nail head rust, tomato fruit worm, cut worm and thrip
(Texas Phenothiazine Co.)

Tribasic Copper sulphate (copper-in basic copper sulphate-expressed as metallic) *	6%
Sevin (1-Naphthyl N-methyl-carbamate) *	5%

'76 Ed.

DR. ROGERS' CHLOR-DUST
Multi-purpose dust for gardens, lawns and farms
(Texas Phenothiazine Co.)

Technical Chlordane *	10.00%

'76 Ed.

Starred ingredients (*) may be responsible for major toxic effects; consult Section II.

DR. ROGERS' DARI-BEEF CATTLE DUST
Control of hornflies
(Texas Phenothiazine Co.)

Technical Methoxychlor	5.00%
Malathion	4.00%
Technical Piperonyl butoxide	1.00%
Pyrethrins	0.10%

'76 Ed.

DR. ROGERS' EZ-12 LINDANE CONCENTRATE
Insecticide
(Texas Phenothiazine Co.)

Xylene *	73.00%
Refined Petroleum oil	10.00%
Gamma isomer of benzene hexachloride from lindane	10.00%

'76 Ed.

DR. ROGERS' MALATHION-50
Insecticide for control of houseflies
(Texas Phenothiazine Co.)

Malathion *	50%
Xylene *	43%

'76 Ed.

DR. ROGERS' MALGORA SPRAY
Controls lice and ticks on beef cattle and goats
(Texas Phenothiazine Co.)

Malathion *	57%
Xylene *	28%

'76 Ed.

DR. ROGERS' MAL-PHENE
Kills ticks, lice, horn flies on beef cattle
(Texas Phenothiazine Co.)

Toxaphene (technical chlorinated camphene)(chlorine content 67-69%) *	45%
Malathion	5%
Xylene *	15%
Refined Petroleum oil	20%

'76 Ed.

DR. ROGERS' TOX-A-DANE
Insecticide
(Texas Phenothiazine Co.)

Toxaphene (technical chlorinated camphene)(chlorine content 67-69%) *	45%
Gamma isomer of benzene hexachloride from lindane	2%
Refined Petroleum oil	28%
Xylene *	15%

'76 Ed.

DR. ROGERS' TOX-ENE
Kills lice, ticks, horn flies on livestock
(Texas Phenothiazine Co.)

Toxaphene (technical chlorinated camphene)(chlorine content 67-69%) *	61.00%
Refined Petroleum oil	16.22%
Xylene	6.78%

'76 Ed.

DR. SCHOLL'S BATH SALTS
(Scholl)

Soda ash *
Sodium perborate *
Borax *

DR. SCHOLL'S BROMIDROSIS POWDER
(Scholl)

Aluminum chlorhydroxide *
Salicylic acid *
Boric acid *

DR. SCHOLL'S CALLOUS SALVE
(Scholl)

Salicylic acid *
Oil eucalyptus *

DR. SCHOLL'S CHLOROPHYLL FOOT LOTION
(Scholl)

Isopropyl alcohol *
Chlorophyll
Menthol *

DR. SCHOLL'S CHLOROPHYLL FOOT POWDER
(Scholl)

Aluminum chlorhydroxide *
Chlorophyllin
Zinc stearate *

DR. SCHOLL'S CORN SALVE
(Scholl)

Salicylic acid *
Oil of eucalyptus *

DR. SCHOLL'S DRY SKIN CREME
(Scholl)

Lanolin
Glyceryl monostearate

DR. SCHOLL'S FOOT BALM
(Scholl)

Lanolin
Methyl salicylate *
Camphor *
Menthol *
Oil of eucalyptus *
Zinc oxide

DR. SCHOLL'S FOOT DEODORANT SPRAY
Aerosol
(Scholl)

Zinc phenolsulfonate *
Methylbenzethonium chloride *
Menthol *
Alcohol

DR. SCHOLL'S FOOT LOTION
(Scholl)

Alcohol
Menthol *
Boric acid *

DR. SCHOLL'S FOOT POWDER
(Scholl)

Salicylic acid *
Boric acid *
Methyl salicylate *

DR. SCHOLL'S FOOT POWDER SPRAY
(Scholl)

Zinc undecylenate *
Aluminum chlorhydrate *
Menthol *
Alcohol

DR. SCHOLL'S FOOT REFRESHER SPRAY
(Scholl)

Zinc phenolsulfonate *
Alcohol
Menthol *

DR. SCHOLL'S ONIXOL
Toe-nail and calloused nail groove softener
(Scholl)

Sodium sulfide *
Urea
Triethanolamine

DR. SCHOLL'S PEDICREME
(Scholl)

Menthol *
Methyl salicylate *
Camphor *

Starred ingredients (*) may be responsible for major toxic effects; consult Section II.

DR. SCHOLL'S PRESTO ATHLETE'S FOOT LIQUID
(Scholl)

Alcohol
Salicylic acid *
Benzoic acid *
Thymol *

DR. SCHOLL'S SHOE DEODORIZER SPRAY
(Scholl)

Undecylenic acid *
Hexachlorophene *
Dichlorophene *
Menthol *

DR. SCHOLL'S SOAP AND SOAK
(Scholl)

Soap powder
Sodium bicarbonate *
Sodium sesquicarbonate *
Sodium borate *

DR. SCHOLL'S SOLVEX ATHLETE'S FOOT OINTMENT
(Scholl)

Salicylic acid *
Benzoic acid *
Thymol *

DR. SCHOLL'S SOLVEX ATHLETE'S FOOT POWDER
(Scholl)

Oxyquinoline sulfate *
Salicylic acid *
Sulfur colloidal
Chlorothymol *

DR. SCHOLL'S SOLVEX ATHLETE'S FOOT SPRAY
(Scholl)

Undecylenic acid *
Dichlorophene
Chlorothymol *
Benzocaine
Propylene glycol
Alcohol

DR. SCHOLL'S SOLVEX LIQUID
(Scholl)

Alcohol
Benzoic acid *
Salicylic acid *
Chlorothymol *
Benzocaine

DR. SCHOLL'S "2" DROP CORN AND CALLOUS REMOVER
(Scholl)

Acetone *
Salicylic acid *
Camphor *
Ether *
Alcohol

DRYCIDE
Insecticide
(Hess & Clark)

Toxaphene * 5%

DRYING AGENT W201L
Commercial dishwashing agent
(Diversey Wyandotte)

Synthetic detergents *

DRYLOCK CEMENT PAINT
(United Gilsonite)

Cement
Hydrated Lime
Lime proof colors

DRYLOCK CEMENT SEALER
(United Gilsonite)

Cement
Hydrated Lime
Lime proof colors

DRYLOK CONCRETE FLOOR PAINT
Covering broad range of colors
(United Gilsonite)

Pigment may include:
　Titanium dioxide
　Iron oxides
　Barium sulfate
　Silicates
　Chrome oxide green
　Tinting colors
Vehicle:
　Synthetic Latex soya alkyd
　　resin 23.0-25.0%
　Volatile: Water 44.7-49.2%

DRYLOK ETCH
(United Gilsonite)

Sulfamic acid *

DRYLOK READY MIXED SEALER (Sage Green, Spice Beige & White)
(United Gilsonite)

Pigment: 62.6-63.5%
　Titanium dioxide 3.8-6.25%
　Portland cement 42.0-43.0%
　Silica & Silicates 51.75-53.2%
Vehicle: 36.5-37.4%
　Vinyl-toluene butadiene
　　resin　　　　　　 20.25%
　Aliphatic hydrocarbons *　79.75%

Tinting colors less than 5%

DRYLOK SILICONE
Water repellent coating for masonry
(United Gilsonite)

Silicone resin 5%
Aliphatic hydrocarbons * 95%

DRY LOOK HAIR SPRAYS

See THE DRY LOOK HAIR SPRAYS

DRYSUM SHAMPOO
(Summers Labs.)

Detergents *
Drying agents

DRYTERGENT
For acne therapy
(C & M Pharmacal)

Purified water
TEA-dodecylbenzenesulfonate *
Boric acid *
Cocamide DEA
Propylene glycol
Fragrance
FD & C Yellow No. 5

DRYTEX
For cleansing oily skin
(C & M Pharmacal)

Salicylic acid * 2%
Hyamine 10X *
Dectol (non-toxic wetting agent)
Acetone *
Isopropyl alcohol * 40%
Purified water
Color
Perfume

DRY THRIP-TOX
Insecticide
(Leffingwell)

Sabadilla alkaloids 0.20%

D-SAN-X
Detergent, deodorant, sanitizer, disinfectant
(Nu-Ball Mfg. Co.)

n-Alkyl (68% C12, 32% C14) dimethyl ethylbenzyl ammonium chloride * 2.25%
n-Alkyl (60% C14, 30% C16, 5% C12, 5% C18) dimethyl benzyl ammonium chloride * 2.25%

D.S. - DE-SCALE (Liquid)
See GUNK D.S. - DE-SCALE (Liquid)

d-SEB
Antiseptic skin cleanser
(CooperCare)

Parachlorometaxylenol 2.0%
Isopropanol 7.6%
Neutral synthetic detergent base

DSMA LIQUID
Postemergence herbicide
(Diamond Shamrock Corp.)

Disodium methanearsonate * 21.8%

DSMA POWDER
Herbicide
(Diamond Shamrock Corp.)

Disodium methanearsonate (anhydrous) * 63%

D-S-S CAPSULES
Stool softener
(Parke-Davis)

Dioctyl sodium sulfosuccinate (U.S.P.) * ..... 50 mg.; 100 mg.

D-S-S PLUS CAPSULES
Stool softener
(Parke-Davis)

Each capsule:
Dioctyl sodium sulfosuccinate * .... 100 mg.
Casanthranol * .... 30 mg.

D-5 TABLETS
See D-5 TABLETS

D TICK DUST
Kills ticks and fleas on dogs
(Hart-Delta, Inc.)

O,O-Diethyl O-(2-isopropyl-6-methyl-4-pyrimidinyl)phosphorothioate *
Technical Piperonyl butoxide
2,2'-Methylenebis(4-chlorophenol)
Pyrethrins
Inert ingred.:
Talc 97.42%

'76 Ed.

D-TRANS INTERMEDIATE 1868
For use in manufacturing household & industrial insecticides
(MGK)

d-trans Allethrin 9.0%
Technical Piperonyl butoxide 18.0%
N-Octyl bicycloheptene dicarboximide (MGK-264) * 30.0%
Petroleum distillate * 43.0%

DUA-CIDE, MUNICHEM
See MUNICHEM DUA-CIDE

DUAL 6E
Herbicide
(Ciba-Geigy Ag. Div.)

Metolachlor * 68.5%

DUAL 8E
Herbicide
(Ciba-Geigy Ag. Div.)

Metolachlor * 86.4%

DUAL-TOX
Insecticide
(Hub States)

Dieldrin * 11.34%
Heptachlor * 23.00%
Xylene * 60.66%

'76 Ed.

DUART HAIR CARE PRODUCTS
Duart Mfg. Co., Ltd.
984 Folsom
San Francisco, Calif. 94107

Phone: 415-986-0260

See COSMETICS, Section VI, General Formulations

DUET INSECTICIDE & LEAF SHINE
(New Plant Life)

Active ingred.:
Pyrethrins 0.01%
Petroleum distillate 0.04%

Inert ingred.:
Isopropanol * 59.37%
Water 40.58%

DU-FOME
Liquid concentrated synthetic detergent
(DuBois Chem.)

Triethanolamine salts of linear alkyl benzene sulfonate *
Diethanolamine condensate of lauric acid
Sodium tripolyphosphate *
Sodium nitrate *

DULARIN SYRUP
Analgesic, antipyretic
(Dooner Labs.)

Each 5 ml.:
Acetaminophen * .... 120 mg.
Non alcoholic syrup

DULARIN TH TABLETS
Tension headaches
(Dooner Labs.)

Each tablet:
Acetaminophen .... 325 mg.
Caffeine .... 30 mg.
Sodium butabarbital * ...... 15 mg.

DULCOLAX (SUPPOSITORIES & TABLETS)
Laxative
(Boehringer Ingelheim)

SUPPOSITORIES:
Bisacodyl (Bis(p-acetoxyphenyl)-2-pyridylmethane) .. 10 mg.

TABLETS:
Bisacodyl (Bis(p-acetoxyphenyl)-2-pyridylmethane) .. 5 mg.

DULZIT
Skin anesthetic cream
(Commerce Drug)

Dibucaine
Benzocaine
Benzalkonium chloride

DUNCAN CERAMICS ANTIQUE GLAZES (AN 300 Series)
(Duncan)

General formula: .... approx. %
Frits #2, 3, 4, 27: Approx. 1/2 PbO *, 1/3 SiO2, remainder oxides of Na, K, Ca, Al, B, Li, Ti   45%
Water 40%
Silica 6%
Kaolin 6%
Carboxymethylcellulose 1%
Tris(hydroxymethyl)nitromethane .... trace
Rutile, ZnO, CuO, ZrSiO4, ZrO   trace

DUNCAN CERAMICS ART GLAZES (AR 600/700 Series)
(Duncan)

General formula:	approx. %
Water	40%
Frit #2: Approx. 44% SiO_2, approx. 31% PbO *, remainder oxides of Na, K, Ca, Al, B	15-22%
Frit #7: Approx. 67% PbO *, approx. 27% SiO_2, approx. 6% CaO	15-20%
Frit #3: approx. 71% PbO *, approx. 25% SiO_2, remainder oxides of Al, and Na	4-8%
Frit #12: Approx. 47% SiO_2, remainder oxides of Na, Ca, B	5%
Kaolin	6%
SiO_2, SnO_2, TiO_2	4-10%
FeO, Fe_2O_3	2%
Carboxymethylcellulose	<1%
Tris(hydroxymethyl)nitromethane	trace

DUNCAN CERAMICS ARTS & CRAFTS ANTIQUING STAINS (AS 200 Series)
(Duncan)

General formula:	approx. %
Linseed oil	38%
Mineral spirits *	25%
Aluminum silicate	16%
Talc	10%
Pigments (non-lead)	8%
Clay	1%
Magnesium oxide	1%
Methanol	trace
Cobalt	trace

DUNCAN CERAMICS ARTS & CRAFTS BASECOATS (BC 100 Series)
Water base vinyl acrylic paint
(Duncan)

General formula:	approx. %
Water	35%
Polyvinyl acetate copolymer	27%
Titanium dioxide	26%
Aluminum silicate	4%
Ethylene glycol	2.5%
Flattening agent	2%
Butyl carbitol acetate	1.5%
Minor components: Methylcellulose, Defoamer, Wetting agent, Dispersing agent, Lecithin, Pigments, Aqua ammonia	

DUNCAN CERAMICS ARTS & CRAFTS GLOSS SEALER (BF 931)
(Duncan)

Vinyl acrylic copolymer	65%
Water	32%
Ethylene glycol	1%
Diethylene glycol monobutylene acetate	<1%
Hydroxyethylcellulose	<1%
Phenylmercuric acetate	0.15%
Dispersant, Defoamer	trace

DUNCAN CERAMICS ARTS & CRAFTS LIQUID METALLICS (LM 400 Series)
Vinyl acrylic paint
(Duncan)

General formula:	approx. %
Water	60%
Vinyl acrylic resin solids	20%
Metallic powder	12%
Ethylene glycol	3%
Butyl carbitol acetate	<2%
Cellosolve	1%
Defoamer, Fumed silicas	trace

DUNCAN CERAMICS ARTS & CRAFTS LIQUID PEARLS (PL 300 Series)
Water base vinyl acrylic paint
(Duncan)

General formula:	approx. %
Acrylic polymer	46%
Water	35%
Pearlescent pigment (non-lead)	13%
Ethylene glycol	3%
Minor components: Methyl cellulose, Surface active agents, Coalescent agents	trace

DUNCAN CERAMICS ARTS & CRAFTS MATTE SEALER (BF 932)
(Duncan)

Vinyl acrylic copolymer	65%
Water	32%
Ethylene glycol	1%
Diethylene glycol monobutylene acetate	<1%
Hydroxymethylcellulose	<1%
Phenylmercuric acetate	0.15%
Flattening agent Dispersant, Defoamer	trace

DUNCAN CERAMICS ARTS & CRAFTS METALLIC ACCENT FINISHES (MA 600 Series)
(Duncan)

Metallic (non-lead) powder	64%
Turpentine *	14%
Varnish	18%
Wax	4%

DUNCAN CERAMICS ARTS & CRAFTS PREP COAT (PA 503)
Vinyl acrylic color
(Duncan)

	approx. %
Vinyl acrylic resin	34.0%
Calcium carbonate and/or Titanium dioxide	34.0%
Water	18.0%
Vinyl acrylic emulsion	8.5%
Methyl cellulose solution 2%	3.5%

DUNCAN CERAMICS ARTS & CRAFTS SPRAY BASECOATS (SB 100 Series)
Aerosol hobby spray
(Duncan)

Ketone and esters *†	57-59%
Aliphatic hydrocarbon propellant	18-23%
Nitrocellulose resin	8-12%
Chlorinated solvent *	7-9%
Pigments	5-10%

†*See* Ketone solvents

DUNCAN CERAMICS ARTS & CRAFTS SPRAYS (SF 900 Series)
Aerosol hobby spray
(Duncan)

Combined amount:	approx. 59%
Aromatic hydrocarbons * Chlorinated solvents *	
Hydrocarbon propellant	approx. 24%
Acrylic resin	approx. 16%
Color	

DUNCAN CERAMICS ARTS & CRAFTS SPRAY STAIN (SS 200 Series)
Aerosol hobby spray
(Duncan)

Aliphatic hydrocarbon solvent *	38-43%
Aliphatic hydrocarbon propellant	18-23%
Ketone *	12-17%
Linseed oil	10%
Aluminum silicate	4%
Talc	3%
Pigments	2%
Clay, Magnesium oxide, Methanol, Cobalt	trace

DUNCAN CERAMICS BISQ-STAIN ACCESSORY ANTIQUING SOLVENT (AS 951)
(Duncan)

Petroleum distillates *	100%

DUNCAN CERAMICS BISQ-STAIN ACCESSORY HAND & BRUSH CLEANER (AS 952)
(Duncan)

Petroleum distillates *	32%
Alkylolamides	15%
Water	53%

DUNCAN CERAMICS BISQ-STAIN ACCESSORY PRODUCT THICKENER AND TEXTURIZER (AS 955)
Paint powder additive
(Duncan)

	approx. %
Powdered Latex polymer	40-50%
Calcium carbonate	20-30%
Diatomaceous Silica	balance

Starred ingredients (*) may be responsible for major toxic effects; consult Section II.

DUNCAN CERAMICS BISQ-STAIN ACCESSORY PRODUCT THIN 'N SHADE (AS 957)
(Duncan)

Propylene glycol	33%
Water	balance

DUNCAN CERAMICS BISQ-STAIN CERAMIC SPRAYS (300 Series)
Aerosol ceramic spray
(Duncan)

Combined amount:	approx. 59%
Aromatic hydrocarbons *	
Chlorinated solvents *	
Hydrocarbon propellant	approx. 24%
Acrylic resin	approx. 16%
Color	

DUNCAN CERAMICS BISQ-STAIN LIQUID GOLDEN PEARL (GP 200 Series)
Water-based vinyl acrylic paint
(Duncan)

General formula	approx. %
Water	60%
Latex acrylic resin	21%
Titanium dioxide coated mica	13%
Ethylene glycol	3%
Ester alcohol	2%
Hydroxypropyl methylcellulose	<1%
Defoamer, Pigment, Aqua ammonia	trace

DUNCAN CERAMICS BISQ-STAIN LIQUID METALLICS (MS 700 Series)
Water base vinyl acrylic paint
(Duncan)

General formula:	approx. %
Water	60%
Vinyl acrylic resin solids	20%
Metallic powder	12%
Ethylene glycol	3%
Butyl carbitol acetate	<2%
Cellosolve	1%
Defoamer, Fumed Silica, Tris(hydroxymethyl)nitromethane	trace

DUNCAN CERAMICS BISQ-STAIN LIQUID PEARLS (PL 100 Series)
Water base vinyl acrylic paint
(Duncan)

General formula:	approx. %
Water	60%
Latex acrylic resin	21%
Titanium dioxide coated mica	13%
Ethylene glycol	3%
Ester alcohol	2%
Hydroxypropyl methylcellulose	<1%
Defoamer, Pigment, Aqua ammonia	trace

DUNCAN CERAMICS BISQ-STAIN METALLIC ACCENT (PS 200 Series)
Hobby metallic paste finishes
(Duncan)

Metallic (non-lead) powder	64%
Turpentine *	14%
Varnish	18%
Wax	4%

DUNCAN CERAMICS BISQ-STAIN OPAQUES (OS 400 Series)
Water base vinyl acrylic paint
(Duncan)

General formula:	approx. %
Water	50%
Calcium carbonate and/or Titanium dioxide	25%
Vinyl acrylic resin	13%
Aluminum silicate	4%
Ethylene glycol	2%
Diatomaceous silicate	2%
Butyl carbitol acetate	1%
Hydroxypropyl methylcellulose, Potassium carbonate, Defoamer, Alkaline surfactant, Isooctyl phenoxypolyethoxy ethanol, Pigments	trace

DUNCAN CERAMICS BISQ-STAIN TRANSLUCENT ANTIQUE (TS 500 Series)
Glaze sealer
(Duncan)

General formula:	approx. %
Mineral spirits *	34%
Aluminum silicate, Magnesium silicate	23%
Polymerized Linseed oil	15%
Polymerized Soya alkyd	11%
Titanium dioxide	11%
Iron oxide pigment	3%
Zr, Co, Ma	trace
Methanol, Organomontmorillonite, Methyl ethyl ketoxime	trace

DUNCAN CERAMICS BISQ-STAIN ULTRA METALLICS (UM-600 Series)
Water base vinyl acrylic paint
(Duncan)

General formula:	approx. %
Water	60%
Latex acrylic resin	21%
Titanium dioxide coated mica	13%
Ethylene glycol	3%
Ester alcohol	2%
Hydroxypropyl methylcellulose	<1%
Defoamer, Pigment, Aqua ammonia	trace

DUNCAN CERAMICS BRUSH-ON GLOSS SEALER (AS 953)
(Duncan)

Vinyl acrylic copolymer	65%
Water	32%
Ethylene glycol	1%
Diethylene glycol monobutylene acetate	<1%
Hydroxyethylcellulose	<1%
Dispersant, Defoamer	trace
Phenylmercuric acetate	0.15%

DUNCAN CERAMICS BRUSH-ON MATTE SEALER (AS 954)
(Duncan)

Vinyl acrylic copolymer	65%
Water	32%
Ethylene glycol	1%
Diethylene glycol monobutylene acetate	<1%
Hydroxymethylcellulose	<1%
Flattening agent, Dispersant, Defoamer	trace
Phenylmercuric acetate	0.15%

DUNCAN CERAMICS COVER COATS (cc 100-cc 161)
(Duncan)

General formula (excluding #cc 137, 138, 139, 145, 146, 153, 158, 160):	approx. %
Water	50%
Clay-talc mixture	32%
Non-lead inorganic pigment mixture	15%
Frit #20 (Silicate glass)	1%
Bentonite	<1%
Carboxymethylcellulose	<1%
Propylene glycol	<1%
Tris(hydroxymethyl)nitromethane	trace
General formula (#cc 137, 138, 139, 145, 146, 153, 158, 160):	approx. %
Water	37%
Non-lead inorganic pigment mixture	35%
Clay-talc mixture	22%
Frit #2 (PbO, 30%)	3%
Carboxymethylcellulose	trace
Propylene glycol	trace
Orthophenylphenol salt	trace

DUNCAN CERAMICS CRACKLETONE GLAZES (CR 800 Series)
(Duncan)

General formula:	approx. %
Frits #4, 11, 20, 24: 50% SiO2, 20% B2O3, 3-6% PbO *, remainder oxides of Na, K, Zn, Al, Ca, Mg, Cd	50%
Water	40-45%
Kaolin	6%
Cryolite	2%
Carboxymethylcellulose	1%
Bentonite, Orthophenylphenol, F2	trace
CR 811, 813, 814 also contain:	
Elemental Cadmium (approx. 1%) *	

Starred ingredients (*) may be responsible for major toxic effects; consult Section II.

DUNCAN CERAMICS CRYSTALTONE GLAZES (20000 Series)
(Duncan)

Most contain up to 20% Lead *
Elemental Cadmium (as the
oxide, silicate, and
sulfoselenide) * .... approx. 1%
is present in the following products:
#20025; 20057; 20058; 20062; 20078;
20079; 20080

See also entries for Duncan Ceramics
Gloss, Matte, and Satintone Glazes for
formulations.

DUNCAN CERAMICS DIPPING GLAZE (DP 400)
(Duncan)

General formula: .... approx. %
  Frit #2: 44% SiO2, 31% PbO *,
    remainder oxides of Na, K, Ca,
    Al, B 41%
  Water 41%
  Frit #3: 71% PbO *, 25% SiO2,
    remainder oxides of Al and Na 10%
  Kaolin 6%
  Frit #4: 60% PbO *, 20% SiO2,
    remainder oxides of Na and B 2%

DUNCAN CERAMICS DUST AWAY GLAZES (Series DA 200)
(Duncan)

General formula: .... approx. %
  Water 60%
  Propylene glycol 11%
  Al2O3 .... 9%
  SiO2 .... 7%
Minor ingred.:
  Kaolin clay, Macaloid, CaO, B2O3,
  Fe2O3, MnO2, Cr2O3, Al2O3

DUNCAN CERAMICS E-Z STROKES (EZ-000 Series)
Water base glaze
(Duncan)

General formula: .... approx. %
  Water 55%
  Inorganic pigment (Sb2O5, Cr2O3,
    TiO2) 33%
  Frit #4: Approx. 59% PbO *, ap-
    prox. 20% SiO2, Approx. 15%
    B2O3, approx. 6% Na2O .... <8%
  Bentonite 3%
  Carboxymethylcellulose .... <1%
  Sodium benzoate .... trace

DUNCAN CERAMICS FIRED ANTIQUES (FA 271-280)
Water base glazes
(Duncan)

General formula (FA 271, 272,
  275, 277, 279, 280): .... approx. %
  Water 67%
  Non-lead inorganic pigment
    mixture 12%
  SiO2 .... 11%
  Bentonite 4%
  Frit #24: Silicate glass 3%
  Carboxymethylcellulose 2%
  Sodium benzoate .... trace
General formula (FA 273, 274,
  276, 278): .... approx. %
  Water 66%
  Leaded inorganic pigment
    mixture 19%
  Frit #4: 59% PbO * 9%
  Bentonite 3%
  Carboxymethylcellulose 2%
  Sodium benzoate .... trace

DUNCAN CERAMICS FROTH GLAZE (SY 549)
(Duncan)

General formula: .... approx. %
  Water 45%
  Frit #12 (approx. 50% silicon diox-
    ide; remainder oxides of Na, Ca,
    B) 29%
  Zirconium silicate 9%
  Calcium phosphate, tribasic 8%
  Silica 4%
  Kaolin 3%
  Non-lead inorganic pigment
    mixture 1%
  Carboxymethylcellulose 1%
  Orthophenylphenol salt .... trace

DUNCAN CERAMICS GLOSS GLAZES (GL-600 Series)
(Duncan)

General formula: .... approx. %
  Frits #1, 2, 3, 4, 11: 40%
    SiO2, 30% PbO*, remain-
    der oxides of Na, B, K,
    Zn, Al 45-55%
  Water 35-45%
  Kaolex 4%
  Silica 1%
  Bentonite 1%
  Carboxymethylcellulose 1%
  Dye, Pigment, Tris(hy-
    droxymethyl)nitromethane .. trace
  Elemental Cadmium (as the
    oxide, silicate, and .... approx.
    sulfoselenide) * 1%
  is present in the following
  products: GL 614; 631; 632;
  637; 657; 658; 659; 660;
  662; 678

DUNCAN CERAMICS GOLDSTONE (AR 727)
Water base glaze
(Duncan)

General formula: .... approx. %
  Water 43%
  Frits #12, 20, 24: Silicate glass,
    Pigments 39%
  Ferric oxide 9%
  Silica 4%
  Kaolin 2%
  Cupric carbonate .... <2%
  Carboxymethylcellulose .... <1%
  Propylene glycol .... trace
  Orthophenylphenol salt .... trace

DUNCAN CERAMICS GRANITE SANDSTONE (SYS550)
(Duncan)

General formula: .... Approx. %
  Frit #4, 15, 22, 23: approx. 1/2
    PbO *, approx. 1/3 SiO2, re-
    mainder oxides of Na, Ba, Ca,
    Zn, Al, K, Ti 40%
  Water 40%
  ZrSiO4, ZnO, TiO2,
    Alumina 10%
  Kaolin 5%
  Carboxymethylcellulose 1%
  Tris nitro .... trace

DUNCAN CERAMICS HIGH GLOSS SEALER (AS 959)
Water-based acrylic clear
(Duncan)

           approx. %
  Vinyl acrylic resin 86.0%
  Water 5.0%
  Propylene glycol 4.0%
  Dibutyl phthalate 1.8%
  Butyl carbitol acetate 1.5%

DUNCAN CERAMICS LEAD FREE GLAZES (LFG, LFS, LFA, LFC, LFW 00 Series)
(Duncan)

Water
Silicon dioxide
Silicate materials
Inorganic colorants

DUNCAN CERAMICS LIQUID CRAYON (LC 100 Series)
Vinyl acrylic crayon paint; ten colors
(Duncan)

           approx. %
  Vinyl acrylic resin 70%
  Wax emulsion 22%
  Propylene glycol 3%
  Petroleum distillate 3%

DUNCAN CERAMICS MATTE GLAZES (MA 700 Series)
(Duncan)

General formula:	approx. %
Water	40-45%
Frit #2, 4, 5, 12: Approx. 1/3 to 1/2 PbO *, remainder non-toxic inorganic oxides	27-35%
CaSiO3, ZnO, ZrO2, SiO2	15-20%
Kaolin	5-10%
SiO2	3-5%
ZnO, ZrO2, Fe2O3	2-3%
Carboxymethylcellulose	1%

DUNCAN CERAMICS PATCH-IT (PA 501)
Hobby repair
(Duncan)

Calcium carbonate	67%
Water	20%
Vinyl acrylic polymer	7%
Aluminum silicate clay	3%
Aliphatic hydrocarbon	2%
Oleic acid, Hydroxypropyl methyl-cellulose, Triethanolamine, Poly-carbonylate dispersant	trace

DUNCAN CERAMICS SATINTONE GLAZES (SA 300 Series)
(Duncan)

General formula:	approx. %
Frit #4, 15, 22, 23: Approx. 1/2 PbO *, approx. 1/3 SiO2, remainder oxides of Na, Ba, Ca, Zn, Al, K, Ti	40%
Water	40%
ZrSiO4, ZnO, TiO2, Alumina	10%
Kaolin	5%
Carboxymethylcellulose	1%
Tris(hydroxymethyl)nitro-methane	trace

DUNCAN CERAMICS SPECIALTY PRODUCT MASK 'N PEEL (SY 548)
Protective rubber coating
(Duncan)

Water base Latex emulsion

DUNCAN CERAMICS SPECIALTY PRODUCT PATCH A TATCH (SY 545)
Ceramic hobby
(Duncan)

Water	75%
Clay	
Carboxymethylcellulose	
Bentonite	
Tris(hydroxymethyl)nitromethane	trace

DUNCAN CERAMICS SPECIALTY PRODUCTS (SY 500)
Water base glazes
(Duncan)

General formula:	approx. %
Frits #2, 4, 12: Approx. 1/3 PbO *, approx. 1/2 SiO2, remainder oxides of Na, K, Ca, Al, B	50%
Water	40%
Kaolin	5%
ZrSiO4, SiO2, Ca3(PO4)2	2%
Carboxymethylcellulose	1%
Tris(hydroxymethyl)nitro-methane	trace

DUNCAN CERAMICS SPECIALTY PRODUCT WAX RESIST (SY 547)
Wax coating
(Duncan)

Water base Paraffin wax emulsion

DUNCAN CERAMICS SPECKLETONE GLAZES (AR 900 Series)
(Duncan)

General formula:	approx. %
Frits #2, 3, 4, 11: 40% PbO *, 40% SiO2, remainder oxides of Na, K, Ca, Al, B, Zn	50%
Water	40%
Kaolin	4%
Bentonite, ZrSiO4	2%
Inorganic pigments	2%
Carboxymethylcellulose	1%
Tris(hydroxymethyl)nitro-methane	trace
Elemental Cadmium (as the oxide, silicate, and sulfoselenide) * is present in products AR 912 and 913	approx. 1%

DUNCAN CERAMICS WHITE FROTH (SY549)
(Duncan)

General formula:	Approx. %
Water	45%
Frit #12: approx. 50% Silicon dioxide, remainder oxides of Na, Ca, B	29%
Zirconium silicate	9%
Calcium phosphate, tribasic	8%
Silica	4%
Kaolin	3%
Non lead, inorganic, pigment mixture	1%
Carboxymethylcellulose	1%
Orthophenylphenol salt	trace

DUNCAN CERAMICS WOODTONE GLAZES (WD-200 Series)
(Duncan)

General formula:	approx. %
Water	40%
Frit #5: 1/3 PbO *, 1/3 SiO2, remainder oxides of K, Ca, Ba, Al, B	32%
CaSiO3, ZrSiO4	17%
Kaolin	6%
Propylene glycol	3%
Inorganic pigments based on ZrO2, SiO2, Fe2O3	2%
Carboxymethylcellulose	trace
Tris(hydroxymethyl)nitro-methane	trace

DUOCIDE CONCENTRATE

See AGWAY DUOCIDE CONCENTRATE

DUOCIDE RAT BAIT STATION

See AGWAY DUOCIDE RAT BAIT STATION

DUOFILM
For warts
(Stiefel Labs.)

Lactic acid *	16.7%
Salicylic acid *	16.7%
Flexible Collodion	

DUO-FLOW
Hard contact lens cleaning and soaking solution
(CooperVision Pharm.)

Alkyl (50% C12, 30% C14, 17% C16, 3% C18) dimethyl benzyl ammonium chloride	0.013%
Poloxamer 188	
Trisodium edetate	0.25%

DUO-KILL EMULSIFIABLE CONCENTRATE

See ROBERTS DUO-KILL EMULSIFIABLE CONCENTRATE

DUOLUBE
Ophthalmic ointment: ocular lubricant
(Muro Pharm.)

White petrolatum	70-90%
Mineral oil	10-20%

DUO-MEDIHALER
Relief of bronchospasm
(Riker Labs.)

Each cc.:
Isoproterenol hydrochloride *	4.0 mg.
Phenylephrine bitartrate *	6.0 mg.

Each inhalation, valve controlled:
Isoproterenol hydrochloride	0.16 mg.
Phenylephrine bitartrate	0.24 mg.

'76 Ed.

DUO-RAA-CO
Embalming fluid
(Embalmers')

Formaldehyde *

DUOSOL
Fecal softener
(Kirkman)

Each tablet:
Dioctyl sodium sulfosuc-cinate *	100 mg.

DUOVENT
Antiasthmatic
(Riker Labs.)

Each tablet:
Theophylline *	130 mg.
Ephedrine HCl	24 mg.
Glyceryl guaiacolate	100 mg.
Phenobarbital	8 mg.

'76 Ed.

DUO-WR (NO. 1 AND NO. 2)
Topical application in the removal of warts
(Whorton)

NO. 1:
Salicylic acid *	25%
Compound tincture Benzoin	

NO. 2:
Formaldehyde *	40%v/v
Compound tincture Benzoin *	

'76 Ed.

DUPHRENE (TABLETS & SYRUP)
Antihistaminic-decongestant
(Vale)

Each tablet or 5 ml.:
Chlorpheniramine maleate	1 mg.
Pyrilamine maleate *	12.5 mg.
Phenylephrine hydrochloride	5 mg.
Alcohol (Syrup only)	5%

DUPLEX SHAMPOO
(C & M Pharmacal)

Purified water
Sodium lauryl sulfate *

DUPLEX T
Anti-dandruff shampoo
(C & M Pharmacal)

Purified water	
Sodium lauryl sulfate	
Solution of Coal tar *	10%
Cocamide DEA	

DUPLI-COLOR PAINT PRODUCTS

Dupli-Color Products
1601 Nicholas Blvd.
Elk Grove Village, Ill. 60007

Phone: 312-439-0600

DU PONT SURFACTANT WK
(Du Pont)

Trimethylnonylpolyoxyethanol *†

†*See* Alkyl polyethylene glycol ether

DURACHLOR
For chlorination of swimming pool water
(Haviland Products Co.)

Sodium dichloro-s-triazine-trione *	98%

'76 Ed.

DURACIDE CONCENTRATE

See WASCO DURACIDE CONCENTRATE

DURADYNE DHC TABLETS
Analgesic
(OJF)

Each tablet:
Hydrocodone bitartrate	5 mg.
Acetaminophen *	150 mg.
Aspirin *	230 mg.
Caffeine	30 mg.

DURAGESIC
Analgesic
(Glaxo Inc.)

Each tablet:
Salicylsalicylic acid *	2.5 gr.
Aspirin *	5 gr.

DURA-GLIT
Brass polish
(French, R. T.)

Kerosene *	<50%
Cotton wadding	25%
Chalk	20%
Fatty acids	6%
Anhydrous Ammonia	<2%
Perfume	trace

DURA-GLOSS WAX
(Consolidated Chem., Inc.)

Acrylic polymers
Polyethylene emulsion

DURATEARS
Ocular lubricant
(Alcon)

Preservatives (each gm.):
Methylparaben	0.05%
Propylparaben	0.01%

Inactive ingred.:
White petrolatum
Anhydrous liquid Lanolin
Mineral oil

DURA-TEX CONCENTRATE
Floor wax
(Nat'l Labs. Div.)

Carnauba or carnauba-type waxes	
Emulsifiers	
Ammonium hydroxide	minor

DURATION NASAL SPRAY
Nasal decongestant
(Plough)

Oxymetazoline hydrochloride	0.05%

DURATITE 2000 ADHESIVE
(DAP)

Hydrocarbon resin	
Rosin ester resin	
Synthetic rubber	
Magnesium silicate	
Hexane *	40%

DURATITE 4000 ADHESIVE
(DAP)

Toluene *	<11%
Hexane	<14%
Lactol spirits	<12%
Isopropyl alcohol	<6%
Synthetic rubber	
Hydrocarbon resin	
Calcium carbonate	
Aluminum silicate	

DURATITE ALL-PURPOSE ADHESIVE
(DAP)

Calcium carbonate	
Hexane *	<30%
Rosin ester resin	
Synthetic Rubber polymer	

DURATITE LATEX WOOD FILLER
(DAP)

Calcium carbonate
Plasticized Polyvinyl acetate emulsion
Sodium benzoate
Water

Starred ingredients (*) may be responsible for major toxic effects; consult Section II.

DURATITE NON-FLAMMABLE CONTACT CEMENT
(DAP)

Acrylic latex emulsion
Rubber latex
Hydrocarbon resin
Water
Polyethoxy ethanol

DURATITE SOLVENT FOR WOOD DOUGH AND SURFACING PUTTY
(DAP)

Phthalate ester
Textile spirits *† .... <25%
Isopropyl alcohol * .... <25%
Ketones * .... <25%
Nitrocellulose
Rosin
Vegetable oil

†See Mineral spirits

DURATITE SURFACING PUTTY
(DAP)

Phthalate ester
Textile spirits .... <10%
Isopropyl alcohol .... <10%
Ketones .... <10%
Nitrocellulose
Rosin
Vegetable oil
Magnesium silicate
Calcium carbonate

DURATITE WATER PUTTY
(DAP)

Calcium sulfate
Silica
Magnesium silicate
Animal glue
Calcium carbonate

DURATITE WHITE GLUE
(DAP)

Plasticized Polyvinyl acetate emulsion

DURATITE WOOD DOUGH
(DAP)

Phthalate ester
Textile spirits .... <10%
Isopropyl alcohol .... <5%
Ketone .... <10%
Nitrocellulose
Rosin
Vegetable oil
Wood fiber
Calcium sulfate
Magnesium silicate

DUR-A-WEAR GYM FINISH
(Uncle Sam)

Polyurethane resins
Petroleum distillate *
Cobalt drier *

DURHAM'S ANATHESIA MOP
For throat irritation
(Durham's)

Benzocaine
Neutral Acriflavine
Alcohol-glycerine menstrum

'76 Ed.

DURHAM'S ANT-KIL POWDER
Insecticide
(Durham's)

Technical Chlordane * 10%

'76 Ed.

DURHAM'S 73% CHLORDANE EMULSIFIABLE CONCENTRATE
Insecticide
(Durham's)

Technical Chlordane * 73%
Petroleum distillates * 22%

'76 Ed.

DURHAM'S 50% MALATHION SPRAY CONCENTRATE
Insecticide
(Durham's)

Malathion * 50%
Methylated naphthalenes 41%

'76 Ed.

DURHAM'S PROLIN RAT-KIL WITH WARFARIN
(Durham's)

Warfarin (3-(a-Acetonylbenzyl)-4-
hydroxycoumarin) 0.025%
Sulfaquinoxaline (N'-(2-Quinoxal-
inyl)sulfanilamide (Prolin)) ... 0.025%

'76 Ed.

DURHAM'S RAT-KIL
Rodenticide
(Durham's)

Warfarin (3-(a-Acetonylbenzyl)-4-
hydroxycoumarin) 0.025%

'76 Ed.

DURHAM'S RED ANT BALLS
(Durham's)

Sodium cyanide * 97%

'76 Ed.

DURHAM'S REUMA-RUB
Liniment
(Durham's)

Oil of wintergreen synthetic *
Camphor *
Menthol *
Oil turpentine *
Acetone *
Chloroform *

'76 Ed.

DURHAM'S SCREW-WORM BOMB
(Durham's)

Gamma isomer of benzene hexa-
chloride (from lindane) 3.0%
Pine oil 17.5%
Xylol * 12.5%

'76 Ed.

DURHAM'S VEGETABLE GARDEN DUST
Insecticide
(Durham's)

Tech. Methoxychlor 5.00%
Rotenone 1.25%
Other cube resins 2.50%

'76 Ed.

"DUROLEAD" BLACK LEADS

See RELIANCE "DUROLEAD" BLACK LEADS

DURSBAN 21D INSECTICIDE
(Dow)

Chlorpyrifos (O,O-Diethyl O-(3,5,6-
trichloro-2-
pyridyl)phosphorothioate) * .. 16.4%
2,2-Dichlorovinyl dimethyl phosphate 7.6%
Related compounds in DDVP 0.6%
Xylene * 65.2%

DURSBAN 1E INSECTICIDE
(Dow)

Active ingred.: 13.0%
  Chlorpyrifos (O,O-Diethyl O-(3,5,6-
  trichloro-2-
  pyridyl)phosphorothioate) *
Inert ingred.: 87.0%
  Petroleum solvent
  Chlorinated solvent *
  Emulsifiers

DURSBAN 2E INSECTICIDE
(Dow)

Chlorpyrifos (O,O-Diethyl O-(3,5,6-
trichloro-2-pyridyl)
phosphorothioate) * 22.4%
Aromatic petroleum derivative
solvent 42.1%
Inert ingred.: 35.5%
  Chlorinated solvent * 25.5%

Starred ingredients (*) may be responsible for major toxic effects; consult Section II.

DURSBAN 24E INSECTICIDE
(Dow)

Active ingred.: 23.7%
  Chlorpyrifos (O,O-Diethyl O-(3,5,6-trichloro-2-pyridyl)phosphorothioate) *
Inert ingred.: 76.3%
  Emulsifiers
  Petroleum derivative solvent *

DURSBAN 6 INSECTICIDAL CONCENTRATE
(Dow)

Active ingred.:
  Chlorpyrifos (O,O-Diethyl O-(3,5,6-trichloro-2-pyridyl)phosphorothioate) *   61.5%
  Aromatic petroleum derivative solvent *   34.5%
Inert ingred.:
  Related compounds in chlorpyrifos 4.0%

DURSBAN 44 INSECTICIDE
(Dow)

Active ingred.:
  Chlorpyrifos (O,O-Diethyl O-(3,5,6-trichloro-2-pyridyl)phosphorothioate) *   43.2%
Inert ingred.:
  Aromatic petroleum derivative solvent * 56.8%

DURSBAN MC INSECTICIDAL CONCENTRATE
(Dow)

Active ingred.: 52.5%
  Chlorpyrifos (O,O-Diethyl O-(3,5,6-trichloro-2-pyridyl)phosphorothioate) *
Inert ingred.: 47.5%
  Methylene chloride
  Related compounds in active ingredient

DURSBAN M INSECTICIDE
(Dow)

Chlorpyrifos (O,O-Diethyl O-(3,5,6-trichloro-2-pyridyl) phosphorothioate) * 41.2%
Xylene * 29.5%
Inert ingred.: 29.3%
  Chlorinated solvent * 22.4%

DURSBAN-XYLENE INSECTICIDAL MIXTURE
(Dow)

Chlorpyrifos (O,O-Diethyl O-(3,5,6-trichloro-2-pyridyl)phosphorothioate) * 65%
Xylene * 35%

DUSTA-CIDE (Dust)
Insecticide
(Research Products Co.)

Malathion * 6.0%

DUST AWAY
Dust mop treatment
(Consolidated Chem., Inc.)

Petroleum distillate *

DUST AWAY GLAZES
See DUNCAN CERAMICS DUST AWAY GLAZES (Series DA 200)

DUST'M
See ROBERTS DUST'M

DUST-MOR LOUSE POWDER
(Hilltop)

Anthracene oil (Carbolineum)
Sulfur
Tech. Methoxychlor 5%
Naphthalene *
Sodium fluoride *
Nicotine sulfate *

                          '76 Ed.

DUST-SEAL
For house dust control
(Green, L.S., Associates)

Mineral oil
Wetting agent derived from a complex alcohol

DU-TER FUNGICIDE WETTABLE POWDER
(Thompson-Hayward)

Triphenyltin hydroxide * 47.5%

DUVELLE'S PERFUME, COLOGNE, TOILET WATER
(Parfums Duvelle)

Alcohol (denatured with diethyl phthalate) *

DUZITALL
Germicidal cleaner
(Uncle Sam)

Soap
Synthetic Phenol *
Isopropanol *
Sodium dodecylbenzene sulfonate *
Tetrasodium ethylenediaminetetraacetate
Sodium tripolyphosphate
Borax *
Propylene glycol
Essential oil
Sodium sulfate
Water

DUZ-KLEEN LIQUID DETERGENT
(Uncle Sam)

Sodium dodecylbenzene sulfonate *
Isopropanol *
Boric acid *
Triethanolamine
Caustic soda *
Propylene glycol
Sequestering agents
Dye
Perfume

DV CREAM
For atrophic vaginitis
(Merrell Dow)

Each tube:
  Dienestrol N.F. 0.01%
  Water-miscible base:
    Lactose
    Propylene glycol
    Stearic acid
    Diglycol stearate
    Trolamine
    Benzoic acid
  Buffered with Lactic acid to an acid pH

D. V. PAIN CAPSULES (Extra Strength)
(Reese Chem.)

Each capsule:
  Acetaminophen * .... 325 mg.
  Salicylamide .... 180 mg.

DV SUPPOSITORIES
For atrophic vaginitis
(Merrell Dow)

Each suppository:
  Dienestrol N.F. .... 0.70 mg.
  Lactose
  In a base of:
    Polyethylene glycol 400
    Polysorbate 80
    Polyethylene glycol 4000
    Glycerin
  Buffered with Lactic acid to an acid pH
  Inert covering:
    Gelatin
    Glycerin
    Water
    Methylparaben
    Propylparaben
    Coloring

D-WEED-O
Non-selective weed killer
(Schneid)

Petroleum oil * 94.94%
2,4-Dichlorophenoxyacetic acid, isooctyl ester *   1.09%
Bromacil (5-Bromo-3-sec-butyl-6-methyluracil) 0.98%
Pentachlorophenol 0.80%
Other chlorophenols 0.09%

                          '76 Ed.

Starred ingredients (*) may be responsible for major toxic effects; consult Section II.

DX 114 FOOT POWDER
(Amlab)

Zinc undecylenate *
Salicylic acid *
Benzoic acid
Ammonium alum
Boric acid *
Zinc stearate
Chlorophyll
Talc
Kaolin
Starch
Calcium silicate
Oil of wormwood

DX 114 LIQUID
Athlete's foot and ringworm
(Amlab)

Undecylenic acid 10%
8-Hydroxyquinoline benzoate
Salicylic acid *
Benzoic acid
Benzocaine
Brilliant green
Extractives from Gum benzoin, Gum
myrrh
Oil of wormwood
Alcohol * 75%

DX 114 OINTMENT
Athlete's foot remedy
(Amlab)

Each gram:
Zinc undecylenate * .... 200 mg.
Undecylenic acid .... 50 mg.
Salicylic acid * .... 25 mg.
Benzocaine .... 25 mg.

DYANAP
Herbicide
(Uniroyal Chem.)

Sodium N-1-naphthylphthalamate 21.2%
Sodium 4,6-dinitro-2-sec-butyl-
phenate * 10.9%
Inerts 67.9%
Including a Ketone and/or an alcohol

DYANSHINE BOOT OIL
(Dyanshine)

Toluene *
Petroleum distillates *

DYANSHINE LEATHER DYE
(Dyanshine)

o-Dichlorobenzene *

DYCILL CAPSULES
Antibiotic therapy
(Beecham Labs.)

Each capsule:
Dicloxacillin sodium . 250 mg.; 500 mg.

DYCLENE "E"
*For cleaning metals for subsequent
metal finishing*
(MacDermid)

Sodium carbonate * .... <40%
Sodium hydroxide * .... <20%
Sodium metasilicate * .... <40%
Complex Phosphates .... <10%

DYCLONE (0.5% SOLUTION & 1.0% SOLUTION)
Topical anesthetic
(Dow Pharm., Dow Chem. Co.)

0.5% SOLUTION (each ml.):
Dyclonine hydrochloride ..... 5 mg.
Chlorobutanol (chloral deriva-
tive) hydrous .... 3 mg.
Hydrochloric acid (if necessary)
Sodium chloride
1.0% SOLUTION (each ml.):
Dyclonine hydrochloride ..... 10 mg.
Chlorobutanol (chloral deriva-
tive) hydrous .... 3 mg.
Hydrochloric acid (if necessary)
Sodium chloride

DYFLEX-G ELIXIR
Relief of asthma
(Econo Med)

Each 15 ml.:
Dyphylline * .... 300 mg.
Guaifenesin .... 300 mg.
Alcohol 20%

DYFLEX-G TABLETS
Relief of asthma
(Econo Med)

Each tablet:
Dyphylline * .... 200 mg.
Guaifenesin .... 200 mg.

DYFLEX TABLETS
Relief of asthma
(Econo Med)

Each tablet:
Dyphylline * .... 200 mg.; 400 mg.

DYLATE SR CAPSULES
Vasodilator
(Elder)

Each capsule:
Papaverine HCl * .... 150 mg.

DYLOX
Insecticide
(Mobay Chemical Corp.)

Trichlorfon (Dimethyl (2,2,2-trichloro-1-
hydroxyethyl)phosphonate) *

DYNA-FOG CONTACT SPRA, EXCELCIDE

See EXCELCIDE DYNA-FOG CON-
TACT SPRA

DYNAKEM
Detergent, disinfectant
(Kem Mfg. Co.)

Active ingred.: 7.63%
Tetrasodium ethylenediamine
tetraacetate 1.58%
Anhydrous Sodium
metasilicate * 4.35%
n-Alkyl (60% C14, 30% C16, 5%
C12, 5% C18)dimethyl ben-
zyl ammonium chlorides .. 0.75%
n-Alkyl (50% C12, 30% C14,
17% C16, 3% C18)dimethyl
ethylbenzyl ammonium
chlorides 0.75%
n-Alkyl (92% C18, 8% C16) N-
ethyl morpholinium ethyl
sulfate 0.10%
3,5-Dibromosalicylanilide ... 0.02%
3,4',5-Tribromosalicylanilide
& other related
bromosalicylanilides 0.08%
Inert ingred.: 92.37%
Cleaning detergents, Wetting agents, Synergizing builders, Chelating agents,
Perfume, Water

DYNALINE PLASTIC PASTE
(Baird Dynamic)

Polyester resins
Mineral fillers

'76 Ed.

DYNALINE UNDERCOATING
(Baird Dynamic)

Aerosol asphaltic

'76 Ed.

DYNAMIC HEAVY DUTY CLEANER
(Paul Koss)

Water .... <85%
Butyl Cellosolve * .... <6%
Monoethanolamine .... <5%
Sodium xylene sulfonate (Anionic surfac-
tant)
Tetrasodium EDTA
Sodium metasilicate
Trisodium phosphate
Fatty amido phosphate
Formalin .... trace
Dye .... trace
pH 11.5-11.9

DYNA-MIGHTY JEWELRY CLEANER
Liquid cleaner
(Kassoy)

Alcohol .... <1%
Ammonia .... <1%

DYNAMO
*Metal cleaner, paint stripper, de-
greaser; industrial use*
(Puritan Chem. Co.)

Sodium hydroxide *

Starred ingredients (*) may be responsible for major toxic effects; consult Section II.

DYNAMO
Liquid laundry detergent
(Colgate-Palmolive)

Nonionic detergent *	approx. 40%
Ethoxylated alcohol sulfate	approx. 10%
Alcohol	approx. 10%
Water	

'76 Ed.

DYNA SPRAY CONCENTRATE
Insecticide
(Kem Mfg. Co.)

Petroleum distillate *	75.60%
Malathion *	22.30%
Beta-butoxy beta'-thiocyano di-ethyl ether	1.60%
N-Octyl bicycloheptene dicarboximide	0.26%
Piperonyl butoxide (technical)	0.16%
Pyrethrins	0.08%

DY-O-DERM
Vitiligo stain
(Owen Labs.)

Purified water
Isopropyl alcohol
Acetone
Dihydroxyacetone
FD & C Yellow No. 6
FD & C Blue No. 1
D & C Red No. 33

DYPAP ELIXIR
Analgesic and antipyretic
(King Pharmaceutical)

Each 5 cc:
Acetaminophen (N-Acetyl-p-aminophenol) *	120 mg.
Ethyl alcohol	10%

DYPAP TABLETS
Analgesic and antipyretic
(King Pharmaceutical)

Each tablet:
Acetaminophen *	300 mg.
Salicylamide	300 mg.
Butabarbital sodium *	15 mg.
Caffeine	30 mg.

DYREEN, HAPPY JACK

See HAPPY JACK DYREEN

DYRENE
Fungicide
(Mobay Chemical Corp.)

4,6-Dichloro-N-(2-chlorophenyl)-1,3,5-triazin-2-amine *

DYREX CAP-TABS
Equine anthelmintic; veterinary
(Fort Dodge)

Each Cap-tab:
Trichlorfon *
#300, 10.9 gm.; #500, 18.2 gm.

DYREX T.F.
Equine anthelmintic; veterinary
(Fort Dodge)

Each #500 bottle:
Trichlorfon *	9.1 gm.
Piperazine HCl	36.9 gm.
Phenothiazine	6.2 gm.

Each #1000 bottle:
Trichlorfon *	18.2 gm.
Piperazine HCl	73.8 gm.
Phenothiazine	12.5 gm.

DYSENAID JR.
Intestinal sedative for diarrhea
(Jenkins Labs.)

Each tablet:
Paregoric (opium 1.32 mg.) *	5 min.
Bismuth subgallate	64.8 mg.
Kaolin	64.8 mg.
Pectin	8.1 mg.

DYTERGE
Nonionic one-bath detergent & leveling agent
(Arkansas Co.)

Ethoxylated fatty alcohol *

'76 Ed.

DYZONE
Insecticide (industrial)
(Barco)

Diazinon	1.00%
Piperonyl butoxide (tech.)	0.414%
Pyrethrins	0.041%
Petroleum distillates *	98.545%

'76 Ed.

D.Z.N. DIAZINON
Insecticide
(Ciba-Geigy Ag. Div.)

Diazinon *

2D (Dust)*	2.0%
14G (Granular)*	14.3%
50W (Wettable powder)*	50.0%

D.Z.N. DIAZINON AG 500
Insecticide
(Ciba-Geigy Ag. Div.)

Diazinon *	48%
Xylene *	36%

D.Z.N. DIAZINON 4E
Insecticide; house and garden
(Ciba-Geigy Ag. Div.)

Diazinon *	47.5%
Aromatic petroleum derivative solvent *	26.2%

D.Z.N. DIAZINON 4S
Insecticide; for control of household pests
(Ciba-Geigy Ag. Div.)

Diazinon *	48.3%
Aromatic petroleum derivative solvent *	43.8%

E

EARDRO
Temporary relief of earache
(Jenkins Labs.)

Benzocaine	0.85%
Antipyrine *	3.2%
Glycerol	q.s.

EAR-DRY
Ear drops
(Scherer Labs.)

Isopropyl alcohol NF	
Boric acid NF	2.75%

EAREX EAR DROPS
(Approved Pharm.)

Benzocaine	0.15 gm.
Antipyrine *	0.70 gm.
Glycerol	q.s

'76 Ed.

EARL'S #6105 ANTI-SEPTIC LOTION HAND SOAP
(Earl, John A., Inc.)

Pure coconut oil soap 100%	18%
Skin conditioners	3%
Cold cream	10%
Hexachlorophene (on soap content)	2%
Cleaner base	33%
Free fatty acids (l mg/g KOH)	

'76 Ed.

pH maximum of 9.4

EARL'S #6301 BOWL CLEANER
(Earl, John A., Inc.)

Active ingredients:	24%
Hydrogen chloride *	
Zinc chloride *	
Oxalic acid *	
Hepta decyl hydroxy ethyl imidazoline	
Inert ingredients:	76%
Water	
Nonylphenoxypoly ethanol	
Polymerized Vinylbenzene	

'76 Ed.

EARL'S #5007 GERMICIDAL CLEANER
(Earl, John A., Inc.)

Combined amount: 18%
  Soap
  Ortho-benzyl-para-chlorophenol *
  Isopropanol *

'76 Ed.

pH maximum of 9

EARL'S #6101 HAND SOAP
(Earl, John A., Inc.)

Saponified pure Coconut oil
Potash
Suitable water softeners

'76 Ed.

EARL'S #5006 HEAVY-DUTY WAX REMOVER
(Earl, John A., Inc.)

Potassium laurate	4.0%
Potassium oleate	7.5%
Synthetic organic detergents	6.0%
Sequestrene compounds	3.0%
Inhibitors	0.3%

'76 Ed.

EARL'S #5022 SANI-CLEAN CLEANER-DISINFECTANT-DEODORANT
(Earl, John A., Inc.)

Tetradecyl dimethyl benzyl ammonium chlorides *	1.60%
Dodecyl dimethyl benzyl ammonium chlorides *	1.28%
Hexadecyl dimethyl benzyl ammonium chlorides	0.32%

'76 Ed.

EARL'S #5002 3-D CLEANER-DISINFECTANT-DEODORANT
(Earl, John A., Inc.)

Active ingredients: 22.64%
  Isopropyl alcohol *
  Potassium soap of coconut fatty acid
  Ortho phenylphenol *
  Sodium salt of linear sodium dodecyl benzene sulfonate
  Potassium xylene sulfonate *
  4-Chloro-2-cyclopentyl phenol
  Ortho benzyl-para-chlorophenol
  Para tertiary amylphenol *
  Trisodium salt of N-hydroxyethylethylene diamine triacetic acid
Inert ingredients: 77.36%
  Water
  Tetrapotassium pyrophosphate *

'76 Ed.

EARL'S #5005 WAX REMOVER & FLOOR CLEANER
(Earl, John A., Inc.)

Potassium soap	
Ammonia (26 Be) *	<4%
Free alkali as KOH	<0.05%

'76 Ed.

pH maximum of 11 & minimum of 8

EARTH BORN SHAMPOOS
(Gillette Co., Personal Care Div.)

The Gillette Co., Personal Care Div., Boston, Mass. 02199 will receive collect phone calls from poison control centers or physicians asking for emergency toxicological information about the company's products.

Phone: 617-421-7000

EARTH CARE PROFESSIONAL PLANT FOOD (Soluble Powder)
(Ciba-Geigy Ag. Div.)

Total Nitrogen	18%
Nitrate nitrogen	3.71%
Ammoniacal nitrogen	1.78%
Urea nitrogen	12.51%
Available Phosphoric acid *	18%
Soluble Potash *	18%
Chlorine	not more than 1%
Iron chelate	0.10%
Manganese chelate	0.05%

EARTH CARE PROFESSIONAL PLANT IRON TONIC (Granules)
(Ciba-Geigy Ag. Div.)

Total Nitrogen	8%
Ammoniacal nitrogen	8%
Available Phosphoric acid *	8%
Soluble Potash *	8%
Chlorine *	not more than 8%
Sulfur	8%
Iron chelate	1.3%

EARTH CARE PROFESSIONAL PLANT IRON TONIC (Soluble Powder)
(Ciba-Geigy Ag. Div.)

Iron chelate *† 10%

†See Iron salts

EAR-TIX-TOX, MARTIN'S

See MARTIN'S EAR-TIX-TOX

EASPRIN
For arthritic and other inflammatory conditions
(Parke-Davis)

Each tablet:
  Aspirin * .... 975 mg.

EASTERDAY MP-45
Cleaner, disinfectant, deodorizer, fungicide
(Easterday)

n-Alkyl (60% C14, 30% C16, 5% C18) dimethyl benzyl ammonium chlorides *	2.25%
n-Alkyl (68% C12, 32% C14) dimethyl ethylbenzyl ammonium chlorides *	2.25%
Sodium carbonate	3.00%
Tetrasodium ethylenediamine tetraacetate	1.00%

EASTERDAY SK-"32"
Concentrated disinfectant, cleaner, deodorant
(Easterday)

Alkyl (60% C14, 30% C16, 5% C12, 5% C18) dimethyl benzyl ammonium chlorides *	1.6%
Alkyl (68% C12, 32% C14) dimethyl ethylbenzyl ammonium chlorides *	1.6%
Sodium carbonate	3.0%
Essential oils	1.0%

EASTERDAY SK-"45"
Concentrated disinfectant, cleaner, fungicide, deodorizer
(Easterday)

Alkyl (60% C14, 30% C16, 5% C12, 5% C18) dimethyl benzyl ammonium chlorides *	2.25%
Alkyl (68% C12, 32% C14) dimethyl ethylbenzyl ammonium chlorides *	2.25%
Sodium carbonate	3.00%
Essential oils *	2.00%

EASY DUSTER INSECTICIDE

See PURINA EASY DUSTER INSECTICIDE

EASY GREASY
Degreaser, motor cleaner
(Lester Labs.)

Solvents *†
Detergents

'76 Ed.

†See Petroleum distillate and Aromatic hydrocarbons

EASY MONDAY CONCENTRATED FABRIC SOFTENER
(Industrial Equities)

Quaternary ammonium compound *	5-10%
Fluorescent whitening agent	<1%
Preservative	<1%
Colorant	<1%
Perfume	<1%
Water	balance

EASY MONDAY FABRIC SOFTENER
(Industrial Equities)

Quaternary ammonium compound *	2-5%
Preservative	<1%
Colorant	<1%
Perfume	<1%
Water	balance

EASY MONDAY HEAVY DUTY LAUNDRY DETERGENT (LIQUID)
(Industrial Equities)

Nonionic surfactant	20-30%
Anionic surfactant	5-10%
Diethanolamine	1-3%
Fluorescent whitening agent	<1%
Colorant	<1%
Perfume	<1%
Water	balance

EASY MONDAY LIQUID BLEACH
(Industrial Equities)

Sodium hypochlorite *	5 1/4%
Sodium chloride	<5%
Water	balance

EASY MONDAY LIQUID DISHWASHING DETERGENT
(Industrial Equities)

Anionic surfactant	6-12%
Hydrotrope	2-4%
Alkanolamide	<1%
Ethyl alcohol	<1%
Opacifier	<1%
Colorant	<1%
Perfume	<1%
Water	balance

EASY MONDAY SPRAY STARCH
(Industrial Equities)

Propellant (Isobutane)	1-10%
Corn starch	1-5%
Preservative	<1%
Silicone	<1%
Fluorescent whitening agent	<1%
Perfume	<1%
Water	balance

EASY-OFF CRAYONS
See CRAYOLA EASY-OFF CRAYONS

EASY-OFF INSTANT MILDEW STAIN REMOVER
(Boyle-Midway)

Sodium hypochlorite *	2.4%
Sodium hydroxide	0.5%
Anionic detergent	<1.0%
Thickener, perfume, water	balance

EASY-OFF OVEN CLEANER (AEROSOL)
(Boyle-Midway)

Sodium hydroxide *	4%
Thickeners	
Detergents	
Propellant	

EASY-OFF OVEN CLEANER (Paste)
(Boyle-Midway)

Sodium hydroxide *	6.0%
Thickeners	

EASY-OFF OVEN CLEANER (Trigger Spray)
(Boyle-Midway)

Sodium hydroxide *	1.8%
Amine	<5%
Detergent	

EASY-OFF WALLPAPER REMOVER
(Klean-Strip)

Organic acid *	24%
Penetrant *†, Wetting agents *	45%
Water	31%

†See Kerosene

EASY-OFF WINDOW CLEANER (Aerosol)
(Boyle-Midway)

Ethylene glycol ether	<5%
Ammonia	trace
Wetting agents	trace
Anti-oxidant	trace
Propellant	

EASY-OFF WINDOW CLEANER (Liquid)
(Boyle-Midway)

Alcohol and Ethylene glycol ether	<10%
Trace amounts of Ammonia, Wetting Agent, Color, Odorant	

EASY-ON SPEED STARCH (Aerosol)
(Boyle-Midway)

Starch
Silicone
Brightener
Perfume
Propellant

EATON'S A-C FORMULA 50
Rodenticide
(Eaton, J.T.)

Pival	0.025%

EATON'S "ALL-WEATHER" BAIT BLOCKS
Rodenticide
(Eaton, J.T.)

Diphacin	0.0025%
Sodium salt of Diphacin	0.0027%

EATON'S POISON PIGEON GRAINS
(Eaton, J.T.)

Strychnine *	0.6%

EATON'S RED SQUILL RAT BAITS
Rodenticide
(Eaton, J.T.)

Fortified Red squill *	10%

EATON'S "SEWER RAT" BAIT BLOCKS
Rodenticide
(Eaton, J.T.)

Diphacin	0.005%

EAU DE PORTUGAL & EAU DE QUININE, PINAUD'S
See PINAUD'S EAU DE PORTUGAL & EAU DE QUININE

EAZYCRETE
Concrete, wood floor resurfacer
(Texas Refinery)

Asphalt	48.0%
Water	45.0%
Asbestos fiber	5.0%
Bentonite clay	2.0%

E.B. - ENGINE BRITE ENGINE CLEANER
See GUNK E.B. - ENGINE BRITE ENGINE CLEANER

Starred ingredients (*) may be responsible for major toxic effects; consult Section II.

EBERHARD FABER PRODUCTS

Eberhard Faber, Inc.
Crestwood
Wilkes-Barre, Pa. 18773

Phone: 717-474-6711

See PENCILS, Section VI, General Formulations

ECHOLS (KINGTEX) ROACH, ANT AND WATERBUG KILLER
Insecticide
(Athena)

o-Isopropoxyphenyl methylcarbamate
(Baygon) * 2%

ECHOLS MOUSE PELLETS
(Athena)

Warfarin 0.025%

ECHOLS ROACH TABLETS
(Athena)

Boric acid * 40%

ECKROAT GOPHER GETTER BAIT
Rodenticide for pocket gophers
(Eckroat Seed Co.)

Strychnine alkaloid * ..... 0.35% by wt.

ECLIPSE
Sunscreen lotion
(Herbert Labs.)

Purified water
Alcohol 5%
Oleth-3 phosphate
Glyceryl PABA 3%
Octyl dimethyl PABA 3%
Petrolatum
Synthetic Spermaceti
Glycerin
Mineral oil
Lanolin alcohol
Cetyl stearyl glycol
Lanolin oil
Triethanolamine
Carbomer-934
Benzyl alcohol 0.5%
Fragrance

ECLIPSE AFTER SUN LOTION
(Herbert Labs.)

Emollient base

ECLIPSE SUNSCREEN LIP AND FACE PROTECTANT
(Herbert Labs.)

Padimate O (Octyl dimethyl PABA)

ECOLASTIC
Roofing
(Tremco)

Water suspension of Aromatic petroleum pitch (Asphalt) 95%
Propylene glycol 3%
Fillers (clay) 2%

ECONOCHLOR
Stabilizer for Durachlor-chlorine in swimming pool water
(Haviland Products Co.)

Di-sodium salt of Cyanuric acid *

'76 Ed.

ECONOCHLOR
Ophthalmic ointment
(Alcon)

Active ingred. (each gm.):
  Chloramphenicol (10 mg./gm.) .. 1.0%
Inactive ingred.:
  White petrolatum
  Anhydrous liquid Lanolin
  Mineral oil

ECONOCHLOR
Ophthalmic solution
(Alcon)

Active ingred. (each ml.):
  Chloramphenicol (5 mg./ml.) ... 0.5%
Preservative:
  Thimerosal 0.01%
Vehicle:
  Hydroxypropyl methylcellulose
Inactive ingred.:
  Boric acid
  Sodium borate (to adjust pH)
  Purified water

ECONOPRED 1/8%
Ophthalmic suspension
(Alcon)

Active ingred. (each ml.):
  Prednisolone acetate 0.125%
Preservative:
  Benzalkonium chloride 0.01%
Vehicle:
  Hydroxypropyl methylcellulose
Inactive ingred.:
  Dried Sodium phosphate
  Edetate disodium
  Polysorbate 80
  Citric acid (to adjust pH)
  Glycerin
  Purified water

ECONOPRED PLUS 1%
Ophthalmic suspension
(Alcon)

Active ingred. (each ml.):
  Prednisolone acetate 1.0%
Preservative:
  Benzalkonium chloride 0.01%
Vehicle:
  Hydroxypropyl methylcellulose
Inactive ingred.:
  Dried Sodium phosphate
  Edetate disodium
  Polysorbate 80
  Citric acid (to adjust pH)
  Glycerin
  Purified water

ECONOSTRIP PAINT STRIPPERS
(Beck Chem.)

Combined amount: .... <10%
  Chloroacetic acid *
  Lactic acid

ECOTRIN
Enteric-coated aspirin
(MenJ Labs.)

Each tablet:
  Aspirin * .... 325 mg.

ECTIBAN EC
Insecticide
(Hess & Clark)

Permethrin 5.7%

ECTIBAN WP
Insecticide
(Hess & Clark)

Permethrin * 25%

ECTOL OINTMENT
Allergy-itching
(Approved Pharm.)

Chlorpheniramine maleate *
Pyrilamine maleate *
Diperodon
Hexachlorophene
Benzalkonium *
Menthol *
Camphor *

'76 Ed.

ECTORAL EMULSIFIABLE CONCENTRATE
For topical application in the treatment of ectoparasite infestation in dogs and cats
(Pitman-Moore)

Ronnel (O,O-Dimethyl O-(2,4,5-trichlorophenyl)
  phosphorothioate) 33.34%
Aromatic petroleum derivatives * 56.32%
Inert ingred.: 10.34%
  Emulsifier

ECTORAL TABLETS
*For systemic treatment of certain ecto-
parasites on dogs and cats*
(Pitman-Moore)

Each tablet:
Ronnel (O,O-Dimethyl O-(2,4,5-trichlo-
rophenyl) phosphorothioate) *
#1: .... 250 mg.
#2: .... 500 mg.
#3: .... 1 gm.

EDWAL ANTI-SCRATCH FILM HARDENER
(Edwal)

Aluminum sulfate *
Acetic acid

EDWAL ANTI-STATIC FILM & GLASS CLEANER
(Edwal)

Isopropanol *
Ammonia

EDWAL COLOR FILM CLEANER (Antistatic, No. 2 Formula)
Photographic supply
(Edwal)

1,1,1-Trichloroethane *
Antistatic agent similar in chemical structure to synthetic detergent

EDWAL COLOR TONERS
Darkroom aids
(Edwal)

Acetic acid
Isopropyl alcohol
Dyes *†
Potassium ferricyanide *

†*See* Toners, photographic products, Section VI, General Formulations

EDWAL-12 DEVELOPER
Photographic supply
(Edwal)

Each quart:
Monomethyl-p-aminophenol .. 90 gr.
Sodium sulfite .... 3 oz.
p-Phenylenediamine * .... 150 gr.
p-Hydroxyphenylglycine ...... 75 gr.

EDWAL-20 DEVELOPER
Photographic supply
(Edwal)

Each quart:
p-Aminophenol * .... 75 gr.
Sodium sulfite .... 3 oz.
p-Phenylenediamine * .... 150 gr.
p-Hydroxyphenylglycine ...... 75 gr.

EDWAL FERROTYPE POLISH
(Edwal)

Petroleum waxes
Petroleum solvent (medium boiling) *
1,1,1-Trichloroethane *

EDWAL FG7
Photographic supply
(Edwal)

Phenidone
Chlorhydroquinone *
Sodium sulfite *
Sodium carbonate *

EDWAL "4 & 1" HYPO ELIMINATOR
For archival work
(Edwal)

Sodium sulfite *
Ammonium sulfite
EDTA (Versene)
Citric acid
Potassium iodide
Ethyl glycol
Isopropyl alcohol

EDWAL "G" DEVELOPER
Developer for photographic papers
(Edwal)

Dimezone S
Hydroquinone
Sodium sulfite *
Potassium carbonate
Sodium bromide
Caustic soda
EDTA (Versene)

EDWAL-20 HIGH ENERGY REPLENISHER
Photographic supply
(Edwal)

Each quart:
Monomethyl-p-aminophenol .. 30 gr.
p-Hydroxyphenylglycine ...... 60 gr.
Sodium sulfite .... 3 oz.
p-Phenylenediamine * .... 150 gr.
p-Aminophenol * .... 75 gr.

EDWAL HI-SPEED LIQUID FIX PHOTO CONC.
Photographic supply
(Edwal)

Ammonium thiosulfate *
Sodium sulfite *
Acetic acid *
Boric acid *

EDWAL HYPO-CHEK
Photographic supply
(Edwal)

Potassium iodide *
Formaldehyde *

EDWAL INDUSTRIAL INDICATING SHORTSTOP
(Edwal)

Acetic acid * 80%
Bromcresol purple

EDWAL LIQUID ORTHAZITE
Darkroom aid
(Edwal)

Benzotriazole
Sodium sulfite *

EDWAL LITHO-F DEVELOPER
Developer for litho films
(Edwal)

Monomethyl-p-amino phenol
Hydroquinone
Sodium sulfite *
Sodium carbonate
Sodium bromide
Benzotriazole

EDWAL NO-SCRATCH
*Hides scratches on films during projec-
tion*
(Edwal)

Turpentine *
Petroleum distillate
1,1,1-Trichloroethane

EDWAL PLATINUM II DEVELOPER
Developer for photographic papers
(Edwal)

Dimezone S
Hydroquinone
Potassium carbonate *
Sodium sulfite
Sodium bromide
EDTA (Versene)

EDWAL QUICK-FIX
Photographic supply
(Edwal)

Ammonium thiosulfate *
Sodium sulfite *
Acetic acid *
Boric acid *

EDWAL SIGNAL SHORTSTOP
Photographic supply
(Edwal)

Acetic acid (equal in strength to 56% acetic
acid) *
Bromcresol purple

EDWAL SINGLE SOLUTION TRAY CLEANER
Cleans photographic trays and processors
(Edwal)

Sodium bisulfate *
Sulfamic acid
Sodium bichromate

EDWAL STABILIZER AND FIXER SYSTEMS CLEANER
Cleans fixer section of processors
(Edwal)

EDTA (Versene)
Sodium hydroxide *
Potassium hydroxide *

EDWAL SUPER-FLAT
Flattens photographic papers
(Edwal)

Polyethylene glycol 400
Stabucell (Condensation product of polyethylene glycols)
Isopropyl alcohol

EDWAL T.S.T.
Photographic supply
(Edwal)

Monomethyl-p-aminophenol
Hydroquinone
Potassium carbonate *†
Sodium sulfite
Potassium bromide
Benzotriazole
Phenidone

†*See* Alkali

E.E.S. CHEWABLE TABLETS AND 400-FILMTAB
Antibiotic
(Abbott)

Each tablet:
  Erythromycin ethyl-
    succinate (USP) ... 200 mg.; 400 mg.

E.E.S. DROPS, GRANULES, AND LIQUID
Antibiotic
(Abbott)

Each 2.5 ml.:
  Erythromycin ethylsuccinate
    (USP) .... 100 mg.

Each 5 ml.:
  Erythromycin ethyl-
    succinate (USP) ... 200 mg.; 400 mg.

EFRICON EXPECTORANT
Antitussive, antihistaminic nasal decongestant
(Lannett)

Each fl. oz.:
  Codeine phosphate * .... 1 gr.
  Phenylephrine HCl .... 30 mg.
  Chlorpheniramine maleate .... 12 mg.
  Ammonium chloride .... 8 gr.
  Potassium guaiacol sulfonate . 8 gr.
  Sodium citrate .... 5 gr.

EHRLICH'S DPS ROACH POWDER
Insecticide
(Ehrlich)

Diazinon * 2.0%
Pyrethrins 0.5%
Amorphous Silica gel 46.0%
Inert (clay) 51.5%

EHRLICH'S PIGEON BAIT
Avicide
(Ehrlich)

Strychnine alkaloid * 0.6%

EHRLICH'S PINE OIL DISINFECTANT
(Ehrlich)

Active ingred. 90%
  Steam-distilled Pine oil *
  Soap
Inert ingred.: 10%
  Water

80-20 GRAIN FUMIGANT
(Industrial Fumigant)

Carbon tetrachloride * 83.5%
Carbon bisulfide 16.5%

80-20 WITH SO2 GRAIN FUMIGANT
(Industrial Fumigant)

Carbon tetrachloride * 82.7%
Carbon bisulfide 16.3%
Sulfur dioxide 1.0%

EISENZUCKER
Hematinic
(Wesley Pharm.)

Each tablet:
  Ferrous fumarate (20.4 mg.
    available iron) * .... 60 mg.
  Thiamine hydrochloride ...... 5 mg.
  Cocoa .... q.s.

EKONO CLEANER

See C-Z EKONO CLEANER

ELAVIL TABLETS
Antidepressant
(MSD)

Each tablet:
  Amitriptyline
    hydrochloride *   10 mg.; 25 mg.;
        50 mg.; 75 mg.;
        100 mg.; or 150 mg.

ELCO CIDE
(Elco Mfg.)

Ronnel 1%
DDVP 1/2%
Petroleum distillate *

ELCO ROACH AND ANT POWDER
(Elco Mfg.)

Sodium fluoride * 40%

ELCO TERMITE KILLER
(Elco Mfg.)

Chlordane * 45.3%
Petroleum distillates * 49.7%

ELDADRYL SYRUP
Expectorant
(Elder)

Each 5 ml.:
  Diphenhydramine
    hydrochloride * .... 13.3 mg.
  Alcohol 7.58%
  Base:
    Menthol
    Sodium citrate
    Ammonium chloride

ELDAMINT
Antacid
(Elder)

Each tablet:
  Calcium carbonate .... 350 mg.
  Aminoacetic acid (Glycine) ... 150 mg.

ELDATAPP
Allergic rhinitis & vasomotor rhinitis and allergic conditions
(Elder)

Each tablet:
  Brompheniramine maleate * 12.0 mg.
  Phenylephrine
    hydrochloride * .... 15.0 mg.
  Phenylpropanolamine
    hydrochloride * .... 15.0 mg.

ELDECORT 1/2% CREAM; 1% CREAM; 2 1/2% CREAM
Allergic, inflammatory or pruritic dermatoses
(Elder)

Hydrocortisone .... 0.5%, 1% or 2.5%

Starred ingredients (*) may be responsible for major toxic effects; consult Section II.

ELDEFED
Antihistaminic
(Elder)

Each tablet:
Triprolidone hydrochloride .. 2.5 mg.
Pseudoephrine
hydrochloride * .... 60.0 mg.

ELDER COLD-TABS
Analgesic-antihistaminic decongestant
(Elder)

Each tablet:
Phenylephrine hydrochloride . 5 mg.
Phenacetin * .... 150 mg.
Pyrilamine maleate * .... 10 mg.
Caffeine .... 15 mg.

ELDER DIAPER RASH OINTMENT
(Elder)

Pramoxine hydrochloride 0.5%
Balsam Peru
Zinc oxide
Zinc stearate

ELDEZINE
Motion sickness and vertigo
(Elder)

Each tablet:
Meclizine hydrochloride * .... 12.5 mg.

ELDIATRIC F.S.
Geriatric B complex with iron & fecal softener
(Elder)

Each 15 ml.:
Vitamin B-1 .... 1.2 mg.
Vitamin B-2 .... 1.7 mg.
Vitamin B-6 .... 1.0 mg.
Vitamin B-12 .... 5.0 mcg.
Niacinamide .... 15.0 mg.
Iron .... 15.0 mg.
Poloxakol .... 200.0 mg.
Alcohol 18.0%

ELDODRAM
Anti-vertigo, motion sickness
(Elder)

Each tablet:
Dimenhydrinate * .... 50 mg.

ELDOPAQUE CREAM
Skin bleach
(Elder)

Hydroquinone * 2%
In an opaque base

ELDOPAQUE FORTE CREAM
Skin bleach
(Elder)

Hydroquinone * 4%
In an opaque base

ELDOQUIN CREAM
Mild bleaching agent
(Elder)

Hydroquinone (1,4-Benzenediol) * .. 2%

ELDOQUIN FORTE CREAM
Skin bleach
(Elder)

Hydroquinone * 4%

ELDOQUIN LOTION
Skin bleach
(Elder)

Hydroquinone * 2%

ELDORADO
Detergent-germicide
(Puritan Chem. Co.)

Active ingred.: 19.92%
Octyl decyl dimethyl am-
monium chloride * 3.750%
Dioctyl dimethyl ammo-
nium chloride * 1.875%
Didecyl dimethyl ammo-
nium chloride * 1.875%
Alkyl (C14, 50%; C12, 40%;
C16, 10%) benzyl dimethyl
ammonium chloride *† .. 5.000%
Tetrasodium ethylenedi-
amine tetraacetate 3.420%
Isopropyl alcohol 3.000%
Ethyl alcohol 1.000%
Inert ingred.: 80.08%

†*See* Benzalkonium chloride

ELECTRA-SOL
Dishwasher detergent
(Economics)

Sodium phosphate *
Sodium silicate
Sodium carbonate
Synthetic wetting agent
Chlorine releasing agent

ELECTROLUX CLEAN SWEEP VACUUM CHIPS
(Electrolux)

Aluminum, iron, & magnesium
silicates 60%
Perfumes (vanilla & lemon) *† 40%

†*See* Volatile oils

ELECTROLUX FLOOR CLEANER AND WAX STRIPPER
(Electrolux)

Nonionic surfactants 1.0%
Anionic surfactants 6.0%
Aqua ammonia 1.5%
Sodium EDTA 0.4%
Sodium xylene sulfonate * 1.0%
Monoethanolamine 2.0%

ELECTROLUX NUVO
Carpet & upholstery cleaner
(Electrolux)

Canadian Formula:
Anionic surfactant 6.0%
Nonionic surfactant 6.0%
Sodium sulfate 5.0%
Sodium EDTA 0.3%
Formaldehyde .... trace
Perfume .... trace
Water .... balance

ELECTROLUX TILE AND TERRAZZO WAX
(Electrolux)

Emulsified Acrylic copolymers . 11.75%
Resin 2.00%
Polyethylene 3.00%
Diethylene glycol monoethyl
ester 2.80%
Dibutyl phthalate 0.30%
Nonionic surfactants .... trace
Tributoxyethyl phosphate 1.20%
Formaldehyde .... trace
Water .... balance

ELECTROLUX TURBO RUG SHAMPOO
(Electrolux)

Ammonium lauryl sulfate 5.7%
Styrene maleic anhydride resin .. 4.1%
Isopropyl alcohol 2.0%
Ammonia * 1.2%
Formaldehyde .... trace
Optical brightener .... trace
Water .... balance

ELECTROLUX TURBO SPOT REMOVER
(Electrolux)

Ammonium lauryl sulfate 0.57%
Styrene maleic anhydride resin .. 0.41%
Isopropyl alcohol 0.20%
Ammonia * 0.12%
Formaldehyde .... trace
Optical brightener .... trace
Stabilizer .... trace
Water .... balance

ELECTROLUX WOOD FLOOR WAX
(Electrolux)

Mineral spirits * 90%
Paraffin wax 5%
Microcrystalline wax 5%

ELECTRO-ZOLE, PURINA

See PURINA ELECTRO-ZOLE

ELEPHANT GLUE
(Sanford Corp.)

Polyvinyl acetate resin emulsion
Water

ELIMINATE, DEL

See DEL ELIMINATE

ELIMSTAPH NO. 2
Germicidal cleaner
(Legge, W.)

Quaternary ammonium compound *

ELIXICON SUSPENSION
Bronchodilator
(Berlex Labs.)

Each 5 ml.:
   Theophylline (anhydrous) * .. 100 mg.

ELIXIRAL
Sedative antispasmodic
(Vita Elixir Co.)

Each 5 cc:
   Phenobarbital * .... 16.20 mg.
   Hyoscyamine sulfate * .... 0.1037 mg.
   Atropine sulfate .... 0.194 mg.
   Hyoscine hydrobromide ... 0.0065 mg.

ELIXOPHYLLIN CAPSULES
Bronchodilator
(Berlex Labs.)

Each capsule:
   Theophylline (anhydrous) * .. 100 mg.
   Polyethylene glycol 400 ...... 124 mg.

ELIXOPHYLLIN CAPSULES 200 mg.
Bronchodilator
(Berlex Labs.)

Each capsule:
   Theophylline (anhydrous) * .. 200 mg.
   Polyethylene glycol 400 ...... 247 mg.

ELIXOPHYLLIN ELIXIR
Bronchodilator
(Berlex Labs.)

Each 15 ml.:
   Theophylline (anhydrous) * .. 80 mg.
   Alcohol 20%

ELIXOPHYLLIN-KI ELIXIR
Bronchodilator, expectorant
(Berlex Labs.)

Each 15 ml.:
   Theophylline (anhydrous) * .. 80 mg.
   Potassium iodide * .... 130 mg.
   Alcohol 10%

ELIXOPHYLLIN SR CAPSULES
Bronchodilator
(Berlex Labs.)

Each sustained-release capsule:
   Theophylline
     (anhydrous) * .... 125 mg.; 250 mg.

ELIZABETH ARDEN COSMETICS

Elizabeth Arden, Inc.
Sub. of Eli Lilly & Co.
1345 Ave. of the Americas
New York, N.Y. 10019

Phone: 212-399-2000

See COSMETICS, Section VI, General Formulations

ELLA BACHE COSMETICS

Ella Bache Beauty Products
8 W. 36th St.
New York, N.Y. 10018

Phone: 212-753-2175

See COSMETICS, Section VI, General Formulations

ELLANAR
Jewel & plastic cement
(L & R)

Nitrocellulose
Plasticizers dissolved in:
   Aromatic hydrocarbons *
   Aliphatic hydrocarbons *

ELLANAR DIP
Silver cleaner
(L & R)

Thiourea
Sulfuric acid *
Dyes
Synthetic wetting agents

ELLANAR JEWELRY CLEANER AND JEWELRY SERVICER
(L & R)

Ammoniated soap
Ammonia *
Isopropyl alcohol *
Perfumes
Dyes

ELLANAR SILVER POLISH
(L & R)

Neutral water base soap
Diatomaceous earth
Cosmetic type mold inhibitor

ELLIOTT PAINT PRODUCTS

Elliott Paint & Varnish Co.
1330 S. Kilbourn Ave.
Chicago, Ill. 60623

Phone: 312-762-7010

See PAINTS, Section VI, General Formulations

ELMER'S CONTACT CEMENT
(Borden, Inc.)

Hydrocarbon-ketone solvent *†
Based rubber-phenolic contact adhesive

†*See* Methyl ethyl ketone

ELMER'S CONTACT CEMENT THINNERS
(Borden, Inc.)

Hydrocarbon-ketone solvent *†

†*See* Methyl ethyl ketone

ELMER'S GLUE ALL
Acetate emulsion adhesive
(Borden, Inc.)

Polyvinyl acetate emulsion

ELMER'S SLIDE-ALL
(Borden, Inc.)

Teflon solution (Aliphatic hydrocarbons including Hexane) *

ELMER'S WATERPROOF GLUE
(Borden, Inc.)

Resorcinol formaldehyde resinous product

EL PICO ALCOHOL STOVE FUEL
(Sta-Lube, Inc.)

S.D. Alcohol * 80%
Isopropanol * 20%

Mixture contains less than 4% methanol

EL PICO ALUMINUM SCREEN CLEANER
(Sta-Lube, Inc.)

Phosphoric acid * 40%
Wetting agent 1%
Water 59%

EL PICO HARD BRUSH CLEANER
(Sta-Lube, Inc.)

Toluene *
Acetone *
Methanol *
Detergent

EL PICO HIGHEST QUALITY PAINT AND VARNISH REMOVER
(Sta-Lube, Inc.)

Methanol * .... 23%/vol.
Methylene chloride * .... 75%/vol.

Starred ingredients (*) may be responsible for major toxic effects; consult Section II.

EL PICO MARINE GRADE PAINT AND VARNISH REMOVER
(Sta-Lube, Inc.)

Methanol *	22%
Methylene chloride *	65%
Chlorothene NU	8%

EL PICO RINSE AWAY PAINT & VARNISH REMOVER
(Sta-Lube, Inc.)

Methanol	10%
Methylene chloride	12%
Acetone	24%
Toluene *	43%
Emulsifier	5%

EL PICO SANDEZE
(Sta-Lube, Inc.)

Acetone	40%
Toluene *	50%
Methanol	10%

ELTAR OINTMENT
Psoriasis and dermatoses
(Elder)

Equiv. to 5% Coal tar: *
   Anthracene
   Phenanthrene
   Naphthalene

ELTRON
For coal tar therapy
(Torch)

Eltar (Crude coal tar, Torch) *	5%
Starch	25%
Zinc oxide	25%

Base:
   Petrolatum & wetting
     agents   qs. ad. 100.0 gm.

'76 Ed.

ELTRON SHAVER CLEANING FLUID
(Eltron)

n-Propanol *	90.0%
Tetrachloroethylene	9.5%
Petroleum distillates	0.5%

EMAGRIN FORTE
Cold relief tablets
(Clapp, Otis)

Phenylephrine hydrochloride	5 mg.
Atropine sulfate	1/1000 gr.
Acetaminophen *	
Caffeine	
Salicylamide	

EMAGRIN PROFESSIONAL STRENGTH
Pain relief
(Clapp, Otis)

Each tablet:
   Aspirin *
   Salicylamide
   Caffeine

EMBEECIDE
Fly kill and insect spray
(Meyer-Blanke Co.)

Pyrethrins	0.075%
Technical Piperonyl butoxide	0.150%
N-Octyl bicycloheptene	
dicarboximide	0.250%
Di-n-propyl isocinchomeronate	0.200%
Petroleum distillate *	99.325%

'76 Ed.

EMDOL TABLETS
For relief of arthritis & rheumatism
(Approved Pharm.)

Each tablet:
   Salicylamide *
   Para aminobenzoic acid sodium *
   Calcium succinate
   Vitamin D   1250 USP units

'76 Ed.

EMETROL
For nausea, vomiting
(Rorer, W.H., Inc.)

Levulose
Dextrose
Orthophosphoric acid

EMILIO PUCCI PERFUMES

Emilio Pucci Perfumes Intl. Inc.
24 E. 64th St.
New York, N.Y. 10021

Phone: 212-752-4777

See COSMETICS, Section VI, General
   Formulations

EMIR DUSTING POWDER (4 oz.) & DELUXE DUSTING POWDER (8 oz.)
(Dana Perfumes)

Essential oils *	>1%
Aromatic chemicals	
Talc	
Zinc stearate	
Magnesium carbonate	

EMIR EAU DE COLOGNE
Sizes - 2 oz., 4 oz., & 8 oz.
(Dana Perfumes)

Essential oils *	>1%
Aromatic chemicals	
Specially denatured Alcohol (39-C) *	
Deionized water	

EMIR SPRAY COLOGNE
Aerosol - 3 oz.
(Dana Perfumes)

Essential oils *	>1%
Aromatic chemicals	
Specially denatured Alcohol (39-C) *	
Dichlorodifluoromethane	
Dichlorotetrafluoroethane	

EMPIRIN ASPIRIN TABLETS
(Burroughs Wellcome)

Each tablet:
   Aspirin *   325 mg.

EMPIRIN WITH CODEINE
Analgesic
(Burroughs Wellcome)

Each tablet:	
Aspirin *	325 mg.
Codeine phosphate *	
No. 2	15 mg.
No. 3	30 mg.
No. 4	60 mg.

EMPRACET WITH CODEINE PHOSPHATE
Analgesic
(Burroughs Wellcome)

Each tablet:	
Codeine phosphate *	30 mg.; 60 mg.
Acetaminophen *	300 mg.

EMPRAZIL-C TABLETS
Nasal decongestant, analgesic, antipyretic, antitussive, anti-inflammatory
(Burroughs Wellcome)

Each tablet:	
Pseudoephedrine	
hydrochloride *	20 mg.
Phenacetin *	150 mg.
Aspirin *	200 mg.
Caffeine	30 mg.
Codeine phosphate *	15 mg.

EMPRAZIL TABLETS
Nasal decongestant, analgesic, antipyretic, anti-inflammatory
(Burroughs Wellcome)

Each tablet:	
Pseudoephedrine	
hydrochloride *	20 mg.
Phenacetin *	150 mg.
Aspirin *	200 mg.
Caffeine	30 mg.

EMRALON
Dry film lubricant
(Acheson Colloids)

Polytetrafluoroethylene

'76 Ed.

Starred ingredients (*) may be responsible for major toxic effects; consult Section II.

EMSOL
Emulsifiable solvent cleaner
(Whitfield Chem.)

Medium flash point Aliphatic petroleum solvent * .... >10%

EMULAVE BAR
For dry skin conditions
(CooperCare)

Aveeno colloidal oatmeal 30%
Vegetable oils
Lanolin derivative
Sudsing & wetting agents

EMUL-O-BALM
Analgesic lotion
(Pennwalt, Pharm. Div.)

Menthol * .... 0.65 gm./fl. oz.
Camphor .... 0.3 gm./fl. oz.
Methyl salicylate * ..... 0.65 gm./fl. oz.

EMULSAMINE BRUSH KILLER
Herbicide
(Amchem)

Alkyl (C12) amine salts of 2,4-
  dichlorophenoxyacetic acid * .. 25.1%
Alkyl (C14) amine salts of 2,4-
  dichlorophenoxyacetic acid 6.3%
Alkyl (C12) amine salts of 2,4,5-
  trichlorophenoxyacetic acid * .. 23.6%
Alkyl (C14) amine salts of 2,4,5-
  trichlorophenoxyacetic acid 5.9%

EMULSAMINE E-3
Herbicide
(Amchem)

Dodecyl amine salts of 2,4-dichlo-
  rophenoxyacetic acid * 50.7%
Tetradecyl amine salts of 2,4-
  dichlorophenoxyacetic acid * .. 12.7%

EMULSAMINE 2,4,5-T
Herbicide
(Amchem)

Alkyl (C12) amine salts of 2,4,5-
  trichlorophenoxyacetic acid * .. 47.1%
Alkyl (C14) amine salts of 2,4,5-
  trichlorophenoxyacetic acid 11.8%

EMULSAVERT 100
Herbicide
(Amchem)

2,4-Dichlorophenoxyacetic acid * . 4.8%
2,4-Dichlorophenoxyacetic acid,
  N,N-dimethyloleylamine salt * . 16.4%
2,4,5-Trichlorophenoxyacetic acid . 3.7%
2,4,5-Trichlorophenoxyacetic acid,
  N,N-dimethyloleylamine salt * . 17.5%

EMULSAVERT 248
Herbicide
(Amchem)

2,4-Dichlorophenoxyacetic acid ... 0.7%
2,4-Dichlorophenoxyacetic acid,
  N,N-dimethyloleylamine salt * . 12.5%
2,4,5-Trichlorophenoxyacetic acid . 6.0%
2,4,5-Trichlorophenoxyacetic acid,
  N,N-dimethyloleylamine salt * . 13.3%

EMULSER CF
Biodegradable nonionic emulsifying agent
(Arkansas Co.)

Polyethylene glycol fatty acid esters *
'76 Ed.

EMULSER OM
Biodegradable nonionic emulsifying agent
(Arkansas Co.)

Alkanolamide-polyglycol-fatty acid condensate *†
'76 Ed.

†*See* Nonionic synthetic detergents

EMULSION "C" DEGREASER
(Consolidated Chem., Inc.)

Tall oil fatty acids
Isopropanol *
Petroleum solvent *
Sodium hydroxide *

EMULSO
Engine cleaner
(Lester Labs.)

Pine oil *
Petroleum solvents *
'76 Ed.

EMULSO DEGREASER
Water-solvent heavy duty cleaner
(National-Purity Soap)

Hard water chelants
Surfactants *

pH of 1% solution, 11

ENCARE
Contraceptive
(Eaton-Merz)

Each insert:
  Nonoxynol-9 .... 2.27%
  Combined amount: .... <12%
    Tartaric acid
    Sodium tartrate
  Sodium lauryl sulfate 2%
  Lactalbumin .... <10%
  Combined amount: .... <5%
    Polypeptide
    Fatty acid condensate
  Sodium bicarbonate 6.69%
  Polyethylene glycol 68%
  Perfume oil .... <0.1%

END-AKE ANALGESIC CREAM
(Columbia Med.)

Methyl nicotinate
Salicylamide *
Histamine dihydrochloride
Dipropyleneglycol salicylate *
Capsicum oleoresin *

END-A-KOFF, JR.
Pediatric cough syrup
(Columbia Med.)

Each 5 ml.:
  Dextromethorphan HBr * ... 5 mg.
  Glyceryl guaiacolate .... 12.5 mg.
  Ammonium chloride .... 60 mg.
  Sodium citrate .... 40 mg.

END-A-KOFF 6-WAY COUGH SYRUP
(Columbia Med.)

Each 10 ml.:
  Dextromethorphan HBr * ... 15 mg.
  Glyceryl guaiacolate .... 50 mg.
  Chlorpheniramine maleate ... 2 mg.
  Phenylephrine HCl .... 5 mg.
  Acetaminophen * .... 120 mg.
  Alcohol 10%

ENDEP
Antidepressant
(Roche)

Each tablet:
  Amitriptyline HCl * . 10 mg.; 25 mg.;
                        50 mg.; 75 mg.;
                        100 mg.; 150 mg.

ENDEW
Stops mildew, ends odors, fights moths
(Clarke, John, & Co.)

Paraformaldehyde * 50%
Naphthalene * 50%

END-O-ALGE 2
See CPC END-O-ALGE 2

END-O-ALGE, SUPER CONCENTRATED
See CPC SUPER CONCENTRATED
END-O-ALGE

ENDOTHAL TURF HERBICIDE
Herbicide
(Pennwalt)

Endothall (as disodium
  salt)(liquid
  concentrate) * .... 1.46 lbs./gal.

Starred ingredients (*) may be responsible for major toxic effects; consult Section II.

ENDOTHAL WEED KILLER
Herbicide
(Pennwalt)

Endothall (as disodium
salt)(liquid
concentrate) * .... 1.46 lbs./gal.

ENDURANCE OIL
(Marathon Oil Co.)

Additives, containing Zinc alkyl
dithiophosphate, Magnesium,
Calcium, Sulfur compounds,
Methacrylate copolymer 1.7%
Mineral oil .... balance

EN-DURE HEAVY DUTY NO RUBBING FLOOR WAX
(Uncle Sam)

Carnauba wax and/or synthetic waxes
Resins (modified phenolics)
Emulsifiers
Ammonia *
Polyethylene
Morpholine *
Potassium hydroxide *
Water

ENDURO CREAM FURNITURE POLISH
(Midwest Mfg.)

Stearic acid
Mineral oil
Bakers emulsion A
Triethanolamine
Water

ENDURO DRY CLEANING FLUID
(Midwest Mfg.)

Naphthol spirits *
Chlorothene *

ENDURON TABLETS
Diuretic
(Abbott)

Each tablet:
　Methyclothiazide * .. 2.5 mg.; or 5 mg.

ENDURONYL FORTE TABLETS
Antihypertensive
(Abbott)

Each tablet:
　Methyclothiazide * .... 5 mg.
　Deserpidine * .... 0.5 mg.

ENDURONYL TABLETS
Antihypertensive
(Abbott)

Each tablet:
　Methyclothiazide * .... 5 mg.
　Deserpidine * .... 0.25 mg.

ENDURO RUG & UPHOLSTERY SHAMPOO
(Midwest Mfg.)

Orvis paste
Isopropyl alcohol *
Ammonia *

ENDURO SPEEDY WAX CLEANER & PRESERVATIVE
(Midwest Mfg.)

Gum tragacanth
Bentonite
Alcohol *
Mineral oil
Sulfonated castor oil *
Glycerine
Filter cell
Wintergreen oil *

ENDURO SPOT REMOVER
(Midwest Mfg.)

Odorless Mineral spirits *
Chlorothene *

ENDURO WIG & TOUPEE CLEANER
(Midwest Mfg.)

Odorless Mineral spirits *
Chlorothene *

ENDUST
Dusting aid, aerosol
(Drackett)

Light mineral oil
1,1,1-Trichloroethane * approx. 20%/wt.
Paraffin hydrocarbon solvent
Hydrocarbon
　propellants .... approx. 30%/wt.
Perfume

ENE-PET SOLUTION
*A ready-to-use enema to relieve consti-
pation in cats and dogs*
(Haver-Lockhart (Brand) Bayvet Div.
Cutter Labs.)

Dioctyl sodium sulfosuccinate * 250 mg.
Glycerine .... 5 ml.

ENERGETIC LIQUID SYNTHETIC DETERGENT
(Armour-Dial, Inc.)

Nonionic active 75-100%
Moisture 10-25%

ENERGINE FIREPROOF CLEANING FLUID
(d-Con)

1,1,1-Trichloroethane * 100%

ENERGINE SPOT REMOVER
(d-Con)

Naphtha * 100%

ENERGIZE COMBUSTION IMPROVER & FUEL OIL TREATMENT
(Uncle Sam)

Heavy Aromatic solvent *
Surfactant
Combustion improver

ENERJETS
To combat drowsiness
(Chilton Labs.)

Each tablet:
　Caffeine * .... 70 mg.
　Sugar .... balance
　Flavoring .... <1%

ENGINE BRITE ENGINE CLEANER (E.B.)

See GUNK E.B. - ENGINE BRITE EN-
GINE CLEANER

ENGINKOOL

See SILOO ENGINKOOL

ENGINSEAL

See SILOO ENGINSEAL

ENGRAN-HP TABLETS
Prenatal vitamin-mineral supplement
(Squibb)

Each tablet:
　Vitamin A acetate ... 4000 USP units
　Ergocalciferol (D) ... 200 USP units
　Iron, elemental (as stabilized
　　ferrous carbonate) .... 9 mg.
　Plus Multivitamins & minerals

ENOVID
Progesten-estrogen combination
(Searle, G.D., & Co.)

Each 5 mg. tablet:
　Norëthynodrel .... 5 mg.
　Mestranol .... 0.075 mg.

Each 10 mg. tablet:
　Norethynodrel .... 9.85 mg.
　Mestranol .... 0.15 mg.

ENOVID-E
Progesten-estrogen combination
(Searle, G.D., & Co.)

Each tablet:
　Norethynodrel .... 2.5 mg.
　Mestranol .... 0.1 mg.

ENOXA LIQUID
Anti-diarrhea
(Direct Div.)

Each 5 ml.:
　Diphenoxylate HCl * ...... 2.5 mg.
　Atropine sulfate .... 0.025 mg.
　Ethyl alcohol 15%

Starred ingredients (*) may be responsible for major toxic effects; consult Section II.

ENOXA TABLETS
Anti-diarrhea
(Direct Div.)

Each tablet:
Diphenoxylate HCl * ...... 2.5 mg.
Atropine sulfate * .... 0.025 mg.

ENSEALS SODIUM SALICYLATE
For minor aches & pains of neuralgic & rheumatic conditions
(Lilly, Eli)

Sodium salicylate * .... 5 gr.

ENTACIDE

See AIRWICK PROFESSIONAL PRODUCTS ENTACIDE

ENTACIDE R

See AIRWICK PROFESSIONAL PRODUCTS ENTACIDE R

ENTERPRISE CLEAR CONCRETE SEALER
(Enterprise Paint Co.)

Xylol *

ENTERPRISE CLEAR MASONRY COATING
(Enterprise Paint Co.)

Petroleum distillates *

ENTERPRISE EPOXY & POOL PRIDE THINNER & BRUSH CLEANER
(Enterprise Paint Co.)

Ethylbenzene *
Cellosolve

ENTERPRISE INSTANT CLEANER AND WAX REMOVER
(Enterprise Paint Co.)

Butyl Cellosolve *
Sodium metasilicate *

ENTEX
Insecticide
(Hub States)

O,O-Dimethyl O-(4-(methylthio)-m-tolyl) phosphorothioate *

Oil soluble concentrate contains 4 lb. of active ingred. per gal.
Spray concentrate contains 4 lb. active ingred. per gal.

'76 Ed.

ENURETROL CHEWABLE TABLETS
Nocturnal enuresis
(Berlex Labs.)

Each tablet:
Ephedrine sulfate * .... 7.5 mg.
Atropine sulfate * .... 0.15 mg.

ENVERT-DT
Herbicide
(Amchem)

2,4-Dichlorophenoxyacetic acid, butoxy ethanol ester * 17.9%
2,4,5-Trichlorophenoxyacetic acid,
butoxy ethanol ester * 17.2%

ENVERT-T
Herbicide
(Amchem)

2,4,5-Trichlorophenoxyacetic acid,
butoxy ethanol ester * 34.0%

ENVIRON, MASTER MIX

See MASTER MIX ENVIRON

ENZIT
Stain remover
(Beautilite Corp.)

Butyl Cellosolve * ...... small amount

'76 Ed.

EPHEDRINE AND NEMBUTAL 25 CAPSULES
Antiallergic, antispasmodic, sedative
(Abbott)

Each capsule:
Ephedrine hydrochloride * ...... 25 mg.
Sodium pentobarbital * ...... 25 mg.

EPHEDROL WITH CODEINE
Antitussive, antispasmodic
(Lilly, Eli)

Each 100 cc:
Codeine sulfate * .... 200 mg.
Ma Huang fluid extract ...... 11 ml.
Potassium guaiacol sulfonate 1.75 gm.
Squill solid extract .... 140 mg.
Tolu balsam .... 120 mg.
Menthol .... 13 mg.

EPHENYLLIN
Antiasthmatic decongestant-sedative
(CMC Research Div.)

Each tablet:
Phenobarbital .... 8 mg.
Theophylline * .... 130 mg.
Ephedrine hydrochloride * ... 24 mg.

E-pHICIENT CLEANER - REGULAR NO. 44
(Polychem Corp.)

Sodium dodecylbenzenesulfonate
Water
Propylene glycol
Linear Alcohol ethoxylate
Coconut diethanolamide
Tetrasodium EDTA
Sodium xylene sulfonate
Quaternium-15
Citric acid

EPIC ARTERIAL
Embalming fluid
(Embalmers')

Formaldehyde *

EPIC BRUSH & ROLLER CLEANER
(Enterprise Paint Co.)

Aliphatic hydrocarbons *
Esters *†

†*See* Solvents and Thinners, Section VI, General Formulations

EPIC CAVITY
Embalming fluid
(Embalmers')

Formaldehyde *

EPIC DRAINAGE
Embalming fluid
(Embalmers')

Methanol *

EPIC GLOSS CUTTER
Prepares surfaces for refinishing
(Enterprise Paint Co.)

Xylol *
Ethanol

EPI*CLEAR ACNE LOTION
For acne; 1 fl. oz. bottle
(Squibb)

Sulfur 10%
Alcohol 10%

EPI*CLEAR ACNE SOAP
(Squibb)

Combined amount: 6.3%
Sulfated surfactants
Hydrocarbon hydrotropes

EPI*CLEAR ANTISEPTIC LOTION
For acne; 1 fl. oz. bottle
(Squibb)

Benzoyl peroxide .... 5% or 10%
In a greaseless water-washable base

Starred ingredients (*) may be responsible for major toxic effects; consult Section II.

EPI*CLEAR SCRUB CLEANSER
For acne
(Squibb)

Aluminum oxide particles in a surfactant cleansing base
Fine: 38%
Medium: 52%
Coarse: 65%

EPIC ODORLESS PAINT THINNER
(Enterprise Paint Co.)

Mineral spirits *
Cellosolve *

EPIC STAIN CONTROL
For use on bare wood before staining & refinishing to control penetration
(Enterprise Paint Co.)

Xylol *
Cellosolve

EPIC STRIP AWAY
Paint and varnish remover
(Enterprise Paint Co.)

Methylene chloride *
Methanol *

EPIFRIN
Ophthalmic solutions
(Allergan Pharm.)

Levo-epinephrine (as the HCl) .... 0.25%; 0.5%; 1.0%; or 2.0%
Benzalkonium chloride
Sodium metabisulfite
Edetate disodium
Purified water
Sodium chloride (in the 0.25% formulation only)

E-PILO OPHTHALMIC SOLUTION
For treatment of glaucoma
(CooperVision Pharm.)

Pilocarpine hydrochloride * .... 1%; 2%; 3%; 4% and 6%
Epinephrine bitartrate 1%
Disodium edetate
Benzalkonium chloride

EPINAL (1/2% and 1/4%)
Ophthalmic solution
(Alcon)

Active ingred.:
　Epinephryl borate (equiv. to epinephrine 0.25% or 0.50%)
Preservative:
　Benzalkonium chloride 0.01%
Vehicle:
　Hydroxypropyl methylcellulose solution
Inactive ingred.:
　Ascorbic acid
　Acetylcysteine
　Boric acid
　Sodium carbonate (to adjust pH)
　Purified water

EPINEPHRICAINE RECTAL OINTMENT
Local anesthetic and antiseptic
(Upjohn)

Epinephrine 0.2%
Secondary-amyltricresols 1.0%
Zinc oxide 2.0%
Benzocaine 2.5%
In a bland base containing vitamins A and D

EPITAPH AEROSOL FOR INSECTS
Insecticide
(Brulin)

Pyrethrins 0.5%
Technical Piperonyl butoxide 1.0%
N-Octyl bicycloheptene dicarboximide 1.0%
Petroleum distillate 8.5%

EPITAPH LIQUID INSECTICIDE
(Brulin)

Technical Piperonyl butoxide 1.0%
Pyrethrins 0.20%
Beta-butoxy-beta-thiocyano-di-ethyl ether * 1.09%
Petroleum distillates * 97.71%

EPN EMULSIFIABLE INSECTICIDE
For use on cotton
(Velsicol)

O-Ethyl, O-p-nitrophenylphenyl-phosphonothioate * 56.00%
Xylene range aromatic solvent .. 31.73%

EPOCA CAVITY
Embalming fluids
(Embalmers')

Formaldehyde *
Methanol *

E-POX-E CEMENT, BALKAMP

See BALKAMP E-POX-E CEMENT

E-POX-E GLUE, BALKAMP

See BALKAMP E-POX-E GLUE

E-POX-E STEEL, BALKAMP

See BALKAMP E-POX-E STEEL

EPOXYBOND PASTE
(Atlas Minerals & Chemicals)

Resin:
　Diglycidyl ether of BPA (Bisphenol A) 30-35%
　1,4 Butane diol diglycidyl ether *† 5-10%
　Calcium carbonate 40-50%
　Organic and inorganic pigments 5-10%
　Fumed Silica 1-5%

Hardener:
　Modified polyamines 30-40%
　Nonyl phenol * 2-5%
　Calcium carbonate 45-55%
　Talc 5-12%
　Fumed Silica 1-5%

†*See* Glycidyl ethers

EPOXYBOND PUTTY
(Atlas Minerals & Chemicals)

Resin:
　Diglycidyl ether of BPA (Bisphenol A) 20-25%
　Pigments 3-10%
　Calcium carbonate 60-75%

Hardener:
　Polyamido amine 10-20%
　Calcium carbonate 80-90%

EPOXYSTRIP
(Beck Chem.)

Combined amount: .... <10%
　Chloroacetic acid *
　Formic acid *
　Cresylic acid * .... <10%

EPPY/N 1/2%
For simple open-angle glaucoma
(Barnes-Hind)

Epinephrine (free base) 0.5%
Isotonic buffered solution
Erythorbic acid
Boric acid
Povidone
Polyoxyl 40 stearate
Benzalkonium chloride 0.01%
Sodium hydroxide (added to adjust pH)

EPPY/N 1%
For simple open-angle glaucoma
(Barnes-Hind)

Epinephrine (free base) 1%
Mildly hypertonic buffered solution
Erythorbic acid
Boric acid
Povidone
Polyoxyl 40 stearate
Benzalkonium chloride 0.01%
Sodium hydroxide (added to adjust pH)

Starred ingredients (*) may be responsible for major toxic effects; consult Section II.

EPRAGEN
Analgesic, sympathomimetic
(Lilly, Eli)

Each Pulvule:
Aspirin *	130 mg.
Phenacetin *	227 mg.
Amobarbital *	50 mg.
Ephedrine hydrochloride *	22 mg.

EPTAM (7-E, 10-G)
Herbicide
(Stauffer)

Eptam (S-Ethyl dipropylthiocarbamate) *

EQUAGESIC-M TABLETS
Relief of musculoskeletal pain accompanied by tension and/or anxiety
(Wyeth Labs.)

Each tablet:
Meprobamate *	200 mg.
Aspirin *	325 mg.

EQUAGESIC TABLETS
Relief of pain accompanied by anxiety and/or tension
(Wyeth Labs.)

Each tablet:
Meprobamate *	150 mg.
Ethoheptazine citrate *	75 mg.
Aspirin *	250 mg.

EQUANIL
Management of anxiety disorders
(Wyeth Labs.)

Capsules (each):
Meprobamate *	400 mg.

Tablets (each):
Meprobamate *	200 mg.; 400 mg.

EQUANIL, WYSEALS
Management of anxiety disorders
(Wyeth Labs.)

Each tablet:
Meprobamate *	400 mg.

EQUANITRATE 10 & 20
Management or treatment of angina pectoris
(Wyeth Labs.)

10 (each tablet):
Pentaerythritol tetranitrate *	10 mg.
Meprobamate	200 mg.

20 (each tablet):
Pentaerythritol tetranitrate *	20 mg.
Meprobamate	200 mg.

EQUICOL
Equine expectorant
(Burns-Biotec)

Each ml.:
Guaifenesin	100 mg.
Thymol (preservative) *	1.66 mg.

EQUI-SHIELD GEL
Insecticide, repellent and coat conditioner for horses
(Carson Chemicals, Inc.)

Pyrethrins	0.1%
Technical Piperonyl butoxide	1.0%
Butoxypolypropylene glycol *	10.0%
Pine oil	2.0%

ERA (Formula 1)
Heavy duty liquid laundry detergent
(Procter & Gamble)

Water	50-74%
Alkyl ethoxylate *	10-24%
Sodium alkyl ethoxylate sulfate	10-24%
Ethanol *	5-9%
Monoethanolamine	1-4%
Minor ingredients, each	trace

pH (as is) - 10.0

ERAMYCIN
Antibiotic-antibacterial
(Wesley Pharm.)

Each tablet:
Erythromycin stearate	250 mg.

ERA PLUS (Formula 2)
Heavy duty liquid laundry detergent
(Procter & Gamble)

Water	50-74%
Alkyl ethoxylate *	10-24%
Sodium alkyl ethoxylate sulfate	10-24%
Ethanol *	10-24%
Enzyme solution (10% enzymes)	1-4%
Sodium formate	1-4%
Minor ingredients, each	trace

pH (as is) - 7.5

ERBON 4 HERBICIDE
(Dow)

Erbon 2-(2,4,5-Trichlorophenoxy)ethyl-2,2-dichloropropionate *	30.5%
Related compounds	10.5%
Inert ingred.:	59.0%
Emulsifiers	
Petroleum solvent *	

ERGONAL
Obstetric use and for menstrual and gynecological disorders
(Vita Elixir Co.)

Each capsule:
Ergot powder N.F. *	259.2 mg.
Aloin, U.S.P.	8.1 mg.
Apiol fluid green	290 mg.
Oil pennyroyal	28 mg.
Cottonseed oil U.S.P.	q.s.ad 10 mins.

ERGOPHENE SKIN OINTMENT
Antiseptic
(Upjohn)

Each oz.:
Fluidextract Ergot *	45 min.
Phenol *	7 1/2 gr.
Zinc oxide	22 1/2 gr.
Sodium borate	1 2/3 gr.

ERGOTAL
Sympatholytic
(Russ Pharm.)

Each capsule:
Phenobarbital *	40.0 mg.
Ergotamine tartrate	0.6 mg.
Belladonna alkaloids	0.2 mg.

ERNO LASZLO ACTIVE SUNBLOCKING LOTION
(Chesebrough-Pond's)

Water	>50%
Octyl methoxycinnamate	>5-10%
Sorbitol	>1-5%
Glyceryl stearate	>1-5%
Benzophenone-3	>1-5%
Cetyl alcohol	>1-5%
Stearic acid	>1-5%
Laureth-23	>0.1-1%
Triethanolamine	>0.1-1%
Quaternium-15	>0.1-1%
Titanium dioxide	>0.1-1%
Methylparaben	>0.1-1%
Carbomer-934	>0.1-1%
Propylparaben	0.1% or less
Simethicone	0.1% or less
Fragrance	0.1% or less
Trisodium EDTA	0.1% or less

ERNO LASZLO BLUSHING CREME (All Shades)
(Chesebrough-Pond's)

Mineral oil	>50%
Titanium dioxide	10-20%
Stearamide MIPA	1-10%
Ceresin	1-10%
Colors	1-10%
Hybrid Safflower oil	1-10%
Silica	0.1-1%
Nonoxynol-4	0.1-1%
Fragrance	0.1-1%
Dioctyl succinate	0.1% or less
Propylene glycol dipelargonate	0.1% or less
Diisopropyl adipate	0.1% or less
Isopropyl palmitate	0.1% or less
Isopropyl myristate	0.1% or less
BHT	0.1% or less
BHA	0.1% or less
Isopropyl stearate	0.1% or less

Starred ingredients (*) may be responsible for major toxic effects; consult Section II.

ERNO LASZLO BLUSHING POWDER (All Shades)
(Chesebrough-Pond's)

Talc	>50%
Bismuth oxychloride	10-20%
Lithium stearate	1-10%
Mineral oil	1-10%
Colors	1-10%
Hybrid Safflower oil	0.1-1%
Silica	0.1-1%
Methylparaben	<0.1%
Quaternium-15	<0.1%
Propylparaben	<0.1%
Dioctyl succinate	<0.1%
Propylene glycol dipelargonate	<0.1%
Diisopropyl adipate	<0.1%
Isopropyl palmitate	<0.1%
Isopropyl myristate	<0.1%
BHT	<0.1%
BHA	<0.1%
Isopropyl stearate	<0.1%

ERNO LASZLO NORMALIZER MAKEUP BASE
(Chesebrough-Pond's)

Water	>50%
Glyceryl stearate	1-5%
Magnesium aluminum silicate	1-5%
Propylene glycol	1-5%
Colors	1-5%
PPG-2 myristal ether propionate	1-5%
Mineral oil	1-5%
Acetylated Lanolin alcohol	1-5%
Stearic acid	1-5%
Lanolin alcohol	0.1-1%
Methylparaben	0.1-1%
Propylparaben	0.1-1%
Fragrance	0.1-1%
Synthetic Spermaceti	0.1-1%
DMDM hydantoin	0.1-1%
Triethanolamine	0.1-1%
Cellulose gum	0.1-1%
Disodium monooleamidosulfosuccinate	0.1-1%

ERNO LASZLO pHELITYL BODYSKIN CREAM
(Chesebrough-Pond's)

Water	>50%
Cetearyl alcohol	>1-5%
Mineral oil	>1-5%
Glyceryl stearate	>1-5%
Acetylated Lanolin alcohol	>1-5%
PEG-8	>1-5%
Cocoa butter	>0.1-1%
PPG-2 myristyl ether propionate	>0.1-1%
Ceteareth-20	>0.1-1%
DMDM hydantoin	>0.1-1%
Trilaneth-4 phosphate	>0.1-1%
Dimethicone	>0.1-1%
Imidazolidinyl urea	>0.1-1%
Sodium hydroxide	0.1% or less
Fragrance	0.1% or less

ERNO LASZLO pHELITYL BODYSKIN LOTION
(Chesebrough-Pond's)

Water	>50%
PEG-8	>1-5%
Mineral oil	>1-5%
Glyceryl stearate	>1-5%
PPG-2 myristyl ether propionate	>1-5%
Trilaneth-4 phosphate	>0.1-1%
Cetearyl alcohol	>0.1-1%
Dimethicone	>0.1-1%
DMDM hydantoin	>0.1-1%
Ceteareth-20	>0.1-1%
Methylparaben	>0.1-1%
Imidazolidinyl urea	>0.1-1%
Lanolin alcohol	>0.1-1%
Carbomer-934	>0.1-1%
Propylparaben	0.1% or less
Sodium hydroxide	0.1% or less
Fragrance	0.1% or less

ERNO LASZLO SPECIAL CONTROLLING LOTION
(Chesebrough-Pond's)

Water	>50%
SD Alcohol 40	>10-25%
Octoxynol-13	>1-5%
Quaternium-26	>0.1-1%
Glycerin	>0.1-1%
Diisopropyl adipate	>0.1-1%
Propylene glycol	>0.1-1%
Allantoin	>0.1-1%
Fragrance	>0.1-1%
Methylparaben	>0.1-1%
Quaternium-33	>0.1-1%
Ethyl hexanediol	>0.1-1%
Trisodium EDTA	0.1% or less

E-R-O EAR DROPS
(Scherer Labs.)

Each fl. oz.:
    Glycerine
    Propylene glycol

ERTINE OINTMENT
First aid & burns
(Approved Pharm.)

Hexachlorophene	0.25%
Diperodon HCl	0.5%
Allantoin	0.2%
Water miscible base:	
Eucalyptol	
Benzyl alcohol	

'76 Ed.

ERUSTICATOR
Rust remover
(Pennwalt)

Hydrofluoric acid *
Ammonium bifluoride

ERUSTORAY
Laundry sour
(Pennwalt)

Silicofluoride *

ERUSTO SALTS SPECIAL
Rust remover
(Pennwalt)

Acid fluorides (Bifluorides) *
Silicofluoride *

ERYTHROCIN STEARATE FILMTAB
Antibiotic
(Abbott)

Erythromycin stearate (USP) .... 125 mg.; 250 mg.; 500 mg.

ERYTHROMAST 36 INTRAMAMMARY SOLUTION
Antibiotic; veterinary
(Syntex Agribusiness)

Each 6 ml. dose:
    Erythromycin .... 300 mg.

ESCAPE STRIPPER

See AIRWICK PROFESSIONAL PRODUCTS ESCAPE STRIPPER

ESCO BEAUTIFYING TINT
Undertakers', embalmers' supplies
(Embalmers')

Chlorinated hydrocarbons *

ESCO DRY SHAMPOO
Undertakers', embalmers' supplies
(Embalmers')

Chlorinated hydrocarbons *

ESCO FLUID COLORING
Undertakers', embalmers' supplies
(Embalmers')

Isopropanol *

ESCO LEAKPROOF SKIN
Undertakers', embalmers' supplies
(Embalmers')

Chlorinated hydrocarbons *
Vinyl resin
Acrylic resin

ESCO LIQUID POWDER
Undertakers', embalmers' supplies
(Embalmers')

Isopropanol *

Starred ingredients (*) may be responsible for major toxic effects; consult Section II.

ESCOT
Antacid
(Direct Div.)

Each capsule:
Bismuth aluminate *† .... 100 mg.
Magnesium trisilicate * ...... 160 mg.
Coprecipitate of Aluminum hy-
droxide and Magnesium
carbonate * .... 130 mg.

†*See* Bismuth salts

E.S. - ESTEAM (Powder)
See GUNK E.S. - ESTEAM (Powder)

ESIDRIX
Diuretic-antihypertensive
(CIBA Pharmaceutical)

Each tablet:
Hydrochlorothiazide * . 25 mg.; 50 mg.

ESKALITH CAPSULES
*Control of manic episodes in manic-de-
pressive psychosis*
(SK&F)

Each capsule:
Lithium carbonate * .... 300 mg.

ESKALITH CR TABLETS
*Control of manic episodes in manic-de-
pressive psychosis*
(SK&F)

Each tablet:
Lithium carbonate * .... 450 mg.

ESKALITH TABLETS
*Control of manic episodes in manic-de-
pressive psychosis*
(SK&F)

Each tablet:
Lithium carbonate * .... 300 mg.

ESOTERICA CREAM (Regu-
lar, Facial, Fortified)
Fade cream
(Norcliff Thayer)

Hydroquinone * 2.0%

ESPOTABS
Laxative
(Combe Inc.)

Yellow Phenolphthalein

ESQUIRE SHOE CARE
PRODUCTS
(Knomark)

Knomark, Inc.
132 Merrick Blvd.
Jamaica, N.Y. 11434

Phone: 212-276-3400

ESTEAM - E.S. (Powder)
See GUNK E.S. - ESTEAM (Powder)

ESTEE LAUDER COSMETIC
PRODUCTS
Estee Lauder Inc.
767 Fifth Ave.
New York, N.Y. 10022

Phone: 212-572-4200

See COSMETICS, Section VI, General
Formulations

ESTEEM, KLENZADE
See KLENZADE ESTEEM

ESTERCOL
For skin irritation
(Torch)

Mercury oleate * 0.45%
Phenol (Carbolic acid) 0.5%
Salicylic acid * 3.0%
Coal tar * 1.2%
Oil emulsion vehicle .... ad. 100.0 cc.

'76 Ed.

ESTERON 76 BE HERBICIDE
(Dow)

2,4-Dichlorophenoxyacetic acid, butyl esters (2,4-dichlorophenoxy-
acetic acid equivalent - 63.2%) * 79.2%
Inert ingred.: 20.8%
Petroleum solvent 16.8%

ESTERON BRUSH KILLER
(Dow)

2,4-D propylene glycol butyl ether
esters * 36.0%
2,4,5-T propylene glycol butyl ether
esters * 34.1%
Inert ingred.: 29.9%
Petroleum solvents * 26.4%

ESTERON 245
CONCENTRATE
Herbicide
(Dow)

2,4,5-Trichlorophenoxy acetic acid,
propylene glycol butyl ether
esters * 92.5%
Inert ingred.: 7.5%
Petroleum solvent 2.5%

ESTERON 6E HERBICIDE
(Dow)

2,4-Dichlorophenoxyacetic acid,
isooctyl ester (2,4-dichlorophen-
oxyacetic acid equivalent -
62.6%) * 94.4%

ESTERON FOUR WEED
KILLER
Herbicide
(Dow)

Active ingred.: 72.8%
2,4-Dichlorophenoxyacetic acid, butoxy
propyl ester *
Inert ingred.: 27.2%
Emulsifiers
Petroleum solvent *

ESTERON 245 HERBICIDE
(Dow)

2,4,5-T butyl ether esters of propylene glycol (2,4,5-T acid equivalent 45.0%) *† 69.2%
Inert ingred.: 30.8%
Petroleum solvent 27.3%

†*See* Trichlorophenoxyacetic acid

ESTERON 44 IMPROVED
WEED KILLER
(Dow)

2,4-Dichlorophenoxyacetic acid, bu-
tyl esters * 51.0%
Inert ingred.: 49.0%
Emulsifiers
Petroleum solvent *

ESTERON 10-10 WEED
KILLER
(Dow)

Active ingred.: 72.8%
2,4-Dichlorophenoxyacetic acid, propyl-
ene glycol butyl ether esters *
Inert ingred.: 27.2%
Emulsifier
Petroleum solvent *

ESTERON 99 WEED KILLER
Herbicide
(Dow)

2,4-Dichlorophenoxyacetic acid,
propylene glycol butyl ether
esters * 41.0%
Inerts: 59.0%
Principally Petroleum solvent *

ESTERON 99 WEED KILLER
CONCENTRATE
Herbicide
(Dow)

2,4-Dichlorophenoxyacetic acid,
propylene glycol butyl ether
esters * 72.8%
Inerts: 27.2%
Principally Petroleum solvent *

ESTES NU-RAL TABLETS
Analgesic
(Estes)

Acetylsalicylic acid * .... 5 gr.
Caffeine .... 1/6 gr.

Starred ingredients (*) may be responsible for major toxic effects; consult Section II.

ESTINYL TABLETS
Estrogen therapy
(Schering)

Each tablet:
Ethinyl estradiol ... 0.02 mg.; 0.05 mg.;
or 0.5 mg.

ESTRACE
Estrogen replacement therapy
(Mead Johnson)

Each tablet:
Estradiol (micronized) ..... 1 or 2 mg.

ETERNAFLEX LATEX
ACRYLIC SEALANT
(Gibson-Homans)

Acrylic latex emulsion .. approx. 35-40%
Plasticizer .... approx. 10%
Whiting .... approx. 45-50%
Petroleum thinner ...... approx. 1%

ETERNAL BLACK WRITING
INK

See HIGGINS ETERNAL BLACK
WRITING INK

ETHIQUE COSMETICS

Ethique Laboratories
P.O. Box 708
Elmhurst, Ill. 60126

Phone: 312-543-9035

See COSMETICS, Section VI, General
Formulations

"ETHYL" ANTIKNOCK
COMPOUND-"MLA"
MOTOR MIX
(Ethyl Corp.)

Mixed Lead alkyls *
Ethylene dibromide *
Ethylene dichloride *
Dye and inerts

"ETHYL" ANTIKNOCK
COMPOUND-TEL
AVIATION MIX
(Ethyl Corp.)

Tetraethyl lead *
Ethylene dibromide *
Ethylene dichloride *
Dye and inerts

"ETHYL" ANTIKNOCK
COMPOUND-"TELMEL"
MOTOR MIX
(Ethyl Corp.)

Tetraethyl lead *
Tetramethyl lead *
Ethylene dibromide *
Ethylene dichloride *
Dye and inerts

"ETHYL" ANTIKNOCK
COMPOUND-TEL MOTOR
MIX
(Ethyl Corp.)

Tetraethyl lead *
Ethylene dibromide *
Ethylene dichloride *
Dye and inerts

"ETHYL" ANTIKNOCK
COMPOUND-TEL MOTOR
33 MIX
(Ethyl Corp.)

Tetraethyl lead *
Methyl cyclopentadienyl manganese tri-
carbonyl
Ethylene dibromide *
Ethylene dichloride *
Dye and inerts

"ETHYL" ANTIKNOCK
COMPOUND-TML MOTOR
MIX
(Ethyl Corp.)

Tetramethyl lead *
Ethylene dibromide *
Ethylene dichloride *
Dye and inerts

"ETHYL" ASHLESS
LUBRICANT ADDITIVE 1
Motor oil additive
(Ethyl Corp.)

Alkylated phenols *†
Organic phosphorus
Nitrogen

†*See* Cresol

"ETHYL" DIESEL IGNITION
IMPROVER
(Ethyl Corp.)

Primary Amyl nitrate *

"ETHYL" OIL SOLUBLE
DYE AUTOMATE (BLUE
LIQUID, BRONZE LIQUID,
ORANGE LIQUID, RED
LIQUID, RED-B LIQUID,
RED-G LIQUID
*Imparts desired color to refinery prod-
ucts*
(Ethyl Corp.)

Organic Azo dye *†
Aromatic solvent *

†*See* Pigments, Section VI, General Formulations

ETRAFON-A TABLETS
Tranquilizer-antidepressant
(Schering)

Each tablet:
Perphenazine .... 4 mg.
Amitriptyline HCl * .... 10 mg.

ETRAFON-FORTE TABLETS
Tranquilizer-antidepressant
(Schering)

Each tablet:
Perphenazine .... 4 mg.
Amitriptyline HCl * .... 25 mg.

ETRAFON 2-10 TABLETS
Tranquilizer-antidepressant
(Schering)

Each tablet:
Perphenazine .... 2 mg.
Amitriptyline HCl * .... 10 mg.

ETRAFON 2-25 TABLETS
Tranquilizer-antidepressant
(Schering)

Each tablet:
Perphenazine .... 2 mg.
Amitriptyline HCl * .... 25 mg.

EUTHROID
Thyroid therapy
(Parke-Davis)

Each tablet:
Sodium levothyroxine and
Sodium
liothyronine * .... 1/2 gr.; 1 gr.;
2 gr.; 3 gr.

EVAC-Q-KIT
Bowel evacuant
(Adria)

Each kit contains:
Evac-Q-Mag (Magnesium cit-
rate oral solution) ...... 10 fl. oz.
Magnesium hydroxide
(USP)(66.8%) ....7.28 gm.
Citric acid (USP) ......26.70 gm.
Potassium bicarbonate
(USP) .... 2.1 gm.
Evac-Q-Tabs
Phenolphthalein (USP) .. 130 mg.
Evac-Q-Sert
Potassium bitartrate ..... 0.962 gm.
Sodium bicarbonate
(USP) .... 0.641 gm.
Polyethylene glycol 400
(NF) .... 1.62 gm.
Polyethylene glycol 1450
(NF) .... 1.40 gm.
Polyethylene glycol 8000
(NF) .... 1.40 gm.

EVAC-Q-KWIK
Bowel evacuant
(Adria)

Each kit contains:
Evac-Q-Mag (Magnesium cit-
rate oral solution) .... 10 fl. oz.
Magnesium hydroxide
(USP)(66.8%) ....7.28 gm.
Citric acid (USP) ......26.7 gm.
Potassium bicarbonate
(USP) .... 2.1 gm.
Evac-Q-Tabs
Phenolphthalein (USP) ... 130 mg.
Evac-Q-Kwik Suppository
Bisacodyl (USP) .... 10 mg.

Starred ingredients (*) may be responsible for major toxic effects; consult Section II.

EVANS QUICK STICK WALL SIZE
(Evans Adhesive Corp.)

Vegetable glue derived from starch

EVELYN MARSHALL COSMETICS

Evelyn Marshall Cosmetics, Ltd.
14 E. 38th St.
New York, N.Y. 10016

Phone: 212-532-6400

See COSMETICS, Section VI, General Formulations

EVE PERM LOTION
Permanent wave lotion
(Bonat)

	percentage range
Water	80.0-90.0%
Ammonium thioglycolate *	6.0-12.0%
Ammonium carbonate	<1.0%
Styrene/acrylamide copolymer	<1.0%
Laureth-23	<1.0%
Fragrance	<1.0%

EVERBLOOM
Cut flower preservative
(Burpee)

Potassium sulfate *
Potassium phosphate, monobasic
Boric acid powder *
Sodium bisulfate, meta
Sodium benzoate
Citric acid
8-Hydroxyquinoline potassium sulfate *
Sugar (fine granulated)

EVERBLUM CLEANING FLUID
(Albatross Chem.)

1,1,1-Trichloroethane *

EVERCIDE 66-OF EMULSIFIABLE
For protection of stored grain
(MGK)

Pyrethrins	6.0%
Technical Piperonyl butoxide	60.0%

EVERCOAT MARINE RESIN & LIQUID HARDENER
Automotive, marine and household use; sealer, surface coating
(Fibre Glass-Evercoat)

Resin:
Polyester resin	100%
Tinting color (<5%)	

Liquid Hardener:
Methyl ethyl ketone peroxide *

EVER-DRY DEODORANTS & ANTIPERSPIRANTS

Ever-Dry Corp.
P.O. Box 400 009
Dallas, Tex. 75240

Phone: 214-233-2800

EVERFAST CEMENT
Adhesive
(Ambroid)

Nitrocellulose type of cement
Alcohols *	20%
Hydrocarbons *†	60%
Ketones *	20%
Allyl isothiocyanate (synthetic oil of mustard)	trace

†See Adhesives, Section VI, General Formulations

EVER GREEN GARDEN SPRAY
Insecticide
(MGK)

Pyrethrins	1.40%
Petroleum distillate	5.60%
Aromatic petroleum distillate *	48.00%

EVER MORE PERM LOTION
Permanent wave lotion
(Bonat)

	percentage range
Water	85.0-95.0%
Ammonium thioglycolate *	5.0-10.0%
Ammonium hydroxide *	<2.0%
Styrene/acrylamide copolymer	<1.0%
Laureth-23	<1.0%
Fragrance	<1.0%
May contain PEG-60 lanolin	<1.0%

EVERSHIELD Mc SEED PROTECTANT
(Gustafson)

Methoxychlor (technical) *	38.0%

EVERSHIELD SEED PROTECTANT
Fungicide, insecticide
(Gustafson)

Captan	29.52%
Malathion	0.34%

EVERSHIELD T SEED PROTECTANT
(Gustafson)

Thiram *	29.52%

EVERSHIELD V SEED PROTECTANT
(Gustafson)

Carboxin *	29.52%

EVERWEAR GYM FINISH
(Uncle Sam)

Modified Phenolic resins
China wood oil
Cobalt driers *
Petroleum distillates *

EVERWEAR GYM FINISH, SUPER

See SUPER EVERWEAR GYM FINISH

EVEX TABLETS
Estrogen replacement
(Syntex Labs.)

Each tablet:
Esterified Estrogens 0.625 mg.; 1.25 mg.

EVIK 80W
Herbicide
(Ciba-Geigy Ag. Div.)

Ametryn *	76%
Related compounds	4%

EVYAN PERFUMES

Evyan Perfumes, Inc.
350 East 35th St.
New York, N.Y. 10016

Phone: 212-532-3800

See COSMETICS, Section VI, General Formulations

EXALGAE L-C (LIQUID CONCENTRATE)
(Koppers)

Alkenyl (90% C18, 10% C16) dimethyl ethyl ammonium bromide *†
n-Alkyl (C14, C16, C12, C18) dimethyl benzyl ammonium chlorides *
n-Alkyl (C12, C14, C16, C18) dimethyl ethylbenzyl ammonium chlorides *
n-Alkyl (C12, C14) dimethyl 1-naphthyl methyl ammonium chlorides *†
Inert ingred.:	60%
Water	
Isopropanol	

†See Cationic surfactants

EXALGAE LIQUI-JEL
(Koppers)

Alkenyl (90% C18, 10% C16) dimethyl ethyl ammonium bromide *†
n-Alkyl (C14, C16, C12, C18) dimethyl benzyl ammonium chlorides *
n-Alkyl (C12, C14, C16, C18) dimethyl ethylbenzyl ammonium chlorides *
n-Alkyl (C12, C14) dimethyl 1-naphthyl methyl ammonium chlorides *†
Inert ingred.:	25%
Water	
Isopropanol	

†See Cationic surfactants

EXALGAE SOLUTION
(Koppers)

Alkenyl (90% C18, 10% C16) dimethyl ethyl
   ammonium bromide *†
n-Alkyl (C14, C16, C12, C18) dimethyl benzyl ammonium chlorides *
n-Alkyl (C12, C14, C16, C18) dimethyl
   ethylbenzyl ammonium chlorides *
n-Alkyl (C12, C14) dimethyl 1-naphthyl
   methyl ammonium chlorides *†
Inert ingred.: 90%
   Water
   Isopropanol

†See Cationic surfactants

EXCEDRIN
Extra-strength pain reliever
(Bristol-Myers)

Each tablet/capsule:
   Acetaminophen * . . . . 250 mg.
   Aspirin * . . . . 250 mg.
   Caffeine * . . . . 65 mg.

EXCEDRIN P.M.
Night time pain reliever
(Bristol-Myers)

Each tablet:
   Acetaminophen * . . . . 500 mg.
   Pyrilamine maleate * . . . . 25 mg.

EXCELCIDE BUG-E-VICT DUST
Insecticide
(Huge')

Pyrethrins *
Inert ingred.:
   Talc
   Diatomaceous earth

EXCELCIDE DYNA-FOG CONTACT SPRA
Insecticide
(Huge')

Petroleum distillate *
Perchloroethylene *
Technical Piperonyl butoxide
Pyrethrins

EXCELCIDE FLY SPRA
Insecticide
(Huge')

Petroleum distillate *
N-Octyl bicycloheptene dicarboximide *
Technical Piperonyl butoxide
Pyrethrins

EXCELCIDE INDUSTRIAL AEROSOL INSECT BOMB
Insecticide
(Huge')

Petroleum distillate * 18.15%
Technical Piperonyl butoxide . . . 1.35%
Pyrethrins 0.5%
Inert ingred.:
   Propellants 80.00%

EXCELCIDE MILL SPRA
Insecticide
(Huge')

Petroleum distillate *
Pyrethrins
Technical Piperonyl butoxide

EXCELCIDE OUTSIDE RESIDUAL
Insecticide
(Huge')

Malathion *
Diazinon *
Inert ingred.:
   Polyoxyethylene sorbitol esters of mixed
     fatty acids
   Lactose
   Milk whey
   Water

EXCELCIDE RESIFUME INSECTICIDE
(Huge')

Vapona *
Diazinon *
Petroleum distillate *

EXCELCIDE SEED & GRAIN WAREHOUSE SPRA
Insecticide
(Huge')

Petroleum distillate *
Beta butoxy beta thiocyanodiethyl ether *
Technical Methoxychlor *
N-Octyl bicycloheptene dicarboximide *
Technical Piperonyl butoxide
Pyrethrins

EXCELCIDE SPECIAL FLY SPRA
Insecticide
(Huge')

Petroleum distillate *
Perchloroethylene *
Technical Piperonyl butoxide
N-Octyl bicycloheptene dicarboximide *
Pyrethrins

EXCELCIDE SURFACE TREATMENT SPRA
Insecticide
(Huge')

Petroleum distillate *
Pyrethrins
Technical Piperonyl butoxide

EXCELCIDE VAPO FLY SPRA INSECTICIDE
(Huge')

Petroleum distillate *
Technical Piperonyl butoxide
N-Octyl bicycloheptene dicarboximide *
Vapona *
Pyrethrins

EXCELLO SQUARES COLORED MOLDED CHALK
(American Crayon Co.)

This product bears the CP Seal issued
by the Crayon, Water Color and Craft Institute, Inc. This seal certifies that the
product contains no materials in sufficient
quantities to be toxic or injurious to the
human body even if ingested.

EXCEL MACHINE DISHWASH
(National-Purity Soap)

Alkaline builders
Water softeners
Buffers
Chlorine *
Antifoam

pH of 1% solution, 11.5

EXCELSIOR CRAYONS
(Reliance Pen & Pencil)

Cellulose gum
Pigment colors (not dyes)
Clay
Talc
Fatty acid ester
Hydrocarbon resin
Hydrogenated fatty acid

EXCLAIM
Cold wave lotion
(Willat)

Ammonium thioglycolate 1-10%

EXELENTO GLOSSINE PRESSING OIL
(Exelento Medicine Co.)

White petroleum jelly
Mineral oil

'76 Ed.

EXELENTO HAIR POMADE
(Exelento Medicine Co.)

Yellow petroleum jelly 2-3%/w
Refined Sulfur
Olive oil NF
Hydrous Lanolin
Methyl salicylate *

'76 Ed.

EX-LAX
Chocolated tablets and unflavored pills
(Ex-Lax)

Yellow Phenolphthalein

EXNA
Diuretic, antihypertensive
(Robins)

Each tablet:
   Benzthiazide * . . . . 50 mg.

Starred ingredients (*) may be responsible for major toxic effects; consult Section II.

EXNA-R
Diuretic, antihypertensive
(Robins)

Each tablet:
Benzthiazide, USP * ...... 50 mg.
Reserpine, USP .... 0.125 mg.

EXPECTORINE VETERINARY COUGH MIXTURE
(Thoroughbred)

Alcohol 7%/v
Fluid ext. Belladonna *
White pine bark
Sanguinaria
Spikenard
Benzocaine
Menthol *
Chloroform * .... 6 m./oz.
Fluid ext. Euphorbia
Wild cherry
Balm gilead buds
Sassafras
Ammonium chloride

EXPO
Dri erase markers
(Sanford Corp.)

Dyes
Resins
Ketones *†
Alcohol *†
Esters *†

†*See* Inks, Section VI, General Formulations

EXPRESSO
Fine, medium, and bold point writing pens
(Sanford Corp.)

Dyes
Glycols
Water
Phenol (as preservative) .... <1%

EXSEL LOTION
For seborrheic dermatitis
(Herbert Labs.)

Selenium sulfide * 2.5%
Edetate disodium
Bentonite
Sodium linear alkylate sulfonate
Alphaolefin sulfonate
Glyceryl monoricinoleate
Silicone
Titanium dioxide
Citric acid monohydrate
Sodium phosphate monobasic, monohydrate
Perfume
Purified water

EXSPEED, FORMULA LC-73

See KLENZADE EXSPEED, FORMULA LC-73

EXTENDAC EXTENDED ACTION COLD CAPSULES
(Vitarine)

Each time release capsule:
Belladonna alkaloids (as 0.25
mg. of the following
salts): .... 0.2 mg.
Atropine sulfate ...... 0.0375 mg.
Scopolamine HBr .. 0.0219 mg.
Hyoscyamine sulfate .. 0.1906 mg.
Phenylpropanolamine
hydrochloride * .... 50 mg.
Chlorpheniramine maleate .. 1 mg.
Pheniramine maleate * ... 12.5 mg.

EXTENDRYL CAPSULES
Decongestant
(Fleming)

JR (each capsule):
Phenylephrine HCl * .... 10 mg.
Chlorpheniramine maleate * 4 mg.
Methscopolamine nitrate * .. 1.25 mg.

SR (each capsule):
Phenylephrine HCl * .... 20 mg.
Chlorpheniramine maleate * 8 mg.
Methscopolamine nitrate * .. 2.5 mg.

EXTENDRYL CHEWABLES
Decongestant
(Fleming)

Each tablet:
Phenylephrine HCl * .... 10 mg.
Chlorpheniramine maleate * 2 mg.
Methscopolamine nitrate * .. 1.25 mg.

EXTENDRYL SYRUP
Decongestant
(Fleming)

Each 5 ml.:
Phenylephrine HCl * .... 10 mg.
Chlorpheniramine maleate * 2 mg.
Methscopolamine nitrate * .. 1.25 mg.

EXTERIOR RUBEROL - EARLY AMERICAN COLORS
(Lehman Bros. Corp.)

Mercury * .... slight

See Paints, Section VI, General Formulations

EXTERMITE
For control of termites & wood boring insect pests
(Biocerta)

Pentachlorophenol * 16.87%
Other chlorophenols & related
compounds 2.98%
Inactive ingred.:
Organic solvents *† 80.15%
'76 Ed.

†*See* Kerosene

EXTRACT ALL
Detergent for carpeting
(Paul Koss)

Water .... >90%
Nonylphenoxypoly(ethyleneoxy)ethanol
(Nonionic surfactant)
Sodium carbonate
Sodium metasilicate
Alkyl dimethyl benzyl ammonium
chloride * .... <2%
Coco amido betaine
Tetrasodium EDTA
Sodium hydroxide
Dye, Optical brightener, Silicone
defoamer .... trace

pH 11.8-12.2

EXTRAMED
Analgesic
(Whitehall Labs.)

Each tablet:
Acetaminophen * .... 7 1/2 gr.

EXTRA STRENGTH SINUTAB CAPSULES
Analgesic-nasal decongestant-antihistamine
(Warner-Lambert)

Each capsule:
Acetaminophen * .... 500.00 mg.
Phenylpropanolamine HCl 18.75 mg.
Chlorpheniramine maleate 2.00 mg.

EXTRA STRENGTH SINUTAB TABLETS
Analgesic-nasal decongestant-antihistamine
(Warner-Lambert)

Each tablet:
Acetaminophen * .... 500 mg.
Phenylpropanolamine HCl .... 25 mg.
Phenyltoloxamine citrate .... 22 mg.

EXZIT CLEANSER, CREME AND LOTION
For treatment of acne
(Dome)

Cleanser:
Colloidal Sulfur 2%
Salicylic acid * 2%

Creme and Lotion:
Colloidal Sulfur 4%
Resorcinol monoacetate * 3%

EYE-SED
Eye lotion
(Scherer Labs.)

Boric acid 2.17%
Zinc sulfate 0.217%
Chlorobutanol 0.25%
Purified water .... q.s.

Starred ingredients (*) may be responsible for major toxic effects; consult Section II.

EYLURE OF LONDON COSMETICS

Eylure of London, Ltd.
410 Eastern Pkwy.
Farmingdale, N.Y. 11735

Phone: 516-752-8833

See COSMETICS, Section VI, General Formulations

E-Z ANT TRAP
(Linck)

Baygon * 0.250%

EZE GARDEN WEED KILLER
Herbicide
(Woolfolk)

Trifluralin (a,a,a-Trifluoro-2,6-dinitro-N,N-dipropyl-p-toluidine) .. 1.75%

EZE-PEEL
Strippable film
(Calgon Corp., Commercial Div.)

Acetone *
Toluol *
Vinyl

E-Z-EST COPPER CLEANER
Liquid cleaner
(E-Z-EST)

Amorphous Silica 325 .... 30.0%
Mineral thickening agent
  (Bentonite) 11.8%
Calcium chloride 7.9%
Sugar 3.9%
Phosphoric acid 2.8%
Water .... balance

E-Z-EST DRIVEWAY CLEANER
Liquid cleaner
(E-Z-EST)

Petroleum solvent * 90%
Oil soluble Emulsifier 10%

E-Z-EST JEWELDIP
Liquid jewelry cleaner
(E-Z-EST)

Ammonium sulfate 5.5%
Organic amine-ammonium sulfonate
  detergent 3.3%
Water

E-Z-EST JEWELUSTER
(E-Z-EST)

Water 91.5%
Sulfuric acid * 2.2%
Nonionic surfactant 0.5%
Thiourea 5.5%
Odorant

E-Z-EST JEWELUSTER FOR COINS
(E-Z-EST)

Water 91.5%
Sulfuric acid * 2.2%
Nonionic surfactant 0.5%
Thiourea 5.5%
Odorant

E-Z-EST LEMON BEE FURNITURE POLISH
(E-Z-EST)

Petroleum solvent * 88%
Wax 12%

E-Z-EST LEMON OIL FURNITURE POLISH
(E-Z-EST)

Petroleum solvent * 66%
Mineral oil * 34%

E-Z-EST MARBLE POLISH
(E-Z-EST)

Water
Thickening gum
Petroleum solvent .... <10%
Wax
Silicone oil
Detergent emulsifier
Mold preventing germicide
Diatomaceous abrasive

E-Z-EST METAL POLISH
(E-Z-EST)

Water
Abrasive ground Silica
Ammonium oxalate * 4.5%
Sodium nitrite * 2.1%
Hexylene glycol 1.2%
Amine oleate soap 3.3%
Ethylene oxide adduct detergent .. 1.3%

E-Z-EST PEARL CLEANER
(E-Z-EST)

Water
Fatty acid ether sulfate detergent *†

†*See* Anionic synthetic detergents

E-Z-EST RUG & UPHOLSTERY SHAMPOO
(E-Z-EST)

Water
Surfactants *
Water conditioner

E-Z-EST SCRATCH CONCEALER
Liquid polish
(E-Z-EST)

Petroleum solvents * 94%
Waxes
Silicone oils
Organic dyes

E-Z-EST SILVER SOAP
(E-Z-EST)

Sodium carbonate
Sodium soap
Diatomaceous earth
Water

E-Z-EST SPEEDIP
Silver tarnish remover
(E-Z-EST)

Water 91.5%
Sulfuric acid * 2.2%
Nonionic surfactant 0.5%
Thiourea 5.5%
Odorant

E-Z-EST SPOT REMOVER
Aerosol dry cleaner
(E-Z-EST)

Petroleum distillates *
Chlorinated hydrocarbons *
Detergent
Propellant

E-Z-EST STEAM IRON CLEANER
(E-Z-EST)

Phosphoric acid (food grade) * 11%
Sodium chloride .... <4%
Water

E-Z-EST STEEL SAVER
Stainless steel cleaner
(E-Z-EST)

Light lubricating oil * 46%
Petroleum thinner * 17%
1,1,1-Trichloroethane * 37%

E-Z-EST STEELUSTER
Metal polish (powder)
(E-Z-EST)

Citric acid 1.9%
Sodium chloride
Detergent
Silica (fine ground)

E-Z-EST TARNISH PREVENTIVE SILVER POLISH
(E-Z-EST)

Stable emulsion of:
  Petroleum solvents * 22%
  Waxes
  Diatomaceous earth
  Emulsifier
  Water

E-Z-EST TILE CLEANER
Liquid basin, tub & tile cleaner
(E-Z-EST)

Muriatic acid * 5.000%
Nonionic nonylphenol 2.000%
Quaternary ammonium chlorides 0.500%
Methyl salicylate 0.025%
Water 92.475%

Starred ingredients (*) may be responsible for major toxic effects; consult Section II.

E-Z-EX WORMER MEDICATED, MOORMAN'S

See MOORMAN'S E-Z-EX WORMER MEDICATED

E-Z GROOM, SERGEANT'S

See SERGEANT'S E-Z GROOM

E-Z-KIL
Rat and mouse killer bait
(E-Z Products Co.)

Warfarin (3(a-Acetonylbenzyl)-4-
  hydroxycoumarin) 0.025%
Sulfaquinoxaline (N'-(2-
  Quinoxalinyl)sulfanilamide) ... 0.025%

'76 Ed.

E-Z STROKES

See DUNCAN CERAMICS E-Z
  STROKES (EZ-000 Series)

E-Z-SYTE POLYCHROMATIC CHALK

See CRAYOLA E-Z-SYTE POLY-
  CHROMATIC CHALK

E-Z WEED "B" HERBICIDE

See PL E-Z WEED "B" HERBICIDE

EZY-12
Insecticide - veterinary
(Pro-Brand Products Co.)

Xylene * 73.00%
Refined Petroleum oil 10.00%
Gamma isomer of benzene hexa-
  chloride from lindane 10.00%

'76 Ed.

EZY-WEED

See J&P EZY-WEED

F

FAB
Detergent
(Colgate-Palmolive)

Alkyl aryl sulfonate * ...... approx. 20%
Combined amount: .... approx. 70%
  Sodium phosphates *
  Sodium sulfate
  Sodium silicate *
Borax .... approx. 1.0%

'76 Ed.

FABERGE BATH PERFUME
(Faberge)

Esters of higher aliphatic acids

FABERGE BATH POWDERS & SACHET
(Faberge)

French Talc
Zinc stearate *
Magnesium carbonate

FABERGE PERFUME, COLOGNES, MEN'S LOTIONS
(Faberge)

Specially Denatured alcohol (Formula No.
  39C) *

FABRIC CRAYONS
Transfer coloring of synthetic fabric
(Binney & Smith)

Major constituent:
  Wax blend
Minor constituents:
  Clay
  Pigments
  Sublimable Dyes

FABULON
Floor finish
(Pierce & Stevens)

Castor polyester
Maleic resin
Chlorinated resin
Cellulose nitrate
Coconut polyester
Esters
Alcohols
Aromatic hydrocarbon *

FABULON EPOXY GYM FINISH
(Pierce & Stevens)

Non-volatile:
  Ester gum modified Phenolic ether resin
Volatile:
  Aromatic hydrocarbons *
  Aliphatic hydrocarbons *

FABULOY
Wood finish
(Pierce & Stevens)

Ester gum modified phenolic ether resin
Modifying acids:
  Palmitic
  Stearic
  Oleic
  Linoleic
  Linolenic
Aromatic hydrocarbons *
Aliphatic hydrocarbons *

FACTOR
*Institutional and industrial cleaning
  product*

Procter & Gamble Co.
Ivorydale Technical Center
Cincinnati, Ohio 45217

Phone: 513-562-1100

FAIR 30
*Prevents growth of tobacco suckers and
  onion and potato sprouting*
(Fairmount Chem. Co.)

Diethanolamine salt of 1,2-Dihydro-
  3,6-pyridazinedione (Maleic
  hydrazide) * 58%

FAIR 85
Tobacco sucker control
(Fairmount Chem. Co.)

Fatty alcohols (C6 0.5%, C8 43%, C10
  56%, C12 0.5%) * 85%

FAIRFIELD AMERICAN FOOD PLANT FOGGING INSECTICIDE (OIL BASE)
(Fairfield American)

Pyrethrins 0.5%
Piperonyl butoxide 5.0%
Petroleum distillate * 94.5%

FAIRFIELD AMERICAN MULTI-PURPOSE PYRENONE INSECTICIDE CONCENTRATE (OIL BASE)
For indoor and outdoor use
(Fairfield American)

Pyrethrins 1.0%
Piperonyl butoxide 10.0%
Petroleum distillate * 79.0%
Emulsifiers 10.0%

FAIR PLUS
Tobacco sucker control
(Fairmount Chem. Co.)

Potassium salt of 1,2-Dihydro-3,6-
  pyridazinedione (Maleic
  hydrazide) * 21.7%

FAIR-TAC
Tobacco sucker control
(Fairmount Chem. Co.)

n-Decanol * 78.5%

FALK'S CAMFO CREME
Soothing skin cream
(Falk)

Camphor *
Glycerin
Turpentine *
Ammonia *
Ammonium carbonate

Starred ingredients (*) may be responsible for major toxic effects; consult Section II.

FALK'S NU SALVE
(Falk)

Pine gum *
Rosin
Beef fat
Beeswax
Linseed oil

FAMILY DOG BRUSHING SPRAY
(Chesebrough-Pond's)

Ethyl alcohol, denatured *	>50%
Fragrance	0.1-1%
Stearalkonium chloride	0.1-1%
Propellant 12/114 (50:50)	25-50%
Oleate ester of Polyoxypropylene glycol	1-5%
Isostearyl alcohol and Lanolin alcohol	1-5%

FANTASTIC
General cleaner concentrate
(Calgon Corp., Commercial Div.)

Complex phosphates *
Soap
Dodecylbenzene sulfonate *†
Diethyleneglycol monobutyl ether *
Water
Sodium silicate

†*See* Alkyl aryl sodium sulfonates

FANTASTIK SPRAY CLEANER

See TEXIZE FANTASTIK SPRAY CLEANER

FARBOIL PAINT PRODUCTS

Farboil Co.
8200 Fischer Rd.
Baltimore, Md. 21222

Phone: 301-477-8200

See PAINTS, Section VI, General Formulations

FAR-GO
Herbicide
(Monsanto)

Triallate (S-(2,2,3-Trichloroallyl)-diisopropylthiocarbamate) *	46.3%

FARNAM HORSE LICE DUSTER
(Farnam Co.)

Rotenone	1.00%
Other cube resins	1.66%
Pyrethrins	0.025%
Piperonyl butoxide, technical	0.25%

'76 Ed.

FARNAM MANE & TAIL WHITENER
For horses and show cattle
(Farnam Co.)

Yellow solution:
Aqua ammonia *
Castile soap

White solution:
Hydrogen peroxide (in aqueous solution) * ...... no more than 8%

'76 Ed.

FARNAM SCREW-WORM EAR-TICK BOMB
Veterinary
(Farnam Co.)

Gamma isomer of benzene hexachloride from lindane	3.0%
Xylol *	12.5%
Mineral oil	30.5%

'76 Ed.

FARNAM STABLE-SPRAY FLY KILLER CONCENTRATE
(Farnam Co.)

Dimethoate (O,O-Dimethyl S-(N-methylcarbamoylmethyl) phosphorodithioate) *	15.912%
2,2-Dichlorovinyl dimethyl phosphate	0.949%
Related compounds	0.071%
Petroleum hydrocarbons	73.068%

'76 Ed.

FASHION FAIR COSMETICS

Fashion Fair Cosmetics
820 S. Michigan Ave.
Chicago, Ill. 60605

Phone: 312-322-9444

See COSMETICS, Section VI, General Formulations

FASHION FRAGRANCES

Fashion Fragrances Inc.
331 Madison Ave.
New York, N.Y. 10017

Phone: 212-687-4147

See COSMETICS, Section VI, General Formulations

FASHION TAN
(Aloe Creme)

Aloe vera plant gel

FASOLV FAT, OIL AND GREASE REMOVER
(Nat'l Labs. Div.)

Sodium silicate	minor
Diethylene glycol monobutyl ether	minor

FAST COURT GYM FINISH
Floor finish
(Lester Labs.)

Petroleum distillates *
Resins

'76 Ed.

FAST CUT (HAND RUBBING COMPOUND)

See PARKO FAST CUT (HAND RUBBING COMPOUND)

FAST CUT (WHEEL POLISHING COMPOUND)

See PARKO FAST CUT (WHEEL POLISHING COMPOUND)

FAST & EASY LATEX WALL PAINT (Y-3080)
(Glidden)

	by weight:
Titanium dioxide	8.4%
Silicates	25.4%
Vinyl acetate/acrylic	5.6%
Glycol ethers, esters	1.5%
Additives (no lead)	1.7%
Water	57.4%

FASTEETH POWDER DENTURE ADHESIVE
(Vicks Toiletry Products Div.)

Karaya gum	88%
Sodium borate *	11%
Flavor	

FASTIN
Anorexiant
(Beecham Labs.)

Each capsule:
Phentermine hydrochloride * . 30 mg.

FAST KILL ANT & ROACH KILLER
Insecticide
(Claire)

Pyrethrins	0.05%
Piperonyl butoxide, tech.	0.1%
MGK 264	0.166%
Diazinon	0.5%
Petroleum distillate *	95.584%

Starred ingredients (*) may be responsible for major toxic effects; consult Section II.

FAST-KILL ROACH & ANT KILLER WITH DIAZINON (AEROSOL)

See SPRAYWAY FAST-KILL ROACH & ANT KILLER WITH DIAZINON (AEROSOL)

FAST PLUG, UGL

See UGL FAST PLUG

FAST WALLPAPER REMOVER (CONCENTRATE)
(Savogran)

Butyl Cellosolve *	<10%
Polyethoxylated linear alcohol (Surface active agent) *†	15-35%

†*See* Nonionic synthetic detergents

FATAL FLY DRY BAIT

See UNICO FATAL FLY DRY BAIT

FATHER JOHN'S MEDICINE
Cough preparation
(Lambda Inc.)

Cod liver oil
Gum arabic
Glycerin
Sugar
Flavoring

FATSCO ANT POISON
Insecticide
(Fatsco)

Sodium arsenate *	3%

F&B CHLORDANE 72% SPRAY
Insecticide; herbicide
(Faesy & Besthoff)

Technical Chlordane *	72.0%
Petroleum distillate *	22.0%

F-B-C TABS
Hematinic
(Elder)

Each tablet:
Ferrous fumarate *	100 mg.
Vitamin C (Ascorbic acid)	10 mg.
Vitamin B1 (Thiamine HCl)	1 mg.
Vitamin B12 (from cobalamin conc.)	1 mcg.

F&B CYTHION (MALATHION) 50% SPRAY

See F&B MALATHION (CYTHION) 50% SPRAY

F&B DORMANT SPRAY
Insecticide
(Faesy & Besthoff)

Petroleum oil *	97%

F&B LAWN AND TURF FUNGICIDE
(Faesy & Besthoff)

Dyrene (2,4-Dichloro-6-(o-chloroanilo)-s-triazine)	4.0%
Maneb (Manganese ethylene bisdithiocarbamate)	4.0%
Zinc, as metallic	0.1%

F&B MALATHION (CYTHION) 50% SPRAY
For home orchards and gardens
(Faesy & Besthoff)

Malathion (O,O-Dimethyl dithiophosphate of diethyl mercaptosuccinate) *	50.0%
Aromatic petroleum derivative solvent *	45.0%

F&B RABBIT & DOG CHASER
(Faesy & Besthoff)

Naphthalene	1 part
F&B dried blood	1 part
F&B tobacco dust (Nicotine 1/2%) *	5 parts

F&B SEVIN FLOWABLE
Insecticide
(Faesy & Besthoff)

Carbaryl (1-Naphthyl N-methylcarbamate) *	41.8%
Water	

F&B SYSTEMIC INSECTICIDE SPRAY
(Faesy & Besthoff)

S-(2-(Ethylsulfinyl)ethyl) O,O-dimethyl phosphorothioate *	13.5%
Aromatic petroleum distillate *	14.5%

F&B TOBACCO DUST
Insecticide
(Faesy & Besthoff)

Nicotine *	0.5%

F&B WEED KILLER
(Faesy & Besthoff)

Sodium arsenite (24.5% arsenic) *	42.5%

FC-50
Floor seal
(Lester Labs.)

Petroleum distillates *
Resins

'76 Ed.

F.C.A.H. CAPSULES
Cold remedy
(Scherer Labs.)

Each capsule:
Methapyrilene hydrochloride *	25 mg.
Phenacetin *	162 mg.
Salicylamide	162 mg.
Atropine sulfate	0.130 mg.

FDS FEMININE DEODORANT SPRAY
(Alberto-Culver)

Isobutane
Methylene chloride
Isopropyl myristate
Mineral oil
Lanolin alcohol
Hydrated Silica
Magnesium stearate
Fragrance

FEBRIN
Analgesic, antipyretic
(Jenkins Labs.)

Each tablet:
Acetophenetidin *	1 1/2 gr.
Acetylsalicylic acid *	2 gr.
Camphor monobromated *	1 gr.
Caffeine	1/4 gr.

FEBRINETTS
Analgesic, antipyretic
(Jenkins Labs.)

Each tablet:
Acetophenetidin *	1/2 gr.
Acetylsalicylic acid *	1 gr.
Camphor monobromated	1/40 gr.
Caffeine	1/20 gr.

FEDAHIST EXPECTORANT
Expectorant formula
(Dooner Labs.)

Each 5 ml.:
Chlorpheniramine maleate	2 mg.
Pseudoephedrine hydrochloride *	30 mg.
Guaifenesin	100 mg.

FEDAHIST GYROCAPS
Allergy, decongestant formula
(Dooner Labs.)

Each timed release capsule:
Chlorpheniramine maleate	10 mg.
Pseudoephedrine hydrochloride *	65 mg.

FEDAHIST SYRUP
Allergy, decongestant formula
(Dooner Labs.)

Each 5 ml.:
Chlorpheniramine maleate	2 mg.
Pseudoephedrine hydrochloride *	30 mg.
Non alcoholic syrup	

Starred ingredients (*) may be responsible for major toxic effects; consult Section II.

FEDAHIST TABLETS
Allergy, decongestant formula
(Dooner Labs.)

Each tablet:
Chlorpheniramine maleate .... 4 mg.
Pseudoephedrine
   hydrochloride * .... 60 mg.

FEDRAZIL
Antihistaminic/nasal decongestant
(Burroughs Wellcome)

Each tablet:
Sudafed (Pseudoephedrine
   HCl) * .... 30 mg.
Perazil (Chlorcyclizine HCl) * . 25 mg.

FEDRITAL
Bronchodilator
(Wesley Pharm.)

Each tablet:
Ephedrine sulfate * .... 3/8 gr.
Phenobarbital .... 1/4 gr.

FEEN-A-MINT
Medicated chewing gum or mints; ca-
*   thartic*
(Plough)

Yellow phenolphthalein

FEILER
For symptomatic relief from bronchial
*   asthma*
(S-K Research Labs.)

Potassium iodide *
Ammoniated glycyrrhizin
Caffeine *

                        '76 Ed.

FELAXIN
For the removal and prevention of hair-
*   balls in cats*
(Burns-Biotec)

White petrolatum .... 47.4% w/w
Malt syrup .... 47.4% w/w
Cod liver oil .... 2.0% w/w
Lecithin .... 2.0% w/w
Vitamin E (dl-alpha Toco-
   pheryl acetate)
   (antioxidant) .... 0.036 IU/gm.
Sodium benzoate .... 0.1% w/w
Caramel
Purified Water

FELCO 99 BUILDING
DISINFECTANT
(Land O'Lakes, Inc.)

Coal tar neutral oils * 63.0%
Soap 17.0%
Phenols * 10.0%

FELCO/LAND O'LAKES AM4
WEED KILLER
Herbicide
(Land O'Lakes, Inc.)

Dimethylamine salt of 2,4-dichlo-
   rophenoxyacetic acid * 49.3%

FELCO/LAND O'LAKES
CHLORDANE
EMULSIFIABLE
CONCENTRATE
Insecticide
(Land O'Lakes, Inc.)

Technical Chlordane 42.00%
Aromatic hydrocarbon * 53.00%

FELCO/LAND O'LAKES
GRAIN FUMIGANT 914
Weevil killer and grain conditioner
(Land O'Lakes, Inc.)

Ethylene dichloride 63.1%
Ethylene dibromide 7.1%
Carbon tetrachloride * 26.9%
Sulfur dioxide * 2.9%

FELCO/LAND O'LAKES
GRAIN GARD
Insecticide
(Land O'Lakes, Inc.)

Malathion * 57%
Xylene range
   aromatic hydrocarbon * 34%

FELCO/LAND O'LAKES HV4
WEED KILLER
Herbicide
(Land O'Lakes, Inc.)

Butyl ester of 2,4-dichlorophenoxy-
   acetic acid * 57.0%

FELCO/LAND O'LAKES
LV400 WEED KILLER
Herbicide - noncrop land
(Land O'Lakes, Inc.)

Isooctyl ester of 2,4-dichlorophen-
   oxyacetic acid * 69.7%

FELCO/LAND O'LAKES 57%
MALATHION
EMULSIFIABLE
CONCENTRATE
Insecticide
(Land O'Lakes, Inc.)

Malathion * 57.0%
Xylene range aromatic
   hydrocarbon * 34.0%

FELCO/LAND O'LAKES
MILL AND FARM BIN
SPRAY
Insecticide
(Land O'Lakes, Inc.)

Technical Piperonyl butoxide .. 0.25%
Pyrethrins 0.025%
Technical Methoxychlor 2.500%
Aromatic petroleum
   hydrocarbons * 97.225%

FELCO/LAND O'LAKES
STOCK-TOX PLUS
Insecticide dip or spray
(Land O'Lakes, Inc.)

Toxaphene (technical chlorinated
   camphene containing 67 to 69%
   chlorine) * 45%
Gamma isomer of benzene hexachloride from lindane 1%
Petroleum hydrocarbon 44%

FELCO/LAND O'LAKES
TOXAPHENE
EMULSIFIABLE
CONCENTRATE
Insecticide
(Land O'Lakes, Inc.)

Toxaphene (technical chlorinated
   camphene) * 58.60%
Xylene range aromatic solvent * 38.40%

FELCO/LAND O'LAKES
VAPONA DAIRY CATTLE
SPRAY
Insecticide
(Land O'Lakes, Inc.)

2,2-Dichlorovinyl dimethyl
   phosphate .... 0.93%/wt.
Related compounds .... 0.07%/wt.
Petroleum distillate * .... 99.00%/wt.

FELOBITS
Vitamin-mineral tablets for cats
(Norden Labs.)

Each tablet:
Vitamin A .... 1500 I.U.
Vitamin D2 .... 150 I.U.
Iron (as ferrous fumarate) .. 5.0 mg.
Plus multivitamins and minerals

FELS NAPHTHA
Laundry soap bar
(Purex Corp.)

Sodium tallow-coconut oil soap   >45%
Clay 30-40%
Sodium silicate (not meta) ..... <5%
Naphtha 1-5%
Titanium dioxide .... <1%
Coloring agent .... <1%
Perfume .... <1%
Water .... balance

Starred ingredients (*) may be responsible for major toxic effects; consult Section II.

FEMGUARD
For vaginal tract infections
(Reid-Provident)

Sulfanilamide *	15.0%
Aminacrine hydrochloride	0.2%
Allantoin	2.0%

FEMIDINE
Cleansing douche
(A.V.P. Pharmaceuticals)

Povidone-iodine

FEMINONE TABLETS
Estrogen supplement
(Upjohn)

Each tablet:
Ethinyl estradiol .... 0.05 mg.

FEMPAIN
For the relief of periodic pain and discomfort
(S.S.S. Co.)

Cinnamyl ephedrine HCl *†	15 mg.
N-Acetyl-p-aminophenol *	3 gr.
Caffeine	1 gr.
Methapyrilene HCl *	12.5 mg.
Homatropine methyl bromide	0.25 mg.

†See Ephedrine

FENAC
Herbicide
(Amchem)

2,3,6-Trichlorophenylacetic acid,
sodium salt * 16.1%

FENAC PLUS
Weed killer for sugar cane
(Amchem)

2,4-Dichlorophenoxyacetic acid, dimethylamine salt *	12.5%
2,3,6-Trichlorophenylacetic acid, dimethylamine salt *	18.5%

FENAMINE
Postemergence weed killer
(Amchem)

Amitrole (3-Amino-1,2,4-triazole)	3.5%
Ammonium salt of 2,3,6-trichlorophenylacetic acid (Fenac)	6.3%
Atrazine (2-Chloro-4-ethylamino-6-isopropylamino-s-triazine) *	10.8%

FEN-ARSENATE DRENCH

See ANCHOR FEN-ARSENATE
DRENCH

FENDOL
Relief of cold symptoms
(Buffington)

Each tablet:
Phenylephrine hydrochloride *	10 mg.
Salicylamide	
Acetaminophen *	
Caffeine	
Atropine sulfate *	1/500 gr.

FENNER'S, DR., PRODUCTS

See DR. FENNER

FENOCIL
Herbicide
(National Chemsearch)

Heavy aromatic naphtha *	86.40%
Bromacil	2.30%
Pentachlorophenol	2.84%
Other Chlorophenols	0.33%

FEOSOL ELIXIR
Hematinic
(MenJ Labs.)

Each 5 ml.:
Ferrous sulfate *	220 mg.
Alcohol	5%

FEOSOL PLUS
Iron plus vitamins
(MenJ Labs.)

Each capsule:
Dried Ferrous sulfate *	200 mg.
Plus multivitamins	

FEOSOL SPANSULE CAPSULES
Hematinic
(MenJ Labs.)

Each capsule:
Dried Ferrous sulfate * ...... 167 mg.

FEOSOL TABLETS
Hematinic
(MenJ Labs.)

Each tablet:
Dried Ferrous sulfate * ...... 200 mg.

FEOSTAT TABLETS
Hematinic
(OJF)

Each tablet:
Ferrous fumarate (Iron - 33.3
mg.) * .... 100 mg.

FERATE-C
Iron supplement
(Vale)

Each tablet:
Ferrous fumarate (equiv. elemental iron 50 mg.) *	150 mg.
Dioctyl sodium sulfosuccinate	25 mg.
Ascorbic acid	200 mg.

FERGON (TABLETS, ELIXIR & CAPSULES)
For iron deficiency anemias
(Breon Labs.)

Each tablet:
Ferrous gluconate * ...... 320 mg.

Each 5 ml.:
Ferrous gluconate * ...... 300 mg.

Each capsule:
Ferrous gluconate * ...... 435 mg.

FERGON PLUS
For iron deficiency and macrocytic anemias
(Breon Labs.)

Each Caplet:
Ferrous gluconate *	500 mg.
Vitamin B12 (with intrinsic factor conc. NF XI)	1/2 unit
Ascorbic acid	75 mg.

FER-IN-SOL
Iron deficiency anemia
(Mead Johnson)

Capsules (each):
Ferrous sulfate (iron-60 mg.) * 190 mg.

Drops (each 0.6 ml.):
Ferrous sulfate (iron-15 mg.) * 75 mg.

Syrup (each 5 ml.):
Ferrous sulfate (iron-18 mg.) * 90 mg.

FERMALOX TABLETS
For iron deficiency anemias
(Rorer, W.H., Inc.)

Each tablet:
Ferrous sulfate *	200 mg.
Magnesium and aluminum hydroxides	200 mg.

FERO-FOLIC-500 FILMTAB
Iron & folic acid supplement
(Abbott)

Each tablet:
Ferrous sulfate *	525 mg.
Vitamin C	500 mg.
Folic acid	0.8 mg.

FERO-GRADUMET FILMTAB & FERO-GRAD-500 FILMTAB
Controlled release iron supplement
(Abbott)

Each tablet:
Ferrous sulfate *	525 mg.
Vitamin C (Fero-Grad-500 Filmtab only)	500 mg.

FERRALYN LANACAPS
Iron therapy
(Lannett)

Time release Ferrous sulfate * . 150 mg.

Starred ingredients (*) may be responsible for major toxic effects; consult Section II.

FERRISOL SOLUTION
Hematinic; veterinary
(Fort Dodge)

Each fl. oz.:
Green Iron and ammonium
citrate .... 1.3 gm.
Copper acetate .... 8.1 mg.
Cobalt sulfate .... 0.23 gm.
Corn sugar
Sodium benzoate
Water

FERROBID
Hematinic
(Glaxo Inc.)

Each Duracap capsule:
Ferrous fumarate (75 mg. ele-
mental iron) * .... 225 mg.
Copper sulfate (U.S.P.) * .... 8 mg.
Ascorbic acid .... 100 mg.

FERRO-COPPERGEN
Oral mineral supplement; veterinary
(Norden Labs.)

Each fl. oz.:
Iron and ammonium citrate .. 1.3 gm.
Manganese citrate soluble .... 65 mg.
Sodium molybdate .... 49 mg.
Copper gluconate .... 33 mg.
Cobalt sulfate .... 16 mg.
Methyl parahydroxybenzoate
(preservative) 0.125%
Propyl parahydroxybenzoate
(preservative) 0.025%

FERROMIN
Heavy-duty steam cleaner; industrial use
(Puritan Chem. Co.)

Sodium hydroxide *

FERRO-SEQUELS
Iron supplement with stool softener
(Lederle)

Each capsule:
Ferrous fumarate (equiv. to approx. 50 mg. of elemental
iron) * .... 150 mg.
Dioctyl sodium
sulfosuccinate * .... 100 mg.

FERRO-TREET
See ANCHOR FERRO-TREET

FERROUS FE-4
*Combustion catalyst for boiler or fur-
nace fuels*
(Ferrous Corp.)

Organo-metallic compound:
Isopropyl alcohol * or Petroleum distillates *

FERROUS FE-6
Combustion catalyst for diesel fuels
(Ferrous Corp.)

Organo-metallic compound:
Isopropyl alcohol * or Petroleum distillates *

FER-SUL CHEMICAL
*Regenerant chemical for oxidizing filter
for removal of iron or sulfur from
water*
(Culligan)

Potassium permanganate * 100%

FER-SUL T.D. CAPSULES
Iron
(Pharmex)

Each capsule:
Ferrous sulfate * .... 150 mg.

FERTILIZER BORATE-48
(U.S. Borax)

Sodium oxide * 21.7%
Boric oxide * 48.8%
Equivalent Boron 15.1%

FERTILIZER BORATE-68
(U.S. Borax)

Sodium oxide * 30.7%
Boric oxide * 68.9%
Equivalent Boron 21.4%

FESOTYME SR CAP
Iron deficiency
(Elder)

Each capsule:
Dried Ferrous sulfate (equiv. to
45 mg. elemental iron) * ... 150 mg.

FESTALAN
Digestive aid
(Hoechst-Roussel)

Each tablet - outer layer:
Atropine methyl nitrate * ...... 1 mg.
Inner core:
Digestive enzymes with bile constituents

FEVER, JR.
Antipyretic
(Jenkins Labs.)

Each tablet:
Acid Acetylsalicylic * .... 1 gr.
Tincture Aconite .... 1/8 m.
Tincture Belladonna .... 1/16 m.
Tincture Bryonia .... 1/10 m.
Tincture Eupatorium .... 1/8 m.

FEVER X (APAPELIXIR)
Analgesic
(Commerce Drug)

Acetaminophen * .... 120 mg/5 ml
Alcohol 9%

F & F COUGH LOZENGES
(F & F)

ORIGINAL FORMULA:
Menthol *
Beechwood creosote *
Eucalyptol *
Horehound
White pine
Wild cherry
Cetyl dimethyl benzyl ammonium chlo-
ride *

CHERRY FLAVORED:
Wild cherry
White pine
Menthol *
Eucalyptol *
Balsam tolu *
Cetyl dimethyl benzyl ammonium chlo-
ride *

LICORICE FLAVORED:
Menthol *
Sodium salicylate *
Eucalyptol *
White pine
Wild cherry
Licorice
Cetyl dimethyl benzyl ammonium chlo-
ride *

'76 Ed.

"F-4-S" FOOD PROCESSOR'S INSECTICIDE
(Weil Chem.)

Refined Mineral oil * 96.95%
Pyrethrins 0.40%
N-Octyl bicycloheptene dicar-
boximide 0.65%
Piperonal bis(2-(butoxyethoxy)-
ethyl)acetal 1.80%
Other related compounds 0.20%

F.H.I.
Food handlers' insecticide
(Puritan Chem. Co.)

Active ingredients: 100%
Petroleum distillate *
N-Octyl bicycloheptene dicarboximide
Technical Piperonyl butoxide
Pyrethrins

FIBERGLASS BOTTOMKOTE PAINT
(International Paint)

Copper *
Mineral spirits *
Aromatics *†
Pigments color code #449, #559, #669,
#779

†*See* Aromatic hydrocarbon solvents

FIBERTONE DIURETIC COMPOUND
(Fibertone)

Each tablet:
Salol * .... 1/2 gr.
Couch grass .... 1/2 gr.
Buchu ext. .... 1/8 gr.
Corn silk .... 1/2 gr.
Oil of juniper * .... 1/20 gr.
Ext. Uva ursi .... 1/4 gr.

FIBRE GLASS-EVERCOAT COLOR AGENT
For polyester and epoxy resins
(Fibre Glass-Evercoat)

Pigments 50%
Plasticizer 50%

FIBRE GLASS-EVERCOAT CREME HARDENER
For hardening auto body plastic fillers
(Fibre Glass-Evercoat)

Benzoyl peroxide * 50%
Butyl benzyl phthalate * 50%

FIBRE GLASS-EVERCOAT LIQUID HARDENER
For hardening polyester resin and plastic filler
(Fibre Glass-Evercoat)

Methyl ethyl ketone peroxide *

FIDDLE STICKS
Fine line drawing and coloring pens
(Sanford Corp.)

Dyes
Glycols
Water
Phenol (as preservative) .... <1%

FIEBING'S ANTIQUE FINISH
Leather polish
(Fiebing)

Candelilla wax
Castile soap
Turpentine *
Mineral spirits *

FIEBING'S BLACK SHOE DYE
(Fiebing)

Denatured alcohol *
Carbitol *
Nigrosine

FIEBING'S BLACK SOLE & HEEL DRESSING
(Fiebing)

Lacca
Borax *
Gelatine adhesive
Sodium oleate
Anhydrous Ammonia *
Terpine hydrate *
Terpenes *

FIEBING'S BOOT POLISH
(Fiebing)

Carnauba wax
Montan wax
Paraffin wax
Turpentine *
Mineral spirits *
Silicone oil

FIEBING'S CARE FOR LEATHER AND SHOES
(Fiebing)

Crown wax
Sodium stearate
Sodium palmitate
Gelatin adhesive
Phenol *
Glycerol
Pine oil *

FIEBING'S FACTORY TYPE BOOT POLISH
(Fiebing)

Carnauba wax
Paraffin wax
Turpentine *
Mineral spirits *
Silicone oil

FIEBING'S LEATHER BALM
Leather polish
(Fiebing)

Carnauba wax
Candelilla wax
Castile soap
Turpentine *
Light naphtha *

FIEBING'S PRIME NEATSFOOT OIL COMPOUND
(Fiebing)

Neatsfoot oil
Paraffin oil
Light naphtha *

FIEBING'S SADDLE SOAP
(Fiebing)

Tallow
Rosin
Sodium carbonate
Borax *
Sodium hydroxide
Japan wax
Carnauba wax
Palm oil
Denatured alcohol
Oil of citronella *

FILIBON
Prenatal dietary supplement
(Lederle)

Vitamin A acetate .... 5000 IU
Vitamin D .... 400 IU
Elemental Iron (as ferrous
   fumarate) .... 30 mg.
Plus multivitamins and minerals

FILIBON F.A.
Prenatal dietary supplement
(Lederle)

Vitamin A acetate .... 8000 IU
Vitamin D .... 400 IU
Elemental Iron (as ferrous
   fumarate) .... 45 mg.
Folic acid .... 1 mg.
Plus multivitamins and minerals

FILIBON FORTE
Prenatal dietary supplement
(Lederle)

Vitamin A acetate .... 8000 IU
Vitamin D .... 400 IU
Elemental Iron (as ferrous
   fumarate) .... 45 mg.
Folic acid .... 1 mg.
Plus multivitamins

FILIBON OT
Prenatal dietary supplement; stool softener
(Lederle)

Vitamin A acetate .... 8000 IU
Vitamin D .... 400 IU
Elemental Iron (as ferrous
   fumarate) .... 30 mg.
Dioctyl sodium sulfosuccinate * 100 mg.
Plus multivitamins and minerals

FILLERITE CURE-IT 6-18 CREME HARDENER
For plastic repairs
(Baird Dynamic)

Benzoyl peroxide * .... <60%
In an ester

'76 Ed.

FILLERITE CURE-IT 4-20 POWDER HARDENER
For plastic filler
(Baird Dynamic)

Benzoyl peroxide * .... <30%
Mineral fillers

'76 Ed.

FILLERITE PLASTIC PASTE
(Baird Dynamic)

Polyester resins
Mineral fillers

'76 Ed.

FILM OFF
Soap film remover
(Sanitek)

Water 52.4%
Tetrasodium EDTA 46.4%
Sodium tripolyphosphate 1.2%

FILTER KOTE
Bacteriostatic; for use on air-conditioning filters in hospitals and nursing homes
(Puritan Chem. Co.)

n-Alkyl (C14, C10, C12, C18) dimethyl benzyl ammonium chlorides
n-Alkyl (C12, C14, C16, C18) dimethyl ethyl benzyl ammonium chlorides
Inert ingredients: 99.7%
   Water
   Triethylene glycol
   Isooctyl phenoxy polyethoxy ethanol

Starred ingredients (*) may be responsible for major toxic effects; consult Section II.

FINAC LOTION
For acne therapy
(C & M Pharmacal)

Sulfur	2%
Hyamine 10X *	
Isopropyl alcohol	8%

In a powder-film forming base

FINAL PELLETED RAT & MOUSE BAIT
(Bell Labs., Inc.)

Warfarin	0.025%
Sulfaquinoxaline	0.025%
Blend of food grade cereals	99.950%

FINAL TOUCH
Liquid fabric softener
(Lever Bros.)

Water	90-95%
Quaternary ammonium compounds	1-5%
Fatty amide	1-5%
Nonionic detergent	<1%
Citric acid	<1%
Perfume	<1%
Optical dye	<1%
Isopropanol	<1%
Sodium citrate	trace
Colorants	trace
Preservatives	nil to trace

FINAST BLEACH
(First National Stores)

Sodium hypochlorite *	5.25%

FIND LEAK DETECTOR
(Lester Labs.)

Synthetic detergents *

'76 Ed.

FINE FARE BLUE LAUNDRY DETERGENT
Dry laundry detergent
(Great Atlantic & Pacific, mfr.; Federated Foods, dist.)

Sodium linear alkyl benzene sulfonate	<17%
Sodium carbonate *	<30%
Sodium silicate	<10%
Sodium carboxymethylcellulose	<2%
Optical brighteners	<1%
Sodium chloride	<10%
Blue dye	trace
Sodium sulfate and moisture	balance

FINE ORGANICS SALICYLANILIDE
Fungicide
(Fine Organics, Inc.)

Salicylanilide *	100%

'76 Ed.

FINESSE
Hospital grade detergent-germicide
(Puritan Chem. Co.)

Coconut oil soap	14.10%
Isopropyl alcohol *	10.58%
o-Benzyl-p-chlorophenol	7.05%

FINIS
Insecticide; professional use
(Malter International)

o-Isopropoxyphenyl methylcarbamate *	10.0%
Methylene chloride	42.5%
Methyl isobutyl ketone	42.5%

FINIS
Aerosol furniture polish
(Scott's Liquid Gold)

Carbon dioxide propellant
Emulsifiers and stabilizers
Silicones
Petroleum naphtha *
Fragrance *
Water (a major component)

FINISH
Detergent
(Economics)

Sodium phosphate *
Sodium silicate
Sodium carbonate
Synthetic wetting agent
Chlorine releasing agent

FINISH RUB

See PARKO FINISH RUB

FINS-UP OXYGEN TABLETS
Provides oxygen for treatment of sick fish or transfer of tropical fish
(Lake Products)

Each tablet:

Barium peroxide *	32.59%
Calcium sulfate	30.17%
Calcium phosphate	29.44%
Manganese dioxide	4.86%
Sodium sulfite	0.03%
Amorphous Carbon	2.92%

FIORINAL TABLETS & CAPSULES
Sedative, analgesic
(Sandoz)

Each tablet or capsule:

Sandoptal (Butalbital USP) *	50 mg.
Caffeine USP	40 mg.
Aspirin USP *	200 mg.
Phenacetin USP *	130 mg.

FIORINAL WITH CODEINE CAPSULES
Sedative, analgesic
(Sandoz)

Each No. 1, No. 2 or No. 3 capsule:

Sandoptal (Butalbital, USP) *	50 mg.
Codeine phosphate, USP *	7.5 mg.; 15 mg.; or 30 mg.
Aspirin, USP *	200 mg.
Phenacetin, USP *	130 mg.
Caffeine, USP	40 mg.

FIRE CHIEF GASOLINE
(Texaco, Inc.; Texaco Canada Ltd.)

Gasoline *
  containing lead antiknock compounds *
Dye

FIRM & DRY
Hair spray
(Bonat)

	percentage range
SD Alcohol 40	45.0-65.0%
Methylene chloride *	10.0-20.0%
Isobutane	6.0-15.0%
Propane	6.0-12.0%
Octylacrylamide/Acrylates/Butylaminoethyl methacrylate polymer	<5.0%
Aminomethyl propanol	<1.0%
Isopropyl myristate	<1.0%
Fragrance	<1.0%

FIRM PERM LOTION
(Halliwell)

	percentage range
Water	75.0-90.0%
Ammonium thioglycolate *	5.0-12.0%
Ammonium hydroxide *	<2.0%
Ammonium carbonate	0.5-3.0%
Potassium coco-hydrolyzed animal protein	1.0-4.0%
Urea	0.5-3.0%
Styrene/Acrylamide copolymer	<1.0%
Sodium hydroxide	<1.0%
Laureth-23	<1.0%
Fragrance	<1.0%
Simethicone	<1.0%

FIRM UP
Hair spray
(Halliwell)

	percentage range
SD Alcohol 40	45.0-65.0%
Methylene chloride *	10.0-20.0%
Isobutane	6.0-15.0%
Propane	6.0-12.0%
Octylacrylamide/Acrylates/Butylaminoethyl methacrylate polymer	<5.0%
Aminomethyl propanol	<1.0%
Isopropyl myristate	<1.0%
Fragrance	<1.0%

1ST AID FOR HEADACHE
(Chex)

Each tablet:
N-Acetyl para-aminophenol * .... 5 gr.

'76 Ed.

"FIRST" DISINFECTANT-DETERGENT SYSTEM
(Advance Chemical Co.)

Active ingredients: 17.80%
Potassium salt of lauric fatty acid
Potassium salt of myristic fatty acid
Potassium ortho-benzylparachlorophen-ate
Isopropanol *
Tetrapotassium-ethylenediaminetetra-acetate
Inactive ingredients: 82.20%
Water
Tetrapotassium pyrophosphate *
Liquid nonionic Surface active agent
(based on dodecyl phenol & ethylene
oxide modified with amylase, protease
& lipase)

FISHSOL FISH EMULSION

See DEXOL FISHSOL FISH EMULSION

FISONS AGROCHEMICAL PRODUCTS

Fisons Corp.
Agrochemical Div.
Two Preston Ct.
Bedford, Mass. 01730

Phone: 617-275-1000

FISONS PHARMACEUTICALS

Fisons Corp.
Pharmaceutical Div.
Two Preston Ct.
Bedford, Mass. 01730

Phone: 617-275-1000

5 DAY ANTIPERSPIRANT
(Williams, J.B.)

Aluminum chlorohydrate
Methylbenzethonium chloride
Alcohol *

FIX CAVITY CHEMICAL
Embalming supply
(Royal Bond)

Formaldehyde * 30%
Methanol *

FIXODENT DENTURE ADHESIVE CREAM
(Vicks Toiletry Products Div.)

Calcium sodium poly(vinylmethylether-maleate)
Mineral oil 26%
Sodium carboxymethylcellulose
Petrolatum
FD & C Red #3

FIZRIN
Antacid
(Glenbrook Labs.)

Each packet:
Aspirin * .... 5.0 gr.
Sodium bicarbonate .... 1825 mg.
Sodium carbonate .... 400 mg.
Citric acid .... 1450 mg.

FLAIR
Insecticide/repellent; dogs and cats
(Jensen-Salsbery Labs.)

Pyrethrins 0.06%
Piperonyl butoxide (technical) .. 0.48%
Malathion 0.50%
Carbaryl 0.50%
Butoxypolypropylene glycol 5.00%
2,3:4,5-Bis(2-butylene)tetrahydro-2-furaldehyde (MGK Repellent 11) 0.14%
Petroleum distillate * 17.85%

FLAIR PENS AND REFILLS
(Gillette Co., Paper Mate Div.)

The Gillette Co., Paper Mate Div.,
Boston, Mass. 02199 will receive collect
phone calls from poison control centers or
physicians asking for emergency toxicological information about the company's
products.

Phone: 617-421-7000

FLAIR THREE WAY LIQUID CLEANER POLISH
(Nat'l Labs. Div.)

Petroleum distillate *
Emulsifiers

FLAIR WOOD AND MULTI-PURPOSE POLISH
(Nat'l Labs. Div.)

Propane-isobutane blend
(propellant) .... minor
Petroleum distillate * .... major

FLAME-GLO COSMETIC PRODUCTS

Flame-Glo Cosmetics
Div. of Del Labs., Inc.
565 Broad Hollow Rd.
Farmingdale, N.Y. 11735

Phone: 516-293-7070

See COSMETICS, Section VI, General
Formulations

FLASH HAND CLEANER
(Skat)

Mild soap base
Cleaned Pennsylvania sand
Soda ash .... small percentage
Silicate of soda
Perfume

FLASHO LIGHTER FLUID
(Norton)

Petroleum distillate *

'76 Ed.

FLAVIHIST
Antihistaminic, analgesic
(Amlab)

Each capsule:
Pheniramine maleate * ..... 6.25 mg.
Pyrilamine maleate * ...... 8.33 mg.
Salicylamide * .... 3.5 gr.
Acetaminophen * .... 2.0 gr.
Atropine sulfate .... 1/600 gr.
Methapyrilene
hydrochloride * .... 8.33 mg.
Ephedrine sulfate * ...... 10.0 mg.
Caffeine .... 0.5 gr.

FLAVIHIST BABY COUGH SYRUP
(Amlab)

Each fl. oz.:
Ammonium chloride .... 300 mg.
Sodium citrate .... 600 mg.
Chloroform .... 3/4 min.
Sodium benzoate 0.1%
Menthol and glycerin in base

FLAVIHIST, EXTRA STRENGTH
Cough syrup
(Amlab)

Each fl. oz.:
Phenylephrine HCl * ...... 10.0 mg.
Pyrilamine maleate * ..... 22.5 mg.
Ephedrine sulfate * ...... 15.0 mg.
d-Methorphan .... 90 mg.
Sodium citrate .... 325.0 mg.
Ammonium chloride .... 650.0 mg.
Chloroform .... 1.5 min.
Menthol and glycerine in base

FLAVIHIST P-A
For relief of symptoms due to colds, sinusitis, allergy and hay fever
(Amlab)

Each prolonged-action capsule:
Phenylpropanolamine HCl * . 50 mg.
Pheniramine maleate ...... 12.5 mg.
Chlorpheniramine maleate .. 1 mg.
Belladonna alkaloids (total): 0.16 mg.
Atropine sulfate .... 0.024 mg.
Scopolamine HBr ..... 0.014 mg.
Hyoscyamine sulfate ... 0.122 mg.

FLAVIHIST THROAT LOZENGES
(Amlab)

Each lozenge:
Cetyl dimethyl benzyl ammonium chloride	2.0 mg.
Benzocaine	5.0 mg.
Phenylephrine HCl	2.5 mg.
Salicylamide	50.0 mg.
Potassium guaiacolsulfonate	15.0 mg.

FLAVOR-FEEN, LIQUID
Anthelmintic; veterinary - livestock
(Clover Chem.)

Each fl. oz.:
Phenothiazine *	7.5 gm.

'76 Ed.

FLAVOR-FEEN, POWDERED
Anthelmintic; veterinary - livestock & poultry
(Clover Chem.)

Phenothiazine NF *	96%/w
Flavoring media	4%/w

'76 Ed.

FLEACOLLAR FOR CATS
(Aceline Products Corp.)

Lindane	0.56%

FLEACOLLAR FOR DOGS
(Aceline Products Corp.)

Lindane	0.63%

FLEA-GO
Insecticidal shampoo
(Fort Dodge)

Oil anise *	2%
Soap anhydrous	37.6%

FLEAVOL SHAMPOO
Veterinary
(Norden Labs.)

Pyrethrins	0.05%
Piperonyl butoxide (tech.)	0.50%
Diisopropyl cresols	0.10%

FLECTO PAINT PRODUCTS
Wood and metal finishes

The Flecto Co., Inc.
1000 45th St.
Oakland, Calif. 94608

Phone: 415-655-2470

See PAINTS, Section VI, General Formulations

FLEECY WHITE BLEACH
Bleach, disinfectant, deodorant
(Purex Corp.)

Sodium hypochlorite *	5 1/4%
Sodium chloride	<5%
Water	Balance

FLEETWOOD COSMETIC PRODUCTS

Fleetwood Co.
1500 Brook Dr.
Downers Grove, Ill. 60515

Phone: 312-495-9300

See COSMETICS, Section VI, General Formulations

FLETCHERS
Adhesive
(Ambroid)

Nitrocellulose type of cement
Alcohols *	20%
Hydrocarbons *†	60%
Ketones *	20%
Allyl isothiocyanate (synthetic oil of mustard)	trace

†See Adhesives, Section VI, General Formulations

FLETCHER'S CASTORIA
Cathartic
(Glenbrook Labs.)

Alcohol	3.5%
Senna extract	equiv. to 6.5%
Flavored syrup	

FLEX HAIR CARE PRODUCTS

Revlon, Inc.
767 Fifth Ave.
New York, N.Y. 10153

Phone: 212-572-5000

Revlon Research Center, Inc.
945 Zerega Ave.
Bronx, N.Y. 10473

Phone: 212-824-9000

See COSMETICS, Section VI, General Formulations

FLEXISEAL SEALANT

See DAP FLEXISEAL SEALANT

FLICK
Control of household insects
(ABCO, Inc.)

Petroleum distillates *	99.622%
Piperonyl butoxide technical	0.303%
Pyrethrins	0.075%

FLIGONE
Insecticide
(Central Chem.)

Petroleum oil *	99.55%
Technical Piperonyl butoxide	0.375%
Pyrethrins	0.075%

'76 Ed.

FLINT, BUFFABLE

See BUFFABLE FLINT

FLINT XL
Liquid floor polish
(Sanitek)

Acrylic polymer emulsion	11.7%
Diethylene glycol monoethyl ether (Cellosolve)	4.0%
Polyethylene wax emulsion	2.4%
Tributoxyethyl phosphate	1.0%
Rosin maleate resin	0.9%
Nonionic surfactants, Formalin, Ammonia, Defoamer, Fluorochemical surfactant	trace
Water	balance

FLO CLEAN
Floor cleaner
(Hillyard Chem.)

Alkaline detergent *†	

'76 Ed.

†See Detergents (synthetic)

FLOC RITE
(Coastal Industries)

Aluminum sulfate *	

FLO-FREE
Drain opener
(Holcomb)

Sulfuric acid *	>10%

'76 Ed.

FLO-MASTER INK
(Faber-Castell)

Xylene * or Xylene * and hi-flash Naphtha (according to color)	73-90%
Aniline dyes	
Resin	

FLOOR-NU, FORMULA HC-62

See KLENZADE FLOOR-NU, FORMULA HC-62

FLO PASTE WAX

See BUTCHER'S FLO PASTE WAX

Starred ingredients (*) may be responsible for major toxic effects; consult Section II.

FLORA-FOG DITHIONE
Insecticide
(Summit Chem. Co.)

Tetraethyl dithiopyrophosphate *	4.75%
Related phosphates	0.25%
Petroleum distillate	95.00%

FLORA-FOG KELTHANE
Insecticide
(Summit Chem. Co.)

1,1-Bis(chlorophenyl)-2,2,2-trichloroethanol	10.0%
Petroleum distillate *	90.0%

FLORA-FOG MALATHION-LINDANE
Insecticide
(Summit Chem. Co.)

Malathion *	10.0%
Gamma isomer of benzene hexachloride *	5.0%
Petroleum distillate *	85.0%

FLORA-FOG PENTAC
Insecticide
(Summit Chem. Co.)

Decachlorobis (2,4-Cyclopentadiene-1-yl) *	10%
Petroleum distillate *	70%
Methylene chloride *	20%

FLORA-FOG VAPONA
Insecticide
(Summit Chem. Co.)

O,O-Dimethyl O-2,2-dichlorovinyl phosphate *	9.3%
Related compounds	0.7%
Petroleum distillate *	90.0%

FLORA-FUME DITHIONE
Greenhouse misting insecticide (liquid)
(Summit Chem. Co.)

Active ingredients:	5.00%
O,O,O,O-Tetraethyl dithiopyrophosphate *	4.75%
Related phosphates	0.25%

FLORA-FUME MALATHION
Insecticide
(Summit Chem. Co.)

Malathion *	10%
Methylene chloride *	90%

FLORA-FUME VAPONA
Insecticide
(Summit Chem. Co.)

2,2-Dichlorovinyl dimethyl phosphate *	9.3%
Related compounds	0.7%
Methylene chloride *	90.0%

FLORALIFE CUT FLOWER PRESERVATIVE (POWDER)
(Floralife, Inc.)

Sugar	>90%/w
Other ingredients	<10%/w

FLORA SEAL
(Uncle Sam)

Modified Phenolic resins
China wood oil
Cobalt driers *
Petroleum distillates *

FLORA-TINT

See GARD FLORA-TINT

FLORIDA FOAM IMPROVED
Cleanser for oily skin or scalp
(Hill Dermaceuticals)

Benzalkonium chloride *
Aluminum acetate basic
Boric acid *
Biodegradable Protein
Nonionic detergent
Base:
    Oat powder

FLOROPRYL OPHTHALMIC OINTMENT
Miotic
(MSD)

Each gram:	
Isofluorophate	0.025%
Polyethylene-mineral oil gel	

FLOWAWAY TABLETS

See DEWITT'S FLOWAWAY TABLETS

FLOWAY
Motor cleaner
(Kano)

Petroleum compounds *†

†*See* Petroleum distillate

F-L-T BOMB
For fleas, lice and ticks on dogs and cats
(Bio-Ceutic)

Carbaryl (1-Naphthyl N-methylcarbamate)	1.00%
2,2'-Methylenebis (4-chloro-phenol) (Dichlorophene)	0.10%
Pyrethrins	0.06%
Technical Piperonyl butoxide	0.60%
Butoxypolypropylene glycol	5.00%
Petroleum distillate *	23.10%

F-L-T POWDER
For control of fleas, lice and ticks on dogs and cats
(Bio-Ceutic)

1-Naphthyl N-methylcarbamate *	5.0%
Technical Piperonyl butoxide	1.0%
Pyrethrins	0.1%
Dichlorophene	0.5%

FLUFFY "all" (Low Phosphate)
Powder laundry detergent
(Lever Bros.)

Sodium sulfate	30-45%
Sodium polyphosphates	25-35%
Nonionic detergent	10-20%
Water	5-15%
Sodium silicate	5-10%
Sodium borates	1-5%
Sodium soap	1-5%
Sodium carbonate	0-5%
Cellulosic	<1%
Perfume	<1%
Optical dye	trace
Colorant	trace

FLUF RINSE

See TEXIZE FLUF RINSE

FLUID CEREFOLIUS
Diuretic
(Walker Pharm.)

Alcohol	25%
Saw palmetto fl. ext.	120 m.
Corn silk tr. (50% drug)	60 m.
Sandalwood fl. ext.	30 m.
Methenamine *	8 gr.

'76 Ed.

FLUONID CREAM 0.01%, 0.025%
Anti-inflammatory for dermatoses
(Herbert Labs.)

Fluocinolone acetonide	0.010%; 0.025%

FLUONID OINTMENT 0.025%
Anti-inflammatory for dermatoses
(Herbert Labs.)

Fluocinolone acetonide	0.025%

FLUONID TOPICAL SOLUTION 0.01%
Anti-inflammatory for dermatoses
(Herbert Labs.)

Fluocinolone acetonide	0.01%

FLUO-PYRE ROACH POWDER
Insecticide
(American Fluoride)

Sodium fluoride *	38.80%
Pyrethrins	0.35%

Starred ingredients (*) may be responsible for major toxic effects; consult Section II.

FLURA DROPS
Aid in the prevention of dental caries
(Kirkman)

Each 0.25 cc.:
  Sodium fluoride (representing
    1.0 mg. of the fluorine ion) . 2.21 mg.

FLURA-LOZ
Prevention of dental caries
(Kirkman)

Each lozenge:
  Sodium fluoride (representing
    1.0 mg. of the fluorine ion) . 2.21 mg.

FLURA-PREN
Prevention of dental caries
(Kirkman)

Each tablet:
  Sodium fluoride (representing
    1.0 mg. of the fluorine ion) . 2.21 mg.
  Polyvitamins

FLURA-TABLET
Prevention of dental caries
(Kirkman)

Each tablet:
  Sodium fluoride (representing
    1.0 mg. of the fluorine ion) . 2.21 mg.

FLURESS
Ophthalmic solution
(Barnes-Hind)

Sodium fluorescein 0.25%
Benoxinate HCl 0.4%
Boric acid buffer containing:
  Povidone
  Purified water
Chlorobutanol 1.0%
Edetate disodium 0.1%

FLY-A-REST
See PURINA FLY-A-REST

FLY-AWAY
Insect repellent
(Miller Chem. & Fert.)

Pyrethrins 0.6%
Butoxy polypropylene glycol * . 89.4%

FLY-AWAY DAIRY SPRAY CONC.
Insect repellent
(Miller Chem. & Fert.)

Pyrethrins 0.54%
Butoxy polypropylene glycol * . 53.29%
Piperonyl butoxide tech. 5.38%
Petroleum distillate * 25.72%

FLY-BATE
See ROBERTS FLY-BATE

FLY BATE
Insecticide
(Corn King)

DDVP 0.32%
Related compounds 0.03%
Ronnel 0.25%

FLY-BYE
See PURINA FLY-BYE

FLYCO BRAND CIODRIN
Insecticide
(F. & W. Enterprises)

Dimethyl phosphate of alpha-
  methylbenzyl-3-hydroxy-cis-
  crotonate (Ciodrin) * 11.94%
Petroleum hydrocarbons 76.06%

'76 Ed.

FLYCO BRAND FLY BAIT
(F. & W. Enterprises)

2,2-Dichlorovinyl dimethyl phosphate 0.5%

'76 Ed.

FLYCO BRAND FLY-CORD
Insecticide-impregnated cotton cord
(F. & W. Enterprises)

Parathion * 13.79%
Diazinon 3.54%

'76 Ed.

FLYCO BRAND VAPONA
Insecticide
(F. & W. Enterprises)

2,2-Dichlorovinyl dimethyl phosphate 10%
High aromatic naphtha * 80%

'76 Ed.

FLY-CORD, FLYCO BRAND
See FLYCO BRAND FLY-CORD

FLY DED INSECT KILLER
(Boyle-Midway)

Resmethrin 0.080%
Related compounds 0.011%
d-trans Allethrin 0.160%
Related compounds 0.012%
Piperonyl butoxide (technical) .. 0.800%
Aromatic petroleum solvent * ... 1.191%
1,1-Trichloroethane * .... <2%
Hydrocarbon propellant and water

'FLY-DIE'
See ROBERTS 'FLY-DIE'

FLY-DU
Insecticide - aerosol
(An-Fo)

Pyrethrins 0.30%
Piperonyl butoxide technical 1.50%
Petroleum hydrocarbons * 18.20%

FLY FOG
Insecticide
(Residex)

Pyrethrins 0.5%
Technical Piperonyl butoxide 3.0%
Petroleum distillate 6.5%
Propellants 90.0%

FLYING COLORS TEMPERA
(Sanford Corp.)

Water
Pigments
Gum arabic or bone glue
Phenol (as preservative) .... <1%

FLY JINX INSECT SPRAY
(Claire)

Methoxychlor, tech. 2.0%
DDVP 0.46%
Related compounds 0.04%
Petroleum distillates * 20.0%

FLY MORT
Insecticide
(Corn King)

2,2-Dichlorovinyl dimethyl phosphate 0.46%
Related compounds 0.04%

FLY PATROL
See PURINA FLY PATROL

FLYS-AWAY REPELLENT SPRAY BOMB
Veterinary
(Farnam Co.)

Butoxy polypropylene glycol * . 26.700%
Pine oil * 21.806%
Citrus oil 5.450%
Rotenone 0.136%
Cube resins other than rotenone . 0.408%

'76 Ed.

FLYS-AWAY REPELLENT "STICK"
Veterinary
(Farnam Co.)

Piperonyl butoxide, technical ... 1.00%
Pyrethrins I & II 0.40%
Petroleum hydrocarbons 3.60%
Butoxy polypropylene glycol 10.00%

'76 Ed.

FLYS-AWAY REPELLENT WIPES
Veterinary
(Farnam Co.)

Pyrethrins	0.20%
Piperonyl butoxide, technical	0.50%
Di-n-propyl isocinchomeronate	1.00%
Oil of citronella	5.00%
Butoxy polypropylene glycol *	20.00%

'76 Ed.

"FOAM N' COMB" DRY SHAMPOO FOR DOGS/CATS

See SERGEANT'S "FOAM N' COMB" DRY SHAMPOO FOR DOGS/CATS

FOAM-NOX, FORMULA LC-81

See KLENZADE FOAM-NOX, FORMULA LC-81

FOAM OFF
Foaming cleaner
(Paul Koss)

Water	>70%
Monoethanolammonium dodecylbenzene sulfonate (Anionic surfactant)	<8%
Tetrapotassium pyrophosphate	<8%
Fatty amido phosphate	<4%
Sodium metasilicate	<3%
Butyl Cellosolve *	<3%
Monoethanolamine	<3%
Sodium xylene sulfonate (Anionic surfactant)	<2%

pH 11.6-11.8

FOAM-TEX

See AIRWICK PROFESSIONAL PRODUCTS FOAM-TEX

FOAMY
Upholstery cleaner
(Lester Labs.)

Detergents *

'76 Ed.

FOG
Liquid steam cleaning compound
(Lester Labs.)

Mild Alkalis *
Detergents *

'76 Ed.

FOG-A-WAY
Insecticide
(Malter International)

Pyrethrins	0.180%
n-Octyl sulfoxide of isosafrole	0.792%
Related compounds	0.108%
Refined Petroleum distillate *	98.920%

FOGERATOR, ARAB

See ARAB FOGERATOR (Aerosol)

FOGICIDE NO. P
Insecticide
(Lorenz)

Piperonyl butoxide
Pyrethrins
Aliphatic hydrocarbons *

FOG-O-MATIC INSECTICIDE
Industrial
(Barco)

Pyrethrins	0.40%
Technical Piperonyl butoxide	0.80%
N-Octyl bicycloheptene dicarboximide	1.33%
Petroleum distillates *	97.47%

'76 Ed.

FOILLE LIQUID
(Blistex)

Benzyl alcohol	4.0%
Benzocaine	2.0%
Base:	balance
Oxyquinoline base	
Sulfur	
Vegetable oil	
Eugenol	

FOILLE OINTMENT
(Blistex)

Benzyl alcohol	4.0%
Benzocaine	2.0%
Base:	balance
Oxyquinoline base	
Vegetable oil	
Eugenol	

FOLEX
Cotton defoliant
(Mobil Chemical Co.)

Merphos (Tributyl phosphorotrithioite) *	72.0%
Related compounds	1.8%

FOMAC FOAM (CLEANSER)
For treatment of acne and oily skin
(Dermik)

Salicylic acid *	2%

Complexed and solubilized with polyvinylpyrrolidone and protein hydrolysate in an anionic-nonionic detergent system

---

FOODGUARD #1
Sanitizing detergent
(Butcher Polish)

approx. % by wt.

Alkyl polyoxyalkalene ether	5%
Tetrapotassium pyrophosphate	5%
Tetrasodium ethylene diamine tetraacetate	3%
Sodium metasilicate	2%
Combined amount:	2%
n-Alkyl dimethyl benzyl ammonium chlorides *	
n-Alkyl dimethyl ethylbenzyl ammonium chlorides *	
Ethyl alcohol	<1%
Water	balance

FOOD SERVICE PACK JOY
Institutional and industrial cleaning product

Procter & Gamble Co.
Ivorydale Technical Center
Cincinnati, Ohio 45217

Phone: 513-562-1100

FOOTLIGHTS CARPET SHAMPOO

See BUTCHER'S FOOTLIGHTS CARPET SHAMPOO

FOOT NOTE

See LARSON'S FOOT NOTE

FORAMBA INSECT SPRAY
Insecticide
(Uncle Sam)

Pyrethrums
Synergists
Petroleum distillates *

FOR BRUNETTES ONLY HAIR COLOR
(Alberto-Culver)

Oleic acid
Isopropyl alcohol
Lauryl alcohol
Propylene glycol
Octoxynol-5
Lauramide DEA
Ethoxydiglycol
Sodium lauriminodipropionate
p-Phenylenediamine
o-Aminophenol
Resorcinol
p-Aminophenol
4-Ethoxy-m-phenylenediamine sulfate
2-Methylresorcinol
1-Naphthol
2-Metoxy-p-phenylenediamine sulfate
4-Nitro-o-phenylenediamine
Hydroquinone
Ammonia
Sodium sulfite
Fragrance
Trisodium EDTA

Starred ingredients (*) may be responsible for major toxic effects; consult Section II.

FORCE'S GOPHER KILLER
Rodenticide
(Carajon Chem.)

Strychnine alkaloid * 0.05%

FORCE'S MOUS-CON NO. 2
Rodenticide
(Carajon Chem.)

Zinc phosphide * 2%

FORCE'S POISON PEANUTS
Rodenticide
(Carajon Chem.)

Strychnine sulphate * 0.5%

FORCE'S RO-DEX
Rodenticide
(Carajon Chem.)

Strychnine alkaloid * 0.5%

FORCOLD
Antitussive-expectorant
(Lemmon Co.)

Each 30 ml.:
Codeine phosphate * . . . . 60 mg.
Chlorpheniramine maleate . . . . 12 mg.
Ephedrine sulfate * . . . . 60 mg.
Sodium citrate . . . . 1 gm.
Menthol . . . . 3 mg.
Alcohol 1%

FORE
Fungicide
(Rohm and Haas)

Coordination product of Zinc ion,
Manganese ethylene
bisdithiocarbamate *† 80%
Inerts 20%

†*See* Maneb and Zineb

FOREMOST 4840 A A FLY SPRAY
Insecticide
(Delta Foremost)

Petroleum distillate *
Technical Piperonyl butoxide . . . . . <1%
Pyrethrins

FOREMOST 1653 AMAZING "IN PLACE" CLEANER - DISINFECTANT
Commercial and industrial use
(Delta Foremost)

Sodium carbonate, anhydrous * . . 26.5%
Sodium metasilicate, anhydrous * . . 24.0%
Potassium dichloro-s-triazinetrione 10.0%

FOREMOST 4565 BOWL CLEANER
Institutional and commercial use
(Delta Foremost)

Hydrogen chloride * 23.0%
Orthodichlorobenzene 2.5%

FOREMOST 1651 CHLOR-DIS PINK
Disinfectant cleaner & deodorizer - dairies and commercial use
(Delta Foremost)

Sodium phosphate (ex-
pressed as Na3PO4-
12H2O) * . . . . 91.75% min.
Sodium hypochlorite . . . . . . 3.25% min.

FOREMOST 1645 CLEANER-SANITIZER
For dairies, and other commercial use
(Delta Foremost)

Sodium carbonate * 35%
N-Alkyl (C12 40%, C14 60%, C16 10%)
dimethyl benzyl ammonium
chloride 5%

FOREMOST 4820 DEL-KILL INSECTICIDE
(Delta Foremost)

o-Isopropoxyphenyl
methylcarbamate 1.00%
Petroleum distillate * 83.94%

FOREMOST 4953-ES ALL SEASON WEED KILLER
Commercial and industrial herbicide
(Delta Foremost)

Mixed Aliphatic hydrocarbons * 96.75%
2,4-Dichlorophenoxyacetic acid
(isooctyl ester)(2,4-D equiv.
0.70%) 1.09%
Pentachlorophenol 0.80%
Other chlorophenols 0.09%
Bromacil (5-Bromo-3-sec-butyl-6-
methyluracil) 0.98%

FOREMOST 4812-ES AMBUSH
Residual insecticide for commercial and industrial use
(Delta Foremost)

Malathion (O,O-Dimethyl dithiophosphate of diethyl
mercaptosuccinate) 2.00%
2,2-Dichlorovinyl dimethyl phosphate (DDVP) 0.51%
Petroleum distillates * 97.00%

FOREMOST 2149-ES MARVEL GERMICIDAL CLEANER
Institutional and commercial use
(Delta Foremost)

N-Alkyl (60% C14, 30% C16, 5%
C12, 5% C18) dimethyl benzyl
ammonium chloride 0.076%
N-Alkyl (50% C12, 30% C14, 17%
C16, 3% C18) dimethyl ethyl-
benzyl ammonium chloride . . 0.076%
Sodium metasilicate 0.240%
Essential oils 0.200%
Inert ingred.: 99.408%
Detergents
Cleaners
Builder
Propellant

FOREMOST 4885 FOOD PLANT INSECT BOMB
(Delta Foremost)

Technical Piperonyl butoxide . . . 1.5%
Pyrethrins 0.3%
Petroleum distillate * 18.2%
Inert ingred.:
Trichloromonofluoromethane . . 40.0%
Dichlorodifluoromethane 40.0%

FOREMOST 2151 GERMICIDAL SPRAY-N-'WIPE CLEANER
Institutional and commercial use
(Delta Foremost)

N-Alkyl (60% C14, 30% C16, 5%
C12, 5% C18) dimethyl benzyl
ammonium chloride 0.076%
N-Alkyl (50% C12, 30% C14, 17%
C16, 3% C18) dimethyl ethyl-
benzyl ammonium chloride . . 0.076%
Sodium metasilicate 0.240%
Inert ingred.: 99.408%
Detergents
Cleaners
Builder
Propellant

FOREMOST 4810 HD 22 INSECT SPRAY
For commercial and industrial use
(Delta Foremost)

Petroleum distillate * 98.9%
Piperonyl butoxide 1.0%
Pyrethrins 0.1%

FOREMOST 4811 HD 55 INSECT SPRAY CONCENTRATE
For commercial and industrial use
(Delta Foremost)

Petroleum distillate *
Technical Piperonyl butoxide
Pyrethrins

FOREMOST 4809-ES INSECT-O-FOG
Insecticide - commercial and industrial use
(Delta Foremost)

Petroleum distillate *
Piperonyl butoxide
Pyrethrins

FOREMOST 4512 LEMON-AIRE
Air freshener, disinfectant for institutional and commercial use
(Delta Foremost)

4-Chloro-2-cyclopentylphenol	0.0256%
Orthophenylphenol	0.1400%
3,4′,5-Tribromosalicylanilide and other related bromo-salicylanilides including:	0.3600%
3,5-Dibromosalicylanilide	
4′,5-Dibromosalicylanilide	
2′,3,4′,5-Tetrabromosalicylanilide	
Essential oils *	2.0000%
Alcohol	54.8100%

FOREMOST 4510 MINTEFFECT
Institutional and commercial germicide
(Delta Foremost)

Active ingred.:	36.11%
Isopropyl alcohol *	
Vegetable oil soaps	
o-Benzyl p-chlorophenol *	
Methyl salicylate *	
Pine oils *	
Inert ingred.:	63.89%
Water	

FOREMOST 4520 PINE OIL DISINFECTANT
Institutional and commercial use
(Delta Foremost)

Active ingredients:	92.6%
Pure steam distilled Pine oil *	
Anhydrous soap	
Isopropyl alcohol *	
Inert ingred.:	7.4%
Water	

FOREMOST 1690 QUAD-DIS
Sanitizer, disinfectant, deodorant for institutional and commercial use
(Delta Foremost)

N-Alkyl (C12 40%, C14 50%, C16 10%) dimethyl ammonium chloride *	10%

FOREMOST 4883 RESID-U-CIDE
Insecticide
(Delta Foremost)

o-Isopropoxyphenyl methylcarbamate	0.67%
Petroleum distillate *	55.96%
Inert ingred.:	
Dichlorodifluoromethane	16.67%
Trichloromonofluoromethane	16.67%

FOREMOST 4555 SANI-TROL
Deodorant for chemical toilets
(Delta Foremost)

Formaldehyde solution *

FOREMOST 4595 SPICE
Room deodorizer, air sanitizer
(Delta Foremost)

Ethanol	32.10%
Triethylene glycol	4.50%
Propylene glycol	3.00%
Diisobutylphenoxyethoxy ethyl dimethyl benzyl ammonium chloride	0.10%
Inert ingred.:	60.30%
Dichlorodifluoromethane	
Trichlorofluoromethane	
Perfume	

FOREMOST 4820 WASP-A-WAY
Kills hornets, wasps
(Delta Foremost)

(5-Benzyl-3-furyl)methyl-2,2-dimethyl-3-(2-methylpropenyl)cyclopropanecarboxylate	0.150% w/w
Related compounds	0.020%
Aromatic petroleum hydrocarbons	0.274%
Petroleum distillate *	11.556%

FOREMOST 4950 WEED KILLER
For commercial and industrial use
(Delta Foremost)

Pentachlorophenol *	6.88%
Other chlorophenols	0.80%
Petroleum distillate *	89.00%

FORFOG-PBPP FOG CONCENTRATE
Insecticide
(Forshaw)

Piperonyl butoxide, technical	1.5%
Pyrethrins	0.15%
Petroleum distillate *	68.35%
Tetrachloroethylene *	30.00%

FORHISTAL LONTABS
Antihistamine
(CIBA Pharmaceutical)

Each Lontab:	
Dimethindene maleate *	2.5 mg.

FOR-JEY
Undertakers', embalmers' supplies
(Embalmers')

Formaldehyde *

FORLIN
Insecticide
(Forshaw)

Lindane *	20%
Petroleum hydrocarbons	75%

FORMADON
Deodorant foot spray
(Gordon Labs.)

Formaldehyde (10% of USP strength) *
Aqueous perfumed base

FOR-MAL 50
Insecticide
(Forshaw)

Malathion *	50%
Petroleum hydrocarbons	45%

FOR-MAL 57
Insecticide
(Forshaw)

Malathion *	57%
Xylene range aromatic petroleum distillate *	35%

FORMAN FORD V805 WOOD SEALER
(Farwell, Ozmun, Kirk)

Active ingred.:	
Pentachlorophenol *	4.4%
Other Chlorophenols	0.6%
Inert ingred.:	
Dipentine	1.5%
Diacetone alcohol	3.5%
Alkyd resin solids	10.4%
Varnish solids	10.4%
Mineral spirits *	68.8%
Calcium naphthenate (6% metal)	0.1%
Lead naphthenate (24% metal)	0.1%
Cobalt naphthenate (6% metal)	0.1%
Antioxidant	0.1%

FORMBY'S ACCENT BLUE WOOD WIPING STAIN
(Formby's)

Low odor exempt Mineral spirits *	50.0%
Isophthalic alkyd	26.0%
Methyl ethyl ketoxime	<0.1%

FORMBY'S ACCENT GREEN WOOD WIPING STAIN
(Formby's)

Low odor exempt Mineral spirits *	50.0%
Isophthalic alkyd	26.0%
Methyl ethyl ketoxime	<0.1%

FORMBY'S ACCENT RED WOOD WIPING STAIN
(Formby's)

Low odor exempt Mineral spirits *	50.0%
Isophthalic alkyd	26.0%
Methyl ethyl ketoxime	<0.1%

Starred ingredients (*) may be responsible for major toxic effects; consult Section II.

FORMBY'S AMERICAN WALNUT WIPING STAIN
(Formby's)

Low odor exempt Mineral spirits *	50.0%
Isophthalic alkyd	26.0%
Methyl ethyl ketoxime	<0.1%

FORMBY'S ANTIQUE CHERRY WOOD WIPING STAIN
(Formby's)

Low odor exempt Mineral spirits *	50.0%
Isophthalic alkyd	26.0%
Methyl ethyl ketoxime	<0.1%

FORMBY'S ANTIQUE WALNUT WOOD WIPING STAIN
(Formby's)

Isophthalic alkyd	26.0%
Low odor exempt Mineral spirits *	24.0%
Xylene	4.0%
Methyl ethyl ketoxime	<0.1%

FORMBY'S DARK WALNUT WOOD WIPING STAIN
(Formby's)

Low odor exempt Mineral spirits *	50.0%
Isophthalic alkyd	26.0%
Methyl ethyl ketoxime	<0.1%

FORMBY'S FRUITWOOD WOOD WIPING STAIN
(Formby's)

Isophthalic alkyd	26.0%
Low odor exempt Mineral spirits *	50.0%
Methyl ethyl ketoxime	<0.1%

FORMBY'S FURNITURE CLEANER
(Formby's)

Mineral spirits *	49%
Mineral seal oil *	49%

FORMBY'S FURNITURE REFINISHER
(Formby's)

Methanol	30%
Methylene chloride	30%
Toluene *	15%
Acetone	30%
Isopropyl alcohol	5%

FORMBY'S LEMON OIL FURNITURE TREATMENT
(Formby's)

Mineral seal oil *	75%
Mineral spirits	25%

FORMBY'S MAPLE WOOD WIPING STAIN
(Formby's)

Low odor exempt Mineral spirits *	50.0%
Isophthalic alkyd	26.0%
Methyl ethyl ketoxime	<0.1%

FORMBY'S MEDITERRANEAN OAK WOOD WIPING STAIN
(Formby's)

Low odor exempt Mineral spirits *	50.0%
Isophthalic alkyd	26.0%
Methyl ethyl ketoxime	<0.1%

FORMBY'S ORIENTAL TEAK WOOD WIPING STAIN
(Formby's)

Low odor exempt Mineral spirits *	50.0%
Isophthalic alkyd	26.0%
Methyl ethyl ketoxime	<0.1%

FORMBY'S PAINT REMOVER
(Formby's)

Methanol	5%
Methylene chloride *	80%
Isopropyl alcohol	10%
Glycol ether	5%

FORMBY'S PAINT REMOVER WASH
(Formby's)

Ethanol	85.0%
Denatured MIBK	0.9%
Approved Hydrocarbon (gasoline, etc.)	0.9%
Ethyl acetate	0.9%

FORMBY'S RED MAHOGANY WOOD WIPING STAIN
(Formby's)

Isophthalic alkyd	26.0%
Low odor exempt Mineral spirits *	47.0%
Methyl ethyl ketoxime	<0.1%

FORMBY'S WALNUT WOOD WIPING STAIN
(Formby's)

Low odor exempt Mineral spirits *	50.0%
Isophthalic alkyd	26.0%
Methyl ethyl ketoxime	<0.1%

FORMCEL FORMALDEHYDE METHYL ALCOHOL SOLUTION
Used in resins for paper, textile treating, plywood, etc.
(Celanese Chem. Co.)

Formaldehyde *	approx. 55%
Methanol *	35%
Water	10-11%

Methoxymethanol is formed in the formaldehyde-methanol solution and will exist in an equilibrium concentration

FORMCEL FORMALDEHYDE NORMAL BUTYL ALCOHOL SOLUTION
Used in resins for paper, textile treating, plywood, etc.
(Celanese Chem. Co.)

Formaldehyde *	approx. 40.0%
Butanol *	55.0%
Water	5.5-6.5%

Butoxymethanol is formed in the formaldehyde-butanol solution and will exist in an equilibrium concentration

FORMICIDE
Hardening compound
(Royal Bond)

Paraformaldehyde *

FORMULA 44 COUGH CONTROL DISCS
See VICKS FORMULA 44 COUGH CONTROL DISCS

FORMULA 44 COUGH MIXTURE
See VICKS FORMULA 44 COUGH MIXTURE

FORMULA 44-D COUGH MIXTURE
See VICKS FORMULA 44-D COUGH MIXTURE

FORMULA 44/40
Gun bluer
(Numrich Arms)

Selenic acid *	7.75%
Nitric acid *	8.58%
Copper sulfate *	6.90%
Aniline dye	0.01%

FORMULA 40 WEED KILLER
Herbicide
(Dow)

2,4-Dichlorophenoxyacetic acid, alkanolamine salts (2,4-dichlorophenoxyacetic acid equivalent 38.6%) *	59.7%

FORMULA 409 ALL PURPOSE CLEANER
(Clorox)

Water	>75%
Ethylene glycol monobutyl ether/ alkyl ether sulfate mixture	5-25%
Sodium metasilicate	0.5-2%
Tetrasodium EDTA	0.5-2%
Green dye	<0.5%

FORMULA 409 BATHROOM CLEANER
(Clorox)

Water	>75%
Propylene glycol isobutyl ether	0.5-5%
Octylphenoxy polyethoxy ethanol	0.5-5%
Tetrasodium EDTA	0.5-5%
Propylene glycol methyl ether	0.5-5%
Quaternary germicide	<0.5%
Fragrance	<0.5%
Propane/isobutane propellant	5-25%

FORNI'S ALPEN KRAUTER
Stimulant laxative
(Fahrney)

Each 30 ml.:
Senna fluid extract *	2 ml.
Water	
Alcohol	16%
Sucrose	
Caramel	

FORNI'S MAGOLO
Antacid
(Fahrney)

Alcohol	20%
Potassium bicarbonate *	
Sodium bicarbonate *	
Peppermint	
Sugar	

FOR OILY HAIR ONLY RINSE
(Gillette Co., Personal Care Div.)

Water	Stearyl alcohol
Ceteth-2	Sodium hydroxide
Citric acid	Extracts of Clover,
Stearalkonium	Chamomile,
chloride	Yarrow, Rose-
Dimethyl steara-	mary, Nettle,
mine	Birch leaf,
Fragrance	Horsetail, and
Glyceryl stearate	Coltsfoot
Phenoxyethanol	
Sodium chloride	

FOR OILY HAIR ONLY SHAMPOO
(Gillette Co., Personal Care Div.)

Ammonium lauryl sulfate
Cocamidopropyl betaine
Propylene glycol
Fragrance
Methylparaben
Color
Extracts of Clover, Chamomile, Yarrow, Rosemary, Nettle, Birch leaf, Horsetail, and Coltsfoot

FORSYN THROID
Insecticide
(Forshaw)

(5-Benzyl-3-furyl)methyl 2,2-dimethyl-3-(2-methylpropenyl)cyclopropane carboxylate	1.500% w/w
Related compounds	0.204%
Aromatic petroleum hydrocarbons	1.986%
Aliphatic petroleum hydrocarbons *	86.250%

FORSYTHE SIGHTSAVING DUSTLESS CHALK
(American Crayon Co.)

This product bears the CP Seal issued by the Crayon, Water Color and Craft Institute, Inc. This seal certifies that the product contains no materials in sufficient quantities to be toxic or injurious to the human body even if ingested.

FORTISSIMO
Hospital grade detergent-germicide
(Puritan Chem. Co.)

Active ingredients:	50.0%
Potassium salt of para tertiary amylphenol *	
Isopropanol *	
Tetrasodium ethylene diamine tetraacetate	
Potassium salt of orthophenylphenol *	
Triethanolamine dodecyl benzene sulfonate	
Inert ingredients:	50.0%
Water	
Disodium 4-dodecyl-2,4' oxydibenzene sulfonate	
Disodium 2,2'-oxybis (4-dodecylbenzene sulfonate)	
Perfume	
Dye	

FORTRESS CREOSOTE WOOD PRESERVER
(Fortress Products Co.)

Coal tar neutral oil *	96.5% min.
Water and free carbon	3.5% max.

FORTRESS CREOSOTE WOOD PRESERVING SOLUTION
(Fortress Products Co.)

Coal tar neutral oil *	14.5%
Petroleum asphalt	35.0%
Petroleum oil *	50.0%
Inert ingredients:	0.5%
Water and free carbon	

FORTRESS PENTA CONCENTRATE
Wood preservative
(Fortress Products Co.)

Pentachlorophenol *	34.4%
Other chlorophenols & related compounds	4.0%
Aromatic petroleum hydrocarbons *	38.2%

FORTRESS PENTA WOOD PRESERVATIVE
(Fortress Products Co.)

Pentachlorophenol *	4.5%
Other chlorophenols and related compounds	0.5%
Petroleum hydrocarbons *	91.9%

FOSTER C.I. MASTIC
Asphaltic coating
(H.B. Fuller, Foster Div.)

Petroleum asphalt *
Petroleum hydrocarbon solvents *
Inorganic pigments *

FOSTER H.I. MASTIC
Coating for use over thermal insulation
(H.B. Fuller, Foster Div.)

Petroleum asphalt *
Colloidal clay
Inorganic pigments *
Water

FOSTEX (CREAM & CAKE)
Acne soapless skin cleansers
(Westwood Pharm.)

Sebulytic (surface active combination of soapless cleansers and wetting agents)
Micropulverized Sulfur	2%
Salicylic acid *	2%

'76 Ed.

FOSTRIL
Acne drying & peeling agent
(Westwood Pharm.)

Liposec (brand of polyoxyethylene lauryl ether)	6%
Micropulverized Sulfur	2%

Greaseless base:
Zinc oxide
Talc
Bentonite

'76 Ed.

FOTOCOL
Special industrial solvent
(IMC Chem.)

Denatured Ethyl alcohol *

FOTOTINT COLORS
Adds color to photographic films
(Edwal)

Acetic acid *
Various dyes

Starred ingredients (*) may be responsible for major toxic effects; consult Section II.

FOULEX
Hoof medication; veterinary
(Troy Chem.)

Pine oil
Cresylic acid *
Linseed oil
Iodine *
Crude oil
Camphor *
Turpentine distillates *

4-POWER
Fuel system cleaner
(Conklin Co.)

Methyl alcohol
Xylol *

FOURSALCO
Antirheumatic
(Jenkins Labs.)

Each tablet:
Salicylic acid *	1/2 gr.
Sodium bicarbonate	3 gr.
Magnesium salicylate *	2 gr.
Strontium salicylate *	2 gr.
Acetophenetidin	1/4 gr.
Methyl salicylate (syn.)	q.s.
Pancreatin	1/40 gr.
Diastase	1/40 gr.

4-WAY COLD TABLETS
(Bristol-Myers)

Each tablet:
Aspirin *	324 mg.
Phenylpropanolamine HCl	12 1/2 mg.
Chlorpheniramine maleate	2 mg.

4-WAY MENTHOLATED NASAL SPRAY
Decongestant, antihistaminic
(Bristol-Myers)

Phenylephrine hydrochloride *
Naphazoline hydrochloride
Pyrilamine maleate *
Buffered isotonic aqueous solution:
Menthol
Camphor
Thimerosal (preservative) 0.005%

4-WAY MOOVIT (Aerosol)
(Cling-Surface)

Kerosene *	13%
Mineral spirits *	50%
Propane/Isobutane	18%

4-WAY NASAL SPRAY
Decongestant, antihistaminic
(Bristol-Myers)

Phenylephrine hydrochloride *
Naphazoline hydrochloride
Pyrilamine maleate *
Buffered isotonic aqueous solution
Thimerosal (preservative) 0.005%

FOY-JOHNSTON PAINT PRODUCTS
Machinery paints

Foy-Johnston, Inc.
1776 Mentor Ave.
Cincinnati, Ohio 45212

Phone: 513-631-4270

See PAINTS, Section VI, General Formulations

FOY-JOHNSTON TRAFFIC PAINT-YELLOW (#9862 and #5062)
(Foy-Johnston)

Pigment:
Chrome yellow *		27.78%
Lead chromate	72.15%	
Silica	27.85%	
Titanium dioxide		7.40%
Aluminum silicate		18.52%
Magnesium silicate		46.30%

Vehicle:
Soya alkyd resin solids	37.10%
Mineral spirits *	10.60%
Naphtha *	48.06%
Suspending aid	2.12%
Dispersing aid	0.71%
Driers (Pb free) *	1.41%

FR-28
Fire retardant
(U.S. Borax)

Disodium octaborate tetrahydrate *

FRAGRANT SUPER
Hair spray
(Bonat)

	percentage range
SD Alcohol 40	55.0-70.0%
Methylene chloride *	9.0-15.0%
Isobutane	8.0-15.0%
Propane	6.0-12.0%
PVP	<5.0%
Fragrance	<1.0%

FRANCES DENNEY COSMETIC PRODUCTS

Frances Denney
437 Madison Ave.
New York, N.Y. 10022

Phone: 212-888-9500

See COSMETICS, Section VI, General Formulations

FRAN-KEM POWDER
Fresh fish and food preservative. Bacteriostat, fungistat, with antioxidant characteristics
(Washington Labs.)

Equal parts:
Fumaric acid
Sodium benzoate *

FRANKLIN BLUE SMEAR SCREWWORM KILLER
(Franklin Labs.)

Ronnel	5%
Xylene *	5%

FRANKLIN BRAND-EM-OL
Cold branding of cattle
(Franklin Labs.)

Barium sulphide (technical) *	14.4%
Sodium hydroxide (technical) *	14.4%
Turpentine	6.2%

FRANKLIN BRICON BACKRUBBER INSECTICIDE
(Franklin Labs.)

Ronnel	30%
Aromatic petroleum derivative solvent *	55%

FRANKLIN CREOFECTANT (Canada Only)
Stock dip; germicide and disinfectant
(Franklin Labs.)

Coal tar hydrocarbons *	64%
Soap	15%
Coal tar acids *	11%

FRANKLIN DAIRY & BEEF CATTLE SPRAY
Insecticide
(Franklin Labs.)

Ciodrin *	1.00%
Vapona	0.25%
Petroleum hydrocarbons *	98.55%

FRANKLIN DEHORNING PASTE
(Franklin Labs.)

Sodium hydroxide *	46.0% w/w
Calcium hydroxide	18.4% w/w

FRANKLIN DURSBAN 44
For control of lice and horn flies on beef breed cattle
(Franklin Labs.)

Chlorpyrifos *	43.2%
Petroleum distillates	56.8%

FRANKLIN FARM & RANCH BRAND ROACH & ANT KILLER
(Franklin Labs.)

Diazinon	0.500%
Pyrethrins	0.052%
Technical Piperonyl butoxide	0.261%
Petroleum distillates *	98.879%

FRANKLIN KILTECT-100 SPRAY

Screwworm killer and fly repellent for horses
(Franklin Labs.)

Petroleum distillate *	15.8%
Pine oil *	16.0%
Ronnel	5.0%
Butoxypolypropylene glycol	5.0%
Chloroform	5.0%
N-Octyl bicycloheptene dicarboximide	0.2%
Di-n-propyl isocinchomeronate	0.4%

FRANKLIN KILTECT-100 (Squirt Bottle)

Screwworm killer and fly repellent
(Franklin Labs.)

Pine oil *	16.0%
Petroleum distillates *	60.8%
Ronnel	5.0%
Butoxypolypropylene glycol	5.0%
Chloroform	5.0%
N-Octyl bicycloheptene dicarboximide	0.2%
Di-n-propyl isocinchomeronate	0.4%

FRANKLIN KILZOL DISINFECTANT

(Franklin Labs.)

Cresylic acid *	15.00%
Coconut fatty acid soap	8.90%
Isopropanol	8.00%
Sodium dodecylbenzene sulfonate	2.55%
4 & 6-Chloro-2-phenylphenol	2.00%
o-Benzyl-p-chlorophenol	1.50%
Tributyltin neodecanoate	0.25%
para-tertiary Amylphenol	0.10%
2,2-Methylenebis(3,4,6-trichlorophenol)	0.05%

FRANKLIN LIVESTOCK INSECTICIDE POWDER

(Franklin Labs.)

Methoxychlor (technical)	5%
Malathion *	4%

FRANKLIN LIVESTOCK INSECTICIDE SPRAY

(Franklin Labs.)

Pyrethrins	0.18%
Piperonyl butoxide (technical)	0.36%
N-Octyl bicycloheptene dicarboximide	0.60%
Di-n-propyl isocinchomeronate	1.20%
Petroleum distillate *	77.56%

FRANKLIN LOUSE-FLY KILLER

(Franklin Labs.)

Rabon	3%

FRANKLIN PROTEC WOUND DRESSING & FLY REPELLENT

(Franklin Labs.)

Pine tar oil *	41.0%
Pine oil *	23.5%
Butoxypolypropylene glycol	5.0%
Diphenylamine	5.0%
Castor oil	5.0%
Urea	5.0%
Benzyl alcohol	2.0%
o-Benzyl-p-chlorophenol	1.0%

FRANKLIN READY-TO-USE STOCK SPRAY

Insecticide
(Franklin Labs.)

2,2-Dichlorovinyl dimethyl phosphate (Vapona)	0.465%
Related compounds	0.035%
Piperonyl butoxide (technical)	0.250%
Pyrethrins	0.025%
Petroleum hydrocarbons *	99.125%
Petroleum distillate	0.100%

FRANKLIN SCREWWORM SPRAY WITH RONNEL

(Franklin Labs.)

Ronnel	2.5%
Xylene *	15.5%

FRANKLIN SPECIAL FARM & RANCH BRAND CRAWLING INSECT KILLER

(Franklin Labs.)

Baygon	0.95%
Related compounds	0.05%
DDVP	0.186%
Related compounds	0.014%
Petroleum distillates *	79.12%

FRANKLIN SPECIAL FARM & RANCH BRAND FLYING INSECT KILLER

(Franklin Labs.)

Resmethrin	0.080%
Related compounds	0.011%
d-trans Allethrin (allyl homolog of Cinerin I)	0.160%
Related compounds	0.012%
Piperonyl butoxide (technical)	0.800%
Aromatic petroleum solvent *	1.191%

FRANKLIN SPINOSE EAR-TICK TREATMENT WITH LINDANE

(Franklin Labs.)

Mineral oil	69.00%
Cottonseed oil	20.00%
Pine oil *	10.25%
Lindane	0.75%

FRANKLIN TOXAPHENE-LINDANE SPRAY MIX

Insecticide
(Franklin Labs.)

Toxaphene *	45%
Lindane	2%
Petroleum solvents	38%

FREART COLORED MOLDED CHALK

(American Crayon Co.)

This product bears the CP Seal issued by the Crayon, Water Color and Craft Institute, Inc. This seal certifies that the product contains no materials in sufficient quantities to be toxic or injurious to the human body even if ingested.

FREEMAN COSMETICS

Freeman Cosmetic Corp.
P.O. Box 17
Hollywood, Calif. 90028

Phone: 213-461-2901

See COSMETICS, Section VI, General Formulations

FREE N' SOFT

Dryer antistat and fabric softener
(Economics)

Blend of Quaternary ammonium salts *

FREERS ELM ARRESTER

Dutch elm disease
(Freers Co.)

Mercuric chloride *	0.12%
Methyl alcohol *	95.65%

FREEZONE

For removal of corns and calluses
(Whitehall Labs.)

Each fl. oz.:

Ether	300 min.
Zinc chloride *	8.75 gr.
Alcohol	20%
Salicylic acid *	
Castor oil	

FRESH CREAM DEODORANT

Deodorant, antiperspirant
(Pharmacraft)

Aluminum chloride Chlorhydrol	7.2% w/w

FRESHETTES

Odor block
(Holcomb)

Paradichlorobenzene *	>10%

'76 Ed.

FRESH ROLL-ON DEODORANT
Deodorant, antiperspirant
(Pharmacraft)

Chlorhydrol (50% sol.) ...... 40.0% w/w
Aluminum chloride
Alcohol .... 13.8 v/v

FRISKY
Disinfectant cleanser paste; hospital grade
(Puritan Chem. Co.)

Active ingredients: 6.41%
  Soap
  Trisodium phosphate *
  3,5,4′ Tribromosalicylanilide *
  5,4′ Dibromosalicylanilide *
Inert ingredients: 93.59%
  Feldspar
  Water
  Perfume and dye

FROST-GUARD
Cold weather skin cream
(Reynes Products, Inc.)

Purified water
TEA stearate
Propylene glycol
Cocoa butter
Dimethicone
Acetylated lanolin
Magnesium stearate
Glyceryl stearate
Mineral oil
Lanolin alcohol
PVP
Methylparaben
Propylparaben

FROST OFF SPRAY DE-ICER
Industrial and institutional use
(Scientific International)

Isopropanol *

FRUIT OF THE LOOM HEAVY DUTY LIQUID LAUNDRY DETERGENT
(Climaco)

Alcohol
Optical brightener
Nonionic surfactant
Anionic surfactant *
Dye
Fragrance
Silicone

FRUITONE A
For control of harvest drop of apples
(Amchem)

2,4,5-Trichlorophenoxy acetic acid *

FRUITONE-N
To control preharvest drop of apples and pears, also used for thinning apples
(Amchem)

Sodium 1-naphthalene acetate 3.5%

FRUITTI-VI-RON
Chewable multiple vitamins plus iron
(Columbia Med.)

Iron * .... 10 mg.
Plus multivitamins

FS AMINE 400 WEED KILLER
(FS Services)

Dimethylamine salts of 2,4-dichloro-
  phenoxyacetic acid * 49%
'76 Ed.

FS 2.0% CIODRIN INSECTICIDE ANIMAL SPRAY SOLUTION
(FS Services)

Dimethyl phosphate of alpha-
  methylbenzyl 3-hydroxy-cis-
  crotonate * 2.00%
Petroleum hydrocarbons 97.64%
'76 Ed.

FS EMULSIFIABLE OIL
Supplemental herbicide carrier
(FS Services)

Refined Petroleum distillate * ... 98.0%
Emulsifier 2.0%
'76 Ed.

FS ESTER 400 WEED KILLER
(FS Services)

Butyl ester of 2,4-dichlorophenoxy-
  acetic acid * 56.5%
'76 Ed.

"FS" FOOD PROCESSOR'S INSECTICIDE
(Weil Chem.)

Refined Mineral oil * 97.57%
Technical Piperonyl butoxide 1.275%
Pyrethrins 0.255%
N-Octyl bicycloheptene
  dicarboximide 0.50%
Allethrin (Allyl homolog of Ci-
  nerin I) 0.20%
Methyl salicylate 0.20%

FS LV 400 WEED KILLER
(FS Services)

Isooctyl ester of 2,4-dichlorophenox-
  yacetic acid * 69%
'76 Ed.

FS SULPHURIZED OIL
For sarcoptic and psoroptic mange on livestock
(FS Services)

Mineral oil * 99.28%
Carbon disulphide 0.52%
Sulphur 0.20%
'76 Ed.

FST-7
Tobacco sucker control
(Fairmount Chem. Co.)

Combination of Fair-Tac and Fair Plus:
  n-Decanol * 38.3%
  Potassium salt of 1,2-Dihydro-
  3,6-pyridazinedione (Maleic
  hydrazide) * 11.1%

FS VAPONA LIVESTOCK SPRAY
For control of flies
(FS Services)

2,2-Dichlorovinyl dimethyl
  phosphate 0.93%
Related compounds 0.07%
Petroleum distillate * 99.00%
'76 Ed.

FUEL TRON
Fuel oil conditioner
(Radiator)

Petroleum distillates *
Tar oil *
'76 Ed.

FULEX A-D-O
Fungicide
(Fuller System)

Hydroxyquinoline sulfate * 25%
'76 Ed.

FULEX APHID SMOKE FUMIGATOR
(Fuller System)

Gamma isomer of benzene
  hexachloride * 5.6%
'76 Ed.

FULEX DDVP FUMIGATOR
(Fuller System)

2,2-Dichlorovinyl dimethyl phosphate (DDVP) * 11.0%
Related compounds 0.8%
'76 Ed.

Starred ingredients (*) may be responsible for major toxic effects; consult Section II.

FULEX-G
Insecticide
(Fuller System)

Mono-, di-, and trichloronaphthalenes *
Gamma isomer of BHC *
Other isomers of BHC

'76 Ed.

FULEX NO. 400 LIQUID
Insecticide
(Fuller System)

Dichloronaphthalene *
Monochloronaphthalene *
Trichlorobenzene *
Naphthalene *
Trichloronaphthalene *

'76 Ed.

FULEX NICOTINE FUMIGATOR
(Fuller System)

Nicotine alkaloid * 14%

'76 Ed.

FULEX PARATHION INSECTICIDAL SMOKE
(Fuller System)

Tech. Parathion (O,O-Diethyl O-p-
nitrophenylthiophosphate) * 9%

'76 Ed.

FULEX SOIL TREATMENT
Fungicide
(Fuller System)

Monchloro-, dichloro- and trichloronaphthalene (all chlorophenols) *   40%
Hydroxyquinoline sulfate 17%
Gamma isomer of benzene
hexachloride * 2.6%
Other isomers of benzene
hexachloride 0.4%

'76 Ed.

FULEX SPIDER-MITE INSECTICIDAL SMOKE
(Fuller System)

2-(p-tert-Butylphenoxy)isopropyl 2-
chloroethyl sulfite 6.7%

'76 Ed.

FULEX TEDION INSECTICIDAL SMOKE
(Fuller System)

Tetradifon (2,4,5,4'-Tetrachlorodi-
phenyl sulphone) 15%

'76 Ed.

FULEX THIODAN INSECTICIDAL SMOKE
(Fuller System)

Endosulfan (Hexachlorohexahydro-
methano-2,4,3-benzodioxathiepin
oxide) * 15%

'76 Ed.

FULLER BRUSH PRODUCTS

The Fuller Brush Co.
2800 Rockcreek Pkwy.
North Kansas City, Mo. 64117

Phone: 816-474-1754

FULLER-O'BRIEN PAINTS

Fuller-O'Brien Div.
The O'Brien Corp.
450 E. Grand Ave.
South San Francisco, Calif. 94080

Phone: 415-761-2300

See PAINTS, Section VI, General Formulations

FUL-SHINE CLEANER
(Fuld-Stalfort)

Potassium soap

'76 Ed.

pH 8.5-8.8

FULVICIN P/G TABLETS
Antifungal antibiotic
(Schering)

Each tablet:
Griseofulvin (ultra
microsize) .... 125 mg.; 250 mg.

FULVICIN U/F TABLETS
Antifungal antibiotic
(Schering)

Each tablet:
Griseofulvin
(microsize) .... 250 mg.; 500 mg.

FUL-VUE WINDSHIELD WASHER ANTI-FREEZE
(Patterson Labs.)

Methanol * 42%

FUMARIN-22
Rodenticide
(Amchem)

3-(alpha-Acetonylfurfuryl)-4-
hydroxycoumarin 0.5%

FUMASOL-A
Rodenticide
(Amchem)

Sodium salt of 3-(alpha-acetonylfurfuryl)-4-hydroxycoumarin 0.5%

FUMATRIN-FORTE
Hematinic-vitamins
(Reid-Provident)

Each tablet:
Ferrous fumarate (equiv. to 100
mg. elemental iron) * ...... 300 mg.
Vitamin B-12 .... 12 mcg.
Ascorbic acid .... 100 mg.
Thiamine mononitrate .... 3 mg.
Desiccated liver .... 100 mg.

FUMAZONE 70E SOIL FUMIGANT
(Dow)

1,2-Dibromo-3-chloropropane & related halogenated C3
aliphatics * 70.6%
Inert ingred.: 29.4%
Petroleum solvent 21.4%

FUMAZONE 86E SOIL FUMIGANT
(Dow)

1,2-Dibromo-3-chloropropane & re-
lated halogenated C3
aliphatics * 84.0%
Inert ingred.: 16.0%
Petroleum solvent 9.0%
Emulsifiers

FUMAZONE 86 FUMIGANT
(Dow)

1,2-Dibromo-3-chloropropane & related halogenated C3
aliphatics * 85.5%
Petroleum solvent 14.5%

FUMEX
Anti-smoking lozenges
(CMC Research Div.)

Silver acetate * .... 6 mg.
Cocarboxylase (Thiamine
pyrophosphate) .... 0.025 mg.
Ammonium chloride .... 25 mg.

FUMI-TROL, SPRAY-TROL BRAND

See SPRAY-TROL BRAND FUMI-
TROL

FUMO-GAS
Fumigant
(Amer. Fumig.)

Ethylene dichloride
Carbon tetrachloride *
Ethylene dibromide *

'76 Ed.

Starred ingredients (*) may be responsible for major toxic effects; consult Section II.

FUMOL-8
Roach repellent concentrate
(Fumol Corp.)

Active ingredients: 90%
  Petroleum distillate *
  N-Octyl bicycloheptene
    dicarboximide *
  2-Hydroxyethyl N-octyl sulfide
Inert ingredients: 10%
  Octyl phenoxy polyethoxy ethanol

'76 Ed.

FUMOL 56
Insect spray
(Fumol Corp.)

Petroleum distillate *
Pyrethrins *
Butyl carbityl propyl piperonyl ether and
  related compounds
N-Octyl bicycloheptene
  dicarboximide *

'76 Ed.

FUMOL "ONE SHOT"
(Aerosol)
Insecticide - industrial
(Fumol Corp.)

Pyrethrins 0.50%
Piperonyl butoxide, technical ... 1.00%
N-Octyl bicycloheptene
  dicarboximide 1.66%
Petroleum distillate * 11.84%

'76 Ed.

FUMOL P-D CONCENTRATE
Insecticide
(Fumol Corp.)

Deodorized Petroleum distillate *   73.8%
O,O-Diethyl O-(2-isopropyl-4-
  methyl-6-pyrimidinyl)
  phosphorothioate * 10.0%
N-Octyl bicycloheptene
  dicarboximide 3.0%
Piperonyl butoxide 1.2%
2-Hydroxyethyl N-octyl sulfide .. 1.0%
Pyrethrins 1.0%
Inert ingredients: 10%
  Octyl phenoxy polyethoxy ethanol

'76 Ed.

FUM-O-MOR INCUBATOR
FUMIGANT
(Hilltop)

Furfuraldehyde * 50%
Formaldehyde * 18.50%
Methyl alcohol 5%

'76 Ed.

FUMO-SPRAY
Fumigant
(Amer. Fumig.)

Refined Hydrocarbons *†
Pyrethrins *
Piperonyl butoxide

'76 Ed.

†*See* Petroleum hydrocarbons

FUNDAL 4EC
Insecticide, ovicide
(NOR-AM)

Chlordimeform * 48.5%/w
Aromatic petroleum distillates * 43.4%/w

FUNDAL S.P.
Insecticide, ovicide
(NCR-AM)

Chlordimeform hydrochloride * ... 97%

FUNGICIN
For fungus infection of external ear
(Pharmex)

Boric acid *
Salicylic acid *
Sodium ethyl mercuri thiosalicylate *
Alcohol 70%

FUNGIDEX CREME
*Fungicide, bactericide, antipruritic;
  veterinary*
(Norden Labs.)

Zinc undecylenate * 12%
Undecylenic acid 5%
Copper undecylenate *† 3%

†*See* Copper and Undecylenic acid

FUNGI-REX
Greaseless fungicide; medical
(Rexall)

Benzoic acid * .... >10%
Salicylic acid * 1-10%
Phenol .... <1%
Thymol * 1-10%

'76 Ed.

FUNGI-REX LIQUID
(Rexall)

Alcohol 40%
Thymol * 1-5%
Salicylic acid * 1-5%
Benzoic acid 1-10%
Glycerin 1-10%

'76 Ed.

FUNGISOL

See MAUGET FUNGISOL

FUNGO 50
(Mallinckrodt, Inc.)

Dimethyl-4,4-O-phenylenebis (3-
  thioallophanate) * 50%

FUNGOID CREME
*Topical treatment for fungus, yeast and
  bacterial infections of the skin*
(Pedinol)

Cetyl pyridinium chloride*
Triacetin
Chloroxylenol
Vanishing creme base

FUNGOID SOLUTION
*Topical treatment for fungus,
  yeast and bacterial infections
  of the skin*
(Pedinol)

Cetyl pyridinium chloride*
Triacetin
Chloroxylenol
Benzalkonium chloride
Nonaqueous vehicle

FUNGOID TINCTURE
*A topical solution for treatment
  of nail fungus, onychomycosis*
(Pedinol)

Cetyl pyridinium chloride*
Triacetin
Chloroxylenol
Glacial Acetic acid
Sodium propionate
Isopropyl alcohol
Acetone

FURACIN DRESSING
VETERINARY
Topical antibacterial agent
(Norden Labs.)

Furacin (brand of Nitrofurazone) .. 0.2%
Water-soluble base

FURACIN SOLUBLE
DRESSING
Topical antibacterial agent
(Norwich-Eaton)

Furacin (brand of nitrofurazone) .. 0.2%
Solubase (Mixture of Polyethylene glycols)

FURACIN SOLUBLE
POWDER
Topical antibacterial agent
(Norwich-Eaton)

Furacin (brand of nitrofurazone) .. 0.2%
Polyethylene glycol 6000

FURACIN SOLUBLE
POWDER VETERINARY
Topical antibacterial agent
(Norden Labs.)

Furacin (brand of Nitrofurazone) .. 0.2%
Water-soluble base

Starred ingredients (*) may be responsible for major toxic effects; consult Section II.

FURACIN TOPICAL CREAM
Topical antibacterial agent
(Norwich-Eaton)

Furacin (brand of nitrofurazone) .. 0.2%
Glycerin
Cetyl alcohol
Mineral oil
Promulgen G
Methylparaben
Propylparaben

FURACIN WATER MIX VETERINARY
Intestinal antibacterial, anticoccidial agent
(Norden Labs.)

Furacin (brand of Nitrofurazone) . 4.59%
Water-soluble stabilizing base

FURADAN
Insecticide, acaricide, nematicide
(Mobay Chemical Corp.)

Carbofuran (2,3-Dihydro-2,2-dimethyl-7-benzofuranol methylcarbamate) *

FURADAN 10 GRANULES

See NIAGARA FURADAN 10 GRANULES

FURADANTIN ORAL SUSPENSION
Urinary tract antibacterial
(Norwich-Eaton)

Furadantin (brand of
nitrofurantoin) * .... 5 mg./ml.

FURADANTIN TABLETS
Urinary tract antibacterial
(Norwich-Eaton)

Each tablet:
Furadantin (brand of
nitrofurantoin) * ... 50 mg.; 100 mg.

FURLOE CHLORO IPC 4EC
Herbicide
(PPG Industries, Chem. Div.)

Isopropyl m-chlorocarbanilate 48%
Xylene * 47%
Emulsifier 5%

FURLOE CHLORO IPC 10G
Herbicide
(PPG Industries, Chem. Div.)

Isopropyl m-chlorocarbanilate * ... 10%
Clay 90%

FURLOE CHLORO IPC 20G
Herbicide
(PPG Industries, Chem. Div.)

Isopropyl m-chlorocarbanilate * ... 20%
Clay 80%

FUROL CREAM
For dandruff scales
(Torch)

Salicylic acid * 3%
Sulfur precipitated 5%

'76 Ed.

FUROX AEROSOL POWDER

See PURINA FUROX AEROSOL POWDER

FUROXONE LIQUID
Intestinal antibacterial agent
(Norwich-Eaton)

Each 15 ml.:
Furoxone (brand of
furazolidone) * .... 50 mg.

FUROXONE SUSPENSION VETERINARY
Intestinal antibacterial agent
(Norden Labs.)

Each 1 ml. dose:
Furoxone (brand of
Furazolidone) * .... 100 mg.

FUROXONE TABLETS
Intestinal antibacterial agent
(Norwich-Eaton)

Furoxone (brand of
furazolidone) * .... 100 mg.

FUTRON 25
Disinfectant, detergent, defilmer, deodorant; hospitals, institutions and industry
(Hysan Corp.)

Tetrasodium salt of ethylene diamine tetraacetic acid 2.2%
N-Alkyl (60% C14, 30% C16, 5% C12, 5% C18) dimethyl benzyl ammonium chloride * 1.5%
N-Alkyl (50% C12, 30% C14, 17% C16, 3% C18) dimethyl ethylbenzyl ammonium chloride * 1.5%
Inert ingred: 94.8%
Detergents *
Wetting, penetrating, water softening, peptizing and emulsifying agents

FYNE-PYNE
Disinfectant, cleaner, deodorizer, degreaser
(Cole, H.A.)

Pine oil * 32.0%
Isopropyl alcohol 9.2%
Soap 11.3%
Inert ingredients (including
coloring) 47.5%

FYRE-FREEZ
Fire extinguisher
(Kidde)

Carbon dioxide in liquefied and gaseous form

FYR-FYTER DRY CHEMICAL RECHARGE
For fire extinguishers
(Norris Industries)

Sodium bicarbonate
Diatomaceous earth
Polysiloxane coating

'76 Ed.

FYR-FYTER KARBALOY LOADED STREAM RECHARGE
For fire extinguishers
(Norris Industries)

Potassium carbonate
Sodium dichromate *
Ethylene glycol

'76 Ed.

FYR-FYTER MULTI-PURPOSE DRY CHEMICAL RECHARGE
For fire extinguishers
(Norris Industries)

Monoammonium phosphate
Diatomaceous earth
Tricalcium phosphate
Polysiloxane coating

'76 Ed.

FYR-FYTER PURPLE K DRY CHEMICAL RECHARGE
For fire extinguishers
(Norris Industries)

Potassium bicarbonate
Diatomaceous earth
Tricalcium phosphate
Polysiloxane coating

'76 Ed.

FYR-FYTER SUPER-KEM DRY CHEMICAL RECHARGE
For fire extinguishers
(Norris Industries)

Potassium chloride
Diatomaceous earth
Tricalcium phosphate
Polysiloxane coating

'76 Ed.

Starred ingredients (*) may be responsible for major toxic effects; consult Section II.

FYTE 60
Solid atmosphere odor control; institutional and commercial use
(Hysan Corp.)

Paradichlorobenzene *	97.15%
Paradiisobutylcresoxyethoxyethyl dimethyl benzyl ammonium chloride	0.25%
Lauryl methacrylate	0.25%
Paraformaldehyde	0.25%
Essential oils	1.00%
Inert ingredients:	1.10%
Nonyl phenoxy polyoxyethylene ethanol	
Synthetic calcium silicate	
Water	

FYTE TB-13
Liquid highly concentrated hospital disinfectant
(Hysan Corp.)

Active ingredients:	38.71%
Isopropyl alcohol *	
Sodium dodecyl benzene sulfonate *	
Ortho benzyl para chlorophenol *	
Ortho phenyl phenol *	
Tetra sodium ethylene diamine tetraacetate	
Para tertiary Amyl phenol *	
Inert ingredients:	61.29%
Water	
Propylene glycol	
Potassium sulphite	
Citrous perfume	

G

GABY GREASELESS SUNTAN LOTION
(Gaby, Inc.)

Gaby, Inc.
1326 Frankford Ave.
Philadelphia, Pa. 19125

Phone: 215-739-7300

See COSMETICS, Section VI, General Formulations

G-63 AEROSOL BURN RELIEF
(Gaby, Inc.)

Gaby, Inc.
1326 Frankford Ave.
Philadelphia, Pa. 19125

Phone: 215-739-7300

GAF PRODUCTS

GAF Corp.
140 W. 51st St.
New York, N.Y. 10020

Phone: 212-621-5000

GAIN (Formula 1)
Granular laundry detergent
(Procter & Gamble)

Sodium sulfate	25-49%
Complex sodium phosphates	10-24%
Sodium silicate	5-9%
Water	5-9%
Sodium alkyl sulfate	5-9%
Sodium alkyl ethoxylate sulfate	5-9%
Sodium alkyl benzene sulfonate	1-4%
Minor ingredients, each	trace

pH (1% solution) - 10.9 max.

GAIN (Formula 2)
Granular laundry detergent
(Procter & Gamble)

Sodium sulfate	25-49%
Sodium carbonate	10-24%
Sodium silicate	10-24%
Sodium alkyl benzene sulfonate	5-9%
Sodium alkyl sulfate	5-9%
Sodium alkyl ethoxylate sulfate	5-9%
Water	1-4%
Minor ingredients, each	trace

pH (1% solution) - 10.9 max.

GAIN (Formula 3)
Granular laundry detergent
(Procter & Gamble)

Sodium sulfate	25-49%
Sodium aluminosilicate	10-24%
Sodium nitrilotriacetate	10-24%
Sodium carbonate	10-24%
Water	5-9%
Sodium alkyl ethoxylate sulfate	5-9%
Sodium alkyl sulfate	5-9%
Sodium silicate	1-4%
Sodium alkyl benzene sulfonate	1-4%
Minor ingredients, each	trace

pH (1% solution) - 10.8 max.

GALAHAD
Detergent-germicide; hospital grade
(Puritan Chem. Co.)

Active ingredients:	39.5%
Isopropanol *	
Para tertiary Amyl phenol *	
Orthophenylphenol *	
Triethanolamine dodecyl benzene sulfonate	
Tetrasodium ethylene diamine tetraacetate	
Inert ingredients:	60.5%
Water	
Disodium 4-dodecyl-2,4'-oxydibenzene sulfonate	
Disodium 2,2'-oxybis (4-dodecylbenzene sulfonate)	
Perfume	
Dye	

GALECRON 4E
Insecticide-ovicide
(Ciba-Geigy Ag. Div.)

Chlordimeform *	48.5%
Aromatic petroleum derivative solvent *	43.4%

GALE LIQUID DAIRY CLEANER
(Paulen Chem.)

Non-ionic detergent and emulsifier (Alkyl phenoxy polyoxyethylene ethanol types) *	>40%
Alcohol	<5%
Organic sequestering agent	<1%

'76 Ed.

GALLEY OVEN-GRILL CLEANER
(Nat'l Labs. Div.)

Potassium hydroxide *	minor
Ethylene glycol monobutyl ether (Butyl Cellosolve)	minor

GALLOTOX CAPTAN FP-700R
Fungicide
(Guard Chem. Co.)

Captan	70%/w

GALLOTOX CAPTAN-METHOXYCHLOR 75-3
Seed treatment
(Guard Chem. Co.)

Captan	75%/w
Methoxychlor (technical)	3%/w

GALOPECTIN TABS.
Antidiarrheal
(Wesley Pharm.)

Each tablet:	
Colloidal Kaolin	5 gr.
Powdered Pectin	1/4 gr.
Mixed Belladonna alkaloids:	1/1000 gr.
Hyoscyamine sulfate	
Atropine sulfate	
Hyoscine hydrobromide	
Bismuth subgallate	1 gr.

GALVA-SHEEN 4899 WHITE PRIME OR FINISH
(Hanna Chemical Coatings Corp.)

Pigment:	42.0%
Titanium dioxide	27.5%
Zinc oxide	8.6%
Calcium carbonate	29.7%
Magnesium silicate	34.2%
Vehicle:	58.0%
Soya modified alkyd	41.4%
Mineral spirits *	58.6%

GAMMA-CIDE RESIDUAL INSECTICIDE
(Weil Chem.)

Pyrethrins	0.050%
Piperonyl butoxide, tech.	0.260%
O,O-Diethyl O-(2-isopropyl-4-methyl-6-pyrimidinyl)phosphorothioate (Diazinon)	0.500%
Aromatic petroleum distillate *	97.190%

Starred ingredients (*) may be responsible for major toxic effects; consult Section II.

GAMMA Rx
Dip or spray for dogs
(Carson Chemicals, Inc.)

Gamma isomer of benzene hexachloride (from lindane) *	8.82%
Methylated naphthalene *	72.00%

GAMOPHEN BRAND HAND CLEANSING LEAVES
(Arbrook)

Hexachlorophene	2%
Sodium carboxymethyl cellulose	
Sodium lauryl sulfate *	
Glycerin	
Methylcellulose	

GANATREX ELIXIR
Dietary supplement
(Merrell Dow)

Each 45 ml.:
Vitamin A	5000 U.S.P. Units
Vitamin D	400 U.S.P. Units
Multivitamins	
Alcohol	15%

GANTANOL (SUSPENSION & TABLETS)
Antibacterial agent for urinary tract infections
(Roche)

Each 5 ml. or tablet:
Sulfamethoxazole *	0.5 gm.

GANTANOL DS TABLETS
Antibacterial
(Roche)

Each double-strength tablet:
Sulfamethoxazole *	1 gm.

GANTRISIN
Antibacterial agent for urinary tract infections
(Roche)

Each tablet:
Sulfisoxazole	0.5 gm.

Pediatric suspension or syrup (each 5 ml. the equivalent of:
Sulfisoxazole in the form of acetyl sulfisoxazole	0.5 gm.

GANTRISIN OPHTHALMIC OINTMENT
Topical antibacterial sulfonamide for eye infections
(Roche)

Sulfisoxazole diolamine	4%
White petrolatum	
Mineral oil	
Phenylmercuric nitrate as preservative	1:50,000

GANTRISIN OPHTHALMIC SOLUTION
Topical antibacterial sulfonamide for eye infections
(Roche)

Each ml.:
Sulfisoxazole diolamine	40 mg.
Phenylmercuric nitrate as preservative	1:100,000

GARAMYCIN CREAM 0.1%
Primary and secondary bacterial infections of the skin
(Schering)

Each gram:
Gentamicin sulfate (equiv. to 1.0 mg. gentamicin base)	1.7 mg.
Methylparaben	1.0 mg.
Butylparaben	4.0 mg.
Base:	
Stearic acid	
Propylene glycol monostearate	
Isopropyl myristate	
Propylene glycol	
Polysorbate 40	
Sorbitol solution	
Purified water	

GARAMYCIN OINTMENT 0.1%
Primary and secondary bacterial infections of the skin
(Schering)

Each gram:
Gentamicin sulfate (equiv. to 1.0 mg. gentamicin base)	1.7 mg.
Methylparaben	0.5 mg.
Propylparaben	0.1 mg.
Petrolatum base	

GARB-O-FLAKES
Diaper and garbage pail deodorant
(Surco Products, Inc.)

Paradichlorobenzene	10%
Perfume	30%
Orthodichlorobenzene *	60%

'76 Ed.

GARDALAX TABLETS
Laxative
(DePree)

Dioctyl sodium sulfosuccinate *
Yellow phenolphthalein

GARD ANTI-RUST
Anti-rust spray
(Gard)

Paraffin oil	13.0%
Chlorinated solvents *	30.5%
Naphtha *	14.0%
Silicone perfume	1.5%
Propellant (Isobutane)	40.0%

'76 Ed.

GARDENADE GRANULES, GOOD-LIFE

See GOOD-LIFE GARDENADE GRANULES

GARDEN BOUQUET SOAP
Toilet soap
(Purex Corp.)

Sodium tallow-coconut oil soap	>80%
Glycerine	<3%
Titanium dioxide	<1%
Sodium chloride	<1%
Emollient	<1%
Coloring agent	<1%
Perfume	<1%
Water	balance

GARDEN-LIFE SOLUBLE PLANT FOOD

See SCIENCE GARDEN-LIFE SOLUBLE PLANT FOOD

GARD FLORA-TINT
Floral paint
(Gard)

Nitrocellulose	8.0%
Plasticizer	2.0%
Ketone solvents *	40.0%
Alcohols	10.0%
Esters	9.0%
Dyes	1.0%
Isobutane propellants	30.0%

'76 Ed.

GARD GLITTER GLUE
(Gard)

Acrylic resin	15.0%
Plasticizer	1.0%
Aliphatic solvents *	54.0%
Propellant	30.0%

'76 Ed.

GARD HAND CLEANER
(Gard)

Combined amount:	68.5%
Aromatic solvent *	
Aliphatic solvent *	
Lanolin ester	1.0%
Perfume	0.5%
Freon "12"	30.0%

'76 Ed.

GARD MR. COLOR (DECORATOR)
Decorative paints
(Gard)

Nitrocellulose	8.0%
Plasticizers	3.0%
Alcohols	10.0%
Ketones *	30.0%
Esters	9.0%
Pigments	10.0%
Isobutane	30.0%

'76 Ed.

GARD MR. COLOR (DESIGNER FORMULA)
Decorative paints
(Gard)

Nitrocellulose	8.0%
Plasticizers	2.0%
Alcohols	10.0%
Ketones *	35.0%
Esters	5.0%
Pigments	10.0%
Isobutane	30.0%

'76 Ed.

GARDONA
Insecticide
(Shell Chem.)

2-Chloro-1-(2,4,5-trichlorophenyl)vinyldimethyl phosphate *

GARD RE-LEASE
Mold release
(Gard)

Silicones	8.0%
Freon propellants	92.0%

'76 Ed.

GARD SPRA-TONE
Floral Paint
(Gard)

Nitrocellulose	9.0%
Plasticizer	2.0%
Ketones *	40.0%
Alcohols	10.0%
Esters	8.0%
Pigments	2.0%
Propellants:	
Freon	15.0%
Isobutane	15.0%

'76 Ed.

GARD SPRAZE
Paint
(Gard)

Nitrocellulose	10.0%
Plasticizers	2.0%
Alcohols	8.0%
Ketones *	40.0%
Esters	5.0%
Pigments	5.0%
Freon "12"	15.0%
Isobutane	15.0%

'76 Ed.

GARD STYRO-WELD
Styrofoam weld
(Gard)

Chlorinated solvent *	55.0%
Combined amount:	45.0%
Freon propellant	
Propane-isobutane	

'76 Ed.

GARD WEATHERPROOF SPRAY
Weatherproofing
(Gard)

Silicones	5.0%
Microcrystalline waxes	2.0%
Resin	2.0%
Chlorinated solvents *	40.0%
Aliphatic solvents	6.0%
Freon & isobutane propellants	45.0%

'76 Ed.

GARFIELD HEADACHE POWDERS
(Lambda Inc.)

Each powder:
Acetaminophen *	5 gr.
Caffeine	

GARFIELD TEA
Natural laxative
(Lambda Inc.)

Senna *
Dandelion
Doggrass

GARFLOR CLEANER
Garage floor cleaner
(National-Purity Soap)

Nonionic surfactant *

pH of 1% solution 12-12.5

GARRY'S CHROME CLEANER
(Garry Labs.)

Wax
Silicone
Diatomaceous earth
Mineral spirits *
Water

GARRY'S CREAM WAX
(Garry Labs.)

Wax
Silicone
Diatomaceous earth
Mineral spirits *
Water

GARRY'S STOP LEAK
Automotive
(Garry Labs.)

Polyethylene glycol
Water

GARRY'S SUPER-WAX
Automotive
(Garry Labs.)

Silicone
Mineral spirits *
Wax
Water

GARRY'S SUPREME
Automotive
(Garry Labs.)

Isopropyl alcohol *
Butyl Cellosolve *
Top cylinder lubricant

GARRY'S UPHOLSTERY CLEANER
(Garry Labs.)

Mixture of Alkaline phosphates

GARRY'S VINYL TOP CLEANER
Automotive
(Garry Labs.)

Silicone
Mineral spirits *
Surfactants
Water

GARRY'S WAX COAT
(Garry Labs.)

Wax
Silicone
Diatomaceous earth
Mineral spirits *
Water

GARTSIDE'S IRON RUST SOAP
(Gartside's)

Oxalic acid *	7%

'76 Ed.

GAS MISER (AS-222P, Formula 2181-52)

See PRESTONE GAS MISER (AS-222P, Formula 2181-52)

GAS-O-CIDE

See MIDLAND GAS-O-CIDE

GATOR ROACH HIVES
Insecticide
(DeSoto Chem.)

Lead arsenate *	16.20%
Total arsenic (as metallic)	3.50%
Water soluble arsenic (as metallic)	0.10%

GAVIOTA LAWN KLEEN
Liquid herbicide
(Brewer Chem.)

Monosodium acid methanearsonate *	2.94%
2-Methoxy-3,6-dichlorobenzoic acid	0.20%
Complex Surfactant - Anionic/Nonionic	<5.00%
Water	>80.00%

GAYPET FLEA, TICK KILLER FOR DOGS & CATS
(Franklin Labs.)

Carbaryl	0.500%
Pyrethrins	0.050%
Piperonyl butoxide (technical)	0.100%
N-Octyl bicycloheptene dicarboximide	0.166%

GAYPET FLEA-TICK POWDER FOR DOGS & CATS
(Franklin Labs.)

Carbaryl *	5%

GAYPET MANGE TREATMENT
(Franklin Labs.)

Benzyl benzoate *	30%

GAYPET PET SHAMPOO
(Franklin Labs.)

Pyrethrins	0.045%
Piperonyl butoxide (technical)	0.090%
N-Octyl bicycloheptene dicarboximide	0.150%
Cedar oil	
Artificial color	

GAYSAL
Antiarthritic
(Geriatric Pharm.)

Each tablet:
Sodium salicylate *	300 mg.
Acetaminophen *	180 mg.
Aluminum hydroxide gel	60 mg.
Butabarbital *	8 mg.
Phenobarbital	4 mg.

GAYSAL-S
Antiarthritic
(Geriatric Pharm.)

Each tablet:
Sodium salicylate *	300 mg.
Acetaminophen *	180 mg.
Aluminum hydroxide gel	60 mg.

GAY VELVET LATEX WALL PAINT
(Akron Paint & Varnish Co.)

Titanium pigment
Latex

GAZE
Liquid machine dishwashing detergent
(Puritan Chem. Co.)

Strong Alkaline components *

GCC-165 WEED KILLER
Industrial use
(Hysan Corp.)

Petroleum oil *	96.10%
2,4-Dichlorophenoxyacetic acid, isooctyl ester	1.09%
Bromacil (5-Bromo-3-sec-butyl-6-methyluracil)	0.61%
Pentachlorophenol	0.80%
Other chlorophenols	0.09%

GCC-425
Brush and broadleaf weed killer
(Hysan Corp.)

Isooctyl ester of 2,4-dichlorophenoxyacetic acid *	26.5%
Isooctyl ester of 2,4,5-trichlorophenoxyacetic acid	6.5%
Isooctyl ester of 2-(2,4,5-trichlorophenoxy)propionic acid	6.3%

GCC-429
Brush and broadleaf weed killer
(Hysan Corp.)

Isooctyl ester of 2,4-dichlorophenoxyacetic acid *	50.32%
Isooctyl ester of 2,4,5-trichlorophenoxyacetic acid	10.32%
Isooctyl ester of 2-(2,4,5-trichlorophenoxy)propionic acid	10.84%

GCC-535
Broadleaf weed killer
(Hysan Corp.)

Dimethylamine salt of 2-(2-methyl-4-chlorophenoxy)propionic acid	4.05%
Dimethylamine salt of 2,4-dichlorophenoxyacetic acid	4.02%

GCC-711
Herbicide
(Hysan Corp.)

Diquat dibromide (6,7-Dihydropyrido(1,2-a:2:1'-C)-pyrazidiinium dibromide) *	1.85%

GCC-712
Non-selective herbicide for broadleaf weeds
(Hysan Corp.)

Paraquat bis(methylsulfate) (1,1'-Dimethyl-4,4'-bipyridinium bis(methylsulfate)) *	2.1%

GC ELECTRONICS CEMENT THINNER (#28 THINNER)
For thinning radio cements
(GC Electronics)

Ethyl acetate	>20%
Acetone	>20%
Butyl acetate	>20%
Toluol *	>20%

GC ELECTRONICS FRENCH VARNISH
(GC Electronics)

Solox *	>10%
Shellac	

GC ELECTRONICS HEAVY POLISH MIXTURE, LIGHT COLOR
(GC Electronics)

Clear Paraffin oil
909-8R Heavy oil

GC ELECTRONICS LIQUID PHONO NON SLIP COMPOUND NO. 86-2
(GC Electronics)

Powdered resin
Solox *

GC ELECTRONICS NON-TOXIC ELECTROTET CLEANER
For cleaning chassis, controls, switches
(GC Electronics)

Mineral spirits (low odor) *	approx. 50%
Chlorothene *	approx. 50%

GC ELECTRONICS VINYLITE CEMENT; NO. 58-8
For plastics, paper, metals
(GC Electronics)

Acetone *	>20%
AYAF Resin	

GC ELECTRONICS WEATHERPROOF SPEAKER CONE DOPE NO. 10-302
(GC Electronics)

Acetone *	>10%
Lucite scrap	
Tricresyl phosphate *	<10%
Toluol *	<10%

GELCOMUL WITH BELLADONNA
For diarrhea
(Commerce Drug)

Each fl. oz.:
Fl. ext. Belladonna leaves (0.03 mg. alkaloids)	0.01 cc.
Kaolin	90 gr.
Pectin	2 gr.
Zinc phenolsulfonate	1 gr.
Sodium methylcarboxycellulose	1/2 gr.

GELDON
For gastric hyperacidity & hypermotility
(Am. Pharmaceutical)

Each 4 tsp.:
Hyoscyamine sulfate	0.0794 mg.
Atropine sulfate	0.0150 mg.
Hyoscine HBr	0.0050 mg.
Magnesium & aluminum hydroxides	

GEL-KAM
Stannous fluoride dental gel - water free
(Scherer Labs.)

Stannous fluoride 0.4%

GELPHETAMINE-4 CAPSULES
Antidepressant, relaxant
(Pharmex)

Each capsule:
D-Amphetamine sulfate *	3 3/4 mg.
dl-Amphetamine sulfate	3 3/4 mg.
D-Desoxyephedrine HCl *	3 3/4 mg.
dl-Desoxyephedrine HCl	3 3/4 mg.
Amobarbital *	1/2 gr.
Gelatin (high protein)	10.00 gr.

GELUMINA WITH MAGNESIUM TRISILICATE
Antacid, adsorbent
(Am. Pharmaceutical)

Each 5 cc.:
Aluminum hydroxide gel	
Magnesium trisilicate	0.5 gm.

GEMNISYN
Analgesic
(Rorer, W.H., Inc.)

Each tablet:
Aspirin *	325 mg.
Acetaminophen *	325 mg.

GEMONIL TABLETS
Anticonvulsant
(Abbott)

Each tablet:
Metharbital *	100 mg.

GEM-SONIC JEWELRY CLEANER
Liquid cleaner
(Standard Products Corp.)

Alcohol	<1%
Ammonia	<1%

GENERAL MOTORS PRODUCTS

General Motors Corp.
GM Toxic Materials Control Activity
3044 W. Grand Blvd.
Detroit, Mich. 48202

Phone numbers:
Business hours: 313-556-1597
Other hours: 313-556-6200

GENERIC AIR FRESHENER - LEMON
Home use air freshener aerosol
(Great Atlantic & Pacific, mfr.; Compass Foods, dist.)

Ethylene oxide condensate of a fatty acid	0.7%
Diethyl phthalate	0.9%
Ethyl alcohol	0.7%
Diglycol laurate (neutral)	0.5%
Perfume oil	0.4%
Petroleum hydrocarbon propellant	30.0%
Water	balance

GENERIC ALL FABRIC BLEACH
(Great Atlantic & Pacific)

Sodium percarbonate	10.0%
Silica gel	0.5%
Sodium carbonate *	35.0%
Sodium chloride	balance
Dye	trace
Perfume	trace
Nonionic surfactant	0.5%

GENERIC ANT & ROACH KILLER
Household aerosol insecticide
(Great Atlantic & Pacific, mfr.; Compass Foods, dist.)

Pyrethrins	0.05%
Piperonyl butoxide	0.10%
N-Octyl bicycloheptene dicarboximide	0.17%
O-Isopropoxyphenyl methylcarbamate	0.50%
Isopropanol	7.50%
Methylene chloride	14.00%
Hydrocarbon propellant	20.00%
Petroleum distillate *	57.70%

GENERIC AUTOMATIC DISHWASHER DETERGENT
(Great Atlantic & Pacific, mfr.; Compass Foods, dist.)

Sodium tripolyphosphate	<30%
Sodium silicate *	<14%
Nonionic surfactant	<3%
Sodium dichloroisocyanurate	<2%
Sodium sulfate and moisture	balance
Anti caking agent	trace

GENERIC BUG KILLER
Household aerosol insecticide
(Great Atlantic & Pacific, mfr.; Compass Foods, dist.)

Petroleum distillate	9.25%
Multicide Intermediate 2084	2.00%
Hydrocarbon propellant	30.00%
Water	balance

GENERIC FLYING INSECT KILLER
Household aerosol insecticide
(Great Atlantic & Pacific, mfr.; Compass Foods, dist.)

Resmethrin	0.325%
Related compounds	0.044%
Aromatic petroleum hydrocarbons	0.430%
Petroleum distillates	6.382%
Hydrocarbon propellant	30.000%
Water	balance

GENERIC GREEN DETERGENT
Liquid dishwashing detergent
(Great Atlantic & Pacific, mfr.; Compass Foods, dist.)

Sodium dodecylbenzene sulfonate	<9.0%
Ammonium alcohol ether sulfonate	<3.0%
Formaldehyde	<0.2%
Citric acid	<0.2%
Perfume	trace
Dyes	trace
Sodium chloride	<1.5%
Urea	<1.0%
Water	balance
Sodium sulfate	<2.0%

GENERIC HEAVY DUTY LAUNDRY DETERGENT
(Great Atlantic & Pacific, mfr.; Compass Foods, dist.)

Sodium sulfate	38.77%
Sodium carbonate *	24.20%
Sodium tridecylbenzene sulfonate	15.00%
Sodium chloride	9.68%
Sodium silicate	7.70%
Water	4.00%
Sodium carboxymethylcellulose	0.50%
Optical brightener	0.15%

pH of a 1% solution - 10.5-11.5

GENERIC HEAVY DUTY LAUNDRY DETERGENT (Liquid)
(Great Atlantic & Pacific, mfr.; Compass Foods, dist.)

Sodium dodecylbenzene sulfonate	<17%
Nonionic surfactant	<7%
Sodium xylene sulfonate	<4%
Sodium citrate	<0.2%
Optical brightener	<0.2%
Perfume	trace
Sodium sulfate	<3%
Caustic soda	trace
Dye	trace
Water	balance to 100%

GENERIC LAUNDRY DETERGENT
Dry laundry detergent
(Great Atlantic & Pacific, mfr.; Federated Foods, dist.; Golden Best Foods, dist.)

Sodium linear alkyl benzene sulfonate	<17%
Sodium carbonate *	<30%
Sodium silicate	<10%
Sodium carboxymethylcellulose	<2%
Optical brighteners	<1%
Sodium chloride	<10%
Sodium sulfate and moisture	balance

GENERIC LEMON DETERGENT
Liquid dishwashing detergent
(Great Atlantic & Pacific, mfr.; Compass Foods, dist.)

Sodium dodecylbenzene sulfonate	<9.0%
Ammonium alcohol ether sulfonate	<3.0%
Formaldehyde	<0.2%
Citric acid	<0.2%
Opacifier	trace
Perfume	trace
Dye	trace
Sodium chloride	<1.5%
Urea	<1.0%
Water	balance
Sodium sulfate	<2.0%

GENERIC LEMON FURNITURE POLISH
(Aerosol)
(Great Atlantic & Pacific, mfr.; Compass Foods, dist.)

Wax	0.2%
Isoparaffinic hydrocarbon	0.4%
Oleic acid	0.1%
Morpholine	0.1%
Perfume	0.2%
Silicone emulsion	2.0%
Hydrocarbon propellant	6.0%
Water	balance

GENERIC PINK DISH DETERGENT
Liquid dish detergent
(Great Atlantic & Pacific, mfr.; Compass Foods, dist.)

Sodium dodecylbenzene sulfonate	7.3000%
Ammonium alcohol ether sulfonate	2.2000%
Sodium sulfate	2.0000%
Sodium xylene sulfonate	0.5000%
Coconut diethanolamide	0.5000%
Sodium citrate	0.2000%
Opacifier	0.2000%
Formaldehyde	0.1000%
Perfume	0.0500%
Dye	0.0002%
Water	26.9500%

pH (as is) - 6.0 to 7.5

GENERIC SHAVE CREAM (Regular and Menthol)
(Great Atlantic & Pacific, mfr.; Compass Foods, dist.)

Stearic acid	5.2%
Glycerine	1.6%
Triethanolamine	1.0%
Sodium lauryl sulfate	1.0%
Stearyl alcohol	0.6%
Menthol (in Menthol)	0.1%
Perfume (in Regular)	0.05%
Propellant - hydrocarbon	4.0%
Water	balance

GENERIC SPRAY STARCH (Aerosol)
(Great Atlantic & Pacific, mfr.; Compass Foods, dist.)

Starch	2.0%
Sodium borate	0.2%
Silicone emulsion	0.1%
Nonionic detergent	trace
Sulfonated Castor oil	trace
Optical brightener	trace
Formaldehyde	trace
Hydrocarbon propellant	5.25%
Water	balance

GENIE INCENSE CONES
(Hindu Incense)

Charcoal	75%
Starch	15%
Combined amount:	10%
Karaya gum	
China clay	
Sodium nitrate	
Essential oils *	
Triethylene glycol	
Aromatic chemicals	

GENOPTIC S.O.P. STERILE OPHTHALMIC OINTMENT
(Allergan Pharm.)

Gentamicin sulfate (equiv. to 3 mg. gentamicin per gram)

GENOPTIC STERILE OPHTHALMIC SOLUTION
(Allergan Pharm.)

Gentamicin sulfate (equiv. to 3 mg. gentamicin per ml.)

GENTLE FELS
For dishwashing, laundering of fine fabrics
(Purex Corp.)

Anionic surfactant *	20-35%
Ethyl alcohol	1-5%
Alkanolamide	1-5%
Lanolin derivative	<1%
Coloring agent	<1%
Perfume	<1%
Water	balance

GENTLE SPRING DOUCHE POWDER
(Block Drug)

Sodium lauryl sulfate *
Sodium chloride
Sodium phosphate, monobasic
Fragrance

GEOCILLIN
Antibiotic
(Roerig)

Each tablet:
Carbenicillin indanyl sodium (equiv. to 382 mg. of carbenicillin) *

GERIBITS
For older pets
(Norden Labs.)

Each tablet:
Vitamin A	1800 I.U.
Vitamin D2	180 I.U.
Elemental Iron (as ferrous fumarate)	9.5 mg.
Plus multivitamins and minerals	

GERILETS FILMTAB
Multiple vitamin supplement with iron
(Abbott)

Each tablet:
Iron *	27 mg.
Multivitamins	

GERITINIC TABLETS
Hematinic with vitamins
(Geriatric Pharm.)

Each tablet:
Ferrous sulfate *	195 mg.
Plus multivitamins and minerals	

GERITOL
Food supplement with iron
(Williams, J.B.)

Each fl. oz.:
Thiamine (B1)	5 mg.
Niacinamide	100 mg.
Pyridoxine (B6)	1 mg.
Methionine	100 gm.
Iron	100 mg.
Riboflavin (B2)	5 mg.
Panthenol	4 mg.
Vitamin B12	3 mcg.
Choline bitartrate	100 mg.
Other vitamin B complex factors as found in yeast ext.	

GERITOL JUNIOR
Food supplement with iron
(Williams, J.B.)

Each fl. oz.:
Vitamin A palmitate . 8,000 USP units
Vitamin D .... 400 USP units
Thiamine (B1) .... 5 mg.
Riboflavin (B2) .... 5 mg.
Niacinamide .... 100 mg.
Panthenol .... 4 mg.
Pyridoxine (B6) .... 1 mg.
Vitamin B12 .... 3 mcg.
Iron .... 100 mg.
Other vitamin B complex factors as
found in yeast ext.

GERITONIC, LIQUID

See LIQUID GERITONIC

GERIX ELIXIR
Dietary supplement of B complex vitamins and iron
(Abbott)

Each 30 ml.:
Iron * .... 15 mg.
B complex vitamins

GERIZYME
Geriatric tonic
(Upjohn)

Each 15 ml.:
Iron (from 43.17 mg. ferrous
gluconate) .... 5 mg.
Plus multivitamins and minerals

GERMAINE MONTEIL COSMETIC PRODUCTS

Germaine Monteil Cosmetiques Corp.
40 W. 57th St.
New York, N.Y. 10019

Phone: 212-582-3010

See COSMETICS, Section VI, General
Formulations

GERMAIN'S ANT, ROACH AND SPIDER SPRAY
(Germain's)

o-Isopropoxyphenyl
methylcarbamate * 0.50%
Petroleum distillate * 68.20%

GERMAIN'S CUTWORM AND LAWN INSECT SPRAY
(Germain's)

O,O-Diethyl O-(2-isopropyl-6-
methyl-4-pyrimidinyl)
phosphorothioate * 25.00%
Aromatic petroleum derivative
solvent * 65.98%

GERMAIN'S FRESH START GRASS & WEED KILLER
(Germain's)

Sodium cacodylate * 9.27%
Dimethylarsinic acid (Cacodylic
acid) 1.60%

GERMAIN'S GRASS AND WEED KILLER
(Germain's)

Aromatic petroleum
hydrocarbon * 94.50%

GERMAIN'S HOME & GARDEN INSECT SPRAY
(Germain's)

d-trans Allethrin (allyl homolog of
Cinerin I) 0.25%
Piperonyl butoxide (technical) 0.80%
N-Octyl bicycloheptene
dicarboximide 0.40%
Petroleum distillate 8.05%

GERMAIN'S IMPROVED CRABGRASS KILLER
(Germain's)

Monosodium acid
methanearsonate * 13.40%

GERMAIN'S IMPROVED MULTI-PURPOSE TOMATO AND VEGETABLE DUST
Insecticide, fungicide
(Germain's)

Endosulfan * 3.0%
Carbaryl * 6.0%
Zineb 6.0%

GERMAIN'S INSECT SPRAY FOR TENDER FOLIAGE PLANTS
(Germain's)

Tetramethrin 0.250%
Related compounds 0.034%
(5-Benzyl-3-furyl)methyl-2,2-
dimethyl-3-(2-methylpropenyl)
cyclopropane carboxylate 0.106%
Related compounds 0.014%
Petroleum distillate* 9.000%

GERMAIN'S NON-SELECTIVE WEED KILLER
(Germain's)

2-Methoxy-4,6-
bis(isopropylamino)-s-triazine . 3.00%
Pentachlorophenol * 2.25%
Other Chlorophenols and related
compounds 0.25%
Petroleum hydrocarbon * 79.80%

GERMAIN'S OXALIS CONTROL FOR DICHONDRA LAWNS
Herbicide
(Germain's)

Monuron * 12.00%

GERMAIN'S ROSE AND FLOWER DUST
Insecticide, fungicide, miticide
(Germain's)

Carbaryl * 5.000%
1,1-Bis(p-chlorophenyl)-2,2,2-
trichloroethanol 3.000%
2,4-Dinitro-6-octyl phenol
crotonate 0.936%
2,6-Dinitro-4-octyl phenol crotonate
Nitrooctyl phenols (principally
dinitro) 0.064%
Zineb 3.000%

GERMAIN'S ROSE & FLOWER SPRAY
Insecticide, fungicide
(Germain's)

Pyrethrins 0.020%
N-Octyl bicycloheptene
dicarboximide 0.300%
Rotenone 0.100%
Other cube resins 0.200%
Methoxychlor (technical) 0.300%
Dichlone 0.120%
2,4-Dinitro-6-octyl phenyl
crotonate 0.091%
2,4-Dinitro-4-octyl phenyl crotonate
Nitrooctyl phenols (principally
dinitro) 0.006%
Petroleum distillate 0.115%

GERMAIN'S ROSE GUARD
Plant food, insecticide, herbicide
(Germain's)

Total Nitrogen 8.00%
Available Phosphoric acid 12.00%
Water soluble Potash 6.00%
Trace minerals
Soil penetrant
Di-Dyston * 1.00%
Trifluralin 0.17%

GERMAIN'S SNAIL, SLUG & INSECT KILLER
(Germain's)

Carbaryl * 5.00%
Metaldehyde * 2.50%

GERMAIN'S SPOT WEEDER
(Germain's)

Diethanolamine salt of 2-(2-
methyl-4-
chlorophenoxy)propionic acid . 0.125%
Diethanolamine salt of 2,4-dichlo-
rophenoxyacetic acid 0.125%
Diethanolamine salt of dicamba
(3,6 Dichloro-o-anisic acid) ... 0.012%

GERMAIN'S SURE-SET FOR TOMATOES
Blossom drop inhibitor
(Germain's)

p-Chlorophenoxyacetic acid 0.005%

GERMAIN'S VITAMIN B1 SOLUTION
Growth stimulant
(Germain's)

1-Naphthaleneacetic acid 0.10%

GERM-ASEPTIC
Disinfectant-detergent
(Barco)

o-Benzyl-p-chlorophenol	4.4%
p-tert-Butylphenol *	3.0%
Isopropyl alcohol	2.4%
Sodium ricinoleate	1.8%
Sodium alkyl benzene sulfonate	0.5%
Nitrilotriacetic acid trisodium salt	0.9%
Potassium hydroxide	0.9%
Perfume	0.5%

'76 Ed.

GERMEX
Disinfectant, deodorizer, poultry drinking water sanitizer
(Salsbury)

n-Alkyl dimethylbenzyl ammonium chlorides (C14, C16, C12, C18) * . 20%

GERMEX
Disinfectant-deodorant
(Kem Mfg. Co.)

Isopropanol *	60.00%
o-Phenylphenol	0.10%
p-tert-Amylphenol	0.05%

GERMEX AEROSOL
Hospital disinfectant, deodorant
(Kem Mfg. Corp.)

o-Phenylphenol	0.10%
p-tert.-Amylphenol	0.05%
Essential oils	0.75%
Alcohol	57.00%

GERMICIN
Disinfectant
(CMC Research Div.)

Benzalkonium chloride (Alkyl benzyl dimethyl ammonium chloride) *

GERM-I-TOL
Germicide
(Fine Organics, Inc.)

Alkyl dimethyl benzyl ammonium chloride * 50%

'76 Ed.

GERMOTOX
See PIONEER GERMOTOX

GER-O-FOAM
Anesthetic analgesic
(Geriatric Pharm.)

Methyl salicylate *	30%
Benzocaine	3%

Volatile oils in a neturalized emulsion base

GERONIAZOL ELIXIR
Circulatory, respiratory & cerebral stimulant
(Philips Roxane Labs.)

Each 5 ml.:
Pentylenetetrazol *	200 mg.
Niacin (as sodium salt)	100 mg.
Alcohol	12%

GERONIAZOL TT TABLETS
Respiratory & circulatory stimulant
(Philips Roxane Labs.)

Each Tempotrol:
Pentylenetetrazol *	300 mg.
Niacin	150 mg.

GET SET HAIR SETTING LOTION
(Alberto-Culver)

Water
SD Alcohol 40
PVP
Formaldehyde
Octoxynol-9
Polysorbate-20
Fragrance

GEVRABON
Vitamin-mineral supplement
(Lederle)

Iron (as ferrous gluconate) ...... 15 mg.
Plus multivitamins and minerals
Alcohol 18%

GEVRAL
Vitamin-mineral supplement
(Lederle)

Each capsule:
Vitamin A acetate	5000 IU
Vitamin D	400 IU
Elemental Iron (as ferrous fumarate)	18 mg.

Plus multivitamins and minerals

GEVRAL T
Vitamin-mineral supplement
(Lederle)

Each capsule:
Vitamin A acetate	5000 IU
Vitamin D	400 IU
Elemental Iron (as ferrous fumarate)	27 mg.

Plus multivitamins and minerals

GG-CEN CAPSULES
Expectorant
(Central Pharmacal Co.)

Each capsule:
Guaifenesin .... 200 mg.

GG-CEN SYRUP
Expectorant
(Central Pharmacal Co.)

Each tsp. (5 ml.):
Glyceryl guaiacolate	100 mg.
Alcohol	10%

GG-TUSSIN COUGH SYRUP
Antitussive and expectorant
(Vitarine)

Each 5 cc:
Guaifenesin	100 mg.
Alcohol (by vol.)	3.5%

GHOST WRITER
Writer and developer - invisible ink
(Sanford Corp.)

Dyes
Glycols
Water
Phenol (as preservative) .... <1%

GIB-SOL
Plant growth regulator
(Elanco Prod.)

Gibberellic acid 2.13%

GIBSON'S PINE OIL
Cleaner, deodorizer
(Dixie Labs.)

Steam distilled Pine oil *	76.0%
Soap	7.6%
Isopropyl alcohol	4.5%

'76 Ed.

GIB-TABS
Plant growth regulator
(Elanco Prod.)

Gibberellic acid 29.6%

GILBERT SPRUANCE PAINT PRODUCTS
See SPRUANCE, GILBERT, PAINT PRODUCTS

GILL DAIRY CATTLE INSECTICIDE
(Gill)

Methoxychlor, technical * 50%

GILLESPIE FURNITURE CLEANER
(Barr, W. M., & Co.)

Odorless Mineral spirits * .... >90%

GILLESPIE OLD FURNITURE REFINISHER
(Barr, W. M., & Co.)

Acetone *	<20%
Methanol	<10%
Methylene chloride *	<20%
Toluol *	<10%

GILLETTE COSMETICS & TOILETRIES
(Gillette Co., Personal Care Div.)

The Gillette Co., Personal Care Div., Boston, Mass. 02199, will receive collect phone calls from poison control centers or physicians asking for emergency toxicological information about the company's products. Phone: 617-421-7000

GILL FLY KILL
(Gill)

2,2-Dichlorovinyl dimethyl phosphate	0.46%
Related compounds	0.04%

GILL PINE OIL
Cleanser, disinfectant, deodorant
(Gill)

Pure steam distilled Pine oil *	
Soap	
Inert ingred.:	
Water	not over 10%

GILL SPRAY "GITSUM"
Insecticide
(Gill)

Perfume oil	0.025%
Pyrethrins	0.100%
Technical Piperonyl butoxide	0.120%
N-Octyl bicycloheptene dicarboximide	0.500%
Petroleum distillates *	99.255%

GILMAN PRODUCTS
Chemical coatings

Gilman Co., Inc.
P.O. Box 1257
Chattanooga, Tenn. 37401

Phone: 615-756-5185

See PAINTS, Section VI, General Formulations

GILSALUME ALUMINUM ROOF COATING
Fibrated aluminum coating
(United Gilsonite)

Pigment:	37.0%	
Aluminum paste-standard fineness	29.9%	
Ceramic fibre	26.9%	
Calcium silicate	43.2%	
Vehicle (Asphalt varnish):	63.0%	
Non volatile	50.8%	
Asphalt		
Volatile	49.2%	
Mineral spirits *		

GILSALUME ALUMINUM ROOF PAINT
(United Gilsonite)

Pigment:	35.40%	
Aluminum paste-standard fineness	100.00%	
Vehicle (Asphalt varnish):	64.60%	
Non volatile:	54.20%	
Asphalt		
Volatile:	45.80%	
Mineral spirits *		

GILT EDGE WOOD SEALER 508
(Farwell, Ozmun, Kirk)

Active ingred.:	
Pentachlorophenol *	4.53%
Other Chlorophenols	0.53%
Inert ingred.:	
Dipentine	1.45%
Diacetone alcohol	5.40%
Alkyd resin solids	10.39%
Varnish solids	10.39%
Mineral spirits *	66.60%
Calcium drier (12% metal)	0.10%
Lead drier (36% metal)	0.19%
Cobalt drier (12% metal)	0.07%
Antioxidant	0.14%
Inert of Pentachlorophenol	0.21%

GINGISOL
Oral antiseptic for gingivitis and pyorrhea
(Gingisol)

Potassium hydroxide	harmless amt.
Rose soluble	
Phenol	1%
Fluorides	trace
Vitamin C	

GITALIGIN TABLETS
Congestive heart failure
(Schering)

Each tablet:	
Gitalin *	0.5 mg.

GITS UM
Insecticide
(Gill)

2,2-Dichlorovinyl O,O-dimethyl phosphate	0.93%
Related compounds	0.07%
Pine oil	2.00%
Petroleum hydrocarbons *	97.00%

GITS UM WASP AND SCORPION BOMB
(Gill)

Pyrethrins	0.150%
Piperonyl butoxide	0.300%
MGK 264	0.500%
Chlordane	2.000%
Petroleum distillate *	62.050%
Inert ingred.:	
Freon 12	35.000%

GIVENCHY GENTLEMAN FOR A MAN'S BATH
(Parfums Givenchy)

Pentasodium triphosphate
Sodium dodecylbenzenesulfonate
Sodium sesquicarbonate
Water
Sodium silicoaluminate
Fragrance

GIVENCHY PERFUMES

Parfums Givenchy, Inc.
Div. Lehn & Fink Products Group
680 Fifth Ave.
New York, N.Y. 10019

Phone: 201-573-5700

See COSMETICS, Section VI, General Formulations

GLAD RAGS
Fabric markers
(Sanford Corp.)

Dyes
Resins
Ketones *†
Alcohol *†
Esters *†

†*See* Inks, Section VI, General Formulations

GLAD RAGS BASE COAT
Fabric marker base coat
(Sanford Corp.)

Titanium dioxide
Resins
Ketones *†
Alcohols *†
Esters *†

†*See* Inks, Section VI, General Formulations

GLAMOUR KITTY CAT LITTER
(Waverly Mineral Products Co.)

Aluminum magnesium silicate	
Iron oxide	small amounts

GLAMOUR KITTY PREMIUM CAT LITTER
(Waverly Mineral Products Co.)

Aluminum-magnesium silicate	
Iron oxide	small amounts
Methyl salicylate	trace amounts
Methylene blue 2B concentrate (diluted)	trace

GLAS-BRITE
(Hillyard Chem.)

Organic solvents *†

'76 Ed.

†*See* Aromatic hydrocarbon solvent

Starred ingredients (*) may be responsible for major toxic effects; consult Section II.

GLASS *PLUS

See TEXIZE GLASS *PLUS

GLAUCON 2%
For treatment of glaucoma
(Alcon)

Active ingred. (each ml.):
 1-Epinephrine hydrochloride (equiv. to
  2% epinephrine base)
Preservative:
 Benzalkonium chloride 0.01%
Inactive ingred.:
  Sodium metabisulfite
  Edetate disodium
  Hydrochloric acid and/or
  Sodium hydroxide (to adjust pH)
  Purified water

GLAZOL
(United Gilsonite)

Vegetable oils
Calcium carbonate

GLEAMETTE
Dishwashing detergent
(Paul Koss)

Active mixture of Anionic
 surfactants * 30%
Sodium dodecylbenzene sulfonate
Sodium xylene sulfonate
Ammonium ether sulfonate
Lauroyl diethanolamide

pH 7.0-7.2

GLEEM
Toothpaste
(Procter & Gamble, Health & Personal
 Care Div.)

Sodium fluoride 0.22%
Calcium pyrophosphate 25-49%
Cellulose gum 1-4%
Sorbitol 10-24%
Glycerin 10-24%
Minor ingredients, each .... <1%
Water 10-24%

GLIDDEN COATINGS & RESINS PAINT PRODUCTS
Paints, coatings, & resins

Glidden Coatings & Resins
Div. of SCM Corp.
Dwight P. Joyce Research Center
Box 8827
Strongsville, Ohio 44136

S.T. Bowell
Phone: Bus. 216-771-5121 Ext. 2285
 Res. 216-777-4061

GLIDDEN COLOR NATURALS (Y-2000)
(Glidden)

	by weight:
Titanium dioxide	19%
Silica and silicates	16%
Acrylic resin	16%
Glycol ethers and esters	2%
Additives	2%
Water	45%

GLIDDEN LATEX LOW LUSTRE TRIM & WALL PAINT (Y-3118 Line)
(Glidden)

	by weight:
Titanium dioxide	19.6%
Vinyl acetate/acrylic resin	20.9%
Glycol ethers, esters	7.4%
Additives (no lead)	2.5%
Water	49.6%

GLID-STRIP PAINT & VARNISH REMOVER (Y-74)
(Glidden)

	by weight:
Methylene chloride *	81.2%
Methanol	3.0%
Alcohols	4.5%
Ketones	6.3%
Additives (no lead)	5.0%

GLIT
Cleaner
(Kano)

Alcohols *

GLO-BRITE WATER COLORS
(Craftint)

Water-soluble, non-toxic Resins
Fluorescent Pigments

GLOSSINE PRESSING OIL

See EXELENTO GLOSSINE PRESS-
ING OIL

GLO-TOX

See PFIZER GLO-TOX

GLOVER'S IMPERIAL FLEA SOAP
(Glover)

Anhydrous Soap	75.7%
Pine tar	8.0%
Petroleum	4.5%
Sulfur	2.0%
Glycerin	0.8%
Pyrethrins	0.034%
Technical Piperonyl butoxide	0.333%
Petroleum distillate	0.133%

GLOVER'S IMPERIAL MEDICATED OINTMENT
*For temporary relief of dry itchy scalp
 and dandruff*
(Glover)

Sulfur	5.0%
Salicylic acid *	3.0%

GLOVER'S IMPERIAL MEDICATED SHAMPOO SOAP
*For temporary relief of oily scalp and
 dandruff*
(Glover)

Pine tar	2.75%
Precipitated Sulfur	2.0%
Crude Petroleum	2.75%
Anhydrous Soap	
Glycerin	

GLOVER'S SARCOPTIC MANGE MEDICINE
*For temporary relief of dry itchy scalp
 and dandruff*
(Glover)

Petroleum *†	89.1%
Rectified tar oil (Pine tar oil)	5.5%
Sulfur	2.5%
Lanolin oil	1.0%
Captan	0.3%

†*See* Petroleum hydrocarbons

GLU-BOND ADHESIVE

See WILHOLD GLU-BOND ADHE-
SIVE

GLUCOVITE
Iron supplement
(Vale)

Each tablet:
Ferrous gluconate *	260 mg.
Thiamine HCl	1 mg.
Riboflavin	0.5 mg.
Ascorbic acid	10 mg.

GLU-ON PANEL ADHESIVE
(Glu-On Fixture)

See WILHOLD GLU-ON PANEL AD-
HESIVE (Glu-On Fixture)

---

l-GLUTAVITE CAPSULES
Dietary supplement for the elderly
(Berlex Labs.)

Each capsule:
Monosodium l-glutamate	580 mg.
Niacin	7.5 mg.
Pyridoxine HCl	0.16 mg.
Thiamine mononitrate	0.16 mg.
Riboflavin	0.32 mg.
Vitamin B12 (Cyanocobalamin)	1 mcg.
Iron (as ferrous sulfate)	1.7 mg.

Starred ingredients (*) may be responsible for major toxic effects; consult Section II.

GLY
Air sanitizer and surface disinfectant
(Hysan Corp.)

Isopropanol *	26.72%
Propylene glycol	14.88%
Diisobutylcresoxyethoxyethyl di-	
methyl benzyl ammonium	
chloride	0.22%
Essential oils	0.68%

GLYCERINE & ROSEWATER BATH BUBBLES
(House of Lowell, Inc.)

TEA-lauryl sulfate *
Lauramide DEA
Modified Polystyrene latex
Perfume *
Formaldehyde
D & C color

GLYCICAL
Antacid
(Cameron Medical Corp.)

Each tablet:
Calcium carbonate	250 mg.
Magnesium glycinate	120 mg.

GLYCOFED
Expectorant & decongestant
(Vale)

Each tablet:
Guaifenesin	100 mg.
Pseudoephedrine	
hydrochloride *	30 mg.

GLYCOLIN
Spray sanitizer, disinfectant, deodorant
(Puritan Chem. Co.)

Active ingredients:	2.30%
Triethylene glycol	
n-Alkyl (C14, C10, C12, C18) dimethyl	
ammonium chlorides	
n-Alkyl (C12, C14, C16, C18) dimethyl	
ethyl benzyl ammonium chlorides	
Essential oils	
Inert ingredients:	97.70%
Water	
Isooctyl phenoxy polyethoxy ethanol *	

GLYCOM
For chronic respiratory conditions of farm animals
(Bio-Ceutic)

Each pound:
Ammonium chloride	226.80 gm.
Glyceryl guaiacolate	36.29 gm.
Ethylenediamine dihy-	
droiodide *	16.60 gm.
Aromatics	
Artificial color	

GLYCO-MIST
Deodorizer, air-sanitizer
(Varley, James)

Active ingred.:	42.5%
Isopropyl alcohol *	28.46%
Triethylene glycol	10.80%
Propylene glycol	3.00%
Para-di-isobutyl phenoxy	
ethoxy ethyl dimethyl	
benzyl ammonium	
chloride	0.24%
Inert ingred.:	57.5%
Water	

GLYCO THYMOLINE
For skin and mucosal irritations
(Kress)

Alcohol	4%
Sodium benzoate	
Menthol *	
Borax *	
Eucalyptol *	
Sodium bicarbonate	
Sodium salicylate *	
Thymol *	
Oil of sweet birch	
Glycerin	
Oil of pine needles	

'76 Ed.

GLYCOTONE
Hematinic
(Wesley Pharm.)

Each tablet:
Calcium glycerophosphate	64.8 mg.
Ferrous fumarate	32.4 mg.
Sodium glycerophosphate	48.6 mg.
Strychnine sulfate *	1/60 gr.
Tr. Gelsemium	1 min.

GLYCOTUSS-dM (TABLETS & SYRUP)
Expectorant, cough suppressant
(Vale)

Each tablet or 5 ml.:
Guaifenesin	100 mg.
Dextromethorphan	
hydrobromide	10 mg.

GLYCO-TUSSIN WITH CODEINE
For coughs due to colds
(Premo)

Each 5 cc.:
Codeine phosphate *	10 mg.
Glyceryl guaiacolate	100 mg.
Pheniramine maleate *	7.5 mg.
Alcohol	3.5%

'76 Ed.

GLYNAZAN EXPECTORANT
Management of non-productive cough due to the common cold
(Scherer Labs.)

Each 5 cc.:
Glynazan (brand of theophyl-	
line-sodium glycinate equiv.	
to 30 mg. of theophylline,	
N.F.) *	60 mg.
Guaifenesin N.F.	50 mg.
Sodium citrate	100 mg.

GLYOPEN N
Biodegradable anionic wetting and emulsifying agent
(Arkansas Co.)

Sodium sulfate of a fatty acid ester *

'76 Ed.

GLY-OXIDE
Cleansing antiseptic for the mouth
(Marion Labs.)

Carbamide peroxide	10%
Anhydrous Glycerol	q.s.
Artificial flavoring	

GLYROL
To reduce intraocular pressure (oral)
(CooperVision Pharm.)

Glycerin v/v	75%

GLYTINIC
For iron deficiency anemia
(Boyle & Co.)

Iron (Ferrous gluconate)	100.0 mg.
Aminoacetic acid (Glycine)	1.3 gm.
Plus multivitamins	

GLY-TRATE META-KAPS
For angina pectoris
(Sutliff & Case)

Each Meta-Kap:
Nitroglycerin *	2.5 mg.

'76 Ed.

GNAWS NO MORE
Rabbit, squirrel & deer repellent
(National B.C. Sales, Inc.)

Aqueous emulsions of Polyolefin	
resin	62%

Starred ingredients (*) may be responsible for major toxic effects; consult Section II.

GODDARD PRODUCTS
(Goddard, J., & Son)

Phone: 414-631-2111

J. Goddard & Son is a Division of S. C. Johnson & Son, Inc. In case of an emergency involving a Goddard product, contact S. C. Johnson & Son, Inc. S. C. Johnson & Son, Inc., Racine, Wisc., will accept collect calls from physicians and Poison Control Centers handling cases involving their products. This emergency telephone service is maintained 24 hours a day, 7 days a week. To insure contact with technically qualified personnel, inform the long distance operator that the call is an emergency. Then request person to person contact with a member of the S. C. Johnson & Son, Inc. emergency call panel.

G.O.F. GARDEN SPRAY
(Techne Corp.)

A Formula:
Captan 16.66%
Malathion * 16.66%

B Formula:
Methoxychlor, tech. * 30.70%
Zineb 25.00%
Attapulgite clay 10.98%

'76 Ed.

GOLD BOND MEDICATED POWDER
(Gold Bond)

Trace amounts:
  Menthol
  Methyl salicylate
  Stearate of zinc
  Salicylic acid
  Thymol
  Eucalyptol
Boric acid * 1-10%
Talc 90%

GOLDEN BELT DRESSING (Non Aerosol)
(Cling-Surface)

Methylene chloride * 30%

GOLDEN CONQUEROR
Hospital disinfectant and deodorizer
(Miller-Norris Co.)

Orthophenylphenol 0.08%
Paratertiaryamylphenol 0.02%
Ethyl alcohol 53.46%

'76 Ed.

GOLDEN MEDICAL DISCOVERY

See DR. PIERCE'S GOLDEN MEDICAL DISCOVERY

GOLDEN ORKIL EMULSIFIABLE CONCENTRATE, PROFESSIONAL

See PROFESSIONAL GOLDEN ORKIL EMULSIFIABLE CONCENTRATE

GOLDEN RELIEF

See DR. FENNER'S GOLDEN RELIEF

GOLDEN TOUCH
No-stick spray for cooking surfaces
(Boyle-Midway)

Vegetable oils
Lecithin of pure vegetable origin
Flavors
Preservatives
Propellant

GOLDEN VENUS COLOGNE

See JAFRA GOLDEN VENUS COLOGNE

GOLDEN YELLOW INSTANT LATHER SHAVING CREAM
Aerosol
(Williams, J.B.)

Triethanolamine soap
Lanolin oil
Propellants

GOLDICIDE CONCENTRATE
Chemical disinfection of surgical and podiatry instruments
(Pedinol)

N-Alkyl dimethyl benzyl ammonium chloride *

GOLD MAGIC SHAVING POWDER
Depilatory to remove beard
(Carson Products)

Calcium thioglycolate * .... <15%
Calcium hydroxide .... <15%

GOLD MEDAL HAIR PRODUCTS

Gold Medal Hair Products, Inc.
15 Hoover St.
Inwood, N.Y. 11696

Phone: 516-371-2600

See COSMETICS, Section VI, General Formulations

GOLDSPECK
Machine dishwashing
(National-Purity Soap)

Meta-silicate *
Soda ash *
Available Chlorine
Non-ionic modified polyethoxy surfactant
Ionized Chromium *†

pH of 1% solution 12.2

†*See* Chromium sulfate

GONESH INCENSE CONES
(Hindu Incense)

Charcoal 75%
Starch 15%
Combined amount: 10%
  Karaya gum
  China clay
  Sodium nitrate
  Essential oils *
  Triethylene glycol
  Aromatic chemicals

GONE SKIN CREME
Reduces brown discoloration of age blemishes
(Bandwagon, Inc.)

Stabilized Hydroquinone 1%

GONIO GEL
To bind gonioscopic lens to eye during examination
(Muro Pharm.)

Methylcellulose 2.500%
Sodium borate .... trace
Boric acid .... trace
Purified water .... qs ad
Methylparaben 0.023%
Propylparaben 0.010%
Propylene glycol .... trace

GOO
Adhesive
(Walthers Specialties)

Synthetic rubber
Acetone solvent *

'76 Ed.

GOODLAX TABLETS, HOFF'S

See HOFF'S GOODLAX TABLETS

GOOD-LIFE ANT AND ROACH KILLER
(Good-Life Chem.)

o-Isopropoxyphenyl methylcarbamate (Baygon) 0.5%
Petroleum distillate * 60.5%

GOOD-LIFE BACK RUBBER COMPOUND
Insecticide
(Good-Life Chem.)

Ronnel (O,O-Dimethyl O-(2,4,5-trichlorophenyl) phosphorothioate)	1.00%
Pine oil	0.50%
Mineral oil *	98.50%

GOOD-LIFE BACK RUBBER CONCENTRATE
Insecticide
(Good-Life Chem.)

Ronnel (O,O-Dimethyl O-(2,4,5-trichlorophenyl) phosphorothioate)	5.00%
Mineral oil *	95.00%

GOOD-LIFE BAG WORM LIQUID
Controls bagworms and mites on ever-greens and ornamentals
(Good-Life Chem.)

Toxaphene (technical chlorinated camphene)(chlorine content 67% to 69%) *	44.775%
Kelthane (1,1-Bis (p-chloro-phenyl)-2,2,2-trichloroethanol)	4.625%
Aromatic petroleum solvent *	45.750%

GOOD-LIFE BAG WORM SPRAY
Kills bag worms and mites
(Good-Life Chem.)

Toxaphene (technical chlorinated camphene)(chlorine content 67% to 69%) *	15.00%
Aramite (2-(p-tert-Butyl-phenoxy)-1-methylethyl-2-chloroethyl sulphite)	0.90%

GOOD-LIFE BUG BUSTER
Garden insecticide
(Good-Life Chem.)

Rotenone *	1.00%
Other cube resins	1.60%

GOOD-LIFE CAPTAN - MALATHION
Fungicide - insecticide dust
(Good-Life Chem.)

Captan (N-Trichloromethylthio-4-cyclohexene-1,2-dicarboximide)	7.50%
Malathion (O,O-Dimethyl dithio-phosphate of diethyl mercaptosuccinate) *	5.00%

GOOD-LIFE CHICKWEED KILLER
(Good-Life Chem.)

Isooctyl ester of silvex (2-(2,4,5-Trichlorophenoxy) propionic acid) *	65.1%

GOOD-LIFE CHLORDANE 8-E
Agricultural insecticide
(Good-Life Chem.)

Chlordane, technical *	71.7%
Petroleum distillate *	22.0%

GOOD-LIFE 45% CHLORDANE SPRAY
Insecticide for lawns and gardens
(Good-Life Chem.)

Technical Chlordane *	46.0%
Petroleum hydrocarbons *	49.0%

GOOD-LIFE CRAB-NO CRABGRASS KILLER
(Good-Life Chem.)

Disodium methanearsonate anhydrous *	12.60%

Total arsenic as elemental, all water soluble, 5.13%

GOOD-LIFE DAIRY COW DUST
Insecticide
(Good-Life Chem.)

Methoxychlor (technical) *	11.00%
Inert ingred.:	89.00%
Talc	

GOOD-LIFE DORMANT OIL SPRAY
Scale - mite control
(Good-Life Chem.)

Ethion (O,O,O',O'-Tetraethyl S,S'-methylene bisphosphorodithioate) *	2.00%
Petroleum oil *	94.00%

GOOD-LIFE E.D.D. IODINE COMPOUND
Veterinary
(Good-Life Chem.)

Ethylene diamine dihydroiodide *	2000 mg./oz.

GOOD-LIFE FRUIT TREE SPRAY
Insecticide - fungicide
(Good-Life Chem.)

Captan (N-Trichloromethylthio-4-cyclohexene-1,2-dicarboximide)	7.50%
Carbaryl (1-Naphthyl-N-methylcarbamate) *	5.00%
Malathion (O,O-Dimethyl dithio-phosphate of diethyl mercaptosuccinate) *	5.00%

GOOD-LIFE FUNGUS SPRAY
Fungicide - ornamentals and vegetable gardens
(Good-Life Chem.)

Folpet (N-(Trichloromethylthio) phthalimide)	25.00%

GOOD-LIFE GARDENADE GRANULES
(Good-Life Chem.)

Dacthal (Dimethyl ester of tetra-chloroterephthalic acid)	2.5%

GOOD-LIFE GARDEN SPRAY OR DUST
Insecticide-fungicide
(Good-Life Chem.)

Methoxychlor (technical)	4.50%
Rotenone *	2.00%
Other cube resins	3.20%
Zineb (Zinc ethylene bisdithiocarbamate)	6.00%

GOOD-LIFE HOG LICE KILLER
(Good-Life Chem.)

Ronnel (O,O-Dimethyl O-(2,4,5-tri-chlorophenyl) phosphorothioate)	5%

GOOD-LIFE HOUSEHOLD BUG KILLER
(Good-Life Chem.)

O,O-Diethyl O-(2-isopropyl-4-methyl-6-pyrimidinyl) phos-phorothioate (Diazinon)	0.500%
Pyrethrins	0.130%
Technical Piperonyl butoxide	1.020%
Petroleum distillate *	98.350%

GOOD-LIFE KORLAN 2E
Control of livestock insects; residual fly spray
(Good-Life Chem.)

Ronnel (O,O-Dimethyl O-(2,4,5-trichlorophenyl)phosphorothioate)	24%
Aromatic petroleum derivative solvent *	71%

GOOD-LIFE LIME SULPHUR FUNGICIDE
(Good-Life Chem.)

Calcium polysulphide *	30%

GOOD-LIFE 57% MALATHION LIQUID
Insecticide
(Good-Life Chem.)

Malathion *	57.68%
Xylene *	37.64%

Starred ingredients (*) may be responsible for major toxic effects; consult Section II.

GOOD-LIFE NO-GRO
Nonselective weed killer
(Good-Life Chem.)

Sodium chlorate * 30%
Sodium metaborate tetrahydrate
(Boron trioxide equiv. 23.3%) 68%

GOOD-LIFE PENTA CONCENTRATE
Wood preservative
(Good-Life Chem.)

Pentachlorophenol * 36.98%
Other chlorophenols and related
compounds 4.30%
Petroleum solvents 22.00%

GOOD-LIFE PENTA-TREET 5%
Wood preservative
(Good-Life Chem.)

Pentachlorophenol * 4.35%
Other chlorophenols and related
compounds 0.65%
Petroleum distillates * 95.00%

GOOD-LIFE PYRO MILL SPRAY
For pests of stored grains and food products
(Good-Life Chem.)

Active ingred.:
Technical Piperonyl butoxide . 1.02%
Pyrethrins 0.13%
Inert ingred.:
Petroleum oil * 98.85%

GOOD-LIFE RAT DUME (FISH BLEND)
Rodenticide
(Good-Life Chem.)

Warfarin (3(a-Acetonylbenzyl)-4-
hydroxycoumarin) 0.025%
N'-2-Quinoxalylsulfanilamide
(Sulfaquinoxaline) 0.025%

GOOD-LIFE RAT DUME (WATER SOLUBLE)
Rodenticide
(Good-Life Chem.)

Sodium salt of warfarin (Sodium salt of (3-(alpha-ace-
tonylbenzyl)-4-
hydroxycoumarin)) .... 0.54% w/w
N'-(2-Quinoxalinyl)-
sulfanilamide
(Sulfaquinoxaline) 0.50%

GOOD-LIFE ROACH 'N ANT KILLER
Insecticide
(Good-Life Chem.)

O,O-Diethyl O-(2-isopropyl-4-
methyl-6-pyrimidinyl)
phosphorothioate 0.50%
Pyrethrins 0.06%
Technical Piperonyl butoxide ... 0.30%
Petroleum distillate * 69.14%

GOOD-LIFE ROSE DUST OR SPRAY
Fungicide and insecticide
(Good-Life Chem.)

Folpet (N-(Trichloromethylthio)
phthalimide) 8.82%
Gamma isomer of benzene hexachloride, from lindane 1.00%
1,1-Bis(chlorophenyl)-2,2,2-
trichloroethanol 4.25%

GOOD-LIFE ROSE SPRAY LIQUID
Insecticide, fungicide, miticide
(Good-Life Chem.)

Petroleum distillate * 63.160%
Karathane (Dinitro (1-methyl-
heptyl) phenyl crotonate) 1.250%
Glyodin (2-Heptadecyl-2-imida-
zoline acetate) 4.500%
Malathion (O,O-Dimethyl dithiophosphate of diethyl
mercaptosuccinate) * 5.300%

GOOD-LIFE TRIM-IT
Herbicide
(Good-Life Chem.)

Sodium cacodylate 1.98%
Cacodylic acid (Dimethylarsinic
acid) 0.34%

GOOD-LIFE VAPONA D.D.V.P. FLY SPRAY
Controls face flies for dairy cows and beef cattle
(Good-Life Chem.)

2,2-Dichlorovinyl dimethyl
phosphate .... 0.93%/wt.
Related compounds .... 0.07%/wt.
Petroleum distillate * ...... 99.00%/wt.

GOOD-LIFE WEED WOE
Lawn weed killer
(Good-Life Chem.)

Diethanolamine salt of 2-(2-methyl-
4-chlorophenoxy)propionic
acid * 13.7%
Diethanolamine salt of 2,4-dichlo-
rophenoxyacetic acid * 13.6%
Diethanolamine salt of dicamba
(3,6-Dichloro-o-anisic acid) 1.3%

GOODWINOL OINTMENT
Mange treatment in dogs
(Goodwinol)

Rotenone *
Orthophenylphenol *
Ethylaminobenzoate

GOODYEAR MILITARY CEMENT
Adhesive retreading cement
(Goodyear)

Natural rubber 5-10%
Rubber solvent naphtha * 90-95%

GOODY'S EXTRA STRENGTH TABLETS
Analgesic
(Goody's Mfg. Corp.)

Each tablet:
Acetophenetidin * .... 130 mg.
Aspirin * .... 260 mg.
Caffeine .... 16.25 mg.

GOODY'S HEADACHE POWDERS
Analgesic
(Goody's Mfg. Corp.)

Each powder:
Acetophenetidin * .... 260 mg.
Aspirin * .... 520 mg.
Caffeine .... 32.5 mg.

GOOP
Multi-purpose hand cleaner
(Critzas Industries)

Petroleum derivative *†
Water
Octadecenoic acid
Surfactant
Triethanolamine oleate
Glycerin
Lanolin
Perfume
Anti-oxidant

†*See* Hand cleaners, Section VI, General
Formulations

GO-PAIN ANALGESIC TABLETS
Analgesic, antihistaminic
(DePree)

Acetaminophen *
Phentoxylamine citrate
Caffeine *

GO PAIN CREAM
External analgesic, counterirritant
(DePree)

Menthol *
Methyl salicylate *
Camphor *
Thymol
Chlorbutanol

GO PAIN GEL
Local anesthetic
(DePree)

Benzocaine

GO PAIN LOTION
External analgesic, counterirritant
(DePree)

Methyl salicylate (Synthetic USP) *
Camphor *
Menthol *
Methyl nicotinate

Starred ingredients (*) may be responsible for major toxic effects; consult Section II.

GO PAIN THROAT LOZENGE
Local anesthetic
(DePree)

Benzocaine

GO PAIN THROAT SPRAY
Local anesthetic
(DePree)

Liquefied Benzocaine
Cetyl pyridinium chloride

GOPHER GASSER

See DEXOL GOPHER GASSER

GOPHER-GO
(Southwest Chem. Co.)

Strychnine *	0.250%
Food coloring	0.010%
Soy bean oil	0.005%
Grain	99.734%
Anise	trace

GORDOBALM
Massage balm
(Gordon Labs.)

Water	
Isopropyl alcohol *	16%/v
Acetone *	
Methyl salicylate *	
Tragicanth	
Menthol *	
Camphor *	
Thymol *	
Eucalyptus oil *	
Color	

GORDOCHOM
For athlete's foot
(Gordon Labs.)

Undecylenic acid *	25%
Dichlorophene	1%
Penetrating, oily base	

GORDOGESIC CREAM
Analgesic
(Gordon Labs.)

Methyl salicylate *	10%

GORDOMATIC CRYSTALS
Foot soak
(Gordon Labs.)

Sodium chloride *
Sodium bicarbonate *
Sodium borate *
Eucalyptus oil *
Menthol *
Thymol *

GORDOMATIC LOTION
Foot spray
(Gordon Labs.)

Isopropyl alcohol *	92%/v
Propylene glycol	
Menthol *	
Camphor *	
Color	

GORDOMATIC POWDER
Aromatic foot powder
(Gordon Labs.)

Talc
Potassium alum
Salicylic acid *
Bentonite
Eucalyptus oil *
Menthol *
Camphor *
Thymol *

GORDON'S DRY SKIN CREME
For skin irritations
(Gordon Labs.)

Cetyl alcohol
Lubricating oils

GORDON'S KIDDIE POWDER
Foot powder
(Gordon Labs)

Italian Talc

GORDON'S PYROGALLIC ACID OINTMENT (25%)
For verrucca therapy
(Gordon Labs.)

Pyrogallic acid *	25%
Chlorobutanol	2%

GORDO-VITE A CREME & LOTION
Dry skin
(Gordon Labs.)

Vitamin A	100,000 U/oz.

GORDO-VITE E CREME
Skin care
(Gordon Labs.)

Vitamin E	1500 I.U./oz.

GORHAM COPPER AND BRASS POLISH, ANTI-TARNISH FORMULA
(Gorham)

Citric acid	4-8%
Salt	4-8%
Amphoterge S wetting agent/tarnish preventative	4-8%
Diatomaceous earth	

GORHAM CREAM SILVER POLISH
(Gorham)

Mild Soap solution
Diatomaceous earth

GORHAM HANDY DISPOSABLE CLOTHS
For polishing silver
(Gorham)

Non-woven rayon fiber cloth impregnated with:
Mild Soap solution
Diatomaceous earth
Isopropanol   approx. 8-10%

GORHAM REGULAR LIQUID SILVER POLISH
(Gorham)

Mild Soap solution
Diatomaceous earth
Isopropanol   approx. 8-10%

GORHAM SILVER POLISH ANTI-TARNISH FORMULA
(Gorham)

Mild Soap solution
Diatomaceous earth
Isopropanol   approx. 8-10%

GORJUS HAIR DRESSING
(Lotshaw)

Lanolin
Stearic acid
Perfume

'76 Ed.

GORMEL CREAM
Treatment of dry skin conditions
(Gordon Labs.)

Urea	20%

GOSHEN LABORATORIES' FOOT ROT LOTION
Veterinary
(Goshen Labs.)

Pine oil *
Petroleum oil *
Turpentine *
Coal tar neutral oils *

GOSHEN LABORATORIES' FOOT ROT OINTMENT
For foot rot in sheep, cattle
(Goshen Labs.)

Methylrosaniline chloride *
Iodine *
Sulfuric acid
Petrolatum base

GOSHEN LABORATORIES' TEAT OINTMENT
Protectant, antiseptic; veterinary
(Goshen Labs.)

Iodine *
Zinc oxide
Lanolin-petrolatum base

GOSHEN LABORATORIES' UDDER OINTMENT
Antiseptic, counterirritant
(Goshen Labs.)

Methyl salicylate *
Iodine *
Lanolin-petrolatum base

GOTAMINE
Migraine therapy
(Vita Elixir Co.)

Each tablet:
  Ergotamine tartrate * .... 1 mg.
  Caffeine * .... 100 mg.

GO-WEST MEAL
See LILLY'S GO-WEST MEAL

GO-WEST SLUG KILLER
See LILLY'S GO-WEST SLUG KILLER

G.P. - GENERAL PURPOSE DEGREASER
See GUNK G.P. - GENERAL PURPOSE DEGREASER

G.P. SOAP
(Royal Bond)

Hexachlorophene

GRAFCO MEDICOPASTE BANDAGE (UNNA'S BOOT DRESSING)
(Graham-Field)

Zinc oxide *
Glycerine
Gelatine

GRAFCO SILVER NITRATE APPLICATORS
Medicated
(Graham-Field)

Each applicator:
  Silver nitrate * 75%
  Potassium nitrate 25%

GRAHAM PAINT AND VARNISH PRODUCTS
Graham Paint and Varnish Co.
4800 S. Richmond Ave.
Chicago, Ill. 60632

Phone: 312-376-7676

GRAIN KEAP
See GROWER SERVICE GRAIN KEAP

GRAMOXONE
Herbicide
(Chipman Inc.)

Paraquat (present as dichloride) * ...... 2 lb./Imperial gal.

GRANDPA'S WONDER PINE TAR TOILET SOAP BAR
(Grandpa)

Vegetable Pine tar *

GRANOL N-M
Seed treatment
(Chipman Inc.)

Maneb 50.00%
Lindane * 18.75%

GRANOX FLOWABLE
Seed treatment
(Chipman Inc.)

Maneb 25%
HCB (Hexachlorobenzene) 5%

GRANOX N-M
Seed treatment
(Chipman Inc.)

Maneb 50%
HCB (Hexachlorobenzene) * 10%

GRANOX P-F-M
Seed treatment
(Chipman Inc.)

Maneb 30.0%
Captan 28.4%
Related derivatives 1.6%

GRANULAR AVADEX
Herbicide
(Monsanto)

Diallate (S-(2,3-Dichloroallyl)-
diisopropylthiocarbamate) * 10%

GRANULAR FAR-GO
Herbicide
(Monsanto)

Triallate (S-(2,2,3-Trichloroallyl)-
diisopropylthiocarbamate) * 10%

GRANULEX
Used externally to relieve pain and promote healing - veterinary
(Bio-Ceutic)

Each 0.82 ml.:
  Trypsin .... 0.1 mg.
  Balsam Peru .... 72.5 mg.
  Castor oil .... 650.0 mg.

GRANULOL LIQUID DRESSING
(Pharmex)

Balsam Peru * 10%
Hydrocortisone 1/4%
Castor oil q.s. 100%

GRAY'S OINTMENT
(Gray, Dr. W.F.)

Zinc oxide
Aluminum oxide
Creosote *
Carbolic acid (Phenol crystals) *
Oil of turpentine *
Menthol crystals *
Pine tar *
Oil of sassafras *

GREASE MONKEY ENGINE CLEANER
(Liquid Glaze, Inc.)

Aromatic hydrocarbon solvent *
Sulfonate of petroleum
Nonyl phenol ethylene oxide condensate
Isopropyl alcohol

GREASE-OFF
Degreasing concentrate for sewage disposal plants
(Scientific International)

Orthodichlorobenzene *

GREASE RELIEF
See TEXIZE GREASE RELIEF

GREAT HOLD PERM LOTION
(Halliwell)

	percentage range
Water	75.0-95.0%
Ammonium thioglycolate	3.0-9.0%
Ammonium hydroxide	<1.0%
Styrene/Acrylamide copolymer	<1.0%
Laureth-23	<1.0%
Fragrance	<1.0%

GREDAG LUBRICANTS
General lubricant
(Acheson Colloids)

Molybdenum disulfide

'76 Ed.

GREEN-DEVIL DUST
Insecticide
(Pearson & Co.)

Malathion *	5%

'76 Ed.

GREEN-DEVIL SPRAY
Insecticide
(Pearson & Co.)

Malathion *	50%
Xylene *	39%

'76 Ed.

GREEN-DEVIL WETTABLE POWDER
Insecticide
(Pearson & Co.)

Malathion *	25%

'76 Ed.

GREEN LEAF PERM LOTION
Permanent wave lotion
(Bonat)

	percentage range
Water	85.0-97.0%
Ammonium thioglycolate	2.0-8.0%
Ammonium hydroxide *	<2.0%
Laureth-23	1.0-3.0%
Fragrance	<1.0%
Azulene	trace
D & C Yellow #10	trace

GREEN LIGHT BORER KILLER
Insecticide
(Green Light)

Lindane (Gamma isomer of benzene hexachloride) *	20%
Xylene *	69%

GREEN LIGHT BUG BAIT AND SNAIL BAIT
(Green Light)

Carbaryl *	5%
Metaldehyde	1%

GREEN LIGHT CAMELLIA, GARDENIA, AZALEA PLANT FOOD
(Green Light)

Total Nitrogen	8%
Ammoniacal nitrogen	8.0%
Available Phosphoric acid *	12%
Soluble Potash *	4%
Total primary plant foods	24%

GREEN LIGHT 74% CHLORDANE EMULSIFIABLE CONCENTRATE
Kills subterranean termites
(Green Light)

Tech. Chlordane *	74%
Petroleum distillates	10.2%

GREEN LIGHT DIAZINON 12-1/2E
Insecticide for lawns and gardens
(Green Light)

O,O-Diethyl O-(2-isopropyl-4-methyl-6-pyrimidinyl) phosphorothioate *	12.5%
Aromatic petroleum derivative solvent *	72.6%

GREEN LIGHT DIAZINON 5 GRANULES
Insecticide for lawns
(Green Light)

O,O-Diethyl O-(2-isopropyl-6-methyl-4-pyrimidinyl) phosphorothioate *	5%

GREEN LIGHT DORMANT SPRAY
Insecticide
(Green Light)

Petroleum oils *	97%

GREEN LIGHT DOWPON M GRASS KILLER
(Green Light)

Sodium salt of Dalapon (2,2-dichloropropionic acid) *	72.5%
Magnesium salt of Dalapon (2,2-dichloropropionic acid) *	12.0%

GREEN LIGHT DURSBAN GRANULES
Insecticide for lawns, flower beds
(Green Light)

Chlorpyrifos	0.5%

GREEN LIGHT FRUIT & NUT TREE SPRAY
(Green Light)

O,O-Diethyl O-(2-isopropyl-6-methyl-4-pyrimidinyl) phosphorothioate *	12.5%
Aromatic petroleum derivative solvent *	72.6%

GREEN LIGHT GENERAL PURPOSE FUNGICIDE
For ornamental flowers, lawns & shrubs
(Green Light)

A co-ordination product of Zinc ion, Manganese ethylene bisdithiocarbamate * 80%

In which the ingredients are:	
Manganese	16%
Zinc	2%
Ethylene bisdithiocarbamate ion	62%

GREEN LIGHT GENERAL SPRAY
Insecticide
(Green Light)

Dimethyl (2,2,2,-trichloro-1-hydroxyethyl) phosphonate *	18.0%
S-(2-(Ethylsulfinyl)ethyl)O,O-dimethyl phosphorothioate	6.0%
Aromatic petroleum distillate *	36.4%

GREEN LIGHT HOUSE PLANT SPRAY
Insecticide
(Green Light)

Pyrethrins	0.25%
Technical Piperonyl butoxide	0.50%
N-Octyl bicycloheptene dicarboximide	0.50%
Petroleum distillate	8.75%

GREEN LIGHT KELTHANE SPRAY
Miticide
(Green Light)

1,1-Bis(chlorophenyl)-2,2,2-trichloroethanol *	18.5%
Xylene *	73.0%

GREEN LIGHT LIQUID EDGER
Herbicide
(Green Light)

Sodium cacodylate	0.6%
Dimethylarsinic acid (Cacodylic acid)	0.1%

GREEN LIGHT LIQUID FLOWABLE SEVIN
Insecticide
(Green Light)

Carbaryl *	28.0%

GREEN LIGHT LIQUID IRON & SOIL ACIDIFIER
(Green Light)

Sulfur	3.9%
Iron (Fe)	4.5%
Copper (Cu)	0.6%
Zinc (Zn)	0.5%
Magnesium (Mg)	0.5%

Starred ingredients (*) may be responsible for major toxic effects; consult Section II.

GREEN LIGHT 50% MALATHION EMULSIFIABLE CONCENTRATE
Insecticide
(Green Light)

Malathion *	50%
Xylene *	39%

GREEN LIGHT PECAN & FRUIT TREE FOOD
(Green Light)

Total Nitrogen	16%
Available Phosphoric acid *	8%
Soluble Potash *	4%
Total primary plant foods	28%

GREEN LIGHT PRUNING PAINT SPRAY
(Green Light)

Asphalt	28.0%
Petroleum distillates *	33.0%

GREEN LIGHT RAT & MOUSE BAIT
Rodenticide
(Green Light)

3-(alpha-Acetonylfurfuryl)-4-hydroxycoumarin	0.025%

GREEN LIGHT ROACH AND ANT KILLER
(Green Light)

2-(1-Methylethoxy)phenol methylcarbamate *	1.0%
Petroleum distillate *	83.7%

GREEN LIGHT ROOT STIMULATOR AND STARTER SOLUTION
(Green Light)

Indolebutyric acid	0.0004%
Ammoniacal nitrogen	not less than 5%
Available Phosphoric acid *	not less than 20%
Water soluble Potash *	not less than 10%
Chlorine	not more than 0.1%

GREEN LIGHT ROSE AND FLOWER DUST
Insecticide, mildew control
(Green Light)

Carbaryl *	5.0%
Rotenone	1.0%
Other cube resins	2.0%
Folpet	5.0%
2,4-Dinitro-6-octyl-phenyl crotonate 2,6-Dinitro-4-octyl-phenyl crotonate	0.94%
Nitrooctyl-phenols (principally dinitro)	0.06%

GREEN LIGHT ROSE FOOD
(Green Light)

Total Nitrogen	6%
Available Phosphoric acid *	10%
Soluble Potash *	4%
Total primary plant foods	20%

GREEN LIGHT SYSTEMIC FUNGICIDE
For roses - to control black spot and powdery mildew
(Green Light)

Benomyl (Methyl 1-(butylcarbamoyl)-2-benzimidazolecarbamate)	50%

GREEN LIGHT TOMATO AND VEGETABLE DUST
Insecticide, fungicide
(Green Light)

Carbaryl *	7.00%
Copper (in basic copper sulfate) expressed as metallic *	6.00%
Rotenone	1.00%
Other cube resins	2.00%

GREEN LIGHT TOMATO BLOOM SPRAY
Fruit drop inhibitor
(Green Light)

p-Chlorophenoxyacetic acid	0.005%
Inert ingred. *†	99.995%

†*See* Isopropyl alcohol

GREEN LIGHT TOMATO DUST
Insecticide & fungicide
(Green Light)

Carbaryl *	7.5%
Basic copper sulfate (expressed as metallic) *	6.0%
Sulfur *	50.0%

GREEN LIGHT VAPAM SOIL FUMIGANT
(Green Light)

Sodium methyl dithiocarbamate anhydrous *	32.7%

GREEN LIGHT VEGETABLE GARDEN DUST
Insecticide
(Green Light)

Carbaryl *	7%
Rotenone	1%
Other cube resins	2%

GREEN LIGHT WASP & HORNET SPRAY
Insecticide
(Green Light)

o-Isopropoxyphenyl methylcarbamate *	1.00%
Pyrethrins	0.10%
Piperonyl butoxide (technical)	0.20%
N-Octyl bicycloheptene dicarboximide	0.33%
Petroleum distillate *	51.73%

GREEN LIGHT WEED & GRASS EPTAM GRANULES
Herbicide
(Green Light)

S-Ethyl dipropylthiocarbamate	2.3%

GREEN LIGHT WIPE-OUT
Broadleaf weed killer
(Green Light)

Dimethylamine salt of 2-(2-methyl-4-chlorophenoxy)propionic acid	7.09%
Dimethylamine salt of 2,4-dichlorophenoxy-acetic acid	2.16%
Dimethylamine salt of Dicamba (3,6-dichloro-o-anisic acid)	0.86%

GREEN MEADOWS CONCENTRATED AIR FRESHENER

See AMWAY GREEN MEADOWS CONCENTRATED AIR FRESHENER

GREEN MINT MOUTHWASH
(Block Drug)

Urea	
Copper chlorophyll	
Sorbitol	
Tween (surface active agent)	
SD Alcohol 38B	12%
Glycine	
Sodium saccharin	
Preservative	
Flavor	

GREEN MT. HOOF SOFTENER
Veterinary ointment
(Dairy Assoc.)

Petrolatum	88%
Lanolin	6%
Pine oil	1.6%
Sanitas	0.9%
Graphite	0.5%
Vegetable oil soap	3%

GREEN POWER
General purpose detergent
(Brewer Chem.)

Sodium alkyl aryl sulfonate *	20-30%
Nonylphenoxy polyethoxy ethanol	approx. 15%
Coconut diethanolamide	<5%

Starred ingredients (*) may be responsible for major toxic effects; consult Section II.

GREEN STRIPE FLOOR WAX

See BUTCHER'S GREEN STRIPE FLOOR WAX

GREEN STUFF
Wax stripper
(Paul Koss)

Water	>85%
Monoethanolamine *	<12%
Monoethanolammonium dodecylbenzene sulfonate (Anionic surfactant)	
Coco diethanolamide	
Ammonium hydroxide	
Dye	trace

pH 10.6-10.9

GREEN THUMB AFRICAN VIOLET PLANT FOOD
(Green Thumb)

Total Nitrogen	4%
Ammoniacal nitrogen	1.1%
Water soluble Urea nitrogen	2.9%
Available Phosphoric acid *	10%
Soluble Potash *	6%
Chlorine	<0.05%

GREEN THUMB ALL-PURPOSE PLANT FOOD
(Green Thumb)

Total Nitrogen	5%
Ammoniacal nitrogen	1.1%
Water soluble Urea nitrogen	3.9%
Available Phosphoric acid *	10%
Soluble Potash *	5%
Chlorine	<0.05%

GREEN THUMB FISH EMULSION FERTILIZER
(Green Thumb)

Total Nitrogen	5%
Ammoniacal nitrogen	0.5%
Water soluble Nitrogen	4.5%
Available Phosphoric acid	1%
Soluble Potash	1%
Chlorine	<0.3%

GREEN THUMB INSECTICIDE
For house plants
(Green Thumb)

Active ingred.:	
Pyrethrins	0.01%
Petroleum distillate	0.04%
Inert ingred.:	
Isopropanol *	59.37%
Water	40.58%

GREEN THUMB LEAF POLISH
(Green Thumb)

Emulsified refined White oil
Nonionic surfactants
Water

GRENALD'S SHUTTLE LOTION
Medicated lotion for the skin
(Amer. Hygienic Labs.)

Menthol	0.5%
Phenol	0.5%
Benzocaine	0.5%
Precipitated Sulfur	
Zinc oxide	
Corn starch	
Glycerin	
Milk of magnesia	
Lime water	
Magma Bentonite	

GRID-10
Dairy cleaner-sanitizer
(Van Waters & Rogers)

n-Alkyl (60% C14, 30% C16, 5% C12, 5% C18) dimethyl benzyl ammonium chloride	5.0%
n-Alkyl (50% C12, 30% C14, 17% C16, 3% C18) dimethyl ethylbenzyl ammonium chloride	5.0%
Phosphoric acid *	30.0%

"GRIDBALL" BRUSH KILLER

See "VELPAR" "GRIDBALL" BRUSH KILLER

GRID DAIRY LIQUID CLEANER #5
(Van Waters & Rogers)

Phosphoric acid *	40%

GRIFFIN ALLWITE LIQUID
Shoe polish
(Boyle-Midway)

Ammonia	trace
Polymers-resins-waxes	
Plasticizers	
Titanium dioxide	
Mineral fillers	
Preservative	trace
Perfume	trace
Surfactant	trace
Thickeners	

GRIFFIN HEEL AND SOLE DRESSING
(Boyle-Midway)

Alcohol *
Vegetable oil
Resins
Cellulose derivative
Dye

GRIFFIN LIQUID WAX SHOE POLISH
(Boyle-Midway)

Polymer resin emulsion
Wax
Plasticizer
Silicone oil
Lanolin derivative
Dyes
Preservative

GRIFFIN SCUFF COVER
Black & Brown Shoe Polish
(Boyle-Midway)

Polymer resin emulsion
Wax
Plasticizer
Silicone oil
Lanolin derivative
Dyes
Preservative

GRIFFIN SCUFF COVER - WHITE
Shoe polish
(Boyle-Midway)

Ammonia	trace
Polymers-resins-waxes	
Plasticizers	
Titanium dioxide	
Mineral fillers	
Preservative	trace
Perfume	trace
Surfactant	trace
Thickeners	

GRIFFIN SHOE DYE
(Boyle-Midway)

Mixed Alcohols *	<50%
Spirit soluble dyes	
Solubilized with Organic and/or mineral acid	<10%

GRIFFIN WAX SHOE POLISH
(Boyle-Midway)

Waxes	
Petroleum distillates *	>10%
Terpenes *	
Lanolin	
Silicone	
Oil-soluble dyes	
Perfume	

GRIFULVIN V ORAL SUSPENSION
Antifungal
(Ortho-Dermatology)

Each 5 ml.:	
Griseofulvin (USP, microsize) *	125 mg.

Starred ingredients (*) may be responsible for major toxic effects; consult Section II.

GRIFULVIN V TABLETS
Antifungal
(Ortho-Dermatology)

Each 125 mg. tablet:
  Griseofulvin (USP,
    microsize) * 81.97%
Each 250 mg. tablet:
  Griseofulvin (USP,
    microsize) * 78.37%
Each 500 mg. tablet:
  Griseofulvin (USP,
    microsize) * 81.95%

GRIMEX
Stove cleaner
(Lester Labs.)

Mild Alkali *
Methylene chloride *

'76 Ed.

GRIMEX HEAVY-DUTY ALKALINE CLEANER & DEGREASER
(Nat'l Labs. Div.)

Potassium hydroxide * .... minor
Phosphates (calculated as elemental phosphorus) 0.85%

GRIPDUST
Treatment for dust cloths, mops, etc.
(Dolge)

Mineral oil 70-75%
1,1,1-Trichloroethane * 26-30%
Isobutane/propane (50/50)
  (Propellant) 20%

GRIPPIT
Paper cement
(Sanford Corp.)

Synthetic rubber polymers
Hexane *

GRIPSHEEN
Liquid floor wax
(Sanitek)

Various Waxes and
  Polyethylenes 9.8%
Rosin maleate resin 2.7%
Dimethylaminoethanol 0.4%
Potassium hydroxide (50% aq.) .. 0.2%
Ammonia .... trace
Water .... balance

GRIPTRED
Nonslip floor surfacing material
(Goodyear)

Phenolic binder
Methyl ethyl ketone *

GRISCOM'S FAMILY LINIMENT
(Aschenbach & Miller)

Ammonia *
Camphor *
Oil of origanum
Turpentine *

'76 Ed.

GRISOWEN
Treatment of ringworm infections
(Owen Labs.)

Each capsule:
  Griseofulvin (microsize) ...... 250 mg.

GRIS-PEG TABLETS
(Dorsey Labs.)

Each 125 mg. tablet:
  Griseofulvin ultramicrosize
    (equiv. to 250 mg. microsize
    griseofulvin) * .... 125 mg.
Each 250 mg. tablet:
  Griseofulvin ultramicrosize
    (equiv. to 500 mg. microsize
    griseofulvin) * .... 250 mg.

GROOM

See CARSON GROOM

GROTAN BROAD SPECTRUM BACTERICIDE
Metal working preservative
(U.S. Professional Labs.)

Hexahydro-1,3,5,-tris(2-hydroxy-
  ethyl)-s-triazine * 78.5%

GROTANOL
Alkaline cleaner
(U.S. Professional Labs.)

Sodium hydroxide * .... minor

GROWER SERVICE ALFALFA WEEVIL SPRAY
Insecticide
(Grower Service Corp.)

Malathion * 23.37%
Methoxychlor, technical * 25.90%

GROWER SERVICE ATRAZINE 4L
Herbicide
(Grower Service Corp.)

Atrazine * 40.8%
Related compounds 2.2%

GROWER SERVICE ATRAZINE 80W
Herbicide
(Grower Service Corp.)

Atrazine * 76%
Related compounds 4%

GROWER SERVICE CYTHION
Insecticide
(Grower Service Corp.)

Malathion * 57%
Xylene * 35%

GROWER SERVICE DIAZINON AG 500
Insecticide
(Grower Service Corp.)

Diazinon * 48%
Xylene * 39%

GROWER SERVICE DINITRO - 3
Herbicide
(Grower Service Corp.)

Dinoseb * 47.35%

GROWER SERVICE DINITRO - 5
Herbicide
(Grower Service Corp.)

Dinoseb * 54.4%

GROWER SERVICE EPN - M PARATHION 3 - 3
Insecticide
(Grower Service Corp.)

EPN * 31%
Methyl parathion * 31%
Xylene 33%

GROWER SERVICE GRAIN KEAP
Fungicide
(Grower Service Corp.)

Propionic acid * 100%

GROWER SERVICE METHYL PARATHION (2E & 4E)
Insecticide
(Grower Service Corp.)

2E:
  O,O-Dimethyl O-p-nitrophenyl
    thiophosphate * 24.9%
  Xylene 68.8%

4E:
  O,O-Dimethyl O-p-nitrophenyl
    thiophosphate * 46.42%
  Xylene 47.46%

GROWER SERVICE METHYL PARATHION 1.5 THIODAN 3 E.C.
Insecticide
(Grower Service Corp.)

O,O-Dimethyl O-p-nitrophenyl
  thiophosphate * 15.9%
Endosulfan 31.9%
Xylene 39.5%

Starred ingredients (*) may be responsible for major toxic effects; consult Section II.

GROWER SERVICE PRIME LEAF TOBACCO SPRAY
Insecticide
(Grower Service Corp.)

Endosulfan *	12.2%
Malathion	12.2%
Xylene *	70.95%

GROWER SERVICE PROPANIL 4
Herbicide
(Grower Service Corp.)

Propanil *	43.48%

GROWER SERVICE SUPERIOR 70 SECOND SPRAY OIL
Insecticide
(Grower Service Corp.)

Refined Petroleum distillate *	98.9%

GROWER SERVICE SUPERKILL PARATHION 1 THIODAN 2 EC
Insecticide
(Grower Service Corp.)

Parathion *	11.5%
Endosulfan *	22.8%
Xylene	60.0%

GROWER SERVICE THIODAN 2 EC
Insecticide
(Grower Service Corp.)

Endosulfan *	24.0%
Xylene *	69.0%

GROWER SERVICE TOXAPHENE 6 E
Insecticide
(Grower Service Corp.)

Toxaphene *	58.57%
Xylene	37.43%

GROWER SERVICE TOX - MP 6 - 3
Insecticide
(Grower Service Corp.)

Toxaphene *	52.00%
Methyl parathion *	26.00%
Xylene *	16.01%

GR-REAT 'N EASY (Aerosol & Liquid)
Bathroom cleaner
(Fiberglass Cleaning)

Dowanol EB *	5%
Sodium xylene sulfonate	5%
Tetrapotassium pyrophosphate	3%
Sodium metasilicate *	3%
Tritan N101	1%
Versene	0.2%
Propellant (Hydrocarbon)	Aerosol only

GR-RIP
(McAleer)

Polyester resin
Talc (Magnesium silicate)

'76 Ed.

GRUMBACHER PRODUCTS
Artists' supplies

M. Grumbacher, Inc.
460 W. 34th St.
New York, N.Y. 10001

24-hour emergency number: 212-279-6406

GTA BAT REPELLENT
(Athelstan)

Paradichlorobenzene *

'76 Ed.

GTA FLY SPRAY
Insecticide
(Athelstan)

O,O-Diethyl O-(2-isopropyl-6-methyl-4-pyrimidyl) phosphorothioate *	1.00%
Xylene *	2.2%

'76 Ed.

GTA RESIDUAL SPRAY CONCENTRATE WM25
Insecticide
(Athelstan)

DDT *	25%

'76 Ed.

G-3 DUST
Insecticide
(FMC Corp., Agricultural Chem. Div.)

O,O-Dimethyl S-4-oxo-1,2,3-benzo-triazin-3(4H)-methyl phosphorodithioate *	3.00%

G-TUSSIN DM SYRUP
Cough suppressant; expectorant
(Columbia Med.)

Each 5 ml.:

Glyceryl guaiacolate	100 mg.
Dextromethorphan HBr *	15 mg.
Alcohol	1.4%

GUAIAHIST TABLETS
Antihistaminic
(Philips Roxane Labs.)

Each tablet:

Glyceryl guaiacolate (Guaifenesin)	100 mg.
Phenylephrine hydrochloride	5 mg.

GUAIAHIST TT TABLETS
Antihistaminic
(Philips Roxane Labs.)

Each Tempotrol:

Glyceryl guaiacolate (Guaifenesin)	300 mg.
Phenylephrine hydrochloride *	20 mg.

GUAIAJEN
For cold symptoms
(Jenkins Labs.)

Each tablet:

Phenylephrine HCl *	5 mg.
Pyrilamine maleate *	12.5 mg.
Glyceryl guaiacolate	100 mg.

GUAIAMEN CREAM
Analgesic cream
(Lannett)

Methyl salicylate *
Guaiacol
Menthol *
Greaseless base

GUAIAMINE CAPSULES
For colds
(Sutliff & Case)

Each capsule:

Caffeine	0.5 gr.
Chlorpheniramine maleate	2.0 mg.
Phenylephrine HCl	5.0 mg.
Glyceryl guaiacolate	50.0 mg.
Salicylamide	3.0 gr.
Acetaminophen *	2.0 gr.

'76 Ed.

GUAIFED CAPSULE
Nasal decongestant & expectorant
(Muro Pharm.)

Each timed release capsule:

Pseudoephedrine HCl *	12 mg.
Guaifenesin	250 mg.
Nu-Pareil	>50%
Hydrogenated Castor oil	<5%
Pharmaceutical glaze	<10%

GUARD ALL
Silicone emulsion polish
(Paul Koss)

Water	>85%
Silicone emulsion	
Formalin	trace

pH 7.0-7.2

Starred ingredients (*) may be responsible for major toxic effects; consult Section II.

GUARDALL X-185
Bactericide, fungicide, viricide
(Bio-Lab)

Coconut fatty acid soap	17.8%
Isopropanol *	16.0%
2,4-,2,5-,2,6-Xylenols *	13.5%
3,5-,2,3-Xylenols *	9.0%
Meta, para-cresol *	6.3%
Sodium dodecylbenzene sulfonate	5.1%
4 and 6-Chloro-2-phenylphenol	4.0%
o-Benzyl-p-chlorophenol	3.0%
Meta, para-isopropylphenol	1.2%
Tributyltin neodecanoate	0.5%
Para-tertiary amylphenol	0.2%
2,2'-Methylenebis(3,4,6-trichlorophenol)	0.1%

GUARDEX ALGAE CONTROL
Swimming pool additive
(Purex Corp.)

n-Alkyl dimethyl benzyl ammonium chloride *	20%
n-Alkyl dimethyl ethylbenzyl ammonium chloride *	20%
Water	balance

GUARDEX CHLORINE CARTRIDGE
Swimming pool additive
(Purex Corp.)

Trichloro-s-triazinetrione *	99.5%
Inert binding material	0.5%

GUARDEX CHLORINE CONCENTRATE TABLETS
Replacement tablets for cartridge
(Purex Corp.)

Trichloro-s-triazinetrione *	99.5%
Inert binding material	0.5%

GUARDEX DRY ACID
Swimming pool additive
(Purex Corp.)

Sodium bisulfate *	90%
Sodium sulfate	10%

GUARDEX DRY CONDITIONER
Swimming pool additive
(Purex Corp.)

Cyanuric acid	98 1/2%
Water	balance

GUARDEX 4-IN-1 TEST KIT
Swimming pool water analysis
(Purex Corp.)

Solution #1:
Orthotolidine	<1%
Hydrogen chloride *	4-5%
Water	Balance

Solution #2:
Phenol red sodium salt	<1%
Water	Balance

Solution #3:
Hydrogen chloride *	<1%
Water	Balance

Solution #4:
Sodium thiosulfate	<1%
Water	Balance

Solution #5:
Bromophenol blue	<1%
Water	Balance

Solution #6:
2-Aminoethanol	30-35%
Hydrochloric acid *	<3%
Water	Balance

Solution #7:
Hydroxyl amine hydrochloride *	4-5%
1-(1-Hydroxy-4-methyl-2-phenylazo) 2-naphthol-4-sulfonic acid	<1%
Isopropanol *	25-35%
Water	Balance

Solution #8:
Ethylenediaminetetraacetic acid, disodium salt	1-3%
Boric acid	<1%
Sodium hydroxide	<1%
Potassium chloride	<1%
Water	Balance

GUARDEX pH STABILIZER
Swimming pool additive
(Purex Corp.)

Sodium sesquicarbonate *	100%

GUARDEX POOL CHLORINE CONCENTRATE
Swimming pool additive
(Purex Corp.)

Sodium dichloro-s-triazinetrione *	95%
Sodium chloride	5%

GUARDEX SUPER CHLORINATOR
Swimming pool additive
(Purex Corp.)

Calcium hypochlorite *	65%
Sodium chloride	15-20%
Calcium hydroxide	<3%
Calcium chloride	<3%
Calcium carbonate	<2%
Water	balance

GUARDEX TILE CLEANER
(Purex Corp.)

Sodium carbonate *	5-8%
Sodium silicate (not meta)	2-4%
Anionic surfactant	<3%
Sodium sulfate	<1%
Silica flour	balance

GUARDEX TILE & VINYL CLEANER
Swimming pool surface cleaner
(Purex Corp.)

Sodium dodecylbenzene sulfonate	<5%
Sodium carbonate	<10%
Sodium silicate (not meta)	<10%
Silica flour	Balance

GUARDSMAN ANTIFREEZE AND SUMMER COOLANT
(Van Waters & Rogers)

Ethylene glycol *

GUARDSMAN BLEACH CONCENTRATE
(Van Waters & Rogers)

Sodium hypochlorite solution *	approx. 14%

GUARDSMAN PAINTS
Specialized industrial product finishes & house paints

Guardsman Chemicals, Inc.
1350 Steele Ave., S.W.
Grand Rapids, Mich. 49507

Phone: 616-452-5181

See PAINTS, Section VI, General Formulations

GUCCI AFTER SHAVE
(Mennen)

SD Alcohol 40 *
Water
Fragrance
Propylene glycol
PEG-60 hydrogenated castor oil

GUCCI COLOGNE POUR HOMME
(Mennen)

SD Alcohol 40 *
Fragrance
Water

GUCCI DUSTING POWDER
(Mennen)

Talc
Magnesium carbonate
Fragrance

GUCCI EAU DE PARFUM
(Mennen)

SD Alcohol 40 *
Fragrance
Water

GUCCI PARFUM 1
(Mennen)

SD Alcohol 40 *
Fragrance
Water

GUCCI SPLASH COLOGNE PARFUM 1
(Mennen)

SD Alcohol 40 *
Fragrance
Water

GUCCI SPLASH COLOGNE POUR HOMME
(Mennen)

SD Alcohol 40 *
Fragrance
Water

GUERLAIN COSMETICS

Guerlain, Inc.
Rte 138
Somers, N.Y. 10589

Phone: 914-232-5015

See COSMETICS, Section VI, General Formulations

GUILLORY'S COAL TAR DIP
(Guillory)

Active ingredients: 90%
　Neutral Coal tar oils *
　Soap
　Phenols *

GUIOSAN SYRUP
Cough syrup
(Vale)

Each fl. oz.:
　Alcohol 0.9%
　Morphine sulfate * .... 14 mg.
　Potassium citrate .... 1.0378 gm.
　Potassium guaiacol
　　sulfonate .... 0.1580 gm.
　White pine & wild cherry .. q.s.

GUISTREY FORTIS (S.C.T. PINK; OVAL)
For cold symptoms
(Bowman Pharm.)

Each tablet:
　Guaifenesin .... 100 mg.
　Phenylephrine HCl * .... 10 mg.
　Chlorpheniramine maleate ... 1 mg.

GULF ACRYLIC LATEX CAULK (ALC-11)
(Gulf Adhesives and Resins)

Ammonia 0.5%
Ethylene glycol 1.0%
Mineral spirits 0.5%

GULF ADHESIVE SOLVENT
(Gulf Adhesives and Resins)

1,1,1-Trichloroethane * 100%

GULF ADHESIVE SOLVENT (AS-21)
(Gulf Adhesives and Resins)

Toluol * 51%
Hexane * 45%
M.E.K. (Methyl ethyl ketone) 2%

GULF ALUMINUM REPAIR (AR-1)
(Gulf Adhesives and Resins)

Methyl ethyl ketone * 37-47%

GULF ARCHITECTURAL GRADE OIL BASE CAULK (AGC-11)
(Gulf Adhesives and Resins)

Asbestos fiber 3%
Mineral spirits 4%

GULF BUTYL CAULK (BC-11)
(Gulf Adhesives and Resins)

Mineral spirits * 10-16%

GULF CONTACT CEMENT (CC-1)
(Gulf Adhesives and Resins)

Methyl ethyl ketone 50%
Toluol * 25%

GULF COVE BASE ADHESIVE (CBA-72)
(Gulf Adhesives and Resins)

Alcohol solvent *†
Resin base

†*See* Alcohols

GULF ECONOMY OIL BASE CAULK (OBC-11)
(Gulf Adhesives and Resins)

Asbestos fiber 2.4%
Mineral spirits 4.3%

GULF FABRIC REPAIR (FR-1)
(Gulf Adhesives and Resins)

Free　Ammonia　(as　ammonium
　hydroxide) 1%

GULF FLOOR GENERAL CONSTRUCTION ADHESIVE
(Gulf Adhesives and Resins)

Toluene * 37.3%
Styrene-Butadiene copolymer 18.7%
Asbestos 1.8%

GULF FOAM AND PANEL ADHESIVE
(Gulf Adhesives and Resins)

n-Heptane * 30%
Acetone...................... 5%

GULF GLAZING COMPOUND (GLC-30)
(Gulf Adhesives and Resins)

Asbestos fiber 2.2%
Mineral spirits .... <1%

GULF HOUSEHOLD CEMENT (HC-1)
(Gulf Adhesives and Resins)

Acetone 40-50%
Toluol * 30-35%
Isophorone .... <5%

GULF LATEX CAULK (LC-11)
(Gulf Adhesives and Resins)

Mineral spirits .... <2%
Ethylene glycol .... <1%

GULF LIQUID SOLDER (LS-1)
(Gulf Adhesives and Resins)

Toluol * 25-30%
Isobutyl acetate 15-20%
Isopropyl alcohol 10-15%

GULFLITE CHARCOAL STARTER
(Gulf)

Petroleum naphtha *

GULFLITE PATIO TORCH FUEL
(Gulf)

Petroleum naphtha *

GULF LUBRICANT 581
(Gulf Adhesives and Resins)

Denatured alcohol .... <10%

GULF PANEL & GENERAL CONSTRUCTION ADHESIVE
(Gulf Adhesives and Resins)

Toluene *	<41%
Asbestos fiber	<4%

GULF PLASTIC RUBBER - WHITE (PRW-1)
(Gulf Adhesives and Resins)

Toluene *	77%

GULF PORCELAIN TOUCH-UP (PTU-1)
(Gulf Adhesives and Resins)

Methyl isobutyl ketone *	50-55%
Normal Propyl alcohol *	15-20%
Isopropyl alcohol	<5%

GULF QUICK REPAIR WOOD FILLER
(Gulf Adhesives and Resins)

Natural glue
Artificial coloring
Water base

GULF RUBBER CEMENT (RC-1)
(Gulf Adhesives and Resins)

Heptane*	65%
Hexane*	28%

GULF SILICONE SEALANT
(Gulf Adhesives and Resins)

Acetic acid derivative	<1%
Fumed Silica	<12%
Organometallic compounds	<2%

GULF STEEL REPAIR (SR-1)
(Gulf Adhesives and Resins)

Methyl ethyl ketone	7-17%
Toluene *	14-24%
Methyl isobutyl ketone	1-11%

GULFTONE
Tonic and appetite stimulant for large animals; veterinary
(Hart-Delta, Inc.)

Each fl. oz.:

Strychnine sulfate *	1 gr.
Arsenic trioxide *	1 gr.
Cobalt sulfate	0.5 gr.
Copper acetate	0.32 gr.
Iron ammonium citrate	1.6 gr.
F.E. Gentian	20 min.

'76 Ed.

GULF VINYL REPAIR (VR-1)
(Gulf Adhesives and Resins)

Tetrahydrofuran *	10%
Methyl ethyl ketone *	10%
Methyl isobutyl ketone	5%

GULF WOOD FILLER (WF-1)
(Gulf Adhesives and Resins)

Acetone *	37.0%
Tributyl phosphate	1.3%
Nitrocellulose	4.6%

GUM MEL
Liquid teething lotion
(VB)

Ethylaminobenzoate
Chlorobutanol *
Hexahydrothymol *

Alcohol	2%

GUMOUT CARBURETOR & FUEL SYSTEM CLEANER
(Pennzoil Co., Gumout Div.)

Polybutene amine inhibitor	<30%
Mixed Xylenes *	<30%

GUMZOR

See DEWITT'S GUMZOR

GUNK A.B.C. - ALUMINUM BODY CLEANER (Liquid)
For use in water solution to clean metal trucks and trailers
(Gunk Labs.)

Acids, organic & inorganic *	<20%
Synthetic wetting agents	>5%
Coupler:	<2%
Glycols	
Water	>70%

GUNK B.O.P. - BRUSH-ON-PARTS CLEANER
For cleaning small mechanical parts; liquid (ready-to-use)
(Gunk Labs.)

Vegetable fatty acid soap	<4%
Synthetic wetting agents	<3%
Phenolic compounds	>5%
Coupler:	<1%
Glycols	
Petroleum distillates	>60%
Aliphatic chlorinated solvents *	<25%
Water	<1%

GUNK C.D. - CORROSION DIGESTER (Powder)
For tank use in water solution
(Gunk Labs.)

Caustic soda *	<70%
Alkaline salts	<6%
Organic chelating agents	<35%

GUNK C.M. - CARBON-MET
(Liquid; Ready to Use)
For solvent degreasing of metals
(Gunk Labs.)

Coal tar distillates *	<65%
Aliphatic chlorinated solvents *	<40%

GUNK CYCLE CARB CLEANER (MC-1)
Carburetor cleaning; aerosol
(Gunk Labs.)

Acetone	<50%
Aromatic hydrocarbons *	<35%
Chlorinated hydrocarbons *	<25%

GUNK CYCLE CARB CLEANER (MC-1A)
Carburetor cleaning; liquid (ready-to-use)
(Gunk Labs.)

Aromatic hydrocarbon *	<70%
Ketone	<35%

GUNK CYCLE CHAIN LUBE (ML-1 AND ML-2)
Lubricant; aerosol
(Gunk Labs.)

Petroleum oil	100%

GUNK CYCLE DEGREASER (MD-1)
Motorcycle degreasing; aerosol
(Gunk Labs.)

Vegetable fatty acid soap	>4%
Synthetic wetting agents	<4%
Petroleum distillates *	>80%
Coupler:	>1%
Glycol	
Water	trace

GUNK CYCLE PLUGS, POINTS AND CHAIN CLEANER (MP-1)
Solvent degreaser; aerosol
(Gunk Labs.)

Chlorinated hydrocarbons *	100%

GUNK D.S. - DE-SCALE (Liquid)
For descaling coils of steam cleaning machines
(Gunk Labs.)

Acids, organic & inorganic *	<30%
Water	>70%

Starred ingredients (*) may be responsible for major toxic effects; consult Section II.

GUNK E.B. - ENGINE BRITE ENGINE CLEANER
For degreasing automobile engines; liquid (ready-to-use)
(Gunk Labs.)

AEROSOL
Vegetable fatty acid soap	>5%
Synthetic wetting agents	<5%
Petroleum distillates *	<90%
Water	trace
Coupler:	<3%
Glycol	

BULK
Vegetable fatty acid soap	>5%
Synthetic wetting agents	<5%
Coupler:	4%
Glycols	
Petroleum distillates *	<70%
Water	<5%

GUNK E.S. - ESTEAM
(Powder)
For use in steam cleaning machines
(Gunk Labs.)

Caustic soda	<9%
Alkaline salts *	<85%
Vegetable fatty acid soap	>2%
Synthetic wetting agents	>4%
Petroleum distillates	<1%

GUNK GARAGE FLOOR, MOWER AND BAR-B-Q CLEANER (FG-1)
General degreasing; aerosol
(Gunk Labs.)

Vegetable fatty acid soap	>5%
Synthetic wetting agents	<5%
Petroleum distillates *	<90%
Coupler:	<2%
Glycol	
Water	trace

GUNK G.P. - GENERAL PURPOSE DEGREASER
Liquid (ready-to-use) degreaser
(Gunk Labs.)

Vegetable fatty acid soap	>5%
Synthetic wetting agents	<5%
Coupler:	<4%
Glycols	
Petroleum distillates *	<70%
Water	<5%

GUNK GXT 1200°F ENGINE AND HEADER PAINT
Aerosol
(Gunk Labs.)

Pigment solids *†	1-15%
Vehicle solids	10-15%
Aliphatic hydrocarbons	20-30%
Aromatic hydrocarbons *	20-30%
Chlorinated hydrocarbons *	35-45%

†*See* Pigments, Section VI, General Formulations

GUNK GXT XTRA TEMP ENGINE ENAMEL
Aerosol
(Gunk Labs.)

Pigment solids *†	1-10%
Vehicle solids	10-15%
Ketones	5-8%
Esters	5-8%
Aliphatic hydrocarbons	15-25%
Aromatic hydrocarbons *	15-25%
Chlorinated hydrocarbons *	35-45%

†*See* Pigments, Section VI, General Formulations

GUNK H.S. - HYDRO-SEAL - DECARBONIZER, DEGREASER AND PAINT STRIPPER
Diphase (Two-Layer) Liquid (Ready-to-Use)
Automotive - heavy duty
(Gunk Labs.)

Vegetable fatty acid soap	12-14%
Synthetic wetting agents	<1%
Phenolic compounds *	16-19%
Aliphatic chlorinated solvents *	45-52%
Soluble chromates	0.2%
Water	14-25%

GUNK I.S. - INDUSTRIAL SHAMPOO AND RUST-RETARDANT CONCENTRATE
For cleaning metal machinery; liquid
(Gunk Labs.)

Vegetable fatty acid soap	<10%
Synthetic wetting agents	>5%
Couplers:	<12%
Glycol ether	
Glycols	
Petroleum distillates	<5%
Water	>70%

GUNK L.H. - LIQUIK HEAVY DUTY (Liquid)
For use in steam cleaning machines
(Gunk Labs.)

Alkaline salts *	<20%
Vegetable fatty acid soap	>1%
Organic chelating agents	<4%
Water	>75%

GUNK L.M. - LIQUIK MEDIUM DUTY (Liquid)
For use in steam cleaning machines
(Gunk Labs.)

Alkaline salts *	<8%
Vegetable fatty acid soap	<9%
Synthetic wetting agents	>1%
Organic chelating agents	<2%
Water	>75%

GUNK MOTOR FLUSH (MF-2)
Engine crankcase cleaning; liquid (ready-to-use)
(Gunk Labs.)

Petroleum distillate *	<90%
Alcohol	>5%
Ester	>5%

GUNK N.M. - NEO-MET BRAKE AND ELECTRIC PARTS DRY CLEANER
Liquid (Ready-to-Use)
General dry-cleaning solvent for metal and fabric
(Gunk Labs.)

Aliphatic chlorinated solvents *	100%

GUNK N.U. - NU-CAST
(Powder)
For tank use in hot water solutions for cleaning of ferrous metal parts
(Gunk Labs.)

Caustic soda *	>50%
Alkaline salts *	>25%
Synthetic wetting agents	>5%
Organic chelating agents	>11%
Petroleum distillates	<2%

GUNK P.R. - PREM-TANK
(Powder)
For tank use in hot water solutions for cleaning of ferrous metal parts
(Gunk Labs.)

Caustic soda *	>45%
Alkaline salts *	<50%
Synthetic wetting agents	>7%
Petroleum distillates	<1%

GUNK S.C. - SUPER CONCENTRATE DEGREASER (Liquid)
(Gunk Labs.)

Synthetic wetting agents	15.0%
Coupler:	0.5%
Glycols	
Petroleum distillates *	84.5%

Never used as is; always reduced with kerosene type aliphatic solvents (usually 1 part SC to 9 parts solvent by/v.).

GUNK S.W. - SWAB CONCRETE CLEANER
(Powder)
Alkaline powder for scrubbing garage floors, driveways & patios
(Gunk Labs.)

Caustic soda	<8%
Alkaline salts *	<80%
Vegetable fatty acid soap	>4%
Synthetic wetting agents	>0.5%
Petroleum distillates	<1%
Clay	>8%

Starred ingredients (*) may be responsible for major toxic effects; consult Section II.

GUNK TAR AND BUG REMOVER (TR-1)
Automobile body degreasing and cleaning; aerosol
(Gunk Labs.)

Vegetable fatty acid soap	>7%
Synthetic wetting agents	<7%
Petroleum distillates *	>80%
Coupler:	<2%
Glycol	
Water	>2%

GUNK V.W. - CAR WASH (Powder)
For washing automobiles and other painted surfaces in water solution
(Gunk Labs.)

Alkaline salts *	<85%
Synthetic wetting agents	>15%

GUNK W.W. - WHITEWALL CLEANER (Liquid)
For scrubbing automobile tires
(Gunk Labs.)

Alkaline salts *	<8%
Vegetable fatty acid soap	<9%
Synthetic wetting agents	>1%
Organic chelating agents	<2%
Water	>75%

GUNK X-7 COMPOUND - DECARBONIZER, DEGREASER AND PAINT STRIPPER FOR TANK USE (Liquid)
Heavy-duty; automotive and industrial
(Gunk Labs.)

Vegetable fatty acid soap	>14%
Synthetic wetting agents	<1%
Phenolic compounds *	<19%
Aliphatic chlorinated solvents *	<52%
Soluble chromates	0.2%
Water	>14%

GUNSMITH'S MAGIC BLUER
Liquid gun blue
(Birchwood Casey)

Selenium *
Nitric acid *
Methanol

GUSTAFSON BOTRAN-30C
Fungicide
(Gustafson)

2,6-Dichloro-4-nitroaniline *	30%
Water	approx. 25%
Oil, emulsifiers, antifreeze, stabilizers, etc.	approx. 45%

GUSTAFSON CAPTAN 300 SEED TREATMENT
Fungicide
(Gustafson)

Captan	30%
Water	approx. 25%
Oil, emulsifiers, antifreeze, stabilizers, etc.	approx. 45%

GUSTAFSON DI-SYSTON SEED TREATMENT INSECTICIDE
(Gustafson)

Disulfoton (O,O-Diethyl S-(2-(ethylthio)ethyl) phosphorodithioate) *	95%

GUSTAFSON FLOWABLE LINDANE 40%
Insecticide
(Gustafson)

Lindane *	40%
Water	approx. 20%
Oil, emulsifiers, antifreeze, etc.	approx. 40%

GUSTAFSON METHOXYCHLOR 300
Insecticide
(Gustafson)

Methoxychlor (technical) *	30%
Water	approx. 25%
Oil, emulsifiers, antifreeze, stabilizers, etc.	approx. 45%

GUSTAFSON 42-S THIRAM FUNGICIDE AND REPELLENT, ORIGINAL FORMULATION
(Gustafson)

Thiram *	40%
Water	approx. 55%
Surfactants	approx. 5%

GUSTAFSON THIRAM-30 FUNGICIDE
(Gustafson)

Thiram *	30%
Water	approx. 35%
Oil, emulsifiers, antifreeze, stabilizers, etc.	approx. 35%

GUSTAFSON VITAVAX-34 SEED TREATMENT
Fungicide
(Gustafson)

Carboxin *	34%
Water	approx. 40%
Oil, emulsifiers, antifreeze, stabilizers, etc.	approx. 26%

GUSTASE PLUS
Gastrointestinal enzymes
(Geriatric Pharm.)

Phenobarbital *	8 mg.
Homatropine methylbromide	2.5 mg.
Gerilase	30 mg.
Geriprotase	6 mg.
Gericellulase	2 mg.

GUTHION
Insecticide
(Mobay Chemical Corp.)

Azinphos-methyl (O,O-Dimethyl S-((4-oxo-1,2,3-benzotriazin-3(4H)-yl)methyl) phosphorodithioate) *

GW PRE-BETA-2 LIQUID
Preplant herbicide for selective control of weeds in sugar beets
(Great Western Sugar Co.)

S-Ethyl cyclohexylethylthiocarbamate (Ro-Neet) *
S-2,3-Dichloroallyl diisopropylthiocarbamate (Avadex)*

GW TELONE II
Soil fumigant for controlling nematodes
(Great Western Sugar Co.)

1,3-Dichloropropene *	92%
Related chlorinated hydrocarbons	

GXT 1200°F ENGINE AND HEADER PAINT
See GUNK GXT 1200°F ENGINE AND HEADER PAINT

GXT XTRA TEMP ENGINE ENAMEL
See GUNK GXT XTRA TEMP ENGINE ENAMEL

GYLANPHEN TABLETS
Expectorant, antitussive
(Lannett)

Phenobarbital *	1/8 gr.
Extract Hyoscyamus	1/10 gr.
Terpin hydrate *	2 gr.
Glyceryl guaiacolate	1 gr.
Calcium lactate	1 gr.

GYNE-LOTRIMIN VAGINAL TABLETS
(Schering/Delbay)

Each tablet:
Clotrimazole	100 mg.
Lactose	
Povidone	
Corn starch	
Magnesium stearate	

Starred ingredients (*) may be responsible for major toxic effects; consult Section II.

GYNERGEN TABLETS
For vascular headaches
(Sandoz)

Each tablet:
Ergotamine tartrate, USP * .. 1.0 mg.

GYNETONE TABLETS (.02 & .04)
Estrogen-androgen therapy
(Schering)

Each tablet:
Ethinyl estradiol,
USP .... 0.02 mg. or 0.04 mg.
Methyltestosterone
NF .... 5 mg. or 10 mg.

H

H-101
Germicide, disinfectant
(Hillyard Chem.)

Quaternary compounds *†
Ethanolamine

'76 Ed.

†*See* Cationic surfactants

HABIT-NIP
Dog and cat repellent
(NIP-CO)

Methyl nonyl ketone 1.9%
Related compounds 0.1%

HAGERTY CARPET SHAMPOO
(Hagerty, W. J.)

Resin, copolymer of styrene and
maleic anhydride 1-10%
Aqueous Ammonium hydroxide * 1-10%
Sodium alkyl sulfate * .... >10%
Sodium salt of sarcosine 1-10%

HAGERTY COPPER AND BRASS POLISH - SWEDISH FORMULA
(Hagerty, W. J.)

Diatomaceous earth .... >10%
Silicon dioxide 1-10%
Isopropanol 1-10%
Combined amount: 1-10%
　Citric acid
　Ammonium chloride
Octyl phenoxy polyethoxy ethanol 1-10%
Mixture of Sulfur compounds
　(organo) 1-10%
Perfume .... trace

HAGERTY FORK CLEANER
(Hagerty, W.J.)

Thiourea 1-10%
Nonionic surfactant 1-10%
Alkyl aryl polyethoxy ethanol 1-10%

HAGERTY JEWEL CLEANER
(Hagerty, W.J.)

Sodium alkyl sulfate plus phos-
　phate builders 1-10%
Ammonium hydroxide .... <1%
Dye mix with EDTA .... trace

HAGERTY PEWTER POLISH
(Hagerty, W.J.)

Phosphate foam builders 1-10%
Glycerine 1-10%
Diatomaceous earth .... >10%
Mixture of ammonium and trieth-
　anolamine fatty acid soaps 1-10%
Sodium alkyl sulfate * .... >10%
Dye .... trace

HAGERTY SILVERSMITHS' POLISH
(Hagerty, W. J.)

Combined amount: .... >10%
　Bentonite
　Diatomaceous earth
Isopropanol 1-10%
Octyl phenoxy polyethoxy ethanol 1-10%
Poly alkylaryl sodium sulphonate .. trace
Polysucrose .... trace
Inorganic pigment .... trace
Formaldehyde .... trace
Organo sulfur compound 1-10%

HAGERTY SILVERSMITHS' WASH
(Hagerty, W.J.)

Sodium salt of a fatty acid 1-10%
Octyl phenoxy polyethoxy ethanol 1-10%
Glycerine 1-10%
Mixture of Organo sulfur
　compounds 1-10%
Diatomaceous earth .... >10%
Perfume .... trace
Dye .... trace

HAGERTY SPRAY CLEAN
(Hagerty, W. J.)

Sodium salt of ethylenediamine tet-
　raacetic acid 1-10%
Phosphate builder * 1-10%
Alkoxy ethanol *† 1-10%
Alkanolamide 1-10%

†*See* Nonionic surfactants

HAIR CONCERN HAIR SHAMPOO
(Sanitek)

Anionic surfactants 11.7%
Nonionic surfactants 8.0%
Potassium-coconut oil soap 6.0%
Sodium EDTA 1.6%
Amphoteric surfactant 1.0%
Isopropyl myristate 1.0%
Peppermint oil, Dow 75, Dye .... trace
Water .... balance

HALAZONE
For disinfection of drinking water
(Abbott)

Each tablet:
Halazone * .... 4 mg.
Sodium borate
Sodium chloride

HALCO GROUT
(Minwax Co.)

Portland cement* 44%
Silicon dioxide 55%
Potassium persulfate .... minor
Sodium perborate .... minor
Melamine formaldehyde resin .. minor

HALDOL (CONCENTRATE & TABLETS)
Psychotherapeutic
(McNeil Pharm.)

TABLET (each):
Haloperidol* .... 1/2 mg.; 1 mg.;
　　　　　　　　　　　2 mg.; 5 mg.;
　　　　　　　　　　　or 10 mg.
CONCENTRATE:
Haloperidol* .... 2 mg./cc

HALEY'S M-O
Laxative
(Winthrop Labs.)

Milk of magnesia 75%
Mineral oil 25%

HALLIWELL B-12 AMINO CREAM CONDITIONER
Hair conditioner
(Halliwell)

	percentage range
Water	85.0-95.0%
Emulsifying wax N.F.	<5.0%
Quaternium-18 *† and Isopropyl alcohol	<5.0%
Stearamidopropyl dimethylamine lactate	<5.0%
PEG-4 stearate	<5.0%
Milk	<5.0%
Keratin amino acid and Sodium chloride	<1.0%
Methylparaben	<1.0%
Wheat germ oil	<1.0%
Fragrance	<1.0%
FD & C Blue No. 1	trace
Propylparaben	<1.0%

†*See* Cationic surfactants

HALLIWELL OIL OF PALM SHAMPOO CONCENTRATE
(Halliwell)

	percentage range
TEA-lauryl sulfate *	40.0-60.0%
Lauramide DEA	15.0-25.0%
Water	15.0-25.0%
SD Alcohol 40	3.0-6.0%
Sodium chloride	<5.0%
Potassium chloride	<5.0%
Laureth-23	<1.0%
Fragrance	<1.0%
Methylparaben	<1.0%
D & C Yellow No. 8	trace

Starred ingredients (*) may be responsible for major toxic effects; consult Section II.

HALLIWELL PRODUCTS
Hair sprays, waving lotions, shampoos

Halliwell Products
250 Lackawanna Ave.
West Paterson, N.J. 07424

Phone: 201-256-3400

See COSMETICS, Section VI, General
Formulations

HALLS COUGH FORMULA
Antitussive
(Warner-Lambert)

Each 10 ml.:
Dextromethorphan HBr ..... 15.0 mg.
Phenylpropanolamine HCl * 37.5 mg.
Menthol .... 14.0 mg.
Eucalyptus oil .... 12.7 mg.
Alcohol 22.0%

HALL'S MENTHO-LYPTUS COUGH DROPS
*Also available in cherry, honey-lemon
and ice blue flavors*
(Warner-Lambert)

Menthol *
Eucalyptol *

HALOG CREAM 0.025%
(Halcinonide Cream 0.025%)
*Anti-inflammatory, antipruritic, vaso-
constrictive*
(Squibb)

Halcinonide
Glyceryl monostearate NF XII
Cetyl alcohol
Synthetic Spermaceti
Polysorbate 60
Propylene glycol
Dimethicone 350
Purified water

HALOG CREAM 0.1%
(Halcinonide Cream 0.1%)
*Anti-inflammatory, antipruritic, vaso-
constrictive*
(Squibb)

Halcinonide
Glyceryl monostearate NF XII
Cetyl alcohol
Synthetic Spermaceti
Isopropyl palmitate
Polysorbate 60
Propylene glycol
Purified water

HALOG OINTMENT
*Anti-inflammatory, antipruritic, and
vasoconstrictive*
(Squibb)

Each gram:
Halcinonide 0.025%; 0.1%
Polyethylene and mineral oil gel base:
  Polyethylene glycol 400
  Polyethylene glycol 6000 distearate
  Polyethylene glycol 300
  Polyethylene glycol 1540
  Butylated hydroxytoluene (preserva-
  tive)

HALOG SOLUTION
(Halcinonide Solution 0.1%)
*Anti-inflammatory, antipruritic, vaso-
constrictive*
(Squibb)

Halcinonide
Edetate disodium
Polyethylene glycol 300
Purified water
Butylated hydroxytoluene

HALORTRON
Antihistamine
(Vita Elixir Co.)

#1 (Yellow Tablet):
  Chlorprophenpridamine * .... 4 mg.

#2 (Green Timed Disintegration Cap.):
  Chlorprophenpridamine * .... 8 mg.

#3 (Green Timed Disintegration Cap.):
  Chlorprophenpridamine * .... 12 mg.

HALO SHAMPOO
(Colgate-Palmolive)

Triethanolamine C12
  sulfate *† .... about 20%
Glycerine
Water
Propylene glycol
Perfume and color
Methylcellulose gum
Fatty acid-diethanolamine condensate

†*See* Alkyl sodium sulfates

'76 Ed.

HALT
Dog repellent
(Animal Repellents)

Capsaicin 0.35%
Light Mineral oil 99.65%
Propellent:
  Nitrogen gas

HAMBLETONIAN POWDER
Tonic; veterinary
(Goshen Labs.)

Arsenic trioxide * 1%
Tartar emetic * 30%
Ferrous sulfate 39%

HAMMOND'S LINIMENT
(Brown Mfg.)

Turpentine *
Linseed oil
Sulfuric acid *

'76 Ed.

HANDI-CALK GUN CONSISTENCY
(Gibson-Homans)

Linseed, soya oils .... >10%
Petroleum thinner 1-10%
Whiting .... >10%
Talc 1-10%

HANDI-CALK WITH NEW STOP-FLO
(Gibson-Homans)

Linseed, soya oils .... >10%
Petroleum thinner 1-10%
Whiting .... >10%
Talc 1-10%

HANDI-GARD ALUMINUM ASBESTOS ROOF COATINGS
(Gibson-Homans)

Asphalt .... >10%
Aluminum pigment .... >10%
Asbestos fiber 1-10%
Calcium silicate 1-10%
Petroleum thinner * .... approx. 50%

HANDI-GARD ALUMINUM NON-FIBRED ROOF COATING
(Gibson-Homans)

Asphalt .... >10%
Aluminum pigment .... >10%
Asbestos fiber 1-10%
Calcium silicate 1-10%
Petroleum thinner * .... approx. 50%

HANDI-GARD ALUMINUM PAINT
(Gibson-Homans)

Asphalt or petroleum resin . approx. 20%
Drying oil .... >10%
Aluminum pigment .... approx. 15%
Petroleum thinner * .... approx. 50%

HANDI-GARD BOWL SETTING COMPOUND
(Gibson-Homans)

Linseed, soya oils .... approx. 10%
Petroleum oils 1-10%
Whiting .... >80%

HANDI-GARD COLD PROCESS ADHESIVE
(Gibson-Homans)

Asphalt .... >55%
Petroleum spirits * .... approx. 40%
Asbestos fiber 1-10%

HANDI-GARD FOUNDATION COATING
(Gibson-Homans)

Asphalt .... >55%
Petroleum spirits * .... approx. 40%
Asbestos fiber 1-10%

Starred ingredients (*) may be responsible for major toxic effects; consult Section II.

HANDI-GARD LEAD SEAL
(Gibson-Homans)

Aluminum silicate	10-15%
Polyvinyl chloride	1-10%
Acetone *	>40%
Wood flour	1-10%
Aromatic solvent (Xylol) *	1-10%
Calcium carbonate	40-50%

HANDI-GARD LIQUID ASBESTOS FIBRED ROOF COATING
(Gibson-Homans)

Asphalt	>55%
Petroleum spirits *	approx. 40%
Asbestos fiber	1-10%

HANDI-GARD LIQUID ASPHALT NON-FIBRED ROOF COATING
(Gibson-Homans)

Asphalt	>55%
Petroleum spirits *	approx. 40%
Asbestos fiber	1-10%

HANDI-GARD PIPE JOINT COMPOUND
(Gibson-Homans)

Linseed, soya oils	approx. 10%
Petroleum oils	1-10%
Whiting	>80%

HANDI-GARD PLASTIC ASBESTOS ROOF COATING
(Gibson-Homans)

Asphalt	>55%
Petroleum spirits *	approx. 40%
Asbestos fiber	1-10%

HANDI-GARD PLUMBERS PUTTY
(Gibson-Homans)

Linseed, soya oils	approx. 10%
Petroleum oils	1-10%
Whiting	>80%

HANDI-GARD SILICONE COATING
(Gibson-Homans)

Silicone resin	5%
Petroleum spirits *	95%

HANDI-GARD TUB & TILE CALK
(Gibson-Homans)

Acrylic resin plasticizers	approx. 10%
Whiting	45-50%
Acrylic latex emulsion	30-40%
Petroleum thinner	<1%

HANDI-GARD VINYL SPACKLING COMPOUND
(Gibson-Homans)

Polyvinyl acetate	>10%
Silica	>10%
Whiting	>10%
Water	>10%
Mercury *	trace

HANDI-GARD WOOD FORMING PLASTIC
(Gibson-Homans)

Cellulose acetate	10-20%
Acetone *	>60%
Wood flour	approx. 10%

HANDI-GLAZE
(Gibson-Homans)

Soya	>10%
Asbestos fiber	2%
Whiting	>80%
Petroleum plasticizer	1-5%

HANDI-GLAZE GUN GRADE GLAZING COMPOUND
(Gibson-Homans)

Linseed and soya oils	10-15%
Water (in emulsion)	5-8%
Whiting	35-40%
Acrylic latex emulsion	10-15%
Silica	35-40%

HANDI-PATCH VINYL SPACKLING COMPOUND
(Gibson-Homans)

Polyvinyl acetate	>10%
Silica	>10%
Whiting	>10%
Water	>10%
Mercury *	trace

HANDI-PUTTI
(Gibson-Homans)

Soya	>10%
Asbestos fiber	2%
Whiting	>80%

HANDLER SHAMPOOS AND CONDITIONERS

See THE HANDLER SHAMPOOS AND CONDITIONERS

HANDS-OFF
Germicidal cleaner
(Kem Mfg. Corp.)

Active ingred.:

Sodium metasilicate	0.214%
Tripotassium ethylenediamine tetraacetate	0.112%
n-Alkyl (60% C14, 30% C16, 5% C12, 5% C18) dimethyl benzyl ammonium chlorides	0.090%
n-Alkyl (68% C12, 32% C14) dimethyl ethylbenzyl ammonium chlorides	0.090%

Inactive ingred.:

Includes detergents, cleaners, builders, water and propellant	99.494%

HANDY KILLER
For killing potato tops
(Adams, Ralph B.)

Sodium arsenite *	40.0%

'76 Ed.

HANDYMATE #1
Cleaner and degreaser
(Sanitek)

Water	79.9%
Sodium silicate pentahydrate	6.9%
Anionic and nonionic surfactants	5.1%
Dipropylene glycol monomethyl ether (Cellosolve)	4.0%
Tetrapotassium pyrophosphate	4.0%
Dye	trace

HANDYMATE #2
Cleaner concentrate
(Sanitek)

Anionic surfactants (30% active)	8.5%
Dipropylene glycol monomethyl ether (Cellosolve)	6.0%
Sodium tripolyphosphate	5.0%
Nonionic surfactants	3.0%
Perfume	1.0%
Pine oil	0.5%
Defoamer and Dye	0.5%
Water	balance

HANDYMATE #3
Glass cleaner
(Sanitek)

Water	balance
Isopropanol	2.0%
Dipropylene glycol monomethyl ether	0.7%
Anionic surfactants	0.2%
Dimethylaminoethanol	0.2%
Ammonia	0.1%
Tetrasodium EDTA	0.1%
Dye	trace

HANFORD'S BALSAM OF MYRRH
Liniment for minor cuts, burns, muscular aches, insect bites
(Hanford, G. C.)

Alcohol (23A, denatured with acetone) *	82%
Myrrh	
Benzoin	
Chlorthymol *	

HANG-N-TOUGH
Acid bowl cleaner
(Paul Koss)

Water	>90%
Hydrogen chloride *	<10%
Isopropanol	
Thickener	trace

HANKSCRAFT VAPORIZER CLEANER TABLETS
(Hankscraft)

Citric acid	approx. 0.50 gm.
Emdex	approx. 0.49 gm.
Sterotex	approx. 0.02 gm.

HANKSCRAFT VAPORIZER FLUID
(Hankscraft)

Alcohol SDA-38B, 190 proof denatured *	57.3%
Deionized water	36.4%
Methyl salicylate U.S.P. (synthetic) *	2.5%
Menthol U.S.P. (racemic) *	2.0%
Eucalyptus oil	1.7%

HANNA PAINT PRODUCTS
Paints

Hanna Chemical Coatings Corp.
1313 Windsor Ave.
Columbus, Ohio 43211

Phone: 614-294-3361

See PAINTS, Section VI, General Formulations

HANNA'S BARN, METAL & ROOF PAINT
(Hanna Chemical Coatings Corp.)

Pigment:	35.0%
Iron oxide	14.4%
Calcium carbonate	38.6%
Barium sulfate	32.0%
Barium metaborate *	15.0%
Vehicle:	65.0%
Soya alkyd	44.3%
Urethane	3.4%
Mineral spirits *	52.3%

HANNA'S CHINO-GLOSS ENAMEL
(Hanna Chemical Coatings Corp.)

Pigment:	32.0%
Titanium dioxide	86.6%
Calcium oxide	13.4%
Vehicle:	68.0%
Soya modified alkyd	48.5%
Mineral spirits *	51.5%

HANNA'S CLEAR GLOSS LACQUER
(Hanna Chemical Coatings Corp.)

Nonvolatile:	24.50%
Nitrocellulose	
Ester gum	
Volatile:	75.50%
Aromatic hydrocarbons *	
Alcohol	
Butyl acetate *	
Ethyl acetate *	

HANNA'S CLEAR SEMI GLOSS LACQUER
(Hanna Chemical Coatings Corp.)

Nonvolatile:	18.50%
Nitrocellulose	
Castor oil	
Ester gum	
Soya oil	
Zinc stearate	
Volatile:	81.50%
Aromatic hydrocarbons *	
Aliphatic hydrocarbons *	
Alcohol	
Butyl acetate *	
Ethyl acetate *	

HANNA'S FARM & RANCH WHITE
(Hanna Chemical Coatings Corp.)

Pigment:	59.0%
Titanium dioxide	17.2%
Calcium carbonate	74.5%
Barium metaborate *	8.3%
Vehicle:	41.0%
Raw and bodied oil	55.8%
Soya alkyd	13.4%
Mineral spirits *	30.8%

HANNA'S GREEN SEAL PAINT
(Hanna Chemical Coatings Corp.)

Pigment:	56.0%
Titanium dioxide	26.2%
Aluminum	20.9%
Magnesium silicate	33.5%
Barium metaborate *	19.4%
Vehicle:	44.0%
Raw and bodied oil	45.7%
Soya alkyd	21.0%
Mineral spirits *	33.3%

HANNA'S K-28 GRAY PRIMER
(Hanna Chemical Coatings Corp.)

Pigment:	41.81%
Titanium dioxide IV	9.43%
Calcium carbonate	10.20%
Silica & silicates	11.70%
Barium metaborate *	7.53%
Zinc oxide	2.95%
Vehicle:	58.19%
Nonvolatile:	
Soya modified alkyd	24.08%
Volatile:	
Mineral spirits (Rule 66) *	31.91%
Driers* and misc. additives	2.20%

Less than 5% tint added

HANNA'S KOAT-ALL QUICK-DRY CLEAR WOOD FINISH
(Hanna Chemical Coatings Corp.)

Nonvolatile:	28.00%
Nitrocellulose-alkyd resin-Damar gum chlorinated diphenyl resin	
Volatile:	72.00%
Aromatic hydrocarbon *	
Amyl acetate *	
Butyl acetate *	
Alcohol	

HANNA'S NO. 4731 LACQUER SEALER
(Hanna Chemical Coatings Corp.)

Nonvolatile:	25.00%
Nitrocellulose	
Rosin	
Castor oil	
Soya oil	
Alkyd resin	
Zinc stearate	
Volatile:	75.00%
Aromatic hydrocarbons *	
Alcohol *	
Ketone *	
Butyl acetate *	

HANNA'S LACQUER THINNER
(Hanna Chemical Coatings Corp.)

Toluol *
Petroleum distillate
Ethyl & butyl acetate

HANNA'S LUSTRO-FINISH VARNISH STAIN
(Hanna Chemical Coatings Corp.)

Vehicle:	100.0%
Soya alkyd	43.8%
Urethane	3.3%
Mineral spirits *	52.9%

HANNA'S ODORLESS THINNER
(Hanna Chemical Coatings Corp.)

Petroleum distillate *

Starred ingredients (*) may be responsible for major toxic effects; consult Section II.

HANNA'S ONE COAT EXTERIOR PAINT
(Hanna Chemical Coatings Corp.)

Pigment:	54.0%
Titanium dioxide	40.6%
Aluminum silicate	15.0%
Magnesium silicate	24.0%
Barium metaborate *	20.4%
Vehicle:	46.0%
Raw and bodied oil	43.2%
Soya alkyd	19.9%
Mineral spirits *	36.9%

HANNA'S ONE COAT SPRAY ENAMEL
(Hanna Chemical Coatings Corp.)

Pigment:	5.33%
Carbon black	15.20%
Calcium carbonate	37.88%
Magnesium silicate	46.92%
Vehicle:	64.67%
Linseed styrene resin	7.24%
Aromatic hydrocarbons *	35.47%
Aliphatic hydrocarbons	18.63%
Halogenated hydrocarbons *	38.66%
Propellant:	30.00%
Aliphatic hydrocarbons *	100%

HANNA'S PERFECT-FLOOR ENAMEL
(Hanna Chemical Coatings Corp.)

Pigment:	34.0%
Titanium dioxide	63.8%
Calcium carbonate	25.1%
Magnesium silicate	11.1%
Vehicle:	66.0%
Soya alkyd	37.7%
Urethane	9.7%
Mineral spirits *	52.6%

HANNA'S POLYURETHANE CLEAR GLOSS
(Hanna Chemical Coatings Corp.)

Vehicle:	100.0%
Soya alkyd	10.6%
Urethane	20.1%
Mineral spirits *	69.3%

HANNA'S READY MIXED ALUMINUM
(Hanna Chemical Coatings Corp.)

Pigment:	10%
Aluminum powder	100%
Vehicle:	90%
Oil modified hydrocarbon	40%
Mineral spirits *	60%

HANNA'S SEMI GLOSS ENAMEL
(Hanna Chemical Coatings Corp.)

Pigment:	49.0%
Titanium dioxide	34.6%
Aluminum silicate	33.8%
Calcium carbonate	31.6%
Vehicle:	51.0%
Soya alkyd	41.5%
Mineral spirits *	58.5%

HANNA'S STREET MARKING PAINT
(Hanna Chemical Coatings Corp.)

Pigment:	59.0%
Titanium dioxide	22.5%
Calcium carbonate	69.5%
Zinc oxide	8.0%
Vehicle:	41.0%
Soya alkyd	31.7%
Mineral spirits *	68.3%

HANNA'S SWAN SPAR VARNISH
(Hanna Chemical Coatings Corp.)

Ester gum modified phenolic ether resin	40.00%
Mineral spirits *	60.00%
Modifying acids: Palmitic, Stearic, Oleic, Linoleic, Linolenic	

HANNA'S SWAN-WHITE ENAMEL
(Hanna Chemical Coatings Corp.)

Pigment:	32.0%
Titanium dioxide	86.5%
Calcium carbonate	13.5%
Vehicle:	68.0%
Soya alkyd	48.5%
Mineral spirits *	51.5%

HANNA'S SWAN-WHITE UNDERCOAT
(Hanna Chemical Coatings Corp.)

Pigment:	39.0%
Titanium dioxide	47.0%
Calcium carbonate	35.6%
Magnesium silicate	9.0%
Zinc stearate	8.4%
Vehicle:	61.0%
Soya alkyd	37.7%
Mineral spirits *	62.3%

HANNA'S XC-80 PRIMER
(Hanna Chemical Coatings Co.)

Pigment:	47.0%
Titanium dioxide	37.2%
Magnesium silicate	60.0%
Diatomaceous Silica	2.8%
Vehicle:	53.0%
Bodied oil	30.4%
Soya alkyd	18.1%
Mineral spirits *	51.5%

HANNA'S XC-3172 SANDING SEALER & FINISH
(Hanna Chemical Coatings Corp.)

Nonvolatile:	36.0%
Vinyl toluene vegetable oil copolymer	90.00%
Zinc stearate	10.00%
Volatile:	64.0%
Aliphatic hydrocarbons *	
Aromatic hydrocarbons *	

HAPONAL
Antispasmodic; sedative
(Jenkins Labs.)

Each capsule:	
Phenobarbital *	50 mg.
Hyoscyamine sulfate *	0.30 mg.
Hyoscine hydrobromide	0.02 mg.
Atropine sulfate	0.06 mg.

HAPPY JACK DYREEN
(Happy Jack)

Each 5 cc.:	
Sulfadiazine	83 mg.
Sulfamethazine	83 mg.
Sulfamerazine	83 mg.
Zinc sulfocarbolate	5 mg.
Salol	10 mg.
Bismuth subsalicylate	40 mg.
Pepsin	20 mg.
Tincture of Belladonna	0.2 cc.

HAPPY JACK EAR CANKER POWDER
(Happy Jack)

Zinc oxide
Boric acid *
Iodoform *

HAPPY JACK FLEA-TICK POWDER FOR DOGS & CATS
Insecticide
(Happy Jack)

1-Naphthyl-N-methylcarbamate *	5%
2,2 Methylene bis (4-chlorophenol) (Dichlorophene)	1%

HAPPY JACK FLEA TICK SPRAY FOR DOGS & CATS
Insecticide
(Happy Jack)

Pyrethrins	0.051%
Tech. Piperonyl butoxide	0.103%
N-Octyl bicycloheptene dicarboximide	0.171%
Rotenone	0.100%
Other cube resins	0.200%
Tech. Methoxychlor	0.500%
Malathion	0.250%
2,3,4,5-Bis (2-butylene tetrahydrofurfural)	0.240%
Petroleum distillates	0.312%

HAPPY JACK KENNEL DIP CONCENTRATE
Insecticide
(Happy Jack)

Gamma isomer of benzene hexachloride *	11.0%
Other isomers of benzene hexachloride	11.0%
Aromatic petroleum distillates *	73.0%

HAPPY JACK KENNEL SPRAY
Insecticide
(Happy Jack)

O,O-Dimethyl O-2,4,5-trichloro-
phenyl phosphorothioate (technical grade) 24%
Aromatic petroleum derivative
solvent * 68%

HAPPY JACK MANGE MEDICINE
Veterinary
(Happy Jack)

Vegetable oils
Sulfur
Fish oil
Turpentine *
Pine tar oil *
Carbolic acid *
Colloidal clay 5%

HAPPY JACK MILKADE
For brood female dogs; veterinary
(Happy Jack)

Salts of sodium and potassium
Calcium gluconate
Lactose
Thiamine hydrochloride .... 16 gr.

HAPPY JACK SKIN BALM
For skin irritation; veterinary
(Happy Jack)

2-Mercaptobenzothiazole 1.5%
Isopropyl alcohol 1.5%

HAPPY JACK TAPE WORM TABLETS FOR DOGS
(Happy Jack)

Each tablet:
2,2'-Dihydroxy-5,5'-
dichlorodiphenylmethane * .. 16 gr.

HAPPY JACK VITACOL
(Happy Jack)

Each capsule:
Vitamin A palmitate 12,500 USP units
Vitamin D (irradi-
ated ergosterol) 1,000 USP units
Iron (from ferrous
sulfate) * .... 30 mg.

HAPPY JACK WORM CAPSULES FOR DOGS
(Happy Jack)

n-Butyl chloride *

HARD HITTER EMULSIFIABLE CONCENTRATE

See PURINA HARD HITTER EMUL-
SIFIABLE CONCENTRATE

HARD HITTER WETTABLE POWDER

See PURINA HARD HITTER WET-
TABLE POWDER

HARD TO HOLD STYLING LOTION CONCENTRATE
(Halliwell)

	percentage range
Water	50.0-70.0%
PVP	20.0-30.0%
Urea	6.0-12.0%
Polysorbate-20	<5.0%
Methylparaben	<5.0%
Aminomethyl propanol	<5.0%
Tetrasodium EDTA	<1.0%
Fragrance	<1.0%
D & C Red No. 19	trace

HARMONYL TABLETS
Tranquilizer, antihypertensive agent
(Abbott)

Each tablet:
Deserpidine * ..... 0.1 mg. or 0.25 mg.

HARRIS FAMOUS ROACH TABLETS
Insecticide
(Harris, P. F.)

Boric acid * 40%

HART-DELTA PET SPRAY
Flea, tick and odor control
(Hart-Delta, Inc.)

Pyrethrins 0.06%
Technical Piperonyl butoxide ... 0.48%
Carbaryl (1-Naphthyl N-
methylcarbamate) 0.50%
2,2'-Thiobis (4-chloro-6-
methylphenol) 0.10%
2,3:4,5-Bis(2-butylene)tetrahydro-
2-furaldehyde 0.24%
Petroleum distillate * 12.50%

'76 Ed.

HASK PRODUCTS
Hair care products

Hask Inc.
277 Northern Blvd.
Great Neck, L.I., N.Y. 11021

Phone: 516-466-0660

See COSMETICS, Section VI, General
Formulations

HAVA-CIDE
For treatment of ear mites in dogs and cats
(Haver-Lockhart (Brand) Bayvet Div.
Cutter Labs.)

Squalene
(Hexamethyltetracosane) 25.00%
Pyrethrins 0.05%
Technical Piperonyl butoxide ... 0.50%

HAV-A-HART
(Carson Chem. Corp.)

Paradichlorobenzene * 99%
Essential oil 1%

'76 Ed.

HAVA-SPAN
For the treatment of shipping fever pneumonia in livestock
(Haver-Lockhart (Brand) Bayvet Div.
Cutter Labs.)

Each bolus:
Sulfamethazine * .... 22.5 gm.

HAVILAND NO. 132 ACID CLEANER
Rust & scale remover
(Haviland Products Co.)

Hydrochloric acid *
Organic corrosion inhibitor

'76 Ed.

HAVILAND NO. 139 ACID CLEANER
Rust remover & metal conditioner
(Haviland Products Co.)

Phosphoric acid *
Iso-propyl alcohol *
Non-ionic surfactant

'76 Ed.

HAVILAND DDVP FLY SPRAY
Liquid insecticide; ready to use
(Haviland Agricultural Chem. Co.)

Dichloro vinyl dimethyl phosphate . 1%
Petroleum distillates * 99%

'76 Ed.

HAVILAND LIQUID BOWL CLEANER
For toilet bowls
(Haviland Products Co.)

Hydrochloric acid *
Non-ionic surfactant

'76 Ed.

HAVILAND MOSQUITO KILLER (Pressurized Spray)
Insecticide
(Haviland Agricultural Chem. Co.)

Benzene hexachloride *
Chlordane *
Pyrethrins
Piperonyl butoxide
Petroleum distillate *
Propellant

'76 Ed.

HAVILAND MOSQUITO SPRAY CONCENTRATE
Insecticide
(Haviland Agricultural Chem. Co.)

Benzene hexachloride *
Chlordane *
Pyrethrins
Piperonyl butoxide
Petroleum distillates *

'76 Ed.

HAVILAND ODORLESS DISINFECTANT
Sanitizer
(Haviland Agricultural Chem. Co.)

Methyl dodecyl benzyl trimethyl am-
　monium chloride * 4%
Methyl dodecyl xylene bis (trimethyl
　ammonium chloride) 1%

'76 Ed.

HAVOLINE MOTOR OIL ION-40
(Texaco Inc.; Texaco Canada Ltd.)

Petroleum lubricating oil
Calcium detergent
Oxidation and corrosion inhibitor *†

†*See* Rust control, Section VI, General
　Formulations

HAWK
Powder detergent
(Kay Chem. Co.)

Sodium carbonate * 40-50%
Sodium tripolyphosphate 20-30%
Anionic detergent 5-15%
Sodium silicate 3-8%

HAWK AFTER SHAVE & COLOGNE
(Mennen)

SD Alcohol 40 *
Water
Fragrance
Propylene glycol
PEG-60 hydrogenated castor oil
Benzophenone-2
FD & C Yellow #5
FD & C Red #4
D & C Green #5

HAZOGEL LOTION
Antipruritic and body rub
(Nortech)

Witch hazel 70.0%
Isopropanol * 20.0%
Water 8.8%
Carbopol Resin 1.0%
Witch hazel fragrance 0.2%

HC-FORM
Dermatitis, pruritus
(Recsei Labs.)

Hydrocortisone 1%
Chlorobutanol 1%
Iodochlorhydroxyquin 3%

HC-JEL
Dermatitis, pruritus
(Recsei Labs.)

Hydrocortisone 1%
Chlorobutanol 1%

H.D. FUNGICIDE
(Dolge)

Active ingred.: 10%
　o-Benzyl-p-chlorophenol
　Soap
Inert ingred.: 90%
　Isopropanol *

HD-7 (Pressurized Spray)
Degreaser-cleaner
(Haviland Agricultural Chem. Co.)

High molecular weight Petroleum sulfo-
　nate
Non-ionic surfactant
Pine oil
Oleic acid
Cresol *
Petroleum distillates *
Propellant

'76 Ed.

HEAD FIRST HAIR CARE PRODUCTS

Head First, Inc.
6430 Sunset Blvd.
Hollywood, Calif. 90028

Phone: 213-461-4058

See COSMETICS, Section VI, General
　Formulations

HEAD & SHOULDERS LOTION
Antidandruff shampoo
(Procter & Gamble, Beauty Care Div.)

Zinc pyrithione 2%
Triethanolammonium lauryl
　sulfate* 15-20%
Triethanolamine 1-4%
Cocamide MEA 1-4%
Magnesium aluminum silicate .. 1-4%
Minor ingredients, each .... <1%
Water .... >50%

HEADS UP CREAM
(Gillette Co., Personal Care Div.)

Water
PEG-8
Petrolatum
Propylene glycol
PEG-6-32
PEG/PPG-35/9 copolymer
PEG-6 stearate
Triethanolamine
Lanolin
Carbomer-940
Sodium lauryl sarcosinate
Fragrance
Methylparaben
Propylparaben

HEAD-TO-TOE SHAMPOO
Baby shampoo
(Sanitek)

Anionic surfactants 9.2%
Potassium-coconut oil soap 8.0%
Nonionic surfactants 7.0%
Isopropyl myristate 1.0%
Sodium EDTA 0.8%
Peppermint, Formalin, Dye .... trace
Water .... balance

HEADWAY

See VICKS HEADWAY

HEATABS
For excessive perspiration
(Amlab)

Each tablet:
　Sodium chloride .... 7 gr.
　Sucrose .... 3 gr.
　Vitamin B1 .... 0.05 mg.
　Vitamin C .... 1.5 mg.

HEATHER COSMETICS
(Whitehall Labs.)

Whitehall Laboratories
Div. American Home Products Corp.
685 Third Ave.
New York, N.Y. 10017

Phone: 212-986-1000

See COSMETICS, Section VI, General
　Formulations

HEAT-REM HEAT RESISTANT PAINT
(Speco)

Chrome *
Iron
Aluminum
Copper *
Titanium
Hydrocarbon vehicle
Resins
Plasticizers
Coal tar solvents *

'76 Ed.

HEATROL
Electrolyte replacement for perspiration losses
(Cross)

Each tablet:
Sodium chloride *
Potassium chloride *
Magnesium carbonate
Tricalcium phosphate

HEAVY BODIED KLEAN-STRIP
Paint remover
(Klean-Strip)

Chlorinated hydrocarbons *	<80%
Alcohols (<4% methanol)	>20%
Thickeners & Inhibitors	<10%

HEDGE-TRIM
See SCIENCE HEDGE-TRIM

HEET
Rubefacient
(Whitehall Labs.)

Alcohol	53%
Capsicum *	
Methyl salicylate *	
Camphor *	

HEET AEROSOL
Counter-irritant analgesic
(Whitehall Labs.)

Methyl salicylate *
Menthol *
Methyl nicotinate
Alcohol
Camphor *

HEIL-OEL
Relief of arthritis and rheumatism pains
(Fahrney)

Alcohol *	72%
Camphor *	
Oil of cloves	
Oil of sassafras *	
Oil of turpentine *	

HEL-CAT
(Calgon Corp., Commercial Div.)

Sodium silicate
Complex phosphate *
Synthetic wetting agents *†
Water

†*See* Synthetic detergents

HELENA RUBINSTEIN COSMETIC PRODUCTS

Helena Rubinstein, Inc.
300 Park Ave.
New York, N.Y. 10022

Phone: 212-935-5300

See COSMETICS, Section VI, General Formulations

HELENE CURTIS HAIR CARE PRODUCTS & TOILETRIES

Helene Curtis Industries, Inc.
4401 W. North Ave.
Chicago, Ill. 60639

Phone: 312-292-2264

See COSMETICS, Section VI, General Formulations

HEMA-C META-KAPS
For iron deficiency anemia
(Sutliff & Case)

Each Meta-Kap:	
Ferrous fumarate *	300 mg.
Ascorbic acid	200 mg.

'76 Ed.

HEMA-COMBISTIX
Urine diagnostic test for occult blood, glucose, protein and for the determination of pH
(Ames)

Protein test area: see ALBUSTIX
pH test area: see BILI-LABSTIX
Glucose test area: see CLINISTIX
Occult blood test area: see HEMASTIX

HEMASTIX
Urine occult blood test reagent strip
(Ames)

Ortho-tolidine
Peroxide
Citrate buffers
Gum arabic
Gelatin
Chloroform
Quinine alkaloid

HEMATRIN
Therapeutic hematinic formula
(Towne, Paulsen)

Each Captab:	
Iron *	50 mg.
Polyvitamins & minerals	

HEMATROL
Topical hemostat for dogs and cats
(Burns-Biotec)

Basic ferric sulfate (equiv. to 22% w/v iron) *

HEMODYNE RECTAL OINTMENT
Anesthetic
(Wesley Pharm.)

Diperodon hydrochloride
Zinc oxide
Bismuth subcarbonate
Pyrilamine maleate *
Cod liver oil
Phenylephrine hydrochloride

HEMOR-RID
Rectal ointment
(Columbia Med.)

Zinc oxide
Diperodon HCl
Bismuth subcarbonate
Pyrilamine maleate *
Phenylephrine HCl *
Cod liver oil-petrolatum base

HEMORRIN RECTAL OINTMENT
For temporary symptomatic relief of hemorrhoids
(Jeffrey Martin, Inc.)

Active ingred. gram:	
Bismuth subgallate	2.25%
Bismuth resorcin compound	1.75%
Peruvian balsam	1.80%
Zinc oxide	11.00%

Also contains:
Benzyl benzoate
Bismuth subiodide
Calcium phosphate
Kaolin
Liquid petrolatum-cocoa butter-polyethylene wax base
Glyceryl monooleate
Glyceryl monostearate

HEMORRIN SUPPOSITORIES
For temporary symptomatic relief of hemorrhoids
(Jeffrey Martin, Inc.)

Each suppository:	
Bismuth subgallate	2.25%
Bismuth resorcin compound	1.75%
Peruvian balsam	1.80%
Zinc oxide	11.00%

Benzyl benzoate
Bismuth subiodide
Calcium phosphate
Coloring
Hydrogenated vegetable oil base

HEMOTONE ARTERIAL FLUID
Embalming supply
(Royal Bond)

| Formaldehyde * | 25% |
| Methanol * | |

HENRY FIELD'S BUG DUST
Insecticide, fungicide
(Henry Field Seed & Nursery Co.)

Methoxychlor (technical)	3.00%
Rotenone	0.75%
Other cube resins	1.50%
Zineb	3.25%
Sulfur	5.00%

HENRY FIELD'S CRAB GRASS CONTROL
Pre-emergence herbicide
(Henry Field Seed & Nursery Co.)

Dacthal (Dimethyl ester of tetrachloroterephthalic acid) 4.16%

HENRY FIELD'S GARDEN WEEDER
Pre-emergence herbicide
(Henry Field Seed & Nursery Co.)

Dacthal granules (Dimethyl ester of
tetrachloroterephthalic acid) 5.0%

HENRY FIELD'S GLADIOLUS AND BULB DUST
Insecticide, fungicide
(Henry Field Seed & Nursery Co.)

Thiram *	5.0%
Zineb	3.9%
Gamma isomer of benzene hexa-chloride from lindane	1.0%

HENRY FIELD'S GRANULAR SOIL INSECTICIDE
(Henry Field Seed & Nursery Co.)

Diazinon * 14.3%

HENRY FIELD'S GREEN THUMB PLANT FOOD
(Henry Field Seed & Nursery Co.)

Total Nitrogen	10%
Phosphoric acid (available P2O5) *	52%
Potash (water soluble)	17%

HENRY FIELD'S LAWN WEED KILLER
Herbicide
(Henry Field Seed & Nursery Co.)

2,4-Dichlorophenoxyacetic acid,
isooctyl ester 2.41%

HENRY FIELD'S MULTI PURPOSE SPRAY
Insecticide & fungicide
(Henry Field Seed & Nursery Co.)

Methoxychlor (technical) *	15.00%
Captan	10.00%
Malathion *	5.00%

HENRY FIELD'S 3.73% PRAMITOL VEGETATION KILLER
(Henry Field Seed & Nursery Co.)

Prometone	3.73%
Petroleum distillate *	80.91%

HENRY FIELD'S TOMATO DUST
Insecticide & fungicide
(Henry Field Seed & Nursery Co.)

Zineb	6.00%
Carbaryl *	4.00%

HEPAHYDRIN TABLETS
Laxative
(Comatic)

Each tablet:
Dehydrocholic acid * .... 3.75 gr.

HEPP-IRON DROPS
Dietary supplement
(Norgine Labs.)

Each cc:
Vitamin B12	25 mcg.
Iron ammonium citrate (equiv. to 20 mg. of iron) *	120 mg.
Thiamine HCl	10 mg.
Pyridoxine HCl	2 mg.
Biotin	2.5 mcg.

HEPTALUBE
Seed treatment
(Techne Corp.)

Heptachlor (Heptachloro-4,7-methanotetrahydroindene) *	25.0%
Related compounds	9.7%

'76 Ed.

HEPTUNA PLUS CAPSULES
Fortified iron supplement
(Roerig)

Each capsule:
Ferrous sulfate, dried, USP * .. 311 mg.
Plus multivitamins and minerals

HERALD TAR SHAMPOO
(Herald Pharm.)

Penetrating surface active cleansers *
Wetting agents *
Purified fraction of Lanolin
Herald tar (equiv. to 2% crude coal tar
USP) *†

†*See* Coal tar

HERB-ALL

See KERR-McGEE HERB-ALL

HERBAL NORFORMS
Feminine hygiene
(Norwich-Eaton)

Each suppository:
Methylbenzethonium chloride	<1%
Lactic acid	trace
Methylparaben	<1%
Fragrance	
In a water-dispersible base

HERBAN 80% WP
Herbicide
(Hercules Incorporated)

Norea (3-(Hexahydro-4,7-methanoindan-5-yl)-1,1-dimethylurea) *	76%
Related reaction products	4%

HERBEX G.O.S. SHAMPOO
(Parker Herbex)

Glycerinated soap solution

HERBEX HAIR CONDITIONER NO. 3
(Parker Herbex)

Glycerin
Sulfonated castor oil *
Chloral hydrate (deriv. of
chloral) .... 0.221 gm./fl.oz.
Alcohol   0.03%/v
Colocynth extract *

HERBEX HAIR & SCALP FRESHENER NO. 1
(Parker Herbex)

Alcohol 14.76%/v
Mullein ext.
Jaborandi ext.
Stoneroot ext.
Figwort herb ext.
Soap bark ext.

HERBEX HAIR & SCALP FRESHENER NO. 2
(Parker Herbex)

Alcohol	14.76%/v
Nux vomica ext.	0.008 gm./fl.oz.
Strychnine alkaloid *	0.6 mg./fl.oz.
Colocynth ext. *	
Capsicum ext. *	

HERBEX HAIR SOFTENER
(Parker Herbex)

Turkey red oil *
Sodium carbonate
Glycerin

HERBEX SHAMPOO
(Parker Herbex)

Mild soap solution

HERBEX S.P. PINK OINTMENT
For dandruff
(Parker Herbex)

Thymol *
Sulfur
Salicylic acid *

HERBEX S.P. YELLOW OINTMENT
Hairdressing, conditioner
(Parker Herbex)

Sulfur
Salicylic acid *
CP Glycerin
Petroleum base

HERBEX TRIPLE X
Hair conditioner
(Parker Herbex)

Chloral hydrate (deriv. of
   chloral) .... 0.11 gm./fl.oz.
Alcohol 36.64%/v
Jaborandi ext.
Colocynth ext. *
Capsicum ext. *
Mullein ext.
Glycerin

HERBEX WHITE OINTMENT
Hairdressing
(Parker Herbex)

Beeswax
Ceresin
Cetyl alcohol

HERBISAN 5
Herbicide
(Fike Chemicals)

Diethyl dithiobis(thionoformate) *

HERBIZOLE
Non-selective weed herbicide
(Fairmount Chem. Co.)

Amitrole (3-Amino-1,2,4-triazole)   21.1%

HERBOLD LOTION
Home permanent wave
(Herbold Lab.)

Ammonium thioglycolate 4-5%
Ammonium hydroxide
Ammonium carbonate
Wetting agent
Perfume oil
Water

                   '76 Ed.

pH 8-9.5

HERCULES BOILER LIQUID
Repairs leaks in heating boilers
(Hercules Chem.)

Tannin extract
Colloidal clay
Wood flour

HERCULES CESSPOOL CLEANER
(Hercules Chem.)

Sodium hydroxide * 100%

HERCULES DRAIN PIPE CLEANER
(Hercules Chem.)

Sodium hydroxide * 70%
Sodium nitrate 25%
Aluminum

HERCULES INK REMOVER
(Kohnstamm)

Denatured Alcohol
Potassium oleate
Hexylene glycol
Toluene *

                   '76 Ed.

HERCULES PENETRATING OIL
(Hercules Chem.)

Mineral spirits * .... >90%
Molybdenum disulphide * 2%

HERCULES R.D. ROOT DESTROYER
Prevents & clears root-blocked sewers
(Hercules Chem.)

Copper sulfate pentahydrate * ... 96.9%

HERCULES TOILET BOWL CLEANER
(Hercules Chem.)

Sodium bisulfate * .... >90%

HERITAGE CLEAR GLOSS
(Touraine Paints, Inc.)

Thinner*† and Drier* 54.5%
Alkyd resin non-volatile 45.5%

                   '76 Ed.

†See Thinners, Section VI, General Formulations

HERITAGE SATIN
(Touraine Paints, Inc.)

Silica 7.6%
Thinner*† and Drier* 58.3%
Alkyd resin non-volatile 34.1%

                   '76 Ed.

†See Thinners, Section VI, General Formulations

HERITAGE SEMI GLOSS
(Touraine Paints, Inc.)

Silica 5.0%
Thinner*† and Drier* 60.4%
Alkyd resin non-volatile 34.6%

                   '76 Ed.

†See Thinners, Section VI, General Formulations

HERPLEX LIQUIFILM
Ophthalmic solution
(Allergan Pharm.)

Idoxuridine 0.1%
Polyvinyl alcohol 1.4%

HERSHEY ESTATES COCOA BUTTER SOAP
(HERCO)

Saponified with Caustic soda:
  Cocoa butter
  Coconut oil
Glycerine 8-10%
Titanium dioxide .... 0.15 to 0.2%
Monsanto Soapanox
  preservative .... 0.010 to 0.015%

HESSBOMB 1382 WITH BIOALLETHRIN
Insecticide
(Hess & Clark)

Water 67.900%
Bio-allethrin 0.200%
Related compounds 0.190%
Aromatic hydrocarbons 0.272%
Aliphatic hydrocarbon
  propellant 30.000%

HESS & CLARK DAIRY & BARN FOGGING SPRAY
Insecticide
(Hess & Clark)

Naled 1%
Petroleum distillates * 96%

HESS & CLARK FARM & HOME DISINFECTANT
(Hess & Clark)

Coal tar phenols (tar acids) * 14%
Neutral Coal tar oils * 56%
Anhydrous soap 20%
Glycerol .... <1%

HESS & CLARK FLY SPRAY
Insecticide
(Hess & Clark)

Petroleum distillate *	99.11%
Pine oil	0.56%
Tech. Piperonyl butoxide	0.30%
Pyrethrins	0.03%

HESS & CLARK INSECT STRIP
(Hess & Clark)

Dichlorvos *	18.6%
Related compounds	1.4%

HESS & CLARK POULTRY SPRAY & LARVICIDE
Insecticide
(Hess & Clark)

Rabon*	23.0%
Dichlorvos and related compounds	5.7%
Xylene*	48.3%

HESS & CLARK PYRENONE DAIRY FLY SPRAY II
Insecticide
(Hess & Clark)

Pyrethrins	0.1%
Piperonyl butoxide (technical)	1.0%
Petroleum distillate	0.4%

HESS & CLARK PYRENONE POULTRY HOUSE & LIVESTOCK SPRAY
Insecticide
(Hess & Clark)

Pyrethrins	5%
Piperonyl butoxide (technical)	25%
Petroleum oil *	70%

HESS & CLARK RAVAP PREMISE & LIVESTOCK SPRAY
Insecticide
(Hess & Clark)

Rabon*	23.0%
Dichlorvos and related compounds	5.7%
Xylene*	48.3%

HESS & CLARK RESIDUAL FLY SPRAY 2 EC
Insecticide
(Hess & Clark)

Dimethoate *	23.40%
Cyclohexanone	32.03%
Heavy Aromatic naphtha	36.82%
Emulsifier	5.10%
Inert ingredients (from dimethoate technical)	2.65%

HESS & CLARK TRICHLORFON POUR-ON
Insecticide
(Hess & Clark)

Trichlorfon *	8%

HESS & CLARK UDDER OINTMENT
(Hess & Clark)

Petrolatum
Lanolin
Methyl salicylate *
Oxyquinoline benzoate

HESS & CLARK VAPONA FEEDLOT 4 EC
Insecticide
(Hess & Clark)

Dichlorvos and related compounds *	43.2%
Petroleum hydrocarbons	51.8%

HESS HAIR MILK
Hair preparation
(Hess Hair)

Alcohol	25%
Lead *	
Glycerin	
Sulfur	
Perfume	

HEVI-DUTY
Highly alkaline soak tank cleaner
(Whitfield Chem.)

Caustic soda *	>10%
Sodium silicates	>10%

HEVO POWDER
Expectorant, bronchial sedative; veterinary
(Goshen Labs.)

Lobelia	2%
Ammonium chloride	10%
Arsenic trioxide *	2%
Nux vomica (strychnine 0.06%)	5%
Ferrous sulfate	5%
Sodium bicarbonate	
Sodium sulfate	

HEXABOIL DRAWING SALVE
(Columbia Med.)

Benzalkonium chloride
Diperodon HCl
Ichthammol
Carbolic acid *
Thymol *
Camphor *
Juniper tar

HEXADROL
Steroid therapy
(Organon)

TABLETS (each):
Hexadrol
(Dexamethasone) 0.50 mg.; 0.75 mg.;
1.50 mg.; 4 mg.

ELIXIR:
Hexadrol
(Dexamethasone)   0.5 mg./5 ml.

Alcohol	5%

HEXADROL CREAM
Adjunctive topical therapy in dermatoses
(Organon)

Hexadrol (Dexamethasone)	0.04%

Base: Cetyl alcohol, Stearyl alcohol, Spermaceti, Liquid petrolatum, Tween 60, Span 60, Glycerin, Sodium bisulfite, Sodium phosphate dibasic, Purified water
Preservatives:

Methylparaben	0.13%
Propylparaben	0.02%

HEXALOL TABLETS
Urinary antiseptic, antispasmodic
(Central Pharmacal Co.)

Each tablet:

Atropine sulfate	0.03 mg.
Hyoscyamine	0.03 mg.
Methenamine *	40.8 mg.
Phenyl salicylate *	18.1 mg.
Benzoic acid *	4.5 mg.
Methylene blue	5.4 mg.

HEXALUBE CREME
Antiseptic creme; veterinary
(Norden Labs.)

Hexachlorophene	0.1%

HEX DIP OR SPRAY
Veterinary - insecticide
(Carson Chemicals, Inc.)

Gamma isomer of benzene hexachloride (from lindane)	11%
Aromatic petroleum derivative solvents *	83.3%

HEXO PHENA

See MARTIN'S HEXO PHENA

HFC HAIR FIBER CONTROL
Setting lotion
(Bonat)

	percentage range
SD Alcohol 40 *	50.0-65.0%
Water	30.0-38.0%
Vinyl acetate/Crotonic acid/ Vinyl neodecanoate polymer	5.0-10.0%
Aminomethyl propanol	<1.0%
Fragrance	<1.0%
Dimethicone copolyol	<1.0%
Benzophenone-4	<1.0%
Methylparaben	<1.0%
Tetrasodium EDTA	<1.0%
Sodium bisulfite	<1.0%
May contain:	
FD & C Yellow No. 5	trace
D & C Red No. 19	trace

H.H.H. MEDICINE
Analgesic
(Aschenbach & Miller)

Oils of camphor *
Wintergreen (artificial) *
Origanum
Camphor *
Soap
Alcohol ... 52%
Ammonia

'76 Ed.

HI-BRITE MINT DISINFECTANT
(Reily Chem.)

Active ingred.: ... 40%
  Isopropyl alcohol *
  Potassium soap
  Ortho-benzyl-para-chlorophenol *
  Methyl salicylate *
  Essential oils *

HI-BRITE PINE SCENT DISINFECTANT
(Reily Chem.)

Active ingred.: ... 34.9%
  Pine oil *
  Anhydrous Potash soap
  Isopropyl alcohol *
  Ortho-benzyl-para-chlorophenol *

HI-COR-1.0, HI-COR-2.5
For relief of inflammatory dermatoses
(C & M Pharmacal)

Hydrocortisone ... 1.0%, 2.5%
Cetyl-stearyl alcohol
Petrolatum
Propylene glycol
Glycerine
Polyoxylstearate
Purified water

HI-COSAN
Hospital disinfectant
(Consolidated Chem., Inc.)

Active ingred.:
  Isopropanol *
  Quaternary ammonium salt *
Inert ingred.:
  Triethylene glycol

HIDE HOUSEHOLD & PATIO SPRAY
Insecticide
(Boord, Clarence)

2,2-Dichlorovinyl dimethyl phosphate	0.46%
Related compounds	0.04%
Petroleum hydrocarbons *	14.50%

'76 Ed.

HIDE PUFF PACK - FOR CRAWLING INSECTS
(Boord, Clarence)

Diazinon ... 1.0%

'76 Ed.

HIDE PUFF PACK - FOR MICE AND RATS
(Boord, Clarence)

Calcium salt of 2-isovaleryl-1,3-indandione * ... 2.18%

'76 Ed.

HIDE ROACH & ANT SPRAY PACK
Insecticide
(Boord, Clarence)

O,O-Diethyl O-(2-isopropyl-6-methyl-4-pyrimidinyl)phosphorothioate	0.500%
Pyrethrins	0.052%
Technical Piperonyl butoxide	0.261%
Petroleum distillate *	99.187%

'76 Ed.

HIDE ROACH & ANT TRAPS
Insecticide
(Boord, Clarence)

Decachlorooctahydro-1,3,4-metheno-2H-cyclobuta(cd)pentalen-2-one ... 0.125%

'76 Ed.

HI-DRI-FOAM RUG SHAMPOO
(National-Purity Soap)

Anionic detergents *
Emulsifiers
Antideposition agents
Brighteners

HI-DRI OIL & GREASE ABSORBENT
(Waverly Mineral Products Co.)

Aluminum-magnesium silicate
Iron oxide ... small amounts

HI-EX FOAM
High expansion fire fighting foam
(Kidde)

Surfactant *
Fatty alcohol

HIGGINS AMERICAN DRAWING INK CARMINE-RED
(Faber-Castell)

Permanent carmine ... 1-10%

HIGGINS AMERICAN WATERPROOF INDIA INK
(Faber-Castell)

Carbon colloid
Arsenic free shellac (small amounts)
Edible gelatin
Buffer elements in aqueous solution

HIGGINS ETERNAL BLACK WRITING INK
(Faber-Castell)

Carbon colloid
Nigrosine *† ... 1-10%

†*See* Aniline

HIGH LIFE, MAX KILL
See MAX KILL HIGH LIFE

HI IMPACT
Broad line marker - permanent
(Sanford Corp.)

Dyes
Resins
Glycol ethers
Alcohol

HIL-BRITE, SUPER
Self-polishing wax
(Hillyard Chem.)

Water wax emulsion

'76 Ed.

HILCOAT, SUPER NO. 503
Floor polish
(Hillyard Chem.)

Water wax emulsion

'76 Ed.

HILCO CLEANER, REGULAR AND TRIPLE STRENGTH
Powdered cleaner
(Hillyard Chem.)

Alkaline detergent *†

'76 Ed.

†*See* Detergents (synthetic)

Starred ingredients (*) may be responsible for major toxic effects; consult Section II.

HILCO LUSTRE, SUPER
Floor preparation
(Hillyard Chem.)

Water wax emulsion

'76 Ed.

HILCRETE SEAL
Floor seal
(Hillyard Chem.)

Aromatic solvent naphtha *

'76 Ed.

HILEX DRYER CYCLE FABRIC SOFTENER SHEETS
(Purex Corp.)

Cationic softener *	50-60%
Nonwoven rayon substrate	37-42%
Perfume	<1%

HILEX FABRIC SOFTENER
(Purex Corp.)

Quaternary ammonium compound *	1-5%
Fluorescent whitening agent	<1%
Preservative	<1%
Colorant	<1%
Perfume	<1%
Water	balance

HILEX-4 ALL FABRIC/ALL COLOR DRY BLEACH
(Purex Corp.)

Sodium percarbonate *†	20-25%
Sodium carbonate *	15-25%
Starch	<1%
Fluorescent whitening agent	<1%
Nonionic surfactant	<1%
Colorant	<1%
Perfume	<1%
Sodium chloride	balance

†*See* Sodium carbonate

HILEX LIQUID BLEACH
(Purex Corp.)

Sodium hypochlorite *	5 1/4%
Sodium chloride	<5%
Water	balance

HILEX LIQUID DISHWASHING DETERGENT
(Purex Corp.)

Anionic surfactant	15-20%
Urea	3-8%
Alkanolamide	<1%
Ethyl alcohol	<1%
Opacifier	<1%
Colorant	<1%
Perfume	<1%
Water	balance

HILEX 6-40 DISINFECTANT BLEACH
(Purex Corp.)

Sodium hypochlorite *	6.40%
Sodium chloride	<6%
Water	balance

HIL-FOAM
Rug shampoo
(Hillyard Chem.)

Liquid detergent *†

'76 Ed.

†*See* Detergents, Section VI, General Formulations

HIL-KOTE
(Hillyard Chem.)

Mineral spirits *

'76 Ed.

HILL CORTAC 0.50 LOTION
For acne
(Hill Dermaceuticals)

Hydrocortisone	0.50%
Sulfur	5.00%
Zinc oxide	20.00%
Isopropyl alcohol	5.00%

Flesh tint vehicle: Methylparaben, Propylparaben, Isopropyl myristate, Oat powder, Sodium propionate, Polymerized sodium salts of Alkylnaphthalene sulfonic acids, Iron oxide, Water

HILL-SHADE LOTION
Sun screen
(Hill Dermaceuticals)

p-Aminobenzoic acid *	
Alcohol	65%
Scented base	

HILLTOP DILATORS
For hard milkers; veterinary
(Hilltop)

Medicated with Tyro Ointment (Hilltop)

'76 Ed.

HILLTOP EGG WASH
Detergent, sanitizer
(Hilltop)

Alkyl(C9-C15) tolyl methyl trimethyl ammonium chloride *	5%
Sodium metasilicate pentahydrate	15%
Sodium carbonate *	20%

'76 Ed.

HILLTOP JELL OINTMENT
Veterinary
(Hilltop)

PLAIN:
Amber petrolatum

CARBOLATED:
Amber petrolatum

Carbolic acid (Phenol) *	2%

'76 Ed.

HILLTOP LINDANE SPRAY
Insecticide
(Hilltop)

Gamma isomer benzene hexachloride from lindane *	12.9%
Refined petroleum derivative *†	83.9%

'76 Ed.

†*See* Petroleum distillate

HILLTOP MAL
Insecticide for control of lice & mites in poultry houses
(Hilltop)

Malathion *	4.0%

'76 Ed.

HILLTOP PHENOTHIAZINE DRENCH WITH LEAD ARSENATE
Veterinary
(Hilltop)

Each fl. oz.:
Phenothiazine	12.5 gm.
Lead arsenate *	0.5 gm.

'76 Ed.

HILLTOP POULTRY HOUSE FUMIGANT
(Hilltop)

Furfuraldehyde *	50.00%
Formaldehyde *	18.50%
Methyl alcohol	5.00%

'76 Ed.

HILLTOP SEVIN
For control of poultry pests
(Hilltop)

Carbaryl (1-Naphthyl N-methylcarbamate) *	5%

'76 Ed.

HILLTOP SODIUM FLUORIDE (Tinted)
Vermifuge; veterinary
(Hilltop)

Sodium fluoride *	95.5%
Sodium silicofluoride	1.5%

'76 Ed.

Starred ingredients (*) may be responsible for major toxic effects; consult Section II.

HILLYARD AMMONIATED FLOOR STRIPPER (NO. 1120 & NO. 2102)
(Hillyard Chem.)

Wax remover *†
Ammonia

'76 Ed.

†*See* Wax removers, Section VI, General Formulations

HILLYARD ASPHALT TILE SEALER
(Hillyard Chem.)

Isopropyl alcohol *

'76 Ed.

HILLYARD CAR WASH NO. 719, POWDER
Cleaner
(Hillyard Chem.)

Alkaline detergent *†

'76 Ed.

†*See* Detergents (synthetic)

HILLYARD CEMENT SEAL NO. 1302
(Hillyard Chem.)

Aromatic solvent naphtha *

'76 Ed.

HILLYARD CLEANER FOR AUTOMATIC SCRUBBERS NO. 2145
(Hillyard Chem.)

Alkaline detergent *†

'76 Ed.

†*See* Detergents, Automatic dishwasher, Section VI, General Formulations

HILLYARD CONDUCTIVE FLOOR CLEANER
(Hillyard Chem.)

Synthetic detergent *

'76 Ed.

HILLYARD DEGREASER
(Hillyard Chem.)

Mineral spirits *

'76 Ed.

HILLYARD DEGREASER NO. 100
(Hillyard Chem.)

Mineral spirits *

'76 Ed.

HILLYARD DISHWASHING COMPOUND, HAND
(Hillyard Chem.)

Synthetic detergent *

'76 Ed.

HILLYARD DISINFECTANT CLEANER (NO. 1103 & NO. 2103)
(Hillyard Chem.)

Quaternary synthetic detergent *†

'76 Ed.

†*See* Cationic surfactants

HILLYARD DRY FOAM RUG SHAMPOO NO. 2105
(Hillyard Chem.)

Liquid detergent *†

'76 Ed.

†*See* Detergents, Section VI, General Formulations

HILLYARD EXTRA STRENGTH WINDOW CLEANER NO. 2106
(Hillyard Chem.)

Organic solvents *†

'76 Ed.

†*See* Aromatic hydrocarbon solvent

HILLYARD FLOOR CLEANER NO. 1100
(Hillyard Chem.)

Synthetic detergent *

'76 Ed.

HILLYARD FLOOR DRESSING NO. 1200
(Hillyard Chem.)

Petroleum oils *

'76 Ed.

HILLYARD FORMULA 777
Cleaner
(Hillyard Chem.)

Oxalic acid *

'76 Ed.

HILLYARD GLASS CLEANER NO. 2104
(Hillyard Chem.)

Organic solvents *†

'76 Ed.

†*See* Aromatic hydrocarbon solvent

HILLYARD GYM FINISH, SUPER
(Hillyard Chem.)

Mineral spirits *

'76 Ed.

HILLYARD LENS CLEANER
(Hillyard Chem.)

Organic solvents *†

'76 Ed.

†*See* Aromatic hydrocarbon solvent

HILLYARD MOP DRESSING NO. 2201
(Hillyard Chem.)

Petroleum oils *

'76 Ed.

HILLYARD NEW FORMULA LAUNDRY DETERGENT
Cleaner
(Hillyard Chem.)

Soap
Alkali *

'76 Ed.

HILLYARD PAINTS
Colortone
Gym Line Marking Enamel
(Hillyard Chem.)

Mineral spirits *

'76 Ed.

HILLYARD PORCELAIN CLEANER, LIQUID
(Hillyard Chem.)

Hydrochloric acid *

'76 Ed.

HILLYARD PORCELAIN CLEANER, RUST REMOVING
Cleaner
(Hillyard Chem.)

Oxalic acid *

'76 Ed.

HILLYARD POWDERED HAND SOAP
Cleaner
(Hillyard Chem.)

Alkali *
Soap

'76 Ed.

Starred ingredients (*) may be responsible for major toxic effects; consult Section II.

HILLYARD RENOVATOR
Cleaner
(Hillyard Chem.)

Soap
Alkali *

'76 Ed.

HILLYARD RESILIENT TILE GYM FINISH
Floor finish
(Hillyard Chem.)

Isopropyl alcohol *

'76 Ed.

HILLYARD SEAL No. 2
Floor seal
(Hillyard Chem.)

Mineral spirits *

'76 Ed.

HILLYARD SOLVENT, SPECIAL NO. 17
Remover
(Hillyard Chem.)

Organic solvent *†

'76 Ed.

†*See* Aromatic hydrocarbon solvent

HILLYARD SOLVENT, SPECIAL NO. 215
Remover
(Hillyard Chem.)

Organic solvent *†

'76 Ed.

†*See* Aromatic hydrocarbon solvent

HILLYARD SYNTHETIC CLEANER NO. 153
Cleaner
(Hillyard Chem.)

Synthetic detergent *

'76 Ed.

HILLYARD TERRAZZO SEAL
Floor sealer
(Hillyard Chem.)

Aromatic solvent naphtha *

'76 Ed.

HILLYARD WAX REMOVER
Cleaner
(Hillyard Chem.)

Liquid detergent *†
Alkali *

'76 Ed.

†*See* Detergents, Section VI, General Formulations

HILLYARD WOOD PRIMER
(Hillyard Chem.)

Mineral spirits *

'76 Ed.

HIL MAID
Cleaner
(Hillyard Chem.)

Alkali *

'76 Ed.

HIL-MIST
(Hillyard Chem.)

Organic solvents *†

'76 Ed.

†*See* Aromatic hydrocarbon solvent

HI-LO
Automatic dishwasher detergent
(Calgon Corp., Commercial Div.)

Caustic soda
Dichloroisocyanurate *
Nonionic detergent
Soda ash *
Complex phosphates *

HILO CAT EAR REMEDY
(Hilo Products)

Sulfathiazole	4.2%
Sulfanilamide	4.2%
Urea	8.4%
Benzyl alcohol	2.95%
Rotenone	0.25%
Other cube resins	0.5%

HILO CAT FLEA POWDER
(Hilo Products)

Rotenone *	1.2%
Other cube resins	2.4%
Dichlorophene (2,2'-Methylenebis (4-chlorophenol))	0.5%
Hexachlorophene (2,2'-Methylenebis (3,4,6-trichlorophenol))	0.5%

HILO CLIPPER CARE
Cools, lubricates electric clippers
(Hilo Products)

Active ingred:
Methyldodecylbenzyl trimethyl ammonium chloride	0.080%
Methyldodecylxylylene bis (trimethyl ammonium chloride)	0.020%
Isopropanol	0.820%
Essential oils	1.000%

Inert ingred:
Oils, Silicones, Propellants	98.080%

HILO DE-WORM TABLETS
Veterinary
(Hilo Products)

Each tablet:
Piperazine eq. (present as piperazine phosphate)	100 mg.

HILO DIP CONCENTRATED RINSE
Kills fleas, lice and ticks on dogs
(Hilo Products)

Rotenone	1%
Other cube resins	2%
Pine oil *	71%
Triethanolamine oleate	9%
Sulfonated castor oil	5%

HILO DOG & CAT REPELLENT TRAINER
(Hilo Products)

Methyl nonyl ketone	1.9%
Related compounds	0.1%

HILO DRY BATH FOR DOGS
Cleans, kills fleas, deodorizes
(Hilo Products)

Technical Piperonyl butoxide	0.880%
Pyrethrins	0.088%
Petroleum oil	0.352%
Inert ingredients:	98.68%
Cleaners	
Deodorants	
Propellent	

HILO DRY-CLEAN FOAM FOR CATS
Cleans, kills fleas, deodorizes
(Hilo Products)

Technical Piperonyl butoxide	0.880%
Pyrethrins	0.088%
Petroleum oil	0.352%
Inert ingredients:	98.68%
Cleaners	
Deodorants	
Propellent	

HILO EAR REMEDY FOR DOGS
(Hilo Products)

Sulfathiazole	4.2%
Sulfanilamide	4.2%
Urea	8.4%
Benzyl alcohol	2.95%
Rotenone	0.25%
Other cube resins	0.50%

HILO FIRST AID SPRAY
Bandage for dogs, cats
(Hilo Products)

Benzocaine	
Benzalkonium chloride *	
Isopropyl alcohol	7%/v

HILO FLEA & FUNGUS POWDER FOR DOGS
(Hilo Products)

Rotenone *	1.2%
Other cube resins	2.4%
Dichlorophene (2,2'-Methylenebis-(4-chlorophenol))	0.5%
Hexachlorophene (2,2'-Methylene-bis(3,4,6-trichlorophenol))	0.5%

HILO FLEA, TICK & INSECT SPRAY FOR DOGS
(Hilo Products)

Pyrethrins	0.025%
Rotenone	0.128%
Other cube extractives	0.236%
Technical Piperonyl butoxide	0.256%
Petroleum distillate	0.101%
Isopropyl alcohol *	24.254%
Butoxypolypropylene glycol *	15.000%

HILO OINTMENT
Medicated ointment for dogs
(Hilo Products)

Dichlorophene (2,2'-Methylenebis (4-chlorophenol))	1.000%
Hexachlorophene (2,2'-Methyl-enebis (3,4,6-trichlorophenol))	1.000%
Camphor oil	0.820%
Rotenone	0.045%
Other cube resins	0.100%

HILO TICK KILLER
(Hilo Products)

Petroleum distillate	0.86%
N-Octyl bicycloheptene dicarboximide	0.60%
Bis(2-butylene) tetrahydro-2-furaldehyde	0.50%
Piperonyl butoxide (technical)	0.36%
Pyrethrins	0.18%

HIL-PHENE
Disinfectant-detergent
(Hillyard Chem.)

Orthophenyl phenol *
Synthetic detergents *

'76 Ed.

HIL-SEAL
(Hillyard Chem.)

Mineral spirits*

'76 Ed.

HIL-SHEEN
Self-polishing wax
(Hillyard Chem.)

Water wax emulsion

'76 Ed.

HIL SUDS
Dish cleaner
(Hillyard Chem.)

Liquid detergent *†

'76 Ed.

†*See* Detergents, Section VI, General Formulations

HIL-TEX II
Masonry seal
(Hillyard Chem.)

Latex emulsion

'76 Ed.

HIL-TONE, SUPER
Mop dressing
(Hillyard Chem.)

Organic solvents *

'76 Ed.

HI-O-DIDE (With Saline Base)
Dietary source of iodine, expectorant; veterinary
(Bio-Ceutic)

Ethylenediamine dihydroiodide *	20 gr.
Saline base & coloring	q.s.

HI-O-DIDE IMPROVED (With Dextrose Base)
Dietary source of iodine, expectorant; veterinary
(Bio-Ceutic)

Ethylenediamine dihydroiodide *	20 gr.
Dextrose base & coloring	q.s.

HI-O-DINE
For foot rot and upper respiratory infections; veterinary
(Corn King)

Ethylenediamine dihydroiodide * 4.83%

HI-POINT 180
(U.S. Peroxygen)

Methyl ethyl ketone peroxide *	60%
Dimethyl phthalate	40%

'76 Ed.

HI-POWER INDOOR INSECT FOGGER
(Chevron)

Active ingred. (by wt.):

Pyrethrins	0.50%
Piperonyl butoxide	1.00%
N-Octyl bicycloheptene dicarboximide	1.67%
Petroleum distillate *	11.83%

Chevron emergency phone number: 415-233-3737

HIPREX
Urinary tract infections
(Merrell Dow)

Each tablet:
Methenamine hippurate * ..... 1 gm.

HIST-A-BALM MEDICATED LOTION
(Columbia Med.)

Phenyltoloxamine dihydrogen citrate	0.75%
Benzalkonium chloride	0.10%
Diperodon HCl	0.25%
Menthol *	
Camphor *	

HISTABID
Antihistamine; decongestant
(Glaxo Inc.)

Each Duracap capsule:

Chlorpheniramine maleate	8 mg.
Phenylpropanolamine hydrochloride *	75 mg.

HISTACOMP SYRUP
Antihistamine compound syrup
(Approved Pharm.)

Each 30 cc.:

Thenylpyramine HCl *	80 mg.
Ammonium chloride	10 gr.
Sodium citrate	5 gr.
Antimony potassium tartrate	1/24 gr.
Menthol & aromatics	q.s.

'76 Ed.

HISTACOMP TABLETS
Allergic symptoms and the common cold
(Approved Pharm.)

Each tablet:

Chloroprophenpyridamine maleate	2 mg.
Salicylamide	3 1/2 gr.
Phenacetin *	2 1/2 gr.
Caffeine	1/2 gr.

'76 Ed.

Starred ingredients (*) may be responsible for major toxic effects; consult Section II.

HISTA-DERFULE
For minor aches and pains due to common cold
(OJF)

Each capsule:
Powdered Opium	2 mg.
Phenacetin *	100 mg.
Atropine sulfate	0.130 mg.
Chlorpheniramine maleate	2 mg.
Salicylamide	100 mg.

HISTAGESIC (D.M. MOTTLED TABS)
(Bowman Pharm.)

Each tablet:
Phenylpropanolamine HCl *	25 mg.
Chlorpheniramine maleate	4 mg.
Dextromethorphan HBr	10 mg.
Acetaminophen	324 mg.

HISTAGESIC MODIFIED (C.T. PINK SPECKLED WITH GREEN)
(Bowman Pharm.)

Each tablet:
Acetaminophen	324 mg.
Phenylpropanolamine hydrochloride *	25 mg.
Chlorpheniramine maleate	4 mg.

HISTAJEN, JR.
Colds and allergies
(Jenkins Labs.)

Each tablet:
Chlorpheniramine maleate	1 mg.
Salicylamide *	105 mg.
Acetophenetidin *	75 mg.
Caffeine	15 mg.

HISTALET-DM SYRUP
Antihistamine, vasoconstrictor
(Reid-Provident)

Each 5 cc.:
Chlorpheniramine maleate	3.0 mg.
Dextromethorphan HBr	15.0 mg.
Pseudoephedrine HCl *	45.0 mg.

HISTALET FORTE
Antihistamine, vasoconstrictor
(Reid-Provident)

Each sustained release tablet:
Phenylpropanolamine HCl *	50 mg.
Pyrilamine maleate *	25 mg.
Chlorpheniramine maleate	4 mg.
Phenylephrine HCl	10 mg.

HISTALETS
For colds, aches & pains
(Columbia Med.)

Each tablet:
Chlorpheniramine maleate *	2 mg.
Salicylamide	3 1/2 gr.
Phenacetin *	2 1/2 gr.
Caffeine	1/2 gr.

HISTALET SYRUP
Antihistamine, vasoconstrictor
(Reid-Provident)

Each 5 cc.:
Chlorpheniramine maleate	3.0 mg.
Pseudoephedrine HCl *	45.0 mg.

HISTALET X SYRUP
Antihistamine, decongestant, expectorant
(Reid-Provident)

Each 5 cc.:
Pseudoephedrine hydrochloride *	45 mg.
Chlorpheniramine maleate	3 mg.
Guaifenesin	200 mg.

HISTALET X TABLETS
Antihistamine, decongestant, expectorant
(Reid-Provident)

Each tablet:
Pseudoephedrine hydrochloride *	120 mg.
Chlorpheniramine maleate	8 mg.
Guaifenesin	200 mg.

HISTAM DECONGESTANT TABLET
(Rawleigh)

Each tablet:
Pyrilamine maleate *	12.5 mg.
Salicylamide	195.0 mg.
Vitamin C (as sodium ascorbate)	25.0 mg.
Phenylephrine hydrochloride	5.0 mg.
Phenacetin *	130.0 mg.
Caffeine, anhydrous	32.0 mg.

'76 Ed.

HISTANA TABLETS
(Approved Pharm.)

Each tablet:
Pyrilamine maleate *	25 mg.

'76 Ed.

HISTAPRIN "C" COLD DECONGESTANT
(Pharmex)

Each capsule:
Phenylephrine HCl	5 mg.
Salicylamide	200 mg.
Chlorpheniramine maleate	2 mg.
Phenacetin *	150 mg.
Caffeine	15 mg.
Vitamin C	200 mg.

HISTAPRIN COLD TABLETS
(Pharmex)

Each tablet:
Chlorpheniramine maleate	2 mg.
Salicylamide	3 1/2 gr.
Phenacetin *	2 1/2 gr.
Caffeine	1/2 gr.

HISTAPRIN COUGH SYRUP
(Pharmex)

Pyrilamine maleate *
Ammonium chloride
Sodium citrate
Antimony potassium tartrate *
Menthol *
Aromatics
Alcohol

HISTA-VADRIN
Antihistaminic - decongestant
(Scherer Labs.)

Each tablet:
Phenylpropanolamine hydrochloride *	40 mg.
Chlorpheniramine maleate	4 mg.
Methapyrilene hydrochloride *	40 mg.
Phenylephrine hydrochloride	5 mg.

HISTA-VADRIN SYRUP
Nasal decongestant - antihistaminic
(Scherer Labs.)

Each 5 cc.:
Alcohol	2%
Phenylpropanolamine hydrochloride *	20 mg.
Chlorpheniramine maleate	2 mg.
Phenylephrine hydrochloride	2.5 mg.

HISTA-VADRIN T D
Nasal congestion
(Scherer Labs.)

Each capsule:
Phenylpropanolamine HCl *	50 mg.
Chlorpheniramine maleate	1 mg.
Pheniramine maleate	12.5 mg.
Atropine sulfate	0.024 mg.
Scopolamine hydrobromide	0.014 mg.
Hyoscyamine sulfate	0.122 mg.
total belladonna alkaloids	0.16 mg.

HISTIVITE-D COUGH SYRUP
(Vitarine)

Each fl. oz.:
Dextromethorphan hydrobromide	30 mg.
Methapyrilene fumarate *	75 mg.
Ammonium chloride	8 gr.
Ephedrine sulfate	3/8 gr.
Menthol	
Alcohol (by volume)	4.8%

HISTJEN CAPSULE
(Jenkins Labs.)

Each capsule:
Phenylpropanolamine HCl *	25 mg.
Pyrilamine maleate *	12.5 mg.
Prophenpyridamine maleate *	12.5 mg.
Phenylephrine HCl	2.5 mg.

HISTOSTAT-50
Feed additive aid in prevention of blackhead in turkeys
(Salsbury)

4-Nitrophenylarsonic acid *	50%

HISTREY (C.T. YELLOW; CREASED)
(Bowman Pharm.)

Each tablet:
Chlorpheniramine maleate * .... 4 mg.

HI STYLE CEILING WHITE PAINT
(Touraine Paints, Inc.)

Titanium dioxide	5.9%
Titanium - calcium	27.3%
Silica & silicates	33.5%
Thinner*† & Drier*	25.5%
Alkyd resin non-volatile	7.8%

'76 Ed.

†See Thinners, Section VI, General Formulations

HI STYLE FLAT BASE PAINTS
(Touraine Paints, Inc.)

BASE "AA":
Titanium calcium	49.8%
Silica	6.1%
Calcium carbonate	6.4%
Thinner*† & Drier*	28.6%
Alkyd resin solution	9.1%

WHITE BASE "B":
Titanium calcium	35.2%
Calcium carbonate	15.7%
Silicates	7.7%
Thinner*† & Drier*	30.5%
Alkyd resin non-volatile	10.9%

NEUTRAL BASE "C":
Titanium calcium	16.1%
Calcium carbonate	14.2%
Silicates	24.9%
Thinner*† & Drier*	33.0%
Alkyd resin non-volatile	11.8%

WHITE (#161):
Titanium calcium	48.5%
Silica	6.2%
Calcium carbonate	7.7%
Thinner*† & Drier*	28.6%
Alkyd resin non-volatile	9.1%

'76 Ed.

†See Thinners, Section VI, General Formulations

HI STYLE GLOSS PAINTS
(Touraine Paints, Inc.)

ALUMINUM GRAY (#275):
Titanium calcium	28.00%
Titanium dioxide	2.53%
Silicates	1.27%
Thinner*† & Drier *	34.40%
Alkyd resin non-volatile	33.80%

AQUA BLUE (#268):
See ALUMINUM GRAY (#275) - same formulation

GREEN MIST (#264):
See ALUMINUM GRAY (#275) - same formulation

PORCELAIN BLUE (#265):
See ALUMINUM GRAY (#275) - same formulation

ROSE PETAL (#274):
See ALUMINUM GRAY (#275) - same formulation

SATINWOOD (#276):
See ALUMINUM GRAY (#275) - same formulation

SUNLITE (#267):
See ALUMINUM GRAY (#275) - same formulation

WARM IVORY (#273):
See ALUMINUM GRAY (#275) - same formulation

WHITE (#261):
Titanium dioxide	19.2%
Titanium calcium	14.4%
Thinner*† & Drier *	26.5%
Alkyd resin non-volatile	37.4%

'76 Ed.

†See Thinners, Section VI, General Formulations

HI STYLE SEMI GLOSS PAINTS
(Touraine Paints, Inc.)

AUTUMN GOLD (#389):
Titanium calcium	48.5%
Silica	6.1%
Calcium carbonate	7.7%
Thinner*† & Drier *	28.6%
Alkyd resin non-volatile	9.1%
Tinting color	<5%

BUCKSKIN BEIGE (#383):
Titanium dioxide	20.1%
Calcium sulphate	5.3%
Calcium carbonate	21.6%
Thinner*† & Drier *	28.9%
Alkyd resin non-volatile	24.1%
Tinting color	<5%

CANDLELIGHT (#385):
Titanium dioxide	23.5%
Calcium sulphate	8.5%
Calcium carbonate	15.0%
Thinner*† & Drier *	28.9%
Alkyd resin non-volatile	24.1%
Tinting color	<5%

CATHAY (#378):
See BUCKSKIN BEIGE (#383) - same formulation

CELERY (#387):
See CANDLELIGHT (#385) - same formulation

CELESTE BLUE (#362):
See BUCKSKIN BEIGE (#383) - same formulation

CONGO IVORY (#370):
See CANDLELIGHT (#385) - same formulation

CORNSILK (#382):
See CANDLELIGHT (#385) - same formulation

(Continued next column)

GREEN MIST (#364):
See BUCKSKIN BEIGE (#383) - same formulation

GREEN VELVET (#384):
See BUCKSKIN BEIGE (#383) - same formulation

OFF WHITE (#379):
See CANDLELIGHT (#385) - same formulation

PARCHMENT WHITE (#388):
See CANDLELIGHT (#385) - same formulation

PORCELAIN BLUE (#365):
Titanium dioxide	16.9%
Calcium carbonate	21.6%
Calcium sulphate	8.5%
Thinner*† & Drier *	28.9%
Alkyd resin non-volatile	24.1%
Tinting color	<5%

PROVINCIAL GOLD (#386):
See AUTUMN GOLD (#389) - same formulation

ROSE PETAL (#374):
See CANDLELIGHT (#385) - same formulation

SATINWOOD (#376):
See PORCELAIN BLUE (#365) - same formulation

SPEARMINT (#381):
See BUCKSKIN BEIGE (#383) - same formulation

SUNLITE (#367):
See CANDLELIGHT (#385) - same formulation

TEAKWOOD (#366):
Titanium dioxide	20.0%
Calcium carbonate	22.6%
Calcium sulphate	6.7%
Thinner*† & Drier *	29.6%
Alkyd resin non-volatile	21.1%
Tinting color	<5%

WARM IVORY (#373):
See CANDLELIGHT (#385) - same formulation

WHITE (#361):
Titanium dioxide	23.5%
Calcium sulphate	8.5%
Calcium carbonate	15.0%
Thinner*† & Drier *	28.9%
Alkyd resin non-volatile	24.1%

'76 Ed.

†See Thinners, Section VI, General Formulations

HI-SUDS
(Calgon Corp., Commercial Div.)

Complex phosphates *
Detergent salts *†
Synthetic detergents *

†See Detergents (synthetic)

HI-T DEGREASOL
(Kleer-Flo Co.)

Petroleum solvents (of the aliphatic type) *	100%

HI-TOR GERMICIDAL DETERGENT
Institutional use
(Huntington Labs.)

Active ingred.:	17.9%
Didecyl dimethyl ammonium chloride *	7.5%
Alkyl (C12 40%, C14 50%, C16 10%) dimethyl benzyl ammonium chloride *	5.0%
Tetrasodium ethylene diamine tetraacetate	5.2%
Essential oils	0.20%

HI-TRI SOLVENT
(Dow)

Trichloroethylene (minimum) *	95%

HI-VIZ F-193 RED-ORANGE ALKYD ENAMEL
Fluorescent brushing color
(Lawter Chem.)

Pigment:	36.1%
Sulphonamide-amine-aldehyde resin (containing less than 3% fluorescent dye (lead free))	88.7%
Silica gel	11.3%
Vehicle:	63.9%
Soya alkyd resin	28.2%
Driers *	2.6%
Aliphatic hydrocarbons *	69.2%

HI-VIZ JET SPRAY
Fluorescent color
(Lawter Chem.)

Nonvolatile:	15.22%
Acrylic resin	
Sulfonamide-amine-aldehyde resin containing less than 3% fluorescent dye (lead free)	
Volatile:	37.78%
Aliphatic hydrocarbons *	
Aromatic hydrocarbons *	
Propellant:	45.00%
Halogenated hydrocarbons *	

HIWOLFIA (S.C.T. RED)
Antihypertensive
(Bowman Pharm.)

Each tablet:	
Rauwolfia serpentina powder root	50 mg.

HIWOLFIA (S.C.T. RED; OVALET)
Antihypertensive
(Bowman Pharm.)

Each tablet:	
Rauwolfia serpentina powder root	100 mg.

H-K POWDER BLEACH
(National Allied Products)

Sodium perborate *	10.0%
Optical brightener	0.2%
Sodium sesquicarbonate	89.8%

H-K RAT BAIT
Rodenticide
(Pipestone Products)

Quinoxalinylsulfanilamide (Sulfaquinoxaline)(N'-(2-quinoxalinyl)sulfanilamide)	0.025%
Warfarin ((3-alpha-Acetonylbenzyl)-4-hydroxycoumarin)	0.025%

HMS LIQUIFILM
Ophthalmic suspension
(Allergan Pharm.)

Medrysone	1.0%
Polyvinyl alcohol	1.4%
Benzalkonium chloride	
Edetate disodium	
Sodium chloride	
Potassium chloride	
Sodium phosphate monobasic, monohydrate	
Sodium phosphate dibasic, anhydrous	
Hydroxypropyl methylcellulose	
Purified water	
Sodium hydroxide or hydrochloric acid if needed to adjust the pH	

HOBBY-CRAFT PLASTER
(Bersted's)

Plaster Paris

HOBBY-CRAFT RUBBER MOLDS
(Bersted's)

Liquid latex

HOFF'S GOODLAX TABLETS
Laxative
(Goodrich-Universal)

Cascara *
Aloin *
Podophyllin *
Gentian *
Ginger

'76 Ed.

HOFF'S LINIMENT
(Goodrich-Universal)

Ammonia *
Camphor *
Turpentine *
Castile soap

'76 Ed.

HOG SARCOPTIC MANGE OIL
Veterinary
(Hilltop)

Crude petroleum oil (containing 0.25%-0.5% sulfur) *	
Creosote oil *	
Gamma isomer of benzene hexachloride	0.1%

'76 Ed.

HOLCOMB'S AEROSOL INSERID
Insecticide
(Holcomb)

Pyrethrins	<1%
Piperonyl butoxide	<1%
Diazinon *	1-10%

'76 Ed.

HOLCOMB'S ALL PURPOSE SEAL COAT
(Holcomb)

Mineral spirits *	>10%
High flash Naphtha *	>10%

'76 Ed.

HOLCOMB'S CONCRETE SEAL
(Holcomb)

Xylene *	>10%
Cyclohexanone	>10%
Methyl isobutyl ketone	>10%

'76 Ed.

HOLCOMB'S METAL LUSTER
(Holcomb)

Denatured alcohol	<10%
Oxalic acid *	1-10%
Aqueous Ammonia *	<10%

'76 Ed.

HOLCOMB'S ODOR CRYSTALS
Odor blocks
(Holcomb)

Paradichlorobenzene *	>10%

'76 Ed.

HOLCOMB'S SEAL REMOVER
(Holcomb)

Methylene chloride *	>10%

'76 Ed.

HOLCOMB'S WINDOW CLEANER
(Holcomb)

Dioxane *	>10%

'76 Ed.

HOLD
4 hour cough suppressant
(Beecham Products)

Each lozenge:	
Dextromethorphan HBr	7.5 mg.

Starred ingredients (*) may be responsible for major toxic effects; consult Section II.

HOLDTU SCHOOL PASTE
(American Crayon Co.)

This product bears the AP Seal issued by the Crayon, Water Color and Craft Institute, Inc. This seal certifies that the product contains no materials in sufficient quantities to be toxic or injurious to the human body even if ingested.

HOLIDAY CONCENTRATED TICK RID
Insecticide
(Pet Chemicals)

Methylated naphthalenes	69%
Ronnel *	16%
O,O-Diethyl O-(2-isopropyl-4-methyl-6-pyrimidinyl) phosphorothioate	5%
Inert ingred.:	10%

Polyoxyethylene sorbitol oleate laurates
Polyoxyethylene sorbitol esters of mixed fatty acids

'76 Ed.

HOLIDAY MEDICATED PET SPRAY FOR ALL DOGS
Insecticide
(Pet Chemicals)

Petroleum distillate *	22.70%
Technical Piperonyl butoxide	1.00%
Hexachlorophene	0.50%
Carbaryl	0.50%
Lanolin	0.50%
Pyrethrins	0.15%
Inert ingred.:	
S.D.A. alcohol	24.65%
Freon 11 and 12 (50-50)	50.00%

'76 Ed.

HOLLYWOOD CHEMISTS COSMETIC PRODUCTS

Hollywood Chemists
7723 Densmore Ave.
Van Nuys, Calif. 91406

Phone: 213-997-7838

See COSMETICS, Section VI, General Formulations

HOMEOPATHIC RHUS TOX 3X PILLS
(Washington Hom.)

Rhus toxicodendron, HPUS (poison ivy extract)

HONOLULU WOOD TREATING CO. PAINT THINNER
(Honolulu Wood Treating Co.)

Petroleum distillate *

HOOFGRO
Dressing, lubricant for horses' hoofs
(Goshen Labs.)

Hydrocarbon oils *†
Coal tar *
Neutral Oils *†
Soap
Phenol *

†*See* Petroleum distillate

HOPKINS AGICIDE ACTIVATOR
Spray tank adjuvant for use with pesticides
(Hopkins Agric.)

Paraffin base Petroleum oil	83%
Polyol fatty acid esters and polyethoxylated derivatives thereof	16%

HOPKINS ALFALFA AND CLOVER SPRAY
Insecticide
(Hopkins Agric.)

Methoxychlor	23.80%
Malathion	23.82%
Xylene-range aromatic solvent *	44.63%

HOPKINS ARBOTECT S
Fungicide for Dutch elm disease
(Hopkins Agric.)

Thiabendazole	1.3%
Aqueous base	98.7%

HOPKINS ARBOTECT 20-S
Fungicide for Dutch elm disease
(Hopkins Agric.)

Thiabendazole *	26.6%

HOPKINS BEAN SEED PROTECTANT
(Hopkins Agric.)

Diazinon *	25.00%
Captan	25.00%
Streptomycin sulfate	6.26%

Contains graphite

HOPKINS CYGON 2-E
Insecticide
(Hopkins Agric.)

Dimethoate *	23.4%
Xylene *	38.4%
Inert ingredients including Cyclohexanone	38.2%

HOPKINS CYTHION
Insecticide
(Hopkins Agric.)

Malathion *	91%

HOPKINS DEFOAMER II
For controlling foam in most aqueous spray systems
(Hopkins Agric.)

Dimethylpolysiloxane	7.5%

HOPKINS DIAZINON-CAPTAN SEED PROTECTANT
Insecticide, nematocide, fungicide
(Hopkins Agric.)

Diazinon *	25%
Captan	25%
Graphite	<20%
Dust base (inert)	<20%

HOPKINS DIAZINON 4 LB. E.C.
Insecticide, nematicide
(Hopkins Agric.)

Diazinon *	48%
Xylene-range aromatic solvent *	39%

HOPKINS DIAZINON SEED PROTECTANT
(Hopkins Agric.)

Diazinon *	33%

Contains Graphite

HOPKINS DICHLONE WETTABLE POWDER FUNGICIDE
(Hopkins Agric.)

Active ingred.:	50%
Dichlone *	
Inert ingred.:	50%
Diluent, surfactant, etc.	

HOPKINS DIMETHOATE 267 E.C. SYSTEMIC INSECTICIDE
(Hopkins Agric.)

Dimethoate *	30.5%
Inert ingredients including Xylene-range aromatic solvent, and Cyclohexanone	69.5%

HOPKINS 'DIOLICE' ANIMAL INSECTICIDE
For control of hornflies and lice on beef and dairy cattle and lice on swine
(Hopkins Agric.)

Coumaphos *	1%

HOPKINS DOZER LIQUID BRUSH AND WEED KILLER
(Hopkins Agric.)

Active ingred.:	32.44%
Fenuron trichloroacetate	
Inert ingred.:	67.56%
Including Petroleum naphtha, Dodecylbenzenesulfonic acid	

HOPKINS DOZER PELLETED BRUSH AND WEED KILLER
(Hopkins Agric.)

Fenuron trichloroacetate 25%

HOPKINS DUO-TOX E.C. INSECTICIDE
(Hopkins Agric.)

Toxaphene * 45%
Gamma isomer of benzene hexachlor-
　ide (from lindane) 2%
Petroleum distillate 44%

HOPKINS DUST'M
Insecticide
(Hopkins Agric.)

Tetrachlorvinphos* 3%

HOPKINS 4% EPN GRANULES
Insecticide
(Hopkins Agric.)

O-Ethyl O-(p-nitrophenyl)
　phenylphosphonothioate * 4.0%

HOPKINS FLY BAIT GRITS
(Hopkins Agric.)

Active ingred.: 1%
　Bomyl *
Inert ingred.: 99%
　Granular mineral base

HOPKINS FLY-DIE LIVESTOCK SPRAY WITH VAPONA
(Hopkins Agric.)

Dichlorvos 0.465%
Related compounds 0.035%
Piperonyl butoxide (technical) . . 0.250%
Pyrethrins 0.025%
Mineral seal oil * 49.563%
Petroleum distillate * 49.662%

HOPKINS HOG MANGE POWDER II (Wet or Dry)
(Hopkins Agric.)

Gamma isomer of benzene hexachlor-
　ide (from lindane) * 1%

HOPKINS HORSE AND STABLE INSECTICIDE
(Hopkins Agric.)

Piperonyl butoxide (technical) . . 0.35%
Pyrethrins 0.07%
Lethane 384 Regular * 1.06%
Mineral oil * 97.30%

HOPKINS LARVACIDE D-1 GRANULAR INSECTICIDE
Broad spectrum insecticide; kills adults & larvae
(Hopkins Agric.)

Chlorpyrifos 1.00%

HOPKINS LAWN AND GARDEN INSECTICIDE E.C.
(Hopkins Agric.)

Diazinon * 25%
Aromatic　petroleum　derivative
　solvent 57%

HOPKINS LAWN GRANULES
Broad spectrum insecticide; kills adults & larvae
(Hopkins Agric.)

Chlorpyrifos 0.50%

HOPKINS LINDANE EMULSIFIABLE CONCENTRATE II
Insecticide
(Hopkins Agric.)

Lindane (Gamma isomer of ben-
　zene hexachloride) * 11.44%
Xylene-range aromatic solvent . . 88.39%

HOPKINS MALATHION 57% EMULSIFIABLE LIQUID
Insecticide
(Hopkins Agric.)

Malathion * 57.00%
Xylene-range aromatic solvent * . . 29.36%

HOPKINS METHOXYCHLOR E.M.-2 E.C.
Broad spectrum insecticide
(Hopkins Agric.)

Methoxychlor 25.2%
Xylene-range aromatic solvent * . . 71.8%

HOPKINS METHOXYCHLOR EMULSIFIABLE CONCENTRATE
Insecticide
(Hopkins Agric.)

Methoxychlor (technical) * 24.8%
Xylene-range aromatic solvent * . . 70.2%
Emulsifier 5.0%

HOPKINS METHYL PARATHION (4 LB./GAL.) E.C.
Insecticide
(Hopkins Agric.)

Methyl parathion * 45.30%
Xylene 48.00%

HOPKINS NEPTUNE
All purpose wetting and spreading agent
(Hopkins Agric.)

Alkylaryl polyoxyethylene glycols
　and Propyl carbinol * 100%

HOPKINS PARATHION (8 LB./GAL.) E.C.
Insecticide
(Hopkins Agric.)

Parathion * 80.20%
Xylene 7.03%

HOPKINS PESTRIN FOGGING SPRAY-C
Space treatment for poultry houses
(Hopkins Agric.)

Pyrethrins 5%
Piperonyl butoxide (technical) 25%
Petroleum distillate * 70%

HOPKINS POULTRY AND GARDEN DUST
(Hopkins Agric.)

Carbaryl * 5%

HOPKINS PROLIN
Rodenticide
(Hopkins Agric.)

Warfarin 0.5%
Sulfaquinoxaline 0.5%

HOPKINS PROLIN PELLETS RAT AND MOUSE KILLER
(Hopkins Agric.)

Warfarin 0.025%
Sulfaquinoxaline 0.025%

HOPKINS QUINTAR 5F
Fungicide
(Hopkins Agric.)

Dichlone * 50%

HOPKINS REVENGE SYSTEMIC HERBICIDE
(Hopkins Agric.)

Sodium salt of Dalapon * 46.7%
Magnesium salt of Dalapon 7.8%
Trichloroacetic acid (sodium salt) . . 30.6%

HOPKINS RODEX BLOX
Rodenticide
(Hopkins Agric.)

Warfarin 0.025%

Starred ingredients (*) may be responsible for major toxic effects; consult Section II.

HOPKINS RODEX PELLETED BAIT
Rodenticide
(Hopkins Agric.)

Warfarin 0.025%

HOPKINS SEVIN CARBARYL BAIT
Insecticide
(Hopkins Agric.)

Carbaryl * 5%

HOPKINS SIXTY-THREE SPECIAL E.C. INSECTICIDE
(Hopkins Agric.)

Parathion * 58%
Methyl parathion * 29%

HOPKINS SLURRY ADDITIVE
(Hopkins Agric.)

Active ingred.: 60%
  Nonionic surfactant *
Inert ingred.: 40%
  Including Acetic acid and Isopropanol

HOPKINS SNAIL AND SLUG PELLETS M-2
Broad spectrum insecticide
(Hopkins Agric.)

Methiocarb * 2%

HOPKINS SODIUM TCA WEED KILLER
Liquid concentrate
(Hopkins Agric.)

Sodium trichloroacetate (trichloroacetic acid equiv. 41.5%) * 47%

HOPKINS SUPERFOAM
Agricultural foam marking agent
(Hopkins Agric.)

Alcohol sulfates *
Alkanolamides *
Butyl alcohol *

HOPKINS THE UNFOAMER
Antifoam-defoaming agent
(Hopkins Agric.)

Dimethylpolysiloxane antifoam
  compound 12.5%

HOPKINS THIODAN 3 E.C.
Insecticide
(Hopkins Agric.)

Endosulfan * 33.72%
Xylene-range aromatic solvent * 56.53%

HOPKINS TOXAPHENE 6 LB. E.C.
Insecticide
(Hopkins Agric.)

Toxaphene * 60.00%
Petroleum oils (Kerosene) 35.00%

HOPKINS UNITE
*A compatibility agent for liquid fertil-
izer-pesticide mixtures*
(Hopkins Agric.)

Acid polyglycols .... >4%
Methyl alcohol * .... <20%

HOPKINS UROX 5.5 WEED KILLER
(Hopkins Agric.)

Active ingred.: 5.5%
  Monuron trichloroacetate *
Inert ingred.: 94.5%
  Granular mineral base

HOPKINS UROX 22 WEED KILLER
(Hopkins Agric.)

Active ingred.: 22%
  Monuron trichloroacetate *
Inert ingred.: 78%
  Granular mineral base

HOPKINS VAPONA LIVESTOCK SPRAY
(Hopkins Agric.)

Dichlorvos * 0.92%
Related compounds 0.08%
Mineral seal oil * 49.50%
Petroleum distillates * 49.50%

HOPKINS VAPONA PLUS SPRAY SOLUTION
Insecticide
(Hopkins Agric.)

Dichlorvos 0.92%
Related compounds 0.08%
Technical Piperonyl butoxide ... 0.10%
Pyrethrins 0.01%
Mineral oil * 49.76%
Petroleum hydrocarbons * 49.13%

HOPKINS ZINC PHOSPHIDE MOUSE BAIT
Rodenticide
(Hopkins Agric.)

Zinc phosphide * 2.00%

HOPPE'S GUN BLUE
(Hoppe, F.)

Selenium dioxide *
Hydrochloric acid
Copper sulfate *

HOPPE'S NO. 9 SOLVENT
For care and cleaning of firearms
(Hoppe, F.)

Denatured alcohol .... about 30%
Hydrocarbon oils * .... about 30%
Aqua ammonia .... about 1%
Essential oils *
Fatty oil base

HORMONIN
Menopausal therapy
(Carnrick Labs.)

Each No. 1 tablet:
  Estriol .... 0.135 mg.
  Estrone .... 0.7 mg.
  Estradiol .... 0.3 mg.

Each No. 2 tablet:
  Estriol .... 0.27 mg.
  Estrone .... 1.4 mg.
  Estradiol .... 0.6 mg.

HOT SHOT ACTIVATED ROACH AND ANT BUG KILLER (LIQUID)
(Conwood Corp., Household Prod. Div.)

d-trans Allethrin (Allyl homolog
  of Cinerin I) 0.030%
Piperonyl butoxide (technical) . 0.060%
N-Octyl bicycloheptene
  dicarboximide 0.100%
O,O-Diethyl O-(2-isopropyl-4-
  methyl-6-
  pyrimidinyl)phosphorothioate 0.500%
Petroleum distillates * 99.235%

HOT SHOT FLY & MOSQUITO INSECT KILLER (LIQUID & PRESSURIZED)
(Conwood Corp., Household Prod. Div.)

Liquid:
  d-trans Allethrin 0.075%
  N-Octyl bicycloheptene
    dicarboximide 0.675%
  Petroleum distillates * 99.100%

Pressurized:
  Tetramethrin 0.250%
  Sumithrin 0.150%
  Petroleum distillates 9.250%

HOT SHOT IMPROVED INDOOR/OUTDOOR FORMULA HOUSE AND GARDEN PEST KILLER (PRESSURIZED)
(Conwood Corp., Household Prod. Div.)

d-trans Allethrin 0.150%
Resmethrin 0.200%
Aromatic petroleum distillate ... 0.272%

HOT SHOT IMPROVED ROACH AND ANT BUG KILLER (PRESSURIZED)
Insecticide
(Conwood Corp., Household Prod. Div.)

d-trans Allethrin	0.050%
Technical Piperonyl butoxide	0.100%
N-Octyl bicycloheptene dicarboximide	0.167%
o-Isopropoxyphenyl methylcarbamate *	0.500%
Petroleum distillates *	86.250%

HOT SHOT OUTDOOR FOGGER
Insecticide
(Conwood Corp., Household Prod. Div.)

d-trans Allethrin (Allyl homolog of Cinerin I)	0.20%
Technical Piperonyl butoxide	1.00%
Technical Methoxychlor	1.00%
2-Hydroxyethyl-n-octyl sulfide	0.95%
Related compounds	0.05%
Petroleum distillate	0.99%

HOT SHOT WASP & HORNET KILLER
(Conwood Corp., Household Prod. Div.)

Resmethrin	0.250%
Related compounds	0.034%
Aromatic petroleum hydrocarbons	0.331%
Petroleum distillate *	20.000%

"HOT-WEATHER" TABLETS
(Pharmex)

Salt	7 gr.
Dextrose	3 gr.
B complex	
Vitamin C	

HOUBIGANT COSMETICS
Perfumes & toilet preparations

Houbigant, Inc.
1135 Pleasant View Terrace West
Ridgefield, N.J. 07657

Phone: 201-941-3400

See COSMETICS, Section VI, General Formulations

HOUSE OF WESTMORE COSMETIC PRODUCTS

House of Westmore, Inc.
Pierce's Rd.
Newburgh, N.Y. 12550

Phone: 914-568-8500

See COSMETICS, Section VI, General Formulations

HOWARD TRESSES COSMETICS

Howard Tresses, Inc.
211 W. Broadway
Inwood, N.Y. 11696

Phone: 516-239-6066

See COSMETICS, Section VI, General Formulations

HP/SILOO OIL ADDITIVE
(Siloo)

Orthodichlorobenzene *
Petroleum distillates *

H-R STERILE LUBRICATING JELLY
(Holland-Rantos)

Propylene glycol
Synthetic water soluble gums
Methyl and propyl parabens

H.S. - HYDRO-SEAL - DECARBONIZER, DEGREASER AND PAINT STRIPPER
See GUNK H.S. - HYDRO-SEAL - DECARBONIZER, DEGREASER AND PAINT STRIPPER

HT 1600 ALUMINUM PAINT
For ovens, stove pipes, furnaces
(United Gilsonite)

Pigment:	17.20%
Aluminum paste - standard lining	100%
Vehicle:	82.80%
Non-volatile: Terpene resin	26.90%
Volatile: Mineral spirits *	73.10%

HTF-273 HEAT TRANSFER FLUID (HTF-273, Formula YA-273 1938-17)
Fluid for solar energy systems
(Union Carbide)

Propylene glycol	94%
Water	3%
Soluble inhibitors	3%

HTH GRANULAR & HTH TABLETS
Bactericides
(Olin Corporation)

Calcium hypochlorite *	65% and 70%

H2OFF NONFLAMMABLE PAINT REMOVER (WATER RINSABLE)
(Savogran)

Methanol *	<20%
Toluol *	<5%
Methylene chloride *	75-95%
Retardants	
Thickeners	

HUBSCO-147
For control of rats and mice
(Hub States)

3-(alpha-Acetonylfurfuryl)-4-hydroxycoumarin	0.025%

'76 Ed.

HUBSCO WEED-TOX
Herbicide
(Hub States)

Ammonium sulfamate *	48.4%

'76 Ed.

HUB STATES AUTOMATIC CLEANOUT FOGGER
Insecticide
(Hub States)

Pyrethrins	0.50%
Technical Piperonyl butoxide	4.00%
Petroleum distillates *	10.50%

'76 Ed.

HUB STATES BUG REPELLENT
(Hub States)

DEET (Diethyl toluamide) *	30%
Deodorant	

'76 Ed.

HUB STATES CONCENTRATED SPACE SPRAY
Insecticide
(Hub States)

Pyrethrins	0.30%
Technical Piperonyl butoxide	1.50%
Petroleum distillates *	18.20%

'76 Ed.

HUB STATES FOGGING INSECTICIDE
(Hub States)

Pyrethrins
Piperonyl butoxide

'76 Ed.

HUB STATES FOG OR SPRAY WITH PYRETHRINS
Insecticide
(Hub States)

Refined Petroleum oil *	98.57%
N-Octyl bicycloheptene dicarboximide	0.75%
Technical Piperonyl butoxide	0.45%
Pyrethrins	0.23%

'76 Ed.

HUB STATES HOUSEHOLD INSECT SPRAY (LIQUID)
Insecticide
(Hub States)

O,O-Diethyl O-(2-isopropyl-4-methyl-6-pyrimidinyl)phosphorothioate	0.500%
Pyrethrins	0.052%
Technical Piperonyl butoxide	0.261%
Petroleum distillate *	99.187%

'76 Ed.

HUB STATES ROACH AND ANT KILLER, PRESSURIZED
Insecticide
(Hub States)

O,O-Diethyl O-(2-isopropyl-6-methyl-4-pyrimidinyl)phosphorothioate	0.500%
Pyrethrins	0.052%
Technical Piperonyl butoxide	0.261%
Petroleum distillates *	69.187%

'76 Ed.

HUB STATES ROACH & ANT KILLER
Insecticide
(Hub States)

Diazinon *
Pyrethrins *
Piperonyl butoxide synergist

'76 Ed.

HUB STATES SELECTIVE WEED AND BRUSH KILLER AMINE FORMULA 400
Weed and brush killer
(Hub States)

Active ingred.:

Diethylethanolamine salt of 2,4-dichlorophenoxyacetic acid (2,4-dichlorophenoxyacetic acid equivalent 12.11%) *	17.54%
Diethylethanolamine salt of 2,-4,5-trichlorophenoxyacetic acid (2,4,5-trichlorophenoxyacetic acid equivalent 6.06%) *	8.84%
Inert ingred.:	73.62%
Petroleum solvents *	
Emulsifiers *	

'76 Ed.

HUB STATES SPACE SPRAY
Insecticide
(Hub States)

Pyrethrins *
Piperonyl butoxide

'76 Ed.

HUB STATES 3-WAY KILL
Residual insect spray
(Hub States)

Diazinon *
Pyrethrins *
Piperonyl butoxide

'76 Ed.

HUB STATES VAPONA FLY BAIT
Kills house flies
(Hub States)

O,O-Dimethyl O-2-2 dichlorovinyl phosphate (DDVP)	0.5%

'76 Ed.

HUB STATES WASP AND HORNET JET SPRAY
Insecticide - for outside use
(Hub States)

O,O-Diethyl O-(2-isopropyl-6-methyl-4-pyrimidinyl)phosphorothioate	0.500%
Pyrethrins	0.052%
Technical Piperonyl butoxide	0.261%
Petroleum distillates *	69.187%

'76 Ed.

HUMI-SORB
Static dehumidification of sealed containers
(Culligan)

Naturally occurring Clay, dehydrated	100%

HUMPHREYS FAMILY REMEDIES
(Humphreys)

Humphreys Pharmacal, Inc.
63 Meadows Rd.
Rutherford, N.J. 07070

Phone: 201-933-7744

HUNTER'S MAGIC MIST AIR SANITIZER
(Hunter Products)

Triethylene glycol	6.00%
Propylene glycol	4.00%
Paradiisobutylphenoxyethoxyethyl dimethyl benzyl ammonium chloride	0.20%
Anhydrous Isopropyl alcohol *	10.80%
Essential oils *	4.00%

'76 Ed.

HUNTER'S MAGIC MIST FLYING INSECT KILLER
(Hunter Products)

Pyrethrins	0.90%
Piperonyl butoxide technical	9.00%
Petroleum hydrocarbons *	10.1%
Inert ingredients:	
Fluorinated hydrocarbons (Freon)	80.00%

'76 Ed.

HUNTOLENE
Bacteriostatic dust control
(Huntington Labs.)

Dilauryl dimethyl ammonium bromide	0.25%
Petroleum distillate *	99.75%

HURRICAINE
Topical anesthetic - oral
(Beutlich, Inc.)

LIQUID or GEL (each 1 oz. bottle):

Ethyl aminobenzoate (Benzocaine)	20%
Polyethylene glycol base	

HURRICAINE SPRAY
Topical anesthetic
(Beutlich, Inc.)

Ethyl aminobenzoate (Benzocaine)	20%
Polyethylene glycol base	

"HUSH" (Pressurized)
Automotive
(Garry Labs.)

Silicone oil
Petroleum distillate *

HUSK OINTMENT
(Blistex)

Phenol	0.29%
Resorcinol	0.32%
Benzocaine	0.26%
Salicylic acid	0.26%
Base:	balance
Zinc oxide	
Bismuth subnitrate	
Vegetable fat	
Beeswax	
Balsam Peru	
Oil of cade	
Propylene glycol	
Starch	
Clove oil	

HYAMINE 10-X
Quaternary germicide
(Rohm and Haas)

Di-isobutyl cresoxy ethoxy ethyl dimethyl benzyl ammonium chloride monohydrate *	98.8%/w

HYAMINE 1622
Quaternary germicide
(Rohm and Haas)

Para-di-isobutyl phen-
oxy ethoxy ethyl di-
methyl benzyl ammo-
nium chloride * 50%/w; 98.8%/w

HYAMINE 2389
Quaternary germicide
(Rohm and Haas)

Methyl dodecyl benzyl trimethyl
ammonium chloride * 40%/w
Methyl dodecyl xylylene bistri-
methyl ammonium chloride ... 10%/w

HYAMINE 3500
Quaternary germicide
(Rohm and Haas)

N-Alkyl(50% C14, 40%
C12, 10% C16)dimethyl
benzyl ammonium
chloride * 50%/w; 80%/w

HYBAR
Sedative, spasmolytic
(Jenkins Labs.)

Each tablet:
Phenobarbital * .... 1/2 gr.
Hyoscine hydrobromide ... 0.0065 mg.
Hyoscyamine hydrobromide 0.0435 mg.

HYBEPHEN (ELIXIR & TABLETS)
Antispasmodic and sedative
(Beecham Labs.)

ELIXIR (each 5 ml.):
Phenobarbital * .... 15 mg.
Hyoscyamine sulfate ...... 0.1277 mg.
Atropine sulfate .... 0.0233 mg.
Scopolamine hydrobromide 0.0094 mg.
Alcohol 16.5%

TABLETS (each):
Phenobarbital * .... 15 mg.
Hyoscyamine sulfate ...... 0.1277 mg.
Atropine sulfate .... 0.0233 mg.
Scopolamine hydrobromide 0.0094 mg.

HYCODAN ORAL TABLETS & SYRUP
Antitussive
(Endo Labs.)

Each tablet and 5 ml.:
Hydrocodone bitartrate * .... 5.0 mg.
Homatropine methylbromide . 1.5 mg.

HYCOMINE PEDIATRIC SYRUP
Antitussive and decongestant
(Endo Labs.)

Each 5 ml.:
Hydrocodone bitartrate * ... 2.5 mg.
Phenylpropanolamine
hydrochloride * .... 12.5 mg.

HYCOMINE SYRUP
Antitussive and decongestant
(Endo Labs.)

Each 5 ml.:
Hydrocodone bitartrate * ..... 5 mg.
Phenylpropanolamine
hydrochloride * .... 25 mg.

HYCOTUSS EXPECTORANT
(Endo Labs.)

Each 5 ml.:
Hydrocodone bitartrate * ..... 5 mg.
Guaifenesin .... 100 mg.
Alcohol .... 10% v/v

HYDE OIL CIODRIN AND VAPONA INSECTICIDE
Ready-to-use animal spray solution
(Hyde Oil)

Dimethyl phosphate of alpha-
methyl-benzyl 3-hydroxy-cis-
crotonate * 1.00%
2,2-Dichlorovinyl dimethyl
phosphate 0.23%
Related compounds 0.02%
Petroleum hydrocarbons * 98.52%

HYDE OIL EMULSIFIABLE CROP OIL
(Hyde Oil)

Specially refined Petroleum
distillate * 98%
Emulsifier 2%

HYDERGINE TABLETS & SUBLINGUAL TABLETS
*Adrenergic blocking agent and vasodi-
lator*
(Sandoz)

Each sublingual tablet:
Dihydroergocor-
nine
mesylate *† .... 0.167 mg.; 0.333 mg.
Dihydroergocris-
tine mesylate *† 0.167 mg.; 0.333 mg.
Dihydroergocryp-
tine mesylate *† 0.167 mg.; 0.333 mg.

Each oral tablet:
Dihydroergocornine
mesylate *† .... 0.333 mg.
Dihydroergocristine
mesylate *† .... 0.333 mg.
Dihydroergocryptine
mesylate *† .... 0.333 mg.

†*See* Ergot

HYDRAMINE-25 & HYDRAMINE-50
Antihistaminic
(Wesley Pharm.)

Each capsule:
Diphenhydramine
hydrochloride * .... 25 or 50 mg.

HYDRA-VALVE KLEEN

See SILOO HYDRA-VALVE KLEEN

HYDRELT CREAM
Dermatoses
(Elder)

Iodochlorhydroxyquin 3%
Hydrocortisone 0.5%

HYDRIC LIQUID BOWL CLEANER
(National-Purity Soap)

Methyl dodecyl xylylene bis trimethyl ammonium chloride ... 0.05%
Methyl dodecyl benzyl (trimethyl
ammonium chloride) 0.20%
Tributyl tin chloride complex of
ethylene oxide condensate of
abietylamine (provides 0.0015%
tin) 0.01%
Hydrochloric acid * 23.90%

pH of 1% solution - less than 1

HYDRISALIC GEL
Keratolytic agent
(Pedinol)

Salicylic acid * 6%
Isopropanol *
Propylene glycol
Hydroxypropyl cellulose

HYDRISEA LOTION
*Topical treatment of hyperkeratotic
and dry skin conditions*
(Pedinol)

Dead Sea Salts concentrate 8%
Sodium
Potassium
Calcium
Magnesium chloride*

HYDRISINOL CREME
Emollient skin softener
(Pedinol)

Sulfonated hydrogenated Castor oil
Hydrogenated Vegetable oil

HYDRISINOL LOTION
*Topical treatment of dry, dehydrated,
scaly skin of feet, hands, or other
parts of body*
(Pedinol)

Sulfonated hydrogenated Castor oil N.F.
IX
Hydrogenated Vegetable oil

HYDROCHLOR
Liquid gas fumigant
(Weil Chem.)

Ethylene dichloride 70%
Carbon tetrachloride * 30%

Starred ingredients (*) may be responsible for major toxic effects; consult Section II.

HYDROCIDE INSECTICIDE
(National Chemsearch)

Petroleum distillates *
Piperonyl butoxide (tech.)
n-Octyl bicycloheptene dicarboximide *
Polyoxyethylene sorbitol mixed ethyl ether
Pyrethrins

HYDRODIURIL
Diuretic/antihypertensive
(MSD)

Each tablet:
  Hydrochlorothiazide *   25 mg.; 50 mg.; or 100 mg.

HYDRO-LITE

See ANCHOR HYDRO-LITE

HYDROPEL
Protective silicone ointment
(C & M Pharmacal)

Silicone 30%
Hydrophobic Starch derivative 10%
Sorbic acid (preservative)
Petrolatum

HYDROPHILIC PETROLATUM
Protective & lubricating dressing
(Torch)

Cholestrol .... 3 gm.
Stearyl alcohol .... 3 gm.
White wax .... 8 gm.
White petrolatum .... 86 gm.

'76 Ed.

HYDROPLUS
Antihypertensive
(Direct Div.)

Each tablet:
  Hydrochlorothiazide * ..... 50 mg.
  Reserpine .... 0.125 mg.

HYDROPRES-25 COMPRESSED TABLETS
Antihypertensive agent
(MSD)

Each tablet:
  Hydrochlorothiazide * ..... 25 mg.
  Reserpine .... 0.125 mg.

HYDROPRES-50 COMPRESSED TABLETS
Antihypertensive agent
(MSD)

Each tablet:
  Hydrochlorothiazide * ..... 50 mg.
  Reserpine .... 0.125 mg.

HYDROSAL LIQUID
For skin irritations
(Hydrosal)

Colloidal Aluminum acetate

'76 Ed.

HYDROSAL OINTMENT
For skin irritations
(Hydrosal)

Colloidal Aluminum acetate
Bland emollient base

'76 Ed.

HYDRO-SEAL - H.S. - DECARBONIZER, DEGREASER AND PAINT STRIPPER

See GUNK H.S. - HYDRO-SEAL - DECARBONIZER, DEGREASER AND PAINT STRIPPER

HYDRO-SERPINE-25 & HYDRO-SERPINE-50
Antihypertensive
(Columbia Med.)

Each tablet:
  Hydrochlorothiazide * . 25 mg.; 50 mg.
  Reserpine .... 0.125 mg.

HYDROSOLVE
Degreaser
(Dolge)

Mineral spirits *

HYDROTHOL 47
Herbicide
(Pennwalt)

Liquid:
  Endothall as dimethylco-coamine salt * .... 1.5 lb./gal.

Granular:
  Endothall as dimethylco-coamine salt * 5%

HYDROTHOL 191
Herbicide
(Pennwalt)

Liquid:
  Endothall as monodimethyl-cocoamine salt * .... 2 lb./gal.

Granular:
  Endothall as monodimethyl-cocoamine salt * 5%

HY-FLOW
Hard contact lens wetting solution
(CooperVision Pharm.)

Polyvinyl alcohol
Hydroxyethylcellulose
Potassium chloride
Sodium chloride
Benzalkonium chloride 0.01%
Disodium edetate 0.025%

HY-FOAM CONCENTRATE
Germicidal, fungicidal, mildewcidal rug & upholstery shampoo
(Barco)

o-Benzyl-p-chlorophenol 3.50%
Inert ingredients: 96.50%
  Surfactants
  Cleaning compounds
  Degreasers

'76 Ed.

HYGA-COLOR
Colored dustless chalkboard chalk
(American Crayon Co.)

This product bears the CP Seal issued by the Crayon, Water Color and Craft Institute, Inc. This seal certifies that the product contains no materials in sufficient quantities to be toxic or injurious to the human body even if ingested.

HYGIEIA WHITE DUSTLESS CHALK
(American Crayon Co.)

This product bears the CP Seal issued by the Crayon, Water Color and Craft Institute, Inc. This seal certifies that the product contains no materials in sufficient quantities to be toxic or injurious to the human body even if ingested.

HY-GRADE LOTION
Hand lotion
(Hy-Grade Labs.)

Isopropyl alcohol *
Glycerin
Camphor *
Ammonia water * 2%

HY-GRO ORCHID PLANT FOOD
(Plantabbs)

Nitrogen (as potassium nitrate, ammonium phosphate, urea) * ...... not less than 18%
Phosphoric acid (as ammonium phosphate, monocalcium phosphate) * ... not less than 18%
Potash (as potassium nitrate) * .... not less than 18%
Chlorine .... not more than 0.5%
Ferrous sulphate 0.15%
Boric acid 0.029%
Magnesium sulfate 0.8%
Manganese sulfate 0.16%
Copper sulfate 0.06%
Zinc sulfate 0.09%
Sodium molybdate 0.009%

See Fertilizers, Section VI, General Formulations

Starred ingredients (*) may be responsible for major toxic effects; consult Section II.

HYGROTON TABLETS
Oral antihypertensive-diuretic
(USV)

Each tablet:
Chlorthalidone (3-Hy-
droxy-3-(4-chloro-3-
sulfamylphenyl)
phthalimidine) * ... 50 mg; 100 mg.

HY-HEX INSECT KILLER
(Hysan Corp.)

Pyrethrins 0.20%
Piperonyl butoxide technical 0.72%
N-Octyl bicycloheptene
dicarboximide 0.40%
Petroleum distillates 8.68%

HYKALOID
(Jenkins Labs.)

Each tablet:
Phenobarbital .... 1/8 gr.
Atropine .... 1/1000 gr.
Kaolin .... 5 gr.
Aluminum hydroxide gel ... 2 1/2 gr.

HYKIL (AEROSOL)
*Insecticide; commercial and institu-
tional use*
(Hysan Corp.)

Petroleum distillate *
N-Octyl bicycloheptene dicarboximide *
Technical Piperonyl butoxide
Pyrethrins
Inert ingredients: 80%
Dichloro difluoro methane
Trichloro monofluoro methane

HY-KIL FLY & ROACH SPRAY
Institutional and commercial use
(Hysan Corp.)

Active ingredients: 100%
Petroleum distillate *
N-Octyl bicycloheptene
dicarboximide *
Technical Piperonyl butoxide
Pyrethrins

HY-KLOR C LIQUID BLEACH CONCENTRATE
(National Allied Products)

Sodium hypochlorite * 12.0%
Salt 10.0%
Water 78.0%

HY-LO
Insecticide
(Sweeney, W.R.)

Pyrethrins 0.5%

HYMOSA
Antirheumatic
(Walker Pharm.)

Alcohol 18 1/2%
Sodium salicylate * .... 16 gr.
Sodium citrate .... 8 gr.
Potassium iodide * .... 4 gr.
Caffeine citrate .... 1/2 gr.
Cimicifuga tr. .... 48 m.
Colchicum fl. ext. .... 5 gr.
Colchicine * .... 1/60 gr.

'76 Ed.

HYMO-SALVA
Counterirritant, local analgesic
(Walker Pharm.)

Methyl salicylate *
Menthol *
Camphor *
Capsicum
Lanolin
Cocoa butter
Petrolatum

'76 Ed.

HY-N.B.P. OINTMENT
(Bowman Pharm.)

Hydrocortisone 1%
Bacitracin
Neomycin
Polymyxin

HY-O-DINE
*Iodine germicide; institutional and
commercial use*
(Hysan Corp.)

Nonyl phenoxy polyethoxyethy-
lene ethanol iodine complex ... 4.375%
Iso-octyl phenoxy polyethoxy
ethanol iodine complex (providing 0.875% titratable iodine) .. 5.245%
Phosphoric acid * 2.338%
Hydrogen chloride * 2.563%

HYPER-ESS
For hypertension
(Jenkins Labs.)

Each tablet:
Potassium nitrate * .... 3 gr.
Ext. Viscus album * .... 1/4 gr.
Ext. Veratrum viride * .... 0.08 gr.
Ext. Hyoscyamus .... 1/4 gr.
Phenobarbital * .... 1/4 gr.

HY-PINE 7
*Disinfectant; institutional and commer-
cial use*
(Hysan Corp.)

Terpineols *
Sodium and potassium 4 and 6 chloro-2-
phenylphenate *
Soap
Pine oil *
Inert ingred.: 76.36%
Water

HYPNOCAINE FIRST AID SPRAY
(Barfred Research Labs.)

Hypnocaine (brand of propasin)
Menthol *
Camphor *
Benzalkonium chloride *
Isopropanol
Aromatic oils *
Freon propellant

'76 Ed.

HYPNOCAINE LOTION
For minor skin pain
(Barfred Research Labs.)

Aluminum acetate
Hypnocaine (brand of propasin)
Benzyl alcohol *
Benzalkonium chloride *
Menthol *
Camphor *

'76 Ed.

HYPNOCAINE OINTMENT
For minor burns
(Barfred Research Labs.)

Hypnocaine (brand of propasin)
Benzyl alcohol *
Menthol *
Lanolin
Petrolatum

'76 Ed.

HYPNOLATE CREAM
Fungistatic ointment
(Barfred Research Labs.)

Sodium caprylate
Zinc caprylate *
Hypnocaine (brand of propasin)
Water soluble base

'76 Ed.

HYPO-CHEK

See EDWAL HYPO-CHEK

HYPOTEARS
Moisturizing eye drops
(CooperVision Pharm.)

Lipiden polymeric system
Benzalkonium chloride 0.01%
Disodium edetate 0.03%

HYPURITY ALL SEASON PERMANENT ANTI-FREEZE
(Hyde Oil)

Ethylene glycol *

Starred ingredients (*) may be responsible for major toxic effects; consult Section II.

HYSAN BERGAMOT DISINFECTANT
(Hysan Corp.)

Isopropyl alcohol * 19.49%
N-Alkyl (60% C14, 30% C16, 5%
C12, 5% C18) dimethyl benzyl
ammonium chlorides 0.50%
N-Alkyl (50% C12, 30% C14, 17%
C16, 3% C18) dimethyl ethyl
benzyl ammonium chlorides .. 0.50%

HYSAN CITRONE
*Disinfectant, deodorant; institutional
and commercial use*
(Hysan Corp.)

Orthophenylphenol 0.176%
Para tertiary Amyl phenol 0.044%
Essential oils 0.300%
Alcohol 53.460%

HYSAN CLEAN MINT
*Disinfectant and deodorant; hospital
use*
(Hysan Corp.)

Orthophenylphenol 0.176%
Paratertiaryamylphenol 0.044%
Essential oils 0.300%
Alcohol 53.460%

HYSAN LEMON 20
*Disinfectant and deodorant; hospital
use*
(Hysan Corp.)

Orthophenylphenol 0.176%
Paratertiaryamylphenol 0.044%
Essential oils 0.300%
Alcohol 53.460%

HYSAN PINE OIL DISINFECTANT
Institutional and commercial use
(Hysan Corp.)

Pine oil *
Soap
Isopropyl alcohol *
Inert ingred.: 10%
Water

HYSAN ROACH POWDER
(Hysan Corp.)

Sodium fluoride * 40.00%
Pyrethrins 0.11%

HYSECT INSECT KILLER
Commercial and industrial use
(Hysan Corp.)

Pyrethrins 0.30%
Piperonyl butoxide technical 0.60%
N-Octyl bicycloheptene
dicarboximide 1.00%
Petroleum distillates 8.10%

HYSPEED GOLD
Lotion skin cleaner
(Calgon Corp., Commercial Div.)

Soap
Emollients
Water
Fatty amide

HYTAKEROL (CAPSULES & SOLUTION)
For hypocalcemic tetany
(Winthrop Labs.)

CAPSULES:
Dihydrotachysterol .... 0.125 mg.

SOLUTION (each ml.):
Dihydrotachysterol .... 0.25 mg.

HY-TEMP
Heat resistant aluminum paint
(Lester Labs.)

Solvents *†
Aluminum
Silicone resins

'76 Ed.

†*See* Xylene

HYTONE CREAM OR OINTMENT
For treatment of many dermatoses
(Dermik)

Microdispersed Hydrocortisone
(U.S.P.) 1/2%; 1%
2 1/2% (Cream only)
Inactive ingred. (Cream):
Ethoxylated saturated & unsaturated
fatty acid esters
Saturated & unsaturated fatty acid es-
ters
Higher molecular weight saturated &
unsaturated alcohols
Free Cholesterol
Propylene glycol
Sorbic acid
Inert ingred. (Ointment):
Mineral oil
White petrolatum
Sorbitan sesquioleate

HY-TOP LAUNDRY DETERGENT
Dry laundry detergent
(Great Atlantic & Pacific, mfr.; Hy-Top
Products, dist.)

Sodium linear alkyl benzene
sulfonate .... <17%
Sodium carbonate * .... <30%
Sodium silicate .... <10%
Sodium carboxymethylcellulose <2%
Optical brighteners .... <1%
Sodium chloride .... <10%
Sodium sulfate and moisture ... balance

HYTROPHEN
Antispasmodic
(Wesley Pharm.)

Each capsule:
Hyoscyamine sulfate ...... 0.1040 mg.
Atropine sulfate .... 0.0195 mg.
Hyoscine hydrobromide ... 0.0065 mg.
Phenobarbital * .... 1/4 gr.

HYVA GENTIAN VIOLET VAGINAL TABLETS
(Holland-Rantos)

Gentian violet * .... 2.0 mg.

"HYVAR" X-L WEED KILLER
(Du Pont)

Lithium salt of Bromacil 21.9%
Lithium hydroxide *
Ethylene glycol
Ethanol
Methanol

"HYVAR" X WEED KILLER
(Du Pont)

Bromacil * 80%

I

IBERET FILMTAB AND IBERET-500 FILMTAB
*Vitamins C and B complex supplement
with iron*
(Abbott)

Each tablet:
Iron * .... 105 mg.
Multivitamins

IBERET-FOLIC-500 FILMTAB
*Vitamins C and B complex with folic
acid supplement and iron*
(Abbott)

Each tablet:
Iron * .... 105 mg.
Multivitamins

IBERET LIQUID AND IBERET-500 LIQUID
*Vitamins C and B complex supplement
with iron*
(Abbott)

Each 5 ml.:
Iron * .... 26.25 mg.
Multivitamins

IBEROL-F FILMTAB
*Vitamins C and B complex with folic
acid supplement and iron*
(Abbott)

Each tablet:
Iron * .... 105 mg.
Multivitamins

IBEROL FILMTAB
Vitamins C and B complex supplement with iron
(Abbott)

Each tablet:
Iron * .... 105 mg.
Multivitamins

I-BOMB INSECTICIDE SPRAY

See PLANT MARVEL I-BOMB INSECTICIDE SPRAY

ICE BITE
Ice and snow melting pellets
(Van Waters & Rogers)

Calcium chloride 97%

ICE-OFF

See SILOO ICE-OFF

ICE REM
Maintenance material
(Speco)

Chloride salts of Aluminum *, Potassium, Calcium
Sodium tripolyphosphate *

'76 Ed.

ICHTHYBALM
Antiseptic, analgesic; veterinary
(Goshen Labs.)

Ichthammol 16%
Balsam Peru 5%
Salicylic acid 1%
Lanolin-petrolatum base

ICKAWAY LIQUID, WARDLEY'S

See WARDLEY'S ICKAWAY LIQUID

ICK & FUNGI-FREE, WARDLEY'S

See WARDLEY'S ICK & FUNGI-FREE

ICTOSTIX
Urine bilirubin test reagent strip
(Ames)

Diazotized 2,4-Dichloraniline

ICTOTEST
Urine bilirubin test reagent tablet
(Ames)

Each tablet:
P-Nitrobenzene diazonium p-toluene sulfonate (bilazo) .... 0.55 mg.
Sulfosalicylic acid * .... 100.00 mg.
Sodium bicarbonate ...... 10.00 mg.
Absorbent asbestos - cellulose mats
Boric acid *

ICY HOT
Topical analgesic balm
(Searle, G.D., & Co.)

Methyl salicylate * 29.0%
Menthol * 7.6%
Petrolatum/paraffin base

IDEAL LIGHTER FLUID
(Classic Chem.)

Petroleum distillates (Naphtha) *

IGAS
Joint sealer; black
(Sika Chem.)

Asphalts
Petroleum resins *†

†*See* Tar oils and Tar acids

IGRAN 80W
Herbicide
(Ciba-Geigy Ag. Div.)

Terbutryn * 76%
Related compounds 4%

I-KLENZE
Cleaner
(Hillyard Chem.)

Hydrochloric acid *

'76 Ed.

I-LITE STERILE EYE DROPS
(Columbia Med.)

Sodium propionate
Sodium chloride
Camphor
Peppermint oil
Benzalkonium chloride
In isotonic solution

ILLINOIS BRONZE PAINT PRODUCTS
Paints and coatings

Illinois Bronze Paint Co.
300 E. Main St.
Lake Zurich, Ill. 60047

Phone: 312-438-8201

See PAINTS, Section VI, General Formulations

ILLUSTRIOUS
Machine dishwashing compound
(Puritan Chem. Co.)

Strong Alkaline components *

IMAVATE TABLETS
Antidepressant
(Robins)

Each tablet:
Imipramine hydrochloride, USP * .... 25 mg.; 50 mg.

IMIDAN
Insecticide, acaricide
(Stauffer)

Imidan (N-(Mercaptomethyl) phthalimide-S-(O,O-dimethyl phosphorodithioate)) *

IMINRES
Outdoor insecticide; for professional use
(Scientific International)

Heavy Aromatic naphtha * 61.10%
Methoxychlor, technical 17.50%
Malathion 11.70%
2,2-Dichlorovinyl dimethyl phosphate 4.37%
Related compounds 0.33%
Inert ingredients:
Emulsifiers 5.00%

IMPACT
Decongestant
(Approved Pharm.)

Each capsule:
Belladonna alkaloids .... 0.16 mg.
  Atropine sulfate
  Scopolamine hydrobromide
  Hyoscyamine sulfate
Phenylpropanolamine hydrochloride * .... 50.0 mg.
Chlorpheniramine maleate ... 1.0 mg.
Pheniramine maleate * ..... 12.5 mg.

'76 Ed.

IMPACT
Broad line marker - permanent
(Sanford Corp.)

Dyes
Resins
Glycol ethers
Alcohol

IMPACT NASAL SPRAY
(Approved Pharm.)

Phenylephrine HCl * 0.5%
Methapyrilene HCl * 0.2%
Cetylpyridinium chloride 0.02%
Thimerosal 0.001%

'76 Ed.

IMPERIAL CLEANING FLUID
(Hubbard's Imperial, Inc.)

Petroleum *†

†See Petroleum distillate

IMPERIAL ROYAL
Cavity fluid & external bleach
(Royal Bond)

Ortho-dichloro-benzene *
Amyl phenol *
Formic acid *
Formaldehyde *
Methanol *

IMPERIAL SEED TREATER
Insecticide
(MFA Oil Co.)

O,O-Diethyl O-(2-isopropyl-6-methyl-4-pyrimidinyl) phosphorothioate * 33.33%

IMPERIAL ZAR
(United Gilsonite)

Oil modified polyurethane 51%
Mineral spirits * 47%
Benzophenone derivative 2%

IMPREGON (Concentrate)
Diaper soak
(Fleming)

Tetrachlorsalicylanilide * 2%

IMPROVED MAXIMUM
Institutional and industrial cleaning product

Procter & Gamble Co.
Ivorydale Technical Center
Cincinnati, Ohio 45217

Phone: 513-562-1100

IMPROVED PRESTONE II WINTER ANTIFREEZE - SUMMER COOLANT (AF-552, Formula Y/354-359 MI-2108)
(Union Carbide)

Ethylene glycol * 95%
Water 3%
Soluble inhibitors 2%

IMPULSE PERFUME DEODORANT BODY SPRAY
(Lever Bros.)

Ethyl alcohol 45-55%
Hydrocarbon propellant-A46 .... 40-50%
Perfume * .... <2%
Propylene glycol .... approx. 4%
Water .... trace

INDIA INCENSE CONES
(Hindu Incense)

Charcoal 75%
Starch 15%
Combined amount: 10%
  Karaya gum
  China clay
  Sodium nitrate
  Essential oils *
  Triethylene glycol
  Aromatic chemicals

INDIAN HERBS TABLETS
Laxative
(Estes)

Ext. Cascara sagrada *
Aloes *
Oil of peppermint
Oleoresin capsicum *

INDIUM FLUOBORATE CONCENTRATE
Making plating solutions
(Indium Corp. of Amer.)

Indium fluoborate *† .... 31.5 oz./gal.
Fluoboric acid (to pH of 1.0) *

†See Potassium fluoborate

INDIUM SULFAMATE PLATING BATH
(Indium Corp. of Amer.)

Indium sulfamate *† .... 105 gm./L.
Sulfamic acid * .... 26 gm./L.

†See Indium and Sulfamic acid

INDOCIN CAPSULES
Anti-inflammatory agent
(MSD)

Each capsule:
  Indomethacin * .... 25 mg.; 50 mg.

INDO SATIN FINISH
(DAP)

Copolymer, a vinyl toluene and polyhydric alcohol ester of Linolenic, Oleic, Linoleic, Palmitic, Stearic acids
VM&P Naphtha * .... <65%
Zinc soap
Cobalt naphthenate
Zinc naphthenate

INDOTHANE
(DAP)

Polyhydric alcohol esterified with fatty acids, modified with toluene diisocyanate (<1%)
Mineral spirits * .... <25%
VM&P Naphtha * .... <35%
Manganese drier

INDUSTROCLEAN
See AMWAY INDUSTROCLEAN

INFANTOL
Diarrhea remedy
(Scherer Labs.)

Each fl. oz.:
  Paregoric (contains 15 mg. opium) * .... 60 min.
  Alcohol 2%
  Pectin N.F.
  Zinc phenolsulphonate *
  Bismuth subsalicylate *
  Ext. Irish moss .... q.s.

INFANTS TYLENOL DROPS
Analgesic-antipyretic
(McNeil Consumer Products Co.)

Each 0.6 ml.:
  Acetaminophen * .... 60 mg.

INFLAMASE FORTE OPHTHALMIC SOLUTION
Steroid
(CooperVision Pharm.)

Prednisolone sodium phosphate .. 1.0%
Benzalkonium chloride 0.01%
Disodium edetate

INFLAMASE OPHTHALMIC SOLUTION
Steroid
(CooperVision Pharm.)

Prednisolone sodium phosphate . 0.125%
Benzalkonium chloride 0.01%
Disodium edetate

INFLATION-KLEEN, FORMULA HC-41
See KLENZADE INFLATION-KLEEN, FORMULA HC-41

INFRARUB
Analgesic
(Whitehall Labs.)

Methyl nicotinate
Histamine dihydrochloride *
Glycol monosalicylate *
Capsicum oleoresin *

INHIBI-TUSSIN SYRUP
For coughs
(Pharmex)

Each 5 cc.:
  d-Methorphan HBr * .... 10 mg.
  Pyrilamine maleate * .... 16 mg.
  Sodium citrate .... 3.3 gr.

INJECT-A-CIDE
See MAUGET INJECT-A-CIDE

INJECT-A-CIDE B
See MAUGET INJECT-A-CIDE B

Starred ingredients (*) may be responsible for major toxic effects; consult Section II.

INK DEVIL
(Lester Labs.)

Chlorinated solvents *

'76 Ed.

INNERCLEAN HERBAL LAXATIVE
(Lambda Inc.)

Senna *
Frangula
Psyllium seed

INNERCLEAN INNER TABS
Laxative
(Lambda Inc.)

Frangula
Senna *
Psyllium seed

INSECT-GUARD
Skin cream - insect repellent
(Reynes Products, Inc.)

Purified water
TEA stearate
N,N-Diethyl-m-toluamide * 20%/w
Glycerin
Cetyl alcohol
Glyceryl stearate
Fragrance
Methylparaben
Propylparaben

INSECTI-SHIELD

See PURINA INSECTI-SHIELD

INSECT-O-FOG, FOREMOST 4809-ES

See FOREMOST 4809-ES INSECT-O-FOG

INSECTOL

See N/S INSECTOL

INSECTRIN EC
Insecticide
(Hess & Clark)

Permethrin 5.7%

INSECTRIN WP
Insecticide
(Hess & Clark)

Permethrin * 25%

INSECTROL LIQUID INSECTICIDE
(Consolidated Chem., Inc.)

Petroleum distillate *
N-Octyl bicycloheptene dicarboximide *
Technical Methoxychlor *
Allethrin (Allyl homolog of cinerin I) *

INSEC-TROL, SPRAY-TROL BRAND

See SPRAY-TROL BRAND INSEC-TROL

INSECTUMCIDE
Fly & insect killer; industrial and institutional use
(Scientific International)

Petroleum distillate * 99.718%
Piperonyl butoxide technical ... 0.251%
Pyrethrins 0.031%

INSEKIL AEROSOL
Insecticide
(Holcomb)

Strobane * 1-10%
Pyrethrins .... <1%
Piperonyl butoxide .... <1%

'76 Ed.

INSEKON 100
Insecticide
(Holcomb)

Pyrethrins .... <1%
Piperonyl butoxide 1-10%

'76 Ed.

INSEKON 1000
Insecticide
(Holcomb)

Pyrethrins .... <1%
Piperonyl butoxide 1-10%

'76 Ed.

INSEMAL 100
Insecticide
(Holcomb)

beta-Butoxy-beta'-thiocyano-di-
ethyl ether * 1-10%
Malathion * 1-10%

'76 Ed.

INSERID 100
Insecticide
(Holcomb)

Pyrethrins .... <1%
Piperonyl butoxide .... <1%
Diazinon .... <1%

'76 Ed.

INSIDOL
Anionic wetting agent
(Arkansas Co.)

Sulfo-dicarboxylic acid ester *†

'76 Ed.

†*See* Anionic synthetic detergents

INSTA-KILL
Insecticide; wasps and hornets
(Kem Mfg. Co.)

Pyrethrins 0.15%
Piperonyl butoxide (technical) .. 0.30%
N-Octyl bicycloheptene
dicarboximide 0.50%
2-(1-Methylethoxy)phenol
methylcarbamate * 0.75%
Petroleum distillate * 78.30%

INSTANT-DIP SILVER CLEANER
(Lewal Industries)

Thiourea 7.37%
Sulphuric acid 66° * 1.62%
Triton 1.00%
Perfume 0.12%
Water 89.89%

INSTANT FELS LAUNDRY DETERGENT
(Purex Corp.)

Sodium carbonate * 20-30%
Anionic surfactant * 10-20%
Sodium silicate (not meta) * ... 5-10%
Sodium tallow-coconut oil soap <2%
Cellulosic .... <2%
Fluorescent whitening agents .. <1%
Coloring agents .... <1%
Perfume .... <1%
Sodium sulfate .... balance

INSTANT FELS LIQUID DISHWASHING SOAP
(Purex Corp.)

Potassium soap 20-30%
Dipotassium dicarboxylic acid . 3-8%
Propylene glycol .... <1%
Isopropyl alcohol .... <1%
Perfume .... <1%
Water .... balance

INSTANT FRESH
Air spray (deodorizer)
(Royal Bond)

Isopropanol *

INSTANT STARTING FLUID

See SOLDER SEAL INSTANT STARTING FLUID

INSTANT VINYL (TRANSPARENT)
Repairs vinyl and leather
(Advance Color Corp.)

Tetrahydrofuran *
Methyl ethyl ketone

Starred ingredients (*) may be responsible for major toxic effects; consult Section II.

INSTITUTIONAL FORMULA TIDE (Phosphate Formula or 0-Phosphate Formula)
Cleaning product

Procter & Gamble Co.
Ivorydale Technical Center
Cincinnati, Ohio 45217

Phone: 513-562-1100

INSTITUTIONAL "LOVE-MY-CARPET" RUG AND ROOM DEODORIZER
(Nat'l Labs. Div.)

Sodium sulfate (anhydrous) ..... major
Alumina .... minor

INSTITUTIONAL LYSOL BRAND DISINFECTANT SPRAY
(Nat'l Labs. Div.)

o-Phenylphenol 0.100%
N-Alkyl (C18 92%; C16 8%)
  N-ethyl morpholinium
  ethylsulfates 0.035%
Ethyl alcohol * 79.000%

INSTITUTIONAL PACK COMET LIQUID
Cleaning product

Procter & Gamble Co.
Ivorydale Technical Center
Cincinnati, Ohio 45217

Phone: 513-562-1100

INSTITUTIONAL PACK COMET (Phosphate Formula or 0-Phosphate Formula)
Cleaning product

Procter & Gamble Co.
Ivorydale Technical Center
Cincinnati, Ohio 45217

Phone: 513-562-1100

INSTITUTION X (Phosphate Formula or 0-Phosphate Formula)
Cleaning product

Procter & Gamble Co.
Ivorydale Technical Center
Cincinnati, Ohio 45217

Phone: 513-562-1100

INTERCLUB RACING BRONZE
Paint
(International Paint)

Copper-bronze powder
Pine tar *
Denatured alcohol 26 *

INTER-COP COPPER PAINT
(International Paint)

Copper *
Color code #150 contains Mercury *
Pigments - no lead

INTERDEX PAINT
Heavy duty marine paint
(International Paint)

Mineral spirits (or turpentine substitute) *
Pigments - no lead

INTEREST
Liquid chlorinated alkaline cleaner
(Diversey Wyandotte)

Potassium hydroxide*
Potassium hypochlorite*

INTERFACE
Soil release polymer coating
(Unelko)

	%/wgt.
Alkyl polysiloxanes (Dimethyl silicone fluids)	10.00%
Sulfuric acid (reagent grade)	1.00%
Isopropanol (Isopropyl alcohol, anhydrous) *	89.00%

INTERLAC PAINT
Heavy duty marine paint
(International Paint)

Mineral spirits (or xylol) *
Pigments - no lead

INTERLUX BOTTOMKOTE
(International Paint)

Mineral spirits *
Color code #49 contains Copper *

INTERLUX BRAND PAINTS
(International Paint)

Mineral spirits (or turpentine substitute) *
Pigments - no lead

INTERLUX CABIN ENAMELS
(International Paint)

Mineral spirits (or turpentine substitute) *

INTERLUX ENGINE ENAMELS
(International Paint)

Mineral spirits *
Pigments - no lead

INTERLUX GREEN PRESERVATIVE
Paint
(International Paint)

Color code #885 contains Copper naphthenate *

INTERLUX SUPERTROP
Paint
(International Paint)

Mineral spirits *
Color code #46 contains Copper oxide *†

†*See* Copper

INTERNATIONAL DIESEL ENGINE ENAMEL
Heavy duty marine paints
(International Paint)

Mineral spirits *
Pigments - no lead

INTERNATIONAL PAINT PRODUCTS
Marine paints, enamels, and varnishes

International Paint Co., Inc.
2270 Morris Ave.
Union, N.J. 07083

Phone: 201-686-1300

See PAINTS, Section VI, General Formulations

INTER-POLY ENAMELS
(International Paint)

Mineral spirits (or turpentine substitute) *
Color codes #260 and #277 contain Copper bronze powder
Pigments - no lead

INTER-TOX PRESERVATIVE WOOD CLEAR
(International Paint)

Color code #1370 contains Zinc naphthenate

INTEX AEROSOL INSECT SPRAY
(Intex)

Pyrethrins 0.2%
Piperonyl butoxide (tech.) 1.0%
Petroleum distillate * 18.8%

INTEX 8302 AROTEX
Disinfectant
(Intex)

Soap 7.65%
4 and 6 Chloro-2-phenylphenol . 1.00%
Isopropanol 10.00%
Ortho-benzyl-para-chlorophenol . 3.00%
2-Chloro-4-phenylphenol 3.30%
Tetrasodium
  ethylenediaminetetraacetate . 1.20%
Sodium tetraphosphate 1.10%

Starred ingredients (*) may be responsible for major toxic effects; consult Section II.

INTEX 806 CLEANER-SANITIZER
(Intex)

Sodium metasilicate anhydrous *	2.4%
Tetrasodium salt of ethylene diamine tetraacetic acid	1.0%
n-Alkyl (C12 58%, C14 32%, C12 5%, C18 5%) dimethyl ethylbenzyl ammonium chloride	0.8%
n-Alkyl (C14 60%, C16 30%, C12 5%, C18 5%) dimethyl benzyl ammonium chloride	0.8%
Tetrapotassium pyrophosphate	5.0%
Nonylphenoxy polyethoxy ethanol	5.0%

INTEX COMMERCIAL DISINFECTANT CLEANER
(Intex)

Sodium carbonate	3.0%
n-Alkyl (C12 50%, C14 30%, C16 17%, C18 3%) dimethyl ethyl benzyl ammonium chlorides *	1.6%
n-Alkyl (C14 60%, C16 30%, C12 5%, C18 5%) dimethyl benzyl ammonium chlorides *	1.6%
Ethanol	0.8%
Inert ingredients:	93.0%
Surfactants	
Builders	

INTEX COMMERCIAL DOUBLE FEATURE
Disinfectant cleaner
(Intex)

Isopropyl alcohol 91%	3.0%
Soda ash *	1.0%
Sodium metasilicate pentahydrate	0.500%
Tetrasodium ethylene diamine tetraacetate dihydrate	2.0%
n-Alkyl (C12 50%, C14 30%, C16 17%, C18 3%) dimethyl ethylbenzyl ammonium chloride	0.128%
n-Alkyl (C14 60%, C16 30%, C12 5%, C18 5%) dimethyl benzyl ammonium chloride	0.128%
Essential oil	0.15%

INTEX 846 CONCENTRATED DISINFECTANT SANITIZER AND DEODORIZER
(Intex)

n-Alkyl (C12 50%, C14 30%, C16 7%, C18 3%) dimethyl ethylbenzyl ammonium chloride *	5.0%
n-Alkyl (C14 60%, C16 30%, C12 5%, C18 5%) dimethyl benzyl ammonium chloride *	5.0%

INTEX 830 DISINFECTANT GERMICIDE
(Intex)

Pine oil steam distilled	7.0%
o-Benzyl-p-chlorophenol	3.5%
Isopropyl alcohol	3.0%
Soap	8.9%

INTEX 8312 GERMICIDAL DETERGENT
Disinfectant
(Intex)

o-Benzyl-p-chlorophenol	2.65%
Isopropanol	0.88%
Tetrasodium ethylenediaminetetraacetate	0.40%
4 and 6 Chloro-2-phenylphenol	0.10%

INTEX 845 PINE OIL DISINFECTANT
(Intex)

Steam distilled Pine oil *	80.0%
Soap	10.0%

INTEX 8051 PORCETEX
(Intex)

Formaldehyde	0.35%
Hydrogen chloride *	15.00%

INTEX STERITEX, 8311
Disinfectant
(Intex)

Isopropanol *	19.80%
Sodium o-benzyl-p-chlorophenate	5.00%
Sodium dodecyl benzene sulfonate	5.20%
Sodium o-phenylphenate	3.00%

INTIMATE TOILETRIES

Revlon, Inc.
767 Fifth Ave.
New York, N.Y. 10153

Phone: 212-572-5000

Revlon Research Center, Inc.
945 Zerega Ave.
Bronx, N.Y. 10473

Phone: 212-824-9000

See COSMETICS, Section VI, General Formulations

IO-CONCENTRATE, PURINA

See PURINA IO-CONCENTRATE

IOCON TAR SHAMPOO CONCENTRATE
(Owen Labs.)

Ethoxylates	
Coal tar solution *	
Cationic conditioner	
Alcohol	1.0%
Benzalkonium chloride	

IODENT PRODUCTS
Dental care products and cosmetics

Iodent Co.
E-4111 Andover
Suite #200
Bloomfield Hills, Mich. 48013

Phone: 313-647-0777

See COSMETICS, Section VI, General Formulations

IODEX
Dairy iodine sanitizer & milk stone remover
(Lester Labs.)

Phosphoric acid *
Complex Iodine detergents *†

'76 Ed.

†*See* Iodine and Detergents

IODEX OINTMENT (Regular Formula)
(Lambda Inc.)

Iodine (USP) *
Petrolatum (NF)
Oleic acid
Aristowax

IODEX OINTMENT (With Methyl Salicylate)
(Lambda Inc.)

Iodine (USP) *
Methyl salicylate *
Petrolatum (NF)
Oleic acid
Aristowax

IODIZED LIME
(Elder)

Each tablet:
    Iodine *
    Potassium iodide *
    Calcium carbonate

IODO-KLEEN

See UNIVERSAL IODO-KLEEN

IODO-NIACIN
Iodotherapy
(OJF)

Each tablet:	
Potassium iodide *	135 mg.
Niacinamide hydroiodide	25 mg.

IODU
Cleaner-sanitizer for the dairy industry
(An-Fo)

Nonyl phenoxy polyethoxy ethanol-iodine complex (providing 1.80% available iodine)	18.0%
Phosphoric acid *	22.0%

IOFEC-20
Disinfectant and detergent-sanitizer
(Whitmoyer)

Alkyl(C12-C15)poly(oxypropylene)poly(oxyethylene)-
iodine complex 14.65%
Phosphoric acid * 5.00%

IOFEC-80
Disinfectant and detergent-sanitizer
(Whitmoyer)

Alkyl(C12-C15)poly(oxypropylene)poly(oxyethylene)-
iodine complex 58.7%
Phosphoric acid * 20.0%

IO-LYTE, PURINA

See PURINA IO-LYTE

IONAMIN '15'
(Phentermine Resin) Anorectic
(Pennwalt, Pharm. Div.)

Each capsule:
Phenyl-tert-butylamine *† .... 15 mg.
  As cation exchange resin complex of
  sulfonated polystyrene

†*See* Amphetamine

IONAMIN '30'
(Phentermine Resin) Anorectic
(Pennwalt, Pharm. Div.)

Each capsule:
Phenyl-tert-butylamine *† .... 30 mg.
  As cation exchange resin complex of
  sulfonated polystyrene

†*See* Amphetamine

IONAX ASTRINGENT CLEANSER
(Owen Labs.)

Isopropyl alcohol 48%
Blend of Polyoxyethylene ethers
Acetone
Salicylic acid
Allantoin

IONAX FOAM
Aerosol oily skin cleanser
(Owen Labs.)

Ethoxylates
Benzalkonium chloride
Nonionic/cationic base

IONAX SCRUB
Abradant cleanser for oily skin, acne
(Owen Labs.)

Microfine Polyethylene granules
Ethoxylates
Alcohol 10%
Benzalkonium chloride
Nonionic/cationic base

IONAX SHAMPOO
(Owen Labs.)

Purified water
Sodium laureth sulfate
Disodium monococamidosulfosuccinate
Amphoteric 12
Lauramide DEA
Quaternium 22
Citric acid
Quaternium 19
Methylparaben
Disodium EDTA
Quaternium 15
D & C Yellow No. 10
Fragrance

IONIL
Antiseborrheic shampoo
(Owen Labs.)

Ethoxylates
Benzalkonium chloride
Salicylic acid *
Alcohol 12%

IONIL RINSE
(Owen Labs.)

Conditioners
Benzalkonium chloride
Purified water base

IONIL T
Antiseborrheic shampoo
(Owen Labs.)

Ethoxylates
Alcohol 12%
Coal tar solution *
Salicylic acid *
Benzalkonium chloride

IOPREP
Antiseptic
(Arbrook)

Iodine complex (combined
  amount): .... 5.5% w/w
  Nonoxynol 4 (Nonylphen-
  oxypolyethyleneoxy (4)
  ethanol)
  Nonoxynol 15 (Nonylphen-
  oxypolyethyleneoxy (15)
  ethanol)
Surfactant: .... approx. 10% w/w
  Nonoxynol 30 (Non-
  ylphenoxypoly-
  ethyleneoxy (30)
  ethanol)

Available iodine 1%

IOSEL 250
Seborrheic dermatitis of the scalp
(Owen Labs.)

Selenium sulfide * 2.5%
Detergent suspension

IO SHEEN DISINFECTANT
*Detergent-sanitizer for hospital, dairy
and industrial use*
(Hart-Delta, Inc.)

Phosphoric acid * 0.60%
Nonylphenoxypoly (ethyleneoxy)
  ethanol-iodine complex (providing 1.75% titratable iodine) 8.75%

'76 Ed.

IO-SHEEN SHAMPOO
*Bacterial and fungicidal shampoo; vet-
erinary*
(Hart-Delta, Inc.)

Polyvinyl pyrrolidone (iodine complex 1%
  in shampoo base, providing 0.1% available iodine)

'76 Ed.

IOWA PAINT PRODUCTS

Iowa Paint Mfg. Co., Inc.
17th St. & Grand Ave.
Des Moines, Iowa 50309

Phone: 515-283-1501

See PAINTS, Section VI, General Formulations

IREX
Iron tonic
(Friendly Labs.)

Ferric chloride *

IREX TABS
Dietary supplement
(Friendly Labs.)

Yeast
Ferrous carbonate *
Thiamine chloride
Copper peptonate

IRISH AIRE "GLYCOLIZED" ROOM DEODORANT, MUNICHEM

See MUNICHEM IRISH AIRE "GLYCOLIZED" ROOM DEODORANT

IRMA SHORELL COSMETIC PRODUCTS

Irma Shorell, Inc.
515 Madison Ave.
New York, N.Y. 10022

Phone: 212-355-6747

See COSMETICS, Section VI, General Formulations

IROLONG
Hematinic
(Direct Div.)

Each capsule:
Ferrous fumarate * .... 300 mg.
Ascorbic acid .... 200 mg.

IRONCLAD CHEX-WEAR ENAMEL (GEORGIAN GREEN 226-41)
(Benjamin Moore)

Pigment:	18.1%
Titanium dioxide (type II)	29.2%
Chromic oxide green	29.0%
Ultramarine blue	12.0%
Calcium carbonate	25.6%
Tinting colors	4.2%
Vehicle:	81.9%
Varnish:	73.4%
Linseed oil, Rosin modified epoxy ether resin	60.5%
Mineral spirits *	39.5%
Mineral spirits *	26.3%
Driers	0.3%

IRONCLAD RETARDO RUST INHIBITIVE PAINT (GREEN 163-40)
(Benjamin Moore)

Pigment:	38.7%
Titanium dioxide (type IV)	13.0%
Zinc yellow	45.6%
Iron blue	6.5%
Silicates	33.4%
Tinting colors	1.5%
Vehicle:	61.3%
Alkyd varnish:	74.6%
Soya modified linseed alkyd resin	54.9%
Mineral spirits*, Aromatics *†	45.1%
Mineral spirits *	24.5%
Driers	0.9%

†*See* Aromatic hydrocarbons

IRONCO-B
Vitamin & iron supplement
(Vale)

Each tablet:

Ferrous sulfate *	194.4 mg.
Plus Multivitamins & minerals	

IRON EASE (Aerosol)
(Sunbeam Appliance)

1000 Centistoke Dimethyl polysiloxane polymer (GE - SF 96)	3.0%/wt.
Propellant 11/12	97.0%/wt.
#11 Trichloromonofluoromethane	
#12 Dichlorodifluoromethane	

'76 Ed.

IRON GO
Water softener and iron remover for swim pool water
(Coastal Industries)

Water	78.6%
Ethylenediaminetetraacetate sodium salt	0.4%
Sodium tripolyphosphate	4.0%
Citric acid	17.0%

IRONIZED YEAST
(Glenbrook Labs.)

Each tablet:

Ferrous sulfate *	56.88 mg.
Vitamin B1	0.37 mg.
Yeast	384.00 mg.

IRONTONE

See DEXOL IRONTONE

IRRIGOL
Douche powder
(Alkalol)

Sodium sulfocarbolate
Sodium bicarbonate
Sodium borate *
Salt
Thymol *
Eucalyptol *
Menthol *

I-SEDRIN PLAIN
Nasal decongestant
(Lilly, Eli)

Ephedrine alkaloid *	1%
Gluconic acid (Glucono delta lactone)	1%
Chlorobutanol (chloroform deriv.)	0.5%
Dextrose	2.7%

I.S. - INDUSTRIAL SHAMPOO AND RUST-RETARDANT CONCENTRATE

See GUNK I.S. - INDUSTRIAL SHAMPOO AND RUST-RETARDANT CONCENTRATE

ISO-BID CAPSULES T.D.
For angina pectoris
(Geriatric Pharm.)

Each capsule:

Isosorbide dinitrate *	40 mg.

ISO-BID SUBLINGUAL TABLETS
For angina pectoris
(Geriatric Pharm.)

Each tablet:

Isosorbide dinitrate *	5 mg.

ISOCLOR EXPECTORANT SYRUP
Cough, colds
(American Critical Care)

Each 5 ml.:

Codeine phosphate *	10 mg.
Pseudoephedrine hydrochloride *	30 mg.
Guaifenesin	100 mg.
Alcohol by vol.	5%

ISOCLOR LIQUID
Colds, hayfever
(American Critical Care)

Each 5 ml.:

Chlorpheniramine maleate	2 mg.
Pseudoephedrine hydrochloride *	30 mg.

ISO CLOR (POWDER - TABLETS)
For swim pools
(Coastal Industries)

Potassium dichloro-s-triazine trione *	60%
Alkyl dimethyl benzyl ammonium chloride	1%
Sodium carbonate *	30%
Tetrasodium pyrophosphate	6%

ISO CLOR SUPER CHLORINE POWDER
Bactericide, algaecide, disinfectant
(Coastal Industries)

Potassium dichloro-s-triazinetrione *	60%
Sodium carbonate *	31%
Alkyl (C14 58%, C16 28%, C12 14%) dimethyl benzyl ammonium chloride	1%
Tetrasodium pyrophosphate	

ISOCLOR TABLETS & TIMESULE CAPSULES
Colds, hayfever
(American Critical Care)

Each tablet:

Chlorpheniramine maleate *	4 mg.
Pseudoephedrine HCl *	60 mg.

Each Timesule capsule:

Chlorpheniramine maleate *	8 mg.
Pseudoephedrine HCl *	120 mg.

ISOHALANT LIQUID
Decongestant
(Elder)

Phenylephrine HCl *	0.5%
Benzyl alcohol (as preservative)	0.5%

ISOLITE

See ANCHOR ISOLITE

ISOLITE, MASTER MIX

See MASTER MIX ISOLITE

Starred ingredients (*) may be responsible for major toxic effects; consult Section II.

ISOPTO CARPINE
Ophthalmic solution
(Alcon)

Active ingred. (each ml.):
Pilocarpine
  hydrochloride *   0.25%; 0.5%; 1%;
                      1.5%; 2%; 3%; 4%;
                      5%; 6%; 8%; 10%
Preservative:
  Benzalkonium chloride 0.01%
Vehicle:
  Hydroxypropyl methylcellulose
Inactive ingred.:
  Boric acid, Sodium citrate, Sodium chlo-
    ride (present in 0.25, 0.5, and 1% only)
  Hydrochloric acid and/or Sodium hy-
    droxide(to adjust pH in 1, 1.5, 2, 3, 4,
    5, 6, 8, and 10%)
  Citric acid, Hydrochloric acid, and/or
    Sodium hydroxide(to adjust pH in
    0.25 and 0.5%)
  Purified water

ISOPTO CETAMIDE
Ophthalmic solution
(Alcon)

Active ingred. (each ml.):
  Sulfacetamide sodium 15%
Preservatives:
  Methylparaben 0.05%
  Propylparaben 0.01%
Vehicle:
  Hydroxypropyl methylcellulose .. 0.5%
Inactive ingred.:
  Sodium thiosulfate 0.3%
  Sodium phosphate (dried) and/or
  Sodium biphosphate (to adjust pH)
  Purified water

ISOPTO CETAPRED
Ophthalmic suspension
(Alcon)

Active ingred. (each ml.):
  Sulfacetamide sodium 10%
  Prednisolone acetate 0.25%
Preservatives:
  Benzalkonium chloride 0.025%
  Methylparaben 0.05%
  Propylparaben 0.01%
Vehicle:
  Hydroxypropyl methylcellulose .. 0.5%
Inactive ingred.:
  Sodium thiosulfate
  Sodium phosphate (dried)
  Sodium biphosphate
  Polysorbate 80
  Edetate disodium
  Hydrochloric acid and/or
  Sodium hydroxide (to adjust pH)
  Purified water

ISOPTO ESERINE
Ophthalmic solution
(Alcon)

Active ingred. (each ml.):
  Physostigmine
    salicylate * .... 0.25% or 0.5%
Preservatives:
  Chlorobutanol (chloral
    derivative) 0.15%
Vehicle:
  Hydroxypropyl methylcellulose . 0.5%
Inactive ingred.:
  Sodium chloride
  Citric acid
  Sodium bisulfite (0.1% in 0.25% strength;
    0.2% in 0.5% strength)
  Purified water

ISO-QUIN
(Cramer Products)

Isopropyl alcohol * 45.000%
Pine Bouquet Perfume #100 ... 0.075%
8-Hydroxyquinoline sulfate 0.125%
Soft water 54.800%

ISORDIL CHEWABLE TABLETS
Coronary vasodilator
(Ives Labs.)

Each tablet:
  Isosorbide dinitrate * .... 10 mg.

ISORDIL ORAL TABLETS
Coronary vasodilator
(Ives Labs.)

Each tablet:
  Isosorbide dinitrate * .. 5 mg.; 10 mg.
                        20 mg.; 30 mg.

ISORDIL SUBLINGUAL TABLETS
Coronary vasodilator
(Ives Labs.)

Each tablet:
  Isosorbide dinitrate * .. 2.5 mg.; 5 mg.;
                            10 mg.

ISORDIL TEMBIDS (SUSTAINED ACTION CAPSULES & TABLETS)
Coronary vasodilator
(Ives Labs.)

Each capsule or tablet:
  Isosorbide dinitrate * .... 40 mg.

ISORDIL WITH PHENOBARBITAL TABLETS
Coronary vasodilator
(Ives Labs.)

Each tablet:
  Isosorbide dinitrate * .... 10 mg.
  Phenobarbital .... 15 mg.

I-SO-SECT
Insecticide
(National Chemsearch)

Xylene * 64.4%
2-(1-Methylethoxy)phenol
  methylcarbamate * 10.0%

ISOTHAN Q-75
Fungicide
(Onyx)

Lauryl isoquinolinium bromide * .. 75%

ISO-THOR FOGGING CONCENTRATE
Insecticide
(Weil Chem.)

Pyrethrins 0.20%
Piperonyl butoxide, tech. 1.00%
Petroleum distillate * 98.80%

ISO-THRICIN THROAT LOZENGES
Relief of minor sore throat pain
(Approved Pharm.)

Each lozenge:
  Hexylresorcinol .... 2.4 mg.
  Benzocaine .... 10 mg.

'76 Ed.

ISOTOX INSECT SPRAY
(Chevron)

Active ingred. (by wt.):
  Carbaryl 5%
  S-(2-(Ethylsulfinyl)ethyl)O,O-di-
    methyl phosphorothioate 5%
  1,1-Bis(p-chlorophenyl)-2,2,2-
    trichloroethanol 2%
  Aromatic petroleum derivative
    solvent * 18%

Chevron emergency phone number: 415-
233-3737

ISOTOX LINDANE SPRAY NO. 200
Insecticide
(Chevron)

Lindane * 20%
Aromatic petroleum derivative
  solvent * 59%

Chevron emergency phone number: 415-
233-3737

ISOTOX SEED TREATER (75)
(Chevron)

Lindane * 75%

Chevron emergency phone number: 415-
233-3737

ISOTOX SEED TREATER (D)
Insecticide, fungicide
(Chevron)

Active ingred. (by wt.):
Captan 10%
O,O-Diethyl O-(2-isopropyl-6-
methyl-4-pyrimidinyl)
phosphorothioate * 30%

Chevron emergency phone number: 415-233-3737

ISOTOX SEED TREATER (F)
Insecticide, fungicide
(Chevron)

Active ingred. (by wt.):
Lindane * 25.0%
Captan 12.5%

Chevron emergency phone number: 415-233-3737

ISOTOX TRANSPLANTER SOLUTION
Insecticide
(Chevron)

Lindane * 7.5%/w

Chevron emergency phone number: 415-233-3737

ISUPREL COMPOUND ELIXIR
Bronchodilator, decongestant
(Breon Labs.)

Each 15 ml.:
Phenobarbital .... 6 mg.
Isoproterenol HCl .... 2.5 mg.
Ephedrine sulfate * .... 12 mg.
Theophylline * .... 45 mg.
Potassium iodide * .... 150 mg.
Alcohol .... 19% v/v

ISUPREL GLOSSETS
For heart block and ventricular arrhythmias; also as bronchodilator
(Breon Labs.)

Each tablet:
Isoproterenol HCl ..... 10 mg.; 15 mg.
Starch
Lactose
Sodium saccharin
Talcum
Sodium bisulfite .... 2 mg.

ISUPREL MISTOMETER
Bronchodilator
(Breon Labs.)

Each nebulizer contains:
Isoproterenol HCl .... 0.25% w/w
Alcohol .... 33% w/w
Fluorohydrocarbons (propellants)
Ascorbic acid

ISUPREL SOLUTIONS
Bronchodilator; for oral inhalation
(Breon Labs.)

Solution 1:100
Isoproterenol HCl 1%
Sodium chloride
Sodium citrate
Citric acid
Saccharin
Chlorobutanol
Sodium bisulfite
Buffered aqueous solution

Solution 1:200
Isoproterenol HCl 0.5%
Sodium chloride
Citric acid
Glycerin
Chlorobutanol
Sodium bisulfite
Buffered aqueous solution

"IT" (Pressurized)
Automotive
(Garry Labs.)

Silicone oil
Petroleum distillate *

ITALIAN BALM
Skin softener
(Campana)

Essential oils *
Alcohol
Methylparaben
Benzoic acid *
Gum tragacanth
Glycerine
Sorbitol
Butylparaben
Propylene glycol
PEG 400 monostearate

ITCHI-KOOL LOTION
Local anesthetic, antihistaminic, antiseptic
(DePree)

Pyrilamine maleate *
Chlorobutanol hemihydrate *
Benzocaine
Camphor *

ITCHI-KOOL OINTMENT
Local anesthetic, antihistaminic, antiseptic
(DePree)

Chlorobutanol hemihydrate *
Benzocaine
Pyrilamine maleate *

ITCHI-KOOL SPRAY
Local anesthetic, antihistaminic
(DePree)

Benzocaine
Pyrilamine maleate *

ITSO INSECT KILLER
Yellow label
(Capitol Chem.)

Tech. Piperonyl butoxide
Pyrethrins

ITT ANTI-RUST
Anti-rust spray
(Gard)

Paraffin oil 3.0%
Chlorinated solvents * 41.6%
Naphtha * 15.0%
Perfume 0.4%
Propellant (Isobutane) 40.0%

'76 Ed.

IVAREST CREAM & LOTION
Antipruritic
(Blistex)

Calamine 14.0%
Pyrilamine maleate * 1.5%
Benzocaine 1.0%
Camphor 0.3%
Menthol 0.7%
Base: .... balance
Propylene glycol
Modified Cellulose
Polymer
Lanolin oil

IVORY BAR
Soap bar
(Procter & Gamble)

Soap from animal and vegetable
fats 75-100%
Water 10-24%
Minor ingredients, each ...... <1%

pH (1% solution) - 10.5

IVORY BEADS
Institutional and industrial cleaning product

Procter & Gamble Co.
Ivorydale Technical Center
Cincinnati, Ohio 45217

Phone: 513-562-1100

IVORY LIQUID (Formula 1)
Dishwashing liquid
(Procter & Gamble)

Water 50-74%
Ammonium alkyl ethoxylate
sulfate * 10-24%
Ethanol 5-9%
Ammonium alkyl sulfate 5-9%
Alkylamine oxide 5-9%
Sodium alkyl glycerol sulfonate . 1-4%
Potassium chloride 1-4%
Opacifier 1-4%
Minor ingredients, each ...... trace

pH (as is) - 7.8

Starred ingredients (*) may be responsible for major toxic effects; consult Section II.

IVORY LIQUID (Formula 2)
Dishwashing liquid
(Procter & Gamble)

Water	50-74%
Ammonium alkyl ethoxylate sulfate *	25-49%
Ethanol	5-9%
Alkylamine oxide	5-9%
Potassium chloride	1-4%
Ammonium xylene sulfonate	1-4%
Opacifier	1-4%
Minor ingredients, each	trace

pH (as is) - 7.0

IVORY SHAMPOO (Normal & Dry Hair)
(Procter & Gamble, Beauty Care Div.)

Ammonium lauryl sulfate	12-18%
Palmitic acid	1-2%
Cocamide MEA	1-2%
Glycol distearate	1-2%
Minor ingredients	<1%
Water	balance

IVORY SHAMPOO (Oily Hair)
(Procter & Gamble, Beauty Care Div.)

Ammonium lauryl sulfate	15-20%
Palmitic acid	1-2%
Cocamide MEA	1-2%
Glycol distearate	1-2%
Minor ingredients	<1%
Water	balance

IVORY SNOW
Light duty soap granules
(Procter & Gamble)

Sodium soap	75-99%
Potassium soap	10-24%
Water	1-4%
Minor ingredients, each	trace

IVY-CHEX
For poison ivy, poison oak & poison sumac
(Bowman Pharm.)

SD Alcohol 40 (89.5%)
Polyvinylpyrrolidone-vinylacetate copolymers
Methyl salicylate *
Benzalkonium chloride

IVY-DRY
Relief from poison ivy
(Ivy Corp.)

Tannic acid	10.0%
Isopropyl alcohol *	12.5%

IVY-DRY CREAM
Poison ivy
(Ivy Corp.)

Tannic acid	
Benzocaine	
Menthol *	
Camphor *	
Methyl and propyl hydroxybenzoates	
Isopropyl alcohol *	7.5%

IVY SUPER DRY
Poison ivy
(Ivy Corp.)

Tannic acid	
Benzocaine	
Menthol *	
Camphor *	
Methyl and propyl hydroxybenzoates	
Isopropyl alcohol *	35%

IXL LIGHTER FLUID
(Classic Chem.)

Petroleum distillates (Naphtha) *

J

J-4 & J-7
Plastic fillers
(Unican)

Polyester resin	50%
Inert mineral Talc	50%

Catalysts:
Solution:

Methyl ethyl ketone peroxide *	60%
Dimethyl phthalate	40%

or
Paste:

Benzoyl peroxide *	50%
Butyl benzyl phthalate	50%

'76 Ed.

JACK AND JILL COUGH SYRUP
(Buckley)

Fluid extract of Ipecac	0.42%
Glycerin	8.4%
Ascorbic acid	0.285%
Benzoic acid	0.133%
Sugar	76.0%

JACQUELINE COCHRAN FRAGRANCES

Jacqueline Cochran, Inc.
630 Fifth Ave.
New York, N.Y. 10111

Phone: 212-489-2430

See COSMETICS, Section VI, General Formulations

JAFRA COSMETICS

Jafra Cosmetics, Inc.
2541 Townsgate Rd.
Westlake Village, Calif. 91359

24-hour emergency phone number: 617-421-7000

JAFRA GOLDEN VENUS COLOGNE
(Jafra Cosmetics)

SD Alcohol 40
Water
Fragrance *

JAFRA MALIBU MIST COLOGNE
(Jafra Cosmetics)

SD Alcohol 40-B
Water
Fragrance *
FD & C Yellow No. 6
FD & C Blue No. 1

JAFRA PRIVATE RESERVE COLOGNE
(Jafra Cosmetics)

Alcohol
Water
Fragrance *
FD & C Yellow No. 6
D & C Yellow No. 10

JAFRA RISQUE' COLOGNE 1/6 DRAM VIAL
(Jafra Cosmetics)

SDA-40 Alcohol
Fragrance *
FD & C Red No. 4
D & C Yellow No. 10

JAFRA RISQUE' 5/16 OUNCE DAB-ON PERFUME
(Jafra Cosmetics)

SDA-40 Alcohol
Fragrance *
Water
FD & C Red No. 4
D & C Yellow No. 10

JAFRA RISQUE' 2 OUNCE SPRAY COLOGNE
(Jafra Cosmetics)

SDA-40 Alcohol
Fragrance *
FD & C Red No. 4
D & C Yellow No. 10

JAFRA RISQUE' SPRAY COLOGNE
(Jafra Cosmetics)

SD-40 Alcohol
Norda CG-074 Fragrance *
Water

JAFRA ROMEO COLOGNE
(Jafra Cosmetics)

SD Alcohol 40
Water
Fragrance *

JAFRA ROYAL KNIGHTS AFTER SHAVE
(Jafra Cosmetics)

SD Alcohol 40-B
Water
Fragrance *
Allantoin
FD & C Yellow No. 5
FD & C Yellow No. 6

JAFRA ROYAL KNIGHTS COLOGNE
(Jafra Cosmetics)

SD Alcohol 40-B
Water
Fragrance *
FD & C Yellow No. 6
FD & C Red No. 4

JAMAICA SPRAY (AEROSOL)
Insecticide
(Fuld-Stalfort)

Active ingred.:
Pyrethrins 0.30%
Technical Piperonyl butoxide .. 0.60%
N-Octyl bicycloheptene
  dicarboximide 1.00%
Petroleum distillates * 18.10%
Inert ingred.:
Propellants 80.00%

              '76 Ed.

JAMES B. DAY PAINT PRODUCTS

See DAY, JAMES B., PAINT PRODUCTS

JANCYN DRYWELL CLEANER (Powder)
Washing machine drywell cleaner
(Jancyn)

Caustic beads * 67%
Sodium nitrate * 27%
Alum whiskers 6%

JANCYN MAIN LINE CLEANER (Powder)
(Jancyn)

Caustic beads * 67%
Sodium nitrate * 27%
Alum whiskers

JANDE' DAB-ON COLOGNE
(Jafra Cosmetics)

SD Alcohol 39-C
Fragrance *
Water
FD & C Yellow No. 6
FD & C Red No. 4
FD & C Blue No. 1

JANDE' SPRAY COLOGNE
(Jafra Cosmetics)

SD Alcohol 39-C
Fragrance *
Water
FD & C Yellow No. 6
FD & C Red No. 4
FD & C Blue No. 1

JANIMINE FILMTAB
Tricyclic antidepressant
(Abbott)

Each tablet:
Imipramine hydrochlo-
  ride (USP) * .... 10 mg.; 25 mg.;
                      50 mg.

JANITOR-IN-A-DRUM

See TEXIZE JANITOR-IN-A-DRUM

JASCO PAINT PRODUCTS

Jasco Chemical Corp.
P.O. Drawer J
Mountain View, Calif. 94042

Phone: 415-968-6005

See PAINTS, Section VI, General Formulations

JAUNDAFLO
Jaundice fluid; embalming supply
(Royal Bond)

Formaldehyde * 18%
Methanol .... <10%

JEAN NATE TOILETRIES

Jean Nate Div.
Lanvin-Charles of the Ritz Inc.
40 W. 57th St.
New York, N.Y. 10019

Phone: 212-621-7300

See COSMETICS, Section VI, General Formulations

JEAN PATOU PRODUCTS
Perfumes & toiletries

Jean Patou, Inc.
Sub. of Borden Inc.
680 Fifth Ave.
New York, N.Y. 10019

Phone: 212-581-1800

See COSMETICS, Section VI, General Formulations

JEAN PIERRE COSMETICS

Jean Pierre Products, Inc.
19750 Magellan Dr.
Torrance, Calif. 90504

Phone: 213-532-3303

See COSMETICS, Section VI, General Formulations

JEN-BALM
Analgesic balm for muscular aches
(Jenkins Labs.)

Each ounce:
Methyl salicylate * 15%
Oil of eucalyptus 3%
Menthol 2%
Greaseless base

JEN-DIRIL
(Jenkins Labs.)

Each tablet:
Hydrochlorothiazide * .... 50 mg.

JEN-I-SOL
Analgesic-antiseptic ointment
(Young, F.E., & Co.)

Benzocaine
Alkyl methyl benzyl-ammonium
  chloride *

JENKINS DOUCHE
(Jenkins Labs.)

Each tablet:
Boric acid *
Borax *
Tannic acid
Sodium salicylate *
Zinc sulphate *
Powdered Alum
Hydrastine hydrochloride *
Thymol *
Sodium bicarbonate
Tartaric acid

JENKINS EPHEDRINE AND PHENOBARBITAL
For symptomatic relief of broncho-spasm in asthma
(Jenkins Labs.)

Each tablet:
Phenobarbital .... 1/4 gr.
Ephedrine hydrochloride * ... 3/8 gr.

JENKINS HEXESTROL & PHENOBARBITAL
Estrogen therapy
(Jenkins Labs.)

Each tablet:
Phenobarbital * .... 1/4 gr.
Hexestrol .... 1 mg.

JENKINS NASAL SPRAY
(Jenkins Labs.)

Each cc:
Hydrocortisone alcohol 0.05%
Naphazoline hydrochloride ... 0.05%
Methapyrilene hydrochloride . 0.2%
Cetyl pyridinium chloride 0.02%
Thimerosal (preservative) 0.005%

JENN-AIR CLEANSER & POLISH
For glass ceramic cook-tops
(SerVaas Labs.)

	by weight
Oxalic acid (as the dihydrate) *	10%
Silica (amorphous)	87%
Sodium carbonate	2%
Nonionic surfactant	<1%
Perfume	trace

JENNY ALL PURPOSE LIQUID CLEANING COMPOUND - APL
(Jenny Div.)

Crystamet (Sodium metasilicate, pentahydrate) *	2.4%
Butyl Cellosolve	1.0%
Tergitol	1.0%
Tetrapotassium pyrophosphate	2.9%
Water	balance

JENNY CAR WASH DETERGENT - COMPOUND CWD
(Jenny Div.)

Sodium tripolyphosphate *	75%
Disodium phosphate, duohydrate	10%
Tetrasodium pyrophosphate	10%
Sterox NJ	5%

JENNY HEAVY-DUTY LIQUID CLEANING COMPOUND - HDL
(Jenny Div.)

Crystamet (Sodium metasilicate, pentahydrate)	4%/w
Caustic potash liquid *	20%/w
TPP (Potassium pyrophosphate)	3%/w
Emcol TS-211 (Phosphate ester acid)	2.5%/w
Tergitol 15-S-12	1%/w
Water	balance

JENSENEX
Geriatric energizer
(Jenkins Labs.)

Each tablet:

Nicotinic acid	50 mg.
Salicylamide *	0.3 gm.
Methamphetamine HCl	2.5 mg.
Cobalamin (vit. B-12 activity)	3 mcg.
Ascorbic acid	15 mg.

JERIS ANTISEPTIC HAIR TONIC
(Jeris)

8-Hydroxyquinoline *
Resorcinol monoacetate *
Tinct. Capsicum
Fixed and volatile oils
Ethyl alcohol

'76 Ed.

JET ACTION BONDO PLASTIC REPAIR COMPOUND
(Bondo Corp.)

Polyester resin
Bondo hardener:

Methyl ethyl ketone peroxide *	60%
Metallic naphthenates & Aniline derivative as promoters	very small amounts

Filler:
Talc

'76 Ed.

JET ACTION FUEL PELLETS
For plastic toy power
(CossCo)

Per pellet:

White: Sodium bicarbonate	92%
Blue: Citric acid	94%

Binders and lubricants

'76 Ed.

JET CONCENTRATED RESIDUAL MILL SPRAY
Insecticide
(Adco)

Petroleum distillate *
(Butyl carbityl)(6-propyl piperonyl) ether and related compounds
Pyrethrins *

JET DEWAXER AND CLEANER
(National-Purity Soap)

Synthetic oil condensate	10%
Active sequestrant	6%
Synthetic surfactant	6%
T.E.A. (Triethanolamine)	8%
Soft, deionized water	70%

JET DRY (LIQUID & SOLID)
Rinse drying agent
(Economics)

Synthetic nonionic wetting agents
Sodium phosphate (solid only) *

JET-WET, MARTIN'S

See MARTIN'S JET-WET

JEWELDIP

See E-Z-EST JEWELDIP

JEWELUSTER

See E-Z-EST JEWELUSTER

JEWELUSTER FOR COINS

See E-Z-EST JEWELUSTER FOR COINS

J-FLEX PLASTIK FILLER
(Unican)

Polyester resin	50%
Inert mineral Talc	49%
Red iron oxide pigment	1%

Catalysts:
Solution:

Methyl ethyl ketone peroxide *	60%
Dimethyl phthalate	40%

or
Paste:

Benzoyl peroxide *	50%
Butyl benzyl phthalate	50%

'76 Ed.

JIFFIX
Photo developer
(Mallinckrodt, Inc.)

Ammonium thiosulfate *

JIFFY TOOTHACHE DROPS
(Block Drug)

SD Alcohol 38B	76%
Benzocaine	5%
Eugenol	9%
Menthol	2%
Glycerine	

JIFOAM OVEN CLEANER
(Clorox)

Propylene glycol	11-25%
Sodium hydroxide *	2-5%
Anionic surfactants	0.5-5%

J.J.
Liquid hard surface cleaner
(Brewer Chem.)

Octylphenoxy polyethoxy ethanol	approx. 5%
Phosphate surfactant, potassium salt	<5%
50% Potassium hydroxide *	10-15%
60% Tetrasodium pyrophosphate	<5%
Potassium silicate	<3%

JO-CUR
Wave set
(Whitehall Labs.)

Karaya gum

JOHNNY ON THE SPOT
Drain opener
(Weil Chem.)

66° Baume' Sulfuric acid *	95%
Coal tar type inhibitor *	5%

Starred ingredients (*) may be responsible for major toxic effects; consult Section II.

JOHNSON & JOHNSON BRAND FIRST AID CREAM ANTISEPTIC
(Johnson & Johnson)

Benzyl alcohol 2.0%
Cetylpyridinium chloride *
Waxes
Oils
Emulsifiers
Water

JOHNSON PRODUCTS COSMETICS
Hair care products

Johnson Products Co., Inc.
8522 S. LaFayette Ave.
Chicago, Ill. 60620

Phone: 312-483-4100

See COSMETICS, Section VI, General
  Formulations

JOHNSON'S ANODYNE LINIMENT
(Etna Chem.)

Alcohol 16%
Ether 6%/v
Gum camphor *
Turpentine *
Spirits of camphor *
Ammonia

                                '76 Ed.

JOHNSON'S ANTISEPTIC
For minor cuts, burns, bruises, sprains
(Martin Drug Co.)

Alcohol *† 70%
Oil of peppermint 0.91%
Menthol 0.38%
Tannic acid .... trace
Benzocaine 0.33%
Color .... trace

                                '76 Ed.

†*See* Ethyl and Isopropyl alcohol

JOHNSON'S BABY CREAM
(Johnson & Johnson Baby Prod. Co.)

Mineral oil
Water
Beeswax
Ceresin
Lanolin
Paraffin
Glyceryl stearate
Sodium borate
Fragrance
Propylparaben

JOHNSON'S BABY LOTION
(Johnson & Johnson Baby Prod. Co.)

Water
Propylene glycol
Sodium stearate
Glyceryl stearate
Sodium oleate
Polysorbate-61
Myristyl myristate
Isopropyl palmitate
Sorbitan stearate
Stearyl alcohol
Beeswax
Cetyl alcohol
Carbomer-934
Benzyl alcohol
Methylparaben
Propylparaben
Butylparaben
BHT
Fragrance
D & C Red No. 33

JOHNSON'S BABY OIL
(Johnson & Johnson Baby Prod. Co.)

Mineral oil
Fragrance

JOHNSON'S BABY POWDER
(Johnson & Johnson Baby Prod. Co.)

Talc
Fragrance

JOHNSON'S BABY SHAMPOO
(Johnson & Johnson Baby Prod. Co.)

Water
Amphoteric-19
Polysorbate-20
PEG-150 distearate
Sorbitan laurate
Boric acid
Fragrance
Benzyl alcohol
D & C Yellow No. 10
FD & C Yellow No. 6

JOHNSON'S BRAND MEDICATED POWDER
(Johnson & Johnson)

Platelet talc, fine grade
Menthol
Perfume

JOHNSON, S. C., PRODUCTS
*Cleaners, polishes, waxes, air fresh-
  eners, cosmetics, insecticides, insect
  repellents*
(Johnson, S. C.)

Phone: 414-631-2111

Product information is regularly sent to
the National Poison Control Network
(Pittsburg, Pa.) and POISINDEX (Denver, Colo.). These organizations review the
information, develop treatment regimens
and make this information available to local poison control centers. S. C. Johnson
& Son, Inc., Racine, Wisconsin, will accept
collect calls from physicians and Poison
Control Centers handling cases involving
their products. This emergency telephone
service is maintained 24 hours a day, 7
days a week. To insure contact with technically qualified personnel, inform the long
distance operator that the call is an emergency. Then request person to person contact with a member of the S. C. Johnson
& Son emergency call panel.

JOHNSON'S NO MORE TANGLES SPRAY-ON CREME RINSE
(Johnson & Johnson Baby Prod. Co.)

Water
Quaternium-18
Benzyl alcohol
PEG-5 stearamine
Isostearyl alcohol
Fragrance

JOHNSTON'S NO-ROACH
Insecticide
(Johnston, Gaston)

Malathion 0.7%
Diazinon 0.3%

                                '76 Ed.

JOHN SUNSHINE PIPE JOINT COMPOUND STICK
(DAP)

Calcium carbonate
Aluminum oxide
Calcium sulfate
Titanium dioxide
Polymerized linseed oil
Micro crystalline wax
Mineral oil
Cobalt naphthenate *

JOLEN CREME BLEACH

Jolen Creme Bleach Corp.
25 Walls Rd.
Fairfield, Conn. 06430

Phone: 203-259-8779

See COSMETICS, Section VI, General
  Formulations

Starred ingredients (*) may be responsible for major toxic effects; consult Section II.

JONES BLAIR PAINT PRODUCTS

Jones Blair Co.
P.O. Box 35286
Dallas, Tex. 75235

Phone: 214-353-1600

JONTUE PERFUMES & TOILETRIES

Revlon, Inc.
767 Fifth Ave.
New York, N.Y. 10153

Phone: 212-572-5000

Revlon Research Center, Inc.
945 Zerega Ave.
Bronx, N.Y. 10473

Phone: 212-824-9000

See COSMETICS, Section VI, General Formulations

JOTUN-BALTIMORE COPPER PAINT CO. PRODUCTS
Marine paints, enamels & varnishes

Jotun-Baltimore Copper Paint Co.
840 Key Highway
Baltimore, Md. 21230

Phone: 301-539-0045

See PAINTS, Section VI, General Formulations

JOVAN COSMETICS

Jovan, Inc.
875 N. Michigan Ave.
Chicago, Ill. 60611

Phone: 312-951-7000

See COSMETICS, Section VI, General Formulations

JOY (Formula 1)
Dishwashing liquid
(Procter & Gamble)

Water	50-74%
Ammonium alkyl ethoxylate sulfate *	10-24%
Ammonium alkyl sulfate	10-24%
Ethanol	5-9%
Alkylamine oxide	1-4%
Ammonium xylene sulfonate	1-4%
Minor ingredients, each	trace

pH (as is) - 7.5

JOY (Formula 2)
Dishwashing liquid
(Procter & Gamble)

Water	50-74%
Magnesium alkyl ethoxylate sulfate	10-24%
Ammonium alkyl ethoxylate sulfate	5-9%
Magnesium alkyl sulfate	1-4%
Ethanol	1-4%
Alkyl ethoxylate	1-4%
Ammonium chloride	1-4%
Alkylamine oxide	1-4%
Ammonium xylene sulfonate	1-4%
Minor ingredients, each	trace

pH (as is) - 7.1

J&P BENOMYL SYSTEMIC FUNGICIDE
(Jackson & Perkins Co.)

Benomyl 50%

J&P EZY-WEED
Preemergence herbicide
(Jackson & Perkins Co.)

Dimethyl ester of tetrachloroterephthalic acid 5%

J&P ROSE & FLOWER DUST OR SPRAY
Insecticide/fungicide
(Jackson & Perkins Co.)

Carbaryl *	3.0%
Malathion	4.0%
Folpet	5.0%
1,1-Bis(chlorophenyl)-2,2,2-trichloroethanol	1.5%

J&P SYSTEMIC ROSE & FLOWER SPRAY
(Jackson & Perkins Co.)

Acephate	0.25%/wt.
Resmethrin	0.10%/wt.
Folpet	0.75%/wt.

JUNICOID
Antihistamine, expectorant
(Jenkins Labs.)

Each 5 cc:
Dextromethorphan HBr *	5 mg.
Cocillana comp., S.E. *	88 mg.
Potassium guaiacolsulfonate	66 mg.
Citric acid	22 mg.
D-Sorbitol	
Pineapple flavoring	

JUNIOR BOWL DEODORANT
(Carson Chem. Corp.)

Paradichlorobenzene *	99%
Essential oil	1%

'76 Ed.

JUST BACTERIOSTATIC DUST CONTROL & FLOOR MAINTAINER
(Fuld-Stalfort)

Alkyl dimethyl benzyl ammonium chloride (contains from 8 to 18 carbon atoms) 0.25%
Petroleum hydrocarbons *

'76 Ed.

JUST CLEANER-DISINFECTANT
(Fuld-Stalfort)

Potassium 2-phenyl-4-chlorophenol
Potassium 2-phenyl-6-chlorophenate
Ethylene diamine tetraacetic acid, sodium salt
Nitrilotri-acetic acid, sodium salt
Di-hexyl sulfosuccinic acid, sodium salt
Tetra potassium pyrophosphate
Polyvinyl pyrrolidone
Potassium o-phenyl phenate
Isopropanol
Sodium sulfite
Essential oils
Glycerin
Soap
Sodium nitrate

'76 Ed.

JUST COLORTEL
Bowl cleaner
(Fuld-Stalfort)

Hydrogen chloride *
Orthophosphoric acid *
Dihydroabietylamine acetate
Nonylphenoxypolyethoxyethanol
Dyes

'76 Ed.

JUSTWAX REMOVER
(Fuld-Stalfort)

Ammoniated soap

'76 Ed.

K

KABO 612 COATING
(Knight, M.A.)

Modified Epoxy resins
Ketones *
Amine curing agents
Pigments, inorganic (no leads)
Fillers
Barytes
Sand
Carbon powder

Starred ingredients (*) may be responsible for major toxic effects; consult Section II.

KAF-TAN
Coffee pot cleaner
(Whitlock, C.G., Process Co.)

Sodium silicate
Sodium perborate *
Sodium carbonate *
Sodium sesquicarbonate *
Sodium citrate

KAMADROX
Antacid
(Elder)

Each tablet:
Magnesium trisilicate ...... 259.2 mg.
Aluminum hydroxide dried
　gel .... 194.4 mg.
Calcium carbonate .... 145.8 mg.

KAMAGEL
For diarrhea & upset stomach
(Towne, Paulsen)

Each fl. oz.:
Opium USP .... 15 mg.
Colloidal Kaolin .... 6 gm.
Pectin .... 300 mg.
Milk of Bismuth .... 5 ml.

KA-NA-BA PASTE WAX FINISH
Spirit wax
(Clean Surface)

Carnauba wax
Naphtha *

'76 Ed.

KA-NA-BA WATER EMULSION
Self-shining wax
(Clean Surface)

Carnauba wax

'76 Ed.

KANALKA TABLETS
Antacid with sedative
(Lannett)

Each tablet:
Phenobarbital sodium * ...... 1/4 gr.
Benzocaine .... 1/4 gr.
Magnesium carbonate .... 2 gr.
Calcium carbonate .... 3 gr.

KANK-A LIQUID
(Blistex)

Cetyl pyridinium chloride 0.5%
Benzocaine 1.0%
Base: .... balance
　Alcohol
　Benzoin compound

KAN-KOR LOTION
For canker sores and irritated gums
(Pharmex)

Benzoin *
Myrrh
Camphor *

KANON AEROSOL DEODORANT
(Mennen)

SD Alcohol 40 *
Water
Butane
Propylene glycol
Fragrance
Benzophenone-3
Myristalkonium chloride
FD & C Red #40
FD & C Blue #1

KANON KONSERVERA FACE CONDITIONER
(Mennen)

Water
Propylene glycol
Synthetic Spermaceti
Isopropyl myristate
Sorbitan oleate
Fragrance
Cetyl alcohol
Stearyl alcohol
Triethanolamine
Carbomer-941
Quaternium-15
FD&C Yellow #5
FD&C Red #4
FD&C Blue #1

KANON KONSERVERA RICH SHAVE FOAM
(Mennen)

Water
TEA-stearate
Glycerin
Isobutane
Potassium stearate
Fragrance
Polysorbate-20
Mixed Isopropanol amine myristate
Propane
Mixed Isopropyl amine lanolate
Butane
TEA-cocoate
Stearic acid
Potassium cocoate
Coconut acid

KANON MAN'S AEROSOL COLOGNE
(Mennen)

SD Alcohol 40 *
Water
Butane
Fragrance
Propylene glycol
Benzophenone-3
D & C Green #5
FD & C Red #4
FD & C Yellow #5

KANON MAN'S COLOGNE
(Mennen)

SD Alcohol 40 *
Water
Fragrance *†
Propylene glycol
PEG-60 hydrogenated castor oil
Benzophenone-3
D&C Green #5
FD&C Red #4
FD&C Yellow #5

†*See* Essential oils

KANON MAN'S TALC
(Mennen)

Talc
Fragrance
Benzethonium chloride

KANON STICK DEODORANT
(Mennen)

Propylene glycol
Water
Sodium stearate
Fragrance
Triclosan

KANTROLL PRESSED CRAYONS
(American Crayon Co.)

This product bears the CP Seal issued by the Crayon, Water Color and Craft Institute, Inc. This seal certifies that the product contains no materials in sufficient quantities to be toxic or injurious to the human body even if ingested.

KANULASE
Digestive enzyme mixture
(Dorsey Labs.)

Each tablet:
Dorase (cellulase) standardized
　to .... 9 mg.
Pancreatin, N.F. .... 500 mg.
Ox bile extract .... 100 mg.
Pepsin .... 150 mg.
Glutamic acid hydrochloride . 200 mg.

KAOCASIL
Adsorbent, for intestinal irritations
(Jenkins Labs.)

Kaolin colloidal .... 1 gr.
Calcium carbonate .... 1 1/2 gr.
Magnesium trisilicate .... 1 gr.
Bismuth subgallate .... 1/4 gr.
Papain .... 1/8 gr.
Atropine sulfate .... 1/2000 gr.

KAOCHLOR-EFF
Hypokalemic-hypochloremic alkalosis
(Adria)

Each tablet:
20 mEq of potassium chloride supplied
by:
Potassium chloride
(USP) * .... 0.596 gm.
Potassium citrate (USP) . 0.216 gm.
Potassium bicarbonate
(USP) .... 1.600 gm.
Betaine hydrochloride ... 1.843 gm.
Saccharin
Artificial citrus fruit flavor and color

KAOCHLOR 10% LIQUID
Hypokalemic-hypochloremic alkalosis
(Adria)

Each 15 ml.:
Potassium and chloride (as po-
tassium chloride 1.5 gm.) .. 20 mEq.
Sugar & Flavoring
Alcohol 5%

KAOCHLOR S-F 10% LIQUID
Hypokalemic-hypochloremic alkalosis
(Adria)

Each 15 ml.:
Potassium and chloride (as potassium chloride 1.5 gm.) .. 20 mEq.
Saccharin and flavoring
alcohol 5%

KAOGORIC
Antidiarrheal
(Wesley Pharm.)

Each tablet:
Paregoric .... 5 min.
Bismuth subgallate .... 120 mg.
Zinc sulfocarbolate .... 15 mg.
Pectin .... 15 mg.
Kaolin .... 120 mg.

KAON CL-10
Hypokalemic-hypochloremic alkalosis
(Adria)

Each tablet:
Potassium chloride
(USP)(equiv. to 10 mEq.) * 746 mg.

KAON-CL 20%
Hypokalemic-hypochloremic alkalosis
(Adria)

Each 15 ml.:
Potassium and chloride (as po-
tassium chloride 3 gm.) *† 40 mEq.
Saccharin & flavoring
Alcohol 5%

†See Potassium salts

KAON-CL TABS
Hypokalemic-hypochloremic alkalosis
(Adria)

Each tablet:
Potassium chloride
(USP)(equiv. to 6.7 mEq.) * 500 mg.

KAON ELIXIR
Potassium therapy
(Adria)

Each 15 ml.:
Potassium (as potassium glu-
conate (USP) 4.68 gm.) * . 20 mEq.
Saccharin, sodium
Aromatics
Alcohol 5%

KAON TABLETS
Potassium therapy
(Adria)

Each tablet:
Potassium (as potassium gluconate (USP) 17 gm.) *† ... 5 mEq.

†See Potassium salts

KAOPECTATE
Relief of diarrhea
(Upjohn)

Each fl. oz.:
Kaolin .... 90 gr.
Pectin .... 2 gr.

KAOPECTATE CONCENTRATE
Relief of diarrhea
(Upjohn)

Each fl. oz.:
Kaolin .... 135 gr.
Pectin .... 3 gr.

KAOPHEN
Intestinal adsorbant & sedative
(Vale)

Each tablet:
Phenobarbital * .... 6.5 mg.
Belladonna extract .... 0.1 mg.
Kaolin .... 388.8 mg.

KAPACK
Adhesive
(Amboid)

Nitrocellulose type of cement
Alcohols * 20%
Hydrocarbons *† 60%
Ketones * 20%
Allyl isothiocyanate (synthetic oil
of mustard) .... trace

†See Adhesives, Section VI, General Formulations

KAPECTIN LIQUID
Diarrhea preparation
(Approved Pharm.)

Kaolin .... 90 gr.
Pectin .... 2 gr.

'76 Ed.

KAPECTIN WITH PAREGORIC
Diarrhea & upset stomach relief
(Approved Pharm.)

Each fl. oz.:
Paregoric (representing 0.25 gr.
granulated opium) * .... 1 fl. dr.
Kaolin .... 90 gr.
Pectin .... 2 gr.

'76 Ed.

KA-PEK
For diarrhea
(Am. Pharmaceutical)

Each fl. oz.:
Kaolin .... 90 gr.
Pectin .... 4 1/2 gr.

KAPINAL
Antacid and adsorbent
(Jenkins Labs.)

Each tablet:
Paregoric (po. opium 0.0375
gr.) .... 10 mins.
Kaolin (colloidal) .... 5 gr.
Aluminum hydroxide .... 2 gr.
Bismuth subcarbonate ...... 1 gr.
Pectin .... 1 gr.
Aromatics .... q.s.

KARATHANE LC
Fungicide and acaricide
(Rohm and Haas)

Combined amount: 35.0%
2,4-Dinitro-6-octyl phenyl crotonate
2,6-Dinitro-4-octyl phenyl crotonate
Nitrooctyl phenols (principally
dinitrophenol) * 2.4%
Inerts 62.6%

KARATHANE TECHNICAL
Fungicide and acaricide
(Rohm and Haas)

Combined amount: 73%
2,4-Dinitro-6-octyl phenyl crotonate
2,6-Dinitro-4-octyl phenyl crotonate
Nitrooctyl phenols (principally
dinitrophenol) * 5%
Inerts 22%

KARATHANE WD
Fungicide and acaricide
(Rohm and Haas)

Combined amount: 18.25%
2,4-Dinitro-6-octyl phenol crotonate
2,6-Dinitro-4-octyl phenyl crotonate
Nitrooctyl phenols (principally
dinitrophenol) * 1.25%
Inerts 80.50%

Starred ingredients (*) may be responsible for major toxic effects; consult Section II.

KARBALOY LOADED STREAM RECHARGE
For fire extinguishers
(Norris Industries)

Potassium carbonate
Sodium dichromate *
Ethylene glycol

'76 Ed.

KARBON KING
Carbon remover
(Lester Labs.)

Mild Alkali *
Emulsifier
Chlorinated solvents *

'76 Ed.

KARBONOFF
Carburetor and automotive parts cleaner
(Clayton Mfg.)

Cresols * .... >20%
Chlorinated solvents * .... >50%
Soaps 1-10%

KARBOUT CONCENTRATE
For peak performance of engines
(Shaler)

Monochloro naphthalene *† 10%
Butyl acetate 2.2%
Tricresyl phosphate 0.9%

'76 Ed.

†*See* Chlorinated naphthalenes

KARGLO AUTO GLAZE
Polish
(Speco)

Gum tragacanth
Alcohol *

'76 Ed.

KARIDIUM LIQUID
Sodium fluoride drops
(Lorvic Corp.)

Each 8 drops (0.5 cc):
Sodium chloride .... 10.0 mg.
Sodium fluoride * .... 2.21 mg.
Distilled water .... q.s.

KARIDIUM TABLETS
Sodium fluoride tablets
(Lorvic Corp.)

Each tablet:
Sodium chloride .... 94.49 mg.
Sodium fluoride * .... 2.21 mg.
Disintegrant .... 0.50 mg.

KARIGEL
Dental caries; acidulated phosphate/ fluoride
(Lorvic Corp.)

Fluoride ion 0.5%

From 1.1% sodium fluoride in a 0.1 molar phosphate aqueous vehicle pH 5.6

KARI-RINSE
Reduction of dental caries
(Lorvic Corp.)

Sodium fluoride (0.02% fluoride ion) 0.05%
Aqueous solution

"KARMEX" WEED KILLER
(Du Pont)

Diuron * 80%

KATONIC IRON TONIC
Veterinary
(Daniels, Dr. A.C.)

Iron pyrophosphate soluble *
Infusion Cascarilla
Infusion Catnip
Alcohol 15%

KAYBIOTIC OINTMENT
(Wesley Pharm.)

Bacitracin .... 500 U
Neomycin .... 3.5 U
Polymixin .... 5000 U

KAY CIEL ORANGE ELIXIR
Potassium chloride supplement
(Berlex Labs.)

Each 15 ml.:
Potassium chloride * . 1.5 gm. (20 mEq.)
Alcohol 4%

KAY CIEL POWDER SOLODOSE
Potassium chloride supplement
(Berlex Labs.)

Each packette:
Potassium chloride * .... 1.5 gm. (20 mEq.)

KAYCORT H.C. CREAM
Anti-inflammatory
(Wesley Pharm.)

Iodochlorhydroxyquin * 3%
Hydrocortisone 1%

KAY DEGREASER R-L
Liquid cleaner
(Kay Chem. Co.)

Anionic & nonionic surfactants . 5-10%
Trisodium phosphate 5-10%
Water .... balance

KAYDERM
Acne treatment
(King Pharmaceutical)

Sulfur ppt.
Sodium borate *
Zinc oxide
Bentonite
Zinc sulfate *
Camphor *
Acetone *

KAYDERM-O
Itching due to minor skin irritations, mild poison ivy and oak and insect bites
(King Pharmaceutical)

Combined amount: 0.25%
Menthol
Phenol
Base:
Zinc oxide
Bentonite
Calcium hydroxide

KAYEXALATE
For treatment of hyperkalemia; powder
(Breon Labs.)

Sodium polystyrene sulfonate

KAY-5 SANITIZER
Powder sanitizer
(Kay Chem. Co.)

Trisodium phosphate 18%
Sodium dichloroisocyanurate 6%

KAY HEAVY DUTY DETERGENT
Powder detergent
(Kay Chem. Co.)

Sodium carbonate * 40-50%
Sodium tripolyphosphate 20-30%
Nonionic surfactant 5-9%
Sodium silicate 3-8%
Anionic surfactant 1-5%

KAY MULTI-PURPOSE CLEANER
Liquid detergent
(Kay Chem. Co.)

Anionic surfactant 10-15%
Nonionic surfactant 5-10%
Chelating agent 1-4%
Water .... balance

KAY-SAN
For skin irritations
(Commerce Drug)

Resorcinol *
Coal tar *

Starred ingredients (*) may be responsible for major toxic effects; consult Section II.

KAY STAINLESS AND PANEL DRESSING
Liquid polish
(Kay Chem. Co.)

Paraffinic oil (105 SUS) *†	30-40%
Emulsifier	5-10%
Water	balance

†See Kerosene

KAYSTRIP
Stripper for oil based paints and enamels
(Clayton Mfg.)

Sodium hydroxide *	>50%
Sodium carbonate	>10%
Sodium phosphate	1-10%
Soap	1-10%

KAYSUL-P
(King Pharmaceutical)

Each 5 cc:
Sulfacetamide *	250 mg.
Methenamine mandelate *	250 mg.

KAY WINDOW CLEANER
Liquid window cleaner
(Kay Chem. Co.)

Water	75-85%
Isopropanol	8-10%
Ammonium hydroxide	1%

KAZ INHALANT
For vaporizers
(Kaz)

Methyl salicylate USP	0.4%
Oil of eucalyptus *	1.0%
Combined amount:	<1.0%
Oil of peppermint USP	
Oil of lavender USP	
Menthol USP	
Camphor USP	
Light mineral oil	96%
Yellow annatto vegetable color	trace amount

KAZON OINTMENT
For skin irritations
(B & B)

B & B Drug Co.
32 Norfolk Ave.
Maplewood, N.J. 07040

Phone: 201-762-3682

KBP/O
For diarrhea
(OJF)

Each capsule:
Powdered Opium *	3 mg.
Bismuth subcarbonate *	60 mg.
Kaolin	350 mg.
Pectin	60 mg.

KEK BOILER CLEANERS
(Kenite)

Tannins *	10-15%
Chromate salts *	
Wood flour	

KELEX
Hematinic
(Nutrition Control)

Each tabseal:
Iron choline citrate in chelated form (40 mg. of elemental iron) *	360 mg.

KELLOGG'S ANT PASTE
(Kellogg's)

Arsenious oxide *	5.0%

'76 Ed.

KELLOGG'S ANT SPRAY & INSECTICIDE
(Kellogg's)

Tech. Chlordane	3%
Petroleum distillate *	97%

'76 Ed.

KELLOGG'S HOUSEHOLD INSECT BOMB (AEROSOL)
(Kellogg's)

Pyrethrins I and II	0.2%
Piperonyl butoxide, tech.	0.5%
Strobane (Camphene, pinene and related terpene polychlorinates) *	2.0%
Petroleum distillates *	37.3%
Propellant	60.0%

'76 Ed.

KELTHANE
Acaracides
(Rohm and Haas)

1,1-Bis(chlorophenyl)-2,2,2-trichloroethanol *
DUST:	30%
EC, W, & AP:	18.5%
35:	35%
MF:	42%
TECH.:	80%

KEMCIDE
Insecticide
(Kem Mfg. Corp.)

Pyrethrins	0.1050%
Technical Piperonyl butoxide	0.2100%
N-Octyl bicycloheptene dicarboximide	0.3500%
Beta-butoxy beta'-thiocyano-diethyl ether	0.1320%
Beta thiocyano ethyl esters of aliphatic acids	0.0812%
Isobornyl thiocyanoacetate	0.2460%
Related terpenes	0.0540%
N-Octyl sulfoxide of isosafrole	0.0175%
Related compounds	0.0025%
Refined Petroleum hydrocarbons *	98.8018%

KEM FD-100
Food processors' insecticide
(Kem Mfg. Co.)

Refined Aliphatic hydrocarbons *	99.728%
N-Octyl bicycloheptene dicarboximide	0.143%
Piperonyl butoxide (technical)	0.086%
Pyrethrins	0.043%

KEM FOGICIDE
Insecticide
(Kem Mfg. Co.)

Pyrethrins	0.30%
Technical Piperonyl butoxide	0.60%
N-Octyl bicycloheptene dicarboximide	1.00%
Petroleum distillates *	98.10%

KEMIKO PRODUCTS
Concrete stains, finishes and sealers

Kemiko, Inc.
4343 Temple City Blvd.
Temple City, Calif. 91780

Phone: 213-579-6270

KEMINT
Bactericide, germicide and disinfectant
(Kem Mfg. Corp.)

Active ingred.:	36.20%
Isopropanol *	27.82%
Anhydrous Vegetable oil soaps	3.96%
4 and 6-Chloro-2-phenylphenol	3.79%
Methyl salicylate	0.63%
Inert ingred.:	63.80%
Water	
Essential oils *	

KEMIST AIR SANITIZER
(Kem Mfg. Co.)

Triethylene glycol	4.5%
Propylene glycol	3.0%
n-Alkyl (50% C14, 40% C12, 10% C16)dimethyl benzyl ammonium chloride	0.1%

KEMIST BUG KILLER
(Kem Mfg. Co.)

Pyrethrins	0.50%
Piperonyl butoxide (technical)	1.00%
N-Octyl bicycloheptene dicarboximide	1.67%
Petroleum hydrocarbons *	16.83%

KEM KILL-B
Insecticide; aerosol
(Kem Mfg. Co.)

Pyrethrins	0.05%
Piperonyl butoxide (technical)	0.10%
N-Octyl bicycloheptene dicarboximide	0.17%
2-(1-Methylethoxy)phenol methylcarbamate	0.50%
Petroleum distillate *	59.50%

Starred ingredients (*) may be responsible for major toxic effects; consult Section II.

KEM KILL-B RESIDUAL INSECTICIDE
(Kem Mfg. Co.)

Pyrethrins	0.05%
Piperonyl butoxide (technical)	0.10%
N-Octyl bicycloheptene dicarboximide	0.17%
2-(1-Methylethoxy)phenol methylcarbamate *	0.50%
Petroleum distillate *	87.50%

KEM KRAB AM
Liquid crabgrass killer
(Kem Mfg. Co.)

Octylammonium methanearsonate *	8.0%
Dodecylammonium methanearsonate	8.0%

KEM LINK COMPATABILITY AGENT

See UNICO KEM LINK COMPATA-BILITY AGENT

KEM NEW FORMULA 7-11
Sanitizing cleanser
(Kem Mfg. Corp.)

Active ingred.:
Sodium oleate	2.62%
Ammonium oleate	2.60%
Ammonium citrate	1.50%
Ammonium ortho-phenylphenate	0.50%
Essential oils	0.49%
Tetrasodium ethylene diamine tetraacetate	0.28%

Inert ingred.:
Polishing, cleaning, brightening, emulsifying, wetting agents, and water	92.01%

KEM PINE 17
Disinfectant
(Kem Mfg. Co.)

Pine oil *	17.00%
Sodium chloro-o-phenylphenate	3.48%
Anhydrous Soaps	12.80%

KEM SCRAM INSECT REPELLENT
(Kem Mfg. Co.)

2-Ethyl-1,3-hexanediol *	20.00%

KEMSECT 15
Insecticide
(Kem Mfg. Co.)

Pyrethrins	1.50%
Piperonyl butoxide (technical)	3.00%
N-Octyl bicycloheptene dicarboximide	5.50%
Petroleum distillates *	90.00%

KEMSOL
Disinfectant for toilet bowls
(Kem Mfg. Co.)

Active ingred.:
Hydrogen chloride *	23.97%
Oxalic acid *	2.12%
Phosphoric acid *	2.10%
Zinc chloride	1.52%
Heptadecyl hydroxyethyl imi-dazolinium chloride	0.31%
Paradiisobutylphenoxyethoxyethyl dimethyl benzyl ammonium chloride	0.09%

Inert ingred.:
Water, Nonylphenoxypolye-thoxyethanol, Polystyrene emulsion, Cleaning agents, Wetting agents, Emulsifiers	69.89%

KEMTREET 850
Algaecide-slimicide for cooling towers
(Kem Mfg. Co.)

n-Alkyl (50% C14, 40% C12, 10% C16) dimethyl benzyl ammonium chloride*	10.0%

KEMTREET 880
Fungicide, bactericide; industrial
(Kem Mfg. Co.)

Sodium dimethyldithiocarbamate *	15%
Nabam *	15%

KEM ZONE FOG
Insecticide
(Kem Mfg. Co.)

Pyrethrins	0.30%
Technical Piperonyl butoxide	0.60%
N-Octyl bicycloheptene dicarboximide	1.00%
Petroleum distillates *	98.10%

KENACORT DIACETATE SYRUP
For adrenocortical deficiency
(Squibb)

Each 5 cc:
Triamcinolone diacetate anhydrous (equiv. to 4 mg. triamcinolone)	4.85 mg.

KENACORT TABLETS
For adrenocortical deficiency
(Squibb)

Each tablet:
Triamcinolone	1 mg.; 2 mg.; 4 mg.; or 8 mg.

KENALOG CREAM 0.1% (Triamcinolone Acetonide Cream USP 0.1%)
Anti-inflammatory, antipruritic, vaso-constrictive
(Squibb)

Triamcinolone acetonide
Propylene glycol
Polyoxyethylene fatty alcohol ether
White petrolatum
Sorbitol solution
Glyceryl monostearate
Polyethylene glycol monostearate
Simethicone
Sorbic acid
Purified water

KENALOG IN ORABASE
Anti-inflammatory, antipruritic, antial-lergic dental paste
(Squibb)

Triamcinolone acetonide	1 mg./gm.

Emollient dental paste:
Gelatin
Pectin
Sodium carboxymethylcellulose
Plastibase (plasticized hydrocarbon gel):
Polyethylene
Mineral oil

KENALOG LOTION
Anti-inflammatory, antipruritic, and vascoconstrictive
(Squibb)

Each ml.:
Triamcinolone acetonide	0.025%; 0.1%

Base:
Propylene glycol
Cetyl alcohol
Stearyl alcohol
Sorbitan monopalmitate
Polysorbate 20
Simethicone
Purified water

KENALOG OINTMENT
Anti-inflammatory, antipruritic and vasoconstrictor; topical use only
(Squibb)

Triamcinolone acetonide	0.1% or 0.025%

Plastibase (plasticized hydrocarbon gel):
Polyethylene
Mineral oil

KENALOG SPRAY
Anti-inflammatory, antipruritic, and vasoconstrictive; topical
(Squibb)

Each gram:
Triamcinolone acetonide	0.147 mg.

Vehicle:
Isopropyl palmitate
Dehydrated Alcohol	10.3%

Isobutane (propellant)

KENCOVE ADHESIVE NO. 3
Resinous base adhesive
(Kentile)

Alcohol *

Starred ingredients (*) may be responsible for major toxic effects; consult Section II.

KENFAST ADHESIVE NO. 2
Resinous base adhesive
(Kentile)

Alcohol *

KENSINGTON SOAP
(Hewitt)

Tallow
Cocoanut oil
Sodium hydroxide

'76 Ed.

KENTILE ACRYLIC FLOOR FINISH
(Kentile)

Ammonia *

KENTILE ADHESIVE NO. 1
Asphalt adhesive
(Kentile)

Clay
Asphalt
Potassium
  dichromate .... very small amount

KENTILE ADHESIVE #9
Epoxy type
(Kentile)

Epoxy resin
Polyamid catalyst (amine-free)
Isopropyl alcohol *

KENTILE VINYL FLOOR FINISH
(Kentile)

Ammonia *
Emulsion of Acrylic resins

KENT STARTING FLUID
(Aerosol)
For diesel and gasoline engines
(Siloo)

Ethyl ether *

KENWOOD ALCO-WIPE PREP PAD
(Searle Medical Products)

Isopropyl alcohol 70%
Ethylene oxide 0.3%
Water

KENWOOD HAND & BODY EMOLLIENT WITH SILICONE
(Searle Medical Products)

Stearic acid 3.17%
Cetyl alcohol 1.10%
Glycerine 1.10%
Methylparaben 0.16%
Triethanolamine 1.30%
Perfume 0.12%
Water

KENWOOD HAND & BODY LOTION
(Searle Medical Products)

Stearic acid 1.33%
Lanolin 0.68%
Petrolatum 1.17%
Mineral oil 1.67%
Triethanolamine 0.49%
Propylene glycol 1.33%
Veegum 0.17%
Perfume 0.13%
Magnesium stearate 0.34%
Methyl and propyl parabens ... 0.36%
Boric acid 0.15%
Menthol 0.08%
Water .... balance

KENWOOD LEMON-GLYCERINE ORAL SWABS
(Searle Medical Products)

Sodium benzoate 0.26%
Lemon-glycerine solution ... 99.74%

KENWOOD LIQUID CASTILE SOAP
(Searle Medical Products)

Coconut fatty acids 14%
Soya fatty acids 14%
Tripolyphosphate 0.28%
Water

KENWOOD LUBRICATING JELLY
(Searle Medical Products)

CMC 5.14%
Glycerine 4.69%
Methyl parasept 0.18%
Propyl parasept 0.05%
Boric acid 0.30%

KENWOOD OIL ENEMA
(Searle Medical Products)

Mineral oil, NF 100%

KENWOOD PHOSPHATE ENEMA
(Searle Medical Products)

Water
Propylene glycol 0.77%
Sodium biphosphate 16.0%
Sodium phosphate 6.00%
Methyl parasept 0.11%
Propyl parasept 0.018%

KENWOOD POVIDONE-IODINE PREP PAD
(Searle Medical Products)

Povidone-iodine 10%
Water

KENWOOD SORBITOL ENEMA
Pre-filled enema
(Searle Medical Products)

Propylene glycol
Triton X-100
Sorbitol solution
Carbowax
Methyl parasept 0.10%
Propyl parasept 0.015%

KERB 50-W
Herbicide
(Rohm and Haas)

3,5-Dichloro-N-(1,1-dimethyl-2-
  propynyl)benzamide 50%

KER-CELL
Commercial laundry detergent
(Diversey Wyandotte)

Sodium metasilicate *
Alkaline salts *

KERFUL
Heavy duty steam cleaning compound
(Clayton Mfg.)

Sodium silicate .... >10%
Sodium carbonate * .... >10%
Sodium phosphate .... >10%
Sodium hydroxide * 20-30%
Soap 1-10%

KERI CREAM
Concentrated emollient for dry skin care
(Westwood Pharm.)

Sorbitol
Isopropyl myristate
Mineral oil
Surface-active multisterols
Nonionic emulsifiers

'76 Ed.

KERID
Earwax remover (drops)
(Blair Labs.)

Urea
Glycerin
Propylene glycol
Chlorbutanol 0.5%

'76 Ed.

Starred ingredients (*) may be responsible for major toxic effects; consult Section II.

KERI LOTION
Skin lubricant-moisturizer
(Westwood Pharm.)

Alpha-Keri combination of Kerohydric brand of dewaxed oil-soluble, keratin-moisturizing fraction of Lanolin, Mineral oil, Nonionic emulsifiers

'76 Ed.

KERIPON NC
Biodegradable nonionic wetting agent
(Arkansas Co.)

Polyethylene glycol fatty acid ester *

'76 Ed.

KERLITE
Light duty steam cleaning compound
(Clayton Mfg.)

Sodium silicate	1-10%
Sodium phosphates *	>50%
Sodium carbonate *	>10%
Soap	1-10%

KERMEED
Steam cleaning compound
(Clayton Mfg.)

Sodium phosphate	>10%
Sodium carbonate *	>10%
Sodium silicate	1-10%
Sodium hydroxide *	10-20%
Soap	1-10%

KERMULSO A
Emulsifying solvent concentrate
(Clayton Mfg.)

Soap	>10%
Pine oil	1-10%
Glycol	1-10%
Petroleum solvent *	>10%

KER-O-JET (Aerosol)
For infectious keratitis of cattle, and for wound dressing
(Bio-Ceutic)

Methyl violet	0.06%
Furfuryl alcohol	0.60%
Tetrahydro furfuryl alcohol	0.03%
Urea	0.60%
Isopropanol *	18.00%
Propylene glycol	20.71%
Inert ingred.:	
Trichlorofluoromethane	30.00%
Dichlorodifluoromethane	30.00%

KERR-McGEE HERB-ALL
Post emergence herbicidal oil
(Kerr-McGee Corp.)

Petroleum solvent *   100%

'76 Ed.

KERR TRIPLE DYE
Umbilical antiseptic for newborns
(Kerr, Frank W., Chemical Co.)

Each ml.:
Proflavin hemisulfate	1.14 mg.
Gentian violet	2.29 mg.
Brilliant green	2.29 mg.

KESTER FLUX NO, 115
(Kester)

W W Gum rosin
Terpene solvent *

KESTER FLUX NO. 196
(Kester)

W W Gum rosin
Aliphatic alcohols *

KESTER FLUX NO. 197
(Kester)

W W Gum rosin
Aliphatic alcohols *

KESTER FLUX NO. 635
(Kester)

Ammonium halide
Polyhydric alcohol
Glycol *†

†*See* Ethylene glycol

KESTER FLUX NO. 715
Soldering flux
(Kester)

Inorganic salts
Zinc chloride *

KESTER FLUX NO. 736
Soldering flux
(Kester)

Inorganic salts
Zinc chloride *

KESTER FLUX NO. 737
Soldering flux
(Kester)

Inorganic salts
Zinc chloride *

KESTER FLUX NO. 751
Soldering flux
(Kester)

Inorganic salts
Zinc chloride *

KESTER FLUX NO. 783
Soldering flux
(Kester)

Inorganic salts
Zinc chloride *

KESTER FLUX NO. 785
Soldering flux
(Kester)

Inorganic salts
Zinc chloride *

KESTER FLUX NO. 815
Soldering flux
(Kester)

Inorganic salts
Zinc chloride *

KESTER FLUX NO. 1015
(Kester)

W W Gum rosin
Terpene solvent *

KESTER FLUX NO. 1429
(Kester)

Ammonium carbamide
Glutamic acid hydrohalide

KESTER FLUX NO. 1544
(Kester)

W W Gum rosin
Short-chain Aliphatic alcohols *

KESTER FLUX NO. 1545
(Kester)

W W Gum rosin
Short-chain Aliphatic alcohols *

KESTER FLUX NO. 1547
(Kester)

W W Gum rosin
Short-chain Aliphatic alcohols *

KESTER FLUX NO. 1571
(Kester)

W W Gum rosin
Short-chain Aliphatic alcohols *

KESTER FLUX NO. 1585
(Kester)

W W Gum rosin
Short-chain Aliphatic alcohols *

KESTER FLUX NO. 1587
(Kester)

W W Gum rosin
Short-chain Aliphatic alcohols *

KESTER FLUX NO. 2000
(Kester)

W W Gum rosin
Aliphatic alcohols *

Starred ingredients (*) may be responsible for major toxic effects; consult Section II.

KESTER FLUX NO. 2211
(Kester)

Amine hydrochloride
Aliphatic alcohols *

KESTER ROSIN RESIDUE REMOVER NO. AP-20
(Kester)

Chlorinated hydrocarbon *
Organic ester

KESTER STAINLESS STEEL FLUX NO. 817
(Kester)

Inorganic salts
Zinc chloride *
Hydrochloric acid *

KETO-DIASTIX
Urine glucose and ketone reagent strip
(Ames)

Glucose area: see DIASTIX
Ketone area: see KETOSTIX

KETOSIN ORAL SOLUTION, MARTIN'S

See MARTIN'S KETOSIN ORAL SOLUTION

KETOSTIX
Urine ketone test reagent strip
(Ames)

Sodium nitroferricyanide
Aminoacetic acid (Glycine)
Sodium phosphate buffer
Dimethylsulfoxide
Chloroform
Dioctyl sodium sulfosuccinate

KEY GRAPHITE PASTE
(W-K-M)

Food grade Corn syrup .... approx. 55%
Amorphous graphite ...... approx. 44%
Sodium pentachlorphenate .... approx. 1%

'76 Ed.

KIDDE CHEMICAL FOAM EXTINGUISHER
Fire extinguisher
(Kidde)

Aluminum sulfate *
Sodium bicarbonate *
Foaming agent

KIDDE DRY CHEMICAL EXTINGUISHER
Fire extinguisher
(Kidde)

Sodium bicarbonate *

KIDDE K
Fire extinguisher
(Kidde)

Potassium bicarbonate *

KIDDE LOADED STREAM
Fire extinguisher
(Kidde)

Potassium carbonate
Ethylene glycol *

KIDDE PUMP TANK EXTINGUISHER
Fire extinguisher
(Kidde)

Calcium chloride (against freezing)

KIDDE SODA-ACID EXTINGUISHER
Fire extinguisher
(Kidde)

Sodium bicarbonate
Sulfuric acid * .... 4 oz.

KIDDE TRI CLASS DRY CHEMICAL FIRE EXTINGUISHER
(Kidde)

Monoammonium phosphate

KIDDE ULTRA-K DRY CHEMICAL EXTINGUISHER
(Kidde)

Potassium chloride *

KIDDE WATER EXTINGUISHER
Fire extinguisher
(Kidde)

Calcium chloride crystals

KIDDIES SIALCO
Analgesic, antihistaminic
(Foy Labs.)

Each tablet:
Chlorpheniramine maleate .. 2.0 mg.
Phenylephrine HCl .... 2.5 mg.
Acetaminophen * .... 62.5 mg.
Salicylamide .... 75.0 mg.

KIDDI-KOFF
(Direct Div.)

Each 5 ml.:
Codeine phosphate (USP) * .. 5 mg.
Pseudoephedrine HCl * ...... 15 mg.
Guaifenesin .... 50 mg.

Free of Sugar, Alcohol, Tartrazine

KID-O
Modeling dough
(Cleveland Cleaner)

Wheat flour 42.0000%
Ammonium alum 0.0060%
Water plus salt solution 55.0000%
Aniline, color certified 0.0002%
Oil (Mineral oil) 2.0000%

'76 Ed.

KILBRUSH

See BONIDE KILBRUSH

KILGORE TOY CAPS
(Kilgore Corp.)

Amorphous Red phosphorus
Potassium chlorate *
Calcium carbonate
Water soluble gum
Lamp black
Antimony sulfide *

KILL-KO PREMISE SPRAY
Insecticide
(Rigo Co.)

Pyrethrins 0.66%
Technical Piperonyl butoxide ... 3.30%
Petroleum distillate 96.04%

KILLMASTER II
Insecticide used on building interiors
(Positive Formulators)

Chlorpyrifos 2.0%
Aromatic petroleum derivative
solvent * 1.2%
Petroleum distillate (Solvent TS-28) * 95.2%
Inerts (Lacquers & Plastics) 1.6%

KILLMICE
Rodenticide
(Twin City Exterminating Co.)

Strychnine alkaloid * 0.1%

'76 Ed.

KILLVERMON CHLORDANE
Roach, water bug, silver fish and ant control
(Twin City Exterminating Co.)

Chlordane 2%
Refined Petroleum distillate * 98%

'76 Ed.

KILLVERMON DIAZINON
Roach, water bug, silverfish and ant control
(Twin City Exterminating Co.)

O,O-Diethyl O-(2-isopropyl-4-methyl 6-pyrimidinyl) phosphorothioate (Diazinon) 0.50%
Refined Petroleum distillate * .. 99.50%

'76 Ed.

Starred ingredients (*) may be responsible for major toxic effects; consult Section II.

KILLVERMON PIVAL RODENTICIDE
(Twin City Exterminating Co.)

2-Pivalyl-1,3-indandione (Pival)	0.025%

'76 Ed.

KIL-MOE
Insecticide
(Halaby, Samuel, Inc.)

Petroleum hydrocarbons *
Piperonyl butoxide
Pyrethrins

KILTECT-100 SPRAY

See FRANKLIN KILTECT-100 SPRAY

KILTECT-100 (Squirt Bottle)

See FRANKLIN KILTECT-100 (Squirt Bottle)

KILZOL DISINFECTANT

See FRANKLIN KILZOL DISINFECTANT

KINDOGRAPH PRESSED CRAYONS
(American Crayon Co.)

This product bears the CP Seal issued by the Crayon, Water Color and Craft Institute, Inc. This seal certifies that the product contains no materials in sufficient quantities to be toxic or injurious to the human body even if ingested.

KING BUG KILLER
Insecticide
(King Pesticides)

Carbaryl *	5%

KING CHLORDANE DUST (ANT & GRUB KILLER)
Insecticide
(King Pesticides)

Tech. Chlordane *	5.0%

KING EXTERIOR FINISH
(King Chem.)

Boiled Linseed oil	60%
Petroleum distillates *	17%
Pentachlorophenol *	10%
Other chlorophenols & related compounds	
Inert ingred.:	13%
Oil colors	
Paraffin wax	
Zinc stearate	

KING FRUIT TREE DUST OR SPRAY
Insecticide, fungicide
(King Pesticides)

Malathion *	4.0%
Methoxychlor	3.0%
Zineb (from Dithane Z-78)	6.5%
Sulfur	40.0%

KING MALATHION DUST
Insecticide
(King Pesticides)

Malathion *	4.0%

KING OF ALL BACTERIA ENZYMES ACTIVATOR
To clean septic tanks, drainfields, dry wells
(King of All)

Enzymes	25%
Monosodium phosphate	5%
Disodium phosphate	5%
Urea	25%
Soya meal	25%
Bicarbonate	5%
Sugar	5%
Yeast	5%

KING OF ALL HEAVY DUTY COMMERCIAL DRAIN KLEENER
(King of All)

Sodium hydroxide (Caustic soda) *	100%

KING OF ALL LIQUID DRAIN KLEENER
(King of All)

50% conc. of 76% Sodium hydroxide (Caustic soda) *	5%
Water	95%
TSP blue dye	trace

KING OF ALL REGULAR DRAIN PIPE KLEENER
(King of All)

Sodium hydroxide (Caustic soda) *	100%

KING OF ALL RUST AND IRON REMOVER
To clean rust and iron from water softeners, sinks, appliances, toilets, etc.
(King of All)

Sodium bisulfite *	60%
Sodium hydrosulfite *	15%
Sodium sulfite *	15%
Soda ash	10%

KING OF ALL SEPTIC TANK AND CESSPOOL KLEENER
(King of All)

Sodium hydroxide (Caustic soda) *	80%
Sodium chloride (Rock salt)	19%
Activated Carbon	1%

KING OF ALL SEWER CLEANER AND ROOT DESTROYER
(King of All)

Sodium hydroxide (Caustic soda) *	80%
Sodium chloride (Rock salt)	20%

KING P.T.V. DUST
Insecticide, fungicide
(King Pesticides)

Carbaryl *	5.0%
Zineb (from Dithane Z-78)	3.9%

KING ROSE DUST
Insecticide & fungicide
(King Pesticides)

Gamma isomer of BHC (from Lindane)	0.5%
Malathion	4.0%
Zineb (from Dithane Z-78)	3.9%
Sulfur *	30.0%
Dinitro capryl phenyl crotonate (from Karathane)	0.9%

KING ROTENONE DUST
Insecticide
(King Pesticides)

Rotenone	1%

KINIZOL
Useful in preventive geriatrics
(King Pharmaceutical)

Each 5 cc:
Pentylenetetrazole *	100 mg.
Nicotinic acid	50 mg.
Alcohol	5%

KIRK'S COCO HARDWATER CASTILE
Soap bar
(Procter & Gamble)

Soap from vegetable fats	50-74%
Water	25-49%
Glycerine	5-9%
Vegetable oil	1-4%
Fatty acid	1-4%
Minor ingredients, each	<1%

pH (1% solution) - 9.7

KITCHEN DRANO (LIQUID)
Drain cleaner
(Drackett)

1,1,1-Trichloroethane *　approx. 75%/wt.
Light mineral oil
Dye

KITTEN & BEAR COOLING TOWER ALGAECIDE
(Stewart Sanitary Supply)

n-Alkyl (50% C14, 40% C12, 10% C16) dimethyl benzyl ammonium chloride *	10%

Starred ingredients (*) may be responsible for major toxic effects; consult Section II.

KITTEN & BEAR CYGON 2-E
Systemic insecticide
(Stewart Sanitary Supply)

Dimethoate * 23.4%/w

KITTEN & BEAR DIAZINON AG-500
Insect control on shade trees, ornamentals and turf
(Stewart Sanitary Supply)

Diazinon * 48%/w
Xylene * 39%/w

KITTEN & BEAR DIAZINON 4E
(Stewart Sanitary Supply)

Diazinon * 47.50%/w
Aromatic petroleum derivative
solvent * 30.40%/w

KITTEN & BEAR DIAZINON 4S
(Stewart Sanitary Supply)

Diazinon * 48.7%/w
Aromatic petroleum derivative
solvent * 39.5%/w

KITTEN & BEAR FILTER FLY CONCENTRATE
(Stewart Sanitary Supply)

Xylene 87%
Alpha isomer of 2-carbomethoxy-1-
methylvinyl dimethyl phosphate
(Phosdrin) * 3%
Related compounds 2%

KITTEN & BEAR FLEA SPRAY
(Stewart Sanitary Supply)

Ronnel 1.00%
2,2-Dichlorovinyl dimethyl
phosphate 0.46%
Related compounds 0.04%
Petroleum distillate * 98.50%

KITTEN & BEAR FLYACIDE 25
Insecticide
(Stewart Sanitary Supply)

Resmethrin 0.250%
Related compounds 0.034%

KITTEN & BEAR ICE MELTING LIQUID
(Stewart Sanitary Supply)

Calcium chloride 33%

KITTEN & BEAR ICE MELTING PELLETS
(Stewart Sanitary Supply)

Calcium chloride 94%

KITTEN & BEAR INSECTICIDE 125
(Stewart Sanitary Supply)

	by weight
Heavy Aromatic naphtha *	61.10%
Methoxychlor (technical)	17.50%
Malathion	11.70%
2,2-Dichlorovinyl dimethyl phosphate	4.37%
Related compounds	0.33%
Emulsifiers	5.00%

KITTEN & BEAR MALATHION 57%
Insecticide
(Stewart Sanitary Supply)

Malathion * 57%
Xylene * 34%

KITTEN & BEAR MOLE FUMIGANT
(Stewart Sanitary Supply)

Paradichlorobenzene 20%
Ethylene dichloride 30%
Carbon tetrachloride * 50%

KITTEN & BEAR MOSQUITO FOG CONCENTRATE
(Stewart Sanitary Supply)

Fenthion 10%
Aromatic petroleum distillate * 90%

KITTEN & BEAR MOSQUITO FOG-1 R.T.U.
(Stewart Sanitary Supply)

Fenthion 1.000%
Aromatic petroleum distillate * . . . 98.925%

KITTEN & BEAR MOSQUITO LARVACIDE 98
(Stewart Sanitary Supply)

Petroleum distillate * 98%

KITTEN & BEAR N-1 NALED FLY SPRAY
(Stewart Sanitary Supply)

Naled 1%/w
Petroleum distillates * 96%/w

KITTEN & BEAR PYRETHRIN-1
Insecticide
(Stewart Sanitary Supply)

Pyrethrins 0.187%/w
Piperonyl butoxide
(technical) 0.757%/w
Isoparaffinic hydrocarbons * 99.056%/w

KITTEN & BEAR PYRETHRIN-3
Insecticide
(Stewart Sanitary Supply)

Petroleum distillate * 98.2%
Technical Piperonyl butoxide 1.5%
Pyrethrins 0.3%

KITTEN & BEAR RAT BURROW FUMIGANT
(Stewart Sanitary Supply)

Paradichlorobenzene 20%
Ethylene dichloride 30%
Carbon tetrachloride * 50%

KITTEN & BEAR RETARD
For controlling growth of grass, trees, shrubs and ivy
(Stewart Sanitary Supply)

1,2-Dihydro-3,6-pyridazinedione
diethanolamine salt * 11.6%

KITTEN & BEAR ROACH AND ANT SPRAY
(Stewart Sanitary Supply)

Petroleum solvents * 99.12%
Diazinon 0.50%
Technical Piperonyl butoxide 0.25%
Pyrethrins 0.05%

KITTEN & BEAR ROACH AND ANT SPRAY - B
(Stewart Sanitary Supply)

Baygon * 1.0%/w
Isoparaffinic hydrocarbons * 83.75%/w

KITTEN & BEAR ROACH AND ANT SPRAY - SPECIAL
(Stewart Sanitary Supply)

Pyrethrins 0.052%
Piperonyl butoxide (technical) 0.260%
Chlorpyrifos 0.500%
Petroleum distillate * 98.736%

KITTEN & BEAR ROACH & ANT BOMB
(Stewart Sanitary Supply)

Diazinon 0.500%
Pyrethrins 0.052%
Piperonyl butoxide (technical) . . 0.261%
Petroleum distillate 8.608%

KITTEN & BEAR ROACH POWDER
(Stewart Sanitary Supply)

Pyrethrins 0.35%
Sodium fluoride * 38.80%

Starred ingredients (*) may be responsible for major toxic effects; consult Section II.

KITTEN & BEAR SNOW PLOW WAX
(Stewart Sanitary Supply)

Petroleum distillates *
and Hydrocarbons

KITTEN & BEAR SPREADER-STICKER
(Stewart Sanitary Supply)

Alkylaryl polyoxyethylene glycols .. 80%

KITTEN & BEAR SUGAR FLY BAIT
(Stewart Sanitary Supply)

2,2-Dichlorovinyl dimethyl
phosphate 0.46%
Related compounds 0.04%

KITTEN & BEAR SWIMMING POOL ALGAECIDE
(Stewart Sanitary Supply)

n-Alkyl (50% C14, 40% C12, 10%
C16) dimethyl benzyl ammonium
chloride * 10%

KITTEN & BEAR T-6 TOXAPHENE
Insecticide
(Stewart Sanitary Supply)

Toxaphene * 60%
Aromatic petroleum hydrocarbons * 34%

KITTEN & BEAR ULV FLUSHING SOLUTION
(Stewart Sanitary Supply)

Dimethyl carbinol * 98%

KITTEN'S MOUSE BAIT
(Stewart Sanitary Supply)

Warfarin 0.025%
Sulfaquinoxaline 0.025%

KITTEN'S RAT BAIT
(Stewart Sanitary Supply)

Warfarin 0.025%
Sulfaquinoxaline 0.025%

KITTEN WAX
(Park Chem.)

Mineral spirits *
Amine soap
Silicone
Abrasive

KIT-TONNE LAXATIVE
A laxative paste for dogs and cats
(Haver-Lockhart (Brand) Bayvet Div.
of Cutter Labs.)

Benzoic acid 0.2%

KITTY BOX CAT LITTER
(Waverly Mineral Products Co.)

Aluminum-magnesium silicate
Iron oxide .... small amounts

KITTY PAN CAT LITTER
(Waverly Mineral Products Co.)

Aluminum-magnesium silicate
Iron oxide .... small amounts

KIWI SHOE POLISHES

The Kiwi Polish Co. PTY, Ltd.
Route 662
Douglassville, Pa. 19518

Phone: 215-326-5800

K KREME
All purpose cleaner
(Paul Koss)

Water .... <90%
Monoethanolammonium dodecyl-
benzene sulfonate (Anionic
surfactant) .... <5%
Fatty amido phosphate
Tetrapotassium pyrophosphate
Monoethanolamine
Perfume .... trace
Dye .... trace

pH 10.4-10.8

KLARON LOTION (DRIES ON CLEAR)
Treatment of acne and seborrhea
(Dermik)

Salicylic acid * .... 2% w/v
Sulfur colloid .... 5% w/v
Greaseless hydro-alcoholic vehicle
S.D. alcohol 13.1%/v

KLEAN AND PRIME

See BALKAMP KLEAN AND PRIME

KLEAN CRETE
Masonry cleaner
(Klean-Strip)

Hydrochloric acid * .... <20%
Acid inhibitors, Emulsifiers ... <5%
Water .... >70%

KLEAN KLAY
Modeling clay
(Art Chem.)

Powdered Kaolloid clay 35-40%
Powdered Gypsum 35-40%
Petrolatum 15%
Wax 10%
Castor oil 1%
Organic pigment .... trace

KLEAN-N-DIS
Detergent-germicide; institutional and industrial use
(Puritan Chem. Co.)

Vegetable oil soap 8.00%
Potassium-o-benzyl-p-
chlorophenate 5.10%
Sodium alkyl (C9) benzene
sulfonate 3.50%
Ethylene diamine tetraacetic acid,
tetrasodium salt 0.08%

KLEAN-STRIP ALL PURPOSE CLEANER
(Klean-Strip)

Water .... >85%
Trisodium phosphate .... <5%
Sodium tripolyphosphate .... <2%
Butyl Cellosolve * .... <5%
Triton X-100 .... <5%

KLEAN-STRIP BLACKBOARD SLATING - BLACK
(Klean-Strip)

Pigment: 35.2%
Lampblack 19.4%
Silica 80.6%

Vehicle: 64.8%
Phenolic resin-linseed oil
(nonvolatile) 71.9%
Petroleum distillates
(volatile) * 28.1%

KLEAN-STRIP BLACKBOARD SLATING - GREEN
(Klean-Strip)

Pigment: 39.2%
Flatting agent 14.5%
Titanium dioxide 19.6%
Calcium carbonate 45.5%
Silica 12.4%
Diatomaceous earth 2.9%
Lampblack 0.1%
Phthalocyanine green 5.9%
Phthalocyanine blue 1.0%
Ferrite yellow 12.6%

Vehicle: 60.8%
Phenolic resin-linseed oil
(nonvolatile) 62.5%
Mineral spirits (volatile) * . 37.5%

KLEAN-STRIP BRUSH CLEANER
(Klean-Strip)

Aliphatic & Aromatic
hydrocarbons * .... >40%
Chlorinated hydrocarbons * .... <20%
Ketones .... <20%
Alcohols (<4% methanol) .... <10%
Liquid soap .... <10%
Glycol ethers & Water .... <10%

Starred ingredients (*) may be responsible for major toxic effects; consult Section II.

KLEAN-STRIP DRIVEWAY CLEANER
(Klean-Strip)

Petroleum distillates *	>80%
Soap	<10%
Emulsifiers & Penetrants	<10%

KLEAN-STRIP FORMULA A
Peels off paint
(Klean-Strip)

Chlorinated hydrocarbons *	>50%
Alcohol	>30%
Petroleum distillates	<10%
Thickeners & Inhibitors	<10%

KLEAN-STRIP FURNITURE FINISH & PAINT REMOVER
(Klean-Strip)

Chlorinated hydrocarbons *	<70%
Alcohol, Petroleum distillates, Ammonia *, & Water (<4% methanol)	>30%
Thickeners & Inhibitors	balance

KLEAN-STRIP GLASS CLEANER
(Klean-Strip)

Alcohols *, Detergents *, Penetrants *†, & Dyes	<30%
Water	>70%

†*See* Kerosene

KLEAN-STRIP HAND CLEANER
(Klean-Strip)

Aliphatic hydrocarbons *	<15%
Glycols & Glycol ethers *	<15%
Emulsifiers, Emollients, Perfume	<10%
Water	>50%
Sodium & amine oleate soap	>15%

KLEAN-STRIP MARINE FINISH REMOVER
(Klean-Strip)

Chlorinated hydrocarbons *	>70%
Alcohol (<4% methanol)	>20%
Thickeners & Inhibitors	<5%

KLEAN-STRIP RUST REMOVER
(Klean-Strip)

Phosphoric acid (75%) *	>20%
Water	>60%
Isopropyl alcohol	<5%

KLEAN-STRIP SPRAY GUN CLEANER
(Klean-Strip)

Caustic potash (45%)	<5%
Water	<20%
Propylene dichloride *	ʾ>25%
Tall oil	<10%
Methylene chloride	>25%
Trisodium phosphate	<5%

KLEAN-STRIP WOOD BLEACH
(Klean-Strip)

Solution A:

Water	<85%
Caustic soda (50%) *	>15%

Solution B:

Hydrogen peroxide *	>25%

KLEAN-STRIP WOOD STAIN REMOVER
(Klean-Strip)

Sodium hypochlorite *	<10%
Water & Stabilizer	>90%

KLEEN-AIR DEODORANT BLOCKS
Industrial and institutional use
(Scientific International)

Paradichlorobenzene *

KLEEN-AIR DEODORANT BLOCKS, HANGER TYPE
Industrial and institutional use
(Scientific International)

Paradichlorobenzene *

KLEEN-AIR DEODORANT BLOCKS, URINAL BLOCK
Industrial and institutional use
(Scientific International)

Paradichlorobenzene *

KLEEN ALL 45
(Paul Koss)

Sulfuric acid *	<95%
Water	

KLEEN GLASS
(Uncle Sam)

Ammonia *
Isopropanol *
Cellosolve *
Sodium nitrite *
Dye

KLEEN GUARD AEROSOL RUB SHAMPOO
(Alberto-Culver)

Water
Detergents
Cleaners & builders
Fragrance
Optical brighteners
Propellants

KLEEN GUARD FURNITURE POLISH WITH LEMON OIL (AEROSOL)
(Alberto-Culver)

Water
Propellant
Silicone emulsion
Mineral spirits *
Oil of almond
Fragrance
Wax
Wax emulsifier
Formaldehyde

KLEENITE
Denture cleanser
(Vicks Toiletry Products Div.)

Sodium chloride	
Trisodium phosphate *	36%
Sodium perborate *	18%
Sucrose	
Sodium dichloroisocyanurate *	
Disodium EDTA	
Flavor	
Sodium lauryl sulfate	
FD & C Green No. 3	

KLEEN-IT FILTER DESCALER & CLEANER

See BIO-GUARD KLEEN-IT FILTER DESCALER & CLEANER

KLEEN KING ALUMINUM CLEANSER
(Faultless Starch/Bon Ami)

Sodium silicofluoride *	<7%
Sulfamic acid	<5%

KLEEN KING RUST & STAIN REMOVER
(Faultless Starch/Bon Ami)

Sodium silicofluoride *	<7%
Sulfamic acid	<5%

KLEEN KING STAINLESS STEEL & COPPER CLEANSER
(Faultless Starch/Bon Ami)

Sodium chloride	<8%
Triton X-100 (non-ionic)	<1%
Octyl phenoxy polyethoxy ethanol	

Starred ingredients (*) may be responsible for major toxic effects; consult Section II.

KLEENKOIL
Inhibited acid solution for coil scale removal
(Clayton Mfg.)

Hydrochloric acid * .... >20%
Coal tar base inhibitor 1-10%

KLEEN-KOW STAINLESS FLY-SPRAY
(Rockland Chem.)

Petroleum distillate *
Di-n-propyl isocinchomeronate
N-Octyl bicycloheptene dicarboximide
Piperonyl butoxide (technical)
Pyrethrins

KLEEN MIST
Deodorant, sanitizer
(C-Z Chemical)

Isopropyl alcohol *
Triethylene glycol
Para di-isobutyl phenoxy ethoxy ethyl di-methyl benzyl ammonium chloride *

'76 Ed.

KLEEN-SHEL, FORMULA 880

See KLENZADE KLEEN-SHEL, FOR-MULA 880

KLEEN STOCK SPRAY OR DIP
Insecticide
(Chevron)

Gamma isomer of benzene hexa-
chloride (from lindane) 1.7%
Toxaphene * 43.4%
Xylene * 14.8%
Petroleum distillate 26.0%

Chevron emergency phone number: 415-233-3737

"KLEENS" WATER BOX BOWL CLEANER TABS
(Curran)

Soda ash *
Cleaners

'76 Ed.

KLEENUP FLOWABLE EMULSION
Insecticide
(Chevron)

Petroleum oils * 80%/w

Chevron emergency phone number: 415-233-3737

KLEEN-UP SOLVENT
Cleaner
(Hillyard Chem.)

Aromatic solvent naphtha *

'76 Ed.

KLEEN WALK WEED KILLER,,UNICO

See UNICO KLEEN WALK WEED KILLER

KLEER BRITE
Dish cleaner
(Burnishine)

Triton-X-100 (Alkylated aryl poly-ether alcohol) *
Ultrawet 60L *
Water

KLEER-BRITE, FORMULA HC-29

See KLENZADE KLEER-BRITE, FORMULA HC-29

KLEER-KLENZ, FORMULA H-32

See KLENZADE KLEER-KLENZ, FORMULA HC-32

KLEER-MOR, HC-1

See KLENZADE KLEER-MOR, HC-1

KLEER PINE

See LEEDSALL KLEER PINE

KLEERWAE COLORED CHALK

See CRAYOLA KLEERWAE COL-ORED CHALK

KLENKLOR

See C-Z KLENKLOR

K-LENS-M ANTI-FOGGING LIQUID AND K-LENS-M CLEANER
For lenses
(Wilkins)

Isopropanol *
Wetting agent

KLENSO
Liquid detergent
(Adco)

Nonionic detergent *†
Anionic synthetic detergent *

†*See* Nonionic synthetic detergents

KLENZADE ACCLEAN, FORMULA HC-500
(Klenzade)

Sodium tripolyphosphate, chlorinated *
Sodium metasilicate *
Sodium carbonate *

KLENZADE 2100 ACID
(Klenzade)

Phosphoric acid *

KLENZADE AIM, FORMULA PL-400
(Klenzade)

Sodium tripolyphosphate, chlorinated *
Sodium metasilicate *
Sodium carbonate *

KLENZADE AUTOMATE 1, FORMULA 2062
(Klenzade)

Potassium hydroxide *
Sodium hypochlorite *

KLENZADE AUTOMATE 2, FORMULA 2124
(Klenzade)

Potassium hydroxide *

KLENZADE AUTOMATE 3, FORMULA 2125
(Klenzade)

Potassium hydroxide *
Sodium hypochlorite *

KLENZADE BEVRO KLENE
(Klenzade)

Butoxy polypropoxy polyethoxy ethanol iodine complex (Iodine - 1.75%)

KLENZADE BRITE-KLENZ (FORMULA HC-19, FORMULA HC-20)
(Klenzade)

Sodium hydroxide *

KLENZADE CHLORINATED KLEER-MOR FORMULA HC-10
(Klenzade)

Linear alkyl benzene sulfonate (biodegrad-able) *
Polyphosphates, chlorinated *†

†*See* Chlorinated sodium tripolyphosphate

Starred ingredients (*) may be responsible for major toxic effects; consult Section II.

KLENZADE CHURN-KLENE
(Klenzade)

Sodium tripolyphosphate *
Alkyl dimethyl dichloro benzyl ammonium chloride * 3.0%
Sodium metasilicate *

KLENZADE DEFOAM ACID, FORMULA 2190
(Klenzade)

Phosphoric acid *

KLENZADE ESTEEM
(Klenzade)

Sodium hydroxide *

KLENZADE EXSPEED, FORMULA LC-73
(Klenzade)

Hydrofluoric acid *
Phosphoric acid *

KLENZADE FLOOR-NU, FORMULA HC-62
(Klenzade)

Chlorinated trisodium phosphate *
Sodium tripolyphosphate

KLENZADE FOAM-NOX, FORMULA LC-81
(Klenzade)

Polyoxyethylene polyoxypropylene glycol

KLENZADE HARD WATER TREATMENT 'A' FORMULA WT-11
(Klenzade)

Polyphosphate compound *

KLENZADE HC-6
(Klenzade)

Sodium tripolyphosphate
Trisodium phosphate *

KLENZADE HC-8
(Klenzade)

Sodium tripolyphosphate
Sodium hypochlorite *

KLENZADE HC-9
(Klenzade)

Sodium tripolyphosphate *
Sodium metasilicate *

KLENZADE HC-22 MECHANICAL CLEANER, FORMULA HC-22
(Klenzade)

Sodium tripolyphosphate *
Sodium metasilicate *

KLENZADE HC-90
(Klenzade)

Sodium tripolyphosphate
Chlorinated trisodium phosphate *

KLENZADE HEAVY-DUTY ACID, FORMULA LC-30
(Klenzade)

Phosphoric acid *

KLENZADE HW-19 ACID MACHINE WASHING COMPOUND
(Klenzade)

Sulfamic acid *
Phosphates *

KLENZADE IM-3
(Klenzade)

Sodium polyphosphates *
Sodium metasilicate *

KLENZADE INFLATION-KLEEN, FORMULA HC-41
(Klenzade)

Sodium hydroxide * . . . . >10%

KLENZADE IODOPHOR, FORMULA ID-11
(Klenzade)

Nonylphenoxypoly ethanol-iodine complex (iodine content - 1.75%)

KLENZADE KLEEN-SHEL, FORMULA 880
(Klenzade)

Sodium tripolyphosphate, chlorinated *
Sodium metasilicate *

KLENZADE KLEER-BRITE, FORMULA HC-29
Bottle washing alkali
(Klenzade)

Sodium hydroxide * . . . . >10%

KLENZADE KLEER-KLENZ, FORMULA HC-32
(Klenzade)

Sodium tripolyphosphate
Sodium hydroxide, chlorinated *

KLENZADE KLEER-MOR, HC-1
(Klenzade)

Linear alkyl benzene sulfonate (biodegradable) *
Sodium tripolyphosphate *

KLENZADE KLENZ-GLIDE 1 AND KLENZ-GLIDE 2
(Klenzade)

Soap
Isopropyl alcohol * 15%

KLENZADE KLENZ-KLOR, FORMULA X-3
For dairy, food plant cleaning
(Klenzade)

Sodium hypochlorite * 3.25%
Sodium phosphate *

KLENZADE KLENZMATION DETERGENT 1, FORMULA AC-1
(Klenzade)

Sodium hydroxide * . . . . >10%

KLENZADE KLENZMATION DETERGENT 2, FORMULA AC-2
(Klenzade)

Potassium hydroxide * . . . . >10%

KLENZADE KLENZMATION DETERGENT 3, FORMULA AC-3
(Klenzade)

Phosphoric acid *

KLENZADE KLENZMATION DETERGENT 6, FORMULA AC-6
(Klenzade)

Polyphosphates *

KLENZADE KLENZMATION DETERGENT 7, FORMULA AC-7
(Klenzade)

Polyphosphates *

KLENZADE KLENZMATION DETERGENT 10, FORMULA AC-10
(Klenzade)

Sodium hydroxide * . . . . >10%

KLENZADE KLENZMATION DETERGENT 30, FORMULA AC-30
(Klenzade)

Phosphoric acid *
Nitric acid *

KLENZADE KLENZ-SCALD, FORMULA 2129
(Klenzade)

Trisodium phosphate *

KLENZADE LAUNDRY DETERGENT SUPER S
(Klenzade)

Sodium tripolyphosphate
Sodium hydroxide * .... >10%
Sodium metasilicate *
Sodium dodecyl benzene sulfonate

KLENZADE 2313 LIQUID ALKALINE CLEANER
(Klenzade)

Potassium hydroxide * .... >10%

KLENZADE LIQUID 'K', FORMULA LC-300
(Klenzade)

Alkyl benzene sulfonate *

KLENZADE MIKROKLENE DF
(Klenzade)

Butoxy polypropoxy polyethoxy ethanol iodine complex (Iodine - 1.75%)

KLENZADE MI-5 MACHINE WASHING COMPOUND
(Klenzade)

Sodium tripolyphosphate, chlorinated *

KLENZADE NU-KLEEN, FORMULA LC-11
(Klenzade)

Glycolic acid
Phosphoric acid *

KLENZADE PASSIV-8, FORMULA PL-8
(Klenzade)

Phosphoric acid *
Nitric acid .... <5%

KLENZADE PIPELINE CLEANER, FORMULA 2048
(Klenzade)

Sodium tripolyphosphate *
Sodium metasilicate, chlorinated *†

†See Chlorinated sodium metasilicate

KLENZADE PL-3
(Klenzade)

Phosphoric acid *

KLENZADE PL-190
(Klenzade)

Sodium tripolyphosphate *
Chlorinated tripolyphosphate *

KLENZADE SPECIAL ALKALI, FORMULA HC-41
(Klenzade)

Sodium hydroxide * .... >10%

KLENZADE SPEED-WASH, FORMULA LC-5
(Klenzade)

Potassium hydroxide * .... >10%

KLENZADE STER-BAC, FORMULA KQ-12
(Klenzade)

Alkyl dimethyl benzyl ammonium chloride * 10%

KLENZADE TRICHLOR-O-CIDE, FORMULA XP-100
(Klenzade)

Potassium dichloroisocyanurate (9.79% available chlorine) *
Sodium tripolyphosphate *

KLENZADE UDDER WASH, FORMULA KDS-33
(Klenzade)

Alkyl dimethyl dichloro benzyl ammonium chloride * 5%
Hydroxyacetic acid

KLENZADE VEGA-KLEEN, FORMULA 1164
(Klenzade)

Sodium tripolyphosphate *

KLENZADE X-4 LIQUID BACTERICIDE
(Klenzade)

Sodium hypochlorite * 6.4%

KLENZADE XY-12 DISINFECTANT & GERMICIDE
(Klenzade)

Sodium hypochlorite * 10.2%

KLENZ-GLIDE 1 AND KLENZ-GLIDE 2

See KLENZADE KLENZ-GLIDE

KLENZ-KLOR, FORMULA X-3

See KLENZADE KLENZ-KLOR, FORMULA X-3

KLENZMATION DETERGENTS

See KLENZADE KLENZMATION

KLENZO
Antiseptic mouthwash
(Rexall)

Alcohol	25%
Zinc chloride	<1%
Benzoic acid	<1%
Ammonium chloride	<1%
Citric acid	<1%
Menthol	<1%
Oil cloves	<1%
Cinnamic aldehyde	<1%
Methyl salicylate	<1%

'76 Ed.

KLENZ-SCALD, FORMULA 2129

See KLENZADE KLENZ-SCALD, FORMULA 2129

KLER
Glass cleaner, de-icer and windshield washer concentrate; industrial and institutional use
(Scientific International)

Isopropyl alcohol *

KLERA-CID
Commercial laundry sour
(Diversey Wyandotte)

Fluoride salts *

KLING-TITE 200 SPRAY
Plant regulator
(Chevron)

Potassium 1-naphthaleneacetate 6.5%/w

Chevron emergency phone number: 415-233-3737

Starred ingredients (*) may be responsible for major toxic effects; consult Section II.

KLING-TITE 800 SPRAY
Plant regulator
(Chevron)

Potassium 1-naphthalene-
acetate * 24.5%/w

Chevron emergency phone number: 415-
233-3737

KLORAMINE
Antihistaminic
(Wesley Pharm.)

Each tablet:
Chlorpheniramine maleate * . . . 4 mg.

KLORASPAN
Antihistaminic
(Wesley Pharm.)

Each tablet:
Chlorpheniramine maleate * . . . 8 mg.

KLORO KOL
Dishwashing machine compound
(DuBois Chem.)

Complex Sodium phosphates *
Sodium hypochlorite *
Sodium carbonate *
Sodium silicates

K-LOR POWDER PACKETS
*Potassium supplement; granules for re-
constitution*
(Abbott)

Potassium chloride for
solution (USP) * . . 15 mEq.; 20 mEq.

KLORVESS EFFERVESCENT
GRANULES
Potassium and chloride supplement
(Dorsey Labs.)

Each packet (2.8 gm.):
Potassium chloride * . . . . . . 1.125 gm.
Potassium bicarbonate . . . . 0.500 gm.
L-Lysine monohydrochloride 0.913 gm.

KLORVESS
(EFFERVESCENT
TABLETS & LIQUID)
Potassium and chloride supplement
(Dorsey Labs.)

Each tablet:
Potassium chloride * . . . . . 1.125 gm.
Potassium bicarbonate . . . . 0.5 gm.
L-Lysine
monohydrochloride . . . . . 0.913 gm.

Each 15 ml.:
Potassium chloride * 1.5 gm. (20 mEq)
Alcohol 1%

K-LYTE
*Therapy or prophylaxis of potassium
deficiency*
(Mead Johnson)

Each effervescent tablet:
Potassium * . . . . 25 mEq.

K-LYTE/CL
Oral potassium supplement
(Mead Johnson)

Each effervescent tablet:
Potassium chloride * . . . . 25 mEq.

K-M
*To disinfect poultry drinking water;
veterinary*
(Hilltop)

Methyl dodecyl benzyl trimethyl
ammonium chloride * 2.64%
Methyl dodecyl xylylene bis trimethyl ammonium chloride . . . 0.66%
Synthetic vitamin K (Menadione
sodium bisulfite) 0.08%

Inactive ingred.:
Water 70.62%
Combined amount: 26.00%
Sodium sulfate (Glauber's salts)
Potassium acetate
Magnesium sulfate (Epsom salts)
Potassium nitrate
Potassium chlorate *
Cert. color

'76 Ed.

KN-48
Chemical toilet deodorant

Zevel Corporation
P.O. Box 112
La Mirada, Calif. 90637

Phone: 714-521-4284

KNIGHT ADHESIVE
PRIMERS NO. 1642
(Knight, M.A.)

Aromatic solvents *
Propyl alcohol *
Phosphoric acid * . . . . to 5%
Acrylonitrile rubber
Other rubber polymers
Silicious, kaolin, calcium fillers

KNIGHTBOND CEMENTS
(SULFUR CEMENTS NO. 6
& NO. 7)
(Knight, M. A.)

Sulfur 50%
Carbon powder or silicious
materials . . . . to 49%
Thiokol . . . . to 1%

KNOCKOUT DRAIN
CLEANER
Professional use
(Internat. Plumb.)

Sulphuric acid *

'76 Ed.

KNOCK-OUT, THE TOTAL
WEED KILLER
Weed killer
(Hub States)

Bromacil (5-Bromo-3-sec-butyl-
methyluracil) 2.00%

'76 Ed.

K.N.O.W
Wart remover
(King Pharmaceutical)

Castor oil
Salicylic acid *
Benzoin *
Aloe *
Storax
Tolu balsam
Camphor *
Alcohol * 50%

K-N-S
Hypnotic, sedative and anticonvulsant
(King Pharmaceutical)

Each fl. oz.:
Sodium bromide * . . . . 120 gr.
Pyridoxine hydrochloride . . . . . 10 mg.
Chloral hydrate * . . . . 1 gr.
Alcohol 4.5%
Base:
Pepsin
Menthol
Aromatics

K.O.

See PYROIL K.O.

KOADONNA GEL
Adsorbent, anticholinergic
(Pharmex)

Kaolin
Pectin
Hyoscyamine *
Hyoscine *
Atropine sulfate *

KOCIDE 101
Agricultural fungicide
(Kocide Chemical)

Copper hydroxide * 77.0%
Surfactants 5.5%

KODAK
Photographic products
(Eastman Kodak)

For emergency information concerning
photographic products of the Eastman Kodak Company which are not listed in this
section, contact the Eastman Kodak Company, Health and Safety Laboratory,
Rochester, New York 14650.

24-hour phone no.: 716-722-5151

Starred ingredients (*) may be responsible for major toxic effects; consult Section II.

KODAK CHROMIUM INTENSIFIER In-4
Photographic
(Eastman Kodak)

Stock solution:
Water to make	1.0 liter
Potassium dichromate *	90.0 gm.
Hydrochloric acid (concentrated) *	64.0 cc.

KODAK DEVELOPER D-8
Photographic
(Eastman Kodak)

Sodium sulfite, desiccated	90.0 gm.
Hydroquinone *	45.0 gm.
Sodium hydroxide (Caustic soda)	37.5 gm.
Potassium bromide	30.0 gm.
Water to make	1.0 liter

KODAK DEVELOPER D-11
Photographic
(Eastman Kodak)

Elon developing agent (p-Methylaminophenol sulfate)	1.0 gm.
Sodium sulfite, desiccated	75.0 gm.
Hydroquinone	9.0 gm.
Sodium carbonate, monohydrated	30.0 gm.
Potassium bromide	5.0 gm.
Water to make	1.0 liter

KODAK DEVELOPER D-19 & DEVELOPER REPLENISHER D-19R
Photographic
(Eastman Kodak)

DEVELOPER D-19:
Elon developing agent (p-Methylaminophenol sulfate)	2.0 gm.
Sodium sulfite, desiccated	90.0 gm.
Hydroquinone	8.0 gm.
Sodium carbonate, monohydrated	52.5 gm.
Potassium bromide	5.0 gm.
Water to make	1.0 liter

DEVELOPER REPLENISHER D-19R:
Elon developing agent (p-Methylaminophenol sulfate)	4.5 gm.
Sodium sulfite, desiccated	90.0 gm.
Hydroquinone *	17.5 gm.
Sodium carbonate, monohydrated	52.5 gm.
Sodium hydroxide *	7.5 gm.
Water to make	1.0 liter

KODAK DEVELOPER D-23
Photographic
(Eastman Kodak)

Elon developing agent (p-Methylaminophenol sulfate)	7.5 gm.
Sodium sulfite, desiccated	100.0 gm.
Water to make	1.0 liter

KODAK DEVELOPER D-25 & DEVELOPER REPLENISHER DK-25R
Photographic
(Eastman Kodak)

DEVELOPER D-25:
Elon developing agent (p-Methylaminophenol sulfate)	7.5 gm.
Sodium sulfite, desiccated	100.0 gm.
Sodium bisulfite	15.0 gm.
Water to make	1.0 liter

DEVELOPER REPLENISHER DK-25R:
Elon developing agent (p-Methylaminophenol sulfate)	10.0 gm.
Sodium sulfite, desiccated	100.0 gm.
Kodalk balanced Alkali	20.0 gm.
Water to make	1.0 liter

KODAK DEVELOPER D-52
Photographic
(Eastman Kodak)

Stock solution:
Elon developing agent (p-Methylaminophenol sulfate)	1.5 gm.
Sodium sulfite, desiccated	22.5 gm.
Hydroquinone	6.0 gm.
Sodium carbonate, monohydrated	17.0 gm.
Potassium bromide	1.5 gm.
Water to make	1.0 liter

KODAK DEVELOPER D-61a & DEVELOPER REPLENISHER D-61R
Photographic
(Eastman Kodak)

DEVELOPER D-61a stock solution:
Elon developing agent (p-Methylaminophenol sulfate)	3.0 gm.
Sodium sulfite, desiccated	90.0 gm.
Sodium bisulfite	2.0 gm.
Hydroquinone	6.0 gm.
Sodium carbonate, monohydrated	14.0 gm.
Potassium bromide	2.0 gm.
Water to make	1.0 liter

DEVELOPER REPLENISHER D-61R:
Stock Solution A:
Elon developing agent (p-Methylaminophenol sulfate)	6.0 gm.
Sodium sulfite, desiccated	180.0 gm.
Sodium bisulfite	4.0 gm.
Hydroquinone *	12.0 gm.
Potassium bromide	3.0 gm.
Water to make	6.0 liters

Stock Solution B:
Sodium carbonate, monohydrated	280.0 gm.
Water to make	2.0 liters

KODAK DEVELOPER D-72
Photographic
(Eastman Kodak)

Elon developing agent (p-Methylaminophenol sulfate)	3.0 gm.
Sodium sulfite, desiccated	45.0 gm.
Hydroquinone *	12.0 gm.
Sodium carbonate, monohydrated	80.0 gm.
Potassium bromide	2.0 gm.
Water to make	1.0 liter

KODAK DEVELOPER D-76 & DEVELOPER REPLENISHER D-76R
Photographic
(Eastman Kodak)

DEVELOPER D-76:
Elon developing agent (p-Methylaminophenol sulfate)	2.0 gm.
Sodium sulfite, desiccated	100.0 gm.
Hydroquinone	5.0 gm.
Borax, granular	2.0 gm.
Water to make	1.0 liter

DEVELOPER REPLENISHER D-76R:
Elon developing agent (p-Methylaminophenol sulfate)	3.0 gm.
Sodium sulfite, desiccated	100.0 gm.
Hydroquinone	7.5 gm.
Borax, granular	20.0 gm.
Water to make	1.0 liter

KODAK DEVELOPER DK-50 & DEVELOPER REPLENISHER DK-50R
Photographic
(Eastman Kodak)

DEVELOPER DK-50 stock solution:
Elon developing agent (p-Methylaminophenol sulfate)	2.5 gm.
Sodium sulfite, desiccated	30.0 gm.
Hydroquinone	2.5 gm.
Kodalk balanced Alkali	10.0 gm.
Potassium bromide	0.5 gm.
Water to make	1.0 liter

DEVELOPER REPLENISHER DK-50R:
Elon developing agent (p-Methylaminophenol sulfate)	5.0 gm.
Sodium sulfite, desiccated	30.0 gm.
Hydroquinone	10.0 gm.
Kodalk balanced Alkali	40.0 gm.
Water to make	1.0 liter

Starred ingredients (*) may be responsible for major toxic effects; consult Section II.

KODAK DEVELOPER DK-60a & DEVELOPER REPLENISHER DK-60aTR
Photographic
(Eastman Kodak)

DEVELOPER DK-60a:

Elon developing agent (p-Methylaminophenol sulfate)	2.5 gm.
Sodium sulfite, desiccated	50.0 gm.
Hydroquinone	2.5 gm.
Kodalk balanced Alkali	20.0 gm.
Potassium bromide	0.5 gm.
Water to make	1.0 liter

DEVELOPER REPLENISHER DK-60aTR:

Elon developing agent (p-Methylaminophenol sulfate)	5.0 gm.
Sodium sulfite, desiccated	50.0 gm.
Hydroquinone	10.0 gm.
Kodalk balanced Alkali	40.0 gm.
Water to make	1.0 liter

KODAK FARMER'S REDUCER R-4a & R-4b
Photographic
(Eastman Kodak)

FARMER'S REDUCER R-4a:
Stock Solution A:

Potassium ferricyanide	37.5 gm.
Water to make	500 cc.

Stock Solution B:

Sodium thiosulfate (Hypo) *	480.0 gm.
Water to make	2.0 liters

FARMER'S REDUCER R-4b:
Solution A:

Potassium ferricyanide	7.5 gm.
Water to make	1.0 liter

Solution B:

Sodium thiosulfate (Hypo) *	200.0 gm.
Water to make	1.0 liter

KODAK FIXING BATH F-5
Photographic
(Eastman Kodak)

Sodium thiosulfate (Hypo) *	240.0 gm.
Sodium sulfite, desiccated	15.0 gm.
Acetic acid, 28%	48.0 cc.
Boric acid, crystals	7.5 gm.
Potassium alum	15.0 gm.
Water to make	1.0 liter

KODAK FIXING BATH F-6
Photographic
(Eastman Kodak)

Sodium thiosulfate (Hypo) *	240.0 gm.
Sodium sulfite, desiccated	15.0 gm.
Acetic acid, 28%	48.0 cc.
Kodalk balanced Alkali	15.0 gm.
Potassium alum	15.0 gm.
Water to make	1.0 liter

KODAK FIXING BATH F-24
Photographic
(Eastman Kodak)

Sodium thiosulfate (Hypo) *	240.0 gm.
Sodium sulfite, desiccated	10.0 gm.
Sodium bisulfite	25.0 gm.
Water to make	1.0 liter

KODAK GOLD PROTECTIVE SOLUTION GP-1
Photographic
(Eastman Kodak)

Gold chloride (1% stock solution)	10.0 cc.
Sodium thiocyanate	15.2 gm.
Water to make	1.0 liter

KODAK GOLD TONER T-21
Photographic
(Eastman Kodak)

Stock Solution A:

Sodium thiosulfate (Hypo) *	960.0 gm.
Potassium persulfate	120.0 gm.
Silver nitrate, crystals	5.0 gm.
Sodium chloride	5.0 gm.
Water	4064.0 cc.

Stock Solution B:

Water	250.0 cc.
Gold chloride	1.0 gm.

KODAK HARDENER F-5a
Photographic
(Eastman Kodak)

Sodium sulfite, desiccated	75.0 gm.
Acetic acid, 28%	235.0 cc.
Boric acid, crystals	37.5 gm.
Potassium alum	75.0 gm.
Water to make	1.0 liter

KODAK HARDENING BATH SB-4
Photographic
(Eastman Kodak)

Water	1.0 liter
Potassium chrome alum	30.0 gm.
Sodium sulfate, desiccated	60.0 gm.

KODAK HYPO ALUM SEPIA TONER T-1a
Photographic
(Eastman Kodak)

Sodium thiosulfate (Hypo) *	480.0 gm.
Potassium alum	120.0 gm.
Silver nitrate, crystals	4.0 gm.
Sodium chloride	4.0 gm.
Water to make	4.0 liters

KODAK HYPO TEST SOLUTION HT-2
Photographic
(Eastman Kodak)

Water	750 cc.
Acetic acid, 28%	125.0 cc.
Silver nitrate	7.5 gm.
Water to make	1.0 liter

KODAK MERCURY INTENSIFIER In-1
Photographic
(Eastman Kodak)

Bleach Solution:

Potassium bromide	22.5 gm.
Mercuric chloride *	22.5 gm.
Water to make	1.0 liter

Solution A:

Water	500 cc.
Sodium cyanide	15.0 gm.

Solution B:

Water	500 cc.
Silver nitrate, crystals	22.5 gm.

KODAK PERSULFATE REDUCER R-15
Photographic
(Eastman Kodak)

Stock Solution A:

Water	1.0 liter
Potassium persulfate	30.0 gm.

Stock Solution B:

Sulfuric acid (dilute solution: 1 part conc. sulfuric acid & 9 parts water)	15.0 cc.
Water to make	500.0 cc.

KODAK POLYSULFIDE TONER T-8
Photographic
(Eastman Kodak)

Polysulfide (Liver of sulfur)	7.5 gm.
Sodium carbonate, monohydrated	2.5 gm.
Water to make	1.0 liter

KODAK PREHARDENER SH-5
Photographic
(Eastman Kodak)

Solution A:

Formaldehyde, about 37% solution by weight *	5 cc.

Solution B:

0.5% Solution of Kodak Anti-Fog No. 2 (6-Nitrobenzimidazole nitrate)	40.0 cc.
Sodium sulfite, desiccated	50.0 gm.
Sodium carbonate, monohydrated	12.0 gm.
Water to make	1.0 liter

Starred ingredients (*) may be responsible for major toxic effects; consult Section II.

KODAK QUINONE-THIOSULFATE INTENSIFIER In-6
Photographic
(Eastman Kodak)

Solution A:
Sulfuric acid (concentrated) *	30.0 cc.
Potassium dichromate *	22.5 gm.
Water to make	1.0 liter

Solution B:
Sodium bisulfite	3.8 gm.
Hydroquinone *	15.0 gm.
Kodak Photo-Flo 200 solution (wetting agent)	3.8 cc.
Water to make	1.0 liter

Solution C:
Sodium thiosulfate (Hypo)	22.5 gm.
Water to make	1.0 liter

KODAK RAPID FIXING BATH F-7
Photographic
(Eastman Kodak)

Sodium thiosulfate (Hypo) *	360.0 gm.
Ammonium chloride	50.0 gm.
Sodium sulfite, desiccated	15.0 gm.
Acetic acid, 28%	48.0 cc.
Boric acid, crystals	7.5 gm.
Potassium alum	15.0 gm.
Water to make	1.0 liter

KODAK RAPID FIXING BATH F-9
Photographic
(Eastman Kodak)

Sodium thiosulfate (Hypo) *	360.0 gm.
Ammonium sulfate	60.0 gm.
Sodium sulfite, desiccated	15.0 gm.
Acetic acid, 28%	48.0 cc.
Boric acid, crystals	7.5 gm.
Potassium alum	15.0 gm.
Water to make	1.0 liter

KODAK REDUCER R-2
Photographic
(Eastman Kodak)

Stock Solution A:
Water	1.0 liter
Potassium permanganate	52.5 gm.

Stock Solution B:
Water	1.0 liter
Sulfuric acid (concentrated)	32.0 cc.

KODAK REDUCER R-5
Photographic
(Eastman Kodak)

Stock Solution A:
Water	1.0 liter
Potassium permanganate	0.3 gm.
Sulfuric acid (dilute solution: 1 part conc. sulfuric acid & 9 parts water)	16.0 cc.

Stock Solution B:
Water	3.0 liters
Potassium persulfate	90.0 gm.

KODAK REDUCER R-8a
Photographic
(Eastman Kodak)

Citric acid	20.0 gm.
Ferric ammonium sulfate (Ferric alum)	45.0 gm.
Potassium citrate	75.0 gm.
Sodium sulfite, desiccated	30.0 gm.
Sodium thiosulfate (Hypo) *	200.0 gm.
Water to make	1.0 liter

KODAK REPLENISHERS
Photographic
(Eastman Kodak)

See KODAK DEVELOPERS

KODAK RESIDUAL SILVER TEST SOLUTION ST-1
Photographic
(Eastman Kodak)

Stock solution:
Water	125 cc.
Sodium sulfide *	2 gm.

KODAK SILVER INTENSIFIER In-5
Photographic
(Eastman Kodak)

Stock Solution No. 1:
Silver nitrate, crystals *	60.0 gm.
Distilled water to make	1.0 liter

Stock Solution No. 2:
Sodium sulfite, desiccated	60.0 gm.
Water to make	1.0 liter

Stock Solution No. 3:
Sodium thiosulfate (Hypo)	105.0 gm.
Water to make	1.0 liter

Stock Solution No. 4:
Sodium sulfite, desiccated	15.0 gm.
Elon developing agent (p-Methylaminophenol sulfate) *	25.0 gm.
Water to make	3.0 liters

KODAK SILVER STAIN REMOVER S-10
Photographic; for removal of fixer stains from clothing
(Eastman Kodak)

Thiourea	75 gm.
Citric acid	75 gm.
Water to make	1 liter

KODAK SPECIAL HARDENER SH-1
Photographic
(Eastman Kodak)

Formaldehyde, about 37% solution by weight	10.0 ml.
Sodium carbonate, monohydrated	6.0 gm.
Water to make	1.0 liter

KODAK STAIN REMOVER S-6
Photographic
(Eastman Kodak)

Stock Solution A:
Potassium permanganate	5.0 gm.
Water to make	1.0 liter

Stock Solution B:
Sodium chloride	75.0 gm.
Sulfuric acid (concentrated)	16.0 cc.
Water to make	1.0 liter

KODAK STOP BATH SB-1 & SB-1a
Photographic
(Eastman Kodak)

SB-1:
Water	1.0 liter
Acetic acid, 28%	48.0 cc.

SB-1a:
Water	1.0 liter
Acetic acid, 28%	125.0 cc.

KODAK STOP BATH SB-5
Photographic
(Eastman Kodak)

Acetic acid, 28%	32.0 cc.
Sodium sulfate, desiccated	45.0 gm.
Water to make	1.0 liter

KODAK SULFIDE SEPIA TONER T-7a
Photographic
(Eastman Kodak)

Stock Bleaching Solution A:
Potassium ferricyanide	75.0 gm.
Potassium bromide	75.0 gm.
Potassium oxalate *	195.0 gm.
Acetic acid, 28%	40.0 cc.
Water	2.0 liters

Stock Toning Solution B:
Sodium sulfide *	45.0 gm.
Water to make	500 cc.

KODAK TRAY CLEANER TC-1
Photographic
(Eastman Kodak)

Water	1.0 liter
Potassium dichromate *	90.0 gm.
Sulfuric acid (concentrated) *	96.0 cc.

KODAK TRAY CLEANER TC-3
Photographic
(Eastman Kodak)

Solution A:
Water	1.0 liter
Potassium permanganate	2.0 gm.
Sulfuric acid (concentrated)	4.0 cc.

Solution B:
Water	1.0 liter
Sodium bisulfite	30.0 gm.
Sodium sulfite, desiccated	30.0 gm.

Starred ingredients (*) may be responsible for major toxic effects; consult Section II.

K.O. DOSE INSECT KILLER
Commercial and institutional use
(Hysan Corp.)

Pyrethrins	0.20%
Technical Piperonyl butoxide	0.720%
N-Octyl bicycloheptene	
dicarboximide	0.40%
Petroleum distillate *	18.68%

KOFF BALLS

See DEWITT'S KOFF BALLS

KOLANTYL (GEL, TABLETS & WAFERS)
Antacid
(Merrell Dow)

GEL (each 5 cc):
Aluminum hydroxide	150 mg.
Magnesium hydroxide	150 mg.

TABLETS (each):
Aluminum hydroxide	300 mg.
Magnesium hydroxide	185 mg.

WAFERS (each):
Aluminum hydroxide	180 mg.
Magnesium hydroxide	170 mg.

KOLMAR CLEANSING CREAM
(Kolmar Labs.)

Water	>50%
Gelling agent	1-5%
Preservative	0.1-1.0%
Epithelizing agent	0.1-1.0%
Bactericide	<0.1%
Moisturizing agent	0.1-1.0%
Nonionic emulsifier	1-5%
Nonionic surfactant	1-5%
Emollient	25-50%
Emulsifier	1-5%
Fragrance	0.1-1.0%

KOLMAR CLEANSING CREAM CONCENTRATE
(Kolmar Labs.)

Water	25-50%
Moisturizing agent	0.1-1.0%
Bactericide	0.1-1.0%
Emollient	25-50%
Nonionic emulsifier	5-10%
Nonionic surfactant	5-10%
Preservative	1-5%

KOLMAR LIQUID MAKEUP WITH POROSITONE (All Shades)
(Kolmar Labs.)

Emollient	10-25%
Emulsifier	1-5%
Preservatives	0.1-1.0%
Co-emulsifier	1-5%
Gelling agent	0.1-1.0%
Powder base	1-5%
Solvent	10-25%
Emulsion stabilizer, thickener	0.1-1.0%
Water	25-50%
Anionic surfactant	0.1-1.0%
Moisturizing agent	<1.0%
Fragrance	0.1-1.0%
Color additives	10-25%

KOLMAR SKIN CLEANSER
(Kolmar Labs.)

Emulsifier	>50%
Emollient	10-25%
Water	5-10%
Fragrance	0.1-1.0%

KOLMAR SKIN FRESHNER
(Kolmar Labs.)

Surfactant	0.1-1.0%
Water	>50%
Solvent	1-5%
Preservative	0.1-1.0%
Fragrance	0.1-1.0%
Color additives	<0.1%

KOLMAR SKIN TONER CONCENTRATE A
(Kolmar Labs.)

Fragrance *	10-25%
Nonionic co-emulsifier	>50%

KOLMAR SKIN TONER CONCENTRATE B
(Kolmar Labs.)

Nonionic co-emulsifier	5-10%
Emollient	10-25%
Stabilizing agent or preservative	1-5%
Water	>50%
Moisturizing agent	0.1-1.0%

KOLO 100

See NIAGARA KOLO 100

KOLODUST

See NIAGARA KOLODUST

KOLODUST 100

See NIAGARA KOLODUST 100

KOLOFOG

See NIAGARA KOLOFOG

KOLOKIL

See NIAGARA KOLOKIL

KOLOTEX

See NIAGARA KOLOTEX

KOLPOSINE
Douche, liquid
(Optimus)

Aluminum ammonium sulfate	
Boric acid *	
Phenol *	<3%
Menthol *	
Glycerin	

KOL-SPANS
Decongestant
(Reese Chem.)

Each capsule:
Total Belladonna alkaloidal salts	0.16 mg.
Atropine sulfate	0.024 mg.
Scopolamine hydrobromide	0.014 mg.
Hyoscyamine sulfate	0.122 mg.
Phenylpropanolamine hydrochloride *	50 mg.
Chlorpheniramine maleate	1 mg.
Pheniramine maleate	12.5 mg.

KOL SUPREME
Machine dishwashing compound
(DuBois Chem.)

Sodium salts of carbonates, silicates and phosphates *†

†*See* Alkali

KOLTAROL
Disinfectant
(Huggins)

Anhydrous soap	18%
Tar acid oil (to a maximum of 20% phenol) *	72%

KOLYNOS TOOTHPASTES
(Whitehall Labs.)

Whitehall Laboratories
Div. American Home Products Corp.
685 Third Ave.
New York, N.Y. 10017

Phone: 212-986-1000

See COSMETICS, Section VI, General Formulations

Starred ingredients (*) may be responsible for major toxic effects; consult Section II.

KOMED HC LOTION (HYDROCORTISONE)
For acne accompanied by inflammation
(Barnes-Hind)

Hydrocortisone acetate	0.5%
Sodium thiosulfate	8%
Salicylic acid *	2%
Menthol	0.1%
Camphor	0.1%
Isopropyl alcohol *	25%
Colloidal alumina	3%

KOMED LOTIONS
For acne
(Barnes-Hind)

MILD:

Sodium thiosulfate	2%
Salicylic acid *	1%
Menthol	0.1%
Camphor	0.1%
Isopropyl alcohol *	25%
Colloidal alumina	3%

REGULAR:

Sodium thiosulfate	8%
Salicylic acid *	2%
Menthol	0.1%
Camphor	0.1%
Isopropyl alcohol *	25%
Colloidal alumina	3%

KONDON'S NASAL JELLY
(Kondon)

Menthol *	1.0%
Oil eucalyptus *	1.9%
Phenol	0.5%
Camphor *	1.0%
Oil of lavender	0.7%

KONDON'S NASAL JELLY WITH EPHEDRINE
(Kondon)

Ephedrine alkaloid *	1.00%
Menthol	0.75%
Oil eucalyptus *	2.00%
Phenol	0.5%
Camphor	0.75%
Oil of pine needles	0.75%

KONSYL
Laxative
(Burton, Parsons & Co.)

Plantago ovata

KOOL-FOOT MEDICATED CREAM
(Blistex)

Zinc undecylenate *	5.0%
Chloroxylenol	0.4%
Base:	balance
Water	
Mineral oil	
Stearic acid	
Isopropyl palmitate	
Isopropyl myristate	
Isopropyl stearate	
Glycerin	

KOOL-O-BALM
Horse liniment
(Carson Chemicals, Inc.)

Menthol *
Camphor *
Methyl salicylate *

KOOL WASH

See AMWAY KOOL WASH

KOPPERSOL MILDEW & FUNGUS SPRAY

See DEXOL KOPPERSOL MILDEW & FUNGUS SPRAY

KOPPERS PAINT PRODUCTS
Coatings, enamels, and water repellents

Koppers Co., Inc.
Koppers Building
Pittsburgh, Pa. 15219

Phone: 412-227-2000

See PAINTS, Section VI, General Formulations

KORE
Germicide, disinfectant, deodorant, cleaner; veterinary
(King Research)

Active ingred.:
  N-Alkyl (C14 50%; C12 40%; C16 10%) dimethyl benzyl ammonium chlorides (Benzalkonium chloride, USP) * ... 5%
Sodium carbonate, monohydrate * ... 45%

Inert ingred.:
  Alkaline detergents
  Nonionic detergents

KORLAN 8 (IMPROVED)
Insecticidal concentrate
(Dow)

O,O-Dimethyl O-2,4,5-trichlorophenyl phosphorothioate *	67.0%
Methylene chloride *	33.0%

KORLAN 24E
Insecticide
(Dow)

O,O-Dimethyl-O-(2,4,5-trichlorophenyl) phosphorothioate	24%
Aromatic petroleum solvent *	61%

KORLAN 2 POUR ON INSECTICIDE FOR LICE
(Dow)

O,O-Dimethyl O-2,4,5-trichlorophenyl phosphorothioate *	24.5%
Inert ingred.:	75.5%
Emulsifiers	
Solvents (including petroleum oil) *†	

†See Petroleum distillate

KOROMEX CONTRACEPTIVE FOAM
(Holland-Rantos)

Nonoxynol-9	12.5%
Propylene glycol	
Propellant 114	
Isopropyl alcohol	
Laureth-4	
Cetyl alcohol	
Propellant 12	
PEG-50 stearate	
Fragrance	

KOROMEX II-A JELLY
Contraceptive jelly
(Holland-Rantos)

Boric acid	2.0%
Nonoxynol-9	2.0%
Perfume	

KOROMEX II CREAM
Contraceptive cream
(Holland-Rantos)

Boric acid	2.0%
Octoxynol	3.0%
Stearic acid	
Perfume	

KOROMEX II JELLY
Contraceptive jelly
(Holland-Rantos)

Boric acid	2.0%
Octoxynol	1.0%
Perfume	

KOTABARB
Sedative
(Wesley Pharm.)

Each tablet:	
Phenobarbital *	1/4 gr.

KOW KARE
Vitamin mineral supplement; veterinary
(Dairy Assoc.)

Peanut hull meal	46.4%
Di-cal phosphate	29.8%
Bone meal	1.4%
Epsom salts	9.3%
Ferrous sulfate	3.4%
Red pepper	0.14%
Iron oxide	7.43%
Ginger	0.07%
Calcium iodate	0.43%
Manganese	0.34%
Yeast-D	0.24%
Cobalt	0.07%
Gentian root	0.68%
Vitamin E	0.07%
Vitamin A	0.16%
Spearmint oil	0.07%

K-PHOS - MODIFIED FORMULA
For urine acidification and recurrent urinary calculi
(Beach Pharm.)

Each tablet:
Potassium acid phosphate *†	155 mg.
Sodium acid phosphate *†	350 mg.

†*See* Phosphates

K-PHOS NEUTRAL TABLETS
Phosphate supplement
(Beach Pharm.)

Each tablet:
Sodium phosphate dibasic, anhydrous *†	852 mg.
Potassium phosphate, monobasic *‡	155 mg.
Sodium phosphate, monobasic *†	130 mg.

†*See* Phosphates
‡*See* Potassium salts

KRAZY GLUE
Adhesive
(Krazy Glue)

Ethyl cyanoacrylate 99.95%

K-R COMPOUND
(Park Chem.)

Kerosene *
Soap
Pine oil *
Abrasives

KREEN
Motor tonic
(Kano)

Petroleum solvents *
Other oils

KREML CORRECTIVE
For dandruff
(Williams, J.B.)

Alcohol *	63.7%
Dihydroxy dichloro diphenyl methane	
Benzalkonium chloride *	
Polyalkalene glycols	

KREML HAIR TONIC
(Williams, J.B.)

Alcohol	19%/v
Benzoic acid	
Dehydroacetic acid	
Methyl dodecyl benzyl trimethyl ammonium chloride *	
Essential oils *	
Mineral oil base	

"KRENITE" BRUSH CONTROL AGENT
(Du Pont)

Fosamine ammonium * 41.5%

"KRENITE" S BRUSH CONTROL AGENT
(Du Pont)

Fosamine ammonium * 41.5%

KRESO DIP
Insecticide - disinfectant - germicide - cleanser
(Kreso)

Coal tar hydrocarbons *	53%
Soap	20%
Coal tar phenols	18%
Water	9%

KRIL
Liquid floor polish
(Sanitek)

Styrene-acrylic copolymer emulsion	11.2%
Diethylene glycol monoethyl ether (Cellosolve)	2.2%
Styrene maleic resin	1.5%
Polyethylene emulsion	1.3%
Tributoxyethyl phosphate	1.0%
Nonionic surfactant	0.2%
Formalin	0.2%
Ammonia, Defoamer, Fluoro-chemical surfactant	trace
Water	balance

KRIPTIN
Antihistamine tablets
(Whitehall Labs.)

Pyrilamine maleate * .... 25 mg.

KROIL
Penetrating oil
(Kano)

Petroleum solvents *
Other oils

KROMAD
Turf fungicide
(Mallinckrodt, Inc.)

Cadmium sebacate *	5.0%
Potassium chromate *	5.0%
Malachite green	1.0%
Auramine	0.5%
Thiram (Tetramethylthiuram disulfide) *	16.0%

"KROVAR" I WEED KILLER
(Du Pont)

Bromacil *	40%
Diuron *	40%

"KROVAR" II WEED KILLER
(Du Pont)

Bromacil *	53%
Diuron *	27%

KRYLON PAINT PRODUCTS

Krylon, Consumer Products
Div. of Borden Chemical
180 E. Broad St.
Columbus, Ohio 43215

Phone: 614-225-4896

KRYOCIDE
Insecticide
(Pennwalt)

Sodium fluoaluminate 96%

KRYZEN
Antispasmodic
(Wesley Pharm.)

Each tablet:
Tr. Gelsemium	3 min.
Salicylamide *	1 gr.
Hyoscyamus	1/8 gr.
Atropine sulfate *	1/500 gr.
Camphor	1/10 gr.

K2r SPOT LIFTER (Aerosol)

See TEXIZE K2r SPOT LIFTER (Aerosol)

K2r SPOT LIFTER (Paste)

See TEXIZE K2r SPOT LIFTER (Paste)

KUDROX (DOUBLE STRENGTH)
Antacid, demulcent
(Kremers-Urban)

Aluminum hydroxide gel
Magnesium hydroxide
d-Sorbitol

KURFEES ALKYD TRAFFIC PAINT 515 (52 Yellow)
(Kurfees Coatings)

Pigment:	56.2%
Chrome yellow (Lead 60%) *	21.8%
Titanium dioxide	1.3%
Calcium carbonate	65.5%
Silicates	11.4%
Vehicle:	43.8%
Soya-alkyd resin	34.8%
Petroleum thinners	65.2%

KURFEES HEAVY BODIED P & V REMOVER 836
Paint and varnish remover
(Kurfees Coatings)

Approximate formulation:

Methylene chloride *	77.0%
Methyl alcohol	3.8%
Other alcohols	8.8%
Emulsifiers	8.2%
Evaporation retardants and thickening agents	2.2%

KURFEES PAINTS
(Kurfees Coatings)

Kurfees Coatings, Inc.
201 E. Market St.
Louisville, Ky. 40201

Phone: 502-584-0151

See PAINTS, Section VI, General Formulations

KURFEES PAINT SOLVENT 388
(Kurfees Coatings)

Petroleum distillate *	100%

KURLASH COSMETIC PRODUCTS

The Kurlash/Diamond Deb Ltd.
175 Great Neck Rd.
Great Neck, N.Y. 11021

Phone: 516-466-6310

See COSMETICS, Section VI, General Formulations

KURL-OFF
Remover
(Hillyard Chem.)

Methylene chloride *

'76 Ed.

KURON HERBICIDE
(Dow)

2-(2,4,5-Trichlorophenoxy) propionic acid propylene glycol butyl ether esters *	69.2%
Inert ingred.:	30.8%
Principally Petroleum solvent *	

KUSTOM KLOR II FORMULATED CHLORINATING GRANULES WITH WATER CONDITIONERS

See BIO-GUARD KUSTOM KLOR II FORMULATED CHLORINATING GRANULES WITH WATER CONDITIONERS

KUT CONCENTRATE
Chemical cleaner; industrial and institutional use
(Scientific International)

Hydrochloric acid *

KUTRASE
Indigestion
(Kremers-Urban)

Each capsule:

Amylolytic enzyme	30 mg.
Proteolytic enzyme	6 mg.
Lipolytic enzyme	75 mg.
Cellulolytic enzyme	2 mg.
Phenyltoloxamine citrate	15 mg.
l-Hyoscyamine sulfate	0.0625 mg.

KUTZIT PAINT REMOVER
(Savogran)

Methanol	20-40%
Toluol *	20-40%
Acetone	20-40%
Methylene chloride	20-40%
Retardants	

KWAL PAINT PRODUCTS

Kwal Paints, Inc.
3900 Joliet St.
Denver, Colo. 80217

Phone: 303-371-5600

See PAINTS, Section VI, General Formulations

KWELL CREAM
For scabies and lice
(Reed & Carnrick)

Lindane	1%
Water dispersible cream:	99%
Lanolin	
Glycerin	
Stearic acid	
2-Amino-2-methyl-1-propanol	
Perfume	
Purified water	

KWELL LOTION
For pediculosis and scabies
(Reed & Carnrick)

Gamma benzene hexachloride	1%
Glyceryl monostearate	
Cetyl alcohol, stearic acid	
Triethanolamine	
2-Amino-2-methyl propanol	
Butyl sodium alginate	
Perfume	

KWELL SHAMPOO
For pediculosis
(Reed & Carnrick)

Gamma benzene hexachloride	1%
Polyoxyethylene sorbitan stearate	
Triethanolamine lauryl sulfate	
Acetone	

KWIKEEZE BRUSH CLEANER
(Savogran)

Methanol	10-30%
Toluol *	40-60%
Acetone	20-40%
Methylene chloride	5-25%
Wetting agent, etc.	

KWIK GRILL CLEANER
Liquid caustic cleaner
(Kay Chem. Co.)

Potassium hydroxide *	20%
Water	balance

KWIK KILL
Insect spray
(McConnon & Co.)

Pyrethrins	0.20%
Technical Piperonyl butoxide	1.00%
Petroleum hydrocarbon *	18.80%

KWIK-KILL BAIT
Insecticide
(Pearson & Co.)

Calcium arsenate *	5.00%
Metaldehyde	2.00%
Arsenic expressed as metallic *	1.88%
Water-soluble arsenic	0.035%

'76 Ed.

KWIK KLEEN DRY SHAMPOO
Embalming supply
(Royal Bond)

Trichloroethane *

KWI KLEEN ACID DETERGENT
Dairy plant use
(National-Purity Soap)

Phosphoric acid *
Organic acid
Nonionic detergent

pH of 1% solution 1.9-2.4

KWI KLEEN ACID DETERGENT (HEAVY DUTY)
Dairy plant use
(National-Purity Soap)

Phosphoric acid *

KWIK-LITE LIGHTER FLUID
(Boyle-Midway)

Naphtha *

KWIK-SEAL

See DAP KWIK-SEAL

KWIT PLUS FERTILIZER
Insecticide
(Scott, O.M.)

Dursban 0.55%
Carrier: Fertilizer 30-5-3

KX-131 HOOD CLEANER
Liquid caustic cleaner
(Kay Chem. Co.)

Potassium hydroxide * 30-40%
Water .... balance

KYANIZE PAINT PRODUCTS
Paints, varnishes & enamels

Kyanize Paints, Inc.
Second & Boston Sts.
Everett, Mass. 02149

Phone: 617-387-5000

See PAINTS, Section VI, General Formulations

K-Y BRAND STERILE LUBRICANT
(Johnson & Johnson)

Sodium carboxymethylcellulose
Sodium alginate
Glycerin
Propylene glycol
Boric acid (less than 1.5%)
Methylparaben

KYLAR-85
Plant growth regulant
(Uniroyal Chem.)

Succinic acid 2,2-dimethyl hydrazide 85%
Inerts 15%
  Surfactant
  Solid diluents

KYMAR OINTMENT IMPROVED
Veterinary
(Burns-Biotec)

Each gram:
  Neomycin palmitate equivalent
    to neomycin .... 3.5 mg.
  Hydrocortisone acetate ...... 2.5 mg.
  Trypsin-chymotrypsin concentrate
    (10,000 Armour units of proteolytic activity)
Base:
  Polyethylene glycols 4000 and 400
  Stearyl alcohol
  Sodium bisulfite
  Tocopherols

L

LABSTIX
Urine pH, protein, glucose, ketones, and blood test reagent strip
(Ames)

pH test area: see BILI-LASTIX
Protein test area: see ALBUSTIX
Glucose test area: see CLINISTIX
Ketone test area: see KETOSTIX
Occult blood test area: see HEMASTIX

LACCO COPPER NAPHTHENATE SOLUTION 2
Fungicide
(Los Angeles Chem.)

Copper (expressed as metallic) 2.0%
Petroleum hydrocarbons * 80.0%

LACCO COPRO 53
Fungicide
(Los Angeles Chem.)

Copper oxychloride sulfate * 94.6%
(Equiv. to 53% copper as metallic)

LACCO CREOSOTE A.W.P.A.
Wood preservative
(Los Angeles Chem.)

Coal tar creosote * 97%

LACCO HI LIN
Insecticide
(Los Angeles Chem.)

Lindane * 12.9%
Xylene * 78.4%

LACCO ISOCARB 100
Insecticide
(Los Angeles Chem.)

Baygon * 1.0%
Petroleum distillate derivative * . 83.8%

LACCO LIN O MULSION 1.7
Insecticide
(Los Angeles Chem.)

Lindane * 20%
Xylene * 62%
Petroleum hydrocarbons 7%

LACCO LIQUID LIME SULPHUR
Fungicide, insecticide
(Los Angeles Chem.)

Calcium polysulfide * 29%
Calcium thiosulfate 2%

LACCO MAGIC SULPHUR
Fungicide, insecticide
(Los Angeles Chem.)

Sulphur * 98%

LACCO MALA MULSION 5
Insecticide
(Los Angeles Chem.)

Malathion * 56.0%
Xylene * 35.0%

LACCO PENTA CONCENTRATE
Wood preservative
(Los Angeles Chem.)

Pentachlorophenol * 36.7%
Other chlorophenols and related
  compounds 4.3%
Petroleum hydrocarbons 40.0%

LACCO PENTA W. R.
Herbicide
(Los Angeles Chem.)

Pentachlorophenol * 4.37%
Other chlorophenols 0.63%
Petroleum hydrocarbons * 81.80%

LACCO SODIUM ARSENITE SOLUTION NO. 4
Insecticide & herbicide
(Los Angeles Chem.)

Sodium arsenite * 43.4%

LACCO SODIUM ARSENITE SOLUTION NO. 6
Insecticide & herbicide
(Los Angeles Chem.)

Sodium arsenite * 52.5%

LACRIL
Artificial tears
(Allergan Pharm.)

Hydroxypropyl methylcellulose ... 0.5%

LACRI-LUBE S.O.P.
Sterile ophthalmic ointment
(Allergan Pharm.)

White petrolatum
Mineral oil
Nonionic lanolin derivatives
Chlorobutanol (chloral derivative as
  a preservative) 0.5%

LA CROSSE VITAMIN A-D DRESSING
Antiseptic and soothing dressing
(La Crosse)

Vitamin A .... 6000 units
Vitamin D .... 600 units
Panthenol 1%
In a base of:
  Lanolin
  Petrolatum

LACTICARE LOTION
For dry skin
(Stiefel Labs.)

Lactic acid *	5.0%
Sodium PCA	2.5%

Purified water
Mineral oil
Isopropyl palmitate
Coceth-6
Sodium hydroxide
Glyceryl stearate
Myristyl lactate
Cetyl alcohol
Carbomer-940
Imidazolidinyl urea
Fragrance
Dehydroacetic acid

L.A. FORMULA
Laxative
(Burton, Parsons & Co.)

Plantago ovata
Dextrose

LA FRANCE
Bluing detergent
(Purex Corp.)

Anionic surfactant	5-10%
Nonionic surfactant	1-5%
Sodium tetraborate (anhydrous)	1-3%
Fluorescent whitening agent	<1%
Enzyme	<1%
Pigment dyes	<1%
Perfume	<1%
Sodium sulfate	balance

LAGERFELD PERFUMES

Parfumes Lagerfeld, Inc.
1345 Ave. of the Americas
New York, N.Y. 10019

Phone: 212-399-2000

See COSMETICS, Section VI, General Formulations

LAGOLINE PAINT
Heavy duty marine paint
(International Paint)

Mineral spirits (or turpentine substitute) *
Pigments - Color codes #1496 & #1746 contain Lead *

LAKE HUMIDIFIER TABLETS
(Lake Products)

Sodium nitrite *

LAMAC'O CEMENT
Re-soling adhesive
(Lamac)

Acetone *
Aromatic solvents *
Nitrated cotton base

LAMAC'O THINNER
Cement thinner
(Lamac)

CP Acetone *

LA MAUR COSMETIC PRODUCTS

La Maur, Inc.
Consumer Products Div.
P.O. Box 1221
Minneapolis, Minn. 55440

Phone: 612-571-1234

See COSMETICS, Section VI, General Formulations

LAMBERT-KAY VETERINARY PRODUCTS

Lambert-Kay
Div. of Carter-Wallace, Inc.
P.O. Box 418
Cranbury, N.J. 08512

Phone: 609-655-6563

LAMINA
Adsorbent antacid for relief of simple scours; veterinary
(Merrick Medicine)

Each 10 ml.:
Bismuth subnitrate	959 mg.
Potassium carbonate	5.9 mg.
Calcium hydroxide	13.3 mg.
Alcohol	5%

LANABAC TABLETS
Analgesic
(Lannett)

Each tablet:
Aspirin *	0.3 gm.
Caffeine	15 mg.
Potassium bromide	15 mg.
Sodium bromide	15 mg.

LANABARB CAPSULES (NO. 1 & NO. 2)
Sedative
(Lannett)

Each No. 1 capsule:
Sodium amobarbital *	3/4 gr.
Sodium secobarbital	3/4 gr.

Each No. 2 capsule:
Sodium amobarbital *	1 1/2 gr.
Sodium secobarbital	1 1/2 gr.

LANABROM ELIXIR
Sleep aid
(Lannett)

Each fl. oz., 60 gr. of the following combined bromides:
Sodium bromide *
Potassium bromide *
Strontium bromide *
Ammonium bromide *

LANABURN OINTMENT
Dressing for burns
(Lannett)

Basic Aluminum acetate
Phenol *
Zinc oxide
Boric acid *
Eucalyptol *
Ichthammol *

LANACANE CREME
Soothes itching & burning
(Combe Inc.)

Benzocaine
Resorcinol *
Chlorothymol *

LANASED TABLETS
Urinary antiseptic
(Lannett)

Each tablet:
Atropine sulfate	0.03 mg.
Hyoscyamine	0.03 mg.
Methenamine	408 mg.
Methylene blue *	5.4 mg.
Phenyl salicylate *	18.1 mg.
Gelsemium *	6.1 mg.
Benzoic acid	4.5 mg.

LANA SOAP
(Hewitt)

Tallow
Cocoanut oil
Sodium hydroxide

'76 Ed.

LANATRATE TABLETS
For relief of migraine and other types of recurrent and throbbing headaches
(Lannett)

Each tablet:
Ergotamine tartrate *	1 mg.
Caffeine alkaloid *	100 mg.

LANATUSS EXPECTORANT
(Lannett)

Each 5 ml.:
Glyceryl guaiacolate	100 mg.
Phenylpropanolamine HCl	5 mg.
Chlorpheniramine maleate	2 mg.
Sodium citrate	197 mg.
Citric acid	60 mg.

LANAURINE
Analgesic ear drops
(Lannett)

Antipyrine *
Benzocaine

LANAZETS
Antibacterial-anesthetic throat lozenges
(Lannett)

Each lozenge:
Cetylpyridinium . . . . 1 mg.
Benzocaine . . . . 5 mg.

LANCOME COSMETIC PRODUCTS
Perfumes and beauty products

Lancome, Div. of Cosmair
530 Fifth Ave.
New York, N.Y. 10036

Phone: 212-697-5115

See COSMETICS, Section VI, General Formulations

LAND O'LAKES CHLORINATED PIPE LINE DETERGENT
(Land O'Lakes, Inc.)

Sodium metasilicate *
Sodium carbonate *
Sodium triazinetrione *

LAND O'LAKES CHLORINE SANITIZER CONCENTRATED
(Land O'Lakes, Inc.)

Sodium hypochlorite * 6.6%

LAND O'LAKES DAIRY DETERGENT
(Land O'Lakes, Inc.)

Chlorine *

LAND O'LAKES/FELCO BACKRUBBER OIL (Korlan)
Insecticide
(Land O'Lakes, Inc.)

Ronnel 1.0%
Mineral oil * 98.5%

LAND O'LAKES/FELCO BACKRUBBER OIL (Malathion)
Insecticide
(Land O'Lakes, Inc.)

Malathion 2.0%
Petroleum hydrocarbons * 98.0%

LAND O'LAKES/FELCO DC&R SPRAY FUMIGANT CONCENTRATE
(Land O'Lakes, Inc.)

2-(Hydroxymethyl)-2-nitro-1,3-propanediol * 19.20%
Formaldehyde 2.02%
Trisodium phosphate 0.29%
Alkyl (C12-67%; C14-25%; C16-7%; C8, C10, C18-1%) dimethyl benzyl ammonium chloride 2.29%

LAND O'LAKES/FELCO DRY DIP (Rabon)
Insecticide
(Land O'Lakes, Inc.)

2-Chloro-1-(2,4,5-trichlorophenyl) vinyl dimethyl phosphate * 3.0%

LAND O'LAKES/FELCO DRY DIP II (Co-Ral)
Insecticide
(Land O'Lakes, Inc.)

O,O-Diethyl O-(3-chloro-4-methyl-2-oxo-2H-1-benzopyran-7-yl) phosphorothioate 1.0%

LAND O'LAKES/FELCO MCP AMINE #4
Herbicide
(Land O'Lakes, Inc.)

Dimethylamine salt of 2-methyl-4-chlorophenoxyacetic acid * 52.2%

LAND O'LAKES/FELCO NO. 4 2,4-D LOW VOLATILE WEED KILLER
(Land O'Lakes, Inc.)

2,4-Dichlorophenoxyacetic acid, butoxy propyl esters *† 72.7%

†*See* 2,4-D esters

LAND O'LAKES/FELCO POUL-DINE
Iodine disinfectant, detergent, sanitizer
(Land O'Lakes, Inc.)

Alkyl (29% C14, 29% C13, 21% C12, 21% C15) poly (oxypropylene) poly (oxyethylene)-iodine complex (provides 1.75% titratable iodine) 14.65%
Phosphoric acid * 5.00%

LAND O'LAKES/FELCO PYRENONE DAIRY CATTLE SPRAY
Insecticide
(Land O'Lakes, Inc.)

Piperonyl butoxide technical 0.30%
Pyrethrins 0.03%
Mineral oil * 99.67%

LAND O'LAKES/FELCO RAT & MOUSE KILLER
Rodenticide
(Land O'Lakes, Inc.)

3-(alpha-Acetonylfurfuryl)-4-hydroxycoumarin 0.025%

LAND O'LAKES/FELCO RONNEL CONCENTRATE
Insecticide dip or spray
(Land O'Lakes, Inc.)

Ronnel 24.0%
Combined amount: 59.0%
Xylene *
Related Hydrocarbons *†

†*See* Aromatic hydrocarbons

LAND O'LAKES/FELCO SWINE-DINE
Iodine disinfectant, detergent, sanitizer
(Land O'Lakes, Inc.)

Alkyl (29% C14, 29% C13, 21% C12, 21% C15) poly (oxypropylene) poly (oxyethylene)-iodine complex (provides 1.75% titratable iodine) 14.65%
Phosphoric acid * 5.00%

LAND O'LAKES/FELCO VAPORIN DAIRY SPRAY
Insecticide
(Land O'Lakes, Inc.)

Dimethyl phosphate of alpha-methylbenzyl 3-hydroxy-cis-crotonate * 1.00%
2,2-Dichlorovinyl dimethyl phosphate 0.23%
Related compounds 0.02%
Petroleum hydrocarbons * 98.50%

LAND O'LAKES HEAVY DUTY CHLORINATED PIPE LINE DETERGENT
(Land O'Lakes, Inc.)

Sodium hydroxide *
Sodium metasilicate *
Sodium carbonate *
Sodium dichloro-s-triazinetrione *

LAND O'LAKES IODINE DETERGENT SANITIZER
(Land O'Lakes, Inc.)

alpha-Alkyl (C11-C15) omega hydroxy poly (oxyethylene)-iodine complex (providing 1.75% titratable iodine) 15.75%
Phosphoric acid * 13.50%

LAND O'LAKES LIQUID PIPE LINE DETERGENT CHLORINATED
(Land O'Lakes, Inc.)

Potassium hydroxide *

LAND O'LAKES MILKSTONE REMOVER CONCENTRATE LO FOAM
(Land O'Lakes, Inc.)

Phosphoric acid *
Glycollic acid

LAND O'LAKES TEAT DIP AND UDDER WASH CONTROLLED IODINE DETERGENT
(Land O'Lakes, Inc.)

alpha-Alkyl (C11-C15) omega hydroxy poly (oxyethylene)-iodine complex 1.00%

LAND & SEA
(Touraine Paints, Inc.)

Soya alkyd resin 31.8%
Modified Urethane alkyd resin ... 21.2%
Thinner*† and driers* 47.0%

'76 Ed.

†See Thinners, Section VI, General Formulations

LANEX FOR PILES
For hemorrhoids
(Carma)

Lanolin
Menthol * .... approx. 1.0%
Petrolatum
Alum
Camphor * 2.0%
Phenol .... <0.5%
Salicylic acid * .... approx. 1.0%
Cocoa butter

LANITOL A
Biodegradable anionic detergent
(Arkansas Co.)

Linear alkyl amine
sulfonate *† .... approx. 30%

'76 Ed.

†See Alkyl sodium sulfonates

LAN-LAY COSMETIC PRODUCTS

Lan-Lay Co.
465 Park Ave.
San Jose, Calif. 95110

Phone: 408-288-9595

See COSMETICS, Section VI, General Formulations

LAN-LIN
Hand cleaner
(Radiator)

Petroleum distillates *
Soaps

'76 Ed.

LANMAN & KEMP-BARCLAY COSMETIC PRODUCTS
Toiletries

Lanman & Kemp-Barclay & Co.
25 Woodland Ave.
Westwood, N.J. 07675

Phone: 201-666-4990

See COSMETICS, Section VI, General Formulations

"LANNATE" INSECTICIDE
(Du Pont)

Methomyl * 90%

"LANNATE" L INSECTICIDE
(Du Pont)

Methomyl * 24%
Contains Methanol

"LANNATE" LV INSECTI-CIDE
(Du Pont)

Methomyl * 29%
Contains Methanol

LANNATES ELIXIR
Tonic
(Lannett)

Each fl. oz.:
Sodium glycerophosphate ... 2 gr.
Calcium glycerophosphate ... 2 gr.
Phosphoric acid .... 1 1/2 m.
Wine base .... q.s.
Alcohol 17%

LANNETT ANALGESIC OINTMENT
(Lannett)

Camphor *
Menthol syn. *
Methyl salicylate *
Lanolin-petrolatum base

LANNETT ANTI-RUST TABLETS
Anti-corrosive for use with benzalkonium aqueous sterilizing solution
(Lannett)

Each tablet:
Sodium carbonate
monohydrate .... 1.15 gm.
Sodium nitrite * .... 0.50 gm.

LANNETT PROMETHAZINE EXPECTORANT DC PLAIN
(Lannett)

Each teaspoonful (5 ml.):
Promethazine hydrochloride   5 mg.
Fluidextract Ipecac .... 0.17 min.
Potassium guaiacolsulfonate   44 mg.
Chloroform .... 0.25 min.
Citric acid, anhydrous ......   60 mg.
Sodium citrate .... 197 mg.
Phenylephrine HCl ....   5 mg.
Alcohol 7%

LANNETT PROMETHAZINE EXPECTORANT DC WITH CODEINE
(Lannett)

Each teaspoonful (5 ml.):
Promethazine hydrochloride   5 mg.
Fluidextract Ipecac .... 0.17 min.
Potassium guaiacolsulfonate   44 mg.
Chloroform .... 0.25 min.
Citric acid, anhydrous ......   60 mg.
Sodium citrate .... 197 mg.
Phenylephrine HCl ....   5 mg.
Codeine phosphate * ....   10 mg.
Alcohol 7%

LANNETT PROMETHAZINE EXPECTORANT DM PEDIATRIC
(Lannett)

Each teaspoonful (5 ml.):
Promethazine hydrochloride   5 mg.
Fluidextract Ipecac .... 0.17 min.
Potassium guaiacolsulfonate   44 mg.
Chloroform .... 0.25 min.
Citric acid, anhydrous ......   60 mg.
Sodium citrate .... 197 mg.
Dextromethorphan
hydrobromide ....   7.5 mg.
Alcohol 7%

LANNETT PROMETHAZINE EXPECTORANT PLAIN
(Lannett)

Each teaspoonful (5 ml.):
Promethazine hydrochloride   5 mg.
Fluidextract Ipecac .... 0.17 min.
Potassium guaiacolsulfonate   44 mg.
Chloroform .... 0.25 min.
Citric acid, anhydrous ......   60 mg.
Sodium citrate .... 197 mg.
Alcohol 7%

LANNETT PROMETHAZINE EXPECTORANT WITH CODEINE
(Lannett)

Each teaspoonful (5 ml.):
Promethazine hydrochloride   5 mg.
Fluidextract Ipecac .... 0.17 min.
Potassium guaiacolsulfonate   44 mg.
Chloroform .... 0.25 min.
Citric acid, anhydrous ......   60 mg.
Sodium citrate .... 197 mg.
Alcohol 7%
Codeine phosphate * ....   10 mg.

Starred ingredients (*) may be responsible for major toxic effects; consult Section II.

LANOFLO ARTERIAL FLUID
Embalming supply
(Royal Bond)

Formaldehyde * 22%
Methanol *
Ethoxylated lanolin

LANO-LO
Antipruritic bath oil
(Whorton)

Dewaxed oil soluble fraction of lanolin
Mineral oil
Emulsifiers
'76 Ed.

LANOLOR CREAM
Perfumed skin protective, powder base
(Squibb)

Deodorized, purified de-waxed lanolin

LANOPHYLLIN ELIXIR
(Lannett)

Each 15 ml.:
Anhydrous Theophylline ..... 80 mg.
Alcohol 20%

LANORINAL (CAPSULES & TABLETS)
Tension headaches
(Lannett)

Each capsule or tablet:
Isobutylallylbarbituric acid * . 50 mg.
Caffeine .... 40 mg.
Aspirin * .... 200 mg.
Phenacetin * .... 130 mg.

LAN-O-SHEEN PRODUCTS
Cleaners

Lan-O-Sheen, Inc.
One W. Water
Saint Paul, Minn. 55107

Phone numbers:
Business hours: 612-224-5681
Other hours: 612-778-1936

LANOTHAL PILLS
(Lannett)

Each pill:
Phenolphthalein .... 1/2 gr.
Aloin * .... 1/4 gr.
Ipecac .... 1/15 gr.
Extract Belladonna * .... 1/12 gr.

LANOXICAPS CAPSULES
Cardiotonic
(Burroughs Wellcome)

Each capsule:
Digoxin (pure crystalline gly-
coside of Digitalis lanata) * 0.05 mg.;
0.1 mg.; 0.2 mg.
Polyethylene glycol
Ethyl alcohol
Propylene glycol
Purified water

LANOXIN ELIXIR PEDIATRIC
Cardiotonic
(Burroughs Wellcome)

Each cc:
Digoxin (pure crystalline gly-
coside of Digitalis lanata) * 0.05 mg.
Alcohol 10%
Methylparaben 0.1%

LANOXIN TABLETS
Cardiotonic
(Burroughs Wellcome)

Each tablet:
Digoxin (pure crys-
talline glycoside
of Digitalis
lanata) * ...... 0.125 mg.; 0.25 mg.;
or 0.5 mg.

LANTEEN JELLY
Vaginal jelly
(Lambda Inc.)

Ricinoleic acid 0.5%
Hexylresorcinol 0.1%
Chlorothymol 0.0077%
Sodium benzoate
Glycerin
Tragacanth base

LANVIN PERFUMES

Lanvin Parfums, Inc.
650 Fifth Ave.
New York, N.Y. 10019

Phone: 212-246-3070

See COSMETICS, Section VI, General
Formulations

LANVISONE CREAM
(Lannett)

Hydrocortisone 1%
Iodochlorhydroxyquin * 3%

LA PINE
Disinfectant
(Therm Processes, Inc.)

Pine oil * 80%
Soap 10%
Water 10%

LARK-64 CARPET STEAM CLEANER
(Nat'l Labs. Div.)

Ethylene glycol monobutyl ether . minor
Isopropyl alcohol .... minor

LARK-32 CONCENTRATED LIQUID CARPET SHAMPOO
(Nat'l Labs. Div.)

Perchlorethylene .... minor
Ethylene glycol monobutyl ether . minor
Isopropyl alcohol .... minor
Tetrasodium
ethylenediaminetetraacetate .... minor

LARO
*General purpose disinfectant and deo-
dorant*
(Whitmoyer)

Active ingred.:
Soap 10%
Isopropanol 10%
4-& 6-Chloro-2-phenylphenol ... 7%
o-Phenylphenol 6%
Tetrasodium ethylenediamine
tetraacetate 1.5%
p-tertiary Amylphenol 1%
Inert ingred.: 64.5%
Water
Sodium hydroxide *
Potassium sulfite

LAROTID
Antibacterial agent
(Roche)

Capsules (each):
Amoxicillin
trihydrate ...... 250 mg.; or 500 mg.

Pediatric Drops (each ml.):
Amoxicillin trihydrate .... 50 mg.

Suspension (each 5 ml.):
Amoxicillin
trihydrate ...... 125 mg.; or 250 mg.

LARSON'S FOOT NOTE
For athlete's foot
(Larson Labs.)

Parachlorometaxylenol
Menthol
Refined Mineral oil
Perfume oil
Isopropyl alcohol 81.08%
Propellant

LARSON'S GENERAL PUR-POSE FUNGICIDE AND DEODORANT
(Larson Labs)

Active ingred.: 46%
Menthol *
Parachlorometaxylenol
Pine oil *
Triethylene glycol melium
Petroleum distillate *
Isopropanol
Propellant

LARSON'S INSECT REPELLENT
(Larson Labs.)

Isopropyl alcohol * 30%
2-Ethyl-1,3-hexanediol * 20%

LARSON'S MINT GLO
Counter-irritant
(Larson Labs.)

Active ingred.: 32%
  Oil of peppermint
  Methyl salicylate (USP) *
  Menthol *
Inert ingred.:
  Greaseless base
  Zephiran chloride

LARSON'S PODIODINE OINTMENT
Antiseptic
(Larson Labs.)

Titratable Povidone-iodine 1%

LARSON'S PODIODINE SOLUTION
Antiseptic
(Larson Labs.)

Titratable Povidone-iodine (USP) .. 1%
Water

LARSON'S PODIODINE SURGICAL SCRUB
Antiseptic
(Larson Labs.)

Titratable Povidone-iodine 0.75%
Water
Surfactants

LARSON'S PODIODINE WHIRLPOOL CONCENTRATE
(Larson Labs.)

Titratable Povidone-iodine 1%
Water

LARSON'S STERIL-IZE
Cold sterilent
(Larson Labs.)

Activated Gluteraldehyde 2%
Water

LARSON'S TAPE ADHERENT, FORMULA JC-5
(Larson Labs)

Abietic anhydride
Parachlorometaxylenol *
Chlorinated solvents *†
Propellant

† See Methylene chloride

LARSON'S TAPE-OFF
Adhesive tape remover
(Larson Labs.)

Active ingredients: 52%
  Chlorinated solvents *
  Petroleum solvents *
  Ethyl alcohol *
Inert ingred.:
  Carbon dioxide

LARVA-LUR
Insecticide
(B&G Co.)

Dimethyl (2,2,2-trichloro-1-hydroxyethyl phosphonate) * ... 5.000%

LASAN UNGUENT
For psoriasis
(Stiefel Labs.)

Anthralin, N.F. 0.4%
Base:
  Cetyl alcohol
  Mineral oil
  White petrolatum
  Sodium lauryl sulfate
Salicylic acid (as preservative)

LASSO
Herbicide
(Monsanto)

Alachlor * 45.1%

LASS-O BLEACH
(Labbco, Inc.)

Sodium hypochlorite * 5 1/4%
Sodium hydroxide ... about 0.2-0.3 of 1%

LASSO EC
Herbicide
(Monsanto)

Alachlor * 43.0%

LASSO II
Granular herbicide
(Monsanto)

Alachlor * 15%

LAUD
Commercial laundry detergent
(Diversey Wyandotte)

Sodium metasilicate *
Alkaline salts *

LAUNCH
Liquid laundry sour
(Diversey Wyandotte)

Fluoride salts *

LAUNDRAMAGIC ALKALINE BUILDER
Laundry alkalinity booster
(Paul Koss)

Water .... <80%
Sodium hydroxide * 20%
Sodium phosphate ester

LAUNDRAMAGIC BLOOD AND PROTEIN REMOVER
Laundry stain remover
(Paul Koss)

Water .... >90%
Tetra triethanolamine salt of EDTA
Sodium docecylbenzene sulfonate (Anionic surfactant)

pH 9.9-10.1

LAUNDRAMAGIC CHLORBRITE
Bleach
(Paul Koss)

Sodium hypochlorite solution * 7%

pH 9.9-10.1

LAUNDRAMAGIC CHLORINE NEUTRALIZER
Laundry bleach neutralizer
(Paul Koss)

Water .... >85%
Sodium sulfite * .... <15%

pH 6.9-7.1

LAUNDRAMAGIC DETERGENT
(Paul Koss)

Water .... >60%
Sodium dodecylbenzene sulfonate
  (Anionic surfactant) * 15-20%
Nonylphenoxypoly(ethyleneoxy)ethanol
  (Nonionic surfactant)
Sodium salt of sulfated linear alcohol
  ethoxylate (Anionic surfactant)
Sodium xylene sulfonate (Anionic surfactant)
Optical brightener .... trace

pH 7.0-7.3

LAUNDRAMAGIC DETERGENT BOOSTER
(Paul Koss)

Water 70%
Tetrapotassium pyrophosphate *† . 30%

pH 10.0-10.2

†See Tetrasodium pyrophosphate

LAUNDRAMAGIC IRON WITE
Laundry stain remover
(Paul Koss)

Water .... <80%
Potassium oxalate * 20%
Potassium salt of a phosphate ester

pH 9.5-10.0

LAUNDRAMAGIC POG REMOVER
Paint, oil, grease remover
(Paul Koss)

Kerosene *	<50%
Methyl isobutyl ketone *	<20%
Butyl acetate *	<15%
Butyl Cellosolve *	10%
Isopropylamine sulfonate	

LAUNDRAMAGIC SOLVENT DEGREASER
(Paul Koss)

Kerosene *	>60%
Butyl acetate *	20%
Nonylphenoxypoly(ethyleneoxy)ethanol (Nonionic surfactant)	
Sodium dodecylbenzene sulfonate (Anionic surfactant)	
Butyl Cellosolve	
Water	

LAUNDRAMAGIC SOUR-SOFTENER
(Paul Koss)

Water	>55%
Glacial acetic acid *	25%
Isopropyl alcohol *	<20%
Dimethyl dihydrogenated tallow ammonium chloride	

pH 3.1-3.3

LAUNDRAMAGIC TANNIN REMOVER
Laundry stain remover
(Paul Koss)

Water	>90%
Citric acid	
Potassium acid oxalate *	<4%

pH 3.4-3.6

LAUNDRAMAGIC WASH-ALL
(Paul Koss)

Water	>55%
Tetrapotassium pyrophosphate	
Sodium xylene sulfonate (Anionic surfactant)	
Sodium dodecylbenzene sulfonate (Anionic surfactant)	
Nonylphenoxypoly(ethyleneoxy)ethanol (Nonionic surfactant)	
Sodium metasilicate	
Sodium salt of a phosphate ester	

pH 10.8-11.0

LAUNETTE SPECIAL
(Phosphate Formula or 0-Phosphate Formula)
Institutional and industrial cleaning product

Procter & Gamble Co.
Ivorydale Technical Center
Cincinnati, Ohio 45217

Phone: 513-562-1100

LAURO
Eye irrigator and drops
(Clapp, Otis)

Berberine hydrochloride
Borax *
Sodium chloride
Boric acid *

LAVA
Soap bar
(Procter & Gamble)

Soap from vegetable fats	25-49%
Pumice	25-49%
Water	10-24%
Glycerine	5-9%
Vegetable oil	1-4%
Fatty acid	1-4%
Minor ingredients, each	<1%

pH (1% solution) - 9.4

LAVACOL
Rubbing alcohol
(Parke-Davis)

Ethyl alcohol *	70%

LAVOGENT
Skin cleansing lotion
(Torch)

Detergent sulfonate *
Stable emulsion of a vegetable oil

'76 Ed.

LAVOPTIK EYE WASH
(Lavoptik)

Each 100 ml.:

Sodium chloride	0.065 gm.
Potassium chloride	0.05 gm.
Calcium chloride	0.015 gm.
Magnesium chloride	0.01 gm.
Sodium acetate	0.35 gm.
Sodium phosphate	0.356 gm.
Edetate disodium	0.10 gm.
Benzalkonium chloride	0.013 gm.
Water	q.s.

LAVORIS FORMULA-Z CONCENTRATE (GREEN)
Mouthwash
(Vicks Toiletry Products Div.)

Water	
SD Alcohol 38-B	20.0%
Glycerin	
Poloxamer 407	
Citric acid	
Sodium hydroxide	
Zinc oxide	<1.0%
Saccharin	
Cetyl pyridinium chloride	
Flavors	
Clove oil	<1.0%
FD & C Blue No. 1	
D & C Yellow No. 10	

LAVORIS FORMULA-Z CONCENTRATE (RED)
Mouthwash
(Vicks Toiletry Products Div.)

Water	
SD Alcohol 38-B	20.0%
Glycerin	
Poloxamer 407	
Citric acid	
Sodium hydroxide	
Zinc oxide	<1.0%
Saccharin	
Cetyl pyridinium chloride	
Flavors	
Clove oil	<0.1%
FD & C Red No. 40	
D & C Red No. 33	

LAVORIS MOUTHWASH & GARGLE
(Vicks Toiletry Products Div.)

Water	
SD Alcohol 38-B	5.0%
Glycerin	
Poloxamer 407	
Saccharin	
Polysorbate 80	
Zinc chloride	<1.0%
Flavors	
Citric acid	
Clove oil	<1.0%
D & C Red No. 6	
D & C Red No. 33	

LAVORIS PROFESSIONAL CONCENTRATE
Mouthwash
(Vicks Toiletry Products Div.)

Water	
SD Alcohol 38-B	20.0%
Glycerin	
Poloxamer 407	
Citric acid	
Sodium hydroxide	
Zinc oxide	
Saccharin	
Cetyl pyridinium chloride	
Flavors	
Clove oil	
FD & C Red No. 40	
D & C Red No. 33	

LAWN-GARD, ARAB
See ARAB LAWN-GARD

LAX-HERB
Cathartic
(Fibertone)

Each tablet:	
Senna powder *	8 gr.

LAX-VAC
Laxative
(Moffet Inc.)

Each chewable tablet:	
Sodium salicylate	1/4 gr.
Bismuth subcarbonate	1/8 gr.
Bismuth subgallate	1/8 gr.
Phenolphthalein, yellow	1 1/2 gr.

Starred ingredients (*) may be responsible for major toxic effects; consult Section II.

LC-65
Hard contact lens cleaning solution
(Allergan Pharm.)

Cleaning agent
Edetate disodium
Thimerosal 1:100,000

LEA COMPOUND
All grades - to satin finish metal
(Lea)

Aluminum oxide or other abrasive
Glue
Oil of wintergreen *

**LEAD WAY BLUE
LAUNDRY DETERGENT**
Dry laundry detergent
(Great Atlantic & Pacific, mfr.; Federated Foods, dist.)

Sodium linear alkyl benzene
  sulfonate . . . . <17%
Sodium carbonate * . . . . <30%
Sodium silicate . . . . <10%
Sodium carboxymethylcellulose . <2%
Optical brighteners . . . . <1%
Sodium chloride . . . . <10%
Blue dye . . . . trace
Sodium sulfate and moisture . . . balance

LEA LIQUABRADE
Liquid buffing medium for metals and plastics; all grades
(Lea)

Abrasives
Greases
Waxes
Fatty acids
Emulsifiers

LEATHER MAGIC
(Choldun; Arrow Labs)

Sodium metasilicate
Isopropanol
Sodium alkyl sulfate *
Triethanolamine lauryl sulfate *
Fatty amide-condensate
Anhydrous fatty acid-amine condensate
Sulfonated ketones
Hydrophilic wax-cyclohexanone-amine
  wax (Vegamin wax)

'76 Ed.

**LE CLAIRE BRASS
CLEANER**
(SerVaas Labs.)

Water 50-55%
Feldspar † 30-35%
Citric acid 5-10%
Cab-O-Sil 1-5%
Nonionic soap 1-5%
Perfume . . . . <1%

†*See* Aluminum silicate

**LECTRIC SHAVE (PRE-
ELECTRIC SHAVING
LOTION)**
(Williams, J.B.)

Alcohol (denatured with colocynth) *
Fatty acid ester (made with and without
  menthol)

LEECH ALUMINUM REPAIR
(Leech)

Plastic and aluminum powder base
Ketone solvents *

LEECH APPLIANCE REPAIR
(Leech)

Nitrocellulose base
Toluol solvent *

LEECH-BOND
(Leech)

Cyanoacrylate *

LEECH-BOND II
(Leech)

Cyanoacrylate *

LEECH BUTYL CAULK
(Leech)

Butyl rubber base
Petroleum distillate *

LEECH CONTACT CEMENT
(Leech)

Rubber base
Ketone solvents *

LEECH EPOXY CEMENT
(Leech)

Resins
Catalyst hardener *†

†*See* Fiberglass & resin plastics, Section
VI, General Formulations

LEECH FABRIC CEMENT
(Leech)

Natural latex
Ammonia *

**LEECH F-26 HEAVY
ADHESIVE**
(Leech)

Rubber base
Acetone *
Petroleum distillate *

**LEECH FOAM & PANEL
ADHESIVE**
(Leech)

Synthetic rubber & resin base
Petroleum distillates *

**LEECH HOUSEHOLD
CEMENT**
(Leech)

Nitrocellulose base
Acetone *
Dineltone
Toluol *

**LEECH LATEX CAULK
(Acrylic)**
(Leech)

Latex base

LEECH LIQUID SOLDER
(Leech)

Plastic cement *†
Aluminum powder

†*See* Plastic cement, Section VI, General
Formulations

LEECH MODEL CEMENT
(Leech)

Nitrocellulose base
Toluol *

**LEECH MULTI-PURPOSE
CEMENT**
(Leech)

Nitrocellulose base
Toluol *
Acetone

**LEECH PANEL-TITE
ADHESIVE**
(Leech)

Synthetic elastomeric polymer
Hexane

LEECH PLASTIC RUBBER
(Leech)

Neoprene rubber base
Toluene *
Acetone

LEECH PUTTI-POXY
(Leech)

Resin
Catalyst hardener

LEECH QUIK-I-POXY
(Leech)

Polyamide resin
Catalyst hardener

Starred ingredients (*) may be responsible for major toxic effects; consult Section II.

LEECH REAL WOODFILLER
(Leech)

Powdered wood
Cellulose plastic cement
Ketone solvents *

LEECH RUBBER CEMENT
(Leech)

Rubber base
Mineral spirits *

LEECH SILACLEAR
(Leech)

Rubber base
Toluene *

LEECH SILAPRENE
(Leech)

Neoprene rubber base
Toluene *

LEECH SPOT-TAK
(Leech)

Rubber base

LEECH STEEL EPOXY
(Leech)

Resins
Catalyst hardener

LEECH STEEL REPAIR
(Leech)

Plastic cement *†
Steel powder
Ketone solvents *

†See Plastic cement, Section VI, General
   Formulations

LEECH SUPER ADHESIVE
(Leech)

Rubber base
Ketone solvents *

LEECH TUB & TILE CAULK
Filler
(Leech)

Polyvinyl acetate

LEECH 507 VINYL REPAIR
(Leech)

Urethane vinyl base
Ketone solvents *

LEECH-WELD CEMENT
(Leech)

Tetrahydrofuran *
Methyl ethyl ketone
Cyclohexanone

LEECH WHITE GLUE
(Leech)

Resins

LEECH WINDSHIELD
   SEALER
(Leech)

Rubber base
Ketone solvents *
Toluol *

LEECH WOODCRAFTER
(Leech)

Aliphatic resin base

LEEDS-ALL GRANULAR
   CYANURIC CHLORINE
Swimming pool treatment
(Alden-Leeds)

Trichloro-s-triazinetrione * 65%
Sodium carbonate * 35%

LEEDSALL KLEER PINE
Pine odor disinfectant
(Leedsall)

Combined amount: 21.9%
   Pine oil *
   Soap
   Potassium chloro-phenyl phenate *
   Isopropyl alcohol *

                                    '76 Ed.

LEEDSALL MINT-O-FECT
Mint disinfectant
(Leedsall)

Active ingredients: 33%
   Isopropyl alcohol *
   Vegetable oil soap
   o-Benzyl p-chlorophenol *
   Methyl salicylate *
   Essential oils *
   Tetra-sodium ethylenediaminetetraace-
   tate

                                    '76 Ed.

LEEDSALL SAN-O-PINE
Pine oil disinfectant
(Leedsall)

Combined amount: 90%
   Steam distilled Pine oil *
   Soap

                                    '76 Ed.

LEEDSALL SUPER
   MAGNACIDE RESIDUAL
   SPRAY

See SUPER MAGNACIDE RESID-
   UAL SPRAY

LEFFINGWELL BASIC
   COPPER CARBONATE
Fungicide
(Leffingwell)

Copper (expressed as metallic) * . 51.0%

LEFFINGWELL FLOWABLE
   60
Insecticide, fungicide
(Leffingwell)

Petroleum oil * 82.0%

LEFFINGWELL FLOWABLE
   75
Insecticide, fungicide
(Leffingwell)

Petroleum oil * 82%/w
Unsulfonated residue, Petroleum oil, minimum 92%

LEFFINGWELL FLOWABLE
   DORMANT
Insecticide, fungicide
(Leffingwell)

Petroleum oil * 82.0%
Unsulfonated residue, Petroleum
   oil, minimum 70.0%

LEFFINGWELL ZINC
   MANGANESE NUTRA-
   SPRAY 18 1/2 - 7
Foliar spray
(Leffingwell)

Zinc-expressed as metallic *† 18.5%
Manganese-expressed as metallic . 7.0%

†See Zinc salts

LEFFINGWELL ZINC
   NUTRA-SPRAY 50
*Foliar or dormant spray for effective
   zinc feeding*
(Leffingwell)

Zinc (expressed as metallic) * 50.0%

Zinc derived from basic zinc sulfate

LEGCLEAN
All-purpose cleaner
(Legge, W.)

Nonionic detergents *

LEGEAR DAIRY & CATTLE
   & HORSE DUST
Insecticide
(LeGear)

Methoxychlor technical 5%
Malathion * 4%

Starred ingredients (*) may be responsible for major toxic effects; consult Section II.

LEGEAR FLEA & TICK POWDER
For use on dogs and cats
(LeGear)

Active ingred.:
Carbaryl *	5.00%
Dichlorophene	0.50%
Aluminum chlorohydroxy allantoinate	0.20%

Inert ingred.:
Pyrophylite	94.30%

LEGEAR FLEA & TICK SPRAY
For use on dogs
(LeGear)

Pyrethrins	0.050%
Piperonyl butoxide, technical	0.100%
N-Octyl bicycloheptene dicarboximide	0.167%
2,3:4,5-Bis(2-butylene)tetrahydro-2-furaldehyde	0.240%
Carbaryl	0.500%
Petroleum distillate	3.843%

LEGEAR LOUSE POWDER WITH RABON
For use on livestock and poultry
(LeGear)

2-Chloro-1-(2,4,5-trichlorophenyl)vinyl dimethylphosphate	3.00%/wt.

LEGEAR MANGE CURE
Veterinary
(LeGear)

Active ingredients:
Benzyl benzoate *	35.94%
Gamma isomer of benzene hexachloride (from lindane)	0.06%

Inert ingredients:
Isopropyl alcohol *	45.00%
Emulsified oil base *†	19.00%

†*See* Emulsifiers and Petroleum distillates

LEGEAR MULTI-PURPOSE DISINFECTANT
(LeGear)

Active ingredients:
Coal tar hydrocarbons *	63%
Soap	17%
Coal tar acids *	10%

Inert ingredients:
Water	10%

LEGEAR SCREW WORM SPRAY
Wound protectant; veterinary
(LeGear)

Ronnel	2.5%
Xylene	0.5%

LEGPHENE
Germicidal cleaner
(Legge, W.)

Phenolics *†

†*See* Disinfectants, Section VI, General Formulations

LEGSURE
Floor polish
(Legge, W.)

A resin-type floor polish containing:
Polystyrene copolymers
Alkali soluble resins

LEG TONE
Veterinary; leg paint for horses
(Haver-Lockhart (Brand) Bayvet Div. Cutter Labs.)

Iodine tincture strong *	20.0%
Camphor	1.0%
Propylene glycol	15.0%
Methyl salicylate	5.0%
Turpentine	1.0%
Ammonium iodide	1.0%
Oil of origanum red	1.0%
Oil of pennyroyal	1.0%
Isopropyl alcohol	45.0%
Alcohol	10.0%

LE GUI PERFUME, COLOGNE, TOILET WATER
(Parfums Duvelle)

Alcohol (denatured with diethyl phthalate) *

LEHMAN BROS. PAINT PRODUCTS
Paints, varnishes, enamels, and tinting colors

Lehman Bros. Corp.
22 Halladay St.
Jersey City, N.J. 07304

Phone: 201-434-1882-3
             212-732-3897-8

See PAINTS, Section VI, General Formulations

LEHN & FINK INSTRUMENT GERMICIDE
(Nat'l Labs. Div.)

Ethyl alcohol	4.640%
Soap	1.180%
o-Phenylphenol	0.518%
o-Benzyl-p-chlorophenol	0.250%
Isopropyl alcohol	0.083%
Tetrasodium ethylenediaminetetraacetate	0.072%
Contains Sodium nitrite	minor

LEMISERP
Hypertension
(Lemmon Co.)

Each tablet:
Reserpine *	0.25 mg.

LEMON-AIRE, FOREMOST 4512

See FOREMOST 4512 LEMON-AIRE

LEMON BEE FURNITURE POLISH

See E-Z-EST LEMON BEE FURNITURE POLISH

LEMON CONCEPT
Disinfectant, deodorant; institutional & commercial use
(Hysan Corp.)

4-Chloro-2-cyclopentylphenol	0.0256%
Orthophenylphenol	0.1400%
3,4',5-Tribromosalicylanilide and other related bromosalicylanilides including:	0.3600%
3,5-Dibromosalicylanilide	
4',5-Dibromosalicylanilide	
2',3,4',5-Tetrabromosalicylanilide	
Essential oils	2.0000%
Alcohol	54.8100%

LEMON JELVYN BEAUTY FRESHNER
(Vicks Toiletry Products Div.)

Water	70–74%
SD Alcohol 40B	25%
Boric acid	1–2%
Fragrance	
FD & C Yellow No. 5	

LEMON JELVYN CLEANSING MILK
Skin lotion
(Vicks Toiletry Products Div.)

Water	
Mineral oil	
Propylene glycol	10%
Glyceryl stearate	
PEG-100 stearate	
Myristyl myristate	
Caprylic/Capric triglyceride	
Polysorbate 85	
Decyl oleate	
Polysorbate 60	
Cetearyl octanoate	
Magnesium aluminum silicate	
Stearic acid	
Fragrance	
Cetyl alcohol	
Methylparaben	
Propylparaben	
Butylparaben	
Myristyl alcohol	
BHA	
FD & C Yellow No. 5	

Starred ingredients (*) may be responsible for major toxic effects; consult Section II.

LEMON MEDICIDE
Disinfectant, deodorant; institutional and commercial use
(Hysan Corp.)

4-Chloro-2-cyclopentylphenol	0.0256%
Orthophenylphenol	0.1400%

3,4′,5-Tribromosalicylanilide
and other related bromosalicylanilides including: 0.3600%
  3,5-Dibromosalicylanilide
  4′,5-Dibromosalicylanilide
  2′3,4′,5-Tetrabromosalicylanilide

Essential oils	2.0000%
Alcohol	54.8100%

LEMON UP COSMETIC PRODUCTS
(Gillette Co., Personal Care Div.)

The Gillette Co., Personal Care Div., Boston, Mass. 02199 will receive collect phone calls from poison control centers or physicians asking for emergency toxicological information about the company's products.

Phone: 617-421-7000

LENSINE EXTRA STRENGTH
Hard contact lens cleaner
(CooperVision Pharm.)

Cleaning agent

Benzalkonium chloride	0.01%
Disodium edetate	0.1%

LENSINE 5
All purpose hard contact lens solution
(CooperVision Pharm.)

Mildly hypertonic solution
Poloxamer 407
Hydroxyethylcellulose
Polyvinyl alcohol
Polyethylene glycol

Benzalkonium chloride	0.01%
Disodium edetate	0.05%

LEOCREME
(Leo Products)

Water
Hydro-protein
Earth wax
Heavy mineral oil
Glycerine
Hydrocarbon emulsifier
Hydrogenated wax
Perfume
Magnesium sulfate
Vitamin D-3 solution
Methylparaben

LEOPILLS
Laxative
(Leo Products)

Extr. Rhubarb
Aloe *
Buckthorn
Olibanum galbanum
Myrrh praep.

LEPAGE'S ALL PURPOSE SUPER PERMAGRIP CEMENT
(LePage's)

Acrylic resin
Acetone *
Isopropyl alcohol *

LEPAGE'S ALL PURPOSE WHITE SCHOOL GLUE
(LePage's)

Polyvinyl acetate
Emulsion

LEPAGE'S EPOXY GLUE
(LePage's)

Resin A contains:
  Epoxy resin

Resin B contains:
  Modified amine

LEPAGE'S EXTRA FAST DRYING MODEL A CEMENT
(LePage's)

Cellulose acetate
Acetone *

LEPAGE'S MUCILAGE
(LePage's)

Dextrine

LEPAGE'S MULTI-PURPOSE HOUSEHOLD CEMENT
(LePage's)

Nitrocellulose
Toluol *

LEPAGE'S NON-METALLIC LIQUID SOLDER
(LePage's)

Nitrocellulose
Acetone *
Aluminum powder

LEPAGE'S ORIGINAL WHITE PASTE
(LePage's)

Starch

LEPAGE'S ORIGINAL WOOD GLUE
(LePage's)

Collagen
Fish skin extractables

LEPAGE'S POLYSTYRENE PLASTIC MODEL CEMENT
(LePage's)

Polystyrene
Toluol *

LEPAGE'S SUPER PERMA-GRIP CONTACT CEMENT
(LePage's)

Elastomer
Petroleum distillates *
Toluene *
Acetone *

L'ERIN COSMETICS

L'Erin Cosmetics
P.O. Box 57
Winston-Salem, N.C. 27102

Phone: 919-744-3526

See COSMETICS, Section VI, General Formulations

LERTON OVULES
Stimulant
(Vita Elixir Co.)

Each capsule:
  Caffeine * .... 250 mg.

LESAN
Fungicide
(Mobay Chemical Corp.)

Sodium (4-(dimethylamino)phenyl) di-azenesulfonate *

LES-SLIP FLOOR GLOSS
Self-polish wax
(Lester Labs.)

Wax
Emulsifiers

'76 Ed.

LESTER HV-7
Hot tank alkali degreaser
(Lester Labs.)

Caustic soda *
Detergents *

'76 Ed.

LESTER PINE OIL DISINFECTANT
(Lester Labs.)

Pine oil *
Soap

'76 Ed.

Starred ingredients (*) may be responsible for major toxic effects; consult Section II.

LESTER WHITE BOWL CLEANER
(Lester Labs.)

Inhibited Muriatic acids
Quaternary ammonium chlorides *

'76 Ed.

LESTOIL
Cleaner

Noxell Corporation
P.O. Box 1799
Baltimore, Md. 21203

Phone: 301-628-7300

LESWEED
Herbicide
(Lester Labs.)

Isopropanol amine salts of 2,4-di-
  chlorophenoxy acetic acid * .. 16.3%

'76 Ed.

LETHALAIRE A-20 AEROSOL
Insecticide
(Va. Chem. Inc.)

Pyrethrins 0.5%
Technical Piperonyl butoxide 4.0%
Petroleum hydrocarbon base *† . 12.5%
Propellant 83.0%

†*See* Petroleum hydrocarbons

LETHALAIRE A-41
Insecticide *
(Va. Chem. Inc.)

2,2-Dichlorovinyl dimethyl phosphate (DDVP) * 18.6%
Related compounds 1.4%

LETHALAIRE V-26
Aerosol insecticide
(Va. Chem. Inc.)

Resmethrin 0.500%
Related compounds 0.068%
Aromatic petroleum
  hydrocarbons 0.662%
Petroleum distillate * 18.750%

LETHANE 384
Organic insecticide
(Rohm and Haas)

Beta-butoxy beta'-thiocyano diethyl ether * 53%/w
Petroleum distillate 47%/w

LEUKERAN TABLETS
Antileukemic
(Burroughs Wellcome)

Each tablet:
  Chlorambucil (p-(Di-2-chlor-
  ethyl)-aminophenylbutyric
  acid) * . . . . 2 mg.

LEVEL BEST - FAST SET FLOOR LEVELER
(Savogran)

Calcium sulfate hemihydrate . . . . . >70%
Vegetable binder

LEVEL-BEST SPACKLING COMPOUND
For repairing plaster
(Savogran)

Calcium sulfate hemihydrate . . . . . >70%
Vegetable binder

LEVO-DROMORAN
Synthetic narcotic-analgesic
(Roche)

Each tablet:
  Levorphanol tartrate * . . . . 2 mg.

LEVOTHROID
Hypothyroidism
(Armour Pharm.)

Each tablet:
  Sodium levothyroxine *† .. 0.025 mg.;
                       0.050 mg.
  0.100 mg.; 0.150 mg.
  0.175 mg.; 0.200 mg.
                     0.300 mg.

†*See* Levothyroxine sodium

LEVSIN DROPS
*Anticholinergic, antispasmodic for in-
fants*
(Kremers-Urban)

Each cc:
  Levsin (l-Hyoscyamine
    sulfate) * . . . . 0.125 mg.
  Alcohol 5%

LEVSIN ELIXIR
Anticholinergic, antispasmodic
(Kremers-Urban)

Each 5 cc:
  Levsin (l-Hyoscyamine
    sulfate) * . . . . 0.125 mg.
  Alcohol 20%

LEVSINEX/ PHENOBARBITAL TIMECAPS
*Anticholinergic, antispasmodic, seda-
tive*
(Kremers-Urban)

Each time release capsule:
  Levsin (l-Hyoscyamine
    sulfate) * . . . . 0.375 mg.
  Phenobarbital * . . . . 45 mg.

LEVSINEX TIMECAPS
Anticholinergic, antispasmodic
(Kremers-Urban)

Each time release capsule:
  Levsin (l-Hyoscyamine
    sulfate) * . . . . 0.375 mg.

LEVSIN-PB DROPS
*Anticholinergic, antispasmodic, seda-
tive for infants*
(Kremers-Urban)

Each cc:
  Levsin (l-Hyoscyamine
    sulfate) * . . . . 0.125 mg.
  Phenobarbital * . . . . 15.0 mg.
  Alcohol 5%

LEVSIN/PHENOBARBITAL ELIXIR
*Anticholinergic, antispasmodic, seda-
tive*
(Kremers-Urban)

Each 5 cc:
  Levsin (l-Hyoscyamine
    sulfate) * . . . . 0.125 mg.
  Phenobarbital * . . . . 15 mg.
  Alcohol 20%

LEVSIN/PHENOBARBITAL TABLETS
*Anticholinergic, antispasmodic, seda-
tive*
(Kremers-Urban)

Each tablet:
  Levsin (l-Hyoscyamine
    sulfate) * . . . . 0.125 mg.
  Phenobarbital * . . . . 15 mg.

LEVSIN TABLETS
Anticholinergic, antispasmodic
(Kremers-Urban)

Each tablet:
  Levsin (l-Hyoscyamine
    sulfate) * . . . . 0.125 mg.

LEXOL
Leather conditioner
(Corona Products)

Sulfated Animal oils 25%

LEXOL LEATHER CLEANER
(Corona Products)

Alpha-olefin sulfonates 20%
Glycerin 10%

"LEXONE" DF WEED KILLER (DRY FLOWABLE)
(Du Pont)

Metribuzin * 75%

"LEXONE" 4L WEED KILLER
(Du Pont)

Metribuzin * 42.8%

"LEXONE" WEED KILLER
(Du Pont)

Metribuzin * 50%

Starred ingredients (*) may be responsible for major toxic effects; consult Section II.

l-GLUTAVITE CAPSULES
Dietary supplement for the elderly
(Berlex Labs.)

Each capsule:
Monosodium l-glutamate	580 mg.
Niacin	7.5 mg.
Pyridoxine HCl	0.16 mg.
Thiamine mononitrate	0.16 mg.
Riboflavin	0.32 mg.
Vitamin B12 (Cyanocobalamin)	1 mcg.
Iron (as ferrous sulfate)	1.7 mg.

L.H. - LIQUIK HEAVY DUTY (Liquid)

See GUNK L.H. - LIQUIK HEAVY DUTY (Liquid)

LIBERTY METAL POLISH
(Scranton Chem.)

Ammonium oxalate *†	4%
Silica	37%
Oleic acid	4%
Alcohol	6%
Ammonia	1.41%
Inert ingredient:	47%
Water	

'76 Ed.

†*See* Oxalate salts

LIBRITABS
Relief of anxiety and tension
(Roche)

Each tablet:
Chlordiazepoxide *	5 mg.; 10 mg.; or 25 mg.

LIBRIUM
Relief of anxiety and tension
(Roche)

Each capsule:
Chlordiazepoxide hydrochloride *	5 mg.; 10 mg.; or 25 mg.

LICE AWAY FOR SWINE

See PURINA LICE AWAY FOR SWINE

LICE-X, UNICO

See UNICO LICE-X

LIDAFORM-HC (CREME & LOTION)
(Dome)

Microdispersed Hydrocortisone acetate	0.5%
Lidocaine	3%
Iodochlorhydroxyquin	3%
Acid pH vehicle:	
Oil-in-water, emulsion-type creme containing a buffered solution of aluminum acetate	

LIDA-MANTLE CREME
Topical anesthetic
(Dome)

Lidocaine	3%
Acid pH vehicle:	
Oil-in-water, emulsion-type creme containing a buffered solution of aluminum acetate	

LIDA-MANTLE-HC CREME
Anti-inflammatory
(Dome)

Lidocaine	3%
Microdispersed Hydrocortisone acetate	0.5%
Acid pH vehicle:	
Oil-in-water, emulsion-type creme containing a buffered solution of aluminum acetate	

LIDEX-E (FLUOCINONIDE) CREAM
Topical anti-inflammatory cream
(Syntex Labs.)

Fluocinonide	0.05%
Water-washable aqueous emollient base:	
Stearyl alcohol	
Cetyl alcohol	
Mineral oil	
Propylene glycol	
Sorbitan monostearate	
Polysorbate 60	
Citric acid	

LIDEX (FLUOCINONIDE) CREAM
Topical anti-inflammatory agent
(Syntex Labs.)

Fluocinonide	0.05%
In a cream base consisting of:	
Stearyl alcohol	
Polyethylene glycol 8000	
Propylene glycol	
1,2,6-Hexanetriol	
Citric acid	

LIDEX (FLUOCINONIDE) OINTMENT
Topical anti-inflammatory agent
(Syntex Labs.)

Fluocinonide	0.05%
In a specially formulated base:	
Amerchol CAB (mixture of sterols and higher alcohols)	
White petrolatum	
Propylene carbonate	
Propylene glycol	

LIFEBUOY
Deodorant bar soap
(Lever Bros.)

Sodium soap	80-90%
Water	10-15%
Perfume	1-2%
Sodium chloride	<1%
Glycerol	<1%
Germicide	<1%
Sodium carbonate or phosphate	<1%
Titanium dioxide	<1%
Sodium sulfate	0-1%
Sodium EDTA	trace
Antioxidant	trace
Colorants	trace
Sodium EHDP	nil to trace

LIFE-GLO CONDITIONER
Hair conditioner
(Bonat)

	percentage range
Water	85.0-95.0%
Emulsifying wax N.F.	<5.0%
Quaternium-18 & Isopropyl alcohol	<2.0%
Stearamidopropyl dimethylamine lactate	<2.0%
PEG-4 stearate	<2.0%
Milk	2.0%
Fragrance	<1.0%
Methylparaben	<1.0%

LIFE GLO SPRAY TINT
Embalming supply
(Royal Bond)

Methanol *

LIFE-GLO TINT
Cosmetic; embalming supply
(Royal Bond)

Isopropanol *
Carbitol *

LIFE LABS. COUGH SYRUP
Expectorant
(Life Labs., Inc.)

Each fl. oz.:
Dextromethorphan HBr *	60 mg.
Pyrilamine maleate *	80 mg.
Chloroform	1 1/2 minims.
Ammonium chloride	10 gr.
Sodium citrate	10 gr.
Alcohol USP	5%

'76 Ed.

LIFE LABS. TERPIN HYDRATE
Expectorant
(Life Labs., Inc.)

Each fl. oz.:
Dextromethorphan HBr *	60 mg.
Terpin hydrate	503 mg.
Alcohol USP	40%

'76 Ed.

Starred ingredients (*) may be responsible for major toxic effects; consult Section II.

LIFE-LIKE FREEZ PAK
(Life-Like)

Water	98.000%
Cellulose	approx. 1.000%
Salt	approx. 1.000%
Blue food color	0.001%

LIFE-LIKE GREASE GUN
(Life-Like)

Mineral oil	93%
Lithium stearate	7%

LIFE-LIKE MODEL TRAIN SMOKE
(Life-Like)

Mineral oil	99.7%
Anise oil	
Violet food coloring	

LIFE-LIKE OIL GUN
(Life-Like)

Mineral oil	99%
Hydraulic oil additive (Nitrogen sulphur phosphorus compound)	1%

LIFE-LIKE TRACK CLEANER
Model train track cleaner
(Life-Like)

Nonionic surfactant (Nonyl phenyl polyethylene glycol ether)	4.5%
Hexylene glycol	4.5%
Diacetone alcohol	2.2%
Water	88.8%

LIGHTNING
Ammoniated general purpose cleaner
(Lester Labs.)

Mild Alkali *	
Synthetic detergents *	
Ammonia *	

'76 Ed.

LIKE-NU
(Lester Labs.)

Soap	
Mild Alkali *	

'76 Ed.

LILLY AMYL NITRITE (No. 2 & No. 3)
Coronary vasodilator in angina pectoris
(Lilly, Eli)

Each Aspirol:
Amyl nitrite *	0.18 ml.; or 0.3 ml.
Diphenylamine	

LILLY AMYTAL AND ACETYLSALICYLIC ACID PULVULES (NO. 1, SCARLET)
Sedative, hypnotic
(Lilly, Eli)

Each tablet:
Amobarbital *	3/4 gr.
Acetylsalicylic acid *	5 gr.

LILLY AMYTAL TABLETS, USP
Sedative
(Lilly, Eli)

Available in tablets containing:
Amobarbital *	1/4 gr.; 1/2 gr.; 3/4 gr.; 1 1/2 gr.

LILLY ANALGESIC BALM OINTMENT
Rubefacient
(Lilly, Eli)

Menthol *	15%
Methyl salicylate *	15%

LILLY BROWN MIXTURE
For relief of coughs
(Lilly, Eli)

Each 30 ml.:
Paregoric (anhydrous morphine 1.44 mg.) *	3.6 ml.
Alcohol 95%	10%
Glycyrrhiza	3.6 ml.
Antimony potassium tartrate	7.2 mg.
Glycerin	
Purified water	
Opium	
Benzoic acid	
Anise oil	
Camphor	

LILLY BUCHU, JUNIPER AND POTASSIUM ACETATE N.F.
(Lilly, Eli)

Alcohol	36%
Buchu solid extract	3.75 gm./100 cc.
Juniper solid extract *†	2.5 gm./100 cc.
Potassium acetate	5 gm./100 cc.

†*See* Juniper tar

LILLY CYANIDE ANTIDOTE PACKAGE
(Lilly, Eli)

Sodium nitrite ampoule:
Sodium nitrite *	300 mg.
Water for injection	10 ml.

Sodium thiosulfate ampoule:
Sodium thiosulfate *	12.5 gm.
Boric acid	
Potassium chloride	
Sodium hydroxide	
Water for injection	50 ml.

Amyl nitrite Aspirol:
Amyl nitrite *	0.3 ml.
Diphenylamine	

LILLY EPHEDRINE SULFATE (Not U.S.P.)
(Lilly, Eli)

Alcohol	12%
Ephedrine sulfate *	226 mg./100 ml.

LILLY ESSENCE PEPSIN (Not N.F.)
(Lilly, Eli)

Alcohol	13%
Pepsin	225 mg./10 ml.
Rennin	180 mg./10 ml.
Wine	1.65 ml./10 ml.
Aromatics	q.s.

LILLY/MILLER BRUSH, BRAMBLE & GRASS KILLER
(Chas. H. Lilly)

Amitrole	21%

LILLY/MILLER CHLORBAN INSECT GRANULES
(Chas. H. Lilly)

Chlorpyrifos *	0.5%

LILLY/MILLER CHLORDANE 8E
Insecticide
(Chas. H. Lilly)

Chlordane (technical) *	72.3%
Petroleum distillate *	21.5%

LILLY/MILLER CONTROL ALL PURPOSE SPRAY
Insecticide/fungicide
(Chas. H. Lilly)

Pyrethrins	0.19%
Rotenone	0.50%
Other Cube resins	0.50%
Copper oleate	8.30%
Petroleum hydrocarbons	3.81%
Xylene *	78.45%

LILLY/MILLER CRABGRASS KILLER & LAWN FOOD
(Chas. H. Lilly)

Nitrogen *†	15%
Phosphate *	4%
Potash *	6%
Sulfur	5%
Iron	1.5%
Dacthal	3%

†*See* Nitrate salts

LILLY/MILLER DIAZINON INSECT SPRAY
(Chas. H. Lilly)

Diazinon *	16.75%
Aromatic petroleum derivative solvents *	75.50%

Starred ingredients (*) may be responsible for major toxic effects; consult Section II.

LILLY/MILLER FEED & WEED
(Chas. H. Lilly)

Nitrogen *†	12%
Phosphoric acid *	2%
Potash *	3%
Calcium	3%
Magnesium	1.5%
Sulfur	8%
Iron	2%
Manganese	0.05%
Zinc	0.05%
2,4-D	0.25%
MCPP	0.15%
Banvel	0.09%

†*See* Nitrate salts

LILLY/MILLER FRUIT & BERRY INSECT SPRAY
(Chas. H. Lilly)

Methoxychlor (technical)	16.70%
Malathion	9.40%
1,1-Bis(p-chlorophenyl)-2,2,2-trichloroethanol	5.00%
Aromatic petroleum derivative solvents *	57.62%

LILLY/MILLER GRANULAR NOXALL VEGETATION KILLER
(Chas. H. Lilly)

Sodium metaborate tetrahydrate (Boron trixode equiv. 22.7%)	66.50%
Sodium chlorate *	30.00%
Diuron	1.25%

LILLY/MILLER HOLLY DIP
To prolong the life of cut holly
(Chas. H. Lilly)

1-Naphthaleneacetic acid, potassium salt	0.65%

LILLY/MILLER HOUSE & PATIO INSECT SPRAY
(Chas. H. Lilly)

Resmethrin	0.250%
Related compounds	0.034%
Aromatic petroleum hydrocarbons	0.332%

LILLY/MILLER HOUSE PLANT INSECT SPRAY
(Chas. H. Lilly)

Tetramethrin	0.250%
Related compounds	0.034%
Resmethrin	0.106%
Related compounds	0.014%
Petroleum distillate	9.000%

LILLY/MILLER LAWN INSECT SPRAY
(Chas. H. Lilly)

Chlorpyrifos	6.79%
Aromatic petroleum derivative solvent *	42.48%
Petroleum distillates	41.48%

LILLY/MILLER LAWN & TURF WEED BOMB
(Chas. H. Lilly)

Dimethylamine salt of 2-(2-Methyl-4-chlorophenoxy) propionic acid	0.130%
Dimethylamine salt of 2,4-Dichlorophenoxyacetic acid	0.287%
Dimethylamine salt of Dicamba	0.029%

LILLY/MILLER LAWN & TURF WEED KILLER
(Chas. H. Lilly)

Dimethylamine 2,4-dichlorophenoxyacetate *†	10.01%
Dimethylamine salt of 2-(2-Methyl-4-chlorophenoxy) propionic acid	4.54%
Dimethylamine salt of Dicamba	1.04%

†*See* 2,4-D

LILLY/MILLER MALATHION
Insecticide
(Chas. H. Lilly)

Malathion *	57%
Aromatic petroleum derivative solvents *	33%

LILLY/MILLER MICROCOP FUNGICIDE
(Chas. H. Lilly)

Copper (expressed as metallic) *	50%

LILLY/MILLER MOSS-KIL
(Chas. H. Lilly)

Zinc, as metallic *†	29.6%

†*See* Zinc chloride

LILLY/MILLER NOXALL VEGETATION KILLER CONCENTRATE
(Chas. H. Lilly)

Prometon	3.6%
2,4-Dichlorophenoxyacetic acid	1.0%
Aromatic petroleum distillates *	76.4%

LILLY/MILLER PET, POULTRY & LIVESTOCK DUST
(Chas. H. Lilly)

Malathion *	4%

LILLY/MILLER POLYSUL SUMMER & DORMANT SPRAY CONCENTRATE
(Chas. H. Lilly)

Calcium polysulfide *	28.7%

LILLY/MILLER PRE-EMERGENT WEED & GRASS KILLER
(Chas. H. Lilly)

Simazine *	4%

LILLY/MILLER PRUNING AID
Protective pruning, sealing paint
(Chas. H. Lilly)

Xylol *	

LILLY/MILLER ROSE & EVERGREEN INSECT SPRAY
(Chas. H. Lilly)

Trichlorfon *	18.0%
S-(2-(Ethylsulfinyl)ethyl) O,O-dimethyl phosphorothioate	6.0%
Xylene *	36.4%

LILLY/MILLER ROSE & FLORAL DUST
Insecticide/miticide/fungicide
(Chas. H. Lilly)

Carbaryl *	5.0%
Rotenone *	1.5%
Other Cube resins	1.5%
Zineb	5.0%

LILLY/MILLER ROSE & FLOWER GARDEN SPRAY
(Chas. H. Lilly)

Pyrethrins	0.026%
Piperonyl butoxide (technical)	0.256%
Rotenone	0.128%
Other Cube extractives	0.238%
Captan	0.504%
2,4-Dinitro-4-octyl phenyl crotonate	0.146%
2,6-Dinitro-4-octyl phenyl crotonate Nitrooctyl phenols (principally dinitro)	0.010%
Petroleum distillate	0.026%

LILLY/MILLER SEVIN INSECT SPRAY
(Chas. H. Lilly)

Carbaryl *	10%

LILLY/MILLER SLUG, SNAIL & INSECT KILLER BAIT
(Chas. H. Lilly)

Metaldehyde *	2%
Carbaryl *	5%

Starred ingredients (*) may be responsible for major toxic effects; consult Section II.

LILLY/MILLER SOIL & BULB DUST
Insecticide, fungicide
(Chas. H. Lilly)

Carbaryl *	5.0%
Rotenone *	1.5%
Other Cube resins	1.5%
Zineb	5.0%

LILLY/MILLER SOIL CLEAN-UP
Soil fumigant solution
(Chas. H. Lilly)

Sodium methyldithiocarbamate (anhydrous) *	32.7%

LILLY/MILLER SPOT WEEDER
(Chas. H. Lilly)

Dimethylamine salt of 2,4-Dichlorophenoxyacetic acid	0.620%
Dimethylamine salt of 2-(2-Methyl-4-chlorophenoxy) propionic acid	0.281%
Dimethylamine salt of Dicamba	0.064%

LILLY/MILLER STA-STUK "m"
Adjuvant for fixed copper sprays
(Chas. H. Lilly)

Potassium resinate	12.0%
Potassium oleate	2.5%

LILLY/MILLER SUPER SPRAY-AID
Spreader-sticker
(Chas. H. Lilly)

Modified Phthalic glycerol alkyd resin	77%

LILLY/MILLER SYSTEMIC ROSE, SHRUB & FLOWER CARE
(Chas. H. Lilly)

O,O-Diethyl S-(2-(ethylthio)ethyl) phosphorodithioate *	1%

LILLY/MILLER TOMATO FRUIT SET
(Chas. H. Lilly)

p-Chlorophenoxyacetic acid	0.005%

LILLY/MILLER TOMATO SET
(Chas. H. Lilly)

Beta-naphthoxyacetic acid	0.0041%

LILLY/MILLER VEGETABLE DUST
Insecticide/fungicide
(Chas. H. Lilly)

Carbaryl *	5%
Rotenone *	1%
Other Cube resins	1%
Zineb	5%

LILLY/MILLER VEGETABLE & FRUIT SPRAY
Insecticide
(Chas. H. Lilly)

Endosulfan *	9.15%
Cottonseed oil	36.60%
Xylene *	49.35%

LILLY/MILLER WASP & HORNET KILLER
(Chas. H. Lilly)

Diazinon	0.500%
Pyrethrins	0.052%
Piperonyl butoxide (technical)	0.261%
Petroleum distillate *	98.608%

LILLY/MILLER WEEDER
(Chas. H. Lilly)

Dimethyl tetrachloroterephthalate	5%

LILLY/MILLER WHACK WASP-HORNET ANT-ROACH KILLER
(Chas. H. Lilly)

Baygon *	0.50%
Petroleum distillate *	64.46%

LILLY RHINITIS, FULL STRENGTH
For relief of symptoms of the common cold
(Lilly, Eli)

Each tablet:	
Belladonna extract *	5.8 mg.
Quinine sulfate *	32.5 mg.
Camphor *	32.5 mg.

LILLY'S GO-WEST MEAL
Kills slugs & snails
(Chas. H. Lilly)

Sodium fluosilicate *	5%
Metaldehyde *	3%

LILLY'S GO-WEST SLUG KILLER
(Chas. H. Lilly)

Metaldehyde *	25%

LILLY'S MOSS-OUT FOR LAWNS
(Chas. H. Lilly)

Ferric sulfate, anhydrous *	35%

LILLY WHITE PINE & AMMONIUM CHLORIDE COMPOUND
(Lilly, Eli)

Each 100 cc:	
Alcohol	7%
White pine bark	8.5 gm.
Wild cherry	8.5 gm.
Sanguinaria	0.8 gm.
Balm Gilead buds	1 gm.
Spikenard	1 gm.
Ammonium chloride	1.75 gm.

LILLY WHITE PINE COMPOUND
(Lilly, Eli)

Each 100 cc:	
Alcohol	7%
White pine bark	8.5 gm.
Wild cherry	8.5 gm.
Sanguinaria	0.8 gm.
Balm Gilead buds	1 gm.
Spikenard	1 gm.
Sassafras *	1 gm.

LILOL
Disinfectant, deodorant
(Navy Brand)

Isopropyl alcohol *	10.03%
Vegetable oil soap	5.50%
o-Phenylphenol	1.48%
4 and 6 Chloro-2-phenylphenol	3.55%
Essential oils	0.44%

LILT (Lotion) "DELUXE"
"Gentle", "Regular", "Super", "Soft-perm", "Special", and "Body Wave"
(Procter & Gamble, Beauty Care Div.)

Monoethylamine thioglycolate *	6-12%
Monoethanolamine	1-4%
Polyoxyethylene lauryl ether	1-4%
Fragrance	1-3%
Mineral oil	1-4%
Minor ingredients, each	1%
Water	50%

LILT (Lotion) "Push Button"
(Procter & Gamble, Beauty Care Div.)

Monoethylamine thioglycolate *	6-12%
Monoethanolamine	1-4%
Polyoxyethylene lauryl ether	1-4%
Isopropyl myristate	3-6%
Fragrance	1-3%
Minor ingredients, each	1%
Water	50%
Propellant	1-4%

Starred ingredients (*) may be responsible for major toxic effects; consult Section II.

LILT (Neutralizer)
Home permanent neutralizer
(Procter & Gamble, Beauty Care Div.)

Hydrogen peroxide	1–4%
Isopropyl palmitate	1–4%
Polyoxyethylene lauryl ether	<1%
Perfume	<1%
Minor ingredients, each	<0.1%
Water	>50%

LIMBITROL TABLETS
Tranquilizer-antidepressant
(Roche)

Each 10-25 tablet:
Chlordiazepoxide	10 mg.
Amitriptyline HCl *	25 mg.

Each 5-12.5 tablet:
Chlordiazepoxide	5 mg.
Amitriptyline HCl *	12.5 mg.

LIME-A-WAY
Lime scale remover
(Economics)

Hydroxyacetic acid
Phosphoric acid *

LIME DROPS BATH OIL
(House of Lowell, Inc.)

TEA-lauryl sulfate *
Lauramide DEA
Laneth-16
Glycerin
Isopropyl palmitate
Perfume *
Formaldehyde
D & C color

LIME FRESH PUREX DISHWASHING LIQUID
(Purex Corp.)

Anionic surfactants *	20-30%
Ethyl alcohol	<3%
Alkanolamide	<3%
Opacifier	<1%
Coloring agent	<1%
Perfume	<1%
Water	balance

LIME SHINE ACID DETERGENT-LIME SOLVENT
(Nat'l Labs. Div.)

Phosphoric acid *
Surfactants

LIMEX LIME REMOVER
For use on porcelain and metal surfaces
(Dorex, Inc.)

Hydroxyacetic acid	18.6%
Nonionic surfactant	0.5%
Citric acid	4.5%
Water	76.4%

LINDANE
Broad spectrum insecticide
(Zoecon Corp.)

Gamma isomer of benzene hexachloride *	99.5% Min.

LINDEX
Insecticide for municipal and institutional use
(ABCO, Inc.)

Petroleum distillates *	99.374%
Gamma isomer of benzene hexachloride from lindane	0.500%
Piperonyl butoxide technical	0.101%
Pyrethrins	0.025%

LINE CLEAN 3

See UNIVERSAL LINE CLEAN 3

LINE TAMER COSMETICS

Line Tamer Inc.
2 Coral Way
Miami, Fla. 33131

Phone: 305-442-4707

See COSMETICS, Section VI, General Formulations

LINICAST
Equine emollient leg bandage
(Burns-Biotec)

Glycerin	36 gm.
Zinc oxide *	16.5 gm.
Calamine	13.2 gm.
Gelatine	
Fumed Silica	
Menthol	
Methylparaben	
Propylparaben	

LINI GEL
Equine liniment gel
(Burns-Biotec)

Isopropyl alcohol *	70% v/v
Methyl salicylate *	8% v/v
Menthol *	1.5% w/v
Camphor *	1.5% w/v

LINITE, DR. NAYLOR'S

See DR. NAYLOR'S LINITE

LINIT PRODUCTS
LINIT FABRIC FINISH
LINIT LAUNDRY STARCH
LINIT LIQUID STARCH
(Best Foods)

Best Foods
CPC International, Inc.
International Plaza
Englewood Cliffs, N.J. 07632

Phone: 201-894-4000

LINSPRAY
Residual insecticidal action; veterinary
(Norden Labs.)

Gamma isomer of benzene hexachloride (from lindane) *	12.0%
Aromatic petroleum derivative solvent *	84.8%

LIP FAST
For sealing lips and eyelids; embalming supply
(Royal Bond)

Scotch Grip Adhesive	
Trichloroethane *	<50%

LIP-GARD
For chapped lips
(Whitehall Labs.)

Live Yeast cell derivative
Camphor *
Menthol *
Lanolin

LIPKOTE, COPPERTONE

See COPPERTONE LIPKOTE

LIPO GANTRISIN
For urinary tract infections
(Roche)

Suspension (each 5 ml.):	
Acetyl sulfisoxazole	1 gm.

LIPSAVER (WILD CHERRY, LIME, ORANGEMINT AND SPEARMINT)
(Sea & Ski)

Mineral oil, heavy (USP)
Microcrystalline Wax
Spermaceti (USP) or Sperm wax
Wecobee-S (with Lecithin)
2-Ethylhexylsalicylate
Sorbic acid (NF)
Lantrol
Allantoin 200 mesh
Anti-Foam "A"
Magnasweet 180
Flavoring

LIQUABRADE

See LEA LIQUABRADE

LIQUA-CLEAN
For hand dishwashing
(Calgon Corp., Commercial Div.)

Dodecylbenzene sulfonate *†
Fatty amide
Water

†*See* Alkyl aryl sodium sulfonates

Starred ingredients (*) may be responsible for major toxic effects; consult Section II.

LIQUA 4 (LIQUID SOAP)
(Armour-Dial, Inc.)

Water and volatiles	75-100%
Lauramide DEA	10-25%
TEA lauryl sulfate	5-10%
Sodium lauroyl sarcosinate	5-10%
Sodium laureth sulfate	5-10%
Minor ingredients (total)	5-10%

LIQUALGINE 3
Antipyretic, analgesic
(Whorton)

Each fl. dr.:
Acetylsalicylic acid *	5 gr.
Salicylic acid	trace
Alcohol	50%/v

'76 Ed.

LIQUALOR CREAM
For dermatitis
(Thomas & Thompson)

Starch
Stearic acid
Anhydrous Lanolin
White wax
Light mineral oil
Potassium carbonate
Triethanolamine
Liquor carbonis detergens *
Borax *
Carbitol *
Menthol *

LIQUAMAR
Anticoagulant
(Organon)

Each tablet:
Phenprocoumon (3-(1'-Phenyl-propyl)-4-hydroxycoumarin) * 3 mg.

LIQUAMELT
Liquid ice & snow melter; municipal & industrial use
(Scientific International)

Ethylene glycol *
Isopropyl alcohol *

LIQUA-SOLV BOWL CLEANER
Bacteriocidal-fungicidal; institutional and industrial use
(Myers, R.A.)

Hyamine 2839	0.20%
Methyl dodecyl xylene bis (tri-methyl ammonium chloride)	0.05%
Tin san provides 0.0015%	0.01%
Hydrochloric acid *	25.00%

LIQUID "all" (Low Phosphate)
Liquid laundry detergent
(Lever Bros.)

Water	55-65%
Potassium and sodium pyrophosphates	20-30%
Nonionic detergents	5-10%
Sodium silicate	1-5%
Anionic detergent	1-5%
Resin	<1%
Cellulosic	<1%
Optical dye	<1%
Perfume	<1%
Colorant	trace

LIQUID "all" (Nonphosphate)
Liquid laundry detergent
(Lever Bros.)

Water	65-75%
Anionic detergent	15-25%
Nonionic detergent	5-10%
Monoethanolamine	1-5%
Sodium soap	<1%
Opacifier	<1%
Perfume	<1%
Optical dyes	trace
Colorants	trace

LIQUID DIRTEX ALL PURPOSE CLEANER (CONCENTRATE)
(Savogran)

Butyl Cellosolve *	<10%
Borax	<5%
Sesquicarbonate of soda *	<10%
Surface active agents, etc.	<20%

LIQUID DRAIN-PEP
Multi-purpose grease and odor remover
(Radiator)

Ortho-dichlorobenzene *

'76 Ed.

LIQUID DRANO
Drain cleaner
(Drackett)

Sodium hydroxide *	1.8%
Sodium ypochlorite *	4.5%
Sodium silicate	1.2%
Emulsifiers	
Water	
Dye	

LIQUIDEMON HEAVY DUTY PF
Liquid steam cleaning compound
(Clayton Mfg.)

Aqueous solution of Potassium hydroxide *	10-20%
Polycarboxylate dispersants	<1%
Synthetic detergents	1-10%

LIQUIDEMON UNIVERSAL PF
Liquid steam cleaning compound for aluminum
(Clayton Mfg.)

Aqueous solution of Sodium silicates *	>10%
Synthetic detergents *	1-10%
Polycarboxylate dispersants	<1%

LIQUID FIRE
Automotive; quick starting fluid
(Radiator)

Ethyl-ether *

'76 Ed.

LIQUID FLUSHOUT
Bowl cleaner
(Dolge)

Hydrogen chloride *	21.5%
Phosphoric acid	6.9%
n-Alkyl dimethyl benzyl ammonium chloride	0.5%
Heptadecyl hydroxyethylimidazo-lium hydrochloride	0.1%
Dehydroabietylamine	0.1%

LIQUID GEL
Rust remover
(Radiator)

Phosphoric acid *

'76 Ed.

LIQUID GERITONIC
Nutrient tonic and stomachic
(Geriatric Pharm.)

Each 5 cc:
Iron (from ferric ammonium citrate) *	20 mg.
Alcohol	20%
Plus multivitamins and minerals	

LIQUID GLAZE ALL PURPOSE CLEANER
(Liquid Glaze, Inc.)

Alkyl sulfonate linear, sodium salt *	
Nitriloacetic acid, trisodium salt	<1.0%
Sodium tripolyphosphate *	
Sodium metasilicate *	
Sodium xylene sulfonate *	
Glycol ether *	
Water	

LIQUID GLAZE DURASHINE GLAZE
(Liquid Glaze, Inc.)

Aliphatic hydrocarbon solvent *
Silicone fluids and resins
Synthetic polymers
Anhydrous Aluminum silicate abrasive
Stearic acid soap

LIQUID GLAZE ELIMINATOR
(Liquid Glaze, Inc.)

Aromatic hydrocarbon solvents *
Aliphatic hydrocarbon solvents *
1,1,1-Trichloroethane *
Butyl acetate *
Glycol ether *
Alkyl sulfonate linear, amine salt *

LIQUID GLAZE GLASS CLEANER
(Liquid Glaze, Inc.)

Water
Glycol ether *
Linear alkyl sulfonate, sodium salt *

LIQUID GLAZE LIQUID CLEANER
(Liquid Glaze, Inc.)

Aliphatic hydrocarbon solvents *
Diatomaceous earth
Amine oleate
Water

LIQUID GLAZE MOTOR WASH
(Liquid Glaze, Inc.)

Alkyl sulfonate linear, amine salt *
Tetrapotassium pyrophosphate *
Aliphatic hydrocarbon solvents *
Glycol ether *
Water

LIQUID GLAZE POLY GLAZE
(Liquid Glaze, Inc.)

Aliphatic hydrocarbon solvents *
Silicone fluid
Polyethylene

LIQUID GLAZE WHITEWALL TIRE CLEANER
(Liquid Glaze, Inc.)

Sodium metasilicate
Caustic soda * .... <2%
Isopropyl alcohol *
Glycol ether *
Alkyl sulfonate linear, sodium salt *
Sodium xylene sulfonate *
Water

LIQUID 'K', FORMULA LC-300

See KLENZADE LIQUID 'K', FORMULA LC-300

LIQUID KOOL
Automotive
(Radiator)

Ethylene glycol *

'76 Ed.

LIQUID-L
Heavy duty liquid laundry detergent
(Shaklee)

Nonionic surfactants
Ethanol .... small amounts
Sodium carbonate ...... small amounts
Brighteners, Perfume,
and Color .... small amounts

LIQUIDOPE NO. 36-2
General purpose coil coating
(GC Electronics)

No. 30 Service cement
Butyl acetate .... <10%

LIQUIDOW
Dust control
(Dow)

Calcium chloride 32-38%
Water .... to 100%

LIQUID PAPER CORRECTION FLUIDS - WHITE AND COLORED
(Liquid Paper)

Methyl chloroform 22.5%
Trichloroethylene * 52.5%
Titanium dioxide
Pigments .... minor conc.
Dyes .... minor conc.
Polymer .... minor conc.
Plasticizer .... minor conc.
Dispersant .... minor conc.

LIQUID PAPER CORRECTION FLUID THINNER
(Liquid Paper)

Methyl chloroform *
Mustard oil .... <0.5%

LIQUID PAPER JUST FOR COPIES
(Liquid Paper)

Titanium dioxide
Water
Polymers
Ethanol .... <12.0%
Methanol .... <2.5%
Pigments .... minor conc.
Plasticizer .... minor conc.
Dispersant .... minor conc.

LIQUID PAPER MISTAKE OUT CORRECTION FLUID
(Liquid Paper)

Titanium dioxide
Water
Polymers
Ethanol .... <12.0%
Methanol .... <2.5%
Pigments .... minor conc.
Plasticizer .... minor conc.
Dispersant .... minor conc.

LIQUID PAPER PEN & INK CORRECTION FLUID
(Liquid Paper)

Methyl chloroform * 52%
Titanium dioxide
Pigments .... minor conc.
Dyes .... minor conc.
Polymer .... minor conc.
Plasticizer .... minor conc.
Dispersant .... minor conc.

LIQUID PLUMR
Drain opener
(Clorox)

Water .... >75%
Sodium hypochlorite * 5-10%
Sodium hydroxide 0.5-2%

LIQUID POWER HEAVY DUTY-LOW SUDS, MULTI-PURPOSE CLEANER-WAX STRIPPER
(Nat'l Labs. Div.)

Sodium metasilicate pentahydrate minor
Tetrasodium
   ethylenediaminetetraacetate ... minor

LIQUID PRESTO
Easter egg dye
(Doxsee Food Corp.)

U.S. certified color 0.7%
Distilled Citrus oil
Resins

LIQUID Q.D.S.
Disinfectant, sanitizer
(Holcomb)

N-Alkyl dimethyl benzyl ammonium chloride * 1-10%
N-Alkyl dimethyl ethylbenzyl ammonium chloride * 1-10%

'76 Ed.

LIQUID THRIP-TOX
Insecticide
(Leffingwell)

Sabadilla alkaloids 0.50%

LIQUID WRENCH
Rust preventative, remover
(Radiator)

Aromatic solvents *
Petroleum oils
Colloidal Graphite

'76 Ed.

LIQUIFILM FORTE
Ocular lubricant
(Allergan Pharm.)

Polyvinyl alcohol 3%
Thimerosal 0.002%
Edetate disodium

Starred ingredients (*) may be responsible for major toxic effects; consult Section II.

LIQUIFILM TEARS
(Allergan Pharm.)

Polyvinyl alcohol	1.4%
Chlorobutanol (chloral deriv.)	0.5%

LIQUIFILM WETTING SOLUTION
(Allergan Pharm.)

Polyvinyl alcohol	
Hydroxypropyl methylcellulose	
Edetate disodium	
Benzalkonium chloride	1:25,000
Sodium chloride	
Potassium chloride	

LIQUIK HEAVY DUTY - L.H. (Liquid)

See GUNK L.H. - LIQUIK HEAVY DUTY (Liquid)

LIQUI-KLENZ
Creme cleanser concentrate
(Hysan Corp.)

2,2'-Methylenebis(3,4,6-trichloro-phenol) (Hexachlorophene)	0.2%

LIQUIK MEDIUM DUTY - L.M. (Liquid)

See GUNK L.M. - LIQUIK MEDIUM DUTY (Liquid)

LIQUI-NOX
Liquid detergent
(Alconox)

Linear alkyl aryl sodium sulfonates (anionic) *
Nonylphenoxypoly(ethyleneoxy)ethanol (non-ionic) *†

†*See* Alkyl phenoxy polyethoxy ethanols

LIQUIPRIN
Analgesic, antipyretic
(Norcliff Thayer)

Each 1.25 ml.:	
Acetaminophen *	60 mg.

LIQUI-RID
Anthelmintic; veterinary
(Hess & Clark)

Each fl. oz.:	
Piperazine base	5.05 gm.

LIQUI-STIK CONCENTRATE

See NIAGARA LIQUI-STIK CONCENTRATE

LIQUIX-C CAPSULES
Analgesic - antipyretic
(Elder)

Each capsule:	
Acetaminophen *	320 mg.
Codeine phosphate *	32 mg.

LIQUOPHYLLINE
For bronchial asthma
(Paddock Labs.)

Each 15 ml.:	
Theophylline *	80 mg.
Alcohol	3 ml.

LIQWEEDATE-2
Herbicide and brush killer
(Brulin)

2-Methoxy-4,6-bis (isopropylamino)-s-triazine	10.0%
Isooctyl ester of 2,4-dichlorophenoxyacetic acid	5.4%

LISTEREX SCRUB
Anti-acne lotion
(Warner-Lambert)

Salicylic acid *	2%

LISTERINE ANTISEPTIC
(Warner-Lambert)

Thymol *	
Eucalyptol *	
Methyl salicylate *	
Menthol *	
Benzoic acid	
Alcohol	25%

LISTERINE ANTISEPTIC THROAT LOZENGES
(Warner-Lambert)

Each lozenge:	
Hexylresorcinol	2.4 mg.

LISTERINE TOOTHPASTE
(Warner-Lambert)

Dicalcium phosphate, dihydrate
Water
Sorbitol
Glycerin
Sodium lauryl sulfate
Titanium dioxide
Sodium carrageenan
Flavor
Cellulose gum
Sodium saccharin
Phosphoric acid

LISTERMINT
Mouthwash
(Warner-Lambert)

Water
SD Alcohol 38-B
Glycerin
Poloxamer 407
Sodium lauryl sulfate
Sodium citrate
Sodium saccharin
Flavoring
Zinc chloride
Citric acid
D & C Yellow #10
FD & C Green #3

LITH-EASE
White lithium lubricant
(American Grease Stick)
(Marketed by: Balkamp, Inc.)

Mineral oil	90-91%
Lithium hydroxy stearate	5-7.5%
Titanium dioxide	3-4%

LITHONATE
Control of manic episodes in manic-depressive psychosis
(Rowell)

Each capsule:	
Lithium carbonate *	300 mg.

LITHOTABS
For control of manic episodes in manic-depressive psychosis
(Rowell)

Each tablet:	
Lithium carbonate *	300 mg.

LITTER-MATE

See ANCHOR LITTER-MATE

LITTLE BOY BLUE BLUING
(Purex Corp.)

Prussian blue	<2%
Oxalic acid	<1%
Perfume	<1%
Water	balance

LIVETTES
To reduce fatigue
(Amlab)

Each tablet:	
Caffeine alkaloid *	100 mg.
Niacin & sodium biphosphate	
Calcium phosphate monobasic	
Dextrose (grape sugar)	
Oleoresin capsicum	
Thiamine mononitrate	

LIVITAMIN CAPSULES
Iron and vitamin deficiency anemias
(Beecham Labs.)

Each capsule:	
Ferrous fumarate (elemental iron 33 mg.) *	100 mg.
Plus multivitamins and minerals	

Starred ingredients (*) may be responsible for major toxic effects; consult Section II.

LIVITAMIN CHEWABLE TABLETS
Iron and vitamin supplement
(Beecham Labs.)

Each tablet:
Ferrous fumarate (elemental
iron 16.4 mg.) .... 50 mg.
Plus polyvitamins & minerals

LIVITAMIN LIQUID
Hematinic
(Beecham Labs.)

Each 15 ml.:
Iron peptonized (elemental iron
35.5 mg.) .... 210 mg.
Plus polyvitamins & minerals

LIVITAMIN PRENATAL TABLETS
(Beecham Labs.)

Each tablet:
Vitamin A acetate ... 6,000 USP units
Vitamin D2 .... 400 USP units
Iron (as ferrous fumarate) .... 50 mg.
Plus polyvitamins & minerals

LIXAMINOL
Antiasthmatic, vasodilator, antitussive
(Ferndale Labs.)

Each 15 cc.:
Aminophylline * .... 250 mg.
Alcohol (20% by volume) ..... 4.5 cc.
Dye free
Sugar free

LIXAMINOL-AT
For asthma
(Ferndale Labs.)

Each tablespoon (15 cc):
Aminophylline (anhydrous) * 250 mg.
Dextromethorphan HBr ..... 20 mg.
Dye free, sugar free

L.M. - LIQUIK MEDIUM DUTY (Liquid)

See GUNK L.M. - LIQUIK MEDIUM
DUTY (Liquid)

LOBANA LOTION
(Ulmer)

Deionized water
Mineral oil
Triethanolamine stearate
Stearic acid
Lanolin
Cetyl alcohol
Potassium stearate
Propylene glycol
Methylparaben
Propylparaben
Fragrance

LOBAX SPECIAL
Chlorine sanitizing agent
(Olin Corporation)

Calcium hypochlorite * 50%

L.O.C. HIGH SUDS

See AMWAY L.O.C. HIGH SUDS

LOCK-EASE
Graphited lock fluid
(American Grease Stick)
(Marketed by: Atlas Supply Co.; Bal-
kamp, Inc.; Chrysler Corp., Parts Div.)

Combined amount: 20%
Mineral oil
Aluminum stearate
Colloidal Graphite (10% dispersion
in mineral oil) 1%
Lead naphthenate .... <1%
Naphtha (aliphatic) * 75%
Tricresyl phosphate (no ortho con-
tent)(synthetic base) 1%
Mixture of: 1%
Organic acids
Lactones
Hydroxyacids
Esters

LOCK N SEAL, BALKAMP

See BALKAMP LOCK N SEAL

LOCORTEN
Anti-inflammatory, antipruritic
(CIBA Pharmaceutical)

Cream, ointment or lotion:
Flumethasone pivalate 0.02%

L.O.C. REGULAR

See AMWAY L.O.C. REGULAR

LOESTRIN 21 1/20
Oral contraceptive
(Parke-Davis)

Each tablet:
Norethindrone acetate .... 1 mg.
Ethinyl estradiol .... 20 mcg.

LOESTRIN 21 1.5/30
Oral contraceptive
(Parke-Davis)

Each tablet:
Norethindrone acetate .... 1.5 mg.
Ethinyl estradiol .... 30 mcg.

LOESTRIN FE 1/20
Oral contraceptive
(Parke-Davis)

Each white tablet:
Norethindrone acetate .... 1 mg.
Ethinyl estradiol .... 20 mcg.

Each brown tablet:
Ferrous fumarate * .... 75 mg.

LOESTRIN FE 1.5/30
Oral contraceptive
(Parke-Davis)

Each green tablet:
Norethindrone acetate .... 1.5 mg.
Ethinyl estradiol .... 30 mcg.

Each brown tablet:
Ferrous fumarate * .... 75 mg.

LOK-GARD
Floor polish
(Hillyard Chem.)

Acrylic water emulsion

'76 Ed.

LOK-UP WINTER ANTIFEEZE

See BIO-GUARD LOK-UP WINTER
ANTIFREEZE

LOK-UP WINTERIZER ALGAECIDE

See BIO-GARD LOK-UP WINTER-
IZER ALGAECIDE

LOK-UP WINTER SHOCK

See BIO-GUARD LOK-UP WINTER
SHOCK

LOK-UP WINTERTROL

See BIO-GUARD LOK-UP WINTER-
TROL

LOMOTIL
Antidiarrheal agent
(Searle, G.D., & Co.)

Each tablet or 5 cc.:
Diphenoxylate
hydrochloride * .... 2.5 mg.
Atropine sulfate .... 0.025 mg.

LONG AID HOT OIL TREATMENT
(Keystone Labs.)

Petrolatum
Lanolin
Mineral oil
Oil of bergamot

LONG AID POMADE
(Keystone Labs.)

Petroleum jelly
Lanolin
Mineral oil (Carnation)
Perfume oil
Isopropyl myristate

Starred ingredients (*) may be responsible for major toxic effects; consult Section II.

LONG AID SHAMPOO
(Keystone Labs.)

Triethanolamine
Lauryl sulfate *†
Ninol AA62
Water softener
Sequesterene
Perfume oil

†See Sodium lauryl sulfate

LONG AID SULPHUR POMADE TREATMENT
(Keystone Labs.)

Petrolatum
Lanolin
Oil of tar rectified
Wettable Sulfur
Salicylic acid *
Isobornyl acetate

LO 'N SLO pH DECREASER

See BIO-GUARD LO 'N SLO pH DE-CREASER

LO/OVRAL TABLETS
Oral contraceptive
(Wyeth Labs.)

Each tablet:
  Norgestrel .... 0.30 mg.
  Ethinyl estradiol .... 0.03 mg.

LO RANGE (Phosphate Formula or 0-Phosphate Formula)
Institutional and industrial cleaning product

Procter & Gamble Co.
Ivorydale Technical Center
Cincinnati, Ohio 45217

Phone: 513-562-1100

L'OREAL OF PARIS HAIR PREPARATIONS & COSMETICS
(Cosmair)

Cosmair, Inc.
530 Fifth Ave.
New York, N.Y. 10036

Phone: 212-840-3900

See COSMETICS, Section VI, General Formulations

LORENZ TOXAPHENE 60% CONC.
Insecticide
(Lorenz)

Toxaphene *
Kerosene
Emulsifier

LOROXIDE LOTION (Flesh tinted)
Treatment of severe acne vulgaris
(Dermik)

Benzoyl peroxide .... 5.5% w/v
Chlorhydroxyquinoline ...... 0.25% w/v
In a greaseless vehicle

"LOROX" L WEED KILLER
(Du Pont)

Linuron * 41%

"LOROX" WEED KILLER
(Du Pont)

Linuron * 50%

LORSBAN 4E INSECTICIDE
(Dow)

Active ingred.:
Chlorpyrifos (O,O-Diethyl O-(3,5,6-trichloro-2-pyridyl)phosphorothioate) * ... 41.2%
Xylene * 29.5%
Inert ingred.: 29.3%
Emulsifiers
Chlorinated solvent *

LORSBAN XYLENE INSECTICIDAL MIXTURE
(Dow)

Active ingred.:
  Chlorpyrifos (O,O-Diethyl O-(3,-5,6-trichloro-2-pyridyl)phosphorothioate) * ... 65%
Inert ingred.:
  Xylene * 35%

LORTAB
Analgesic
(Russ Pharm.)

Each tablet:
  Acetaminophen * .... 325.000 mg.
  Promethazine HCl .... 3.125 mg.
  Hydrocodone bitartrate .. 2.500 mg.

LORTAB 7
(Russ Pharm.)

Each tablet:
  Hydrocodone bitartrate ...... 7 mg.
  Acetaminophen * .... 500 mg.

LOSAPAN
Laxative
(Leo Products)

Active ingred.:
  Frangula bark
  Chelidonium
Also contains:
  Boldo leaves
  Agrimony
  Peppermint leaves
  Carduus benedictus
  Centaury hypericum
  Hedera leaves

LO-SHUN
Commercial laundry softener
(Diversey Wyandotte)

Quaternary ammonium compound *

LO-TOX SPRAY
Insecticide; commercial and industrial use
(Schneid)

Petroleum distillate * 99.37%
N-Octyl bicycloheptene
  dicarboximide 0.33%
Technical Piperonyl butoxide ... 0.20%
Pyrethrins 0.10%

'76 Ed.

LOTRIMIN CREAM 1%
Dermatologic use; antifungal
(Schering/Delbay)

Clotrimazole .... 10 mg.
Base:
  Sorbitan monostearate
  Polysorbate 60
  Cetyl esters wax
  Cetostearyl alcohol
  2-Octyldodecanol
  Purified water
  Benzyl alcohol 1%

LOTRIMIN SOLUTION 1%
Dermatologic use; antifungal
(Schering/Delbay)

Clotrimazole .... 10 mg.
Nonaqueous vehicle:
  Polyethylene glycol 400

LOTSHAW BODY RUB
(Lotshaw)

Glycerin
Olive oil
Lanolin
Hexachlorophene
Menthol *
Carbamide
Oxyquinoline sulfate *
Homogeneous cream base

'76 Ed.

LOTSHAW HAIR DRESS FOR MEN
(Lotshaw)

Lanolin
Mineral oil
Stearic acid composition
Perfume

'76 Ed.

LOTSHAW PELLENT
Repellent
(Lotshaw)

N,N-Diethyl-metatoluamide * . 15%/wt.

'76 Ed.

LOTUSATE CAPLETS
Hypnotic
(Winthrop Labs.)

Each Caplet:
   Talbutal (5-Allyl-5-sec.-butyl-
     barbituric acid) * .... 120 mg.

LO-TUSSIN
(Direct Div.)

Each 5 ml.:
   Codeine phosphate (USP) * ..... 10 mg.
   Pseudoephedrine HCl * ..... 30 mg.
   Guaifenesin .... 100 mg.

Free from Sugar, Alcohol, Tartrazine

LOUANGEL TOILETRIES

Louangel Corp.
70 Franklin Ave.
Brooklyn, N.Y. 11205

Phone: 212-625-0114

See COSMETICS, Section VI, General
   Formulations

LOUSE X
Insecticide
(Techne Corp.)

Ronnel (O,O-Dimethyl O-2,4,5-tri-
   chlorophenyl phosphorothioate) .. 5%

'76 Ed.

LOVE-LONGER
Desensitizing lubricant
(Youngs Drug Products)

Benzocaine 7.5%
Polyethylene glycol 400
Carbomer 940
Fragrance
Water
Sodium hydroxide (5% solution to adjust
   pH)

LOVE-MY-CARPET RUG AND ROOM DEODORIZER (Regular, Floral, and Citrus Fresh)
(Lehn & Fink)

Sodium sulfate (anhydrous) 68.5%
Sodium bicarbonate (USP) 26.0%
Hydrated Sodium aluminosilicate   minor
Dipropylene glycol .... minor
Fragrance .... minor

LO-VOL 4D
Herbicide
(Diamond Shamrock Corp.)

Isooctyl ester of 2,4-dichlorophen-
   oxyacetic acid * 66.8%

LO-VOL 6D
Herbicide
(Diamond Shamrock Corp.)

Isooctyl ester of 2,4-dichlorophen-
   oxyacetic acid * 87.3%

LOWILA CAKE
Soap-free, nonirritant efficient skin cleanser
(Westwood Pharm.)

Sodium lauryl sulfoacetate
Corn dextrin base

'76 Ed.

LOW TEMPERATURE DETERGENT F101
Commercial laundry detergent
(Diversey Wyandotte)

Sodium metasilicate *
Alkaline salts *

LOW TEMPERATURE LIQUID DETERGENT L101
Commercial laundry detergent
(Diversey Wyandotte)

Sodium hydroxide *
Synthetic detergents

L.S.C.
Lubricant, rust preventative
(Radiator)

Petroleum distillates *

'76 Ed.

L-S-D LOW SUDSING DETERGENT
(National Chemicals, Inc.)

Modified Polyethoxylated straight chain
   alcohol
Anionic phosphate ester (hydrotropes) *
Hydroxyacetic acid
Tetrapotassium pyrophosphate

L-7 LOOSENER & LUBRICANT (Aerosol)
(American Grease Stick)

Combined amount: 97.7%
   Petroleum distillate *
   2-Butyl alcohol
   Glycerol mono-oleate
   1,1,1-Trichloroethane *
Carbon dioxide 2.3%

LSR
For removal of scale from equipment
(DuBois Chem.)

Phosphoric acid *
Glycolic acid
Muriatic acid *
Nonionic surfactants

LTS LOTION SOAP
For industrial use
(Calgon Corp., Commercial Div.)

Soap
Triclosan
Water

LUB-A-CABLE

See BALKAMP LUB-A-CABLE

LUBAFAX
Surgical lubricant
(Burroughs Wellcome)

Methylparaben 0.07%
Propylparaben 0.03%

LUB-A-GRAPH

See BALKAMP LUB-A-GRAPH

LUBATH
Bath oil
(Warner-Lambert)

Mineral oil
PPG-15 stearylether
Oleth-2
Nonoxynol-5
Fragrance
D & C Green #6

LUBRIDERM CREAM
Extreme dry skin moisturizer
(Warner-Lambert)

Water
Mineral oil
Petrolatum
Glycerin
Glyceryl stearate
PEG-100 stearate
Squalane
Lanolin
Lanolin alcohol
Lanolin oil
Cetyl alcohol
Sorbitan laurate
Fragrance (for scented formula only)
Methylparaben
Butylparaben
Propylparaben
Quaternium-15

LUBRIDERM LOTION
Dry skin moisturizer
(Warner-Lambert)

Water
Mineral oil
Petrolatum
Sorbitol
Lanolin
Lanolin alcohol
Stearic acid
Triethanolamine
Cetyl alcohol
Fragrance (scented formula only)
Butylparaben
Methylparaben
Propylparaben
Sodium chloride

Starred ingredients (*) may be responsible for major toxic effects; consult Section II.

LUCILLE BOUCHARD COSMETICS
(Lucille Bouchard)

Lucille Bouchard Mink Oil
　Cosmetiques, Inc.
P.O. Box 46
Circleville, N.Y. 10919

Phone: 914-692-2777

See COSMETICS, Section VI, General
　Formulations

LUCKY HEART COSMETIC PRODUCTS

Lucky Heart Cosmetics
390 Mulberry
Memphis, Tenn. 38101

Phone: 901-526-7658

See COSMETICS, Section VI, General
　Formulations

LUCKY TIGER DANDRUFF TREATMENT
(York, L.T.)

Alcohol-water solution
Oxyquinoline phosphate *
Sodium salicylate *

LUCKY TIGER HAIR TONIC
(York, L.T.)

Alcohol-water solution
Oxyquinoline phosphate *
Sodium salicylate *
Ucon (by-product of petroleum cracking)

LUCKY TIGER OINTMENT
Fungicide, antiseptic agent
(York, L.T.)

Sulfur base
Oxyquinoline phosphate *

LUCKY TIGER SPECIAL FORMULA WITHOUT OIL
Health aid
(York, L.T.)

Alcohol 50%
Sodium salicylate *
Oxyquinoline phosphate *

LUCKY TIGER 3 PURPOSE HAIR TONIC
Health aid
(York, L.T.)

Alcohol 55%
Sodium salicylate *
Oxyquinoline phosphate *

LUDENE
Bowl cleaner & disinfectant (concentrated)
(Hysan Corp.)

Hydrogen chloride * 23.70%
Heptadecyl hydroxyethylimidazo-
　linium chloride 0.10%
Inert ingredients: 76.20%
　Detergents
　Emulsifiers
　Acrylic copolymers
　Inhibitors

LU LU LOTION
Acne remedy
(Sheraton Labs.)

Water
Ethanol (190 proof)
Zinc oxide (USP)
Sodium borate (USP) *
Acetone (NF) *
Zinc sulfate (USP) *
Sulfur (precipitated USP)
Magnesium aluminum silicate
Camphor (USP) *

'76 Ed.

LUMBER LAST WOOD PRESERVATIVE #10
(Elco Mfg.)

Pentachlorophenol * 5%
Petroleum distillate *

LUMINAL OVOIDS
Sedative, antispasmodic, hypnotic
(Winthrop Labs.)

Luminal (Phenobarbital) *

　Each yellow tablet: .... 16 mg.
　Each light green tablet: .... 32 mg.

LUPERSOL DDM-9
Catalyst
(Lucidol Div.)

Methyl ethyl ketone peroxide (as
　a mixture of $C_4H_{10}O_4$ and
　$C_8H_{18}O_6$) * 40%
Oxygen (active) .... 9% max.

LURIDE DROPS
Fluoride supplement
(Hoyt Labs.)

Each drop:
　Fluoride ion (from 0.275 mg.
　　sodium fluoride) * .... 0.125 mg.

LURIDE LOZI-TABS
Fluoride supplement
(Hoyt Labs.)

Each full-strength tablet:
　Fluoride (from 2.2 mg. sodium
　　fluoride) .... 1.0 mg.

Each half-strength tablet:
　Fluoride (from 1.1 mg. sodium
　　fluoride) .... 0.5 mg.

Each quarter-strength tablet:
　Fluoride (from 0.55 mg. sodium
　　fluoride) .... 0.25 mg.

LURIDE PROPHYLAXIS PASTE
To clean, polish, and apply fluoride to the teeth
(Hoyt Labs.)

Fluoride (from ammonium silico-
　fluoride in an M/10 phosphoric
　acid solution equivalent to 1.2%
　fluoride) 0.4%
Silicon dioxide

LURIDE-SF (Special Formula) LOZI-TABS
Fluoride supplement
(Hoyt Labs.)

Each tablet:
　Fluoride (from 2.2 mg. sodium
　　fluoride) .... 1.0 mg.

No artificial color or flavor

LURIDE TOPICAL GEL OR SOLUTION
(Hoyt Labs.)

Fluoride (from sodium fluoride and
　hydrogen fluoride) * 1.2%
M/10 Phosphoric acid solution or gel (pH
　3-4)

LURON (With Lanolin)
Powdered hand soap
(U. S. Borax)

Toilet soap
Borax *
Lanolin
Perfume

LUST-O-WITE
Porcelain bowl cleaner
(Hillyard Chem.)

Sodium bisulfate *

'76 Ed.

LUSTRA BOWL
Bowl cleaner
(National Chemsearch)

Hydrochloric acid *
Citric acid
Nonyl phenol ethylene oxide condensate
Dehydroabietylamine ethylene oxide condensate
Methyldodecylbenzyltrimethyl ammonium chloride *
Methyldodecylxylene bis(trimethyl ammonium chloride) *†

†*See* Cationic surfactants

LUSTRASILK COSMETIC PRODUCTS

Lustrasilk Corp.
P.O. Box 334
Minneapolis, Minn. 55440

Phone: 612-425-1377

See COSMETICS, Section VI, General Formulations

LUSTRE CREME LIQUID SHAMPOO
(Colgate-Palmolive)

Triethanolammonium lauryl sulfate *
Fatty-acid diethanolamine condensate
Methylcellulose gum
Sodium chloride
Water and Alcohol
Perfume, color and preservative

'76 Ed.

LUSTRE CREME LOTION SHAMPOO
(Colgate-Palmolive)

Sodium lauryl sulfate * ..... about 20%
Isostearic acid
Glycol stearates
Fatty-acid diethanolamine condensate
Lanolin
Sodium chloride
Citric acid
Perfume, color and preservative

'76 Ed.

LUSTRE GLEEM SUPER GLOSS
Non-wax wax finish for resilient floors
(American-Lincoln)

Emulsified Acrylic resins -
nonvolatile 14%

LUSTRE-GLOSS
Self polishing wax
(Hillyard Chem.)

Water wax emulsion

'76 Ed.

LUVABLE
Floor finish
(Paul Koss)

Water .... >80%
Emulsion of oligomers and polymers, primarily acrylic
Emulsion of Polyethylene
Fluorochemical surfactant .... trace
Formalin .... trace

pH 7.7-8.0

LUX BEAUTY BAR SOAP
(Lever Bros.)

Sodium soap 80-90%
Water 10-15%
Perfume 1-5%
Sodium chloride .... <1%
Glycerol .... <1%
Sodium carbonate or phosphate . <1%
Titanium dioxide .... <1%
Sodium sulfate .... <1%
Sodium EDTA .... trace
Antioxidant .... trace
Colorants .... trace
Sodium EHDP .... nil to trace

LUX LIQUID
Liquid dishwashing detergent
(Lever Bros.)

Water 50-60%
Anionic detergents 30-40%
Fatty alkanolamides 1-5%
Ethanol .... <1%
Opacifier .... <1%
Perfume .... <1%
Colorant .... trace

LUXURY BUBBLES
(House of Lowell, Inc.)

TEA-lauryl sulfate *
Lauramide DEA
Perfume *
Formaldehyde
D & C color

LUXURY SHAVING TABLET
(Williams, J.B.)

Sodium and potassium soap

LUZIER COSMETICS

Luzier, Inc.
P.O. Box 496
Kansas City, Mo. 64141

Phone: 816-531-8338

See COSMETICS, Section VI, General Formulations

LYDIA E. PINKHAM TABLETS
(CooperVision Pharm.)

Iron *† 24%
Extract of: 40%
 Pleurisy root
 Jamaica dogwood
 Licorice

†*See* Iron salts

LYDIA E. PINKHAM VEGETABLE COMPOUND
Uterine sedative
(CooperVision Pharm.)

Extract of:
 Jamaica dogwood
 Pleurisy root
 Black cohosh
 Life root
 Licorice
 Dandelion
 Gentian
 Alcohol 13%

LYDIA O'LEARY COSMETIC PRODUCTS

Lydia O'Leary, Inc.
575 Madison Ave.
New York, N.Y. 10022

Phone: 212-753-4600

See COSMETICS, Section VI, General Formulations

LYNSOL
Shellac thinner, stove fuel, printing press cleaner
(Sterling-Clark-Lurton)

Methanol .... <4%
Ethyl alcohol (190 Proof) * approx. 93%
Ketones & esters .... approx. 3%
Hydrocarbon .... <1%

LYON DENATURED ALCOHOL SOLVENT
(Van Waters & Rogers)

Methyl (wood) alcohol 5%

LYON'S, DR., TOOTH POWDER (REGULAR)

See DR. LYON'S TOOTH POWDER (REGULAR)

LYSOFF POUR-ON FOR LICE
For beef and dairy cattle
(Cutter (Brand) Bayvet Div. Cutter Labs.)

Fenthion 7.6%
Petroleum distillate 56.7%
Xylene * 20.0%

LYSOL BRAND AEROSOL DEODORIZING CLEANER
(Lehn & Fink)

Tetrapotassium pyrophosphate	minor
Diethylene glycol monobutyl ether	minor
Ethyl alcohol	minor
Isobutane	minor
o-Phenylphenol	minor

LYSOL BRAND BASIN, TUB, TILE CLEANER
(Lehn & Fink)

Active ingredients:
Tetrasodium ethylenediamine tetraacetate	1.52%
Sodium metasilicate anhydrous	0.06%
Alkyl (67% C12, 25% C14, 7% C16, 1% C8-C10-C18) dimethyl benzyl ammonium chlorides	0.08%
Alkyl (50% C14, 40% C12, 10% C16) dimethyl benzyl ammonium chlorides	0.02%
Inert ingredients:	98.32%

Includes detergents and other grease-cutting agents

LYSOL BRAND BATHROOM CLEANER
(Lehn & Fink)

Sodium metasilicate	minor
Ethylene glycol monobutyl ether	minor
Tetrasodium ethylenediaminetetraacetate	minor
Alkyl (C14 50%, C12 40%, C16 10%) dimethyl benzyl ammonium chloride	minor

LYSOL BRAND DEODORIZING CLEANER
(Lehn & Fink)

Active ingredients:
Soap	5.5%
o-Benzyl-p-chlorophenol	3.2%
Isopropanol	1.1%
Inert ingredients:	90.2%

Includes detergents, certified colors and other grease-cutting agents

LYSOL BRAND DEODORIZING CLEANER II
(Lehn & Fink)

Quaternary ammonium compounds	2.70%
Tetrasodium ethylenediaminetetraacetate	1.00%
Ethyl alcohol	0.34%

LYSOL BRAND DISINFECTANT - PINE SCENT
(Lehn & Fink)

Soap	16.5%
Pine oil	5.0%
o-Benzyl-p-chlorophenol	4.5%
Isopropyl alcohol	1.5%
Tetrasodium ethylenediamine tetraacetate	0.9%

LYSOL BRAND DISINFECTANT - REGULAR
(Lehn & Fink)

Soap	16.5%
o-Phenylphenol	2.8%
o-Benzyl-p-chlorophenol	2.7%
Alcohol	1.8%
Xylenols	1.5%
Isopropyl alcohol	0.9%
Tetrasodium ethylenediamine tetraacetate	0.9%

LYSOL BRAND DISINFECTANT SPRAY, SCENT II
(Lehn & Fink)

Ethyl alcohol *	79.6%
Carbon dioxide	minor
o-Phenylphenol	minor
N-Alkyl (C18 92%, C16 8%) N-ethyl morpholinium ethyl sulfates	minor

LYSOL BRAND LIQUID DISINFECTANT TOILET BOWL CLEANER
(Lehn & Fink)

Hydrogen chloride *	8.50%
Alkyl (67% C12, 25% C14, 7% C16, 1% C8-C10-C18) dimethyl benzyl ammonium chlorides	1.00%

LYSOL BRAND PINE ACTION
Cleans, disinfects, deodorizes
(Lehn & Fink)

Pine oil *	15.0%
Isopropyl alcohol	11.7%
o-Phenylphenol	0.78%

Includes cleaning agents, color and water

LYSOL BRAND SPRAY DISINFECTANT
(Lehn & Fink)

o-Phenylphenol	0.1%
N-Alkyl (C18 92%; C16 8%)-N-ethyl morpholinium ethylsulfates	0.035%
Alcohol *	67.748%

LYSTADS CONCENTRATED AEROSOL INSECT KILLER
(Lystads)

Pyrethrins I & II *	1.0%
Technical Piperonyl butoxide	2.0%
N-Octyl bicycloheptene dicarboximide	3.34%
Petroleum hydrocarbon	13.66%

LYSTADS ENTROL
(Lystads)

Petroleum distillate *
N-Octyl bicycloheptene dicarboximide *
Technical Piperonyl butoxide
Pyrethrins *

LYSTADS FLY SPRAY FOR CATTLE & FOGGING
Insecticide
(Lystads)

2,2-Dichlorovinyl dimethyl phosphate	0.93%
Related compounds	0.07%
Petroleum hydrocarbons *	99.00%

LYSTADS RAT & MOUSE KILLER
Rodenticide
(Lystads)

Fumarin (3-(a-Acetonylfurfuryl)-4-hydroxycoumarin)	0.025%

LYSTADS RAT & MOUSE KILLER WATER SOLUBLE
Rodenticide
(Lystads)

3-(a-Acetonylfurfuryl)-4-hydroxy-coumarin, sodium salt	0.14%

LYSTADS SUGAR BAIT FOR FLIES
Insecticide
(Lystads)

2,2-Dichlorovinyl dimethyl phosphate	0.093%
Related compounds	0.007%
Ronnel *	0.250%

LYTEERS
Simulates natural tears
(Barnes-Hind)

Sodium chloride	0.65%
Potassium chloride	0.15%
Cellulosic derivative	0.25%
Benzalkonium chloride	0.01%
Edetate disodium	0.05%

M

MAALOX NO. 1 TABLETS
Antacid
(Rorer, W.H., Inc.)

Each tablet:
Magnesium-aluminum hydroxides	0.4 gm.

MAALOX NO. 2 TABLETS
Antacid
(Rorer, W.H., Inc.)

Each tablet:
Magnesium-aluminum hydroxides	0.8 gm.

Starred ingredients (*) may be responsible for major toxic effects; consult Section II.

MAALOX PLUS
Antacid/antiflatulent
(Rorer, W.H., Inc.)

Tablets (each):
Magnesium hydroxide .... 200 mg.
Aluminum hydroxide .... 200 mg.
Simethicone .... 25 mg.

Suspension (each 5 ml.):
Magnesium hydroxide .... 200 mg.
Aluminum hydroxide .... 225 mg.
Simethicone .... 25 mg.

MAALOX SUSPENSION
Antacid
(Rorer, W.H., Inc.)

Each 12 fl. oz.:
Magnesium-aluminum
hydroxides .... 355 ml.

MAAS & WALDSTEIN PAINT PRODUCTS
Lacquers & enamels

Maas & Waldstein Co.
2121 McCarter Hwy.
Newark, N.J. 07104

Phone: 201-484-1600

See PAINTS, Section VI, General Formulations

MACE
Liquid formulation contained in Chemical Mace
(Smith & Wesson/General Ordnance)

2-Chloroacetophenone (Phenylchloromethyl ketone) * .. 0.9% w/w
Inert carriers

MACHINE WASH WOOLITE
Laundry detergent for fine washables
(Boyle-Midway)

Anionic surface active agent *
Builders

MACKLANBURG-DUNCAN ACRYLIC LATEX CAULK
(Macklanburg-Duncan)

Calcium carbonate (Ground
limestone) .... <60.0%
Acrylic latex rubber emulsion
(55% solids in water) .... <35.0%
Butyl-benzyl phthalate .... <10.0%
Mineral spirits (mixture of aliphatic hydrocarbons with BP
300°–360°) .... <3.0%
Water .... <3.0%
Titanium dioxide pigment ..... <3.0%
Dispersant (Sodium and zinc
hexametaphosphate) .... <1.0%
Nonionic surfactant (Alkylaryl
polyether alcohol) .... <1.0%
Ethylene glycol (1,2-Ethanediol) <1.0%
Pigment dispersant, Tamol 850 <0.2%
Glycidoxy-propyltrimethoxy
silane .... <0.1%
Ammonium hydroxide 26°Be' . <0.5%

MACKLANBURG-DUNCAN ARCHITECTURAL GRADE ALUMINUM
(Macklanburg-Duncan)

Calcium carbonate .... <80.00%
Soybean oil (mixed triglyceride
oils) .... <13.00%
Polybutene .... <7.00%
Mineral spirits (mixture of aliphatic hydrocarbons) ...... <6.00%
Aluminum paste (metal leaflets) <0.30%
Vegetable acids (oleic and
linoleic) .... <1.00%
Processed mineral fibers (Calcium alumino silicates) ..... <1.00%
Cobalt naphthenate (12% metal) <0.05%
Manganese drier (12% metal) .. <0.05%

MACKLANBURG-DUNCAN ARCHITECTURAL WHITE AND WHITE SPEEDLOAD
(Macklanburg-Duncan)

Calcium carbonate .... <80.0%
Soybean oil (mixed triglyceride
oils) .... <15.0%
Polybutene .... <10.0%
Processed mineral fibers (Calcium alumino silicates) ...... <1.0%
Cobalt naphthenate * .... <0.5%
Manganese .... <0.5%
Mineral spirits .... <5.0%
Titanium dioxide .... <1.0%
Phthalocyanine blue pigment . <0.1%
Vegetable acids, Soya (primarily
linoleic) .... <1.0%

MACKLANBURG-DUNCAN BEIGE LATEX CAULKING
(Macklanburg-Duncan)

Calcium carbonate (Ground
limestone) .... <60.0%
Acrylic latex rubber emulsion
(55% solids in water) .... <35.0%
Butyl-benzyl phthalate .... <10.0%
Mineral spirits (mixture of aliphatic hydrocarbons with BP
300°–360°F) .... <3.0%
Water .... <3.0%
Burnt umber pigment (nonionic
dispersed iron oxide) .... <0.1%
Dispersant (Sodium and zinc
hexametaphosphate) .... <1.0%
Nonionic surfactant (Alkylaryl
polyalcohol) .... <1.0%
Ethylene glycol (1,2-Ethanediol) <1.0%
Pigment dispersant (Tamol 850) <0.2%
Glycidoxy-propyltrimethoxy
silane .... <0.1%
Ammonium hydroxide 26°Be' . <0.5%

MACKLANBURG-DUNCAN BLACK LATEX
(Macklanburg-Duncan)

Calcium carbonate .... <60.0%
Acrylic latex rubber emulsion .. <35.0%
Butyl-benzyl phthalate .... <10.0%
Mineral spirits (mixture of aliphatic hydrocarbons) ...... <3.0%
Tinting black (nonionic dispersed carbon black) .... <2.0%
Sodium & zinc
hexametaphosphate .... <1.0%
Nonionic surfactant (Alkylaryl
polyether alcohol) .... <1.0%
Ethylene glycol (1,2-Ethanediol) <1.0%
Glycidoxy propyltrimethoxy
silane .... <1.0%
Ammonium hydroxide 26°Be' <0.5%
Pigment dispersant (Tamol 850) <0.2%

MACKLANBURG-DUNCAN BRONZE ACRYLIC LATEX
(Macklanburg-Duncan)

Calcium carbonate .... <60.0%
Acrylic latex rubber emulsion .. <35.0%
Butyl-benzyl phthalate .... <10.0%
Mineral spirits (mixture of aliphatic hydrocarbons) ...... <3.0%
Burnt umber (nonionic dispersed iron oxide) .... <0.5%
Tinting black (nonionic dispersed carbon black) .... <1.0%
Sodium & zinc
hexametaphosphate .... <1.0%
Nonionic surfactant (Alkylaryl
polyether alcohol) .... <1.0%
Ethylene glycol (1,2-Ethanediol) <1.0%
Glycidoxy propyltrimethoxy
silane .... <0.1%
Ammonium hydroxide 26°Be' <0.5%
Tamol 850 .... <0.2%

MACKLANBURG-DUNCAN BROWN ACRYLIC LATEX CAULKING
(Macklanburg-Duncan)

Calcium carbonate (Ground
limestone) .... <60.0%
Acrylic latex rubber emulsion
(55% solids in water) .... <35.0%
Butyl-benzyl phthalate .... <10.0%
Mineral spirits (mixture of aliphatic hydrocarbons with BP
300°–360°F) .... <3.0%
Burnt umber pigment (nonionic
dispersed iron oxide) .... <1.0%
Black pigment (nonionic dispersed carbon black) .... <0.2%
Dispersant (Sodium and zinc
hexametaphosphate) .... <1.0%
Nonionic surfactant (Alkylaryl
polyether alcohol) .... <1.0%
Ethylene glycol (1,2-Ethanediol) <1.0%
Pigment dispersant (Tamol 850) <0.2%
Glycidoxy-propyltrimethoxy
silane .... <0.1%
Ammonium hydroxide 26°Be' <0.5%

Starred ingredients (*) may be responsible for major toxic effects; consult Section II.

MACKLANBURG-DUNCAN CEDAR TAN ACRYLIC LATEX
(Macklanburg-Duncan)

Calcium carbonate	<60.0%
Acrylic latex rubber emulsion	<35.0%
Butyl-benzyl phthalate	<10.0%
Mineral spirits (mixture of aliphatic hydrocarbons)	<3.0%
Burnt umber (nonionic dispersed iron oxide)	<5.0%
Sodium & zinc hexametaphosphate	<1.0%
Nonionic surfactant (Alkylaryl polyether alcohol)	<1.0%
Ethylene glycol (1,2-Ethanediol)	<1.0%
Tamol 850	<0.2%
Glycidoxy propyltrimethoxy silane	<0.1%
Ammonium hydroxide 26°Be'	<0.5%

MACKLANBURG-DUNCAN GRAY ACRYLIC LATEX
(Macklanburg-Duncan)

Calcium carbonate	<60.00%
Acrylic latex rubber emulsion	<35.00%
Butyl-benzyl phthalate	<10.00%
Mineral spirits (mixture of aliphatic hydrocarbons)	<3.00%
Phthalocyanine blue pigment	<0.01%
Tinting black (nonionic dispersed carbon black)	<0.01%
Nonionic surfactant (Alkylaryl polyether alcohol)	<1.00%
Ethylene glycol (1,2-Ethanediol)	<1.00%
Tamol 850	<0.20%
Glycidoxy propyltrimethoxy silane	<0.10%
Ammonium hydroxide 26°Be'	<0.50%
Sodium & zinc hexametaphosphate	<1.00%

MACKLANBURG-DUNCAN MORTAR PATCH
(Macklanburg-Duncan)

Calcium carbonate	<60.00%
Acrylic latex rubber emulsion	<35.00%
Butyl-benzyl phthalate	<10.00%
Mineral spirits (mixture of aliphatic hydrocarbons)	<3.00%
Burnt umber (nonionic dispersed iron oxide)	<0.10%
Tinting black (nonionic dispersed carbon black)	<0.01%
Sodium & zinc hexametaphosphate	<1.00%
Nonionic surfactant (Alkylaryl polyether alcohol)	<1.00%
Ethylene glycol (1,2-Ethanediol)	<1.00%
Glycidoxy propyltrimethoxy silane	<0.10%
Ammonium hydroxide 26°Be'	<0.50%
Tamol 850	<0.20%

MACKLANBURG-DUNCAN OLIVE GREEN ACRYLIC LATEX
(Macklanburg-Duncan)

Calcium carbonate	<60.0%
Acrylic latex rubber emulsion	<35.0%
Butyl-benzyl phthalate	<10.0%
Mineral spirits (mixture of aliphatic hydrocarbons)	<3.0%
Burnt umber (nonionic dispersed iron oxide)	<0.5%
Phthalocyanine green pigment	<0.1%
Sodium & zinc hexametaphosphate	<1.0%
Nonionic surfactant (Alkylaryl polyether alcohol)	<1.0%
Ethylene glycol (1,2-Ethanediol)	<1.0%
Glycidoxy propyltrimethoxy silane	<0.1%
Ammonium hydroxide 26°Be'	<0.5%
Tamol 850	<0.2%

MACKLANBURG-DUNCAN REDWOOD ACRYLIC LATEX CAULK
(Macklanburg-Duncan)

Calcium carbonate (Ground limestone)	<60.0%
Acrylic latex rubber emulsion (55% solids in water)	<35.0%
Butyl-benzyl phthalate	<10.0%
Mineral spirits (mixture of aliphatic hydrocarbons with BP 300°–360°F)	<3.0%
Water	
Red iron oxide pigment (nonionic dispersed)	<3.0%
Burnt umber pigment (nonionic dispersed)	<2.0%
Dispersant (Sodium and zinc hexametaphosphate)	<1.0%
Nonionic surfactant (Alkylaryl polyalcohol)	<1.0%
Ethylene glycol (1,2-Ethanediol)	<1.0%
Pigment dispersant (Tamol 850)	<0.2%
Glycidoxy-propyltrimethoxy silane	<0.1%
Ammonium hydroxide 26°Be'	<0.5%

MACKLANBURG-DUNCAN SPACKLING COMPOUND
(Macklanburg-Duncan)

Calcium carbonate	<75.00%
Water	<17.00%
Polyvinyl acetate emulsion (56% solids in water)	<13.00%
Mineral spirits (mixture of aliphatic hydrocarbons with BP 300°-360°F)	<3.00%
Ethylene glycol (1,2-Ethanediol)	<1.00%
Sodium carboxymethyl cellulose	<1.00%
Ammonium hydroxide 26°Be'	<0.05%
Alkylaryl polyalcohol nonionic surfactant	<0.25%
Bis-tributyl tin oxide	<0.30%

MACKLANBURG-DUNCAN TUB AND TILE CAULK
(Macklanburg-Duncan)

Calcium carbonate (Ground limestone)	<60.0%
Acrylic latex rubber emulsion (55% solids in water)	<35.0%
Butyl-benzyl phthalate	<10.0%
Mineral spirits (mixture of aliphatic hydrocarbons with BP 300°–360°F)	<6.0%
Water	<3.0%
Titanium dioxide pigment	<3.0%
Dispersant (Sodium and zinc hexametaphosphate)	<1.0%
Nonionic surfactant (Alkylaryl polyether alcohol)	<1.0%
Ethylene glycol (1,2-Ethanediol)	<1.0%
Bis-tributyltin oxide	<0.5%
Pigment dispersant (Tamol 850)	<0.2%
Glycidoxy-propyltrimethoxy silane	<0.1%
Ammonium hydroxide 26°Be'	<0.5%

MACKLANBURG-DUNCAN WHITE VINYL ADHESIVE CAULK
(Macklanburg-Duncan)

Polyvinyl acetate emulsion (56% solids in water)	<48.0%
Calcium carbonate	<48.0%
Butyl-benzyl phthalate	<8.0%
Normal-amyl acetate	<4.0%
Ethylene glycol (1,2-Ethanediol)	<2.0%
Trisodium phosphate dodecahydrate	<0.5%
Titanium dioxide	<0.5%
Sodium carboxymethylcellulose	<0.5%

MACKLANBURG-DUNCAN WHITE VINYL PAINTER'S LATEX SEALANT
(Macklanburg-Duncan)

Polyvinyl acetate emulsion	<48.0%
Calcium carbonate	<43.0%
Mineral spirits (mixture of aliphatic hydrocarbons BP 300°–360°F)	<7.0%
Butyl-benzyl phthalate	<7.0%
Ethylene glycol (1,2-Ethanediol)	<3.0%
Water	<1.0%
Nonionic surfactant (Alkylaryl polyether alcohol)	<1.0%
Trisodium phosphate dodecahydrate	<0.5%
Sodium carboxymethylcellulose	<0.5%

MACKWIN FOREST PINE DISINFECTANT
(Mackwin)

Pine oil *	20.0%
Soap	7.3%
Orthobenzyl para chloro phenol	3.0%
Inert ingredients:	
Water	64.7%
Hexylene glycol	5.0%

Starred ingredients (*) may be responsible for major toxic effects; consult Section II.

MAC-O-LAC PAINT PRODUCTS

Mac-O-Lac Paints Inc.
5400 E. Nevada
Detroit, Mich. 48234

Phone: 313-892-1900

See PAINTS, Section VI, General Formulations

MACRODANTIN CAPSULES
Urinary tract antibacterial
(Norwich-Eaton)

Each capsule:
  Macrodantin (brand of
    nitrofurantoin
    macrocrystals) * .... 25 mg.; 50 mg.;
                        or 100 mg.

MAGAN TABLETS
Analgesic
(Adria)

Each tablet:
  Magnesium salicylate (salicylate equivalent 500 mg.) * .. 545 mg.

MAGCYL
Relief of occasional constipation
(Elder)

Each capsule:
  Danthron .... 25.0 mg.
  Dioctyl sodium
    sulfosuccinate * .... 100.0 mg.

MAGDROX
Gastric antacid
(Vita Elixir Co.)

Suspension of:
  Magnesium hydroxide
  Aluminum hydroxide

MAGIC AFTER SHAVE CREAM #22
(Carson Products)

Water
Stearic acid
Propylene glycol
Cetyl alcohol
Sorbitan sesquioleate
Isopropyl myristate
Polysorbate 60
Mineral oil
Fragrance
Potassium stearate
Menthol
Methylparaben
Propylparaben
FD & C Yellow #5

MAGIC AFTER SHAVE SKIN CONDITIONER #24
(Carson Products)

Water
Propylene glycol
Dimethicone
Fragrance
Methylparaben
Allantoin
Carbomer-941
Triethanolamine
Menthol
Propylparaben
Cyclohexanediamine tetraacetic acid
FD & C Blue #1

MAGIC AMERICAN CLEANING PRODUCTS

Magic American Chemical Corp.
23700 Mercantile Rd.
Cleveland, Ohio 44122

Phone: 216-464-2353

MAGIC CIRCLE DEER REPELLENT
(State College Labs.)

Bone tar oil 93.75%
Surfactant 6.25%

MAGIC CIRCLE FOG SPRAY CONC.
Insecticide
(Ehrlich)

Pyrethrins 0.4%
Piperonyl butoxide 1.0%
Petroleum distillate * 98.6%

MAGIC CIRCLE HOUSEHOLD INSECT SPRAY
(Ehrlich)

o-Isopropoxyphenyl
  methylcarbamate * 1%
Petroleum distillate * 84%

MAGIC CIRCLE INSECT KILLER
(Ehrlich)

Diazinon 0.5%
Pyrethrins 0.052%
Piperonyl butoxide 0.261%
Petroleum distillate * 99.187%

MAGIC CIRCLE MILL INSECTICIDE
(Ehrlich)

Pyrethrins 0.12%
Piperonyl butoxide 0.60%
2,2-Dichlorovinyl dimethyl
  phosphate 0.46%
Related compounds 0.04%
Petroleum hydrocarbons * 98.78%

MAGIC CIRCLE RABBIT REPELLENT
(Ehrlich)

Thiram * 20%

MAGIC CIRCLE RAT & MOUSE KILLER
(Ehrlich)

Warfarin 0.025%

MAGIC CIRCLE ROACH & ANT KILLER #2
(Ehrlich)

Pyrethrins 0.052%
Piperonyl butoxide 0.260%
Chlorpyrifos 0.500%
Petroleum distillate * 98.736%

MAGIC EXTRA CRISP SIZING AEROSOL
(Armour-Dial, Inc.)

Water 75-100%
Propellant 5-10%
Starch 1-5%
Sodium borate 1-5%
Minor ingredients (total) 1-5%

MAGIC FILM AND SCUM REMOVER
(Paul Koss)

Water .... >70%
Tetrapotassium pyrophosphate
Tetrasodium EDTA
Benzalkonium chloride * 2%
Coco amido betaine

pH 10.7-10.9

MAGIC GLOSS
Waxless floor treatment
(Adco)

Polyethylene wax
Alkali soluble resin
Co-polymer of acrylic and styrene

MAGIC HOUSEHOLD BLEACH
Bleach, disinfectant, deodorant
(Purex Corp.)

Sodium hypochlorite * 5 1/4%
Sodium chloride .... <5%
Water .... Balance

MAGICLEAN
Cleaner, sanitizer
(Lester Labs.)

Detergents
Quaternary ammonium compounds *

'76 Ed.

MAGIC MARKER INK, PERMANENT
(Magic Marker Corp.)

Solids: 15%
   Consisting of nontoxic synthetic resins
   and aniline dyestuff combination
Solvents: 85%
   Aromatic hydrocarbon (of medium boiling point range; contains no benzene,
   carbon tetrachloride, toluene or fusel
   oil) *

MAGIC MARKER, OVERHEAD PROJECTION INK (OPI)
(Magic Marker Corp.)

Solids: 10%
   Non-toxic film-forming resins
   Aniline dyestuffs *
Solvents: 90%
   Water
   Ethanol

MAGIC MARKER, PERMANENT, ODORLESS
(Magic Marker Corp.)

Solids: 15%
   Non-toxic synthetic resins & aniline
   dyestuff combination *†
Solvents: 85%
   Ethanol *
   Glycol ethers *

†See Aniline

MAGIC MARKER, WATER COLOR
(Magic Marker Corp.)

Solids: 8%
   Acid dyes
Solvents: 92%
   Water
   Glycol

MAGIC MIST AIR SANITIZER

See HUNTER'S MAGIC MIST AIR
   SANITIZER

MAGIC MIST FLYING INSECT KILLER

See HUNTER'S MAGIC MIST
   FLYING INSECT KILLER

MAGICOLOR BRUSH & ROLLER CLEANER
(Magicolor)

Aliphatic hydrocarbons *

MAGICOLOR CLEAR CONCRETE & STONE SEALER
(Magicolor)

Petroleum distillates *
Esters *†

†See Solvents and Thinners, Section VI,
   General Formulations

MAGICOLOR EPOXY THINNER
(Magicolor)

Xylol *
Cellosolve

MAGICOLOR GLOSS REMOVER
Prepares surfaces for refinishing
(Magicolor)

Xylol *
Ethanol

MAGICOLOR PAINT THINNER
*For oil-base paints and varnish; cleans
   brushes and rollers*
(Magicolor)

Mineral spirits *
Cellosolve *

MAGICOLOR PAINT & VARNISH REMOVER
(Magicolor)

Methylene chloride *
Methanol *

MAGICOLOR WOOD SEALER
(Magicolor)

Ethyl cellulose 5.4%
Varnish solution † 15.4%
Xylol * 79.2%

† Varnish solution
   Non volatile: 42.5%
      Perta rosin ester
      Tricresyl phosphate
   Volatile: 57.5%
      Cellosolve

MAGIC PREWASH AEROSOL
(Armour-Dial, Inc.)

Water 50-75%
Petroleum distillate * 10-25%
Propellant 5-10%
Minor ingredients (total) 10-25%

MAGIC RAIN COLD WAVE, PIN-CURL, PORT, SAPPHIRE & SPECIAL LOTIONS
(Willat)

Ammonium thioglycerol 1-10%

MAGIC RAIN RUBY, CLEAR & OPAL LOTIONS
(Willat)

Ammonium thioglycolate 1-10%

MAGIC REMOVER

See CHOLDUN'S MAGIC REMOVER

MAGIC SHAVING POWDER
(Red Label and Blue Label)
(Carson Products)

Barium sulfide * . . . . <15%
Calcium hydroxide . . . . <15%
Fillers:
   Starch
   Calcium carbonate

MAGIC SPRAY SIZING AEROSOL
(Armour-Dial, Inc.)

Water 75-100%
Propellant 5-10%
Minor ingredients (total) 1-5%

MAGIC STARCH AEROSOL
(Armour-Dial, Inc.)

Water 75-100%
Propellant 5-10%
Starch 1-5%
Sodium borate 1-5%
Minor ingredients (total) 1-5%

MAGIKIL
Insecticide
(Lethelin)

o-Isopropoxyphenyl methylcarbamate
   (Baygon) * 1%

MAGIKIL ANT TRAP
(Lethelin)

Borax 5.4%

MAGIKIL JELLY
Insecticide
(Lethelin)

o-Isopropoxyphenyl methylcarbamate
   (Baygon) * 1%

MAGIKIL ROACH TRAP
(Lethelin)

Baygon *

Starred ingredients (*) may be responsible for major toxic effects; consult Section II.

MAGNACIDE H
Aquatic herbicide
(Magna Corp.)

Acrolein * 92%

MAGNA MIST VAPO FLUID
For colds, coughs, bronchitis
(Magna, Inc.)

Camphor * 7%
Menthol * 7%
Oil cedar leaf 3%
Isobornyl acetate 10%
Eucalyptus oil * 73%

'76 Ed.

MAGNOLIA CRAYONS
(Reliance Pen & Pencil)

Cellulose gum
Pigment colors (not dye)
Clay
Talc
Synthetic Petroleum waxes
Fatty acid esters
Fatty acid

MAGONATE TABS
Magnesium deficiency
(Fleming)

Each tablet:
Magnesium gluconate .... 500 mg.

MAHDEEN COSMETIC PRODUCTS

Mahdeen Laboratories
P.O. Box 1959
Fort Worth, Tex. 76101

Phone: 817-293-0450

See COSMETICS, Section VI, General
Formulations

MAIDEN LANE
Cold wave lotion
(Willat)

Ammonium thioglycolate 1-10%

MAJESTIC METAL CLEANER
(Majestic Wax Co.)

Hydrocarbons *† 63%
Water 37%

†*See* Aliphatic hydrocarbons

MAJESTIC PLASTIC CLEANER
(Majestic Wax Co.)

Hydrocarbons *† 64%
Water 36%

†*See* Aliphatic hydrocarbons

MAJESTIC STAINLESS STEEL POLISH
(Majestic Wax Co.)

Hydrocarbons *† 100%

†*See* Aliphatic hydrocarbons

MAJESTIC WHITE GLOVE FURNITURE POLISH
(Majestic Wax Co.)

Hydrocarbons *† 100%

†*See* Aliphatic hydrocarbons

MAJESTIC WHITE GLOVE GENERAL PURPOSE POLISH
(Majestic Wax Co.)

Hydrocarbons *† 100%

†*See* Aliphatic hydrocarbons

MAJIC-ADE
Tonic, carminative
(Humco)

Alcohol * 33%
Camphor *
Capsicum *
Menthol *
Alcohol
Peppermint
Black catechu
Ammonia, 28%
Methyl salicylate *

MAJOR ACCENT
Broad line water color markers
(Sanford Corp.)

Dyes
Glycols
Water
Phenol (as preservative) .... <1%

MAL
See HILLTOP MAL

MALACIDE GRAIN PROTECTANT NO. 2
Insecticide
(Techne Corp.)

Malathion * 57%
Xylol * 43%

'76 Ed.

MALACOAT
See MFA MALACOAT

MALAFOG
Insecticide
(Brulin)

beta-Butoxy beta'-thiocyano di-
ethyl ether * 1.6%
Malathion 2.5%
Petroleum hydrocarbons * 95.9%

MALA-SPRAY
See MFA MALA-SPRAY

MALATHION ULV CONCENTRATE
Insecticide
(Amer. Cyanamid, Agric. Div.)

O,O-Dimethyl phosphorodithioate of diethyl
mercaptosuccinate * 91.0%/w

MAL-A-TOX LIVESTOCK SPRAY & DIP
Insecticide
(Hess & Clark)

Toxaphene * 43.0%
Malathion 4.3%
Heavy Aromatic naphtha 42.7%

MALATOX-XL
Insecticide
(Dolge)

Petroleum distillates * 95-98%
Malathion 3-4%
Essential oils .... <0.2%

MALA-TROL, SPRAY-TROL BRAND
See SPRAY-TROL BRAND MALA-
TROL

MALGORA SPRAY
See DR. ROGERS' MALGORA
SPRAY

MALIBU MIST COLOGNE
See JAFRA MALIBU MIST CO-
LOGNE

MALLINCKRODT MERCURIAL OINTMENT
For use against crab lice
(Mallinckrodt, Inc.)

Mercury (Hg) * 9%

MAL-PHENE
See DR. ROGERS' MAL-PHENE

MALTER INTERNATIONAL MALATHION W.E.
Concentrated insecticide
(Malter International)

Malathion (O,O-Dimethyl dithiophosphate of diethyl mercaptosuccinate)	10.00%
Aromatic petroleum solvents (Xylene) *	84.80%

MAMMOL OINTMENT
Dressing for nipples of nursing mothers
(Abbott)

Bismuth subnitrate *	40%
Castor oil	30%
Lanolin, anhydrous	22%
Ceresin wax	7%
Balsam Peru	1%

MANALAX
Laxative
(Jenkins Labs.)

Each tablet:
Phenolphthalein	2 gr.
Atropine sulphate	1/500 gr.
Mannitol	
Sodium glycocholate	
Sodium taurocholate	
Extract of Cascara *	

MANDELAMINE GRANULES
Urinary tract antiseptic
(Parke-Davis)

Each packet:
Methenamine mandelate *	0.5 gm.; 1.0 gm.

MANDELAMINE SUSPENSION
Urinary tract antiseptic
(Parke-Davis)

Each 5 ml.:
Methenamine mandelate *	250 mg.

MANDELAMINE SUSPENSION FORTE
Urinary tract antiseptic
(Parke-Davis)

Each 5 ml.:
Methenamine mandelate *	500 mg.

MANDELAMINE TABLETS
Urinary tract antiseptic
(Parke-Davis)

Each tablet:
Methenamine mandelate *	0.5 gm.; 1.0 gm.

MANDEX
Urinary antiseptic
(Vale)

Each tablet:
Methenamine mandelate *	250 mg.
Salicylamide *	120 mg.
Belladonna extract	5 mg.

MANGEX
For mange in dogs
(Carson Chemicals, Inc.)

Benzyl benzoate *	30.0% w/w
Soap (anhydrous)	7.5% w/w

MANHATTAN CAVITY FLUID
Embalming supply
(Royal Bond)

Formaldehyde *
Methanol *

MANHATTAN FIRM ARTERIAL FLUID
Embalming supply
(Royal Bond)

Formaldehyde *	34%
Methanol *	

MANPOWER AEROSOL DEODORANT
(Armour-Dial, Inc.)

Propellant	50-75%
SD Alcohol - 40	25-50%
Antimicrobial active	0.1-1%
Minor ingredients (total)	1-5%

MANPOWER SOLID DEODORANT
(Armour-Dial, Inc.)

SD Alcohol-40	50-75%
Propylene glycol	10-25%
Water	10-25%
Sodium stearate	5-10%
Minor ingredients (total)	0.1-1%
Antimicrobial active	0-0.1%

MANTADIL CREAM
Antipruritic, anti-inflammatory, anesthetic
(Burroughs Wellcome)

Chlorcyclizine hydrochloride *	2%
Hydrocortisone acetate	0.5%
Inactive ingred.:	
Liquid petrolatum	
White petrolatum	
Emulsifying wax	
Purified water	
Methylparaben (preservative)	0.25%

"MANZATE" D FUNGICIDE
(With a zinc salt added)
(Du Pont)

Maneb *	80%

"MANZATE" FUNGICIDE
(Du Pont)

Maneb *	80%

"MANZATE" 200 FUNGICIDE
(Du Pont)

Coordination product of zinc ion and manganese ethylenebisdithiocarbamate *	80%

MAPO
Bath oil - for dry, flaky, itchy skin
(Herald Pharm.)

Mineral oil
Lanolin
Nonionic emulsifier *

MAPROFIX 563
Detergent, foaming
(Onyx)

Sodium lauryl sulfate *	99%

MAPROFIX TLS-65
Detergent, foaming
(Onyx)

Triethanolamine lauryl sulfate *	65%

MAPROFIX WA
Detergent, foaming
(Onyx)

Sodium lauryl sulfate *	30%

MARAFLUID SUPER HT
(Marathon Oil Co.)

Additive, containing Calcium and sulfur compounds, Zinc alkyl dithiophosphate, Polymer	10%
Mineral oil	balance

MARANOX
Analgesic
(Dent, C.S.)

Each tablet:
Acetaminophen *	325 mg.

MARATHON ANTIFREEZE AND COOLANT
(Marathon Oil Co.)

Additives, containing Inhibitor and Dye	2.5%/wt.
Water	2.5%/wt.
Ethylene glycol *	balance

MARATHON ANTI-WEAR HYDRAULIC OIL
(Marathon Oil Co.)

Additives, containing Zinc alkyl dithiophosphate, Inhibitor, Detergent, Methacrylate copolymer	1%
Mineral oil	balance

Starred ingredients (*) may be responsible for major toxic effects; consult Section II.

MARATHON GAS LINE ANTIFREEZE
(Marathon Oil Co.)

Methanol * 100%

MARATHON GEAR LUBRICANT (550 Series)
(Marathon Oil Co.)

Additives, containing Methacrylate copolymer	1%
Mineral oil	balance

MARATHON H.F. OIL (287)
(Marathon Oil Co.)

Mineral oil *

MARATHON LEAD-FREE GASOLINE
(Marathon Oil Co.)

Dye and Additives	0.02%
Petroleum hydrocarbons (mixed) *	balance

MARATHON MILE MAKER GASOLINE
(Marathon Oil Co.)

Dye and Additives	0.02%
Organo-Lead additives	0.10%
Petroleum hydrocarbons (mixed) *	balance

MARATHON MULTI-PURPOSE GEAR COMPOUND (570 Series)
(Marathon Oil Co.)

Additives, containing Methacrylate copolymer, Sulfur and Phosphorus compounds	6.3%
Mineral oil	balance

MARATHON NO. 1 FUEL OIL
(Marathon Oil Co.)

Petroleum hydrocarbons (mixed) * 100%

MARATHON NO. 2 FUEL OIL
(Marathon Oil Co.)

Petroleum hydrocarbons (mixed) * 100%

MARATHON SCL LUBRICANT
(Marathon Oil Co.)

Additive, containing Sulfur, Chlorine *, Lead *	5%
Mineral oil	balance

MARATHON TYPE F AUTOMATIC TRANSMISSION FLUID
(Marathon Oil Co.)

Additive, containing Zinc alkyl dithiophosphate, Boron, Nitrogen, and Sulfur compounds ..	8%
Mineral oil	balance

MARATHON WINDSHIELD WASHER SOLVENT
(Marathon Oil Co.)

Additives, containing Detergent and Dye	<0.03%
Methanol *	40%
Water	balance

MARAX-DF SYRUP
Bronchodilator, expectorant
(Roerig)

Each 5 ml.:
Ephedrine sulfate *	6.25 mg.
Theophylline	32.50 mg.
Atarax (Hydroxyzine HCl) .	2.5 mg.
Alcohol (Ethyl alcohol)	5% v/v
Free of all coal tar dyes	

MARAX TABLETS & SYRUP
Bronchodilator
(Roerig)

Each tablet:
Ephedrine sulfate *	25 mg.
Theophylline *	130 mg.
Atarax (Hydroxyzine HCl)	10 mg.

Each 5 ml. (Syrup):
Ephedrine sulfate *	6.25 mg.
Theophylline	32.50 mg.
Atarax (Hydroxyzine HCl)	2.5 mg.
Alcohol (Ethyl alcohol)	5% v/v

MARBLEN (LIQUID & TABLETS)
Antacid
(Fleming)

Calcium carbonate
Magnesium carbonate
Peach/Apricot flavor
Unflavored (Liquid only)

MARCELLE COSMETICS

Professional Cosmetic Corp.
Clinton Air Industrial Park
Plattsburgh, N.Y. 12901

Phone: 518-561-8600

See COSMETICS, Section VI, General Formulations

MARCHAND'S GOLDEN HAIR WASH
(Marchand)

Liquid:
Hydrogen peroxide *	1-10%

Powder:
Sodium ammonium phosphate .	>10%
Sodium carbonate *	>10%
Sodium lauryl sulfate *	1-10%

MAREZINE TABLETS
Antiemetic, anticholinergic, antihistaminic
(Burroughs Wellcome)

Each tablet:
Cyclizine hydrochloride *	50 mg.

MARFAK AP GREASE
(Texaco Canada Ltd.)

Mineral oil *
Lithium-lead soap *

MARFAK GREASE
(Texaco Inc.; Texaco Canada Ltd.)

Mineral oil *
Sodium soap

MARFAK HD GREASE
(Texaco Inc.; Texaco Canada Ltd.)

Mineral oil *
Sodium soap

MARFAK MP GREASE
(Texaco Canada Ltd.)

Mineral oil *
Lithium soap

MARFONYL COUGH SYRUP
(Wesley Pharm.)

Each fl. oz.:
Antimony potassium tartrate .	1/12 gr.
Ammonium chloride	8 gr.
Cocillana tincture	40 min.
In a vehicle containing Syrup, Honey, Glucose and Aromatics	

MARGON WOOD PUTTY AND CRACK FILLER
(United Gilsonite)

Plaster
Calcium carbonate
Dextrine
Wood flour

MAR-HYDE
Vinyl lacquer
(Talsol)

Methyl ethyl ketone	55%
Cellosolve acetate	15%
Toluene *	14%
Cyclohexanone	3%
Resin, pigment, plasticizer	13%

Starred ingredients (*) may be responsible for major toxic effects; consult Section II.

MAR-HYDE AEROSOL
Vinyl lacquer
(Talsol)

Methyl ethyl ketone *	52%
Cellosolve acetate *	12%
Toluene *	9%
Resin, pigment, plasticizer	6%
Propellant (Propane-butane)	21%

MARIN COUNTY GOPHER BAIT
For mechanical application only
(Marin)

Strychnine *	2.63%

MARIN COUNTY GOPHER POISON GRAIN BAIT
Rodenticide
(Marin)

Strychnine *	0.29%

MARIN COUNTY RAT & MOUSE BAIT (Wax Form & Grain Form)
Rodenticide
(Marin)

Diphacinone	0.005%

MARIN COUNTY SPARROW POISON BAIT
(Marin)

Strychnine *	0.25%

MARIN COUNTY ZINC PHOSPHIDE POISON GRAIN
Rodenticide
(Marin)

Zinc phosphide *	1.00%

MARINE MASTER OUTBOARD MOTOR OIL
(Marathon Oil Co.)

Additive, Detergent	10%
Stoddard solvent *	20%
Mineral oil	balance

MARKET BASKET PINE OIL
Disinfectant, deodorant, cleanser
(Ritchie Grocer Co.)

Steam distilled Pine oil *	80%
Combined amount:	10%
Soap	
Isopropyl alcohol	

'76 Ed.

MARKS-A-LOT
Marking ink
(Carter's Ink)

Aromatics
Plasticizer
Resin
Dyes

'76 Ed.

MARK V
Plastic paste
(Baird Dynamic)

Polyester resins
Mineral fillers

'76 Ed.

MAR-PIPER

See MARTIN'S MAR-PIPER

MARRACH COSMETICS

Marrach, Inc.
3060 Valleywood Dr.
Dayton, Ohio 45429

Phone: 513-293-2026

See COSMETICS, Section VI, General Formulations

MARS COLORS

See WEBER MARS COLORS

MARSON'S BLACK SOLDER
Plastic filler
(Marson)

Resin component:	
Styrene monomer	10-14%
Polyester (100% solids)	26-31%
Pigment & filler	50-60%
Di-methyl aniline	0.1-0.4%
Catalyst component:	
Benzoyl peroxide *	48-52%
Phthalate plasticizer	48-52%

MARTIN'S AMINE-IODINE MEDICATED
Expectorant, dietary source of iodine; veterinary
(Martin, C.J.)

Ethylenediamine dihydroiodide *	4.6%
Inactive ingredients:	
Salt (NaCl) *	95.4%

MARTIN'S ANTI-PICK
For poultry cannibalism
(Martin, C.J.)

Sulfur	5.52%
Aluminum ammonium sulfate	11.04%
Oil red	0.55%
Inert ingredients:	
Petrolatum	77.37%
Paraffin	5.52%

MARTIN'S ARSEPHENO CATTLE DRENCH
For tape worms; veterinary
(Martin, C.J.)

Each oz.:	
Phenothiazine	10 gm.
Lead arsenate *	5 gr.

MARTIN'S ARSEPHENO SHEEP & GOAT DRENCH
For tape worms; veterinary
(Martin, C.J.)

Each oz.:	
Phenothiazine	12 1/2 gm.
Lead arsenate *	7 1/2 gr.

MARTIN'S BEEF CATTLE DUST
Insecticide
(Martin, C.J.)

Chlorinated camphene containing 67 to 69% chlorine (Toxaphene) *	5%
Gamma isomer of benzene hexachloride (Lindane)	1%

MARTIN'S BOMBANE JET STREAM

See BOMBANE JET STREAM

MARTIN'S BRANDING FLUID
Veterinary
(Martin, C.J.)

Caustic soda *
Oil of tar *
Water

MARTIN'S CANINE CAPS
Anthelmintic; veterinary
(Martin, C.J.)

Tetrachlorethylene *	97.68%
Arecoline hydrobromide	0.39%
Ethyl cellulose	1.51%
Mineral oil	0.42%

MARTIN'S CARBOLIN OIL
Wood preservative, insecticide, repellent
(Martin, C.J.)

Petroleum distillate *	80%
Anthracene oil *	20%

MARTIN'S CHINCH BUG KILLER
Insecticide
(Martin, C.J.)

Chlorpyrifos (O,O-Diethyl O-(3,5,6-trichloro-2-pyridyl) phosphorothioate) *	2.85%
Petroleum distillate *	85.00%

MARTIN'S 74% CHLORDANE CONCENTRATE
Insecticide
(Martin, C.J.)

Technical Chlordane *	74%
Petroleum hydrocarbons	20%

MARTIN'S COAT DRESSING WITH LANOLIN FOR SHOW ANIMALS
(Martin, C.J.)

Combined amount:	100%
Mineral oil	
Lanolin	

MARTIN'S COW & CALF DUST
Insecticide
(Martin, C.J.)

Methoxychlor (technical)	5.00%
Malathion	4.00%
Piperonyl butoxide (technical)	0.51%
Pyrethrins	0.06%

MARTIN'S CREOSOTE DIP
Disinfectant, deodorizer, cleanser; veterinary
(Martin, C.J.)

Coal tar neutral oils *	56%
Soap	15%
Phenols *	19%

MARTIN'S CUBE POWDER
Insecticide
(Martin, C.J.)

Rotenone *	5%
Other cube resins	10%

MARTIN'S DAIRY DUST
Insecticide; veterinary
(Martin, C.J.)

Methoxychlor (technical)	5.00%
Malathion	4.00%
Piperonyl butoxide (technical)	0.51%
Pyrethrins	0.06%

MARTIN'S DEHORNING PROTECTIVE DRESSING
(Martin, C.J.)

Coal tar oil *	75%
Pine tar oil *	25%

MARTIN'S DIAZINON 12.5E LAWN & GARDEN INSECT CONTROL
(Martin, C.J.)

O,O-Diethyl O-(2-isopropyl-6-methyl-4-pyrimidinyl) phosphorothioate *	12.50%
Aromatic petroleum derivative solvent *	79.00%

MARTIN'S DIAZINON GARDEN DUST
Insecticide
(Martin, C.J.)

O,O-Diethyl O-(2-isopropyl-6-methyl-4-pyrimidinyl) phosphorothioate *	4.0%

MARTIN'S DIAZINON GRANULAR LAWN INSECT CONTROL
(Martin, C.J.)

O,O-Diethyl O-(2-isopropyl-6-methyl-4-pyrimidinyl) phosphorothioate *	2.0%

MARTIN'S DIAZINON HOUSEHOLD INSECT SPRAY
(Martin, C.J.)

O,O-Diethyl O-(2-isopropyl-6-methyl-4-pyrimidinyl) phosphorothioate	0.500%
Pyrethrins	0.052%
Technical Piperonyl butoxide	0.260%
Petroleum distillates *	98.540%

MARTIN'S DIAZINON PECAN AND FRUIT TREE SPRAY
Insecticide
(Martin, C.J.)

O,O-Diethyl O-(2-isopropyl-6-methyl-4-pyrimidinyl) phosphorothioate *	12.50%
Aromatic petroleum derivative solvent *	79.00%

MARTIN'S EAR-TIX-TOX
Ear tick control; veterinary
(Martin, C.J.)

Ronnel (O,O-Dimethyl O-(2,4,5-trichlorophenyl)phosphorothioate)	5.00%
Petrolatum	12.5%
Pine oil *	50.0%
Petroleum distillate *	30.0%

MARTIN-SENOUR PAINT PRODUCTS

The Martin-Senour Co.
Division of The Sherwin-Williams Co.
1370 Ontario St.
Cleveland, Ohio 44113

Phone: 216-566-3108

See PAINTS, Section VI, General Formulations

MARTIN-SENOUR UNIVERSAL PAINT THINNER
(Martin-Senour)

Petroleum distillates (volatile) *	
Mineral spirits *	

'76 Ed.

MARTIN'S FLEA & TICK SPRAY
Insecticide
(Martin, C.J.)

Pyrethrins	0.06%
Piperonyl butoxide	0.48%
Methoxychlor (technical)	0.50%
2,2-Thiobis(4-chlor-6-methylphenol)	0.10%
2,3,4,5,-Bis(2-butylene)tetrahydro-2-furaldehyde	0.24%
Petroleum distillate *	23.12%

MARTIN'S GOPHER BAIT
Rodenticide
(Martin, C.J.)

Strychnine alkaloid *	0.30%

MARTIN'S HEXACHLOROETHANE
For liver flukes; veterinary
(Martin, C.J.)

Each 30 cc.:	
Hexachloroethane *	15 1/3 gm.
Bentonite and water	

MARTIN'S HEXO PHENA
Two-way drench for liver flukes; veterinary
(Martin, C.J.)

Each oz.:	
Hexachloroethane *	10 gm.
Phenothiazine	10 gm.
Bentonite	

MARTIN'S HORSE FLY BOMB
Insecticide
(Martin, C.J.)

Butoxypolypropylene glycol *	16.47%
Pyrethrins	0.17%
Piperonyl butoxide (technical)	1.66%
Petroleum distillate *	11.70%
Dichlorodifluoromethane	70.00%

MARTIN'S HOUSEHOLD AND PATIO BUG BOMB
Insecticide
(Martin, C.J.)

Petroleum distillate *	51.70%
Butoxypolypropylene glycol *	16.47%
Pyrethrins	0.17%
Technical Piperonyl butoxide	1.66%
Inert ingredients:	30.00%
Propellant	

Starred ingredients (*) may be responsible for major toxic effects; consult Section II.

MARTIN'S HOUSEHOLD ANT & ROACH BOMB
Insecticide
(Martin, C.J.)

O,O-Diethyl O-(2-isopropyl-4-
  methyl-6-pyrimidinyl)
  phosphorothioate 0.500%
Pyrethrins 0.052%
Technical Piperonyl butoxide .. 0.261%
Petroleum distillate * 69.187%
Inert ingred.:
  Propellent 30%

MARTIN'S JET-WET
Spreader-sticker
(Martin, C.J.)

Ethoxylated polymethylated nonal alcohol *†
1,2-Ethanediol *

†*See* Alkyl ethoxylate

MARTIN'S KETOSIN ORAL SOLUTION
Control of acetonemia in dairy cattle
(Martin, C.J.)

Propylene glycol USP 99.5%

MARTIN'S LARGE CANINE CAPSULES
Anthelmintic-veterinary
(Martin, C.J.)

Each capsule:
  Tetrachloroethylene * .... 4 cc.
  Arecoline hydrobromide * .... 0.4 gr.
  Mineral oil .... 0.03 cc.

MARTIN'S LICE KILLER
Insecticide
(Martin, C.J.)

Carbaryl (1-Naphthyl
  methylcarbamate) * 5%

MARTIN'S LIVESTOCK DUST
Insecticide
(Martin, C.J.)

Technical Methoxychlor * 11.00%
Technical Piperonyl butoxide ... 0.51%
Pyrethrins 0.06%
Petroleum distillate 0.43%
Inert ingred.:
  Talc 88.00%

MARTIN'S LIVESTOCK WOUND PROTECTANT
(Martin, C.J.)

Ronnel (O,O-Dimethyl O-2(2,4,5-
  trichlorophenyl)phosphorothio-
  ate) 2.5%
Pine oil * 15.0%
Xylene 0.5%

MARTIN'S 50% MALATHION CONCENTRATE
Insecticide
(Martin, C.J.)

Malathion * 50%
Aromatic petroleum derivative
  solvent * 44%

MARTIN'S MAR-PIPER
*Liquid wormer for poultry, horses,
  swine; veterinary*
(Martin, C.J.)

Piperazine (eq. of 17 gm. piperazine
  base per 100 cc.) 17%

MARTIN'S PENTA-CON "1 TO 10 CONCENTRATE"
Wood preservative and soil poison
(Martin, C.J.)

Pentachlorophenol * 35.3%
Other chlorophenols 4.1%
Aromatic petroleum solvent * 14.0%

MARTIN'S PET-D-TICK
*Controls lice, ticks and fleas on cats &
  dogs*
(Martin, C.J.)

Carbaryl (1-Naphthyl N-methyl-
  carbamate) * 5.00%
Inert ingredient: 95.00%
  Talc

MARTIN'S PHENOTHIAZINE REGULAR DRENCH
Anthelmintic; veterinary
(Martin, C.J.)

Each oz.:
  Phenothiazine * .... 12.5 gm.

MARTIN'S PINK EYE WOUND DRESSING
Veterinary
(Martin, C.J.)

Sulfanilamide 1.2500%
Sulfathiazole 3.7500%
Urea 0.2500%
Methyl violet 0.0025%
Benzyl alcohol * 13.4975%
Propylene glycol 66.2500%
Dichlorodifluoromethane 15.0000%

MARTIN'S PROLIN RATBAIT PELLETS
Rodenticide
(Martin, C.J.)

Warfarin 0.025%
N-(2-Quinoxalinyl) sulfanilamide
  (Sulfaquinoxaline) 0.025%

MARTIN'S QUAMM DISINFECTANT
(Martin, C.J.)

Combined amount: 10%
  Methyldodecylbenzyl trimethyl ammo-
    nium chloride *
  Methyldodecylxylylene bis (trimethyl
    ammonium chloride) *†

†*See* Cationic surfactants

MARTIN'S ROKIL
Insecticide
(Waltham Chem. Co.)

O,O-Diethyl O-(2-isopropyl-4-
  methyl-6-pyrimidinyl)
  phosphorothioate 0.500%
Pyrethrins 0.052%
Technical Piperonyl butoxide ... 0.261%
Petroleum distillate * 99.187%

MARTIN'S ROOM DEODORANTS (FLORAL, SPICE)
(Martin, C.J.)

Triethylene glycol 5.0%
Propylene glycol 5.0%

MARTIN'S SCARLET OIL SMEAR
Antiseptic dressing; veterinary
(Martin, C.J.)

Mineral oil 85.4%
Methyl salicylate * 3.0%
Menthol 0.5%
Eucalyptus oil * 3.0%
Pine oil 2.0%
Phenol * 2.0%
Biebrich scarlet red 0.1%
Inert ingredients:
  Colloidal silica 4.0%

MARTIN'S SMEAR INSECTICIDE
*Kills screw worms, ear ticks, blowfly
  maggots on livestock*
(Martin, C.J.)

Ronnel (O,O-Dimethyl-O-(2,4,5-
  trichlorophenyl)phosphorothio-
  ate) 5.0%
Pine oil * 35.0%
Xylene * 3.0%

MARTIN'S 25'S PHENOTHIAZINE BOLUSES
*Removal of common stomach worms;
  veterinary*
(Martin, C.J.)

Each bolus:
  Phenothiazine * .... 25 gm.

MARTIN'S 50'S PHENOTHIAZINE BOLUSES
Removal of common stomach worms; veterinary
(Martin, C.J.)

Each bolus:
Phenothiazine * .... 12 1/2 gm.

MARTIN'S STOCK TOX
Livestock spray to control lice, ticks & hornflies
(Martin, C.J.)

Toxaphene *	62.0%
Petroleum hydrocarbons	32.0%

MARTIN'S SUPER STOCK TOX
Livestock spray to control lice, ticks, and hornflies
(Martin, C.J.)

Toxaphene *	62.0%
Gamma isomer of benzene hexachloride from lindane	2.5%
Petroleum solvents	29.5%

MARTIN'S SWEET PHENOTHIAZINE CRUMBLES MEDICATED
Removal of worms; veterinary
(Martin, C.J.)

Phenothiazine (12 1/2 gm. phenothiazine per ounce) * 42.68%

MARTIN'S UDDER OINTMENT
Antiseptic ointment
(Martin, C.J.)

Methyl dodecyl benzyl trimethyl ammonium chloride	0.075%
Cetyl alcohol	6.0%
Menthol	0.075%
Camphor *	3.0%
Methyl salicylate *	2.0%
Zinc oxide	5.0%
Inactive ingredients (base):	83.85%
Lanolin	
Petrolatum	

MARTIN'S U.S.-E.Q. 335
Screw worm remedy for calves
(Martin, C.J.)

Mineral oil *	42%
Pine oil *	35%
Gamma isomer of benzene hexachloride (from lindane) *	3%

MARTIN'S U.S. FORMULA NO. 62
Screw worm smear
(Martin, C.J.)

Diphenylamine	35.0%
Benzene *	35.0%
Sulfonated castor oil	7.5%

MARTIN'S UTERINE BOLUS
Veterinary
(Martin, C.J.)

Each bolus:
Urea	207 gr.
Sulfanilamide *	33 gr.
Sulfathiazole *	5 gr.

MARTIN'S VEGETABLE DUST
Insecticide
(Martin, C.J.)

Carbaryl *	5%
Rotenone	1%
Other cube resins	2%

MARTIN'S VIOLET WOUND DRESSING
Antiseptic treatment for livestock
(Martin, C.J.)

Isopropyl alcohol *	52.32%
Methyl salicylate *	3.51%
Tannic acid	1.46%
Eugenol	0.58%
Methyl violet	0.29%
Inert ingredients:	41.84%
Dichlorodifluoromethane	

MARTIN'S WOUND DRESSING
Antiseptic treatment for minor cuts and abrasions on livestock
(Martin, C.J.)

Methyl violet	0.5%
Tannic acid	2.5%
Methyl salicylate *	6.0%
Isopropyl alcohol *	90.0%
Eugenol	1.0%

MARVEL-BAC CONCENTRATED GERMICIDE

See C-Z MARVEL-BAC CONCENTRATED GERMICIDE

MARVEL CLEANING FLUID
(Barco Chem. Products Co.)

Carbon tetrachloride *

'76 Ed.

MARVEL GERMICIDAL CLEANER, FOREMOST 2149-ES

See FOREMOST 2149-ES MARVEL GERMICIDAL CLEANER

MARVEL LUBRICATING OIL
General all purpose lubricating oil
(Marvel Oil)

Solvent extracted Naphthenic petroleum oil
Mineral spirits *
Tricresyl phosphate *
Methyl salicylate *
Chlorinated aromatic hydrocarbon *
Red Aniline petroleum dye
Industrial grade fatty oil

MARVEL MYSTERY OIL
Additive to fuel and crankcase oil of internal combustion engines
(Marvel Oil)

Solvent extracted Naphthenic petroleum oil
Mineral spirits *
Tricresyl phosphate *
Methyl salicylate *
Chlorinated aromatic hydrocarbon *
Red Aniline petroleum dye
Industrial grade fatty oil

MARY KAY COSMETICS

Mary Kay Cosmetics
8787 Stemmons Frwy.
Dallas, Tex. 75247

Phone: 214-630-8787

See COSMETICS, Section VI, General Formulations

MARY QUANT COSMETICS

Mary Quant Cosmetics Ltd.
655 Madison Ave.
New York, N.Y. 10021

Phone: 212-758-1072

See COSMETICS, Section VI, General Formulations

MASK 'N PEEL

See DUNCAN CERAMICS SPECIALTY PRODUCT MASK 'N PEEL (SY 548)

MASOTEN 80% SOLUBLE POWDER
For control of parasites on fish
(Cutter (Brand) Bayvet Div. Cutter Labs.)

Trichlorfon * 80%

MASSACRE - SP
Roach and ant bomb
(ABCO, Inc.)

O,O-Diethyl O-(2-isopropyl-6-methyl-4-pyrimidinyl)phosphorothioate	0.500%
Pyrethrins	0.052%
Piperonyl butoxide (technical)	0.261%
Petroleum distillate *	69.187%

MASSE CREAM
Nipple care; diaper rash
(Ortho)

Allantoin

MASSENGILL DOUCHE POWDER
(Beecham Products)

Sodium chloride
Ammonium alum
Phenol
Methyl salicylate

MASSENGILL MEDICATED DOUCHE
(Beecham Products)

Active ingred.:
Povidone-iodine 0.23%

MASTER MIX BLUE DEATH RAT AND MOUSE BAIT HIDE-A-PACK
Rodenticide
(Central Soya)

3-(alpha-Acetonylfurfuryl)-4-
hydroxycoumarin 0.025%

MASTER MIX BLUE DEATH RAT BAIT
Rodenticide
(Central Soya)

3-(alpha-Acetonylfurfuryl)-4-
hydroxycoumarin 0.025%

MASTER MIX CYGON 2-E
Systemic insecticide
(Central Soya)

Dimethoate (O,O-Dimethyl S-(N-
methylcarbamoylmethyl)
phosphorodithioate) * 23.4%

MASTER MIX ENVIRON
Disinfectant
(Central Soya)

o-Phenylphenol 3.9%
4-Chloro-2-phenylphenol * 3.6%
6-Chloro-2-phenylphenol * 1.1%
p-Tertiary amylphenol 0.8%

MASTER MIX FLY SPRAY
For dairy and beef cattle
(Central Soya)

Petroleum hydrocarbons * 98.57%
Dimethyl phosphate of alpha-
methylbenzyl 3-hydroxy-cis-
crotonate (Ciodrin) * 1.00%
2,2-Dichlorovinyl dimethyl
phosphate 0.23%
Related compounds 0.02%

MASTER MIX HOG LICE GRANULES
(Central Soya)

Ronnel (O,O-Dimethyl O-(2,4,5-
trichlorophenyl)phosphorothioate) 5%

MASTER MIX ISOLITE
Drinking water medication; veterinary
(Central Soya)

Each oz.:
Sodium sulfathiazole * .... 0.67 oz.
Ethylenediamine dihydriodide   7 gr.
Inert ingred.: 31.4%
Electrolytes
Colloidal silica (anticaking agent)
Color added

MASTER MIX MALATHION 50% EMS
Insecticide
(Central Soya)

Malathion * 50%
Aromatic petroleum hydrocarbons * 45%

MASTER MIX MASTER SPRAY
Dairy, stock and space insecticide
(Central Soya)

Petroleum distillate * 95.070%
Butoxypolypropylene glycol 4.750%
Pyrethrins 0.030%
Technical Piperonyl butoxide . 0.150%

MASTER MIX PIPERAZINE WATER WORMER
Veterinary
(Central Soya)

Piperazine base ...... 17.0 grams/100 ml.

MASTER MIX SULMET DRINKING WATER SOLUTION
All purpose sulfa-drug; veterinary
(Central Soya)

Sodium sulfamethazine * 12.5%

MASTER MIX SULMET OBLETS
All purpose sulfa-drug; veterinary
(Central Soya)

Sulfamethazine * .... 2.5 gm.

MASTIMIN
Dairy cattle teat dip
(Diversey Wyandotte)

Nonionic detergent - Iodine complex
Titratable Iodine * 1%

MASURY-COLUMBIA FLOOR CARE PRODUCTS AND INDUSTRIAL GERMICIDES

Masury-Columbia Co.
1502 N. 25th Ave.
Melrose Park, Ill. 60160

Phone: 312-345-9202

MASURY PAINT PRODUCTS

Masury Paint Co.
1403 Severn
Baltimore, Md. 21230

Phone: 301-837-5150

MATAR GERMICIDAL DETERGENT
(Huntington Labs.)

Sodium o-phenylphenate 6.00%
Sodium o-benzyl-p-chlorophenate 9.50%
Sodium p-tertiary amyl phenate .. 3.00%
Tetrasodium ethylene diamine
tetraacetate 2.00%
Sodium xylene sulfonate 5.93%
Isopropyl alcohol 3.16%

MATCHABELLI BODY TONIC
(Chesebrough-Pond's)

Ethyl alcohol, denatured * ...... >50%
Propylene glycol .... 0.1% or less
Color .... 0.1% or less
Water 25-50%
Fragrance 1-5%
Quaternium-22 .... 1-5%

MATCHABELLI DEODORANT STICK
(Chesebrough-Pond's)

Propylene glycol .... >50%
Water .... >25-50%
Sodium stearate .... >5-10%
Fragrance .... >0.1-1%
Triclosan .... 0.1% or less
Color .... 0.1% or less

MATCH LIGHT
Instant lighting charcoal briquets
(Kingsford)

Saturated Aliphatic petroleum
hydrocarbons * 10-15%
Charcoal briquets 85-90%

MATTRESS FRESH
Bactericide, mold and mildew preventative
(Cardinal Products Corp.)

Hyamine 1622 * 10%

'76 Ed.

MAUGET FUNGISOL
Systemic fungicide for tree injection
(Mauget, J. J., Co.)

DEBC (2-(2-Ethoxyethoxy)ethyl-2-
benzimidazolecarbamate) 1.7%
2-MBC (Methyl 2-
benzimidazolecarbamate) 0.3%
Inert: Diethylene glycol ethyl
ether * 98.0%

MAUGET INJECT-A-CIDE
Systemic insecticide for tree injection
(Mauget, J. J., Co.)

Metasystox-R * 50%

MAUGET INJECT-A-CIDE B
Systemic insecticide for tree injection
(Mauget, J. J., Co.)

Technical Bidrin * 82%

MAUTZ PAINT PRODUCTS

Mautz Paint Co.
939 E. Washington Ave.
Madison, Wis. 53703

Phone: 608-255-1661

See PAINTS, Section VI, General Formulations

MAXAFIL
Sunscreen for sun sensitive skin
(CooperCare)

Cinnoxate 4%
Menthyl anthranilate 5%
Colorless

MAX FACTOR COSMETICS & TOILETRIES

Max Factor & Co.
1655 N. McCadden Pl.
Hollywood, Calif. 90028

Phone: 213-856-6000

See COSMETICS, Section VI, General
Formulations

MAX 80-20 FIA
Pesticide
(Dow)

Active ingred.:
Carbon tetrachloride * 82.9%
Carbon disulfide 16.5%
Inert ingred.:
Inhibitor 0.6%

MAX HIGH LIFE
Pesticide
(Dow)

Active ingred.:
Carbon tetrachloride * 82.9%
Carbon disulfide 16.5%
Inert ingred.:
Inhibitor 0.6%

MAXIBOLIN
Anabolic steroid
(Organon)

TABLETS (each):
Ethylestrenol .... 2 mg.
ELIXIR (each 5 ml.):
Ethylestrenol .... 2 mg.
Alcohol 10%

MAXIDEX
Ophthalmic suspension
(Alcon)

Active ingred. (each ml.):
Dexamethasone (Dexametha-
sone 21 Alcohol) 0.1%
Preservative:
Benzalkonium chloride 0.01%
Vehicle:
Hydroxypropyl methylcellulose 0.5%
Inactive ingred.:
Sodium chloride
Sodium phosphate (dried)
Polysorbate 80
Edetate disodium
Citric acid and/or
Sodium hydroxide (to adjust pH)
Purified water

MAXIDEX
Ophthalmic ointment
(Alcon)

Active ingred. (each gm.):
Dexamethasone sodium phosphate
(equiv. to Dexamethasone phosphate
0.05%)
Inactive ingred.:
Mineral oil
White petrolatum

MAXIM BALM
Analgesic ointment
(Maxim Chem.)

Thymol *
Cedar leaf *
Eucalyptus *
Oil of nutmeg *
Camphor *
Menthol *
Steam distilled Wood turpentine *

'76 Ed.

MAXIMUM STRENGTH SINUTAB II NO DROWSINESS FORMULA (Tablets and Capsules)
Analgesic-nasal decongestant
(Warner-Lambert)

Each dosage unit:
Acetaminophen * .... 500 mg.
Pseudoephedrine HCl .... 30 mg.

MAXIMUM STRENGTH SUCRETS
Throat lozenges
(Beecham Products)

Each lozenge:
Hexylresorcinol .... 4 mg.

MAXITROL
Ophthalmic ointment
(Alcon)

Active ingred. (each gm.):
Neomycin sulfate (equiv. to neomycin
3.5 mg./gm.)
Polymyxin B sulfate ...... 6000 units
Dexamethasone 0.1%
Preservatives:
Methylparaben 0.05%
Propylparaben 0.01%
Inactive ingred.:
White petrolatum
Anhydrous liquid Lanolin

MAXITROL
Ophthalmic suspension
(Alcon)

Active ingred. (each ml.):
Neomycin sulfate (equiv. to
neomycin 3.5 mg./ml.)
Polymyxin B sulfate ...... 6000 units
Dexamethasone 0.1%
Preservative:
Benzalkonium chloride 0.004%
Vehicle:
Hydroxypropyl
methylcellulose 0.5%
Inactive ingred.:
Sodium chloride
Polysorbate 20
Hydrochloric acid and/or
Sodium hydroxide (to adjust pH)
Purified water

MAX KILL HIGH LIFE
Liquid grain fumigant
(Research Products Co.)

Carbon tetrachloride * 82.9%
Carbon bisulfide 16.5%
Aliphatic hydrocarbons 0.6%

MAX KILL MALATHION 57-WE
Insecticide
(Research Products Co.)

Malathion * 57.0%
Aromatic petroleum derivative
solvent * 34.0%

MAX KILL MILL & BIN SPRAY
Insecticide
(Research Products Co.)

Technical Methoxychlor 3.0%
Pyrethrins 0.025%
Technical Piperonyl butoxide .. 0.063%
Aromatic petroleum derivative
solvent * 20.0%
Petroleum distillate 76.912%

MAX-KILL SPOT 59
Fumigant
(Research Products Co.)

Ethylene dibromide * 59.0%
Carbon tetrachloride 29.5%
Ethylene dichloride 10.0%
Carbon disulfide 1.5%

MAYBELLINE COSMETICS

Maybelline Co.
3030 Jackson Ave.
Memphis, Tenn. 38151

Phone: 901-320-2011

See COSMETICS, Section VI, General
Formulations

MAYFIELD, DR., PRODUCTS

See DR. MAYFIELD

MAYFLOWER PAINTS

Mayflower Paint Co.
201 E. Market St.
Louisville, Ky. 40201

Phone: 502-584-0151

See PAINTS, Section VI, General Formulations

M$B AUTOMATIC DISH DETERGENT
(Wakefern; supplier, Korex Co.)

Sodium tripolyphosphate *
Sodium carbonate
Nonionic surfactant
Chlorinated isocyanurate
Sodium silicate
Sodium chloride

M$B BLUE LAUNDRY DETERGENT
(Wakefern; supplier, Witco Chem.)

Anionic surfactant *
Sodium carbonate
Sodium silicate (not meta)
Cellulosic
Fluorescent whitening agent
Colorant
Fragrance
Sodium sulfate

MBC CONCENTRATE SOIL FUMIGANT
(Hendrix and Dail)

Methyl bromide * 98%
Chloropicrin * 2%

M$B CLEANSER
(Wakefern; supplier, Fitzpatrick Bros.)

Silica sand
Soda ash
ACL 85
Sulframin 85

MBC SOIL FUMIGANT
(Hendrix and Dail)

Methyl bromide * 68.6%
Chloropicrin * 1.4%
Petroleum hydrocarbons 30.0%

MBC-33 SOIL FUMIGANT
(Hendrix and Dail)

Methyl bromide 67%
Chloropicrin * 33%

M$B DRY BLEACH
(Wakefern; supplier, Stanson Detergents)

Sodium chloride
Sodium carbonate . . . . trace
Sodium percarbonate
Sodium perborate *
Color . . . . trace
Surfactant . . . . trace

M$B LEMON LIQUID DISH DETERGENT
(Wakefern; supplier, J. L. Prescott Co.)

Water
Sodium dodecyl benzene sulfonate
Sodium lauryl ether sulfate
Sodium xylene sulfonate
Coconut diethanolamide
Sodium sulfate
Fragrance
Formalin
Tetrasodium EDTA

M$B PINE OIL CLEANER
(Wakefern; supplier, Howland Chem.)

Pine oil *
Tall oil soap
Isopropyl alcohol
Chelating agent
Water

M$B PINK FABRIC SOFTENER
(Wakefern; supplier, Laundry Aids)

Quaternary ditallow
Diamido * 2.7%
Soft water (10 ppm's) 97.3%

M$B PINK LIQUID DISH DETERGENT
(Wakefern; supplier, J. L. Prescott Co.)

Water
Sodium dodecyl benzene sulfonate
Sodium lauryl ether sulfate
Sodium xylene sulfonate
Coconut diethanolamide
Sodium sulfate
Latex opacifier
Fragrance
Formalin
Tetrasodium EDTA
Color dye

McALEER POLISH & CLEANER
Automotive
(McAleer)

Proprietary Ethanol
Vegetable gums
Glycerin
Mineral oils
Mahogany soap
Diatomaceous earth
Amyl acetate *
Formaldehyde *

'76 Ed.

McALEER QUICK WAX
Automobiles, furniture, floors
(McAleer)

Mineral spirits *
Vegetable and petroleum waxes

'76 Ed.

MC-3 CLEANER
(Pennwalt)

Polyphosphate *
Sodium carbonate *
Sodium metasilicate
Alkyl aryl sulfonate *

McCLOSKEY VARNISH PRODUCTS
Varnishes, wood finishes and sealers

McCloskey Varnish Company
7600 State Road
Philadelphia, Pa. 19136

Phone: 215-624-4400

See PAINTS, Section VI, General Formulations

McCONNON INSECTICIDAL DUST
(McConnon & Co.)

Rotenone * 0.75%
Other cube extractives 1.50%

McCONNON PHENOL-5
Disinfectant
(McConnon & Co.)

Pine oil * 20.0%
Soap 7.3%
Orthobenzyl para chloro phenol . . . 3.0%
Inert ingredients:
Water 64.7%
Hexylene glycol 5.0%

McCONNON WHITE LINIMENT
(McConnon & Co.)

Camphor * 5.50%
Turpentine * 51.00%
Ammonia (26° Be) * 12.70%

Starred ingredients (*) may be responsible for major toxic effects; consult Section II.

McD ALL PURPOSE CONCENTRATE
Liquid detergent
(Kay Chem. Co.)

Anionic surfactant *	25-30%
Nonionic surfactant	10-15%
Chelating agent	2-4%
Water	balance

McD DRIVE-THRU & LOT CLEANER
Cleaning concrete and asphalt pavements
(Kay Chem. Co.)

Nonionic detergent	5-10%
Chelating agent	5-10%
Tripotassium phosphate	5-15%
Water	balance

McD FRYER BOIL-OUT COMPOUND
Liquid caustic cleaner
(Kay Chem. Co.)

Potassium hydroxide *	30-40%
Water	balance

McD GRILL CLEANER
Liquid caustic cleaner
(Kay Chem. Co.)

Potassium hydroxide *	20%
Water	balance

McD GRILL CLEANER NF
(Kay Chem. Co.)

Sodium carbonate *	2-5%
Anionic and nonionic detergent	4-10%

McD LAUNDRY & LOT CLEANER
Powder detergent
(Kay Chem. Co.)

Sodium carbonate *	40-50%
Sodium tripolyphosphate	20-30%
Sodium silicate	5-10%
Nonionic surfactant	5-9%
Anionic surfactant	1-3%

McD POWDER BLEACH
(Kay Chem. Co.)

Sodium dichloroisocyanurate *	35-45%
Sodium tripolyphosphate	5-10%

McD SANITIZER
Powder sanitizer
(Kay Chem. Co.)

Trisodium phosphate	18%
Sodium dichloroisocyanurate	6%

McD STAINLESS CLEANER DRESSING
Liquid polish
(Kay Chem. Co.)

Paraffinic oil (105 SUS) *†	30-40%
Emulsifier	5-10%
Water	balance

†*See* Kerosene

McKAY'S MAXLIN LINIMENT
For horses
(Spohn)

Menthol USP *	
Strong tincture Iodine NF *	
Oil of wormwood	
Ether USP	45 gr./fl. oz.
Camphor *	
Soap liniment NF	
Alcohol	56%

'76 Ed.

McKESSON'S COLD SORE LOTION
(McKesson)

Ethyl alcohol	70%/v
Benzyl alcohol	5%/v
t-Amyl phenol *	
s-Octyl phenol *	
n-Heptyl phenol *	
Camphor *	
Synthetic gum benzoin	
Benzoic acid	
Methyl salicylate *	

McKESSON'S POISON IVY CREAM
(McKesson)

Zirconium oxide (carbonated hydrous zirconia)	4%
Benzocaine	
Pyrilamine maleate *	
Polyvinylpyrrolidone	

McNESS CRYSTAL CLEANSER
(Furst-McNess Co.)

Trisodium phosphate *	72.7%
Sodium sesquicarbonate	27.3%

MCP AMINE 4
Herbicide
(Diamond Shamrock Corp.)

Dimethylamine salt of 2-methyl-4-chlorophenoxyacetic acid *	52%

MCP GREASE
(Texaco, Inc.)

Mineral oil *
Lithium soap
Dye

MCPP + 2,4-D AMINE
Herbicide
(Fallek-Lankro Corp.)

Diethanolamine salt of 2-(2-Methyl-4-chlorophenoxy) propionic acid *	31.0%
Diethanolamine salt of 2,4-Dichlorophenoxyacetic acid *	15.35%

MCPP K-4
Herbicide
(Fallek-Lankro Corp.)

Potassium salt of 2-(2-Methyl-4-chlorophenoxy) propionic acid *	48.3%

MC-3 CLEANER
(Pennwalt)

Polyphosphate *
Sodium carbonate *
Sodium metasilicate
Alkyl aryl sulfonate *

MD-7
Powdered hand soap
(U.S. Borax)

Toilet soap
Lanolin
Urea
Emollients
Hexachlorophene

MEASURIN
Analgesic
(Breon Labs.)

Each tablet:	
Aspirin *	10 gr.

MEBARAL
Sedative and anticonvulsant
(Breon Labs.)

Each tablet:	
Mephobarbital *	32 mg.; 50 mg.; 100 mg. or 200 mg.

MECHOLYL OINTMENT
Minor muscular aches, simple neuralgia
(Gordon Labs.)

Methacholine chloride	0.25%
Methyl salicylate *	10%

MECK LIQUID CHLORINATED CLEANER
Institutional and industrial use
(Yale Chem. Co.)

Caustic potash (Potassium hydroxide) *	>17%
Polyphosphates	>16%
Sodium hypochlorite	<2%

MECLAN CREAM
Topical antibiotic
(Ortho-Dermatology)

Meclocycline sulfosalicylate	1%

MEDACHE
For non-vascular headaches
(Organon)

Each tablet:
Phenyltoloxamine dihydrogen
citrate * .... 44 mg.
Salicylamide .... 150 mg.
Acetaminophen * .... 150 mg.
Caffeine .... 32 mg.

MEDICIDE (SCENTED AND UNSCENTED)
Hospital disinfectant deodorant
(Hysan Corp.)

Orthophenylphenol 0.176%
Paratertiaryamylphenol 0.044%
Essential oils (scented only) 0.300%
Alcohol 53.460%

MEDICONE DRESSING (CREAM)
*For minor burns, wounds, raw skin sur-
faces, diaper rashes, sunburns*
(Medicone)

Each gram:
Benzocaine .... 5.0 mg.
Oxyquinoline sulfate .... 0.5 mg.
Cod liver oil .... 125.0 mg.
Zinc oxide .... 125.0 mg.
Menthol .... 1.8 mg.
Petrolatum
Lanolin
Talcum
Paraffin
Perfume

MEDICONET
*Medicated antiseptic, anti-pruritic, as-
tringent hygienic cloth wipe*
(Medicone)

Benzalkonium chloride 0.02%
Ethoxylated lanolin 0.5%
Methylparaben 0.15%
Hamamelis water 50%
Glycerin 10%
Purified water USP
Perfume .... q.s

MEDICOPASTE BANDAGE (UNNA'S BOOT DRESSING)

See GRAFCO MEDICOPASTE
BANDAGE (UNNA'S BOOT
DRESSING)

MEDIGEN, DR. NAYLOR'S

See DR. NAYLOR'S MEDIGEN

MEDIHALER-EPI
*Oral inhalation therapy; asthma and
emphysema*
(Riker Labs.)

Epinephrine bitartrate * .... 7.0 mg./ml.
Inert propellent

'76 Ed.

MEDIHALER-ERGOTAMINE
For relief of migraine
(Riker Labs.)

Each cc:
Ergotamine tartrate (in fine
particle suspension) * ...... 9.0 mg.

'76 Ed.

Each inhalation: valve controlled, limited
to 6 inhalations per 24 hrs.

MEDIHALER-ISO
*Oral inhalation therapy; asthma, em-
physema and chronic bronchitis*
(Riker Labs.)

Isoproterenol sulfate * ...... 2.0 mg./ml.
Inert propellent

'76 Ed.

MEDI-KOOL-PAK
Veterinary
(Thoroughbred)

Camphor *
Aluminum sulfate *
Spirits turpentine *
Tannic acid *
Methyl salicylate *
Boric acid *
Eucalyptus oil *
Myrbane oil *
Cedarleaf *
Tansy *
Menthol *
Tinct. of Cantharides *
Calcium acetate
Tinct. Arnica
Ethyl aminobenzoate
Peppermint oil
Cedarwood oil
Wormwood oil *†

†See Volatile oils

MEDI-KOOL-TITENER
Veterinary leg tightener
(Thoroughbred)

Gum camphor *
Methyl salicylate *
Tannic acid *
Spirits turpentine *
Oil peppermint
Oil myrbane *
Oil cedarleaf *
Oil eucalyptus *
Menthol *
Ethyl aminobenzoate
Tinct. Cantharides *
Tinct. Arnica
Oil cedarwood
Oil wormwood *†
Oil tansy *

†See Volatile oils

MEDI-MYCIN LOTION
For sunburn, insect bites, etc.
(Approved Pharm.)

Zirconium oxide
Pyrilamine maleate *
Benzocaine
Calamine
Actamer
Alcohol
Veegum
Glycerine

'76 Ed.

MEDI-QUIK FIRST AID SPRAY (AEROSOL)
Skin antiseptic and anesthetic
(Glenbrook Labs.)

Isobutane 35%
Benzalkonium chloride .... minor
Lidocaine .... minor
Camphor .... minor
Benzyl alcohol .... minor

MEDI-QUIK FIRST AID SPRAY (PUMP)
Skin antiseptic and anesthetic
(Glenbrook Labs.)

Polyethylene glycol 600 .... minor
Benzalkonium chloride .... minor
Lidocaine hydrochloride .... minor
Benzyl alcohol .... minor

MEDROL ACETATE TOPICAL
*Allergic dermatoses and inflammatory
skin diseases*
(Upjohn)

Each gm.:
Medrol acetate (Meth-
ylprednisolone
acetate) .... 2.5 mg. (0.25%);
10 mg. (1.0%)
Methylparaben .... 4 mg.
Butylparaben .... 3 mg.

MEDROL ENPAK
*Enema for adjunctive treatment of ul-
cerative colitis*
(Upjohn)

Each unit (reconstituted):
Medrol acetate (Methylprednis-
olone acetate) .... 40 mg.
Sodium chloride
Polysorbate 80

MEDROL TABLETS
Anti-inflammatory corticosteroid
(Upjohn)

Each tablet:
Medrol
(Methylpredniso-
lone) .... 2 mg.; 4 mg.; 8 mg.;
16 mg.; 24 mg.;
32 mg.

Starred ingredients (*) may be responsible for major toxic effects; consult Section II.

MEGACE
Antineoplastic
(Mead Johnson)

Each tablet:
Megestrol acetate .... 20 or 40 mg.

MELFIAT 105
Anorectic
(Reid-Provident)

Each capsule:
Phendimetrazine tartrate * .. 105 mg.

MELFIAT TABLETS
Anorectic
(Reid-Provident)

Each tablet:
Phendimetrazine tartrate * ... 35 mg.

MELLARIL (CONCENTRATE & TABLETS)
Tranquilizer
(Sandoz)

Concentrate (each ml.):
Thioridazine hydro-
chloride USP * ... 30 mg.; 100 mg.
Tablets (each):
Thioridazine hydro-
chloride USP * .... 10 mg.; 15 mg.;
25 mg.; 50 mg.;
100 mg.; 150 mg.;
or 200 mg.

MELLARIL-S SUSPENSION
(Sandoz)

Each 5 ml.:
Thioridazine * .... 25 mg.; 100 mg.

MELOIDS
Throat lozenges
(Cunningham Distributors)

Licorice
Menthol *
Capsicum

MELT
Anti-freeze
(Garry Labs.)

Ethylene glycol *

MEM TOILETRIES

Mem Co., Inc.
Northvale, N.J. 07647

Phone: 201-767-0100

See COSMETICS, Section VI, General
Formulations

MENEST
Estrogen therapy
(Beecham Labs.)

Each tablet:
Esterified estrogens,
U.S.P. .... 2.5 mg.; 1.25 mg.;
0.625 mg.; 0.3 mg.

MENESTREX
Relief of menstrual pain & tension
(Rex Laboratory, Inc.)

REGULAR (each capsule):
Quinine sulfate * .... 100 mg.
Salicylamide .... 125 mg.
Pyrilamine maleate .... 15 mg.
Caffeine .... 30 mg.
Ferric-o-phosphate .... 16 mg.
Niacin .... 5 mg.

EXTRA STRENGTH (each capsule):
Quinine sulfate * .... 130 mg.
Salicylamide .... 150 mg.
Pyrilamine maleate .... 15 mg.
Caffeine .... 30 mg.
Ferric-o-phosphate .... 16 mg.
Niacin .... 5 mg.

'76 Ed.

MENIC
For mental confusion of senility
(Geriatric Pharm.)

Each tablet:
Pentylenetetrazole * .... 100 mg.
Nicotinic acid .... 50 mg.

MENNEN ANTIPERSPIRANT SPRAY DEODORANT
(Mennen)

Active ingred.:
Aluminum chlorohydrate
Benzethonium chloride *
24% SD Alcohol 40
Other ingred.:
Water
Propylene glycol
Polysorbate-20
Fragrance

MENNEN BATH TALC
(Mennen)

Talc
Fragrance
Benzethonium chloride

MENNEN BRUSHLESS SHAVE (REGULAR & MENTHOL-ICED)
(Mennen)

Water
Stearic acid
Mineral oil
Potassium stearate
Glycerin
TEA-stearate
Mixed Isopropanol amine myristate
Titanium dioxide
Fragrance
Menthol (Menthol-Iced only)
Mixed Isopropanol amine lanolate
Methylparaben

MENNEN LATHER SHAVE MENTHOL ICED
(Mennen)

Water
Potassium stearate
Glycerin
Sodium stearate
Coconut oil
Potassium cocoate
Stearic acid
Sodium cocoate
Menthol
SD Alcohol 40
Boric acid
Sodium silicate
Camphor
Fragrance

MENNEN LATHER SHAVE REGULAR
(Mennen)

Water
Potassium stearate
Glycerin
Sodium stearate
Coconut oil
Potassium cocoate
Stearic acid
Sodium cocoate
Boric acid
Sodium silicate
Fragrance

MENNEN MEDICATED FACE CONDITIONER
(Mennen)

Active ingred.:
Salicylic acid *
SD Alcohol 40 * 59%
Other ingred.:
Water
Propylene glycol
Fragrance
Benzophenone-3
FD & C Red #4
FD & C Yellow #5

Starred ingredients (*) may be responsible for major toxic effects; consult Section II.

MENNEN PUSHBUTTON DEODORANT
(Mennen)

SD Alcohol 40 *
Isobutane
Propane
Dipropylene glycol
Fragrance
Benzethonium chloride

MENNEN SHAVE TALC
(Mennen)

Talc
Titanium dioxide
Fragrance
Iron oxides
Benzethonium chloride

MENRIUM 5-2
For management of emotional and somatic components of the menopausal syndrome
(Roche)

Each tablet:
Chlordiazepoxide * .... 5 mg.
Water-soluble esterified
   Estrogens .... 0.2 mg.

MENRIUM 5-4
For management of emotional and somatic components of the menopausal syndrome
(Roche)

Each tablet:
Chlordiazepoxide * .... 5 mg.
Water-soluble esterified
   Estrogens .... 0.4 mg.

MENRIUM 10-4
For management of emotional and somatic components of the menopausal syndrome
(Roche)

Each tablet:
Chlordiazepoxide * .... 10 mg.
Water-soluble esterified
   Estrogens .... 0.4 mg.

MENSTRA-EZE
Pre-menstrual tension; menstrual pain; replenish body iron
(Reese Chem.)

Each capsule:
Ferrous fumarate .... 55 mg.
Salicylamide .... 260 mg.
Ephedrine sulfate * .... 8 mg.
Quinine sulfate .... 16 mg.
Acetanilid .... 32 mg.

MENSTRESS CAPSULES
For cramps
(Pharmex)

Each capsule:
Cinnamyl ephedrine HCl *† ... 15 mg.
N-Acetyl-p-aminophenol * .. 3 gr.
Caffeine .... 1 gr.
Methapyrilene HCl * .... 12.5 mg.
Homatropine methyl bromide 0.25 mg.

†*See* Ephedrine

MENTHODERM
Liniment in a tube
(Barfred Research Labs.)

Methyl salicylate *
Menthol *
Eucalyptol *
Camphor *

'76 Ed.

MENTHOLATUM DEEP HEATING LOTION
Rubefacient, counterirritant
(Mentholatum)

Lanolin
Methyl salicylate * 20%
Menthol 6%

MENTHOLATUM DEEP HEATING RUB
Rubefacient, counterirritant
(Mentholatum)

Lanolin
Methyl salicylate * 12.7%
Menthol 5.9%
Oil eucalyptus *
Oil turpentine *

MENTHOLATUM OINTMENT
Rubefacient, nasal decongestant
(Mentholatum)

Menthol * 1.35%
Camphor * 9.00%
Petrolatum
Combined amount: .... <1%
   Oil sweet birch
   Oil pine
   Oil eucalyptus

MENTHOLATUM STICK
For chapped lips
(Mentholatum)

Octyl dimethyl PABA * 1.4%
Menthol
Camphor
Mixed Essential oils
Petrolatum

MENTROLZ TABLETS
Pre-menstrual tension, cramps, headache
(Mayer Labs.)

Each tablet:
Mayercin .... 300.5 mg.
Homatropine methyl
   bromide .... 0.5 mg.
Ammonium chloride ..... 300 mg.
Caffeine alk. .... 32 mg.
Acetophenetidin * .... 150 mg.
Salicylamide * .... 225 mg.

'76 Ed.

MEPERGAN FORTIS
Analgesic and sedative for moderate pain
(Wyeth Labs.)

Each capsule:
Meperidine hydrochloride * ... 50 mg.
Promethazine hydrochloride .. 25 mg.

MEPHOHAB (C.T. WHITE)
Anticonvulsant, sedative
(Bowman Pharm.)

Each tablet:
Mephobarbital * .... 32.4 mg.

MEPHYTON
Hemostatic agent
(MSD)

Each tablet:
Phytonadione (Vitamin K-1) ... 5 mg.

MEPRIAM
Tranquilizer
(Lemmon Co.)

Each tablet:
Meprobamate * .... 400 mg.

MEPROCON CMC
Tranquilizer
(CMC Research Div.)

Each tablet:
Meprobamate USP * .... 400 mg.

MEPROSPAN CAPSULES
Relief of anxiety and tension
(Wallace Labs.)

Each sustained release capsule:
Meprobamate * ... 200 mg. or 400 mg.

'76 Ed.

Starred ingredients (*) may be responsible for major toxic effects; consult Section II.

MERCODOL WITH DECAPRYN
Cough syrup
(Merrell Dow)

Each 5 cc.:
Codeine phosphate * .... 10 mg.
Nethamine (Etafedrine
  hydrochloride) .... 10 mg.
Phenylephrine hydrochloride * 5 mg.
Decapryn (Doxylamine
  succinate) * .... 6 mg.
Alcohol 5%
Syrup: Thyme, Tolu, Menthol, Sodium
  citrate

MERCO DUST MOP TREATMENT
(National-Purity Soap)

Petroleum distillate *
Cationic emulsifier *
Petroleum paraffin

MERC-O-DUST P
Seed disinfectant
(Seed-Treet)

Mercury pentanedione *† 2.0%

'76 Ed.

†*See* Mercury compounds

MERCOLIZED CREAM
Bleach cream
(Blistex)

Hydroquinone * 2.0%
Base: .... balance
  Water
  Mineral oil
  Propylene glycol
  Petrolatum
  Hydroxyethyl cellulose
  Sodium meta bisulfite
  Cetearyl alcohol
  Ceteareth 20

MERCRESIN TINCTURE
Antiseptic
(Upjohn)

Secondary-amyltricresols 1/10%
Orthohydroxyphenylmercuric
  chloride 1/10%
Acetone * 10%
Alcohol 50%

MERGAMMA N-M
Seed treatment
(Chipman Inc.)

Maneb 37.5%
Gamma BHC (from lindane) * .. 18.75%

MERLE NORMAN COSMETIC PRODUCTS
Beauty preparations & cosmetics

Merle Norman Cosmetics
9130 Bellanca Ave.
Los Angeles, Calif. 90045

Phone: 213-641-3000

See COSMETICS, Section VI, General
  Formulations

MEROPA LUBRICANTS
(Texaco Canada Ltd.)

Petroleum lubricating oil
Lead soap *
Sulfurized fatty oil

MESANTOIN TABLETS (Mephenytoin)
Anticonvulsant
(Sandoz)

Each tablet:
Mephenytoin USP * .... 100 mg.

MESUROL
Insecticide, bird repellent, molluscicide
(Mobay Chemical Corp.)

3,5-Dimethyl-4-(methylthio)phenol methylcarbamate *

META HENNA HAIR CARE PRODUCTS

Meta Henna Intl., Inc.
850 Nicholas Blvd.
Elk Grove Village, Ill. 60007

Phone: 312-593-3044

See COSMETICS, Section VI, General
  Formulations

METAHYDRIN
Diuretic
(Merrell Dow)

Each tablet:
Trichlormethiazide
  Pink .... 2 mg.
  Blue .... 4 mg.

METALENE
(Lester Labs.)

Synthetic detergents *

'76 Ed.

METAL KLEAN
(Sunbeam Appliance)

Methylene chloride * .... 70.0%/wt.
Methocel HB (Hydroxy-butyl
  methyl cellulose) .... 1.0%/wt.
Toluene * .... 2.4%/wt.
Paraffin wax .... 1.7%/wt.
Methanol .... 3.6%/wt.
Isopropyl alcohol .... 4.0%/wt.
Dowanol DPM (Dipropylene
  glycol methyl ether) .... 3.8%/wt.
Ammonium hydroxide 26° * 5.7%/wt.
Alkyl aryl sulfonate (bio-de-
  gradable detergent) .... 7.0%/wt.
Sodium chromate .... 0.02%/wt.

'76 Ed.

METAL TREAT CONCENTRATE
(Klean-Strip)

Phosphoric acid (75%) * .... >50%
Water .... >40%
Alcohols, Penetrants, & Rust
  inhibitors .... <10%

METANDREN
Androgen therapy
(CIBA Pharmaceutical)

Linguets:
  Methyltestosterone .... 5 mg.; 10 mg.

Tablets:
  Methyltestosterone .... 10 mg.; 25 mg.

METAQUAT GERMICIDAL CLEANER

See SPARTAN METAQUAT GERMI-
  CIDAL CLEANER

META SUDS
Detergent
(Pittsburgh Chem. Lab.)

Trisodium phosphate * 40%
Snow Flake Crystals 40%
Wetting agent 20%

'76 Ed.

METASYSTOX-R
Insecticide
(Mobay Chemical Corp.)

Oxydemeton methyl (S-(2-
  (Ethylsulfinyl)ethyl) O,O-dimethyl
  phosphorothioate) *

METATENSIN
Diuretic/antihypertensive
(Merrell Dow)

Each yellow tablet:
  Trichlormethiazide .... 2 mg.
  Reserpine .... 0.1 mg.

Each violet tablet:
  Trichlormethiazide .... 4 mg.
  Reserpine .... 0.1 mg.

Starred ingredients (*) may be responsible for major toxic effects; consult Section II.

METED SHAMPOO
Helps control oily dandruff
(CooperCare)

Sulfur 3%
Salicylic acid * 2%
Combination of highly concentrated detergents

METED-2 SHAMPOO
Helps control dry, scaly dandruff
(CooperCare)

Colloidal Sulfur 2.3%
Salicylic acid * 1.0%
Combination of detergents

METER DESCALER
(Consolidated Chem., Inc.)

Hydrochloric acid *

METHACIDE
Anthelmintic; dogs, cats
(Beecham Labs.)

Methylbenzene * ..... 0.1 gm.; 0.25 gm.;
0.50 gm.; 1.0 gm.;
3.0 gm.

METHAGUAL
Relief of minor muscular pains
(Gordon Labs.)

Methyl salicylate *
Guaiacol
Petrolatum base

METHAMPEX
CNS Stimulant; anorexiant
(Lemmon Co.)

Each tablet:
Methamphetamine
hydrochloride * .... 10 mg.

METHANOX PLUS
Residual fly spray concentrate
(Farnam Co.)

Methoxychlor, technical 21.0%
Butoxypolypropylene glycol 10.0%
Dimethyl phthalate 10.0%
Aromatic petroleum solvent * 57.0%

'76 Ed.

METHERGINE TABLETS
For prevention and control of postpartum hemorrhage
(Sandoz)

Each tablet:
Methylergonovine maleate
USP .... 0.2 mg.

METH-O-GAS
Fumigant
(Great Lakes Chem. Corp.)

Methyl bromide * 100%

"METHOMYL" COMPOSITION
Insecticide
(Du Pont)

Methomyl * 90%

METHOXONE-ESTER 500
Herbicide
(Chipman Inc.)

Butyl ester formulation of 2-methyl-4-chlorophenoxyacetic acid (MCP) *

MCPA equiv. 500 gm. per liter (present as butyl ester)

METHOXONE SODIUM 300
Herbicide
(Chipman Inc.)

MCPA equiv. (Sodium potassium salts of MCPA) * .... 300 gm. per liter

METHYL FUME
(Industrial Fumigant)

Methyl bromide * 100%

METICORTEN TABLETS
Anti-inflammatory
(Schering)

Each tablet:
Prednisone .... 1 mg.; 5 mg.

METI-DERM AEROSOL
Treatment of dermatoses
(Schering)

Prednisolone
50 mg./150 gm. container

METI-DERM CREAM 0.5%
Treatment of dermatoses
(Schering)

Each gram:
Prednisolone .... 5 mg.
Aluminum
chlorhydroxyallantoinate ... 2.5 mg.
Methylparaben .... 0.2 mg.
Butylparaben .... 1.8 mg.
Emulsion-type vehicle:
Propylene glycol monostearate
Stearic acid
Polyoxyethylene sorbitan monopalmitate
Isopropyl myristate
Propylene glycol
Purified water

METI-DERM w/NEOMYCIN AEROSOL
Treatment of dermatoses
(Schering)

Each 150 gm. container:
Prednisolone .... 50 mg.
Neomycin sulfate .... 50 mg.
Vehicle:
Isopropyl myristate
Propellant mixture:
Trichloromonofluoromethane
Dichlorodifluoromethane

METI-DERM w/NEOMYCIN OINTMENT
Treatment of dermatoses
(Schering)

Each gram:
Prednisolone .... 5 mg.
Neomycin sulfate (equiv. to 3.5
mg. neomycin base) .... 5 mg.
Methylparaben .... 0.2 mg.
Butylparaben .... 1.8 mg.
Petrolatum base

METIMYD OPHTHALMIC OINTMENT
Anti-inflammatory, antibacterial
(Schering)

Each gram:
Prednisolone acetate .... 5 mg.
Sodium sulfacetamide .... 100 mg.
Methylparaben .... 0.5 mg.
Propylparaben .... 0.1 mg.
Base:
Mineral oil
White petrolatum

METIMYD OPHTHALMIC SUSPENSION
Anti-inflammatory, antibacterial
(Schering)

Each cc:
Prednisolone acetate .... 5 mg.
Sodium sulfacetamide .... 100 mg.
Phenylethyl alcohol .... 5 mg.
Benzalkonium chloride ..... 0.25 mg.
Disodium hydrogen phosphate
Sodium dihydrogen phosphate
Tyloxapol
Sodium thiosulfate
Disodium edetate
Purified water

MET-L-RAX
Liquid floor polish
(Sanitek)

Acrylic polymer emulsion 12.2%
Diethylene glycol monoethyl
ether (Cellosolve) 3.1%
Polyethylene emulsion 1.7%
Tributoxyethyl phosphate 1.0%
Styrene maleic resin 0.8%
Dibutyl phthalate 0.5%
Nonionic surfactant 0.3%
Formalin 0.2%
Defoamer, Ammonia, Fluoro-
chemical surfactant .... trace
Water .... balance

Starred ingredients (*) may be responsible for major toxic effects; consult Section II.

METRA-FOG
Insecticide; flies, mosquitoes
(National Chemsearch)

Aromatic petroleum derivative solvent *	95.10%
Fenthion	3.25%
2,2-Dichlorovinyl dimethyl phosphate	1.30%
Related compounds	0.10%

METRATE TABLETS
Treatment of acid urinary tract infections of horses
(Daniels, Dr. A.C.)

Each tablet:
Hexamethylenamine *	40 gr.
Potassium nitrate *	40 gr.

METRAZOL (TABLETS & LIQUIDUM)
CNS stimulant
(Knoll Pharm.)

Each tablet or 5 cc:
Metrazol (Pentylenetetrazol) *	100 mg.
Alcohol (Liquidum only)	15%

MEVANIN-C
Vitamin & mineral supplement
(Beutlich, Inc.)

Each capsule:
Ferrous sulfate *	65 mg.
Vitamin A	3000 USP units
Vitamin D	300 USP units
Plus polyvitamins & minerals	

MEVATINIC-C
Hematinic
(Beutlich, Inc.)

Ferrous sulfate (exsiccated) *	200 mg.
Ascorbic acid	225 mg.
Folic acid	0.1 mg.
Copper (from copper sulfate)	0.33 mg.
Plus polyvitamins and minerals	

MEXSANA MEDICATED POWDER
(Plough)

Zinc oxide
Cornstarch
Kaolin
Irgasan DP-300

MEYER'S BEATSALL CRYSTALS
Fumigant, insecticide
(Meyer, T.)

Paradichlorobenzene *	100%

'76 Ed.

MEYER'S BEATSALL FOG SPRAY
Insecticide
(Meyer, T.)

Petroleum distillate *	98.206%
Tech. Piperonyl butoxide	1.496%
Pyrethrins	0.298%

'76 Ed.

MEYER'S CHLORDANE EMULSION CONCENTRATE
Insecticide
(Meyer, T.)

Chlordane, tech. *	46.0%
Petroleum distillate *	43.5%

'76 Ed.

MEYER'S LINDANE SPRAY
Insecticide
(Meyer, T.)

Gamma isomer of benzene hexachloride (from lindane)	0.5%
Petroleum distillate *	99.5%

'76 Ed.

MEYER'S MIX POWDER
Insecticide - for roaches, house fleas, silverfish
(Meyer, T.)

Pyrethrins	not less than 0.15%
Sodium fluoride *	not less than 39.0%

'76 Ed.

MFA BACKRUBBER OIL
Insecticide
(MFA Oil Co.)

Ronnel	1.00%
Mineral oil	49.21%
Deodorized Kerosene *	49.21%

MFA CHICKEN DUSTER
Insecticide
(MFA Oil Co.)

Malathion *	4%

MFA CIODRIN E.C. INSECTICIDE
For use on livestock
(MFA Oil Co.)

Dimethyl phosphate of alpha-methylbenzyl 3-hydroxy-cis-crotonate *	25.5%
Petroleum hydrocarbons	59.7%

MFA CTC
Prevents termites
(MFA Oil Co.)

Technical Chlordane *	74.35%
Petroleum hydrocarbons	17.65%

MFA DAIRY CATTLE DUST
Insecticide
(MFA Oil Co.)

Methoxychlor (technical) *	50%

MFA 2,4-D AMINE WEED KILLER
Herbicide
(MFA Oil Co.)

Dimethylamine salt of 2,4-dichlorophenoxyacetic acid *	49.4%

MFA DISINFECTANT AND DEODORANT
Disinfectant, deodorant
(MFA Oil Co.)

Coal tar neutral oils *	63.0%
Soap	17.0%
Phenols *	10.0%

MFA DRY DIP
Louse control on swine, cattle, & horses
(MFA Oil Co.)

Co-Ral	1.0%

MFA EVERGREEN SPRAY
Insecticide
(MFA Oil Co.)

Toxaphene *	49.73%
1,1-Bis(p-chlorophenyl)-2,2,2, trichloroethanol	5.07%
Other isomers & reaction products	1.27%
Petroleum hydrocarbons	33.93%

MFA GARDEN DUST
Insecticide-fungicide
(MFA Oil Co.)

Methoxychlor (technical)	5.0%
Captan	5.0%
Malathion *	4.0%

MFA GARDEN WEEDER
(MFA Oil Co.)

Dimethyl ester of tetrachloroterephthalic acid	2.5%

MFA GARDEN WEED PREVENTER
(MFA Oil Co.)

Dimethyl ester of tetrachloroterephthalic acid *	75%

MFA LAWN WEED KILLER
Herbicide
(MFA Oil Co.)

Dimethylamine salt of 2,4-dichlorophenoxyacetic acid *	13.52%
Dimethylamine salt of dicamba (3,6-Dichloro-o-anisic acid)	6.76%
Dimethylamine salt of related acids	1.19%

Starred ingredients (*) may be responsible for major toxic effects; consult Section II.

MFA LIVESTOCK DUST
Insecticide
(MFA Oil Co.)

O,O-Diethyl O-(3-chloro-4-methyl-2-
oxo-(2H)-1-benzopyran-7-yl)
phosphorothioate 1.0%

MFA LIVESTOCK TOXAPHENE
Insecticide
(MFA Oil Co.)

Toxaphene * 59.0%
Petroleum hydrocarbons 28.5%

MFA LO-V SUPER BRUSH KILLER
Herbicide
(MFA Oil Co.)

Mixed Octyl ester of 2,4-dichloro-
phenoxyacetic acid * 34.2%
Mixed Octyl ester of 2,4,5-trichlo-
rophenoxyacetic acid * 32.6%

MFA LO-V 2,4,5-T
Herbicide
(MFA Oil Co.)

Mixed Octyl ester of 2,4,5-trichlo-
rophenoxyacetic acid * 65.2%

MFA MALACOAT
*Protection of stored grain against in-
sects*
(MFA Oil Co.)

Malathion * 57%
Xylene * 32%

MFA MALA-SPRAY
Insecticide
(MFA Oil Co.)

Malathion * 57%
Aromatic petroleum derivative
solvent * 35%

MFA MALATHION E.C.
For controlling field crop insects
(MFA Oil Co.)

Malathion * 57%
Aromatic petroleum derivative
solvent * 35%

MFA METHOXYCHLOR E.C.
Insecticide
(MFA Oil Co.)

Methoxychlor (technical) 24.0%
Aromatic petroleum
hydrocarbon * 72.5%

MFA MULTI SPRAY - FORMULA A
Insecticide
(MFA Oil Co.)

Malathion * 30.00%
Captan 16.66%

MFA MULTI SPRAY - FORMULA B
Insecticide
(MFA Oil Co.)

Methoxychlor (technical) * 30.7%
Zineb 25.0%

MFA PYRENONE E.C.
Insecticide
(MFA Oil Co.)

Petroleum solvents * 83%
Technical Piperonyl butoxide 10%
Pyrethrins 1%

MFA RAT & MOUSE KILLER (READY TO USE)
Rodenticide
(MFA Oil Co.)

3-(Alpha-acetonylfurfuryl)-4-hy-
droxy-coumarin 0.025%

MFA RONNEL GRANULES
Controls lice on swine
(MFA Oil Co.)

Ronnel 5%

MFA RON-PONA FLY BAIT
Insecticide
(MFA Oil Co.)

Ronnel 0.500%
2,2-Dichlorovinyl dimethyl
phosphate 0.228%
Related compounds 0.022%

MFA ROSE AND FLORAL DUST
Insecticide
(MFA Oil Co.)

Zineb 3.9%
Dinitro (1-methyl heptyl) phenyl
crotonate 0.9%
Related compounds 0.1%
Gamma isomer of benzene hexachloride from lindane 1.0%
Methoxychlor 5.0%
1,1-Bis(chlorphenyl)-2,2,2-
trichloroethanol 1.48%

MFA ROTENONE DUST
Insecticide
(MFA Oil Co.)

Rotenone 1.66%
Other cube resins 3.34%

MFA TOMATO DUST
Insecticide-fungicide
(MFA Oil Co.)

Toxaphene * 5.0%
Zineb 5.0%

MFA NO. 6 TOXAPHENE E.C.
Insecticide for field crops
(MFA Oil Co.)

Toxaphene * 58.98%
Petroleum hydrocarbons 38.02%

MFA NO. 4 WEED KILLER
Herbicide
(MFA Oil Co.)

Butyl ester of 2,4-dichlorophenoxy-
acetic acid * 57.6%

MFA NO. 6 WEED KILLER
Herbicide
(MFA Oil Co.)

Butyl ester of 2,4-dichlorophenox-
yacetic acid * 77.48%

MGK ALLETHRIN CONC. 2.5%
Insecticide
(MGK)

Petroleum distillate * 97.28%
Allethrin (Allyl homolog of Ci-
nerin I) 2.50%
Related compounds 0.22%

MGK ALLETHRIN CONC. 20%
Insecticide
(MGK)

Petroleum distillate * 78.25%
Allethrin (Allyl homolog of Ci-
nerin I) * 20.00%
Related compounds 1.75%

MGK BIG GAME REPELLENT - BGR-W
For protection of conifer seedlings
(MGK)

Putrescent whole egg solids 5%
Inert ingredients 95%

MGK BIG GAME REPELLENT CONCENTRATE
For protection of conifer seedlings
(MGK)

Putrescent whole egg solids 15%
Inert ingredients 85%

Starred ingredients (*) may be responsible for major toxic effects; consult Section II.

MGK DIETHYL TOLUAMIDE
For use in manufacturing repellents for personal use
(MGK)

N,N-Diethyl toluamide *	100%
Meta isomer	95% (min.)
Other isomers	5% (max.)

MGK DOG AND CAT REPELLENT
(MGK)

Methyl nonyl ketone *†

†*See* Ketone solvents

MGK INSECT LOOSENER
Insecticide
(MGK)

Oil *†	36%
Pyrethrins	9%

†*See* Kerosene

MGK PYROCIDE BOOSTER O
Insecticide
(MGK)

Petroleum distillate *	94.75%
Tech. Piperonyl butoxide	3.75%
Pyrethrins	1.50%

MGK REPELLENT 11
For use in manufactuing repellents for personal use and in pet sprays
(MGK)

2,3:4,5-Bis(2-butylene)tetrahydro-2-furaldehyde *	100%

MGK REPELLENT 326
For use in manufacturing repellents for personal use and in cattle sprays
(MGK)

Di-n-propyl isocinchomeronate *	100%

MGK REPELLENT 874
Repellent
(MGK)

2-Hydroxyethyl-n-octyl sulfide	95%
Other related compounds	5%

MH-30
Plant growth regulant
(Uniroyal Chem.)

Maleic hydrazide *	30%
Diethanolamine	28%
Inerts	42%
Surfactant	
Water	

M H - 30 LIQUID MALEIC HYDRAZIDE
Herbicide & plant growth inhibitor
(FMC Corp., Agricultural Chem. Div.)

Diethanolamine salt of 1,2-dihydropyridazine-3,6-dione *	58.00%

MICATIN CREAM AND LOTION
Antifungal
(Ortho-Dermatology)

Miconazole nitrate	2%

MICRIN PLUS BRAND MOUTHWASH
(Johnson & Johnson)

Ethyl alcohol	16%
Menthol	
Thymol	
Eucalyptol	
Oil of peppermint	
Methyl salicylate	
Cetylpyridinium chloride	
Water	
Emollients	
Wetting agents	
Certified dyes	
Saccharin	

MICROCOP FUNGICIDE

See LILLY/MILLER MICROCOP FUNGICIDE

MICRO-GEN PRODUCTS
(Micro-Gen Equipment Corp.)

Phone: 414-631-2111

In case of an emergency involving a Micro-Gen product, contact S. C. Johnson & Son, Inc.; S. C. Johnson will accept collect calls from physicians and Poison Control Centers handling cases involving their products. This emergency telephone service is maintained 24 hours a day, 7 days a week. To insure contact with technically qualified personnel, inform the long distance operator that the call is an emergency. Then request person to person contact with a member of the S. C. Johnson & Son, Inc., emergency call panel.

MICROIL
Lubricant
(Kano)

Refined Petroleum oil *

MICRO-K EXTENCAPS
Potassium supplement
(Robins)

Each capsule:	
Potassium chloride *	600 mg.

MICRO-KIL 10
Hospital disinfectant
(Varley, James)

Isopropyl alcohol *	25.29%
o-Phenyl phenol *	2.94%
o-Benzyl-p-chlorophenol *	7.05%
Potassium hydroxide	2.71%
Sodium dodecylbenzene sulfonate	1.48%
p-tertiary Amyl phenol	0.10%
Essential oils	0.25%
Sodium lauryl alcohol sulfate	0.20%
Sodium tripolyphosphate	0.13%

MICRONOR TABLETS
Oral contraceptive
(Ortho)

Each tablet:	
Norethindrone	0.35 mg.

MICROPORE
(Carter's Ink)

PRC resin
Plasticizers
Solvent (1-5 Pentane diol) *†
Surfactant
Dyes

'76 Ed.

†*See* Inks, Section VI, General Formulations

MICROSTIX
Nitrite, total bacteria and gram negative bacteria test reagent strip
(Ames)

Nitrite test area:
  p-Arsinilic acid
  N-(1-Naphthyl)ethylenediamine dihydrochloride acid buffer

Total Bacteria test area:
  Bovine brain/heart infusion
  Triphenyltetrazolium chloride

Gram Negative test area:
  Bovine brain/heart infusion
  Triphenyltetrazolium chloride
  Sodium desoxycholate

MIDLAND GAS-O-CIDE
Liquid gas fumigant
(Midland Labs.)

Ethylene dichloride
Carbon tetrachloride *

MIDLAND MILL-O-CIDE 100
Contact insecticide
(Midland Labs.)

Refined Mineral oil *
N-Octyl bicycloheptene dicarboximide
Methyl salicylate *
Technical Piperonyl butoxide
Pyrethrins
Allethrins *

Starred ingredients (*) may be responsible for major toxic effects; consult Section II.

MIDLAND WARE-O-SPRAY
Space spray
(Midland Labs.)

Refined Mineral oil
Aromatic petroleum derivatives *
Malathion *
Piperonyl butoxide, technical
Pyrethrins

MIDOL
Antispasmodic-analgesic
(Glenbrook Labs.)

Aspirin *	454 mg.
Cinnamedrine	14.9 mg.
Caffeine	32.4 mg.

MIDRAN DECONGESTANT TABLETS
(Columbia Med.)

Each tablet:
Phenylephrine HCl *	5 mg.
Chlorpheniramine maleate *	2 mg.
Salicylamide *	1 1/2 gr.
Acetaminophen *	1/2 gr.
Caffeine *	1/2 gr.

MIKROKLENE DF

See KLENZADE MIKROKLENE DF

MILDEWCIDE
Protection against mildew and musty odors
(Vapor Products)

Paraformaldehyde * 100%

'76 Ed.

MILDEWDISK
Mildew preventive
(Vapor Products)

Biphenyl *	95%
Paper disk	5%

'76 Ed.

MILDEW STOP
Mildew preventive
(Cardinal Products Corp.)

Paraformaldehyde * 100%

'76 Ed.

MILDEW STOP SPRAY
Mold-mildew and musty odor preventative
(Cardinal Products Corp.)

Propellant (Freon 11-12 (50/50))	55.0%
1,1,1-Trichloroethene *	25.9%
Isopropyl alcohol (anhydrous)	17.8%
Perfume oil	0.4%

'76 Ed.

MILDU-CURE

See MORGRO MILDU-CURE

MILES NERVINE CAPSULE-SHAPED TABLET
Nighttime sleep aid
(Miles Labs., Inc.)

Each tablet:
Pyrilamine maleate * .... 25 mg.

MILKADE, HAPPY JACK

See HAPPY JACK MILKADE

MILKINOL
Laxative
(Kremers-Urban)

Liquid petrolatum
Dioctyl sodium sulfosuccinate *

MILKY BATH BUBBLES
(House of Lowell, Inc.)

TEA-lauryl sulfate *
Lauramide DEA
Modified Polystyrene latex
Perfume *
Formaldehyde
D & C color

MILLERHAUS' FAMOUS LINIMENT
Rubefacient, counterirritant
(C.T.S. Labs.)

Oil eucalyptus *
Turpentine *
Oil mustard (syn.) *
Methyl salicylate (syn.) *
Oil sassafras (imitation) *
Pine oil *
Camphor *
Refined Kerosene *
Certified color

MILLER LIME SULFUR SOLUTION
Fungicide
(Miller Chem. & Fert.)

Calcium polysulphide * 29%

MILLER "8" LIQUID MALATHION
Insecticide
(Miller Chem. & Fert.)

Malathion * 79%

MILLER LIQUID "55" MALATHION
Insecticide
(Miller Chem. & Fert.)

Malathion *	55%
Xylene range aromatic solvent *	36%

MILLER MYLONE 25-D MICO-FUME
Fungicide
(Miller Chem. & Fert.)

3,5-Dimethyltetrahydro-1,3,5-2H-
thiadiazine-2-thione * 25.5%

MILLER-NORRIS PREMIUM FOAM SPRAY & WIPE CLEANER
Germicidal and surface deodorant
(Miller-Norris Co.)

N-Alkyl (60%, C14; 30%, C16; 5%, C12; 5%, C18) dimethyl benzyl ammonium chloride	0.076%
N-Alkyl (50%, C12; 30%, C14; 17%, C16; 3%, C18) dimethyl ethyl-benzyl ammonium chloride	0.076%
Sodium metasilicate	0.24%
Essential oils	0.20%
Inert ingred.:	99.408%
Detergents	
Cleaners	
Builder and propellant	

'76 Ed.

MILLER PARATHION "8" LIQUID
Insecticide
(Miller Chem. & Fert.)

Parathion * 79%

MILLER'S #4 ESTER
Herbicide
(Miller Chem. Co.)

Butyl ester of 2,4-dichloro phenoxy
acetic acid * 56.5%

'76 Ed.

MILLER'S #6 ESTER
Herbicide
(Miller Chem. Co.)

Butyl ester of 2,4-dichloro phenoxy
acetic acid * 78%

'76 Ed.

MILLER SEVIN #2 AQUA
Insecticide
(Miller Chem. & Fert.)

Carbaryl (1-Naphthyl N-
methylcarbamate) * 21.50%

MILLER SEVIN #5 AQUA
Insecticide
(Miller Chem. & Fert.)

Carbaryl (1-Naphthyl N-
methylcarbamate) * 53.68%

MILLER'S LO VOL #4 2,4-D ESTER
Herbicide
(Miller Chem. Co.)

Iso-octyl ester of 2,4-dichloro phenoxy acetic acid * 69%

'76 Ed.

MILLER'S RAT & MOUSE BAIT
(Chas. H. Lilly)

Warfarin 0.025%
Sulfaquinoxaline 0.025%

MILLER'S WASPTRAP
(Chas. H. Lilly)

N-Pentyl-valerate 100%

MILLIONAIRE AFTER SHAVE & COLOGNE
(Mennen)

SD Alcohol 40 *
Water
Fragrance
Propylene glycol
PEG-60 hydrogenated castor oil
Benzophenone-3
FD & C Yellow #5
FD & C Red #4
D & C Green #5

MILLIONAIRE STICK DEODORANT
(Mennen)

Propylene glycol
Water
Sodium stearate
Fragrance
Triclosan
FD & C Yellow #5
FD & C Red #4
D & C Green #5

MILL-O-CIDE 100

See MIDLAND MILL-O-CIDE 100

MILL-O-CIDE SUPER STRENGTH
Contact insecticide
(Midland Labs.)

Active ingredients: 100%
  Refined Mineral oil *
  N-Octyl bicycloheptene
    dicarboximide *
  Piperonyl butoxide, technical
  Methyl salicylate *
  Pyrethrins
  Allethrin (Allyl homologue of
    Cinerin I) *

MIL-NOR CRYSTAL CLEAR DUST MOP TREATMENT
(Miller-Norris Co.)

Petroleum distillate *

'76 Ed.

MIL-NOR LEMON DISINFECTANT
(Miller-Norris Co.)

Active ingredients: 7.1%
  Alkyl (C14, 58%; C16, 28%; C12, 14%)
    dimethyl benzyl ammonium
    chloride *
  Isopropanol
  Essential oils *

'76 Ed.

MIL-NOR SPRAY 66
*Universal heavy duty cleaner & de-
greaser*
(Miller-Norris Co.)

Contains Alkali *

'76 Ed.

MILOCEP
Herbicide
(Ciba-Geigy Ag. Div.)

Metolachlor * 36.3%
Propazine * 18.7%

MILOGARD 4L
Herbicide
(Ciba-Geigy Ag. Div.)

Propazine * 43%

MILOGARD 80W
Herbicide
(Ciba-Geigy Ag. Div.)

Propazine * 80%

MILPATH (200 & 400)
For gastrointestinal disorders
(Wallace Labs.)

Each tablet:
  Meprobamate * .... 200 mg. or 400 mg.
  Tridihexethyl chloride *† .... 25 mg.

'76 Ed.

†*See* Atropine

MILPREM (200 & 400)
*For physiological & emotional symp-
toms of the menopause*
(Wallace Labs.)

Each tablet:
  Meprobamate * .... 200 mg. or 400 mg.
  Conjugated estrogens .... 0.45 mg.

'76 Ed.

MILTON BRADLEY TOYS AND SCHOOL SUPPLIES

See BRADLEY, MILTON, TOYS AND
SCHOOL SUPPLIES

MILTOWN
Relief of anxiety and tension
(Wallace Labs.)

Each tablet:
  Meprobamate * ..... 200 mg.; 400 mg.

'76 Ed.

MILTRATE-10
Prophylaxis of pain in angina pectoris
(Wallace Labs.)

Each tablet:
  Meprobamate .... 200 mg.
  Pentaerythritol tetranitrate *   10 mg.

'76 Ed.

MILTRATE-20
Prophylaxis of pain in angina pectoris
(Wallace Labs.)

Each tablet:
  Meprobamate .... 200 mg.
  Pentaerythritol tetranitrate *   20 mg.

'76 Ed.

MINICAPS
Vitamin supplement
(Wesley Pharm.)

Each capsule:
  Vitamin A .... 5000 U.S.P. Units
  Vitamin D .... 400 U.S.P. Units
  Plus multivitamins

MINI-LIX
For asthma
(Ferndale Labs.)

Each tablespoon (15 cc):
  Aminophylline (anhydrous) *   100 mg.
  Alcohol 20%/v
  Sugar free

MINI-MIST INSTANT HAIR REFRESHANT
(Block Drug)

Glyceryl starch
SD Alcohol 40
Fragrance
Isobutane
Methylene chloride

MINIPLEX
Vitamin supplement
(Wesley Pharm.)

Each capsule:
  Vitamin A (1.4 mg.) .... 5,000 I.U.
  Vitamin D (10 mcg.) .... 400 I.U.
  Iron .... 13.4 mg.
  Plus multivitamins and minerals

Starred ingredients (*) may be responsible for major toxic effects; consult Section II.

MINI-POO DRY SHAMPOO
(Block Drug)

Talc
Magnesium carbonate
Fragrance

MINIT-RUB
Analgesic ointment
(Bristol-Myers)

	by weight
Anhydrous Lanolin	4.5%
Camphor *	2.3%
Menthol *	3.5%
Methyl salicylate *	15.0%

MINK DIFFERENCE HAIR SPRAYS
(Gillette Co., Personal Care Div.)

The Gillette Co., Personal Care Div., Boston, Mass. 02199 will receive collect phone calls from poison control centers or physicians asking for emergency toxicological information about the company's products.

Phone: 617-421-7000

MINNETONKA COSMETIC PRODUCTS

Minnetonka, Inc.
Jonathan Industrial Center
Chaska, Minn. 55318

Phone: 612-448-4181

See COSMETICS, Section VI, General Formulations

MINOTAL
Analgesic
(Carnrick Labs.)

Each tablet:
Acetaminophen *	325 mg.
Sodium butabarbital	15 mg.

MINTEFFECT, FOREMOST 4510

See FOREMOST 4510 MINTEFFECT

MINTENE
Disinfectant; institutional and commercial use
(Hysan Corp.)

Isopropyl alcohol *	17.65%
Soap	11.00%
Terpineol	6.45%
Methyl salicylate *	4.14%
Ortho-benzyl para-chlorophenol	3.74%
Oil of peppermint USP	0.01%
Oil of spearmint USP	0.01%

MINTENE-5
Germicide, fungicide, disinfectant and deodorant
(Puritan Chem. Co.)

4-Chloro-2-cyclopentyl phenol	2.0%
Isopropyl alcohol *	15.3%
Sodium dodecyl benzene sulfonate	3.5%
Orthophenyl phenol	2.0%

MINTERENE
Disinfectant cleaner; institutional and industrial use
(Schneid)

Active ingredients:	23.20%

Isopropanol *
Methyl salicylate *
N-Alkyl (60% C14, 30% C16, 5% C12, 5% C18) dimethyl benzyl ammonium chlorides *
N-Alkyl (50% C12, 30% C14, 17% C16, 3% C18) dimethyl ethylbenzyl ammonium chlorides *
Mint essential oils

Inert ingredients:	76.80%

Water
Polyethoxylated nonyl phenol

'76 Ed.

MINTEX WATERLESS HAND CLEANER (PASTE TYPE)
(Savogran)

Mineral spirits *	35-55%
Oleic acid	<10%
Surface active agents, etc.	<20%

MINTEZOL CHEWABLE TABLETS
Anthelmintic
(MSD)

Each tablet:
Thiabendazole *	500 mg.

MINTEZOL SUSPENSION
Anthelmintic
(MSD)

Each 5 cc:
Thiabendazole *	500 mg.

MINT GLO

See LARSON'S MINT GLO

MINTIDE-5 DISINFECTANT
(Weil Chem.)

Active ingred.:	28.56%

Isopropyl alcohol *
Vegetable oil soap
o-Benzyl-p-chlorophenol *
Methyl salicylate *

MINTO-CHLOR SYRUP
Expectorant
(Vale)

Each fl. oz.:
Alcohol	2%
Potassium citrate	1.296 gm.
Tolu syrup	q.s.

MINTO-CHLOR SYRUP WITH CODEINE
Cough suppressant
(Vale)

Each fl. oz.:
Alcohol	2%
Codeine sulfate *	59.1 mg.
Potassium citrate	1.296 gm.
Tolu syrup	q.s.

MINT-O-DIS
Disinfectant
(Schneid)

Isopropyl alcohol *	18.44%
Potassium coconut soap	6.02%
Sodium orthobenzylparachlorophenate	3.76%
Methyl salicylate *	2.00%
Essential oils	0.32%

'76 Ed.

MINT-O-FECT

See LEEDSALL MINT-O-FECT

MINT-O-GREEN, PL

See PL MINT-O-GREEN

MINTOL
Disinfectant
(Dolge)

Isopropanol	6%
o-Benzyl-p-chlorophenol	5%
Potassium castor oil soap	4%
Water	
Dyestuff	trace

MINTOL-128
Disinfectant
(Dolge)

Isopropanol *	18-19%
Potassium ricinoleate	7-8%
o-Phenylphenol	5%
o-Benzyl-p-chlorophenol	3%
p-tert-Amylphenol	2%
Tetrasodium ethylenediaminetetraacetate	1-2%
Essential oils	trace
Propargyl alcohol	trace
Dyestuff	trace

Starred ingredients (*) may be responsible for major toxic effects; consult Section II.

MINT-O-SOL
Germicide, disinfectant, deodorant
(Consolidated Chem., Inc.)

Sodium carbonate *
Nonionic surfactant
Quaternary ammonium salt *
Sodium tripolyphosphate *
Water
Essential oils
Color

MIRACID
Soil acidifier & plant food
(Stern's Garden Products)

Nitrogen	30.0%
Phosphoric acid *	10.0%
Soluble Potash *	10.0%
Polyminerals	

MIRACLE
Germicidal disinfectant and odor neutralizer; industrial and institutional use
(Scientific International)

Active ingredients:	59.80%
Isopropyl alcohol *	
Triethylene glycol	
Essential oils *	
N-Alkyl (C14, C12, C16) dimethyl benzyl ammonium chloride *	
Inert ingredients:	40.20%
Dichlorodifluoromethane	
Water	
Diethanolamine salts of the fatty acids of coconut oil	

MIRACLE ALGAE KILLER
Home aquarium use
(Miracle Pet Products)

3-(p-Chlorophenyl)-1,1-dimethylurea	1.6%
Deionized water	98.4%

'76 Ed.

MIRACLE ANCHOR ADHESIVE (HT4620)
(Miracle Adhesives)

Neoprene rubber
Pigments
Resins
Aromatic hydrocarbon *

MIRACLE AQUARIUM CLEANER DISINFECTANT
(Miracle Pet Products)

Potassium permanganate *	8.0%
Copper sulfate *	2.5%
Deionized water	89.5%

'76 Ed.

MIRACLE CERAMIC TILE CEMENT (MA-200)
(Miracle Adhesives)

Synthetic latex
Resins
Clay
Water 35%
Wetting agents

MIRACLE CHLORINE/FLUORINE REMOVER
Water conditioner for aquarium use
(Miracle Pet Products)

Each tablet:	
Subsulfites and rhodonides of sodium and iron	7.0%
Sodium perborate *	5.0%
Polyvinyl-pyrrolidone	0.5%
Sodium chloride *	87.5%

'76 Ed.

MIRACLE CLEAR-ICH MARINE
Aquarium use
(Miracle Pet Products)

Copper chelate	0.12%
Distilled water from copper-free stills	99.88%

'76 Ed.

MIRACLE DRY WALL ADHESIVE
(Miracle Adhesives)

Rubber
Resin
Pigments
Aliphatic petroleum hydrocarbon *

MIRACLE FISH STERILIZER
General antiseptic; aquarium use
(Miracle Pet Products)

Sodium chloride	10.00%
Methylene blue	1.00%
Malachite green	0.10%
Acriflavine	0.05%
Deionized water	88.85%

'76 Ed.

MIRACLE-GRO
Plant food
(Stern's Garden Products)

Nitrogen	15.0%
Phosphoric acid *	30.0%
Soluble Potash *	15.0%
Polyminerals	

MIRACLE-GRO FOR ROSES
Plant food
(Stern's Garden Products)

Nitrogen	18.0%
Phosphoric acid *	24.0%
Soluble Potash *	16.0%
Polyminerals	

MIRACLE-GRO FOR TOMATOES
(Stern's Garden Products)

Total Nitrogen (N)	18%
4.4% Ammoniacal nitrogen	
6.0% Nitrate nitrogen	
7.6% Nitrogen derived from urea	
Available Phosphoric acid (P2O5) *	18%
Soluble Potash (K2O) *	21%
Polyminerals	

MIRACLE ICH REMEDY
Treatment of ichthyophthirius; aquarium use
(Miracle Pet Products)

Malachite green	0.40%
Acriflavine	0.05%
Quinine sulfate	0.04%
Deionized water	99.51%

'76 Ed.

MIRACLE PLANT FERTILIZER
Aids plant growth in aquariums
(Miracle Pet Products)

Potassium nitrate	5.0%
Calcium phosphate	5.0%
Calcium sulfate	2.5%
Magnesium sulfate	2.5%
Sodium chloride	2.5%
Trace elements	1.0%
Water	81.5%

'76 Ed.

MIRACLE PLASTICS BIRD SPRAY MIST
To control lice and mites of pet birds
(Miracle Plastics)

Pyrethrins	0.090%
Technical Piperonyl butoxide	0.180%
N-Octyl bicycloheptene dicarboximide	0.300%
Petroleum distillates	0.430%
Triethylene glycol	0.075%
Propylene glycol	0.075%

'76 Ed.

MIRACLE PLASTICS CAT FLEA & TICK SPRAY
(Miracle Plastics)

Pyrethrins	0.070%
Technical Piperonyl butoxide	0.140%
N-Octyl bicycloheptene dicarboximide	0.230%
Methoxychlor (technical)	0.500%
2:3:4:5-Bis(2-butylene)tetrahydro-2-furaldehyde	0.200%
Petroleum distillates	6.360%

'76 Ed.

Starred ingredients (*) may be responsible for major toxic effects; consult Section II.

MIRACLE PLASTICS FLEA & TICK SPRAY FOR DOGS
(Miracle Plastics)

Pyrethrins	0.070%
Technical Piperonyl butoxide	0.140%
N-Octyl bicycloheptene dicarboximide	0.230%
Methoxychlor (technical)	0.500%
2:3:4:5-Bis(2-butylene)tetrahydro-2-furaldehyde	0.200%
Petroleum distillates	6.360%

'76 Ed.

MIRACLE PLASTICS HAMSTER SPRAY
Kills fleas, deodorizes
(Miracle Plastics)

Pyrethrins	0.045%
Technical Piperonyl butoxide	0.090%
N-Octyl bicycloheptene dicarboximide	0.150%
Petroleum distillates	0.215%
Propylene glycol	0.075%
Triethylene glycol	0.075%

'76 Ed.

MIRACLE STARTR-WATR
Makes tap water suitable for aquariums
(Miracle Pet Products)

Sodium thiosulfate *	24.00%
Methylene blue	0.02%
Potassium permanganate	0.25%
Deionized, copper-free water	75.73%

'76 Ed.

MIRACLE TONIC
For fungus, ich, finrot; aquarium use
(Miracle Pet Products)

Methylene blue	1.50%
Malachite green	0.10%
Acriflavine	0.05%
Quinine sulfate	0.04%
Distilled water	98.31%

'76 Ed.

MIRACLE TUB CAULK
(Miracle Adhesives)

Synthetic resins
Calcium carbonate
Vinyl acrylic resin

MIRACLE TURTLE BATH
Anti-bacterial turtle medication; aquarium use
(Miracle Pet Products)

Sodium sulfaquinoxaline	0.40%
Sodium sulfathiazole	0.30%
Sodium sulfamethazine	0.30%
Sodium sulfamerazine	0.30%
Neomycin sulfate	0.20%
Distilled water	98.50%

'76 Ed.

MIRACLE TURTLE EYE MEDICATION
Aquarium use
(Miracle Pet Products)

Tetracycline hydrochloride	1.50%
Distilled water	98.50%

'76 Ed.

MIRACLE WALLBOARD ADHESIVE
(Miracle Adhesives)

Rubber
Resinous materials
Pigments
Aliphatic petroleum hydrocarbon *

MIRACLE WATER AGER
Aquarium use; removes chlorine from tap water
(Miracle Pet Products)

Sodium thiosulfate *	24.00%
Quinine sulfate	0.04%
Distilled water	75.96%

'76 Ed.

MIRACLE WATER CLEAR
Aquarium use; makes cloudy water clear
(Miracle Pet Products)

Potassium permanganate *	4.0%
Deionized water	96.0%

'76 Ed.

MIRACLE WHITE ALL FABRIC BLEACH (POWDER)
Laundry bleach
(Drackett)

Sodium perborate *	<10%
Sodium silicate	<10%
Anionic surfactant	<5%
Sodium sulfate	
Minor ingredients: Optical brighteners, Enzyme, Dye	

MIRACLE WHITE EGO LAUNDRY DETERGENT (LIQUID)
Heavy duty laundry detergent and pre-spotter
(Drackett)

Nonionic surfactant	<20%
Anionic surfactants	<10%
Triethanolamine	<10%
Glassy phosphate	<1%
Water	

MIRACLE WHITE LAUNDRY DETERGENT WITH BALSAM (POWDER)
(Drackett)

Sodium carbonate *	25-35%
Anionic surfactant *	15-20%
Sodium silicate	<10%
Sodium sulfate	
Minor amounts of Clay, Optical brighteners, Perfume	

MIRACLE WHITE SOIL AND STAIN REMOVER (LIQUID)
Pump spray laundry prespotter
(Drackett)

Nonionic surfactant	<10%
Triethanolamine	<5%
Water	
Minor amounts of Anionic surfactant, Ethanol, Glassy phosphate	

MIRACLE WHITE SUPER CLEANER
Laundry prespotter and detergent additive
(Drackett)

Anionic and nonionic surfactants	<5%
Sodium citrate	
Water	
Minor amounts of Soil suspending agent, Preservative	

MIRADON TABLETS
Anticoagulant
(Schering)

Each tablet:
Miradon (Anisindione) *	50 mg.

MIRASECT
Insecticide
(Lorenz)

Diazinon	0.25%
Lindane	0.25%
Piperonyl butoxide	0.30%
Pyrethrins	0.03%
Aliphatic hydrocarbons *	99.17%

MISALOID
(Jenkins Labs.)

Each tablet:
N-Acetyl-p-aminophenol *	5.0 gr.
Salicylamide	3.0 gr.
d-Methamphetamine HCl	2.5 mg.
Triple barb (representing 33 1/3% each) Pentobarbital sodium, Butabarbital sodium, Phenobarbital sodium	8.0 mg.

MI-31 SOLUTION

See REXALL MI-31 SOLUTION

MISTLETOE PERFUME, COLOGNE, TOILET WATER
(Parfums Duvelle)

Alcohol (denatured with diethyl phthalate) *

MISTOCIDE

See SUMMIT MISTOCIDE

MISTOCIDE-B

See SUMMIT MISTOCIDE-B

MISTOCIDE-D

See SUMMIT MISTOCIDE-D

MISTOCIDE-D PLUS

See SUMMIT MISTOCIDE-D PLUS

MISTOCIDE PLUS

See SUMMIT MISTOCIDE PLUS

MIST-O-MATIC DRILL BOX TREATMENT
Seed treatment
(Gustafson)

Phenylmercuric acetate (mercury equivalent 0.86%) * 1.44%

MIST-O-MATIC LIQUID SEED DISINFECTANT
Seed treatment
(Gustafson)

Phenyl mercuric ammonium acetate (mercury equivalent 2.0%) * 3.5%

MITECIDE OTIC SOLUTION
Ear mites in dogs and cats
(Elanco Prod.)

Mineral oil 90.05%
Technical Methoxychlor 1.0%
Technical Piperonyl butoxide ... 1.0%
2,2'-Methylenebis(3,4,6-trichloro-phenol) (Hexachlorophene) ... 0.5%
Pyrethrins 0.1%

MITEE DARK THREAD CUTTING OIL
(DAP)

Petroleum lubricating oil * ...... >50%
Organically bound Sulfur
Chlorine

MITEE DRIPLESS PIPE JOINT COMPOUND
(DAP)

Calcium carbonate
Clay
Carbon black
Mineral oil
Vegetable oil
Phospholipid
Phthalate ester

MITEE LIGHT THREAD CUTTING OIL
(DAP)

Petroleum lubricating oil * ...... >50%
Organically bound Sulfur
Chlorine

MITEE PENETRATING OIL
(DAP)

Petroleum oil * .... <55%
Kerosene * .... <20%
Mineral spirits * .... <30%

MITEE PIPE JOINT COMPOUND
(DAP)

Calcium carbonate
Aluminum silicates
Polymerized Linseed oil
Petroleum lubricating oil .... <10%

MITEE SOLDERING PASTE
(DAP)

Zinc chloride * .... <15%
Ammonium chloride
Petrolatum
Water
Micro crystalline wax

MITEE STAINLESS PLUMBERS PUTTY
(DAP)

Calcium carbonate
Vegetable oil
Hydrocarbon plasticizer
Organic thickener
Water
Mineral oil * .... <2%

MI-31 SOLUTION

See REXALL MI-31 SOLUTION

MITONE
Mange treatment for dogs
(Beecham Labs.)

Isopropanol * 73.9%
Benzyl benzoate * 20.0%
Benzocaine 2.0%
Rotenone 0.3%

MITOX
Otitis medication; veterinary
(Norden Labs.)

Neomycin base (as the sulfate) ... 0.5%
Sulfacetamide 9.0%
Sevin 1.0%
Tetracaine hydrochloride 0.5%
Chlorophyll and base 89.0%

MITY-QUIN CREAM
Antifungal, antibacterial, anti-inflammatory, antipruritic
(Reid-Provident)

Each gram:
Iodochlorhydroxyquin (3%) ... 30 mg.
Hydrocortisone (0.5%) .... 5 mg.

MIX-R-MYCIN CONCENTRATE

See PURINA MIX-R-MYCIN CONCENTRATE

M.L.D. BOWL CLEANSE

See SPARTAN M.L.D. BOWL CLEANSE

MME. C. J. WALKER HAIR & SCALP PREPARATIONS
(Walker, Mme.)

Mme. C. J. Walker Mfg. Co., Inc.
617 Indiana Ave.
Indianapolis, Ind. 46202

Phone: 317-631-7143

See COSMETICS, Section VI, General Formulations

M NOSCOTUSS
Antitussive, antihistaminic, expectorant, decongestant
(Life Labs., Inc.)

Each 5 cc:
Noscapine * .... 10 mg.
Phenylephrine hydrochloride * 5 mg.
Chlorpheniramine maleate ... 1 mg.
Potassium guaiacol sulfonate . 75 mg.
Alcohol USP 5%
Menthol .... 0.5 mg.

'76 Ed.

MOBAN & MOBAN CONCENTRATE
For management of manifestations of schizophrenia
(Endo Labs.)

Each tablet:
Molindone
hydrochloride * ..... 5 mg.; 10 mg.; 25 mg.
Each ml. (Concentrate):
Molindone hydrochloride * ... 20 mg.

Starred ingredients (*) may be responsible for major toxic effects; consult Section II.

MOBIDIN
Anti-inflammatory-analgesic
(Ascher, B.F.)

Each tablet:
  Magnesium salicylate * .... 600.0 mg.

MOBISYL
Antiarthritic creme
(Ascher, B.F.)

Each tube:
  Triethanolamine salicylate * 20.0%

MOCAP
Nematocide, insecticide
(Mobil Chemical Co.)

Ethoprop (O-Ethyl S,S-dipropyl phosphorodithioate) *

  Granular 10%
  Liquid 70.6%

MODANE
Laxative therapy
(Warren-Teed)

Liquid (each 5 ml.):
  Danthron, USP * .... 37.5 mg.
  Alcohol 5%

Mild Tablets (each):
  Danthron, USP * .... 37.5 mg.

Tablets (each):
  Danthron, USP * .... 75 mg.

MODANE SOFT
Stool softener
(Warren-Teed)

Each capsule:
  Docusate sodium, USP * .... 120 mg.

MODERIL TABLETS
Hypotensive agent, tranquilizer
(Pfizer)

Crystalline Rescinnamine
Each tablet:
  Yellow .... 0.25 mg.
  Salmon .... 0.50 mg.

MODERN MAID CERAMIC CLEANER
Cleaner for glass top stoves
(SerVaas Labs.)

	by weight
Oxalic acid (as the dihydrate) *	10%
Silica (amorphous)	87%
Sodium carbonate	2%
Nonionic surfactant	<1%
Perfume	trace

MODICON TABLETS
Oral contraceptive
(Ortho)

Each tablet:
  Norethindrone .... 0.5 mg.
  Ethinyl estradiol .... 0.035 mg.

MODOWN (Emulsifiable Concentrate)
Herbicide
(Mobil Chemical Co.)

Bifenox (Methyl 5-(2,4-dichlorophenoxy)-2-nitrobenzoate) 21%
Also contains
  Monochlorobenzene

MODOWN (Wettable Powder)
Herbicide
(Mobil Chemical Co.)

Bifenox (Methyl 5-(2,4-dichlorophenoxy)-2-nitrobenzoate) 80%

MOFFET ANALGESIC CREME
(Moffet Inc.)

Camphor *	5%
Menthol *	5%
Methyl salicylate *	10%
Aqueous base	

MOGUL A-492
Microbiocide; industrial use
(Mogul Div., Dexter Corp.)

Calcium hypochlorite * 30%

MOGUL A-495
Microbiocide; industrial use
(Mogul Div., Dexter Corp.)

Calcium hypochlorite * 65%

MOGUL AG-411 (also known as 6411 and 7411)
Microbiocide; industrial use
(Mogul Div., Dexter Corp.)

Didecyl dimethyl ammonium
  chloride 20%
Isopropanol 8%

MOGUL AG-412
Microbiocide; industrial use
(Mogul Div., Dexter Corp.)

Didecyl dimethyl ammonium
  chloride 50%
Isopropanol 20%

MOGUL AG-414 (also known as 7414)
Microbiocide; industrial use
(Mogul Div., Dexter Corp.)

Poly (oxyethylene(dimethyliminio)
ethylene (dimethyliminio) ethylene dichloride) * 3.6%

MOGUL AG-415 (also known as 6415)
Microbiocide; industrial use
(Mogul Div., Dexter Corp.)

Poly (oxyethylene(dimethyliminio)
ethylene (dimethyliminio) ethylene dichloride) * 15%

MOGUL AG-431
Microbiocide; industrial use
(Mogul Div., Dexter Corp.)

Active ingred.:
  Copper as elemental * 7.1%
Inert ingred.:
  Triethanolamine and water 92.9%

MOGUL AG-441 (also known as 6441)
Microbiocide; industrial use
(Mogul Div., Dexter Corp.)

Disodium ethylene bis
  (dithiocarbamate) * 15%
Sodium dimethyl dithiocarbamate . 15%

MOGUL AG-451 (also known as 6451)
Microbiocide; industrial use
(Mogul Div., Dexter Corp.)

2,2-Dibromo-3-nitrilopropionamide * 5%

MOGUL AG-452
Microbiocide; industrial use
(Mogul Div., Dexter Corp.)

2,2-Dibromo-3-nitrilopropionamide * 20%

MOGUL AG-460 (also known as 6460)
Microbiocide; industrial use
(Mogul Div., Dexter Corp.)

Methylene bis (thiocyanate) * 2.55%
Dimethyl formamide 5.95%

MOGUL AG-461
Microbiocide; industrial use
(Mogul Div., Dexter Corp.)

Methylene bis (thiocyanate) * 5.1%
Dimethyl formamide 11.9%

MOGUL AG-471 (also known as 6471 and 7471)
Microbiocide; industrial use
(Mogul Div., Dexter Corp.)

n-Alkyl (60% C14, 30% C16, 5% C12,
  5% C18) dimethyl benzyl ammonium chlorides * 3.0%
Bis(tri-n-butyltin)oxide 0.6%

Starred ingredients (*) may be responsible for major toxic effects; consult Section II.

MOGUL AG-472
Microbiocide; industrial use
(Mogul Div., Dexter Corp.)

n-Alkyl (60% C14, 30% C16, 5% C12,
 5% C18) dimethyl benzyl ammonium chlorides * 25%
Bis(tri-n-butyltin)oxide 5%

MOGUL EG-5311
Oxygen scavenger; industrial use
(Mogul Div., Dexter Corp.)

Hydrazine * 8.8%

MOGUL OS-306
Oxygen scavenger; industrial use
(Mogul Div., Dexter Corp.)

Hydrazine * 17.5%

MOGUL OS-307
Oxygen scavenger; industrial use
(Mogul Div., Dexter Corp.)

Hydrazine * 34.6%

MOI-STIR (Manual Pump Spray)
*Mouth moistening solution for relief of
 xerostomia/artificial saliva*
(Kingswood Labs.)

Water 90%
Sorbitol 5%
Sodium carboxymethylcellulose 5%
Parabens 1%
All Electrolytes 1%

MOISTURE MAGNET
Mildewcide
(Chemical Processors)

Calcium chloride *

MOLE-NOTS
Rodenticide
(Nott)

Strychnine sulfate * 0.35%

MOLETOX II POISON BAIT MOLE & GOPHER KILLER

See BONIDE MOLETOX II POISON
 BAIT MOLE & GOPHER KILLER

MOLETOX POISON PEANUTS MOLE & GOPHER KILLER

See BONIDE MOLETOX POISON
 PEANUTS MOLE & GOPHER
 KILLER

MOLINARD PERFUMES

Molinard Perfumes U.S.A.
P.O. Box 164
Lake Forest, Ill. 60045

Phone: 312-295-1426

See COSMETICS, Section VI, General
 Formulations

MOL-IRON CHRONOSULE SUSTAINED RELEASE CAPSULES
Iron-deficiency anemia
(Schering)

Each capsule:
 Ferrous sulfate (78 mg. elemental iron) * .... 390 mg.

MOL-IRON PANHEMIC CHRONOSULE SUSTAINED RELEASE CAPSULES
Iron-deficiency anemia
(Schering)

Each capsule:
 Ferrous sulfate (78 mg. elemen-
  tal iron) * .... 390 mg.
Plus polyvitamins

MOL-IRON TABLETS & LIQUID
For iron-deficiency anemias
(Schering)

TABLETS or LIQUID (each tablet or 4
 cc):
 Ferrous sulfate * .... 195 mg.
 Alcohol (Liquid only) 4.75%

MOL-IRON WITH VITAMIN C CHRONOSULE SUSTAINED RELEASE CAPSULES
Iron-deficiency anemia
(Schering)

Each capsule:
 Ferrous sulfate (78 mg. elemen-
  tal iron) * .... 390 mg.
 Ascorbic acid .... 150 mg.

MOL-IRON WITH VITAMIN C TABLETS
Iron-deficiency anemia
(Schering)

Each tablet:
 Ferrous sulfate (39 mg. elemen-
  tal iron) * .... 195 mg.
 Ascorbic acid .... 75 mg.

MOLLIMENTUM
Hoof dressing; veterinary
(Troy Chem.)

Cottonseed oil
Beeswax
Spirits turpentine *
Rosin

MOLY DRY FILM (Aerosol)
(Cling-Surface)

Methylene chloride 58%
Toluol * 20%
Propane/Isobutane 18%

MOLYNOCTIN L
Soybean seed treatment/inoculant
(Kalo)

Sodium molybdate

MOLY T
Soybean seed treatment
(Kalo)

Thiram*
Sodium molybdate

MOMENTUM
Muscular low backache
(Whitehall Labs.)

Each tablet:
 Phenyltoloxamine .... 12.5 mg.
 Salicylsalicylic acid * .... 5 gr.
 Microfined Aspirin * .... 2 1/2 gr.

MONACET APC COMPOUND
Analgesic
(Rexall)

Each tablet:
 Aspirin * .... 3 1/2 gr.
 Phenacetin * .... 2 1/2 gr.
 Caffeine .... 1/2 gr.

        '76 Ed.

MONAM SOIL FUMIGANT
(Chemical Formulators)

Sodium methyldithiocarbamate * .. 29%

        '76 Ed.

MONITOR
Insecticide-acaricide
(Mobay Chemical Corp.)

O,S-Dimethyl phosphoramidothioate *

MONITOR 4 SPRAY
Insecticide
(Chevron)

Monitor (O,S-Dimethyl
 phosphoramidothioate) * 40.0%

Chevron emergency phone number: 415-
 233-3737

MONOBASE
Emollient
(Torch)

Wax
Fatty alcohols
Propylene glycol
Emulsifying agent

'76 Ed.

MONOCETE SOLUTION
Verruca cauterant
(Pedinol)

Monochloracetic acid * 80%
Coloring agent

MONOSULPH
(Diamond Shamrock, Process Chemicals Div.)

Sulfated castor oil *

MONSIEUR DE GIVENCHY FOR A MAN'S BATH
(Parfums Givenchy)

Pentasodium triphosphate
Sodium dodecylbenzenesulfonate
Sodium sesquicarbonate
Water
Sodium silicoaluminate
Fragrance

MONSTER MULTIPLE VITAMINS
(Bristol-Myers)

Each tablet:
Vitamin A .... 3500 USP units
Vitamin D .... 400 USP units
Plus Multivitamins

MONSTER MULTIPLE VITAMINS PLUS IRON
(Bristol-Myers)

Vitamin A .... 3500 USP units
Vitamin D .... 400 USP units
Iron (Ferrous fumarate) .... 10 mg.
Plus Multivitamins

MONTGOMERY WARD HYDRO FLOW DEFOAMER
To decrease foam in extractor cleaning machines recovery tanks
(Scot Labs.; dist., Montgomery Ward)

Silicone emulsion 5–6%
Preservative .... trace
Water .... balance

MONTGOMERY WARD HYDRO FLOW TRAFFIC SPOTTER
Spot pretreatment for use before extraction shampooing
(Scot Labs.; dist., Montgomery Ward)

Glycol ether 4–7%
Amphoteric surfactant 9–11%
Water .... balance

MONTGOMERY WARD RUG SHAMPOO
(Scot Labs.; dist., Montgomery Ward)

Acrylic polymer emulsion 2–4%
Anionic surfactant 45%
Preservative .... trace
Water .... balance

MOON BRITE
Restorer for floors
(Paul Koss)

Water .... >85%
Pine oil
Tributoxyethyl phosphate (plasticizer)
Polyethylene emulsion
Nonylphenoxypoly(ethyleneoxy)ethanol (Nonionic surfactant)
Isopropylamine sulfonate
Fatty amido phosphate
Optical brightener .... trace
Fluorosurfactant .... trace

pH 7.0-7.2

MOON DROPS COSMETICS & TOILETRIES
(Revlon)

Revlon, Inc.
767 Fifth Ave.
New York, N.Y. 10153

Phone: 212-572-5000

Revlon Research Center, Inc.
945 Zerega Ave.
Bronx, N.Y. 10473

Phone: 212-824-9000

See COSMETICS, Section VI, General Formulations

MOONSHINE
Floor cleaner
(Paul Koss)

Water .... >95%
Carbitol solvent (Diethylene glycol monoethyl ether)
Nonylphenoxypoly(ethyleneoxy)ethanol (Nonionic surfactant)
Ethylene oxide condensate
Fatty amido phosphate
Sodium xylene sulfonate (Anionic surfactant)
Modified Acrylic emulsion
Dye

pH 7.8-8.0

MOORE, BENJAMIN, PAINT PRODUCTS
Paints, varnishes & enamels

Benjamin Moore & Co.
Chestnut Ridge Rd.
Montvale, N.J. 07645

Phone: 201-573-9600

See PAINTS, Section VI, General Formulations

MOORE'S ALKYD DULAMEL SEMI-GLOSS ENAMEL (WHITE 207-01)
(Benjamin Moore)

Pigment: 36.0%
  Titanium dioxide (type II) .. 62.8%
  Silicates 37.2%
Vehicle: 64.0%
  Alkyd varnish: 82.5%
    Soya alkyd resin 48.9%
    Mineral spirits * 51.1%
  Driers 0.5%
  Mineral spirits * 17.0%

MOORE'S HOUSE PAINT (OUTSIDE WHITE 110-01)
(Benjamin Moore)

Pigment: 44.5%
  Titanium dioxide (type II) .. 38.6%
  Zinc oxide 23.6%
  Calcium carbonate 30.7%
  Silicates 7.1%
Vehicle: 55.5%
  Alkyd varnish: 66.9%
    Linseed modified castor alkyd resin 76.8%
    Mineral spirits*, Aromatic hydrocarbons * 23.2%
  Mineral spirits * 31.6%
  Driers 0.6%
  N-(Trichloromethylthio) phthalimide 0.9%

MOORE'S HOUSE PAINT (TUDOR BROWN 110-63)
Exterior use
(Benjamin Moore)

Pigment: 14.5%
  Iron oxide (Class II) 74.8%
  Silicates 25.2%
Vehicle: 85.5%
  Alkyd varnish: 73.8%
    Soya modified linseed alkyd resin 66.0%
    Mineral spirits*, Aromatics *† 34.0%
  Mineral spirits * 25.4%
  Driers 0.5%
  N-(Trichloromethylthio) phthalimide 0.3%

†*See* Aromatic hydrocarbons

Starred ingredients (*) may be responsible for major toxic effects; consult Section II.

MOORE'S IMPERVO ENAMEL (SUN YELLOW 133-12)
(Benjamin Moore)

Pigment:	18.8%
Titanium dioxide (type IV)	39.9%
Monoazo yellow	56.9%
Silicates	3.2%
Vehicle:	81.2%
Alkyd varnish:	79.2%
Soya alkyd resin	54.4%
Mineral spirits *	45.6%
Mineral spirits *	20.2%
Driers	0.6%

MOORE'S IMPERVO ENAMEL (WHITE 133-01)
(Benjamin Moore)

Pigment:	29.4%
Titanium dioxide (type IV)	91.8%
Zinc oxide	8.2%
Vehicle:	70.6%
Alkyd varnish:	79.9%
Safflower modified alkyd resin	55.2%
Mineral spirits*, Aromatics *†	44.8%
Mineral spirits *	19.4%
Driers	0.7%

†See Aromatic hydrocarbons

MOORE'S PORCH & FLOOR ENAMEL (DECK GRAY 112-71)
(Benjamin Moore)

Pigment:	26.4%
Titanium dioxide (type IV)	15.5%
Calcium carbonate	81.2%
Silicates	1.7%
Tinting colors	1.6%
Vehicle:	73.6%
Alkyd varnish:	85.3%
Phenolic, Petroleum resin, Modified linseed alkyd resin	58.0%
Mineral spirits*, Aromatics *†	42.0%
Mineral spirits *	13.6%
Driers	1.1%

†See Aromatic hydrocarbons

MOORE'S PORCH & FLOOR ENAMEL (GREEN 112-40)
Alkyd enamel for wood, concrete or metal
(Benjamin Moore)

Pigment:	14.0%
Titanium dioxide (type IV)	2.7%
Yellow iron oxide	46.4%
Phthalocyanine blue	3.1%
Copper phthalocyanine green	2.3%
Calcium carbonate	38.9%
Silicates	3.9%
Tinting colors	2.7%
Vehicle:	86.0%
Alkyd varnish:	87.1%
Phenolic, petroleum resin modified linseed alkyd resin	57.8%
Mineral spirits*, Aromatics *†	42.2%
Mineral spirits *	11.8%
Driers	1.1%

†See Aromatic hydrocarbons

MOORGARD LATEX HOUSE PAINT (BRILLIANT WHITE 103-01)
(Benjamin Moore)

Pigment:	32.5%
Titanium dioxide (type II)	69.9%
Zinc oxide	12.0%
Silicates	18.1%
Vehicle:	67.5%
Vinyl acetate/acrylic emulsion:	40.5%
Vinyl acetate/acrylic resin	50.0%
Water	50.0%
Alkyd resin emulsion:	59.4%
Linseed modified castor alkyd resin	18.8%
Water, Glycols, Aromatic hydrocarbons *	81.2%
2-N-Octyl-4-isothiazolin-3-one	0.1%

MOORGARD LATEX HOUSE PAINT (NEWPORT BLUE 103-35)
(Benjamin Moore)

Pigment:	20.4%
Titanium dioxide (type IV)	16.4%
Zinc oxide	11.7%
Silica	70.5%
Tinting colors	1.4%
Vehicle:	79.6%
Vinyl acetate/acrylic emulsion:	42.0%
Vinyl acetate/acrylic resin	50.0%
Water	50.0%
Alkyd resin emulsion:	57.9%
Linseed modified castor alkyd resin	17.2%
Water, Glycols, Aromatic hydrocarbons *	82.8%
2-N-Octyl-4-isothiazolin-3-one	0.1%

MOORGLO LATEX HOUSE & TRIM PAINT (PROVINCIAL OLIVE 096-45)
(Benjamin Moore)

Pigment:	17.1%
Titanium dioxide (type IV)	27.9%
Zinc oxide	13.9%
Chromic oxide green	34.5%
Yellow iron oxide	4.3%
Silicates	16.7%
Tinting colors	2.7%
Vehicle:	82.9%
Acrylic emulsion:	46.5%
Acrylic resin	46.5%
Water	53.5%
Alkyd resin emulsion:	53.4%
Linseed modified soya alkyd resin	20.3%
Water, Glycols, Mineral spirits *	79.7%
2-N-Octyl-4-isothiazolin-3-one	0.1%

MOORGLO LATEX HOUSE & TRIM PAINT (WHITE 096-01)
(Benjamin Moore)

Pigment:	27.5%
Titanium dioxide (type II)	92.3%
Zinc oxide	7.7%
Vehicle:	72.5%
Acrylic emulsion:	47.2%
Acrylic resin	46.5%
Water	53.5%
Alkyd resin emulsion:	52.7%
Linseed alkyd resin	20.8%
Water, Glycols, Mineral spirits*, Aromatics *†	79.2%
2-N-Octyl-4-isothiazolin-3-one	0.1%

†See Aromatic hydrocarbons

MOORMAFUME
See MOORMAN'S MOORMAFUME

MOORMAKLEEN 1 STROKE ENVIRON
See MOORMAN'S MOORMAKLEEN 1 STROKE ENVIRON

MOORMAN'S DUST WITH CO-RAL INSECTICIDE
(Moorman)

Coumaphos	1.0%

MOORMAN'S E-Z-EX WORMER MEDICATED
Veterinary
(Moorman)

Thiabendazole *	3.3%

MOORMAN'S FLY BAIT PLUS
Insecticide
(Moorman)

Methomyl *	1.000%
(z)-9-Tricosene	0.025%

MOORMAN'S FLY SPRAY
Insecticide
(Moorman)

Combined amount:	100.0%
Refined Petroleum distillate *	
Technical Piperonyl butoxide	
Pyrethrins	

MOORMAN'S INSECTICIDE CONCENTRATE
(Moorman)

Aromatic petroleum derivative *	74.4%
Ronnel	20.0%

Starred ingredients (*) may be responsible for major toxic effects; consult Section II.

MOORMAN'S INSECTICIDE DUST
(Moorman)

Technical Methoxychlor	3.0%

MOORMAN'S INSECT KILLER
Aerosol insecticide
(Moorman)

Resmethrin	0.200%
Related compounds	0.028%
d-trans Allethrin	0.150%
Related compounds	0.012%
Aromatic petroleum hydrocarbons	0.272%
Propellant A-46 (hydrocarbon)	30.000%
Water	68.000%

MOORMAN'S LIVESTOCK SPRAY
Insecticide
(Moorman)

Dimethyl phosphate of alpha-methylbenzyl 3-hydroxy-cis-crotonate *	1.00%
2,2-Dichlorovinyl dimethyl phosphate	0.23%
Related compounds	0.02%
Petroleum hydrocarbons *	96.47%

MOORMAN'S MOORMAFUME
Insecticide
(Moorman)

Lindane *	6.0%

MOORMAN'S MOORMAKLEEN 1 STROKE ENVIRON
Disinfectant; detergent
(Moorman)

Sodium o-phenylphenate *	11.3%
Sodium o-benzyl-p-chlorophenate *	9.4%
Sodium p-tertiary-amylphenate *	2.3%

MOORMAN'S RA-MO-CIDE
Rodenticide
(Moorman)

Warfarin	0.025%

MOORMAN'S WORM-A-CIDE
Veterinary
(Moorman)

Each 54.6 gm. packet: 2,2-Dichlorovinyl dimethyl phosphate *	11.5 gm.

MOORMAN'S WORM-DOZE
Veterinary
(Moorman)

Piperazine (as piperazine dihydrochloride)	52.0%

MOORWHITE PRIMER (WHITE 100-00)
For exterior use
(Benjamin Moore)

Pigment:		51.2%
Titanium dioxide (type II)	24.0%	
Silicates	76.0%	
Vehicle:		48.8%
Alkyd varnish:	62.0%	
Soya-linseed modified castor alkyd resin	85.4%	
Mineral spirits*, Aromatic hydrocarbons *	14.6%	
Mineral spirits *	35.9%	
Driers	0.9%	
N-(Trichloromethylthio)-pthalimide	1.2%	

MOORWOOD SOLID COLOR STAIN (REDWOOD 080-20)
For exterior use
(Benjamin Moore)

Pigment:		51.9%
Iron oxide - Class 1	28.4%	
Silica	71.6%	
Vehicle:		48.1%
Alkyd varnish:	34.1%	
Soya alkyd resin	94.1%	
Mineral spirits	5.9%	
Mineral spirits *	65.0%	
Driers	0.4%	
N-(Trichloromethylthio)-phthalimide	0.5%	

MOOVIT SUPER PENETRATING OIL (Aerosol)
(Cling-Surface)

Perchloroethylene *	30%
1,1,1-Trichloroethane *	30%

MOOVIT SUPER PENETRATING OIL (Non-aerosol)
(Cling-Surface)

Stoddard solvent *	30%

MOPAR DOOR-EASE
(Chrysler Corp., MoPar Div.)

See DOOR-EASE

MOPAR SIL-GLYDE
(Chrysler Corp., MoPar Div.)

See SIL-GLYDE

MOP & GLO
Floor shine cleaner
(Lehn & Fink)

Acrylic copolymer	15%
Glycol ether derivatives	4%
Alkyl phenyl ethoxylates	2%
Styrene copolymer	1%
Ethylene glycol	trace
Ammonium hydroxide	trace
PMA	trace
Water	77%

MOP MAGIC
Soapless detergent
(Consolidated Chem., Inc.)

Synthetic detergents
Alkaline phosphates

MOR-EEN POWDER
Anthelmintic; veterinary, avian
(Hilltop)

Phenothiazine	25%
Copper sulfate *	20%
Nicotine sulfate *	1%
Kamala	
Tobacco powder	
Nux vomica	9%
Guaiacol	
Iron sulfate	
Capsicum	
Areca nut	
Iron oxide	
Sulfur	
Oil of anise	
Mineral oil	

'76 Ed.

MORESTAN
Acaricide, insecticide, fungicide
(Mobay Chemical Corp.)

6-Methyl-1,3-dithiolo(4,5-b)quinoxalin-2-one *

MORGRO ALL IN ONE DUST
Insecticide, miticide, fungicide
(Morgro)

Carbaryl (1-Naphthyl N-methylcarbamate) *	5.0%
Rotenone *	1.5%
Other cube resins	1.5%
Zineb	5.0%

MORGRO BENOMYL SYSTEMIC FUNGICIDE
(Morgro)

Benomyl (Methyl(1-butylcarbamoyl)-2-benzimindazolecarbamate)	50%

MORGRO CRABGRASS SPRAY
Herbicide
(Morgro)

Monosodium acid methanearsonate *	8.4%

MORGRO FRUIT AND BERRY SPRAY
Insecticide
(Morgro)

Diazinon (O,O-Diethyl O-(2-isopropyl-4-methyl-6-pyrimidinyl) phosphorothioate) *	8.30%
Kelthane (1,1-Bis(chlorophenyl)-2,-2,2-trichloroethanol)	3.20%

Starred ingredients (*) may be responsible for major toxic effects; consult Section II.

MORGRO HOUSE AND PATIO SPRAY
Insecticide
(Morgro)

o-Isopropoxyphenyl methylcarbamate *	1.0%
Petroleum distillate *	83.0%

MORGRO INSECTICIDE-MITICIDE
(Morgro)

Carbaryl (1-Naphthyl N-methylcarbamate) *	12.5%
1,1-Bis(p-chlorophenyl)-2,2,2-trichloroethanol	9.2%
Xylene *	54.5%

MORGRO JOINT GRASS & WEED KILLER
Herbicide
(Morgro)

Sodium cacodylate	1.98%
Dimethylarsenic acid (Cacodylic acid)	0.34%

MORGRO KELTHANE MITICIDE
(Morgro)

1,1-Bis(p-chlorophenyl)-2,2,2-trichloroethanol	9.5%
Petroleum distillates *	

MORGRO LIQUID SEVIN
Insecticide; aqueous suspension
(Morgro)

Carbaryl *	22.5%

MORGRO LIQUID WEED & GRASS KILLER
(Morgro)

Prometon (2,4-Bis(isopropylamino)-6-methoxy-s-triazine)	2.00%
Pentachlorophenol *	1.00%
Other Chlorinated phenols	0.15%

MORGRO MALATHION 57 SPRAY
Insecticide for fruit trees and ornamentals
(Morgro)

Malathion *	57.0%
Xylol *	35.0%

MORGRO MILDU-CURE
Controls powdery mildew & spider mites on ornamentals, flowers, shrubs & fruit crops
(Morgro)

Dinitro (1-methylheptyl)phenyl crotonate	2.44%
(1-Methylheptyl) phenol and related compounds	0.69%

MORGRO MITICIDE
(Morgro)

1,1-Bis(chlorophenyl)-2,2,2-trichloroethanol *	9.5%

MORGRO ORNAMENTAL SPRAY
Insecticide
(Morgro)

Carbaryl	6.00%
S-(2-(ethylsulfinyl)ethyl)O,O-dimethyl phosphorothioate	6.00%
1,1-Bis(p-chlorophenyl)-2,2,2-trichloroethanol	2.40%
Aromatic petroleum derivative solvent *	50.00%

MORGRO PEST PELLETS
Pesticide for slugs, snails, ants & earwigs
(Morgro)

Carbaryl (1-Naphthyl N-methylcarbamate) *	4.00%
Metaldehyde	1.00%

MORGRO PLUS FUNGICIDE
(Morgro)

Thiram (Tetramethyl thiuram disulfide)	1.00%
Cadmium chloride *	0.50%

MORGRO ROOT BORER CONTROL
(Morgro)

Paradichlorobenzene *	99.00%

MORGRO ROSE FOOD PLUS SYSTEMIC INSECTICIDE
(Morgro)

O,O-Diethyl S-(2(ethylthio) ethyl) phosphorodithioate *	1.0%

MORGRO SOIL & BULB DUST
Insecticide, fungicide, miticide
(Morgro)

Carbaryl (1-Naphthyl N-methylcarbamate) *	5.0%
Rotenone *	1.5%
Other cube resins	1.5%
Zineb	5.0%

MORGRO SYSTEMIC INSECTICIDE
For ornamental trees, shrubs, flowers and tomatoes
(Morgro)

O,O-Diethyl S-(2(ethylthio) ethyl) phosphorodithioate *	2%

MORGRO VEGETABLE & TOMATO DUST
Insecticide, fungicide
(Morgro)

Carbaryl (1-Naphthyl N-methylcarbamate) *	5.0%
Rotenone *	1.5%
Other cube resins	5.0%
Zineb	5.0%

MOR-O LIQUID
For control of coccidiosis in chickens
(Hilltop)

Sodium arsanilate *
Quebracho liquid extract *
Sodium hydroxide

'76 Ed.

MORTICIDE
Insecticide
(Royal Bond)

Pyrethrins *
Kerosene *
Piperonyl butoxide

MORUGUENT OINTMENT
For minor burns and other skin irritations
(Beecham Labs.)

Cod-liver oil concentrate (Vitamins A and D)
Lanolin-petrolatum base

MORUSAN OINTMENT
For minor burns and other skin irritations
(Beecham Labs.)

Benzocaine	2%

Cod-liver oil concentrate (Vitamins A and D)
Lanolin-petrolatum base

MORWEAR PAINT PRODUCTS
Morwear Paint Co.
2431 Peralta St.
Oakland, Calif. 94607

Phone: 415-444-6516

See PAINTS, Section VI, General Formulations

MOSCO CORN AND CALLUS REMOVER
(Moss Chemical Co.)

Salicylic acid *	>50%
Methyl salicylate *	<10%

MOSQUITO BEATER
(Bonide)

Methylated naphthalenes *	16.0%
Naphthalene *	4.5%
b-Butoxy-b-thiocyanodiethyl ether *	1.0%
Butoxy polypropylene glycol	0.5%
Petroleum distillate	9.0%

MOSQUITO LARVAECIDE
Mosquito control chemical
(National Chemsearch)

Coal tar neutral oils *
Soap
Phenols *

MOSS-KIL

See LILLY/MILLER MOSS-KIL

MOSS-OUT FOR LAWNS

See LILLY'S MOSS-OUT FOR LAWNS

MOTA CAR WASH
Powdered car wash
(Lester Labs.)

Detergents *

'76 Ed.

MOTH BLOCKETTE
(Carson Chem. Corp.)

Naphthalene *	99%
Essential oil	1%

'76 Ed.

MOTHER'S FRIEND
Rubefacient
(S.S.S. Co.)

Alcohol	6 1/2%
Winter pressed Cottonseed oil	
Soft liquid soap	
Camphor *	
Menthol *	

MOTH SCENT-INEL
(Carson Chem. Corp.)

Paradichlorobenzene *	99%
Essential oil	1%

'76 Ed.

MOTOMCO DIPHACINONE CONCENTRATE
Rodenticide
(Motomco)

Diphacinone (2-Diphenylacetyl-1,3-indandione) *	0.1%

MOTOMCO TRACKING POWDER
Rodenticide
(Motomco)

Calcium salt of 2-isovaleryl-1,3-indandione *

MOTOMCO WARFARIN CONCENTRATE
Rodenticide
(Motomco)

Warfarin (3-(a-Acetonylbenzyl)-4-hydroxycoumarin)	0.5%

MOTOMCO WARFARIN-S CONCENTRATE
Rodenticide
(Motomco)

Warfarin (3-(a-Acetonylbenzyl)-4-hydroxycoumarin)	0.5%
N'-(2-Quinoxalinyl)sulfanilamide (Sulfaquinoxaline)	0.5%

MOTOMCO WATER SOLUBLE DIPHACINONE CONCENTRATE
Rodenticide
(Motomco)

Sodium salt of diphacinone (2-Diphenylacetyl-1,3-indandione) *	0.106%

MOTOR MEDIC NO. 1
Automotive
(Radiator)

Petroleum distillates *	
Isopropanol *	

'76 Ed.

MOUSE MAIZE
Rodenticide
(B&G Co.)

Strychnine alkaloid *	0.35%/wt.

MOUSE-NOTS SPECIAL
Rodenticide
(Nott)

Warfarin	0.025%

MOUSE SEED
Rodenticide
(Reardon, W.G.)

Warfarin	0.025%

MOW-POWER

See BURNISHINE MOW-POWER

MP-10
Mildewcide
(Chemical Processors)

Paraformaldehyde *
Paradichlorobenzene *

M-P SEALANT
For automotive coolant systems
(Radiator)

Petroleum distillates *

'76 Ed.

MR. CHAMP, PYROIL

See PYROIL MR. CHAMP

MR. CLEAN (Non-Phosphate)
Liquid household cleaner
(Procter & Gamble)

Water	75-100%
Sodium citrate	5-9%
Sodium cumene sulfonate	5-9%
Sodium carbonate	5-9%
Sodium alkyl benzene sulfonate	1-4%
Minor ingredients, each	<1%

pH (undiluted) - 10.5
pH (1% solution) - 9.7

MR. COLOR (DECORATOR)

See GARD MR. COLOR (DECORATOR)

MR. COLOR (DESIGNER FORMULA)

See GARD MR. COLOR (DESIGNER FORMULA)

MR. FOG
Insecticide; municipal use
(Navy Brand)

Petroleum distillate *	96.26%
Malathion	1.80%
Vapona	1.30%
Related compounds	0.10%
Mineral seal oil	0.40%
Inert ingredients:	
Epichlorohydrin	0.14%

MR. MELT
Ice melter
(Miller, Frank)

Calcium chloride	94-97%

MR. MUSCLE
Aerosol and non-aerosol oven cleaners
(Drackett)

Monoethanolamine .... <10%/wt.
Caustic soda * .... <2%
Siliceous clay
Soap
Water
Perfume
Hydrocarbon propellant (aerosol only)
Corrosion inhibitor

MR. PEP FATIGUE CHASERS
(Chex)

Each tablet:
  Caffeine * .... 3 gr.
  Citric acid .... 3 gr.
                   '76 Ed.

MR. SHHHHH, PYROIL
See PYROIL MR. SHHHHH

MR. SKETCH
Broad line water color markers
(Sanford Corp.)

Dyes
Glycols
Water
Phenol (as preservative) .... <1%

MRS. STEWART'S BLUING
(Ford, L.)

Each fl. oz.:
  Ferric-ferrocyanide .... 1/3 gr.
  Oxalic acid .... 0.035 gr.

MR. ZIP KABLE-EASE
Speedometer cable lubricant
(American Grease Stick)

Colloidal Graphite dispersion in mineral oil 48%
Mineral oil 50%
Sorbitan fatty acid ester 2%

MSA ALGICIDE
See BIO-GUARD MSA ALGICIDE

MSA FEND A-2 WATER-SOLUBLE PROTECTIVE CREAM
(M-S-A)

2-Amino-2-methyl-1,3-propanediol *
Surface active agents:
  Arlacel 60
  Tween 60
Butyl stearate
Magnesium stearate
Stearic acid
Citric acid
Methyl cellulose
Methyl Aseptoform (Methylparaben)
Perfume
Titanium dioxide
Tween 60

MSA FEND E-2 PROTECTIVE CREAM
(M-S-A)

Castor oil
Ceresin (Paraffin hydrocarbons)
Diethylene glycol monostearate
Aldo MSD (Glyceryl stearate)
Lanolin
Methyl Aseptoform (Methylparaben)
Perfume
Titanium dioxide
Citric acid
Methyl cellulose

MSA FEND S-2 SILICONE PROTECTIVE CREAM
(M-S-A)

Arlacel 60
Carbopol 934
Castor oil
Magnesium stearate
Methyl Aseptoform (Methylparaben)
Propyl Aseptoform (Propylparaben)
Perfume
Silicone
Sorbitol
Stearic acid
Thixcin
Titanium dioxide
Tween 60

MSA FEND 1-2 WATER-INSOLUBLE CREAM
Protective cream
(M-S-A)

Aluminum hydroxide, powder
Castor oil
Paraffin hydrocarbons (Ceresin)
Kaolin
Lanolin
Mineral oil
Methyl Aseptoform (Methylparaben)
Protopet No. 1 (White petrolatum)
Starch
Titanium dioxide
Triton
Perfume

MT. HOOD C-20 LAUNDRY POWDER
(Mt. Hood Chemical Corp.)

Tallow-base soap
Sodium metasilicate pentahydrate
Sodium tripolyphosphate *
Sodium sesquicarbonate

It has free alkalinity approx. 9%-11%

MUCOMYST - MUCOMYST-10
Mucolytic agent
(Mead Johnson)

MUCOMYST:
  Acetylcysteine 20%

MUCOMYST-10
  Acetylcysteine 10%

Available in vials of 10 ml. and 30 ml.

MUDRANE
Bronchodilator, mucolytic
(Poythress, Wm. P.)

Each tablet:
  Potassium iodide .... 195 mg.
  Aminophylline anhydrous * .. 130 mg.
  Phenobarbital .... 16 mg.
  Ephedrine HCl * .... 8 mg.

MUDRANE-2
For emphysema, asthma, bronchitis
(Poythress, Wm. P.)

Each tablet:
  Potassium iodide .... 195 mg.
  Aminophylline anhydrous * .. 130 mg.

MUDRANE ELIXIR
Antiasthmatic
(Poythress, Wm. P.)

Each 5 cc:
  Guaifenesin .... 26 mg.
  Theophylline * .... 20 mg.
  Ephedrine HCl * .... 4 mg.
  Phenobarbital .... 2.5 mg.
  Alcohol (v/v) 20%

MUDRANE-GG
For bronchial asthma
(Poythress, Wm. P.)

Each tablet:
  Guaifenesin .... 100 mg.
  Aminophylline anhydrous * .. 130 mg.
  Ephedrine HCl * .... 16 mg.
  Phenobarbital .... 8 mg.

MUDRANE GG-2
For emphysema
(Poythress, Wm. P.)

Each tablet:
  Guaifenesin .... 100 mg.
  Aminophylline anhydrous * .. 130 mg.

Starred ingredients (*) may be responsible for major toxic effects; consult Section II.

MUFFIN BOWL DEODORANT
(Carson Chem. Corp.)

Paradichlorobenzene * 99%
Essential oil 1%

'76 Ed.

MUG SOAP
(Williams, J.B.)

Sodium & potassium soap

"MULE KICK" CLOSET BOWL CLEANER
(Sexauer, J.A.)

Sodium bisulphate *

'76 Ed.

"MULE KICK" LIQUID DRAIN CLEANER
(Sexauer, J.A.)

Sulphuric acid *

'76 Ed.

"MULE KICK" WASTE PIPE CLEANER
(Sexauer, J.A.)

Caustic soda (Sodium hydroxide) *

'76 Ed.

MULSOL
Rust inhibitor cleaner
(Whitfield Chem.)

High flash Petroleum solvents * .. >10%

MULTICAINE OINTMENT
Anesthetic-antiseptic ointment
(Barfred Research Labs.)

Butyl p-amino benzoate
Hypnocaine (brand of propasin)
Benzyl alcohol *

'76 Ed.

MULTI-CIDE II
Kills resistant flies and mosquitoes
(Certified Labs.)

Heavy aromatic naphthas * 86.75%
Methoxychlor (technical) 7.50%
2,2-Dichlorovinyl dimethyl phosphate (and related compounds) 0.75%

MULTIFAK 2 GREASE
(Texaco Inc.)

Mineral oil *
Lithium soap

MULTI-FILM L
Water dispersible spreader-activator for agricultural sprays
(Kalo)

Alkylaryl sulfonates *
Free fatty acids
Isopropanol *
Aliphatic petroleum oils *

MULTIFORT
Multiple vitamin capsules
(Eastern Research Labs.)

Each capsule:
Vitamin A
(palmitate) ...... 10,000 USP units
Plus polyvitamins

'76 Ed.

MULTIGEAR EP LUBRICANT
(Texaco Inc.; Texaco Canada Ltd.)

Petroleum lubricating oil
Sulfur-phosphorus additive

MULTIPOWER-3 MOTOR OIL (10W through 50W, Straight Grades)
(Marathon Oil Co.)

Additives, containing Zinc alkyl
dithiophosphate, Sulfonate,
Methacrylate copolymer 9.5%
Mineral oil .... balance

MULTIPOWER-3 MOTOR OIL (15W-40)
(Marathon Oil Co.)

Additives, containing Zinc alkyl
dithiophosphate, Inhibitor,
Dispersant, Detergent, Methacrylate copolymer, Olefin
copolymer 28%
Mineral oil .... balance

MULTI-PURPOSE INSECT SPRAY
(C-Z Chemical)

Pyrethrins 0.150%
Piperonyl butoxide technical ... 0.750%
Petroleum oil * 99.100%

'76 Ed.

MULTI SCRUB EVERYDAY SCRUBBING LOTION
For acne and oily skin
(Bristol-Myers)

Active ingred.:
Polyethylene granules
Sulfur
Also contains:
Water, Sodium laureth sulfate, Carbomer 940, Propylene glycol, Fragrance, Lauramide DEA, Sodium hydroxide, Citric acid, Thymol, Formaldehyde

MULTI SCRUB MEDICATED CLEANSING SCRUB
For acne and oily skin
(Bristol-Myers)

Active ingred.:
Polyethylene granules
Sulfur
Salicylic acid *
Also contains:
Water, Sodium nonoxynol-1 sulfate,
Poloxamer 184, Dioctyl sodium sulfo-
succinate, Methylcellulose, Corn
starch, Sodium lauryl sulfoacetate,
Fragrance, EDTA

MULTISTIX
*Urine, pH, protein, glucose, ketone, bil-
irubin, occult blood, and urobilinogen
test strip*
(Ames)

pH area: see BILI-LABSTIX
Protein area: see ALBUSTIX
Glucose area: see CLINISTIX
Ketone area: see KETOSTIX
Bilirubin area: see ICTOSTIX
Occult blood area: see HEMASTIX
Urobilinogen area: see UROBILISTIX

MUM GENTLE FORMULA CREAM DEODORANT
(Bristol-Myers)

Aluminum chlorohydrate
Water
Glyceryl stearate
Propylene glycol
Stearyl alcohol
Isopropyl palmitate
Ceteareth-20
Isopropyl myristate
Fragrance
Titanium dioxide
Isopropyl stearate
Quaternium-15

MUNICHEM AL-CON
*Control of algae in swimming pools;
municipal, professional and industrial use*
(MuniChem Corp.)

N-Alkyl (50% C14, 40% C12, 10%
C16) dimethyl benzyl ammonium chlorides * 10.00%

'76 Ed.

MUNICHEM AQUA KILL
*Aquatic herbicide; municipal, profes-
sional and industrial use*
(MuniChem Corp.)

Diquat dibromide * 4.35%

'76 Ed.

Starred ingredients (*) may be responsible for major toxic effects; consult Section II.

MUNICHEM CHLOR-MAL 96
Insecticide for municipal, professional and industrial use
(MuniChem Corp.)

Technical Chlordane *	12.00%
Malathion	3.16%
Mixed Aliphatic hydrocarbons *	80.84%

'76 Ed.

MUNICHEM DEAD LINE BUG KILLER
Surface spray insecticide
(MuniChem Corp.)

Pyrethrins	0.050%
Technical Piperonyl butoxide	0.100%
N-Octyl bicycloheptene dicarboximide	0.166%
O,O-Diethyl O-(2-isopropyl-6-methyl-4-pyrimidinyl) phosphorothioate	0.500%
Petroleum distillate *	74.184%
Inert ingredients: Dichlorodifluoromethane	25.000%

'76 Ed.

MUNICHEM DEODORANT BLOCKS
Bacteriostatic odor killer; institutional and municipal use
(MuniChem Corp.)

n-Alkyl (60% C14, 30% C16, 5% C12, 5% C18) dimethyl benzyl ammonium chloride	0.125%
n-Alkyl (50% C12, 30% C14, 17% C16, 3% C18) dimethyl ethyl benzyl ammonium chloride	0.125%
Lauryl methacrylate	0.250%
Paraformaldehyde	0.250%
Inactive ingredients:	99.250%
Paradichlorobenzene	
Essential oils	
Nonyl phenoxy polyoxyethylene ethanol	
Synthetic calcium silicate, water	

'76 Ed.

MUNICHEM DUA-CIDE
Fogging oil insecticide concentrate for municipal, professional and industrial use
(MuniChem Corp.)

Aromatic petroleum solvent *	57.6%/wt.
Beta-butoxy beta'-thiocyano diethyl ether *	23.6%/wt.
Malathion	18.8%/wt.

'76 Ed.

MUNICHEM FILTER FLY CONTROL
For use in sewage plants
(MuniChem Corp.)

Mixed Aliphatic hydrocarbons *	73.00%
Malathion	3.00%

'76 Ed.

MUNICHEM GERM AWAY
Germicidal sanitizer, deodorizer; institutional and municipal use
(MuniChem Corp.)

Active ingredients:	59.80%
Isopropyl alcohol *	
Triethylene glycol	
Essential oils	
N-Alkyl (C14, C12, C16) dimethyl benzyl ammonium chloride *	
Inert ingredients:	40.20%
Dichlorodifluoromethane	
Water	
Diethanolamine salts of the fatty acids of coconut oil	

'76 Ed.

MUNICHEM IRISH AIRE "GLYCOLIZED" ROOM DEODORANT
(MuniChem Corp.)

Alcohol *	32.33%
Triethylene glycol	7.5%

'76 Ed.

MUNICHEM LEMON "GLYCOLIZED" ROOM DEODORANT
Air sanitizer
(MuniChem Corp.)

Alcohol	32.33%
Triethylene glycol	7.50%

'76 Ed.

MUNICHEM MUNI-FOG
Concentrated insecticide for municipal, professional and industrial use
(MuniChem Corp.)

Technical Chlordane *	12.00%
Malathion	3.16%
Mixed Aliphatic hydrocarbons *	80.84%

'76 Ed.

MUNICHEM MUNI-KILL
Herbicide; municipal, professional and industrial use
(MuniChem Corp.)

Mixed Aliphatic hydrocarbons *	94.97%
2,4-Dichlorophenoxyacetic acid, isooctyl ester	1.09%
Bromacil (5-Bromo-3-sec-butyl-6-methyluracil)	0.98%
Pentachlorophenol	0.80%
Other chlorophenols	0.09%

'76 Ed.

MUNICHEM MUNI S A
Concentrated weed killer; municipal, professional and industrial use
(MuniChem Corp.)

Sodium arsenite *	44.0%

'76 Ed.

MUNICHEM MUNI-X
Concentrated insecticide; municipal, professional and industrial use
(MuniChem Corp.)

Petroleum distillate *	99.525%
N-Octyl bicycloheptene dicarboximide	0.250%
Technical Piperonyl butoxide	0.150%
Pyrethrins	0.075%

'76 Ed.

MUNICHEM MYCOBAC
Surface disinfectant-deodorizer for hospital use
(MuniChem Corp.)

Sodium ethylmercurithiosalicylate	0.002%
Tributyltin linoleate	0.012%
Tributyltin isopropyl succinate	0.024%
Tributyltin benzoate	0.036%
N-Alkyl (60% C14, 30% C16, 5% C12, 5% C18) dimethyl benzyl ammonium chloride	0.486%
Isopropanol *	39.025%

'76 Ed.

MUNICHEM PACEMAKER
Germicidal cleaner for municipal, industrial and professional use
(MuniChem Corp.)

Isopropyl alcohol	1.0000%
Tetrasodium ethylene diamine tetraacetate	0.9500%
Alkyl (50% C12, 30% C14, 17% C16, 3% C18) dimethyl ethyl-benzyl ammonium cyclohexyl sulfamate	0.3000%

'76 Ed.

MUNICHEM PORCELAIN CLEANER
Municipal, professional and industrial use
(MuniChem Corp.)

Hydrogen chloride *	7.50%
Alkyl (C14 50%, C12 40%, C16 10%) dimethyl benzyl ammonium chloride	0.05%

'76 Ed.

MUNICHEM POSITIVE WEED CONTROL
Liquid weed killer; municipal, professional and industrial
(MuniChem Corp.)

Mixed Aliphatic hydrocarbons *	96.10%
Bromacil (5-Bromo-3-sec-butyl-6-methyluracil)	0.97%
Pentachlorophenol	0.79%
Other chlorophenols	0.09%

'76 Ed.

Starred ingredients (*) may be responsible for major toxic effects; consult Section II.

MUNICHEM REPEL
Insect repellent
(MuniChem Corp.)

N,N-Diethyl-meta-toluamide	4.200%
N-Octyl bicycloheptene dicarboximide	1.200%
2,3:4,5-Bis(2-butylene)tetrahydro-2-furaldehyde	0.300%
Di-n-propyl isocinchomeronate	0.300%

'76 Ed.

MUNICHEM SLEDGE
Insecticide for municipal, industrial and professional use
(MuniChem Corp.)

Pyrethrins	0.15%
Tech. Piperonyl butoxide	0.30%
N-Octyl bicycloheptene dicarboximide	0.53%
Tech. Chlordane	2.00%
Petroleum distillate *	62.02%

'76 Ed.

MUNICHEM STRIKE INSECTICIDE
Municipal, industrial and professional use
(MuniChem Corp.)

Pyrethrins	0.3%
Technical Piperonyl butoxide	0.6%
N-Octyl bicycloheptene dicarboximide	1.0%
Petroleum distillate *	13.1%
Inert ingredients:	
Dichlorodifluoromethane	42.5%/wt.
Trichloromonofluoromethane	42.5%/wt.

'76 Ed.

MUNICHEM SUPER WEED AND BRUSH CONTROL
Municipal, professional and industrial use
(MuniChem Corp.)

Ammonium sulfamate *	48.4%

'76 Ed.

MUNICHEM TETRA 25
Disinfectant, defilmer, deodorant, detergent; municipal, professional and industrial use
(MuniChem Corp.)

Tetrasodium salt of ethylene diamine tetraacetic acid	2.2%
Sodium tripolyphosphate	2.0%
n-Alkyl (60% C14, 30% C16, 5% C12, 5% C18) dimethyl benzyl ammonium chloride *	1.5%
n-Alkyl (50% C12, 30% C14, 17% C16, 3% C18) dimethyl ethylbenzyl ammonium chloride *	1.5%

'76 Ed.

MUNICIDE, DEL
See DEL MUNICIDE

MUNI-FOG, MUNICHEM
See MUNICHEM MUNI-FOG

MUNI-KILL, MUNICHEM
See MUNICHEM MUNI-KILL

MUNI S A, MUNICHEM
See MUNICHEM MUNI S A

MUNI-X, MUNICHEM
See MUNICHEM MUNI-X

MURCIL
Tranquilizer
(Direct Div.)

Each capsule:
Chlordiazepoxide HCl * 10 mg.; 25 mg.

MURINE FOR YOUR EYES
Eyewash
(Abbott)

Potassium bicarbonate	
Potassium carbonate	
Berberine hydrochloride	
Boric acid	<2%
Glycerin	
Hydrastine hydrochloride	
Merthiolate (Thimerosal, Lilly)	0.001%
Benzalkonium chloride	0.004%

MURIPSIN TABLETS
For gastric subacidity
(Norgine Labs.)

Each tablet:
Glutamic acid hydrochloride	500 mg.
Pepsin	35 mg.

MUROCEL
Ophthalmic solution: ocular lubricant
(Muro Pharm.)

Methylcellulose	1.000%
Boric acid	<2.000%
Sodium borate	trace
Sodium chloride	trace
Propylene glycol	trace
Methylparaben	0.023%
Propylparaben	0.010%
Purified water	qs ad

MUROCOLL-2
Ophthalmic solution for mydriasis, cycloplegia and to break posterior synechiae in iritis
(Muro Pharm.)

Phenylephrine HCl *	10.00%
Scopolamine HBr	0.30%
Disodium EDTA	trace
Sodium metabisulfite	trace
Disodium phosphate	<2.00%
Citric acid	<2.00%
Purified water	qs ad
Benzalkonium chloride	0.01%

MUROCOLL-19
Ophthalmic solution: used to produce mydriasis and cycloplegia for refraction
(Muro Pharm.)

Scopolamine HBr *	0.30%
Sodium chloride	<1.00%
Disodium EDTA	trace
Boric acid	<2.00%
Benzalkonium chloride	0.01%
Sodium acetate	trace
Purified water	qs ad

MURO 128 OINTMENT
Hypertonic ophthalmic ointment: for corneal edema
(Muro Pharm.)

White petrolatum	40-60%
Mineral oil	5-10%
Lanolin	15-20%
Sodium chloride	5%
Purified water	qs ad

MURO 128 SOLUTION
Hypertonic ophthalmic solution: for corneal edema
(Muro Pharm.)

Sodium chloride	5.000%
Hydroxypropyl methylcellulose	<3.000%
Boric acid	<2.000%
Sodium borate	trace
Propylene glycol	trace
Methylparaben	0.023%
Propylparaben	0.010%
Purified water	qs ad

MURO'S OPCON
Ophthalmic solution: ocular vasoconstrictor
(Muro Pharm.)

Naphazoline HCl *	0.10%
Hydroxypropyl methylcellulose	<1.00%
Disodium EDTA	trace
Boric acid	trace
Sodium carbonate	trace
Sodium chloride	trace
Potassium chloride	trace
Benzalkonium chloride	0.01%
Purified water	qs ad

MURO'S OPCON-A
Ophthalmic solution: ocular antihistamine and decongestant
(Muro Pharm.)

Naphazoline HCl *	0.025%
Pheniramine maleate *	0.300%
Hydroxypropyl methylcellulose	<1.000%
Disodium EDTA	trace
Boric acid	trace
Sodium borate	trace
Sodium chloride	trace
Benzalkonium chloride	0.010%
Purified water	qs ad

Starred ingredients (*) may be responsible for major toxic effects; consult Section II.

MURO TEARS
Ophthalmic solution: artificial tears
(Muro Pharm.)

Hydroxypropyl methylcellulose	0.50%
Dextran 40	<1.00%
Sodium chloride	<1.00%
Potassium chloride	<1.00%
Disodium EDTA	trace
Benzalkonium chloride	0.01%
Purified water	qs ad

MURPHY'S #824-C DETERGENT
Deodorizer, disinfectant, sanitizer, cleaner
(Murphy-Phoenix)

N-Alkyl (C12 50%, C14 30%, C16 17%, C18 3%) dimethyl ethylbenzyl ammonium chloride *	1.6%
N-Alkyl (C14 60%, C16 30%, C12 5%, C18 5%) dimethyl benzyl ammonium chloride *	1.6%
Trisodium phosphate	5.0%
Sodium metasilicate anhydrous	4.8%
Ethylenediaminetetraacetic acid tetrasodium salt	2.3%

MURPHY'S LAUNDRY AID
Spot cleaner
(Murphy-Phoenix)

Tetrahydro 1,4 oxazine vegetable oil compound *
Tetra sodium salt of ethylene diamine acetate

MURPHY'S OIL SOAP
Cleaner
(Murphy-Phoenix)

Vegetable oil soap

MUSTARINE
Counterirritant
(Brown Mfg.)

Oleoresin capsicum	1 3/4%
Turpentine	3 1/10%
Camphor	3/4%
Menthol	3/8%
Various oils	
Petrolatum base	

'76 Ed.

MUSTEROLE
Analgesic rub
(Plough)

Wax	
Mineral oil	
Glycol monosalicylate *	1.90% w/w
Methyl salicylate	0.63% w/w
Volatile oil of mustard *	2.85% w/w

MUSTEROLE, DEEP STRENGTH
See DEEP STRENGTH MUSTEROLE

MYAMBUTOL TABLETS
For treatment of pulmonary tuberculosis
(Lederle)

Each tablet:
Myambutol (Ethambutol hydrochloride)	100 mg.; 400 mg.

MY-B-DEN SUBLINGUAL TABLETS
For treatment of varicose vein complications, bursitis, etc.
(Dome)

Each tablet:
Adenosine phosphate	20 mg.

MYCELEX 1% CREAM
Treatment of dermal infections
(Dome)

Each gram:
Clotrimazole	10 mg.
Sorbitan monostearate	
Polysorbate 60	
Cetyl esters wax	
Cetostearyl alcohol	
2-Octyldodecanol	
Purified water	
Preservative (Benzyl alcohol)	1%

MYCELEX-G 1% VAGINAL CREAM
Candidal vulvovaginitis
(Dome)

Each applicatorful:
Clotrimazole	50 mg.
Sorbitan monostearate	
Polysorbate 60	
Cetyl esters wax	
Cetostearyl alcohol	
2-Octyldodecanol	
Purified water	
Preservative (Benzyl alcohol)	1%

MYCELEX-G VAGINAL TABLETS
Treatment of vulvovaginal candidiasis
(Dome)

Each tablet:
Clotrimazole	100 mg.
Lactose	
Povidone	
Corn starch	
Magnesium stearate	

MYCELEX 1% SOLUTION
Treatment of dermal infections
(Dome)

Each ml.:
Clotrimazole	10 mg.
Polyethylene glycol 400	

MYCHEL
Broad and medium spectrum antibiotic
(Rachelle Labs.)

Each capsule:
Chloramphenicol	250 mg.

MYCOBAC, MUNICHEM
See MUNICHEM MYCOBAC

MYCOLOG CREAM
Anti-inflammatory, antipruritic, antiallergic; topical use
(Squibb)

Each gm.:
Nystatin	100,000 units
Neomycin sulfate (equiv. to 2.5 mg. neomycin base)	
Gramicidin	0.25 mg.
Triamcinolone acetonide	1 mg.
Polysorbate 60	
Alcohol	
Aluminum hydroxide concentrated wet gel	
Titanium dioxide	
Glyceryl monostearate	
Polyethylene glycol monostearate	
Simethicone	
Sorbic acid	
Propylene glycol	
Ethylenediamine hydrochloride	
White petrolatum	
Polyoxyethylene fatty alcohol ether	
Methylparaben	
Propylparaben	
Sorbitol solution	

MYCOLOG OINTMENT
Anti-inflammatory, antipruritic, antiallergic; topical use
(Squibb)

Each gm.:
Nystatin	100,000 units
Neomycin sulfate (equiv. to 2.5 mg. neomycin base)	
Gramicidin	0.25 mg.
Triamcinolone acetonide	1 mg.
Plastibase (plasticized hydrocarbon gel):	
Polyethylene	
Mineral oil	

MYCOMIST
Fungicidal deodorant spray for shoes
(Gordon Labs.)

Chlorophyll	
Formalin *	
Benzalkonium chloride *	

MYCOQUIN OINTMENT
Antibacterial-antifungal
(Elder)

Iodochlorhydroxyquin *	3.0%

Starred ingredients (*) may be responsible for major toxic effects; consult Section II.

MYCOSTATIN CREAM
Antifungal, antibiotic
(Squibb)

Each gram:
Nystatin (USP) .... 100,000 units
Base:
Aluminum hydroxide concentrated wet
gel
Titanium dioxide
Propylene glycol
Cetearyl alcohol
Ceteareth-20
White petrolatum
Sorbitol solution
Glyceryl monostearate
Polyethylene glycol monostearate
Sorbic acid
Simethicone

MYCOSTATIN OINTMENT
Antifungal antibiotic
(Squibb)

Each gm.:
Nystatin U.S.P. .... 100,000 units
Plastibase (plasticized hydrocarbon gel):
Polyethylene
Mineral oil

MYCOSTATIN ORAL (SUSPENSION & TABLETS)
Antifungal antibiotic
(Squibb)

SUSPENSION (each cc):
Nystatin U.S.P. .... 100,000 units
Vehicle containing 50% Sucrose

TABLETS (each):
Nystatin U.S.P. .... 500,000 units

MYCOSTATIN TOPICAL POWDER
Antifungal antibiotic
(Squibb)

Each gm.:
Nystatin U.S.P. .... 100,000 units
Talc U.S.P.

MYCOSTATIN VAGINAL TABLETS
Antifungal antibiotic
(Squibb)

Each tablet:
Nystatin U.S.P. .... 100,000 units
Lactose
Ethyl cellulose
Stearic acid
Starch

MYDRIACYL
Ophthalmic solution
(Alcon)

Active ingred. (each ml.):
Tropicamide .... 0.5% or 1.0%
Preservative:
Benzalkonium chloride 0.01%
Inactive ingred.:
Sodium chloride
Disodium edetate
Hydrochloric acid and/or Sodium hy-
droxide (to adjust pH)
Purified Water

MY FOLLY PERFUME, COLOGNE, TOILET WATER
(Parfums Duvelle)

Alcohol (denatured with diethyl phthalate) *

MYLEPSIN
Canine anticonvulsant
(Fort Dodge)

Each tablet:
Primidone * .... 250 mg.

MYLONE 50D EASY TO USE SOIL FUMIGANT
(Hopkins Agric.)

Active ingred.: 50%
Tetrahydro-3,5,-dimethyl-2H-1,3,5-thia-
diazine-2-thione *
Inert ingred.: 50%
Dispersing and sticking agents, and inert
carrier

MYOFLEX CREME
*Topical analgesic, antirheumatic ad-
junct*
(Warren-Teed)

Triethanolamine salicylate * 10%

MYOTALIS
Digitalis therapy
(Vita Elixir Co.)

Each tablet:
Digitalis * .... 1 1/2 gr.

MYOTOXIN TABLETS
Cardiotonic glycoside
(Vita Elixir Co.)

Digitoxin *
Tablet #1 .... 0.1 mg.
Tablet #2 .... 0.2 mg.

MYRINGACAINE
For treatment of ear infections
(Upjohn)

Benzocaine 4%
Ephedrine hydrochloride 0.44%
Orthohydroxyphenylmercuric
chloride 0.05%
In a glycerin and propylene glycol base

MYRTLEWOOD PERFUME
(Parfums Duvelle)

Alcohol (denatured with diethyl phthalate) *

MYRURGIA COSMETIC PRODUCTS
Perfumes & soaps

Myrurgia Perfumes, Inc.
1370 Ave. of the Americas
New York, N.Y. 10019

Phone: 212-541-5410

See COSMETICS, Section VI, General
Formulations

MYTAB
Germicide
(Fine Organics, Inc.)

Myristyl trimethyl ammonium
bromide * 100%

'76 Ed.

MYZIN SMEAR (E.Q. 335)
Screwworm control - veterinary
(Fort Dodge)

Gamma isomer of benzene hexachlor-
ide from lindane * 3%
Pine oil * 35%
Inert ingred.:
Mineral oil 42%
Santocel 10%
Emulsives 10%

N

NAA 0.2 DUST (Double Strength)
Fungicide
(FMC Corp., Agricultural Chem. Div.)

Naphthaleneacetic acid 0.2%

NACAP
Corrosion inhibitor
(Vanderbilt, R.T.)

Sodium mercaptobenzothiazole * .. 50%

NA-CHURS LIQUID FERTILIZER 3-18-18
(Na-Churs)

Total Nitrogen (from aqua ammonia-
urea) 3%
Available Phosphoric acid (from 75%
phosphoric acid) * 18%
Water soluble Potash (from 45% potassium hydroxide) * 18%

Starred ingredients (*) may be responsible for major toxic effects; consult Section II.

NA-CHURS LIQUID FERTILIZER 3-18-18 (With Sulfur)
(Na-Churs)

Total Nitrogen (from aqua ammonia-urea-ammonium thiosulfate)	3%
Available Phosphoric acid (from 75% phosphoric acid) *	18%
Soluble Potash (from 45% potassium hydroxide) *	18%
Sulfur (from ammonium thiosulfate)	1%

NA-CHURS LIQUID FERTILIZER 9-18-9
(Na-Churs)

Total Nitrogen (from aqua ammonia-urea)	9%
Available Phosphoric acid (from 75% phosphoric acid) *	18%
Water soluble Potash (from 45% potassium hydroxide) *	9%

NA-CHURS LIQUID FERTILIZER 9-18-9 (With Sulfur)
(Na-Churs)

Total Nitrogen (from aqua ammonia-urea-ammonium thiosulfate)	9%
Available Phosphoric acid (from 75% phosphoric acid) *	18%
Soluble Potash (from 45% potassium hydroxide) *	9%
Sulfur (from ammonium thiosulfate)	1%

NA-CHURS LIQUID FERTILIZER 10-10-10
(Na-Churs)

Total Nitrogen (from aqua ammonia-urea)	10%
Available Phosphoric acid (from 75% phosphoric acid) *	10%
Water soluble Potash (from 45% potassium hydroxide) *	10%

NA-CHURS LIQUID FERTILIZER 10-10-10 (With Sulfur)
(Na-Churs)

Total Nitrogen (from aqua ammonia-urea-ammonium thiosulfate)	10%
Available Phosphoric acid (from 75% phosphoric acid) *	10%
Soluble Potash (from 45% potassium hydroxide) *	10%
Sulfur (from ammonium thiosulfate)	1%

NA-CHURS LIQUID FERTILIZER 16-4-4 (With Sulfur)
(Na-Churs)

Total Nitrogen (from aqua ammonia-urea-ammonium thiosulfate)	16%
Available Phosphoric acid (from 75% phosphoric acid) *	4%
Water soluble Potash (from 45% potassium hydroxide) *	4%
Sulfur (from ammonium thiosulfate)	8%

NACO AMINE 4D-2 WEED KILLER
Herbicide
(Grace, W.R.)

Dimethylamine salt of 2,4-D *	49%

NACO COPPER "53" BASIC COPPER SULFATE
Fungicide
(Grace, W.R.)

Copper expressed as metallic *	53%

NACO COPPER CARB NO. 20
Seed treatment
(Grace, W.R.)

Metallic Copper *	20.00%

NACO LV-4D WEED KILLER
Herbicide
(Grace, W.R.)

Isooctyl ester of 2,4-D *	69.0%

NACO MICRONIZED WETTABLE SULFUR
Fungicide
(Grace, W.R.)

Sulfur *	95.00%

NACO SULPHUR - COPPER 65-4 DUST
Fungicide
(Grace, W.R.)

Sulphur *	65.00%
Copper expressed as metallic *	4.00%

NACO 70 SUPREME A 70 SECOND SUPERIOR OIL
Insecticide
(Grace, W.R.)

Petroleum oils *	99.2%

NACREM
Nasal decongestant cream
(Jenkins Labs.)

Ammonium chloride	1.5%
Menthol *	q.s.
Methyl salicylate (syn.) *	q.s.
Camphor *	q.s.
Oil eucalyptus *	q.s.

NAIL-A-CAIN
Relief of pain of ingrown nails
(Lambda Inc.)

Benzocaine	
Tannic acid *	
Isopropyl alcohol	61%
Diethyl ether	20%

NAIR AEROSOL FOAM
Depilatory
(Carter Products)

Combined amount:	<10%
Calcium and sodium thioglycolates	
Free Calcium hydroxide	
Nonionic emulsifiers	
Cetyl alcohol	
Mineral oil	
Water	
Perfume	
Hydrocarbons (propellant)	

NAIR AEROSOL SPRAY
Depilatory
(Carter Products)

Combined amount:	<10%
Calcium and sodium thioglycolates	
Free Calcium hydroxide	
Nonionic emulsifiers	
Mineral oil	
Petrolatum	
Hydrocarbons (propellant)	
Water	
Perfume	

NAIR CREAM AND LOTION
Depilatory
(Carter Products)

Calcium thioglycolate	<10%
Free Calcium hydroxide	
Mineral oil	
Nonionic emulsifiers	
Water	
Perfume	

NALKIL 2701 LIQUID WITH ENDRIFT
Herbicide
(Nalco Chem.)

Petroleum oil *	96.00%
2,4-Dichlorophenoxyacetic acid, isooctyl ester	1.10%
Bromacil	0.61%
Pentachlorophenol	0.79%
Other chlorophenols	0.09%

NALKIL 2702 LIQUID WITH ENDRIFT
Herbicide
(Nalco Chem.)

Petroleum oil *	96.07%
Bromacil	0.97%
Pentachlorophenol	0.79%
Other chlorophenols	0.09%

NALKIL 2703 LIQUID WITH ENDRIFT
Herbicide
(Nalco Chem.)

Petroleum oil *	94.94%
2,4-Dichlorophenoxyacetic acid, isooctyl ester	1.09%
Bromacil	0.98%
Pentachlorophenol	0.80%
Other chlorophenols	0.09%

NALKIL 2726 LIQUID WITH ENDRIFT
Herbicide
(Nalco Chem.)

Petroleum oil *	73.62%
2,4-Dichlorophenoxyacetic acid, isooctyl ester *	8.65%
Bromacil	4.79%
Pentachlorophenol *	6.18%
Other Chlorophenols	0.72%

NALKIL 2727 LIQUID WITH ENDRIFT
Herbicide
(Nalco Chem.)

Petroleum oil *	82.17%
Bromacil	5.78%
Pentachlorophenol *	4.71%
Other Chlorophenols	0.55%

NALKIL 2728 LIQUID WITH ENDRIFT
Herbicide
(Nalco Chem.)

Petroleum oil *	75.88%
2,4-Dichlorophenoxyacetic acid, isooctyl ester	6.46%
Bromacil	5.66%
Pentachlorophenol *	4.61%
Other Chlorophenols	0.54%

NAMIDE
Vitamins
(Kirkman)

PLAIN & BUFFERED (each tablet):
Niacinamide, USP * .... 500 mg.

NAMIDE-C
Vitamins
(Kirkman)

Each tablet:
Niacinamide, USP *	500 mg.
Vitamin C, USP	500 mg.

NAPA BALKAMP ANTI-SEIZE COMPOUND
Sealant and anti-seize compound for threaded fittings and gaskets
(Balkamp, Inc.; Mfr., Armite Labs.)

Pure metallic Lead powder *	72%
Petroleum oil *	20%
Petroleum grease (Barium soap 15%)	8%

NAPA BALKAMP FORMULA 12/34 AEROSOL/BULK
Penetrant, lubricant, corrosion inhibitor
(Balkamp, Inc.; Mfr., Armite Labs.)

Mineral spirits *	70%
Mineral oil *	21%
Petrolatum	6%
Emulsifiers	3%
Carbon dioxide (Aerosol)	

NAPHCON
Decongestant eye drops
(Alcon)

Each ml.:
Naphazoline hydrochloride	0.012%
Benzalkonium chloride (as preservative)	0.01%

NAPHCON - A
Ophthalmic solution
p (Alcon)

Active ingred. (each ml.):
Naphazoline hydrochloride	0.025%
Pheniramine maleate	0.3%

Preservative:
Benzalkonium chloride	0.01%

Inactive ingred.:
Boric acid
Sodium borate
Edetate disodium
Sodium chloride
Sodium hydroxide and/or Hydrochloric acid (to adjust pH)
Purified water

NAQUA TABLETS
Diuretic and antihypertensive
(Schering)

Each tablet:
Trichlormethiazide * .... 2 mg.; 4 mg

NAQUIVAL TABLETS
Diuretic and antihypertensive
(Schering)

Each tablet:
Trichlormethiazide *	4 mg
Reserpine	0.1 mg

NARDIL
Antidepressant
(Parke-Davis)

Each tablet:
Phenelzine sulfate (equiv. to 15 mg. of phenelzine base) *

NARINE GYROCAPS
Nasal congestion, rhinnorhea
(Dooner Labs.)

Each timed-release capsule:
Chlorpheniramine maleate	8.0 mg
Phenylephrine hydrochloride *	20.0 mg
Methscopolamine nitrate	2.5 mg

NASAFED
Decongestant - expectorant
(Russ Pharm.)

Each capsule:
Pseudoephedrine HCl *	120 mg
Brompheniramine maleate	12 mg

NASAPAP
Decongestant - analgesic
(Russ Pharm.)

Each tablet:
Acetaminophen	325 mg
Pseudoephedrine HCl *	30 mg

NASDRO
Nose and throat drops
(Jenkins Labs.)

Ephedrine sulphate *	1%
Chlorobutanol *	5%
Menthol *	
Camphor *	
Oil eucalyptus *	
Thymol *	
Oil red thyme *†	
Isotonic dextrose saline solution	

†*See* Thyme oil

NASO-DEX CAPSULES
Cold & hay fever capsules
(Commerce Drug)

Each capsule:
Belladonna alkaloidal salts	0.16 mg.
Phenylpropanolamine HCl *	50 mg.
Pheniramine maleate	12.5 mg.
Chlorpheniramine maleate	1 mg.

NASO-MIST SPRAY
Antibacterial, antihistamine, nasal decongestant
(Vitarine)

Methapyrilene hydrochloride	0.15%
Phenylephrine hydrochloride *	0.5%
Benzalkonium chloride	0.02%

NASOPHEN
Treatment of rhinitis and sinusitis
(Premo)

0.25% Strength:
Phenylephrine hydrochloride, USP

1% Strength:
Phenylephrine hydrochloride, USP *

'76 Ed.

NATIONAL PAINT PRODUCTS
Paints & varnishes

National Paint & Varnish Co., Inc.
2835 E. Washington Blvd.
Los Angeles, Calif. 90023

Phone: 213-268-2823

See PAINTS, Section VI, General Formulations

NATPIRIN
Analgesic
(Schiff)

Sodium salicylate (from natural sources) *	7.5 gr.
Kelp from Pacific sea kelp	
Calcium carbonate	
Oil wintergreen (from natural sources) *	

Starred ingredients (*) may be responsible for major toxic effects; consult Section II.

NATSYN
General purpose rubber
(Goodyear)

Polyisoprene

NATURE'S REMEDY (Film Coated)
Laxative
(Norcliff Thayer)

Aloe * .... 100 mg.
Cascara sagrada .... 150 mg.

NATURETIN
Diuretic and antihypertensive agent
(Squibb)

Each tablet:
Bendroflumethiazide * 2.5 mg.; 5.0 mg.
or 10.0 mg.

NAVANE CAPSULES
Psychotropic agent
(Roerig)

Each capsule:
Thiothixene * .... 1 mg., 2 mg., 5 mg.,
10 mg. and 20 mg.

NAVANE CONCENTRATE
Psychotropic agent
(Roerig)

Thiothixene hydrochloride
(equivalent to
thiothixene) * .... 5 mg./ml.
Alcohol, U.S.P .... 7.0% v/v

NAVY BRAND BAKERY RESIDUAL
All purpose residual insecticide spray;
industrial use
(Navy Brand)

Petroleum distillate *
2-Butoxyethanol *
Baygon (o-Isopropoxyphenyl methylcarbamate) *
Pyrethrins

NAVY BRAND BLS
Broadleaf weed killer for turf and
lawns
(Navy Brand)

Dimethylamine salt of 2-(methyl-4-
chlorophenoxy) propionic acid * 16.2%
Dimethylamine salt of 2,4-dichlo-
rophenoxyacetic acid * 16.1%

NAVY BRAND FOGGING MIST
Insecticide; municipal use
(Navy Brand)

Petroleum distillate * 96.26%
Malathion 1.80%
Vapona 1.30%
Related compounds 0.10%
Mineral seal oil 0.40%
Inert ingredients:
Epichlorohydrin 0.14%

NAVY BRAND LIQUID TRIM
Herbicide
(Navy Brand)

Diquat dibromide * 1.85%

NAVY BRAND MILL SPRAY
Insecticide; industrial and institutional
use
(Navy Brand)

Pyrethrins 0.104%
Piperonyl butoxide, technical .. 0.850%
Petroleum hydrocarbons * 99.046%

NAVY BRAND WK-70
Herbicide; concentrate
(Navy Brand)

Sodium metaborate (anhydrous) 9.07%
Sodium chlorate * 18.00%

NAVY BRAND WKB-15
Weed and brush killer
(Navy Brand)

2,4-Dichlorophenoxyacetic acid
isooctyl esters * 23.8%
2,4,5-Trichlorophenoxyacetic acid
isooctyl esters * 11.4%

NAVYPINE
Disinfectant
(Navy Brand)

Isopropyl alcohol * 10.70%
Soap 5.55%
Pine oil 5.00%
o-Phenylphenol 3.00%
o-Benzyl-p-chlorophenol 2.25%

NAYLOR'S, DR., PRODUCTS

See DR. NAYLOR'S

NAZAC CONTINUOUS ACTION DECONGESTANT CAPSULES
For nasal congestion due to colds or
hay fever
(Columbia Med.)

Each capsule:
Belladonna alkaloids .... 0.16 mg.
Phenylpropanolamine HCl * 50 mg.
Chlorpheniramine maleate ... 1 mg.
Pheniramine maleate .... 12.5 mg.

N-B3 (PLAIN & BUFFERED)
B Vitamin
(Kirkman)

Each tablet:
Niacin NF * .... 500 mg.

ND-150
Water soluble safety solvent
(National Chemsearch)

Sodium alkyl aryl sulfonate *
Tetra sodium ethylenediamine tetra ace-
tate
Sodium metasilicate
Ethylene glycol monobutyl ether *

N-DIT
Detergent/disinfectant
(Holcomb)

N-Alkyl dimethyl benzyl ammonium chloride * 1-10%

'76 Ed.

NEET (CREAM AND LOTION)
Odorless hair remover
(Whitehall Labs.)

Calcium thioglycolate *

NEGABOT PASTE
Equine anthelmintic
(Cutter (Brand) Bayvet Div. Cutter
Labs.)

Trichlorfon * 40%

NEGUVON POUR-ON
Insecticide for cattle
(Cutter (Brand) Bayvet Div. Cutter
Labs.)

Trichlorfon * 8%

NELLITE 90 NEMATICIDE
(Dow)

Active ingred.: 90.0%
Phenyl N,N'-dimethyl phosphorodiami-
date *
Inert ingred.: 10.0%
Silicon dioxide
Wetting agent

NELLITE TG NEMATICIDE
(Dow)

Phenyl N,N'-dimethyl phosphorodiamidate (minimum) * 97%

NELLITE WS NEMATICIDE
(Dow)

Active ingred.:
Phenyl N,N'-dimethyl
phosphorodiamidate * 2.7%
Inert ingred.:
Primarily water 97.3%

NEMACUR
Nematicide
(Mobay Chemical Corp.)

Ethyl 3-methyl-4-(methylthio)phenyl(1-
methylethyl)phosphoramidate *

NEMA WORM CAPSULES
Anthelmintic; veterinary
(Parke-Davis)

Tetrachlorethylene *

NEMBUTAL ELIXIR
Sedative, hypnotic, antispasmodic
(Abbott)

Each 5 ml.:
Pentobarbital * .... 18.2 mg.
Alcohol 18%

NEMBUTAL SODIUM CAPSULES
Sedative, hypnotic, antispasmodic
(Abbott)

Each capsule:
Pentobarbital sodium *
  Yellow with yellow cap .... 30 mg.
  Clear with yellow cap ...... 50 mg.
  Yellow or clear with orange
    cap .... 100 mg.

NEMBUTAL SODIUM SUPPOSITORIES
Sedative & hypnotic
(Abbott)

Each suppository:
Pentobarbital
  sodium * .... 30 mg.; 60 mg.;
      120 mg.; or 200 mg.

NEOBACIMYX
Ophthalmic ointment; dogs and cats
(Burns-Biotec)

Each gram:
Bacitracin zinc .... 400 units
Neomycin sulfate (equiv. to
  3.5 mg./gm. of neomycin
  base) 0.5%
Polymyxin B sulfate ...... 5,000 units
In a base of White petrolatum and Mineral oil

NEOBACIMYX-H
Ophthalmic ointment; dogs and cats
(Burns-Biotec)

Each gram:
Bacitracin zinc .... 400 units
Neomycin sulfate (equiv. to
  3.5 mg./gm. of neomycin
  base) 0.5%
Polymyxin B sulfate ...... 5,000 units
Hydrocortisone acetate 1.0%
In a base of White petrolatum and Mineral oil

NEO-CAFOTAN TABLETS
Analgesic, antipyretic, antihistaminic
(Premo)

Each tablet:
Chlorpheniramine maleate .. 2 mg.
Aspirin * .... 0.32 gm.
Caffeine .... 0.03 gm.

NEOCASTADERM
Dermatological preparation for fungus infections
(Lannett)

Resorcin *
Boric acid *
Acetone

NEOCET
Cold tablets
(Vale)

Each tablet:
Pyrilamine maleate * .... 25 mg.
Phenacetin * .... 130 mg.
Salicylamide .... 130 mg.
Hyoscyamus .... 10 mg.
Caffeine (anhydrous) .... 16 mg.

NEOCET JUNIOR
Analgesic, antihistaminic
(Vale)

Each tablet:
Pyrilamine maleate * .... 12.5 mg.
Phenacetin * .... 64.8 mg.
Salicylamide .... 64.8 mg.
Hyoscyamus .... 5.4 mg.
Caffeine (anhydrous) .... 8.1 mg.

NEOCHOLAN
Hydrocholeretic
(Dow Pharm., Dow Chem. Co.)

Each tablet:
Dehydrocholic acid * .... 250 mg.

NEOCIN
Antibacterial analgesic sore throat lozenges
(Commerce Drug)

Each lozenge:
Acetaminophen * .... 1 1/2 gr.
Benzocaine .... 10 mg.
Cetyl pyridinium chloride .... 2 mg.

NEO-COROVAS TYMCAPS
Coronary vasodilator
(Amfre-Grant)

Each Tymcap:
Pentaerythritol tetranitrate * .. 30 mg.

NEO-CORT-DOME CREME & LOTION
(Dome)

Microdispersed Hydro-
  cortisone alcohol 0.25%; 0.5%; 1.0%
Neomycin sulfate
  (equiv. 0.35% neomycin base) ... 0.5%
Acid pH vehicle:
  Oil-in-water, emulsion-type creme containing a buffered solution of aluminum acetate

NEO-CORTICIN
Ophthalmic ointment - veterinary
(Burns-Biotec)

Each gram:
Hydrocortisone acetate 0.5%
Neomycin sulfate (equiv. to 3.5
  mg./gm. neomycin base) 0.5%
Sulfacetamide sodium 10%
White petrolatum and Mineral oil base

NEOCURTASAL
Salt substitute
(Winthrop Labs.)

Potassium chloride
Glutamic acid
Potassium glutamate
Calcium silicate
Tribasic calcium phosphate
Potassium iodide 0.01%

NEOCYLATE TABLETS
Analgesic
(Central Pharmacal Co.)

Each tablet:
Potassium salicylate * .... 280 mg.
Aminobenzoic acid .... 250 mg.

NEO-DARBAZINE SPANSULE CAPSULES
Antibiotic therapy for control of gastroenteritis; veterinary
(Norden Labs.)

Each No. 1 capsule:
Prochlorperazine maleate
  (equiv. to 3.33 mg.
  prochlorperazine) * .... 5.40 mg.
Isopropamide iodide (equiv. to
  1.67 mg. isopropamide) * .. 2.27 mg.
Neomycin sulfate (equiv. to 25
  mg. neomycin base) .... 35.7 mg.

Each No. 3 capsule:
Prochlorperazine maleate
  (equiv. to 10 mg.
  prochlorperazine) * .... 16.2 mg.
Isopropamide iodide (equiv. to
  5 mg. isopropamide) * ..... 6.8 mg.
Neomycin sulfate (equiv to 75
  mg. neomycin base) .... 107 mg.

NEOFED
Decongestant
(Vale)

Each tablet:
Pseudoephedrine
  hydrochloride * .... 60 mg.

'76 Ed.

Starred ingredients (*) may be responsible for major toxic effects; consult Section II.

NEOGEN SUPPOSITORIES (FULL STRENGTH & HALF STRENGTH)
For bronchial asthma
(Premo)

FULL STRENGTH (each suppository):
Pentobarbital *	1 gr.
Aminophylline *	4 gr.
Theophylline *	3 gr.
Ephedrine sulfate *	3/8 gr.
Benzocaine	3 gr.

HALF STRENGTH (each suppository):
Pentobarbital *	1/2 gr.
Aminophylline *	2 gr.
Theophylline *	1 1/2 gr.
Ephedrine sulfate *	3/16 gr.
Benzocaine	1 1/2 gr.

'76 Ed.

NEO-GERM-I-TOL SPECIAL 80%
Biocide
(Fine Organics, Inc.)

n-Alkyl (C12 40%, C14 50%, C16 10%) dimethyl benzyl ammonium chloride *	80%
Ethyl alcohol	20%

'76 Ed.

NEOGESIC
Analgesic
(Vale)

Each tablet:
Salicylamide	194.4 mg.
Phenacetin *	129.6 mg.
Caffeine anhydrous	16.2 mg.

NEOLAX TABLETS
Cholagogue, fecal softener
(Central Pharmacal Co.)

Each tablet:
Dehydrocholic acid	240 mg.
Dioctyl sodium sulfosuccinate *	50 mg.

NEOLITE ALL PURPOSE ADHESIVE
(Goodyear)

Synthetic rubber (Polychloroprene)	10-20%
Rubber solvent naphtha *	25-30%
Acetone *	25-30%
Methyl ethyl ketone *	20-25%
Toluene *	5-10%

NEOLOZ-B
Relief of minor sore throat
(Cameron Medical Corp.)

Each lozenge:
Benzocaine	10 mg.
Cetyl dimethyl benzyl ammonium chloride	1 mg.

NEOMARK LOTION
For seborrheic dermatoses
(C & M Pharmacal)

Salicylic acid *	1.6%
LCD	2.0%
Beta-Naphthol	1.0%
Resorcin monoacetate	1.0%
Castor oil	
Isopropyl alcohol *	68.0%
Ethyl alcohol	1.6%
Purified water	

NEO-MET BRAKE AND ELECTRIC PARTS DRY CLEANER - N.M.

See GUNK N.M. - NEO-MET BRAKE AND ELECTRIC PARTS DRY CLEANER

NEOMIDE
Antibacterial ophthalmic ointment - veterinary
(Burns-Biotec)

Each gram:
Neomycin sulfate (equiv. to 3.5 mg./gm. neomycin base)	0.5%
Sulfacetamide sodium	10%
White petrolatum and Mineral oil base	

NEO-MIST 1/2% NASAL SPRAY
Decongestant, antiseptic
(Am. Pharmaceutical)

Phenylephrine HCl *	0.50%
Cetalkonium chloride	0.02%

NEOPAP SUPPRETTES
Antipyretic & analgesic
(Webcon)

Each suppository:
Acetaminophen *	2 gr.

NEO-PINE
Pine oil disinfectant
(Puritan Chem. Co.)

Pine oil *	12.0%
Isopropanol	10.0%
Soap	6.5%
Sodium salt of orthobenzylparachlorophenol	3.5%

NEOQUESS
(OJF)

Each tablet:
Phenobarbital *	16.2 mg.
Hyoscyamine sulfate	0.1037 mg.
Hyoscine hydrobromide	0.0065 mg.
Atropine sulfate	0.0194 mg.

NEO-128 SOLUBLE POWDER
Drinking water medication for swine and poultry
(Salsbury)

Neomycin base (from neomycin sulfate)	25 gm.

NEOSORB PLUS
Antacid
(Lemmon Co.)

Each tablet:
Dried Aluminum hydroxide gel	300 mg.
Magnesium hydroxide	150 mg.

NEOSPECT
Bronchodilator and expectorant
(Lemmon Co.)

Each tablet:
Neothylline (Dyphylline) *	100 mg.
Ephedrine sulfate *	25 mg.
Phenobarbital *	15 mg.
Glyceryl guaiacolate	100 mg.

NEOSPORIN AEROSOL
Bacterial skin infections
(Burroughs Wellcome)

Each 90 gm. aerosol:
Polymyxin B sulfate	100,000 units
Bacitracin zinc	8,000 units
Neomycin sulfate (equiv. to 70 mg. neomycin base)	100 mg.
Dichlorodifluoromethane	
Trichloromonofluoromethane	

NEOSPORIN-G CREAM
Antibiotic
(Burroughs Wellcome)

Each gram:
Polymyxin B sulfate	10,000 units
Neomycin sulfate (equiv. to 3.5 mg. neomycin base)	5 mg.
Gramicidin	0.25 mg.
Liquid petrolatum	
White petrolatum	
Purified water	
Propylene glycol	
Polyoxyethylene polyoxypropylene compound	
Emulsifying wax	
Methylparaben (preservative)	0.25%

NEOSPORIN OINTMENT OPHTHALMIC
Bacterial infections of the eye
(Burroughs Wellcome)

Each gram:
Aerosporin (Polymixin B sulfate)	10,000 units
Bacitracin zinc	400 units
Neomycin sulfate (equiv. to 3.5 mg. neomycin base)	5 mg.
White petrolatum	

NEOSPORIN OINTMENT (TOPICAL)
Antibiotic
(Burroughs Wellcome)

Each gram:
Polymyxin B sulfate	5,000 units
Bacitracin zinc	400 units
Neomycin sulfate (equiv. to 3.5 mg. neomycin base)	5 mg.
Special white petrolatum	q.s.

NEOSPORIN OPHTHALMIC SOLUTION
Bacterial infections of the eye
(Burroughs Wellcome)

Each cc:
Polymyxin B sulfate ..... 10,000 units
Neomycin sulfate (equiv. to
   1.75 mg. neomycin base) .. 2.5 mg.
Gramicidin .... 0.025 mg.
Thimerosal 0.001%
Alcohol 0.5%
Propylene glycol
Polyoxyethylene polyoxypropylene
   compound
Sodium chloride
Water for injection

NEOSPORIN POWDER
Antibiotic
(Burroughs Wellcome)

Each gram:
Polymyxin B sulfate ..... 5,000 units
Bacitracin zinc .... 400 units
Neomycin sulfate (equiv. to 3.5
   mg. neomycin base) .... 5 mg.
Special lactose base

NEO-SYNALAR CREAM
Topical anti-inflammatory, antibacterial agent
(Syntex Labs.)

Fluocinolone acetonide 0.025%
Neomycin sulfate (equivalent to
  0.35% neomycin base) 0.5%
Aqueous base:
  Stearic acid
  Propylene glycol
  Sorbitan monostearate and monooleate
  Polysorbate 60
  Methylparaben
  Propylparaben

NEO-SYNALAR CREAM VETERINARY
Anti-inflammatory, antibacterial agent
(Syntex Labs.)

Fluocinolone acetonide 0.025%
Neomycin sulfate (equiv. to 0.35%
  neomycin base) 0.5%

NEO-SYNEPHRINE COMPOUND COLD TABLETS
Decongestant, analgesic, antipyretic & antihistaminic
(Winthrop Labs.)

Each tablet:
Neo-synephrine
  hydrochloride * .... 5 mg.
Acetaminophen (N-Acetyl-p-
  aminophenol) * .... 150 mg.
Thenfadil hydrochloride *† .. 7.5 mg.
Caffeine .... 15 mg.

†*See* Antihistaminics

NEO-SYNEPHRINE HYDROCHLORIDE
Intranasal use
(Winthrop Labs.)

SOLUTION:
Phenylephrine hy-
  drochloride,
  USP * 0.125%; 0.25%; 0.5%;
                        or 1.0%
SPRAY:
Phenylephrine hydrochloride, USP *
  For children & adults: 0.25%
  For adults: 0.5%
JELLY:
Phenylephrine hydrochloride,
  USP * 0.5%

NEO-TEARS
Ocular lubricant
(Barnes-Hind)

Polyvinyl alcohol
Hydroxyethylcellulose
Sodium chloride
Potassium chloride
Sodium phosphate
Sodium biphosphate
Polyethylene glycol 300
Sodium hydroxide (to adjust pH)
Purified water
Thimerosal 0.004%
Edetate disodium 0.02%

NEOTEP
Decongestant
(Direct Div.)

Each capsule:
Chlorpheniramine maleate * .. 9 mg.
Phenylephrine HCl * .... 21 mg.

NEOTHYLLINE (TABLETS & ELIXIR)
Bronchodilator
(Lemmon Co.)

TABLETS (each):
Dyphylline * .... 200 mg. and 400 mg.

ELIXIR (each 15 ml.):
Dyphylline * .... 160 mg.
Glycerin 10%
Alcohol 18%

NEOTHYLLINE-GG (TABLETS & ELIXIR)
Bronchodilator-expectorant
(Lemmon Co.)

Each tablet or 30 ml.:
Neothylline (Dyphylline) * .. 200 mg.
Guaifenesin .... 200 mg.
Alcohol (Elixir only) 10%

NEOTUSSIN
Expectorant & antitussive
(Moffet Inc.)

Each 30 cc:
Codeine phosphate * .... 60 mg.
Potassium guaiacol sulfonate . 0.5 gm.
Citric acid .... 0.3 gm.

NEOVICAPS T.R.
Stress formula
(Scherer Labs.)

Each capsule:
Thiamine mononitrate (Vi-
  tamin B-1) .... 15 mg.
Riboflavin (Vitamin B-3) .... 10 mg.
Pyridoxine HCl (Vitamin B-6) .. 5 mg.
Niacinamide .... 50 mg.
Ascorbic acid (Vitamin C) .... 300 mg.
Zinc .... 15 mg.

NEOWAX
Self-polishing, high-gloss wax
(Lester Labs.)

Wax
Emulsifiers

                             '76 Ed.

NEOZYL
Treatment of cold symptoms
(Direct Div.)

Each 5 ml.:
Codeine phosphate * .... 10 mg.
Phenylpropanolamine HCl * 18.75 mg.
Alcohol 5%

NEPHRON BENZOCAINE-N
Topical anesthetic ointment
(Nephron)

Benzocaine 18%
In a water soluble base of Polyethylene
glycols

NEPHRON INHALANT
(Nephron)

Racemic Epinephrine hydrochloride 2.25%
Chlorobutanol (Chloroform deriv.) 0.5%

NEPHROX
Antacid
(Fleming)

Each 5 cc:
Aluminum hydroxide .... 320 mg.
Mineral oil 10%/v

NEPO
Broad and fine line needlepoint markers
(Sanford Corp.)

Dyes
Resins
Glycol ethers
Alcohol

"NEPOLON" COATINGS, BIRD

See BIRD "NEPOLON" COATINGS

Starred ingredients (*) may be responsible for major toxic effects; consult Section II.

NERO ANTI-MATING SPRAY
Protection for female dogs
(Nero Pet Products)

Oil of lemongrass	2%
Propellent and other inert ingredients	98%
	'76 Ed.

NERO COAT GLOSS & DEODORANT
Dog grooming
(Nero Pet Products)

Essential oils *
Methylene bis trichlorophenol (Hexachlorophene)
Isopropanol *

'76 Ed.

NERO DOGGIE DRY BATH
(Nero Pet Products)

Sodium lauryl sulfate *
Coconut oil, amine condensate

'76 Ed.

NERO INDOOR DOG REPELLENT
(Nero Pet Products)

Methyl nonyl ketone	1.9%
Related compounds	0.1%
	'76 Ed.

NERO OUTDOOR DOG REPELLENT
(Nero Pet Products)

Methyl nonyl ketone	1.9%
Related compounds	0.1%
	'76 Ed.

NERO PUPPY HOUSEBREAK TRAINER
(Nero Pet Products)

Ammonium carbonate
Aqua Ammonia *

'76 Ed.

NERVINE CAPSULE-SHAPED TABLET

See MILES NERVINE CAPSULE-SHAPED TABLET

NER-VITA
Tonic
(Etna Chem.)

Strychnine sulphate	0.006 gm./100 cc.
Calcium	
Sodium	
Potassium	
Iron & manganese glycerophosphates	
Sodium formate	
Citric, formic, lactic & glycerophosphoric acids	
	'76 Ed.

NESACAINE
Local anesthetic
(Pennwalt, Pharm. Div.)

1% SOLUTION:
Nesacaine (Chloroprocaine hydrochloride)	10 mg./ml.

2% SOLUTION:
Nesacaine (Chloroprocaine hydrochloride)	20 mg./ml.

NESACAINE CE
Local anesthetic without preservative
(Pennwalt, Pharm. Div.)

Chloroprocaine HCl	2%; 3%

NESTLE COLORTINT
(Nestle-LeMur)

Purified basic colors	<1%
Sodium pyrophosphate	1-10%
Sodium sulfate	>10%

NESTLE-LEMUR COSMETIC PRODUCTS
Cosmetics, toiletries, permanent wave supplies

Nestle-LeMur Co.
66 E. 34th St.
New York, N.Y. 10016

Phone: 212-679-0900

See COSMETICS, Section VI, General Formulations

NESTLE POMADE HONGROISE
(Nestle-LeMur)

Beeswax	>10%
Soap	>10%
Inorganic colors	1-10%
Perfume essence	<1%

NETTIE ROSENSTEIN PERFUMES & EAUX DE PARFUMS
(Rosenstein, N.)

Nettie Rosenstein, Inc.
220 E. 23rd St.
New York, N.Y. 10010

Phone: 212-371-6300

NEURABALM
Liniment, antiseptic
(S.S.S. Co.)

Alcohol SD 27	54%
Methyl salicylate *	
Oil of eucalyptus *	
Camphor *	
Menthol *	
Chlorothymol *	
Acetone *	
Oil of cajuput *	
Benzocaine	

NEUROVAL ELIXIR
Sedative
(Vale)

Each fl. oz.:
Alcohol	10%
Sodium phenobarbital *	129.6 mg.
Sodium bromide *	1.944 gm.
Potassium bromide *	1.944 gm.

NEUTONE
Floor dressing
(Hillyard Chem.)

Mineral spirits *

'76 Ed.

NEUTRACOMP
Nonalkaline antacid
(CMC Research Div.)

Each tablet:
Aluminum hydroxide	260 mg.
Magnesium trisilicate	488 mg.

NEUTRALODOR AIR FRESHENER

See AMWAY NEUTRALODOR AIR FRESHENER

NEUTRALOX (TABLETS & LIQUID)
Antacid-adsorbent-protective
(Lemmon Co.)

Each tablet & 5 ml.:
Aluminum hydroxide	300 mg.
Magnesium hydroxide	150 mg.

NEUTRODOR DEODORIZING BLOCS
(Nat'l Labs. Div.)

Paradichlorobenzene *	major

Starred ingredients (*) may be responsible for major toxic effects; consult Section II.

NEUTROGENA ACNE DRYING GEL
(Neutrogena Corp.)

Witch hazel
Isopropyl alcohol *
Propylene glycol
Carbomer 940
Triethanolamine
EDTA
Methylparaben
Propylparaben
Benzophenone-2
Color

NEUTROGENA ACNE SOAP
(Neutrogena Corp.)

Triethanolamine
Stearic acid
Tallow
Water
Glycerin
Coconut oil
Castor oil
TEA-lauryl sulfate
Sodium hydroxide
Oleic acid
Acetylated lanolin alcohol
Cocamide DEA
SD Alcohol 3-A
Fragrance

NEUTROGENA BABY SOAP
(Neutrogena Corp.)

Triethanolamine
Stearic acid
Tallow
Glycerin
Water
Coconut oil
Castor oil
Sodium hydroxide
Oleic acid
Laneth-10 acetate
Cocamide DEA
Nonoxynol-14 and PEG-4 octoate
Fragrance

NEUTROGENA BODY OIL
(Scented and Unscented)
(Neutrogena Corp.)

Isopropyl myristate
Sesame oil
PEG-40 sorbitan peroleate
Fragrance (Scented only)

NEUTROGENA DRY SKIN SOAP (Scented and Unscented)
(Neutrogena Corp.)

Triethanolamine
Stearic acid
Tallow
Glycerin
Water
Coconut oil
Castor oil
Sodium hydroxide
Oleic acid
Laneth-10-acetate
Nonoxynol-14 and PEG-4 octoate
Cocamide DEA
Fragrance (Scented only)
BHT

NEUTROGENA HAND CREAM (Scented and Unscented)
(Neutrogena Corp.)

Water
Glycerin
Cetearyl alcohol
Sodium cetearyl sulfate
Fragrance (Scented only)
Stearic acid
Methylparaben
Propylparaben
Sodium sulfate
Dilauryl thiodipropionate

NEUTROGENA IMPERIAL SOAP (Scented and Unscented)
(Neutrogena Corp.)

Triethanolamine
Stearic acid
Tallow
Glycerin
Water
Coconut oil
Castor oil
Sodium hydroxide
Oleic acid
Cocoamide DEA
Fragrance (Scented only)

NEUTROGENA LOTION FOR HAND & SKIN (Scented and Unscented)
(Neutrogena Corp.)

Water
Glyceryl stearate and PEG-100 stearate
Isopropyl myristate
Butylene glycol
Cetyl alcohol
Carbomer 934
Imidazolidinyl urea
Fragrance (Scented only)
Methylparaben
Triethanolamine
Propylparaben
Sodium lauryl sulfate

NEUTROGENA RAINBATH DRY SKIN BATH GEL (Scented and Unscented)
(Neutrogena Corp.)

Water
Sodium laureth sulfate
Oleyl betaine (Velvetex OLB-50)
Lauramide DEA
Polysorbate 20
Fragrance (Scented only)
Propylene glycol
Methylparaben
Propylparaben
Sodium chloride
Citric acid
Color

NEUTROGENA REGULAR SOAP (Scented and Unscented)
(Neutrogena Corp.)

Triethanolamine
Stearic acid
Tallow
Water
Glycerin
Coconut oil
Castor oil
Sodium hydroxide
Oleic acid
Cocamide DEA
Fragrance (Scented only)

NEUTROGENA SOLID SHAMPOO
(Neutrogena Corp.)

Triethanolamine
Stearic acid
Water
Tallow
Coconut oil
Olive oil
Glycerin
Sodium hydroxide
Oleic acid
Lauric acid
Castor oil
Lanolin linoleate
TEA-lauryl sulfate
Hydrolyzed animal protein
Fragrance
EDTA
BHT
D&C Green No. 8
FD&C Green No. 3

NEVAROT
Wood preserver
(Texas Refinery)

Petroleum distillate *	78.1%
Aromatic solvents *	9.0%
Pentachlorophenol *	4.4%
Other chlorophenols	0.6%
Petroleum resins	6.9%
Petroleum waxes	1.0%

NEVER-LITE STOCK SPRAY

See CEN-PE-CO NEVER-LITE
STOCK SPRAY

Starred ingredients (*) may be responsible for major toxic effects; consult Section II.

NEVER-MIST
Eyeglass cleaner and anti-fogger
(Schnapp Enterprises)

Sipex S (American Alcohol's lauryl
  sulfate) 8%
Isopropyl alcohol 12%
Turquoise dye

NEVER-TEL DEODORANT
(York, L.T.)

Perfumed solution of Alcohol *
Gum Benzoin

NEVR-DULL MAGIC WADDING POLISH
Metal polish
(Basch, George)

The George Basch Co., Inc.
19 Hanse Ave.
Freeport, N.Y. 11520

Phone: 516-378-8100

NEVROTOSE, CAPSUTABS NO. 2
Sedative
(Vale)

Each tablet:
  Barbital * .... 64.8 mg.
  Hyoscyamus .... 8.1 mg.
  Valerian extract .... 16.2 mg.
  Passiflora extract .... 64.8 mg.

NEVROTOSE, CAPSUTABS NO. 3
Sedative
(Vale)

Each tablet:
  Phenobarbital * .... 32.4 mg.
  Hyoscyamus .... 16.2 mg.
  Camphor monobromated * .. 8.1 mg.
  Passiflora extract .... 16.2 mg.
  Valerian extract .... 16.2 mg.

NEW CAR PREP
(Garry Labs.)

Wax
Silicone
Diatomaceous earth
Mineral spirits *
Water

NEW DAWN CONDITIONING SHAMPOO-IN HAIR COLOR
(Alberto-Culver)

Water
Oleic acid
Isopropyl alcohol
Lauryl alcohol
Propylene glycol
Octoxynol-5
Ammonium lauryl sulfate
Glycerin
PEG-3 lauramide
PEG-5 tallow amine
Sodium lauriminodipropionate
Ethoxydiglycol
p-Phenylenediamine
Resorcinol
p-Aminophenol
4-Ethoxy-m-phenylenediamine sulfate
2-Nitro-p-phenylenediamine
o-Aminophenol
2-Methoxy-p-phenylenediamine sulfate
Hydroquinone
1-Naphthol
4-Nitro-o-phenylenediamine
4-Ethoxy-m-phenylenediamine
Ammonia
Sodium sulfite
Fragrance
BHA

NEW DAWN CREAM LOTION DEVELOPER
(Alberto-Culver)

Water
Hydrogen peroxide
PEG-6 stearate
Polysorbate-60
Phenacetin
Phosphoric acid

NEW EASY GREASY
Degreaser, mortar cleaner
(Lester Labs.)

Solvents *†
Detergents

'76 Ed.

†*See* Aromatic hydrocarbon solvent

NEW FORMULA KEM 77
Industrial cleaner and disinfectant
(Kem Mfg. Corp.)

Potassium oleate and linoleate .. 9.20%
Isopropyl alcohol 5.88%
Ethyl alcohol 2.90%
o-Benzyl-p-chlorophenol 2.62%
Tetrasodium ethylene diamine
  tetraacetate 2.28%
o-Phenylphenol 2.00%
p-tert.-Amylphenol 1.00%

NEW K.I.L. 6
For commercial laundry use; sanitizing fabric treatment
(M. D. Industries)

n-Alkyl (60% C14, 30% C16, 5% C12,
  5% C18) dimethyl benzyl ammonium chlorides * 20%
n-Alkyl (68% C12, 32% C14) dimethyl
  ethylbenzyl ammonium
  chlorides * 20%

NEW K.I.L. 9
Germicide, disinfectant, sanitizer, deodorizer
(M. D. Industries)

n-Alkyl (60% C14, 30% C16, 5% C12,
  5% C18) dimethyl benzyl ammonium chlorides * 20%
n-Alkyl (68% C12, 32% C14) dimethyl
  ethylbenzyl ammonium
  chlorides * 20%

NEW LOOK FINISH RESTORER (AS-988, Formula 8653-71)

See SIMONIZ NEW LOOK FINISH
  RESTORER (AS-988, Formula 8653-
  71)

NEW PLANT LIFE FISH EMULSION FERTILIZER 5-1-1
(New Plant Life)

Total Nitrogen 5.0%
  Nitrate nitrogen 0%
  Ammoniacal nitrogen 0.5%
  Other water soluble nitrogen .. 4.0%
  Water insoluble nitrogen 0.5%
Available Phosphoric acid 1.0%
Soluble Potash 1.0%

NEW PLANT LIFE LEAF SHINE AND CLEANER
(New Plant Life)

Mineral oil 12.4%
Nonionic surfactant 0.1%
Water 87.5%

NEW PLANT LIFE PLANT FOOD 5-10-5
(New Plant Life)

Total Nitrogen 5%
  Ammoniacal nitrogen 1.1%
  Water soluble urea nitrogen .. 3.9%
Available Phosphoric acid * 10%
Soluble Potash 5%

NEW SKIN
Liquid bandage
(Lambda Inc.)

Pyroxylin solution *
Oil of cloves (USP) *
8-Hydroxyquinoline

Starred ingredients (*) may be responsible for major toxic effects; consult Section II.

NEW TRU FLEX PAINTS
(Touraine Paints, Inc.)

BAMBOO CREAM (#682):
Titanium dioxide	14.36%
Calcium carbonate	8.16%
Silica	16.28%
100% Alkyd resin emulsion	2.45%
Acrylic polymer resin	17.87%
Water	40.90%

BISCAYNE GREEN (#681):
See BAMBOO CREAM (#682) - same formulation

CHARCOAL BROWN (#683):
Brown iron oxide	8.9%
Silica	24.4%
100% Alkyd resin emulsion	2.54%
Acrylic polymer resin	18.85%
Water	45.30%

COLONIAL YELLOW (#684):
See BAMBOO CREAM (#682) - same formulation

DOESKIN BEIGE (#687):
See BAMBOO CREAM (#682) - same formulation

PLATINUM GRAY (#685):
See BAMBOO CREAM (#682) - same formulation

RANCH BROWN (#695):
See CHARCOAL BROWN (#683) - same formulation

STURBRIDGE GRAY (#696):
See BAMBOO CREAM (#682) - same formulation

SUBURBAN RED (#692):
Red iron oxide *	11.11%
Silica	22.20%
100% Alkyd resin emulsion	2.54%
Acrylic polymer resin	18.85%
Water	45.30%

'76 Ed.

---

nf-180 SUSPENSION
Treatment of scours in baby pigs
(Hess & Clark)

Furazolidone * .... 100 mg./cc.

NFZ PUFFER
Antiseptic powder
(Hess & Clark)

Nitrofurazone 0.2%

NFZ SOLUBLE
Water medicate for poultry, swine
(Hess & Clark)

Nitrofurazone 4.59%

NFZ SWINE SCOUR SOLUBLE
Water medication for swine
(Hess & Clark)

Nitrofurazone 4.59%

NIACAL (C.T. BLUE-GREEN; OVAL)
(Bowman Pharm.)

Each tablet:
Calcium lactate	324 mg.
Niacin	25 mg.
Peppermint flavor	

NIAGARA AGRICULTURAL PRODUCTS
(FMC Corp., Agricultural Chem. Div.)

In any emergency situation involving spills, transportation accidents, or human intoxication, technical assistance may be had by calling the following: Department of Health and Safety FMC Corporation Agricultural Chemical Division Middleport, N.Y. 14105

Phone: 716-735-3761

NIAGARA APPLE & PEACH KOLOFORM
Fungicide
(FMC Corp., Agricultural Chem. Div.)

Sulfur *	53%
2,3-Dichloro-1,4-naphthoquinone	1.25%

NIAGARA AQUA ETHION 8 INSECTICIDE
(FMC Corp., Agricultural Chem. Div.)

Ethion (O,O,O',O'-Tetraethyl S,S'-methylene bisphosphorodithioate) * 81.0%

NIAGARA AQUA PHOS KIL 6
Miticide-insecticide
(FMC Corp., Agricultural Chem. Div.)

Parathion * 64.5%

NIAGARA CARBAMATE DUST
Fungicide
(FMC Corp., Agricultural Chem. Div.)

Ferbam 7%

NIAGARA C-O-C-S COPODUST
Fungicide
(FMC Corp., Agricultural Chem. Div.)

Copper expressed as metallic (Copper oxychloride sulfate) * 6%

NIAGARA D-D SOIL FUMIGANT
Fumigant
(FMC Corp., Agricultural Chem. Div.)

Chlorinated C3 hydrocarbons: .. 100.00%
1,2-Dichloropropene
1,2-Dichloropropane *
Other related chlorinated hydrocarbons

NIAGARA DEFOLIANT "L"
Defoliant
(FMC Corp., Agricultural Chem. Div.)

Sodium chlorate (NaClO3) * 18.20%

NIAGARA DIBROM 8 MISCIBLE
Insecticide
(FMC Corp., Agricultural Chem. Div.)

Dimethyl 1,2-dibromo-2,2-dichloroethylphosphate *	64.5%
Xylene *	17.0%

NIAGARA DICHLONE
Fungicide
(FMC Corp., Agricultural Chem. Div.)

2,3-Dichloro-1,4-naphthoquinone * 50%

NIAGARA DINITRO DRY (WETTABLE)
Insecticide
(FMC Corp., Agricultural Chem. Div.)

Dinitro-ortho-cresol * 40%/w

NIAGARA EAR-TICK-OIL
Insecticide
(FMC Corp., Agricultural Chem. Div.)

Gamma isomer of benzene hexachloride	0.72%
Other isomers of benzene hexachloride	4.75%

NIAGARA ETHION 67
Miticide-insecticide
(FMC Corp., Agricultural Chem. Div.)

O,O,O',O'-Tetraethyl S,S'-methylene bisphosphorodithioate *	8.9%
Petroleum oil *	82.5%

NIAGARA ETHION DORMANT OIL
Miticide-insecticide
(FMC Corp., Agricultural Chem. Div.)

O,O,O',O'-Tetraethyl S,S'-methylene bisphosphorodithioate *	2.65%
Petroleum oil *	95%

NIAGARA ETHION 4 MISCIBLE
Miticide-insecticide
(FMC Corp., Agricultural Chem. Div.)

Ethion *	46.5%
Petroleum distillate	45.0%

NIAGARA ETHION .67 OIL
Insecticide
(FMC Corp., Agricultural Chem. Div.)

Ethion *	9.0%
Petroleum oil *	75.0%

NIAGARA ETHION 92 OIL
Miticide-insecticide
(FMC Corp., Agricultural Chem. Div.)

O,O,O',O'-Tetraethyl S,S'-methylene bisphosphorodithioate *	2.2%
Petroleum oil *	95%

Starred ingredients (*) may be responsible for major toxic effects; consult Section II.

NIAGARA ETHION SUPERIOR OIL
Miticide-insecticide
(FMC Corp., Agricultural Chem. Div.)

O,O,O′,O′-Tetraethyl S,S′-methylene
  bisphosphorodithioate * 2%
Petroleum oil (superior type, 100
  Sec.) * 93%

NIAGARA ETHION SUPERIOR 70 OIL
Miticide-insecticide
(FMC Corp., Agricultural Chem. Div.)

O,O,O′,O′-Tetraethyl S,S′-methylene
  bisphosphorodithioate * 2%
Petroleum oil (superior type, 70
  Sec.) * 94%

NIAGARA ETHION 1 THIODAN 2 EC
Miticide-insecticide
(FMC Corp., Agricultural Chem. Div.)

O,O,O′,O′-Tetraethyl S,S′-methyl-
  ene bisphosphorodithioate * ... 11.4%
Endosulfan
  (Hexachlorohexahydromethano-
  2,4,3-benzodioxathiepin
  oxide) * 22.9%
Xylene * 57.5%

NIAGARA FERBAM SPRAY
Fungicide
(FMC Corp., Agricultural Chem. Div.)

Ferbam * 76.0%

NIAGARA FOLPET 50 WETTABLE
Fungicide
(FMC Corp., Agricultural Chem. Div.)

N-(Trichloromethylthio)phthalimide 50%

NIAGARA FURADAN 10 GRANULES
Insecticide
(FMC Corp., Agricultural Chem. Div.)

Carbofuran (2,3-Dihydro-2,2-di-
  methyl-7-benzofuranyl
  methylcarbamate) * 10.0%

NIAGARA INSTANT LAUNDRY STARCH
(Best Foods)

Best Foods
CPC International, Inc.
International Plaza
Englewood Cliffs, N.J. 07632

Phone: 201-894-4000

NIAGARA KOLO 100
Fungicide, insecticide
(FMC Corp., Agricultural Chem. Div.)

Sulfur * 75.40%
Phygon (2,3-Dichloro-1,4-
  naphthoquinone) 3.50%

NIAGARA KOLODUST
Insecticide, fungicide
(FMC Corp., Agricultural Chem. Div.)

Sulfur * 84%

NIAGARA KOLODUST 100
Fungicide
(FMC Corp., Agricultural Chem. Div.)

Sulfur * 83.16%
Phygon 0.05%

NIAGARA KOLOFOG
Fungicide
(FMC Corp., Agricultural Chem. Div.)

Fused bentonite Sulfur *

NIAGARA KOLOKIL
Insecticide
(FMC Corp., Agricultural Chem. Div.)

Fused bentonite Sulfur
Lead arsenate * 15%

NIAGARA KOLOTEX
Fungicide
(FMC Corp., Agricultural Chem. Div.)

Sulfur 73.70%
Standard Lead arsenate * 10%

NIAGARA LEAF DROPPER DEFOLIANT
(FMC Corp., Agricultural Chem. Div.)

Sodium chlorate (NaClO3) * 18.20%

NIAGARA LIQUI-STIK CONCENTRATE
(FMC Corp., Agricultural Chem. Div.)

Naphthalene acetic acid 5.70%

NIAGARA M C P (Amine Weed Killer)
Herbicide
(FMC Corp., Agricultural Chem. Div.)

Diethanolamine salt of chlorotoloxyacetic acid * 49.50%

NIAGARA METHOXCIDE 5 DUST
Insecticide
(FMC Corp., Agricultural Chem. Div.)

Methoxychlor tech. 5%

NIAGARA METHYL PARATHION 1 THIODAN 2 C.O. EC
Insecticide
(FMC Corp., Agricultural Chem. Div.)

O,O-Dimethyl O-p-nitrophenyl
  thiophosphate * 11.2%
Endosulfan
  (Hexachlorohexahydromethano-
  2,4,3-benzodioxathiepin
  oxide) 22.4%

NIAGARA MISCIBLE CITRUS OIL
Insecticide
(FMC Corp., Agricultural Chem. Div.)

Petroleum oil * 99.20%

NIAGARA MYLONE 50
Fungicide and pre-planting control of weeds
(FMC Corp., Agricultural Chem. Div.)

3,5-Dimethyltetrahydro-1,3,5,2H-
  thiadiazine-2-thione * 50.00%

NIAGARA PEANUT DUST 34-80
Fungicide
(FMC Corp., Agricultural Chem. Div.)

Sulfur 80.00%
Copper (from basic copper sulfate)
  expressed as metallic * 3.40%

NIAGARA PERTHANE 5 MALATHION 4 DUST
Insecticide
(FMC Corp., Agricultural Chem. Div.)

Diethyl diphenyl dichloroethane .. 4.75%
Related reaction products 0.25%
Malathion 4.00%

NIAGARA PHOSKIL 1 DUST
Insecticide
(FMC Corp., Agricultural Chem. Div.)

Parathion * 1%

NIAGARA PHOSPHAMIDON 4 SPRAY
Insecticide
(FMC Corp., Agricultural Chem. Div.)

Active ingred.:
  Phosphamidon * 49.0%

NIAGARA POLYRAM 80 WP
Fungicide
(FMC Corp., Agricultural Chem. Div.)

Mixture of Ethylenebis (dithiocarbamate)zinc and (Dithiobis-
  (thiocarbonyl)iminoethylene)bis-
  (dithiocarbamoto)zinc 80%

Starred ingredients (*) may be responsible for major toxic effects; consult Section II.

NIAGARA RO-KILL 100 DUST
Insecticide
(FMC Corp., Agricultural Chem. Div.)

Rotenone 1%
Other cube extractives 2%

NIAGARA SPRAY STARCH
(Best Foods)

Best Foods
CPC International, Inc.
International Plaza
Englewood Cliffs, N.J. 07632

Phone: 201-894-4000

NIAGARA-STIK
For thinning apples
(FMC Corp., Agricultural Chem. Div.)

Naphthaleneacetic acid (sodium salt) 7.10%

NIAGARA TEDION 1.0 MISCIBLE
Miticide
(FMC Corp., Agricultural Chem. Div.)

Tetradifon (2,4,5,4'-Tetrachlorodiphenylsulfone)   12.30%
Xylene base, aromatic petroleum solvent * 35.00%

NIAGARA TEPP
Insecticide
(FMC Corp., Agricultural Chem. Div.)

Tetraethyl pyrophosphate * 40%
Other related organic phosphate esters 60%

NIAGARA THIODAN 4 DUST
Insecticide
(FMC Corp., Agricultural Chem. Div.)

Hexachloro-hexahydro-methano-2,-4,3-benzodioxathiepin oxide * ... 4.0%

NIAGARA THIODAN MISCIBLE
Insecticide
(FMC Corp., Agricultural Chem. Div.)

Endosulfan (Hexachloro-hexahy-dromethano-2,4,3-benzodiox-athiepin oxide) * 24.00%
Xylene base, aromatic petroleum solvent * 69.00%

NIAGARA THIRAM DUST
Fungicide
(FMC Corp., Agricultural Chem. Div.)

Thiram (Tetra-methylthiuramdisulfide) * ... 4.875%

NIAGARA THIRAM 65 WETTABLE POWDER
Fungicide
(FMC Corp., Agricultural Chem. Div.)

Thiram (Tetra-methylthiuramdisulfide) * ... 65.00%

NIAGARA TOXAKIL 20 DUST
Insecticide
(FMC Corp., Agricultural Chem. Div.)

Toxaphene * 20%

NIAGARA TRIONA
Light Soluble, Light Medium Soluble, Medium Soluble, Heavy Medium Soluble & Heavy Soluble
Insecticide
(FMC Corp., Agricultural Chem. Div.)

Petroleum oil * 99.3%

NIAGARA Z-C DUST
Fungicide
(FMC Corp., Agricultural Chem. Div.)

Ziram * 7%

NIAGARA Z-C SPRAY
Fungicide
(FMC Corp., Agricultural Chem. Div.)

Ziram * 70%

NIASCORB
Vitamins
(Kirkman)

Each tablet:
  Niacin NF * .... 500 mg.
  Vitamin C, USP .... 500 mg.

NIAZOLE IMPROVED
Analeptic
(Wesley Pharm.)

Each tablet:
  Pentylene tetrazole * .... 100 mg.
  Niacin .... 50 mg.

N'ICE
Cough lozenges - sugarless
(Beecham Products)

Each lozenge:
  Menthol .... 3 mg.
  In sorbitol base

NICE 'N EASY ALUMINUM SIDING, AWNING, AND MOBILE HOME CLEANER
(Alumin-Nu)

Hydrofluoric acid * .... <1.1%

NICE 'N EASY EXTERIOR VINYL SIDING, AWNING, MOBILE HOME, DOOR & WINDOW CLEANER
(Alumin-Nu)

Hydrofluoric acid * .... <1.1%

NICKEL-ITCH OINTMENT
For skin irritations
(Wambaugh)

Zinc oxide *
Calamine
Glycerin
Phenol .... >1%
Petrolatum base

'76 Ed.

NICOCAP
Pellagra therapy
(ICN Pharm.)

Each time-release capsule:
  Nicotinic acid .... 400 mg.

NICO-METRAZOL (ELIXIR & TABLETS)
CNS stimulant, vasodilator
(Knoll Pharm.)

Each tablet or 5 cc:
  Metrazol (original brand of pentylenetetrazol) * .... 100 mg.
  Nicotinic acid .... 50 mg.
  Alcohol (Elixir only) 15%

NICONYL
Tuberculosis
(Parke-Davis)

Isoniazid (U.S.P.) * .... 100 mg.

NICOTINEX
Niacin elixir
(Fleming)

Each 5 cc:
  Nicotinic acid .... 50 mg.
  Sherry wine, alcohol base 15%

N-2 IDEAL STENCIL INK
(Ideal Stencil)

Stoddard solvent * 90%
Black dye
Toluol * 3%
Xylol * 7%

Starred ingredients (*) may be responsible for major toxic effects; consult Section II.

NIFEREX
Hematinic
(Central Pharmacal Co.)

ELIXIR (each 5 ml.):
Iron (elemental) (as a polysac-
charide-iron complex) * ... 100 mg.
Alcohol * 10%

TABLETS (each):
Iron (elemental) (as a polysac-
charide-iron complex) * ... 50 mg.

NIFEREX-150 CAPSULES (each):
Iron (elemental) (as a polysac-
charide-iron complex) * ... 150 mg.

NIFEREX-150 FORTE CAPSULES
Hematinic
(Central Pharmacal Co.)

Each capsule:
Iron (elemental)(as a polysac-
charide-iron complex) * ... 150 mg.
Folic acid .... 1 mg.
Cyanocobalamin (Vitamin
B12) .... 25 mcg.

NIFEREX FORTE ELIXIR
Hematinic
(Central Pharmacal Co.)

Each 5 ml.:
Iron (elemental)(as a polysac-
charide-iron complex) * ... 100 mg.
Folic acid .... 1 mg.
Cyanocobalamin (Vitamin
B12) .... 25 mcg.
Alcohol 10%

NIFEREX-PN
Prenatal vitamin mineral supplement
(Central Pharmacal Co.)

Each tablet:
Iron (elemental) (as a polysac-
charide-iron complex) * ... 60 mg.
Vitamin A .... 4000 I.U.
Vitamin D2 .... 400 I.U.
Plus multivitamins and minerals

NIFEREX WITH VITAMIN C TABLETS
Hematinic
(Central Pharmacal Co.)

Each tablet:
Iron (elemental) (as a poly-
saccharide-iron
complex) * .... 50 mg.
Ascorbic acid activity ..... 250 mg.
Present as:
Ascorbic acid USP ...... 100 mg.
Sodium ascorbate ...... 168.75 mg.

NIGHT OF OLAY BEAUTY CREAM
(Vicks Toiletry Products Div.)

Water
Mineral oil
Potassium stearate
Sodium stearate
Cetyl palmitate
Cetyl alcohol
Cholesterol
Butylparaben
Sodium carbomer 934
Potassium carbomer 934
Propylparaben
Sodium laurate
Potassium laurate
Castor oil
Sodium myristate
Potassium myristate
Myristyl alcohol
Sodium palmitate
Potassium palmitate
Stearyl alcohol
Fragrance
FD & C Red No. 4

NIGLYCON
Coronary dilator, slow release
(CMC Research Div.)

Each tablet:
Nitroglycerin * .... 2.4 mg.

NIKOBAN
Smoking deterrent
(Williams, J.B.)

Each lozenge:
Lobeline sulfate * .... 0.5 mg.

NILAIN
Analgesic
(A.V.P. Pharmaceuticals)

Each capsule:
Aspirin * .... 5 gr.
Acetaminophen * .... 2 1/2 gr.
Caffeine .... 1/2 gr.

NILODOR DEODORIZERS

Nilodor Co., Inc.
7740 Freedom Ave., N.W.
North Canton, Ohio 44720

Phone: 216-499-4321

NILPRIN 7 1/2
Analgesic
(A.V.P. Pharmaceuticals)

Each tablet:
Acetaminophen * .... 7 1/2 gr.

NINA RICCI PERFUMES

Nina Ricci Parfums
630 Fifth Ave.
New York, N.Y. 10111

Phone: 212-489-2430

See COSMETICS, Section VI, General
Formulations

"99 PLUS"
Insecticide
(Brilco Labs.)

Petroleum distillate *
Technical Piperonyl butoxide
Pyrethrins *
Ether & related compounds

90-PAR
Insecticide
(Leffingwell)

Petroleum oil * 98.0%
Unsulfonated residue, petroleum oil, min. 93.0%

NIORIC TABLETS & ELIXIR
Geriatric stimulant
(Ascher, B.F.)

Each tablet or 5 ml.:
Pentylenetetrazol * .... 100 mg.
Alcohol (Elixir only) 15%

NIP-ET BREATH FRESHENER (Mint and Cinnamon Flavors)
(Stanback)

Alcohol, SDA #38-B .... >40%
Propylene glycol .... <40%
Flavors .... <1%
Water .... >15%
Colors: .... trace
FD & C Yellow #5
FD & C Blue #1
FD & C Red #40

NIPHEN
For athlete's foot or ringworm of hands
(Torch)

Paranitrophenol * 1%
Vehicle:
Isopropyl alcohol *
Wetting agent

'76 Ed.

NIPIRIN CAPSULES
Sedative, hypnotic, analgesic
(Elder)

Each capsule:
Aspirin * .... 324.0 mg.
Pentobarbital acid * .... 32.4 mg.

NITE-BRITE
(United Gilsonite)

Calcium/strontium sulphide * 24%
Alkyd resin 22%
Mineral spirits * 32%

Starred ingredients (*) may be responsible for major toxic effects; consult Section II.

NITE LIFT CONCENTRATE
(Kolmar Labs.)

Emollient	>50%
Emulsifier	10-25%
Nonionic emulsifier	10-25%
Nonionic surfactant	5-10%
Epithelizing agent	1-5%
Preservative	0.1-1.0%
Bactericide	0.1-1.0%

NITE LIFT CREAM
(Kolmar Labs.)

Water	>50%
Preservative	0.1-1.0%
Gelling agent	0.1-1.0%
Bactericide	<0.1%
Emollient	10-25%
Moisturizing agents	10-25%
Epithelizing agent	0.1-1.0%
Emulsifier	1-5%
Nonionic emulsifier	1-5%
Nonionic surfactant	1-5%
Solvent	1-5%
Humectant	0.1-1.0%
Fragrance	0.1-1.0%
Color additives	0.1-1.0%

NITRODINE
(Cramer Products)

10% Povidone iodine solution

NITRO-DUR
Vasodilator, anti-anginal
(Key Pharmaceuticals, Inc.)

Nitroglycerin * ..... 2% w/w

NITROFORM
Fertilizer
(Hercules Incorporated)

Urea formaldehyde polymer (releasing 25-27% water insoluble nitrogen)

NITROGLYN
For prophylactic management of angina pectoris
(Key Pharmaceuticals, Inc.)

Each sustained action tablet:
Nitroglycerin * ..... 1/10 gr.; 1/25 gr.; or 1/50 gr.

NITROL OINTMENT
Topical vasodilator
(Kremers-Urban)

Nitroglycerin * 2.0%
Lanolin-petrolatum base

NITROSTAT
Management of angina pectoris
(Parke-Davis)

Each tablet:
Nitroglycerin * ..... 0.15 mg.; 0.3 mg.; 0.4 mg.; 0.6 mg.
Polyethylene glycol 4000

NITROTAN (Liquid)
(Cramer Products)

Soft water	79.65%
Isopropyl alcohol *	16.25%
Benzyl alcohol (NF)	3.25%
Picric acid	0.10%
Tannic acid	0.75%

N-L CONCENTRATE ALL PURPOSE CLEANER
(Nat'l Labs. Div.)

Phosphates (calculated as elemental phosphorus) 0.93%
Surfactants

N-L DEGREASER 101
(Nat'l Labs. Div.)

Aromatic solvents *
Petroleum distillate *

N-L 500 DEODORIZING CLEANER
(Nat'l Labs. Div.)

Soap	5.5%
o-Benzyl-p-chlorophenol	3.2%
Isopropanol	1.1%

N-L WAX STRIPPER
(Nat'l Labs. Div.)

Ammonium hydroxide *	minor
Ethylene glycol monobutyl ether (Butyl Cellosolve)	minor
Diethanolamine	minor
Triethylenetetramine	minor

N.M. - NEO-MET BRAKE AND ELECTRIC PARTS DRY CLEANER

See GUNK N.M. - NEO-MET BRAKE AND ELECTRIC PARTS DRY CLEANER

N-N COUGH SYRUP
(Vitarine)

Each fl. oz.:

Dextromethorphan hydrobromide	60 mg.
Potassium guaiacolsulfonate	390 mg.
Ammonium chloride	390 mg.
Chlorpheniramine maleate *	3 mg.
Alcohol (by volume)	5%

NO ASPIRIN
Analgesic
(Rexall)

Each tablet:
Acetaminophen * ..... 5 gr.

'76 Ed.

NO-BAC BACTERIACIDE
Disinfectant; cleaner
(Navy Brand)

Isopropyl alcohol *	25.94%
Soap	5.69%
o-Benzyl-p-chlorophenol	4.90%
Methyl salicylate *	1.22%
o-Phenylphenol	0.75%
Essential oils	0.50%

NOBACCO LOZENGES
To combat tobacco habit
(Approved Pharm.)

Each lozenge:

Lobeline sulfate *	1/64 gr.
Dextrose	3 gr.
Oil of peppermint	

'76 Ed.

NO BUGS M'LADY SHELF & DRAWER PAPER
(Paper Products Inc.)

Lindane

NOC-OUT (Aerosol Bomb)
Insecticide
(C-Z Chemical)

Technical Piperonyl butoxide	0.72%
n-Octyl bicycloheptene dicarboximide	0.40%
Pyrethrins	0.2%
Petroleum distillate *	18.68%
Propellant	80.00%

'76 Ed.

NOCTEC (CAPSULES & SYRUP)
Sedative, hypnotic
(Squibb)

Each capsule or 5 cc:

Chloral hydrate (2,2,2-Trichloro-1,1-ethanediol) *	
Capsules	250 mg.; 500 mg.
Syrup	500 mg.

NOCULATE SYSTEMIC INSECTICIDE GRANULAR

See PRATT NOCULATE SYSTEMIC INSECTICIDE GRANULAR

NOCULATE 3 INSECT SPRAY

See PRATT NOCULATE 3 INSECT SPRAY

NODOZ KEEP ALERT TABLETS
Stimulant
(Bristol-Myers)

Each tablet:
Caffeine * ..... 100 mg.

Starred ingredients (*) may be responsible for major toxic effects; consult Section II.

NODS
Sedative
(CMC, Inc.)

Each capsule:
Methapyrilene hydrochloride * 25 mg.
Scopolamine aminoxide
hydrobromide * .... 0.2 mg.

NOFEX-NP
Disinfectant
(Dolge)

approx. %
n-Alkyl dimethyl benzyl ammonium
chlorides * 5%
Soda ash dense 3%
Hampene 100 .... 1%

NO-FLAME REMOVER
(Reliable Paste)

Methylene chloride * .... >75%
Methanol * .... >10%

NO GERM DISINFECTANT

See C-Z NO GERM DISINFECTANT

NO-GRO, GOOD-LIFE

See GOOD-LIFE NO-GRO

NO ITCH, SERGEANT'S

See SERGEANT'S NO ITCH

NO-KOLOR COLOR REMOVER, PUTNAM

See PUTNAM NO-KOLOR COLOR REMOVER

NOKORODE SOLDERING PASTE
(Dunton)

Aqueous solution of:
Zinc chloride *
Ammonium chloride *
Petrolatum carrier

NO-KOTIN
To combat tobacco habit
(Walker Pharm.)

Lobeline sulfate * .... 1/16 gr.
'76 Ed.

NOLAMINE
Oral nasal decongestant
(Carnrick Labs.)

Each timed-release tablet:
Chlorpheniramine maleate * .. 4 mg.
Phenindamine tartrate * ...... 24 mg.
Phenylpropanolamine
hydrochloride * .... 50 mg.

NOLUDAR
Hypnotic
(Roche)

Each tablet:
Methyprylon * .... 50 mg.; or 200 mg.

NOLUDAR 300
Hypnotic
(Roche)

Each capsule:
Methyprylon * .... 300 mg.

NOLVASAN OINTMENT
Germicidal - veterinary
(Fort Dodge)

Chlorhexidine diacetate 1%

NOLVASAN SOAPLESS SHAMPOO
For dogs & cats
(Fort Dodge)

Chlorhexidine diacetate 0.5%

NOLVASAN SOLUTION
Disinfectant solution - veterinary
(Fort Dodge)

1,1'-Hexamethylenebis-
(5-(p-chlorophenyl)biguanide)-
diacetate * 2%

NO MALE
Veterinary - mating repellent
(Carson Chemicals, Inc.)

Chlorophyll
Essential oils *
Aromatic chemicals *
Propellants

NO-MITE SPRAY
Kills lice and mites on canaries, parakeets and all caged birds
(Geisler Pet Products)

Pyrethrins 0.06%
Technical Piperonyl butoxide ... 0.12%
N-Octyl bicycloheptene
dicarboximide 0.20%
Petroleum distillate 0.29%
Triethylene glycol 0.075%
Propylene glycol 0.075%

NO MORE TANGLES SPRAY-ON CREME RINSE

See JOHNSON'S NO MORE TANGLES SPRAY-ON CREME RINSE

NO-MO-STANE LIQUID
Liquid fungicide for fresh cut lumber and timber
(Forshaw)

Sodium pentachlorophenate * .. 19.75%
Sodium salts of other
chlorophenols 2.75%
Sodium metaborate (anhyd) 0.29%
Phenyl mercuric lactate 0.40%

NO-MOTH
(Reefer-Galler)

Paradichlorobenzene *
'76 Ed.

NON-ROACH
For roaches, water bugs
(Twin City Exterminating Co.)

Sodium fluoride * 50%
'76 Ed.

NON-TOX NO. 1 INSECTICIDE
(Barco)

Piperonyl butoxide technical ... 0.698%
Pyrethrins 0.080%
Synergist 0.035%
Petroleum distillates * 99.187%
'76 Ed.

NOPALCOL 4-O
Emulsifier
(Diamond Shamrock, Process Chemicals Div.)

Polyglycol oleate

NOPALCOL 6-L
Textile lubricant
(Diamond Shamrock, Process Chemicals Div.)

Polyglycol laurate

NOPCOGEN 14-L
Detergent
(Diamond Shamrock, Process Chemicals Div.)

Diethyl amido laurate

NO-PEST PRODUCTS

See TEXIZE NO-PEST PRODUCTS

NORDETTE TABLETS
Oral contraceptive
(Wyeth Labs.)

Each tablet:
Levonorgestrel .... 0.15 mg.
Ethinyl estradiol .... 0.03 mg.

Starred ingredients (*) may be responsible for major toxic effects; consult Section II.

NORFLEX
Skeletal muscle spasm
(Riker Labs.)

Each tablet:
Orphenadrine citrate * ...... 100 mg.

'76 Ed.

NORFORMS ORIGINAL FEMININE SUPPOSITORIES
Feminine hygiene
(Norwich-Eaton)

Each suppository:
Methylbenzethonium chloride .. <1%
Lactic acid .... trace
Methylparaben .... <1%
In a water-dispersible base

NO-RINSE BODY-BATH
(N/R Labs.)

Deionized water
Triethanolamine lauryl sulfate .. 13.64%
Lauramide DEA
Propylene glycol
Perfume
Formaldehyde
Sodium benzoate

NO-RINSE SHAMPOO
(N/R Labs.)

Deionized water
Triethanolamine lauryl sulfate ... 3.05%
Lauramide DEA
Propylene glycol
Formaldehyde
Perfume
Sodium benzoate

NORINYL 1 + 35 (21-DAY AND 28-DAY)
Oral contraceptive agent
(Syntex F.P.)

Each active tablet (21 per package):
Norethindrone .... 1 mg.
Ethinyl estradiol .... 0.035 mg.

28-Day package also contains 7 inert tablets

NORINYL 1 + 50 (21-Day and 28-Day)
Oral contraceptive agent
(Syntex F.P.)

Each active tablet (21 per package):
Norethindrone .... 1 mg.
Mestranol .... 0.05 mg.

28-Day package also contains 7 inert tablets

NORINYL 1 + 80 (21-Day and 28-Day)
Oral contraceptive agent
(Syntex F.P.)

Each active tablet (21 per package):
Norethindrone .... 1 mg.
Mestranol .... 0.08 mg.

28-Day package also contains 7 inert tablets

NORINYL-2 mg. TABLETS
Oral contraceptive agent (20 day regimen)
(Syntex F.P.)

Each tablet:
Norethindrone .... 2 mg.
Mestranol .... 0.1 mg.

NORISODRINE AEROTROL
Bronchial asthma
(Abbott)

Each 15 ml. Aerotrol (controlled-dose nebulizer):
Norisodrine (Isoproterenol) hydrochloride 0.25%
Sodium saccharin
Artificial flavor
Distilled water
Alcohol 22.0%
Ascorbic acid 0.1%
Propellant

NORISODRINE SULFATE FOR ORAL INHALATION
For asthma, bronchitis
(Abbott)

Each 10% cartridge:
Isoproterenol sulfate .... 10 mg.
Lactose .... 90 mg.
Each 25% cartridge:
Isoproterenol .... 25 mg.
Lactose .... 75 mg.

NORISODRINE WITH CALCIUM IODIDE SYRUP
Asthma
(Abbott)

Each tsp. (5 ml.):
Isoproterenol sulfate .... 3 mg.
Calcium iodide, anhydrous ... 150 mg.
Alcohol 6%

NORKEM 450
Spot-weeder; aerosol
(Kem Mfg. Co.)

Diethanolamine salt of 2-(2-methyl-4-chlorophenoxy)-propionic acid 0.178%
Diethanolamine salt of 2,4-dichlorophenoxyacetic acid 0.177%
Diethanolamine salt of Dicamba 0.016%

NORKEM 500
Herbicide
(Kem Mfg. Co.)

Diquat dibromide * 2.16%

NORKEM 1200
Plant growth inhibitor
(Kem Mfg. Co.)

Diethanolamine salt of 1,2-dihydro 3,6-pyridazinedione * 58%

NORKEM 600C
Herbicide
(Kem Mfg. Co.)

Petroleum oil * 97.19%
Bromacil 0.61%
Pentachlorophenol 0.80%
Other Chlorophenols 0.09%

NORKEM 400T
Herbicide
(Kem Mfg. Co.)

Dimethylamine salt of 2-(2-methyl-4-chlorophenoxy)propionic acid 2.77%
Dimethylamine salt of 2,4-dichlorophenoxyacetic acid 6.10%
Dimethylamine salt of Dicamba .. 0.64%
Dimethylamine salt of related compounds 0.08%

NORKON TABLETS
Relief of minor pain of arthritis & rheumatism
(Norkon Pharm.)

Aspirin * .... 324 mg.
Ascorbic acid
Calcium glutamate .... 130 mg.

NORLAC
Prenatal nutritional supplement
(Rowell)

Each tablet:
Vitamin A acetate ... 8000 USP units
Calciferol (D-2) ..... 400 USP units
Ferrous fumarate (elemental iron, 60 mg.) * .... 180 mg.
Plus multi-vitamins & minerals

NORLAC RX
Prenatal supplement for high risk of folic acid deficiency
(Rowell)

Vitamin A acetate ..... 8000 USP units
Calciferol (D-2) ..... 400 USP units
Ferrous fumarate (Elemental iron 60 mg.) * ....180 mg.
Folic acid .... 1 mg.
Plus multivitamins and minerals

NORLESTRIN Fe TABLETS
Oral contraceptive
(Parke-Davis)

Each 1 mg. tablet:
Norethindrone acetate .... 1 mg.
Ethinyl estradiol .... 50 mcg.
Ferrous fumarate (7 tablets) .. 75 mg.

Each 2.5 mg. tablet:
Norethindrone acetate .... 2.5 mg.
Ethinyl estradiol .... 50 mcg.
Ferrous fumarate (7 tablets) .. 75 mg.

Starred ingredients (*) may be responsible for major toxic effects; consult Section II.

NORLESTRIN TABLETS
Oral contraceptive
(Parke-Davis)

Each 1 mg. tablet:
Norethindrone acetate .... 1 mg.
Ethinyl estradiol .... 50 mcg.

Each 2.5 mg. tablet:
Norethindrone acetate .... 2.5 mg.
Ethinyl estradiol .... 50 mcg.

NORM-EVAC TABLETS
Constipation aid
(Premo)

Each tablet:
Dioctyl sodium
sulfosuccinate * . 60 mg.; 100 mg.; or
120 mg.

'76 Ed.

NO RO
Insecticide
(Meyer, T.)

Tech. Chlordane 2%
Petroleum distillate * 98%

'76 Ed.

NO-ROACH

See JOHNSTON'S NO-ROACH

NO ROOST (GELATIN & SPRAY)
Bird control
(Aegis Labs.)

Polybutene (Polybutylene) . 50.00% Min.
2-5 Ditert. hydroquinone (2-5
Ditertiary-amyl
hydroquinone) .... 1.00% Min.
Refined Mineral oil .... 45.00% Ave.
Lithium stearate .... 4.00% Ave.

'76 Ed.

NORPHYL TABLETS
Bronchial asthma, myocardial infarction
(Vita Elixir Co.)

Each tablet:
Aminophylline * .... 1 1/2 gr.

NORPRAMIN
Antidepressant
(Merrell Dow)

Each tablet:
Desipramine HCl *
Yellow .... 25 mg.
Green .... 50 mg.
Orange .... 75 mg.
Peach .... 100 mg.
White .... 150 mg.

NOR-Q.D. TABLETS
Oral contraception (continuous regimen, 42 tablets/card)
(Syntex F.P.)

Each tablet:
Norethindrone .... 0.35 mg.

NORTHLAND BEEF CATTLE CHEMICAL
Control of hornflies on cattle
(Northland Products Co.)

Ronnel 1.0%
Mineral oil (unsulfonated residue
80% or better) * 98.9%

NORTHLAND COA CROP OIL
Post-emergence treatment; supplemental carrier for herbicides
(Northland Products Co.)

Refined Petroleum distillate * 98.0%/wt.
T-MULZ AO2 emulsifier .... 2.0%/wt.

NO-RUB FLOOR WAX

See WILBERT'S NO-RUB FLOOR WAX

NO-RUB FURNITURE CREAM

See WILBERT'S NO-RUB FURNITURE CREAM

NORWICH-EATON PRODUCTS

Norwich-Eaton Pharmaceuticals
Div. of MortonNorwich
P.O. Box 191
Norwich, N.Y. 13815

For round-the-clock medical consultation on Norwich-Eaton Products: Phone: (607) 335-2565

NOSALT
Salt alternative
(Norcliff Thayer)

Potassium chloride*

NO SAND SURFACE PREPARATION
(Klean-Strip)

Petroleum distillates * .... >25%
Alcohols (no methanol) * .... >50%
Ketones * .... <20%

NO SCALD DPA
For control of storage scald on apples
(Chemley Prod.)

Diphenylamine * 83%
(specially purified)

NO SCALD DPA LIQUID CONCENTRATE 160
For control of storage scald on apples
(Chemley Prod.)

Diphenylamine (specially purified)* 31%

NOSECT
Insect repellent
(Dro)

Dimethyl phthalate 18.0%
Butyl dimethyl dihydro gamma pyrone carboxylate 6.0%
2-Ethylhexanediol-1,3 .... 6.0%

'76 Ed.

NOSECT 50 D BOMB
Insecticide
(Dro)

Petroleum distillates * 70.913%
Malathion 2.500%
Chlordane, tech. 1.500%
Pyrethrins 0.025%
Piperonyl butoxide, tech. 0.062%
Propellant 25.000%

'76 Ed.

NO SHOCK STATIC RETARDER
Antistat for rugs
(Uncle Sam)

Surfactants *
Acetic acid
Isopropanol *
Water

NOSKOTE, COPPERTONE (Jar and Tube)

See COPPERTONE NOSKOTE (Jar and Tube)

NOSQUITO
Mosquito and gnat repellent; veterinary
(Farnam Co.)

N,N-Diethyl-m-toluamide 8.313%
Other isomers 0.437%
N-Octyl bicycloheptene
dicarboximide 2.500%
2,3:4,5-Bis(2-butylene)tetrahydro-
2-furaldehyde 0.625%
Di-n-propyl isocinchomeronate .. 0.625%

'76 Ed.

NOSTAIN
Deck and tile cleaner for swimming pools
(Modern Pool Products)

Oxalic acid *

NOT ON THE CARPET (Aerosol)

See BISSELL NOT ON THE CARPET (Aerosol)

Starred ingredients (*) may be responsible for major toxic effects; consult Section II.

NOTT ANT TRAPS
Insecticide
(Nott)

Baygon * 1.0%

NOVAFED
Decongestant
(Dow Pharm., Dow Chem. Co.)

Each 5 ml.:
Pseudoephedrine
hydrochloride * .... 30 mg.
Alcohol 7.5%

NOVAFED A
Decongestant-antihistaminic
(Dow Pharm., Dow Chem. Co.)

Each 5 ml.:
Pseudoephedrine
hydrochloride * .... 30 mg.
Chlorpheniramine maleate .... 2 mg.
Alcohol 5%

NOVAFED A CAPSULES
*Controlled-release decongestant-anti-
histaminic*
(Dow Pharm., Dow Chem. Co.)

Each capsule:
Pseudoephedrine
hydrochloride * .... 120 mg.
Chlorpheniramine maleate * . 8 mg.

NOVAFED CAPSULES
Controlled-release decongestant
(Dow Pharm., Dow Chem. Co.)

Each capsule:
Pseudoephedrine
hydrochloride * .... 120 mg.

NOVAHISTINE COUGH FORMULA
(Dow Pharm., Dow Chem. Co.)

Each 5 ml.:
Dextromethorphan HBr * .... 10 mg.
Guaifenesin .... 100 mg.
Alcohol 7.5%

NOVAHISTINE DH
Antitussive-decongestant
(Dow Pharm., Dow Chem. Co.)

Each 5 ml.:
Codeine phosphate * ...... 10 mg.
Phenylpropanolamine
hydrochloride * .... 18.75 mg.
Chlorpheniramine maleate .. 2 mg.
Alcohol 5%

NOVAHISTINE DMX
Antitussive-decongestant
(Dow Pharm., Dow Chem. Co.)

Each 5 ml.:
Dextromethorphan
hydrobromide .... 10 mg.
Pseudoephedrine
hydrochloride * .... 30 mg.
Guaifenesin (Glyceryl
guaiacolate) .... 100 mg.
Alcohol 10%

NOVAHISTINE ELIXIR
Decongestant-antihistaminic
(Dow Pharm., Dow Chem. Co)

Each 5 ml.:
Phenylpropanolamine
hydrochloride * .... 18.75 mg.
Chlorpheniramine maleate .. 2 mg.
Alcohol 5%

NOVAHISTINE EXPECTORANT
Antitussive-decongestant
(Dow Pharm., Dow Chem. Co.)

Each 5 ml.:
Codeine phosphate * ...... 10 mg.
Phenylpropanolamine
hydrochloride * .... 18.75 mg.
Guaifenesin (Glyceryl
guaiacolate) .... 100 mg.
Alcohol 7.5%

NOVAHISTINE FORTIS CAPSULES
For relief of respiratory congestion
(Dow Pharm., Dow Chem. Co.)

Each capsule:
Phenylephrine hydrochloride * 10 mg.
Chlorpheniramine maleate .... 2 mg.

NOVAHISTINE LP TABLETS
For relief of respiratory congestion
(Dow Pharm., Dow Chem. Co.)

Each tablet:
Phenylephrine hydrochloride * 20 mg.
Chlorpheniramine maleate .... 4 mg.

NOVAHISTINE MELET TABLETS
For relief of respiratory congestion
(Dow Pharm., Dow Chem. Co.)

Each tablet:
Phenylephrine hydrochloride * 10 mg.
Chlorpheniramine maleate .... 2 mg.

NOVATEX GREASE
(Texaco Inc.)

Mineral oil *
Calcium soap

NOVIN TABLETS
*An analgesic, antipyretic and antispas-
modic for horses, dogs and cats*
(Haver-Lockhart (Brand) Bayvet Div.
Cutter Labs.)

Each tablet:
Dipyrone * .... 5 gr.

NOVRAD (PULVULES & SUSPENSION)
Antitussive
(Lilly, Eli)

PULVULES (each):
Levopropoxyphene
napsylate * .... 100 mg.

SUSPENSION (each 5 ml.):
Levopropoxyphene
napsylate * .... 50 mg.

NOXALL VEGETATION KILLER CONCENTRATE

See LILLY/MILLER NOXALL VEG-
ETATION KILLER CONCEN-
TRATE

NOXELL CORPORATION PRODUCTS

Noxell Corporation
P.O. Box 1799
Baltimore, Md. 21203

Phone: 301-628-7300

NOXFISH
For control of rough fish
(Penick)

Rotenone * 5%
Other cube extractives 10%

NOXIT TABLETS
Analgesic
(C.T.S. Labs.)

Acetophenetidin * .... 2 1/2 gr.
Aspirin *
Caffeine

NOXON METAL POLISH
(Boyle-Midway)

Oxalic acid * 1-10%
Silica powder
Aqueous Ammonia * 1-10%
Vegetable fatty acids
Alcohols 1-10%
Petroleum distillate .... <1%
Water

NOXON QUIK-DIP SILVER CLEANER
(Boyle-Midway)

Thiourea .... <10%
Sulfuric acid * .... <2%
Detergent .... trace
Perfume
Water

Starred ingredients (*) may be responsible for major toxic effects; consult Section II.

NOX-TOX
Insecticide
(Carpenter, W.D.)

Petroleum distillates *	99.718%
Piperonyl butoxide tech.	0.251%
Pyrethrins	0.031%

NOXZEMA PRODUCTS

Noxell Corporation
P.O. Box 1799
Baltimore, Md. 21203

Phone: 301-628-7300

NP-27 CREAM
Anti-dermatophytosis pedis
(Norwich-Eaton)

8-Hydroxyquinoline benzoate	2.50%
Propylparaben	<1%
Methylparaben	1-10%
Salicylic acid	<1%
Benzoic acid	trace
Eucalyptol, thymol, menthol	<1%

NP-27 LIQUID
Anti-dermatophytosis pedis
(Norwich-Eaton)

Undecylenic acid*	10%
Isopropyl alcohol*	56%

NP-27 POWDER
Anti-dermatophytosis pedis
(Norwich-Eaton)

Boric acid *	10%
Propylparaben	1.75%
Salicylic acid*	1.5%
Benzoic acid	0.75%
Eucalyptol	0.25%
Thymol	0.175%
Menthol	0.125%
Chlorothymol	0.125%

NP-27 POWDER AEROSOL
Anti-dermatophytosis pedis
(Norwich-Eaton)

Zinc undecylenate*	20.0%
Alcohol	20.5%
Talc	

NPS ACID TRUCK CLEANER
(National-Purity Soap)

Hydrofluoric acid *
Hydrochloric acid *
Sulfuric acid *
Nonionic detergent

NPS ANTISTAT
Antistat agent for carpets
(National-Purity Soap)

Quaternary ammonium compound *

NPS 80/20 POWDERED SOAP #144
For use in commercial laundries
(National-Purity Soap)

Anhydrous soap	92%
Vegetable oil	
Animal tallow	

pH 1% solution, 9.5 - 9.8

NPS JET SPRAY DEGREASER
Hard surface cleaner
(National-Purity Soap)

T.E.A. (Triethanolamine)
Wetting agent
Synthetic biodegradable detergent
Grease saponifier

NPS J-OIL SOAP
All purpose gel type cleaner
(National-Purity Soap)

Anhydrous Potash soap	50%
Water conditioning agents	
Sequestering agents	

NPS #20 LIQUID HAND SOAP
(National-Purity Soap)

Anhydrous Potash soap	20%

NPS #40 LIQUID HAND SOAP
(National-Purity Soap)

Anhydrous Potash soap	40%

NPS MECHANICS HAND SOAP
Powdered hand soap; institutional & industrial use
(National-Purity Soap)

Vegetable bleach soap
Borax *
Emollients
Lanolin
Methyl salicylate *

pH 1%, 10 - 10.5

NPS ODOR NEUTRALIZER
Deodorizing cleaner; institutional use
(National-Purity Soap)

Deodorizing Essential oils
Surfactant *

NPS 100 FLOOR CLEANER
Masonry cleaner
(National-Purity Soap)

Grease emulsifying Surfactants *
Phosphatic cleaners *

pH of use solution 12.1

NPS PREMIUM HEAVY DUTY HANDSOAP
(National-Purity Soap)

Blend of vegetable and tallow soaps
Vegetable cleaners and emollients

NPS SANITIZING AGENT
Disinfectant and sanitizer; commercial and industrial use
(National-Purity Soap)

n-Alkyl (60% C14, 30% C16, 5% C12, 5% C18) dimethyl benzyl ammonium chlorides *	5%
n-Alkyl (50% C12, 30% C14, 17% C16, 3% C18) dimethyl ethylbenzyl ammonium chlorides *	5%

NPS SOLUBLE PINE OIL
Disinfectant deodorizer cleaner; institutional and industrial use
(National-Purity Soap)

Pine oil *
Soap (Anionic detergent)
Alcohol
Emulsifying agents

NPS SPRAY ON SPOT CLEANER
(National-Purity Soap)

Inorganic builders
Water soluble solvents
Water conditioners
Dyes
Perfumes
Nonionic synthetic surfactants *

pH of 1% solution, 12 - 12.2

NPS SUPER WHIP
Soapless detergent
(National-Purity Soap)

Detergent builders
Water conditioning Sequestrants
Wetting agents
Synthetic detergents *

NPS WATERLESS HAND CLEANER
(National-Purity Soap)

Hydrocarbon solvent *†
Emulsifying system

†See Petroleum distillate

NPS WIG-WASH
(National-Purity Soap)

Nonionic and anionic detergents *
Brighteners
Solubilizers

Starred ingredients (*) may be responsible for major toxic effects; consult Section II.

NP-27 CREAM
Anti-dermatophytosis pedis
(Norwich-Eaton)

8-Hydroxyquinoline benzoate	2.50%
Propylparaben	<1%
Methylparaben	1-10%
Salicylic acid	<1%
Benzoic acid	trace
Eucalyptol, thymol, menthol	<1%

NP-27 LIQUID
Anti-dermatophytosis pedis
(Norwich-Eaton)

Undecylenic acid *	10%
Isopropyl alcohol *	56%

NP-27 POWDER
Anti-dermatophytosis pedis
(Norwich-Eaton)

Boric acid *	10%
Propylparaben	1.75%
Salicylic acid *	1.5%
Benzoic acid	0.75%
Eucalyptol	0.25%
Thymol	0.175%
Menthol	0.125%
Chlorothymol	0.125%

NP-27 POWDER AEROSOL
Anti-dermatophytosis pedis
(Norwich-Eaton)

Zinc undecylenate *	20.0%
Alcohol	20.5%
Talc	

NR (Film Coated)

See NATURE'S REMEDY (Film
Coated)

N/S INSECTOL
Wood preservative and disinfectant
(Northern States Labs.)

Pentachlorophenol *	15.35%
2,3,4,6-Tetrachlorophenol *	15.35%
4 and 6 Chloro-2-phenylphenols	5.00%
Other chlorophenols	4.40%
Aromatic petroleum derivative solvent *	40.00%
Inert ingred.:	19.90%
Diacetone alcohol	

'76 Ed.

N/S IODINE DISINFECTANT
Cleaner, disinfectant, deodorizer
(Northern States Labs.)

Nonyl phenoxypoly (ethylene oxy) ethanol-iodine complex (min. available iodine 1.75%)	8.75%
Phosphoric acid *	8.50%

'76 Ed.

N/S MANGE OIL
(Northern States Labs.)

Toxaphene *	45.00%
Gamma isomer of benzene hexachloride (from lindane)	2.00%
Methylated naphthalenes	10.00%
Petroleum distillate	27.00%

'76 Ed.

N/S SEVICIDE (5 AND 50)
For control of poultry and livestock pests
(Northern States Labs.)

Carbaryl (1-Naphthyl N-methylcarbamate) *	5%/wt.; 50%/wt.

'76 Ed.

N-2 IDEAL STENCIL INK
(Ideal Stencil)

Stoddard solvent *	90%
Black dye	
Toluol *	3%
Xylol *	7%

NTZ NASAL SPRAY
Decongestant nasal spray
(Winthrop Labs.)

Neo-Synephrine HCl *	0.5%
Thenfadil HCl	0.1%
Zephiran chloride	1-5000

NuAIR SPACE DEODORIZER
(Lester Labs.)

Ammonia	
Formaldehyde *	

'76 Ed.

NU BOL LIQUID TOILET BOWL KLEENER
(King of All)

Hydrogen chloride *	23%
Dimethyl benzyl ammonium chloride (N-alkyl (C12 40%, C14 50%, C16 10%))	0.005%
Bis(tributyltin)oxide	0.01%
Inert ingred.:	76.94%
Water	70%
Surfactant	6.94%

NU-BRO RAT BAIT
Rodenticide
(B&N Products)

Warfarin (3(a-Acetonylbenzyl)-4-hydroxycoumarin)	0.025%
N'-2-Quinoxalinylsulfanilamide (Sulfaquinoxaline)	0.025%

'76 Ed.

NU-CAST - N.U. (Powder)

See GUNK N.U. - NU-CAST (Powder)

NU-CLO 85 DESERT GRANULES
Swimming pool treatment
(Alden-Leeds)

Trichloro-s-triazinetrione *	100%

NU-CLO HIT HARD SHOCK
Swimming pool treatment
(Alden-Leeds)

Calcium hypochlorite *	70%

NU-CLO QUICK KILL ALGAE DESTROYER
Swimming pool treatment
(Alden-Leeds)

Trichloro-s-triazinetrione *	100%

NU-CLO 7-DAY CHLORINATING TABLETS
Swimming pool treatment
(Alden-Leeds)

Trichloro-s-triazinetrione *	100%

NU-CLO SHOCK
Swimming pool treatment
(Alden-Leeds)

Trichloro-s-triazinetrione *	81%
Inert ingred.:	19%
Sodium carbonate *	

NU-CLO STABILIZED CHLORINE TABLETS
Swimming pool treatment
(Alden-Leeds)

Trichloro-s-triazinetrione *	66%
Inert ingred.:	
Sodium carbonate *	34%

NUCOFED CAPSULES
Antitussive, decongestant
(Beecham Labs.)

Each capsule:	
Codeine phosphate *	20 mg.
Pseudoephedrine HCl *	60 mg.

NUCOFED EXPECTORANT SYRUP
(Beecham Labs.)

Each 5 ml.:	
Codeine phosphate	20 mg.
Pseudoephedrine HCl *	60 mg.
Guaifenesin	200 mg.
Flavoring	q.s.
Alcohol	12.5%

NUCOFED SYRUP
For coughs
(Beecham Labs.)

Each 5 ml.:	
Codeine phosphate *	20 mg.
Pseudoephedrine HCl *	60 mg.
Flavoring	q.s.

Starred ingredients (*) may be responsible for major toxic effects; consult Section II.

NUDECK ROOF CEMENT & COATING
(United Gilsonite)

Asphalt
Mineral spirits * 18%
Inert fillers

NU-FILM-17
Extender, sticker-spreader
(Miller Chem. & Fert.)

Pinolene (Di-1-p-menthene)

NU-FILM-P
Sticker-spreader
(Miller Chem. & Fert.)

Pinolene (Di-1-p-menthene)

NU-FLOW
Medicated shampoo
(CooperCare)

Parachlorometaxylenol 2.0%
Isopropanol 7.5%
Neutral, emollient complex; soapless

NU-FLOW D FLOWABLE CHLORONEB FUNGICIDE
Seed treatment
(Wilbur-Ellis Co.)

Chloroneb (1,4-Dichloro-2,5-
dimethoxybenzene) 30%

NU-FLOW ND
Fungicide; seed treatment
(Wilbur-Ellis Co.)

Chloroneb (1,4-Dichloro-2,5-
dimethoxybenzene) 23.5%
2-(Thiocyanomethylthio)
benzothiazole 9.0%

NUGANIA
Cold wave lotion
(Willat)

Mono-thioglycerol 1-10%

NU-GLO
See C-Z NU-GLO

NU-GLO
Rubber mat refinisher
(Lester Labs.)

Detergents *
Alcohol

'76 Ed.

NU-GLU
(Carter's Ink)

Vinyl acetate emulsion
Polyvinyl alcohol

'76 Ed.

NU-IRON
For nutritional deficiencies of crops
(Cities Service Co.)

Fe *† 29%

†*See* Iron salts

NUJOL
Laxative
(Plough)

Extra heavy Mineral oil .... 100.0% w/w

NU-KLEEN, FORMULA LC-11

  See KLENZADE NU-KLEEN, FORMULA LC-11

NUMORPHAN
Narcotic analgesic
(Endo Labs.)

Each suppository:
  Oxymorphone hydrochloride * . 5 mg.

NUMOTIZINE
Rubefacient
(Hobart)

Each 100 gm.:
  Guaiacol .... 0.260 gm.
  Beechwood creosote * .... 1.302 gm.
  Methyl salicylate .... 0.260 gm.
  Polyols .... 51.260 gm.
  Aluminum silicate .... 46.888 gm.
  Coloring .... 0.030 gm.

'76 Ed.

NUMOTIZINE COUGH SYRUP
Antitussive
(Hobart)

Each fl. oz.:
  Glyceryl guaiacolate .... 0.324 gm.
  Ammonium chloride .... 0.324 gm.
  Sodium citrate .... 1.296 gm.
  Menthol .... 2.6 mg.
  Dioctyl sodium
    sulfosuccinate 1-20,000

'76 Ed.

N.U. - NU-CAST (Powder)

  See GUNK N.U. - NU-CAST (Powder)

NUPERCAINAL ANESTHETIC OINTMENT
(CIBA Pharmaceutical)

Dibucaine (NF) 1%
Acetone bisulfite (preservative) ... 1/2%

NUPERCAINAL PAIN-RELIEF CREAM
(CIBA Pharmaceutical)

Dibucaine (NF) 0.5%
Water-washable base
Acetone sodium bisulfite
  (preservative) 0.37%

NUPERCAINAL PAIN-RELIEF SPRAY
(CIBA Pharmaceutical)

Dibucaine hydrochloride (NF) 0.25%
Alcohol 46%

NUPERCAINAL SUPPOSITORIES
Hemorrhoids
(CIBA Pharmaceutical)

Each suppository:
  Dibucaine (NF) .... 2.5 mg.
  Zinc oxide
  Bismuth subgallate
  Acetone sodium bisulfite
    (preservative) 0.05%
  Cocoa butter

NU POWER TOP OIL
Automotive
(Radiator)

Petroleum distillates *

'76 Ed.

NU-Q
Disinfectant-sanitizer-deodorizer-concentrate
(Nu-Ball Mfg. Co.)

n-Alkyl (68% C12, 32% C14) dimethyl
ethylbenzyl ammonium
chloride * 5.0%
n-Alkyl (60% C14, 30% C16, 5% C12,
5% C18) dimethyl benzyl ammonium chloride * 5.0%

NU-RAL TABLETS

  See ESTES NU-RAL TABLETS

N-URISTIX
Urine glucose, nitrite and protein test strip
(Ames)

Protein area: see ALBUSTIX
Glucose area: see CLINISTIX
Nitrite area: see MICROSTIX

Starred ingredients (*) may be responsible for major toxic effects; consult Section II.

NUROPATHIC DROPS
Counterirritant; internal and external
(Osgood)

Alcohol 86%
Capsicum *
Lobelia *
Camphor *
Oils of:
   Spearmint
   Cassia
   Spruce
   Wormwood *†

'76 Ed.

†See Volatile oils

NURSE BRAND ANTI-DIARRHEA COMPOUND
(DePree)

Kaolin (colloidal grade)
Pectin

NU SALVE

See FALK'S NU SALVE

NUSAN
Chemical filter backwash
(Modern Pool Products)

Sulphuric acid *

NUSOFT FABRIC SOFTENER

Best Foods
CPC International, Inc.
International Plaza
Englewood Cliffs, N.J. 07632

Phone: 201-894-4000

NU-TONE HORMONE SPRAY
Plant hormone
(Miller Chem. & Fert.)

alpha-Naphthalene acetic acid ... 3.62%

NUTRACORT CREAM
(Owen Labs.)

Hydrocortisone 0.25%; 0.50%
Fatty alcohols
Emulsifiers
Liquid petrolatum

NUTRACORT GEL
(Owen Labs.)

Hydrocortisone 1%
Alcohol 22%
Propylene glycol

NUTRACORT LOTION
(Owen Labs.)

Hydrocortisone 0.25%; 0.50%;
   1.0%
Fatty alcohols
Emulsifiers
Liquid petrolatum

NUTRA-PHOS 17
Foliar spray
(Leffingwell)

Zinc-expressed as metallic *† 7.0%
Manganese-expressed as metallic . 8.0%
Phosphoric acid (P2O5)
   available * 17.0%

†See Zinc salts

NUTRA-PHOS 24
Foliar spray for effective zinc and phosphoric acid feeding
(Leffingwell)

Zinc expressed as metallic * 12.0%
Phosphoric acid (P2O5 available) .. 24.0%
Inert ingred.: 64.0%
   Zinc derived from hydrate basic sulphate complex
   Available Phosphoric acid derived from metal phosphates

NUTRA-PHOS 3-15
Foliar spray
(Leffingwell)

Phosphoric acid (P2O5)
   available * 15.0%
Zinc-expressed as metallic *† 15.0%
Manganese-expressed as metallic . 15.0%

†See Zinc salts

NUTRA-PHOS Fe
Foliar nutrient spray
(Leffingwell)

Nitrogen (ammoniacal) 3.0%
Available Phosphoric acid * 27.0%
Iron (expressed as elemental) 21.0%

NUTRA-PHOS K
Foliar spray
(Leffingwell)

Zinc potassium phosphate *†

†See Zinc salts and Phosphates

NUTRA-PHOS Mg 0-25-0
Foliar nutrient spray
(Leffingwell)

Available Phosphoric acid * 25.0%
Calcium 10.0%
Magnesium 5.5%
Zinc 5.5%

NUTRA-PHOS SUPER-K 7-13-34
Plant food
(Leffingwell)

Nitrogen 7.0%
Available Phosphoric acid * 13.0%
Soluble Potash * 34.0%
Zinc *† 12.5%

†See Zinc salts

NUTRA-PHOS TEN
Spray dried product for use as a foliar nutritional spray
(Leffingwell)

Phosphoric acid (phosphate derived from complex metal
   phosphates) * 10.0%
Zinc (as elemental) (zinc derived from complex phosphate and carbonate salts) * 14.0%
Manganese (as elemental) (manganese derived from basic and normal carbonates) 7.0%

NUTRA-PHOS ZMC 0-4-0
Foliar nutrient spray
(Leffingwell)

Available Phosphoric acid * 4.0%
Calcium 9.0%
Sulfur 8.0%
Copper * 6.0%
Manganese 10.0%
Zinc *† 10.0%

†See Zinc salts

NUTRASPA
Bath oil
(Owen Labs.)

Mineral oil
Emulsifiers

NUTRA-SPRAY 17 1/2-4-4
For zinc, manganese and copper deficiencies in citrus trees and field crops
(Leffingwell)

Zinc (expressed as metallic) * 17.5%
Manganese (expressed as metallic) . 4.0%
Copper (expressed as metallic) ... 4.0%

NUTRA-SPRAY COPPER BORDEAUX 22
Fungicide
(Leffingwell)

Copper (as elemental) (copper derived from basic copper
   sulfate) * 22.0%

NUTRA-SPRAY Mn 35
Foliar spray-micronutrient fertilizer
(Leffingwell)

Manganese (as elemental) (manganese derived from manganese carbonate) * 35.0%

Starred ingredients (*) may be responsible for major toxic effects; consult Section II.

NUTRA-SPRAY ZM 25-25
Foliar spray
(Leffingwell)

Zinc-expressed as metallic *† 25.0%
Manganese-expressed as metallic . 25.0%

†*See* Zinc salts

NUTRA-SPRAY ZMC 12-2-10
Fungicide and foliar spray
(Leffingwell)

Copper (as elemental) (copper derived from basic copper
sulfates) * 10.0%
Zinc (as elemental) (zinc derived
from oxides and basic sulfates) * 12.0%
Manganese (as elemental) (manganese derived from the
carbonate) 2.0%

NUTRI-TONIC HOME PERMANENT
(Del Labs.)

Active ingredients:
Thioglycolic acid *
Ammonia *
Emulsifiers

NUTRI-TONIC PERMANENT SOLUTION
Waving solution
(Del Labs.)

Ammonium thioglycolate * . about 7.5%
Nonionic emulsifiers .... about 5.0%
Lanolin and lanolin deriv. 0.5%
Mineral oil and deriv. ...... about 5.0%
pH 9

NUVAC '60' CAPSULES
Stool softener
(La Crosse)

Each capsule:
Dioctyl sodium sulfosuccinate * 60 mg.
Casanthranol * .... 30 mg.

NUVETTE SHAMPOO
For fabrics
(W-B Chem.)

Sodium-n-methyl-n-oleyl taurate *
Sodium lauryl sulphate *
Sodium N-lauryl sarcosinate

NUZINE OINTMENT
For anorectal irritations
(Hobart)

Guaiacol 1.66%
Oxyquinoline sulfate 0.42%
Zinc oxide 2.50%
In a smooth base with lanolin

'76 Ed.

NYLO-BOND (SPRAY AND BRUSH)
Adhesive retreading cement
(Goodyear)

Natural rubber 5-10%
Rubber solvent naphtha * 90-95%

NYLON DIP
(Smith, Robert)

Sulfonated fatty acid amides *†
'76 Ed.

†*See* Alkyl sodium sulfonates

NYOMIN
Hypertension
(Elder)

Each tablet:
Potassium nitrate .... 150 mg.
Sodium nitrite * .... 30 mg.

NYQUIL NIGHTTIME COLDS MEDICINE
(Vicks Health Care Div.)

Active ingred. (each fl. oz. or 30 ml.):
Acetaminophen * .... 600 mg.
Doxylamine succinate ...... 7.5 mg.
Ephedrine sulfate .... 8 mg.
Dextromethorphan HBr ..... 15 mg.
Inactive ingred.:
Alcohol 25%

NYRAL LOZENGES
Throat lozenges
(Vale)

Each lozenge:
Cetyl pyridinium chloride .... 0.5 mg.
Benzocaine .... 5.0 mg.
Methylparaben .... 2.0 mg.
Propylparaben .... 0.5 mg.

NYSTAFORM-HC OINTMENT
Dermatoses in infants
(Dome)

Nystatin (100,000 units/gm.)
Iodochlorhydroxyquin 3%
Microdispersed Hydrocortisone
alcohol 1%
Water-dispersible emulsified white petrolatum base containing octylphenoxyethanol

NYSTAFORM OINTMENT
(Dome)

Nystatin, USP ...... 100,000 units/gm.
Iodochlorhydroxyquin 1%
Water-dispersible, emulsified White petro-
latum base containing
Octylphenoxyethanol

NYTILAX
Laxative
(Leeming Div.)

Each tablet:
Sennosides A and B .... 12 mg.

NYTOL CAPSULES AND TABLETS
Sleep-aid
(Block Drug)

Each tablet:
Pyrilamine maleate * .... 25 mg.

Each capsule:
Pyrilamine maleate * .... 50 mg.

O

OAKITE PRODUCTS
Household and industrial cleaners

Oakite Products, Inc.
50 Valley Rd.
Berkeley Heights, N.J. 07922

Phone: 201-464-6900

See CLEANERS, Section VI, General Formulations

OBALAN TABLETS
Treatment of obesity
(Lannett)

Each tablet:
Phendimetrazine tartrate
USP * .... 35 mg.

O.B. CREAM
(Blistex)

Water
Cocoa butter
Stearic acid
Petrolatum
Glycerin
Triethanolamine
Glyceryl stearate

OBESTAT
Appetite suppressant (timed-release)
(Lemmon Co.)

Each capsule:
Phenylpropanolamine
hydrochloride * .... 75 mg.

OBSOL
Liquid concrete cleaner
(Lester Labs.)

Phosphates *
Detergents *

'76 Ed.

Starred ingredients (*) may be responsible for major toxic effects; consult Section II.

OBTUNDIA CALAMINE CREAM
Antipruritic
(Clapp, Otis)

Metacresolated camphor *†
Zinc oxide
Calamine

†*See* Cresols and Camphor

OBTUNDIA CREAM
Burn and wound ointment
(Clapp, Otis)

Metacresolated camphor *†
In bland emulsified petrolatum base

†*See* Cresols and Camphor

OBTUNDIA SPRAY
Burn and wound treatment
(Clapp, Otis)

Metacresolated camphor *†

†*See* Cresols and Camphor

OBTUNDIA SURGICAL DRESSING
(Clapp, Otis)

Metacresolated camphor *†

†*See* Cresols and Camphor

OCEAN
Isotonic saline mist
(Fleming)

Each 45 ml. bottle:
 Sodium chloride 0.65%
 Benzyl alcohol (as preservative)

OCEAN PINE OIL
Disinfectant, deodorant, cleanser
(Ocean Coffee Co.)

Steam distilled Pine oil * 80%
Combined amount: 10%
 Soap
 Isopropyl alcohol

'76 Ed.

OCEAN SPRAY INSECTICIDE
Household use
(Ocean Coffee Co.)

Beta-butoxy beta'-thiocyano diethyl ether * 3.57%
Petroleum distillate * 96.43%

'76 Ed.

OCTAGON
Bar laundry soap
(Colgate-Palmolive)

Soap
Sodium silicate
Combined amount: .... approx. 5%
 Sodium phosphate *
 Sodium carbonate *

'76 Ed.

OCTAGON LIQUID DETERGENT
(Colgate-Palmolive)

Alkyl aryl sulfonate * ..... approx. 12%
Organic foam builders
Sodium sulfate
Ethyl alcohol .... <3%
Ethoxylated alcohol sulfate approx. 10%

'76 Ed.

OCTAGON LIQUID SOAP
(Colgate-Palmolive)

Sodium soap .... approx. 25%
Ethyl alcohol .... approx. 9%
Water .... approx. 65%
Perfume, color

'76 Ed.

OCTAGON SOAP POWDER
(Colgate-Palmolive)

Sodium soap .... >60%
Combined amount: ..... approx. 25%
 Sodium carbonate *
 Sodium chloride
 Sodium silicate *

'76 Ed.

OCU-BATH
*Sterile, isotonic eye lotion with propio-
 nate*
(Commerce Drug)

Sodium propionate
Borax
Boric acid
Sodium chloride
Rose and camphor waters
Distilled ext. of Witch hazel
Glycerine
Berberine bisulphate
Benzalkonium chloride

OCU-DROP
Isotonic eye drops
(Commerce Drug)

Ephedrine-hydrochloride
Sodium propionate
Borax
Boric acid
Sodium chloride
Camphor
Extract of Witch hazel
Berberine acid sulfate
Chlorobutanol

ODIN CR
(Foy Labs.)

Each tablet:
 Purified Hesperidin .... 100 mg.
 Ascorbic acid .... 100 mg.
 Rutin .... 20 mg.

ODOL
Mouth wash
(Odol)

Alcohol * 80%

'76 Ed.

ODOR-BAN DEODORANT
(Haver-Lockhart (Brand) Bayvet Div.
 Cutter Labs.)

Biphenyl and Perfume * 3.7%
Ethyl alcohol (190 proof,
 denatured) * 96.3%

ODOR-CON (Liquid Concentrate)
Odor counteractant
(Bio-Cide)

Chlorine dioxide * 2%
Sodium carbonate 3%
De-ionized Water 95%

ODORID-DRY (Dry Powder)
*Odor neutralizer for closed spaces, re-
 frigerators, etc.*
(Bio-Cide)

Chlorine dioxide * 0.25%
Inert non-toxic mineral fillers ... 99.75%

ODORID (Liquid Ready to Use)
Household deodorizer and bacteriostat
(Bio-Cide)

Chlorine dioxide * 0.10%
Sodium carbonate 0.15%
De-ionized Water 99.75%

ODORLESS ZEEN
Dry cleaner
(Cleveland Cleaner)

Mineral spirits, odorless *

'76 Ed.

ODOR-TROL
Control of urine odor
(Haver-Lockhart (Brand) Bayvet Div.
 Cutter Labs.)

Each tablet:
 Methionine * .... 200 mg.

ODRINIL
Diuretic
(Fox Pharmacal)

Each tablet:
Pwd. ext. of Buchu
Pwd. ext. of Uva Ursi
Pwd. ext. of Corn silk
Pwd. ext. of Juniper *
Caffeine *

OEM ANTIFREEZE COOLANT (AF-335G, Formula YA-335 (8697-87))
(Union Carbide)

Ethylene glycol * 95%
Water 3%
Soluble inhibitors 2%

OFF
Asphalt remover
(Consolidated Chem., Inc.)

Toluene *
Ortho dichlorobenzene *
Mineral spirits *
Tall oil amide

OFF-EZY CORN REMOVER
Keratolytic
(Commerce Drug)

Benzocaine
Flexible Collodion *
Salicylic acid *
Lactic acid
Camphor *

OFLYO LIQUID SPRAY
Insecticide
(Adco)

Petroleum distillate *
Tech. Piperonyl butoxide
Pyrethrins *

OGEN TABLETS
Oral estrogen
(Abbott)

Each tablet:
Piperazine estrone
sulfate .... 0.75 mg.; 1.5 mg.;
3.0 mg.; or 6.0 mg.

OGEN VAGINAL CREAM
Treatment of atrophic vaginitis or kraurosis vulvae
(Abbott)

Each gram:
Piperazine estrone sulfate .... 1.5 mg.

OGILVIE COSMETIC PRODUCTS

Ogilvie Products, Inc.
Div. Lehn & Fink Products Group
225 Summit Ave.
Montvale, N.J. 07645

Phone: 201-573-5700

See COSMETICS, Section VI, General Formulations

OGILVIE HOME PERMANENT WAVE LOTION, CREME
(Ogilvie)

Water
Ammonium thioglycolate *
Ammonium hydroxide
Mineral oil
Potassium coco-hydrolyzed protein
Potassium oleate
Lanolin
Glycol
Lanolin oil
Laureth-23

OGILVIE ON-THE-ROD NEUTRALIZER
(Ogilvie)

Water
PEG-150 disterate
Hydrogen peroxide *
Phosphoric acid
Tetrasodium pyrophosphate
Sodium stannate

OGILVIE PRECISELY RIGHT BODY AND STYLING WAVE FOR COLOR TREATED HAIR
Heat activator - Part A, Waving lotion - Part B
(Ogilvie)

The mixture of Part A and Part B contains:
Water
Ammonium thioglycolate *
Ammonium dithiodiglycolate
Laureth-23
Potassium coco-hydrolyzed animal protein
Fragrance
Ammonium hydroxide
Styrene/acrylate copolymer
Methylparaben
Ammonium phosphate
Disodium phosphate

OGILVIE PRECISELY RIGHT BODY AND STYLING WAVE FOR COLOR TREATED HAIR - NEUTRALIZER
(Ogilvie)

Water
Hydrogen peroxide *
Quaternium-40
Cetearyl alcohol
Sodium lauryl sulfate
Ceteth-20
Methylparaben
Fragrance
Disodium phosphate
Phosphoric acid

OGILVIE PRECISELY RIGHT BODY AND STYLING WAVE FOR REGULAR HAIR
Heat activator - Part A, Waving lotion - Part B
(Ogilvie)

The mixture of Part A and Part B contains:
Water
Ammonium thioglycolate *
Ammonium dithiodiglycolate
Laureth-23
Ammonium hydroxide
Potassium coco-hydrolyzed animal protein
Fragrance
Styrene/acrylate copolymer
Methylparaben
Ammonium phosphate
Disodium phosphate
D & C Yellow No. 10
Carmine

OGILVIE PRECISELY RIGHT BODY AND STYLING WAVE FOR REGULAR HAIR - NEUTRALIZER
(Ogilvie)

Water
Hydrogen peroxide *
Quaternium-52
Cetearyl alcohol
Sodium lauryl sulfate
Ceteth-20
Methylparaben
Fragrance
Disodium phosphate
Phosphoric acid

OILATUM SOAP
For dry skin
(Stiefel Labs.)

Polyunsaturated vegetable oil 7.5%

OIL BOOTTOPPING
Heavy duty marine paint
(International Paint)

Mineral spirits (or turpentine substitute) *
Pigments - no lead

OIL-DRI NON-SLIP PAINT
(Oil-Dri)

Magnesium silicate	57.88%
Lithopone	6.00%
Silica	31.72%
Asbestos	2.40%
Carbon black	2.00%
Lead	<1%/gal.
Resin plus oil	27.44%
Mineral spirits	54.57%
Toluol *	15.05%

'76 Ed.

OIL-I-CIDE
Insecticide; also shines, cleans foliage
(International Lubricant)

Petroleum oil *

OIL OF OLAY BEAUTY FLUID
(Vicks Toiletry Products Div.)

Water
Mineral oil
Potassium stearate
Sodium stearate
Cholesterol
Cetyl palmitate
Butylparaben
Sodium carbomer 934
Potassium carbomer 934
Propylparaben
Methylparaben
Sodium laurate
Potassium laurate
Castor oil
Sodium myristate
Potassium myristate
Myristyl alcohol
Cetyl alcohol
Sodium palmitate
Potassium palmitate
Stearyl alcohol
Fragrance
FD & C Red No. 4

OIL-O-SOL
Inhibitory antiseptic for wet dressing
(Mosso)

Linseed oil
Oil of turpentine *
Natural Camphor *
Oil of spearmint *
Oil of eucalyptus *

'76 Ed.

O.K.
Cleaning fluid
(Albatross Chem.)

1,1,1-Trichloroethane *	
Sovasol No. 4	<10%

OLAY VITALIZING CREAM
(Vicks Toiletry Products Div.)

Mineral oil	
Water	
Beewax	
Microcrystalline wax	
Sodium borate	<1.0%
Cholesterol	
Fragrance	
D & C Red No. 30 - Alumina lake	

OLD BLUE
Laundry aid
(Climaco)

Sodium dichlorocyanurate *

OLD DUTCH CLEANSER
Household cleanser
(Purex Corp.)

Siliceous abrasive	>85%
Alkaline builder	1-10%
Anionic surfactant	1-3%
Chlorine bleaching agent	<2%
Coloring agent	<1%
Perfume	<1%

OLD ENGLISH LEMON CREAM WAX
Furniture polish
(Boyle-Midway)

Silicone oils	<5%
Polishing oils	<1%
Isoparaffinic solvent	<5%
Waxes	
Wetting agents	
Preservative	

OLD ENGLISH LEMON FURNITURE POLISH (Aerosol)
(Boyle-Midway)

Waxes	<20%
Silicone oils	<5%
Isoparaffinic solvent	<25%
Wetting agent	<1%
Propellant	

OLD ENGLISH LEMON FURNITURE POLISH (Trigger pump)
(Boyle-Midway)

Polishing oil	<1%
Silicone oil	<5%
Isoparaffinic solvent	<5%
Nonionic surface active agent	
Thickener	
Waxes	
Preservatives	

OLD ENGLISH LEMON OIL FURNITURE POLISH
(Boyle-Midway)

Polishing oils *†

†*See* Petroleum distillate

OLD ENGLISH RED OIL FURNITURE POLISH
(Boyle-Midway)

Petroleum polishing oil *†	
Oil of cedarwood	trace
Turpentine	trace

†*See* Mineral seal oil

OLD ENGLISH SCRATCH COVER
(Boyle-Midway)

Petroleum polishing & staining oils *

OLD HI SPORTSMAN
Adhesive
(Ambroid)

Nitrocellulose type of cement
Alcohols *	20%
Hydrocarbons *†	60%
Ketones *	20%
Allyl isothiocyanate (synthetic oil of mustard)	trace

†*See* Adhesives, Section VI, General Formulations

OLEON
Dishwashing detergent
(Lester Labs.)

Synthetic detergents *
Softeners

'76 Ed.

"OLE TIME" WOODSMAN JUNGLE FORMULA
Insect repellent
(Ole Time Woodsman)

Active ingred.:
N,N,-Diethyl-meta-toluamide *	71.25%
Other Diethyl toluamides	3.75%

Inert ingred.:
Denatured Ethanol *	25.00%

"OLE TIME" WOODSMAN JUNGLE FORMULA (Aerosol)
Insect repellent
(Ole Time Woodsman)

N,N,-Diethyl-meta-toluamide*	57%
Other Isomers	3%

Starred ingredients (*) may be responsible for major toxic effects; consult Section II.

"OLE TIME" WOODSMAN KAMPERS LOTION
Suntan lotion, insect repellent
(Ole Time Woodsman)

Isoparaffinic hydrocarbons *	42.0%
N,N,-Diethyl-meta-toluamide *	40.4%
Other Isomers	2.1%
Mineral oil	8.9%
Camphor *	2.9%
2-Ethoxyethyl p-methoxycin-	
namate	1.8%
Canadian balsam	1.5%
Isobornyl acetate	0.4%

"OLE TIME" WOODMAN'S LIQUID FLY DOPE
Fly repellent
(Ole Time Woodsman)

Rectified Oil of pine tar *	35.0%
N,N,-Diethyl-meta-toluamide and other isomers *	27.0%
Mineral oil	25.0%
Citronella	4.7%
Penny Royal	4.7%
Camphor *	2.9%
Oil of bay	0.7%

† *See* Pine tar oils

OLIN PRODUCTS

Olin Corporation
120 Long Ridge Rd.
Stamford, Conn. 06904

Emergency response phone: 203-356-2345

OLIVCREME
(Aschenbach & Miller)

Aschenbach & Miller
245 Race St.
Philadelphia, Pa. 19106

Phone: 215-627-4363

OLYMPIC STAIN PRODUCTS
(Olympic Stain)

OLYMPIC STAIN
Div. of The Clorox Co.
2233 112th Ave., N.E.
Bellevue, Wash. 98004

Phone: 206-453-1700

OMAR WALLPAPER CLEANER
(Clean Prod.)

Clean Products Co.
7275 Neville St.
Columbus, Ohio 44102

Phone: 614-252-1104

OMEGA

See AIRWICK PROFESSIONAL PRODUCTS OMEGA

OMEGA CHALKBOARD CHALK IN COLOR
(Weber Costello)

Calcium carbonate	95%
Vegetable binder	5%
Nontoxic pigments	

OMEGA OIL
Rubefacient
(Block Drug)

Isopropyl alcohol	50.00%
Methyl salicylate *	23.00%
Mineral oil	
Histamine dihydrochloride	0.02%
Methyl nicotinate	0.30%
Capsicum oleoresin	0.25%

OMNIBUS SOAP
(Hewitt)

Tallow
Coconut oil
Sodium hydroxide

'76 Ed.

OMNIPAK

See AIRWICK PROFESSIONAL PRODUCTS OMNIPAK

OMNIPEN CAPSULES
Antibiotic therapy
(Wyeth Labs.)

Each capsule:
Ampicillin
(anhydrous) ...... 250 mg.; 500 mg.

OMNIPEN SUSPENSION
Antibiotic therapy
(Wyeth Labs.)

Each 5 ml.:
Ampicillin ...... 125 mg.; 250 mg.; 500 mg.

OMNI-TUSS SUSPENSION
Antitussive, bronchodilator, expectorant, antihistaminic
(Pennwalt, Pharm. Div.)

Each 5 ml.:
Codeine *	10 mg.
Phenyltoloxamine	5 mg.
Chlorpheniramine	3 mg.
Ephedrine *	25 mg.
All as cation exchange resin complexes of sulfonated polystyrene	
Guaiacol carbonate	20 mg.

ONCE AROUND
Acid type cleaner
(Paul Koss)

Water	>70%
Hydrogen chloride *	20%
Hydrogen fluoride *	<10%
Nonionic surfactant	
Dye	trace

101 LIQUID BLEACH
(Gardiner Mfg.)

Sodium hypochlorite *	5.25%

'76 Ed.

ONE SHOT
Liquid laundry detergent
(Brewer Chem.)

Soil suspension agent	<5%
Nonylphenoxy polyethoxy ethanol	approx. 20%
Fluorescent whitening agent	<1%

ONE STEP CARPET CLEANER (Aerosol)

See BISSELL ONE STEP CARPET CLEANER (Aerosol)

ONE STEP FIBERGLASS & BATHROOM CLEANER (Aerosol)

See BISSELL ONE STEP FIBERGLASS & BATHROOM CLEANER (Aerosol)

ONE STEP OVEN CLEANER (Aerosol)

See BISSELL ONE STEP OVEN CLEANER (Aerosol)

ONE STEP SPOT LIFTER (Aerosol)

See BISSELL ONE STEP SPOT LIFTER (Aerosol)

ONE STROKE
Bacteriostatic compound for dustless cleaning & sweeping of floors; institutional & commercial use
(Hysan Corp.)

Heptadecyl hydroxyethylimidazolinium chloride	0.250%
N-Alkyl (60% C14, 30% C10, 5% C12, 5% C18) dimethyl benzyl ammonium chlorides	0.125%
N-Alkyl (50% C12, 30% C14, 17% C16, 3% C18) dimethyl ethylbenzyl ammonium chlorides	0.125%
Isopropyl alcohol	0.060%
Essential oils	0.200%
Petroleum distillate *	

1-STROKE VES-PHENE
Germicidal detergent
(Vestal)

o-Phenylphenol *	10.0%
o-Benzyl p-chlorophenol *	8.5%
p-Tertiary amylphenol	2.0%

'76 Ed.

Starred ingredients (*) may be responsible for major toxic effects; consult Section II.

110 WARM WAVE LOTION
(Willat)

Mono-thioglycolate 1-10%

120 DAY AUTOMATIC BOWL CLEANER
Toilet bowl cleaner
(Twinoak Products)

Calcium hypochlorite * 38.0%

ONEX SEAL II
Floor sealer
(Hillyard Chem.)

Mineral spirits *

'76 Ed.

ONEX SEAL II, COLORED
Floor sealer
(Hillyard Chem.)

Mineral spirits *

'76 Ed.

ONEX SEAL, SPECIAL
Floor sealer
(Hillyard Chem.)

Mineral spirits *

'76 Ed.

ONIXOL, DR. SCHOLL'S
See DR. SCHOLL'S ONIXOL

O-N MEN-THO-SOTE
For colds
(Owen Drug)

Owen Drug Co.
1700 S. First St.
Salisbury, N.C. 28144

Phone: 803-636-0951

ON'N OFF (Pressurized Spray)
All purpose cleaning compound
(Haviland Agricultural Chem. Co.)

Sodium tripolyphosphate *
Cocoanut oil soap
Sodium metasilicate
Ethylene glycol *
N-Butyl ether
Propellant

'76 Ed.

ONOX
Prevents athlete's foot
(Onox)

Zinc chloride *
Sodium chloride
Sodium nitrate *
Sodium silicofluoride *
Boric acid *

O-N SKIN-ITCH ANTISEPTIC
Fungicide; medical
(Owen Drug)

Owen Drug Co.
1700 S. First St.
Salisbury, N.C. 28144

Phone: 803-636-0951

ONYX WHITE LEATHER DRESSING
Shoe dressing
(Zoes, C.A.)

Pigment:
   Titanium dioxide
Liquid solvent:
   Water

Non-toxic per manufacturer - does not contain lead pigment.

OPACEDRIN
Analgesic, antihistaminic, antisecretory, antipyretic
(Elder)

Each capsule:
   Acetaminophen (N-Acetyl-p-
     aminophenol) * .... 50 mg.
   Salicylamide * .... 200 mg.
   Chlorpheniramine maleate ... 2 mg.
   Caffeine .... 8 mg.
   Phenylephrine
     hydrochloride * .... 5 mg.

OPASAL
Analgesic-decongestant
(Elder)

Each capsule:
   Acetaminophen * .... 325.0 mg.
   Phenylpropanolamine
     hydrochloride * .... 18.0 mg.

OPENUP
Plumbing cleaner
(Ampion)

Sodium hydroxide * 99%
Aluminum 1%

OPHTHETIC
Ophthalmic solution
(Allergan Pharm.)

Proparacaine HCl 0.5%

OPTAURAL
Local analgesic and decongestant for ear
(Optimus)

Atropine sulfate .... 1/40 gr.
Benzocaine .... 2 gr.
Antipyrine * .... 8 gr.
Glycerin .... q.s. ad 1/2 fl. oz.

OP-THAL-ZIN
Astringent eye drops
(Alcon)

Each ml.:
   Zinc sulfate 0.25%
   Benzalkonium chloride (as
     preservative) 0.01%

OPTILETS-M-500 FILMTAB
Therapeutic multiple vitamins with minerals
(Abbott)

Each tablet:
   Iron * .... 20 mg.
   Multivitamins and minerals

OPTIMYD OPHTHALMIC SOLUTION
Anti-inflammatory, antibacterial
(Schering)

Each cc:
   Prednisolone sodium phosphate (equiv.
     to 5.0 mg. of prednisolone phosphate)
   Sodium sulfacetamide .... 100 mg.
Inactive ingredients:
   Sodium thiosulfate
   Tyloxapol
   Disodium edetate
   Monobasic Sodium phosphate
   Dibasic anhydrous Sodium phosphate
   Sodium hydroxide (to adjust pH)
   Benzalkonium chloride, USP . 0.025%
   Phenylethyl alcohol, NF 0.5%
   Purified water

OPTIPRIME OPHTHAKOTE OPHTHALMIC SOLUTION
Anti-inflammatory, antibacterial agent; veterinary
(Syntex Agribusiness)

Neomycin sulfate (equivalent to
   0.35% neomycin base) 0.5%
Polymixin B sulfate .... 10,000 units/cc
In a Hydroxypropyl methylcellulose vehicle containing:
   Polyethylene glycol 4000
   Propylene glycol
   Methylparaben
   Propylparaben
   Citric acid
   Sodium hydroxide, and/or Sulfuric acid
    to adjust pH

OPTIVET DURACOAT OPHTHALMIC SOLUTION
For use in dogs
(Burns-Biotec)

Each ml.:
   Gentamicin sulfate (equiv. to 3 mg. gentamicin base)
   Betamethasone acetate (equiv. to 0.89
    mg. betamethasone alcohol)
   Polyoxyl 40 stearate
   Polyoxyethylated vegetable oil
   Edetate disodium
   Phenylmercuric nitrate (as
    preservative) .... 0.02 mg.
   Purified Water .... q.s.

Starred ingredients (*) may be responsible for major toxic effects; consult Section II.

OPTIVET OPHTHALMIC OINTMENT-STERILE
For use in dogs and cats
(Burns-Biotec)

Each gram:
Gentamicin sulfate (equiv. to 3 mg. gentamicin)
Methylparaben .... 0.5 mg.
Propylparaben .... 0.1 mg.
White petrolatum

OPTIVET OPHTHALMIC SOLUTION-STERILE
For use in dogs and cats
(Burns-Biotec)

Each ml.:
Gentamicin sulfate (equiv. to 3 mg. gentamicin)
Disodium phosphate .... 2.9 mg.
Monosodium phosphate ...... 0.1 mg.
Sodium chloride .... 7.4 mg.
Benzalkonium chloride (as preservative) .... 0.1 mg.
Purified Water .... q.s.

OPTOLOW
Ophthalmic liquid
(Wesley Pharm.)

Sodium propionate
Sodium chloride
Camphor
Peppermint oil
Benzalkonium chloride
Propionic acid

OPTOZINE
Ophthalmic liquid
(Wesley Pharm.)

Phenylephrine hydrochloride 0.12%
Methylcellulose 0.5%
Isotonic base:
Boric acid
Potassium chloride

ORABASE
For minor irritations of the mouth and gums
(Hoyt Labs.)

Pectin
Gelatin
Sodium carboxymethylcellulose
Plasticized Hydrocarbon gel (polyethylene and mineral oil gel base)

ORABASE HCA ORAL PASTE
For oral lesions
(Hoyt Labs.)

Each gram:
Hydrocortisone acetate .... 5 mg.
Pectin
Gelatin
Sodium carboxymethylcellulose
Plasticized hydrocarbon gel (5% polyethylene in mineral oil)
Imitation Vanilla flavoring

ORABASE WITH BENZOCAINE
Analgesic oral protective paste
(Hoyt Labs.)

Benzocaine
Pectin
Gelatin
Sodium carboxymethylcellulose
Plasticized hydrocarbon gel (in a polyethylene and mineral oil gel base)

ORACIN
Throat lozenge
(Vicks Health Care Div.)

Each lozenge:
Benzocaine .... 6.25 mg.
Menthol 0.1%
In a cooling sorbitol sugars base

ORACIN CHERRY FLAVORED
Throat lozenge
(Vicks Health Care Div.)

Each lozenge:
Benzocaine .... 6.25 mg.
Menthol 0.08%
In a cooling sorbitol sugars base

ORADEX-C
Throat troches
(Commerce Drug)

Each troche:
Cetylpyridinium chloride .... 2.5 mg.
Benzocaine .... 10.0 mg.

ORAHEMA SOLU-CAPS
Basic iron with supplemental vitamins
(Sutliff & Case)

Each Solu-Cap:
Ferrous fumarate * .... 200 mg.
Folic acid .... 0.5 mg.
Polyvitamins and minerals

'76 Ed.

ORA-JEL
For teething pain, toothache, denture irritations
(Commerce Drug)

Benzocaine in a special base

ORAL-AID JEL
For the relief of teething pains, toothaches & denture irritations
(Columbia Med.)

Benzocaine

ORALPHYLLIN
Antiasthmatic, bronchial & coronary dilator
(CMC Research Div.)

Each 15 cc:
Theophylline .... 80 mg.
Alcohol .... 20%/vol.

ORAPHEN-PD SYRUP
Analgesic, antipyretic
(Comatic)

Each 5 ml.:
Acetaminophen * .... 120 mg.

Additive free product

ORASEPT
Orifice antiseptic - embalming supply
(Royal Bond)

Phenyl phenol *

ORASONE
Oral corticosteroid therapy
(Rowell)

Prednisone .... 1 mg., 5 mg., 10 mg., 20 mg.

Film-coated Prednisone .... 50 mg.

ORDRAM (8-E, 10-G)
Herbicide
(Stauffer)

Ordram (S-Ethyl hexahydro-1H-azepine-1-carbothioate) *

ORETIC TABLETS
Diuretic
(Abbott)

Each tablet:
Hydrochlorothiazide * 25 mg.; or 50 mg.

ORETICYL FORTE, TABLETS
Antihypertensive
(Abbott)

Each tablet:
Hydrochlorothiazide * ...... 25 mg.
Deserpidine .... 0.25 mg.

ORETICYL (25 or 50) TABLETS
Antihypertensive
(Abbott)

Each tablet:
Hydrochlorothiazide * 25 mg.; or 50 mg.
Deserpidine .... 0.125 mg.

ORETON METHYL BUCCAL TABLETS
Androgen therapy
(Schering)

Each tablet:
Methyltestosterone .... 10 mg.

ORETON METHYL TABLETS
Androgen therapy
(Schering)

Each tablet:
Methyltestosterone .... 10 mg.; 25 mg.

Starred ingredients (*) may be responsible for major toxic effects; consult Section II.

ORETON PROPIONATE BUCCAL TABLETS
Androgen therapy
(Schering)

Each tablet:
Testosterone propionate ...... 10 mg.

ORGANIC-QUAT DETERGENT/ DISINFECTANT
(Nat'l Labs. Div.)

n-Alkyl (60% C14, 30% C16, 5% C12,
5% C18) dimethyl benzyl ammonium chlorides * 4.5%
n-Alkyl (68% C12, 32% C14) dimethyl
ethylbenzyl ammonium
chlorides * 4.5%
Sodium carbonate .... minor
Tetrasodium ethylenediamine
tetraacetate .... minor

ORIGINAL ECLIPSE SUNSCREEN GEL
(Herbert Labs.)

Padimate O (Octyl dimethyl PABA)
Glyceryl PABA

ORIGINAL FLEACOLLAR FOR CATS

See FLEACOLLAR FOR CATS

ORIGINAL FLEACOLLAR FOR DOGS

See FLEACOLLAR FOR DOGS

ORIOLE IODOPHOR
Germicide-detergent
(Oriole Equipment & Supply)

Nonylphenoxy polyethoxy ethanol
iodine complex 18.00%
Phosphoric acid * 5.00%
'76 Ed.

ORKIL CHLOROHEPTON CONCENTRATE NO. 2, PROFESSIONAL

See PROFESSIONAL ORKIL CHLO-
ROHEPTON CONCENTRATE
NO. 2

ORKIN-AIRE INDUSTRIAL BOMB
Insecticide
(Orkin)

Pyrethrins 0.50%
Technical Piperonyl butoxide ... 1.00%
N-Octyl bicycloheptene
dicarboximide 1.00%
Petroleum distillate * 17.50%
Inert ingred.: 80.00%
Propellants
'76 Ed.

ORKIN-AIRE INSECT BOMB
Insecticide
(Orkin)

Pyrethrins 0.50%
Technical Piperonyl butoxide ... 1.00%
N-Octyl bicycloheptene
dicarboximide 1.00%
Petroleum distillate * 17.50%
Inert ingred.: 80.00%
Propellants
'76 Ed.

ORKINCIDE ANTI-COAGULANT RODENT BAIT, PROFESSIONAL

See PROFESSIONAL ORKINCIDE
ANTI-COAGULANT RODENT
BAIT

ORKIN PRODUCTS

See PROFESSIONAL ORKIN PROD-
UCTS

ORKINTROL FORMULA W/ E 1-31 CONCENTRATE, PROFESSIONAL

See PROFESSIONAL ORKINTROL
FORMULA W/E 1-31 CONCEN-
TRATE

ORLANE/JEAN D'ALBRET COSMETICS

Orlane/Jean d'Albret
499 Park Ave.
New York, N.Y. 10022

Phone: 212-757-4200

See COSMETICS, Section VI, General
Formulations

ORNACOL
*Relieves nasal coughing and nasal
congestion*
(MenJ Labs.)

Phenylpropanolamine HCl * ... 18 mg.
Acetaminophen .... 325 mg.

ORNADE SPANSULE CAPSULES
Decongestant, antihistamine
(SK&F)

Each capsule:
Phenylpropanolamine
hydrochloride * .... 75 mg.
Chlorpheniramine maleate .... 12 mg.

OR-NON
For coughs
(Ortega Pharm.)

Each 30 cc:
Dextromethorphan HBr * ... 60 mg.
Phenylephrine HCl * .... 30 mg.
Potassium guaiacol-sulfonate . 500 mg.
Chlorpheniramine maleate ... 2 mg.

ORTEGA-OTIC-M
Relief of pain and infection of the ear
(Ortega Pharm.)

Each cc:
Hydrocortisone free alcohol 0.25%
Polymyxin B sulfate, USP . 2000 units
Neomycin base (as neomy-
cin sulfate) .... 3.5 mg.
Diperodon hydrochloride .. 0.5%
Propylene glycol & glycerine base

ORTHAZITE, LIQUID

See EDWAL LIQUID ORTHAZITE

ORTHENE INSECT SPRAY
(Chevron)

Acephate (O,S-Dimethyl
acetylphosphoramidothioate) * 15.6%

Chevron emergency phone number:
415-233-3737

ORTHO ANT, ROACH & SPIDER SPRAY
(Chevron)

Active ingred. (by wt.):
2-(1-Methylethoxy)phenyl
methylcarbamate * 1.0%
Petroleum distillate * 82.3%

Chevron emergency phone number:
415-233-3737

ORTHO AQUATIC WEED KILLER NO. 60
Herbicide
(Chevron)

Aromatic petroleum distillate * .. 95.0%

Chevron emergency phone number:
415-233-3737

ORTHO BRUSH KILLER A
(Chevron)

Ammonium sulfamate * 43%/w

Chevron emergency phone number:
415-233-3737

Starred ingredients (*) may be responsible for major toxic effects; consult Section II.

ORTHO CHICKWEED & CLOVER KILLER
Herbicide
(Chevron)

Isooctyl ester of silvex (2-(2,4,5-
Trichlorophenoxy)propionic
acid) * 13.8%

Chevron emergency phone number:
415-233-3737

ORTHO CHICKWEED, SPURGE & OXALIS KILLER
(Chevron)

Silvex (isooctyl ester) * 15.1%/w

Chevron emergency phone number:
415-233-3737

ORTHO CHINCH BUG AND SOD WEBWORM CONTROL
(Chevron)

O,O,O,O-Tetrapropyl
dithiopyrophosphate 3.2%/w

Chevron emergency phone number:
415-233-3737

ORTHO CHINCH BUG SPRAY
(Chevron)

Active ingred. (by wt.):
O,O,O,O-Tetrapropyl
dithiopyrophosphate 13%
Aromatic petroleum derivative
solvent * 81.2%

Chevron emergency phone number:
415-233-3737

ORTHOCIDE-BOTRAN SULFUR 10-5-40 DUST
Fungicide-insecticide
(Chevron)

Captan 10%/w
2,6-Dichloro-4-nitroaniline * 5%/w
Sulfur 40%/w

Chevron emergency phone number:
415-233-3737

ORTHOCIDE 7.5 DUST
Fungicide
(Chevron)

Captan 7.5%

Chevron emergency phone number:
415-233-3737

ORTHOCIDE 4 FLOWABLE
Fungicide
(Chevron)

Captan 38%/w

Chevron emergency phone number:
415-233-3737

ORTHOCIDE GARDEN FUNGICIDE
(Chevron)

Captan 50%

Chevron emergency phone number:
415-233-3737

ORTHOCIDE 75 SEED PROTECTANT
(Chevron)

Captan 75%/w

Chevron emergency phone number:
415-233-3737

ORTHOCIDE SOIL TREATER "X"
Fungicide
(Chevron)

Captan 10%
Pentachloronitrobenzene * 10%

Chevron emergency phone number:
415-233-3737

ORTHO CITRUS INSECT SPRAY
(Chevron)

Active ingred. (by wt.):
Ethion * 10%
Petroleum oil * 75%

Chevron emergency phone number:
415-233-3737

ORTHO CRAB GRASS & DANDELION KILLER
(Chevron)

Active ingred. (by wt.):
Dodecylammonium
methanearsonate * 8.0%
Octylammonium
methanearsonate * 8.0%
2,4-Dichlorophenoxyacetic acid
(octylammonium salt) 8.16%

Chevron emergency phone number:
415-233-3737

ORTHO CRAB GRASS KILLER
Herbicide
(Chevron)

Octyl ammonium methanearsonate * 8%
Dodecyl ammonium
methanearsonate * 8%

Chevron emergency phone number:
415-233-3737

ORTHO-CREME
Contraceptive cream
(Ortho)

Nonoxynol 9 .... 2.00%
Ricinoleic acid 0.75%
Boric acid 3.00%
Sodium lauryl sulfate 0.28%

ORTHO DAIRY & HORSE FLY SPRAY R
(Chevron)

Active ingred. (by wt.):
Pyrethrins 0.03%
Technical Piperonyl butoxide . 0.25%
Di-n-propyl isocinchomeronate . 0.20%
Petroleum distillate * 99.49%

Chevron emergency phone number:
415-233-3737

ORTHO DIAZINON INSECT SPRAY
For use on lawns and gardens
(Chevron)

Active ingred. (by wt.):
O,O-Diethyl O-(2-isopropyl-6-
methyl-4-pyrimidinyl)
phosphorothioate 25%
Aromatic petroleum derivative
solvent * 57%

Chevron emergency phone number:
415-233-3737

ORTHO DIAZINON SOIL & TURF INSECT CONTROL
(Chevron)

O,O-Diethyl O-(2-isopropyl-6-methyl-
4-pyrimidinyl)phosphorothioate * 5%

Chevron emergency phone number:
415-233-3737

ORTHO DIBROM 8 EMULSIVE
Insecticide
(Chevron)

Active ingred.:
Naled * 58%
Light Aromatic petroleum
distillate * 20%

Chevron emergency phone number:
415-233-3737

ORTHO DIBROM FLY & MOSQUITO SPRAY
(Chevron)

Naled 1%/w
Petroleum distillates * 96%/w

Chevron emergency phone number:
415-233-3737

ORTHO DIBROM 235 SPRAY
Insecticide
(Chevron)

Naled * 26%/w
Aromatic petroleum derivative
solvent * 61%/w

Chevron emergency phone number:
415-233-3737

Starred ingredients (*) may be responsible for major toxic effects; consult Section II.

ORTHO DIBROM-TOXAPHENE 1.5-6 EMULSIVE
Insecticide
(Chevron)

Naled * 11.8%/w
Toxaphene * 54.4%/w
Aromatic petroleum derivative
  solvent * 23.0%/w

Chevron emergency phone number:
  415-233-3737

ORTHO DIENESTROL CREAM
Estrogen, vaginal
(Ortho)

Dienestrol 0.01%

ORTHO DIFOLATAN BOTRAN 35-35 SEED PROTECTANT
Fungicide
(Chevron)

Captafol * 35%/w
2,6 -Dichloro-4-nitroaniline * 35%/w

Chevron emergency phone number:
  415-233-3737

ORTHO DIFOLATAN BOTRAN 60-20 SEED PROTECTANT
Fungicide
(Chevron)

Captafol * 60%/w
2,6-Dichloro-4-nitroaniline * 20%/w

Chevron emergency phone number:
  415-233-3737

ORTHO DIQUAT 2 SPRAY
Herbicide
(Chevron)

Diquat dibromide * 35.3%/w

Chevron emergency phone number:
  415-233-3737

ORTHO DIQUAT WATER WEED KILLER
Herbicide
(Chevron)

Diquat dibromide (6,7-Dihydrodi-
  pyrido(1,2-a:2′,1′-c)pyrazidiinium
  dibromide) * 35.3%

Chevron emergency phone number:
  415-233-3737

ORTHO DOWPON M GRASS KILLER
(Chevron)

Active ingred. (by wt.):
  Sodium salt of Dalapon * 72.5%
  Magnesium salt of Dalapon 12.0%

Chevron emergency phone number:
  415-233-3737

ORTHO DRILL BOX WHEAT SEED PROTECTANT
Fungicide
(Chevron)

Active ingred. (by wt.):
  Captan 20%
  Hexachlorobenzene * 20%

Chevron emergency phone number:
  415-233-3737

ORTHO DYRENE LAWN DISEASE CONTROL
(Chevron)

Dyrene (4,6-Dichloro-N-(2-chlo-
  rophenyl)-1,3,5-triazine-2-
  amine) * 50%/w

Chevron emergency phone number:
  415-233-3737

ORTHO EARWIG & ROACH BAIT
(Chevron)

Active ingred. (by wt.):
  2-(1-Methylethoxy)phenyl
    methylcarbamate * 2%

Chevron emergency phone number:
  415-233-3737

ORTHO FENCE & GRASS EDGER
Herbicide
(Chevron)

Active ingred. (by wt.):
  Erbon 4.9%
  Related compounds 1.7%

Chevron emergency phone number:
  415-233-3737

ORTHO FLY KILLER D
Insecticide
(Chevron)

Naled (Dibrom) * 36%
Aromatic petroleum derivative
  solvent * 49%

Chevron emergency phone number:
  415-233-3737

ORTHO FOGGING INSECTICIDE
(Chevron)

Active ingred. (by wt.):
  (5-Benzyl-3-furyl)methyl 2,2-
    dimethyl-3-(2-methylpro-
    penyl)cyclopro-
    panecarboxylate 0.200%
  Related compounds 0.027%
  Aromatic petroleum
    hydrocarbons 0.265%
  Petroleum distillate * 99.500%

Chevron emergency phone number:
  415-233-3737

ORTHO FRUIT & VEGETABLE INSECT CONTROL
(Chevron)

Active ingred. (by wt.):
  O,O-Diethyl O-(2-isopropyl-6-
    methyl-4-pyrimidinyl)
    phosphorothioate * 25%
  Aromatic petroleum derivative
    solvent * 57%

Chevron emergency phone number:
  415-233-3737

ORTHO GRAIN FUMIGANT (73)
(Chevron)

Ethylene dibromide * 70.0%
Methyl bromide * 30.0%

Chevron emergency phone number:
  415-233-3737

ORTHO-GYNOL
Contraceptive jelly
(Ortho)

p-Diisobutylphenoxypolyethoxy-
  ethanol 1.00%

ORTHO HCB 4 FLOWABLE SEED PROTECTANT
Fungicide
(Chevron)

Hexachlorobenzene * 37%/w

Chevron emergency phone number:
  415-233-3737

ORTHO HOME AND GARDEN SPRAY
Insecticide
(Chevron)

Active ingred. (by wt.):
  (5-Benzyl-3-furyl)methyl-2,2-di-
    methyl-3-(2-
    methylpropenyl)cyclopro-
    panecarboxylate 0.250%
  Related compounds 0.034%
  Aromatic petroleum
    hydrocarbons 0.331%
  Petroleum distillate 6.500%

Chevron emergency phone number:
  415-233-3737

Starred ingredients (*) may be responsible for major toxic effects; consult Section II.

ORTHO HOME ORCHARD SPRAY
Insecticide
(Chevron)

Captan	15.0%
Malathion *	7.5%
Methoxychlor, technical *	15.0%

Chevron emergency phone number:
415-233-3737

ORTHO HOME PEST CONTROL
(Chevron)

Pyrethrins	0.05%
Piperonyl butoxide (technical)	0.26%
O,O-Diethyl O-(2-isopropyl-6-methyl-4-pyrimidinyl)phosphorothioate	0.50%
Petroleum distillates *	99.12%

Chevron emergency phone number:
415-233-3737

ORTHO HORNET & WASP JET SPRAY
(Chevron)

	by wt.:
Pyrethrins	0.10%
Piperonyl butoxide (technical)	0.20%
N-Octyl bicycloheptene dicarboximide	0.33%
2-(1-Methylethoxy)phenyl methylcarbamate *	0.50%
Isoparaffinic hydrocarbons *	83.87%

Chevron emergency phone number:
415-233-3737

ORTHO HOUSEHOLD INSECT CONTROL
(Chevron)

Active ingred. (by wt.):

(5-Benzyl-3-furyl)methyl-2,2-di-methyl-3-(2-methylpropenyl)cyclopro-panecarboxylate	0.250%
Related compounds	0.034%
Aromatic petroleum hydrocarbons	0.331%
Petroleum distillate	6.500%

Chevron emergency phone number:
415-233-3737

ORTHO INDOOR PLANT INSECT SPRAY
Insecticide
(Chevron)

Pyrethrins	0.02%
Rotenone	0.13%
Other cube resins	0.13%
Technical Piperonyl butoxide	0.25%
Petroleum distillate	0.08%

Chevron emergency phone number:
415-233-3737

ORTHO INSTANT BLUESTONE
Fungicide
(Chevron)

Copper sulfate pentahydrate *	94.3%

Chevron emergency phone number:
415-233-3737

ORTHO-KLOR 44 CHLORDANE SPRAY
Ant and soil insect control
(Chevron)

Active ingred. (by wt.):

Technical Chlordane *	44%
Petroleum distillate *	51%

Chevron emergency phone number:
415-233-3737

ORTHO-KLOR 72 CHLORDANE SPRAY
Insecticide
(Chevron)

Technical Chlordane *	72.0%
Petroleum distillate *	21.0%

Chevron emergency phone number:
415-233-3737

ORTHO LAWN FUNGICIDE
(Chevron)

Pentachloronitrobenzene *	24.0%/w

Chevron emergency phone number:
415-233-3737

ORTHO LAWN INSECT SPRAY
(Chevron)

Active ingred. (by wt.):

Chlorpyrifos ((O,O-Diethyl O-3,-5,6-trichloro-2-pyridyl) phosphorothioate) *	5.3%
Aromatic petroleum derivative solvent *	3.0%
Petroleum distillate *	87.0%

Chevron emergency phone number:
415-233-3737

ORTHO LINDANE BORER & LEAF MINER SPRAY
Insecticide
(Chevron)

Lindane, gamma isomer of benzene hexachloride *	20%
Aromatic petroleum derivative solvent *	59%

Chevron emergency phone number:
415-233-3737

ORTHO LIQUID COTTON DEFOLIANT
(Chevron)

Sodium chlorate *	18%

Chevron emergency phone number:
415-233-3737

ORTHO MALATHION 50 INSECT SPRAY
(Chevron)

Active ingred. (by wt.):

Malathion	50%
Aromatic petroleum derivative solvent *	33%

Chevron emergency phone number:
415-233-3737

ORTHO MALATHION 8 SEED PROTECTANT
(Chevron)

Malathion *	81%/w

Chevron emergency phone number:
415-233-3737

ORTHO MCP 4 WEED KILLER
(Chevron)

Diethanolamine salt of 2-methyl-4-chlorophenoxy acetic acid *	52%

Chevron emergency phone number:
415-233-3737

ORTHO MOLE CRICKET BAIT
Insecticide
(Chevron)

2-(1-Methylethoxy)phenol methylcarbamate *	2%/w

Chevron emergency phone number:
415-233-3737

ORTHO MOSQUITO & FLY INSECT SPRAY
(Chevron)

Active ingred. (by wt.):

(5-Benzyl-3-furyl)methyl-2,2-di-methyl-3-(2-methylpropenyl)cyclopro-panecarboxylate	0.250%
Related compounds	0.034%
Aromatic petroleum hydrocarbons	0.331%
Petroleum distillate	6.500%

Chevron emergency phone number:
415-233-3737

Starred ingredients (*) may be responsible for major toxic effects; consult Section II.

ORTHO-NOVUM 1/35 TABLETS
Oral contraceptive
(Ortho)

Each tablet:
Norethindrone .... 1.000 mg.
Ethinyl estradiol .... 0.035 mg.

ORTHO-NOVUM 1/50 TABLETS
Oral contraceptive
(Ortho)

Each tablet:
Norethindrone 1.00%
Mestranol 0.05%

ORTHO-NOVUM 1/80 TABLETS
Oral contraceptive
(Ortho)

Each tablet:
Norethindrone .... 1.00 mg.
Mestranol .... 0.08 mg.

ORTHO-NOVUM TABLETS, 2 mg.
Oral contraceptive
(Ortho)

Each tablet:
Norethindrone .... 2.00 mg.
Mestranol .... 0.10 mg.

ORTHO OUTDOOR INSECT FOGGER
(Chevron)

Active ingred. (by wt.):
(5-Benzyl-3-furyl)methyl-2,2-di-
methyl-3-(2-
methylpropenyl)cyclopro-
panecarboxylate 0.250%
Related compounds 0.034%
2-Hydroxyethyl-n-octyl sulfide 0.950%
Related compounds 0.050%
Aromatic petroleum
hydrocarbons 0.331%
Petroleum distillate 7.000%

Chevron emergency phone number:
415-233-3737

ORTHO PARAQUAT CL
Herbicide
(Chevron)

Paraquat dichloride * 29.1%/w

Chevron emergency phone number:
415-233-3737

ORTHO PERTHANE 4 EMULSIVE
Insecticide
(Chevron)

Diethyl diphenyl dichloroethane .. 40.0%
Related compounds 5.5%
Aromatic petroleum derivative
solvent * 35.0%

Chevron emergency phone number:
415-233-3737

ORTHO PHALTAN ROSE & GARDEN FUNGICIDE
(Chevron)

Folpet 75%

Chevron emergency phone number:
415-233-3737

ORTHO PLICTRAN 50 WETTABLE
Miticide
(Chevron)

Tricyclohexyltin hydroxide * 50%/w

Chevron emergency phone number:
415-233-3737

ORTHO POISON OAK & POISON IVY KILLER
Herbicide
(Chevron)

Diethanolamine salt of 2,4-Dichlo-
rophenoxyacetic acid 0.75%
Diethanolamine salt of 2-(2-methyl-
4-chlorophenoxy)propionic acid 0.75%

Chevron emergency phone number:
415-233-3737

ORTHO PRODUCTS

Standard Oil Co. of California
Environmental Health Center
P.O. Box 1272
Richmond, CA 94802

Emergency medical consultation
concerning Chevron or Ortho products
may be obtained on a 24-hour basis from
Chevron's Poison Information Center.

Emergency phone number: 415-233-3737

ORTHO PRUNING PAINT
(Chevron)

Active ingred. (by wt.):
Asphalt solids 21%
Petroleum distillates * 23%

Chevron emergency phone number:
415-233-3737

ORTHORIX FOLIAGE SPRAY
Fungicide-miticide
(Chevron)

Calcium polysulfides * 27.5%

Chevron emergency phone number:
415-233-3737

ORTHORIX SPRAY
Fungicide
(Chevron)

Calcium polysulfides * 26%/w

Chevron emergency phone number:
415-233-3737

ORTHO ROSE & FLORAL SPRAY
Insecticide, fungicide
(Chevron)

Active ingred. (by wt.):
Carbaryl 1.000%
Folpet 0.700%
Pyrethrins 0.025%
Technical Piperonyl butoxide 0.256%
Rotenone 0.128%
Other Cube resins 0.237%
Petroleum distillate 0.025%

Chevron emergency phone number:
415-233-3737

ORTHO ROSE & FLOWER JET DUSTER
Insecticide, fungicide
(Chevron)

Carbaryl * 2.4%
Malathion 3.2%
Folpet 4.0%
1,1-Bis(p-chlorophenyl)-2,2,2-
trichloroethanol 1.2%

Chevron emergency phone number:
415-233-3737

ORTHO ROSE MILDEW CONTROL
Fungicide
(Chevron)

a,a-Bis(p-chlorophenyl)-3-pyri-
dine methanol 1.3%/w

Chevron emergency phone number:
415-233-3737

ORTHO SEPTIC SEEP
To correct soils from seepage
(Chevron)

Calcium polysulfides * 26%
Iso-octyl phenoxy polyethoxy
ethanol 10%

Chevron emergency phone number:
415-233-3737

Starred ingredients (*) may be responsible for major toxic effects; consult Section II.

ORTHO SEVIN GARDEN DUST
Insecticide for the garden; to control fleas and ticks on dogs and cats
(Chevron)

Carbaryl * 5%/w

Chevron emergency phone number:
415-233-3737

ORTHOSIL
Detergent
(Pennwalt)

Sodium orthosilicate

ORTHO SOD WEBWORM CONTROL
Insecticide
(Chevron)

Active ingred. (by wt.):
O,O,O,O-Tetrapropyl
dithiopyrophosphate 13.0%
Aromatic petroleum derivative
solvent * 81.2%

Chevron emergency phone number:
415-233-3737

ORTHO SOIL TREATER 3X WITH GRAPHITE
Fungicide
(Chevron)

Captan 30%/w
Pentachloronitrobenzene * 30%/w

Chevron emergency phone number:
415-233-3737

ORTHO SOYBEAN SEED PROTECTANT
(Chevron)

Captan 25%

Chevron emergency phone number:
415-233-3737

ORTHO SPOT WEED & GRASS KILLER
(Chevron)

Active ingred. (by wt.):
Paraquat bis (methylsulfate) *   0.44%
Aliphatic petroleum derivative
solvent * 15.00%

Chevron emergency phone number:
415-233-3737

ORTHO THIODAN 2 EMULSIVE
Insecticide
(Chevron)

Endosulfan 23.5%
Aromatic petroleum derivative
solvent * 68.5%

Chevron emergency phone number:
415-233-3737

ORTHO TOMATO BLOSSOM-FRUIT SET
(Chevron)

Beta naphthoxy acetic acid .. 0.0042%/w

Chevron emergency phone number:
415-233-3737

ORTHO TOMATO VEGETABLE DUST
Insecticide, fungicide
(Chevron)

Captan 5.00%
Methoxychlor, technical 5.00%
Rotenone from cube 0.75%
Other resins from cube 0.75%

Chevron emergency phone number:
415-233-3737

ORTHO TOMATO & VEGETABLE INSECT SPRAY
(Chevron)

Active ingred. (by wt.):
Pyrethrins 0.030%
Technical Piperonyl butoxide   0.160%
Rotenone 0.128%
Other Cube resins 0.238%
Petroleum distillate 0.120%

Chevron emergency phone number:
415-233-3737

ORTHO TOXAPHENE 6 EMULSIVE
Insecticide
(Chevron)

Toxaphene * 58%/w
Petroleum distillate 29%/w

Chevron emergency phone number:
415-233-3737

ORTHO TOXAPHENE 8 EMULSIVE
Insecticide
(Chevron)

Toxaphene * 71%
Petroleum distillate 16%

Chevron emergency phone number:
415-233-3737

ORTHO TRIFORINE EC
Fungicide
(Chevron)

Triforine (N,N'-(1,4-Piperazinediyl-
bis(2,2,2-
trichloroethylidene))bis(formamide)) 18.2%

Chevron emergency phone number:
415-233-3737

ORTHO VOLCK SUPREME-DIAZINON COMBINATION
Insecticide-miticide
(Chevron)

Petroleum oil * 92.5%/w
O,O-Diethyl O-(2-isopropyl-6-
methyl-4-pyrimidinyl)-
phosphorothioate * 4.5%/w

Chevron emergency phone number:
415-233-3737

ORTHO WEED KILLER "D"
(Chevron)

Diquat dibromide * 4.35%/w

Chevron emergency phone number:
415-233-3737

ORTHO WHEAT SEED PROTECTANT
Fungicide
(Chevron)

Captan 40%/w
Hexachlorobenzene * 40%/w

Chevron emergency phone number:
415-233-3737

ORTHO WHEAT SEED PROTECTANT FLOWABLE
Fungicide
(Chevron)

Captan 18%/w
Hexachlorobenzene * 18%/w

Chevron emergency phone number:
415-233-3737

OR-TOPTIC-M
Ophthalmic
(Ortega Pharm.)

Each cc:
Sodium sulfacetamide * ..... 100 mg.
Prednisolone acetate .... 5 mg.
Phenylephrine hydrochloride .   0.12%
Base:
Sodium borate
Boric acid *
Carboxymethylcellulose
Polysorbate 80
Sodium thiosulfate
Chlorobutanol 0.2%
Methyl paraben 0.015%
Propyl paraben 0.015%

ORVUS EXTRA GRANULAR

Procter & Gamble Co.
Ivorydale Technical Center
Cincinnati, Ohio 45217

Phone: 513-562-1100

Starred ingredients (*) may be responsible for major toxic effects; consult Section II.

ORVUS HIGH TEMP.
(Phosphate Formula or 0-Phosphate Formula)
Institutional and industrial cleaning product

Procter & Gamble Co.
Ivorydale Technical Center
Cincinnati, Ohio 45217

Phone: 513-562-1100

ORVUS K LIQUID
Institutional and industrial cleaning product

Procter & Gamble Co.
Ivorydale Technical Center
Cincinnati, Ohio 45217

Phone: 513-562-1100

ORVUS WA PASTE
Institutional and industrial cleaning product

Procter & Gamble Co.
Ivorydale Technical Center
Cincinnati, Ohio 45217

Phone: 513-562-1100

OSMOBAND
Wood preservative bandage
(Osmose Wood Preserving)

Sodium fluoride *	20.0%
Pentachlorophenol	8.9%
Other Chlorophenols and related compounds	1.1%
Creosote	15.0%

OSMOPLASTIC
Wood preserving compound
(Osmose Wood Preserving)

Sodium fluoride *	43.70%
Creosote	40.00%
Potassium bichromate *	3.10%
2,4-Dinitrophenol *	2.00%

OSPHO
Metal primer and rust treatment
(Skybryte)

Phosphoric acid *	32.00%
Wetting agent	0.50%
Sodium dichromate *	0.50%
Water	67.25%

OSTERCAL-A
Dietary supplement
(Jenkins Labs.)

Each tablet:
Calcium (from oyster shell)	750 mg.
Vitamin A	1600 Int. Units
Vitamin D	400 Int. Units

OSTI-DERM LOTION
Antiperspirant, astringent, antipruritic
(Pedinol)

Liquefied Phenol *
Glycerin
Zinc oxide
Magnesium carbonate
Aluminum acetate solution
Camphor water
Hydrated Aluminum silicate gel

O-SYL DISINFECTANT-DETERGENT
(Nat'l Labs. Div.)

o-Phenylphenol	5.00%
o-Benzyl-p-chlorophenol	4.50%
Tetrasodium ethylenediaminetetraacetate	3.04%
Isopropyl alcohol	1.50%
p-tert-Amylphenol	1.00%

OTIC DOMEBORO SOLUTION
Relief of otitis externa
(Dome)

Acetic acid	2%
Aluminum acetate solution	

OTIC NEO-CORT-DOME SUSPENSION
External otitis
(Dome)

Microdispersed Hydrocortisone alcohol	1%
Acetic acid	2%
Neomycin sulfate (equiv. 0.35% neomycin base)	0.5%
Acid pH vehicle: Oil-in-water, emulsion-type creme containing a buffered solution of aluminum acetate	

OTIC TRIDESILON SOLUTION 0.05%
Anti-inflammatory, antipruritic, vaso-constrictive
(Dome)

Desonide	0.05%
Acetic acid	2%
Purified water	
Propylene glycol	
Sodium acetate	
Citric acid	

OTOBIONE OTIC SUSPENSION
Anti-inflammatory, antibacterial
(Schering)

Each ml.:
Polymixin B sulfate	10,000 units
Hydrocortisone	10 mg.
Aqueous vehicle: Disodium edetate, Povidone, Polysorbate 80, Propylene glycol, Glycerin, Distilled water, Sulfuric acid or Sodium hydroxide to adjust pH when necessary	

OTOBIOTIC OTIC SOLUTION
Antibacterial
(Schering)

Each cc:
Neomycin sulfate (equiv. to neomycin 3.5 mg.)	5 mg.
Sodium propionate	50 mg.
Perfume vehicle: Glycerin	
Isopropanol	20%
Water	
Sodium metabisulfite	0.1%
Propionic acid (to adjust pH to 6)	

OTO C-B-A DROPS
Removal of ear wax
(Elder)

Benzalkonium chloride	0.09%
Acetic acid	2.0%
Chloroxylenol	0.12%

OTOCORT
Treatment of otitis externa
(Lemmon Co.)

Each ml.:
Neomycin (as neomycin sulfate)	3.5 mg.
Polymyxin B sulfate	2000 U.
Hydrocortisone	0.1%
Antipyrine	5%
Dibucaine hydrochloride	0.25%
Methyl and propyl parabens	
Sodium bisulfite	
Glycerin	
Purified water	

OTOMITE
Treatment of ear mites in dogs and cats
(Carson Chemicals, Inc.)

Squalane (Hexamethyltetracosane)	25.00%
Pyrethrins	0.05%
Technical Piperonyl butoxide	0.50%

OTOMYXIN LIQUID
Bacterial infections of external auditory canal
(Elder)

Neomycin (from neomycin sulfate)	3.5 mg.
Polymixin B sulfate	2000 Units
Hydrocortisone	0.1%
Antipyrine	5.0%
Dibucaine hydrochloride	0.25%

OTOREID-HC
Ear drops
(Reid-Provident)

Each cc.:
Hydrocortisone (free alcohol)	10.0 mg.
Polymixin B sulfate	10,000 units
Neomycin (as neomycin sulfate)	3.5 mg.
Propylene glycol and Glycerine	q.s.

Starred ingredients (*) may be responsible for major toxic effects; consult Section II.

O-TWO
Oxygen tablets for minnow buckets and fish
(Lake Products)

Each tablet:
Barium peroxide *	32.59%
Calcium sulfate	30.17%
Calcium phosphate	29.44%
Manganese dioxide	4.86%
Sodium sulfite	0.03%
Amorphous Carbon	2.92%

OUT
Bowl, porcelain cleaner
(Fuld-Stalfort)

Hydrogen chloride *
Dihydroabietylamine
Polyethylene glycol ether of alkylated phenol *
Perfume

'76 Ed.

OUT DAMNED SPOT
Carpet spot remover
(Paul Koss)

Water	>90%

Triethanolamine
Trisodium salt of EDTA
Sodium dodecylbenzene sulfonate (Anionic surfactant)
Fatty amido phosphate
Isopropyl alcohol

pH 9.4-9.6

OUTGRO
For ingrown nails
(Whitehall Labs.)

Each fl. oz.:
Chlorobutanol *
Tannic acid *
Isopropyl alcohol *

OVCON-35
Oral contraceptive
(Mead Johnson)

Each peach tablet:
Norethindrone	0.4 mg.
Ethinyl estradiol	0.035 mg.

Available in packages of 21 tablets, or packages of 28 tablets which include 7 green inert tablets.

OVCON-50
Oral contraceptive
(Mead Johnson)

Each yellow tablet:
Norethindrone	1.0 mg.
Ethinyl estradiol	0.05 mg.

Available in packages of 21 tablets, or packages of 28 tablets which include 7 green inert tablets.

OVEN ART
Broad line marker for "Shrink Art"
(Sanford Corp.)

Dyes
Resins
Glycol ethers
Alcohol

OVEN 'N' GRILL
See AMWAY OVEN 'N' GRILL

OVERTIME
Long acting premise insecticide
(Bio-Ceutic)

Permethrin *	10%

OVRAL TABLETS
Oral contraceptive
(Wyeth Labs.)

Each tablet:
Norgestrel	0.5 mg.
Ethinyl estradiol	0.05 mg.

OVRETTE TABLETS
Oral contraceptive
(Wyeth Labs.)

Each tablet:
Norgestrel	0.075 mg.

OVULEN
Progestogen-estrogen combination
(Searle, G.D., & Co.)

Each tablet:
Ethynodiol diacetate	1.0 mg.
Mestranol	0.1 mg.

OXINE (Liquid Concentrate)
Bacteriostat and sanitizer
(Bio-Cide)

Chlorine dioxide *	2%
Sodium carbonate	3%
De-ionized Water	95%

OXIPHEN
Cathartic
(Webcon)

Each tablet:
Sodium glycocholate	16.2 mg.
Sodium taurocholate	16.2 mg.
Phenolphthalein	32.4 mg.
Extract Cascara	32.4 mg.
Aloin	8.1 mg.

OXIPOR V.H.C.
For treatment of psoriasis
(Whitehall Labs.)

Liquor carbonis detergens *
Salicylic acid *
Benzocaine
Alcohol *

OX-LINE EXTERIOR RUBEROL HOUSE PAINT
(Lehman Bros. Corp.)

Mercury *

See Paints, Section VI, General Formulations

OXO
Rust, scale and tarnish remover; industrial and institutional use
(Scientific International)

Phosphoric acid *

OXOIDS
Autonomic regulator
(Lemmon Co.)

Each tablet:
Phenobarbital *	20 mg.
Ergotamine tartrate *	0.3 mg.
Belladonna extract (equiv. to 0.1 mg. belladonna alkaloids) *	8 mg.

OXY-5
Acne-pimple medication
(Norcliff Thayer)

Benzoyl peroxide	5%

OXY-10
Acne-pimple medication
(Norcliff Thayer)

Benzoyl peroxide	10%

OXY-10 COVER
Acne-pimple medication
(Norcliff Thayer)

Benzoyl peroxide	10%

OXYDOL (Formula 1)
Granular laundry detergent
(Procter & Gamble)

Sodium sulfate	25-49%
Complex sodium phosphates	10-24%
Sodium carbonate	10-24%
Sodium aluminosilicates	10-24%
Water	5-9%
Sodium alkyl ethoxylate sulfate	5-9%
Sodium alkyl sulfate	5-9%
Sodium alkyl benzene sulfonate	1-4%
Sodium perborate	1-4%
Sodium silicate	1-4%
Minor ingredients, each	trace

pH (1% solution) - 10.9 max.

Starred ingredients (*) may be responsible for major toxic effects; consult Section II.

OXYDOL (Formula 2)
Granular laundry detergent
(Procter & Gamble)

Sodium sulfate	25-49%
Sodium carbonate	10-24%
Sodium silicate	10-24%
Sodium alkyl benzene sulfonate	10-24%
Water	5-9%
Sodium alkyl ethoxylate sulfate	5-9%
Sodium perborate	1-4%
Minor ingredients, each	trace

pH (1% solution) - 10.9 max.

OXYDOL (Formula 3)
Granular laundry detergent
(Procter & Gamble)

Sodium sulfate	25-49%
Sodium carbonate	10-24%
Sodium silicate	10-24%
Sodium alkyl benzene sulfonate	10-24%
Water	5-9%
Sodium alkyl ethoxylate sulfate	5-9%
Sodium perborate	1-4%
Sodium alkyl sulfate	1-4%
Minor ingredients, each	trace

pH (1% solution) - 10.9 max.

OXYDOL (Formula 4)
Granular laundry detergent
(Procter & Gamble)

Sodium sulfate	25-49%
Complex sodium phosphates	10-24%
Sodium silicate	10-24%
Sodium alkyl benzene sulfonate	5-9%
Sodium alkyl sulfate	5-9%
Water	5-9%
Sodium alkyl ethoxylate sulfate	5-9%
Sodium perborate	1-4%
Minor ingredients, each	trace

pH (1% solution) - 10.5 max.

OXYDOL (Formula 5)
Granular laundry detergent
(Procter & Gamble)

Sodium sulfate	25-49%
Sodium aluminosilicate	10-24%
Sodium carbonate	10-24%
Sodium nitrilotriacetate	10-24%
Sodium alkyl sulfate	5-9%
Sodium alkyl ethoxylate sulfate	5-9%
Water	5-9%
Sodium silicate	1-4%
Sodium perborate	1-4%
Sodium alkyl benzene sulfonate	1-4%
Minor ingredients, each	trace

pH (1% solution) - 10.9 max.

OXY MONOBOR-CHLORATE
Herbicide
(Occidental Chem. Co.)

Sodium metaborate tetrahydrate *	68%
Sodium chlorate *	30%

OXY UREABOR
Herbicide
(Occidental Chem. Co.)

Sodium metaborate tetrahydrate *	66.5%
Sodium chlorate *	30.0%
Bromacil	1.5%

OXY-WASH
Medicated acne cleanser
(Norcliff Thayer)

Benzoyl peroxide	10%

OXYZAL WET DRESSING
Antiseptic
(Gordon Labs.)

Oxyquinoline sulfate *	
Benzalkonium chloride	1:2000

OZ
Industrial deodorant for air conditioning systems
(Lester Labs.)

Petroleum distillates *
Isopropyl alcohol *
Perfume

'76 Ed.

OZ EXTERIOR WHITE PRIMER
(Osmose Wood Preserving)

Active ingred.:
Bis(tri-n-butyltin)oxide	0.3%
Petroleum solvents *	57.5%

Inert ingred.:
Titanium dioxide
Others

OZ REDWOOD FINISH WOOD PRESERVER
(Osmose Wood Preserving)

Bis(tri-n-butyltin)oxide	0.3%
Petroleum distillate *	81.2%

OZ WOOD PRESERVER CLEAR
(Osmose Wood Preserving)

Bis(tri-n-butyltin)oxide	0.300%
Petroleum solvents *	94.385%

P

P-2000
Alkali cleaner
(Calgon Corp., Commercial Div.)

Caustic soda *
Wetting agents
Alkaline salts *

P-2003
Alkali cleaner
(Calgon Corp., Commercial Div.)

Caustic *
Organic sequesterant

P-3504
Solvent cleaner-stripper
(Calgon Corp., Commercial Div.)

Methylene chloride *
Cresol *
Soap
Sodium chromate *

P-3576
Solvent
(Calgon Corp., Commercial Div.)

1,1,1-Trichloroethane *

PAARLAN
Herbicide
(Elanco Prod.)

Isopropalin	68.6%

PAAS DYE TABLETS
(Plough)

Salt
Sodium bicarbonate powder
Polyethylene glycol
Talc
FD & C colors

PABAFILM
Sunscreen gel
(Owen Labs.)

Amyl dimethyl PABA	2.5%
Ethyl alcohol	70%
Isopropyl alcohol	3.5%

PABAGEL
Sunscreen gel
(Owen Labs.)

Para-aminobenzoic acid	5%
Alcohol	57%

PABALATE
Antirheumatic, antiarthritic
(Robins)

Each tablet:
Sodium salicylate, USP *	0.3 gm.
Sodium aminobenzoate	0.3 gm.
Ascorbic acid	50 mg.

PABALATE-SF
Analgesic, antirheumatic, antiarthritic
(Robins)

Each tablet:
Potassium salicylate *	0.3 gm.
Potassium aminobenzoate	0.3 gm.
Ascorbic acid	50 mg.

PABANOL LOTION
Sunburn preventative
(Elder)

Para aminobenzoic acid	5%
Alcohol, SDA 40-A *	70%

Starred ingredients (*) may be responsible for major toxic effects; consult Section II.

PABIRIN
Analgesic
(Dorsey Labs.)

Each tablet:
Aspirin * .... 300 mg.
Aminobenzoic acid .... 300 mg.
Aluminum hydroxide gel, dried 100 mg.

P-A-C COMPOUND TABLETS
Analgesic
(Upjohn)

Each tablet:
Phenacetin * .... 2 1/2 gr.
Aspirin * .... 3 1/2 gr.
Caffeine (anhydrous) .... 1/2 gr.

P-A-C COMPOUND WITH CODEINE SULFATE TABLETS
Analgesic
(Upjohn)

Each tablet:
Codeine sulfate * ..... 1/4 gr.; 1/2 gr.
Phenacetin * .... 2 1/2 gr.
Aspirin * .... 3 1/2 gr.
Caffeine (anhydrous) .... 1/2 gr.

PACE FLUORIDE TOOTHPASTE (Spearmint or Peppermint)
(Procter & Gamble, Health & Personal Care Div.)

Sodium fluoride 0.22%
Hydrated Silica 25-40%
Sorbitol 15-29%
Glycerin 15-29%
Sodium alkyl sulfate 1-6%
Minor ingredients, each 1%
Water 15-30%

PACEMAKER, MUNICHEM

See MUNICHEM PACEMAKER

PACER LATEX CAULK

See DAP PACER LATEX CAULK

PACER PANEL AND DRYWALL ADHESIVE

See DAP PACER PANEL AND DRY-WALL ADHESIVE

PACKER'S PINE TAR SHAMPOO
For dandruff and itchy scalp
(CooperCare)

Shampoo base
Propylene glycol
Isopropyl alcohol
Perfume
Pine tar *

PACKER'S PINE TAR SOAP
Toilet soap with pine tar
(CooperCare)

Soap
Natural Pine tar *

PAC LOTION
Soap for industrial and office use
(Calgon Corp., Commercial Div.)

Soap
Triclosan
Water

PACO SOLVENT TR 590 FORMULA NO. 2
Fuel, metal cleaner, shellac thinner
(Publicker)

S.D.A No. 1 (20 parts ethyl alcohol, 0.8 part C.P. methanol, &
0.2 part methyl isobutyl
ketone) * .... 100 gal.
Methyl isobutyl ketone .... 1 gal.
Ethyl acetate .... 1 gal.
Gasoline .... 1 gal.

'76 Ed.

PACO SOLVENT TR 590 FORMULA NO. 4
Fuel, metal cleaner, shellac thinner
(Publicker)

S.D.A. No. 1 (20 parts ethyl alcohol, 0.8 part C.P. methanol, &
0.2 part methyl isobutyl
ketone) * .... 100 gal.
Ethyl acetate .... 5 gal.
Gasoline (aviation grade) ...... 1 gal.

'76 Ed.

PACO SOLVENT TR 590 FORMULA NO. 5
Fuel, metal cleaner, shellac thinner
(Publicker)

S.D.A. No. 1 (20 parts ethyl alcohol, 0.8 part C.P. methanol, &
0.2 part methyl isobutyl
ketone) * .... 100 gal.
Ethyl acetate .... 1 gal.
Methyl isobutyl ketone .... 1 gal.
Stoddard solvent .... 1 gal.

'76 Ed.

PACO SOLVENT TR 590 FORMULA NO. 6
(Publicker)

S.D.A. No. 1 (20 parts ethyl alcohol, 0.8 part C.P. methanol, &
0.2 part methyl isobutyl
ketone) * .... 100 gal.
Methyl isobutyl ketone .... 5 gal.
Stoddard solvent .... 1 gal.

'76 Ed.

PACO SOLVENT TR 600
(Publicker)

S.D.A. No. 1 (20 parts ethyl alcohol, 0.8 part C.P. methanol, &
0.2 part methyl isobutyl
ketone) * .... 100 gal.
Isopropyl alcohol (99%) * ...... 10 gal.
Methyl isobutyl ketone .... 1 gal.

'76 Ed.

PACO SOLVENT TR 601
For Rotogravure printing operations
(Publicker)

S.D.A. No. 1 (20 parts ethyl alcohol, 0.8 part C.P. methanol, &
0.2 part methyl isobutyl
ketone) * .... 100 gal.
Isopropyl alcohol (99%) .... 5 gal.
Methanol .... 5 gal.
Methyl isobutyl ketone .... 1 gal.

'76 Ed.

PACQUIN EXTRA DRY SKIN HAND CREAM
(Pacquin Div.)

Stearic acid
Cetyl alcohol
Glycerine
Emollient base

PACQUIN MEDICATED HAND CREAM
(Pacquin Div.)

Stearic acid
Orthophenyl phenol
Emollient base

PACQUIN SKIN CREAM WITH ALOE
(Pacquin Div.)

Aloe juice
Isopropyl palmitate
Mineral oil
Petrolatum
Synthetic beeswax
Cetyl alcohol
Dimethicone
Triethanolamine stearate
Glyceryl stearate

PACRITE APPLE WAX WITH THIABENDAZOLE
Fungicide; apple coating
(American Machinery Corp.)

Active ingred.: 0.1%
Thiabendazole
Inert ingred.: 99.9%
Soybean protein
Shellac
Wood rosin
Oleic acid
Water

PAD KOTE
Astringent, external; veterinary
(Happy Jack)

Cod liver oil
Juniper tar
Balsam Peru *
Tannic acid *
Turpentine .... <2%
Gentian violet *
Brilliant green
Phenol .... <1%
Alcohol isopropyl * 60%

PADLOCK SEALER

See AIRWICK PROFESSIONAL
PRODUCTS PADLOCK SEALER

PAGEANT
Liquid dishwashing detergent
(Diversey Wyandotte)

Synthetic detergents

PAINT-OFF B160
(Beck Chem.)

Methylene chloride * .... >50%
Isopropyl alcohol .... <10%

PAINT-OFF BRUSH TYPE PAINT & VARNISH REMOVER
(Beck Chem.)

Mixed amines .... <10%
Methylene chloride * .... >50%

PALADIS
Disinfectant-sanitizer-deodorizer-concentrate
(Basic Chemicals Inc.)

n-Alkyl (68% C12, 32% C14) dimethyl
ethylbenzyl ammonium
chloride * 5.0%
n-Alkyl (60% C14, 30% C16, 5% C12,
5% C18) dimethyl benzyl ammonium chloride * 5.0%

PALCO DAIRY AND BEEF CATTLE INSECTICIDE OIL
Face rubber and back rubber
(Palco, Inc.)

Dimethyl phosphate of alpha-
methylbenzyl 3-hydroxy-cis-
crotonate * 1.00%
Petroleum hydrocarbons * 99.00%

PALGARD METAL PRIMER
(Pratt & Lambert)

May contain more than 1% Lead *

PALL MALL SOAP
(Hewitt)

Tallow
Coconut oil
Sodium hydroxide

'76 Ed.

PALM BEACH COSMETICS

Palm Beach Beauty Products Co.
950 Xenia Ave. S.
Minneapolis, Minn. 55416

Phone: 612-546-0322

See COSMETICS, Section VI, General
Formulations

PALMOLIVE BRUSHLESS SHAVE CREAM
(Colgate-Palmolive)

Mineral oil
Stearic acid
Olive oil
Propylene glycol
Triethanolamine
Water
Perfume and preservative

'76 Ed.

PALMOLIVE CRYSTAL CLEAR
Granular dishwasher detergent
(Colgate-Palmolive)

Sodium tripolyphosphate
6H2O * .... approx. 30%
Silicated sodium
carbonate * .... approx. 15%
Sodium sulfate .... approx. 15%
Boric acid * .... approx. 2%
Sodium chloride .... approx. 10%
Sodium metasilicate .... <10%
Perfume, dye, chlorinated oxidant, moisture and conditioning agent

'76 Ed.

PALMOLIVE DISHWASHING LIQUID
Light-duty liquid detergent
(Colgate-Palmolive)

Combined amount: .... approx. 35%
Ethoxylated alcohol sulfate *†
Alkylaryl sulfonate *
Plus conventional organic foam builders
and stabilizers
Ethyl alcohol 6%
Water .... approx. 50%

†*See* Alcohol sulfate salts

'76 Ed.

PALMOLIVE LATHER SHAVING CREAM
(Colgate-Palmolive)

Super-fatted soap
Water
Glycerine
Preservative
Perfume and color

'76 Ed.

PALMOLIVE RAPID SHAVE
(Colgate-Palmolive)

Super-fatted soap
Fatty-acid diethanolamine condensate
Glycerine
Water
Perfume
Propellant gas

'76 Ed.

PALMOLIVE TOILET SOAP
(Colgate-Palmolive)

Soap
Perfume and color
Moisture

'76 Ed.

PALS SUPPLEMENTAL VITAMINS
(Bristol-Myers)

Vitamin A .... 3500 USP units
Vitamin D .... 400 USP units
Plus multivitamins

PALS SUPPLEMENTAL VITAMINS PLUS IRON
(Bristol-Myers)

Vitamin A .... 3500 USP units
Vitamin D .... 400 USP units
Iron (Ferrous fumarate) .... 12 mg.

PAM (Aerosol)
No-stick spray for cooking surfaces
(Boyle-Midway)

Lecithin of pure vegetable origin
Hydrogenated vegetable oil
Ethyl alcohol
Hydrocarbon propellant

PAM (Pump)
No-stick spray for cooking surfaces
(Boyle-Midway)

Lecithin of pure vegetable origin
Hydrogenated vegetable oil
Ethyl alcohol

PAMELOR (CAPSULES AND SOLUTION)
Antidepressant
(Sandoz)

Each capsule:
Nortriptyline hydrochloride USP * .... 10 mg.; 25 mg.

Solution (each 5 ml.):
Nortriptyline hydrochloride
USP * .... 10 mg.

PAMINE TABLETS
Antispasmodic
(Upjohn)

Each tablet:
Methscopolamine bromide * . 2.5 mg.

Starred ingredients (*) may be responsible for major toxic effects; consult Section II.

PANAFIL OINTMENT
For enzymatic debridement of wounds,
ulcers, burns
(Rystan)

Papain powder 10%
Urea USP 10%
Water-soluble Chlorophyll 0.5%
Hydrophilic base

PANALGESIC
Analgesic/counterirritant - topical
(Poythress, Wm. P.)

Salicylates * 58%
Aspirin
Menthyl salicylate
Combined amount: 4%
Camphor
Menthol
Emollient oils 20%
Alcohol (by volume 22%) 18%/w
Green dye

PANALGESIC
Analgesic
(Wesley Pharm.)

Each tablet:
Acetaminophen * .... 300 mg.

PAN-DERMA MEDICATED SKIN LOTION AND OINTMENT
(Pan Derma)

Ethyl aminobenzoate (Benzocaine)
Phenol *
Menthol *
Camphor *
Zinc tannate

PANEL NU (AEROSOL)

See DAP PANEL NU (AEROSOL)

PANEL-TITE ADHESIVE

See LEECH PANEL-TITE ADHE-
SIVE

PANELWOOD 6039

See WELDWOOD PANELWOOD 6039

PANITOL
Tension headaches
(Wesley Pharm.)

Each tablet:
Butalbital .... 15 mg.
Panitone (Wesley brand of
Acetaminophen) * .... 325 mg.

PANITONE "500"
Analgesic
(Wesley Pharm.)

Each tablet:
Acetaminophen * .... 500 mg.

PANIVON
Analgesic
(Wesley Pharm.)

Each capsule:
Propoxyphene
hydrochloride * .... 65 mg.
Aspirin .... 227 mg.
Phenacetin .... 162 mg.
Caffeine .... 32.4 mg.

PANOL
Rubefacient
(Watkins Products, Inc.)

Alcohol 62%
Oil wintergreen *
Oil clove *
Menthol *
Camphor *
Oil peppermint *
Oil eucalyptus *
Safrol *

PANOXYL (5 & 10) GEL
Acne treatment
(Stiefel Labs.)

Benzoyl peroxide .... 5% or 10%
Polyoxyethylene lauryl ether 6%
Ethyl alcohol 40%
In a gel base of:
Colloidal Magnesium aluminum silicate
Hydroxypropylmethylcellulose
Citric acid
Purified water

PANSCOL LOTION
Treatment of dermatitis
(Baker-Cummins)

Salicylic acid * 3%
Lactic acid * 2%
Phenol .... <1%
Emollients

PANSCOL OINTMENT
Treatment of dermatitis
(Baker-Cummins)

Salicylic acid * 3%
Lactic acid * 2%
Phenol .... <1%

PANTEK II
Disinfectant for equipment and poultry
and livestock buildings
(Whitmoyer)

Cresylic acid * 50%
Soap emulsifier 38%

PANTENE COSMETIC PRODUCTS
Hair care preparations & toiletries

Pantene Co.
340 Kingsland Ave.
Nutley, N.J. 07110

Phone: 201-235-4133

See COSMETICS, Section VI, General
Formulations

PANTHER RINSE
Wash additive
(Edwal)

Sodium sulfite *
Ammonium sulfite
EDTA (Versene)
Citric acid
Ethylene glycol
Isopropyl alcohol

PAN ULTRA STICK
Sun protective
(Baker-Cummins)

Benzophenone (oil soluble)
Moisturizers
Lipids

PAN ULTRA SUN LOTION
(Baker-Cummins)

Benzophenone (water soluble)
Moisturizers
Lipids

PANWARFIN TABLETS
Prothrombin depressant
(Abbott)

Each tablet:
Warfarin sodium *
Lavender .... 2 mg.
Orange .... 2 1/2 mg.
Peach .... 5 mg.
Yellow .... 7 1/2 mg.
White .... 10 mg.

P.A.P. NO. 1
Sedative and anodyne
(Jenkins Labs.)

Each tablet:
Phenobarbital .... 1/4 gr.
Acetophenetidin * .... 2 1/2 gr.
Acetylsalicylic acid * .... 3 1/2 gr.

PAPACON
For the relief of cerebral and peripheral
ischemia
(CMC Research Div.)

Each timed release capsule:
Papaverine hydrochloride,
N.F. * .... 150 mg.

PAPER MATE PENS & REFILLS
(Gillette Co., Paper Mate Div.)

The Gillette Co., Paper Mate Div.,
Boston, Mass. 02199, will receive collect
phone calls from poison control centers or
physicians asking for emergency toxicological information about the company's
products.

Phone: 617-421-7000

Starred ingredients (*) may be responsible for major toxic effects; consult Section II.

PAP-KAPS-150
Relief of cerebral and peripheral ischemia
(Sutliff & Case)

Each Meta-Kap:
Papaverine hydrochloride * ... 150 mg.

'76 Ed.

PARA BAN INSECTICIDE FOGGER
(Haver-Lockhart (Brand) Bayvet Div. Cutter Labs.)

2,2-Dichlorovinyl dimethyl
phosphate 0.47%

PARA BOMB-M-1
Insecticide and repellent for use on dogs and cats
(Haver-Lockhart (Brand) Bayvet Div. Cutter Labs.)

Pyrethrins 0.06%
Piperonyl butoxide (technical) .. 0.48%
Malathion 0.50%
2,3:4,5-Bis(2-butylene)tetrahydro-
2-furaldehyde 0.24%
Petroleum distillate * 23.67%

PARACIDE CAPSULES NO. 1
Anthelmintic; small animals
(Norden Labs.)

Each capsule:
2,2'-Methylenebis(4-
chlorophenol) .... 125 mg.
Toluene * .... 150 mg.

PARACIDE CAPSULES NO. 2 1/2
Anthelmintic; small animals
(Norden Labs.)

Each capsule:
2,2'-Methylenebis(4-
chlorophenol) .... 250 mg.
Toluene * .... 300 mg.

PARACIDE CAPSULES NO. 5
Anthelmintic; small animals
(Norden Labs.)

Each capsule:
2,2'-Methylenebis(4-
chlorophenol) .... 500 mg.
Toluene * .... 600 mg.

PARACIDE CAPSULES NO. 10
Anthelmintic; small animals
(Norden Labs.)

Each capsule:
2,2'-Methylenebis(4-
chlorophenol) .... 1.0 gm.
Toluene * .... 1.2 gm.

PARACIDE CAPSULES NO. 25
Anthelmintic; small animals
(Norden Labs.)

Each capsule:
2,2'-Methylenebis(4-
chlorophenol) .... 2.5 gm.
Toluene * .... 3.0 gm.

PARACIDE CAPSULES NO. 40
Anthelmintic; small animals
(Norden Labs.)

Each capsule:
2,2'-Methylenebis(4-
chlorophenol) .... 4.0 gm.
Toluene * .... 4.8 gm.

PARADE DETERGENT (POWDER)
(Safeway Stores)

Alkyl aryl sodium sulfonate * ... 18%
Sodium tripolyphosphate * 25%
Sodium silicate 10%
Sodium sulfate 36%
Combined amount: 1%
Carboxymethyl cellulose
Optical brighteners
Perfume
Moisture 9%
Sodium carbonate 2%

PARA-DI MOTH CRYSTALS

See PATTERSON'S PARA-DI MOTH CRYSTALS

PARA DIP
Pesticidal dip for dogs
(Haver-Lockhart (Brand) Bayvet Div. Cutter Labs.)

Carbaryl 8.0%
Gamma isomer of benzene hexa-
chloride (from lindane) 3.9%
Captan 1.0%
Aromatic solvents * 65.0%

PARADOW
Insecticide; deodorant block
(Dow)

Paradichlorobenzene *

PARADUST
Kills ticks, fleas and lice on dogs and cats
(Hart-Delta, Inc.)

Carbaryl (1-Naphthyl N-methylcarbamate) *
2,2-Methylenebis(4-chlorophenol) (Dichlorophene)
Aluminum chlorohydroxy allantoinate
Inert ingred.:
Pyrophyllite 94.3%

'76 Ed.

PARAGON PAINT PRODUCTS
Paints & varnishes

Paragon Paint & Varnish Corp.
5-49 46th Ave.
Long Island City, N.Y. 11101

Phone: 212-729-7420

See PAINTS, Section VI, General Formulations

PARA-JEL
Teething, toothache jel
(Approved Pharm.)

Combined amount: 5%
Benzocaine
Cetyl dimethyl benzyl ammonium chloride *

'76 Ed.

PARA NUGGETS & CRYSTALS
Insecticide
(Uncle Sam)

Paradichlorobenzene * 100%

PARA POWDER
For use on dogs or cats - kills ticks, fleas and lice
(Haver-Lockhart (Brand) Bayvet Div. Cutter Labs.)

Carbaryl * 5%

PARA-S-1 AEROSOL
Insecticide and repellent for use on dogs and cats
(Haver-Lockhart (Brand) Bayvet Div. Cutter Labs.)

Pyrethrins 0.06%
Piperonyl butoxide (technical) .. 0.48%
Methoxychlor (technical) 0.50%
Carbaryl 0.50%
2,3:4,5-Bis(2-butylene)tetrahydro-
2-furaldehyde 0.24%
Petroleum distillate * 22.84%

PARA-TOX
Treatment of body lice
(DePree)

Pyrethrum
Piperonyl butoxide

PARCO COLD CLEANER 450
Various industrial uses
(Parker Div.)

Solution containing:
Sulfuric acid * 30%

PARCOLENE 1, 2A, 3, 8A, and 10
Various industrial uses
(Parker Div.)

Solutions containing:
Chromic acid *

Starred ingredients (*) may be responsible for major toxic effects; consult Section II.

PAR DETERGENT POWDER
(Safeway Stores)

Linear alkyl aryl sulfonate *	20%
Sodium carbonate *	32%
Sodium sulfate	30%
Sodium silicate	12%
Combined amount:	1%
Carboxymethylcellulose	
Optical brightener	
Perfume	
Water	5%

PAREPECTOLIN
Symptomatic relief of diarrhea
(Rorer, W.H., Inc.)

Each fluid oz.:
Paregoric (equivalent) *	3.7 ml.
Contains opium 15 mg./fl. oz.	
Pectin	162 mg.
Kaolin (specially purified)	5.5 gm.
Alcohol	0.69%

PAR FABRIC SOFTENER
(Safeway Stores)

Ditallow dialkyl ammonium methosulfate	4%
Isopropyl alcohol	1%
Other: Nonionic surfactant, Perfume, Dye	1%
Water	balance

pH, undiluted 5

PARID BOMB
Repellent, antiseptic & local anesthetic; veterinary
(Carson Chemicals, Inc.)

Sevin *	2.5%
Pyrethrins	0.06%
Piperonyl butoxide	0.6%
Butoxypolypropylene glycol	5%

PARKE-DAVIS ASPIRIN COMPOUND TABLETS
Analgesic
(Parke-Davis)

Each tablet:
Aspirin *	3 1/2 gr.
Phenacetin *	2 1/2 gr.
Caffeine	1/2 gr.

PARKE-DAVIS ASPIRIN COMPOUND WITH CODEINE PHOSPHATE TABLETS NO. 2 AND NO. 3
(Parke-Davis)

Each No. 2 tablet:
Codeine phosphate *	1/4 gr.
Aspirin *	3 1/2 gr.
Phenacetin *	2 1/2 gr.
Caffeine	1/2 gr.

Each No. 3 tablet:
Codeine phosphate *	1/2 gr.
Aspirin *	3 1/2 gr.
Phenacetin *	2 1/2 gr.
Caffeine	1/2 gr.

PARKE-DAVIS MENTHOLATED EXPECTORANT
(Parke-Davis)

Each fluid oz.:
Chloroform	2 gr.
Wild cherry	24 gr.
Marrubium	8 gr.
Inula	8 gr.
Poplar bud	4 gr.
Sanguinaria	3 gr.
Menthol	q.s.
Honey	q.s.
Rectified Tar oil	q.s.

PARKER ACCELERATOR 130
Various industrial uses
(Parker Div.)

Sodium nitrite *

PARKER ACCELERATOR 131
Various industrial uses
(Parker Div.)

Sodium nitrite (40% solution) *

PARKER ACCELERATOR 170
Various industrial uses
(Parker Div.)

Sodium bifluoride *

PARKER NEUTRALIZER 1
Various industrial uses
(Parker Div.)

Sodium bisulfite *

PARKER PERMANENT SUPER QUINK
Inks - Blue, Blue-black, Black
(Parker Pen)

Dyes
Iron salts
Organic acids

PARKER PERMANENT SUPER QUINK
Inks - Turquoise, green
(Parker Pen)

Dyes
Chelated copper
Organic acids

PARKER PERMANENT SUPER QUINK RED INK
(Parker Pen)

Dyes
Chelated chromium
Organic acids

PARKER'S LEMON OIL
Polish
(Parker, C.W., Co.)

D & C Yellow	1%
American White Oil 10 NF (Mineral oil)	99.5%
Lemon Bouquet #5265	<1%

PARKER'S PERFECT POLISH
(Parker, C.W., Co.)

Antimony trichloride solution *　1-10%

PARKER WASHABLE SUPER QUINK
Inks
(Parker Pen)

Dyes
Organic acids

PARKO ANTI-STATIC PLASTIC POLISH
(Park Chem.)

Paraformaldehyde *
Wax
Mineral oil
Wetting agent
Diatomaceous earth
Water

PARKO FABRIC CLEANER
(Park Chem.)

Aromatic hydrocarbons *
Chlorinated hydrocarbons *

PARKO FAST CUT (HAND RUBBING COMPOUND)
(Park Chem.)

Kerosene *
Soap
Pine oil *
Abrasives

PARKO FAST CUT (WHEEL POLISHING COMPOUND)
(Park Chem.)

Kerosene *
Sulfonated oil *
Abrasives

PARKO FINISH RUB
Synthetic enamel repair
(Park Chem.)

Kerosene *
Soap
Pine oil *
Abrasives

Starred ingredients (*) may be responsible for major toxic effects; consult Section II.

PARKO GLOSS POLISH AND CLEANER AND LIQUID POLISHES
(Park Chem.)

Alcohol
Glycerine
Mineral oil
Wetting agents
Diatomaceous earth
Water

PARKO PENETRATING OIL
(Park Chem.)

Aromatic solvents *

PARKO POLISHING PASTE
(Park Chem.)

Kerosene *

PARKO TAR, SILICONE & WAX REMOVER
(Park Chem.)

Petroleum solvent *

PARKO WINDSHIELD WASHER SOLUTION
(Park Chem.)

Methanol *

PARK'S PASTE WAX
(Park Chem.)

Silicone
Wax
Mineral spirits *
Diatomaceous earth
Pigments

PAR LIQUID DETERGENT
(Safeway Stores)

Alkyl aryl sodium sulfonate *	25%
C12-14 Alcohol ethoxy sulfate (NH4)	3%
Ethoxylated C12-14 alcohol	3%
Sodium xylene sulfonate urea	4%
Water	balance

PARMETOL D
Antimicrobial for metalworking fluids
(U.S. Professional Labs.)

2,2-Dibromo-3-nitrilopropionamide *	20%

PARNON (LIQUID CONCENTRATE)
Fungicide for roses, zinnias, apple trees and grapevines
(Elanco Prod.)

a,a-Bis(p-chlorophenyl)-3-pyridine-methanol (Parnon)	4.0%

PARSONS' ABRASIVE CLEANSER (Institutional)
(Armour-Dial, Inc.)

Silica flour	75-100%
NaLAS (active)	1-5%
Na2CO3 (Sodium carbonate)	5-10%
Potassium dichloro-iso-cyanurate	0.1-1%
Minor ingredients (total)	0.1-1%

PARSONS' ACRYLIC FOR WOOD
(Armour-Dial, Inc.)

Rule 66 Mineral spirits *	75-100%
Neocryl B-705	5-10%
Piccotex 120	1-5%
Minor ingredients (total)	0.1-1%

PARSONS' ALL PURPOSE CLEANER (Institutional)
(Armour-Dial, Inc.)

Water	75-100%
Alkyl aryl sulfonic acid	1-5%
Triton X-100	1-5%
Marsamide #10	1-5%
Sodium hydroxide	0.1-1%
Minor ingredients (total)	1-5%

PARSONS' AMMONIA - Clear, Lemon, Pine, and Sudsy
(Armour-Dial, Inc.)

Water	75-100%
Ammonia *	1-5%
Nonionic active (Clear, Lemon, Sudsy only)	0.1-5%
Anionic active (Pine, Sudsy, Lemon only)	1-5%
Minor ingredients (total)	0.1-1%

PARSONS' BOWL CLEANER (Institutional)
(Armour-Dial, Inc.)

Water	75-100%
Hydrochloric acid *	10-25%
Nonionic surfactant	1-5%
Minor ingredients (total)	1-5%

PARSONS' GLASS AND WINDOW CLEANER (Institutional)
(Armour-Dial, Inc.)

Water	75-100%
Dipropylene glycol methyl ether	1-5%
Isopropyl alcohol	1-5%
Methyl alcohol	1-5%
Nonionic surfactant	0.1-1%
Minor ingredients (total)	0.01-0.1%

PARSONS' LIQUID SOAP 40% - Green and Natural
(Armour-Dial, Inc.)

Moisture and volatile	50-75%
Potash soap *	25-50%
Glycerin	1-5%
Minor ingredients (total)	0.1-1%

PARSONS' RUG SHAMPOO (Institutional)
(Armour-Dial, Inc.)

Water	75-100%
Sodium lauryl sulfate	5-10%
Sulfonates	5-10%
Ammonia	0.1-1%
Minor ingredients (total)	1-5%

PART-EASE
Loosener & lubricant
(American Grease Stick)
(Marketed by: Balkamp, Inc.)

Colloidal Graphite dispersion in aliphatic naphtha	5.0%
Oxygenated organic acids	20.0%
Naphtha (aliphatic) *	64.5%
Tricresyl phosphate (synthetic base) *	10.0%
Nonylphenoxy acetic acid	0.5%

PARTIAL ECLIPSE SUNTAN LOTION
(Herbert Labs.)

Padimate O (Octyl dimethyl PABA)

PARTSITE

See ALSOL PARTSITE

PASIBAR
Analgesic
(Jenkins Labs.)

Each tablet:	
Acetylsalicylic acid *	3 1/2 gr.
Acetophenetidin *	2 1/2 gr.
Caffeine alkaloid	1/4 gr.
Phenobarbital	1/4 gr.

PASSIV-8, FORMULA PL-8

See KLENZADE PASSIV-8, FORMULA PL-8

PASTELLO COLORED DUSTLESS CHALK
(American Crayon Co.)

This product bears the CP Seal issued by the Crayon, Water Color and Craft Institute, Inc. This seal certifies that the product contains no materials in sufficient quantities to be toxic or injurious to the human body even if ingested.

PATCH A TATCH

See DUNCAN CERAMICS SPECIALTY PRODUCT PATCH A TATCH (SY 545)

PATCH-IT

See DUNCAN CERAMICS PATCH-IT (PA 501)

Starred ingredients (*) may be responsible for major toxic effects; consult Section II.

PATERSON ACUCOLOR 2 BLEACH FIX: PART A
(Braun North America)

Acetic acid 2%

PATERSON ACUCOLOR 3 BLEACH FIX: PART A
(Braun North America)

Ammonium thiocyanate * .... <10%

PATERSON ACUCOLOR 2 BLEACH FIX: PART B
(Braun North America)

Acetic acid 3.5%

PATERSON ACUCOLOR 3 BLEACH FIX: PART B
(Braun North America)

Sodium bisulfite .... <2%

PATERSON ACUCOLOR 3 DEVELOPER: PART A
(Braun North America)

Triethylene glycol .... <35%

PATERSON ACUCOLOR 2 DEVELOPER: PART B
(Braun North America)

Sodium bisulfite .... <1%

PATERSON ACUCOLOR 3 DEVELOPER: PART B
(Braun North America)

Diethylene glycol .... <5%

PATERSON ACUCOLOR 3 STABILIZER
(Braun North America)

Acetic acid 1.0%

PATH-O-CIDE
Hospital disinfectant, cleaner
(Weil Chem.)

Active ingred.: 8.5%
  Methyl dodecyl benzyl trimethyl ammonium chloride *
  Methyl dodecyl xylylene bis (trimethyl ammonium chloride) *
  Trisodium phosphate
  Sodium metasilicate
  Sodium carbonate
Inert ingred.: 91.5%
  Water
  Nonyl phenyl polyethylene glycol ether
  Sodium hexametaphosphate *
  Tetrapotassium pyrophosphate *

PATIOLIFE 8009

See WELDWOOD PATIOLIFE 8009

PATTERSON'S AEROSOL INSECT KILLER
(Patterson Chem.)

2,2-Dichlorovinyl dimethyl
  phosphate 0.46%
Related compounds 0.04%
Petroleum hydrocarbons * 14.50%

'76 Ed.

PATTERSON'S ALGAECIDE
(Patterson Chem.)

Di-isobutyl phenoxy ethoxy ethyl
dimethyl benzyl ammonium
chloride * 10.0%

'76 Ed.

PATTERSON'S BAG WORM SPRAY
Insecticide
(Patterson Chem.)

Toxaphene * 40%
Malathion 18%
Aliphatic petroleum hydrocarbons . 22%
Aromatic petroleum hydrocarbons * 13%

'76 Ed.

PATTERSON'S BHC EMULSION CONCENTRATE
Insecticide
(Patterson Chem.)

Gamma isomer of benzene
  hexachloride * 11%
Other isomers of benzene
  hexachloride 16%
Petroleum solvent * 66%

'76 Ed.

PATTERSON'S CAPTAN GARDEN SPRAY
Fungicide
(Patterson Chem.)

Captan 50%

'76 Ed.

PATTERSON'S CATTLE GRUB CONTROL DUST
Insecticide
(Patterson Chem.)

Rotenone * 1.5%
Other cube resins 2.5%

'76 Ed.

PATTERSON'S CHICKWEED KILLER
Herbicide
(Patterson Chem.)

2-Ethyl hexyl ester of silvex (2(2,4,5-
trichlorphenoxy) propionic
acid) * 13.3%

'76 Ed.

PATTERSON'S 20% CHLORDANE CONCENTRATE
Insecticide
(Patterson Chem.)

Chlordane, tech. * 20%
Petroleum distillate * 80%

'76 Ed.

PATTERSON'S 45% CHLORDANE EMULSIFIABLE CONCENTRATE
Insecticide
(Patterson Chem.)

Chlordane, tech. * 45%
Aliphatic petroleum hydrocarbons * 50%

'76 Ed.

PATTERSON'S CORN EARWORM DROPS
Insecticide
(Patterson Chem.)

Pyrethrins 0.1%
Technical Piperonyl butoxide 0.8%

'76 Ed.

PATTERSON'S CREOSOTE DIP & DISINFECTANT
(Patterson Chem.)

Coal tar neutral oils * 55.1%
Soap 23.9%
Phenols * 11.0%

'76 Ed.

PATTERSON'S DAIRY BACKRUBBER CONCENTRATE
Insecticide
(Patterson Chem.)

Methylated naphthalenes *
Butoxy polypropylene glycol *
Methoxychlor, tech. *

'76 Ed.

PATTERSON'S DAIRY CATTLE DUST
Insecticide
(Patterson Chem.)

Methoxychlor, tech. 5%

'76 Ed.

Starred ingredients (*) may be responsible for major toxic effects; consult Section II.

PATTERSON'S 2,4-D AMINE WEED KILLER
Herbicide
(Patterson Chem.)

Dimethylamine salt of 2,4-dichlorophenoxyacetic acid * 50.4%

'76 Ed.

PATTERSON'S DORMANT SPRAY OIL
(Patterson Chem.)

Petroleum oil * 99.0%

'76 Ed.

PATTERSON'S FACE FLY SPRAY
Insecticide
(Patterson Chem.)

Pyrethrins	0.075%
Piperonyl butoxide, technical	0.600%
Butoxypolypropylene glycol	5.300%
Mineral oil *	93.875%

'76 Ed.

PATTERSON'S FOGGING CONCENTRATE PYRENONE TYPE
Insecticide
(Patterson Chem.)

Pyrethrins	0.30%
Piperonyl butoxide, tech.	1.50%
Deodorized petroleum oil *	98.20%

'76 Ed.

PATTERSON'S GARDEN DUST
Insecticide-fungicide
(Patterson Chem.)

Zineb	3.9%
Captan	2.5%
Carbaryl (1-Naphthyl-N methyl carbamate) *	2.0%
Rotenone	1.0%
Other cube extractives	1.6%

'76 Ed.

PATTERSON'S GARDEN WEED PREVENTER
(Patterson Chem.)

Dimethyl tetrachloroterephthalate (Dacthal) 2.5%

'76 Ed.

PATTERSON'S GENERAL WEED KILLER
(Patterson Chem.)

Sodium arsenite (arsenic as metallic 23.1%) * 40%

'76 Ed.

PATTERSON'S GRAIN FUMIGANT NO. 925
(Patterson Chem.)

Ethylene dichloride	68.5%
Carbon tetrachloride *	29.0%
Sulphur dioxide	2.5%

'76 Ed.

PATTERSON'S GREENHOUSE SPRAY
Insecticide
(Patterson Chem.)

Xylene range aromatic petroleum distillate *
Methoxychlor, tech. *
Malathion *
1,1-Bis-(p-chlorophenyl)-2,2,2-trichloroethanol *
N-Trichloro-methylthiophthalimide
Sodium dodecyl benzene sulfonate
Iso-octylphenoxypolyethoxyethanol
Petroleum distillate *
Tributyltin chloride complex of polyethylene oxide with abietylamine

'76 Ed.

PATTERSON'S HI-TEST BUTYL ESTER 2,4-D WEED KILLER
(Patterson Chem.)

Butyl ester of 2,4-dichlorophenoxyacetic acid (2,4-D equiv. 46%) * 57.4%

'76 Ed.

PATTERSON'S HOG OIL
Insecticide
(Patterson Chem.)

Petroleum oils *	92.8%
Pine tar oils *	1.7%
Sulphurized oil	5.5%

'76 Ed.

PATTERSON'S HOUSEHOLD INSECTICIDE
(Patterson Chem.)

O,O-Diethyl O-(2-isopropyl-6-methyl-4-pyrimidinyl) phosphorothioate	0.50%
Pyrethrins	0.05%
Piperonyl butoxide, tech.	0.25%
Petroleum solvent *	99.20%

'76 Ed.

PATTERSON'S IRON SULPHATE (Copperas)
(Patterson Chem.)

Iron, as ferrous *	20%
Sulphur	11%

'76 Ed.

PATTERSON'S KELTHANE EMULSIFIABLE CONCENTRATE
Insecticide
(Patterson Chem.)

Kelthane	18.5%
Xylene *	70.0%

'76 Ed.

PATTERSON'S LAWN WEED KILLER
(Patterson Chem.)

2,4,5-Trichlorophenoxyacetic acid, iso-octyl ester	4.4%
2,4-Dichlorophenoxyacetic acid, iso-octyl ester *	9.3%

'76 Ed.

PATTERSON'S 5% LINDANE SPRAY
Insecticide
(Patterson Chem.)

Gamma isomer of benzene hexachloride from lindane	5%
Xylol *	88%

'76 Ed.

PATTERSON'S LINDANE SPRAY CONCENTRATE
(Patterson Chem.)

Gamma isomer of benzene hexachloride from lindane *	12.5%
Aromatic petroleum derivative solvent *	82.5%

'76 Ed.

PATTERSON'S LIQUID CRABGRASS & CHICKWEED KILLER
Herbicide
(Patterson Chem.)

Disodium methyl arsonate (anhydrous) * 12.6%

'76 Ed.

PATTERSON'S LIVESTOCK FLY SPRAY
(Patterson Chem.)

Petroleum distillate *	97.75%
beta-Butoxy-beta'-thiocyano diethyl ether *	2.25%

'76 Ed.

PATTERSON'S LIVESTOCK FLY SPRAY WITH CRAG FLY REPELLENT
(Patterson Chem.)

Butoxypolypropylene glycol	6.09%
beta-Butoxy-beta'-thiocyano diethyl ether	0.60%
Methoxychlor, tech.	1.00%
Methylated naphthalenes	1.18%
Petroleum distillate *	91.13%

'76 Ed.

PATTERSON'S MALATHION GRAIN PROTECTANT
Insecticide
(Patterson Chem.)

Malathion *	55%
Aromatic petroleum derivative solvents *	40%

'76 Ed.

PATTERSON'S MALATHION LIVESTOCK SPRAY (PREMIUM GRADE)
Insecticide
(Patterson Chem.)

Malathion *	55%
Aromatic petroleum solvents *	40%

'76 Ed.

PATTERSON'S 25% METHOXYCHLOR EMULSIFIABLE CONCENTRATE
Insecticide
(Patterson Chem.)

Methoxychlor, tech.	25%
Methylated aromatic petroleum derivatives *	69%

'76 Ed.

PATTERSON'S MILL & PLANT FOOD SPRAY
Insecticide
(Patterson Chem.)

Pyrethrins	0.15%
Piperonyl butoxide, tech.	1.20%
Deodorized petroleum oil *	98.65%

'76 Ed.

PATTERSON'S MOLE KILLER POISON PEANUTS
Rodenticide
(Patterson Chem.)

Strychnine alkaloid *	0.3%

'76 Ed.

PATTERSON'S MULTIPURPOSE FUNGICIDE
(Patterson Chem.)

Captan	22%
Zineb (zinc as metallic, 5%)	21%

'76 Ed.

PATTERSON'S PARA-DI MOTH CRYSTALS
(Patterson Chem.)

Paradichlorobenzene *	100%

'76 Ed.

PATTERSON'S PENTACHLOROPHENOL CONCENTRATE 1 TO 10
Insecticide, wood preservative
(Patterson Chem.)

Pentachlorophenol *	37%
Other chlorophenols and related compounds	3%
Aromatic petroleum solvents *	30%
Special solvents	30%

'76 Ed.

PATTERSON'S PENTACHLOROPHENOL PRESERVATIVE
Wood preservative
(Patterson Chem.)

Pentachlorophenol *	5.00%
Petroleum hydrocarbons *	94.80%

'76 Ed.

PATTERSON'S PET FLEA KILLER & DEODORANT
(Patterson Chem.)

Pyrethrins	0.06%
Piperonyl butoxide, tech.	0.48%
Malathion	0.50%
Methoxychlor, tech.	0.50%
2,2-Thiobis-(4-chloro-6-methylphenol)	0.10%
Petroleum distillate *	23.36%

'76 Ed.

PATTERSON'S PINE OIL DISINFECTANT
Germicide-deodorant
(Patterson Chem.)

Steam distilled Pine oil *
Anhydrous soap

'76 Ed.

PATTERSON'S PLANT SPRAY
Insecticide, fungicide
(Patterson Chem.)

Methoxychlor, tech.	13.50%
1,1-Bis-(p-chlorophenyl)-2,2,2-trichloroethanol	2.88%
Gamma isomer of benzene hexa-chloride from lindane	2.75%
Copper oleate	2.00%
Xylene-range aromatic petroleum distillate *	58.35%

'76 Ed.

PATTERSON'S PYRENONE DAIRY SPRAY
Insecticide
(Patterson Chem.)

Pyrethrins	0.5%
Piperonyl butoxide, tech.	4.0%
Petroleum distillate *	85.5%

'76 Ed.

PATTERSON'S PYRENONE EMULSION CONCENTRATE
Insecticide
(Patterson Chem.)

Petroleum solvents *	74%
Piperonyl butoxide, tech.	10%
Pyrethrins	1%
Inert ingredients (emulsifier)	15%

'76 Ed.

PATTERSON'S PYRENONE GRAIN SPRAY CONCENTRATE
Insecticide
(Patterson Chem.)

Pyrethrins	1%
Piperonyl butoxide, tech.	8%
Petroleum distillate *	71%

'76 Ed.

PATTERSON'S PYRENONE 20 NEW
Insecticide
(Patterson Chem.)

Piperonyl butoxide, tech.	5.03%
Pyrethrins	0.62%
Petroleum oil *	94.35%

'76 Ed.

PATTERSON'S RENEW HERBICIDE
(Patterson Chem.)

Sodium cacodylate *	11.30%
Dimethylarsinic acid (Cacodylic acid) *	1.95%
Total arsenic (as elemental) all in water soluble form	6.35%

'76 Ed.

Starred ingredients (*) may be responsible for major toxic effects; consult Section II.

PATTERSON'S ROOT AND CROWN ROT CONTROL
Fungicide
(Patterson Chem.)

p-Dimethylaminobenzenediazo sodium sulfonate *	5.0%
Pentachloronitrobenzene (PCNB) *	69.0%

'76 Ed.

PATTERSON'S ROSE SPRAY
Insecticide
(Patterson Chem.)

Xylene *
Methoxychlor, tech. *
Malathion *
Kelthane *
N-Trichloromethylthiophthalimide
Tributyltin compound *

'76 Ed.

PATTERSON'S ROSE SPRAY FLOWER BOMB
Insecticide & fungicide
(Patterson Chem.)

Pyrethrins	0.0255%
Tech. Piperonyl butoxide	0.2560%
Rotenone	0.1280%
Other cube extractives	0.2360%
Captan	0.5035%
Dinitro (1-methylheptyl)phenyl crotonate	0.1560%
Dinitro (1-methylheptyl) phenol & related compounds	0.0440%
Petroleum distillate	0.0880%

'76 Ed.

PATTERSON'S 1% ROTENONE
Insecticide
(Patterson Chem.)

Rotenone	1.000%
Other cube extractives	1.224%
Methylated naphthalenes *	92.776%

'76 Ed.

PATTERSON'S 5% ROTENONE EMULSION CONCENTRATE
Insecticide
(Patterson Chem.)

Rotenone *	5.00%
Other cube extractives	6.12%
Methylated naphthalenes *	78.88%

'76 Ed.

PATTERSON'S SCREWWORM & EAR TICK BOMB
Insecticide
(Patterson Chem.)

Gamma isomer of benzene hexachloride from lindane *	3%
Pine oil *	15%
Mineral oil	15%
Emulsifier, Atlox 1045A	3%
Propellant, Freon 11-12	64%

'76 Ed.

PATTERSON'S SODIUM ARSENITE SOLUTION
Herbicide
(Patterson Chem.)

Sodium arsenite (arsenic as metallic, 23.1%) *	40%

'76 Ed.

PATTERSON'S SOD WEBWORM SPRAY
Insecticide
(Patterson Chem.)

O,O-Diethyl O-(2-isopropyl-6-methyl-4-pyrimidinyl) phosphorothioate (Diazinon) *	12.50%
Pyrethrins	0.03%
Piperonyl butoxide, tech.	0.25%
Petroleum solvent *	82.22%

'76 Ed.

PATTERSON'S SPREADER-STICKER
For increased effectiveness of insecticide, fungicide, herbicide sprays
(Patterson Chem.)

Emulsifiable A-C polyethylene
Fatty acid-amine condensate
Alkyl aryl sulfonate *

'76 Ed.

PATTERSON'S STORED GRAIN DUST
Insecticide
(Patterson Chem.)

Methoxychlor, tech.	5%

'76 Ed.

PATTERSON'S TOBACCO DUST
Insecticide, fertilizer
(Patterson Chem.)

Nitrogen	2.0%
Phosphoric acid	2.0%
Potash	3.0%
Nicotine *	0.9%

'76 Ed.

PATTERSON'S TOMATO DUST
Insecticide-fungicide
(Patterson Chem.)

Zineb	3.9%
Captan	2.5%
Carbaryl ((1-Naphthyl-N methyl) carbamate) *	2.0%
Rotenone	1.0%
Other cube extractives	1.6%

'76 Ed.

PATTERSON'S TOXAPHENE-LINDANE LIVESTOCK SPRAY & DIP
Insecticide
(Patterson Chem.)

Toxaphene *	45.00%
Gamma isomer of benzene hexachloride from lindane	2.50%
Methylated naphthalene	12.12%
Petroleum distillate	22.50%

'76 Ed.

PATTERSON'S TURF FUNGICIDE
Fungicide
(Patterson Chem.)

Cycloheximide (Beta-(2-(3,5-dimethyl-2-oxocyclohexyl)-2-hydroxyethyl)-glutarimide)	0.75%
Thiram *	75.00%

'76 Ed.

PATTERSON'S TURF INSECT KILLER EMULSIFIABLE
Concentrate
(Patterson Chem.)

Toxaphene *	36.00%
Pyrethrins	0.03%
Piperonyl butoxide, tech.	0.25%
Petroleum distillate	58.72%

'76 Ed.

PATTERSON'S WARFARIN RAT & MOUSE KILLER
(Patterson Chem.)

Warfarin	0.025%

'76 Ed.

PATTERSON'S WEEVIL KILLER & GRAIN CONDITIONER IMPROVED EDB
(Patterson Chem.)

Ethylene dichloride	63.1%
Carbon tetrachloride *	26.9%
Ethylene dibromide	7.1%
Sulfur dioxide	2.9%

'76 Ed.

Starred ingredients (*) may be responsible for major toxic effects; consult Section II.

PATTY-O-CANDLE
Insecticide
(Empire Mfg. Co.)

Oil of citronella	3%
Petroleum wax	97%

'76 Ed.

PAUL KOSS DEFOAMER
(Paul Koss)

Water	>60%
Silicone emulsion (10% active)	
Isopropyl alcohol *	<20%

PAUL KOSS HEAVY DUTY INDUSTRIAL CLEANER
(Paul Koss)

Water	>80%
Butyl Cellosolve *	5%
Monoethanolamine	
Sodium xylene sulfonate (Anionic surfactant)	
Tetrasodium EDTA	
Sodium metasilicate	
Trisodium phosphate	
Fatty amido phosphate	
Formalin	trace
Dye	trace

pH 11.5-11.9

PAUL KOSS HEAVY DUTY STEAM CLEANER LIQUID
(Paul Koss)

Potassium hydroxide *	15.0%
Sodium metasilicate pentahydrate *	5.0%
Tetrasodium EDTA	
Tetrasodium pyrophosphate	
Coco amido alkyl betaine	

pH approx. 13.5-13.8

PAUL KOSS LATHER LOTION HAND SOAP
(Paul Koss)

Water	>80%
Triethanolamine coco soap	
Tetrasodium EDTA	
Glycerine	
Latex opacifier	
Perfume	
Dye	

PAUL KOSS LIQUID RUG SHAMPOO
(Paul Koss)

Water	>70%
Isopropyl alcohol *	15%
Sodium lauryl sulfate	
Lauroyl diethanolamide	
Tetrasodium EDTA	
Optical brightener	trace
Formalin	trace

PAUL KOSS PINE ODOR CLEANER
(Paul Koss)

Water	>85%
Nonylphenoxypoly(ethyleneoxy)ethanol (Nonionic surfactant)	
Tetrapotassium pyrophosphate	
Alkyl dimethyl benzyl ammonium chloride *	<3%
Pine perfume	
Dye	trace

pH 10.2-10.4

PAUL KOSS RUG SPOTTER
(Paul Koss)

Water	>90%
Butyl carbitol acetate	
Isopropyl alcohol	
Coco amido betaine	
Tetrasodium EDTA	
Perfume	trace
Dye	trace

pH 7.0-7.2

PAUL KOSS SAFETY SOLVENT
(Paul Koss)

Stoddard solvent (Petroleum distillate) *	70%
Methylene chloride *	25%
Perchloroethylene	

PAUL KOSS SHOWER WASH
Acid scale remover
(Paul Koss)

Water	>85%
Phosphoric acid *	<10%
Hydrogen chloride *	<5%
Nonionic surfactant	

pH 1.2-1.4

PAUL KOSS STEAM CONCENTRATE
Extractor detergent
(Paul Koss)

Water	>85%
Butyl Cellosolve *	5%
Tetrapotassium pyrophosphate	
Sodium carbonate	
Coco amido betaine	
Optical brightener	trace
Formalin	trace

pH 10.9-11.2

PAUL KOSS SUPER SEAL
Water emulsion floor seal
(Paul Koss)

Water	>80%
Mixed emulsion of oligomers and polymers, primarily acrylic	
Fluorosurfactant	trace
Formalin	trace

pH 7.8-8.0

PAUL KOSS TRAFFIC LANE CLEANER
Carpet cleaner
(Paul Koss)

Water	>90%
Butyl Cellosolve *	5%
Tetrapotassium pyrophosphate	
Sodium carbonate	
Coco amido betaine	
Optical brightener	trace
Formalin	trace

pH 11.0-11.1

PAUL KOSS WATER SOLUBLE DEODORANT
(Paul Koss)

Water	>85%
Alkyl dimethyl benzyl ammonium chloride *	<6%
POE (20) sorbitan monolaurate (Nonionic surfactant)	
Floral fragrance	

pH 7.0-7.2

PAUL KOSS WINTERGREEN WATER SOLUBLE DEODORANT
(Paul Koss)

Water	>90%
POE (20) sorbitan monolaurate (Nonionic surfactant)	
Alkyl dimethyl benzyl ammonium chloride *	3%
Methyl salicylate *	<2%

pH 7.0-7.2

PAVACEN CENULES
Cerebral vasodilator
(Central Pharmacal Co.)

Each Cenule (timed release capsule):
Papaverine hydrochloride *	150 mg.

PAVEROLAN LANACAPS
Muscle relaxant
(Lannett)

Each time release capsule:
Papaverine hydrochloride USP *	150 mg.

PAX ACTION WEED'N FEED 18-4-4
Herbicide & fertilizer
(PAX Co.)

Alkanolamine salt of 2,4-dichlorophenoxyacetic acid	0.870%
Dimethylamine salt of dicamba (3,6-Dichloro-o-anisic acid)	0.125%
Total nitrogen	18.0%
4.0% Ammoniacal nitrogen 14.0% from Urea	
Available Phosphoric acid *	4.0%
Soluble Potash *	4.0%

Starred ingredients (*) may be responsible for major toxic effects; consult Section II.

PAXFARIN
Rodenticide
(Biocerta)

Warfarin (3-(a-Acetonylbenzyl)-4-
  hydroxycoumarin) 0.025%
                        '76 Ed.

PAXIDE POWDER
Insecticide
(Biocerta)

Pyrethrins 0.90%
Inert ingred.:
  Pyrethrum other than
    pyrethrins 99.10%
                        '76 Ed.

PAXIDE TYPE B
Insecticide
(Biocerta)

Tech. Piperonyl butoxide 1.00%
Pyrethrins 0.40%
Odorless petroleum * 98.60%
                        '76 Ed.

PAXIDE TYPE R
Insecticide
(Biocerta)

Pyrethrins 0.5%
Oil *† 99.5%
                        '76 Ed.

†*See* Kerosene

PAXIT (SKIN CLEANSER)
Waterless; for industrial use
(Calgon Corp., Commercial Div.)

Aliphatic hydrocarbons *
Emulsifying agents
Water

PAX-LANO-SAV HEAVY
DUTY
Industrial skin cleanser
(Calgon Corp., Commercial Div.)

Vegetable scrubbers
Soap
Emollients
Detergent salts *†

†*See* Detergents (synthetic)

PAX-SOLV
For industrial use
(Calgon Corp., Commercial Div.)

Aliphatic hydrocarbons *
Emulsifying agents
Emollients
Water

PAYLOAD
(Calgon Corp., Commercial Div.)

Sodium silicates
Complex phosphates *
Synthetic wetting agents *†
Diethylene glycol monobutyl ether *

†*See* Synthetic detergents

PAYONS EXTRUDED
WATER COLOR WAX
CRAYONS
(American Crayon Co.)

This product bears the CP Seal issued by
the Crayon, Water Color and Craft Institute, Inc. This seal certifies that the product contains no materials in sufficient
quantities to be toxic or injurious to the
human body even if ingested.

PAZO HEMORRHOID
OINTMENT
(Bristol-Myers)

                       by weight
Benzocaine 0.80%
Ephedrine sulfate * 0.24%
Zinc oxide 4.00%
Camphor * 2.18%
Emollient base 92.78%

PAZO HEMORRHOID
SUPPOSITORIES
(Bristol-Myers)

Each suppository: .... by weight
Benzocaine .... 15.44 mg.
Ephedrine sulfate * ...... 4.63 mg.
Zinc oxide .... 72.20 mg.
Camphor * .... 42.07 mg.
Emollient base .... 1790.65 mg.

PBZ
Antihistamine
(Geigy Pharmaceuticals)

Each tablet:
  Tripelennamine HCl * . 25 mg.; 50 mg.

PBZ ELIXIR
Antihistamine
(Geigy Pharmaceuticals)

Each 5 ml.:
  Tripelennamine citrate * .... 37.5 mg.

PBZ EXPECTORANT WITH
CODEINE AND
EPHEDRINE
(Geigy Pharmaceuticals)

Each 4 ml.:
  Tripelennamine citrate * ..... 30 mg.
  Codeine phosphate * .... 8 mg.
  Ephedrine sulfate * .... 10 mg.
  Ammonium chloride .... 80 mg.

PBZ EXPECTORANT WITH
EPHEDRINE
(Geigy Pharmaceuticals)

Each 4 ml.:
  Tripelennamine citrate * .... 30 mg.
  Ephedrine sulfate * .... 10 mg.
  Ammonium chloride .... 80 mg.

PBZ LONTABS
Antihistamine
(Geigy Pharmaceuticals)

Each tablet:
  Tripelennamine HCl * .... 50 mg.

PBZ OINTMENT AND
CREAM
Antihistamine
(Geigy Pharmaceuticals)

Ointment:
  Tripelennamine HCl * 2%
  Petrolatum base

Cream:
  Tripelennamine HCl * 2%
  Water-washable base

PBZ-SR
Antihistamine
(Geigy Pharmaceuticals)

Each tablet:
  Tripelennamine HCl * .... 100 mg.

PBZ TABLETS WITH
EPHEDRINE
Antihistamine
(Geigy Pharmaceuticals)

Each tablet:
  Tripelennamine HCl * .... 25 mg.
  Ephedrine sulfate * .... 12 mg.

PCNB 10 DUST
Fungicide
(FMC Corp., Agricultural Chem. Div.)

Pentachloronitrobenzene 10%

PCQ RAT & MOUSE BAIT
(Bell Labs., Inc.)

Diphacinone 0.005%
Blend of food grade cereals 99.995%

PDA DAIRY AEROSOL
Insecticide
(Hess & Clark)

Pyrethrins 0.50%
Technical Piperonyl butoxide 1.00%
N-Octyl bicycloheptene
  dicarboximide 1.00%
Refined Petroleum oil 8.00%

PDQ

See SILOO PDQ

Starred ingredients (*) may be responsible for major toxic effects; consult Section II.

PEACOCK WATER COLORS
(Binney & Smith)

Water-soluble base
Organic plasticizer *
Non-toxic pigments

PEAK ANTIFREEZE AND COOLANT
(Northern Petrochemical)

Ethylene glycol *	95%
Alkaline metal earths	2.5%
Water	2.5%

PEARL DROPS
Dentifrice
(Carter Products)

Metal hydroxides & metal salts	<50%
Water	
Thickeners	
Saccharin	
Polyalcohol	
Preservative	
Flavor	

PEARSON'S BORER SPRAY & STOCK DIP
Insecticide
(Pearson & Co.)

Lindane (Gamma isomer of benzene hexachloride) *	20%
Xylene *	65%

'76 Ed.

PEARSON'S BUG SPRAY
Insecticide
(Pearson & Co.)

Pyrethrins	0.050%
Technical Piperonyl butoxide	0.125%
O,O-Diethyl O-(2-isopropyl-4-methyl-6-pyrimidinyl)phosphorothioate	0.500%
Petroleum distillate *	99.325%

'76 Ed.

PEARSON'S 45% CHLORDANE E.C.
Insecticide
(Pearson & Co.)

Technical Chlordane *	45.0%
Petroleum hydrocarbons *	45.0%

'76 Ed.

PEARSON'S 75% CHLORDANE E.C.
Insecticide
(Pearson & Co.)

Technical Chlordane *	75.0%
Petroleum hydrocarbons *	15.0%

'76 Ed.

PEARSON'S 18.6% DIELDRIN E.C.
Insecticide
(Pearson & Co.)

Dieldrin *	18.60%
Petroleum hydrocarbons	73.40%

'76 Ed.

PEARSON'S DIEL-RAM
Seed treatment - insecticide and fungicide
(Pearson & Co.)

Dieldrin *	30%
Thiram *	40%
Aluminum powder	4%

'76 Ed.

PEARSON'S EASY-EDGER
Herbicide
(Pearson & Co.)

Sodium cacodylate	5.650%
Dimethylarsinic acid (Cacodylic acid)	0.975%

'76 Ed.

PEARSON'S FUMIGRAIN P-75
Insecticide
(Pearson & Co.)

Ethylene dichloride	67.49%
Carbon tetrachloride *	32.51%

'76 Ed.

PEARSON'S GOPHER KILLER
Rodenticide
(Pearson & Co.)

Strychnine alkaloid *	0.3%

'76 Ed.

PEARSON'S GREEN LAWN FUNGICIDE
(Pearson & Co.)

Pentachloronitrobenzene *	24%

'76 Ed.

PEARSON'S INSTITUTIONAL BUG KILLER
Insecticide
(Pearson & Co.)

Piperonyl butoxide, technical	0.50%
Pyrethrins	0.06%
Petroleum oil *	99.44%

'76 Ed.

PEARSON'S KLEEN-GRO
Herbicide
(Pearson & Co.)

Dimethyl ester of tetrachloroterephthalic acid	2.5%

'76 Ed.

PEARSON'S MELON & PINE SEED PROTECTANT
Seed treatment - insecticide and fungicide
(Pearson & Co.)

Thiram (Tetramethylthiuram disulfide) *	64.27%
Aldrin *	7.14%

'76 Ed.

PEARSON'S MOLY-STAND
Seed treatment stimulant & fungicide
(Pearson & Co.)

Thiram (Tetramethylthiuram disulfide) *	25.00%
Molybdenum	4.75%

'76 Ed.

PEARSON'S 5% NEMA-KILL
Nematocide
(Pearson & Co.)

1,2-Dibromo-3-chloropropane *	4.85%
Other halogenated C3 compounds	0.10%

'76 Ed.

PEARSON'S 10% NEMA-KILL
Nematocide
(Pearson & Co.)

1,2-Dibromo-3-chloropropane *	9.70%
Related brominated and/or chlorinated C3 hydrocarbons	0.20%

'76 Ed.

PEARSON'S POISON PASTE
Insecticide & rodenticide
(Pearson & Co.)

Phosphorus *	2.00%

'76 Ed.

PEARSON'S POISON PEANUT PELLETS
Rodenticide
(Pearson & Co.)

Strychnine alkaloid *	0.5%

'76 Ed.

PEARSON'S RAT POISON
(Pearson & Co.)

Zinc phosphide *	2.0%

'76 Ed.

Starred ingredients (*) may be responsible for major toxic effects; consult Section II.

PEARSON'S RED-I-CAT CONCENTRATE
Rodenticide
(Pearson & Co.)

Warfarin (3-(a-Acetonylbenzyl)-4-hydroxycoumarin)	0.5%
Sulfaquinoxaline (N'-(2-Quinoxalinyl) sulfanilamide)	0.5%

'76 Ed.

PEARSON'S RED-I-CAT READY MIXED BAIT
Rodenticide
(Pearson & Co.)

3(a-Acetonylbenzyl)-4-hydroxycoumarin	0.025%
N'-(2-Quinoxalinyl) sulfanilamide	0.025%

'76 Ed.

PEARSON'S RED-I-CAT W.S.
Rodenticide
(Pearson & Co.)

Sodium salt of warfarin (Sodium salt of 3-(a-Acetonylbenzyl)-4-hydroxycoumarin)	0.54%
Inert ingred.:	99.46%
Silica	

'76 Ed.

PEARSON'S ROACH POISON
(Pearson & Co.)

Sodium fluoride *	59.00%
Powdered stems of Ryania speciosa	18.00%
Sodium silicofluoride	1.00%
Pyrethrins	0.18%

'76 Ed.

PEARSON'S ROSE DUST & ROSE SPRAY
Fungicide, insecticide
(Pearson & Co.)

Sulfur	20.00%
Copper (as metallic) *	3.70%
Dichloro diphenyl trichloroethane *	5.00%
Rotenone	0.75%
Other cube resins	1.50%

'76 Ed.

PEARSON'S SEED-SAVER
Bird repellent; insecticide
(Pearson & Co.)

Aldrin *	20.53%
Hardwood oil	9.00%

'76 Ed.

PEARSON'S SPEEDY-WEEDER
Herbicide
(Pearson & Co.)

Monosodium acid methanearsonate *	34.8%

'76 Ed.

PEARSON'S THERMO-FOG
Insecticide
(Pearson & Co.)

2,2-Dichlorovinyl dimethyl phosphate	0.92%
Related compounds	0.08%
Petroleum distillate *	99.00%

'76 Ed.

PEARSON'S TOMATO DUST
Fungicide, insecticide
(Pearson & Co.)

Zineb	3.9%
Sevin *	3.0%

'76 Ed.

PEARSON'S TOMATO FIXER
Plant regulator
(Pearson & Co.)

Beta-naphthoxyacetic acid (98%)	0.1417%

'76 Ed.

PEARSON'S WATERBUG & ROACH KILLER
Insecticide
(Pearson & Co.)

Decachlorooctahydro-1,3,4-metheno-2H-cyclobuta(cd)pentalen-2-one	0.125%

'76 Ed.

PEARSON'S ZEBRA DUST
Insecticide, fungicide
(Pearson & Co.)

Rotenone	1.00%
Other cube resins	2.00%
Zineb	3.25%

'76 Ed.

PECORA AC-20 ACRYLIC LATEX CALK
(Pecora)

Acrylic latex	>32%
Dipropylene glycol dibenzoate	>9%
Alkylaryl polyether alcohol	trace
Titanium dioxide	>1%
Calcium carbonate	<53%
Sodium phosphate	trace
2-(Hydroxy methyl amino) ethanol	trace
Tributyl tin oxide	trace
G-Glycidoxypropyl trimethoxysilane	trace
Sodium carboxylate	trace
Mineral spirits	>2%
Ethylene glycol	<2%

PECORA ACOUSTICAL SEALANT BA-98
(Pecora)

Butyl rubber polymer	>20%
Mineral spirits	<7%
Bentonite clay	<3%
Talc	>25%
Calcium carbonate	<25%
Titanium dioxide	>3%
Denatured ethyl alcohol	<2%
Polybutene	<15%

PECORA A-103 MASTIC
(Pecora)

Asphalt	>50%
Asbestos fiber	<24%
Mineral spirits *	>13%
Xylol *	<13%

PECORA AQUAPOXY
Epoxy mortar grout system
(Pecora)

Part A:	
Polyamide	>28%
Xylol *	<2%
Ethoxylated non-ionic emulsifier	<2%
Ethylene glycol monobutyl ether acetate *	>2%
Water	>50%
Polyvalent metallic soap in Aliphatic hydrocarbon	trace
Part B:	
Epoxy resin	>39%
Ethoxylated non-ionic emulsifier	<2%
Methyl cellulose	trace
Calcium carbonate	>18%
Water	<41%
Aggregate:	
Portland cement	<29%
Silicone dioxide	<70%
Chrysotile asbestos	>1%

PECORA ASBESTOS FURNACE CEMENT (24WR2)
(Pecora)

Water	>5%
Sodium silicate *	>22%
Asbestos fiber	>1%
Lamp black	trace
Clay	<19%
Silica sand	<53%

Starred ingredients (*) may be responsible for major toxic effects; consult Section II.

PECORA BC-158 ONE-PART BUTYL RUBBER SEALANT
(Pecora)

Butyl rubber	<27%
Polyisobutylene	<8%
Asbestos fiber	<3%
Talc	>15%
Calcium carbonate	>20%
Titanium dioxide	>7%
Hydrogenated Rosin	trace
Vegetable oil blend (linseed-soya)	<9%
Mineral spirits	<8%
Bentonite clay	trace
Denatured ethyl alcohol	trace
24% Lead tallate (0.017 lead as metal)	trace
6% Cobalt tallate	trace
Tall oil fatty acid	trace

PECORA 600 CLEAR ACRYLIC JOINT SEALANT
(Pecora)

Acrylic terpolymer	>64%
Powdered Castor oil	>6%
Xylene *	>10%
Toluene *	<20%

PECORA DURAMEM H-550
Elastomeric membrane waterproofing system
(Pecora)

Base:

Coal tar *	<50%
Dipropylene glycol dibenzoate	<10%
Calcium oxide	>3%
Carbon black pigment	>10%
Silicone oil	trace
Xylol *	<5%
Polypropylene glycol	>10%
Dibutyl tin laurate	trace
Lead octoate (12% lead as metal)	trace

Activator:

Aromatic process oil *†	>13%
Polymethylene polyphenylisocyanate	<2%
Coal tar oil	<10%
Polyether polyurethane	>31%
Coal tar	>40%
Calcium oxide	<3%

†*See* Aromatic hydrocarbon solvent

PECORA DYNATROL II POLYURETHANE RUBBER SEALANT
(Pecora)

Base:

Polypropylene glycol	>42%
Polyoxypropylene polyol	<3%
Dipropylene glycol dibenzoate	<2%
P,P'-Methylenedianaline	trace
16% NCO Polyisocyanate prepolymer	trace
Butyl methylphenol	trace
Isocyanate-silane	trace
Dehydrated Castor oil	<5%
Titanium dioxide	>4%
Magnesium silicate	<40%
Phenyl mercury acetate-10%	trace
Sodium alumino silicate	trace

Activator:

7% NCO Polyether prepolymer	100%

PECORA FF-3 BLACK ASBESTOS ROOF CEMENT
(Pecora)

Asphalt	>31%
Asbestos fiber	<16%
Talc	>28%
Mineral spirits *	<25%

PECORA MARK 200 SOLVENT RUBBER EMULSION CERAMIC WALL TILE ADHESIVE
(Pecora)

Water	>24%
Potassium hydroxide	trace
Polyoxyethylated fatty alcohol	>2%
Triethanolamine	trace
Calcium carbonate	<27%
Suprex clay	>5%
Mineral spirits	<7%
Pentaerythritol ester of rosin	>8%
Hydrocarbon resin	<9%
Tall oil fatty acid	trace
Carboxyl vinyl polymer	>1%
Ethylene glycol	<3%
2-(Hydroxy methyl amino) ethanol	trace
Tributyl tin oxide	trace
Carboxylated latex	<11%

PECORA M-242 ELASTIC GLAZING COMPOUND
(Pecora)

Calcium carbonate	<85%
Asbestos fiber	<3%
Bentonite clay	trace
24% Lead tallate (0.0216 lead as metal)	trace
Soya oil	>9%
Tall oil fatty acid	trace
Polybutene	>1%
Denatured ethyl alcohol	trace
Mineral spirits	>1%
Modified Polyester (FDA approved)	trace

PECORA M241 ELASTIC GLAZING COMPOUND
(Pecora)

Soya oil	8%
Tall oil fatty acid	trace
Polybutene	<5%
Mineral spirits	trace
Asbestos fiber	2%
Calcium carbonate	>75%
Titanium dioxide	2%
Talc	7%
Alkyl aldoxim	trace

PECORA P-53 CHLORINATED RUBBER BASE PRIMER
(Pecora)

Toluol *	<50%
Chlorinated rubber	>25%
Mercapto-silane	<3%
Chlorinated paraffin	<22%
Epichlorohydrin	trace

PECORA P-200 EPOXY PRIMER
(Pecora)

Part A:

Xylene *	>18%
Epoxy resin	>55%
Toluene *	<27%

Part B:

Polyamide resin	<32%
2,4,6-Tri(dimethylaminoethyl) phenol	<5%
Anhydrous Isopropanol *	>63%

PECORA P-75 POLYURETHANE PRIMER
(Pecora)

Toluol *	<50%
Polyisocyanate	>30%
Ethyl glycol acetate	>12%
Xylene *	>7%

PECORA P-37 SILICONE WATER REPELLENT
(Pecora)

Silicone polymer	>5%
Mineral spirits *	<95%

PECORA 200R2 ARCHITECTURAL CALKING COMPOUND
(Pecora)

Vegetable oil blend (linseed-soya)	>27%
Petrolatum	<5%
Asbestos fiber	<8%
Calcium carbonate	<52%
Titanium dioxide	<2%
Bentonite clay	trace
Lead tallate (0.08% lead as metal)	trace
Cobalt tallate (0.003% cobalt as metal)	trace
Tall oil fatty acid	trace
Denatured ethyl alcohol	trace
Mineral spirits	<5%

PECORA SPECIAL 7HR4 BLACK BEDDING COMPOUND
Mirror mastic
(Pecora)

Asphalt	<47%
Asbestos fiber	<32%
Mineral spirits *	>21%

Starred ingredients (*) may be responsible for major toxic effects; consult Section II.

PECORA SYNTHACALK GC-5
Two-part polysulfide sealant
(Pecora)

Base:
Thiokol liquid polysulfide polymer	>40%
Calcium carbonate	>28%
Stearic acid	trace
Chlorinated paraffin	<16%
Titanium dioxide	>12%
Acetone	trace
Toluene *	<2%
Water	trace

Activator:
Epoxy resin	>21%
Silica dioxide	<2%
Dipropylene glycol dibenzoate	<22%
Zinc peroxide *	<47%
Dibutyl tin oxide	<8%

PECORA SYNTHACALK GC-9
One-part polysulfide base synthetic rubber sealant
(Pecora)

Thiokol liquid polysulfide polymer	>35%
2-Mercaptoethanol	trace
Epoxy resin	trace
Toluol *	>3%
Alkyl benzyl phthalate *†	>18%
Dehydrated Castor oil	<2%
Titanium dioxide	>4%
Barium oxide *‡	<3%
Calcium carbonate	>30%
Calcium peroxide * ‡	<4%
Amino silane	trace

†*See* Phthalic acid esters
‡*See* Barium salts (soluble)
‡*See* Hydrogen peroxide

PECORA TUB & TILE CALK (BRILLIANT WHITE) A116A VINYL LATEX
(Pecora)

Polyvinyl acetate polymer	>22%
Arylsulfonamideformaldehyde resin	<6%
Xylol *	>2%
Ethylene glycol	<3%
Dipropylene glycol dibenzoate	>2%
Ultramarine blue	trace
Clay	<10%
Calcium carbonate	>25%
Titanium dioxide	>5%
Hydroxyethylcellulose	trace
Water	>25%

PECORA 60 UNICRYLIC
One-part acrylic polymeric sealant
(Pecora)

Acrylic terpolymer	>34%
Monocyclic terpenes	trace
Tall oil fatty acid	trace
Propylene carbonate	>4%
Cellosolve acetate	>3%
Bentonite clay	>6%
Calcium carbonate	<33%
Talc	<8%
Titanium dioxide	>3%
Xylene *	<7%

PECORA UREXPAN NR-200 URETHANE SELF-LEVELING SEALANT
(Pecora)

Base:
Polypropylene glycol *	>40%
Butyl methylphenol	>1%
Talc	<45%
Titanium dioxide	>4%
Carbon black	trace
Dipropylene glycol dibenzoate	<6%
Bentonite clay	>1%
Propylene carbonate	trace
Phenyl mercury acetate (10% metal)	trace
Sodium alumino silicate	<2%

Activator:
4% NCO Polyether urethane	100%

PECTOCOMP
For diarrhea
(Lannett)

Each fl. oz.:
Pectin	4 gr.
Kaolin	90 gr.
Zinc phenolsulfonate	1 1/8 gr.
Aromatized aqueous vehicle	qs ad

PEDAMETH
For acidifying urine
(OJF)

Each capsule:
Methionine *	200 mg.

PEDENEX OINTMENT
For athlete's foot
(Approved Pharm.)

Caprylic acid
Zinc undecylenate *
Sodium propionate

'76 Ed.

PEDIACOF
Decongestant and cough syrup for children
(Breon Labs.)

Each 5 ml.:
Codeine phosphate	5.0 mg.
Phenylephrine HCl	2.5 mg.
Chlorpheniramine maleate	0.75 mg.
Potassium iodide *	75.0 mg.
Sodium benzoate	0.2%
Alcohol	5%

PEDIAFLOR DROPS
Prevention of dental caries
(Ross Labs.)

Each cc:
Fluoride (as sodium fluoride) *	0.5 mg.

PEDIAMYCIN CHEWABLE TABLETS
Antibiotic
(Ross Labs.)

Each tablet:
Erythromycin ethylsuccinate (USP)	200 mg.

PEDIAMYCIN DROPS, LIQUID, 400-LIQUID AND SUSPENSION
Antibiotic
(Ross Labs.)

Each 2.5 ml.:
Erythromycin ethyl-succinate (USP)	100 mg.

Each 5 ml.:
Erythromycin ethyl-succinate (USP)	200 mg.; 400 mg.

PEDIAQUIL LIQUID
Cough preparation
(Philips Roxane Labs.)

Each 5 ml.:
Phenylephrine hydrochloride	2.5 mg.
Guaifenesin	50 mg.
Alcohol	5%

PEDI-BATH
Foot bath and soak
(Pedinol)

Colloidal sulfur *
Balsam Peru *

PEDI-BORO SOAK PAKS
Astringent wet dressing
(Pedinol)

Aluminum sulfate
Calcium acetate
Coloring agent

PEDI-CORT V CREME
Antibacterial, antifungal, antipruritic
(Pedinol)

Iodochlorhydroxyquin	3%
Hydrocortisone	1%

PEDICRAN WITH IRON
Iron deficiency
(Scherer Labs.)

Each 5 cc:
Cyanocobalamin	25 mcg.
Ferric pyrophosphate *	250 mg.
Thiamine mononitrate (B1)	10 mg.
Nicotinamide	10 mg.
Alcohol	1%

PEDICREME, DR. SCHOLL'S
See DR. SCHOLL'S PEDICREME

Starred ingredients (*) may be responsible for major toxic effects; consult Section II.

PEDI-DRI FOOT POWDER
Antiperspirant, deodorant, fungicide
(Pedinol)

Aluminum chlorohydroxide *
Zinc undecylenate *
Menthol *
Formaldehyde *

PEDINOL CASTELLANI PAINT
Local antifungal agent and drying agent for macerations and ulcerations
(Pedinol)

Basic Fuchsin
Phenol *
Resorcinol *
Acetone
Alcohol

PEDINOL CASTELLANI PAINT (Colorless)
Local antifungal agent and drying agent for macerations and ulcerations
(Pedinol)

Phenol *
Resorcinol *
Acetone
Alcohol

PEDINOL SALICYLIC ACID CREME 25%
Keratolytic agent for the removal of verrucae
(Pedinol)

Salicylic acid * 25%

PEDINOL SALICYLIC ACID CREME 60%
Keratolytic agent for removal of verrucae
(Pedinol)

Salicylic acid * 60%

PEDI-PRE-TAPE
Spray adherent
(Pedinol)

Gum rosin
1,1,1-Trichloroethane *
Propellants

PEDI-SKIN ADHERENT NO. 2
Adheres dressing, protects skin, promotes easy tape removal
(Pedinol)

Gum rosin
1,1,1-Trichloroethane *

PEDI-VIT A CREME
Aids the healing process of the skin
(Pedinol)

Vitamin A .... 100,000 u./oz.

PEDI-WHIRL CONCENTRATE
To clean, sanitize, and deodorize whirlpools and whirlpool drains
(Pedinol)

Triton X-100
Benzalkonium chloride

PEDRIC ELIXIR
Analgesic
(Vale)

Each 5 ml.:
   Acetaminophen * .... 120 mg.
   Alcohol 10%

PEDRIC SENIOR
Analgesic
(Vale)

Each tablet:
   Acetaminophen * .... 320 mg.

PEDRIC WAFERS
Analgesic
(Vale)

Each wafer:
   Acetaminophen * .... 120 mg.

PEELZ WALLPAPER RELEASE COATING
(Zinsser, Wm., & Co.)

Non-volatile: 25.75%
Volatile: 74.25%
   Water
   Glycol *†

†See Ethylene glycol

PEKTAMALT
Antidiarrheal
(Warren-Teed)

Pectin, USP
Kaolin, USP
Potassium, as Kaon (brand of potassium gluconate, USP) *†
Sodium citrate, USP
Alcohol 7%

†See Potassium salts

PELADOW
Dust control and ice melting chemical air drier
(Dow)

Calcium chloride .... 94.0% min.

PELLENT
See LOTSHAW PELLENT

PELLITOL OINTMENT
Antiseptic - protective
(Pitman-Moore)

Resorcinol * 5%
Bismuth subgallate 1%
Bismuth subnitrate 9%
Zinc oxide 17%
Calamine 10%
Juniper tar 1%

PENA GYM SEALER HEAVY DUTY
See C-Z PENA GYM SEALER HEAVY DUTY

PENASEAL
See C-Z PENASEAL

PENA SEAL
(Uncle Sam)

Modified Phenolic resins
China wood oil
Cobalt driers *
Petroleum distillates *

PENEPHITE
Penetrating oil
(Kano)

Petroleum solvents *
Graphite

PENETROLIN A CONC.
Anionic wetting agent
(Arkansas Co.)

Sodium alkylnaphthalene sulfonate *†

'76 Ed.

†See Alkyl aryl sodium sulfonates

PENGUIN
Freezer wrap marker - permanent
(Sanford Corp.)

Dyes
Resins
Glycol ethers
Alcohol

PENGUIN FEET TREAT CREAM
See DEWITT'S PENGUIN FEET TREAT CREAM

PENGUN
Tear gas pen
(Penguin Industries)

Alphachloracetophenone *

Starred ingredients (*) may be responsible for major toxic effects; consult Section II.

PENICK PURIFIED PYRETHRUM EXTRACT
Insecticide
(Penick)

Pyrethrins *	20%
Petroleum distillate *	80%

PENICK PYRETHRUM POWDER
Insecticide
(Penick)

Pyrethrins	1.3%

PENICK SBP-1382 AEROSOL INSECTICIDE
Control of house flies
(Penick)

(5-Benzyl-3-furyl)methyl 2,2-dimethyl-3-(2-methylpropenyl)cyclopropane-carboxylate	0.440% w/w
Related compounds	0.060%
Aromatic petroleum hydrocarbons	1.000%
Petroleum distillate *	18.480%

PENIT INK
Water based ink
(Sanford Corp.)

Water	
Dyes	
Phenol (as preservative)	<1%

PENLIN
Penetrating liniment
(Truett Labs.)

Oil wormwood *†	4.00%
Menthol *	2.28%
Oil sassafras *	1.44%
Methyl salicylate *	1.44%
Chlorothymol	0.1%
Acetone *	90.74%

†*See* Essential oils

PENNAMINE D7
Herbicide
(Pennwalt)

2,4-D acid as heptylamine salt (liquid concentrate) *	4 lbs./gal.

PENNCLEAN
(Pennwalt)

Phosphoric acid *

PENNWALT CLEANER
(Pennwalt)

Sodium orthosilicate
Caustic soda *
Phosphates
Wetting agents

PENNWALT DESICCANT L-10
(Pennwalt)

Arsenic acid *	11.75 lbs./gal.

PENNWALT HERBICIDE 273
(Pennwalt)

Endothall (as dipotassium salt) *	3 lbs./gal.

PENNWALT HERBICIDE 283
(Pennwalt)

Endothall as dimethyltridecyl mono salt (liquid conc.) *	2 lbs./gal.

PEN-O-PAKE
Opaquing pen for negatives
(Sanford Corp.)

Dyes
Resins
Glycol ethers
Alcohol

PENSAL M
Detergents
(Pennwalt)

Sodium orthosilicate
Sodium carbonate *
Soap or detergents

PEN. SEAL NO. 21
Floor seal
(Hillyard Chem.)

Mineral spirits *

'76 Ed.

PEN-SONIC TECHNICAL PEN CLEANER
Liquid cleaner
(Alvin & Co.)

Alcohol	<1%
Ammonia	<1%

PENTA-CARE CONCENTRATE 1-10
Wood preservative
(Sonford Products)

Pentachlorophenol *	35.3%
Other chlorophenols	4.1%
Aromatic petroleum solvent *	14.0%

PENTA-CARE READY-TO-USE
Wood preservative
(Sonford Products)

Pentachlorophenol	4.48%
Other chlorophenols	0.52%
Aromatic petroleum derivative *	94.8%

PENTACON-40
Wood preservative
(Forshaw)

Pentachlorophenol *	33.20%
Other chlorophenols & related compounds	6.80%
Petroleum solvents	35.00%

PENTA-CON "1 TO 10 CONCENTRATE," MARTIN'S

See MARTIN'S PENTA-CON "1 TO 10 CONCENTRATE"

PENTACRESOL INSTRUMENT DISINFECTING SOLUTION
(Upjohn)

Secondary-amyltricresols	0.22% w/w
Isopropyl alcohol *	86.76% w/w
Inert ingredients	13.02% w/w
Contains Sodium nitrate	

PENTACRESOL ORAL 1:1000
Antiseptic mouth wash
(Upjohn)

Each 100 ml.:
Secondary-amyltricresols	100.0 mg.
Sodium chloride	861.0 mg.
Calcium chloride	33.0 mg.
Potassium chloride	29.9 mg.
Alcohol	30%

PENTA-CURE
Wood preservative
(Apperson Chemicals)

Pentachlorophenol *	5%
Petroleum solvent *	95%

PENTAC WP 50
Miticide
(Zoecon Corp.)

Bis(pentachloro-2,4-cyclopentadien-1-yl) *	50%

PENTA-E CAPSULES
Angina pectoris
(Recsei Labs.)

Each capsule:
Pentaerythritol tetranitrate *	10 mg.; 20 mg.; or 30 mg.

PENTA-PENN
Wood preservative
(Rockland Chem.)

Pentachlorophenol *	5.20%
Petroleum hydrocarbons *	94.80%

Starred ingredients (*) may be responsible for major toxic effects; consult Section II.

PENTARCORT
Treatment of a wide variety of dermatoses
(Dalin)

Hydrocortisone alcohol (micronized)	1/2%
Solution of Coal tar	2%
Iodochlorhydroxyquinoline	3%
Diperodon hydrochloride	1/4%
Vitamin A	850 units/gm.
Vitamin D	85 units/gm.

Dalicreme base:
Stearic acid
Cetyl alcohol
Propylene glycol
Dibasic potassium phosphate
Monobasic potassium phosphate
Glyceryl monostearate
Polyoxyethylene sorbitan monostearate
Sorbitan monostearate
Acetylated lanolin
Lanolin-alcohol extract
Sorbitol
D & C Red #19

'76 Ed.

PENTASAN 20
Wood preservative
(Ambroid)

Pentachlorophenol *	5%
Inert ingredients	13%
Hydrocarbons *†	82%

†*See* Wood preservatives, Section VI, General Formulations

PENTA-TREET 5%, GOOD-LIFE

See GOOD-LIFE PENTA-TREET 5%

PENTA WOOD PRESERVATIVE CONC.
(Wood Treating Chemicals Co.)

Pentachlorophenol *	36.98%
Other chlorophenols & related compounds	4.30%
Petroleum solvents	22.00%

PENTA WOOD PRESERVATIVE RTU
(Wood Treating Chemicals Co.)

Pentachlorophenol *	4.35%
Other chlorophenols & related compounds	0.65%
Petroleum solvents	95.00%

PENTA-WOOD-SEAL, CABOT'S

See CABOT'S PENTA-WOOD-SEAL

PENTIDE

See BONIDE PENTIDE

PENTRAX TAR SHAMPOO
Medicated tar shampoo
(CooperCare)

Fractar (equiv. to 4.3% crude Coal tar) *
Blend of highly concentrated detergents

PENTRITOL
Coronary vasodilator
(Armour Pharm.)

Each capsule:
Pentaerythritol tetranitrate (PETN) * ... 30 mg. or 60 mg.

PEN-VEE K
Antibiotic therapy
(Wyeth Labs.)

Oral solution (each 5 ml.):
Potassium phenoxymethyl penicillin .. 125 mg.; 250 mg.
Tablets:
Potassium phenoxymethyl penicillin .. 125 mg.; 250 mg.; or 500 mg.

PENWAR
Wood preservative
(Forshaw)

Pentachlorophenol *	4.40%
Other chlorinated phenols	0.60%
Petroleum hydrocarbons *	89.80%

PENWAR 1-5
Wood preservative
(Forshaw)

Pentachlorophenol *	22.53%
Other chlorinated phenols	2.05%

PEPPETS
Laxative
(Peppet Labs.)

Yellow Phenolphthalein

'76 Ed.

PEPSIN ESSENCE, LILLY (Not N.F.)

See LILLY ESSENCE PEPSIN (Not N.F.)

PEPSODENT DENTIFRICE
(Lever Bros.)

Water	30-40%
Hydrogenated Starch hydrolyzate	20-30%
Aluminum oxide	10-20%
Hydrated Silica	10-20%
Glycerin	1-10%
Polyethylene glycol	1-5%
Sodium alkyl sulfate	1-5%
Dicalcium phosphate	<1%
Cellulose gum	<1%
Flavor	<1%
Titanium dioxide	<1%
Sodium saccharin	<1%
Sodium benzoate	trace

PEPTO-BISMOL
For gastrointestinal upset
(Norwich-Eaton)

Bismuth subsalicylate
Methyl salicylate *
Salicylic acid *
Sodium salicylate *

263 mg. salicylic acid per 30 ml. (fl. oz.)

PEPTO-BISMOL TABLETS
For gastrointestinal upset
(Norwich-Eaton)

Bismuth subsalicylate
Calcium carbonate
Mannitol
Methylsalicylate *

118.6 mg. salicylate/tablet

PEPTO MANGAN
Iron tonic w/vitamins
(Lambda Inc.)

Each 4 tablespoonfuls:
Vitamin B1 (Thiamine hydrochloride)	6 mg.
Vitamin B2 (Riboflavin)	4 mg.
Niacinamide	40 mg.
Iron (as ferrous chloride)	100 mg.
Calcium (as hypophosphite & chloride)	188 mg.
Phosphorous (as hypophosphite)	188 mg.
Manganese (as hypophosphite)	4 mg.
Alcohol	12%

PERAZINE
Anthelmintic
(Wesley Pharm.)

Each 5 cc (1 tsp.):
Piperazine citrate (Eq. to 500 mg. piperazine hexahydrate) 550 mg.

PERCHLOR
Drycleaning & degreasing solvent
(PPG Industries, Chem. Div.)

Stabilized Tetrachloroethylene * . 100%

PERCOBARB
Narcotic analgesic and sedative
(Endo Labs.)

Each capsule:
Oxycodone hydrochloride *	4.50 mg.
Oxycodone terephthalate	0.38 mg.
Hexobarbital *	100 mg.
Aspirin *	224 mg.
Phenacetin *	160 mg.
Caffeine	32 mg.

PERCODAN TABLETS
Analgesic
(Endo Labs.)

Each tablet:
Oxycodone hydrochloride *	4.50 mg.
Oxycodone terephthalate	0.38 mg.
Aspirin *	325.00 mg.

Starred ingredients (*) may be responsible for major toxic effects; consult Section II.

PERCORTEN LINGUETS
Adrenal cortex replacement therapy
(CIBA Pharmaceutical)

Each Linguet:
Desoxycorticosterone acetate .... 5 mg.

PERCY MEDICINE
Antacid-astringent for simple diarrhea and gastric discomfort
(Merrick Medicine)

Each 10 ml.:
Bismuth subnitrate .... 959 mg.
Potassium carbonate .... 5.9 mg.
Calcium hydroxide .... 21.9 mg.
Alcohol 5%

PERDIEM
Laxative granules
(Rorer, W.H., Inc.)

Psyllium (Plantago hydrocolloid) ... 82%
Senna (Cassia pod concentrate) * .. 18%

PERI-COLACE (CAPSULES & SYRUP)
Laxative and stool softener
(Mead Johnson)

Capsules (each):
Casanthranol * .... 30 mg.
Docusate sodium * .... 100 mg.

Syrup (each 15 cc.):
Casanthranol * .... 30 mg.
Docusate sodium * .... 60 mg.

PERIDIN-C
Dietary supplement
(Beutlich, Inc.)

Each tablet:
Ascorbic acid .... 200 mg.
Hesperidin complex .... 150 mg.
Hesperidin methyl chalcone .. 50 mg.

PERITROL-10 AND PERITROL-20
Vasodilator
(Wesley Pharm.)

Each tablet:
Pentaerythritol
tetranitrate * ..... 10 mg. or 20 mg.

PERITROL WITH PHENOBARBITAL
Vasodilator
(Wesley Pharm.)

Each tablet:
Pentaerythritol tetranitrate * . 10 mg.
Phenobarbital .... 1/4 gr.

PERK BEAUTY FRESHENER FOR NO-WAX FLOORS
(Lehn & Fink)

Water 88%
Acrylic copolymer 10%
Glycol ether derivatives 1%
Plasticizers 1%
Ammonium hydroxide .... trace

PERK PELLETS
(Armour-Dial, Inc.)

Sodium soap 75-100%
Moisture 5-10%
Minor ingredients (total) 1-5%

PERK SOAP POWDER
(Armour-Dial, Inc.)

Sodium soap 75-100%
Moisture 5-10%
Minor ingredients (total) 1-5%

PERMA BLUE LIQUID GUN BLUE
(Birchwood Casey)

Selenium *
Nitric acid *
Methanol

PERMA BLUE PASTE GUN BLUE
(Birchwood Casey)

Selenium *
Phosphoric acid *
Methanol

PERMABOND
(GC Electronics)

Ethyl cyanoacrylate monomer

PERMACIDE
See SUMMIT PERMACIDE

PERMACIDE PLUS
See SUMMIT PERMACIDE PLUS

PERMA CRAYONS
(Binney & Smith)

Wax blend
Non-toxic pigments

PERMA-FLEX-IT
Plastic paste
(Baird Dynamic)

Polyester resins
Mineral fillers

PERMA-GYM-FINISH
Gymnasium coating
(Consolidated Chem., Inc.)

Phenolic resins in solvents *

PERMANITE
Resin
(Knight, M.A.)

Furfuryl alcohol polymer
Formaldehyde *
Furfuraldehyde *
Mixed amines

PERMANITE ACCELERATOR NO. 3 CONCENTRATE
(Knight, M.A.)

Phosphoric acid * 33%
Propyl alcohol *

PERMA-SEAL
Seals the pores to the surface
(Consolidated Chem., Inc.)

Phenolic resins in solvents *

PERMA-STA
Permanent anti-freeze
(Chemcentral)

Ethylene glycol base * .... >90%

PERMATOX 155
See CHAPMAN PERMATOX 155

PERMATOX 10-S
See CHAPMAN PERMATOX 10-S

PERMEATRATE SOLUTION
Pet care; treatment of constipation
(Haver-Lockhart (Brand) Bayvet Div. Cutter Labs.)

Dioctyl sodium sulfosuccinate 5%

PERMICIDE
Algicide
(Coastal Industries)

Copper sulfate * 6.5%
Citric acid 13.0%
EDTA 0.1%
Water

PERMITIL CHRONOTAB TABLETS
Psychopharmacologic agent
(Schering)

Each tablet:
Fluphenazine hydrochloride * .. 1 mg.

'76 Ed.

Starred ingredients (*) may be responsible for major toxic effects; consult Section II.

PERMITIL ORAL CONCENTRATE
Psychopharmacologic agent
(Schering)

Each cc.:
Fluphenazine hydrochloride * . . 5 mg.

PERMITIL TABLETS
Psychopharmacologic agent
(Schering)

Each tablet:
Fluphenazine
hydrochloride * . . 0.25 mg.; 2.5 mg.;
5 mg.; or 10 mg.

PERMOPLAST MODELING CLAY
(American Art Clay Co.)

This product bears the CP Seal issued by the Crayon, Water Color and Craft Institute, Inc. This seal certifies that the product contains no materials in sufficient quantities to be toxic or injurious to the human body even if ingested.

PERNOX
Lathering scrub cleanser for black-heads, oily skin & acne
(Westwood Pharm.)

Desquamex (brand of abradant microfine granules of polyethylene) with:
Sulfur 2%
Salicylic acid * 1.5%
Sebulytic (brand of penetrating, surface-active combination of soapless cleansers & wetting agents)

'76 Ed.

PEROXYL MOUTHRINSE
For cleansing minor oral lesions
(Hoyt Labs.)

Hydrogen peroxide * 1.5%

PERSA-GEL
Acne treatment
(Ortho-Dermatology)

Benzoyl peroxide 5%; 10%

PERT (Normal & Dry Hair)
Shampoo
(Procter & Gamble, Beauty Care Div.)

Sodium laureth sulfate * 20-25%
Cocamide MEA 1-5%
Myristic acid 1-5%
Glycol distearate 1-5%
Minor ingredients . . . . <1%
Alcohol SD-40 . . . . 1-5%
Water . . . . balance

PERT (Oily Hair)
Shampoo
(Procter & Gamble, Beauty Care Div.)

Sodium lauryl sulfate 8-10%
Sodium laureth sulfate * 8-10%
Cocamide MEA 1-5%
Myristic acid 1-5%
Glycol distearate 1-5%
Minor ingredients . . . . <1%
Alcohol SD-40 . . . . 1-5%
Water . . . . balance

PERTOFRANE CAPSULES
Treatment of depression
(USV)

Each capsule:
Desipramine   hydrochloride
(10,11-Dihydro-5(3-methyl-aminopropyl)-5H-dibenz(b,f)azepine
hydrochloride) * . . . . 25 mg.
or 50 mg.

PERTUSSIN 8 HOUR COUGH FORMULA
(Chesebrough-Pond's)

Each 100 ml.:
Alcohol (95%) . . . . 9.5 ml.
Dextromethorphan
hydrobromide* . . . . 150.0 mg.
Sodium citrate . . . . 1.5 gm.
Ammonium chloride . . . . 0.5 gm.
Chloroform (loss
unavoidable) . . . . 0.3 gm.

PERTUSSIN PLUS NIGHT-TIME COLD MEDICINE
Cough/cold symptomatic relief
(Chesebrough-Pond's)

Each fl. oz. (30 ml.):
Dextromethorphan
hydrobromide* . . . . 30 mg.
Acetaminophen* . . . . 600 mg.
Phenylephrine hydrochloride . . 10 mg.
Chlorpheniramine maleate . . . 2 mg.
Base:
Sucrose 45%
Glycerine 10%
Alcohol (by vol.)* 25%

PERTUSSIN WILD BERRY COUGH SYRUP
(Chesebrough-Pond's)

Each 100 ml.:
Dextromethorphan
hydrobromide* . . . . 70 mg.
Ammonium chloride . . . . 0.5 gm.
Sodium citrate . . . . 1.5 gm.
Chloroform (loss unavoidable) 0.2 gm.
Alcohol . . . . 9 ml.

PERUNA
Antitussive
(Consolid. Royal)

Alcohol 15%
Potassium iodide *
Iron citrate *
Ammonium citrate
Extr. Gentian
Extr. Boneset
Extr. Cascara sagrada
Oleoresin Ginger
USP Malt syrup
USP Extr. Licorice
USP Menthyl parasept
USP Riboflavin
USP Niacinamide
USP Citric acid
USP Calcium panothenate
USP Thiamine hydrochloride
USP Pyridoxine hydrochloride

'76 Ed.

PER-VAD
Low foaming acid sanitizer
(Diversey Wyandotte)

Sulfonated Oleic acid 2.6%
Phosphoric acid* 15.0%

PERVO PAINT PRODUCTS

The Pervo Paint Co.
6624 Stanford Ave.
Los Angeles, Calif. 90001

Phone: 213-758-1147

See PAINTS, Section VI, General Formulations

PER-ZENE-34
For use in drinking water-anthelmintic for hogs and poultry
(Texas Phenothiazine Co.)

Piperazine monohydrochloride . . . 44.1%

'76 Ed.

PEST-A-FOG
Insecticide
(Hess & Clark)

1,1,1-Trichloroethane * 68.5%
Baygon 1.0%
Dichlorvos and related compounds 0.5%
Propellant A-70 . . . . 30.0%

PES-TA-REST

See COLONIAL PES-TA-REST

PEST-B-GON INSECT BAIT
(Chevron)

2-(1-Methylethoxy)phenyl
methylcarbamate * 2%/w

Chevron emergency phone number:
415-233-3737

Starred ingredients (*) may be responsible for major toxic effects; consult Section II.

PETAL CLOSET FRESHNER
(Carson Chem. Corp.)

Paradichlorobenzene *	99%
Essential oil	1%

'76 Ed.

"PETALIFE"
Cut flower preservative
(Ampco Chem. Div.)

d-Glucose	95%
Combined amount:	5%
Detergent	
Trace elements	

PetDent
Canine dentifrice; veterinary
(Burns-Biotec)

Dibasic calcium phosphate
Potassium bitartrate
Sodium bicarbonate
Sodium lauryl sulfate *
Methylparaben (as preservative)
Propylparaben (as preservative)
Flavoring
Certified food coloring

PET-D-TICK, MARTIN'S

See MARTIN'S PET-D-TICK

PETERSON'S OINTMENT
For hemorrhoids; itching irritations
(Peterson)

Carbolic acid *	2.5%
Camphor *	
Tannic acid *	
Zinc oxide	
Beeswax	
Oil of lavender	
Petrolatum	

PET-GUARD GEL
Insecticide-repellent
(Carson Chemicals, Inc.)

Pyrethrins	0.1%
Technical Piperonyl butoxide	1.0%
Butoxypolypropylene glycol *	10.0%
Pine oil	2.0%

PETROGALAR, PHENOLPHTHALEIN
Laxative
(Wyeth Labs.)

Phenolphthalein	0.3%
In an aqueous suspension of Mineral oil	65%

PETROGALAR, PLAIN
Laxative
(Wyeth Labs.)

Aqueous suspension of Mineral oil	65%

PETRO-PHYLIC LIQUID SOAP
Antiseptic, skin cleanser, shampoo; veterinary
(Goshen Labs.)

Lecithin
Hexachlorophene
Coconut oil base

PETRO-SORB OIL & GREASE ABSORBENT
(Waverly Mineral Products Co.)

Aluminum-magnesium silicate	
Iron oxide	small amounts

PETROSYLLIUM NO. 1
Laxative
(Whitehall Labs.)

Mineral oil
Psyllium seed

PETROSYLLIUM NO. 2 WITH PHENOLPHTHALEIN
Cathartic
(Whitehall Labs.)

Each fl. oz.:	
Phenolphthalein	3 3/4 gr.
Mineral oil	
Psyllium jelly	

PETTIT PAINT PRODUCTS
Marine paints, varnishes, & specialties

Pettit Paint Co., Inc.
36 Pine St.
Rockaway, N.J. 07866

Phone: 201-625-3100

See PAINTS, Section VI, General Formulations

PFD HEAVY DUTY LAUNDRY DETERGENT (DRY)
(Industrial Equities)

Sodium chloride *	45-50%
Sodium carbonate *	30-35%
Nonionic surfactant	5-10%
Sodium silicate (not meta)	5-10%
Cellulosic	<2%
Fluorescent whitening agent	<1%
Perfume	<1%

PFIKLOR 10% LIQUID
Potassium supplement
(Pfizer)

Each 15 cc:	
Potassium chloride	1.5 gm.

PFIZER BLUE LOTION (Pump Spray)
Antiseptic; veterinary
(Pfizer Inc., Agricultural Div.)

Methylbenzenethonium chloride	0.50%
Menthol, Camphor, Chlorothymol	0.20%
Isopropyl alcohol	12.48%
Octoxynol	
Propylene glycol	
FD & C Blue #1	

PFIZER GLO-TOX
Insecticide
(Pfizer Inc., Agricultural Div.)

Toxaphene *	43.0%
Malathion	4.3%

PFIZER LIVESTOCK SPRAY (AEROSOL)
Insecticide
(Pfizer Inc., Agricultural Div.)

Pyrethrins	0.20%
Technical Piperonyl butoxide	0.40%
N-Octyl bicycloheptene dicarboximide	0.67%
Di-n-propyl isocinchomeronate	2.0%

PFIZER PINK EYE & WOUND DRESSING SPRAY (Pump Spray)
Veterinary
(Pfizer Inc., Agricultural Div.)

Sulfacetamide	8.0%
Sulfanilamide	1.0%
Sulfathiazole	0.3%
Azosulfamide	0.14%
Urea	

P&G BLUE DETERGENT
Institutional and industrial cleaning product

Procter & Gamble Co.
Ivorydale Technical Center
Cincinnati, Ohio 45217

Phone: 513-562-1100

pH 6.9
For chemical burns
(Bullard)

Monobasic Potassium phosphate *	68%
Dibasic Sodium phosphate USP *	13.4%
Benzalkonium chloride	1:5000
Disodium EDTA	1:2000

PHACID SHAMPOO
(Baker-Cummins)

Amphoteric surfactants

PHARMEX BLISTER CREAM
For chapped lips and fever blisters
(Pharmex)

Camphor *
Menthol *
Benzoin
Allantoin
Lanolin-petrolatum base

PHARMEX EAR DROPS
(Pharmex)

Benzocaine	0.15 gm.
Antipyrine *	0.70 gm.
Glycerol	q.s.

PHARMEX FIRST AID CREAM
Antiseptic, antihistamine, antibiotic cream
(Pharmex)

Tyrothricin *
Pyrilamine maleate *
Vitamins A & D
Bithionol
Benzocaine
Menthol *
Camphor *

PHARMEX FLU CAPSULES
(Pharmex)

Each two capsules:
Salicylamide *	10 gr.
Phenacetin *	2 1/2 gr.
Caffeine	1/2 gr.
Quinine *	2 gr.
Ascorbic	50 mg.

PHARMEX RECTAL SUPPOSITORIES
(Pharmex)

Bismuth subgallate
Bismuth oxyiodide
Peru balsam *
Resorcin *
Zinc oxide
Boric acid *

PHASE III
Deodorant bar
(Lever Bros.)

Acyl isethionate	45-55%
Fatty acids	15-25%
Sodium soap	10-15%
Water	5-10%
Sodium isethionate	1-5%
Anionic detergent	1-5%
Sodium chloride	<2%
Perfume	<1%
Germicide	<1%
Titanium dioxide	<1%
Colorants	trace

PHAZYME 95
Gastrointestinal gas relief
(Reed & Carnrick)

Outer layer:
Specially-activated Simethicone	25 mg.

Core:
Pancreatin	240 mg.
Specially-activated Simethicone	70 mg.

PHAZYME WITH PHENOBARBITAL
Relief of discomforts due to gastrointestinal gas
(Reed & Carnrick)

Each tablet:
Pancreatin, NF	240 mg.
Specially activated Simethicone	60 mg.
Phenobarbital *	15 mg.

PHENALGIN POWDER
Analgesic
(Etna Chem.)

Acetanilid *	50%
Ammonium carbonate	
Sodium bicarbonate	

'76 Ed.

PHENALGIN TABLETS
Analgesic
(Etna Chem.)

Each tablet:
Acetanilid *	1.25 gr.
Ammonium carbonate	
Sodium bicarbonate	

'76 Ed.

PHENAPHEN CAPSULES
Analgesic, antipyretic
(Robins)

Each capsule:
Acetaminophen, USP *	325 mg.

PHENAPHEN CAPSULES WITH CODEINE
Analgesic
(Robins)

Each capsule:
Acetaminophen, USP *	325 mg.
Codeine phosphate *	
No. 2 (black and yellow)	15 mg.
No. 3 (black and green)	30 mg.
No. 4 (green and white)	60 mg.

PHENAPHEN-650 WITH CODEINE
Analgesic
(Robins)

Each tablet:
Codeine phosphate, USP *	30 mg.
Acetaminophen, USP *	650 mg.

PHENATIN TD CAPSULE
(Jenkins Labs.)

Each capsule:
Phenylpropanolamine HCl *	50 mg.
Chlorpheniramine maleate	1 mg.
Pheniramine maleate	12.5 mg.
Atropine sulfate	0.025 mg.
Scopolamine hydrobromide	0.014 mg.
Belladonna alkaloids (total)	0.16 mg.
Hyoscyamine sulfate	0.122 mg.

PHENCASET IMPROVED
Analgesic-antipyretic
(Elder)

Each tablet:
Phenacetin *	150 mg.
Aspirin *	225 mg.
Caffeine	30 mg.
Aluminum hydroxide, dried gel	100 mg.

PHENDOFF
Antihistamine-decongestant
(Cameron Medical Corp.)

Each capsule:
Chlorpheniramine maleate	2 mg.
Phenylephrine HCl	5 mg.
Salicylamide *	200 mg.
Acetaminophen *	150 mg.
Caffeine	30 mg.

PHENE-O-CLEAN
Toilet bowl cleaner
(Hillyard Chem.)

Hydrochloric acid *

'76 Ed.

PHENERGAN COMPOUND
Nasal allergies, hay fever, sinusitis associated with pain or fever
(Wyeth Labs.)

Each tablet:
Promethazine hydrochloride	6.25 mg.
Pseudoephedrine hydrochloride *	60 mg.
Aspirin *	600 mg.

PHENERGAN-D
Nasal allergies, hay fever, sinusitis
(Wyeth Labs.)

Each tablet:
Promethazine hydrochloride	6.25 mg.
Pseudoephedrine hydrochloride *	60 mg.

PHENERGAN EXPECTORANT PEDIATRIC, WITH DEXTROMETHORPHAN
(Wyeth Labs.)

Each 5 ml.:
Dextromethorphan
  hydrobromide * .... 7.5 mg.
Promethazine hydrochloride ... 5 mg.
Fluidextract Ipecac .... 0.17 min.
Potassium guaiacolsulfonate ... 44 mg.
Citric acid, anhydrous ...... 60 mg.
Sodium citrate .... 197 mg.
Alcohol 7%

PHENERGAN EXPECTORANT PLAIN
(Wyeth Labs.)

Each 5 ml.:
Promethazine hydrochloride ... 5 mg.
Fluidextract Ipecac .... 0.17 min.
Potassium guaiacolsulfonate ... 44 mg.
Citric acid, anhydrous ...... 60 mg.
Sodium citrate .... 197 mg.
Alcohol 7%

PHENERGAN EXPECTORANT WITH CODEINE
(Wyeth Labs.)

Each 5 ml.:
Promethazine hydrochloride ... 5 mg.
Fluidextract Ipecac .... 0.17 min.
Potassium guaiacolsulfonate ... 44 mg.
Citric acid, anhydrous ...... 60 mg.
Sodium citrate .... 197 mg.
Codeine phosphate (1/6
  gr.) * .... 10 mg.
Alcohol 7%

PHENERGAN SUPPOSITORIES
Antihistaminic, antiemetic, sedative
(Wyeth Labs.)

Each suppository:
Promethazine
  hydrochloride * ... 12.5 mg.; 25 mg.;
                                  50 mg.
Ascorbyl palmitate
Silicon dioxide
White wax
Cocoa butter

PHENERGAN SYRUP
Antihistaminic, antiemetic, sedative
(Wyeth Labs.)

Each 5 ml.:
Promethazine
  hydrochloride * .... 6.25 mg.
Alcohol 1.5%

PHENERGAN SYRUP FORTIS
Antihistaminic, antiemetic, sedative
(Wyeth Labs.)

Each 5 ml.:
Promethazine hydrochloride * ... 25 mg.
Alcohol 1.5%

PHENERGAN TABLETS
Antihistaminic, antiemetic, sedative
(Wyeth Labs.)

Each tablet:
Promethazine
  hydrochloride * ... 12.5 mg.; 25 mg.;
                              or 50 mg.

PHENERGAN VC EXPECTORANT PLAIN
(Wyeth Labs.)

Each 5 ml.:
Promethazine hydrochloride ... 5 mg.
Phenylephrine
  hydrochloride * .... 5 mg.
Fluidextract Ipecac .... 0.17 min.
Potassium guaiacolsulfonate ... 44 mg.
Citric acid, anhydrous ...... 60 mg.
Sodium citrate .... 197 mg.
Alcohol 7%

PHENERGAN VC EXPECTORANT WITH CODEINE
(Wyeth Labs.)

Each 5 ml.:
Promethazine hydrochloride ... 5 mg.
Phenylephrine
  hydrochloride * .... 5 mg.
Fluidextract Ipecac .... 0.17 min.
Potassium guaiacolsulfonate ... 44 mg.
Citric acid, anhydrous ...... 60 mg.
Sodium citrate .... 197 mg.
Codeine phosphate (1/6
  gr.) * .... 10 mg.
Alcohol 7%

PHENETRON COMPOUND TABLETS
Antihistaminic
(Lannett)

Each tablet:
Aspirin * .... 390 mg.
Caffeine .... 32.4 mg.
Chlorprophenpyridamine
  maleate .... 2 mg.

PHENETRON SYRUP
Antihistaminic
(Lannett)

Each teaspoonful (5 ml.):
Chlorpheniramine maleate ..... 2 mg.

PHENISTIX
Urine phenylpyruvic acid test reagent strip
(Ames)

Ferric ammonium sulfate
Magnesium sulfate
Cyclohexylsulfamic acid

PHENO-BAR PINE DISINFECTANT
(Barco)

Pure steam distilled Pine oil *
Fatty acid emulsifier
Isopropanol *
Ortho-benzyl-para-chlorophenol *

'76 Ed.

PHENO-CEN
Germicidal detergent
(Central Chem.)

Isopropyl alcohol 10.0%
Ortho-benzyl-para-chlorophenol .. 7.20%
Para-tertiary amyl phenol * 4.30%
Ortho-phenolphenate 6.28%
4 Chloro 2 cyclo-pentylphenate ... 0.47%
4 Chloro 2 phenylphenate 0.31%

'76 Ed.

PHENOLAX WAFERS
Laxative
(Upjohn)

Each wafer:
Phenolphthalein .... 64.8 mg.
Sugar
Aromatics

PHENO-NUX
Sedative & digestive aid
(Vale)

Each tablet:
Phenobarbital * .... 16.2 mg.
Nux vomica extract * .... 8.1 mg.
Calcium carbonate .... 194.4 mg.

PHENO-NUX AND PEPSIN
Antiemetic
(Wesley Pharm.)

Each tablet:
Phenobarbital * .... 1/8 gr.
Ext. Nux vomica * .... 1/8 gr.
Saccharated Pepsin .... 1 gr.

PHENOPTIC 2.5%
Ophthalmic solution: used as an ocular decongestant and vasoconstrictor
(Muro Pharm.)

Phenylephrine HCl * 2.50%
Disodium EDTA .... trace
Monobasic sodium phosphate .... trace
Disodium sodium phosphate ..... trace
Sodium metabisulfite .... trace
Benzalkonium chloride 0.01%
Purified water .... qs ad

PHENOTROPINE #2
Antispasmodic, sedative
(Moffet Inc.)

Each tablet:
Phenobarbital * .... 15 mg.
Atropine sulfate .... 0.20 mg.

Starred ingredients (*) may be responsible for major toxic effects; consult Section II.

PHENSPRAY NASAL SPRAY
Decongestant-antiallergic
(Lannett)

Phenylephrine HCl *	0.25%
Pyrilamine maleate *	0.15%
Cetyl-dimethyl benzyl ammonium chloride	1:2000
Thimerosal (as preservative)	0.001%

PHENTERSPAN
Anorexiant
(Wesley Pharm.)

Each capsule:
  Phentermine * .... 30 mg.

PHENYLZIN OPHTHALMIC SOLUTION
Astringent, antiseptic, decongestant
(CooperVision Pharm.)

Zinc sulfate	0.25%
Phenylephrine HCl	0.12%
Boric acid *	
Sodium carbonate	
Potassium chloride	
Hydroxypropyl methylcellulose	
Sodium bisulfite	0.01%
Benzalkonium chloride	0.01%
Disodium edetate	0.01%

PHEOCAL PASTE
P.C.P. paste
(Torch)

Phenol (Carbolic acid)	1.0 gm.
Calomel (Mercurous chloride) *	3.0 gm.
Lassar's paste	ad 100.0 gm.

'76 Ed.

PHILLIPS' MILK OF MAGNESIA (REGULAR, FLAVORED)
Antacid-laxative
(Glenbrook Labs.)

Magnesium hydroxide .... 8.0 %

PHILLIPS' TABLETS
Antacid-laxative
(Glenbrook Labs.)

Each 4.8 gr. tablet:
  Phillips' Milk of Magnesia (1 tsp. or 4 ml.) in concentrated form equivalent to 311 mg. of magnesium hydroxide

pHisoAc
For acne
(Winthrop Labs.)

Colloidal Sulfur	6%
Resorcinol *	1.5%
Alcohol	10%

pHisoDan SHAMPOO
For dandruff
(Winthrop Labs.)

Sulfur	5%
Sodium salicylate	0.5%
Entsufon (Sodium octylphenoxyethoxy-ethyl ether sulfonate)	
Lanolin cholesterols	
Petrolatum	

pHisoDerm
Cleanses skin and scalp; detergent
(Winthrop Labs.)

Entsufon
Lanolin cholesterols
Petrolatum

pHisoHex
Antibacterial detergent
(Winthrop Labs.)

Entsufon (Sodium octylphenoxyethoxy-ethyl ether sulfonate)	
Hexachlorophene *	wt. basis 3%
Lanolin cholesterols	
Petrolatum	

pH MINUS
Reduces alkalinity (pH) in swim pool water
(Coastal Industries)

Sodium bisulphate *

PHOENIX CONCENTRATED DEGREASER AND MOTOR CLEANER
(Phoenix Oil)

Nonyl phenyl polyethylene glycol ether	7%
Petroleum hydrocarbon *	93%

PHOME #40
Liquid toilet soap
(National-Purity Soap)

Anhydrous Potash soap	40%
Vegetable oils, saponified	

PHOS-FLUR
Oral rinse supplement
(Hoyt Labs.)

Each 5 ml.:
  Fluoride (from 2.2 mg. sodium fluoride) .... 1.0 mg.
  M/10 Phosphate solution at a pH of 4

PHOS-FLUR CHEWABLE TABLETS
(Hoyt Labs.)

Each tablet:
  Fluoride (from 2.2 mg. sodium fluoride) * .... 1.0 mg.
  Acidulated phosphate

PHOSKIL 1 DUST

See NIAGARA PHOSKIL 1 DUST

PHOSKLEEN
Acid phosphate cleaner
(Whitfield Chem.)

Sodium or ammonium dihydrogen phosphate *† .... >10%

†*See* Sodium phosphate, monobasic

PHOSPHO-SODA (FLAVORED & UNFLAVORED)
(Fleet)

Each 100 ml.:
Sodium biphosphate	48 gm.
Sodium phosphate *	18 gm.

PHOSTOXIN FUMIGANT
New coated tablets
Coated pellets
(Phostoxin Sales)

Aluminum phosphide * 55%

pH PLUS
Raises pH in swim pool water
(Coastal Industries)

Sodium carbonate *

PHRENILIN
Analgesic
(Carnrick Labs.)

Each tablet:
Acetaminophen *	325 mg.
Sodium butabarbital	15 mg.
Caffeine	40 mg.

PHYLDROX
Bronchodilator
(Lemmon Co.)

Each tablet:
Neothylline (Dyphylline) *	100 mg.
Ephedrine sulfate *	25 mg.
Phenobarbital *	15 mg.

PHYLEX
Nasal spray
(Friendly Labs.)

Phenylephrine hydrochloride USP	1/4%
Methylparaben	0.02%
Propylparaben	0.01%
Sodium bisulfite	0.2%

PHYLORINOL
Oral antiseptic
(Schaffer)

Boric acid	0.60%
Viscarin	0.48%
Phenol	0.53%
Iodine (NF) *	0.60%
Chlorophyll	0.45%

Starred ingredients (*) may be responsible for major toxic effects; consult Section II.

PHYSAN 20
Disinfectant, sanitizer, deodorizer
(Consan Pacific)

n-Alkyl (60% C14, 30% C16, 5% C12,
  5% C18) dimethyl benzyl ammonium chlorides * 10%
n-Alkyl (68% C12, 32% C14) dimethyl
  ethylbenzyl ammonium
  chlorides * 10%

PHYSPAN & PHYSPAN-130
*For symptoms of asthma and broncho-
  spasm*
(Savage Labs.)

Each sustained release capsule:
  Theophylline (USP
    anhydrous) * ... 260 mg. or 130 mg.

PIC ANT TRAP
(Pic)

Borax 5.00%
Peanut butter 89.75%
Sugar 5.00%
Sodium benzoate 0.25%

PICFUME
Insecticide
(Dow)

Chloropicrin * 99%

PIC INSECT REPELLENT LOTION
(Pic)

Deet * 22.82%
Related Toluamides 1.20%
N-Octyl bicycloheptene
  dicarboximide 1.72%
Tetrahydro-2-furaldehyde ... 1.43%
Di-N-propyl isocinchomeronate 1.43%
Distilled water 71.40%

PIC INSIDE OUTSIDE BUG KILLER
(Pic)

Tetramethrin 0.20%
D-Phenothrin 0.20%
Petroleum distillate *

PIC MOSQUITO COILS
(Pic)

D-Allethrin 0.5%

PICTOL
Photo developer
(Mallinckrodt, Inc.)

Monomethyl-para-aminophenol sulfate *

PIC X-100 INSECT REPELLENT
(Pic)

Deet * 95%
Related Toluamides 5%

PIERCE II (Phosphate Formula or 0-Phosphate Formula)
*Institutional and industrial cleaning
  product*

Procter & Gamble Co.
Ivorydale Technical Center
Cincinnati, Ohio 45217

Phone: 513-562-1100

PIERCE & STEVENS PRODUCTS
*Coatings, floor finishes, & "Hybond"
  Contact Adhesive*

Pierce & Stevens Chemical Corp.
P.O. Box 1092
Buffalo, N.Y. 14240

Phone: 716-856-4910

See PAINTS, Section VI, General Formulations

PIERRE CARDIN PERFUMES

Pierre Cardin Parfums
630 Fifth Ave.
New York, N.Y. 10111

Phone: 212-489-2430

See COSMETICS, Section VI, General
  Formulations

PIG BOOSE SOLUBLE MEDICATED

See PURINA PIG BOOSE SOLUBLE
  MEDICATED

PIGEON-9
Pigeon control - municipal & farm use
(B&G Co.)

Strychnine alkaloid * .... 0.6%/wt.

PIGGLY WIGGLY LAUNDRY DETERGENT
Dry laundry detergent
(Great Atlantic & Pacific, mfr.; Piggly
  Wiggly Corp., dist.)

Sodium linear alkyl benzene
  sulfonate .... <17%
Sodium carbonate * .... <30%
Sodium silicate .... <10%
Sodium carboxymethylcellulose <2%
Optical brighteners .... <1%
Sodium chloride .... <10%
Blue dye .... trace
Sodium sulfate and moisture ... balance

PIK-UP
Dust mop and dust cloth treatment
(Hysan Corp.)

Isopropyl alcohol 5.00%
2,2'-Methylene bis(3,4,6-
  trichlorophenol) 0.25%
Ortho-benzyl para-chlorophenol 0.1125%
Petroleum distillate *

PILOCAR DROPPERETTES OPHTHALMIC SOLUTION
For treatment of glaucoma
(CooperVision Pharm.)

Pilocarpine
  hydrochloride * ...... 1%; 2% and 4%
Benzalkonium chloride 0.005%

PILOCAR OPHTHALMIC SOLUTION
For treatment of glaucoma
(CooperVision Pharm.)

Pilocarpine
  hydrochloride * 0.5%; 1%; 2%; 3%;
                        4% and 6%
Hydroxypropyl methylcellulose .. 0.33%
Benzalkonium chloride 0.01%
Disodium edetate 0.01%

PILODYNE OINTMENT
(International Chem.)

Each oz.:
  Benzocaine 3%
  Carbolic acid 1%
  Camphor 1%
  Menthol 1%
  Eucalyptus oil 0.1%
  Zinc oxide 5%
  Sulfur 5%
  Boric acid * 5%
  Balsam Peru 3%
  Petrolatum .... q.s.

'76 Ed.

PILOMIOTIN OPHTHALMIC SOLUTION
Miotic
(CooperVision Pharm.)

Each 15 ml.:
  Pilocarpine HCl * 1%; 2%; 4%
  Aqueous sol. of Boric acid
  Sodium carbonate
  Potassium chloride
  Benzalkonium chloride 0.01%
  Disodium edetate 0.01%

PIMA SYRUP
Expectorant
(Fleming)

Each teaspoon:
  Potassium iodide * .... 5 gr.

PIMPLEX MORNING SCRUB
Skin cleanser; for acne control
(Jeffrey Martin, Inc.)

Active ingred.:
Polyethylene granules	18.0%
Sulfur	1.4%
p-Chloro-m-xylenol	0.5%
Allantoin calcium pantothenate	0.10%

Also contains:
Purified water
Sodium laureth sulfate
Cetearyl alcohol
Lauryl betaine
Cocamide DEA
Ceteareth-20
Glycol stearate
Sodium sulfite
Fragrance *†
Ext. D & C Yellow #7

†*See* Essential oils

PIMPLEX NIGHTIME GEL
Drying aid for acne
(Jeffrey Martin, Inc.)

Active ingred.:
p-Chloro-m-xylenol	0.5%
Allantoin calcium pantothenate	0.1%
Ethyl alcohol	67.7%/v

Also contains:
Purified water
Laneth-10 acetate
Diisopropanolamine
Carbomer-940
Fragrance *†
FD & C Blue #1

†*See* Essential oils

PIMPLEX SKIN CLEANSING LOTION
For acne control; skin cleanser
(Jeffrey Martin, Inc.)

Each 4 and 8 oz. bottle:
Purified water
Alcohol-SD40
Witch hazel
Polysorbate-80
Benzoic acid
Fragrance *†
Boric acid *
p-Chloro-m-xylenol
Allantoin calcium pantothenate
FD & C Blue #1

†*See* Essential oils

PINALENE DISINFECTANT
See C-Z PINALENE DISINFECTANT

PINAUD'S EAU DE PORTUGAL & EAU DE QUININE
(Pinaud)

Denatured ethyl alcohol *	>10%
Perfume essence	1-10%

PINCOTAL
Antacid, sedative, spasmolytic combination
(King Pharmaceutical)

Each 5 cc:
Calcium aluminum carbonate di-amino acetate	0.5 gm.
Calcium carbonate	1 mg.
Mephobarbital sodium	8 mg.
Hyoscyamine sulfate	0.0519 mg.
Atropine sulfate	0.0097 mg.
Hyoscine hydrobromide	0.0032 mg.

PINEL
Disinfectant, deodorant
(Consolidated Chem., Inc.)

Steam-distilled Pine oil *
Soap
Inorganic phosphates *
Isopropanol *
Ortho-benzyl-para-chlorophenol *

PINE-O-CIDE
Cleaner
(Hillyard Chem.)

Pine oil *

'76 Ed.

PINE-OLA PLUS
Disinfectant cleaner
(Holcomb)

Caustic potash *	1-10%
Santophen	1-10%

'76 Ed.

PINE PLUS
Pine oil cleaner and deodorizer
(Cole, H.A.)

Pine oil *	32.0%
Soap	11.3%
Isopropyl alcohol	9.2%
Water	47.5%

PINEUTUSS DM SYRUP
Cough syrup
(Elder)

Each 15 ml.:
Ammonium chloride	324.0 mg.
Dextromethorphan hydrobromide	15.0 mg.
Alcohol	5.0%

PINEX CONCENTRATE
Cough syrup for reconstitution
(Alvin Last)

Dextromethorphan hydrobromide	<1%
Alcohol (USP)	3%

PINEX REGULAR
Cough syrup
(Alvin Last)

Dextromethorphan hydrobromide	<0.2%
Alcohol (USP)	3.0%

PINK BLISTER
Counterirritant, analgesic, anti-inflammatory; veterinary
(Goshen Labs.)

Red mercuric iodide *	3.75%
Iodine *	1.87%
Menthol *	
Methyl salicylate *	
Oil of cedarwood *	
Oil of origanum *	
Alcohol	82.00%

PINK LADY AUTOMATIC DISHWASHER DETERGENT
(Industrial Equities)

Sodium chloride *	45-55%
Sodium tripolyphosphate	30-40%
Sodium silicate (not meta)	5-10%
Nonionic surfactant	1-3%
Sodium dichloro-s-triazinetrione	1-3%

PINK LADY CONCENTRATED FABRIC SOFTENER
(Industrial Equities)

Quaternary ammonium compound *	5-10%
Fluorescent whitening agent	<1%
Preservative	<1%
Colorant	<1%
Perfume	<1%
Water	balance

PINK LADY HEAVY DUTY LAUNDRY DETERGENT (DRY)
(Industrial Equities)

Sodium chloride *	45-50%
Sodium carbonate *	30-35%
Nonionic surfactant	5-10%
Sodium silicate (not meta)	5-10%
Cellulosic	<2%
Fluorescent whitening agent	<1%
Perfume	<1%

PINK LADY LIQUID DISHWASHING DETERGENT
(Industrial Equities)

Anionic surfactant	6-12%
Hydrotrope	1-3%
Alkanolamide	<1%
Ethyl alcohol	<1%
Opacifier	<1%
Colorant	<1%
Perfume	<1%
Water	balance

PINK STUFF
Liquid hand soap
(Paul Koss)

Potassium coco soaps
Tetrasodium EDTA
Dye
Perfume
Formalin
Water

Starred ingredients (*) may be responsible for major toxic effects; consult Section II.

PINTOFF PAINT & VARNISH REMOVER
(International Paint)

Methylene chloride *
Color code #199 contains Methanol *

PIONEER ACTION GERMICIDAL CLEANER
Disinfectant for hospital use
(Pioneer)

n-Alkyl (60% C14, 30% C16, 5% C12, 5% C18) dimethyl benzyl ammonium chlorides *	2.25%
n-Alkyl (68% C12, 32% C14) dimethyl ethylbenzyl ammonium chlorides *	2.25%
Sodium carbonate	3.00%
Tetrasodium ethylenediamine tetraacetate	1.00%

PIONEER CONTROL-35 GERMICIDAL CLEANER
Disinfectant for hospital use
(Pioneer)

Didecyl dimethyl ammonium chloride *	4.5%
Tetrasodium ethylenediamine tetraacetate	2.0%
Sodium carbonate	1.0%
Sodium metasilicate	0.5%

PIONEER GERMOTOX
Disinfectant deodorant; hospital grade
(Pioneer)

Soap	0.05%
Sodium o-phenylphenate	0.05%
4-Chloro-2-cyclopentylphenol	0.03%
p-tert.-Amylphenol	0.01%
Isopropyl alcohol	0.10%
Essential oils	0.80%
Tetrasodium ethylenediamine tetraacetate	0.07%

PIPCIDE TABLETS
An anthelmintic for dogs and cats
(Haver-Lockhart (Brand) Bayvet Div. Cutter Labs.)

Piperazine citrate (anhydrous) . . 7.5 gm.

PIPERSOL
Anthelmintic; dogs and cats
(Burns-Biotec)

Each ml.:
Piperazine citrate (equiv. to 100 mg. piperazine hexahydrate, equiv. to 44 mg. piperazine base) . . . . 110 mg.
In a flavored syrup preserved with Methylparaben and Propylparaben

PIPERTAB-2 & PIPERTAB-10
Wormer for dogs and cats
(Burns-Biotec)

Each #2 tablet:
Piperazine dihydrochloride (equiv. to 50 mg. piperazine base)

Each #10 tablet:
Piperazine dihydrochloride (equiv. to 250 mg. piperazine base)

PIPRA-POWDER "53"
See ANCHOR PIPRA-POWDER "53"

PIRIMOR 50W
Insecticide for the control of aphids
(ICI Americas)

Pirimicarb * 50%

piSEC
Drying gel for acne
(Owen Labs.)

Ethoxylate
Colloidal Sulfur

PIT STOP
Odor control of poultry and animal wastes
(Salsbury)

Norwegian seaweed extract
Natural steroid Saponins

PITTCLOR CALCIUM HYPOCHLORITE
For water purification
(PPG Industries, Chem. Div.)

Calcium hypochlorite *	65%
Sodium chloride *	30%
Inactive calcium compounds	

PITTS CARMINATIVE
(Commerce Drug)

Blackberry root	
Jamaica ginger	
Oil anise	
Oil nutmeg *	
Refined sugar	
Alcohol	2%

PIVAL CONCENTRATE
Rodenticide
(Motomco)

2-Pivalyl-1,3-indandione 0.5%

PIVALYN CONCENTRATE WATER SOLUBLE
Rodenticide
(Motomco)

Sodium salt of 2-pivalyl-1,3-indandione * 1.5%

PIVALYN, WATER SOLUBLE
Rodenticide
(Motomco)

Sodium salt of 2-pivalyl-1,3-indandione 0.14%

PK GLASS CLEANER
(Paul Koss)

Water	>99%
Isopropyl alcohol	
Wetting agent	

PK OIL BREAK
Carpet spotter
(Paul Koss)

Butyl Cellosolve *	15%
Tall oil fatty acid	
Kerosene	5%
Tetrasodium EDTA	
Monoethanolamine	
Sodium sulfite	<1%
Water	balance

pH 9.0-9.2

P.K.P. LIQUID
Antidiarrheal
(Wesley Pharm.)

Each fl. oz.:
Opium	16 mg.
Kaolin	90 gr.
Pectin	2 gr.

PL-200
Construction adhesive
(Goodrich, B.F.)

Rubber solvent *	15-25%/vol.
Hexane *	30-40%/vol.
Isopropanol	10% max./vol.

PL-400
Construction adhesive
(Goodrich, B.F.)

Hexane *	30-40%/vol.
Toluene *	10-20%/vol.

PLA
See TESTOR'S PLA

PLACE PACK RAT CONTROL
See PURINA PLACE PACK RAT CONTROL

PLACIDYL
Sedative, hypnotic
(Abbott)

Each capsule:
Ethchlorvynol * . . . . 100 mg.; 200 mg.; 500 mg.; or 750 mg.

PLANTABBS AQUARIUM PLANT FOOD
(Plantabbs)

Nitrate nitrogen	7.25%
Ammoniacal nitrogen	3.75%
Total available Nitrogen	11.00%
Available Phosphoric acid	15.00%
Potash, water soluble	20.00%

PLANTABBS LIQUID PLANT FOOD
(Plantabbs)

Nitrogen (as urea)	10%
Phosphoric acid (as phosphoric acid, di potassium phosphate)	10%
Potash (as di potassium phosphate)	10%
Chlorine	not more than 0.05%

PLANTABBS SOLUBLE PLANT FOOD (POWDER & TABLETS)
(Plantabbs)

Nitrate nitrogen	7.25%
Ammoniacal nitrogen	3.75%
Total available Nitrogen	11.00%
Available Phosphoric acid	15.00%
Potash, water soluble	20.00%
Chlorine	not more than 0.05%

PLANTAMUCIN GRANULES
Gastro-intestinal
(Elder)

Mucinoid fraction of blond Psyllium seed (Plantago ovata)
Gum karaya
Brewer's yeast

PLANTFUME 103 SMOKE GENERATOR
Insecticide
(Plant Prod.)

Tetraethyl dithionopyrophosphate * 15%

PLANT MARVEL AFRICAN VIOLET INSECTICIDE SPRAY
(Plant Marvel)

Pyrethrins	0.0255%
Rotenone	0.128%
Other cube extractives	0.236%
Technical Piperonyl butoxide	0.256%
Petroleum hydrocarbon	0.102%

PLANT MARVEL I-BOMB INSECTICIDE SPRAY
Insecticide
(Plant Marvel)

Pyrethrins	0.0255%
Rotenone	0.128%
Other cube extractives	0.236%
Technical Piperonyl butoxide	0.256%
Petroleum hydrocarbon	0.102%

PLANT O-TWO
Provides oxygen for plant water & soil conditioning
(Lake Products)

Each 7 gr. tablet:

Barium peroxide *	32.59%
Calcium sulfate	30.17%
Calcium phosphate	29.44%
Manganese dioxide	4.86%
Sodium sulfite	0.03%
Amorphous carbon	2.92%

PLANT PRODUCTS NICOTINE PRESSURE FUMIGATOR
(Plant Prod.)

Nicotine (expressed as alkaloid 14%) *

PLANT PRODUCTS TEDION-DITHIO PRESSURE FUMIGATOR
(Plant Prod.)

O,O,O,O-Tetraethyl dithio-pyrophosphate *	12.5%
Tetradifon (p-Chlorophenyl 2,4,5 trichlorophenyl sulfone)	15.0%

"PLANT SHINE"
(Schultz Co.)

Water
Waxes
Resins
Emulsifiers

PLANTVAX-5L
Systemic fungicide
(Uniroyal Chem.)

Oxycarboxin	5%
Inerts	95%
Mainly Diacetone alcohol (acetone free) *	

PLANTVAX 75W
Systemic fungicide
(Uniroyal Chem.)

Oxycarboxin *	75%
Inerts	25%
Related compounds	
Wetting agents	

PLAQUENIL SULFATE
For malaria, lupus erythematosus, and rheumatoid arthritis
(Winthrop Labs.)

Each tablet:

Hydroxychloroquine sulfate, USP (equiv. to 155 mg. of base) *	200 mg.

PLASTIC GLOSS
Chemical cleaner, synthetic detergent
(National-Purity Soap)

Nonionic and anionic surface active agents *

PLASTIC PAINT PRODUCTS

Plastic Co. of America
6542 N. Sheridan Rd.
Chicago, Ill. 60626

Phone: 312-274-0800

See PAINTS, Section VI, General Formulations

PLASTIC WOOD
(Boyle-Midway)

Nitrocellulose	
Wood flour	
Combined amount:	>10%
Aliphatic ketones *	
Toluene *	
Alcohol	
Resin	
Plasticizers	
Dyes for colored wood	

PLASTIC WOOD SOLVENT
(Boyle-Midway)

Mixture of:	100%
Aliphatic ketone *	
Toluene *	

PLASTI-GLAZE
(Gibson-Homans)

Linseed, soya & fish oils	>10%
Petroleum thinner	1-5%
Whiting	>80%
Asbestos fiber	2%

PLASTI-KOTE AUTO TOP GUARD (CLEAR SATIN FINISH 404-1404)
Protects car tops against stains and fading
(Plasti-Kote)

Pigment:	0.65%
Zinc stearate	100.0%
Vehicle, non-volatile:	7.49%
Vinyl resin	52.0%
Acrylic resin	32.0%
Dioctyl phthalate	16.0%
Vehicle, volatile:	72.86%
Aromatic hydrocarbons *	
Ketones *	
Propellant:	19.00%
Propane hydrocarbons	100.0%

PLASTI-KOTE AUTO TOP SPRAY (BLACK 401-1401)
Restores vinyl car tops
(Plasti-Kote)

Pigment:	1.38%
Carbon black	70.0%
Silicates	30.0%
Vehicle, non-volatile:	6.97%
Acrylic resin	25.5%
Vinyl copolymer resin	61.8%
Plasticizer	12.7%
Vehicle, volatile:	72.65%
Aromatic hydrocarbon *	3.4%
Aliphatic hydrocarbon	2.3%
Ketones *	94.1%
Perfume	0.2%
Propellant:	19.00%
Aliphatic hydrocarbon	100.0%

Starred ingredients (*) may be responsible for major toxic effects; consult Section II.

PLASTI-KOTE AUTO TOP SPRAY (FLAT BLACK 405-1405)
Restores vinyl car tops
(Plasti-Kote)

Pigment:	2.19%
Carbon black	33.0%
Silicates	67.0%
Vehicle, non-volatile:	7.98%
Acrylic resin	25.5%
Vinyl copolymer resin	61.8%
Plasticizer	12.7%
Vehicle, volatile:	70.83%
Aromatic hydrocarbon *	3.4%
Ketones *	96.4%
Perfume	0.2%
Propellant:	19.00%
Aliphatic hydrocarbon	100.0%

PLASTI-KOTE CHOKE AND CARBURETOR CLEANER
(Plasti-Kote)

Xylol *
Methylene chloride *
Petroleum distillates *

PLASTI-KOTE COMPETITION COLORS (CANDY APPLE BLUE 301-1301)
(Plasti-Kote)

Pigment:	0.46%
Phthalo blue	100.0%
Vehicle, non-volatile:	13.32%
Cellulose nitrate	
Maleic resin	
Castor oil alkyd	
Dioctyl phthalate	
Vehicle, volatile:	67.22%
Aromatic hydrocarbons *	
Esters	
Alcohol	
Ketones *	
Propellant:	19.00%
Propane hydrocarbons	100.0%

PLASTI-KOTE COMPETITION COLORS (CANDY APPLE GOLD 306-1306)
(Plasti-Kote)

Pigment:	10.01%
Gold bronze powder *	100.0%
Vehicle, non-volatile:	6.16%
Acrylic resin	100.0%
Vehicle, volatile:	60.83%
Aliphatic hydrocarbons *	91.0%
Ketones	9.0%
Propellant:	23.0%
Propane hydrocarbons	100.0%

PLASTI-KOTE COMPETITION COLORS (CANDY APPLE RED 300-1300)
(Plasti-Kote)

Pigment:	0.50%
Scarlet toner	100.0%
Vehicle, non-volatile:	13.90%
Cellulose nitrate	
Maleic resin	
Non-oxidizing Castor oil alkyd	
Dioctyl phthalate	
Vehicle, volatile:	66.60%
Esters and Ketones *	94.5%
Aromatic hydrocarbons *	5.5%
Propellant:	19.00%
Propane hydrocarbons	100.0%

PLASTI-KOTE COMPETITION COLORS METAL FLAKE (RED 310-1310)
(Plasti-Kote)

Pigment:	0.91%
Standard lining Aluminum powder	44.5%
Scarlet toner	55.5%
Vehicle, non-volatile:	13.90%
Cellulose nitrate	
Maleic resin	
Castor oil alkyd	
Dioctyl phthalate	
Vehicle, volatile:	66.19%
Aromatic hydrocarbons *	
Esters	
Ketones	
Alcohols	
Propellant:	19.00%
Propane hydrocarbons	100.0%

PLASTI-KOTE DEGREASER AND MOTOR CLEANER
(Plasti-Kote)

Non-volatile:	
Nonionic surface active agent	6.80%
Volatile:	
Aromatic hydrocarbons *	78.20%
Propellant:	
Aliphatic hydrocarbons	15.00%

PLASTI-KOTE EASY WAY RUST NOT (RED OXIDE PRIMER 243-1243)
Metal paint
(Plasti-Kote)

Pigment:	12.71%
Red iron oxide	36.0%
Titanium dioxide	5.0%
Magnesium silicate	58.7%
Anti-settling agent	0.3%
Vehicle, non-volatile:	10.78%
Medium Soya alkyd resin	100.0%
Vehicle, volatile:	53.51%
VM&P naphtha	28.0%
Xylol *	65.0%
Acetone	7.0%
Propellant:	23.00%
Aliphatic hydrocarbon	100.0%

PLASTI-KOTE EASY WAY RUST NOT (SHAMROCK GREEN 258-1258)
Metal paint
(Plasti-Kote)

Pigment:	1.66%
Phthalo green	33.0%
Ferrite yellow	42.0%
Titanium dioxide	18.0%
Benzidine yellow	7.0%
Vehicle, non-volatile:	14.78%
Modified Tall oil alkyd	100.0%
Vehicle, volatile:	60.56%
Aromatic hydrocarbon *	25.0%
Ketones and Esters	75.0%
Propellant:	23.00%
Aliphatic hydrocarbons	100.0%

PLASTI-KOTE ENGINE ENAMEL (ALUMINUM 207)
(Plasti-Kote)

Pigment:	4.39%
Standard Aluminum lining paste	100.0%
Vehicle, non-volatile:	6.93%
Acrylic alkyd resin	100.0%
Vehicle, volatile:	65.68%
Aromatic hydrocarbon *	77.0%
Ketones	23.0%
Propellant:	23.00%
Aliphatic hydrocarbon	100.0%

PLASTI-KOTE ENGINE ENAMEL (FORD RED 206)
(Plasti-Kote)

Pigment:	2.74%
Toluidine red	38.0%
Molybdate orange *	62.0%
Vehicle, non-volatile:	14.44%
Modified Tall oil alkyd resin	100.0%
Vehicle, volatile:	59.82%
Aromatic hydrocarbon *	24.4%
Ketones *	66.3%
Esters	8.3%
Alcohol	1.0%
Propellant:	23.00%
Propane hydrocarbon	100.0%

PLASTI-KOTE ENGINE ENAMEL (UNIVERSAL BLACK 203)
(Plasti-Kote)

Pigment:	0.59%
Carbon black	100.0%
Vehicle, non-volatile:	13.64%
Modified Tall oil alkyd	100.0%
Vehicle, volatile:	62.77%
Aromatic hydrocarbons *	24.0%
Esters	8.0%
Ketones *	68.0%
Propellant:	23.00%
Propane hydrocarbons	100.0%

Starred ingredients (*) may be responsible for major toxic effects; consult Section II.

PLASTI-KOTE ENGINE ENAMEL (UNIVERSAL GRAY 202)
(Plasti-Kote)

Pigment:	3.67%
Titanium dioxide	95.0%
Carbon black	4.0%
Phthalo green	1.0%
Vehicle, non-volatile:	13.64%
Modified Tall oil alkyd	100.0%
Vehicle, volatile:	59.69%
Aromatic hydrocarbons *	
Ketones *	
Propellant:	23.00%
Propane hydrocarbons	100.0%

PLASTI-KOTE ENGINE ENAMEL (UNIVERSAL RED 209)
(Plasti-Kote)

Pigment:	2.11%
Toluidine red	54.0%
Molybdate orange *	35.0%
Titanium dioxide	11.0%
Vehicle, non-volatile:	14.35%
Modified Tall oil alkyd resin	100.0%
Vehicle, volatile:	60.54%
Aromatic hydrocarbon *	23.7%
Ketones *	67.3%
Esters	8.0%
Alcohol	1.0%
Propellant:	23.00%
Propane hydrocarbon	100.0%

PLASTI-KOTE FAST DRY SPRAY PAINT (GLOSS BLACK T-1)
(Plasti-Kote)

Pigment:	0.59%
Carbon black	100.0%
Vehicle, non-volatile:	13.64%
Modified Tall oil alkyd	100.0%
Vehicle, volatile:	62.77%
Aromatic hydrocarbons *	24.0%
Esters	8.0%
Ketones	68.0%
Propellant:	23.00%
Propane hydrocarbons	100.0%

PLASTI-KOTE FAST DRY SPRAY PAINT (GRAY METAL PRIMER T-18)
(Plasti-Kote)

Pigment:	12.94%
Titanium dioxide	43.0%
Magnesium silicate	56.0%
Lampblack	0.7%
Anti-settling agent	0.3%
Vehicle, non-volatile:	10.67%
Medium Soya alkyd resin	100.0%
Vehicle, volatile:	53.39%
VM&P naphtha	26.0%
Xylol *	67.0%
Acetone	7.0%
Propellant:	23.00%
Aliphatic hydrocarbon	100.0%

PLASTI-KOTE HAMMER FINISH SPRAY PAINT (COPPER HAMMER FINISH 216)
(Plasti-Kote)

Pigment:	3.55%
Non-leafing Aluminum	37.3%
Yellow iron oxide	37.6%
Red iron oxide	25.1%
Vehicle, non-volatile:	23.75%
Soya alkyd resin	100.0%
Vehicle, volatile:	53.70%
Aromatic hydrocarbons *	46.0%
Aliphatic hydrocarbons	22.1%
Chlorinated solvents	15.9%
Ketones	6.0%
Propellant:	19.00%
Propane hydrocarbons	100.0%

PLASTI-KOTE HOT PAINT (BLACK HP-1/11)
Heat resistant paint
(Plasti-Kote)

Pigment:	5.60%
Black iron oxide	50.0%
Silicates	31.0%
Suspended agents	19.0%
Vehicle, non-volatile:	2.24%
Silicone resin	65.0%
Acrylic resin	35.0%
Vehicle, volatile:	62.16%
Aromatic hydrocarbon *	66.0%
M C L	34.0%
Propellant:	30.00%
Aliphatic hydrocarbon	100.0%

PLASTI-KOTE HOT PAINT (RED HP-3/13)
Heat resistant paint
(Plasti-Kote)

Pigment:	3.21%
Cadmium red	59.0%
Diatomaceous earth	32.9%
Suspending agent	2.2%
Vehicle, non-volatile:	4.20%
Silicone acrylic resin	100.0%
Vehicle, volatile:	62.59%
Aromatic hydrocarbons *	65.0%
Methylene chloride	35.0%
Propellant:	30.00%
Aliphatic hydrocarbons	100.0%

PLASTI-KOTE HOT PAINT (WHITE HP-2/12)
Heat resistant paint
(Plasti-Kote)

Pigment:	13.03%
Titanium dioxide	65.75%
Diatomaceous earth	38.80%
Suspending agent	1.35%
Vehicle, non-volatile:	2.05%
Silicone resin	100.00%
Vehicle, volatile:	54.92%
Aromatic hydrocarbons *	67.00%
Methylene chloride	33.00%
Propellant:	30.00%
Aliphatic hydrocarbon	100.00%

PLASTI-KOTE RUST PENETRANT AND DEMOISTURANT
(Plasti-Kote)

Xylol *
Methylene chloride *

PLASTI-KOTE SILVER FAST DRY SPRAY PAINT
(Plasti-Kote)

Pigment:	4.39%
Standard Aluminum lining paste	100.0%
Vehicle, non-volatile:	6.93%
Acrylic alkyd resin	100.0%
Vehicle, volatile:	65.68%
Aromatic hydrocarbon *	77.0%
Ketones	23.0%
Propellant:	23.00%
Aliphatic hydrocarbon	100.0%

PLASTI-KOTE SPRA-CLEAR
Clear acrylic spray
(Plasti-Kote)

Vehicle, non-volatile:	6.28%
Acrylic resin	100.0%
Vehicle, volatile:	70.72%
Aromatic hydrocarbons *	44.0%
Methylene chloride	26.2%
Ketones	29.8%
Propellant:	23.00%
Propane hydrocarbon	100.0%

PLASTI-KOTE SPRA-WAY PAINT & VARNISH REMOVER
(Plasti-Kote)

Non-volatile:	1.2%
Crude scale wax	
Ethyl cellulose	
Volatile:	73.8%
Esters	
Alcohol	
Halogenated solvents *†	
Propellant:	25.0%
Propane hydrocarbons *	

†*See* Chlorinated solvents

PLASTI-KOTE VINYL SPRAY (BLACK 411-1411)
(Plasti-Kote)

Pigment:	1.38%
Carbon black	70.0%
Silicates	30.0%
Vehicle, non-volatile:	6.97%
Acrylic resin	25.5%
Vinyl copolymer resin	61.8%
Plasticizer	12.7%
Vehicle, volatile:	72.65%
Aromatic hydrocarbon *	3.4%
Aliphatic hydrocarbon	2.3%
Ketones *	94.1%
Perfume	0.2%
Propellant:	19.00%
Aliphatic hydrocarbon	100.0%

Starred ingredients (*) may be responsible for major toxic effects; consult Section II.

PLASTI-KOTE VINYL SPRAY (GOLD 418-1418)
(Plasti-Kote)

Pigment:	2.94%
Lampblack	0.28%
Phthalo green	0.06%
Brown iron oxide	0.99%
Standard Aluminum lining	8.25%
Yellow iron oxide	66.02%
Titanium dioxide	3.77%
Silicates	20.63%
Vehicle, non-volatile:	6.13%
Acrylic resin	26.40%
Vinyl copolymer resin	60.40%
Plasticizer	13.20%
Vehicle, volatile:	71.93%
Aromatic hydrocarbon *	3.38%
Aliphatic hydrocarbon	2.25%
Ketones *	94.20%
Perfume	0.17%
Propellant:	19.00%
Propane hydrocarbon	100.00%

PLASTI-MEND
Liquid plastic - repairs, seals vinyls
(NIP-CO)

Methyl ethyl ketone *
Cyclohexanone *

PLASTOID FURNACE CEMENT
(Gibson-Homans)

Sodium silicate *	>10%
Asbestos fiber	1-10%
Whiting	>10%
Water	>10%

PLASTOID PUTTY
(Gibson-Homans)

Linseed, soya oils	2-5%
Petroleum thinner	1-10%
Whiting	>80%

PLATINE SPRAY COLOGNE
Aerosol - 3 oz.
(Dana Perfumes)

Essential oils *	>1%

Aromatic chemicals
Specially denatured Alcohol (39-C) *
Distilled water
Dichlorofluoromethane
Dichlorotetrafluoroethane

PLAYTIME WATER COLORS
(Binney & Smith)

Water-soluble base
Organic plasticizer
Non-toxic pigments

PL CHAIN & CABLE LUBRICANT (Aerosol)
For use in industry and municipalities
(Precision Labs.)

Petroleum distillates *

PL-350 DEOXIDIZING CLEANER
Institutional, municipal and industrial use
(Precision Labs.)

Hydrogen chloride *

PL DEVASTATE 1 NON-SELECTIVE WEED KILLER
(Precision Labs.)

Petroleum oil *	96.64%
2,4-Dichlorophenoxyacetic acid, isooctyl ester	1.10%
Bromacil	0.61%
Pentachlorophenol	0.79%
Other chlorophenols	0.09%

PL DI-KILL
General and aquatic weed control
(Precision Labs.)

Diquat dibromide *	1.85%

PLEASANT PELLETS, DR. PIERCE'S

See DR. PIERCE'S PLEASANT PELLETS

PLEASANT RELIEF

See RAWLEIGH PLEASANT RELIEF

PLEASE CAR CLEANER CONCENTRATE
(Arrow Labs.)

Sodium alkyl aryl sulfate *
Triethanolamine lauryl sulfate *
Fatty amide-condensate
Anhydrous fatty acid-amine condensate
Sulfonated ketones
Hydrophilic wax-cyclohexanone-amine wax

'76 Ed.

PLEASE LEATHER CLEANER
(Arrow Labs.)

Mineral spirits *

'76 Ed.

PLEASE WHITE WALL TIRE CLEANER
(Arrow Labs.)

Sodium metasilicate
Isopropyl alcohol *

'76 Ed.

PLEXADINE SHAMPOO
For dogs and horses; antibacterial, antifungal
(Bio-Ceutic)

Nonylphenoxypoly (ethyleneoxy) ethanol-iodine complex *	5%
Inert ingred.:	95%

Lauryldimethylamine oxide
Lauric acid-diethanolamine condensate
Polyethylene glycol ether of linear alcohol
Modified Oxyethylated straight chain alcohol
Distilled water

PLEXADINE SOLUTION
Topical antiseptic; veterinary
(Bio-Ceutic)

Nonylphenoxypoly (ethyleneoxy) ethanol-iodine complex *	12.5%
Isopropyl alcohol *	65.0%

PLEXONAL TABLETS
Sedative, hypnotic
(Sandoz)

Each tablet:	
Sodium barbital *	45.00 mg.
Sodium butalbital *	25.00 mg.
Sodium phenobarbital USP *	15.00 mg.
Dihydroergotamine mesylate USP	0.16 mg.
Scopolamine hydrobromide USP	0.08 mg.

PLEXTONE PAINT PRODUCTS

Plextone Corp. of America
2141 McCarter Hwy.
Newark, N.J. 07104

Phone: 201-484-4443

See PAINTS, Section VI, General Formulations

PL E-Z WEED "B" HERBICIDE
(Precision Labs.)

Dimethylamine salt of 2-(2-methyl-4-chlorophenoxy)propionic acid *	16.2%
Dimethylamine salt of 2,4-dichlorophenoxyacetic acid *	16.1%

PL FAST STARTING FLUID
(Aerosol)
For all gasoline and diesel engines
(Precision Labs.)

Ethyl ether *
Petroleum hydrocarbons *

Starred ingredients (*) may be responsible for major toxic effects; consult Section II.

PL GRANULAR SOIL STERILANT
Herbicide; municipal and industrial use
(Precision Labs.)

Sodium chlorate *	40.0%
Sodium metaborate *	55.2%
Monuron	2.4%

PLIAGEL
Cleaning solution for soft (hydrophyllic) contact lenses
(CooperVision Pharm.)

Poloxamer 407
Sorbic acid (preservative)
Trisodium edetate (preservative)

PLICTRAN 50W MITICIDE
(Dow)

Tricyclohexyltin hydroxide *	50%

PLINE CHLORINATED CLEANER
Dairy use
(Yale Chem. Co.)

Sodium tripolyphosphate	>35%
Soda ash *	>35%
Sodium metasilicate *	<15%
Sodium dichloroisocyanurate	<3%

PL INSECT REPELLENT
Institutional & industrial use
(Precision Labs.)

N,N-Diethyl-meta-toluamide	3.78%
Other isomers	0.42%
N-Octyl bicycloheptene dicarboximide	1.20%
2,3:4,5-Bis (d-2-butylene) tetrahydro-2-furaldehyde	0.30%
Di-n-propyl isocinchomeronate	0.30%

PL INSTANT BANDAGE (Aerosol)
Institutional and industrial use
(Precision Labs.)

Alcohol
Polyvinylpyrrolidone/vinyl acetate copolymer
Benzocaine
Di-isobutyl cresoxy ethoxy ethyl dimethyl benzyl ammonium chloride, monohydrate *†

†*See* Cationic surfactants

PLIOBOND (20, 30 and 40 series)
Adhesive
(Goodyear)

Synthetic rubber copolymer of:	10-20%
Butadiene	
Acrylonitrile *	
Synthetic resins (phenolic)	5-10%
Methyl ethyl ketone *	60-80%

PLIOLITE (S-SERIES RESINS)
Synthetic copolymer resins used in paints, latices, etc.
(Goodyear)

High styrene/butadiene copolymers

PL MINT-O-GREEN
Disinfectant, deodorant, cleaner; institutional, municipal and industrial use
(Precision Labs.)

Isopropyl alcohol *	17.65%
Soap	11.00%
Terpineol	6.45%
Methyl salicylate *	4.14%
Potassium orthobenzyl parachlorophenol	3.74%
Oil of peppermint U.S.P.	0.01%
Oil of spearmint U.S.P.	0.01%

PL RESPOND DETERGENT
Cleaner, disinfectant; institutional, municipal and industrial use
(Precision Labs.)

Tetrasodium ethylenediamine tetraacetate	1.58%
Anhydrous Sodium metasilicate	4.35%
N-Alkyl (60% C14, 30% C16, 5% C12, 5% C18) dimethyl benzyl ammonium chlorides	0.75%
N-Alkyl (50% C12, 30% C14, 17% C16, 3% C18) dimethyl ethylbenzyl ammonium chlorides	0.75%
N-Alkyl (C18 92%, C16 8%) N-ethyl morpholinium ethyl sulfate	0.10%
3,5-Dibromosalicylanilide	0.02%
3,4',5-Tribromosalicylanilide	0.08%
Other related bromosalicylanilides	
Inert ingredients:	92.37%
Cleaning detergents *†	
Wetting agents	
Synergizing builders	
Chelating agents	
Perfume	
Water	

†*See* Detergents, Section VI, General Formulations

PL RHINO GREASE DISSOLVER
(Precision Labs.)

Potassium hydroxide *
Potassium carbonate
Potassium chloride
Ferric acid
Sodium oxide

PL-345 RUST, CORROSION AND TARNISH REMOVER
(Precision Labs.)

Mineral acids *

PL-100 SAFETY SOLVENT
Industrial solvent degreaser
(Precision Labs.)

Chlorothene *

PL SANACLEAN PORCELAIN CLEANER
Institutional, municipal and industrial use
(Precision Labs.)

Hydrogen chloride *	9.45%
Dehydroabietylamine	2.50%
Inert ingredients:	88.05%
Detergents	
Cleaners	
Emulsifiers	
Deodorants	

PL S-523 CONCENTRATED INSECTICIDE
(Precision Labs.)

Beta-butoxy-beta-thiocyano-diethyl ether *	10.7%
Malathion *	10.0%
Petroleum distillates *	78.8%

PL SLUG WASP & HORNET SPRAY
(Precision Labs.)

o-Isopropoxyphenyl methylcarbamate *	0.50%
Petroleum distillate *	51.87%

PL SMASH ROACH'N ANT KILLER (Aerosol)
(Precision Labs.)

O,O-Diethyl O-(2-isopropyl-4-methyl-6-pyrimidinyl)phosphorothioate	0.500%
Pyrethrins	0.050%
Technical Piperonyl butoxide	0.262%
Petroleum distillate *	95.238%

PL SPRAY AND WIPE GERMICIDAL CLEANER AND SURFACE DEODORANT
(Precision Labs.)

N-Alkyl (60% C14, 30% C16, 5% C12, 5% C18) dimethyl benzyl ammonium chloride	0.076%
N-Alkyl (50% C12, 30% C14, 17% C16, 3% C18) dimethyl ethylbenzyl ammonium chloride	0.076%
Sodium metasilicate	0.24%
Essential oils	0.20%
Inert ingredients:	99.408%
Detergents	
Cleaners	
Builder	
Propellant	

PL SUBMERGE PAINT STRIPPER, DEGREASER & CLEANER
Immersion-type vat cleaner; industrial
(Precision Labs.)

Methylene chloride *

PL SUPER SANACLEAN BOWL CLEANER
(Precision Labs.)

Hydrogen chloride *	23.70%
Heptadecyl hydroxyethylimidazo- linium chloride	0.10%
Compatible Detergents, Emulsifiers, Acrylic copolymers, Inhibitors	

PL TOPICAL ANESTHETIC (Aerosol)
Institutional and industrial use
(Precision Labs.)

Dipropylene glycol
Polyethylene glycol dioleate
Benzocaine
Methyl parasept
Di-isobutyl phenoxy ethoxy ethyl di-methyl benzyl ammonium chloride, monohydrate *

PL TRAFFIC PAINT
Municipal and industrial use
(Precision Labs.)

Petroleum distillates *
Lead compounds *

PL ULTIMATE II
Insect killer
(Precision Labs.)

Tetramethrin ((1-Cyclohexene- 1,2-dicarboximido)methyl-2,2- dimethyl-3- (methylpropenyl)cyclopropane carboxylate)	0.200%
3-Phenoxybenzyl d-cis and trans 2,2-dimethyl-3-(2-methylpro- penyl)cyclopropane- carboxylate	0.191%
Other isomers	0.009%
Petroleum distillate *	9.250%

PL ULTIMATE SUPER FOGGING INSECT KILLER (Aerosol)
(Precision Labs.)

Pyrethrins	0.30%
Piperonyl butoxide technical	0.60%
N-Octyl bicycloheptene dicarboximide	1.00%
Petroleum distillates	8.10%

PLUMBER SAVER DRAIN OPENER

See DAYS EASE PLUMBER SAVER DRAIN OPENER

PLUNGE
Drain cleaner
(Drackett)

Sodium hydroxide *	9.5%/wt.
Wetting agents	
Ammonium hydroxide	<1.0%/wt.
Dye	
Water	

PLUS ANT & ROACH KILLER
Household aerosol insecticide
(Great Atlantic & Pacific, mfr.; Plus Discount Foods, dist.)

Pyrethrins	0.05%
Piperonyl butoxide	0.10%
N-Octyl bicycloheptene dicarboximide	0.17%
O-Isopropoxyphenyl methylcarbamate	0.50%
Isopropanol	7.50%
Methylene chloride	14.00%
Hydrocarbon propellant	20.00%
Petroleum distillate *	57.70%

PLUS AUTOMATIC DISHWASHER DETERGENT
(Great Atlantic & Pacific, mfr.; Plus Discount Foods, dist.)

Sodium tripolyphosphate	35%
Sodium silicate *	16%
Nonionic surfactant	2%
Chlorinated isocyanurate	2%
Anti caking	1%
Perfume	trace
Sodium sulfate and moisture	balance

PLUS BUG KILLER
Household aerosol insecticide
(Great Atlantic & Pacific, mfr.; Plus Discount Foods, dist.)

Petroleum distillate	9.25%
Multicide Intermediate 2084	2.00%
Hydrocarbon propellant	30.00%
Water	balance

PLUS FLYING INSECT KILLER (Aerosol)
(Great Atlantic & Pacific, mfr.; Plus Discount Foods, dist.)

Resmethrin	0.325%
Related compounds	0.044%
Aromatic petroleum hydrocarbons	0.430%
Petroleum distillates	6.382%
Hydrocarbon propellant	30.000%
Water	balance

PLUS HEAVY DUTY BLUE ALL TEMPERATURE LAUNDRY DETERGENT
(Great Atlantic & Pacific, mfr.; Plus Discount Foods, dist.)

Sodium linear alkyl benzene sulfonate	<20%
Sodium carbonate *	<30%
Sodium silicate	<12%
Sodium carboxymethylcellulose	<2%
Optical brighteners	<1%
Sodium chloride	<15%
Dye	trace
Sodium sulfate and moisture	balance

pH of 0.1% solution - 10.0-10.9

PLUS HEAVY DUTY LAUNDRY DETERGENT
(Great Atlantic & Pacific, mfr.; Plus Discount foods, dist.)

Sodium linear alkyl benzene sulfonate	<20%
Sodium carbonate *	<30%
Sodium silicate	<12%
Sodium carboxymethylcellulose	<2%
Optical brighteners	<1%
Sodium chloride	<15%
Sodium sulfate and moisture	balance

pH of 0.1% solution - 10.0-10.9

PLUS LEMON FURNITURE POLISH (Aerosol)
(Great Atlantic & Pacific, mfr.; Plus Discount Foods, dist.)

Silicone emulsion	<10.00%
Hydrocarbon propellant (Isobu- tane 85%-Propane 15%)	<5.00%
Isoparaffinic hydrocarbon	<0.75%
Wax	<0.50%
Perfume	<0.50%
Morpholine	trace
Oleic acid	trace
Water	balance

PLUS PINK DETERGENT
(Great Atlantic & Pacific, mfr.; Plus Discount Foods, dist.)

Sodium linear alkyl benzene sulfo- nate (52% active) *	27.0%
Ammonium ethoxylated primary alcohol sulfate	5.0%
Sodium xylene sulfonate (50% active)	2.5%
Urea	0.5%
Formaldehyde (37%)	0.3%
Dye, perfume	trace
Opacifier	trace

pH - 6.5-7.5

PLUS WHITE TOOTHPASTE
(L.T. Labs.)

Organic thickeners
Organic sweeteners
Polyhydric glycols
Inorganic abrasives
Surface active agents
Certified dye
Flavor

'76 Ed.

PL VICTORY PINE ODOR
Disinfectant, cleaner, deodorizer
(Precision Labs.)

Soap	8.00%
Pine oil	7.00%
Ortho-benzyl-para-chlorophenol, sodium salt	5.00%

PMC DISPOSABLE DOUCHE
(Thomas & Thompson)

Menthol *
Boric acid *
Eucalyptus oil *
Alum
Phenol *
Oil of peppermint
Thymol *
Water

PMC POWDER
Douche powder for feminine hygiene
(Thomas & Thompson)

Menthol *
Boric acid *
Eucalyptus oil *
Alum
Phenol *
Oil of peppermint
Thymol *

PMP PRESERVATIVE POWDER
Embalming supply
(Royal Bond)

Paraformaldehyde *

P N S SUPPOSITORIES
Rectal
(Winthrop Labs.)

Each suppository:
    Pontocaine (brand of tetra-
        caine) hydrochloride .... 10 mg.
    Neo-synephrine (brand of
        phenylephrine) HCl * ..... 5 mg.
    Superinone (brand of
        tyloxapol) .... 25 mg.
    Bismuth subcarbonate * ..... 100 mg.

PNS UNNA BOOT (Non-Sterile)
To reduce swelling of sprains and strains
(Pedinol)

Glycerine
Gum acacia
Zinc oxide
White petrolatum
Amylum
Oil base

POCKET ACCENT
Medium line water color markers
(Sanford Corp.)

Dyes
Glycols
Water
Phenol (as preservative) .... <1%

PODIASPRAY (SPRAY-ON POWDER)
For athlete's foot & superficial fungus infections of the skin
(Dalin)

Undecylenic acid *
Salicylic acid *
Dichlorophene
Hexachlorophene
Aromatized base

'76 Ed.

PODOGEL
Aromatic cooling lotion
(Gordon Labs.)

Menthol *
Camphor *
Isopropyl alcohol *
Propylene glycol

POD PINE SCENT DISINFECTANT
(Standard Coffee Co., Inc.)

Active ingred.: 34.90%
    Steam distilled Pine oil *
    Anhydrous cocoanut oil soap
    Isopropyl alcohol *
    Ortho-benzyl-para-chlorophenol *

Inert ingred.: 65.10%
    Water
    Optical brightener

POINTS NORTH AFTER SHAVE
See AMWAY POINTS NORTH AFTER SHAVE

POINT-TWO DENTAL RINSE
(Hoyt Labs.)

Sodium fluoride * 0.2%

POLARAMINE EXPECTORANT
For coughs
(Schering)

Each 5 cc.:
    Dexchlorpheniramine maleate   2 mg.
    d-Isoephedrine sulfate * ..... 20 mg.
    Glyceryl guaiacolate .... 100 mg.
    Alcohol 7.2%

POLARAMINE REPETABS
Antihistamine therapy
(Schering)

Each Repetab:
    Dexchlorpheniramine
        maleate * .... 4 mg.; 6 mg.

POLARAMINE SYRUP AND TABLETS
Relief of certain allergic manifestations
(Schering)

Each tablet or 5 cc:
    Dexchlorpheniramine maleate * 2 mg.
    Alcohol (syrup only) 6%/v

POLAROID FILM: PROCESSING REAGENT JELLY
Alkaline jelly serving as medium for film development
(Polaroid Corp.)

Alkali metal hydroxides (pH
    14) *† .... <10%
Inert liquid plastic

†*See* Sodium hydroxide

POLAROID PRINT COATER
To make photographic print permanent
(Polaroid Corp.)

Acetic acid .... approx. 5%
Isopropanol * 25-50%
Nontoxic liquid plastic

POLIDENT DENTU-GRIP
Denture adhesive
(Block Drug)

Sodium carboxymethylcellulose
Ethylene oxide homopolymer
Monosodium phosphate
Dicalcium phosphate
Flavor

POLIDENT POWDER
Denture cleanser
(Block Drug)

Flavor
Surfactant
Sodium bicarbonate
Soda ash *
Sodium perborate *
Potassium dichloroisocyanurate *
Potassium monopersulfate *
Sodium tripolyphosphate
Micronized Silica

POLIDENT TABLETS
Denture cleanser
(Block Drug)

Soda ash
Sodium monopersulfate *
Potassium monopersulfate *
Sodium bicarbonate
Surfactant
Citric acid
Flavor

POLI-GRIP
Denture adhesive
(Block Drug)

Petrolatum
Mineral oil
Karaya gum
Preservative
Flavors
Magnesium oxide

POLISHED AMBERS COSMETICS

Revlon, Inc.
767 Fifth Ave.
New York, N.Y. 10153

Phone: 212-572-5000

Revlon Research Center, Inc.
945 Zerega Ave.
Bronx, N.Y. 10473

Phone: 212-824-9000

See COSMETICS, Section VI, General Formulations

POL-NU

See CHAPMAN POL-NU

POL-NU 15-15

See CHAPMAN POL-NU 15-15

POL-NU PAK

See CHAPMAN POL-NU PAK

POLY 250
Floor polish
(Hillyard Chem.)

Latex

'76 Ed.

POLYBOR-3
Insecticide
(U.S. Borax)

Disodium octaborate tetrahydrate * 98%

POLYBOR-CHLORATE WEED & GRASS KILLER
(U.S. Borax)

Disodium octaborate tetrahydrate * 73%
Sodium chlorate * 25%

POLY-CHIP TOP COAT
Floor paint
(Tremco)

Xylene * .... <65%
Polyurethane prepolymer .... <45%

POLYCHROMATIC ALPHASITE CHALKBOARD CHALK
(Weber Costello)

Calcium carbonate 95%
Vegetable binder 5%

POLYDERM CREAM
For the treatment of dermatitis
(Russ Pharm.)

Iodochlorhydroxyquin (NF) * 3%
Hydrocortisone (USP) 1%

POLY GLAZE

See LIQUID GLAZE POLY GLAZE

POLYGLYCOAT LUSTERIZING SEALANT
(Polyglycoat)

Solvents * 77.6%

POLYGLYCOAT TEXTILE SEALANT
(Polyglycoat)

Petroleum naphtha * .... >85%
Copolymer resin .... <15%

POLYGLYCOAT VINYL CLEANER STEP 1
(Polyglycoat)

Trisodium phosphate 2%
Butyl Cellosolve * 4%
Bleach 0.5%
Metasilicate 2%

POLYGLYCOAT VINYL FINISH
(Polyglycoat)

Ammonia 0.600%
Formaldehyde 0.002%
Dipropylene glycol monomethyl . 1.200%

POLYGLYCOAT VINYL STRIPPER
(Polyglycoat)

Trisodium phosphate 2%
Butyl Cellosolve * 4%
Bleach 0.5%
Metasilicate 2%

POLY-KOTE, IMPROVED
Floor polish
(Hillyard Chem.)

Latex

'76 Ed.

POLY-KOTE, REGULAR
Floor polish
(Hillyard Chem.)

Latex

'76 Ed.

POLYMAGMA PLAIN TABLETS
Treatment of diarrhea
(Wyeth Labs.)

Each tablet:
Claysorb (activated
attapulgite) .... 500 mg.
Pectin .... 45 mg.
Hydrated Alumina powder ... 50 mg.

POLY-PRED LIQUIFILM
(Allergan Pharm.)

Each ml.:
Prednisolone acetate 0.5%
Neomycin sulfate 0.5%
Polymyxin B sulfate .... 5000 units
Polyvinyl alcohol 1.4%

POLY-PRO SHAMPOO
(House of Lowell, Inc.)

TEA-lauryl sulfate *
Lauramide DEA
Hydrolyzed animal protein (and) oleylam-
   idoamine
Sodium chloride
Citric acid
Formaldehyde
Methylparaben
Propylparaben
Modified Polystyrene latex
Perfume *
D & C color

POLYSEPT
Effective in pseudomonas and staphy-
   lococcal infections
(Dalin)

Each gram:
Polymyxin B sulfate ...... 5000 units
Bacitracin .... 400 units
Neomycin sulfate (equiva-
   lent to 3.5 mg. of neomycin
   base) .... 5 mg.
Diperodon hydrochloride
   (1%) .... 10 mg.
White petrolatum base

'76 Ed.

POLYSORB HYDRATE
For dry skin conditions
(Fougera)

Sorbitan sesquioleate
Wax and petrolatum base

POLYSPORIN OINTMENT
Bactericidal
(Burroughs Wellcome)

Each gram:
Polymyxin B sulfate ..... 10,000 units
Bacitracin zinc .... 500 units
Special white petrolatum .... q.s.

Starred ingredients (*) may be responsible for major toxic effects; consult Section II.

POLYSPORIN OINTMENT OPHTHALMIC
Bacterial infections of the eye
(Burroughs Wellcome)

Each gram:
Aerosporin (Polymixin
  sulfate) .... 10,000 units
Bacitracin zinc .... 500 units
White petrolatum .... q.s.

POLYSTAT
Feed additive aid in prevention of coccidiosis, large roundworms & tapeworms in chickens and turkeys
(Salsbury)

Sulfanitran (Acetyl-(para-nitro-
  phenyl)-sulfanilamide) 30%
Butynorate (Dibutyltin dilaurate) .. 20%
Dinsed
  (Dinitrodiphenylsulfonylethylene-
  diamine) * 20%

POLYSTAT-3
Feed additive aid in prevention of coccidiosis, large roundworms & tapeworms in chickens and turkeys
(Salsbury)

Sulfanitran (Acetyl-(para-nitro-
  phenyl)-sulfanilamide) 30%
Butynorate (Dibutyltin dilaurate) .. 20%
Dinsed
  (Dinitrodiphenylsulfonylethylene-
  diamine) * 20%
Roxarsone (3-Nitro-4-hydroxyphen-
  ylarsonic acid) 5%

POLYSUL SUMMER & DORMANT SPRAY CONCENTRATE

See LILLY/MILLER POLYSUL SUMMER & DORMANT SPRAY CONCENTRATE

POLYTAR BATH
For eczema, psoriasis, pruritic dermatoses
(Stiefel Labs.)

Polytar: Blend of Juniper tar *, Pine
  tar *, Coal tar solution *, Polyunsaturated vegetable oil, Water-dispersible solubilized crude Coal
  tar * 25%
Butyl stearate 25%

POLYTAR SHAMPOO
For seborrhea, dandruff
(Stiefel Labs.)

Polytar: Juniper tar *, Pine tar *,
  Coal tar solution *, Polyunsaturated vegetable oil, Water-dispersible solubilized crude Coal tar * ... 1%
Surfactant shampoo base

POLYTAR SOAP
For eczema, psoriasis, seborrhea
(Stiefel Labs.)

Polytar: Juniper tar *, Pine tar *,
  Coal tar solution *, Polyunsaturated vegetable oil, Water-dispersible solubilized crude Coal tar * ... 1%

POLY-TEX ALL FABRIC LIQUID BLEACH
(Purex Corp.)

Hydrogen peroxide * 5-10%
Nonionic surfactant .... <3%
Coloring agent .... <1%
Water .... balance

POLYURETHANE GLOSS
(Pierce & Stevens)

Non-volatile:
  Polyhydric alcohol partially esterified with linolenic, oleic, linoleic, palmitic, stearic acid (modified with tolylene diisocyanate)
Volatile:
  Mineral spirits *

POLYURETHANE SATIN
(Pierce & Stevens)

Non-volatile:
  Polyhydric alcohol partially esterified with linolenic, oleic, linoleic, palmitic, stearic acid (modified with tolylene diisocyanate, modified alkyd resin)
Volatile:
  Mineral spirits *

POLY-ZAG
Bowl sanitizer & cleaner
(Hysan Corp.)

Hydrogen chloride * 23.70%
Heptadecyl hydroxyethylimidazo-
  linium chloride 0.10%
Inert ingredients: 76.20%
  Detergents
  Emulsifiers
  Acrylic copolymers
  Inhibitors

POMADE HONGROISE, NESTLE

See NESTLE POMADE HONGROISE

POMATEX DOUBLE-DUTY HAIR CREAM
(Pomatex)

Mineral oil, USP
Petrolatum, USP
Spermaceti, a vegetable dye, USP
Perfume

'76 Ed.

PONDIMIN TABLETS
Anorexiant
(Robins)

Each tablet:
  Fenfluramine hydrochloride * . 20 mg.

POND'S CREAM & COCOA BUTTER SKIN SOFTENING CREAM
(Chesebrough-Pond's)

Water .... >50%
Glyceryl stearate .... >1-5%
PEG-8 .... >1-5%
PPG-2 myristyl ether
  propionate .... >1-5%
Cetearyl alcohol .... >1-5%
Isopropyl lanolate .... >0.1-1%
Cocoa butter .... >0.1-1%
Myristyl myristate .... >0.1-1%
PPG-10 cetyl ether .... >0.1-1%
Ceteareth-20 .... >0.1-1%
Petrolatum .... >0.1-1%
Dimethicone .... >0.1-1%
Hydrogenated Lanolin .... >0.1-1%
Fragrance .... >0.1-1%
Methylparaben .... >0.1-1%
Quaternium-15 .... >0.1-1%
Carbomer-934 .... >0.1-1%
Stearyl alcohol .... 0.1% or less
Propylene glycol .... 0.1% or less
Caramel .... 0.1% or less
Colors .... 0.1% or less
Magnesium aluminum
  silicate .... 0.1% or less
Hydrogenated Coconut oil .. 0.1% or less
Propylparaben .... 0.1% or less
Sodium hydroxide .... 0.1% or less
Sorbitan sesquioleate ...... 0.1% or less
Disodium EDTA .... 0.1% or less
Cetyl alcohol .... 0.1% or less

PONTOCAINE CREAM
Topical anesthetic
(Breon Labs.)

Tetracaine (base) 1%
Methylparaben
Sodium bisulfite

PONTOCAINE EYE OINTMENT
Anesthetic ointment
(Breon Labs.)

Each gm.:
  Tetracaine (base) .... 5 mg.
  White petrolatum
  Light mineral oil

PONTOCAINE OINTMENT
Topical anesthetic
(Breon Labs.)

Tetracaine (base) 0.5%
Menthol
White petrolatum
White wax

PONTOCAINE TOPICAL SOLUTION
For surface anesthesia of eye, nose, and throat
(Breon Labs)

Solution 0.5%—each ml.:
Tetracaine *	5 mg.
Sodium chloride	7.5 mg.
Chlorobutanol *	4 mg.

Solution 2%—each ml.: *
Tetracaine *	20 mg.
Chlorobutanol	4 mg.

* This solution is colored with FD & C Blue #1 to prevent its accidental use for injection.

POOL AID LIQUID
(Coastal Industries)

Alkyl dimethyl benzyl ammonium chloride *	7.5%
Complexed Copper	0.1%
Trisodium phosphate	2.4%
Water	

POOL-COTE, TURQUOISE ROYALE
Swimming pool paint
(Modern Pool Products)

Pigment:	26%
Titanium dioxide	37%
Calcium carbonate	63%
Vehicle:	74%
Chlorinated rubber	17%
Soya alkyd resin	6.8%
Chlorinated resin	8.7%
Aromatic solvent *	67.5%

Tinting materials <5%

POOL DEODOR
Winter deodorizer for swim pool water
(Coastal Industries)

Alkyl dimethyl benzyl ammonium chloride *	10%
Water	

POOL SAFE
Swimming pool conditioner, concentrated
(Marmet Supply Co.)

Sodium dichloro-s-triazinetrione *	95%

'76 Ed.

PORCELANA MEDICATED CREAM
Helps lighten discolored or darkened skin areas
(Jeffrey Martin, Inc.)

Active ingred.:
Hydroquinone *
Also contains:
Purified water
Myristyl myristate
PEG-8
Glyceryl monostearate
Cetyl alcohol
Magnesium aluminum silicate
Dioctyl sodium sulfosuccinate
Dimethicone
Choleth-24
Fragrance
Locust bean gum
Sodium sulfite
Citric acid
Sodium bisulfite
Sorbic acid

PORCETEX 8051
See INTEX 8051 PORCETEX

POREEN
Concentrating drying agent
(Diversey Wyandotte)

Synthetic detergents *

POR-ROK ANCHORING CEMENT
(Minwax Co.)

Calcium sulfate	70%
Silicon dioxide	30%

POR-ROK CONCRETE REPAIR KIT - CEMENT
(Minwax Co.)

Portland cement	30%
Calcium carbonate	70%

PORSO-WHITE
Porcelain & stainless steel cleaner
(Weil Chem.)

Phosphoric acid *
Citric acid
Nonionic surfactant
Acrylic emulsion - small amt. to create opacity
Camphor oil perfume *

PORTION-PAC GERMICIDAL DETERGENT
(Earl, John A., Inc.)

n-Alkyl (C12-40%, C14-50%, C16-10%) dimethyl benzyl ammonium chlorides *	10.00%
Tetra sodium salt of ethylene diamine tetraacetic acid	0.25%

'76 Ed.

POSNER'S COSMETIC PRODUCTS

Posner Laboratories Inc.
301 Helen St.
South Plainfield, N.J. 07080

Phone: 201-753-0900

See COSMETICS, Section VI, General Formulations

POSTACNE LOTION (FLESH TINTED)
Treatment of mild acne & oily skin
(Dermik)

Microsize Sulfur	2.0% w/v
Hydro-alcoholic vehicle	
S.D. alcohol	29% v/v

POSTENE SURFACE PRESERVATIVE
Embalming supply
(Royal Bond)

Formaldehyde *
Methanol *
Ortho-dichlorobenzene *

POSTER PASTELLO COLORED DUSTLESS CHALK
(American Crayon Co.)

This product bears the CP Seal issued by the Crayon, Water Color and Craft Institute, Inc. This seal certifies that the product contains no materials in sufficient quantities to be toxic or injurious to the human body even if ingested.

POTASSINE
For potassium deficiency
(Recsei Labs.)

Potassium chloride	7.5% or 10%

POULAX
Laxative; veterinary, avian
(Hilltop)

Epsom salts	15%
Potassium chlorate *	
Saltpeter	
Potassium dichromate *	

'76 Ed.

POWDER-ENE II
Rug cleaner

Von Schrader Co.
1600 Junction Ave.
Racine, Wis. 53403
Attention: Mr. Geoff Rench

Phone: 414-634-1956

See RUG CLEANERS, Section VI, General Formulations

POWER
Powdered hand soap; industrial and institutional use
(Scientific International)

Lanolin
Borax *

POWER BOND #190

See ROSS POWER BOND #190 &
SUPER GLUE #190

POWER GEL
Heavy duty cleaner
(Paul Koss)

Water	>70%
Potassium tall oil soap	
Pine oil	
Fatty amido phosphate	
Trisodium phosphate dodecahydrate	
Tetrasodium EDTA	
Sodium metasilicate	
Dye	trace
Formalin	trace

pH 11.8-11.9

POWER GUARD LEMON 16
Household and commercial disinfectant
(Snee, W.G., Co.)

Quaternary ammonium compound *	
Essential oils *	4.60%
Isopropanol *	

POWER GUARD R D 10 DISINFECTANT-SANITIZER-DEODORANT
(Snee, W.G., Co.)

Quaternary ammonium compound *	
Ethanol	12.5%

POWERJET STEAM CLEANER & PRESSURE WASHER CONCENTRATE
(Nat'l Labs. Div.)

Detergent	
Wetting agents	
Emulsifiers	
Phosphates (calculated as elemental phosphorus)	1.37%
Potassium hydroxide *	minor
Silicates	minor

POWERMIX
Lubricating oil
(Texaco Canada Ltd.)

Mineral oil *
Methacrylate copolymer
Additive package containing:
  Nitrogen
  Dye

POWERPAKT
Cavity fluid; embalming supply
(Royal Bond)

Formaldehyde index *	45%
Methanol *	

POWER "PLUS" CONCENTRATE EMULSION BOWL CLEANER
(Schneid)

Active ingred.:	30.11%
Hydrogen chloride *	
Zinc chloride *	
Phosphoric acid *	
Anhydrous Oxalic acid	
Para diisobutyl phenoxy ethoxy ethyl dimethyl benzyl ammonium chloride *	
Heptadecyl hydroxy ethyl imidazoline	
Inert ingred.:	69.89%
Nonylphenoxypolyethoxy-ethanol	
Polymerized vinyl benzene	
Water	

'76 Ed.

POWERTONE
Arterial fluid; embalming supply
(Royal Bond)

Formaldehyde index *	36%
Methanol *	

POW POWER, WATKINS

See WATKINS POW POWER

POWRITE
Detergent, rust control agent
(Whitfield Chem.)

Phosphate *	>10%
Carbonate *	>10%
Silicate neutral salts	>10%
May contain:	
Free Caustic *	>10%
Chromium salts (trace)	

PQ-8

See CHAPMAN PQ-8

PQ-10

See CHAPMAN PQ-10

P&Q ALL FABRIC BLEACH
For household laundry
(Great Atlantic & Pacific)

Sodium percarbonate	10.0%
Silica gel	0.5%
Sodium carbonate *	35.0%
Sodium chloride	balance to 100%
Dye	trace
Nonionic surfactant	0.5%

P&Q AUTOMATIC DISHWASHER DETERGENT
(Great Atlantic & Pacific)

Sodium tripolyphosphate	<30%
Sodium silicate *	<14%
Nonionic surfactant	<3%
Sodium dichloroisocyanurate	<2%
Sodium sulfate and moisture	balance
Anti caking agent	trace

P&Q GREEN DETERGENT
Liquid dishwashing detergent
(Great Atlantic & Pacific)

Sodium dodecylbenzene sulfonate	<9.0%
Ammonium alcohol ether sulfonate	<3.0%
Formaldehyde	<0.2%
Citric acid	<0.2%
Perfume	trace
Dyes	trace
Sodium chloride	<1.5%
Urea	<1.0%
Water	balance
Sodium sulfate	<2.0%

P&Q HEAVY DUTY LAUNDRY DETERGENT
Home liquid laundry detergent
(Great Atlantic & Pacific)

Sodium dodecylbenzene sulfonate *	<17%
Nonionic surfactant	<7%
Sodium xylene sulfonate	<4%
Sodium citrate	<0.2%
Optical brightener	<0.2%
Perfume	trace
Sodium sulfate	<3%
Caustic soda	trace
Dye	trace
Water	balance to 100%

P&Q LEMON DETERGENT
Liquid dishwashing detergent
(Great Atlantic & Pacific)

Sodium dodecylbenzene sulfonate	<9.0%
Ammonium alcohol ether sulfonate	<3.0%
Formaldehyde	<0.2%
Citric acid	<0.2%
Opacifier	trace
Perfume	trace
Dye	trace
Sodium chloride	<1.5%
Urea	<1.0%
Water	balance
Sodium sulfate	<2.0%

Starred ingredients (*) may be responsible for major toxic effects; consult Section II.

P&Q PINK DISH DETERGENT
Liquid dish detergent
(Great Atlantic & Pacific)

Sodium dodecylbenzene sulfonate	7.3000%
Ammonium alcohol ether sulfate	2.2000%
Sodium sulfate	2.0000%
Sodium xylene sulfonate	0.5000%
Coconut diethanolamide	0.5000%
Sodium citrate	0.2000%
Opacifier	0.2000%
Formaldehyde	0.1000%
Perfume	0.0500%
Dye	0.0002%
Water	26.9500%

pH (as is) 6.0 to 7.5

PR 1760
Floor polish stripper
(Sanitek)

Dimethylaminoethanol	2.0%
Dipropylene glycol monomethyl ether (Cellosolve)	1.5%
Sodium tripolyphosphate	1.3%
Anionic surfactants	1.0%
Nonionic surfactants	0.8%
Defoamer, Dye	trace
Water	balance

PRAGMATAR OINTMENT
(MenJ Labs.)

Cetyl alcohol-coal tar distillate	4%
Precipitated Sulfur	3%
Salicylic acid *	3%

PRAGMATAR OINTMENT
Skin disorders; veterinary
(Norden Labs.)

Combined amount:	4%
Cetyl alcohol	
Coal tar distillate (providing colorless fractions of crude coal tar 0.35%) *	
Special Sulfur	3%
Salicylic acid *	3%
Base	q.s.

PRAGMATAR SHAMPOO
Dermatological use; veterinary
(Norden Labs.)

Combined amount:	0.5%
Cetyl alcohol	
Coal tar distillate (provides fractions of crude coal tar 0.044%)	
Lauryl isoquinolinium bromide	0.2%
Hexachlorophene	2.0%
Isopropyl alcohol *	19.0%
Special shampoo base	q.s.

PRAMET FA FILMTAB
Prenatal vitamin and mineral supplement
(Ross Labs.)

Each tablet:
Iron *	60 mg.
Multivitamins and minerals	

PRAMILET FA FILMTAB
Prenatal vitamin and mineral supplement
(Ross Labs.)

Each tablet:
Iron *	40 mg.
Multivitamins and minerals	

PRAMITOL 25E
Herbicide
(Ciba-Geigy Ag. Div.)

Prometon *	25%

PRAMITOL 5PS
Pelleted herbicide
(Ciba-Geigy Ag. Div.)

Prometon	5.00%
Simazine	0.75%
Sodium chlorate *	40.00%
Sodium metaborate	50.00%

PRAMITOL 80 WP
Herbicide
(Ciba-Geigy Ag. Div.)

Prometon *	80%

PRANG CAKE TEMPERA
(American Crayon Co.)

This product bears the CP Seal issued by the Crayon, Water Color and Craft Institute, Inc. This seal certifies that the product contains no materials in sufficient quantities to be toxic or injurious to the human body even if ingested.

PRANG FINGER PAINT
(American Crayon Co.)

This product bears the CP Seal issued by the Crayon, Water Color and Craft Institute, Inc. This seal certifies that the product contains no materials in sufficient quantities to be toxic or injurious to the human body even if ingested.

PRANG FLUORESCENT LECTURERS COLORED MOLDED CHALK
(American Crayon Co.)

This product bears the CP Seal issued by the Crayon, Water Color and Craft Institute, Inc. This seal certifies that the product contains no materials in sufficient quantities to be toxic or injurious to the human body even if ingested.

PRANG LECTURERS COLORED MOLDED CHALK
(American Crayon Co.)

This product bears the CP Seal issued by the Crayon, Water Color and Craft Institute, Inc. This seal certifies that the product contains no materials in sufficient quantities to be toxic or injurious to the human body even if ingested.

PRANG LIQUID TEMPERA
(American Crayon Co.)

This product bears the CP Seal issued by the Crayon, Water Color and Craft Institute, Inc. This seal certifies that the product contains no materials in sufficient quantities to be toxic or injurious to the human body even if ingested.

PRANG MEDIA MIXERS
(American Crayon Co.)

This product bears the CP Seal issued by the Crayon, Water Color and Craft Institute, Inc. This seal certifies that the product contains no materials in sufficient quantities to be toxic or injurious to the human body even if ingested.

PRANG MODELING CLAY
(American Crayon Co.)

This product bears the CP Seal issued by the Crayon, Water Color and Craft Institute, Inc. This seal certifies that the product contains no materials in sufficient quantities to be toxic or injurious to the human body even if ingested.

PRANG POWDER TEMPERA
(American Crayon Co.)

This product bears the CP Seal issued by the Crayon, Water Color and Craft Institute, Inc. This seal certifies that the product contains no materials in sufficient quantities to be toxic or injurious to the human body even if ingested.

PRANG SEMI-MOIST WATER COLORS
(American Crayon Co.)

This product bears the CP Seal issued by the Crayon, Water Color and Craft Institute, Inc. This seal certifies that the product contains no materials in sufficient quantities to be toxic or injurious to the human body even if ingested.

PRANG TEXTILE COLORS
(Inmont Corp.)

Petroleum solvents of the Mineral spirits type *
Organic or inorganic pigments (no lead or chromates)
Alkyd resins
Melamine resins

'76 Ed.

PRANG WATER COLOR MARKERS
(American Crayon Co.)

This product bears the CP Seal issued by the Crayon, Water Color and Craft Institute, Inc. This seal certifies that the product contains no materials in sufficient quantities to be toxic or injurious to the human body even if ingested.

PRANG WATER SOLUBLE BLOCK PRINTING INKS
(American Crayon Co.)

This product bears the CP Seal issued by the Crayon, Water Color and Craft Institute, Inc. This seal certifies that the product contains no materials in sufficient quantities to be toxic or injurious to the human body even if ingested.

PRATT ANT & ROACH KILLER
(Pratt-Gabriel Div.)

Baygon *	0.5%
Petroleum distillate *	80.8%

PRATT BORDO-MIX (BORDEAUX MIXTURE)
Fungicide
(Pratt-Gabriel Div.)

Copper *	12.75%
Hydrated Lime *	87.25%

PRATT CHLORDANE-74 INSECT SPRAY
(Pratt-Gabriel Div.)

Chlordane *	74.0%
Isoparaffinic hydrocarbons *	20.0%
Emulsifier	6.0%

PRATT CRABGRASS & BROADLEAF WEED KILLER
(Pratt-Gabriel Div.)

Dodecyl ammonium methanearsonate *	8.00%
Octyl ammonium methanearsonate *	8.00%
Octyl ammonium salt of 2,4-dichlorophenoxyacetic acid	5.44%

PRATT CYGON 2E SYSTEMIC INSECTICIDE
(Pratt-Gabriel Div.)

Dimethoate *	23.4%
Cyclohexanone	32.0%
Aromatic petroleum solvent *	38.4%

PRATT DANDELION DESTROYER
(Pratt-Gabriel Div.)

Dimethylamine salt of 2,4-dichlorophenoxyacetic acid *	17.22%
Dimethylamine salt of dicamba *	3.43%
Water base	

PRATT DP-2 SPECIAL INSECT SPRAY
(Pratt-Gabriel Div.)

Isoparaffinic hydrocarbons *	98.411%
Diazinon	0.500%
Pyrethrins	0.100%
Piperonyl butoxide	0.200%
N-Octyl bicycloheptene dicarboximide	0.700%

PRATT DURSBAN 135 EC LAWN & ORNAMENTAL PLANT INSECTICIDE
(Pratt-Gabriel Div.)

Dursban *	13.5%
Xylene *	80.5%
Emulsifier	5.0%

PRATT D-X INSECT SPRAY
(Pratt-Gabriel Div.)

Piperonyl butoxide	2.0%
Pyrethrins	0.28%
Rotenone	0.75%
Pine oil	20.0%
Aromatic petroleum solvent *	30.47%

PRATT 6E OIL SPRAY
Insecticide
(Pratt-Gabriel Div.)

Ethion *	2.0%
Petroleum oil *	96.35%

PRATT FRUIT TREE SPRAY
Insecticide & fungicide
(Pratt-Gabriel Div.)

Captan	6%
Methoxychlor *	10%
Malathion *	6%
Sulfur	25%

PRATT HOUSE PLANT SPRAY BOMB
(Pratt-Gabriel Div.)

Pyrethrum	0.056%
Rotenone	0.008%
Other cube resins	0.016%
Pine oil	0.900%
Petroleum distillate	0.406%

PRATT 505 K INSECT SPRAY
(Pratt-Gabriel Div.)

Methoxychlor	24.0%
Malathion	13.0%
Kelthane	3.0%
Xylene *	51.17%

PRATT & LAMBERT PAINT PRODUCTS
Paints, varnishes, & epoxy coatings

Pratt & Lambert, Inc.
75 Tonawanda
Buffalo, N.Y. 14207

Mailing address:
Box 22
Buffalo, N.Y. 14240

Phone: 716-873-6000

See PAINTS, Section VI, General Formulations

PRATT & LAMBERT RED LEAD PRIMER
(Pratt & Lambert)

Lead *	>1%

PRATT 5% LINDANE BORER SPRAY
Insecticide
(Pratt-Gabriel Div.)

Lindane	5%
Aromatic 100 *†	90%
Emulsifier	5%

†*See* Aromatic hydrocarbon solvent

PRATT MALATHION-50 SPRAY
Insecticide
(Pratt-Gabriel Div.)

Malathion *	50%
Xylene *	43.3%

PRATT METHOXYCHLOR-25 INSECT SPRAY
Insecticide
(Pratt-Gabriel Div.)

Methoxychlor	25.00%
Xylene *	72.00%

PRATT MITE SPRAY
Miticide
(Pratt-Gabriel Div.)

Kelthane *	18.5%

PRATT NA WEED KILLER
(Pratt-Gabriel Div.)

Prometon	3.5%
Iso-octyl ester of 2,4-dichlorophenoxyacetic acid	1.5%
Xylene *	79.36%
Emulsifier	2.5%

PRATT NOCULATE SYSTEMIC INSECTICIDE GRANULAR
(Pratt-Gabriel Div.)

Disyston *	1%

Starred ingredients (*) may be responsible for major toxic effects; consult Section II.

PRATT NOCULATE 3 INSECT SPRAY
(Pratt-Gabriel Div.)

Meta-Systox-R (S-(2-(Ethyl-sulfinyl)ethyl) O-O-dimethyl phosphorothioate)	6.0%
Kelthane	0.9%
Methoxychlor (technical)	5.0%
Methyl isobutyl ketone	20.0%
Aromatic petroleum distillate *	49.6%

PRATT PRUNING BOMB AND PRUNING DRESSING
(Pratt-Gabriel Div.)

Asphalt
Light aromatic solvent *†

†*See* Aromatic hydrocarbon solvent

PRATT PYRETHRUM FOGGING SPRAY
Insecticide
(Pratt-Gabriel Div.)

Isoparaffinic hydrocarbons *	99.15%
Pyrethrum	0.10%
Piperonyl butoxide	0.75%

PRATT ROOM FOGGER
(Pratt-Gabriel Div.)

Pyrethrins	0.50%
Technical Piperonyl butoxide	1.00%
N-Octyl bicycloheptene dicarboximide	1.68%
Petroleum distillates *	11.82%

PRATT ROSE & FLOWER DUST
Fungicide & insecticide
(Pratt-Gabriel Div.)

Sevin *	3%
Folpet	5%
Malathion	4%
Kelthane	1.5%

PRATT SPREADER STICKER
(Pratt-Gabriel Div.)

Emulsified beta-Pinene polymer	96%

PRATT TOMATO & VEGETABLE DUST OR SPRAY
Insecticide, fungicide
(Pratt-Gabriel Div.)

Rotenone	0.75%
Other cube resins	1.50%
Copper (in basic copper sulfate), as metallic copper *	7.00%

PRATT TURF FUNGICIDE 50% WETTABLE POWDER
(Pratt-Gabriel Div.)

Dyrene *	50.0%

PRATT TURF HERBICIDE 6,000
(Pratt-Gabriel Div.)

Dimethylamine salt of 2-(2-methyl-4-chlorophenoxy)propionic acid	2.77%
Dimethylamine salt of 2,4-dichlorophenoxyacetic acid	6.10%
Dimethylamine salt of dicamba	0.63%
Dimethylamine salts of related compounds	0.08%

PRATT 2 SEVIN
Insecticide
(Pratt-Gabriel Div.)

Carbaryl *	22.5%

PRATT WASP & HORNET SPRAY
(Pratt-Gabriel Div.)

Pyrethrins	0.10%
Piperonyl butoxide	0.20%
N-Octyl bicycloheptene dicarboximide	0.33%
Baygon	0.50%
Isoparaffinic hydrocarbons *	83.87%

PRATT WHITEFLY SPRAY
Insecticide
(Pratt-Gabriel Div.)

Resmethrin	0.250%

PRECARE FA
For treatment of vitamin and mineral deficiencies
(Russ Pharm.)

Each tablet:
Ferrous fumarate (32.87% Fe) *	66 mg.
Potassium iodine (76.45% I)	150 mcg.
Vitamin A acetate	8000 I.U.
Vitamin D2	400 I.U.
Plus multivitamins and minerals	

PRECURSOR
Embalming supply
(Royal Bond)

Ethylene diamine tetraacetic acid, sodium salt

PRED FORTE
Ophthalmic suspension
(Allergan Pharm.)

Prednisolone acetate	1.0%
Benzalkonium chloride	
Polysorbate 80	
Boric acid	
Sodium citrate	
Sodium bisulfite	
Sodium chloride	
Edetate disodium	
Hydroxypropyl methylcellulose	
Purified water	

PRED MILD
Ophthalmic suspension
(Allergan Pharm.)

Prednisolone acetate	0.12%
Benzalkonium chloride	
Polysorbate 80	
Boric acid	
Sodium citrate	
Sodium bisulfite	
Sodium chloride	
Edetate disodium	
Hydroxypropyl methylcellulose	
Purified water	

PREDNICEN-M TABLETS
Anti-inflammatory
(Central Pharmacal Co.)

Each tablet:
Prednisone	5 mg.

PREE-ZERV
Christmas tree preserver
(Lake Products)

Lake Products Co., Inc.
P.O. Box 498
Ballwin, Mo. 63011

Phone: 314-536-1600

PREFAR (4-E)
Herbicide
(Stauffer)

Prefar (S-(O,O-Diisopropyl phosphorodithioate) of N-(2-mercaptoethyl) benzenesulfonamide) *

PREFLEX
Cleaning solution for soft contact lenses
(Burton, Parsons & Co.)

Sodium phosphates	
Sodium chloride	
Tyloxapol	
Hydroxyethylcellulose	
Polyvinyl alcohol	
Thimerosal (as preservative)	0.004%
Disodium edetate (as preservative)	0.2%

PREFRIN-A
Ophthalmic solution
(Allergan Pharm.)

Pyrilamine maleate	0.1%
Phenylephrine HCl	0.12%

PREFRIN LIQUIFILM
Ophthalmic solution
(Allergan Pharm.)

Phenylephrine HCl	0.12%
Polyvinyl alcohol	1.4%
Antipyrine	0.1%

Starred ingredients (*) may be responsible for major toxic effects; consult Section II.

PREFRIN-Z LIQUIFILM
Ophthalmic solution
(Allergan Pharm.)

Zinc sulfate	0.25%
Phenylephrine HCl	0.12%
Polyvinyl alcohol	1.4%
Thimerosal	0.005%

PREGENT
Prenatal supplement
(Beutlich, Inc.)

Each tablet:
Calcium carbonate	300 mg.
Vitamin D	300 I.U.
Ferrous sulfate (dried) *	130 mg.
Ascorbic acid	100 mg.
Hesperidin complex	10 mg.
Folic acid	0.1 mg.

PRE-LAC DAIRY WORMER

See PURINA PRE-LAC DAIRY WORMER

PRELL CONCENTRATE (GEL)
Shampoo
(Procter & Gamble, Beauty Care Div.)

Triethanolamine alkyl sulfate *	25-35%
Coconut monoethanolamide	1-7%
Hydroxypropyl methylcellulose	1-4%
Triethanolamine	1-4%
Ethanol	3-5%
Sodium tripolyphosphate	1-4%
Perfume	1-2%
Minor ingredients, each	<1%
Water	>50%

PRELL ENRICHED FORMULA CONCENTRATE (GEL)
Shampoo
(Procter & Gamble, Beauty Care Div.)

Ammonium lauryl sulfate	8-14%
Sodium lauryl sulfate	4-8%
Coconut diethanolamide	5-10%
Alcohol	0-5%
Minor ingredients, each	<1%
Water	50%

PRELL ENRICHED FORMULA LIQUID
Shampoo
(Procter & Gamble, Beauty Care Div.)

Ammonium lauryl sulfate	5-10%
Sodium lauryl sulfate	3-5%
Coconut diethanolamide	1-3%
Alcohol	<1%
Minor ingredients, each	<1%
Water	50%

PRELL LIQUID
Shampoo
(Procter & Gamble, Beauty Care Div.)

Triethanolamine alkyl sulfate *	10-24%
Coconut monoethanolamide	1-6%
Hydroxypropyl methylcellulose	<1%
Triethanolamine	1-4%
Ethanol	5-9%
Perfume	1-2%
Minor ingredients, each	<1%
Water	>50%

PRELUDIN ENDURETS
Prolonged-action appetite suppressant
(Boehringer Ingelheim)

Each tablet:
Phenmetrazine hydrochloride (2-Phenyl-3-methyl-tetrahydro-1,4-oxazine hydrochloride) *	50 mg.; 75 mg.

PRELUDIN TABLETS
Appetite suppressant
(Boehringer Ingelheim)

Each tablet:
Phenmetrazine hydrochloride (2-Phenyl-3-methyl-tetrahydro-1,4-oxazine hydrochloride) *	25 mg.

PREMERGE 3 DINITRO AMINE HERBICIDE
(Dow)

Active ingred.:	50.7%
2-sec-Butyl-4,6-dinitrophenol, alkanolamine salts *	
Inert ingred.:	49.3%
Sequestering agents	
Methanol	
Water	

PREMO ALKALINE AROMATIC TABLETS
Antiseptic mouth wash
(Premo)

Each tablet:
Sodium bicarbonate	5 gr.
Sodium borate *	5 gr.
Sodium chloride	5 gr.
Sodium benzoate	7/24 gr.
Sodium salicylate	7/24 gr.
Oil eucalyptol	
Thymol	
Menthol	
Oil wintergreen *	

'76 Ed.

PREMO ANALGESIC BALM
(Premo)

Methyl salicylate *
Menthol *
Lanolin

'76 Ed.

PREMO ANTI-HISTAMINE TABLETS
(Premo)

Each tablet:
Pyrilamine maleate N.F. *	25 mg.

'76 Ed.

PREMO CASCARA COMPOUND (DR. HINKLES) TABLETS
Laxative
(Premo)

Each tablet:
Extract Cascara	1/4 gr.
Aloin *	1/4 gr.
Podophyllin *	1/6 gr.
Extract Belladonna	1/8 gr.
Oleoresin ginger	1/16 gr.

'76 Ed.

PREMOCONES
Hemorrhoidal suppositories
(Premo)

Tyrothricin *
Bismuth subgallate *
Bismuth oxyiodide *
Peruvian balsam *
Benzocaine
Zinc oxide

'76 Ed.

PREMO EAR ANODYNE
Ear drops
(Premo)

Each 15 cc.:
Antipyrine *	0.8 gm.
Benzocaine	0.2 gm.
Glycerine anhydrous	q.s.

'76 Ed.

PREMO EYE DROPS
(Premo)

Chlorobutanol
Berberine sulfate *
Boric acid *
Zinc sulfate

'76 Ed.

PREMO HEMORRHOIDAL SUPPOSITORIES
(Premo)

Bismuth subnitrate *
Balsam Peru *
Tannic acid *
Resorcinol *
Zinc oxide
Benzocaine

'76 Ed.

Starred ingredients (*) may be responsible for major toxic effects; consult Section II.

PREMO ORAL-DENTAL JELLY
(Premo)

Benzocaine
Glycerine
Menthol *

'76 Ed.

PREMOTRATE TABLETS
(Premo)

Each tablet:
Pentaerythritol
tetranitrate * .... 10 mg.; 20 mg.

'76 Ed.

PREM-TANK - P.R. (Powder)

See GUNK P.R. - PREM-TANK (Powder)

PRENTOX ALLETHRIN FOGGING & CONTACT SPRAY
Insecticide
(Prentiss)

Allethrin (allyl homolog of Cinerin I) 0.250%
Piperonyl butoxide (technical) ... 0.500%
N-Octyl bicycloheptene
dicarboximide 0.825%
Petroleum distillates * 98.425%

PRENTOX ALLETHRIN MOSQUITO ADULTICIDE FOR ULV FOGGERS
(Prentiss)

Allethrin * 12.00%
Related compounds 1.34%
Piperonyl butoxide (technical) .. 60.00%
Mineral oil 26.66%

PRENTOX BERRY BUSH SPRAY CONCENTRATE
(Prentiss)

Malathion 5.5%
Heavy Aromatic naphtha * 89.2%

PRENTOX D.D.V.P. FIVE
Insecticide
(Prentiss)

2,2-Dichlorovinyl dimethyl
phosphate * 4.65%
Related compounds 0.35%
Petroleum distillates * 15.00%

PRENTOX DIAZINON AG500
Insecticide
(Prentiss)

Diazinon * 48%
Xylene 39%

PRENTOX DIAZINON 1E INSECTICIDE
(Prentiss)

Diazinon * 13.20%
Aromatic petroleum derivative
solvent 72.32%

PRENTOX DIAZINON 4E INSECTICIDE
Control of roaches, ants, silverfish, other pests
(Prentiss)

Diazinon * 47.5%
Aromatic petroleum derivative
solvent * 30.0%

PRENTOX DIAZINON 6E INSECTICIDE
Control of roaches, ants, silverfish, other pests
(Prentiss)

Diazinon * 68.0%
Aromatic petroleum derivative
solvent 6.6%

PRENTOX DIAZINON 6.25 E INSECTICIDE
(Prentiss)

Diazinon * 6.25%
Aromatic petroleum derivative
solvent 80.25%

PRENTOX DIAZINON EMULSIFIABLE CONCENTRATE
Insecticide
(Prentiss)

Diazinon * 6.25%
Aromatic petroleum derivative
solvent 80.25%

PRENTOX DIAZINON 12-1/2 EMULSIFIABLE CONCENTRATE
Lawn and garden insect control
(Prentiss)

Diazinon * 12.5%
Aromatic petroleum derivative
solvent * 73.0%

PRENTOX DIAZINON 25% EMULSIFIABLE CONCENTRATE
Lawn and garden insect control
(Prentiss)

Diazinon * 25.0%
Aromatic petroleum derivative
solvent * 55.7%

PRENTOX DIAZINON 4S INSECTICIDE
For control of cockroaches and other household pests
(Prentiss)

Diazinon * 48.7%
Aromatic petroleum derivative
solvent * 43.6%

PRENTOX DIAZINON 1% SOLUTION
Control of roaches and ants
(Prentiss)

Diazinon 1.0%
Kerosene * 99.0%

PRENTOX DIMETHOATE 2E
Insecticide
(Prentiss)

Dimethoate * 23.4%

PRENTOX DPBM CONCENTRATE #4425
Insecticide for use in mechanical sprayers
(Prentiss)

2,2-Dichlorovinyl dimethyl
phosphate 0.46%
Other related compounds 0.04%
Pyrethrins 2.00%
Piperonyl butoxide (technical) .. 4.00%
N-Octyl bicycloheptene
dicarboximide 4.00%
Petroleum distillates * 89.50%

PRENTOX DUAL PYRIFOS RESIDUAL 50
Insecticide
(Prentiss)

Dursban 0.500%
Pyrethrins 0.060%
Piperonyl butoxide (technical) . 0.120%
N-Octyl bicycloheptene
dicarboximide 0.200%
Petroleum distillates * 99.088%

PRENTOX DURSBAN 2E INSECTICIDE
Controls pests of household, turf and ornamentals
(Prentiss)

Chlorpyrifos * 22.4%
Aromatic petroleum derivative
solvent * 46.2%

PRENTOX DURSBAN 4E INSECTICIDE
Controls pests of household, turf and ornamentals
(Prentiss)

Chlorpyrifos * 44.8%
Xylene * 46.3%

Starred ingredients (*) may be responsible for major toxic effects; consult Section II.

PRENTOX EMULSIFIABLE DUAL PRO-PYRIFOS
Insecticide
(Prentiss)

Chlorpyrifos *	31.99%
Piperonyl butoxide (technical)	4.44%
N-Octyl bicycloheptene dicarboximide	7.40%
Pyrethrins	2.22%
Xylene range aromatic solvent	22.12%
Petroleum distillates	26.83%

PRENTOX EMULSIFIABLE SPRAY CONCENTRATE #96
Insecticide
(Prentiss)

Pyrethrins	0.96%
Piperonyl butoxide (technical)	9.60%
Petroleum distillates *	81.44%

PRENTOX EMULSIFIABLE SPRAY CONCENTRATE #101
For control of roaches, waterbugs and silverfish
(Prentiss)

Pyrethrins	1.20%
Piperonyl butoxide (technical)	9.60%
Petroleum distillates *	81.20%

PRENTOX FOGGING CONCENTRATE #1
Insecticide
(Prentiss)

Pyrethrins	0.3%
Piperonyl butoxide (technical)	0.6%
N-Octyl bicycloheptene dicarboximide	1.0%
Petroleum distillates *	98.1%

PRENTOX FOGGING CONCENTRATE #2
Insecticide
(Prentiss)

Pyrethrins	0.45%
Piperonyl butoxide (technical)	0.90%
N-Octyl bicycloheptene dicarboximide	1.50%
Petroleum distillates *	97.15%

PRENTOX FOGGING INSECTICIDE PF
(Prentiss)

Pyrethrins	0.5%
Piperonyl butoxide (technical)	5.0%
Petroleum distillate *	94.5%

PRENTOX GRAIN PROTECTANT DUST NO. 101
(Prentiss)

Pyrethrins	0.06%
Technical Piperonyl butoxide	1.00%

PRENTOX HOUSEHOLD FLY-DI INSECT SPRAY
(Prentiss)

Pyrethrins	0.2%
Petroleum distillate *	99.8%

PRENTOX INSECT FOGGING SPRAY CONCENTRATE F-102
(Prentiss)

Pyrethrins	0.15%
Piperonyl butoxide (technical)	1.50%
Deodorized Kerosene *	98.35%

PRENTOX INSECT SPRAY "A"
For the control of flies, roaches, silver-fish and other pests
(Prentiss)

Pyrethrins	0.075%
Piperonyl butoxide (technical)	0.150%
N-Octyl bicycloheptene dicarboximide	0.250%
Petroleum distillates *	99.525%

PRENTOX INSECT SPRAY "B"
For the control of flies, mosquitoes, roaches, silverfish, fleas, and other pests
(Prentiss)

Pyrethrins	0.15%
Piperonyl butoxide (technical)	0.30%
N-Octyl bicycloheptene dicarboximide	0.50%
Petroleum distillates *	99.05%

PRENTOX INSECT SPRAY "C"
For the control of flies, mosquitoes, roaches, silverfish, beetles, and other pests
(Prentiss)

Pyrethrins	0.30%
Piperonyl butoxide (technical)	0.60%
N-Octyl bicycloheptene dicarboximide	1.00%
Petroleum distillates *	98.10%

PRENTOX INSECT SPRAY "D"
For the control of flies, mosquitoes, roaches, silverfish, and other pests
(Prentiss)

Pyrethrins	0.45%
Piperonyl butoxide (technical)	0.90%
N-Octyl bicycloheptene dicarboximide	1.50%
Petroleum distillates *	97.15%

PRENTOX 5 LB. MALATHION SPRAY
Insecticide
(Prentiss)

Malathion *	57%
Methylated naphthalenes	35%

PRENTOX 2 LB. METHOXYCHLOR SPRAY
Insecticide
(Prentiss)

Active ingred.:	93%
Methoxychlor (technical) *	24%
Methylated naphthalenes *	69%
Inert ingred.:	7%
Emulsifier - a blend consisting of:	
Emcol 300	90%
Emcol 500	10%

PRENTOX LINDANE 20% EMULSIFIABLE CONCENTRATE
Insecticide
(Prentiss)

Lindane	20.00%
Xylene range aromatic solvent *	67.05%
Cyclohexanone	5.00%

PRENTOX LIQUID HOUSEHOLD INSECT SPRAY #1
(Prentiss)

Pyrethrins	0.05%
Piperonyl butoxide (technical)	0.26%
Diazinon	0.50%
Petroleum distillates *	99.12%

PRENTOX MALATHION 50% EMULSIFIABLE INSECTICIDE
(Prentiss)

Malathion *	50.0%
Aromatic solvents	27.0%
Petroleum distillates	17.3%

PRENTOX MALATHION 5 LB. EMULSIFIABLE CONCENTRATE PREMIUM GRADE
Insecticide
(Prentiss)

Malathion *	57%
Methylated naphthalenes	34%

PRENTOX MALATHION 5 LB. EMULSIFIABLE INSECTICIDE
(Prentiss)

Malathion *	55.0%
Heavy Aromatic naphtha	35.6%

PRENTOX MALATHION 57% PREMIUM GRADE EMULSIFIABLE INSECTICIDE
(Prentiss)

Malathion *	57%
Xylene	40%

Starred ingredients (*) may be responsible for major toxic effects; consult Section II.

PRENTOX 80% MALATHION SPRAY
For aphids, mites, scale insects
(Prentiss)

Malathion *	80%
Methylated naphthalenes	5%

PRENTOX METHOXYCHLOR 25% SPRAY
Insecticide
(Prentiss)

Methoxychlor (technical)	25.4%
Xylene *	71.6%

PRENTOX MILL SPRAY CONCENTRATE #562
For control of roaches, silverfish and insect pests of stored fruit
(Prentiss)

Pyrethrins	0.62%
Piperonyl butoxide (technical)	5.03%
Petroleum hydrocarbons *	94.35%

PRENTOX MOSQUITO FOG CONCENTRATE
(Prentiss)

Fenthion	9.3%
Aromatic petroleum distillates *	90.0%

PRENTOX MOSQUITO FOGGING CONCENTRATE F103
(Prentiss)

Petroleum oil *	97.09%
Technical Piperonyl butoxide	2.64%
Pyrethrins	0.27%

PRENTOX MOSQUITO YARD SPRAY CONCENTRATE
(Prentiss)

Aromatic petroleum derivative solvent *	75%
Malathion	12%
Methoxychlor (technical)	10%

PRENTOX PB CONCENTRATE #20
Insecticide
(Prentiss)

Pyrethrins	0.62%
Piperonyl butoxide (technical)	5.03%
Petroleum distillates *	94.35%

PRENTOX PB CONCENTRATE #125
Insecticide
(Prentiss)

Pyrethrins	1.25%
Piperonyl butoxide (technical)	5.05%
Petroleum distillates *	93.70%

PRENTOX POMATO TOMATO POTATO DUST OR SPRAY
(Prentiss)

Methoxychlor (technical) *	10%
Captan	6%

PRENTOX PRENCHLOR 8-LB. EMULSIFIABLE CONCENTRATE INSECTICIDE
For control of subterranean termites
(Prentiss)

Technical Chlordane *	72.0%
Petroleum distillate *	21.0%

PRENTOX PRENFISH TOXICANT
Liquid-emulsifiable
(Prentiss)

Rotenone *	5.0%
Other cube extractives *	10.0%

PRENTOX PYRETHRUM 1%
Insecticide for spraying or fogging
(Prentiss)

Pyrethrins	1%
Refined Petroleum distillates *	99%

PRENTOX PYRIFOS RESIDUAL 25
Insecticide
(Prentiss)

Pyrethrins	0.030%
Piperonyl butoxide (technical)	0.060%
N-Octyl bicycloheptene dicarboximide	0.100%
Chlorpyrifos	0.250%
Petroleum distillates *	99.544%

PRENTOX PYRONYL CROP SPRAY
Insecticide
(Prentiss)

Pyrethrins	6.00%
Piperonyl butoxide (technical)	60.00%
Petroleum distillates *	14.00%

PRENTOX PYRONYL - DIAZINON EMULSIFIABLE CONCENTRATE
Insecticide
(Prentiss)

Diazinon	10.0%
Pyrethrins	1.0%
Piperonyl butoxide (technical)	5.0%
Petroleum distillates *	72.4%

PRENTOX PYRONYL 1.2-2.4-4.0 EMULSIFIABLE CONCENTRATE
Insecticide to control pests infesting grain and food storage plants
(Prentiss)

Petroleum distillates *	80.4%
N-Octyl bicycloheptene dicarboximide	4.0%
Piperonyl butoxide (technical)	2.4%
Pyrethrins	1.2%

PRENTOX PYRONYL FOGGING AND CONTACT SPRAY
Insecticide
(Prentiss)

Pyrethrins	0.250%
Piperonyl butoxide (technical)	0.500%
N-Octyl bicycloheptene dicarboximide	0.825%
Petroleum distillates *	98.425%

PRENTOX PYRONYL LIVESTOCK SPRAY CONCENTRATE
Insecticide
(Prentiss)

Petroleum distillates *	78.80%
Piperonyl butoxide (technical)	12.00%
Pyrethrins	1.20%

PRENTOX PYRONYL MOSQUITO ADULTICIDE FOR ULV FOGGERS
(Prentiss)

Pyrethrins *	12%
Piperonyl butoxide (technical)	60%
Mineral oil	28%

PRENTOX PYRONYL OIL CONCENTRATE #525
Insecticide for use in spray equipment
(Prentiss)

Pyrethrins	5.00%
Piperonyl butoxide (technical)	25.00%
Petroleum distillates *	70.00%

PRENTOX PYRONYL OIL CONCENTRATE #1229-A
Insecticide
(Prentiss)

Pyrethrins	1.00%
Piperonyl butoxide (technical)	2.00%
N-Octyl bicycloheptene dicarboximide	2.94%
Petroleum distillates *	94.06%

Starred ingredients (*) may be responsible for major toxic effects; consult Section II.

PRENTOX PYRONYL OIL CONCENTRATE #1233
Insecticide
(Prentiss)

Pyrethrins	1.00%
Piperonyl butoxide (technical)	2.00%
N-Octyl bicycloheptene dicarboximide	3.33%
Petroleum distillates *	93.67%

PRENTOX PYRONYL OIL CONCENTRATE #1530
Insecticide for use in spray equipment
(Prentiss)

Pyrethrins	1.50%
Piperonyl butoxide (technical)	3.00%
N-Octyl bicycloheptene dicarboximide	5.50%
Petroleum distillates *	90.00%

PRENTOX PYRONYL OIL CONCENTRATE #3610
Insecticide for use in spray equipment
(Prentiss)

Pyrethrins	3.00%
Piperonyl butoxide (technical)	6.00%
N-Octyl bicycloheptene dicarboximide	10.00%
Petroleum distillates *	81.00%

PRENTOX PYRONYL OIL CONCENTRATE #12294
Insecticide
(Prentiss)

Pyrethrins	1.00%
Piperonyl butoxide (technical)	2.00%
N-Octyl bicycloheptene dicarboximide	2.94%
Mineral oil *	90.06%
Petroleum distillates	4.00%

PRENTOX PYRONYL OIL CONCENTRATE OR-3610-A
Insecticide for use in spray equipment
(Prentiss)

Pyrethrins	3.00%
Piperonyl butoxide (technical)	6.00%
N-Octyl bicycloheptene dicarboximide	10.00%
Petroleum distillates *	81.00%

PRENTOX PYRONYL POULTRY HOUSE & BARN FLY SPRAY
(Prentiss)

Pyrethrins	2.00%
Piperonyl butoxide (technical)	4.00%
N-Octyl bicycloheptene dicarboximide	6.66%
Petroleum distillates *	87.34%

PRENTOX PYRONYL POULTRY HOUSE & BARN FLY SPRAY "A"
(Prentiss)

Pyrethrins	0.62%
Piperonyl butoxide (technical)	5.03%
Petroleum hydrocarbons *	94.35%

PRENTOX RAX TRACKING POWDER
Rodenticide
(Prentiss)

Warfarin	1.00%

PRENTOX RAX WATER SOLUBLE WARFARIN RTU
Rodenticide
(Prentiss)

Active ingred.:	
Warfarin, sodium salt	0.54%
Inert ingred.:	
Silica	99.46%

PRENTOX READY-TO-USE MOSQUITO FOG CONTAINS BAYTEX
(Prentiss)

Fenthion	0.93%
Aromatic petroleum distillates *	99.00%

PRENTOX REDI-USE MOUSE & RAT BAIT
(Prentiss)

Warfarin	0.025%

PRENTOX RESIDUAL CONCENTRATE DV-ONE
Control of cockroaches
(Prentiss)

Chlorpyrifos *	13.00%
2,2-Dichlorovinyl dimethyl phosphate	4.82%
Related compounds	0.37%
Xylene *	76.81%

PRENTOX RESIDUAL CONCENTRATE DV-TWO
Control of cockroaches
(Prentiss)

Chlorpyrifos *	24.00%
2,2-Dichlorovinyl dimethyl phosphate	8.32%
Related compounds	0.68%
Xylene *	62.00%

PRENTOX RESIDUAL INSECT SPRAY #2
(Prentiss)

Dursban	0.5%
Pyrethrins	0.1%
Piperonyl butoxide (technical)	0.2%
N-Octyl bicycloheptene dicarboximide	0.3%
Aromatic petroleum derivative solvent	1.0%
Petroleum distillates *	97.9%

PRENTOX RESIDUAL PYRIFOS 25
Insecticide
(Prentiss)

Chlorpyrifos	0.25%
Piperonyl butoxide (technical)	0.25%
Pyrethrins	0.05%
Petroleum distillates *	99.11%

PRENTOX RESIDUAL SPRAY w/BAYGON
Insecticide
(Prentiss)

Baygon *	1.00%
Petroleum distillates *	83.75%

PRENTOX RESIDUAL SPRAY w/DIAZINON
To control cockroaches and ants
(Prentiss)

Diazinon	0.5%
Petroleum distillates *	99.5%

PRENTOX ROACH, ANT AND SILVERFISH POWDER
(Prentiss)

Pyrethrins	0.9%

PRENTOX SEVIN 4F
Insecticide
(Prentiss)

Carbaryl *	42.6%

PRENTOX SPRAY CONCENTRATE #625
For control of roaches, waterbugs and silverfish
(Prentiss)

Pyrethrins	0.62%
Piperonyl butoxide (technical)	5.03%
Petroleum hydrocarbons *	94.35%

PRENTOX SPRAY CONCENTRATE #1575
For control of roaches, waterbugs and silverfish
(Prentiss)

Pyrethrins	1.50%
Piperonyl butoxide (technical)	7.50%
Petroleum hydrocarbons *	91.00%

Starred ingredients (*) may be responsible for major toxic effects; consult Section II.

PRENTOX SYNPREN-FISH TOXICANT
Liquid-emulsifiable
(Prentiss)

Rotenone *	2.5%
Other cube extractives	5.0%
Piperonyl butoxide (technical)	2.5%

PRENTOX SYNPY-DIAZINON EMULSIFIABLE CONCENTRATE
For control of cockroaches, ants, silverfish, spiders
(Prentiss)

Diazinon *	20.0%
Pyrethrins	2.0%
Piperonyl butoxide (technical)	10.0%
Petroleum distillates	55.0%

PRENTOX TFL KILLER
For ticks, fleas and lice on dogs
(Prentiss)

Pyrethrins	0.25%
Piperonyl butoxide (technical)	2.15%
Petroleum distillates *	97.20%

PRENTOX 3 WAY DUST GARDEN INSECTICIDE
(Prentiss)

Sulfur *	10%
Rotenone	1%
Other cube resins	2%

PRENTOX VAPON 2
Emulsifiable concentrate insecticide
(Prentiss)

Aromatic petroleum derivatives *	68.10%
2,2-Dichlorovinyl dimethyl phosphate *	22.69%
Related compounds	1.71%

PRENTOX VAPON 20%
Insecticide
(Prentiss)

2,2-Dichlorovinyl dimethyl phosphate	18.6%
Related compounds	1.4%
Heavy Aromatic naphtha	1.5%
Xylene range aromatic solvent *	73.5%

PRE-PAIR INSTRUMENT CLEANER
(Polychem Corp.)

Sodium dodecylbenzenesulfonate
Water
Propylene glycol
Linear Alcohol ethoxylate
Coconut diethanolamide
Tetrasodium EDTA
Sodium xylene sulfonate
Quaternium-15
Citric acid

PRE-PAIR 2 LOW FOAM INSTRUMENT CLEANER
(Polychem Corp.)

Water
Polyoxypropylene-polyoxyethylene block copolymer
Sodium xylene sulfonate
Anionic phosphate ester, potassium salt
Tetrasodium EDTA
Quaternium-15
Citric acid
FD & C Yellow #5

PRE-PAIR LUBRICANT
(Polychem Corp.)

Water
Polybutene
Propylene glycol
Oleth-2
Oleth-20
Triethanolamine oleate
Sulfated Castor oil
DMDM hydantoin
Methylparaben
Propylparaben

PREPARATION H
Suppositories & ointment for hemorrhoid relief
(Whitehall Labs.)

Live yeast cell deriv. (skin respiratory factor)	2,000 units/oz.
Shark liver oil	3.0%
Phenyl mercuric nitrate	1:10,000

PREPARATION H CLEANSING PADS
Rectal cleansing pads
(Whitehall Labs.)

Glycerine
Hamamelis water
Methylparaben

PREPARATION H STOOL SOFTENER
(Whitehall Labs.)

Dioctyl sodium sulfosuccinate *

PREP SURFACE BONDING PRIMER
(Reliable Paste)

Xylol *	<8%
Aliphatic hydrocarbons (Rule 66 type) *	
Alkyd resin	10%
Driers *	
Isobutyl alcohol	about 10%

PRE-SAN
Herbicide
(Mallinckrodt, Inc.)

S-(O,O-Diisopropyl phosphorodithioate) of N-(2-mercaptoethyl) benzenesulfonamide *	45.2%

PRE-SERT
Hard contact lens cushioning solution
(Allergan Pharm.)

Polyvinyl alcohol	3.0%
Benzalkonium chloride	1:25,000

PRESTO ATHLETE'S FOOT LIQUID, DR. SCHOLL'S
See DR. SCHOLL'S PRESTO ATHLETE'S FOOT LIQUID

PRESTO, LIQUID
See LIQUID PRESTO

PRESTO MULTICOLOR
Easter egg dye
(Doxsee Food Corp.)

U.S. certified color	1.0%
Edible waxes	
Edible gums	

PRESTONE CARB & CHOKE CLEANER (AS-217N, Formula 1936-68)
(Union Carbide)

Aromatic hydrocarbons *	71%
Ketones	29%
Hydrocarbon propellant	

PRESTONE DE-ICER (AS-243, Formula 1543-19)
Pressurized windshield de-icer
(Union Carbide)

Methyl alcohol *	45%
Water	40%
Ethylene glycol *	15%
Carbon dioxide propellant	

PRESTONE ENGINE STARTING FLUID (AS-236, Formula MI-2238)
(Union Carbide)

Unrefined Ether *	63%
Aliphatic hydrocarbon	36%
Mineral oil	1%
Carbon dioxide propellant	

PRESTONE FOAMING ACTION GREASE EATER (AS-186N, Formula 2219-11)
(Union Carbide)

Water	52%
Petroleum distillates *	40%
Anionic surfactant	6%
Sodium metasilicate	2%
Hydrocarbon propellant	

PRESTONE GAS LINE ANTI-FREEZE (AS-131 - Formula MI-2273; AS-132 - Formula MI-2274)
(Union Carbide)

Methyl alcohol * 100%

PRESTONE GAS MISER (AS-222P, Formula 2181-52)
Automotive gasoline additive
(Union Carbide)

Petroleum distillates * 96%
Polyalkylamine 4%

PRESTONE HEAVY DUTY BRAKE FLUID (AS-400, 401, 402, 403, Formula PM-5822)
(Union Carbide)

Mixed Polyglycol ethers * 73%
Polyalkylene glycol 26%
Inhibitors 1%

PRESTONE HEAVY DUTY COOLING SYSTEM CLEANER (AS-100, Formula MI-2223)
(Union Carbide)

Cleaner:
  Oxalic acid * 95%
  Clay 4%
  Nonionic surfactants 1%
Neutralizer:
  Sodium carbonate * 95%
  Clay 4%
  Nonionic surfactants 1%

PRESTONE HEAVY DUTY SILICONE CAR WAX & CLEANER (AS-149, Formula MI-2233)
(Union Carbide)

Petroleum distillates * 40%
Water 39%
Inorganic polishing agents 11%
Silicone fluids 5%
Emulsifier 3%
Wax 2%

PRESTONE HIGH PERFORMING OIL TREATMENT (AS-220, Formula MI-2202)
(Union Carbide)

Hydrocarbon (high molecular
  weight) * 100%

PRESTONE PRE-SOFTENED PASTE WAX (AS-155, Formula 2221-76)
(Union Carbide)

Water 44%
Petroleum distillates* 31%
Inorganic polishing agents 12%
Waxes 7%
Silicone fluids 5%
Emulsifier 1%

PRESTONE PRIME GAS DRYER (AS-130, Formula MI-2218)
(Union Carbide)

Methyl alcohol * 100%

PRESTONE RADIATOR ANTI-RUST AND WATER PUMP LUBRICANT (AS-110/111, Formula 2017-44)
(Union Carbide)

Water 64–67%
Mineral oil * 25–27%
Surfactants and emulsifiers 8–9%

PRESTONE SQUEEZE DE-ICER (AS-244, Formula 2138-66)
(Union Carbide)

Water 50%
Methyl alcohol * 35%
Ethylene glycol 15%

PRESTONE SUPER FLUSH (AS-107, Formula 2017-29A)
(Union Carbide)

Water 78%
Sodium citrate 10%
Anionic and Nonionic surfactants .. 7%
Isopropyl alcohol 5%

PRESTONE SUPER HEAVY DUTY BRAKE FLUID (AS-600, 601, 602, 603, Formula PM-5830)
(Union Carbide)

Mixed Polyglycol ethers * 79%
Polyalkylene glycol 20%
Inhibitors 1%

PRESTONE 10-MINUTE RADIATOR FLUSH (AS-105 (Solvent), Formula 2017-20A)
(Union Carbide)

Petroleum distillates * 74%
n-Butyl alcohol 18%
Nonionic surfactants 8%

PRESTONE 10-MINUTE RADIATOR FLUSH (AS-105 (Aqueous)/AS-106 Formula 8623-49)
(Union Carbide)

Water 84–85%
Sodium citrate 7%
Anionic and Nonionic
  surfactants 5%
Isopropyl alcohol 3–4%

PRESTONE TRANS STOP LEAK (AS-225N, Formula MI-2235)
(Union Carbide)

Refined Mineral oil * 100%

PRESTONE II WINTER ANTIFREEZE - SUMMER COOLANT (AF-532, Formula Y/354-359 MI-2108), IMPROVED

See IMPROVED PRESTONE II WIN-TER ANTIFREEZE - SUMMER COOLANT (AF-552, Formula Y/354-359 MI-2108)

PRESTONE II WINTER-SUMMER ANTIFREEZE - ANTIBOIL (AF-542, Formula YA-238-243)
(Union Carbide)

Ethylene glycol * 95%
Water 3%
Soluble inhibitors 2%

PRESTONE VINYL HARDTOP CLEANER (AS-148, Formula 1372-145R)
(Union Carbide)

Water 91%
Glycol ether * 3%
Anionic and nonionic surfactants ... 3%
Inorganic detergent builder 3%

PRESTONE VINYL HARDTOP WAX & CONDITIONER (AS-146, Formula MI-2210)
(Union Carbide)

Water 86%
Waxes and Resins 12%
Glycol ether * 1%
Emulsifier 1%

PRESTONE WINDSHIELD WASHER ANTIFREEZE & CLEANER (AS-141, Formula MI-2232)
(Union Carbide)

Methyl alcohol * 68%
Water 27%
Ethylene glycol 5%

Starred ingredients (*) may be responsible for major toxic effects; consult Section II.

PRESTONE WINDSHIELD WASHER CONCENTRATE (AS-142, Formula 1945-85B)
(Union Carbide)

Methyl alcohol * 64%
Water 36%

PRESTO PATCH SPACKLING PASTE
(Savogran)

Calcium carbonate .... <80%
Acrylic latex .... <20%
Glycols .... <5%

PRESTO WATER BATH TREATMENT
(National Presto Ind.)

Sodium hypochlorite 0.5%

PRESUN
Sunscreen lotion
(Westwood Pharm.)

Para-aminobenzoic acid (PABA) ... 5%
Ethyl alcohol 55%
Special skin emollients

'76 Ed.

PREVENTION PLUS LIQUID DRAIN OPENER
(Dorex, Inc.)

Sulfuric acid * 93.2%

PRIMAQUINE PHOSPHATE
For vivax malaria
(Winthrop Labs.)

Each tablet:
  Primaquine phosphate, USP
  (equiv. to 15 mg. base) * .. 26.3 mg.

PRIMATENE MIST
Asthmatic anti-spasmodic
(Whitehall Labs.)

Epinephrine *

PRIMATENE TABLETS M
Asthmatic bronchodilator
(Whitehall Labs.)

Theophylline *
Ephedrine *
Methapyrilene *

PRIMATENE TABLETS P
Asthmatic bronchodilator
(Whitehall Labs.)

Theophylline *
Ephedrine *
Phenobarbital *

PRIME ANTIFREEZE COOLANT (AF-562, Formula YA-335 (8697-87))
(Union Carbide)

Ethylene glycol * 95%
Water 3%
Soluble inhibitors 2%

PRIME LEAF TOBACCO SPRAY

See GROWER SERVICE PRIME LEAF TOBACCO SPRAY

PRINCEP 4G
Granular herbicide
(Ciba-Geigy Ag. Div.)

Simazine 4%

PRINCEP 4L
Herbicide
(Ciba-Geigy Ag. Div.)

Simazine * 41.9%

PRINCEP 80W
Herbicide
(Ciba-Geigy Ag. Div.)

Simazine * 80%

PRINCESS MARCELLA BORGHESE COSMETICS

Princess Marcella Borghese, Inc.
Sub. of Revlon, Inc.
767 Fifth Ave.
New York, N.Y. 10153

Phone: 212-572-5000

See COSMETICS, Section VI, General Formulations

PRIVATE RESERVE COLOGNE

See JAFRA PRIVATE RESERVE COLOGNE

PRIVINE SOLUTION & SPRAY
Nasal decongestant
(CIBA Pharmaceutical)

Naphazoline hydrochloride 0.05%

PRIZE WINNER DOG SPRAY
Insecticide
(Dro)

Isobornyl thiocyanoacetate 1.640%
Related terpenes 0.360%
Allethrin (Allyl homolog of Cinerin I) 0.075%
N-Octyl bicycloheptene dicarboximide 0.500%
Methoxychlor, tech. 1.000%
Rotenone 0.033%
Other cube resins 0.067%
Butoxypolypropylene glycol 6.000%
2,2-Thiobis-(4-chloro-6-methyl phenol) 0.100%
Petroleum distillate * 59.975%

'76 Ed.

PROBATE TABLETS
Antianxiety and muscle-relaxant properties
(Vita Elixir Co.)

Each tablet:
  Meprobamate * .... 400 mg.

PROBE
Heavy duty liquid organic drain cleaner; professional use
(Scientific International)

Sulfuric acid *

PROBEX
Liquid drain & sewer maintainer; municipal, industrial and institutional use
(Scientific International)

Sulfuric acid *

PRO-BRAND BLUE-LOTION BOMB
Drying dressing for superficial wounds, cuts and abrasions for livestock
(Pro-Brand Products Co.)

Methyl violet 1.0%
Tannic acid 1.0%
Carbolic acid 1.0%
Methyl salicylate * 2.5%
Eugenol 0.5%
Propylene glycol 5.0%
Isopropyl alcohol * 39.0%
Inert ingred.:
  Propellent 50.0%

'76 Ed.

PRO-BRAND PRO-TOX-L
Insecticide - veterinary
(Pro-Brand Products Co.)

Toxaphene (technical chlorinated camphene)(chlorine content 67-69%) * 45%
Gamma isomer of benzene hexachloride from lindane 2%
Refined Petroleum oil 28%
Xylene * 15%

'76 Ed.

Starred ingredients (*) may be responsible for major toxic effects; consult Section II.

PRO-BRAND PRO-TOX-M
For ticks, hornflies and lice on cattle and sheep; residual surface spray
(Pro-Brand Products Co.)

Toxaphene (technical chlorinated camphene)(chlorine content 67-69%) * 45%
Malathion 5%
Xylene * 15%
Refined Petroleum oil 20%

'76 Ed.

PROCAN SR
Treatment of ventricular tachycardia, atrial fibrillation and paroxysmal atrial tachycardia
(Parke-Davis)

Each tablet:
  Procainamide
    hydrochloride* .. 250 mg.; 500 mg.; 750 mg.

PRO-CAP 65
Analgesic
(Foy Labs.)

Each capsule:
  Propoxyphene HCl * .... 65 mg.

PRO-CIDE
Professional-grade insecticide - aerosol
(Va. Chem. Inc.)

Pyrethrins 0.5%
Technical Piperonyl butoxide 4.0%
Petroleum hydrocarbon oil base * 12.5%

PROCTOCORT CREAM
For treatment of severe anorectal inflammation
(Rowell)

Hydrocortisone 1%
In a water-miscible base

PROCTODON CREAM
Anesthetic cream
(Rowell)

Diperodon HCl 1%
In a water-miscible base

PROCYST TABLETS
Antispasmodic-sedative
(Moffet Inc.)

Each tablet:
  Sodium bromide * .... 0.15 gm.
  Sodium benzoate .... 0.15 gm.
  Extract Belladonna .... 8 mg.
  Extract Hyoscyamus .... 8 mg.

PROFEDRIN TABLETS
Nasal decongestant
(Bio-Factor Labs.)

Each tablet:
  Phenylpropanolamine
    hydrochloride * .... 25 mg.

'76 Ed.

PROFESSIONAL BHC 12 EMULSIFIABLE CONCENTRATE
Insecticide
(Dettelbach Pesticide Corp.)

Gamma isomer of benzene
  hexachloride * 12.0%
Other isomers of benzene hexachloride and related compounds 18.0%
Xylene * 65.0%

'76 Ed.

PROFESSIONAL 30% DDT CONCENTRATE
Insecticide
(Dettelbach Pesticide Corp.)

Xylene * 70.0%
Dichlorodiphenyltrichloroethane . 30.0%

'76 Ed.

PROFESSIONAL DELNAV 25 INSECTICIDE EMULSIFIABLE CONCENTRATE
Insecticide
(Dettelbach Pesticide Corp.)

Dioxathion (2,3-p-Dioxanedithiol
  S,S-bis(O,O-diethyl
  phosphorodithioate)) * 17.5%
Related compounds (Delnav) 7.5%
Aromatic petroleum derivative * 65.0%

'76 Ed.

PROFESSIONAL DIELDRIN 18 EMULSIFIABLE CONCENTRATE
Insecticide
(Dettelbach Pesticide Corp.)

Dieldrin * 18.6%
Xylene * 73.9%

'76 Ed.

PROFESSIONAL GOLDEN ORKIL EMULSIFIABLE CONCENTRATE
Insecticide
(Dettelbach Pesticide Corp.)

Technical Chlordane *
Petroleum distillates *
Heptachlor *
Related compounds
Inert ingredients:
  Nonylphenoxypolyethoxyethanol   14%

'76 Ed.

PROFESSIONAL "L-D" 46% CHLORDANE EMULSIFIABLE CONCENTRATE
Insecticide
(Dettelbach Pesticide Corp.)

Technical Chlordane * 46.0%
Refined Petroleum distillates * .. 40.0%

'76 Ed.

PROFESSIONAL "L-D" 20% CHLORDANE SOLUTION IN OIL
Insecticide
(Dettelbach Pesticide Corp.)

Technical Chlordane * 20%
Refined Petroleum distillates * 80%

'76 Ed.

PROFESSIONAL "L-D" 25% DDT CONCENTRATE EMULSIFIABLE
Insecticide
(Dettelbach Pesticide Corp.)

Xylene * 70.0%
Dichlorodiphenyltrichloroethane . 25.0%

'76 Ed.

PROFESSIONAL NO. 20 LINDANE EMULSION CONCENTRATE
Insecticide
(Dettelbach Pesticide Corp.)

Gamma isomer of benzene hexachloride from lindane * 20.0%
Xylene * 75.0%

'76 Ed.

PROFESSIONAL MALATHION 50 EMULSIFIABLE LIQUID
Insecticide
(Dettelbach Pesticide Corp.)

Malathion * 50%
Aromatic petroleum derivatives * .. 40%

'76 Ed.

PROFESSIONAL MALATHION FLY BAIT WITH D.D.V.P.
Insecticide
(Dettelbach Pesticide Corp.)

Malathion (O,O-Dimethyl dithiophosphate of diethyl
  mercaptosuccinate) 1.00%
DDVP (0.93% 2,2-Dichlorovinyl dimethyl phosphate and 0.07% related compounds) * 1.00%

'76 Ed.

Starred ingredients (*) may be responsible for major toxic effects; consult Section II.

PROFESSIONAL ORKIL CHLOROHEPTON CONCENTRATE NO. 2
Insecticide
(Dettelbach Pesticide Corp.)

Technical Chlordane *	23.65%
Heptachlor *	8.51%
Related compounds	3.31%
Petroleum hydrocarbons *	54.53%

'76 Ed.

PROFESSIONAL ORKIN BOOSTER CONCENTRATE H EMULSIFIABLE
Insecticide
(Dettelbach Pesticide Corp.)

Petroleum distillates *	80.4%
N-Octyl bicycloheptene dicarboximide	4.0%
Technical Piperonyl butoxide	2.4%
Pyrethrins	1.2%

'76 Ed.

PROFESSIONAL ORKINCIDE ANTI-COAGULANT RODENT BAIT
Rodenticide
(Dettelbach Pesticide Corp.)

Diphacinone (2-Diphenylacetyl-1,3-indandione)	0.005%

'76 Ed.

PROFESSIONAL ORKIN CONCENTRATE 399
Insecticide
(Dettelbach Pesticide Corp.)

N-Octyl bicycloheptene dicarboximide	5.0%
Technical Piperonyl butoxide	3.0%
Pyrethrins	1.5%
Petroleum distillate *	90.5%

'76 Ed.

PROFESSIONAL ORKIN FORMULA 1-19 RODENTICIDE CONCENTRATE
(Dettelbach Pesticide Corp.)

Diphacinone (2-Diphenylacetyl-1,3-indandione) *	0.1%

'76 Ed.

PROFESSIONAL ORKIN SPECIAL FOG SPRAY
Insecticide
(Dettelbach Pesticide Corp.)

Piperonyl butoxide, technical	5.0%
Pyrethrins	0.5%
Deodorized Kerosene *	44.5%
Tetrachloroethylene *	50.0%

'76 Ed.

PROFESSIONAL ORKIN SPECIAL FORMULA CHLORDANE 75% EMULSIFIABLE CONCENTRATE
Insecticide
(Dettelbach Pesticide Corp.)

Technical Chlordane *	75%
Petroleum distillates *	18%

'76 Ed.

PROFESSIONAL ORKIN SPECIAL FORMULA FOR FOOD PROCESSING PLANT
Insecticide
(Dettelbach Pesticide Corp.)

Pyrethrins	0.33%

'76 Ed.

PROFESSIONAL ORKIN SPECIAL FORMULA PFT
Insecticide
(Dettelbach Pesticide Corp.)

Sodium fluoride *	33.33%
Pyrethrins	0.33%

'76 Ed.

PROFESSIONAL ORKIN SPECIAL FORMULA-R-333 D D GRADE
Insecticide
(Dettelbach Pesticide Corp.)

Sodium fluoride *	33.33%
Piperonyl butoxide, technical	1.67%
Pyrethrins	0.13%

'76 Ed.

PROFESSIONAL ORKIN SPECIAL FORMULA RD-98 ROACH POWDER WITH DIAZINON
Insecticide
(Dettelbach Pesticide Corp.)

O,O,-Diethyl O-(2-isopropyl-4-methyl-6-pyrimidinyl) phosphorothioate (Diazinon)	1.333%
Pyrethrins	0.333%

'76 Ed.

PROFESSIONAL ORKIN'S SOIL FUMIGANT
(Dettelbach Pesticide Corp.)

Ethylene dibromide *	15%

'76 Ed.

PROFESSIONAL ORKINTROL FORMULA W/E 1-31 CONCENTRATE
Insecticide
(Dettelbach Pesticide Corp.)

4-Isopropoxyphenyl methylcarbamate *	18.3%
Aromatic petroleum derivatives *	69.7%

'76 Ed.

PROFESSIONAL SUPREME SHAMPOO
(House of Lowell, Inc.)

TEA-lauryl sulfate *
Lauramide DEA
Sodium chloride
Citric acid
Perfume *
Formaldehyde
D & C color

PROFUME A FUMIGANT
(Dow)

Methyl bromide *	99.75%
Chloropicrin	0.25%

PROGRESS PAINT PRODUCTS

Progress Paint Mfg. Co.
P.O. Box 33188
Louisville, Ky. 40232

Phone: 502-587-8685

See PAINTS, Section VI, General Formulations

PROKETAZINE TABLETS
Antipsychotic
(Wyeth Labs.)

Each tablet:
Carphenazine maleate * .... 25 mg.; or 50 mg.

PROLAMINE CAPSULES
Appetite control
(Thompson Med.)

Each capsule:
Phenylpropanolamine HCl *	35 mg.
Caffeine *	140 mg.

PROLATE (50-WP)
Insecticide
(Stauffer)

Prolate (N-(Mercaptomethyl) phthalimide-S-(O,O-dimethyl) phosphorodithioate) *

PROLIN REDI-NIPS
Rodenticide
(NIP-CO)

Warfarin (3(a-Acetonylbenzyl)-4-
    hydroxycoumarin) 0.025%
Quinoxalinylsulfanilamide
    (Sulfaquinoxaline) 0.025%

PROLIXIN (ELIXIR & TABLETS)
For psychotic disorders
(Squibb)

Elixir (each 5 ml.):
    Fluphenazine hydrochloride *   2.5 mg.
    Alcohol 14%/v

Tablets (each):
    Fluphenazine
        hydrochloride *   1 mg.; 2.5 mg.;
            5 mg. and 10 mg.

PROMETHYASUL, WARDLEY'S

See WARDLEY'S PROMETHYASUL

PROMIST
Expectorant - antitussive - decongestant
(Russ Pharm.)

Each 5 ml.:
    Hydrocodone bitartrate ....   2.5 mg.
    Pseudoephedrine
        hydrochloride * .... 30.0 mg.
    Guaifenesin (Glyceryl
        guaiacolate) .... 100.0 mg.
    Alcohol 5%

PROMIST TABLETS
Decongestant
(Russ Pharm.)

Each tablet:
    Pseudoephedrine
        hydrochloride * .... 30 mg.
    Guaifenesin .... 250 mg.

PROMPT BENZOCAINE CREME
Local anesthetic
(DePree)

Resorcinol *
Chlorothymol *
Benzocaine

PROMPT TABLETS & ELIXIR
Analgesic
(DePree)

Acetaminophen *

PRONESTYL CAPSULES
Treatment of ventricular arrhythmias & related cardiac conditions
(Squibb)

Each capsule:
    Procainamide hydro-
        chloride U.S.P. *   250 mg.; 375 mg.;
            or 500 mg.

PRO-NOXFISH
Fish toxicant
(Penick)

Rotenone * 2.5%
Other cube extractives 5.0%
n-Octyl sulfoxide of isosafrole
    (Sulfoxide) 2.2%
Related compounds 0.3%

PRONTO-GEL
Greaseless analgesic jelly
(Commerce Drug)

Methyl nicotinate
Methyl salicylate *
Camphor *
Menthol *
Glycol monosalicylate
Isopropanol * 50%

PROPADRINE (CAPSULES & ELIXIR)
Nasal decongestant
(MSD)

CAPSULES (each):
    Phenylpropanolamine
        hydrochloride *   25 mg.; 50 mg.

ELIXIR (each fl. oz.):
    Phenylpropanolamine
        hydrochloride * .... 0.12 gm.
    Alcohol 16%

PROP ELECTRIC PRE-SHAVE
(Mennen)

SD Alcohol 40 *
Myristyl propionate
Water
Isopropyl myristate
Fragrance
Menthol *
D&C Green #5
FD&C Blue #1

PROPHYLLIN (OINTMENT & POWDER)
Antipruritic
(Rystan)

POWDER (per packet when dissolved in
    8 oz. of water):
    Sodium propionate 1.0000%
    Water-soluble Chlorophyll ... 0.0025%

OINTMENT:
    Sodium propionate 5%
    Water-soluble Chlorophyll ... 0.0125%

PROSECA
Acne dry-wash, drying agent & antiseborrheic shampoo
(Westwood Pharm.)

Liposec (brand of polyoxyethylene
    lauryl ether) 3%
Sulfur 4%
Wetting agents
Surface active cleansers *
                              '76 Ed.

PROSOL
Ear eczema
(Torch)

Mercury oleate * 0.25%
Coal tar 0.60%
Salicylic acid * 1.50%
Phenol 0.25%
p-Nitrophenol 0.25%
Combined amount: .... ad 100.0 cc
    Oil emulsion
    Isopropyl alcohol *

                              '76 Ed.

PROTECTO
(Kester)

W W Gum rosin
Organic esters

PROTECTOR SCREW WORM AEROSOL
Wound spray
(Hess & Clark)

Ronnel 2.5%
Xylene * 15.5%

PROTEC WOUND DRESSING & FLY REPELLENT

See FRANKLIN PROTEC WOUND
    DRESSING & FLY REPELLENT

PROTEIN 21 CONDITIONER FOR DRY OR DAMAGED HAIR
(Mennen)

Water
SD Alcohol 40 *
Quaternium-23 *†
Hydrolyzed animal Protein
Stearalkonium chloride *
Dimethicone copolyol
Fragrance
Isosteareth-10
Methylparaben
Propylparaben

†*See* Cationic surfactants

Starred ingredients (*) may be responsible for major toxic effects; consult Section II.

PROTEIN 21 CONDITIONER FOR FINE, THIN, LIMP HAIR
(Mennen)

Water
SD Alcohol 40 *
Quaternium-19 *†
Hydrolyzed animal Protein
Fragrance
Dimethicone copolyol
Stearalkonium chloride *

†*See* Cationic surfactants

PROTEIN 21 HAIR SPRAY EXTRA HOLD (SCENTED)
(Mennen)

SD Alcohol 40 *
Isobutane
Propane
Butyl ester of PVM/MA copolymer
Amino methyl propanol
Fragrance
PPG-12-PEG-50 lanolin
Myristoyl hydrolyzed animal protein
Dimethicone copolyol

PROTEIN 21 HAIR SPRAY EXTRA HOLD (UNSCENTED)
(Mennen)

SD Alcohol 40 *
Isobutane
Propane
Butyl ester of PVM/MA copolymer
Amino methyl propanol
PPG-12-PEG-50 lanolin
Myristoyl hydrolyzed animal protein
Dimethicone copolyol
Fragrance

PROTEIN 21 HAIR SPRAY REGULAR HOLD (SCENTED)
(Mennen)

SD Alcohol 40 *
Isobutane
Propane
Butyl ester of PVM/MA copolymer
Fragrance
Amino methyl propanol
PPG-12-PEG-50 lanolin
Myristoyl hydrolyzed animal protein
Dimethicone copolyol

PROTEIN 21 HAIR SPRAY REGULAR HOLD (UNSCENTED)
(Mennen)

SD Alcohol 40 *
Isobutane
Propane
Butyl ester of PVM/MA copolymer
Amino methyl propanol *
Myristoyl hydrolyzed animal protein
Fragrance
Dimethicone copolyol

PROTEIN 21 SHAMPOO FOR DRY HAIR
(Mennen)

Water
TEA-lauryl sulfate *
Lauramide DEA
Linoleamide DEA
Hydrolyzed animal Protein
Tetrasodium EDTA
Citric acid
Laneth-10 acetate
Fragrance
Methylparaben
Quaternium-15
Propylparaben

PROTEIN 21 SHAMPOO FOR NORMAL HAIR & PROTEIN 21 SHAMPOO FOR OILY HAIR
(Mennen)

Water
TEA-lauryl sulfate *
Lauramide DEA
Hydrolyzed animal Protein
Linoleamide DEA
Tetrasodium EDTA
Citric acid
Laneth-10 acetate
Fragrance
Methylparaben
Quaternium-15
Propylparaben

PROTEIN 21 SHAMPOO FOR OILY HAIR
(Mennen)

Water
TEA-lauryl sulfate *
Lauramide DEA
Hydrolyzed animal protein
Linoleamide DEA
Tetrasodium EDTA
Citric acid
Laneth-10 acetate
Fragrance
Methylparaben
Quaternium-15
Propylparaben

PROTEIN 29 CLEAR GEL HAIR GROOM
(Mennen)

Water
Mineral oil
Oleth-10
Glycerin
Propylene glycol
Oleth-3 phosphate
Lanolin alcohol
Oleth-20
Triethanolamine
Hydrolyzed animal protein
Methylparaben
Quaternium-15
Fragrance
FD & C Green #3

PROTEIN 29 CREME HAIR GROOM
(Mennen)

Water
Mineral oil
Glycerin
Beeswax
Saccharated lime
Hydrolyzed animal Protein
Fragrance
Quaternium-15
Sodium pyrithione

PROTEIN 29 DRY CONTROL
(Mennen)

SD Alcohol 40 *
Isobutane
Propane
Butyl ester of PVM/MA copolymer
Fragrance
Amino methyl propanol
PPG-12-PEG-50 lanolin
Dimethicone copolyol
Myristoyl hydrolyzed animal protein

PROTEIN 29 HAIR GROOM (AEROSOL)
(Mennen)

SD Alcohol 40 *
Isobutane
Propane
PPG-26 oleate
Butyl ester of PVM/MA copolymer
Lanolin oil
Dimethicone copolyol
Myristoyl hydrolyzed animal protein
Fragrance
Oleth-3
Amino methyl propanol

PROTEIN 29 HAIR GROOM (LIQUID)
(Mennen)

SD Alcohol 40 *
Water
PPG-33-buteth-45
PPG-33-butyl ether
Propylene glycol
Citric acid
Hydrolized animal protein
Benzophenone-11
Fragrance
Myristalkonium chloride
FD & C Green #3

PROTEIN 29 PUMP HAIR SPRAY EXTRA HOLD
(Mennen)

SD Alcohol 40
Water
Butyl ester of PVM/MA copolymer
Aminomethyl propanol
Dimethyl phthalate
Myristoyl hydrolyzed animal Protein
Fragrance

Starred ingredients (*) may be responsible for major toxic effects; consult Section II.

PROTEIN 29 PUMP HAIR SPRAY REGULAR HOLD
(Mennen)

SD Alcohol 40
Water
Butyl ester of PVM/MA copolymer
Aminomethyl propanol
Fragrance
Myristoyl hydrolyzed animal Protein
Dimethyl phthalate

PRO-TEX

See AIRWICK PROFESSIONAL
PRODUCTS PRO-TEX

PROTEXAL
Antibacterial
(Nat'l Milling)

o-Benzyl-p-chlorophenol 0.75%

PRO-TOX-L
See PRO-BRAND PRO-TOX-L

PRO-TOX-M
See PRO-BRAND PRO-TOX-M

PROTURF BROAD SPECTRUM FUNGICIDE
(Scott, O.M.)

Phenylmercuric acetate * 0.69%
Thiram * 4.65%
Carrier base: Vermiculite

PROTURF FERTILIZER PLUS DICOT WEED CONTROL II
(Scott, O.M.)

2,4-Dichlorophenoxyacetic acid ... 1.37%
2-(4-Chloro-2-methylphenoxy) propionic acid 1.37%
Carrier: Fertilizer 36-0-0

PROTURF FERTILIZER PLUS INSECTICIDE III
(Scott, O.M.)

Dursban 0.55%
Carrier: Fertilizer 30-5-3

PROTURF FERTILIZER PLUS 101 BROAD SPECTRUM FUNGICIDE
(Scott, O.M.)

Daconil 11.25%
Carrier: Fertilizer 18-5-5

PROTURF FF II
(Scott, O.M.)

Pentachloronitrobenzene 15.40%
Carrier: Fertilizer 14-3-3

PROTURF FUNGICIDE II
(Scott, O.M.)

Chloroneb 6.25%

PROTURF FUNGICIDE III
(Scott, O.M.)

Dyrene * 8.70%
Carrier base: Vermiculite

PROTURF HD FERTILIZER WITH WEEDGRASS PREVENTER
(Scott, O.M.)

Bensulide 7.80%
Carrier: Fertilizer 26-0-11

PROTURF INSECTICIDE ONE
(Scott, O.M.)

Diazinon * 4.5%
Carrier base: Corncobs

PROTURF INSECTICIDE III
(Scott, O.M.)

O,O-Diethyl O-(3,5,6-trichloro-2-
pyridyl) phosphorothioate * ... 1.34%
Carrier base: Corncobs

PROTURF K-O-G WEED CONTROL
(Scott, O.M.)

Dicamba * 0.70%
Carrier base: Corncobs

PROTURF NEMATOCIDE
(Scott, O.M.)

Mocap * 5.00%
Carrier base: Corncobs

PROTURF 101V FUNGICIDE
(Scott, O.M.)

Daconil 9.50%
Carrier: Vermiculite

PROTURF SYSTEMIC FUNGICIDE
(Scott, O.M.)

Thiophanate-M 2.30%
Carrier: Corncobs

PROTURF WEEDGRASS PREVENTER
(Scott, O.M.)

Bensulide 8.50%
Carrier: Corncobs

PROVAL #3
Analgesic
(Reid-Provident)

Each capsule:
  Codeine phosphate * .... 30 mg.
  Acetaminophen * .... 325 mg.

PROX
Rust preventative
(Kano)

Resinous compounds

PROXAGESIC COMPOUND-65
Analgesic
(Direct Div.)

Each capsule:
  Propoxyphene HCl * .... 65 mg.
  Aspirin * .... 227 mg.
  Phenacetin * .... 162 mg.
  Caffeine .... 32.5 mg.

P.R. - PREM-TANK (Powder)

See GUNK P.R. - PREM-TANK (Powder)

PRUCARA
Laxative
(ICN Pharm.)

Each tablet:
  Prune concentrate .... 162 mg.
  Cascarin * .... 162 mg.

PRUNICODEINE
For relief of coughs
(Lilly, Eli)

Each 30 ml.:
  Codeine sulfate * .... 60 mg.
  Wild cherry bark .... 1.58 gm.
  White pine bark .... 1.05 gm.
  Sanguinaria .... 262 mg.
  Terpin hydrate .... 175 mg.

PRURILO
Pruritis
(Whorton)

REGULAR:
  Menthol 1/2%
  Phenol 1/2%
  Calamine lotion
PEDIATRIC:
  Menthol 1/4%
  Phenol 1/4%
  Calamine lotion

'76 Ed.

PRUVO
(Pruvo Pharmacal Co.)

Each tablet:
  Aspirin * .... 5 gr.
  Salicylamide .... 1/2 gr.
  Ascorbic acid .... 3 mg.

'76 Ed.

Starred ingredients (*) may be responsible for major toxic effects; consult Section II.

PRYME
Wood lightener
(Pierce & Stevens)

Non-volatile:
Polyester resin
Vinyl resin
Maleic modified soybean oil
Siliceous pigment
Dibutylamine pyrophosphate
Volatile:
Alcohols
Aromatic hydrocarbon *

P.S.C. IMPROVED FORMULA
Peptic ulcer and other conditions with gastric hyperacidity
(King Pharmaceutical)

Each ounce:
Phenobarbital sodium * ....   3 gr.
Powdered extract of
  Belladonna * ....   1.5 gr.
Bismuth subcarbonate ......   1.2 gm.
Magnesium oxide, light ..... 10.3 gm.
Calcium carbonate ....   5.1 gm.
Magnesium carbonate ......   3.8 gm.
Sodium bicarbonate ..... q.s. 1 ounce
Oil of peppermint

PSORELIEF
For the treatment of psoriasis
(Columbia Med.)

Coal tar solution *
Allantoin
Isopropyl myristate
Psorilan

PSOREX MEDICATED CREAM
For the temporary relief of psoriasis symptoms
(Jeffrey Martin, Inc.)

Active ingred./each 2 oz. tube:
Coal tar (USP) 1.00%
Allantoin 0.25%

PSOREX MEDICATED SHAMPOO
Antidandruff
(Jeffrey Martin, Inc.)

Active ingred.:
Coal tar (USP) 1.00%
Allantoin 0.25%

PSORIGEL TAR CONCENTRATE
Treatment of psoriasis and eczema
(Owen Labs.)

Coal tar solution * 7.5%
Alcohol 33%
Hydroalcoholic gel vehicle

P & S SHAMPOO
Antiseborrheic shampoo
(Baker-Cummins)

Salicylic acid * 2.0%
Lactic acid 0.5%

PT 555 ALLETHRIN
Insect fogger
(Whitmire Research)

Allethrin (Allyl homolog of Cinerin
  I) 0.5%
Technical Piperonyl butoxide 4.0%
Refined Petroleum oil 8.0%

PT 576 D-TRANS ALLETHRIN AND PHENOTHRIN
Insect fogger
(Whitmire Research)

d-trans Allethrin (Allyl homolog
  of Cinerin I) 0.300%
Related compounds 0.023%
Phenothrin 0.191%
Other isomers 0.009%
Petroleum distillate * 14.477%

PT 110 RESMETHRIN
Insecticide; aerosol generator
(Whitmire Research)

Resmethrin 1%

PT 585 SEVIN-ROTENONE PYRETHRUM
Flea and tick fogger
(Whitmire Research)

Carbaryl 0.50%
Rotenone 0.10%
Rotenoids and other cube
  extractives 0.20%
Pyrethrins 0.50%
Technical Piperonyl butoxide 0.25%
Butoxypolypropylene glycol 2.50%

PT 1300 WITH ORTHENE
Insecticide
(Whitmire Research)

Acephate 3%

PULSAPHEN
Sedative w/antispasmodic
(Wesley Pharm.)

Each tablet:
Phenobarbital * .... 15 mg.
Passiflora extract .... 1 mg.
Hyoscyamus extract * .... 22 mg.

PUNCH
Laundry detergent
(Colgate-Palmolive)

Combined amount: 14%
Alkyl benzene sulfonate *
Soap
Nonionic surfactant
Inorganic builders 74.6%
Phosphate *
Silicate *
Sodium sulfate
Color, perfume and minor
  ingredients 1.8%
Moisture 9.5%

'76 Ed.

PURA-MYCIN, PURINA
See PURINA PURA-MYCIN

PURA-MYCIN SOLUBLE POWDER CONCENTRATE
See PURINA PURA-MYCIN SOLUBLE POWDER CONCENTRATE

PURE
Liquid machine dishwashing compound; industrial and institutional use
(Scientific International)

Very concentrated Alkalis *

PUREEN
Liquid bowl cleaner, disinfectant, deodorant - hospital grade
(Puritan Chem. Co.)

Hydrogen chloride * 9.8%
Phosphoric acid * 5.0%
Sulfamic acid 4.0%
n-Alkyl (60% tetradecyl, 30% hexadecyl, 5% dodecyl, 5% octadecyl)
  dimethyl benzyl ammonium
  chlorides 0.1%
n-Alkyl (50% dodecyl, 30% tetradecyl, 17% hexadecyl, 3% octadecyl)
  dimethyl benzyl ammonium
  chlorides 0.1%

PURE LEMON ODOR 7
Household and commercial disinfectant
(Snee, W.G., Co.)

Quaternary ammonium compound *
Essential oils 2.25%

PURE LEMON ODOR 15
Household and commercial disinfectant
(Snee, W.G., Co.)

Quaternary ammonium compound *
Isopropanol *
Essential oils * 6.5%

PURE MINT DISINFECTANT
(Snee, W.G., Co.)

Active ingredients: 46%
Isopropyl alcohol *
o-Benzyl-p-chlorophenol *
Soap
Methyl salicylate *

PURE MINT ODOR 7
Household and commercial disinfectant
(Snee, W.G., Co.)

Quaternary ammonium compound *
Isopropanol *
Methyl salicylate * 4.5%

Starred ingredients (*) may be responsible for major toxic effects; consult Section II.

PURE MINT ODOR 15
Household and commercial disinfectant
(Snee, W.G., Co.)

Quaternary ammonium compound *
Isopropanol *
Methyl salicylate * 9%

PURE-MOR
Disinfectant
(Hilltop)

Pine oil * 80%
Soap 10%

'76 Ed.

PURE PINE
Pine oil disinfectant
(Snee, W.G., Co.)

Combined amount: 90%
Steam distilled Pine oil *
Soap

PURE PINE ODOR 6
Household and commercial disinfectant
(Snee, W.G., Co.)

Isopropanol *
Pine oil *
Quaternary ammonium
compound * 10.67%

PURE PINE ODOR 13
Household and commercial disinfectant
(Snee, W.G., Co.)

Isopropanol *
Pine oil *
Quaternary ammonium
compound * 21.35%

PUREX ALL FABRIC/ALL COLOR DRY BLEACH
(Purex Corp.)

Sodium percarbonate *† 20-25%
Sodium carbonate * 15-25%
Starch .... <1%
Fluorescent whitening agent ... <1%
Nonionic surfactant .... <1%
Perfume .... <1%
Colorant .... <1%
Sodium chloride * .... balance

†*See* Sodium carbonate

PUREX BLEACH
(Purex Corp.)

Sodium hypochlorite * 5 1/4%
Sodium chloride .... <5%
Water .... balance

PUREX DRY CHLORINE BLEACH (NO PHOSPHATE)
(Scientific Packaging)

Sodium carbonate * 15-25%
Sodium silicate (not meta) .... <5%
Potassium salt of chlorinated
Triazinetrione .... <5%
Anionic surfactant .... <2%
Perfume .... <1%
Sodium sulfate .... balance

PUREX HEAVY DUTY LIQUID LAUNDRY DETERGENT
(Purex Corp.)

Soil release agent .... <5%
Nonionic surfactant 5-15%
Anionic surfactant 20-30%
Fluorescent whitening agent ... <1%
Perfume .... <1%
Colorant .... <1%
Water .... balance

PUREX HEAVY DUTY NO-PHOSPHATE DRY DETERGENT
(Purex Corp.)

Sodium carbonate * 20-35%
Anionic surfactant * 10-20%
Sodium silicate (not meta) * ... 5-15%
Cellulosic .... <2%
Fluorescent whitening agent ... <1%
Perfume .... <1%
Sodium sulfate .... balance

PUREX SOFT
Fabric softener
(Purex Corp.)

Quaternary ammonium
compound * 7-14%
Sodium chloride .... <1%
Preservative .... <1%
Coloring agent .... <1%
Perfume .... <1%
Water .... balance

PURGE
Purgative/laxative
(Fleming)

Each 2 oz.:
Castor oil 95%
In sweetened lemon flavored base

PURGE II CONCENTRATED AEROSOL INSECT KILLER
For use in Automizer
(Cline-Buckner, Inc.)

Pyrethrins 1.00%
Piperonyl butoxide technical 2.00%
N-Octyl bicycloheptene
dicarboximide 3.34%
Petroleum hydrocarbons * 13.66%

PURGIT
Drain cleaner
(Haviland Products Co.)

Sodium hydroxide *
Sodium nitrate
Metallic zinc aluminum alloy

'76 Ed.

PURGITE
Cooling system cleaner
(Choldun; Arrow Labs.)

Oxalic acid *
Sodium bisulfite

'76 Ed.

PURGITE, HEAVY DUTY
Acid cleaner
(Choldun; Arrow Labs.)

Oxalic acid *

'76 Ed.

PURICIDE ALGICIDE
Swimming pool algae inhibitor
(Snee, W.G., Co.)

Quaternary ammonium compound * 10%

PURIDINE
See PURINA PURIDINE

PURINA ACID CLEANER
(Ralston)

Phosphoric acid * .... >30%
Hydroxyacetic acid .... <10%

PURINA ANIMAL SHAMPOO
(Ralston)

Pyrethrins 0.075%
Piperonyl butoxide 0.750%
Sodium lauryl sulfate 8.500%

PURINA AS-700 ETTS
Antibiotic
(Ralston)

Each lb.:
Chlortetracycline .... 2 gm.
Sulfamethazine * .... 2 gm.

PURINA BACK SCRATCH CONC.
Insecticide
(Ralston)

Toxaphene * 65.00%
Lindane 0.65%

PURINA CALF SCOURS CONTROL
(Ralston)

Neomycin sulfate (139 milligrams of neomycin base per ml.)*
Vitamins

PURINA CATTLE DUST
Insecticide
(Ralston)

Methoxychlor, technical * 10%

PURINA CATTLE LICE-CHEK
(Ralston)

Fenthion 7.6%
Petroleum distillate 56.7%
Xylene * 20.0%

PURINA CHECK-FLY AND WORM CONTROL
Insecticide-wormer
(Ralston)

Phenothiazine * 17.8%

PURINA CHEK-R-FURAN
Medicated Premix for poultry & swine
(Ralston)

Furazolidone (NF 180) 2.2%
Corn meal 97.8%

PURINA CHEK-R-MYCIN
Antibiotic
(Ralston)

Each 6.4 oz.:
  Chlortetracycline
    hydrochloride .... 25.6 gm.

PURINA C & S POWDER
Detergent
(Ralston)

Sodium carbonate * 35%
N-Alkyl dimethyl ammonium
  chlorides * 5%
Sodium tripolyphosphate * 50%
Nonylphenol polyethylene glycol
  ether 5%
Water and odorant 5%

PURINA CYGON INSECTICIDE
(Ralston)

Dimethoate * 23.4%

PURINA DAIRY CLEANER
(Ralston)

Sodium carbonate * .... >20%
Sodium tripolyphosphate .... >30%
Available chlorine .... >1%

PURINA DAIRY SPRAY
Insecticide
(Ralston)

Pyrethrins 0.06%
Technical Piperonyl butoxide 0.48%
Petroleum oils * 99.46%

PURINA DAIRY SPRAY CONCENTRATE
Insecticide
(Ralston)

Ciodrin * 21.5%
Xylene * 67.4%

PURINA DAIRY SPRAY SPECIAL
Insecticide
(Ralston)

Ciodrin * 1%
Vapona 0.25%

PURINA DIAZINON INSECTICIDE 25-E
Insecticide
(Ralston)

Diazinon * 25.0%
Xylene * 40.0%
Petroleum distillate 25.7%

PURINA DIAZINON SPRAY 12 1/2%
Yard and lawn insecticide
(Ralston)

Diazinon * 12.5%
Xylene * 40.0%

PURINA DISINFECTANT
(Ralston)

Quaternary ammonium
  compounds * 5.8%

PURINA DISINFECTANT CONCENTRATE 4X
(Ralston)

Quaternary ammonium
  compounds * 23.6%

PURINA DOG DIP
Insecticide
(Ralston)

Lindane 6.50%
Xylene * 45.45%
Aromatic petroleum derivative
  solvent 40.05%

PURINA DOG & HOUSE SPRAY
(Ralston)

Carbaryl 0.500%
Rotenone 0.100%
Rotenoids & other cube
  extractives 0.200%
Pyrethrins I & II 0.050%
Technical Piperonyl butoxide ... 0.250%
Butoxypolypropylene glycol 2.500%

PURINA DOG SHAMPOO
(Ralston)

Pyrethrins 0.075%
Technical Piperonyl butoxide ... 0.075%
Sodium lauryl sulfate 8.500%
Combined amount: 8.675%
  Foam builders
  Detergents
  Lanolin
  Deodorant
  FD&C colors

PURINA DOG WORMER (LIQUID)
(Ralston)

Piperazine monohydrochloride ... 4.77%

PURINA EASY DUSTER INSECTICIDE
(Ralston)

Co-Ral * 1%

PURINA EGG CLEANER
(Ralston)

Sodium metasilicate * .... <15%
Sodium carbonate * .... >20%
Trisodium phosphate .... >20%
Tetrasodium pyrophosphate ..... >35%

PURINA ELECTRO-ZOLE
Medication via drinking water for large animals
(Ralston)

Sodium sulfathiazole * 90%

PURINA FACEFLY BOMB
Insecticide
(Ralston)

Pyrethrins 0.18%
Piperonyl butoxide, technical .. 0.36%
N-Octyl bicycloheptene
  dicarboximide 0.60%
Di-n-propyl isocinchomeronate .. 1.20%
Petroleum distillate * 77.66%

Starred ingredients (*) may be responsible for major toxic effects; consult Section II.

PURINA FARM & HOME WASP KILLER
(Ralston)

Tetrachloroethylene *	32.00%
Trichloromonofluoromethane	20.00%
Dichlorodifluoromethane	20.00%
Petroleum distillate	13.75%
Methylene chloride	11.00%
Pine oil	2.80%
Rotenone	0.12%
Other related Cube resins	0.28%
Pyrethrins I & II	0.05%

PURINA FLEA COLLAR FOR DOGS
Insecticide
(Ralston)

Carbaryl *	16%

PURINA FLY-A-REST
Insecticide
(Ralston)

Pyrethrins	0.500%
Technical Piperonyl butoxide	1.000%
N-Octyl bicycloheptene dicarboximide	1.000%
Refined Petroleum oil	8.000%

PURINA FLY-BYE
Insecticide
(Ralston)

Pyrethrins	0.20%
Piperonyl butoxide	0.40%
N-Octyl isocinchomeronate 2,3:4,5-bis (2-butylene) tetrahydro-2-furaldehyde	0.50%
Petroleum distillate *	77.40%

PURINA FLY LARVICIDE BLOCK
Insecticide
(Ralston)

Rabon *	1%

PURINA FLY LARVICIDE
(Feed Premix)
Insecticide
(Ralston)

Rabon *	7.76%

PURINA FLY PATROL
Insecticide
(Ralston)

Methomyl *	1.0%

PURINA FRUIT TREE SPRAY
Insecticide-fungicide
(Ralston)

Methoxychlor, technical *	16.67%
Malathion *	8.33%
Captan	16.67%

PURINA FUROX AEROSOL POWDER
Antibiotic
(Ralston)

Furazolidone *	10%

PURINA HARD HITTER EMULSIFIABLE CONCENTRATE
Insecticide
(Ralston)

Permethrin	5.7%

PURINA HARD HITTER WETTABLE POWDER
Insecticide
(Ralston)

Permethrin *	25%

PURINA HOG & CATTLE DUSTING POWDER
Insecticide
(Ralston)

Malathion	4.0%
Sulfur	10.0%

PURINA HOG WORMER-D
(Ralston)

Dichlorvos *	20%
Plastic base	

PURINA HORSE SHAMPOO
(Ralston)

Sodium lauryl sulfate	8.5%

PURINA HORSE SPRAY CONCENTRATE
Insecticide
(Ralston)

Methoxychlor, technical	5%
Butoxy polypropylene glycol	50%
Aromatic petroleum derivative solvent *	36.75%
Emulsifiers	

PURINA HORSE WORMER
Anthelmintic
(Ralston)

Thiabendazole (equiv. to 20 gm./lb.)	4.4%

PURINA HOUSEHOLD INSECT KILLER
Insecticide
(Ralston)

Tetramethrin	0.250%
Fenothrin	0.143%
Petroleum distillate *	9.250%

PURINA INSECTICIDE MIST
(Ralston)

Pyrethrins	0.1%
Piperonyl butoxide	1.0%

PURINA INSECTI-SHIELD
Insecticide
(Ralston)

Fenvalerate *	8.0%

PURINA IO-CONCENTRATE
General purpose disinfectant
(Ralston)

Iodophor (surfactant-iodine complex providing 3.5% available iodine)	
Phosphoric acid *	9.0%

PURINA IO-LYTE
Organic iodine treatment for drinking water; veterinary
(Ralston)

Ethylenediamine dihydroiodide *	14.1%
Sodium chloride *	
Potassium chloride *	

PURINA IRON PLUS II
Hematinic
(Ralston)

Iron sulfate *	not less than 10.0%

PURINA LICE AWAY FOR SWINE
Insecticide
(Ralston)

Fenthion	3%
Dipropylene glycol monomethyl ether *	>50%

PURINA LICE & FLY KILLER CR
Insecticide
(Ralston)

Co-Ral *	1%

PURINA LIQUID DETERGENT
(Ralston)

Sodium dodecyl benzene sulfonate *	
Other surfactants	
Total surfactants >25%	

PURINA LIQUID WORMER
Veterinary
(Ralston)

Piperazine monohydrochloride	22.77%

Starred ingredients (*) may be responsible for major toxic effects; consult Section II.

PURINA LIQUID WORMER CONCENTRATE 3X
Veterinary
(Ralston)

Dipiperazine sulfate .... 80.0 gm./100 cc

PURINA LIVESTOCK PLUS
(Feed Mix)
Antibiotic
(Ralston)

Each lb.:
Chlortetracycline * .... 20 gm.

PURINA MALATHION SPRAY
Insecticide
(Ralston)

Malathion * 54.60%
Xylene * 35.00%

PURINA MANGE CONTROL
(Ralston)

Lindane * 6.5%

PURINA MIX-R-MYCIN CONCENTRATE
Antibiotic
(Ralston)

Each lb.:
Oxytetracycline * .... 20 gm.

PURINA MOUSE CONTROL PELLETS
Rodenticide
(Ralston)

Warfarin 0.025%

PURINA NEOMYCIN FEED MIX
Antibiotic
(Ralston)

Each lb.:
Neomycin * .... 14 gm.

PURINA NEOMYCIN PLUS SOLUBLE POWDER
Antibiotic
(Ralston)

Each 4 oz. packet:
Neomycin sulfate (equiv. to
8.75 gm. neomycin base) ... 12.5 gm.
Methscopolamine bromide * . 62.4 mg.

PURINA NEOMYCIN SOLUBLE CONCENTRATE
Antibiotic
(Ralston)

Each 50 gm. packet:
Neomycin sulfate * .... 35.7 gm.

PURINA ODOR CONTROL
(Ralston)

Quaternary ammonium salts * 5%
Isopropanol * 15%
Ethanol 2.5%

PURINA PIG BOOSE SOLUBLE MEDICATED
Antibiotic
(Ralston)

Each lb.:
Neomycin sulfate (providing
8 gm. neomycin base per
lb.)* .... 11.43 gm.

PURINA PIG PLUS
Antibiotic
(Ralston)

Each lb.:
Chlortetracycline * .... 2.50 gm.
Penicillin (from procaine
penicillin) .... 1.25 gm.
Sulfamethazine 0.55%

PURINA PIG & POULTRY WORMER SUPER CONCENTRATE
(Ralston)

Piperazine phosphate
monohydrate 53.57%

PURINA PIG SCOURS CONTROL
(Ralston)

Each cc.:
Neomycin sulfate * .... 13.9 mg.

PURINA PIG WORMER (LIQUID)
(Ralston)

Piperazine monohydrochloride ... 18.22%

PURINA PLACE PACK RAT CONTROL
Rodenticide
(Ralston)

Warfarin 0.025%

PURINA POULTRY DUSTING POWDER
(Ralston)

Sevin * 5%
Sulfur 10%

PURINA POULTRY INSECTICIDE
(Ralston)

Malathion 4.00%
Xylene * 25.00%
Petroleum oil 65.75%
Emulsifiers 5.25%

PURINA PRE-LAC DAIRY WORMER
Anthelmintic
(Ralston)

Thiabendazole (equiv. to 42 gm./
lb.) 9.2%

PURINA PURA-MYCIN
Antibiotic treatment via water; veterinary
(Ralston)

Per cc.:
Terramycin .... 25 mg.
Propylene glycol

PURINA PURA-MYCIN SOLUBLE POWDER CONCENTRATE
Antibiotic
(Ralston)

Each 4 oz. packet:
Oxytetracycline
hydrochloride * .... 25.6 gm.

PURINA PURIDINE
Sanitizer
(Ralston)

Titratable Iodine 1%

PURINA RANGE CATTLE SPRAY
Insecticide
(Ralston)

Toxaphene * 45.00%
Gamma isomer of benzene hexa-
chloride (from lindane) 0.45%
Aromatic petroleum derivative
solvents * 41.55%
Xylene 5.00%

PURINA RAT CONTROL PELLETS
Rodenticide
(Ralston)

Warfarin 0.025%

PURINA ROACH & ANT INSECTICIDE
(Ralston)

Dursban 0.50%
Petroleum oils * 88.76%

PURINA ROACH, ANT & SPIDER SPRAY
(Ralston)

Dursban 0.50%
Pyrethrins 0.05%
Piperonyl butoxide 0.10%
N-Octyl bicycloheptene
dicarboximide 0.17%
Petroleum oils * 58.66%

Starred ingredients (*) may be responsible for major toxic effects; consult Section II.

PURINA RUB ON HORSE INSECTICIDE
(Ralston)

Pyrethrins	0.10%
Fly repellents	1.05%
Petroleum distillate *	93.4%

PURINA SANITIZER
(Chlorinated)
(Ralston)

Sodium dichloro-s-triazinetrione	65%
Available Chlorine *	40%

PURINA 6-DAY WORM KILL CONCENTRATE 11.2%
Anthelmintic
(Ralston)

Coumaphos *	11.2%

PURINA 6-DAY WORM KILL ETTS
Anthelmintic
(Ralston)

Coumaphos	0.32%

PURINA 6-DAY WORM KILL FEED PREMIX
Anthelmintic
(Ralston)

Coumaphos *	1.12%

PURINA SPRAY AND DIP
Insecticide, emulsifiable
(Ralston)

Ronnel	24.0%
Xylene *	59.6%

PURINA STARLICIDE COMPLETE
Avicide
(Ralston)

3-Chloro-p-toluidine hydrochloride	0.1%

PURINA STOCK SPRAY-D
Animal insecticide
(Ralston)

Dioxathion *	11.9%
Xylene *	50.0%
Petroleum solvent	27.9%

PURINA STOCK SPRAY LIQUID
Insecticide
(Ralston)

Toxaphene *	45.0%
Gamma isomer of benzene hexachloride	2.7%
Aromatic petroleum derivative solvents *	20.0%
Petroleum hydrocarbons	19.3%
Xylene	5.0%

PURINA STOCK SPRAY SPECIAL
Insecticide
(Ralston)

Methoxychlor	22%
Toxaphene *	22%

PURINA SULFA
(Ralston)

Sodium sulfamethazine *	12.5%

PURINA SULFA NOX
Sulfonamide; veterinary
(Ralston)

CONCENTRATE:

Sulfaquinoxaline sodium *	12.85%

LIQUID:

Sulfaquinoxaline sodium	3.44%

PURINA SWINE PLUS
Antibiotic
(Ralston)

Each lb.:

Oxytetracycline	2.5 gm.
Furazolidone *	5.0 gm.
Arsanilic acid	0.5%

PURINA TOMATO AND VEGETABLE DUST
Insecticide, fungicide
(Ralston)

Sevin *	3%
Zineb	3.9%
Pyrethrins	0.05%
Piperonyl butoxide	0.50%

PURINA UDDER OINTMENT
(Ralston)

Methanol	0.50%
Methylsalicylate	1.00%
Benzocaine	2.00%
Emollient ointment	96.50%

PURINA WORM KILL MEDICATED
Anthelmintic
(Ralston)

Thiabendazole	9.9%

PURINA WORM KILL PASTE 43%
Anthelmintic
(Ralston)

Each dose:

Thiabendazole *	7.5 gm.

PURINA WOUND PROTECTOR
Veterinary
(Ralston)

Ronnel	2.5%
Petroleum oils *	<45%
Propellants	25%
Dipropyl isocinchomeronate	0.40%

PURITAN CARPET-FOAM
Dry foam carpet shampoo
(Puritan Chem. Co.)

Sodium lauryl sulfate	5.70%
o-Benzyl-p-chlorophenol	0.60%
Inert ingredients:	93.70%
Synthetic organic detergents *	
Other cleaning and brightening compounds	

PURITAN CHEMICAL COMPANY PRODUCTS

Puritan Chemical Company
916 Ashby St., N.W.
Atlanta, Ga. 30318

Collect phone calls received on 24-hour basis from physicians requesting toxicological information.
Mr. Eddie Lomax, Jr.
Technical Director Atlanta, Ga.

Office: 404-872-0721
Residence: 404-696-3427

PURITY #22 SOAP POWDER
Floor cleaner
(National-Purity Soap)

Anhydrous soap	22%
Alkaline builders *†	

pH of 1% solution, 11.0-11.5

†*See* Builders (detergents)

PURODIGIN TABLETS
Treatment of congestive heart failure
(Wyeth Labs.)

Each tablet:
Crystalline
Digitoxin * ...... 0.1 mg.; 0.15 mg.; 0.2 mg.

PUROGENE (Liquid Concentrate)
Potable water treatment
(Bio-Cide)

Chlorine dioxide *	2%
Sodium carbonate	3%
De-ionized Water	95%

Starred ingredients (*) may be responsible for major toxic effects; consult Section II.

PURO PINE OIL DISINFECTANT
(United Chemical Co., Inc.)

Active ingredients: 90%
  Steam distilled Pine oil *
  Vegetable oil soap
Inert ingredient: . . . . not more than 10%
  Water

'76 Ed.

PURPLE K DRY CHEMICAL RECHARGE
For fire extinguishers
(Norris Industries)

Potassium bicarbonate
Diatomaceous earth
Tricalcium phosphate
Polysiloxane coating

'76 Ed.

PURPLE MAGIC
See CHOLDUN'S PURPLE MAGIC

PURPLE SPARKLE
All purpose cleaner & degreaser
(Haviland Products Co.)

Sodium phosphates *
Sodium metasilicate
Sodium xylene sulfonate *
Polyethylene glycol
Tert-dodecyl thioether

'76 Ed.

PURPOSE BRAND SHAMPOO
(Johnson & Johnson)

Sorbitan esters
Amphoteric surfactants *
Polyethylene glycol esters
Benzyl alcohol
Boric acid
Perfume

PURPOSE BRAND SOAP
(Johnson & Johnson)

Sodium and potassium salts of fatty acids
Glycerin
Perfume
Certified dye

PUTNAM FADELESS DYES
(Putnam Color & Dye)

Aniline dyestuff (direct and acid type) *
Salt

PUTNAM NO-KOLOR COLOR REMOVER
(Putnam Color & Dye)

Sodium hydrosulphite *
Sodium tetra pyrophosphate

PUTTI-POXY
See LEECH PUTTI-POXY

P.V. CARPINE LIQUIFILM
Ophthalmic solutions
(Allergan Pharm.)

Pilocarpine nitrate * . 1/2%; 1.0%; 2.0%;
          3.0%; 4.0%; or 6.0%
Polyvinyl alcohol 1.4%
Chlorobutanol (chloral derivative as
  a preservative) 0.5%
Sodium acetate
Sodium chloride
Citric acid
Menthol
Camphor
Phenol
Eucalyptol
Purified water

P-V-TUSSIN
Antihistamine, antitussive, decongestant, expectorant
(Reid-Provident)

Each 5 cc:
  Hydrocodone bitartrate . . . . . . 2.5 mg.
  Phenylephrine HCl * . . . . 5 mg.
  Ammonium chloride . . . . 50 mg.
  Pyrilamine maleate * . . . . 6 mg.
  Chlorpheniramine maleate . . . 2 mg.
  Phenindamine tartrate * . . . . . 5 mg.
  Alcohol 5%

P.V. TUSSIN TABLETS
Antitussive, antihistamine, expectorant
(Reid-Provident)

Each tablet:
  Hydrocodone bitartrate . . . . . . 5 mg.
  Phenindamine tartrate * . . . . . 25 mg.
  Guaifenesin . . . . 200 mg.

PY-BU-TOX INSECTICIDE
(Weil Chem.)

Pyrethrins 0.075%
Piperonyl butoxide, tech. 0.375%
Petroleum distillate * 99.550%

PYCOPAY TOOTH POWDER
(Block Drug)

Sodium chloride
Sodium bicarbonate
Tricalcium phosphate
Calcium carbonate
Magnesium carbonate
Flavors

PYNAMITE STOVE CLEANER
(Pine, Morton S.)

Pine oil *
Vegetable oil soap
Tripoli

'76 Ed.

PYNO
Pine oil disinfectant
(Miller-Norris Co.)

Active ingredients: 90%
  Pure Pine oil *
  Soap

'76 Ed.

PYOCIDIN OTIC SOLUTION
Steroid/antibacterial
(Berlex Labs.)

Each ml.:
  Polymyxin-B sulfate . . . . . 10,000 units
  Hydrocortisone . . . . 5 mg.
  Water
  Propylene glycol

PYOTANNIC BLUE
Wound dressing - veterinary
(Fort Dodge)

Aniline methyl violet *
Tannic acid *
Oil cloves *
Glycerine
Alcohol base

PYRADYNE
Analgesic-antihistaminic
(Lemmon Co.)

Each tablet:
  Salicylamide . . . . 210 mg.
  Phenacetin * . . . . 150 mg.
  Caffeine . . . . 30 mg.
  Pyrilamine maleate * . . . . 15 mg.

PYRADYNE COMP.
Analgesic-antihistaminic
(Lemmon Co.)

Each tablet:
  Ipecac & opium powder
    (Dover's Powder) . . . . 15 mg.
  Salicylamide . . . . 120 mg.
  Phenacetin * . . . . 100 mg.
  Caffeine . . . . 8 mg.
  Pyrilamine maleate * . . . . 10 mg.
  Atropine sulfate . . . . 0.12 mg.
  Camphor monobromated . . . . 8 mg.

PYREFUME SUPER 20 HR
Insecticide
(Penick)

Pyrethrins 2.5%
Petroleum distillate * 97.5%

PYRENE DRY CHEMICAL RECHARGE
For fire extinguishers
(Norris Industries)

Sodium bicarbonate
Diatomaceous earth
Polysiloxane coating

'76 Ed.

Starred ingredients (*) may be responsible for major toxic effects; consult Section II.

PYRENE KARBALOY LOADED STREAM RECHARGE
For fire extinguishers
(Norris Industries)

Potassium carbonate
Sodium dichromate *
Ethylene glycol

'76 Ed.

PYRENE MULTI-PURPOSE DRY CHEMICAL RECHARGE
For fire extinguishers
(Norris Industries)

Monoammonium phosphate
Diatomaceous earth
Tricalcium phosphate
Polysiloxane coating

'76 Ed.

PYRENE PURPLE K DRY CHEMICAL RECHARGE
For fire extinguishers
(Norris Industries)

Potassium bicarbonate
Diatomaceous earth
Tricalcium phosphate
Polysiloxane coating

'76 Ed.

PYRENE SUPER-KEM DRY CHEMICAL RECHARGE
For fire extinguishers
(Norris Industries)

Potassium chloride
Diatomaceous earth
Tricalcium phosphate
Polysiloxane coating

'76 Ed.

PYRENONE CROP SPRAY (OIL BASE)
Insecticide (garden, agricultural, and livestock)
(Fairfield American)

Pyrethrins	6.0%
Piperonyl butoxide	60.0%
Petroleum distillate *	24.0%
Emulsifiers	10.0%

PYRENONE DIAZINON DUAL USE E.C. (OIL BASE)
Insecticide (indoors & outdoors)
(Fairfield American)

Pyrethrins	3.33%
Piperonyl butoxide	16.64%
Diazinon *	32.02%
Aromatic petroleum derivative *	24.91%
Petroleum distillate	13.32%
Emulsifiers	5.00%
From Diazinon	4.78%

PYRENONE DIAZINON RESIDUAL SPRAY (OIL BASE)
Insecticide (indoors and outdoors)
(Fairfield American)

Pyrethrins	0.052%
Piperonyl butoxide	0.261%
Diazinon	0.500%
Petroleum distillate *	98.608%
From Diazinon	0.079%
Solvent	0.500%

PYRENONE DURSBAN DUAL USE E.C. (OIL BASE)
Insecticide (indoors and outdoors)
(Fairfield American)

Pyrethrins	3.33%
Piperonyl butoxide	16.64%
Petroleum distillate	13.32%
Chlorpyrifos (Dursban) *	31.99%
Aromatic petroleum distillate *	27.64%
Emulsifiers	5.00%
From Dursban	2.08%

PYRENONE DURSBAN ROACH & ANT SPRAY (OIL BASE)
Insecticide (indoors and outdoors)
(Fairfield American)

Pyrethrins	0.052%
Piperonyl butoxide	0.260%
Chlorpyrifos (Dursban)	0.500%
Petroleum distillate *	98.736%
From Dursban	0.452%

PYRENONE FOOD PLANT FOGGING INSECTICIDE (OIL BASE)
(Fairfield American)

Pyrethrins	0.5%
Piperonyl butoxide	5.0%
Petroleum distillate *	94.5%

PYRENONE INDUSTRIAL SPRAY E.C. (OIL BASE)
Insecticide (indoors)
(Fairfield American)

Pyrethrins	1.0%
Piperonyl butoxide	10.0%
Petroleum distillate *	79.0%
Emulsifiers	10.0%

PYRENONE MAGC 5-1 (OIL BASE)
Insecticide (indoors and outdoors)
(Fairfield American)

Pyrethrins	1.0%
Piperonyl butoxide	5.0%
Petroleum distillate *	94.0%

PYRENONE MAGC 12.5-2.5 (OIL BASE)
Insecticide (indoors and outdoors)
(Fairfield American)

Pyrethrins	2.5%
Piperonyl butoxide	12.5%
Petroleum distillate *	85.0%

PYRENONE 25-5 MAGC (OIL BASE)
Insecticide (indoor and outdoor)
(Fairfield American)

Pyrethrins	5.0%
Piperonyl butoxide	25.0%
Petroleum oil *	70.0%

PYRENONE PCO ROACH CONCENTRATE (OIL BASE)
Indoor and outdoor use
(Fairfield American)

Pyrethrins	1.5%
Piperonyl butoxide	7.5%
Petroleum distillate *	91.0%

PYRICAIN
For temporary relief of sore throat
(Jenkins Labs.)

Each tablet:
Sodium propionate	10 mg.
Benzocaine	5 mg.

PYRIDIUM
Urinary tract analgesic
(Parke-Davis)

Each tablet:
Phenazopyridine hydrochloride *	100 mg.; 200 mg.

PYRIN-AID LIQUID
Kills head, body and crab lice and their eggs
(Columbia Med.)

Pyrethrins	0.2%
Piperonyl butoxide, technical	2.0%
Deodorized Kerosene	0.8%

PYROCIDE BOOSTER CONCENTRATE E
Insecticide
(MGK)

Pyrethrins	1.5%
Tech. Piperonyl butoxide	7.5%
Petroleum distillate *	91.0%

PYROCIDE DRY
Insecticide
(MGK)

Oil *†	45.8%
Pyrethrins	2.2%

†*See* Kerosene

Starred ingredients (*) may be responsible for major toxic effects; consult Section II.

PYROCIDE FOGGING CONCENTRATE 5628
Insecticide for industrial use
(MGK)

Pyrethrins	3%
Technical Piperonyl butoxide	6%
N-Octyl bicycloheptene dicarboximide (MGK-264)	10%
Petroleum distillate *	81%

PYROCIDE FOGGING FORMULA 7067 FOR ULV MOSQUITO ADULTICIDING
(MGK)

Pyrethrins	5%
Technical Piperonyl butoxide	25%
Petroleum distillate *	20%
Mineral oil	50%

PYROCIDE GROWERS SPRAY
Insecticide
(MGK)

Pyrethrins	1.40%
Mineral oil	5.60%
Aromatic petroleum distillate *	48.00%

PYROCIDE INTERMEDIATE 57
(MGK)

Pyrethrins	10.0%
Tech. Piperonyl butoxide	50.0%
Petroleum distillate *	40.0%

PYROCIDE INTERMEDIATE NO. 5192
(MGK)

Pyrethrins	9.0%
Tech. Piperonyl butoxide	18.0%
N-Octyl bicycloheptene dicarboximide (MGK 264) *	30.0%
Petroleum distillate *	43.0%

PYROCIDE MOSQUITO ADULTICIDING CONCENTRATE FOR ULV FOGGING, F-7088
(MGK)

Pyrethrins *	12%
Technical Piperonyl butoxide	60%
Mineral oil	28%

PYROFOG
Insecticide for fogging machines
(Carpenter, W.D.)

Pyrethrins	0.15%
Piperonyl butoxide (technical)	0.30%
N-Octyl bicycloheptene dicarboximide	0.50%
Petroleum distillate *	99.05%

PYROGESIC
Analgesic-antipyretic
(Elder)

Each tablet:	
Acetaminophen *	325.0 mg.

PYROIL "A"
Gasoline additive
(Pyroil)

High molecular weight esters	1-10%
Mixture of oxygenated unsaponifiable hydrocarbons	1-10%
Alkyl aryl phosphate, low percentage	
Mineral oil *	>90%

'76 Ed.

PYROIL "B"
Motor oil additive
(Pyroil)

Combined amount:	>10%
High molecular weight esters of the acids produced in oxidation	
Barium soaps of the oxidate *†	
Mineral oil *	80%

'76 Ed.

†*See* Barium salts, soluble

PYROIL BRAKE FLUID
(Pyroil)

Combined amount:	100%
Poly-oxy-alkylene glycols *†	
Tri-glycol-ethers *†	

'76 Ed.

†*See* Brake fluids, Section VI, General Formulations

PYROIL CARBURETOR CLEANER (AEROSOL)
(Pyroil)

Mixture of Petroleum distillates	>40%
Xylol *	>50%

'76 Ed.

PYROIL CARBURETOR CLEANER (NON-AEROSOL)
(Pyroil)

Combined amount:	>30%
High molecular weight esters	
Mixture of oxygenated unsaponifiable hydrocarbons	
Alkyl aryl phosphate, low percent	
Aromatic solvents *	
Mineral oil *	>60%

'76 Ed.

PYROIL DIESEL FUEL CONDITIONER
(Pyroil)

Mixture of Petroleum distillates *	>10%
Mineral oil *	>80%

'76 Ed.

PYROIL GASLINE ANTIFREEZE
(Pyroil)

Combined amount:	<1%
High molecular weight esters	
Mixture of oxygenated unsaponifiable hydrocarbons	
Methanol *	>90%

'76 Ed.

PYROIL K.O.
(Pyroil)

White spirits *	>50%
Ethylene glycol monobutyl ether *	1-10%
Petroleum oxydates with minor amounts of barium *†	1-10%
Propellant	>30%

'76 Ed.

†*See* Barium salts, soluble

PYROIL MR. CHAMP
Penetrating oil
(Pyroil)

NON-AEROSOL:

Amine salt of an acid	>10%
Mineral spirits *	>20%
Mineral oils *	>60%
Graphite	<1%

AEROSOL:

Amine salt of an acid	>10%
Mineral spirits *	>20%
Mineral oil *	>60%

'76 Ed.

PYROIL MR. SHHHHH
Household oil
(Pyroil)

Combined amount:	1-10%
High molecular weight esters of the acids produced in oxidation	
Mixture of oxygenated unsaponifiable hydrocarbons	
Barium soaps of the oxidate *†	
Mineral oil *	>90%

'76 Ed.

†*See* Barium salts, soluble

PYROIL RADIATOR FAST FLUSH
(Pyroil)

Mineral spirits *	>50%
N-Butanol *	>20%
Alkyl phenol ethoxylate	>10%

'76 Ed.

Starred ingredients (*) may be responsible for major toxic effects; consult Section II.

PYROIL RADIATOR RUST INHIBITOR
(Pyroil)

Amine salt of an acid .... >20%
Water .... >70%

'76 Ed.

PYROIL RADIATOR STOP LEAK
(Pyroil)

Amine salt of an acid 1-10%
Ginger root 1-10%
Water .... >80%

'76 Ed.

PYROIL RX-1
Fast engine purge
(Pyroil)

Combined amount: .... >30%
  High molecular weight esters
  Mixture of oxygenated unsaponifiable
    hydrocarbons
  Alkyl aryl phosphate, low percent
Mineral oil * .... >60%

'76 Ed.

PYROIL RX-2
Additive for worn motors
(Pyroil)

Combined amount: .... >30%
  High molecular weight esters of the
    acids produced in oxidation
  Barium soaps of the oxidate *†
Mineral oil * .... >60%

'76 Ed.

†*See* Barium salts, soluble

PYROIL RX-3
Additive for transmissions
(Pyroil)

Combined amount: .... >30%
  Amine salt of an acid
  Chlorinated hydrocarbons, low percent
Mineral oil * .... >60%

'76 Ed.

PYROIL STARTING FLUID
(Pyroil)

Combined amount: .... <1%
  High molecular weight esters
  Mixture of oxygenated unsaponifiable
    hydrocarbons
Ethyl ether * .... >90%

'76 Ed.

PYROIL WINDSHIELD DE-ICER (AEROSOL)
(Pyroil)

Methanol * .... >70%
Mixture of Glycols .... trace

'76 Ed.

PYROIL WINDSHIELD WASHER ANTIFREEZE
(Pyroil)

CONCENTRATE:
  Methanol * .... >70%
  Mercapto ethoxylate .... <1%
  Water .... >10%

PREMIX:
  Methanol * .... >40%
  Mercapto ethoxylate 1-10%
  Water .... >50%

'76 Ed.

PYROIL WINDSHIELD WASHER CLEANER AND BUG REMOVER
(Pyroil)

Isopropyl alcohol 1-10%
Mercapto ethoxylate .... <1%
Water .... >90%

'76 Ed.

PYROIL WINTER OIL TREATMENT
(Pyroil)

Combined amount: .... >20%
  Mixture of derivatives of polyisobutenyl
    succinimide, esters of oleic acid and
    substituted polyamines
  Hydrocarbon solvent *
Mineral oil * .... >70%

'76 Ed.

PYRO-JET
Heavy duty steam cleaner; industrial use
(Puritan Chem. Co.)

Sodium hydroxide *

PYROLUBE
High temperature lubricant
(Kano)

Graphited base
Blended oils

PYRO MILL SPRAY, GOOD-LIFE

See GOOD-LIFE PYRO MILL SPRAY

PYRRALAN EXPECTORANT
(Lannett)

Each fl. oz.:
  Thenylpyramine fumerate *   80 mg.
  Ephedrine hydrochloride ..... 30 mg.
  Ammonium chloride .... 500 mg.
  Special expectorant base ..... q.s.a.d.

PYRRALAN EXPECTORANT "DM"
(Lannett)

Each fl. oz.:
  Thenylpyramine fumerate *   80 mg.
  Ephedrine hydrochloride .... 30 mg.
  Ammonium chloride .... 500 mg.
  D-Methorphan
    hydrobromide .... 10 mg./5 ml.
  Special expectorant base ..... q.s.a.d.

PY-VONA STOCK FLY SPRAY, UNICO

See UNICO PY-VONA STOCK FLY SPRAY

PZAZZ
Cream cleanser; institutional & industrial use
(Puritan Chem. Co.)

2,2'-Methylenebis(3,4,6-
  trichlorophenol) 0.25%
Inert ingredients: 99.75%
  Includes cleaning, brightening, emulsi-
    fying and wetting agents

Q

Q.A. CONCENTRATED SOLUTION
(National Chemicals, Inc.)

Active ingred.: 10%
  N-Alkyl dimethyl benzyl ammonium
    chlorides *
  N-Alkyl dimethyl ethylbenzyl ammo-
    nium chlorides *
Inert ingred.: 90%
  Water

Q-DOPE
Polystyrene coil dope
(GC Electronics)

Polystyrene resin
Toluene * .... >10%

Q.D.S., LIQUID

See LIQUID Q.D.S.

QMF
Motor flush
(Radiator)

Aromatic solvents *

'76 Ed.

Starred ingredients (*) may be responsible for major toxic effects; consult Section II.

Q-NARY
Disinfectant, sanitizer, deodorizer
(United Chemical Co., Inc.)

n-Alkyl (50% C12, 30% C14, 17% C16,
3% C18) dimethyl ethylbenzyl ammonium chlorides * 5%
n-Alkyl (60% C14, 30% C16, 5% C12,
5% C18) dimethyl benzyl ammonium chlorides * 5%

'76 Ed.

Q-SAN CONCENTRATE 1 TO 3

See CHAPMAN Q-SAN CONCEN-
TRATE 1 TO 3

QS4 LIQUID CONCENTRATE
*Cleaner, disinfectant, sanitizer, deodor-
ant, fungicide*
(Brulin)

n-Alkyl (60% C14, 30% C16, 5% C12,
5% C18) dimethyl benzyl ammonium chlorides * 1.6%
n-Alkyl (68% C12, 32% C14) dimethyl
ethylbenzyl ammonium
chlorides * 1.6%
Sodium carbonate * 3.0%

QUAALUDE-150
Hypnotic
(Lemmon Co.)

Each tablet:
Methaqualone * .... 150 mg.

QUAALUDE-300
Hypnotic
(Lemmon Co.)

Each tablet:
Methaqualone * .... 300 mg.

QUAD-DIS, FOREMOST 1690

See FOREMOST 1690 QUAD-DIS

QUADETTS
Sulfonamide therapy
(Elder)

Each tablet:
Sulfamethazine * .... 167 mg.
Sulfamerazine * .... 167 mg.
Sulfadiazine * .... 167 mg.

QUADRAHIST TABLETS
Antihistamine
(Pharmex)

Each tablet:
Pyrilamine maleate * .... 6.25 mg.
Phenyltoloxamine di-hydrogen
citrate .... 6.25 mg.
Prophenpyridamine maleate . 6.25 mg.
Methapyrilene
hydrochloride * .... 6.25 mg.

QUADRAMIN
Mineral supplement
(Wesley Pharm.)

Each 3 tablets:
Calcium .... 312 mg.
Zinc .... 200 mg.
Magnesium .... 132 mg.
Potassium .... 99 mg.

QUADRAMOID LIQUID
Sulfonamide therapy
(Elder)

Each 5 cc:
Sulfamethazine * .... 167 mg.
Sulfamerazine * .... 167 mg.
Sulfadiazine * .... 167 mg.
Alcohol 5%

QUADRINAL
Bronchodilator-expectorant
(Knoll Pharm.)

TABLETS (each):
Ephedrine hydrochloride * ... 24 mg.
Phenobarbital .... 24 mg.
Theophylline calcium
salicylate * .... 130 mg.
Potassium iodide .... 320 mg.
SUSPENSION (each 5 cc.):
Ephedrine hydrochloride * ... 12 mg.
Phenobarbital .... 12 mg.
Theophylline calcium
salicylate * .... 65 mg.
Potassium iodide .... 160 mg.

QUAD-SULFAS
*For control of coccidiosis, coryza in
chicken, turkey flocks; veterinary*
(Hilltop)

Sulfamerazine sodium 1.2%
Sulfamethazine sodium 1.7%
Sulfaquinoxaline sodium 2.2%
Sulfathiazole sodium 3.9%
Inactive ingred.:
Sodium hydroxide 0.5%
Water 90.498%
D & C coloring 0.002%

'76 Ed.

QUAKER SALVE
(C.T.S. Labs.)

Eucalyptus *
Phenol *
Petrolatum

QUAMM DISINFECTANT, MARTIN'S

See MARTIN'S QUAMM DISINFEC-
TANT

QUANTO GERMICIDAL DETERGENT
Institutional use
(Huntington Labs.)

Active ingred.: 8.95%
Didecyl dimethyl ammonium
chloride * 3.75%
Alkyl (C12 40%, C14 50%, C16
10%) dimethyl benzyl am-
monium chloride * 2.50%
Tetrasodium ethylene diamine
tetraacetate 2.60%
Essential oils 0.10%

QUARTETS COUGH AND COLD TABLETS
*Decongestant, antihistaminic, antitus-
sive*
(DePree)

Pseudoephedrine HCl *
d-Methorphan HBr *
Guaiphenesin

QUAT 42
Germicidal cleaner
(Banner Mfg. Co.)

n-Alkyl (60% C12, 30% C14, 5%
C16, 5% C18) dimethyl benzyl
ammonium chlorides * 2.25%
Alkyl (68% C12, 32% C14) di-
methyl ethylbenzyl ammonium
chlorides * 2.25%
Sodium carbonate * 3.00%
Inert ingredients contain compat-
ible, Non-ionic detergents *,
Builders 92.50%

'76 Ed.

QUATRA-D, DEL

See DEL QUATRA-D

QUATRAMINE A
*Germicide, sanitizing agent; institu-
tional & industrial use*
(Puritan Chem. Co)

n-Alkyl (60% tetradecyl, 30% hexadecyl, 5% octadecyl)
dimethyl benzyl ammonium
chlorides * 5.0%
n-Alkyl (50% dodecyl, 30% tetradecyl, 17% hexadecyl, 3% octadecyl)
dimethyl benzyl ammonium
chlorides * 5.0%

QUATSYL-256 CLEANER DISINFECTANT
(Nat'l Labs. Div.)

Octyl decyl dimethyl ammonium
  chloride *† 3.750%
Dioctyl dimethyl ammonium
  chloride *† 1.875%
Didecyl dimethyl ammonium
  chloride * 1.875%
Alkyl (C14, 50%; C12, 40%; C16,
  10%) benzyl dimethyl ammonium chloride * 5.000%
Tetrasodium
  ethylenediaminetetraacetate .. 3.420%
Isopropyl alcohol 3.000%
Ethyl alcohol 1.000%

†*See* Cationic surfactants

QUEEN ANN SHAMPOO
(Uncle Sam)

Vegetable oils
Potassium hydroxide
Tetrasodium ethylene diamine tetraace-
tate
Propylene glycol
Water

QUEEN OF DIAMONDS
Cold wave lotion
(Willat)

Ammonium thioglycolate 1-10%

QUELIDRINE SYRUP
*Non-narcotic antihistaminic cough
  suppressant*
(Abbott)

Each tsp. (5 ml.):
  Dextromethorphan
    hydrobromide * .... 10 mg.
  Chlorpheniramine maleate .. 2 mg.
  Ephedrine hydrochloride * . 5 mg.
  Phenylephrine
    hydrochloride * .... 5 mg.
  Ammonium chloride .... 40 mg.
  Ipecac fluidextract .... 0.005 ml.
  Alcohol 2%

QUEST GERMICIDE CLEANER

See BUTCHER'S QUEST GERMI-
  CIDE CLEANER

QUIBRON CAPSULES & LIQUID
Bronchodilator-expectorant
(Mead Johnson)

Each capsule or 15 ml.:
  Theophylline * .... 150 mg.
  Glyceryl guaiacolate .... 90 mg.

QUIBRON PLUS ELIXIR & CAPSULES
Bronchodilator
(Mead Johnson)

Each capsule or 15 ml.:
  Theophylline (anhydrous) * .. 150 mg.
  Glyceryl guaiacolate .... 100 mg.
  Ephedrine HCl * .... 25 mg.
  Butabarbital * .... 20 mg.
  Alcohol (Elixir) 15%

QUICK
*Heavy duty degreaser and motor
  cleaner; industrial and institutional
  use*
(Scientific International)

Petroleum distillate *

QUICK AID DRY CHEMICAL EXTINGUISHER
Fire extinguisher
(General Fire Extinguisher)

Sodium bicarbonate * .... over 98%
Zinc stearate
Silicate

"QUICK CLEAN"
(Ziebart)

Stoddard solvent *

QUICK DEATH INSECTICIDE
*Bed bugs, roaches, moths, water bugs,
  ants, fleas & mosquitoes*
(Victory Chem.)

Petroleum distillates *
Diethyl diphenyl dichloroethane
Related compounds
Beta'-butoxy beta'-thiocyano-diethyl
  ether *
Beta-thiocyanoethyl esters (of mixed fatty
  acids containing 10 to 18 carbon
  atoms) *
Essential oils *

'76 Ed.

QUICK DRY ZAR
(United Gilsonite)

Non-volatile: 40%
  Polyhydric alcohol partially esterified
    with Linolenic, Oleic, Linoleic, Pal-
    mitic, Stearic acids, modified with To-
    lylene diisocyanate
Volatile: 60.00%
  Aliphatic hydrocarbons *

QUICK-FIX
See EDWAL QUICK-FIX

QUICK PEP TABLETS
(Thompson Med.)

Each tablet:
  Caffeine alkaloid *
  Dextrose
  Sodium biphosphate
  Niacin
  Calcium phosphate monobasic
  Thiamine mononitrate

QUICK POLISHING COMPOUND
(McAleer)

Kerosene *
Sodium oleate
Paraffin oil
Pine oil *
Tripoli

'76 Ed.

QUICKSET
(U.S. Peroxygen)

Methyl ethyl ketone peroxide * 60%
Dimethyl phthalate 40%

'76 Ed.

QUICK STICK WALL SIZE, EVANS

See EVANS QUICK STICK WALL
  SIZE

QUIDE TABLETS
Treatment of schizophrenic reactions
(Dow Pharm., Dow Chem. Co.)

Each tablet:
  Piperacetazine * ...... 10 mg.; 25 mg.

QUIETABS
Tranquilizing aid
(Commerce Drug)

Pyrilamine maleate *

QUIET NITE COUGH SYRUP
(Rexall)

Chlorpheniramine maleate .... <1%
Ephedrine sulfate * .... <1%
Dextromethorphan hydrobromide .. <1%
Acetaminophen * 1-10%
Alcohol 26%

'76 Ed.

QUIET WORLD TABLETS
Sedative
(Whitehall Labs.)

Aspirin *
Acetaminophen *
Methapyrilene *
Scopolamine *

QUIKCIDE
Insecticide; aerosol
(Kem Mfg. Co.)

Pyrethrins	0.30%
Technical Piperonyl butoxide	1.50%
Petroleum distillate *	18.20%

QUIKCIDE INSECTICIDE CONCENTRATE
(Kem Mfg. Co.)

N-Octyl bicycloheptene dicarboximide	0.336%
Piperonyl butoxide (technical)	0.203%
Pyrethrins I and II	0.101%
Refined Petroleum distillates *	99.360%

QUIKCIDE REPELLENT
Insecticide and repellent for horses
(Kem Mfg. Co.)

Active ingred.:
Pyrethrins	0.50%
Technical Piperonyl butoxide	1.00%
N-Octyl bicycloheptene dicarboximide	1.67%
Dipropyl isocinchomeronate	2.00%
Petroleum distillate *	84.83%

Inert ingred.:
Emulsifier (Polyoxyethylene sorbate)	10.00%

QUIK-I-POXY
See LEECH QUIK-I-POXY

QUIK-KIL
Insecticide - institutional
(Miller-Norris Co.)

Pyrethrins	0.3%
Technical Piperonyl butoxide	0.6%
N-Octyl bicycloheptene dicarboximide	1.0%
Petroleum distillate *	13.1%
Inert ingredients:	85.0%
Dichlorodifluoromethane	42.5%/wt.
Trichloromonofluoromethane	42.5%/wt.

'76 Ed.

QUIK 'N EASY SPOT LIFTER
(Penn-Champ)

1,1,1-Trichloroethane *	70%
Propellent	approx. 25%
Silica	approx. 5%

QUIK-O-MATIC
Granular automatic dishwasher detergent (institutional)
(Colgate-Palmolive)

Combined amount:	approx. 98%
Pentasodium tripolyphosphate *	
Sodium metasilicate *	
Sodium carbonate *	
Organic low-foam wetting agent	about 2%

'76 Ed.

QUIK-TROL, SPRAY-TROL BRAND
See SPRAY-TROL BRAND QUIK-TROL

QUINAGLUTE DURA-TABS
Cardiac antiarrhythmia agent
(Berlex Labs.)

Each tablet (Prolonged Release):
Quinidine gluconate *	5 gr.

QUINAMM
Specific therapy for night leg cramps
(Merrell Dow)

Each tablet:
Quinine sulfate *	260 mg.

QUINE CAPSULES
Antimalarial
(Rowell)

Quinine sulfate *	200 mg.; 300 mg.

QUINIDEX EXTENTABS
For cardiac arrhythmias
(Robins)

Each Extentab:
Quinidine sulfate, USP *	300 mg.

QUINITE
Antihypertensive, diuretic
(Direct Div.)

Each tablet:
Quinine sulfate *	260 mg.

QUINOLOR COMPOUND OINTMENT
For infections of skin
(Squibb)

Chlorhydroxyquinolin	0.5%
Benzoyl peroxide	10.0%

Plastibase with:
Menthol *
Methyl salicylate *
Eugenol *

QUINSANA DEODORANT FOOT POWDER
(Mennen)

Talc
Silica
Fragrance
Triclosan

QUINSANA PLUS MEDICATED FOOT POWDER
(Mennen)

Active ingred.:
Zinc undecylenate *
Undecylenic acid
Other ingred.:
Talc
Silica
Fragrance

QUOTANE OINTMENT
Topical anesthetic
(MenJ Labs.)

Dimethisoquin hydrochloride *	0.5%

QUSEPTIC
Disinfectant, deodorant
(Norden Labs.)

n-Alkyl (C14, C12, C16) dimethyl benzyl ammonium chloride *	10.0%
Ethyl alcohol	2.5%

QWIK STRIP PAINT STRIPPERS (-DT, -E, -P, -R, -V)
(ABCO, Inc.)

Methanol *
Methylene chloride *

R

RACET
Antibacterial, anti-fungal, anti-inflammatory, anti-pruritic
(Lemmon Co.)

Iodochlorhydroxyquin	3%
Hydrocortisone	0.5%

Stearic acid, Cetyl alcohol, Petrolatum, Polyoxyl 40 stearate, Sorbitol, Propylene glycol, Methylparaben, Propylparaben, Purified water, Perfume

RACET - 1% CREAM
Antibacterial, antifungal, anti-inflammatory, antipruritic
(Lemmon Co.)

Iodochlorhydroxyquin *	3%
Hydrocortisone	1%

Also contains: Stearic acid, Cetyl alcohol, Petrolatum, Polyoxyl 40 stearate, Sorbitol, Propylene glycol, Methylparaben, Propylparaben, Purified water, Perfume

RACET LCD CREAM
Antibacterial, anti-fungal, anti-inflammatory, anti-pruritic
(Lemmon Co.)

Iodochlorhydroxyquin 3%
Hydrocortisone 0.5%
Coal tar solution * 5%
Stearic acid, Cetyl alcohol, Petrolatum, Polyoxyl 40 stearate, Sorbitol, Propylene glycol, Methylparaben, Propylparaben, Purified water, Perfume

RACING BRONZE ANTIFOULING
Paint
(International Paint)

Copper-bronze powder
Pine tar *
Mineral spirits 24 *

RAD-E-CATE 25
Herbicide
(Vineland Chem.)

Sodium dimethylarsinate * 23.4%
Dimethylarsinic acid 4.0%

RADIANT BLEACH
(Radiant Wash Solution Corp.)

Sodium hypochlorite * 5.25%

'76 Ed.

RADIANT JELL
(Uncle Sam)

Plastic resins
Waxes
Petroleum distillates *
Borax *
Surfactants
Water
Emulsifiers

RADIATOR'S LIQUID BLOCK SEAL
(Radiator)

Alkaline salts of silicic acid *†

'76 Ed.

†*See* Sodium silicate

RADIATOR'S LIQUID BOILER SOLDER SEAL
(Radiator)

Alkaline salts of silicic acid *†

'76 Ed.

†*See* Sodium silicate

RAD INSTANT CLEANER
All purpose cleaner; white powder
(RAD, Inc.)

Soda ash * 42%
Bicarbonate of soda 41%
Sodium metasilicate pentahydrate * 12%
Liquid Surfactant 4%
Pine oil 1%

RAID INSECTICIDE PRODUCTS
(Johnson, S. C.)

Phone: 414-631-2111

RAID is the trademark for a line of insecticide formulations. It is important that the specific RAID product be identified by specific name such as RAID HOUSE & GARDEN BUG KILLER, RAID ANT & ROACH KILLER or RAID FLYING INSECT KILLER, etc., and by the ingredients listed on the label. As with all insecticide products, active ingredients are declared on the container label. Product information is regularly sent to the National Poison Control Network (Pittsburg, Pa.) and POISINDEX (Denver, Colo.). These organizations review the information, develop treatment regimens and make this information available to local poison control centers. S. C. Johnson & Son, Inc., Racine, Wisconsin, will accept collect calls from physicians and Poison Control Centers handling cases involving their products. This emergency telephone service is maintained 24 hours a day, 7 days a week. To insure contact with technically qualified personnel, inform the long distance operator that the call is an emergency. Then request person to person contact with a member of the S. C. Johnson & Son emergency call panel.

RAIN-COTE
Masonry water repellent
(Lester Labs.)

Petroleum distillates *
Silicone
Oils

'76 Ed.

RAIN REM
Maintenance material
(Speco)

Silicone compound in
Aromatic solvent *

'76 Ed.

RAINSEAL
Water repellent transparent coating
(Texas Refinery)

Combined amount: 95.0%
Aromatic hydrocarbons *
Aliphatic hydrocarbons *
Silicone resin 5.0%

RAIN-X AUTOMOTIVE GLASS TREATMENT
Repellent coating for windshields and windows
(Unelko)

%/wgt.
Alkyl polysiloxanes (Dimethyl silicone fluids) 10.00%
Sulfuric acid (reagent grade) 1.00%
Isopropanol (Isopropyl alcohol, anhydrous) * 89.00%

RALSTON RAT KILL (WATER SOLUBLE)
Rodenticide
(Ralston)

Sodium salt of 2-pivalyl-1,3-
indandione 0.14%

RAMA INCENSE CONES
(Hindu Incense)

Charcoal 75%
Starch 15%
Combined amount: 10%
Karaya gum
China clay
Sodium nitrate
Essential oils *
Triethylene glycol
Aromatic chemicals

RAMEX
For stopped up drains
(ABCO, Inc.)

Sulfuric acid *

RA-MO-CIDE, MOORMAN'S

See MOORMAN'S RA-MO-CIDE

RAMON'S BROWNIE PILLS
Diuretic
(Brown Mfg.)

Each pill:
Theobromine sodio-
salicylate * .... 100 mg.
Ext. Uva ursi
Methylene blue

'76 Ed.

RAMON'S COVAC
Antihistamine, analgesic
(Brown Mfg.)

Each tablet:
Pyranisamine maleate * .... 12.50 mg.
Acetophenetidin * .... 1.50 gr.
Sodium salicylate * .... 1.50 gr.
Caffeine .... 0.25 gr.

'76 Ed.

Starred ingredients (*) may be responsible for major toxic effects; consult Section II.

RAMON'S HERBS
Laxative
(Brown Mfg.)

Compound of Senna leaves	44%
Jalap	25%
Mandrake roots *	10%
Aromatic and flavoring herbs	21%

'76 Ed.

RAMON'S MILD LAXATIVE WITH BILE SALTS
(Brown Mfg.)

Yellow Phenolphthalein, not USP	1/2 gr.
Cascara ext.	2/3 gr.
Oleoresin capsicum	1/40 gr.
Salts of bile	1 gr.
Sodium glycocholate	
Sodium taurocholate	

'76 Ed.

RAMON'S PINK PILLS
Laxative
(Brown Mfg.)

Aloin	1/4 gr.
Podophyllin *	1/6 gr.
Yellow Phenolphthalein, not USP	
Ext. Cascara sagrada	2 gr.

'76 Ed.

RAMON'S TABS
Analgesic
(Brown Mfg.)

Aspirin *	5 gr.
Caffeine	1/4 gr.

'76 Ed.

RAMROD & ATRAZINE WETTABLE POWDER
Herbicide
(Monsanto)

2-Chloro-N-isopropylacetanilide *	48.1%
Atrazine *	20.9%

RAMROD 20 GRANULAR
Herbicide
(Monsanto)

2-Chloro-N-isopropylacetanilide *	20%

RAMROD WETTABLE POWDER
Herbicide
(Monsanto)

2-Chloro-N-isopropylacetanilide *	65%

RANDO HD OILS
(Texaco Canada Ltd.)

Petroleum lubricating oil
Oxidation and corrosion inhibitor *†
Barium detergent *

†*See* Rust control, Section VI, General Formulations

RANDOX
Herbicide
(Monsanto)

Emulsifiable Conc.:
N,N-Diallyl-2-chloroacetamide *	47.1%

Granules:
N,N-Diallyl-2-chloroacetamide *	20%

RANI INCENSE CONES
(Hindu Incense)

Charcoal	75%
Starch	15%
Combined amount:	10%
Karaya gum	
China clay	
Sodium nitrate	
Essential oils *	
Triethylene glycol	
Aromatic chemicals	

RAPHON
Antiseptic hemostat
(Nephron)

Racemic Epinephrine hydrochloride	1:525
Chlorobutanol	0.3%
Zephiran chloride (Alkyl-dimethyl-benzyl-ammonium chlorides)	1:2000
Saline	

RA-PID-GRO
Soluble plant food for foliar or root feeding
(Ra-Pid-Gro Corp.)

Total Nitrogen *†	23%
Ammoniacal nitrogen	4%
Nitrate nitrogen	5%
Other water soluble nitrogen	14%
Water insoluble nitrogen	0%
Available Phosphoric acid *	19%
Soluble Potash	17%

†*See* Fertilizers, Section VI, General Formulations

RA-PID-GRO ACID-GRO
Fertilizer
(Ra-Pid-Gro Corp.)

Total Nitrogen *†	30%
Ammoniacal nitrogen	2.3%
Nitrate nitrogen	3.2%
Urea nitrogen	24.5%
Water-insoluble nitrogen	0%
Available Phosphoric acid *	12%
Soluble Potash	11%
Boron	0.02%
Copper	0.05%
Iron	0.10%
Manganese	0.05%
Zinc	0.05%

†*See* Fertilizers, Section VI, General Formulations

RAPID-KILL, DEL
See DEL RAPID-KILL

RAPID SEWER SOLVENT
(Consolidated Chem., Inc.)

Sodium hydroxide *

RASP BABY AND CHILDREN'S COUGH SYRUP
(Commerce Drug)

Alcohol	2%
Wild cherry	
Sanguinaria (Bloodroot)	
Ammonium chloride	
Honey	
Menthol *	

RAT-BEGONE
Rat bait; industrial and institutional use
(Scientific International)

Warfarin (3(a-Acetonylbenzyl)-4-hydroxycoumarin)	0.025%
Sulfaquinoxaline (N'-2-Quinoxalinylsulfanilamide)	0.025%

RAT DUME (FISH BLEND), GOOD-LIFE
See GOOD-LIFE RAT DUME (FISH BLEND)

RAT DUME (WATER SOLUBLE), GOOD-LIFE
See GOOD-LIFE RAT DUME (WATER SOLUBLE)

RATIO TABLETS
Antacid
(Warren-Teed)

Each tablet:	
Calcium carbonate, USP	400 mg.
Magnesium carbonate, USP	50 mg.

Starred ingredients (*) may be responsible for major toxic effects; consult Section II.

RAT-KIL

See DURHAM'S RAT-KIL

RAT NIP
Rodenticide
(NIP-CO)

Extractives of Red squill
(fortified) * 10%

RAT-NOTS
Rodenticide
(Nott)

Red squill powder (fortified) * 10%

RAT-O-CIDE
(Amer. Fumig.)

Prolin *

'76 Ed.

RAT-O-CIDE NO. 2
Rodenticide
(Amer. Fumig.)

Diphacin *

'76 Ed.

RAT-OLA
Rodenticide; prepared dry meal bait pellets
(Rockland Chem.)

Prolin 0.025%

RAT-O-MICE
Rodenticide - ready to use pellets
(McConnon & Co.)

Warfarin (3-(alpha-Acetonylben-
zyl)-4-hydroxycoumarin) 0.025%
Quinoxalinylsulfanilamide
(Sulfaquinoxaline) 0.025%

RATOPAX
Rodenticide
(Biocerta)

Convallaria 6.5%
Maritima scilla *† 3.5%
Digitalis * 2%

'76 Ed.

†*See* Squill

RATOREX WITH PROLIN
Rodenticide
(Mackwin)

Warfarin 0.025%
Quinoxalinylsulfanilamide
(Sulfaquinoxaline) 0.025%

RAT SAX
Rodenticide
(South Omaha Supply)

Warfarin (3-(a-Acetonylbenzyl)-4-
hydroxycoumarin) 0.025%

'76 Ed.

RAT-TAT-TAT
Rodenticide
(National Chemsearch)

Warfarin (3-(a-Acetonylbenzyl)-4-
hydroxycoumarin) 0.025%

RAUDIXIN
Antihypertensive, tranquilizer
(Squibb)

Each tablet:
Rauwolfia serpentina,
powdered whole root 50 mg.; 100 mg.

RAU-SED TABLETS
Tranquilizer
(Squibb)

Each tablet:
Reserpine * .... 0.25 mg.

RAUSERP
Antihypertensive
(Bio-Factor Labs.)

Each tablet:
Rauwolfia serpentina . 50 mg.; 100 mg.

'76 Ed.

RAUSERPA
Hypotensive
(Direct Div.)

Each tablet:
Rauwolfia serpentina . 50 mg.; 100 mg.

RAUTENSIN
Antihypertensive
(Dorsey Labs.)

Each tablet:
Alseroxylon (Fraction of Rauwolfia serpentina) .... 2 mg.

RAUVAL
Antihypertensive
(Vale)

Each tablet:
Rauwolfia serpentina . 50 mg.; 100 mg.

RAUWESLIN
Antihypertensive
(Wesley Pharm.)

Each tablet:
Rauwolfia serpentina ... 50 or 100 mg.

RAUWICON
Tranquilizer
(CMC Research Div.)

Rauwolfia serpentina *

RAUWILOID
Hypertension
(Riker Labs.)

Each tablet:
Rauwiloid (Alseroxylon fraction
of Rauwolfia serpentina) ... 2.0 mg.

'76 Ed.

RAUZIDE
Antihypertensive
(Squibb)

Each tablet:
Rauwolfia serpentina .... 50 mg.
Bendroflumethiazide * .... 4 mg.

RAVE BODY WAVE AEROSOL FOAM
(Chesebrough-Pond's)

Water .... >50%
Sodium bisulfite * .... >5-10%
Hydrofluorocarbon 152A ...... >5-10%
Sodium borate * .... >1-5%
Diethanolamine .... >1-5%
Sodium carbonate .... >1-5%
Cocoamphoglycinate .... >0.1-1%
Butane .... >0.1-1%
Disodium EDTA .... 0.1% or less

RAVE BODY WAVE FINISHING RINSE
(Chesebrough-Pond's)

Water .... >50%
Hydrogen peroxide * .... >1-5%
Mineral oil .... >0.1-1%
Stearyl alcohol .... >0.1-1%
Ceteth-20 .... >0.1-1%
Cetearyl alcohol .... >0.1-1%
Quaternium-7 .... >0.1-1%
Sodium lauryl sulfate .... >0.1-1%
Phosphoric acid .... 0.1% or less
Ceteareth-20 .... 0.1% or less
Phenacetin .... 0.1% or less

RAVE CONDITIONER (NORMAL/DRY FORMULA)
(Chesebrough-Pond's)

Water .... >50%
Cetyl alcohol .... >1-5%
Emulsifying wax .... >1-5%
Quaternium-31 .... >1-5%
Stearamidopropyl
dimethylamine .... >0.1-1%
PEG-8 stearate .... >0.1-1%
Hydrolyzed animal protein .... >0.1-1%
Fragrance .... >0.1-1%
Methylparaben .... >0.1-1%
DMDM hydantoin .... >0.1-1%
Propylparaben .... 0.1% or less
Citric acid .... 0.1% or less
Disodium EDTA .... 0.1% or less

Starred ingredients (*) may be responsible for major toxic effects; consult Section II.

RAVE CONDITIONER (OILY HAIR)
(Chesebrough-Pond's)

Water	>50%
Cetyl alcohol	>1-5%
Emulsifying wax	>1-5%
Quaternium-31	>1-5%
PEG-8 stearate	>0.1-1%
Hydrolyzed animal protein	>0.1-1%
Stearamidopropyl dimethylamine	>0.1-1%
Acetylated Lanolin alcohol	>0.1-1%
Fragrance	>0.1-1%
Methylparaben	>0.1-1%
DMDM hydantoin	>0.1-1%
Propylparaben	0.1% or less
Propylene glycol	0.1% or less
Citric acid	0.1% or less
Disodium EDTA	0.1% or less
Color	0.1% or less

RAVE DETERGENT BOOSTER (POWDER)
(Drackett)

Complex sodium phosphate *†	25-35%
Sodium tetraborate *	20-30%
Sodium carbonate *	15-25%
Sodium sulfate	
Sodium chloride	
Secondary alcohol ethoxylate	1%
Brighteners, Perfume, Dye, Other minor ingredients	

†See Complex phosphates

RAVE SOFT STYLER HEAT STYLING MIST
(Chesebrough-Pond's)

Water	>50%
SD Alcohol 40 *	>5-10%
Polyquaternium-4	>0.1-1%
Cetearyl octanoate	>0.1-1%
Ceteth-20	>0.1-1%
Quaternium-7	>0.1-1%
Hydrolyzed animal protein	0.1% or less
Fragrance	0.1% or less
Ceteareth-20	0.1% or less
Sodium lauryl sulfate	0.1% or less
Propylene glycol	0.1% or less
Magnesium nitrate	0.1% or less
Chloromethyl isothiazolinone	0.1% or less
Colors	0.1% or less
Methyl isothiazolinone	0.1% or less

RAWFOLA
Antihypertensive
(Foy Labs.)

Each tablet:
Rauwolfia serpentina	50 mg.

RAWLEIGH AEROSOL FURNITURE POLISH & CLEANER
(Rawleigh)

Silicone
Wax

'76 Ed.

RAWLEIGH AEROSOL HOUSEHOLD INSECTICIDE
(Rawleigh)

Beta-butoxy-beta-thiocyano-diethyl ether	1.000%
Pyrethrins	0.100%
Methoxychlor, tech.	1.000%
Piperonyl butoxide, tech.	0.166%
Petroleum hydrocarbons	7.38%

'76 Ed.

RAWLEIGH AUTO WAX
(Rawleigh)

Wax
Oleic acid
Silicone
Morpholine *
Petroleum distillate *

'76 Ed.

RAWLEIGH CALF SCOUR TREATMENT
(Rawleigh)

Each tablet:
Dihydrostreptomycin	0.25 gm.
Sulfathiazole *	50.00 gr.
Kaolin	

'76 Ed.

RAWLEIGH CLEANSER
(Rawleigh)

Trisodium phosphate *	75%
Soda ash *	25%

'76 Ed.

RAWLEIGH DIURETIC TABLETS
(Rawleigh)

Each tablet:
Sodium benzoate	2 gr.
Potassium bicarbonate	1 gr.
Powd. ext. Triticum	1 gr.
Powd. ext. Uva ursi	1/2 gr.
Powd. ext. Cornsilk	1/4 gr.
Urea	1/4 gr.

'76 Ed.

RAWLEIGH INSECT DUST NO. 3
(Rawleigh)

Rotenone	0.50%
Zinc ethylenebisdithiocarbamate	3.90%

'76 Ed.

RAWLEIGH INSECT REPELLENT
(Rawleigh)

2-Ethylhexanediol-1,3 *	20%

'76 Ed.

RAWLEIGH LAXATIVE TABLETS
(Rawleigh)

Each tablet:
Phenolphthalein	1 1/2 gr.

'76 Ed.

RAWLEIGH LOZENGES
(Rawleigh)

Each lozenge:
Powd. ext. Licorice	2.37 gr.
Benzoic acid	0.066 gr.
Tincture Capsicum	0.039 gr.
Oleoresin cubeb	0.020 gr.
Oil anise	0.049 gr.
Oil eucalyptus	0.033 gr.
Menthol	0.026 gr.

'76 Ed.

RAWLEIGH MALATHION INSECTICIDE
(Rawleigh)

Malathion *	5%

'76 Ed.

RAWLEIGH MUSTARD COMPOUND APPLICATION
(Rawleigh)

Each oz.:
Methyl salicylate *	21.00 gr.
Camphor *	12.66 gr.
Oleoresin capsicum	9.4 gr.
Turpentine	8.5 gr.
Oil eucalyptus	8.5 gr.
Oil camphor	8.5 gr.
Oil mustard, synthetic	6.2 gr.

'76 Ed.

RAWLEIGH NASAL SPRAY, DECONGESTANT
(Rawleigh)

Phenylephrine hydrochloride *	0.50%
Pheniramine maleate (Prophenpyridamine)	0.15%
Cetalkonium chloride	0.055%

'76 Ed.

RAWLEIGH PINE OIL TYPE DISINFECTANT
(Rawleigh)

Pine oil *	20%
Isopropanol	10%
Soap	10%
Ortho-benzyl-para-chlorophenol	3.5%

'76 Ed.

Starred ingredients (*) may be responsible for major toxic effects; consult Section II.

RAWLEIGH PLEASANT RELIEF
For hyperacidity
(Rawleigh)

Each fl. oz.:
Bismuth subsalicylate	8.0 gr.
Salol	1.5 gr.
Zinc phenolsulfonate	0.8 gr.

'76 Ed.

RAWLEIGH POULTRY/ SWINE WORMER
Veterinary
(Rawleigh)

Piperazine hexahydrate base	34%

'76 Ed.

RAWLEIGH PREMIUM FLY KILLER
Insecticide
(Rawleigh)

Petroleum hydrocarbons *	99.44%
Technical Piperonyl butoxide	0.50%
Pyrethrins	0.06%

'76 Ed.

RAWLEIGH RAT AND MOUSE KILLER (DRY BAIT)
Rodenticide
(Rawleigh)

2-Pivalyl-1,3-indandione	0.025%

'76 Ed.

RAWLEIGH READY RELIEF
(Rawleigh)

Each fl. oz.:
Oil lavender *	83.0 gr.
Menthol *	61.8 gr.
Camphor *	19.2 gr.
Oil dwarf pine needles	3.1 gr.
Oil juniper berries	1.6 gr.
Oil eucalyptus	0.4 gr.

'76 Ed.

RAWLEIGH RUMEN-ETTES
(Rawleigh)

Each lb.:
Phenothiazine *	240 gm.

'76 Ed.

RAWLEIGH SELTZER
Laxative
(Rawleigh)

Each oz.:
Sodium bicarbonate	210 gr.
Tartaric acid	179 gr.
Sodium citrate	295 gr.

'76 Ed.

RAWLEIGH SEVIN GARDEN DUST
(Rawleigh)

Sevin (Carbaryl (1-naphthyl N-methylcarbamate)) *	5%
Sulfur	3%

'76 Ed.

RAWLEIGH SPRAY ROACH & ANT KILLER
(Rawleigh)

Diazinon	0.500%
Pyrethrins	0.052%
Piperonyl butoxide, tech.	0.261%
Petroleum distillate *	74.187%
Propellant	25.000%

'76 Ed.

RAWLEIGH SUPER CLEANER CONCENTRATE
(Rawleigh)

Tetrapotassium pyrophosphate	12.529%/w
Butyl Cellosolve *	2.955%/w

'76 Ed.

RAWLEIGH UDDER BALM
Veterinary
(Rawleigh)

Glycerin	73.30%
Resorcinol *	2.10%
Pine oil	1.70%
Camphor	0.85%
Methyl salicylate	0.85%
Guaiacol	0.85%
Oleoresin capsicum	0.25%

'76 Ed.

RAWLEIGH VAPONA INSECTICIDE CATTLE & BARN SPRAY
(Rawleigh)

2,2-Dichlorovinyl dimethyl phosphate	0.930%
Related compounds	0.070%
Pyrethrins	0.002%
Tech. Piperonyl butoxide	0.017%
Petroleum distillate *	98.981%

'76 Ed.

RAWLEIGH VAPONA INSECTICIDE FLY BAIT
(Rawleigh)

2,2-Dichlorovinyl dimethyl phosphate	0.46%
Related compounds	0.04%

'76 Ed.

RAYDEX
Cleaner
(Pennwalt)

Soda ash *
Alkaline phosphate *
Wetting agent

RAYLENE
Commercial laundry sour
(Diversey Wyandotte)

Fluoride salts *

RAY-NOX
Sun screen for acne, etc.
(Torch)

Para-aminobenzoic acid	12.5 gm.
Hydrophilic vehicle ad	100.0 gm.

'76 Ed.

RAZE
Roach and ant spray
(ABCO, Inc.)

Pyrethrins	0.05%
Technical Piperonyl butoxide	0.125%
Malathion	2.000%
Aromatic petroleum derivative solvent *	6.210%
Petroleum distillate *	91.615%

RAZE RAT & MOUSE BAIT
(Bell Labs., Inc.)

Microencapsulated Warfarin	0.025%
Sulfaquinoxaline	0.025%
Blend of food grade cereals	99.950%

R/C PREINJECTION CO-INJECTION FLUID
Embalming supply
(Royal Bond)

Propylene glycol

R & C SPRAY
Insecticide
(Reed & Carnrick)

Active ingred.:	7.4%
Pyrethrins	0.3%
Piperonyl butoxide (technical)	1.5%
Petroleum distillate	5.6%
Inert ingred.:	92.6%
Includes Alcohol SDA #23A *	

RD HAIRDRESSING
(L.T. Labs.)

Fatty alcohols
Mineral oil USP
Anionic detergents
Glycols
Polyhydric glycols
Sulfur USP
Lead acetate NF *
Perfume

'76 Ed.

R.D. ROOT DESTROYER

See HERCULES R.D. ROOT DE-
STROYER

RD SHAMPOO
(L.T. Labs.)

Surface active agent *	<10%
Lanolin derivatives	
Alkanolamines	
Certified dyes	
Perfume	

'76 Ed.

READY RELIEF

See RAWLEIGH READY RELIEF

REAL-KILL ANT & ROACH KILLER
(Realex Corp.)

d-trans Allethrin (allyl homolog of Cinerin I)	0.030%
Piperonyl butoxide (technical)	0.060%
N-Octyl bicycloheptene dicarboximide	0.100%
O,O-Diethyl O-(2-isopropyl-6-methyl-4-pyrimidinyl) phosphorothioate (Diazinon)	0.500%
Petroleum distillate *	96.235%

REAL-KILL AUTOMATIC INDOOR FOGGER
Insecticide
(Realex Corp.)

d-trans Allethrin (allyl homolog of Cinerin I)	0.300%
Related compounds	0.023%
3-Phenoxybenzyl d-cis and trans 2,2-dimethyl-3-(2-methylpropenyl) cyclopropanecarboxylate	0.191%
Other isomers	0.009%
Petroleum distillate *	14.277%

REAL-KILL DO IT YOURSELF BUG CONTROL
(Realex Corp.)

Chlorpyrifos	0.50%
Aromatic petroleum derivative solvent	0.28%
Petroleum distillate *	99.19%

REAL-KILL EXTRA-STRENGTH ROACH & ANT KILLER
Insecticide
(Realex Corp.)

Pyrethrins	0.030%
Technical Piperonyl butoxide	0.150%
Chlorpyrifos	0.500%
Essential oil	1.000%
Petroleum distillate *	95.287%

REAL-KILL FLORIDA FORMULA ROACH & ANT KILLER
Insecticide
(Realex Corp.)

Pyrethrins	0.030%
n-Octyl bicycloheptene dicarboximide	0.250%
Chlorpyrifos	0.500%
Petroleum distillate *	96.187%

REAL-KILL FLYING INSECT KILLER
(Realex Corp.)

Resmethrin	0.200%
Related compounds	0.027%
d-trans Allethrin (allyl homolog of Cinerin I)	0.150%
Aromatic petroleum hydrocarbon	0.265%
Petroleum distillate	1.150%

REAL-KILL HOUSE & GARDEN PLUS
Insecticide
(Realex Corp.)

d-trans Allethrin (allyl homolog of cinerin I)	0.150%
Resmethrin	0.350%
Related compounds	0.048%
Aromatic petroleum distillate	0.464%

REAL-KILL LIQUID ANT & ROACH KILLER
(Realex Corp.)

Pyrethrins	0.030%
Technical Piperonyl butoxide	0.150%
O,O-Diethyl O-(2-isopropyl-6-methyl-4-pyrimidinyl) phosphorothioate (Diazinon)	0.500%
Petroleum distillate *	99.245%

REAL-KILL ROSE & GARDEN INSECT SPRAY
(Realex Corp.)

Pyrethrins	0.02%
Piperonyl butoxide	0.02%
Petroleum distillate	0.08%

REAL-KILL SPOT WEED KILLER
(Realex Corp.)

Amine salts of:

2,4-D	0.260%
Dicamba	0.025%
MCPP (2-(2-Methyl-4-chlorophenoxy)propionic acid)	0.261%

REAL-KILL VEGETATION KILLER
(Realex Corp.)

Diquat dibromide	0.23%

REAL-KILL YARD & PATIO OUTDOOR FOGGER
Insecticide
(Realex Corp.)

d-trans Allethrin (allyl homolog of cinerin I)	0.100%
Resmethrin	0.150%
Related compounds	0.020%
2-Hydroxyethyl-n-octyl sulfide	0.950%
Related compounds	0.050%
Aromatic petroleum hydrocarbons	0.198%

REBOUND
Institutional and industrial cleaning product

Procter & Gamble Co.
Ivorydale Technical Center
Cincinnati, Ohio 45217

Phone: 513-562-1100

REBUFF
Personal repellent
(Animal Repellents)

Capsaicin	0.35%
NF grade White mineral oil	85%
Pressurized with Nitrogen gas	

RECOFEN "D"
Cough suppressant and expectorant
(Reese Chem.)

Each oz.:

Dextromethorphan hydrobromide *	60 mg.
Terpin hydrate	55 mg.
Sodium citrate	330 mg.
Menthol	3 mg.
Alcohol	10%

RECSEI-TUSS (ELIXIR AND TABLETS)
Expectorant
(Recsei Labs.)

Each tablet or 5 cc:

Guaifenesin	100 mg.

RECTAL MEDICONE-HC SUPPOSITORIES
Temporary relief of severe anorectal inflammation, pruritus and pain
(Medicone)

Each suppository:

Hydrocortisone acetate	10 mg.
Benzocaine	2 gr.
Oxyquinoline sulfate	1/4 gr.
Zinc oxide	3 gr.
Menthol	1/7 gr.
Balsam Peru	1 gr.
Cocoa butter	
Vegetable & petroleum oil base	
Color	

Starred ingredients (*) may be responsible for major toxic effects; consult Section II.

RECTAL MEDICONE SUPPOSITORIES
For relief of pain, burning, and itching in simple hemorrhoids
(Medicone)

Each suppository:
Benzocaine	2 gr.
Oxyquinoline sulfate	1/4 gr.
Menthol	1/7 gr.
Zinc oxide	3 gr.
Balsam Peru	1 gr.
Cocoa butter base	
Vegetable & petroleum oil base	
Color	

RECTAL MEDICONE UNGUENT
Temporary relief of simple hemorrhoids and anorectal discomfort
(Medicone)

Each gram:
Benzocaine	20 mg.
Oxyquinoline sulfate	5 mg.
Menthol	4 mg.
Balsam Peru	12.5 mg.
Zinc oxide	100.0 mg.
Petrolatum	625 mg.
Lanolin	210 mg.
Color	

RED ARROW INSECT SPRAY
(Pratt-Gabriel Div.)

Pyrethrins	0.50%
Rotenone	1.50%
Cube resins	3.00%
Technical Piperonyl butoxide	3.00%
Xylene *	85.00%

RED BAND FLOOR WAX
Heavy duty grade
(McAleer)

Morpholine oleate *
Vegetable waxes
Terpene phenolic resins *†
Shellac
Borax *
Ammonia *
Colloidal silica

'76 Ed.

†*See* Terpenes and Phenol

RED CEDAR SHINGLE & SHAKE PRESERVATIVE
Water repellent preservative
(Honolulu Wood Treating Co.)

Copper-8-quinolinolate	0.35%
Petroleum hydrocarbons *	89.40%

Made exclusively for Red Cedar Shingle & Shake Co.

RED CROSS NURSE SPRAY DISINFECTANT
(Hubbard, J.)

Alcohol *	69.30%
Mixture of: Oil lavender, Oil rosemary *, Terpinyl acetate, Oil eucalyptus *, Oil pine, Thymol *, 3,4,6-Trichlorophenol	1.58%

RED CROSS TOOTHACHE DROPS
(Mentholatum)

Eugenol (USP) *	85%
Alcohol	15%

RED DEVIL ALUMINUM POLISH
(Marine Elect.)

Stearic acid
Oleic acid
Kerosene *
Water
Triethanolamine
Alumina
Tergitol NPX

'76 Ed.

RED DEVIL DRY WEED KILLER
(Marine Elect.)

2,4-Dichlorophenoxyacetic acid	6%

'76 Ed.

RED-DEVIL DUST
Insecticide
(Pearson & Co.)

Sabadilla alkaloids *
  Derived from 20% sabadilla seed, powdered and activated

'76 Ed.

RED DEVIL POWER GEL TILE & GROUT CLEANER
(Red Devil)

Phosphoric acid *

'76 Ed.

RED DEVIL SOOT & CARBON REMOVER
Powder form
(Marine Elect.)

Copper chloride *

'76 Ed.

RED DEVIL SOOT REMOVER
Liquid
(Marine Elect.)

Lead naphthenate *
F. O. dispersant
Kerosene *

'76 Ed.

RED DEVIL TILE AND GROUT CLEANER
(Red Devil)

Sulfamic acid *

'76 Ed.

RED HAND BOAT COPPER
(International Paint)

Copper *
Mineral spirits *
Aromatics *†
Pigments color code #48, #50, #72

†*See* Aromatic hydrocarbon solvent

REDKEN LABS. COSMETICS

Redken Labs., Inc.
6625 Variel Ave.
Canoga Park, Calif. 91303

Phone: 213-992-2700

See COSMETICS, Section VI, General Formulations

RED-KOTE, DR. NAYLOR'S (Dauber Bottle or Spray Bomb)

See DR. NAYLOR'S RED-KOTE (Dauber Bottle or Spray Bomb)

RED ROBIN DUST
Insecticide
(Pearson & Co.)

Rotenone	1.0%
Other cube resins	2.0%

'76 Ed.

RED ROCKET DEGREASER

See BUTCHER'S RED ROCKET DEGREASER

RED STAVE WALL SIZE
(Hercules Incorporated)

Starch	
Phenolphthalein	0.03%
Benzoic acid	0.25%
Sodium acid fluoride	0.50%

RED STAVE WHEAT PASTE
(Hercules Incorporated)

Starch
Dowicide A 0.3%

RED STUFF
Cleaner/degreaser
(Paul Koss)

Water .... >80%
Monoethanolamine * .... >10%
Butyl Cellosolve * .... >4%
Monoethanolamine sulfonate (Anionic surfactant)
Coco diethanolamide
Dye .... trace
Perfume .... trace

pH 10.7-10.9

RED-TOP BOTRAN 6 CAPTAN 10 SULFUR 25 DUST
Fungicide; agricultural
(Wilbur-Ellis Co.)

2,6-Dichloro-4-nitroaniline 6%
Captan 10%
Sulfur * 25%

RED-TOP CONTACT WEEDKILLER
Herbicide; agricultural
(Wilbur-Ellis Co.)

Dinoseb * 30%

RED-TOP CRYOLITE 30 SULFUR 30 DUST
Insecticide, fungicide; agricultural
(Wilbur-Ellis Co.)

Sodium fluoaluminate 30%
Sulfur * 30%

RED-TOP LINDANE 75 SEED COAT
Seed treatment insecticide; agricultural
(Wilbur-Ellis Co.)

Lindane * 75%

RED-TOP METHYL PARATHION 5 SPRAY
Insecticide; agricultural
(Wilbur-Ellis Co.)

Methyl parathion * 54.5%
Xylene range aromatic solvent ... 40.5%

RED-TOP PREMIUM GRADE MALATHION GRAIN PROTECTANT
Insecticide; agricultural
(Wilbur-Ellis Co.)

Malathion * 57%
Xylene range aromatic solvent * ... 38%

RED-TOP SEVIN 10 DUST
Insecticide; agricultural
(Wilbur-Ellis Co.)

Carbaryl * 10%

RED-TOP SEVIN 5 PELLETS
Insecticide; agricultural
(Wilbur-Ellis Co.)

Carbaryl * 5%

RED-TOP STRIKE
For control of algae
(Wilbur-Ellis Co.)

Copper sulfate pentahydrate * 25.8%

RED-TOP TOXAPHENE 8 SPRAY
Insecticide; agricultural
(Wilbur-Ellis Co.)

Toxaphene * 73%
Xylene range aromatic solvents * .. 15%

RED-TOP WIL-O-MITE DUST
Insecticide; agricultural
(Wilbur-Ellis Co.)

2-(p-tert-Butylphenoxy)cyclohexyl 2-propynyl sulfite 4%

RED-TOP WOOD PRESERVATIVE CONCENTRATE
Insecticide, fungicide; agricultural
(Wilbur-Ellis Co.)

Pentachlorophenol * 32%
Other Chlorophenols & related compounds 4%

REDU

See AMWAY REDU

REDUCETS (IMPROVED FORMULA)
(Columbia Med.)

Each capsule:
Vitamin A .... 2,000 USP Units
Vitamin D .... 200 USP Units
Calcium .... 87 mg.
Phosphorus .... 45 mg.
Iron .... 10 mg.
Methylcellulose .... 100 mg.
Benzocaine .... 5 mg.
Plus multivitamins

RED & WHITE BLUE LAUNDRY DETERGENT
Dry laundry detergent
(Great Atlantic & Pacific, mfr.; Red & White International, dist.)

Sodium linear alkyl benzene
  sulfonate .... <17%
Sodium carbonate * .... <30%
Sodium silicate .... <10%
Sodium carboxymethylcellulose <2%
Optical brighteners .... <1%
Sodium chloride .... <10%
Blue dye .... trace
Sodium sulfate and moisture ... balance

RED & WHITE LAUNDRY DETERGENT
Dry laundry detergent
(Great Atlantic & Pacific, mfr.; Red & White International, dist.)

Sodium linear alkyl benzene
  sulfonate .... <17%
Sodium carbonate * .... <30%
Sodium silicate .... <10%
Sodium carboxymethylcellulose <2%
Optical brighteners .... <1%
Sodium chloride .... <10%
Sodium sulfate and moisture ... balance

REDY-MASTIC ACOUSTICAL SEALANT No. 4045
(Bogert, A.Z.)

Butyl rubber 20%
Mineral spirits * 11%
Inert fillers 61%
Asbestos 7%
Soya oil .... <1%
Oleic acid .... <1%

REDY-MASTIC CEILING TILE ADHESIVE No. 43
(Bogert, A.Z.)

Resinous binder (derived from
  rosin and/or modified rosin) .. 39-45%
Petroleum naphtha 8%
Clay 43-49%
Isopropanol 4%

REDY-MASTIC COVE BASE ADHESIVE No. 72
(Bogert, A.Z.)

Resinous binder (derived from
  rosin and/or modified rosin) .. 37-43%
Isopropanol * 14%
Clay 43-49%

REDY-MASTIC PANEL ADHESIVE (Waterproof) No. P-150
(Bogert, A.Z.)

Hexane * 32%
Toluene * .... <2%
Isopropanol .... <2%
SBR Rubber/hydrocarbon resin
  binder 34%
Inert filler 32%

REDY-MASTIC PANEL DRYWALL CONSTRUCTION ADHESIVE No. PDC-100
(Bogert, A.Z.)

Hexane *	34%
Toluene *	<5%
Mineral spirits	<5%
Isopropanol	2%
SBR rubber/hydrocarbon resin binder	29%
Inert fillers	27%

REDY-MASTIC STAIR TREAD ADHESIVE (Rubber base) No. 490
(Bogert, A.Z.)

Hexane *	45%
Toluene *	1%
SBR rubber/wood rosin & hydrocarbon resin binder	40%
Inert fillers	14%

REDY-MASTIC SUBFLOOR CONSTRUCTION ADHESIVE No. SFC-200
(Bogert, A.Z.)

Toluene *	37%
SBS rubber/coumarone resin binder	28%
Inert filler	33%
Asbestos	2%

REDY-MASTIC TILE AND CARPET ADHESIVE No. 404
(Bogert, A.Z.)

Resinous binder (derived from rosin and/or modified rosin)	42-48%
Clay	40-46%
Petroleum naphtha	3%
Methanol	7%
Isopropanol	2%

REDY-MASTIC WHITE BUTYL CAULK No. 763
(Bogert, A.Z.)

Butyl rubber	19%
Mineral spirits *	26%
Hydrocarbon resin	<5%
Titanium dioxide	<5%
Inert fillers	47%

REESE'S PEDIATRIC FORMULA
Children's cough & cold treatment
(Reese Chem.)

Each 5 ml.:

Dextromethorphan hydrobromide	3.75 mg.
Pseudoephedrine hydrochloride *	15.00 mg.
Guaifenesin	50.00 mg.

REFRANE
Laundry detergent
(Diversey Wyandotte)

Sodium metasilicate *	
Alkaline salts *	

REGAL AQUAGLO (NON-YELLOWING WHITE 333-01)
Interior enamel paint
(Benjamin Moore)

Pigment:		24.4%
Titanium dioxide (type II)	95.2%	
Silicates	4.8%	
Vehicle:		75.6%
Acrylic/vinyl acetate emulsion:	58.8%	
Acrylic/vinyl acetate resin	48.0%	
Water	52.0%	
Acrylic emulsion:	41.2%	
Acrylic resin	10.6%	
Water, Glycols *†	89.4%	

†See Paints, Section VI, General Formulations

REGAL AQUAVELVET (WHITE 319-01)
Interior flat paint
(Benjamin Moore)

Pigment:		30.0%
Titanium dioxide (type II)	87.8%	
Calcium carbonate	12.2%	
Vehicle:		70.0%
Acrylic emulsion:	100%	
Acrylic resin	30.7%	
Water, Glycols *†	69.3%	

†See Paints, Section VI, General Formulations

REGAL LIQUID SOAP
(Armour-Dial, Inc.)

Water	25-50%
SD Alcohol	10-25%
Ammonium laureth sulfate active	10-25%
Sodium dodecylbenzene sulfonate active	10-25%
Minor ingredients (total)	1-5%

REGAL WALL SATIN DECORATORS WHITE (215-01)
Interior flat paint
(Benjamin Moore)

Pigment:		34.4%
Titanium dioxide (type III)	65.2%	
Silicates	34.8%	
Vehicle:		65.6%
Vinyl acetate/acrylic emulsion:	100%	
Vinyl acetate/acrylic resin	24.8%	
Water, Glycols *†	75.2%	

†See Paints, Section VI, General Formulations

REGATTA 250 - BALTIMORE RED COPPER
For use on pleasure craft
(Jotun-Baltimore Copper Paint Co.)

Pigment:		38%
Iron oxide	7%	
Cuprous oxide *	20%	
Calcium carbonate	4%	
Aluminum silicate	7%	
Vehicle:		62%
Processed Rosin	22%	
Petroleum hydrocarbon resin	15%	
Cresol *	4%	
Aromatic hydrocarbons *	5%	
Aliphatic hydrocarbons	16%	

REGATTA 3803 - BALTOCOP GREEN
For use on pleasure craft
(Jotun-Baltimore Copper Paint Co.)

Vehicle:		100%
Copper naphthenate *	26%	
Mineral spirits *	74%	

REGATTA 3021 - BALTOGUARD ANTIFOULING RED
For use on pleasure craft
(Jotun-Baltimore Copper Paint Co.)

Pigment:		60%
Cuprous oxide *	48%	
Tributyltin fluoride	2%	
Zinc oxide	3%	
Iron oxide	7%	
Vehicle:		40%
Chlorinated rubber resin	7%	
Rosin	5%	
Epoxidized Soya bean oil	1%	
Tricresyl phosphate	3%	
Aromatic hydrocarbons	24%	

This type of product is also produced in Blue and Green

REGATTA 3400 - BALTO-POLLY EGRET WHITE
For use on pleasure craft
(Jotun-Baltimore Copper Paint Co.)

Pigment:		28%
Titanium dioxide	27%	
Aluminum silicate	1%	
Vehicle:		72%
Alkyd resin	19%	
Polyurethane modified alkyd	18%	
Aliphatic hydrocarbons *	29%	
Aromatic hydrocarbons *	5%	
Driers and Antiskinning agent	1%	

This type of product also produced in Penguin Black, Curlew Buff, Puffin Ivory, Loon Gray, Heron Blue, Teal Green, Kingfisher Blue, Mallard Green, Crane Red, Kittiwake Blue, Grebe Yellow, Widgeon Green and Petrel Gray.

REGATTA 3811 - BALTO-TIN
For use on pleasure craft
(Jotun-Baltimore Copper Paint Co.)

Vehicle:		100%
Tributyltin oxide *	2%	
Mineral spirits *	98%	

Starred ingredients (*) may be responsible for major toxic effects; consult Section II.

REGATTA 3280 - BALTO-WHITE GLOSS
For use on pleasure craft
(Jotun-Baltimore Copper Paint Co.)

Pigment:		34%
	Titanium dioxide	34%
Vehicle:		66%
	Soya alkyd resin	34%
	Processed Soya bean oil	3%
	Mineral spirits *	27%
	Driers * and Antiskinning agent	2%

REGATTA 3000 COPPER BRONZE
For use on pleasure craft
(Jotun-Baltimore Copper Paint Co.)

Pigment:		34%
	Metallic Copper	34%
Vehicle:		66%
	Rosin modified Vinyl-butyral resin	8%
	Pine oil	6%
	Alcohol, denatured	52%

REGATTA 3630 - EPOXYDUR BLACK MASTIC BASE
For use on pleasure craft
(Jotun-Baltimore Copper Paint Co.)

Pigment:		50%
	Lampblack	3%
	Silicon dioxide	2%
	Magnesium silicate	45%
Vehicle:		50%
	Liquid Epoxy resin	23%
	Petroleum tar *†	21%
	Butanol	3%
	Xylol *	3%

†*See* Tar oils and Tar acids

REGATTA 3631 - EPOXYDUR MASTIC CONVERTER
For use on pleasure craft
(Jotun-Baltimore Copper Paint Co.)

Vehicle:		100%
	Polyamide resin	71%
	2,4,6-Tri(dimethyl-aminomethyl)phenol	6%
	Butanol	8%
	Toluol *	15%

REGATTA 3017 - F.A.F. RED ANTIFOULING
For use on pleasure craft
(Jotun-Baltimore Copper Paint Co.)

Pigment:		65%
	Cuprous oxide *	49%
	Iron oxide	7%
	Magnesium silicate	7%
	Silicon dioxide	2%
Vehicle:		35%
	Processed Rosin	16%
	Petroleum hydrocarbon resin	5%
	Tributyltin oxide	2%
	Aromatic and Aliphatic hydrocarbons	12%

This type of product also produced in Blue and Green

REGATTA 3231 - MANHASSETT GREEN
For use on pleasure craft
(Jotun-Baltimore Copper Paint Co.)

Pigment:		15%
	Titanium dioxide	12%
	Phthalocyanine green	1%
	Yellow Iron oxide	1%
	Aluminum silicate	1%
Vehicle:		85%
	Soya alkyd resin	45%
	Mineral spirits *	38%
	Driers * and Antiskinning agent	2%

This type of product also produced in Gloss White, Semi-gloss White, Flat White, Flat Black, Gloss Black, Aluminum Miami Gray, Chrome Gray, Stanchion Brown, Pine Green, Arizona Buff, Medium Buff, Cape Breton Green, Flag Blue, Mist Blue, Caribbean Blue, Oyster White, Arctic Green, Cream, Vermillion, Mahogany, International Orange, Lakewood Green

REGATTA 3260 - SEAGLAZE GLOSS WHITE
For use on pleasure craft
(Jotun-Baltimore Copper Paint Co.)

Pigment:		29%
	Titanium dioxide	29%
Vehicle:		71%
	Soya alkyd resin	23%
	Silicone modified alkyd resin	13%
	Mineral spirits *	34%
	Driers	1%

REGATTA 3100 - SPAR VARNISH
For use on pleasure craft
(Jotun-Baltimore Copper Paint Co.)

Vehicle:		100%
	Soya alkyd resin	12%
	Phenolic modified rosin ester	6%
	Zinc resinate	1%
	Treated Linseed oil	40%
	Mineral spirits *	40%
	Driers and Antiskinning agent	1%

REGATTA 3015 - TRITOX RED ANTIFOULING
For use on pleasure craft
(Jotun-Baltimore Copper Paint Co.)

Pigment:		46%
	Cuprous oxide *	20%
	Iron oxide	14%
	Calcium carbonate	4%
	Aluminum silicate	8%
Vehicle:		54%
	Processed Rosin	21%
	Petroleum hydrocarbon resin	14%
	Aliphatic and Aromatic hydrocarbons *	19%

REGATTA VINYLTEX-60 BLACK ANTIFOULING WITH BIO MET (TBTO)
For use on pleasure craft
(Jotun-Baltimore Copper Paint Co.)

Pigment:		25%
	Lampblack	4%
	Magnesium silicate	21%
Vehicle:		75%
	Vinyl resin	7%
	Rosin	12%
	Tricresyl phosphate	1%
	Tributyltin oxide	8%
	Aromatic hydrocarbons *	24%
	Ketones	23%

This type of product also produced in Bright Green, White, Scarlet and Blue

REGATTA VINYLTEX-55 FAST RED ANTIFOULING WITH CUPROUS OXIDE
For use on pleasure craft
(Jotun-Baltimore Copper Paint Co.)

Pigment:		56%
	Cuprous oxide *	47%
	Red Iron oxide	5%
	Aluminum silicate	4%
Vehicle:		44%
	Vinyl resin	5%
	Rosin	7%
	Tricresyl phosphate	2%
	Tributyltin fluoride	3%
	Aromatic hydrocarbons *	10%
	Ketones	17%

This type of product also produced in Green and Blue

REGENT
Full firming arterial fluid
(Royal Bond)

Formaldehyde index *		27%
Methanol *		

REGLONE
Herbicide
(Chipman Inc.)

Diquat (present as dibromide) (1:1'-Ethylene-2:2'-dipyridylium cation) * ...... 200 gm. per liter

REGROTON TABLETS
Oral antihypertensive
(USV)

Each tablet:
Chlorthalidone (3-Hydroxy-3-(4-chloro-3-sulfamylphenyl)phthalimidine) *	50 mg.
Reserpine USP, pure crystalline alkaloid from the root of Rauwolfia serpentina *	0.25 mg.

REGUL-AIDS CAPSULES
For relief, prevention of constipation
(Columbia Med.)

Dioctyl sodium sulfosuccinate * 100 mg.

REGUTOL
Constipation relief, prevention
(Plough)

Dioctyl sodium sulfosuccinate *   100 mg.

REJOICE (Test Market)
Liquid skin cleanser
(Procter & Gamble)

Water	75-100%
Ammonium laureth sulfate	10-24%
Glycerine	1-4%
Cocamide MEA	1-4%
Glycol distearate	1-4%
Quaternium 19	1-4%
Coconut acid	1-4%
Minor ingredients, each	<1%

REJUVATONE
Embalming supply
(Royal Bond)

Methanol *
Formaldehyde .... <1%

RE-JUV-NAL
Disinfectant-detergent
(Hillyard Chem.)

Quaternary compounds *
Synthetic detergents *

'76 Ed.

RELA TABLETS
Analgesic and muscle relaxant
(Schering)

Each tablet:
  Carisoprodol * .... 350 mg.

RELAX-U-CAPS
For the relief of insomnia
(Columbia Med.)

Methapyrilene HCl * .... 25 mg.

RELDAN MC INSECTICIDAL CONCENTRATE
(Dow)

Active ingred.: 50.5%
  Chlorpyrifos-Methyl (O,O-Dimethyl O-(3,5,6-trichloro-2-pyridyl)phosphorothioate) *
Inert ingred.: 49.5%
  Methylene chloride
  Related compounds in active ingredient

RELIABLE PASTE ANTIQUE REFINISHERS REMOVER
(Reliable Paste)

Acetone *	approx. 60%
Methanol *	approx. 30%
Toluol *	approx. 10%

RELIABLE PASTE #1776 COLD PROCESS STRIPPER
(Reliable Paste)

Methylene chloride *	>75%
Methanol *	>10%

RELIABLE PASTE LACQUER THINNERS
(Reliable Paste)

Acetone and other ketones
n-Butyl acetate and other esters
Isopropyl alcohol
Toluol * .... <20%
Aliphatic hydrocarbons 30%

RELIABLE PASTE MARINE REMOVER
(Reliable Paste)

Methylene chloride *	>75%
Methanol *	>10%

RELIABLE PASTE SHELLAC SOLVENT
(Reliable Paste)

Methanol *

RELIABLE PASTE WATER WASH NoFLAME
(Reliable Paste)

Methylene chloride *	>75%
Methanol *	>10%

RELIANCE "DUROLEAD" BLACK LEADS
(Reliance Pen & Pencil)

Graphite
Clay
Natural waxes, such as Japan and candelilla waxes
Synthetic waxes

RELIANCE UNIVERSAL PAINT PRODUCTS

Reliance Universal, Inc.
1600 Watterson Towers
1930 Bishop Lane
Louisville, Ky. 40218

Phone: 502-459-9110

See PAINTS, Section VI, General Formulations

RELY-ON

See DAP RELY-ON

RELY-ON LATEX CAULK

See DAP RELY-ON LATEX CAULK

REMINGTON ELECTRIC SHAVER SAVER
Head cleaner lubricant
(Remington Products)

Alcohol *	86%
Silicone and fatty acid ester	q.s.
Sustain (blend of antioxidants)	trace

'76 Ed.

REMOVE
Inhibited chemical cleaner for the construction industry
(Scientific International)

Hydrochloric acid *

REMOVE FABRIC SPOT CLEANER

See AMWAY REMOVE FABRIC SPOT CLEANER

REMSED
Sedative, antiemetic, antihistamine
(Endo Labs.)

Promethazine
  hydrochloride * ..... 25 mg. or 50 mg.

RENESE-R TABLETS
Edema, hypertension
(Pfizer)

Each tablet:
  Polythiazide * .... 2.0 mg.
  Reserpine * .... 0.25 mg.

RENESE TABLETS
Edema, hypertension
(Pfizer)

Each tablet:
  Polythiazide * .... 1 mg.; 2 mg.; 4 mg.

RENEW HERBICIDE

See PATTERSON'S RENEW HERBICIDE

REN-O-SAL
For stimulating growth of chickens & turkeys
(Salsbury)

Each tablet:
  3-Nitro-4-hydroxyphenylarsonic
    acid * .... 36 mg.

RENO-SED TABLETS
Genito-urinary antisepsis and sedation
(Vita Elixir Co.)

Each tablet:
Methenamine *	2 gr.
Salol *	1/2 gr.
Methylene blue	1/10 gr.
Benzoic acid	1/8 gr.
Atropine SO4	1/1000 gr.
Hyoscyamine SO4	1/2000 gr.

Starred ingredients (*) may be responsible for major toxic effects; consult Section II.

RENOVET AIR FRESHENER
(Consolidated Chem., Inc.)

Isopropanol *
Triethylene glycol
Propylene glycol
Dichlorodifluoromethane
Trichloromonofluoromethane
Essential oils *
Orthophenylphenol *

RE-NU
Tile refinisher
(Lester Labs.)

Detergents *

'76 Ed.

RENUZIT AIR FRESHENER
Aerosol space spray
(Drackett)

Petroleum distillate .... <10%/wt.
Emulsifiers
Water
Preservative .... <0.1%/wt.
Hydrocarbon propellant
Perfume
Corrosion inhibitor

RENUZIT DEPENDABLE CLEANER
Home dry cleaner
(Drackett)

Petroleum distillate * 100%

RENUZIT SOFT STARCH
Spray fabric sizing - aerosol
(Drackett)

Starch
Sodium carboxymethyl cellulose
Sodium borate .... <0.5%/wt.
Preservative .... <0.1%/wt.
Silicone oil
Perfume
Water
Hydrocarbon propellant

RENUZIT SOLID AIR FRESHENER
Gel air freshener
(Drackett)

Carrageenan
Sodium carboxymethyl cellulose
Potassium chloride
Water
Dye or pigment
Perfume
Preservative .... <0.1%

REP BOILER REPAIR
(Kenite)

Tannins * 35%
Wood flour
Wood particles
Ground mica

REPCON
Rain repellent & surface conditioner
(Unelko)

	%/wgt.
Alkyl polysiloxanes (Dimethyl silicone fluids)	10.00%
Sulfuric acid (reagent grade)	1.00%
Isopropanol (Isopropyl alcohol, anhydrous) *	89.00%

REPELLEX "L"
Cattle spray and repellent
(ABCO, Inc.)

Pyrethrins	00.06%
Piperonyl butoxide (technical) ..	00.12%
N-Octyl bicycloheptene dicarboximide	00.20%
Di-n-propyl isocinchomeronate ..	00.40%
Petroleum distillate *	99.22%

REPEL-X FLY SPRAY CONCENTRATE
Veterinary
(Farnam Co.)

Piperonyl butoxide, technical ...	1.00%
Pyrethrins I and II	0.40%
Petroleum hydrocarbons	3.60%
Butoxypolypropylene glycol * ...	50.00%
Mineral oil *	40.00%

'76 Ed.

REPOSANS-10
Tranquilizer
(Wesley Pharm.)

Each capsule:
  Chlordiazepoxide hydrochloride * .... 10 mg.

REPRIEVE
Fast pain relief
(Mayer Labs.)

Each tablet:
Homatropine methyl bromide	0.5 mg.
Caffeine, alk.	32 mg.
Salicylamide *	225 mg.
Thiamine mononitrate	50 mg.

'76 Ed.

REQUA'S STYPTIC PENCIL
(Requa)

Aluminum sulfate * 90%

RESA TABLETS
Tranquilizing and antihypertensive agent
(Vita Elixir Co.)

Each tablet:
  Reserpine (alkaloid of Rauwolfia serpentina) * .... 0.25 mg.

RESERJEN
(Jenkins Labs.)

Each tablet:
  Reserpine * .... 0.25 mg.

RESERPAL
(Bio-Factor Labs.)

Each tablet:
  Reserpine * .... 1 mg.

'76 Ed.

RESERPOID TABLETS
Antihypertensive and tranquilizing agent
(Upjohn)

Each tablet:
  Reserpine * .... 0.25 mg.

RESIBOND POWDERS FOR MORTARS
(Knight, M.A.)

Silicious fillers
Barytes
Kaolin
Catalysts added may be one or more of the following:
  Methyl ethyl ketone peroxide *
  Cyclohexanone peroxide *
  Dicumyl peroxide
  Benzoyl peroxide *

RESIBOND SOLUTION
(Knight, M.A.)

Modified Polyester resins and fillers
Styrene monomer
Cobalt naphthenate *
Dimethyl aniline *

RESICIDE CONCENTRATE, SUPER

See SUPER RESICIDE CONCENTRATE

RESICIDE EMULSION CONCENTRATE
Insecticide
(Residex)

Pyrethrins	1.35%
Technical Piperonyl butoxide ...	2.70%
N-Octyl bicycloheptene dicarboximide	4.46%
Petroleum distillates *	79.49%

RESICIDE FOGGING COMPOUND
Insecticide
(Residex)

Pyrethrins	0.30%
Technical Piperonyl butoxide ...	0.60%
N-Octyl bicycloheptene dicarboximide	1.00%
Petroleum distillates *	98.10%

RESIDEX DIAZINON 4E INSECTICIDE
(Residex)

Diazinon *	47.5%
Aromatic petroleum derivative solvent *	26.2%

Starred ingredients (*) may be responsible for major toxic effects; consult Section II.

RESIDEX DIAZINON 4S INSECTICIDE
(Residex)

Diazinon * 48.7%
Aromatic petroleum derivative
  solvent * 39.5%

RESIDEX DURSBAN ROACH CONCENTRATE
(Residex)

Chlorpyrifos * 16.00%
Petroleum distillate 73.96%

RESIDEX HOUSEHOLD INSECT SPRAY
Insecticide
(Residex)

O,O-Diethyl O-(2-isopropyl-4-
  methyl-6-pyrimidinyl)
  phosphorothioate 0.50%
Pyrethrins 0.05%
Technical Piperonyl butoxide ... 0.10%
N-Octyl bicycloheptene
  dicarboximide 0.17%
Petroleum distillates * 99.18%

RESIDEX LINDANE 20% EMULSIFIABLE
Insecticide
(Residex)

Gamma isomer of benzene hexachloride from lindane * 20.0%
Aromatic petroleum derivative
  solvent * 51.8%

RESIDEX MALATHION 5 LB. EMULSIFIABLE CONC.
Insecticide
(Residex)

Malathion * 57%
Aromatic petroleum solvent * 35%

RESIDEX PROLIN RESRATTUS
Rodenticide
(Residex)

Warfarin 0.025%
Quinoxalinyl sulfanilamide (Sulfaquinoxaline) (N)-(2-quinoxali-
  nyl sulfanilamide) 0.025%

RESIDEX RESIVAP ROACH CONCENTRATE
(Residex)

Chlorpyrifos * 16.40%
2,2-Dichlorovinyl dimethyl
  phosphate 7.60%
Related compounds 0.60%
Petroleum distillates 60.20%
Xylene 5%

RESIDEX ROACH POWDER
Insecticide
(Residex)

Sodium fluoride * 38.8%
Pyrethrins 0.35%

RESIDEX WARFARIN RESRATTUS
Rodenticide
(Residex)

Warfarin 0.025%

RESIFUME INSECTICIDE, EXCELCIDE

See EXCELCIDE RESIFUME INSEC-
  TICIDE

RES-I-KILL
*Insecticide; industrial and institutional
use*
(Scientific International)

Pyrethrins 0.050%
Technical Piperonyl butoxide ... 0.100%
N-Octyl bicycloheptene
  dicarboximide 0.166%
O,O-Diethyl (O-2-isopropyl-6-
  methyl-4-pyrimidinyl)
  phosphorothioate 0.500%
Petroleum distillate * 74.184%
Inert ingred.:
  Propellant 25.000%

RESINOL GREASELESS CREAM
For minor skin irritations
(Mentholatum)

Resorcinol * 2.0%
Zinc oxide 4.5%
Calamine 3.5%

RESINOL OINTMENT
Antipruritic
(Mentholatum)

Zinc oxide 12%
Calamine 6%
Resorcinol * 2%
In a base of:
  Lanolin
  Petrolatum

RESIPOWDER (P-D)
Insecticide
(Residex)

O,O-Diethyl O-(2-isopropyl-4-
  methyl-6-pyrimidinyl)
  phosphorothioate * 2.00%
Pyrethrins 0.35%

RESISTO NO RUBBING FLOOR WAX
(Uncle Sam)

Resins (modified phenolic)
Carnauba wax
Emulsifiers
Ammonia *
Colloidal Silica
Polyethylene
Water

RESIVAP ROACH CONCENTRATE

See RESIDEX RESIVAP ROACH
  CONCENTRATE

RES-N-GEL

See WEBER RES-N-GEL

RESOLVE
Automatic dishwasher detergent
(Calgon Corp., Commercial Div.)

Chlorinated trisodium phosphate *
Complex phosphates *

RESOURCE
Liquid alkaline cleaner
(Diversey Wyandotte)

Sodium hydroxide *

RESPECT
Liquid laundry cleaner
(Diversey Wyandotte)

Synthetic detergents *

RESPITAL TABLETS
(Premo)

Each tablet:
  Reserpine, USP * .... 0.1 mg.; 0.25 mg.

'76 Ed.

RESPOND DETERGENT, PL

See PL RESPOND DETERGENT

RESULFOLIN
(Torch)

Resorcinol monoacetate * 3%
Sulfur precipitated (dispersed) ... 5%
Flesh-tinted hydrophilic vehicle ad 100%

'76 Ed.

RESULTS
Insecticide
(Dyna Systems)

Petroleum distillates * 18.20%
Technical Piperonyl butoxide ... 0.50%
N-Octyl bicycloheptene
  dicarboximide 0.50%
Pyrethrins I & II 0.20%
Petroleum distillates propellant 80.60%

Starred ingredients (*) may be responsible for major toxic effects; consult Section II.

RETIN-A BRAND (TRETINOIN) ACNE TREATMENT
(Johnson & Johnson)

Tretinoin (Vitamin A acid)	0.05%
Polyethylene glycol 400	approx. 50%
Ethyl alcohol	approx. 55%
Butylated hydroxytoluene	

RETIN-A CREAM
Acne treatment
(Ortho-Dermatology)

Tretinoin	0.05%; 1%

RETIN-A GEL
Acne treatment
(Ortho-Dermatology)

Tretinoin	0.01%; 0.025%

RETIN-A LIQUID
Acne treatment
(Ortho-Dermatology)

Tretinoin	0.05%

REUMA-RUB

See DURHAM'S REUMA-RUB

REVELL PLASTIC MODEL CEMENT
(Revell)

Polystyrene resin	27.00%
Toluene *	72.75%
Oil of mustard	0.25%

REVLON COSMETIC PRODUCTS
Cosmetics and toiletries

Revlon, Inc.
767 Fifth Ave.
New York, N.Y. 10153

Phone: 212-572-5000

Revlon Research Center, Inc.
945 Zerega Ave.
Bronx, N.Y. 10473

Phone: 212-824-9000

See COSMETICS, Section VI, General Formulations

REX 925
Granular soap
(National-Purity Soap)

Tallow soap
Nonionic detergent *
Silicate builders
pH modifiers
Phosphate (equiv. to 7% P2O5) *

pH of 1% solution: 11.5-12

REXALL COLDSORE LOTION
(Rexall)

Benzoin	1-10%
Camphor *	1-5%
Menthol	<1%
Alcohol *	90%

'76 Ed.

REXALL DIURETIC PILLS
(Rexall)

Each tablet:

Extract of Buchu	12.15 mg.
Uva Ursi	48.6 mg.
Cascara sagrada	4.05 mg.
Potassium nitrate *	48.6 mg.
Podophyllin *	1.85 mg.
Oil juniper	0.4 mg.
Kaolin	20.63 mg.

'76 Ed.

REXALL EAR WAX DROPS
(Rexall)

Carbolic acid	<1%
Potassium chloride	<1%
Glycerin	>90%
Urea	1-10%

'76 Ed.

REXALL LIP AID SALVE
(Rexall)

Camphor *	1-5%
Phenol	<1%
Menthol *	1-5%
Mineral oil	>10%

'76 Ed.

REXALL MI-31 SOLUTION
(Rexall)

Alcohol	25%
Eucalyptol	<1%
Methyl salicylate	<1%
Oil of thyme	<1%
Benzoic acid	<1%
Boric acid *	1-5%

'76 Ed.

REXALL MOUTHWASH W/ CHLOROPHYLL
(Rexall)

Alcohol	25%
Chlorophyll	<1%
Polysorbate 80	<1%
Glycerin	1-10%
Sodium citrate	<1%
Oil spearmint	<1%
Oil peppermint	<1%
Menthol	<1%

'76 Ed.

REXALL THRU PENETRATING ANALGESIC
(Rexall)

Salicylamide	1-10%
Menthol *	1-10%
Camphor *	1-5%
Benzocaine	1-5%
Methyl salicylate *	1-10%
Isopropyl alcohol *	66%

'76 Ed.

REXALL TIMED ACTION COLD CAPSULES
(Rexall)

Each capsule:

Chlorpheniramine maleate *	4 mg.
Phenylephrine hydrochloride *	20 mg.

'76 Ed.

REX INSTANT PRE-SIZED PASTE
For hanging wallpaper
(Patent)

Processed wheat material	
Vancide 51Z	trace
Dextrine	
Animal glue	
Bicarbonate of soda	
Bentonite	
Aluminum sulfate	

REX LOW SUDS
Laundry detergent
(National-Purity Soap)

Synthetic nonionic surfactants *
Buffering salts
Water conditioners
Optical brighteners

pH of 1% solution: 11.5

REX PASTE
For hanging wallpaper
(Patent)

Processed wheat material	
Vancide 51Z	trace

REX SOLUTION
Athlete's foot, poison oak and poison ivy
(Rex Laboratory, Inc.)

Chlorobutanol	1 1/2 gr./oz.
Salicylate acid *	
Benzoic acid	
Thymol *	
Gentian violet *	
Alcohol *	70%/vol.

'76 Ed.

REX VINYL PASTE
For hanging light weight cloth and paperback vinyl
(Patent)

Processed wheat material	
Vancide 51Z	trace

Starred ingredients (*) may be responsible for major toxic effects; consult Section II.

REX WALL SIZE
(Patent)

Dextrine
Animal glue
Bicarbonate of soda
Aluminum sulfate
Bentonite

REZAMID LOTION (FLESH TINTED)
Antiseptic, anti-seborrheic; for treatment of acne
(Dermik)

Resorcinol *	2% w/v
Sulfur	5% w/v
Parachlorometaxylenol	0.5% w/v
Hydro-alcoholic vehicle	
S.D. alcohol	28.5% v/v

REZAMID SHAMPOO (SUSPENSION)
Anti-seborrheic, anti-bacterial shampoo
(Dermik)

Sulfur colloid	2% w/v
Salicylic acid *	2% w/v
Foaming cleanser	

R.H. COSMETICS
R.H. Cosmetics Corp.
736 Parkside Ave.
Brooklyn, N.Y. 11226

Phone: 212-856-2222

See COSMETICS, Section VI, General Formulations

RHEUMASAL
Relief of rheumatic & arthritic pains & aches
(Jenkins Labs.)

Each tablet:
Sodium salicylate *	5 gr.
Potassium iodide	1 gr.
Ext. Gelsemium *	1/4 gr.
Ext. Cimicifuga	1/8 gr.

RHINALL
Nasal decongestant
(Scherer Labs.)

Phenylephrine HCl, USP	0.25%
Chlorobutanol	0.15%
Sodium bisulfite	0.03%
Benzalkonium chloride	1:10000
Isotonic saline solution base	

RHINEX
Decongestant-buffered analgesic
(Lemmon Co.)

Each tablet:
Aspirin *	150 mg.
Chlorpheniramine maleate	1.25 mg.
Phenylephrine HCl	2.5 mg.
Dried Aluminum hydroxide gel and magnesium hydroxide	

RHINEX D-LAY
Analgesic-decongestant (timed-release)
(Lemmon Co.)

Each tablet:
Acetaminophen *	300 mg.
Salicylamide	300 mg.
Phenylpropanolamine HCl *	60 mg.
Chlorpheniramine maleate	4 mg.

RHINEX DM
Antitussive/expectorant/antihistamine/decongestant
(Lemmon Co.)

Each tsp.:
Dextromethorphan hydrobromide	7.5 mg.
Chlorpheniramine maleate	1 mg.
Glyceryl guaiacolate	50 mg.
Phenylpropanolamine hydrochloride *	12.5 mg.
Ammonium chloride	100 mg.
Alcohol	5%

RHINIDRIN TABLETS
Antihistamine, analgesic, decongestant
(Central Pharmacal Co.)

Each tablet:
Acetaminophen *	150 mg.
Phenacetin *	150 mg.
Phenylpropanolamine hydrochloride *	25 mg.
Phenyltoloxamine citrate	25 mg.

RHINIHAB JR. (C.T. SALMON)
(Bowman Pharm.)

Each tablet:
Phenylephrine hydrochloride *	2.5 mg.
Chlorpheniramine maleate	1.0 mg.
Fruit flavoring	

RHINOGESIC
Analgesic, antihistaminic
(Vale)

Each tablet:
Phenylephrine hydrochloride *	5 mg.
Chlorpheniramine maleate	2 mg.
Salicylamide	250 mg.
Acetaminophen *	150 mg.

RHINOGESIC-GG
Analgesic, antihistaminic
(Vale)

Each tablet:
Phenylephrine hydrochloride *	5 mg.
Chlorpheniramine maleate	2 mg.
Salicylamide	250 mg.
Acetaminophen *	150 mg.
Guaifenesin	100 mg.

RHINOGESIC JUNIOR
Analgesic, antihistaminic, decongestant
(Vale)

Each tablet:
Acetaminophen *	60 mg.
Salicylamide	90 mg.
Phenylephrine hydrochloride	2 mg.
Chlorpheniramine maleate	1 mg.

RHINO GREASE DISSOLVER, PL
See PL RHINO GREASE DISSOLVER

RHINOSYN CAPSULES
Antihistamine, decongestant
(Comatic)

Each capsule:
Chlorpheniramine maleate *	10 mg.
Pseudoephedrine HCl *	120 mg.

RHINOSYN-DM SYRUP
Antitussive, antihistamine, decongestant
(Comatic)

Each 5 ml.:
Dextromethorphan HBr *	15 mg.
Chlorpheniramine maleate *	2 mg.
Pseudoephedrine HCl *	30 mg.

Additive free product

RHINOSYN-DMX SYRUP
Antitussive, expectorant
(Comatic)

Each 5 ml.:
Dextromethorphan HBr *	10 mg.
Guaifenesin	100 mg.

Additive free product

RHINOSYN-PD SYRUP
Antihistamine, decongestant
(Comatic)

Each 5 ml.:
Chlorpheniramine maleate *	2 mg.
Pseudoephedrine HCl *	30 mg.

Additive free product

RHINOSYN SYRUP
Antihistamine, decongestant
(Comatic)

Each 5 ml.:
Chlorpheniramine maleate *	4 mg.
Pseudoephedrine HCl *	60 mg.

Additive free product

Starred ingredients (*) may be responsible for major toxic effects; consult Section II.

RHINOSYN-X SYRUP
Expectorant, antitussive, decongestant
(Comatic)

Each 5 ml.:
Guaifenesin	100 mg.
Dextromethorphan HBr *	10 mg.
Pseudoephedrine HCl *	30 mg.

Additive free product

RHINSPEC
Cough and cold treatment
(Lemmon Co.)

Each tablet:
Acetaminophen *	300 mg.
Glyceryl guaiacolate	100 mg.
Phenylephrine hydrochloride	5 mg.

RHODIA 2,4-D AMINE NO. 4
Herbicide
(Rhone-Poulenc)

Dimethylamine salt of 2,4-dichlo-
rophenoxyacetic acid * 47.29%

RHODIA 2,4-D AMINE NO. 6
Herbicide
(Rhone-Poulenc)

Dimethylamine salt of 2,4-dichlo-
rophenoxyacetic acid * 66.81%

RHODIA 2,4-D BUTYL ESTER 4E
Herbicide
(Rhone-Poulenc)

Butyl ester of 2,4-dichlorophenox-
yacetic acid * 56.88%

RHODIA 2,4-D BUTYL ESTER 6E
Herbicide
(Rhone-Poulenc)

Butyl ester of 2,4-dichlorophenox-
yacetic acid * 76.29%

RHODIA 2,4-D GRAN 20
Herbicide
(Rhone-Poulenc)

Isooctyl ester of 2,4-dichlorophen-
oxyacetic acid * 29.50%

RHODIA 2,4-D LOW VOLATILE ESTER 4L
Herbicide
(Rhone-Poulenc)

Isooctyl ester of 2,4-dichlorophen-
oxyacetic acid * 68.17%

RHODIA 2,4-D LOW VOLATILE ESTER 6L
Herbicide
(Rhone-Poulenc)

Isooctyl ester of 2,4-dichlorophen-
oxyacetic acid * 90.87%

RHOMENE
Herbicide
(Rhone-Poulenc)

Dimethylamine salt of 2-methyl-4-
chlorophenoxyacetic acid * 52.2%

RHONOX
Herbicide
(Rhone-Poulenc)

Isooctyl ester of 2-methyl-4-chloro-
phenoxyacetic acid * 74.4%

RHULICREAM
For skin irritations
(Lederle)

Zirconium oxide	1.00%
Benzocaine	1.00%
Menthol	0.70%
Camphor	0.30%
Isopropyl alcohol	8.80%
Methylparaben	0.08%
Propylparaben	0.02%

RHULIHIST LOTION
Analgesic-anesthetic
(Lederle)

Tripelennamine HCl USP *	1%
Calamine USP	3%
Zirconium oxide	1%
Benzocaine	1%
Camphor	0.1%
Menthol	0.1%
Methylparaben	0.08%
Propylparaben	0.02%

RHULISPRAY
Analgesic-anesthetic
(Lederle)

Active ingred. (percent w/w):	35.582%
Phenylcarbinol	0.674%
Menthol	0.025%
Camphor	0.253%
Calamine	4.710%
Benzocaine	1.153%
Isopropyl alcohol *	28.767%
Inactive ingred. and propellant	64.418%

RICHCO SC-64 DISINFECTANT RINSE
(Richardson Chem.)

Monosodium phosphate anhydrous *†	>40%
Sodium dodecyl benzene sulfonate *	>10%
Trichloromelamine	>10%
Citric acid anhydrous	>10%

'76 Ed.

†*See* Phosphates

RID-A-BIRD 1100
Pest bird control
(Rid-A-Bird)

Fenthion *	11%
Aromatic petroleum distillate *	11%
Amolite #8 oil (dewaxed paraffin-type oil)	78%

RID-A-BIRD CONTROL LIQUID
Pest bird control
(Rid-A-Bird)

Endrin *	9.4%
Amolite #8 oil (dewaxed paraffin-type oil)	90.40%

RID-ITCH
Antiseptic, fungicide; medical
(Thomas & Thompson)

Alcohol	65%
Glycerin	
Salicylic acid *	
Resorcinol *	
Chlorothymol *	
Benzoic acid *	
Biebrich scarlet red (medicinal)	
Boric acid *	

RID-O DUST MOP TREATMENT
(National-Purity Soap)

Petroleum distillate *

RIDSECT HOUSE & GARDEN PRESSURIZED SPRAY
Insecticide
(Chipman Inc.)

Methoxychlor	2.0%
Pyrethrins	0.22%
Technical Piperonyl butoxide	1.10%

RID-WEED WEED KILLER
Herbicide
(Consolidated Chem., Inc.)

Sodium arsenite * 27.36%

RIGHT GUARD ANTIPERSPIRANTS AND DEODORANTS
(Gillette Co., Personal Care Div.)

The Gillette Co., Personal Care Div., Boston, Mass. 02199 will receive collect phone calls from poison control centers or physicians asking for emergency toxicological information about the company's products.

Phone: 617-421-7000

RIGWASH COMPOUND
Institutional and industrial cleaning product

Procter & Gamble Co.
Ivorydale Technical Center
Cincinnati, Ohio 45217

Phone: 513-562-1100

Starred ingredients (*) may be responsible for major toxic effects; consult Section II.

RINADE B.I.D. CAPS
Decongestant
(Econo Med)

Each capsule:
Chlorpheniramine maleate ... 8 mg.
d-Isoephedrine
hydrochloride * .... 120 mg.

RING GONE
(Paul Koss)

Water .... >80%
Hydrogen chloride * .... <10%
Phosphoric acid * 7%
Nonionic surfactant
Nonylphenoxypoly(ethyleneoxy)ethanol
iodine complex

RINSE AWAY AFTER SHAMPOO DANDRUFF RINSE
(Alberto-Culver)

Active ingred.:
Benzalkonium chloride
Lauryl isoquinolinium bromide
Other ingred.:
Water
Oleamide MIPA
Polysorbate-20
Fragrance
PVP
Trisodium EDTA
D & C Green No. 5
FD & C Yellow No. 5

RINSO (Low Phosphate)
Powder laundry detergent
(Lever Bros.)

Sodium sulfate 20-45%
Sodium polyphosphate 20-30%
Anionic detergent 10-20%
Sodium silicate 5-15%
Water 5-10%
Sodium carbonate 0-5%
Cellulosic .... <1%
Perfume .... <1%
Optical dye .... trace
Colorants .... trace

RINSO (Nonphosphate)
Powder laundry detergent
(Lever Bros.)

Sodium carbonate * 30-40%
Sodium sulfate 10-30%
Anionic detergent 10-20%
Sodium silicate 10-20%
Water 1-5%
Cellulosic .... <1%
Perfume .... <1%
Optical dye .... trace
Colorants .... trace

RISE SHAVING CREAM
(Carter Products)

Soap
Water
Nonionic emulsifiers
Fragrance (Regular, Menthol, Lime, Baby Face, Heavy)
Humectant
Hydrocarbons (propellant)

RISQUE' COLOGNE 1/6 DRAM VIAL

See JAFRA RISQUE' COLOGNE 1/6 DRAM VIAL

RISQUE' 5/16 OUNCE DAB-ON PERFUME

See JAFRA RISQUE' 5/16 OUNCE DAB-ON PERFUME

RISQUE' 2 OUNCE SPRAY COLOGNE

See JAFRA RISQUE' 2 OUNCE SPRAY COLOGNE

RISQUE' SPRAY COLOGNE

See JAFRA RISQUE' SPRAY CO-LOGNE

RITALIN
Psychomotor stimulant
(CIBA Pharmaceutical)

Each tablet:
Methylphenidate
hydrochloride * ..... 5 mg.; 10 mg.; or 20 mg.

RIT COLOR REMOVER
(Best Foods)

Best Foods
CPC International, Inc.
International Plaza
Englewood Cliffs, N.J. 07632

Phone: 201-894-4000

RIT FABRIC DYES
(Best Foods)

Best Foods
CPC International, Inc.
International Plaza
Englewood Cliffs, N.J. 07632

Phone: 201-894-4000

"RIT dyes have been found not to require labeling under the Federal Hazardous Substances Act except for the purpose of indicating their content of ordinary table salt (NaCl)" - per manufacturer.

RIT NYLON WHITENER & FABRIC BRIGHTENER
(Best Foods)

Best Foods
CPC International, Inc.
International Plaza
Englewood Cliffs, N.J. 07632

Phone: 201-894-4000

RIVERSIDE 120 HERBICIDE
(Riverside/Terra)

Monosodium acid
methanearsonate * 51.3%

RIVERSIDE 612 HERBICIDE
(Riverside/Terra)

Monosodium acid
methanearsonate * 35.5%

RIVERSIDE 912 HERBICIDE
(Riverside/Terra)

Monosodium acid
methanearsonate * 48.0%

RIVERSIDE MALATHION 5
Insecticide
(Riverside/Terra)

Malathion * 56.8%
Aromatic petroleum solvent * 36.2%

RIVERSIDE METHYL PARATHION 4
Insecticide
(Riverside/Terra)

O,O-Dimethyl O-p-nitrophenyl
phosphorothioate * 45.4%
Aromatic petroleum solvent 50.6%

RIVERSIDE METHYL PARATHION 7.2
Insecticide
(Riverside/Terra)

O,O-Dimethyl O-p-nitrophenyl
phosphorothioate * 71.7%
Aromatic petroleum solvent 15.9%

RIVERSIDE PARATHION 4
Insecticide
(Riverside/Terra)

Parathion * 46.8%
Aromatic petroleum solvent 48.4%

RIVERSIDE PARATHION 8
Insecticide
(Riverside/Terra)

Parathion * 80.6%
Aromatic petroleum solvent 10.2%

RIVERSIDE RAIDER 33
Insecticide
(Riverside/Terra)

O,O-Dimethyl O-p-nitrophenyl
phosphorothioate * 31.6%
O-Ethyl O-p-nitrophenyl
phenylphosphonothioate * 31.6%
Aromatic petroleum solvent 27.4%

Starred ingredients (*) may be responsible for major toxic effects; consult Section II.

RIVERSIDE RAIDER 42
Insecticide
(Riverside/Terra)

O,O-Dimethyl O-p-nitrophenyl phosphorothioate *	42.0%
O-Ethyl O-p-nitrophenyl phenylphosphonothioate *	21.0%
Aromatic petroleum solvent	27.6%

RIVERSIDE SODIUM CHLORATE
Defoliant-desiccant
(Riverside/Terra)

Sodium chlorate *	29.5%

RIVERSIDE TOXAPHENE 6
Insecticide
(Riverside/Terra)

Toxaphene *	58.7%
Aromatic petroleum solvent *	38.3%

RIZ
Disinfectant
(Holcomb)

Santophen (Sodium orthobenzyl-parachlorophenol) *	>10%

'76 Ed.

RLR LAUNDRY TREATMENT
Laundry additive; white powder
(RAD, Inc.)

Soda ash *	52%
CMC	18%
EDTA	3%
Optical brightener	2%
Liquid Surfactant *	25%

ROACHES' LAST MEAL
(Maas, A.G.)

Sodium fluoride *	40%
Inert ingredient: Soda ash *	60%

ROACH TABZ
Kills roaches and water bugs
(Bandwagon, Inc.)

O,O-Dimethyl O-(2,4,5-trichloro-phenyl) phosphorothioate *	1.20%
2,2-Dichlorovinyl dimethyl phosphate	0.20%
Related compounds	0.02%

ROBAXIN
Skeletal muscle relaxant
(Robins)

Each tablet:
Methocarbamol, USP *	500 mg.

ROBAXIN-750
Skeletal muscle relaxant
(Robins)

Each tablet:
Methocarbamol, USP *	750 mg.

ROBAXISAL
Muscle relaxant-analgesic
(Robins)

Each tablet:
Methocarbamol, USP *	400 mg.
Aspirin, USP *	325 mg.

ROBERTS 0167
Carpet gripper adhesive
(Roberts Consolidated Ind.)

Toluene *	approx. 16%
Ketone solvents	approx. 14%
Petroleum distillates	approx. 45%

ROBERTS 0308
Brushable contact cement, natural
(Roberts Consolidated Ind.)

Toluene *	approx. 10%
Ketone solvents *	approx. 14%
Petroleum distillates *	approx. 45%

ROBERTS 0901
Carpet gripper solvent
(Roberts Consolidated Ind.)

Toluene *	approx. 10%
Ketone solvents *	approx. 20%
Petroleum distillates *	approx. 70%

ROBERTS 0911
Universal cushion back seam solvent
(Roberts Consolidated Ind.)

1,1,1-Trichloroethane *	100%

ROBERTS 4000
Carpet pad adhesive, regular
(Roberts Consolidated Ind.)

Petroleum distillates *	approx. 78%

ROBERTS 4001
Carpet pad adhesive, non-flammable
(Roberts Consolidated Ind.)

1,1,1-Trichloroethane *	approx. 90%

ROBERTS 4015
Cushion back seam adhesive
(Roberts Consolidated Ind.)

1,1,1-Trichloroethane *	approx. 60%

ROBERTS ALL-WEATHER OUTDOOR CARPET ADHESIVE 6037
(Roberts Consolidated Ind.)

Toluene *	approx. 5%
Petroleum distillates *	approx. 20%

ROBERTS CYGON 2E CONCENTRATE
Insecticide
(Roberts Labs.)

Dimethoate *	23.4%
Aromatic petroleum derivatives *	38.4%

ROBERTS DUO-KILL EMULSIFIABLE CONCENTRATE
Insecticide
(Roberts Labs.)

Ciodrin *	10.0%
Vapona	2.3%
Related compounds	0.2%
Petroleum hydrocarbons	77.0%

ROBERTS DUST'M
Insecticide
(Roberts Labs.)

Rabon *	3.0%

ROBERTS FLY-BATE
Insecticide
(Roberts Labs.)

2,2-Dichlorovinyl dimethyl phosphate	0.46%/wt.
Related compounds	0.04%/wt.

ROBERTS 'FLY-DIE'
Livestock spray
(Roberts Labs.)

O,O-Dimethyl 2,2-dichlorovinyl phosphate	0.500%
Piperonyl butoxide	0.250%
Pyrethrins	0.025%
Mineral oil	49.613%
Petroleum distillates *	49.612%

ROBERTS HOG MANGE POWDER
Sarcoptic mange and lice control
(Roberts Labs.)

Gamma isomer of benzene hexa-chloride from lindane	1.00%

ROBERTS HORSE AND STABLE INSECTICIDE
Insecticide
(Roberts Labs.)

Piperonyl butoxide (technical)	0.35%/wt.
Pyrethrins	0.07%/wt.
Beta-butoxy beta'-thiocyano diethyl ether	1.06%/wt.
Mineral oil *	98.52%/wt.

ROBERTS HOUSE & GARDEN AEROSOL
Insecticide
(Roberts Labs.)

Resmethrin (SBP-1382)	0.350%
Related compounds	0.048%
Aromatic petroleum hydrocarbons	0.464%

Starred ingredients (*) may be responsible for major toxic effects; consult Section II.

ROBERTS LINDANE EMULSIFIABLE CONCENTRATE
Insecticide
(Roberts Labs.)

Lindane (Gamma isomer of benzene hexachloride) *	11.14%
Petroleum derivative solvent *	84.39%

ROBERTS MALATHION 57%
Insecticide
(Roberts Labs.)

Malathion *	57%
Aromatic petroleum derivative solvent *	35%

ROBERTS POULTRY DUST
Insecticide
(Roberts Labs.)

Sevin (Carbaryl) *	5.0%

ROBERTS PROLIN ANTICOAGULANT CONCENTRATE
Rodenticide
(Roberts Labs.)

Warfarin	0.5%
Sulfaquinoxaline	0.5%

ROBERTS PROLIN PELLETED RAT & MOUSE BAIT
(Roberts Labs.)

Warfarin	0.025%
Sulfaquinoxaline	0.025%

ROBERTS PYRENONE DAIRY AEROSOL
Insecticide
(Roberts Labs.)

Pyrethrins	0.5%
Piperonyl butoxide	5.0%

ROBERTS PYRENONE DAIRY & FOOD PLANT SPRAY
Insecticide
(Roberts Labs.)

Pyrethrins	0.25%
Piperonyl butoxide	2.50%

ROBERTS ROACH & ANT SPRAY
Insecticide
(Roberts Labs.)

Diazinon	0.500%
Pyrethrins	0.052%
Piperonyl butoxide	0.261%

ROBERTS RODEX COATED WARFARIN RAT & MOUSE BAIT (Pelleted)
(Roberts Labs.)

Warfarin	0.025%

ROBERTS VAPONA-PLUS
Insecticide
(Roberts Labs.)

2,2-Dichlorovinyl dimethyl phosphate	0.92%/wt.
Related compounds	0.08%/wt.
Beta-butoxy beta'-thiocyano diethyl ether	0.53%/wt.
Petroleum hydrocarbons *	98.41%/wt.

ROBERTS VAPORA
Insecticide
(Roberts Labs.)

2,2-Dichlorovinyl dimethyl phosphate *	17.173%
Related compounds	1.327%
Xylene *	74.000%

ROBICILLIN VK
Anti-infective agent
(Robins)

Each tablet:
Penicillin V potassium, USP .... 250 mg.; 500 mg.

Each 5 ml. for oral solution:
Penicillin V potassium, USP .... 125 mg.; 250 mg.

RO-BILE
Comprehensive digestant
(Rowell)

Each tablet:
Outer coating:

Pepsin	260 mg.

Enteric-coated core:

Enzyme concentrate	75 mg.
Ox bile extract	100 mg.
Dehydrocholic acid	30 mg.
Belladonna extract *	8 mg.

ROBIMYCIN
Anti-infective agent
(Robins)

Each tablet:
Erythromycin, USP .... 250 mg.

ROBIN CONCENTRATED FABRIC SOFTENER
(Industrial Equities)

Quaternary ammonium compound *	5-10%
Fluorescent whitening agent	<1%
Preservative	<1%
Colorant	<1%
Perfume	<1%
Water	balance

ROBINETTS
Vitamin supplement
(Wesley Pharm.)

Each capsule:
Vitamin A (Palmitate) 5000 USP Units
Vitamin D .... 400 USP Units
Iron (Ferrous sulfate, dried) . 13.4 mg.
Plus multivitamins & minerals

ROBIN FABRIC SOFTENER
(Industrial Equities)

Quaternary ammonium compound *	2-5%
Preservative	<1%
Colorant	<1%
Perfume	<1%
Water	balance

ROBIN LIQUID DISHWASHING DETERGENT
(Industrial Equities)

Anionic surfactant	6-12%
Hydrotrope	1-3%
Alkanolamide	<1%
Ethyl alcohol	<1%
Opacifier	<1%
Colorant	<1%
Perfume	<1%
Water	balance

ROBITET 250 & 500
Anti-infective agent
(Robins)

Each capsule:
Tetracycline hydrochloride, USP .. 250 mg.; or 500 mg.

ROBITUSSIN
Antitussive-expectorant
(Robins)

Each 5 ml.:

Guaifenesin, NF	100 mg.

In aromatic syrup

Alcohol	3.5%

ROBITUSSIN A-C SYRUP
Expectorant, antitussive
(Robins)

Each 5 ml.:

Guaifenesin, USP	100.0 mg.
Codeine phosphate, USP *	10.0 mg.
Alcohol	3.5%

ROBITUSSIN-CF
Expectorant, nasal decongestant, cough suppressant
(Robins)

Each 5 ml.:

Guaifenesin, USP	100.0 mg.
Phenylpropanolamine hydrochloride, USP *	12.5 mg.
Dextromethorphan hydrobromide, USP *	10.0 mg
Alcohol	4.75%

Starred ingredients (*) may be responsible for major toxic effects; consult Section II.

ROBITUSSIN-DAC
Expectorant, nasal decongestant, anti-tussive
(Robins)

Each 5 ml.:
Guaifenesin, USP .... 100 mg.
Pseudoephedrine hydrochlo-
ride, USP * .... 30 mg.
Codeine phosphate, USP * ... 10 mg.
Alcohol 1.4%

ROBITUSSIN-DM
Antitussive, expectorant
(Robins)

Each 5 ml.:
Guaifenesin, NF .... 100 mg.
Dextromethorphan hydrobro-
mide, NF * .... 15 mg.
Alcohol 1.4%

ROBITUSSIN-DM COUGH CALMERS (Lozenge)
Antitussive, expectorant
(Robins)

Each lozenge:
Guaifenesin, NF .... 50 mg.
Dextromethorphan hydrobro-
mide, NF * .... 7.5 mg.

ROBITUSSIN-PE
Decongestant, expectorant
(Robins)

Each 5 ml.:
Guaifenesin, USP .... 100 mg.
Pseudoephedrine hydrochlo-
ride, USP * .... 30 mg.
Alcohol 1.4%

ROCCAL BRAND SANITIZING AGENT
(Winthrop Products Inc.)

Quaternary ammonium compounds *

ROCCAL MIST AIR SANITIZER (HOSPITAL TYPE)
(Nat'l Labs. Div.)

Triethylene glycol 8.0%
Dipropylene glycol 2.0%
Alkyl dimethyl benzyl ammonium
chloride 0.1%
Essential oils 0.5%
Ethyl alcohol 16.0%

ROCCAL 10 SPA
Disinfectant-sanitizer-deodorant
(Stewart Sanitary Supply)

Alkyl (C14, 50%; C12, 40%; C16,
10%) dimethyl benzyl ammonium chloride * 10.0%
Ethanol 2.5%

ROCCAL II 10% SANITIZING AGENT/GERMICIDE-ALGICIDE DEODORIZER
(Nat'l Labs. Div.)

Alkyl (C14, 50%, C12 40%, C16
10%) dimethyl benzyl ammonium chloride * 10.00%
Ethyl alcohol 1.25%

ROCHE MEDICAL EMERGENCY TELEPHONE NUMBER
24-hour a day assistance

Roche Laboratories
Nutley, N.J. 07110

Phone: 201-235-2355

ROCKLAND HOUSEHOLD AEROSOL
Insecticide
(Rockland Chem.)

Pyrethrins 0.45%
Tech. Piperonyl butoxide 1.125%
Refined Petroleum distillate * .. 13.425%
Propellant 85.000%

ROCKLAND MALATHION 50
Insecticide
(Rockland Chem.)

Malathion * 57%
Xylene * 33%

ROCKLAND SUGAR FLY BAIT
Insecticide
(Rockland Chem.)

DDVP 0.46%

ROCKLAND WEED KILLER
(Rockland Chem.)

Ammonium sulfamate * 48.4%

RO-DENT
Rodenticide
(Mackwin)

Diphacinone (2-Diphenylacetyl-
1,3-indandione) 0.005%

RODEN-TROL, SPRAY-TROL BRAND
See SPRAY-TROL BRAND RODEN-TROL

RODEX
Rodenticide
(ABCO, Inc.)

Warfarin (3-(a-Acetonylbenzyl)-4-
hydroxycoumarin) 0.5%

ROFFLER HAIR CARE PRODUCTS

Roffler Industries
400 Chess St.
Coraopolis, Pa. 15108

Phone: 412-771-4333

See COSMETICS, Section VI, General Formulations

ROGENIC TABLETS
Hematinic
(OJF)

Each tablet:
Iron (as ferrous fumarate, fer-
rous sulfate, ferrous
gluconate) *† .... 60 mg.
Ascorbic acid .... 100 mg.
Pyridoxine HCl .... 6 mg.
Vitamin B-12 .... 25 mcg.
Dessicated Liver .... 25 mg.

†*See* Iron salts

ROGERS C-100-C LIVESTOCK INSECTICIDE
(Rogers Chemical Co.)

Mineral oil
Aromatic petroleum derivative solvent *
Methoxychlor (technical) *
Piperonyl butoxide (technical)
Pyrethrins

ROGERS', DR., PRODUCTS
See DR. ROGERS

RO-KILL 100 DUST
See NIAGARA RO-KILL 100 DUST

RO-KIL SPRAY
Insecticide
(FMC Corp., Agricultural Chem. Div.)

Rotenone * .... 5.00%/wt.
Other cube resins or
extractives .... 5.00%/wt.

ROLAIDS
Antacid
(Warner-Lambert)

Each tablet:
Dihydroxy aluminum sodium
carbonate .... 334 mg.

ROMAN CLEANSER BLEACH
Laundry bleach; household sanitizer
(Roman Cleanser Co.)

Sodium hypochlorite * .. 5.25%
Sodium hydroxide .... equiv. to 0.1%

Starred ingredients (*) may be responsible for major toxic effects; consult Section II.

ROMAZINE EXPECTORANT WITH CODEINE
(Wesley Pharm.)

Each tsp. (5 cc):
Codeine phosphate * ...... 10 mg.
Promethazine hydrochloride 5 mg.
Fl. ext. Ipecac .... 0.17 min.
Potassium guaiacolsulfonate 44 mg.
Citric acid .... 60 mg.
Sodium citrate .... 197 mg.
Alcohol 7%

ROMAZINE PEDIATRIC
Antitussive
(Wesley Pharm.)

Each tsp. (5 cc):
Dextromethorphan
hydrobromide .... 7.5 mg.
Promethazine hydrochloride 5 mg.
Fl. ext. Ipecac .... 0.17 min.
Potassium guaiacolsulfonate 44 mg.
Citric acid .... 60 mg.
Sodium citrate .... 197 mg.
Alcohol 7%

ROMAZINE, PLAIN
Antihistaminic
(Wesley Pharm.)

Each tsp. (5 cc):
Promethazine hydrochloride 5 mg.
Fl. ext. Ipecac .... 0.17 min.
Potassium guaiacolsulfonate 44 mg.
Citric acid .... 60 mg.
Sodium citrate .... 197 mg.
Alcohol 7%

ROMAZINE VC EXPECTORANT
Antihistaminic, antitussive
(Wesley Pharm.)

Each tsp. (5 cc):
Promethazine hydrochloride 5 mg.
Phenylephrine
hydrochloride * .... 5 mg.
Fl. ext. Ipecac .... 0.17 min.
Potassium guaiacolsulfonate 44 mg.
Citric acid .... 60 mg.
Sodium citrate .... 197 mg.
Alcohol 7%

ROMAZINE VC EXPECTORANT WITH CODEINE
(Wesley Pharm.)

Each tsp. (5 cc):
Codeine phosphate * ...... 10 mg.
Promethazine hydrochloride 5 mg.
Phenylephrine
hydrochloride * .... 5 mg.
Fl. ext. Ipecac .... 0.17 min.
Potassium guaiacolsulfonate 44 mg.
Citric acid .... 60 mg.
Sodium citrate .... 197 mg.
Alcohol 7%

ROMEO COLOGNE

See JAFRA ROMEO COLOGNE

ROMILAR CF
Cough medicine
(Block Drug)

Dextromethorphan
hydrobromide * 0.25%
Alcohol 20.00%
Sugar base
Glycerine
Sodium saccharin
Preservative
Sodium citrate
Sodium chloride
Citric acid
Ammonium chloride
Flavors

ROMILAR CHILDREN'S
Cough medicine
(Block Drug)

Dextromethorphan hydrobromide 0.04%
Sugar base
Glycerine
Preservative
Sodium citrate
Citric acid
Flavors

ROMILAR III
Cough medicine
(Block Drug)

Dextromethorphan hydrobromide 0.08%
Phenylpropanolamine
hydrochloride * 0.22%
Alcohol 20.00%
Sugar base
Glycerine
Sodium saccharin
Preservative
Sodium citrate
Sodium chloride
Citric acid
Ammonium chloride
Flavors

RONDOMYCIN
Broad-spectrum antibiotic
(Wallace Labs.)

CAPSULES (each):
Methacycline HCl
equiv. to 140 mg. of methacycline base .... 150 mg.
equiv. to 280 mg. of methacycline base .... 300 mg.

SYRUP (each 5 cc):
Methacycline HCl
equiv. to 70 mg./5 cc of methacycline base .... 75 mg.

'76 Ed.

RO-NEET (6-E, 10-G)
Herbicide
(Stauffer)

Ro-neet (S-Ethyl cyclohexylethylthiocarbamate) *

RONIACOL
Vasodilator
(Roche)

Each tablet:
Nicotinyl alcohol tartrate * .. 50 mg.

Each Timespan tablet:
Nicotinyl alcohol tartrate * .. 150 mg.

Elixir (each 5 ml.):
Nicotinyl alcohol * .... 50 mg.

RONSONOL LIGHTER FLUID
(Ronson)

Hydrocarbon naphtha solvents *†

†*See* Petroleum naphtha

ROOST NO MORE
Bird repellent liquid
(National B.C. Sales, Inc.)

Mineral oil 60%

Non-toxic per manufacturer

ROOTO (NOS. 1, 2, 3 & 4)
For clogged drains, grease traps; clears sluggish & root-blocked sewers
(Rooto)

Sodium hydroxide *

ROOTONE WITH FUNGICIDE, IMPROVED
For better rooting, to control damping-off of cuttings
(Amchem)

Thiram * 4.000%
Ingred. active as growth promoters:
Naphthylacetamide 0.067%
2-Methyl-1-naphthylacetic acid 0.033%
2-Methyl-1-naphthylacetamide 0.013%
Indole-3-butyric acid 0.057%

ROOTO'S CLOSET BOWL CLEANER (DRY)
(Rooto)

Sodium bisulfate * 84%
Sodium carbonates 10%

ROOTO'S COMMERCIAL DRAIN CLEANER
(Rooto)

Potassium hydroxide *

ROOTO'S COMMERCIAL ENZYMATIC DRAIN CLEANER
(Rooto)

Commercial Enzyme, nonpathogenic mi-
crobial source
Sodium phosphate buffering system *†
Non-ionic wetting agents

†*See* Phosphates

Starred ingredients (*) may be responsible for major toxic effects; consult Section II.

ROOTO'S CONCRETE CLEANER
(Rooto)

Phosphates *
Surfactants *

ROOTO'S LIQUID BOWL CLEANER
(Rooto)

Hydrochloric acid *

ROOTO'S LIQUID DRAIN CLEANER REGULAR
(Rooto)

Potassium hydroxide *

ROOT OUT
Root destroyer
(Popular Products, Inc.)

Copper sulphate pentahydrate *   99%

ROOT RAIDER

See BLUE SEAL ROOT RAIDER

ROOTSOL

See DEXOL ROOTSOL

ROSE BOQUET THEATRE SPRAY
Deodorant
(Central Chem.)

Essential oils *

'76 Ed.

ROSE BOWL CLEANER
Institutional and industrial use
(Dalco Corp.)

Di-isobutyl phenoxy ethyl dimethyl benzyl ammonium chloride	1%
Phosphoric acid *	24.2%
Combined amount:	7.9%
Sulfamic acid	
Oxalic acid	

ROSELIFE
Cut flower preservative
(Ampco Chem. Div.)

d-Glucose	93%
Combined amount:	7%
Detergent	
Trace element	

ROSE MILK SKIN CARE CREAM
(Williams, J.B.)

Mineral oil
Lanolin oil
Stearic acid
Cetyl alcohol
Emulsifiers
Perfume

ROSS CONTACT CEMENT #139
(Ross Chem.)

Chloroprene rubber	25.0%
Toluol *	35.0%
Aliphatic hydrocarbons	35.0%
Resins	5.0%

ROSS EPOXY GLUE #178 AND #179
(Ross Chem.)

Mixture of:
Epoxy resin
Polyamide resin

ROSS GREAT GRIPPER #145
(Ross Chem.)

Synthetic rubber resin dispersion in water

ROSS HOUSEHOLD CEMENT #107
(Ross Chem.)

Nitrocellulose resin solution in:	
Isopropyl acetate	18.6%
Butyl acetate	13.7%
Toluol *	55.8%
Isopropyl alcohol	11.9%

ROSS JEWELRY CLEANER #400
(Ross Chem.)

Ammonium hydroxide	1.0%
Blue dye	
Water	99.0%

ROSS LIQUID PORCELAIN #172
(Ross Chem.)

Acrylic resin	40.0%
Toluol *	25.0%
Xylol *	25.0%
Pigment	10.0%

ROSS LIQUID RUBBER #158
(Ross Chem.)

Black pigment dispersed in a Chloroprene rubber-resin solution dissolved in:
Toluol *
Aliphatic hydrocarbons *

ROSS LIQUID SOLDER #102
(Ross Chem.)

Nitrocellulose resin solution in:	
Isopropyl acetate	20.0%
Butyl Cellosolve	4.0%
Toluol *	11.0%
Isopropyl alcohol	45.0%

ROSS METAL MENDER #152
(Ross Chem.)

Pigments dispersed in
Polyvinyl chloride resin solution dissolved in
Methyl ethyl ketone *

ROSS MUCILAGE #33
(Ross Chem.)

Potato dextrine	26.0%
Water	64.0%
Urea	5.0%
Borax	4.0%
Sodium bisulfite	0.1%
Sodium carbonate	0.6%
Sodium ortho-phenyl phenolate	0.1%
Trisodium ethylenediaminetetra-acetic acid trihydrate	0.2%

ROSS POLYSTYRENE PLASTIC CEMENT #63 AND #64
(Ross Chem.)

Polystyrene resin solution in:	
Toluol *	70.0%
Oil of mustard	0.25%

ROSS POWER BOND #190 & SUPER GLUE # 190
(Ross Chem.)

Cyanoacrylate resin solution *

ROSS RUBBER CEMENT #44
(Ross Chem.)

Natural rubber	12.0%
Ethyl alcohol	1.0%
Ester gum	1.0%
Aliphatic hydrocarbons *	86.0%

ROSS SCHOOL GLUE #1
(Ross Chem.)

Polyvinyl alcohol polymer	5.2%
Polyvinyl acetate polymer	27.2%
Water	65.6%
Butyl benzyl phthalate	1.4%
Formaldehyde	3.4%
Anionic defoaming agent	0.2%

ROSS SNIF-PROOF PLASTIC CEMENT #65 and #66
(Ross Chem.)

Polystyrene resin	26.0%
d-Limonene *	74.0%

Starred ingredients (*) may be responsible for major toxic effects; consult Section II.

ROSS SYSTEMIC INSECTICIDE CARTRIDGES
For roses, shrubs, trees, evergreens
(Daniels, Ross)

O,O-Diethyl-S-(2-
(ethylthio)ethyl)phosphoro-
dithioate * 2%

ROSS TERMITE CONTROL CARTRIDGES
For control of subterranean termites
(Daniels, Ross)

Technical Chlordane *	12%
Related compounds	8%
Petroleum hydrocarbons	1%

ROSS THINNER FOR RUBBER CEMENT #242
(Ross Chem.)

Aliphatic hydrocarbons * 100.0%

ROSS WHITE GLUE #111
(Ross Chem.)

Polyvinyl acetate emulsion (in water)
Polyvinyl acetate polymer	55.0%
Water	45.0%

ROSS WHITE PASTE #20
(Ross Chem.)

Corn starch	32.0%
Water	67.7%
Benzoic acid	0.2%
Sodium benzoate	0.05%
Sodium ortho-phenyl phenolate	0.1%
Methyl salicylate	trace

ROTATE PLUS
Liquid machine dishwashing detergent
(Diversey Wyandotte)

Potassium hydroxide *
Potassium hypochlorite *

ROTENOX LIVESTOCK SPRAY CONCENTRATE
Insecticide
(Farnam Co.)

Rotenone *	1.19%
Other cube resins	2.38%
Piperonyl butoxide, technical	0.20%
Butoxypolypropylene glycol *	32.13%
Mixed mono and diphosphate esters of ethoxylated alkylphenol	5.00%
Petroleum distillate *	59.10%

'76 Ed.

ROTO-FLO 5OR
Insecticide
(Leffingwell)

Petroleum oil *	82.00%/w
Rotenone	0.20%
Other extractives of cube and/or derris	0.40%

ROTOSYN INSECT DUST
See BONIDE ROTOSYN INSECT DUST

ROTT-FYTER CLEAR 985
Water-repellent wood preservative
(McCloskey Varnish Co.)

Active ingred.:	5.6%
Pentachlorophenol *	5.0%
Other chlorophenols	0.6%
Inert ingred. *†	94.4%

†*See* Petroleum distillate

ROUGH ON RATS
Anticoagulant
(Brown Mfg.)

3-(alpha-Acetonylfurfuryl)-4-
hydroxycoumarin 0.025%

'76 Ed.

ROUNDUP
Herbicide
(Monsanto)

Glyphosate, isopropylamine salt * 41.0%

ROUX HAIR CARE PRODUCTS
(Roux)

Roux Laboratories, Inc.
Sub. of Revlon, Inc.
3733 University Blvd. W.
Jacksonville, Fla. 32217

Phone: 904-731-3050

See COSMETICS, Section VI, General Formulations

ROYAL BOND ANTISEPTIC SOAP
Liquid antiseptic soap
(Royal Bond)

Amyl phenol *

ROYAL BOND CAVITY FLUID
Cavity fluid
(Royal Bond)

Formaldehyde *
Methanol *

ROYAL BOND CLEANING LIQUID FOR INSTRUMENTS
(Royal Bond)

Phenyl phenol *
Isopropanol *
Detergent
Diethylene glycol *

ROYAL BOND LAVENDER SMELLING SALTS
(Royal Bond)

Ammonia *

ROYAL BOND LIQUID TISSUE
Tissue builder
(Royal Bond)

Methanol *

ROYAL BOND ODORLESS CAVITY
Embalming supply
(Royal Bond)

Formaldehyde	<10%
Phenol *	>15%
Methanol	

ROYAL BOND PLASTIC SPRAY ADHESIVE & SEALER
Embalming supply
(Royal Bond)

Acrylic resin
Acetone *

ROYAL BOND REGULAR HARD ARTERIAL FLUID
Embalming supply
(Royal Bond)

Formaldehyde *	30%
Methanol *	

ROYAL BOND SOLVENT
All purpose solvent
(Royal Bond)

Acetone *

ROYAL BOND STERILE DISINFECTANT
(Royal Bond)

Alkyl benzyl ammonium chloride *†	4.5%
Isopropanol *	

†*See* Alkyl dimethyl benzyl ammonium chloride

ROYAL CROWN MUCILAGE
(Sanford Corp.)

Water	
Gum arabic or potato dextrine	
Phenol (as preservative)	<1%

ROYALE CLEANER/WAX
(AS-930, Formula 2104-150)

See SIMONIZ ROYALE CLEANER/WAX (AS-930, Formula 2104-150)

Starred ingredients (*) may be responsible for major toxic effects; consult Section II.

ROYALE MARINE BOAT CLEANER (MS-310, Formula 2206-66)

See SIMONIZ ROYALE MARINE BOAT CLEANER (MS-310, Formula 2206-66)

ROYALE MARINE FIBERGLASS CLEANER/ WAX (MS-300, Formula 2175-47)

See SIMONIZ ROYALE MARINE FIBERGLASS CLEANER/WAX (MS-300, Formula 2175-47)

ROYALE MARINE FIBERGLASS RUBBING COMPOUND (MS-320, Formula LOS-1944)

See SIMONIZ ROYALE MARINE FIBERGLASS RUBBING COMPOUND (MS-320, Formula LOS-1944)

ROYALE MARINE INSTANT GLAZE (MS-305, Formula 8622-27-2)

See SIMONIZ ROYALE MARINE INSTANT GLAZE (MS-305, Formula 8622-27-2)

ROYAL KNIGHTS AFTER SHAVE

See JAFRA ROYAL KNIGHTS AFTER SHAVE

ROYAL KNIGHTS COLOGNE

See JAFRA ROYAL KNIGHTS COLOGNE

ROYAL LINE TOILET SYSTEM TREATMENT
(Earl, John A., Inc.)

Active ingredients: 34.16%
  Phosphoric acid *
  Hydrogen chloride *
  Isopropyl alcohol *
  Toluene *
  Sulfonic acid
  Oxalic acid anhydrous *
  p-Diisobutylphenoxyethoxyethyl dimethyl benzyl ammonium chloride *
  Hepta decyl hydroxyethyl imidazoline
Inert ingredients: 65.84%
  Nonylphenoxypolyethoxyethanol
  Polymerized Vinyl benzene
  Water

'76 Ed.

ROYAL MH-30
Plant growth regulant
(Uniroyal Chem.)

Maleic hydrazide * 21.7%
Inerts 78.3%
  Surfactant
  Water

ROYAL OIL SOAP #50
Multi-purpose cleaner or industrial conveyor lubricant
(National-Purity Soap)

Saponified vegetable oils
Sequesterants

ROYAL SATIN
Automotive
(Garry Labs.)

Wax
Silicone
Diatomaceous earth
Mineral spirits *
Water

ROYAL SLO-GRO
Plant growth regulant
(Uniroyal Chem.)

Maleic hydrazide * 21.7%
Inerts 78.3%
  Surfactant
  Water

ROYALTAC
Plant growth regulant
(Uniroyal Chem.)

n-Decanol * 78.4%
n-Octanol 0.4%
Inert 21.2%
  Surfactant

ROZOL CANARY SEED MOUSE BAIT
(Chempar)

2-((p-Chlorophenyl)phenylacetyl)-1,3-indandione 0.005%

ROZOL MINERAL OIL CONCENTRATE
Rodenticide
(Chempar)

2-((p-Chlorophenyl)phenylacetyl)-1,3-indandione
(Chlorophacinone) * 0.28%

ROZOL PARAFFINIZED PELLETS
Rodenticide
(Chempar)

2-((p-Chlorophenyl)phenylacetyl)-1,3-indandione 0.005%

ROZOL READY-TO-USE RAT AND MOUSE BAIT
(Chempar)

2-((p-Chlorophenyl)phenylacetyl)-1,3-indandione 0.005%

ROZOL RODENTICIDE 0.1% DRY CONCENTRATE
(Chempar)

2-((p-Chlorophenyl)phenylacetyl)-1,3-indandione 0.1%

ROZOL RODENTICIDE 2% DRY CONCENTRATE
(Chempar)

2-((p-Chlorophenyl)phenylacetyl)-1,3-indandione * 2.00%

ROZOL TRACKING POWDER
Rodenticide
(Chempar)

2-((p-Chlorophenyl)phenylacetyl)-1,3-indandione * 0.2%

RP SUPER FILTER COAT CONCENTRATE
Air filter coating
(Research Products Corp.)

Soluble Hydrocarbon oil *† ... 96%
o-Benzyl-p-chlorophenol 1%
Polyethylene thickener 3%

†See Adhesives, Section VI, General Formulations

R.S. LOTION NO. 2
Drying antiseptic
(Hill Dermaceuticals)

Sulfur 8%
Resorcinol monoacetate 4%
Oil absorbing oat protein jell base

"RS" RESIDUAL INSECTICIDE
For use in warehouses
(Weil Chem.)

o-Isopropoxyphenyl methylcarbamate * 1.00%
Pyrethrins 0.03%
Piperonyl butoxide 0.236%
Odorless base oil * 83.734%
Inert ingredients:
  Isopropyl alcohol 9.98%
  Methylene chloride 5.00%
  Essential oil 0.02%

RTU-1010
Seed treatment fungicide
(Cargill)

Carboxin 10%
Thiram * 10%
Ethylene glycol 10-20%

Starred ingredients (*) may be responsible for major toxic effects; consult Section II.

RTU-PCNB
Seed treatment fungicide
(Cargill)

Pentachloronitrobenzene * 24.5%
Ethylene glycol 10-20%

RUB-A-DUB
Laundry marking pen - permanent
(Sanford Corp.)

Dyes
Resins
Glycol ethers
Alcohol

RUBEROL FLOOR ENAMEL
(Lehman Bros. Corp.)

Mercury * .... trace

See Paints, Section VI, General Formulations

RUBEROL GLOSS ENAMEL
(Lehman Bros. Corp.)

Mercury * .... trace

See Paints, Section VI, General Formulations

RUB-R-KLEEN

See ALSOL RUB-R-KLEEN

RUELENE 35D SYSTEMIC INSECTICIDE
(Dow)

4-tert-Butyl-2-chlorophenyl methyl
methylphosphoramidate * 35.7%
Inert ingred.: 64.3%
  Alcohol
  Emulsifier
  Petroleum solvents
  Xylene *
  Isopropyl alcohol

RUELENE 25 E
Cattle insecticide
(Dow)

4-tert Butyl-2-chlorophenyl
methyl methyl-
phosphoramidate * 25.0%
Inert ingred., primarily: 75.00%
  Mineral seal oil
  Isopropyl benzene *

RUELENE 8 R
Cattle insecticide
(Dow)

4-tert Butyl-2-chlorophenyl methyl
methyl-phosphoramidate * 13.5%
Inert ingred., primarily: 86.5%
  Isopropyl alcohol
  Castor oil

RUELENE 12R SYSTEMIC INSECTICIDE
(Dow)

4-tert-Butyl-2-chlorophenyl methyl
methylphosphoramidate * 13.4%
Inert ingred.: 86.6%
  Oil
  Alcohol

RUFOLEX CAPSULES
Iron & vitamin deficiencies
(Lannett)

Each capsule:
  Ferrous fumerate * .... 200 mg.
  Plus Multivitamins

RuGLYDE
Rubber lubricant
(American Grease Stick)

Potassium vegetable oil soap ... 7.0%
Ethylene glycol 1.3%
Corrosion inhibitors .... <1.0%
Water 91.7%

RUMEN-ETTES

See RAWLEIGH RUMEN-ETTES

RUM-K
Potassium replacement
(Fleming)

Each 10 cc:
  Potassium chloride * 1.5 gm. (20 mEq)
  Butter/Rum flavored base

RUN ROACH
Roach killer and repellent
(Lester Labs.)

Petroleum distillates *
Piperonyl butoxide, tech.
Pyrethrins *

'76 Ed.

RUST-GO
Rust/scale remover
(Holcomb)

Hydrochloric acid * .... >10%

'76 Ed.

RUSTICIDE
Rust remover
(Skybryte)

Phosphoric acid * 32.00%
Wetting agent 0.25%
Water 67.75%

RUST JELLY
(Sheffield Bronze Paint)

Phosphoric acid *

RUST-OFF
Descaler, deruster, destrainer, defilmer - industrial use
(Puritan Chem. Co.)

Hydrochloric acid *

RUST OFF
Multi-purpose rust & oxide film remover
(Conklin Co.)

Phosphoric acid *

RUST-OLEUM
Rust preventive coating
(Rust-Oleum)

Processed fish oil
Essential rust-inhibiting
pigments *† .... >10%

†See Rust control, Section VI, General Formulations

RUST-OLEUM ACID RESISTING COATING SYSTEMS
(Rust-Oleum)

Solvent type vinyl based 1-10%
Essential rust-inhibiting
pigmentation *† 1-10%

†See Rust control, Section VI, General Formulations

RUST-OLEUM CHEMICAL & WATER RESISTANT COATING SYSTEM
(Rust-Oleum)

Polyamide epoxy resin .... >10%
Essential rust-inhibiting
pigmentation *† .... >10%

†See Rust control, Section VI, General Formulations

RUST-OLEUM GENERAL PURPOSE RUST-PREVENTIVE PRIMERS AND FINISH COATINGS
(Rust-Oleum)

Combined amount: .... >10%
  Processed fish oil
  Alkyd resin
Essential rust-inhibiting
pigmentation *† .... >10%

†See Rust control, Section VI, General Formulations

RUST-OLEUM HEAT RESISTANT COATINGS
(Rust-Oleum)

Silicone & modified silicone resins >10%
Essential rust-inhibiting
pigmentation *† .... >10%

†See Rust control, Section VI, General Formulations

Starred ingredients (*) may be responsible for major toxic effects; consult Section II.

RUSTO LOTION
(Washington Hom.)

Grindelia robusta
Camphor *
Isopropanol *

RUST PROOF COMPOUND H
(Texaco Inc.)

Petrolatum
Corrosion inhibitor *†

†See Rust control, Section VI, General
Formulations

RUST PROOF COMPOUND L
(Texaco Inc.; Texaco Canada Ltd.)

Petrolatum
Corrosion inhibitor *†
Stoddard solvent *

†See Rust control, Section VI, General
Formulations

RUST PROOF COMPOUND LB
(Texaco Inc.)

Petrolatum
Corrosion inhibitor *†
Stoddard solvent *
Carbon black

†See Rust control, Section VI, General
Formulations

RUSTPRUF
Automotive
(Garry Labs.)

Sodium silicate
Sodium chromate *
Soda ash
Water

RUSTREM ANTI-RUST PAINT
(Speco)

Metallic pigments of: Chrome *,† Iron,
Aluminum, Copper *, Titanium
Lampblack
Resins
Plasticizers
Coal tar solvents *

'76 Ed.

†See Chromate salts

RUSTREM SOLVENT & THINNER
(Speco)

Coal tar aromatics *

'76 Ed.

RVPABA STICK
Topical sunscreen and cosmetic protective
(Elder)

p-Aminobenzoic acid *
In neutral red petrolatum wax base

RVP OINTMENT
Topical sunscreen
(Elder)

Red veterinary Petrolatum (Elder)

R-W LOTION
Relief of athlete's foot and ringworm
(Elmira Drug & Chem. Co.)

Benzoic acid *
Salicylic acid *
Isopropanol * 69%

RYLON HARD GLOSS PAINTS
(Touraine Paints, Inc.)

BLACK (#901):
  Carbon black 3.35%
  Soya alkyd resin solution (50%
    solids) 80.25%
  Thinner*† and drier* 16.40%
CHINESE RED (#925):
  Toluidine red 6.3%
  Dinitraniline orange 4.7%
  Soya alkyd resin solution (52.5%
    solids) 83.5%
  Thinner*† and drier* 5.5%
  Tinting color - less than 5%
DULL BLACK:
  Carbon black 2.16%
  Silica & silicates 6.64%
  Soya (maleic modified) alkyd
    resin solution (50% solids) .. 66.00%
  Thinner*† and drier* 25.20%
EMERALD (#919):
  Yellow iron oxide 3.31%
  Hansa yellow 3.31%
  Phthalocyanine blue 1.00%
  Soya alkyd resin solution (56.5%
    solids) 83.00%
  Thinner*† and drier* 9.24%
  Tinting color - less than 5%
HAZEL GREEN (#929):
  Titanium dioxide 12.85%
  Calcium carbonate 12.85%
  Soya alkyd resin solution (56.3%
    solids) 67.74%
  Thinner*† and drier* 7.06%
  Tinting color - less than 5%
IVORY (#913):
  Titanium dioxide 24.0%
  Soya alkyd resin solution (56.5%
    solids) 67.5%
  Thinner*† and drier* 8.5%
  Tinting color - less than 5%
MANDARIN RED (#911):
  Toluidine red 10.8%
  Soya alkyd resin solution (53.8%
    solids) 83.4%
  Thinner*† and drier* 5.8%
MAPLE (#920):
  Yellow iron oxide 12.11%
  Hansa yellow 2.52%
  Dinitraniline orange 3.97%
  Soya alkyd resin solution (56.5%
    solids) 73.26%
  Thinner*† and drier* 8.14%

(Continued next column)

Tinting color - less than 5%
PARAKEET YELLOW (#931):
  Titanium dioxide 21.2%
  Hansa yellow 5.3%
  Soya alkyd resin solution (56.6%
    solids) 66.1%
  Thinner*† and drier* 7.4%
  Tinting color - less than 5%
PRINCESS BLUE (#918):
  Titanium calcium 15.3%
  Calcium carbonate 3.1%
  Phthalcyanine blue 3.1%
  Soya alkyd resin solution (56.5%
    solids) 70.6%
  Thinner*† and drier* 7.9%
  Tinting color - less than 5%
ROB ROY BLUE (#927):
  See IVORY (#913) - same formulation
SILVER GRAY (#916):
  Titanium dioxide 15.8%
  Calcium carbonate 10.6%
  Soya alkyd resin solution (56.5%
    solids) 66.2%
  Thinner*† and drier* 7.4%
  Tinting color - less than 5%
STARDUST BLUE (#926):
  Titanium dioxide 7.33%
  Calcium carbonate 15.43%
  Silicates 6.54%
  Soya alkyd resin solution (55.4%
    solids) 64.77%
  Thinner*† and drier* 5.93%
  Tinting color - less than 5%
TURQUOISE (#932)
  See IVORY (#913) - same formulation
WALNUT BROWN (#912):
  Iron oxide 13.6%
  Calcium carbonate 4.9%
  Soya alkyd resin solution (56.5%
    solids) 73.3%
  Thinner*† and drier* 8.2%
  Tinting color - less than 5%
WHITE (#900):
  Titanium dioxide 30.0%
  Soya alkyd resin solution (56.5%
    solids) 60.2%
  Thinner*† and drier* 9.8%

'76 Ed.

†See Thinners, Section VI, General Formulations

RYNO-TOX
Insecticide
(Leffingwell)

Ryanodine alkaloid 0.08%

RYPLEX CEILING WHITE PAINT
(Touraine Paints, Inc.)

Titanium dioxide 17.2%
Silica & silicates 22.8%
Vinyl latex non-volatile 11.2%
Water 48.8%

'76 Ed.

RYPLEX PAINTS
(Touraine Paints, Inc.)

AUTUMN GOLD (#589):
Titanium dioxide	16.05%
Calcium carbonate	7.43%
Silica & silicates	14.80%
Vinyl latex non-volatile	11.53%
Water	50.14%

BLACK:
Lamp black	2.35%
Silica & silicates	13.10%
Calcium carbonate	23.65%
Vinyl latex non-volatile	11.05%
Water	49.85%

BUCKSKIN BEIGE (#583):
See AUTUMN GOLD (#589) - same formulation

CANDLELIGHT (#585):
Titanium dioxide	16.87%
Silica & silicates	22.93%
Vinyl latex non-volatile	11.26%
Water	49.01%

CATHAY (#578):
See AUTUMN GOLD (#589) - same formulation

CELERY (#587):
See CANDLELIGHT (#585) - same formulation

CELESTE BLUE (#564):
See AUTUMN GOLD (#589) - same formulation

CONGO IVORY (#572):
See CANDLELIGHT (#585) - same formulation

CORNSILK (#582):
See CANDLELIGHT (#585) - same formulation

GREEN MIST (#571):
Titanium dioxide	13.7%
Calcium carbonate	13.7%
Silica & silicates	11.2%
Vinyl latex non-volatile	11.48%
Water	49.90%

GREEN VELVET (#584):
See AUTUMN GOLD (#589) - same formulation

OFF WHITE (#579):
See CANDLELIGHT (#585) - same formulation

PARCHMENT WHITE (#588):
See CANDLELIGHT (#585) - same formulation

PORCELAIN BLUE (#570):
See GREEN MIST (#571) - same formulation

PROVINCIAL GOLD (#586):
See AUTUMN GOLD (#589) - same formulation

ROSE PETAL (#563):
See CANDLELIGHT (#585) - same formulation

SATINWOOD (#576):
See GREEN MIST (#571) - same formulation

SPEARMINT (#581):
See AUTUMN GOLD (#589) - same formulation

SUNLITE (#569):
See CANDLELIGHT (#585) - same formulation

TEAKWOOD (#568):
Titanium dioxide	9.95%
Calcium carbonate	15.15%
Silica & silicates	11.70%
Vinyl latex non-volatile	13.8%
Water	49.4%

WARM IVORY (#566):
See CANDLELIGHT (#585) - same formulation

WHITE (#561):
See CANDLELIGHT (#585) - same formulation

'76 Ed.

RYPLEX SAND FINISH PAINT
(Touraine Paints, Inc.)

Titanium dioxide	16.0%
Silica & silicates	27.6%
Vinyl latex non-volatile	10.7%
Water	45.7%

'76 Ed.

RYPLEX SEMI GLOSS PAINTS
(Touraine Paints, Inc.)

BLACK (#1060):
Carbon black	1.00%
Vinyl acrylic non-volatile	34.00%
Water	65.00%

BUCKSKIN BEIGE (#1083):
Titanium dioxide	18.8%
Silicates	4.7%
Vinyl acrylic non-volatile	25.4%
Water	51.1%

CATHAY (#1078):
See BUCKSKIN BEIGE (#1083) - same formulation

CELESTE BLUE (#1064):
See BUCKSKIN BEIGE (#1083) - same formulation

CORNSILK (#1082):
See BUCKSKIN BEIGE (#1083) - same formulation

GREEN VELVET (#1084):
See BUCKSKIN BEIGE (#1083) - same formulation

OFF WHITE (#1079):
See BUCKSKIN BEIGE (#1083) - same formulation

ROSE PETAL (#1063):
See BUCKSKIN BEIGE (#1083) - same formulation

SATINWOOD (#1076):
See BUCKSKIN BEIGE (#1083) - same formulation

SPEARMINT (#1081):
See BUCKSKIN BEIGE (#1083) - same formulation

WARM IVORY (#1066):
See BUCKSKIN BEIGE (#1083) - same formulation

WHITE (#1061):
Titanium dioxide	18.8%
Silicates	4.7%
Vinyl acrylic non-volatile	25.4%
Water	51.1%

'76 Ed.

RYTE RAT-25
Rodenticide
(Wright Rodent & Pest Control)

3-(alpha-Acetonylfurfuryl)-4-hydroxycoumarin	0.025%

RYTRON B
Hematinic
(Wesley Pharm.)

Each tablet:
Ferrous sulfate U.S.P. *	3 gr.
Thiamine hydrochloride	1 mg.
Riboflavin	1 mcg.

S

S-33
Acid cleaner
(Calgon Corp., Commercial Div.)

Sulfamic acid *

S-44
Detergent
(Calgon Corp., Commercial Div.)

Complex phosphates *
Sodium silicates
Ethylene oxide adducts
Alkaline salts *

S-49
Solvent
(Calgon Corp., Commercial Div.)

Petroleum distillate *
Chlorinated hydrocarbon solvents *

S-88
Steam cleaner
(Calgon Corp., Commercial Div.)

Caustic soda *
Alkaline salts *
Synthetic detergents

S-250
Stimulant
(Direct Div.)

Each capsule:
Caffeine *	250 mg.

S-406
Solvent cleaner, stripper
(Calgon Corp., Commercial Div.)

Methylene chloride *
Orthodichlorobenzene
Cresylic acid salts *
Petroleum distillate *
Emulsifiers

SABRE
Cold wave lotion
(Willat)

Ammonium thioglycolate	1-10%

S.A.C. COLD CAPSULES
(Towne, Paulsen)

Each capsule:
Pheniramine maleate *	5 mg.
Methapyrilene HCl *	5 mg.
Pyrilamine maleate *	10 mg.
Vitamin C	200 mg.
Hesperidin complex	100 mg.
Atropine sulfate	0.1 mg.
Salicylamide	250 mg.
Caffeine	30 mg.

Starred ingredients (*) may be responsible for major toxic effects; consult Section II.

S.A.C. COLD CAPSULES WITH PHENYLEPHRINE
(Towne, Paulsen)

Each capsule:
Pheniramine maleate *	5 mg.
Methapyrilene HCl *	5 mg.
Pyrilamine maleate *	10 mg.
Vitamin C	200 mg.
Hesperidin complex	40 mg.
Salicylamide	250 mg.
Caffeine	30 mg.
Phenylephrine HCl	5 mg.

S.A.C. MEDICATED THROAT LOZENGES
For relief of minor throat irritations
(Towne, Paulsen)

Each lozenge:
Benzocaine	10 mg.
Terpin hydrate	100 mg.
Phenylpropanolamine *	10 mg.
Cetyl pyridinium chloride	1:1500

S.A.C. NASAL SPRAY
Decongestant
(Towne, Paulsen)

Pheniramine maleate	0.03%
Methapyrilene HCl	0.03%
Pyrilamine maleate	0.04%
Phenylephrine HCl *	0.5%
Cetyl dimethyl benzyl ammonium chloride	0.05%
Thimerosal	0.001%

S-A-8 LIMITED PHOSPHATE (JAPAN)

See AMWAY S-A-8 LIMITED PHOSPHATE (JAPAN)

S-A-8 LIQUID LAUNDRY DETERGENT

See AMWAY S-A-8 LIQUID LAUNDRY DETERGENT

S-A-8 NO PHOSPHATE

See AMWAY S-A-8 NO PHOSPHATE

S-A-8 PLUS - MODIFIED

See AMWAY S-A-8 PLUS - MODIFIED

SAFE
Embalming powder, preservative, mold and mildew preventative
(Royal Bond)

Paraformaldehyde *
Paradichloro-benzene *

SAFECT AEROSOL
Insecticide
(Dro)

Pyrethrins	0.15%
Allethrin (Allyl homolog of cinerin I)	0.15%
N-Octyl bicycloheptene dicarboximide	0.75%
Tech. Piperonyl butoxide	0.50%
Tech. Methoxychlor	1.00%
Methylated naphthalenes	5.00%
Petroleum distillates	7.45%

'76 Ed.

SAFECT SPRAY
Insecticide
(Dro)

Petroleum distillate *	98.33%
N-Octyl bicycloheptene dicarboximide	1.08%
Tech. Methoxychlor	0.54%
Allethrin (Allyl homolog of cinerin I)	0.05%

'76 Ed.

SAFEGUARD
Antibacterial soap bar
(Procter & Gamble)

Soap from animal and vegetable fats	75-100%
Water	10-24%
Fatty acid	5-9%
Sodium chloride	1-4%
Perfume	1-4%
3,4,4'-Trichlorocarbanilide	1-4%
Minor ingredients, each	<1%

pH (1% solution) - 10.5

SAFE 'N SURE
Soap for industrial, hospital and office use
(Calgon Corp., Commercial Div.)

Soap
Water

SAFER AGRO-CHEM'S INSECTICIDAL SOAP
(Concentrate)
(Safer Agro-Chem)

Potassium salts of Fatty acids	50.50%
Water	16.16%
Alcohol (Ethanol) *	30.10%
Alcohol (Methanol)	3.24%

SAFE-T-SOLV SOLVENT CLEANER
(Consolidated Chem., Inc.)

Methylene chloride *
Perchloroethylene *
Mineral spirits *

SAF-T-FOG BRAND INSECTICIDE
(Puritan Chem. Co.)

Active ingredients:	100%
Petroleum distillate *	
N-Octyl bicycloheptene dicarboximide	
Technical Piperonyl butoxide	
Pyrethrins	

SAIL HEAVY DUTY BLUE ALL TEMPERATURE LAUNDRY DETERGENT
(Great Atlantic & Pacific)

Sodium linear alkyl benzene sulfonate	<20%
Sodium carbonate *	<30%
Sodium silicate	<12%
Sodium carboxymethylcellulose	<2%
Optical brighteners	<1%
Sodium chloride	<15%
Dye	trace
Sodium sulfate and moisture	balance

pH of 0.1% solution - 10.0-10.9

SAIL HEAVY DUTY LAUNDRY DETERGENT
(Great Atlantic & Pacific)

Sodium linear alkyl benzene sulfonate	<20%
Sodium carbonate *	<30%
Sodium silicate	<12%
Sodium carboxymethylcellulose	<2%
Optical brighteners	<1%
Sodium chloride	<15%
Sodium sulfate and moisture	balance

pH of 0.1% solution - 10.0-10.9

SAIL LIQUID LAUNDRY DETERGENT
(Great Atlantic & Pacific)

Sodium dodecylbenzene sulfonate	15.00%
Nonionic surfactant	10.00%
Sodium xylene sulfonate	4.00%
Sodium sulfate	3.00%
Opacifier	0.25%
Optical brightener	0.20%
Sodium citrate	0.10%
Perfume	0.09%
Dye	0.02%
Sodium hydroxide	0.01%
Water	balance

SALACID 25% AND SALACID 60%
Keratolytic ointment for removal of verrucae
(Gordon Labs.)

Salicylic acid *	25% or 60%

SALACTIC FILM
Keratolytic agent for the removal of verrucae
(Pedinol)

Salicylic acid (USP) *	16.7%
Lactic acid (USP) *	16.7%
Flexible Collodion (USP)	
Coloring agent	

Starred ingredients (*) may be responsible for major toxic effects; consult Section II.

SALAGEN TABLETS
Analgesic
(Lannett)

Aspirin * . . . . 10 gr.
Aluminum hydroxide
Magnesium hydroxide

SALASED
Urinary antiseptic, antispasmodic
(Wesley Pharm.)

Each tablet:
Methenamine . . . . 2 gr.
Salol * . . . . 1/2 gr.
Methylene blue . . . . 1/10 gr.
Benzoic acid . . . . 1/8 gr.
Atropine sulfate . . . . 1/1000 gr.
Hyoscyamine sulfate . . . . . 1/2000 gr.

SALATAR CREAM
Dermatological
(Lannett)

Solution of Coal tar 5%
Salicylic acid * 3%

SALETO
Analgesic
(Mallard)

Each tablet:
Aspirin * . . . . 210 mg.
Acetaminophen * . . . . 115 mg.
Salicylamide . . . . 65 mg.
Caffeine anhydrous . . . . 16 mg.

SAL HEPATICA
Laxative
(Bristol-Myers)

Monosodium phosphate *

SALIBAR, JR.
Analgesic, sedative
(Jenkins Labs.)

Each tablet:
Acetylsalicylic acid * . . . . 2 gr.
Phenobarbital (barbituric acid
derivative) * . . . . 1/8 gr.
Aromatics . . . . q.s.

SALIGEL
Acne gel
(Stiefel Labs.)

Salicylic acid * 5.0%
Alcohol 40.0%

SALIMEPH FORTE
Analgesic
(Kremers-Urban)

Each tablet:
Salicylamide * . . . . 600 mg.
Acetaminophen * . . . . 250 mg.

SALINEX
*Buffered isotonic saline nasal mist for
dry nasal membranes*
(Muro Pharm.)

Sodium chloride 0.4%
Propylene glycol . . . . <1%
Polyethylene glycol . . . . trace
Disodium EDTA . . . . trace
Hydroxypropyl methylcellulose . . . trace
Monosodium phosphate
monohydrate . . . . trace
Disodium phosphate anhydrous . . trace
Benzalkonium chloride 0.1%
Purified water . . . . qs ad

SALIVART
Synthetic saliva
(Westport Pharm.)

Each 100 ml.:
Carboxymethylcellulose
sodium . . . . 1.000 gr.
Sorbitol . . . . 3.000 gr.
Sodium chloride . . . . 0.084 gr.
Potassium chloride . . . . 0.120 gr.
Calcium chloride (2 HOH) . . 0.015 gr.
Magnesium chloride (6 HOH) 0.005 gr.
Potassium monohydrogen
phosphate . . . . 0.034 gr.
Propellant: Carbon dioxide (CO_2)

SALOMENTH OINTMENT
(Vale)

Menthol *
Methyl salicylate *

SALONIL
Keratolytic
(Torch)

Salicylic acid * 40%
Lanolin ad 100%

'76 Ed.

SALOXIUM
Analgesic
(Whitehall Labs.)

Each tablet:
Salicylsalicylic acid * . . . . 7 1/2 gr.

SALSBURY HOG & CATTLE SULFA WITH VITAMINS, ELECTROLYTES & EDDI
Drinking water medication
(Salsbury)

Sodium sulfathiazole
sesquihydrate * 68.65%
Ethylenediamine dihydroiodide,
Potassium chloride *, Sodium
chloride *, Sodium carbonate,
Sucrose, Vitamin A (1,000,000
I.U.) *, Vitamin D3 (800,000
I.C. units) * 31.35%

SALSBURY MALATHION DRY INSECTICIDE
Premium grade with deodorant
(Salsbury)

Malathion * 5%

SALSBURY MANGE & LICE CONTROL
Insecticide
(Salsbury)

Malathion * 57%
Solvent, Aromatic petroleum
derivative * 35%

SALSBURY 90-90-60 SULFA BOLUSES (WITH ELECTROLYTES)
For individual administration to live-stock
(Salsbury)

Each bolus:
Sulfathiazole * . . . . 90 gr.
Sulfanilamide * . . . . 90 gr.
Sulfamethazine * . . . . 60 gr.

SALSBURY TRIPLE SULFA SOLUBLE POWDER WITH VITAMINS & ELECTROLYTES
Water medication for poultry and live-stock
(Salsbury)

Sulfamerazine sodium * 27.20%
Sulfamethazine sodium * 27.20%
Sodium sulfathiazole
sesquihydrate * 29.85%
Vitamin A * . . . . 1,250,000 I.U.
Vitamin D3 * . . . . . . 625,000 I.C. units

SALSBURY TRIPLE SULFA SOLUTION
*Water medication with electrolytes for
poultry and livestock*
(Salsbury)

Each 100 cc:
Sulfathiazole sodium 3.65%
Sulfamethazine sodium 4.26%
Sulfamerazine sodium 3.13%

SAL-SEPT CREAM
For use in skin disorders
(Bio-Factor Labs.)

Each 100 gm.:
Salicylic acid * . . . . 3 gm.
Mixed Parasepts (Esters of p-hy-
droxybenzoic acid) * . . . . . . 12 gm.

Base:
Propylene glycol
Polyethylene glycol
Zinc stearate

'76 Ed.

SAL-SUDS
Cleaner
(Sanitek)

Anionic surfactants 8%
Nonionic surfactant 7%
Potassium-coconut oil soap 5%
Oleic acid 3%
Sodium EDTA 2%
Amphoteric surfactant 1%
Isopropyl myristate 1%
Water . . . . balance

Starred ingredients (*) may be responsible for major toxic effects; consult Section II.

SALUTE
Commercial dishwashing detergent
(Diversey Wyandotte)

Sodium metasilicate *
Sodium hypochlorite releasing agent

SALVASOL
Safety solvent and electric motor cleaner; industrial use
(Puritan Chem. Co.)

Petroleum distillates *
Chlorinated hydrocarbons *

SALVO WEED KILLER
Herbicide
(Olin Corporation)

Isooctyl ester of 2,4-dichlorophen-
oxyacetic acid * 81.8%
Petroleum distillates .... <10.0%

SAMSON DRAIN PIPE CLEANER
(Internat. Plumb.)

Sodium hydroxide *

'76 Ed.

SAMUEL CABOT PAINT PRODUCTS

See CABOT, SAMUEL, PAINT PROD-
UCTS

SANABALM EMOLLIENT SKIN CREAM
(Sanabalm)

Allantoin
Isopropyl myristate
Wax
Lanolin fractions
Liquid petrolatum
Sorbitan sesquioleate
Water

SANABALM POWDER
Medicated foot and body powder
(Sanabalm)

Talc
Boric acid *
Salicylic acid *
Zinc stearate
Thymol .... trace
Eucalyptol .... trace
Camphor .... trace
Formaldehyde .... trace

SANA-BOLE EMULSION TOILET BOWL CLEANER
Industrial and institutional use
(Puro Chem. Co.)

Hydrogen chloride * 26%

SANA-BOLE LIQUID DRAIN PIPE CLEANER & MAINTAINER
Industrial and institutional use
(Puro Chem. Co.)

Caustic soda (Sodium hydroxide) *

SANACLEAN PORCELAIN CLEANER, PL

See PL SANACLEAN PORCELAIN
CLEANER

SANAMINE DEODORANT GERMICIDE CLEANER
(Rochester Germicide)

n-Alkyl (60% C14, 30% C16, 5% C12,
5% C18) dimethyl benzyl ammonium chlorides * .... <10%
n-Alkyl (68% C12, 32% C14) dimethyl ethylbenzyl ammonium
chlorides * .... <10%
Sodium sesquicarbonate * .... <10%
Sodium carbonate * .... <10%
Tetrasodium ethylenediamine
tetraacetate .... <1%
Octyl phenoxy polyethoxy ethanol <10%
Water .... >80%

SAN-A-MOR
To sanitize poultry drinking water
(Hilltop)

Alkyl tolyl methyl trimethyl ammonium chloride * 5.2%
Propylene glycol solution 94.8%

'76 Ed.

SAN-A-MOR CONCENTRATE
*To disinfect and sanitize poultry drink-
ing water*
(Hilltop)

Alkyl tolyl methyl trimethyl ammonium
chloride *
Tetra sodium salt of ethylene diamine te-
tra-acetic acid
Trisodium phosphate *
Water and Sodium bicarbonate 74.4%

'76 Ed.

SANCAP 80W
Herbicide
(Ciba-Geigy Ag. Div.)

Dipropetryn (2-Ethylthio-4,6-
bis(isopropylamino)-s-triazine) * . 80%

SANCHIA SILICONE PROTECTIVE CREAM
For skin
(Clapp, Otis)

Silicone (Polydimethyl siloxane)

SAN-CURA OINTMENT
For skin and scalp irritations
(Thompson Med.)

Chlorobutanol (chloral derivative) .. 1%
Hexachlorophene
Benzocaine
Chlorothymol *
Benzoic acid *
Salicylic acid *
Benzyl alcohol
Cod liver oil
Lanolin
Petrolatum washable base

SANDEZE, EL PICO

See EL PICO SANDEZE

SANDRA LEE HEALTH & BEAUTY PRODUCTS

Sandra Lee Products
13165 N.W. 47th Ave.
Miami, Fla. 33054

Phone: 305-685-6089

See COSMETICS, Section VI, General
Formulations

SANDRIL TABLETS
Tranquilizer
(Lilly, Eli)

Reserpine *
Each tablet:
Green: .... 0.25 mg.
Orange: .... 0.1 mg.

SANFORD CASE SEALER
(Sanford Corp.)

Water
Gum arabic (or potato dextrine)
Phenol (as preservative) .... <1%

SANFORD CHECKWRITER NUMBERING MACHINE INK
(Sanford Corp.)

Pigments
Castor oil

SANFORD DELUXE MARKERS
Chisel point marker - permanent
(Sanford Corp.)

Aromatic solvent:
Xylene *
Toluene *
Dyes
Resins

SANFORD DRAWING INK
Water based ink
(Sanford Corp.)

Water
Dyes
Phenol (as preservative) .... <1%

Starred ingredients (*) may be responsible for major toxic effects; consult Section II.

SANFORD GOLD DECORATOR FLUID
Pigmented ink
(Sanford Corp.)

Pigments
Aromatic solvents:
  Contains Xylene *
Synthetic polymers

SANFORD HOT COLORS FLUORESCENT COLORS
(Sanford Corp.)

Pigments
Gum arabic (or bone glue)
Phenol (as preservative) .... <1%

SANFORD INDELIBLE INK, BLACK
(Sanford Corp.)

Nigrosine
Benzyl alcohol *
Butyl Cellosolve *

SANFORD KING SIZE MARKERS
Chisel point marker - permanent
(Sanford Corp.)

Aromatic solvent:
  Xylene *
  Toluene *
Dyes
Resins

SANFORD LIBRARY PASTE
(Sanford Corp.)

Water
Potato dextrine adhesive
Phenol (as preservative) .... <1%

SANFORD RECORDER PENS
(Sanford Corp.)

Glycerine
Glycols
Dyes

SANFORD RUBBER CEMENT
(Sanford Corp.)

Natural creppe rubber
Hexane *

SANFORD SILVER DECORATOR FLUID
Pigmented ink
(Sanford Corp.)

Pigments
Aromatic solvent:
  Contains Xylene *
Synthetic polymers

SANFORD STAMP PADS AND STAMP PAD INKS
(Sanford Corp.)

Glycerine
Glycols
Dyes

SANFORD TEMPERA
(Sanford Corp.)

Water
Pigments
Gum arabic (or bone glue)
Phenol (as preservative) .... <1%

SANFORD THINNER FOR RUBBER CEMENT
(Sanford Corp.)

Aliphatic solvents *

SANFORD WHITE DECORATOR FLUID
Pigmented ink
(Sanford Corp.)

Pigments
Aromatic solvent:
  Contains Xylene *
Synthetic polymers

SAN - HEAVY DUTY CLEANER & VARNISH CLEANER
(Savogran)

Trisodium phosphate * .... >50%
Sodium tetraborate * .... <20%
Sodium perborate * .... <20%
Soda ash * .... <20%

SANI-BANANA
Floor cleaner
(Sanitek)

Nonionic surfactants 5.0%
Acrylic copolymer emulsion, po-
  tassium salt 0.7%
Banana perfume, Dow 75, Dye . trace
Water .... balance

SANI-BOWL INDUSTRIAL BOWL CLEANER
(Uncle Sam)

Hydrogen chloride *
Inhibitors
Dye
Water

SANICIDE, SASCO

See SASCO SANICIDE

SANICO #600
Porcelain, enamel and metal cleaner
(Navy Brand)

Hydrogen chloride *
Ammonium chloride

SANI-DU
Sanitizer
(An-Fo)

Sodium dichloro-s-triazinetrione
  dihydrate * 20.25%
Sodium carbonate * 12.50%

SANI-FLUSH 4-MONTH AUTOMATIC BOWL CLEANER
(Boyle-Midway)

Calcium hypochlorite (as
  100%) * .... <20%
Calcium carbonate (and other
  inerts) .... balance

SANI-FLUSH TANK II AUTOMATIC TOILET BOWL CLEANER
(Boyle-Midway)

Blue Cake:
  Nonionic and anionic
    detergents .... <45%
  Sodium chloride and Sodium
    sulfate * .... <55%
  Dye .... <5%

White Tablet:
  Trichloroisocyanurate * 85-95%
  Boric acid .... <10%
  Sodium stearate .... <5%

SANI-FLUSH TOILET BOWL CLEANER (GRANULAR)
(Boyle-Midway)

Sodium bisulfate * 62%
Inerts including Sodium carbonate,
  Sodium chloride, Colorant,
  Fragrance 38%

SANI-FLUSH TOILET BOWL CLEANER (LIQUID)
(Boyle-Midway)

Hydrochloric acid * 7.00%
Oxalic acid * 2.00%
Alkyl trimethyl-ammonium
  chloride 0.25%

SANI-FLUSH TOILET CLEANER AND DEODORIZER (Liquid)
(Boyle-Midway)

Triclosan 0.970%
Sodium xylene sulfonate 1.000%
Essential oils 1.250%

SANI-FLUSH TOILET CLEANER & DEODORIZER (Solid)
(Boyle-Midway)

Nonionic detergents * .... >25%
Fragrance *†
Colorant

†*See* Essential oils

Starred ingredients (*) may be responsible for major toxic effects; consult Section II.

SANI-MIST (LIQUID)
Athletes foot treatment
(Sani-Mist, Inc.)

Undecylenic acid	<10%
Salicylic acid *	<5%
Menthol	<1%

SANI-POOL
(Austin, J.)

Sodium hypochlorite *	12%

SANI-SOAP
Veterinary
(Hilltop)

Vegetable oil base liquid soap
Fortified with Hexachlorophene   '76 Ed.

SANISPOT
Spot remover
(Sanitek)

Dipropylene glycol monomethyl ether (Cellosolve)	5%
Anionic surfactant	2%
Water	balance

SANISTRIP XL
Floor polish stripper
(Sanitek)

Dipropylene glycol monomethyl ether (Cellosolve)	2.9%
Sodium tripolyphosphate	2.4%
Nonionic surfactants	1.5%
Dimethylaminoethanol	1.5%
Anionic surfactants	1.2%
Perfume, Dye, Defoamer, Pine oil	trace
Water	balance

SANIT
Cleaner, disinfectant, deodorant, sanitizer; institutional use
(ABCO, Inc.)

Ortho-benzyl-para-chlorophenol	1.03%
Soap	5.05%
Trisodium phosphate	1.33%
Isopropyl alcohol	0.973%
Sodium xylene sulfonate	1.98%
Coconut diethanolamides	4.64%

SANITATE
Detergent, deodorant, sanitizer, disinfectant
(Basic Chemicals Inc.)

n-Alkyl (68% C12, 32% C14) dimethyl ethylbenzyl ammonium chloride *	2.25%
n-Alkyl (60% C14, 30% C16, 5% C12, 5% C18) dimethyl benzyl ammonium chloride *	2.25%

SANI-T-10 DISINFECTANT-SANITIZER-ALGICIDE

See SPARTAN SANI-T-10 DISINFECTANT-SANITIZER-ALGICIDE

SANITEK 18
Liquid floor wax
(Sanitek)

Various Waxes and Polyethylenes	14.6%
Rosin maleate resin	3.6%
Dimethylaminoethanol	0.7%
Potassium hydroxide (50% aq.)	0.3%
Dow 75 (Dow Chemical Co.)	trace
Ammonia	trace
Water	balance

SANITEK 40% COCO SOAP
Hand soap concentrate
(Sanitek)

Potassium-coconut oil soap	39%
Sodium EDTA	
Water	

SANITEK CONVEYOR CHAIN LUBRICANT
Conveyor belt lubricant
(Sanitek)

Potassium-tall oil-coconut oil soap	26.6%
Sodium EDTA	1.2%
Trisodium phosphate	1.0%
Water	balance

SANITEK CREME HAND LOTION
(Sanitek)

Propylene glycol	15.2%
Mineral oil	11.6%
Stearic acid	5.0%
Triethanolamine	1.9%
Lanolin	1.8%
Isopropanol	1.2%
Xanthan gum, Perfume, Dye	trace
Water	balance

SANITEK 40 OIL SOAP
Lubricant
(Sanitek)

Potassium-soybean oil soap	39%
Water	balance

SANITEK STAINLESS STEEL CLEANER
Liquid pump spray cleaner
(Sanitek)

Isopropanol *	57%
Mineral oil	25%
Dipropylene glycol monomethyl ether (Cellosolve)	17%
Silicone fluid	1%

SANITEK, T.C.M.
Hard surface cleaner
(Sanitek)

Isopropyl alcohol *	20%
Dipropylene glycol methyl ether (Cellosolve)	5%
Dye, Silicone	trace
Water	balance

SANITEK WAX WASH
Liquid floor cleaner
(Sanitek)

Potassium-soybean oil soap	14.0%
Waxes and Polyethylene	2.2%
Trisodium phosphate	1.4%
Pine oil	1.4%
Rosin maleate resin	0.6%
Lemon oil, Ammonia, Dimethylaminoethanol, Potassium hydroxide	trace
Water	balance

SANITIZ DISINFECTANT & GERMICIDE
(Lester Labs.)

Benzalkonium chloride (high molecular alkyl dimethyl benzyl ammonium chlorides) *	10%

'76 Ed.

SANITIZE
For sanitizing dishes, utensils
(Consolidated Chem., Inc.)

Methyldodecylbenzyl trimethyl ammonium chloride *	10%

SANITROL
Germicide and sanitizing agent
(Kem Mfg. Co.)

n-Alkyl (C14 50%, C12 40%, C16 10%)dimethyl benzyl ammonium chlorides *	10.00%
Ethanol	2.25%

SANI-TROL, FOREMOST 4555

See FOREMOST 4555 SANI-TROL

SANI-WAX PRODUCTS
Polishes & cleaners

Sani-Wax Inc.
P.O. Box 5126
Arlington, Tex. 76011

Phone: 817-461-1823

SANI-WHITE
Shoe polish
(Hollywood Shoe Polish)

Hollywood Shoe Polish, Inc.
7 East 43rd St.
New York, N.Y. 10017

Phone: 212-490-3163

SANMETTO
Urinary sedative
(Lambda Inc.)

Saw palmetto	
Sandalwood	
Corn silk	
Alcohol	20.6%

SAN-O-CAN GARBAGE CAN DEODORIZER
(ABCHEM)

Paradichlorobenzene * 99%

SAN-O-DIS
Disinfectant, sanitizer, deodorizer
(Stein Chemical Co.)

n-Alkyl (50% C12, 30% C14, 17% C16, 3% C18) dimethyl ethylbenzyl ammonium chloride * 5.0%
n-Alkyl (60% C14, 30% C16, 5% C12, 5% C18) dimethyl benzyl ammonium chloride * 5.0%

'76 Ed.

SAN ODORANT POWDER
Embalmers' supply
(Embalmers')

Zinc peroxide *
Paraformaldehyde *

SAN-O-FEC 2
Disinfectant, deodorant, sanitizer
(Whitmoyer)

Didecyl dimethyl ammonium chloride * 15%

SAN-O-FEC 5
Disinfectant, deodorant, sanitizer
(Whitmoyer)

Didecyl dimethyl ammonium chloride * 37.5%

SANOGENE (Liquid Concentrate)
Bacteriostat and sanitizer
(Bio-Cide)

Chlorine dioxide * 2%
Sodium carbonate 3%
De-ionized Water 95%

SAN-O-GENT, STEIN'S
See STEIN'S SAN-O-GENT

SAN-O-MINT, DEL
See DEL SAN-O-MINT

SAN-O-PINE
See LEEDSALL SAN-O-PINE

SANOX
Cleaner-disinfectant for hospital and institutional use
(Conklin Co.)

Didecyl dimethyl ammonium chloride * 4.5%
Tetrasodium ethylenediamine tetraacetate 2.0%
Sodium carbonate 1.0%
Sodium metasilicate (anhydrous) . . . 0.5%

SAN PHENO X
Germicide, disinfectant & deodorant
(Huntington Labs.)

Active ingred.: 21.6%
  Soap 9.0%
  Alcohol 6.0%
  Sodium salt of o-benzyl-p-chlorophenol 3.6%
  o-Benzyl-p-chlorophenol 3.0%
Inert ingred.: 78.4%
  Water 77.3%
  Glycerine 1.0%
  Sodium sulfite 0.1%

SANSERT TABLETS
Prophylactic agent for migraine headaches
(Sandoz)

Each tablet:
  Methysergide maleate USP * . . 2 mg.

SAN SOLVENT
Cesspool cleaner
(Vega)

Sodium hydroxide *

'76 Ed.

SANTA BARBARA FERAL PIGEON AND CROW BAIT - STARLICIDE TREATED GRAIN
(Santa Barbara)

Starlicide (3-Chloro-p-toluidine) . . 0.37%

SANTA BARBARA GOPHER POISON
Rodenticide
(Santa Barbara)

Rolled barley
Strychnine alkaloid * 0.2%

SANTA BARBARA GOPHER POISON STRYCHNINE BAIT
Rodenticide; for mechanical application only
(Santa Barbara)

Strychnine alkaloid * . . . . . . 1.3% or 2.6%

SANTA BARBARA PROLIN RAT BAIT
Rodenticide
(Santa Barbara)

3(a-Acetonylbenzyl)-4-hydroxycoumarin 0.25%
Sulfaquinoxalint (N'-(2-Quinoxalinyl)sulfanilamide) 0.25%

SANTA BARBARA RABBIT POISON
Rodenticide
(Santa Barbara)

Rolled barley
Strychnine alkaloid * 0.4%

SANTA BARBARA RODENT BAIT DIPHACINONE TREATED GRAIN
(Santa Barbara)

Diphacinone . . . . 0.005% or 0.01%

SANTA BARBARA RODENT BAIT ZINC PHOSPHIDE TREATED GRAIN
(Santa Barbara)

Zinc phosphide * 1.00%

SANTA BARBARA STARLING AND BLACKBIRD BAIT - STARLICIDE TREATED GRAIN
(Santa Barbara)

Starlicide (3-Chloro-p-toluidine hydrochloride) 0.92%

SANTA BARBARA STRYCHNINE BIRD POISON
(Santa Barbara)

Strychnine alkaloid * 0.55%

SANTA BARBARA STRYCHNINE HORN LARK POISON BAIT
(Santa Barbara)

Strychnine alkaloid * 0.65%

SANTA BARBARA STRYCHNINE LINNET POISON BAIT
(Santa Barbara)

Strychnine alkaloid * 0.43%

SANTA BARBARA STRYCHNINE SPARROW POISON BAIT
(Santa Barbara)

Strychnine alkaloid * 0.3%

SANTA BARBARA WARFARIN P TREATED GRAIN
(Santa Barbara)

Warfarin 0.025%
Sulfaquinoxaline 0.025%

Starred ingredients (*) may be responsible for major toxic effects; consult Section II.

SANTA FE NEUTRAL CLEANER
Floor cleaner
(Hillyard Chem.)

Liquid detergent *†

'76 Ed.

†*See* Detergents, Section VI, General Formulations

SANTI-DISH
Machine dishwashing compound
(Lester Labs.)

Phosphate *
Silicates
Detergents *

'76 Ed.

SAN VEINO
Embalmers' supply
(Embalmers')

Chlorinated hydrocarbons *

SAPOLIN PAINT PRODUCTS

Sapolin Paints, Inc.
1250 Broadway
New York, N.Y. 10001

Phone: 212-947-3070

See PAINTS, Section VI, General Formulations

SARAKA
Laxative
(Plough)

Frangula *
Gum karaya

SARCOMUL
Scabicide; veterinary
(Goshen Labs.)

Sulfur	2.25%

Cresols *
Pine oil *

SARGENT ART CRAYONS
(Sargent Art)

Waxes (paraffin, stearic acid and/or others)	65-95%
Colored pigments (non-toxic per manufacturer)	5-35%

SARGENT ART PAINTS
(Sargent Art)

Water solution containing gums and other non-toxic materials	60-90%
Color pigments (non-toxic per manufacturer)	10-40%

S.A.S.-500
Ulcerative colitis
(Rowell)

Each tablet:
Sulfasalazine *	500 mg.

SASCO COAL TAR DISINFECTANT
(S and S Co.)

Coal tar neutral oils *
Phenols *
Soap

SASCO PINE ODOR DISINFECTANT
(S and S Co.)

Alkyl (C14 58%, C16 28%, C12 14%) dimethyl benzyl ammonium chloride *	1.97%
Isopropanol	4.75%
Pine oil	3.95%
Water	89.33%

SASCO PINE OIL DISINFECTANT
(S and S Co.)

Pine oil *
Soap
Isopropyl alcohol *

SASCO ROACH & INSECT SPRAY
(S and S Co.)

Petroleum distillate *
Tech. Chlordane *

SASCO SANICIDE
Insecticide
(S and S Co.)

Petroleum distillates *
Tech. Piperonyl butoxide
Pyrethrins

SASCO-SOL LIQUID BOWL CLEANER
(S and S Co.)

Hydrogen chloride *	30.11%

para-Diisobutyl phenoxyethoxy-ethyl dimethyl benzyl ammonium chloride *

SASCO STERITONE
Disinfectant
(S and S Co.)

Soap
Orthobenzyl parachlorophenol *
Tetrasodium ethylene diamine tetraacetate *

SASTID (AL)
Acne scrub cleanser
(Stiefel Labs.)

Sulfur	1.6%
Salicylic acid *	1.6%
Aluminum oxide particles	20%

Base:
Soapless Surfactants

SASTID (PLAIN)
Acne scrub cleanser
(Stiefel Labs.)

Sulfur	1.6%
Salicylic acid *	1.6%

Base:
Soapless Surfactants

SASTID SOAP
For acne
(Stiefel Labs.)

Precipitated Sulfur	10.0%
Salicylic acid *	3.0%

SATE ARTERIAL AND CAVITY
Embalming fluid
(Embalmers')

Formaldehyde *

SATIN GLOSS NO RUBBING FLOOR WAX
(Uncle Sam)

Carnauba wax and/or synthetic waxes
Resins (modified phenolic)
Emulsifiers
Ammonia *
Polyethylene
Water

SATIN IMPERVO LOW LUSTRE ENAMEL (WHITE 235-01)
(Benjamin Moore)

Pigment:		43.0%
Titanium dioxide (type II)	67.0%	
Calcium carbonate	8.9%	
Silicates	24.1%	
Vehicle:		57.0%
Alkyd varnish:	79.3%	
Soya alkyd resin	48.7%	
Mineral spirits *	51.3%	
Mineral spirits *	20.2%	
Driers	0.5%	

SATINIQUE HAIR SPRAY WITH PROTEIN

See AMWAY SATINIQUE HAIR SPRAY WITH PROTEIN

SATIN-7
Plastic filler
(Unican)

Polyester resin	50%
Inert mineral Talc	49%
Black iron oxide pigment	1%

Catalysts:
  Solution:

Methyl ethyl ketone peroxide *	60%
Dimethyl phthalate	40%

    or
  Paste:

Benzoyl peroxide *	50%
Butyl benzyl phthalate	50%

'76 Ed.

SATINTONE GLAZES

See DUNCAN CERAMICS SATIN-TONE GLAZES (SA 300 Series)

SATIN ZAR
(United Gilsonite)

Oil modified polyurethane	43%
Mineral spirits *	55%
Colloidal silica	2%

SAUSALITO CREAM DEODORANT
(Mayer Labs.)

Aluminum chlorohydroxyallantoin

'76 Ed.

SAV-A-BRUSH BRUSH CLEANER
(Schalk)

Trisodium phosphate *

'76 Ed.

SAV-A-BRUSH, SUPER

See SUPER SAV-A-BRUSH

SAV-A-BRUSH, WATER RINSE

See WATER RINSE SAV-A-BRUSH

S A VAGINAL CREAM
(Wesley Pharm.)

Sulfanilamide *	15%
9-Aminoacridine hydrochloride	0.2%
Allantoin	2.0%

Dispersible base:
  Stearic acid
  Diglycol stearate
  Triethanolamine
  Propylene glycol
  Lactic acid
  Water

SAV-COTE PAINT PRODUCTS

Sav-Cote Chemical Labs., Inc.
P.O. Box 770
Lakewood, N.J. 08701

Phone: 201-364-4700

SAV-I OINTMENT
Treatment of irritation & minor infections of the eye lids
(Columbia Med.)

Mercuric oxide *	1%
Mineral oil-petrolatum base	

SAVOGRAN CRACK FILLER WATER PUTTY
(Savogran)

Calcium sulfate	>70%
Vegetable binder	

SAVOGRAN DEGLOSSER (BONDER-CLEANER)
(Savogran)

Mineral spirits *	50-70%
Methylene chloride *	20-40%
Methanol	<4%

SAVOGRAN DRIVEWAY CLEANER & DEGREASER
(Savogran)

Mineral spirits	<10%
Sodium metasilicate *	<10%
Surface active agents, etc.	<20%

SAVOGRAN TILE GROUT (READY TO USE)
(Savogran)

Calcium carbonate	<80%
Acrylic latex	<30%
Glycols	<5%

SAVOGRAN TILE GROUT (WATER MIX)
(Savogran)

Portland cement	45-65%
Flour sand	30-50%
Titanium pigment	<10%
Binders	

SAVOGRAN WOOD PUTTY
(Savogran)

Calcium sulfate hemihydrate	>70%
Wood flour	<20%
Vegetable binder	

SAVOL
Antiseptic-disinfectant, deodorant
(Savol)

Soap
Cresylic acid *
Oil of eucalyptus *
Oil of cassia *

SAVOL-CREAM
For skin irritations
(Savol)

Oil of camphor *
Betanaphthol *
Oil of eucalyptus *
Camphor gum *
Menthol *
Zinc oxide

SAV-ON DEODORIZING BLOCKS
(Uncle Sam)

Paradichlorobenzene *
Essential oils *

SAV-ON PINE ODOR DIS COEF 3 & 5
(Uncle Sam)

Alcohol *
Pine oil *
Soap
Synthetic Phenol *
Ethylenediaminetetraacetate
Water

SAV-ON PINE SCRUB SOAP
(Uncle Sam)

Pine oil *
Vegetable oil soap
Water

SAVOSS
Counterirritant; veterinary
(Troy Chem.)

Isopropyl alcohol *	15%

Oil wormwood *†
Iodine *
Camphor *
Tar *
Cedar *
Pine *
Turpentine distillates *

†*See* Volatile oils

SAWYER'S CRYSTAL AMMONIA
(Wright, J.A.)

Ammonium hydroxide (15°BE) *

SAWYER'S CRYSTAL BLUE
(Wright, J.A.)

Water	
Dye	
Oxalic acid	<1%

S.B.P. PLUS
Sedative-hypnotic
(Lemmon Co.)

Each tablet:

Sodium secobarbital *	50 mg.
Sodium butabarbital *	30 mg.
Phenobarbital	15 mg.
Homatropine methylbromide	2.5 mg.

Starred ingredients (*) may be responsible for major toxic effects; consult Section II.

SBS-50 CLEANER-DISINFECTANT
(Sugar Beet)

Ethoxylated linear alcohol-type of non-ionic detergent
Hyamine 3500 (see quaternary ammonium compounds) *
Phosphates and other alkaline salts *

'76 Ed.

SBS-60 CREAM DEODORANT SOAP
(Sugar Beet)

Cellulose and alginate gums
Lanolin
Synthetic detergent
Soap compatible germicide (Chlorinated xylenol type) *
Fatty acid-ethanolamine soap

'76 Ed.

SBS-221 HEAVY DUTY ALL-SOLUBLE BORAX HAND SOAP
(Sugar Beet)

Soda soap
Borax *

'76 Ed.

SBS-71 HEAVY DUTY LOTION DEODORANT SKIN CLEANSER
(Sugar Beet)

Cellulose gum	0.5-1.0%
Synthetic detergents *	15-20%
Germicide (chlorinated xylenol type)	0.5-5.0%
Polyglycol esters	1-5%
Lanolin	0.5-1.0%
Scent & dye (D&C #19 Red)	<0.3%

'76 Ed.

SBS-61 HEAVY DUTY LOTION DEODORANT SOAP
(Sugar Beet)

Fatty acid - ethanolamine soap	20-25%
Germicide (chlorinated xylenol type)	0.5-5%
Synthetic detergents	0-6%
Perfume	0.1-0.5%
Dye	0.03-0.1%
Lanolin	0.5-1.0%

'76 Ed.

SBS-72 LIGHT DUTY LOTION DEODORANT SKIN CLEANSER
(Sugar Beet)

Synthetic detergents *	10-20%
Lanolin	0.5-1%
Perfume and dye (D&C Blue #1)	<0.3%
Germicide (chlorinated xylenol type)	0.5-5%
Polyglycol esters	3-5%
E.D.T.A. acid	<0.5%
Sodium nitrite	<0.5%

'76 Ed.

SBS-40 MEDICATED SKIN CREAM
(Sugar Beet)

Polyethylene glycol ether
Fatty acid ester
Wax ester
Germicide, chlorinated xylenol type *†
Petrolatum
Synthetic detergent *
Lanolin
Glyoxyl diureide
Carboxy vinyl polymer

'76 Ed.

†See 4-Chloro-3,5-xylenol

SBS-41 MEDICATED SKIN LOTION
(Sugar Beet)

Polyethylene glycol ether	1-5%
Fatty acid ester	1-5%
Wax ester	5%
Germicide (chlorinated xylenol type)	0.5-1%
Petrolatum	1-5%
Cellulose gum	<0.5%
Lanolin	0.5-1.0%
Glyoxyl diureide	<0.5%
Carboxy vinyl polymer	<0.5%
Hydroxybenzoic acid esters	<0.5%
Scent	0.1-0.5%

'76 Ed.

SBS-11 SKIN CLEANSER
(Sugar Beet)

Soda soaps
Corn meal
Cob
Rice hulls

'76 Ed.

SBS-30 WATERLESS HAND CLEANER
(Sugar Beet)

Paraffin type hydrocarbon *
Fatty acid-alkolamine soap
Synthetic detergent *
Polyglycol
Lanolin
Cellulose gum
Perfume
Para chloro meta xylenol (bacteriostat)

'76 Ed.

SCADAN
Scalp lotion
(Dome)

Cetyl trimethyl ammonium bromide (Cetab)	1%
Stearyl dimethyl benzyl ammonium chloride	0.1%

SCALECIDE
Ovicide
(Pratt-Gabriel Div.)

Petroleum oil * ... 98%

SCALE GON
Descaler
(Calgon Corp., Commercial Div.)

Phosphoric acid *
Emulsifiers
Water

SCALE KING
Rust & scale remover
(Lester Labs.)

Sulfamic acid *
Corrosion inhibitors

'76 Ed.

SCALE-LAX
To open clogged drains & pipes
(Radiator)

Hydrochloric acid *

'76 Ed.

SCALE-OFF
Concentrated inhibited chemical cleaner; industrial and institutional use
(Scientific International)

Hydrochloric acid *

SCALE-RID
Insecticide
(Agway)

Ethion *	2.0%/wt.
Petroleum oil (Superior type 60 second oil) *	95.0%/wt.

SCALE-TOX
Insecticide
(Miller Chem. & Fert.)

Petroleum oil * ... 97%

SCANNON PERFUMES & TOILETRIES

Scannon Ltd.
650 Fifth Ave.
New York, N.Y. 10019

Phone: 212-246-3070

See COSMETICS, Section VI, General Formulations

SCAN-X
Surface disinfectant · deodorizer · air refreshener
(ABCO, Inc.)

Active ingred.:	53.7%
n-Alkyl (60% C14, 30% C16, 5% C12, 5% C18) dimethyl benzyl ammonium chloride	0.1%
n-Alkyl (68% C12, 32% C14) dimethyl ethylbenzyl ammonium chloride	0.1%
Isopropanol *	53.0%
Essential oils	0.5%
Inert ingred.:	46.3%
Dichlorodifluoromethane	
Water	
Triethylene glycol	
Sodium nitrite	

SCATTER PERM PRODUCTS
(Gillette Co., Personal Care Div.)

The Gillette Co., Personal Care Div., Boston, Mass. 02199 will receive collect phone calls from poison control centers or physicians asking for emergency toxicological information about the company's products.

Phone: 617-421-7000

S.C.C. LIQUID CLEANER CONCENTRATE
(Solvit)

Liquid wetting agents *†	
Sodium carbonate	small amount
Chelating agent:	small amount
NA4EDTA (Tetrasodium EDTA)	

†*See* Synthetic detergents

SCENE WINDOW, GLASS AND MULTI-PURPOSE CLEANER
(Nat'l Labs. Div.)

Ammonium hydroxide	minor
Isobutane (propellant)	minor
Ethyl alcohol	major

SCENT-AWAY DEODORIZER
Controls odors in septic tanks, cesspools, land fill areas; industrial and institutional use
(Scientific International)

Orthodichlorobenzene *

SCENT-OFF PELLETS
Dog and cat repellent
(Johnson Nurseries, Div. of Plantabbs)

Oil of lemongrass	2%
Oil of citronella	1.2%
Allyl isothiocyanate (Imitation oil of mustard)	0.2%
Blend of Oil of orange, Methyl salicylate, Geraniol, Ionone alpha, Oil of bergamot	0.2%
Inert ingredients:	
Paraffin wax	96.1%
Coal tar dye	0.3%

SCENT-OFF "TWIST-ONS"
Dog and cat repellent
(Johnson Nurseries, Div. of Plantabbs)

Oil of lemongrass	2%
Oil of citronella	1.2%
Allyl isothiocyanate (Imitation oil of mustard)	0.2%
Blend of Oil of orange, Methyl salicylate, Geraniol, Ionone alpha, Oil of bergamot	0.2%
Inert ingredients:	
Paraffin wax	96.1%
Coal tar dye	0.3%

SCENT O' LEMON
Disinfectant, sanitizer, cleaner
(Weil Chem.)

N-Alkyl (C12, C14, C16, C18) dimethyl benzyl ammonium chlorides *
N-Alkyl (C14, C16, C12, C18) dimethyl ethylbenzyl ammonium chlorides *
Tetrasodium ethylenediamine tetraacetate
Tetrapotassium pyrophosphate
Isopropyl alcohol
Nonyl phenyl polyethylene glycol ether

SCHALK'S DEGLOSSER
(Schalk)

Xylene *
Acetone
Petroleum distillate
Ethanol

'76 Ed.

SCHALK'S PATCH PASTE
(Schalk)

Mineral spirits *

'76 Ed.

SCHALK'S SPOT DRY CLEANER
(Schalk)

Perchlorethylene *

'76 Ed.

SCHALK'S WATERLESS HAND CLEANER
(Schalk)

Petroleum distillate *

'76 Ed.

SCHAMBERG'S LOTION
Temporary relief of itching
(C & M Pharmacal)

Menthol	0.15%
Phenol	1.0%
Zinc oxide	
Peanut oil	
Lime water	
Dispersant	

SCHNEID'S ALGAECIDE 1250
Swimming pool algaecide and germicide
(Schneid)

Active ingredients:	10.00%
N-Alkyl (C14, C16, C12, C18) dimethyl benzyl ammonium chlorides *	
N-Alkyl (C12, C14, C16, C18) dimethyl ethylbenzyl ammonium chlorides *	
Inert ingredients:	90.00%
Water	
Isopropanol	

'76 Ed.

SCHNEID'S BLACK DISINFECTANT
Phenol coefficient 2
(Schneid)

Active ingredients:	90%
Coal tar neutral oils *	
Sodium soap	
Coal tar acids *	
Inert ingredients:	10%
Water	

'76 Ed.

SCHNEID'S BLACK DISINFECTANT
Available in phenol coefficients 3, 5 or 6
(Schneid)

Active ingredients:	90%
Coal tar neutral oils *	
Sodium soap	
Coal tar acids *	
Cresylic acid *	
Inert ingredients:	10%
Water	

'76 Ed.

SCHNEID'S BOWL KLEAN
(Schneid)

Hydrochloric acid *

'76 Ed.

SCHNEID'S FOGGING SPRAY CONCENTRATE
Insecticide
(Schneid)

Petroleum distillate *	99.02%
N-Octyl bicycloheptene dicarboximide	0.52%
Technical Piperonyl butoxide	0.31%
Pyrethrins	0.15%

'76 Ed.

Starred ingredients (*) may be responsible for major toxic effects; consult Section II.

SCHNEID'S LEMON DISINFECTANT
(Schneid)

Potassium coconut soap	8.05%
Sodium orthobenzylparachlorophenate	3.34%
Isopropyl alcohol	3.02%
Terpineols	1.91%
Essential oils	0.32%

'76 Ed.

SCHNEID'S PINE OIL DISINFECTANT
Institutional and industrial use
(Schneid)

Pine oil *	80%
Soap	10%
Water	10%

'76 Ed.

SCHNEID'S POWDER CONCENTRATE BOWL CLEANER
(Schneid)

Hydrogen chloride *	24%

'76 Ed.

SCHNEID'S ROACH AND ANT SPRAY
(Schneid)

Petroleum distillate *	98.19%
Aromatic petroleum derivatives	1.00%
Technical Dieldrin	0.50%
N-Octyl bicycloheptene dicarboximide	0.16%
Technical Piperonyl butoxide	0.10%
Pyrethrins	0.05%

'76 Ed.

SCHOLL DRY ANTI-PERSPIRANT SPRAY
(Scholl)

Aluminum chlorhydrate *

SCHOLL'S, DR., PRODUCTS
See DR. SCHOLL

SCHULTZ INSTANT LIQUID PLANT FOOD
(Schultz Co.)

Urea
Potassium phosphates *
Potassium nitrates *
Water

SCHULTZ INSTANT SOLUBLE PLANT FOOD
(Schultz Co.)

Urea
Potassium phosphates *
Potassium nitrates *

SCIENCE BENOMYL
Systemic fungicide for lawn diseases
(Science Prod.)

Benomyl	50%

SCIENCE BERRY-SET
Hormone-type spray for bigger berries
(Science Prod.)

Beta-naphthoxyacetic acid	2.67%

SCIENCE BLOSSOM-SET
Plant growth regulator
(Science Prod.)

Beta-naphthoxyacetic acid	
4 fl. oz. container	0.1389%
8 fl. oz. container (concentrate)	3.6575%
8 and 12 oz. spray containers	0.0042%

SCIENCE CLOVER MITE & RED SPIDER SPRAY (AEROSOL & PUMP-TYPE)
(Science Prod.)

1,1-Bis(chlorophenyl)-2,2,2-trichloroethanol	0.25%

SCIENCE CRAB GRASS KILLER
(Science Prod.)

Octylammonium methanearsonate *	8%
Dodecylammonium methanearsonate *	8%

SCIENCE DIAZINON SPRAY
Multi-purpose insecticide
(Science Prod.)

O,O,-Diethyl O-(2-isopropyl-4-methyl-6-pyrimidinyl) phosphorothioate *	12.5%
Aromatic petroleum derivative solvent *	72.6%

SCIENCE DURSBAN INSECTICIDE
(Science Prod.)

Chlorpyrifos	6.0%
Aromatic petroleum derivative solvent *	3.4%
Xylene *	84.5%

SCIENCE EPTAM GARDEN WEED CONTROL
Herbicide
(Science Prod.)

S-Ethyl dipropylthiocarbamate	2.3%

SCIENCE FORE LAWN AND ORNAMENTAL FUNGICIDE
(Science Prod.)

Co-ordination product of Zinc ion and Manganese ethylene bisdithiocarbamate *†	80%

†*See* Maneb and Zineb

SCIENCE FRUIT, NUT & GARDEN SPRAY
(Science Prod.)

O,O-Diethyl O-(2-isopropyl-4-methyl-6-pyrimidinyl) phosphorothioate	8.30%
1,1-Bis(chlorophenyl)-2,2,2-trichloroethanol	3.20%
Xylene *	79.26%

SCIENCE FRUIT-TREE AND BERRY SPRAY
(Science Prod.)

Technical Methoxychlor *	19.75%
Malathion *	7.50%
Captan	15.00%

SCIENCE GARDEN INSECT SPRAY
(Science Prod.)

Malathion	12.5%
Methoxychlor (technical)	12.5%
Xylene *	69.0%

SCIENCE GARDEN-LIFE SOLUBLE PLANT FOOD
(Science Prod.)

Total Nitrogen	10%
Available Phosphoric acid *	52%
Water soluble Potash	17%

SCIENCE GARDEN WEEDER
(Science Prod.)

Dacthal	5%

SCIENCE GLADIOLUS AND BULB DUST
Controls storage rot and thrips
(Science Prod.)

Thiram *	50%
Methoxychlor (technical)	5%

SCIENCE GRASS & WEED TOP-KILLER
(Science Prod.)

Sodium cacodylate *	12.6%
Dimethylarsinic acid (Cacodylic acid)	2.2%

Starred ingredients (*) may be responsible for major toxic effects; consult Section II.

SCIENCE HEDGE-TRIM
Plant growth regulator
(Science Prod.)

Diethanolamine salt of 1,2-dihydro-
3,6-pyridazinedione (equiv. to 30%
Maleic hydrazide) * 58%

SCIENCE HORNET & WASP BOMB
(Science Prod.)

Malathion	3.00%
2,2-Dichlorovinyl dimethyl phosphate	0.46%
Related compound	0.04%
Xylene *	15.00%
Petroleum distillate	43.00%

SCIENCE HOUSEHOLD INSECT BOMB
(Science Prod.)

Baygon	0.5%
Petroleum distillate *	69.00%

SCIENCE HOUSE PLANT INSECTICIDE
(Science Prod.)

Pyrethrins	0.025%
Rotenone	0.140%
Other Cube resins	0.280%
Technical Piperonyl butoxide	0.250%
Petroleum distillate	0.100%

SCIENCE KELTHANE EC
Miticide
(Science Prod.)

1,1-Bis(chlorophenyl)-2,2,2-trichloroethanol	18.5%
Xylene *	73.0%

SCIENCE LAWN WEED-KILLER
(Science Prod.)

Dimethylamine salt of dicamba	3.42%
Dimethylamine salt of related acids	0.56%
Dimethylamine salt of 2,4-dichlorophenoxyacetic acid *	17.12%

SCIENCE LIQUID FERTILIZER 12-6-6
(Science Prod.)

Total Nitrogen (N)	12%
Available Phosphoric acid (P2O5) *	6%
Soluble Potash (K2O) *	6%

SCIENCE 57% MALATHION SPRAY
Insecticide
(Science Prod.)

Malathion *	57%
Xylene *	31%

SCIENCE 25% METHOXYCHLOR SPRAY
Insecticide
(Science Prod.)

Methoxychlor (technical)	25%
Xylene *	72%

SCIENCE MULTI-PURPOSE GARDEN DUST OR SPRAY
(Science Prod.)

Technical Methoxychlor	5%
Malathion *	5%
Captan	5%

SCIENCE RABBIT AND DEER REPELLENT
(Science Prod.)

Thiram *	20%

SCIENCE ROSE AND FLORAL DUST
Insecticide-fungicide
(Science Prod.)

Carbaryl *	3%
Malathion	4%
Folpet	5%
1,1-Bis(chlorophenyl)-2,2,2-trichloroethanol	1.5%

SCIENCE ROSE AND FLORAL SPRAY
Insecticide-fungicide-miticide
(Science Prod.)

Pyrethrins	0.0258%
Piperonyl butoxide (technical)	0.2582%
Rotenone	0.1286%
Other Cube resins	0.1930%
Captan	0.5136%
2,4-Dinitro-6-octyl phenyl crotonate and 2,6-Dinitro-4-octyl phenyl crotonate	0.1465%
Nitrooctyl phenols (principally dinitro)	0.0100%
Petroleum distillate	0.2015%

SCIENCE ROSE AND GARDEN FUNGICIDE
(Science Prod.)

Folpet	75%

SCIENCE SEED PROTECTANT
(Science Prod.)

Thiram *	50%

SCIENCE SEVIN LIQUID
Insecticide for lawns, gardens, ornamentals
(Science Prod.)

Carbaryl *	22.5%

SCIENCE SPREADER-STICKER
Makes chemical sprays more effective
(Science Prod.)

Modified Phthalic glyceryl alkyd
resin *† 77%

†*See* Polyester resins

SCIENCE STOP-GRASS
Chemical grass edger
(Science Prod.)

Diethanolamine salt of 1,2-dihydro-
3,6-pyridazinedione (equiv. to 30%
Maleic hydrazide) * 58%

SCIENCE STUMP REMOVER
(Science Prod.)

Potassium nitrate *

SCIENCE SYSTEMIC INSECTICIDE GRANULES
(Science Prod.)

O,O-Diethyl S-(2-(ethylthio)ethyl)
phosphorodithioate * 1%

SCIENCE SYSTEMIC SPRAY
Insecticide
(Science Prod.)

S-(2-(Ethylsulfinyl)ethyl) O,O-dimethyl phosphorothioate	6.0%
Methoxychlor (technical)	5.0%
1,1-Bis(p-chlorophenyl)-2,2,2-trichloroethanol	0.9%
Xylene *	49.6%

SCIENCE THURICIDE
Insecticide
(Science Prod.)

Bacillus thuringiensis Berliner, 4000 I.U. per mg.	0.8%
Petroleum hydrocarbon solvent	3.0%

SCIENCE TOMATO-GRO
Plant food
(Science Prod.)

Total Nitrogen (N)	10%
Available Phosphoric acid (P2O5) *	52%
Soluble Potash (K2O) *	17%

SCIENCE TOMATO SAVER
Plant growth regulator
(Science Prod.)

Calcium (derived from 21.0% calcium chloride) 7.58%

SCIENCE TOMATO & VEGETABLE DUST
Insecticide, fungicide
(Science Prod.)

Carbaryl *	5.0%
Zineb (metallic zinc equiv. 1.65%)	7.0%

Starred ingredients (*) may be responsible for major toxic effects; consult Section II.

SCIENCE VAPAM SOIL FUMIGANT SOLUTION
(Science Prod.)

Sodium methyldithiocarbamate
　(anhydrous) * 32.7%

SCIENCE ZINEB GARDEN FUNGICIDE
(Science Prod.)

Zineb (metallic zinc equiv. 17.7%) .. 75%

SCODONNAR (ELIXIR & TABLETS)
Antispasmodic
(Vitarine)

Each 5 cc or tablet:
Phenobarbital (1/4 gr.) ...... 16.2 mg.
Hyoscyamine sulfate ...... 0.1037 mg.
Atropine sulfate .... 0.0194 mg.
Hyoscine hydrobromide ... 0.0065 mg.

S-523 CONCENTRATED INSECTICIDE

See PL S-523 CONCENTRATED IN-
　SECTICIDE

SCOOT
*Cleaner and brightener for aluminum
and stainless steel; industrial use*
(Puritan Chem. Co.)

Hydrofluoric acid *
Phosphoric acid *

SCOPE
Mouthwash and gargle
(Procter & Gamble, Health & Personal
Care Div.)

Cetylpyridinium chloride 0.045%
Domiphen bromide 0.005%
Ethyl alcohol .... 16% w/w
Glycerol 10-20%
Minor ingredients, each ...... <1%
Water .... >50%

SCORE
Gym finish
(Holcomb)

Mineral spirits * .... >10%
High flash naphtha * .... >10%
　　　　　　　　　　　'76 Ed.

SCORE HAIR GROOM
(Bristol-Myers)

Water
Mineral oil
Glycerin
Lauramide DEA
Sodium laureth-4 phosphate
Sodium oleth-7 phosphate
Steareth-20
Lanolin alcohol
Isopropyl myristate
MDM hydantoin
Fragrance
D & C Green No. 6
D & C Violet No. 2

SCOTCH HEATHER
Air deodorizer
(Barco)

Isopropyl alcohol 9.00%
Triethylene glycol 7.50%
Propylene glycol 3.00%
Methyldodecylbenzyl trimethyl
　ammonium chloride 0.40%
Essential oil aromatic 0.25%
　　　　　　　　　　　'76 Ed.

SCOTCH WAX
Automotive
(McAleer)

Mineral spirits *
Waxes
Silicone oils
Diatomaceous earth
Amyl acetate *
　　　　　　　　　　　'76 Ed.

SCOTTS CRABGRASS PREVENTER AND DANDELION CONTROL PLUS FERTILIZER
(Scott, O.M.)

Bensulide 5.10%
2,4-Dichlorophenoxyacetic acid .. 0.76%
2-(4-Chloro-2-methylphenoxy) pro-
　pionic acid 0.76%
Fertilizer formula: 20-6-6

SCOTT'S EMULSION
Vitamin A & D food supplement
(Beecham Products)

Each 4 teaspoons:
Vitamin A .... 5000 I.U.
Vitamin D .... 400 I.U.

SCOTTS GOOSEGRASS/ CRABGRASS
Control for Bermuda grass
(Scott, O.M.)

Bensulide 5.25%
Oxadiazon 1.31%
Carrier base: Corncobs

SCOTTS LAWN DISEASE PREVENTER
Fungicide
(Scott, O.M.)

Pentachloronitrobenzene * 16.9%
Carrier: Vermiculite

SCOTTS LAWN INSECT CONTROL
(Scott, O.M.)

Diazinon * 4.5%
Carrier: Corncobs

SCOTTS LAWN INSECT CONTROL PLUS FERTILIZER
(Scott, O.M.)

Diazinon * 3.60%
Carrier: Fertilizer 28-6-4

SCOTTS LAWN WEED CONTROL
(Scott, O.M.)

2,4-Dichlorophenoxyacetic acid ... 2.95%
Dicamba 0.48%
Carrier: Vermiculite

SCOTT'S LIQUID GOLD
Wood cleaner
(Scott's Liquid Gold)

Fragrance 1%/v
Naphtha * .... approx. 15%/v
1,1,1-Trichloroethane * .. approx. 10%/v
Corvus or equivalent *† .. approx. 75%/v

†*See* Mineral oils (unspecified)

SCOTTS ORNAMENTAL HERBICIDE I
(Scott, O.M.)

Oxadiazon 2%
Carrier base: Clay

SCOTTS STARTER FERTILIZER WITH CRABGRASS PREVENTER
(Scott, O.M.)

Siduron 3.10%
Fertilizer formula: 16-21-5

SCOTTS SUMMER CRABGRASS CONTROL
(Scott, O.M.)

Disodium methanearsonate * 2.90%
Carrier: Vermiculite

SCOTTS WESTERN LAWN INSECT CONTROL
(Scott, O.M.)

Dursban * 1.35%
Carrier: Vermiculite

SCOTTS WESTERN LAWN INSECT CONTROL PLUS FERTILIZER
(Scott, O.M.)

Dursban 0.55%
Carrier: Fertilizer 30-5-3

SCRAM
Dog repellent spray
(Chevron)

Bone oil 0.50%
Paradichlorobenzene 1.00%
Allyl isothiocyanate 0.30%
Oil sassafras (artificial) * 0.50%

Chevron emergency phone number:
415-233-3737

SCREWLOOSE

See SILOO SCREWLOOSE

SCRIPTO BUTANE LIGHTER FUEL
(Scripto)

Lower aliphatic hydrocarbon mixture consisting primarily of Isobutane *

SCRIPTO ERASABLE BALL PEN INKS
(Scripto)

Pigments *
Mineral oil
Aliphatic hydrocarbons
Fatty acids
Natural or synthetic rubber

SCRIPTO FIBER TIPPED PEN OR ROLLING PEN INK
(Scripto)

Aqueous solutions of water soluble dyestuffs
Glycols (small quantities)
Phenolic and/or acidic preservatives (trace amounts)

SCRIPTO INKS, BALL PEN
(Scripto)

Dyestuffs
Alcoholic, glycolic or glycolic ether solvents
Fatty acids and/or other surface active agents

S.C. - SUPER CONCENTRATE DEGREASER (Liquid)

See GUNK S.C. - SUPER CONCENTRATE DEGREASER (Liquid)

SCULPTAMOLD
Powdered sculpting and modeling media
(American Art Clay Co.)

This product bears the CP Seal issued by the Crayon, Water Color and Craft Institute, Inc. This seal certifies that the product contains no materials in sufficient quantities to be toxic or injurious to the human body even if ingested.

SCUM-A-WAY SCUM REMOVER
(Uncle Sam)

Surfactants *
Chelaters
Wetting agent
Water

SEA BREEZE ANTISEPTIC FOR THE SKIN
(Sea Breeze)

Alcohol 43%/v
Synthetic Camphor .... <1%
Oil of peppermint .... <1%
Oil of cloves .... <1%
Benzoic acid .... <1%
Eugenol .... <1%
Oil of eucalyptus .... <1%
Boric acid .... <1%

SEA BREEZE COMPLEXION BAR
(Sea Breeze)

Anhydrous Soap 82-87%
Water 10-14%
Fragrance .... <2%
Glycerine .... <2%
Sodium chloride .... <1%
Titanium dioxide .... <1%
O-Tolyl biguanide .... <1%

SEA BREEZE MEDICATED SHAVE LOTION
(Sea Breeze)

Alcohol 43%/v
Synthetic Camphor .... <1%
Oil of peppermint .... <1%
Oil of cloves .... <1%
Benzoic acid .... <1%
Eugenol .... <1%
Oil of eucalyptus .... <1%
Boric acid .... <1%
Polyox WSR-205 .... <1%
D&C Green #5 .... trace

SEA BREEZE PROFESSIONAL HAND CREAM
(Sea Breeze)

Allantoin .... <1%
Chloroxylenol .... <1%
Water .... >50%
Synthetic Spermaceti .... <5%
Petrolatum .... <5%
Isopropyl palmitate .... <5%
Carbomer 934 .... <1%
Triethanol amine .... <1%
Stearyl alcohol .... <1%
Ceteareth-20 .... <1%
Fragrance .... <1%
Lanolin .... <1%
Methylparaben .... <1%
Propylparaben .... <1%
BHT .... <1%

SEALA-FLOR

See C-Z SEALA-FLOR

SEALBRITE 74
Fungicide; citrus coating
(American Machinery Corp.)

Active ingred.: 0.1%
  Thiabendazole
Inert ingred.: 97%
  Starch
  Surfactants
  Water

SEALBRITE LUSTRE-DRY WITH THIABENDAZOLE
Fungicide; citrus coating
(American Machinery Corp.)

Active ingred.: 0.1%
  Thiabendazole
Inert ingred.: 99.9%
  Soybean protein
  Shellac
  Wood rosin
  Oleic acid
  Isopropyl alcohol
  Water

SEALBRITE PRIME SHINE WITH THIABENDAZOLE
Fungicide; citrus coating
(American Machinery Corp.)

Active ingred.: 0.1%
  Thiabendazole
Inert ingred.: 99.9%
  Soybean protein
  Shellac
  Wood rosin
  Oleic acid
  Soybean oil
  Water

Starred ingredients (*) may be responsible for major toxic effects; consult Section II.

SEALBRITE 561 WITH THIABENDAZOLE
Fungicide; citrus, pineapple and cuke coating
(American Machinery Corp.)

Active ingred.:	0.1%
Thiabendazole	
Inert ingred.:	99.9%
Polyethylene beads	
Shellac	
Oleic acid	
Water	

SEALE'S LOTION - MODIFIED
Acne therapy
(C & M Pharmacal)

Sulfur	6.4%
Sodium borate	
Zinc oxide	
Acetone *	
Bentonite	
Purified water	

SEAL-OFF
Sealer & paint remover
(Sanitek)

Methylene chloride *	91.2%
Methanol	6.0%
Paraffin wax	2.0%
Hydroxypropyl methylcellulose	0.8%

SEAL-TITE
Floor polish
(Hillyard Chem.)

Latex

'76 Ed.

SEAL-TOX
Wood preservative
(Forman Ford)

Pentachlorophenol *	5%

SEAL TREAT WOOD PRESERVATIVE
(Klean-Strip)

Pentachlorophenol *	5%
Petroleum hydrocarbons *	94%
Water repellents	1%

SEAPROOF 4225 - INTERNATIONAL ORANGE
Marine paint
(Jotun-Baltimore Copper Paint Co.)

Pigment:	32%
Dinitraniline orange	6%
Calcium carbonate	26%
Vehicle:	68%
Soya alkyd resin	36%
Mineral spirits *	31%
Driers	1%

This type of product is also produced in Gloss White, Semi-gloss White, Flat White, Gloss Black, Pearl Gray, Ocean Gray, Leather Brown, Cream, Pine Green, Fairbanks Buff, Meadow Green, Chesapeake Blue, Sea Blue, Signal Red and Olympic Green.

SEA-PROOF X-253 EVERTOX RED COPPER
Marine paint
(Jotun-Baltimore Copper Paint Co.)

Pigment:	46%
Cuprous oxide *	20%
Iron oxide	14%
Calcium carbonate	4%
Aluminum silicate	8%
Vehicle:	54%
Processed Rosin	22%
Petroleum hydrocarbon resin	14%
Aromatic hydrocarbons *	6%
Aliphatic hydrocarbons	12%

This type of product also produced in Green and Blue

SEARS, ROEBUCK PRODUCTS

Poison Control Coordinator, D/817
Sears, Roebuck and Co.
925 S. Homan Ave.
Chicago, Ill. 60607

Information about Sears, Roebuck products is offered on a 24-hour basis to physicians and poison control centers.

Phone: 303-623-5827

SEA & SKI BLOCK OUT CLEAR LOTION
(Sea & Ski)

Escalol 507 (Octyl dimethyl PABA)
Oxybenzone (USP)
Purified water (USP)
Ucon Lubricant LB1715 (cosmetic grade)
Ceraphyl 50 (Myristyl lactate)
Klucel G (Hydroxypropyl cellulose)
FD & C Blue #1
Daphne #7
SD40-1 Alcohol *

SEA & SKI BLOCK OUT CREAM LOTION
(Sea & Ski)

Escalol 507 (Octyl dimethyl PABA)
Oxybenzone (USP)
Amerchol L101
Cerasynt 840
Mineral oil, heavy (USP)
Cocoa butter (USP)
Carbopol 940
Silicone fluid #556
Triethanolamine (USP)
Propylparaben (USP)
Methylparaben (USP)
Germall-115
Tenox 6
Daphne #7
Purified water (USP)

SEA & SKI DARK TANNING BUTTER
(Sea & Ski)

Modulan
Amerlate W
Ozokerite #4, Sno-White
N-5 Mineral oil
Tween 60
Cocoa butter (USP)
Cobee 76
White petrolatum (USP)
Tenox 6
Butylparaben, purified
Fragrance #561

SEA & SKI DARK TANNING OIL
(Sea & Ski)

Escalol 507 (Octyl dimethyl PABA)
Kaydol Mineral oil, heavy (USP)
Carnation Mineral oil 65/75
Isopropyl palmitate
Butylparaben (USP)
Benzoic acid (USP)
Menthol (USP)
Daphne #7

SEA & SKI GOLDEN TAN LOTION
(Sea & Ski)

Escalol 507 (Octyl dimethyl PABA)
Amerchol L101
Cerasynt 840
Mineral oil, heavy (USP)
Cocoa butter (USP)
Carbopol 940
Triethanolamine (USP)
Propylparaben (USP)
Methylparaben (USP)
Germall-115
Tenox 6
Daphne #7
FD & C Yellow #6
FD & C Yellow #5
Purified water (USP)

SEA & SKI LOTION
(Sea & Ski)

Escalol 507 (Octyl dimethyl PABA)
Amerchol L101
Cerasynt 840
Mineral oil, heavy (USP)
Cocoa butter (USP)
Carbopol 940
Triethanolamine (USP)
Propylparaben (USP)
Methylparaben (USP)
Germall-115
Tenox 6
Daphne #7
Brilliant Blue #1
FD & C Yellow #6
FD & C Yellow #10
Purified water (USP)

SEBAQUIN
Antiseborrheic shampoo
(Summers Labs.)

Diiodohydroxyquin 3%

SEBASORB
Medicated skin lotion for acne
(Summers Labs.)

Attapulgite	10%
Hexachlorophene	1%
Polysorbate 80	
Salicylic acid *	2%
Colloidal Sulfur	2%
In a grease-free vanishing base	

SEBASUM
Dermatologic skin cleanser
(Summers Labs.)

Polysorbate 80	
Acetone *	
Isopropanol *	50%

SEBAVEEN SHAMPOO
For seborrhea
(CooperCare)

Aveeno colloidal oatmeal	5%
Sulfur	2%
Salicylic acid *	2%
Emollients	4%
Sudsing & wetting agents	
Soap-free	

SEBESTA'S POCKET GOPHER BAIT
Rodenticide
(Sebesta Bait)

Strychnine * 0.31%

SEBESTA'S PRAIRIE DOG, GROUND SQUIRREL, FIELD MICE AND KANGAROO RAT BAIT
Rodenticide
(Sebesta Bait)

Strychnine * 0.44%

SEBISOL
Anti-dandruff shampoo
(C & M Pharmacal)

Orthobenzylparachlorophenol	0.1%
Betanaphthol	1%
Salicylic acid *	2%
Alkyl-aryl surfactant shampoo base *† with Polyethylene glycol and Alkanolamide conditioners	

†*See* Alkyl aryl sodium sulfonates

SEBIZON LOTION
Antiseborrheic preparation
(Schering)

Each gm.:
Sulfacetamide sodium *	100 mg.
Methylparaben	1 mg.
Emulsion: Trisodium ethylenediamine tetraaceate, Propylene glycol, Isopropyl myristate, Propylene glycol monostearate, Water, Sodium thiosulfate	

SEBORID
Antiseborrheic shampoo
(Herald Pharm.)

Polyoxyethylene lauryl ethers	
Ethoxylated alkylolamide	
Modified alcohol sulfate	
Salicylic acid *	2%

SEBUCARE
Antiseborrheic - grooming scalp lotion
(Westwood Pharm.)

Liposec (brand of polyoxyethylene lauryl ether)	5%
Salicylic acid *	2%
Capitrol (brand of penetrating water-dispersible hair grooming base containing 60%/v alcohol)	

'76 Ed.

SEBULEX
Antiseborrheic shampoo
(Westwood Pharm.)

Sebulytic (brand of penetrating surface-active combination of soapless cleansers & wetting agents)	
Micropulverized Sulfur	2%
Salicylic acid *	2%

'76 Ed.

SEBUTONE
Antiseborrheic tar shampoo
(Westwood Pharm.)

Tar (equiv. to 0.5% crude coal tar USP)	
Sebulytic (brand of penetrating surface-active combination of soapless cleansers & wetting agents)	
Kerohydric (brand of dewaxed, oil-soluble, keratin-moisturizing fraction of lanolin)	
Sulfur	2%
Salicylic acid *	2%

'76 Ed.

SECODRIN 'ENCORE' TABLETS
(Premo)

Each tablet:
Secobarbital *	60 mg.
d-Methamphetamine HCl *	10 mg.

'76 Ed.

SECODRIN TABLETS
(Premo)

Each tablet:
Secobarbital *	30 mg.
d-Methamphetamine HCl * ...	5 mg.

'76 Ed.

SECONAL SODIUM PULVULES, U.S.P. CAPSULES
Sedative, hypnotic
(Lilly, Eli)

Available in capsules containing:
Secobarbital sodium * .. 1/2 gr.; 3/4 gr.; or 1 1/2 gr.

SECONAL SODIUM SUPPOSITORIES
(Lilly, Eli)

Each suppository:
Secobarbital sodium *
Pink-colored foil	1/2 gr.
Light-blue-colored foil	1 gr.
Gold-colored foil	2 gr.
Silver-colored foil	3 gr.

2ND DEBUT CEF 600
(Kolmar Labs.)

Water	>50%
Fragrance	0.1-1.0%
Color	0.1-1.0%
Bactericide	<0.1%
Anionic emulsifier	5.0-10%
Emollient	0.1-1.0%
Moisturizing agent	0.1-1.0%
Preservatives	0.1-1.0%
Solvent	1.0-5.0%

2ND DEBUT CEF 1200
(Kolmar Labs.)

Water	>50%
Fragrance	0.1-1.0%
Color	0.1-1.0%
Bactericide	<0.1%
Anionic emulsifier	5-10%
Emollient	0.1-1.0%
Moisturizing agent	0.1-1.0%
Preservatives	0.1-1.0%
Solvent	1.0-5.0%

2ND DEBUT CEF 600 CONCENTRATE
(Kolmar Labs.)

Bactericide	0.1-1.0%
Emollient	25-50%
Preservatives	1.0-5.0%
Anionic emulsifier	10-25%
Moisturizing agent	1.0-5.0%

Starred ingredients (*) may be responsible for major toxic effects; consult Section II.

2ND DEBUT CEF 1200 CONCENTRATE
(Kolmar Labs.)

Bactericide	0.1-1.0%
Emollient	25-50%
Preservatives	1.0-5.0%
Anionic emulsifier	10-25%
Moisturizing agent	1.0-5.0%

SECRAN/FE ELIXIR
Iron deficiency anemia
(Scherer Labs.)

Each 5 cc:
Ferric pyrophosphate *	250 mg.

Plus Polyvitamins

SECRAN LIQUID
B-Vitamins supplement
(Scherer Labs.)

Each 5 cc.:
Cyanocobalamin	25 mcg.
Thiamine mononitrate (B1)	10 mg.
Nicotinamide	10 mg.
Alcohol	17%

SECRET (Cream)
Antiperspirant
(Procter & Gamble, Health & Personal Care Div.)

Aluminum hydroxychloride	5-9%
Zirconyl hydroxychloride	3-6%
Glycine	1-4%
Paraffin wax	1-4%
Isopropyl palmitate	1-4%
Glyceryl monostearate	1-4%
Polyoxyethylene stearate	1-4%
Glycerol	1-4%
Diethyleneglycol monostearate	1-4%
Minor ingredients, each	<1%
Water	>50%

SECRET DEODORANT (Aerosol)
(Procter & Gamble, Health & Personal Care Div.)

Zinc phenolsulfonate	1-4%
Propylene glycol	1-4%
Alcohol SD-40	45-55%
Water	1-5%
Minor ingredients	<1%
Propellant (Isobutane)	35-45%

SECRET (Dry Formula)
Aerosol antiperspirant
(Procter & Gamble, Health & Personal Care Div.)

Aluminum chlorohydrate*	10–15%
Isopropyl myristate	3–8%
Quaternium-18 hectorite	1–5%
Cyclomethicone	5–10%
Dimethicone	1–5%
Propylene carbonate	<1%
Bentone	0.5–2%
Minor ingredients	<1%
Propellant (Isobutane)	>50%

SECRET (Roll-on)
Antiperspirant
(Procter & Gamble, Health & Personal Care Div.)

Aluminum hydroxychloride	10-15%
Zirconyl hydroxychloride	5-9%
Glycine	1-4%
Paraffin wax	1-4%
Isopropyl palmitate	1-4%
Glyceryl monostearate	5-10%
Polyoxyethylene stearate	5-9%
Glycerol	1-4%
Magnesium aluminum silicate	1-4%
Minor ingredients, each	<1%
Water	>50%

SECTILIN SHAMPOO
For the eradication of fleas, lice and ticks on dogs
(Bio-Ceutic)

Gamma isomer of benzene hexachloride (from lindane)	0.097%
Inert ingred.:	99.903%

    Sodium lauryl sulfate *
    Triethanolamine lauryl sulfate *
    Lanolin alcohols
    Ammonium lauryl sulfate *
    Dewaxed lanolin
    Lauric acid diethanolamine condensate
    Perfume oil
    Hydrogen chloride
    Methylparaben
    Propylparaben
    Disodium salt of 1-p-sulfaphenylazo-2-naphthol-6-sulfonic acid
    Certified color
    Water

SECURITY ANTIROT - 10X
Wood preservative
(Woolfolk)

Pentachlorophenol *	33.2%
Other chlorophenols & related compounds	6.8%
Aromatic petroleum derivative solvent *	40.0%

SECURITY BENZEX
Insecticide
(Woolfolk)

Gamma isomer of benzene hexachloride (BHC) *	6.00%
Other isomers of benzene hexachloride (BHC) *	7.48%

SECURITY BHC CONCENTRATE EMUL.
Insecticide
(Woolfolk)

Gamma isomer of benzene hexachloride *	11.7%
Other isomers of benzene hexachloride *	15.7%
Aromatic petroleum derivative solvent *	68.6%

SECURITY BIG 10 DUST
Insecticide
(Woolfolk)

Carbaryl (1-Naphthyl N-methylcarbamate) *	10.0%

SECURITY BOTRAN-CAPTAN PEACH DUST 6-7 1/2
Fungicide
(Woolfolk)

2,6-Dichloro-4-nitroaniline	6.0%
Captan	7.5%

SECURITY 6% BOTRAN PEACH DUST
Fungicide
(Woolfolk)

2,6-Dichloro-4-nitroaniline	6.0%

SECURITY BOTRAN-SULPHUR PEACH DUST 6-78
Fungicide
(Woolfolk)

2,6-Dichloro-4-nitroaniline	6.0%
Sulphur, as elemental *	78.0%

SECURITY BOTRAN 75 W
Fungicide
(Woolfolk)

2,6-Dichloro-4-nitroaniline *	75.0%

SECURITY BSZ BASIC ZINC SULPHATE
Fungicide
(Woolfolk)

Zinc, as metallic, from basic zinc sulphate *	20.0%

SECURITY CALCIUM ARSENATE
Insecticide
(Woolfolk)

Tricalcium arsenate *	70.0%

SECURITY 7 1/2% CAPTAN PEACH DUST
Fungicide
(Woolfolk)

Captan	7.5%

SECURITY COPPER-SULPHUR-10% SEVIN
Insecticide, fungicide
(Woolfolk)

Sulfur, as elemental *	72.5%
Copper, as metallic, from copper oxide *	3.4%
Carbaryl (1-Naphthyl N-methylcarbamate) *	10.0%

SECURITY 20-40 COTTON DUST
Insecticide, fungicide
(Woolfolk)

Toxaphene *	20.0%
Sulfur, as elemental	40.0%

Starred ingredients (*) may be responsible for major toxic effects; consult Section II.

SECURITY EPN - 5 EC
Insecticide
(Woolfolk)

O-Ethyl O-p-nitrophenyl
phenylphosphonothioate * 55.0%
Aromatic petroleum derivative
solvent 32.1%

SECURITY EPN - SULPHUR 1 1/2-6
Insecticide, fungicide
(Woolfolk)

O-Ethyl O-p-nitrophenyl
phenylphosphonothioate * 5.00%
Sulfur 73.50%

SECURITY EPN 25-W
Insecticide
(Woolfolk)

O-Ethyl O-p-nitrophenyl
phenylphosphonothioate * 25.0%

SECURITY FERBAM DUST
Fungicide
(Woolfolk)

Ferbam * 11.4%

SECURITY FISH TOX 5
Insecticide
(Woolfolk)

Rotenone 5.0%
Other cube' resins 9.8%
Heavy aromatic naphtha * 68.2%

SECURITY FLAC
Insecticide
(Woolfolk)

Calcium arsenate * 70.0%

SECURITY GRAIN FUMIGANT
Insecticide
(Woolfolk)

Ethylene dichloride .. 70%/wt., 75%/vol.
Carbon
tetrachloride * .... 30%/wt., 25%/vol.

SECURITY GRAIN PROTECTANT
Insecticide
(Woolfolk)

Malathion 1.0%

SECURITY KELTHANE EMUL. CONC.
Miticide
(Woolfolk)

1,1-Bis(p-chlorophenyl)-2,2,2-
trichloroethanol * 18.5%

SECURITY LAWN WEED KILLER
Herbicide
(Woolfolk)

N-Oleyl 1,3-propylene diamine salt
of 2,4-dichlorophenoxy acetic
acid * 33.0%

SECURITY LIME SULPHUR
Fungicide
(Woolfolk)

Calcium polysulphide * 30.0%

SECURITY 20% LINDANE EMUL. CONC.
Insecticide
(Woolfolk)

Gamma isomer of benzene hexachloride from lindane * 20.0%
Aromatic petroleum derivative
solvent * 65.6%

SECURITY MALATHION 5-E
Insecticide
(Woolfolk)

Malathion * 56.1%
Aromatic petroleum derivative
solvent * 35.2%

SECURITY METHYL PARATHION EC 4
Insecticide
(Woolfolk)

O,O-Dimethyl O-p-nitrophenyl
thiophosphate * 45.0%
Aromatic petroleum derivative
solvent 38.6%
Petroleum hydrocarbons 9.0%

SECURITY METHYL PARATHION-ENDRI-SOL
Insecticide
(Woolfolk)

Endrin * 17.7%
O,O-Dimethyl O-p-nitrophenyl
thiophosphate * 17.8%
Heavy Aromatic naphtha * 55.6%

SECURITY METHYL PARATHION-EPN 4-2 COTTON SPRAY
Insecticide
(Woolfolk)

O-Ethyl O-p-nitrophenyl
phenylphosphonothioate * 21.0%
O,O-Dimethyl O-p-nitrophenyl
thiophosphate * 42.0%
Aromatic petroleum derivative
solvent 23.7%

SECURITY MILL SPRAY
Insecticide
(Woolfolk)

Technical Piperonyl butoxide 1.50%
Pyrethrins 0.15%
Petroleum hydrocarbons * 98.35%

SECURITY MOTOX 63 COTTON SPRAY
Insecticide
(Woolfolk)

Toxaphene 53.2%
O,O-Dimethyl O-p-nitrophenyl
thiophosphate * 26.6%
Aromatic petroleum derivative
solvent 14.9%

SECURITY NUTONEX SULPHUR WETTABLE
Fungicide
(Woolfolk)

Sulfur, as elemental * 96.0%

SECURITY ORNAMENTAL & FRUIT SPRAY OIL
Insecticide
(Woolfolk)

Petroleum oil * 98.0%

SECURITY PAN PEACH SPRAY
Insecticide-fungicide
(Woolfolk)

Zinc, as metallic (equiv. to 55% basic
sulphate of zinc, as
ZnSO4Zn(OH)2) * 11.0%
Sulphur, as elemental 39.0%

SECURITY PAN-THION SPRAY
Insecticide-fungicide
(Woolfolk)

Parathion * 1.8%
Zinc, in the form of basic sulphate,
as metallic 10.0%
Sulfur, as elemental 38.5%

SECURITY PARA-NEX PEACH SPRAY 2-8
Insecticide-fungicide
(Woolfolk)

Parathion * 3.00%
Sulphur 76.00%

SECURITY PARATHION-CAPTAN
Insecticide, fungicide
(Woolfolk)

Captan 25.0%
Parathion * 7.5%

Starred ingredients (*) may be responsible for major toxic effects; consult Section II.

SECURITY PARATHION-EC4
Insecticide
(Woolfolk)

Parathion *	45.3%
Aromatic petroleum derivative solvent	48.0%

SECURITY PARATHION-SULPHUR 2-6
Insecticide, fungicide
(Woolfolk)

Parathion *	3.75%
Sulfur	76.25%

SECURITY POWDERED CUBE
Insecticide
(Woolfolk)

Rotenone *	5.0%
Other cube resins	10.0%

SECURITY POWERTOX COTTON SPRAY
Insecticide
(Woolfolk)

O-Ethyl O-p-nitrophenyl phenylphosphonothioate *	31.6%
O,O-Dimethyl O-p-nitrophenyl thiophosphate *	31.6%
Aromatic petroleum derivative solvent	19.2%

SECURITY QUIK TREM
Chemical edger
(Woolfolk)

Ammonium sulfamate	11.36%

SECURITY ROACH & ANT KILL
(Woolfolk)

Chlorpyrifos (O,O-Diethyl O-(3,-5,6-trichloro-2-pyridyl) phosphorothioate)	0.50%
Pyrethrins	0.10%
Piperonyl butoxide	0.20%
N-Octyl bicycloheptene dicarboximide	0.30%
Aromatic petroleum derivative solvent	0.29%
Petroleum distillate *	95.58%

SECURITY ROSE AND TURF FUNGICIDE
(Woolfolk)

Benomyl (Methyl 1-(butylcarbamoyl)2-benzimidazolecarbamate)	50%

SECURITY ROSE, FLOWER, ORNAMENTAL DUST
Insecticide-fungicide
(Woolfolk)

Zinc ethylene bisdithiocarbamate (Zineb)	6.00%
1-Naphthyl N-methylcarbamate *	5.00%
1,1-Bis(chlorophenyl)-2,2,2-trichloroethanol	2.00%
Gamma isomer of benzene hexachloride from lindane	1.00%
Dinitro (1-methyl heptyl) phenyl crotonate	0.90%
Other nitro phenols & derivatives chiefly dinitro (1-methyl heptyl) phenol	0.10%

SECURITY SEVIN BEAN DUST
Insecticide
(Woolfolk)

Carbaryl (1-Naphthyl N-methylcarbamate) *	1.75%

SECURITY SEVIN-SULPHUR 2-6
Insecticide, fungicide
(Woolfolk)

Carbaryl (1-Naphthyl N-methylcarbamate) *	12.50%
Sulfur, as elemental	69.75%

SECURITY SPREADER-STICKER
(Woolfolk)

Combined amount:	35.0%
Emulsifiable A-C Polyethylene	
Fatty acid-amine condensate	
Alkyl aryl sulfonate *	

SECURITY STERACIDE
Herbicide
(Woolfolk)

Sodium chlorate *	41.0%
Sodium metaborate	51.0%
Bromacil (5-Bromo-3-sec-butyl-6-methyluracil)	1.6%

SECURITY SUPERIOR OIL-70
Insecticide
(Woolfolk)

Petroleum oil *	98.0%

SECURITY THIODAN EMUL. CONC.
Insecticide
(Woolfolk)

Endosulfan *	22.3%
Heavy aromatic solvent *†	71.0%

†See Aromatic hydrocarbon solvent

SECURITY THIODAN-PARATHION 2-1
Insecticide
(Woolfolk)

Endosulfan	22.8%
Parathion (O,O-Diethyl O-p-nitrophenyl thiophosphate) *	11.4%

SECURITY THREE WAY COTTON SPRAY 6-3
Insecticide
(Woolfolk)

Parathion *	58.11%
O,O-Dimethyl O-p-nitrophenyl thiophosphate	29.12%
Xylene range aromatic solvent	7.30%

SECURITY TOMATO & VEGETABLE DUST
Insecticide, fungicide
(Woolfolk)

Maneb	6.0%
Carbaryl *	5.0%

SECURITY TOX-MP COTTON SPRAY 6-1 1/2
Insecticide
(Woolfolk)

Toxaphene	55.4%
O,O-Dimethyl O-p-nitrophenyl phosphorothioate *	13.8%
Aromatic petroleum derivative solvent	17.2%

SECURITY TOX-SOL-6
Insecticide
(Woolfolk)

Toxaphene *	59.0%
Petroleum hydrocarbons	31.8%
Xylene	4.8%

SECURITY WET-AID
Wetting agent
(Woolfolk)

Dodecyl ether of polyethylene glycol *	90.0%

SECURITY ZINEB DUST
Fungicide, insecticide
(Woolfolk)

Zineb (Zinc ethylenebis(dithiocarbamate))	6.5%

SEDACAPS SLEEP AID CAPSULES
(Vitarine)

Each capsule:
Methapyrilene hydrochloride * 25 mg.

Starred ingredients (*) may be responsible for major toxic effects; consult Section II.

SEDADROPS
Pediatric sedative & hypnotic
(Merrell Dow)

Each 1.0 ml.:
Phenobarbital * .... 16 mg.
Oil of peppermint

SEDAGEST TABLETS
For gastric hyperacidity
(Approved Pharm.)

Each tablet:
Aluminum hydroxide gel
USP .... 5 gr.
Magnesium trisilicate ...... 4 gr.
Magnesium phosphate
tribasic * .... 2 gr.
Pectin .... 1/4 gr.
Total Belladonna alkaloids . 0.054 mg.
Flavor & color .... q.s.

'76 Ed.

SEDAJEN
Sedative
(Jenkins Labs.)

Each tablet:
Phenobarbital * .... 5/16 gr.
Passiflora .... 1 1/2 gr.
Hyoscyamus (total alkaloids
0.0003 gr.) .... 3/4 gr.

SEDAMINE ANTI-NAUSEA LIQUID
(Life Labs., Inc.)

Each 15 cc.:
Pyridoxine hydrochloride USP 10 mg.
Thiamine hydrochloride USP 10 mg.
Buffered phosphorated solution of levu-
lose and dextrose

'76 Ed.

SEDAMYL
Daytime sedation
(Riker Labs.)

Each tablet:
Acetylcarbromal * .... 250 mg.

'76 Ed.

SEDASTAT-T
Hypnotic
(Wesley Pharm.)

Each tablet:
Dimenhydrinate * .... 50 mg.

SEDATUSSIN
Antitussive
(Lilly, Eli)

Each 100 cc:
Cephalin hydrochloride .... 0.007 gm.
Sodium benzoate .... 0.875 gm.
Sanguinaria solid extract ... 0.21 gm.
Squill .... 0.25 gm.
Tolu balsam and menthol .. q.s.

SEDDO CAPS
Insomnal capsules
(Friendly Labs.)

Each capsule:
Methapyrilene hydrochloride * 25 mg.

SEDRAL
*Treatment of bronchial asthma, hay fe-
ver*
(Vita Elixir Co.)

Each tablet:
Phenobarbital .... 1/8 gr.
Theophylline * .... 2 gr.
Ephedrine * .... 3/8 gr.

SED-TENS SE
Anticholinergic
(Lemmon Co.)

Each tablet:
Homatropine methylbromide * 10 mg.

SEED SILK
Insecticide
(Lorenz)

Heptachlor * 25.0%
Graphite 10.0%
Kaolin 65.0%

SEE SPRAY WINDOW CLEANER

See AMWAY SEE SPRAY WINDOW
CLEANER

SELETOC (CAPSULES & MINICAPS)
*For acute symptoms of arthritic condi-
tions in dogs*
(Burns-Biotec)

CAPSULES (each):
Sodium selenite (equiv. to selenium 1 mg.) * .... 2.19 mg.
Vitamin E (as d-alpha tocopheryl acid succinate) ..... 56.2 mg.

MINICAPS (each):
Sodium selenite (equiv. to selenium 0.25 mg.) * .... 0.55 mg.
Vitamin E (as d-alpha tocopheryl acid succinate) ..... 14 mg.

SELSUN BLUE LOTION SHAMPOO
Antiseborrheic
(Abbott)

Selenium sulfide * 1%

SELSUN CREAM SHAMPOO
Antiseborrheic
(Abbott)

Selenium sulfide * 1.0%

SELSUN SUSPENSION
Antiseborrheic agent
(Abbott)

Selenium sulfide * .... 2 1/2% w/v

SEMETS (TROCHES)
Relief of minor throat irritations
(Beecham Labs.)

Each troche:
Cetylpyridinium chloride 1:1500
Benzocaine .... 3 mg.
Cherry-flavored candy base ... q.s

SENCO ALL-PURPOSE PAINT THINNER
(Senn, Geo., Inc.)

Aliphatic hydrocarbon *
Masking agents

'76 Ed.

SENCOR
Herbicide
(Mobay Chemical Corp.)

Metribuzin (4-Amino-6-(1,1-dimethyle-
thyl)-3-(methylthio)-1,2,4,-triazin-
5(4H)-one) *

SENDRAN INSECTICIDAL SHAMPOO
For control of fleas on dogs and cats
(Haver-Lockhart (Brand) Bayvet Div.
Cutter Labs.)

o-Isopropoxyphenyl
methylcarbamate 0.125%

SENDRAN TICK AND FLEA COLLAR FOR DOGS
(Haver-Lockhart (Brand) Bayvet Div.
Cutter Labs.)

o-Isopropoxyphenyl
methylcarbamate * 9.4%

SENDRAN TICK AND FLEA DAB-ON
For use on dogs and cats
(Haver-Lockhart (Brand) Bayvet Div.
Cutter Labs.)

o-Isopropoxyphenyl
methylcarbamate * 1%

SENDRAN 50% WETTABLE POWDER
*For control of fleas and ticks; veteri-
nary*
(Haver-Lockhart (Brand) Bayvet Div.
Cutter Labs.)

o-Isopropoxyphenyl
methylcarbamate * 50%

SENECA DL
(Diversey Wyandotte)

Sodium hydroxide *

Starred ingredients (*) may be responsible for major toxic effects; consult Section II.

SENILEX
Psychotonic in geriatrics
(OJF)

Each tablet:
Pentylenetetrazol * .... 100 mg.
Niacin .... 50 mg.

SENSODYNE TOOTHPASTE
(Block Drug)

Strontium chloride 10%
Sodium saccharin
Surfactant
Micronized Silica
Polishing agents
Sorbitol
Glycerine
Hydroxyethylcellulose
Guar gum
Flavors
Preservative

SENTINEL SOLID HOUSEHOLD INSECTICIDE
(Miller-Morton)

Naled * 25%

SENTOL
Liquid acid cleaner
(Diversey Wyandotte)

Phosphoric acid *

SENTRY
Pressurized irritating stream; personal protection
(Penguin Industries)

Capsaicin (derived from oleoresin capsicum) 0.35%

SENTRY
Disinfectant, sanitizer
(Pennwalt)

Calcium hypochlorite * 65%

SENTRY IV COLLAR - CATS, SERGEANT'S

See SERGEANT'S SENTRY IV COLLAR - CATS

SENTRY IV COLLAR - DOGS, SERGEANT'S

See SERGEANT'S SENTRY IV COLLAR - DOGS

SENTRY LIQUID

See AIRWICK PROFESSIONAL PRODUCTS SENTRY LIQUID

SENTRY SOLID

See AIRWICK PROFESSIONAL PRODUCTS SENTRY SOLID

SEPO THROAT LOZENGES
(Clapp, Otis)

Each lozenge:
Benzocaine

SEPTO
Germicidal and antiseptic liquid
(Vita Elixir Co.)

Methylbenzethonium chloride *
Ethanol 2%
Menthol

SEPT-X
Clears, activates home sewage systems
(Rooto)

Aluminum hydroxide
Ferric hydroxide
Calcium sulfate

SEQUESTRENE COPPER
Copper chelate plant nutrient
(Ciba-Geigy Ag. Div.)

Tech. Disodium cupric ethylenediamine tetraacetate trihydrate (13% copper as metallic) *†

†*See* Copper

SEQUESTRENE 138Fe
Iron chelate - plant nutrient
(Ciba-Geigy Ag. Div.)

Tech. Sodium ferric ethylenediamine di(o-hydroxy-phenylacetate) (6% iron as metallic)

SEQUESTRENE 330Fe
Iron chelate - plant nutrient
(Ciba-Geigy Ag. Div.)

Tech. Sodium ferric diethylenetriamine pentaacetate (10% iron as metallic) *

SEQUESTRENE LIQUID MANGANESE
(Ciba-Geigy Ag. Div.)

Technical Disodium manganous ethylenediamine tetraacetate dihydrate .... 5.0% Mn.

SEQUESTRENE LIQUID ZINC
Zinc chelate - plant nutrient
(Ciba-Geigy Ag. Div.)

Tech. Disodium zinc ethylenediamine tetraacetate dihydrate (6% zinc as metallic) *

SEQUESTRENE MANGANESE
Manganese chelate plant nutrient
(Ciba-Geigy Ag. Div.)

Tech. Disodium manganous ethylenediamine tetraacetate dihydrate (12% manganese as metallic) *

SEQUESTRENE ZINC
Zinc chelate - plant nutrient
(Ciba-Geigy Ag. Div.)

Tech. Disodium zinc ethylenediamine tetraacetate dihydrate (14.2% zinc as metallic) *

SERAX
Management of anxiety disorders
(Wyeth Labs.)

Capsules:
Oxazepam * .... 10 mg.; 15 mg.; or 30 mg.

Tablets:
Oxazepam * .... 15 mg.

SEREEN
Sedative
(Foy Labs.)

Each capsule:
Chlordiazepoxide HCl * 5 mg.; 10 mg.

SERENE CAPSULES
Tranquilizer
(Approved Pharm.)

Each capsule:
Methapyrilene HCl * ...... 25 mg.
Salicylamide .... 2 gr.
Scopolamine aminoxide hydrobromide * .... 0.20 mg.
'76 Ed.

SERENTIL
Tranquilizer
(Boehringer-Ingelheim)

Mesoridazine besylate * ...... 10 mg.; 25 mg.; 50 mg. or 100 mg.

SERENTIL CONCENTRATE
Tranquilizer
(Boehringer-Ingelheim)

Each cc.:
Mesoridazine besylate * ...... 25 mg.

SERGEANT'S CAT FLEA POWDER
Insecticide
(Miller-Morton)

Technical Methoxychlor 2.50%
Pyrethrins 0.06%
Piperonyl butoxide technical 0.60%

SERGEANT'S E-Z GROOM
Foam shampoo for dogs and cats - kills fleas
(Miller-Morton)

Technical Piperonyl butoxide .. 0.44%
Pyrethrins 0.044%
Inert ingred.: 99.516%
Cleaners
Deodorant
Propellant

Starred ingredients (*) may be responsible for major toxic effects; consult Section II.

SERGEANT'S FLEA & TICK DIP
(Miller-Morton)

Malathion	24.0%
Methoxychlor (technical)	16.8%
Pine oil	16.0%
Petroleum distillate	9.4%
Xylene *	25.0%

SERGEANT'S FLEA & TICK POWDER
Insecticide
(Miller-Morton)

Sevin *	5.0%

SERGEANT'S FLEA & TICK SPRAY FOR CATS
(Miller-Morton)

O-Isopropoxyphenyl methylcarbamate	0.25%

SERGEANT'S FLEA & TICK SPRAY FOR DOGS
(Miller-Morton)

O-Isopropoxyphenyl methylcarbamate	0.25%

SERGEANT'S "FOAM N' COMB" DRY SHAMPOO FOR DOGS/CATS
(Miller-Morton)

Technical Piperonyl butoxide	0.44%
Pyrethrins	0.044%
Inert ingred.:	99.516%
Cleaners	
Deodorant	
Propellant	

SERGEANT'S NO ITCH
For dogs
(Miller-Morton)

Parfentjev's yeast fraction	
Soap	
Benzyl alcohol	1.5%

SERGEANT'S "ONE SHOT" INDOOR FOGGER
(Miller-Morton)

Ronnel	2.00%
2,2-Dichlorovinyl dimethyl phosphate	0.47%
Related compounds	0.03%
Petroleum distillate	1.94%

SERGEANT'S PUMP CAT FLEA & TICK SPRAY
(Miller-Morton)

Carbaryl	0.50%

SERGEANT'S PUMP DOG FLEA & TICK SPRAY
(Miller-Morton)

Carbaryl	0.50%
2,3:4,5-Bis(2-butylene)tetrahydro-2-furaldehyde	0.25%

SERGEANT'S PUPPY WORM CAPSULES
(Miller-Morton)

n-Butyl chloride *	272 mg./capsule

SERGEANT'S SARCOPTIC MANGE MEDICINE
Ectoparasiticide; veterinary
(Miller-Morton)

Paraffin oil base	24.94%
Kerosene	22.00%
Petroleum crude oil	23.16%
Pine tar oil *	26.23%
Sulphur	0.40%

SERGEANT'S SENTRY IV COLLAR - CATS
(Miller-Morton)

Naled *	10.0%

SERGEANT'S SENTRY IV COLLAR - DOGS
(Miller-Morton)

Naled *	15.0%

SERGEANT'S SENTRY V FLEA & TICK COLLAR FOR CATS
(Miller-Morton)

Naled *	7.0%
O-Isopropoxyphenyl methylcarbamate *	2.4%

SERGEANT'S SENTRY V FLEA & TICK COLLAR FOR DOGS
(Miller-Morton)

Naled *	15.0%
O-Isopropoxyphenyl methylcarbamate *	4.2%

SERGEANT'S SKIP-FLEA SHAMPOO
Insecticide
(Miller-Morton)

Tech. Piperonyl butoxide	0.5%
Pyrethrins or d-trans Allethrin	0.05%

SERGEANT'S SKIP-FLEA SOAP
(Miller-Morton)

Anhydrous soap	84%
Beta naphthol *	3%
Oil of pennyroyal	1%

SERGEANT'S SURE SHOT WORM CAPSULES
Veterinary
(Miller-Morton)

n-Butyl chloride *	816 mg./capsule

SERGEANT'S TAPEWORM MEDICINE
Veterinary
(Miller-Morton)

Arecoline hydrobromide *	1.25% (4 mg./tab.)

SERGEANT'S TICK KILLER
(Miller-Morton)

o-Isopropoxyphenyl methylcarbamate	0.25%

SERGEANT'S WORM-AWAY - CATS
(Miller-Morton)

Piperazine (as citrate)	140 mg./capsule

SERGEANT'S WORM-AWAY - DOGS
(Miller-Morton)

Each capsule:	
Piperazine (as citrate)	140 mg.

SERPASIL
Hypotensive & tranquilizing agent
(CIBA Pharmaceutical)

Tablets:	
Reserpine *	1 mg.; 0.25 mg.; or 0.1 mg.
Elixir (each 4 ml.):	
Reserpine *	0.2 mg.

SERPASIL-ESIDRIX
Antihypertensive agent
(CIBA Pharmaceutical)

Each #1 tablet:	
Reserpine *	0.1 mg.
Hydrochlorothiazide *	25 mg.
Each #2 tablet:	
Reserpine *	0.1 mg.
Hydrochlorothiazide *	50 mg.

SERPICON
Tranquilizer, antihypertensive
(CMC Research Div.)

Each tablet:	
Reserpine	0.1 or 0.25 mg.

SERUTAN
Laxative
(Williams, J.B.)

Vegetable hemicellulose derived from Plantago ovata
Sodium carboxymethylcellulose
Specially refined powdered oatmeal
Defatted wheat germ

Starred ingredients (*) may be responsible for major toxic effects; consult Section II.

SERVAC
Liquid acid cleaner
(Diversey Wyandotte)

Phosphoric acid *

SERVANT
Institutional and industrial cleaning product

Procter & Gamble Co.
Ivorydale Technical Center
Cincinnati, Ohio 45217

Phone: 513-562-1100

SETTELZ
Digestant
(Watkins Products, Inc.)

Bismuth subsalicylate
Salol *
Zinc phenolsulfonate *

7-ACTION COLD CAPSULES
(Approved Pharm.)

Each capsule:
Salicylamide *	1 3/4 gr.
Camphor, monobromated	1/2 gr.
Caffeine *	1/4 gr.
Phenolphthalein	1/5 gr.
Atropine sulfate *	1/1000 gr.
Quinine sulfate *	1/4 gr.

'76 Ed.

SEVENTEEN COSMETIC PRODUCTS

Seventeen Inc.
33 Virginia Ave.
West Nyack, N.Y. 10994

Phone: 914-358-2426

See COSMETICS, Section VI, General Formulations

SEVICIDE (5 AND 50)

See N/S SEVICIDE (5 AND 50)

SEVIN-AIR-LV
Insecticide
(Techne Corp.)

Carbaryl (1-Naphthyl N-
methylcarbamate) * 24.4%

'76 Ed.

SEYMOUR OF SYCAMORE PAINT PRODUCTS
Paints & spray paints

Seymour of Sycamore, Inc.
917 Crosby Ave.
Sycamore, Ill. 60178

Phone: 815-895-9101

See PAINTS, Section VI, General Formulations

SEYMOUR SPRAY PAINT BOWLING BALL BLACK GLOSS LACQUER (16-815)
(Seymour)

Non-volatile:	13.2%
Carbon black	0.4%
Nitrocellulose, Dioctylphthalate, Maleic resins, Coconut alkyd resin	12.8%
Volatile:	86.8%
Ketones, * Alcohols *, Acetates *†	53.5%
Aromatic hydrocarbons *	11.3%
Propellant (Propane-isobutane)	22.0%

†*See* Paints, Section VI, General Formulations

SEYMOUR SPRAY PAINT CARRIAGE BLACK GLOSS ENAMEL (16-115)
(Seymour)

Non-volatile:	14.6%
Carbon black	0.9%
Synthetic Petroleum resins, Soya and Vinyl toluene linseed alkyd resins	13.7%
Volatile:	85.4%
Ketones	4.9%
Halogenated hydrocarbons *, Aromatic hydrocarbons *, Aliphatic hydrocarbons *, Driers *	50.5%
Propellant (Propane-isobutane)	30.0%

SEYMOUR SPRAY PAINT CLEAR ACRYLIC GLOSS LACQUER (RECON CLEAR) (16-121)
(Seymour)

Non-volatile:	10.7%
Acrylic ester resin, Castor oil alkyd resins	10.7%
Volatile:	89.3%
Ketones *	24.7%
Aromatic hydrocarbons *, Aliphatic hydrocarbons *	34.6%
Propellant (Propane-isobutane)	30.0%

SEYMOUR SPRAY PAINT DOVE WHITE GLOSS ENAMEL (16-113)
(Seymour)

Non-volatile:	21.0%
Titanium dioxide	10.0%
Soya and Vinyl toluene linseed alkyd resins	11.0%
Volatile:	79.0%
Ketones	5.3%
Halogenated hydrocarbons *, Aromatic hydrocarbons *, Aliphatic hydrocarbons *, Driers *	43.7%
Propellant (Propane-isobutane)	30.0%

SEYMOUR SPRAY PAINT INK BLACK FLAT ENAMEL (16-133)
(Seymour)

Non-volatile:	14.9%
Carbon black	0.4%
Calcium carbonate	5.4%
Silicates	2.5%
Soya and Vinyl toluene linseed alkyd resins	6.6%
Volatile:	85.1%
Ketones	4.5%
Halogenated hydrocarbons *, Aromatic hydrocarbons *, Aliphatic hydrocarbons *, Driers *	50.6%
Propellant (Propane-isobutane)	30.0%

SEYMOUR SPRAY PAINT LIGHT HOUSE WHITE FLAT ENAMEL (16-134)
(Seymour)

Non-volatile:	26.2%
Titanium dioxide	5.7%
Calcium carbonate	6.6%
Silicates	4.2%
Soya and Vinyl toluene linseed alkyd resins	9.7%
Volatile:	73.8%
Ketones	8.3%
Aromatic hydrocarbons *, Aliphatic hydrocarbons *, Driers *	35.5%
Propellant (Propane-isobutane)	30.0%

SEYMOUR SPRAY PAINT METALLIC BRIGHT ALUMINUM (16-811)
(Seymour)

Non-volatile:	12.5%
Aluminum powder	3.3%
Acrylic ester resin	9.2%
Volatile:	87.5%
Ketones	10.5%
Aromatic hydrocarbons *, Aliphatic hydrocarbons *	47.0%
Propellant (Propane-isobutane)	30.0%

SEYMOUR SPRAY PAINT METALLIC COPPER PENNY (16-809)
(Seymour)

Non-volatile:	16.4%
Copper bronze powder	7.6%
Acrylic ester resin	8.8%
Volatile:	83.6%
Ketones	8.9%
Aromatic hydrocarbons *	44.7%
Propellant (Propane-isobutane)	30.0%

SEYMOUR SPRAY PAINT METALLIC GOLD CREST
(Seymour)

Non-volatile:	17.0%
Gold bronze powder	7.4%
Acrylic ester resin	9.6%
Volatile:	83.0%
Ketones	19.4%
Aromatic hydrocarbons *	33.6%
Propellant (Propane-isobutane)	30.0%

SEYMOUR SPRAY PAINT PALM GREEN GLOSS ENAMEL (16-126)
(Seymour)

Non-volatile:	14.1%
Titanium dioxide	1.1%
Azo anisidine yellow	0.6%
Phthalo green	0.3%
Synthetic Petroleum resins, Soya and Vinyl toluene linseed alkyd resins	12.1%
Volatile:	85.9%
Ketones	5.1%
Halogenated hydrocarbons *, Aromatic hydrocarbons *, Aliphatic hydrocarbons *, Driers *	50.8%
Propellant (Propane-isobutane)	30.0%

SEYMOUR SPRAY PAINT RACING RED GLOSS LACQUER (16-823)
(Seymour)

Non-volatile:	15.3%
Watchtung red	0.8%
Lt. Toluidine red	0.7%
Nitrocellulose, Maleic resins, Coconut alkyd resin	13.8%
Volatile:	84.7%
Ketones *, Alcohols *, Acetates *†	53.8%
Aromatic hydrocarbons *, Aliphatic hydrocarbons	8.9%
Propellant (Propane-isobutane)	22.0%

†See Paints, Section VI, General Formulations

SEYMOUR SPRAY PAINT RAVEN BLACK FLAT LACQUER (16-806)
(Seymour)

Non-volatile:	12.0%
Carbon black	0.5%
Silicates	3.1%
Nitrocellulose, Dioctylphthalate, Maleic resins, Coconut alkyd resin	8.4%
Volatile:	88.0%
Ketones *, Alcohols *, Acetates *†	57.5%
Aromatic hydrocarbons *, Aliphatic hydrocarbons	8.5%
Propellant (Propane-isobutane)	22.0%

†See Paints, Section VI, General Formulations

SEYMOUR SPRAY PAINT REBUILDER BLACK SEMI-GLOSS LACQUER (16-838)
(Seymour)

Non-volatile:	13.6%
Carbon black	0.5%
Silicates	1.7%
Nitrocellulose, Dioctylphthalate, Maleic resins, Coconut alkyd resin	11.4%
Volatile:	86.4%
Ketones *, Alcohols *, Acetates *†	55.1%
Aromatic hydrocarbons *	9.3%
Propellant (Propane-isobutane)	22.0%

†See Paints, Section VI, General Formulations

SEYMOUR SPRAY PAINT ROAR'N RED GLOSS ENAMEL (16-123)
(Seymour)

Non-volatile:	16.4%
Titanium dioxide	1.2%
Lithol-Rupine red	1.0%
Pure yellow Iron oxide	0.8%
Azo anisidine yellow	0.7%
Synthetic Petroleum resins, Soya and Vinyl toluene linseed alkyd resins	12.7%
Volatile:	83.6%
Ketones	4.8%
Halogenated hydrocarbons *, Aromatic hydrocarbons *, Aliphatic hydrocarbons *, Driers *	4.8%
Propellant (Propane-isobutane)	30.0%

SEYMOUR SPRAY PAINT SHINY DOLLAR METALLIC ALUMINUM (16-111)
(Seymour)

Non-volatile:	10.5%
Aluminum powder	1.8%
Styrene resin	8.7%
Volatile:	89.5%
Aromatic hydrocarbons *, Aliphatic hydrocarbons *	59.5%
Propellant (Propane-isobutane)	30.0%

SEYMOUR SPRAY PAINT SUN YELLOW GLOSS ENAMEL (16-119)
(Seymour)

Non-volatile:	14.9%
Titanium dioxide	1.8%
Azo anisidine yellow	1.1%
Synthetic Petroleum resins, Soya and Vinyl toluene linseed alkyd resin	12.0%
Volatile:	85.1%
Ketones	5.0%
Halogenated hydrocarbons *, Aromatic hydrocarbons *, Aliphatic hydrocarbons *, Driers *	50.1%
Propellant (Propane-isobutane)	30.0%

SEYMOUR SPRAY PAINT SUN YELLOW GLOSS LACQUER (16-819)
(Seymour)

Non-volatile:	16.3%
Titanium dioxide	1.9%
Azo anisidine yellow	0.4%
Nitrocellulose, Dioctylphthalate, Maleic resins	14.0%
Volatile:	83.7%
Ketones *, Alcohols *, Acetates *†	52.4%
Aromatic hydrocarbons *, Aliphatic hydrocarbons	9.3%
Propellant (Propane-isobutane)	22.0%

†See Paints, Section VI, General Formulations

SEYMOUR SPRAY PAINT SWAN WHITE GLOSS LACQUER (16-813)
(Seymour)

Non-volatile:	19.6%
Titanium dioxide	6.7%
Nitrocellulose, Dioctylphthalate, Maleic resins, Coconut alkyd resin	12.9%
Volatile:	80.4%
Ketones *, Alcohols *, Acetates *†	48.2%
Aromatic hydrocarbons *	10.2%
Propellant (Propane-isobutane)	22.0%

†See Paints, Section VI, General Formulations

SEYMOUR VINYL COAT HIGH SHEEN BLACK (16-403)
(Seymour)

Non-volatile:	11.5%
Carbon black	0.4%
Vinyl and vinyl acrylic resins, Dibutylphthalate	11.1%
Volatile:	88.5%
Ketones *	70.5%
Propellant (Propane-isobutane)	18.0%

SEYMOUR VINYL COAT SATIN BLACK (16-420)
(Seymour)

Non-volatile:	9.7%
Carbon black	0.4%
Silicates	0.5%
Vinyl and vinyl acrylic resins, Dibutylphthalate	8.8%
Volatile:	90.3%
Ketones *	72.3%
Propellant (Propane-isobutane)	18.0%

SEYMOUR VINYL COAT SOFT OFF-WHITE (16-422)
(Seymour)

Non-volatile:	12.7%
Titanium dioxide	4.1%
Silicates	0.5%
Vinyl and vinyl acrylic resins, Dibutylphthalate	8.1%
Volatile:	87.3%
Ketones *	69.3%
Propellant (Propane-isobutane)	18.0%

SF-77
Cleaner and degreaser
(Damon Chemical Co.)

Alkaline compounds *

SHADOTONE PRODUCTS

See COOK'S SHADOTONE PRODUCTS

SHAKLEE BASIC-D
Granulated automatic dishwashing compound
(Shaklee)

Sodium carbonate *, Silicate, Other alkaline salts
Wetting agents . . . .   small amounts
Chlorine releasing agents   small amounts

SHAKLEE BASIC-H
Liquid all purpose household cleaner
(Shaklee)

Non-ionic surfactants *
Water

pH of concentrated product - essentially neutral

SHAKLEE BASIC-I
Liquid heavy duty industrial and household cleaner
(Shaklee)

Non-ionic surfactants
Organic and inorganic bases *†
Water

†*See* Lye

SHAKLEE BASIC-L
Powdered laundry concentrate
(Shaklee)

Non-ionic surfactants
Sodium carbonate *
Sodium silicate
Suspending agents, brighteners, perfume and color

SHARPIE
Fine line permanent marker
(Sanford Corp.)

Dyes
Resins
Glycol ethers
Alcohol

SHARPIE LITHO
Fine line permanent marker
(Sanford Corp.)

Aromatic solvent:
   Xylene *
   Toluene *
Dyes
Resins

SHAVER SAVER, REMINGTON ELECTRIC

See REMINGTON ELECTRIC SHAVER SAVER

SHAVINE
Depilatory to remove beard
(Carson Products)

Barium sulfide * . . . .   <15%
Calcium hydroxide . . . .   <15%
Fillers:
   Starch
   Calcium carbonate

SHEAFFER BALL PEN INKS
In refills only
(Sheaffer Eaton)

Synthetic dyes . . . .   up to 50%
Polyhydric alcohols 0-55%
Aromatic alcohols 0-55%
Glycol ethers 0-55%

SHEAFFER INKS FOR SPLIT NIB FOUNTAIN PENS (In Bottles and Cartridges)
(Sheaffer Eaton)

Synthetic Dyes 1-5%
Humectant . . . .   <2%
Iron compounds 0-1%
Tannic acid 0-0.5%
Phenolic compounds . . . .   <0.5%
Solvent (Water) . . . .   balance

SHEAFFER ROLLING BALL MARKER INKS (In Refills Only)
(Sheaffer Eaton)

Synthetic Dyes 7-9%
Mixture of Glycols and Glycol
   ethers * 10-40%
Surfactants . . . .   <0.5%
Synthetic Resins . . . .   <2.0%
Phenolic compounds . . . .   <0.5%
Cosolvent (proprietary) 15-20%
Solvent (Water) . . . .   balance

SHEAFFER "SOFTSTROKE" FIBER TIP MARKER INKS (In Throwaway Markers Only)
(Sheaffer Eaton)

Synthetic Dyes 2-5%
Mixture of Glycols and Glycol
   ethers * 15-25%
Surfactant 0-0.5%
Phenolic compounds . . . .   <0.5%
Solvent (Water) . . . .   balance

SHEAFFER "TEKTOR" PLASTIC TIP MARKER INKS (In Refills Only)
(Sheaffer Eaton)

Synthetic Dyes 2-5%
Mixture of Glycols and Glycol
   ethers * 15-25%
Surfactant 0.5%
Phenolic compounds 0.05%
Solvent (Water) . . . .   balance

SHEFFIELD BRONZE PAINT PRODUCTS
Aluminum paint and paint specialties

Sheffield Bronze Paint Corp.
17814 Waterloo Rd.
Cleveland, Ohio 44119

Phone: 216-481-8330

See PAINTS, Section VI, General Formulations

SHEFFIELD RED LEAD PRIMER
(Sheffield Bronze Paint)

Red lead * 28.98%

SHELLACOL
Proprietary solvent
(IMC Chem.)

Ethyl alcohol (denatured) *

SHELLZONE
Antifreeze
(Shell Oil)

Ethylene glycol * 95%

SHERRY-JEN TONIC
Appetite stimulant
(Jenkins Labs.)

Each fluid oz.:
   Alcohol 9%
   Thiamine hydrochloride . . . . . .   8 mg.
   Riboflavin . . . .   4 mg.
   Cyanocobalamin . . . .   4 mcg.
   Nicotinamide . . . .   20 mg.
   Calcium pantothenate . . . .   5 mg.
   Pyridoxine hydrochloride . . . . .   1 mg.
   Inositol . . . .   30 mg.
   Choline bitartrate . . . .   60 mg.
   Ferric ammonium citrate . . . . .   60 mg.
   d-Sorbitol, genuine sherry wine vehicle

SHERWIN-WILLIAMS PAINT PRODUCTS
Paints, varnishes, lacquers, enamels, and stains

The Sherwin-Williams Co.
101 Prospect Ave., N.W.
Cleveland, Ohio 44115

Phone: 216-566-2000

See PAINTS, Section VI, General Formulations

SHIELD (Liquid)
(C-Z Chemical)

Amphoteric wetting agent 40% . .   10%
4,6-Chloro-2-phenyl phenol *† . .   10%
Diethanolamine 2%
Tetra potassium pyrophosphate .   6%
Sodium hydroxide * 2.16%
Water 69.84%

'76 Ed.

†*See* Chloro-2-phenyl phenol

Starred ingredients (*) may be responsible for major toxic effects; consult Section II.

SHIELD
Deodorant bar
(Lever Bros.)

Sodium soap	80-90%
Water	5-10%
Free Fatty acids	3-10%
Perfume	1-5%
Sodium chloride	0.5-5%
Germicide	<1%
Sodium phosphate	<1%
Glycerin	<1%
Sodium sulfate	<1%
Sodium EDTA	trace
Sodium EHDP	trace
Antioxidant	trace
Titanium dioxide	trace
Colorants	trace

SHIELD DISINFECTANT DEODORANT (Aerosol Bomb)
(C-Z Chemical)

Lauryl methacrylate	08.50%
Ortho phenyl phenol	00.10%
Hepta decyl hydroxy ethyl imidazoline	00.10%
Polyvinyl pyrrolidinone	00.10%
Isopropyl alcohol *	28.80%
Inert ingred.:	
Dichloro difluoro methane	
Trichloro monofluoro methane	
Perfume	

'76 Ed.

SHIFT-EZE
For all transmissions
(Radiator)

Petroleum distillates *

'76 Ed.

SHILOH FOR COUGHS
Antitussive
(Brown Mfg.)

Chloroform	3 m./fl. oz.
Terpin hydrate	1 1/4%
Benzocaine	
Ammonium chloride	
Oil of peppermint	
Licorice	
Sodium citrate	
Sodium salicylate *	1%
Oil of tar *	2 1/5%
Glycerin	
Syrup	

'76 Ed.

SHILOH THROAT TABLETS
(Brown Mfg.)

Each tablet:
Cetylkonium chloride (Cetyl dimethyl benzylammonium chloride)	5 mg.
Benzocaine	5 mg.

'76 Ed.

SHIMMER MULTI-PURPOSE CLEANER-POLISH (AEROSOL)
(Nat'l Labs. Div.)

Mineral oil *	major
Petroleum distillate *	major
Isobutane/Propane (propellant)	

SHINE-ALL, REGULAR
Floor cleaner
(Hillyard Chem.)

Liquid detergent *†

'76 Ed.

†*See* Detergents, Section VI, General Formulations

SHINE-ALL, SUPER
Cleaner
(Hillyard Chem.)

Liquid detergent *†

'76 Ed.

†*See* Detergents, Section VI, General Formulations

SHINES LIKE THE SUN AUTOMOTIVE VINYL CONDITIONER (AS-967, Formula 2146-134)

See SIMONIZ SHINES LIKE THE SUN AUTOMOTIVE VINYL CONDITIONER (AS-967, Formula 2146-134)

SHINES LIKE THE SUN LIQUID CAR WAX (AS-966, Formula 2080-102)

See SIMONIZ SHINES LIKE THE SUN LIQUID CAR WAX (AS-966, Formula 2080-102)

SHINES LIKE THE SUN PASTE CAR WAX (AS-965, Formula 2106-61)

See SIMONIZ SHINES LIKE THE SUN PASTE CAR WAX (AS-965, Formula 2106-61)

SHISEIDO COSMETICS

Shiseido Cosmetics (America) Ltd.
540 Madison Ave.
New York, N.Y. 10022

Phone: 212-752-2644

See COSMETICS, Section VI, General Formulations

SHOCKAWAY
Antistatic for carpets
(Paul Koss)

Solution of Benzalkonium chloride   <1%

pH 7.0

SHOK 'N LOK CHLORINATED STABILIZER

See BIO-GUARD SHOK 'N LOK CHLORINATED STABILIZER

SHONTEX HAIR CARE PRODUCTS

Shontex Products Co.
1221 Ocean Ave.
Santa Monica, Calif. 90401

Phone: 213-451-8121

See COSMETICS, Section VI, General Formulations

SHOPRITE ACTIVATED BORAX
(Wakefern; supplier, Stanson Detergents)

Sodium chloride
Sodium carbonate (trace)
Borax *

SHOPRITE AFTER BATH FRICTION LOTION
(Wakefern; supplier, B. H. Krueger)

SD Alcohol 40
Water
Fragrance
Benzophenone-2
Menthol
Dye

SHOPRITE AFTER SHAVE LOTION
(Wakefern; supplier, B. H. Krueger)

SD Alcohol 40
Water
Fragrance
Menthol
Dye

SHOPRITE ALL FABRIC DRY BLEACH
(Wakefern; supplier, Purex Corp.)

Sodium carbonate *
Sodium perborate
Alkyl phenoxy ethoxy ethanol
Sodium silicate
Sodium linear dodecyl benzene sulfonate
Fluorescent whitening agents
Sodium sulfate
Dye and perfume

Starred ingredients (*) may be responsible for major toxic effects; consult Section II.

SHOPRITE ALL-PURPOSE DETERGENT (White and Blue)
(Wakefern; supplier, Witco Chem.)

Sodium sulfate
Sodium tripolyphosphate
Sodium tridecyl benzene sulfonate
Sodium silicate (1:2.4 ratio)
Sodium carboxymethylcellulose
Sodium chloride
Protein (partially hydrolyzed)
Moisture, Fluorescent whiteners
Perfume
Blue coloring (in Blue product)

SHOPRITE AMMONIA (Clear, Cloudy, and Lemon)
(Wakefern; supplier, Laundry Aids)

Clear:
  Ammonium hydroxide (3.3% solution) *
  Water (soft)

Cloudy:
  Ammonium hydroxide (3.3% solution) *
  Water (soft)
  Opacifier
  Clarifying agent

Lemon:
  Ammonium hydroxide solution *
  Water (soft)
  Alkylate sulfonate
  Clarifying agent
  Color
  Perfume

SHOPRITE AUTOMATIC BOWL CLEANER
(Wakefern; supplier, Neptune Chem.)

Nonyl phenol methoxylate
Triphenolmethane dye
Lemon perfume
Sodium borate *
Water

SHOPRITE AUTOMATIC DISH DETERGENT
(Wakefern; supplier, Korex Co.)

Sodium tripolyphosphate *
Sodium carbonate
Nonionic surfactant
Chlorinated isocyanurate
Sodium silicate
Sodium chloride

SHOPRITE BATH OIL CONCENTRATE
(Wakefern; supplier, B. H. Krueger)

Mineral oil
PEG-4 dilaurate
PEG-40 sorbitan peroleate
Lanolin oil
Fragrance
Benzophenone-3
Dye

SHOPRITE BLEACH
(Wakefern; supplier, J. L. Prescott Co.)

Sodium hypochlorite solution *
Sodium hydroxide *

SHOPRITE BUBBLING BATH OIL
(Wakefern; supplier, Abolition Products)

Water
Sodium C14-16 olefin sulfonate
Sodium laureth sulfate
Sodium chloride
Cocamide DEA
Coco-betaine
Formalin
Fragrance
Dye

SHOPRITE CHILDREN'S CHEWABLE COLD TABLETS
(Wakefern; supplier, Pennex Products)

Each tablet:
  Aspirin * . . . . 81.00 mg.
  Phenylephrine HCl . . . . 1.25 mg.

SHOPRITE CLEANSER
(Wakefern; supplier, Fitzpatrick Bros.)

Silica sand
Soda ash
ACL 85
Sulframin 85
Green dye

SHOPRITE CLEAR ACRYLIC FLOOR FINISH
(Wakefern; supplier, Howland Chem.)

Ammonia *
Alkali soluble resin
Plasticizers
Polymer
Water

SHOPRITE CLEAR DISH DETERGENT
(Wakefern; supplier, J. L. Prescott Co.)

Water
Sodium xylene sulfonate
Sodium dodecyl benzene sulfonate
Sodium lauryl ether sulfate
Coconut diethanolamide
Preservative
Chelating agent
Perfume

SHOPRITE CLEAR FLOOR WAX
(Wakefern; supplier, Howland Chem.)

Ammonia *
Alkali soluble resin
Plasticizers
Polymer
Polyethylene emulsion
Formaldehyde
Water

SHOPRITE COLD WATER LAUNDRY DETERGENT
(Wakefern; supplier, J. L. Prescott Co.)

Water
Sodium xylene sulfonate
Sodium dodecyl benzene sulfonate
Ethoxylated dodecyl alcohol
TEA dodecyl benzene sulfonate
Chelating agent
Optical brightener
Sodium carbonate
Opacifier
Perfume
Color dye

SHOPRITE CONTINUOUS COLD CAPSULES
(Wakefern; supplier, Pennex Products)

Each capsule:
  Phenylpropanolamine HCl * . . 75 mg.
  Chlorpheniramine maleate . . . . 8 mg.

SHOPRITE CONTROLLED SUDS DETERGENT-FLUFFY
(Wakefern; supplier, North American Chem. Corp.)

Complex phosphates *
Surfactants
Sodium silicates
Sodium sulfate
Sodium carbonate
Active Borax
Carboxymethyl cellulose
Optical brighteners
Perfume
Water

SHOPRITE COUGH SYRUP DM
(Wakefern; supplier, Pennex Products)

Each 5 ml.:
  Ethyl alcohol 1.4%
  Guaifenesin . . . . 100 mg.
  d-Methorphan HBr * . . . . 15 mg.

SHOPRITE CREAM DEODORANT
(Wakefern; supplier, B. H. Krueger)

Water
Aluminum chlorohydrate complex
Glycol stearate
Spermaceti
Propylene glycol
Coceta-6
Acetylated lanolin
Mineral oil
Lanolin alcohol
Urea
Propylparaben
Butylparaben

Starred ingredients (*) may be responsible for major toxic effects; consult Section II.

SHOPRITE C.W. LAUNDRY DETERGENT
(Wakefern; supplier, Witco Chem.)

Sodium sulfate
Sodium tripolyphosphate
Anionic surfactant (Sodium tridecyl benzene sulfonate)
Sodium silicate (1:2.4 ratio)(not meta)
Moisture
Sodium chloride
Sodium carboxymethylcellulose
Protein (partially hydrolyzed)
Fluorescent whiteners
Perfume
Coloring (if applicable)

SHOPRITE DANDRUFF SHAMPOO
(Wakefern; supplier, Abolition Products)

Water
Sodium C14-16 olefin sulfonate
Sodium laureth sulfate
Cocamide DEA
Coco-betaine
p-Chloro-m-xylenol
Formalin
Styrene acrylic latex
Sodium bicarbonate
Fragrance
Dye

SHOPRITE DECONGESTANT TABLETS
(Wakefern; supplier, Pennex Products)

Each tablet:
Aspirin * .... 325 mg.
Caffeine .... 20 mg.
Aluminum hydroxide .... 60 mg.
Magnesium carbonate .... 60 mg.
Phenylephrine HCl .... 5 mg.
Chlorpheniramine maleate ... 2 mg.

SHOPRITE DENTURE ADHESIVE
(Wakefern; supplier, Iodent Co.)

Karaya gum
Propylparaben
Magnesium oxide
Peppermint oil
Petrolatum blend
Dye

SHOPRITE DENTURE CLEANSER TABLETS
(Wakefern; supplier, Iodent Co.)

Sodium bicarbonate
Polyvinylpyrollidone
Isopropyl alcohol
Peppermint oil
Sodium acid pyrophosphate
Sorbitol crystals
Pluronic F68 (polyoxyalkylene derivative of propylene glycol)
Sodium lauryl sulfate
Citric and tartaric acids
Oxone
Sodium perborate
Trisodium phosphate
Silica
Preservatives

SHOPRITE DRYER CYCLE FABRIC SOFTENER SHEETS
(Wakefern; supplier, J. L. Prescott Co.)

Dimethyl di(hydrogenated tallow) ammonium methyl sulfate *†
Perfume

†See Dialkyl dimethyl ammonium chloride

SHOPRITE EXTRA STRENGTH COUGH SYRUP
(Wakefern; supplier, Pennex Products)

Each 5 ml.:
Dextromethorphan HBr ..... 5 mg.
Chlorpheniramine maleate .. 1 mg.
Ethyl alcohol .... 10% v/v
Sodium citrate .... 250 mg.

SHOPRITE FLUFFY CONTROLLED SUDS PHOSPHATE LAUNDRY DETERGENT, Formulation A
(Wakefern; supplier, Witco Chem.)

Sodium carbonate *
Sodium tripolyphosphate
Sodium sulfate
Sodium silicate (1:2.4 ratio)(not meta)
Nonionic surfactant
Anionic surfactant (Sodium dodecyl benzene sulfonate)
Sodium perborate, Borax, Sodium carboxymethylcellulose, Protein (partially hydrolyzed), Fluorescent whitener, Anticaking agent, Perfume, and Water

SHOPRITE FLUFFY CONTROLLED SUDS PHOSPHATE LAUNDRY DETERGENT, Formulation B
(Wakefern; supplier, Witco Chem.)

Sodium carbonate *
Sodium sulfate
Sodium tripolyphosphate
Nonionic surfactant
Sodium silicate (1:2.4 ratio)(not meta)
Anionic surfactant (Sodium dodecyl benzene sulfonate)
Sodium perborate, Borax, Sodium carboxymethylcellulose, Protein (partially hydrolyzed), Fluorescent whitener, Anticaking agent, Perfume, and Water

SHOPRITE FOAM RUG CLEANER
(Wakefern; supplier, Zoe Chem.)

Surfactants *
Sodium nitrite
Formaldehyde solution 1.0% 0.1%
Ammonia
Water

SHOPRITE GREEN ALL PURPOSE CLEANER
(Wakefern; supplier, J. L. Prescott Co.)

Water
Sodium xylene sulfonate
Sodium dodecyl benzene sulfonate
Ethoxylated dodecyl alcohol
Sodium sulfate
Ammonium hydroxide solution
Latex opacifier
Perfume
Color dye

SHOPRITE GREEN DISH DETERGENT
(Wakefern; supplier, J. L. Prescott Co.)

Water
Sodium xylene sulfonate
Sodium dodecyl benzene sulfonate
Sodium lauryl ether sulfate
Coconut diethanolamide
Preservative
Chelating agent
Perfume
Color dye

SHOPRITE HEAVY DUTY LAUNDRY DETERGENT
(Wakefern; supplier, J. L. Prescott Co.)

Water
Sodium xylene sulfonate
Sodium dodecyl benzene sulfonate
Ethoxylated dodecyl alcohol
TEA dodecyl benzene sulfonate
Chelating agent
Optical brightener
Sodium carbonate
Opacifier
Perfume
Color dye

SHOPRITE INSECT REPELLENT
(Wakefern; supplier, Zoe Chem.)

N,N-Diethyl-meta-toluamide *
Isopropyl alcohol *
Essential oil
Propellent

SHOPRITE LAUNDRY DETERGENT (White and Blue)
(Wakefern; supplier, Witco Chem.)

Sodium sulfate
Sodium tripolyphosphate
Anionic surfactant (Sodium tridecyl benzene sulfonate)
Sodium silicate (1:2.4 ratio)(not meta)
Moisture
Sodium chloride
Sodium carboxymethylcellulose
Protein (partially hydrolyzed)
Fluorescent whiteners
Perfume
Coloring (if applicable)

Starred ingredients (*) may be responsible for major toxic effects; consult Section II.

SHOPRITE LEMON CONCENTRATED FABRIC SOFTENER
(Wakefern; supplier, J. L. Prescott Co.)

Water
Quaternary ammonium sulfate (complex difatty compound) *
Optical brightener
Antifoam
Preservatives
Perfume
Color dye

SHOPRITE LEMON DISH DETERGENT
(Wakefern; supplier, J. L. Prescott Co.)

Water
Sodium xylene sulfonate
Sodium dodecyl benzene sulfonate
Sodium lauryl ether sulfate
Coconut diethanolamide
Preservative
Chelating agent
Perfume

SHOPRITE LEMON FABRIC SOFTENER RINSE
(Wakefern; supplier, J. L. Prescott Co.)

Water
Quaternary ammonium sulfate (complex difatty compound) *
Optical brightener
Antifoam
Preservatives
Perfume
Color dye

SHOPRITE LEMON REFRESH CLEANER
(Wakefern; supplier, Howland Chem.)

Sodium metasilicate
Sodium carbonate *
Modified Coconut diethanolamide
Chelating agent
Sodium xylene sulfonate
Lemon perfume
Water
Coloring . . . .   trace

SHOPRITE LIME DISH DETERGENT
(Wakefern; supplier, J. L. Prescott Co.)

Water
Sodium xylene sulfonate
Sodium dodecyl benzene sulfonate
Sodium lauryl ether sulfate
Coconut diethanolamide
Preservative
Chelating agent
Perfume
Opacifier
Color dye

SHOPRITE LIQUID CLEANSER WITH MILD ABRASIVE
(Wakefern; supplier, Barcolene Co.)

Water
Calcium carbonate
Surfactants
Chelating agent
Suspension agent
Preservative
Fragrance compound

SHOPRITE LIQUID DETERGENT
(Wakefern)

Sodium N-dodecyl benzene sulfonate *
Sodium xylene sulfonate
Alcohol ether sulfate

SHOPRITE MALDROXAL
Antacid
(Wakefern; supplier, L. Perrigo Co.)

Aluminum hydroxide gel
Magnesium hydroxide
Sodium saccharin
Propylene glycol
Methylparaben
Propylparaben
Butylparaben
Peppermint oil
Sorbitol
Magnesium aluminum silicate
Water

SHOPRITE MEDICATED BLUE SHAMPOO
(Wakefern; supplier, National Pharmaceuticals)

Selenium sulfide (1%) *
Water
Amphoteric-2
Sodium lauryl sulfate
Bentonite
Lauramide DEA
Citric acid
Ethylene glycol monostearate
Titanium dioxide
Sodium phosphate
Captan
Glyceryl ricinoleate
Perfume
Artificial coloring:
    FD & C Blue #1
    D & C Yellow #10

SHOPRITE MEDICATED CHEST RUB
(Wakefern; supplier, Pennex Products)

Petrolatum 80%
Paraffin 9%
Perfume * 16%

SHOPRITE NAIL POLISH REMOVER - OILY
(Wakefern; supplier, HABA International)

Acetone *
Water
PEG-15 tallow polyamine
D & C Yellow #11
D & C Red #33
Green #5

SHOPRITE NASAL SPRAY D
(Wakefern; supplier, L. Perrigo Co.)

Water
Sodium bisulfite
Pheniramine maleate 0.02%
Benzalkonium chloride
Thimerosal
Potassium phosphate monobasic
Sodium phosphate monobasic
Phenylephrine hydrochloride * 0.50%

SHOPRITE NI-CALM
(Wakefern; supplier, Pennex Products)

Each oz.:
    Ethyl alcohol 25%
    d-Methorphan HBr . . . .   15 mg.
    Acetaminophen * . . . .   600 mg.
    Chlorpheniramine maleate . .   1 mg.
    Ephedrine sulfate . . . .   24.3 mg.

SHOPRITE NON-AEROSOL SPRAY FURNITURE POLISH
(Wakefern; supplier, Howland Chem.)

Wax emulsion
Silicones *
Water
Lemon perfume

SHOPRITE NON-ASPIRIN EXTRA STRENGTH CAPSULES
(Wakefern; supplier, Pennex Products)

Each capsule:
    Acetaminophen * . . . .   500 mg.

SHOPRITE NON-ASPIRIN EXTRA STRENGTH TABLETS
(Wakefern; supplier, Pennex Products)

Each tablet:
    Acetaminophen * . . . .   500 mg.

SHOPRITE NON-ASPIRIN PAIN RELIEVER
(Wakefern; supplier, Pennex Products)

Each tablet:
    Acetaminophen * . . . .   325 mg.

Starred ingredients (*) may be responsible for major toxic effects; consult Section II.

SHOPRITE NO PHOS BLUE AND BRAVE NO PHOS WHITE DETERGENT
(Wakefern; supplier, Witco Chem.)

Washing soda *
Sodium sulfate
Sodium tridecyl benzene sulfonate
Sodium silicate (1:2.4 ratio)
Sodium carboxymethylcellulose
Protein (partially hydrolyzed)
Sodium chloride
Moisture, Fluorescent whiteners
Perfume
Blue coloring in Blue product and Anti-caking agents

SHOPRITE NO PHOS LAUNDRY DETERGENT
(Wakefern; supplier, Witco Chem.)

Sodium carbonate *
Sodium sulfate
Anionic surfactant (Sodium tridecyl benzene sulfonate)
Sodium silicate (1:2.4 ratio)(not meta)
Sodium chloride
Moisture
Sodium carboxymethylcellulose
Anti-caking agents
Fluoresecent whiteners
Perfume
Blue coloring (if applicable)

SHOPRITE NO PHOSPHATE DETERGENT
(Wakefern; supplier, Theobald Industries)

Linear alkyl benzene sulfonate *
Sodium sulfate
Sodium carbonate
Sodium silicate (1:2.4 ratio)
Sodium chloride
Sodium carboxymethyl cellulose
Optical whitener
Perfume
Colorant

pH of a 1% solution is 10.7 to 11.0

SHOPRITE NO SOIL
(Wakefern; supplier, Howland Chem.)

Sodium metasilicate *
Sodium carbonate
Chelating agent
Tall oil soap
Modified Coconut diethanolamine
Pine oil
Coloring .... trace
Water

SHOPRITE NO WAX FLOOR CLEANER/FINISH
(Wakefern; supplier, Howland Chem.)

Ammonia *
Alkali soluble resin
Plasticizers
Polymer
Water
Surfactants (nonionic)

SHOPRITE PAIN RELIEVER TABLETS
(Wakefern; supplier, Pennex Products)

Aspirin * .... 180 mg.
Acetaminophen .... 90 mg.
Salicylamide .... 90 mg.
Caffeine .... 30 mg.

SHOPRITE PEARLIZED DISH DETERGENT
(Wakefern; supplier, J. L. Prescott Co.)

Water
Sodium xylene sulfonate
Sodium dodecyl benzene sulfonate
Sodium lauryl ether sulfate
Coconut diethanolamide
Preservative
Chelating agent
Perfume
Ethylene gylcol monostearate

SHOPRITE PINE AMMONIA
(Wakefern; supplier, J. L. Prescott Co.)

Ammonium hydroxide solution *
Ethoxylated alcohol
Perfume
Color dye

SHOPRITE PINK DISH DETERGENT
(Wakefern; supplier, J. L. Prescott Co.)

Water
Sodium xylene sulfonate
Sodium dodecyl benzene sulfonate
Sodium lauryl ether sulfate
Coconut diethanolamide
Preservative
Chelating agent
Perfume
Opacifier
Color dye

SHOPRITE PINK FABRIC SOFTENER RINSE
(Wakefern; supplier, J. L. Prescott Co.)

Water
Quaternary ammonium sulfate (complex difatty compound) *
Optical brightener
Antifoam
Preservatives
Perfume
Color dye

SHOPRITE POUR N' MOP
(Wakefern; supplier, Howland Chem.)

Ammonia *
Alkali soluble resin
Plasticizers
Polymer
Anionic polyethylene emulsion
Formaldehyde
Water
Blue dye .... trace

SHOPRITE RINSE AID
(Wakefern; supplier, Manstan Chem.)

Nonionic surfactant (Terminated alkyl aryl ether)
Water

SHOPRITE SAL SODA
(Wakefern; supplier, Stanson Detergents)

Sodium carbonate *
Sodium chloride

SHOPRITE "SCRUNCHY BEAR" BUBBLE SOLUTION
Bubble bath
(Wakefern; supplier, Manhattan Products)

Water
Alkylate sulfonate
Alkylolamide
Cellosize
Sodium chloride
Dye stuff (color)

SHOPRITE SCRUNCHY BUBBLE FUN
(Wakefern; supplier, Purex Corp.)

Anionic surfactant *
Foam stabilizer (alkanolamide)
Fragrance
Colorant
Water

SHOPRITE SHAMPOO PRODUCTS
(Wakefern; supplier, Abolition Products)

General formula:
Water
Sodium C14-16 olefin sulfonate
Sodium laureth sulfate
Cocoamide DEA
Coco-betaine
Sodium chloride
Color
Perfume
Preservatives
Humectants
Thickeners

SHOPRITE SOLID AIR FRESHENER (Berry, Lemon and Floral Scents)
(Wakefern; supplier, Blue Cross Labs.)

Carrageen
Perfume
Water

SHOPRITE SOLID BOWL FRESHENER
(Wakefern; supplier, Neptune Chem.)

Linear aliphatic ethoxylate
Sodium sulfate
Sodium borate *
Perfume

Starred ingredients (*) may be responsible for major toxic effects; consult Section II.

SHOPRITE SPOT FREE
Spot and soil remover
(Wakefern; supplier, Manstan Chem.)

Nonionic surfactant (Terminated alkyl
aryl ether)
Sodium hydroxide (used for neutralization
only)

SHOPRITE SPRAY ALL PURPOSE CLEANER
(Wakefern; supplier, J. L. Prescott Co.)

Water
2-Butoxyethanol (Butyl Cellosolve) *
Diethanolamine
Coconut diethanolamide
Sodium lauryl ether sulfate
Formalin
Ethoxylated dodecyl alcohol
Perfume
EDTA
Dye

SHOPRITE SPRAY DISINFECTANT
(Wakefern; supplier, Cello Chem.)

Ethyl alcohol
Triethylene glycol
Alkyldimethyl benzene ammonium chlo-
rides *
Bromo salicylanilides
Surfactant
Corrosion inhibitor
Propellant - propane-butane

SHOPRITE SPRAY GLASS CLEANER
(Wakefern; supplier, J. L. Prescott Co.)

Water
Isopropyl alcohol
2-Butoxyethanol (Butyl Cellosolve) *
Formalin
Ammonium hydroxide
Ethoxylated dodecyl alcohol
Perfume
EDTA
Dye

SHOPRITE SPRAY SPOT AND STAIN REMOVER
(Wakefern; supplier, J. L. Prescott Co.)

Water
Ethoxylated dodecyl alcohol *
Formalin
Perfume
EDTA
Dye

SHOPRITE SPRAY & WAX - REGULAR
(Wakefern; supplier, Zoe Chem.)

Silicone
Emulsifying agents
Wax
Perfume - regular scent
Water

SHOPRITE SPRAY & WIPE - LEMON
(Wakefern; supplier, Zoe Chem.)

Silicone
Emulsifying agents
Wax
Perfume - lemon
Water

SHOPRITE SS COUGH SYRUP
(Wakefern; supplier, Pennex Products)

Each 10 ml.:
　　Ethyl alcohol 10%
　　d-Methorphan HBr * .... 15 mg.
　　Cetyl pyridinium chloride 0.01%
　　Doxylamine succinate .... 7.5 mg.

SHOPRITE TOILET BOWL CLEANER
(Wakefern; supplier, Contract Packaging)

Sodium bisulfate *
Sodium carbonate
Octyl phenoxy polyethoxy ethanol
Sodium sulfate
Methyl salicylate
Sodium silico aluminate
Dye

SHOPRITE WATER CONDITIONER
(Wakefern; supplier, Stanson Detergents)

Sodium chloride
Sodium carbonate *

SHOPRITE WAX REMOVER
(Wakefern; supplier, Howland Chem.)

Sodium metasilicate
Modified Coconut diethanolamide
Aqua ammonia *
Monoethanolamine
Mint perfume .... trace
Water

SHOPRITE WHITE ALL PURPOSE CLEANER
(Wakefern; supplier, J. L. Prescott Co.)

Water
Sodium xylene sulfonate
Sodium dodecyl benzene sulfonate
Ethoxylated dodecyl alcohol
Sodium sulfate
Ammonium hydroxide solution
Latex opacifier
Perfume

SHOPRITE WINDOW WASH
(Wakefern; supplier, Diversified Packaging)

Ammonia (26% NH4OH) ...   0.5%
Isopropanol ....   about 5.0%
Nonionic surfactant (Octylphenoxy polye-
thoxy ethanol)
Dye

SHORT STOP
(Lester Labs.)

Petroleum distillates *
Chlorinated solvents *

'76 Ed.

SHOWER TO SHOWER BRAND BODY POWDER
(Johnson & Johnson)

Fine grade platelet Talc
Sodium bicarbonate
Perfume

SHOWEY PORCELAIN CLEANER & METAL POLISH
(Fuld-Stalfort)

Aqua ammonia (26° Be) * 3.5%
Oxalic acid * 1.6%
Pine oil 2.5%
Fine silica abrasive
Soap
Water

'76 Ed.

SHOW SHINE (HOOF & HORN)
(SerVaas Labs.)

Silica (amorphous) 60%/w
Cade oil 20%/w
Paraffin oil 10%/w
Stearic acid 10%/w

SHREDDI-MIX MODELING MACHE
(Bersted's)

Paper
Plaster
Salt
Glue

SHUR-KILL
Insecticidal spray; industrial
(Barco)

2,2-Dichlorovinyl dimethyl
　　phosphate 0.46%
Related compounds 0.04%
　　Octachloro-4,7-methanotetra-
　　hydroindane 1.80%
Related compounds 1.20%
Petroleum distillates * 96.50%

'76 Ed.

SHUTTLE BLEMISH DISCS
Medicated pads for teenage acne
(Unique Products)

Deionized water
Cetyl trimethyl ammonium bro-
　　mide 1%
Stearyl dimethyl benzyl ammonium
　　chloride 0.1%
Propylene glycol
Methyl parasept
Cosmetic grade IPA

SIALCO
For relief of allergy, cold, sinus symptoms
(Foy Labs.)

Each tablet:
Chlorpheniramine maleate *	4 mg.
Salicylamide	150 mg.
Acetaminophen *	125 mg.
Phenylephrine hydrochloride *	5 mg.

SICCATIFF DE COURTRAY
Japan quick dryer
(Weber, F.)

Manganese *†
Cobalt *‡
Zirconium *‡†

†See Manganese salts
‡See Cobalt driers
‡See Zirconium oxide
†

SICK-'EM
Remove sewer line stoppage - municipal use
(ABCO, Inc.)

Sodium hydroxide (Caustic soda) *

SIDONNA
For irritable bowel syndrome
(Reed & Carnrick)

Each tablet:
Specially activated Simethicone	25 mg.
Hyoscyamine sulfate, N.F.	0.1037 mg.
Atropine sulfate USP	0.0194 mg.
Hyoscine hydrobromide USP (equiv. to belladonna alkaloids (as bases) 0.1049 mg.)	0.0065 mg.
Sodium butabarbital N.F. *	16 mg.

SIERRA PINE TOILET SOAP-BAR
(Los Angeles Soap)

Sodium soap made from tallow and coconut oil
Perfume
Deodorant
Dye

SIGHT SAVERS SILICONE EYEGLASS CLEANER
(Dow Corning Corp.)

Silicone glycol	2.0%
Detergent	2.5%
Isopropyl alcohol *	10.0%
Dipropylene glycol methyl ether	2.0%
Water	83.5%
Perfume and colorant	trace

SIGHT SAVERS SPRAY LENS CLEANER
(Dow Corning Corp.)

Methyl polysiloxane	0.5%
Isopropyl alcohol *	36.5%
Mineral spirits	3.0%
Freon propellant	60.0%

SIGNAL MOUTHWASH
(Lever Bros.)

Water	80-90%
Ethyl alcohol	10-15%
Hydrogenated Starch hydrolyzate	1-5%
Sodium alkyl sulfate	<1%
Polysorbate-20	<1%
Flavor	<1%
Sodium saccharin	trace
Sodium chloride	trace
Sodium acetate	trace
Acetic acid	trace
Colorants	trace

SIGNAL MOUTHWASH CONCENTRATE
(Lever Bros.)

Water	40-50%
Ethyl alcohol	30-40%
Hydrogenated Starch hydrolyzate	10-15%
Sodium alkyl sulfate	<1%
Polysorbate-20	<1%
Flavor	<1%
Sodium saccharin	<1%
Sodium chloride	<1%
Sodium acetate	trace
Acetic acid	trace
Colorants	trace

SIGTAB TABLETS
Vitamin supplement
(Upjohn)

Each tablet:
Vitamin A	5000 I.U.
Vitamin D	400 I.U.
Plus multivitamins	

SIGUNIT
(Sika Chem.)

Caustic powder *

SIKADUR HI-MOD, GEL & REGULAR
(Sika Chem.)

A Component:
Epoxy resin

B Unit:
Alkaline amine *†

†See Coatings, Section VI, General Formulations

SIKADUR HI-MOD LV
(Sika Chem.)

A Component:
Epoxy resins
Butyl glycidal ether

B Component:
Alkaline amine *†

†See Coatings, Section VI, General Formulations

SIKADUR LO-MOD, REGULAR, GEL & LV
(Sika Chem.)

A Unit:
Epoxy resin

B Unit:
Alkaline amine *†

†See Coatings, Section VI, General Formulations

SIKA EPOXY THINNER
(Sika Chem.)

Methyl ethyl ketone *
Toluene *
Isobutyl acetate

SIKA EQUIPMENT CLEANER
(Sika Chem.)

Petroleum solvent (Solvesso 150) *
Cellosolve *

SIKAFLEX 1A
(Sika Chem.)

Isocyanates *
Xylol *

SIKAFLEX MEMBRANE
(Sika Chem.)

Coal tar *
Isocyanates *

SIKAFLEX PRIMER
(Sika Chem.)

Isocyanate
Toluene *
Methyl ethyl ketone *

SIKAFLEX-T68
(Sika Chem.)

A Unit:
Coal tar *
Polyester resins
Xylol *

B Unit:
Isocyanates
Tin mercaptan

SIKAGARD 670
(Sika Chem.)

A Unit:
Epoxy resins
Glycol ethers *

B Unit:
Acrylic amine

Starred ingredients (*) may be responsible for major toxic effects; consult Section II.

SIKAGARD 694
(Sika Chem.)

A Unit:
Epoxy resin

B Unit:
Polyamide

C Unit:
Portland cement
Lead silica chromate *†

†See Lead & Chromate salts

SIKAGARD AQUA TOP
(Sika Chem.)

A Unit:
Epoxy resins

B Unit:
Acrylic amines

SIKAGARD HI-BILD
(Sika Chem.)

A Unit:
Epoxy resins

B Unit:
Alkaline amines *†

†See Coatings, Section VI, General Formulations

SIKA SEAL
Solvent solution
(Sika Chem.)

Asphalt
Gilsonite resin
Petroleum resin
Xylol *
Mineral spirits *

SIKA TRANSPARENT
Water repellent impregnation
(Sika Chem.)

Siliconates
Xylol *

SILACLEAR

See LEECH SILACLEAR

SILAIN-GEL LIQUID
Antacid, antiflatulent
(Robins)

Each 5 ml.:
Simethicone, NF .... 25 mg.
Aluminum hydroxide (equivalent to dried aluminum hydroxide gel, USP) .... 282 mg.
Magnesium hydroxide, NF ... 285 mg.

SILAIN TABLETS
Antiflatulent
(Robins)

Each tablet:
Simethicone, NF .... 50 mg.

SILA-LUX SILICONE ALKYD ENAMELS
(International Paint)

Mineral spirits (or turpentine substitute) *
Pigments - no lead

SILAPRENE

See LEECH SILAPRENE

SILA-SLIDE
Multi-purpose silicone lubricant; industrial and institutional use
(Scientific International)

1,1,1-Trichloroethane *

SILEXIN
Cough tablets
(Clapp, Otis)

Each tablet:
Dextromethorphan hydrobromide *
Benzocaine

SILEXIN COUGH SYRUP
Antitussive and expectorant
(Clapp, Otis)

Each tsp.:
Dextromethorphan hydrobromide *
Guaifenesin

SIL-GLYDE
Lubricating compound
(American Grease Stick)
(Marketed by: Balkamp, Inc.; Chrysler Corp., Parts Div.; Chrysler Corp., MoPar Div.)

Castor oil 40%
Polypropylene glycol * 47%
Silicone fluid 1%
Silicone dioxide 10%
Inhibitors & film strength additives (each less than 1%)

SILIKROIL
Lubricant
(Kano)

Petroleum solvents *
Silicone
Other oils

SILKIENCE COSMETIC PRODUCTS
(Gillette Co., Personal Care Div.)

The Gillette Co., Personal Care Div., Boston, Mass. 02199 will receive collect phone calls from poison control centers or physicians asking for emergency toxicological information about the company's products.

Phone: 617-421-7000

SILK & SATIN COSMETICS

Silk & Satin Hair Products
P.O. Box 432
Durham, N.C. 27702

Phone: 919-471-4919

See COSMETICS, Section VI, General Formulations

SILKTEX
Embalming supply
(Royal Bond)

Diethylene glycol *

SILKY ACRYLIC LATEX FLAT BASE PAINTS
(Touraine Paints, Inc.)

BASE "AA":
  Titanium dioxide 24.6%
  Silica & silicates 18.5%
  Vinyl acrylic latex non-volatile 11.1%
  Water 45.7%
BASE "B":
  Titanium dioxide 15.35%
  Calcium carbonate 6.10%
  Silica & silicates 14.35%
  Vinyl acrylic latex non-volatile 14.70%
  Water 49.50%
BASE "C":
  Titanium dioxide 6.65%
  Calcium carbonate 13.35%
  Silica & silicates 15.50%
  Vinyl acrylic latex non-volatile 12.9%
  Water 51.6%
BASE "D":
  Titanium dioxide 3.2%
  Barium sulfate 19.4%
  Silicates 6.5%
  Vinyl acrylic latex non-volatile 21.2%
  Water 59.7%

'76 Ed.

SILKY ACRYLIC LATEX SEMI GLOSS BASE PAINTS
(Touraine Paints, Inc.)

WHITE BASE "A" & "B":
  Titanium dioxide 18.67%
  Barium sulfate 2.33%
  Acrylic resin non-volatile 26.00%
  Water 53.00%
NEUTRAL BASE "C":
  Titanium dioxide 7.75%
  Barium sulfate 5.15%
  Acrylic resin non-volatile 28.60%
  Water 58.40%
BASE "D":
  Titanium dioxide 3.7%
  Barium sulfate 12.3%
  Acrylic resin non-volatile 27.5%
  Water 56.5%

'76 Ed.

Starred ingredients (*) may be responsible for major toxic effects; consult Section II.

SILKY FLAT PAINTS
(Touraine Paints, Inc.)

AQUA MIST (#957):
Titanium dioxide	23.7%
Silica & silicates	18.5%
Vinyl acrylic latex	10.9%
Water	46.9%

AVOCADO (#970):
Titanium dioxide	21.5%
Silica & silicates	20.7%
Vinyl acrylic latex	10.9%
Water	46.9%

BERMUDA PINK (#956):
See AQUA MIST (#957) - same formulation

BLACK (#949):
Carbon black	1.27%
Calcium carbonate	12.68%
Silica and silicates	23.25%
Vinyl acrylic latex	12.78%
Water	50.10%

BLUE HAZE (#954):
See AQUA MIST (#957) - same formulation

BONE WHITE (#961):
Titanium dioxide	24.6%
Silica and silicates	18.5%
Vinyl acrylic latex	11.1%
Water	45.7%

CHAMPAGNE (#953):
See AQUA MIST (#957) - same formulation

CONFETTI (#955):
See AQUA MIST (#957) - same formulation

DUCKLING (#966):
Titanium dioxide	21.55%
Silica and silicates	20.65%
Vinyl acrylic latex	10.90%
Water	46.91%

HOLIDAY GREEN (#952):
See AQUA MIST (#957) - same formulation

SAND DUNE (#960):
See DUCKLING (#966) - same formulation

SEA SHELL (#965):
See BONE WHITE (#961) - same formulation

SPANISH GOLD (#964):
See DUCKLING (#966) - same formulation

TUMBLEWEED (#951):
See DUCKLING (#966) - same formulation

WHISPER (#967):
See DUCKLING (#966) - same formulation

WHITE (#950):
Titanium dioxide	24.55%
Silica and silicates	18.55%
Vinyl acrylic latex	11.10%
Water	45.71%

'76 Ed.

SILKY LATEX UNDERCOATER PAINT
(Touraine Paints, Inc.)

Titanium dioxide	21.8%
Silica & silicates	3.2%
Water	57.3%
Acrylic latex non-volatile	17.7%

'76 Ed.

SILKY SAND TEXTURE PAINT
(Touraine Paints, Inc.)

Titanium dioxide	9.4%
Calcium carbonate	28.3%
Silica & silicates	12.3%
100% Alkyd resin	2.8%
Acrylic latex non-volatile	12.4%
Water	34.8%

'76 Ed.

SILKY SEMI GLOSS
(Touraine Paints, Inc.)

AQUA MIST (#757):
Titanium dioxide	20.6%
Barium sulphate	2.3%
Acrylic resin non-volatile	25.9%
Water	51.2%

BLACK (#749):
Carbon black	1.0%
Acrylic resin non-volatile	34.0%
Water	65.0%

The following colors have the same formulation as AQUAMIST:
AVOCADO (#770), BERMUDA PINK (#756), BLUE HAZE (#754), BONE WHITE (#761), CHAMPAGNE (#753), CONFETTI (#755), DUCKLING (#766), HOLIDAY GREEN (#752), SAND DUNE (#760), SEA SHELL (#765), SPANISH GOLD (#764), TUMBLEWEED (#751), WHISPER (#767), WHITE (#750)

'76 Ed.

SILOO AIR BRAKE CONDITIONER
Anti-freeze and anti-rust
(Siloo)

Methanol *

SILOO BATTERY CLEANER (Aerosol)
(Siloo)

Phosphate detergents *†
Wetting agents
Emulsifiers
Water

†*See* Metal cleaners, Section VI, General Formulations

SILOO BATTERY TERMINAL PROTECTOR (Aerosol)
(Siloo)

Petroleum distillates *

SILOO BELT DRESSING (Aerosol)
(Siloo)

Chlorinated solvents *
Rosin esters

SILOO BRAKE PARTS CLEANER (Aerosol)
(Siloo)

Perchloroethylene *

SILOO CARB-LIFE
Carburetor cleaner
(Siloo)

Xylol *
Glycol ethers

SILOO CAR WASH CONCENTRATE
(Siloo)

Alkylbenzene sulfonate *

SILOO COPPER GASKET SPRAY (Aerosol)
(Siloo)

Petroleum distillates *

SILOO DIESEL FUEL ANTI-GEL
(Siloo)

Petroleum distillates *
Chlorinated hydrocarbons *

SILOO DIESEL FUEL CONDITIONER
(Siloo)

Petroleum distillates *

SILOO ENGINE SHAMPOO (Aerosol)
Degreaser-cleaner; aerosol
(Siloo)

Petroleum distillates *
Xylol *

SILOO ENGINKOOL
Liquid; for prevention of engine overheating
(Siloo)

Sodium nitrite *

SILOO ENGINSEAL
Stops leaks in main bearing seals
(Siloo)

Petroleum distillates *
Chlorinated hydrocarbons *

SILOO FAST MOTOR FLUSH
Cleans car engines before oil change
(Siloo)

Petroleum distillates *
Glycol ethers *
Ketone solvents *

SILOO FOR GAS TANKS
Liquid; for use in gasoline and diesel fuel tanks
(Siloo)

Propanol
Xylol *

SILOO GASKET AND DECAL REMOVER (Aerosol)
(Siloo)

Methylene chloride *

SILOO GAS LINE ANTI-FREEZE
(Siloo)

Methanol * 100%

SILOO GAS TREATMENT
Multi-purpose concentrate
(Siloo)

Xylol *
Petroleum distillates *

SILOO GLASS CLEANER AND LABEL REMOVER (Aerosol)
(Siloo)

Ammonia 1%
Nonionic detergent 1%
Isopropyl alcohol 10%
Glycol ether 5%
Hydrocarbon propellant 6%

SILOO HYDRA-VALVE KLEEN
Concentrated solvent additive for crankcase oil
(Siloo)

Xylol *

SILOO ICE-OFF
Aerosol de-icer for car windows
(Siloo)

Isopropanol *

SILOO IGNITION SEALER
Protective coating for ignitions; aerosol
(Siloo)

Petroleum distillates *

SILOO OCTANE TREATMENT
(Siloo)

Methanol 15%
Petroleum distillates * 60%
Phosphate esters 10%
Glycol ether 15%

SILOO PDQ
Penetrates, lubricates & loosens rusted parts
(Siloo)

Petroleum distillates *

SILOO PRESSURIZED LOCK DE-ICER AND LUBRICATOR
(Siloo)

Isopropyl alcohol *

SILOO SAHARA GAS
Liquid gas line anti-freeze and conditioner
(Siloo)

Methanol * 100%

SILOO SCREWLOOSE
Penetrating solvent
(Siloo)

Petroleum distillates *
Xylene *

SILOO SILICONE LUBRICANT (Aerosol)
(Siloo)

Silicones
Chlorinated solvents *

SILOO SMOKE-STOP
Concentrated oil treatment
(Siloo)

Blend of:
Petroleum compounds *†
Viscosity improving polymer

†*See* Petroleum distillate

SILOO STARTING FLUID (Aerosol)
For diesel and gasoline engines
(Siloo)

Ethyl ether *

SILOO SY-COOL
Cooling system treatment
(Siloo)

Alkali *†

†*See* Radiator cleaners, Section VI, General Formulations

SILOO TRANS-KLEEN
Liquid transmission additive
(Siloo)

Petroleum distillates *
Xylene *

SILOO TRANSMISSION LEAK-STOP
(Siloo)

Petroleum distillates *

SILOO TUNE-UP AND PVC SOLVENT
Automotive
(Siloo)

Orthodichlorobenzene *

SILOO VINYL TOP CLEANER & WAX (Aerosol)
(Siloo)

Petroleum distillates *

SILOO WINDSHIELD WASHER ANTI-FREEZE & CLEANER
(Siloo)

Methanol *

SILOO WINDSHIELD WASHER "READY-MIX" ANTI-FREEZE & CLEANER
(Siloo)

Methanol *

SILVACOL TABLETS
Expectorant
(Moffet Inc.)

Each tablet:
Iodized calcium (available iodine 10%) .... 1/6 gr.
Guaiacol N.F. .... 1/8 minims

SILVER CURL HOME WAVE (TWIN CONDITIONING) WAVING LOTION
(Gillette Co., Personal Care Div.)

Water
Diisopropanolamine *
Ammonium thioglycolate *
Steareth-20
Quaternium-40
Fragrance
Potassium coco-hydrolyzed animal protein
Sodium styrene/PEG-10 maleate/Nonoxynol-10 maleate/Acrylate copolymer
EDTA
Ammonium nonoxynol-4 sulfate
D & C Yellow No. 10
D & C Red No. 19

SILVI-RHAP LV-4TP
Herbicide
(Vertac)

2-Ethylhexyl ester of silvex (2-(2,-4,5-trichlorophenoxy)propionic acid) * 65.2%

SILVO
Silver polish
(French, R. T.)

Chalk	20%
Ethyl alcohol (denatured)	25%
Fatty acids	<2%
Anhydrous Ammonia	0-0.5%
Perfume	0-0.06%

SIMBOL
Chlorinated alkaline cleaner
(Diversey Wyandotte)

Sodium hydroxide *
Sodium hypochlorite releasing agent

SIMECO SUSPENSION
Antacid, antiflatulant
(Wyeth Labs.)

Each tsp. (5 ml.):

Aluminum hydroxide gel (equiv. to 365 mg. of dried aluminum hydroxide gel)	365 mg.
Magnesium hydroxide	300 mg.
Simethicone	30 mg.

Sodium content   0.3-0.6 mEq. per tsp.

SIMICHROME POLISH
(Competition Chem.)

Stearic acid
Oleic acid
Diatomaceous earth
Ammonia

SIMONIZ AUTOMOTIVE HEAVY DUTY CLEANER/ DEGREASER (AS-970, Formula 2069-44)
(Union Carbide)

Water	86%
Anionic surfactant	6%
Glycol ether *	5%
Alkaline detergent builders	3%

SIMONIZ BODYGARD EXPRESS CAR WAX (AS-954, Formula 9811-48B)
(Union Carbide)

Water	79%
Silicone fluids	10%
Siliceous powders	10%
Wax	1%

SIMONIZ BODYGARD LIQUID WAX (AS-953, Formula 9795-71)
(Union Carbide)

Petroleum distillates *	40%
Water	39%
Inorganic polishing agents	11%
Silicone fluids	5%
Emulsifiers	3%
Wax	2%

SIMONIZ BODYGARD PASTE WAX (AS-951, Formula 9769-75)
(Union Carbide)

Water	54%
Petroleum distillates *	22%
Siliceous powders	14%
Silicone fluids	4%
Ethylene glycol	3%
Waxes	2%
Emulsifiers	1%

SIMONIZ CAR INTERIOR CLEANER (AS-919, Formula TPS-159)
(Union Carbide)

Water	93%
Nonionic and anionic surfactants	6%
Inorganic detergent builders	1%
Hydrocarbon propellant	

SIMONIZ CAR WASH (AS-928, Formula 2167-63)
(Union Carbide)

Water	67%
Anionic and nonionic surfactants	22%
Isopropanol	8%
Glycol ether	1%
Borax	1%
Thickener	1%

SIMONIZ CHROME CLEANER (AS-915, Formula MI-2307)
(Union Carbide)

Water	56%
Mineral filler	24%
Petroleum distillates	11%
Emulsifiers	6%
Oxalic acid *	3%

SIMONIZ DRYING AGENT (ACL-605, Formula 9736-84D) (ACL-615, Formula 9736-84B) (ACL-620, Formula 9736-84A)
Commercial car wash chemical concentrate
(Union Carbide)

Water	86%
Hydrocarbon oil *	6%
Alkyl amine	3%
Quaternary amine	2%
Glycol ether	2%
Isopropanol	1%

SIMONIZ HEAVY DUTY RUBBING COMPOUND (AS-923, Formula MI-2311)
Automotive paint cleaner paste
(Union Carbide)

Inorganic polishing agents	42%
Water	25%
Petroleum distillates *	23%
Vegetable oils	5%
Detergents	5%

SIMONIZ HEAVY DUTY WHITEWALL TIRE & MAT CLEANER (AS-909, Formula 2069-44)
(Union Carbide)

Water	86%
Anionic surfactant	6%
Glycol ether *	5%
Alkaline detergent builders	3%

SIMONIZ LIQUID CAR WAX (AS-906S, Formula 2050-6; 2050-27)
(Union Carbide)

Petroleum distillates *	39%
Water	38%
Inorganic polishing agents	11%
Silicone fluids	6%
Emulsifiers	3%
Wax	2%
Thickener	1%

SIMONIZ LIQUID MASTER WAX (AS-942, Formula MI-2315)
(Union Carbide)

Water	59%
Petroleum distillates *	25%
Inorganic polishing agents	8%
Silicone fluids	4%
Waxes	3%
Emulsifier	1%

SIMONIZ LIQUID WAX (AS-907, Formula 2148-118)
(Union Carbide)

Petroleum distillates *	39%
Water	38%
Inorganic polishing agents	11%
Silicone fluids	6%
Emulsifiers	3%
Wax	2%
Thickener	1%

SIMONIZ MASTER WAX (AS-944, Formula 8652-24)
(Union Carbide)

Water	54%
Petroleum distillates *	22%
Inorganic polishing agents	14%
Silicone fluids	4%
Ethylene glycol	3%
Waxes	2%
Emulsifiers	2%

SIMONIZ NEW LOOK FINISH RESTORER (AS-988, Formula 8653-71)
Liquid car cleaner
(Union Carbide)

Petroleum distillates *	39%
Water	39%
Inorganic Polishing agents	11%
Silicone fluids	6%
Emulsifiers	3%
Waxes	2%

Starred ingredients (*) may be responsible for major toxic effects; consult Section II.

SIMONIZ NEW LOOK PROTECTANT (AS-989, Formula 2146-134)
Automotive vinyl dressing
(Union Carbide)

Water	50%
Silicone fluids	22%
Petroleum distillates *	18%
Emulsifiers	7%
Ethylene glycol	3%

SIMONIZ NO BUFF CAR WAX (AS-936, Formula MI-2314)
(Union Carbide)

Water	75%
Petroleum distillates *	20%
Waxes	2%
Emulsifiers	2%
Silicone fluids	1%

SIMONIZ ORIGINAL FINE CAR WAX (AS-962, Formula MI-2319)
(Union Carbide)

Petroleum distillates *	72%
Waxes	28%

SIMONIZ PRE-SOFTENED PASTE WAX (AS-902/904, Formula 8652-24)
(Union Carbide)

Water	53%
Petroleum distillates *	22%
Inorganic polishing agents	14%
Silicone fluids	4%
Ethylene glycol	3%
Waxes	2%
Emulsifiers	2%

SIMONIZ PRE-WAX LIQUID CLEANER (AS-921, Formula MI-2310)
(Union Carbide)

Water	69%
Mineral filler	18%
Petroleum distillates *	13%

SIMONIZ PROFESSIONAL CLEANER WAX (AS-908W, Formula 2221-107)
(Union Carbide)

Petroleum distillates *	65%
Inorganic polishing agents	20%
Waxes	11%
Silicone fluid	4%

SIMONIZ ROYALE CLEANER/WAX (AS-930, Formula 2104-150)
(Union Carbide)

Water	55%
Petroleum distillates *	22%
Inorganic polishing agents	15%
Silicone fluids	5%
Waxes	2%
Emulsifiers	1%

SIMONIZ ROYALE MARINE BOAT CLEANER (MS-310, Formula 2206-66)
(Union Carbide)

Water	86%
Isopropanol *	10%
Glycol ether	3%
Surfactants	1%

SIMONIZ ROYALE MARINE FIBERGLASS CLEANER/WAX (MS-300, Formula 2175-47)
Marine paste wax
(Union Carbide)

Water	38%
Petroleum distillates *	34%
Inorganic Polishing agents	11%
Silicone fluids	8%
Waxes	7%
Emulsifiers	2%

SIMONIZ ROYALE MARINE FIBERGLASS RUBBING COMPOUND (MS-320, Formula LOS-1944)
Boat cleaner paste
(Union Carbide)

Inorganic Polishing agents	40%
Water	30%
Petroleum distillate *	25%
Emulsifiers	5%

SIMONIZ ROYALE MARINE INSTANT GLAZE (MS-305, Formula 8622-27-2)
Liquid boat polish
(Union Carbide)

Water	92%
Isopropanol	5%
Silicone fluids	3%

SIMONIZ SHINES LIKE THE SUN AUTOMOTIVE VINYL CONDITIONER (AS-967, Formula 2146-134)
(Union Carbide)

Water	50%
Silicone fluids	22%
Petroleum distillates *	18%
Emulsifiers	7%
Ethylene glycol	3%

SIMONIZ SHINES LIKE THE SUN LIQUID CAR WAX (AS-966, Formula 2080-102)
(Union Carbide)

Petroleum distillates *	50%
Water	28%
Inorganic polishing agents	10%
Silicone fluids	6%
Waxes	4%
Emulsifier	2%

SIMONIZ SHINES LIKE THE SUN PASTE CAR WAX (AS-965, Formula 2106-61)
(Union Carbide)

Petroleum distillates *	50%
Water	23%
Inorganic polishing agents	10%
Silicone fluids	8%
Waxes	7%
Emulsifiers	2%

SIMONIZ SILICONE GLAZE (AS-986, Formula 2138-65)
Automotive liquid polish
(Union Carbide)

Water	92%
Isopropanol *	5%
Silicone fluids	3%

SIMONIZ SPRAY SUPERPOLY (AS-984, Formula 9795-48)
Automotive spray-on wax
(Union Carbide)

Petroleum distillates *	39%
Water	34%
Inorganic polishing agents	11%
Silicone fluids	7%
Resin	4%
Emulsifiers	3%
Wax	2%

SIMONIZ SUPERPOLY CAR WASH (AS-928, Formula 2167-63)
(Union Carbide)

Water	67%
Anionic and Nonionic surfactants	22%
Isopropanol	8%
Glycol ether	1%
Borax	1%
Thickener	1%

SIMONIZ SUPERPOLY LIQUID (AS-982, Formula 2206-104; 8691-36)
Automotive liquid polish
(Union Carbide)

Petroleum distillates *	40-45%
Water	30-32%
Inorganic polishing agents	9-10%
Silicone fluids	7-9%
Waxes	2-5%
Emulsifiers	2-3%

SIMONIZ SUPERPOLY PASTE (AS-981, Formula 2206-33; 2206-14; 8691-50)
Automotive paste polish
(Union Carbide)

Petroleum distillates *	40%
Water	24-29%
Inorganic polishing agents	12-17%
Silicone fluids	10-11%
Waxes	5-7%
Emulsifiers	2-3%

SIMONIZ SUPERPOLY POLY GLAZE (AS-983, Formula 2138-65, 8622-27-2)
Automotive liquid polish
(Union Carbide)

Water	92%
Isopropanol	5%
Silicone fluids	3%

SIMONIZ SUPERPOLY 10-MINUTE PRE-WAX/PRE-POLY CLEANER (AS-987, Formula 2206-66)
Automotive liquid pre-wax cleaner
(Union Carbide)

Water	86%
Isopropanol *	10%
Glycol ether	3%
Surfactants	1%

SIMONIZ ULTRA ROYALE (AS-930U, Formula 2079-68)
Automotive soft paste wax
(Union Carbide)

Water	52%
Petroleum distillates *	22%
Inorganic polishing agents	14%
Silicone fluids	6%
Ethylene glycol	3%
Waxes	2%
Emulsifiers	1%

SIMONIZ VINYL HARDTOP CLEANER (AS-912, Formula 1957-127B)
(Union Carbide)

Water	93%
Glycol ether *	5%
Nonionic surfactant	1%
Sodium metasilicate	1%

SIMONIZ VINYL TOP CLEANER/WAX (AS-914, Formula MI-2306)
(Union Carbide)

Water	59%
Resins	33%
Emulsifiers	5%
Glycol & Glycol ether *	3%
Hydrocarbon propellant	

SIMONIZ VISTA ONE STEP CLEANER/WAX (AS-956, Formula MI-2318)
(Union Carbide)

Petroleum distillates *	65%
Inorganic polishing agents	20%
Waxes	11%
Silicone fluids	4%

SIMONIZ VISTA SOFT AND EASY WAX (AS-952, Formula MI-2317)
(Union Carbide)

Water	44%
Petroleum distillates *	31%
Inorganic polishing agents	12%
Waxes	7%
Silicone fluids	5%
Emulsifier	1%

SIMONIZ WHITE POLISHING COMPOUND (AS-925, Formula MI-2312)
Automotive paint cleaner paste
(Union Carbide)

Water	40%
Inorganic polishing agents	35%
Petroleum distillates *	19%
Emulsifiers	4%
Waxes	2%

SIMRON
Oral hematinic
(Merrell Dow)

Each capsule:
Elemental iron (as ferrous gluconate)	10 mg.

SIMRON PLUS
Oral hematinic
(Merrell Dow)

Each capsule:
Elemental iron (as ferrous gluconate)	10 mg.
Ascorbic acid	50 mg.
Pyridoxine hydrochloride	1.0 mg.
Folic acid	0.1 mg.
Vitamin B12 activity	3.33 mcg.

SINACIN TABLETS
For treatment of sinusitis
(Pharmex)

Each tablet:
Phenacetin *	150 mg.
Acetaminophen *	150 mg.
Phenylpropanolamine HCl *	25 mg.
Phenyltoloxamine cit.	22 mg.

SINACON
Analgesic, antipyretic, decongestant
(Glaxo Inc.)

Each tablet:
Acetaminophen *	325 mg.
Pseudoephedrine hydrochloride *	15 mg.

SINADRIN
Sinus congestion and headache
(Reese Chem.)

Each tablet:
Salicylamide	227 mg.
Acetaminophen *	162 mg.
Caffeine	32.5 mg.
Phenylephrine hydrochloride *	5 mg.
Phenylpropanolamine hydrochloride *	5 mg.
Phenyltoloxamine dihydrogen citrate	25 mg.

SINADRIN (Super Strength)
Sinus headache & congestion
(Reese Chem.)

Each tablet:
Acetaminophen	500 mg.
Phenylpropanolamine hydrochloride *	25 mg.
Phenyltoloxamine citrate	22 mg.

SINAL TABLETS
Relief of sinus headaches, common cold and nasal congestion
(Approved Pharm.)

Each tablet:
Phenacetin *	150 mg.
Acetaminophen *	150 mg.
Phenyltoloxamine citrate	22 mg.
Phenylpropanolamine hydrochloride *	25 mg.

'76 Ed.

SINAREST NASAL SPRAY
Decongestant
(Pharmacraft)

Phenylephrine HCl	0.5%

SINAREST TABLETS
Decongestant, analgesic, antihistaminic
(Pharmacraft)

Each tablet:
Acetaminophen *	325 mg.
Chlorpheniramine maleate	2 mg.
Phenylpropanolamine HCl *	18.7 mg.

SINA-SPANS
Decongestant
(Reese Chem.)

Each capsule:
Total Belladonna alkaloidal salts		0.16 mg.
Atropine sulfate	0.024 mg.	
Scopolamine hydrobromide	0.014 mg.	
Hyoscyamine sulfate	0.122 mg.	
Phenylpropanolamine hydrochloride		50 mg.
Chlorpheniramine maleate		1 mg.
Pheniramine maleate		12.5 mg.

"SINBAR" WEED KILLER
(Du Pont)

Terbacil *	80%

Starred ingredients (*) may be responsible for major toxic effects; consult Section II.

SINE-AID TABLETS
Analgesic-decongestant
(McNeil Consumer Products Co.)

Each tablet:
Acetaminophen * .... 325 mg.
Phenylpropanolamine
    hydrochloride * .... 25 mg.

SINE-OFF ONCE-A-DAY SINUS SPRAY
Relief from sinus and nasal congestion
(MenJ Labs.)

Xylometazoline HCl 0.1%
Thimerosal 0.001%
Aromatics:
    Menthol
    Eucalyptol
    Camphor
    Methyl salicylate

SINE-OFF TABLETS EXTRA STRENGTH ACETAMINOPHEN FORMULA
Relief of sinus headache and congestion
(MenJ Labs.)

Each tablet:
Chlorpheniramine maleate   2.0 mg.
Phenylpropanolamine HCl *   18.75 mg.
Acetaminophen * ....   500.0 mg.

SINE-OFF TABLETS WITH ASPIRIN (ADDED STRENGTH)
Relief of sinus headache and congestion
(MenJ Labs.)

Each tablet:
Chlorpheniramine maleate   2.0 mg.
Phenylpropanolamine HCl *   18.75 mg.
Aspirin * ....   325.0 mg.

SINEQUAN CAPSULES
Anxiety, depression
(Roerig)

Each capsule:
Doxepin HCl * ..... 10 mg.; 25 mg.;
    50 mg.; 75 mg.; 100 mg.; 150 mg.

SINEXIN (BLACK-YELLOW; TWO PIECE)
(Bowman Pharm.)

Each capsule:
Salicylamide .... 226.8 mg.
Phenacetin * .... 162.0 mg.
Phenylephrine hydrochloride   5.0 mg.
Chlorpheniramine maleate .   2.0 mg.
Caffeine ....   32.4 mg.

SINEX LONG-ACTING DECONGESTANT NASAL SPRAY
See VICKS SINEX LONG-ACTING
    DECONGESTANT NASAL SPRAY

SINEX NASAL SPRAY
See VICKS SINEX NASAL SPRAY

SINGLET TABLETS
For relief of respiratory congestion
(Dow Pharm., Dow Chem. Co.)

Each tablet:
Phenylephrine
    hydrochloride * .... 40 mg.
Chlorpheniramine maleate ...   8 mg.
Acetaminophen * .... 500 mg.

SINO-DRANE TABLETS
Nasal decongestant
(International Chem.)

Each tablet:
Dextromethorphan HBr * ... 10 mg.
Salicylamide .... 227 mg.
Phenacetin * .... 100 mg.
Caffeine .... 10 mg.
Ascorbic acid .... 20 mg.
Phenylephrine HCl ....   5 mg.
Chlorpheniramine maleate ..   2 mg.

'76 Ed.

SINOZE, IMPROVED (C.T. BLUE SCORED)
(Bowman Pharm.)

Each tablet:
Acetaminophen * .... 325 mg.
Phenylpropanolamine HCl ... 25 mg.
Phenyltoloxamine citrate ... 22 mg.

SINU-LETS
Relief from sinus headaches
(Columbia Med.)

Each tablet:
Phenacetin * .... 150 mg.
Acetaminophen * .... 150 mg.
Phenylpropanolamine HCl *   25 mg.
Phenyltoloxamine citrate ... 22 mg.

SINULIN
Sinus headache
(Carnrick Labs.)

Each tablet:
Phenylpropanolamine
    hydrochloride * .... 37.5 mg.
Chlorpheniramine maleate ...   2 mg.
Acetaminophen * .... 325 mg.
Salicylamide .... 250 mg.
Homatropine methylbromide 0.75 mg.

SINUREX
For relief of sinus headaches
(Rexall)

Each tablet:
Phenylpropanolamine
    hydrochloride * .... 25.00 mg.
Chlorpheniramine maleate ... 0.50 mg.
Methapyrilene fumarate * .   6.26 mg.
Salicylamide .... 300.00 mg.

'76 Ed.

SINUSEZE
Sinus pain relief
(Amlab)

Each tablet:
Acetaminophen * .... 150.0 mg.
Salicylamide .... 150.0 mg.
Phenylpropanolamine HCl *   25.0 mg.
Phenyltoloxamine citrate ... 22.0 mg.

SINUSTAT TABLETS, IMPROVED
Relief from pain of sinus headaches and common cold
(Vitarine)

Each tablet:
Acetaminophen * .... 325 mg.
Phenylpropanolamine
    hydrochloride * .... 25 mg.
Phenyltoloxamine citrate .... 22 mg.

SINUTAB
Analgesic-nasal decongestant-antihistamine
(Warner-Lambert)

Each tablet:
Acetaminophen * .... 325 mg.
Phenylpropanolamine HCl ... 25 mg.
Phenyltoloxamine citrate ... 22 mg.

SINUTAB CAPSULES EXTRA STRENGTH
See EXTRA STRENGTH SINUTAB
    CAPSULES

SINUTAB TABLETS EXTRA STRENGTH
See EXTRA STRENGTH SINUTAB
    TABLETS

SINUTAB II
Analgesic-nasal decongestant
(Warner-Lambert)

Each tablet:
Acetaminophen * .... 325 mg.
Phenylpropanolamine HCl ... 25 mg.

SINUTAB II NO DROWSINESS FORMULA MAXIMUM STRENGTH (Tablets and Capsules)
See MAXIMUM STRENGTH SINU-
    TAB II NO DROWSINESS FOR-
    MULA (Tablets and Capsules)

S.I.R.-AID SEWER COMPOUND
For sewers and drains; industrial and institutional use
(Scientific International)

Sodium hydroxide *

Starred ingredients (*) may be responsible for major toxic effects; consult Section II.

S.I.R. BAND
Instant spray bandage; industrial and institutional use
(Scientific International)

Alcohol
Polyvinylpyrrolidone/vinyl acetate copolymer
Benzocaine
Di-isobutyl cresoxy ethoxy ethyl dimethyl benzyl ammonium chloride monohydrate *

S.I.R. DE-LIMER
For deliming dishwashing machines, steam tables, etc.; industrial and institutional use
(Scientific International)

Phosphoric acid *

S.I.R. DEO-GRAIN
Cleaner, deodorizer; industrial and institutional use
(Scientific International)

Orthodichlorobenzene *

SIREN
Indoor space and surface spray; insecticide
(Puritan Chem. Co.)

Active ingredients: 90%
  Petroleum distillate *
  N-Octyl bicycloheptene dicarboximide
  Technical Piperonyl butoxide
  Pyrethrins
Inert ingredient: 10%
  Dipentene

S.I.R. FRY & GRILL CLEANER
Industrial and institutional use
(Scientific International)

Very strong Alkalis *

S.I.R. GIANT DEODORANT BLOCKS
For industrial and institutional use
(Scientific International)

Paradichlorobenzene *

SIR JOHN
Toilet bowl cleaner
(C-Z Chemical)

Hydrogen chloride * 12.4%
Phosphoric acid (H3PO4) * 7.5%
Inert ingred.:
  Water 28%
  Methyl salicylate 1%
  Non-ionic wetting agent 15%
  Amine-o 6%

'76 Ed.

SIR-KILL
Vaporizing insecticide; industrial and institutional use
(Scientific International)

Petroleum distillate * 98.955%
Piperonyl butoxide tech. 0.330%
Pyrethrins 0.165%
N-Octyl bicycloheptene
  dicarboximide 0.550%

S.I.R. LAUNDRY DETERGENT
For automatic washer; industrial and institutional use
(Scientific International)

Alkalis *

S.I.R. MS-11 SAFETY SOLVENT
Cleaner, degreaser for metal machinery parts
(Scientific International)

Ether *
Alcohol (ethyl)
Kerosene *
Paraffin oil

SIR-PHENE
Disinfectant and deodorant; industrial and institutional use
(Scientific International)

Active ingred.: 31.10%
  Isopropanol *
  Vegetable oil soap
  Ortho-benzyl-para-chlorophenol *
  Methylsalicylate *

S.I.R. SAFETY SOLVENT
Degreaser and cleaner for electrical and mechanical equipment
(Scientific International)

Perchlorethylene *

S.I.R. START
Engine starting fluid, industrial and institutional use
(Scientific International)

Ethyl ether *
Petroleum hydrocarbons *

S.I.R. WEED AND VEGETATION KILLER
Industrial and institutional use
(Scientific International)

Bromacil   (5-Bromo-3-sec-butyl-6-
  methyluracil) 1.0%

SIX
Insecticide
(Hess & Clark)

Malathion 3%

SIXOPINE
Cleanser, deodorant, disinfectant
(West Chem. Prod.)

Pine oil *
Soap
Alcohol
Propylene glycol *

6-12 PLUS INSECT REPELLENT LIQUID
(d-Con)

2-Ethyl-1,3-hexanediol * 80.00%
N,N-Diethyl-meta-toluamide ... 9.50%
Other isomers 0.50%

6-12 PLUS INSECT REPELLENT SPRAY
(d-Con)

2-Ethyl-1,3-hexanediol * 25.00%
N,N-Diethyl-meta-toluamide ... 4.75%
Other isomers 0.25%

6-12 PLUS INSECT REPELLENT STICK
(d-Con)

2-Ethyl-1,3-hexanediol * 56.00%
N,N-Diethyl-meta-toluamide ... 8.65%
Other isomers 0.45%

60-40-20
Skin mask
(Vicks Toiletry Products Div.)

Water
Phosphate starch
SD Alcohol 40
Bentonite
Zinc oxide
Propylene glycol
Glycerin
Titanium dioxide
Octylhydroxy stearate
Methylparaben
Propylparaben
Fragrance

61 CLEANER

See ALSOL 61 CLEANER

SKALZOL
Dry acid scale remover
(Stiles-Kem)

Aquadene *
Sulfamic acid *

SK-AMITRIPTYLINE TABLETS
Antidepressant
(SK&F)

Each tablet:
  Amitriptyline
    hydrochloride * ...   10 mg.; 25 mg.;
      50 mg.; 75 mg.; 100 mg.; 150 mg.

Starred ingredients (*) may be responsible for major toxic effects; consult Section II.

SK-AMPICILLIN CAPSULES
Treatment of infections
(SK&F)

Each capsule:
Ampicillin .... 250 mg.; 500 mg.

SK-AMPICILLIN FOR ORAL SUSPENSION
Treatment of infections
(SK&F)

Each 5 ml.:
Ampicillin .... 125 mg.; 250 mg.

SKAN COSMETICS
(Skan)

Skan Laboratories, Inc.
767 W. Woodbury Rd.
Altadena, Calif. 91001

Phone: 213-681-6749

See COSMETICS, Section VI, General Formulations

SK-65 APAP TABLETS
Analgesic
(SK&F)

Each tablet:
Propoxyphene hydrochloride * 65 mg.
Acetaminophen .... 650 mg.

SK-APAP WITH CODEINE TABLETS
Analgesic
(SK&F)

Each tablet:
Acetaminophen * .... 300 mg.
Codeine phosphate * .. 15 mg.; 30 mg.; 60 mg.

SKAT HAND SOAP, PASTE HAND SOAP
(Skat)

Mild soap base
Cleaned Pennsylvania sand
Soda ash .... small percentage
Silicate of soda
Perfume

SKAZE
Descaler, deruster, destainer, defilmer; industrial use
(Puritan Chem. Co.)

Hydrochloric acid *
Phosphoric acid *
Sulfamic acid

SK-CHLORAL HYDRATE CAPSULES
Sedative and hypnotic
(SK&F)

Each capsule:
Chloral hydrate * .... 500 mg.

SK-CHLOROTHIAZIDE TABLETS
Diuretic, antihypertensive
(SK&F)

Each tablet:
Chlorothiazide * .... 250 mg.; 500 mg.

SK DAIRY CATTLE SPRAY WITH DDVP
Insecticide
(Mutual Products)

Pyrethrins	0.05%
Technical Piperonyl butoxide	0.10%
N-Octyl bicycloheptene dicarboximide	0.15%
Di-n-propyl isocinchomeronate	0.20%
2,2-Dichlorovinyl dimethyl phosphate	0.465%
Related compounds	0.035%
Petroleum distillate *	99.000%

'76 Ed.

SK-DEXAMETHASONE TABLETS
Anti-inflammatory
(SK&F)

Each tablet:
Dexamethasone .... 0.5 mg.; 0.75 mg.; 1.5 mg.

SK-DIPHENHYDRAMINE CAPSULES
Antihistaminic
(SK&F)

Each capsule:
Diphenhydramine hydrochloride * ... 25 mg.; 50 mg.

SK-DIPHENHYDRAMINE ELIXIR
Antihistaminic
(SK&F)

Each 5 ml.:
Diphenhydramine hydrochloride * .... 12.5 mg.
Alcohol 14.5%

SK-DIPHENOXYLATE TABLETS
Diarrhea
(SK&F)

Each tablet:
Diphenoxylate hydrochloride * .... 2.500 mg.
Atropine sulfate .... 0.025 mg.

SKEETA-FOG
Insecticide concentrate; flies and mosquitoes
(National Chemsearch)

Aromatic petroleum derivative solvent *	84.50%
Methoxychlor (technical)	12.50%
2,2-Dichlorovinyl dimethyl phosphate	2.32%
Related compounds	0.18%

SKEET-AWAY
For mosquito control
(Agway)

Methoxychlor (technical)	23.8%
Malathion	23.8%
Xylene *	43.5%

SKELAXIN
Skeletal muscle relaxant
(Robins)

Each tablet:
Metaxalone (5-(3,5-Dimethyl-phenoxymethyl)-2-oxazolidinone) * .... 400 mg.

SKELLITE
For cooking, lighting
(Getty)

Household Naphtha *

SKELLYSOLVE-S STODDARD CLEANING SOLVENT
(Getty)

Refined petroleum industrial naphthas *

SKETCHO OIL PASTEL CRAYONS
(American Crayon Co.)

This product bears the CP Seal issued by the Crayon, Water Color and Craft Institute, Inc. This seal certifies that the product contains no materials in sufficient quantities to be toxic or injurious to the human body even if ingested.

SK-HYDROCHLOROTHIAZIDE TABLETS
Diuretic, antihypertensive
(SK&F)

Each tablet:
Hydrochlorothiazide * 25 mg.; 50 mg.

SKIDPROOF
Floor polish
(Consolidated Chem., Inc.)

Water emulsion of synthetic resins
Acrylic polymers

Starred ingredients (*) may be responsible for major toxic effects; consult Section II.

SKIFF
Chilled water cooling system treatment
(Stiles-Kem)

Aquadene *
Water
Biocide
Inhibitor *†
Antifoam

†See Rust Control, Section VI, General Formulations

SKIN BRACER AFTER SHAVE
(Mennen)

Water
SD Alcohol 40 *
Propylene glycol
Fragrance
Menthol *
Benzoic acid
FD&C Yellow #5
FD&C Blue #1

SKIN BRACER BURNISHED LEATHER AFTER SHAVE
(Mennen)

SD Alcohol 40 *
Water
Propylene glycol
Fragrance
Benzophenone-3
FD&C Red #4
FD&C Yellow #5
D&C Green #5

SKIN BRACER DRY LIME AFTER SHAVE
(Mennen)

SD Alcohol 40 *
Water
Propylene glycol
Fragrance
Benzophenone-3
FD&C Red #4
FD&C Yellow #5
D&C Green #5

SKIN BRACER ELECTRIC PRE-SHAVE
(Mennen)

SD Alcohol 40 *
Myristyl propionate
Water
Fragrance
Menthol *
D&C Green #5
FD&C Blue #1

SKIN BRACER LIME ELECTRIC PRE-SHAVE
(Mennen)

SD Alcohol 40 *
Myristyl propionate
Water
Fragrance
Benzophenone-2
Menthol *
FD&C Yellow #5
FD&C Blue #1

SKIN BRACER SPICE AFTER SHAVE
(Mennen)

SD Alcohol 40 *
Water
Propylene glycol
Fragrance
PEG-60 hydrogenated castor oil
Benzophenone-3
FD & C Yellow #5
FD & C Red #4
D & C Green #5

SKIN BRACER WILD MOSS AFTER SHAVE
(Mennen)

SD Alcohol 40 *
Water
Propylene glycol
Fragrance
Benzophenone-3
FD&C Red #4
FD&C Yellow #5
D&C Green #5

SKIN EASE
For skin infections; veterinary
(Goshen Labs.)

Menthol *
Salicylic acid *
Resorcinol *

SKIN-LUBE
(Cramer Products)

Petrolatum (NF) 87.9800%
Silicone SF-96 .... 1.7500%
D & C Green #6 .... 0.0015%
Zinc stearate (USP) * 10.2500%
Preservatol 0.0200%

SKIP-FLEA SHAMPOO, SERGEANT'S

See SERGEANT'S SKIP-FLEA SHAMPOO

SKIP-FLEA SOAP, SERGEANT'S

See SERGEANT'S SKIP-FLEA SOAP

SKIPS
Anti-smoking lozenge
(Chex)

Sugar 85.0%
Molasses 4.0%
Cocoa 4.0%
Licorice extract 1/2%
Cubeb berries 1 1/2%
Elm bark 4.0%
St. John's bread 1/2%
Herbal spices 1/2%

'76 Ed.

SK-LYGEN CAPSULES
Relief of anxiety and tension
(SK&F)

Each capsule:
Chlordiazepoxide
hydrochloride * ..... 5 mg.; 10 mg.;
25 mg.

SK-METHOCARBAMOL TABLETS
Relief of acute painful musculoskeletal conditions
(SK&F)

Each tablet:
Methocarbamol * .. 500 mg.; 750 mg.

SKOGO
Industrial powdered hand soap
(Lester Labs.)

Soap
Borax *

'76 Ed.

SKOPE
Hot water heating system treatment
(Stiles-Kem)

Aquadene *
Water
Inhibitor *†

†See Rust Control, Section VI, General Formulations

SKORTEX
Commercial laundry detergent
(Diversey Wyandotte)

Alkaline salts *
Synthetic detergents *

SKOW'R POW'R
Scale remover
(Paul Koss)

Water .... >70%
Hydrogen chloride * .... <25%
Benzalkonium chloride
Nonionic surfactant
Diethyl thiourea

SK-PENICILLIN G TABLETS
Antibiotic
(SK&F)

Each tablet:
Penicillin G potassium   400,000 units
or 800,000 units

SK-PENICILLIN VK FOR ORAL SOLUTION
Antibiotic
(SK&F)

Each 5 ml.:
Penicillin V potassium
(equiv. to Penicillin
V) .... 125 mg.; 250 mg.

Starred ingredients (*) may be responsible for major toxic effects; consult Section II.

SK-PENICILLIN VK TABLETS
Antibiotic
(SK&F)

Each tablet:
Penicillin V potassium
(equiv. to Penicillin
V) . . . . 250 mg.; 500 mg.

SK-PHENOBARBITAL TABLETS
Sedative, hypnotic
(SK&F)

Each tablet:
Phenobarbital * . . . . 15 mg.; 30 mg.

SK-PRAMINE TABLETS
Antidepressant
(SK&F)

Each tablet:
Imipramine
hydrochloride * . . . . 10 mg.; 25 mg.;
50 mg.

SK-PREDNISONE TABLETS
Anti-inflammatory
(SK&F)

Each tablet:
Prednisone . . . . 5 mg.

SK-PROBENECID TABLETS
Treatment of hyperuricemia associated with gout
(SK&F)

Each tablet:
Probenecid * . . . . 500 mg.

SK-QUINIDINE SULFATE TABLETS
Anti-arrhythmic
(SK&F)

Each tablet:
Quinidine sulfate * . . . . 200 mg.

SKRAM PRESSURIZED INSECT REPELLENT
(Conwood Corp., Household Prod. Div.)

N,N-Diethyl-meta-toluamide * . 14.25%
Other isomers of diethyl
toluamide 0.75%

SKRAM UNSCENTED INSECT REPELLENT
(Conwood Corp., Household Prod. Div.)

N,N-Diethyl-meta-toluamide * . 14.25%
Other isomers of diethyl
toluamide 0.75%

SK-RESERPINE TABLETS
Hypertension
(SK&F)

Each tablet:
Reserpine . . . . 0.25 mg.

SK-SOXAZOLE TABLETS
Urinary tract infections
(SK&F)

Each tablet:
Sulfisoxazole . . . . 500 mg.

SK-TETRACYCLINE CAPSULES
Antibiotic
(SK&F)

Each capsule:
Tetracycline
hydrochloride . . . . . 250 mg.; 500 mg.

SKY CHIEF GASOLINE
(Texaco Inc.)

Gasoline
Containing Lead anti-knock compounds *
Dye

SLASH
Sanitizer, detergent
(Fergusson, Alex. C., Co.)

N-Alkyl (C14, C12, C16) dimethyl
benzyl ammonium chlorides * . . 5.0%
Inert ingred.: 95.0%
Water
Octyl phenoxy polyethoxy ethanol *

SLEDGE, MUNICHEM

See MUNICHEM SLEDGE

SLEEK CLEANER AND DEODORANT
Institutional and commercial use
(Hysan Corp.)

N-Alkyl (60% C14, 30% C16, 5%
C12, 5% C18) dimethyl benzyl
ammonium chloride 0.076%
N-Alkyl (50% C12, 30% C14, 17%
C16, 3% C18) dimethyl ethyl-
benzyl ammonium chloride . . 0.076%
Sodium metasilicate 0.24%
Essential oils 0.20%
Inert ingredients: 99.408%
Detergents *
Cleaners
Builder *
Propellant

SLEEPAWAY
For euthanasia of any animal
(Fort Dodge)

Sodium pentobarbital * 26%
Isopropyl alcohol 10%
Propylene glycol 20%

SLEEP CAPS TABLETS
(Thompson Med.)

Each tablet:
Methapyrilene HCl * . . . . 25 mg.
Salicylamide *

SLEEP-ETTES
Sleep aid
(Reese Chem.)

Each capsule:
Pyrilamine maleate * . . . . 25 mg.
Salicylamide . . . . 150 mg.

SLEEP-EZE
For insomnia
(Whitehall Labs.)

Each tablet:
Methapyrilene
hydrochloride * . . . . 25 mg.
SP-8 (Scopolamine
hydrobromide) * . . . . 0.125 mg.

SLEEP TABS
Sedative
(Towne, Paulsen)

Each tablet:
Methapyrilene
hydrochloride * . . . . 25.0 mg.
Scopolamine aminoxide
hydrobromide . . . . 0.2 mg.
Salicylamide . . . . 250.0 mg.

SLIM-MINT CHEWING GUM
Aid to appetite control
(Thompson Med.)

Benzocaine
Methylcellulose
Oil of anise
Dextrose
Oil of peppermint
Oil of wintergreen
Oil of cinnamon
Oil of clove

SLINGSHOT
Wasp & hornet insect spray
(Hysan Corp.)

Pyrethrins 0.15%
Tech. Piperonyl butoxide 0.30%
N-Octyl bicycloheptene
dicarboximide 0.53%
Tech. Chlordane 2.00%
Petroleum distillate * 62.02%

SLIPICONE RELEASE
(Dow Corning Corp.)

Methyl polysiloxane 7.0%
Propellant 11 . . . . 56.0%
Propellant 12 . . . . 37.0%

Starred ingredients (*) may be responsible for major toxic effects; consult Section II.

SLOAN'S LINIMENT
(Warner-Lambert)

Capsicum *
Methyl salicylate *
Oil camphor *
Turpentine *
Oil pine *

SLO-FEDRIN A 30 GYROCAPS
Decongestant, asthma (with sedative)
(Dooner Labs.)

Each timed-release capsule:
  Ephedrine sulfate * .... 30 mg.
  Amobarbital .... 15 mg.

SLO-FEDRIN A 60 GYROCAPS
Decongestant, asthma (with sedative)
(Dooner Labs.)

Each timed release capsule:
  Ephedrine sulfate * .... 60 mg.
  Amobarbital .... 30 mg.

SLO-FEDRIN 30 GYROCAPS
Decongestant, asthma
(Dooner Labs.)

Each timed release capsule:
  Ephedrine sulfate * .... 30 mg.

SLO-FEDRIN 60 GYROCAPS
Decongestant, asthma
(Dooner Labs.)

Each timed release capsule:
  Ephedrine sulfate * .... 60 mg.

SLO-GRO
Plant growth regulant
(Uniroyal Chem.)

Maleic hydrazide * 30%
Diethanolamine 28%
Inerts 42%
  Surfactant
  Water

SLO-PHYLLIN GG CAPSULE
Asthma, bronchitis, emphysema
(Dooner Labs.)

Each capsule:
  Theophylline (anhydrous) * .. 150 mg.
  Guaifenesin .... 90 mg.

SLO-PHYLLIN GG SYRUP
Asthma, bronchitis, emphysema
(Dooner Labs.)

Each 15 ml.:
  Theophylline (anhydrous) * .. 150 mg.
  Guaifenesin .... 90 mg.

SLO-PHYLLIN 60 GYROCAPS
Asthma, bronchitis, emphysema
(Dooner Labs.)

Each timed release capsule:
  Theophylline (anhydrous) * .. 60 mg.

SLO-PHYLLIN 125 GYROCAPS
Asthma, bronchitis, emphysema
(Dooner Labs.)

Each timed release capsule:
  Theophylline (anhydrous) * .. 125 mg.

SLO-PHYLLIN 250 GYROCAPS
Asthma, bronchitis, emphysema
(Dooner Labs.)

Each timed release capsule:
  Theophylline (anhydrous) * .. 250 mg.

SLO-PHYLLIN 80 SYRUP
Asthma, bronchitis, emphysema
(Dooner Labs.)

Each 15 ml.:
  Theophylline (anhydrous) * .. 80 mg.
  Non alcoholic syrup

SLO-PHYLLIN TABLET 100 MG.
Asthma, bronchitis, emphysema
(Dooner Labs.)

Each tablet:
  Theophylline (anhydrous) * .. 100 mg.

SLO-PHYLLIN TABLET 200 MG.
Asthma, bronchitis, emphysema
(Dooner Labs.)

Each tablet:
  Theophylline (anhydrous) * .. 200 mg.

SLOW-K
Potassium supplement
(CIBA Pharmaceutical)

Potassium chloride *

SLOW RELEASE ALGIMYCIN PLL-C
For algae control in ponds, lakes and lagoons
(Great Lakes Biochemical)

Copper sulfate pentahydrate (copper as metallic 5.00%) * 19.91%

SLOWS-IT
To retard plant growth
(Navy Brand)

Diethanolamine salt of 1,2-dihydro 3,6-pyridazinedione (Maleic hydrazide) * 58%

SLUG-GETA SNAIL & SLUG BAIT
(Chevron)

3,5-Dimethyl-4-(methylthio)phenyl methylcarbamate * 2%/w

Chevron emergency phone number: 415-233-3737

SLUGIT
Slug and snail killer
(McHutchison & Co.)

Metaldehyde * .... 20% w/v

SLUG-KILL
Insecticide
(Plant Prod.)

Metaldehyde dust * 15%

SLUG WASP & HORNET SPRAY

See PL SLUG WASP & HORNET SPRAY

SMASHING WHITE LAUNDRY BOOSTER

See AMWAY SMASHING WHITE LAUNDRY BOOSTER

SMASH ROACH'N ANT KILLER, PL (Aerosol)

See PL SMASH ROACH'N ANT KILLER (Aerosol)

SMILE
Sewer and drain opener; municipal-industrial
(ABCO, Inc.)

Sulfuric acid *

SMOKE-STOP

See SILOO SMOKE-STOP

SNAP
Solvent degreaser & cleaner
(National Chemsearch)

Aromatic petroleum solvents *
Aliphatic petroleum solvents
Nonionic wetting agents
Anionic emulsifiers

SNAROL MEAL
Snail and slug killer
(Boyle-Midway)

Metaldehyde * 3.0%

Starred ingredients (*) may be responsible for major toxic effects; consult Section II.

SNAROL PELLETS
Snail and slug killer
(Boyle-Midway)

Metaldehyde * 3.3%

SNEE BOWL CLEANER
For cleaning toilet bowls and porcelain urinals
(Snee, W.G., Co.)

Hydrochloric acid *

SNEE CHC-15
Chlorine sanitizing agent
(Snee, W.G., Co.)

Calcium hypochlorite * 15%
Sodium carbonate * 85%

SNEE HOUSEHOLD AMMONIA
(Snee, W.G., Co.)

Active ingred.: 33%
  Aqua ammonia *

SNEE MURIATIC ACID
For bowl and swimming pool cleaning
(Snee, W.G., Co.)

20° Commercial Hydrochloric acid *

SNEE PINE ODOR DISINFECTANT & CLEANER
(Snee, W.G., Co.)

Active ingredients: 50%
  Isopropyl alcohol *
  Steam distilled pine oil *
  Soap
  o-Benzyl-p-chlorophenol *

SNIF-PROOF PLASTIC CEMENT #65 and #66

See ROSS SNIF-PROOF PLASTIC CEMENT #65 and #66

SNO-BALL
Plastic filler
(Unican)

Polyester resin 50%
Inert mineral Talc 47%
Titanium dioxide pigment 3%

Catalysts:
  Solution:
    Methyl ethyl ketone peroxide * 60%
    Dimethyl phthalate 40%
  or
  Paste:
    Benzoyl peroxide * 50%
    Butyl benzyl phthalate 50%

'76 Ed.

SNO BOL
Bowl cleaner
(Staley)

A. E. Staley Mfg. Co.
2200 E. Eldorado St.
Decatur, Ill. 62525

Phone: 217-423-4411

SNOBOY BLEACH
(Moore, A.F.)

Sodium hypochlorite * 5.25%

'76 Ed.

SNO-CLEANG
Porcelain cleaner (concentrate)
(Hysan Corp.)

Hydrogen chloride * 9.45%
Dehydroabietylamine (and other stabilized amines) 2.50%
Inert ingredients: 88.05%
  Detergents
  Cleaners
  Emulsifiers
  Deodorants

SNOOTIE
(Sea & Ski)

Silicone fluid
Stearic acid (USP)
Escalol 507
Propylparaben (USP)
Water, purified (USP)
Triethanolamine (USP)
Glycerin (USP)
Daphne #7 Fragrance
Methylparaben (USP)
Germall 115

SNOW-WHITE (CRYSTALS & NUGGETS)
(Reefer-Galler)

Paradichlorobenzene *

'76 Ed.

SNUDS
Car wash
(Help)

Sodium alkyl aryl type wetting agent *† 40%

'76 Ed.

†*See* Alkyl aryl sodium sulfate

SNUDSY SUDS
(Help)

Sodium phosphates *
Sesquicarbonate of soda
Sodium alkyl aryl type wetting agent *

'76 Ed.

SOACLENS
Antiseptic soaking & wetting solution for hard contact lenses
(Burton, Parsons & Co.)

Thimerosal (Lilly) 0.004%
EDTA 0.1%

SOAKARE
Hard contact lens soaking solution
(Allergan Pharm.)

Benzalkonium chloride 0.01%
Edetate disodium 0.25%

SOAKOFF WALLPAPER REMOVER
(Reliable Paste)

Sulfonated oils *
Methylene chloride *
Soda ash *

SOAP AND SOAK, DR. SCHOLL'S

See DR. SCHOLL'S SOAP AND SOAK

SO CLENE
Chalk board cleaner
(Hysan Corp.)

2,2'-Methylene bis(3,4,6-trichlorophenol) 0.2500%
Ortho benzyl para chlorophenol 0.1125%
Essential oils 0.2700%
Petroleum distillate *

SODANUX
Stomachic
(Vale)

Each tablet:
  Nux vomica * .... 6.5 mg.
  Sodium bicarbonate * ..... 324.0 mg.

SODIUM ETHALYL CAPSULES
Analgesic, hypnotic
(Premo)

Each capsule:
  Sodium pentobarbital * ...... 65 mg.
  Sodium butabarbital * .... 40 mg.
  Sodium phenobarbital .... 25 mg.

'76 Ed.

SODIUM SULAMYD OPHTHALMIC OINTMENT 10% - STERILE
Ophthalmic sulfonamide preparation
(Schering)

Each gm.:
  Sulfacetamide sodium .... 100 mg.
  Methylparaben .... 0.5 mg.
  Propylparaben .... 0.1 mg.
  Benzalkonium chloride ..... 0.25 mg.
  Sorbitan monolaurate
  Bland unctuous petrolatum base
  Water

Starred ingredients (*) may be responsible for major toxic effects; consult Section II.

SODIUM SULAMYD OPHTHALMIC SOLUTION 10% - STERILE
Ophthalmic sulfonamide preparation
(Schering)

Each cc:
Sulfacetamide sodium .... 100 mg.
Methylcellulose .... 5 mg.
Methylparaben .... 0.5 mg.
Propylparaben .... 0.1 mg.
Sodium thiosulfate .... 3.1 mg.
Sodium dihydrogen phosphate

SODIUM SULAMYD OPHTHALMIC SOLUTION 30% - STERILE
Ophthalmic sulfonamide preparation
(Schering)

Each cc:
Sulfacetamide sodium * ..... 300 mg.
Methylparaben .... 0.5 mg.
Propylparaben .... 0.1 mg.
Sodium thiosulfate .... 1.5 mg.
Sodium dihydrogen phosphate

SO-E-Z
Bowl cleaner & disinfectant
(Weil Chem.)

Hydrogen chloride
n-Alkyl (C14, C16, C12, C18) dimethyl benzyl ammonium chlorides *
n-Alkyl (C12, C14, C16, C18) dimethyl ethylbenzyl ammonium chlorides *

SO FAST ALCOHOL
(Southland Paint Co., Inc.)

Methanol *

SO FAST BRUSH CLEANER
(Southland Paint Co., Inc.)

Butyl Cellosolve *
Toluene *
Petroleum distillates

SO FAST LACQUER THINNER
(Southland Paint Co., Inc.)

Methyl ethyl ketone
Isopropyl alcohol
Methyl amyl alcohol
Isobutyl isobutyrate
Toluene *
Aliphatic hydrocarbons

SO FAST LIQUID SANDER AND DEGLOSSER
(Southland Paint Co., Inc.)

Isopropyl alcohol
Xylene *
Petroleum distillates

SO FAST PAINT AND VARNISH REMOVER
(Southland Paint Co., Inc.)

Toluene *
Acetone
Methanol

SO FAST PAINT THINNER
(Southland Paint Co., Inc.)

Petroleum distillates *
Mineral spirits *

SOFLENS ENZYMATIC CONTACT LENS CLEANER
(Allergan Pharm.)

Stabilized Papain

SOFNER
Undertakers', embalmers' supplies
(Embalmers')

Sequestrene *

SOFNER-GARD CHEMICAL
To dissolve iron: normally used as an additive to water softener regenerants
(Culligan)

Sodium dithionite * 65%
Sodium bisulfite 35%
Sulpho rhodamine-B (dye) .... trace

SOFSKIN HAND CREAM

Sofskin, Inc.
575 Madison Ave.
New York, N.Y. 10022

Phone: 212-753-4600

See COSMETICS, Section VI, General Formulations

SOF' STROKE (REGULAR & MENTHOL ICED)
(Mennen)

Water
TEA-stearate
Isobutane
Potassium stearate
Glycerin
Polysorbate-20
Mixed Isopropanol amine myristate
Propane
Mixed Isopropanol amine lanolate
Fragrance
Menthol (Menthol Iced only)
Butane
TEA-cocoate
Stearic acid
Potassium cocoate
Coconut acid
FD&C Blue #1 (Menthol Iced only)

SOFT AND DRI ROLL-ON ANTIPERSPIRANT, BABY POWDER
(Gillette Co., Personal Care Div.)

Aluminum-Zirconium tetrachlorohydrex gly
Water
Cyclomethicone
Steareth-2
Aluminum starch octenylsuccinate
PPG-15 stearyl ether
Steareth-21
Butylparaben
Methylparaben

SOFT AND DRI ROLL-ON ANTIPERSPIRANT, SCENTED
(Gillette Co., Personal Care Div.)

Aluminum-Zirconium tetrachlorohydrex gly
Water
Cyclomethicone
Steareth-2
Aluminum starch octenylsuccinate
PPG-15 stearyl ether
Steareth-21
Butylparaben
Methylparaben

SOFT AND DRI ROLL-ON ANTIPERSPIRANT, UNSCENTED
(Gillette Co., Personal Care Div.)

Aluminum-Zirconium tetrachlorohydrex gly
Water
Cyclomethicone
Steareth-2
Aluminum starch octenylsuccinate
PPG-15 stearyl ether
Steareth-21
Butylparaben
Methylparaben

SOFTENER-TABS
Stool-softener
(Fibertone)

Each tablet:
Dioctyl sodium
sulfosuccinate * .... 100 mg.

SOFTENER THAN SOFT
Liquid fabric softener/conditioner
(Shaklee)

Cationic fabric softener
Sodium sulfate .... small amounts

SOFTEZ
Stool softener
(Wesley Pharm.)

Each capsule:
Dioctyl sodium
sulfosuccinate * .... 100 mg.

SOFT & FADE
Laundry aid
(Climaco)

Sodium dichlorocyanurate *

SOFT SCRUB
Liquid cleanser
(Clorox)

Calcium carbonate	50-75%
Water	25-50%
Linear alkylbenzene sulfonate (Anionic surfactant)	0.5-5%
Amine oxide (Nonionic surfactant)	0.5-5%
Sodium (or potassium) citrate	0.5-5%
Fragrance	<0.5%
Dowicil 200 (antimicrobial)	<0.5%
Sodium hypochlorite solution	<0.5%

"SOFTSTROKE" FIBER TIP MARKER INKS (In Throwaway Markers Only)

See SHEAFFER "SOFTSTROKE" FIBER TIP MARKER INKS (In Throwaway Markers Only)

SO HELP ME HANNAH OINTMENT
For poison oak, ivy
(So Help Me Hannah Labs.)

Zinc oxide
Endothermic hectorite
Iron oxide
Calamine
Glycerin

SOILAX
Cleaner
(Economics)

Sodium carbonate *
Sodium sesquicarbonate *
Ammonium chloride
Anionic wetting agents *

SOILBROM-90
Fumigant
(Great Lakes Chem. Corp.)

Ethylene dibromide * 92.8%

SOLACEN
Anxiety and tension relief in psychoneurotic disorders
(Wallace Labs.)

Each capsule:
Solacen (Tybamate) * 250 mg.; 350 mg.

'76 Ed.

SOLARCAINE LOTION
First aid lotion
(Plough)

Mineral oil	
Benzocaine	0.5% w/w
Irgasan Dp-300	0.2% w/w
Propylparaben	0.1% w/w
Propylene glycol	
Methylparaben	0.2% w/w
Camphor *	
Menthol *	
Germall 115 (Imidazolidinyl urea)	0.3% w/w
Hydrogen peroxide solution, 35%	0.2% w/w
Phosphoric acid, 85%	0.02% w/w

SOLDAX
Adhesive
(Ambroid)

Nitrocellulose type of cement	
Alcohols *	20%
Hydrocarbons *†	60%
Ketones *	20%
Allyl isothiocyanate (synthetic oil of mustard)	trace

†*See* Adhesives, Section VI, General Formulations

SOLDER SEAL GAS TREATMENT
Automotive
(Radiator)

Petroleum distillates *

'76 Ed.

SOLDER SEAL INSTANT STARTING FLUID
For use in diesel & gasoline engines
(Radiator)

Ethyl-ether *

'76 Ed.

SOLDER SEAL RADIATOR REPAIR
(Radiator)

Vegetable fibers
Aluminum oxides

'76 Ed.

SOLDER SEAL WATER PUMP LUBE
Automotive; lubricant & rust preventive
(Radiator)

Petroleum distillates *

'76 Ed.

SOLDER SEAL WINDSHIELD WASHER SOLVENT
(Radiator)

Isopropanol *

'76 Ed.

SOLFOTON
Mild sustained sedation
(Poythress, Wm. P.)

Each tablet or capsule:
Phenobarbital * .... 16 mg.
Blended with Bensulfoid ...... 65 mg.

SOLIDAIRE

See AIRWICK PROFESSIONAL PRODUCTS SOLIDAIRE

SOLIDAIRE PLUS

See AIRWICK PROFESSIONAL PRODUCTS SOLIDAIRE PLUS

SOLO (Formula 1)
Heavy duty liquid laundry detergent
(Procter & Gamble)

Water	50-74%
Alkyl ethoxylate *	10-24%
Ethanol *	10-24%
Ditallow dimethyl ammonium chloride	5-9%
Minor ingredients, each	trace

pH (as is) - 7.5

SOLO (Formula 2)
Heavy duty liquid laundry detergent
(Procter & Gamble)

Water	50-74%
Alkyl ethoxylate *	10-24%
Ethanol *	5-9%
Alkylamine oxide	1-4%
Ditallow dimethyl ammonium chloride	1-4%
Minor ingredients, each	trace

pH (as is) - 6.9

SOLTEX
Anti-dandruff shampoo
(C & M Pharmacal)

o-Benzyl-p-chlorophenol 0.1%
Alkyl-aryl surfactant
Polyethylene glycol
Alkanolamide conditioners

SOLTICE HI-THERM
For colds, muscular soreness
(Chattem)

Camphor *
Menthol *
Methyl salicylate *
Eucalyptus oil *

Starred ingredients (*) may be responsible for major toxic effects; consult Section II.

SOLTICE QUICK RUB
For colds, muscular soreness
(Chattem)

Camphor *
Menthol *
Methyl salicylate *
Eucalyptus oil *

SOLUBOR
Boron supplement; agricultural
(U.S. Borax)

Boric oxide * 66.0%
Equivalent Boron 20.5%

SOLV-CLEAN LIQUID GLASS AND DAIRY CLEANER
(Solvit)

Phosphoric acid * 25%
Non-ionic surface active agent 10%

SOLVENE TYPE CLEANER
(Sanford Corp.)

1,1,1-Trichloroethane *

SOLVENTOL
All purpose cleaner
(Rooto)

Phosphates *
Sodium carbonates *
Sodium sesquicarbonates *

SOLVEX 3139
(Texaco Canada Ltd.)

Petroleum distillate *

SOLVEX PRODUCTS
See DR. SCHOLL'S SOLVEX

SOLVIT
Cleaner
(Solvit)

Steam-distilled Pine oil *
Wetting agents *
Sodium carbonate
Sesquicarbonate of soda
Chelating agent:
  Na4EDTA (Tetrasodium EDTA)
Borax

SOLVIT AIR SANITIZER AND DEODORANT BOMB
(Solvit)

Isopropanol *
Triethylene glycol
Propylene glycol
p-Diisobutyl phenoxy-ethoxy ethyl dimethyl benzyl ammonium chloride *

SOLVIT CD 4.5
*Cleaner, disinfectant, deodorizer, fun-
gicide - hospital and institutional use*
(Solvit)

Alkyl (60% C14, 30% C16, 5% C12,
  5% C18) dimethyl benzyl ammonium chlorides * 2.25%
Alkyl (68% C12, 32% C14) dimethyl
  ethylbenzyl ammonium
  chlorides * 2.25%
Sodium carbonate 3.00%

SOLVIT CLEAN-ALL
*Machine dishwashing compound - com-
mercial*
(Solvit)

Complex Phosphates
Sodium metasilicate *
Sodium carbonate *
Sodium tripolyphosphate
Surfactants
Chlorinated isocyanurate *

SOLVIT INDUSTRIAL AEROSOL INSECTICIDE
(Solvit)

Pyrethrins 0.7%
Technical Piperonyl butoxide 2.0%
Petroleum solvent 7.3%
Inert ingredients: 90.0%
  Propellents

SOLVIT PROFESSIONAL RAT & MOUSE KILLER
Rodenticide
(Solvit)

2-Pivalyl-1,3 indandione 0.025%
Inert ingred.: 99.975%
  Coarse ground grain

SOLVIT RESIDUAL INSECT SPRAY
(Solvit)

Active ingredients: 99.43%
  O,O-Diethyl O-(2-isopropyl-
    4-methyl-6-pyrimidinyl)
    phosphorothioate * 0.500%
  Pyrethrins 0.052%
  Technical Piperonyl
    butoxide 0.261%
  Petroleum distillates * 98.617%

SOLVIT SPACE SPRAY INSECTICIDE
(Solvit)

Technical Piperonyl butoxide 1.50%
Pyrethrins 0.15%
Refined Petroleum oil * 98.35%

SOLVIT SUPER FOG
Insecticide
(Solvit)

Beta butoxy beta'thiocyano di-
  ethyl ether * 3.00%
Malathion 3.00%
Petroleum distillate * 94.00%

SOLVO BOWL KLEAN
(Consolidated Chem., Inc.)

Hydrochloric acid *

SOLVO CLEANER
Floor polish (wax) remover
(Consolidated Chem., Inc.)

Soap
Detergent containing Alkaline phosphates *†

†*See* Trisodium phosphate

SOLVOL
Powdered steam cleaner
(Lester Labs.)

Phosphates *
Detergents *

'76 Ed.

SOLVOWAY RUG SHAMPOO
(Uncle Sam)

Synthetic detergents and surfactants *
Optical brightener
Tetrachloroethylene * .... <10%
Butyl Cellosolve * .... <10%
Dye (Palatine Blue) .... trace
Water

SOMA (CAPSULES & TABLETS)
*Relief of pain from skeletal muscle
  spasms*
(Wallace Labs.)

CAPSULES (each):
  Soma (Carisoprodol) * ...... 250 mg.

TABLETS (each):
  Soma (Carisoprodol) * ...... 350 mg.

'76 Ed.

SOMA COMPOUND
*Relief of pain & stiffness in various
  conditions affecting muscle & joints*
(Wallace Labs.)

Each tablet:
  Carisoprodol * .... 200 mg.
  Phenacetin * .... 160 mg.
  Caffeine .... 32 mg.

'76 Ed.

SOMA COMPOUND + CODEINE
*Relief of pain & stiffness in various
  conditions affecting muscle & joints*
(Wallace Labs.)

Each tablet:
  Carisoprodol * .... 200 mg.
  Phenacetin * .... 160 mg.
  Caffeine .... 32 mg.
  Codeine phosphate * .... 16 mg.

'76 Ed.

Starred ingredients (*) may be responsible for major toxic effects; consult Section II.

SOMBULEX
Hexobarbital hypnotic
(Riker Labs.)

Each tablet:
N-Methyl cyclohexenyl methyl
barbituric acid * .... 250 mg.
'76 Ed.

SOMINEX (CAPSULES & TABLETS)
Aid to sleep
(Williams, J.B.)

CAPSULES (each):
Scopolamine aminoxide
HBr * .... 0.5 mg.
Methapyrilene HCl * .... 50 mg.
Salicylamide .... 200 mg.

TABLETS (each):
Scopolamine aminoxide
HBr * .... 0.25 mg.
Methapyrilene HCl * .... 25 mg.
Salicylamide .... 200 mg.

SOMNICAPS
For the relief of insomnia
(Am. Pharmaceutical)

Each capsule:
Methapyrilene hydrochloride * 25 mg.

SONFORD BHC ONE
Insecticide
(Sonford Products)

Benzene hexachloride, gamma
isomer * 12.8%
Benzene hexachloride, other
isomers * 13.3%
Petroleum distillate 70.65%

SONIC SILVER CLEANER
Silver detarnisher
(Standard Prods.; Invento; Mfr., Winfield Brooks)

Ethylene thiourea .... <10%
Sulfuric acid * .... <5%
Detergents, Dye, Perfume ..... <10%
Water .... balance

SONOMA COUNTY'S DIPHACINONE RAT & MOUSE BAIT
Rodenticide
(Sonoma)

Diphacinone (2-Diphenylacetyl-
1,3-indanedione) 0.005%

SONOMA COUNTY'S RED SQUILL RAT BAIT
Rodenticide
(Sonoma)

Extractives of Red squill * 4.50%

SONOMA COUNTY'S STRYCHNINE GOPHER POISON GRAIN BAIT
Rodenticide
(Sonoma)

Strychnine alkaloid * 2.6%

SONOMA COUNTY'S STRYCHNINE JACK RABBIT POISON GRAIN BAIT
Rodenticide
(Sonoma)

Strychnine alkaloid * 0.29%

SONOMA COUNTY'S STRYCHNINE LINNET POISON
(Sonoma)

Strychnine alkaloid * 0.43%

SONOMA COUNTY'S STRYCHNINE POISON GRAIN BAIT FOR GOPHERS, SQUIRRELS & MICE
Rodenticide
(Sonoma)

Strychnine alkaloid * 0.29%

SONOMA COUNTY'S STRYCHNINE SPARROW POISON
(Sonoma)

Strychnine alkaloid * 0.25%

SONTOX
Wood preservative
(Sonford Products)

Pentachlorophenol * 86.0%
Other chlorophenols & related
compounds 10.0%

SONTOX-S
Wood preservative
(Sonford Products)

Sodium pentachlorophenate * 79%
Sodium salts of other chlorophenols 11%

SOOTHE
Eye decongestant
(Burton, Parsons & Co.)

Each cc:
Camphor 0.01%
Phenylephrine HCl 0.15%
Thimerosal 0.004%

SOOTHIE

See WATKINS SOOTHIE

SOOTHOGEL CREAM
(Vale)

Calamine
Zinc oxide
Camphor-phenol 1%

SOPOR - 150 & 300 mg.
Hypnotic, sedative
(American Critical Care)

Each tablet:
Methaqualone * .... 150 mg.; 300 mg.

SOPP SOAP
Post-harvest fungicide
(American Machinery Corp.)

Active ingred.: 18.9%
Anhydrous Sodium ortho-
phenylphenate (26% sodium
ortho-phenyl-phenate
tetrahydrate) *
Inert ingred.: 81.1%
Hexamethylenetetramine *
Sodium hydroxide *
Petro AA
Water

SOPRONOL OINTMENT
Fungicide; medical
(Wyeth Labs.)

Sodium propionate 12.3%
Sodium caprylate 10.0%
Zinc caprylate * 5.0%

SOPRONOL POWDER
Fungicide; medical
(Wyeth Labs.)

Sodium propionate 5%
Zinc propionate * 5%
Sodium caprylate 10%

SOPRONOL SOLUTION
Fungicide; medical
(Wyeth Labs.)

Sodium propionate 12.3%
Sodium caprylate 10%
Dioctyl sodium sulfosuccinate 0.1%
n-Propyl alcohol * 13%

SORBACIDE
Herbicide adjuvant
(Leffingwell)

Anionic surfactants 3.0%/w
Phosphoric acid * 11.0%/w
Metallic sulfates and chlorides .. 11.0%/w

SORBA-SPRAY Cu 0-10-0
Foliar nutrient spray
(Leffingwell)

Available Phosphoric acid * 10.0%
Copper * 4.0%
Zinc 1.0%

SORBA-SPRAY Mg 0-10-0
Soluble nutrient spray, spreader and buffering agent
(Leffingwell)

Phosphoric acid *	10.0%
Zinc (as elemental)	1.0%
Magnesium (as elemental)	3.0%
Alkylbenzenesulfonate	2.0%

SORBA-SPRAY MIP 0-10-0
Foliar nutrient spray
(Leffingwell)

Available Phosphoric acid *	10.0%
Iron	2.0%
Manganese	2.0%

SORBA-SPRAY Mn 0-12-0
Soluble nutrient spray, spreader and buffering agent
(Leffingwell)

Zinc sulfate	5.5%
Phosphoric acid *	17.0%
Manganese (as elemental)	2.0%
Alkylbenzenesulfonate	2.0%

SORBA-SPRAY ZIP 0-8-0
Soluble nutrient spray, spreader and buffering agent
(Leffingwell)

Phosphoric acid *	8.0%
Iron (elemental)	3.0%
Zinc sulfate	2.4%
Alkylbenzenesulfonate	4.0%

SORBA-SPRAY ZKP 0-16-9
Soluble nutrient spray, spreader & buffering agent
(Leffingwell)

Nutrient spray:

Phosphoric acid, available (as potassium phosphate, phosphoric acid)	16.0%
Potash, water soluble (as potassium phosphate)	9.0%
Zinc, as elemental (as zinc sulphate)	1.0%

Spray adjuvant:

Zinc sulphate *	3.0%
Phosphoric acid *	17.6%
Alkyl benzene sulfonate	2.0%

SORBA-SPRAY ZNP 10-12-0
Soluble nutrient spray, spreader & buffering agent
(Leffingwell)

Nutrient spray:

Nitrogen (as ammonium phosphate, urea)	10.0%
Phosphoric acid, available (as ammonium phosphate, phosphoric acid)	12.0%
Zinc, as elemental (as zinc sulphate) *	2.0%

Spray adjuvant:

Zinc sulfate *	6.0%
Phosphoric acid, available *	12.0%
Alkyl benzene sulfonate	1.5%

SORB-IT
Adsorbent
(Hillyard Chem.)

Calcined clay

'76 Ed.

SORBUTUSS
Antitussive, expectorant, demulcent
(Dalin)

Each 5 cc:

Dextromethorphan hydrobromide *	10 mg.
Glyceryl guaiacolate	100 mg.
Ipecac fluid extract	0.05 min.
Potassium citrate	85 mg.
Citric acid	35 mg.
Mint-flavored, glycerine-sorbitol vehicle	

'76 Ed.

SORETTS LOZENGES
Anesthetic throat lozenge
(Lannett)

Each lozenge:

Benzocaine	1/2 gr.
Extract Licorice	1/8 gr.
Menthol	1/200 gr.

SOS MALATHION BACK RUBBER OIL
Insecticide
(South Omaha Supply)

Malathion	2.000%
Rotenone	0.030%
Other cube resins	0.045%
Pine oil	1.250%
Mineral oil *	96.675%

'76 Ed.

SOS TOXAPHENE BACK RUBBER OIL
Insecticide
(South Omaha Supply)

Toxaphene *	5.00%
Petroleum oil *	95.00%

'76 Ed.

SOUTHERN COATINGS PRODUCTS

Southern Coatings, Inc.
P.O. Box 160
Sumter, S.C. 29150

Phone: 803-775-6351

SOVASOL No. 5
(Mobil Oil)

Aliphatic petroleum solvent *
Boiling range: .... 300-400° F

SOWECO LARVACIDE
(Soweco)

Chloropicrin *

SOXA-FORTE TABLETS
Sulfonamide therapy
(Vita Elixir Co.)

Each tablet:

Sulfisoxazole *	0.5 gm.
Phenazopyridine *	50 mg.

SOXA TABLETS
Sulfonamide therapy
(Vita Elixir Co.)

Each tablet:

Sulfisoxazole *	0.5 gm.

SOYALOID COLLOID BATH POWDER PACKETS
For treatment of dermatoses and dermatitis
(Dome)

Combined amount:	2%
Soya protein complex	
Polyvinylpyrrolidone	

SOY-DOME
Soapless skin lotion cleanser
(Dome)

Hexachlorophene *	3%
Soya protein complex	
Polyvinylpyrrolidone (PVP)	1%
Acid pH vehicle:	
Oil-in-water, emulsion-type creme containing a buffered solution of aluminum acetate	

SOY-SITZ
Colloid bath
(Dome)

Polyvinylpyrrolidone (PVP)
Aluminum sulfate
Calcium acetate
Soya protein complex

SPALIX
Antispasmodic, sedative
(Reid-Provident)

Each tablet:

Phenobarbital *	16 mg.
Hyoscyamine sulfate	0.1037 mg.
Atropine sulfate	0.0194 mg.
Scopolamine (hyoscine) hydrobromide	0.0065 mg.

SPARINE CONCENTRATE
Antipsychotic
(Wyeth Labs.)

Each ml.:

Promazine hydrochloride *	30 mg.

SPARINE (TABLETS & SYRUP)
Antipsychotic
(Wyeth Labs.)

Tablets (each):
Promazine
  hydrochloride *   ...   10 mg.; 25 mg.;
                        50 mg.; 100 mg.

Syrup (each 5 ml.):
  Promazine hydrochloride * ... 10 mg.

SPARKETTE
Alkaline detergent
(Pennwalt)

Sodium orthosilicate
Sodium carbonate *
Soap or detergents

SPARKLE
Liquid bowl cleaner
(Puritan Chem. Co.)

Hydrogen chloride * 24%

SPARKLE
Alkaline detergent
(Pennwalt)

Sodium orthosilicate
Sodium carbonate *
Soap or detergents

SPARKLE EMULSION BOWL CLEANER
(Uncle Sam)

Hydrogen chloride *
Quaternary ammonium compound *
Corrosion inhibitor
Styrene
Surfactants
Water

SPARKLE PINE CLEANER AND DISINFECTANT
(Funk, A. J.)

Pine oil * 30%
Isopropyl alcohol 10%
Coconut fatty acid amide soap 15%
Glycol ether 3%
Water 42%

SPARKL-X AMMONIA
(Purex Corp.)

Ammonia * 1-5%
Nonionic surfactant .... <1%
Water .... balance

SPARQUAT 256 GERMICIDAL CLEANER

See SPARTAN SPARQUAT 256 GERMICIDAL CLEANER

SPARROW-CRACKS
English sparrow control
(B&G Co.)

Strychnine alkaloid * .... 0.6%/wt.

SPARTAN GERMICIDAL BOWL CLEANSE
(Spartan)

Hydrogen chloride * 23.00%
n-Alkyl (C14, 50%; C12, 40%; C16,
  10%) dimethyl benzyl ammonium chlorides 0.05%

SPARTAN METAQUAT GERMICIDAL CLEANER
(Spartan)

n-Alkyl (C14, 50%; C12, 40%; C16,
  10%) dimethyl benzyl ammonium
  chlorides * 3.50%
Sodium metasilicate * 2.65%
Tetrasodium
  ethylenediaminetetraacetate ... 1.84%

SPARTAN M.L.D. BOWL CLEANSE
(Spartan)

Phosphoric acid * 25.00%
n-Alkyl (C14, 50%; C12, 40%; C16,
  10%) dimethyl benzyl ammonium chloride 0.05%

SPARTAN PD-64 PHENOLIC BASE CLEANER-DISINFECTANT
(Spartan)

Isopropyl alcohol * 10.30%
Sodium xylene sulfonate 10.30%
Orthophenylphenol * 6.18%
Potassium ricinoleate * 6.13%

SPARTAN SANI-T-10 DISINFECTANT-SANITIZER-ALGICIDE
(Spartan)

n-Alkyl (60% C14, 30% C16, 5% C12,
  5% C18) dimethyl benzyl ammonium chlorides * 5.0%
n-Alkyl (68% C12, 32% C14) dimethyl
  ethylbenzyl ammonium
  chlorides * 5.0%

SPARTAN SPARQUAT 256 GERMICIDAL CLEANER
(Spartan)

Octyl decyl dimethyl ammonium
  chloride *† 3.750%
Dioctyl dimethyl ammonium
  chloride *† 1.875%
Didecyl dimethyl ammonium
  chloride * 1.875%
Alkyl (C14, 50%; C12, 40%; C16,
  10%) dimethyl benzyl ammo-
  nium chloride * 5.000%
Tetrasodium
  ethylenediaminetetraacetate .. 3.420%
Isopropyl alcohol 3.000%
Ethyl alcohol 1.000%
Perfume 0.300%

†*See* Cationic surfactants

SPARTAN STERIGENT GERMICIDAL CLEANER
(Spartan)

n-Alkyl (C14, 50%; C12, 40%; C16,
  10%) dimethyl benzyl ammonium
  chlorides * 4.5%

SPASMED
Antispasmodic & sedative
(Jenkins Labs.)

Each tablet:
  Hyoscyamine hydrobromide 0.1037 mg.
  Atropine sulfate .... 0.0194 mg.
  Hyoscine hydrobromide ... 0.0065 mg.
  Tri-bar (33 1/3% each): .... 16.2 mg.
    Butabarbital sodium *
    Pentobarbital sodium *
    Phenobarbital sodium *

SPASMED (ELIXIR)
(Jenkins Labs.)

Each 5 cc:
  Alcohol * 15%
  Hyoscyamine hydrobromide 0.1037 mg.
  Hyoscine hydrobromide ... 0.0065 mg.
  Atropine sulfate .... 0.0194 mg.
  Tri-bar (representing 33
    1/3% each): .... 16.2 mg.
    Butabarbital sodium *
    Pentobarbital sodium *
    Phenobarbital sodium *

SPASMED, JR.
Sedative
(Jenkins Labs.)

Each tablet:
  Homatropine methylbromide . 1/96 gr.
  Phenobarbital sodium * ..... 1/8 gr.
  Lactose .... q.s.
  Special mint flavor .... q.s.

SPASMOPHEN ELIXIR & TABLETS
Antispasmodic, sedative
(Lannett)

Elixir, each 5 ml.:
Phenobarbital	15 mg.
Hyoscyamine sulfate	0.1037 mg.
Atropine sulfate	0.0194 mg.
Hyoscine hydrobromide	0.0065 mg.

Each tablet:
Phenobarbital *	15 mg.
Hyoscyamine sulfate *	0.1037 mg.
Atropine sulfate *	0.0194 mg.
Hyoscine hydrobromide	0.0065 mg.

SPASMOSED
Antispasmodic, sedative
(Wesley Pharm.)

Each tablet:
Phenobarbital *	8 mg.
Atropine sulfate	0.06 mg.
Bismuth subnitrate	0.12 gm.

SPD
Drain and sewer opener
(Damon Chemical Co.)

Potassium hydroxide *	75.00%
Sodium hydroxide *	19.25%
Cupric carbonate	0.75%
Pine oil	2.00%
Sodium dodecyl benzene sulfonate	0.40%

Inactive ingredients:
Sodium bicarbonate	2.00%
Sodium sulphate	0.60%

SPD ANALGESIC CREAM
For arthritis, rheumatism, neuralgia
(Am. Pharmaceutical)

Methyl salicylate *
Methyl nicotinate
Dipropyleneglycol salicylate *
Oleoresin capsicum
Camphor *
Menthol *

SPEAK EASY
Non-aerosol (pump) breath freshener
(Amer. Safety Razor Co.)

Ethyl alcohol	37%
Deionized water	22%
Peppermint oil	approx. 1%
Honey	40%

SPECKLETONE GLAZES

See DUNCAN CERAMICS SPECK-LETONE GLAZES (AR 900 Series)

SPECO SOLVENT & THINNER
(Speco)

Coal tar aromatic solvent *

'76 Ed.

SPECS PAINT THINNER
(Sunnyside)

Aliphatic & aromatic hydrocarbons (Petroleum distillates) *

SPEC-TAK 1000
Alkaline cleaner
(Diversey Wyandotte)

Sodium hydroxide *

SPECTINOMYCIN TABLETS AND ORAL LIQUID
Antibacterial agent; veterinary
(Syntex Agribusiness)

Each tablet:
Spectinomycin base (as spectinomycin dihydrochloride)	100 mg.

Each ml.:
Spectinomycin (from spectinomycin dihydrochloride pentahydrate)	50 mg.

SPECTRACIDE ANT AND ROACH CONTROL
(Ciba-Geigy Ag. Div.)

Diazinon	0.500%
Pyrethrins	0.052%
Technical Piperonyl butoxide	0.261%
Petroleum distillate *	95.862%

SPECTRACIDE CRAWLING INSECT CONTROL (Granules)
(Ciba-Geigy Ag. Div.)

Diazinon *	5%

SPECTRACIDE GARDEN INSECT DUST
(Ciba-Geigy Ag. Div.)

Diazinon *	4%

SPECTRACIDE GARDEN ROSE & HOUSEPLANT SPRAY
Insecticide
(Ciba-Geigy Ag. Div.)

Diazinon	0.5%
Chlorofluorocarbons 11 & 12	

SPECTRACIDE LAWN & GARDEN INSECT CONTROL
(Ciba-Geigy Ag. Div.)

Diazinon *	25.0%
Aromatic petroleum derivative solvent *	54.4%

SPECTRACIDE LAWN INSECT CONTROL (Granular)
(Ciba-Geigy Ag. Div.)

Diazinon *	2%

SPECTRACIDE PROFESSIONAL HOME PEST CONTROL
(Ciba-Geigy Ag. Div.)

Diazinon	0.500%
Pyrethrins	0.052%
Technical Piperonyl butoxide	0.261%
Aromatic petroleum derivative solvent *	98.617%

SPECTRACIDE PROFESSIONAL HOME PEST CONTROL (Pressurized)
(Ciba-Geigy Ag. Div.)

Diazinon	0.500%
Pyrethrins	0.052%
Technical Piperonyl butoxide	0.261%
Petroleum distillate *	68.608%

SPECTRACIDE ROSE AND FLOWER SPRAY
Insecticide, fungicide
(Ciba-Geigy Ag. Div.)

Diazinon	0.500%
Pyrethrins	0.025%
Technical Piperonyl butoxide	0.250%
Folpet	0.500%

SPECTRACIDE 6000 LAWN AND GARDEN INSECT CONTROL
(Ciba-Geigy Ag. Div.)

Diazinon *	5%

SPECTRO-JEL
Soapless skin cleanser
(Recsei Labs.)

Methyl cellulose	0.88%
Carboxypolymethylene	0.05%
Cetyl alcohol	1.75%
Sorbitan mono-oleate	1.0%
Fumed Silica	0.15%
Triethanolamine stearate	0.750%
Glycol polysiloxane	0.80%

SPECTRUM LIQUID TEMPERA
(Avalon Industries)

This product bears the AP Seal issued by the Crayon, Water Color and Craft Institute, Inc. This seal certifies that the product contains no materials in sufficient quantities to be toxic or injurious to the human body even if ingested.

Starred ingredients (*) may be responsible for major toxic effects; consult Section II.

SPECTRUM POWDER TEMPERA
(Avalon Industries)

This product bears the AP Seal issued by the Crayon, Water Color and Craft Institute, Inc. This seal certifies that the product contains no materials in sufficient quantities to be toxic or injurious to the human body even if ingested.

SPE-DE-WAY WOOD BLEACH UNIT "A"
(Spe-De-Way)

Hydrogen peroxide 0.205%

SPE-DE-WAY WOOD BLEACH UNIT "B"
(Spe-De-Way)

Sodium hydroxide 0.03%
Borax 0.015%
Sodium silicate 0.015%

SPEED DEMON FLAMMABLE PAINT REMOVER
(Schalk)

Acetone
Toluene *
Methylene chloride

'76 Ed.

SPEED DEMON HAND CLEANER
(Schalk)

Petroleum distillate *

'76 Ed.

SPEED DEMON NON FLAMMABLE PAINT REMOVER
(Schalk)

Methylene chloride *

'76 Ed.

SPEED DEMON PANEL AND CONSTRUCTION ADHESIVE
(Schalk)

Petroleum distillate *

'76 Ed.

SPEEDIE-RUB
Hand rubbing compound
(McAleer)

Kerosene *
Sodium oleate
Paraffin oil
Pine oil *
Tripoli

'76 Ed.

SPEEDIP

See E-Z-EST SPEEDIP

SPEEDI-SEAL
(Touraine Paints, Inc.)

Titanium dioxide 15.1%
Calcium carbonate 15.1%
Silicates 2.1%
Vinyl latex non-volatile 13.9%
Water 53.8%

'76 Ed.

SPEEDKIL
Indoor space and surface spray; insecticide
(Puritan Chem. Co.)

Active ingredients: 100%
   Petroleum distillate *
   2,2-Dichlorovinyl dimethyl phosphate and related compounds (DDVP) *
   N-Octyl bicycloheptene dicarboximide
   Technical Piperonyl butoxide
   Pyrethrins

SPEEDRIN TABLETS
Antacid-analgesic
(Columbia Med.)

Aspirin * . . . . 5 gr.
Aluminum hydroxide-glycine
Magnesium carbonate

SPEEDSOL
Solvent
(Oklahoma Refining)

Paraffins * 50%
Naphthenes * 42%
Aromatics * 7%
Olefins 1%

SPEED STICK ANTIPERSPIRANT STICK (FRESH & SPICE)
(Mennen)

Active ingred.:
   Aluminum chlorohydrate *
Other ingred.:
   Cyclomethicone
   Stearyl alcohol
   Glyceryl stearate
   PEG-100 stearate
   Fragrance

SPEED STICK ANTIPERSPIRANT STICK (UNSCENTED)
(Mennen)

Active ingred.:
   Aluminum chlorohydrate *
Other ingred.:
   Cyclomethicone
   Stearyl alcohol
   Glyceryl stearate
   PEG-100 stearate

SPEED STICK DEODORANT
(Mennen)

Propylene glycol
Water
Sodium stearate
Fragrance
Triclosan
FD&C Blue #1
FD&C Yellow #5

SPEED STICK DRY LIME DEODORANT
(Mennen)

Propylene glycol
Water
Sodium stearate
Fragrance
Triclosan
FD&C Yellow #5
FD&C Blue #1

SPEED STICK HERBAL DEODORANT
(Mennen)

Propylene glycol
Water
Sodium stearate
Fragrance
Triclosan
D&C Green #5
FD&C Yellow #5

SPEED STICK SPICE SCENT DEODORANT
(Mennen)

Propylene glycol
Water
Sodium stearate
Fragrance
Triclosan
FD&C Red #4
D&C Orange #4
D&C Green #5
FD&C Yellow #5

SPEED-WASH, FORMULA LC-5

See   KLENZADE   SPEED-WASH, FORMULA LC-5

Starred ingredients (*) may be responsible for major toxic effects; consult Section II.

SPEEDY
Liquid scale remover
(Lester Labs.)

Hydrochloric acid *
Corrosion inhibitors

'76 Ed.

SPERTI
Skin ointment
(Whitehall Labs.)

Live yeast-cell deriv.
Shark liver oil 3.0%
Phenylmercuric nitrate 1-10,000
Lanolin
Mineral jelly

SPIC & SPAN (Formula 1)
Household cleaner
(Procter & Gamble)

Sodium sesquicarbonate * 50-74%
Tetrasodium pyrophosphate 10-24%
Sodium tripolyphosphate 1-4%
Sodium alkyl benzene sulfonate . 1-4%
Sodium sulfate 1-4%
Minor ingredients, each .... <1%

pH (1% solution) - 9.8

SPIC & SPAN (Formula 2)
Household cleaner
(Procter & Gamble)

Sodium sesquicarbonate * 50-74%
Tetrasodium pyrophosphate 10-24%
Sodium tripolyphosphate 1-4%
Sodium alkyl benzene sulfonate . 1-4%
Sodium silicate 1-4%
Sodium sulfate 1-4%
Minor ingredients, each .... <1%

pH (1% solution) - 9.8

SPIC & SPAN (Non-Phosphate Formula) (Formula 1)
Household cleaner
(Procter & Gamble)

Sodium sesquicarbonate * 25-49%
Sodium sulfate 25-49%
Sodium carbonate 10-24%
Sodium citrate 5-9%
Sodium alkyl benzene sulfonate . 1-4%
Minor ingredients, each .... <1%

pH (10% solution) - 10.1

SPIC & SPAN (Non-Phosphate Formula) (Formula 2)
Household cleaner
(Procter & Gamble)

Sodium sesquicarbonate * 75-99%
Sodium carbonate 10-24%
Sodium sulfate 1-4%
Sodium silicate 1-4%
Sodium alkyl benzene sulfonate . 1-4%
Minor ingredients, each .... <1%

pH (10% solution) - 10.1

SPIDER-sMITE

See DEXOL SPIDER-sMITE

SPIF
Liquid drain pipe opener
(Navy Brand)

Sulphuric acid *

SPIK D-5 HEAVY DUTY FLOOR CLEANER
For use in automatic scrubbing machines
(National-Purity Soap)

Nonionic surfactant *
Diethanolamine coconut oil condensate
Surface active soap
Sequestrant (liquid Versene)
Defoaming agent

SPIK D-6 HEAVY DUTY LIQUID
Detergent floor cleaner & odor counteractant; institutional use
(National-Purity Soap)

Nonionic surfactant *
Quaternary ammonium compound *
Defoamer
Perfume

SPIKE 80W
Herbicide
(Elanco Prod.)

1-(5-tert-butyl-1,3,4-thiadiazol-2-yl)-
1,3-dimethylurea * 80%

SPINOSE EAR-TICK TREATMENT WITH LINDANE

See FRANKLIN SPINOSE EAR-TICK TREATMENT WITH LINDANE

SPIREX OINTMENT
Fungicidal ointment
(International Chem.)

Undecylenic acid 5%
Zinc undecylenate * 20%

'76 Ed.

SPIRIT (Refreshment Bar Soap)
(Armour-Dial, Inc.)

Sodium soap 75-100%
Moisture (water) 10-25%
Perfume 1-5%
Minor ingredients (total) 1-5%

SPIT SHINE
Pump spray for floors
(Sanitek)

Mineral spirits * 35.0%
Carnauba wax 1.6%
Nonionic surfactant 1.6%
Formalin 0.3%
Benzaldehyde 0.2%
Xanthan gum .... trace
Water .... balance

SPIX
Insecticide
(Dolge)

Petroleum distillate *
Piperonyl butoxide, tech.
Essential oils *
Pyrethrins *

SPIX AEROSOL
Insecticide
(Dolge)

Petroleum distillate *
Piperonyl butoxide, technical
Pyrethrins *
N-Octyl bicycloheptene dicarboximide *
Essential oils *
Isobutane/propane
(Propellant) .... 35% max.

SPLURGE
Water thinned texture paint
(United Gilsonite)

Silicates 73%
Calcium carbonate 13%
Soya protein 13%
Sodium pentachlorophenate ...... <1%
Sodium chloride .... <1%

SPOHN'S COMPOUND
Antitussive; veterinary
(Spohn)

Sulfur
Creosote *
Oil of tar *
Turpentine *

'76 Ed.

SPOOX
Residual roach liquid
(Hysan Corp.)

O,O-Diethyl O-(2-isopropyl-4-
methyl-6-
pyrimidinyl)phosphorothioate 0.500%
Pyrethrins 0.052%
Technical Piperonyl butoxide
(equiv. to 0.209% (butylcarbi-
tyl)(6-propylpiperonyl) ether
and 0.052% other related
compounds) 0.261%
Petroleum distillate * 99.187%

SPORTS*RUB
(Cramer Products)

Stearic acid (USP)	12.50%
Cetyl alcohol	2.97%
Isopropyl myristate	1.00%
Glycerine (USP)	3.75%
Triethanolamine	0.78%
Soft water	61.00%
Methyl salicylate (USP) *	15.00%
Menthol (USP)	3.00%

SPOT BALM FOR DOGS
For skin irritations; veterinary
(Happy Jack)

Glycerin	
Salicylic acid *	
Tannic acid	
Sulfanilamide	5%
Brilliant green	
Isopropyl alcohol *	60%

SPOT DANDELION CONTROL
Spray can
(Scott, O.M.)

Alkanolamine salts (ethanol and isopropanol series) of 2,4-Dichlorophenoxyacetic acid	1.66%
Dimethylamine salt of Dicamba	0.31%

SPOT GUARD
Dishwashing rinse additive
(Calgon Corp., Commercial Div.)

Anionic wetting agents *
Nonionic wetting agents

SPOT-KIL
Herbicide
(Malter International)

Sodium cacodylate	7.5%
Dimethylarsinic acid (Cacodylic acid)	1.3%

Total elemental arsenic in water soluble form 4.2%

SPOT KILL
Algicide for swimming pools
(Bio-Lab)

Sodium dichloro-s-triazinetrione *	100%

SPOT KILL SUPER ALGAE DESTROYER

See BIO-GUARD SPOT KILL SUPER ALGAE DESTROYER

SPOTRETE
Turf fungicide
(Cleary)

Thiuram *	75%

'76 Ed.

SPOT-TAK

See LEECH SPOT-TAK

SPOTTON CATTLE INSECTICIDE
For control of cattle grubs and lice
(Cutter (Brand) Bayvet Div. Cutter Labs.)

Fenthion *	20%

SPRA-CLEAR

See PLASTI-KOTE SPRA-CLEAR

SPRA-GON ANT & ROACH KILLER
(Rempel)

Tech. Chlordane	2.5%

'76 Ed.

SPRA-GON DAIRY & STOCK SPRAY
Insecticide
(Rempel)

Petroleum oil *	
Pine oil *	
Tech. Piperonyl butoxide	
Pyrethrins *	

'76 Ed.

SPRA-GON DROSOPHILA SPRAY
Insecticide
(Rempel)

Petroleum oil *	97.75%
Technical Piperonyl butoxide	2.00%
Pyrethrins	0.25%

'76 Ed.

SPRA-GON INDUSTRIAL FLY SPRAY
Insecticide
(Rempel)

Petroleum oil *	98.90%
Technical Piperonyl butoxide	1.00%
Pyrethrins	0.10%

'76 Ed.

SPRA-TONE

See GARD SPRA-TONE

SPRA-WAY PAINT & VARNISH REMOVER

See PLASTI-KOTE SPRA-WAY PAINT & VARNISH REMOVER

SPRAY B-I-N PRIMER SEALER
(Zinsser, Wm., & Co.)

Pigment:	15.90%
Titanium dioxide	52.0%
Silicates	48.0%
Non-volatile vehicle:	9.10%
Shellac resin	100.0%
Volatile vehicle:	60.60%
Alcohols *	46.5%
Ketones *	53.5%
Propellant:	14.40%
Propane-Isobutane	

SPRAY DIRTEX CLEANER (AEROSOL PACK)
For windows, mirrors, porcelain
(Savogran)

Butyl Cellosolve *	<20%
Ammonia	trace
Propellant	<5%

SPRAY FLO
Cleaner
(Pennwalt)

Sodium orthosilicate
Phosphate *
Soda ash *
Wetting agent

SPRAY-N-GLUE 0099

See WELDWOOD SPRAY-N-GLUE 0099

SPRAY NOX INSECT SPRAY
(Claire)

Pyrethrins	0.20%
Piperonyl butoxide, tech.	1.0%
Petroleum distillates *	18.8%

SPRAY 'N STARCH

See TEXIZE SPRAY 'N STARCH

SPRAY 'N WASH (Aerosol)

See TEXIZE SPRAY 'N WASH (Aerosol)

SPRAY 'N WASH (Liquid Spray)

See TEXIZE SPRAY 'N WASH (Liquid Spray)

SPRAYTEC REPELLENT CONCENTRATE
Roach repellent
(Summit Chem. Co.)

2-Hydroxyethyl-N-octyl sulfide	4.75%
Other related compounds	0.25%
N-Octyl bicycloheptene dicarboximide	10.00%
Petroleum distillate *	75.00%
Inert ingredients:	10.00%
Non-ionic emulsifiers	

Starred ingredients (*) may be responsible for major toxic effects; consult Section II.

SPRAY-TROL BRAND CONCEN-TROL
Insecticide
(Coyne)

Petroleum hydrocarbon oil base *
Tech. Piperonyl butoxide
Pyrethrins

SPRAY-TROL BRAND CONTAC-TROL
Insecticide
(Coyne)

Petroleum hydrocarbon oil base *
Tech. Piperonyl butoxide
Pyrethrins

SPRAY-TROL BRAND DIAZI-TROL
Insecticide
(Coyne)

Petroleum hydrocarbon oil base *
Diazinon *
Piperonyl butoxide
Pyrethrins

SPRAY-TROL BRAND FUMI-TROL
Fumigant
(Coyne)

Ethylene dichloride *
Carbon tetrachloride *

SPRAY-TROL BRAND INSEC-TROL
Insecticide
(Coyne)

Petroleum hydrocarbon oil base *
Tech. Piperonyl butoxide
Pyrethrins

SPRAY-TROL BRAND MALA-TROL
Insecticide
(Coyne)

Aromatic petroleum solvent *
Malathion *
Emulsifier

SPRAY-TROL BRAND QUIK-TROL
Insecticide
(Coyne)

Petroleum hydrocarbon oil base *
Tech. Piperonyl butoxide
Pyrethrins

SPRAY-TROL BRAND RODEN-TROL
Rodenticide
(Coyne)

Warfarin (3-(a-Acetonylbenzyl)-4-
hydroxycoumarin) 0.5%

SPRAY-TROL BRAND SUPER-TROL
Insecticide
(Coyne)

Petroleum hydrocarbon oil base *
Tech. Piperonyl butoxide
Pyrethrins

SPRAY-TROL BRAND SURE-TROL
Insecticide
(Coyne)

Petroleum hydrocarbon oil base *
Tech. Piperonyl butoxide
Pyrethrins

SPRAY-TROL BRAND TOXI-TROL
Insecticide
(Coyne)

Petroleum hydrocarbon oil base *
Methoxychlor *
Lindane *

SPRAYWAY AIR SANITIZER & DEODORIZER (ALL FRAGRANCES) (AEROSOL)
(Sprayway)

Triethylene glycol 7.5%

SPRAYWAY FAST-KILL ROACH & ANT KILLER WITH DIAZINON (AEROSOL)
(Sprayway)

Pyrethrins 0.050%
Technical Piperonyl butoxide .. 0.100%
N-Octyl bicycloheptene
   dicarboximide 0.166%
Diazinon 0.500%
Petroleum distillate * 95.584%

SPRAYWAY P-51 INSECT SPRAY (AEROSOL)
(Sprayway)

Technical Methoxychlor 2.00%
2,2-Dichlorovinyl dimethyl phosphate (DDVP) 0.46%
Related compounds 0.04%
Petroleum distillates * 20.00%

SPRAYWAY TRU-NOX INSECTICIDE (AEROSOL)
(Sprayway)

Petroleum solvent * 18.80%
Technical Piperonyl butoxide ... 1.00%
Pyrethrins 0.20%

SPRAYZON MAGIC CLEANER
(Uncle Sam)

Butyl Cellosolve * .... <10%
Sodium metasilicate *
Surfactants *
Ethylenediaminetetraacetate
Soda ash *
Inhibitors
Dye
Water

SPRAZE

See GARD SPRAZE

SPRECTO WITH REPELLENT
Insecticide & repellent
(Pitman-Moore)

Pyrethrins .... 0.05% w/w
Technical Piperonyl butoxide   0.1% w/w
Carbaryl (1-Naphthyl N-
   methylcarbamate) .... 0.5% w/w
2,3:4,5-bis(2-
   Butylene)tetrahydro-2-
   furaldehyde .... 0.2% w/w
N-Octyl bicycloheptene
   dicarboximide .... 0.4% w/w
Petroleum distillate .... 3.35% w/w

SPRED ANTIQUE GLAZE (Y-508)
(Glidden)

Silica & silicates 13.0%
Combined amount: 37.5%
   Linseed
   Safflower
   Urethane oil
Mineral spirits * 23.4%
Kerosene * 23.7%
Additives (no lead) 2.4%

SPRED BRUSH & ROLLER CLEANER (Y-60)
(Glidden)

Aromatic hydrocarbons * 57.7%
Isopropyl alcohols 8.8%
Surfactant 21.3%
Amines & phosphates 12.2%

SPRED DECORATOR ENAMEL - WHITE (Y-525)
(Glidden)

Titanium dioxide 21.5%
Vinyl acetate/acrylic resin 20.0%
Glycol ethers, esters 5.8%
Additives (no lead) 2.3%
Water 50.4%

Starred ingredients (*) may be responsible for major toxic effects; consult Section II.

SPRED GEL-FLO HOUSE PAINT (Y-1900 Line)
(Glidden)

Titanium dioxide	25.7%
Combined amount:	40.3%
Soya	
Tall oil alkyd	
Mineral spirits *	26.5%
N-(Trichloromethylthio)phthal-imide	2.1%
Kerosene	4.1%
Additives (no lead)	1.3%

SPRED GLIDE-ON (Y-3500 Line)
(Glidden)

	by weight:
Titanium dioxide	16.2%
Silicates	21.9%
Acrylic resin	11.4%
Glycol ethers, esters	4.2%
Additives	2.1%
Water	44.2%
Di(phenylmercuric) dodecenyl succinate	0.06%

SPRED GLOSS ALUMINUM (Y-992)
(Glidden)

Aluminum paste	11.0%
Combined amount:	32.8%
Linseed oil	
Resin	
Driers *	
Aliphatic hydrocarbons *	56.2%

SPRED GLOSS ENAMEL - WHITE (Y-900)
(Glidden)

Titanium dioxide	24.8%
Tall oil alkyd	39.9%
Mineral spirits *	34.6%
Additives (no lead)	0.7%

SPRED GLOSS SPRAY ENAMEL - LIMEQUAT (Y-1060)
(Glidden)

Titanium dioxide	5.8%
Tall oil alkyd	14.0%
Acetone	33.8%
Toluene *	17.9%
Methylene chloride	11.1%
Glycol ethers, esters	2.4%
Propane	15.0%

SPRED LATEX ENAMEL UNDERCOAT (Y-300)
(Glidden)

Titanium dioxide	13.6%
Silicates	19.8%
Acrylic/vinyl acetate resin	15.6%
Glycol ethers & esters	5.2%
Additives (no lead)	1.9%
Water	43.9%

SPRED LATEX ENAMEL (Y-3700 Line)
(Glidden)

Silicates	6.6%
Titanium dioxide	16.4%
Vinyl acetate/acrylic resin	28.0%
Glycol ethers, esters	5.2%
Additives (no lead)	3.2%
Water	40.6%

SPRED LATEX GLOSS ENAMEL (Y-3300 Line)
(Glidden)

Titanium dioxide	20.6%
Acrylic resin	26.2%
Glycol, ethers, esters *†	10.7%
Additives (no lead)	2.5%
Water	38.9%
Silicates	1.1%

†See Ethylene glycol alkyl (and aryl) ethers

SPRED LATEX HOUSE PAINT PRIMER (Y-3651)
(Glidden)

Titanium dioxide	12.1%
Silicates	36.1%
Combined amount:	25.4%
Linseed oil	
Tall alkyd	
Kerosene	7.3%
Mineral spirits	16.3%
Additives (no lead)	2.8%

SPRED LATEX HOUSE PAINT (Y-3600 Line)
(Glidden)

Titanium dioxide	18.7%
Zinc oxide	7.7%
Silicates	9.7%
Tall oil alkyd	5.6%
Acrylic resin	12.9%
Additives (no lead)	2.4%
Water	40.4%
2-n-Octyl-4-isothiazolin-3-one	0.04%
Glycol ethers, esters	2.6%

SPRED LATEX HOUSE & TRIM (Y-3900)
(Glidden)

	by weight
Titanium dioxide	24%
Acrylic resin	23%
Glycol ethers and esters	7%
Additives	2%
Water	44%
Di-iodomethyl-p-tolyl sulfone and Di(phenylmercuric) dodecenyl succinate	0.3%

SPRED LATEX INTERIOR STAINS (Y-600 Line)
(Glidden)

Oxides & colors	8.0%
Vinyl acetate/acrylic resin	3.0%
Diethylene glycol *	20.0%
Additives (no lead)	2.0%
Water	67.0%

SPRED LATEX STAINS (Y-420 Line)
(Glidden)

Titanium dioxide	4.9%
Silicates	10.1%
Acrylic resin	19.2%
Glycol ethers & esters	3.7%
Additives (no lead)	2.7%
Water	59.1%
Di-iodomethyl-p-tolyl sulfone	0.3%

SPRED LUSTRE SEMI-GLOSS ENAMEL (Y-4600 Line)
(Glidden)

	by weight
Titanium dioxide	22.9%
Calcium carbonate	9.9%
Silicates	3.5%
Combined amount:	29.2%
Soya	
Tall oil alkyd	
Driers (no lead) *	
Mineral spirits *	34.5%

SPRED PREP (Y-66)
(Glidden)

Aliphatic hydrocarbons *	58.7%
Glycol ethers	30.7%
Ketone	5.8%
Isopropyl alcohol	4.8%

SPRED PRIMER SEALER (Y-3416)
(Glidden)

Titanium dioxide	8.3%
Silicates	22.5%
Butadiene-styrene resin	18.2%
Additives (no lead)	2.0%
Water	49.0%

SPRED SATIN LATEX WALL PAINT (Y-3400 Line)
(Glidden)

Titanium dioxide	11.2%
Silicates	21.0%
Vinyl acetate/acrylate resin	13.8%
Glycol ethers, esters	3.6%
Additives (no lead)	2.0%
Water	48.4%

SPRED SPAR VARNISH (Y-40)
(Glidden)

Combined amount:	52.4%
Phenolic castor tung oil *†	
Driers (no lead) *	
Mineral spirits *	43.0%
Esters	1.0%
Isopropyl alcohol	3.6%

†See Tung oil

Starred ingredients (*) may be responsible for major toxic effects; consult Section II.

SPRED URETHANE FLORENAMEL (Y-800)
(Glidden)

Titanium dioxide	25.7%
Soya, tung polyurethane	16.2%
Tall oil alkyd	18.4%
Mineral spirits *	34.7%
Additives (no lead)	1.4%
Silicates	3.6%

SPRED URETHANE LIQUID PLASTIC (Y-10)
(Glidden)

Soya, tung urethane oil	19.6%
Tall oil alkyd	19.8%
Mineral spirits *	53.5%
Additives (no lead)	1.3%
Silicates	5.8%

SPRED URETHANE LIQUID PLASTIC (Y-20)
(Glidden)

Soya, tung urethane oil	23.4%
Tall oil alkyd	23.4%
Mineral spirits *	52.7%
Additives (no lead)	0.5%

SPRED WOOD UNDERCOATER (Y-555)
(Glidden)

Titanium dioxide	15.3%
Calcium carbonate	33.3%
Silicates	7.9%
Soya, Tall oil alkyd	15.6%
Mineral spirits *	27.4%
Additives (no lead)	0.5%

SPREDZIT
Spreader for insecticide & weed killer
(Dolge)

Modified Phthalic glycerol alkyd resin	77%

SPRITE BOUQUET
Air sanitizer deodorizer
(Hysan Corp.)

Triethylene glycol	3.50%
Propylene glycol	3.00%
Methyldodecylbenzyl trimethylammonium chloride	0.16%
Methyldodecylxylylene bis(trimethylammonium chloride)	0.04%

SPRITE CONCENTRATED FABRIC SOFTENER
(Industrial Equities)

Quaternary ammonium compound *	5-10%
Fluorescent whitening agent	<1%
Preservative	<1%
Colorant	<1%
Perfume	<1%
Water	balance

SPRITE FABRIC SOFTENER
(Industrial Equities)

Quaternary ammonium compound *	2-5%
Preservative	<1%
Colorant	<1%
Perfume	<1%
Water	balance

SPRITE LIQUID DISHWASHING DETERGENT
(Industrial Equities)

Anionic surfactant	6-12%
Hydrotrope	1-3%
Alkanolamide	<1%
Ethyl alcohol	<1%
Opacifier	<1%
Colorant	<1%
Perfume	<1%
Water	balance

SPRITZ

See AIRWICK PROFESSIONAL PRODUCTS SPRITZ

SPROUT NIP POTATO SPROUT INHIBITOR
(PPG Industries, Chem. Div.)

Emulsifiable concentrate:	
Isopropyl m-chlorocarbanilate *	36%
Vegetable oil	36%
Surfactant & emulsifier	15%
Alcohol *	13%
Aerosol grade:	
Isopropyl m-chlorocarbanilate *	46.5%
Alcohol *	8.0%
Propylene glycol	45.5%

SPRUANCE, GILBERT, PAINT PRODUCTS

The Gilbert Spruance Co.
Tioga & Richmond
Philadelphia, Pa. 19134

Phone: 215-739-6172

See PAINTS, Section VI, General Formulations

SPRUCE PRIME-IT-ALL HOT ROD PRIMER PLATINUM GRAY (98-15)
(Seymour)

Non-volatile:	15.5%
Titanium dioxide	3.2%
Silicates	4.0%
Nitrocellulose, Dioctylphthalate, Maleic resins, Coconut alkyd resin	8.3%
Volatile:	84.5%
Ketones *, Alcohols *, Acetates *†	55.5%
Aromatic hydrocarbons *	7.0%
Propellant (Propane-isobutane)	22.0%

†*See* Paints, Section VI, General Formulations

SPRUCE PRIME-IT-ALL METAL PRIMER RED IRON OXIDE (98-26)
(Seymour)

Non-volatile:	16.4%
Pure yellow Iron oxide	1.2%
Carbon black	0.2%
Silicates	5.1%
Pure red Iron oxide	4.1%
Linseed alkyd resins and additives	5.8%
Volatile:	83.6%
Ketones *	23.6%
Aromatic hydrocarbons *, Aliphatic hydrocarbons *, Driers *	30.0%
Propellant (Propane-isobutane)	30.0%

SPRUCE SPRAY PAINT EVERGREEN GLOSS ENAMEL (98-8)
(Seymour)

Non-volatile:	14.1%
Titanium dioxide	0.7%
Azo anisidine yellow	0.9%
Phthalo blue	0.3%
Synthetic Petroleum resins, Soya and Vinyl toluene linseed alkyd resins	12.2%
Volatile:	85.9%
Ketones *	5.0%
Halogenated hydrocarbons *, Aromatic hydrocarbons *, Aliphatic hydrocarbons *, Driers *	50.9%
Propellant (Propane-isobutane)	30.0%

SPRUCE SPRAY PAINT FLAT BLACK ENAMEL (98-10)
(Seymour)

Non-volatile:	14.9%
Carbon black	0.4%
Calcium carbonate	5.4%
Silicates	2.5%
Soya and Vinyl toluene linseed alkyd resins	6.6%
Volatile:	85.1%
Ketones *	4.5%
Halogenated hydrocarbons *, Aromatic hydrocarbons *, Aliphatic hydrocarbons *, Driers *	50.6%
Propellant (Propane-isobutane)	30.0%

SPRUCE SPRAY PAINT FLAT WHITE ENAMEL (98-12)
(Seymour)

Non-volatile:	26.2%
Titanium dioxide	5.7%
Calcium carbonate	6.6%
Silicates	4.2%
Soya and Vinyl toluene linseed alkyd resins	9.7%
Volatile:	73.8%
Ketones *	8.3%
Aromatic hydrocarbons *, Aliphatic hydrocarbons *, Driers *	35.5%
Propellant (Propane-isobutane)	30.0%

Starred ingredients (*) may be responsible for major toxic effects; consult Section II.

SPRUCE SPRAY PAINT GLITTERING BLACK GLOSS LACQUER (98-18)
(Seymour)

Non-volatile:	13.2%
Carbon black	0.4%
Nitrocellulose, Dioctylphthalate, Maleic resins, Coconut alkyd resin	12.8%
Volatile:	86.8%
Ketones *, Alcohols *, Acetates *†	53.5%
Aromatic hydrocarbons *	11.3%
Propellant (Propane-isobutane)	22.0%

†See Paints, Section VI, General Formulations

SPRUCE SPRAY PAINT GLOSS BLACK ENAMEL (98-3)
(Seymour)

Non-volatile:	14.6%
Carbon black	0.9%
Synthetic Petroleum resins, Soya and Vinyl toluene linseed alkyd resins	13.7%
Volatile:	85.4%
Ketones	4.9%
Halogenated hydrocarbons *, Aromatic hydrocarbons *, Aliphatic hydrocarbons *, Driers *	50.0%
Propellant (Propane-isobutane)	30.0%

SPRUCE SPRAY PAINT GLOSS WHITE ENAMEL (98-2)
(Seymour)

Non-volatile:	21.0%
Titanium dioxide	10.0%
Soya and Vinyl toluene linseed alkyd resins	11.0%
Volatile:	79.0%
Ketones	5.3%
Halogenated hydrocarbons *, Aromatic hydrocarbons *, Aliphatic hydrocarbons *, Driers *	43.7%
Propellant (Propane-isobutane)	30.0%

SPRUCE SPRAY PAINT METALLIC CHROME ALUMINUM (98-1)
(Seymour)

Non-volatile:	10.5%
Aluminum powder	1.8%
Styrene resin	8.7%
Volatile:	89.5%
Aromatic hydrocarbons *, Aliphatic hydrocarbons *	59.5%
Propellant (Propane-isobutane)	30.0%

SPRUCE SPRAY PAINT ROCKET RED GLOSS ENAMEL (98-4)
(Seymour)

Non-volatile:	15.6%
Lt. Paratoner red	1.9%
Synthetic Petroleum resins, Soya and Vinyl toluene linseed alkyd resins	13.7%
Volatile:	84.4%
Ketones	4.9%
Halogenated hydrocarbons *, Aromatic hydrocarbons *, Aliphatic hydrocarbons *, Driers *	49.5%
Propellant (Propane-isobutane)	30.0%

SPRUCE SPRAY PAINT SPACE BLUE GLOSS ENAMEL (98-35)
(Seymour)

Non-volatile:	15.4%
Titanium dioxide	3.1%
Phthalo blue	0.2%
Synthetic Petroleum resins, Soya and Vinyl toluene linseed alkyd resins	12.1%
Volatile:	84.6%
Ketones	5.5%
Halogenated hydrocarbons *, Aromatic hydrocarbons *, Aliphatic hydrocarbons *, Driers *	49.1%
Propellant (Propane-isobutane)	30.0%

SPRX-1 and SPRX-2
Anorexiant
(Direct Div.)

Each tablet:	
Phendimetrazine tartrate *	35 mg.

SPRX-3
Anorexiant
(Direct Div.)

Each capsule:	
Phendimetrazine tartrate *	35 mg.

SPRX-105
Anorexiant
(Direct Div.)

Each capsule:	
Phendimetrazine tartrate *	105 mg.

S-P-T
Hypothyroidism
(Fleming)

U.S.P. pork Thyroid (desiccated) *	
Green:	1 gr.
Brown:	2 gr.
Red:	3 gr.
Black:	5 gr.

SP-10 HARDENER
(Baird Dynamic)

Methyl ethyl ketone peroxide *	60%
In an ester	

'76 Ed.

SP-10 PLASTIC SEALER
(Baird Dynamic)

Polyester resin
Mineral fillers

'76 Ed.

SPUR-TEX SUPREME DISINFECTANT CLEANER-DEODORANT
Bactericidal and fungistatic
(Spurrier Chem.)

N-Alkyl (C14 60%; C16 30%; C12 5%; C18 5%) dimethylbenzylammonium chloride *	2.50%
Methyl salicylate *	1.65%
Tetrasodium salt of ethylenediaminetetraacetic acid	0.25%
Inert ingredients:	
Water	92.35%
Sodium tripolyphosphate	0.25%
Nonylphenoxypoly (ethyleneoxy) ethanol	2.50%
Sodium nitrite	0.50%

SPUR-TEX SUPREME DISINFECTANT RINSE
For glassware, dishes, etc.
(Spurrier Chem.)

N-Alkyl (C14 60%; C16 30%; C12 5%; C18 5%) dimethylbenzylammonium chloride *	5.0%
Inert ingredients:	
Nonylphenoxypoly (ethyleneoxy) ethanol	2.5%
Water	92.5%

SQUELCH INSECTICIDE
Insecticide
(ABCO, Inc.)

Petroleum distillate *	99.6285%
Technical Piperonyl butoxide	0.3300%
Pyrethrins	0.0415%

SSKI
(Upsher-Smith)

Potassium iodide solution, N.F. (saturated) *

SSS BOUQUET ROOM DEODORANT
(Standardized Sanitation Systems)

Isopropyl alcohol *
Triethylene glycol
Propylene glycol
Dipropylene glycol
Inert ingredients: 70.35%
  Trichloromonofluoromethane
  Dichlorodifluoromethane
  Essential oil USDA Reg. #4584-65
  Methylene chloride *
  Isobutane
  Propylene oxide

SSS CRAWLING INSECT KILLER WITH .25% SBP-1382
(Standardized Sanitation Systems)

(5-Benzyl-3-furyl) methyl-2,2-di-
  methyl-3-(2-methylpropenyl)
  cyclopropanecarboxylate 0.250%
Related compounds 0.034%
Aromatic petroleum
  hydrocarbons 0.331%
Petroleum distillate * 86.375%

SSS D-TRANS FLYING INSECT KILLER
(Standardized Sanitation Systems)

d-trans Allethrin (Allyl homolog of
  cinerin I) 0.30%
Piperonyl butoxide (technical) 0.60%
N-Octyl bicycloheptene
  dicarboximide 1.00%
Petroleum distillate 8.10%

SSS HOSPITAL STRENGTH DISINFECTANT-DEODORANT
(Standardized Sanitation Systems)

Isopropanol * 59.16%
Orthophenylphenol 0.10%
Ortho-benzyl para-chlorophenol .. 0.10%
4-Chloro-3,5-xylenol 0.10%

SSS MINT ROOM DEODORANT
(Standardized Sanitation Systems)

Isopropanol * 12.350%
Propylene glycol 6.175%
Triethylene glycol 6.175%

SSS SBP-1382 WASP & HORNET JET SPRAY
(Standardized Sanitation Systems)

(5-Benzyl-3-furyl) methyl 2,2-di-
  methyl-3-(2-methylpropenyl)
  cyclopropanecarboxylate 0.250%
Related compounds 0.034%
Aromatic petroleum
  hydrocarbons 0.331%
Petroleum distillate * 26.375%

SSS SPICE ROOM DEODORANT
(Standardized Sanitation Systems)

Isopropyl alcohol * 12.350%
Triethylene glycol 6.175%
Propylene glycol 6.175%
Inert ingredients: 75.30%
  Trichloromonofluoromethane
  Dichlorodifluoromethane
  Essential oil USDA Reg. #4584-24

S.S.S. TONIC (Liquid)
Iron & vitamin therapy
(S.S.S. Co.)

Each 3 tablespoons:
  Iron (as the ammonium
    citrate) *† .... 100 mg.
  Niacinamide .... 20 mg.
  Polyvitamins
  Alcohol 12%

†*See* Iron salts

S.S.S. TONIC (Tablets)
Iron & vitamin therapy
(S.S.S. Co.)

Each 2 tablets:
  Iron (Ferrous fumarate) * .... 100 mg.
  Niacinamide .... 60 mg.
  Plus polyvitamins and minerals

STĀ
Antifreeze
(Chemcentral)

Methanol * .... >95%

STA-BRITE
Wood preservative
(Sonford Products)

Sodium pentachlorophenate * 32.0%
Sodium salts of other chlorinated
  phenols 4.4%
Sodium tetraborate decahydrate .. 58.0%

STA-DED
Insecticide
(Dyna Systems)

Petroleum distillates * 74%
2-(1-Methylethoxy)phenol
  methylcarbamate * 1%
Petroleum distillates propellant ... 25%

STA-FLO SPRAY STARCH
(Staley)

A. E. Staley Mfg. Co.
2200 E. Eldorado St.
Decatur, Ill. 62525

Phone: 217-423-4411

STAIN-AID
Cleaner
(Lewis Research Labs.)

Sodium perborate * 33.3%
Sodium tripolyphosphate 25%
Sodium metasilicate 15%

'76 Ed.

STA-LEMON
Disinfectant-deodorant-cleaner
(Reily Chem.)

Active ingredients: 4.25%
  Isopropyl alcohol 1.55%
  n-Alkyl (C14 50%, C12 40%,
    C16 10%) dimethyl benzyl
    ammonium chlorides * .. 1.47%
  Essential oils 0.67%
  Ethanol 0.36%
  Trisodium salt of N-(2-hy-
    droxyethyl) ethylene dia-
    mine triacetic acid 0.20%
Inert ingredients: 95.75%
  Water 94.92%
  Octylphenoxy polyethoxy
    ethanol 0.83%

STAM F-34
Herbicide
(Rohm and Haas)

3',4'-Dichloropropionanilide * 35%

STA-MINT
Disinfectant-deodorant-cleaner
(Reily Chem.)

Isopropyl alcohol 3.05%
n-Alkyl (C14 50%, C12 40%, C16
  10%) dimethyl benzyl ammonium
  chlorides * 1.60%
Methylsalicylate * 1.25%
Trisodium hydroxyethyl ethylene
  diamine triacetic acid 0.30%

STAM LV-10
Herbicide
(Rohm and Haas)

3',4'-Dichloropropionanilide * 35%

STAMPEDE 3E
Herbicide
(Rohm and Haas)

Propanil* 33.8%

STANBACK POWDERS
Analgesic, antipyretic
(Stanback)

Aspirin * .... 648 mg.
Caffeine .... 15 mg.
Salicylamide .... 194.4 mg.
Potassium chloride, Tricalcium
  phosphate, DSS Granular
  (Cyanamid) .... <70 mg.

Starred ingredients (*) may be responsible for major toxic effects; consult Section II.

STANBACK TABLETS
Analgesic, antipyretic
(Stanback)

Aspirin * .... 324 mg.
Starch .... <85 mg.

STANCHEM PRODUCTS
Fire retardant paints & coatings

Stanchem Inc.
401 Berlin St.
East Berlin, Conn. 06023

Phone: 203-828-0571

See Paints, Section VI, General Formulations

STANDARD DRY WALL PRODUCTS
Protective coatings for masonry

Standard Dry Wall Products, Inc.
7800 N.W. 38th St.
Miami, Fla. 33166

Phone: 305-592-2081

STANDFAST SCRUBBABLE FLOOR FINISH
(Uncle Sam)

Polyacrylate (metal cross-linked)
Resin (modified phenolic)
Polyethylene
Surfactants *
Plasticizers
Glycol ethers *
Emulsifiers
Fluorocarbons
Water

STAND-UP
Soybean seed treatment
(Kalo)

Thiram *

STAND-UP PLUS
Soybean seed treatment
(Kalo)

Thiram *
Sodium molybdate

STANLEY HOME PRODUCTS
(Stanley Home Products)

Stanley Home Products, Inc.
333 Western Ave.
Westfield, Mass. 01085

Phone: 413-562-3631

STANLEY'S CROW REPELLENT (Liquid)
(Borderland Prod.)

Refined Coal tar * 94%
Inert ingred.:
    Water 2.7%
    Carbon 3.3%

S.T. 37 ANTISEPTIC SOLUTION
(Beecham Products)

Hexylresorcinol .... 1:1000 solution

STAPH-TROLE ANTISEPTIC CLEANER
(Multi-Clean Products)

N-Alkyl (C14, C12, C16) dimethyl
    benzyl ammonium chlorides * .. 2.76%
Trisodium phosphate 0.77%
Ethylenediaminetetraacetic acid,
    tetrasodium salt 0.59%
Inert ingredients:
    Water
    Octyl phenoxy polyethoxy ethanol
    Sodium tripolyphosphate
    Dye-D&C 19 (FDA approved for food
    use)
                                '76 Ed.

STA-PINE
Deodorant-cleaner
(Reily Chem.)

Isopropyl alcohol 1.53%
n-Alkyl (C14 50%, C12 40%, C16
    10%) dimethyl benzyl ammonium
    chlorides * 1.46%
Essential oils 0.42%
Trisodium salt of N-(2-hydroxy-
    ethyl) ethylene diamine triacetic
    acid 0.25%

STA-PUF FABRIC SOFTENER
(Staley)

A. E. Staley Mfg. Co.
2200 E. Eldorado St.
Decatur, Ill. 62525

Phone: 217-423-4411

STA PUT NON SKID SPRAY FOR RUGS (Aerosol)
(Cling-Surface)

Methylene chloride * 83%
Propane/Isobutane 30%

STAR
Aluminum brightener; industrial use
(Puritan Chem. Co.)

Hydrofluoric acid *
Phosphoric acid *

STAR BRONZE PAINT PRODUCTS
Clear wood finishes and touch-up enamels

Star Bronze Company
Alliance, Ohio 44601

Phone: 216-823-1550

See PAINTS, Section VI, General Formulations

STAR GYM FINISH
Floor finish
(Hillyard Chem.)

Mineral spirits *

                                '76 Ed.

STA-RITE
Wood preservative
(Sonford Products)

Pentachlorophenol * 4.48%
Other chlorophenols 0.52%
Petroleum distillate * 86.00%

STA-RITE 1-4
Wood preservative
(Sonford Products)

Pentachlorophenol * 18.7%
Other chlorophenols 2.17%
Petroleum distillate * 43.1%

STARLICIDE COMPLETE

See PURINA STARLICIDE COMPLETE

STARTEX ANTIFREEZE
(Texaco Inc.)

Ethylene glycol *
Sodium nitrites *
Dye

STARTR-WATR, MIRACLE

See MIRACLE STARTR-WATR

START TO FINISH CLEANER-POLISH
(Liquid Glaze, Inc.)

Silicone fluid and resin
Diatomaceous earth
Aliphatic hydrocarbon solvent *
Aromatic hydrocarbon solvent *
Amine oleate
Water

STA-STUK "m"

See LILLY/MILLER STA-STUK "m"

STATE CHEMICALS PINE OIL
Disinfectant-deodorant cleaner
(State Chemicals)

Combined amount: 82%
 Pine oil *
 Soap

STATIC GUARD (Antistatic Spray)
(Alberto-Culver)

Alcohol
Propellants
Dimethyl ditallow ammonium chloride
Other ingredients

STATOBEX-G
Anorexiant
(Lemmon Co.)

Each tablet:
 Phendimetrazine tartrate * .... 35 mg.

STATOBEX (TABLETS & CAPSULES)
Anorexiant
(Lemmon Co.)

Each tablet or capsule:
 Phendimetrazine tartrate * .... 35 mg.

STATROL
Ophthalmic ointment
(Alcon)

Active ingred. (each gm.):
 Neomycin sulfate (equiv. to 3.5 mg. neo-
 mycin)
 Polymyxin B sulfate ...... 6000 units
Preservatives:
 Methylparaben 0.05%
 Propylparaben 0.01%
Inactive ingred.:
 White petrolatum
 Anhydrous liquid Lanolin

STATROL
Ophthalmic solution
(Alcon)

Active ingred. (each ml.):
 Neomycin sulfate (equiv. to 3.5 mg. neo-
 mycin)
 Polymyxin B sulfate ..... 16,250 units
Preservative:
 Benzalkonium chloride 0.004%
Vehicle:
 Hydroxypropyl methylcellulose   0.5%
Inactive ingred.:
 Boric acid
 Sodium chloride
 Hydrochloride acid and/or
 Sodium hydroxide (to adjust pH)
 Purified water

STAUFFER CAPTAN (50-WP, 80-WP)
Fungicide
(Stauffer)

Captan (N-((Trichloromethyl)thio)-4-cy-
 clohexene-1,2-dicarboximide)

STAUFFER FOLPET (50-WP)
Fungicide
(Stauffer)

Folpet (N-(Trichloromethylthio)-
 phthalimide)

STA-WAKE DEXTABS
(Approved Pharm.)

Each tablet:
 Caffeine * .... 1 1/2 gr.
 Dextrose .... 3 gr.
                                '76 Ed.

STAX, BLUE
See BLUE STAX

STAX, REGULAR
Hairdressing & conditioner
(King Research)

Petrolatum
Mineral oil
Lanolin
Paraffin
Isopropyl myristate
PEG-8 dilaurate
Oleyl alcohol
Fragrance
Captan

STAY AWAKE TABLETS
(Towne, Paulsen)

Each tablet:
 Caffeine alkaloid * .... 200 mg.
 Niacin .... 10 mg.
 Thiamine .... 10 mg.
 Dextrose
 Sodium biphosphate
 Calcium phosphate monobasic
 Oleoresin capsicum

STAY-CLEAN ALUMINUM FLUX
(Harris, J.W.)

Fluoride derivatives * 27%

STAY-CLEAN FLUX
(Harris, J.W.)

Methanol
Glycerine
Zinc chloride
Hydrochloric acid *
Ammonium chloride
Water

STAY-CUT
Deglosser
(Reliable Paste)

Solvents
Naphtha *
Acetone *
Isobutyl acetate *

STAY-FLO TABLETS
(Stayner)

Each tablet:
 Sodium fluoride * .... 2.21 mg.
 Copper sulfate .... 0.25 mg.

STAYNER ANTISPASMODIC COMPOUND
(Stayner)

Each tablet:
 Atropine sulfate .... 0.0194 mg.
 Hyoscyamine sulfate * ... 0.1037 mg.
 Hyoscine hydrobromide .. 0.0065 mg.
 Phenobarbital * .... 16.2000 mg.

STAYNER ANTISPASMODIC COMPOUND ELIXIR
(Stayner)

Each 5 cc.:
 Phenobarbital * .... 16.2000 mg.
 Hyoscyamine sulfate * ... 0.1037 mg.
 Atropine sulfate .... 0.0194 mg.
 Hyoscine hydrobromide .. 0.0065 mg.
 Alcohol 23%

STAYNER BROMPHENIRAMINE COMPOUND D.C. EXPECTORANT
(Stayner)

Each 5 ml.:
 Codeine phosphate * .... 10 mg.
 Brompheniramine maleate * ..   2 mg.
 Glyceryl guaiacolate .... 100 mg.
 Phenylephrine HCl * ....   5 mg.
 Phenylpropanolamine HCl * ..   5 mg.
 Alcohol 3.5%

STAYNER BROMPHENIRAMINE COMPOUND ELIXIR
(Stayner)

Each 5 cc.:
 Brompheniramine maleate * ... 4 mg.
 Phenylephrine HCl * .... 5 mg.
 Phenylpropanolamine HCl * ... 5 mg.
 Alcohol 2.3%

Starred ingredients (*) may be responsible for major toxic effects; consult Section II.

STAYNER BROMPHENIRAMINE COMPOUND EXPECTORANT
(Stayner)

Each 5 cc.:
Brompheniramine maleate *	2 mg.
Phenylephrine HCl *	5 mg.
Phenylpropanolamine HCl *	5 mg.
Glyceryl guaiacolate	100 mg.
Alcohol	3.5%

STAYNER BROMPHENIRAMINE COMPOUND TABLETS S.A.
(Stayner)

Each sustained action tablet:
Brompheniramine maleate *	12 mg.
Phenylephrine HCl *	15 mg.
Phenylpropanolamine HCl *	15 mg.

STAYNER CHLORPHENIRAMINE COMPOUND T.D. CAPSULES
(Stayner)

Each time release capsule:
Chlorpheniramine maleate *	8 mg.
Phenylpropanolamine HCl *	50 mg.
Isopropamide iodide (equiv. to 2.5 mg. of Isopropamide) *	

STAYNER DECONGESTANT TABLETS
(Stayner)

Each tablet:
Phenylpropanolamine HCl *	40 mg.
Phenylephrine HCl *	10 mg.
Phenyltoloxamine citrate	15 mg.
Chlorpheniramine maleate *	5 mg.

STAYNER DIPHENOXYLATE COMPOUND TABLETS
Antidiarrheal
(Stayner)

Each tablet:
Diphenoxylate hydrochloride *	2.500 mg.
Atropine sulfate *	0.025 mg.

STAYNER DOXYLAMINE COMPOUND TABLETS
(Stayner)

Each tablet:
Doxylamine succinate *	10 mg.
Pyridoxine hydrochloride	10 mg.

STAYNER D.S.S. PLUS CAPSULES
(Stayner)

Each capsule:
Dioctyl sodium sulfosuccinate *	100 mg.
Casanthranol	30 mg.

STAYNER ERGOTAMINE COMPOUND TABLETS
(Stayner)

Each tablet:
Ergotamine tartrate	1 mg.
Caffeine *	100 mg.

STAYNER E.T.H. COMPOUND SYRUP
(Stayner)

Each 5 ml.:
Ephedrine sulfate *	6.25 mg.
Theophylline	32.50 mg.
Hydroxyzine hydrochloride	2.50 mg.
Alcohol	5% v/v
Dye free	

STAYNER E.T.H. COMPOUND TABLETS
(Stayner)

Each tablet:
Ephedrine sulfate *	25 mg.
Theophylline *	130 mg.
Hydroxyzine HCl	10 mg.

STAYNER PROMETHAZINE COMPOUND WITH CODEINE
(Stayner)

Each 5 cc.:
Promethazine HCl	5 mg.
Codeine phosphate *	10 mg.
Fluidextract Ipecac	0.17 min.
Potassium guaiacolsulfonate	44 mg.
Alcohol	7%

STAYNER PROMETHAZINE COMPOUND WITH PHENYLEPHRINE AND CODEINE
(Stayner)

Each 5 cc.:
Promethazine HCl	5 mg.
Phenylephrine HCl	5 mg.
Codeine phosphate *	10 mg.
Fluidextract Ipecac	0.17 min.
Potassium guaiacolsulfonate	44 mg.
Alcohol	7%

STAYNER PROMETHAZINE HCL EXPECTORANT
(Stayner)

Each 5 cc.:
Promethazine HCl	5 mg.
Fluidextract Ipecac	0.17 min.
Potassium guaiacolsulfonate	44 mg.
Alcohol	7%

STAYNER PROMETHAZINE VC EXPECTORANT
(Stayner)

Each 5 cc.:
Promethazine HCl	5 mg.
Phenylephrine HCl *	5 mg.
Fluidextract Ipecac	0.17 min.
Potassium guaiacolsulfonate	44 mg.
Alcohol	7%

STAYNER PROMETHAZINE W/DEXTRO-METHORPHAN
(Stayner)

Each 5 cc.:
Dextromethorphan HBr *	7.5 mg.
Promethazine HCl	5.0 mg.
Fluid ext. Ipecac	0.17 min.
Potassium guaiacolsulfonate	44.0 mg.
Citric acid, anhydrous	60.0 mg.
Sodium citrate, hydrous	197.0 mg.
Alcohol	7%

STAYNER PROPOXYPHENE COMPOUND-65 CAPSULES
(Stayner)

Each capsule:
Propoxyphene HCl (USP) *	65.0 mg.
Aspirin (USP)	227.0 mg.
Phenacetin	162.0 mg.
Caffeine anhydrous (USP)	32.4 mg.

STAYNER SINUS TABLETS
(Stayner)

Each tablet:
Acetaminophen *	325 mg.
Phenylpropanolamine HCl *	25 mg.
Phenyltoloxamine citrate	22 mg.

STAYNER T.E.P. COMPOUND TABLETS
(Stayner)

Each tablet:
Theophylline *	2 gr.
Ephedrine HCl *	3/8 gr.
Phenobarbital	1/8 gr.

STAYPUT
Semi-paste remover
(Reliable Paste)

Toluol *	approx. 10%
Acetone *	approx. 60%
Methanol *	approx. 30%

STAY-SILV 20
Brazing alloy
(Harris, J.W.)

Silver	20%
Copper	45%
Zinc	30%
Cadmium *	5%

Starred ingredients (*) may be responsible for major toxic effects; consult Section II.

STAY-SILV 30
Brazing alloy
(Harris, J.W.)

Silver	30%
Copper	27%
Zinc	23%
Cadmium *	20%

STAY-SILV 31
Brazing alloy
(Harris, J.W.)

Silver	31.5%
Copper	34.0%
Zinc	15.5%
Cadmium *	19.0%

STAY-SILV 35
Brazing alloy
(Harris, J.W.)

Silver	35%
Copper	26%
Zinc	21%
Cadmium *	18%

STAY-SILV 40
Brazing alloy
(Harris, J.W.)

Silver	40%
Copper	18%
Zinc	15%
Cadmium *	27%

STAY-SILV 41
Brazing alloy
(Harris, J.W.)

Silver	41%
Copper	17%
Zinc	18%
Cadmium *	24%

STAY-SILV 45
Brazing alloy
(Harris, J.W.)

Silver	45%
Copper	15%
Zinc	16%
Cadmium *	24%

STAY-SILV 50
Brazing alloy
(Harris, J.W.)

Silver	50.0%
Copper	15.5%
Zinc	16.5%
Cadmium *	18.0%

STAY-SILV 50n
Brazing alloy
(Harris, J.W.)

Silver	50.0%
Copper	15.5%
Zinc	15.5%
Cadmium *	16.0%
Nickel	3.0%

STAY-SILV 60
Brazing alloy
(Harris, J.W.)

Silver	60%
Copper	20%
Zinc	7%
Cadmium *	10%

STAY-SILV FLUX BLACK & WHITE
(Harris, J.W.)

Boric acid *
Potassium bifluoride
Potassium fluoborate
Tetraborate
Water
Elemental Boron (black only)

STAY-WET REMOVER
(Reliable Paste)

Toluol *	approx. 10%
Acetone *	approx. 60%
Methanol *	approx. 30%

STAZON CALK
(Gibson-Homans)

Linseed, soya oils	>10%
Petroleum thinner	1-10%
Whiting	>65%
Talc	1-10%

STEAM-IT-SPECIAL
Steam cleaner
(Calgon Corp., Commercial Div.)

Caustic potash *
Sodium silicate
Wetting agents

STEAMSAFE
Steam cleaning compound for aluminum
(Clayton Mfg.)

Sodium bicarbonate	1-10%
Sodium carbonate *	>10%
Sodium silicate *	>20%
Sodium polyphosphate *	>10%
Synthetic detergent	1-10%
Soap	1-10%

STEARNS' ELECTRIC BRAND PASTE
Rodenticide and roach killer
(Stearns' Electric Paste Co.)

Phosphorus *	2 1/2%

STEDBAC
Germicide
(Fine Organics, Inc.)

Stearyl dimethyl benzyl ammonium chloride *	100%

'76 Ed.

STEDYTABS DELFETAMINE
For obesity
(Eastern Research Labs.)

Each tablet:
Delfetamine (dl-N-Methylamphetamine hydrochloride) * . 30 mg.

'76 Ed.

STEDYTABS DELFETA-SED
For obesity
(Eastern Research Labs.)

Each tablet:
Delfetamine (dl-N-Methylamphetamine hydrochloride) * 30 mg.
Sedafax (special micronized grade of amobarbital) * .... 120 mg.

'76 Ed.

STEELCOTE PAINT PRODUCTS

Steelcote Mfg. Co.
3418 Gratiot St.
St. Louis, Mo. 63103

Phone: 314-771-8053

See PAINTS, Section VI, General Formulations

STEEL SAVER

See E-Z-EST STEEL SAVER

STEELUSTER

See E-Z-EST STEELUSTER

STEEM-UP
Cleans steam irons
(Lake Products)

Amidosulfonic acid *	98%
Lauroylisoquinolinium bromide	2%

STEER-SEAL
Power-steering conditioner & sealer
(Radiator)

Petroleum distillates *

'76 Ed.

STEIN'S SAN-O-GENT
Detergent, deodorant, sanitizer, disinfectant
(Stein Chemical Co.)

n-Alkyl (50% C12, 30% C14, 17% C16, 3% C18) dimethyl ethylbenzyl ammonium chloride *	1.6%
n-Alkyl (60% C14, 30% C16, 5% C12, 5% C18) dimethyl benzyl ammonium chloride *	1.6%

'76 Ed.

Starred ingredients (*) may be responsible for major toxic effects; consult Section II.

STELAZINE CONCENTRATE & TABLETS
Antianxiety, antipsychotic
(SK&F)

Each ml.:
Trifluoperazine * . . . . 10 mg.

Each tablet:
Trifluoperazine * 1 mg.; 2 mg.; 5 mg.;
or 10 mg.

STEM-AX
Granular systemic insecticide
(National Chemsearch)

O,O-Diethyl-S-(2-
(ethylthio)ethyl)phos-
phorodithioate * 2%

STEMITE GRANULES
Systemic insecticide
(Chemical Formulators)

O,O-Diethyl-O (and S)-2-(ethyl-
mercapto)-ethyl
thiophosphate * 1.890%
Related organic compounds 0.095%

'76 Ed.

STEPHAN TOILETRIES

The Stephan Co.
1850 W. McNab Rd.
Fort Lauderdale, Fla. 33309

Phone: 305-971-0600

See COSMETICS, Section VI, General
Formulations

STEP 2 VINYL SHIELD
(Polyglycoat)

Ammonia 0.600%
Formaldehyde 0.002%
Dipropylene glycol monomethyl . 1.200%

STERA-SHEEN ALL DAIRY SANITIZER (Blue Label)
(Purdy, N.B.)

Sodium dichloro-S-triazinetrione . 10%
Sodium dodecyl benzene sulfonate 0.5%
Tetrasodium ethylenediamine
tetraacetate 3.50%
Sodium tripolyphosphate *
Sodium chloride

'76 Ed.

pH between 7 and 8

STERA-SHEEN LAST RINSE SANITIZER (Blue Label)
(Purdy, N.B.)

Sodium dichloro-S-triazinetrione   5%
Sodium dodecylbenzene sulfonate 0.5%
Tetrasodium ethylenediamine
tetraacetate 3.50%
Sodium tripolyphosphate *
Tetra sodium pyrophosphate *

'76 Ed.

pH between 8 and 9

STERA-SHEEN SANITIZER & CLEANER (Green Label)
(Purdy, N.B.)

Sodium dichloro-S-triazinetrione . . . 3%
Trisodium phosphate * 20%
Tetrasodium ethylenediamine
tetraacetate 2%
Sodium tripolyphosphate
Light soda ash *

'76 Ed.

pH between 9 and 10

STER-BAC, FORMULA KQ-12

See KLENZADE STER-BAC, FOR-
MULA KQ-12

STERIBALM

See UNIVERSAL STERIBALM

STERIBULB
For use in commercial gas sterilizer
(Ben Venue Labs.)

Ethylene oxide * 20%/w
Trichloromonofluoromethane . . . 80%/w

STERIGENT GERMICIDAL CLEANER

See SPARTAN STERIGENT GER-
MICIDAL CLEANER

STERI-KLEEN, FORMULAE #33
Disinfectant, deodorant
(Barco)

Alkyl dimethyl-benzyl-ammonium
chlorides (high molecular) * . . . 2.50%
Alkyl aryl polyether alcohol 1.00%
Essential oils 0.25%

'76 Ed.

STERIL-AIDE CLEANER
(Advance Chemical Co.)

Active ingred.: 1.85%
Ammonium oxalate
2,2'-Methylenebis(3,4,6-trichlorophenol)
Ammonium ethylene diamine tetraace-
tate
Ammonium ortho phenyl phenate
Inert ingred.: 98.15%
Cleaners
Brighteners
Emulsifiers
Wetting agents

STERILE DISINFECTANT CLEANER
(Advance Chemical Co.)

Active ingred.: 11.62%
Sulfuric acid *
Ortho phosphoric acid *
Nonylphenoxypoly (ethyleneoxy)
Ethanol-iodine complex
Methyl dodecyl benzyl trimethyl am-
monium chloride
Methyl dodecyl xylylene bis (trimethyl
ammonium chloride) *

Inert ingred.: 88.38%
Water
Perfume
Inhibitor
Color

STERIL-IZE

See LARSON'S STERIL-IZE

STERITEX, 8311

See INTEX STERITEX, 8311

STERITONE, SASCO

See SASCO STERITONE

STERI-UNNA BOOT (Sterile)
*For the treatment of sprains, strains
and leg ulcers*
(Pedinol)

Zinc oxide
Glycerine
White petrolatum
Gum arabic
Amylum

STERIZONE
*Hospital type bowl, porcelain & shower
stall cleaner*
(Hysan Corp.)

Hydrogen chloride * 9.5%
Nonylphenoxypolyethoxyethanol-
iodine complex (provides 0.3% titratable iodine) 3.0%
Essential oils 1.2%

Starred ingredients (*) may be responsible for major toxic effects; consult Section II.

STERL-AID DISINFECTANT
Disinfectant, germicide, deodorant
(An-Fo)

N-Alkyl dimethyl benzyl ammonium chlorides * 10.2%

Inert ingred.: 89.8%
   Water
   Ethanol

STERLING-CLARK-LURTON LACQUER THINNER (CLEAN AIR, PAINTERS')
(Sterling-Clark-Lurton)

Aromatic hydrocarbons * .. approx. 15%
Aliphatic hydrocarbons .... approx. 20%
Ketones .... approx. 30%
Alcohols .... approx. 30%
Keto-alcohols .... <5%

STERLING HALITE MELTING CRYSTALS
Rock salt
(International Salt)

Typical analysis:
  Sodium chloride * 97.788%
  Moisture 0.030%
  Water insolubles 0.564%
  Calcium sulfate 1.613%
  Calcium chloride 0.005%
  Magnesium chloride 0.000%

STERNO CANNED HEAT
(Sterno)

Ethyl alcohol
Methanol .... <4%
                             '76 Ed.

STERO-DARVON WITH A.S.A.
Analgesic - rheumatoid arthritis
(Lilly, Eli)

Each tablet:
  Aspirin * .... 500 mg.
  Paramethasone acetate ...... 0.25 mg.
  Propoxyphene
    hydrochloride * .... 32 mg.

STER-O-KEM NO. 3
Disinfectant cleaner
(Damon Chemical Co.)

Active ingredients: 7.0%
  Potassium dichloro-s-triazinetrione
  Tetrasodium ethylene diamine tetraac-
  etate

STEWART DE-SCALE
Removes rust, scale, corrosion
(Stewart Sanitary Supply)

Hydrochloric acid *

STEWART POLYPHOSPHATE GLASS
Inhibits formation of scale, corrosion and "red water" in small air conditioning systems
(Stewart Sanitary Supply)

Graham's salt * 99.699%

STEWART'S, MRS., BLUING
See MRS. STEWART'S BLUING

STICK IT
Adhesive
(Ambroid)

Nitrocellulose type of cement
  Alcohols * 20%
  Hydrocarbons *† 60%
  Ketones * 20%
  Allyl isothiocyanate (synthetic oil
    of mustard) .... trace

†*See* Adhesives, Section VI, General Formulations

STIKCOL
Control of premature drop of apples
(FMC Corp., Agricultural Chem. Div.)

Triethanolamine salt of silvex (2-
  (2,4,5-Trichlorophenoxy) propionic acid) 5.3%

STIKCOL-D
Control of premature drop of apples
(FMC Corp., Agricultural Chem. Div.)

Triethanolamine salt of silvex (2-
  (2,4,5-Trichlorophenoxy) propionic acid) * 10.4%

STIK DUST
For drop control of apples & pears
(FMC Corp., Agricultural Chem. Div.)

Naphthaleneacetic acid 0.1%

STILLMAN'S CREAM
(Stillman)

Hydroquinone *
Zinc oxide
Inert ingredients:
  Mineral oil
  Snow white Petrolatum
  Ceresin wax
  Silicones
Stabilizers:
  Propyl hydroxybenzoate
  Sodium metabisulphite

STIMULAX CAPSULES
Bowel stimulant/stool softener
(Geriatric Pharm.)

Each capsule:
  Geri-casagra (Casanthranol) * 30 mg.
  Dioctyl sodium
    sulfosuccinate * .... 250 mg.

STIM-U-PLANT
Plant food tablets
(Stim-U-Plant)

Nitrogen 11%
Phosphoric acid (available) * 12%
Potash * 15%
Vitamin B1

STIM-U-PLANT AFRICAN VIOLET FOOD
(Stim-U-Plant)

Urea nitrogen 4%
Ammonia nitrogen 1%
Total nitrogen 5%
Available Phosphoric acid * 8%
Potash water sol. * 7%
Total primary plant food 20%

STIM-U-PLANT ALL PURPOSE LIQUID PLANT FOOD
(Stim-U-Plant)

Urea nitrogen 6%
Ammonia nitrogen 1%
Total nitrogen 7%
Available Phosphoric acid * 7%
Potash water sol. * 7%

STIM-U-PLANT ALL PURPOSE PLANT FOOD POWDER
(Stim-U-Plant)

Nitrate nitrogen 4.5%
Ammonia nitrogen 10.5%
Available Phosphoric acid * 30%
Potash water sol. * 15%

STIM-U-PLANT FISH EMULSION
(Stim-U-Plant)

Total nitrogen 5.0%
  Nitrate nitrogen 0.1%
  Ammoniacal nitrogen 0.5%
  Other water soluble nitrogen ... 4.0%
  Water insoluble nitrogen 0.4%
Available Phosphoric acid 1.0%
Soluble Potash 1.0%

STIM-U-PLANT HOUSE PLANT & AFRICAN VIOLET SPRAY (Aerosol)
Insecticide
(Stim-U-Plant)

Pyrethrins 0.025%
Piperonyl butoxide, tech. 0.256%
Rotenone 0.128%
Other cube extractives 0.236%
Petroleum distillate 0.102%

STIM-U-PLANT INSECT SPRAY FOR HOUSEPLANTS
(Stim-U-Plant)

Pyrethrins 0.02%
Piperonyl butoxide (technical) 0.20%
Petroleum distillate 0.08%

Starred ingredients (*) may be responsible for major toxic effects; consult Section II.

STIM-U-PLANT IVY-PHILODENDRON PLANT FOOD
(Stim-U-Plant)

Nitrogen . . . . not less than 11%
Phosphoric acid
  (avail.) * . . . . not less than 12%
Potash water soluble
  (derived from potassium nitrate, mono-ammonium,
  phosphate) * . . . . . . not less than 15%

STIM-U-PLANT LEAF POLISH
(Stim-U-Plant)

Silicone alkyd resin base
Methylene chloride *
Aliphatic hydrocarbons *

STIMURUB
Analgesic cream
(Clapp, Otis)

Menthol *
Methyl salicylate *
Oleoresin of capsicum

STINGER
*Pressurized irritating stream; personal
  protection*
(Penguin Industries)

Capsaicin (derived from oleoresin
  capsicum) 0.35%

"STING 'N ITCH" BALM
*For sting and itch of all insect bites,
  allergies, etc.*
(Pharmex)

Menthol *
Camphor *
Methyl nicotinate
Methyl salicylate *
Benzocaine
Quaternary ammonium compound
Oleoresin Cassia
Oleoresin Capsicum
Lanolin

STINGY STICK

See BIO-GUARD STINGY STICK

STIXIT SCHOOL PASTE
(American Crayon Co.)

This product bears the CP Seal issued by
the Crayon, Water Color and Craft Institute, Inc. This seal certifies that the product contains no materials in sufficient quantities to be toxic or injurious to the human body even if ingested.

ST. JOSEPH COUGH SYRUP FOR CHILDREN
(Plough)

Each 5 ml.:
  Dextromethorphan
    hydrobromide * . . . . 7.5 mg.
  Sodium citrate
  Citric acid
  Sodium benzoate
  Caramel color
  190 Proof Alcohol 0.5%
  Menthol *
  Raspberry flavor

ST. JOSEPH FEVER REDUCER ELIXIR & DROPS FOR CHILDREN
(Plough)

Elixir:
  Acetaminophen * . . . . . 120 mg./5 cc.
  Alcohol 7%

Drops:
  Acetaminophen * . . . . . 60 mg./0.6 cc.
  Alcohol 9.5%

ST. JOSEPH NOSE DROPS FOR CHILDREN
(Plough)

Sodium chloride
Zephiran chloride . . . . 0.02% w/w
Phenylephrine
  hydrochloride * . . . . 0.25% w/w

STOCKADE BAR-FLY & WORM CONTROL BLOCK
Medicated feeding block for cattle
(Harvest Brand)

Phenothiazine 2.00%
Plus Salt (NaCl) and feed supplements

STOCKADE HI-Q KIL-A-PEST FLY & WORM CONTROL BLOCK
Medicated feeding block for cattle
(Harvest Brand)

Phenothiazine 2.00%
Plus Salt (NaCl) and feed supplements

STOCKADE KIL-A-PEST 12 FLY CONTROL BLOCK
Medicated feeding block for cattle
(Harvest Brand)

Phenothiazine 1.25%
Plus Salt (NaCl) and feed supplements

STOCKADE WORMER MINERAL
*Control of common stomach worms in
  livestock*
(Harvest Brand)

Phenothiazine 3.00%
Plus Salt (NaCl) and feed supplements

STOCKADE WORMER MINERAL BLOCK
*Control of common stomach worms in
  livestock*
(Harvest Brand)

Phenothiazine 4.00%
Plus Salt (NaCl) and feed supplements

STOCK TOX, MARTIN'S

See MARTIN'S STOCK TOX

STOMAL
(Foy Labs.)

Each tablet:
  Atropine sulfate . . . . 0.0194 mg.
  Hyoscyamine sulfate . . . . . 0.1037 mg.
  Phenobarbital * . . . . 16.2000 mg.
  Scopolamine
    hydrobromide . . . . 0.0065 mg.

STOMASEPTINE
Douche powder
(Berlex Labs.)

Sodium chloride
Sodium bicarbonate
Sodium borate *
Sodium perborate
Fragrance

STONO
Cleans monuments
(Dolge)

Ammonium bifluoride *

STOP
Liquid floor polish
(Sanitek)

Acrylic polymer emulsion 11.0%
Diethylene glycol monoethyl
  ether (Cellosolve) 3.5%
Polyethylene emulsion 1.6%
Rosin maleate resin 1.3%
Tributoxyethyl phosphate 0.9%
Nonionic surfactant 0.2%
Formalin, Ammonia, Defoamer,
  Fluorochemical surfactant . . . trace
Water . . . . balance

STOPAIN TABLETS
Analgesic
(Columbia Med.)

Each tablet:
  Acetyl-p-aminophenol * . . . . . 1 1/2 gr.
  Salicylamide . . . . 2 gr.
  Aspirin * . . . . 3 1/2 gr.
  Caffeine . . . . 1 gr.

STOP-A-LEAK, DR. NAYLOR'S

See DR. NAYLOR'S STOP-A-LEAK

Starred ingredients (*) may be responsible for major toxic effects; consult Section II.

STOPSHOK
Antistatic agent
(Hillyard Chem.)

Liquid detergent *†

'76 Ed.

†*See* Detergents, Section VI, General Formulations

STOP SLIP BELT DRESSING
For automotive fan and v-belts
(Radiator)

Petroleum distillates *

'76 Ed.

STRAWBERRY OINTMENT
(Cramer Products)

Petrolatum (NF)	82.50%
Boric acid (NF)	7.75%
Sulfur (USP)	5.00%
Benzocaine (NF)	2.00%
Camphor (USP) *	2.50%
8-Hydroxyquinoline base	0.25%

STREMA
For treatment of nocturnal systremma and other muscular cramps
(Foy Labs.)

Each capsule:
Quinine sulfate * .... 260 mg.

STREPCILLIN F-25
Antibiotic feed additive for poultry and swine
(Salsbury)

Penicillin (from procaine penicillin)	3.75 gm./lb.
Streptomycin (from streptomycin sulfate)	18.75 mg./lb.
Wheat middlings	
Soybean oil	

STRESSTABS 600 WITH IRON
Dietary supplement
(Lederle)

Each tablet:
Elemental Iron (as ferrous fumarate) .... 27 mg.
Plus multivitamins

STRICKLAND COSMETIC PRODUCTS

J. Strickland & Co.
1400 Ragan
Memphis, Tenn. 38106

Phone: 901-774-9023

See COSMETICS, Section VI, General Formulations

STRI-DEX B.P. 10%
For treatment of acne
(Glenbrook Labs.)

Benzoyl peroxide * 10%

STRI-DEX MEDICATED LOTION
For treatment of acne
(Glenbrook Labs.)

Ethyl alcohol	28%
Salicylic acid	minor
Citric acid	minor
Sulphonated alkyl benzenes, sodium salts	minor

STRI-DEX MEDICATED PADS
For treatment of acne
(Glenbrook Labs.)

Ethyl alcohol	28%
Salicylic acid	minor
Citric acid	minor
Sulphonated alkyl benzenes, sodium salts	minor

STRIKE
Wasp & hornet insecticide
(Hysan Corp.)

Pyrethrins	0.10%
Piperonyl butoxide (technical)	0.20%
N-Octyl bicycloheptene dicarboximide	0.33%
o-Isopropoxyphenyl methylcarbamate *	0.50%
Petroleum distillate	6.84%

STRIKE

See RED-TOP STRIKE

STRIKE INSECTICIDE, MUNICHEM

See MUNICHEM STRIKE INSECTICIDE

STRIP-ALL
Heavy duty stripper; industrial and institutional use
(Scientific International)

Methanol *
Methylene chloride *
Propylene dichloride *

STRIP-ALL
(Hillyard Chem.)

Wax remover *†
Ammonia

'76 Ed.

†*See* Wax removers, Section VI, General Formulations

STRIP-COTE
Gelled paint stripper
(Whitfield Chem.)

Methylene chloride *	>10%
Organic acid similar to acetic acid	1-10%
Methanol	1-10%

STRIP EASE
Adhesive remover
(Lambda Inc.)

Trichloroethane (modified) and Aromatics
Mineral spirits
Chlorothymol 0.04%
Methyl salicylate *
Isoamyl acetate
Ethylcellulose

STRIP-EZE
Nonflammable seal remover for varnish, paints
(Consolidated Chem., Inc.)

Methylene chloride *
Caustic soda *
Propylene dichloride *
Methanol *

STRIP-IT-SPECIAL
Paint stripper
(Calgon Corp., Commercial Div.)

Methylene chloride *
Methyl alcohol *
Wax

STRIP OFF
Wax stripper
(Paul Koss)

Water	>80%
Monoethanolamine *	<15%
Monoethanolammonium dodecylbenzene sulfonate (Anionic surfactant)	
Coco diethanolamide	

pH 11.0-11.1

STRIP-TEE
Alkaline-solvent cleaner and degreaser
(Calgon Corp., Commercial Div.)

Butyl Cellosolve *
Complex phosphates *
Caustic soda *
Water

STRIP-X PAINT REMOVER
(Klean-Strip)

Aromatic hydrocarbons *	>30%
Chlorinated hydrocarbons *	>20%
Alcohols (no methanol)	<20%
Ketones	<20%
Soap, Thickeners, & Inhibitors	<10%

STRYPEEZE SEMI-PASTE PAINT REMOVER
(Savogran)

Toluol *	20-40%
Methanol	20-40%
Acetone	10-20%
Methylene chloride	10-20%
Retardants	
Wetting agents	

S.T. 37 ANTISEPTIC SOLUTION
(Beecham Products)

Hexylresorcinol .... 1:1000 solution

STUART PHARMACEUTICALS

Stuart Pharmaceuticals
Div. ICI Americas, Inc.
Concord Pike & Murphy Rd.
Wilmington, Del. 19897

Phone: 302-575-2231

STUK
Adhesive
(Ambroid)

alpha-Cyano-acrylate *† 100%

†*See* n-Alkyl-a-cyanoacrylates

STULEX (S.C.T. YELLOW)
(Bowman Pharm.)

Each tablet:
　Docusate sodium (Dioctyl sodium sulfosuccinate) .... 100 mg.

STURMAN'S DRY CLEANER & SPOT REMOVER
(Crestwood Products)

1,1,1-Trichloroethane *	33 1/3%
Methylene chloride *	33 1/3%
Petroleum distillate *	33 1/3%

'76 Ed.

S2 INHALANT
For asthma
(Nephron)

Racemic Epinephrine hydrochloride	2.25%
Chlorbutanol (chloroform deriv.)	0.5%

STYLE WRITER

See CARTER'S STYLE WRITER

STYPTO-CAINE SOLUTION
Hemostatic solution
(Pedinol)

Hydroxyquinoline sulfate *†
Tetracaine HCl
Aluminum chloride *
Aqueous Glycol base

†*See* Hydroxyquinoline salts

STYRO-WELD

See GARD STYRO-WELD

STYX CONCENTRATE
Insecticide
(Bartlett, F.A.)

Rotenone	3.19%
Other cube extractives	6.37%
Methylated naphthalene *	28.48%
Pyrethrin	1.00%
Petroleum distillate	3.97%

SUBMERGE PAINT STRIPPER, DEGREASER & CLEANER, PL

See PL SUBMERGE PAINT STRIPPER, DEGREASER & CLEANER

SUBTRACK
Strips tire marks and rubber burns from concrete floors; industrial use
(Puritan Chem. Co.)

Petroleum distillates *

SUBURBAN SPAR VARNISH
(Touraine Paints, Inc.)

Thinner*† & Drier *	54.4%
Non-volatile alkyd resin	45.6%

'76 Ed.

†*See* Thinners, Section VI, General Formulations

SUCARYL (SODIUM FORM)
Liquid sweetener
(Abbott)

Sodium saccharin	1.6%
Benzoic acid	0.1%
Methylparaben	0.05%

SUCRETS (CHILDREN'S) SORE THROAT LOZENGES
(Beecham Products)

Each lozenge:
　Hexylresorcinol .... 2.4 mg.

SUCRETS COUGH CONTROL FORMULA
(Beecham Products)

Each lozenge:
　D-Methorphan .... 7.5 mg.

SUCRETS DECONGESTANT LOZENGES
(Beecham Products)

Each lozenge:
　Phenylpropanolamine HCl *　25.0 mg.

SUCRETS MAXIMUM STRENGTH

See MAXIMUM STRENGTH SUCRETS

SUCRETS SORE THROAT LOZENGES
(Beecham Products)

Each lozenge:
　Hexylresorcinol .... 2.4 mg.

SUDAFED COUGH SYRUP
Decongestant/cough suppressant/expectorant
(Burroughs Wellcome)

Each 5 ml.:
Pseudoephedrine hydrochloride *	30 mg.
Dextromethorphan hydrobromide	10 mg.
Guaifenesin	100 mg.
Alcohol	2.4%

SUDAFED PLUS TABLETS/ SYRUP
Decongestant plus antihistamine
(Burroughs Wellcome)

Each tablet:
Pseudoephedrine HCl *	60 mg.
Chlorpheniramine maleate	4 mg.

Each 5 ml.:
Pseudoephedrine HCl *	30 mg.
Chlorpheniramine maleate	2 mg.

SUDA-PROL SYRUP & TABLETS
(Columbia Med.)

Syrup (each 5 ml.):
Tripolidine HCl	1.25 mg.
Pseudoephedrine HCl *	30 mg.

Tablets (each):
Tripolidine HCl	2.5 mg.
Pseudoephedrine HCl *	60 mg.

SUDDEN ACTION
Breath freshener
(Whitehall Labs.)

Spearmint oil *
Peppermint oil *

Starred ingredients (*) may be responsible for major toxic effects; consult Section II.

SUDDEN BEAUTY COSMETICS
(Whitehall Labs.)

Whitehall Laboratories
Div. American Home Products Corp.
685 Third Ave.
New York, N.Y. 10017

Phone: 212-986-1000

See COSMETICS, Section VI, General
Formulations

SUDRIN (C.T. WHITE; SCORED)
(Bowman Pharm.)

Each tablet:
Pseudoephedrine HCl * ...... 30 mg.

SUFAMAL VAGINAL CREME
(Milex)

Sulfanilamide 15%
Aminacrine HCl 0.2%
Allantoin 2.0%

SUL-BLUE ANTI-DANDRUFF SHAMPOO
(Columbia Med.)

Selenium sulfide * 1%

SULFACET-R LOTION (FLESH TINTED)
Treatment of pustular inflammatory acne and seborrheic dermatitis
(Dermik)

Sodium sulfacetamide .... 10% w/v
Sulfur .... 5% w/v

SULFA NOX, PURINA

See PURINA SULFA NOX

SULFAQUIN-O-MOR
For coccidiosis, acute fowl cholera; veterinary
(Hilltop)

Each 100 cc:
Sulfaquinoxaline sodium (2-sulfanilamidoquinoxaline sodium in excess sodium hydroxide solution) (equiv. to 3.2 g. sulfaquinoxaline per 100 cc.) ..... 3.44 g.
'76 Ed.

SULFAQUIN-O-MOR CONCENTRATE (33.3%)
To control coccidiosis in chickens, turkeys; veterinary
(Hilltop)

Each 100 cc:
Sulfaquinoxaline * in excess
Hydroxide * .... 33.3 g.
'76 Ed.

SULFASOX (C.T. WHITE)
(Bowman Pharm.)

Each tablet:
Sulfasoxazole .... 500 mg.

SULFATONIC, WARDLEY'S

See WARDLEY'S SULFATONIC

SULFA-TRIACET
Antibiotic-antibacterial
(Wesley Pharm.)

Each tablet:
Sulfadiazine * .... 2 1/2 gr.
Sulfamerazine * .... 2 1/2 gr.
Sulfacetamide * .... 2 1/2 gr.

SULF-10 DROPPERETTE OPHTHALMIC SOLUTION
Antibacterial
(CooperVision Pharm.)

Sodium sulfacetamide 10%
Thimerosal 0.005%

SULFIZIN
Anti-infective
(Direct Div.)

Each tablet:
Sulfisoxazole * .... 500 mg.

SULFODENE SCRATCHEX DOG AND CAT SPRAY
Insecticide
(Combe Inc.)

Pyrethrins 0.07%
Carbaryl 0.50%
Petroleum distillate 0.28%

SULFOIL
For cleansing skin and hair
(C & M Pharmacal)

Sulfonated Castor oil
Propylene glycol
Purified water

SULFO-LO
Antiseptic
(Whorton)

Sulfur compounds of potassium and zinc *†
Calamine
Alcohol 30%/v
Colloidal Sulfur

'76 Ed.

†*See* Zinc salts

SULF-10 OPHTHALMIC SOLUTION
Antibacterial
(CooperVision Pharm.)

Sodium sulfacetamide 10%
Thimerosal 0.01%
Hydroxypropyl methylcellulose ... 0.1%

SULFOXIDE PYREXCEL 20
Insecticide
(Penick)

Pyrethrins 0.62%
n-Octyl sulfoxide of isosafrole 4.38%
Related compounds 0.60%
2-Butoxy ethanol * 9.96%

SULKAMYCIN-S BOLETTES
For calf scours
(Norden Labs.)

Each Bolette:
Sulfamethazine * .... 2.0 gm.
Neomycin sulfate (equiv. to neomycin base 175 mg.) .. 250.0 mg.

SULKAMYCIN-S POWDER
Scours; veterinary
(Norden Labs.)

Each 21.7 gm.:
Sulfamethazine * .... 8.0 gm.
Powd. ext. Belladonna (equiv. to 0.7 mg. belladonna alkaloids) .... 64 mg.
Neomycin sulfate (equiv. to 700 mg. neomycin base) .... 1.0 gm.

SUL-LITE

See ANCHOR SUL-LITE

SULMET DRINKING WATER SOLUTION, MASTER MIX

See MASTER MIX SULMET DRINKING WATER SOLUTION

SULMET OBLETS, MASTER MIX

See MASTER MIX SULMET OBLETS

SULPHO-LAC
For treatment of acne and seborrhea
(Lambda Inc.)

Sulfur
Sulfurated lime *
Zinc sulfate *

SULPHO-LAC SOAP
For oily skin and acne
(Lambda Inc.)

Precipitated Sulfur 9%
Zinc oxide 1%

SULPHRIN
Ophthalmic suspension: for ocular in-fections
(Muro Pharm.)

Each ml.:
Sodium sulfacetamide *	100 mg.
Prednisolone acetate	5 mg.
Phenylephrine HCl	0.12%
Sodium borate	trace
Boric acid	<1.00%
Hydroxypropyl methylcellulose	<1.00%
Polysorbate 80	<1.00%
Sodium metabisulfite	<1.00%
Disodium EDTA	<1.00%
Propylene glycol	<1.00%
Sodium thiosulfate	<1.00%
Methylparaben	0.05%
Propylparaben	0.01%
Purified water	qs ad

SULQUIN 6-50 CONCENTRATE
Anti-bacterial; veterinary
(Salsbury)

Each 100 cc:
Sulfaquinoxaline sodium *	28.62 grams

SULRAY MINERAL BATHS
(Lambda Inc.)

Sodium sesquicarbonates *
Sodium chloride *
Colloidal Sulfur *
Alkyl aryl sulphonate *

SULRAY SOAP
For acne pimples, oily skin and black-heads
(Lambda Inc.)

Sopanox
Zinc oxide
Sulfur

SULTAR
Laxative, tonic
(Friendly Labs.)

Flowers of Sulfur
Cream of tartar
Sugar
Flavoring

SULTRIN
Triple sulfa cream and vaginal tablets
(Ortho)

Cream:
Sulfathiazole	3.42%
Sulfacetamide	2.86%
Sulfabenzamide	3.7%
Urea	0.64%

Each tablet:
Sulfathiazole *	172.5 mg.
Sulfacetamide *	143.75 mg.
Sulfabenzamide *	184.0 mg.

SUL-TROL-E
Drinking water medication for cattle, sheep and swine
(Hess & Clark)

Sodium sulfathiazole (as hexahydrate) *	67%

SUM
Triple action detergent
(Help)

Non-ionic wetting agent
Sodium carbonate
Sodium phosphate (sometimes metasili-cate) *

'76 Ed.

SUMMIT CANNERS' SPECIAL INSECTICIDE
(Summit Chem. Co.)

Pyrethrins	0.4%
Piperonyl butoxide (tech.)	1.0%
N-Octyl bicycloheptene dicarboximide	1.0%
Petroleum distillate *	97.6%

SUMMIT DIBROM ULV INSECTICIDE
(Summit Chem. Co.)

Naled *	15%
Heavy Aromatic naphtha *	83%

SUMMIT FOGGING INSECTICIDE
(Summit Chem. Co.)

Naled	1.00%
Petroleum distillate *	98.89%
Inert ingredients (from Naled 90)	0.11%

SUMMIT MISTOCIDE
(Summit Chem. Co.)

Pyrethrins	0.4%
Piperonyl butoxide (tech.)	0.5%
N-Octyl bicycloheptene dicarboximide	0.5%
Petroleum distillate *	98.6%

SUMMIT MISTOCIDE-B
Insecticide
(Summit Chem. Co.)

S-Bioallethrin	0.325%
Other isomers	0.025%
Technical Piperonyl butoxide	0.700%
N-Octyl bicycloheptene dicarboximide	1.168%
Petroleum distillate *	97.782%

SUMMIT MISTOCIDE-D
Insecticide
(Summit Chem. Co.)

d-trans Allethrin (allyl homolog of Cinerin I)	0.250%
Technical Piperonyl butoxide	0.500%
N-Octyl bicycloheptene dicarboximide	0.825%
Petroleum distillate *	98.425%

SUMMIT MISTOCIDE-D PLUS
Insecticide
(Summit Chem. Co.)

d-trans Allethrin (allyl homolog of Cinerin I)	0.60%
Technical Piperonyl butoxide	1.20%
N-Octyl bicycloheptene dicarboximide	2.00%
Petroleum distillate *	96.20%

SUMMIT MISTOCIDE PLUS
Insecticide
(Summit Chem. Co.)

Pyrethrins	0.50%
Technical Piperonyl butoxide	1.00%
N-Octyl bicycloheptene dicarboximide	1.67%
Petroleum distillate *	96.83%

SUMMIT MUSHROOM HOUSE FOGGING INSECTICIDE
(Summit Chem. Co.)

O,O-Dimethyl O-2,2 dichlorovinyl phosphate *	9.3%
Related compounds	0.7%
Petroleum distillate *	90.0%

SUMMIT PERMACIDE
(Summit Chem. Co.)

Diazinon	1.0%
Pyrethrins	0.05%
N-Octyl bicycloheptene dicarboximide	0.20%
Petroleum distillate *	98.75%

SUMMIT PERMACIDE PLUS
Insecticide
(Summit Chem. Co.)

o-Isopropoxyphenyl methylcarbamate *	1%
Petroleum distillate *	83%

SUMMIT POULTRY HOUSE FOGGING CONCENTRATE
Insecticide
(Summit Chem. Co.)

Pyrethrins	0.6%
Technical Piperonyl butoxide	3.0%
Petroleum distillate *	96.4%

Starred ingredients (*) may be responsible for major toxic effects; consult Section II.

SUMMIT PRODUCTS
Hair care products

Summit Laboratories, Inc.
1335 W. 47th St.
Chicago, Ill. 60609

Phone: 312-927-8202

See COSMETICS, Section VI, General Formulations

SUMMIT PYRETHRINS CONCENTRATE FOR TOBACCO WAREHOUSES
Insecticide
(Summit Chem. Co.)

Pyrethrins	1.0%
Petroleum distillate *	99.0%

SUMMIT PYRETHRINS FOGGING CONCENTRATE
Insecticide
(Summit Chem. Co.)

Pyrethrins	3%
Technical Piperonyl butoxide	6%
N-Octyl bicycloheptene dicarboximide	10%
Petroleum distillate *	81%

SUMMIT PYRETHRINS FOGGING CONCENTRATE II
Insecticide
(Summit Chem. Co.)

Pyrethrins	2.0%
Piperonyl butoxide (technical)	2.5%
N-Octyl bicycloheptene dicarboximide	2.5%
Petroleum distillate *	93.0%

SUMMIT SBP-1382-2 LB. E.C.
Control of roaches, flies, mosquitoes, etc.
(Summit Chem. Co.)

Resmethrin	24.30% w/w
Related compounds	3.30% w/w
Aromatic petroleum hydrocarbons *	66.40% w/w

SUMMIT SUMITHRIN GREENHOUSE SPRAY
(Summit Chem. Co.)

Sumithrin *	25.990%
Other isomers	1.210%
Petroleum distillate *	60.788%

SUMMIT SUPER PERMACIDE
Insect spray; ready-to-use liquid
(Summit Chem. Co.)

Active ingredients:	99.97%
Chlorpyrifos (O,O-Diethyl O-(3,5,6-trichloro-2-pyridyl)phosphoro-thioate)	0.50%
Pyrethrins	0.05%
N-Octyl bicycloheptene dicarboximide	0.20%
Petroleum distillate *	99.22%

SUMMIT TOBACCO WAREHOUSE FOGGING INSECTICIDE
(Summit Chem. Co.)

2,2-Dichlorovinyl dimethyl phosphate *	9.3%
Related compounds	0.7%
Petroleum distillate *	90.0%

SUNBEAM COFFEE MAKER CLEANER
(Sunbeam Appliance)

Sodium metasilicate
Sodium tripolyphosphate *
Sodium dichloro-s-triazine-2,4,6-trione *

'76 Ed.

SUNBEAM STEAM IRON CLEANER
(Sunbeam Appliance)

Versene 100 (Tetra sodium salt of ethylene diamine te-tra acetic acid (tech.)) *	18.0%/wt.
Benax 2-A (Anionic sulfo-nate wetting agent)	0.2%/wt.
Nalco 1695 (inhibitor)	0.0011%/wt.
Phosphoric acid (85%)	1.68%/wt.
Water	
Dye - pontamine turquoise	0.02%/wt.

'76 Ed.

SUNBEAM SUPER FINE LUBRICANT
(Sunbeam Appliance)

Humble oil #36 (Spinistic oil) *†	100.0%/wt.

'76 Ed.

†*See* Petroleum oil

SUNBEAM TEFLON CLEANER
(Sunbeam Appliance)

Sodium metasilicate
Sodium perborate *

'76 Ed.

SUN CONDITIONER/ STABILIZER
Swimming pool water disinfectant sta-bilizer
(FMC Corp., Sun Swimming Pool Products)

s-Triazinetrione *	94%
Water	6%

SUNDARE CLEAR LOTION
Sunscreen
(CooperCare)

Cinnoxate	1.75%
Alcohol	51.8%
Polypropylene glycol	
Methylcellulose	
Perfume	
Water	

SUNDARE CREAMY LOTION
Sunscreen
(CooperCare)

Cinnoxate (in water and glycerin)
Triethanolamine stearate
Isopropyl myristate
Lanolin oil
Cetyl alcohol
Methyl, butyl and propyl parabens
FD & C Yellow #6
Fragrance

SUN DETERGENT
(Los Angeles Soap)

Sodium alkyl aryl sulfonate
Sodium carbonate *
Sodium silicate
Sodium sulfate
Sodium carboxymethylcellulose
Optical whitener
Perfume

SUN FAST TABS (Tablets)
Swimming pool water disinfectant and sanitizer
(FMC Corp., Sun Swimming Pool Products)

Trichloro-s-triazinetrione *	70%
Sodium carbonate *	30%

SUN FRESH
Mildewcide
(Chemical Processors)

Paraformaldehyde *
Paradichlorobenzene *

SUNGARD LOTION
Sunscreen
(Dome)

Padimate-O	2.5%
Dioxybenzone	3.0%
Alcohol (contained in vehicle)	55%

Starred ingredients (*) may be responsible for major toxic effects; consult Section II.

SUNLIGHT LIQUID
Liquid dishwashing detergent
(Lever Bros.)

Water	40-50%
Anionic detergents	40-50%
Lemon juice	5-15%
Magnesium chloride	0.5-5%
Ethanol	1-5%
Perfume	<1%
Colorants	trace

SUNLIGHT POWDER
Low phosphate powder automatic dishwashing detergent
(Lever Bros.)

Sodium carbonate *	30-40%
Sodium polyphosphates	20-30%
Sodium sulfate	10-20%
Sodium silicate	10-20%
Water	5-10%
Nonionic detergent	1-5%
Sodium dichlorisocyanurate	<2%
Perfume	<1%
Monostearyl acid phosphate	trace
Colorants	trace

SUN LIQUID CHLORINE SANITIZER
Swimming pool disinfectant and sanitizer
(FMC Corp., Sun Swimming Pool Products)

Sodium hypochlorite *	10%
Water	90%

SUN MINUS (Granular Solid)
Swimming pool water pH reducer
(FMC Corp., Sun Swimming Pool Products)

Sodium bisulfate *	100%

SUNNYSIDE CHARCOAL LIGHTER FLUID
(Sunnyside)

Petroleum distillate *

SUNNYSIDE DENATURED ALCOHOL SOLVENT
Shellac thinner, cleaning solvent, liquid fuel
(Sunnyside)

Ethyl alcohol (denatured) *

SUNNYSIDE GASOLINE STOVE & LANTERN FUEL
(Sunnyside)

Petroleum distillate *

SUNNYSIDE LAMP OIL
For use in wick-type kerosene lamps
(Sunnyside)

Odorless Petroleum distillate *
Various scents and colorants

SUNNYSIDE LIQUID BRUSH CLEANER
(Sunnyside)

Toluol *
Acetone *
Methylene chloride *
Triethanolamine
Amine salt (surfactant)

SUNNYSIDE NON-FLAMMABLE PAINT & VARNISH REMOVER
(Sunnyside)

Methylene chloride *
Methanol *
Aromatic hydrocarbon *
Methyl cellulose
Wax
Emulsifier

SUNNYSIDE ODORLESS PAINT THINNER
(Sunnyside)

Petroleum distillate *

SUNNYSIDE PENTA PRESERVATIVE
Wood preservative
(Sunnyside)

Pentachlorophenol *
Petroleum distillate *

SUNNYSIDE PENTA WATER REPELLENT
Wood preservative
(Sunnyside)

Pentachlorophenol *	4.37%
Other chlorinated phenols	0.51%
Petroleum hydrocarbons *	86.10%

SUNNYSIDE SHELLAC
(Sunnyside)

Shellac
Denatured Ethyl alcohol *

SUNNY SOL "100"
For swimming pool chlorination and sanitizing
(Jones Chemicals)

Sodium hypochlorite *	9.2%
Sodium chloride	9.6%
Water	80.6%
Sodium hydroxide *	0.6%

SUNNY SOL "150"
For swimming pool chlorination and sanitizing
(Jones Chemicals)

Sodium hypochlorite *	12.5%
Sodium chloride	9.6%
Water	77.1%
Sodium hydroxide *	0.8%

SUNNY SOL BLEACH
(Jones Chemicals)

Sodium hypochlorite *	5.25%
Sodium chloride	8.65%
Water	85.44%
Sodium hydroxide *	0.66%

SUN-O-CAINE
For skin irritations, burns
(VB)

Zinc oxide
Menthol *
Ethyl aminobenzoate

SUN PAC
Mildewcide
(Chemical Processors)

Paraformaldehyde *

SUN PLUS (Granular Solid)
Swimming pool water pH increaser
(FMC Corp., Sun Swimming Pool Products)

Sodium carbonate (Soda ash) *	100%

SUN POOL CHLORINATING CONCENTRATE (Tablets and Sticks)
Swimming pool water disinfectant and sanitizer
(FMC Corp., Sun Swimming Pool Products)

Trichloro-s-triazinetrione *	99.5%
Water	0.5%

SUN POOL CHLORINATING CONCENTRATE, GRANULAR & BOOSTER (Granular Solid)
Swimming pool water disinfectant and sanitizer
(FMC Corp., Sun Swimming Pool Products)

Sodium dichloro-s-triazinetrione dihydrate *	100%

SUNSHINE NEUTRAL CLEANER
(Uncle Sam)

Vegetable oils
Synthetic detergents *
Water softener
Ethylenediaminetetraacetate

SUN-SOFT FABRIC SOFTENER
(Barcolene)

Complex difatty Quaternary sulfate *†	3-5%
Polyoxyethylated vegetable oil	trace
Fragrance	trace
Optical brightener	trace

†*See* Cationic detergents

SUN SOLAR ALGAECIDE CONCENTRATE (Liquid)
Swimming pool water algaecide
(FMC Corp., Sun Swimming Pool Products)

Alkyl dimethyl benzyl ammonium chloride (C14, 60%; C12, 25%; C16, 15%) *	50%
Ethanol	10%
Water	40%

SUN SOLAR ALGAECIDE "10" (Liquid)
Swimming pool water algaecide
(FMC Corp., Sun Swimming Pool Products)

Alkyl dimethyl benzyl ammonium chloride (C14, 60%; C12, 25%; C16, 15%) *	10%
Water	90%

SUNSTICK
Lip and face protectant
(CooperCare)

Digalloyltrioleate
Emollient
Colorless lubricating base

SUN SWIMMING POOL PRODUCTS

FMC CORPORATION
2000 Market St.
Philadelphia, PA 19103

Emergency information may be obtained at 215-299-5800

SUNTAN RESEARCH & DEVELOPMENT PRODUCTS

Suntan Research & Development, Inc.
P.O. Box 2734
Daytona Beach, Fla. 32015

Phone: 904-258-7396

See COSMETICS, Section VI, General Formulations

SUNTONE
Arterial fluid; embalming supply
(Royal Bond)

Methanol *	
Formaldehyde index *	18%

SUN WEATHER-GUARD (Liquid)
Swimming pool winterizing algaecide
(FMC Corp., Sun Swimming Pool Products)

Alkyl dimethyl benzyl ammonium chloride (C14, 60%; C12, 25%; C16, 15%) *	5%
Water	95%

SUPER ANAHIST NASAL SPRAY
(Warner-Lambert)

Phenylephrine HCl *	0.25%
Alcohol	0.038%
Thimerosal (preservative)	0.002%

SUPER ANAHIST TABLETS
(Warner-Lambert)

Each tablet:

Phenylpropanolamine HCl *	25 mg.
Acetaminophen *	325 mg.

SUPER ANAPAC COLD TABLETS AC (ANTI-COUGH)
(Rexall)

Each tablet:

Phenylpropanolamine hydrochloride	7.5 mg.
Salicylamide	5 gr.
Acetaminophen *	1.25 gr.
Dextromethorphan hydrobromide	3.75 mg.
Chlorpheniramine maleate	1 mg.
Caffeine	0.25 gr.
Vitamin C	20 mg.

'76 Ed.

SUPER ANAPAC TABLETS
(Rexall)

Each tablet:

Chlorpheniramine maleate	1.0 mg.
Salicylamide *	5.0 gr.
Acetaminophen *	1.25 gr.
Caffeine	0.25 gr.
Phenylpropanolamine HCl *	7.5 mg.
Vitamin C	20 mg.

'76 Ed.

SUPER ARSONATE
Postemergence herbicide
(Diamond Shamrock Corp.)

Monosodium acid methanearsonate *	58.2%

SUPER BAINICIDE
Insect spray
(Lester Labs.)

Petroleum distillates *
Piperonyl butoxide
Pyrethrins *
Essential oils *

'76 Ed.

SUPER BLUE
(Birchwood Casey)

Selenium *
Nitric acid *
Phosphoric acid *

SUPER BLUE DRAGON GARDEN DUST
Insecticide & fungicide
(Dragon)

Carbaryl *	5%

SUPER BONUS FOR DICHONDRA
Herbicide/insecticide
(Scott, O.M.)

Diphenamid *	3.50%
Neburon	1.06%
Monuron	0.17%
Dursban	0.26%
Fertilizer base: 25-0-0	

SUPER BONUS 7
Herbicide
(Scott, O.M.)

Atrazine	2.00%
Carrier base: Fertilizer 21-3-3	

SUPER BREAK III
Liquid laundry builder
(Brewer Chem.)

50% Potassium hydroxide *	40-50%
50% Sodium hydroxide	30-40%
Potassium silicate	15-25%

SUPER BRITE II
Liquid cleaner
(Kay Chem. Co.)

Anionic and nonionic surfactants	5-10%
Trisodium phosphate	5-10%
Water	balance

SUPER "C" DEODORANT
Liquid air freshener
(Continental Mfg. Co.)

Terpinyl acetate *†	10-30%
Turpentine *	5-25%
Terpineol *	5-25%
Boise de rose	5-25%
Lemon oil 340	10-30%
d'Limonene *	10-30%
Geraniol S *	1-15%
Benzaldehyde	1-10%
Diphenyl oxide	1-10%
Phenyl ethyl alcohol	1-10%
Amyl salicylate *	5-25%
L-Carvone	1-10%
Isobornyl acetate *‡	1-10%
Eucalyptus *	1-10%
Benzyl acetate	1-10%
Citral	1-10%
Eugenol	1-10%
Coumarin *	1-10%
Vanillin	1-10%
Musk ambrette	1-10%
Lime oil	1-10%
Netgtk acetiogebibe	1-10%
Ocotea cymbarum	1-10%
Amyl acetate	1-10%
Oil lemongrass	1-10%
Oil clove	1-10%
Oil peppermint	1-10%
Methyl salicylate *	1-10%
Cinnamic aldehyde *	5-25%
Diethyl phthalate *	15-50%

†*See* Terpenes
‡*See* Borneol

SUPER CHLOR, WARDLEY'S

See WARDLEY'S SUPER CHLOR

SUPERCITIN SUGAR-FREE COUGH SYRUP
Antitussive, antihistamine expectorant
(Vitarine)

Each 10 cc:
Dextromethorphan hydrobromide *	20 mg.
Chlorpheniramine maleate	2 mg.
Sodium citrate	100 mg.
Acetaminophen *	120 mg.

SUPERCOLD COUGH MEDICINE

See WATKINS SUPERCOLD COUGH MEDICINE

SUPER COLD TABS
(Reese Chem.)

Each tablet:
Acetaminophen	500 mg.
Phenylpropanolamine hydrochloride *	25 mg.
Phenyltoloxamine citrate	22 mg.

SUPER DAL-E-RAD + 2
Herbicide
(Vineland Chem.)

Dodecylammonium methanearsonate	8.0%
Octylammonium methanearsonate *	8.0%
Octylammonium salt of 2,4-dichlorophenoxyacetic acid *	8.16%

SUPER DAL-E-RAD "CALAR"
Herbicide
(Vineland Chem.)

Calcium acid methanearsonate *	10.3%

SUPER-DECON CAPSULES
Decongestant, antihistaminic, analgesic
(Vitarine)

Each capsule:
Salicylamide *	250 mg.
Caffeine (anhydrous)	32 mg.
Phenylephrine hydrochloride	5 mg.
Methapyrilene hydrochloride *	12.5 mg.
Vitamin C (Ascorbic acid)	50 mg.

SUPER DIE-FLY SUGAR-BASE FLY-KILLER
(Farnam Co.)

Dimethyl (2,2,2-trichloro-1-hydroxyethyl) phosphonate *	1.0%

'76 Ed.

SUPER DISIT "N-1"
Germicidal detergent-deodorizer concentrate
(ABCO, Inc.)

Active ingred.:	7.583%
n-Alkyl (60% C14, 30% C16, 5% C12, 5% C18) dimethyl benzyl ammonium chlorides *	1.758%
n-Alkyl (68% C12, 32% C14) dimethyl ethylbenzyl ammonium chlorides *	1.758%
Sodium metasilicate *	2.216%
Sodium hydroxide *	1.050%
Ethylene diamine tetraacetic acid tetrasodium salt	0.573%
Essential oils	2.228%
Inert ingred.:	92.417%
Water	
Polyoxyethylene nonylphenol	
Hexylene glycol	
Artificial color	

SUPER DISIT P
Cleaner, disinfectant, deodorant, sanitizer
(ABCO, Inc.)

Ortho-benzyl-para-chlorophenol	3.1%
Soap	15.1%
Isopropyl alcohol	2.91%

SUPER D PERLES
Vitamin therapy
(Upjohn)

Each perle:
Vitamin A	10,000 I.U.
Vitamin D	400 I.U.

SUPER D WEEDONE
Herbicide
(Amchem)

Diethanol amine salt of 2,4-dichlorophenoxyacetic acid *	20.1%
Diethanol amine salt of dicamba	1.9%

SUPERDYNE
Concentrated cold-process iodine containing detergent for cleansing and disinfecting
(Salsbury)

Glycolic acid *	44.1%
p-(Nonylphenyl)-omega-hydropoly-(oxyethylene)-iodine complex (82,500 ppm titratable iodine)	34.2%

SUPER EVERWEAR GYM FINISH
(Uncle Sam)

Epoxy resins
Cobalt driers *
Petroleum distillates *

SUPER GLOSS NO RUBBING FLOOR WAX
(Uncle Sam)

Synthetic waxes
Resins (modified phenolic)
Emulsifiers
Ammonia
Polyethylene
Water

SUPER HISTA-C CAPSULES
Analgesic, decongestant, antihistaminic, antitussive
(DePree)

Acetaminophen *
Phenylpropanolamine *
Dextromethorphan *
Pyrilamine maleate *

SUPER HISTA-C SYRUP
Analgesic, decongestant, antitussive, antihistaminic
(DePree)

d-Methorphan HBr *
Phenylpropanolamine HCl *
Chlorpheniramine maleate *
Acetaminophen *

Starred ingredients (*) may be responsible for major toxic effects; consult Section II.

SUPER HY-KIL INSECT KILLER
Commercial and institutional use
(Hysan Corp.)

Pyrethrins	0.5%
Technical Piperonyl butoxide	1.0%
N-Octyl bicycloheptene dicarboximide	1.0%
Petroleum distillate	8.5%

SUPER HY-KIL LIQUID INSECTICIDE
Institutional and commercial use
(Hysan Corp.)

Pyrethrins	0.165%
Technical Piperonyl butoxide	0.330%
N-Octyl bicycloheptene dicarboximide	0.550%
Beta-butoxy beta'-thiocyano di-ethyl ether	0.106%
n-Octyl sulfoxide of isosafrole	0.0175%
Related compounds	0.0025%
Petroleum distillate *	98.829%

SUPER IODEX
Dairy iodine sanitizer & milk stone remover
(Lester Labs.)

Phosphoric acid *
Complex Iodine detergents *†

'76 Ed.

†*See* Iodine and Detergents

SUPERIOR ALL-SEASON MOTOR OIL (10W-40)
(Marathon Oil Co.)

Additives, containing Zinc alkyl dithiophosphate, Olefin copolymer	30%
Mineral oil	balance

SUPERIOR NU-OIL #70
Insecticide & fungicide
(Miller Chem. & Fert.)

Petroleum oil * 98.8%

SUPER-KEM DRY CHEMICAL RECHARGE
For fire extinguishers
(Norris Industries)

Potassium chloride
Diatomaceous earth
Tricalcium phosphate
Polysiloxane coating

'76 Ed.

SUPER-KILL INSECT SPRAY
Insecticide
(Rawleigh)

2,2-Dichlorovinyl dimethyl phosphate	0.46%
Related compounds	0.04%
Pyrethrins	0.25%
Technical Piperonyl butoxide	1.00%
Petroleum distillates *	13.25%

'76 Ed.

SUPER-KILL ROACH COMPOUND
Insecticide
(Maco Labs.)

Sodium fluoride *	40%
O,O-Diethyl O-(2-isopropyl-4-methyl-6-pyrimidinyl)phosphorothioate	1%
Inert ingredients:	59%
Sodium borate	

'76 Ed.

SUPER MAGNACIDE RESIDUAL SPRAY
Insecticide; kills waterbugs, ants, silverfish, carpet beetles & bed bugs
(Leedsall)

Piperonyl butoxide (technical)	1.27%
Pyrethrins	0.13%
Chlordane (technical)	2.00%

'76 Ed.

SUPERM LOTION
Permanent wave lotion
(Bonat)

	percentage range
Water	75.0-95.0%
Ammonium thioglycolate *	6.0-18.0%
Ammonium hydroxide *	<2.0%
Sodium hydroxide *	<1.0%
Styrene/acrylamide copolymer	<1.0%
Laureth-23	<1.0%
Fragrance	<1.0%

SUPER ODRINEX
Appetite suppressant
(Fox Pharmacal)

Each tablet:	
Phenylpropanolamine hydrochloride *	33 1/3 mg.
Caffeine *	100 mg.

SUPER 100 BARN & STOCK SPRAY
Insecticide
(Central Petroleum)

Pyrethrins	0.10%
Piperonyl butoxide, technical	0.20%
N-Octyl bicycloheptene dicarboximide	0.33%
Di-n-propyl isocinchomeronate	0.40%
Petroleum distillate *	98.97%

SUPER PLUMB DRAIN OPENER
(Plumb Craft)

Potassium hydroxide * 100%

'76 Ed.

SUPER POLI-GRIP
Denture adhesive
(Block Drug)

Petrolatum
Mineral oil
Sodium carboxymethylcellulose
Ethylene oxide homopolymer
Sodium phosphate (monobasic)
Preservative
Flavors

SUPERPOLY CAR WASH (AS-928, Formula 2167-63)

See SIMONIZ SUPERPOLY CAR WASH (AS-928, Formula 2167-63)

SUPERPOLY LIQUID (AS-982, Formula 2206-104; 8691-36)

See SIMONIZ SUPERPOLY LIQUID (AS-982, Formula 2206-104; 8691-36)

SUPERPOLY PASTE (AS-981, Formula 2206-33; 2206-14; 8691-50)

See SIMONIZ SUPERPOLY PASTE (AS-981, Formula 2206-33; 2206-14; 8691-50)

SUPERPOLY POLY GLAZE (AS-983, Formula 2138-65, 8622-27-2)

See SIMONIZ SUPERPOLY POLY GLAZE (AS-983, Formula 2138-65, 8622-27-2)

SUPERPOLY 10-MINUTE PRE-WAX/PRE-POLY CLEANER (AS-987, Formula 2206-66)

See SIMONIZ SUPERPOLY 10-MINUTE PRE-WAX/PRE-POLY CLEANER (AS-987, Formula 2206-66)

SUPER POR-ROK CEMENT
(Minwax Co.)

Portland cement *	38%
Silicon dioxide	55%
Calcium aluminate	minor
Potassium persulfate	minor
Sodium perborate	minor
Melamine formaldehyde resin	minor

Starred ingredients (*) may be responsible for major toxic effects; consult Section II.

SUPER RESICIDE CONCENTRATE
Insecticide
(Residex)

Pyrethrins	3.0%
Technical Piperonyl butoxide	6.0%
N-Octyl bicycloheptene dicarboximide	10.0%
Deodorized Petroleum distillate *	81.0%

SUPER-RINGGO POLY BOWL CLEANER
(United Chemical Co., Inc.)

Hydrogen chloride *	24.82%
Para di-isobutyl phenoxy ethoxy ethyl dimethyl benzyl ammonium chloride	0.20%

'76 Ed.

SUPER ROYAL
Arterial fluid; embalming supply
(Royal Bond)

Formaldehyde *
Methanol *

SUPER RYPLEX LATEX SATIN SHEEN BASE PAINTS
(Touraine Paints, Inc.)

BASE "AA":	
Titanium dioxide	27.6%
Barium sulfate	2.2%
Vinyl acrylic non-volatile	21.0%
Water	49.2%
BASE "B":	
Titanium dioxide	15.2%
Barium sulfate	6.5%
Silicates	6.5%
Vinyl acrylic non-volatile	22.4%
Water	49.4%
BASE "C":	
Titanium dioxide	6.5%
Barium sulfate	15.1%
Silicates	6.5%
Vinyl acrylic non-volatile	22.4%
Water	49.5%
BASE "D":	
Titanium dioxide	3.2%
Barium sulfate	19.4%
Silicates	6.5%
Vinyl acrylic non-volatile	21.2%
Water	49.7%

'76 Ed.

SUPER RYPLEX LATEX SATIN SHEEN PAINTS
(Touraine Paints, Inc.)

AUTUMN GOLD (#1289):	
Titanium dioxide	19.76%
Silicates	3.95%
Calcium carbonate	7.90%
Vinyl acrylic non-volatile	20.40%
Water	48.00%

The following colors have the same formulation as AUTUMN GOLD:
BLACK (#1260), BUCKSKIN BEIGE (#1283), CANDLELIGHT (#1285), CATHY (#1278), CELERY (#1287), CELESTE BLUE (#1264), CORNSILK (#1282), GREEN HAZE (#1292), GREEN MIST (#1271), MINT ICE (#1290), OFF-WHITE (#1279), PARCHMENT (#1288), WHITE (#1288), PINK DAWN (#1291), PORCELAIN BLUE (#1270), PROVINCIAL GOLD (#1286), SPEARMINT (#1281), SUNLITE (#1269), WARM IVORY (#1266), WHITE

'76 Ed.

SUPER RYPLEX LATEX SEMI GLOSS BASE PAINTS
(Touraine Paints, Inc.)

WHITE BASE "A" & "B":	
Titanium dioxide	18.7%
Barium sulfate	2.3%
Vinyl acrylic non-volatile	26.0%
Water	53.0%
NEUTRAL BASE "C":	
Titanium dioxide	7.74%
Barium sulfate	5.16%
Vinyl acrylic non-volatile	28.7%
Water	58.4%
ACCENT BASE "D":	
Titanium dioxide	2.6%
Barium sulfate	10.5%
Vinyl acrylic non-volatile	29.3%
Water	57.6%

'76 Ed.

SUPER RYPLEX LATEX UNDERCOATER PAINT
(Touraine Paints, Inc.)

Titanium dioxide	17.7%
Calcium carbonate	13.3%
Vinyl acrylic non-volatile	15.6%
Water	53.4%

'76 Ed.

SUPER SAV-A-BRUSH
(Schalk)

Xylene *
Acetone

'76 Ed.

SUPER SCOOT
Cleaner and brightener for aluminum and stainless steel; industrial use
(Puritan Chem. Co.)

Hydrofluoric acid *

SUPER SOFT
Laundry softener
(Brewer Chem.)

Fluorescent whitening agent	<1%
Complex difatty Quaternary softener concentrate	10-15%

SUPER SOLVENT
Automotive, heavy duty cooling system cleaner
(Radiator)

Oxalic acid *
Aminosulfonic acids *

'76 Ed.

SUPER-SOLV PAINT THINNER & CONDITIONER
(Barr, W. M., & Co.)

Aliphatic hydrocarbons	75%
Aromatic hydrocarbons *	25%

SUPER STOCK TOX, MARTIN'S
See MARTIN'S SUPER STOCK TOX

SUPER-STRIP NONFLAMMABLE PAINT REMOVER
(Savogran)

Methanol *	<20%
Toluol *	<5%
Methylene chloride *	75-95%
Retardants	
Thickeners	

SUPER SUDS
Granular detergent
(Colgate-Palmolive)

Alkyl aryl sulfonate *	approx. 20%
Combined amount:	approx. 70%
Sodium silicate *	
Sodium sulfate	
Pentasodium tripolyphosphate *	

'76 Ed.

SUPER-TROL, SPRAY-TROL BRAND
See SPRAY-TROL BRAND SUPER-TROL

SUPERTROP PAINT
(International Paint)

Copper *
Color code #46

Starred ingredients (*) may be responsible for major toxic effects; consult Section II.

SUPER TURF BUILDER PLUS HALTS
Fertilizer with herbicide
(Scott, O.M.)

Bensulide 5.75%
Carrier: Fertilizer 30-5-3

SUPER TURF BUILDER PLUS 2
Herbicide/fertilizer
(Scott, O.M.)

2,4-Dichlorophenoxyacetic acid ... 1.10%
2-(4-Chloro-2-methylphenoxy) propionic acid 1.10%
Fertilizer formula: 32-4-4

SUPER TURF BUILDER PLUS 2 FOR GRASS (W/S)
Herbicide/fertilizer
(Scott, O.M.)

2,4-Dichlorophenoxyacetic acid ... 0.55%
2-(4-Chloro-2-methylphenoxy) propionic acid 0.55%
Fertilizer formula: 26-5-3
Iron (FAS) 1.10%

SUPER TURF BUILDER PLUS 2 FOR IRON DEFICIENT SOIL (I)
Herbicide/fertilizer
(Scott, O.M.)

2,4-Dichlorophenoxyacetic acid ... 0.60%
2-(4-Chloro-2-methylphenoxy) propionic acid 0.60%
Fertilizer formula: 22-3-3
Iron (FS.M) 1.10%

SUPER WERNET'S POWDER
Denture adhesive
(Block Drug)

Sodium carboxymethylcellulose
Ethylene oxide homopolymer
Monosodium phosphate
Dicalcium phosphate
Flavor

SUPPRESS TRI-MINT DEODORANT SPRAY
Industrial and institutional use
(Scientific International)

Active ingredients: 43.0%
Isopropyl alcohol *
Triethylene glycol
Propylene glycol *
Essential oils: *
  Spearmint
  Peppermint
  Wintergreen

SUPPRESS WITH SPEARMINT AND DOUBLEMINT
*Odor suppressant, air sanitizer, virus-
cide; industrial and institutional use*
(Scientific International)

Active ingredients: 20%
Isopropyl alcohol *
Triethylene glycol
Essential oils *
Inert ingredients: 80%
Dichlorodifluoromethane
Trichloromonofluoromethane

SUPRA
Car polish
(Calgon Corp., Commercial Div.)

Emulsifiers
Petroleum distillate *

SUPURB DETERGENT (POWDER)
(Safeway Stores)

Linear alkyl aryl sulfonate * 15%
Fatty acid sodium soap 5%
Sodium tripolyphosphate * 24%
Sodium silicate 8%
Sodium sulfate 38%
Combined amount: 1%
  Carboxymethylcellulose
  Optical brightener
  Perfume
Moisture 9%

SUPURB LIQUID DETERGENT
(Safeway Stores)

Surfactant mixture: 40%
Alkyl benzene sulfonate (NaLAS) *†
C12-C15 Alcohol ethoxysulfate (Na)
C12-C15 Alcohol ethoxylate *
Coconut oil diethanolamide
Xylene sulfonate (Na) 8%
Ethyl alcohol (SDA 3A) 5%
Other: Citrate,   Polystyrene,
  Na2SO4, NaCl, Dye, Perfume .. 2%
Water .... balance

pH, undiluted 7.1

†See Alkyl aryl sodium sulfonates

SURBEX-750 WITH IRON FILMTAB
*Vitamins B complex, C and E supple-
ment with iron*
(Abbott)

Each tablet:
Iron * .... 27 mg.
Multivitamins

SURBEX-750 WITH ZINC FILMTAB
*Vitamins B complex, C and E supple-
ment with zinc*
(Abbott)

Each tablet:
Zinc * .... 22.5 mg.
Multivitamins

SURE-BUFF BUFFABLE FLOOR FINISH
(Uncle Sam)

Vegetable wax
Acrylic polymers (metal cross-linked)
Resin (synthetic maleic anhydride & mod-
ified phenolic)
Polyethylene
Ammonia *
Glycol ethers *
Plasticizers
Surfactants
Water

SURE (Roll-on)
Antiperspirant
(Procter & Gamble, Health & Personal
Care Div.)

Aluminum hydroxychloride 10-15%
Zirconyl hydroxychloride 5-9%
Glycine 1-4%
Paraffin wax 1-4%
Isopropyl palmitate 1-4%
Glyceryl monostearate 5-10%
Polyoxyethylene stearate 5-9%
Glycerol 1-4%
Magnesium aluminum silicate 1-4%
Minor ingredients, each .... <1%
Water .... >50%

SURE (Super Dry)
Aerosol antiperspirant and deodorant
(Procter & Gamble, Health & Personal
Care Div.)

Aluminum chlorohydrate * 10-15%
Isopropyl myristate 3-8%
Quarternium-18 hectorite 1-5%
Cyclomethicone 5-10%
Dimethicone 1-5%
Propylene carbonate .... <1%
Bentone 0.5-2%
Minor ingredients .... <1%
Propellant (Isobutane) .... >50%

SURE SHOT 2.2
*Control of insects in fruit trees and veg-
etable gardens*
(Terminal Grain)

Sevin (Carbaryl) * 11.5%
Malathion * 11.5%
Aromatic petroleum distillates * .. 9.4%

'76 Ed.

SURE SHOT WORM CAPSULES, SERGEANT'S

See SERGEANT'S SURE SHOT
WORM CAPSULES

SURE-SLEEP
To induce restful sleep
(Amlab)

Each capsule:
Methapyrilene HCl * .... 25.0 mg.
Salicylamide .... 200.0 mg.
Scopolamine aminoxide
  HBr * .... 0.25 mg.

Starred ingredients (*) may be responsible for major toxic effects; consult Section II.

SURE-TROL, SPRAY-TROL BRAND

See SPRAY-TROL BRAND SURE-TROL

SURFACAINE
(Cyclomethycaine, Lilly)
Rectal and vaginal anesthetic
(Lilly, Eli)

Each suppository:
3-(2-Methylpiperidino)-propyl-
para-cyclohexyloxy benzoate
sulfate .... 10 mg.

SURFACTANT 705
Nonionic emulsifier
(Rohm and Haas)

Ethoxylated alcohol *

SURFACTANT DN-65
Nonionic detergent
(Rohm and Haas)

Modified Ethoxylated alcohol *

SURFADIL LOTION
Allergic dermatitis
(Lilly, Eli)

Each 100 cc.:
Diphenhydramine HCl * ..... 1 gm.
Surfacaine .... 0.5 gm.
Titanium dioxide .... 5 gm.

SURF COAT
Floor finish
(Hillyard Chem.)

Mineral spirits *

'76 Ed.

SURFISAN SPRAY
Embalming supply - surface disinfection, preservation and deodorizing
(Royal Bond)

Chloroform *
Methanol *
Thymol *
Amyl phenol *

SURFLAN
Herbicide
(Elanco Prod.)

Oryzalin 75%

SURFOL
Post-immersion bath oil
(Stiefel Labs.)

Mineral oil
Isopropyl myristate
Isostearic acid
PEG-40 sorbitan peroleate
Fragrance
2-(2'-Hydroxy-5'-
methylphenyl)benzotriazole
D & C Green #6

SURF ROACH & ANT KILLER
Insecticide
(Miller-Norris Co.)

Pyrethrins 0.050%
Technical Piperonyl butoxide .. 0.100%
N-Octyl bicycloheptene
dicarboximide 0.166%
O,O-Diethyl(O-2-isopropyl-6-
methyl-4-
pyrimidinyl)phosphorothioate
(Diazinon) 0.500%
Petroleum distillate * 74.184%
Inert ingred.:
Propellant 25.000%

'76 Ed.

SURGE K.O. DYNE
Iodine detergent-sanitizer
(Babson Bros. Co.)

Nonylphenoxypoly(ethyleneoxy)-
ethanol-iodine complex 13.75%
Phosphoric acid 75% * 6.00%
Glycolic acid 7.00%

SURGE LIQUATONE BACTERICIDE
(Babson Bros. Co.)

N-Alkyl (50% C14, 40% C12, 10%
C16) dimethyl benzyl ammonium chlorides * 20%/w

SURGE MITROCIN-PLUS
Detergent-sanitizer
(Babson Bros. Co.)

N-Alkyl (60% C14, 30% C16, 5% C12,
5% C18) dimethyl benzyl ammonium chlorides 5.0%
N-Alkyl (50% C12, 30% C14, 17%
C16, 3% C18) dimethyl ethylbenzyl ammonium chlorides 5.0%
Phosphoric acid * 26.2%

SURGE POWDERED CHLORINE
Dairy equipment sanitizer
(Babson Bros. Co.)

Sodium dichloro-S-triazinetrione * 15.0%

SURGE TEAT-KOTE
Iodophor bactericide - an aid in the control of mastitis
(Babson Bros. Co.)

Butoxy monoether of polyoxypropylene glycol - iodine complex .. 4.01%
Phosphoric acid * 0.32%

SURGE ZINICIN
Concentrated bactericide, disinfectant
(Babson Bros. Co.)

Sodium hypochlorite * 10 1/2%/w

SURGI-CREAM
Depilatory
(Gambine Products, Inc.)

Calcium thioglycolate *

SURG-I-SOAP
Medicated liquid hand soap
(Scientific International)

Cocoanut oils handsoap &
emollients 10%
Triclosan 0.25%

SURIN
Rubefacient
(McKesson)

Methacholine chloride 0.25%
Camphor *
Menthol *
Methyl salicylate *

SUR-KLEEN, DEL

See DEL SUR-KLEEN

SURMONTIL CAPSULE
Anti-depressant
(Ives Labs.)

Each capsule:
Trimipramine male-
ate * .... 25 mg.; 50 mg.

SUSTAIRE SUSTAINED RELEASE TABLETS
Bronchodilator
(Roerig)

Each tablet:
Anhydrous
Theophylline * 100 mg. and 300 mg.

SU-TUSS
Expectorant, antitussive
(Moffet Inc.)

Alcohol 20%
Each fl. oz.:
Codeine phosphate * .... 1 gr.
Terpin hydrate .... 2 gr.

SW-3
Hot or cold tank paint stripper
(Calgon Corp., Commercial Div.)

Caustic *
Nonionic detergent
Alkaline salts

SWAB CONCRETE CLEANER - S.W. (Powder)
See GUNK S.W. - SWAB CONCRETE CLEANER (Powder)

S W AERO SPRAY FOAM WOUND TREATMENT
For use on livestock
(Haver-Lockhart (Brand) Bayvet Div. Cutter Labs.)

Coumaphos * 3.0%

SWAMP ROOT
See DR. KILMER'S SWAMP ROOT

SWAT
Fly and insect killer
(Agway)

Pyrethrins 0.30%
Piperonyl butoxide (technical) 0.60%
N-Octyl bicycloheptene
  dicarboximide 1.00%
Petroleum distillate 8.10%

SWAT, DEL
See DEL SWAT

SWEENEY'S ANT-GO
Insecticide
(Sweeney, W.R.)

Sodium arsenate * 2.3%

SWEENEY'S POISON PEANUTS
Rodenticide
(Sweeney, W.R.)

Strychnine alkaloid * 0.3%

SWEENEY'S POISON WHEAT WITH ROZOL
Rodenticide; natural colored wheat
(Sweeney, W.R.)

2-((p-
  Chlorophenyl)phenylacetyl)-
  1,3-indandione 0.005%

SWEENEY'S POISON WHEAT WITH STRYCHNINE SULFATE
Rodenticide; dark red colored wheat
(Sweeney, W.R.)

Strychnine sulfate * 0.5%

SWEENEY'S RAT KILLER READY MIXED
(Sweeney, W.R.)

Warfarin (3-(alpha-Acetonyl-
  benzl)-4-hydroxycoumarin) 0.025%
N'-(2-Quinoxalinyl)sulfanilamide
  (Sulfaquinoxaline) 0.025%

SWEENEY'S SODIUM FLUORIDE INSECTICIDE
(Sweeney, W.R.)

Sodium fluoride * 40%

SWEEP
Municipal insecticide
(ABCO, Inc.)

Pyrethrins 0.050%
Piperonyl butoxide (technical) .. 0.125%
Malathion 2.000%
Aromatic petroleum derivative
  solvent * 7.625%
Petroleum distillate * 90.200%

SWEET ADELINE PERFUME, COLOGNE, TOILET WATER
(Parfums Duvelle)

Alcohol (denatured with diethyl phthal-ate) *

SWEETHEART CONCENTRATED FABRIC SOFTENER
(Purex Corp.)

Quaternary ammonium
  compound * 5-10%
Fluorescent whitening agent .... <1%
Preservative .... <1%
Sodium chloride .... <1%
Perfume .... <1%
Water .... balance

SWEETHEART FABRIC SOFTENER
(Purex Corp.)

Quaternary ammonium
  compound * 2-5%
Preservative .... <1%
Sodium chloride .... <1%
Perfume .... <1%
Water .... balance

SWEETHEART LIQUID DISHWASHING DETERGENT
(Purex Corp.)

Anionic surfactant * 10-15%
Alkanolamide .... <1%
Hydrotrope .... <3%
Ethyl alcohol 2-5%
Coloring agent .... <1%
Perfume .... <1%
Opacifier .... <1%
Water .... balance

SWEETHEART TOILET SOAP
(Purex Corp.)

Sodium tallow-coconut oil soap   >80%
Glycerine .... <3%
Titanium dioxide .... <1%
Sodium chloride .... <1%
Coloring agent .... <1%
Perfume .... <1%
Water .... balance

SWEET KILL
See CP SWEET KILL

SWEET PEA PERFUME & COLOGNE
(Parfums Duvelle)

Alcohol (denatured with diethyl phthal-ate) *

SWEL
(Lester Labs.)

Chlorinated solvents *

'76 Ed.

SWIM-EAR
For the prevention of swimmer's ear
(Fougera)

Boric acid * 2.75%
Isopropyl alcohol *

SWIMTRINE
Algaecide for swimming pools
(Applied Biochemists)

Copper as elemental (from mixed
  copper ethanolamine
  complexes) * 7.41%

SWINGER
Detergent sanitizer; institutional and commercial use
(Hysan Corp.)

Tetrasodium ethylenediamine
  tetraacetate 1.58%
Anhydrous Sodium
  metasilicate * 4.35%
N-Alkyl (60% C14, 30% C16, 5%
  C12, 5% C18) dimethyl benzyl
  ammonium chlorides 0.75%
N-Alkyl (50% C12, 30% C14, 17%
  C16, 3% C18) dimethyl ethyl-
  benzyl ammonium chlorides .. 0.75%
N-Alkyl (C18-92%, C16-8%) N-
  ethyl   morpholinium   ethyl
  sulfate 0.10%
3,5-Dibromosalicylanilide 0.02%
3,4',5-Tribromosalicylanilide 0.08%
Other related bromosalicylanilides
Inert ingredients: 92.37%
  Cleaning detergents *
  Wetting agents
  Synergizing builders
  Chelating agents
  Perfume
  Water

Starred ingredients (*) may be responsible for major toxic effects; consult Section II.

SWISH
Heavy duty all purpose cleaner
(Haviland Products Co.)

Sodium phosphates *
Cocoanut oil soap
Sodium metasilicate
Ethylene glycol n-butyl ether *

'76 Ed.

SWISH TOILET BOWL CLEANER
(Burnishine)

Hydrochloric acid *

SWISS KRISS
Laxative
(Modern Products)

Dried leaves of Senna
Licorice root
Fennel
Anise
Caraway seed
Dandelion
Peppermint
Papaya
Strawberry, peach and lemon verbena
Cyani flowers
Parsley
Juniper berries

SWITER EMULSION DETERGENT FOR TOILET BOWLS
(Fuld-Stalfort)

Hydrogen chloride *
Perfume
Polyethylene glycol ether of alkylated phenol *

'76 Ed.

S.W. - SWAB CONCRETE CLEANER (Powder)

See GUNK S.W. - SWAB CONCRETE CLEANER (Powder)

S.W.T. TABLETS
Nighttime sleep aid
(Ray Drug)

Each tablet:
  Pyrilamine maleate * .... 25 mg.

SYBIL IVES HAIR CARE PRODUCTS

Sybil Ives, Inc.
635 W. 18th St.
Hialeah, Fla. 33010

Phone: 305-885-1911

See COSMETICS, Section VI, General Formulations

SY-COOL

See SILOO SY-COOL

SYMMETREL
Antiparkinson; antiviral
(Endo Labs.)

Each capsule:
  Amantadine hydrochloride * . 100 mg.

Each 5 ml.:
  Amantadine hydrochloride * . 50 mg.

SYMPADIL
Decongestant
(Cameron Medical Corp.)

Each capsule:
  Phenylephrine HCl .... 5 mg.
  Acetaminophen * .... 325 mg.
  Caffeine .... 30 mg.

SYNA-CLEAR
Decongestant
(Pruvo Pharmacal Co.)

Each tablet:
  Phenylpropanolamine
    hydrochloride * .... 50 mg.
  Pheniramine maleate * .... 12 1/2 mg.
  Pyrilamine maleate * ..... 12 1/2 mg.
  Vitamin C .... 25 mg.

'76 Ed.

SYNALAR CREAM 0.025% AND 0.01%
Topical anti-inflammatory agent
(Syntex Labs.)

Fluocinolone acetonide 0.025% and 0.01%
Aqueous base:
  Stearic acid
  Propylene glycol
  Sorbitan monostearate and monooleate
  Polysorbate 60
  Citric acid
  Methylparaben
  Propylparaben

SYNALAR CREAM VETERINARY
Anti-inflammatory agent
(Syntex Labs.)

Fluocinolone acetonide 0.025%

SYNALAR-HP CREAM
Topical anti-inflammatory agent
(Syntex Labs.)

Fluocinolone acetonide 0.2%
Aqueous base:
  Stearyl alcohol
  Cetyl alcohol
  Mineral oil
  Propylene glycol
  Sorbitan monostearate
  Polysorbate 60
  Citric acid
  Methylparaben
  Propylparaben

SYNALAR OINTMENT
Topical anti-inflammatory agent
(Syntex Labs.)

Fluocinolone acetonide 0.025%
In a base of:
  White petrolatum, USP

SYNALAR SOLUTION
Topical anti-inflammatory agent
(Syntex Labs.)

Fluocinolone acetonide 0.01%
In a base of:
  Propylene glycol
  Citric acid

SYNALAR SOLUTION VETERINARY
Anti-inflammatory agent
(Syntex Labs.)

Fluocinolone acetonide 0.01%

SYNALGOS CAPSULES
Analgesic relaxant
(Ives Labs.)

Each capsule:
  Promethazine
    hydrochloride .... 6.25 mg.
  Acetylsalicylic acid * ..... 356.40 mg.
  Caffeine .... 30.00 mg.

SYNALGOS-DC CAPSULES
Analgesic relaxant
(Ives Labs.)

Each capsule:
  Dihydrocodeine bitar-
    trate * .... 16.00 mg.
  Promethazine
    hydrochloride .... 6.25 mg.
  Acetylsalicylic acid * ..... 356.40 mg.
  Caffeine .... 30.00 mg.

SYNALTRANS-D INSECTICIDE

See AERO-MASTER SYNALTRANS-D INSECTICIDE

SYNEMOL CREAM
Topical anti-inflammatory agent
(Syntex Labs.)

Fluocinolone acetonide 0.025%
Aqueous emollient base:
  Stearyl alcohol
  Cetyl alcohol
  Mineral oil
  Propylene glycol
  Sorbitan monostearate
  Polysorbate 60
  Citric acid

SYNKAYVITE
For vitamin K deficiency and hypo-prothrombinemia
(Roche)

Each tablet:
  Menadiol sodium diphosphate .. 5 mg.

Starred ingredients (*) may be responsible for major toxic effects; consult Section II.

SYNKOLOID PAINT PRODUCTS

Synkoloid Co.
P.O. Box 60937
Los Angeles, Calif. 90060

Phone: 213-263-7121

See PAINTS, Section VI, General Formulations

SYNOPHYLATE ELIXIR
Bronchodilator
(Central Pharmacal Co.)

Each 15 ml.:
Theophylline sodium glycinate
(equiv. to 165 mg.
theophylline) * .... 330 mg.
Alcohol 20%

SYNOPHYLATE-GG SYRUP & TABLETS
Bronchodilator, expectorant
(Central Pharmacal Co.)

Each 15 ml. or tablet:
Theophylline sodium glycinate
(equiv. to 150 mg.
theophylline) * .... 300 mg.
Glyceryl guaiacolate .... 100 mg.
Alcohol (syrup only) 10%

SYNOPHYLATE TABLETS
Bronchodilator
(Central Pharmacal Co.)

Each tablet:
Theophylline sodium glycinate
(equiv. to 165 mg.
theophylline) * .... 330 mg.

SYNOSTAN CAPSULES
For cold symptoms, sinus congestion
(Premo)

Salicylamide *
Pyrilamine maleate *
Ascorbic acid (Vitamin C)
Phenylephrine hydrochloride *
Caffeine
Bioflavinoids

'76 Ed.

SYNOTIC
Otic solution for the relief of pruritus and inflammation in the dog; veterinary
(Syntex Agribusiness)

Fluocinolone acetonide 0.01%
Dimethyl sulfoxide 60%

SYNOVEX-H IMPLANTS VETERINARY
Heifer finishing implants
(Syntex Agribusiness)

Each cartridge:
Testosterone propionate ..... 200 mg.
Estradiol benzoate .... 20 mg.

SYNOVEX-S IMPLANTS VETERINARY
Steer finishing implants
(Syntex Agribusiness)

Each cartridge:
Progesterone .... 200 mg.
Estradiol benzoate .... 20 mg.

SYN-REZ SHIELD COAT
Floor sealer
(Consolidated Chem., Inc.)

Water emulsion latex

SYN SOL
Sanitizer
(Calgon Corp., Commercial Div.)

Chlorinated trisodium phosphate *

SYNTHA D2B
Detergent and chemical cleaner
(National-Purity Soap)

Combination of nonionic and anionic Synthetic detergents *
Sequestering agent

pH of 1% solution, 9.8

SYNTHALOIDS
Anesthetic-antiseptic throat lozenges
(Buffington)

Each lozenge:
Benzocaine
Calcium iodized

SYNTHETAR CREAM
(Vale)

Synthetic Coal tar * 3%
Zinc oxide 10%

SYNTHRIN INDUSTRIAL SPRAY 0.25 (OIL BASE)
Insecticide, indoors
(Fairfield American)

(5-Benzyl-3-furyl)methyl-2,2-dimethyl-3-(2-methylpropenyl)
cyclopropanecarboxylate 0.250%
Related compounds 0.034%
Aromatic petroleum
hydrocarbons 0.329%
Petroleum distillate * 99.375%
Solvents 0.012%

SYNTHROID
Thyroid deficiencies
(Flint Labs.)

Each tablet:
Levothyroxine sodium, USP * ... 25 mcg.; 50 mcg.; 100 mcg.; 150 mcg.; 200 mcg.; 300 mcg.
Lactose, USP
Sugar, powdered, USP (corn starch)
Acacia, USP
Povidone, USP
Polysorbate 80, USP
Magnesium stearate, USP
Talc, USP
Gelatin, USP

SYS-TEM
Insecticide for ornamentals and trees
(Malter International)

Meta-Systox-R (S-
2(Ethylsulfinyl)ethyl O,O-dimethyl phosphorothioate) 2.0%
Aromatic petroleum distillate * .. 51.0%
Methyl isobutyl ketone 40.0%

SYSTOSECT
Systemic insecticide
(Certified Labs.)

O,O-Diethyl-S-(2-
(ethylthio)ethyl)phosphorodithioate * 2%

SYSTOX
Insecticide
(Mobay Chemical Corp.)

Demeton (O,O-Diethyl O-(2-
(ethylthio)ethyl) phosphorothioate mixture with O,O-diethyl S-(2-
(ethylthio)ethyl) phosphorothioate) *

T

TABEX CHLORINE SWIMMING POOL TABLETS
(Pool Equipment, Inc.; Aspen Industries, mfr.)

Trichloro-s-triazinetrione (available chlorine, 85.5%) * 95%

'76 Ed.

TABGARD CHLORINATING TABLETS

See BIO-GUARD TABGARD CHLORINATING TABLETS

Starred ingredients (*) may be responsible for major toxic effects; consult Section II.

TABLOID BRAND A.P.C. WITH CODEINE
Analgesic
(Burroughs Wellcome)

Each tablet:
Aspirin *	227 mg.
Phenacetin *	162 mg.
Caffeine	32 mg.
Codeine phosphate *	
No. 2	15 mg.
No. 3	30 mg.
No. 4	60 mg.

TABU BATH OIL
Sizes - 1/2 oz., & 1 oz.
(Dana Perfumes)

Essential oils *	>1%
Aromatic chemicals	
Isopropyl myristate	

TABU DRY PERFUME
Sachet - 1 oz.
(Dana Perfumes)

Essential oils *	>1%
Aromatic chemicals	
Talcs	
Magnesium silicate	
Iron oxide	

TABU DUSTING POWDER (4 oz.), SHAKER BATH POWDER (2 oz.), & DELUXE DUSTING POWDER (8 oz.)
(Dana Perfumes)

Essential oils *	>1%
Aromatic chemicals	
Talc	
Zinc stearate	
Magnesium carbonate	

TABU EAU DE COLOGNE
Sizes - 2 oz., 4 oz., 8 oz., & 32 oz.
(Dana Perfumes)

Essential oils *	>1%
Aromatic chemicals	
Specially denatured Alcohol (39-C) *	
FD & C Yellow #6	
Deionized water	

TABU LIPSTICK
(Dana Perfumes)

Essential oils	<1%
Aromatic chemicals	
Fatty alcohols	
Fatty acids	
Oils	
Waxes	

TABU MIST CONCENTRATE (Glass Bottle)
Aerosol - 1/2 oz., 1 oz.
(Dana Perfumes)

Essential oils *	>1%
Aromatic chemicals	
Specially denatured Alcohol (39-C) *	
D & C Red #17	
Dichlorotetrafluoroethane	

TABU PERFUME
Sizes - 1/8, 1/4, 1/2, & 1 oz.
(Dana Perfumes)

Essential oils *	>1%
Aromatic chemicals	
Specially denatured Alcohol (39-C) *	
FD & C Yellow #6	

TABU PERFUME MIST (Glass Bottle)
Aerosol - 1/4 oz.
(Dana Perfumes)

Essential oils *	>1%
Aromatic chemicals	
Specially denatured Alcohol (39-C) *	
Azulene	
D & C Red #17	
Dichlorotetrafluoroethane	

TABU PERFUME OIL
Size - 1/4 oz.
(Dana Perfumes)

Essential oils *	>1%
Aromatic chemicals	
Isopropyl myristate	

TABU SKIN PERFUME OIL
Size - 1/4 oz.
(Dana Perfumes)

Essential oils *	>1%
Aromatic chemicals	
Isopropyl myristate	

TABU SOAP
(Dana Perfumes)

Essential oils	>1%
Aromatic chemicals	
Tallow	
Coconut oil	
Glycerine	
Lanolin	
Water	

TABU SOLID COLOGNE
Size - 2 oz.
(Dana Perfumes)

Essential oils *	>1%
Aromatic chemicals	
Specially denatured Alcohol (39-C) *	
Deionized water	
Sodium stearate	
Propylene glycol	
Cetyl alcohol	

TABU SPRAY COLOGNE
Aerosol - 3 oz.
(Dana Perfumes)

Essential oils *	>1%
Aromatic chemicals	
Specially denatured Alcohol (39-C) *	
Distilled water	
Dichlorofluoromethane	
Dichlorotetrafluoroethane	

TABU SPRAY COLOGNE (COLORED)
(Dana Perfumes)

Essential oils *	>1%
Specially denatured Alcohol (39-C) *	
Distilled water	
Dichlorotetrafluoroethane	
D & C Red #17	

T.A.C. CAPSULES
(Towne, Paulsen)

Each capsule:
Pheniramine maleate *	12.5 mg.
Chlorpheniramine maleate	1 mg.
Belladonna alkaloids (total)	0.16 mg.
Phenylpropanolamine HCl *	50 mg.

TACE CAPSULES
Synthetic estrogen
(Merrell Dow)

Green soft gelatin capsule:
Chlorotrianisene in vegetable oil	12 mg.

Hard gelatin capsule:
Chlorotrianisene in tristearin	25 mg.

Green and yellow soft gelatin capsule:
Chlorotrianisene in emulsifiable vehicle	72 mg.

TAGAFED SYRUP
Antihistaminic
(Direct Div.)

Each 5 ml.:
Triprolidine HCl *	1.25 mg
Pseudoephedrine HCl	30 mg.
Sodium benzoate	0.1%
Methyl paraben	0.1%

TAGAFED TABLETS
Antihistaminic
(Direct Div.)

Each tablet:
Triprolidine HCl *	2.5 mg.
Pseudoephedrine HCl	60 mg.

Starred ingredients (*) may be responsible for major toxic effects; consult Section II.

TAGAMET TABLETS & LIQUID
Treatment of duodenal ulcer and gastrointestinal diseases
(SK&F)

Each tablet:
Cimetidine * .... 200 mg.; 300 mg.

Each 5 ml.:
Cimetidine hydrochloride
(equiv. to Cimetidine) * .... 300 mg.
Alcohol 2.8%

TAGATAP SYRUP
Antihistaminic
(Direct Div.)

Each 5 ml.:
Brompheniramine maleate * ... 4 mg.
Phenylephrine HCl * ... 5 mg.
Phenylpropanolamine HCl * ... 5 mg.
Alcohol 2.3%

TAGATAP TABLETS
Antihistaminic
(Direct Div.)

Each tablet:
Brompheniramine maleate * .. 12 mg.
Phenylephrine HCl * .... 15 mg.
Phenylpropanolamine HCl * .. 15 mg.

TAKE NOTICE INSTANT TEMPORARY HAIR COLORING - WINTER WHITE
(Bonat)

	percentage range
Water	90.0-99.0%
Isopropyl alcohol	<1.0%
Sodium borate	<1.0%
Benzyl alcohol	<1.0%
DMHF	<1.0%
Carbomer-940	<1.0%
PED-6 isopalmitate	<1.0%
Cellulose gum	<1.0%
Sodium benzoate	<1.0%
Fragrance	<1.0%
Acid violet 43	trace
Sodium bisulfite	trace

TALBOT'S FABRIC COLOR AEROSOL
Vinyl lacquer
(Talsol)

Methyl ethyl ketone *	54%
Cellosolve acetate *	13%
Toluene *	8%
Resin, Pigment, Plasticizer	4%
Propellant (Propane-butane)	21%

TALLY
Penetrating seal
(Holcomb)

Mineral spirits *	>10%
High flash naphtha *	>10%

'76 Ed.

TALOIN OINTMENT
Diaper rash protective ointment
(Warren-Teed)

Methylbenzethonium chloride *
Zinc oxide, USP
Calamine, USP
Eucalyptol, USP *
Siliconized water-repellent tallow base

TAL-STRIP
Paint stripper
(Talsol)

Methylene chloride *	83%
Methanol	<4%

TALWIN 50
Analgesic for oral use
(Winthrop Labs.)

Each tablet:
Pentazocine HCl (equiv. to 50 mg. base) *

TALWIN COMPOUND
For relief of moderate pain
(Winthrop Labs.)

Each Caplet:
Pentazocine HCl (equivalent to 12.5 mg. base) *
Aspirin .... 325 mg.

TAME HAIR PRODUCTS
(Gillette Co., Personal Care Div.)

The Gillette Co., Personal Care Div., Boston, Mass. 02199 will receive collect phone calls from poison control centers or physicians asking for emergency toxicological information about the company's products.

Phone: 617-421-7000

TAMMS PRODUCTS

Tamms Industries Co.
1222 Ardmore Ave.
Drawer Box C
Itasca, Ill. 60143

Phone: 312-773-2350

TAMOL N
Dispersant
(Rohm and Haas)

Sodium salt of a condensed aryl sulfonic acid *†

†*See* Alkyl aryl sodium sulfonates

TANAC, TANAC STICK & TANAC ROLL-ON
For cracked lips, cold sores & fever blisters
(Commerce Drug)

Tannic acid
Benzocaine
Benzalkonium chloride *

TANDEARIL TABLETS
Anti-inflammatory agent
(Geigy Pharmaceuticals)

Each tablet:
Oxyphenbutazone * .... 100 mg.

TANGLEFOOT TREE PAINT (Liquid)
(Tanglefoot)

Copper naphthenate *
Asphaltum
Petroleum naphtha *

TANIPENT
Vasodilator
(Moffet Inc.)

Each tablet:
Pentaerythritol tetranitrate * .... 10 mg.; 20 mg.

TANUROL OINTMENT
Topical and rectal
(OJF)

Tannic acid	3%
Benzocaine	1%
Phenol	0.75%
Petrolatum base	q.s.

TAPAR
Analgesic
(Parke-Davis)

Each tablet:
Acetaminophen (U.S.P.) * ... 325 mg.

TAPE-OFF, LARSON'S

See LARSON'S TAPE-OFF

TAPE-TAB POWDER
Anthelmintic; veterinary, avian
(Hilltop)

Nicotine alkaloid *
Phenothiazine
2,2'-Dihydroxy-5,5'-dichlorodiphenyl methane
Nux vomica * 6.61%
Anise

'76 Ed.

TAPE-TABS
Anthelmintic; veterinary, avian
(Hilltop)

Nicotine alkaloid *	2.64%
Phenothiazine	19.80%
2,2'-Dihydroxy-5,5'-dichlorodiphenyl methane	14.85%

'76 Ed.

Starred ingredients (*) may be responsible for major toxic effects; consult Section II.

TAPULINE
Antidiarrheal
(Wesley Pharm.)

Each tablet:
Activated Attapulgite .... 600 mg.
Pectin .... 60 mg.
Homatropine methylbromide .. 0.5 mg.

TARACTAN
Management of manifestations of psychotic disorders
(Roche)

Each tablet:
Chlorprothixene * ...... 10 mg.; 25 mg.;
50 mg.; or 100 mg.

Concentrate (each 5 ml.):
Chlorprothixene * .... 100 mg.

TARBONIS CREAM
For eczemas, dermatoses
(Reed & Carnrick)

Special Coal tar extract * 5%

TARCORTIN (Cream and Lotion)
For acute, subacute & chronic dermatoses
(Reed & Carnrick)

Special Coal tar extract
(Tarbonis) * 5.0%
Hydrocortisone, free alcohol 0.5%
Hydrophilic base .... q.s.

TARGET FLOOR FINISH
(Zinsser, Wm., & Co.)

Non-volatiles: 34%
Urea resin & poly non-hydroxy and aldehydic acid condensates
Volatiles: 66%
Alcohols
Aromatic hydrocarbons *

TARLA-DIPHAS RED
Rodenticide
(B&G Co.)

Diphacinone, sodium salt (2-Diphenylacetyl-1,3-indandione, sodium salt) 0.005%

TAR-OFF
Dissolves and emulsifies tar and asphalt; industrial and institutional use
(Scientific International)

Petroleum distillates *
Solvents
Emulsifiers

TARRY
Swim pool disinfectant
(Coastal Industries)

Trichloro-s-triazine *† 100%

†*See* Trichlorotriazinetrione

TARSUM
Shampoo
(Summers Labs.)

Coal tar solution * 10%
Salicylic acid * 5%

TARZOFF
Tar remover
(Holcomb)

Xylene * .... >10%
Dipentene 1-10%

'76 Ed.

TAT ANT TRAP
(Linck)

Baygon * 0.250%

TAT LIQUID ROACH AND ANT KILLER (With Power Spout)
(Linck)

Pyrethrins 0.050%
Piperonyl butoxide, technical .. 0.100%
N-Octyl bicycloheptene
dicarboximide 0.166%
o-Isopropoxyphenyl
methylcarbamate 0.500%
Petroleum distillate * 84.700%

TAT ROACH TRAP
Insecticide
(Linck)

Baygon * 2%

TAYSTRON
Dietary supplement
(Vale)

Each chewable tablet:
Elemental Iron (as ferrous
fumarate) .... 15 mg.
Multivitamins

TCL CHLORINE SANITIZER
Dairy use
(Yale Chem. Co.)

Sodium dichloro-s-triazinetrione
(Sodium
dichloroisocyanurate) * 20.84%

T-D-C (DETERGENT)
(National Chemicals, Inc.)

Nonylphenol polyglycol ether (Nonylphenoxypoly (ethyleneoxy) ethanol) *
Hydroxyacetic acid *
Isopropanol *

T & E 10/02
Estrogen-androgen therapy
(Bio-Factor Labs.)

Each tablet:
Methyltestosterone .... 10 mg.
Ethinyl estradiol .... 0.02 mg.

'76 Ed.

TEAC CLEANING KIT TZ-275
Tape recorder head cleaner
(TEAC Corp.)

Trichlorotrifluoroethane ... approx. 80%
Isopropyl alcohol * .... approx. 20%

TEAC HEAD CLEANER HC-1 (Consumer Version)
Liquid tape recorder head cleaner
(TEAC Corp.)

Trichlorotrifluoroethane 90%
1,1,1-Trichloroethane * 10%

TEAC HEAD CLEANER HC-2 (Professional Version)
Liquid tape recorder head cleaner
(TEAC Corp.)

Trichlorotrifluoroethane 90%
1,1,1-Trichloroethane * 10%

TEAC RUBBER CLEANER RC-1 (Consumer Version)
Liquid tape recorder cleaner
(TEAC Corp.)

Petroleum distillate (Aromatic
naphtha) * 100%

TEAC RUBBER CLEANER RC-2 (Professional Version)
Liquid tape recorder cleaner
(TEAC Corp.)

Petroleum distillate (Aromatic
naphtha) * 100%

TEAC STAINLESS POLISH SP-1 (Consumer Version)
Stereo equipment polish
(TEAC Corp.)

Trichlorotrifluoroethane 88%
Mineral spirits * 10%
Silicone 2%

TEAC STAINLESS POLISH SP-2 (Professional Version)
Stereo equipment polish
(TEAC Corp.)

Trichlorotrifluoroethane 88%
Mineral spirits * 10%
Silicone 2%

Starred ingredients (*) may be responsible for major toxic effects; consult Section II.

TEAR-EFRIN EYE DROPS
Emollient, decongestant
(CooperVision Pharm.)

Hydroxypropyl methylcellulose	0.5%
Phenylephrine HCl	0.12%
Sodium chloride	
Sodium bisulfite	0.05%
Benzalkonium chloride	0.01%
Disodium edetate	0.01%

TEARISOL EYE DROPS
Ocular lubricant, emollient
(CooperVision Pharm.)

Hydroxypropyl methylcellulose	
Sodium & potassium chlorides	
Benzalkonium chloride	0.01%
Disodium edetate	0.01%

TEARS PLUS ARTIFICIAL TEARS
(Allergan Pharm.)

Polyvinyl alcohol	1.4%
Povidone	

TECHNA-SOLVE
Multipurpose safety solvent; heavy duty cleaner and degreaser
(Dolge)

Perchloroethylene *	
Mineral spirits *	

TECHNE BACK RUBBER CONCENTRATE
Insecticide
(Techne Corp.)

Ronnel	6.78%
2,2-Dichlorovinyl dimethyl phosphate	1.58%
Related compounds	0.12%
Petroleum distillate *	91.52%

'76 Ed.

TECHNE 40% BUTYL ESTER TYPE WEEDKILLER
Herbicide
(Techne Corp.)

2,4-D, butyl ester (2,4-D actual acid 32%) *	40%
Aliphatic petroleum solvent *	60%

'76 Ed.

TECHNE BUTYL ESTER WEEDKILLER NO. 4
Herbicide
(Techne Corp.)

2,4-D, butyl ester (equiv. to 46% 2,4-D actual acid) *	57.4%
Aliphatic petroleum solvent *	

'76 Ed.

TECHNE BUTYL ESTER WEEDKILLER NO. 6
Herbicide
(Techne Corp.)

2,4-D, butyl ester (equiv. to 62.5% 2,4-D actual acid) *	79%
Aliphatic petroleum solvent	

'76 Ed.

TECHNE CATTLE GRUB DUST
(Techne Corp.)

Rotenone *	1.67%
Other cube resins	3.33%
Attapulgite clay	95.00%

'76 Ed.

TECHNE CHLORDANE EMULSION CONCENTRATE
Insecticide
(Techne Corp.)

Technical Chlordane *	45%
Aliphatic petroleum solvent *	45%

'76 Ed.

TECHNE CHLORDANE WE 8
Insecticide
(Techne Corp.)

Technical Chlordane *	72%
Aliphatic petroleum solvent *	23%

'76 Ed.

TECHNE COPPER CARBONATE
Fungicide
(Techne Corp.)

Metallic Copper (in basic copper carbonate) *	20.0%

'76 Ed.

TECHNE DAIRY DUST
(Techne Corp.)

Methoxychlor, tech.	10.99%
Piperonyl butoxide, tech.	0.60%
Pyrethrins	0.06%
Wheat flour	88.35%

'76 Ed.

TECHNE DAIRY SPRAY
Insecticide
(Techne Corp.)

Piperonyl butoxide, tech.	0.40%
Pyrethrins	0.04%
Pine oil	1.00%
Petroleum hydrocarbons *	98.56%

'76 Ed.

TECHNE DAIRY SPRAY OIL TYPE
Insecticide
(Techne Corp.)

Mineral oil *	99.67%
Piperonyl butoxide tech.	0.30%
Pyrethrins	0.03%

'76 Ed.

TECHNE 2,4-D AMINE WEEDKILLER
Herbicide
(Techne Corp.)

2,4-D, dimethylamine salt (equiv. to 2,4-D actual acid 41%) *	49.4%

'76 Ed.

TECHNE DSMA CRABGRASS KILLER
Herbicide
(Techne Corp.)

Disodium methyl arsonate, anhydrous (equiv. to 20% disodium methyl arsonate hexahydrate) *	12.6%

'76 Ed.

TECHNE EMULSIFIABLE LINDANE 12-1/2%
Insecticide
(Techne Corp.)

Gamma isomer of benzene hexachloride (from lindane) *	12.50%
Methylated naphthalenes	9.34%
Mesityl oxide	18.41%
Xylene *	48.00%
Cyclohexanone	6.25%

'76 Ed.

TECHNE GRAIN BIN SPRAY
Insecticide
(Techne Corp.)

Methoxychlor, tech.	5%
Petroleum hydrocarbons *	95%

'76 Ed.

TECHNE GRAIN SURFACE SPRAY
Grain treatment
(Techne Corp.)

Deodorized base oil *	97.8%
Piperonyl butoxide technical	2.0%
Pyrethrins	0.2%

'76 Ed.

Starred ingredients (*) may be responsible for major toxic effects; consult Section II.

TECHNE HEPTACHLOR WE 3 LF
Insecticide
(Techne Corp.)

Heptachlor *	31.0%
Related compounds	12.1%
Petroleum distillate	47.9%

'76 Ed.

TECHNE LAWN WEEDKILLER
Herbicide
(Techne Corp.)

2-Ethyl 4-methyl pentanol ester of 2,4-dichlorophenoxyacetic acid *	7.66%
2-Ethyl hexanol ester of 2,4-dichlorophenoxyacetic acid	3.28%
2-Ethyl 4-methyl pentanol ester of 2,4,5-trichlorophenoxypropionic acid	1.83%
2-Ethyl hexanol ester of 2,4,5-trichlorophenoxypropionic acid	0.79%

'76 Ed.

TECHNE LIME SULFUR
(Techne Corp.)

Calcium polysulfides (total combined sulfur not more than 23%) *	29.0%

'76 Ed.

TECHNE LINDANE SEED TREATER
For agricultural use
(Techne Corp.)

Gamma isomer of benzene hexachloride (from lindane) *	15%

'76 Ed.

TECHNE LOW-VOL 2,4-D NO. 4
Herbicide
(Techne Corp.)

2,4-D, 2-ethyl pentanol ester *	
2,4-D, 2-ethyl hexanol ester *	
Aliphatic petroleum hydrocarbons *	30.5%

'76 Ed.

TECHNE MALATHION WE 5
Insecticide
(Techne Corp.)

Malathion (O,O-Dimethyl dithiophosphate of diethyl mercaptosuccinate) *	55%
Xylol *	35%

'76 Ed.

TECHNE METHOXYCHLOR EMULSION CONCENTRATE
Insecticide
(Techne Corp.)

Methoxychlor, tech. *	24%
Methylated naphthalene *	63%
Dimethyl phthalate	10%

'76 Ed.

TECHNE MILLFUME NO. 1
Fumigant
(Techne Corp.)

Carbon tetrachloride *
Carbon bisulfide
Sulfur dioxide

'76 Ed.

TECHNE MILLFUME "66"
Grain treatment
(Techne Corp.)

Carbon tetrachloride *	80.99%
Carbon disulphide	12.02%
Ethylene dibromide	6.60%
Petroleum ether	0.39%

'76 Ed.

TECHNE OILER INSECTICIDE
Insecticide
(Techne Corp.)

Petroleum hydrocarbons *	87.94%
Butoxypolypropylene glycol	7.00%
Toxaphene (tech. chlorinated camphene chlorine content 67% to 69%) *	5.00%
Gamma isomer of benzene hexachloride from lindane	0.06%

'76 Ed.

TECHNE PENTA 10-1 WOOD PRESERVATIVE
(Techne Corp.)

Pentachlorophenol *	34%
Other chlorophenols and related compounds	6%
Aromatic hydrocarbon solvent *	60%

'76 Ed.

TECHNE PYRENONE WHEAT PROTECTANT
Grain treatment
(Techne Corp.)

Technical Piperonyl butoxide	1.10%
Pyrethrins	0.08%

'76 Ed.

TECHNE RAT & MOUSE KILLER
(Techne Corp.)

2-Pivalyl-1,3-indandione	0.025%
Rolled oats	99.975%

'76 Ed.

TECHNE ROTENONE GARDEN DUST
Insecticide
(Techne Corp.)

Rotenone	1.0%
Other cube resins	1.6%
Attapulgite clay	97.4%

'76 Ed.

TECHNE ROTENONE WETTABLE POWDER
Insecticide
(Techne Corp.)

Rotenone *	5%
Other cube resins	10%

'76 Ed.

TECHNE SILVEX E-C NO. 4
Herbicide
(Techne Corp.)

Silvex (2-(2,4,5-Trichlorophenoxy)propionic acid, isooctyl esters) *	71.7%

'76 Ed.

TECHNE 2,4,5-T CONCENTRATE NO. 4
Herbicide
(Techne Corp.)

2,4,5-T, butyl ester *	54.2%
Aliphatic petroleum hydrocarbons *	45.8%

'76 Ed.

TECHNE TOXAPHENE EMULSION CONCENTRATE
Insecticide
(Techne Corp.)

Toxaphene (tech. chlorinated camphene with 67-69% chlorine) *	60%
Aliphatic petroleum solvent *	35%

'76 Ed.

TECHNE VAPONA 2-E
Insecticide
(Techne Corp.)

2,2-Dichlorovinyl dimethyl phosphate *	22.0%
Related compounds	1.7%
Aromatic petroleum solvent *	71.3%

'76 Ed.

Starred ingredients (*) may be responsible for major toxic effects; consult Section II.

TECHNE VAPONA INSECTICIDE 50 OS CONCENTRATE
Insecticide
(Techne Corp.)

2,2-Dichlorovinyl dimethyl
  phosphate * 46.5%
Related compounds 3.5%
Petroleum hydrocarbons 50.0%

'76 Ed.

TEDRAL-25
Bronchodilator
(Parke-Davis)

Each tablet:
  Theophylline * .... 130 mg.
  Ephedrine hydrochloride * .. 24 mg.
  Butabarbital * .... 25 mg.

TEDRAL SA
Bronchodilator
(Parke-Davis)

Each tablet:
  Theophylline * .... 180 mg.
  Ephedrine hydrochloride * .. 48 mg.

TEEBACIN
Antituberculosis agent
(CMC Research Div.)

Each tablet:
  Sodium
    aminosalicylate * . 500 mg.; 690 mg.;
      or 1.0 gm.

TEEBACIN ACID (PAS)
Antituberculosis agent
(CMC Research Div.)

Each tablet:
  p-Aminosalicylic
    acid * .... 500 mg.; or 1000 mg.

Each buffered tablet:
  p-Aminosalicylic acid * ...... 500 mg.
  Buffered with Magnesium glycinate,
    Magnesium carbonate

TEEBACONIN
Antituberculosis agent
(CMC Research Div.)

Each tablet:
  Isoniazid (INH) * .... 50 mg.; 100 mg.;
    or 300 mg.

TEEBACONIN & VITAMIN B6
Antituberculosis agent
(CMC Research Div.)

Each 100 mg. tablet:
  Isoniazid (INH) * .... 100 mg.
  Pyridoxine hydrochloride
    (Vitamin B6) .... 5 mg.; 10 mg.;
      or 50 mg.

Each 300 mg. tablet:
  Isoniazid (INH) * .... 300 mg.
  Pyridoxine hydrochloride (Vi-
    tamin B6) .... 30 mg.

TEENAC CREAM
For acne
(Elder)

Colloidal Sulfur 1.5%
Red mercuric sulfide * 0.5%
Urea

TEGA BARB #1
Relief of pain and tension
(Ortega Pharm.)

Each tablet:
  Aspirin * .... 5 gr.
  Phenobarbital .... 1/4 gr.

TEGA-BRON ELIXIR
(Ortega Pharm.)

Each 15 ml.:
  Theophylline anhydrous * .... 80 mg.
  Alcohol 20%

TEGA-PAP
Analgesic and antipyretic
(Ortega Pharm.)

Each 5 cc:
  Acetaminophen * .... 120 mg.
  Alcohol 10%

TEGA-PAP IMPROVED
*Analgesic, duo-decongestant, antihis-
taminic*
(Ortega Pharm.)

Each tablet:
  N-Acetyl-p-aminophenol * .... 5 gr.
  Phenylpropanolamine HCl * .. 25 mg.
  Phenylephrine HCl .... 10 mg.
  Chlorpheniramine maleate .... 2 mg.

TEGA-TINIC TABLETS
For secondary anemias
(Ortega Pharm.)

Each tablet:
  Vitamin B-12 .... 10 mcg.
  Gastric substance .... 50 mg.
  Thiamine HCl .... 10 mg.
  Ascorbic acid .... 75 mg.
  Folic acid .... 0.033 mg.
  Ferrous sulfate * .... 195 mg.

TEGA-TUSSIN
*Relief of cough and nasal stuffiness due
to common cold*
(Ortega Pharm.)

Each 30 cc:
  Dihydrocodeinone-bitartrate * 25 mg.
  Chlorpheniramine maleate ... 2 mg.
  Potassium guaiacol-sulfonate . 500 mg.
  Phenylephrine HCl * .... 30 mg.

TEGA-ZOL ELIXIR
*For mental and physical depression of
the aged*
(Ortega Pharm.)

Each 5 cc:
  Pentylenetetrazol (Metrazol) * 100 mg.
  Nicotinic acid .... 50 mg.
  d-Amphetamine HCl .... 1.5 mg.

TEGRIN CREAM & SOAP
(Block Drug)

Cream:
  Allantoin 1.7%
  Refined Coal tar extract * 5.0%
  Emollient cream base
  Preservative
  SD Alcohol 23-A 4.0%
  Fragrance

Soap:
  Refined Coal tar extract 2.0%
  Soap base
  Fragrance

TEGRIN LOTION
(Block Drug)

Allantoin 1.7%
Refined Coal tar * 5.0%
Lotion base
Preservative
SD Alcohol 23-A 4.0%
Fragrance

TEGRIN SHAMPOO (CREAM)
(Block Drug)

Refined Coal tar extract * 5%
Sodium lauryl sulfate *
Stearic acid
Preservative
SD Alcohol 23-A 3%
Fragrances

TEGRIN SHAMPOO (LOTION)
(Block Drug)

Refined Coal tar extract * 5%
Sodium lauryl sulfate *
Alkanolamide
Preservative
SD Alcohol 23-A 4.6%
Fragrances

"TEKTOR" PLASTIC TIP MARKER INKS (In Refills Only)

See SHEAFFER "TEKTOR" PLAS-
TIC TIP MARKER INKS (In Refills
Only)

TELDRIN
Timed-release allergy capsules
(MenJ Labs.)

Each capsule:
  Chlorpheniramine maleate * .. 8 mg.
  Maximum strength .... 12 mg.

TELES SUSPENSION
For seborrheic dermatitis
(Torch)

Sulfated suspension of Tellurium
  dioxide * 2.5%

'76 Ed.

Starred ingredients (*) may be responsible for major toxic effects; consult Section II.

TELONE C-17 SOIL FUNGICIDE AND NEMATICIDE
(Dow)

Active ingred.:
　1,3-Dichloropropene 76.3%
　Chloropicrin * 17.1%
Inert ingred.:
　Related Chloropropenes and
　　chloropropanes 6.6%

TEMARIL-P SPANSULE CAPSULES
Relief of pruritus and coughs in dogs and cats
(Norden Labs.)

Each No. 1 capsule:
　Trimeprazine tartrate (equiv. to
　　3.75 mg. trimeprazine) * . . . 4.7 mg.
　Prednisolone . . . . 1 mg.

Each No. 2 capsule:
　Trimeprazine tartrate (equiv. to
　　7.5 mg. trimeprazine) * . . . . 9.4 mg.
　Prednisolone . . . . 2 mg.

TEMARIL-P TABLETS
Relief of pruritus and coughs; dogs
(Norden Labs.)

Each tablet:
　Trimeprazine (as the tartrate) * 5 mg.
　Prednisolone . . . . 2 mg.

TEMASEPT I
Germicide
(Fine Organics, Inc.)

Dibromsalan 50%
Tribromsalan * 50%

'76 Ed.

TEMASEPT IV (TBS)
Bacteriostatic & deodorizing component
(Fine Organics, Inc.)

3,4',5-Tribromosalicylanilide * . . . 99.1%

'76 Ed.

TEMPLAR COPY PENCIL
(Reliance Pen & Pencil)

Cellulose gum
Water-soluble dye
Pigment colors (not dye)
Fatty acid esters
Talc

TEMPRA
Analgesic, antipyretic
(Mead Johnson)

Drops (each 0.6 ml.):
　Acetaminophen * . . . . 60 mg.

Syrup (each 5 ml.):
　Acetaminophen * . . . . 120 mg.

TEM-PRA-TONE TEMPERA
(Binney & Smith)

Soluble Starches
Glycerine
Preservative
Non-toxic pigments

TENALATE OINTMENT
Antifungal
(Wesley Pharm.)

Undecylenic acid 5%
Zinc undecylenate 20%

10° BELOW
Automotive
(Garry Labs.)

Methyl alcohol *
Water

TENDER LEAF HOUSE PLANT FOOD

See DEXOL TENDER LEAF HOUSE
　PLANT FOOD

TENDER-LEAF PLANT SPRAY

See DEXOL TENDER-LEAF PLANT
　SPRAY

TENDER LEAF PLANT STARTER

See DEXOL TENDER LEAF PLANT
　STARTER

"10-4" CHEMICAL BILLY
Pressurized CN stream; personal protection
(Penguin Industries)

CN (Chloracetophenone) * . . . . . . <0.9%

10 MINUTE FLUSH
Automotive, cooling system cleaner
(Radiator)

n-Butanol *
Olefins *

'76 Ed.

10-MINUTE RADIATOR FLUSH (AS-105 (Aqueous)/ AS-106 Formula 8623-49)

See PRESTONE 10-MINUTE RADIA-
　TOR FLUSH (AS-105 (Aqueous)/
　AS-106 Formula 8623-49)

10-MINUTE RADIATOR FLUSH (AS-105 (Solvent), Formula 2017-20A)

See PRESTONE 10-MINUTE RADIA-
　TOR FLUSH (AS-105 (Solvent), For-
　mula 2017-20A)

TENORAN 50WP
Herbicide
(Ciba-Geigy Ag. Div.)

Chloroxuron * 50%

TEN-SET
Epoxy adhesive & putty; general use
(Fibre Glass-Evercoat)

Tube A:
　Epoxy resin

Tube B:
　Amine hardeners *

TENSE-X
Analgesic, sedative
(Wesley Pharm.)

Each tablet:
　Panitone (Wesley brand of
　　Acetaminophen) * . . . . 300 mg.
　Methapyrilene
　　hydrochloride * . . . . 25 mg.

TEN-SOL LEG PAINT
Veterinary
(Thoroughbred)

Alcohol 59.17%
Potassium iodide *
Menthol *
Oils of wormwood *
Peppermint *
Methyl salicylate *
Ethyl aminobenzoate

TENUATE
For hunger control
(Merrell Dow)

Each tablet:
　Diethylpropion hydrochloride * 25 mg.

TENUATE DOSPAN
For hunger control
(Merrell Dow)

Each controlled-release tablet:
　Diethylpropion hydrochloride * 75 mg.

TERA-SEAL
Floor seal
(Hillyard Chem.)

Aromatic solvent naphtha *

'76 Ed.

TERCODRYL SYRUP
For allergic & asthmatic coughs, etc.
(Approved Pharm.)

Each fl. oz.:
　Codeine phosphate * . . . . 3/4 gr.
　Pyrilamine maleate * . . . . 25 mg.
　Terpin hydrate *
　Sodium citrate
　Menthol *
　Glycerin
　Honey
　Sugar syrup

'76 Ed.

TERCOL JUNIOR COUGH SYRUP
For children
(Commerce Drug)

D-Methorphan hydrobromide *
Cocillana *
Potassium guaiacol sulfonate *
Ammonium chloride
Alcohol 2%

TERFONYL (SUSPENSION & TABLETS)
(Squibb)

Each 5 cc. tsp. & each tablet:
Squibb Triple Sulfas (Trisulfapyrimi-
dines, USP)
Sulfadiazine * .... 0.167 gm.
Sulfamerazine * .... 0.167 gm.
Sulfamethazine * .... 0.167 gm.

TERG-A-ZYME
Laboratory detergent
(Alconox)

Hydrocarbon sulfonates (derived from lin-
ear alkylates, biodegradable) *†
Complex Phosphates *
Protease enzyme

†*See* Alkyl aryl sodium sulfonates

TERGIQUAT GERMICIDAL CLEANER
(Nat'l Labs. Div.)

Alkyl (50% C14, 40% C12, 10% C16)
dimethyl benzyl ammonium
chloride * 2.3%
Tetrasodium
ethylenediaminetetraacetate ... 1.9%
Didecyl dimethyl ammonium
chloride 0.7%
Sodium carbonate .... minor
Sodium bicarbonate .... minor
Ethoxylated Alcohol .... minor

TERGISYL PREMEASURED DETERGENT DISINFECTANT
(Nat'l Labs. Div.)

Potassium o-benzyl-p-
chlorophenate 0.45%
Tetrasodium
ethylenediaminetetraacetate 0.97%
Sodium carbonate .... minor
Sodium bicarbonate .... minor

TERIDOL JR. COUGH SYRUP
(Approved Pharm.)

Terpin hydrate *
Cocillana *
Potassium guaiacol sulfonate *
Ammonium chloride

'76 Ed.

TERMACIDE
Water repellent wood preservative
(Honolulu Wood Treating Co.)

Pentachlorophenol * 5.0%
Petroleum hydrocarbons * 88.9%

TERMICIDE 5-15
Herbicide
(Terminal Grain)

2,4-Dichlorophenoxyacetic acid
triethanolamine salt (equiv. to
3.43% 2,4-dichlorophenoxy-
acetic acid) 5.75%
Triethanolamine
methanearsonate * 15.80%

'76 Ed.

TERM-I-KILL
Control of subterranean termites
(ABCO, Inc.)

Technical Chlordane 2.00%
Petroleum distillates * 23.00%

TERMINIX A4
Insecticide
(Terminix)

Aldrin * 42%
Aromatic petroleum derivative
product * 50%

TERMINIX 3A3B
Insecticide, wood preservative
(Terminix)

Mineral spirits *
Trichlorobenzene *
Beta naphthol *
Butoxyethanol *
Diacetone alcohol *
Pine oil *
Technical Chlordane *

TERMINIX AERO TERM
Industrial insecticide
(Terminix)

Pyrethrins I & II 0.700%
Technical Piperonyl butoxide ... 1.000%
Rotenoids & other cube resins .. 0.067%
Rotenone 0.033%
Butoxypolypropylene glycol 4.000%
Refined Petroleum oil * 14.200%

Inactive ingred.: 80.000%
Propellent gas

TERMINIX BTL
Insecticide
(Terminix)

Mineral spirits * 99.50%
Lindane 0.50%

TERMINIX C8
Insecticide
(Terminix)

Technical Chlordane * 72%
Petroleum distillate 21%

TERMINIX GP-MAL CONCENTRATE
Insecticide
(Terminix)

Malathion * 55.0%
Xylene * 32.2%

TERMINIX H3
Insecticide
(Terminix)

Heptachlor * 27.70%
Related compounds 10.80%
Aromatic petroleum derivative
solvents * 56.50%

TERMINIX INSIDE RESIDUAL DUST
Insecticide
(Terminix)

Carbaryl (1-Naphthyl N-
methylcarbamate) * 2.0%
Technical Piperonyl butoxide 1.0%
Pyrethrins 0.1%
Inert ingredients: 96.9%
Pyrophylite

TERMINIX MFG CONCENTRATE
Insecticide
(Terminix)

Deodorized Kerosene * 81.5%
Technical Piperonyl butoxide 5.0%
Pyrethrins 1.0%

TERMINIX PROFESSIONAL FLY KILLER
Insecticide
(Terminix)

2,2-Dichlorovinyl dimethyl
phosphate * 0.46%
Related compounds 0.04%

TERMINIX PROFESSIONAL INSECTICIDE
(Terminix)

Hydrogenated rotenone and
other cube resins 0.302%
Pyrethrins I and II 0.201%
Alpha terpineol 5.035%
1-Limonene 0.907%
Petroleum distillate refined * .. 13.760%
1,1,1-Trichloroethane 7.667%
N-Octyl sulfoxide of isosafrol ... 0.675%
Related compounds 0.092%
Butoxypolypropylene glycol 3.833%
Isopropyl alcohol 0.766%
Para diisobutyl phenoxyethoxy-
ethyl dimethyl benzyl ammo-
nium chloride 0.096%

TERMINIX PROFESSIONAL RAT KILL
Rodenticide
(Terminix)

3-(alpha-Acetonylfurfuryl) 4-hydroxycou-
marin
Corn meal or similar products

TERMINIX WP
Insecticide, wood preservative
(Terminix)

Mineral spirits *
Pentachlorophenol *
2-Butoxyethanol *
Beta naphthol *
Tetrachlorophenols *

TERMITE-I-CIDE 500
Insecticide
(Terminal Grain)

Technical Chlordane (equivalent to
14.4% octochloro-4,7-methanote-
trahydroindane and 9.6% related
compounds) 24%
Aldrin * 12%

'76 Ed.

TERPACOF
Cough sedative & expectorant
(Jenkins Labs.)

Each 5 ml.:
  Codeine phosphate * .... 10 mg.
  Terpin hydrate .... 88 mg.
  Alcohol 42%

TERPEX JR. COUGH SYRUP
(Approved Pharm.)

D-Methorphan * .... 25 mg.
Terpin hydrate *
Potassium guaiacol sulfonate
Cocillana *
Ammonium chloride

'76 Ed.

TERPHAN ELIXIR
Expectorant & cough suppressant
(Vale)

Each 5 ml.:
  Alcohol 40%
  Terpin hydrate .... 85 mg.
  Dextromethorphan
    hydrobromide .... 10 mg.

TERRACHLOR 2 LBS. EMULSIFIABLE
Fungicide
(Olin Corporation)

Pentachloronitrobenzene 24%
Aromatic petroleum
  distillates * .... approx. 70%

TERRACLOR SUPER-X EMULSIFIABLE
Soil fungicide
(Olin Corporation)

Pentachloronitrobenzene 23.2%
5-Ethoxy-3-(trichloromethyl)-
  1,2,4-thiadiazole 5.8%
Aromatic petroleum
  distillates * .... approx. 65%

TERRACLOR TECHNICAL
Soil fungicide
(Olin Corporation)

Pentachloronitrobenzene * 99.0%
Related compounds 1.0%

TERRA-COAT LT-2 SEED TREATMENT FUNGICIDE
(Olin Corporation)

Pentachloronitrobenzene 24%
Aromatic petroleum
  distillates * .... approx. 70%

TERRADRESS TERRAZZO MAINTAINER
(Uncle Sam)

Surfactants *
Chelaters
Polymers
Resins (modified phenolics)
Polyethylene
Ammonia *
Glycol ethers *
Plasticizers
Dye
Water

TERRA-FLO 2 FLOWABLE SEED TREATMENT FUNGICIDE
(Olin Corporation)

Pentachloronitrobenzene 20%
Petroleum distillates * .... approx. 40%

TERRAZZINE
Floor polish
(Hillyard Chem.)

Mineral spirits *

'76 Ed.

TERRAZZO SEAL
Floor sealer
(Sanitek)

Blend of: 88.7%
  Toluene *
  Xylene *
Polystyrene resin 10.4%
Chlorinated paraffin resin 0.9%

TERRO ANT KILLER
Insecticide
(Senoret)

Sodium arsenate * 2.27%

TERR-O-CIDE 15
For control of soil pests
(Great Lakes Chem. Corp.)

Ethylene dibromide 40%
Chloropicrin * 15%
Inert: 45%
  Solvent (equiv. Diesel #2)

TERR-O-CIDE 54-45
Fumigant
(Great Lakes Chem. Corp.)

Ethylene dibromide 54%
Chloropicrin * 45%

TERR-O-CIDE 72-27
Fumigant
(Great Lakes Chem. Corp.)

Ethylene dibromide 72%
Chloropicrin * 27%

TERR-O-GAS 67
Fumigant
(Great Lakes Chem. Corp.)

Methyl bromide 67%
Chloropicrin * 32%

TERRO ROACH KILLER
Insecticide
(Senoret)

Sodium fluoride * 32%
Sodium fluosilicate 8%

"TERSAN" LSR TURF FUNGICIDE
(Du Pont)

Maneb * 80%

"TERSAN" 75 TURF FUNGICIDE
(Du Pont)

Thiram * 75%

"TERSAN" 1991 TURF FUNGICIDE
(Du Pont)

Benomyl 50%

TESTOR'S CEMENT FOR PLASTIC MODELS
(Testor)

High molecular weight Polystyrene resin
Petroleum toluol *
Allyl isothiocyanate 0.25%

TESTOR'S ENGINE FUEL
(Testor)

Methanol *
Nitromethane *
Carbide and Carbon's Ucon oil

TESTOR'S HOUSEHOLD CEMENT
(Testor)

Cellulose nitrate
Di-octyl phthalate
Isopropyl alcohol *
Isopropyl acetate *
Acetone *
Butyl acetate *
Allyl isothiocyanate 0.25%

TESTOR'S MODEL CEMENT FORMULA A
(Testor)

Cellulose acetate
Alkyl phosphate (Santicizer 141, Monsanto) *
Acetone *
Allyl isothiocyanate 0.25%

TESTOR'S MODEL CEMENT FORMULA B
(Testor)

Cellulose nitrate
Di-octyl phthalate
Isopropyl alcohol *
Isopropyl acetate *
Acetone *
Butyl acetate *
Allyl isothiocyanate 0.25%

TESTOR'S PLA
Paint for plastics
(Testor)

Vinyl-toluene alkyd
Mineral spirits *
Driers *
Pigments:
WHITE:
  Titanium dioxide
BLACK:
  Lampblack
BLUES:
  Phthalocyanine blue *†
  Titanium dioxide
BROWNS:
  Iron oxide *
  Titanium dioxide
REDS:
  Calcium 2 B red
  Benzidine orange
YELLOWS:
  Benzidine yellows
  Titanium dioxide
GREENS:
  Phthalocyanine green *†
  Benzidine yellows
ORANGE:
  Benzidine orange
  Titanium dioxide
SILVER:
  Aluminum powder
GOLD:
  Bronze powder
COPPER:
  Copper powder *
PINKS:
  Calcium 2 B red
  Benzidine orange
  Titanium dioxide
PURPLES:
  Maroon toner (Pigment red 52)
  Titanium dioxide
  Phthalocyanine blue *†

†*See* Pigments, Section VI, General Formulations

TESTOR'S SPRAY PLA (AEROSOL)
Spray paint for plastics
(Testor)

Vinyl-toluene alkyd
Mineral spirits *
Methylene chloride *
Hydrocarbon propellant
  70% Propane
  30% Isobutane
Driers *
Pigments:
WHITE:
  Titanium dioxide
BLACK:
  Lampblack
BLUES:
  Phthalocyanine blue *†
  Titanium dioxide
BROWNS:
  Iron oxide *
  Titanium dioxide
REDS:
  Calcium 2 B red
  Benzidine orange
YELLOWS:
  Benzidine yellows
  Titanium dioxide
GREENS:
  Phthalocyanine green *†
  Benzidine yellows
ORANGE:
  Benzidine orange
  Titanium dioxide
SILVER:
  Aluminum powder
GOLD:
  Bronze powder
COPPER:
  Copper powder *
PINKS:
  Calcium 2 B red
  Benzidine orange
  Titanium dioxide
PURPLES:
  Maroon toner (Pigment red 52)
  Titanium dioxide
  Phthalocyanine blue *†

†*See* Pigments, Section VI, General Formulations

TETLES
(Lester Labs.)

Chlorinated solvents *

'76 Ed.

TETRA 25, MUNICHEM

See MUNICHEM TETRA 25

TETRACAINE HYDROCHLORIDE DROPERETTE
Topical anesthetic
(CooperVision Pharm.)

Tetracaine hydrochloride 0.5%
Chlorobutanol 0.4%

Starred ingredients (*) may be responsible for major toxic effects; consult Section II.

TETRA CAPSULES
Decongestant, analgesic
(Reese Chem.)

Each capsule:
Phenylpropanolamine
hydrochloride * .... 18 mg.
Acetaminophen .... 325 mg.

TETRACHEL
Broad and medium spectrum antibiotic
(Rachelle Labs.)

Each capsule:
Tetracycline
hydrochloride ..... 250 mg.; 500 mg.

TETRALATE MULTI-PURPOSE INSECTICIDE E.C. (OIL BASE)
Indoor and outdoor use
(Fairfield American)

Tetramethrin 2.50%
Related compounds 0.34%
Resmethrin 2.50%
Related compounds 0.46%
Aromatic petroleum
hydrocarbons * 20.00%
Petroleum distillate * 10.00%
Emulsifiers * 60.00%
Solvents 4.20%

TETRANOL
Biodegradable anionic wetting agent
(Arkansas Co.)

Sodium sulfate of a fatty acid ester *

'76 Ed.

TETRA-SOL SPOT REMOVER
(Midwest Mfg.)

Odorless Mineral spirits *
Chlorothene *

TETROX
Powdered hand dishwashing cleaner
(Economics)

Sodium tripolyphosphate *
Sodium bicarbonate
Alkyl aryl sodium sulfonate *
Sodium sulfate

pH is 8.5

TETTERINE OINTMENT, POWDER & SOAP
(Shuptrine)

Shuptrine Co.
P.O. Box 22127
Savannah, Ga. 31403

Phone: 912-232-8303

See COSMETICS, Section VI, General
Formulations

TEXACO ANTIFREEZE AND SUMMER COOLANT
(Texaco Canada Ltd.)

Ethylene glycol *
Sodium arsenite *
Dye

TEXACO BRAKE FLUID SUPER HEAVY DUTY
(Texaco Canada Ltd.)

Glycols *†
Glycol ethers *

†*See* Ethylene glycol

TEXACO CARBURETOR CLEANER AND ENGINE TUNE-UP
(Texaco Canada Ltd.)

Petroleum distillate *
Aromatic solvent *
Diacetone alcohol

TEXACO CHARCOAL LIGHTER FLUID
(Texaco Canada Ltd.)

Petroleum distillate *

TEXACO COTTON PICKER OIL R & O 150
(Texaco Inc.)

Petroleum lubricating oil
Oxidation and corrosion inhibitor *†

†*See* Rust control, Section VI, General
Formulations

TEXACO CUP GREASE
(Texaco Inc.)

Mineral oil *
Calcium soap

TEXACO FUEL SYSTEM DE-ICER
(Texaco Canada Ltd.)

Methanol *
Morpholine *

TEXACO HOUSEHOLD CLEANING SOLVENT
(Texaco Canada Ltd.)

Petroleum distillate (mineral spirit type) *

TEXACO MOTOR OIL
(Texaco Inc.)

Petroleum lubricating oil
Calcium detergent *†
Oxidation and corrosion inhibitor *‡

†*See* Detergents (synthetic)
‡*See* Rust Control, Section VI, General
Formulations

TEXACO OUTBOARD GEAR OIL EP 90
(Texaco Inc.; Texaco Canada Ltd.)

Petroleum lubricating oil
Phosphorous and Sulfur inhibitor *†

†*See* Rust Control, Section VI, General
Formulations

TEXACO RADIATOR ANTI-RUST AND WATER PUMP LUBRICANT
(Texaco Canada Ltd.)

Emulsifiers
Corrosion inhibitors *†
Water

†*See* Rust control, Section VI, General
Formulations

TEXACO RADIATOR FAST FLUSH
(Texaco Canada Ltd.)

Ethylene glycol *
Sodium bichromate *
Alkaline buffers
Water

TEXACO RADIATOR STOP LEAK
(Texaco Canada Ltd.)

Cellulose
Clays
Mineral oil *
Sulfonates *†
Water

†*See* Alkyl sodium sulfonates

TEXACORT SCALP LOTION
Topical steroid/anti-inflammatory
(CooperCare)

Hydrocortisone 1%
Alcohol 33%
Propylene glycol
Polysorbate 20
Benzalkonium chloride
Water

TEXACO SUPER CAR CLEANER AND WAX
(Texaco Canada Ltd.)

Waxes
Petroleum distillate *
Silicon dioxide

TEXACO SUPER MOTOR DETERGENT
(Texaco Canada Ltd.)

Ashless Detergent
Calcium detergent
Mineral oil *

TEXACO TDH OIL
(Texaco Inc.)

Petroleum lubricating oil
Calcium detergent
Oxidation and corrosion inhibitor *†
Dye

†See Rust control, Section VI, General
Formulations

TEXACO TIRE MOUNTING FLUID CONCENTRATE
(Texaco Canada Ltd.)

Ethylene glycol *
Surfactants *
Alkaline buffer
Water
Perfume

TEXACO TORQUE FLUID C-2
(Texaco Inc.)

Petroleum lubricating oil
Corrosion and oxidation inhibitor *†

†See Rust Control, Section VI, General
Formulations

TEXACO TRACK ROLL LUBRICANT
Grease
(Texaco Inc.)

Mineral oil *
Calcium soap

TEXAMATIC FLUID
(Texaco Inc.; Texaco Canada Ltd.)

Petroleum lubricating oil
Oxidation and corrosion inhibitor *†
Dye

†See Rust Control, Section VI, General
Formulations

"TEXASPHALTIC"
Preservative for commercial fishing nets and gear, and wood
(Texasphaltic Co.)

Copper naphthenate (equiv. to 2% of copper expressed as metallic)	25%
Ester gums	10%
Petroleum distillate *	65%

TEXAS REFINERY PAINT PRODUCTS

Texas Refinery Corp.
P.O. Box 711
Ft. Worth, Texas 76101

Phone: 817-332-1161

See PAINTS, Section VI, General Formulations

TEXAS STAR FLY REPELLANT & WOUND DRESSING
(Pearson & Co.)

Pine tar *	38%
Bone oil (anhydrous)	23%
Mineral oil	8%
Pine oil	5%
Turkey red oil	2%

'76 Ed.

TEXAS STAR SCREWWORM KILLER
Insecticide
(Pearson & Co.)

Benzol *	47.5%
Pine tar *	47.5%
Pine oil	5.0%

'76 Ed.

"TEXAS-T" CATTLE OIL
Control of hornflies
(McConnell Equipment Corp.)

Ronnel (O,O-Dimethyl O-(2,4,5-trichlorophenyl)-phosphorothioate)	1.0%
Pine oil	2.0%
Refined Mineral oil *	97.0%

'76 Ed.

"TEXAS-T" CATTLE OIL FORMULA NO. 2
Control of lice and hornflies
(McConnell Equipment Corp.)

Malathion	2%
Pine oil	2%
Refined Mineral oil *	96%

'76 Ed.

"TEXAS-T" DAIRY OIL
Control of hornflies and face flies
(McConnell Equipment Corp.)

Ciodrin (Dimethyl phosphate of alpha-methylbenzyl 3-hydroxy-cis-crotonate) *	1.0%
Pine oil	2.0%
Refined Mineral oil *	97.0%

'76 Ed.

TEXINOL
Liquid cleaner
(Legge, W.)

Pine oil *
Surfactants *

TEXIZE BATHROOM FANTASTIK
Household cleaner/disinfectant
(Texize)

Sodium dodecylbenzenesulfonate	0.6%
Sodium o-benzyl-p-chlorophenate	0.5%

TEXIZE FANTASTIK SPRAY CLEANER
Household cleaner
(Texize)

Glycol ether	2.0-3.0%
Synthetic detergents	0.4-0.6%
Inorganic builders, dye, chelating agents	
Water	95.0-96.0%

TEXIZE FLUF RINSE
(Texize)

Quaternary ammonium compound *	1-3%
Synthetic detergents	<1%
Isopropanol	<1%
Water	97-98%

TEXIZE GLASS *PLUS
Glass cleaner
(Texize)

Ammonia as NH3	<1%
Isopropanol	
Glycol ether	
Synthetic detergent	5-8%
Water	92-96%

TEXIZE GREASE RELIEF
Grease remover
(Texize)

Synthetic nonionic and anionic detergents & amides	9-10%
Inorganic builders, perfume, dye, and preservatives	4-5%
Water	85-86%

TEXIZE JANITOR-IN-A-DRUM
Household cleaner
(Texize)

Synthetic detergents	2-5%
Builders, stabilizers, dye, perfume	<1%
Pine oil	<1%
Water	94-95%

TEXIZE K2r SPOT LIFTER (Aerosol)
Spot remover for fabrics
(Texize)

Combined amount:	40-45%
Aliphatic hydrocarbons *	
Petroleum hydrocarbons *	
Chlorinated hydrocarbons *	
Propellant	45-50%

TEXIZE K2r SPOT LIFTER (Paste)
Spot remover for fabrics
(Texize)

Combined amount:	85-95%
Aliphatic petroleum solvents *	
Aromatic petroleum solvents *	
Isopropyl alcohol *	

Starred ingredients (*) may be responsible for major toxic effects; consult Section II.

TEXIZE NO-PEST FARM STRIP INSECTICIDE
(Texize)

2,2-Dichlorovinyl dimethyl phosphate *	19.2%
Related compounds	0.8%

TEXIZE NO-PEST FLEA AND TICK KILLER
(Texize)

Chlorpyrifos *	0.50%
Aromatic solvent	0.33%

TEXIZE NO-PEST GARDEN INSECT SPRAY
(Texize)

Pyrethrins	0.02%
Piperonyl butoxide (technical)	0.20%
Petroleum distillate	0.08%

TEXIZE NO-PEST HOME INSECT CONTROL
(Texize)

O,O-Diethyl-O-(2-isopropyl-6-methyl-4-pyrimidinyl) phosphorothioate	0.500%
Piperonyl butoxide (technical)	0.260%
Petroleum distillate	0.208%
Pyrethrins	0.052%

TEXIZE NO-PEST INDOOR FOGGER
(Texize)

d-trans Allethrin (allyl homolog of Cinerin I)	0.300%
Related compounds of the above	0.023%
3-Phenoxybenzyl d-cis and trans 2,2-dimethyl-3-(2-methylpropenyl) cyclopropanecarboxylate	0.191%
Other isomers of the above	0.009%
Petroleum distillate *	14.477%

TEXIZE NO-PEST INDUSTRIAL STRIP INSECTICIDE
(Texize)

2,2-Dichlorovinyl dimethyl phosphate *	19.2%
Related compounds	0.8%

TEXIZE NO-PEST PROFESSIONAL STRENGTH ANT AND ROACH KILLER
(Texize)

2,2-Dichlorovinyl dimethyl phosphate *	19.2%
Related compounds	0.8%
Chlorpyrifos	0.500%
Petroleum distillate *	95.848%

TEXIZE NO-PEST STRIP
(Texize)

2,2-Dichlorovinyl dimethyl phosphate *	19.2%
Related compounds	0.8%

TEXIZE PINE HOUSEHOLD CLEANER
(Texize)

Sulfated and nonionic detergents and amides	10-15%
Pine oil	5-7%
Water	75-80%
Combined amount:	1-5%
Glycol ethers	
Inorganic salts	
Dyes	

TEXIZE PINE POWER DISINFECTANT
(Texize)

Pine oil *	19.9%
Combined amount:	12-13%
Isoproponal *	
Denatured Ethanol	
Anionic surfactants, Ethylenediamine tetraacetic acid	13-14%
Water	52-54%

TEXIZE PINK LOTION FOR DISHES
Dish detergent
(Texize)

Sulfated and sulfonated synthetic detergents *†	20-25%
Dye, Perfume, Preservative, & Inorganic salts	1-3%
Water	72-77%

†See Anionic synthetic detergents

TEXIZE SPRAY 'N STARCH
(Texize)

Cellulose gum	1.0–2.0%
Ironing aids, Preservatives, and Perfume	0.3–0.5%
Water	98.0–99.0%

TEXIZE SPRAY 'N WASH (Aerosol)
Laundry soil and stain remover
(Texize)

Aliphatic petroleum distillate *	18.0–19.0%
Synthetic detergents, Solubilizers, and Perfume	27.0–28.0%
Water	45.0–46.0%
Propellant (hydrocarbon)	6.5–7.5%

TEXIZE SPRAY 'N WASH (Liquid Spray)
Laundry soil and stain remover
(Texize)

Nonionic and anionic surfactants	10-15%
Dye, perfume, and preservative	<1%
Water	88-92%

TEXIZE SPRING SCENT CLEANER
Household cleaner
(Texize)

Anionic and nonionic synthetic detergents	5-7%
Water	93-95%
Combined amount:	<1%
Sodium silicate	
Perfume	
Dye	

TEXIZE WOOD PLUS
Furniture cleaner and polish
(Texize)

Silicone and Anionic synthetic detergents	3-5%
Denatured Ethanol, Preservatives, Perfume, and Emulsifiers	2-4%
Water	93-96%

TEXIZE YES
Liquid laundry detergent and softener
(Texize)

Synthetic detergents, * Amides, and Soap	30-40%
Dyes, Preservatives, and Perfume	1% max.
Water	62-67%

TEXOFF II
Stain remover
(ABCO, Inc.)

Hydrofluoric acid *

T-F-7
Insecticide - veterinary
(Carson Chemicals, Inc.)

Sevin *	5%

TFE DRY FILM (Aerosol)
(Cling-Surface)

Methylene chloride *	30%
Toluol *	7%
1,1,1-Trichloroethane *	17%
Propane/Isobutane	30%

THALFED TABLETS
Antiasthmatic
(Beecham Labs.)

Each tablet:

Phenobarbital	8 mg.
Theophylline, hydrous *	0.12 gm.
Ephedrine hydrochloride *	25 mg.

Starred ingredients (*) may be responsible for major toxic effects; consult Section II.

THANTIS LOZENGES
Local analgesic & antiseptic for throat
& mouth irritations
(Hynson, Westcott & Dunning, Inc.)

Each lozenge:
Merodicein (Disodium salt of
monohydroxymercuridiio-
doresorcinsulfonphthalein) .. 1/8 gr.
Saligenin (Orthohydroxy-ben-
zyl-alcohol) .... 1 gr.
'76 Ed.

T-H DED-WEED BE-4D
Herbicide
(Thompson-Hayward)

2,4-D, butyl ester * .... 4 lb./gal.
Kerosene *

T-H DED-WEED BE-6D
Herbicide
(Thompson-Hayward)

2,4-D, butyl ester * .... 6 lb./gal.
Kerosene *

T-H DED-WEED LV-4T
Herbicide
(Thompson-Hayward)

2,4,5-T * .... 4 lb./gal.
Kerosene *

T-H DED-WEED LV-6T
Herbicide
(Thompson-Hayward)

2,4,5-T * .... 6 lb./gal.
Kerosene *

THE DRY LOOK HAIR SPRAYS
(Gillette Co., Personal Care Div.)

The Gillette Co., Personal Care Div.,
Boston, Mass. 02199 will receive collect
phone calls from poison control centers or
physicians asking for emergency toxicological information about the company's
products.

Phone: 617-421-7000

THE HANDLER SHAMPOOS AND CONDITIONERS
(Gillette Co., Personal Care Div.)

The Gillette Co., Personal Care Div.,
Boston, Mass. 02199 will receive collect
phone calls from poison control centers or
physicians asking for emergency toxicological information about the company's
products.

Phone: 617-421-7000

THEOBID
Bronchodilator
(Glaxo Inc.)

Each Duracap capsule:
Theophylline (anhydrous) * .. 260 mg.

THEOBID JR.
Bronchodilator
(Glaxo Inc.)

Each Duracap capsule:
Theophylline * .... 130 mg.

THEOCLEAR L.A.-130 AND -260 CENULES
Bronchodilator
(Central Pharmacal Co.)

Each time-release capsule:
Theophylline
(anhydrous) * .... 130 mg.; 260 mg.

THEOCLEAR-80 SYRUP
Bronchodilator
(Central Pharmacal Co.)

Each 15 ml.:
Theophylline (anhydrous) * .. 80 mg.

THEOCLEAR-100 and -200 TABLETS
Bronchodilator
(Central Pharmacal Co.)

Each tablet:
Theophylline
(anhydrous) * .... 100 mg.; 200 mg.

THEO-COL CAPSULES & ELIXIR
(Columbia Med.)

Each capsule or 15 ml.:
Theophylline * .... 150 mg.
Glyceryl guaiacolate .... 90 mg.
Alcohol (Elixir) 15%

THEO-DUR
Bronchodilator
(Key Pharmaceuticals, Inc.)

Theophylline * .... 100 mg.; 200 mg.;
or 300 mg.
Lactose 15%
Starch 12%
Sucrose 15%

THEOFED TABLETS
Bronchial asthma therapy
(Sutliff & Case)

Each tablet:
Phenobarbital .... 8 mg.
Theophylline (anhydrous) * .. 130 mg.
Ephedrine HCl * .... 24 mg.
Atropine sulfate .... 1/300 gr.
Pyrilamine maleate * .... 25 mg.
Glyceryl guaiacolate .... 50 mg.
Magnesium trisilicate .... 130 mg.
'76 Ed.

THEO-GUAIA
For asthmatic conditions
(Sutliff & Case)

CAPSULES (each):
Theophylline * .... 100 mg.
Glycerol guaiacolate .... 100 mg.

LIQUID (each 5 cc.):
Theophylline * .... 50 mg.
Glycerol guaiacolate .... 35 mg.
Alcohol (approx.) 20%
'76 Ed.

THEOKIN ELIXIR & TABLETS
Bronchodilator, expectorant
(Knoll Pharm.)

Each 15 cc or tablet:
Theophylline calcium salicylate
(provides 225 mg. theophyl-
line, anhydrous) * .... 448 mg.
Potassium iodide .... 450 mg.
Alcohol (Elixir only) 9.5%

THEO-LIX
Spasmolytic, bronchodilator, relaxant
(Vale)

Each 15 ml.:
Theophylline * .... 80 mg.
Alcohol 20%

THEOPHENEDRINE TABLETS T.P.E.
(Premo)

Each tablet:
Theophylline * .... 2 gr.
Phenobarbital .... 1/8 gr.
Ephedrine HCl * .... 3/8 gr.
'76 Ed.

THEOPHYL CHEWABLE TABLETS
Bronchodilator
(Knoll Pharm.)

Each tablet:
Theophylline (anhydrous) * .. 100 mg.

THEOPHYL-SR CAPSULES
Bronchodilator
(Knoll Pharm.)

Each sustained release capsule:
Theophylline
(anhydrous) * ... 125 mg. or 250 mg.

THEOPHYL-225 (TABLETS & ELIXIR)
Bronchodilator
(Knoll Pharm.)

Each tablet:
Theophylline (anhydrous) * .. 225 mg.

Each 30 ml.:
Theophylline (anhydrous) * .. 225 mg.
Alcohol 5%
Calcium salicylate .... <1%

THERABRAKERS
Cough & cold relief
(Reese Chem.)

Each capsule:
Vitamin C .... 200 mg.
Dextromethorphan
  hydrobromide .... 5 mg.
Phenyltoloxamine citrate .... 10 mg.
Phenylephrine
  hydrochloride * .... 5 mg.
Caffeine .... 30 mg.
Acetaminophen * .... 100 mg.
Salicylamide .... 50 mg.

THERAC LOTION
Acne therapy
(C & M Pharmacal)

Colloidal Sulfur 4.0%
Salicylic acid * 2.35%
Aqueous Bentonite base

THERACOF MULTIPLE ACTION MEDICINE
Antitussive, antihistaminic, decongestant
(Reese Chem.)

Each oz.:
Carbetapentane citrate ...... 45 mg.
Phenylpropanolamine
  hydrochloride * .... 30 mg.
Pheniramine maleate * .... 15 mg.
Pyrilamine maleate * .... 20 mg.
Guaiafenesin .... 300 mg.
Acetaminophen * .... 360 mg.
Alcohol 10%

THERACORT
For acne therapy
(C & M Pharmacal)

Hydrocortisone 0.25%
Colloidal Sulfur 4.00%
Salicylic acid * 2.35%
Magnesium aluminum silicate
Acacia
Propylene glycol
Methyl paraben
Purified water

THERA-FLUR (Acidulated) TOPICAL GEL-DROPS
Fluoride applications to control caries
(Hoyt Labs.)

Each gel-drop:
Fluoride ion (from 1.1% sodium
  fluoride) * 0.5%
0.1 Molar phosphate
Aqueous vehicle (at pH 4.5)

THERA-FLUR-N (Neutral) TOPICAL GEL-DROPS
Fluoride applications to control caries
(Hoyt Labs.)

Each gel-drop:
Fluoride ion (from 1.1% sodium
  fluoride) * 0.5%
Aqueous vehicle at neutral pH

THERAGRAN
Multivitamin therapy
(Squibb)

Each 5 cc tsp.:
Vitamin A palmitate (10,000
  U.S.P.u.) .... 3 mg.
Vitamin D (400 U.S.P.u.)
  (Cholecalciferol) .... 10 mcg.
Plus multivitamins

THERAGRAN HEMATINIC
Multivitamin therapy with hematinics
(Squibb)

Each tablet:
Vitamin A acetate (8,333
  U.S.P.u.) .... 2.5 mg.
Vitamin D (133 U.S.P.u.)
  (Ergocalciferol) .... 3.3 mcg.
Iron, elemental (as stabilized
  ferrous carbonate) * ...... 66.7 mg.
Plus multivitamins and minerals

THERAGRAN-M
Multivitamin & minerals therapy
(Squibb)

Each tablet:
Vitamin A (as acetate) (10,000
  U.S.P.u.) .... 3 mg.
Vitamin D (400 U.S.P.u.)
  (Ergocalciferol) .... 10 mcg.
Iron, elemental (as stabilized
  ferrous carbonate) .... 12 mg.
Plus multivitamins and minerals

THERALAX SUPPOSITORIES
Laxative
(Beecham Labs.)

Each suppository:
Bisacodyl .... 10 mg.
Synthetic Triglycerides base

THERALAX TABLETS
Laxative
(Beecham Labs.)

Each tablet:
Bisacodyl .... 5 mg.

THERAPAV CAPSULES
Oral papaverine
(Berlex Labs.)

Each capsule:
Papaverine
  hydrochloride * .... 75 mg.; 150 mg.
Polyethylene glycol

THERAPOGEN
Antiseptic; veterinary
(Meyer, T.)

Active ingred.:
Alcohol 14.30%
Soap 11.10%
Terpineol 6.10%
Safrole 1.70%
Naphthalene 1.00%
2,2′-Methylenebis(3,4,6-trichloro-
  rophenol) (Hexachlorophene) 0.70%
Thymol 0.35%
Inert ingred. 64.75%
  Water
  Thymene substitute
  Glycerine

      '76 Ed.

THEREVAC DISPOSABLE ENEMA
(Bowman Pharm.)

Each tube capsule:
Docusate potassium (Dioctyl potassium
  sulfosuccinate) *
Benzocaine
Medicinal soft soap in a base of
  Polyethylene glycol 400 and glycerine

THERMA-KOOL
Hot or cold compress
(Nortech)

Water 72.23%
Propylene glycol (USP) 25.90%
Carbopol Resin 1.35%

THERMODENT TOOTHPASTE
(Leeming Div.)

Strontium chloride hexahydrate ... 10%
Diatomaceous earth
Silica
Guar gum
Hydroxy ethyl cellulose

THERMO-GESIC CONCENTRATE
Cream analgesic
(Pharmex)

Methyl nicotinate
Methyl salicylate *
Camphor *
Ginger
Menthol *
Cassia
Capsicum

THERMOTABS
Buffered heat fatigue tablets
(Beecham Products)

Sodium chloride .... 0.45 gm./wt.
Potassium chloride .... 30 mg./wt.
Calcium carbonate .... 18 mg./wt.
Dextrose .... 0.2 gm./wt.

THEROPHYLLIN
Control of body odors in the dog
(Burns-Biotec)

Each tablet:
Potassium sodium copper
chlorophyllin * .... 12.5 mg.

T-H FUMIGANT NO. 2
(Thompson-Hayward)

Carbon tetrachloride * 81.3%
Carbon bisulfide 12.1%
Ethylene dibromide 6.6%

T-H FUMIGANT 82FR
Fumigant
(Thompson-Hayward)

Carbon bisulfide 16.5%
Carbon tetrachloride * 83.1%
n-Pentane 0.4%

T-H GRAIN CONDITIONER & WEEVIL KILLER
Insecticide-fungicide
(Thompson-Hayward)

Carbon tetrachloride * 27.4%
Ethylene dibromide 5%
Ethylene dichloride 64.6%
Sulfur dioxide 3%

THIABENDAZOLE CONCENTRATE
Post-harvest fungicide
(American Machinery Corp.)

Active ingred.: 3%
2-(4-Thiazolyl) benzimidazole *
Inert ingred.: 97%
Starch
Surfactants
Water

THIACIDE
For urine acidification & recurrent urinary calculi & infection
(Beach Pharm.)

Each tablet:
Potassium acid phosphate .... 250 mg.
Methenamine mandelate * .... 500 mg.

THI-CIN
Mouthwash concentrate
(Warren-Teed)

Sodium bicarbonate, USP
Sodium chloride, USP
Sodium borate, NF *
Sodium benzoate, NF
Sodium salicylate, USP *
Thymol, NF *
Menthol, USP *
Methyl salicylate *
Oil eucalyptus, NF *

THIMET 15-G SOIL AND SYSTEMIC INSECTICIDE
(Amer. Cyanamid, Agric. Div.)

Phorate (O,O-Diethyl S-
((ethylthio)methyl)
phosphorodithioate) * 15%
Inert (largely clay carrier) 85%

THIN 'N SHADE

See DUNCAN CERAMICS BISQ-STAIN ACCESSORY PRODUCT THIN 'N SHADE (AS 957)

THINOLENE
(Reliable Paste)

Mineral spirits *

Aromatic content less than 8%

THIN-X
Paint thinner
(Sterling-Clark-Lurton)

Mineral spirits *

THIOSPERSE SLUDGE INHIBITOR
(Stewart Sanitary Supply)

Barium sulfonate * 21.25%

THIRAMAD
Turf fungicide
(Mallinckrodt, Inc.)

Thiram (Tetramethylthiuram
disulfide) * 75%

33 PLUS LAWN WEED KILLER
(Ciba-Geigy Ag. Div.)

Dimethylamine salt of 2,4-Dichlo-
rophenoxyacetic acid * 6.25%
Dimethylamine salt of 2-(2-
Methyl-4-chlorophenoxy) pro-
pionic acid * 10.83%
Dimethylamine salt of Dicamba 1.20%

THISTROL
Herbicide
(Amchem)

Sodium salt of 4-(2-methyl-4-chlo-
rophenoxy) butyric acid * 23.5%

THOMAS HAIR CARE PRODUCTS

Thomas Hair & Scalp Corp.
4034 W. Lawrence Ave.
Chicago, Ill. 60630

Phone: 312-282-2377

See COSMETICS, Section VI, General
Formulations

THOMPSON'S WATER SEAL
(Thompson, E.A.)

Hydrocarbon resins
Mineral spirits *

THORAZINE
Tranquilizer, antiemetic
(SK&F)

Chlorpromazine hydrochloride *
Tablets: .... 10 mg.; 25 mg.;
50 mg.; 100 mg.;
or 200 mg.
'Spansule' capsules: . 30 mg.; 75 mg.;
150 mg.; 200 mg.;
or 300 mg.
Syrup: .... 10 mg./5 cc.
Concentrate: .... 30 mg./cc.;
or 100 mg./cc.

THORAZINE SUPPOSITORIES
Tranquilizer, antiemetic
(SK&F)

Each suppository:
Chlorpromazine
hydrochloride * .... 25 mg.; 100 mg.
Glycerin
Glyceryl monopalmitate
Glyceryl monostearate
Hydrogenated coconut oil fatty acids
Hydrogenated palm kernel oil fatty acids

THOR COUGH & COLD SYRUP
(Towne-Paulsen)

Each fl. oz.:
Dextromethorphan HBr ..... 75 mg.
Chlorpheniramine maleate ... 2 mg.
Methapyrilene HCl ...... 20 mg.
Pheniramine maleate .... 10 mg.
Phenylephrine HCl .... 10 mg.
Glyceryl guaiacolate .... 200 mg.
Vitamin C .... 100 mg.
Alcohol 5%

THOR LOZENGES
(Towne-Paulsen)

Each lozenge:
Dextromethorphan HBr ...... 7.5 mg.
Phenylpropanolamine HCl * . 10 mg.
Cetyl pyridinium chloride .... 2 mg.
Benzocaine .... 10 mg.

THOROBRED "H-P" SPRAY, UNICO

See UNICO THOROBRED "H-P" SPRAY

THORO CLEANSING AMMONIA
Cleaning ammonia
(Thoro)

Distilled water
Aqua ammonia *
Dow 9N9 (Nonylphenols)

Starred ingredients (*) may be responsible for major toxic effects; consult Section II.

THORO DRY CLEANER
(Thoro)

Ether *
Chloroform *
Methanol *
Naphtha base *

THOROKIL
Herbicide
(Holcomb)

2,4-D * 1-10%
Bromacil .... <1%
Pentachlorophenol .... <1%

'76 Ed.

THOROUGHBRED HEEL OINTMENT
Veterinary
(Thoroughbred)

Zinc oxide
Camphor *
Benzoin
Lanolin
Balsam Peru *
Menthol *
Oil of eucalyptus *

THOROUGHBRED VETERINARY COLIC ANODYNE
(Thoroughbred)

Alcohol * 67.8%/v
Fl. ext. Hyoscyamus *
Salicylic acid *
Aromatic base *
Chloroform .... 6 m./oz.
Capsicum *
Ammonium salicylate *

THORZETTES LOZENGES
(Towne-Paulsen)

Each lozenge:
  Dextromethorphan HBr ...... 3 mg.
  Cetylpyridinium chloride ..... 1.5 mg.
  Benzocaine .... 5 mg.

T-H PERMAGARD CONCENTRATE NO. 10
Wood preservative
(Thompson-Hayward)

Pentachlorophenol * 40%
Petroleum distillate

3-IN-1 BOLT LOOSENER
(Boyle-Midway)

Petroleum oils * .... >10%
Petroleum/solvent system .... >10%
Colloidal Graphite

3-IN-1 BOLT LOOSENER SPRAY
(Boyle-Midway)

Petroleum oils * .... >10%
Petroleum/solvent system .... >10%
Colloidal Graphite
Propellant

3-IN-1 HOUSEHOLD OIL
(Boyle-Midway)

Petroleum lubricating oil * ...... >10%
Corrosion inhibitor 1-10%
Fragrance

3-IN-1 HOUSEHOLD OIL SPRAY
(Boyle-Midway)

Combined amount: .... >10%
  Petroleum lubricating oil *
  Rust inhibitor
Fragrance
Propellant

3-IN-1 MOTOR OIL SAE-20
(Boyle-Midway)

Petroleum oil * .... >10%
Corrosion inhibitor *† 1-10%
Fragrance

†*See* Rust control, Section VI, General
  Formulations

3M PRODUCTS

3M
3M Center
St. Paul, Minn. 55144

Phone: 612-733-1110

3-NITRO-10
Feed additive - veterinary
(Salsbury)

3-Nitro-4-hydroxyphenylarsonic
  acid * 10%

3-NITRO-20
Feed additive - veterinary
(Salsbury)

3-Nitro-4-hydroxyphenylarsonic
  acid * 20%

3-NITRO-50
Feed additive - veterinary
(Salsbury)

3-Nitro-4-hydroxyphenylarsonic
  acid * 50%

3-NITRO-80
Feed additive - veterinary
(Salsbury)

3-Nitro-4-hydroxyphenylarsonic
  acid * 80%

3-NITRO W
Water medication - veterinary
(Salsbury)

One-oz. pouch:
  Monosodium 3-nitro-4-
    hydroxyphenylarsonate *   21.7 gm.

3 PAK BOWL FRESHNER
(Carson Chem. Corp.)

Paradichlorobenzene * 99%
Essential oil 1%

'76 Ed.

3 PAK CEDAR SCENTED MOTH CAKE
(Carson Chem. Corp.)

Paradichlorobenzene * 99%
Essential oil 1%

'76 Ed.

3 PAK HEARTS
(Carson Chem. Corp.)

Paradichlorobenzene * 99%
Essential oil 1%

'76 Ed.

3 PAK SANITIZER
(Carson Chem. Corp.)

Paradichlorobenzene * 99%
Essential oil 1%

'76 Ed.

3V LIQUID DETERGENT
(National-Purity Soap)

Blend of Nonionic and anionic surface ac-
  tive agents *
Sequestrants
Brighteners
Lanolin
Perfume
Emollients

3-WAY AIR FRESHENER
(Reefer-Galler)

Mineral spirits 6.0%
Perfume
Propellant
Water

'76 Ed.

3-WAY KILL

See HUB STATES 3-WAY KILL

THRIFTY ANTI-COAGULANT RAT AND MOUSE BAIT
(Thrifty Rat & Mouse Bait Co.)

Fumarin 22 (3-(alpha-Acetonyl-furfuryl)-4-hydroxycoumarin) . 0.025%

'76 Ed.

THRIOCAINE
Throat lozenge
(Lemmon Co.)

Each lozenge:
Cetylpyridinium chloride ..... 0.5 mg.
Benzocaine .... 5 mg.

THRIP-TOX, DRY

See DRY THRIP-TOX

THRIP-TOX, LIQUID

See LIQUID THRIP-TOX

THRU PENETRATING ANALGESIC, REXALL

See REXALL THRU PENETRATING ANALGESIC

THRUSH-X
Bactericide - veterinary
(Farnam Co.)

Dichlorphene * 10.00%
Parachlorometaxylenol 0.50%

'76 Ed.

THRUST STARTING FLUID
For gasoline & diesel engines
(Radiator)

Ethyl-ether *

'76 Ed.

T-H SUPER FUMIGAS
Fumigant-insecticide
(Thompson-Hayward)

Carbon bisulfide 16.34%
Carbon tetrachloride * 82.2%
n-Pentane 0.36%
Sulfur dioxide 1%

THUBAN LUBRICANT
(Texaco Inc.)

Petroleum lubricating oil

T-H WEEVIL KILL
Insecticide
(Thompson-Hayward)

Carbon tetrachloride * 63.6%
Ethylene dibromide 7.2%
Ethylene dichloride 29.2%

THYMOLAC
Fungicide; medical
(Thymolac)

Thymol .... <1%
Salicylic acid * 1-10%
Benzoic acid 1-10%
Acetone * .... >10%
Water 10%
Isopropyl alcohol * .... approx. 52%

THYROLAR
Thyroid hormone replacement
(Armour Pharm.)

Each 1/2 gr. tablet:
Sodium levothyroxine * ....   25 mcg.
Sodium l-triiodothyronine * 6.25 mcg.

Each 1 gr. tablet:
Sodium levothyroxine * ....   50 mcg.
Sodium l-triiodothyronine * 12.5 mcg.

Each 2 gr. tablet:
Sodium levothyroxine * ....   100 mcg.
Sodium l-triiodothyronine *   25 mcg.

Each 3 gr. tablet:
Sodium levothyroxine * ....   150 mcg.
Sodium l-triiodothyronine * 37.5 mcg.

Each 5 gr. tablet:
Sodium levothyroxine * ....   250 mcg.
Sodium l-triiodothyronine * 62.5 mcg.

TICKLE
Anti-perspirant deodorant
(Bristol-Myers)

Aluminum chlorohydrate *

TICK TOCK
Vitreous cleaner
(Holcomb)

Hydrochloric acid * 19.5%

'76 Ed.

TIC TOC FLORAL DEODORETTES
Perfumed cakes
(Curran)

Paradichlorobenzene *

'76 Ed.

TIDE (Formula 1)
Granular laundry detergent
(Procter & Gamble)

Complex sodium phosphates 10-24%
Sodium sulfate 10-24%
Sodium aluminosilicate 10-24%
Sodium carbonate 10-24%
Water 5-9%
Sodium alkyl sulfate 5-9%
Sodium alkyl ethoxylate sulfate 5-9%
Sodium alkyl benzene sulfonate . 1-4%
Sodium silicate 1-4%
Minor ingredients, each .... trace

pH (1% solution) - 10.9 max.

TIDE (Formula 3)
Granular laundry detergent
(Procter & Gamble)

Complex sodium phosphates 10-24%
Sodium sulfate 10-24%
Sodium aluminosilicate 10-24%
Sodium carbonate 10-24%
Water 5-9%
Sodium alkyl sulfate 1-4%
Sodium alkyl ethoxylate sulfate 5-9%
Sodium alkyl benzene sulfonate 5-9%
Sodium silicate 1-4%
Minor ingredients, each .... trace

pH (1% solution) - 10.9 max.

TIDE (Formula 4)
Granular laundry detergent
(Procter & Gamble)

Sodium sulfate 25-49%
Sodium aluminosilicate 10-24%
Sodium carbonate 10-24%
Sodium alkyl sulfate 5-9%
Sodium alkyl ethoxylate sulfate 5-9%
Sodium alkyl benzene sulfonate . 5-9%
Water 5-9%
Polyacrylate 1-4%
Sodium silicate 1-4%
Minor ingredients, each .... trace

pH (1% solution) - 10.9 max.

TIDE (Formula 7)
Granular laundry detergent
(Procter & Gamble)

Sodium sulfate 25-49%
Sodium aluminosilicate 10-24%
Sodium nitrilotriacetate 10-24%
Sodium carbonate 10-24%
Sodium alkyl sulfate 5-9%
Sodium alkyl ethoxylate sulfate 5-9%
Water 5-9%
Sodium silicate 1-4%
Sodium alkyl benzene sulfonate . 1-4%
Minor ingredients, each .... trace

TIFFAN "E"
Cosmetic moisturizing cream
(D'Lanerg)

Mineral oil Kaydol
Stearic acid XXX
Palm kernal oil
Isopropyl myristate
Clindrol 868 (Stearamide DEA)
Vitamin E
Quaternium-15
Imidazolidinyl urea
Water
FD & C Yellow #5
Methyl paraben
Germall
Protein WSPX-250
Perfume Norda

TIGUVON POUR-ON ANIMAL INSECTICIDE
(Cutter (Brand) Bayvet Div. Cutter Labs.)

Fenthion * 3%

Starred ingredients (*) may be responsible for major toxic effects; consult Section II.

TIHIST-DP SYRUP
Cough syrup
(Vita Elixir Co.)

Each 5 cc.:
d-Methorphan HBr .... 10 mg.
Pyrilamine maleate * .... 16 mg.
Sodium citrate .... 3.3 gr.

TIHIST NASAL DROPS
(Vita Elixir Co.)

Each 30 cc:
Pyrilamine maleate 0.1%
Phenylephrine HCl * 0.25%
Sodium bisulfite (isotonic soln.) 0.2%
Methylparaben 0.02%
Propylparaben 0.01%

TIJA FILM-COATED TABLETS
Antimicrobial
(Vita Elixir Co.)

Each tablet:
Oxytetracycline hydrochloride 250 mg.

TIJA SYRUP
Antimicrobial
(Vita Elixir Co.)

Each 5 cc:
Oxytetracycline hydrochloride 125 mg.

TILCON II
Dairy cattle teat dip
(Diversey Wyandotte)

Synthetic detergent-Iodine complex
Titratable Iodine * 0.25%

TILE-MITE
Bathroom cleaner
(Sanitek)

Phosphoric acid * 18.2%
Nonionic surfactant 3.6%
Dye .... trace
Water .... balance

TILLAM (6-E, 10-G)
Herbicide
(Stauffer)

Pebulate (S-Propylbutylethylthiocarba-
mate) *

TIMBRETONE PRODUCTS

See COOK'S TIMBRETONE PROD-
UCTS

TIMELY
Disinfectant, cleaner, deodorant
(Barco)

Octylphenoxypoly (ethyleneoxy)
ethanol 5.00%
Nitrilo triacetic acid, trisodium salt 2.20%
Alkyl dimethyl dichlorobenzyl ammonium chloride * 2.50%

'76 Ed.

TIME-MIST METERED AEROSOL INSECTICIDE
(Time-Mist Div.)

Pyrethrins 1.76%
Technical Piperonyl butoxide ... 17.54%
Petroleum distillate * 19.67%

TIME-MIST METERED AIR SANITIZER
(Time-Mist Div.)

Triethylene glycol 9.15%
Dipropylene glycol 3.43%
Alkyl dimethyl benzyl ammonium
chloride 0.17%
Essential oils 0.86%
Alcohol 31.99%
Inert ingred.: 54.40%
Propellants

"TIME SAVER"

See W-W "TIME SAVER"

TIME SAVER BLEACH
Bleach, disinfectant, deodorant
(Wallace Chemical Co.)

Sodium hypochlorite * 5 1/4%
Sodium chloride .... <5%
Water .... Balance

TIMPREG

See CHAPMAN TIMPREG

TIMPREG B

See CHAPMAN TIMPREG B

TIMPREG B (SPECIAL)

See CHAPMAN TIMPREG B (SPE-
CIAL)

TIMPREG PAK

See CHAPMAN TIMPREG PAK

TINACTIN CREAM 1%
*Treatment of superficial fungous infec-
tions of the skin*
(Schering)

Each gm.:
Tolnaftate .... 10 mg.
Solubilized in:
Polyethylene glycol-400
Propylene glycol
With:
Carboxypolymethylene
Monoamylamine
Titanium dioxide
Butylated hydroxytoluene

TINACTIN POWDER 1%
*Treatment of superficial fungous infec-
tions of the skin*
(Schering)

Each gram:
Tolnaftate .... 10 mg.
Corn starch
Talc

TINACTIN POWDER (1%) AEROSOL
*Treatment of superficial fungous infec-
tions of the skin*
(Schering)

Tolnaftate .... 72 mg.
Butylated hydroxytoluene
Talc
Polyethylene-polypropylene glycol mono-
butyl ether
Propellant: .... to make 120 gm.
Trichloromonofluoromethane
Dichlorodifluoromethane

TIN-ALL
Soldering paint
(Damon Chemical Co.)

Zinc chloride *

TINASTAT LOTION
Keratolytic lotion
(Vita Elixir Co.)

Each 2 oz.:
Equal parts of:
Sodium hyposulfite (sat. soln.) *
Benzethonium chloride (3% soln.) *
Preservative

TINDAL TABLETS
Tranquilizer
(Schering)

Each tablet:
Acetophenazine maleate * .... 20 mg.

TING (AEROSOL, CREAM, AND POWDER)
Germicidal, fungicidal, antiseptic
(Pharmacraft)

Benzoic acid
Boric acid *
Zinc oxide
Zinc stearate *
Alcohol (Cream) 20.0%

TING MEDICATED SOAP
Antifungal
(Pharmacraft)

Undecylenic acid 2.0%

TINIQUAD
Antibiotic-antibacterial
(Wesley Pharm.)

Each tablet:
Sulfadiazine *		25 mg.
Sulfamerazine *		25 mg.
Sulfamethazine *		25 mg.
Sulfacetamide *		50 mg.

TINK
For clogged drains
(Dolge)

Sodium hydroxide *

TINOSTAT
*Feed additive aid in prevention of coc-
cidiosis and hexamitiasis in turkeys*
(Salsbury)

Butynorate (Dibutyltin dilaurate) *   25%

TINS-TYTER PERFECT BOND TINNING FLUID, BALKAMP

See BALKAMP TINS-TYTER PER-
FECT BOND TINNING FLUID

TINTEX DYES
Fabric dyes and colors
(Knomark)

Knomark, Inc.
132 Merrick Blvd.
Jamaica, N.Y. 11434

Phone: 212-276-3400

TINTZ CREME COLOR SHAMPOO
(Fleetwood)

Sodium lauryl sulfate *		>40%
Glyceryl stearate		
Protein		
p-Phenylenediamine *		3%
o-Aminophenol *†		3%
p-Aminophenol *		0.1-2%
p-o-Nitrophenol *‡		
Resorcinol *		0.2-2%

†*See* p-Aminophenol
‡*See* p-Nitrophenol

TINVER
For treatment of tinea versicolor
(Barnes-Hind)

Sodium thiosulfate *		25.0%
Salicylic acid *		1.0%
Isopropyl alcohol		10.0%
Propylene glycol		
Menthol *		
Edetate disodium		
Colloidal Alumina		

TIP TONI
Waving lotion
(Gillette Co., Personal Care Div.)

Water
Diisopropanolamine *
Ammonium thioglycolate *
Potassium coco-hydrolyzed animal protein
Steareth-20
Fragrance
EDTA
D & C Red No. 19

TIP TONI SILKWAVE TOUCH-UP WAVING LOTION (TOTAL CONDITIONING)
(Gillette Co., Personal Care Div.)

Water
Diisopropanolamine *
Ammonium thioglycolate *
Steareth-20
Quaternium-40
Fragrance
Potassium coco-hydrolyzed animal protein
Sodium styrene/PEG-10 maleate/Nonox-
  ynol-10 maleate/Acrylate copolymer
EDTA
Ammonium nonoxynol-4 sulfate
D & C Yellow No. 10
D & C Red No. 19

TIP TONI TWENTY-CURL HOME WAVE (TWIN CONDITIONING) WAVING LOTION
(Gillette Co., Personal Care Div.)

Water
Diisopropanolamine *
Ammonium thioglycolate *
Steareth-20
Quaternium-40
Fragrance
Potassium coco-hydrolyzed animal protein
Sodium styrene/PEG-10 maleate/Nonox-
  ynol-10 maleate/Acrylate copolymer
EDTA
Ammonium nonoxynol-4 sulfate
D & C Yellow No. 10
D & C Red No. 19

TITAN BULK LIQUID FOGGING INSECTICIDE
(Nat'l Labs. Div.)

Petroleum distillate *		98.15%
Essential oils		0.69%
N-Octyl bicycloheptene dicarboximide		0.61%
Technical Piperonyl butoxide		0.37%
Pyrethrins		0.18%

TITAN CONCENTRATE RESIDUAL INSECTICIDE
(Nat'l Labs. Div.)

Ronnel *		24.0%
Aromatic petroleum derivative solvent *		58.9%

TITAN DUAL ACTION CONTACT & RESIDUAL INSECTICIDE SPRAY
(Nat'l Labs. Div.)

(5-Benzyl-3-furyl)methyl-2,2-dimethyl-3-(2-methylpro-penyl) cyclopropanecarboxylate		0.350% w/w
Related compounds		0.048%
Aromatic petroleum hydrocarbons		0.464%

TITAN FLY BAIT (BLUE)
(Nat'l Labs. Div.)

2,2-Dichlorovinyl dimethyl phosphate		0.093%
Related compounds		0.007%
Ronnel		0.250%

TITAN INSECT KILLER
(Nat'l Labs. Div.)

Pyrethrins		0.25%
Technical Piperonyl butoxide		0.90%
N-Octyl bicycloheptene dicarboximide		0.50%
Propane/Isobutane (propellant)		major

TITAN LONG SHOT WASP & HORNET KILLER WITH SBP 1382
(Nat'l Labs. Div.)

(5-Benzyl-3-furyl)methyl-2,2-dimethyl-3-(2-methylpro-penyl) cyclopropanecarboxylate		0.250% w/w
Related compounds		0.034%
Aromatic petroleum hydrocarbons		0.332%
Petroleum distillate *		98.884%

TITAN MIST INSECTICIDE MODULE
(Nat'l Labs. Div.)

Pyrethrins		0.9%
Piperonyl butoxide (technical)		1.8%
N-Octyl bicycloheptene dicarboximide		3.0%
Petroleum distillates *		14.3%
Propane/Isobutane (propellant)		major

TITESEALS
Sealing compound
(Radiator)

Polymerized vegetable oils
Inert mineral fillers
Resins

'76 Ed.

T.L.C. BABY LOTION
(Polychem Corp.)

Water
Stearic acid
Polysorbate-60
Mineral oil
PEG-2 stearate
Glycerin
Sorbitan stearate
Cetyl alcohol
PEG-20 lanolate
PVP
Magnesium stearate
Dimethicone
Sorbic acid
Propylparaben
Urea
Fragrance
Allantoin

T.L.C. CLEANSING BATH OIL
(Polychem Corp.)

Mineral oil
PEG-4 mono/dilaurate
Lanolin oil
Fragrance

T.L.C. CONTINEX
Skin cleanser
(Polychem Corp.)

Water
Disodium monooleamidosulfosuccinate
Sodium lauryl sulfate
Cocoamide DEA
Laneth-10 acetate
Fragrance
Propylene glycol
Methylparaben
Propylparaben
Citric acid

T.L.C. HOSPITAL BATH
(Polychem Corp.)

Water
Disodium monooleamidosulfosuccinate
Sodium lauryl sulfate
Cocoamide DEA
Laneth-10 acetate
Fragrance
Propylene glycol
Methylparaben
Propylparaben
Citric acid

T.L.C. HOSPITAL LOTION
(Polychem Corp.)

Water
Stearic acid
Polysorbate-60
Mineral oil
PEG-2 stearate
Glycerin
Sorbitan stearate
Cetyl alcohol
PEG-20 lanolate
PVP
Magnesium stearate
Dimethicone
Sorbic acid
Propylparaben
Urea
Fragrance
Allantoin
Menthol

T.L.C. MOUTH RINSE
(Polychem Corp.)

Water
Sorbitol
Glycerin
Cetylpyridinium chloride
Polysorbate 20
Polysorbate 80
Flavor

TNT ANT FREE
Insecticide
(TNT Chem.)

Sodium arsenate * 1.66%

TNT HOUSE AND GARDEN
Insecticide
(TNT Chem.)

Technical Piperonyl butoxide 1.25%
Pyrethrins 0.25%
Oil 1.00%

TNT INSECT BOMB
Insecticide
(TNT Chem.)

Allethrin 0.015%
Pyrethrins 0.035%
DDVP 0.5%
Petroleum distillates * 79.450%
Propellant 20.00%

TNT TRIPLE ACTION INSECT KILLER
Insecticide
(TNT Chem.)

Petroleum distillates * 99.240%
Diazinon (O,O-Diethyl O-(2-iso-
   propyl-4-methyl-6-
   pyrimidinyl)phosphorothioate) 0.500%
Essential oils 0.120%
Technical Piperonyl butoxide .. 0.100%
Pyrethrins 0.040%

TNT TRIPLE ACTION ROACH & ANT KILLER
Insecticide
(TNT Chem.)

Allethrin 0.03%
DDVP 0.3%
Baygon 0.5%
Petroleum distillates * 88.670%

TOFRANIL-PM
Antidepressant
(Geigy Pharmaceuticals)

Each capsule:
  Imipramine
    pamoate * ...... 75 mg.; 100 mg.;
        125 mg. or 150 mg.

TOFRANIL TABLETS
Antidepressant
(Geigy Pharmaceuticals)

Each tablet:
  Imipramine
    hydrochloride * .... 10 mg.; 25 mg.;
        or 50 mg.

TOK (E-25 & WP-50)
Herbicides
(Rohm and Haas)

E-25:
  2,4-Dichlorophenyl p-nitrophenyl
    ether * 25%

WP-50:
  2,4-Dichlorophenyl p-nitrophenyl
    ether * 50%

TOL-C
Hematinic
(Ascher, B.F.)

Each tablet:
  Ferrous fumerate * .... 300 mg.
  Ascorbic acid .... 500 mg.

TOLFRINIC
Hemopoietic
(Ascher, B.F.)

Each tablet:
  Ferrous fumerate * .... 600 mg.
  Ascorbic acid .... 100 mg.
  Vitamin B12 w/intrinsic factor concen-
    trate 1.0 N.F. XI Unit (oral)

TOLU-SED COUGH SYRUP
Temporary relief of cough due to colds
(Scherer Labs.)

Each 5 cc.:
  Codeine phosphate * .... 10 mg.
  Guaifenesin N.F. .... 100 mg.
  Alcohol 10%

  Contains no sugar

Starred ingredients (*) may be responsible for major toxic effects; consult Section II.

TOLU-SED DM COUGH SYRUP
Temporary relief of cough due to common cold
(Scherer Labs.)

Each 5 cc.:
Alcohol	10%
Dextromethorphan hydrobromide *	10 mg.
Guaifenesin N.F.	100 mg.

Contains no sugar

TOMATO-GRO

See SCIENCE TOMATO-GRO

TOM CAT

See BONIDE TOM CAT

TOMELLEM'S DEHORNING PASTE
Veterinary
(Tomellem)

Calcium hydroxide *	40%
Sodium hydroxide *	30%

TOM FIELDS APPLE BLOSSOM COLOGNE
(Tom Fields)

SD Alcohol 40B	62.35%
Fragrance oil *	2.23%
Water (deionized)	35.23%
Color	trace

TOM FIELDS CRAZY CREME
Skin moisturizer
(Tom Fields)

Polawax	5.00%
Stearic acid	1.00%
Tegosept P	trace
Crodafos N3 Neutral (DEA-oleth-3-phosphate)	1.00%
Lanolin	1.00%
Mineral oil	2.00%
Silicone-225 (Dimethicone)	trace
Carbopol 934 (Carbomer 934)	trace
Water (deionized)	77.86%
Glycerine	10.00%
Tegosept M	trace
Triethanolamine 85%	1.20%
Fragrance	1.00%
Color	trace

TOM FIELDS FLAVORED LIP GLOSS
(Tom Fields)

Petrolatum	82.9%
Lanolin alcohol	5.0%
Microcrystalline wax	8.0%
Carnauba wax	1.0%
Safflower oil	3.0%
Propylparaben	trace
Fragrance	trace
Color	trace

TOM FIELDS FLAVORED STICK POMADE
(Tom Fields)

Castor oil	53.92%
Acetylated Lanolin alcohol	12.00%
Beeswax	12.00%
Candelilla wax	7.00%
Fragrance	4.00%
Carnauba wax	1.50%
Paraffin wax	2.00%
Hydrogenated Tallow glyceride	2.50%
Ozokerite	2.00%
Mineral oil	1.00%
Lanolin oil	trace
Isopropyl myristate	trace
Stearic acid	trace
Propylene glycol	trace
BHA	trace
Propyl gallate	trace
Aluminum hydroxide	trace
Color	trace
Titanium dioxide	trace

TOM FIELDS JUST DESSERTS
Flavored lip cosmetic
(Tom Fields)

White petrolatum	73.95%
Beeswax	15.00%
Safflower oil	4.00%
Candelilla wax	5.00%
Fragrance *	2.00%
Propyl gallate	trace
Color	trace

TOM FIELDS LILY OF THE VALLEY COLOGNE
(Tom Fields)

SD Alcohol 40B	62.35%
Fragrance oil *	2.23%
Water (deionized)	35.35%
Color	trace

TOM FIELDS LIPS & LOTION
Flavored lip moisturizer
(Tom Fields)

Polawax	2.00%
Stearic acid	1.00%
Tegosept P	trace
Crodofos N3 Neutral (DEA-oleth-3-phosphate)	1.00%
Lanolin (anhydrous)	1.00%
Mineral oil	2.00%
Silicone 225 (Dimethicone)	trace
Carbopol 934 (Carbomer 934)	trace
Water (deionized)	81.44%
Propylene glycol	10.00%
Tegosept M	trace
Triethanolamine 85%	trace
Fragrance	trace

TOM FIELDS MERRY LIPS POMADE
(Tom Fields)

Castor oil	49.25%
Octyl dodecanol	20.00%
Candelilla wax	8.00%
Isopropyl lanolate	7.50%
Ozokerite	5.00%
Fragrance	2.00%
Microcrystalline wax	4.00%
Cetyl alcohol	3.50%
Corn starch	trace
Wheat germ glycerides	trace
Propylene glycol	trace
BHA	trace
Propyl gallate	trace
Aluminum hydroxide	trace
Titanium dioxide	trace
Color	trace

TOM FIELDS NAIL POLISH REMOVER
(Tom Fields)

Ethyl alcohol *	99%
Castor oil	trace
Perfume	trace
Color	trace

TOM FIELDS NATIONAL HAND LOTION
(Tom Fields)

Polawax	2.00%
Stearic acid	1.00%
Tegosept P	trace
Crodafos N3 Neutral (DEA-oleth-3-phosphate)	1.00%
Lanolin	1.00%
Mineral oil	2.00%
Silicone-225 (Dimethicone)	trace
Carbopol 934 (Carbomer 934)	trace
Water (deionized)	80.64%
Propylene glycol	10.00%
Tegosept M	trace
Triethanolamine 85%	trace
Fragrance oil	1.00%

TOM FIELDS NATURAL LIP POMADE
(Tom Fields)

Mineral oil	43.40%
Ceresin	27.00%
Lanolin	12.50%
Beeswax	11.75%
Petrolatum	2.50%
Fragrance	1.00%
Carnauba	1.00%
Propylene glycol	trace
BHA	trace
Propyl gallate	trace
Citric acid	trace
Color	trace

Starred ingredients (*) may be responsible for major toxic effects; consult Section II.

TOM FIELDS NATURAL NAIL POLISH
(Tom Fields)

Nitrocellulose	15.0%
Polyester resin	15.0%
Dibutyl phthalate	5.0%
Camphor	1.0%
Tolulol	24.0%
Ethyl acetate	16.0%
Butyl acetate *	23.9%
Color	trace

TOM FIELDS PINK NAIL POLISH
(Tom Fields)

Nitrocellulose	15.00%
Polyester resin	15.00%
Dibutyl phthalate	5.00%
Camphor	1.00%
Tolulol	24.00%
Ethyl acetate	15.00%
Butyl acetate *	23.90%
Purified Titanium dioxide	1.00%
Color	trace

TOM FIELDS PINK & PRETTY LIPSTICK
(Tom Fields)

Castor oil	63.68%
Candelilla wax	7.00%
Beeswax	4.00%
Ozokerite	4.00%
Carnauba wax	3.50%
Butyl myristate	2.50%
Mineral oil	2.50%
Paraffin	1.50%
Fragrance	1.00%
Aluminum hydroxide	trace
Propylene glycol	trace
BHA	trace
Propyl gallate	trace
Titanium dioxide	trace
Color	trace

TOM FIELDS SOFT SPORT LOTION
Skin freshener
(Tom Fields)

Solulan 98 (Laneth-10 acetate)	2.84%
Cetyl alcohol	trace
Arlacel 165 (Glyceryl stearate & PEG-100 stearate)	1.90%
Water (deionized)	84.90%
Tegosept M/Methylparaben	trace
Carbopol 934 (Carbomer 934)	trace
Triethanolamine 85%	trace
SD Alcohol 40B	8.61%
Menthol (USP)	trace
Fragrance	trace

TOM FIELDS TEA ROSE COLOGNE
(Tom Fields)

SD Alcohol 40B	62.36%
Fragrance oil *	2.23%
Water (deionized)	35.18%
Color	trace

TOM FIELDS TINKERBELL BUBBLE BATH
(Tom Fields)

Water (deionized)	70.86%
Equex (Ammonium lauryl ether sulfate & Alkanolamide)	23.77%
Fragrance	trace
SD Alcohol 40B	4.76%
Color	trace

TOM FIELDS TINKERBELL BUBBLE BATH CRYSTALS
(Tom Fields)

Sodium sesquicarbonate *	74.5%
Sodium lauryl sulfoacetate	25.0%
Silica	trace

TOM FIELDS TINKERBELL COLOGNE
(Tom Fields)

SD Alcohol 40B	62.36%
Fragrance oil *	2.21%
Water (deionized)	35.27%
Color	trace

TOM FIELDS TINKERBELL COLOR BATH CRYSTALS
(Tom Fields)

Sodium sesquicarbonate *	74.5%
Sodium lauryl sulfoacetate	25.0%
Silica	trace
Color	trace

TOM FIELDS TINKERBELL DUSTING POWDER
(Tom Fields)

Talc #1615	99.52%
Fragrance oil	trace
Irgasan DP 300 (Triclosan)	trace

TOM FIELDS TINKERBELL HAND LOTION
(Tom Fields)

Polawax (Emulsifying wax)	2.00%
Stearic acid	1.00%
Tegosept "P"	trace
Crodafos N3 Neutral (DEA oleth-3 phosphate)	1.00%
Lanolin	1.00%
Mineral oil	2.00%
Silicone #225 (Dimethicone)	trace
Carbopol #934 (Carbomer 934)	trace
Water (deionized)	8.25%
Propylene glycol	10.00%
Tegosept "M"	trace
Triethanolamine 85%	trace
Fragrance	trace
Color	trace

TOM FIELDS TINKERBELL PERFUME
(Tom Fields)

SD Alcohol 40B	72.36%
Water (deionized)	17.48%
Fragrance oil *	10.00%
Color	trace

TOM FIELDS TINKERBELL PRESSED POWDER
(Tom Fields)

Talc	81.72%
Zinc stearate	5.00%
Laureth-4	4.25%
Methylparaben	trace
Propylparaben	trace
Sodium dihydroacetate	trace
Fragrance	trace
Titanium dioxide	6.25%
Iron oxides	1.40%

TOM FIELDS TINKERBELL SHAMPOO
(Tom Fields)

2MCAS Modified	35%
Lanamide 55 (Cocamide DEA)	5%
Polyethylene glycol 6000 distearate (PEG 150 distearate)	1%
Tween 20 (Polysorbate 20)	1%
Color	trace
Fragrance	1%
Water (deionized)	57%

TONECOL
Cough syrup
(A.V.P. Pharmaceuticals)

Each 5 cc:

Dextro-methorphan hydrobromide *	10 mg.
Chlorpheniramine maleate	1 mg.
Phenylephrine HCl	5 mg.
Sodium citrate	15 mg.
Glyceryl guaiacolate	25 mg.
Alcohol	7%

TO-NE-KA BRAND HERBS AND MEDICINE BALL
Cathartic
(C.T.S. Labs.)

Buckthorn
Senna
Cascara sagrada *
Aloe

TO-NE-KA BRAND OINTMENT
For skin
(C.T.S. Labs.)

Methyl salicylate *
Oil Pine tar *
Balsam Peru *
Petroleum base

TO-NE-KA CORN REMOVER
(C.T.S. Labs.)

Salicylic acid *
Pyroaxin
Acetone *

Starred ingredients (*) may be responsible for major toxic effects; consult Section II.

TO-NE-KA FOOT BALM CREAM
(C.T.S. Labs.)

Eucalyptus *
Peppermint *
Thymol *
Menthol *
Camphor *
Phenol *
Lanolin
Glycerin
Salicylic acid *
Benzoic acid *
Special base

TO-NE-KA INHALANT & RUBBING OIL
(C.T.S. Labs.)

Eucalyptus oil *
Menthol *
Peppermint oil *
Thymol *
Camphor *

TONELAX
Peristaltic stimulant
(A.V.P. Pharmaceuticals)

Each tablet:
Danthron * .... 75 mg.
Calcium pantothenate .... 25 mg.

TONE SOAP (Bar Soap)
(Armour-Dial, Inc.)

Sodium soap 75-100%
Moisture (water) 10-25%
Glycerin 1-5%
Cocoa butter 1-5%
Perfume 1-5%
Minor ingredients (total) 1-5%

TONETTE CHILDREN'S HOME WAVE (TWIN CONDITIONING) WAVING LOTION
(Gillette Co., Personal Care Div.)

Water
Diisopropanolamine *
Ammonium thioglycolate *
Steareth-20
Quaternium-40
Fragrance
Potassium coco-hydrolyzed animal protein
Sodium styrene/PEG-10 maleate/Nonoxynol-10 maleate/Acrylate copolymer
EDTA
Ammonium nonoxynol-4 sulfate
D & C Yellow No. 10
D & C Red No. 19

TONETTE SILKWAVE FOR CHILDREN (TOTAL CONDITIONING) WAVING LOTION
(Gillette Co., Personal Care Div.)

Water
Diisopropanolamine *
Ammonium thioglycolate *
Steareth-20
Quaternium-40
Fragrance
Potassium coco-hydrolyzed animal protein
Sodium styrene/PEG-10 maleate/Nonoxynol-10 maleate/Acrylate copolymer
EDTA
Ammonium nonoxynol-4 sulfate
D & C Yellow No. 10
D & C Red No. 19

TONGA AFTER SHAVE

See AMWAY TONGA AFTER SHAVE

TONGA COLOGNE

See AMWAY TONGA COLOGNE

TONGA SPRAY DEODORANT

See AMWAY TONGA SPRAY DEODORANT

TONI BODY HOME WAVE (TWIN CONDITIONING) WAVING LOTION
(Gillette Co., Personal Care Div.)

Water
Diisopropanolamine *
Ammonium thioglycolate *
Steareth-20
Quaternium-40
Fragrance
Potassium coco-hydrolyzed animal protein
Sodium styrene/PEG-10 maleate/Nonoxynol-10 maleate/Acrylate copolymer
EDTA
Ammonium nonoxynol-4 sulfate

TONI GENTLE CONDITIONING WAVING LOTION
(Gillette Co., Personal Care Div.)

Water
Diisopropanolamine *
Ammonium thioglycolate *
Ammonium sulfate
Steareth-20
Quaternium-40
Potassium coco-hydrolyzed animal protein
Fragrance
Sodium styrene/PEG-10 maleate/Nonoxynol-10 maleate/Acrylate copolymer
EDTA
Ammonium nonoxynol-4 sulfate
D & C Yellow No. 10
D & C Red No. 19

TONI GENTLE HOME WAVE (TWIN CONDITIONING) WAVING LOTION
(Gillette Co., Personal Care Div.)

Water
Diisopropanolamine *
Ammonium thioglycolate *
Steareth-20
Ammonium sulfate
Quaternium-40
Fragrance
Potassium coco-hydrolyzed animal protein
Sodium styrene/PEG-10 maleate/Nonoxynol-10 maleate/Acrylate copolymer
EDTA
Ammonium nonoxynol-4 sulfate
D & C Yellow No. 10
D & C Red No. 19

TONI REGULAR CONDITIONING WAVING LOTION
(Gillette Co., Personal Care Div.)

Water
Diisopropanolamine *
Ammonium thioglycolate *
Steareth-20
Quaternium-40
Potassium coco-hydrolyzed animal protein
Fragrance
Sodium styrene/PEG-10 maleate/Nonoxynol-10 maleate/Acrylate copolymer
EDTA
Ammonium nonoxynol-4 sulfate
D & C Yellow No. 10
D & C Red No. 19

TONI REGULAR HOME WAVE (TWIN CONDITIONING) WAVING LOTION
(Gillette Co., Personal Care Div.)

Water
Diisopropanolamine *
Ammonium thioglycolate *
Steareth-20
Quaternium-40
Fragrance
Potassium coco-hydrolyzed animal protein
Sodium styrene/PEG-10 maleate/Nonoxynol-10 maleate/Acrylate copolymer
EDTA
Ammonium nonoxynol-4 sulfate
D & C Yellow No. 10
D & C Red No. 19

TONI SILKWAVE BODY (TOTAL CONDITIONING) WAVING LOTION
(Gillette Co., Personal Care Div.)

Water
Diisopropanolamine *
Ammonium thioglycolate *
Steareth-20
Quaternium-40
Fragrance
Potassium coco-hydrolyzed animal protein
Sodium styrene/PEG-10 maleate/Nonoxynol-10 maleate/Acrylate copolymer
EDTA
Ammonium nonoxynol-4 sulfate

TONI SILKWAVE GENTLE (TOTAL CONDITIONING) WAVING LOTION
(Gillette Co., Personal Care Div.)

Water
Diisopropanolamine *
Ammonium thioglycolate *
Steareth-20
Ammonium sulfate
Quaternium-40
Fragrance
Potassium coco-hydrolyzed animal protein
Sodium styrene/PEG-10 maleate/Nonoxynol-10 maleate/Acrylate copolymer
EDTA
Ammonium nonoxynol-4 sulfate
D & C Yellow No. 10
D & C Red No. 19

TONI SILKWAVE REGULAR (TOTAL CONDITIONING) WAVING LOTION
(Gillette Co., Personal Care Div.)

Water
Diisopropanolamine *
Ammonium thioglycolate *
Steareth-20
Quaternium-40
Fragrance
Potassium coco-hydrolyzed animal protein
Sodium styrene/PEG-10 maleate/Nonoxynol-10 maleate/Acrylate copolymer
EDTA
Ammonium nonoxynol-4 sulfate
D & C Yellow No. 10
D & C Red No. 19

TONI SILKWAVE SILVER CURL (TOTAL CONDITIONING) WAVING LOTION
(Gillette Co., Personal Care Div.)

Water
Diisopropanolamine *
Ammonium thioglycolate *
Steareth-20
Quaternium-40
Fragrance
Potassium coco-hydrolyzed animal protein
Sodium styrene/PEG-10 maleate/Nonoxynol-10 maleate/Acrylate copolymer
EDTA
Ammonium nonoxynol-4 sulfate
D & C Yellow No. 10
D & C Red No. 19

TONI SILKWAVE SUPER (TOTAL CONDITIONING) WAVING LOTION
(Gillette Co., Personal Care Div.)

Water
Diisopropanolamine *
Ammonium thioglycolate *
Steareth-20
Quaternium-40
Fragrance
Potassium coco-hydrolyzed animal protein
Sodium styrene/PEG-10 maleate/Nonoxynol-10 maleate/Acrylate copolymer
EDTA
Ammonium nonoxynol-4 sulfate
D & C Yellow No. 10
D & C Red No. 19

TONI SUPER CONDITIONING WAVING LOTION
(Gillette Co., Personal Care Div.)

Water
Diisopropanolamine *
Ammonium thioglycolate *
Steareth-20
Quaternium-40
Potassium coco-hydrolyzed animal protein
Fragrance
Sodium styrene/PEG-10 maleate/Nonoxynol-10 maleate/Acrylate copolymer
EDTA
Ammonium nonoxynol-4 sulfate
D & C Yellow No. 10
D & C Red No. 19

TONI SUPER HOME WAVE (TWIN CONDITIONING) WAVING LOTION
(Gillette Co., Personal Care Div.)

Water
Diisopropanolamine *
Ammonium thioglycolate *
Steareth-20
Quaternium-40
Fragrance
Potassium coco-hydrolyzed animal protein
Sodium styrene/PEG-10 maleate/Nonoxynol-10 maleate/Acrylate copolymer
EDTA
Ammonium nonoxynol-4 sulfate
D & C Yellow No. 10
D & C Red No. 19

TOPANEST
Dental anesthetic
(Barfred Research Labs.)

Hypnocaine (brand of propasin)
Benzyl alcohol *
Benzalkonium chloride *

'76 Ed.

TOPAZONE AEROSOL POWDER
Topical antibacterial agent
(Norden Labs.)

Topazone (brand of Furazolidone) *
3-oz. can .... 3.4 gm.
7-oz. can .... 7.9 gm.

TOPCARE CLEANER/ SHINER FORMULA
(Nat'l Labs. Div.)

Petroleum distillate *

TOPCO ALL PURPOSE CLEANER
(Topco)

Tetrasodium phosphate *† 17.5%

'76 Ed.

†*See* Trisodium phosphate

TOPCO AMMONIA
(Topco)

Ammonium hydroxide * ..... 6.2 - 7.0%

'76 Ed.

TOPCO AUTOMATIC DISHWASH
(Topco)

Sodium tripolyphosphate 36%
Sodium metasilicate * 12%
Sodium carbonate * 49%
Trichloro-s-triazinetrione 1%

'76 Ed.

TOPCO BLEACH
(Topco)

Sodium hypochlorite * ...... 5.25 - 6.0%

'76 Ed.

TOPCO BLUE DETERGENT
(Topco)

Sodium alkyl aryl sulfonate * 10%
Sodium silicate 15%
Sodium tripolyphosphate * 27%
Sodium sulfate 48%

'76 Ed.

TOPCO BUG KILLER
(Topco)

Pyrethrins 0.25%
Piperonyl butoxide 1.25%
Petroleum distillate 1.00%

'76 Ed.

TOPCO CLEANSER
(Topco)

Sodium dodecyl benzene sulfonate . 3.0%
Trisodium phosphate * 6.5%
Tetrasodium phosphate 1.5%
Trichloro-s-triazinetrione 0.5%

'76 Ed.

TOPCO FLYING INSECT KILLER
(Topco)

Pyrethrin 0.2%
Piperonyl butoxide 1.0%
N-Octyl bicycloheptene
 dicarboximide 1.0%
Petroleum distillate 0.8%

'76 Ed.

Starred ingredients (*) may be responsible for major toxic effects; consult Section II.

TOPCO HEAVY DUTY DETERGENT
(Topco)

Sodium alkyl aryl sulfonate	10%
Sodium silicate	15%
Sodium carbonate *	40%
Sodium sulfate	25%

'76 Ed.

TOPCO OVEN CLEANER
(Topco)

Sodium metasilicate *	5.0%
Sodium hydroxide *	3.0%
Ammonium hydroxide	0.6%

'76 Ed.

TOPCO PHOSPHATE FREE DETERGENT
(Topco)

Sodium metasilicate pentahydrate *	22%
Sodium carbonate *	40%
Sodium sesquicarbonate *	25%

'76 Ed.

TOPCO SPRAY DISINFECTANT
(Topco)

o-Phenylphenol	0.10%
n-Alkyl-n-ethyl morpholinium ethyl sulfates	0.035%
Isopropyl alcohol *	67.10%

'76 Ed.

TOPCO SUDSY AMMONIA
(Topco)

Ammonium hydroxide *	6.2 - 7.0%

'76 Ed.

TOPCO VALIANT APC'S
(Topco)

Acetylsalicylic acid *	3 1/2 gr.
Phenacetin *	2 1/2 gr.
Caffeine	1/2 gr.

'76 Ed.

TOPCO VALIANT RUBBING ALCOHOL
(Topco)

Isopropyl alcohol *	70%

'76 Ed.

TOPCO VALIANT RUBBING ALCOHOL WITH WINTERGREEN
(Topco)

Isopropyl alcohol *	70%
Methyl salicylate *	2%

'76 Ed.

TOPEX BUFFERED ACNE MEDICATION
(Vicks Toiletry Products Div.)

Benzoyl peroxide *	10.0%
Propylene glycol	
Stearic acid	
PEG-20 stearate	
Glyceryl stearate	
Isopropyl palmitate	
Zinc laurate	
Benzoic acid	

TOPIC
Antipruritic
(Syntex Labs.)

Benzyl alcohol *	5%
Gel base:	
Camphor	<1%
Menthol	<1%
Isopropyl alcohol *	30%
Purified water	
Hectorite	
Propylene glycol	
Sodium laureth sulfate	
Perfume	
Color	

TOPICAINE OINTMENT
Topical anesthetic; veterinary
(Goshen Labs.)

Dibucaine	1%
Lanolin-petrolatum base	

TOPICORT EMOLLIENT CREAM 0.25%
Relief of corticosteroid responsive dermatosis
(Hoechst-Roussel)

Each gram:	
Desoximetasone	2.5 mg.
Base:	
Isopropyl myristate	
Cetylstearyl alcohol	
White petrolatum	
Mineral oil	
Lanolin alcohol	
Purified water	

TOP JOB (Formula 1)
Liquid household cleaner
(Procter & Gamble)

Water	50-74%
Tetrapotassium pyrophosphate	10-24%
Sodium cumene sulfonate	5-9%
Sodium bicarbonate	1-4%
Sodium carbonate	1-4%
Sodium alkylethoxylate sulfate	1-4%
Ammonia	<1%
Minor ingredients, each	<1%

pH (undiluted) - 10.5
pH (1% solution) - 9.9

TOP JOB (Formula 2)
Liquid household cleaner
(Procter & Gamble)

Water	50-74%
Tetrapotassium pyrophosphate	10-24%
Sodium cumene sulfonate	5-9%
Sodium bicarbonate	1-4%
Sodium carbonate	1-4%
Potassium soap	1-4%
Sodium linear alkylate sulfonate	1-4%
Ammonia	<1%
Minor ingredients, each	<1%

pH (undiluted) - 10.5
pH (1% solution) - 10.0

TOP JOB (Non-Phosphate Formula) (Formula 1)
Liquid household cleaner
(Procter & Gamble)

Water	50-74%
Sodium carbonate	5-9%
Sodium cumene sulfonate	5-9%
Sodium linear alkylate sulfonate	5-9%
Sodium citrate	5-9%
Alkyl ethoxylate	1-4%
Ammonia	<1%
Minor ingredients, each	<1%

pH (undiluted) - 10.2
pH (1% solution) - 9.8

TOP JOB (Non-Phosphate Formula) (Formula 2)
Liquid household cleaner
(Procter & Gamble)

Water	50-74%
Sodium cumene sulfonate	10-24%
Sodium citrate	5-9%
Sodium carbonate	1-4%
Alkyl ethoxylate	1-4%
Sodium alkylethoxylate sulfate	1-4%
Ammonia	<1%
Minor ingredients, each	<1%

pH (undiluted) - 10.2
pH (1% solution) - 9.8

TOPOL TOOTHPOLISH - REGULAR
For removing stains from cigarette tar
(Jeffrey Martin, Inc.)

Water
Dicalcium phosphate dihydrate
Dicalcium phosphate
Sorbitol
Propylene glycol
Sodium lauryl sulfate
Magnesium aluminum silicate
Sodium saccharin
Methylparaben
Propylparaben
Cellulose gum
Flavor

Starred ingredients (*) may be responsible for major toxic effects; consult Section II.

TOPOL TOOTHPOLISH W/FLUORIDE
For removing stains from cigarette tar
(Jeffrey Martin, Inc.)

Sodium fluoride
Insoluble Sodium metaphosphate
Water
Sorbitol
Glycerin
Sodium lauryl sulfate
Dicalcium phosphate
Sodium carrageenan
Magnesium aluminum silicate
Flavor
Silica
Cellulose gum
Sodium saccharin
Methylparaben
Propylparaben
Titanium dioxide

TOPS TABLETS
Analgesic
(Premo)

Acetaminophen * .... 5 gr.

'76 Ed.

TOPSYN GEL
Topical anti-inflammatory agent
(Syntex Labs.)

Fluocinonide 0.05%
Base:
  Propylene glycol
  Propyl gallate
  Disodium edetate
  Carbopol 940 (Carboxypolymethylene)
  Sodium hydroxide and/or Hydrochloric
    acid to adjust pH

TOPTIC OINTMENT
Topical antibiotic for dogs and cats
(Elanco Prod.)

Each gram:
  Cephalonium .... 10 mg.
  Polymyxin B sulfate ..... 5,000 units
  Flumethasone .... 0.25 mg.
  Iodochlorhydroxyquin .... 30 mg.
  Piperocaine hydrochloride .... 40 mg.
  Mineral oil (heavy) ....300 mg.
  Petrolatum (white) .... q.s.

TOP TONE II DANDRUFF SHAMPOO AND SCALP REVITALIZER
(House of Lowell, Inc.)

Castor oil
TEA-lauryl sulfate
Potassium hydroxide
Lauramide DEA
Methyl salicylate
Eucalyptus oil
Pine tar
Siberian fir oil
Menthol

TOR
Germicidal cleaner
(Huntington Labs.)

Active ingred.: 7.2%
  Sodium carbonate 3.0%
  N-Alkyl (60% C14, 30% C16, 5%
    C12, 5% C18) dimethyl benzyl
    ammonium chlorides *† 1.6%
  N-Alkyl (50% C12, 30% C14, 17%
    C16, 3% C18) dimethyl ethyl-
    benzyl ammonium
    chlorides *‡ 1.6%
  Sodium metasilicate * 1.0%
Inert ingred.: 92.8%
  Water
  2-Alkanoxy polyethoxy ethanol
  Tetrapotassium pyrophosphate *

†*See* Alkyl dimethyl benzyl ammonium chloride
‡*See* Alkyl dimethyl ethylbenzyl ammonium chloride

TORA
Anorexiant
(Direct Div.)

Each tablet:
  Phentermine HCl * .... 8 mg.

TORAK, EMULSIFIABLE CONCENTRATE
Insecticide
(Hercules Incorporated)

Dialifor (O,O-Diethyl S-(2-chloro-1-
  phthalimidoethyl) phosphorodithioate) *

TORBIDAN 2-8 SPRAY
Insecticide
(Chevron)

Active ingred. (by wt.):
  Toxaphene 66.0%
  O,O-Dimethyl O-(p-nitrophenyl)
    thiophosphate * 16.5%
  Aromatic petroleum derivative
    solvent 11.0%

Chevron emergency phone number:
  415-233-3737

TORCH GLOW
Lamp fuel
(Sunnyside)

Petroleum distillate *

TORDON BEADS
Herbicide
(Dow)

4-Amino-3,5,6-trichloro picolinic
  acid, potassium salt 2.3%
Disodium tetraborate
  pentahydrate * 79.2%
Disodium tetraborate
  decahydrate * 16.5%

TORDON 225E MIXTURE HERBICIDE
(Dow)

Active ingred.:
Picloram ((4-Amino-3,5,6-trichloro-
  picolinic acid), triisopropanolamine salt) * 20.1%
2,4,5-Trichlorophenoxyacetic acid,
  propylene glycol butyl ether
  esters * 17.2%
Inert ingred.: 62.7%
  Ethylene glycol ethyl ether
  Xylene
  Emulsifiers

TORDON 40 HERBICIDE
(Dow)

Active ingred.:
Picloram ((4-Amino-3,5,6-trichloro-
  picolinic acid), isooctyl esters) * 62.4%
Inert ingred.: 37.6%
  Heavy Aromatic naphtha
  Methanol

TORDON 225 HERBICIDE
(Dow)

4-Amino-3,5,6-trichloropicolinic
  acid, triethylamine salt * 15.2%
2,4,5-Trichlorophenoxyacetic acid,
  triethylamine salt * 14.9%
Inert ingred.: 69.9%
  Sequestering agents
  Isopropanol
  Water

TORDON 472 HERBICIDE
(Dow)

Active ingred.:
Picloram ((4-Amino-3,5,6-trichloro-
  picolinic acid), dimethylamine
  salt) 2.4%
2,4-Dichlorophenoxyacetic acid, di-
  methylamine salt * 38.8%
Inert ingred.: 58.8%
  Isopropyl alcohol
  Water
  Sequestrants

TORDON 22K
(Dow)

4-Amino-3,5,6-trichloropicolinic
  acid, potassium salt * 24.9%
Inert ingred.: 75.1%
  Isopropanol
  Water
  Dispersing agents

TORDON K HERBICIDE
(Dow)

Active ingred.: 24.0%
  Picloram ((4-Amino-3,5,6-trichloro-
    picolinic acid), potassium salt) *
Inert ingred.: 76.0%
  Glycol ether
  Water

Starred ingredients (*) may be responsible for major toxic effects; consult Section II.

TORDON 10K PELLETS
Brush killer
(Dow)

Picloram (4-Amino-3,5,6-trichloro-picolinic acid, potassium salt) *	11.6%
Inert ingred.:	88.4%
Clay	

TORDON 101 MIXTURE
Weed and brush killer
(Dow)

4-Amino-3,5,6-trichloropicolinic acid, triisopropanolamine salt *	10.2%
2,4-Dichlorophenoxyacetic acid, triisopropanolamine salt *	39.6%
Inert ingred.:	50.2%
Sequestering agents	
Water	
Isopropanol	

TORDON 155 MIXTURE
Brush killer
(Dow)

4-Amino-3,5,6-trichloropicolinic acid, isooctyl esters *	15.1%
2,4,5-Trichlorophenoxyacetic acid, propylene glycol butyl ether esters *	63.4%
Inert ingred.:	21.5%
Aromatic petroleum solvent	
Methanol	

TORDON 212 MIXTURE
Herbicide
(Dow)

4-Amino-3,5,6-trichloropicolinic acid, triisopropanolamine salt *	18.1%
2,4-Dichlorophenoxyacetic acid, triisopropanolamine salt *	37.7%
Inert ingred.:	44.2%
Surfactants	
Water	

TORDON 101R FORESTRY HERBICIDE
(Dow)

Active ingred.:	
Picloram ((4-Amino-3,5,6-trichloro-picolinc acid), triisopropanola-mine salt)	5.4%
2,4-Dichlorophenoxyacetic acid, triisopropanolamine salt *	20.9%
Inert ingred.:	73.7%
Sequestering agents	
Water	
Isopropanol	

TORECAN
Antiemetic
(Boehringer-Ingelheim)

Each tablet:	
Thiethylperazine maleate *	10 mg.

TORECAN SUPPOSITORIES
Antiemetic
(Boehringer-Ingelheim)

Each suppository:	
Thiethylperazine maleate *	10 mg.
Theobroma oil	

TORPEDO
Acid scale remover
(Stiles-Kem)

Blend of Inorganic acids *

TOSS'N SOFT
Dryer cycle fabric softener sheet
(Purex Corp.)

Cationic softener *	70–75%
Ether foam	25–30%
Perfume	<1%

TOTACILLIN CAPSULES
Antibiotic therapy
(Beecham Labs.)

Each capsule:	
Ampicillin trihydrate	250 mg.; 500 mg.

TOTACILLIN FOR ORAL SUSPENSION
Antibiotic therapy
(Beecham Labs.)

Each 5 ml.:	
Ampicillin trihydrate	125 mg.; 250 mg.

TOTAL ECLIPSE SUNSCREEN LOTION COOLING ALCOHOL BASE
(Herbert Labs.)

Oxybenzone (Benzophenone-3)	
Padimate O (Octyl dimethyl PABA)	
Glyceryl PABA	
Alcohol	80.9%

TOTAL ECLIPSE SUNSCREEN LOTION RICH, MOISTURIZING BASE
(Herbert Labs.)

Padimate O (Octyl dimethyl PABA)
Oxybenzone (Benzophenone-3)

TOTAL FINISH BATHROOM CARE
Coating to clean, seal & polish surfaces
(Unelko)

	%/wgt.
Alkyl polysiloxanes (Dimethyl silicone fluids)	10.00%
Sulfuric acid (reagent grade)	1.00%
Isopropanol (Isopropyl alcohol, anhydrous) *	89.00%

TOTAL HARD CONTACT LENS SOLUTION
(Allergan Pharm.)

Polyvinyl alcohol
Edetate disodium
Benzalkonium chloride

TOTA-VI-CAPS GELATIN CAPSULE
Vitamin supplement
(Elder)

Each capsule:	
Vitamin A	5000 Units
Vitamin D	400 Units
Vitamin E	2 Int'l. Units
Plus multivitamins	

TOTE
Herbicide
(Dolge)

Urox liquid oil concentrate	18-20%
Heavy aromatic naphtha *	80-82%

TOTIL
Sanitizer/detergent
(Calgon Corp., Commercial Div.)

Ethylene oxide adduct
Quaternary ammonium chloride *
Alkaline salts *
Complex phosphates *

TOUCH OF SCENT (AEROSOL)
Air freshner
(Scott's Liquid Gold)

Denatured Ethyl alcohol
Scent
Hydrocarbon propellant (A-70)

TOUCH OF SWEDEN HAND LOTION
(Dow)

Emollients	16.5%
Water	81.0%

TOUCH-UP
Liquid cleaner
(Kay Chem. Co.)

Water	78-85%
Isopropanol *	8-10%
Ammonium hydroxide *	1-3%

TOUCH-UP LACQUER
Acrylic lacquer
(Talsol)

Cellosolve acetate	<25%
Isopropyl alcohol	<10%
Methyl ethyl ketone	<10%
Methyl isobutyl ketone	<10%
Toluene *	<30%
Xylene	<5%
Lead	<6%

TOURAINE CAL COTER PAINT
(Touraine Paints, Inc.)

Titanium pigment	37.6%
Calcium carbonate	30.3%
Silica	3.8%
Processed Linseed oil	26.7%
Thinner *† & Drier *	1.6%

'76 Ed.

†See Thinners, Section VI, General Formulations

TOURAINE EXTERIOR BASE PRIMERS
(Touraine Paints, Inc.)

#449:
Titanium dioxide	13.55%
Basic silicate white lead *	16.85%
Basic lead carbonate *	3.35%
Calcium carbonate	8.40%
Magnesium silicate	23.60%
Linseed oil	12.30%
Thinner & drier	14.80%
Soya alkyd resin	7.20%

CREAM (#446):
See #449 - same formulation

GREEN (#442):
Titanium dioxide	1.60%
Basic silicate white lead *	16.30%
Basic lead carbonate *	3.26%
Calcium carbonate	16.30%
Magnesium silicate	26.40%
Linseed oil	13.80%
Thinner & drier	10.80%
Soya alkyd resin	11.70%

RED (#445):
See GREEN (#442) - same formulation

'76 Ed.

TOURAINE FLOOR AND TRIM
(Touraine Paints, Inc.)

Thinner * & Drier *	54.5%
Non-volatile maleic modified soya alkyd resin	45.5%

'76 Ed.

†See Thinners, Section VI, General Formulations

TOURAINE FLOOR LATEX PAINTS
(Touraine Paints, Inc.)

BLENDING WHITE (#215):
Titanium dioxide	9.9%
Calcium carbonate	12.3%
Acrylic latex non-volatile	26.3%
Water	51.5%

CANYON RED (#203):
Iron oxide *	12.1%
Calcium carbonate	9.7%
Acrylic latex non-volatile	25.9%
Water, coalescing solvents	52.3%

HOLLY GREEN (#202):
Titanium dioxide	2.5%
Calcium carbonate	19.7%
Acrylic latex non-volatile	26.3%
Water, coalescing solvents	51.5%
Tinting color	approx. 5%

QUAKER GRAY (#206):
Titanium dioxide	7.4%
Calcium carbonate	14.8%
Acrylic latex non-volatile	26.3%
Water, coalescing solvents	51.5%
Tinting color	approx. 5%

SLATE GRAY (#201):
See QUAKER GRAY (#206) - same formulation

TERRACE GREEN (#204):
See QUAKER GRAY (#206) - same formulation

WHITE (#200):
Titanium dioxide	20.0%
Calcium carbonate	2.5%
Acrylic latex non-volatile	26.6%
Water	50.9%

WOODLAND BROWN (#205):
Iron oxide	9.9%
Calcium carbonate	12.3%
Acrylic latex non-volatile	26.3%
Water, coalescing solvents	51.5%
Tinting color	<5%

'76 Ed.

TOURAINE FLOOR, PORCH AND DECK ENAMELS
(Touraine Paints, Inc.)

BLACK (#815):
Carbon black	3.31%
Silicates	0.49%
Soya alkyd resin solution (41% solids)	78.90%
Thinner*† & Drier *	17.30%

BROWN (#805):
Iron oxide	5.40%
Calcium carbonate	10.80%
Bon maroon	0.57%
Silicates	0.57%
Lamp black	0.65%
Soya alkyd resin solution (57% solids)	73.00%
Thinner*† & Drier *	9.01%

BROWN MAHOGANY (#804):
Iron oxide *	74.70%
Lamp black	2.49%
Bon maroon	2.90%
Silicates	2.90%
Soya alkyd resin solution (57% solids)	15.11%
Thinner*† & Drier *	1.87%

DARK GRAY (#810):
Titanium dioxide	8.00%
Calcium carbonate	16.00%
Silicates	1.00%
Soya alkyd resin solution (57% solids)	66.75%
Thinner*† & Drier *	8.25%

(Continued next column)

FLAGSTONE GRAY (#809):
See DARK GRAY (#810) - same formulation

GOLDEN OAK (#802):
Iron oxide *	10.71%
Titanium dioxide	2.56%
Calcium carbonate	5.12%
Silicates	0.57%
Soya alkyd resin solution (57% solids)	72.10%
Thinner*† & Drier *	8.90%

LIGHT GRAY (#808):
See DARK GRAY (#810) - same formulation

MAROON (#813):
Iron oxide *	22.08%
Bon maroon	1.44%
Silicates	0.48%
Soya alkyd resin solution (57% solids)	67.64%
Thinner*† & Drier *	8.36%

SANDUST (#816):
See DARK GRAY (#810) - same formulation

TERRACE GRAY (#803):
Titanium dioxide	15.55%
Calcium carbonate	7.78%
Silicates	0.98%
Soya alkyd resin solution (57% solids)	67.31%
Thinner*† & Drier *	8.33%

TILE RED (#811):
Iron oxide *	19.40%
Silicates	0.60%
Soya alkyd resin solution (57% solids)	71.20%
Thinner*† & Drier *	8.80%

WALNUT (#801):
Iron oxide *	11.10%
Calcium carbonate	7.88%
Lampblack	0.42%
Soya alkyd resin solution (57% solids)	71.20%
Thinner*† & Drier *	8.80%

WHITE (#814):
Titanium dioxide	24.8%
Calcium carbonate	15.2%
Soya alkyd resin solution (57% solids)	54.3%
Thinner*† & Drier *	6.7%

'76 Ed.

†See Thinners, Section VI, General Formulations

TOURAINE LATEX EXTERIOR BASE PRIMER WHITE
(Touraine Paints, Inc.)

Titanium dioxide	15.14%
Lead silicate *	11.66%
Magnesium silicate	5.83%
Dibasic Lead phosphate *	4.06%
Barium compound *	3.50%
Acrylic polymer resin	21.10%
Water	38.80%

'76 Ed.

TOURAINE PAINT PRODUCTS
Interior and exterior paints and varnishes

Touraine Paints, Inc.
1760 Revere Beach Pkwy
Everett, Mass. 02149

Phone: 617-387-4690

See PAINTS, Section VI, General Formulations

TOURAINE POLYURETHANE SATIN GLOSS
(Touraine Paints, Inc.)

Silica	12.5%
Polyhydric alcohol partially esterified with linolenic, oleic, linoleic, palmitic, and stearic acids (modified with tolylene diisocyanate)	37.5%
Combined amount:	50.0%
Mineral spirits *	
Drier *	

'76 Ed.

TOURAINE POLYURETHANE SUPER GLOSS
(Touraine Paints, Inc.)

Polyhydric alcohol partially esterified with linolenic, oleic, linoleic, palmitic, and stearic acids (modified with tolylene diisocyanate)	50%
Combined amount:	50%
Mineral spirits *	
Drier *	

'76 Ed.

TOURAINE #32 PRIMER & SEALER
(Touraine Paints, Inc.)

Titanium dioxide	8.8%
Titanium calcium	17.7%
Calcium carbonate	19.9%
Silicates	2.9%
Thinner*† & Driers *	28.3%
Non-volatile alkyd resin	22.4%

'76 Ed.

†*See* Thinners, Section VI, General Formulations

TOURAINE REDWOOD WOOD FINISH
(Touraine Paints, Inc.)

Boiled linseed oil	67.9%
Combined amount:	19.1%
Petroleum distillates *	
Driers *	
Pentachlorophenol *	5.8%
Inert ingredients:	
Iron oxide pigment	3.3%
Paraffin wax	2.9%
Silicates	0.7%
Zinc stearate	0.3%

'76 Ed.

TOURAINE TRIM PAINTS
(Touraine Paints, Inc.)

BLACK (#510):
Carbon black	3.3%
Silicates	1.3%
Soya alkyd resin solution	76.2%
Thinner*† & Drier *	19.2%

CAPE COD BLUE (#512):
Titanium dioxide	4.2%
Phthalocyanine blue	5.3%
Silicates	1.0%
Soya alkyd resin solution	71.6%
Processed Linseed oil	11.5%
Thinner*† & Drier *	6.4%
Tinting color	<5%

CARDINAL RED (#505):
Toluidine red	11.8%
Silicates	1.2%
Soya alkyd resin solution	67.0%
Processed Linseed oil	10.9%
Thinner*† & Drier *	9.1%

FERN GREEN (#519):
Titanium dioxide	17.4%
Zinc oxide	2.9%
Silicates	2.9%
Soya alkyd resin solution	40.1%
Processed Linseed oil	27.7%
Thinner*† & Drier *	9.0%
Tinting color	10%

MAROON (#508):
Iron oxide *	26.1%
Silicates	1.7%
Soya alkyd resin solution	57.8%
Processed Linseed oil	9.5%
Thinner*† & Drier *	4.9%
Tinting color	<5%

TOBACCO BROWN (#509):
Iron oxide *	22.2%
Silicates	1.2%
Maroon oxide	1.0%
Alkyd resin solution	60.5%
Processed Linseed oil	10.0%
Thinner*† & Drier *	5.1%
Tinting color	<5%

TULIP YELLOW (#520):
Titanium dioxide	24.4%
Zinc oxide	1.3%
Silicates	2.2%
Soya alkyd resin solution	37.6%
Processed Linseed oil	26.1%
Thinner*† & Drier *	8.4%
Tinting color	<5%

TURQUOISE (#521):
Titanium dioxide	17.4%
Zinc oxide	2.9%
Silicates	2.9%
Soya alkyd resin solution	40.1%
Processed Linseed oil	27.7%
Thinner*† & Drier *	9.0%
Tinting color	<5%

WHITE (#500):
Titanium dioxide	38.1%
Silicates	1.4%
Zinc oxide	5.5%
Soya alkyd resin solution	37.2%
Processed Linseed oil	9.1%
Thinner*† & Drier *	8.7%

'76 Ed.

†*See* Thinners, Section VI, General Formulations

Starred ingredients (*) may be responsible for major toxic effects; consult Section II.

TOWER OF POWER
Insecticide
(Hub States)

Active ingredients:	12.50%
Pyrethrins	0.50%
Technical Piperonyl butoxide	4.00%
Petroleum distillates	8.00%

'76 Ed.

TOWLE SILVERSMITHS TARNISH PREVENTIVE SILVER POLISH
(E-Z-EST)

Stable emulsion of:	
Petroleum solvents *	22%
Waxes	
Diatomaceous earth	
Emulsifier	
Water	

TOWNE-PAULSEN'S BABY COUGH SYRUP
(Towne, Paulsen)

Each fl. oz.:	
Vitamin C	150 mg.
Potassium guaiacolsulfonate	100 mg.
Sodium citrate	600 mg.
Ammonium chloride	300 mg.
Chloroform	1 m.
Alcohol	2%

TOWNE-PAULSEN'S CHILDREN'S COLD TABLETS
(Towne, Paulsen)

Each tablet:	
Chlorpheniramine maleate	0.75 mg.
Vitamin C	35 mg.
Phenylephrine HCl	1 mg.
Salicylamide *	100 mg.
Caffeine *	16.25 mg.

TOWNE-PAULSEN'S CHILDREN'S COUGH SYRUP
(Towne, Paulsen)

Each fl. oz.:	
Dextromethorphan HBr	45 mg.
Chlorpheniramine maleate	4 mg.
Ammonium chloride	520 mg.
Potassium guaiacolsulfonate	520 mg.
Antimony potassium citrate	5 mg.
Chloroform	2 min.
Alcohol	5%

TOWNE-PAULSEN'S PERIODIC CAPSULES
For periodic pain
(Towne, Paulsen)

Each capsule:	
Cinnamyl ephedrine HCl *	15 mg.
Acetaminophen (APAP) *	180 mg.
Caffeine *	60 mg.
Methapyrilene HCl *	12.5 mg.
Homatropine methyl bromide	0.25 mg.

TOWNE-PAULSEN'S T.E.P.
For bronchial asthma, hay fever
(Towne, Paulsen)

Each tablet:	
Theophylline *	2 gr.
Ephedrine HCl *	3/8 gr.
Phenobarbital	1/8 gr.

TOX-A-DANE

See DR. ROGERS' TOX-A-DANE

TOXAKIL 20 DUST

See NIAGARA TOXAKIL 20 DUST

TOXALIN
Insecticide
(Techne Corp.)

Toxaphene (technical chlorinated camphene with 67% to 69% chlorine) *	45.0%
Gamma isomers of benzene hexachloride from lindane	2.0%
Aliphatic petroleum solvent	43.0%

'76 Ed.

TOXANE
Insecticide
(Cotton States Chem.)

Toxaphene *	45%
Malathion, tech.	5%
Aromatic petroleum distillate *	42%

TOXANOX PLUS
Insecticide; veterinary
(Farnam Co.)

Toxaphene *	45.00%
Gamma isomer of benzene hexachloride from lindane	1.80%
Petroleum distillate	47.70%

'76 Ed.

TOXAPHENE SOLUTION
Insecticide
(Hercules Incorporated)

Toxaphene (Chlorinated camphene containing 67-69% chlorine) *	90%
Xylene	10%

TOX-ENE

See DR. ROGERS' TOX-ENE

TOX-EOL "WH" CONCENTRATE
Insecticide
(Cre-O-Tox)

Heptachlor *	32.9%
Related compounds	11.5%
Petroleum distillate	50.3%

TOX-EOL WH 5 CONCENTRATE
Termite soil poisoning agent
(Cre-O-Tox)

Petroleum distillate	62.2%
Technical Chlordane	23.2%
Heptachlor *	11.4%

TOX-EOL WH 95 CONCENTRATE
Termite soil poisoning agent
(Cre-O-Tox)

Petroleum distillate	42%
Technical Chlordane	32.8%
Heptachlor *	16%
Related products	5.2%

TOX-HID

See UNICO TOX-HID

TOXIC-GUARD
To help neutralize effect of plant poisons on skin
(Reynes Products, Inc.)

Purified water
TEA stearate
Propylene glycol
Acetylated lanolin alcohol
Dimethicone
Magnesium stearate
PVP
Glyceryl stearate
Mineral oil
Lanolin alcohol
Methylparaben
Propylparaben

TOXI-FOG

See WEEVIL-CIDE TOXI-FOG

TOXI-TROL, SPRAY-TROL BRAND

See SPRAY-TROL BRAND TOXI-TROL

TOX - MP 6 - 3

See GROWER SERVICE TOX - MP 6 - 3

TOX-R
Insecticide
(Leffingwell)

Rotenone *	4.0%
Other chloroform extractives	7.0%

Starred ingredients (*) may be responsible for major toxic effects; consult Section II.

TPC BACK RUBBER CONCENTRATE
Controls hornflies on dairy cattle
(Texas Phenothiazine Co.)

Ronnel (O,O-Dimethyl O-(2,4,5-tri-
chlorophenyl)
phosphorothioate) * 34%

'76 Ed.

TPC BLUE-LOTION BOMB
Drying dressing for all livestock
(Texas Phenothiazine Co.)

Methyl violet 1.0%
Tannic acid 1.0%
Carbolic acid 1.0%
Methyl salicylate * 2.5%
Eugenol 0.5%
Propylene glycol 5.0%
Isopropyl alcohol * 39.0%
Inert ingred.: 50.0%
Propellent

'76 Ed.

TPC HOUSEHOLD ROACH SPRAY
(Texas Phenothiazine Co.)

O,O-Diethyl O-(2-isopropyl-4-
methyl-6-pyrimidinyl)
phosphorothioate 0.33%
Pyrethrins 0.06%
Technical Piperonyl butoxide ... 0.15%
N-Octyl bicycloheptene
dicarboximide 0.20%
Technical Chlordane 1.00%
Refined Petroleum oil * 48.26%

'76 Ed.

TPC LIVESTOCK INSECTICIDE DUSTER
*For spot treatment of livestock to con-
trol screw worms and ear ticks*
(Texas Phenothiazine Co.)

Ronnel (O,O-Dimethyl O-(2,4,5-tri-
chlorophenyl) phosphorothioate) * 5%

'76 Ed.

TPC LIVESTOCK SMEAR
*Kills screw-worms, ear ticks, ear mites,
blowfly maggots*
(Texas Phenothiazine Co.)

Ronnel (O,O-Dimethyl O-(2,4,5-
trichlorophenyl)phosphorothioate) 5%
Mineral oil * 35%
Xylene * 3%

'76 Ed.

TPC LIVESTOCK WOUND PROTECTANT BOMB
*Kills screw worms, ear ticks and blowfly
maggots on livestock*
(Texas Phenothiazine Co.)

Ronnel (O,O-Dimethyl O-(2,4,5-
trichlorophenyl)phosphorothio-
ate) 2.5%
Mineral oil * 15.0%
Xylene 0.5%

'76 Ed.

TPC WASP JET SPRAY
(Texas Phenothiazine Co.)

Pyrethrins 0.15%
Technical Piperonyl butoxide .. 0.30%
N-Octyl bicycloheptene
dicarboximide 0.53%
Technical Chlordane 2.00%
Petroleum distillate * 62.02%

'76 Ed.

TRAC II SHAVE CREAM
(Gillette Co., Personal Care Div.)

Water
Potassium stearate
Peanut oil
Isobutane
Laureth-23
Sorbitol
Mineral oil
Stearic acid
Propane
Cetyl alcohol
Fragrance
Carbomer-941
PEG-15 cocamine
Butane
BHA
BHT

TRAILWAY 4D
Herbicide
(Diamond Shamrock Corp.)

N-Oleyl-1,3-propylenediamine salt of
2,4-Dichlorophenoxyacetic acid * 57%

TRANCOPAL
Mild anxiety and tension
(Breon Labs.)

Each Caplet:
Chlormezanone * .... 100 mg.; 200 mg.

TRANMEP
Tranquilizer
(Reid-Provident)

Each tablet:
Meprobamate USP * .... 400 mg.

TRANQUIL-AID
(Thompson Med.)

Glycerol guaiacolate
Methapyrilene HCl *
Salicylamide
Magnesium trisilicate

TRANQUILIB
Relaxant
(Reese Chem.)

Each capsule:
Phenyltoloxamine citrate .... 5 mg.
Pyrilamine maleate * .... 20 mg.
Salicylamide .... 180 mg.

TRANQUILIUM CAPSULES
Tranquilizing aid
(Vitarine)

Each capsule:
Methapyrilene
hydrochloride * .... 25 mg.
Sodium salicylate * .... 60 mg.
Salicylamide * .... 160 mg.
Thiamine hydrochloride .... 2.5 mg.
Riboflavin .... 0.5 mg.
Pyridoxine hydrochloride ... 0.5 mg.
Niacinamide .... 20 mg.

TRANQUOIDS
Tranquilizer
(Pharmex)

Each tablet:
Methapyrilene
hydrochloride * .... 25 mg.
Salicylamide .... 250 mg.
P. E. Valerian .... 15 mg.
P. E. Passiflora .... 15 mg.

TRANSACT
Medicated acne gel
(Westwood Pharm.)

Liposec (brand of polyoxyethylene
lauryl ether) 6%
Micropulverized Sulfur 2%
Alcohol 40%
Greaseless base

'76 Ed.

TRANS-AID
*Additive for use with Brushkiller 170
& Weedone 2,4,5-T on winged elm,
mixed oak brush & mesquite*
(Amchem)

Ammonium thiocyanate *

TRANSAMINE OA-3D
Herbicide
(Vertac)

N,N-Dimethyloleyl-linoleyl amine
salt of 2,4-dichlorophenoxyacetic
acid (equiv. to 35.2% 2,4-D
acid) * 61.5%

TRANSAMINE OA-1.5D-1.5T
Herbicide
(Vertac)

N,N-Dimethyloleyl-linoleyl amine
salt of 2,4-dichlorophenoxyacetic
acid (equiv. to 17.3% of 2,4-D
acid) * 30.5%
N,N-Dimethyloleyl-linoleyl amine
salt of 2,4,5-trichlorophenoxy-
acetic acid (equiv. to 17.4% 2,4,5-
T acid) * 30.0%

TRANSAMINE OA-3T
Herbicide
(Vertac)

N,N-Dimethyloleyl-linoleyl amine salt of 2,4,5-trichlorophenoxy-acetic acid (equiv. to 33.1% of 2,-4,5-T acid) * 57.5%

TRANSEAL
Automatic transmission sealer & conditioner
(Radiator)

Petroleum distillates *

'76 Ed.

TRANSFLUSH
See ALSOL TRANSFLUSH

TRANS-KLEEN
See SILOO TRANS-KLEEN

TRANS-MEDIC
Transmission treatment
(Radiator)

Chlorinated hydrocarbons *

'76 Ed.

TRANSPORT
Bullet point markers - permanent
(Sanford Corp.)

Aromatic solvent:
　Xylene *
　Toluene *
Dyes
Resins

TRANS STOP LEAK (AS-225N, Formula MI-2235)
See PRESTONE TRANS STOP LEAK (AS-225N, Formula MI-2235)

TRANS-VERT
Additive for improving the activity of Envert and Emulsavert products on resistant species
(Amchem)

Monosodium acid
　methanearsonate * 51.19%

TRANXENE CAPSULES & TABLETS
Tranquilizer
(Abbott)

Each capsule or tablet:
　Clorazepate dipotassium * .. 3.75 mg.;
　　　　　　　　　　7.5 mg.; or 15 mg.

TRANXENE-SD TABLETS
Tranquilizer
(Abbott)

Clorazepate dipotassium *
　Tablets .... 22.5 mg
　Half-Strength Tablets ...... 11.25 mg.

TRATES
Coronary dilator
(Direct Div.)

Each capsule:
　Nitroglycerin * ...... 2.5 mg.; 6.5 mg.

TRAV-AREX TABLETS
For travel and motion sickness
(Columbia Med.)

Each tablet:
　Dimenhydrinate * .... 50 mg.

TRAVEL-EZE TABLETS
For motion sickness
(Approved Pharm.)

Each tablet:
　Pyrilamine maleate * ...... 25 mg.
　Hyoscine hydrobromide .... 0.325 mg.

'76 Ed.

TRAV MAR
See X-PANDO TRAV MAR

TRC ALUMINUM ROOF COATING
(Texas Refinery)

Asphalt 22.84%
Aliphatic and Aromatic
　hydrocarbons * 49.46%
Aluminum paste 27.70%

TRC ANTI-OXIDENE COATING
Rust protector
(Texas Refinery)

Blown asphalt 60%
Combined amount: 40%
　Aliphatic hydrocarbons *
　Aromatic hydrocarbons *

TRC SUREBRITE SUPER ALUMINUM PAINT
(Texas Refinery)

Petroleum hydro resin 7.5%
Phenolic resin 2.0%
Linseed oil 10.0%
Aliphatic and Aromatic
　hydrocarbons * 50.0%
Driers 0.5%
Aluminum paste 19.5%

TRE BIEN FURNITURE CREME
(Trewax)

Mineral oil 50%
Water 50%

TREE SEAL
For grafting or pruning
(Morrison's Orchard Supply)

Siliceous materials 13.040%

'76 Ed.

TREE TANGLEFOOT (Bulk)
Tree banding compound
(Tanglefoot)

Castor oil
Natural gum resins
Vegetable wax

TREE-TOX
See BONIDE TREE-TOX

TREFLAN E.C.
Selective herbicide
(Elanco Prod.)

Trifluralin (a,a,a-Trifluoro-2,6-dinitro-N,N-dipropyl-p-toluidine) * 44.5%

TREFLAN GRANULAR
Selective herbicide
(Elanco Prod.)

Trifluralin (a,a,a-Trifluoro-2,6-dinitro-N,N-dipropyl-p-toluidine) ... 5.0%

TRE-HOLD
Controls regrowth of sprouts after trimming
(Amchem)

1-Naphthaleneacetic acid, ethyl ester 1%

TREMCO FLOOR SEAL
(Tremco)

Xylene * .... <65%
Polyurethane prepolymer .... <45%

TREMIN TABLETS
Antispasmodic for parkinsonism
(Schering)

Each tablet:
　Trihexyphenidyl
　　hydrochloride * ...... .2 mg.; 5 mg.

TREMPRIME QUICK DRY
Roofing primer
(Tremco)

Blend of high flash Aliphatic and aromatic petroleum naphthas * ... 77%
Asphalt 13%
Petroleum hydrocarbon resin 10%

TREMSTRIP 20
Paint remover
(Tremco)

Methylene chloride *	<90%
Methanol	<10%
Detergent	<5%

TRENDAR TABLETS
Analgesic-diuretic for menstrual symptoms
(Whitehall Labs.)

Acetaminophen *
Pamabrom (2-Amino-2-methyl-1-propanol 8-bromotheophyllinate) *†
Phenindamine *

†*See* 2-Amino-2-methyl-1-propanol & Theophylline

TREND HEAVY DUTY LAUNDRY DETERGENT
(Purex Corp.)

Sodium carbonate *	20-30%
Anionic surfactant *	10-15%
Sodium silicate (not meta) *	5-15%
Cellulosic	<2%
Fluorescent whitening agent	<1%
Perfume	<1%
Sodium sulfate	balance

TREND HEAVY DUTY LIQUID LAUNDRY DETERGENT
(Purex Corp.)

Nonionic surfactant	15-25%
Anionic surfactant	5-10%
Fluorescent whitening agent	<1%
Coloring agent	<1%
Perfume	<1%
Hydrotrope	<1%
Water	balance

TREND LIQUID
For dishwashing, laundering of fine fabrics
(Purex Corp.)

Anionic surfactants *	10-25%
Alkanolamide	<2%
Hydrotrope	<2%
Ethyl alcohol	<2%
Opacifier	<1%
Coloring agent	<1%
Perfume	<1%
Water	balance

TRESS CARE
(Smith, Robert)

Tertiary amine salt
Ethoxylated fatty alcohol *

'76 Ed.

TREWAX BEAUTY SEALER
For slate, flagstone, stone & brick
(Trewax)

Solvent base acrylics *†	100%

†*See* Sealing compounds, Section VI, General Formulations

TREWAX CAR CLEANER
(Trewax)

Cleaning compounds	20%
Water	80%

TREWAX CAR FINISH
(Trewax)

Odorless Mineral spirits *	75%
Vegetable waxes	25%

TREWAX CLEANING WAX
(Trewax)

Vegetable waxes	15%
Odorless Mineral spirits *	85%

TREWAX CLEAR PASTE WAX
(Trewax)

Odorless Mineral spirits *	75%
Vegetable waxes	25%

TREWAX COLORED PASTE WAX
(Trewax)

Vegetable waxes	25%
Odorless Mineral spirits *	75%

TREWAX CONCENTRATED INSTANT WAX STRIPPER & FLOOR CLEANER
(Trewax)

Water	90%
Phosphates *	10%

TREWAX GOLD LABEL "SELF-POLISHING" WAX
(Trewax)

Acrylic polymers	18%
Water	82%

TREWAX HARDWOOD FLOOR FINISHING KIT
(Trewax)

Trewax Wood Cleaner:
Odorless Mineral spirits *	99%

Trewax Indian Sand:
Vegetable waxes	25%
Odorless Mineral spirits *	75%

TREWAX INDIAN SAND
(Trewax)

Vegetable waxes	25%
Odorless Mineral spirits *	75%

TREWAX LIQUID FLOOR WAX
(Trewax)

Waxes and acrylic polymers	16%
Water	84%

TREWAX SLATE WAX
(Trewax)

Vegetable waxes	25%
Odorless Mineral spirits *	75%

TREWAX WOOD CLEANER
(Trewax)

Odorless Mineral spirits *	99%

TRIACILLIN-250
Antibiotic-antibacterial
(Wesley Pharm.)

Each capsule:
    Ampicillin trihydrate (equivalent to 250 mg. ampicillin)

TRIALENE HAND SOAP
(Beck Chem.)

Solvents:
Xylol *	10%
Aromatics	trace

Cocoanut oil soap base

TRIAMINIC-DM COUGH FORMULA
Antitussive, decongestant
(Dorsey Labs.)

Each 5 ml.:
Phenylpropanolamine hydrochloride *	12.5 mg.
Dextromethorphan hydrobromide	10.0 mg.

TRIAMINIC EXPECTORANT
Decongestant, expectorant, antihistaminic
(Dorsey Labs.)

Each 5 ml.:
Phenylpropanolamine hydrochloride *	12.5 mg.
Guaifenesin (Glyceryl guaiacolate)	100 mg.
Alcohol	5%

Starred ingredients (*) may be responsible for major toxic effects; consult Section II.

TRIAMINIC EXPECTORANT DH
Antitussive, decongestant, antihistaminic, expectorant
(Dorsey Labs.)

Each 5 ml.:
Hydrocodone bitartrate * ... 1.67 mg.
Phenylpropanolamine
  hydrochloride * .... 12.50 mg.
Pheniramine maleate * ... 6.25 mg.
Pyrilamine maleate * ...... 6.25 mg.
Guaifenesin .... 100.00 mg.
Alcohol 5%

TRIAMINIC EXPECTORANT WITH CODEINE
Antitussive, decongestant, antihistaminic, expectorant
(Dorsey Labs.)

Each 5 ml.:
Codeine phosphate * ...... 10 mg.
Phenylpropanolamine
  hydrochloride * .... 12.5 mg.
Guaifenesin .... 100.0 mg.
Alcohol 5%

TRIAMINICIN
Analgesic, decongestant, antihistaminic
(Dorsey Labs.)

Each tablet:
Phenylpropanolamine
  hydrochloride * .... 25 mg.
Chlorpheniramine maleate .... 2 mg.
Aspirin .... 450 mg.
Caffeine .... 30 mg.

TRIAMINICIN ALLERGY TABLETS
Decongestant, antihistamine
(Dorsey Labs.)

Each tablet:
Phenylpropanolamine
  hydrochloride * .... 37.5 mg.
Chlorpheniramine maleate .... 4 mg.

TRIAMINICIN CHEWABLES
Decongestant & antihistaminic
(Dorsey Labs.)

Each chewable tablet:
Phenylpropanolamine
  hydrochloride * .... 6.25 mg.
Chlorpheniramine maleate .... 0.5 mg.

TRIAMINICOL DECONGESTANT COUGH SYRUP
Decongestant, antihistaminic, antitussive
(Dorsey Labs.)

Each 5 ml.:
Phenylpropanolamine
  hydrochloride * .... 12.5 mg.
Pheniramine maleate * ...... 6.25 mg.
Pyrilamine maleate * .... 6.25 mg.
Dextromethorphan
  hydrobromide * .... 15 mg.
Ammonium chloride .... 90 mg.

TRIAMINIC (ORAL INFANT DROPS & SYRUP)
Nasal decongestant, antihistaminic
(Dorsey Labs.)

Oral Infant Drops (each ml.):
Phenylpropanolamine
  hydrochloride * .... 20.0 mg.
Pheniramine maleate * ..... 10.0 mg.
Pyrilamine maleate * ...... 10.0 mg.

Syrup (each 5 ml.):
Phenylpropanolamine
  hydrochloride * .... 12.5 mg.
Chlorpheniramine maleate .... 2.0 mg.

TRIAMINIC-12 TABLETS
Nasal decongestant, antihistamine (12-hour)
(Dorsey Labs.)

Each tablet:
Phenylpropanolamine
  hydrochloride * .... 75 mg.
Chlorpheniramine maleate .... 12 mg.

TRIAMINIC (TABLETS & JUVELETS)
Nasal decongestant, antihistaminic
(Dorsey Labs.)

TABLETS (each):
Phenylpropanolamine
  hydrochloride * .... 50 mg.
Pheniramine maleate * ...... 25 mg.
Pyrilamine maleate * .... 25 mg.

JUVELETS (each tablet):
Phenylpropanolamine
  hydrochloride * .... 25.0 mg.
Pheniramine maleate * ...... 12.5 mg.
Pyrilamine maleate * .... 12.5 mg.

TRI-ANAMINE
Expectorant, decongestant, antihistaminic
(Life Labs., Inc.)

Each 5 ml.:
Phenylpropanolamine
  hydrochloride * .... 12.5 mg.
Pheniramine maleate ...... 6.25 mg.
Pyrilamine maleate .... 6.25 mg.
Glyceryl guaiacolate .... 100 mg.
Alcohol 5%

'76 Ed.

TRIANOL PAINT STRIPPERS
(Beck Chem.)

Combined amount: .... >10%
  Phenol *
  Cresylic acid *
Methylene chloride

TRIAVIL-2-10 TABLETS
Psychotropic
(MSD)

Each tablet:
Perphenazine .... 2 mg.
Amitriptyline hydrochloride * . 10 mg.

TRIAVIL-2-25 TABLETS
Psychotropic
(MSD)

Each tablet:
Perphenazine .... 2 mg.
Amitriptyline hydrochloride * . 25 mg.

TRIAVIL-4-10 TABLETS
Psychotropic
(MSD)

Each tablet:
Perphenazine .... 4 mg.
Amitriptyline hydrochloride * . 10 mg.

TRIAVIL-4-25 TABLETS
Psychotropic
(MSD)

Each tablet:
Perphenazine .... 4 mg.
Amitriptyline hydrochloride * . 25 mg.

TRIAVIL-4-50 TABLETS
Psychotropic
(MSD)

Perphenazine .... 4 mg.
Amitriptyline HCl * .... 50 mg.

TRIBARB CAPSULES
Sedative
(Lannett)

Each capsule:
Sodium secobarbital * ...... 1/2 gr.
Sodium butabarbital * ...... 1/2 gr.
Phenobarbital * .... 1/2 gr.

TRIBUCIDE
Water repellent preservative
(Honolulu Wood Treating Co.)

Bis(tri-n-butyltin)oxide * 2.0%
Petroleum hydrocarbons * 88.0%

TRI-CALSATE
Granular effervescent for temporary relief of gastric discomfort
(Paxton, F.H.)

Tri-basic calcium phosphate
Di-basic sodium phosphate special *
Bicarbonate of soda
Citric acid

TRICARBAMIX
Fungicide
(Pennwalt)

Zineb 45%
Maneb * 15%
Ferbam * 15%

TRICARBAMIX Zn
Fungicide
(Pennwalt)

Ziram * 45%
Ferbam 15%
Maneb 15%

Starred ingredients (*) may be responsible for major toxic effects; consult Section II.

TRI-CEN GERMICIDAL DETERGENT
(Central Chem.)

Isopropyl alcohol	7.79%
Ortho-benzyl-para-chlorophenate	4.40%
Ortho-phenylphenate	2.82%
Para-tertiary-amylphenate *	2.49%

'76 Ed.

TRICHLOR
Solvent
(PPG Industries, Chem. Div.)

Stabilized Trichlorethylene *	100%

TRICHLOREX TABLETS
Diuretic
(Lannett)

Each tablet:
Trichlormethiazide *	4 mg.

TRICHLOR-O-CIDE, FORMULA XP-100

See KLENZADE TRICHLOR-O-CIDE, FORMULA XP-100

TRICHOTINE-D
Disposable douche
(Reed & Carnrick)

Sodium chloride
Sodium lauryl sulfate
Silica
Tetrasodium EDTA

TRICHOTINE LIQUID CONCENTRATE
Vaginal cleanser
(Reed & Carnrick)

Sodium lauryl sulfate *	
Sodium borate *	
Aromatics	
Ethyl alcohol (SDA 23A)	8%

TRICHOTINE POWDER
Vaginal cleanser
(Reed & Carnrick)

Sodium lauryl sulfate
Sodium perborate *
Sodium chloride
Aromatics

TRICIDIN
First aid ointment
(Amlab)

Each gram:
Polymyxin B sulfate	5000 units
Bacitracin	400 units
Neomycin sulfate (equiv. to 3.5 mg. neomycin base)	5 mg.
Diperodon hydrochloride	10 mg.
In a White petrolatum base	

TRICO TABS
Analgesic, sedative
(Moffet Inc.)

Each tablet:
Phenobarbital *	8 mg.
Aspirin *	0.18 gm.
Phenacetin *	0.12 gm.

TRI-ETHANE
Solvent
(PPG Industries, Chem. Div.)

Stabilized 1,1,1-Trichlorethane *	100%

TRI-FLOW
Lubricant
(Formby's)

1,1,1-Trichloroethane *	20-30%
n-Amyl acetate	3-4%

TRIGESIC TABLETS
Analgesic, antipyretic agent
(Squibb)

Each tablet:
Acetyl-p-aminophenol *	125 mg.
Acetylsalicylic acid *	230 mg.
Caffeine	30 mg.

TRI-GRAIN PAIN TABLETS
(Pharmex)

N-Acetyl p-aminophenol *	1 1/2 gr.
Salicylamide	2 1/2 gr.
Aspirin *	2 1/2 gr.
Caffeine	1/2 gr.

TRIHEMIC 600 HEMATINIC TABLETS
(Lederle)

Each tablet:
Vitamin C (Ascorbic acid)	600 mg.
Vitamin B12 (Cobalamin concentrate, N.F.)	25 mcg.
Intrinsic factor concentrate	75 mg.
Folic acid	1 mg.
Vitamin E (d-alpha Tocopheryl acid succinate)	30 Int. Units
Elemental Iron (as present in 350 mg. of ferrous fumarate) *	115 mg.
Dioctyl sodium sulfosuccinate U.S.P.	50 mg.

TRIHISTA-COD ELIXIR
Expectorant
(Recsei Labs.)

Each 5 cc:
Codeine phosphate (1 gr. fl. oz.) *	10 mg.
Guaifenesin	20 mg.
Phenylpropanolamine *	7.5 mg.
Phenylephrine HCl *	2.5 mg.
Pyrilamine maleate *	5 mg.
Chlorpheniramine maleate	0.5 mg.
Sodium citrate	100 mg.

TRIHISTA-PHEN 25
Decongestant
(Recsei Labs.)

Each tablet:
Phenylpropanolamine HCl *	12.5 mg.
Pyrilamine maleate *	10.0 mg.
Pheniramine maleate *	7.5 mg.
Chlorpheniramine maleate *	1.0 mg.
Calcium lactate	250 mg.

TRIHISTA-PHEN CAPSULES
Relief of respiratory tract congestion
(Recsei Labs.)

Each capsule:
Chlorpheniramine maleate *	8 mg.
Phenylephrine HCl *	20 mg.
Scopolamine methylnitrate *	2.5 mg.

TRIHISTA-PHEN LIQUID
Relief of excessive cough & nasal congestion
(Recsei Labs.)

Each 5 cc:
Phenylpropanolamine HCl *	12.5 mg.
Tri-Histin (triple antihistamine) *	10 mg.
Guaifenesin	50 mg.

TRILAFON
Tranquilizer, antiemetic
(Schering)

CONCENTRATE:
Perphenazine *	16 mg./5 cc.

REPETABS:
Perphenazine *	8 mg.

TABLETS:
Perphenazine *	2 mg.; 4 mg.; 8 mg.; or 16 mg.

TRILIUM
Analgesic (aspirin free)
(Whitehall Labs.)

Each tablet:
Acetaminophen *	325 mg.

TRI-LUX WIDE SPECTRUM PAINTS
(International Paint)

Copper *
Ketone solvents *
Aromatics *†
Bis(tri-n-butyltin)fluoride *
Pigments color code #61, #63, #64, #65, #66, #67, #68

†*See* Aromatic hydrocarbon solvent

TRIMAGEL TABLETS
For the relief of gastric hyperacidity
(Columbia Med.)

Each tablet:
Magnesium trisilicate	0.5 gm.
Dried Aluminum hydroxide gel	0.25 gm.

Starred ingredients (*) may be responsible for major toxic effects; consult Section II.

TRIM-ELIM WATER PILLS
(Reese Chem.)

Each tablet:
P. E. Uva ursi leaves	....	30 mg.
P. E. Buchu leaves	....	30 mg.
Potassium citrate	....	60 mg.
Theobromine and Sodium salicylate *	....	50 mg.

TRIMETTE A TABS & CAPSULES
Decongestant
(Wesley Pharm.)

Each tablet or capsule:
Caffeine (anhydrous) *	......	140 mg.
Phenylpropanolamine hydrochloride *	....	40 mg.

TRIMETTE F TABS & CAPSULES
Decongestant
(Wesley Pharm.)

Each tablet or capsule:
Caffeine (anhydrous) *	......	100 mg.
Phenylpropanolamine hydrochloride *	....	25 mg.

TRIMETTE T TABS & CAPSULES
Decongestant
(Wesley Pharm.)

Each tablet or capsule:
Caffeine (anhydrous) *	......	180 mg.
Phenylpropanolamine hydrochloride *	....	50 mg.

TRIM-IT, GOOD-LIFE

See GOOD-LIFE TRIM-IT

TRIMO-SAN VAGINAL JELLY
(Milex)

Oxyquinoline sulfate	....	0.025%
Boric acid	....	1.00%
Borax		0.700%
Carboxypolymethylene (Carbomer), NF	....	2.33%

TRIMOX 250 & 500 CAPSULES
Antibiotic
(Squibb)

Amoxicillin trihydrate
Magnesium stearate
FD&C Blue #2
D&C Yellow #10
Titanium dioxide
Gelatin

TRIMOX 125 & 250 FOR ORAL SUSPENSION
Antibiotic
(Squibb)

Amoxicillin trihydrate
Sodium citrate
Sodium benzoate
Color, FD&C Red #40
Flavor, imitation wild cherry
Sugar

TRIM TIP
(Carter's Ink)

Glycol *†
Dyes *
Sodium benzoate

'76 Ed.

†*See* Ethylene glycol

TRIND-DM
Decongestant, analgesic, expectorant
(Mead Johnson)

Each 5 ml.:
Phenylephrine HCl	....	2.75 mg.
Acetaminophen *		120 mg.
Dextromethorphan HBr	.....	7.5 mg.
Guaifenesin	....	50 mg.
Alcohol	....	15%

TRIND SYRUP
Decongestant, analgesic, expectorant
(Mead Johnson)

Each 5 ml.:
Guaifenesin	....	50 mg.
Phenylephrine hydrochloride		2.75 mg.
Acetaminophen *	......	120 mg.
Alcohol	....	15%

TRINOXOL
Herbicide
(Amchem)

2,4,5-Trichlorophenoxyacetic acid, butoxy ethanol ester * 59.7%

TRINSITRATE CAPSULES
Hematinic
(Columbia Med.)

Two capsules contain:
Dessicated liver	....	350 mg.
Vitamin B12 activity (Cobalamine)	....	25 mcg.
Ferrous sulfate exsiccated *	..	800 mg.
Vitamin C (Ascorbic acid)	....	150 mg.

TRIO-BAR
Sedative
(Jenkins Labs.)

Each tablet:
Butabarbital sodium *	....	1/2 gr.
Phenobarbital *	....	1/2 gr.
Phenobarbital sodium *	......	1/2 gr.

TRIONA

See NIAGARA TRIONA

TRI-ORTHENE
Municipal sewer deodorant
(Puritan Chem. Co.)

Chlorinated hydrocarbons *

TRIOSULF
Antibacterial
(Jenkins Labs.)

Each tablet:
Sulfadiazine *	....	2.5 gr.
Sulfamerazine *	....	2.5 gr.
Sulfamethazine *	....	2.5 gr.

TRIOX LIQUID VEGETATION KILLER
Herbicide
(Chevron)

Prometon	....	1.86%
Pentachlorophenol *	....	0.68%
Other chlorinated phenols	......	0.08%

Chevron emergency phone number:
415-233-3737

TRIPHED
Antihistaminic/decongestant
(Lemmon Co.)

Each tablet:
Triprolidine hydrochloride *	.	2.5 mg.
Pseudoephedrine hydrochloride *	....	60 mg.

TRIPLE C
Concentrated car wash detergent
(Calgon Corp., Commercial Div.)

Alkyl aryl sulfonate *
Fatty amide
Water

TRIPLE D
Soapless detergent, disinfectant & deodorant
(Consolidated Chem., Inc.)

Nonionic surfactant
Sodium ethylene diamine acetic acid
Sodium oxybis (4 dodecylbenzene sulfonate) *†
Sodium tripolyphosphate *
Essential oils *
Soda ash *
Quaternary ammonium salt *

†*See* Alkyl aryl sodium sulfonates

TRIPLE-NOCTIN L
Soybean seed treatment/inoculant
(Kalo)

Thiram *
Sodium molybdate

TRIPLE-NOCTIN II
Soybean seed treatment/inoculant
(Kalo)

Thiram *
Sodium molybdate

TRIPLE PASTE
(Torch)

Burow's solution .... 1 part
Absorption base .... 2 parts
Lassar's zinc oxide paste .... 3 parts

'76 Ed.

TRIPLE X
Pediculosis control; kills lice and eggs
(Youngs Drug Products)

Pyrethrins 0.3%
Piperonyl butoxide, technical 3.0%
Petroleum distillate 1.2%
Benzyl alcohol 2.4%

TRIP-L-KIL

See BONIDE TRIP-L-KIL

TRISEM (SUSPENSION & TABLETS)
Triple sulfonamide therapy
(Beecham Labs.)

Each 5 ml. & tablet:
  Sulfamerazine * .... 0.167 gm.
  Sulfadiazine * .... 0.167 gm.
  Sulfamethazine * .... 0.167 gm.

TRISILOBARB TABLETS
Antacid
(Wesley Pharm.)

Each tablet:
  Magnesium trisilicate .... 5 gr.
  Dried Aluminum hydroxide
    gel .... 2 1/2 gr.
  Phenobarbital .... 1/12 gr.

TRISOGEL
Antacid
(Lilly, Eli)

Each fl. oz.:
  Magnesium trisilicate .... 3.5 gm.
  Aluminum hydroxide .... 0.9 gm.

TRITHION (4-E, 8-E)
Insecticide
(Stauffer)

Trithion (S-((p-Chlorophenylthio)methyl)
O,O-diethyl phosphorodithioate) *

TRITON B-1956
Spreader-sticker
(Rohm and Haas)

Phthalic glycerol alkyd resin, modified

TRITON CF-10
Low foam nonionic detergent
(Rohm and Haas)

Ethoxylated benzyl ether of
  octylphenol *†

†*See* Nonionic surfactants

TRITON CF-21
Nonionic low foam surfactant
(Rohm and Haas)

Modified Alkyl aryl polyether alcohol *

TRITON CF-32
Low foam nonionic detergent
(Rohm and Haas)

Amine polyglycol condensate *†

†*See* Nonionic surfactants

TRITON CF-54
Nonionic low foam detergent
(Rohm and Haas)

Modified Polyethoxy adduct *†

†*See* Nonionic surfactants

TRITON DF-12 & DF-16
Nonionic low foam surfactants
(Rohm and Haas)

Modified Alcohol ethoxylate *

TRITON GR-5
Anionic surfactant
(Rohm and Haas)

Sulfonated alkyl ester in isopropanol *

TRITON GR-7
Anionic surfactant
(Rohm and Haas)

Sulfonated alkyl ester in petroleum distillate *

TRITON H-55 & H-66
Anionic surfactant
(Rohm and Haas)

Phosphate ester supplied in the free acid
form

TRITON N-57 & N-101
Nonionic detergents
(Rohm and Haas)

Alkylated aryl polyether alcohol *

TRITON QS-15
Nonionic surfactant compatible in strong alkaline solutions
(Rohm and Haas)

Sodium salt of an oxyethylated surfactant
  containing anionic & cationic centers *

TRITON QS-30 & QS-44
Anionic surfactant
(Rohm and Haas)

Phosphate ester supplied in the free acid
form

TRITON 770 CONCENTRATE
Anionic industrial & household detergent
(Rohm and Haas)

Sodium alkyl aryl polyether sulfate *

TRITON X-15, X-35, X-45, X-100, X-102, X-114, X-120 (Powder), X-165, X-305, X-363, X-405
Nonionic detergents
(Rohm and Haas)

Alkylated aryl polyether alcohol *

TRITON X-151, X-152, X-161, X-171, X-172, X-180, X-190, X-193, X-700, X-800
Pesticide emulsifiers
(Rohm and Haas)

Alkyl aryl polyether alcohols *
  with organic sulfonates

TRITON X-155
Acid stable detergent
(Rohm and Haas)

Alkyl phenoxy polyethoxy ethanol *

TRITON X-200
Anionic detergent for industrial & household formulations
(Rohm and Haas)

Sodium salt of an alkyl aryl polyether sulfonate *

TRITON X-207 & X-363M
Cleaning compound & emulsifier
(Rohm and Haas)

Alkyl aryl polyether alcohols *
Nonionic solubilizing agent

TRITON X-301
Anionic industrial & household detergent
(Rohm and Haas)

Sodium alkyl aryl polyether sulfate *

TRITON X-400
Cationic hair & fabric softener
(Rohm and Haas)

Stearyl dimethyl benzyl ammonium chloride *

Starred ingredients (*) may be responsible for major toxic effects; consult Section II.

TRITUSSIN COUGH SYRUP
(Towne, Paulsen)

Each fl. oz.:
Codeine phosphate *	58 mg.
Pyrilamine maleate	40 mg.
Prophenpyridamine maleate	10 mg.
Methapyrilene HCl	10 mg.
Ammonium chloride	520 mg.
Potassium guaiacolsulfonate	520 mg.
Vitamin C	100 mg.
Hesperidin methyl chalcone	50 mg.
Chloroform	2 m.
Alcohol	5%

Menthol and glycerin in a flavored syrup base

TRIUMPH BOWL CLEANER
(Navy Brand)

Hydrogen chloride *	24.82%
Para di-isobutyl-phenoxy ethoxy ethyl, dimethyl benzyl ammonium chloride	0.20%

TRIUMPH WATER EMULSION PASTE WAX
(Uncle Sam)

Waxes
Emulsifiers
Surfactants
Resins
Ammonia
Water

TRIZYME

See AMWAY TRIZYME

TRO-K
Germicide-local anesthetic
(Moffet Inc.)

Each lozenge:
Phenylmercuric borate *	0.3 mg.
Benzocaine	3.0 mg.
Aromatics	q.s.

TROLENE 18 INSECTICIDE
(Dow)

Ronnel (O,O-Dimethyl O-(2,4,5-trichlorophenyl)phosphorothioate) *	18.0%
Inert ingred. (major):	82.0%
Salt	
Diatomaceous earth	

TROLENE 20 L INSECTICIDE
(Dow)

Active ingred.:	20.0%
Ronnel *	
Inert ingred.:	80.0%
Soybean oil	
Emulsifiers	

TRONIC
Spreader-activator for herbicide sprays
(Kalo)

Alkylarylpolyoxyethylene glycols *†
Mixed Petroleum distillates *
Alkyl amine acetate
Alkylaryl sulfonates *
Polyhydric alcohol

†*See* Alkyl aryl polyoxyethylene

TRONOTHANE HYDROCHLORIDE CREAM OR JELLY
(Abbott)

Pramoxine hydrochloride	1%

TROPH-IRON LIQUID
(MenJ Labs.)

Each 5 ml.:
Thiamine hydrochloride (Vitamin B1)	10 mg.
Cyanocobalamin (Vitamin B12)	25 mcg.
Iron (present as soluble pyrophosphate)	30 mg.

TROPH-IRON TABLETS
Vitamins B1, B12, iron
(MenJ Labs.)

Each tablet:
Thiamine hydrochloride (Vitamin B1)	10 mg.
Cyanocobalamin (Vitamin B12)	25 mcg.
Iron (present as soluble pyrophosphate)	30 mg.

TROPHY GYM FINISH
Floor seal & finish
(Hillyard Chem.)

Mineral spirits *

'76 Ed.

TROPHY SEAL
Floor seal & finish
(Hillyard Chem.)

Mineral spirits *

'76 Ed.

TROUTMAN'S COUGH SYRUP
(G. E. Labs.)

Each 5 ml.:
Dextromethorphan hydrobromide *	10 mg.

Vehicle:
Corn syrup
Water
Sucrose
Ammonium chloride
Caramel
Flavors (Horehound, Menthol and Peppermint)
Alcohol	5%

TROXYMITE
(Texas Refinery)

Epoxy resin	10.7%
Fatty amide	5.8%
Sand	83.1%
Titanium dioxide and lampblack	0.4%

TROYCO OINTMENT
Analgesic; veterinary
(Troy Chem.)

Lanolin
Pine oil *
Wax
Cedar leaf oil *

TRU FLEX ACRYLIC LATEX HOUSE PAINT
(Touraine Paints, Inc.)

WHITE BASE "A" & "B":
Titanium dioxide	16.2%
Silica	16.2%
Calcium carbonate	6.0%
100% Alkyd resin emulsion	2.8%
Acrylic polymer resin	18.1%
Water	40.7%

NEUTRAL BASE "C":
Titanium dioxide	6.2%
Silica	22.7%
Calcium carbonate	8.2%
100% Alkyd resin emulsion	2.8%
Acrylic polymer resin	18.4%
Water	41.6%

ACCENT BASE "D":
Titanium dioxide	3.2%
Silica	25.2%
Calcium carbonate	8.2%
100% Alkyd resin emulsion	2.8%
Acrylic polymer resin	18.5%
Water	42.0%

CLEAR BASE "E":
Silica	25.3%
Calcium carbonate	10.5%
100% Alkyd resin emulsion	2.9%
Acrylic polymer resin	18.8%
Water	42.6%

EXTERIOR YELLOW BASE "H":
Titanium dioxide	9.9%
Titanium yellow *	9.9%
Silica	15.9%
Calcium carbonate	4.0%
100% Alkyd resin emulsion	2.7%
Acrylic polymer resin	17.7%
Water	40.0%

'76 Ed.

Starred ingredients (*) may be responsible for major toxic effects; consult Section II.

TRU FLEX ACRYLIC LATEX TRIM PAINTS
(Touraine Paints, Inc.)

ADRIATIC BLUE (#304):
Titanium dioxide	13.87%
Barium sulfate	4.63%
Acrylic polymer resin	27.30%
Water	54.20%

BERKSHIRE GREEN (#301):
Chromium oxide green	7.87%
Phthalo green	2.63%
Acrylic polymer resin	30.85%
Water	58.65%

BLACK (#310):
Carbon black	1.0%
Acrylic polymer resin	33.3%
Water	65.7%

BRILLIANT WHITE (#300):
Titanium dioxide	25.00%
Acrylic polymer resin	25.50%
Water	49.50%

ENSIGN BLUE (#303):
Titanium dioxide	5.32%
Phthalo blue	2.68%
Acrylic polymer resin	31.30%
Water	60.70%

MOHAWK BROWN (#306):
Iron oxide *	10.3%
Acrylic polymer resin	30.5%
Water	59.2%

PIONEER GREEN (#305):
See BERKSHIRE GREEN (#301) - same formulation

ROYAL RED (#302):
Toluidine red	7.0%
Acrylic polymer resin	33.4%
Water	59.6%

'76 Ed.

TRU FLEX PAINTS
(Touraine Paints, Inc.)

BLACK:
Black Iron oxide	6.72%
Silica	26.88%
100% Alkyd resin emulsion	2.72%
Acrylic polymer resin	20.00%
Water	43.60%

BLENDING WHITE (#677):
Titanium dioxide	16.12%
Calcium carbonate	8.06%
Silica	16.12%
100% Alkyd resin emulsion	2.62%
Acrylic polymer resin	18.95%
Water	38.05%

BUCKINGHAM GREEN (#697):
Titanium dioxide	4.42%
Chromium oxide	2.19%
Yellow Iron oxide	2.23%
Calcium carbonate	13.28%
Silica	13.28%
100% Alkyd resin emulsion	2.72%
Acrylic polymer resin	19.40%
Water	42.60%

CEDAR GREEN (#693):
Titanium dioxide	6.56%
Chromium oxide	4.38%
Calcium carbonate	13.10%
Silica	13.05%
100% Alkyd resin emulsion	2.70%
Acrylic polymer resin	19.10%
Water	41.10%

CHARCOAL (#689):
Titanium dioxide	4.10%
Calcium carbonate	12.30%
Silica	20.50%
100% Alkyd resin emulsion	2.64%
Acrylic polymer resin	19.30%
Water	41.05%

Continued next column

COACH RED (#699):
Toluidine red	4.77%
Iron oxide	4.77%
Silica	21.45%
100% Alkyd resin emulsion	2.62%
Acrylic polymer resin	19.54%
Water	46.84%

COLONIAL GREEN (#698):
See BUCKINGHAM GREEN (#697) - same formulation

COLONY GOLD (#670):
Titanium dioxide	8.07%
Calcium carbonate	10.10%
Silica	20.30%
100% Alkyd resin emulsion	2.52%
Acrylic polymer resin	18.90%
Water	40.20%

GEORGIA BEIGE (#674):
See COLONY GOLD (#670) - same formulation

ONYX GRAY (#694):
See CHARCOAL (#689) - same formulation

PINE NEEDLE GREEN (#686):
See CHARCOAL (#689) - same formulation

REPUBLIC GOLD (#671):
See COLONY GOLD (#670) - same formulation

STORM CLOUD GRAY (#691):
See CHARCOAL (#689) - same formulation

VERMONT MOSS(#675):
See COLONY GOLD (#670) - same formulation

VIRGINIA BROWN (#672):
See CHARCOAL (#689) - same formulation

WHITE (#666):
Titanium dioxide	23.8%
Silicate	12.9%
100% Alkyd resin emulsion	4.94%
Vinyl acrylic resin	15.9%
Water	42.5%

'76 Ed.

TRU FLEX PRIMERS
(Touraine Paints, Inc.)

CREAM (#610):
Titanium dioxide	17.9%
Lead silicate *	11.9%
Silicates	6.0%
Barium salts *	4.2%
100% Alkyd resin emulsion	2.7%
Acrylic polymer resin	18.84%
Water	38.36%

GREEN (#609):
Titanium dioxide	4.10%
Lead silicate *	12.42%
Calcium carbonate	8.21%
Silicates	6.17%
Chromium oxide	4.10%
Barium salts *	4.10%
100% Alkyd resin emulsion	2.74%
Acrylic polymer resin	19.18%
Water	38.92%

GRAY (#608):
Titanium dioxide	4.02%
Lead silicate *	12.06%
Calcium carbonate	12.06%
Silicates	8.04%
Barium salts *	4.02%
100% Alkyd resin emulsion	2.69%
Acrylic polymer resin	18.80%
Water	38.30%

RED (#611):
Red oxide	8.1%
Silica & silicates	16.4%
Calcium carbonate	10.3%
Barium salts *	4.2%
Acrylic polymer emulsion	22.7%
Water	38.3%

'76 Ed.

TRU-GLO

See ALSOL TRU-GLO

TRULY FINE CREME RINSE
(Safeway Stores)

Stearyl dimethyl benzyl ammonium chloride	4%
Cetyl alcohol	2%
Propylene glycol monostearate	1%
Other: Perfume, Nonionic surfactant, Potassium chloride, Dye	1%
Water	92%

pH, undiluted 4

TRULY FINE SHAMPOO
(Safeway Stores)

Triethanolamine lauryl sulfate *	15%
Fatty amide	8%
Collagen protein hydrolysate	2%
Other	2%
Water	73%

pH, undiluted 7.5

Starred ingredients (*) may be responsible for major toxic effects; consult Section II.

TRULY FINE TOILET BAR SOAP
(Safeway Stores)

Tallow/Coconut oil soap (Na)	84%
Trichlorocarbanilide	1%
Other: Perfume, Sodium chloride, Glycerine, Silicate, EDTA, Titanium dioxide, Surfactant (LAS), Dye	3%
Water	12%

TRU-MINT
Disinfectant
(Miller-Norris Co.)

Active ingredients:	28%
Isopropyl alcohol *	
Soap	
Ortho-benzyl para-chlorophenol *	
Methyl salicylate *	

'76 Ed.

TRU-NOX INSECTICIDE (AEROSOL)

See SPRAYWAY TRU-NOX INSECTICIDE (AEROSOL)

TRUST
All-purpose detergent
(Essential Chem.)

Sodium dodecyl benzene sulfonate *	18.6%
3,5-Dimethyl-4 chlorophenol	2.0%

TRYAD
Detergent disinfectant cleaner
(Whitmoyer)

n-Alkyl (50% C14, 40% C12, 10% C16) dimethyl benzyl ammonium chloride *	5.00%
Sodium hydroxide *	3.00%
Tetrasodium salt of EDTA	0.88%
Inert ingred.:	91.12%
Contains detergents	

TRYPZYME AEROSOL
External wound dressing; veterinary
(Burns-Biotec)

Each gram:	
Trypsin (crystallized)	0.1 mg.
Oil Balsam peru	72.5 mg.
Castor oil	800.0 mg.
Emulsifier (Igepal CO-530)	
Propellant (Propane and Isobutane)	

TSG CROUP LIQUID
Bronchospasmic conditions of asthma
(Elder)

Each 30 ml.:	
Theophylline sodium glycinate *	600 mg.
Potassium iodide	200 mg.
Ephedrine hydrochloride *	50 mg.
Codeine phosphate *	30 mg.
Alcohol	15%

TSG-KI ELIXIR
Bronchospasmic conditions of asthma
(Elder)

Each 15 ml.:	
Theophylline sodium glycinate, N.F. (Theophylline equiv. 150 mg.) *	300 mg.
Potassium iodide	100 mg.
Alcohol	15%

TSP - HEAVY DUTY CLEANER
(Savogran)

Trisodium phosphate *	>80%
Sodium sesquicarbonate	<20%

TUCKO
Fungus infections of the skin - athlete's foot/ringworm
(Tucko Sales Co.)

Salicylic acid *	1-10%
Benzoic acid	1-10%
Oil of tar *	1-10%
Benzocaine	<1%
Glycerine	<1%
Camphor	<1%
Menthol	<1%
Isopropyl alcohol *	58%

TUCO AGRICULTURAL PRODUCTS

TUCO
Div. of The Upjohn Co.
7171 Portage Rd.
Kalamazoo, Mich. 49001

Phone: 616-385-6613

TUFF-BOND GENERAL PURPOSE ADHESIVE
(Moore, G.E.)

Ethyl alcohol	0.40%
Petroleum distillate *	40%
Reclaimed rubber	
Resin	
Inert filler	

TUFF-BOND QUIK-SET ADHESIVE
(Moore, G.E.)

Acetone *	15%
Methyl ethyl ketone *	18%
Toluol *	3%
Petroleum distillate *	35%
Neoprene rubber	
Resin	
Inert filler	

TUFF-JOB
Liquid steam cleaning compound; industrial and institutional use
(Scientific International)

Very strong Alkalis *

TUFF JOB OIL
(Stewart Sanitary Supply)

Petroleum distillate *	100%

TUFF KOTE FURNITURE POLISH & WAX
(McAleer)

Mineral spirits *
Waxes
Silicone oils
Diatomaceous earth
Amyl acetate *

'76 Ed.

TUFF KOTE WAX
Floor wax
(McAleer)

Morpholine oleate *
Polyethylene vinyl polymers
Shellac *
Borax *
Ammonia *

'76 Ed.

TUF-FOOT
For tender feet of dogs; veterinary
(Bonaseptic)

Balsam Peru	
Balsam Tolu	
Balsam Styrax	
Aloe *	
Benzoin	
Alcohol *	80%

TUFFSHEEN
Liquid floor wax
(Sanitek)

Various Waxes and Polyethylenes	13.0%
Rosin maleate resin	3.6%
Dimethylaminoethanol	0.5%
Potassium hydroxide (50% aq.)	0.3%
Ammonia	trace
Water	balance

TUFFSHEEN II
Liquid floor polish
(Sanitek)

Acrylic polymer emulsion	10.4%
Diethylene glycol monoethyl ether (Cellosolve)	4.0%
Polyethylene emulsion	3.3%
Rosin maleate resin	1.5%
Tributoxyethyl phosphate	0.9%
Nonionic surfactant	0.3%
Formalin, Ammonia, Fluorochemical surfactant	trace
Water	balance

TUFF-STRIP 911
Ammoniated wax stripper
(Sanitek)

Ammonia	4.9%
Isopropanol	3.0%
Anionic surfactants (30% active)	2.2%
Dipropylene glycol monomethyl ether (Cellosolve)	1.5%
Sodium tripolyphosphate	1.3%
Nonionic surfactants, Dye, Defoamer	trace
Water	balance

TUFF STUFF ENGINE SCOUR (AS-186, Formula 2028-74)
Pressurized automobile engine block cleaner
(Union Carbide)

Petroleum distillates *	95%
Nonionic surfactants	5%
Carbon dioxide propellant	

TUFFY "C"
Corrosion resistant finish
(Lester Labs.)

Epoxy resins

'76 Ed.

TUF SKIN (COLORLESS) LIQUID
(Cramer Products)

Isopropyl alcohol *	70%
W.W. Gum rosin	20%
Benzoin tincture 10%	10%

TUF-SKIN (ORIGINAL) LIQUID
(Cramer Products)

Isopropyl alcohol *	69.99%
D & C Yellow #11	0.01%
W.W. Gum rosin	20.00%
Benzoin tincture 10%	10.00%

TUFTHANE TOP COAT
Floor paint
(Tremco)

Xylene *	<65%
Polyurethane prepolymer	<45%

TUINAL PULVULES (NOS. 2, 3, & 4)
(Blue body, orange cap)
Sedative, hypnotic
(Lilly, Eli)

No. 2 (F66) (each Pulvule):
Secobarbital sodium	1 1/2 gr.
Amobarbital sodium *	1 1/2 gr.

No. 3 (F65) (each Pulvule):
Secobarbital sodium	3/4 gr.
Amobarbital sodium *	3/4 gr.

No. 4 (F64) (each Pulvule):
Secobarbital sodium	3/8 gr.
Amobarbital sodium *	3/8 gr.

TULVEX
For ringworm, fungus, infections, athlete's foot
(Commerce Drug)

Benzethonium chloride *	
Benzalkonium chloride *	
Undecylenic acid *	
Tannic acid	
Isopropyl alcohol *	70%

TUMS EXTRA STRENGTH
Antacid
(Norcliff Thayer)

Each tablet:
Precipitated Calcium carbonate	750 mg.
Sugar/Starch	1,146 mg.
Wintergreen flavoring	<1%

TUMS (ORANGE, LEMON OR CHERRY)
Antacid
(Norcliff Thayer)

Each tablet:
Precipitated Calcium carbonate	500 mg.
Sugar/Starch	750-753 mg.
Flavoring - orange, lemon or cherry	approx. 1%

TUMS, PEPPERMINT
Antacid
(Norcliff Thayer)

Each tablet:
Precipitated Calcium carbonate	500 mg.
Sugar/Starch	714 mg.
Peppermint flavoring	<1%

TUMS, WINTERGREEN
Antacid
(Norcliff Thayer)

Each tablet:
Precipitated Calcium carbonate	500 mg.
Sugar/Starch	764 mg.
Wintergreen flavoring	<1%

"TUPERSAN" WEED KILLER
(Du Pont)

Siduron * ... 50%

"TUPERSAN" 70 WEED KILLER
(Du Pont)

Siduron ... 70%

TURF BUILDER (I)
Fertilizer
(Scott, O.M.)

Fertilizer formula: 22-3-3
Iron (Fe)	1.26%
Carrier: Vermiculite	

TURF BUILDER PLUS HALTS
Herbicide
(Scott, O.M.)

Bensulide ... 4.78%; 3.58%; 2.98%
Carrier base: Fertilizer 20-6-6

TURF BUILDER PLUS LAWN DISEASE PREVENTER
Fungicide/fertilizer
(Scott, O.M.)

Pentachloronitrobenzene ... 9.95%
Fertilizer formula: 18-6-6

TURF BUILDER PLUS 2
Herbicide
(Scott, O.M.)

2,4-Dichlorophenoxyacetic acid	0.99%
2-(4-Chloro-2-methylphenoxy) propionic acid	0.99%
Carrier: Fertilizer 26-3-3	

TURF BUILDER PLUS 2 FOR GRASS
Fertilizer with herbicide
(Scott, O.M.)

2,4-Dichlorophenoxyacetic acid	0.60%
2-(4-Chloro-2-methylphenoxy) propionic acid	0.60%
Carrier: Fertilizer 22-3-3	

TURF BUILDER PLUS 2 (W/S)
Herbicide/fertilizer
(Scott, O.M.)

2,4-Dichlorophenoxyacetic acid	0.60%
2-(4-Chloro-2-methylphenoxy) propionic acid	0.60%
Fertilizer: 22-3-3	
Iron (FS.M)	1.10%

TURF BUILDER WITH HALTS
Herbicide
(Scott, O.M.)

Dacthal ... 6.30%
Carrier base: Fertilizer 20-5-5

TURF BUILDER WITH MOSS CONTROL
Herbicide/fertilizer
(Scott, O.M.)

Ferrous sulfate heptahydrate * ... 10.9%
Carrier fertilizer: 19-3-3

TURFICIDE EMULSIFIABLE FUNGICIDE
(Olin Corporation)

Pentachloronitrobenzene	24%
Aromatic petroleum distillates *	approx. 70%

TURFICIDE 10% GRANULAR FUNGICIDE
(Olin Corporation)

Pentachloronitrobenzene * 10%

TURPATINE
Thinner
(Barr, W. M., & Co.)

Pinene hydrocarbons * 100%

TURTLE WAX (LIQUID)
(Turtle Wax, Inc.)

Genuine and oxidized waxes
Silicone fluids and resins
Aliphatic solvents (no kerosene or aromatic solvents) *
Abrasives
Very small amounts of perfume, dye, emulsifying agents

'76 Ed.

TUSSACOL
For cold symptoms
(Jenkins Labs.)

Each tablet:
Dextromethorphan
  hydrobromide .... 7.5 mg.
Pyrilamine maleate * .... 8.0 mg.
Chlorpheniramine maleate .. 0.3 mg.
Phenylephrine
  hydrochloride * .... 5.0 mg.
Acetaminophen * .... 100.0 mg.
Glyceryl guaiacolate ...... 50.0 mg.

TUSSAGESIC SUSPENSION
Decongestant, antihistaminic, analgesic, antitussive
(Dorsey Labs.)

Each 5 ml.:
Phenylpropanolamine
  hydrochloride * .... 12.5 mg.
Pheniramine maleate ...... 6.25 mg.
Pyrilamine maleate * ...... 6.25 mg.
Dextromethorphan
  hydrobromide * .... 15 mg.
Terpin hydrate .... 90 mg.
Acetaminophen * .... 120 mg.

TUSSAGESIC TABLETS
Decongestant, antihistaminic, analgesic, antitussive
(Dorsey Labs.)

Each tablet:
Phenylpropanolamine
  hydrochloride * .... 25 mg.
Pheniramine maleate ...... 12.5 mg.
Pyrilamine maleate * ...... 12.5 mg.
Dextromethorphan
  hydrobromide * .... 30 mg.
Terpin hydrate .... 180 mg.
Acetaminophen * .... 325 mg.

TUSSAR-2
Cough syrup
(Armour Pharm.)

Each 5 ml.:
Codeine phosphate USP * ... 10 mg.
Carbetapentane citrate NF ... 7.5 mg.
Chlorpheniramine maleate
  USP .... 2.0 mg.
Glyceryl guaiacolate NF ..... 50 mg.
Sodium citrate USP .... 130 mg.
Citric acid USP .... 20 mg.
Methylparaben USP 0.1%
Alcohol 5%

TUSSAR DM
Cough syrup
(Armour Pharm.)

Each 5 ml.:
Dextromethorphan hydrobromide (NF) .... 15 mg.
Chlorpheniramine maleate
  (USP) .... 2 mg.
Phenylephrine hydrochloride
  (USP) * .... 5 mg.
Methylparaben (USP) 0.1%

TUSSAR SF
Cough syrup
(Armour Pharm.)

Each 5 ml.:
Codeine phosphate USP * ... 10 mg.
Carbetapentane citrate NF ... 7.5 mg.
Chlorpheniramine maleate
  USP .... 2.0 mg.
Glyceryl guaiacolate NF ..... 50 mg.
Sodium citrate USP .... 130 mg.
Citric acid USP .... 20 mg.
Methylparaben USP 0.1%
Alcohol 12%

TUSSEND
Antitussive-decongestant
(Dow Pharm., Dow Chem. Co.)

Each 5 ml. or tablet:
Hydrocodone bitartrate * ..... 5 mg.
Pseudoephedrine
  hydrochloride * .... 30 mg.
Alcohol (Liquid only) 5%

TUSSEND EXPECTORANT
Antitussive-decongestant
(Dow Pharm., Dow Chem. Co.)

Each 5 ml.:
Hydrocodone bitartrate * .... 5 mg.
Pseudoephedrine
  hydrochloride * .... 30 mg.
Guaifenesin (Glyceryl
  guaiacolate) .... 200 mg.
Alcohol 15%

TUSSIONEX (SUSPENSION, CAPSULES & TABLETS)
Antitussive
(Pennwalt, Pharm. Div.)

Each tablet, capsule or 5 ml.:
Hydrocodone *† .... 5 mg.
Phenyltoloxamine .... 10 mg.

†*See* Hydrocodone bitartrate

TUSSTROL
Antitussive, antihistaminic, expectorant, decongestant
(Reid-Provident)

Each 5 cc:
Codeine phosphate * .... 10 mg.
Pyrilamine maleate * .... 5 mg.
Phenylpropanolamine HCl * .. 15 mg.
Potassium guaiacolsulfonate .. 100 mg.

TUTAG FELINE LAXATIVE
(Direct Div.)

Each 2 oz:
Cod liver oil
Caramel USP
Lecithin
Malt syrup
White petrolatum (USP)
Sodium benzoate (USP) 0.1%
Vitamin E (dl-alpha-Tocopheryl acetate NF) . 0.036 IU/gm.
Purified water

TUTTLE'S ELIXIR
Counterirritant; veterinary liniment
(Tuttle's Elixir Div.)

Alcohol 30%
Gum camphor *
P.G.S. Turpentine *
Oil of hemlock *
Ox gall
Ammonia solution *
Distilled water

TUVACHE PERFUMES & COLOGNES
(Tuvache Inc.)

Perfume oil * 20%
S.D. Alcohol 39c * 80%

'76 Ed.

#12D CONCENTRATE SUPER FOG-O-MATIC INSECTICIDE
Industrial use only
(Barco)

Diazinon 1.00%
Malathion * 8.00%
Petroleum distillates * 91.00%

'76 Ed.

12-HOUR COLD CAPSULES
(Pharmex)

Each capsule:
Belladonna alkaloidal salts . 0.16 mg.
Atropine sulfate .... 0.024 mg.
Scopolamine hydrobromide . 0.014 mg.
Hyoscyamine sulfate ...... 0.122 mg.
Phenylpropanolamine
  hydrochloride * .... 50 mg.
Chlorpheniramine maleate . 1 mg.
Pheniramine maleate ...... 12.5 mg.

Starred ingredients (*) may be responsible for major toxic effects; consult Section II.

20 CARATS DUSTING POWDER (4 oz.)
(Dana Perfumes)

Essential oils	>1%
Aromatic chemicals	
Talc	
Zinc stearate	
Magnesium carbonate	

20 CARATS EAU DE PARFUM
Sizes - 2 oz., 4 oz.
(Dana Perfumes)

Essential oils *	>1%
Aromatic chemicals	
Specially denatured Alcohol (39-C) *	
Deionized water	

20 CARATS EAU DE PARFUM SPRAY
Sizes - 2 oz., 3.5 oz., 4 oz.
(Dana Perfumes)

Essential oils *	>1%
Aromatic chemicals	
Specially denatured Alcohol (39-C) *	
Dichlorotetrafluoroethane	

20 CARATS PERFUME
Size - 1 oz.
(Dana Perfumes)

Essential oils *	>1%
Aromatic chemicals	
Specially denatured Alcohol (39-C) *	

20 CARATS SPRAY PERFUME PURSER
Size - 1/3 oz.
(Dana Perfumes)

Essential oils *	>1%
Aromatic chemicals	
Specially denatured Alcohol (39-C) *	
Dichlorotetrafluoroethane	

20 CARATS ULTRA SMOOTHING HAND AND BODY LOTION
(Dana Perfumes)

Essential oils *
Aromatic chemicals
Water
Acetylated lanolin
Mineral oil
Stearic acid
Triethanolamine
Cetyl alcohol
Methylparaben
Propylene glycol
BHA
Propyl gallate
Citric acid

20 MULE POWER BATHROOM CLEANER
(U.S. Borax)

Tetrasodiummethylenediamine- tetraacetate	4.56%
Isopropanol	2.40%
o-Benzyl-p-chlorophenol	0.14%

20 MULE TEAM
Borax
(U.S. Borax)

Sodium tetraborate decahydrate *	

20/20 CONTACT LENS WETTING SOLUTION
(S.S.S. Co.)

Benzalkonium chloride	0.004%
Methylcellulose	0.500%
Chlorbutanol	0.150%
Borated-potassium buffered base solution	

20/20 GLASS CLEANER CONCENTRATE
Glass cleaner
(Sanitek)

Isopropanol *	40.3%
Dipropylene glycol monomethyl ether (Cellosolve) *	14.2%
Anionic surfactants	4.1%
Dimethylaminomethanol	3.0%
Ammonia	1.8%
Tetrasodium ethylenediamine- tetraacetic acid	1.0%
Dye	trace
Water	balance

TWINKLE COPPER CLEANER (PASTE)
(Drackett)

Citric acid	<10%/wt.
Sodium chloride	
Surfactants	
Water	
Abrasive	
Dye & perfume	
Humectant	

TWINKLE CREAM FOR SILVER (PASTE)
(Drackett)

Abrasive
Soap
Nonionic surfactant
Water
Humectants
Tarnish inhibitor
Dye and Perfume

TWIN LIGHT BENOMYL FUNGICIDE
(Seacoast)

Benomyl	50%

TWIN LIGHT CRABGRASS PREVENTER WITH TUPERSAN
(Seacoast)

Tupersan	4.7%

TWIN LIGHT DIAZINON 5% GRANULAR
Insecticide
(Seacoast)

Diazinon *	5%

TWIN LIGHT DIAZINON 14% GRANULAR
Insecticide
(Seacoast)

Diazinon *	14%

TWIN LIGHT DIAZINON SPRAY
Insecticide
(Seacoast)

Diazinon emulsion *	10%

TWIN LIGHT DUSTALL 1%
Insecticide
(Seacoast)

Rotenone	1%

TWIN LIGHT GARDEN SPRAY
Insecticide
(Seacoast)

Malathion *	15.0%
Kelthane	5.0%
Methoxychlor	7.5%

TWIN LIGHT GRANULAR BENOMYL TURF FUNGICIDE
(Seacoast)

Benomyl	1.5%

TWIN LIGHT GRANULAR CHLORONEB SNOW MOLD TURF FUNGICIDE
(Seacoast)

Chloroneb	7.5%

TWIN LIGHT GRANULAR LAWN FUNGICIDE
(Seacoast)

Thiram	5.00%
Cadmium chloride *	0.75%

Starred ingredients (*) may be responsible for major toxic effects; consult Section II.

TWIN LIGHT GRANULAR SNOWMOLD TURF FUNGICIDE
(Seacoast)

Thiram	2.50%
Cadmium chloride *	0.38%

TWIN LIGHT GRANULAR TURF FUNGICIDE W/ CHLOROTHALONIL
(Seacoast)

Chlorothalonil (Daconil)	5%

TWIN LIGHT GRANULAR TURF FUNGICIDE W/ DYRENE
(Seacoast)

Dyrene *	5%

TWIN LIGHT LAWN INSECTICIDE WITH DURSBAN
(Seacoast)

Dursban *	1.16%

TWIN LIGHT METHOXYCHLOR SPRAY
Insecticide
(Seacoast)

Methoxychlor emulsion *	25%

TWIN LIGHT MULTI-PURPOSE SPRAY
Insecticide/fungicide
(Seacoast)

Sevin *	10.0%
Malathion	8.0%
Folpet	14.5%
Kelthane	1.5%

TWIN LIGHT PROFESSIONAL CRABGRASS PREVENTER WITH BALAN
(Seacoast)

Balan	1.9%

TWIN LIGHT PROFESSIONAL DACTHAL CRABGRASS PREVENTER
(Seacoast)

Dacthal	4.7%

TWIN LIGHT PROFESSIONAL DURSBAN LAWN INSECT KILLER
(Seacoast)

Dursban *	2.32%

TWIN LIGHT ROSE & FLOWER DUST OR SPRAY
Insecticide/fungicide
(Seacoast)

Malathion	4%
Folpet	5%
Sevin *	3%

TWIN LIGHT SPRAYALL FOR FRUIT
Insecticide/fungicide
(Seacoast)

Malathion	4.0%
Captan	7.5%
Sevin *	5.0%

TWIN LIGHT TOMATO-VEGETABLE DUST OR SPRAY
Insecticide/fungicide
(Seacoast)

Sevin *	5.0%
Zineb	4.5%

"2" DROP CORN AND CALLOUS REMOVER, DR. SCHOLL'S

See DR. SCHOLL'S "2" DROP CORN AND CALLOUS REMOVER

2/G
Expectorant
(Dow Pharm., Dow Chem. Co.)

Each tsp. (5 ml.):
Guaifenesin (Glyceryl guaiacolate)	100 mg.
Alcohol	3.5%
Corn derivatives	

2G/DM
Expectorant-antitussive
(Dow Pharm., Dow Chem. Co.)

Each tsp. (5 ml.):
Guaifenesin (Glyceryl guaiacolate)	100 mg.
Dextromethorphan hydrobromide *	15 mg.
Alcohol	5%
Corn derivatives	

TWO-IN-ONE GRAIN FUMIGANT
(Industrial Fumigant)

Carbon tetrachloride *	81.3%
Carbon bisulfide	12.1%
Ethylene dibromide	6.6%

TYBATRAN
Tranquilizer
(Robins)

Each capsule:
Tybamate *	250 mg.; 350 mg.

TYDEE-TABS
Toilet bowl cleaner
(Lake Products)

Potassium dichloroisocyanurate *	10%

TYLAN 10
Premix/medicated; antibiotic
(Elanco Prod.)

Each pound:
Tylosin (as tylosin phosphate) *	10 gm.

TYLAN 40
Premix/medicated; antibiotic
(Elanco Prod.)

Each pound:
Tylosin (as tylosin phosphate) *	40 gm.

TYLAN PLUS NEOMYCIN EYE POWDER
Topical antibiotic; veterinary
(Elanco Prod.)

Each 20 gram:
Tylosin activity (as the base)	2%
Neomycin as neomycin sulfate	0.25%
Metycaine (Piperocaine hydrochloride)	1%
Acriflavine neutral (coloring agent)	0.5%
Boric acid *	q.s.

TYLAN 10 PLUS SULFA
Premix/medicated; antibiotic
(Elanco Prod.)

Each pound:
Tylosin (as tylosin phosphate) *	10 gm.
Sulfamethazine	2.2% (10 gm.)

TYLAN 40 PLUS SULFA
Premix/medicated; antibiotic
(Elanco Prod.)

Each pound:
Tylosin (as tylosin phosphate) *	40 gm.
Sulfamethazine	8.8% (40 gm.)

TYLAN PLUS VITAMINS
Control and treatment of swine dysentery
(Elanco Prod.)

Each gallon of treated water:
Tylosin	250 mg.
Vitamin A	6,000 I.U.
Vitamin D2	750 I.U.
Plus multivitamins	

TYLAN SOLUBLE
Antibiotic; veterinary
(Elanco Prod.)

Tylosin (as the tartrate) *	100 gm.

Starred ingredients (*) may be responsible for major toxic effects; consult Section II.

TYLENOL EXTRA-STRENGTH ADULT LIQUID PAIN RELIEVER
Analgesic-antipyretic
(McNeil Consumer Products Co.)

Each 30 ml.:
Acetaminophen * .... 1000 mg.

TYLENOL EXTRA-STRENGTH CAPSULES/TABLETS
Analgesic-antipyretic
(McNeil Consumer Products Co.)

Each capsule:
Acetaminophen * .... 500 mg.

Each tablet:
Acetaminophen * .... 500 mg.

TYLENOL REGULAR STRENGTH CAPSULES/TABLETS
Analgesic/antipyretic
(McNeil Consumer Products Co.)

Each capsule or tablet:
Acetaminophen * .... 325 mg.

TYLENOL WITH CODEINE ELIXIR
Analgesic - antipyretic
(McNeil Pharm.)

Each 5 ml.:
Codeine phosphate * .... 12 mg.
Acetaminophen * .... 120 mg.
Alcohol 7%

TYLENOL WITH CODEINE TABLETS
Analgesic, antipyretic, antitussive
(McNeil Pharm.)

Each tablet:
Acetaminophen * .... 300 mg.
Codeine phosphate *
No. 1 .... 7.5 mg.
No. 2 .... 15 mg.
No. 3 .... 30 mg.
No. 4 .... 60 mg.

TYLOCINE SULFA 50 TABLETS
Antibiotic for cats and dogs
(Elanco Prod.)

Each tablet:
Tylosin .... 50 mg.
Sulfamethazine * .... 25 mg.
Sulfamerazine * .... 25 mg.
Sulfadiazine * .... 25 mg.

TYLOCINE SULFA 200 TABLETS
Antibiotic for cats and dogs
(Elanco Prod.)

Each tablet:
Tylosin .... 200 mg.
Sulfamethazine * .... 100 mg.
Sulfamerazine * .... 100 mg.
Sulfadiazine * .... 100 mg.

TYLOCINE TABLETS
Antibiotic for dogs and cats
(Elanco Prod.)

Each tablet:
Tylosin * .... 200 mg.

TYLOX CAPSULES
Analgesic
(McNeil Pharm.)

Each capsule:
Oxycodone hydrochloride * .... 4.5 mg.
Oxycodone terephthalate .... 0.38 mg.
Acetaminophen * .... 500 mg.

TYMATRO THROAT TROCHES (C.T. GREEN; FLAVORED)
(Bowman Pharm.)

Each lozenge:
Cetylpyridinium chloride ..... 1.5 mg.
Benzocaine .... 5.0 mg.

TYMPAGESIC
Analgesic ear drops
(Adria)

Phenylephrine hydrochloride, USP * 0.25%
Antipyrine, USP * 5%
Benzocaine, USP 5%
In Propylene glycol, NF

TYROHIST CREAM
Antihistamine, antibacterial, analgesic
(Columbia Med.)

Pyrilamine maleate *
Benzalkonium chloride
Benzocaine
Camphor
Menthol
Neo-Calamine

TYROHIST NASAL SPRAY
(Columbia Med.)

Pyrilamine maleate *
Phenylephrine HCl *
Cetalkonium chloride
Preservatives

TYRO OINTMENT
For superficial cuts, chaps, bruises of all domestic animals; veterinary
(Hilltop)

Tyrothricin 1:10,000
Base:
Lanolin anhydrous
Paraffin
Petrolatum
Liquid petrolatum
Methyl salicylate *
Guaiacol
Cyclonol (Meta homo menthol)
Certified F & D color

'76 Ed.

TYROSUM
Skin cleanser for acne
(Summers Labs.)

Acetone *
Polysorbate 80
Isopropanol * 50%

TYROSUM PACKETS
Skin cleanser for acne
(Summers Labs.)

Each packet (3 cc Tyrosum on cotton pad):
Acetone *
Polysorbate
Isopropanol * 50%

TYZINE 0.1% NASAL SOLUTION
(Pfizer)

Tetrahydrozoline hydrochloride 0.1%

TYZINE 0.05% PEDIATRIC NASAL DROPS
(Pfizer)

Tetrahydrozoline hydrochloride .. 0.05%

U

UAA TABLETS
Urinary antiseptic, antispasmodic
(Econo Med)

Each tablet:
Atropine sulfate .... 0.03 mg.
Hyoscyamine (as the sulfate) 0.03 mg.
Methylene blue .... 5.50 mg.
Methenamine .... 50.00 mg.
Phenyl salicylate * .... 20.00 mg.
Benzoic .... 5.00 mg.

UCAR ANTIFREEZE COOLANT (AF-572, Formula YA-335 (8697-87))
(Union Carbide)

Ethylene glycol * 95%
Water 3%
Soluble inhibitors 2%

Starred ingredients (*) may be responsible for major toxic effects; consult Section II.

U-C MULTI-PURPOSE SPRAY
Insecticide for institutional and industrial use
(United Chemical Co., Inc.)

Piperonyl butoxide technical	1.27%
Pyrethrins	0.13%
Petroleum oil *	98.60%

'76 Ed.

UCO-PHENE
Disinfectant for hospital and institutional use
(United Chemical Co., Inc.)

Active ingredients:	39%
Isopropyl alcohol *	
Vegetable oil soaps	
o-Benzyl p-chlorophenol *	
Methyl salicylate *	
Essential oils	
Inert ingredients:	61%
Water	

'76 Ed.

UDDER-BAC
Dairy farm udder wash and sanitizer
(Diversey Wyandotte)

Polyethylene glycolether of linear secondary alcohol-iodine complex (providing 1.75% of titratable iodine) *	13.45%
Phosphoric acid *	6.75%
Citric acid	4.00%

UDDER-DU
Iodine sanitizer & udder wash for dairy cows
(An-Fo)

Nonyl phenoxy polyethoxy ethanol-iodine complex (providing 1.67% available iodine)	8.35%
Nonylphenoxypoly (ethyleneoxy) ethanol	7.00%
Phosphoric acid *	12.00%

U-DO-IT TERMITE CONTROL CONCENTRATE, ARAB
See ARAB U-DO-IT TERMITE CONTROL CONCENTRATE

UGL ASPHALT DRIVEWAY FILLER
(United Gilsonite)

Acrylic latex	18%
Polymeric plasticizer	7%
Surfactants	1.5%
Mineral spirits	2%
Calcium carbonate	56.5%
Water	15%
Silane	<1%
Tinting colors	<5%

UGL ASPHALT PAINT
(United Gilsonite)

Asphalt
Mineral spirits *
Inert fillers

UGL BUTYL CAULK
(United Gilsonite)

Cured Butyl rubber	
Vegetable oil	
Hydrocarbon resin	
Mineral spirits *	22%
Calcium carbonate	
Silica	

UGL CAULKING COMPOUND
(United Gilsonite)

Soya oil
Petroleum resin
Mineral spirits *
Inert fillers

UGL FAST PLUG
(United Gilsonite)

Cement
Hydrated lime

UGL FOUNDATION COATING
Paint product
(United Gilsonite)

Asphalt
Mineral spirits *

UGL GOLD PAINT
(United Gilsonite)

Pigment:	20.00%
Gold bronze powder *	100.00%
Vehicle:	80.00%
Polystyrene resin	25.00%
Aromatic hydrocarbons *	75.00%

UGL JOINT CEMENT
(United Gilsonite)

Casein
Soya protein
Hydrated lime
Soda ash *
Inert fillers

UGL LATEX CAULK
(United Gilsonite)

Acrylic latex	18%
Polymeric plasticizer	7%
Surfactants	1.5%
Mineral spirits	2%
Calcium carbonate	56.5%
Water	15%
Silane	<1%
Tinting colors	<5%

UGL LATEX CONCRETE CRACK FILLER
(United Gilsonite)

Acrylic latex	18%
Polymeric plasticizer	7%
Surfactants	1.5%
Mineral spirits	2%
Calcium carbonate	56.5%
Water	15%
Silane	<1%
Tinting colors	<5%

UGL PLASTER PATCH
(United Gilsonite)

Plaster
Calcium carbonate
Dextrine

UGL SUPER ONE HOUSE PAINT (WHITE)
(United Gilsonite)

Titanium dioxide	24.6%
Zinc oxide	4.0%
Calcium sulfate	11.4%
Silicates	11.4%
Linseed-soya alkyd resin	23.6%
Linseed oil	8.4%
Mineral spirits* and driers	16.5%
Thiazolyl-benzimidazole	0.1%

UGL TILE GROUT
(United Gilsonite)

Portland cement
Calcium carbonate
Plaster
Polyvinyl alcohol
Glue

UGL TUB & TILE CAULK
(United Gilsonite)

Acrylic latex	18.5%
Polymeric plasticizer	7.5%
Surfactants	1.5%
Calcium carbonate	55.5%
Water	17%
Silane	<1%
Tinting colors	<5%

UKG DETERGENT GERMICIDE
Institutional and industrial use
(Dalco Corp.)

n-Alkyl (50% C12, 30% C14, 17% C16, 3% C18) dimethyl ethyl benzyl ammonium chloride *	3.2%
n-Alkyl (60% C14, 30% C16, 5% C12, 5% C18) dimethyl benzyl ammonium chloride *	3.2%
Sodium carbonate (Soda ash) *	4%

Starred ingredients (*) may be responsible for major toxic effects; consult Section II.

ULO SYRUP
Acute cough associated with respiratory infections, inflammations
(Riker Labs.)

Each 5 ml.:
Chlophedianol HCl * .... 25 mg.

'76 Ed.

ULTIMA COSMETICS
(Revlon)

Revlon, Inc.
767 Fifth Ave.
New York, N.Y. 10153

Phone: 212-572-5000

Revlon Research Center, Inc.
945 Zerega Ave.
Bronx, N.Y. 10473

Phone: 212-824-9000

See COSMETICS, Section VI, General Formulations

ULTIMATE II
See PL ULTIMATE II

ULTIMATE SUPER FOGGING INSECT KILLER, PL (Aerosol)
See PL ULTIMATE SUPER FOGGING INSECT KILLER (Aerosol)

ULTRA BAN
Anti-perspirant lotion
(Bristol-Myers)

Aluminum chlorohydrate *

ULTRA BAN II (Fresh, Regular & Neutral Scents)
Anti-perspirant deodorant spray
(Bristol-Myers)

Active ingred.:
Aluminum chlorohydrate *
Other ingred.:
Isobutane
Isopropyl palmitate
Isopropyl myristate
SD Alcohol 40
Quaternium-18 hectorite
Isopropyl stearate
Fragrance

ULTRA BLEACH & GLOW
(Keystone Labs.)

Hydroquinone * 2%
Myristal lactate
Mineral oil (Kaydol)
Stearic acid
Glyceryl monostearate
Triethanolamine
Sodium sulfite

ULTRA-BRITE TOOTHPASTE
(Colgate-Palmolive)

Insoluble Calcium
phosphate .... approx. 50%
Glycerine .... approx. 20%
Carboxy methyl cellulose
Combined amount: .... approx. 2%
Sodium n-lauroyl sarcosinate
Sodium lauryl sulfate
Flavor (Essential oils and chloroform)
Preservative

'76 Ed.

ULTRA BURNISHING COMPOUND
(Brewer Chem.)

Sodium tripolyphosphate .... <5%
Modified Ethoxylate .... <5%
50% Potassium hydroxide * 15-25%
Potassium silicate 10-20%

ULTRA DERM BATH OIL
(Baker-Cummins)

Nonionic emulsifiers
Lipids

ULTRA DERM MOISTURIZER
(Baker-Cummins)

Oil-in-water emulsion

ULTRA-D PART SYNTHETIC MOTOR OIL
(Marathon Oil Co.)

Additives, containing Zinc alkyl
dithiophosphate, Sodium and
Sulfur compounds, Styrene ester polymer 17.3%
Polyolefin 21.0%
Mineral oil .... balance

ULTRA GLOW SKIN TONE CREAM
(Keystone Labs.)

Hydroquinone * 2%
Water
Glyceryl stearate and Sodium lauryl sulfate
Glyceryl stearate and Isopropyl myristate,
Stearyl stearate
Propylene glycol
Isopropyl myristate
Cetyl alcohol
Fragrance
Sodium bisulfite
Steareth-20
Methylparaben and Propylparaben, Benzylparaben
BHA
Sodium sulfite
Disodium EDTA
Propyl gallate
Citric acid

ULTRAMAR CLE
Emulsifier and wetting agent
(Brewer Chem.)

Triethanolamine alkyl aryl
sulfonate * 100%

ULTRAMAR NI
Agricultural wetting agent
(Brewer Chem.)

Nonylphenoxy polyethoxy
ethanol 80-90%
Pine oil .... <5%
Isopropyl alcohol .... <20%

ULTRA MIDE LOTION
Moisturizer
(Baker-Cummins)

Urea 25%
Emollients
Humectants

ULTRAQU
Sanitizer
(Brewer Chem.)

n-Alkyl (50% C14, 40% C12, 10%
C16) dimethyl benzyl ammonium
chloride * 5-6%
Sodium metasilicate * 3.0%
Tetra sodium salt of ethylene
diamine tetraacetic acid 1.5-2.0%
Octylphenoxy polyethoxy
ethanol (nonionic) .... approx. 5%
Water 80-90%

ULTRA ROYALE (AS-930U, Formula 2079-68)
See SIMONIZ ULTRA ROYALE (AS-930U, Formula 2079-68)

ULTRASAN
Sanitizer
(Brewer Chem.)

n-Alkyl (50% C14, 40% C12, 10%
C16) dimethyl benzyl ammonium chloride * 8-12%
Water 88-92%

ULTRATHANE FINISH
Floor finish
(Hillyard Chem.)

Mineral spirits *

'76 Ed.

ULTRATHANE SEAL
Floor seal
(Hillyard Chem.)

Mineral spirits *

'76 Ed.

ULTRA-VAC CAPSULES
Stool softener
(Pharmex)

Each capsule:
Dioctyl sodium
succinate * .... 100 mg.; 250 mg.

ULTRA-VIOLET AUTOMOTIVE LEAK DETECTION ADDITIVES
(Ultra-Violet)

Oil soluble Dyes *† 0-40%
Water soluble Dyes *† 0-30%
Mineral oil 0-70%
Ethylene glycol * 0-17%

†*See* Pigments, Section VI, General Formulations

ULTRA-VIOLET TRACER CONCENTRATES
(Ultra-Violet)

Coumarin derivative dyes *† 0-10%
Other dyes .... <5%
Alcohols * 0-90%
Xylene * 0-95%

†*See* Coumarin

ULTRA WHITE BLEACH
(Brewer Chem.)

Sodium hypochlorite * 6.0%

ULTRA WHITE BLEACH (Extra-Strength)
(Brewer Chem.)

Sodium hypochlorite * 9.2%

UMBRELLA
Surface treatment
(Barr, W. M., & Co.)

Aliphatic and aromatic
hydrocarbons * 90%
Silicone, Metallic soap, Resins 10%

UNCLE SAM'S CREME GLOSS FURNITURE POLISH
(Uncle Sam)

Sulfonated castor oil *
Paraffin based oil
Emulsifier
Water

UNCLE SAM'S LEMON OIL POLISH
(Uncle Sam)

Mineral oil (paraffin based)
Citronella *

UNCLE SAM'S ODORLESS DISINFECTANT
(Uncle Sam)

Quaternary ammonium compound *
Tetrasodium ethylene diamine tetraacetate
Surfactants
Water

UNCLE SAM'S VAPORIZER INSECT SPRAY (#2 1/2, 375, 5 & 8)
Insecticide
(Uncle Sam)

Pyrethrum
Synergists
Petroleum distillates *

UNCLE SAM'S WINTERGREEN GERMICIDE
(Uncle Sam)

Methyl salicylate *
Emulsifiers
Synthetic Phenols *
Soap
Alcohol
Water

UNDECILLIN LIQUID
For athlete's foot
(Pharmex)

Para-nitrophenol *

UNDELENIC OINTMENT
For itching & discomfort of athlete's foot
(Gordon Labs.)

Undecylenic acid *
Zinc undecylenate *

UNDELENIC TINCTURE
For itching and discomfort of athlete's foot
(Gordon Labs.)

Undecylenic acid *
Isopropyl alcohol * 79%/v
Propylene glycol
Triethanolamine

UNGUENTINE AEROSOL
Topical anesthetic and antiseptic
(Norwich-Eaton)

Benzocaine
Benzalkonium chloride *
Parachlorometaxylenol
Phenol *
Menthol *
Alcohol .... 6.6% w/v

UNGUENTINE OINTMENT FOR BURNS
Topical anesthetic and antiseptic
(Norwich-Eaton)

Phenol * 1.0%
Parahydrecin (brand of Isomerol) . 0.01%
Zinc oxide
Aluminum hydroxide
Zinc carbonate *
Zinc acetate *
Eucalyptus oil *
Thyme oil *
Oleostearin
Petrolatum

UNGUENTINE PLUS
Antiseptic and anesthetic
(Norwich-Eaton)

Lidocaine hydrochloride
Parachlorometaxylenol *
Aluminum hydroxide
Zinc carbonate *
Zinc acetate *
Zinc oxide
Phenol *
Oil eucalyptus *
Oil thyme *
Menthol *
Eugenol

UNICAP CAPSULES
Vitamin therapy
(Upjohn)

Each capsule:
Vitamin A .... 5000 I.U.
Vitamin D .... 400 I.U.
Plus multivitamins

UNICAP CHEWABLE TABLETS
Vitamin therapy
(Upjohn)

Each tablet:
Vitamin A .... 5000 I.U.
Vitamin D .... 400 I.U.
Plus multivitamins

UNICAP M TABLETS
Vitamin therapy
(Upjohn)

Each tablet:
Vitamin A .... 5000 I.U.
Vitamin D .... 400 I.U.
Iron .... 18 mg.
Plus multivitamins and minerals

UNICAP PLUS IRON TABLETS
Vitamin therapy
(Upjohn)

Each tablet:
Vitamin A .... 5000 I.U.
Vitamin D .... 400 I.U.
Iron .... 18 mg.
Plus multivitamins

Starred ingredients (*) may be responsible for major toxic effects; consult Section II.

UNICAP SENIOR TABLETS
Vitamin therapy
(Upjohn)

Each tablet:
Vitamin A .... 5000 I.U.
Iron .... 10 mg.
Plus multivitamins and minerals

UNICAP TABLETS
Vitamin therapy
(Upjohn)

Each tablet:
Vitamin A .... 5000 I.U.
Vitamin D .... 400 I.U.
Plus multivitamins

UNICAP T TABLETS
Vitamin therapy
(Upjohn)

Each tablet:
Vitamin A .... 5000 I.U.
Vitamin D .... 400 I.U.
Iron .... 18 mg.
Plus multivitamins and minerals

UNI-CHLOR

See UNIVERSAL UNI-CHLOR

UNICIDE 60
Insecticide, fungicide
(Leffingwell)

Petroleum oil * 99.0%/w
Unsulfonated residue, petroleum oil
minimum 92%

UNICO ALFALFA WEEVIL SPRAY
Insecticide
(Universal Cooperatives)

Malathion 22.4%
Methoxychlor, technical 22.6%
Aromatic petroleum derivative
solvent * 50.3%

UNICO ANT AND ROACH KILLER
(Universal Cooperatives)

Baygon * 1.0%
Petroleum distillate * 83.8%

UNICO ANT, ROACH & SPIDER INSECT SPRAY
(Universal Cooperatives)

Baygon 0.50%
Petroleum distillate * 82.19%

UNICO AQUAGENE-1 SPRAY ADJUVANT
(Universal Cooperatives)

Alkyl aryl polyoxyethylene glycols
(biodegradable) 80%

UNICO BAN AMINE WEED KILLER
(Universal Cooperatives)

Dimethylamine salt of Dicamba
(3,6-Dichloro-o-anisic acid) * .. 15.3%
Dimethylamine salt of related
acids 2.4%
Dimethylamine salt of 2,4-Dichlo-
rophenoxyacetic acid * 30.5%

UNICO BEAN DUST
Insecticide
(Universal Cooperatives)

Rotenone 1.0%
Other cube resins 1.6%

UNICO 1% CIODRIN INSECTICIDE
Back rubber solution
(Universal Cooperatives)

Dimethyl phosphate of alpha-methylbenzyl 3-hydroxy-cis-
crotonate * 1%
Petroleum base oil * 99%

UNICO COPPER-ROTENONE 7-1 DUST
Insecticide-fungicide
(Universal Cooperatives)

Copper, expressed as metallic (in basic
copper sulfate) * 7%
Rotenone 1%
Other cube resins 2%

UNICO CRABGRASS KILLER
Herbicide
(Universal Cooperatives)

Octylammonium methylarsonate * .. 8%
Dodecylammonium methyl-
arsonate * 8%

UNICO CRABGRASS KILLER B
(Universal Cooperatives)

S-(O,O-Diisopropyl phosphorodithioate) ester of N-(2-mercaptoethyl)
benzenesulfonamide 3.6%

UNICO CYGON 2-E SYSTEMIC INSECTICIDE
Controls houseflies
(Universal Cooperatives)

Dimethoate * 23.4%

UNICO DAIRY AND STOCK FLY SPRAY
Insecticide
(Universal Cooperatives)

Ciodrin * 1.00%
2,2-Dichlorovinyl dimethyl
phosphate 0.23%
Related compounds 0.02%
Petroleum hydrocarbons * ... 98.48%

UNICO 2,4-D AMINE WEED KILLER
Herbicide
(Universal Cooperatives)

Dimethylamine salt of 2,4-dichlo-
rophenoxyacetic acid * 47.2%

UNICO DIAZINON 4E
Insecticide
(Universal Cooperatives)

O,O-Diethyl O-(2-isopropyl-6-
methyl-4-pyrimidinyl)
phosphorothioate * 48%
Xylene * 36%

UNICO DIAZINON EMULSIFIABLE LAWN AND GARDEN INSECTICIDE
(Universal Cooperatives)

O,O-Diethyl O-(2-isopropyl-6-
methyl-4-pyrimidinyl)
phosphorothioate * 25%
Aromatic petroleum derivative
solvents * 57%

UNICO DINITRO "T"
Herbicide
(Universal Cooperatives)

Triethanolamine salt of Dinoseb * ... 51%

UNICO 2,4-D LO-V ESTER WEED KILLER
Herbicide
(Universal Cooperatives)

2-Ethyl hexyl ester of 2,4-dichloro-
phenoxyacetic acid * 65.1%

UNICO FATAL FLY DRY BAIT
(Universal Cooperatives)

O-Isopropoxyphenyl
methylcarbamate 0.125%
(Z)-9-Tricosene 0.125%

UNICO FENTHION FLY AND MOSQUITO SPRAY
(Universal Cooperatives)

Fenthion * 25.20%
Aromatic petroleum distillate * .. 67.98%

UNICO "51" DUST COPPER-ROTENONE
Insecticide/fungicide
(Universal Cooperatives)

Copper, expressed as metallic (in cop-
per oxide) * 5%
Rotenone * 1%
Other Cube resins 2%

Starred ingredients (*) may be responsible for major toxic effects; consult Section II.

UNICO FRUIT SPRAY TREE-TRELLIS-GARDEN
Insecticide/fungicide/miticide
(Universal Cooperatives)

Carbaryl *	17.5%
1,1-Bis(p-chlorophenyl)-2,2,2-trichloroethanol	6.0%
Captan	17.5%

UNICO GARDEN DUST
Insecticide/fungicide
(Universal Cooperatives)

Carbaryl *	3.0%
Zineb	3.2%
Ziram	3.8%
Rotenone *	1.0%
Other Cube resins	1.6%

UNICO GARDEN SPRAY POWDER
Insecticide
(Universal Cooperatives)

Carbaryl *	12.50%
Rotenone	2.50%
Other cube resins	4.00%
Zineb	6.25%
Ziram	6.25%

UNICO GARDEN WEED KILLER GRANULES
Preemergence herbicide
(Universal Cooperatives)

Dimethyl ester of tetrachloroterephthalic acid	2.5%

UNICO HOUSE & GARDEN INSECT SPRAY
Insecticide
(Universal Cooperatives)

Pyrethrins	0.25%
Piperonyl butoxide, technical	1.00%
Petroleum distillate	1.00%

UNICO HOUSEHOLD A-TWO MIST INSECTICIDE
(Universal Cooperatives)

Tetramethrin	0.250%
Related compounds	0.034%
Resmethrin	0.250%
Related compounds	0.034%
Petroleum distillate	8.800%

UNICO INSECT SPRAY
Household insecticide
(Universal Cooperatives)

Petroleum distillate *	99.465%
2,2-Dichlorovinyl dimethyl phosphate (DDVP)	0.180%
Related compounds	0.020%
Piperonyl butoxide, technical	0.300%
Pyrethrins	0.035%

UNICO KELTHANE EMULSIFIABLE
Miticide
(Universal Cooperatives)

1,1-Bis(p-chlorophenyl)-2,2,2,-trichloroethanol	18.5%
Xylene *	73.0%

UNICO KEM LINK COMPATABILITY AGENT
For liquid fertilizer/pesticide mixtures
(Universal Cooperatives)

Principal functioning agents:	70%
Alkyl aryl polyoxyethylene glycol phosphate ester surfactants	

UNICO KLEEN WALK WEED KILLER
For non-selective control of weeds
(Universal Cooperatives)

Prometon	1.49%
Pentachlorophenol	0.86%
Other chlorophenols and related compounds	0.10%
Aromatic petroleum derivative solvent *	91.00%

UNICO LAWN BUG BLASTER
(Universal Cooperatives)

Chlorpyrifos *	25.4%
Aromatic petroleum derivative solvent *	43.2%

UNICO LAWN WEED KILLER
Herbicide
(Universal Cooperatives)

Dimethylamine salt of 2,4-dichlorophenoxyacetic acid *	13.8%

UNICO LICE-X
Granular insecticide - control of hog lice
(Universal Cooperatives)

Ronnel	5%

UNICO LINDANE EMULSIFIABLE CONCENTRATE
Insecticide
(Universal Cooperatives)

Lindane	12.7%
Xylene *	84.2%

UNICO LIVESTOCK & BARN FOGGING SPRAY
Insecticide
(Universal Cooperatives)

Technical Piperonyl butoxide	1.0%
Pyrethrins	0.1%
Petroleum base oil *	98.9%

UNICO LIVESTOCK PRESSURIZED SPRAY
Insecticide
(Universal Cooperatives)

Ronnel	2.5%
Xylene	0.5%

UNICO LOUSE AND FLEA POWDER
(Universal Cooperatives)

Malathion	5%

UNICO LO-V BRUSH KILLER
Herbicide
(Universal Cooperatives)

2-Ethyl hexyl ester of 2,4,5-trichlorophenoxyacetic acid *	31.5%
2-Ethyl hexyl ester of 2,4-dichlorophenoxyacetic acid *	33.0%

UNICO LO-V BRUSH KILLER 1-2
(Universal Cooperatives)

2-Ethylhexyl ester of 2,4,5-Trichlorophenoxyacetic acid *	15.75%
2-Ethylhexyl ester of 2,4-Dichlorophenoxyacetic acid *	33.75%

UNICO LO V ESTER 33 WEED KILLER
(Universal Cooperatives)

Isooctyl ester of 2,4-Dichlorophenoxyacetic acid *	55.80%

UNICO MALATHION-4 CATTLE AND POULTRY DUST
Insecticide
(Universal Cooperatives)

Malathion	4%

UNICO MALATHION-5 EMULSIFIABLE CONCENTRATE
Insecticide
(Universal Cooperatives)

Malathion *	57.0%
Xylene *	39.0%

UNICO MALATHION GRAIN SPRAY, PREMIUM GRADE
Insecticide
(Universal Cooperatives)

Malathion *	57%
Xylene *	32%

Starred ingredients (*) may be responsible for major toxic effects; consult Section II.

UNICO MALATHION 51 SPRAY
Insecticide
(Universal Cooperatives)

Malathion *	51.3%
Xylene *	40.8%

UNICO METHOXYCHLOR EMULSIFIABLE CONCENTRATE
Insecticide
(Universal Cooperatives)

Methoxychlor, technical	23.8%
Aromatic petroleum derivative solvent *	70.8%

UNICO ORNAMENTAL & GARDEN FUNGICIDE
(Universal Cooperatives)

Chlorothalonil	75%

UNICO PENTA CONCENTRATE
Wood preservative
(Universal Cooperatives)

Pentachlorophenol *	35.26%
Other chlorophenols & related compounds	4.10%
Petroleum hydrocarbons	41.00%

UNICO PRAMITOL 5PS
Herbicide
(Universal Cooperatives)

Prometon	5.00%
Simazine	0.75%
Sodium chlorate *	40.00%
Sodium metaborate	50.00%

UNICO PREMIUM GRAIN FUMIGANT NO. 2
(Universal Cooperatives)

Carbon disulfide	16.3%
Carbon tetrachloride *	82.3%
Sulfur dioxide	1.0%
Pentane	0.4%

UNICO PRESSURIZED DAIRY FLY SPRAY-V
Insecticide
(Universal Cooperatives)

Pyrethrins	0.5%
Technical Piperonyl butoxide	1.0%
N-Octyl bicycloheptene dicarboximide	1.0%
Petroleum distillates *	12.5%

UNICO PROLIN "READY-TO-USE" PELLETS
Rodenticide
(Universal Cooperatives)

Warfarin	0.025%
N′-(2-Quinoxalyl)sulfanilamide (Sulfaquinoxaline)	0.025%

UNICO PROLIN RODENTICIDE CONCENTRATE
(Universal Cooperatives)

Warfarin	0.5%
N′-(2-Quinoxalinyl) sulfanilamide (Sulfaquinoxaline)	0.5%

UNICO PY-VONA STOCK FLY SPRAY
Insecticide
(Universal Cooperatives)

Petroleum base oil *	99.52%
2,2-Dichlorovinyl dimethyl phosphate (DDVP)	0.18%
Related compounds	0.02%
Technical Piperonyl butoxide	0.25%
Pyrethrins	0.03%

UNICO RONNEL-2 EMULSIFIABLE CONCENTRATE
Insecticide
(Universal Cooperatives)

Ronnel	23.8%
Aromatic petroleum derivative solvent *	60.2%

UNICO ROSE AND FLORAL DUST NO. 2
Insecticide, fungicide
(Universal Cooperatives)

Carbaryl *	5.00%
Zineb	5.00%
Sulfur	20.00%

UNICO ROSE AND FLORAL SPRAY POWDER NO. 2
Insecticide, fungicide
(Universal Cooperatives)

Carbaryl *	12.5%
Zineb	12.5%
Sulfur	25.0%

UNICO ROTENONE SPRAY POWDER
Insecticide
(Universal Cooperatives)

Rotenone *	5%
Other cube resins	10%

UNICO SEVIN ZINEB 3-5.2 DUST
Insecticide, fungicide
(Universal Cooperatives)

Carbaryl *	3.0%
Zineb	5.2%

UNICO SNAIL & SLUG PELLETS-M
(Universal Cooperatives)

Mesurol *	2.0%

UNICO SPREADER STICKER G
Nonionic surfactant-adjuvant for pesticide sprays
(Universal Cooperatives)

Alkyl polyoxyethylene ether	20.0%
Inert ingredients:	80.0%
3.5% Isopropyl alcohol	

UNICO STOCK SPRAY CONCENTRATE
Insecticide
(Universal Cooperatives)

Dimethyl phosphate of alpha-methylbenzyl 3-hydroxy-cis-crotonate *	12.6%
Petroleum hydrocarbons	79.3%

UNICO TERMITE KILL
(Universal Cooperatives)

Technical Chlordane *	45.00%
Kerosene *	50.57%

UNICO THIODAN EMULSIFIABLE CONCENTRATE
Insecticide
(Universal Cooperatives)

Endosulfan *	22.8%
Aromatic petroleum derivative solvent *	70.2%

UNICO THOROBRED "H-P" SPRAY
Fly spray for horses
(Universal Cooperatives)

Petroleum base oil *	98.9%
Technical Piperonyl butoxide	1.0%
Pyrethrins	0.1%

UNICO 2,4,5-T LO-V ESTER BRUSH KILLER
Herbicide
(Universal Cooperatives)

Isooctyl ester of 2,4,5-trichlorophenoxyacetic acid *	63%

Starred ingredients (*) may be responsible for major toxic effects; consult Section II.

UNICO TOMATO-POTATO & VEGETABLE DUST
Insecticide/fungicide
(Universal Cooperatives)

Carbaryl * 5%
Copper, expressed as metallic (in copper oxide) * 7%

UNICO 5% TOXAPHENE BACK RUBBER SOLUTION
Insecticide
(Universal Cooperatives)

Toxaphene * 5%
Petroleum distillate * 95%

UNICO TOXAPHENE EMULSIFIABLE CONCENTRATE
Insecticide
(Universal Cooperatives)

Toxaphene * 60%
Petroleum distillate 35%

UNICO TOXAPHENE LIVESTOCK SPRAY CONCENTRATE
Insecticide
(Universal Cooperatives)

Toxaphene * 59.0%
Petroleum distillate 31.0%

UNICO TOX-HID
Rodenticide
(Universal Cooperatives)

Warfarin 0.025%

UNICO TURF TREETER "T"
Herbicide
(Universal Cooperatives)

Dimethylamine salt of 2,4-Dichlorophenoxyacetic acid 3.23%
Dimethylamine salt of 2-(2-Methyl-4-chlorophenoxy) propionic acid * 10.59%
Dimethylamine salt of Dicamba (3,6-Dichloro-o-anisic acid) ... 1.28%

UNICO WASP & HORNET SPRAY
(Universal Cooperatives)

Pyrethrins 0.10%
Piperonyl butoxide, technical 0.20%
N-Octyl bicycloheptene dicarboximide 0.33%
o-Isopropoxyphenyl methylcarbamate 0.50%
Isoparaffinic hydrocarbons * 83.87%

UNICO WOOD SAVER
Wood preservative
(Universal Cooperatives)

Pentachlorophenol * 4.32%
Other chlorinated phenols 0.63%
Petroleum hydrocarbons * 92.55%

UNICO ZIPCIDE CATTLE DUST BAG
Control of horn flies and lice on beef and dairy cattle
(Universal Cooperatives)

Co-ral (Coumaphos) 1%

UNION CARBIDE CARB & CHOKE CLEANER (AS-217, Formula 1936-68)
(Union Carbide)

Aromatic hydrocarbons * 71%
Ketones 29%
Hydrocarbon propellant

UNION CARBIDE CARBURETOR & FUEL SYSTEM CLEANER (AS-224, Formula 1936-68)
(Union Carbide)

Aromatic hydrocarbons * 71%
Ketones 29%

UNION CARBIDE SILICONE SPRAY LUBRICANT (AS-196/193, Formula 1912-148A)
(Union Carbide)

Trichloroethane * 94%
Silicone fluid 4%
Vegetable oil 2%
Hydrocarbon propellant

UNION CARBIDE TRANSMISSION STOP LEAK AND FLUID CONDITIONER (AS-255, Formula MI-2235)
(Union Carbide)

Refined Mineral oil * 100%

UNIPEN CAPSULES, SOLUTION AND TABLETS
Antibiotic
(Wyeth Labs.)

Capsules:
    Nafcillin sodium as the monohydrate .... 250 mg.

Solution (each 5 ml.):
    Nafcillin sodium as the monohydrate .... 250 mg.

Tablets:
    Nafcillin sodium as the monohydrate .... 500 mg.

UNISET BLOW STYLING LOTION
(Bonat)

	percentage range
Water	40.0-55.0%
SD Alcohol 40	35.0-45.0%
Vinyl acetate/crotonic acid/vinyl neodecanoate polymer	<5.0%
Vinyl acetate/crotonic acid copolymer	<1.0%
Butylene glycol	<1.0%
Aminomethyl propanol	<1.0%
Tetrasodium EDTA	<1.0%
Dimethicone copolyol	<1.0%
Methylparaben	<1.0%
Fragrance	<1.0%
Sodium bisulfite	<1.0%

UNISOL
Preservative-free saline solution for soft contact lens use
(CooperVision Pharm.)

A non-preserved, isotonic, buffered Salt solution

UNISOM
Sleep aid
(Leeming Div.)

Each tablet:
    Doxylamine succinate .... 25 mg.

UNISTAT-3
Feed additive aid in prevention of coccidiosis in chickens
(Salsbury)

Nitromide (3,5-Dinitrobenzamide) . 25%
Sulfanitran (Acetyl-(para-nitrophenyl)-sulfanilamide) 30%
Roxarsone (3-Nitro-4-hydroxyphenyl-arsonic acid) * 5%

UNITED GILSONITE PAINT PRODUCTS
Cement paints, paint sundries, and clear finishes

United Gilsonite Laboratories
P.O. Box 70
Scranton, Pa. 18501

Phone: 717-344-1202

See PAINTS, Section VI, General Formulations

UNITED STATES GYPSUM CO.
Paints, adhesives, sealers; building construction materials

United States Gypsum Co.
101 S. Wacker Dr.
Chicago, Ill. 60606

Phone: 312-321-4000

Starred ingredients (*) may be responsible for major toxic effects; consult Section II.

UNIVERSAL ANTISTONE
Organic detergent, liquid dairy cleaner
(Universal Milking Machine)

Phosphoric acid *

'76 Ed.

UNIVERSAL CHLOR-O-SAN
Disinfectant, germicide
(Universal Milking Machine)

Sodium hypochlorite * 6.4%

'76 Ed.

UNIVERSAL DRAIN PIPE CLEANER
(Internat. Plumb.)

Sodium hydroxide *

'76 Ed.

UNIVERSAL IODO-KLEEN
Detergent sanitizer
(Universal Milking Machine)

Nonylphenoxy poly (ethyleneoxy)
ethanol-iodine complex (1.75%
available iodine) 15.75%
Phosphoric acid * 13.50%

'76 Ed.

UNIVERSAL LINE CLEAN 3
*Prevents lime formation, removes milk-
stone*
(Universal Milking Machine)

Phosphoric acid *

'76 Ed.

UNIVERSAL STERIBALM
Udder wash
(Universal Milking Machine)

N-Alkyl (C14-50%, C12-40%, C16-
10%) dimethyl benzyl ammonium
chloride * 10%

'76 Ed.

UNIVERSAL UNI-CHLOR
Dairy equipment sanitizer
(Universal Milking Machine)

Sodium dichloroisocyanurate (available chlorine 20%) * 36%

'76 Ed.

UNNA'S BOOT DRESSING

See GRAFCO MEDICOPASTE
BANDAGE (UNNA'S BOOT
DRESSING)

UNPROCO
Antitussive, expectorant
(Direct Div.)

Each capsule:
Guaifenesin .... 200 mg.
Dextromethorphan hydro-
bromide * .... 30 mg.

UPJOHN ZINC SULFIDE COMPOUND LOTION IMPROVED
Treatment of acne
(Upjohn)

Each fl. oz.:
Zinc * .... approx. 12.3 gr.
Sulfur (present as sul-
fide, polysulfides, and
thiosulfate) * ...... approx. 22 gr.
Sodium borate
Boric acid
Aluminum hydroxide
Aromatic

URACID CAPSULES
*Management of diaper rash in children,
control of odor*
(Wesley Pharm.)

Each capsule:
dl-Methionine .... 0.2 mg.

URATIN
Urinary antiseptic, antispasmodic
(Wesley Pharm.)

Each tablet:
Methenamine * .... 40.8 mg.
Atropine sulfate * .... 0.03 mg.
Hyoscyamine sulfate * ...... 0.03 mg.
Salol * .... 18.1 mg.
Benzoic acid .... 4.5 mg.
Methylene blue * .... 5.4 mg.

UREACIN-20 CREME
*Treatment of hyperkeratotic dry skin
conditions*
(Pedinol)

Urea * 20%

UREACIN-40 CREME
*Treatment of nail destruction and dis-
solution*
(Pedinol)

Urea * 40%

UREACIN-10 LOTION
*Treatment of simple dry skin resulting
from aging, exposure to sun, wind,
soap, & detergents*
(Pedinol)

Urea * 10%
Lactic acid

URI-BLU TABLETS
For urinary infections
(Pharmex)

Each tablet:
Methenamine * .... 2 gr.
Salol * .... 1/2 gr.
Methylene blue .... 1/10 gr.
Benzoic acid .... 1/8 gr.
Atropine sulfate .... 1/1000 gr.
Hyoscyamine sulfate ...... 1/2000 gr.

URIDIUM TABLETS
Genito-urinary use
(Pharmex)

Each tablet:
Phenylazodiaminopyridine
HCl * .... 100 mg.

URISAL
Urinary antiseptic, antispasmodic
(Wesley Pharm.)

Each tablet:
Methenamine * .... 40.8 mg.
Atropine sulfate * .... 0.03 mg.
Hyoscyamine * .... 0.03 mg.
Phenyl salicylate * .... 18.1 mg.
Benzoic acid .... 4.5 mg.

URISEP
Urinary antiseptic
(Direct Div.)

Each tablet:
Atropine sulfate * .... 0.03 mg.
Hyoscyamine * .... 0.03 mg.
Methenamine * .... 40.8 mg.
Methylene blue .... 5.4 mg.
Phenyl salicylate * .... 18.1 mg.
Benzoic acid .... 4.5 mg.

URISTAT
Urinary antispasmodic and antiseptic
(Lemmon Co.)

Each tablet:
Atropine sulfate .... 0.03 mg.
Hyoscyamine (as the sulfate) 0.03 mg.
Methenamine .... 50 mg.
Methylene blue .... 5.5 mg.
Phenyl salicylate * .... 20 mg.
Benzoic acid .... 5 mg.

URISTIX
*Urine glucose and protein test reagent
strip*
(Ames)

Protein test area: see ALBUSTIX
Glucose test area: see CLINISTIX

URITRAL CAPSULES
Urinary antiseptic, analgesic
(Central Pharmacal Co.)

Each capsule:
Methenamine mandelate ..... 250 mg.
Phenazopyridine
hydrochloride * .... 50 mg.

Starred ingredients (*) may be responsible for major toxic effects; consult Section II.

UROBILISTIX
Urine urobilinogen test reagent strip
(Ames)

Dimethylaminobenzaldehyde
Dimethyl sulfoxide
Stannic chloride
Chloroform
Sodium phosphate

UROBIOTIC-250 CAPSULES
Urinary tract infections
(Roerig)

Each capsule:
Oxytetracycline hydrochloride   250 mg.
Sulfamethizole *   250 mg.
Phenazopyridine
   hydrochloride *   50 mg.

UROLATE
Urinary antiseptic
(Wesley Pharm.)

Each tablet:
Methenamine mandelate *   0.5 gm.

URO-PHOSPHATE
Keeps the urine acid
(Poythress, Wm. P.)

Each tablet:
Sodium acid phosphate *†   500 mg.
Methenamine *   300 mg.

†*See* Sodium phosphate, monobasic

UROQID-ACID
For urine acidification & chronic urinary tract infection
(Beach Pharm.)

Each tablet:
Methenamine mandelate *   350 mg.
Sodium acid phosphate   200 mg.

UROQID-ACID NO. 2
For urine acidification & chronic urinary tract infection
(Beach Pharm.)

Each tablet:
Methenamine mandelate *   500 mg.
Sodium acid phosphate   500 mg.

UROSTAT FORTE
(Elder)

Each tablet:
Methenamine   81.6 mg.
Sodium biphosphate   40.8 mg.
Phenyl salicylate (Salol) *   36.2 mg.
Methylene blue   10.8 mg.
Hyoscyamine, alkaloid *   0.12 mg.

UROX 'B' WATER SOLUBLE CONCENTRATE WEED KILLER
(Hopkins Agric.)

Bromacil *   40.8%
Inert ingredients (including an ethanol amine)   59.2%

UROX 'HX' GRANULAR WEED KILLER
Herbicide for non-crop use
(Hopkins Agric.)

Active ingred.:
   Bromacil   4%
Inert ingred.:
   Granular mineral base   96%

UROX LIQUID OIL CONCENTRATE WEED KILLER
(Hopkins Agric.)

Monuron trichloroacetate (Monuron 17.69% minimum, trichloroacetate acid 14.56% minimum) *   32.25%
Aromatic petroleum solvent *   20-30%
Dodecylbenzenesulfonic acid, Corrosion inhibitor, and Inert ingredients   35-45%

URSA OIL HEAVY DUTY
(Texaco Inc.)

Petroleum lubricating oil
Oxidation & corrosion inhibitor *†
Calcium detergent *‡

†*See* Rust Control, Section VI, General Formulations
‡*See* Detergents (synthetic)

URSA OILS S-3
(Texaco Inc.)

Petroleum lubricating oil
Calcium detergent *†
Oxidation and corrosion inhibitor *‡

†*See* Detergents (synthetic)
‡*See* Rust Control, Section VI, General Formulations

URSA SUPER PLUS
Lubricating oil
(Texaco Canada Ltd.)

Mineral oil *
Methacrylate copolymer
Additive package containing:
   Zn, P, Ca, S, N
   Silicone anti-foamant

URSATEX OILS
(Texaco Inc.)

Petroleum lubricating oil
Calcium detergent
Oxidation and corrosion inhibitor *†

†*See* Rust control, Section VI, General Formulations

URSINUS INLAY TABS
Analgesic, decongestant, antihistaminic
(Dorsey Labs.)

Calurin (Calcium carbaspirin) equivalent to 300 mg. aspirin *
Phenylpropanolamine
   hydrochloride *   25 mg.
Pheniramine maleate *   12.5 mg.
Pyrilamine maleate *   12.5 mg.

U-SAN-O MOTHPROOFING SOLUTION
(Laidlaw Corp.)

Methoxychlor (technical) *   34%
Aromatic petroleum solvent *   66%

U-SAN-O MOTH SPRAY
(Laidlaw Corp.)

Ammonium silico fluoride 98% *   14.0%
Wetting agent   0.4%
Water   85.6%

U.S. BORAX LOTION SOAP
Powdered hand soap
(U.S. Borax)

Toilet soap
Urea
Lanolin
Emollients

USCO TROPICAL ROACHKIL INSECT SPRAY
(Uncle Sam)

Diazinon *
Pyrethrums
Synergists
Perfume
Petroleum distillates *

U.S.-E.Q. 335

   See MARTIN'S U.S.-E.Q. 335

U.S. MARINE COATINGS PRODUCTS

U.S. Marine Coatings, Inc.
P.O. Box 5425
Sarasota, Fla. 33579

Phone: 813-921-2244

U. S. METAL POLISH
(SerVaas Labs.)

Silica (amorphous)   60%/w
Cade oil   20%/w
Paraffin oil   10%/w
Stearic acid   10%/w

Starred ingredients (*) may be responsible for major toxic effects; consult Section II.

UTICILLIN VK FLAVORED GRANULES
Penicillin susceptible infections
(Upjohn)

Each 5 ml. of reconstituted solution:
Penicillin V potassium
(equiv. to penicillin
V) .... 125 mg.; 250 mg.

UTICILLIN VK TABLETS
Penicillin susceptible infections
(Upjohn)

Each tablet:
Penicillin V potassium
(equiv. to penicillin
V) .... 250 mg.; 500 mg.

UTILITY THINNING SPIRITS

See COOK'S UTILITY THINNING SPIRITS

V

VACON
Nasal decongestant
(Scherer Labs.)

Phenylephrine HCl, USP	0.2%
Chlorobutanol	0.15%
Sodium bisulfite	0.03%
Benzalkonium chloride	1:10000
Isotonic saline solution base	

VAGIDINE
Relief of symptoms of vulvo-vaginitis
(Elder)

Cream:
Sulfanilamide *	15%
Aminacrine hydrochloride	0.2%
Allantoin	2%

Suppository (each):
Sulfanilamide	1.05 gm.
Aminacrine hydrochloride	0.014 gm.
Allantoin	0.14 gm.

VAGILIA CREAM
Vaginal anti-infective
(Lemmon Co.)

Each gm.:
Sulfisoxazole	10%
Aminacrine hydrochloride	0.2%
Allantoin	2.0%

Also contains:
Stearic acid, Mineral oil, Polysorbate 60, Sorbitan monostearate, Sorbitol, Methylparaben, Propylparaben, Purified water

VAGILIA SUPPOSITORIES
Vaginal anti-infective
(Lemmon Co.)

Each suppository:
Sulfisoxazole	600 mg.
Aminacrine hydrochloride	12 mg.
Allantoin	120 mg.

Also contains:
Lactose, Polyethylene glycol 400, Polyethylene glycol 4000, Glycerin, Polysorbate 80, Lactic acid
Inert covering:
Gelatin, Glycerin, Water, Methylparaben, Propylparaben, Coloring

VAGIMINE CREAM
Anti-infective
(Direct Div.)

Sulfanilamide *	15%
9-Aminoacridine	0.2%
Allantoin	2%

VAGISEC LIQUID
Treatment of trichomonal vaginal infections
(Schmid Labs.)

Polyoxyethylene nonyl phenol *†
Sodium ethylenediaminetetraacetate
Sodium dioctyl sulfosuccinate

'76 Ed.

†See Alkyl phenoxy polyethoxy ethanols

VAGITRIC
Treatment of trichomoniasis
(Elder)

Each tablet:
9-Aminoacridine hydrochloride *	25.0 mg.

VAGITRIC CREAM
Treatment of trichomoniasis
(Elder)

9-Aminoacridine hydrochloride 0.25%

VALACET JUNIOR
Analgesic
(Vale)

Each tablet:
Phenacetin *	64.8 mg.
Hyoscyamus	5.4 mg.
Aspirin *	64.8 mg.
Caffeine (anhydrous)	8.1 mg.

VALACET (Tablets & Capsules)
Analgesic
(Vale)

Each tablet or capsule:
Phenacetin *	129.6 mg.
Hyoscyamus	10.8 mg.
Aspirin *	129.6 mg.
Caffeine (anhydrous)	16.2 mg.
Gelsemium extract	0.6 mg.

VALADOL
Antipyretic and analgesic
(Squibb)

TABLETS (each):
Acetaminophen *	325 mg.

LIQUID (each 5 cc):
Acetaminophen	120 mg.
Alcohol	9%

VALAX
Laxative
(Vale)

Each tablet:
Dioctyl sodium sulfosuccinate *	100 mg.
Danthron	37.5 mg.

VALAY TOILET BOWL DEODORANT
(Curran)

Paradichlorobenzene *
'76 Ed.

VALCAINE OINTMENT
(Vale)

Benzocaine	5%
Menthol *	
Phenol *	
Zinc oxide	
Camphor *	
Petrolatum base	

VALDEINE
Analgesic
(Vale)

Each tablet:
Codeine phosphate *	16.2 mg.
Aspirin *	227.0 mg.
Phenacetin *	162.0 mg.
Caffeine	32.4 mg.

VALDRENE EXPECTORANT SYRUP
(Vale)

Each fl. oz.:
Alcohol	5%
Diphenhydramine hydrochloride *	80.0 mg.
Ammonium chloride	778.0 mg.
Sodium citrate	324.0 mg.
Menthol	6.5 mg.

VALE ALKALINE AROMATIC
Gargle
(Vale)

Each tablet:
Sodium chloride *	324.0 mg.
Sodium bicarbonate *	324.0 mg.
Sodium borate *	324.0 mg.
Sodium benzoate	18.9 mg.
Sodium salicylate *	18.9 mg.
Oil of wintergreen, * Thymol *, Oil of Eucalyptus *	q.s.

VALERIANETS-DISPERT
Sedative
(Lambda Inc.)

Each tablet:
Extract Valerian * .... 0.05 gm.

VALESIN
Analgesic
(Vale)

Each tablet:
Acetaminophen * .... 150 mg.
Aspirin * .... 150 mg.
Salicylamide .... 150 mg.

VALE SULFUR AND RESORCIN COMP. OINTMENT
(Vale)

Sulfur
Resorcin *
Juniper tar *
Thymol *
Zinc oxide
Boric acid *

VALIANT
Detergent, germicide; hospital grade
(Puritan Chem. Co.)

Active ingredients: 37.0%
Isopropanol *
Sodium dodecyl benzene sulfonate *
Ortho secondary amylphenol *
Orthophenylphenol *
Inert ingredients: 63.0%
Water
Hydroxyethyl cellulose
Perfume
Dye

VALIANT APC'S, TOPCO
See TOPCO VALIANT APC'S

VALIANT RUBBING ALCOHOL, TOPCO
See TOPCO VALIANT RUBBING AL-
COHOL

VALIANT RUBBING ALCOHOL WITH WINTERGREEN, TOPCO
See TOPCO VALIANT RUBBING AL-
COHOL WITH WINTERGREEN

VALIHIST
Antihistaminic-decongestant
(Clapp, Otis)

Each capsule:
Phenylephrine hydrochloride   10 mg.
Chlorpheniramine maleate   1.0 mg.
Pyrilamine maleate .... 12.5 mg.
Caffeine
Acetaminophen *

VALIMENT
Liniment
(Vale)

Each 100 ml.:
Menthol ....   1 gm.
Camphor * ....   2 gm.
Methyl salicylate * ....   5 ml.
Eucalyptol * ....   2 ml.
Oil of mustard ....   0.1 ml.
Turpentine ....   1 ml.

VALISONE AEROSOL
Acute contact dermatitis
(Schering)

Betamethasone valerate (equiv. to
7.5 mg. betamethasone) .... 9.1 mg.
Mineral oil
Fractionated coconut oil
Propellant: .... to make 85 gm.
Trichloromonofluoromethane
Dichlorodifluoromethane

VALISONE CREAM 0.1%
Dermatologic use
(Schering)

Each gram:
Betamethasone valerate (equiv.
of 1.0 mg. of betamethasone) 1.2 mg.
Emollient cream contains:
Mineral oil
Petrolatum
Polyethylene glycol 1000 monocetyl
ether
Cetostearyl alcohol
Monobasic sodium phosphate
Phosphoric acid
4-Chloro-m-cresol
Water

VALISONE LOTION 0.1%
Dermatologic
(Schering)

Each gram:
Betamethasone valerate (equiv. to 1.0
mg. betamethasone)
Isopropyl alcohol 47.5%
Water
Carboxy vinyl polymer
Sodium hydroxide (to adjust pH to 4.7)

VALISONE OINTMENT 0.1%
Dermatologic
(Schering)

Each gram:
Betamethasone valerate (equiv.
to 1.0 mg. of betamethasone) 1.2 mg.
Base:
Liquid and white Petrolatum
Hydrogenated Lanolin

VALIUM
*Aids in the relief of tension, anxiety and
skeletal muscle spasm*
(Roche)

Each tablet:
Diazepam * ...... 2 mg.; 5 mg.; 10 mg.

VALMID
Nonbarbiturate sedative
(Dista)

Each Pulvule:
Ethinamate * .... 500 mg.

VALOBAR
Analgesic & sedative
(Vale)

Each tablet:
Phenobarbital ....   16.2 mg.
Phenacetin * .... 162.0 mg.
Aspirin * .... 226.8 mg.
Caffeine anhydrous ....   32.4 mg.

VALOPHEN
Analgesic
(Vale)

Each tablet:
Phenacetin * .... 162.0 mg.
Aspirin * .... 226.8 mg.
Caffeine (anhydrous) ....   32.4 mg.
Gelsemium extract ....   4.0 mg.

VALORIN
Pain relief
(Clapp, Otis)

Each tablet:
Acetaminophen * ....   325 mg.

VALSPAR ALKYD EXTERIOR PRIMER WHITE (55001)
(Valspar Corp.)

Pigment: 49.2%
Titanium dioxide type IV ..   30.4%
Barium sulfate 19.2%
Silica & silicates 49.6%
Folpet 0.8%
Vehicle: 50.8%
Linseed soya alkyd resin ..   32.4%
Raw linseed oil 3.4%
Combined amount: 64.2%
Aliphatic hydrocarbons *
Driers *

VALSPAR ANTI-FOULING BOTTOM PAINT ESCOLUX BRONZE (3594)
Marine finish
(Valspar Corp.)

Pigment: 35.2%
Copper bronze *† 100.0%
Vehicle: 64.8%
Tung phenolic petroleum
resin   29.5%
Hydrogenated rosin ester ..   7.5%
Aromatic hydrocarbon * ..   49.0%
Aliphatic hydrocarbons ...   14.0%

†*See* Copper

VALSPAR ANTI-FOULING BOTTOM PAINT "98" RED COPPER (3589)
(Valspar Corp.)

Pigment:	44.9%
Cuprous oxide *	19.00%
Inerts from Cu2O	1.21%
Red iron oxide	8.08%
Magnesium silicate	16.57%
Vehicle:	55.1%
Pine tar oil *	18.18%
Pine oil	0.64%
Rosin	13.66%
Mineral spirits *	22.66%

VALSPAR FOULGARD ANTI-FOULING VINYL BOTTOM PAINT BRIGHT RED (3548)
Marine finish
(Valspar Corp.)

Pigment:	20.9%
Bon maroon - pyrotone red	7.7%
Silicates	13.2%
Vehicle:	79.1%
Vinyl resin	9.4%
Gum rosin	6.0%
Tributyltin fluoride *	12.9%
Ketones	22.2%
Esters	18.5%
Aromatic hydrocarbons *	10.1%

VALSPAR FOULGARD ANTI-FOULING VINYL BOTTOM PAINT COHO BLUE (3537)
Marine finish
(Valspar Corp.)

Pigment:	28.3%
Phthalocyanine blue	2.5%
Zinc oxide	6.7%
Titanium dioxide type IV	7.1%
Silicates	12.0%
Vehicle:	71.7%
Vinyl resin	8.5%
Gum rosin	5.6%
Tributyltin fluoride *	11.7%
Ketones	20.0%
Esters	17.1%
Aromatic hydrocarbons *	8.8%

VALSPAR FOULGARD ANTI-FOULING VINYL BOTTOM PAINT WHITE (3505)
Marine finish
(Valspar Corp.)

Pigment:	32.6%
Titanium dioxide type IV	14.6%
Zinc oxide	6.7%
Silicates	11.3%
Vehicle:	67.4%
Vinyl resin	8.7%
Rosin	5.8%
Ketones	18.7%
Esters	14.6%
Aromatic hydrocarbons *	8.1%
Tributyltin fluoride *	11.5%

VALSPAR HOUSE PAINT-- 215 NON-CHALKING WHITE
(Valspar Corp.)

Pigment:	61.3%
Titanium dioxide	20.1%
Zinc oxide	22.9%
Calcium carbonate	28.3%
Magnesium silicate	28.3%
Folpet	0.4%
Vehicle:	38.7%
Bodied linseed oil	19.0%
Refined linseed oil	58.3%
Combined amount:	22.7%
Aliphatic hydrocarbons *	
Driers *	

VALSPAR HOUSE PAINT-- 217 WHITE 4 EVR
(Valspar Corp.)

Pigment:	57.9%
Titanium dioxide type III	24.9%
Zinc oxide	24.9%
Calcium carbonates	18.6%
Silicates	31.1%
1,2-Bis (n-propylsulfonyl) ethene (Vancide PA)	0.5%
Vehicle:	42.1%
Refined linseed oil	54.5%
Bodied linseed oil	20.5%
Aliphatic hydrocarbons* & Driers	25.0%

VALSPAR LOW LUSTRE HOUSE PAINT--315 WHITE
(Valspar Corp.)

Pigment:	44.9%
Titanium dioxide	20.0%
Silica & Silicates	24.5%
1,2 Bis (n-propylsulfonyl) ethene (Vancide PA)	0.4%
Vehicle:	55.1%
Raw linseed oil	5.7%
Linseed oil alkyd	14.9%
Aliphatic hydrocarbons* & Driers	34.5%

VALSPAR PAINT PRODUCTS
Paints, varnishes, enamels

The Valspar Corporation
1101 Third St. S.
Minneapolis, Minn. 55415

Phone: 612-332-7371

See PAINTS, Section VI, General Formulations

VAL-TEP
Bronchodilator
(Vale)

Each tablet:	
Phenobarbital	8 mg.
Theophylline *	130 mg.
Ephedrine hydrochloride *	24 mg.

VALVE-MEDIC
Automotive, cleaner & lubricant
(Radiator)

Aromatic solvents *

'76 Ed.

VAM-O
Rodenticide
(Dro)

Warfarin	0.025%

'76 Ed.

VAN BRITE SELF POLISHING WAX
(Adco)

Carnauba wax
Petroleum oxidized wax
Resin
Emulsifier

VANCARE ALGAECIDE CONCENTRATED
For control of algae growth in swimming pools
(Van Waters & Rogers)

Alkyl (50% C12, 30% C14, 17% C16, 3% C18) dimethyl dichlorobenzyl ammonium chloride *	20%

VANCARE DRY ACID
For pH control in chemically balanced swimming pools
(Van Waters & Rogers)

Sodium bisulfate *	93.5%

VANCARE DRY CHLORINE CONCENTRATE
Cyanurate type
(Van Waters & Rogers)

Sodium dichloro-s-triazinetrione *	100%

VANCIDE 51
Fungicide
(Vanderbilt, R.T.)

Sodium dimethyldithiocarbamate *	27.6%
Sodium 2-mercaptobenzothiazole	2.4%

VANCIDE 89
Fungicide
(Vanderbilt, R.T.)

N-Trichloromethylthio-4-cyclohexene-1,2-dicarboximide (Captan) *
Powder:	90%
Liquid:	45%

VANCIDE MZ-96
Fungicide
(Vanderbilt, R.T.)

Zinc dimethyldithiocarbamate
  (Ziram) * 96%

VANCIDE 89RE
Fungicide, bacteriostat
(Vanderbilt, R.T.)

N-Trichloromethylthio-4-cyclohex-
  ene-1,2-dicarboximide (Captan) *   97%

VANCIDE 51Z
Fungicide/bactericide
(Vanderbilt, R.T.)

WETTABLE POWDER:
  Zinc dimethyldithiocarbamate * 87.0%
  Zinc 2-mercaptobenzothiazole .. 7.5%

DISPERSION:
  Zinc dimethyldithiocarbamate * 46.0%
  Zinc 2-mercaptobenzothiazole .. 4.0%

VANI-BLOCS REST ROOM DEODORANT
(Nat'l Labs. Div.)

Paradichlorobenzene * .... major

VANISH SOLID, AUTOMATIC

See AUTOMATIC VANISH SOLID

VANISH TOILET BOWL CLEANER, AUTOMATIC (LIQUID)

See AUTOMATIC VANISH TOILET
  BOWL CLEANER (LIQUID)

VANISH TOILET BOWL CLEANER (GRANULAR)
(Drackett)

Sodium bisulfate * .... 62.0%/wt.
Monopotassium peroxysulfate 0.04%/wt.
Sodium carbonate
Sodium chloride
Anionic surfactant, Dye, Perfume

VANISH TOILET BOWL CLEANER (LIQUID)
(Drackett)

Hydrochloric acid * 9.25%
Cationic surfactants .... approx. 2%
Nonionic surfactant
Water
Dye and Perfume

VANI-SOL BOWL CLEANSE
(Nat'l Labs. Div.)

Hydrochloric acid * 23%
Methyldodecyl benzyl ammonium
  chloride .... minor
Methyldodecylxylene
  bis(trimethylammonium)
  chloride .... minor
o-Benzyl-p-
  chlorophenol .... minor

VANI-SOL BULK DISINFECTANT WASHROOM CLEANER
(Nat'l Labs. Div.)

Tetrasodium
  ethylenediaminetetra-
  acetate 1.52%
Sodium metasilicate 0.06%
Alkyl (67% C12, 25% C14, 7% C16,
  1% C8-C16-C18) dimethyl ben-
  zyl ammonium chlorides 0.08%
Alkyl (50% C14, 40% C12, 10%
  C16) dimethyl benzyl ammo-
  nium chlorides 0.02%
Ethylene glycol monobutyl ether minor
Ethoxylated Alcohol .... minor

VANI-SOL DISINFECTANT WASHROOM CLEANER
(Nat'l Labs. Div.)

Sodium metasilicate 0.06%
Ethylene glycol monobutyl ether minor
Ethoxylated alcohol .... minor
Alkyl (67% C12; 25% C14; 7% C16;
  1% C8-C10-C18) dimethyl benzyl
  ammonium chlorides 0.08%
Alkyl (50% C14; 40% C12; 10% C16)
  dimethyl benzyl ammonium
  chloride 0.02%
Tetrasodium
  ethylenediaminetetraacetate .. 1.52%

VANI-SOL PER DIEM
Toilet bowl cleaner
(Nat'l Labs. Div.)

Hydrochloric acid * 8%
Alkyl (67% C12, 25% C14, 7% C16, 1%
  C8-C10-C18) dimethyl benzyl am-
  monium chloride 1%

VANI-SOL WASHROOM DRAIN OPENER
(Nat'l Labs. Div.)

Sodium hydroxide * .... major

VANITY CARE
Liquid soap
(Smith, Robert)

Alkyl sodium sulfonates *

'76 Ed.

VANOBID (VAGINAL OINTMENT AND TABLETS)
*Antifungal antibiotic for treatment of
  vaginitis*
(Merrell Dow)

OINTMENT:
  Candicidin .... 0.6 mg./gm.
  Petrolatum U.S.P.

TABLETS (each):
  Candicidin .... 3 mg.
  Starch
  Lactose
  Magnesium stearate

VANO LIQUID STARCH
(Purex Corp.)

Corn starch 5-10%
Sodium chloride 5-10%
Sulfonated oil .... <1%
Preservative .... <1%
Emulsifying agent .... <1%
Coloring agent .... <1%
Fluorescent whitening agent ... <1%
Water .... Balance

VANO SPRAY STARCH
(Purex Corp.)

Propellant .... <10%
Corn starch 1-5%
Preservative .... <1%
Silicone .... <1%
Fluorescent whitening agent ... <1%
Perfume .... <1%
Water .... >85%

VANOXIDE LOTION (VANISHES)
Treatment of severe acne vulgaris
(Dermik)

Benzoyl peroxide .... 5% w/v
Chlorhydroxyquinoline 0.25%
In a greaseless vehicle

VANQUISH
Analgesic
(Glenbrook Labs.)

Each tablet:
  Aspirin * .... 227 mg.
  Acetaminophen * .... 194 mg.
  Caffeine .... 33 mg.
  Dried Aluminum hydroxide gel 25 mg.
  Magnesium hydroxide .... 50 mg.

VANSEB
Dandruff shampoo; cream and lotion
(Herbert Labs.)

Sulfur 2%
Salicylic acid * 1%

VANSEB-T
Tar shampoo; cream and lotion
(Herbert Labs.)

Sulfur 2%
Salicylic acid * 1%
Coal tar solution, USP * 5%

Starred ingredients (*) may be responsible for major toxic effects; consult Section II.

VANTAGE
Detergent
(Calgon Corp., Commercial Div.)

Complex phosphates *
Caustic soda *
Sodium silicates
Wetting agents *

VAN WATERS' DRY ACID
For pH control in chemically balanced swimming pools
(Van Waters & Rogers)

Sodium bisulfate * 93.5%

VAN WATERS' DRY CHLORINE CONCENTRATE
Cyanurate type
(Van Waters & Rogers)

Sodium dichloro-s-triazinetrione * 100%

VAN WATERS' DRY CHLORINE GRANULAR
(Van Waters & Rogers)

Calcium hypochlorite * 70%

VAN WATERS' DRY CHLORINE TABLETS
(Van Waters & Rogers)

Calcium hypochlorite * 70%

VAPAM
Soil fumigant
(Stauffer)

Vapam (Sodium methyl dithiocarbamate) *

VAP*A*ROMA DEODORIZER
For deodorizing diaper pails & garbage pails
(Victory Chem.)

Combined amount: 100%
  Paradichlorobenzene *
  Perfume oils *

'76 Ed.

VAPO AEROSOL
Insecticide
(Pet Chemicals)

DDVP *
Ronnel *
Deodorized Kerosene *
Xylol *
Freon 11 & 12 (50-50)

'76 Ed.

VAPO-AIR MEDICATED VAPORIZER SPRAY
Relief from stuffiness of colds, sinus, hayfever
(Approved Pharm.)

Dipropylene glycol
Triethylene glycol
Eucalyptol *
Menthol *

'76 Ed.

VAPO-CIDE
Insecticide
(Research Products Co.)

2,2-Dichlorovinyl dimethyl
  phosphate 4.65%
Related compounds 0.35%
Petroleum distillates * 95.00%

VAP-O-CLEAN

See DeVILBISS VAP-O-CLEAN

VAPO-CRESOLENE MEDICATED VAPOR INHALANT
Liquid
(Vapo-Cresolene)

Cresylic acid (fraction of coal tar) *

VAPO FLY SPRA INSECTICIDE, EXCELCIDE

See EXCELCIDE VAPO FLY SPRA INSECTICIDE

VAPO FOR COLDS
For use with electric vaporizers
(Approved Pharm.)

Methyl salicylate *
Menthol *
Camphor *
Oil of eucalyptus *
Oil of peppermint *
Oil of lavender

'76 Ed.

VAPOL
Counterirritant, colds; veterinary
(Thoroughbred)

Camphor *
Thymol *
Oil of eucalyptus *
Methyl salicylate *
Menthol *
Oil of turpentine *
Oil of cedar wood *
Petrolatum

VAPO-MIST 500
Insecticide
(Industrial Fumigant)

2,2-Dichlorovinyl dimethyl
  phosphate * 4.650%
Related compounds 0.350%
Petroleum distillates 14.724%
Inert ingredients 80.276%

VAPO-MIST INHALANT
For temporary relief of spasms of bronchial asthma
(S-K Research Labs.)

Racemic epinephrine (solution)
Chlorobutanol (chloroform
  derivative) 0.5%

'76 Ed.

VAPON WIG CLEANER
(Vapon)

Isopropyl alcohol *

VAPORA

See ROBERTS VAPORA

VAPOR GARD
Anti-transpirant
(Miller Chem. & Fert.)

Pinolene (Di-1-p-menthene)

VAPORKILL SPRAY
Insecticide
(Gill)

2,2-Dichlorovinyl dimethyl
  phosphate 0.465%
Related compounds 0.035%
Pyrethrins 0.030%
Technical Piperonyl butoxide .. 0.060%
N-Octyl bicycloheptene
  dicarboximide 0.102%
Petroleum distillate * 14.308%

VAPOROOTER
For root growth control in sewers; fumigant
(Airrigation)

Sodium methyldithiocarbamate
  (anhydrous) * 28.8%

VAPORUB

See VICKS VAPORUB

VAPOSECTOR
Insecticide
(West Chem. Prod.)

Petroleum hydrocarbons *
Technical Piperonyl butoxide
N-Octyl bicycloheptene dicarboximide *
Pyrethrins

Starred ingredients (*) may be responsible for major toxic effects; consult Section II.

VAPOSTEAM

See VICKS VAPOSTEAM

VAPO-TOX
Insecticide
(Techne Corp.)

Toxaphene (chlorinated camphene with 67-69% chlorine) *	60.0%
2,2-Dichlorovinyl dimethyl phosphate	2.30%
Related compounds	0.20%
Aliphatic petroleum distillate	33.5%

'76 Ed.

VAPSOL
Fast drying safety solvent
(Lester Labs.)

Chlorinated solvents *

'76 Ed.

VASAL
Smooth muscle spasmolytic
(Direct Div.)

Each capsule:
Papaverine HCl * .... 150 mg.

VASELINE DERMATOLOGY FORMULA CREAM
(Chesebrough-Pond's)

Water	>50%
Petrolatum	>10-25%
Myreth-3 myristate	>1-5%
Glycerin	>1-5%
Triethanolamine	>0.1-1%
Dimethicone	>0.1-1%
Carbomer-934	>0.1-1%
Methylparaben	>0.1-1%
Fragrance	>0.1-1%
Propylparaben	0.1% or less
Imidazolidinyl urea	0.1% or less

VASELINE DERMATOLOGY FORMULA LOTION
(Chesebrough-Pond's)

Water	>50%
Glycerin	>1-5%
Petrolatum	>1-5%
Mineral oil	>1-5%
Stearic acid	>1-5%
Glycol stearate and other ingred.	>1-5%
Acetylated Lanolin alcohol	>1-5%
Glyceryl stearate	>1-5%
Dimethicone	>0.1-1%
Magnesium aluminum silicate	>0.1-1%
PEG-40 stearate	>0.1-1%
Cetyl alcohol	>0.1-1%
Methylparaben	>0.1-1%
Fragrance	>0.1-1%
Propylparaben	0.1% or less
Carbomer-934	0.1% or less
Disodium EDTA	0.1% or less
DMDM hydantoin	0.1% or less

VASOCIDIN OPHTHALMIC SOLUTION
Antibacterial/steroid
(CooperVision Pharm.)

Prednisolone sodium phosphate	0.25%
Phenylephrine hydrochloride	0.125%
Sodium sulfacetamide	10%

VASOCLEAR OPHTHALMIC SOLUTION
Ocular decongestant
(CooperVision Pharm.)

Naphazoline HCl	0.02%
Lipiden polymeric system	
Benzalkonium chloride	0.01%
Disodium edetate	0.03%

VASOCON-A OPHTHALMIC SOLUTION
Antihistaminic/decongestant
(CooperVision Pharm.)

Antazoline phosphate	0.5%
Naphazoline hydrochloride	0.05%
Phenylmercuric acetate	0.002%

VASOCON REGULAR OPHTHALMIC SOLUTION
Decongestant
(CooperVision Pharm.)

Naphazoline hydrochloride	0.1%
Phenylmercuric acetate	0.002%

VASODRINE
Topical sympathomimetic agent
(Premo)

Epinephrine, USP 1:1000

'76 Ed.

VASOMINIC - T.D.
Antihistaminic decongestant
(A.V.P. Pharmaceuticals)

Each tablet:
Phenylpropanolamine hydrochloride *	50 mg.
Pheniramine maleate *	25 mg.
Pyrilamine maleate *	25 mg.

VASOSULF OPHTHALMIC SOLUTION
Antibacterial
(CooperVision Pharm.)

Sodium sulfacetamide	15%
Phenylephrine hydrochloride	0.125%

VASO-80 UNICELLES
For angina pectoris
(Reid-Provident)

Each sustained release capsule:
Pentaerythritol tetranitrate * . 80 mg.

V.A. TILE ADHESIVE NO. 10
(Kentile)

Water dispersion of:
Latex
Asphalt

V.A. TILE ADHESIVE NO. 711
(Kentile)

Water dispersion of:
Latex
Petroleum resin

VA-TRO-NOL NOSE DROPS

See VICKS VA-TRO-NOL NOSE DROPS

VEDS
Cathartic
(Friendly Labs.)

Each 1 1/4 gr. pill:
Aloe *	3/4 gr.
Podophyllin *	1/16 gr.
Total alkaloids	0.00078 gr.
Oleoresin ginger	q.s.
Jalap	1/4 gr.
Ext. Belladonna	1/16 gr.

VEGADEX
Herbicide
(Monsanto)

Emul. Conc.:
2-Chloroallyl-diethyldithiocarbamate *	46.4%

Granules:
2-Chloroallyl-diethyldithiocarbamate *	20%

VEGA-KLEEN, FORMULA 1164

See KLENZADE VEGA-KLEEN, FORMULA 1164

VEGAT-OX 100
Chemical trimmer solution
(Stewart Sanitary Supply)

Ammonium sulfamate 8.2%*

VEGAT-OX B
Herbicide
(Stewart Sanitary Supply)

Lithium salt of Bromacil 3%

VEGAT-OX D
Herbicide
(Stewart Sanitary Supply)

Diquat dibromide * 1.85%

Starred ingredients (*) may be responsible for major toxic effects; consult Section II.

VEGAT-OX LWK C-2
Herbicide
(Stewart Sanitary Supply)

Monuron trichloroacetate	3.15%
Heavy Aromatic naphtha *	91.35%

VEGAT-OX V.K.C.
Nonselective weed control
(Stewart Sanitary Supply)

Prometon	4.66%
Petroleum distillate *	77.35%

VEG-GO
General weed and aquatic weed killer
(Scientific International)

Diquat dibromide ((6,7-Dihydro-pyrido)(1,2-a:2:1'-c)pyrazidiinium dibromide) *	1.85%

VEGIBEN
Preemergence weed killer for vegetable crops
(Amchem)

Ammonium salt of 3-Amino-2,5-dichlorobenzoic acid (Amiben) *	23.4%

VEGIBEN GRANULAR
Preemergence weed killer for vegetable crops
(Amchem)

Ammonium salt of 3-Amino-2,5-dichlorobenzoic acid (Amiben) *	10.8%

VEG-I-KILL
Non-selective herbicide; industrial and institutional use
(Scientific International)

Petroleum solvent *	96.10%
2,4-Dichlorophenoxyacetic acid, isooctyl ester	1.09%
Bromacil (5-Bromo-3-sec-butyl-6-methyluracil)	0.61%
Pentachlorophenol	0.80%
Other chlorophenols	0.09%

VEGTROL-DRY
Herbicide; industrial use
(Malter International)

Sodium chlorate *	58%
Sodium metaborate	42%

VEL LOTION DETERGENT
(Colgate-Palmolive)

Alkyl aryl sulfonate *	approx. 25%
Sodium sulfate	
Phosphates	small amount
Ethoxylated alcohol sulfate	approx. 10%
Builders, stabilizers	approx. 3%
Alcohol	approx. 5%

'76 Ed.

"VELPAR" "GRIDBALL" BRUSH KILLER
(Du Pont)

Hexazinone *	10%

"VELPAR" L WEED KILLER
(Du Pont)

Hexazinone *	25%

"VELPAR" WEED KILLER
(Du Pont)

Hexazinone *	90%

VELSICOL CHLORDANE 4EC
Termite control
(Velsicol)

Technical Chlordane *	45.3%
Petroleum distillate *	49.7%

VELSICOL CHLORDANE 8EC
Termite control
(Velsicol)

Technical Chlordane *	72%
Petroleum distillate *	21%

VELSICOL ENDRIN 1.6
Agricultural insecticide
(Velsicol)

Endrin *	19.7%
Xylene range aromatic solvent	74.5%

VELSICOL HEPTACHLOR 2EC
Insecticide for seed treatment
(Velsicol)

Heptachlor *	23.29%
Related compounds	8.18%
Xylene range aromatic solvent *	63.53%

VELSICOL HEPTACHLOR 3EC
Insecticide for seed treatment
(Velsicol)

Heptachlor *	32.1%
Related compounds	12.5%
Xylene range aromatic solvent *	50.4%

VELTANE EXPECTORANT
(Lannett)

Each 5 ml.:

Brompheniramine maleate	2 mg.
Phenylephrine HCl	5 mg.
Phenylpropanolamine HCl	5 mg.
Glyceryl guaiacolate	100 mg.
Alcohol	3.5%

VELTANE TABLETS
Antihistaminic
(Lannett)

Each tablet:

Brompheniramine maleate *	4 mg.

VELTAP ELIXIR
For use in upper respiratory infections
(Lannett)

Each 5 ml.:

Brompheniramine maleate	4 mg.
Phenylephrine HCl	5 mg.
Phenylpropanolamine HCl	5 mg.
Alcohol	2.3%

VELVACAIN A & D OINTMENT
Soothing burn ointment
(Commerce Drug)

Dichlorophene
Benzocaine
Cod liver oil
Benzalkonium chloride (50% USP)

VELVA-SHEEN
Mop treatment
(Majestic Wax Co.)

Petroleum hydrocarbons *	100%

VELVA-SHEEN FOR HOSPITALS
Mop treatment
(Majestic Wax Co.)

Combined amount:	99.99%
Petroleum hydrocarbons * Emulsifier	
Tri-N-butyl tin oxide	0.01%

VELVATEX SIGHTSAVING DUSTLESS CHALK
(American Crayon Co.)

This product bears the CP Seal issued by the Crayon, Water Color and Craft Institute, Inc. This seal certifies that the product contains no materials in sufficient quantities to be toxic or injurious to the human body even if ingested.

VELVEEN

See C-Z VELVEEN

VELVET GLOVE CREAM
Dermatologic
(Elder)

Allantoin

Starred ingredients (*) may be responsible for major toxic effects; consult Section II.

VELVET PEACH HAND LOTION
(House of Lowell, Inc.)

Mineral oil
Glycerin
Isopropyl palmitate
Stearic acid
Glyceryl stearate
Lanolin
Polysorbate-60
Cetyl alcohol
Modified Polystyrene latex
Perfume
Methylparaben
Propylparaben
Formaldehyde
D & C color

VEON 245
Herbicide
(Dow)

Triethylamine salt of 2,4,5-trichlo-
rophenoxyacetic acid * 57.2%

V.E.P. HEAVY DUTY MOTOR OIL
(Marathon Oil Co.)

Additives, Zinc alkyl dithiophosphate, Methacrylate
copolymer 6.2%
Mineral oil .... balance

VEREQUAD
Bronchodilator, expectorant
(Knoll Pharm.)

Suspension (each 5 cc):
  Phenobarbital .... 4 mg.
  Theophylline calcium
    salicylate * .... 65 mg.
  Ephedrine hydrochloride * .. 12 mg.
  Guaifenesin .... 50 mg.

Tablets (each):
  Phenobarbital * .... 8 mg.
  Theophylline calcium
    salicylate * .... 130 mg.
  Ephedrine hydrochloride * .. 24 mg.
  Guaifenesin .... 100 mg.

VERMED
For the treatment of vertigo
(Russ Pharm.)

Each capsule:
  Pentylenetetrazol .... 25.0 mg.
  Pheniramine maleate * ...... 12.5 mg.
  Nicotinic acid .... 50.0 mg.

VERMINGO
Insecticide
(Consolidated Chem., Inc.)

Petroleum distillate *
N-Octyl bicycloheptene dicarboximide *
Technical Piperonyl butoxide
Pyrethrins

VERNAM (7-E, 10-G)
Herbicide
(Stauffer)

Vernam (S-Propyl dipropylthiocarbamate) *†

†*See* Vernolate

VERNATE II
Antihistaminic
(Direct Div.)

Each capsule:
  Chlorpheniramine maleate * . 8 mg.
  Phenylpropanolamine HCl * . 50 mg.
  Isopropamide * .... 2.5 mg.

VERNAX
(Hagerty, W.J.)

Beeswax 1-10%
Turpentine * .... >10%
Potassium soap .... <1%
Mixture of perfumes .... <1%

VERNOX INSECT KILLER
Commercial and institutional use
(Hysan Corp.)

Pyrethrins 0.20%
Technical Piperonyl butoxide ... 0.720%
N-Octyl bicycloheptene
  dicarboximide 0.40%
Petroleum distillate * 18.68%

VERREX
For removal of benign epithelial growths such as common warts
(C & M Pharmacal)

Salicylic acid * 30.0%
Podophyllin * 10.0%
Penederm 0.5%
Ethylcellulose
Cellosolve
Collodion
Castor oil
Acetone

VERRUSOL
For the removal of warts
(C & M Pharmacal)

Salicylic acid * 30.0%
Podophyllin 5.0%
Cantharidin 1.0%
Penederm 0.5%
Ethylcellulose
Cellosolve
Collodion
Castor oil
Acetone

VERSAL HEMORRHOIDAL
(Suppositoria Labs.)

Each suppository:
  Bismuth subgallate
  Bismuth resorcin comp.
  Balsam Peru *
  Zinc oxide
  Boric acid *

VERSENOL 120
Chelating agent
(Dow)

N-(Carboxymethyl)-N'-(2-hydroxy-
ethyl)-N,N'-ethylene diglycine, trisodium salt *† 48%

†*See* Versene

VERTIFUME
Fumigant
(Dow)

Carbon tetrachloride * 82.9%
Carbon bisulfide 16.5%

VERTON CE HERBICIDE
(Dow)

2,4-Dichlorophenoxy acetic acid
  propylene glycol (C3H6O to
  C9H18O3) butyl ether esters * . 36.0%
2,4,5-Trichlorophenoxyacetic acid
  (same esters) * 34.1%
Inert ingred., primarily: 29.9%
  Petroleum solvent *

VERTON 2D
Weed and brush killer
(Dow)

2,4-Dichlorophenoxyacetic acid,
  propylene glycol butyl ether esters (2,4-Dichlorophenoxyacetic
  acid equivalent 24.5%) 39.6%
Inert ingred., primarily: 60.4%
  Xylene *

VERTON 2T HERBICIDE
(Dow)

2,4,5-Trichlorophenoxyacetic acid,
  propylene glycol butyl ether
  esters 37.2%
Inert ingred.: 62.8%
  Emulsifiers
  Xylene *

VERUX
Wart ointment; veterinary
(Burns-Biotec)

Castor oil 38%
Salicylic acid * 18%
Hydrogenated Castor oil 7%
Special base 37%

VERV ALERTNESS CAPSULES
Timed disintegration capsules
(Am. Pharmaceutical)

Each capsule:
  Caffeine * .... 200 mg.

VER-VAR
Chemical removal of common warts
(Owen Labs.)

Podophyllum resin * 10%
Salicylic acid 10%
Vinyl resin, acetone vehicle

Starred ingredients (*) may be responsible for major toxic effects; consult Section II.

VES-PHENE
Germicidal detergent
(Vestal)

o-Phenylphenol 3.9%
o-Benzyl p-chlorophenol 3.3%
p-Tertiary amylphenol 0.8%

'76 Ed.

VESPRIN ORAL SUSPENSION
Tranquilizer, antiemetic, adjuvant in anesthesia
(Squibb)

Each 5 cc tsp.:
Triflupromazine hydrochloride
(10-(3-
Dimethylaminopropyl)-2-(trifluoromethyl) phenothiazine
hydrochloride) * .... 50 mg.

VESPRIN TABLETS
Tranquilizer, antiemetic, adjuvant in anesthesia
(Squibb)

Each tablet:
Triflupromazine hy-
drochloride (10-(3-
Dimethylamino-
propyl)-2-(trifluo-
romethyl) pheno-
thiazine
hydrochloride) * . 10, 25, and 50 mg.

VETROLIN, THE GREEN LINIMENT
Veterinary
(Thoroughbred)

Alcohol * 57%/v
Camphor *
Methyl salicylate *
Oils of Cedarwood *, Sassafras *, Art,
Spike, Origanum, Rosemary *
Castile soap

VETS MANGE & LICE
Livestock control
(Spencer Vet Supply Co.)

Gamma isomer of benzene hexachloride (from lindane) * 12.5%
Xylol * 82.5%

V-H POWDER
Vaginal douche
(Optimus)

Boric acid *
Carbolic acid *
Ammonium alum
Menthol *
Methyl salicylate *
Benzoic acid *
Salicylic acid *
Magnesium sulfate
Thymol *

VICKS BLUE COUGH DROPS
(Vicks Health Care Div.)

Menthol .... <1%
In a soothing Vicks sugars base

VICKS COUGH SILENCERS
Cough drop
(Vicks Health Care Div.)

Each lozenge:
Dextromethorphan (equiv. to
dextromethorphan HBr) ... 2.5 mg.
Benzocaine .... 1 mg.
Special Vick Medication: 0.35%
Menthol
Anethole
Peppermint oil

VICKS COUGH SYRUP
(Vicks Health Care Div.)

Each 5 ml.:
Active ingred.:
Dextromethorphan HBr * . 3.5 mg.
Guaifenesin .... 25.0 mg.
Sodium citrate .... 200.0 mg.
Inactive ingred.:
Alcohol 5%

VICKS DAYCARE DAYTIME COLDS MEDICINE, CAPSULES
(Vicks Health Care Div.)

Each capsule:
Acetaminophen * .... 325.0 mg.
Dextromethorphan HBr .... 10.0 mg.
Phenylpropanolamine HCl * 12.5 mg.

VICKS DAYCARE DAYTIME COLDS MEDICINE, LIQUID
(Vicks Health Care Div.)

Each fl. oz.:
Active ingred.:
Acetaminophen * .... 600 mg.
Dextromethorphan HBr .... 20 mg.
Phenylpropanolamine HCl ... 25 mg.
Inactive ingred.:
Alcohol 7.5%

VICKS FORMULA 44 COUGH CONTROL DISCS
Cough drop
(Vicks Health Care Div.)

Each 2.25 gm. Disc:
Dextromethorphan (equiv. to
dextromethorphan HBr) .. 5.0 mg.
Benzocaine .... 1.25 mg.
Special Vick Medication: 0.35%
Menthol
Anethole
Peppermint oil

VICKS FORMULA 44 COUGH MIXTURE
(Vicks Health Care Div.)

Each 10 ml.:
Active ingred.:
Dextromethorphan HBr * 15.0 mg.
Doxylamine succinate .... 7.5 mg.
Sodium citrate .... 500.0 mg.
Inert ingred.:
Alcohol 10%

VICKS FORMULA 44-D COUGH MIXTURE
(Vicks Health Care Div.)

Each 10 ml.:
Active ingred.:
Dextromethorphan HBr * ... 20 mg.
Phenylpropanolamine HCl * 25 mg.
Guaifenesin .... 100 mg.
Inert ingred.:
Alcohol 10%

VICKS HEADWAY
Relief of colds, sinus, allergies
(Vicks Health Care Div.)

Each capsule or tablet:
Acetaminophen * .... 325.00 mg.
Phenylpropanolamine
HCl * .... 18.75 mg.
Chlorpheniramine maleate 2.00 mg.

VICKS INHALER
Decongestant nasal inhaler
(Vicks Health Care Div.)

Each inhaler:
1-Desoxyephedrine * .... 50 mg.
Special Vick Medication: .... 150 mg.
Camphor *
Menthol *
Methyl salicylate *
Bornyl acetate *

VICKS MEDICATED COUGH DROPS - LEMON FLAVOR
(Vicks Health Care Div.)

Menthol .... <1%
Flavored with:
Lemon oil
Citric acid
In a soothing Vick sugars base

VICKS MEDICATED COUGH DROPS - REGULAR FLAVOR
(Vicks Health Care Div.)

Special Vick Medication: .... <1%
Menthol
Thymol
Eucalyptus oil
Camphor
Tolu balsam
Benzyl alcohol
In a soothing Vick sugars base

Starred ingredients (*) may be responsible for major toxic effects; consult Section II.

VICKS MEDICATED COUGH DROPS - WILD CHERRY FLAVOR
(Vicks Health Care Div.)

Special Vick Medication: .... <1%
  Menthol
  Thymol
  Eucalyptus oil
  Camphor
  Tolu balsam
  Benzyl alcohol
In a soothing Vick sugars base

VICKS SINEX LONG-ACTING DECONGESTANT NASAL SPRAY
(Vicks Health Care Div.)

Oxymetazoline HCl 0.050%
Thimerosal (preservative) 0.001%

VICKS SINEX NASAL SPRAY
(Vicks Health Care Div.)

Phenylephrine HCl 0.500%
Cetyl pyridinium chloride 0.04%
Special Vick Medication:
  Menthol *
  Eucalyptol *
  Camphor *
  Methyl salicylate *
Preservative: Thimerosal 0.001%

VICKS THROAT LOZENGE
(Vicks Health Care Div.)

Each lozenge:
  Benzocaine .... 5 mg.
  Cetylpyridinium chloride ..... 1.6 mg.
  Special Vick Medication: ..... <1%
    Menthol
    Camphor
    Eucalyptus oil

VICKS VAPORUB
External rub for colds
(Vicks Health Care Div.)

Special Vick Medication: 14%
  Camphor *
  Menthol *
  Spirits of turpentine *
  Oil of eucalyptus *
  Oil of cedar leaf *
  Myristica oil
  Thymol *

VICKS VAPOSTEAM
Liquid medication for hot steam
(Vicks Health Care Div.)

Active ingred.:
  Polyoxyethylene dodecanol 1.8%
  Aromatics 12.4%
    Eucalyptus oil
    Camphor *
    Menthol *
  Tincture of benzoin 5.0%
Inactive ingred.:
  Alcohol 55.0%

VICKS VA-TRO-NOL NOSE DROPS
(Vicks Health Care Div.)

Ephedrine sulfate * 0.5%
Special Vick aromatic blend: 0.060%
  Menthol
  Eucalyptol
  Camphor
  Methyl salicylate
Preservative: Thimerosal 0.001%

VICKS VICTORS
Cough lozenge
(Vicks Health Care Div.)

Special Vick Medication: .... <1%
  Menthol
  Eucalyptus oil
In a soothing Vick sugars base

VICKS VICTORS - CHERRY FLAVORED
Cough lozenge
(Vicks Health Care Div.)

Special Vick Medication: .... <1%
  Menthol
  Eucalyptus oil
In a soothing Vick sugars base

VICODIN TABLETS
Narcotic analgesic
(Knoll Pharm.)

Each tablet:
  Hydrocodone bitartrate * .... 5 mg.
  Acetaminophen .... 500 mg.

VICON
Emulsion bowl cleaner
(ABCO, Inc.)

Hydrogen chloride * 23.29%
Orthodichlorobenzene 2.50%

VICON-C
Therapeutic vitamins and minerals
(Glaxo Inc.)

Each capsule:
  Ascorbic acid .... 300 mg.
  Niacinamide .... 100 mg.
  Zinc sulfate, USP * .... 80 mg.
  Magnesium sulfate, USP .... 70 mg.
  Thiamine mononitrate ...... 20 mg.
  d-Calcium pantothenate ..... 20 mg.
  Riboflavin .... 10 mg.
  Pyridoxine hydrochloride .... 5 mg.

VICON PLUS
Vitamins and minerals
(Glaxo Inc.)

Each capsule:
  Vitamin A acetate .... 4000 I.U.
  Vitamin E .... 50 I.U.
  Ascorbic acid .... 150 mg.
  Zinc sulfate USP * .... 80 mg.
  Magnesium sulfate USP .... 70 mg.
  Niacinamide .... 25 mg.
  Thiamine mononitrate ..... 10 mg.
  d-Calcium pantothenate .... 10 mg.
  Riboflavin .... 5 mg.
  Manganese chloride .... 4 mg.
  Pyridoxine HCl .... 2 mg.

VI-CO-TUSS CAPSULES
Cold remedy
(International Chem.)

Atropine sulfate .... 0.024 mg.
Scopolamine HBr .... 0.014 mg.
Hyoscyamine sulfate .... 0.122 mg.
Phenylpropanolamine HCl * ... 50.0 mg.
Chlorpheniramine maleate ... 1.0 mg.
Pheniramine maleate * ...... 12.5 mg.

'76 Ed.

VI-CO-TUSS COUGH SYRUP
(International Chem.)

Each 10 cc:
  Pyrilamine maleate * ...... 12.5 mg.
  Chlorpheniramine maleate .. 1.0 mg.
  Dextromethorphan * ...... 15.0 mg.
  Phenylephrine HCl * ...... 5.0 mg.
  Guayanesin .... 60.0 mg.
  Potassium guaiacosulfonate 100.0 mg.
  Acetaminophen * .... 60 mg.

'76 Ed.

VI-CO-TUSS NASAL SPRAY
(International Chem.)

Pyrilamine maleate * 0.15%
Phenylephrine HCl 0.25%
Benzalkonium chloride 0.05%
Aqueous isotonic solution

'76 Ed.

VI-CO-TUSS PEDIATRIC COUGH SYRUP
(International Chem.)

Each fl. oz.:
  Sodium citrate .... 2.35 gm.
  Ascorbic acid .... 0.94 gm.
  Ipecac .... 0.07 gm.
  Citric acid .... 0.07 gm.
  Plasdone (emulsifier) ...... 0.47 gm.
  Sorbitol sol. .... 17.86 gm.

'76 Ed.

VICTORS

See VICKS VICTORS

VICTORS - CHERRY FLAVORED

See VICKS VICTORS - CHERRY FLAVORED

VICTORY AROMA
Insecticide, deodorizer
(Victory Chem.)

Paradichlorobenzene *
Perfume oils *

'76 Ed.

VICTORY AROMA KRYSTALS
Insecticide, deodorizer
(Victory Chem.)

Paradichlorobenzene *
Perfume oils *

'76 Ed.

VICTORY AROMA RING BLOCK
Insecticide, deodorizer
(Victory Chem.)

Paradichlorobenzene *
Perfume oils *

'76 Ed.

VICTORY DISINFECTANT 5
Institutional and commercial use
(Hysan Corp.)

Soap
Pine oil *
Sodium salt of 4 and 6-chloro-2-phenyl-
phenol *
Inert ingred.: 80%
Water

VICTORY PINE ODOR

See PL VICTORY PINE ODOR

VIDAL SASSOON HAIR CARE PRODUCTS & COSMETICS

Vidal Sassoon, Inc.
2049 Century Park E.
Century City, Calif. 90067

Phone: 213-553-6100

See COSMETICS, Section VI, General
Formulations

VI-DAYLIN WITH FLUORIDE CHEWABLE TABLETS
Dietary supplement
(Ross Labs.)

Each tablet:
Fluoride (as sodium fluoride) ... 1 mg.
Multivitamins

VIDDEN D SOIL FUMIGANT
(Dow)

Combined amount: 99%
1,3-Dichloropropene *
1,2-Dichloropropane *
Related chlorinated aliphatics

VIDECON
(Vita Elixir Co.)

Each capsule:
Vitamin D .... 50,000 units

VIGATE BOUQUET AIR SANITIZER
(Hysan Corp.)

Triethylene glycol 3.50%
Propylene glycol 3.00%
Methyl dodecyl benzyl trimethyl
ammonium chloride 0.16%
Methyl dodecyl xylylene bis (tri-
methyl ammonium chloride) ... 0.04%

VIGILANCE ALGAECIDE
Germicide, disinfectant, deodorant, sanitizer
(Fergusson, Alex. C., Co.)

Tetra sodium salt ethylene diamine
tetra acetic acid 0.5%
Methyl dodecyl benzyl trimethyl ammonium chloride * 8.0%
Methyl dodecyl xylylene bis trimethyl ammonium chloride 2.0%

VIGILANCE B.C.D. CLEANER
Bactericide, disinfectant
(Fergusson, Alex. C., Co.)

Sodium hypochlorite * .... >3.25%
Sodium phosphate * .... >91.75%
Inert ingred.:
Sodium chloride .... <5.00%

VIGILANT CLEANING PRODUCTS
(Vigilant Products)

Vigilant Products Co., Inc.
27 Main St.
Ogdensburg, N.J. 07439

Phone: 201-827-3333

VIGRAN
Multivitamins
(Squibb)

Each tablet:
Vitamin A as palmitate (5000
U.S.P. u.) .... 1.5 mg.
Vitamin D (400 U.S.P. u.)
(Ergocalciferol) .... 10 mcg.
Plus multivitamins

VIGRAN WITH IRON
Prevention of vitamin-iron deficiencies
(Squibb)

Each tablet:
Vitamin A (as
acetate) .... 5000 USP Units
Vitamin D
(Ergocalciferol) ... 400 USP Units
Iron (as dried ferrous sulfate) . 27 mg.

VI-JON COSMETICS
(Vi-Jon)

Vi-Jon Laboratories, Inc.
6300 Etzel Ave.
St. Louis, Mo. 63133

Phone: 314-721-2990

See COSMETICS, Section VI, General
Formulations

VIKING HOOD CLEANER
Liquid caustic cleaner
(Kay Chem. Co.)

Potassium hydroxide * 50-90%

VILIVA
Iron therapy - deficiency anemia
(Vita Elixir Co.)

Ferrous fumarate * .... 3 gr.

VI-MIN-CO
Dietary supplement
(Jenkins Labs.)

Each capsule:
Vitamin A .... 5,000 U.S.P. Units
Vitamin D .... 400 U.S.P. Units
Iron (from ferrous sulphate) . 13.4 mg.
Plus multivitamins and minerals

VINELAND ASCORBISOL-K
Antihemorrhagic for drinking water; poultry
(Vineland Laboratories, Inc.)

Ascorbic acid
Stabilized Menadione sodium bisulfite *

VINELAND COPPER-K
Antihemorrhagic for drinking water; poultry
(Vineland Laboratories, Inc.)

Copper sulfate *
Stabilized Menadione sodium bisulfite *

VINELAND FORMALDEGEN
For fumigating poultry equipment
(Vineland Laboratories, Inc.)

Paraformaldehyde * 91%

Starred ingredients (*) may be responsible for major toxic effects; consult Section II.

VINELAND SANI-SQUAD
Germicide, disinfectant
(Vineland Laboratories, Inc.)

Formaldehyde *
5 Methyl-2-isopropyl-1-phenol *
Methyldodecylbenzyltrimethyl ammo-
nium chloride *
Methyldodecylxylylene bis(trimethyl am-
monium chloride) *
Ethyl alcohol
Methyl alcohol *

VINELAND THIAZOLE SODIUM
*Treatment of bacterial scours caused by
E. coli in swine
Treatment of bacterial pneumonia as-
sociated with Pasteurella spp. in
swine*
(Vineland Laboratories, Inc.)

Sodium sulfathiazole * 100%

VINELAND UDDER MAGIC
(Vineland Laboratories, Inc.)

Lanolin
Petrolatum
Glycerin
Methyl salicylate *

VINELAND VI-LYTE
*Treatment of bacterial pneumonia and
bacterial scours in swine
Aid in control of infectious coryza in
chickens*
(Vineland Laboratories, Inc.)

Sodium sulfathiazole * 67.0%
Ethylene diamine
  dihydroiodide 1.6%
Electrolytes: Sodium, Potassium,
  Calcium, Magnesium, Iron * .. 30.0%
Vitamin A .... 1,000,000 Units
Vitamin D-3 .... 500,000 Units

VINELAND VIMETHAZINE
Coccidiosis, coryza pullorum, poultry
(Vineland Laboratories, Inc.)

Sodium sulfamethazine * 100%

VINE-O-MITE
Vinyl cleaner
(Paul Koss)

Water .... >85%
Isopropyl alcohol * .... <11%
Glycerine
Trisodium phosphate dodecahydrate
Silicone emulsion
Fluorochemical surfactant

VINIZOL
*Cerebral stimulant, vasodilator and
nutritional supplement*
(King Pharmaceutical)

Each 10 cc:
  Pentylenetetrazol * .... 200 mg.
  Nicotinic acid .... 100 mg.
  Vitamin B-12 .... 25 mcg.
  Vitamin B1 .... 10 mg.
  Alcohol 5%

VINYL-RUB RUBBING ALCOHOL
(Bowman Pharm.)

Absolute Alcohol 70%/v

VINYLTEX 51 - WASH PRIMER ACTIVATOR
(Jotun-Baltimore Copper Paint Co.)

Vehicle: 100%
  Isopropanol 65%
  Water 16%
  Phosphoric acid * 19%

VINYLTEX 50 - WASH PRIMER BASE
(Jotun-Baltimore Copper Paint Co.)

Pigment: 11%
  Zinc tetroxychromate 9%
  Magnesium silicate 1%
  Lampblack 1%
Vehicle: 89%
  Vinyl butyral resin 9%
  Isopropanol * 58%
  Water 2%
  Butanol * 20%

VINYLTEX 53 ZINC CHROMATE ANTICORROSIVE
(Jotun-Baltimore Copper Paint Co.)

Pigment: 14%
  Basic Zinc chromate 8%
  Lampblack 1%
  Magnesium silicate 5%
Vehicle: 86%
  Vinyl chloride resin 16%
  Tricresyl phosphate 1%
  Methyl isobutyl ketone 40%
  Toluol * 29%

VINY-LUX ANTIFOULING
Paint
(International Paint)

Ketones *
Aromatics *†
Color codes #339, #340, and #350 contain
  Copper *

†*See* Aromatic hydrocarbon solvent

VINY-LUX PRIMER
Paint
(International Paint)

Ketones *
Aromatics *†
Pigments - no lead

†*See* Aromatic hydrocarbon solvent

VINYZENE BP-5
Industrial bactericide
(Ventron)

10,10′ Oxybisphenoxarsine in epoxidized soybean oil (dilute
formulation) *† 1%

†*See* Arsenic

VIOFORM
Antifungal, antibacterial
(CIBA Pharmaceutical)

Ointment:
  Iodochlorhydroxyquin * 3%
  Petrolatum base

Cream:
  Iodochlorhydroxyquin * 3%
  Water-washable base

VIOFORM-HYDROCORTISONE
*Antibacterial, antifungal, antipruritic,
anti-inflammatory*
(CIBA Pharmaceutical)

Cream, ointment or lotion:
  Iodochlorhydroxyquin 3%
  Hydrocortisone 1%

Mild cream or ointment:
  Iodochlorhydroxyquin 3%
  Hydrocortisone 0.5%

VIO-GERIC
Vitamin & mineral supplement
(Rowell)

Vitamin A .... 5000 I.U.
Vitamin D .... 400 I.U.
Iron .... 18 mg.
Plus multi-vitamins & minerals

VIOTAG CREAM
Anti-inflammatory, antiseptic
(Direct Div.)

Hydrocortisone acetate 1%
Iodochlorhydroxyquin 3%

VI-PENTA F
Vitamins with fluoride
(Roche)

Chewables (each tablet):
  Fluoride (as sodium fluoride) . 1 mg.
  Multivitamins

Multivitamin Drops & Infant Drops (each
0.6 ml.):
  Fluoride (as sodium fluoride) . 0.5 mg.
  Multivitamins

Starred ingredients (*) may be responsible for major toxic effects; consult Section II.

VIRACIL COLD CAPSULES
(Approved Pharm.)

Each capsule:
Phenylephrine HCl	5 mg.
Hesperidin	50 mg.
Thenylene HCl *	12 1/2 mg.
Pyrilamine maleate *	12 1/2 mg.
Vitamin C	50 mg.
Salicylamide	2 1/2 gr.
Caffeine	1/2 gr.
Sodium salicylate *	1 1/4 gr.

'76 Ed.

VIRCHEM BEE-WASP
Insecticide
(Va. Chem. Inc.)

Tetrachloroethylene *	32%
Trichloromonofluoromethane	20%
Dichlorodifluoromethane	20%
Petroleum distillate	13.75%
Methylene chloride	11%
Pine oil	2.80%
Rotenone	0.12%
Other related cube resins	0.28%
Pyrethrins I & II	0.05%

VIRCHEM EIGHT
Aerosol insecticide
(Va. Chem. Inc.)

2,2-Dichlorovinyl dimethyl phosphate (DDVP) *	2.74%
Related compounds	0.21%
Chlorofluorocarbon-12	

VIRCHEM ONE
Aerosol insecticide
(Va. Chem. Inc.)

Pyrethrins	0.5%
Technical Piperonyl butoxide	1.0%
N-Octyl bicycloheptene dicarboximide	1.0%
Petroleum distillates *	12.5%

VIRCHEM ONE-SHOT
Aerosol insecticide
(Va. Chem. Inc.)

Pyrethrins	0.5%
Technical Piperonyl butoxide	4.0%
Petroleum distillate *	12.5%

VIRCHEM THREE HUNDRED
Hi-pressure aerosol insect killer
(Va. Chem. Inc.)

Pyrethrins	0.5%
Tech. Piperonyl butoxide	1.0%
N-Octyl dichloroheptene dicarboximide	1.0%
Butoxy polypropylene glycol	5.0%
Petroleum distillates *	12.5%

VIRCHEM TWENTY-FOUR
Aerosol insecticide
(Va. Chem. Inc.)

Pyrethrins	0.5%
Technical Piperonyl butoxide	1.0%
N-Octyl bicycloheptene dicarboximide	1.0%
Petroleum distillates *	12.5%

VIRCHEM TWENTY-THREE
Aerosol insecticide
(Va. Chem. Inc.)

Pyrethrins	0.5%
Technical Piperonyl butoxide	1.0%
N-Octyl bicycloheptene dicarboximide	1.0%
Petroleum distillates *	12.5%

VIRCHEM TWO-THIRTY-TWO
Aerosol insecticide
(Va. Chem. Inc.)

Pyrethrins	1.95%
Technical Piperonyl butoxide	3.00%
N-Octyl bicycloheptene dicarboximide	2.00%
Petroleum distillates *	18.05%

VIRIDIUM TABLETS
Genito-urinary tract antisepsis
(Vita Elixir Co.)

Each tablet:
Phenylazodiaminopyridine hydrochloride (Azo dye) *	100 mg.

VIRMIST B CONCENTRATED AEROSOL INSECT KILLER
(Va. Chem. Inc.)

Pyrethrins	1.07%
Technical Piperonyl butoxide	2.14%
N-Octyl bicycloheptene dicarboximide	2.14%
Petroleum hydrocarbons *	11.60%

VIROMED
Symptomatic relief of flu miseries
(Whitehall Labs.)

Each tablet:
Aspirin *	5 gr.
Chlorpheniramine maleate	1 mg.
Pseudoephedrine HCl *	15 mg.
Dextromethorphan HBr	7.5 mg.
Glyceryl guaiacolate	50 mg.

VIRO-PHENE
Air sanitizer, deodorizer
(Kem Mfg. Co.)

Isopropyl alcohol *	60.00%
Propylene glycol	5.00%
o-Phenylphenol	0.10%
p-tert-Amylphenol	0.05%

VIROSAN CONCENTRATE TEAT DIP
(Bio-Ceutic)

Chlorhexidine digluconate	4%
Glycerin	48%

VIROSAN SOLUTION
Virucide fungicide; veterinary
(Bio-Ceutic)

Chlorhexidine digluconate	2.0%
Isopropyl alcohol	1.0%

VIRO-TEC HOSPITAL SPRAY
Disinfectant, deodorant
(American Hospitex)

2-Phenylphenol	0.143%
2-Chloro-4-phenylphenol	0.029%
Ethanol	67.646%

VISALENS SOAKING/ CLEANING SOLUTION
For cleaning contact lenses
(Leeming Div.)

Phenylmercuric nitrate	1:25,000
Benzalkonium chloride	0.02%
Disodium edetate	0.10%

VISALENS WETTING SOLUTION
Contact lens wetting solution
(Leeming Div.)

Polyvinyl alcohol	
Methyl cellulose	
Disodium edetate	
Sodium chloride	
Potassium chloride	
Benzalkonium chloride	1:25,000

VIS-A-VIS
Broad and fine overhead projector markers; nonpermanent inks
(Sanford Corp.)

Dyes	
Glycols	
Water	
Phenol (as preservative)	<1%

VISINE AC
(Leeming Div.)

Tetrahydrozoline hydrochloride	0.05%
Zinc sulfate	0.25%
Benzalkonium chloride	0.01%
Disodium edetate	0.10%
Sodium chloride	
Boric acid	
Sodium citrate	

Starred ingredients (*) may be responsible for major toxic effects; consult Section II.

VISINE EYE DROPS
Decongestant for minor eye irritations
(Leeming Div.)

Tetrahydrozoline hydrochloride	0.05%
Sodium chloride	
Boric acid	approx. 1.20%
Sodium borate	
Benzalkonium chloride	0.01%
Disodium edetate	0.10%

VISKO-RHAP INVERTING OIL
For pesticide sprays
(Rhone-Poulenc)

Combined ingredients:	100%
Water-in-oil emulsifiers *†	
Solvents *‡	

†*See* Alkyl phenoxy polyethoxy ethanols
‡*See* Petroleum distillate

VISKO-RHAP LOW VOLATILE ESTER 2D
Herbicide
(Rhone-Poulenc)

2-Ethylhexyl ester of 2,4-dichloro-phenoxyacetic acid (isooctyl ester) *	35.64%

VISKO-RHAP OIL-SOLUBLE AMINE A-3D
Herbicide
(Rhone-Poulenc)

N,N-Dimethyl oleyl-linoleyl amine salt of 2,4-dichlorophen-oxyacetic acid *	61.07%

VI-SORBITS
Vitamin-iron tablets for pets
(Norden Labs.)

Each tablet:
Elemental Iron	9.5 mg.
Vitamin A	1250 I.U.
Vitamin D2	125 I.U.
Plus multivitamins and minerals	

VISTA ONE STEP CLEANER/WAX (AS-956, Formula MI-2318)

See SIMONIZ VISTA ONE STEP CLEANER/WAX (AS-956, Formula MI-2318)

VISTARIL (CAPSULES & ORAL SUSPENSION)
For anxiety & tension
(Pfizer)

CAPSULES (each 25 mg.):
Hydroxyzine pa-moate equiv. to hydroxyzine hydrochloride	25 mg.

CAPSULES (each 50 & 100 mg.):
Hydroxyzine pa-moate equiv. to hydroxyzine hydrochloride *	50 mg.; or 100 mg.

ORAL SUSPENSION (each 5 ml.):
Hydroxyzine pa-moate equiv. to hydroxyzine hydrochloride	25 mg.

VISTA SOFT AND EASY WAX (AS-952, Formula MI-2317)

See SIMONIZ VISTA SOFT AND EASY WAX (AS-952, Formula MI-2317)

VIT
Liquid bowl cleaner
(ABCO, Inc.)

Muriatic acid *

VITABATH HAND & BODY LOTION (All Shades)
(Kolmar Labs.)

Water	>50%
Emulsion stabilizer, thickener	0.1-1.0%
Preservative	0.1-1.0%
Emollient	5-10%
Emulsifier	1-5%
Co-emulsifier	1-5%
Fragrance	0.1-1.0%
Color	0.1-1.0%

VITACOL

See HAPPY JACK VITACOL

VITADYE LOTION
Covermark
(Elder)

Dihydroxyacetone *	5.0%

VITA ELIXIR
(Vita Elixir Co.)

Each 45 cc:
Alcohol	25%
Vitamin A palmitate	5,000 Units
Vitamin D-2	500 Units
Iron (as sulfate)	10 mg.
Plus multi-vitamins and minerals	

VITA FLUFF HAIR CARE PRODUCTS

Vita Fluff Products
Div. of Duon, Inc.
P.O. Box 422
Forest Park Branch
Dayton, Ohio 45405

Phone: 513-268-6873

See COSMETICS, Section VI, General Formulations

VITALIS DRY CONTROL (Regular)
Hair spray
(Bristol-Myers)

SD Alcohol 40 *
Carbon dioxide
Ethyl ester of PVM/MA copolymer
Fragrance
Triisopropanolamine
PPG-26 oleate
Dimethicone
Laureth-4
BHT

VITALIS DRY TEXTURE
Hair groom
(Bristol-Myers)

Water
SD Alcohol 40
PPG-10 glyceryl ether
PPG-40 butyl ether
Myristyl lactate
Triisopropanolamine
MDM hydantoin
PEG-15 cocamine
PVP
Carbomer 940
Fragrance
Sodium bisulfite
FD & C Green No. 3
D & C Yellow No. 10

VITALIS REGULAR HOLD
Non-aerosol hair spray
(Bristol-Myers)

SD Alcohol 40 *
Ethyl ester of PVM/MA copolymer
Fragrance
Aminomethyl propanol
Laureth-23
PPG-26 oleate
BHT

VITALIS SUPER HOLD
Non-aerosol hair spray
(Bristol-Myers)

SD Alcohol 40 *
Water
Ethyl ester of PVM/MA copolymer
Fragrance
Aminomethyl propanol
Laureth-23
PPG-26 oleate
BHT

Starred ingredients (*) may be responsible for major toxic effects; consult Section II.

VITALIS WITH V7
Hair groom
(Bristol-Myers)

SD Alcohol 40
PPG-40 butyl ether
Water
Benzyl benzoate
Fragrance
Dihydroabietyl alcohol
D & C Yellow No. 10
FD & C Yellow No. 6

VITA-METRAZOL ELIXIR
CNS stimulant; vitamins
(Knoll Pharm.)

Each 5 cc.:
Pentylenetetrazol * .... 100 mg.
Niacinamide .... 10 mg.
Thiamine HCl .... 1 mg.
Riboflavin-5'-phosphate
    sodium .... 1.4 mg.
Pyridoxine HCl .... 1 mg.
Alcohol 15%

VITA-METRAZOL TABLETS
CNS stimulant; vitamins
(Knoll Pharm.)

Each tablet:
Pentylenetetrazol * .... 100 mg.
Niacinamide .... 10 mg.
Thiamine mononitrate .... 1 mg.
Pyridoxine HCl .... 1 mg.
Riboflavin .... 1 mg.
Ascorbic acid .... 25 mg.

VITAON THERAPEUTIC ELIXIR
(Vita Elixir Co.)

Each 5 cc.:
Vitamin B12 .... 25 mcg.
Thiamine hydrochloride ..... 10 mg.
Ferric pyrophosphate
    (soluble) * .... 250 mg.

VITA PINE
Disinfectant
(Schneid)

Pine oil * 13.54%
Isopropanol * 10.20%
Potassium coconut oil soap 5.44%
Sodium salt of
    orthobenzylparachlorophenol . 4.05%

'76 Ed.

VITARINE TRANQUILIZER CAPSULES
(Vitarine)

Each capsule:
Methapyrilene
    hydrochloride * .... 25 mg.
Sodium salicylate * .... 160 mg.
Salicylamide * .... 160 mg.
Thiamine hydrochloride ..... 2.5 mg.
Riboflavin .... 0.5 mg.
Pyridoxine hydrochloride .... 0.5 mg.
Niacinamide .... 20 mg.

VITATONE SORBA-SPRAY 5-14-4
Foliar nutrient spray
(Leffingwell)

Total nitrogen 5.0%
    Ammoniac nitrogen 1.0%
    Urea nitrogen 4.0%
Phosphoric acid * 14.0%
Potash 4.0%
Zinc 1.5%

VITAVAX
Fungicide
(Uniroyal Chem.)

Carboxin * 75%
Inerts 25%
    Wetting agents
    Solid diluents

VITAVAX 3F FLOWABLE FUNGICIDE
(Uniroyal Chem.)

Carboxin * 34%
Inerts 66%
    Suspending agents
    Diluents
    Ethylene glycol *
    Water

VITAVAX FLOWABLE FUNGICIDE
(Uniroyal Chem.)

Carboxin * 34%
Inerts 66%
    Suspending agents
    Diluents
    Ethylene glycol *
    Water

VITAVAX 17 FLOWABLE FUNGICIDE
(Uniroyal Chem.)

Carboxin * 17%
Inerts 83%
    Suspending agents
    Diluents
    Ethylene glycol *
    Water

VITAVAX 200 FLOWABLE FUNGICIDE
(Uniroyal Chem.)

Carboxin 17%
Thiram * 17%
Inerts 66%
    Suspending agents
    Diluents
    Ethylene glycol
    Water

VITAVAX 200 FUNGICIDE
(Uniroyal Chem.)

Carboxin 37.5%
Thiram * 37.5%
Inerts 25.0%
    Wetting agents
    Diluents

VITAVAX 300 FUNGICIDE
(Uniroyal Chem.)

Carboxin * 37.5%
Captan 37.5%
Inerts 25%
    Wetting agents
    Diluents

VITAVAX-10G
Fungicide
(Uniroyal Chem.)

Carboxin 10%
Inerts 90%
    Whiting
    Starch
    Related materials

VITA ZINC
(Russ Pharm.)

Each capsule:
Ascorbic acid .... 300 mg.
Niacinamide .... 100 mg.
Thiamine mononitrate .... 20 mg.
d-Calcium pantothenate ..... 20 mg.
Riboflavin .... 10 mg.
Pyridoxine hydrochloride .... 5 mg.
Magnesium sulfate .... 70 mg.
Zinc sulfate .... 80 mg.

VIVACTIL TABLETS
Antidepressant
(MSD)

Each tablet:
Protriptyline
    hydrochloride * ...... 5 mg.; 10 mg.

VIVARIN
Stimulant tablets
(Williams, J.B.)

Each tablet:
Caffeine alkaloid * .... 200 mg.
Dextrose .... 150 mg.

VLEM-DOME LIQUID CONCENTRATE
For treatment of various types of acne
(Dome)

Calcium polysulfide *
Calcium thiosulfate *

Starred ingredients (*) may be responsible for major toxic effects; consult Section II.

VL NEUTRAL CONCENTRATE
General purpose cleaner
(Lester Labs.)

Synthetic detergents *
Mild Alkali *

'76 Ed.

V-M CAPSULES

See DR. DANIELS' V-M CAPSULES

VM PREPARATION
Liquid vitamin and mineral supplement
(Alvin Last)

Calcium hypophosphite	<0.5%
Calcium chloride	1.0%
Manganese hypophosphite	<0.05%
Quinine sulfate	<0.05%
Sugar	22%
Alcohol (USP)	12%
Liver concentrate	<0.05%
Benzaldehyde	<0.002%
Fluid extract Hops	<0.03%
Glycerin	<6.0%
Corn syrup	<6.0%
Hypophosphorous acid	<0.5%
Ferrous chloride	<1.0%
Niacinamide	<0.10%
Thiamine hydrochloride	<0.05%
Riboflavin	<0.05%
Dry Dimolt Siastalic	<0.5%
Sodium hypophosphite	<1.0%

VOLAXIN
Analgesic, mild tranquilizer
(Elder)

Each tablet:
Salicylamide *	500 mg.
Phenyltoloxamine citrate	25 mg.

VOLAXIN-A
Analgesic, mild tranquilizer
(Elder)

Each tablet:
Salicylamide *	500 mg.
Phenyltoloxamine citrate	25 mg.
Methscopolamine nitrate *	0.8 mg.

VON'S PINK TABLETS
Antacid
(New York Von)

Calcium carbonate
Magnesium trisilicate
Magnesium hydroxide

VOO DOO 42 KILLS RATS & MICE
Rodenticide
(Xterminator)

Warfarin (3-(a-Acetonylbenzyl)-4-hydroxycoumarin)	0.025%

'76 Ed.

VOO DOO MAGIC MIST ROACH & ANT AEROSOL
Insecticide
(Xterminator)

O,O-Diethyl O-(2-isopropyl-4-methyl-6-pyrimidinyl) phosphorothioate	0.500%
Pyrethrins	0.050%
Piperonyl butoxide, tech.	0.100%
N-Octyl bicycloheptene dicarboximide	0.166%
Petroleum distillate *	96.184%
Inert propellent	3.000%

'76 Ed.

VOO DOO NEW-ROACH-MAGIC
Kills resistant roaches
(Xterminator)

O,O-Diethyl O-(2-isopropyl-4-methyl-6-pyrimidinyl) phosphorothioate	0.5000%
Pyrethrins	0.0625%
Piperonyl butoxide, tech.	0.1250%
N-Octyl bicycloheptene dicarboximide	0.2080%
Petroleum distillate *	99.1045%

'76 Ed.

VOO DOO ROACH POWDER
Insecticide
(Xterminator)

Pyrethrins	1.00%
Piperonyl butoxide (technical)	10.00%
Amorphous silica gel	40.00%
Petroleum hydrocarbons *	49.00%

'76 Ed.

VOO DOO WHITE MAGIC INSECTICIDE
Insecticide
(Xterminator)

Tech. Chlordane	2%

'76 Ed.

VORLEX
Soil fumigant
(NOR-AM)

Chlorinated C3 hydrocarbons including Dichloropropenes *, Dichloropropane *, Related chlorinated hydrocarbons	80.0%/w
Methyl isothiocyanate *	20.0%/w

VORTEX
Liquid steam cleaner; industrial use
(Puritan Chem. Co.)

Synthetic detergents *

VOS-BAN
Insecticide
(Certified Labs.)

Chlorpyrifos (O,O-Diethyl O-(3,-5,6-trichloro-2-pyridyl) phosphorothioate)	3.00%
2,2-Dichlorovinyl dimethyl phosphate	2.60%
Related compounds	0.20%
Aromatic petroleum derivative solvent *	90.00%

VOUCH
Commercial laundry detergent
(Diversey Wyandotte)

Sodium hydroxide *
Alkaline salts

VOXIN-PG
Decongestant
(Norwich-Eaton)

Phenylpropanolamine hydrochloride *	75 mg.
Guaifenesin	400 mg.

VPI 260
Vapor phase inhibitor
(Shell Oil)

Dicyclohexyl ammonium nitrite *

VROOM BOWL CLEANER
Industrial and institutional use
(Scientific International)

Alkyl (C14 50%, C12 40%, C16 10%) dimethyl benzyl ammonium chloride	0.05%
Hydrogen chloride *	23.50%
Inert ingred.:	76.45%
Water	
Styrene carboxylic acid copolymer opacifier	
Octyl phenoxy polyethoxy ethanol	
Nonyl phenoxy polyethoxy ethanol	

VULCAN FC-30 CLOROFUME GRAIN FUMIGANT
(Vulcan Materials)

Chloroform *	72.2%
Carbonbisulfide *	20.4%
Ethylene dibromide *	7.4%

VULCAN FC-1 FORMULA 72 GRAIN FUMIGANT
(Vulcan Materials)

Ethylene dichloride	70.2%
Carbon tetrachloride *	29.8%

VULCAN FC-2 FORMULA 635 GRAIN FUMIGANT
(Vulcan Materials)

Carbon tetrachloride *	63.6%
Ethylene dichloride	29.2%
Ethylene dibromide	7.2%

Starred ingredients (*) may be responsible for major toxic effects; consult Section II.

VULCAN FC-3 FORMULA 815 GRAIN FUMIGANT
(Vulcan Materials)

Carbon tetrachloride *	81.3%
Carbon disulfide	12.1%
Ethylene dibromide	6.6%

VULCAN FC-14 FORMULA 82-H GRAIN FUMIGANT
(Vulcan Materials)

Carbon tetrachloride *	83.1%
Carbon bisulfide	16.5%

VULCAN FC-7 GRAIN FUMIGANT
(Vulcan Materials)

Ethylene dibromide	7.9%
Ethylene dichloride	64.7%
Carbon tetrachloride *	27.4%

VULCAN FC-4 GRAIN STORAGE FUMIGANT
(Vulcan Materials)

Ethylene dibromide	5.0%
Ethylene dichloride	64.6%
Carbon tetrachloride *	27.4%
Sulfur dioxide	3.0%

VULCAN FC-13 MILL MACHINERY FUMIGANT
(Vulcan Materials)

Ethylene dibromide *	20.5%
Ethylene dichloride	19.6%
Carbon tetrachloride *	59.9%

VULCAN FC-15 TERMINAL GRAIN FUMIGANT
(Vulcan Materials)

Carbon tetrachloride *	82.3%
Carbon bisulfide	16.3%
Sulfur dioxide	1.0%
Pentane	0.4%

V.V.S. SPECIAL FORMULA
Vaginal suppository capsules
(Econo Med)

Each suppository:
Sulfisoxazole	700 mg.
Allantoin	140 mg.
Aminacrine hydrochloride	14 mg.
In a water miscible, absorptive base

V.W. - CAR WASH (Powder)

See GUNK V.W. - CAR WASH (Powder)

"VYDATE" CONCENTRATE 42 INSECTICIDE/ NEMATICIDE
(Du Pont)

Oxamyl *	42%

"VYDATE" L INSECTICIDE/ NEMATICIDE
(Du Pont)

Oxamyl *	24%
Contains Methanol

W

WAGNER BRAKE FLUIDS
(Wagner Div.)

Polypropylene glycol *	20%
Propylene or dipropylene glycol *	10%
Mixture of Glycol ethers *	70%
Diethylene glycol monoethyl ether	
Triethylene glycol monoethyl ether	
Triethylene glycol monomethyl ether	

WAGNOL 40
Insecticide
(Wagnol, Inc.)

O,O-Diethyl-O-(2-isopropyl-4-methyl-6-pyrimidinyl) phosphorothioate *	25.2%
Aromatic petroleum derivative solvent *	54.3%

'76 Ed.

WAKOZ TABLETS
Stimulant; for mental alertness
(Jeffrey Martin, Inc.)

Each tablet:
Caffeine *	200 mg.

WALDEX
Paint cleaner
(Lester Labs.)

Detergents *	
Phosphates *	

'76 Ed.

WALGREENS HOUSE & GARDEN INSECT SPRAY
(Walgreen Labs.)

Pyrethrins	0.25%
Piperonyl butoxide, technical	1.00%
Isoparaffinic petroleum distillate	1.00%
Inert ingredients:	
Polyethylene glycol oleate	0.75%
Perfume	0.10%
1,1,1-Trichloroethane *	20.00%
Sodium nitrite	0.10%
Sodium benzoate	0.10%
Deionized water	61.70%
Propellant (hydrocarbon blend of 8.52% propane and 6.48% isobutane)	15.00%

'76 Ed.

WALGREENS INSECT FOGGER
Outdoor spray
(Walgreen Labs.)

Pyrethrins	0.25%
Technical Piperonyl butoxide	1.00%
Petroleum distillate	1.00%
Inert ingredients:	
Polyethylene glycol oleate	0.75%
Perfume	0.10%
1,1,1-Trichloroethane *	20.00%
Sodium nitrite	0.10%
Sodium benzoate	0.10%
Deionized water	61.70%
Propellant (hydrocarbon blend of 8.52% propane and 6.48% isobutane)	15.00%

'76 Ed.

WALGREENS INSECT REPELLENT SPRAY
(Walgreen Labs.)

2-Ethylhexanediol-1,3 (Ethohexadiol, U.S.P.) *	20.000%
Inert ingred.:	
Isopropyl alcohol *	29.875%
Perfume oil	0.125%
Freon No. 11	25.000%
Freon No. 12	25.000%

'76 Ed.

WALL TO WALL RUG SHAMPOO

See BISSELL WALL TO WALL RUG SHAMPOO

WALTHAM WHITE MOLDED CHALK
(American Crayon Co.)

This product bears the CP Seal issued by the Crayon, Water Color and Craft Institute, Inc. This seal certifies that the product contains no materials in sufficient quantities to be toxic or injurious to the human body even if ingested.

WALVET
Wallpaper cleaner
(Cleveland Cleaner)

Wheat flour	42.0000%
Ammonium alum	0.0060%
Water and salt solution	55.0000%
Aniline, color not certified	0.0002%
Kerosene oil	2.0000%

'76 Ed.

WANDA
Cold wave lotion
(Willat)

Ammonium thioglycolate 1-10%

WANS NO. 1 SUPPRETTES
Anti nausea
(Webcon)

Each suppository:
Pyrilamine maleate * .... 50 mg.
Sodium pentobarbital * ...... 50 mg.

WANS NO. 2 SUPPRETTES
Anti nausea
(Webcon)

Each suppository:
Pyrilamine maleate * .... 50 mg.
Sodium pentobarbital * ..... 100 mg.

WANS SUPPRETTES (CHILDREN)
Anti nausea
(Webcon)

Each suppository:
Pyrilamine maleate * .... 25 mg.
Sodium pentobarbital * ...... 30 mg.

WARBICIDE 5
Insecticide
(Chipman Inc.)

Rotenone * 5%

WARDLEY'S ALLCLEAR
Aquarium algicide
(Wardley Products)

Each tablet:
Active ingredients: 6.719%
Monuron (3-(p-Chlorophenyl)-1,1-di-
methylurea)
Dehydroabietylamine acetate
Dichlone (2,3-Dichloro-1,4-naphthoqui-
none)
Inert ingredients: 93.281%
Lactose
Sodium bicarbonate
Microcrystalline cellulose
Tartaric acid
Stearic acid

'76 Ed.

WARDLEY'S ANTICHLORINE COMPOUND
Aquarium remedy for instant chlorine removal
(Wardley Products)

Anhydrous Sodium thiosulfate
Sodium carbonate *
Inert ingredients: 98.98%
Demineralized water

'76 Ed.

WARDLEY'S AQUA PURER
Clears cloudy aquarium water
(Wardley Products)

Potassium permanganate 0.005%
Inert ingredients:
Demineralized water 99.995%

'76 Ed.

WARDLEY'S AQUA TONIC
Aquarium remedy; tropical fish disorders
(Wardley Products)

Sodium chloride (Salt)
Acriflavine (neutral)
Tetra-methylthionine chloride
Quinine hydrochloride
Magnesium sulfate
Inert ingredients: 97.75%
Demineralized water

'76 Ed.

WARDLEY'S FUNGUS REMEDY
Aquarium remedy; for disorders of tropical fish
(Wardley Products)

Sodium chloride (Salt)
9-Aminoacridine hydrochloride
Inert ingredients: 98.97%
Demineralized water

'76 Ed.

WARDLEY'S ICKAWAY LIQUID
Aquarium remedy
(Wardley Products)

Merbromin N.F. *
Sodium chloride
Inert ingredients: 97.523%
Distilled water

'76 Ed.

WARDLEY'S ICK & FUNGI-FREE
Aquarium remedy
(Wardley Products)

Malachite green (zinc free) 0.75%
Inert ingredients: 99.25%
Sodium chloride
Water

'76 Ed.

WARDLEY'S PROMETHYASUL
Treatment of most disorders of tropical fish
(Wardley Products)

Active ingredients: 2.47%
Sulfamylon (Mafenide hydrochloride)
9-Aminoacridine HCl
Tetramethylthionine chloride
Malachite green
Inert ingredients: 97.53%
Demineralized water
Sodium lauryl sulfate

'76 Ed.

WARDLEY'S SULFATONIC
Aquarium remedy; treatment of common diseases of tropical fish
(Wardley Products)

Sodium chloride (Salt)
Sulfathiazole sodium, U.S.P.
Inert ingredients: 98.84%
Demineralized water

'76 Ed.

WARDLEY'S SUPER CHLOR
Aquarium remedy
(Wardley Products)

Anhydrous Sodium thiosulfate * ... 22%
Inert ingredients: 78%
Demineralized water
Sodium carbonate *

'76 Ed.

WARDLEY'S SUPERTONIC
Aquarium remedy; for mild and severe infections
(Wardley Products)

Proflavine dihydrochloride (3,6-Diamino
acridinium hydrochloride)
Tetra-methylthionine chloride
Inert ingredients: 99.710%
Demineralized water

'76 Ed.

WARE-O-SPRAY

See MIDLAND WARE-O-SPRAY

WARFAR-MOR
With or without Prolin
(Hilltop)

Warfarin (3-(a-Acetonylbenzyl)-4-
hydroxycoumarin) 0.025%

'76 Ed.

Starred ingredients (*) may be responsible for major toxic effects; consult Section II.

WARNER WESTERN FRAGRANCES

Warner Western Fragrances
767 Fifth Ave.
New York, N.Y. 10022

Phone: 212-935-8600

See COSMETICS, Section VI, General
Formulations

WART-AWAY
Treatment of warts
(DePree)

Salicylic acid *
Camphor *
Glacial acetic acid *

WART FIX
Wart remover
(Alvin Last)

Castor oil	99.9%
D & C Red #17	<0.01%

WASATCH FOGGING CONCENTRATE
Insecticide
(Morgro)

Pyrethrins	0.30%
Piperonyl butoxide	1.50%
Petroleum hydrocarbons *	98.20%

WASATCH GRAIN FUMIGANT
(Morgro)

Carbon tetrachloride *	83.3%
Carbon disulphide	16.7%

WASATCH METHYL PARATHION 47% EMULSIBLE
Insecticide
(Morgro)

O,O-Dimethyl O-p-nitrophenyl phosphorothioate *	47.0%
Petroleum hydrocarbons	47.0%

WASATCH PARATHION 25% EMULSIBLE
Insecticide
(Morgro)

Parathion *	25.0%
Aromatic petroleum derivative solvent	70.0%

WASATCH PARATHION 50% EMULSION CONCENTRATE
Insecticide
(Morgro)

Parathion *	50%
Aromatic petroleum solvent	42%

WASATCH PHOSDRIN 4 EMULSIBLE
Insecticide
(Morgro)

Alpha isomer of 2-carbomethoxy-1-methylvinyl phosphate *	30.4%
Related compounds	20.4%
Petroleum hydrocarbons	43.2%

WASCO DAIRY CATTLE SPRAY
Insecticide
(Morgro)

2,2-Dichlorovinyl dimethyl phosphate	0.93%
Related compounds	0.07%
Petroleum hydrocarbons *	99.00%

WASCO DARI DIP
Post milking iodine dip
(Morgro)

Nonylphenoxypolyethoxyethanol-iodine complex (titratable iodine 1.0%)	17.0%

WASCO DDVP
Insecticide
(Morgro)

2,2-Dichlorovinyl dimethyl phosphate *	22.0%
Related compounds	1.7%
Aromatic petroleum solvent *	71.3%

WASCO DURACIDE CONCENTRATE
Wood preservative
(Morgro)

Pentachlorophenol *	33.6%
Other Chlorophenols and related compounds	5.0%
Methanol	approx. 30.0%

WASCO ETHION 2.2 SUPERIOR OIL
Insecticide
(Morgro)

Ethion (O,O,O',O'-Tetraethyl S,S'-methylene bisphosphorodithioate) *	2.2%
Petroleum oil *	95.0%

WASCO LINDANE EMULSIBLE
Insecticide
(Morgro)

Gamma isomer of benzene hexa-chloride (from lindane) *	20.00%
Petroleum hydrocarbons	76.87%

WASCO MALATHION 5
Insecticide
(Morgro)

Malathion *	57%
Aromatic petroleum derivatives *	35%

WASCO PYRENONE 10-1
Insecticide
(Morgro)

Pyrethrins	1%
Piperonyl butoxide (technical)	10%
Petroleum oil *	82%

WASCO PYRENONE INSECT SPRAY
Insecticide
(Morgro)

Piperonyl butoxide technical	1.27%
Pyrethrins	0.13%
Petroleum hydrocarbons *	98.60%

WASCO WATER WEED KILLER
Herbicide; irrigation and drainage ditches
(Morgro)

Aromatic hydrocarbons (consisting primarily of xylenes) *	95.0%

WASP-A-WAY, FOREMOST 4820

See FOREMOST 4820 WASP-A-WAY

WASP LONG RANGE JET SPRAY
Insecticide
(Miller-Norris Co.)

Pyrethrins	0.15%
Tech. Piperonyl butoxide	0.30%
N-Octyl bicycloheptene dicarboximide	0.53%
Tech. Chlordane	2.00%
Petroleum distillate *	62.02%

'76 Ed.

WASP NOT
Kills hornets, yellow jackets & wasps
(Nott)

Beta-butoxy beta'-thiocyano diethyl ether *	1.75%
Pine oil	2.00%
Dichloroethyl ether *	1.25%

Starred ingredients (*) may be responsible for major toxic effects; consult Section II.

WASP-STOPPER
Insecticide
(Whitmire Research)

Methylene chloride *	11.00%
Perchloroethylene *	32.00%
Trichloromonofluoromethane	20.00%
Pyrethrins I & II	0.05%
Rotenone	0.12%
Other related cube resins	0.28%
Dichlorodifluoromethane	20.00%
Petroleum distillate *	13.75%
Pine oil	2.80%

WASPTRAP

See MILLER'S WASPTRAP

WATCO-DENNIS PAINT PRODUCTS
Finishes, stains, and sealers

Watco-Dennis Corp.
1756 22nd. St.
Santa Monica, Calif. 90404

Phone: 213-829-2226

See PAINTS, Section VI, General Formulations

WATERENE
Water conditioner, algaecide, for air-conditioning systems
(Lester Labs.)

Sequestrants
Chlorophenol *
Corrosion inhibitors

'76 Ed.

WATER RINSE SAV-A-BRUSH
(Schalk)

Xylene *
Petroleum distillate
Glycol ether
Lanolin

'76 Ed.

WATER WOR-MOR
Drinking water anthelmintic; veterinary
(Hilltop)

Piperazine citrate base	32.3%
Magnesium sulfate	5%

'76 Ed.

WATKINS ANALGESIC BALM
Medicated cream
(Watkins Products, Inc.)

Methyl salicylate *	7.0%
Menthol *	
Oleoresin capsicum *	

WATKINS ANTACID
(Watkins Products, Inc.)

Aluminum hydroxide
Magnesium hydroxide

WATKINS ANT & ROACH SPRAY
Insecticide
(Watkins Products, Inc.)

O,O-Diethyl O-(2-isopropyl-4-methyl-6-pyrimidinyl)thiophosphate (Diazinon)	0.500%
Pyrethrins	0.050%
Piperonyl butoxide, tech.	0.125%
Petroleum distillate *	71.325%
Inert ingred.:	
Dichlorodifluoromethane	28.000%

WATKINS COUGH SYRUP
Antitussive
(Watkins Products, Inc.)

Camphor *	
Extracts:	
White pine	
Wild cherry	
Balm gilead	
Spikenard	
Blood root	
Alcohol	10.25%

WATKINS CREAM OF CAMPHOR LINIMENT
Rubefacient - counter irritant
(Watkins Products, Inc.)

Camphor *
Ammonium chloride
Turpentine *
Oil thyme *
Ammonia *

WATKINS DEODORANT BLOCKS
Spring Rose
French Lilac
(Watkins Products, Inc.)

Paradichlorobenzene *	99.6%

WATKINS DUSTER SPRAY
(Watkins Products, Inc.)

Propellants 11 & 12	
Mineral oil	
Petroleum distillates *	26%

WATKINS FIRST AID CREAM
Medicated cream
(Watkins Products, Inc.)

Phenol	1.0%
Benzocaine	
Camphor *	
Menthol *	
Oil of cloves *	
Eucalyptol *	

WATKINS FOOT POWDER SPRAY
Antiseptic powder
(Watkins Products, Inc.)

Dichlorophene	0.02%
Menthol	
Freon propellants	

WATKINS FURNITURE CREAM
Furniture & appliance cream
(Watkins Products, Inc.)

Wax emulsion	
Silicone emulsion	
Methyl salicylate	0.05%

WATKINS GUARD WAX
(Watkins Products, Inc.)

Polyethylene emulsion
Acrylic and styrene emulsions
Resin
Ammonia
Carbitol

WATKINS INHALANT
(Watkins Products, Inc.)

Alcohol	80%
Menthol *	
Eucalyptus *	
Lavender	

WATKINS INSECTICIDE
(Aerosol)
(Watkins Products, Inc.)

(5-Benzyl-3-furyl)methyl-2,2-di-methyl-3-(2-methylpropenyl)cyclopropane-carboxylate	0.250%
Related compounds	0.034%
Aromatic solvents	0.341%
Petroleum distillates *	59.357%
Inert ingred.:	
Dichlorodifluoromethane	40.018%

WATKINS INSECT REPELLENT
(Watkins Products, Inc.)

N,N-Diethyl metatoluamide & related compounds *	15.00%
Inert ingred.:	
Isopropyl alcohol *	25.00%
Dichloro-difluoromethane	30.00%
Trichloro-monofluoromethane	30.00%

WATKINS LEMON FURNITURE POLISH
(Aerosol)
(Watkins Products, Inc.)

Propellent 12	
Isoparaffinic hydrocarbon *	17%
Wax emulsion	
Silicone emulsion	

Starred ingredients (*) may be responsible for major toxic effects; consult Section II.

WATKINS LINIMENT
Rubefacient - counter irritant
(Watkins Products, Inc.)

Alcohol	47%

Camphor *
Safrol *
Capsicum *
Oil spruce

WATKINS MENTHOL CAMPHOR OINTMENT
Rubefacient
(Watkins Products, Inc.)

Menthol *
Camphor *
Ointment base

WATKINS PETROCARBO SALVE
Medicated ointment
(Watkins Products, Inc.)

Phenol *	1.75%

Oil cajeput *
Oil hemlock *
Safrol *
Oil camphor *†
Ointment base

†See Camphor oil

WATKINS PINE OIL DISINFECTANT
(Watkins Products, Inc.)

Pine oil *	73.77%
Potash soap	21.11%

WATKINS POW POWER
Industrial strength household cleaner
(Watkins Products, Inc.)

Ethylene glycol monobutyl ether	3.5%

Ethoxylated alcohol *
Sodium xylene sulfonate
Sodium silicate *

WATKINS RAT-MOUSE KILLER BAIT STATION
Rodenticide
(Watkins Products, Inc.)

Warfarin	0.025%

WATKINS SOOTHIE
(Watkins Products, Inc.)

Camphor *
Menthol *
Carbolic acid *
Oil of cloves *
Eucalyptol *

WATKINS SUPERCOLD COUGH MEDICINE
Antitussive
(Watkins Products, Inc.)

Each 5 ml.:
Dextromethorphan hydrobromide	7.5 mg.

Potassium guaiacolsulfonate
Sodium citrate

WATKINS TOILET BOWL CLEANSER
(Watkins Products, Inc.)

Hydrochloric acid *	23%
N-Alkyl dimethyl benzyl ammonium chloride	0.05%
Tri-butyl tin oxide	0.01%

WATSON-STANDARD PAINT PRODUCTS
Paints, finishes and coatings

Watson-Standard Co.
P.O. Box 11250
Pittsburgh, Pa. 15238

Phone: 412-362-8300

See PAINTS, Section VI, General Formulations

WAXOFF
(Schalk)

Trisodium phosphate *

'76 Ed.

WAZINE-34 (LIQUID)
Removal of large roundworms from chickens & turkeys
(Salsbury)

Each 100 cc:
Piperazine (present as sulfate)	34%

WAZINE SOLUBLE
Piperazine wormer for poultry, swine and horses
(Salsbury)

Piperazine dihydrochloride, piperazine base (240 grams per lb.)	53%

WD-40
Light lubricant, penetrant, water displacing corrosion preventive
(WD-40 Co.)

Bulk:
Petroleum distillate (Stoddard solvent) *	>70%
Petroleum base oil *	>20%
Proprietary corrosion inhibitors & wetting agents	balance

Aerosol:
Petroleum distillate (Stoddard solvent) *	>50%
Petroleum base oil *	>15%
Hydrocarbon propellant (LPG)	25%
Proprietary corrosion inhibitors & wetting agents	balance

WEAPON 4-E
Insecticide
(Techne Corp.)

O-Ethyl O-p-nitrophenyl phenylphosphonothioate *	46.7%
Xylene	47.3%

'76 Ed.

WEATHERPROOF ALUMINUM PAINT (137-00)
(Benjamin Moore)

Pigment:	12.1%
Aluminum paste (type II), Class B	100.0%
Vehicle:	87.9%
Varnish:	100%
Linseed, Coumarone-indene resin	31.6%
Mineral spirits*, Aromatics *†	68.4%

†See Aromatic hydrocarbons

WEBCO POWDER TEMPERA
Art material
(Weber Costello)

Earth oxides or nontoxic organic pigments

WEBER COBALT BLUE
Artists' color
(Weber, F.)

Cobalt oxide *
Aluminum oxide

WEBER DAMAR VARNISH
Artists' material
(Weber, F.)

Singapore white Damar gum
Turpentine *

WEBER ETCHERS' PRINTING INK
(Weber, F.)

Frankfort, vine and lamp blacks

Starred ingredients (*) may be responsible for major toxic effects; consult Section II.

WEBER INTENSE BLUE, INTENSE CERULEAN BLUE, INTENSE GREEN
Artists' color
(Weber, F.)

Copper phthalocyanine *

WEBER LEMON YELLOW
Artists' color
(Weber, F.)

Zinc chromate *

WEBER LIGHT DRYING OIL
Artists' supply
(Weber, F.)

Linseed oil
Turpentine *
Drying oil

WEBER MARS COLORS
Artists' color
(Weber, F.)

Hydrate and oxide of iron *

WEBER MASTIC VARNISH, FULL STRENGTH
Artists' material
(Weber, F.)

Gum mastic
Turpentine *

WEBER OXIDE OF CHROMIUM (OPAQUE & TRANSPARENT)
Artists' color
(Weber, F.)

Sesquioxide of Chromium *

WEBER PAINTING OIL NO. 1
Artists' material
(Weber, F.)

Gum damar
Refined oil
Turpentine *

WEBER PRUSSIAN BLUE
Artists' color
(Weber, F.)

Ferric ferrocyanide *

WEBER RAW UMBER
Artists' color
(Weber, F.)

Iron oxide *
Manganese oxide *

WEBER RES-N-GEL
Mixing medium in oil painting
(Weber, F.)

Colloidal synthetic resin gel

WEBER STAND OIL, DUTCH TYPE
Artists' material
(Weber, F.)

Polymerized Linseed oil

WEBER WATER-PROOF DRAWING INK BLACK
Artists' material
(Weber, F.)

Carbon ink

WEBER ZINC WHITE
Artists' color
(Weber, F.)

Oxide of zinc *

WEBER ZINC YELLOW
Artists' color
(Weber, F.)

Zinc chromate *

WEEDAR 64
Herbicide
(Amchem)

Dimethylamine salt of 2,4-dichlo-
rophenoxyacetic acid * 49.5%

WEEDAR 64A
Herbicide
(Amchem)

Dimethylamine salt of 2,4-dichlo-
rophenoxyacetic acid * 57.4%

WEEDAR AMINE BRUSH KILLER
(Amchem)

Dimethylamine salt of 2,4-dichlo-
rophenoxyacetic acid * 24.5%
Triethylamine salt of 2,4,5-trichlo-
rophenoxyacetic acid * 28.5%

WEEDAR MCPA
Herbicide
(Amchem)

Dimethylamine salt of 2-methyl-4-
chlorophenoxyacetic acid * 27.6%

WEEDAR SODIUM MCPA
Herbicide
(Amchem)

Sodium salt of 2-methyl-4-chloro-
phenoxyacetic acid * 23.9%

WEEDAR 2,4,5-T
Herbicide
(Amchem)

Triethylamine salt of 2,4,5-trichlo-
rophenoxyacetic acid * 52.2%

WEEDAZOL
Herbicide
(Amchem)

3-Amino-1,2,4-triazole 50%

WEED-B-GON
Herbicide
(Chevron)

Isooctyl ester of 2,4-dichlorophen-
oxyacetic acid * 17.8%
Isooctyl ester of silvex (2-(2,4,5-
Trichlorophenoxy)propionic
acid) 8.4%

Chevron emergency phone number:
415-233-3737

WEED-B-GON BAR
Lawn weed control
(Chevron)

2,4-Dichlorophenoxyacetic acid
(triethylamine salt) * 18.0%/w

Chevron emergency phone number:
415-233-3737

WEED-B-GON JET WEEDER
(Chevron)

Active ingred. (by wt.):
2,4-Dichlorophenoxyacetic acid
(diethanolamine salt) 0.75%
2-(2-Methyl-4-chlorophenoxy)
propionic acid (diethanolamine
salt) 0.75%

Chevron emergency phone number:
415-233-3737

WEED-B-GON LAWN WEED KILLER
(Chevron)

Active ingred. (by wt.):
2,4-Dichlorophenoxyacetic acid
(butoxy propyl esters) 21.4%
Silvex (butoxy propyl esters) . . . 10.0%

Chevron emergency phone number:
415-233-3737

WEED-B-GON M
Controls lawn weeds
(Chevron)

Active ingred. (by wt.):
2,4-Dichlorophenoxyacetic acid
(diethanolamine salt) * 14.2%
2-(2-Methyl-4-chlorophenoxy)
propionic acid (diethanolamine
salt) * 14.3%

Chevron emergency phone number:
415-233-3737

Starred ingredients (*) may be responsible for major toxic effects; consult Section II.

WEEDETH
Herbicide
(Miller Chem. Co.)

Dimethylamine salt of 2,4-dichloro-
   phenoxyacetic acid * 49%

'76 Ed.

WEED-FREE G

See CHAPMAN WEED-FREE G

WEED GO 20-2-1
Herbicide; industrial use
(Malter International)

Sodium pentachlorophenate * .. 17.10%
Sodium salts of other
   chlorophenols 2.96%

WEED-HOE 120
Herbicide
(Vineland Chem.)

Monosodium acid
   methanearsonate * 51.19%

WEEDMASTER HERBICIDE
(Velsicol)

Dimethylamine salt of Dicamba * 12.4%
Dimethylamine salt of related
   acids 3.1%
Dimethylamine salt of 2,4-dichlo-
   rophenoxyacetic acid * 35.7%

WEED-O-KIL COMPLETE WEED KILLER

See CHACON WEED-O-KIL COM-
PLETE WEED KILLER

WEEDONE 638
Herbicide
(Amchem)

2,4-Dichlorophenoxyacetic acid * . 31.0%

WEEDONE AERO-CONCENTRATE E
Herbicide
(Amchem)

Butyl ester of 2,4-dichlorophenoxy-
   acetic acid * 76.0%

WEEDONE BRUSH KILLER 32
Herbicide
(Amchem)

Butoxy ethanol ester of 2,4,5-tri-
   chlorophenoxyacetic acid * 10.8%
Butoxy ethanol ester of 2,4-dichlo-
   rophenoxyacetic acid * 22.6%

WEEDONE BRUSH KILLER 64
Herbicide
(Amchem)

Butoxy ethanol ester of 2,4,5-tri-
   chlorophenoxyacetic acid * 19.7%
Butoxy ethanol ester of 2,4-dichlo-
   rophenoxyacetic acid * 41.3%

WEEDONE CONCENTRATE 48
Herbicide
(Amchem)

Ethyl ester of 2,4-dichlorophenoxy-
   acetic acid * 38.6%

WEEDONE CRABGRASS KILLER, LIQUID
(Amchem)

Calcium acid methyl arsonate *† . 10.3%

†*See* Calcium acid methanearsonate

WEEDONE CRABGRASS KILLER SODAR
Herbicide
(Amchem)

Disodium methylarsonate
   hexahydrate * 50%

WEEDONE INDUSTRIAL BRUSH KILLER
Herbicide
(Amchem)

Butoxy ethanol ester of 2,4,5-tri-
   chlorophenoxyacetic acid * 29.6%
Butoxy ethanol ester of 2,4-dichlo-
   rophenoxyacetic acid * 30.9%

WEEDONE LV4
Herbicide
(Amchem)

Butoxy ethanol ester of 2,4-dichlo-
   rophenoxyacetic acid * 62.5%

WEEDONE LV6
Herbicide
(Amchem)

Butoxy ethanol ester of 2,4-dichlo-
   rophenoxyacetic acid * 88.1%

WEEDONE SPOT GRASS KILLER
(Amchem)

3-Amino-1,2,4-triazole 1.0%

WEEDONE 2,4,5-TP
Herbicide
(Amchem)

Butoxyethanol ester of silvex (2-
   (2,4,5-Trichlorophenoxy)
   propionic acid) * 58.9%

WEEDONE 2,4,5-T SPECIAL AIR SPRAY FORMULA
Herbicide
(Amchem)

2,4,5-Trichlorophenoxyacetic acid,
   butoxy ethanol ester * 58.3%

WEED-OX 115
Herbicide
(Stewart Sanitary Supply)

2,4-Dichlorophenoxyacetic acid, dimethylamine salt * 13.2%

WEED-OX 230
Herbicide
(Stewart Sanitary Supply)

2,4-Dichlorophenoxyacetic acid, dimethylamine salt * 26.4%

WEED-OX CRABGRASS KILLER
(Stewart Sanitary Supply)

Disodium methanearsonate
   (anhydrous) * 12.6%

WEED-RHAP A-4D
Herbicide
(Vertac)

Dimethylamine salt of 2,4-dichlo-
   rophenoxyacetic acid (equiv. to
   41.1% of 2,4-dichlorophenoxy-
   acetic acid) * 49.5%

WEED-RHAP A-4-MCPA
Herbicide
(Vertac)

Dimethylamine salt of 2-methyl-4-
   chlorophenoxyacetic acid (equiv.
   to 42.6% of MCPA) * 52.2%

WEED-RHAP B-4D
Herbicide
(Vertac)

Butyl ester of 2,4-dichlorophenoxy-
   acetic acid (equiv. to 46.9% of 2,4-
   dichlorophenoxyacetic acid) * .. 58.8%

WEED-RHAP B-6D
Herbicide
(Vertac)

Butyl ester of 2,4-dichlorophenoxy-
   acetic acid (equiv. to 63.1% of 2,4-
   dichlorophenoxyacetic acid) * .. 79.1%

Starred ingredients (*) may be responsible for major toxic effects; consult Section II.

WEED-RHAP LV-4D
Herbicide
(Vertac)

2-Ethylhexyl ester of 2,4-dichloro-
phenoxyacetic acid (equiv. to
46.3% of 2,4-dichlorophenoxy-
acetic acid) * 69.9%

WEED-RHAP LV-6D
Herbicide
(Vertac)

2-Ethylhexyl ester of 2,4-dichloro-
phenoxyacetic acid (equiv. to
62.5% of 2,4-dichlorophenoxy-
acetic acid) * 94.2%

WEEDRITE GRANULES
Herbicide
(Chipman Inc.)

Diquat * 2.5%
Paraquat * 2.5%

WEED-TOX

See HUBSCO WEED-TOX

WEED WOE, GOOD-LIFE

See GOOD-LIFE WEED WOE

WEEVIL-CIDE FORMULA 1
Grain fumigant
(Dow)

Carbon tetrachloride * 81.7%
Carbon bisulfide 16.2%
Sulfur dioxide 1.5%

WEEVIL-CIDE FORMULA 1A
Grain fumigant
(Dow)

Carbon bisulfide 16.5%
Carbon tetrachloride * 82.9%

WEEVIL-CIDE GRAIN FUMIGANT
(Weevil-Cide)

Carbon tetrachloride * 81.54%
Carbon disulfide 16.16%
Sulfur dioxide 1.54%

WEEVIL-CIDE TOXI-FOG
Fogging insecticide
(Weevil-Cide)

Malathion 3.90%
Technical Methoxychlor 2.45%
Pyrethrins 0.33%
Technical Piperonyl butoxide ... 0.57%
Carbon tetrachloride 0.52%
Aromatic petroleum derivative
solvent 4.52%
Petroleum distillate * 87.51%

WEEVIL GO MILL SPRAY
Insecticide
(Adco)

Petroleum distillate *
Tech. Piperonyl butoxide
Pyrethrins *

WEEVIL-TOX
Fumigant
(Miller Chem. & Fert.)

Carbon disulphide * 100%

WELADOL DISINFECTANT
Veterinary
(Pitman-Moore)

Polyethoxy polypropoxypolyethox-
yethanol-iodine complex 7.9%
Nonyl phenoxy polyethoxy ethanol-
iodine complex 7.6%
Hydrogen chloride 0.1%
Inert - water & perfume 84.4%

WELDIT
Undertakers', embalmers' supplies
(Embalmers')

Toluol *
Methyl ethyl ketone

WELDWOOD ACOUSTICAL TILE ADHESIVE 6041
(Roberts Consolidated Ind.)

Isopropyl alcohol .... approx. 5%
Petroleum distillates .... approx. 5%

WELDWOOD ACRYLIC CAULK 6048
(Roberts Consolidated Ind.)

Acrylic latex resins .... approx. 60%
Inert fillers .... approx. 35%
Water .... approx. 5%

WELDWOOD BIG STICK PANEL & FOAM ADHESIVE 6018
(Roberts Consolidated Ind.)

Latex resins .... approx. 40%
Inert fillers .... approx. 10%
Water .... approx. 50%

WELDWOOD BUTYL RUBBER CAULK 6049
(Roberts Consolidated Ind.)

Butyl rubber .... approx. 80%
Petroleum distillate * ..... approx. 20%

WELDWOOD CARPET CEMENT 0504
(Roberts Consolidated Ind.)

Petroleum distillate * 10%

WELDWOOD CERAMIC WALL & COUNTER TILE ADHESIVE 6053
(Roberts Consolidated Ind.)

Latex resins .... approx. 37%
Water .... approx. 20%
Fillers .... approx. 43%

WELDWOOD CLEANER & THINNER 1005
(Roberts Consolidated Ind.)

Methylene chloride * 10-25%
Petroleum distillate * 50-75%

WELDWOOD CONTACT CEMENT 2047
(Roberts Consolidated Ind.)

Toluene * .... approx. 20%
Ketone solvents .... approx. 10%
Petroleum distillates ..... approx. 50%

WELDWOOD FLOOR TILE CEMENT 3057
(Roberts Consolidated Ind.)

Petroleum distillate 5%

WELDWOOD HHR BRUSHABLE CONTACT CEMENT 0308 (NATURAL)
(Roberts Consolidated Ind.)

Toluene * .... approx. 10%
Ketone solvents * .... approx. 14%
Petroleum distillates * .... approx. 45%

WELDWOOD HHR BRUSHABLE CONTACT CEMENT 0309 (RED)
(Roberts Consolidated Ind.)

Toluene * .... approx. 10%
Ketone solvents * .... approx. 14%
Petroleum distillates * .... approx. 45%

WELDWOOD HHR SPRAY CONTACT CEMENT 0306 (NATURAL)
(Roberts Consolidated Ind.)

Toluene * .... approx. 10%
Ketone solvents * .... approx. 14%
Petroleum distillates * .... approx. 45%

WELDWOOD HHR SPRAY CONTACT CEMENT 0307 (RED)
(Roberts Consolidated Ind.)

Toluene * .... approx. 10%
Ketone solvents * .... approx. 14%
Petroleum distillates * .... approx. 45%

WELDWOOD LATEX CAULK 6047
(Roberts Consolidated Ind.)

Latex resins	approx. 50%
Inert fillers	approx. 20%
Water	approx. 30%

WELDWOOD MARINE WOODLIFE READY TO USE 1409-22
Wood preservative
(Roberts Consolidated Ind.)

Copper naphthenate *	10%
Petroleum solvents *	80%

WELDWOOD MULTI-PURPOSE FLOOR ADHESIVE 3055
(Roberts Consolidated Ind.)

Toluene *	approx. 5%
Petroleum distillates	approx. 4%

WELDWOOD NONFLAMMABLE BRUSH CONTACT CEMENT 2000
(Roberts Consolidated Ind.)

1,1,1-Trichloroethane *	approx. 86%

WELDWOOD NONFLAMMABLE SOLVENT 0911
(Roberts Consolidated Ind.)

1,1,1-Trichloroethane *	100%

WELDWOOD PANEL ADHESIVE 6017
(Roberts Consolidated Ind.)

Methyl ethyl ketone *	approx. 25%
Toluol *	approx. 5%
Naphtha *	approx. 30%

WELDWOOD PANEL ADHESIVE, NON-FLAMMABLE 6034
(Roberts Consolidated Ind.)

1,1,1-Trichloroethane *	approx. 70%

WELDWOOD PANEL AND DRYWALL ADHESIVE 6031
(Roberts Consolidated Ind.)

Petroleum distillates *	approx. 30%
Ethyl alcohol	approx. 1%

WELDWOOD PANELWOOD 6039
(Roberts Consolidated Ind.)

General purpose construction mastic

Ethyl alcohol	approx. 5%
Petroleum distillate *	approx. 30%

WELDWOOD P.A.R. (Clear and Redwood) (8023-8022)
Water repellent finish for wood
(Roberts Consolidated Ind.)

Inert Water repellent solids	approx. 19%
Petroleum distillates *	approx. 80%

WELDWOOD PATIOLIFE 8009
Stain finish, sealer, water repellent for wood
(Roberts Consolidated Ind.)

Pigment	3%
Water repellent resins	45%
Petroleum distillate *	52%

WELDWOOD PENTACHLOROPHENOL CONCENTRATE 10-1 1409-07
(Roberts Consolidated Ind.)

Pentachlorophenol *	34.4%
Other chlorophenols	4.0%
Ketone solvents	60.0%

WELDWOOD PENTACHLOROPHENOL READY TO USE 1409-10
(Roberts Consolidated Ind.)

Pentachlorophenol *	4.3%
Other chlorophenols	0.5%
Petroleum distillates *	90.0%

WELDWOOD PLASTIC RESIN GLUE 7047
(Roberts Consolidated Ind.)

Urea formaldehyde resin	80%
Cellulose flour	18%

WELDWOOD PLUS-10 CONTACT CEMENT
(Roberts Consolidated Ind.)

Synthetic Resin & natural polymers and inert fillers	47%
Water	53%

WELDWOOD RESORCINOL GLUE, WATERPROOF W256
Adhesive; 2 components
(Roberts Consolidated Ind.)

Liquid

Resorcinol resin	approx. 54%
Alcohol *	approx. 34%

Powdered catalyst

Paraformaldehyde *	approx. 88%

WELDWOOD SPRAY-N-GLUE 0099
Aerosol adhesive
(Roberts Consolidated Ind.)

Petroleum distillates *	approx. 50%
Methylene chloride *	approx. 10%
Propane	approx. 15%

WELDWOOD STANDARD SOLVENT 0901
(Roberts Consolidated Ind.)

Toluene *	approx. 10%
Ketone solvents *	approx. 20%
Petroleum distillates *	approx. 70%

WELDWOOD SUB FLOOR AND CONSTRUCTION ADHESIVE
Two types
(Roberts Consolidated Ind.)

1) Solvent based 6043:

Petroleum distillate *	approx. 30%
Ethyl alcohol	trace

2) Latex based 6016:

Latex	approx. 75%
Ethanol	approx. 8%
Water	approx. 9%

WELDWOOD WATERPROOF CEMENT 6013
(Roberts Consolidated Ind.)

Toluene *	approx. 1%
Petroleum distillates *	approx. 15%

WELDWOOD WATERPROOFING SEALER W178
(Roberts Consolidated Ind.)

Petroleum distillates *	approx. 80%

WELDWOOD WHITE GLUE W204
Adhesive
(Roberts Consolidated Ind.)

Polyvinyl acetate resin	approx. 50%

WELDWOOD WOODLIFE CONCENTRATE CLEAR 1409-12
Wood preservative
(Roberts Consolidated Ind.)

Pentachlorophenol *	14.6%
Other chlorophenols	1.7%
Petroleum solvents *	39.0%

Starred ingredients (*) may be responsible for major toxic effects; consult Section II.

WELDWOOD WOODLIFE READY TO USE - CLEAR 1409-14
Wood preservative
(Roberts Consolidated Ind.)

Pentachlorophenol * 4.3%
Other chlorophenols 0.5%
Petroleum solvents * 85.0%

WELDWOOD WOODWORKERS GLUE 3097
White glue
(Roberts Consolidated Ind.)

Polyvinyl acetate resin . . . . approx. 50%

WELDWOOD WOODYOUTH 8028
Water repellent for wood
(Roberts Consolidated Ind.)

Inert Water repellent solids . approx. 12%
Petroleum distillates * . . . . approx. 88%

WELLA COSMETIC PRODUCTS
Hair preparations

The Wella Corp.
524 Grand Ave.
Englewood, N.J. 07631

Phone: 201-569-1020

See COSMETICS, Section VI, General
Formulations

WERNET'S POWDER
Denture adhesive
(Block Drug)

Ethylene oxide homopolymer
Gum karaya
Flavor

WESCALDRIN
Vitamin and mineral supplement
(Wesley Pharm.)

Each capsule:
  Ferrous fumarate
    (supplying iron 49.3
    mg.) * . . . . .150 mg.
  Vitamin A (acetate) . . . 4000 USP Units
  Vitamin D
    (Ergocalciferol) . . . . . .400 USP Units
  Plus multivitamins & minerals

WESCILLIN 250 & WESCILLIN 400
Antibiotic-antibacterial
(Wesley Pharm.)

Each tablet:
  Penicillin G potassium
    (buffered) . . . . 250,000 or
                   400,000 Units

WESCODYNE
Disinfectant, sanitizer
(West Chem. Prod.)

Polyethoxypolypropoxypolyethoxyethanol
  -iodine complex
Nonylphenoxypoly(ethyleneoxy)ethanol-
  iodine complex

WESCOHEX ANTIBACTERIAL SURGICAL SCRUB
(Vitarine)

Westron (brand of sulfonated anionic and
  nonionic detergent) *
Lanolin
Petrolatum
Hexachlorophene * 3%
Polyethylene glycol 400
Lauric myristic monoethanolamide
Dimethoxane *
Sodium citrate
Water

WESCOID
Anorexic
(Wesley Pharm.)

Each tablet:
  Phendimetrazine * . . . . 35 mg.

WESCOL
Cleaning, disinfecting cutting oil systems
(West Chem. Prod.)

Coal tar neutral oils *
Soap
Homologs of Phenol *
Phenol *
Chlorinated phenols *

WESCOLATES
Laxative
(Wesley Pharm.)

Each tablet:
  Sodium glycocholate
  Sodium taurocholate . . . . 1 1/2 gr.
  Sodium succinate . . . . 1 1/2 gr.
  Phenolphthalein . . . . 1/2 gr.
  Cascara sagrada . . . . 1/2 gr.

WESCOPHEN-S
Sedative w/antispasmodic
(Wesley Pharm.)

Each tablet:
  Phenobarbital * . . . . 30 mg.
  Hyoscyamus extract * . . . . 46 mg.
  Valerian powder . . . . 30 mg.
  Passiflora extract . . . . 30 mg.

WESDEX-T
Anorexic
(Wesley Pharm.)

Each tablet:
  Phendimetrazine * . . . . 35 mg.

WESLEY ALKALINE GARGLE
(Wesley Pharm.)

Each tablet:
  Sodium bicarbonate
  Sodium biborate
  Sodium benzoate
  Sodium salicylate
  Sodium chloride
  Eucalyptus
  Menthol
  Menthyl salicylate

WESLEY FLATULENCE TABLETS
Cathartic
(Wesley Pharm.)

Each tablet:
  Nux vomica ext. (0.185 gr.
    Strychnine) * . . . . 1/4 gr.
  Ginger . . . . 3/4 gr.
  Pancreatin . . . . 1/20 gr.
  Cascara sagrada ext. . . . . 1/4 gr.
  Capsicum . . . . 1/8 gr.

WESLIN OINTMENT
(Wesley Pharm.)

Methyl salicylate *
Eucalyptus oil *
Menthol *

WESMATIC, FORTE
Bronchial asthma
(Wesley Pharm.)

Each tablet:
  Phenobarbital . . . . 1/8 gr.
  Ephedrine sulfate * . . . . 1/4 gr.
  Theophylline * . . . . 120 mg.
  Chlorpheniramine maleate . . . 2 mg.
  Glyceryl guaiacolsulfonate . . . 100 mg.

WESMATIC TABLETS
Bronchial asthma
(Wesley Pharm.)

Each tablet:
  Phenobarbital . . . . 1/8 gr.
  Ephedrine sulfate * . . . . 1/4 gr.
  Theophylline * . . . . 120 mg.
  Chlorpheniramine maleate . . . 2 mg.

WESMYCIN CAPSULES
Antibiotic-antibacterial
(Wesley Pharm.)

Each capsule:
  Tetracycline hydrochloride . . . 250 mg.

WESPER-C
Analgesic
(Wesley Pharm.)

Acetylsalicylic acid * . . . . 5 gr.
Ascorbic acid . . . . 55 mg.
Aluminum hydroxide gel . . . . 35 mg.

WESPRIN BUFFERED
Analgesic
(Wesley Pharm.)

Each tablet:
Aspirin * .... 5 gr.
Buffered with Aluminum and Magnesium complex

WESPRIN REGULAR
Analgesic
(Wesley Pharm.)

Each tablet:
Aspirin * .... 3 1/2 gr.
Phenacetin * .... 2 1/2 gr.
Caffeine .... 1/2 gr.

WESPRIN w/GELSEMIUM
Analgesic
(Wesley Pharm.)

Each tablet:
Phenacetin * .... 2 gr.
Hyoscyamus .... 1/6 gr.
Aspirin * .... 2 gr.
Caffeine (anhydrous) .... 1/4 gr.
Ext. Gelsemium .... 1/100 gr.

WESTASEPT
Concentrated surgical soap
(West Chem. Prod.)

Hexachlorophene *
Potassium coconut oil soap
Lecithin

WEST BEND HUMIDIFIER BACTERIA TREATMENT #1971
(West Bend; Mfr., R. P. S. Products, Inc.)

n-Alkyl (60% C14, 30% C16, 5% C12, 5% C18) dimethyl benzyl ammonium chlorides * 2.25%
n-Alkyl (68% C12, 32% C14) dimethyl ethylbenzyl ammonium chlorides * 2.25%

WEST BEND HUMIDIFIER TREATMENT (LIQUID) #1960 AND #2060
Prevents lime scale build-up in humidifiers
(West Bend; Mfr., Whink Products Co.)

Sodium hexametaphosphate 1.05%
EDTA (Disodium ethylenediaminetetraacetate dihydrate) 0.04%
Algaecide (Alkyl dimethyl benzyl ammonium chloride) 0.01%
Perfume - Lilac D-93, #J79-144V 0.20%
Water 98.70%

WEST BEND HUMIDIFIER WATER TREATMENT TABLETS #1942
(West Bend; Mfr., Elco Chemical, Inc.)

Benzoic acid * 31.0%
Adipic acid 24.0%
EDTA (Ethylenediaminetetraacetic acid) 14.0%
APAP (Acetyl-p-aminophenol) ... 1.5%
Tris(hydroxymethyl)nitromethane 12.5%
Microcrystalline Cellulose 17.0%

WESTERN ELECTRIC METAL PASTE POLISH
(SerVaas Labs.)

Silica (amorphous) 60%/w
Cade oil 20%/w
Paraffin oil 10%/w
Stearic acid 10%/w

WESTROL
Anorexiant
(Wesley Pharm.)

Each tablet:
Phentermine * .... 8 mg.

WES-TUSSIN
Antitussive
(Wesley Pharm.)

Each tsp. (5 cc):
Glyceryl guaiacolate .... 100 mg.
Alcohol 3.5%
Palatable aromatic syrup

WEST-WARD ACETAMINOPHEN ELIXIR N.F.
Analgesic
(West-ward)

Each tsp. (5 ml.):
Acetaminophen N.F. * ...... 120 mg.
Alcohol (by volume) 8%
'76 Ed.

WEST-WARD ANTIHISTAMINE NASAL SPRAY
(West-ward)

Pyrilamine maleate * 0.15%
Phenylephrine HCl 0.25%
Cetyl dimethyl benzyl ammonium chloride 0.05%
'76 Ed.

WEST-WARD ANTIHISTAMINE WITH SPC TABLETS
Analgesic & antipyretic
(West-ward)

Each tablet:
Pyrilamine maleate .... 25 mg.
Salicylamide .... 3 1/2 gr.
Phenacetin * .... 2 1/2 gr.
Caffeine .... 1/2 gr.

'76 Ed.

WEST-WARD ATHLETE'S FOOT SPRAY
(West-ward)

Undecylenic acid 5%
Benzoic acid 4%
Salicylic acid * 2%
Benzocaine 1%
Propylparaben 0.01%
Isopropyl alcohol * 50%

'76 Ed.

WEST-WARD COLD CAPSULES
Timed disintegration
(West-ward)

Each capsule:
Total Belladonna alkaloids (total belladonna alkaloid salts 0.16 mg.) .... 0.128 mg.
Atropine sulfate .... 0.024 mg.
Scopolamine hydrobromide .... 0.014 mg.
Hyoscyamine sulfate ... 0.122 mg.
Phenylpropanolamine hydrochloride * .... 50 mg.
Chlorpheniramine maleate . 1 mg.
Pheniramine maleate ..... 12.5 mg.

'76 Ed.

WEST-WARD COUGH SYRUP DM-PLUS
(West-ward)

Each 5 ml.:
Dextromethorphan hydrobromide * .... 15 mg.
Chlorpheniramine maleate .. 1 mg.
Phenylephrine hydrochloride .. 5 mg.
Glyceryl guaiacolate .... 50 mg.
Alcohol (by volume) 3.5%

'76 Ed.

WEST-WARD DIOCTYL WITH CASANTHRANOL CAPSULES
For constipation
(West-ward)

Each capsule:
Dioctyl sodium sulfosuccinate * .... 100 mg.
Casanthranol * .... 30 mg.

'76 Ed.

WEST-WARD DIOCTYL WITH DANTHRON CAPSULES
For constipation
(West-ward)

Each capsule:
Dioctyl sodium sulfosuccinate *   50 mg.
Danthron (1,8-
Dihydroxyanthraquinone)   .. 25 mg.

'76 Ed.

WEST-WARD HEMORRHOIDAL SUPPOSITORIES
(West-ward)

Each suppository:
Bismuth subgallate *
Zinc oxide
Boric acid *
Tannic acid *
Resorcin *
Benzocaine
Peruvian balsam *

'76 Ed.

WEST-WARD NASAL DECONGESTANT TABLETS
(West-ward)

Phenylephrine hydrochloride   ...   5 mg.
Chlorpheniramine maleate   .....   2 mg.
Salicylamide .... 227 mg.
Phenacetin * .... 100 mg.
Caffeine .... 10 mg.
Ascorbic acid .... 20 mg.

'76 Ed.

WEST-WARD THEOPHYLLINE ELIXIR
Bronchodilator
(West-ward)

Each tbs. (15 ml.):
Theophylline (anhydrous) *   ..   80 mg.
Alcohol (by volume) 20%

'76 Ed.

WEST-WARD THEOPHYLLINE, EPHEDRINE & PHENO TABLETS N.F.
Antiasthma
(West-ward)

Each tablet:
Theophylline * .... 130 mg.
Ephedrine hydrochloride * ... 24 mg.
Phenobarbital * .... 8 mg.

'76 Ed.

WEST-WARD TRIPLE ANTIBIOTIC OINTMENT
(West-ward)

Each gm.:
Polymyxin B sulfate ...... 5,000 units
Bacitracin .... 400 units
Neomycin sulfate .... 5 mg.

'76 Ed.

WEST-WARD URINARY ANTISEPTIC TABLETS
(West-ward)

Each tablet:
Methenamine * .... 2 gr.
Salol .... 1/2 gr.
Methylene blue .... 1/10 gr.
Benzoic acid .... 1/8 gr.
Atropine sulfate .... 1/1000 gr.
Hyoscyamine sulfate ...... 1/2000 gr.

'76 Ed.

WET-EGE SPIRITS
Paint thinner
(Oklahoma Refining)

Paraffins * 47%
Naphthenes * 42%
Aromatics * 9%
Olefins 2%

WET-N-SOAK WETTING AND SOAKING SOLUTION FOR HARD CONTACT LENSES
(Allergan Pharm.)

Polyvinyl alcohol

WET ONES
Pre-moistened towelettes
(Lehn & Fink)

Alcohol 10%
Propylene glycol 1%
Lanolin, ethoxylated .... trace
Oleyl alcohol, ethoxylated ..... trace
Aromatic phosphate ester ..... trace
Citric acid .... trace
Disodium phosphate .... trace
Sorbic acid .... trace
Perfume .... trace
Water .... balance

WHACK WASP-HORNET ANT-ROACH KILLER

See LILLY/MILLER WHACK WASP-
HORNET ANT-ROACH KILLER

WHAM
*Cleaner, deodorizer for drain lines, sep-
tic tanks, grease traps*
(Hercules Chem.)

Orthodichlorobenzene,
emulsifiable * .... >80%

WHEATON FABRIC SOFTENER
Laundry compound
(Wheaton Chemical Co.)

Quaternary ammonium chloride salt *

'76 Ed.

WHEATON SAFETY DISINFECTANT
Sanitizer
(Wheaton Chemical Co.)

Sodium orthophenyl phenate *

'76 Ed.

WHIFF WITH CHLOROPHYLL & X-ON

See C-Z WHIFF WITH CHLORO-
PHYLL & X-ON

WHINK RUST STAIN REMOVER
(Whink)

Combined amount: ..... 6%-8% solution
Hydrofluoric acid *
Water

WHIRL
Chlorinated alkaline cleaner
(Diversey Wyandotte)

Sodium hydroxide *
Sodium hypochlorite releasing agent

WHIRL
Cold wave lotion
(Willat)

Ammonium thioglycolate 1-10%

WHIRLWIND
Machine polishing compound
(McAleer)

Kerosene *
Paraffin wax
Ethylethanolamine oleate
Pine oil *
Tripoli

'76 Ed.

WHISK-AWAY BATHTUB RUST REMOVER
(W. W. Stewart Div., Zephyr Mfg. Co.)

Hydrochloric acid * .... approx. 4%
Ammonium chloride
Citric acid
Water

WHISK-AWAY COFFEEMAKER & PLASTICWARE CLEANER
Stain remover
(W. W. Stewart Div., Zephyr Mfg. Co.)

Sodium hypochlorite *	16%
Water	84%

WHISK-AWAY FABRIC RUST REMOVER
To remove rust from fabrics, carpeting, etc.
(W. W. Stewart Div., Zephyr Mfg. Co.)

Hydrofluoric acid *	4%
Water	96%

WHISK-AWAY LEMON OIL POLISH
(W. W. Stewart Div., Zephyr Mfg. Co.)

Base oil #2 *	96.5%
Paraffin oil	2.5%
Lemon oil	1.0%

WHISK-AWAY PANEL CARE
Cleans and polishes
(W. W. Stewart Div., Zephyr Mfg. Co.)

Base oil #2 *	92%
Perchlorethylene	approx. 5%
Paraffin oil	2%
Cedar forest Perfume oil	<1%

WHISK-AWAY STEAM IRON CLEANER
(W. W. Stewart Div., Zephyr Mfg. Co.)

Phosphoric acid *
Water

WHISTLE CLEAN RINSE
Floor neutralizing rinse
(Paul Koss)

Water	>80%
Glacial acetic acid *	<7%
Isopropyl alcohol	<7%
POE sorbitan monolaurate	
Artificial Oil of cassia	
Dye	

pH 3.4-3.6

WHIT-CIDE
Bactericide
(Whitfield Chem.)

Hexahydro-1,3,5-tris(2-hydroxy-ethyl)-s-triazine *	>10%

WHITE CAP PINE DISINFECTANT
(White Cap, Inc.)

Pine oil *	60%
Soap *	15%
Isopropanol *	15%
Water	10%

WHITE DIAMOND BOWLING ALLEY WAX
See BUTCHER'S WHITE DIAMOND BOWLING ALLEY WAX

WHITE FROTH (SY549)
See DUNCAN CERAMICS WHITE FROTH (SY549)

WHITE GLOVE FURNITURE POLISH
See MAJESTIC WHITE GLOVE FURNITURE POLISH

WHITE GLOVE GENERAL PURPOSE POLISH
See MAJESTIC WHITE GLOVE GENERAL PURPOSE POLISH

WHITEHALL ARTHRITIS PAIN FORMULA
Analgesic
(Whitehall Labs.)

Aspirin *
Aluminum hydroxide
Magnesium hydroxide

WHITE KING CLEANSER
(Los Angeles Soap)

Silica
Alkyl aryl type detergent *
Sodium phosphate *
Trichloroisocyanuric acid (bleach) *
Perfume

WHITE KING COLD CREAM TOILET SOAP BAR
(Los Angeles Soap)

Sodium soap made from tallow & coconut oil
Perfume
Dye
Titanium dioxide

WHITE KING "D" DETERGENT
(Los Angeles Soap)

Sodium alkyl aryl sulfonate
Sodium polyphosphate
Sodium carbonate *
Sodium sulfate
Sodium silicate
Perfume
Optical whitener
Carboxymethylcellulose

WHITE KING SOAP
(Los Angeles Soap)

Sodium soap made from tallow & coconut oil
Perfume
Sodium sesquicarbonate
Sodium silicate
Sodium carbonate
Optical whitener
Carboxymethylcellulose

WHITE KING WATER SOFTENER
(Los Angeles Soap)

Sodium polyphosphate
Sodium sesquicarbonate
Sodium carbonate *
NTA (Nitrilotriacetic acid)

WHITE LIGHTNIN'
Plastic filler
(Marson)

Resin component:	
Styrene monomer	10-14%
Polyester (100% solids)	26-31%
Pigment & filler *	50-60%
Di-methyl aniline	0.1-0.4%
Catalyst component:	
Benzoyl peroxide *	48-52%
Phthalate plasticizer	42-48%
Pigment	3-5%

WHITE MAGIC ALL PURPOSE CLEANER (LIQUID)
(Safeway Stores)

Complex phosphated amide	13.0%
Tetra potassium phosphate *	13.0%
Ammonium xylene sulfonate	6.0%
Polystyrene polymer, perfume	0.4%
Water	balance

WHITE MAGIC AMMONIA WATER
(Safeway Stores)

Ammonia (NH3) *	4%
Surfactants	1%
Water	95%

WHITE MAGIC AUTOMATIC DISHWASHING (POWDER)
(Safeway Stores)

Sodium tripolyphosphate	42%
Sodium polysilicate (anhydrous basis)	20%
Chlorinated trisodium phosphate (anhydrous) *	9%
Ethoxylated alcohol	2%
Water (hydrate)	27%

WHITE MAGIC CLEANSER, SCOURING POWDER
(Safeway Stores)

Alkyl aryl sodium sulfonate	2%
Chlorinated trisodium phosphate *	13%
Silica flour	85%

Starred ingredients (*) may be responsible for major toxic effects; consult Section II.

WHITE MAGIC DETERGENT (POWDER)
(Safeway Stores)

Linear Alkyl aryl sulfonate *	20%
Sodium tripolyphosphate *	24%
Sodium silicate	10%
Sodium sulfate	35%
Combined amount:	2%
Perfume	
Carboxymethylcellulose	
Optical brightener	
Moisture	9%

WHITE MAGIC FLOOR WAX
(Safeway Stores)

An Acrylic polymer	15%
Emulsifiable Polyethylene	3%
Styrene maleic anhydride resin	1%
Diethylene glycol ethyl ether (Carbitol)	5%
Plasticizers:	2%
Tributoxy ethyl phosphate	
Dibutyl phthlate	
Other: Surfactants, Preservatives, Defoamer	1%
Water	balance

WHITE MAGIC GLASS CLEANER (Liquid)
(Safeway Stores)

Isopropyl alcohol	4%
Ethylene glycol dibutyl ether (Butyl Cellosolve) *	3%
Other: Nonionic surfactant, Ammonia, EDTA, Perfume, Dye	1%
Water	balance

pH, undiluted 10

WHITE MAGIC HEAVY DUTY LIQUID DETERGENT
(Safeway Stores)

Alcohol ethoxylate *	35%
Alkyl aryl sulfonate *	12%
Triethanolamine	4%
Ethyl alcohol (SDA-3A)	6%
Other: Fluorescent whitener, Inorganic salts, Perfume, Dye	1%
Water	42%

WHITE MAGIC LIQUID BLEACH
(Safeway Stores)

Sodium hypochlorite *	5.5%
Sodium hydroxide	0.2%
Sodium chloride and chlorate *	5.3%
Water	balance

WHITE MAGIC LIQUID DETERGENT
(Safeway Stores)

Linear alkyl aryl sulfonate (Na) *	20%
Linear alcohol ethoxy sulfate (NH4)	11%
Lauric diethanolamide	4%
Sodium xylene sulfonate	9%
Perfume, dye, polystyrene polymer	0.5%
Water	balance

WHITE MAGIC LOW SUDS DETERGENT (Powder)
(Safeway Stores)

Linear Alkyl aryl sulfonate *	12%
Fatty acid sodium soap	5%
Sodium tripolyphosphate *	33%
Sodium silicate	12%
Combined amount:	2%
Carboxymethylcellulose	
Optical brightener	
Perfume	
Sodium sulfate	27%
Water	9%

WHITE MAGIC SWIMMING POOL ACID
(Safeway Stores)

Hydrogen chloride (by weight) *	32%
Water and small amounts of inerts	balance

WHITE MAGIC SWIMMING POOL CHLORINE
(Safeway Stores)

Sodium hypochlorite *	13%
Sodium hydroxide	0.5%
Sodium chloride and chlorate *	15%
Water	balance

WHITE MONDAY LIQUID BLEACH
(Industrial Equities)

Sodium hypochlorite *	5 1/4%
Sodium chloride	<5%
Water	balance

WHITE RAIN HAIR PRODUCTS
(Gillette Co., Personal Care Div.)

The Gillette Co., Personal Care Div., Boston, Mass. 02199 will receive collect phone calls from poison control centers or physicians asking for emergency toxicological information about the company's products.

Phone: 617-421-7000

WHITE STAR AUTOBODY FILLER & CREME HARDENER
(Fibre Glass-Evercoat)

Filler:

Polyester resin	50%
Magnesium silicate	50%

Creme Hardener:

Benzoyl peroxide *	50%
Butyl benzyl phthalate *	50%

WHITE STUFF
Floor finish
(Paul Koss)

Water	>80%
Emulsion of oligomers and polymers, primarily acrylic	
Emulsion of Polyethylene	
Fluorochemical surfactant	trace
Formalin	trace

pH 7.7-8.0

WHITE TIRE MAGIC

See CHOLDUN'S WHITE TIRE MAGIC

WHITMIRE PT 250 BAYGON
Insecticide
(Whitmire Research)

Baygon *	1%

WHITMIRE PT 260 DIAZINON
Insecticide
(Whitmire Research)

Diazinon *	1.0%

WHITMIRE PT 270 DURSBAN
Insecticide
(Whitmire Research)

Chlorpyrifos	0.50%

WHITMIRE PT 150 PYRETHRUM
Insecticide
(Whitmire Research)

Pyrethrins I & II	0.25%
Piperonyl butoxide, technical	0.25%

WHITMIRE PT 565 PYRETHRUM
Insect fogger
(Whitmire Research)

Pyrethrins	0.5%
Piperonyl butoxide, technical	1.0%
N-Octyl bicycloheptene dicarboximide	1.0%
Refined petroleum oil	8.0%

Starred ingredients (*) may be responsible for major toxic effects; consult Section II.

WHITMIRE PT 575 PYRETHRUM
Insect fogger
(Whitmire Research)

Pyrethrins I & II	0.5%
Piperonyl butoxide, technical	4.0%
Refined petroleum oil	8.0%
Chlorofluorocarbon 11 & 12	

WHITMIRE PT 140 RESMETHRIN
Insecticide
(Whitmire Research)

Resmethrin	0.50%

WHITMIRE PT 550 RESMETHRIN
Insect fogger
(Whitmire Research)

Resmethrin	0.50%

WHITMIRE PT 1200 RESMETHRIN
Adult whitefly control in greenhouses
(Whitmire Research)

Resmethrin	1.00%

WHITMIRE PT 515 WASP-FREEZE
(Whitmire Research)

Tetrachloroethylene *	32%
Trichloromonofluoromethane	20%
Dichlorodifluoromethane	20%
Petroleum distillate *	13.75%
Methylene chloride *	11%
Pine oil	2.80%
Rotenone	0.12%
Other related cube resins	0.28%
Pyrethrins I & II	0.05%

WHITMIRE'S TICKS-OFF INSECT REPELLENT BOMB
(M-S-A)

Combined amount:	0.408%
Rotenone	0.136%
Other cube resins	0.272%
Butoxypolypropylene glycol	9.592%
Dimethyl phthalate	8.000%
N,N-Diethyl-meta-toluamide	1.900%
Other isomers	0.100%

WHITMOYER PIPERAZINE-34
Anthelmintic; veterinary
(Whitmoyer)

Piperazine (from piperazine monohydrochloride)	34%
Water	66%

WHITMOYER PIPERAZINE A/M
Wormer for poultry and swine
(Whitmoyer)

Piperazine (as piperazine dihydrochloride)	44.00%
Other ingredients:	56.00%
Electrolytes including Citric acid, Sodium bicarbonate, Sodium acetate, Potassium chloride, Magnesium chloride, Calcium acetate	
Artificial color and flavor added	

WHITMOYER PIPERAZINE DIHYDROCHLORIDE
For control of large round worms - veterinary
(Whitmoyer)

Piperazine (as piperazine dihydrochloride)	52%

WHITMOYER PIPERAZINE WORMER PRE-MIX
For control of large round worms - veterinary
(Whitmoyer)

Piperazine (as piperazine dihydrochloride)	22.2%

WHITMOYER PIPERAZINE WORMER SOLUTION
Anthelmintic; veterinary
(Whitmoyer)

Piperazine (from piperazine monohydrochloride)	17%
Water	83%

WHIT-PEEL "S"
Strippable protective coatings
(Whitfield Chem.)

Ketones	>10%
Toluene *	>10%
Methylene chloride	>10%

WHITSPHILL
For fungus infections of the glabrous skin
(Torch)

FULL STRENGTH:

Salicylic acid *	6 gm.
Benzoic acid	12 gm.
Hydrophilic vehicle ad	100 gm.

HALF STRENGTH:

Salicylic acid *	3 gm.
Benzoic acid	6 gm.
Hydrophilic vehicle ad	100 gm.

'76 Ed.

WHITSYN-S
For coccidiosis; veterinary, avian
(Whitmoyer)

Pyrimethamine (2,4-Diamino-5-(p-chlorophenyl)-6-ethylpyrimidine)	0.91%
Sulfaquinoxaline	3.00%
Monoethanolamine	
Polyoxyethylene alkyl aryl ether	
Propylene glycol	
Sorbitol	

WHIZ FAST-EASY CARBURETOR CLEANER
(Classic Chem.)

Petroleum distillates *	>10%/w

WHIZ GASLINE ANTIFREEZE
(Classic Chem.)

Methanol *	>10%/w

WHIZ LOOSEN-ALL
(Classic Chem.)

Petroleum distillates *	>10%/w

WHIZ PREMIXED WINDSHIELD WASHER FLUID
(Classic Chem.)

Methanol *	>10%/w

WHIZ WINDSHIELD DE-ICER
(Classic Chem.)

Methanol *	>10%/w

WHIZ WINDSHIELD WASHER SOLVENT AND ANTI-FREEZE
(Classic Chem.)

Methanol *	>10%/w

WIBI
Dry skin lubricator
(Owen Labs.)

Emulsified blend of Polyglycol
Menthol (small amount)

WICK N' LOCK

See BALKAMP WICK N' LOCK

WIGRAINE (TABLETS & SUPPOSITORIES)
For migraine headache
(Organon)

Each tablet & suppository:
Ergotamine tartrate *	1.0 mg.
Caffeine *	100.0 mg.
Belladonna alkaloids (levorotatory)	0.1 mg.
Phenacetin *	130.0 mg.

WILBERT'S FRESH-PINE DISINFECTANT CLEANER & DEODORANT
(Wilbert)

Steam-distilled Pine oil *
Isopropanol *
Liquid soap

WILBERT'S LEMON OIL FURNITURE POLISH
(Wilbert)

Refined paraffinic crude oil *
Perfume

WILBERT'S NO-RUB FLOOR WAX
(Wilbert)

Synthetic polymers
Synthetic waxes
Synthetic resins
Morpholine *
Oleic acid (Red oil)
Ammonia

WILBERT'S NO-RUB FURNITURE CREAM
(Wilbert)

Refined Paraffinic oil *
Emulsifier

WILBERT'S SILVER DIP
(Wilbert)

Mineral acid *
Synthetic detergent
Thiourea

WILBUR-ELLIS BUSAN 30 E.C.
Seed treatment fungicide; agricultural
(Wilbur-Ellis Co.)

Busan (2-(Thiocyanomethylthio) benzothiazole) *	30%

WILBUR-ELLIS DIBROM 8 SPRAY
Insecticide; agricultural
(Wilbur-Ellis Co.)

Naled *	60%

WILBUR-ELLIS MALATHION 8 SPRAY
Insecticide; agricultural
(Wilbur-Ellis Co.)

Malathion *	81.2%

WILBUR-ELLIS PARATHION 8 FLOWABLE
Insecticide; agricultural
(Wilbur-Ellis Co.)

Parathion *	80%

WILBUR-ELLIS PHOSPHAMIDON 8 SPRAY
Insecticide; agricultural
(Wilbur-Ellis Co.)

Phosphamidon *	74.5%
Related compounds	3.5%

WILDROOT CREAM OIL HAIR DRESSING
(Colgate-Palmolive)

Mineral oil and wax	about 35%
Beeswax	
Lanolin	about 5%
Emulsifier	
Water	about 50%
Perfume and preservative	

'76 Ed.

WILHOLD BUILDERS ADHESIVE
(Wilhold Glues, Inc.)

Vinyl acetate
Alkyd resins
Plasticizers	approx. 1%
Portland cement	
Other fibers	

WILHOLD BUILDERS CONSTRUCTION ADHESIVE
(Wilhold Glues, Inc.)

Styrene butyrate rubber and resin	20%
Petroleum distillates *	80%

WILHOLD CLEAR EPOXY GLUE
(Wilhold Glues, Inc.)

Epoxy resins
Amide resins
Amine resins

WILHOLD CONCRETE ADHESIVE
(Wilhold Glues, Inc.)

Polyvinyl acetate polymer
Plasticizers	approx. 1%
Hydrocarbons	approx. 1%

WILHOLD CONTACT CEMENTS (Smooth Spread; Professional)
(Wilhold Glues, Inc.)

Neoprene rubber and resins	20%
Butanone	20%
Toluol *	20%
Isopropyl acetate	5%
Petroleum distillates	35%

WILHOLD CONTACT CEMENT "21"
(Wilhold Glues, Inc.)

Neoprene rubber and resins	20%
1,1,1-Trichloroethane *	80%

WILHOLD EPOXY CEMENT FOR CONCRETE
(Wilhold Glues, Inc.)

Epoxy with amine and amide hardeners and fillers

WILHOLD FLASH GLUE
(Wilhold Glues, Inc.)

alpha-Cyanoacrylate *†	18%

†*See* n-Alkyl-a-cyanoacrylates

WILHOLD GLU-BOND ADHESIVE
(Wilhold Glues, Inc.)

Nitrile rubber *	20%
Phenolic resin	80%

WILHOLD GLUE (Glu-Bird; Decorator's; Heavy Body Craft)
(Wilhold Glues, Inc.)

Polyvinyl acetate polymer
Plasticizers	approx. 1%
Hydrocarbons	approx. 1%

WILHOLD GLU-ON PANEL ADHESIVE (Glu-On Fixture)
(Wilhold Glues, Inc.)

Neoprene rubber and resin	55%
Toluol *	20%
Butanone	10%
Petroleum distillates	15%

WILHOLD PLASTIC MODEL CEMENT
(Wilhold Glues, Inc.)

Styrene resin	20%
Butanone *	60%
Petroleum distillates *	20%

WILHOLD PLASTIC RESIN GLUE
(Wilhold Glues, Inc.)

Urea resin
Paraformaldehyde *

WILHOLD VINYL PLASTIC CEMENT
(Wilhold Glues, Inc.)

Vinyl resin	20%
Butanone *	70%
Toluol *	10%

WILHOLD WATERPROOF GLUE
(Wilhold Glues, Inc.)

Phenol-resorcinol resin
Paraformaldehyde *

WILLIAMS GOLDEN YELLOW LATHER SHAVING CREAM
(Williams, J.B.)

Potassium soap
Glycerin
Boric acid *
Lanolin derivatives

WILLIAMS SHAVING STICK
(Williams, J.B.)

Sodium and potassium soaps

WIL-O-MITE DUST

See RED-TOP WIL-O-MITE DUST

WILPOWR
Anorexiant
(Foy Labs.)

Each capsule:
  Phentermine HCl * .... 30 mg.

WILSON-IMPERIAL PAINT PRODUCTS
Paint removers, brush cleaners, finishes

Wilson-Imperial Co.
115 Chestnut
Newark, N.J. 07105

Phone: 201-589-6050

WINDEX (LIQUID & AEROSOL)
Window cleaner
(Drackett)

Isopropanol & glycol ether solvents	<10%/wt.
Anionic surfactant	<0.5%/wt.
Ammonium hydroxide	very small amount
Water	

WIND-GUARD
Skin cream for chapping, drying skin
(Reynes Products, Inc.)

Purified water
TEA stearate
Mineral oil
Glycerin
Propylene glycol
Dipropylene glycol
Dimethicone
Acetylated lanolin
Hydroxyethyl cellulose
Methyl paraben
Propyl paraben
FD & C Yellow #5
FD & C Yellow #6

WIND 'N WEATHER HAND CREAM
(House of Lowell, Inc.)

Stearic acid
Glycerin
Isopropyl palmitate
Cetyl alcohol
Glyceryl stearate
Lanolin
Modified Polystyrene latex
Potassium hydroxide
Sodium hydroxide
Formaldehyde
Methylparaben
Propylparaben
Perfume
D & C color

WINDO CLEAN, DOUBLE STRENGTH
Cleaner
(Hillyard Chem.)

Organic solvents *†

'76 Ed.

†See Aromatic hydrocarbon solvent

WIND-O-SHINE AEROSOL
Window cleaner
(Dolge)

Isopropyl alcohol *	
Ammonia	
Isobutane/propane (50/50) (Propellant)	20%

WINDOW-LITE GLASS POLISH
(Patterson Labs.)

Patterson Labs., Inc.
11930 Pleasant Ave.
Detroit, Mich. 48217

Phone: 313-843-4500

WINGS'M AEROSOL
Insecticide
(Dro)

Butoxypolypropylene glycol *	12.55%
Tech. Piperonyl butoxide	0.80%
N-Octyl bicycloheptene dicarboximide	0.50%
Pyrethrins	0.20%
Allethrin (allyl homolog of cinerin I)	0.15%

'76 Ed.

WINK H. D.
Car & truck wash
(National-Purity Soap)

Detergents *

pH of 1% solution, 12.0

WINSTROL
Anabolic steroid
(Winthrop Labs.)

Each tablet:
  Stanozolol, NF .... 2 mg.

WINTERFECT
Disinfectant, deodorant
(Damon Chemical Co.)

n-Alkyl (50% C14, 40% C12, 10% C16) dimethyl benzyl ammonium chloride *	2.5%
Ethanol *	0.5%
Isopropanol *	35.0%
Inert ingredients:	62.0%
Wetting agents	
Deodorants	
Water	

WINTER-PHENE
Disinfectant, germicide
(Varley, James)

Active ingred.:	39%
Isopropyl alcohol *	25.94%
Vegetable oil soaps	5.69%
o-Benzyl p-chlorophenol	4.90%
Methyl salicylate *	1.22%
o-Phenyl phenol	0.75%
Essential oils	0.50%
Inert ingred.:	61%
Water	

WINTERSET
Swimming pool treatment
(Modern Pool Products)

Disodium copper ethylenediaminetetraacetate *†

†See Copper

WINTHROP ANTI-RUST TABLETS
Anticorrosive
(Winthrop Labs.)

Each tablet:
Sodium carbonate (monohydrate)	1.16 gm.
Sodium nitrite *	500 mg.

Starred ingredients (*) may be responsible for major toxic effects; consult Section II.

WINT MINT
Disinfectant, cleaner, deodorizer; institutional and commercial use
(Hysan Corp.)

Isopropyl alcohol *	11.00%
Terpineol	3.00%
Methyl salicylate *	2.00%
N-Alkyl (60% C14, 30% C16, 5% C12, 5% C18) dimethyl benzyl ammonium chloride	0.50%
N-Alkyl (50% C12, 30% C14, 17% C16, 3% C18) dimethyl ethyl-benzyl ammonium chloride	0.50%
Oil of peppermint USP	0.05%
Oil of spearmint USP	0.05%

WIPE FLY PROTECTANT
Veterinary
(Farnam Co.)

Pyrethrins	0.20%
Piperonyl butoxide, technical	0.50%
Di-n-propyl isocinchomeronate	1.00%
Oil of citronella	5.00%
Butoxypolypropylene glycol *	20.00%

'76 Ed.

WIPE 'N SPRAY
Insecticide
(Hess & Clark)

Pyrethrins	0.06%
Piperonyl butoxide (technical)	0.12%
N-Octyl bicycloheptene dicarboximide	0.20%
Di-n-propyl isocinchomeronate	0.40%
Mineral oil *	99.22%

WIPE-OUT
Windshield washer anti-freeze and solvent
(Van Waters & Rogers)

Methanol *	37%
Ammonia	0.1%

WIPE-OUT

See GREEN LIGHT WIPE-OUT

WISK (Low Phosphate)
Liquid laundry detergent
(Lever Bros.)

Water	50-60%
Potassium and sodium pyrophosphates	10-20%
Anionic detergent	10-20%
Sodium silicate	1-5%
Fatty alkanolamides	1-5%
Potassium soap	1-5%
Cellulosics	<1%
Perfume	<1%
Optical dye	trace
Colorants	trace

WISK (Nonphosphate)
Liquid laundry detergent
(Lever Bros.)

Water	50-60%
Anionic detergents	10-30%
Sodium citrate	5-20%
Nonionic detergent	5-10%
Monoethanolamine	1-5%
Sodium soap	0-2%
Cellulosic	<1%
Perfume	<1%
Optical dyes	trace
Opacifier	trace
Colorants	trace

WITCO 8% COPPER NAPHTHENATE
Fungicide
(Witco)

Copper expressed as metallic	8%
Copper naphthenate *	Typically 70-80%
Petroleum distillate *	Typically 20-30%

WITCO 8% ZINC NAPHTHENATE
Fungicide
(Witco)

Zinc naphthenate	Typically 55-60%
Petroleum distillate *	Typically 40-45%
Zinc, expressed as metallic	8%

WIZ
Concentrated foaming cleaner; industrial and institutional use
(Scientific International)

N-Alkyl (C12 40%, C14 50%, C16 10%) dimethyl benzyl ammonium chloride	0.384%
Essential oil	0.480%
Ethylene diamine tetraacetic acid	0.960%
Trisodium phosphate	1.920%
Isopropyl alcohol	5.760%
Inert ingred.:	90.496%
Detergents *	
Builders	
Cleaners	
Propellant	

WIZARD AIR FRESHENER (Aerosol, various fragrance types)
(Boyle-Midway)

Deodorant oil (essential oil type)	<1%
Emulsifiers	
Propellant	

WIZARD AIR FRESHENER (Solid, various fragrance types)
(Boyle-Midway)

Gelling agents	<5%
Denatured alcohol	<2%
Fragrance *†	<2%
Preservatives	

†See Essential oils

WIZARD CAT LITTER DEODORIZER
(Boyle-Midway)

Sodium sulfate	<70%
Sodium bicarbonate *	<25%
Corn starch	<15%
Fragrance	trace

WIZARD CHARCOAL LIGHTER
(Boyle-Midway)

Petroleum distillate *	>90%
Dye	

WIZARD DECORATIVE AIR FRESHENER (Various Shapes and Fragrances)
(Boyle-Midway)

Essential oils *	approx. 10%
Dyes, pigment, and color stabilizers	trace
Waxes	
Petrolatum	

WIZARD RUG & ROOM DEODORIZER
(Boyle-Midway)

Sodium sulfate	<70%
Sodium bicarbonate *	<25%
Corn starch	<15%
Fragrance	trace

WIZARD SUPER RUG AND ROOM DEODORIZER
(Boyle-Midway)

Sodium sulfate	<70%
Sodium bicarbonate *	<25%
Corn starch	<15%
Fragrance	<2%

WIZARD WICK DEODORIZER (Various fragrance types)
(Boyle-Midway)

Emulsifiers of fatty acid, polyoxyethylene oleyl esters (nonionic types)	1-5%
Deodorant oils (essential oil type) *	1-5%
Alcohol	1-5%
Formaldehyde	trace
Antioxidant	trace

WIZ-KLEEN
Porcelain and bowl cleaner; industrial and institutional use
(Scientific International)

Alkyl (C14 50%, C12 40%, C16 10%) dimethyl benzyl ammonium chloride	0.05%
Hydrogen chloride *	7.50%
Inert ingred.:	92.45%
Water	
Styrene-carboxylic acid copolymer	
Octyl phenoxy polyethoxy ethanol	
Nonyl phenoxy polyethoxy ethanol	

WOLMANAC SOLUTION
Wood preservative
(Honolulu Wood Treating Co.)

Active ingred.:	
Chromium trioxide *	2.7%
Copper oxide	1.1%
Arsenic pentoxide *	2.0%
Inert ingred.:	94.2%
Pyradine	trace
Dye coloring	trace
Water soluble elemental Arsenic	1.3%

WONDER BAR OIL POLISH
(Uncle Sam)

Paraffin based oil
Wax
Dye

WONDER BASE LATEX SEALER
Wall primer
(Zinsser, Wm., & Co.)

Pigment (Silicates)	7.5%
Acrylic resin	10.0%
Water	82.5%

WONDER-BREL
Plant growth stimulant
(Science Prod.)

Gibberellic acid (potassium salt)	
Liquid:	0.08570%
Push-button spray:	0.00502%

WONDER BRONZE OIL
(Uncle Sam)

Paraffin based oil

WONDER DRIP FLUID (PINE)
(Uncle Sam)

Pine oil *
Mineral oil *

WONDER FLOOR OIL
(Uncle Sam)

Paraffin base oil

WONDER FLUFF
Bubble bath for dogs
(8 in 1 Pet Products)

Pyrethrins	0.050%
Technical Piperonyl butoxide	0.100%
N-Octyl bicycloheptene dicarboximide	0.167%
Petroleum distillates	0.243%
2,2-Methylenebis(3,4,6-trichlorophenol)	1.000%

'76 Ed.

WONDER LIQUID SOAPS
(Uncle Sam)

Vegetable oils
Potassium hydroxide
Propylene glycol
Perfume
Tetrasodium ethylene diamine tetraacetate
Water

WONDER METAL POLISH
(Uncle Sam)

Oleic acid
Oxalic acid *
Alcohol *
Ammonia *
Silica in water

Contains no free acid

WONDER MIST

See AMWAY WONDER MIST

WONDER PINE AROMA DISINFECTANT COEF. 2
(Uncle Sam)

Pine oil *
Soap
Isopropanol *
Dye
Water

WONDER PINE OIL DISINFECTANT COEF. 3
(Uncle Sam)

Pine oil *
Soap
Isopropanol *
Dye
Water

WONDER PINE OIL DISINFECTANT COEF. 5
(Uncle Sam)

Pine oil *
Soap
Water

WONDER PREPARED PASTE & LIQUID WAX
(Uncle Sam)

Waxes (vegetable & mineral)
Petroleum distillates *
Dye

WONDER RUG & UPHOLSTERY CLEANER
(Uncle Sam)

Vegetable oils
Potassium hydroxide
Synthetic detergent *
Naphtha *
Water

WONDER WAX CLEANER
(Uncle Sam)

Soap
Surfactants *
Ammonia *
Tetrasodium ethylenediaminetetraacetate
Silicates
Water

WONDRA (Scented & Unscented)
Skin conditioning lotion
(Procter & Gamble, Beauty Care Div.)

Glycerin	1-5%
Cetyl alcohol	1-5%
Cetyl palmitate	1-5%
Myreth-3 palmitate	1-5%
Minor ingredients, each	<1%
Water	>50%

WOODBURY TOILETRIES
(Jergens, A.)

Andrew Jergens Co.
2535 Spring Grove Ave.
Cincinnati, Ohio 45214

Phone: 513-421-1400

See COSMETICS, Section VI, General Formulations

WOODIE PENTA WOOD PRESERVATIVE
(Savogran)

Mineral spirits *	85%
Pentachlorophenol *	5%

WOODKILL ESTER CONCENTRATE
Herbicide
(Techne Corp.)

Butyl ester of 2,4-D *	42.67%
Butyl ester of 2,4,5-T *	42.20%
Aliphatic petroleum hydrocarbons *	15.13%

'76 Ed.

WOOD-KOTE ANTIQUE BASE (Regal Blue)
(Spe-De-Way)

Pigment:	18.8%/wt.
Titanium dioxide	26.90%
Thalo blue	4.40%
Raw umber	1.50%
Calcium carbonate	67.20%
Vehicle:	81.2%/wt.
Vinyl acrylic emulsion	58.00%
Water & surfactant	34.11%
Polyols & glycol ethers	7.89%

Starred ingredients (*) may be responsible for major toxic effects; consult Section II.

WOOD-KOTE BRUSH CLEANER
(Spe-De-Way)

Ketones .... 29.0%/wt.
Esters .... 30.5%/wt.
Aromatics *† .... 40.5%/wt.

†See Aromatic hydrocarbon solvent

WOOD-KOTE CLEAR DULL-SATIN FINISH
Eggshell Luster
(Spe-De-Way)

Polyhydric alcohol partially esterified with linolenic, oleic,
linoleic, palmitic, stearic acids
(modified   with   tolylene
diisocyanate) .... 36%/wt.
Combined amount: .... 59%/wt.
  Aliphatic hydrocarbons *
  Driers *
Colloidal silica .... 5%/wt.

WOOD-KOTE CRYSTAL CLEAR FINISH FOR WOOD
(Spe-De-Way)

Nitro-cellulose .... 5.1955%/wt.
Dioctyl phthalate plasticized
  alkyd resin .... 12.8%/wt.
Dry Zinc .... 0.004%/wt.
Benzophenone .... 0.0005%/wt.
Glycol ethers * .... 15.0%/wt.
Ketones * .... 13.0%/wt.
Alcohols .... 15.0%/wt.
Aromatic hydrocarbons * .. 8.0%/wt.
Naphthas * .... 31.0%/wt.

WOOD-KOTE GELLED WOOD STAIN
(Spe-De-Way)

V. T. Alkyd resin 10-15%
Inorganic pigments 10-15%
Organic pigments *† 5%
Aliphatic hydrocarbons * 40-50%
Aromatic hydrocarbons * 15-20%
Drier .... trace

†See Paints, Section VI, General Formulations

WOOD-KOTE LIQUID PLASTIC POLYURETHANE CLEAR HIGH GLOSS FINISH
*For exterior and interior wood and
  metal surfaces*
(Spe-De-Way)

Polyhydric alcohol partially es-
terified with Linolenic, Oleic,
Linoleic, Palmitic, Stearic
acids, modified with Tolylene
diisocyanate .... 49%/wt.
Combined amount: .... 51%/wt.
  Aliphatic hydrocarbons *
  Driers *

WOOD-KOTE LIQUID PLASTIC POLYURETHANE CLEAR SATIN FINISH
*For exterior and interior wood and
  metal surfaces*
(Spe-De-Way)

Polyhydric alcohol partially es-
terified with Linolenic, Oleic,
Linoleic, Palmitic, Stearic
acids, modified with Tolylene
diisocyanate .... 40%/wt.
Combined amount: .... 54%/wt.
  Aliphatic hydrocarbons *
  Driers *
Colloidal silica .... 6%/wt.

WOOD-KOTE MARINE FINISH HIGH GLOSS
(Spe-De-Way)

Polyhydric alcohol partially es-
terified with Linolenic, Oleic,
Linoleic, Palmitic, Stearic
acids, modified with Tolylene
diisocyanate .... 49%/wt.
Combined amount: .... 51%/wt.
  Aliphatic hydrocarbons *
  Driers *

WOOD-KOTE MARINE FINISH SATIN FINISH
(Spe-De-Way)

Polyhydric alcohol partially es-
terified with Linolenic, Oleic,
Linoleic, Palmitic, Stearic
acids, modified with Tolylene
diisocyanate .... 40%/wt.
Combined amount: .... 54%/wt.
  Aliphatic hydrocarbons *
  Driers *
Colloidal silica .... 6%/wt.

WOOD-KOTE MARINE FINISH WHITE
(Spe-De-Way)

Polyhydric alcohol partially es-
terified with Linolenic, Oleic,
Linoleic, Palmitic, Stearic
acids, modified with Toly-
lene diisocyanate .... 39.3%/wt.
Combined amount: .... 34.2%/wt.
  Aliphatic hydrocarbons *
  Driers *
Color pigment .... 26.5%/wt.

WOODLIFE CONCENTRATE CLEAR 1409-12

See WELDWOOD WOODLIFE CON-
CENTRATE CLEAR 1409-12

WOODLIFE READY TO USE - CLEAR 1409-14

See WELDWOOD WOODLIFE
READY TO USE - CLEAR 1409-14

WOODLIFE WOOD PRESERVATIVE 1409-14
(Roberts Consolidated Ind.)

Pentachlorophenol * 4.3%
Other chlorophenols 0.5%
Petroleum solvents * 85.0%

WOOD LORE
Wood finish
(Pierce & Stevens)

Modified Alkyd resins
Modifying acids: palmitic, stearic, oleic,
  linoleic, linolenic, oleostearic
Aromatic hydrocarbons *
Aliphatic hydrocarbons *

WOOD PLUS

See TEXIZE WOOD PLUS

WOOD-REM
Wood preservative
(Speco)

Hydrocarbon vehicle *
Resins
Plasticizers
Coal tar solvents *†
Creosote *

'76 Ed.

†See Aromatic solvent naphtha

WOODTOX PREPRIME RTU
Water repellent & wood preservative
(Wood Treating Chemicals Co.)

Pentachlorophenol * 4.5%
Other chlorophenols & related
  compounds 0.5%
Mineral spirits * 86.7%

WOODVALE
Air sanitizer
(Holcomb)

N-Alkyl dimethyl benzyl ammonium
  chloride .... <1%

'76 Ed.

WOODWARD-WANGER'S DRAIN CLEAN
(Woodward-Wanger)

Sodium hydroxide *

'76 Ed.

WOODWARD-WANGER'S DRAIN-PIPE CLEANER
(Woodward-Wanger)

Sodium hydroxide *

'76 Ed.

WOODYOUTH 8028

See WELDWOOD WOODYOUTH 8028

WOOLITE COLD WATER WASH (Liquid)
Wool and delicate fabric detergent
(Boyle-Midway)

Anionic and nonionic detergents *	<30%
Fragrance	trace
Optical brightener	trace

WOOLITE COLD WATER WASH (Powder)
Wool and delicate fabric detergent
(Boyle-Midway)

Anionic detergents *	<25%
Sodium carbonate *	<15%
Fragrance	trace
Optical brightener	trace

WOOLITE GENTLE CYCLE
Cold water wash for machine use
(Boyle-Midway)

Sodium alkyl aryl sulfonate *	<30%
Other Anionic and nonionic surfactants	
Sodium sulfate	
Sodium chloride	
Fragrance	
Dye	

WOOLITE SELF-CLEANING RUG CLEANER
(Boyle-Midway)

Anionic detergents	<5%
Corrosion inhibitor	
Optical brighteners	
Propellants	

WOOLITE SPRAY FOAM RUG CLEANER
(Boyle-Midway)

Anionic and nonionic detergents	<5%
Corrosion inhibitors	
Propellant	

WOOLITE UPHOLSTERY CLEANER
(Boyle-Midway)

Anionic and nonionic detergents	<5%
Glycol ether solvent	
Optical brighteners	
Corrosion inhibitors	
Propellant	

WOOL WASH
(Smith, Robert)

Sulfonated fatty acid amides *†

'76 Ed.

†*See* Alkyl sodium sulfonates

WOOL WASH
In packets
(Reefer-Galler)

Combined amount:	75%
Sodium phosphate *	
Sodium sulfate	
Sodium silicate *	
Linear alkyl benzene sulfonate, *	
Nonionic detergent, Soap	14%
Perfume, brightener, suspending and	
preservative agents	2%
Moisture	9%

'76 Ed.

WORLD'S BEST URN CLEANER
(CFS Continental)

Trisodium phosphate *	>95%

WORM-A-CIDE, MOORMAN'S

See MOORMAN'S WORM-A-CIDE

WORMAL
Feed additive for worming chickens & turkeys
(Salsbury)

Granules:

Butynorate (Dibutyltin dilaurate) *	7.0%
Piperazine base (present as sulfate)	5.5%
Phenothiazine *	29.0%
Fuller's earth	

Tablets (each):

Butynorate (Dibutyltin dilaurate) *	125 mg.
Piperazine base (present as sulfate)	50 mg.
Phenothiazine *	500 mg.

WORM-AWAY - CATS, SERGEANT'S

See SERGEANT'S WORM-AWAY - CATS

WORM-AWAY - DOGS, SERGEANT'S

See SERGEANT'S WORM-AWAY - DOGS

WORM-DOZE

See MOORMAN'S WORM-DOZE

WORTH PARFUMS PRODUCTS

Worth Parfums Corp.
5 E. 57th St.
New York, N.Y. 10022

Phone: 212-752-4150

See COSMETICS, Section VI, General Formulations

WRIGHT'S ANTI-TARNISH SILVER CREAM
(Wright, J.A.)

Water	
Diatomaceous earth	
Polyethylene glycol	<7%
Dithio-bis (stearyl propionate)-62	
Alkyl polyoxyethylene ether	
n-Fatty or n-alkyl trimethyl quaternary ammonium chlorides *†	<2%
Isooctyl phenyl polyethoxy ethanol	
Essential oil	
Citric acid	
Sodium citrate	
Dye	

†*See* Cationic surfactants

WRIGHT'S BRASS CLEANER
(Wright, J.A.)

Water	
Silica	
Aqua ammonia 26° BE	<6%
Oleic acid	
Isopropyl alcohol	<4%
Oxalic acid	3%

WRIGHT'S COPPER CLEANER
(Wright, J.A.)

Water	
Diatomaceous earth	
Stearoyl ethylene cycloimido, Hydroxyethylene sodium alcoholate, Methylene sodium carboxylate	
Salt (NaCl)	
Mono- and Diglycerides	
Polypropylene glycol 1025	<3%
Oxalic acid	<3%
Glycerol monostearate and Polyoxyethylene stearate blend	

WRIGHT'S SILVER CREAM
(Wright, J.A.)

Water	
Diatomaceous earth	
Soap	
Sodium carbonate *	<3%
Essential oil	

Starred ingredients (*) may be responsible for major toxic effects; consult Section II.

WRITE BROS. PENS
(Gillette Co., Paper Mate Div.)

The Gillette Co., Paper Mate Div., Boston, Mass. 02199, will receive collect phone calls from poison control centers or physicians asking for emergency toxicological information about the company's products.

Phone: 617-421-7000

WRM RID
Dewormer for dogs, cats
(Bingman Labs.)

Arecoline hydrobromide *	0.125%
Piperazine dihydrochloride	8.800%
Magnesia oxide	
Calcium carbonate	
Carob flour	
Sugar	
Mineral oil	

"WS" FOGGING CONCENTRATE
Contact insecticide
(Weil Chem.)

Refined Mineral oil *	86.74%
Aromatic petroleum derivative *	10.00%
Malathion	2.00%
Technical Piperonyl butoxide	1.05%
Pyrethrins	0.21%

W-W ROOT DESTROYER
Opens clogged sewers
(Woodward-Wanger)

Sodium hydroxide (Caustic soda) *	>10%
	'76 Ed.

W-W SEPTIC TANK AND CESSPOOL CLEANER
(Woodward-Wanger)

Sodium hydroxide (Caustic soda) *	>10%
	'76 Ed.

W-W SEPTIC TANK ENERGIZER
Aids bacterial action
(Woodward-Wanger)

Sodium bisulfate *	>10%
	'76 Ed.

W-W "TIME SAVER"
Liquid drain opener & cleaner
(Woodward-Wanger)

Potassium hydroxide *	>10%
	'76 Ed.

W.W. - WHITEWALL CLEANER (Liquid)

See GUNK W.W. - WHITEWALL CLEANER (Liquid)

WYANOID OINTMENT
For relief of hemorrhoids
(Wyeth Labs.)

Zinc oxide
Ephedrine sulfate *
Balsam Peru *
Boric acid *
Benzocaine
Emollient base

WYANOIDS
Suppositories for hemorrhoids
(Wyeth Labs.)

Ext. Belladonna (0.19 mg. equiv. total alkaloids)	15 mg.
Zinc oxide	
Bismuth oxyiodide *	
Balsam Peru *	
Ephedrine sulfate	3 mg.
Boric acid *	
Bismuth subcarbonate *	
Cocoa butter	
Beeswax	

WYANOIDS HC
Rectal suppositories
(Wyeth Labs.)

Each suppository:
Hydrocortisone acetate	10 mg.
Extract Belladonna (0.19 mg. equiv. total alkaloids)	15 mg.
Ephedrine sulfate	3 mg.
Zinc oxide	176 mg.
Boric acid *	543 mg.
Bismuth oxyiodide	30 mg.
Bismuth subcarbonate	146 mg.
Peruvian balsam	30 mg.
Cocoa butter	
Beeswax	

WYGESIC TABLETS
Analgesic
(Wyeth Labs.)

Each tablet:
Propoxyphene hydrochloride *	65 mg.
Acetaminophen *	650 mg.

WYNN'S CARBURETOR CLEANER (Aerosol)
(Wynn Oil Co.)

	approx. %
Xylene *	35%
Acetone	35%
Diacetone alcohol	12%
Propane propellant	18%

WYNN'S ENGINE TUNE-UP
Solvent cleaner to be added to engine oil
(Wynn Oil Co.)

Naphthenic oil *	approx. 90%
Mixture of solvents:	approx. 10%
Butyl carbitol	
Butyl Cellosolve	
Methyl isobutyl carbinol	
Diacetone alcohol	
Cyclohexanone	

WYNN'S X-TEND CARBURETOR CLEANER (Aerosol)
(Wynn Oil Co.)

	approx. %
Xylene *	35%
Acetone	35%
Diacetone alcohol	12%
Propane propellant	18%

WYNN'S X-TEND ENGINE TUNE-UP
Solvent cleaner to be added to engine oil
(Wynn Oil Co.)

Naphthenic oil *	approx. 90%
Mixture of solvents:	approx. 10%
Butyl carbitol	
Butyl Cellosolve	
Methyl isobutyl carbinol	
Diacetone alcohol	
Cyclohexanone	

X

X-ALL
Herbicide
(Amchem)

3-Amino-1,2,4-triazole	4.2%
2-Chloro-4,6-bis(ethylamino)-s-triazine *	12.6%

X-ALL CONCENTRATE
Herbicide
(Amchem)

3-Amino-1,2,4-triazole	15.0%
2-Chloro-4,6-bis(ethylamino)-s-triazine *	45.0%

X-DRIN CAPSULES
Aid in appetite control
(Pharmex)

Each capsule:
Vitamin A	1333 USP units
Vitamin D	133 USP units
Iron (as fumarate)	3.33 mg.
Benzocaine	6.5 mg.
Plus polyvitamins and minerals	

X-DRIN TABLETS
Aid in appetite control
(Pharmex)

Each tablet:
Carboxymethylcellulose ..... 7 1/2 gr.
Phenylpropanolamine * ..... 25 mg.
Benzocaine .... 1/12 gr.

XORU-OX LIQUID OIL CONCENTRATE WEED KILLER
(Stewart Sanitary Supply)

Monuron trichloroacetate * 32.25%

XORU-OX MANUFACTURING CONCENTRATE FOR MANUFACTURING USE ONLY
(Stewart Sanitary Supply)

Monuron trichloroacetate * 32.25%

X-OTAG S.R.
Skeletal muscle relaxant
(Direct Div.)

Each tablet:
Orphenadrine citrate * ...... 100 mg.

XOX BLEACH
Sodium hypochlorite solution
(Thoro)

Water 94.75%
Sodium hypochlorite * 5.25%

X-PANDO NO. 77 MOSAIC CEMENT
(X-Pando)

Magnesium oxysulfate *

X-PANDO PIPE JOINT COMPOUND
(X-Pando)

Magnesium oxychloride *

X-PANDOSEAL, STANDARD FORMULA
(X-Pando)

Hydrocarbons *†
Gums
Resins

†*See* Petroleum hydrocarbons

X-PANDOTITE
(X-Pando)

Magnesium oxychloride *

X-PANDO TRAV MAR
Waterproofing basement walls; general adhesive
(X-Pando)

Epoxy resin
Ethylene diamine

X-PECTORINE
For emphysema, chronic bronchitis & bronchial asthma
(Recsei Labs.)

Each tablet:
Potassium iodide * .... 500 mg.
Guaifenesin .... 100 mg.

XPERT SATIN SHEEN POLYURETHANE CLEAR (Y-4035)
Protective coating for finishing wood surfaces
(Glidden)

Pigment:
Silica aerogel 0.6%
Vehicle:
Linseed urethane resin (Type I) 13.0%
Mineral spirits * and Driers * . 18.8%
Ketone 16.5%
Halogenated hydrocarbon * ... 26.6%
Propellant: 24.5%
Isobutane
Propane

XSEB SHAMPOO
(Baker-Cummins)

Salicylic acid * 4%

XSEB-T SHAMPOO
(Baker-Cummins)

Coal tar solution * 10%
Salicylic acid * 4%

X-SECT INSECTICIDE
(National Chemsearch)

Petroleum distillates *
Essential oils *
N-Octyl bicycloheptene dicarboximide *
Piperonyl butoxide technical
Pyrethrins

X-7 COMPOUND - DECARBONIZER, DEGREASER AND PAINT STRIPPER FOR TANK USE (Liquid)

See GUNK X-7 COMPOUND - DECARBONIZER, DEGREASER AND PAINT STRIPPER FOR TANK USE (Liquid)

X-TEND CARBURETOR CLEANER (Aerosol)

See WYNN'S X-TEND CARBURETOR CLEANER (Aerosol)

X-TEND ENGINE TUNE-UP

See WYNN'S X-TEND ENGINE TUNE-UP

X-TERM 50
Insecticide
(Cotton States Chem.)

Heptachlor * 22.68%
Related compounds 8.82%
Aromatic petroleum distillates * 64.50%

X-WAX
For removal of wax from ear canals and prevention of cerumen build-up
(CMC Research Div.)

Allantoin
Ethoxylated lanolin
Water
Polysorbate 60
Polysorbate 80
Benzethonium chloride *
Methyl paraben sorbic acid

XYLOCAINE JELLY
Local anesthetic
(Astra Pharm.)

Each ml.:
Lidocaine hydrochloride ..... 20 mg.
Methyl-p-hydroxybenzoate ... 0.7 mg.
Propyl-p-hydroxybenzoate .... 0.3 mg.
Sodium hydroxide ...... to adjust pH
Sodium carboxymethylcellulose

XYLOCAINE OINTMENT 2.5%
Topical anesthetic
(Astra Pharm.)

Lidocaine 2.5%
In a water miscible ointment:
Polyethylene glycols
Propylene glycol

XYLOCAINE OINTMENT 5%
Topical anesthetic
(Astra Pharm.)

Lidocaine 5%
In a water miscible ointment:
Polyethylene glycols
Propylene glycol

XYLOCAINE SUPPOSITORIES
For pain of hemorrhoids
(Astra Pharm.)

Each suppository:
Lidocaine .... 100 mg.
Bismuth subgallate .... 115 mg.
Zinc oxide .... 375 mg.
Aluminum subacetate .... 75 mg.
Peruvian balsam .... 100 mg.
Neutral glycerides of saturated
vegetable fatty acids q.s.-ad 2.6 gm.

Starred ingredients (*) may be responsible for major toxic effects; consult Section II.

XYLOCAINE VISCOUS
Topical anesthetic; for mouth and pharynx
(Astra Pharm.)

Lidocaine HCl 2%
Sodium carboxymethylcellulose
Flavoring

Y

YAGER'S LINIMENT
For relief of minor aches and pains
(Yager)

Active ingred.:
Camphor * 3.1%
Oil of turpentine 8.0%
Inactive ingred.:
Clove oil (fragrance)
Castor oil (emollient)
Ammonium oleate (penetrant base, less than 0.5% free ammonia)

YALE BULK TANK CLEANER
Dairy use
(Yale Chem. Co.)

Sodium tripolyphosphate .... >35%
Soda ash * .... >35%
Sodium metasilicate * .... <20%
Sodium dichloroisocyanurate ..... >2%
Alkyl aryl sulfonate .... <4%

YALE'S IODE UDDER WASH
Cleaner sanitizer
(Yale Chem. Co.)

Nonylphenoxypoly (ethyleneoxy) ethanol-iodine complex (providing 1.75% titratable iodine) 14.25%
Phosphoric acid * 12.50%

YARDLEY COSMETICS & TOILETRIES

Yardley of London, Inc.
875 N. Michigan Ave.
Chicago, Ill. 60611

Phone: 312-951-7100

See COSMETICS, Section VI, General Formulations

YATES-ASTRO ROACH KILLER CONCENTRATE
Insecticide
(Yates-Astro)

O,O-Diethyl O-(2-isopropyl-4-methyl-6-pyrimidinyl)phosphorothioate * 18.50%
Piperonyl butoxide, technical ... 3.08%
Pyrethrins 0.31%
Aromatic petroleum derivative solvent * 63.11%

YELLOW STUFF
Neutral cleaner
(Paul Koss)

Water .... >80%
Monoethanolammonium dodecylbenzene sulfonate (Anionic surfactant)
Butyl Cellosolve * .... <6%
Fatty amido phosphate
Perfume .... trace
Dye .... trace
Formalin .... trace
pH 7.6-7.8

YES

See TEXIZE YES

YOUNGER THAN SPRINGTIME
Dermophilic moisture cream
(Aquamint Labs.)

Each ingredient less than 10%/w.:
Mineral oil
Glycerin
Cosmetic lanolin (trace)
Stearyl dimethyl benzyl ammonium chloride *
Stearyl alcohol
Glyceryl monostearate
Stearic acid diethanolamine
Benzoic acid

YVES ROCHER COSMETICS

Yves Rocher Inc.
2909 MacArthur Blvd.
Northbrook, Ill. 60062

Phone: 312-498-6115

See COSMETICS, Section VI, General Formulations

YVES SAINT LAURENT PERFUMES

Yves Saint Laurent Parfums
40 W. 57th St.
New York, N.Y. 10019

Phone: 212-621-7327

See COSMETICS, Section VI, General Formulations

Z

ZACTANE TABLETS
Analgesic
(Wyeth Labs.)

Each tablet:
Ethoheptazine citrate * ...... 75 mg.

ZACTIRIN COMPOUND - 100
Analgesic
(Wyeth Labs.)

Each tablet:
Ethoheptazine citrate * ...... 100 mg.
Aspirin * .... 227 mg.
Phenacetin .... 162 mg.
Caffeine .... 32.4 mg.

ZACTIRIN TABLETS
Analgesic
(Wyeth Labs.)

Each tablet:
Ethoheptazine citrate * ...... 75 mg.
Aspirin (5 gr.) * .... 325 mg.

ZAR
(United Gilsonite)

Oil modified polyurethane 52%
Mineral spirits * 48%

ZAR REDWOOD STAIN-FINISH
(United Gilsonite)

Pigment: 5.00%
Iron oxide * 85.0%
Silicates 15.0%
Vehicle: 95.00%
Vinyl acetate copolymer ... 5.8%
Safflower alkyd 5.8%
Fungicidal ingredients: 0.1%
Thiazolyl-benzimidazole . 100%
Water 88.3%

ZARUMIN
Relief of joint aches, pains
(Williams, J.B.)

Each tablet:
Salicylamide .... 4.0 gr.
Potassium salicylate * .... 3.5 gr.

Z-C DUST

See NIAGARA Z-C DUST

Z-C SPRAY

See NIAGARA Z-C SPRAY

ZEASORB
Highly absorbent medicated powder
(Stiefel Labs.)

Para-chloro-meta-xylenol 0.5%
Allantoin salts 0.2%
Microporous cellulose

ZEEN, ODORLESS

See ODORLESS ZEEN

Starred ingredients (*) may be responsible for major toxic effects; consult Section II.

ZEMO LOTION
(Plough)

Specially denatured alcohol #38B	37.00% w/w
Boric acid *	1.80% w/w
Borax	0.37% w/w
Potassium nitrate	0.37% w/w
Sodium salicylate	0.45% w/w
Benzoic acid	0.45% w/w
Glycerine	
Phenol 90% solution *	

ZEMO OINTMENT
(Plough)

D & C Red No. 17	
Wax	
Irgasan DP-300	0.1% w/w
ortho Iodobenzoic acid	0.266% w/w
Zinc oxide	5.36% w/w
Bismuth subnitrate	3.99% w/w
Sodium salicylate	0.851% w/w
Boric acid *	1.72% w/w
Benzoic acid	0.31% w/w
Menthol *	
Methyl salicylate *	2.25% w/w
Aromatic oils *†	

†See Essential oils

ZEN
Vitreous cleaner
(Holcomb)

Hydrochloric acid *	20.0%

'76 Ed.

ZEPHIRAN CHLORIDE
Antiseptic, germicide
(Winthrop Labs.)

High molecular, Alkyl dimethyl-benzyl ammonium chlorides *

ZEPINE
Antihypertensive
(Foy Labs.)

Each tablet:	
Reserpine	0.25 mg.

ZEP MANUFACTURING CO. PRODUCTS

Zep Manufacturing Co.
1310 Seaboard Industrial Blvd., N.W.
P.O. Box 2015
Atlanta, Ga. 30301

In emergency, after business hours:
Dr. Fineman: 404-252-1587
Dan Padgett: 404-435-2973
Bob Beach: 404-351-2952
Wayne Canady: 404-971-3367

In emergency, during business hours:
Dr. Fineman: 404-352-1680
Dan Padgett: 404-352-1680
Bob Beach: 404-352-1680
Wayne Canady: 404-352-1680

"006" WEED KILLER
(Hysan Corp.)

Petroleum oil *	96.10%
2,4-Dichlorophenoxyacetic acid, isooctyl ester	1.09%
Bromacil (5-Bromo-3-sec-butyl-6-methyluracil)	0.61%
Pentachlorophenol	0.80%
Other chlorophenols	0.09%

ZEST
Soap-synthetic detergent bar
(Procter & Gamble)

Soap from animal and vegetable fats	50-74%
Anionic synthetic detergent	25-49%
Sodium sulfate and Sodium chloride	5-9%
Water	5-9%
3,4,4'-Trichlorocarbanilide	<1%
Minor ingredients, each	<1%

pH (1% solution) - 10.0

ZETAR EMULSION (For the Bath and for Rx Compounding)
Generalized recalcitrant dermatoses
(Dermik)

Whole Coal tar *	300 mg./ml.
Inactive ingred.:	
Ethoxylated saturated & unsaturated fatty acid esters	

ZETAR SHAMPOO
For relief of scalp conditions
(Dermik)

Colloidal whole Coal tar	1%
p-Chloro-m-xylenol	0.5%

ZIDE
Diuretic
(Direct Div.)

Each tablet:	
Hydrochlorothiazide *	50 mg.

ZINCFRIN
For minor ocular irritations
(Alcon)

Each ml.:	
Zinc sulfate	0.25%
Phenylephrine HCl	0.12%
Benzalkonium chloride	0.01%

ZINCOFAX SOOTHING SKIN CREAM
(Burroughs Wellcome)

Zinc oxide	15%
Lanolin	

ZINCON
Dandruff shampoo
(Lederle)

Zinc pyrithione	1%

ZINSSER, WM., PAINTS PRODUCTS
Primer sealers, shellacs, floor finishes and wallpaper strippers

William Zinsser & Co., Inc.
39 Belmont Dr.
Somerset, N.J. 08873

Phone: 201-469-8100

See PAINTS, Section VI, General Formulations

ZIP
Fire starter
(French, R. T.)

Kerosene *	<85%
Resin	<10%
Emulsifier (Sodium sulfonates)	<1%
Hydrochloric acid	<1%
Chalk	<1%
Water	

ZIPCIDE CATTLE DUST BAG
Insecticide
(Hess & Clark)

Coumaphos *	1%

ZIPCIDE CATTLE DUST BAG, UNICO

See UNICO ZIPCIDE CATTLE DUST BAG

ZIPCIDE 1% CO-RAL DUST
Insecticide
(Hess & Clark)

Coumaphos *	1%

ZIPCIDE GREEN BAG
Insecticide
(Hess & Clark)

Coumaphos *	1%

ZIPCIDE REFILL CARTRIDGE
Insecticide
(Hess & Clark)

Coumaphos *	1%

ZIPCIDE "R" REFILL BAG
Insecticide
(Hess & Clark)

Coumaphos *	1%

Starred ingredients (*) may be responsible for major toxic effects; consult Section II.

ZIP-KLEEN
Brush cleaner
(Star Bronze)

Methylene chloride *
Mineral spirits *
Ethyl alcohol
Methanol .... <4%
Pine oil *
Acetone *

ZIP MECHANIC'S BORATED HAND SOAP

See C-Z ZIP MECHANIC'S BORATED HAND SOAP

ZIPOLA
Zipper lubricant
(High Chem.)

Petroleum waxes
Perchlorethylene base *

'76 Ed.

ZIPPO LIGHTER FLUID
(Zippo Mfg. Co.)

Paraffins *
Naphthenes *
Aromatics *† .... <10%

†*See* Aromatic hydrocarbons

ZIP-STRIP
(Star Bronze)

Methylene chloride *
Mineral spirits *
Ethyl alcohol
Methanol .... <4%

ZIP-ZORB OIL & GREASE ABSORBENT
(Waverly Mineral Products Co.)

Aluminum-magnesium silicate
Iron oxide .... small amounts

ZIRADRYL LOTION
For poison ivy or oak
(Parke-Davis)

Benadryl hydrochloride * 1%
Zirconium oxide (as the carbonate) .. 2%
Camphor
Alcohol 2%

ZIZO, LIQUID
Drain cleaner
(Hillyard Chem.)

Potassium hydroxide *

'76 Ed.

ZNLIN
For poison ivy, poison oak, sunburn and skin allergies
(Herald Pharm.)

Zinc oxide *
Calcium hydroxide
Mineral oil
Nonionic emulsifiers *

ZOALENE COCCIDIOSTAT
Poultry parasiticide
(Dow)

3,5-Dinitro-o-toluamide
(minimum) * 98%

ZOAMIX
Medicated premix for poultry
(Dow)

3,5-Dinitro-o-toluamide * 25%
Inert ingredients: 75%
Soybean oil
Soybean meal

ZOAMIX N COCCIDIOSTAT PREMIX
Poultry parasiticide
(Dow)

Active ingred.:
3,5-Dinitro-o-toluamide * 25%
3-Nitro-4-hydroxyphenylarsonic
acid * 10%
Inert ingred.: 65%
Soybean meal
Soybean oil
Pyrogenic Silica

ZODEAC-100 TABLETS
Vitamins
(Econo Med)

Each tablet:
Zinc sulfate (dried)(zinc 15
mg.) .... 41.55 mg.
Ferrous fumarate (iron 60
mg.) .... 192.00 mg.
Vitamin A palmitate ...... 8000 I.U.
Vitamin D (Ergocalciferol) 400 I.U.
With multivitamins and minerals

ZOES BLACK LEATHER DYE
(Zoes, C.A.)

o-Dichlorobenzene *

ZOES SUEDE DYE AND DRESSING
For shoes
(Zoes, C.A.)

Water base
Proprietary solvent alcohol

ZOKON PAINT REMOVER
(Lester Labs.)

Mild Alkali *
Methylene chloride *

'76 Ed.

ZONIUM CHLORIDE CONCENTRATE
Antiseptic
(Lannett)

Benzalkonium
chloride * .... 12.8%, 17% and 50%

ZONIUM CHLORIDE SOLUTION
Antiseptic
(Lannett)

Benzalkonium chloride 1:1000

ZONK
Cleaner/degreaser/deodorizer
(Paul Koss)

Water .... >90%
Nonylphenoxypoly(ethyleneoxy)ethanol
(Nonionic surfactant)
Sodium carbonate
Sodium metasilicate
Alkyl dimethyl benzyl ammonium
chloride * .... <2%
Coco amido betaine
Tetrasodium EDTA
Sodium hydroxide
Dye .... trace
Optical brightener .... trace
Silicone defoamer .... trace

ZON-KIL, DEL

See DEL ZON-KIL

ZOOM SPRAY CLEANER CONCENTRATE

See AMWAY ZOOM SPRAY CLEANER CONCENTRATE

ZORATOR TOILET BOWL DEODORANT
Floral or pine scented
(Curran)

Paradichlorobenzene * 100%

'76 Ed.

ZOREX PERFUMED PARA MOTH PAD (Rose & Pine)
(Curran)

Paradichlorobenzene *

'76 Ed.

Starred ingredients (*) may be responsible for major toxic effects; consult Section II.

ZOTOS HAIR CARE PRODUCTS

Zotos International, Inc.
100 Tokeneke Rd.
Darien, Conn. 06820

Phone: 203-655-8911

See COSMETICS, Section VI, General Formulations

ZP RODENT BAIT
(Bell Labs., Inc.)

Zinc phosphide *	2%
Blend of food grade cereals	98%

ZP RODENT BAIT AG
(Bell Labs., Inc.)

Zinc phosphide *	2%
Blend of food grade cereals	98%

ZP TRACKING POWDER
Rodenticide
(Bell Labs., Inc.)

Zinc phosphide *	10%
Carriers	90%

ZUD
Cleanser for removing rust and stains
(Boyle-Midway)

Silica (abrasives)

Oxalic acid *	1-10%

ZURD
Rodenticide
(Murd Co.)

Warfarin	0.025%

Sulfaquinoxaline

'76 Ed.

ZYMACAP CAPSULES
Vitamin deficiencies
(Upjohn)

Each capsule:

Vitamin A	5000 I.U.
Vitamin D	400 I.U.

Plus multivitamins

ZYMALIXIR
Hematinic
(Upjohn)

Each 5 ml.:

Iron (from 130 mg. ferrous gluconate)	15 mg.
Liver concentrate	65 mg.
Alcohol	1.5%

Plus multivitamins

ZYMASYRUP
Dietary supplement
(Upjohn)

Each 5 ml.:

Vitamin A	5000 I.U.
Vitamin D	400 I.U.
Alcohol	2%

Plus multivitamins

ZYMOLE TROKEYS
(Consolid. Royal)

Menthol *
Oil of eucalyptus *
Oil of red thyme *
Oil of peppermint *
Gum acacia

'76 Ed.

ZYNOLYTE PAINT PRODUCTS

Zynolyte Products Co.
15700 S. Avalon Blvd.
Compton, Calif. 90224

Phone: 213-321-6964

SECTION VI

General Formulations

Compiled with the assistance of Carol Glasgow, M.S., Jean Braddock, Patricia Greeno, and Kathleen McNamara. Other acknowledgments are given below.

INTRODUCTION

In this section are given in alphabetical order several hundred formulas for products and preparations commonly found in households and on farms. These formulas are offered as a guide to the probable composition of any product that is not specially listed by brand name in the Trade Name Index (Section V). A precise statement is not important; formulas are needed only to orient the physician. His questions are:

What kinds of material are usually employed? Are there any highly toxic components? About what percentage of the product is the toxic component? What can be said about its toxic nature?

Directions for Use

1. Use Section VI when ingredients are unknown.
   a. If the category of use is known but the trade name is unknown; cᴀ
   b. Specifically, if the trade name is known and the category of use (furniture polish, laundry bleach) is known but ingredients are not listed in the Trade Name Index. Note that addresses of manufacturers are listed in Section VII.
2. Consult Table of Contents on p. VI-7, the alphabetical listing of categories of use.
3. Consult appropriate formula.
   a. Note toxicity rating.
   b. Note ingredients starred (asterisks). The starred ingredient may be responsible for major toxic effects.
4. Consult Ingredients Index, Section II.

The Table of Contents

The key to the General Formulations Section lies on p. VI-7. This thoroughly cross-indexed list should be examined for the common name, category of use, or type of product responsible for the poisoning. The index category refers by page number to a statement of composition.

Here are given a formula and a list of constituents.

The Formula

The formula is a "typical" or "basic" or "representative" one. In many formulas, the percentage of each constituent is indicated; these are at best only approximations. The formulas obviously cannot literally describe all products, but they can illustrate for each category something of the proportions that are frequently employed. The formulas do give considerable guidance when ingredients are not known or cannot easily be found; for example, specific ingredients are not listed for some products in the Trade Name Index (Section V). A number of reasons may be cited for these omissions. Sometimes the coverage is incomplete, and the product is not listed. In some cases the composition is a trade secret, and information is deliberately withheld; in others the composition varies with the availability or the market price of raw materials, and the manufacturer cannot vouch for the formula a month, a year, or even a few days hence and therefore says nothing.

As presented here the "formulations" are heterogeneous; some merely list "standard" or well known ingredients (for example, *modeling clay*: kaolin, gypsum, petrolatum, wax, castor oil, vegetable dye); others give a prototype formula (*e.g., wood polish, cream type*: mineral oil, 55%; emulsifying agent, 3%; isopropanol, 4%; water, 38%); still others indicate, for each constituent, ranges of composition sometimes quite wide which reflect the variability of current practice (*e.g., granular detergents (light-duty/delicate fabrics)*: anionic surfactant, 14–36%; sodium sulfate, 25–42%; sodium tripolyphosphate, 0–33%; sodium silicate, 0–18%; sodium chloride, 0–14%; sodium perborate, 0–6%; polyethylene glycol, 0–1%; soap, 0–1%; sodium xylene sulfonate or sodium toluene sulfonate, 0–1%). There is no guarantee that any of these formulas in use contains all of the ingredients. Many were adapted from correspondence with manufacturers, some from encyclopedias, reference books, textbooks, and the scientific literature. Some are composites made from scanning the product formulas in the Trade Name Index. In a number of categories, ingredients of these products were tabulated in the order of their use frequency; these statistics were used as guides for the general formulations ultimately proposed.

The "May Contain" List

In addition to the formula or list under each category title, there is a second list headed "may contain." These substances have been compiled from many sources: (a) product labels, (b) letters from manufacturers, (c) reference books and (d) personal communications. No consistent screening has been applied to remove obsolescent, rare, or experimental materials. There is no guarantee on the other hand that the lists are exhaustively complete. Imperfect as they are, no better source of readily available information is known to us. On occasion, data may be found here to explain a puzzling reaction; for instance, these lists should be of help to allergists.

Toxicity Ratings in Section VI

Each general formulations category has been given a toxicity rating to assist the physician in making a prognosis when his patient has ingested some product for which knowledge of the precise composition is unobtainable. If the toxicity rating is low (1 or 2), the hazard is low. For certain formulations, one or more ingredients are starred (asterisk). Starred ingredients may be found in the Ingredients Index (Section II). References are provided in the Ingredients Index (Section II) to the Therapeutic Index (Section III) for a description of toxic symptoms and of recommended treatment for poisonings by selected substances.

In assignment of a toxicity rating, the point of view has been conservative. By this is meant that the toxicity rating describes the most toxic of several alternative formulations. As an example, the toxicity rating of cutting oils, insoluble type, may be considered. These mixtures of mineral oils, fatty oils, sulfur, chlorinated hydrocarbons and phosphates, except for the chlorinated hydrocarbons and phosphates, might be given a toxicity rating of 2. The phosphates are present in small percentages so that only if the percentage of the chlorinated hydrocarbons is high enough will a higher toxicity rating be required. For example, if the oil contains 1–10% chlorinated hydrocarbons, the product would be given a toxicity rating of 3. Therefore, the toxicity rating 2 or 3 is given to this category. The toxicity rating may thus be interpreted as "probably not more toxic than" the estimate given. A corollary is that a product may have a toxicity less than that listed for the category. Although this may appear to be a discrimination against the safer formula, caution demands such advice. Since our intent is solely to assist the doctor in planning emergency treatment, a con-

servative position is the only defensible one. In the "may contain" lists are certain ingredients whose toxicity would be sufficient to increase the toxicity rating of the product above that assigned (if that ingredient is present in sufficient or usual percentages). We have stated the toxicity rating of the product *in that case* at the right of the same line with the ingredient responsible. For example, the toxicity rating for the category of "Abrasive cleaners" is 2; in the "may contain" list is sodium perborate which in sufficient percentage would give the product a toxicity rating of 3.

In certain categories, no general toxicity rating is given, *e.g.*, "chlorinated solvents"; instead, toxicity ratings are listed for each solvent. It is obviously difficult to guess the toxicity of a mixture for which the percentage composition is not given; the difficulty is heightened for mixtures in which the percentage of one component may vary widely (*e.g.*, the alcohol content in cleaning fluids). In fact, the uncertainties are so great that we have been repeatedly tempted to omit the toxicity ratings in this section. The decision to offer them is based on day-to-day experience. When calls come from the emergency department, the toxicologist is always asked to evaluate the toxicity of ingested material regardless of acknowledged imperfections in his knowledge.

In general, toxicity ratings are not given for agricultural products because the active components are usually known from the label. (See also trade names and chemical names under Pesticides in this section.) Many of the active components are listed in the Ingredients Index (Section II).

How to Assign Toxicity Ratings to Products

The following remarks are designed to guide the physician or toxicologist who proposes to assign an appropriate toxicity rating to any commercial product. As described in detail in the introduction to Section II, toxicity ratings are estimates of lethality and reflect the approximate amount of any "poison" that must be ingested per kilogram of body weight to kill a typical victim. The exact but arbitrary limits that define each numerical toxicity class are specified in Table VI-1. The techniques outlined below were used to select the ratings in Section VI, as well as all unpublished ratings in our files. See also: R. E. Gosselin, *Journal of the American Medical Association, 163*: 1333, 1957.

Two ways are available for assessing the toxicity of commercial mixtures (when the most meaningful data—the effects of known doses in the human—are unknown). First, the product itself can be given to laboratory animals to esti-

Table VI-1

Toxicity Rating or Class	Probable Oral LETHAL Dose (Human)	
	Dose (mg./kg.)	For 70-kg. Person (150 lb.)
6 Super toxic	<5	A taste (less than 7 drops)
5 Extremely toxic	5–50	Between 7 drops and 1 tsp.
4 Very toxic	50–500	Between 1 tsp. and 1 oz.
3 Moderately toxic	0.5–5	Between 1 oz. and 1 pt. (or 1 lb.)
2 Slightly toxic	5–15	Between 1 pt. and 1 qt.
1 Practically nontoxic	>15	More than 1 qt. (2.2 lb.)

mate (a) the lethal dose, (b) the nature of the toxic syndrome, and (c) the target organ sustaining damage if any. Manufacturers secure these data about their own merchandise, and increasing numbers furnish this information to us. Second, most toxicity ratings in our files, however, are based on another method of estimation, which requires a toxicological appraisal of each ingredient in the commercial mixture. Ideally the identity of every constituent and the complete composition should be known; in practice, full information is seldom available and seldom essential. Whenever Section II contains information about the lethality of single ingredients when tested separately, the probable lethal dose of a commercial product can be inferred if one is willing to assume that all constituents act independently and have neither additive nor antagonistic effects. Except when two or more ingredients are chemically related, this simplifying assumption is believed to be permissible in most cases because the final estimates are not intended to be precise. Another way of stating our working hypothesis is this: **the presumptive lethal dose of a commercial mixture may be gauged as the smallest quantity which contains a fatal amount of any <u>one</u> of its constituents.** By this operational definition, the toxicity of a mixture is determined solely by one of its ingredients (or one group of chemically related ingredients), all others being regarded as diluents. This critical ingredient is designated in Sections V and VI by an asterisk, but only if the ingredient is present in sufficient concentration to give the product an overall toxicity rating of 3 or more.

To illustrate these remarks, hypothetical examples are useful. Because of inadequate data for man, the acute toxicity of 2,4-dichlorophenol cannot be specified precisely, but the lethal dose is generally believed to lie somewhere within range of 50 to 500 mg./kg., *i.e.*, within the toxicity class 4. Any product containing dichlorophenol as the only significant toxic ingredient would be assigned (a) a toxicity rating of 4 if the concentration of propylene dichloride were

greater than 10%, (b) a rating of 3 if the concentration lay between 1 and 10%, and (c) a toxicity rating of 2 if the concentration lay between 0.1 and 1%. In other words, a factor of 10 is used in going from one toxicity rating to another. Obviously these limits are arbitrary, but a convention of this kind is an operational necessity in most cases. Where the acute toxicity lies near the border of toxicity ranges 3 and 4, which is the case for xylene, the toxicity rating of 4 would be given if the concentration of xylene were 20% or more; a rating of 3, for concentrations between 2 and 20%; or a rating of 2, for concentrations between 0.2 and 2%. Boundary values are unnecessary whenever the lethal dose of the only starred ingredient is comparatively well established (*e.g.*, 0.4 gm./kg. for aspirin). As another example, a product composed half of benzene and half of carbon tetrachloride would be assigned a rating of 4, and both components would receive an asterisk. A product made half of benzene and half of kerosens would also be rated 4, but only the benzene would be starred, since the rating of pure kerosene is 3, *i.e.*, approximately ¹⁄₁₀ as toxic as benzene.

For products of unknown percentage composition, the assignment of toxicity rating becomes an elaborate guess. If the most toxic ingredient is thought to be present in substantial amounts (perhaps 20% or more), the product is rated as though that ingredient were present in pure form. Whenever it is obvious that the most toxic substance is a minor constituent, the rating is lowered as seems best to fit the circumstances. Doubt is always resolved in favor of the higher rating.

When ratings are established for products in which the "dangerous" ingredient is one with long and widespread human experience, *e.g.*, ethyl alcohol or sulfur, the toxicity ratings are assigned by utilizing available information of the effects on man. In these cases the systems described above based on limits of 100-10-1-0.1% or of 100-20-2-0.2% may not be followed rigorously.

We believe that these toxicity ratings can be

useful devices for designating the lethality of bulk products, such as powders, solutions, emulsions, ointments, etc., where the composition is commonly stated as percentages. For products marketed as single units—tablets, pills, capsules, suppositories, troches, etc.—the composition often is not fully described. For example, the composition of a tablet is commonly designated by the number of milligrams of active ingredient per tablet, without stating the nature or amounts of active binders, fillers, etc. Both the physician and the layman are conditioned to specify the dose by the number of tablets, and this is true of toxic as well as therapeutic doses. From the number of tablets and the quantity of drug in each, the total dose is revealed; this can be compared with the lethal dose published in Section II for several of the commoner drugs. In this scheme a toxicity rating is unnecessary and awkward, but for the purpose of product research it was thought worthwhile to assign toxicity ratings to these unit-dose medicaments. To do this it was necessary first to estimate the total weight of each pill, tablet, capsule, etc., so that the concentrations of active ingredients could be calculated. C. J. Latiolais, the former chief pharmacist at the Strong Memorial Hospital, reported the unit sizes that are usually encountered in standard pharmaceuticals, and selected an average or typical unit weight for each item. These values are presented in Table VI-2. By pretending, for example, that all capsules weigh the same (0.25 gm. according to the average in Table VI-2), toxicity ratings were assigned to all drug products in this compilation.

To summarize: the toxicity rating of a product is intended to describe its degree of acute lethality when ingested. Any rating assigned by the methods described here is necessarily provisional and should never be treated as a constant or a known value. At least three kinds of uncertainty are commonly encountered, viz., unknown are (1) the exact and complete composition of the product, (2) the precise toxicity of each separate ingredient, and (3) the possibility of chemical or biological interactions between the various constituents. As with all judgment values, honest differences of opinion are inevitable, and most borderline products could readily be upgraded or downgraded by one toxicity class. Obviously one must avoid the error of pretending that all products with the same rating are equally toxic. Toxicity ratings are only guideposts, intended to supplement but never to substitute for special knowledge, common sense, or sound clinical judgment.

Acknowledgments

Ideally these formulations should be prepared by well qualified technologists who authoritatively cite ranges of composition based on types of materials and select the formulas most characteristic of products in each category. Ideally the toxicity ratings should then be made by equally expert industrial toxicologists who could draw on special privileged information. For this edition, at our request about 130 leading manufacturers of various categories of products reviewed the formulations given in the fourth edition and characterized them as up-to-date and adequate or, on the other hand, as obsolete or needing additional formulas. Many sent sample formulas which in their expert opinions represented those most likely to be used currently. In a number of instances they gave either specific percentage compositions or ranges of compositions frequently encountered. Several of these lists are incorporated almost as received. It is a pleasure to acknowledge the assistance of James M. McNerny of the Cosmetics, Toiletries and Fragrances Association (CTFA) for assistance in preparing the section on the general formulations of cosmetics. We were permitted to draw on a compendium of formulations recently developed by the CTFA. It is a pleasure also to acknowledge the assistance of Peter Hay, Sandoz Colors & Chemicals; J. Laurence Robinson, Dry Color Manufacturers' Association; Laurence D. Gill, Mobay Chemical Corporation; Ala-

Table VI-2[a]

	Weight Range (gm.)	Average (gm.)
Capsules	0.1–1.4	0.25
Tablets (compressed)	0.04–2.4	0.35
Tablets (enteric coated)	0.1–1.7	0.80
Tablets (sugar coated)	0.1–1.0	0.40
Pills	0.15–0.4	0.32
Troches	1.0–2.5	1.5
Suppositories		2.0
Granules, effervescent contain 80% inert ingredients		

[a] Values assigned by C. J. Latiolais.

dar Burgyan, Ferro Corporation; and Philip L. Flor, Magruder Tartan Colors, for the many revisions in the section on Pigments which has been divided into two parts, Pigments and Dyes, at their suggestion; of Elmer A. Bannan, Jack Griffith, and James Weaver of Proctor and Gamble for the sections on detergents and soaps; of Carol Glasgow who labored diligently to compile the list of Common Formulations of Pesticides.

Many manufacturers sent us useful information; to our regret it is impossible to mention each contributor individually. Their letters often included critically valuable data, e.g., unpublished toxicity measurements of products or constituents, as well as advice on their experience with accidental misuse of their products, or names and telephone numbers of responsible members of their staffs who can be reached in an emergency.

The following men and women and the companies they represent have also given valuable information and advice:

Joan E. Young, Corporate Regulatory Affairs and Product Safety, Airwick Industries; Robert J. Hillerman, Production Development Manager, Allied Materials Corp.; Al Furman, Vice President, Alsol Products, Inc.; Bipin Patol, Chemist, American Art Clay Co. Inc.; W. C. Helmgren, Technical Director, American Greasestick Co.; Richard D. Snodgrass, Chief Chemist, The Anderson Co.; James Schmitt, Applied Biochemists; Roger C. Steinhauer, Textiles, Household Products Research & Development Dept., Armour-Deal, Inc.; Arrow Laboratories; H. J. Matson, Manager Product Specifications, Atlantic Richfield Co.; Yale Gressel, Manager, Toxicology, Avon Products, Inc.; James B. Backes, President, M. Backes Sons, Inc.; Arthur J. Kiehn, Chief Chemist, Bardahl Mfg. Corp.; M. W. Rosenthal, Vice President, Research & Development, Block Drug Co., Inc.; Dr. R. Golden, Borden Chemical; Gene F. Tappan, Boyle-Midway; Joseph A. Corrandono, Carbona Products Co.; Fred J. Landolf, General Manager, Carbona Products Co.; G. Conlon, The Carter's Ink Co.; Saul Bell, Cheseborough-Pond's, Inc., C. R. Biesel, Biomedical Research Coordinator, Clairol Research Laboratories; G. Spangler, Cling Surface Co.; Dean M. Coons, Manager Research Service, The Clorox Co.; Alexander W. Bouchal, Ph.D., Medical Service, Colgate-Palmolive Co.; J. A. Monick, Ph.D., Colgate Palmolive Co.; Norm Estrin, The Cosmetic, Toiletry & Fragrance Association; Mr. Charles H. Wulf, President, Coughlin Products, Inc.; Elizabeth Clarkson, Executive Vice-President, The Crayon, Water Color & Craft Institute; Allen B. Reed, Vice President, CRC Chemicals; Thomas Mulrane, Chemist, Darworth, Inc.; J. D. Bonfiglio, Technical Director, Research, Dap, Inc.; Robert Davis, Davis Dresel Development, Del

Chemical Corp.; Arthur Marshall, Delco Moraine Division, General Motors Corp.; Fred A. Simpson, Delco Products, General Motors Corp.; Stanley J. Radknowski, Diamond International Corp.; John J. Healy, Joseph Dixon Crucible Co.; R. J. Pokorny, C. B. Dolge Co.; Charles L. Groh, Toxicology, Dow-Corning Corp.; C. A. Lesinski, Designed Products, Dow Chemical; Thomas B. Hilton, Director, Product Development, The Drackett Co.; Melvin Stonebraker, Director of Product Development, The Drackett Co.; Barbara M. Schwieter, The Drackett Co.; W. J. Corbett, Manager, Regulatory Compliance Service, Dubois Chemicals; Harris J. Kenner, M. W. Dunton Co.; Sandra Beckwith, Perry Polss, Supervisor, Petroleum Products Division, E. I. du Pont de Nemours & Co., Inc.; F. F. Ehrick, Technical Services Lab., E. I. du Pont de Nemours & Co.; Carl Briegen, E-Z-EST Products Co.; Warren H. Jones, M.D., Clinical Services, Health & Safety Lab, Eastman Kodak Co.; Thomas Fairman, Eppert Oil Co.; Ted Narabara, Flamort Chemical Co.; Dr. Frank Weber, Technical Research, R. T. French Co.; Kenneth J. Kohnle, Technical Director, The Fuller Brush Co.; Michael G. Norton, Technical Service, Fuller-O'Brien Corp.; F. J. Schumaker, G. C. Electronics, Division of Hydrometals, Inc.; Nancy C. Smith, Executive Vice President, Gard Industries; John Nair, Staff Toxicologist, General Electric Co.; George E. S. Thompson, Golden Gate Paint & Coatings Co.; E. B. Katzenmeyer, Jr., Manager, Industrial Hygiene, B. F. Goodrich Co.; Dr. W. E. McCormick, Environmental Control Dept., B. F. Goodrich Co.; E. L. Fareri, Gulf Research & Development Co.; Tech. Director, Hercules, Inc.; Paul L. Kiefer, Kenner Creative Products; Donald M. Gibson, Gibson Paint Co.; Robert J. Kirkpatrick, Jr., Director of Research, Gibson-Homans Co.; Arthur L. Grindell, The A. C. Gilbert Co.; Dr. C. J. Goldwater; John G. Martyn, Automotive Division, Grow Chemical Corp.; Wm. J. Hagerty, W. J. Hagerty & Sons, Ltd., Inc.; Wm. Perlberg, Vice President, Research & Development, The Hartz Mountain Corp.; Jerry W. Hillyard, Vice President, Hillyard Chemical Co.; Gary Hutton, President, Hub States Corp.; R. W. Worland, S. C. Johnson & Son, Inc.; L. D. Dromgold, Manager, Kendall Amalie Refining; Robert Pugh, Kentile Floors, Inc.; Robert Thomann, Manager Materials & Processes, Kidde Belleville; Robert Miller, The Klean-Strip Co., Inc.; Jack Richmond, Technical Director, Knomark, Inc.; Daniel Kaufman, Vice President, H. Kohnstamm & Co.; Gary G. Altman, Ph.D., Lester Laboratories, Inc.; Frederick Freeland, Manager of Engineering, Lionel; Joe Dwyer, Marine Electrolysis Eliminator Co.; Dr. Raoul Desjarins, Medical Consultant, The Mennen Co.; D. S. Sears, Mobil Chemical Co.; Phillip S. Landis, Mobil Oil Corp.; W. A. Kennedy,

Manager, Mobile Oil Corp.; Gerald Cooper, Manager, Food Product Development, Morton Salt Co.; Technical Director, Namrich Arms; David G. Ashton, National Purity Soap & Chemical; A. B. Levine, Adhesive Division, National Starch & Chemical Corp.; W. W. Soderlund, National Starch & Chemical Corp.; Thomas P. Yates, Tech. Manager, Automotive Chemicals, Northern Petrochemical Co.; W. E. O'Malley, Ph.D., M.D., Director U.S. Medical Affairs, Parke, Davis & Co.; Technical Director, Parks Rockets; Arthur R. Ray, Patent Cereals Sales Corp.; John R. Benson, Penguin Industries; Dr. David Heeren, Phamacare Services; Jack P. Cannon, Vice President, Hamilton Scotch Division, Platner Industries,; John Williams, Director of Research, Phoenix Oil Co.; Technical Director, Pittsburgh Plate Glass Co.; F. Kirk Nelson, Plough, Inc.; Don Corkill, Lester C. Leenerts, Technical Copy Control, Purex Corp.; N. A. McLelland, Purex Corp.; Dr. C. G. Kologiski, Chief Chemist, Radiator Specialty Co.; R. E. Broyles, Director Federal Regulatory Compliance, Ralston Purina Co.; Raymond L. Balfour, Chief Legal Officer, Ray-O-Vac; Dale O. Bender, Research Products Corp.; Joseph Sterne, Reynolds Metals; Dr. G. A. Karkar, Rochester Germicide Co.; Roy A. Carlston, Jr., Field Technical Services, Rust-Oleum Corp.; Shirley J. Wasson, Chief Chemist, Rutland Products, Rutland Fire & Clay Co.; Olson, President, The Savogran Co.; Stephen Sichak, Scholl, Inc.; Abraham Y. Schultz, President, Schultz Co.,; Technical Information Center, SCM Corp.; Howard J. Smith, Pemco Products; Wm. Neuberg, Shamrock Chemicals; Irving Skeist, President, Skeist Laboratories, Inc.; Charles E. Watkins, Jr., Standard Chemical Co.; Ralph T. Ulery, Star Bronz Co.; R. L. Peake, Chemical Systems Division, Stauffer Chemical Division; R. A. Greenberg, Swift & Co.; David T. Stebbins, Talsol Corporation; Ronald T. Richards, Industrial Hygiene & Toxicology, Texaco, Inc.; Charles W. Ellis, Analytical Section, Texise; Herman Schwartz, General Manager, Uncle Sam Chemical Co; Unelko Corp.; C. U. Dernehl, M.D., Assoc. Medical Director, Union Carbide Corp.; W. G. Whitehead, Manager of Products Safety & Regulatory Affairs, Home & Automotive Products Division; U.S. Borax & Chemical Corp.; John C. Middleton, Supervisor, Product Safety, U.S. Borax Research Corp.; Kenneth S. Freeman, Consumer Products Safety, U.S. Gypsum Co.; Al Rogers, USM Corp.; Thomas Blake, Vick Division Research & Development; James Schmitt, Applied Biochemists, Inc.; Albert Katz, West Chemical Products, Inc.; G. C. Whitlock, President, C. G. Whitlock Process Co.; Dr. Robert Dickey, Chemist, Wilhold Glues, Inc.; Carl M. Irwin, Willert Home Products, Inc.; A. E. Foster, Chief Chemist, Winsor & Newton; Sandra E. Reiss, Industrial Toxicologist, BASF Wyandotte Corp.; P. C. Zoes, Zoes Mfg. Co., Inc.

Contents

ABRASIVES	ADHESIVES (Cont.)

ABRASIVES

Abrasives contain silicon carbide, aluminum oxide, ferric oxide or silicon dioxide .... Toxicity rating 1

ALUMINUM OXIDE (alumina, corundum, emery, some white rouges)
Special synthetic corundum:

SiO_2	0–2.5%
Fe_2O_3	0–0.5%
TiO_2	2–4%
Na_2O	0–1%
Al_2O_3	93–98%

May contain traces of magnesium

ALUMINUM ZIRCONIA ABRASIVE

ZrO_2	10–45%
SiO_2	0–1.7%
Fe_2O_3	0–0.5%
TiO_2	2–3%
Na_2O	0–1%
Al_2O_3	52–83%

LAPPING COMPOUNDS
Abrasive (silicon carbide)
Petroleum grease

RED ROUGE
Iron oxide (ferric oxide, Fe_2O_3)

RUBY ABRASIVE (synthetic ruby)

SiO_2	0–0.5%
TiO_2	0–0.5%
Fe_2O	0–1%
Cr_2O_3	2–5%
Al_2O_3	94–97%

SILICON CARBIDE (carborundum)

WHITE ROUGES .... Toxicity rating 1

Silica	96–97%
Alumina	1.3%
Iron oxide	0.2%
Magnesia	0.1%
Potassium hydroxide	0.0–0.3%
Sodium carbonate	0.1%
Calcium oxide	0.01%
Barium stearate	0.7%

ADHESIVES

There are hundreds of formulas for adhesives. These few listed comprise the selection by experts in the trade of representative formulas. Various formulas appear again and again under various categories; thus, despite the classifications, most adhesives are multipurpose.

AIR FILTER ADHESIVES OR
  COATING .... Toxicity rating 3

Soluble hydrocarbon oil	96%

(About 25% soap-type additive)
See Kerosine

Polyethylene thickener	3%
Sodium o-phenylphenate	1%

May contain in propellant container:
  Methylene chloride and carbon dioxide

ASPHALT .... Toxicity rating 3

Asphalt	50–60%
Petroleum solvent*	30–50%
Asbestos fiber	0–15%
Limestone or other fillers	0–20%

ADHESIVES (Cont.)

BUILDERS .... Toxicity rating 2

Polyvinyl acetate	80%
Dibutyl phthalate	15%
Silicone	0.01%
Methylcellulose	0.10%
Phenol	0.10%

Hardener:
  Portland cement
  Asbestos or sand
May contain:
  Fungicides
  See also Furniture Cements 1 and 2;
    Tile Adhesives 3; Metal Cements;
    Marine Glue 1; Pipe Joint Cement;
    Wall sizes.

CANVAS
1. Polyvinyl acetate .... Toxicity rating 2

Polyvinyl acetate emulsion	79.89%
Diethyl phthalate	15.00%
Silicone defoamer	0.01%
Methylcellulose	0.10%
Water	4.9%
Phenol	1.0%

2. Nitrocellulose cement .... Toxicity rating 3

Nitrocellulose	20.0%
Acetone*	39%
Methyl acetate*	39%
Camphor	2%

3. Neoprene latex adhesive .... Toxicity rating 2?

Neoprene latex (50%)	90.0%
Casein	1.0%
Ammonia (28%)	0.2%
Dowicide (pentachlorophenol)	0.1%
Water	8.7%

May contain:
  Pentachlorphenol*
  Petroleum solvents*
  Resins
See also Tile Adhesives 2; Resinous 1.

CASEIN GLUES .... Toxicity rating 2

Casein	15%
Urea	10%
Zinc oxide	1%
Ammonium hydroxide	1%
Sodium o-phenylphenate	0.25%
Water	72.25%

CHINA CEMENT .... Toxicity rating 2
1. Water emulsion type

Polyvinyl acetate emulsion	85–100%
Dibutyl phthalate	0–15%

2. Solvent type .... Toxicity rating 3

Cellulose nitrate	15–25%
Isopropyl alcohol	5–20%
Acetone	20–40%
Toluol*	20–30%
Butyl acetate	0–5%
Dibutyl phthalate	0–5%

May also contain:
  Methyl ethyl ketone
  Butyl alcohol
  Hexane
  Isopropyl acetate
  Ethyl acetate
  Camphor
  Methyl acetate
  Ethyl alcohol
  Heptane
  Methyl isobutyl ketone

Starred ingredients (*) may be responsible for major toxic effects; consult Section II.

ADHESIVES (Cont.)

CONTACT CEMENT

1. Resin latex type	Toxicity rating 2
Neoprene latex	50%
Resin gum emulsion	33.7%
Water	14.25%
Casein	1.2%

    Trace (less than 0.5%):
      Ammonium hydroxide
      Sodium o-phenylphenate
      Sodium pentachlorophenate
      2,2-Methylenebis(4-methyl-6-ter-
        tiary-butylphenol)

2. Rubber cement	Toxicity rating 2
Hexane*	90%
Rubber	10%

    Solvents may also contain:
      Toluene*
      Ketone (acetone)*
      Chloroethene*

3. Solvent type	
Neoprene rubber	16%
Modified phenolic resin	8%
Magnesium oxide	1%
Zinc oxide	0.5%
Solvent blend	75%

      Blend of toluene,* hexane-type al-
        iphatic* cut, methyl ethyl ke-
        tone*
    May contain:
      1,1,1-Trichloroethane* for non-
        flammable adhesives

DENTAL PLATE CEMENT (to mend	
broken plates)	Toxicity rating 3
Methylmethacrylate polymer	30%
Methylmethacrylate monomer	70%

DENTURE ADHESIVES (see NONPRESCRIPTION DRUGS

FABRIC CEMENTS	Toxicity rating 2
1. Natural rubber latex	98.0%
Sulphur	0.5%
Zinc	0.5%

    May also contain:
      Toluene, xylene, petroleum distillate

	Toxicity rating 2
2. Polyvinyl acetate emulsion	79.89%
Diethyl phthalate	15%
Silicone	0.01%
Methylcellulose	0.10%
Water	4.9%
Phenol	0.10%
	Toxicity rating 3
3. Nitrocellulose	20%
Acetone*	39%
Ethyl acetate*	39%
Camphor*	2%
	Toxicity rating 2?
4. Neoprene latex (50%)	90.00%
Water	8.70%
Casein	1%
Dowicide	0.01%
Ammonia (28%)	0.2%

FILM CEMENT	Toxicity rating 3
Cotton base†	12–18%
Acetone*	18–24%
Methanol	0.5–1%
Methyl Cellosolve acetate	18–24%
Ethylene dichloride*	34–40%

ADHESIVES (Cont.)

FILM CEMENT (Cont.)

    May contain:
      Esters, ketones, acetates* (amyl, bu-
        tyl, ethyl)
      Dioxane*
      Methylene chloride*
      Butyrolactone

†Cotton base contains:	
Nitrocellulose	16%
Ethanol	7%
Secondary butyl acetate	30%
Methyl ethyl ketone	40%
Isopropanol	7%

FISHING ROD CEMENTS	Toxicity rating 2?
1. Epoxy resin	65%
Polyamide resin	35%

    These resins are liquid and should be
      mixed just before using

	Toxicity rating 3
2. Nitrocellulose	20%
Acetone*	39%
Methyl acetate	39%
Camphor*	2%
	Toxicity rating 3
3. Neoprene	
Methyl ethyl ketone*	

FURNACE CEMENT	Toxicity rating 3
1. Sodium silicate solution (37.6% solids)	40–60%
Abestos fiber	4–6%
Clay or other filler	30–60%
Carbon black	0–2%
Caustic	1–2%

FURNITURE CEMENT	
1. Animal wood glue	Toxicity rating 2
Water	59.8%
Animal glue	40.0%
Dowicide A	0.2%
2. Viny wood glue	Toxicity rating 2
Polyvinyl acetate emulsion	97%
Dibutyl phthalate	3%
3. Dry casein glue	Toxicity rating 4
Casein	72%
Calcium hydroxide	19%
Sodium fluoride*	8%
Kerosene	1%

GASKET CEMENTS	Toxicity rating 2
1. Epoxy resin	~65%
Polyamide resin	~35%
	Toxicity rating 3
2. Natural resins	60%
Denatured alcohol*	40%

    May contain:
      Blown vegetable oil
      Isopropyl alcohol*

3. Oil-resistant synthetic rubber	~15%
Oil-resistant phenol aldehyde resin	~15%
Solvent*	~70%

GLUE, GENERAL PURPOSE	
1. Dextrin mucilage	Toxicity rating 3
Dextrin	30.0%
Borax*	5.0%
Phenol	0.2%
Water	64.8%
2. Nitrocellulose cements	Toxicity rating 3
Nitrocellulose	20%
Acetone*	39%

Starred ingredients (*) may be responsible for major toxic effects; consult Section II.

| ADHESIVES (Cont.) | | ADHESIVES (Cont.) | |

GLUE, GENERAL PURPOSE (Cont.)

Methyl acetate*	39%
Camphor*	2%
3. Polyvinyl acetate wood glue	Toxicity rating 2
Polyvinyl acetate emulsion	79.89%
Dibutyl phthalate	15.0%
Silicone defoamer	0.01%
Methylcellulose	0.10%
Water	4.9%
Formalin	0.1%
May contain:	
Diethylene glycol dibenzoate	
4. Gum arabic mucilage	Toxicity rating 2
Gum arabic	30.00%
Formaldehyde	0.20%
Phenol	0.10%
Glycerin	3.00%
Oil of wintergreen	0.01%
Water	6.69%
5. Sodium silicate (water glass)*	Toxicity rating 3
6. Flexible glue type	Toxicity rating 2
Animal glue	33%
Sucrose	33%
Polyethylene glycol	0.3%
Sodium o-phenylphenate	0.1%
Phenol	0.1%
Methyl salicylate	0.01%
Water	to 100%
May contain:	
Alkali	
	Toxicity rating 2?
7. Polychloroprene latex (50%)	90.00%
Water	8.70%
Casein	1.00%
Sodium o-phenylphenate	0.01%
Ammonia (28%)	0.2%

LEATHER GLUE   Toxicity rating 4

1. Rubber—resin solids	25%
Toluene*	45%
Hexane	25%
Ethyl acetate	5%
	Toxicity rating 2
2. Polyvinyl acetate	50%
Emulsion in water	
3. Nitrocellulose cements	Toxicity rating 3
4. Polystyrene base adhesives	Toxicity rating 4?

LINOLEUM CEMENT (see TILE ADHESIVE)

MARINE GLUES

1. Dry casein glue	Toxicity rating 4
Casein	72.0%
Calcium hydroxide	19.0%
Sodium fluoride*	8.0%
Kerosene	1.0%
2. Epoxy adhesive	Toxicity rating 2–3
A. Epoxy resin with butyl glycidyl ether	65%
B. Polyamine* (diethylene triamine, tetraethylene pentamine, or triethylene tetramine)	35%
May contain:	
Polyamide resin with polyamine	
These resins are both liquid and should be mixed just before using.	
3. Resorcinol—formaldehyde resin	Toxicity rating 2?

METAL CEMENTS   Toxicity rating 3

Inert ingredients	55–75%
Vinyl plastic	5–10%
Ketone solvents* (see acetone)	15–25%
Diethyl phthalate	0.5–1%
Butyl acid phosphate	0.5–1%
May contain:	
Epoxy resin compounds*	
Iron powder	

MICROFILM CEMENT   Toxicity rating 4

Cotton base	70–80%
Acetic acid* (see acid)	1–3%
Cotton base contains:	
Nitrocellulose	16.0%
Ethanol	8.5%
Isopropyl alcohol	7.0%
Secondary butyl acetate	30.5%
Toluene*	38.0%
May contain:	
Acetone	
Aliphatic hydrocarbons	
Methyl ethyl ketone	
Methyl isobutyl ketone	
Phthalates	
Xylene	

MODEL CEMENTS   Toxicity rating 3

May contain:	
Nitrocellulose	15%
Acetone*	30–85%
Cellulose acetate	8–15%
Isopropanol	12%
Dibutyl phthalate	3%
Hexane	30%
Ethyl (isopropyl, amyl, butyl) acetate	30%
Toluol*	20–25%
Naphtha*	15–20%
Ethanol	5–10%
Camphor*	2%
May also contain:	
Polystyrene	
See Plastic Cements	

MUCILAGE, GENERAL PURPOSE (see GLUE, GENERAL PURPOSE)

PASTE, LIBRARY   Toxicity rating 1–2

1. Corn, wheat, or potato dextrin	35%
Glucose	5%
Phenol or sodium o-phenylphenate	0.2%
Oil of wintergreen	0.01%
Glycerine	trace
Water	60%
May contain:	
Borax	
Trisodium phosphate	
	Toxicity rating 1–2
2. Starch gum	45%
Glycerin	5%
Defoamer	0.1%
Formaldehyde	0.2%
Phenol	0.1%
Water	to 100%
May also contain:	
Dowicide and other preservatives	
Sodium nitrate	
Mineral spirits	
Sodium pentachlorophenate	
Animal glue	
Sodium bicarbonate	

Starred ingredients (*) may be responsible for major toxic effects; consult Section II.

ADHESIVES (Cont.)

PASTE, LIBRARY (Cont.)

Aluminum sulfate
Benzoate
Bentonite
Sodium fluosilicate

PATCHING CEMENT .... Toxicity rating 1
1. Sand 60–70%
   Portland cement 20–30%
   Thermoplastic resin 2–5%
   Also contains emulsifiers and stabiliz-
   ers.
2. Patching plaster
   Limestone 50–70%
   Plaster of Paris 30–50%
   Calcium proteinate .... trace
3. Plastic putty
   Plaster of Paris 50–60%
   Limestone 40–50%
   Polyvinyl alcohol 0.1–1%
   Methylcellulose polymer 0.5–1%
   Wood flour 0.5–1%
   May contain thickeners and pigments.

PIPE JOINT CEMENT .... Toxicity rating 1
1. Linseed oil 25–35%
   Lithopone 5–15%
   Slate filler 40–60%
   May contain antiskin agent

Toxicity rating 1–2
2. Black strap molasses 40–50%
   Amorphous graphite 40–50%
   Vermiculite 0–30%
   Bentonite 0–15%
   Lithopone 0–15%
   Sodium pentachlorophenate 1%
   May contain:
   Slate
   Titanium dioxide

PLASTIC CEMENT .... Toxicity rating 2
1. Polyvinyl acetate 79.8%
   Clay (kaolin) 15.5%
   Polyvinyl alcohol 5.0%
   Sodium o-phenylphenate 0.1%
   Colloid (sanctioned by FDA) 0.1%
2. Nitrocellulose cement .... Toxicity rating 3
   Nitrocellulose 20%
   Acetone* 39%
   Methyl acetate* 39%
   Camphor* 2%
3. Rubber cement .... Toxicity rating 3
   Hexane* 93%
   Rubber 7%
   Toxicity rating 4
4. Polystyrene 21%
   Benzene* 43%
   Toluene* 24%
   Acetone 8%
   Naphtha 4%

RESINOUS .... Toxicity rating 2
1. Polyvinyl acetate emulsion with
   poly(vinyl acetate-ethylene)
   emulsion 79.89%
   Dibutyl phthalate 15.00%
   Silicone defoamer 0.01%
   Methylcellulose 0.10%
   Water 4.90%
   Formalin 0.10%

ADHESIVES (Cont.)

RESINOUS (Cont.)

May contain:
Diethylene glycol dibenzoate
2. Synthetic rubber latex
   Polystyrene butadiene 50%
   Glycerol ester of hydrogenated rosin
   emulsion 33.7%
   Casein 1.2%
   2,2-Methylenebis(4-methyl-6-tertiary-
   butylphenol) 0.25%
   Sodium o-phenylphenate 0.1%
   Ammonium hydroxide 0.2%
   Sodium pentachlorophenate 0.1%
   Solubilized copper-8-quinolinolate 0.1%
   Defoamer 0.1%
   Water .... to 100%
3. Polyvinyl butyral 13.3%
   Rosin 25.0%
   Castor oil, hydrogenated 44.0%
   Mixture of stearamide, palmitamide,
   oleamide 4.4%
   Titanium dioxide 1.9%
   Clay (kaolin) 10.4%
   May contain:
   Alcohol
   Paraffin wax
   Polyvinyl chloride

ROOFING CEMENT .... Toxicity rating 3
   Petroleum asphalt 25–35%
   Petroleum solvents* 15–25%
   Asbestos fiber 5–15%
   Limestone, clay other filler 35–45%

RUBBER CEMENT .... Toxicity rating 3
1. Hexane,* gasoline,* benzol,* naphtha,*
   alcohol (solvents) 93%
   Rubber—natural, SBR 7%
   May contain:
   Rosin
   Ester gum
   Antioxidants

Toxicity rating 2
2. Butadiene styrene latex 50.0%
   Rosin gum emulsion 33.7%
   Water 14.25%
   Ammonium hydroxide 0.2%
   2,2-Methylenebis(4-methyl-6-tertiary-
   butylphenol) 0.25%
   Sodium o-phenylphenate 0.1%
   Sodium pentachlorophenate 0.1%
   Cunilate 2778-I 0.1%
   Colloid 581-B 0.1%
   Toxicity rating 3
3. Centrifuged natural latex 50–75%
   Black color (carbon) 0.2–0.6%
   Ethylene glycol* 5–10%
   Dispersed sulfur 0.05–0.1%
   Trisodium phosphate 0.2–0.5%
   Creosote 0.03–0.1%
   Stabilizer 0.3–1.5%
   Ammonium 1–3%
   Inert (earths, flours, etc.) 20–40%

SHOE CEMENTS .... Toxicity rating 3
1. Hexane,* gasoline,* naphtha* (sol-
   vents)
   Rubber—natural, SBR
   May contain:
   Rosin

Starred ingredients (*) may be responsible for major toxic effects; consult Section II.

ADHESIVES (Cont.)	

SHOE CEMENTS (Cont.)

Ester gum
Antioxidants

	Toxicity rating 4
2. Cellulose nitrate	
Acetone	
Aromatic hydrocarbon solvents*	
	Toxicity rating 2
3. Butadiene styrene latex (40% solids)	50.0%
Rosin gum emulsion	33.7%
Water	14.25%
Casein	1.2%
Ammonium hydroxide	0.2%
Sodium o-phenylphenate	0.1%
Sodium pentachlorophenate	0.1%
Cunilate 2778-I	0.1%
2,2-Methylenebis(4-methyl-6-tertiary-	
butylphenol)	0.25%
Colloid 581-B	0.1%
	Toxicity rating 2
4. Polyvinyl butyral	13.3%
Rosin	25.0%
Caster oil, hydrogenated	44.0%
Oleamide, stearamide, palmitamide	
mixture	4.4%
Titanium dioxide	1.9%
Clay (kaolin)	10.4%
Alcohol	

THERMOPLASTIC ... Toxicity rating 2

1. Polyvinyl acetate emulsion with	
poly(vinyl acetate-ethylene)	
emulsion	79.89%
Dibutyl phthalate	15.00%
Silicone defoamer	0.01%
Methylcellulose	0.10%
Water	4.90%
Formalin	0.10%
May contain:	
Diethylene glycol dibenzoate	
	Toxicity rating 2
2. Polyvinyl acetate emulsion	97%
Dibutyl phthalate	3%
	Toxicity rating 2
3. Polyvinyl butyral	13.3%
Rosin	25.0%
Castor oil, hydrogenated	44.0%
Oleamide, palmitamide, stearamide	
mixture	4.4%
Titanium dioxide	1.9%
Clay (kaolin)	10.4%
	Toxicity rating 2
4. Synthetic rubber latex (Polystyrene	
butadiene)	50%
Glyceral ester of hydrogenated rosin	
emulsion	33.7%
Casein	1.2%
Ammonium hydroxide	0.2%
Sodium o-phenylphenate	0.1%
Sodium pentachlorophenate	0.1%
Cunilate 2778-I	0.1%
2,2-Methylenebis(4-methyl-6-tertiary-	
butylphenol)	0.25%
Water	14.25%
5. "Hot melt"	Toxicity rating 2
Polyvinyl acetate-ethylene	35%
Wax	35%
Glycerol ester of hydrogenated rosin	29.5%
BHT (antioxidant)	0.5%

TILE ADHESIVES ... Toxicity rating 2

1. Rubber/resin emulsion	
Resin-tackified rubbers	
Rosin gum emulsion	33.7%
Butadiene styrene latex	50%
Water	14.25%
Casein	1.2%
Ammonium hydroxide	0.2%
Sodium o-phenylphenate	0.1%
Sodium pentachlorophenate	0.1%
2,2-Methylenebis(4-methyl-6-tertiary-	
butylphenol)	0.25%
Cunilate 2778-I, Colloid 581-G	1.2% each
2. Rubber/resin solvent	Toxicity rating 3
Inert rubbers and resins	30–35%
Inert mineral fillers	40–50%
Petroleum solvents* or alcohol	
solvents*	15–30%
3. Asphalt emulsion	Toxicity rating 1–2
Inert asphalt	40%
Inert mineral fillers	30%
Water	30%
4. Water base	Toxicity rating 1–2
Waste sulfite liquor	50%
Preservative	0.05%
Inert mineral filler	50%
	Toxicity rating 2?
5. Epoxy resin	65%
Polyamide amino resin	35%
These are both liquid, come in sepa-	
rate containers, and should be	
mixed just before using.	
	Toxicity rating 2–3
5a.Epoxy resin	90%
Diethylenetriamine*	10%
	Toxicity rating 2
6. Butadiene styrene latex (40% solids)	50%
Rosin gum emulsion	33.7%
Casein	1.2%
2,2-Methylenebis(4-methyl-6-tertiary-	
butylphenol)	0.25%
Ammonium hydroxide	0.2%
Sodium o-phenylphenate	0.1%
Sodium pentachlorophenate	0.1%
Cunilate 2778-I	0.1%
Colloid 581-B (FDA-approved)	0.1%
Water	14.25%
7. Rubber cement	Toxicity rating 3
Hexane*	93%
Rubber	7%
8. Portland cement	Toxicity rating 3
May contain:	
Calcium carbonate	
China clay	
Dryer (containing lead)*	
Magnesium oxide	
Magnesium silicate	
Mercuric oxide (red or yellow)*	
Mineral thinner*	
Phenyl mercurial oleate*	
Titanium calcium pigment	
Vegetable oil	
Organic monoamines or polya-	
mines	

WALL SIZES ... Toxicity rating 2 or 3
Dextrin
Animal glue
Sodium bicarbonate
Aluminum sulfate

Starred ingredients (*) may be responsible for major toxic effects; consult Section II.

ADHESIVES (Cont.)

WALL SIZES (Cont.)

Bentonite
May also contain:
    Methyl alcohol*
    Vinyl acetate

WATERPROOF ADHESIVES

1. Rubber cement		Toxicity rating 3
Hexane*	90%	
Rubber	10%	
		Toxicity rating 1
2. Casein	15.00%	
Urea	10.00%	
Zinc oxide	1.00%	
Ammonium hydroxide	1.00%	
Sodium o-phenylphenate	0.25%	
Water	72–75%	
		Toxicity rating 2?
3. Epoxy resin	65%	
Polyamide resin	35%	

  Both liquid—come in separate containers and should be mixed just before using.

4. Resorcinol—formaldehyde resin ..... Toxicity rating 2?

AGRICULTURAL PRODUCTS

BRANDING FLUID
Barium sulfide
Sodium hydroxide
Turpentine

DEBARKING COMPOUND
Sodium arsenite

DEHORNING PASTE
Antimony trichloride
Calcium hydroxide
Potassium hydroxide
Salicylic acid
Sodium hydroxide

EGG DETERGENT
Alkyl (C_9 to C_{16}) tolyl trimethyl ammonium chloride
Calcium hypochlorite
Dodecyl dimethyl benzyl ammonium chloride
Potassium dichloro-S-triazinetrione
Sodium carbonate
Sodium metasilicate, pentahydrate
Trisodium phosphate

FERTILIZERS
1. Commercial fertilizers (bulk—for farmer)

	Toxicity rating
Anhydrous ammonia	4 or 5
Ammonia-ammonium nitrate solution	4
Ammonium solution	4
Ammoniated superphosphate†	3
Ammonium nitrate	3
Ammonium nitrate solution	3
Ammonium phosphate	3
Ammonium phosphate-nitrate	3
Ammonium phosphate-sulfate	3
Ammonium sulfate	3
Blood meal	1
Bone meal	1
Boron salts	4
Calcium ammonium nitrate solution	3

AGRICULTURAL PRODUCTS (Cont.)

FERTILIZERS (Cont.)

Calcium cyanamide	3
Calcium nitrate	3
Cobalt salts	4
Copper salts	4
Fish emulsion	1
Fish meal	1
Hoof and horn meal	1
Iron salts	3
Liquid phosphoric acid (concentrated)	5?
Mixed fertilizers, dry	3?
Mixed fertilizers, liquid	2 or 3?
Potassium chloride	3
Potassium sulfate	3
Seed meal, castor (see Ricin, Section II)	4 or 5
Seed meal, other than castor	2?
Sewage sludge, activated	2?
Sodium nitrate	3
Superphosphate, normal (50% calcium sulfate)†	1 or 2
Superphosphate, treble (all calcium as calcium phosphate)†	2
Tankage††	1
Urea	1

2. Dry mixed (small package—as sold to the home gardner) .... Toxicity rating 3
Ammonium phosphate*
Ammonium sulfate*
Potassium chloride*
Seeds meals (other than castor)
Superphosphate, normal†
Urea
May contain:
  Ammonium superphosphate†
  Ammonium nitrate*
  Ammonium phosphate-nitrate*
  Ammonium phosphate-sulfate*
  Blood meal } usually in small amounts
  Bone meal }
  Calcium cyanamide*
  Calcium nitrate*
  Fish meal
  Hoof and horn meal
  Potassium sulfate*
  Seed meal, castor*
  Sewage sludge, activated
  Sodium nitrate*
  Superphosphate treble†
  Tankage††

3. Liquid mixtures (saturated solution) .... Toxicity rating 2 or 3
Ammonium phosphate*
Ammonium sulfate*
Fish emulsion
Potassium chloride*
Urea
May contain:
  Ammonium solution*
  Ammonium nitrate*
  Ammonium phosphate-nitrate*
  Ammonium phosphate sulfate*
  Calcium ammonium nitrate*
  Calcium nitrate*
  Phosphate acid*

Starred ingredients (*) may be responsible for major toxic effects; consult Section II.

AGRICULTURAL PRODUCTS (Cont.)

FERTILIZERS (Cont.)

Potassium sulfate*
Sodium nitrate*
4. Natural products (day) . . . . Toxicity rating 1 or 2
Blood meal
Bone meal
Cotton seed meal
Fish meal
Horn and hoof meal
Manure
Sewage sludge, activated
Tankage††
May contain trace amounts of the following:
Boron salts
Cobalt salts
Copper salts
Iron salts
Magnesium salts
Manganese salts
Molybdenum salts
Zinc salts

† Superphosphate is phosphate rock treated with sulfuric acid, calcium hydrogen phosphate, calcium phosphate and calcium sulfate: $[Ca_3(PO_4)_2]_3 \cdot CaE_2$. Usually contains 3 to 4% calcium fluoride in final product.
†† Tankage is the rendered, dried, and ground by-product from slaughterhouses. It is largely meat and bone.
† Superphosphate is phosphate rock treated with sulfuric acid, calcium hydrogen phosphate, calcium phosphate and calcium sulfate: $[Ca_3(PO_4)_2]_3 \cdot CaE_2$. Usually contains 3 to 4% calcium fluoride in final product.
†† Tankage is the rendered, dried, and ground by-product from slaughterhouses. It is largely meat and bone.

FRUIT DROP INHIBITOR
Gibberellic acid
Potassium salt of naphthalene acetic
acid
Triethanolamine salt of silvex

NEST LITTER
Carbaryl
Magnesium aluminum sulfate*
Malathion

ROOST PAINT
Anthracene oil
BHC
BHC, other isomers of
Creosote oil
Cyclohexanone
DDT
O'O-Diethyl-O-(2-isopropyl-4-methyl-6-pyrimidinyl)phosphorothioate
Lindane
Malathion
Methylated naphthalene
Nicotine
Nicotine alkaloid
Oil
Paraffin hydrocarbons
Petroleum distillate
Petroleum hydrocarbons
Petroleum oil
Phenols
Pine oil
Pyridine

AGRICULTURAL PRODUCTS (Cont.)

SOIL CONDITIONER
Aluminum sulfate
Ammonium sulfate
Disodium tetraborate decahydrate
Disodium tetraborate pentahydrate
Gibberellic acid
Monuron
Polyacrylonitrile
Sequestered trace element mixture
Sulfur

SPREADER ACTIVATOR (1974 List):
Ag. Foam
Alkyl aryl polyether alcohol
Alkyl aryl polyoxyethylene
Ortho X-77
Tronic

SPREADER ACTIVATOR (1969 List):
Alkyl aryl polyoxyethylene glycols
Casein
Ethylene glycol
Ethylene oxide acetate
Fatty acids, free
Hydrated lime
Isopropanol
Paraffinic ketone
Petroleum oil
Petroleum sulfonates
Phthalic glycerol alkyd resin
Potassium abietate
Potassium oleate
Sodium dodecylbenzene sulfonate
Synthetic resins

SPREADERS, STICKERS (1974 List):
Alky oletin aromatic polymers
Citowett Plus
Triton

SPREADERS, STICKERS (1969 List):
Acrylic polymer
Alkyl aryl polyether alcohols
Casein
Ethylene oxide
Hydrated lime
Paraffinic ketone
Phthalic glycerol alkyd resins
Sulfonated oil
Vegetable oil

ANTISTATIC PRODUCTS

ANTISTATIC LIQUIDS (Carpeting; spray)
1. Cationic type
   Alkyl dimethyl benzyl ammonium
   chloride, 0.1–0.5%
   Remainder water
2. Nonionic type
   N-Acetylethanolamine, 1–3%
   Remainder water

ARTS AND CRAFTS PRODUCTS

Most materials in this group carry appreciable quantities of pigment which are responsible for any toxicity. (See Pigments.)

The danger of poisoning due to the ingestion of coloring matter is greatest in artists' materials for two reasons:

(1) The pigment material is applied directly and no matter what the media—oil, water color, pastel, etc.—the actual coloring material itself is a very high percentage of the mix.

(2) Artists are prone to use the pigments the Old Masters used, some of which were very toxic, e.g., emerald green (Paris

ARTS AND CRAFTS PRODUCTS (Cont.)

green) which is cupric aceto-arsenite. In contrast, commercial paint manufacturers are much more apt to use modern organic colors which are as good or better than the older colors and usually much less toxic.

The above hazards are compounded when one considers that painting as a hobby is becoming increasingly common, and therefore the chance of concentrated color mixes being present and accessible in the home is becoming greater every day. On the other hand, it is becoming a practice to list ingredients on labels and to replace the more toxic pigments with new, less toxic ones as they are developed.

Although a few pigments are listed under each media, it is well to refer to Pigments (in this section) which is as comprehensive as knowledge and space can make it.

AEROGRAPH COLORS .... Toxicity rating 3–4
Pigment	13–41%
Reducer	0–30%
Gums	12–19%

Among the pigments are chrome lemon ($PbCrO_4$ and PbS), chrome yellow ($PbCrO_4$), chrome orange ($PbCrO_4 \cdot PbSO_4$).

ANTIQUING AGENTS
1. Antiquing glaze .... Toxicity rating 3

Magnesium carbonate	3.8–4.5%
Silica	4.0–4.6%
Silicates	5.0–5.3%
Linseed oil modified polyurethane resin	10.0–11.0%
Alkydized synthetic oil	32.0–34.0
Petroleum distillates	0.8–1.2%
Drier	
Tinting colors less than 5%	

2. Antiquing base coat .... Toxicity rating 2

Titanium dioxide, type II	11.0–12.0%
Phthalocyanine blue	1.0–1.3%
Red iron oxide, class A	0.2–0.5%
Calcium carbonate	7.0–8.0%
Vinyl acrylic copolymer resin	22.0–23.0%
Additives	0.5–1.3%
Ethylene glycol	1.5–1.8%
Phenyl mercuric acetate	0.1–0.2%
Water	54.0–55.0%

Mercury as metallic mercury is 0.012% of total weight of contained solids.

CASTING COMPOUND .... Toxicity rating 2
Calcium sulfate
Talc
Hydrous aluminum silicate
Calcium carbonate
Silicone dioxide
Sodium silicate

CRAYONS
Crayons here are separated into two major categories: Children's, which are subdivided into Wax and Pressed which are nontoxic, especially those which carry the CP or AP Seal of The Crayon, Water Color and Craft Institute, Inc.; and Industrial, which may be toxic.

1. Children's crayons .... Toxicity rating 1–2
A. Wax

Paraffin and other waxes	60–98%
Pigments	1–40%

B. Pressed

Paraffin and other waxes	10–50%
Pigments and extenders	10–95%

CRAYONS (Cont.)
2. Industrial crayons .... Toxicity rating 4
The following pigment is to be suspected:
Lead chromate
Other pigments are nontoxic

FABRIC PAINT .... Toxicity rating 3–4
Pigments* (organic and inorganic, lead)	40–80%
Self-drying oils of linseed type	20–45%
Varnish	0–20%
Naphtha	
Aluminum hydrate	

Among the pigments are medium yellow (Pb), primrose (Pb), terra cotta (Pb).

FINGER PAINT .... Toxicity rating 1
Bentonite (colloidal hydrated aluminum silicate or
Titanium oxide
Nontoxic colors (vegetable, inorganic or synthetic)

Preservatives	trace amounts

Formaldehyde, benzoic acid sales, Dowicil 100 (a hexaminium chloride), dimethoxane, hydroxyethyl carbinolamine

Nontoxic if the product bears the AP or CP seal of The Crayon, Water Colo r and Craft Institute (originally assured by conformance with NBS Standard CS 130-461).

GLITTERING DECORATIVE COLOR Toxicity rating 3
Petroleum solvent*
Coated metallic flake of aluminum

MODELING CLAY .... Toxicity rating 1
Kaolin
Gypsum
Petrolatum
Wax
Castor oil
Vegetable dye
May contain:
    Aluminum silicate
    Ammonium alum
    Borax
    Dextrin
    Fatty acids
    Glycerine
    Gum arabic
    Polyvinyl acetate
    Preservatives
    Methylcellulose
    Sulfur
Sulfur dioxide*
    Turpentine*

OIL PAINT (see Pigments) .... Toxicity rating 3–4
Pigment	30–90%
Stabilizer	0–20%
Self-drying oils of the linseed type	10–50%

Only the toxic forms of pigment are listed below. For further information see Pigments section.

COMMON NAME	TOXIC ELEMENT	REFERENCE LISTING IN PIGMENT SECTION
Cadmium lemon	Cadmium	Cadmium sulfide
Cadmium orange	Cadmium	Cadmium orange
Cadmium red	Cadmium	Cadmium red

Starred ingredients (*) may be responsible for major toxic effects; consult Section II.

ARTS AND CRAFTS PRODUCTS (Cont.)		

COMMON NAME	TOXIC ELEMENT	REFERENCE LISTING IN PIGMENT SECTION
Cadmium yellow	Cadmium	Cadmium yellow
Cobalt violet	Arsenic	Cobalt violet
Cremnitz white	Lead	Basic lead carbonate
Emerald greenn	Arsenic, copper	(Paris green) emerald green
Flake white	Lead	Basic lead carbonate and ZnO
Flesh tint	Lead	Naples yellow, basic lead carbonate and ZnO
		Genuine rose madder
Foundation white	Lead	Variety of basic lead carbonate
Jaune brilliant	Lead	Naples yellow, basic lead carbonate, ZnO, HgS
Magenta	Arsenic	
Mauve blue shade	Arsenic	
Mauve red shade	Arsenic	
Naples yellow	Lead, cadmium	Naples yellow
Chrome green	Lead	Lead chromate and Prussian blue
Chrome lemon	Lead	Lead chromate and Prussian blue
Chrome yellow	Lead	Lead chromate and Prussian blue
Chrome orange	Lead	Lead chromate and Prussian blue
Chrome deep	Lead	Lead chromate, Prussian blue and raw sienna
Transparent oxide of chromium	Arsenic	Green, transparent oxide of chromium

PASTELS . . . . Toxicity rating 1
1. School pastels
    Calcium carbonate
    Aluminum silicate
    Calcium sulfate
    Organic and inorganic pigments (nontoxic)
    Water-soluble binder (nontoxic)
2. Artist's pastels . . . . Toxicity rating 3–4
    Aluminum silicate
    Magnesium carbonate
    Calcium carbonate
    Cellulose type binder
    Organic and inorganic pigment* including chrome colors (oranges, yellow and greens) in competitive grades

PENCILS
1. Lead pencils . . . . Toxicity rating 1
    Clay 26%
    Graphite 66%
    Wax 8%
    (Fats, stearic acid, paraffins)
2. Indelible pencils or copying pencils . . . Toxicity rating 3
    Methyl or crystal violet*, small amounts likely to be taken orally; hazard small
3. Colored leads . . . . Toxicity rating 2–4
    Pigments: see Industrial crayons above

ARTS AND CRAFTS PRODUCTS (Cont.)		

PENCILS (Cont.)
    Others: water-soluble acid dyestuff which are usually comparatively harmless
    The following are of low toxicity:
    Binders: natural gums and cellulose
    Inerts: clay and talc, $CaCO_3$, silica
    Waxes: natural and synthetic (Carbowax-polyethylene glycol)
    Surfactants: trace

PORCELAIN ENAMEL POWDER . . . . Toxicity Rating 4
For copper (or hobbyist) use
    Sand 30–40%
    Lead oxide* (see Lead salts) 30–40%
    Alkaline carbonates 5–15%
    Boron 5–15%
    Antimony oxide* (see Antimony salts)
    Tin oxide
    Titanium dioxide   0–5%
    Arsenic oxide* (see Arsenic)
    Zinc oxide
    Barium oxide
    Metallic oxides (cobalt, copper, iron, chrome, etc.) 0–5%
    Enamels for iron and steel are lead-, antimony- and arsenic-free

POSTER COLORS . . . . Toxicity rating 3–4
    Pigment* 8–60%
    Reducer 0–50%
    Gums 2.5–13%
    Phenolic preservatives

TEMPERA PAINT . . . . Toxicity rating 3–4
    Tempera employs albuminous, colloidal or synthetic media instead of oil, e.g., vinyl, acrylic, or copolymer resins together with cellulose thickening agents, wetting agents, preservatives. Tempera is generally prepared as cylinders or crayons.
1. Pigments* 10–40%
    Gum or dextrines 5–10%
    Water 30–50%
    May contain:
    Aluminum silicate
    Barium sulfate
    Barium sulfate-zinc sulfide compounds
    Calcium carbonate
    Calcium sulfate
    Glucose
    Glues (animals)
    Glycerine
    Preservatives (phenol, formaldehyde)
    Wetting agents
2. Formula for artists . . . . Toxicity rating 3–4
    Pigments*
    Egg emulsion (from egg white)
    Linseed oil

WATER COLOR . . . . Toxicity rating 3–5
    Pigments* 15–50%
    Hydroxy ethyl celulose 0–35%
    Gums or dextrines 18–32%
    Wetting agent 0–2%
    Reducer 0–15%
    Water . . . .   to 100%
    May contain:
    Barium sulfate
    Calcium sulfate
    Glucose

Starred ingredients (*) may be responsible for major toxic effects; consult Section II.

ARTS AND CRAFTS PRODUCTS (Cont.)

WATER COLOR (Cont.)

Phenolic preservatives
Phenyl mercury preservatives
Plasticizer
Polyethylene glycol

COMMON NAME	REFERENCE LISTING IN PIGMENTS SECTION
Aureolin	Potassium cobaltinitrite
Cadmium yellow	Cadmium sulfide, cadmium sulfoselenide and barium sulfate
Maganese blue	Barium manganate and barium sulfate, or barium nitrate
Mineral blue	Basic copper carbonate
Emerald green	Paris green

AUTOMOTIVE PRODUCTS

ANTIFREEZE/COOLANT . . . . Toxicity rating 3
1. Glycols* (95% monoethylene glycol, 5% diethylene glycol) 95%
   Alkali metal borates and phosphates   2–3%
   Water 2–3%
   Dye . . . . trace
2. Miscellaneous
   Calcium chlorite, sodium chloride and inhibited propylene glycol are used for refrigeration brines
   Calcium chloride solutions are also used in tractor tires for added weight.
   Glycerol and ethyl alcohol are used as antifreezes for cosmetics
   Lubricating oils have been used as cooling agents in specially prepared engines.

ANTIKNOCK (see FUELS, MOTOR FUEL ADDITIVES)

AUTOMOTIVE CLEANERS AND CAR WASH COMPOUNDS . . . . Toxicity rating 3
  These are usually made up of alkyl aryl sodium sulfonate, particularly sodium dodecylbenzene sulfonate with emulsifiers and creams which may contain toxic amounts of petroleum ether derivatives.
1. General purpose:
   Petroleum naphthas* 50–60%
   o-Benzyl-p-chlorophenol   0.1%
   Petroleum and synthetic waxes 40–50%
   Emulsifying agents
2. Alkyl aryl sodium sulfonate* 40%
   Sodium sulfate 60%
   May contain:
   Diethanolamine
   Lauryl diethanolamide
3. Solid:
   Sodium dodecylbenzene sulfonate (alkyl aryl sodium sulfonate)* 40–100%
   Sodium sulfate 15–25%
   May contain:
   Alkyl diethanolamine 2%
   Nonionic detergents, such as phenolethylene oxide type 10–15%
4. Liquid:
   Dodecyl benzene sulfonate 6%
   Coconut oil amine 2%
   Water 92%
   May contain:
   Benzene
   Fatty amide condensate

AUTOMOTIVE PRODUCTS (Cont.)

AUTOMOTIVE CLEANERS AND CAR WASH COMPOUNDS (Cont.)
Hydrochloric acid
Hydrophilic wax
Polyphosphates
Silicone
Sulfonated ketones
Triethanolamine lauryl sulfonate

AUTOMATIC TRANSMISSION FLUIDS . . . . . . Toxicity rating 2
Mineral oils 75–100%
Oxidation inhibitors and detergents . . .   0–20%
  Zinc dialkyl dithiophosphate
  Phosphorous pentasulfide-terpene and addition products
  Barium and calcium petroleum sulfonates
  Barium and calcium alkyl phenolates
  Ashless detergents
Pour depressants and viscosity improvers   0–5%
  Polymethacrylate esters
  Polyisobutylenes
Hydrocarbon wax—naphthalene condensation products
Antiwear agents 0–2%
  Organic borates
Antifoam agents . . . . less than 200 p.p.m.
  Polysiloxanes
Sealant 0–5%
  Triarylphosphate
May contain:
Dyes . . . . 0–200 p.p.m.

BRAKE FLUIDS . . . . Toxicity rating 3
Lubricant 20–25%
  Castor oil
  Castor oil soap
  Butyl or glyceryl ether of polyoxyethylene propylene glycol
  Polypropylene glycol
Solvent 80–85%
  Methyl, ethyl and butyl ethers of ethylene glycol* and related glycols
  Brake fluids may contain:
    Butylene glycol*
    Diethylene glycol*
    Ethylene glycol*
    Hexylene glycol*
    Polyethylene glycol*
Inhibitors
  Amine soaps
  Potash soaps
  Borax
Antioxidants
  Bisphenol A
  Hydroquinone
Dyes

BRAKE SYSTEM FLUSHING FLUIDS   Toxicity rating 3
Methyl, ethyl or isopropyl alcohol*

CARBURETOR CLEANERS . . . . Toxicity rating 3
1. Tall oil 5–18%
   Cresol* 10–25%
   Potassium hydroxide 1–4%
   Ethylene dichloride* 15–50%
   Sodium chromate* 0.5–5%
   Ammonium oxalate 0.3–3%
   Alcohol 1–10%

Starred ingredients (*) may be responsible for major toxic effects; consult Section II.

AUTOMOTIVE PRODUCTS (Cont.)

CARBURETOR CLEANERS (Cont.)

Water	10–40%
2.	Toxicity rating 3
Ethylene dichloride*	63%
(Other chlorinated hydrocarbons may be substituted, such as o-dichloroben- zene,* dichloropentane* and methyl- ene dichloride*)	
Cresol (low-boiling cresylic acids may be substitued)	25%
Oleic acid	7.2%
Potassium hydroxide (sodium hydroxide)	1.4%
Water	3.4%
3. "Odorless" carbon removers	Toxicity rating 3–4
Aliphatic* or aromatic* hydrocarbon solvents with oil-soluble wetting agents	

CORROSION INHIBITORS

1. Chromate type:	Toxicity rating 3
Sodium chromate*	10–20%
Borax	0–4%
Phosphates	0–4%
Silicates	0–1%
Water	to 100%
Some inhibitors have potassium bi- chromate* (toxicity rating 4)	
2. Soluble oil type:	Toxicity rating 3
Mineral oil* (see kerosene)	80–90%
Potash rosin soap	9–16%
Mineral oil sulfonates	0–10%
Alkaline salts (borax, phosphates)	0–2%
May contain:	
Oxidized petroleum waxes	
Organic metallic salts (calcium)	
Waxes	
3. Sodium nitrate type:	Toxicity rating 3
Sodium nitrate*	20–100%
Alkaline salts	0–5%
Water	
4. "Straight" alkali type:	Toxicity rating 3
Borax	
Borates*	
Sodium carbonate	
Sodium metasilicates	
Sodium phosphates	
5. Organic type:	Toxicity rating 3–4
a. Organic amine nitrites, e.g., diisopro- pyl ammonium nitrite* (see Ni- trites), dicyclohexyl ammonium nitrite* (see Ammonium Salts)	0–100%
Sodium mercaptobenzothiazol* (LD$_{50}$ (rat) 1.6 gm./kg. as 10% aqueous solution)	0–50%
Alkaline salts (borax, phosphates)	0–5%
Water	
b. Polyoxyethylene glycol ether of a high-molecular-weight organic amine	
Quaternary ammonium salt	
Acetylenic alcohol	

DRESSINGS

1. Convertible top dressing	Toxicity rating 3
Petroleum naphtha* or	
Stoddard solvent*	
Dowicide A	2%
Resin	
Wax	

AUTOMOTIVE PRODUCTS (Cont.)

DRESSINGS (Cont.)

2. Leather or rubber coating	Toxicity rating 3
a. Titanium dioxide	13%
Aluminum stearate	1%
Calcium carbonate	13%
Mineral spirits*	33%
Cobalt (6%)	0.5%
Lead (24%)	0.5%
Wax or resin	
b.	Toxicity rating 4
Acrylic resin	10%
Plasticizer	1%
Aromatic ketone solvent*	89%
(see Aromatic Hydrocarbon Solvent)	
c.	Toxicity rating 2
Latex polymer acrylic resin	10%
Plastic	1%
Water	89%

ENGINE AND MOTOR CLEANERS

ENGINE AND MOTOR CLEANERS	Toxicity rating 4
1. Ethylene dichloride*	63%
(or other chlorinated hydrocarbons, such as o-dichlorobenzene,* dichlo- ropentane,* methylene dichloride,* 1,1,1,-trichloroethylene*)	
Cresol* (low-boiling, cresylic acids* may be substituted)	25%
Oleic acid	7.2%
Potassium (or sodium) hydrozide	1.4%
Water	3.0%
	Toxicity rating 3
2. Methylene chloride*	0.25%
Perchloroethylene*	5–60%
Stoddard solvent*	40–70%
	Toxicity rating 3
3. Perchloroethylene*	0–60%
Trichloroethane*	0–60%
Methylene chloride*	0–25%
Petroleum solvents*	40–70%
Chlor-aromatic solvents* (see o-dichlo- robenzene, chlorinated naphthalenes	0–100%
Detergent	
Emulsifier	
May contain:	
Alkali	
Corrision inhibitors	
Essential oils	
Lubricating oils*	
Pine oil	
Versene	

FLUSHES (Radiator) (see under RADIATOR CLEANERS below)

FOAM SUPPRESSORS

Antifoams, defoamers, foam preventive
Alcohols (* if >10%)
Alkyl lactates
Amyl alcohol*
Calcium acetate
Calcium ricinoleate
Castor oil soap
Dibutyl phthalate
Ethyl oleate
Phenyl stearate
Polyglycols (* if >50%)
Silicone compounds
Sulfones (* if >10%)
Surfactants (anionic—* if >50%; cationic—* if >20%)
Vegetable oils

Starred ingredients (*) may be responsible for major toxic effects; consult Section II.

AUTOMOTIVE PRODUCTS (Cont.)

FOAM SUPPRESSORS (Cont.)

Volatile solvents (toxicity rating 3 if >10% alkyl; toxicity rating 4 if >10% aryl)

FROST REMOVER

1. Spray type: .... Toxicity rating 3
   - Isopropyl alcohol 25%
   - Ethylene glycol* 50%
   - Water 25%
   - Propellant, CO_2
2. Alcohol .... Toxicity rating 3
   - Isopropyl alcohol* 30–100%
   - N-Propyl alcohol* 15–30%
   - Propylene glycol
   - Ethylene glycol*
   - Water 5–15%

May contain:
   - Tetrahydrofurfuryl alcohol (see Alcohols, higher*)

FUEL TANK DRIERS (see DRIERS)

OILS (see under OILS)

POLISH (see under POLISHES)

RADIATOR CLEANERS (FLUSHES)

1. Alkaline .... Toxicity rating 3–4
   - Sodium orthosilicate 9%
   - Sodium tripolyphosphate 4%
   - Sodium dichromate 2%
   - May contain:
     - Sodium chromate* 16%
2. Acid .... Toxicity rating 4
   - Oxalic acid* 40%
   - Boric acid* 60%
   - May contain:
     - Hydrochloric acid*
     - Sodium bisulfite*
3. Mixed .... Toxicity rating 4
   - a. Oxalic acid* 40–100%
     - Boric acid* 60%
     - Detergent
   - b. .... Toxicity rating
     - Sodium carbonate 85%
     - Potassium dichromate* 15%
4. Solvent .... Toxicity rating 3–4
   - Mainly petroleum ethers*
   - May be chlorinated hydrocarbons* (e.g., o-dichlorobenzenes)
5. Liquid fast flushes may contain: ...... Toxicity rating 3
   - n-Butanol*
   - Olefins*
   - Isopropanol*
6. Heavy duty powders may contain: ... Toxicity rating 4?
   - Oxalic acid*
   - Sulfamic acid*

1. RADIATOR STOP LEAK .... Toxicity rating 2
   - Dextrin 5–10%
   - Cellulose gum 0.5%
   - Asbestos 5%
   - Soda ash 0.8%
   - Isopropanol 10–15%
   - Water .... to 100%
   - May contain:
     - Aluminum oxide
2. Soluble oil type .... Toxicity rating 3
   - Asbestos
   - Clays
   - Mineral oil* (see Kerosene)

AUTOMOTIVE PRODUCTS (Cont.)

RADIATOR STOP LEAK (Cont.)

   - Wood flour
   - Sulfonates
   - Water

RUBBING COMPOUND (see POLISHES)

SHOCK ABSORBER FLUIDS

1. Delco type: .... Toxicity rating 3
   - Naphthenic or paraffinic petroleum oil* (see Kerosene)
2. Houdaille type .... Toxicity rating 2
   - Glycerin
   - Alcohol
   - Glucose
   - Water

3. Petroleum ether* .... Toxicity rating 3 .... 97%
   - Kerosene 3%
4. Shock absorber oils .... Toxicity rating 2
   - Mineral oils 90–100%
   - Fatty oils 0–5%
   - May contain:
     - Viscosity improvers 0–5%
     - Polymethacrylate esters
     - Dyes .... 0–150 p.p.m.

TIRE CLEANERS .... Toxicity rating 2–3

1. Potassiuim hydroxide*
   - Metasilicates } .... about 20%
   - Alkyl aryl sulfonate
   - Water 80%
   - May contain:
     - Isopropyl alcohol
     - Glycol ethers
     - Xylene*
     - Monoethanolamine
2. Aerosol whitewall cleaner .... Toxicity rating 3
   - Anionic detergents*
   - Phosphates
   - Aliphatic solvent (trace)
   - Aerosol propellant

3. Trisodium phosphate or sodium ... Toxicity rating 3
   - tripolyphosphate 5%
   - Metasilicate 5%
   - Alkyl aryl sulfonates 5%
   - Butyl cellosolve* 10%
   - EDTA 1%
   - Perfume 1%
   - Fluorescein .... trace

TIRE PAINT

1. Black tire paint .... Toxicity rating 3
   - Aliphatic solvents* 35–45%
   - Resins 40–50%
   - Pigments 5–10%
2. White tire paint .... Toxicity rating 3–4
   - Pigments (10–25%)
     - Titanium dioxide 50–100%
     - Calcium carbonate 0–50%
     - Silicates 0–50%
   - Vehicles (75–90%)
     - Synthetic rubber 10–25%
     - Plasticizers 10–25%
     - Aromatic hydrocarbons* 25–75%
     - Aliphatic hydrocarbons 0–25%

TIRE REPAIR .... Toxicity rating 3–4

1. Adhesive
   - Rubber, synthetic

Starred ingredients (*) may be responsible for major toxic effects; consult Section II.

AUTOMOTIVE PRODUCTS (Cont.)	BATTERIES (Cont.)

TIRE REPAIR (Cont.)

Rubber, or polymer resin
Volatile solvent* 85–95%
  Benzene, toluene, chlorinated hydrocarbon, or petroleum distillate
Self-vulcanizing cements also contain small amounts of rubber accelerators and vulcanizing agents.
  May contain
    Ammonia
    Sulfur
    Chlorinated hydrocarbons*
    Trichloroethylene*
2. Tubeless bonding compound .... Toxicity rating 4
   Toluol* .... over 80%

TRANSMISSION FLUIDS (see AUTOMATIC TRANSMISSION FLUIDS)

UNDERCOATINGS .... Toxicity rating 4
1. Pigment (15–50%)
   Iron oxide 0–50%
   Silicates 0–50%
   Lead or lead salts* 0–50%
   Zinc and zinc salts* 0–50%
   May contain:
     Titanium dioxide 0–50%
   Vehicle (50–85%)
   Alkyd resin 0–50%
   Phenolic resin 0–50%
   Fish oil 0–25%
   Vegetable oil 0–25%
   Aromatic hydrocarbons* 0–50%
   Aliphatic hydrocarbons* 0–50%
2. Pigments .... Toxicity rating 4
   Iron oxide
   Titanium oxide
   Red lead
   Lead silicochromate
   Vehicle
   Phenolic ether resin
   Polyamid resin
   Aromatic hydrocarbon
   Cellosolve or methyl isobutyl ketone
3. Asphaltic material
   Solvent
   If aliphatic hydrocarbon—toxicity rating is 3; if aromatic hydrocarbon–toxicity rating is 4.

UPPER CYLINDER LUBRICANTS .... Toxicity rating 3
   Mineral oils* 85–100%
   C1.S P Compounds 0–10%
   Isobutylene polymers 0–5%

WAX (see POLISHES)

WINSHIELD DEICERS (see under FROST REMOVERS)

BATTERIES

DRY CELL BATTERIES, fully charged .... Toxicity rating 2
1. Conventional "D" size battery (carbon-zinc) contains:
   Carbon .... 4 gm.
   Manganese dioxide .... 23 gm.
   Ammonium chloride .... 6 gm.
   Zinc chloride .... 3 gm.
   Cornstarch .... 0.02 gm.
   Zinc (container) .... 13 gm.
   Mercuric chloride .... 0.01 gm.
   Water .... Balance

DRY CELL BATTERIES (Cont.)

High-performance battery contains:
   Carbon .... 5 gm.
   Manganese dioxide .... 27 gm.
   Zinc chloride .... 6 gm.
   Cornstarch .... 0.02 gm.
   Zinc (container) .... 16 gm.
   Magnesium oxide .... 0.12 gm.
   Mercuric oxide .... 0.01 gm.
   Water .... balance
Even if the whole battery were swallowed, only 20 mg. of mercury chloride would be ingested which is at least a fifth of the MLD for a child. The fountain pen-typed battery is one-fifth this size, so there is a sufficient margin of error to be perfectly safe even if several were swallowed, a highly improbable situation.
2. Alkaline manganese "D" cell: .... Toxicity rating 2
   Zinc metal .... 18.5 gm.
   Mercury metal .... 1.3 gm.
   Potassium hydroxide .... 8.5 gm.
   Carboxymethyl cellulose .... 0.5 gm.
   Zinc oxide .... 0.8 gm.
   Manganese dioxide .... .49 gm.
   Carbon .... 5 gm.
   Water .... balance
3. Mercury cell battery, largest size, (for hearing aids, pen lights, and small transistor radios—a potential hazard .... Toxicity rating 5
   Mercury (metallic) .... 0.1 gm.
   Mercuric oxide* .... 4 gm.
   Zinc .... 1.2 gm.
   Potassium hydroxide .... 0.4 gm.
   Zinc oxide .... 0.07 gm.
   Carbon .... 0.24 gm.
   Manganese sesquioxide .... 0.5 gm.
   Water .... balance
   If the nickel case should be ruptured or dissolved on ingestion, 4 gm. of mercuric oxide would be lethal.
4. Silver button cell for hearing aide use (largest size) .... Toxicity rating 2
   Zinc metal .... 0.25 gm.
   Mercury metal .... 0.02 gm.
   Potassium hydroxide .... 0.1 gm.
   Silver oxide .... 1 gm.
   Zinc oxide .... 0.01 gm.
   Manganese dioxide .... 0.06 gm.
   Graphite .... 0.01 gm.
   Water .... balance

DRY CELL BATTERIES, completely discharged
1. Conventional "D" size:
   Some discharge products: $MnOOH, Mn_2O_3 \cdot ZnO \cdot Mn_2O_3$, Mn^{2+}, $ZnCl_2 \cdot 2 NH_3$.
   Instead of $ZnCl_2 \cdot 2 NH_3$, a new product is formed—$ZnCl_2 \cdot 4 Zn(OH)_2 \cdot 5 H_2O$.
2. Alkaline manganese "D" cell:
   Similar products: $MnOOH$, $Mn_2O_3 \cdot Mn_3O_4 \cdot Zn$, mostly ZnO.
3. Mercury cell battery, largest size:
   Now: Mercury (metallic)   3.9 gm.
     Mercuric oxide
     Zinc
     Zinc oxide   1.6 gm.
   Otherwise little change.
4. Silver button cell for hearing aid use (large size)
   Now: Zinc metal
     Silver oxide
     Zinc oxide

Starred ingredients (*) may be responsible for major toxic effects; consult Section II.

BATTERIES (Cont.)

DRY CELL BATTERIES (Cont.)

Silver (metal)	0.3 gm.

Otherwise little change.

BLEACHES

NAIL BLEACH (see COSMETICS)

SKIN BLEACH (see COSMETICS)

WOOD BLEACHES	No rating
1. Caustic soda*	8%
Sodium silicate	2.5%
Water	to 100%
	No rating
2. Hydrogen peroxide*	30–35% solution

In practice, 1 may be applied before 2. If bleaching calls for use of powdered oxalic acid or borax, toxicity rating is 4.

	Toxicity rating 3
3. Sodium hydrosulfite (see sodium sulfite)	10%
Water	90%
4. Oxalic acid,* supersaturated	No rating
5. Paint stripper	Toxicity rating 3
Methylene chloride*	70–75%
Methanol*	10–20%
Ammonia	2–3%

CANDLES

CHURCH	Toxicity rating 1
Beeswax	
Paraffin	

The candle wick is treated with:
Ammonium chloride
Ammonium phosphate
Ammonium sulfate
Borax
Boric acid
Potassium nitrate

HOUSEHOLD	Toxicity rating 1
Stearic acid	
Paraffin	
Dye (minute amount)	

INSECT REPELLENT (see HOUSE and GARDEN PESTICIDES)

CAULKING COMPOUNDS

In early 1974, barium oxide and titanium dioxide were in short supply. Restrictions have been placed on asbestos usage. Substitutions and changes are frequent. Manufacturers must be contacted directly in case of doubt.

CAULKING COMPOUNDS

1.	Toxicity rating 3
Styrenated alkyd resin ⎫	
Titanium dioxide ⎪	
Calcium carbonate ⎬	40%
Asbestos fiber ⎭	
Xylene*	20%
2.	Toxicity rating 1
Polyvinyl acetate	
Titanium dioxide	
Calcium carbonate	
3.	Toxicity rating 3

CAULKING COMPOUNDS (Cont.)

CAULKING COMPOUNDS (Cont.)

Vegetable oils (edible)
Mineral thinner*
Drier (cobalt)* (see Cobalt salts)
Titanium dioxide
Calcium carbonate
Asbestos fiber
May contain:
Aluminium or calcium stearate
Asphalt
Chromium*
Iron oxide
Petroleum sulfonate
Wax
Zinc oxide
Lead*

4.	Toxicity rating 1
Soybean oill	15–20%
Polybutene	6–10%
Fatty acid	0.5–1%
Mineral spirits	2–4%
Marble dust	45–55%
Talc	15–20%
Cobalt drier*	

Aluminum caulking compound contains aluminum flake; white contains titanium dioxide; black contains carbon black.

5. Termite destroying	Toxicity rating 3
Asphalt	30–45%
Petroleum distillate*	15–20%
Asbestos	5–15%
Mineral dust (e.g., soap stone)	25–35%
Dieldrin* or aldrin*	0.75–2%
6. Asphalt cements or caulking compounds	Toxicity rating 3
Asphalt	45–70%
Mineral spirits*	10–25%
Kerosene	0–20%
Asbestos fiber	5%
Ground rock dust (minus 100 mesh)	0–25%

7. Cement sealer
Portland cement
Titanium dioxide
Silicates
Resins
May contain:
Aromatic hydrocarbons
Aliphatic hydrocarbons
Ethylene glycol
Hydrated lime
Mica
Colors

8. Polysulfide caulking compound	Toxicity rating 3
Liquid polysulfide polymer	100 parts
Titanium dioxide	20%
Calcium carbonate	25–75%
Polychlorinated polyphenols	0–50%
Molecular sieve	2%
Calcium peroxide	8–12%
Barium peroxide*	0–4%
Potassium phosphate	2–4%
Liquid epoxy resin	2–6%
9. Silicone rubber caulking	Toxicity rating 2?
Polydimethylsiloxane	85%
Silica	15%
May contain as pigments	
Aluminum flake	
Carbon black	

Starred ingredients (*) may be responsible for major toxic effects; consult Section II.

| CAULKING COMPOUNDS (Cont.) | CLEANERS (Cont.) |

CAULKING COMPOUNDS (Cont.)

Titanium dioxide	
10. Hypalon caulk	Toxicity rating 3
Hypalon (chlorosulfonated polyethylene polymer)	20%
Elastomeric binder	
Chlorinated paraffin plasticizer	20%
Asbestos or silicon dioxide extenders	10%
Titanium dioxide pigment	12%
Talc (extender)	8%
Tribasic lead maleate	6%
Rosin, MBTS and Thiuram	0.5%
Xylene*	10%
Tributyl phosphate	9%
Fractal A	3%
Isopropyl alcohol	2%

CHALK

CHALKS	Toxicity rating 1 or 2
1. Calcium carbonate	50–80% minimum
Pigments	
"Other essential materials"	
2. Calcium sulfate	90% minimum
Pigments	
"Other essential material"	
May contain:	
Inert filler	

CLEANERS

ABRASIVE CLEANER	Toxicity rating 2
Largely abrasive (silica, pumice) soap and sometimes fillers (clay usually about)	70–90%
Phosphates (trisodium, tripoly, pyro)	5–25%
Sodium sulfate	0–5%
Alkyl aryl sodium sulfonates	2–4%
Trichloroisocyanuric acid	0.3–5%
Water	0.5–10%

May contain:
- Caustic soda
- Chlorinated trisodium phosphate
- Citric acid
- Kerosene
- Potassium persulfate
- Sodium alkylbenzene sulfonate
- Sodium carbonate
- Sodium hypochlorite
- Sodium perborate* (in which case toxicity rating is 3)
- Sodium perchlorate
- Sodium stearate

ACID AND ALKALINE CLEANERS

Most acid and alkaline cleaners are listed under the intended use, *e.g.*, toilet bowl, metal, etc. Some individual metal cleaners, *e.g.*, copper, silver, stainless steel, aluminum, are also listed.

ALKALINE CLEANERS (see also ALKALI, Section III)

1.	No rating
Ammonium hydroxide*	3–29%
Water	71–97%
2.	No rating
Sodium hydroxide*	94%
Sodium carbonate	2%
Soap	

ALKALINE CLEANERS (Cont.)

Nonionic surfactant
Sometimes contain:
- Borax
- Calcium hydroxide*
- Sodium silicates
- Trisodium phosphate

ALUMINUM CLEANERS (see also Metal Cleaners below)

For ecological reasons, phosphates may be reduced and different detergents added, *e.g.*, or nonionics, ethoxylated alcohols, nonylphenol.

1.	Toxicity rating 3
Sodium metasilicate*	45%
Sodium tripolyphosphate*	30%
Sodium bicarbonate	20–25%
Sodium lignosulfate or alkyl aryl sodium sulfonate	3%
Nonionic surfactants (high in ethylene dioxide)	1%
2.	Toxicity rating 3
Oxalic acid crystals* (see Acid)	6%
Sodium fluoride*	4%
Soap	4%
Feldspar	85%
Wetting agent	1%

May contain
- Caustic soda* (see Alkali)
- Citric acid
- Ethylenediaminetetraacetic acid (Versene)
- Phosphoric acid
- Stearic acid

3. Silicofluoride or hydrofluoric acid
Anionic or nonionic detergents
Water
Dye
May contain:
- Sulfuric acid

4. Acid
Emulsifiers
Surface active agents
Organic solvents
May contain:
- Phosphoric acid

AUTOMOTIVE CLEANERS (see Automotive this section)

BOILER CLEANERS

Liquid (see Acid)	Toxicity rating 3
Hydrochloric acid	
Phosphoric	
Oxalic acid*	
Sulfamic acid	
Citric acid	
Ammonium or sodium fluoride*	
Powder	Toxicity rating 3
Asbestine	50%
Sodium carbonate*	25%
Trisodium phosphate	15%
Potassium dichromate*	5%
Quebracho	5%

BOILER TREATMENTS

Liquid	Toxicity rating 3
Sodium carbonate	6%
Trisodium phosphate	4%
Sodium dichromate*	2%

Starred ingredients (*) may be responsible for major toxic effects; consult Section II.

CLEANERS (Cont.)	CLEANERS (Cont.)

BOILER TREATMENTS (Cont.)

Sodium borate*	2%
Isopropanol	18%
Water	68%
Dispersant (sludge conditioner), *e.g.*, tannin, lignin sulfonates, low-molecular-weight polyacrylamides	
Powder	Toxicity rating 3
Chromates and dichromates*	
Nitrites	
Complex organic amines	
Inorganic ammonia compounds	
Dispersant (sludge conditioner), *e.g.*, tannin, lignin sulfonates, low-molecular-weight polyacrylamides	

CESSPOOL CLEANERS (see SEWER, CESSPOOL, SEPTIC TANK CLEANERS)

CHROME CLEANERS .... Toxicity rating 3 or 4

1. Abrasive
   Ammonium hydroxide* (see Alkali)
   Ammonium oxalate*
2. Abrasive
   Alcohol
   Naphtha*
   Petroleum oil
   Water
3. Oxalic acid*
   Hydrochloric acid* (see Acid)
   May contain:
   Emulsifiers

COFFEE POT CLEANERS

1.	Toxicity rating 3
Tripolyphosphate*	65%
Sodium metasilicate	30%
Alkyl aryl sodium sulfonate	5%
Ethoxylated tridecyl alcohol	0.05%
Sodium bicarbonate	

2.	Toxicity rating 3 or 4
Sodium phosphates*	
Sodium silicate	
Sodium perborate*	
Sodium carbonate*	
Surfactant	

3.	Toxicity rating 3
Silicate of soda	52.5%
"Santocel"	1.0%
Sodium sesquicarbonate	16.5%
Soda ash*	12.5%
Sodium perborate*	10.0%
CF-10	5.0%
Sodium citrate	2.5%

COIN (see JEWELRY CLEANERS)

COPPER CLEANERS (see also Metal Cleaners, below) ...... Toxicity rating 2–3

Sulfamic, citric, tartaric acid	5–10%
Sodium chloride	5–10%
Anionic synthetic surfactant	1–3%
Siliceous abrasive	to 100%
May contain:	
Fatty acid amide	
Petroleum solvents*	
Waxy tarnish preventitive	

DAIRY CLEANERS

1. Alkaline	Toxicity rating 4
Isooctylphenylpolyethoxy ethanol	1–5%
Sodium carbonate	30–35%

DAIRY CLEANERS (Cont.)

Sodium tripolyphosphate	35% maximum
Sodium bicarbonate	15–25%
Anionic surfactant	5–15%

2. Acid	Toxicity rating 4
Quaternary ammonium compounds*	15–20%
Phosphoric acid (75%)* (see Acid)	30%
Reso P-150	5%
Water	50%
May contain:	
Iodine	

3. Sanitizers	Toxicity rating 3
Quaternary ammonium compounds*	10–20%
Nonionic surfactants	5–10%
Water	to 100%
May contain:	
Sodium carbonate	
Sodium tripolyphosphate	

DENTURE CLEANERS (see NONPRESCRIPTION DRUGS)

DETERGENTS (SYNTHETIC)

The term "detergent" meaning originally "cleaner," is now widely used to specify the nonsoap cleaners referred to as synthetic detergents which are used in greater amounts than soap products today. There are three types of these surface active agents: cationic, anionic and nonionic in descending toxicity. Cationic and anionic surfactants are listed as such in Section II, nonionic surfactants have so many varied classes that they cannot be listed under a single prototype; fortunately they are *usually* of low toxicity. Examples in common use are the alkyl aryl polyether alcohols which are listed in Section II. Although the make-up of these synthetic detergents seem infinite, examples of various types are listed. The hazard is related to the degree of alkalinity (see Lye).

1. Granular detergents, laundry/general purpose	Toxicity rating 2–3
Anionic surfactant* (ammonium, sodium, potassium or magnesium salts of linear alkylbenzene sulfonate, alkyl sulfate, or alkyl ethoxylate sulfate)	0–23%
Nonionic surfactant (alkyl ethoxylate)	0–20%
Sodium carbonate*	0–68%
Sodium tripolyphosphate	0–62%
Sodium sulfate	0–51%
Sodium aluminosilicate	0–25%
Trisodium nitrilotriacetate	0–25%
Sodium silicate	2–20%
Sodium sesquicarbonate*	0–17%
Sodium tetraborate*	0–14%
Montmorillonite clay	0–10%
Sodium perborate*	0–6%
Soap	0–6%
Dialkyldimethylammonium salts	0–3%
Dextrin	0–2%
Polyethylene glycol	0–1%
Sodium carboxymethyl cellulose	0–1%
Cornstarch	0–1%
Sodium toluene sulfonate	0–1%
Tallow alcohol	0–1%
Sodium chloride	0–1%
May contain:	
Colorant	
Perfume	
Fluorescent whitening agent	
Methylcellulose	
Sodium polymeric metaphosphate	

CLEANERS (Cont.)	CLEANERS (Cont.)

DETERGENTS (SYNTHETIC) (Cont.)

Enzyme

2. Granular detergents, light-duty/delicate
   fabric .... Toxicity rating 2
   Anionic surfactant* (ammonium, so-
   dium, potassium or magnesium
   salts of linear alkylbenzene sulfo-
   nate, alkyl ethoxylate sulfate, or al-
   kyl sulfate) 14–36%
   Sodium sulfate 25–42%
   Sodium tripolyphosphate* 0–33%
   Sodium silicate* 0–18%
   Sodium chloride 0–14%
   Sodium perborate* 0–6%
   Polyethylene glycol 0–1%
   Soap 0–1%
   Sodium xylene sulfonate or sodium tol-
   uene sulfonate 0–1%
   May contain:
   Nonionic surfactant (alkyl ethoxy-
   late)
   Colorant
   Perfume
   Sodium carboxylmethyl cellulose
   Fluorescent whitening agent
   Sodium polymeric metaphosphate

3. Liquid detergents, heavy-duty laun-
   dry .... Toxicity rating 2–3
   Anionic surfactant* (ammonium, so-
   dium, potassium or magnesium
   salts of linear alkylbenzene sulfo-
   nate, or alkyl ethoxylate sulfate) 0–22%
   Nonionic surfactant (allkyl ethoxylate,
   ethoxylated alkyl phenol) 5–32%
   Tetrapotassium pyrophosphate* ... 0–33%
   Ethanol* 0–15%
   Sodium citrate 0–10%
   Soap 0–6%
   Fatty acid alkanol amide 0–5%
   Potassium or sodium toluene sulfonate,
   or potassium or sodium xylene
   sulfonate 0–3%
   Sodium silicate 0–3%
   Citric acid 0–2%
   Isopropanol 0–2%
   Propylene glycol 0–2%
   Water 34–83%
   May contain:
   Colorant
   Perfume
   Sodium carboxymethyl cellulose
   Sodium chloride
   Detergent-fabric softener combination
   also may contain in addition to the
   above:
   Dialkyldimethylammonium salt
   Alkyltrimethylammonium salt
   Alkyldiethylmethylammonium salt

4. Liquid detergents, hand dishwashing/
   delicate fabrics .... Toxicity rating 2
   Anionic surfactant* (ammonium, so-
   dium, potassium or magnesium
   salts of linear alkylbenzene sulfonate, alkyl sulfate, alkyl ethoxylate
   sulfate, alkyl glyceryl sulfonate) .. 0–29%
   Ethanol 0–11%
   Nonionic surfactant (alkyl ethoxylate,
   alkyl amine oxide) 0–15%

DETERGENTS (SYNTHETIC) (Cont.)

Sodium or potassium toluene sulfonate
   or xylene sulfonate 0–7%
Fatty acid alkanol amide 0–6%
Ammonium, potassium and sodium
   chloride 0–5%
Alkyldiethylmethylammonium salt ... 0–5%
Hydroxyethylcellulose 0–1%
Isopropanol 0–1%
Water 44–89%
May contain:
   Gelatin protein
   Fluorescent whitening agent
   Ammonium sulfate
   Ammonium citrate
   Perfume
   Colorant

5. Liquid detergent, hard-surface cleaner/
   organic solvent base .... Toxicity rating 2
   Organic solvent* (isopropanol, petroleum naphtha, ethanol, butoxyethanol diethyleneglycol monoethyl ether) 0–35%
   Pine oil* 0–30%
   Anionic surfactant* (sodium, potassium, ammonium or magnesium
   salt of linear alkylbenzene
   sulfonate) 0–15%
   Nonionic surfactant (ethoxylated alkyl
   phenol, alkyl ethoxylate) 0–6%
   Sodium carbonate* 0–15%
   Ammonia 0–5%
   Tetrasodium pyrophosphate 0–2%
   Disinfectant* (mixed quaternary am-
   monium salts, o-benzyl-p-
   chlorophenol) 0–4%
   Soap 0–10%
   Water 50%

6. Liquid detergent, hard-surface
   cleaner/surfactant base .... Toxicity rating 3
   Tetrapotassium pryophosphate ... 10–15%
   Anionic surfactant* (sodium, potas-
   sium, ammonium or magnesium
   salts of linear alkylbenzene sulfo-
   nate, or alkyl ethoxylate sulfate) . 0–15%
   Nonionic surfactant (alkyl ethoxylate) 0–10%
   Fatty acid alkanol amide 0–5%
   Sodium or potassium carbonate* ... 0–15%
   Sodium citrate 0–10%
   Water 75%

**DETERGENTS, AUTOMATIC
   DISHWASHER** .... Toxicity rating 3

1. Household, low alkalinity
   Sodium tripolyphosphate 10–40%
   Sodium silicate, hydrated 15–30%
   Trisodium phosphate* 10–20%
   Nonionic surfactant 3%
   Sodium hypochlorite 1%

2. Household, high alkalinity ...... Toxicity rating 4
   Sodium metasilicate, anhydrous* .. 10–20%
   Sodium tripolyphosphate 10–40%
   Sodium carbonate* 10–40%
   Surfactant (nonionic or anionic) ... 1–6%
   Potassium dichloro-s-triazinetrione . 0–1%

3. Commercial, high alkalinity
   May contain:
   Alkyl aryl sodium sulfonate

Starred ingredients (*) may be responsible for major toxic effects; consult Section II.

CLEANERS (Cont.)	CLEANERS (Cont.)

DETERGENTS, AUTOMATIC DISHWASHER (Cont.)

Chlorinated trisodium phosphate
Polyalkalene glycol
Sodium sulfate

DETERGENTS, HAND WASHING (liquid), light-duty, dishes and delicate fabrics

Anionic surfactant (sodium or ammonium salts of alkylbenzene sulfonate, alkyl sulfate, alkyl polyethoxy sulfate, alkyl aryl polyether sulfonate, alkyl glycerol ether sulfonate)	20–40%
Noninic surfactant (alkyl phenyl polyethoxyethanol, polyalkalene glycol, fatty acid alkanolamine amide)	0–8%
Soap	0–2%
Na or K toluene sulfonate or xylene sulfonate	0–10%
Tetrapotassium pyrophosphate	0–25%
Fatty acid, alkanolamine amide	0–2%
Denatured ethyl alcohl	0–10%
Isopropyl alcohol (* if >10%)	0–12%
Water	40–70%
Pine oil*	0–38%
Propylene glycol	0–10%
Naphtha*	0–30%

May contain:
o-Benzyl-p-chlorophenol†
Chloro-o-phenylphenol†
Diethanolamine
Dyes
Ethylene glycol (* if >10%)
Optical brightener
Perfumes
Petroleum solvents (* if >10%)
Sodium carboxymethyl cellulose— trace
Sodium nitrate
Sodium or ammonium sulfate
Sodium salts of ethylenediaminetetraacetic acid
Sodium tripolyphosphate
Trisodium phosphate (* if >10%)

DIAPER CLEANERS .... Toxicity rating 3

1. Quaternary ammonium compounds*	0–20%
Sodium metasilicate	0–5%
Trisodium phosphate	0–5%
Triethanolamine oleate	0–1%
Sodium sesquicarbonate	
Sodium perborate*	
Sodium tripolyphosphate	
Anionic detergents	
2. Paradichlorobenzene*	
Essential oils	

DISINFECTANT CLEANERS

1. Quaternary ammonium compounds*	Toxicity rating 2
Alkyl (C₈–C₁₈) dimethylbenzyl ammonium chloride	0.5–2.5%
Octyl or nonyl phenoxy polyethoxyethanol (see Alkyl)	2–5%
Sodium carbonate	0.1–0.3%
Sodium salt of ethylenediaminetetraacetic acid (see Versene)	0.1–1.0%
Sodium sulfite or nitrite	0.05–1.0%
Water	90–98%
May contain:	

DISINFECTANT CLEANERS (Cont.)

Alkyl phenoxy polyethoxy alcohol
Alkyl dimethyl amyl ammonium chlorides

2. Substituted phenolic	Toxicity rating 2
Coconut oil soap (anhydrous)	10–15%
Alkyl aryl sodium sulfonate	
Isopropyl alcohol	6–15%
Propylene glycol	6–10%
Substituted phenols (e.g., o-benzyl-p-chlorophenol)	3–10%
Potassium hydroxide or sodium hydroxide	0.2–0.8%
Sodium sulfite or nitrite	0.05–1.0%
Water	70–80%
3. Substituted phenolics and pine oil	Toxicity rating 2
Coconut oil soap (anhydrous)	4–10%
Substituted phenols (e.g., o-benzyl-p-chlorophenol)	3–5%
Isopropyl alcohol	5–10%
Pine oil	5–10%
Water	70–80%
4. Pine oil disinfectant	Toxicity rating 3
Pine oil*	60–80%
Vegetable oil soap (anhydrous)	20–30%
Water	10–20%

Germicides of pine type or mint type may contain anhydrous soap (10–12%), steam distilled pine oil or methyl salicylate* (3–15%), alcohol (5–10%), o-benzyl-p-chlorophenol (3–5%) and water (to make 100%).

DRAIN AND PIPE, POWDER ....   No rating

Sodium or potassium hydroxide* (see alkali)	90–100%
Sodium nitrate	0–30%
Aluminum particles (metal)	2–5%
Sodium chloride	0–10%
Sodium carbonate	2–5%
Talc	
May contain:	
Trichlorobenzene	1%
Kerosene	1%
Urea	5%
Sodium chloride	10–20%
Pine oil	0.25%
Methyl salicylate	0.25%
Corrosion inhibitor (thiourea)	0.1%
Nonionic surfactant	0.5%

DRAIN AND PIPE, LIQUID ....   No rating

1. Hydrochloric acid* (see Acid)	
Sulfuric acid	
1,3-Dichloro-5,5-dimethylhydantoin* (see Hypochlorite)	3–5%
May contain:	
Enzymes	
Saprophytic, nonpathogenic bacteria	
2. Sodium or potassium hydroxide solutions	5–10%
3. 1,1,1-Trichloroethane	70–100%
May contain:	
Surfactants	
Corrosion inhibitors	

DRY CLEANERS

Once, carbon tetrachloride was considered the dry cleaner par excellence, in a large part due to its nonflammability. Now, because of its toxic action, especially on liver and kidneys, it has been banned from household products. Methyl chloroform is sometimes used.

Starred ingredients (*) may be responsible for major toxic effects; consult Section II.

CLEANERS (Cont.)		CLEANERS (Cont.)	

DRY CLEANERS (Cont.)

1. 1,1,1-Trichloroethane* . . . . Toxicity rating 3
   100%

2. 1,1,1-Trichloroethane* . . . . Toxicity rating 3
   less than 100%
   Combined with:
   Perchloroethylene*
   Petroleum solvents (Stoddard solvent)*
   Surfactants
   Emulsifiers
   Toluene
   May contain:
   Ethylene dichloride
   o-Dichlorobenzene
   Xylene
   If xylene, toluene, or o-dichlorobenzene are present, in appreciable quantities, the toxicity rating is 4.

EGG CLEANSER . . . . Toxicity rating 3
Sodium tripolyphosphate* 50%
Sodium metasilicate 15%
Quaternary ammonium compounds . . . 10%
Soda ash 20%
Isooctylphenylpolyethoxy ethanol 5%
Antifoam 1%
May contain:
Sodium carbonate

ENGINE AND MOTOR (see AUTOMOTIVE CLEANERS)

FIREARM . . . . Toxicity rating 3
Denatured ethanol 30%
Kerosene* 30%
Saponifiable animal oil 25%
Aqua ammonia 2%
Oil mirbane (nitrobenzene)* 2%
Essential oils 11%
May contain:
Emulsifiers
Lubricating oil

FLOOR CLEANERS . . . . Toxicity rating 3
1. Pine oil* 0–10%
   Fatty acid soap 5–30%
   Synthetic anionic* or nonionic surfactant 0–20%
   Sodium polyphosphates 0–15%
   Amines 0–5%
   Ammonia 0–5%
   Toxicity rating 3
2. Petroleum solvents* 85–100%
   Waxes 4–12%
   Synthetic nonionic surfactant 0–10%
   May contain:
   Dyes, trace
   Nitrobenzene*
   Perfumes, trace
   Sodium perborate*
   Sodium metasilicate
   Trisodium phosphate
   Alkyl aryl sodium sulfonate
   Carboxymethyl cellulose
   Glycol ether
   Potassium hydroxide

FURNACE AND FIREPLACE (soot destroyers)
1. . . . . Toxicity rating 2

FURNACE AND FIREPLACE (Cont.)

Charcoal
Potassium nitrate
2. . . . . Toxicity rating 3
   Sodium chloride 74.0%
   Ammonium chloride 10.0%
   Copper sulfate* 3.5%
   Wood flour 10.0%
   Red iron oxide 1.5%
   Magnesium carbonate 1.0%
3. Liquid . . . . Toxicity rating 3
   Kerosene* 65%
   Copper 6% liquid linoresinate 14%
   Zinc 8% liquid linoresinate 2%
   o-Dichlorobenzene* 14%
   Morpholine 3%
   Petronate 0.1%
   Butyl alcohol 1%
   Flake naphthalene 0.6%
   Camphor 0.05%
   May contain:
   Copper chloride*

GENERAL CLEANER
Powder (all purpose) . . . . Toxicity rating 3
Trisodium phosphate* 10–90%
Sodium carbonate* (see Alkali) 10–60%
Sodium sesquicarbonate* 20–30%
Sodium pyrophosphate* 0–20%
Sodium tripolyphosphate* 5–50%
Sodium silicate 0–5%
Alkyl aryl sodium sulfonate 5–20%
May contain:
Pine oil* 10%
Sodium perborate (* if >1%)
Liquid (all purpose) . . . . Toxicity rating 2–3
Synthetic anionic surfactant (or nonionic surfactant) 5–10%
Fatty acid amides 1–5%
Water 50–70%
May contain:
Stoddard solvent* or naphtha* . . . 25%
Complex phosphates (pyrophosphate or tripolyphosphate) 10%
Pine oil* 10–30%
Alkali* (caustic potash, carbonates and metasilicates) 10–30%
Detergents should also be consulted in this section.

GERMICIDAL (see DISINFECTANT)

GLASS (window cleaners) . . . . Toxicity rating 2
1. Butyl cellosolve 3–5%
   Alcohol 3–5%
   Wetting agent 0.5–1%
   Isopropanol 0–15%
   Dyes . . . . trace
   Silicone . . . . trace
   Water . . . . to 100%
   May contain:
   Alkali
   Ammonia
   Bentonia
   Celite
   Essential oils
   Naphthas
   Nonyl phenoxy polyethoxy ethanol-iodine complex
   Organic solvents

Starred ingredients (*) may be responsible for major toxic effects; consult Section II.

CLEANERS (Cont.)		CLEANERS (Cont.)	

GLASS WINDOW CLEANERS (Cont.)

Phosphoric acid
Sodium polyphosphate
Turkey red oil
Waxes (carnauba, Japan)

2.	Toxicity rating 2
Isopropyl alcohol	6–25%
Glycol ether	10–11%
Ethylene glycol	1%
Surfactant (usually an anionic but occasionally a nonionic, such as Triton X-200 or Turkey red oil)	
Water	60–85%

3.	Toxicity rating 2
If a spray, a small amount of hydrocarbon propellants	3–5%

May contain:

Dyes	small amount
Perfumes	
Phosphates	
Freon	each 6%
Fillers	

4.	Toxicity rating 2 or 3
Window waxes	
Silica abrasive	
Amine soaps	
Waxes	
Petroleum solvent*	
Ammonium hydroxide	trace

HAND CLEANERS, POWDERED

a.	Toxicity rating 2
Pumice	40–70%
Soap	20–35%
Sodium phosphate	0–5%
Colloidal clay	0–25%
Sodium carbonate	0–5%
b.	Toxicity rating 4
Borax*	60–80%
Soap	20–40%

HAND CLEANERS, WATERLESS .... Toxicity rating 3

Soap (sodium, potassium, ammonium or triethanolamine)	10–30%
Solvent (high flash naphtha*)	20–60%
Anionic surfactant	0–10%

May contain:
Mild abrasive
Water
Cream base
Perfume

INDUSTRIAL: GENERAL

This category has been covered under the subheads: Dairy, Automotive, etc. In general, the cleaners are much the same as in other categories except stronger. For example, the surfactant may be a quarternary ammonium compound, toxic rating 4. Concentrated strong acids or alkalis are apt to be present. If fluorides or borates are present, they are apt to be there in toxic amounts. If what is needed is not under a more specific category, the ingredients mentioned above are those to be considered toxicologically.

JEWELRY CLEANERS .... Toxicity rating 2

Animal fatty acid	5–15%
Aqua ammonia*	5–25%
Isopropanol	10–15%
Dye	traces
Perfume	traces
Water	to 100%

JEWELRY CLEANERS (Cont.)

May contain:
Cyanide* (if present, toxicity rating 5)
Thiourea
Sulfuric acid*
Polyethylene glycols

LEATHER CLEANERS

Saddle soaps are probably the most widely used home cleaners for leather, although they are far from being the only products used.

1. Saddle soap	Toxicity rating 2
a. Palm oil	21.4%
Rosin (light)	1.8%
Caustic soda (°Bé 38) (33%)	11.4%
Water	51.4%
Glycerine	7.7%
Talc	0.3%
May contain:	
Cyclohexanol	3%
Wax	1.5%
b.	Toxicity rating 2
Powdered soap	15.0%
Beeswax	8%
Neatsfoot oil	5.0%
Water	72.0%
c.	Toxicity rating 3
Carnauba wax	40.9%
Soap flakes	15.2%
Tallow	19.7%
Turpentine*	15.9%
Sperm oil	4.5%
Water	3.8%
d.	Toxicity rating 2
Triethanolamine oleate	3.8%
Alcohol	3.8%
Potassium carbonate	0.5%
Water	q.s. 100%
2.	Toxicity rating 3
Mineral oil* (see Kerosene)	45–55%
Nonionic surfactant	45–55%
3.	Toxicity rating 3
Sulfonated oils*	20–30%
Mineral spirits*	35–40%
Water	35–40%
4.	Toxicity rating 2
Alkyl aryl sodium sulfonate	7%
Water	93%

May contain:
Fatty amide condensate
Isopropanol
Hydrophylic wax-cyclohexanoneamine wax
Sodium metasilicate
Sulfonated ketones

LENS CLEANERS   Toxicity rating 2

1. Surfactant } Phosphate salt }	4%
Water	96%
2. Isopropyl alcohol	12%
Wetting agent	2–4%
Water	82–86%

May contain:
Silicones

LIME MORTAR CLEANER .... Toxicity rating 3

Sulfamic acid*	97%

LIPSTICK (see STAIN, SPOT, etc.)

CLEANERS (Cont.)   CLEANERS (Cont.)

MASONRY CLEANER (CONCRETE)

		No rating
Phosphoric acid* (see Acid)	25%	
Isopropanol	maximum 5%	
Anionic surfactant	maximum 3%	
Dye		
Water		

May contain:
  Alkyl sodium phosphate
  Hydrochloric acid*
  Trisodium phosphate*

METAL CLEANERS

For ecological reasons, phosphates may be reduced and different detergents added, *e.g.*, anionics or nonionics, ethoxylated alcohols, nonylphenol.

1. Alkaline type .... Toxicity rating 3
    Caustic soda or potash*
      (see alkali) 0–50%
    Trisodium phosphate* 25–75%
    Sodium metasilicate 10–75%
    Soap or detergent (alkyl aryl sodium
      sulfoante) 5–20%
2. Solvent type .... Toxicty rating 3
  a. Perchloroethylene* 1–100%
     Trichloroethylene* 1–100%
     1,1,1-Trichloroethane* 1–100%
  b. .... Toxicity rating 3
     Kerosene* 5–80%
     Potassium soap of oleic acid 5–25%
     Glycol ether 5–20%
     Surfactant 5–20%
3. Acid type* (see Acid) .... Toxicity rating 4
  a. Hydrochloric acid or one or more of
     the following 5–25%
     Sulfuric acid 10–20%
     Chromic acid* 5–20%
     Phosphoric acid 10–25%
     Citric acid 10–25%
    Surfactant 5–10%
    May contain:
      Cedarwood oil
      Kerosene*
      Sodium carbonate
      Tripolyphosphates
  b. .... Toxicity rating 2
     Phosphoric acid 40–80%
     Water 40–80%
     Surfactant 0–5%
  c. .... Toxicity rating 2
     Citric acid 5–50%
     Ammonium citrate 0–20%
     Water 0–50%
     Surfactant 0–5%
  See under the individual metal if listed, such as aluminum, copper, silver, stainless steel, etc.

MONUMENT CLEANERS

1. Granite .... Toxicity rating 4
    Ammonium or sodium bifluoride*
     (see sodium fluoride) 100%
2. Marble
  a. Sodium hydrosulfate .... Toxicity rating 3?
  b. Mixture of alcohol and ketone
  c. Hydrogen peroxide, 50%*
  d. See under porcelain cleaners
3. For iron and mill stain
    Muriatic acid*

MONUMENT CLEANERS (Cont.)

  Phosphoric acid*
  Oxalic acid*

OVEN CLEANER

1. .... Toxicity rating 3
    Potassium or sodium hydroxide* (see
     Alkali) .... maximum 10%
    Starch, glue, etc. 5–15%
    Nonionic synthetic surfactant 1–5%
    May contain:
     N-Acetyl ethanolamine 0–2%
     Butyl Cellosolve 0–2%
     Glycols
     Jellifying agents
     Methylene chloride*
     Oleic acid
     Petroleum distillates* 0–25%
     Pine oil*
     Silica
     Sodium orthosilicate 10%
     Sodium xylene sulfonate 0–0.5%
     Whiting 0–2%
2. Oven cleaners .... No rating
    Sodium hydroxide base* (see Alkali)
3. .... Toxicity rating 2
    Sodium orthosilicate 11.0%
    Whiting (chalk) 2.0%
    Cellulose 2.5%
    N-Acetyl ethanolamine 2.0%
    Butyl cellosolve 2.0%
    Sodium xylene sulfonate 0.5%
    Water .... q.s.
4. Spray-type .... Toxicity rating 2–3
    Amines
    Detergents
    Ether-type solvents
    Propellants
    Sodium hydroxide* .... maximum 5%
    Thickeners

PAINT BRUSH CLEANERS

Painters still use turpentine* (toxicity rating 4) for cleaning paint brushes, followed by washing in ordinary soap. Therefore, turpentine is still recommended as such. However, there are paint brush cleaners on the market, usually a mixture of aromatic hydrocarbons, methyl alcohol and acetone. Sample formulas are:

	Toxicity rating 4
1. Benzene (and toluene, xylene)*	25–90%
Acetone	10–40%
Methyl alcohol	10–15%
Naphtha or Stoddard solvent	0–5%

Naphthas* and related compounds (kerosene) if present as principal constituents would have toxicity rating 3.

	Toxicity rating 3
2.	
Kerosene*	57%
Oleic acid	29%
Ammonia (strong)	7%
Alcohol (denatured)	7%

PAINT AND VARNISH CLEANERS

1. Liquid	Toxicity rating 2
a. Soap	2%
Anionic surfactant	1%
Water	q.s.
b.	Toxicity rating 2
Sulfated fatty alcohol	10%

Starred ingredients (*) may be responsible for major toxic effects; consult Section II.

CLEANERS (Cont.)

PAINT AND VARNISH CLEANERS (Cont.)

Ammonia	20%
Water	70%
c.	Toxicity rating 2–3
Soap	6%
Kerosene*	17%
Colloidal clay	7%
Water	70%
Borax*	
Isopropyl alcohol	
Tetrasodium pyrophosphate	
2. Paste type	Toxicity rating 2–3
Soap	20–30%
Kerosene*	0–40%
Trisodium phosphate	0–15%
Water	50–75%
May contain:	
Filler (silica, kaolin)	10–40%
Sodium carbonate* (see Alkali)	0–40%
Perfume	less than 1%
3. Powdered	Toxicity rating 3
Trisodium phosphate*	30–50%
Soda ash (sodium carbonate*) (see Alkali)	25–50%
Soap	0–8%
May contain:	
Sodium bicarbonate	25%
Ammonium chloride	5%
4. Miscellaneous	Toxicity rating 3
Dichloromethane*	49.0%
Ethylene dichloride*	30.0%
Alcohol	3.5%
Naphthalene*	8.5%
Paraffin	7.0%
Resin	1.4%
Rubber	0.5%
Acetophenol	0.1%

PAINT AND VARNISH REMOVERS

1. Flammable	Toxicity rating 4
Benzene*	15–50%
Methanol	10–25%
Acetone	10–25%
Paraffin wax	1–5%
Toluene*	0–75%
Ethylcellulose	1–2%
May contain:	
Alkyl aryl sodium sulfonate	
Borax	
Ethanol or proprietary solvent	
Isopropanol	0–5%
Mineral spirits	
Phenol*	
Potassium bitartrate or citrate	
Sodium sesquicarbonate	
1,1,1-Trichloroethane	0–55%
Triethyl ammonium phosphates	
Trisodium phosphate	
2. Nonflammable	Toxicity rating 3
Methylene chloride*	70–90%
Methanol	5–15%
Toluene*	1–3%
Methyl cellulose or ethyl cellulose	0.75–1.0%
Paraffin wax	2–5%
May contain:	
Carbon tetrachloride* (if present, toxicity rating 4)	40%
Isopropanol	0–9%
Mineral spirits	0–3%

CLEANERS (Cont.)

PAINT AND VARNISH REMOVERS (Cont.)

Nonionic surfactants } Potassium oleate }	3–6%
Ethylene dichloride	
3. Stripping agents, paint remover	Toxicity rating 3–4
Phenols*	
Cresols*	
Methylene chloride*	
Organic acid catalyst (acetate, formate)	
Concentrated alkali*	

PAINT CLEANER	Toxicity rating 2
Waxes	
Resins	
Emulsifiers	
Water	

PLANT CLEANER	Toxicity rating 2
Waxes	
Resins	
Emulsifiers	
Water	

PORCELAIN, MARBLE, TILE AND ENAMEL CLEANERS

1.	Toxicity rating 2
Abrasive	88%
Sodium tripolyphosphate	5%
Alkyl aryl sodium sulfonate	5%
Trisodium sulfonate	2%
2.	Toxicity rating 3
Stoddard solvent*	0–31%
Morpholine	0–2%
Trisodium phosphate	0–3%
Soap	0–3%
Wetting agent	0–1%
Silica	0–65%
Water	to 100%

RADIATOR CLEANERS (see AUTOMOTIVE PRODUCTS)

RUBBING COMPOUND (see AUTOMOTIVE PRODUCTS)

RUG AND UPHOLSTERY CLEANERS

Like so many cleaners, the permutations and combinations are legion. Formulas may be varied to suit various needs. Those listed here are examples only with an attempt to cover most of the ingredients apt to be met. The formulas may be used for carpets, rugs and upholstery.

1. Synthetic detergent	Toxicity rating 3

Solid types contain anionic (sodium lauryl sulfate) and nonionic sufactants* up to 40–50% with fillers, *e.g.*, sodium silicate, sodium sulfate. The liquid types are similar except that the active ingredients are much more dilute, *e.g.*:

Fatty alcohol sulfate	2.0%
Trisodium phosphate	1.5%
Alcohol	10.5%
Water	86.0%
2. Alkaline cleaners	Toxicity rating 2–3
Soda soap	55–75%
Trisodium phosphate	6–15%
Sodium carbonate	0–15%
Borax*	0–30%
Naphthalene*	0–1%
Oils, essential	0–1.5%

Starred ingredients (*) may be responsible for major toxic effects; consult Section II.

CLEANERS (Cont.)	CLEANERS (Cont.)

RUG AND UPHOLSTERY CLEANERS (Cont.)

May contain:
Sodium lauryl sulfate (see Alkyl sodium sulfate*)

3. Soap-solvent combination . . . . Toxicity rating 2
Butyl Cellosolve 2.5–3.5%
Ethylene dichloride 7.5–8.5%
Oleic acid 7.5–11.0%
Ammonia (28%) 0.7–5%
Triethanolamine 0–8%
Soap 0–2%
Borax 0–2%
Denatured alcohol 0–10%
Isopropyl alcohol 0–7%
Water 45–95%

4. Upholstery (mainly for) . . . . Toxicity rating 3
Perchloroethylene*   or   1,1,1-
trichloroethane* . . . . up to 50%
Petroleum solvent (Stoddard*) . . . . up to 50%
Alkaline salts 10–20%
Butane propellant, for sprays only
Water
May contain:
Ammonia
Borax, small amount
Ethylene dichloride
Lanolin
o-Dichlorobenzene
Perfume
Pine oil, up to 10%
Soap
Sodium bicarbonate
Sodium chloride
Sodium sulfate

5. Absorbent type (for rugs) . . . . Toxicity rating 4
a. Sawdust
Trichloroethylene*
b. Buckwheat or bentonite 60–70%
Petroleum distillate* (*light) 25%
Wood flour 5%
May contain:
Salicylic acid 1%

SEWER, CESSPOOL, SEPTIC TANK
CLEANERS . . . .   No rating
1. Sodium and potassium hydroxide* (see
alkali) 90–100%
Aluminum particles (metal) 2–5%
Sodium carbonate 2–5%
Talc 2–5%
Trichlorobenzene 1%
Kerosene . . . . 1% -
Urea 5%
2. Sodium bisulfate* (see Acid) 80–100%
Sodium chloride 10–20%
Enzymes
Dried yeast
Peat moss
Copper sulfate
Sugar
Aluminum sulfate
Lime
Note: By far the most common cleaner in this category is
strong sodium hydroxide (up to 100%). Alkalis of this strength
are extremely dangerous if splashed in the eye. Blindness may
result.
3. . . . . Toxicity rating 2
Cerelose dextrose 80%

SEWER, CESSPOOL, SEPTIC TANK CLEANERS (Cont.)

Enzymes 15%
Yeast 5%

SHAVER CLEANER
1. . . . . Toxicity rating 3
1,1,1-Trichloroethane* 95%
Petroleum lubricant
Perfume . . . . trace
Dye . . . . trace
2. . . . . Toxicity rating 2
Ethyl alcohol 85–87%
Pelargonic, stearic, palmitic or myristic
acid esters 10–13%
Silicone 0.5–1.0%
Dye . . . . trace
May contain:
n-Alkyl dimethyl benzyl* ammonium
chloride 0.06%
Captan

SHOE CLEANERS (see also Saddle Soap under Leather
cleaners, and Shoe polishes)
For white shoes . . . . Toxicity rating 2 or 3
Titanium dioxide
Trisodium phosphate*

SILVER CLEANERS (see POLISHES)

SKIN CLEANERS (see under DETERGENTS above; also
SOAPS)

STAINLESS STEEL CLEANERS (also
see Metal Cleaners) . . . . Toxicity rating 2
Sulfamic, citric, tartaric acid 5–10%
Sodium chloride 5–10%
Anionic synthetic surfactant 1–3%
Corrosion inhibitor (e.g., sodium acid
phosphates, borax, etc.) 0–1%
Siliceous abrasive . . . . to 100%

STAIN, SPOT, LIPSTICK, RUST REMOVERS
1. Bleach type . . . . Toxicity rating 2
Sodium hypochlorite 2–8%
Water 92–98%
2. Solvent type . . . . Toxicity rating 3–4
Perchloroethylene* or trichloro-
ethane 20–50%
Naphtha* 10–30%
Isopropanol 10–30%
Acetic acid 5–10%
3. General type . . . .   No rating
Ammonium hydroxide*
May contain:
Amyl, butyl and ethyl acetate*
Benzene*
Essential oils
Oxalic acid*
p-Hydroxybenzoic acid
Soap
Sodium sulfate
Surfactants (alkyl aryl sodium sul-
fonate)
Tetrapotassium pyrophosphate
Toluene*
4. Bleach type (coffee stain removers) . . . Toxicity rating 3
Sodium hypochlorite* 8%
Water 92%
5. Iodine stain remover . . . . Toxicity rating 2
Sodium thiosulfate 10%
Water 90%

Starred ingredients (*) may be responsible for major toxic effects; consult Section II.

CLEANERS (Cont.)

STAIN, SPOT, LIPSTICK, RUST REMOVERS (Cont.)

6. Lipstick removers .... Toxicity rating 3
   a. Isopropyl alcohol*
   b. Isoamyl acetate* .... Toxicity rating 3
      Petroleum hydrocarbons*
   c. Butyl Cellosolve* .... Toxicity rating 4
      Chloroform*
      Alcohol
7. Rust and ink removers .... Toxicity rating 3 or 4
   Oxalic acid
   Methyl alcohol*
   Water
8. Rust remover .... No rating
   Phosphoric acid* 30–50%
   Penetrant 1–5%
   Alcohols 1–5%
   Water 40%
   Corrosion inhibitors .... trace

STEAM (IRON)* CLEANERS   Toxicity rating 3
Caustic soda* (see Alkali) 15–25%
Anionic detergents* (see akyl aryl sodium sulfonate)
Trisodium phosphate* 75–85%

STOVE AND OVEN CLEANERS (see OVEN CLEANERS)

TAR REMOVERS .... Toxicity rating 4
Xylene*
Chlorinated hydrocarbons*
Mineral spirits
May contain:
   Isopropyl alcohol
   Surfactants

TEFLON CLEANER .... Toxicity rating 3
Sodium perborate
Sodium metasilicate
Inorganic salts
Synthetic organic detergents

TIRE CLEANERS (see AUTOMOTIVE PRODUCTS)

TOILET BOWL CLEANERS (ACID CLEANERS)

1. Solid .... Toxicity rating 3–4
   Sodium acid sulfate* 70–100%
   Octyl or nonyl phenoxy polyethoxy
      ethanol ....
   Sodium sulfate 0–3%
   Sodium acid oxalate* 0–2%
   1,3-Dichloro-5,5-dimethylhydantoin*
      (probably similar to chlorinated
      isocyanurates) 0–95%
   Sodium chloride 0–10%
   Sodium carbonate 0–10%
   Perfume (pine oil, methyl salicylate
      etc.) 0–1%
   May contain:
      Alkyl aryl sodium sulfonate ... 0–2%
2. Liquid .... Toxicity rating 3–4
   Hydrochloric acid* 8–30%
   Octyl or nonyl phenoxy poly ethoxy
      ethanol
   Quaternary ammonium compounds .. 0–3%
   Kerosene 0–3%
   (Chlorinate phenols* (e.g., o-benzyl-p-
      chlorophenol, 1-3-dichloro-5-
      dimethylhydantoin) 0–1%
   Perfume }
   Dye   } 0–0.5%

CLEANERS (Cont.)

TOILET BOWL CLEANERS (ACID CLEANERS) (Cont.)

May contain:
   Alkyl aryl sodium sulfonate
   o- or p-Dichlorobenzene
   Hepta decyl hydroxyethyl imidazo-
      line
   Iodine
   Soda ash*
   Sodium metasilicate*
   Sodium nitrate
   Sodium tripolyphosphate
   Turbifying agents, e.g.,
      Polystyrene resin
      Polyacrylate resin
   Tetrasodium pyrophosphate
   2,2'-Thiobis(4,6-dichlorophenol)
   Tris(hydroxymethyl)nitromethane   0.1–0.5%
   Versene
   Zinc chloride*

TYPEWRITER CLEANER .... Toxicity rating 3
1,1,1-Trichloroethane (methyl chloroform)*

WALL CLEANERS (see also Paint, Floor,
or Wallpaper Cleaners) .... Toxicity rating 3
Ammonium hydroxide*
Borax
Colloidal clay
Diglycol stearate
Kerosene*
Powdered dry soap
Silica
Soda ash
Sodium lauryl sulfate
Sulfated fatty alcohol
Trisodium phosphate*
Nonionic surfactants 0.5–5.0%

WALLPAPER CLEANER .... Toxicity rating 2
1. Wheat flour 42%
   Water and salt solution 55%
   Kerosene 2%
   Ammonium alum 0.006%
   Aniline or vegetable dye .... trace
2. Kaolin 79%
   100 Octane DC naphtha* 20%
   Carbon tetrachloride* 1%
   May contain:
      Alkali metal salts as perservatives
         (slight amount)
      Ammonium hydroxide*
      Borax*
      Coconut oil soap
      Ethyl ether*
      Ethylene dichloride*
      Ethylene glycol monobutyl ether
      Glycerin
      Kerosene (slight amount)
      Naphthalene*
      Nonionic surfactant
      Oleic acid
      Potash
      Sawdust
      Soda ash
      Triethanolamine
      Trisodium phosphate

WALLPAPER REMOVER .... Toxicity rating 3
1. Cellosolve* (ethylene glycol monoethyl
      ether) 25%

Starred ingredients (*) may be responsible for major toxic effects; consult Section II.

CLEANERS (Cont.)	

WALLPAPER REMOVER (Cont.)

Water	to 100%
May contain:	
Butyl Cellosolve*	
Soda ash	5%
Sodium tetradecyl sulfate (alkyl sodium sulfate)*	
2. Hydroxyacetic acid*	30%
Penetrant	40%
Water	30%

3. Either organic or mineral acids in different proportions.
Penetrant* (see Kerosene)
Water

WINDSHIELD WASHER SOLVENTS ... Toxicity rating 3

1. Concentrate:

Methyl alcohol	90%
Water	9.8%
Surfactant	0.2%
Dye	trace

To be diluted 1:1 with water

2. Ready to use:

a. Ethylene glycol*	10–45%
Isopropyl alcohol	50–85%
Potassium phosphate	0–1%
Water	4–20%
Dye	trace
b. Propylene glycol	0–10%
Ethylene glycol*	10–15%
Isopropyl alcohol*	50–85%
Dye } Surfactant }	0–2%
c. Isopropyl alcohol*	30–85%
Water	5–50%
Surfactant	0–5%
Dye	trace
d. Methyl alcohol*	5–25%
Isopropyl alcohol*	25–50%
Water	0–30%
Surfactant } Dye }	small amounts

COATINGS

ASPHALT	Toxicity rating 3–4
Asphalt	55–65%
	(up to 70%)
Mineral spirits*	25–35%
Asbestos fiber	6–12%
May contain:	
Aluminum pigment	
Aromatic solvents*	
Silicates and carbonates	0–20%

Use of asbestos is diminishing.

BOILER COVERING	Toxicity rating 1
Asbestos fiber	
Clay	
Marble	

METAL COATINGS

1. Zinc	Toxicity rating 2–3
Pigment	80.8%
Metallic zinc (100%) or	
Zinc 80%, zinc oxide 20%	
Vehicle	19.2%
Sodium silicate	
Potassium silicate	
Sodium and potassium silicate	

COATINGS (Cont.)	

METAL COATINGS (Cont.)

Ethyl silicate
Ammonium silicate
Chlorinated rubber
Styrene-butadiene rubber
Other rubbers
Epoxy and epoxy polysulfides*
(see Resin plastics, Section VI or Polysulfides)

2. Aluminum coating	Toxicity rating 3–4
Pigment	10–12%
Aluminum powder (100%)	
Vehicle:	88–90%
Vegetable oil or marine oil	25.0%
Polyindenes and terpenes	
Phenolic resin solids	25.0%
Aliphatic* or aromatic* hydrocarbons	60–77%
May contain:	
Driers	

RUBBER BASE COATINGS	Toxicity rating 3
Pigment	36.4%
Titanium dioxide	18.9%
Zinc oxide	3.1%
Magnesium silicate	14.4%
Also see Pigments	
Vehicle:	63.6%
Chlorinated rubbers and alkyd resin solids, or	25.4%
Chlorinated resins, chlorinated bisphenols	
Blended hydrocarbons* (see Petroleum distillate)	38.2%
Rubbers, synthetic and natural	Toxicity rating 3–4

Aromatic hydrocarbon solvents*
Lower alcohols (e.g., isopropyl*)
Siliceous fillers
May contain:
Methyl isobutyl ketone*
Methyl ethyl ketone*
Dibutyl phthalate
Dioctyl phthalate

SILICONE COATINGS	Toxicity rating 3–4
Silicone resin	3–5% (or more)
Aliphatic* or aromatic solvents*	95–97%

Often resins, such as epoxy, polyamide, nitrocellulose, alkyd, phenolic, etc., may be used similarly to silicone.

CORN REMOVERS (see NONPRESCRIPTION DRUGS)

COSMETICS

ANTIPERSPIRANTS (see DEODORANTS)

ASTRINGENTS (see SKIN FRESHENERS)

BABY PREPARATIONS

1. Baby cream	Toxicity rating 1
Mineral oil, light	15.0%
Petrolatum	5.0%
Amerchol L 101†	15.0%
Mineral wax, microcryst, (175° F.)	10.0%
Glyceryl monostearate	5.0%
Methyl and propyl parabens	0.2%
Water	49.8%

† Amerchol L 101 is a mineral extract of lanolin sterols and higher alcohols.
May contain:
Beeswax

Starred ingredients (*) may be responsible for major toxic effects; consult Section II.

| COSMETICS (Cont.) | COSMETICS (Cont.) |

BABY PREPARATIONS (Cont.)

Hydrogenated fatty oils	
Spermaceti	
2. Baby lotion (nonionic emulsion type) .	Toxicity rating 1
a. Mineral oil, light	35.0%
Lanolin	2.0%
Cetyl alcohol	2.0%
Tween 80†	5.0%
Arlacel 80†	2.0%
Methyl and propyl parabens†	0.2%
Water	53.8%

† Tween 80 and Arlacel 80 are nonionic surfactants (emulsifying agents), the former a polyoxyethylene sorbitan monooleate, the latter a sorbitan mono-oleate (both have toxicity rating 1). The parabens (esters of *p*-hydroxybenzoic acid) are preservatives and antioxidants.

May contain:
Antimicrobials
Emulsifiers (glyceryl monostearate)
Humectants (propylene glycol, glycerol, sorbitol)
Lanolin isolates or derivatives (see under Baby Oil, below)
Thickeners (sodium alginate)

It can almost be taken for granted that cosmetic products contain traces of perfume (except where noted).

b. Baby lotions, creams, oils	Toxicity rating 1
Oils, fats and waxes	25–>50%
Emulsifiers	0.1–1%
Humectants	1–5%
Preservatives	0.1–1%
Thickeners	0.1–1%
Essential oil (fragrance)	0.1–1%
Water	>50%
Color	0.1–1%
3. Baby oil	Toxicity rating 1
Mineral oil, light	80.0%
Isopropyl myristate (palmitate)	14.0%
Lanolin	5.5%

May contain vegetable oils, also one or more of lanolin isolates or derivatives, such as:
Lantrol
Lanosel
Medulan
Isopropylan

4. Baby powder	Toxicity rating 1
a. Talc	93.0%
Kaolin	5.0%
Zinc oxide	2.0%
b. Rice starch	100%
c. Talc	50.0%
Dry-Flo†	50.0%

† Dry-flo is the aluminum salt of a low-substituted alkenyl half-ester of starch.

May contain boric acid*, if so	Toxicity rating 2
Magnesium carbonate	5%
Perfume oil	trace
5. Baby soap	Toxicity rating 1
Sodium soaps of coconut and palm oil	

BARRIER CREAMS (PROTECTIVE)

1.	Toxicity rating 1
Stearic acid	10.0%
Beeswax	1.5%
Glycerin	5.0%
Casein	0.3%

BARRIER CREAMS (PROTECTIVE) (Cont.)

Ammonium hydroxide	0.5%
Water, *q.s.*	100.0%
2.	Toxicity rating 2
Zinc oxide	10.0%
Zinc stearate	5.0%
Titanium dioxide	10.0%
Butyl stearate	5.0%
Liquid petrolatum	10.0%
White petrolatum	60.0%
3.	Toxicity rating 2
Silicone, high viscosity	25.0%
White petrolatum	75.0%
4.	Toxicity rating 2
Polyethylene glycol 1540 monostearate	5.0%
Butyl stearate	5.0%
Petrolatum	3.0%
Diglycol stearate (neutral)	4.0%
Paraffin	3.0%
Potassium hydroxide	7.0%
Magnesium stearate	15.0%
Water	58.0%

Barrier creams may contain:
Aluminum compounds*
Benzoic acid
Borates
Calamine
Ceresin
Lanolin
Salicylates*
Sodium silicate
Talc
Triethanolamine

BATH PREPARATIONS

1. Bath oils	Toxicity rating 2
a. Emulsifiable type:	
Perfume* (see Oils, essential)	10.0%
Sulfated castor oil* (50%) (see Turkey red oil)	50.0%
Water	40.0%
b. Insoluble type:	
Perfume* (see Oils, essential)	10.0%
Isopropyl myristate (palmitate)	90.0%

May contain:
Alcohol
Castor oil
Coloring
Lanolin

c. Mineral oil type:	
Mineral oil	40–80%
Perfume oils*	2–50%
Isopropyl myristate (sebacate palmitate)	0–27%
Isostearic acid	0–2%
Benzyl alcohol	0–1%
Color	
d. Mineral or vegetable oils	>50%
Perfumes	1–5%
Preservatives	0.1–1%
Surfactants/emulsifiers	1–5%
Water	*q.s.*
2. Bath salts, effervescent	Toxicity rating 2
Sodium bicarbonate	60.0%
Tartaric acid	39.0%
Perfume	1.0%
3. Bath salts, plain	Toxicity rating 2
Trisodium phosphate* (see Alkali)	50.0%
Sodium chloride	48.0%

Starred ingredients (*) may be responsible for major toxic effects; consult Section II.

COSMETICS (Cont.)	COSMETICS (Cont.)

BATH PREPARATIONS (Cont.)

Perfume	2.0%

Bath salts may contain:
Borax*
Coloring
Sodium hexametaphosphate
Starch

4. Bubble bath, liquid		Toxicity rating 2
Triethanolamine dodecylbenzene sulfonate—linear*		20–33%
Fatty acid alkanolamides		5–12%
Perfume		1–5%
Water		40.8–73.9%
Methyl paraben		0.1–0.2%
5. Bubble bath, powdered		Toxicity rating 2
Sodium lauryl sulfate* (see Alkyl sodium sulfate)		30.0%
Sodium chloride		68.0%
Perfume		2.0%

Bubble bath may contain:
Alcohol
Alkyl benzene sodium sulfonate*
Coloring
Dioctyl sodium sulfosuccinate
Propylene glycol
Sodium hexametaphosphate
Sodium sulfate
Sodium tripolyphosphate

BLEACH AND FRECKLE CREAMS AND OINTMENTS .... Toxicity rating 3

The excipients of these preparations are either simple ointment bases (consisting of petrolatum, mineral oil, lanolin) or vanishing creams (stearate types). As active ingredients they may contain:

Ammoniated mercury†
Bismuth subnitrate
Hydroquinone*
Mercuric chloride†
Mercuric oxide†
Mercurous chloride (calomel)†
Monobenzone (hydroquinone monobenzyl ether)
Oxalic acid*
Zinc oxide
Zinc peroxide
† See Mercury, Section III

1. Bleach lotions	Toxicity rating 3
Hydrogen peroxide (5%)*	64.0%
Tincture of benzoin	4.0%
Water, q.s.	100.0%
2. Freckle lotions	Toxicity rating 3
a. Potassium chlorate*	2.0%
Potassium carbonate	6.0%
Sodium borate	1.0%
Sugar	6.0%
Glycerin	16.0%
Rose water, q.s.	100.0%
b.	Toxicity rating 2
Acetic acid (dilute)	4.0%
Alcohol	4.0%
Citric acid	6.0%
Glycerin	6.0%
Water, q.s.	100.0%
3. Skin lighteners	
Water	>50%
Essential oil (fragrance)	0–3%
Glyceryl monostearate	5–25%
Glycerin	5–10%

BLEACH AND FRECKLE CREAMS AND OINTMENT (Cont.)

Hydroquinone	1–5%
Stearic acid	1–5%

BLEMISH COVERS (cream)	Toxicity rating 1
Fats, oils, waxes	5–>50%
Colors and other additives	0–50%
Fillers (e.g., calcium carbonate)	0–20%
Humectants	0–10%
Thickeners and emulsifiers	0–10%
Preservatives	0.1–1%
Essential oil (fragrance)	0.1–1%

CLEANSING CREAMS, GRAINS AND LOTIONS

1. Cleansing grains		
Fillers (e.g., talc and calcium carbonate)		>50%
Foam booster		10–25%
Anionic surfactant		5–10%
Thickener		1–5%
Abradants (e.g., pumice, corn meal, plastic beads)		1–5%
Color and additives		1–5%
Essential oils (fragrance)		0.1–1%
2. Cleansing lotion (emulsion)		Toxicity rating 2
Mineral oil, light		35.0%
Triethanolamine stearate		10.0%
Water		55.0%
3. Cold cream type		Toxicity rating 2
Mineral oil, light		50.0%
Beeswax		17.0%
Borax		1.0%
Water		32.0%
4. Fats, oils, waxes		5–>50%
Water		25–>50%
Emulsifiers		1–25%
Humectants		1–5%
Color		0.1–1%
Essential oils (fragrances)		0.1–1%
Preservatives		0.1–1%
5. Liquefying cream type		Toxicity rating 2
Mineral oil, light		65.0%
Petrolatum		15.0%
Paraffin F125–127		20.0%
6. Nonionic emulsion, cream type		Toxicity rating 2
Mineral oil, light		50.0%
Beeswax		7.0%
Atlas G-1726†		6.0%
Tween 40†		2.0%
Water		33.0%

† Atlas G-1726 is a polyoxyethylene sorbitol derivative of beeswax. Tween 40 is a polyoxyethylene sorbitan monopalmitate.

Cleansing creams and lotions may contain:
Alcohol
Alkanolamines (see monoethanol amines, diethanolamines, triethanolamines)
Allantoin
Antibacterials and preservatives (hexachlorophene, bithionol, methyl and propyl parabens)
Fatty alcohols (cetyl, stearyl, oleyl)
Lanolin, its isolates and derivatives
Perfume
Polyols (glycerol, propylene glycol)
Synthetic "fatty" oils (isopropyl myristate-palmitate, diglycol laurate)

Starred ingredients (*) may be responsible for major toxic effects; consult Section II.

COSMETICS (Cont.)	COSMETICS (Cont.)

CLEANING CREAMS, GRAINS, AND LOTIONS (Cont.)

Thickeners (stearic acid, glyceryl monostearate)
Waxes (beeswax, spermaceti)

CONDITIONING (EMOLLIENT) CREAMS

1. Conditioning cream, anhydrous ...... Toxicity rating 1
    Lanolin 70.0%
    Petrolatum 18.0%
    Oil of sweet almond 12.0%
2. Conditioning cream, emulsified
    Lanolin 25.0%
    Lanolin alcohols 15.0%
    Mineral oil 25.0%
    Water 35.0%
3. Conditioning cream (USP "hydrophilic
   ointment"), anionic
    Stearyl alcohol 25.0%
    Petrolatum 25.0%
    Propylene glycol 12.0%
    Sodium lauryl sulfate (see alkyl so-
      dium sulfate) 1.0%
    Water 37.0%
4. Conditioning cream ("moisturizing")
   nonionic
    Mineral oil 20.0%
    Stearic acid 15.0%
    Lanolin 5.0%
    Beeswax 2.0%
    d-Sorbitol (70%) 13.0%
    Arlacel 85† 1.0%
    Tween 85† 1.0%
    Water 43.0%
  † Arlacel 85 is sorbitan trioleate, Tween 85 is polyoxyethylene sorbitan trioleate.
    Conditioning creams may contain:
    Natural fatty oils (olive, coconut, corn, peach kernel, peanut, sesame) also in hydrogenated form.
    Natural fats (cocoa butter, lard)
    Synthetic "fatty" oils (butyl stearate, diglycol laurate)
    Hydrocarbon solids (paraffin, ozokerite, microcrystalline waxes)
    Waxes (beeswax, spermaceti)
    Fatty alcohols (cetyl, stearyl, oleyl)
    Lanolin isolates and derivatives
    Anionic, cationic* and nonionic emulsifiers
    Polyols (propylene glycol, glycerol, sorbitol)
    Synthetic esters (glyceryl monostearate, polyethylene glycol stearates)
    Preservatives and oxidants (parabens, tocopherol, alkyl gallates)
    Antibacterials (hexachlorophene, bithionol)
    Perfume (especially menthol and camphor)

DENTIFRICES (see NONPRESCRIPTION DRUGS)

DENTURE ADHESIVES (see NONPRESCRIPTION DRUGS)

DENTURE CLEANERS .... Toxicity rating 4

1. Sodium perborate* 32.4%
    Sodium chloride 60.0%
    Magnesium sulfate 2.5%
    Calcium chloride 2.5%
    Sodium carbonate 2.5%
    Perfume
    May contain:
      Trisodium phosphate
2. Liquid
    Potassium monopersulfate 25–50%

DENTURE CLEANERS (Cont.)

    Sodium perborate 0.1–0.25%
    Sodium carbonate 25–50%
    Essential oil (fragrance) 0.1–1%
    Trisodium phosphate 10–25%
The above is a typical formula derived from the following groups:

Soaking Denture Cleaners

Oxygen source, 10–30%
  Sodium perborate
  Sodium carbonate peroxide
  Potassium monopersulfate
  Sodium peroxide (rare)
Alkaline agents, 20–70%
  Trisodium phosphate
  Sodium carbonate
Hypochlorite formers, 1–50%
  Chlorinated trisodium phosphate
  Chlorcyanuric acid derivatives
  Calcium hypochlorites
Fillers and extenders, 0–50%
  Sodium chloride
  Sodium sulfate
  Sodium sesquicarbonate
  Sodium bicarbonate
Anticaking agents, 0.2–2.0%
  Micronized silica
  Calcium phosphates
  Alkyl sulfonates
Detergents, 0.1–2.0%
Flavors, colors, q.s.

DEODORANTS AND ANTIPERSPIRANTS

1. Cream antiperspirant (with deodorant
   action) .... Toxicity rating 2
    Aluminum chlorhydroxide 20.0%
    Sorbitan monostearate (Span 60) .. 5.0%
    Polyoxyethylene sorbitan monos-
      tearate (Tween 60) 5.0%
    Stearic acid 15.0%
    Propylene glycol 5.0%
    Water 50.0%
2. Deodorant and antiperspirant cream Toxicity rating 2 or
    Aluminum sulfate, anhydrous 9–10%
    Spermaceti 9.5%
    Glyceryl monostearate 9.5%
    Chondrus 1.0%
    Sodium lauryl sulfate 1.0%
    Glycerine 5.0%
    Cetyl alcohol 1.0%
    Perfume 0.4–0.75%
    Water 63–65%
3. Deodorants, stick .... Toxicity rating 2
    Alcohol (ethyl) .... >50%
    Essential oil (fragrance) 0.1–1%
    Soap 5–10%
    Water 5–10%
    Other (chelating agents, waxes, hu-
      mectants, color) 5–10%
    Deodorant agent 0–5%
4. Liquid antiperspirant (with deodorant
   action) .... Toxicity rating 2–3
    Aluminum chloride 15.0%
    Urea 5.0%
    Propylene glycol 5.0%
    Water 75.0%
5. Roll-on and cream deodorant,
   antiperspirant .... Toxicity rating 2
   a. Lotion type (emulsified)

Starred ingredients (*) may be responsible for major toxic effects; consult Section II.

COSMETICS (Cont.)	

DEODORANTS AND ANTIPERSPIRANTS (Cont.)

Antiperspirant salts (e.g., aluminum salts)	10–25%
Emulsifiers, thickeners, preservatives	>10–25%
Essential oil (fragrance)	0.1–1%
Emollients	0.1–5%
b. Roll-on deodorant antiperspirant, lotion type (emulsified)	Toxicity rating 2
Cetyl alcohol	3.0%
Polyoxytheylene (20) cetyl ether	4.5%
Polyoxyethylene sorbitan monolaurate	1.0%
Aluminum chlorhydroxide complex	20.0–24.0%
Urea	2.0%
Trisodium salt of hydroxyalkylethylene diamine triacetic acid	0.05%
Perfume	0.2%
Water	45.1–49.1%
6. Roll-on deodorant, clear	Toxicity rating 2
Alcohol 40	20.0%
Polyoxylated nonyl phenol (Igepal CO-630)	1.0%
Methyocel 65 Hg. (4000 c.p.s.)	0.75%
Urea	2.0%
Aluminum chlorhydroxide complex	20.0%
Water	56.25%
Spray deodorant (with antiperspirant action)	Toxicity rating 3
Aluminum phenolsulfonate	10.0%
Propylene glycol	5.0%
Alcohol*	85.0%
Perfume	q.s.
7. Spray deodorant with antiperspirant action	Toxicity rating 2
Alcohol (ethyl)	0–>50%
Propellant	>50%
Antiperspirant salts (e.g., aluminum chlorhydroxide)	0–10%
Deodorant agents	0–5%
Other (oils, humectants, suspending agents (e.g., bentonite))	0–10%
8. Spray deodorants—feminine	Toxicity rating 1
Propellant	>50%
Talc and fillers	0–10%
Alcohol (ethyl)	0–5%
Essential oil (fragrance)	0.1–1%
Humectants	0.1–1%

DEPILATORIES

1. Cream depilatories	Toxicity rating 2
Thioglycolate (calcium or ammonium)	5–10%
Hydroxide (calcium or sodium)	2–6%
Emulsifiers, humectants, waxes	0.1–1%
Water	>50%
2. Wax depilatory	Toxicity rating 1
Rosin	50.0%
Beeswax	25.0%
Paraffin	15.0%
Petrolatum	10.0%

EMOLLIENT CREAMS (see CONDITIONING CREAMS)

EYE MAKEUP

1. Eyebrow pencils	Toxicity rating 1
Lampblack	10.0–20.0%
Petrolatum	40.0%
Paraffin, q.s.	100.0%

EYE MAKEUP (Cont.)

May contain:	
Aluminum silicate	
Stearates	
2. Eyebrow plucking creams	Toxicity rating 2
Benzocaine	2.0%
Cold cream	98.0%
3. Eye creams (eye tissue creams, eye wrinkle creams)	Toxicity rating 1
Lecithin	6.0%
Cholesterin	2.0%
Beeswax	24.0%
Lanolin	6.0%
Sodium benzoate	1.0%
Boric acid*	
Mineral oil	
Ascorbyl palmitate	
Almond oil, q.s.	100.0%
4. Eyelash and eyebrow dyes	Toxicity rating 2
Brown, black and blue certified oil soluble dyes	
5. Eyebrow colorant (cake)	Toxicity rating 1
Fillers (e.g., talc)	>50%
Inorganic color and other additives	10–25%
Binders (oily esters)	1–5%
Preservatives	0.1–1%
6. Eyelash creams	Toxicity rating 3
Lanolin	5.0%
Cocoa butter	4.0%
Paraffin	10.0%
Cetyl alcohol	2.0%
Peach kernel oil,* q.s.	100.0%
7. Eyelash oils	Toxicity rating 1
Lanolin	8.0%
Cocoa butter	4.0%
Cetyl alcohol	8.0%
Alcohol	2.0%
Water	100.0%
Olive oil, q.s.	100.0%
8. Eye liner (liquid)	Toxicity rating 1
Water	>50%
Film formers (e.g., acrylic resins)	5–10%
Inorganic color and other additives	10–25%
Humectants	5–10%
Other: (emulsifiers, film formers, thickeners)	0–5%
Preservatives	0.1–1%
May contain:	
Alkanolamine stearate	
Higher fatty alcohol	
Polyvinylpyrrolidone	
Cellulose ether	
Methylparaben	
Polyol	
Antioxidant	
Perfume	
Titanium dioxide	
9. Eye shadow (powder)	
a. Fillers (e.g., talc)	25 > 50%
Inorganic colors and additives	10 > 50%
Zinc stearate	1–10%
Oils	1–10%
Others (water, humectants)	0–10%
Preservatives	0.1–1%
b. Eye shadow (stick)	
Fats, oils, waxes	>50%
Inorganic colors and other additives	5–50%
Essential oil (fragrance)	0.1–1%

Starred ingredients (*) may be responsible for major toxic effects; consult Section II.

COSMETICS (Cont.)	COSMETICS (Cont.)

EYE MAKEUP (Cont.)

c. Eye shadow (cream)

Water	25–50%
Pearlescent agents	0–50%
Inorganic colors and other additives	1–25%
Humectants	10–25%
Oils and waxes	1–10%
Emulsifiers	1–15%
Thickeners	1–5%
Essential oil (fragrance)	0.1–1%
Preservatives	0.1–1%

10. Mascara .... Toxicity rating 1

a.
Triethanolamine stearate	50.0%
Carnauba wax	25.0%
Paraffin	15.0%
Lanolin	5.0%
Pigments (insoluble)	5.0%

b.
Waxes (beeswax, carnauba wax)	10–25%
Thickeners (other than wax)	1–5%
Color	1–5%
Preservatives	0.1–1%
Water	>50%

The pigments in eye make-up cosmetics are of an inert character (carbon black, iron oxides, chromium oxide, ultramarine, carmine).

The excipients may contain:
Beeswax
Cetyl alcohol
Glyceryl monostearate
Gums (tragacanth)
Mineral oil
Perfume
Preservatives (p-hydroxybenzoates)
Propylene glycol
Spermaceti
Synthetics (isopropyl myristate)
Vegetable oils

11. Eye makeup remover .... Toxicity rating 1

Oils (mineral and/or vegetables)	>50%
Pigments	0–5%
Waxes	1–10%
Essential oil (fragrance)	0–0.1%
Preservatives	0.1–1%

FACE MASKS

1. Beauty clays .... Toxicity rating 1

Purified siliceous earth	10.0%
Kaolin	40.0%
Glycerin	6.0%
Water, q.s.	100.0%

2. Face packs .... Toxicity rating 2

Zinc stearate	4.0%
Zinc oxide	4.0%
Glycerin	8.0%
Tragacanth	4.0%
Alcohol	10.0%
Limewater, q.s.	100.0%

May contain:
Acacia
Balsam of Peru
Glyceryl monostearate
Hexachlorophene
Magnesium carbonate
Mercurized wax
Salicylic acid
Spermaceti
Sulfonated castor oil
Talc
Titanium oxide

FACE MASKS (Cont.)

Zinc sulfocarbolate

3. Paste masks (facial and mud packs)

Hydroxyethyl cellulose	10–25%
Alcohol (ethyl)	5–10%
Bentonite	1–5%
Water	>50%

FACE POWDER (see POWDERS)

FINGERNAIL PREPARATIONS (see NAIL COSMETICS)

FOUNDATION CREAMS

1. Foundation (vanishing) cream ...... Toxicity rating 1

Stearic acid	15.0%
Arlacel 60†	2.0%
Tween 60†	1.5%
d-Sorbitol (70%)	7.5%
Water	74.0%

† Arlacel 60 is sorbitan monostearate, Tween 60 is polyoxyethylene sorbitan monostearate.

2. "Tinted" (pigmented) foundation and make-up cream .... Toxicity rating 1

Mineral oil	15.0%
Stearic acid	10.0%
Lanolin	7.0%
Cetyl alcohol	2.0%
Propylene glycol	5.0%
Triethanolamine	1.3%
Borax	0.5%
Pigments (insoluble)	3.0%
Water	56.0%

Foundation creams (and hand creams and lotions) may contain:
Emulsifiers (anionic, cationic* and nonionic surfactants)
Humectants (propylene glycol, glycerol, sorbitol)
Lanolin isolates and derivatives
Perfume
Preservatives (parabens)
Special barrier agents (zinc stearate, cellulose derivatives, silicones)
Synthetic esters (glyceryl, glycol, polyethylene glycol monostearate)
Thickeners (sodium alginate, gum tragacanth, quince seed, mucilage)
Waxes (beeswax, spermaceti)

FRECKLE CREAMS AND OINTMENTS (see BLEACH AND FRECKLE CREAMS)

HAIR PREPARATIONS

1. Brilliantines and hair dressings

a. Cream type dressing .... Toxicity rating 1

Mineral oil	25.0%
Beeswax	5.0%
Triethanolamine stearate	5.0%
Water	65.0%

b. Conditioners (nonalcoholic) .... Toxicity rating 1

Oils and waxes	5–10%
Polymers and resins	0–10%
Essential oil (fragrance)	0.1–1%
Preservatives	0.1–1%
Emulsifiers	0.1–1%
Water	>50%
Protein	1–5%

c. Cream rinses, creme rinses .... Toxicity rating 2

Cationic surfactants	5–10%
Water	>50%

Starred ingredients (*) may be responsible for major toxic effects; consult Section II.

COSMETICS (Cont.)	COSMETICS (Cont.)

HAIR PREPARATIONS (Cont.)

Other:

Emollients, conditioners, bodying agents, resins	1–10%
Preservatives	0.1–1%
Essential oil (fragrance)	0.1–1%

d. Hair dressings and other grooming aids (includes hair gels, hair creams, hair pomades, not tonic or lotions) .... Toxicity rating 1

Mineral oil	0->50%
Lanolin	0–25%
Emulsifiers	5–10%
Surfactants	0–3%
Color, essential oil, preservatives	trace
Water	0–50%
Other (humectants, resins, petrolatum, waxes, borax, propellant)	0–70%

e. Liquid brilliantine .... Toxicity rating 1

Mineral oil	75.0%
Isopropyl myristate	25.0%

f. Solid brilliantine .... Toxicity rating 1

Mineral oil	50.0%
Petrolatum	40.0%
Paraffin	10.0%

g. "Two-layer" dressings .... Toxicity rating 1

Mineral oil	25.0%
Alcohol	25.0%
Water	50.0%

Brilliantines and hair dressings may contain:

Antiseptics
Cetyl alcohol
Cholesterol
Gums (e.g., tragacanth)
Lanolin
Oil of bergamot (and other essential oils)
Olive oil (and other vegetable oils)
Synthetic oils (e.g., butyl stearate)
Synthetic thickeners (polyglycols, cellulose derivatives)
Tars

2. Dyes, colors and tints .... Toxicity rating 2

a. Essential oil (fragrance)	trace–0.5%
p-Phenylenediamine and other color intermediates	trace–4%
Alcohol (ethyl)	0–11%
Isopropyl alcohol	0–1%
Ammonium hydroxide	0–3%
Carbitol	0–4%
Humectants	0–5%
Fatty acids, fatty acid alcohols	0–60%
Hair color base (see below)	40%
Water	17–20%

Hair color base

Solubilizer	4.9%
Nonionic surfactant	16%
Foam booster	20%
Oils (mineral and/or vegetable)	5%
Cationic surfactant	trace
Leveling agent	3%
Water	50%

Cream developer

Hydrogen peroxide	11%
Emulsifiers	2%

HAIR PREPARATIONS (Cont.)

Waxes	1.8%
Stabilizer	trace
Water	84.0%

b. Oxidation type (blond) .... Toxicity rating 2

p-Phenylenediamine	0.30%
p-Methylaminophenol	0.50%
p-Aminodiphenylamine	0.15%
o-Aminophenol	0.15%
Pyrocatechol	0.25%
Resorcinol	0.25%
Inert base	98.40%

Oxidation hair dyes may contain (depending upon shade)

p-Aminophenol
2,4-Diaminoanisol
2,4-Diaminophenol
4-Nitro-o-phenylenediamine
2-Nitro-p--phenylenediamine
Pyrogallol
Sodium sulfite
p-Toluylenediamine

c. Metallic type (two bottles) .... Toxicity rating 3

(a) Silver nitrate*	10.0%
Ammonia (10%)	30.0%
Water	60.0%
(b) Pyrogallol*	5.0%
Water	95.0%

Other metal based hair colorings may contain:

Acetic acid
Bismuth acetate
Cadmium chloride*
Cobalt chloride*
Cupric chloride*
Ferric chloride
Lead acetate*
Manganese sulfate
Nickel sulfate
Sodium sulfite
Sodium thiosulfate

d. Hair rinses, (color rinses, dyes, toners .... Toxicity rating 2

Fatty acid and fatty acid alcohols	>40%
Dyes	0.1–1%
Emulsifiers	1–5%
Water	>40%

May contain:
Perfume
Glycols
Thickening agents

e. Hair lighteners with color .... Toxicity rating 3

Part 1

Hydrogen peroxide	>50%

Part 2

Water	>50%
Alcohol (ethyl) and propylene glycol	>50%
Anionic surfactant	5–10%
Alkali (ammonia pH 8.5–10)	1–5%
Oxidation dyes (p-phenylenediamine derivatives)	0.1–1%
Preservatives	0.1–1%
Sequestrant	0.1–1%
Antioxidant	0.1–1%

Part 3

Potassium persulfate	>50%

Starred ingredients (*) may be responsible for major toxic effects; consult Section II.

COSMETICS (Cont.)

HAIR PREPARATIONS (Cont.)

  f. *Part 1.* Bleach base

Fats, oils, gels, (long fatty acid alcohols)	10–25%
Nonionic surfactants, humectants	10–25%
Ammonia (free of salts) persulfate	10–25%
Other	0–5%
Water	q.s.

     Part 2

      Hydrogen peroxide

      Note: Parts 1 and 2 are usually mixed before use.

3. Wave sets (alcoholic)	Toxicity rating 1
Water	25–>50%
Alcohol	1–>50%
Other ingredients (combined to form)	0–25%
Surfactants, emulsifiers, resins, protein	
Color	0.1–1%
Preservatives	0.1–1%
Essential oil (fragrance)	0.1–1%
4. Hair Spray	Toxicity rating 2
a. Pressurized	
Lacquers and wave sets (see above)	50%
Propellant	50%
b. One of the following as a base	Toxicity rating 2
(1) Resinous plastic in alcohol	50%
(2) Polyvinylpyrrolidone	50%
(3) Carboxylated polyvinyl alcohol	50%

    All may contain:

      Cety alcohol

      Ethoxylated lanolin (hygroscopic)

      Isopropyl laurate

      Lanolin

      Oleyl alcohol

  c. Hair color sprays (aerosol)

Fatty acid and fatty acid alcohols and phenols	30–>50%
Dyes	0.1–1%
Emulsifiers	1–5%
Water	30–>50%
Isopropanol	1–5%
Ammonium hydroxide	1–5%
Propylene glycol	1–5%
Propellant	5–10%
5. Permanent waves—waving lotion	Toxicity rating 3
Ammonium thioglycolate	5–10%
Water	>50%
Alkalies (e.g., ammonia or amines)	1–5%
Dye-colorants	0.1–1%
Essential oil (fragrance)	0.1–1%
Other salts	0–5%
Permanent waves-neutralizers for home permanents	Toxicity rating 3–5
a. Hydrogen peroxide	1–6%
Cationic surfactants	0–1%
Water	>50%
Phosphates	0–1%
Emulsifiers	0–5%
Clouding agents	0–5%
Protein	0–2%
b. Sodium perborate	>50%
Water	>50%
Other (magnesium carbonate, sodium hexametaphosphate)	0–trace

COSMETICS (Cont.)

HAIR PREPARATIONS (Cont.)

c. Sodium (or potassium) bromate	10–25%
Surfactants	0–1%
Phosphates	0–1%
Protein	0–2%
Clouding agents	0–5%
Water	>50%
6. Straighteners	Toxicity rating 2
Polyethylene glycol 6000	2.1%
Cetyl alcohol	13.0%
Stearyl alcohol	8.6%
Triethanolamine lauryl sulfate	1.1%
Propylene glycol	16.0%
Ammonium thioglycolate (53%)	10.5%
Ammonium hydroxide (28%)	3.3%
Perfume	2.0%
Water	43.4%
7. Shampoos	
a. Baby shampoo	Toxicity rating 1
Nonionic surfactants	0–10%
Anionic surfactants	0–25%
Amphoteric surfactants	0–25%
Color	0.1–1%
Essential oil (fragrance)	0.1–1%
Preservatives	0.1–1%
Water	>50%
Other (chelating agents, thickeners, humectants)	0–5%
b. Coloring hair shampoos	
Nonionic surfactants	0–10%
Anionic surfactants	0–25%
Amphoteric surfactants	0–25%
Color	0.1–1%
Color additives	1–5%
Essential oil (fragrance)	0.1–1%
Preservatives	0.1–1%
Water	>50%
Other (chelating agents, thickeners, humectants)	0–5%
c. Dandruff shampoo	Toxicity rating 2
Antidandruff agent (e.g., colloidal sulfur, zinc pyridinethione, selenium sulfide, coal tar derivatives, salicylic acid, resorcin)	1–5%
Nonionic surfactants	0–10%
Anionic surfactants	0–25%
Color	0.1–1%
Essential oil (fragrance)	0.1–1%
Preservatives	0.1–1%
Water	>50%
Other (chelating agents, thickeners, humectants)	0–5%
d. General shampoo	Toxicity rating 2
Nonionic surfactants	0–10%
Anionic surfactants	0–25%
Amphoteric surfactants	0–25%
Color	0.1–1%
Essential oil (fragrance)	0.1–1%
Preservatives	0.1–1%
Water	>50.0%
Other (chelating agents, thickeners, humectants)	0–5%
e. Soap shampoos	Toxicity rating 2
Potassium coconut oil soap	25.0%
Potassium olive oil soap	5.0%
Alcohol	15.0%
Glycerol	5.0%
Water	50.0%

Starred ingredients (*) may be responsible for major toxic effects; consult Section II.

COSMETICS (Cont.)	COSMETICS (Cont.)

HAIR PREPARATIONS (Cont.)

f. Soapless shampoo, cream type .... Toxicity rating 3

Sodium lauryl sulfate* (see alkyl sodium sulfate)	50.0%
Sodium stearate	10.0%
Water	40.0%

g. Soapless shampoo, liquid type .... Toxicity rating 3

Triethanolamine dodecyl sulfate* (see alkyl sodium sulfate)	40.0%
Ethanolamide of lauric acid	15.0%
Water	45.0%

Shampoos may contain:
- Antibacterials
- Cholesterol
- Egg powder
- Ethylenediaminetetraacetic acid
- Lanolin
- Nonionic surfactants ("Tweens")
- Other anionic surfactants ("Tergitols")
- Perfume
- Polyols (propylene glycol, glycerol)
- Preservatives (p-hydroxybenzoates)
- Sodium hexametaphosphate
- Tars*
- Trisodium phosphate
- Vegetable gum (e.g., karaya)

8. Tonics .... Toxicity rating 2

Hair tonics and hair lotions (alcoholic)

Alcohol	25->50%
Oils (mineral, vegetable, castor)	5–10%
Essential oil (fragrance)	0.1–1%
Water	0->50%

Hair tonics may contain:
- Benzalkonium chloride*
- β-Naphthol
- Bithionol
- Camphor*
- Cantharides tincture
- Chloral hydrate*
- Menthol*
- Parachlorometaxylenol
- Perfume
- Phosphoric acid
- Pilocarpine
- Polyalkylene glycols
- Quinine*
- Resorcinol*
- Sorbitan derivative
- Salicylic acid*
- Tars
- Thymol

HAND CLEANERS (see CLEANERS)

HAND CREAMS

Composition of hand cream generally resembles that of foundation (vanishing) cream.

HAND LOTIONS .... Toxicity rating 1

Stearic acid	5.0%
Lanolin	1.0%
Arlacel 80	0.5%
Tween 60	2.5%
d-Sorbitol (70%)	3.5%
Water	87.5%

May contain other ingredients (see under Foundation cream)

HORMONE CREAMS AND LOTIONS   Toxicity rating 1

These hormone cosmetics are conditioning preparations containing substances of estrogen or progesterone character or both. Their estrogenic potency as a rule corresponds to not more than 10,000 International Units of estrone per ounce; the progesterone content is not more than 5 mg. per ounce.

Oils, fats, and waxes	5–25%
Emulsifiers	0.1–1%
Humectants	1–5%
Preservatives	0.1–1%
Thickeners	0.1–1%
Essential oil (fragrance)	0.1–1%
Water	>50%
Color	0.1–1%

May contain:

Hormone	trace

LIPSTICKS .... Toxicity rating 1–2

Castor oil	25–50%
Beeswax	1–5%
Essential oil (fragrance)	0.1–1%
Color (FDA approved) including "pearlescent" agents	25–50%
Antioxidants and preservatives	0.1–1%
Lanolin	1–5%
Other (oils, waxes, fats, and flavoring agents)	25–50%

Color

Certified dyes (soluble)	2–5% of base
Certified color lakes (insoluble)	10–15% of base

Lipstick base may contain:
- Cetyl alcohol
- Cocoa butter
- Hydrogenated fats and oils
- Mineral waxes (e.g., ceresine)
- Perfume
- Polyethylene glycol ethers
- Preservatives (p-hydroxybenzoates)
- Propylene glycol monoesters
- Spermaceti
- Tetrahydrofurfuryl acetate
- Waxes (candelilla)

LIQUEFYING CREAMS .... Toxicity rating 1

Paraffin	6.0%
White wax	12.0%
Liquid petrolatum	54.0%
Stearic acid	1.0%
Sodium borate	1.0%
Water	26.0%

LIQUID MAKEUPS

1. Liquid cosmetic stockings .... Toxicity rating 2

Propylene glycol monostearate	4.0%
Oleic acid	2.0%
Liquid petrolatum	1.0%
Bentonite suspension (5%)	20.0%
Color pigments	14.0%
Triethanolamine	1.5%
Propylene glycol	6.0%
Methyl p-hydroxybenzoate	0.2%
Water, q.s.	100.0%

2. Liquid powders .... Toxicity rating 1

a.

Titanium dioxide	2.0%
Talc	1.0%
Stearic acid	10.0%
Liquid petrolatum	12.0%
Triethanolamine	3.0%
Water, q.s.	100.0%
Perfume	q.s.

b. .... Toxicity rating 2

Starred ingredients (*) may be responsible for major toxic effects; consult Section II.

COSMETICS (Cont.)	COSMETICS (Cont.)

LIQUID MAKEUPS (Cont.)

Cetyl alcohol	0.2%
Lanolin, anhydrous	0.2%
Glyceryl stearate	0.8%
Sodium hydroxide	0.2%
Stearic acid	7.5%
Propylene glycol	15.0%
Titanium dioxide	5.0%
Color pigments	5.0 to 12.0%
Water, q.s.	100.0%

Liquid powders may contain:
Alcohol
Boric acid
Calcium carbonate
Candelilla wax
Carnauba wax
Clay
Essential oils
Esters
Ethyl parasept
Glycerin
Glycols
Iron oxide
Lecithin
Magnesium carbonate
Magnesium oleate
Oils
Sorbitol
Spermaceti
Waxes
Zinc oxide
Zinc stearate

3. Liquid leg and body paints	Toxicity rating 2–3
Water	25–>50%
Alcohol	0–50%
Color additives	1–25%
Humectants	5–10%
Film formers (e.g., acrylic resins)	5–10%
Propellant	0–10%
Essential oil (fragrance)	0.1–1%
Others: emulsifiers, fillers	5–10%
4. Makeup fixatives	Toxicity rating 1
Water	>50%
Film former (e.g., PVP)	1–5%
Preservatives	>1%
Humectant	0.1–1%
Alkanolamines	0.1–1%
Thickener	0.1–1%
Other (ultraviolet absorber and chelating agents)	>1%

MASCARA (see EYE MAKEUP)

MOUTHWASHES AND BREATH FRESHENERS (Not Concentrated)

1. Alkaline mouthwash	Toxicity rating 1 or 2
Sodium bicarbonate	2.0%
Sodium chloride	0.5%
Sodium cyclamate	0.2%
Flavor oils, mixed	0.3%
Alcohol	25.0%
Water	72.5%
Color certified	q.s.
2. Alcohol (ethyl)	10–25%
Humectants (e.g., glycerol, sorbitol, propylene glycol)	0–25%
Astringents	0–0.3%
Antiseptics	0–3%
Color preservatives	0.1–1%

MOUTHWASHES AND BREATH FRESHENERS (NOT CONCENTRATED) (Cont.)

Flavor	0.1–1%
Water	>50%
3. Astringent mouthwash	Toxicity rating 1 or 2
Zinc chloride	0.2%
Saccharine sodium	0.1%
Flavor oils, mixed†	0.2%
Alcohol	25.0%
Water	74.5%
Color, certified	q.s.

† See under NONPRESCRIPTION DRUGS, DENTIFRICES.

4. Mouthwashes and breath fresheners (concentrated)	Toxicity rating 2
Alcohol (ethyl)	>70%
Water	>50%
Flavors and sweeteners	10–25%
Glycerin	1–5%
Color, preservative	<0.1%
Astringent	<0.1%

Mouthwashes may contain:
Ammonium phosphate (dibasic)
Benzalkonium chloride*
Benzoic acid
Cetyl pyridinium chloride*
Chlorophyllin (copper derivative)
Decamethylene-bis-(4-aminoquinaldinium acetate)
Glycerol
Hexyl resorcinol
Methyl salicylate
Povidone-iodine†
Propylene glycol
Sorbitol
Urea (carbamide)
Zinc chloride
† See Polyvinylpyrrolidone (Section II).

NAIL COSMETICS

1. Cuticle softener	Toxicity rating 2
Humectants (e.g., glycerin)	5–10%
Potassium hydroxide	1–3%
Essential oil (fragrance)	0.1–1%
Water	>50%
2. Nail bleaches	Toxicity rating 2
Citric acid	4.0%
Potassium binoxalate	1.0%
Water, q.s.	100.0%
3. Nail enamel	Toxicity rating 3
Nitrocellulose	11.4%
Tricresyl phosphate*	8.3%
Dibutyl phthalate	13.5%
Ethyl acetate*	31.5%
Butyl acetate*	30.0%
Ethyl alcohol	4.9%
D & C Red No. 19	0.1%
D & C Red No. 31	0.2%
Oil pink	0.1%
4. Nail finishes	Toxicity rating 3
Celluloid	6.0%
Amyl acetate*	75.0%
Acetone,* q.s.	100.0%
5. Nail basecoats and polishes	Toxicity rating 3 or 4
Solvents (e.g., aromatic solvents, xylene,* toluene,* acetone,* ethyl acetate,* ethanol)	>50%
Plasticizers (butyl acetate, dibutyl phthalate, camphor)	10–25%

Starred ingredients (*) may be responsible for major toxic effects; consult Section II.

COSMETICS (Cont.)

NAIL COSMETICS (Cont.)

Cellulose nitrate	5–15%
Resins	0–15%
Other:	
Methyl alcohol	0–5%
Natural pearlescents	0–5%

May contain:
Alkyl esters (*e.g.*, amyl acetate, ethyl lactate)
Dyes (soluble)
Glycol ethers
Gums (*e.g.*, dammar, sandarac)
Hydrocarbons, aromatic (xylene)* and aliphatic (hexane)
Ketones (*e.g.*, acetone, methyl ethyl ketone)
Lakes (insoluble)
Phosphoric acid esters (*e.g.*, tricresyl phosphate)
Resins, synthetic (methyl methacrylate)

6. Nail polish and enamel removers (oily nail polish and enamel removers)	Toxicity rating 3 or 4
Solvents (acetone,* ethyl acetate*	>50%
Essential oil (fragrance)	0.1–1%
Water	10–20%
Lanolin, oils, cetyl alcohol (oily products)	2–10%

May contain:
Solvents (acetone,* ethyl acetate* butyl acetate)
Benzene*
Castor oil
Olive oil
Spermaceti
Ethyl oleate
Butyl stearate

7. Nail whites	
Cream	Toxicity rating 1
Titanium dioxide	2.0%
Beeswax	12.0%
Cetyl alcohol	4.0%
Oxycholesterin	16.0%
Petrolatum	24.0%
Cocoa butter	4.0%
Sodium borate	0.6%
Tincture of benzoin	6.0%
Water, *q.s.*	100.0%
Liquid	Toxicity rating 1
Titanium dioxide	1.0%
Glyceryl monostearate	4.0%
Beeswax	1.0%
Almond oil	10.0%
Petrolatum	6.0%
Water, *q.s.*	100.0%

PERFUMES, TOILET WATERS AND COLOGNES

1. Perfumes	Toxicity rating 3
Perfume essence* (concentrate) (see Oils, essential)	1–25%
Alcohol*	75–99%
2. Stick perfumes	Toxicity rating 3
Sodium soap	11.0%
Benzyl alcohol	15.0%
Propylene glycol	29.0%
Triethylene glycol	34.8%

COSMETICS (Cont.)

PERFUMES, TOILET WATERS AND COLOGNES (Cont.)

Brij 92 (polyoxyethylene 2 oleylether)	5.0%
Perfume oil*	5.0%
Dye solutions, *q.s.*	100.0%
3. Toilet waters and colognes	Toxicity rating 3
Perfume essence* (concentrate) (see oils, essential)	3–10%
Alcohol* (plus water)	90–97%

The perfume essence (concentrate may contain as many as 50 or even more components from the classes of:
Essential oils (from leaves, needles, roots, peels)
Floral oils (from petals or whole flowers)
Gums, resins and balsams (tree exudates)
Animal perfumery materials (musks, ambergris)
Isolates (individual components of natural oils and their chemical conversion products)
Synthetics (odorous substances of nonphysiological or other artificial origin)

4. Solid colognes	Toxicity rating 3
Sodium stearate	10%
Sorbitol	5%
Cologne essence	2%
Alcohol*	80%
Water	3%
5. Gel colognes	Toxicity rating 3
Alcohol 40* (see Alcohol, ethyl)	60.0–70.0%
Perfume oils	3.0–5.0%
Carbopol 640	0.5–0.8%
Diisopropanolamine	0.4–0.6%
Water	23.4–36.1%
6. Sachets	
a. Gels and creams	Toxicity rating 1
Emollients	5–10%
Emulsifiers	5–10%
Essential oils	1–5%
Water	>50%
b. Powders	Toxicity rating 3?
(1) Essential oil (fragrance)	1–5%
(2) Talc	70%
Magnesium carbonate	20%
Essential oil	8%
7. Pomades	Toxicity rating 3?
Essential oil (fragrance)	8%
Emollients	50%

POWDERS

1. Body (dusting, talcum, excluding after shave)	Toxicity rating 1
Talc	>50%
Calcium carbonate	0–10%
Magnesium carbonate	0–10%
Zinc stearate	1–5%
Essential oil (fragrance)	1–5%
Kaolin	1–5%
Preservatives	0.1–1%
2. Face powder	Toxicity rating 2
Talc	25–>50%
Color and other additives	10–50%
Kaolin	5–25%
Zinc stearate	5–10%

Starred ingredients (*) may be responsible for major toxic effects; consult Section II.

COSMETICS (Cont.)		COSMETICS (Cont.)	

POWDERS (Cont.)

Fatty acid esters		0–5%
Magnesium carbonate		0–5%
Essential oil (fragrance)		0.1–1%

May contain:
- Barium sulfate
- Boric acid* (if substantial percentages, toxicity rating 4)
- Cetyl alcohol
- Hydrolyzed silk fibroin
- Stearates (of magnesium, aluminum)
- Starch (rice, corn)
- Titanium dioxide

3. Men's talcum (after shave) .... Toxicity rating 2

Talc	>50%
Calcium carbonate	0–10%
Magnesium carbonate	5–10%
Zinc stearate	1–5%
Essential oil (fragrance)	1–5%
Kaolin	1–5%
Preservatives	0.1–1%

4. Powder compact .... Toxicity rating 1 to 2

Composition similar to that of face powder, except for the use of "binders," such as gum mucilage. Cake make-up employs an emulsifiable binder (e.g., nonionic surfactant).

May contain:
- Glyceryl or glycol stearate
- Mineral oil
- Synthetic oil (e.g., ethyl stearate)
- Wax

ROUGES

1. Cake (solid cake) .... Toxicity rating 2

Talc	>50%
Clay, chalk, starch	10–25%
Zinc (oxide, stearate)	5–10%
Color	1–5%

May contain:
- Liquid petrolatum
- Tragacanth mucilage
- Perfume

2. Liquid or cream .... Toxicity rating 2

Mineral and/or vegetable oils	10–25%
Color	1–5%
Essential oil (fragrance)	0.1–1%
Water	>50%
Thickeners	1–5%

May contain:
- Stearic acid
- Cetyl alcohol
- Potassium hydroxide
- Glycerin
- Sorbitan sesquioleate
- Lanolin
- Sorbital
- Ammonium hydroxide
- Ethyl alcohol
- Ethyl cellulose
- Oleic monoglyceride
- Beeswax
- Cocoa butter

3. Liquid .... Toxicity rating 2

Carmine	4.0%
Ammonium hydroxide (28%)	6.0%
Glycerin	12.0%

ROUGES (Cont.)

Water, q.s.	100.0%
4. Liquid lip rouges	Toxicity rating 2
Ethyl alcohol	88.0%
Ethyl cellulose	3.5%
Oleic acid monoglyceride	3.5%
Red color pigment	5.0%
5. Paste	Toxicity rating 2
Carmine	4.0%
Ammonium hydroxide	4.0%
Beeswax	6.0%
Cetyl alcohol	4.0%
Stearic acid	8.0%
Cocoa butter	4.0%
Petrolatum, q.s.	100.0%

SACHETS (see PERFUMES)

SHAVING CREAMS AND LOTIONS

1. Shaving cream (brushless type) ...... Toxicity rating 2

Stearic acid	25.0%
Mineral oil	10.0%
Triethanolamine	0.5%
Borax	0.5%
Water	64.0%
Perfume	q.s.

Brushless Shave creams may contain:
- Propylene glycol
- Maleic anhydride
- Olive oil

2. Shaving cream (lather type) .... Toxicity rating 2

Sodium and potassium stearine soap	30.0%
Sodium and potassium coconut oil soap	15.0%
Glycerol	10.0%
Water	45.0%
Perfume	q.s.

May contain:
- Alcohol
- Borax
- Lard
- Linseed oil
- Menthol
- Phenol
- Silicate
- Soap
- Sodium alginate
- Sodium salicylate
- Tallow
- Zinc compounds

3. Shaving cream (aerosols) .... Toxicity rating 2

Fatty acid alcohol and amine soaps	10–25%
Essential oil (fragrance)	0.1–1%
Water	>50%
Propellant	0–10%

Other:

Emulsifiers	0.1–1%
Humectants	1–5%
Sodium or potassium stearate	

4. Shaving lotions

a. Aftershave lotion .... Toxicity rating 2

Menthol	0.1%
Camphor	0.1%
Sorbitol	2.0%
Perfume oil	1.0%
Alcohol*	50.0–90%
Water	q.s.

Aftershave lotions may contain:
- Bay rum*

Starred ingredients (*) may be responsible for major toxic effects; consult Section II.

COSMETICS (Cont.)

SHAVING CREAMS AND LOTIONS (Cont.)

Benzalkonium chloride*
Benzoic acid
Bithionol
Boric acid*
Ethyl *p*-aminobenzoate (benzo-
    caine)
Glycerol
Jamaica rum
Aluminum chlorhydroxy allan-
    toinate
Menthol
Potassium alum
Propylene glycol
Quaternary ammonium com-
    pounds
Ultraviolet ray absorbers
Witch hazel
Zinc phenolsulfonate

b. Preshave lotions, astringent type .. **Toxicity rating 2**

Aluminum phenolsulfonate	2.0%
Alcohol*	55.0%
Water	42.5%
Perfume	0.5%

c. Preshave lotions, oily type ...... **Toxicity rating 2**

Isopropyl myristate-palmitate ...	25.0%
Alcohol*	74.5%

Preshave lotions may contain most of the ingredients listed under Aftershave Lotions, above.

5. Shaving caps (cakes, sticks, etc.) ..... **Toxicity rating 3**

Surfactants	>50%
Essential oil (fragrance)	1–5%
Humectants and oils	0–10%
Stannous chloride	
Titanium dioxide	
Water	5–10%
Antibacterial agents	0–5%
Color	0.1–1%
Other:	
Abradant (*e.g.*, pumice)	0–5%
Optical brighteners	0.1–1%

SKIN BLEACHES (see BLEACH AND FRECKLE CREAMS)

SKIN FRESHENERS .... Toxicity rating 2

1. Astringent (*e.g.*, zinc salts) 0–2%

Alcohol	25–>50%
Fats and oils	0–10%
Essential oil (fragrance)	1–5%
Water	0–>50%
Witch hazel extract	0–35%

2. Hamamelis water 60.0%

Camphorated alcohol (10%)	15.0%
Citric acid	1.0%
Alcohol	24.0%

May contain:

Arnica
Bay rum
Boric acid
Brucine sulfate
Chamomile
Esters
Floral waters
Glycerin
Lactic acid
Magnesia

COSMETICS (Cont.)

SKIN FRESHENERS (Cont.)

Menthol
Oil of lavender
Phosphoric acid
Talc
Tincture of benzoin

STYPTIC PENCIL .... Toxicity rating 2

Potassium aluminum sulfate (12 H$_2$O).	90.0%
Glycerol	5.0%
Talc	5.0%

SUNTAN PREPARATIONS

1. Suntan cream (emulsion) .... **Toxicity rating 2**

a. Water	>50%
Fats, oils, waxes	10–25%
Emulsifiers	1–10%
Humectants	0–10%
Preservatives	0.1–1%
Essential oil (fragrance)	0.1–1%
Sunscreen agent	1–5%
b. Monoglyceryl *p*-aminobenzoate	3.0%
Mineral oil	25.0%
Sorbitan monostearate	4.0%
Polyoxyethylene sorbitan mono-stearate	6.0%
Water	62.0%

2. Suntan gels and oils .... **Toxicity rating 2**

Oils (*e.g.*, mineral)	>50%
Emollient	1–10%
Thickeners	1–10%
Sunscreen agent	1–5%
Preservatives	0.1–1%
Color	0.1–1%
Essential oil (fragrance)	0.1–1%

3. Suntan lotion (alcoholic) .... **Toxicity rating 3**

Menthyl anthranilate	5.0%
Propylene glycol ricinoleate	10.0%
Glycerol	10.0%
Alcohol*	65.0%
Water	10.0%

4. Suntan oil .... **Toxicity rating 3**

2-Ethyl hexyl salicylate*	5.0%
Sesame oil	40.0%
Mineral oil	55.0%

5. Indoor tanning preparation .... **Toxicity rating 2**

Lanolin, deodorized	25–50%
Vegetable oil (*e.g.*, sesame oil)	10–25%
Mineral oil	10–25%
Water	10–25%
Essential oil (fragrance, color and antoxidant)	0.1–1%
Tanning agents (dihydroxy acetone)	1–5%
Sunscreen agent	1–5%

TALCUM POWDERS (see POWDERS)

TOILET WATERS (see PERFUME)

TOOTHPASTES AND POWDERS (see DENTIFRICES, under NONPRESCRIPTION DRUGS)

VANISHING CREAMS (see FOUNDATION CREAM)

VITAMIN CREAMS .... Toxicity rating 1

Cod liver oil	20.0%
Lanolin, anhydrous	30.0%
Petrolatum	50.0%

Starred ingredients (*) may be responsible for major toxic effects; consult Section II.

DECORATIONS

CHRISTMAS SPRAYS .... Toxicity ratings 2–3
  May contain:
    Distearyl dimethyl benzyl ammonium
      chloride
    Ethyl cellulose
    Fatty acids (primarily stearic)
    Lucite
    Methylene chloride*
    Perfume
    Polyvinyl acetate resin

CHRISTMAS TREE ORNAMENTS   Toxicity rating 3 or 4
  Christmas tree ornaments of the "bubble
    light" variety frequently contain such
    substances as ethyl alcohol,* methyl
    chloride,* methylene chloride,* or
    ethyl ether*

CHRISTMAS SNOW SPRAY ...... Toxicity rating 3 or 4
  Waxes
  Fatty acids
  Perfume
  Chlorinated hydrocarbon solvents*
  Petroleum distillates*
  Nitrocellulose or hydrocarbon resins
  Isobutane propellant

DEGREASERS

DEGREASERS (see also Cleaners)
Household liquid: .... Toxicity rating 2
1. Combinations of anionic and nonionic
    synthetic surfactants, usually
    about 15 to 20%. Balance water.
  Example:
    Alkyl phenol polyethylene glycol⎫
      ether)   ⎬ 20%
    Alkyl aryl sodium sulfonate)⎭
  Water softener⎫
    Color   ⎬
    Perfume ⎬ q.s.–100%
    Water   ⎭
2. Water solutions of coconut fatty acids
    in combination with the above
    mentioned surfactants
3. Terpene distillates* (see Terpenes) ... Toxicity rating 3
  Petroleum distillates*
  May contain:
    Methyl polysiloxane
    Tall oil fatty acids (see rosin and
      rosin oil)
4. Powder .... Toxicity rating 3
  Carbon tetrachloride*
  Kaolin
  Naphtha
5. Vapor .... Toxicity rating 3
  Perchloroethylene (100%)
  Carbon tetrachloride (100%) .... Toxicity rating 4
  Trichloroethylene (100%) .... Toxicity rating 4

GREASE REMOVERS .... Toxicity rating 3
  Mineral spirits* 60–70%
  Oleic acid 5–10%
  Caustic potash (30% solution) 5–10%
  Butyl alcohol 5–10%
  Butyl Cellosolve 5–10%
  Methyl chloroform 0–5%
  Alkyl aryl sulfonate (10% solution) 0–5%
  Methyl ethyl ketone

DEGREASERS (Cont.)

GREASE REMOVERS (Cont.)

  May contain:
    Alkaline soap
    Alkalis (trisodium phosphate, sodium
      carbonate)
    Isophorone
    Isopropanol
    Phosphoric acid

TAR REMOVERS .... Toxicity rating 4
  Xylene*
  Chlorinated hydrocarbons*
  May contain:
    Isopropyl alcohol*
    Mineral spirits*
    Surfactants

WAX REMOVERS (see GREASE REMOVERS, above)

DEICERS

DEICERS, REFRIGERATORS AND
    AUTOMOTIVE .... Toxicity rating 2–3
1. Propylene glycol 0–100%
  Ethylene glycol* 0–50%
  Isopropyl alcohol 0–25%
  Water 0–25%
  May contain:
    n-Propyl alcohol
2. Methanol 0–50%

DEICERS, FUEL SYSTEM
    ANTIFREEZE .... Toxicity rating 4
1. Isopropanol or propanol* 60%
  Toluene* 30%
  Acetone 10%
2. .... Toxicity rating 3
  Isopropanol or propanol* 20%
  Methanol* 80%
3. .... Toxicity rating 4
  Methanol* 70%
  Xylene* 30%
4. Methanol 96%
  Trace materials 4%
  Additives are either water-freezing point depressants, such
as ethanol, isopropanal, dimethyl formamide, hexylene gly-
col, dipropylene glycol, or surface-active agents.

FROST REMOVER
1. Spray type: .... Toxicity rating 3
  Isopropyl alcohol 25%
  Ethylene glycol* 50%
  Water 25%
  Propellant, CO_2
2. Alcohol .... Toxicity rating 3
  Isopropyl alcohol* 30–100%
  N-Propyl alcohol*
  Propylene glycol 15–30%
  Ethylene glycol*
  Water 5–15%
  May contain:
    Tetrahydrofurfuryl alcohol (see
      higher alcohols)

DEODORIZERS

BATHROOM DEODORANT
1. Naphthalene* .... Toxicity rating 4
2. Paradichlorobenzene* .... Toxicity rating 3

Starred ingredients (*) may be responsible for major toxic effects; consult Section II.

DEODORIZERS (Cont.)	DEODORIZERS (Cont.)

BATHROOM DEODORANT (Cont.)

3. Sodium bisulfate* .... Toxicity rating 3
These compounds may or may not contain a trace of perfume

CLEANSER TYPE	Toxicity rating 3
1. Pine oil* 60% minimum)	always
Anhydrous soap 30% maximum)	90%
Water	10%
2. Quaternary ammonium compound* ..	2.5–10%
Nonionic surfactant	0.6–2.5%
Phosphates, carbonates, or	
metasilicates	2–3%
EDTA	0.5–1%
For metal surfaces add sodium nitrite	
3. Synthetic phenols	3.5–5%
	maximum
Isopropanol	2–3%
Anhydrous soap	5–15%
EDTA	0.5–1%
Water to make	100%
Trace amounts of color and fragrance	
May contain:	
Magnesium sulfate	

DEODORANT BLOCKS	Toxicity rating 3
1. p-Dichlorobenzene*	99%
Essential oils	1%
2.	Toxicity rating 4
Naphthalene*	80%
Cedar wood	0–20%
3.	Toxicity rating 4
Paraformaldehyde*	85%

GARBAGE CAN	Toxicity rating 3
1. o-Dichlorobenzene*	20–60%
Petroleum distillate	10%
Pine oil	5%
May contain:	
Methylated aromatic petroleum	
derivatives*	14–15%
Dichlorodiphenyltrichloroethane ...	5%
2,2'-Thiobis(4-chloro-6-	
methylphenol)	0.25%
Propellants if spray	60%
2.	No rating
Sodium chloride	90%
Lime* (see Alkali)	10%
3.	Toxicity rating 3
p-Dichlorobenzene*	95%
Pine oil	1.5%
Essentials oils, small amounts	
4.	Toxicity rating 4
Naphthalene*	85%
Methyl salicylate	5%
5. Sodium hypochlorite*	No rating

ICE BOX OR REFRIGERATOR	
DEODORIZERS	Toxicity rating 1
Activated charcoal	100%

SPRAY TYPE DEODORIZERS	Toxicity rating 2
1. Ethyl or isopropyl alcohol	<30%
Glycol ethers	<8%
Surfactant (quaternary ammonium	
salts)	
Perfume	
Water	
Propellants	

SPRAY TYPE DEODORIZERS (Cont.)

2.	Toxicity rating 2 or 3
Metazene	4.0%
Petroleum distillates	6.0%
Propellants	up to 90.0%
May contain:	
Aluminum chlorhydrol	
Bromsalicylanilide	
2,3,4,5-Bis(2-	
butylene)tetrahydrofurfural	
Cellosolve acetate	
Dichlorodifluoromethanol	
Ethanol	
Fatty esters	
Formaldehyde	
Lauryl methacrylate	
Methoxychlor	
Methylene chloride	
o-Phenylphenol	
p-Dichlorobenzene*	
Pine oil	up to 10%
Piperonyl butoxide	
Pyrethrin	
Synthetic surfactants	
Trichloromonofluoromethane	
Wax	
Zinc phenolsulfonate	
3. See DISINFECTANTS, SPRAY	
TYPE	

WICK TYPE DEODORIZERS	Toxicity rating 3
Formaldehyde (37%)	2–3%
Water-soluble perfume	2–3%
Coloring	trace
Water	to 100%
Emulsifiers	
Essential oils	
Aromatic chemicals* (see Xylene Section II)	
Chlorophyll	

DISINFECTANTS

ALKALINE DISINFECTANTS	
1. Quaternary ammonium compounds*	3–25%
Inert ingredients, may contain:	
Builders	
Chelating agents	
Perfume	
Water	
Wetting agents	
2. Chlorine type	
Hypochlorite (dry or liquid form)	
Chlorine (from isocyanuric acids)	

DAIRY DISINFECTANTS	No rating
1.	Toxicity rating 2
Iodophor disinfectants (provides 1.6%	
available iodine)	
Polyethoxy polypropoxy ethanol-iodine complex	7–10%
Nonyl phenyl ether of polyethylene glycol-iodine complex	7–10%
Hydrochloric, phosphoric, citric or butyronic acid	0–10%
Dairies mostly use organic acids.	
2.	Toxicity rating 3
Calcium or sodium hypochlorite*	3–35%
Sodium chloride	0–64%
Phosphates*	1–91%

Starred ingredients (*) may be responsible for major toxic effects; consult Section II.

DISINFECTANTS (Cont.)

DAIRY DISINFECTANTS (Cont.)

Anionic wetting agents	0–5%
Potassium permanganate	0.01%
3.	Toxicity rating 3
Alkyl (C₈ to C₁₈) dimethyl benzyl ammonium chloride*	to 10–11%
May contain:	
Low level of color	
Water	
Ethyl alcohol	possible trace

HALOGENS

1. Liquid	No rating
Sodium hypochlorite*	5–16%
Sodium hydroxide	0.1–1.0%
Sodium chloride	5–10%
Water	84–90%
2. Powder:	Toxicity rating 3–4
Organic chlorine compound,* *e.g.,*	50–100%
Hexachlorobenzene*	
Dichlorobenzene*	
Dichloroisocyanurate*	0–92%
Pelletizing binders, etc.	0.50%
3.	No rating
Calcium hypochlorite* (see hypochlorite)	50–100%
May contain:	
Trisodium phosphate	0–92%
Halazone	
Pine oil	
Soap	
Soda ash	
Sodium borate*	

MISCELLANEOUS DISINFECTANTS

	Toxicity rating 3
Formaldehyde*	20%
May contain:	
Mercury compounds	small amount

PHENOL DISINFECTANTS

PHENOL DISINFECTANTS	Toxicity rating 4
Chlorophenols, *e.g.,* o-benzyl-p-chlorophenol or chloro-2-phenylphenol (also sodium salts)	3–8%
Phenols* (often from coal tar)	
Phenol	
Tertiary amyl phenol	
Cresol	20–50%
o-Phenylphenol	
Versene	1–3%
	0–20%
Complex phosphates, *e.g.,* tetrapyrophosphate, tripolyphosphate, as K and Na salts	1–3%
Glycerine	1%
Soap	4–30%
Isopropyl alcohol	1–20%
Surfactants, *e.g.,* sodium dodecyl benzyl sulfonate	
Water	
May contain:	
Aromatic hydrocarbon solvents* ("Coal tar hydrocarbons or coal tar neutral oils")	44–58%

PINE OIL

PINE OIL	Toxicity rating 3
1. Pine oil*	60–90%
Soap	10–30%
Water	10%
Nearly all of this type.	
2. Pine oil	5–10%

DISINFECTANTS (Cont.)

PINE OIL (Cont.)

Phenols*	2–6%
Soap	5–10%
Alcohol	5–10%
May contain:	
Dye	
Isopropanol*	
Potassium o-benzyl-p-chlorophenate	
Potassium tetrapyrophosphate	
Propylene glycol	
Versene	

QUATERNARY AMMONIUM COMPOUNDS

1.	Toxicity rating 4
Quaternary ammonium compounds*	20–50%
Mostly derivatives of dimethyl benzyl ammonium chloride	
Water	to 100%
2.	Toxicity rating 3
Quaternary ammonium compounds*	3–6%
Ethylene oxide condensate	6–10%
Sodium carbonate	2–3%
Versene	0–2%
Inert ingredients, probably liquid	
Glycerine	1%
Soap	4–30%
Isopropanol	7–20%
Sodium dodecyl benzyl sulfonate	
May contain:	
Dyes	
Essential oils	
Ethanol	
Nonyl phenol polyethylene glycol ether	
Nonyl phenoxy polyoxyethylene ethanol	
Sodium tripolyphosphate	

SPRAY TYPE DISINFECTANTS

SPRAY TYPE DISINFECTANTS	Toxicity rating 3
o-Phenylphenol	1%
N-Alkyl (C₁₈ 92%, C₁₆ 8%)	
N-Ethyl morpholinium ethylsulfates	0.035%
Alcohol	67–70%
Inert ingredients (including propellant)	32%

DRIERS

AIR DEHUMIDIFIERS

1.	Toxicity rating 2
Calcium chloride	100%
2.	Toxicity rating 1
Diatomaceous earth impregnated with calcium chloride	20%

FUEL TANK (to absorb water in gasoline)

FUEL TANK (to absorb water in gasoline)	Toxicity rating 3
Methyl alcohol*	100%

PAINT DRIERS (see PAINT)

DUST CONTROL

DUST CONTROL

1. Floor sweep	Toxicity rating 1
Sand and sawdust (one to one) coated with paraffin oil	
2.	Toxicity rating 3
Mineral oil* (see kerosene)	
Nonionic surfactant	

Starred ingredients (*) may be responsible for major toxic effects; consult Section II.

DUST CONTROL (Cont.)	DYES (Cont.)

DUST CONTROL (Cont.)

Alkyl dimethyl benzyl ammonium chloride	0.25%
Propellants	
3.	Toxicity rating 1
Mineral oil (edible grade)	
Perfume	
Propellants	
4.	Toxicity rating 3
Sanitizing dust control	
Mineral oil	20–96%
Petroleum distillate*	0–100%
Trichlorethylene	

May contain:
1,1,1-Trichloroethane*
4- and 6-Chloro-o-phenylphenol*
o-Phenylphenol
Quaternary ammonium compounds*
Nonionic surfactants
Silicones
Propellants

DYES

For toxicity information on the dyestuff see PIGMENTS, this section.

EASTER EGG DYES	Toxicity rating 1 or 2
U.S. certified color	0.5–5%
Edible gums	trace
Edible waxes	trace
Citric acid	trace
Phosphoric acid	trace
Resins	
Salt	
Essential oils (citrus)	
Lactose and dextrose	to 100%

May contain:
Sodium bicarbonate
Polyethylene glycol
Talc

EYELASH AND EYEBROW (see COSMETICS)

FABRIC (see under DYES, RUG)

HAIR (see COSMETICS)

LEATHER	Toxicity rating 3–4
Methyl,* ethyl or isopropyl alcohol	30%
Xylene*	
Aniline dye	

May contain:
Nitrobenzene*
Tannic acid
o-Dichlorobenzene*
1-1-1-Trichloroethane*

RUG

1. Rug dyes	Toxicity rating 3
Aniline dye	
Acetic acid	
Citric acid	
Diethylene glycol*	
Sodium chloride	
2. Fabric dyes	Toxicity rating 2–4
Dyestuff*—direct or direct and acid	14% av. (3.35–40.4%)
Alkyl amyl sodium sulfate (40% active)	8%
Sodium chloride	78%

RUG (Cont.)

May contain:	
Soap	
Sodium sulfate	
Toluol*	up to 60%
Isopropyl alcohol	up to 40%
SHOE DYES	Toxicity rating 3
Denatured ethanol* or isopropanol*	50–98%
Aniline dyes	0–3%
o-Dichlorobenzene*	15–20%
Diethylene glycol monomethyl ether	0–3%
Acetic acid	1–10%
Water	1–10%

May contain:
Butadiene/styrene resin
Emulsified wax
Chlorinated solvents*
Nitrobenzene*
Hexylene glycol
Terpenes (pine oil)
Glycerine
Mineral spirits*
Xylene*

FIBERGLASS AND RESIN PLASTICS

The resin component, the glass fiber material and the finished products are considered to be nontoxic, but the hardeners (or "catalysts") are toxic in the following degree:
HARDENERS

1. Methyl ethyl ketone peroxide* (30–100%)	Toxicity rating 3
2. Cyclohexanone	Toxicity rating 2
3. Benzoyl peroxide (8–50%)	Toxicity rating 2
4. Dialkylaniline* (see Aniline) (trace to 100%)	Toxicity rating 3
5. Toluene sulfonic acid	Toxicity rating ?
6. 2,2-Diaminodiethylamine*	Toxicity rating 3

A particular hazard is present when the hardener is packaged in small plastic bottles, closely resembling the nursing bottles found in toy baby kits.

FILLERS

CONCRETE PATCHER
Sand
Portland cement

DRY JOINT COMPOUND	Toxicity rating 2
Casein	4–7%
Ammonium oxalate	1%
Ammonium borate	1%
or	
Sodium pentachlorphenate	0.2%
Asbestos	4–10%
Mica	15–40%
Calcium carbonate	
FURNACE CEMENT	Toxicity rating 2
Clay	
Asbestos fiber	
Sodium silicate*	
Caustic*	
Carbon black	
PATCHING PLASTER	Toxicity rating 1

1. Ground marble
   Plaster
2. Rutland Kex
   Plaster (calcium sulfate)

Starred ingredients (*) may be responsible for major toxic effects; consult Section II.

FILLERS (Cont.)		FILLERS (Cont.)	

PATCHING PLASTER (Cont.)

Ground marble
Mica
Glue
3. Plaster of Paris
Retarder

PLASTIC FILLERS

Polyester resin	Toxicity rating 2
Styrene monomer	15-20%
Alkyd resin	30-35%
Talc filler	45-55%
Dialkyl aniline	0.1-0.4%
Hardener	Toxicity rating 3
Methyl ethyl ketone peroxide*	60%
or	
Benzoyl peroxide	35%
or	
Dimethyl aniline* (see Aniline) in di-butyl phthalate	100%

Calcium phosphate
May contain:
Metallic naphthenates
Milled fiberglass
Red dye

PUTTIES

1. Crack filler	Toxicity rating 2
Calcium sulfate	80-90%
Dextrin	10-20%
Silica	10-15%
2. Glazing compound	Toxicity rating 1
Fish oil	7-12%
Soybean oil	5-10%
Marble dust	40-50%
Fatty acid	0-4%
Mineral spirits	1%
Asbestos	3-5%

May contain:
Titanium dioxide
Polybutene
Safflower oil, fish oil, inert fillers
Linseed oil, lard oil

3. Wood putties	Toxicity rating 1
Calcium sulfate	80-90%
Dextrin	10-15%
Wood flour	3-5%

READY MIXED JOINT COMPOUND	Toxicity rating 2
Plasticized polyvinyl acetate emulsion	6% (nonvolatile basis)
Diethylene glycol monoethyl ether	1%
Phenyl mercury acetate	0.015%
Mica	15-40%
Asbestos	3-6%
Calcium carbonate to make	100% (nonvolatile basis)
Water (wet weight basis)	about 40%

SPACKLING COMPOUND	Toxicity rating 2
Calcium sulfate	92%
Mica	5%
Glue	3%

May contain:
Calcium carbonate
Acetate resin emulsion
Plasticized polyvinol

STOVE LINING	Toxicity rating 3

Clay
Asbestos
Borax*

WALLBOARD JOINT CEMENT	Toxicity rating 1

Ochre
Clay
Ground marble
Casein
Mica
Asbestos
May contain:
Methyl cellulose
Polyvinyl acetate
Polyvinyl alcohol
Talc
Sodium acetate

WHITE LEAD PUTTIES .... Toxicity rating 3 or 4

Note: 5, 10, 20 and 30% putties have been sold. The percentages refer to the weight percentage of basic lead carbonate* in the pigment. New federal regulations appear to forbid the sale of products containing more than 0.5% lead.

Ground limestone ⎫	
Asbestos fiber	
Talc ⎬	90%
Titanium dioxide ⎭	
Linseed oil ⎫	8%
Soybean oil ⎭	
Mineral spirits	2%

May contain:
Fish oil
Bentonite
See also Glazing Compound under Putties above

FIRE EXTINGUISHERS

CARBON DIOXIDE	No rating
Compressed carbon dioxide gas	80-100%
Compressed nitrogen gas	0-20%

FOAM FIRE EXTINGUISHERS

1. Mechanical foams	Toxicity rating 2
Hydrolyzed protein	25-45%
Ethylene glycol	3-6%
Cellosolve	3-6%
Heavy metal salts (Fe, Zn)	0.5-2%
Bactericide	1% maximum
2. Powder foams	Toxicity rating 2

a. Single generator powders with all ingredients in one system
b. Dual generator powders with aluminium sulfate and soda-stabilizer in separate systems

Sodium bicarbonate	40-45%
Aluminum sulfate	40-100%
Metal stearates (Zn, Al, Mg)	2-6%
Stabilizers (licorice extracts, lignums, glues, egg albumen, dry hydrolyzed protein)	2-6%
Clay	

3. Liquid foams	Toxicity rating 2

Charge "A"
Aluminum sulfate-saturated solution
Charge "B"

Sodium bicarbonate	5-7%
Water	to 100%

Starred ingredients (*) may be responsible for major toxic effects; consult Section II.

| FIRE EXTINGUISHERS (Cont.) | FIREPLACE COLORS (Cont.) |

FOAM FIRE EXTINGUISHERS (Cont.)

Stabilizer (licorice extracts, lignums, egg albumen, glues, dry hydrolyzed protein)	4–6%

LIQUID FIRE EXTINGUISHERS
1. Chlorobromoethane*	Toxicity rating 4
(see chlorobromopropene)	100%
2. Halons	Toxicity rating 2
a. Bromotrifluoromethane	100%
b. Dichlorodifluoromethane	100%
c. Dichlorotrifluoroethane	100%
d. Trichloromonofluoromethane	100%
For deep-seated fires	Toxicity rating 3
Triton X-100	
Sodium hydroxide* (see Alkali)	
Sodium dichromate*	

MISCELLANEOUS FIRE
EXTINGUISHERS	Toxicity rating 4
Methyl bromide*	100%

POWDER EXTINGUISHERS
1.	Toxicity rating 2
Sodium and/or potassium bicarbonate	85–99%
Metal stearates (Zn, Al, Mg)	1–2%
Treated with silicones	0.5–3%
Flowing agents (mica, alumina, aerogels, tricalcium phosphate)	1–15%
Vegetable coloring matter	
2.	Toxicity rating 2
Ammonium monophosphate	70–85%
Potassium sulfate	10–25%
Flowing agent (aerogel)	3–10%
Silicones	0.5–3%
May contain:	
Diammonium phosphate	
3. Miscellaneous dry	
a. Borax compounds (90–100%)	Toxicity rating 4
b. Clays (bentonite) (100%)	Toxicity rating 1
c. Pitch (100%)	Toxicity rating 1
d. Graphite (100%)	Toxicity rating 1

SODA ACID
Sodium bicarbonate	97.5%
Sulfuric acid* (see Acid)	2.5%

WATER BASE
WATER BASE	Toxicity rating 3
1. Calcium chloride	30–40%
Sodium dichromate* or chromate* ...	0.5–2%
Water	q.s.
	Toxicity rating 3
2. Potassium carbonate	35–45%
Ethylene glycol	1–3%
Sodium dichromate* or chromate* ...	0.5–2%
Water	q.s.

FIREPLACE COLORS

FIREPLACE COLORS	
1.	Toxicity rating 3
Copper chloride* (see Copper oxychloride*)	10–25%
Coke dust, sawdust	60–90%
Organic ash	
2. Flame colorations	Toxicity rating
Violet	
Potassium compounds	3
May contain:	
Rubidium compounds	3?
Cesium compounds	3?

FIREPLACE COLORS (Cont.)

FIREPLACE COLORS (Cont.)	
Blue	
Copper chloride, bromide, sulfate	4
May contain:	
Lead compounds	5
Arsenic compounds	5
Selenium compounds	6
Green	
Copper sulfate or chloride	4
May contain:	
Copper compounds	4
Thallium compounds	5
Tellurium compounds	5?
Barium compounds	4 or 5
Molybdenum compounds	5?
Antimony compounds	5
Zinc compounds	4
Borates	4
Phosphates	3
Ammonium compounds	?
Red	
Strontium nitrate	2
May contain:	
Calcium compounds	2
Lithium compounds	3
Yellow	
Sodium compounds	?

FIREPROOFING COMPOUNDS

FIREPROOFING COMPOUNDS	Toxicity rating 2
Ammonium chloride	
Boric acid	
Ammonium phosphate	

FIREWORKS

FIREWORKS	
Oxidizing agents	Toxicity rating 4
Potassium nitrate*	
Potassium chlorate*	
Barium nitrate*	
Potassium perchlorate*	
Fuel and binders	
Charcoal	
Fossil gums	
Gelatin	
Glue	
Iron powder	
Lampblack	
Lead nitrate* (see Lead salts)	
Magnesium	
Milk sugar	
Petroleum	
Resins	
Shellac	
Starch	
Stearin	
Sugar	
Surfur	
Zinc powder	
Colors	Toxicity rating 4 or 5
Phosphorus,* mercury,* sulfocyanate, antimony,* copper,* salts, e.g., arsenate,* carbonate, oxalate,* oxide, sulfate, sulfide,* and chloride.	

Starred ingredients (*) may be responsible for major toxic effects; consult Section II.

FLAVORS	FLUXES (Cont.)

FLAVORS

1. Vanilla extract .... Toxicity rating 2
   Vanilla oleoresin,
   Concentrated vanilla flavoring or
     concentrated vanilla extract
   Ethyl alcohol, not less than 35%
   May contain:
     Glycerin
     Propylene glycol
     Sugar (including invert sugar)
     Dextrose
     Corn syrup (including dried corn
       syrup)
2. Lemon extract .... Toxicity rating 2?
   Oil of lemon, not less than 5%
   Ethyl alcohol 80%
   Water 15%
   Flavors may contain: .... Toxicity rating:
     Cloves 1
     Ginger 1
     Horseradish 1
     Mustard 1
     Nutmeg 1
     Pepper (cayenne, black) 1
     Sage (ground) 2
     Wintergreen (essence) 2
3. Many of the flavors are Essential Oils.
   The Ingredients Index (Section II)
   lists them under Oils and under Essential Oils.
4. Almond extract .... Toxicity rating 2?
   Oil of bitter almonds free from hy-
     drocyanic acid, not less than 1%

FLUXES

SOLDERING FLUXES
   Aluminum, lead, stainless steel and tin   Toxicity rating 4
   a. Liquid
      Chlorides—Zn,* NH$_4$, Sn and Li—
        (mainly zinc + a much smaller
        amount of NH$_4$) 10–35%
      HCl* (see Acid) 0–40%
      Stainless steel flux has and needs
        the highest content of HCl
      Wetting agent
      Water .... to 100%
   b. Organic ....Toxicity rating 2–3
      Organic salts (hydrochlorides of an-
        iline, glutamic acid, betaine,
        salicylic acid*) 7–10%
      Urea 4–6%
      Water 84–89%
   c. Pastes (all metals except
        aluminum) .... Toxicity rating 4
      Zinc chloride* 20–30%
      Ammonium chloride 5%
      Petrolatum 65–75%
   d. Rosin   Toxicity rating 3
      Mixtures of solutions of rosin (col-
        ophony) in organic solvents (ali-
        phatic alcohols,* terpenes,* hy-
        drocarbons*)
      e.g., Rosin 10–20%

SOLDERING FLUXES (Cont.)

      Ethylamine hydrochloride 1–2%
      Alcohol* 80–90%
   e. Silver solder (also used for brazing
      ferrous and nonferrous metals
      including titanium) .... Toxicity rating 4
      e.g., Boric acid* 40–50%
      Cadmium
      Potassium fluoroborate 10–20%
      Potassium bifluoride* (see
        Fluorides) 20–30%

WELDING FLUXES .... Toxicity rating 4
   Alkaline fluorides*
   Alkaline earth metals

FOAMS

POLYURETHANE FOAMS .... Toxicity rating ?
   The foams consist of a diisocyanate, a polyol, a
blowing agent, and frequently a catalyst accelerator.
1. Diisocyanate—often toluene diisocyan-
   ate (sensitization)
2. Polyol .... Toxicity rating 2
3. Catalyst—sometimes aliphatic amines,
   e.g., morpholines, triethyl diamine,
   tetramethyl butane diamine ...... Toxicity rating 4
4. Blowing agent—a fluocarbon, halon or
   a chlorinated hydrocarbon*
5. Catalyst accelerator—frequently organic tin compounds (irritant) and
   toxic (see Stannous salts)
   Foams are not reactive. Some of the components are reactive; one (TDI) can produce severe pulmonary effects and
sensitization.

FUELS

CHARCOAL LIGHTERS .... Toxicity rating 3
   naphtha* .... up to 100%
   Perfume 0.1%
   May contain:
   Aromatics

COOKING FUELS .... Toxicity rating 3
1. Petroleum hydrocarbons (kerosene,*
   naphtha*) 100%
2. Denatured ethanol* 70%
   Methanol 3%
   Acetone 3%
   Nitrocellulose 2.5%
   Water .... q.s.
3. Ethanol 95%
   Methanol 4%
   Ethyl acetate 4%
   Perfume
   Denatonium benzoate
   Fuchsine

FIRE KINDLERS .... Toxicity rating 3–4
   Kerosene* 89%
   Dyes* 11%
   May contain:
     Copper naphthenate
     Isopropyl alcohol
     Perfume hickory
     Halon propellant

Starred ingredients (*) may be responsible for major toxic effects; consult Section II.

FUELS (Cont.)	FUELS (Cont.)

FIRE KINDLERS (Cont.)

Tablets .... Toxicity rating 4
  Potassium chlorate*
  Small amounts of
    Graphite
    Clay
    Manganese dioxide
    Nitrocellulose cement
Flares used for lighting fires, so called "kindle flares," are made from bagasse of sugar cane, petrolatums, and candle wax.

LIGHTER FLUID .... Toxicity rating 3
Petroleum hydrocarbons (naphthas*) . 100%
Perfume .... trace

MODEL AIRPLANE FUELS
1. Alcohol type .... Toxicity rating 3
  Methanol* 70%
  Nitromethane* 10%
  Ucon synthetic oil (#PM5651) 20%
2. Diesel type .... Toxicity rating 3
  Kerosine* 40–60%
  Diethyl ether* .... >30%
  Castor oil/synthetic (glycol or ether
    based) .... <25%
  Hexyl nitrate .... <2%
3. Glow power
  Methanol* 60–70%
  Synthetic oil 20–28%
  Nitromethane 5%
  Propylene oxide
    May contain:
      Amyl acetate
      Nitroethane
4. Race Power
  Methanol* 10–50%
  Castor oil
  Synthetic oil 10–20%
  Nitromethane* 30–70%

MOTOR FUEL .... Toxicity rating 3
1. Tetraethyl lead* (see Lead, Section
    III) 0–0.1%
  Petroleum hydrocarbons (gasoline)* .. 99–100%
  Additives .... trace
  May contain:
    N,N'-Alkyl-aryl- and
      di-alkyl-phenylenediamines
    N,N'-Di-sec-butyl-p-phenylenediamine
    N,N'-Disalicylidene-1,2-propanedi-
      amine
    Oil-soluble dyes
2. Racing .... Toxicity rating 3
    Methanol* 30–70%
    Isopropanol* 0–70%
    Castor oil 0–30%
    Nitromethane* 0–30%
3. Diesel fuel .... Toxicity rating 3
  Kerosene*

MOTOR FUEL ADDITIVE .... Toxicity rating 3
Mineral oil (see Kerosene*) 90%
Mixture of oxygenated, unsaponifiable
  hydrocarbons 8%
Isopropyl alcohol .... trace
High-molecular-weight esters

MOTOR FUEL ADDITIVE (Cont.)

Rust inhibitor (see Automotive Prod-
  ucts)
N,N'-Disalicylidine-1,2-propanediamine
N,N'-Di-sec-butyl-p-phenylene diamine
N,N'-Alkyl-aryl-
  and di-alkyl-phenylenediamines
Ethylene dichloride
Ethylene dibromide
Tetraethyl lead* (see Lead, Section III)
Dye 0.0003%
  Blue: Essentially 1,4-
        di(isopropylamino anthra-
        quinone)
  Yellow: Essentially p-diethylaminoa-
        zobenzene
  Red: Essentially methyl deriva-
        tives of azobenzene-4-azo-
        2-naphththol
  Chemical additives in petroleum fuels:
1. Oxidation inhibitors
2. Copper deactivators
3. Corrosion inhibitors
4. Combustion chamber deposit modifiers
5. Anti-icing compounds
6. Antiknock agents
7. Antistatic additives

ICE SUBSTITUTE

ICE SUBSTITUTE .... Toxicity rating 2
Roccal 65%
Trisodium phosphate 15%
Water 99.20%

INCENSE

INCENSE (PUNK) .... Toxicity rating 2
Charcoal 75%
Starch 15%
Karaya gum
China clay
Essential oils 10%
Triethylene glycol
Aromatic chemicals

INKS

The ratings given for inks do not include pigments which in most cases are relatively nontoxic. However, some pigments are toxic, and the Pigments section should be consulted.

BALL PEN .... Toxicity rating 2
Glycols* and/or glycol ethers 40–70%
Spirit soluble dyes and/or basic dyes .. 5–40%
Resins .... up to 40%
May contain:
  Benzyl alcohol, probably nontoxic in
    amounts available.

COLORED PIGMENTED INKS ...... Toxicity rating 3–4
White: Titanium dioxide and zinc oxide   10–20%
Gold: Bronze powders* (see Copper
  salts) 10–20%
Silver: Aluminum powder 10–20%
Colors: pigments (see Pigments) 5–10%
Solution used:
  Resin: Styrene copolymers 10–20%

Starred ingredients (*) may be responsible for major toxic effects; consult Section II.

INKS (Cont.)

COLORED PIGMENTED INKS (Cont.)

Solvent: Aromatic naphthas	80–90%

May contain:
- Alcohols
- Naphthas, petroleum
- Odor-masks
- Phenols*
- Wetting agents

DRAWING OR INDIA INKS — Toxicity rating 2–3

Carbon black	2–10%
Dyes or pigments (see Pigments)*	2–10%
Shellac	2–5%
Water	80–90%

May contain:
- Acetone
- Alcohols
- Ammonia
- Camphor
- Preservatives
- Synthetic resins

DUPLICATING INKS — Toxicity rating 3?

Dyes (see Pigments)	2–10%
Alcohols*	40–50%
Glycol ethers (see Ethylene glycol, Section III)	40–50%
Water	10–30%

May contain:
- Glycols
- Oils
- Resins

EMULSION INKS — Toxicity rating 3

Carbon black	5–10%
Dye (see Pigments)	0–2%
Mineral oil* (see Kerosene)	40–90%
Emulsifier	2–20%
Water	5–60%

FIBER TIPPED INKS — Toxicity rating 2

Water	70–95%
Water-soluble dyes	1–12%
Glycols or glycerin	0–20%
Soluble gums	0–3%

FLUORESCENT INKS — Toxicity rating 3

Fluorescent pigments* (see Pigments)
Alkyd resin vehicle
May contain:
- Esters*
- Ketones*
- Urea

HEKTOGRAPH INKS — Toxicity rating 3

Mineral acids	2%
Dye (see pigments)	5–10%
Solvents (water, glycerine, glycols,* alcohol,* glycol ethers*)	75–85%

INDELIBLE INKS — Toxicity rating 3–4

Nigrosine dyes (see Pigments (black))	5–20%
Solvents (aniline oil,* cresol,* glycolethers*)	80–90%

May contain:
- Carbon black or lampblack
- Naphthas
- Toluene
- Xylene*

INK REMOVERS, ERADICATORS

Ink eradicators usually contain bleaches.

INKS (Cont.)

INK REMOVERS, ERADICATORS (Cont.)

1. Acid solution — No rating
Tartaric acid	
Phosphoric acid	1–4% in water solution
Citric acid	
Mineral acid (see Acid)	

2. Alkaline solution — Toxicity rating 2
Sodium hypochlorite	3–4%
Water	96%

   May contain:
   - Sodium chloride
   - Sodium phosphates

3. — Toxicity rating 3
Ammonium sulfide*	5%
Oxalic acid*	5%

   Separate solutions applied alternately to ink stains

4. — Toxicity rating 2
Citric acid* (see Acid)	50%
Alum	50%

   Dry rubbed into stain followed by water

5. Ballpoint — Toxicity rating 3
   - Alcohols*
   - Glycol ethers*
   - Surfactants*
   - Naphthas*
   - Chlorinated hydrocarbons*
   - Emulsifiers

MARKING INKS

1. Permanent — Toxicity rating 3 or 4
Dyes (see Pigments)	2–8%
Solvents (naphthas,* aromatic hydrocarbons* (xylene, toluene)	80–90%
Resins (rosin, rosin derivatives of synthetic resin)	2–5%

   May contain:
   - Alcohols*
   - Cresol*
   - Glycol ethers*
   - Oils, oleic acid

2. Water-soluble — Toxicity rating 2
Water	70–80%
Dyes	3–10%
Glycerin or glycol	6–20%
Water-soluble gums	0–3%

MIMEOGRAPH CORRECTION FLUID

1. Ether type — Toxicity rating 3
Diethyl ether*	40–75%
Plasticizers	5–15%
Ethanol	0–15%
Nitrocellulose	3–8%
Pigments, dyes or toners (see Pigments)	0–5%

2. Nonether type — Toxicity rating 3
Ethyl acetate* (or other ketone or ester)	20–40%
Ethanol*	20–50%
Plasticizer	5–15%
Nitrocellulose	3–8%
Pigments, dye or toner (see Pigments)	0–5%

MIMEOGRAPH INKS

1. Oil base — Toxicity rating 3
Carbon black	5–10%
Dye (see Pigments)	0–2%
Mineral oil* (see Kerosene)	60–80%

Starred ingredients (*) may be responsible for major toxic effects; consult Section II.

INKS (Cont.)	INKS (Cont.)

MIMEOGRAPH INKS (Cont.)

Rosin and rosin derivatives	0–20%
2. Water base	Toxicity rating 3
Carbon black	0–5%
Dye (see Pigments)	0–5%
Ethylene glycol* or other polyhy-	
droxy compounds	10–30%
Surface active agents	0–2%
Water-soluble thickener	2–8%
Water	50–70%
3. Emulsion inks	Toxicity rating 3
Carbon black	5–10%
Dye	0–2%
Mineral oil	40–90%
Water	5–60%
Emulsifier	2–20%

MUSIC INKS ... Toxicity rating 3

Chromic acid*	<10%
Pigments (see Pigments)	<10%
Phenol	trace
Organic acids	
Copper (chemically bound)	
Varnish	
Kerosene	
Iron salts	
Glycols	
Fatty acids	
Surfactants	

OPAQUE INKS ... Toxicity rating 3–4

Dyes, pigments (see Pigments)	8–30%
Alcohols*	20–40%
Glycol ethers*	20–40%
Resins	<10%
May contain:	
Acetone*	
Cresol*	
Lacquer solvents*	

REDUCERS AND THINNERS, INKS Toxicity rating 2

May contain:
- Driers containing very small amounts of lead, manganese, or cobalt
- Lanolin
- Petrolatum
- Petroleum oils
- Waxes

SILK SCREEN INKS ... Toxicity rating 2–3
- Alkyd resin
- Organic and inorganic pigments* (see Pigments)

SOLUBLE MARKING INKS ... Toxicity rating 2

Water	70–95%
Water-soluble dyes	1–12%
Glycols or glycerin	0–20%
Soluble gums	0–3%

STAMPING INKS ... Toxicity rating 3

Pigments (see Pigments)	7–30%
Alcohol	20–40%
Glycol ether*	10–40%
Glycols*	20–40%
Glycerine	40–50%
May contain:	
Acetone	
Aniline*	
Cresol	
Lacquer solvents	

STAMPING INKS (Cont.)
- Phenol*
- Resins

STENCIL INKS ... Toxicity rating 3–4

Pigments (see Pigments)	10–30%
Solvents (naphthas* often used, oils, toluene,* xylene,* alcohol*)	40–60%
Resins (rosin or rosin derivatives, synthetic resins)	5–15%

WRITING AND FOUNTAIN PEN INKS ... Toxicity rating 2

Synthetic dyes (see Pigments)	0.5–5%
Water	90–95%
May contain:	
Alcohol	
Gallic acid	
Glycols	
Iron salts	
Mineral acid	0.1%
Oxalic, tartaric, citric acid	not more than 0.15%
Sodium hydroxide	not less than 1%
Surfactants	
Tannic acid	
Thymol, phenol	not less than 1%

LAUNDRY PRODUCTS

COMMERCIAL BLEACHES (Laundry) Toxicity rating 3 or 4

May contain:
- Oxalic acid*
- Sodium dithionite (sodium hydrosulfite)
- Sodium perborate*
- Sodium peroxide* (see also Hydrogen peroxide)
- Trisodium phosphate

1. Liquid	Toxicity rating 3
a. Sodium hypochlorite*	3–16%
Sodium hydroxide and/or sodium carbonate	0.2–0.5%
Sodium chloride	3–12%
Water	80–95%
b. Hydrogen peroxide*	3–20%
Water	80–97%
2. Tablets	Toxicity rating 3
* Potassium salt of chlorinated isocyanuric acid* (see Trichloroisocyanuric acid)	3–50%
Starch	50–97%

HOUSEHOLD BLEACHES, LIQUID Toxicity rating 1–3

1. Sodium hypochlorite*	3–10%
Sodium chloride	3–8%
Sodium hydroxide and/or sodium carbonate	0.01–0.5%
Water	85–95%
2. Hydrogen peroxide*	3%
Water	

HOUSEHOLD BLEACHES, POWDER

1. Chlorine type:	Toxicity rating 3
Organic chlorine (salts of di- or trichloroisocyanuric acid,* etc.)	2–20%
Sodium tripolyphosphate*	0–20%
Sodium silicate	0–5%

Starred ingredients (*) may be responsible for major toxic effects; consult Section II.

LAUNDRY PRODUCTS (Cont.)	LAUNDRY PRODUCTS (Cont.)

HOUSEHOLD BLEACHES, POWDER (Cont.)

Alkyl aryl sodium sulfonate or sodium alkyl sulfate	0–10%
Optical brightener	0–0.5%
Bluing	0–0.5%
Sodium sulfate	0–90%
2. Oxygen type:	Toxicity rating 3 or 4
Sodium perborate* or sodium carbonate perhydrate	5–40%
Sodium sesquicarbonate* or sodium carbonate*	0–70%
Sodium silicate	0–5%
Sodium tripolyphosphate*	0–40%
Alkyl aryl sodium sulfonate	2–10%
Sodium sulfate	0–70%
Fluorescent dye	0.2–0.4%
Bluing	0–0.5%

LAUNDRY BLUING

1. Detergent type:	Toxicity rating 3
Alkyl aryl sodium sulfonate*	10–25%
Sodium sulfate	40–75%
Sodium tripolyphosphate	10–30%
Blue dye	less than 1%
Fluorescent dye	less than 1%
Germicide	0.5–2%
2. Liquid type:	Toxicity rating 2
Blue dye (aniline blue)	1–2%
Water	98–99%
3. Ball, block or cube bluing:	Toxicity rating 2
Ultramarine blue	40–50%
Sodium bicarbonate	30–40%
Glucose	10–30%

May contain:
  Acetic acid
  Corn syrup
  Dextrin
  If oxalic acid* or borax* toxicity
    rating 3
  Prussian blue
  Soap

LAUNDRY RINSES

1. Fabric rinse and softener	Toxicity rating 2
Dialkyl (C_{16}–C_{18}) dimethyl ammonium compounds	2–8%
Isopropanol	1–2%
Water	90–93%

May contain:
  Sulfonated fatty acid amides
  Optical bleaching agent
  Dye
  Nonionic surfactants (alkyl phenyl
    polyethoxyethanol, polyoxyethylene ether)

2. Fabric rinse and softener	Toxicity rating 2
Dialkyl (C_{16}–C_{18}) dimethyl ammonium compounds	2–4%
Methyl (C_{16}–C_{18}) alkylamidoethyl (C_{16}–C_{18}) alkyl imidazolinium compounds	2–4%
Isopropanol	1–2%
Water	89–92%

May contain:
  Nonionic surfactants (nonylphenyl
    polyethylene glycol ether, poly-
    ethylene glycol ether of a linear
    alcohol)
  Opacifier (polystyrene latex)

LAUNDRY RINSES (Cont.)

Dye
Perfume

3. Laundry rinsing aid	Toxicity rating 2
Nonionic surfactant	2%
Sodium carboxymethylcellulose	9%
Water	

LAUNDRY STARCH

1. Liquid:	Toxicity rating 2
Corn starch	7–10%
Sodium carboxymethyl cellulose	2–3%
Sodium chloride	3–4%
Borax	0–2%
Formaldehyde	0–0.2%
Phenolic preservatives	0–0.3%
Water	to 100%

May contain:
  Bluing
  Dye
  Emulsifying agents
  p-Methylbenzoic acid
  Perfume
  Phenyl mercuric acetate
  Sodium hexameta phosphate
  Sodium tripolyphosphate
  Sulfated and sulfonated oils
  Terpineol
  Tricresyl phosphate
  Wheat flour

2. Powder:	Toxicity rating 2
Corn starch	0–95%
Borax	2%
Vinyl acetate copolymer resin	0–20%
o-Phenylphenol, sodium salt	0.1%
Pentachlorophenol, sodium salt	0.1%
Wax	

3. Spray:
  Corn starch
  Silicone
  Propellant

LAXATIVES (see NONPRESCRIPTION DRUGS)

LINIMENTS (see NONPRESCRIPTION DRUGS)

LUBRICANTS

CONVEYER LUBRICANT	Toxicity rating 3

1. Soap (may be liquid)
  Versene* (see EDTA)
2. Alkanolamides

GEAR LUBRICANTS (see OILS, this section)

GRAPHITE LUBRICANTS	Toxicity rating 1
Carbon	70–98%
Inert ingredients	5–30%
Silica	0–0.5%
Alumina	trace

May contain:
  Iron oxide

GRAPHITE LUBRICANTS, LIQUID	Toxicity rating 3

Graphite
Blended oils* (see Kerosene)

GREASES	Toxicity rating 2

Petroleum oils
Soap (Na, Li, Ca, Al, Ba)
May contain:
  Borax

Starred ingredients (*) may be responsible for major toxic effects; consult Section II.

LUBRICANTS (Cont.)		LUBRICANTS (Cont.)	

GREASES (Cont.)

    Chromate
    Dye
    Graphite
    Lead compounds
    Molybdenum disulfide
    Talc
    Zinc salt

LUBRICATING PENCILS	Toxicity rating 1
Paraffin wax and oil	
Petrolatum	small amount
Coloring	trace
Mica	
Film strength additives	

PUMP LUBRICANTS	Toxicity rating 2
Emulsifying cutting oil	20–25%
Water	80%
May contain:	
Coupling agents	
Inhibitors	
Petroleum sulfonate	
Soap	

RUBBER LUBRICANTS .... Toxicity rating 2 or 3
1. Isopropyl alcohol*
    Grease
    Wetting agents
    Defoaming agents
    Rust inhibitors
    May contain:
      Potassium soap
      Butylene glycol
2. Potassium vegetable oil
    Ethylene glycol
    Rust inhibitors
    Chelating agent
    Defoaming agent

SILICONE LUBRICANTS	Toxicity rating 3
Lubricating oil* (see Kerosene)	78–80%
Paraffin wax	14–15%
Defoamer	5–6%
Silicone oil	0.4–0.5%

THREAD LUBRICANTS (A.P.I. GREASE)	Toxicity rating 3 or 4
1. Aluminum stearate grease	20.5%
Silicone compound	12.8%
Silicone fluid	2.6%
Graphite	18.0%
Lead*	30.5%
Copper	3.3%
Zinc*	12.3%
2. Colloidal graphite dispersion in aliphatic naphtha	
1. Aliphatic naphtha*	Approx. 60%
2. Oxygenated organic acids*†	Approx. 20%
3. Colloidal graphite dispersion in aliphatic naphtha	
4. Tricresyl phosphate*	
† See Acid, Section II.	

WIRE DRAWING COMPOUNDS .. Toxicity rating 2 or 3
1. Sodium and/or potassium soaps (high titer)
   Strong alkalies in slight excess (trisodium phosphate, sodium metasilicate, etc.)
   Water

WIRE DRAWING COMPOUNDS (Cont.)

2. Sodium and/or potassium soaps, modified with small additions of calcium soaps, aluminum soaps, magnesium soaps
  May contain:
    Water
3. Sodium and/or potassium soaps, with or without calcium, aluminum, magnesium, etc., soaps.
  Pigments (whiting, mica, talc, etc.)
  May contain:
    Water
All these formulas may be modified by the addition of borax,* special synthetic lubricants, oils, etc.

ZIPPER LUBRICANT	Toxicity rating 3
Petroleum wax	
In perchloroethylene base*	
Lubricants may contain:	
Carnauba wax: other waxes	
Lacquer solvents*	
Microcrystalline waxes	
Petroleum oils (naphthenic)	
Pour point depressant (polymeric type)	
Trichloroethylene*	
Varnish	

MATCHES

HEAD	Toxicity rating 2
Glue (animal)	10–12%
Potassium chlorate	40–60%
Sulfur	3–6%
Wood rosin (or synthetic resins)	0–5%
Silica flour (or ground glass)	15–40%
Phosphorus sesquisulfide (strike-anywhere matches only)	1–10%
Coloring dyes	0.05–0.3%
May contain:	
Corn starch	1–3%
Infusorial earth	3–8%
Formaldehyde	negligible
Gums (tragacanth or arabic)	0–2%
Plaster of Paris	0–5%
Potassium dichromate	0.2–0.5%
Pumice	0–5%
Zinc oxide	0–5%

Full book of 20 matches contains about 200 mg. potassium chlorate; 20 kitchen matches contain about 300 mg.

STICK	
Paraffin (crude scale or slack wax)	0.005–0.015 gm./stick
Ammonium phosphate	negligible

STRIKING SURFACE	Toxicity rating 2
Binder (synthetic resins or latex, or a natural gum arabic)	15–40%
Red phosphorus	40–60%
Silica flour (or ground glass)	20–40%
Coloring dyes or pigments	0.1–5%

MILDEW PROOFING

	Toxicity rating 3

1. Water soluble: commonest are lactic acid, salicylic acid* and sodium salts of chlorinated phenols* in

---

Starred ingredients (*) may be responsible for major toxic effects; consult Section II.

MILDEW PROOFING (Cont.)	MILDEW PROOFING (Cont.)

concentrations of 0.25 to 0.75%.
Quaternary ammonium com-
pounds such as dimethyl benzyl
ammonium chloride are used in
concentrations of 2.0 to 3.0%.
An available product for the laundry-
dry cleaning industry, approved
by U.S. Dept. Agriculture, contains up to 19% sodium pentachlorophenate.*

                           Toxicity rating 3–4
2. Solvents* (see Solvents and Thinners,
this section) or oil carrier; chlorinated phenols,* zinc or copper
naphthenates 0 to 8%, salicylanilide* 0 to 1%, 8-hydroxyquinoline
usually at concentrations of 0.5 to
1.0%.
(See Fungicides, under Pesticides)
3. . . . . Toxicity rating 3–4

Aliphatic* (see Kerosene) or aromatic hydrocarbon solvents*	30–75%
Pentachlorophenol	2–6%
Diatomaceous earth	0–25%
Methylene chloride or 1, 1, 1-trichloroethane	0–30%
Methoxychlor	0–2%

May contain:
  Benzoic acid
  Beta-naphthol
  Bismuth benzoate
  Borates*
  Calcium propionate
  Chloronaphthalene*
  Chloroxylenols*
  Chloro-2-phenylphenol*
  Copper oleate
  Copper-8-quinolinolate
  Copper resinate
  m-, *o*-, and *p*-Cresol*
  Cuprammonium* (see Copper)
  Dichlorodimethyl succinate
  2,2′-Dihydroxy-5′,5′-dichlorodi-
    phenyl-methane
  Di-(phenylmercuric)dodecenyl succi-
    nate
  Ethylmercuric phosphate*
  Formaldehyde*
  Hexyl resorcinol
  8-Hydroxyquinoline
  Mercuric benzoate* (see Mercury
    compounds)
  Mercuric chloride*
  Mercuric salicylate (see Mercury
    compounds)
  Mercurophen (see Mercury com-
    pounds)
  2,2′-Methylenebis(4-chlorophenol)
  Monobromobenzene
  p-Nitrophenol*
  Paraformaldehyde
  Phenylmercuric acetate*
  Phenylmercury acetoxy octodeca-
    noic acid* (see Phenylmercury
    salts)
  Phenylmercury oleate* (see Phenyl-
    mercury salts)
  Phenylmercury saccharinate* (see
    Phenylmercury salts)

  o-Phenylphenol
  Phenyl salicylate*
  Sodium silicofluoride* (see Silico-
    fluoride salts)
  Tetrachloroethane*
  Tetrachlorophenol* (see Pentachlo-
    rophenol)
  Tetrabromo-*o*-cresol
  Tribromonaphthol (no data; 4?)
  Trichlorophenol*
  Zinc chloride* (see Zinc salts)
  Zinc dimethyldithiocarbamate*
  Zinc oleate (see Zinc salts)
  Zinc resinate (see Zinc salts)
  Zinc sulfate (see Zinc salts)
4. Powder. U.S. Dept. Agriculture limits
industrial laundry and dry clean-
ing products to 7.5% pentachloro-
phenol*

NONPRESCRIPTION DRUGS

ACNE REMEDIES/ANTIACNE AIDS

1. Cake, stick	Toxicity rating 2
Sulfur	8%
Resorcinol	1%
Salicylic acid	2%
May contain:	
Bentonite	4%
Soapless detergents	
2. Cleanser	Toxicity rating 2
a. Sulfur	4%
Salicylic acid	2%

May contain:
  Aluminum oxide (fine, medium or
    rough)
  Alrosal
  Coconut, castor or pine oils
  Detergents
  Edetate sodium
  Emulsifiers
  Lanolin cholesterols
  Lecithin
  Lubricants

p-Chloro-*m*-xylenol	2%
Petrolatum	
Polyethylene granules	
Polyoxyethylene lauryl ether	3%
b. PVP-I 7.5% (available I 0.75%)	
3. Cream	Toxicity rating 2–3
Sulfur	2–8%
Salicylic acid	0–2%
Resorcinol*	0–2%
May contain:	
Alcohol	10%
Allantoin	
Benzalkonium chloride	0.2%
Camphor*	
Detergents	
Menthol*	
p-Chloro-*m*-xylenol	0.375%
Phenol*	
Polyoxyethylene lauryl ether	6%
Zinc oxide	

Starred ingredients (*) may be responsible for major toxic effects; consult Section II.

ACNE REMEDIES/ANTIACNE ACIDS (Cont.)

4. Foam .... Toxicity rating 2–3
   Soap
   Pumice
   May contain:
      Alcohol 40%
      Benzalkonium chloride 0.2%
      Benzoyl peroxide 5–10%
      Polyoxyethylene lauryl ether 6%
      Surfactant
5. Gel .... Toxicity rating 2–3
   Sulfur 0–5%
   Resorcinol 0–2%
   May contain:
      Alcohol 9–44%
      Allantoin 0.2%
      Benzoyl peroxide 5–10%
      Benzyl alcohol 1%
      Menthol 0.2%
      Mercuric sulfide* 0.5%
      Polyoxyethylene lauryl ether 6%
      Urea
6. Liquids, pads, solutions .... Toxicity rating 3
   Salicylic acid* 0.5–3%
   May contain:
      Boric acid* 2%
      Cetyl alcohol 0.5%
      Citric acid
      Hyamine 10X 0.08%
      Isopropyl alcohol* 70%
      Polysorbate 80
      Sodium alkyl aryl polyether
      Sulfonated alkyl benzenes
7. Lotions .... Toxicity rating 3?
   a. Benzoyl peroxide 5–10%
   b. Sulfur 2–10%
      Resorcinol* 1–4%
      Salicylic acid* 1–2%
   Either may contain:
      Alrosal
      Benzoyl peroxide 5%
      Calcium hydroxide
      Camphor*
      Castor oil
      Chlorohydroxyquinoline 0.25%
      Cholesterols
      Coconut oil
      Coal tar solution 2%
      Colloidal alumina
      Isopropyl alcohol* 30%
      Lanolin
      Lecithin
      Menthol*
      p-Chloro-m-xylenol 0.5%
      Pine oil
      Sodium edetate
      Sodium thiosulfate 8%
      Sulfurated potash
      Thymol 0.5%
      Zinc oxide 10%
      Zinc sulfate 1%

ANALGESICS (EXTERNAL)

1. Analgesic ointment-like products .... Toxicity rating 3–4
   a. Menthol* 1–15%
      Methyl salicylate* 10–22%
   May contain:
      Boric acid* 9%
      Camphor* 3–9%

ANALGESICS (EXTERNAL) (Cont.)

   Capsicum oleoresin 0.5%
   Chloral hydrate 2%
   Eucalyptus oil* 1.5%
   Eugenol*
   Glycol monosalicylate
   Histamine dihydrochloride
   Hydrocarbon waxes
   Lanolin
   Methacholine chloride 0.25%
   Methyl nicotinate 1%
   Mustard oil
   Petrolatum
   Pine oil
   Sorbitan sesquioleate
   Thymol 1%
   Turpentine oil
   Water-soluble base
  b. .... Toxicity rating 2
   Butamben picrate 1%
   Nitromersol 1:5000
  c. .... Toxicity rating 2–3
   Trithamalamine salicylate* 10%
   Greaseless-base
2. Analgesic liquids .... Toxicity rating 3–4
   Methyl salicylate* 2–50%
   Menthol* 0–10%
   Camphor* 0–5%
   May contain:
      Acetone*
      Aspirin* 8%
      Benzocaine 3%
      Capsicum oleoresin 1.8%
      Chloroform* 40%
      Eucalyptus oil* 2%
      Glycerin
      Greaseless emulsion base
      Hard soap 6%
      Histamine dihydrochloride
      Isopropyl alcohol* 64%
      Kerosine*
      Lanolin
      Methyl nicotinate
      Pine oil 0.85%
      Rosemary oil 1%
      Turpentine* 45%
3. Analgesic balms
   See 2 above.
4. Analgesic creams
   See 1 above.
5. Analgesic lotions
   See 2 above.

ANALGESICS (INTERNAL)

1. Analgesic liquids .... Toxicity rating 4
   a. Acetaminophen* .... 120–500 mg./5 cc.
      Alcohol 7–10%
   b. Choline salicylate* .... 870 mg./5 cc.
      (equivalent to 648 mg. aspirin)
2. Analgesic capsules and tablets
   a. .... Toxicity rating 4
      Acetaminophen* .... 5–486 mg.
   May contain:
      Phenyltoloxamine citrate ..... 30 mg.
      Potassium salicylate* .... 325 mg.
   b. .... Toxicity rating 3–4
      Acetaminophen* .... 0–325 mg.
      Aspirin* .... 0–421 mg.

Starred ingredients (*) may be responsible for major toxic effects; consult Section II.

| NONPRESCRIPTION DRUGS (Cont.) | NONPRESCRIPTION DRUGS (Cont.) |

ANALGESICS (INTERNAL) (Cont.)

Caffeine*	0–75 mg.
Phenacetin*	0–162 mg.
Salicylamide*	0–230 mg.

May contain:

Aluminum hydroxide	25 mg.
Calcium carbonate	100 mg.
Magnesium hydroxide	50 mg.
Methapyrilene fumarate* (see Antihistamines)	25 mg.
Milk powder	50 mg.
Phenyltoloxamine dihydrogen citrate	44 mg.

c.	Toxicity rating 4
Aspirin	75–650 mg.

May contain:

Aluminum glycinate	73.5 mg.
Aluminum hydroxide	150 mg.
Citric acid	1055 mg.
Magnesium hydroxide	150 mg.
Magnesium carbonate	140 mg.
Monocalcium phosphate	200 mg.
Orange flavor	
Phenylephrine HCl	1.25 mg.
Salicylsalicylic acid*	486 mg.
Sodium bicarbonate	1900 mg.

3. Analgesic granules and powders	Toxicity rating 3–4
Acetaminophen*	0–195 mg.
Aspirin*	0–648 mg.
Caffeine*	0–33 mg.
Phenacetin*	0–130 mg.
Salicylamine*	0–194 mg.

May contain:

Citric acid	to make 2.8
Sodium bi-	gm.
carbonate	sodium citrate
Potassium chloride	96 mg.
Sodium carbonate	

ANTACIDS

This general listing includes antacid capsules, chewing gum, liquids, powders and tablets. Quantities are per solid dosage unit or 15 cc. liquid.

Consists of one or more of the acid neutralizers:	Toxicity rating 2
Aluminum hydroxide or phosphate	1500 mg.
Calcium carbonate or phosphate	3000 mg.
Dihydroxyaluminum aminoacetate	1500 mg.
Magaldrate	1200 mg.
Magnesium oxide, hydroxide, trisilicate or carbonate	1250 mg.
Sodium bicarbonate	2680 mg.

May also contain:

Alginates	
Amylase, protease	
Aspirin*	325 mg.
Bismuth subcarbonate	600 mg.
Cellulose	0.75 mg.
Charcoal	40 mg.
Chloroform	30 mg.
Citric acid	1055 mg.
Cream and milk powder	500 mg.
Glycine	900 mg.
Mannitol, sorbitol, lactose	
Papain	32.5 mg.
Peppermint and cherry flavorings	
Simethicone	75 mg.

ANTHELMINTICS

1. Tablets	Toxicity rating 3–4
Methylrosaniline chloride* (gentian violet)	9.6 or 25 mg.
2. Capsule (liquid filled)	Toxicity rating 3
Tetrachlorethylene*	0.2 ml., 1 ml., 5 ml.

ANTIBACTERIAL PREPARATIONS, TOPICAL ORAL

1. Liquids	Toxicity rating 3–4

Contains one or more of the following antibacterial agents:

Boric acid*	
Carbamide peroxide	11%
Cetalkonium chloride	870 mg./5 cc.
Cetylpyridinium chloride	
Chloramine-T	5%
Cresol*	
Domiphen bromide	0.005%
Hexylresorcinol	0.1%
Methylbenzethonium chloride	
Monoxychlorosene	(available chlorine) 6%
Phenol*	2%
Potassium chlorate	
Povidone-iodine	0.5%
Zinc chloride	

May contain:

Alcohol
Benzocaine
Benzoin
Camphor*
Cassia oil
Chlorophyll
Choline salicylate
Eucalyptol*
Glycerin
Menthol
Methyl salicylate*
Pine oil
Potassium iodide
Spearmint oil
Sweet birch oil
Tannic acid
Thymol

2. Troches and lozenges	Toxicity rating 2

Contains one or more of the following:

Benzocaine	10 mg.
Cetalkonium chloride	4 mg.
Cetylpyridinium chloride	3 mg.
Hexylresorcinol	2.4 mg.
Meralein sodium	8 mg.
Phenol*	33 mg.
Tyrothricin	2 mg.

May contain:

Ascorbic acid	100 mg.
Benzyl alcohol	4 mg.
Butyl-p-hydroxybenzoate	0.5 mg.
Diperodon · HCl	1 mg.
Ethyl-p-hydroxybenzoate	1.5 mg.
Eucalyptol	
Glycerin	
Menthol	
Methyl salicylate*	
Methyl-p-hydroxybenzoate	3 mg.
Sodium borate	
Thymol	

Starred ingredients (*) may be responsible for major toxic effects; consult Section II.

ANTIBIOTIC OINTMENTS/CREAMS
Toxicity rating 2
Consists of one or more of the antibiotics:
Bacitracin	5000 U
Gramicidin	0.25 mg.
Neomycin	5 mg.
Oxytetracycline	30 mg.
Polymyxin B	10,000 U

ANTIHISTAMINES
As constituent of combination products, see Cold remedies, Sleep aids, Poison ivy and Poison oak remedies.
Tablets (swallow or chew) .... Toxicity rating 2
a. Cyclizine · HCl	50 mg.
b. Dimenhydrinate	50 mg.
c. Meclizine · HCl	50 mg.

ANTIPURITICS (see POISON IVY AND POISON OAK REMEDIES)

ANTISEBORRHEIC PREPARATIONS
1. Shampoo, tar-containing .... Toxicity rating 2–3
Tar as one of the following:
Coal tar	1–2.5%
Fractar-5	8.75%
Juniper tar	1–4%
Tar	equipotent to 5% LCD†

† Liquor carbonis detergens.
2. Povidone-iodine† (0.75% available
iodine)	7.5%
Base available as: shampoo	92.5%

3. Triclosan 0.1–0.2%
Base, available as: shampoo 99.8–99.9%
May contain:
Alcohol	13%
Allantoin	0.2%
Benzalkonium chloride	0.2%

Coconut oil
EDTA sodium
Detergents, highly concentrated
Lanolin, de-waxed, oil-soluble pulverized keratin-moisturizing fraction
p-Chloro-m-xylenol	0.5%
Salicylic acid	0.5–2%

Sulfonated castor oil
Sulfur, micropulverized 2%
Surfactants
Triethanolamine
Water
† See Polyvinylpyrrolidone (Section II).
4. Creams and lotions, tar-containing ... Toxicity rating 2
Tar, cetyl .... coal 4–5%
May contain:
Allantoin	0.2%

Emulsion base
Sulfur, colloidal 3%
5. Creams and lotions, nontar-containing
a. .... Toxicity rating 2
Cetyl trimethyl ammonium bromide	1%
Stearyl dimethyl benzyl ammonium chloride	0.1%

b. .... Toxicity rating 3
Resorcinol monoacetate*	1.5–2%
Alcohol	28–81%

May contain:
Ammonium chloride
Bromide
Castor oil 1.5%

ANTISEBORRHEIC PREPARATIONS (Cont.)
p-Chloro-m-xylenol	<0.5%
Lauryl isoquinolinium	
Salicylic acid	0.5–3%
Sulfur, colloidal	0–5%

c. .... Toxicity rating 2
Salicylic acid*	2%
Sulfur, colloidal	2–5%

May contain:
Alcohol	13–60%
p-Chloro-m-xylenol	0.5%

lauryl ether
d. .... Toxicity rating 2
Anionic surfactants/base	99–99.5%
Zinc pyrithione	0.5–1%

Available as: cream, dressing, lotion, shampoo

ANTITUSSIVES (see COUGH REMEDY MIXTURES)

ASPIRIN PREPARATIONS FOR CHILDREN
1. Liquids and drops .... Toxicity rating 4
a. Acetaminophen*	120–500 mg./5 cc.
Alcohol	7–10%

b. .... Toxicity rating 3
Choline salicylate* .... 105 mg./0.6 cc.
(equivalent to 81 mg. aspirin)
2. Tablets, chewable .... Toxicity rating 3–4
a. Aspirin* .... 75–81 mg.
Flavorings
b. .... Toxicity rating 3–4
Acetaminophen* .... 120 mg.
Flavorings

ATHLETE'S FOOT REMEDIES (See FUNGICIDES)

BLEACHING PREPARATIONS (see HAIR PREPARATIONS)

BURN REMEDIES
Available as aerosol, cream, foam, liquid, lotion, ointment, impregnated pads and soap.
Toxicity rating 3
Contains one or two of the following local anesthetics:
Benzocaine	2–20%
Lidocaine	
Benzyl alcohol	4%
Butamben picrate	1%
Chlorobutanol	0.75%
Dibucaine	1%
Phenol	1%
Pontocaine	1%
Pramoxine · HCl	0.5%
Tetracaine · HCl	0.5%

and one or more of the following antiseptics:
Bacitracin	200 U/gm.
Benzalkonium Cl	0.5%
Benzethonium Cl	0.1–0.5%
Cetyltrimethylammonium Br	
p-Chloro-m-xylenol	
8-Hydroxyquinoline sulfate	0.5%
Methylbenzethonium Cl	0.5%
Neomycin	0.3%
Nitromersol	1:5000
Orthohydroxyphenyl mercuric chloride	0.056%
Oxyquinoline benzoate	0.025%
Parhydracin	
Polymyxin B	4000 U/gm.

Starred ingredients (*) may be responsible for major toxic effects; consult Section II.

NONPRESCRIPTION DRUGS (Cont.)	NONPRESCRIPTION DRUGS (Cont.)

BURN REMEDIES (Cont.)

Povidone-iodine	10%
Triclosan	

May contain:

Acetone*	
Allantoin	
Camphor	
Castor bean	
Cod liver oil	70%
Isopropyl alcohol*	7–46%
Lanolin	
Menthol	
Methyl salicylate*	
Oils of bay	
Salicylic acid*	
Spearmint	
Sulfur	
Thyme	
Thymol	0.5%
Zinc oxide	2%

CALLUS, CORN AND WART REMEDIES

1. Creams and ointments .... Toxicity rating 3–4
   a. Salicylic acid*
      Castor oil
      Triethanolamine
      Methyl salicylate*
      Sodium salicylate*
   b. Pancin (a special formulation of
         calcium pantothenate, ascorbic
         acid and starch)
2. External liquids

a. .... Toxicity rating 3–4	
Salicylic acid*	11–18%
Benzoic acid	
Glacial acetic acid*	2–11%
Pyroxylin	0–7%

May contain:

Acetone	17–75%
Alcohol	1.5–70%
Benzocaine	
Castor oil	3–22%
Camphor	1.3–1.8%
Chlorobutanol	1%
Collodion	2%
Diperodon · HCl	1%
Ether*	32–67%
Ferric chloride tincture	
Menthol	2%
Zinc chloride	1.9–2.7%
b. .... Toxicity rating 4	
Cantharidin*	0.7%
Acetone	
Collodion	
c. .... Toxicity rating 4	
Phenoxyethanoic acid*	
Pyroxylin	
Acetone	
d. .... Toxicity rating 4	
Cresol*	5%
Resorcinol	0.17%
Isoporopyl alcohol	15%
Ether	5%

May contain:
   Acetone
   Anethinex
   Balsam
   Beeswax
   Belladonna

CALLUS, CORN AND WART REMEDIES (Cont.)

Benzocaine
Benzyl alcohol
Boric acid*
Bismuth subcarbonate
Calamine
Camphor*
Chlorabutanol
Castor oil
Collodion
Eugenol
Geraniol
Glacial acetic acid*
Isopropyl alcohol
Lactic acid
Lanolin
Lard
Menthol
Metaphen
Methyl salicylate*
Mineral oil
Oil of cadeberry
Oil of cassia
Oil of eucalyptus
Oil of turpentine
Paraffin
Petrolatum
Phenol*
Pine oil
Procaine
Salol
Trichloroacetic acid*
Zinc chloride*

e. Ammonium salt of sulfated alkyl	
phenopolyglycol ether	5%
Cresol	5%
Isopropyl alcohol	
Resorcinol	0.17%
Base	

3. Medicated pads and plasters ..... Toxicity rating 3–4?	
a. Salicylic acid*	
b. Phenoxyethanoic acid* .... Toxicity rating 4?	

CALLUS REMEDIES (see CALLUS, CORN AND WART
   REMEDIES)

CALLUS REMOVERS (see CALLUS, CORN AND WART
   REMEDIES)

CANKER AND COLD SORE REMEDIES

Liquid or semisolid preparations

1. Benzocaine .... Toxicity rating 2	
2. .... Toxicity rating 3	
Chloroform*	1–30%
3. Phenol* .... Toxicity rating 3–4	

Either may contain:
   Aluminum dehydroxyallantoinate
   Aluminum hydrate
   Benzalkonium chloride
   Benzyl alcohol
   Benzoin
   Camphor
   Chlorothymol
   Eucalyptol
   Ethyl alcohol
   Isopropyl alcohol*
   Lanolin
   Magnesium trisilicate
   Menthol
   Methylbenzethonium chloride

Starred ingredients (*) may be responsible for major toxic effects; consult Section II.

NONPRESCRIPTION DRUGS (Cont.)	NONPRESCRIPTION DRUGS (Cont.)

CANKER AND COLD SORE REMEDIES (Cont.)

Methyl salicylate*
Sodium acid carbonate
Tannic acid
Thymol

CHAFING AND CHAPPING (see ANALGESICS, EXTERNAL)

CHEST RUBS .... Toxicity rating 4
May contain:
Camphor*
Menthol*
Turpentine spirits
Eucalyptus oil*† 16%
Cedar leaf oil*†
Myristica oil
Thymol*
Oleagenous base 84%
† See Essential oils.

CHEWABLE VITAMINS (see CHILDREN'S VITAMINS)

CHILDREN'S VITAMINS
1. Vitamin drops .... Toxicity rating 2
   a. Ascorbic acid .... 100/mg./cc.
      Propylene glycol
   b. Cod liver oil concentrate .... Toxicity rating 2
      Vitamin A .... 1560 U/drop
      (16.5 mg./gm. drops)
      Vitamin D .... 312 U/drop
      (0.27 mg./gm. drops)
   c. Iron preparations .... Toxicity rating 2–3
      Biotin .... 2.5 μg.
      Iron* .... 20 mg.
      Vitamin B-1 (thiamine) .... 10 mg.
      Vitamin B-6 (pyridoxine) .... 2 mg.
      Vitamin B-12 (cyanocobalamin) . 25 μg.
   d. Multiple vitamins (per 1 cc.) .... Toxicity rating 2
      Vitamin A 1500–8000
                                    USP
                                    U (0.45–2.4
                                    mg)
      Vitamin B-1 (thiamine) .... 0.6–1 mg.
      Vitamin B-2 (riboflavin) .... 0.7–1.2 mg.
      Vitamin B-6 (pyridoxine) .... 0.6–2 mg.
      Vitamin C (ascorbic acid) .... 60 mg.
      Vitamin D (calciferol) .... 400–650 USP
                                    U (10–16 μg)
      May contain:
      Fluoride (as NaF) .... 0.5–1.0 mg.
      Iron (as Fe-sulfate) .... 10 mg.
      Niacinamide .... 16 mg.
      Pantothenic acid .... 10 mg.
      Vitamin B-12 (cyanocobalamin) . 5 μg.
      Vitamin E (tocopherol) .... 5 μg.
2. Vitamin capsules and tablets .... Toxicity rating 2–3
   a. Iron supplement
      Ascorbic acid .... 150 mg.
      Iron* (as Fe-fumarate) .... 67 mg.
   b. Cod liver oil concentrate capsules . Toxicity rating 2
      Vitamin A .... 12,000 U
      Vitamin D .... 1250 U
   c. Cod liver oil concentrate tablets ... Toxicity rating 2
      Vitamin A .... 4000 U
      Vitamin D .... 400 U
      Vitamin C .... 0–50 mg.
   d. Multiple vitamin chewable tablets . Toxicity rating 2
      Vitamin A .... 4000 USP U
                                    (1.2 mg.)

CHILDREN'S VITAMINS (Cont.)

Vitamin D (calciferol) .... 400 USP U
                                (10 μg.)
Vitamin E (tocopherol) .... 0–4 IU
Vitamin C (ascorbic acid) ...... 60–100 mg.
Vitamin B-1 (thiamine) .... 0.8–2 mg.
Vitamin B-2 (riboflavin) .... 1–2.5 mg.
Vitamin B-6 (pyridoxine) .... 1–10 mg.
Vitamin B-12 (cyanocobalamine) . 2–5 μg.
Niacinamide .... 10–20 μg.
May contain:
Calcium .... 250 mg.
Fluoride (as 1.1–2.2 mg. NaF) ... 0.5–1 mg.
Iron .... 10–30 mg.
Pantothenic acid .... 2–7 mg.

COLD REMEDIES FOR CHILDREN
1. Liquids (per 5 cc.)
   a. .... Toxicity rating 2?
      Chlorpheniramine maleate .... 2 mg./5 cc.
      May contain:
      Phenylephrine · HCl* .... 25 mg./5 cc.
      Chloroform .... 13.5 mg./5 cc.
      Alcohol 5%
   b. .... Toxicity rating 2
      Phenylpropanolamine HCl* ...... 12.5 mg.
      Dextromethorphan · HBr* ...... 30 mg.
      Chloroform 0.2%
      Alcohol 8%
      Pheniramine maleate* .... 6.25 mg.
      Phenylpropanolamine · HCl* .... 12.5 mg.
      Pyrilamine maleate* .... 6.25 mg.
2. Tablets, chew and swallow .... Toxicity rating 3–4
   Chlorpheniramine maleate .... 0.5–2 mg.
   May contain:
   Ascorbic acid .... 30 mg.
   Aspirin* .... 80 mg.
   Methapyrilene fumarate .... 2.5 mg.
   Phenylephrine · HCl* .... 2.5 mg.
   Phenylpropanolamine · HCl* .... 12.5 mg.
   Salicylamide* .... 80 mg.

COLD REMEDIES
Capsules, liquids (per 5 cc.), tablets, and time-release units
                                Toxicity rating 4
Contains one of the sympathomimetics:
Ephedrine sulfate* .... 10 mg.
Phenylephrine · HCl .... 2.5–20 mg.
Phenylpropanolamine · HCl .... 10–50 mg.
                                Toxicity rating 3–4
and one or two of the antihistamines:*
Chlorpheniramine maleate .... 1–4 mg.
Methapyrilene fumarate .... 5–10 mg.
Methapyrilene · HCl .... 9 mg.
Phenindamine tartrate .... 10 mg.
Pheniramine maleate .... 6.25–12.5 mg.
Phenyltoloxamine citrate .... 6.25–25 mg.
Pyrilamine maleate .... 15 mg.
Thenyldiamine · HCl .... 7.5 mg.
Thonzylamine · HCl .... 6.25 mg.
May contain:
Acetaminophen* .... 120–325 mg.
Alcohol 8%
Aluminum hydroxide .... 65 mg.
Ascorbic acid .... 30–200 mg.
Aspirin* .... 390 mg.
Atropine sulfate*
Belladonna alkaloids .... 0.2 mg.
Caffeine .... 15–33 mg.

Starred ingredients (*) may be responsible for major toxic effects; consult Section II.

NONPRESCRIPTION DRUGS (Cont.)

COLD REMEDIES (Cont.)

Calcium ascorbate	38 mg.
Chloretone	0.5%
Chloroform	14 mg.
Dextromethorphan · HBr*	30 mg.
Glyceryl guaiacolate	13 mg.
Magnesium hydroxide	125 mg.
Phenacetin*	160 mg.
Salicylamide*	200–365 mg.
Yellow phenolphthalein	15 mg.

COLD SORE AIDS (see CANKER AND COLD SORE REMEDIES

CONSTIPATION AIDS (see LAXATIVES)

CONTACT LENS PRODUCTS .... Toxicity rating 2
1. Cleaning solution
   May contain:

Benzalkonium chloride	0.02%
EDTA	0.1%
nonionic detergent Thimerosal	0.001%

2. Soaking solution

Benzalkonium chloride	0.005–0.01%

   May contain:

Benzethonium chloride	4%
Buffers	
Chlorobutanol	0.4%
EDTA	0.25%
Phenylmercuric nitrate	0.004%
Thimerosal	0.8%

3. Wetting solution

Benzalkonium chloride	0.004–0.01%

   May contain:

Buffers	
Chlorobutanol	0.5%
EDTA	0.02–0.1%
Phenylmercuric nitrate	0.013%
Thimerosal	0.004%

CORN REMEDIES (see CALLUS, CORN AND WART REMEDIES)

CORN REMOVERS (see CALLUS, CORN AND WART REMEDIES)

COUGH DROPS .... Toxicity rating 2

Dextromethorphan	7.5 mg.

   May contain:

Benzocaine	5 mg.
Benzyl alcohol	0.5%
Glyceryl guaiacolate	50 mg.
Honey flavor	
Menthol	
Anethole	0.39%
Peppermint oil	

COUGH EXPECTORANTS (see COUGH REMEDY MIXTURES)

COUGH REMEDY MIXTURES
Contains (quantities per 5 cc. or tablet)

one of the antitussives:	Toxicity rating 3
Codeine phosphate*	15 mg.
Dextromethorphan · HBr*	30 mg.
Noscapine	10 mg.

and one or more of the expectorants:

Ammonium chloride	200 mg.
Chloroform	30 mg.
Glyceryl guaiacolate	100 mg.
Sodium citrate	100 mg.
Terpin hydrate*	180 mg.

NONPRESCRIPTION DRUGS (Cont.)

COUGH REMEDY MIXTURES (Cont.)

May contain one of the sympathomimetics:	Toxicity rating 3–4
Ephedrine · HCl*	8–30 mg.
Methoxyphenamine	17 mg.
Phenylephrine · HCl	10 mg.
Phenylpropanolamine · HCl	17.5 mg.
May contain one of the antihistamines:*	Toxicity rating 3–4
Chlorpheniramine maleate	2 mg.
Doxylamine succinate	7.5 mg.
Methapyrilene fumarate	81 mg.
Pheniramine maleate	10 mg.
Phenyltoloxamine citrate	12.5 mg.
Pyrilamine maleate	4–13 mg.
Thenyldiamine · HCl	4 mg.

May contain:

Acetaminophen	120 mg.
Alcohol	25%
Antimony potassium tartrate	1 mg.
Benzocaine	3 mg.
Creosote	0.2 mg.
Eriodictyon	172 mg.
Ipecac	
Menthol	
Thymol	

COUGH SYRUPS FOR CHILDREN .. Toxicity rating 2–3

Dextromethorphan*	2.5–7.5 mg.

May contain one of the sympathomimetics:

Phenylephrine · HCl*	2.5 mg.
Phenylpropanolamine · HCl*	12.5 mg.

May contain one or two of the antihistamines:

Chlorpheniramine maleate*	1 mg.
Pheniramine maleate*	6.25 mg.
Pyrilamine maleate*	6.25 mg.

May contain one or more of the expectorants:

Ammonium chloride	32–84 mg.
Bark	
Chloroform	0.25%
Euphorbia	
Extracts cocillana	
Glyceryl guaiacolate	100 mg.
Ipecac	0.1 mg.
Menthol	
Potassium guaiacolsulfonate	
Senega root	
Sodium citrate	100 mg.
Terpin hydrate	
White squill*	
Wild cherry	
Wild lettuce leaves	

May contain:

Alcohol	5%
Ascorbic acid	20 mg.
Benzocaine	2 mg.
Sodium salicylate*	108 mg.

DANDRUFF REMOVERS (see Shampoos, Dandruff, under COSMETICS, HAIR PREPARATIONS)

DANDRUFF SHAMPOOS (see Shampoos, Dandruff, under COSMETICS, HAIR PREPARATIONS)

DECONGESTANTS
1. Tablets   Toxicity rating 4

a. Phenyl propanolamine*	50 mg.
b. Pseudoephedrine · HCl*	30 mg.†

Starred ingredients (*) may be responsible for major toxic effects; consult Section II.

NONPRESCRIPTION DRUGS (Cont.)

NONPRESCRIPTION DRUGS (Cont.)

DECONGESTANTS (Cont.)

2. Liquids .... Toxicity rating 4
 Pseudoephedrine · HCl* .... 30 mg.†
 † See Ephedrine.
3. Combination liquids, capsules and tablets
 See Sympathomimetic amines under cold remedies
4. Inhalants, nasal sprays and nose drops
 See under individual headings.

DENTRIFICES

1. Liquid dentrifices .... Toxicity rating 2
 Sodium alginate 0.8%
 Saccharin sodium 0.1%
 Flavor 1.5%
 Alcohol 20.0%
 Glycerin 8.0%
 Sodium lauryl sulfate 4.0%
 Amaranth solution (5%) 0.2%
 Water, q.s. 100.0%
2. Gel .... Toxicity rating 2–3
 Humectant (e.g., sorbitol) 60–75%
 Abradant (e.g., silica) 15–20%
 Surfactant
 Color
 Flavor
 Fluoride* 0.5–1.23%
3. Paste and liquid .... Toxicity rating 2
 Abradant (e.g., silica) 25–50%
 Humectants 30–40%
 Binder (gum) 1–5%
 Flavor 0.5–5%
 Color .... >0.1%
 Anionic surfactant 1–5%
 Water 10–50%
4. Tooth paste .... Toxicity rating 1
 Dicalcium phosphate 40.0%
 Sodium lauryl sulfate 1.5%
 Glycerol 20.0%
 Gum tragacanth 1.5%
 Saccharin 0.1%
 Fluoride 0.1%
  (as sodium fluoride or monofluoro phosphate)
 Flavor oils 0.9%
 Water 36.0%
5. Tooth powder .... Toxicity rating 1
 Dicalcium phosphate 15–20%
 Sodium metaphosphate
  (insoluble) 70–75%
 Sodium lauryl sulfoacetate 2.0%
 Saccharin 0.2%
 Flavor oils 1.8%
 Dentifrices may contain:
  Aluminum hydrate
  Ammonium phosphate, dibasic
  Calcium carbonate
  Calcium pyrophosphate
  Calcium sulfate
  Chlorophyllin (copper derivative)
  Chlorothymol
  Dioctyl sodium sulfosuccinate
  Eucalyptol
  Gum karaya
  Hexachlorophene
  p-Hydroxybenzoate
  Irish moss
  Magnesium carbonate

DENTRIFICES (Cont.)

 Magnesium oxide
 Magnesium phosphate (tri-)
 Menthol
 Methylcellulose
 Oil of anise
 Oil of caraway
 Oil of cinnamon
 Oil of cloves
 Oil of eucalyptus
 Oil of peppermint
 Oil of spearmint
 Oil of thyme
 Oil of wintergreen (methyl salicylate)
 Potassium chlorate
 Soap, neutral
 Sodium alginate
 Sodium benzoate
 Sodium bicarbonate
 Sodium carboxymethylcellulose
 Sodium fluoride (0.1% as fluoride)
 Sodium N-lauroyl sarcosinate
 Sodium monofluorophosphate
  (0.1% as fluoride)
 Sorbitol
 Stannous fluoride (0.1% as fluoride)
 Thymol
 Urea (carbamide)

DENTURE ADHESIVES

1. Dental adhesive powders
 a. Karaya-based formula .... Toxicity rating 1
  Gum karaya 99–100%
  Flavor (peppermint, spearmint, wintergreen) 0–1%
 b. Karaya borax formula .... Toxicity rating 3
  Gum karaya 90–99%
  Sodium borate* 1–10%
  Flavor 0–1%
The following may be used to neutralize karaya gum:
 Magnesium hydroxide (or oxide)
 c. .... Toxicity rating 1
  Pectin 2–20%
  Gelatin 5–20%
  Carboxymethyl cellulose 30–70%
  Flavor 0–1%
 d. .... Toxicity rating 1
  Carboxymethyl cellulose 30–70%
  Hydroxyethylcellulose 30–70%
  Flavor 0–1%
2. Denture adhesive creams .... Toxicity rating 1
 a. Gum karaya 30–60%
  Petrolatum 40–70%
  Flavor 0–1%
 b. Gum karaya 30–60%
  Petrolatum 40–70%
  Benzocaine 1–5%
  Hydrocortisone 0–1%
  Flavor 0–1%
 c. Pectin 2.5–10%
  Gelatin 2.5–10%
  Carboxymethyl cellulose 30–45%
  Polyethylene-gelled mineral oil ... 30–60%
  Flavor 0–1%

Starred ingredients (*) may be responsible for major toxic effects; consult Section II.

DENTURE ADHESIVES (Cont.)

d. Calcium-sodium salt of poly (vinyl
methyl ether-maleate)
copolymer .... ?
or
Polyethylene oxide, high molecular
weight 5–10%
Petrolatum 40–70%
Flavor 0–1%
May also contain:
Magnesium oxide
Magensium carbonate
Gum acacia
Gum tragacanth

DEPILATORIES

1. Powder .... Toxicity rating 4
    Barium sulfide*
    Calcium hydroxide
    Base
2. Cream, lotion .... Toxicity rating 2
    Calcium carbonate, light 0–21%
    Calcium hydroxide 0–1.5%
    Calcium thioglycolate trihydrate ... 2.2–6%
    Cetyl alcohol, flakes 0–4.5%
    Perfume 0–0.5%
    Sodium lauryl sulfate 0–0.5%
    Sodium silicate solution 0–3.5%
    Distilled or deionized water *q.s.* 100%
3. Aerosol
    Same as cream and lotion with addi-
    tion of propellant.

DIAPER RASH, AND PRICKLY HEAT REMEDIES

1. Creams, ointments and pastes .... Toxicity rating 2
    a. Aluminum acetate, buffered ..... Toxicity rating 2
    b. Vitamin A .... 850 U/gm.
       Vitamin D .... 85 U/gm.
    c. .... Toxicity rating 2
       Bacitracin .... 200 U/gm.
       Neomycin .... 3 mg.
       Polymyxin B .... 4000 U
       Benzalkonium chloride .... 5 mg.
    d. .... Toxicity rating 2–3
       Salicylic acid* 2%
    e. .... Toxicity rating 2
       Undecylenate 15%
    f. .... Toxicity rating 2
       Zinc oxide 15–25%
       Benzethonium chloride 0.1%
All may contain:
    Allantoin
    Amino acids
    Balsam of Peru
    Benzoin
    Boric acid* 5%
    Calamine 3%
    Cetyl alcohol
    Diperodon-HCl 1%
    Methylphenylpolysiloxane
    Parabens
    Phenol
    Zinc oxide 25%
Base materials contain:
    Beeswax
    Glycerin
    Lanolin
    Liquid petrolatum
    Paraffin

DIAPER RASH, AND PRICKLY HEAT REMEDIES (Cont.)

Silicone
    Starch 25%
    Talc
    White petrolatum 50%
    Wool fat
    Zinc oxide paste 98%
2. Lotion
    a. Aluminum acetate .... Toxicity rating 2?
    b. Benzalkonium chloride* ..... Toxicity rating 2–3?
    Either may contain:
       Allantoin
       Balsam of Peru
       Cetyl alcohol
       Lanolin
       Methylbenzethonium chloride 1:1500
       Methylphenylpolysiloxane
       Mineral oil
       Refined sterols
       Silicone
3. Powder
    a. Benzalkonium chloride* .... Toxicity rating 2–3
    b. Methylbenzethonium chloride ...... Toxicity rating 2
                                            1:1800
    c. Oatmeal derivatives .... Toxicity rating 1
    d. .... Toxicity rating 1
       Povidone 2%
    e. .... Toxicity rating 2
       Undecylenate 15%
    f. .... Toxicity rating 2?
       Zinc oxide
       Talc
       Starch
All may contain:
    Aromatic oils
    Balsam of Peru
    Boric acid* .... <4.4%
    Colloidal soya complex
    Corn starch
    Diaphen
    Edetate disodium
    Menthol
    Orthophenylphenol
    Phenol .... <0.25%
    Salicylic acid 0.5%
    Talc
    Triclosane 0.1%

DIARRHEA REMEDIES

1. Capsules, granules and tablets
    a. .... Toxicity rating 1
       Activated wood charcoal .... 324 mg.
    b. .... Toxicity rating 2–3
       Lactobacillus acidophilus .... 2×10^9 organ-
                                            isms
    Either may contain:
       Bismuth .... 324 mg.
       Carboxycellulose .... 100 mg.
       Lactobacillus bulgaricus
       Opium* .... 3.24 mg.
2. Liquids and suspensions (per 30 cc.) .. Toxicity rating 1
    a. Kaolin .... 0–12 gm
                                    (average
                                    5–6 gm:)
       Pectin .... 0–600 mg.
                                    (average
                                    150 mg.)
    May contain:
       Alcohol 10%

Starred ingredients (*) may be responsible for major toxic effects; consult Section II.

DIARRHEA REMEDIES (Cont.)

Alumina gel
Atropine sulfate .... 0.0194 mg.
Bismuth subgallate .... 300 mg.
Bismuth subsalicylate* .... 525 mg.
Carboxymethyl cellulose
Codeine phosphate* .... 32.4 mg.
Eucalyptus oil
Homatropine methylbromide ... 0.9 mg.
Hyoscine-HBr .... 0.0065 mg.
Hyoscyamine sulfate .... 0.1037 mg.
Menthol
Methyl salicylate
Opium* .... 24 mg.
Paregoric .... 4.5 ml.
Salol .... 105 mg.
Sodium benzoate .... 60 mg.
Zinc phenolsulfonate .... 53 mg.
b. Activated attapulgite .... 300 mg.
Colloidal attapulgite .... 900 mg.

ECZEMA AND PSORIASIS REMEDIES
1. Emollient preparations .... Toxicity rating 2
Includes cake, cream, liquid, lotion,
   ointment, powder and spray
May contain one or more of the fol-
   lowing:
Aliphatic alcohol
Aluminum sulfate
Calcium acetate
Cetyl alcohol
p-Chloro-m-xylenol 0.5%
Cholesterol
Colloidal oatmeal
Corn dextran
Glycerin
Isopropyl myristate
Isopropyl palmitate
Isopropyl sebacate
Lanolin, dewaxed oil-soluble keratin
   moisturizing fraction
Lecithin phospholipids
Menthol
Mineral oil
Nonionic emulsifier
Olive oil
Polyether alcohols
Polyethylene glycol 400 dioleate
Sodium lauryl sulfoacetate
Sorbitol
Triethanolamine stearate
Vegetable oil, polyunsaturated
2. Preparations containing therapeutic
   agents
a. Bar .... Toxicity rating 2
  (a) Juniper, pine and coal tars ... 1%
  (b) Vegetable oils and dewaxed
       lanolin 25%
     Colloidal oatmeal 22%
b. Bath oil .... Toxicity rating 2-3
Tar distillates* 25-33%
c. Cream .... Toxicity rating 2-3
  (a) Allantoin 2%
     Coal tar extract* 5%
  (b) Coal tar solution* 5.8%
  (c) Vitamin A 200,000 U/33
                  cc.

ECZEMA PSORIASIS REMEDIES (Cont.)

Dexpanthenol 2%
(d) Urea 20%
    Nonlipid base
(e) Iodochlorhydroxyquin 3%
    Acid mantle (aluminum ace-
      tate) in cream base
(f) Methapyrilene-HCl 2%
    Benzocaine 3%
d. Gel .... Toxicity rating 3
Camphor*
Menthol*
Benzyl alcohol 9%
Isopropyl alcohol* 30%
e. Liquids .... Toxicity rating 3
  (a) crude coal tar 2.5%
  (b) coal tar* 18-25%
Either may contain:
  Isopropyl myristate
  Lanolin, keratin-moisturizing frac-
    tion
  Mineral oil
  Nonionic surfactant 10%
  Salicylic acid* 3%
f. Lotions .... Toxicity rating 2-3
  (a) Tar distillate* 5%
    May contain:
     Allantoin 2%
     Zinc oxide
     Talc
     Hydrophilic base
  (b) Phenol 1%
  (c) Phenyltoloxamine citrate 1%
  (d) Benzocaine 2%
  (e) Dexpanthenol 2%
    (b), (c), (d) and (e) may contain
    Calamine .... 2 gm./30 cc.
    Cresol 0.75%
    Glycerin
    Menthol 0.1%
    Mercury* 0.45%
    Zinc oxide .... 2 gm./30 cc.
g. Ointment, tar containing
  (a) Crude coal tar 2.88%
    Starch 53.75%
  (b) Ichthammol 1.54%
    Ext. hamamelis 0.25%
    Either may contain:
    Ammoniated mercury 21.6 mg./30
                gm.
    Benzoic acid
    Resorcinal
    Salicylic acid* 3%
    Sodium borate 0.1%
    Sodium stearate
    Starch
    Sulfur 4%
    Zinc oxide 15.17%
h. Ointment, nontar containing
  (a) Zinc bacitracin .... 400 U/gm.
    Neomycin .... 3 mg./gm.
    Polymyxin B .... 8000 U/gm.
  (b) Phenol .... <1%
    Salicylic acid 1%
  (c) Dimethisoquin HCl 0.5%
  (d) Iodochlorhydroxyquin 3%

EYE DROPS (see OPHTHALMIC PRODUCTS)

EYE WASHES (see OPHTHALMIC PRODUCTS)

Starred ingredients (*) may be responsible for major toxic effects; consult Section II.

NONPRESCRIPTION DRUGS (Cont.)   NONPRESCRIPTION DRUGS (Cont.)

FOOT OINTMENTS (see FUNGICIDES)

FOOT POWDERS (see FUNGICIDES)

FOOT SPRAYS (see FUNGICIDES)

FUNGICIDES
1. .... Toxicity rating 3
    Copper undecylenate 0-.5%
    Undecylenic acid 2-5%
    Zinc undecylenate* 0-20%
    Available as:
      a. Cream with 77.5% base
      b. Foam with 34.65% base
      c. Gel with 95% base
      d. Ointment with 75% base
      e. Powder with 78% base
    Foam (aerosol) also contains:
      Ethyl alcohol 60%
      Menthol 0.25%
      Methylbenzethonium chloride .. 0.1%
2. .... Toxicity rating 2
    Bismuth crystal violet 0.5-1%
    Available as:
      a. Liquid with 81-89.5% base
      b. Ointment with 99% base
    May contain:
      Alcohol .... up to 70%
      Benzoic acid .... up to 6%
      Glycerin .... up to 10%
      Salicylic acid* .... up to 5%
3. .... Toxicity rating 1
    Glyceryl triacetate 25-33.3%
    Available as:
      a. Cream with 75% base
      b. Liquid with 70% base
      c. Powder with 66.7% base
      d. Spray with 75% base/propel-
        lants
4. .... Toxicity rating 4
    Boric acid* 5-15%
    Hydroxyquinoline sulfate 0.5%
    Base 84.5%
    Available as:
      Powder
5. .... Toxicity rating 3
    Camphor* 4-10%
    Phenol* 2-4.5%
    Available as:
      a. Liquid with 85.5-88% base
      b. Powder with 94% base
6. .... Toxicity rating 3-4
    Benzoic acid 1-5%
    Boric acid* 0-15%
    Salicylic acid* 1-3%
    Thymol 0-1%
    Available as:
      a. Ointment with 76-97.9% base
      b. Powder with 80-92% base
      c. Spray with 80-92% base
7. .... Toxicity rating 2
    Alcohol 36-50%
    Benzethonium 0.5%
    Available as:
      Spray with 50-63% base/propel-
        lant
    May contain
      Salicylanilide 2.5%
8. .... Toxicity rating 2
    Caprylic acid 0.2%
    Caprylate salts of sodium/zinc 0-10%

FUNGICIDES (Cont.)

    Propionic acid 0-3%
    Propionate salts of sodium/zinc 0-12.3%
    Salicylic acid* 0-3%
    Available as:
      a. Cream with 91-92% base
      b. Liquid with 77.7% base
      c. Ointment with 72.7% base
      d. Powder with 81% base
    All may contain:
      Castor oil
      Cholesterol 1%
      Liquid petrolatum
      Polyethylene glycol distearate
      Resorcinol 5%
      Synthetic glyceride wax
      Turpentine
9. Shampoo
    a. .... Toxicity rating 3
      Coal tar extract* 5%
    b. .... Toxicity rating 3
      Liquid carbonis detergens
        (LCD)* 10%
    c. .... Toxicity rating 2-3
      Tar distillate* 3%
10. Solution ....Toxicity rating 4?
    Coal tar solution* 100%

HAYFEVER REMEDIES (see COLD REMEDIES)

HEADACHE REMEDIES (see ANALGESICS (INTER-
    NAL))

HEMORRHOIDAL PREPARATIONS
These products contain one or more of the
    following:
    Anesthetic
      Benzocaine 0-20%
      Dibucaine 0-1%
      Diperodon 0-1%
      Pontocaine 0-1%
      Pramoxine 0-1%
2. Antiseptic .... Toxicity rating 3-4
    Benzalkonium chloride 0-0.1%
    Boric acid* 0-20%
    Cetylpyridinium chloride 0-0.5%
    Menthol 0-0.5%
    Methylparaben 0-2%
    Oxyquinolone benzoate 0-0.1%
    Oxyquinolone sulfate 0-0.3%
    Phenol 0-0.1%
    Phenylmercuric nitrate 0-0.1%
3. Astringent .... Toxicity rating 2
    Bismuth carbonate 0-2%
    Bismuth subgallate 0-2.5%
    Hamamelis water 0-70%
    Witch hazel 0-50%
    Zinc oxide 0-10%
4. Emollient and/or lubricant ...... Toxicity rating 1-2
    Cocoa butter
    Cod liver oil 0-0.1%
    Glycerine 0-10%
    Lanolin
    Petrolatum
    Shark liver oil 0-3%
    Water soluble-lanolin derivatives ... 0-20%
    All may contain:
      Acetone sodium bisulfate 0-0.5%
      Alcohol 0-70%

Starred ingredients (*) may be responsible for major toxic effects; consult Section II.

HEMORRHOIDAL PREPARATIONS (Cont.)

Allantoin	0–0.3%
Balsam of Peru	0–1.8%
Benzyl benzoate	0–1.2%
Dexapanthenol	0–2%
Ephedrine sulfate	0–0.2%
Extract belladonna*	
Methyl paraben	
Soya bean oil	

Available as:
   Cleansing tissues, creams, foam, liquid, ointment, pads, rectal cleanser, suppositories.

INHALANTS, STEAM

Toxicity rating 3

Each teaspoonful (5 cc.) contains:

Camphor*	20–310 mg.
Methyl salicylate*	0–75 mg.

Inhalers may contain:

2-Aminoheptane	325 mg.
Aromatics	
Bornyl acetate	150 mg.
Camphor	150 mg.
p-Desoxyephedrine	250 mg.
Menthol	150 mg.
Methylhexaneamine	250 mg.
Methyl salicylate	150 mg.
Propylhexedrine*	250 mg.

A single inhaler probably contains less than 1% of a lethal dose of any ingredient.

INSECT REPELLENTS

Toxicity rating 3

Butopyronoxyl	0–2%
Diethyltoluamide	2.85–47.5%
Dimethyl phthalate	0–1.25%
Ethohexadiol	0–80%
m-Homomenthyl salicylate	0–5.1%
Other isomers	0–8.5%
Di-n-propyl isocinchomeronate N-Octyl bicycloheptene dicarboximide	
Base	20–86%

Available as:
   Aerosol, cream, foam, liquid, lotion, stick.

INSECTICIDES

Toxicity rating 3

1.
N-Octyl bicycloheptene dicarboximide	0–1.67%
Petroleum distillate*	0–99.28%
Pyrethrins	0.075%–0.5%
Technical piperonyl butoxide	0–2%
Base	0–99.8%

Available as:
   Aerosol, liquid and powder.

2. Toxicity rating 3
DDVP	0–0.186%
O-Isopropoxyphenyl methylcarbamate	0.5–0.665%
Petroleum distillates*	83–89.6%
Base propellents	10–15%

Available as:
   Aerosol, liquid

3. Toxicity rating 3–4?
DDVP*	0.5–18.6%
Related compounds	0–1.4%
Base	80–99.5%

Available as:
   Granules and strip

4. Toxicity rating 2

INSECTICIDES (Cont.)

Carbaryl	0.5%
Dichlorophen	0.4%
Malathion	0.25%
2,3,4,5-Bis(2-butylene)tetrahydro-2-furaldehyde	98.6%
Base	

Available as:
   Aerosol

5. Toxicity rating 2
Technical chlordane	2%
Base	98%

Available as:
   Liquid

LAXATIVES

1. Bulk producing laxatives .... Toxicity rating 1–2
   Sodium carboxymethyl cellulose
   Methylcellulose
   Plantago loeflingii
   Irish moss concentrate
   Prune powder
   Agar
   Plantago hemicellulose
   Psyllium muciloid
   Plantago ovata
   Gum karaya
   Pectin
   Sterculia gum
   Acacia gum
   Calcium alginate, sodium alginate

2. Emollient laxatives .... Toxicity rating 1
   Petrolatum liquid (mineral oil)

3. Enema, suppository .... Toxicity rating 2
Bisacodyl	10 mg./suppository
Dioctyl sodium sulfosuccinate	0–5%
Glycerin	0–76%
Mineral oil	0–130 mg.
Sodium diphosphate	0–17.8%
Sodium phosphate*?	0–48%

4. Fecal softeners .... Toxicity rating 2–3
   Dioctyl sodium sulfosuccinate*
   Calcium dioctylsulfosuccinate*
   Dioctyl potassium sulfosuccinate*
   Polyoxyalkol (oxyethylene oxypropylene polymer (propethylene oxides)

5. Irritant or stimulant laxatives .... Toxicity rating 2–3
   Cascara sagrada, extract, fluid-extract,
   Danthron, NF
   Cassia acutifolia extract (senna)
   Sennosides A + B
   Isatin
   Bisacodyl
   Aloes*
   Aloin*
   Castor oil
   Casanthrol
   Oxyphenisatin
   Di(acetylhydroxyphenyl)isatin
   May contain:
   Calomel
   Frangula
   Jalap
   Podophyllum
   Rhubarb

6. Saline laxatives .... Toxicity rating 2
   Magnesium sulfate, Epsom salts

Starred ingredients (*) may be responsible for major toxic effects; consult Section II.

NONPRESCRIPTION DRUGS (Cont.)

LAXATIVES (Cont.)

Sodium phosphate	
Sodium biphosphate	
Potassium sulfate	
Milk of magnesia	
7. Simple purgative	Toxicity rating 2
Phenolphthalein in gum, chocolate, pill, emulsion, tablet, wafer	15–142 mg./dose
8. Tablet, capsule	Toxicity rating 2
Calcium dioctyl sulfosuccinate	0–240 mg.
Casanthranol	0–30 mg.
Cascara sagrada extract	0–65%
Danthron	0–75%
Dioctyl sodium sulfosuccinate	0–100 mg.
Sodium carboxymethyl cellulose	0–400%
Yellow phenolphthalein	0–100 mg.

LAXATIVES FOR CHILDREN

Aloes*	Toxicity rating 3–4
Cascara sagrada	42 mg.
Available as a tablet	

LINIMENTS

Most have approximately 50 to 85% ethyl alcohol, occasionally isopropyl or amyl alcohol is used.

1. Chloroform liniment	Toxicity rating 3
CHCl₃*	25–30%
Alcohol	45%
2. Other formulas frequently contain several of the following:	Toxicity rating 4
Camphor*	1.0–2.5%
Oil of wintergreen (methyl salicylate)*	5–35%
Pine oil*	up to 87%
Turpentine*	2–15%
Menthol	1–2%
Oil of eucalyptus (including oil of cajeput and eucalyptol)	1–3%
Oleo resin capsicum	1% or less
Phenols (various)	1% or less
May contain:	
Essential oils* in addition to those mentioned (especially mustard, wormwood, peppermint, pine, cedar, sassafras)	up to 5%
Chloroform* and related compounds (e.g., chloral)*	1–30%
Occasionally iodine, ammonia or acids (mineral and organic)	small amounts usually less than 2%

MULTIPLE VITAMINS (see VITAMINS, CHILDREN)

NASAL DECONGESTANTS (see DECONGESTANTS)

NASAL SPRAYS

NASAL SPRAYS	Toxicity rating 2–3
Methapyrilene hydrochloride	0–0.2%
Naphazoline hydrochloride	0–0.5%
Pheniramine maleate	0–0.125%
Phenylephrine hydrochloride*	0–1%
Phenylpropanolamine hydrochloride*	0–0.75%
Pyrilamine maleate	0–0.125%
May contain:	
Benzalkonium chloride	0.02%
Cetylpyridinium	0.02%
Thimerosal	0.011%

NOSE DROPS

NOSE DROPS	Toxicity rating 2–3
Cyclopentamine·HCl	0–0.1%
Ephedrine lactate*	0–1%
Naphazoline	0–0.05%

NONPRESCRIPTION DRUGS (Cont.)

NOSE DROPS (Cont.)

Phenylephrine sulfate*	
Cyclopentamine	0–0.35%
May contain:	
Camphor	<0.1%
Eucalyptol	<0.1%
Menthol	<0.1%
Methyl salicylate	<0.1%
Thimerosal	<0.1%

OBESITY CONTROL (see WEIGHT CONTROL PREPARATIONS)

OPHTHALMIC OINTMENT

These ointments have a suitable bland base.

1. Mercuric oxide ointment	Toxicity rating 3
Mercuric oxide*	1–2%
Thimerosal (merthiolate)	0.1%
May contain mild anesthetic, e.g.:	
Piperocaine, benzocaine	0.5–5%
Boric acid	5%
2. Cortisone ointments	Toxicity rating 2
Cortisone derivatives	0.5–2.5%
May contain antibiotics, e.g.:	
Neomycin	0.5–3.5%
3. Antibiotics	Toxicity rating 2
Terramycin	0.1%
or Polymixin B	10,000 units
Bacitracin	500 units
Neomycin	0.3%
4. Miscellaneous	Toxicity rating 4
Antihistamics,* e.g.:	
Thenylpyramine (see methapyrilene hydrochloride)	0.5 (for children)–5%

OPHTHALMIC PRODUCTS

1. Artificial tears	Toxicity rating 2
Contains one or more of the viscosity agents:	
Carboxymethyl cellulose	
Gelatin	
Hydroxypropyl methylcellulose	0.5–1%
Methylcellulose	0.45–0.5%
Propylvinyl alcohol	1.4%
and one of the following preservatives:	
Benzalkonium chloride	0.004–0.01%
Chlorobutanol	0.1–0.05%
EDTA	0.01–0.05%
May contain:	
Calcium chloride	
Dextrose	
Glycerine	
Parabens	
Polysorbate 80	
Potassium chloride	
Magnesium chloride	
Sodium acetate, borate, chloride, citrate, hydroxide	
2. Decongestant drops	Toxicity rating 2
Contains one of the viscosity agents:	
Hydroxypropyl methylcellulose	0.5%
Methylcellulose	0.45%
Polyvinyl alcohol	1.4%
and one or two of the preservatives:	
Benzalkonium chloride	0.004–0.01%
Chlorobutanol	0.10%
EDTA	0.01–0.1%

Starred ingredients (*) may be responsible for major toxic effects; consult Section II.

NONPRESCRIPTION DRUGS (Cont.)

NONPRESCRIPTION DRUGS (Cont.)

OPHTHALMIC PRODUCTS (Cont.)

Thimerosal	0.001–0.005%
and one or two of the vasoconstrictors:	Toxicity rating 2?
Naphazoline·HCl	0.012%
Phenylephrine·HCl	0.2%
Tetrahydrozoline·HCl	0.05%
Zinc	0.25%

and may contain:
Antipyrine
Barbital*?
Benzethonium
Berberine
Boric acid*?
Camphor
Ephedrine*?
Glycerine
Hydrastine
Electrolytes: potassium or sodium bicarbonate, borate, chloride, carbonate, citrate, sulfate, phosphate.

3. Eye washes	Toxicity rating 2

Contain one of the preservatives:

Benzalkonium chloride	0.006–0.01%
Cetylpyridinium chloride	
Edetate sodium	0.05%
Thimerosal	0.002–0.005%

and one or more of the buffers:
Sodium borate
Sodium carbonate
Sodium biphosphate
Sodium phosphate
and may contain:
Alcohol

Antipyrine	0.4%
Berberine·HCl	
Camphor	
Electrolytes	
Hydrastine·HCl	
Phenylephrine	
Sodium salicylate	0.056%

PEPTIC ULCER REMEDIES (see ANTACIDS)

PERIODIC PAIN REMEDIES (MENSTRUAL) (see ANALGESICS INTERNAL)

POISON IVY AND POISON OAK REMEDIES

1.	Toxicity rating 2
Benzocaine	0–3%
Calamine	0–10%
Camphor	0–1%
Menthol	0–0.7%
Zirconium oxide	0–4%

Available as:
a. Cream with 81–98% base
b. Ointment with 88% base
   May contain:

Benzalkonium·Cl	0.01%
Diphenhydramine·HCl	1%
Pyrilamine maleate	1.5%

c. Spray with 80% base
   May contain:

Zinc oxide	2%
Isopropyl alcohol	9%
d. Lotion, liquid with 50–70% base	Toxicity rating 3

   May contain:

Acetanilide	0.02%
Diperodon·HCl	0.25%

POISON IVY AND POISON OAK REMEDIES (Cont.)

Diphenhydramine·HCl	0.1%
Isopropyl alcohol	0.35%
Methyl paraben	0.08%
Phenyltoloxamine dihydrogen citrate	0.1%
Propyl paraben	0.02%
Pyrilamine maleate*	1.5%
Tannic acid	0.10%
Tripelennamine·HCl	0.1%
2.	Toxicity rating 1?
Tetracaine·HCl	1%
Base	99%

Available as:
Cream

3.	Toxicity rating 1?
Paramoxine	1%
Base	99%

Available as:
Cream or lotion

PRICKLY HEAT REMEDIES (see DIAPER RASH AND PRICKLY HEAT REMEDIES)

PSORIASIS REMEDIES (see ECZEMA AND PSORIASIS REMEDIES)

RASH REMEDIES (see DIAPER RASH AND PRICKLY HEAT REMEDIES)

REDUCING AIDS (see WEIGHT CONTROL PRODUCTS)

RUBEFACIENTS	Toxicity rating 4

These ointments are similar to the liniments but with usually a lanolin or petrolatum base and containing three or more of the following:

Camphor	2%
Oil wintergreen (methyl salicylate)*	15–40%
Turpentine	2–15%
Menthol*	5–15%
Capsicum	less than 1%
Essential oils*	
Oil of eucalyptus (with oil of cajeput and eucalyptol)	1–3%
Phenols (various)	1% or less
May contain various essential oils* other than listed: (Especially pine, sassafras, cloves, mustard, cedar)	2–3%
Croton oil	small amounts

SEBORRHEA REMEDIES (see ANTISEBORRHEIC PREPARATIONS)

SEDATIVES (see SLEEP AIDS)

SINUS REMEDIES (see DECONGESTANTS)

SLEEP AIDS

1. Tablets and capsules	Toxicity rating 3–5?
Methapyrilene*	10–50 mg.
or	
Pyrilamine maleate	6–18 mg.
plus hydrochloride	14–19 mg.
Scopolamine (aminoxide HBr)	0.125–0.450 mg.
b. Methapyrilene*	10–50 mg.
Potassium bromide	195–518 mg.

Either may contain:

Ext. passion flower	22.5 mg.
Niacin	4–5 mg.
Niacinamide	5–60 mg.

Starred ingredients (*) may be responsible for major toxic effects; consult Section II.

NONPRESCRIPTION DRUGS (Cont.)

SLEEP AIDS (Cont.)

Potassium salicylate*	85–195 mg.
Riboflavin	6 mg.
Salicylamide*	200–325 mg.
Thiamine	1–15 mg.

STOMACH DISTRESS AIDS (see ANTACIDS)

STOOL SOFTENERS (see LAXATIVES)

SUNBURN REMEDIES (see BURN REMEDIES)

SUPPOSITORIES

1. Rectal .... Toxicity rating 3–4
   These usually contain zinc oxide .. 2.5–14% (usually 10%)

Bismuth salts (usually subgallate)	2–7%
Catecholamines (usually ephedrine but also epinephrine derivatives)*	0.14–2%
Anesthetics (benzocaine, nupercaine, diperodon)	0.2–6.5%
Balsam	3%
Base:	
Cocoa butter or Carbowax or hydrogenated vegetable oils	to 100%

2. Vaginal suppositories. .... Toxicity rating 2–3
   Popular modern forms are usually compressed tablets made with lactose as a base.
   Prescriptions may contain:
   Gentian violet*
   Hydrocortisone
   Antibiotics
   Chemotherapeutic agents

SWEETENERS (see WEIGHT CONTROL PREPARATIONS)

TEETHING AIDS (see CANKER AND COLD SORE REMEDIES)

THROAT LOZENGES (see ANTIBACTERIAL PREPARATIONS, TOPICAL ORAL)

THROAT TROCHES (see ANTIBACTERIAL PREPARATIONS, TOPICAL ORAL

TOOTHACHE REMEDIES (see CANKER AND COLD SORE REMEDIES)

VAGINAL DOUCHES

1. Vaginal douches, liquid .... Toxicity rating 2–3?
   a.

Lactose	0–>50%
Essential oil (fragrance)	1–5%
Phenol	<0.1%
Menthol	<0.1%
Water	0–>50%
May contain	
Acetone	up to 10%
Alcohol	up to 50%
Alum	1–5%
Peroxyhydrate	
Phenyl mercuric acetate	0.2%
Sodium borate	
Sodium chloride	
Soap	

   b. Povidone-iodine†
   † See Polyvinylpyrrolidone (Section II).
2. Vaginal douches, powdered
   These douches may be divided in several classes: those that contain boric acid and/or anionic detergents in generous amounts; those that are relatively benign; and those that contain metallic disinfectants.

NONPRESCRIPTION DRUGS (Cont.)

VAGINAL DOUCHES (Cont.)

a.	Toxicity rating 4
Boric acid*	25–85%
Zinc salts*—sulfate	4–12.5%
In addition usually contain:	
Phenlsulfonate (sulfocarbolate)*	2–5%
Alum	1–14%
Phenols	less than 1%
Essential oils (menthol, eucalyptol, lavender and methyl salicylate)	less than 1%
Organic acids (citric, salicylic)	
b. Generally contain	Toxicity rating 3
Zinc salts—sulfate	4–5%
Phenolsulfonate (sulfocarbolate)*	7%
Oxyquinoline sulfate or citrate	2–15%
Na bicarbonate	12–90%
Organic acids (tartaric, lactic, citric)	15–25%
Carbohydrates	10–25%
Phenols	less than 1%
Anionic detergent	2–3%
Essential oils	1–2%
c. Miscellaneous	
1. Sodium caprylate	Toxicity rating 1
2. Alkylarylsulfate (see alkyl aryl sodium sulfates)*	Toxicity rating 3
	35%
Na₂SO₄	53%
Oxyquinoline sulfate dispersant	

VITAMINS (see CHILDREN'S VITAMINS)

VITAMINS AND MINERALS (see VITAMINS, CHILDREN)

WART REMOVERS (see CALLUS, CORN AND WART REMEDIES)

WEIGHT CONTROL PREPARATION

1. Artificial sweeteners .... Toxicity rating 1–2

Calcium saccharin	0–5%
Sodium saccharin	0–0.1%
Available as:	
Liquids, powder and tablets	

2. Benzocaine preparations .... Toxicity rating 2

Benzocaine	5 mg.
Carboxymethyl cellulose	
Methylcellulose	100 mg.
Vitamins/minerals	
Available as:	
Capsules, gum and tablets	

3. Bulk increasers .... Toxicity rating 1

Dextrose	0–50%
Methylcellulose	0–100%
Psyllium mucilloid	
Sodium bicarbonate (equivalent to 250 mg. sodium)	
May contain:	
Citric acid	
Flour	
Sugar	

4. Glucose preparations .... Toxicity rating 1
   Corn syrup
   Sweetened, condensed whole milk
   Vegetable oils
   Vitamins
   Available as:
   Candy, tablets
   May contain:
   Citric acid
   Dried yeast

Starred ingredients (*) may be responsible for major toxic effects; consult Section II.

NONPRESCRIPTION DRUGS (Cont.)

WEIGHT CONTROL PREPARATIONS

Guar flour
Minerals
Soy flour
Starch

5. Phenylpropanolamine preparations ... Toxicity rating 3
   Benzocaine
   Caffeine
   Methylcellulose
   Phenylpropanolamine*
   Available as:
   Tablets

NONSKID PRODUCTS

NONSKID PRODUCTS

1. Fan and belt ... Toxicity rating 3
   Stoddard solvent* or petroleum naphtha* ... 30%
2. Floor ... Toxicity rating 3
   Methyl ethyl ketone*
   Phenolic binder
3. Rug ... Toxicity rating 3
   Propellant
   Methylene chloride*

NOVELTIES, ADULTS

CIGARETTE JOKE TABLET ... Toxicity rating 3
Calcium carbonate
Metaldehyde*

COCKTAIL GLASS FROSTER
Liquid CO_2
Propellant

SCROLL ART (kit for oil paints on wall panels) ... Toxicity rating 4
Artist's oil paints* (see Arts and Crafts Products, this section)
Turpentine*
(No lead)

NOVELTIES, CHILDREN

ART KIT ... Toxicity rating 1 or 2
Azo pigments
Diarylide yellows
Hansa yellow
Iron oxides
Lithol toners
Phthalocyanine
Ultramarine
LD_{50} values are greater than 10 gm./kg., thus are defined as "nontoxic" by the Federal Hazardous Substances Act.

BOUNCING PUTTY ... Toxicity rating 1

Silicone	82.0%
Boron oxide	3.5%
Ammonium carbonate	3.9%
Aluminum stearate	3.9%
Glycerine	3.0%
Iron salts	0.22%
Titanium dioxide	2.6%
Silicon dioxide	0.8%

CHEMICAL UNDERWATER FLOWERS ... Toxicity rating 2
Metal salts: manganese, cobalt, nickel, copper, iron, etc.)

NOVELTIES, CHILDREN (Cont.)

CHEMICAL UNDERWATER FLOWERS (Cont.)
Sodium silicate
Water ... to 100%

CHEMI-LUME LIGHTS ... Toxicity rating 2
Fluorescein rhodamine B
Methyl cellulose

CHEMISTRY SETS

The following ingredients may be found in one or more of three popular chemistry sets. The substances have been grouped into three categories: (1) those from which no toxicity is expected, (2) those of moderate toxicity, and (3) those which could produce more severe toxic effects when taken in the available quantities. In general a container in a chemistry set holds 15 gm. of an ingredient, but this is not constant and cannot be counted on in any individual case of ingestion.

1. Ingredients of very low toxicity
   Bean seed
   Calcite
   Calcium carbonate
   Cochineal
   Calcium sulfate
   Copper wire
   Diatomaceous earth
   Epoxidized soybean oil
   Granulated zinc
   Graphite
   Gum arabic
   Iron metal (powdered)
   Logwood
   Muscovite
   Nichrome wire
   Nickel steel wire
   Phenolphthalein solution
   Polyvinyl alcohol (in small amounts)
   Powdered charcoal
   Powdered iron
   Rhodamine B; Triphenylmethane dye
   Sodium sulfate
   Starch
   Sulfur
   Thionine (in dilute solution)
   Zinc metal
2. Ingredients of low toxicity. (Ingestion of large amounts would be required before symptoms appeared. The acetic acid would be corrosive if in a concentrated form.)
   Acetic acid (dilute)
   Acetyl-tributyl citrate (plasticizer)
   Ammonium chloride
   Bronze powder
   Calcium chloride
   Calcium monophosphate
   Chrome alum (chromium potassium sulfate)
   Giberellic acid
   Gypsum (calcium sulfate, hydrous)
   Magnesium sulfate
   Manganese sulfate
   Mineral oil
   Oregon balsam (see Balsam of Peru)
   Shellac
   Sodium bicarbonate
   Sodium bisulfite
   Sodium chloride
   Sodium ferrocyanide

Starred ingredients (*) may be responsible for major toxic effects; consult Section II.

| NOVELTIES, CHILDREN (Cont.) | NOVELTIES, CHILDREN (Cont.) |

CHEMISTRY SETS (Cont.)

    Sodium iodide
    Sodium thiosulfate
    Strontium chloride
3. Potentially toxic ingredients. (Although considered more toxic than the first two groups, each ingestion must be evaluated according to the actual amount and concentration involved. With the acids, for example, the concentration is more critical than the volume, and the local effect is usually more grave than the systemic. Treatment of this last group of chemicals, therefore must be individualized. In every case, more comprehensive toxicity data (Section II) should be sought, since this outline is not intended to furnish complete information.)

    Aluminum sulfate
    Ammonium hydroxide
    Azodicarbonamide
    Azurite (basic copper carbonate)
    Benedicts solution (alkaline copper sulfate)
    Borates
    Calcium hypochlorite
    Calcium nitrate
    Calcium oxide
    Cedarwood oil redistilled
    Cobalt chloride
    Diglycolstearate
    Ethanol
    Ferric ammonium sulfate
    Ferrous ammonium sulfate
    Gold solution (last appeared in chemistry sets in 1962)
    8-Hydroxyquinoline
    Melamine formaldehyde
    Nickel ammonium sulfate
    Ninhydrin
    Potassium chloride
    Sodium bisulfate
    Sodium carbonate
    Sodium salicylate
    Sodium silicate solution
    Sodium tetraborate
    Stilbene
    Strontium nitrate
    Tannic acid
    Tartaric acid
    Trisodium phosphate
    Zinc sulfate

FLYING MISSILES .... Toxicity rating 2

Sodium bicarbonate	52.5%
Citric acid (anhydrous)	37.0%
Starch	5.0%
Talc	2.5%
Magnesium stearate	0.5%
Calcium pyrophosphate	2.5%

FOTO FUN KIT .... Toxicity rating 3

Silver nitrate*	1.03%
Ammonia water	0.5%

PLAY DOUGH .... Toxicity rating 1

1. Water
    Wheat flour
    Sodium chloride
    Calcium chloride
    Highly refined mineral spirits low odor
    Titanium dioxide
    Aluminum sulfate
    Borax
    Color (food dyes)
    Preservative (sodium benzoate)
    Perfume
2. Day Glo Play Dough
    Same as above except day glo pigments are used in place of dyes.

SMOKE FLUID FOR TOY ELECTRIC TRAINS

Pure white mineral oil U.S.P. grade viscosity	85 sec. 1000 parts
Hexahydrothymol U.S.P.	1 part
Fractol (minerol oil)	1 part

SMOKE PELLETS FOR TOY ELECTRIC TRAINS

Santo Wax-M	1 part
Santo Wax-P	0.15 part
J. Solvent	(approx. 0.2 part)

May contain:
    Tetramethylbenzene
    Xylene
    Ethyl toluene
    Propyl benzene
    Cumene
    Trimethylbenzene
    Ethyl benzene
    Naphthalene

TOY CAPS .... Toxicity rating 4

    Amorphous red phosphorus
    Potassium chlorate*
    Antimony trisulfide* (see Antimony salts)
    Water-soluble gum
    Inert abrasive

OILS

AROMATIC (see ESSENTIAL OILS, Section II)

BABY (see COSMETICS)

CUTTING OILS

1. Cutting oils—chemical coolants ...... Toxicity rating 3

Water	50–90%
Rust inhibitors	1–10%
Sodium nitrite*	
Ethanol amines	
Potassium or sodium soaps	
Lubricity agents	20–50%
Polyether glycols	
Alkyl-phenol-ethylene oxide condensation products	
Bactericides	0–1%
Chlorophenols	
Organic mercurials* (see Methyl mercuric chloride)	
Iodine compounds	
Formaldehyde releasers	
Quaternary ammonium compounds	

Note: Chemical coolants are usually diluted with from 50 to 150 parts of water to 1 part of the coolant to form the products used in metal-working operations.

Starred ingredients (*) may be responsible for major toxic effects; consult Section II.

OILS (Cont.)	OILS (Cont.)

CUTTING OILS (Cont.)

2. Cutting oils—insoluble type .... Toxicity rating 2 or 3
   - Mineral oils (including sulfurized mineral oils) 80–100%
   - Fatty oils (including sulfurized fatty oils) 1–40%
   - Sulfur (combined and suspended) .. 0–10%
   - Chlorine (chlorinated paraffins rarely chlorinated aromatics) 0–10%
   - Phosphorus (organic phosphates and phosphites) 0–1%
3. Cutting oils—soluble type .... Toxicity rating 2 or 3
   - Mineral oils 60–90%
   - Water 1–5%
   - Emulsifiers 5–30%
     - Sodium and amine soaps
     - Sodium sulfonates, naphthenates, rosinates
   - Coupling agents 1–2%
     - Alcohols
     - Glycol ethers
     - Glycols
   - Rust inhibitors 1–10%
     - Amines
     - Fatty oils
     - Sulfurized fatty oils
   - Bactericides 0–1%
     - Chlorophenols
     - Organic mercurials*
     - Iodine compounds
     - Formaldehyde releasers
     - Quaternary ammonium compounds

Note: Soluble cutting oils are usually diluted with from 10 to 75 parts of water to 1 part of the oil to form emulsions that are used in metal-working operations.

ESSENTIAL OILS (see Section II under OILS and under ESSENTIAL OILS)

FURNACE OILS .... Toxicity rating 3
   - Petroleum distillates*

GEAR OILS .... Toxicity rating 2 or 3
   - Mineral oils 70–100%
   - Lubricity agents, extreme pressure agents, antiwear agents 0–20%
     - CI, S.P. compounds
     - Fatty oils
     - Sulfurized fatty oils
     - Chlorinated paraffins*
     - Lead soaps, lead naphthenate*
     - Tricresyl and other organic phosphates
   - Oxidation and corrosion inhibitors 0–5%
     - Barium and calcium petroleum sulfonates
     - Barium and calcium phenolates*
     - 2,6-Ditertiary butyl-*p*-cresol
     - Amines, diphenylamine
     - Zinc dialkyl dithiophosphates
   - Pour depressants and viscosity improvers 0–5%
     - Polymethacrylate esters
     - Polyisobutylenes
     - Alkylstyrene polymers
     - Hydrocarbon wax-naphthalene condensation products
   - Antifoam agents .... 0–150 p.p.m.
     - Polysiloxanes

GEAR OILS (Cont.)
   - May contain:
     - Trichloethylene* (as cut-back solvent 0–25%

GENERAL PURPOSE OILS
   (household, electric motors) ..... Toxicity rating 2 or 3
   - Mineral oils 90–100%
   - May contain:
     - Rust inhibitors (sulfonates, amines, fatty oils, fatty acids) 0–10%
     - Odorants 0–trace
     - Silicone

GREASES .... Toxicity rating 2
   - Petroleum oils
   - Soap (Na, Li, Ca, Al)
   - May contain:
     - Barium compounds
     - Borax
     - Chromate
     - Dye
     - Graphite
     - Lead compounds
     - Molybdenum disulfide
     - Talc
     - Zinc salt

METAL PROTECTIVE OILS
1. Slushing type .... Toxicity rating 3
   - Mineral oil 40–60%
   - Stoddard solvent* 40–60%
   - Kerosene* 40–60%
   - May contain:
     - Sodium sulfonates 0–5%
     - Petroleum oxidates 0–5%
2. Protective coating type .... Toxicity rating 2 or 3
   - Asphalts 40–60%
   - Light petroleum distillates* 40–60%
   - May contain:
     - Fatty oils 0–5%
     - Mineral oils 35–60%
     - Petrolatum 30–50%
     - Petroleum wax 0–20%
     - Stoddard solvent* 0–25%
     - Soaps 0–3%

MISCELLANEOUS OILS .... Toxicity rating 3 or 4
   - Mineral oils
   - Additives
   - Xylene*
   - Alkaline salts of organic acids
   - Rust inhibitors
   - Kerosene
   - Silicone
   - Propellant
   - Phosphorus .... trace
   - Zinc .... trace
   - Barium .... trace
   - Citronella (home) .... trace

MOTOR OILS .... Toxicity rating 2
   - Mineral oils 75–100%
   - Oxidation inhibitors and detergents ... 0–20%
     - Zinc dialkyl dithiophosphate
     - Phosphorus pentasulfide-terpene addition products
     - Barium and calcium petroleum sulfonate
     - Barium and calcium phenolates
     - Ashless detergents

Starred ingredients (*) may be responsible for major toxic effects; consult Section II.

OILS (Cont.)	PAINT (Cont.)

OILS (Cont.)

MOTOR OILS (Cont.)

Pour depressants and viscosity improvers	0–5%
Polymethacrylate esters	
Polyisobutylenes	
Alkyl styrene polymers	
Hydrocarbon wax-naphthalene condensation products	
Antifoam agents	0–150 ppm
Polysiloxanes	

PENETRATING OILS	Toxicity rating 2 or 3
Mineral oils	40–80%
Kerosene*	20–60%

May contain:

Surface active agents	0–3%
Fatty oils and fatty acids	0–5%
Xylene*	0–10%
Tributyl phosphate	0–3%
Butyl alcohol	
Chlorinated hydrocarbons* (CCl₄)	

SHOCK ABSORBER OILS (see AUTOMOTIVE PRODUCTS)

TOP CYLINDER LUBRICANTS (see AUTOMOTIVE PRODUCTS)

OINTMENT (see NONPRESCRIPTION DRUGS)

PAINT

AEROSOL PAINT PRODUCTS
Aerosol packaged paint products of wide variety are available in almost all of the categories given below. In addition to the listed ingredients for the base paint product there will be present the propellant, *e.g.*, propane or combinations.

ANTIALGAE PAINTS	Toxicity rating 4
Cuprous oxide*	copper as metal 7%
Copper soap	
Arsenic oxide* (see Arsenic pentoxide) arsenic as metal 7%	
Copper sulfate pentahydrate*	
Mercury soap	mercury as metal 0.3%
2,2 Dihydroxy 5,5-dichlorodiphenyl-methane* or 2,2-methylenebis (4-chlorophenol)*	

ANTICORROSION PAINTS	Toxicity rating:

Pigment:

Zinc chromate*	4
Lead chromate*	4
Red lead oxide*	3
Basic lead carbonate*	4
Zinc oxide	2 or 3
Lead monoxide*	3

Vehicle:

Rosin	2
Pine oil*	3
Coal tar*	4
Petroleum ether*	3

Anticorrosion paints may contain:

Ammonium hydroxide*	3
Arsenic*	5
Cuprous oxide*	4
Ethyl alcohol	3
Kerosene*	3
Mercuric oxides*	5
Metallic soap	?
Methylene chloride*	3
Paraffin	
Plastic thickener	

ANTICORROSION PAINTS (Cont.)

Rust retardant	
bis(Tributyl tin)oxide	

DRIERS	Toxicity rating:
Vanadium compounds*	3 or 4
Manganese compounds*	3
Zinc compounds*	4
Iron compounds*	3
Cobalt compounds*	4
Potassium hydroxide*	4
Lead naphthenate*	3?
Lead octoate* (see Lead acetate)	3?
Lead tallate*	3?
Other lead compounds*	4

FINGER PAINTS (see ARTS AND CRAFTS PRODUCTS)

LACQUERS	Toxicity rating 2 or 3

Nitrocellulose	
Ester gum (glyceryl, methyl and ethyl esters of resin acids)	
Cottonseed oil	
Synthetic resins made from cotton and oil	
Synthetics made from soya beans	
Pigments	
Nitric acid	
Lead oxide	
Magnesium oxide	

LACQUER THINNERS	Toxicity rating 4
Ethyl alcohol	0–5%
Ethyl acetate*	20–21%
Butyl alcohol*	10–11%
Butyl acetate*	20–23%
Toluene*	25–28%
Aliphatic hydrocarbons*	16–20%

May contain:

Amyl acetate*	
Isopropyl acetate*	
Isopropyl alcohol*	
Pigment	
Xylene*	

OILS	Toxicity rating 2
Linseed oil	
Soybean oil	
Fish oil	
Castor oil	
Synthetic oil	
Tung oil	
Perilla oil	
Oiticica oil	

PAINT REMOVERS (see CLEANERS)

PLASTICIZERS	Toxicity rating 3
Tricresyl phosphate*	
Diethyl phthalate	
Diamyl phthalate	
Dibutyl phthalate	
Linseed oil	
Soy oil	
Camphor*	
Castor oil	

SOLVENTS AND THINNERS (see under SOLVENTS AND THINNERS, this section)

STAINS	Toxicity rating 3
Oleo resinous varnishes	
Mineral spirits*	

Starred ingredients (*) may be responsible for major toxic effects; consult Section II.

| PAINT (Cont.) | PAINT (Cont.) |

SURFACE CONDITIONER (see also Paint and Varnish removers, and Cleaners)

1. Chlorinated hydrocarbons*	25–80%
2. Alcohols	5–15%
3. Ketones	2–10%
4. Glycol ether	0–10%
5. Mineral spirits	0–10%
6. Naphtha	0–5%
7. Detergents	0–3%
8. Cellulose derivatives	0–2%
9. Wax	0–2%
10. Amines (triethylamine)	0–1%

TIRE PAINTS (see AUTOMOTIVE PRODUCTS)

TYPICAL ANALYSIS OF PAINTS

1. Aluminum, bronze and other metallic
    paints ...... Toxicity rating 3
Aluminum pigment	7–15%
Petroleum resin	0–40%
Vegetable oil varnish	0–40%
Linseed oil	0–30%
Aromatic thinners* (if over 25%, toxicity rating 4)	0–50%
Mineral spirits*	0–30%
Coumarone indene resin	0–15%

    Bold bronze contains copper or copper-tin alloy pigment.
    See Note 5 below

2. Asphalt paints, including screen
    enamel, stove enamel ...... Toxicity rating 3
Asphalt or gilsonite	20–50%
Oil or varnish	0–20%
Mineral spirits*	45–70%
Carbon black	0–15%

    See Note 5 below

3. Flat wall paint oil, primers and
    sealers ...... Toxicity rating 3
Titanium dioxide	0–20%
Titanium calcium	0–40%
Lithopone*	0–40%
Inert filler pigments	10–50%
Alkyd resin or oil varnish	9–25%
Mineral spirits*	25–35%

    See Notes 1, 5, and 6 below

4. Gloss enamel and floor enamels ...... Toxicity rating 3
Titanium dioxide	0–35%
Titanium calcium	0–35%
Inert pigments	0–20%
Alkyd resin or oil varnish	30–40%
Mineral spirits*	30–40%

    See Notes 1, 5, and 6 below

5. House paint, trim paint, exterior oil,
    exterior primers ...... Toxicity rating 3
Titanium dioxide	0–20%
Titanium calcium	0–35%
Zinc oxide	0–25%
White lead* (Note 2)	0–20%
Inert filler pigments	0–40%
Linseed oil	0–35%
Alkyd resin	0–30%
Mineral spirits*	5–30%

    See Notes 1, 3, 4, 5, and 6 below

6. Latex house paint ...... Toxicity rating 2
Titanium dioxide	10–20%
Inert filler pigments	20–55%
Polyvinyl acetate elastomer ⎫ Acrylic elastomer ⎬ Styrene butadiene elastomer ⎭	10–25%
Ethylene glycol	0–2%

TYPICAL ANALYSIS OF PAINT (Cont.)

Emulsifying agents	0–1%
Zinc oxide	5–10%
Alkyd resin	5–30%
Chlorinated phenols (or o-phenyl phenols)	0.1–0.5%
Water	20–35%
Vegetable oils or resins	0–10%

    See Notes 2 and 6 below
    Latex house paints may contain higher quantities of mercury fungicides than latex wall paints, but not exceeding 0.2% as mercury without special labeling.

7. Latex wall paint, texture coatings,
    fillers ...... Toxicity rating 2
Titanium dioxide	10–20%
Inert filler pigments	15–55%
Polyvinyl acetate elastomer ⎫ Acrylic elastomer ⎬ Styrene butadiene elastomer ⎭	10–25%
Lithopone	0–5%
Ethylene glycol	0–2%
Emulsifying agents	0–1%
Chlorinated phenols (or o-phenyl phenols)	0.1–0.5%
Water	25–60%
Vegetable oils or resins	0–10%

    See Notes 2 and 6 below

8. Semigloss, satin or eggshell enamel ...... Toxicity rating 3
Titanium dioxide	10–25%
Titanium calcium	0–40%
Lithopone*	0–40%
Inert filler pigments	5–25%
Alkyd resin or oil varnish	25–30%
Mineral spirits*	20–30%

    See Notes 1, 5, and 6 below

9. Stains, penetrating or wiping; wood
    fillers ...... Toxicity rating 3

    It is often difficult to determine by percentage composition whether a product is a stain or a varnish. At times the only way to decide is on the basis of usage.
Gilsonite or asphalt	0–25%
Aniline dyes* (see introduction to Pigments)	0–3%
Vegetable oil varnish	0–25%
Alkyd resin	0–25%
Mineral spirits*	50–80%

    Blonding or wiping contain 0–30% pigments plus fillers
    See Notes 1 and 5 below
    Some stain products contain wood preservatives, usually pentachlorophenol in the range of 3–5%. The presence of materials of this nature should be shown on the label.

10. Varnish, gloss, flat (satin); varnish
    stains ...... Toxicity rating 3
Alkyd resin	0–50%
Vegetable oil varnish	0–55%
Mineral spirits*	45–65%

    Colored varnishes contain similar coloring materials indicated in stains.
    See Note 5 below

Starred ingredients (*) may be responsible for major toxic effects; consult Section II.

| PAINT (Cont.) | PESTICIDES |

TYPICAL ANALYSIS OF PAINT (Cont.)

Fillers and pigments	0–5%
Polyurethane resin	0–55%
Phenolic resin	0–15%

NOTE 1: Typical formula applies to white and pastel colors with less than 5% tinting color added. In deeper colors, color pigments replace part or all the titanium pigment. If these color pigments contain lead compounds a warning statement should appear on the label. In these cases the formula may show content of the following lead compounds:

Chrome Yellow*—Lead chromate
Chrome Orange*—Basic lead chromate
Molybdate Orange*—Lead chromate molybdate
Chrome Green*—Ferric ferrocyanide and lead chromate

NOTE 2: Latex paints usually do not contain lead compounds, or color pigments containing lead. Exterior latex paints may contain mercury fungicides (see Note 4).

NOTE 3: White lead may occur in white and colored house paints in the following forms. Each requires lead warning statement on label. Formula may show the following lead compounds:

Basic carbonate white lead—Basic lead carbonate
Basic sulfate white lead—Basic lead sulfate
Basic silicate white lead—Basic lead silicate
Leaded zinc oxide—Zinc oxide and lead sulfate
Lead titanate
"Fume-Proof" or "Fume-Resistant" house paints denote NO lead content.

NOTE 4: "Mildew-Resistant" house paints usually contain mercury compounds, such as phenyl mercury oleate, phenyl mercury acetate, or phenyl mercury succinate. Label formula would indicate content and label should carry special warning statement of mercury compounds. If there is less than 0.2% of mercury compound in the coating, special warning labeling is not required.

NOTE 5: Paints containing mineral spirits, petroleum distillates and aromatic hydrocarbons are particularly dangerous if material enters lungs. Proper label warning indicates "Do not induce vomiting" if ingested. See Kerosene and Xylene in Section III.

NOTE 6: Inert filler pigments include typical compounds:

Asbestine (talc)	Toxicity rating 1
Calcium carbonate (whiting)	1
Calcium sulfate	1
China clay (alumino silicate)	1
Silica and silicates	1
Magnesium silicate (talc)	1
Talc (magnesium silicate)	1
Whiting (calcium carbonate)	1

NOTE 7: See Pigments; Dyes.

VARNISHES AND SHELLACS .... Toxicity rating 3 or 4

Resins
Methyl alcohol*
Ethyl alcohol*
Gasoline*
Benzene*
Sodium hydroxide
Turpentine*
Lead*

WATER REPELLANTS (see SPORTS PRODUCTS, WATERPROOFING COMPOUNDS)

PESTICIDES

Pesticides on the market in the recent past are listed alphabetically by product name. Alternate names also used are cited. The chemical formulas have not been included; they are frequently displayed on product labels. The principal use is indicated by a code (see the table below). The manufacturer can be identified by the number referring to that in the alphabetical list of manufacturers immediately following this list. Note: this list is separate from the manufacturers of the products in the Trade Name Index (V) listed in the final section (VII) of this volume.

The following sources were used for this compilation by Carol Glasgow of the Pharmacology Department, UCSF.

Gosselin, R. E., Hodge, H. C., Smith, R. P. and Gleason, M. N., *Clinical Toxicology of Commercial Products*, Williams & Wilkins, Baltimore, 1976.

Thomson, W. T., *Agricultural Chemicals*, Books I-IV, Thomson Publications, Fresno, Calif., 1976/1977.

Farm Chemicals Handbook, Meister Publishing Co., Willoughby, Ohio, 1981.

Nanogen Index, A Dictionary of Pesticides, compiled and edited by Kingsley Packer, published by Nanogens International, Freedom, Calif., 1975.

The original listings came from the Thomson series, additional pesticides and alternate names were added from Farm Chemicals Handbook, Nanogen Index and CTCP. If two different chemicals or products have the same name, they are identified by either their use, *e.g.* herbicide or insecticide, or by the producer. Mrs. Jean Braddock prepared and organized these lists in computerized form.

Key to Uses

Ac – Acaricide
Ad – Synergist
Al – Algicide
An – Anthelmintic
Aq – Aquatic
Av – Avicide
B – Bactericide
Ct – Cut flowers preservative
Df – Defoliant
F – Fungicide
Fm – Fumigant
Ft – Fish toxicant
H – Herbicide
I – Insecticide
M – Molluscicide
Mp –Mildew proofing
N – Nematocide
Pg – Plant growth regulator
R – Rodenticide
Re – Repellant
Sl – Slimicide
St – Seed treatment
Wp – Wood preservative

Starred ingredients (*) may be responsible for major toxic effects; consult Section II.

PESTICIDES (Cont.)			
PRODUCT NAME	ALTERNATE NAME	PRINCIPAL USE	MANU- FACTURER
A 363	Aminocarb	I	115, 488
AA	Allyl Alcohol	H /F	
AAtack	Thiram	F /St	
AAteck	Tec	F	
AAterra	Ethazol	F	
AAtram		H	190
AAtrex	Atrazine	H	190, 193
2-AB	Frucote	F	
Abar	Leptophos	I	
Abat	Abate	I	
Abate		I	046
Abathion	Abate	I	
2-AB Deccotane	Frucote	F	
AC 3422	Parathion	I	046
AC 3911	Phorate	I	046
AC 5223	Cyprex	F	046
AC 18682	Dimethoate	I /Ac	046
AC 26691	Cythioate	I	046
AC 84777	Difenzoquat	H	046
AC 92390	(see American Cyanamid Co.)	H	046
AC 92553	(see American Cyanamid Co.)	H	046
Acaraben	Chlorobenzilate	Ac	190
Acaralate	Chloropropylate	I /Ac	190
Acarin	Kelthane	Ac	439
Acarol	Bromopropylate	I /Ac	190, 193
Acaron	Chlordimeform	I /Ac	652
Accel	SD 8339	Pg	
Accelerate	Endothall	H	566
Accothion	Fenitrothion	I	046
Acephate		I	187
Acephate-Met	Methamidophos	I	187, 488
Acid Lead Arsenate	Lead Arsenate	I	
ACP 322	N-1-Naphthylphthalamic Acid	H	
Acquimite	Chloropicrin	Fm	
Acquinite (fumigant)	Chloropicrin	Fm	
Acquinite (herbicide)	Acrolein	H	
Acrex	Dinobuton	F /Ac	403
Acricid	Binapacryl	F /Ac	346
Acritet	(see Stauffer Chemical Co.)	Fm	697
Acrolein		Aq/H	661, 757
Acrylaldehyde	Acrolein	H	
Actellic		I /Ac	364
Acti-Aid	Cycloheximide	Pg	754
Acti-Dione	Cycloheximide	F	754
Action	Methamidophos	I	
Actispray	Cycloheximide	F	295
Activol	Gibberellic Acid	Pg	370
Actril	Ioxynil	H	457
Afalon	Linuron	H	346
Afesin	Monolinuron	H	
Aflix	Formothion	I /Ac	
Afnor	Chlorophacinone	R	
Afos	Mecarbam	I /Ac	
Afugan	Pyrazophos	F	346
Agrimycin 17	Streptomycin	B	574
Agrisil	Trichloronate	I	115
Agri-Strep	Streptomycin	B	466
Agritol		I	004
Agritox (herbicide)	MCPA	H	
Agritox (insecticide)	Trichloronate	I	115
A-Gro	Methyl Parathion	I	
Agrocide 6G	Lindane	I	
Agrosan	(see ICI Plant Protection Division)	St	370
Agrosol S		St	364
Agrotec	2,4-D	H	475
Agrothion	Fenitrothion	I /Ac	370
Agroxone	MCPA	H	370
Agrox 2-Way		St	364
Agrox 3-Way		St	364

Starred ingredients (*) may be responsible for major toxic effects; consult Section II.

	PESTICIDES (Cont.)		
PRODUCT NAME	ALTERNATE NAME	PRINCIPAL USE	MANU-FACTURER
Agualine	Acrolein	H	
Akar	Chlorobenzilate	Ac	193
Akton		I	661
Alachlor		H	496
Alanap	N-1-Naphthylphthalamic Acid	H	760
Alanap-1	N-1-Naphthylphthalamic Acid	H	760
Alar	Daminozide	Pg	760
Alboleum	Albolineum	I	
Albolineum	(see ICI Plant Protection Division)	I	370
Aldicarb		I /Ac	757
Aldrin		I	667
Aldrite 4	Aldrin	I	667
Aldrosol	Aldrin	I	
Alfacron	Iodofenphos	I	193
Alfa-Tox		I	190
Alfol-10	Off-Shoot-T	Pg	
Algae-Rhap CU 7 Liquid Copper Algaecide		Al	785
Algaetrol 76	(see Thompson-Hayward Chemical Co.)	H	736
Algimycin PLL-C	(see Great Lakes Biochemical Co.)	Al	316
Alicep		H	109
Alipur		H	109
Alkron	Parathion	I	
Alleron	Parathion I		
Allethrin		I	460, 718
Allidochlor	CDAA	H	496
Allisan	Dicloran	F	127
Allyl Al	Allyl Alcohol	H /F	
Allyl Alcohol		H /F	661, 295
Allyxycarb		I	115
Alon	Isoproturon	H	
Alphachloralose		R	571, 619
Alphakil	Alphachloralose	R	619
Alpha-Naphthaleneacetic Acid	1-Naphthaleneacetic Acid	Pg	
Alpha-Naphthylacetic Acid	1-Naphthaleneacetic Acid	Pg	
Alpha-Naphthyl Thiourea	ANTU	R	
Alphaspra	1-Naphthaleneacetic Acid	Pg	
Alsol	Etacelasil	Pg	193
Altosid	Methoprene	I	820
Altozar		I	820
Aluminum Phosphide	Phosphine	I /Fm	038, 262
AMA		H	199, 787
Ambithion		I	046
Ambox	Binapacryl	Ac	346
Ambush	Aldicarb	I /Ac	364
Amchem 3-CP	(see Amchem Products, Inc.)	Pg	757
Amcide	Ammonium Sulfamate	H	
Amdom	Picloram	H	043
Amerol	3-Amino-1,2,4-Triazole	H	
Ametrex	Ametryne	H	439
Ametryn	Ametryne	H	
Ametryne		H	190
Amex 820	Butralin	H	757, 691
Amiben	Chloramben	H	757
Amid-Thin W	NAD	Pg	757
Amilon WP		H	757
Amine Methanearsonates	AMA	H	199, 787
2-Aminobutane	Frucote	F	
Aminocarb		I	115, 488
Aminopyridine	Avitrol	Re	097
Aminotriazole	3-Amino-1,2,4-Triazole	H	
3-Amino-1,2,4-Triazole		H	046, 757
Amiphos	DAEP	I	532
Amitraz		I /Ac	127, 754
Amitril-T		H	046
Amitril T.L.	Amitril-T	H	046
Amitrol	3-Amino-1,2,4-Triazole	H	
Amitrole	3-Amino-1,2,4-Triazole	H	
Amitrol-T	Amitril-T	H	757
Amizine		H	757

Starred ingredients (*) may be responsible for major toxic effects; consult Section II.

PRODUCT NAME	ALTERNATE NAME	PRINCIPAL USE	MANU- FACTURER
	PESTICIDES (Cont.)		
Amizol	3-Amino-1,2,4-Triazole	H	757
Ammate	Ammonium Sulfamate	H	247
Ammate X	Ammonium Sulfamate	H	247
Ammonium Fluosilicate	Dri-Die	I	
Ammonium Methanearsonate	AMA	H	199, 787
Ammonium Polysulfide		F	031
Ammonium Sulfamate		H	247
Amobam	(see Roberts Chemicals, Div. of Security Chemicals, Inc.)	F	631
Amoxone	2,4-D	H	
AMS	Ammonium Sulfamate	H	
Amthio	(see Mallinckrodt, Inc.)	H	442
ANA	1-Naphthaleneacetic Acid	Pg	
Anabasine		I	
Ancrack	Dyanap	H	241
Ancymidol		Pg	259
Anilazine	2,4-Dichloro-6-o-Chloroanilino-s-Triazine	F	488
Anilinocadmium Dilactate		F	
Anilix	Chlorfensulphide	Ac	
Animert V-101		Ac	580
Aniten	Flurenol	H	145
Annalos	Petroleum Distillate	H	
Anofex	DDT	I	
Ansar 170 HC	MSMA	H	232
Ansar 529 HC	MSMA	H	232
Ansar 8100	Disodium Methylarsonate	H	232
Antak	Off-Shoot-T	Pg	241
Anthio	Formothion	I	646
Anthionix	Formothion	I	
Anthon	Trichlorfon	I	115
Anthraquinone		Re	115, 340
Anti-Carie	Hexachlorobenzene	St	
Anti-K	Sulfaquinoxaline	Ad	466
Antimilace	Metaldehyde	M	
Antimony Potassium Tartrate		I	337, 442
Antimycin-A	(see Ayerst Laboratories)	Ab	100
Antor		H	128
Antracol	Propineb	F	115
Antrol	AMA	H	
ANTU		R	049
Anturat	ANTU	R	
4-AP	Avitrol	Re	
Aphamite	Parathion	I	
Aphidan		I	349
Aphox	Pirimicarb	I	364
Apl-Luster	Thiabendazole	F	566
Apl-Luster-T	Thiabendazole	F	566
Appa	Imidan	I	
Appex	Tetrachlorvinphos	I	
Apple-Set	1-Naphthaleneacetic Acid	Pg	
Aquacide	Diquat Dibromide	H	
Aquaflo	Aromatic Hydrocarbon Solvent	Aq/H	
Aqualin	Acrolein	Aq/H	661
Aqualine	Acrolein	H	
Aquathol	Endothal	H	566
Aqua-Vex	Silvex	H	566
Aquazine	Simazine	H	190
Aquinite	Chloropicrin	Fm	
Arasan	Thiram	F /St	247
Arasan 42-S	Thiram	F /Re	247
Arbortrine	Benomyl	F	073
Areginal		Fm/I	
Arelon	Isoproturon	H	346
Aresin	Monolinuron	H	346
A-Rest	Ancymidol	Pg	259
Aretan	Methoxyethylmercuric Chloride	F	115
Aretit	Dinoseb Acetate	H	346
Arisan	Eptapur	H	
Arkotine DDT	DDT	I	664

PESTICIDES (Cont.)			
PRODUCT NAME	ALTERNATE NAME	PRINCIPAL USE	MANU-FACTURER
Aromatic Compounds	Aromatic Hydrocarbon Solvent	H	
Aromatic Hydrocarbon Solvent		H	160, 208
Aromatic Oils	Aromatic Hydrocarbon Solvent	H	
Aromatic Solvents	Aromatic Hydrocarbon Solvent	H	
Arprocarb	2-Isopropoxyphenyl N-Methylcarbamate	I	115, 488
Arresin	Monolinuron	H	
Arrhenal	Disodium Methylarsonate	H	
Arsan	Cacodylic Acid	H	
Arsenate of Lead	Lead Arsenate	I	
Arsenic Acid		H	202, 566
Arsinette	Lead Arsenate	H	
Arsinyl	Disodium Methylarsonate	H	
Arsonate Liquid	MSMA	H	232
Asazol	MSMA	H	
Asilan	Asulam	H	
Asozin	Rhizoctol	F /St	
ASP-51	Chlordane	I	
Aspon	Tetra-n-Propyl Dithionopyrophosphate	I	697
Aspor	Zineb	F	499
Asulam		H	457, 626
Asulox	Asulam	H	457
Asuntol	Coumaphos	I	
ATA	3-Amino-1,2,4-Triazole	H	
Atgard	Dichlorvos	An	232
Atlacide	Sodium Chlorate	H	370
Atlas 'A'	Sodium Arsenite	I	626
Atranex	Atrazine	H	439
Atratol	Sodium Chlorate	H	190
Atratol A	Atrazine	H	190
Atratol 8P		H	190
Atratol 80W		H	190
Atrazine		H	661, 785
Atrinal	Dikegulac-Sodium	Pg	434
Aules	Thiram	F /St	
Auragreen	Basic Copper Carbonate	F	442
A & V-70 Algaecide	(see A & V Inc.)	Al	094
Avadex	Diallate	H	496
Avadex BW	Triallate	H	496
Avenge	Difenzoquat	H	046
Avicol	Pentachloronitrobenzene	F /St	
Avirosan	Dimethametryn	H	193
Avirosan 500		H	193
Avitrol		Re	097
Avlothane	Hexachloroethane	An	367
Axiom	Akton	I	
Azak	2,6-Di-tert-Butyl-p-Tolyl-N-Methylcarbamate	H	343
Azide		H /I	595
Azidithion	Menazon	I	
Azinos	Azinphos-Ethyl	I	
Azinphos-Ethyl		I	115, 439
Azinphos-Methyl	Guthion	I	
Aziprotryn		H	193
Aziprotryne	Aziprotryn	H	
Azobenzene		Ac	250
Azobenzide	Azobenzene	Ac	250
Azodrin	Monocrotophos	I /Ac	661
Azolan	3-Amino-1,2,4-Triazole	H	439
Azole	3-Amino-1,2,4-Triazole	H	
B-995	Daminozide	Pg	
Baam	Amitraz	I	754
Bacillus Thuringiensis Berliner	Agritol	I	004, 116
Bacticin		F	754
Bactospeine	Agritol	I	116
Bakthane	Agritol	I	
Balan	Benefin	H	259
Baldex	Paraquat	H	
Balfin	Benefin	H	259
Banafine	Benefin	H	259

Starred ingredients (*) may be responsible for major toxic effects; consult Section II.

PESTICIDES (Cont.)

PRODUCT NAME	ALTERNATE NAME	PRINCIPAL USE	MANU-FACTURER
Banair	(see ICI Australia Limited)	H	367
Banarat	Prolin	R	
Bandane		H	781
Bandock		H	664
Banex	Dicamba	H	
Banfine	Benefin	H	
Ban-Hoe	(see Shellstar Ltd.)	H	670
Banrot	(see Mallinckrodt, Inc.)	F	442
Bantrol	Ioxynil	H	
Bantu	ANTU	R	
Banvel	Dicamba	H	781
Banvel D	Dicamba	H	781
Banvel K		H	781
Banvel M	MCPA	H	781
Baran	Fluoroacetamide	R	727
Barbamate	Chlorobutynyl Chlorocarbanilate	H	
Barban	Chlorobutynyl Chlorocarbanilate	H	
Barbasco	Rotenone	Ft	
Barium Carbonate		R	103, 106
Barium Fluosilicate		I	106
Barium Silicofluoride	Barium Fluosilicate	I	
Barnon		H	667
Baron	Erbon	H	238
Barquat MB-50	Benzalkonium Chloride	B	430
Barquat MB-80	Benzalkonium Chloride	B	430
Barricade		I	781
BAS 0660 W		Pg	109
BAS 2350		I	109
BAS 2903 H	Prynachlor	H	109
BAS 3170	Benodanil	F	109
BAS 3191	Furcarbanil	F	109
BAS 3460	Carbendazim	F	109
BAS 08300 W		Pg	112
Basagran	Bentazon	H	109, 112
Basagran-DP		H	109, 112
Basagran-KV		H	109, 112
Basagran-M		H	109, 112
Basalin	Fluchloralin	H	112
Basamaize	Prynachlor	H	
Basamid	Mylone	N	109
Basanite	4,6-Dinitro-2-sec-Butyl Phenol	H	112
Basanite-Five	4,6-Dinitro-2-sec-Butyl Phenol	H	112
Basfapon	Dalapon	H	109, 112
Basfungin	Methylmetiram	F	109
Basic Copper Carbonate		F	196
Basic Copper Chloride	Cupric Chloride, Basic	F	
Basic Copper Sulfate	Tribasic Copper Sulfate	F	
Basic Lead Arsenate	Lead Arsenate	I	
Basicop	Tribasic Copper Sulfate	F	
Basic Zinc Sulfate	Zinc Sulfate, Basic	B	
Bassa		I	418
Basudin	Diazinon	I /N	193
Batasan	Fentinacetate	F /Al	
Bavistin	Carbendazim	F	109
Bay 2352	Niclosamide	An	115
Bay 5072	p-Dimethylaminobenzenediazo Sodium Sulfonate	F /St	115
Bay 5212	Tolylfluanid	F	115
Bay 10756	Demeton	I /Ac	115
Bay 15080	Benquinox	F	115
Bay 16259	Azinphos-Ethyl	I	115
Bay 17147	Guthion	I	115
Bay 18510	Phenthoate	I /Ac	115
Bay 19639	Disulfoton	I /Ac	115
Bay 21097	Oxydemeton-Methyl	I /Ac	115
Bay 22555	p-Dimethylaminobenzenediazo Sodium Sulfonate	F /St	115
Bay 23323	Disyston S	I /Ac	115
Bay 23655	Metasystox S	I /Ac	115

Starred ingredients (*) may be responsible for major toxic effects; consult Section II.

	PESTICIDES (Cont.)		
PRODUCT NAME	ALTERNATE NAME	PRINCIPAL USE	MANU- FACTURER
Bay 25141	Fensulfothion	I /N	115
Bay 25634	Coumatetralyl	R	115
Bay 25648	Clonitralid	M	115
Bay 29493	Fenthion	I	115
Bay 30130	Propanil	H	115
Bay 30686	Eradex	F /Ac	115
Bay 33051	Phenthoate	I /Ac	115
Bay 33172	Fuberidazole	F	115
Bay 36205	Chinomethionat	I /Ac	115
Bay 37289	Trichloronate	I	115
Bay 37344	Methiocarb	I	115
Bay 39007	2-Isopropoxyphenyl N-Methylcarbamate	I	115
Bay 41831	Fenitrothion	I /Ac	115
Bay 44646	Aminocarb	I	115
Bay 45432	Omethoate	I /Ac	115
Bay 46131	Propineb	F	115
Bay 47531	Dichlofluanid	F	115
Bay 49854	Tolylfluanid	F	115
Bay 50282	Allyxycarb	I	115
Bay 60618	Benzthiazuron	H	115
Bay 68138	Phenamiphos	N	115
Bay 70142	Carbofuran	I /Ac	115
Bay 70533	Chlorfenprop-Methyl	H	115
Bay 71628	Methamidophos	I	115
Bay 74283	Methabenzthiazuron	H	115
Bay 77049	Diethchinalphion	I	115
Bay 77488	Phoxim	I	115
Bay 78418	Edifenphos	F	115
Bay 79770	Chloraniformethan	F	115
Bay 94337	Metribuzin	H	115
Bay 105807	Isoprocarb	I	115
Baycarb	Bassa	I	115
Baycid	Fenthion	I	115
Bayclean	Dimanin A	Al/B	115
Bay-Dam 18654		F	115
Baygon	2-Isopropoxyphenyl N-Methylcarbamate	I	115, 488
Bay-Hox 1901		I	115
Bayleton	Bay-Meb 6447	F	115, 488
Bayluscide	Clonitralid	M	115, 488
Bay-Meb 6447		F	115
Bay-Met 1486		H	115
Baymix	Coumaphos	I	
Bay NTN 6867		H	115
Bay NTN 9306		I	115, 488
Bayrusil	Diethchinalphion	I	115
Baytan	Methoxyethylmercuric Chloride	F	115
Baytex	Fenthion	I	115, 488
Baythion	Phoxim	I	115
BBC 12	DBCP	Fm	547
BCM	Carbendazim	F	
BCPE		Ac	532
Beet-Kleen		H	664
Belt	Chlordane	I	781
Ben 30	Benazolin	H	
Benachlor	Aromatic Hydrocarbon Solvent	H	
Benalan	Benefin	H	259
Benazolin		H	127
Bencornox	Benazolin	H	
Bendex	Fenbutatin-Oxide	Ac	
Bendiocarb		I	291, 292
Bendioxide	Bentazon	H	
Benefin		H	259
Benfluralin	Benefin	H	
Benlate	Benomyl	F	247
Benochlor	Aromatic Hydrocarbon Solvent	H	
Benodanil		F	109
Benomyl		F	247
Benopan	Benazolin	H	
Benquinox		F	115

PESTICIDES (Cont.)

PRODUCT NAME	ALTERNATE NAME	PRINCIPAL USE	MANU-FACTURER
Bensecal	Benazolin	H	
Bensulide	Betasan	H	
Bentazon		H	109, 112
Benthiocarb		H	187, 418
Bentrazone	Bentazon	H	
Benzabor	2,3,6-Trichlorobenzoic Acid	H	766
Benzac 1281	2,3,6-Trichlorobenzoic Acid	H	757
Benza-Chlor	Aromatic Hydrocarbon Solvent	H	
Benzadox		H	334
Benzahex	BHC	I	
Benzalkonium Chloride		B /F	430
Benzar	Benazolin	H	
Benzene Hexachloride	BHC	I	
Benzex	BHC	I	817
Benzilan	Chlorobenzilate	Ac	439
Benzomarc	Phenobenzuron	H	568
Benzomate		Ac	532
Benzoylprop Ethyl		H	667
Benzoxamate	Benzomate	Ac	
Benzphos	Phosalone	I /Ac	
Benzthiazuron		H	115
Benzyfuroline	Resmethrin	I	
Benzyl Benzoate		Ac	082, 103
Beosit	Thiodan	I /Ac	
Berelex	Gibberellic Acid	Pg	370
Bermat	Chlordimeform	I /Ac	610
Betanal	Phenmedipham	H	538, 652
Betanal-AM	Desmedipham	H	652
Betanex	Desmedipham	H	538, 652
Betasan		H	697
Bethrodine	Benefin	H	
Bexane	4-(2-Methyl-4-Chlorophenoxy) Butyric Acid	H	
Bexton	Propachlor	H	238
BFV	Formaldehyde Solution	F /Ge	
BHC		I	233, 625
Bichloride of Mercury	Mercuric Chloride	F /I	574
Bidisan	Chlorfenprop-Methyl	H	115
Bidrin		I	193. 661
Bifenox		H	490
Big Dipper	DPA	H	046
Binapacryl		Ac	346
Bine-Trol	MCPA	H	622
Binnell	Benefin	H	259
Bioallethrin	Pyrethroids	I	460, 601
Biocide	Acrolein	H	
Bioguard	Thiabendazole	F	
Bioquin 1	8-Hydroxyquinoline	F	
Bioresmethrin	Pyrethroids	I	
Biothion		I	046
Biotrol	Agritol	I	544
Biotrol-Plus		I	544
Biotrol VHZ	(see Nutrilite Products, Inc.)	I	544
Biotrol XK	Agritol	I	544
BIPC	Chlorbufam	H	
Biphenyl	Diphenyl	F	
Birlane	Chlorfenvinphos	I	664
2,3,4,5-Bis(2-Butylene) Tetrahydrofural		Re	460
Bisethyl xanthogen		H	631
Bismuth Subsalicylate		F	103, 565
Bis(Tri-n-Butyltin) Oxide		F	514
Bitemol	Simazine	H	
Black Leaf 40	Nicotine	I	118
Bladafume	Sulfotepp	I	115
Bladan	Parathion	I	115
Bladan	Tetraethyl Pyrophosphate	I	283
Bladan-M	Methyl Parathion	I	
Bladex	Cyanazine	H	661, 667
Blagal		H	664
BLA-S	Blasticidin	F	523

Starred ingredients (*) may be responsible for major toxic effects; consult Section II.

PESTICIDES (Cont.)

PRODUCT NAME	ALTERNATE NAME	PRINCIPAL USE	MANU-FACTURER
Blasticidin		F	523
Blasticidin-S	Blasticidin	F	
Blattanex	2-Isopropoxyphenyl N-Methylcarbamate	I	115
Bleaching Powder	Calcium Hypochlorite	F /B	
Blex	Actellic	I /Ac	364
Blitox	Cupric Chloride, Basic	F	
Blue Copperas	Copper Salts, (Cupric)	F	
Bluestone	Copper Salts, (Cupric)	F	
Blue Vitriol	Copper Salts, (Cupric)	F	
Blulan	Benefin	H	259
B-Nine	Daminozide	Pg	760
Bo-Ana	Famphur	I	046
Bolero	Benthiocarb	H	187, 418
Bolls-Eye	Cacodylic Acid	H	211
Bolstar	Bay NTN 9306	I	115, 488
Bomyl		I	355
Bonalan	Benefin	H	259
Bone Oil		I /Re	
Bone Tar Oil	Bone Oil	I	
Bonide Blue Death Ratkiller	Phosphorus	R	124
Borascu	Borax	H	766
Borax		H	406, 766
Bordeaux		F	166
Bordo Mixture	Bordeaux	F	
Borer Sol	Ethylene Dichloride	I /Fm	229
Borlin	Picloram	H	
Borocil		H	547
Borolin	Picloram	H	766
Boron	Borax	H	
Boro-Spray	Borax	H	406
BOTEC Peanut Seed Protectant	Dicloran	F	754
Botran	Dicloran	F	754
Botrilex	Pentachloronitrobenzene	F /St	115
Bovinox	Trichlorfon	I	
BPMC	Bassa	I	
Brasoran	Aziprotryn	H	
Brassicol	Pentachloronitrobenzene	F /St	346
Bravo	Chlorothalonil	F	232
Brellin	Gibberellic Acid	Pg	
Brestan	Fentinacetate	F /Al	346
Brimestone	Sulfur	F /Ac	
Brimstone	Sulfur	F /Ac	
Briton	Trichlorfon	I	
Broadside	(see The Ansul Co.)	H	067
Brocide	Ethylene Dichloride	I /Fm	
Brofene	Bromophos	I /Ac	
Bromacil		H	247, 439
Bromclophos	Naled	I /Ac	
Bromex (herbicide)	Chlorbromuron	H	538
Bromex (insecticide)	Naled	I	439
Brominal	Bromoxynil	H	757
Brominil	Bromoxynil	H	
Bromodine	(see C and R Products Development, Inc.)	Df/Mp	139
Bromofenoxim	Bromophenoxime	H	
Bromo-Fume	1,2-Dibromoethane	Fm	
Brom-O-Gas	Methyl Bromide	Fm	319
Bromomethane	Methyl Bromide	Fm	
Bromophenoxime		H	193
Bromophos		I /Ac	145
Bromophos-Ethyl		I /Ac	145
Bromopropylate		Ac	190, 193
Bromo-O-Sol		I /N	319
Bromoxynil		H	457, 757
Bronate	Bromoxynil	H	626
Bronocot	Bronopol	B	
Bronopol		B	127
Bronox	(see Fisons Limited, Agrochemical Div.)	H	292
Brophene	Bromophos	I /Ac	
Brown Copper Oxide	Cuprous Oxide	F	

Starred ingredients (*) may be responsible for major toxic effects; consult Section II.

PESTICIDES (Cont.)			
PRODUCT NAME	ALTERNATE NAME	PRINCIPAL USE	MANU-FACTURER
Brozone		N /H	238
Brulan	Tebuthiuron	H	
Brush Buster	Dicamba	H	781
Brush Killers	Trichlorophenoxyacetic Acid	H	
Brush-Rhap	(see Vertac Chemical Corp.)	H	785
BSZ	Zinc Coposil	F	
BT	Indar	F	
BTB	Agritol	I	
BTC	Benzalkonium Chloride	B /F	
BTS 27419	Amitraz	I /Ac	
BTV	Agritol	I	
Bualta		Pg	130
Buban 37		H	130
Buctril	Bromoxynil	H	626
Buctril Industrial	Bromoxynil	H	626
Bueno	MSMA	H	232
Bufencarb		I	187
Bunema		B /F	130
Bunt-No-More	Hexachlorobenzene	St	
Buntosan		St	367
Bupirimate		F	370
Busan 30	Busan 72	F /St	130
Busan 30A	Busan 72	F /St	130
Busan 72		F /St	130
Busan 72A	Busan 72	St	130
Butacarb		I	127
Butacarbe	Butacarb	I	
Butachlor		H	439, 496
Butacide	Piperonyl Butoxide	Ad	275
Butafume	Frucote	F	
Buthidazole	Ravage	H	781
Butoxone	2,4-DB	H	626
Butoxy Polypropylene Glycol		Re	757
beta-Butoxy-beta-Thiocyanodiethyl Ether		I	634
Butralin		H	691, 757
Butter of Zinc	Zinc Chloride	Wp	
Buturon	Eptapur	H	
Butylamine	Frucote	F	
Butylate		H	697
n-Butyl Phthalate		Re	253
Butyrac 118	2,4-DB	H	757
Butyrac 175	2,4-DB	H	757
Butyron	Eptapur	H	
BUX	Bufencarb	I	187
C 570	Phosphamidon	I /Ac	
C 709	Bidrin	I	193
C 1414	Monocrotophos	I /Ac	193
C 1983	Chloroxuron	H	193
C 2059	Fluometuron	H	193
C 2242	Chlortoluron	H	193
C 3126	Patoran	H	193
C 3470	Lironion	H	193
C 6313	Chlorbromuron	H	193
C 7019	Aziprotryn	H	193
C 8353	Dioxacarb	I	193
C 8514	Chlordimeform	I /Ac	193
C 8949	Chlorfenvinphos	I	193
C 9122	Bromophenoxime	H	193
C 9491	Iodofenphos	I	193
C 18898	Dimethametryn	H	193
C 19490	Piperophos	H	193
Cacodylic Acid		H	211, 787
Caddy	Cadmium Chloride	F	199
Cadminate		F	442
Cadmium Chloride		F	199
Cadmium Sulfate		F	199
Cad-Trete		F	199
CAID	Chlorophacinone	R	427
Calar		H	787

Starred ingredients (*) may be responsible for major toxic effects; consult Section II.

PESTICIDES (Cont.)			
PRODUCT NAME	ALTERNATE NAME	PRINCIPAL USE	MANU-FACTURER
Calcium Acid Methylarsenate	Calar	H	787
Calcium Arsenate		I /H	433, 817
Calcium Arsenite		I	181
Calcium Cyanamide		H /F	776
Calcium Cyanide		F	038, 776
Calcium Hypochlorite		F /B	550, 566
Calcium Polysulfide		F /I	187, 475
Calcium Sulfide		F	
Cal-Cop 10	Copper Ammonium Carbonate	F	
Calcyanide	Calcium Cyanide	Fm	
Caldon	4,6-Dinitro-2-sec-Butyl Phenol	H	346
Calirus	Benodanil	F	109
Calixin	Tridemorph	F	109
Calo-Clor		F	442
Calocure	Mercuric Chloride	F /I	442
Calo-Gran		F	442
Calomel	Mercurous Chloride	F	
CAMA	Calar	H	
Camphechlor	Toxaphene	I	
Can-Trol	MCPB	H	626
Caparol	Prometryne	H	190
Caprane	Karathane	F /Ac	
Capryl	Karathane	F /Ac	
Caprylic Alcohol		Pg	
Captafol		F	187, 691
Captan		F	187, 355
Captane	Captan	F	
Capthion		I /F	367
Caragard	Terbumeton	H	193
Carbam	Vapam	N /F	109, 697
Carbamate	Ferbam	F	295
Carbamult	Promecarb	I	652
Carbanolate	Aldicarb	I	
Carbaryl		I	109, 757
Carbatene	Metiram	F	
Carbendazim		F	109, 346
Carbetamex	Carbetamide	H	457, 625
Carbetamide		H	457, 625
Carbicron	Bidrin	I	193
Carbofos	Malathion	I	
Carbofuran		I /N	295
Carbon Bisulfide	Carbon Disulfide	Fm	—
Carbon Disulfide		Fm	295, 595
Carbon Tet	Carbon Tetrachloride	Fm	
Carbon Tetrachloride		Fm	697, 793
Carbophenothion		I /Ac	697
Carbophos	Malathion	I	
Carboxin		F /St	760
Carbyne	Chlorobutynyl Chlorocarbanilate	H	
Carfene	Guthion	I	
Carpene	Cyprex	F	499
Carpidor	Benefin	H	259
Cartap		I	724
Carzol	Formetanate	I	538, 652
Casoron	Dichlobenil	H	736
Casoron 133	Dichlobenil	H	580
Castrix		R	115
Catechol	Pyrocatechol	St	250
CBBP	Chlorphonium	Pg	
CCC	Chlormequat	Pg	
CDAA		H	496
CDEC	Vegadex	H	
Ceca	Udonkor	F	532
CeCeCe	Chlormequat	Pg	
Cekiuron	Diuron	H	157
Cekufon	Trichlorfon	I	157
Cekugib	Gibberellic Acid	Pg	157
Cekusan	Dichlorvos	I	157
Cekuzina	Simazine	H	157

Starred ingredients (*) may be responsible for major toxic effects; consult Section II.

PESTICIDES (Cont.)			
PRODUCT NAME	ALTERNATE NAME	PRINCIPAL USE	MANU- FACTURER
Celamerck S-2957	Chlorthiophas	I /Ac	145
Cela S-1942	Bromophos	I /Ac	145
Cela S-2225	Bromophos-Ethyl	I /Ac	145
Celathion	Chlorthiophas	I /Ac	145
Cela W-524	Triforine	F	145
Celdion	Fentiazon	F	724
Celfume	Methyl Bromide	Fm	262
Cellu-Quin	Copper Quinolinolate	F	
Celmer	Methoxyethylmercuric Chloride	F	262
Celmide	1,2-Dibromoethane	Fm	262
Celmone	1-Naphthaleneacetic Acid	Pg	262
Celphos	Phosphine	I /Fm	262
Cepha	Ethephon	Pg	307
Cercobin	Thiophanate	F	
Cercobin-M	Thiophanate Methyl	F	
Cercobin Methyl	Thiophanate Methyl	F	
Ceredon	Benquinox	F	115
Ceregam	(see Societe pour la Protection de l'Agriculture)	I /F	691
Cereline	Benquinox	F	
Ceresan Universal	Phenylmercuric Esters	F /St	115
Certan	Metoxuron	H	646
Certox	Strychnine	R	
Certrol	Ioxynil	H	
CET	Simazine	H	
Cevadine	Sabadilla	I	
CF 125	Chlorflurenol	Pg	145, 766
CFNP		H	
CFV	Chlorfenvinphos	I	
CGA 10832	Profluralin	H	190
CGA 12223		I /N	193
CGA 13586	Etacelasil	Pg	193
CGA 15324		I /Ac	190, 193
CGA 18762	Procyazine	H	193
CGA 24705		H	190, 193
CGA 30599	(see Ciba-Geigy Limited)	F	193
CHE 8728		Pg	488
Check-Mate	(see Vineland Chemical Co.)	H	787
Chem-Bam	Nabam	F	166
Chemform	Streptomycin	B	
Chem-Hoe	Propham	H	595
Chem Neb	Maneb	F	
Chem-O-Bam	Amobam	F	
Cyanamid	Calcium Cyanamide	H /F	805
Cyanamide	Calcium Cyanamide	H /F	
Cyanazine		H	661, 664
Cyanides		R /Fm	046, 370
Cyanofenphos		I	718
Cyanogas	Calcium Cyanide	Fm	046
Cyanophenphos	Cyanofenphos	I	
Cyanophos		I	718
Cyanox	Cyanophos	I	718
CYAP	Cyanophos	I	
Cycle	Procyazine	H	190
Cycloate		H	697
Cyclodan	Thiodan	I /Ac	
Cycloheximide		F /Pg	754
Cyclomorph	Dodemorph	F	
Cyclon	Hydrocyanic Acid	Fm	
Cyclone B	Hydrocyanic Acid	Fm	
Cycloprate	ZR-856	Ac	
Cycluron	(see BASF Aktiengesellschaft)	H	109
Cycocel	Chlormequat	Pg	046
Cycogan	Chlormequat	Pg	439
Cycogan Extra	Chlormequat	Pg	109
Cyfen	Fenitrothion	I /Ac	
Cyflee	Cythioate	I	046
Cygon	Dimethoate	I	046
Cyhexatin		Ac	238

Starred ingredients (*) may be responsible for major toxic effects; consult Section II.

PESTICIDES (Cont.)			
PRODUCT NAME	ALTERNATE NAME	PRINCIPAL USE	MANU- FACTURER
Cylan	Phosfolan	I	046
Cymag	Cyanides	R	370
Cyolan	Phosfolan	I	
Cyolane	Phosfolan	I	046
CYP	Cyanofenphos	I	718
Cypendazole	Bay-Dam 18654	F	
Cyperquat		H	334
Cyprazine		H	334
Cyprex		F	046
Cytel	Fenitrothion	I /Ac	046
Cythioate		I	046
Cythion	Malathion	I	046
Cytrol	Amitril-T	H	
Cytrol Amitrole-T	Amitril-T	H	046
Cytrolane	Mephosfolan	I	046
2,4-D		H	238, 785
D 50	2,4-D	H	664
D 735	Carboxin	F /St	760
D 1221	Carbofuran	I	
DAC 893	Dimethyl-2,3,5,6-Tetrachloroterephthalate	H	232
Dacamine	2,4-D	H	232
Dacamine 4T	Trichlorophenoxyacetic Acid	H	232
Dacamox	Thiofanox	I	232, 664
Daconate	MSMA	H	232
Daconil 2787	Chlorthalonil	F	232
Dacthal	Dimethyl-2,3,5,6-Tetrachloroterephthalate	H	232
Dacthalor	Dimethyl-2,3,5,6-Tetrachloroterephthalate	H	
DAEP		I	532
Dagadip	Carbophenothion	I /Ac	
Dailon	Diuron	H	
Dalapon		H	232, 238
Dal-E-Rad	Disodium Methylarsonate	H	787
Dal-E-Rad 100	Disodium Methylarsonate	H	787
Dal-E-Rad 120	MSMA	H	787
Dalf	Methyl Parathion	I	115
Dalmatian Insect Flowers	Pyrethrum	I	
Daminozide		Pg	760
Danex	Trichlorfon	I	439
Daninon	Chlorfensulphide	Ac	
DAPA	p-Dimethylaminobenzenediazo Sodium Sulfonate	F /St	
Dapacryl	Binapacryl	Ac	346
Daphene	Dimethoate	I /Ac	
Dasanit	Fensulfothion	I /N	115, 488
DATC	Diallate	H	496
Dazomet	Mylone	N	109, 697
Dazzel	Diazinon	I /N	
2,4-DB		H	127, 736
DBCP		Fm	062
2,6-DBN	Dichlobenil	H	580, 736
DBP	n-Butyl Phthalate	Re	625
2,4-D Butyric	2,4-DB	H	
DCB	o-Dichlorobenzene	H /I	238
DCMO	Carboxin	F /St	760
DCMOD	Oxycarboxin	F	760
DCMU	Diuron	H	
DCNA	Dicloran	F	127, 754
d-Con	Warfarin	R	226
DCPA	Dimethyl-2,3,5,6-Tetrachloroterephthalate	H	
DCPC	DMC	Ac	
DCR-1339	Starlicide	Av	
D-D		Fm	661, 667
DDPP	Pyridinitril	F	
DDT		I	233, 502
DDVF	Dichlorvos	I	
DDVP	Dichlorvos	I	
Decanol	Off-Shoot-T	Pg	
Deccotane	Frucote	F	
Dechloran	Mirex	I	

Starred ingredients (*) may be responsible for major toxic effects; consult Section II.

PESTICIDES (Cont.)			
PRODUCT NAME	ALTERNATE NAME	PRINCIPAL USE	MANU-FACTURER
Dechlorane	Mirex	I	031
De-Cut	Maleic Hydrazide	Pg	280
Dedelo	DDT	I	
Dedevap	Dichlorvos	I	115
Ded-Weed	(see Thompson-Hayward Chemical Co.)	H	736
Deet	N,N-Diethyl-m-Toluamide	Re	460
DEF	S,S,S-Tributyl Phosphorotrithioate	Df/H	488
De-Fend	Dimethoate	I	736
De-Fol-Ate	Sodium Chlorate	H	566
De-Green	S,S,S-Tributyl Phosphorotrithioate	Df/H	697
Deiquat	Diquat Dibromide	H	
Delan	Dithianon	F	145
Delan-Col	Dithianon	F	145
Deleaf Defoliant	Tributyl Phosphorotrithioite	Df/H	490
Delicia	Phosphine	Fm	
Delnav	Navadel	I	128
Delphene	N,N-Diethyl-m-Toluamide	Re	343
Delta	Chlorophacinone	R	
Demeton		I /Ac	115, 488
Demeton-S-Methyl Sulfoxide	Oxydemeton-Methyl	I /Ac	115, 488
Demosan	Chloroneb	F	247
Demos-L40	Dimethoate	I /Ac	499
Demox	Demeton	I /Ac	
Denapon	Carbaryl	I	
Derosal	Carbendazim	F	346
Derribante	Dichlorvos	I	610
Derrin	Derris	I	
Derris		I /Ft	121, 275
Des-I-Cate	Endothall	H	566
Desmedipham		H	538, 652
Desmetryn		H	193
De-Sprout	Maleic Hydrazide	Pg	280
Dessin	Dinobuton	Ac/F	475
Destun	Perfluidone	H	739
Destun Cotton Herbicide	Perfluidone	H	739
Detamide	N,N-Diethyl-m-Toluamide	Re	
Dethdiet	Red Squill	R	565
Dethmor	Warfarin	R	565
Dethmore	Warfarin	R	565
Dethnel	Warfarin	R	
Detia	Phosphine	Fm	
Devrinol	Napropamide	H	697
DEX	Bisethylxanthogen	H	631
Dexon	p-Dimethylaminobenzenediazo Sodium Sulfo-nate	F /St	115, 488
Dextrone	Diquat Dibromide	H	188
Dextrone-X	Paraquat	H	
Dialifor		I /Ac	128
Diallate		H	496
Diama	AMA	H	
Diamidfos	Nellite	N	
Dianat	Dicamba	H	
Diazacosterol Hydrochloride	Ornitrol	Av	
Diazajet	Diazinon	I	
Diazatol	Diazinon	I	
Diazide	Diazinon	I	
Diazinon		I	190, 355
Diazoben	p-Dimethylaminobenzenediazo Sodium Sulfo-nate	F /St	
Diazol	Diazinon	I	439
Dibam	Sodium Dimethyl Dithiocarbamate	F	631
Dibrom	Naled	I /Ac	187
1,2-Dibromoethane		Fm	238, 319
Dibutalin	Butralin	H	
Dibutyl Phthalate	n-Butyl Phthalate	Re	
Dibutyl Succinate	Di-n-Butyl Succinate	Re	
Di-n-Butyl Succinate		Re	310
2,6-Di-tert-Butyl-p-Tolyl-N-Methylcarba-mate		H	343

	PESTICIDES (Cont.)		
PRODUCT NAME	ALTERNATE NAME	PRINCIPAL USE	MANU- FACTURER
DIC 1577	Tantizon	H	115
Dicamate		F	
Dicamba		H	781
Dicarbam	Carbaryl	I	109
Dicarzol	Formetanate	I /Ac	538
Dichlobenil		H	580, 736
Dichlofenthion	VC-13 Nemacide	N /I	
Dichlofluanid		F	115
Dichlofluanide	Dichlofluanid	F	
Dichlone		F	355
Dichlor	Propylene Dichloride	Fm	
Di-Chlor Emulsion	Ethylene Dichloride	Fm	
Dichlorfenidim	Diuron	H	
o-Dichlorobenzene		H /I	238
p-Dichlorobenzene		Fm	595
2,4-Dichloro-6-o-Chloroanilino-s-Triazine		F	488
Dichloroethyl Ether	sym-Dichloroethyl Ether	Fm/I	
sym-Dichloroethyl Ether		Fm/I	757
Dichlorofenthion	VC-13 Nemacide	N /I	
Dichlorophen	Dichlorophene	F /B	
Dichlorophene		F /B	685
Dichlorophenoxyacetic Acid	2,4-D	H	
Dichloropropane	Propylene Dichloride	Fm	
Dichloropropane Dichloropropene Mixture	D-D	Fm/N	
Dichloropropene	1,3-Dichloropropene	Fm	
1,3-Dichloropropene		Fm	238
Dichloropropionic Acid	Dalapon	H	
Dichlorphos	Dichlorvos	I	
Dichlorprop		H	109, 115
Dichlorvos		I	115, 661
Dicloran		F	127, 754
Dicofol	Kelthane	Ac	
Dicontal		I	115
Dicrotophos	Bidrin	I	
Dicuran	Chlortoluron	H	193
Didigam	(see ICI Plant Protection Division)	I	370
Didigam S		I	691
Didimac 25	DDT	I	370
Dieldrex	Dieldrin	I	667
Dieldrin		I	667
Dieldrine	Dieldrin	I	
Dieldrite	Dieldrin	I	667
Dienochlor		Ac	352
Diesel Oil		H	265, 493
Diethchinalphion		I	115
Diethion	Ethion	I /Ac	
Diethquinalphione	Diethchinalphion	I	
N,N-Diethylbenzamide		?	
Diethyltoluamide	N,N-Diethyl-m-Toluamide	Re	
N,N-Diethyl-m-Toluamide		Re	460
Di-Farmon	(see Farm Protection Ltd.)	H	286
Difenoxuron	Lironion	H	
Difenson	Ovotran	Ac	
Difenthos	Abate	I	
Difenzoquat		H	046
Diflubenzuron		Ig	580, 736
Difluron	Diflubenzuron	I	
Difolatan	Captafol	F /St	187
Difosan	Captafol	F	
Dikar		F /Ac	634
Dikegulac-Sodium		Pg	434
Dikotex	MCPA	H	
Dimanin A		Al/B	115
Dimanin C		Al/B	115
Dimaz	Disulfoton	I /Ac	
Dimecron	Phosphamidon	I /Ac	187
Dimefox		Ac/I	517, 796
Dimephenthoate	Phenthoate	I /Ac	
Dimet	Disodium Methylarsonate	H	

Starred ingredients (*) may be responsible for major toxic effects; consult Section II.

PESTICIDES (Cont.)			
PRODUCT NAME	ALTERNATE NAME	PRINCIPAL USE	MANU- FACTURER
Dimethenthoate	Phenthoate	I /Ac	
Dimethirimol		F	370
Dimethoate		I /Ac	046, 112
Dimethoate-Met	Omethoate	I /Ac	115
Dimethogen	Dimethoate	I /Ac	
Dimethrin		I	460
p-Dimethylaminobenzenediazo Sodium Sulfo- nate		F /St	115, 488
Dimethyl Arsinic Acid	Cacodylic Acid	H	
Dimethyl Phthalate	Methyl Phthalate	Re	
Dimethyl-2,3,5,6-Tetrachloroterephthalate		H	232
m-(3,3-Dimethylureido) Phenyl-tert-Butylcar- bamate		H	295
Dimexan	Tri-P.E.	H	
Dimexano	Tri-P.E.	H	
Dimilin	Diflubenzuron	I	580, 736
Dimite	DMC	Ac	673
Dinitramine		H	766
Dinitro	4,6-Dinitro-2-sec-Butyl Phenol	H	
Dinitrobutylphenol	4,6-Dinitro-2-sec-Butyl Phenol	H	
4,6-Dinitro-2-sec-Butyl Phenol		H	238
Dinitrocresol	4,6-Dinitro-o-Cresol	I /F	
4,6-Dinitro-o-Cresol		I /F	121, 448
Dinitrophenol	2,4-Dinitrophenol	I /Ac	
2,4-Dinitrophenol		I /Ac	454
Dinobuton		Ac/F	403
Dinocap	Karathane	F /Ac	
Dinofen	Dinobuton	Ac/F	
Dinoseb	4,6-Dinitro-2-sec-Butyl Phenol	H	
Dinoseb Acetate		H	346
Dinoseb Methacrylate	Binapacryl	Ac/F	
Dinoterb Acetate		H /N	517
Di-On	Diuron	H	439
Dioxacarb		I	193
Dioxathion	Navadel	I	128
Dipel (Bacillus Thuringiensis)	Agritol	I	004
Dipel (Heliothis Polyhedrosis Virus)	(see Abbott Laboratories)	I	004
Diphacin	Diphenadione	R	
Diphacinone	Diphenadione	R	
Diphenadione		R	781
Diphenamid		H	754
Diphenyl		F	238, 496
Dipher	Zineb	F	
Dippel's Oil	Bone Oil	I /Re	
Dipram	Propanil	H	
Dipropalin		H	
Dipropetryn	Dipropetryne	H	
Dipropetryne		H	190, 193
Di-n-Propyl Isocinchomerate		Re	460
Dipterex	Trichlorfon	I	115
Diquat	Diquat Dibromide	H	
Diquat Dibromide		H	187, 370
Direz	2,4-Dichloro-6-o-Chloroanilino-s-Triazine	F	
Dirimal	Oryzalin	H	259
Disan	Betasan	H	697
Disodium Methanearsonate	Disodium Methylarsonate	H	
Disodium Methylarsonate		H	199, 232
Disomar	Disodium Methylarsonate	H	
Disulfoton		I /Ac	115, 488
Di-Syston	Disulfoton	I /Ac	115, 488
Disyston S		I /Ac	115
Disyston Sulphoxide	Disyston S	I	115
Di-Systox	Disulfoton	I /Ac	
Di-Tac	Disodium Methylarsonate	H	
Ditalimfos		F	238
Dithane A-40	Nabam	F	634
Dithane D-14	Nabam	F	634
Dithane M-22	Maneb	F	634
Dithane M-22 Special	Maneb	F	634

Starred ingredients (*) may be responsible for major toxic effects; consult Section II.

PRODUCT NAME	ALTERNATE NAME	PRINCIPAL USE	MANU-FACTURER
	PESTICIDES (Cont.)		
Dithane M-45	Mancozeb	F	634
Dithane R-24	Indar	F	634
Dithane Z-78	Zineb	F	634
Dithianon		F	145
Dithio	Sulfotepp	I /Ac	
Dithiodemeton	Disulfoton	I /Ac	
Dithiomethon	Thiometon	I	
Dithione	Sulfotepp	I /Ac	
Dithiosystox	Disulfoton	I /Ac	
Ditranil	Dicloran	F	
Di-Trapex	Vorlex	Fm	538, 652
Diumate	Diuron	H	211
Diurex	Diuron	H	439
Diurol	Diurol 5030	H	439
Diurol 5030		H	439
Diuron		H	247, 355
Divipan	Dichlorvos	I	439
Dixon	Phosphamidon	I /Ac	610
DMA	Disodium Methylarsonate	H	
DMA-4	2,4-D	H	238
DMA-100	Disodium Methylarsonate	H	
DMAA	Cacodylic Acid	H	
DMC (acaricide)		Ac	532
DMC (plant growth regulator)	BAS 0660W	Pg	
DMDT	Methoxychlor	I	
DMP	Methyl Phthalate	Re	
DMSP	Fensulfothion	N /I	
DMTT	Mylone	N /Sl	
DMU	Diuron	H	
DN-289	4,6-Dinitro-2-sec-Butyl Phenol	H	
DNBP	4,6-Dinitro-2-sec-Butyl Phenol	H	
DNC	4,6-Dinitro-o-Cresol	I /F	
DNOC	4,6-Dinitro-o-Cresol	I /F	
DNOCP	Karathane	F /Ac	
DNOSBP	4,6-Dinitro-2-sec-Butyl Phenol	H	
Dodemorfe	Dodemorph	F	
Dodemorph		F	109
Dodine	Cyprex	F	
Doguadine	Cyprex	F	
Dojyopicrin	Chloropicrin	Fm/I	
Dokirin	Copper Quinolinolate	F	
Dol Granule	Lindane	I	523
Dolmix Granule	(see Nihon Nohyaku Co., Ltd.)	I	523
Dolochlor	Chloropicrin	Fm/I	
Doom	Milky Disease Spores	I	274
Doquadine	Cyprex	F	
Dorlone		Fm	238
Dormant Oils		I /H	187, 265
Dormone	2,4-D	H	231
Dosanex	Metoxuron	H	646
Dosanex FL	Metoxuron	H	646
Dosater	Metoxuron	H	646
Double-Noctin		F /St	391
Dovip (livestock insecticide)	Famphur	I	
Dovip (vegetation insecticide)	Phosphamidon	I	
Dowco 132	Ruelene	I	238
Dowco 163	Nitrapyrin	B	238
Dowco 179	Dursban	I	238
Dowco 186	Fentin Hydroxide	F	238
Dowco 199	Ditalimfos	F	238
Dowco 213	Cyhexatin	Ac	238
Dowco 214	Chlorpyrifos-Methyl	I	238
Dowco 233	Triclopyr	H	238
Dowco 269	Pyroxychlor	?	238
Dowco 275		?	238
Dowco 290		H	238
Dowfume 59		Fm	238
Dowfume 75		Fm	238
Dowfume C		Fm	238

Starred ingredients (*) may be responsible for major toxic effects; consult Section II.

PESTICIDES (Cont.)

PRODUCT NAME	ALTERNATE NAME	PRINCIPAL USE	MANU-FACTURER
Dowfume EB-5		Fm	238
Dowfume EB-15 Inhibited		Fm	238
Dowfume F		Fm	238
Dowfume MC-2		Fm	238
Dowfume MC-33		Fm	238
Dowfume N		Fm	238
Dowfume V		Fm	238
Dowfume W-85	1,2-Dibromoethane	Fm	238
Dow General	4,6-Dinitro-2-sec-Butyl Phenol	H	238
Dow General Weed Killer	4,6-Dinitro-2-sec-Butyl Phenol	H	238
Dowicide 1	Phenylphenol	F /Di	238
Dowicide 2	Trichlorophenol	F /B	238
Dowicide 2S	Trichlorophenol	F /B	238
Dowicide 4		F /B	238
Dowicide 6	2,3,4,6-Tetrachlorophenol	F	238
Dowicide 6 Conc.	2,3,4,6-Tetrachlorophenol	F	238
Dowicide 7	Pentachlorophenol	H /Wp	238
Dowicide 31		F /B	238
Dowicide 32		F /B	238
Dowicide A		F	238
Dowicide B	Trichlorophenol	F /B	238
Dowicide F		F /Wp	238
Dowicide G		I /F	238
Dowpon	Dalapon	H	238
Dow Selective	4,6-Dinitro-2-sec-Butyl Phenol	H	238
Dow Selective Weed Killer	4,6-Dinitro-2-sec-Butyl Phenol	H	238
2,4-DP	Dichlorprop	H	
DPA		H /I	046
Drat	Chlorophacinone	R	457
Drawinol	Dinobuton	Ac/F	
Draza	Methiocarb	I	115
Drazoxolon		F	370
DRB	Nirit	F	
Drepamon		H	499
Drexel Defol	Sodium Chlorate	Df	241
Drexel Sucker-Agent 504	Off-Shoot-T	Pg	241
Dri-Die		I	295
Drifene AP		I	562
Drinox	Aldrin	I	
Drinox H-34	Heptachlor	I	
Drop Leaf	Sodium Chlorate	Df	
DRW 1139	Goltix	H	
DS 5328	(see Diamond Shamrock)	H	232
DS 15647	Thiofanox	I	
DSE	Nabam	F	
DSMA	Disodium Methylarsonate	H	
DU 112307	Diflubenzuron	I	
Dual	(see Ciba-Geigy Corp.)	H	190
Dualweed	Chlorobutynyl Chlorocarbanilate	H	292
Duphar	Tetradifon	Ac	580
Duraset	N-m-Tolylphthalamic Acid	Pg	760
Durotox	Pentachlorophenol	Wp	694
Dursban		I	238
Du-Sprex	Dichlobenil	H	580
Du-Ter	Fentin Hydroxide	F	580, 736
Dyanacide	Phenylmercuric Esters	F	
Dyanap		H	760
Dybar	Fenuron	H	247
Dyfonate	Fonofos	I	697
Dygun		I	
Dylox	Trichlorfon	I	115, 488
Dymid	Diphenamid	H	421
Dynex	Diuron	H	211
Dynone	Prothiocarb	F /St	
Dypar	Methyl Parathion	I	
Dyrene	2,4-Dichloro-6-o-Chloroanilino-s-Triazine	F	488
E 500	Ambithion	I	
E 605	Parathion	I	
E 1059	Demeton	I /Ac	

Starred ingredients (*) may be responsible for major toxic effects; consult Section II.

PESTICIDES (Cont.)

PRODUCT NAME	ALTERNATE NAME	PRINCIPAL USE	MANU-FACTURER
Earthcide	Pentachloronitrobenzene	F /St	
Easy Off-D	Tributyl Phosphorotrithioite	Df	490
Eau Grison	Calcium Polysulfide	F	
Ectoral	Ronnel	I	589
EDB	1,2-Dibromoethane	Fm	
E-D-Bee	1,2-Dibromoethane	Fm	
EDC	Ethylene Dichloride	Fm	
EDCO	Methyl Bromide	Fm	
ED/CT	Ethylene Dichloride	Fm	
EDDP	Edifenphos	F	
Edifenphos		F	115, 523
Eerex	Monuron	H	
EGT	Glytac	H	
Ekalux	Diethchinalphion	I	646
Ekamet		I	646
Ekatex	Methyl Parathion	I	
Ekatin	Thiometon	I	646
Ekatin WF	Thiometon	I	646
Ekatox	Parathion	I	
Ektafos	Bidrin	I	193
El-103	Tebuthiuron	H	259
El-119	Oryzalin	H	259
El-131	Prosulfalin	H	259
El-161	Ethalfluralin	H	259
El-179	Isopropalin	H	259
El-241	Parnon	F	259
El-291	Tricyclazole	F	259
El-531	Ancymidol	Pg	259
El-620	Emulphor	Ad	259
El-719	Emulphor	Ad	259
Elancolan	Trifluralin	H	259
Elbanil	Chlorpropham	H	
Elcar	(see Sandoz, Inc.)	I	643
Elgetol	4,6-Dinitro-o-Cresol	I /F	
Elgetol 30	4,6-Dinitro-o-Cresol	I /F	
Elgetol 318	4,6-Dinitro-2-sec-Butyl Phenol	H	
Elocron	Dioxacarb	I	193
Elsan	Phenthoate	I /Ac	535
Elvaron	Dichlofluanid	F	115
Embark	(see 3M Co.)	Pg	739
Embathion	Ethion	I /Ac	
Emblem	Benefin	H	442
Embutox	2,4-DB	H	457
Emerald Green	Copper Acetoarsenite	I	
Emmatos	Malathion	I	
Emmatos Extra	Malathion	I	
Emulphor		Ad	307
Emulsamine E-3		H	757
Endaven	Benzoylprop Ethyl	H	
Endosan	Binapacryl	Ac	346
Endosulfan	Thiodan	I /Ac	
Endothal	Endothall	H	566
Endothall		H /Df	566
Endox	Coumatetralyl	R	
Endrex	Endrin	I	
Endrin		I	667, 781
Endrocid	Coumatetralyl	R	
Enide	Diphenamid	H	754
Enide Dinitro EC		H	754
Enovit	Thiophanate	F	
Enovit-Super	Thiophanate-Methyl	F	
Enstar	Kinoprene	Ig	820
ENT 15108	Parathion	I	
ENT 17510	Allethrin	I	
ENT 20218	N,N-Diethyl-m-Toluamide	Re	
ENT 20871	Sesamex	Ad	
ENT 21170	Dimethrin	I	
ENT 27164	Carbofuran	I /Ac	
ENT 27226	Propargite	Ac	

Starred ingredients (*) may be responsible for major toxic effects; consult Section II.

PESTICIDES (Cont.)			
PRODUCT NAME	ALTERNATE NAME	PRINCIPAL USE	MANU- FACTURER
ENT 27300	Promecarb	I	
ENT 27566	Formetanate	I /Ac	
ENT 27967	Amitraz	I /Ac	
ENT 70531	Kinoprene	Ig	
Entex	Fenthion	I	115
Envert-T	Trichlorophenoxyacetic Acid	H	
EP-316	Promecarb	I	
EP-332	Formetanate	I /Ac	
EP-333	Chlordimeform	I /Ac	
EP-452	Phenmedipham	H	
EP-475	Desmedipham	H	
EPBP		I	535
Ephirsulphonate	Ovotran	Ac	
EPN		Ac/I	247, 781
EPN (pin)	EPN	I /Ac	
Epoxyethane	Ethylene Oxide	Fm	
Epoxypropane	Propylene Oxide	Fm	
Eptam	Ethyl Di-n-Propylthiolcarbamate	H	697
Eptapur		H	109
EPTC	Ethyl Di-n-Propylthiolcarbamate	H	
Equigard	Dichlorvos	I	232
Equino-Aid	Trichlorfon	I	
Erade	Chinomethionat	I /Ac	
Eradex		Ac/F	115
Eradicane		H	697
Erazidon (MU)	Chinomethionat	F /Ac	
Erazidon (MU)	Eradex	Ac/F	
Erbon		H	238
Erbotan	Thiazfluron	H	
Esteron	2,4-D	H	238
Esteron 245	Trichlorophenoxyacetic Acid	H	238
Eston	Metasystox-S	I /Ac	
Estone	2,4-D	H	
Estonmite	Ovotran	Ac	
Estox	Metasystox-S	I /Ac	115
Etacelasil		Pg	190
Etazine	Secbumeton	H	193
ETCMTB	Ethazol	F	
Ethalfluralin		H	259
Ethazol		F	550
Ethephon		Pg	307, 757
Ethiofencarb		I	
Ethiofencarp	Ethiofencarb	I	115
Ethiolate	(see Gulf Oil Chemicals Co.)	H	334
Ethion		I /Ac	295, 625
Ethirimol		F	370
Ethoate-Methyl	Fitios B/77	I /Ac	
Ethodan	Ethion	I	
Ethofumasate		H	291, 292
Ethohexadiol	2-Ethyl-1,3-Hexanediol	Re	
Ethoprop		N /I	490
Ethoprophos	Ethoprop	N /I	
Ethoxyquin		F /Pg	496
Ethrel	Ethephon	Pg	
Ethyl Di-n-Propylthiolcarbamate		H	697
Ethylene		Pg	496, 661
Ethylene Bromide	1,2-Dibromoethane	Fm	
Ethylene Dibromide	1,2-Dibromoethane	Fm	
Ethylene Dichloride		Fm	232, 238
Ethylene Oxide		Fm	112, 757
Ethyl Formate		Fm	205, 304
Ethyl Guthion	Azinphos-Ethyl	I	115
2-Ethyl-1,3-Hexanediol		Re	757
Ethyl Parathion	Parathion	I	
Ethyl Pyrophosphate	Tetraethyl Pyrophosphate	I	
Ethyl Xanthogen Disulfide	Bisethylxanthogen	H	
Etilon	Parathion	I	
ETO	Ethylene Oxide	Fm	
Etridiazol	Ethazol	F	

Starred ingredients (*) may be responsible for major toxic effects; consult Section II.

PRODUCT NAME	ALTERNATE NAME	PRINCIPAL USE	MANU-FACTURER
	PESTICIDES (Cont.)		
Etrimfos	Ekamet	I	
Etrofol		I	115
Etrofolan	Isoprocarb	I	115
Etrolene	Ronnel	I	238
Euparen	Dichlofluanid	F	115
Euparene	Dichlofluanid	F	115
Euparen-M	Tolylfluanid	F	115
Evik	Ametryne	H	190
Evital	Norflurazon	H	643
Evitol	Norflurazon	H	
EXD	Bisethylxanthogen	H	
Exhalt 4-10	(see Kay-Fries Chemicals, Inc., Crop Protection Div.)	At	394
Exotherm	Chlorothalonil	F	232
Exotherm Termil	Chlorothalonil	F	232
Exporsan	Betasan	H	
Extrax	Rotenone	I	
E-Z-Off D	S,S,S-Tributyl Phosphorotrithioate	Df	
FAC	Prothoate	I /Ac	499
FAC Super		Ac	691
Fair-Tac	Off-Shoot-T	Pg	280
FAM	MNFA	I /Ac	
Famfos (vegetation insecticide)	Phosphamidon	I	
Famfos (livestock insecticide)	Famphur	I	
Famid	Dioxacarb	I	193
Famophos	Famphur	I	
Famphur		I	046
Faneron	Bromophenoxime	H	193
Fanfos	Famphur	I	
Far-Go	Triallate	H	496
Farmon Condox	(see Farm Protection Ltd.)	H	286
Fatal	Dimethyl-2,3,5,6-Tetrachloroterephthalate	H	064
FBHC	BHC	I	352
Fenaben	(see Amchem Products)	H	043
Fenac	2,3,6-Trichlorophenylacetic Acid	H	
Fenac Plus		H	757
Fen-All	2,3,6-Trichlorobenzoic Acid	H	733
Fenamin	Atrazine	H	
Fenaminosulf	p-Dimethylaminobenzenediazo Sodium Sulfonate	F /St	
Fenamiphos	Phenamiphos	N	
Fenatrol		H	757
Fenavar		H	757
Fenbutatin-Oxide		Ac	661
Fence Rider	Trichlorophenoxyacetic Acid	H	232
Fenchlorfos	Ronnel	I	
Fenchlorphos	Ronnel	I	
Fenidin	Fenuron	H	
Fenitrothion		I /Ac	038, 115
Fenizon	Fenson	Ac	
Fenolovo	Fentin Hydroxide	F	
Fenolovo Acetate	Fentinacetate	F /Al	
Fenophosphon	Trichloronate	I	
Fenoprop	Silvex	H	
Fenormone	Silvex	H	
Fenson		Ac	499
Fensulfothion		N /I	115, 488
Fenthion		I	115, 488
Fentiazon		F	724
Fentin	Fentinacetate	F /Al	
Fentinacetate		F /Al	346
Fentin Acetate	Fentinacetate	F /Al	
Fentine Acetate	Fentinacetate	F /Al	
Fentin Hydroxide		F	580, 736
Fenulon	Fenuron	H	
Fenuron		H	247
Fenuron-TCA	Urab	H	
Ferbam		F	295
Ferbame	Ferbam	F	

Starred ingredients (*) may be responsible for major toxic effects; consult Section II.

PESTICIDES (Cont.)

PRODUCT NAME	ALTERNATE NAME	PRINCIPAL USE	MANU- FACTURER
Ferberk	Ferbam	F	
Fermate	Ferbam	F	247
Fermide	Thiram	F /St	
Fermide 850	Thiram	F /St	
Fermocide	Ferbam	F	
Fernacol	Thiram	F /St	
Fernasan	Thiram	F /St	370
Fernesta	2,4-D	H	370
Fernimine	2,4-D	H	370
Fernoxone	2,4-D	H	370
Ferrous Sulfate		H /Wp	
Ferxone	2,4-D	H	091
Ficam	Bendiocarb	I	292
Field Clean Weed Killer	2,4-D	H	
Filariol	Bromophos-Ethyl	I /Ac	145
Finaven	Difenzoquat	H	
Finidim	Fenuron	H	
Fintrol	Antimycin-A	Ft	100
Fire Ant Bait	Mirex	I	031
Fish-Tox	Rotenone	Ft	
Fitios B/77		I /Ac	499
Flac	Calcium Arsenate	I /H	
Flavensomycin	(see Montedison S.p.A.)	B	499
Flit MLO	(see Exxon Company)	L	265
Floraltone	TIBA	Pg	757
Florel	Ethephon	Pg	757
Florencol	Flurenol	H	
Flotation Sulfur	Sulfur	F /Ac	
Flowers of Sulfur	Sulfur	F /Ac	
Fluchloralin		H	110, 112
Flufenprop-Isopropyl	Barnon	H	667
Fluometuron		H	190, 193
Fluorakil 100	Fluoroacetamide	R	
Fluoretoxuron		H	346
Fluoridamid		Pg	781
Fluoroacetamide		I	010
Fluoroacetanilide		R	277
Fluoroacetate		R	010
Fluoromidine	Ethofumasate	H	
Flurecol	Flurenol	H	
Flurecol-n-Butylester	Flurenol	H	
Flurenol		H	145
FMC 5273	Piperonyl Butoxide	Ad	295
FMC 9102	Metiram	F	295
FMC 9260	Tetramethrin	I	295
FMC 10242	Carbofuran	I /N	295
FMC 11092	m-(3,3-Dimethylureido) Phenyl-tert-Butylcar-bamate	H	295
FMC 17370	Resmethrin	I	295
Folbex	Chlorobenzilate	Ac	193
Folcid	Captafol	F	
Folcidin	Bay-Dam 18654	F	115
Folex	Tributyl Phosphorotrithioite	H	490
Folidol	Parathion	I	115
Folidol E-605	Parathion	I	115
Folidol M	Methyl Parathion	I	115
Folimat	Omethoate	I /Ac	115
Folithion	Fenitrothion	I /Ac	115
Folosan	Fusarex	F /Pg	
Folpan	Folpet	F	439
Folpet		F	187, 697
Fonofos		I	697
Fore	Mancozeb	F	634
Forlin	Lindane	I	298
For-Mal 50	Malathion	I	298
Formaldehyde	Formaldehyde Solution	F /B	
Formaldehyde Solution		F /B	247, 496
Formalin	Formaldehyde Solution	F /B	
Formetanate		Ac/I	538, 652

Starred ingredients (*) may be responsible for major toxic effects; consult Section II.

PESTICIDES (Cont.)

PRODUCT NAME	ALTERNATE NAME	PRINCIPAL USE	MANU-FACTURER
Formetanate Hydrochloride	Carzol	I /Ac	
Formothion		I /Ac	646
Formula 40	2,4-D	H	238
Forron	Trichlorophenoxyacetic Acid	H	
Forstan	Chinomethionat	I /Ac	
For-Syn	Resmethrin	I	298
Fortified Oils	Petroleum Distillate	I /H	
Fortrol	Cyanazine	H	664
Forturf	Chlorothalonil	F	
Fos-Fall A	S,S,S-Tributyl Phosphorotrithioate	Df	488
Fosfamid	Dimethoate	I /Ac	
Fosferno	Parathion	I	370
Fosferno 50	Parathion	I	370
Fosferno M 50	Methyl Parathion	I	370
Fospirate	Chlorpyrifos-Methyl	I	238
Fostion	Prothoate	I /Ac	499
Fostion MM	Dimethoate	I /Ac	046
Fosvex	Tetraethyl Pyrophosphate	I	
Fratol	Fluoroacetate	R	
French Green	Copper Acetoarsenite	I	
Frenock		H	718
Frescon	Triphenmorph	M	667
Frucote		F	259
Fruitdo	Copper Quinolinolate	F	
Fruitone A	Trichlorophenoxyacetic Acid	H	757
Fruitone N	1-Naphthaleneacetic Acid	Pg	757
Fruitone T	Silvex	H	757
Frumin Al	Disulfoton	I /Ac	646
Fuberidazol	Fuberidazole	F /St	
Fuberidazole		F /St	115
Fuel Oil		I /H	187, 265
Fuklasin	Ziram	F	652
Fulcin	Griseofulvin	F /B	
Fulvicin	Griseofulvin	F /B	
Fumagon	DBCP	Fm	
Fumarin	Coumafuryl	R	757
Fumasol	Coumafuryl	R	757
Fumazone 86	DBCP	Fm	238
Fumazone 86E	DBCP	Fm	238
Fumette	(see Bayer AG)	Fm	115
Fumigant-1	Methyl Bromide	Fm	781
Fumo-Gas	1,2-Dibromoethane	Fm	052
Fundal	Chlordimeform	I /Ac	538, 652
Fundex	Chlordimeform	I /Ac	
Fungchex	Mercuric Chloride	F	784
Fungiclor	Pentachloronitrobenzene	F /St	
Funginex	Triforine	F	145
Fungi-Rhap CU 6 Liquid Copper Fungicide	(see Transvaal, Inc.)	F	745
Fungo	Thiophanate Methyl	F	442
Fungo 50	Thiophanate Methyl	F	442
Furadan	Carbofuran	I /N	295, 488
Furcarbanil		F	109
Furidazol	Fuberidazole	F /St	
Furloe	Chlorpropham	H	595
Furmarin	Coumafuryl	R	
Fussol	Fluoroacetamide	R	649
FW 293	Kelthane	Ac	
FW 734	Propanil	H	
Fyfanon	Malathion	I	175
Fylene	Metoxuron	H	646
Fytolan	Cupric Chloride, Basic	F	
G 23992	Chlorobenzilate	Ac	
G 24163	Chloropropylate	Ac	
G 24480	Diazinon	I /N	
G 27692	Simazine	H	
G 27901	Trietazine	H	
G 28029	Phencapton	Ac	
G 30027	Atrazine	H	
G 30028	Propazine	H	

Starred ingredients (*) may be responsible for major toxic effects; consult Section II.

	PESTICIDES (Cont.)		
PRODUCT NAME	ALTERNATE NAME	PRINCIPAL USE	MANU- FACTURER
G 30044	Simetone	H	
G 30130	Propanil	H	
G 30344	Simazine	H	
G 32911	Simetryn	H	
G 34161	Prometryne	H	
G 34162	Ametryne	H	
G 36393	Methoprotryne	H	
G.A.	Gibberellic Acid	Pg	
Galecron	Chlordimeform	I	190
Galipan	Benazolin	H	
Gallotox	Phenylmercuric Esters	F /H	751
Gamaphex	Lindane	I	
Gamma BHC	Lindane	I	
Gammagof	Lindane	I	
Gamma HCH	Lindane	I	
Gammalin	Lindane	I	370
Gammalin 20	Lindane	I	370
Gammex	Lindane	I	
Gammexane	Lindane	I	370
Ganocide	Drazoxolon	F	370
Gardcide	Tetrachlorvinphos	I	
Gardentox	Diazinon	I /N	
Gardona	Tetrachlorvinphos	I	667
Gardoprim		H	193
Garlon	Silvex	H	238
Garrathion	Carbophenothion	I /Ac	697
Garvox	Bendiocarb	I	292
Gatnon	Benzthiazuron	H	115
GC 1189	Kepone	I	
GC 1283	Mirex	I	
GC 2466	Mucochloric Anhydride	F	
GC 3703	Bomyl	I	
GCC 711		H	361
GCP 1634	Cyperquat	H	
Gearphos	Methyl Parathion	I	
Gebutox	4,6-Dinitro-2-sec-Butyl Phenol	H /F	346
Genitox	DDT	I	031
Gerdoprim	Terbuthylazine	H	
Germ-Mate		St	391
Gerox	Streptomycin	B	
Gesabal	Heptazine	H	193
Gesadural	Simetone	H	193
Gesafloc	Trietazine	H	193
Gesafram	Methoxy Propazine	H	193
Gesagard	Prometryne	H	193
Gesamil	Propazine	H	193
Gesapax	Ametryne	H	193
Gesapon	DDT	I	193
Gesaprim	Atrazine	H	193
Gesaran	Methoprotryne	H	193
Gesarex	DDT	I	193
Gesarol	DDT	I	193
Gesatop	Simazine	H	193
Gesoran	Simazine	H	
Gestatop	Simazine	H	
Gibberellic Acid		Pg	004, 574
Gibberellin	Gibberellic Acid	Pg	
Gibrel	Gibberellic Acid	Pg	466
Gib-Sol	Gibberellic Acid	Pg	259
Gib-Tabs	Gibberellic Acid	Pg	259
Glucochloralose	Alphachloralose	Re	
Glyodex	(see Agway Inc.)	F	025
Glyodin		F /Ac	025
Glyoxime		Pg	190
Glyphosate		H	496
Glyphosine		Pg	496
Glytac		H	547
Golden Decoy		I	559
Goltix		H	115

Starred ingredients (*) may be responsible for major toxic effects; consult Section II.

PESTICIDES (Cont.)

PRODUCT NAME	ALTERNATE NAME	PRINCIPAL USE	MANU- FACTURER
Goodrite ZAC	(see Goodrich)	F	313
Gotnion	Guthion	I	
Grain Storer P	(see Cenex)	F	151
Grain Treet	(see Kemin Industries)	F	397
Grainwet	(see Kalo Laboratories, Inc.)		391
Gramevin	Dalapon	H	
Gramoxone	Paraquat	H	370
Gramoxone S	Paraquat	H	370
Granol NM		F /St	364
Granox Liquid		F /St	364
Granox NM	Granox Liquid	St	364
Granox PFM		F /St	364
Grascide	Propanil	H	
Grassland Weedkiller	Benazolin	H	127
Green Vitriol	Ferrous Sulfate	H /Wp	
Gresfeed	Griseofulvin	F	
Grex	Benomyl	F	
Grifulvin	Griseofulvin	F	463
Griseofulvin		F /B	028, 466
Grisetin	Griseofulvin	F	
Grocel	Gibberellic Acid	Pg	
GS 13005	Methidathion	I /Ac	
GS 13529	Terbuthylazine	H	
GS 14254	Secbumiton	H	
GS 14259	Terbumeton	H	
GS 14260	Terbutryne	H	
GS 16068	Dipropetryne	H	
GS 19851	Bromopropylate	Ac	
GS 29696	Thiazfluron	H	
Guanidine	Cyprex	F	
Guanoctine	Guazatine	F	
Guazatine		F	403
Gusathion	Guthion	I	115
Gusathion A	Azinphos-Ethyl	I	115
Gusathion A-M		I	115
Gusathion M	Guthion	I	115
Guthion		I	115, 488
Gypsine	Lead Arsenate	I	
Gypsum	(see U.S. Gypsum Co., Chemicals Div.)	C	769
Gyron	DDT	I	
H 321	Methiocarb	I	
H 1313	Dichlobenil	H	
Haiari	Rotenone	I /Ft	
Halizan	Metaldehyde	M	727
Halts	Bandane	H	
Hanane	Dimefox	Ac/I	
HC 1281	2,3,6-Trichlorobenzoic Acid	H	
HCB	Hexachlorobenzene	F /St	
HCCH	BHC	I	
HCH	BHC	I	
HCN	Hydrocyanic Acid	Fm	
Hedonal	2,4-D	H	115
Heliothis Polyhedrosis Virus	Biotrol VHZ	I	
Heliotropin Acetal	Tropital	Ad	
HEOD	Dieldrin	I	
Heptachlor		I	781
Heptamul	Heptachlor	I	
Heptazine		H	193
Heptenophos		I	346
Herbatim	Vapam	F /H	
Herbazin	Simazine	H	
Herbazolin	Benazolin	H	
Herbicide 273	Endothall	H	566
Herbicide 283	Endothall	H	566
Herbiol	Petroleum Distillate	I /H	
Herbisan	Bisethylxanthogen	H	631
Herbit	Phenothiol	H	349
Herbitox	VM & P Naphthas	H	
Herbizole	3-Amino-1,2,4-Triazole	H	280

Starred ingredients (*) may be responsible for major toxic effects; consult Section II.

PESTICIDES (Cont.)			
PRODUCT NAME	ALTERNATE NAME	PRINCIPAL USE	MANU- FACTURER
Hercules 9753	2,6-Di-tert-Butyl-p-Tolyl-N-Methylcarba-mate	H	343
Hercules 14503	Dialifor	I /Ac	343
Hercules 22234	Antor	H	343
Hercules AC 528	Navadel	I	343
Hercules AC 5727	UC 10854	I	343
Herkol	Dichlorvos	I	
Hexa C.B.	Hexachlorobenzene	F	
Hexachlor	BHC	I	
Hexachloran	BHC	I	
Hexachloride	BHC	I	
Hexachlorobenzene		St	364
Hexachloroethane		An	367
Hexachlorophene		F /B	391
Hexadrin	Endrin	I	
Hexaferb	Ferbam	F	
Hexafor	BHC	I	625
Hexa-Nema	VC-13 Nemacide	N /I	
Hexapoudre	BHC	I	625
Hexasul	Sulfur	F /Ac	
Hexathane	Zineb	F	
Hexathir	Thiram	F /St	
Hexavin	Carbaryl	I	
Hexazir	Ziram	F	
Hexide	Hexachlorophene	F /B	391
Hexyclan	BHC	I	
Hexyclan Soprocide	BHC	I	
Hexylthiocarbam	Cycloate	H	
HHDN	Aldrin	I	
Hibrom	Naled	I /Ac	
Hinosan	Edifenphos	F	115, 523
Hizarocin	Cycloheximide	F /B	
HOCH	Formaldehyde Solution	F /B	
Hoe 2671	Thiodan	I /Ac	346
Hoe 2747	Monolinuron	H	346
Hoe 2784	Binapacryl	Ac/F	346
Hoe 2873	Pyrazophos	F	346
Hoe 2904	Dinoseb Acetate	H	346
Hoe 2960	Triazophos	I /N	346
Hoe 2982	Heptenophos	I	346
Hoe 2989	Pyracarbolid	F	346
Hoe 2991	Fluoretoxuron	H	346
Hoe 6052	Pyracarbolid	F	346
Hoe 6053	Pyracarbolid	F	346
Hoe 13764	Pyracarbolid	F	346
Hoe 16410	Isoproturon	H	346
Hoe 17411	Carbendazim	F	346
Hoe 22870		H	346
Hoe 23408		H	346
Hokko-Mycin	Streptomycin	B	
Hokmate	Ferbam	F	
Holtox		H	664
Homai		F /St	532
Hong Nien	Phenylmercuric Esters	F /H	
Hopcide	Etrofol	I	418
Hopcin	Bassa	I	
Horbadox	Penoxalin	H	
Hormex Rooting-Powder	Indolebutyric Acid	Pg	
Hormodin	Indolebutyric Acid	Pg	466
Hormotuho	MCPA	H	400
Hosdon		I	523
Hosdon Granule	Hosdon	I	523
Hostaquick	Heptenophos	I	346
Hostathion	Triazophos	I /N	346
HOX	Ethiofencarb	I	
HRS-16	Dienochlor	Ac	
Hydout	Endothall	H	566
Hydram	Molinate	H	697
Hydrocyanic Acid		Fm	046, 247

Starred ingredients (*) may be responsible for major toxic effects; consult Section II.

PESTICIDES (Cont.)

PRODUCT NAME	ALTERNATE NAME	PRINCIPAL USE	MANU-FACTURER
Hydrogen Cyanide	Hydrocyanic Acid	Fm	
Hydrol	Allyxycarb	I	115
Hydroprene	Altozar	Ig	
Hydrothal	Endothall	H	
Hydrothol	Endothall	H	566
Hydroxydiphenyl	Phenylphenol	F /Di	
2-Hydroxyethyl-n-Octyl Sulfide		Re	460
Hydroxyisoxazole	Tachigaren	F/Pg	
8-Hydroxyquinoline		F /B	
Hykil	Petroleum Distillate	I /H	361
Hymexazole	Tachigaren	F /Pg	
Hytox	Etrofolan	I	590
Hyvar	Bromacil	H	247
Hyvar XL	Bromacil	H	247
Hyvar XP	Bromacil	H	247
IBA	Indolebutyric Acid	Pg	
IBP	Kitazin	F	
IFC	Propham	H	
Igran	Terbutryne	H	190
Ikurin	Ammonium Sulfamate	H	
Imidan		I	697
Imugan	Chloraniformethan	F	115
Inakor	Atrazine	H	
Incco	Valone	R	
Indar		F	634
Indolebutyric Acid		Pg	466, 722
Inezin	(see Nissan Chemical Industries, Ltd.)	F	535
INPC	Propham	H	
Insectophene	Thiodan	I /Ac	
Inverton 245	Trichlorophenoxyacetic Acid	H	
Iodofenphos		I	193
Iotox	Ioxynil	H	
Ioxynil		H	457
IPC	Propham	H	595
IPPC	Propham	H	
IPSP	Aphidan	I	
Iron Sulfate	Ferrous Sulfate	H /Wp	
Iscothan	Karathane	F /Ac	
Iscothane	Karathane	F /Ac	
Isobac	Hexachlorophene	F	391
Isobac 20	Hexachlorophene	F	391
Isobenzan		I	667
Isocarb		I	433
Isocarbamid	Merpelan AZ	H	
Iso-Cornox	Mecoprop	H	127
Isofenphos	Oftanol	I	
Isomethiozin	Tantizon	H	
Isoprocarb		I	115
Isopropalin		H	259
Isopropoxyphenyl N-Methylcarbamate		I	115, 488
Isoproturon		H	193, 346
Isothan	Lauryl Isoquinolinium Bromide	F	553
Isothioate	Hosdon	I	
Isotox	Lindane	I	187
Isoval	Valone	R	
Isoxathion		I	649
IT 3233	Flurenol	H	
IT 3456	Chlorflurenol	Pg	
Itopaz	Ethion	I /Ac	
Ivoset	Dinoseb Acetate	H	
Ivosit	Dinoseb Acetate	H	109
Ixodex	DDT	I	
Japidemic	Milky Disease Spores	I	274
Jiffy Grow	Indolebutyric Acid	Pg	
Jodfenphos	Iodofenphos	I	
Jolt	Ethoprop	N /I	781
Jon-Trol	Disodium Methylarsonate	H	626
Kaken	Cycloheximide	Pg	
Kalo	Calcium Arsenate	I	

Starred ingredients (*) may be responsible for major toxic effects; consult Section II.

PESTICIDES (Cont.)

PRODUCT NAME	ALTERNATE NAME	PRINCIPAL USE	MANU-FACTURER
Kanepar	Chlorfenac	H	181
Karamate		F	
Karathane		F	634
Karbaspray	Carbaryl	I	
Karbation	Vapam	F /Fm	
Karbofos	Malathion	I /Ac	
Karbutilate	m-(3,3-Dimethylureido)Phenyl-tert-Butylcar-bamate	H	
Karmex	Diuron	H	247
Karphos	Isoxathion	I	649
Karsan	Formaldehyde Solution	F /B	
Kasugamycin	Kasumin	F	
Kasumin		F	349
Kathon LP	(see Rohm and Haas Co.)	F	634
Kathon 893 SP	(see Rohm and Haas Co.)	F /St	634
Kauritil	Cupric Chloride, Basic	F	109
Kayafume	Methyl Bromide	Fm	
Kazoe		H /F	595
K-Cop Liquid Agricultural Fungicide	(see Kocide Chemical Corp.)	F	412
Kelthane		I /Ac	439, 634
Kemate	2,4-Dichloro-6-o-Chloroanilino-s-Triazine	F	
Kenapon	Dalapon	H	238
Kepone		I	031
Kerb	Pronamide	H	634
Kerosene		H	265, 295
Kerosine	Kerosene	H	
Kildip	Dichlorprop	H	
Killex	Trimec	H	
Kill Kantz	ANTU	R	
Kilmag	Calcium Arsenate	I /H	031
Kilmite-40	Tetraethyl Pyrophosphate	I	475
Kiloseb	4,6-Dinitro-2-sec-Butyl Phenol	H	
Kilprop	Mecoprop	H	
Kilrat	Zinc Phosphide	R	
Kilsem	MCPA	H	
Kilval	Vamidothion	I /Ac	625
Kinoprene		I	820
Kitazin		F	418
Kitazin-P	Kitazin	F	418
Klean-Krop	Dyanap	H	736
Klean-Up	(see Thompson-Hayward Chemical Co.)	H	736
Kleen-Krop	Dyanap	H	
Kleer-Lot		H	757
Kloben	Neburon	H	247
Klorex	Sodium Chlorate	H	403
K-Lox	(see Sandoz, Inc.)	Al	643
K-Lox S	K-Pool	Al	412
KMH	Maleic Hydrazide	Pg	
Knockbal		I	349
Knockmate	Ferbam	F	
Knoxweed		H	697
Koban	Ethazol	F	442
Kobu	Pentachloronitrobenzene	F /St	
Kobutol	Pentachloronitrobenzene	F /St	
Kocide	Copper Hydroxide	F	412
Kocide 101	Copper Hydroxide	F	412
Kocide 220	Copper Hydroxide	F	412
Kocide 404	Copper Hydroxide	F	412
Kolofog	Sulfur	F /Ac	295
Kolospray	Sulfur	F /Ac	295
Komeen	(see Sandoz, Inc.)	H	643
Kopfume	1,2-Dibromoethane	Fm	
Kop-Fume	1,2-Dibromoethane	Fm	
Kop Karb	Basic Copper Carbonate	F	
Kopmite	Chlorobenzilate	Ac	
Kop-Mite	Chlorobenzilate	Ac	
Korlan	Ronnel	I	238
Kotol	BHC	I	664
K-Pin	Picloram	H	

Starred ingredients (*) may be responsible for major toxic effects; consult Section II.

PRODUCT NAME	ALTERNATE NAME	PRINCIPAL USE	MANU- FACTURER
K-Pool	(see Kocide Chemical Corp.)	Al	412
Krecalvin	Dichlorvos	I	
Krenite		H	247
Krenite Brush Control Agent	Krenite	H /Pg	247
Krezone	MCPA	H	
Kroma-Clor	(see Mallinckrodt, Inc.)	F	442
Kromad	(see Mallinckrodt, Inc.)	F	442
Krotiline	2,4-D	H	
Krovar		H	247
Krumkil	Coumafuryl	R	754
Kryocide	Cryolite	I	566
Krysid	ANTU	R	
KSM	Kasumin	F	
KUE 2079 A	Clearcide	H	
KUE 13032 c	Dichlofluanid	F	
KUE 13183 b	Tolylfluanid	F	
Kumiai	Metacrate	I	
Kumulus	Sulfur	F /Ac	109
Kumulus S	Sulfur	F /Ac	109
Kuprite	Cuprous Oxide	F	
Kuron	Silvex	H	238
Kurosal	Silvex	H	
Kusakira	Credazine	H	649
Kusatol	Sodium Chlorate	H	
Kwik-Kil	Strychnine	R	
Kwit	Ethion	I /Ac	655
Kylar	Daminozide	Pg	760
Kypchlor	Chlordane	I	
Kypfarin	Warfarin	R	
Kypfos	Malathion	I	
Kypman	Maneb	F	
Kypzin	Zineb	F	
Labilite		F	532
Lamprecide		Ft	346
Landrin		I	661
Lanex	Fluometuron	H	538
Lannate	Methomyl	I	247
Larvacide	Chloropicrin	Fm/I	
Larvatrol	Agritol	I	445
Lasso	Alachlor	H	496
Lauryl Isoquinolinium Bromide		?	
Lauxtol A	Pentachlorophenol	H /Wp	
Lazo	Alachlor	H	
Lead Arsenate (Acid or Basic)		I	433, 817
Lebaycid	Fenthion	I	115
Legumex	4-(2-Methyl-4-Chlorophenoxy)Butyric Acid	H	291
Leguminez Extra	Benazolin	H	127
Legurame	Carbetamide	H	
Lemonene	Diphenyl	F	
Lenacil		H	247
Leptophos		I	781
Lethalaire G-52	Tetraethyl Pyrophosphate	I	790
Lethalaire G-54	Parathion	I	790
Lethane 384	B-Butoxy-B-Thiocyanodiethyl Ether	I	634
Lethox	Carbophenothion	I /Ac	590
Leymin	Benazolin	H	
Lexone	Metribuzin	H	247
Ley-Cornox	Benazolin	H	127
Leytosan	Phenylmercuric Esters	F	
LH 3012	Propineb	F	
Lilly-36352	Trifluralin	H	
Lime Sulfur	Calcium Polysulfide	F /I	
Lindafor	Lindane	I	625
Lindagam	Lindane	I	
Lindamul	Lindane	I	625
Lindane		I	352, 625
Lindol 6G	Lindane	I	
Line Rider	Trichlorophenoxyacetic Acid	H	232
Linormone	MCPA	H	562

Starred ingredients (*) may be responsible for major toxic effects; consult Section II.

PESTICIDES (Cont.)			
PRODUCT NAME	ALTERNATE NAME	PRINCIPAL USE	MANU-FACTURER
Lintox	Lindane	I	697
Linurex	Linuron	H	439
Linuron		H	247, 346
Liphadione	Chlorophacinone	R	
Liquiphene	Phenylmercuric Esters	F	
Liranox	Mecoprop	H	
Lironion		H	193
LM-91	Chlorophacinone	R	
Lolop Granule		H	523
Lonacol	Zineb	F	115
Lonchocarpus	Cube Extract	I /Ft	
Lonocol M	Maneb	F	
Lorox	Linuron	H	247
Lorsban	Dursban	I	238
Lorvec	Pyroxychlor	F	
Lucel	Chlorquinox	F	292
Lumeton	Methoprotryne	H	193
Luprosil	(see BASF Aktiengesellschaft)	F	109
Lurat	Coumafuryl	R	
Lutrol	Edifenphos	F	
M 40	MCPA	H	
M 74	Disulfoton	I /Ac	
M 81	Thiometon	I	
M 3432	Drepamon	H	
Macbal		I	349
Machete	Butachlor	H	496
Macondray	2,4-D	H	
Mad		H	736
MAFA	Neo-Asozin	F	
MAFU	Dichlorvos	I	115
Magic Circle Repellents	Bone Oil	Re	696
Magnetic 70	Sulfur	F /Ac	
Maintain-3	Maleic Hydrazide	Pg	766
Maintain-CF125	Chlorflurenol	Pg	766
Malachite	Basic Copper Carbonate	F	
Malamar	Malathion	I	
Malaphos	Malathion	I	
Malariol	(see Shell International Chemical Co.)	L	667
Malaspray	Malathion	I	
Malathion		I	046, 626
Maleic Hydrazide		Pg	241, 760
Maleic Hydrazine	Maleic Hydrazide	Pg	
Malix	Thiodan	I /Ac	346
Maloran	Chlorbromuron	H	190, 193
Malphos	Malathion	I	
MAMA		H	067
Mancofol	Mancozeb	F	
Mancozeb		F	247, 634
Maneb		F	247, 634
Maneba	Maneb	F	
Manebgan	Maneb	F	439
Manesan	Maneb	F	625
Manoc	Maneb	F	
Manzate 200	Mancozeb	F	247
Manzate 200 Fungicide	Mancozeb	F	247
Manzeb	Mancozeb	F	
Maposol	Vapam	Fm	601
Mar-Frin	Warfarin	R	451
Marlate	Methoxychlor	I	247
Marmer	Diuron	H	
Marpelon		H	
Marvex	Dichlorvos	I	
MAS	Rhizoctol	F /St	
Matacil	Aminocarb	I	115, 488
Mataven	Difenzoquat	H	667
Maygon		H	664
MB	Methyl Bromide	Fm	
MB 9057	Asulam	H	457
MB 10064	Bromoxynil	H	457

Starred ingredients (*) may be responsible for major toxic effects; consult Section II.

PRODUCT NAME	ALTERNATE NAME	PRINCIPAL USE	MANU-FACTURER
	PESTICIDES (Cont.)		
MBC	Sodium Chlorate Borate	H	547
MBR-6033	Fluoridamid	Pg	739
MBR-8251	Perfluidone	H	739
MBR-12325		Pg/H	739
MBX	Methyl Bromide	Fm	
MC 25	Guazatine	F	517
MC 474	Mecarbam	I /Ac	517
MC 1053	Dinobuton	Ac/F	517
MC 1108	Dinoterb Acetate	H /N	517
MC 2188	Chlormephos	I	517
MC 4379	Bifenox	H	517
MCP	MCPA	H	
MCPA		H	231, 785
MCPB	4-(2-Methyl-4-Chlorophenoxy)Butyric Acid	H	
4-MCPB	4-(2-Methyl-4-Chlorophenoxy)Butyric Acid	H	
MCP-Butyric	4-(2-Methyl-4-Chlorophenoxy)Butyric Acid	H	
MCPP	Mecoprop	H	
M-Diphar	Maneb	F	
MEB	Maneb	F	
MEB 6046		I	115
MEB 6447	Bay-Meb 6447	F	115
Mebenil	Methylmetiram	F	
MeBr	Methyl Bromide	Fm	
Mecarbam		I /Ac	517, 724
Mecoper	Mecoprop	H	538
Mecopex	Mecoprop	H	505
Mecoprop		H	199, 231
Mediben	Dicamba	H	
Meldane	Coumaphos	I	
Melprex	Cyprex	F	046
Meltatox	Dodemorph	F	109
MEMA	Panogen	F /St	
MEMC	Methoxyethylmercuric Chloride	F	
Menazon		I	370
Mencs	Vorlex	Fm	
Mendok		Pg	
Menite	Phosdrin	I /Ac	
Meobal		I	718
MEP	Fenitrothion	I /Ac	
Mepaton	Methyl Parathion	I	
Mephanac	MCPA	H	
Mephosfolan		I	046
Mepro	Mecoprop	H	
Meptox	Methyl Parathion	I	
Mercaptodimethur	Methiocarb	I	
Mercaptofos	Demeton	I /Ac	
Mercaptophos	Demeton	I /Ac	
Mercaptothion	Malathion	I	
Mercuram	Thiram	F	787
Mercuric Chloride		F /I	574
Mercuric Oxide	Mercury Compounds	F	
Mercurous Chloride		F	442
Mercury Bichloride	Mercuric Chloride	F /I	
Mercury Compounds		I /F	
Merge 823	MSMA	H	736
Merkazin	Prometryne	H	
Merpan	Captan	F	439
Merpelan AZ		H	115
Merphos	Tributyl Phosphorotrithioite	H	490
Mersolite	Phenylmercuric Esters	F /H	784
Mertect	Thiabendazole	F	466
Mesamate	MSMA	H	211
Mesoranil	Aziprotryn	H	193
Mesurol	Methiocarb	I	115, 488
MET 1486	Ustilan	H	
Meta	Metaldehyde	M	
Metacetaldehyde	Metaldehyde	M	
Metacide	Methyl Parathion	I	115
Metacil	Aminocarb	I	

Starred ingredients (*) may be responsible for major toxic effects; consult Section II.

PESTICIDES (Cont.)			
PRODUCT NAME	ALTERNATE NAME	PRINCIPAL USE	MANU-FACTURER
Metacrate		I	718
Metadelphene	N,N-Diethyl-m-Toluamide	Re	343
Metafos	Methyl Parathion	I	
Metaldehyde		M	205
Metalkamate	Bufencarb	I	
Metam	Vapam	Fm	
Metam-Fluid BASF	Vapam	Fm	109
Metamitron	Goltix	H	
Metam-Sodium	Vapam	Fm	
Metaphos	Methyl Parathion	I	
Metasystemox	Oxydemeton-Methyl	I /Ac	
Metasystox-R	Oxydemeton-Methyl	I /Ac	115, 488
Metasystox-S	Oxydemeton-Methyl	I /Ac	115
Metaxon	MCPA	H	
Methabenzthiazuron		H	115
Methachlorphenprop	Chlorfenprop-Methyl	H	
Metham	Vapam	Fm	
Methamidophos		I	187, 488
Metham-Sodium	Vapam	Fm	
Methanal	Formaldehyde Solution	F /B	
Methanearsonate	AMA	H	
Methar (W.A. Cleary Corp.)	Disodium Methylarsonate	H	199
Methar (MU)	AMA	H	
Methazole		H	781
Methidathion		I /Ac	190, 193
Methiocarb		I	115, 488
Meth-O-Gas	Methyl Bromide	Fm	319
Methomyl		I /N	247, 661
Methoprene		Ig	820
Methoprotryne		H	193
Methoxcide	Methoxychlor	I	
Methoxo	Methoxychlor	I	
Methoxone (ICI Plant Protection Division)	Mecoprop	H	370
Methoxone (MU)	MCPA	H	
Methoxychlor		I	247, 355
Methoxyethylmercuric Chloride		F	115, 262
Methoxyethylmercury Chloride	Methoxyethylmercuric Chloride	F	
Methoxyethylmercury Silicate	Ceregam	I /F	
Methoxy Propazine		H	190
Methyl Bromide		Fm	238, 319
4-(2-Methyl-4-Chlorophenoxy)Butyric Acid		H	457, 626
Methylene Chloride		F	238, 352
Methyl Fosferno	Methyl Parathion	I	
Methyl Guthion	Guthion	I	
Methyl-Mercaptophos Teolovy	Demeton	I /Ac	
Methylmetiram		F	109
Methyl Niran	Methyl Parathion	I	
Methyl Nonyl Ketone		Re	460
Methyl Parathion		I	406, 496
Methyl Phthalate		Re	253
Methylthiophanate	Thiophanate Methyl	F	
Methylthiotriazine	Desmetryn	H	
Metilmercaptofosoksid	Oxydemeton-Methyl	I /Ac	
Metilmerkaptofosoksid	Oxydemeton-Methyl	I /Ac	
Metiltriazotion	Azinphos-Ethyl	I	
Metiram		F	109
Metmercapturon	Methiocarb	I	
Metobromuron	Patoran	H	
Metoprotryn	Methoprotryne	H	
Metoxuron		H	646
Metribuzin		H	247, 488
Metron	Methyl Parathion	I	406
Mevinphos	Phosdrin	I /Ac	
Mexide	Rotenone	I	817
Mezene	Ziram	F	499
MGK 264		Ad	460
MGK Dog and Cat Repellent	Methyl Nonyl Ketone	Re	460
MGK R-326	Di-n-Propyl Isocinchomerate	Re	460
MGK Repellent 11	2,3,4,5-Bis(2-Butylene)Tetrahydrofurfural	Re	460

Starred ingredients (*) may be responsible for major toxic effects; consult Section II.

PESTICIDES (Cont.)

PRODUCT NAME	ALTERNATE NAME	PRINCIPAL USE	MANU-FACTURER
MGK Repellent 326	Di-n-Propyl Isocinchomerate	Re	460
MGK Repellent 874	2-Hydroxyethyl-n-Octyl Sulfide	Re	460
MH	Maleic Hydrazide	Pg	
MH-30	Maleic Hydrazide	Pg	760
MH-40	Maleic Hydrazide	Pg	760
MIC	Vorlex	Fm	
Micofume	Mylone	N	475
Microbiocide 4200	(see Rohm and Haas Co.)	F	634
Micro-Flotox	Sulfur	F	187
Microzul	Chlorophacinone	R	
Midox	p-Chlorobenzyl p-Chlorophenyl Sulfide	Ac	127
Milbam	Ziram	F	
Milbex	Chlorfensulphide	Ac	532
Mil-Col	Drazoxolon	F	370
Milcurb	Dimethirimol	F	370
Milcurb Super	Ethirimol	F	370
Mildex	Karathane	F /Ac	
Mildothane	Thiophanate Methyl	F	457
Milfaron	Chloraniformethan	F	115
Milgo	Ethirimol	F	370
Milky Disease Spores		I	274
Miller 531	(see Miller Chemical & Fertilizer Corp.)	F	475
Miller 658	(see Miller Chemical & Fertilizer Corp.)	F	475
Milmer	Copper Quinolinolate	F	
Milogard	Propazine	H	190, 193
Milsar	Chlorfensulphide	Ac	
Milstem	Ethirimol	F	370
Miltox	(see Sandoz, Ltd.)	F	646
Mineral Spirits	VM & P Naphthas	H	265, 758
MIPC	Isoprocarb	I	
Mipcin	Isoprocarb	I	
Mirex		I	031
Misasin	Chlorfensulphide	Ac	
Mitac	Amitraz	I /Ac	127
MITC	Vorlex	Fm	
Mitemate	(see Nihon Nohyaku Co., Ltd.)	I	523
Mitigan	Kelthane	Ac	439
Mitis Green	Copper Acetoarsenite	I	
Mitran		I	532
2M-4Kh-M	4-(2-Methyl-4-Chlorophenoxy)Butyric Acid	H	
MLT	Malathion	I	718
MMA	MSMA	H	
MNFA		Ac/I	532
MNF O 166	Merpelan AZ	H	
MO		H	487, 676
MO-500	CFNP	H	
Mobilawn	VC-13 Nemacide	N /I	490
Mobilnix	Petroleum Distillate	H	490
Mocap	Ethoprop	I	490
Modown	Bifenox	H	490
Mole Death	Strychnine	R	301
Molinate		H	697
Monalide		H	652
Monam	Vapam	Fm	
Mondak	Dicamba	H	781
Monitor	Methamidophos	I	187, 488
Monkil WP	Rhizoctol	F /St	
Monoammonium Methanearsonate	MAMA	H	
Monobor-Chlorate		H	547
Mono-Calcium Arsenite	Calcium Arsenite	I	
Monocron	Monocrotophos	I /Ac	439
Monocrotophos		I /Ac	193, 661
Monolinuron		H	346
Monosodium Methanearsonate	MSMA	H	211, 232
Monox	(see Nihon Nohyaku Co., Ltd.)	F	523
Monoxone		H	370
Monurex	Monuron	H	439
Monuron		H	355, 439
Monuron-TCA	Monuron	H	

Starred ingredients (*) may be responsible for major toxic effects; consult Section II.

PESTICIDES (Cont.)

PRODUCT NAME	ALTERNATE NAME	PRINCIPAL USE	MANU-FACTURER
Monzet	Urbacide	F	
Mor-Cran	N-1-Naphthylphthalamic Acid	H	760
Morestan	Chinomethionat	I /Ac	115, 488
Morkit	Anthraquinone	Re	115
Morocide	Binapacryl	Ac/F	346
Morphactin	Chlorflurenol	Pg	
Morrocid	Binapacryl	Ac/F	346
Motox	Toxaphene	I	817
Motox 6-3 Cotton Spray		I	817
Mous-Con	Zinc Phosphide	R	142
Mouse-Nots	Strychnine	R	541
Mouse-Tox	Strychnine	R	
Mous-Rid	Strychnine	R	142
Moxie	Methoxychlor	I	
MPMC	Meobal	I	
MSAMA	MSMA	H	
MSMA		H	211, 232
MTMC	Metacrate	I	
Mucochloric Anhydride		F	031
Multimet	Bendiocarb	I	652
Murfotox	Mecarbam	I /Ac	
Murfulvin	Griseofulvin	F	
Muriol	Chlorophacinone	R	
Murotox	Mecarbam	I /Ac	
Murvesco	Fenson	Ac	517
Muscatox	Coumaphos	I	
Muscotox	Coumaphos	I	
Mycozol	Thiabendazole	F /An	
Mylone		N	355
1-Naphthaleneacetic Acid	Pg		NAA
NAAM	NAD	Pg	
Nabac	Hexachlorophene	F /B	391
Nabac 25 EC	Hexachlorophene	F /B	391
Nabam		F	166, 634
Nabame	Nabam	F	
Nac	Carbaryl	I	
NAD		Pg	328, 757
Nafusaku	1-Naphthaleneacetic Acid	Pg	
Naled		I /Ac	187, 439
Nalkil	Bromacil	H	520
Namate	Disodium Methylarsonate	H	211
Namekil	Metaldehyde	M	
Namilan		I	727
Nankor	Ronnel	I	238
Naphthalene-Acetamide	NAD	Pg	328, 757
Naphthalene Acetic Acid	1-Naphthaleneacetic Acid	Pg	
1-Naphthaleneacetic Acid		Pg	295, 757
a-Naphthylacetic Acid	1-Naphthaleneacetic Acid	Pg	370
N-l-Naphthylphthalamic Acid		H	211, 760
Naphthylthiourea	ANTU	R	
Naptalam	N-1-Naphthylphthalamic Acid	H	
Napropamide		H	697
Naptox	Copper Naphthenates	F	694
Naramycin	Cycloheximide	F	
NATA	TCA	H	346
NATCA	TCA	H	
Navadel		I	128
Navon	Chlorpropham	H	
NC 6897	Bendiocarb	I	291
NC 8438	Ethofumasate	H	291
NC 9634		Pg	291
Neburea	Neburon	H	
Neburex	Neburon	H	439
Neburon		H	247, 439
Nedcidol	Diazinon	I	
Neguvon	Trichlorfon	I	115
Nellite		N	238
Nemacur	Phenamiphos	N /I	115, 488
Nemafene	D-D	Fm	661, 667

Starred ingredients (*) may be responsible for major toxic effects; consult Section II.

PESTICIDES (Cont.)

PRODUCT NAME	ALTERNATE NAME	PRINCIPAL USE	MANU-FACTURER
Nemafume	DBCP	Fm	
Nemagon	DBCP	Fm	661
Nemanax	DBCP	Fm	
Nemaset	DBCP	Fm	
Nemex		Fm/I	
Nendrin	Endrin	I	
Neo-Asozin		F	
Neobor	Borax	H /I	
Neobyne	Chlorobutynyl Chlorocarbanilate	H	292
Neocid	DDT	I	193
Neocidol	Diazinon	I /N	193
Neo-Nicotine	Anabasine	I	
Neo-Pynamin	Tetramethrin	I	275, 718
Neoron	Bromopropylate	Ac	193
Neo So Sin Gin-S	Neo-Asozin	F	676
Nephis	1,2-Dibromoethane	Fm	
Nephocarp	Carbophenothion	I /Ac	
Nerkol	Dichlorvos	I	
Nettle-Ban		H	664
Neutrocop	Copper Sulfate Monohydrate	F	
Nexagan	Bromophos-Ethyl	I /Ac	145
Nexion	Bromophos	I /Ac	145
Nexit	Lindane	I	
Nexoval	Chlorpropham	H	
N.F. 48	Thiophanate	F	
NIA 1240	Ethion	I /Ac	295
NIA 5488	Tetradifon	Ac	295
NIA 5996	Dichlobenil	H	295
NIA 9044	Binapacryl	Ac/F	295
NIA 9102	Metiram	F	295
NIA 9260	Tetramethrin	I	295
NIA 10242	Carbofuran	I	295
NIA 10637		H	295
NIA 11092	m-(3,3-Dimethylureido)Phenyl-tert-Butylcarbamate	H	295
NIA 17370	Resmethrin	I	295
Niacide	Ferbam	F	295
Niagara-Stik	1-Naphthaleneacetic Acid	Pg	295
Niagaratran	Ovotran	Ac	295
Niagrathal	Endothall	H /Pg	295
Nialate	Ethion	I /Ac	
Niclosamide		An	115, 488
Nicotine		I	166
Niklor	Chloropicrin	Fm	
Niletar	Methyl Parathion	I	
Nimitex	Biothion	I	
Nimitox	Abate	I	
Nimrod	Bupirimate	F	370
NIP	Nitrofen	H	634
Niran (Tamogen Ltd.)	Chlordane	I	727
Niran (Monsanto Agricultural Products Co.)	Parathion	I	496
Nirit		F	346
Nissol	MNFA	Ac/I	532
Nitrador	4,6-Dinitro-o-Cresol	I /F	
Nitralin		H	667
Nitrapyrin		B	238
Nitrochloroform	Chloropicrin	Fm	
Nitrofen		H	634, 676
Nitrolime	Calcium Cyanamide	H /F	
Nitrophen	Nitrofen	H	
Nitropone C	4,6-Dinitro-2-sec-Butyl Phenol	H	
Nitrox	Methyl Parathion	I	163
Nix-Scald	Ethoxyquin	F	
N-m-t	N-m-Tolylphthalamic Acid	Pg	
No-Bunt	Hexachlorobenzene	St	754
No Bunt 40	Hexachlorobenzene	St	754
Nogos	Dichlorvos	I	193
Nomersan	Thiram	F /St	370
No-Pest	Dichlorvos	I	734

Starred ingredients (*) may be responsible for major toxic effects; consult Section II.

PESTICIDES (Cont.)

PRODUCT NAME	ALTERNATE NAME	PRINCIPAL USE	MANU- FACTURER
Norbormide		R	464, 730
Norex	Chloroxuron	H	538
Norflurazon		H	643, 646
Nortran	Ethofumasate	H	
Nortron	Ethofumasate	H	291, 292
No-Scald	DPA	F	178
Novathion	Fenitrothion	I /Ac	175
Novege	Erbon	H	
Novigam	Lindane	I	
Noxfish	Rotenone	Ft	565
NPA	N-1-Naphthylphthalamic Acid	H	
NPA-3	N-1-Naphthylphthalamic Acid	H	
NPD	Tetra-n-Propyl Dithionopyrophosphate	I	
NRDC 104	Resmethrin	I	
N-Serve	Nitrapyrin	B	238
Nucidol	Diazinon	I /N	
Nu-Cop	Copper Sulfate Monohydrate	F	
Nudrin	Methomyl	I	661
Nu-Lawn Weeder	Bromoxynil	H	757
Nurelle	Pyroxychlor	F	
Nu Set	Silvex	H	475
Nu-Tone	1-Naphthaleneacetic Acid	Pg	475
Nuvacron	Monocrotophos	I /Ac	193
Nuvan	Dichlorvos	I	193
Nuvanal N	Iodofenphos	I	
Nuvanol	Fenitrothion	I /Ac	
Nuvanol N	Iodofenphos	I	193
Oatax	Chlorobutynyl Chlorocarbanilate	H	664
Octachlor	Chlordane	I	781
Octacide 264	MGK 264	Ad	
Octalene	Aldrin	I	781
Octalox	Dieldrin	I	781
Octamethyl Pyrophosphoramide		I /Ac	292
Octanol	Caprylic Alcohol	Pg	
ODB	o-Dichlorobenzene	H /I	
OFF	N,N-Diethyl-m-Toluamide	Re	388
Off-Shoot-O		Pg	129
Off-Shoot-T		Pg	129
Ofnack		I	487
Ofnak	Ofnack	I	487
Oftanol		I	115
Ofunack	(see Mitsui Chemical Industry Co., Ltd.)	I	487
Ohric		F	718
Oko	Dichlorvos	I	115
Oleocuivre	Cuprous Oxide	F	601
Oleofac	Prothoate	I /Ac	
OM-2424	Ethazol	F	
Omethoate		I /Ac	115
Omite	Propargite	I	760
OMPA	Octamethyl Pyrophosphoramide	I /Ac	
OMS 658	Bromophos	I /Ac	
OMS 659	Bromophos-Ethyl	I /Ac	
OMS 716	Promecarb	I	
OMS 771	Aldicarb	I /Ac	
OMS 1342	CMS 2957	I /Ac	
OMS 1804	Diflubenzuron	I	
OMU	Cycluron	H	
Ontracic 800	Methoxy Propazine	H	190
Ontrack WE-1		H	190
Ontrack WE-2	Methoxy Propazine	H	190
Onyxide 172		F	553
Orchex	Petroleum Distillate	I /H	265
Ordram	Molinate	H	697
Ornitrol		Av	097
Orthene	Acephate	I	187
Ortho 5353	Bufencarb	I	187
Ortho 9006	Methamidophos	I	187
Orthoarsenic Acid	Arsenic Acid	H	202, 566
Ortho Chlorobenzene	Hydrocarbon Solvent	H	

Starred ingredients (*) may be responsible for major toxic effects; consult Section II.

PESTICIDES (Cont.)

PRODUCT NAME	ALTERNATE NAME	PRINCIPAL USE	MANU-FACTURER
Orthocide	Captan	F /St	187
Ortho Dichlorobenzene	o-Dichlorobenzene	H /I	
Ortho-Klor	Chlordane	I	187
Ortho-Phenylphenol	Phenylphenol	B/F	
Orthophos	Parathion	I	
Ortho Phosphate Defoliant	S,S,S-Tributyl Phosphorotrithioate	B	
Orthorix	Calcium Polysulfide	F	
Orthoxenol	Phenylphenol	F /B	
Ortran	Acephate	I	187
Oryzalin		H	259
OS-2046	Phosdrin	I /Ac	
Osbac	Bassa	I	115, 418
Oust (Preemergence herbicide)	Dimethyl-2,3,5,6-Tetrachloroterephthalate	H	247
Oust (Postemergence herbicide)	Disodium Methylarsonate	H	247
Outfox	Cyprazine	H	334
Ovatran	Ovotran	Ac	
Ovex	Ovotran	Ac	
Ovotran		Ac	238
Ovochlor	Ovotran	Ac	
Oxadiazon		H	625, 626
Oxamyl		I /Ac	247
Oxime-Copper	Copper Quinolinate	F	
Oxine	8-Hydroxyquinoline	F /B	
Oxine-Copper	Copper Quinolinolate	F	
Oxine-Cu	Copper Quinolinolate	F	
Oxirane	Ethylene Oxide	Fm	
Oxycarboxin		F	760
Oxycil	Sodium Chlorate	H	547
Oxy Cop 8L	Copper Ammonium Carbonate	F	547
Oxydemeton-Methyl		I /Ac	115, 488
Oxydiazol	Methazole	H	
Oxydisulfoton	Disyston S	I /Ac	
Oxyquinoline	8-Hydroxyquinoline	F /B	
Oxyquinoline Citrate	(see Merck Chemical Div., Merck & Co., Inc.)	Ct	466
Oxyquinolinoleate de Cuivre	Copper Quinolinate	F	
Oxythioquinox	Chinomethionat	I /Ac	
Oxytril	Ioxynil	H	457
Paarlan	Isopropalin	H	259
Padan	Cartap	I	724
Paint Thinners	Petroleum Distillate		
Pallethrine	Allethrin	I	
Pamosol 2 Forte	Zineb	F	
Pamosol Z	Zineb	F	
Panoctine	Guazatine	F	403
Panogen	(see KenoGard AB)	F	403
Panoram		F	403
Panoram D-31	Dieldrin	I /St	
Panthion	Parathion	I	
Papthion	Phenthoate	I /Ac	
Paracide	p-Dichlorobenzene	Fm	
Paracrystals	p-Dichlorobenzene	Fm	
Paradichlorobenzene	p-Dichlorobenzene	Fm	595
Paradow	p-Dichlorobenzene	Fm	238
Paraform	Paraformaldehyde	Fm	
Paraformaldehyde		Fm	172
Parahep		I	490
Paramar	Parathion	I	
Para-Nuggets	p-Dichlorobenzene	Fm	
Parapest M-50	Methyl Parathion	I	590
Paraphos	Parathion	I	
Paraquat		H	187, 370
Paraquat Chloride	Paraquat	H	
Paraquat CL	Paraquat	H	
Parathene	Parathion	I	
Parathion		I	115, 496
Parathion-Methyl	Methyl Parathion	I	
Parawet	Parathion	I	
Parazene	p-Dichlorobenzene	Fm	
Parexan	(see M/S Riedel de Haen)	I	511

Starred ingredients (*) may be responsible for major toxic effects; consult Section II.

PESTICIDES (Cont.)

PRODUCT NAME	ALTERNATE NAME	PRINCIPAL USE	MANU-FACTURER
Parexan Neu	(see M/S Riedel de Haen)	I	511
Parinol	Parnon	F	
Paris Green	Copper Acetoarsenite	I	
Parmone	1-Naphthaleneacetic Acid	Pg	
Parnon		F	259
Partron-M	Methyl Parathion	I	
Parzate (Sodium salt)	Nabam	F	247
Parzate (Zinc salt)	Zineb	F	247
Pathclear	Paraquat	H	370
Patoran		H	109, 193
Paxilon	Methazole	H	
Pay-Off	Penoxalin	Pg	046
PCA	Pyrazon	H	
PCNB	Pentachloronitrobenzene	F /St	
PCP	Pentachlorophenol	H /Wp	
PCPA		Pg	
PCPBS	Fenson	Ac	
PCP-Na	Pentachlorophenol	H	
PDB	p-Dichlorobenzene	Fm	
PDC	Propylene Dichloride	Fm	
PDQ	4-(2-Methyl-4-Chlorophenoxy)Butyric Acid	H	
PDU	Fenuron	H	
PEBC	S-Propyl Butylethylthiocarbamate	H	
Pebulate	S-Propyl Butylethylthiocarbamate	H	
Pelt-44	Thiophanate Methyl	F	
Pelt Sol	Thiophanate	F	
Pencal	Calcium Arsenate	I /H	566
Penchlorol	Pentachlorophenol	H /Wp	
Penite	Sodium Arsenite	H /I	566
Pennamine D	2,4-D	H	566
Penncap-M	Methyl Parathion	I	566
Penncapthrin	(see Pennwalt Corp.)	?	566
Penoxalin		H	046
Penta	Pentachlorophenol	H /Wp	
Pentac	Pentachlorophenol	Ac	352
Pentachlorin	DDT	I	
Pentachloronitrobenzene		F /St	346, 550
Pentachlorophenol		H /Wp	238, 433
Pentacon	Pentachlorophenol	H /Wp	298
Pentagen	Pentachloronitrobenzene	F /St	
Penta-Kil	Pentachlorophenol	H /Wp	
Pentanol	Pentachlorophenol	H /Wp	
Pentaphenate	Pentachlorophenol	H /Wp	
Pentasol	Pentachlorophenol	H /Wp	
Penwar	Pentachlorophenol	H /Wp	298
Peprothion		I	
Peratox	Pentachlorophenol	H /Wp	
Perchlorobenzene	Hexachlorobenzene	St	
Perchloromethane	Carbon Tetrachloride	Fm	
Perecot	Cuprous Oxide	F	370
Perenox	Cuprous Oxide	F	370
Perfekthion	Dimethoate	I /Ac	109
Perfluidone		H	739
Perfmide	Tebuthiuron	H	
Permacide	Pentachlorophenol	H /Wp	721
Permite	Pentachlorophenol	H /Wp	694
Perselect		H	664
Perthane		I	634
Pescombi		I /Ac	
Pestan	Mecarbam	I /Ac	724
Pestmaster (MU)	1,2-Dibromoethane	Fm	
Pestmaster (Velsicol Chemical Corp.)	Methyl Bromide	Fm	781
Pestmaster EDB-85	1,2-Dibromoethane	Fm	
Pestox III	Octamethyl Pyrophosphoramide	I /Ac	292
Pestox XIV	Dimefox	I /Ac	292
Pestox XV	(see Fisons Ltd.)	I	292
Pest Strip	Dichlorvos	I	
PETD	Metiram	F	
Petroleum Distillate		I /H	187, 265

Starred ingredients (*) may be responsible for major toxic effects; consult Section II.

	PESTICIDES (Cont.)		
PRODUCT NAME	ALTERNATE NAME	PRINCIPAL USE	MANU- FACTURER
Petroleum Naphtha		H	187, 265
Petroleum Oil	Dormant Oils	I /H	
Petroleum Solvents	Petroleum Distillate	I /H	
PH 60-40	Diflubenzuron	I	580
Phaltan		F	187
Phenacide	Toxaphene	I	
Phenador-X	Diphenyl	F	
Phenamiphos		N	115, 488
Phenatox	Toxaphene	I	
Phenazin		F	523
Phencapton		Ac	193
Phenisobromolate	Bromopropylate	Ac	
Phenkapton	Phencapton	Ac	
Phenmad	Phenylmercuric Esters	F /H	442
Phenmedipham		H	
Phenobenzuron		H	568
Phenotan	Dinoseb Acetate	H	
Phenothiazine		I /An	799
Phenothiol		H	349
Phenox	2,4-D	H	445
Phenoxylene Plus	(see Fisons Ltd., Agrochemical Div.)	H	292
Phenthoate		I /Ac	499, 535
Phentinacetate	Fentinacetate	F /Al	
Phentinoacetate	Fentinacetate	F /Al	
Phenylbenzene	Diphenyl	F	
Phenylmercuric Esters		F /H	157, 751
Phenylmercury Acetate	Phenylmercuric Esters	F /H	
Phenylphenol		B/F	238
Phix	Phenylmercuric Esters	F	178
Phorate		I	038, 046
Phortox	Trichlorophenoxyacetic Acid	H	
Phosalone		Ac/I	625, 626
Phosdrin		I /Ac	661, 667
Phosfene	Phosdrin	I /Ac	
Phosfolan		I	046
Phosfon	Chlorphonium	Pg	490
Phoskil	Parathion	I	295
Phosmet	Imidan	I	
Phosphamidon		I /Ac	187, 193
Phosphine (gas)		Fm	038, 228
Phosphine (solid)		Fm	038, 228
Phosphorus		I /R	352, 697
Phostoxin	Phosphine	Fm/I	227, 228
Phosvel	Leptophos	I	781
Phosvin	Zinc Phosphide	R	352
Phosvit	Dichlorvos	I	532
Phoxim		I	115
Phoxime	Phoxim	I	
Phthalic Acid	Dimethyl-2,3,5,6-Tetrachloroterephthalate	H	
Phthalophos	Imidan	I	
Phthalthrin	Tetramethrin	I	
Phygon	Dichlone	F	760
Phyomone	1-Naphthaleneacetic Acid	Pg	370
Physan-HC	MSMA	H	067
Phytar 560	Cacodylic Acid	H	211
Phytomycin	Streptomycin	B	
Phytosol	Trichloronate	I	
Pic-Clor	Chloropicrin	Fm	626
Picfume	Chloropicrin	Fm	238
Picloram		H	238
Pid	Diphenadione	R	
Pik-Off	Glyoxime	Pg	190
Pimacol	1-Naphthaleneacetic Acid	Pg	
Pimacol-Sol	1-Naphthaleneacetic Acid	Pg	
Pindone	2-Pivalyl-1,3-Indandione	R	
Pinethylene	Exhalt 4-10	At	394
Pine Oil		I	616
Pinoran	Lironion	H	
Pio	Piomy	F	

Starred ingredients (*) may be responsible for major toxic effects; consult Section II.

PRODUCT NAME	ALTERNATE NAME	PRINCIPAL USE	MANU-FACTURER
	PESTICIDES (Cont.)		
Piomy		F /Ab	349
Piomycin	Piomy	F	
Piperalin		F	259
Piperazine		Pc	385
Piperonyl Butoxide		Ad	460, 598
Piperophos		H	193
Pipron	Piperalin	F	259
Piprotal		Ad	460
Piran	(see Tamogan Ltd.)	I	727
Pirimicarb		I	364
Pirimiphos-Ethyl		I	364
Pirimiphosethyl	Pirimiphos-Ethyl	I	
Pirimiphos-Methyl	Actellic	I /Ac	364
Pirimor	Pirimicarb	I	364
Pivacin	2-Pivalyl-1,3-Indandione	R	
Pival	2-Pivalyl-1,3-Indandione	R	508
Pivaldione	2-Pivalyl-1,3-Indandione	R	
2-Pivalyl-1,3-Indandione		R	508
Pivalyl Valone	2-Pivalyl-1,3-Indandione	R	
Pivalyn	2-Pivalyl-1,3-Indandione	R	
PKhNB	Pentachloronitrobenzene	F /St	
Planavin	Nitralin	H	667
Planotox	2,4-D	H	457
Plantgard	2,4-D	H	
Plantvax	Oxycarboxin	F	760
Plictran	Cyhexatin	I /Ac	238
Plondrel	Ditalimfos	F	239
Plucker	1-Naphthaleneacetic Acid	Pg	
Plus de Riz	Propanil	H	
PMA	Phenylmercuric Esters	F /H	
PMAC	Phenylmercuric Esters	F /H	
Pmacetate	Phenylmercuric Esters	F /H	
PMAS	Phenylmercuric Esters	F /H	199
P.M.P. (rodenticide)	Valone	R	
PMP (insecticide)	Imidan	I	
Podox-L	(see Mineral Research and Development Corp.)	F	481
Polaris	Glyphosine	Pg	496
Polisin	Prometryne	H	
Polybor	Borax	H	766
Polybor 3	Borax	H	766
Polybor-Chlorate		H	766
Polyhedrosis Virus	Biotrol VHZ	I	
Polymone 60		H	691
Polynox		F	523
Polyoxin		F	349, 418
Polyoxymethylene	Paraformaldehyde	F	
Polyram	Metiram	F	109
Polyram-Combi	Metiram	F	109
Polyram-M	Maneb	F	109
Polyram-Ultra	Thiram	F /St	109
Polyram-Z	Zineb	F	109
Pomarsol	Thiram	F /St	115
Pomarsol Forte	Thiram	F /St	115
Pomarsol Z Forte	Ziram	F	115
Po-San (Th)		Pg	442
Po-San (FCH)		Pg	442
Po-San Turf Fungicide		F	442
Potablan	Monalide	H	652
Potassium Antimonyl Tartrate	Antimony Potassium Tartrate	I	
Potassium Azide	Azide	H /F	
Potassium Gibberellate	Gibberellic Acid	Pg	
Powertox		I	817
PP-062	Pirimicarb	I	370
PP-149	Ethirimol	F	370
PP-211	Pirimiphos-Ethyl	I	370
PP-511	Actellic	I /Ac	370
PP-588	Bupirimate	F	370
PP-675	Dimethirimol	F	370

Starred ingredients (*) may be responsible for major toxic effects; consult Section II.

PRODUCT NAME	ALTERNATE NAME	PRINCIPAL USE	MANU-FACTURER
	PESTICIDES (Cont.)		
PP-781	Drazoxolon	F	370
Pramitol	Methoxy Propazine	H	190
Pramitol 5PS		H	190
Prebane	Terbutryne	H	
Pre-Beta 1		H	322
Pre-Beta 2		H	322
Preeglone Extra	Paraquat	H	
Prefalon	Linuron	H	
Prefar	Betasan	H	697
Prefix	Chlorthiamid	H	667
Preflan	Tebuthiuron	H	
Prefmid	Tebuthiuron	H	
Prefox		H	334
Pregard	Profluralin	H	
Premalox	(see May & Baker Ltd.)	H	457
Premerge	4,6-Dinitro-2-sec-Butyl Phenol	H	238
Premerge 3	4,6-Dinitro-2-sec-Butyl Phenol	H	238
Prep		H /Df	757
Pre-San	Betasan	H	442
Prethlene	Chlordimeform	I /Ac	
Prethylene	Chlordimeform	I /Ac	
Prevanol	Chlorpropham	H	
Preventol	Dichlorophene	F /B	685
Previcur	Prothiocarb	F /St	538, 652
Prezervit	Mylone	?	
Priglone	Paraquat	H	
Primagram		H	193
Primatol	Methoxy Propazine	H	193
Primatol A	Atrazine	H	193
Primatol M80	Terbuthylazine	H	193
Primatol P	Propazine	H	193
Primatol Q	Prometryne	H	193
Primatol S	Simazine	H	193
Primaze	Atrazine	H	190
Primextra	Primagram	H	193
Primicid	Pirimiphos-Ethyl	I	364
Princep	Simazine	H	190, 193
Printop	Simazine	H	
Proban (insecticide)	Cythioate	I	046
Proban (herbicide)	(see David Chemical Co.)	H	220
Probe	Methazole	H	781
Procyazine		H	190
Prodan	(see Tamogan Ltd.)	I	727
Profluralin		H	190
Profume	Methyl Bromide	Fm	238
Pro-Gibb	Gibberellic Acid	Pg	004
Pro-Gibb 47	Gibberellic Acid	Pg	004
Prolan		I	
Prolate	Imidan	I	697
Prolin		R	598, 632
Promar	Diphenadione	R	781
Promecarb		I	652
Promecarbe	Promecarb	I	
Prometon	Methoxy Propazine	H	
Prometone	Methoxy Propazine	H	
Prometrex	Prometryne	H	439
Prometryn	Prometryne	H	
Prometryne		H	190, 193
Pronamide		H	634
Pro-Nox Fish	Rotenone	Ft	565
Propachlor		H	496, 671
Propanex	Propanil	H	211
Propanid	Propanil	H	
Propanil		H	634, 785
Propargite		Ac	760
Propazine		H	190, 193
Propenal	Acrolein	H	
Propenol	Allyl Alcohol	H /F	
Propenyl Alcohol	Allyl Alcohol	H /F	

Starred ingredients (*) may be responsible for major toxic effects; consult Section II.

PRODUCT NAME	ALTERNATE NAME	PRINCIPAL USE	MANU-FACTURER
	PESTICIDES (Cont.)		
Propetamiphos	Safrotin	I	
Propham		H	567, 595
Prophos	Ethoprop	N /I	
Propineb		F	115, 499
Propinebe	Propineb	F	
Propionic Acid Grain Preserver	(see Union Carbide Corp., Agricultural Products)	F	757
Propi-Rhap	Dichlorprop	H	
Prop-Job	Propanil	H	067
Propon	Silvex	H	
Proponex D		H	661
Proponex-Plus	Mecoprop	H	664
Propoxur	2-Isopropoxyphenyl N-Methylcarbamate	I	
Proprop	Dalapon	H	
S-Propyl Butylethylthiocarbamate		H	697
Propylene Dichloride		Fm	238
Propylene Oxide	(see Jefferson Chemical Co., Inc.)	Fm	385
Propyzamide	Pronamide	H	
Prosulfalin		H	259
Protect		St	334
Protector-3L Seed Treatment	(see Agway Inc.)	F	025
Prothiocarb		F /St	538, 652
Prothoate		I /Ac	499
Prowl	Penoxalin	H	046
Proxol	Trichlorfon	I	754
Prussic Acid	Hydrocyanic Acid	Fm	
Prynachlor		H	109
PSP	Aphidan	I	
PTF	Metiram	F	
Purasan-SC-10	Phenylmercuric Esters	F	331
Puraturf No. 10	Phenylmercuric Esters	F	331
Puraturf 117	(see Guard Chemical Co.)	F	331
Purivel	Metoxuron	H	646
Pynamin	Allethrin	I	718
Pyracarbolid		F	346
Pyramin	Pyrazon	H	109, 112
Pyramin Plus		H	109
Pyramin RB	Pyrazon	H	112
Pyrazon		H	109, 112
Pyrazophos		F	346
Pyrenone		I	275
Pyresyn	Pyrethrin I	I	
Pyrethrin I		I	460, 598
Pyrethroids		I	460, 598
Pyrethrum		I	460, 598
Pyrexcel	Pyrethrin I	I	
Pyridinitril		F	145
Pyrobor	Borax	H	406
Pyrocatechol		St	250
Pyrocide	Pyrethrin I	I	460
Pyroxychlor		F	238
Qikron		Ac	532
Quel	Ancymidol	Pg	
Queletox	Fenthion	Av	115
Quick	Chlorophacinone	R	
Quicksan 20	Phenylmercuric Esters	Sl	700
Quilan	Benefin	H	259
Quinalphos	Diethchinalphion	I	
8-Quinolinol	8-Hydroxyquinoline	F /B	
Quinomethionate	Chinomethionat	I /Ac	
Quinondo	Copper Quinolinolate	F	
Quinophenol	8-Hydroxyquinoline	F /B	
Quintex	(see Murphy Chemical Ltd.)	H	517
Quintozene	Pentachloronitrobenzene	F /St	
R1303	Carbophenothion	I /Ac	
R1504	Imidan	I	
R1513	Azinphos-Ethyl	I	
R1582	Guthion	I	
R2061	S-Propyl Butylethylthiocarbamate	H	

Starred ingredients (*) may be responsible for major toxic effects; consult Section II.

PESTICIDES (Cont.)			
PRODUCT NAME	ALTERNATE NAME	PRINCIPAL USE	MANU- FACTURER
R2063	Cycloate	H	
R2170	Oxydemeton-Methyl	I /Ac	
R7465	Napropamide	H	
Rabcide		F	
Rabon	Tetrachlorvinphos	I	232
Rabond	Tetrachlorvinphos	I	
Racumin	Coumatetralyl	R	115
Radapon	Dalapon	H	238
Radazin	Atrazine	H	
Rad-E-Cate	(see Vineland Chemical Co.)	H	787
Ramik	Diphenadione	R	781
Rampart	Phorate	I	
Ramrod	Propachlor	H	496
Ramucide	Chlorophacinone	R	
Randox	CDAA	H	496
Raphone	MCPA	H	
Rapid	Pirimicarb	I	364
Rasikal	Sodium Chlorate	H	
Ratafin	Coumafuryl	R	
Rat-A-Way	Coumafuryl	R	
Raticate	Norbormide	R	
Ratilan	Coumachlor	R	
Rat-Nip	Phosphorus	R	529
Ratomet	Chlorophacinone	R	
Ratorex	Warfarin	R	436
Ratox	Thallium Sulfate	R	
Rattract	ANTU	R	
Rat-Tu	ANTU	R	
Rattunal	Warfarin	R	
Ravage	(see Velsicol Chemical Corp.)	H	781
Raviac	Chlorophacinone	R	
Ravicac	Chlorophacinone	R	
Ravion	Carbaryl	I	
Ravyon	Carbaryl	I	439
Rax Water Soluble	Warfarin	R	598
RE 4355	Naled	I /Ac	
Readex	Eradex	Ac/F	
Rebelate	Dimethoate	I	112
Reddon	Trichlorophenoxyacetic Acid	H	238
Red Squill		R	643, 703
Reducymol	Ancymidol	Pg	
Regim-8	TIBA	Pg	376
Region	Diquat Dibromide	H	
Reglone	Diquat Dibromide	H	370
Reglox	Diquat Dibromide	H	370
Regulox	Maleic Hydrazide	Pg	231
Reldan	Chlorpyrifos-Methyl	I	238
Remasan	Maneb	F	625
Remtal	(see Fisons Limited, Agrochemical Div.)	H	292
Residuren Extra	(see Farm Protection Ltd.)	H	286
Resisan	Dicloran	F	
Resistox	Coumaphos	I	
Resitox	Coumaphos	I	
Resmethrin		I	275, 565
Res-Q	(see PBI - Gordon Corp.)	St	559
Retard	Maleic Hydrazide	Pg/H	241
RH-124	Indar	F	634
RH-787	Vacor	R	634
RH-2512		H	634
RH-2915		H	634
RH-8817		?	634
Rhizoctol		F /St	115
Rhodiatox	Parathion	I	626
Rhomenc	MCPA	H	
Rhomene	MCPA	H	626
Rhonox	MCPA	H	626
Ricetrine	(see Applied Biochemists, Inc.)	Al	073
Rilof	Piperophos	H	
Rimocidin	Streptomycin	B	

Starred ingredients (*) may be responsible for major toxic effects; consult Section II.

PESTICIDES (Cont.)

PRODUCT NAME	ALTERNATE NAME	PRINCIPAL USE	MANU-FACTURER
Ripenthall	Endothall	H /Pg	
RO-7-6145	Dikegulac-Sodium	Pg	
Roccal	Benzalkonium Chloride	B /F	808
Rodene	Red Squill	R	
Ro-Dex	Strychnine	R	
Rodine	Red Squill	R	
Rogor	Dimethoate	I /Ac	499
Rogue	Propanil	H	
Ro-Ko	Rotenone	I /Ft	
Ro-Neet	Cycloate	H	697
Ronnel		I	238
Ronstar	Oxadiazon	H	625, 626
Rootnone	NAD	Pg	
Rootone	Indolebutyric Acid	Pg	757
Rootone (Union Carbide Agricultural Products Co., Inc.)	1-Naphthaleneacetic Acid	Pg	757
Rosetone	NAD	Pg	
Rosex	Warfarin	R	
Rospan	Chloropropylate	Ac	
Rospin	Chloropropylate	Ac	193
Rotefive	Rotenone	I /Ft	
Rotenone		I /Ft	275, 565
Rotessenol	Rotenone	I /Ft	
Rot-Not	Copper Naphthenates	F	
Rotox	Methyl Bromide	Fm	289
Roundup	Glyphosate	H	496
Rowmate		H	757
Rowtate	Cisanilide	H	
Roxion	Dimethoate	I /Ac	145
Royal MH-30	Maleic Hydrazide	Pg	760
Royal Slo-Gro	Maleic Hydrazide	Pg	760
Royaltac	Off-Shoot-T	Pg	760
Rozol	Chlorophacinone	R	181, 427
RP2929	(see Rhone-Poulenc, Inc.)	H	626
RP11974	Phosalone	Ac/I	
RP17623	Oxadiazon	H	
RP26019		F	625, 626
RPH	Thiabendazole	F /An	637
R-55 Repellent		Re	583
Rubitox	Phosalone	Ac/I	
Ruelene		I /An	238
Rukseam	DDT	I	
Rumetan	Zinc Phosphide	R	
Runcatex	Mecoprop	H	
Ruphos	Navadel	I	
Rutgers 612	2-Ethyl-1,3-Hexanediol	Re	
Ryania		I	565
Rycelan	Oryzalin	H	
Rycelon	Oryzalin	H	
Ryzelan	Oryzalin	H	259
Ryzelon	Oryzalin	H	
S-7	EPBP	I	
S276	Disulfoton	I /Ac	
S410	Metasystox-S	I /Ac	
S767	Fensulfothion	N /I	
S1752	Fenthion	I	
S2940	Phenthoate	I /Ac	
S4084	Cyanophos	I	
S4087	Cyanofenphos	I	
S4400	Agritox	I	
S5660	Fenitrothion	I /Ac	
S6176	Ethiolate	H	
S6876	Omethoate	I /Ac	
S9115	Cyprazine	H	
S10165	Propanil	H	
S15076	Ethiolate	H	
S22012	Benzthiazuron	H	
S25128	Methabenzthiazuron	H	
Sabadilla		I	598

Starred ingredients (*) may be responsible for major toxic effects; consult Section II.

PESTICIDES (Cont.)

PRODUCT NAME	ALTERNATE NAME	PRINCIPAL USE	MANU- FACTURER
SADH	Daminozide	Pg	
Safeguard	(see Rothwell Plant Health, Ltd.)	St	637
Safrotin		I	646
Salicylanilide		F	377
Salithion		I	718
Salsan	Drazoxolon	F	
Salvo	2,4-D	H	211
Samuron	Desmetryn	H	193
SAN 9789	Norflurazon	H	
SAN 197 I	Ekamet	I	
SAN 52139 I	Safrotin	I	
Sanaseed	Strychnine	R	124
Sancap	Dipropetryne	H	190
Sandothion	Formothion	I /Ac	646
Sandoz 6626	Diethchinalphion	I	
Sanocide	Hexachlorobenzene	St/F	
Sanspor	Captafol	F	370
Sanspor	(see ICI Plant Protection Division)	F	370
Santobrite	Pentachlorophenol	H /Wp	496
Santocel C	Dri-Die	I	
Santochlor	p-Dichlorobenzene	Fm	496
Santophen	Pentachlorophenol	H /Wp	496
Santophen I Germicide	(see Monsanto Co.)	B	496
Santoquin	Ethoxyquin	F	
Sapecron	Chlorfenvinphos	I	193
Saphicol	Menazon	I	
Saphi-Col	Menazon	I	370
Saphizon	Menazon	I	370
Saphos	Menazon	I	
Sappiran	Ovotran	Ac	532
Saprol	Triforine	F	145
Sarclex	Linuron	H	
Sarolex	Diazinon	I	190
Saturn	Benthiocarb	H	418
Saturno	Benthiocarb	H	418
Savirad	Metoxuron	H	646
Sayfor 4	Menazon	I	370
Sayfos	Menazon	I	370
Sayphos	Menazon	I	
SBP-1382	Resmethrin	I	565
SC-12937	Ornitrol	Av	
Scaldip	DPA	F	
Scal-Dip	DPA	F	
Schradan	Octamethyl Pyrophosphoramide	I /Ac	
Schweinfurt Green	Copper Acetoarsenite	I	
Scogal		H	664
SD 3562	Bidrin	I	661
SD 4294	Bidrin	I	661
SD 7859	Chlorfenvinphos	I	661
SD 8339		Pg	661
SD 9129	Monocrotophos	I /Ac	661
SD 11831	Nitralin	H	661
SD 14114	Fenbutatin-Oxide	Ac	661
SD 15418	Cyanazine	H	661
Secbumeton		H	190, 193
Seedrin Liquid	Aldrin	I	626
Selektin	Prometryne	H	
Selinon	4,6-Dinitro-o-Cresol	I /F	
Semeron	Desmetryn	H	193
Semeron 25	Desmetryn	H	193
Semparol	Atrazine	H	193
Sencor	Metribuzin	H	115, 488
Sencoral	Metribuzin	H	115
Sencorex	Metribuzin	H	115
Sendran	2-Isopropoxyphenyl N-Methylcarbamate	I /M	214
Sentry Grain Preserver	Propionic Acid Grain Preserver	F	757
Septene	Carbaryl	I	
Serafume	(see The Dow Chemical Co.)	Fm	238
Seritox 50	Dichlorprop	H	457

Starred ingredients (*) may be responsible for major toxic effects; consult Section II.

PESTICIDES (Cont.)

PRODUCT NAME	ALTERNATE NAME	PRINCIPAL USE	MANU-FACTURER
		Ad	679
Sesamex	Sesamex	Ad	679
Sesoxane	(see Union Carbide Corp., Agricultural Products)	I	757
Sevidol			
Sevimol	Carbaryl	I	757
Sevin	Carbaryl	I	757
SG-67	Dri-Die	I	
Shed-A-Leaf	Sodium Chlorate	H	626
Shimmerex	Phenylmercuric Esters	F	
Shirlan	Salicylanilide	F	377
Shortstop	Terbutryne	H	190
Shortstop E	Terbutryne	H	190
Shoxin	Norbormide	R	
SI 6505	Tachigaren	F /Pg	
SI 6711	Isoxathion	I	
Sicarol	Pyracarbolid	F	346
Siduron		H	247
Silica Aerogel	Dri-Die	I	223
Silikil	Dri-Die	I	
Silmurin	Red Squill	R	
Silosan	Actellic	I /Ac	364
Silvanol	Lindane	I	
Silvex		H	238, 785
Silvi-Rhap	Silvex	H	785
Silvisar 510	Cacodylic Acid	H	067
Silvisar 550	MSMA	H	067
Simadex	Simazine	H	292
Simanex	Simazine	H	439
Simazine		H	190, 193
Simetone		H	193
Simetryn		H	193
Sinbar	Terbacil	H	247
Sindone	(see Union Carbide Agricultural Products Co., Inc.)	H	757
Sinituho	Pentachlorophenol	H /Wp	
Sinox	4,6-Dinitro-o-Cresol	I /F	295
Sinox General	4,6-Dinitro-2-sec-Butyl Phenol	H	295
Sirmate	Rowmate	H	
Slimicide	Acrolein	Sl	
Slo-Gro	Maleic Hydrazide	Pg	760
Slow Release Algimycin PLL-C	Algimycin PLL-C	Al	316
SMA	Monoxone	H	
SMDC	Vapam	F /H	
Smite	Azide	F	760
Smut-Go	Hexachlorobenzene	St	
SN 4075	Phenmedipham	H	652
SN 34615	Promecarb	I	652
SN 35830	Monalide	H	652
SN 36056	Formetanate	Ac/I	652
SN 36268	Chlordimeform	I /Ac	652
SN 38107	Desmedipham	H	652
SN 38584	Phenmedipham	H	652
SN 41703	Prothiocarb	F /St	652
SNP	Parathion	I	
Sodar	Disodium Methylarsonate	H	
Sodium Aluminofluoride	Cryolite	I	
Sodium Arsenate		I	601
Sodium Arsenite		H /I	121, 271
Sodium Azide	Azide	H /I	
Sodium Borate	Borax	H	
Sodium Chlorate		H	406, 547
Sodium Chlorate Borate		I	547, 766
Sodium Cyanide	Cyanides	R	
Sodium Dimethyl Dithiocarbamate	(see Roberts Chemicals Div. of Security Chemicals, Inc.)	F	631
Sodium Fluoaluminate	Cryolite	I	
Sodium Fluoroacetate	Fluoroacetate	R	
Sodium Methyldithiocarbamate	Vapam	Fm	
Sodium Monochloroacetate	Monoxone	H	

Starred ingredients (*) may be responsible for major toxic effects; consult Section II.

PESTICIDES (Cont.)

PRODUCT NAME	ALTERNATE NAME	PRINCIPAL USE	MANU-FACTURER
Sodium Monofluoroacetate	Fluoroacetate	R	
Sodium Pentachlorophenate		H	238
Sodium Phenylphenate	Dowicide A	F	
Sodium Polyborates	(see U.S. Borax & Chemical Corp.)	H /L	766
Sodium TCA	Sodium Trichloroacetate	H	
Sodium TCA Inhibited	Sodium Trichloroacetate	H	
Sodium Tetraborate Decahydrate	Borax	H	
Sodium Trichloroacetate		H	238, 346
Sofril	Sulfur	F /Ac	
Soilbrom	1,2-Dibromoethane	Fm	319
Soilbrom-40	1,2-Dibromoethane	Fm	319
Soilbrome-85	1,2-Dibromoethane	Fm	319
Soilbrom-90 EC	1,2-Dibromoethane	Fm	319
Soilfume	1,2-Dibromoethane	Fm	295
Solfarin	Warfarin	R	
Sol Kop 10	Copper Ammonium Carbonate	F	
Solo	N-1-Naphthylphthalamic Acid	H	760
Solvent Naphthas	VM & P Naphthas	H	
Solvirex (MU)	Demeton	I /Ac	
Solvirex (Sandoz, Ltd.)	Disulfoton	I /Ac	646
Somilan	Ethalfluralin	H	
Sonalan	Ethalfluralin	H	259
Sonalen	Ethalfluralin	H	
Sopp	Dowicide A	F	
Soprabel	Lead Arsenate	I	
Sopracol	Drazoxolon	F	
Sopracol 781	Drazoxolon	F	
Sopragam		I	691
Sopranebe	Maneb	F	691
Soprathion	Parathion	I	691
Soprocide	BHC	I	
Sorgoprim	Terbuthylazine	H	
SP-1103	Tetramethrin	I	
Spanon	Chlordimeform	I /Ac	
Spectracide	Diazinon	I	190
Spergon	Chloranil	F /St	760
Sperlox-S	Sulfur	F	550
Sperlox-Z	Zineb	F	550
Spersul Thiovit	Sulfur	F /Ac	550
Spike	Tebuthiuron	H	259
Spotrete	Thiram	F	199
Spra-Cal	Calcium Arsenate	I /H	566
Spray-Cop	Copper Sulfate Monohydrate	F	
Spring-Bak	Nabam	F	442
Sprotive Dust SG-67	Dri-Die	I	
Sprout-Nip	Chlorpropham	H	595
Sprout-Off		Pg	280
Sprout-Off	Maleic Hydrazide	Pg	
Sprout Stop	Maleic Hydrazide	Pg	241
Spud-Nic	Chlorpropham	Pg	
Sput-Nic	Chlorpropham	Pg	
Squill	Red Squill	R	
SR 73	Clonitralid	M	
SR 406	Captan	F	
SRA 5172	Methamidophos	I	
SRA 7312	Diethchinalphion	I	
SRA 12869	Oftanol	I	
SS 1451	Eradex	Ac/F	
SS 2074	Chinomethionat	I /Ac	
S-Seven	EPBP	I	535
Stabilene Fly Repellent	Butoxy Polypropylene Glycol	Re	757
Stafast	1-Naphthaleneacetic Acid	Pg	
Stam F-34	Propanil	H	634
Stam LV-10	(see Rohm and Haas Co.)	H	634
Stam M-4	Propanil	H	634
Standard Lead Arsenate	Lead Arsenate	I	
Starlicide		Av	
Sta-Set	Silvex	H	
Stathion	Parathion	I	

Starred ingredients (*) may be responsible for major toxic effects; consult Section II.

PRODUCT NAME	ALTERNATE NAME	PRINCIPAL USE	MANU-FACTURER
	PESTICIDES (Cont.)		
STCA	Sodium Trichloroacetate	H	
Steriweed		H	367
Stikcol-D	Silvex	H	295
Stocktrine	(see Applied Biochemists, Inc.)	Al	073
Stoddard Solvent		H	187, 583
Stomp	Penoxalin	H	046
Stop-Drop	1-Naphthaleneacetic Acid	Pg	
Stop Scald	Ethoxyquin	F /Pg	496
Stove Oil	Petroleum Distillate	H	
Strathion	Parathion	I	
Strepcen	Streptomycin	B	
Streptomycin		B	466, 574
Streycin Sulfate	Streptomycin	B	
Strobane-T	Toxaphene	I	733
Strychnine		R	298, 598
Strychnos	Strychnine	R	
Stunt-Man	Maleic Hydrazide	Pg	
Subitex	Dinoseb	H	346
Sucker Plucker	Off-Shoot-T	Pg	241
Sucker-Stuff	Maleic Hydrazide	Pg	241
Suffix	Benzoylprop Ethyl	H	664, 667
Sulfallate	Vegadex	H	
Sulfamate	Ammonium Sulfamate	H	
Sulfaquinoxaline		R	466
Sulfasin	Bisethylxanthogen	H	
Sulfodiazol	Ustilan	H	
Sulfonimide	Captafol	F	
Sulforon	Sulfur	F /Ac	238
Sulfotep	Sulfotepp	I /Ac	
Sulfotepp		I /Ac	115
Sulfox-Cide	Sulfoxide	Ad	
Sulfoxide		Ad	565
Sulfoxyl	Sulfoxide	Ad	
Sulfur		F /Ac	295, 643
Sulfuryl Fluoride		I /Fm	238
Sulkol	Sulfur	F /Ac	
Sulsol	Sulfur	F /Ac	
Sumithion	Fenitrothion	I /Ac	718
Sumitol	Secbumeton	H	190, 193
Summer Oils	Dormant Oils	I /H	
Suncide	2-Isopropoxyphenyl N-Methylcarbamate	I	115
Super Cosan	Sulfur	F /Ac	
Super Crab-E-Rad	AMA	H	787
Super Crab-E-Rad AMA	AMA	H	787
Super Crab-E-Rad Calar	Calar	H	787
Super Dal-E-Rad	AMA	H	787
Super Dal-E-Rad	Calar	H	787
Super Dal-E-Rad Calar	Calar	H	787
Super-Desprout	Maleic Hydrazide	Pg	280
Supernox	Propanil	H	
Super Sucker-Stuff	Maleic Hydrazide	Pg	241
Supona	Chlorfenvinphos	I	667
Supracide	Methidathion	I	190, 193
Sup'r-Flo (herbicide)	Diuron	H	626
Sup'r-Flo (fungicide)	Maneb	F	626
Sup'r-Flo Diuron Flowable	Diuron	H	626
Surcopur	Propanil	H	115
Surecide	Cyanofenphos	I	718
Sure-Set	PCPA	Pg	
Surflan	Oryzalin	H	259
Surpur	Propanil	H	115
Su Seguro Carpidor	Trifluralin	H	
Sustar-2-S	Fluoridamid	Pg	
Susvin	Monocrotophos	I /Ac	610
Sutan	Butylate	H	697
Suzu	Fentinacetate	F /M	
Suzu H	Fentin Hydroxide	F	
Sward	Prosulfalin	H	259
Swat	Bomyl	I	031

Starred ingredients (*) may be responsible for major toxic effects; consult Section II.

PESTICIDES (Cont.)

PRODUCT NAME	ALTERNATE NAME	PRINCIPAL USE	MANUFACTURER
Swebate	Biothion	I	
Swep		H	535
Syllit	Cyprex	F	403
Synklor	Chlordane	I	781
Synthrin	Resmethrin	I	275
Systemox	Demeton	I /Ac	115
Systox	Demeton	I /Ac	115, 488
Sytam	Octamethyl Pyrophosphoramide	I /Ac	
Sytasol	Dinobuton	Ac/F	
Sytemp		I	628
2,4,5-T	Trichlorophenoxyacetic Acid	H	
Tabatrex	Di-n-Butylsuccinate	Re	310
Tabutrex	Di-n-Butylsuccinate	Re	310
Tachigaren		F /Pg	649
Tag	Phenylmercuric Esters	F /H	
Taktic	Amitraz	I /Ac	
Talan	Dinobuton	Ac/F	
Talbot Lead Arsenate	Lead Arsenate	I	464
Tamaron	Methamidophos	I	115
Tandex	m-(3,3-Dimethylureido)Phenyl-tert-Butylcarbamate	H	295
Tanone	Phenthoate	I /Ac	499
Tantizon		H	115
Task	Dichlorvos	I	232
Taterpex	Chlorpropham	H	484
Tayssato	Methoxyethylmercuric Chloride	F	400
Taytox	Copper Ammonium Carbonate	F	
TBA	2,3,6-Trichlorobenzoic Acid	H	
2,3,6-TBA	2,3,6-Trichlorobenzoic Acid	H	
TBCS-53	Tribasic Copper Sulfate	F	
TBPMC	Knockbal	I	
TBTO	Bis(Tri-n-Butyltin)Oxide	F	514
TBZ	Thiabendazole	An/F	
TCA	Trichloroacetic Acid	H	
2,3,6-TCA	Chlorfenac	H	
TCB	Trichlorobenzene	H	
TCBA	2,3,6-Trichlorobenzoic Acid	H	
TCBC	Trichlorobenzyl Chloride	H	
TCMTB	Busan 72	St	
Tear Gas	Chloropicrin	Fm	
Tebulan	Tebuthiuron	H	
Tebuthiuron		H	259
TEC		F	001
Tecoram	TEC	F	
Tecto	Thiabendazole	F /An	466
Tecto RPH	Thiabendazole	F /An	637
Tedion	Tetradifon	Ac	379, 580
Tekkam	1-Naphthaleneacetic Acid	Pg	
Tekwaisa	Methyl Parathion	I	
Telefos	Prothoate	I /Ac	
Telone	1,3-Dichloropropene	Fm	238
Telone C		Fm	238
Telvar	Monuron	H	247
Telvar-ML	Monuron	H	247
Temephos	Biothion	I	
Temik	Aldicarb	I /Ac	757
Temophos	Abate	I	
Ten-Eighty	Fluoroacetate	R	
Ten-Eighty-One	Fluoroacetamide	R	
Tenoran	Chloroxuron	H	190, 193
TEPP	Tetraethyl Pyrophosphate	I	
Terbacil		H	247
Terbufos		I	046
Terbumeton		H	193
Terbuthylazine		H	193
Terbutrol	2,6-Di-tert-Butyl-p-Tolyl-N-Methylcarbamate	H	
Terbutryn	Terbutryne	H	
Terbutryne		H	190, 439

Starred ingredients (*) may be responsible for major toxic effects; consult Section II.

PRODUCT NAME	ALTERNATE NAME	PRINCIPAL USE	MANU-FACTURER
	PESTICIDES (Cont.)		
Termil	Chlorothalonil	F	232
Termitkil	o-Dichlorobenzene	Fm	
Term-I-Trol	Pentachlorophenol	Wp	
Terraclor	Pentachloronitrobenzene	F	550
Terraclor Super-X	Ethazol	F	550
Terracoat	Ethazol	St	550
Terracur		N /F	115
Terracur-P	Fensulfothion	N /I	115
Terraklene	Paraquat	H	370
Terra-Sytam	Dimefox	Ac/I	
Terrazole	Ethazol	F	550
Terr-O-Cide	(see Great Lakes Chemical Corp.)	Fm/N	319
Terr-O-Gas	(see Great Lakes Chemical Corp.)	N /I	319
Terr-O-Gas 100	Methyl Bromide	Fm	319
Terr-O-Gel	(see Great Lakes Chemical Corp.)	Fm	319
Tersan 75	Thiram	F	247
Tersan 1991	Benomyl	F	247
Tersan LSR	Maneb	F	247
Tersan SP	Chloroneb	F	247
Tetrachloromethane	Carbon Tetrachloride	Fm	
2,3,4,6-Tetrachlorophenol		Wp	238
Tetrachlorvinphos		I	661, 667
Tetradifon		Ac	379, 580
Tetradiphon	Tetradifon	Ac	
Tetraethyl Pyrophosphate		I	475
Tetrafluoron	Fluoretoxuron	H	
Tetralex Plus		H	664
Tetramethrin		I	275, 718
Tetrapion	Frenock	H	718
Tetra-n-Propyl Dithionopyrophosphate		I	697
Tetrasul	Animert V-101	Ac	
Tetron	Tetraethyl Pyrophosphate	I	
Tetroxone	(see ICI Plant Protection Division)	H	370
TFN	Lamprecide	Ft	
TH 6040	Diflubenzuron	I	
Thallium Sulfate		I /R	115
Thanite		I	460
Thiabendazole		F /An	466
Thiadiazinthion	Terracur	N /F	
Thiazfluron		H	193
Thibenzole	Thiabendazole	F /An	466
Thifor	Thiodan	I /Ac	
Thimer		F	199
Thimet	Phorate	I	046
Thimul	Thiodan	I /Ac	
Thiochloroethyl	Clearcide	H	
Thiodan		I /Ac	295, 781
Thiodemeton	Disulfoton	I /Ac	
Thiodiphenylamine	Phenothiazine	I /An	
Thiofanox		I	231, 664
Thioknock	Thiram	F /St	
Thiolux	Sulfur	F /Ac	643, 646
Thiometan	Metasystox-S	I /Ac	115
Thiometon		I	646
Thionax	Thiodan	I /Ac	439
Thionazin	Zinophos	I /N	
Thioneb	Metiram	F	
Thionex	Thiodan	I /Ac	439
Thiophal	Folpet	F	
Thiophanate		F	532, 566
Thiophanate Methyl		F	532, 566
Thiophos	Parathion	I	046
Thioquinox	Eradex	Ac/F	
Thiosan	Thiram	F /St	
Thiosulfan Tionel	Thiodan	I /Ac	
Thiotepp	Sulfotepp	I /Ac	
Thiotex	Thiram	F /St	
Thiovit	Sulfur	F /Ac	646
Thiram		F /St	247, 566

Starred ingredients (*) may be responsible for major toxic effects; consult Section II.

PESTICIDES (Cont.)			
PRODUCT NAME	ALTERNATE NAME	PRINCIPAL USE	MANU- FACTURER
Thiramad	Thiram	F /St	442
Thirasan	Thiram	F /St	
Thistrol	4-(2-Methyl-4-Chlorophenoxy)Butyric Acid	H	757
Thitrol	4-(2-Methyl-4-Chlorophenoxy)Butyric Acid	H	757
Thiuramin	Thiram	F /St	
Thuricide	Agritol	I	643
Thylate	Thiram	F	247
Thylpar M-50	Methyl Parathion	I	
Thynon	Dithianon	F	
Tiazon	Mylone	N /Sl Pg	757
TIBA			
Tiezene	Zineb	F	499
Tiguvon	Fenthion	I	115
Tilcarex	Pentachloronitrobenzene	F /St	115
Tillam	S-Propyl Butylethylthiocarbamate	H	697
Tillantox	Benquinox	F	
Tillex	(see Sandoz)	F /St	643
Tilt 60 WP		F	193
Timbo	Rotenone	I /Ft	
Timet	Phorate	I	
Tinox	(see VEB Elektro Chemisches Kombinat)	I	778
Tiovel	Thiodan	I /Ac	781
Tip-Off	1-Naphthaleneacetic Acid	Pg	244
Tippon	Trichlorophenoxyacetic Acid	H	238
Tirampa	Thiram	F /St	
Tirpate	(see 3M Co.)	N	739
Tiurolan	Tebuthiuron	H	
TMTD	Thiram	F /St	
TMTDS	Thiram	F /St	
TNCS 53	Tribasic Copper Sulfate	F	
To-2	CMPT	H	
Tobacco Sucker Control Agent 148	Off-Shoot-T	Pg	
Tobacco Sucker Control Agent 504	Off-Shoot-T	Pg	
Tobaz	Thiabendazole	F	466
TOK	Nitrofen	H	634, 676
Tolban	Profluralin	H	190
Tolkan	Isoproturon	H	625
Toll	Methyl Parathion	I	
Tolylfluanid		F	115
N-m-Tolylphthalamic Acid		Pg	439, 760
Tomarin	Coumafuryl	R	
Tomaset	N-m-Tolylphthalamic Acid	Pg	439
Tomato Fix	PCPA	Pg	
Tomatotone	PCPA	Pg	
Tomorin	Coumachlor	R	193
Topane	Dowicide A	F	
Topcide	Benzadox	H	334
Topiclor	Chlordane	I	
Topitox	Chlorophacinone	R	
Topsin	Thiophanate	F	532
Topsin-M	Thiophanate Methyl	F	532, 566
Topsin Wettable Powder	Thiophanate	F	532, 566
Topsin WP Methyl	Thiophanate Methyl	F	566
Topusyn	Desmetryn	H	
Topzol	Red Squill	R	124
Torak	Dialifor	I /Ac	128
Torbidan EC		I	
Tordon	Picloram	H	238
Torque	Fenbutatin-Oxide	Ac	667
Torsite	Phenylphenol	F	
Tota-Col	Paraquat	H	370
Totril	Ioxynil	H	457
Toxakil	Toxaphene	I	295
Toxaphene		I	373, 785
2,4,5-TP	Silvex	H	
TPTA	Fentinacetate	F /Al	
TPTH	Fentin Hydroxide	F	
TPTOH	Fentin Hydroxide	F	
Tramat	Ethofumasate	H	652

Starred ingredients (*) may be responsible for major toxic effects; consult Section II.

PESTICIDES (Cont.)

PRODUCT NAME	ALTERNATE NAME	PRINCIPAL USE	MANU- FACTURER
Trametan	Thiram	F /St	
Transamine		H	785
Transplantone		Pg	757
Trapex	Vorlex	Fm	
Trasan	MCPA	H	
Trefanocide	Trifluralin	H	259
Treficon	Trifluralin	H	
Treflam	Trifluralin	H	
Treflan	Trifluralin	H	259
Treflanocide Elancolan	Trifluralin	H	259
Trefmid		H	259
Tre-Hold	1-Naphthaleneacetic Acid	Pg	757
Trevin	Thiophanate Methyl	F	
Trex-San	(see Mallinckrodt, Inc.)	H	442
Trex-San Bent	(see Mallinckrodt, Inc.)	H	442
Triadimefon	Bay-Meb 6447	F	
Triallate		H	496
Triasyn	Anilazine	F	
Triatox	Amitraz	I /Ac	
Triazophos		I /N	346
Triazotion	Azinphos-Ethyl	I	
Tribac	2,3,6-Trichlorobenzoic Acid	H	
Tribactur	Agritol	I	567
Tri-Ban	2-Pivalyl-1,3-Indandione	R	
Tri-Basic	Tribasic Copper Sulfate	F	
Tribasic Copper Sulfate		F	196, 206
Tribrome	Methyl Bromide	Fm	
Tribunil	Methabenzthiazuron	H	115
Tributon		H	115
S,S,S-Tributyl Phosphorotrithioate		B/H	488
Tributyl Phosphorotrithioite		B/H	490
Tricalcium Arsenate	Calcium Arsenate	I /H	
Tricarbamix	Ziram	F	567
Tricarbasul	(see Pennwalt Holland B.V.)	F	567
Tricarnam	Carbaryl	I	
Tri-Chlor	Chloropicrin	Fm/I	
Trichlorfenson	Ovotran	Ac	
Trichlorfon		I	488, 754
Trichloroacetic Acid		H	085, 346
Trichlorobenzene		H	
2,3,6-Trichlorobenzoic Acid		H	291, 292
Trichlorobenzyl Chloride		H	496
Trichloromethane	Chloroform	Fm	
Trichloronat	Trichloronate	I	
Trichloronate		I	115
Trichlorophenol		F /B	238
Trichlorophenoxyacetic Acid		H	238, 785
2,3,6-Trichlorophenylacetic Acid		H	757
Trichlorphon	Trichlorfon	I	
Triclopyr		H	238
Tri-Clor	Chloropicrin	Fm/I	526
Tricornox	Benazolin	H	127
Tricyclazole		F	259
Tricyclohexyl Hydroxytin	Cyhexatin	Ac	238
Tridemorph		F	109, 110
Tridex		H	
Tri-Endothal	Endothall	H	566
Trietazine		H	291, 292
Triethanolamine-Copper Complex	A & V-70 Algaecide	H	
Tri-Fen	Chlorfenac	H	
Tri-Fene	Chlorfenac	H	733
Trifenmorph	Triphenmorph	M	
Trifenson	Fenson	Ac	
Trifluralin		H	259, 499
Triflurex	Trifluralin	H	439
Trifocide	4,6-Dinitro-o-Cresol	I /F	567
Trifolex-Tra	(see Shell Chemicals U.K. Ltd.)	H	664
Triforine		F	145
Triformol	Paraformaldehyde	Fm	

Starred ingredients (*) may be responsible for major toxic effects; consult Section II.

PESTICIDES (Cont.)

PRODUCT NAME	ALTERNATE NAME	PRINCIPAL USE	MANU-FACTURER
Trifungol	Ferbam	F	567
Triherbide	Propham	H	
Triherbide-CIPC	Chlorpropham	H	567
Triherbide-IPC	Propham	H	567
Tri-Iodobenzoic Acid	TIBA	Pg	
Trim	Trifluralin	H	
Trimangol	Maneb	F	567
Trimanoc	Maneb	F	567
Trimanzone	(see Pennwalt Holland B.V.)	F	567
Trimastan		F	567
Trimaton	Vapam	Fm	567
Trimec	(see PBI-Gordon Corp.)	H	559
Trimetion	Dimethoate	I /Ac	
Trinex	Trichlorfon	I	
Trinox	Trichlorfon	I	
Trinoxol	Trichlorophenoxyacetic Acid	H	757
Tri-PCNB	Pentachloronitrobenzene	F /St	
Tri-P.E.		H	567
Tripece		Pg	567
Tripene	ZR-619	Ig	
Triphenmorph		M	667
Triphenyltin Acetate	Fentinacetate	F /Al	
Triphenyltin Hydroxide	Fentin Hydroxide	F	
Triple-Noctin		F	391
Tripomol	Thiram	F /St	567
Triquintam		F	567
Trirodazeen	Nirit	F	567
Tri-Rodazene	Nirit	F	
Triscabol	Ziram	F	567
Trithion	Carbophenothion	I /Ac	697
Tritisan	Pentachloronitrobenzene	F /St	346
Tritofterol	Zineb	F	567
Tritrol	4-(2-Methyl-4-Chlorophenoxy)Butyric Acid	H	
Tri-VC-13	VC-13 Nemacide	N /I	567
Trixabon		H	567
Trixan		H	567
Triziman	(see Pennwalt Holland B.V.)	F	567
Triziman D	Vondozeb	F	567
Trolene	Ronnel	I	238
Tronabor	Borax	H	406
Tropital		Ad	460
Tropotox	4-(2-Methyl-4-Chlorophenoxy)Butyric Acid	H	457
Trotox	4-(2-Methyl-4-Chlorophenoxy)Butyric Acid	H	
Truban	Ethazol	F	442
Trucidor	Vamidothion	I	
Trysben	2,3,6-Trichlorobenzoic Acid	H	247
Trysben 200	2,3,6-Trichlorobenzoic Acid	H	247
Tserenox	Benquinox	F	
Tsitrex	Cyprex	F	
Tsumacide	Metacrate	I	523
Tuads	Thiram	F /St	
Tuberite	Propham	H	
Tubothane	Maneb	F	457
Tubotin	Fentinacetate	F	457
Tugon	Trichlorfon	I	115
Tugon Fliegenkugel	2-Isopropoxyphenyl N-Methylcarbamate	I	115
Tumbleleaf	Sodium Chlorate	H	406
Tumex	8-Hydroxyquinoline	F	
Tunic	Methazole	H	
3336 Turf Fungicide	Thiophanate	F	
Tuscopper	Copper Naphthenates	F	
Tutane	Frucote	F	259
Tuzet	Urbacide	F	115
U-27267	(see TUCO, Div. of the Upjohn Co.)	H	754
U-36059	Amitraz	I /Ac	
UBI-N252		B/Df	760
UBI-P293		Pg	760
UC 7744	Carbaryl	I	757
UC 10854		I	757

Starred ingredients (*) may be responsible for major toxic effects; consult Section II.

PRODUCT NAME	ALTERNATE NAME	PRINCIPAL USE	MANU- FACTURER
UC 19786	Dinobuton	Ac/F	757
UC 20299	Prep	H	757
UC 21149	Aldicarb	I /Ac	757
UC 22463	Rowmate	H	757
Udonkor		F	532
Ultracide	Methidathion	I /Ac	193
Ultra-Sofril	Benomyl	F	
Ulvair	Monocrotophos	I /Ac	193
Umbethion	Coumaphos	I	610
Unden	2-Isopropoxyphenyl N-Methylcarbamate	I	115
Unidol	Methyl Parathion	I	
Unipon	Dalapon	H	
Uniroyal D014	Propargite	Ac	760
Urab		H	355
Urbacid	Urbacide	F	115
Urbacide		F	115
Urbasulf	Rhizoctol	F /St	
Ureabor		H	547
Ureabor 8D		H	547
Urifume	1,2-Dibromoethane	Fm	
Urox	Monuron	H	355
Urox B	Bromacil	H	355
Urox HX	Bromacil	H	355
USB-3584	Dinitramine	H	
Uspulum	(see Bayer AG)	F	115
Ustilan		H	115
Vacor		R	634
Valexon	Phoxim	I	634
Validacin	Validamycin	F	724
Validamycin		F	724
Validamycin A	Validamycin	F	
Valone		R	508
Vamidoate	Vamidothion	I	
Vamidothion		I	625
Vancide 51	(see R.T. Vanderbilt Co., Inc.)	F	775
Vancide FE-95	Ferbam	F	775
Vancide MZ-96	Ziram	F	775
Vancide TM-95	Thiram	F /St	775
Vancide TM-Flowable	Thiram	F /St	775
Vancide-Zineb 85	Zineb	F	775
Van Dyk 264	MGK 264	Ad	
Vantal	(see Montedison S.p.A.)	I	499
Vapam		Fm	697
Vapona	Dichlorvos	I	661, 667
Vaponite	Dichlorvos	I	661
Vaporooter	Vapam	Fm	697
Vapotone	Tetraethyl Pyrophosphate	I	187
Varitox	Trichloroacetic Acid	H	457
VC-13	VC-13 Nemacide	I /N	
VC-13 Nemacide		I /N	490
VCS 438	Methazole	H	
Vectal	Atrazine	H	292
Vegabate I		H	715
Vegadex		H	496
Vegedex	Vegadex	H	
Vegfru	Phorate	I	
Vegiben	Chloramben	H	757
Vel 4283	Safrotin	I	
Vel 5026	Ravage	H	
Vel 5052		H	781
Velpar		H	247
Velpar Weed Killer	Velpar	H	247
Velsicol 1068	Chlordane	I	781
Vendex	Fenbutatin-Oxide	I /Ac	661, 667
Ventox	Acritet	Fm	228
Venzar	Lenacil	H	247
Veon	Trichlorophenoxyacetic Acid	H	238
Veon 245	Trichlorophenoxyacetic Acid	H	238
Veratridine	Sabadilla	I	

Starred ingredients (*) may be responsible for major toxic effects; consult Section II.

	PESTICIDES (Cont.)		
PRODUCT NAME	ALTERNATE NAME	PRINCIPAL USE	MANU-FACTURER
Veratrin	Sabadilla	I	
Vergemaster	2,4-D	H	231
Vernam	Vernolate	H	697
Vernolate		H	697
Vertifume		Fm	238
Verton	2,4-D	H	238
Verton 2D	2,4-D	H	238
Verton 2T	Trichlorophenoxyacetic Acid	H	238
Vi-Cad	Cadmium Chloride	F	
Vidden-D	D-D	Fm	238
Vikane Fumigant	Sulfuryl Fluoride	Fm	238
Vinyl Carbinol	Allyl Alcohol	H /F	
Vinylphate	Chlorfenvinphos	I	
Viozene	Ronnel	I	
Vi-Par	Mecoprop	H	787
Vi-Pex	Mecoprop	H	787
Viricuivre	Cupric Chloride, Basic	F	625
Viron/H	Biotrol VHZ	I	646
Vitigran Blue	Cupric Chloride, Basic	F	346
Vitigran Concentrate	Cupric Chloride, Basic	F	346
VM & P Naphthas		H	187, 493
Volaton	Phoxim	I	115
Volck Oils	Dormant Oils	I	187
Vomiting Gas	Chloropicrin	Fm	
Vondalhyde	Maleic Hydrazide	Pg	567
Vondcaptan	Captan	F	567
Vondodine	Cyprex	F	567
Vondozeb		F	567
Vondrax	Maleic Hydrazide	Pg	567
Vonduci	Diuron	H	567
Vonduron	Diuron	H	567
Vorlex		Fm	652
Voronit		F /St	115
Vorox	Simazine	H	
VPM	Vapam	Fm	
Vydate	Oxamyl	I	247
Vydate L Oxamyl	Oxamyl	I	247
W 5769	Chlorfenprop-Methyl	H	
Wacker S14/10	Dimefox	Ac/I	796
Warbex	Famphur	I	046
Warf	Warfarin	R	118
Warfarat	Warfarin	R	
Warfarin		R	598, 781
Warficide	Warfarin	R	
Weedall	Petroleum Distillate	H	
Weedar (NI, FCH)	2,4-D	H	757
Weedar (NI)	MCPA	H	757
Weedar (FCH)	Trichlorophenoxyacetic Acid	H	757
Weedar-64	2,4-D	H	757
Weedar-At	3-Amino-1,2,4-Triazole	H	757
Weedazol	3-Amino-1,2,4-Triazole	H	757
Weedazol T	3-Amino-1,2,4-Triazole	H	757
Weedbeads	Sodium Pentachlorophenate	H	238
Weed-B-Gon (NI, FCH, Th)	2,4-D	H	187
Weed-B-Gon (FCH, NI)	Silvex	H	187
Weed Broom		H	626
Weed Drench	Allyl Alcohol	H	
Weed-E-Rad (Th, FCH)	Disodium Methylarsonate	H	787
Weed-E-Rad (Th, FCH, NI)	MSMA	H	787
Weedex	Simazine	H	
Weedez Wonder Bar	2,4-D	H	626
Weed-Hoe (FCH)	Disodium Methylarsonate	H	787
Weed-Hoe (Th, FCH)	MSMA	H	787
Weedmaster		H	781
Weed Oils	Petroleum Distillate	H	
Weedol	Paraquat	H	370
Weedone	Calar	H	757
Weedone (Th, FCH, NI)	2,4-D	H	757
Weedone (FCH)	Pentachlorophenol	H	757

Starred ingredients (*) may be responsible for major toxic effects; consult Section II.

PESTICIDES (Cont.)			
PRODUCT NAME	ALTERNATE NAME	PRINCIPAL USE	MANU- FACTURER
Weedone (FCH)	Trichlorophenoxyacetic Acid	H	757
Weedone (NI)	Silvex	H	757
Weedone Crabgrass Killer	Calar	H	757
Weedone-2,4,5-TP	Silvex	H	757
Weed-Rhap	2,4-D	H	785
Weedrite	Diquat Dibromide	H	754
Weedtrine		H /Aq	187
Weedtrine-D		H	073
Weevil-Tox	Carbon Disulfide	Fm	475
Wettable Sulfur	Sulfur	F /Ac	
White Oils	Dormant Oils	I /H	
White Phosphorus	Phosphorus	I /R	
Wittox C	Copper Naphthenates	F	811
WL 17731	Benzoylprop Ethyl	H	
WL 19805	Cyanazine	H	
WL 29762	Barnon	H	
Wofatox	Methyl Parathion	I	
X-52		H	523
Xylene			208, 758
Xylol	Xylene		
Yaltox	Carbofuran	I /N	
Yamaclean		H	535
Yanock	Fluoroacetamide	R	
Yasoknock	Fluoroacetate	R	
Yellow Oxide of Mercury	(see Sandoz Ltd.)	F	646
Yellow Phosphorus	Phosphorus	I /R	
Yomesan	Niclosamide	An	214
ZAC	Goodrite ZAC	F	
Zaclondiscoids	Hydrocyanic Acid	Fm	
Zardex	ZR-856	Ac	820
Z-C	Ziram	F	295
Z-C Spray	Ziram	F	295
Zeapur	Simazine	H	
Zeazin	Atrazine	H	
Zebtox	Zineb	F	
Zeidane	DDT	I	
Zelan	MCPA	H	
Zelio	Thallium Sulfate	R /I	115
Zephiran	Benzalkonium Chloride	B /F	808
Zerdane	DDT	I	
Zerlate	Ziram	F	247
Zidan	Zineb	F	439
Ziman-Dithane	Mancozeb	F	
Zimate	Zineb	F	
Zinc Chloride	(see E.I. du Pont de Nemours & Co., Inc.)	Wp	247
Zinc Coposil		F	187
Zinc Copro	Zinc Coposil	F	
Zincmate	Ziram	F	
Zinc Metiram	Metiram	F	
Zinc Phosphide		R	262, 352
Zinc Sulfate	(see Cities Service Co., Industrial Chemicals Div.)	Wp	196
Zinc Sulfate, Basic	(see Woolfolk Chemical Works, Inc.)	B	817
Zineb		F	295, 634
Zinkcarbamate	Ziram	F	
Zinosan	Zineb	F	625
Ziram		F	295, 566
Zirberk	Ziram	F	
Ziride	Ziram	F	
Zithiol	Malathion	I	625
Zitox	Ziram	F	
Zolone	Phosalone	Ac/I	625, 626
Zoocoumarin	Warfarin	R	
Zorial	Norflurazon	H	643
Zotox Crab Grass Killer	Arsenic Acid	H	
ZR-512	Altozar	Ig	
ZR-515	Methoprene	Ig	
ZR-619		Ig	820
ZR-777	Kinoprene	Ig	

Starred ingredients (*) may be responsible for major toxic effects; consult Section II.

PESTICIDES (Cont.)

PRODUCT NAME	ALTERNATE NAME	PRINCIPAL USE	MANU-FACTURER
ZR-856		Ac	820
6-12	2-Ethyl-1,3-Hexanediol	Re	226
666	BHC	I	
1080	Fluoroacetate	R	
1081	Fluoroacetamide	R	
3956	Toxaphene	I	

PESTICIDES (Cont.)

001
AAGRUNOL, N.V., CHEMICAL WORKS
OosterKade 10
Groningen, Holland

004
ABBOTT LABORATORIES
Chemical & Agricultural Products Div.
14th and Sheridan Rds.
North Chicago, IL 60064
(312) 937-5171

007
ABCO INC.
230 Industry Blvd.
North Huntingdon, PA 15642
(412) 864-1900

010
**ACETO AGRICULTURAL CHEMICAL
CORP.**
126-02 Northern Blvd.
Flushing, NY 11368
(212) 898-2300

013
AGCHEM DIVISION
See PENNWALT CORP.

016
AGRICO CHEMICAL CO.
One Williams Center
Tulsa, OK 74103
(918) 538-3641

019
**AGRICOLA CHEMICALS LTD. (Great
Britain)**
2 Stratford Place
London W1N9AE, England

022
**AGRICULTURAL & INDUSTRIAL
CHEMICALS, INC.**
665 Fifth Ave.
New York, NY 10022
(212) 335-1140

025
AGWAY INC.
P.O. Box 4933
Syracuse, NY 13221
(315) 477-6145

028
ALDRICH CHEMICAL CO., INC.
940 S. St. Paul Ave.
Milwaukee, WI 53233
(414) 273-3850

031
ALLIED CHEMICAL CORP.
Agricultural Div.
P.O. Box 1000-R
Morristown, NJ 07960
(201) 455-3984

034
ALLIED CHEMICAL CORP.
Industrial Chemicals Div.
Box 1139-R
Morristown, NJ 07960
(201) 538-8000

037
ALLIED CHEMICAL CORP.
Specialty Chemicals Div.
P.O. Box 1087R
Morristown, NJ 07960
(201) 455-4338

038
ALL INDIA MEDICAL CORP.
185 Princess St.
P.O. Box 2398
Bombay, 400 002, India

040
ALPHA LABORATORIES, INC.
1685 S. Fairfax St.
P.O. Box 22223
Denver, CO 80222
(303) 756-1338

043
AMCHEM PRODUCTS, INC.
See UNION CARBIDE AGRICULTURAL PRODUCTS
CO., INC.

046
AMERICAN CYANAMID CO.
Agricultural Div.
P.O. Box 400
Princeton, NJ 08540
(609) 799-0400

049
AMERICAN FLUORIDE CORP.
17 Huntington Pl.
New Rochelle, NY 10801
(914) 633-7005

PESTICIDES (Cont.)

052
AMERICAN FUMIGATING CO.
9A S. Florissant Rd.
St. Louis, MO 63135
(314) 521-1300

055
AMERICAN HOECHST CORP.
Agricultural Div.
Route 202-206 North
Somerville, NJ 08876
(201) 685-2000

058
AMOCO OIL CO.
200 E. Randolph Dr.
Chicago, IL 60601
(312) 856-5111

061
AMSCO DIVISION
Union Oil Co. of California
3100 S. Meacham Rd.
Palatine, IL 60067
(312) 885-5450

062
AMVAC CHEMICAL CORP.
4100 E. Washington Blvd.
Los Angeles, CA 90023
(213) 264-3910

064
THE ANDERSONS
P.O. Box 119
Maumee, OH 43537
(419) 893-5050

067
ANSUL CO.
One Stanton St.
Marinette, WI 54143
(715) 735-7411

070
APPERSON CHEMICALS, INC.
P.O. Box 2555
Jacksonville, FL 32203
(904) 389-6671

073
APPLIED BIOCHEMISTS, INC.
5300 W. County Line Rd.
Mequon, WI 53092
(414) 242-5870

076
ARAPAHOE CHEMICALS, INC.
2075 N. 55th St.
P.O. Box 511
Boulder, CO 80301
(303) 442-1926

079
ASGROW FLORIDA CO.
P.O. Drawer D
Plant City, FL 33566
(813) 752-1177

082
ASHLAND CHEMICAL CO.
P.O. Box 2219
Columbus, OH 43216
(614) 889-3333

085
ATANOR S.A.M.
Lavalle 348 2o Piso
Buenos Aires, Argentina

088
ATLANTIC RICHFIELD CO.
515 S. Flower St.
Los Angeles, CA 90071
(213) 486-3511

091
ATUL PRODUCTS LTD.
Post Atul, Dist. Valsad
Gujarat State, Pin 396020, India

094
A & V, INC.
850 Hickory St.
Pewaukee, WI 53072
(414) 691-4540

097
AVITROL CORP.
P.O. Box 45141
Tulsa, OK 74145
(918) 663-1063

100
AYERST LABORATORIES
685 Third Ave.
New York, NY 10017
(212) 986-1000

103
BAKER, J.T., CHEMICAL CO.
222 Red School Lane
Phillipsburg, NJ 08865
(201) 859-2151

PESTICIDES (Cont.)

106
BARIUM AND CHEMICALS, INC.
P.O. Box 218
Steubenville, OH 43952
(614) 282-9776

109
BASF AKTIENGESELLSCHAFT
Carl-Bosch-Str. 38
D-6700 Ludwigshafen
Federal Republic of Germany

110
BASF INDIA LTD.
Agrochemical Div.
Maybaker House, Sudam Kalu Ahire Marg.
Bombay 400 025, India

112
BASF WYANDOTTE CORP.
Agricultural Chemicals Div.
100 Cherry Hill Rd.
P.O. Box 181
Parsippany, NJ 07054
(201) 263-0200

115
BAYER AG
Pflanzenschutz Anwendungstechnik Beratung
509 Leverkusen Bayerwerk
Federal Republic of Germany

116
BIOCHEM PRODUCTS AG
Lange Gasse 33
4010 Basel, Switzerland

118
BLACK LEAF PRODUCTS CO.
667 N. State St.
Elgin, IL 60120
(312) 697-4400

121
BLUE SPRUCE CO.
50 Division Ave.
Millington, NJ 07946
(201) 647-4570

124
BONIDE CHEMICAL CO., INC.
2 Wurz Ave.
Yorkville, NY 13495
(315) 736-8231

127
THE BOOTS CO., LTD.
Agro Chemical Div.
1 Thane Rd. West
Nottingham, England

128
BOOTS HERCULES AGROCHEMICALS CO.
3411 Silverside Rd.
Box 7489
Wilmington, DE 19803
(302) 575-7850

129
BUCKEYE CELLULOSE CORP.
Agricultural Specialties Dept.
1355 Lynnfield Rd.
Memphis, TN 38138
(901) 761-2500

130
BUCKMAN LABORATORIES, INC.
1256 N. McLean Blvd.
Memphis, TN 38108
(901) 278-0330

133
BURTS & HARVEY LTD.
Crabtree Manorway
Belvedere, Kent DA17 6BQ
England

136
CALBIOCHEM
P.O. Box 12087
San Diego, CA 92112
(714) 453-7331

139
C AND R PRODUCTS DEVELOPMENT, INC.
Address unknown

142
CARAJON CHEMICAL CO., INC.
P.O. Box 167
Fremont, MI 49412
(612) 924-3900

145
CELAMERCK GmbH & CO., KG
P.O. Box 202
6507 Ingelheim/Rhein
Federal Republic of Germany

PESTICIDES (Cont.)

148
CELANESE CORP.
1211 Ave. of the Americas
New York, NY 10036
(212) 764-7640

151
CENEX, INC.
P.O. Box 43089
St. Paul, MN 55164
(612) 451-5151

154
CENTERCHEM, INC.
475 Park Ave.
New York, NY 10016
(212) 725-5665

157
CEQUISA
Muntaner 322, 1o 2a
Barcelona, Spain

160
CHARTER CHEMICALS
Charter International Oil Co.
P.O. Box 5008
Houston, TX 77012
(713) 923-3300

163
CHEMAGRO AGRICULTURAL DIVISION
See MOBAY CHEMICAL CORP.

166
CHEMICAL FORMULATORS, INC.
3260 Powers Ferry Rd., SE
Marietta, GA 30067
(404) 952-6132

169
CHEMICAL INSECTICIDE CORP.
Address unknown

172
CHEMICAL SUPPLY CO., LTD.
AMP House
Dingwall Rd.
Croyden, CR9 3QU England

175
CHEMINOVA
P.O. Box 9
DK 7620 Lemvig, Denmark

178
CHEMLEY PRODUCTS CO.
P.O. Box 14, Northtown Sta.
Chicago, IL 60659
(312) 674-8033

181
CHEMPAR CHEMICAL CO., INC.
60 E. 42nd St.
New York, NY 10065
(212) 687-3990

184
CHEMSERVICE CO.
8-20 Merry Lane
East Hanover, NJ 07936
(201) 386-0171

187
CHEVRON CHEMICAL CO.
Agricultural Pesticides Div.
575 Market St.
San Francisco, CA 94105
(415) 894-7800

188
CHIPMAN CHEMICALS, INC.
P.O. Box 128
River Rouge, MI 48218
(313) 842-6200

190
CIBA-GEIGY CORP.
Agricultural Division
P.O. Box 11422
Greensboro, NC 27409
(919) 292-7100

193
CIBA-GEIGY LTD.
P.O. Box CH 4002
Basle 7, Switzerland

196
CITIES SERVICE CO.
Box 50360
Atlanta, GA 30302
(404) 261-9100

199
CLEARY, W.A., CHEMICAL CORP.
1049 Somerset St.
Somerset, NJ 08873
(201) 247-8000

PESTICIDES (Cont.)

200
COMLETS CHEMICAL INDUSTRIAL CO.,
LTD.
61 Shinping Rd.
Taiping Hsiang 406
Taichung Hsien
Taiwan, Republic of China

202
COMMERCIAL CHEMICALS CO.
P.O. Box 7415
Memphis, TN 38107

205
COMMERCIAL SOLVENTS CORP.
245 Park Ave.
New York, NY 10017
(212) 661-5454

206
CP CHEMICALS, INC.
Arbor St.
P.O. Box 158
Sewaren, NJ 07077
(201) 636-4300

208
CROWLEY TAR PRODUCTS CO., INC.
261 Madison Ave.
New York, NY 10016
(212) 682-1200

211
CRYSTAL CHEMICAL CO.
1525 N. Post Oak Rd.
Houston, TX 77055
(713) 682-1221

214
CUTTER ANIMAL HEALTH
LABORATORIES
Div. of Bayvet Corp.
P.O. Box 390
Shawnee Mission, KA 66201
(913) 631-4800

217
DARWORTH CO.
Tower Lane
Avon, CT 06001
(203) 677-7721

220
DAVID CHEMICAL CO.
Address unknown

223
DAVISON CHEMICAL DIVISION
See GRACE, W.R., & CO.

226
The d-CON CO., INC.
225 Summit Ave.
Montvale, NJ 07645
(201) 573-5700

227
DEGESCH AMERICA, INC.
P.O. Box 116
Weyers Cave, VA 24486
(703) 234-9281

228
DEGESCH, GmbH
Address unknown

229
DEXOL INDUSTRIES, INC.
1450 W. 228th
Torrance, CA 90501
(213) 326-8373

231
DIAMOND SHAMROCK
AGROCHEMICALS LTD.
Bayheath House
4, The Fairway, Petts Wood
Kent BR5 1EG, England

232
DIAMOND SHAMROCK CORP.
Agricultural Chemicals Div.
1100 Superior Ave.
Cleveland, OH 44114
(216) 694-5222

233
DIAMOND SHAMROCK DE MEXICO, S.A.
Melchor Ocampo, 436-80-piso
Mexico 5, D.F.

235
DOVER CHEMICAL CORP.
Sub. of I.C.C. Industries, Inc.
15th & Davis Sts.
Dover, OH 44622
(216) 343-7711

239
DOW CHEMICAL LTD.
Swan Office Center
1508 Coventry Rd.
Yardley, Birmingham B25 8AD
England

PESTICIDES (Cont.)

238
DOW CHEMICAL U.S.A.
P.O. Box 1706
Midland, MI 48640
(517) 636-1000

241
DREXEL CHEMICAL CO.
P.O. Box 9306
Memphis, TN 38109
(901) 744-4370

244
DUPHAR-MIDOX, LTD.
Smarden, Kent TN 278QL
England

247
DU PONT, E.I., DE NEMOURS & CO., INC.
1007 Market St.
Wilmington, DE 19898
(302) 774-2421

250
EASTERN CHEMICAL CORP.
Div. of Guardian Chemical Corp.
230 Marcus Blvd.
Hauppauge, NY 11787
(516) 273-0900

253
EASTMAN CHEMICAL PRODUCTS, INC.
200 S. Wilcox Dr.
Kingsport, TN 37662
(615) 247-0411

256
EHRLICH, J.C., CHEMICAL CO., INC.
840 William Lane
Reading, PA 19612
(215) 921-0641

259
ELANCO PRODUCTS CO.
Div. of Eli Lilly & Co.
P.O. Box 1750
Indianapolis, IN 46206
(317) 261-3000

262
EXCEL INDUSTRIES LIMITED
Jogeshwari (West)
Bombay 400 060 India

265
EXXON COMPANY, U.S.A.
P.O. Box 2180
Houston, TX 77001
(713) 656-3636

268
FABRIEK VAN CHEMISCHE
PRODUCTEN
 VONDELINGENPLAAT B.V.
P.O. Box 7120
Rotterdam 3031, Netherlands

271
FAESY & BESTHOFF, INC.
143 River Road
Edgewater, NJ 07020
(201) 945-6200

274
FAIRFAX BIOLOGICAL LABORATORY
Electronic Rd., P.O. Box 242
Clinton Corners, NY 12514
(914) 266-3705

275
FAIRFIELD AMERICAN CORP.
3932 Salt Rd.
Medina, NY 14103
(716) 798-2141

277
FAIRFIELD CHEMICAL CO.
P.O. Box 20-A
Blythewood, SC 29016
(803) 754-3856

280
FAIRMOUNT CHEMICAL CO., INC.
Agri-Specialties Div.
2317 Versailles Rd.
Lexington, KY 40504
(606) 233-7399

I.G. FARBEN
Address unknown

286
FARM PROTECTION LTD.
Great Britain
Address unknown

289
FERGUSON FUMIGANTS, INC.
93 Ford Lane
Hazelwood, MO 63042
(314) 731-0414

PESTICIDES (Cont.)

291
FISONS INC.
Agricultural Chemicals Div.
2 Preston Court
Bedford, MA 01730
(617) 275-1000

292
FISONS LTD.
Agrochemical Div.
Hauxton, Cambridge CB2 5HU
England

295
FMC CORP.
Agricultural Chemical Div.
2000 Market St.
Philadelphia, PA 19103
(215) 299-6000

298
FORSHAW CHEMICALS, INC.
650 State St.
Charlotte, NC 28208
(704) 372-6790

301
FORT DODGE LABORATORIES, INC.
P.O. Box 518
Fort Dodge, IA 50501
(515) 573-3131

304
FRITZCHE DODGE & OLCOTT INC.
76 Ninth Ave.
New York, NY 10011
(212) 929-4100

307
GAF CORP.
Chemical Div.
140 W. 51st St.
New York, NY 10020
(212) 621-5000

310
GLENN CHEMICAL CO., INC.
4149 N. Milwaukee
Chicago, IL 60641

313
GOODRICH, B.F., CHEMICAL CO.
Div. of the B.F. Goodrich Co.
6100 Oak Tree Blvd.
Cleveland, OH 44131
(216) 524-0200

223
GRACE, W.R., & CO.
Agricultural Chemicals Group
100 N. Main St.
Memphis, TN 38103
(901) 522-2000

316
GREAT LAKES BIOCHEMICAL CO., INC.
6120 W. Douglas Ave.
Milwaukee, WI 53218
(414) 464-1200

319
GREAT LAKES CHEMICAL CORP.
P.O. Box 2200
West Lafayette, IN 47906
(317) 463-2511

322
THE GREAT WESTERN SUGAR CO.
P.O. Box 5308
Denver, CO 80217
(303) 893-4600

325
GREEN CROSS PRODUCTS
Address unknown

328
GREENWOOD CHEMICAL CO.
P.O. Box 26, Hwy. 690
Greenwood, VA 22943
(703) 456-6832

331
GUARD CHEMICAL CO.
One Ave. L
Newark, NJ 07105
(201) 589-6330

250
GUARDIAN CHEMICAL CORP.
230 Marcus Blvd.
Hauppauge, NY 11787
(516) 273-0900

334
GULF OIL CHEMICALS CO.
Industrial and Specialty Chemicals Div.
9009 W. 67th St.
Shawnee Mission, KS 66202
(913) 722-3200

PESTICIDES (Cont.)

337
HARSHAW CHEMICAL CO.
1945 E. 97th St.
Cleveland, OH 44106
(216) 721-8300

340
HENRY, J.F., CHEMICAL CO., INC.
245 Park Avenue
East Rutherford, NJ 07073
(201) 939-7100

343
HERCULES INC.
910 Market St.
Wilmington, DE 19899
(302) 575-6500

344
HINDUSTAN INSECTICIDES LTD.
Bahadur Shah Zafar Marg.
New Delhi 110 002, India

346
HOECHST AKTIENGESELLSCHAFT
6230 Frankfurt (Main)-80
Federal Republic of Germany

349
HOKKO CHEMICAL INDUSTRY CO., LTD.
Mitsui Bldg. No. 2
4-2, Nihonbashi Hongoku-cho
Chuo-ku, Tokyo, Japan

352
HOOKER CHEMICALS AND PLASTICS CORP.
P.O. Box 344
Niagara Falls, NY 14302
(716) 278-7000

355
HOPKINS AGRICULTURAL CHEMICAL CO.
P.O. Box 7532
Madison, WI 53707
(608) 222-0624

358
HUMMEL CHEMICAL CO.
P.O. Box 250
South Plainfield, NJ 07080
(201) 754-1800

361
HYSAN CORP.
919 W. 38th St.
Chicago, IL 60609
(312) 376-8900

364
ICI AMERICAS, INC.
Wilmington, DE 19897
(302) 575-3000

367
ICI AUSTRALIA LTD.
ICI House, 1 Nicholson St.
P.O. Box 4311
Melbourne, Victoria, 3001
Australia

370
ICI PLANT PROTECTION DIVISION
Fernhurst, Haslemere
Surrey, England

373
IDACON, INC.
10611 Harwin
Houston, TX 77036
(713) 988-9252

376
IMC CHEMICAL GROUP, INC. (BOSTON)
2000 Prudential Tower
Boston, MA 02199
(617) 266-8100

377
IMPERIAL CHEMICAL INDUSTRIES, LTD.
Imperial Chemical House
Millbank, London SW1, England

378
INVENTA CORP.
Ready Money Terrace, 167
Besant Rd., Worli
Bombay 400 018, India

379
I. PI. CI. S.P.A.
Industria Prodetti Chimici
Via F. Beltrami, 11
20026 Novate Milanese, Italy

382
ISHIHARA SANGYO KAISHA, LTD.
11, Edobori-Kamidori
1-chome, Nishi-Ku, Osaka, Japan

PESTICIDES (Cont.)

385
JEFFERSON CHEMICAL CO., INC.
P.O. Box 430
Bellaire, TX 77401
(713) 529-4471

386
JEWNIN-JOFFE CHEMICALS LTD.
Shalom Tower 9, Ahad Haam St.
P.O. Box 29511
Tel-Aviv, Israel

388
JOHNSON, S.C., & SON, INC.
1525 Howe St.
Racine, WI 53403
(414) 554-2111

391
KALO LABORATORIES, INC.
9233 Ward Pkwy.
Kansas City, MO 64114
(816) 363-1800

394
KAY-FRIES, INC.
Crop Protection Div.
Stony Point, NY 10980
(914) 942-0400

396
KEMICHROM, S.A.
Caracas, 15
Barcelona 30, Spain

397
KEMIN INDUSTRIES, INC.
2100 Maury St.
P.O. Box 70
Des Moines, IA 50301
(515) 266-2111

400
KEMIRA OY
Box 330
00101 Helsinki 10, Finland

403
KENOGARD AB
P.O. Box 11033
S-100 61 Stockholm
Sweden

406
KERR-McGEE CHEMICAL CORP.
Kerr-McGee Center
P.O. Box 25861
Oklahoma City, OK 73125
(405) 270-1313

409
KLIPFONTEIN ORGANIC PRODUCTS CORP., LTD.
P.O. Box 150
Kempton Park, Transvaal, Republic of South Africa

412
KOCIDE CHEMICAL CORP.
12701 Almeda Rd.
Houston, TX 77045
(713) 433-6404

415
KOPPERS CO., INC.
2100 Koppers Bldg.
Pittsburgh, PA 15219
(412) 227-2000

418
KUMIAI CHEMICAL INDUSTRY CO., LTD.
4-26 Ikenohata
1-chome Taitoh-ku
Tokyo 110, Japan

421
LILLY, ELI, & CO.
307 E. McCarty St.
Indianapolis, IN 46206
(317) 261-2000

424
LINCK, O.E., CO.
Div. of Walco-Linck Corp.
Routes 3 and 46
Clifton, NJ 07015
(201) 471-1070

427
LIPHA (LYONNAISE INDUSTRIELLE PHARMACEUTIQUE)
115 Avenue Lacassagne Blite postale 106 RP
69212 Lyon Cedex I, France

430
LONZA INC.
22-10 Rt. 208
Fair Lawn, NJ 07410
(201) 796-4200

PESTICIDES (Cont.)

433
LOS ANGELES CHEMICAL CO.
4545 Ardine St.
South Gate, CA 90280
(213) 583-4761

434
MAAG AGROCHEMICALS MARKETING
Hoffman-La Roche, Inc.
340 Kingsland St.
Nutley, NJ 07110
(201) 235-3633

436
THE MACKWIN CO.
McConnon & Co.
25 McConnon Dr.
Winona, MN 55987
(507) 452-2910

439
MAKHTESHIM-AGAN
P.O. Box 60
Beer-Sheva, Israel

442
MALLINCKRODT, INC.
P.O. Box 5439
St. Louis, MO 63147
(314) 895-5034

445
MANTEK CORP.
P.O. Box 22263
Dallas, TX 75207

448
MARKS, A.H., & CO., LTD.
Wyke Lane
Bradford BD12 9EJ, West Yorkshire, England

451
MARTIN, C.J., CO.
P.O. Box 1089
Nacogdoches, TX 75961
(713) 564-1413

454
MARTIN MARIETTA CHEMICALS
Sodyeco Div.
P.O. Box 10098
Charlotte, NC 28237
(704) 827-4351

457
MAY & BAKER LTD.
37-39 Manor Rd.
Romford, Essex, England RM1 2TL

460
McLAUGHLIN GORMLEY KING CO.
8810 - 10th Ave. North
Minneapolis, MN 55427
(612) 544-0341

463
McNEIL LABORATORIES, INC.
Camp Hill Rd.
Fort Washington, PA 19034
(215) 248-4500

464
MECHEMA LTD.
Talbot Wharf Chemical Works
Port Talbot
West Glamorgan SA13 IRL U.K.

466
MERCK CHEMICAL DIV.
Merck & Co., Inc.
126 Lincoln Ave., P.O. Box M
Rahway, NJ 07065
(201) 574-4000

469
MFA OIL CO.
200 S. Seventh St.
Columbia, MO 65201
(314) 442-0171

472
MICHIGAN CHEMICAL CORP.
2 N. Riverside Plaza
Chicago, IL 60606
(312) 454-7900

475
MILLER CHEMICAL & FERTILIZER CORP.
P.O. Box 333
Hanover, PA 17331
(717) 632-8921

478
MILLMASTER CHEMICAL CO.
Div. Millmast Onyx Corp.
99 Park Ave.
New York, NY 10016
(212) 687-2757

481
MINERAL RESEARCH AND DEVELOPMENT CORP.
4 Woodlawn Green
Charlotte, NC 28210
(704) 525-2771

PESTICIDES (Cont.)

484
MIRFIELD AGRICULTURAL CHEMICALS LTD.
P.O. Box 1
Mirfield, Yorkshire, England

487
MITSUI TOATSU CHEMICALS, INC.
2-5, Kamsumigaseki 3-chome chiyodu-ku
Tokyo, Japan

488
MOBAY CHEMICAL CORP.
Agricultural Chemicals Div.
P.O. Box 4913
Kansas City, MO 64120
(816) 242-2000

490
MOBIL CHEMICAL CO.
Phosphorus Division
P.O. Box 26683
Richmond, VA 23261
(804) 798-4291

493
MOBIL OIL CORP.
150 E. 42nd St.
New York, NY 10017
(212) 883-4242

496
MONSANTO AGRICULTURAL PRODUCTS CO.
800 N. Lindbergh Blvd.
St. Louis, MO 63166
(314) 694-1000

499
MONTEDISON S.P.A.
Agricultural Products Div.
Via Bonfadini, 148
20138 Milano, Italy

502
MONTROSE CHEMICAL CORP. OF CALIFORNIA
P.O. Box E, 2401 Morris Ave.
Union, NJ 07083
(201) 964-3250

505
MORTON CHEMICAL CO.
See NOR-AM AGRICULTURAL PRODUCTS, INC.

508
MOTOMCO, INC.
267 Vreeland Ave.
Paterson, NJ 07543
(201) 345-6200

511
M/S RIEDEL DE HAEN
West Germany
Address unknown

514
M & T CHEMICALS INC.
Rahway, NJ 07065
(201) 499-0200

517
MURPHY CHEMICALS LTD.
Wheathampstead
St. Albans, Herts, England

520
NALCO CHEMICAL CO.
2901 Butterfield Rd.
Oak Brook, IL 60521
(312) 887-7500

523
NIHON NOHYAKU CO., LTD.
Export Division
2-5 Nihonbashi, 1-chome Chuo-Ku
Tokyo, Japan

526
NIKLOR CHEMICAL CO., INC.
2060 E. 220th St.
Long Beach, CA 90810
(213) 830-2253

529
NIP-CO MANUFACTURING, INC.
P.O. Box 368
Glenford, NY 12433
(914) 657-8100

530
NIPPON KAYAKU CO., LTD.
New Kaijo Bldg., 2-1
1-Chome, Marunouchi, Chiyoda-ku
Tokyo, Japan

532
NIPPON SODA CO., LTD.
Fine Chemicals Div.
Shin-Ohtemachi Bldg.
2-1, 2-chome Ohtemachi
Chiyoda-ku Tokyo, Japan

PESTICIDES (Cont.)

535
NISSAN CHEMICAL INDUSTRIES, LTD.
Kowa-Hitotsubashi Bldg.
7-1, 3-chome, Kanda-Nishiki-cho
Chiyoda-ku, Tokyo, Japan

538
NOR-AM AGRICULTURAL PRODUCTS, INC.
350 W. Shuman Blvd.
Naperville, IL 60540
(312) 961-5600

541
NOTT MANUFACTURING CO., INC.
Pleasant View Rd.
Pleasant Valley, NY 12569
(914) 635-3243

544
NUTRILITE PRODUCTS, INC.
5600 Beach Blvd.
Buena Park, CA 90620
(714) 521-3900

547
OCCIDENTAL CHEMICAL CO.
P.O. Box 198
Lathrop, CA 95330
(209) 858-2511

550
OLIN CORP.
P.O. Box 991
Little Rock, AR 72203
(501) 378-3600

553
ONYX CHEMICAL CO.
Millmaster Onyx Group
190 Warren St.
Jersey City, NJ 07302
(201) 434-1700

187
ORTHO DIVISION
Chevron Chemical Co.
575 Market St.
P.O. Box 3744
San Francisco, CA 94105
(415) 894-7800

556
OSMOSE WOOD PRESERVING CO.
980 Ellicott St.
Buffalo, NY 14209
(716) 882-5905

559
PBI GORDON CORP.
300 S. 3rd St.
Kansas City, KS 66118
(913) 342-8780

562
PECHINEY-PROGIL
7, rue Lamennais
Paris, 8, France

565
PENICK CORP.
1050 Wall St. West
Lyndhurst, NJ 07071
(201) 935-6600

566
PENNWALT CORP.
Agchem Div.
3 Parkway
Philadelphia, PA 19102
(215) 587-7000

567
PENNWALT HOLLAND B.V.
Sub. of Pennwalt Corp.
P.O. Box 7120
3000 HC Rotterdam, Holland

568
PEPRO
Centre de Recherches de la Dargoire
Quartier de la Dargoire
69 Lyon 9
France

571
PFANSTIEHL LABORATORIES, INC.
1219 Glen Rock Ave.
Waukegan, IL 60085
(312) 623-0370

574
PFIZER, INC.
235 E. 42nd St.
New York, NY 10017
(212) 573-2323

577
PHELPS DODGE REFINING CORP.
300 Park Ave.
New York, NY 10022
(212) 940-6554

PESTICIDES (Cont.)

580
PHILIPS-DUPHAR B.V.
Appollolaan 151
1077 AR Amsterdam, Holland

583
PHILLIPS PETROLEUM CO.
511 TRW Bldg.
Bartlesville, OK 74004
(918) 661-4130

586
PHOSTOXIN SALES, INC.
P.O. Box 495
Alhambra, CA 91802
(213) 283-2761

589
PITMAN-MOORE, INC.
P.O. Box 344
Washington Crossing, NJ 08560
(609) 737-3700

590
PLANTERS PRODUCTS, INC.
Esteban St., Legaspi Village
Makati, Meto Manila, Philippines

592
POLYSCIENCES, INC.
Paul Valley Industrial Park
Warrington, PA 18976
(215) 343-6484

595
PPG INDUSTRIES, INC.
Chemical Div.
One Gateway Center
Pittsburgh, PA 15222
(412) 434-2252

598
PRENTISS DRUG & CHEMICAL CO., INC.
363 Seventh Ave.
New York, NY 10001
(212) 736-6766

601
PROCIDA S.A.
5, rue Bellini
92 806 Puteaux, France
or:
Saint-Marcel
13367 Marseille Cedex 4, France

604
PROCTER & GAMBLE CO.
Ivorydale Technical Center
Cincinnati, OH 45201
(513) 562-1100

607
PRODUITS CHIMIQUES UGINE
KUHLMANN
Tour Manhattan Cedex 21
92087 Paris la DeFense, France

610
QUIMICA ESTRELLA S.A.C.I.e.I.
Agrochemical and Veterinary Dept.
Av. Constituyentes 2995
Buenos Aires, Argentina 1427

613
RALSTON PURINA CO.
13001 St. Charles Rock Rd.
St. Louis, MO 63188
(314) 291-6724

616
REICHHOLD CHEMICALS, INC.
525 N. Broadway
White Plains, NY 10603
(914) 682-5700

619
RENTOKIL LABORATORIES
Felcourt, East Grinstead
Sussex, England

622
RHODIA INC.
See RHONE-POULENC CHEMICAL CO.

625
RHONE-POULENC AGROCHIMIE
14-20 rue Pierre Baizet
BP 9163-69263 Lyon, France

626
RHONE-POULENC CHEMICAL CO.
Agrochemical Div.
P.O. Box 125
Monmouth Junction, NJ 08852
(201) 297-0100

628
RING AROUND PRODUCTS
Address unknown

PESTICIDES (Cont.)

**631
ROBERTS CHEMICALS, INC.**
Div. of Security Chemicals, Inc.
P.O. Box 546
Nitro, WV 25143
(304) 755-3336

**632
ROBERTS LABORATORIES**
4995 N. Main St.
Rockford, IL 61103
(815) 877-6076

**634
ROHM AND HAAS CO.**
Agricultural Division
Independence Mall West
Philadelphia, PA 19105
(215) 592-3000

**637
ROTHWELL PLANT HEALTH, LTD.**
Rothwell, Lincoln
England

**640
RUMIANCA S.P.A.**
via Grazioli 27
20161 Milano, Italy

**643
SANDOZ, INC.**
480 Camino Del Rio South
San Diego, CA 92108
(714) 298-4343

**646
SANDOZ, LTD.**
Agro Div
Lichtstrasse
CH-4002 Basle, Switzerland

**649
SANKYO CO. LTD.**
No. 7-12, Ginza 2-chome
Chuo-ku, Tokyo 104, Japan

**652
SCHERING AKTIENGESELLSCHAFT**
Postfach 650311
D-100 Berlin 65
Federal Republic of Germany

**655
SCOTT, O. M., & SONS CO.**
333 N. Maple St.
Marysville, OH 43041
(513) 644-0011

**658
SEARLE AGRICULTURE INC.**
Algonquin Rd.
Cary, IL 60013
(312) 639-2141

**661
SHELL CHEMICAL CO.**
Agricultural Chemicals
P.O. Box 3871
Houston, TX 77001
(713) 241-6161

**664
SHELL CHEMICALS U.K. LTD.**
Agricultural Div.
39/41 St. Mary's St.
Ely, Cambridgeshire, CB7 4HG
England

**667
SHELL INTERNATIONAL CHEMICAL CO.,
LTD.**
Shell Centre
London SE1 7PG
England

**670
SHELLSTAR LTD.**
Address unknown

**671
SHEN HONG AGRICULTURAL
CHEMICAL CO., LTD.**
6F, 25, Nanking East Rd. Sec. 3
P.O. Box 46-209
Taipei, Taiwan
Republic of China

**673
SHERWIN-WILLIAMS CO.**
Chemicals Div.
P.O. Box 6506
Cleveland, OH 44101
(216) 566-2344

**676
SHING NUNG CHEMICAL CO., LTD.**
Shing Nung Bldg.
45 Wu Chuan Center St.
Taichung, Taiwan, R. O. C.

**679
SHULTON INC.**
697 Route 46
Clifton, NJ 07015
(201) 546-7000

PESTICIDES (Cont.)

682
SIGMA CHEMICAL CO.
P.O. Box 14508
St. Louis, MO 63178
(314) 771-5765

685
SINDAR CORP.
Address unknown

688
SNIA VISCOSA S.p.A.
Chemical Division
Via Montebello 18
20121 Milano, Italy

376
SOBIN CHEMICALS, INC.
See IMC CHEMICAL GROUP, INC. (BOSTON)

691
SOCIETE POUR LA PROTECTION DE
L'AGRICULTURE (SOPRA)
8 Avenue Reaumer
92-Clamart
Paris, France

694
SPEEKMAN, F.M., CO.
241 Quint St.
San Francisco, CA 94124
(415) 826-7200

696
STATE COLLEGE LABORATORIES
See ERLICH, J.C., CHEMICAL CO., INC.

697
STAUFFER CHEMICAL CO.
Agricultural Chemical Div.
Nyala Farm. Rd.
Westport, CT 06880
(203) 222-3000

700
STECKER CHEMICALS, INC.
P.O. Box 326
Ridgefield, NJ 07657
(201) 445-0433

703
STEPHENSON CHEMICAL CO., INC.
2444 West Point Rd.
College Park, GA 30337
(404) 762-0194

706
STERLING ORGANICS
Div. of Sterling Drug Inc.
90 Park Ave.
New York, NY 10016
(212) 972-2632

709
STERWIN CHEMICALS, INC.
Fine Chemicals Div.
Subs. Sterling Drug Inc.
90 Park Ave.
New York, NY 10016
(212) 972-4141

712
STORY CHEMICAL CORP.
500 Agard Rd.
Muskegon, MI 49445
(616) 766-3011

715
STULL CHEMICAL CO.
1006 Paulsun Dr.
San Antonio, TX 78219
(512) 227-5255

718
SUMITOMO CHEMICAL CO., LTD.
15, 5-chome, Kitahama
Higashi-ku, Osaka, Japan

721
SUMMIT CHEMICAL CO.
117 W. 24th St.
Baltimore, MD 21218
(301) 467-1233

722
SYNTEX S.A.
Chemical Div.
Apartado Postal 517
Cuernanaca, Morelos, Mexico

724
TAKEDA CHEMICAL INDUSTRIES, LTD.
12-10 Nihonbashi 2-Chome
Chou-ku Tokyo 103, Japan

727
TAMOGAN CHEMICALS LTD.
3-5 Hakhashmal St.
P.O. Box 2438
Tel-Aviv, Israel

730
TAVOLEX LABORATORIES
Address unknown

PESTICIDES (Cont.)

733
TENNECO CHEMICALS, INC.
Park 80 Plaza West-1
Saddle Brook, NJ 07662
(201) 646-3800

734
TEXIZE
P.O. Box 368
Greenville, SC 29602
(803) 963-4261

736
THOMPSON-HAYWARD CHEMICAL CO.
5200 Speaker Rd.
Kansas City, KS 66110
(913) 321-3131

739
3M CO.
3M Center
St. Paul, MN 55101
(612) 733-1110

742
TOWER CHEMICAL CO.
P.O. Box 1103
Clermont, FL 32711
(305) 656-2333

745
TRANSVAAL, INC.
See VERTAC CHEMICAL CORP.

748
TRIANGLE CHEMICAL CO.
P.O. Box 4528
Macon, GA 31208

751
TROY CHEMICAL CORP.
One Avenue L
Newark, NJ 07105
(201) 589-2500

754
TUCO, DIV. OF THE UPJOHN CO.
7000 Portage Rd.
Kalamazoo, MI 49001
(616) 385-6613

757
UNION CARBIDE AGRICULTURAL PRODUCTS CO., INC.
P.O. Box 17610
Jacksonville, FL 32216
(904) 731-4250

758
UNION CHEMICALS DIV.
Union Oil Co. of California
P.O. Box 60455, Union Oil Center
Los Angeles, CA 90060
(213) 486-7600

760
UNIROYAL CHEMICAL
Div. of Uniroyal, Inc.
Emic Bldg., Spencer St.
Naugatuck, CT 06770
(203) 723-3525

763
UNIVERSAL CROP PROTECTION LTD.
Park House, Maidenhead Rd.
Cookham, Berkshire, England SI6 9DS

766
U.S. BORAX & CHEMICAL CORP.
3075 Wilshire Blvd.
Los Angeles, CA 90010
(213) 381-5311

769
U.S. GYPSUM CO.
Chemicals Div.
101 S. Wacker Dr.
Chicago, IL 60606
(312) 321-4399

772
USS AGRI-CHEMICALS
Div. of U.S. Steel Corp.
P.O. Box 1685
Atlanta, GA 30301
(404) 572-4000

775
VANDERBILT, R.T., CO., INC.
30 Winfield St.
Norwalk, CT 06855
(203) 853-1400

776
VAN WATERS & ROGERS
P.O. Box 5932
San Mateo, CA 94403
(415) 573-8000

778
VEB CHEMIEKOMBINAT BITTERFELD
44 Bitterfeld, Zorbiger Strass 1
German Democratic Republic

PESTICIDES (Cont.)

781
VELSICOL CHEMICAL CORP.
341 E. Ohio St.
Chicago, IL 60611
(312) 670-4500

784
VENTRON CORP.
Chemicals Div.
Congress St.
Beverly, MA 01915
(617) 922-1875

785
VERTAC CHEMICAL CORP.
5100 Poplar Ave.
Memphis, TN 38137
(901) 767-6851

787
VINELAND CHEMICAL CO., INC.
West Wheat Rd., P.O. Box 745
Vineland, NJ 08360
(609) 691-3535

790
VIRGINIA CHEMICALS, INC.
3340 W. Norfolk Rd.
Portsmouth, VA 23703
(804) 483-7000

268
VONDELINGEN PLAAT B.V.,
  FABRIEK VAN CHEMISCHE PRODUCTEN
P.O. Box 7120
Rotterdam, 3031, Netherlands

793
VULCAN MATERIALS CO.
Chemicals Div.
P.O. Box 7689
Birmingham, AL 35223
(205) 877-3000

796
WACKER-CHEMIE GmbH
Prinzregentenstrasse 22
8000 Munchen 22, West Germany

799
WEST AGRO-CHEMICAL, INC.
P.O. Box 1386
Shawnee Mission, KS 66222
(913) 384-1660

802
WILLOW CREEK CO.
Address unknown

805
WILSON & GEO. MEYER & CO.
270 Lawrence Ave.
South San Francisco, CA 94080
(415) 871-1770

808
WINTHROP LABORATORIES
90 Park Ave.
New York, NY 10016
(212) 972-4141

811
WITCO CHEMICAL CORP.
Organics Div.
277 Park Ave.
New York, NY 10017
(212) 872-4200

814
WITCO CHEMICAL CORP.
Pioneer Division
277 Park Ave.
New York, NY 10017
(212) 644-6300

817
WOOLFOLK CHEMICAL WORKS, INC.
P.O. Box 938
Fort Valley, GA 31030
(912) 825-5511

820
ZOECON CORP.
975 California Ave.
Palo Alto, CA 94304
(415) 857-1130

PET CARE

AQUARIUM PRODUCTS
Aquarium algicide
  Monuron* plus one or more of the
    following:
    Simazine*   Toxicity rating 3 if > 10%
    Atrazine*
    Dichlone*
    Dehydroabietylamine acetate
Aquarium cleaner-disinfectant . . . . Toxicity rating 3
    Potassium permanganate* 8.0%
    Copper sulfate* 7.5%
    Water 84.5%
Aquarium medications for fish and tur-
    tles . . . . Toxicity rating 2? or 3?
Dilute solutions (water 97.5–99.8%) of
    the following single or in combi-
    nation:
    Acryflavine
    9-Aminoacridine hydrochloride
    3,6-Diamino acridinium hydrochlo-
      ride
    Malachite green (*if > 1%)
    Merbromin N.F. (*if > 1%)

Starred ingredients (*) may be responsible for major toxic effects; consult Section II.

PET CARE (Cont.)	PET CARE (Cont.)

AQUARIUM PRODUCTS (Cont.)

Neomycin sulfate	
Quinine hydrochloride (*if > 1%)	
Sodium sulfaquinoxaline	
Sodium sulfamethazine	
Sodium sulfamerazine	
Sulfathiazole sodium	
Tetracycline hydrochloride	
Tetramethylthionine chloride (*if > 1%)	

Aquarium plant fertilizer

Potassium nitrate	5.0%
Calcium phosphate	5.0%
Calcium sulfate	2.5%
Magnesium sulfate	2.5%
Sodium chloride	2.5%
Trace elements	1.0%
Water	81.5%
Aquarium sealer	Toxicity rating 2?
Methyl polysiloxane†	84.5%
Acetoxy functional siloxane	5.5%
Inert filler and pigment	10.0%

†See Silicone oils.

Aquarium water conditioner	Toxicity rating 3?

1. Dechlorination
   a. Sodium thiosulfate* 24%
   May contain:
   Methylene blue (*if > 1%)
   Potassium phosphate, permanganate (0.25%)
   Quinine sulfate 0.04%
   Sodium carbonate, (*if > 10%), chloride, phosphate
   b. Tablet, each contains .... Toxicity rating 3
   Subsulfites and rhodanides* of sodium and iron 7.0%
   Sodium perborate* 5.0%
   Polyvinyl-pyrrolidone 0.5%
   Sodium chloride* 87.5%
2. To clear cloudy water .... Toxicity rating 2 or 3
   Potassium permanganate 0.005-4%
   Water .... 96-99+%

CAT BOX LITTER	Toxicity rating 1-2
Aluminum-magnesium silicate	
Iron oxide	small amount

DEODORANTS	Toxicity rating 3? or 4?
Perfumes* 4 if 40% of some essential oils (e.g., Pine oil*)	0-40%
May contain:	
Isopropyl alcohol*	0-60%
Formalin	0-0.5%
Fatty acids	
Hexetidine	5 mg.
Chlorhexidine	0.5%
Nonionic detergents	

DOG AND CAT REPELLENTS
1. Liquid .... Toxicity rating 3

Isopropyl alcohol*	80%
Water	14%
Lemon grass oil	3%
Eucalyptus oil*	3%
Diethyl phthalate	1%
May contain:	
Ammonium carbonate	
Aqua ammonia	
Aromatic hydrocarbons*	10%
Bone oil	

DOG AND CAT REPELLENTS (Cont.)

Diethyl phthalate*	80%
Mineral oil* (see Kerosene)	80%
Nicotine* (if present, toxicity rating 5)	ca. 6%
Oil of allspice	
Oil of mustard	
Phenols	ca. 1%
Pine tar*	ca. 12%
Soap	ca. 1%
Wood creosote* (see Creosote)	ca. 10%

2. Spray .... Toxicity rating 4

Lemon grass oil	2-11%
Citronella oil	
Synthetic oil of mustard (allyl isothiocyanate)	0.05-0.5%
Propellants and inert ingredients	93-98%

3. .... Toxicity rating 3-4
   Methyl nonyl ketone* .... ca. 2%

DOG DENTIFRICE	Toxicity rating 1-2
Potassium bitartrate	
Sodium bicarbonate	
Sodium lauryl sulfate	
Dicalcium phosphate	
Methylparaben	
Prophylparaben	
Saccharin	
Oil of cassia, of wintergreen	
Food color	

DRY CLEANERS, DOG AND CAT
1. .... Toxicity rating 2
   Sodium lauryl sulfate
   Coconut oil, amine condensate
2. .... Toxicity rating 3? or 4?
   Naphthalene*
   Calcium carbonate
   Magnesium carbonate
   Sulfur
   Aluminum silicate
   May contain:
   Borax*
   Degreased starch
   Glycerine
   Kerosene
   Phenol*
   Pine oil
   Sodium carbonate (*if > 10%)
   Wetting agents
   Zinc oxide
   Pesticides (see below)
3. Insecticidal .... Toxicity rating 2

a. Chlordane	0.25%
or	
Methoxychlor	0.5%
May contain:	
Isoctyl phenoxy polyethoxy ethanol	1%
Petroleum distillate	ca. 4%
Pine oil	2%
b. Foam	Toxicity rating 2
Piperonyl butoxide	0.4-0.9%
Pyrethrins	0.04-0.08%
Petroleum oil	ca. 0.3%
Inert ingredients	98- > 99%
Cleaners	
Deodorants	
Propellants	

Starred ingredients (*) may be responsible for major toxic effects; consult Section II.

PET CARE (Cont.)	

EAR MITES

1. .... Toxicity rating 2
   - Methoxychlor 1%
   - Piperonyl butoxide 1%
   - Pyrethrins 0.05%
   - Mineral oil 90%
2. .... Toxicity rating 2
   - Pyrethrins 0.05%
   - Squalene 25%
   - Piperonyl butoxide 0.5%
3. .... Toxicity rating 3–4
   - Rotenone (*if > 1.5%)
   - Chloroform (*if > 10%)
   - Oil (coon, mineral, olive)

FLEA COLLAR

1. .... Toxicity rating 2–3?
   - 2,2-Dichlorovinyl dimethyl phosphate   4–19%
   - Related compounds 0.3–1.5%
2. .... Toxicity rating 2
   - Gamma isomer of benzene hexachloride
     (from lindane) 0.6–1%

FLEA POWDER

1. .... Toxicity rating 3–4
   - Carbaryl (1-naphthyl N-methylcar-
     bamate) 3–12.5%
   - Dichlorophene 0.5–1%
   - May contain:
     - Aluminum chlorohydroxy allantoin-
       ate
     - Amorphous silica gel 2%
     - Butoxy polypropylene glycol 4%
     - Piperonyl butoxide 0.5%
     - Pyrethrins 0.1%
     - Pyrophyllite 0–95%
     - Talc 0–95%
2. .... Toxicity rating 2
   - Methoxychlor .... 2.5% or
   - Chlordane 1%
     or
   - Benzene hexachloride 0.5%
     or
   - Hexachlorophene 2%
     or
   - Dichlorophene 0.5%
   - May contain:
     - Piperonyl butoxide 0.6%
     - Pyrethrins 0.06%
     - Rotenone 1.2%
     - Other cube resins 2.4%
     - Sulfur 2%
     - Propylene glycol 2%
     - Malathion 0.5–4%

FLEA TABLETS .... Toxicity rating 3–4?
   - Ronnel* .... 0.25–1 gm.

MANGE

1. Liquid .... Toxicity rating 3
   - Benzyl benzoate 20–36%
   - Isopropyl alcohol 45–60%
   - May contain:
     - Acetone (*if > 10%)
     - Benzene hexachloride 0.06%
     - Chloroform (*if > 10%)
     - Emulsified oil base .... ca. 20%
2. Salve .... Toxicity rating 2–3
   - May contain:
     - Benzene hexachloride 0.1%
     - Benzocaine

PET CARE (Cont.)	

MANGE (Cont.)

   - Carbolic acid (*if > 1%)
   - Dichlorophene 0.5%
   - Ethylaminobenzoate
   - Oil (coon, wintergreen) (*if > 1%)
   - Orthophenylphenol (*if > 10%)
   - Petroleum base
   - Rotenone 0.12%
   - Salicyclic acid (*if > 1%)
   - Sulfur

PESTICIDES FOR PETS

See Section II for toxicity ratings (asterisks and toxicity ratings are based here on the ingredient being present in >10%).

   - Allethrin* 3
   - Ammonium lauryl dodecyl benzene
     sulfonate
   - Ammonium lauryl sulfate
   - BHC* 4
   - Boric acid* 4
   - Butoxypolypropylene glycol
   - Camphor oil* 4
   - Captan
   - Carbaryl* 4
   - Chloranil* 3
   - bis(5-Chloro-2-hydroxyphenyl)-meth-
     ane (Dichlorvos)* 3
   - Copper (* depending on the compound)
   - Cube resins
   - DDD* 3
   - DDVP* 4
   - Di-butyl succinate
   - Dichlorophene* 4
   - p-Di-isobutyl phenoxy ethoxy ethyldi-
     methyl benzyl ammonium chloride
     (Benzethonium chloride)* 4
   - Dimethyl phthalate* 3
   - Dipentene* 3
   - Essential oil* 4
   - Ethyl alcohol
   - Ethylene glycol* 3
   - Eugenol* 3
   - Glycerin
   - Isobornyl thiocyanoacetate (Thanite)*
     3
   - Isopropanol (Isopropyl alcohol)* 3
   - Korlan (Ronnel)* 3
   - Lanolin
   - Lindane* 4
   - Malathion* 4
   - Methoxychlor* 3
   - Methylenebischlorophenol
     (Dichlorophene)* 3
   - Naphthalene* 4?
   - N-Octyl bicycloheptene dicarboximide*
     3
   - Oil anise* 4
   - Para-cymene (Xylene)* 4
   - Para-methane
   - Petroleum* 3
   - Petroleum distillate* 3
   - Petroleum oil* 3
   - Pine oil* 3
   - Pine tar* 4
   - Piperonyl butoxide
   - Piperonyl cyclonene* 3
   - Propylene glycol
   - Pyrethrins* 3

Starred ingredients (*) may be responsible for major toxic effects; consult Section II.

PET CARE (Cont.)	PET CARE (Cont.)

PESTICIDES FOR PETS (Cont.)

Pyrethrum
Pyridinium chloride
Rotenone* 4
Soap anhydrous
Sodium arsenite* 6
Sodium carboxymethyl cellulose (see Carboxycellulose)
Sodium cresylate* 4
Sulfur
Terpene hydrocarbon* (see Terpenes)
Toxaphene* 4
Vegetable oil

SOAPS

1.	Toxicity rating 3
Anhydrous	29–84%
May contain:	
Acetone	0–2%
β-Butoxy β-thiocyano diethyl ether	0–1%
β-Naphthol	0–3%
Glycerin	
Lanolin	1%
Methanol	0–10%
Neutralized cresylic acid	0–0.5%
Petroleum hydrocarbons	0–5%
Rotenone	0.06–0.3%
Other cube resins	0.6%
Sulfur	0–2%
2. Shampoo, insecticidal (see Cosmetics)	Toxicity rating 3
May contain:	
Benzene hexachloride	0–0.1%
Captan	0–2%
p-Chloro-m-xylenol	0–2%
Color, certified	
Diisopropyl cresols	0–0.1%
Isobornyl thiocyanoacetate	0–5%
Other related terpenes	0–1%
Lindane	0–0.3%
Malathion	0–1%
Methoxychlor	
Perfume	
Piperonyl butoxide	0.5–1.2%
Preservatives (methylparaben, propylparaben)	
Pyrethrins	0.05–0.1%
Salicyclic acid (*if > 1%)	0–2%
	Toxicity rating 2
3. Coconut oil soap	100%
	Toxicity rating 2
4. Olive oil soap	30–83%
5. Bubble bath (see Cosmetics)	Toxicity rating 2
May contain:	
MGK 264	0.17%
Piperonyl butoxide	0.1%
Pyrethrins	0.05%
6. The insecticidal preparations may contain (see also notation on Pesticides for Pets, above):	
Benzyl benzoate* 3	
Bithionol* 3–4	
Citrus oil	
Dichlorodiphenyl dichloroethane	0.75%
Dipentene	0.5–2.3%
Ethylene dichloride* 3	
Isoborneol propionate, isobornyl thiocyanoacetate and related terpenes	0.02%–2.0%
Isopropyl alcohol* 3	

SOAPS (Cont.)

Methylene bis(trichlorophenol)	0.5%
MGK repellant 11* 3	
Naphthalene* 3–4	0.5–15%
Other cube resins	0.2–2.1%
Para-cymene	0.5–0.8%
Petroleum oils	0.2–0.3%
Pine oil	0.5–1.0%
Piperonyl butoxide	0.5–0.9%
Pyrethrins	0.02–0.09%
Rotenone	0.1–0.7%
Siberian pine needle oil	1.0–2.0%
Terpenes	

SPRAYS

May contain (see notation on Pesticides for Pets, above):	
Allethrin	0.075%
Benzene hexachloride* 3	0–9%
Butoxypolypropylene glycol* 3	6.0–15%
2,3,4,5 bis(2-Butylene-tetra-hydrofurfural) (MGK Repellant 11)	0.3%
Captan	0.1%
Dichlorophene	0.5%
Isopropyl alcohol* 3	0–25%
Isobornyl thiocyanoacetate	1.64%
Isopropyl myristate and palmitate	
Malathion	0.25%
Menthols* 4	
Methoxychlor	1.0%
Menthylated naphthalene* 4 (see Naphthalene)	0–72%
1-Naphthyl-N-methylcarbamate	0–1.0%
N-Octyl bicycloheptene dicarboximide	0.5%
Other cube resins	0.07–0.24%
Petroleum distillates* 3	0.1–60%
Piperonyl butoxide	0.26%
Propellant	to 100%
Pyrethrins	0.025%
Related terpenes	0.36%
Rotenone	0.03–0.13%
May also contain:	
Lindane* 3–4	
Malathion* 3–4	
Perfume	
Propylene glycol	
Salicylic acid* 3–4	
Sodium lauryl sulfate	
Sulfur	
Spray, bird; for lice, mites	Toxicity rating 2
Pyrethrins	0.06–0.09%
Piperonyl butoxide	0.12–0.18%
N-Octyl bicycloheptene dicarboximide	0.2–0.3%
Petroleum distillates	0.075–0.3%
Triethylene glycol	0.075%
Propylene glycol	0.075%
Spray, hamster; insecticide, deodorant	Toxicity rating 2
Pyrethrins	0.045%
Piperonyl butoxide	0.09%
N-Octyl bicycloheptene dicarboximide	0.15%
Petroleum distillates	0.2%
Propylene glycol	0.8%
Triethylene glycol	0.8%

Starred ingredients (*) may be responsible for major toxic effects; consult Section II.

PET CARE (Cont.)

TICKS

1. .... Toxicity rating 3
Piperonyl butoxide	0.5–6%
Pyrethrins	0.6%
May contain:	
Benzene hexachloride*	0–2%
Carbaryl*	0–5%
Nonylphenoxypolyethoxyethanol	0–20%

2. .... Toxicity rating 3
Rotenone	0–1%
Other cube resins	0–2%
Pine oil*	71%
Triethanolamine oleate	9%
Sulfonated castor oil	5%

3. Organic phosphate .... Toxicity ratings as indicated
   See Navadel, Delnav (3.5%)* 3, Malathion (24%)* 4, Dichlorovinyl dimethyl phosphate (1%), Ronnel (5%)

   May contain (toxicity ratings if > 10%):
1,1-Dichloro-2,2-bis(p-ethylphenyl)ethane	0–10%
Methoxychlor* 3	0–24%
Petroleum distillate* 3	0–50%
Pine oil* 3	0–25%
Xylene* 4	0–75%

WORMERS

1. .... Toxicity rating 2
   Piperazine adipate, phosphate, hydrochloride, citrate
Tablet or capsule	ca. 40–400 mg. (as base)
Liquid	ca. 50 mg–5 gm. per oz.

2. .... Toxicity rating 3–4
   Arecoline hydrobromide* 4
   Tetrachlorethylene* 3
   May contain:
   Mineral oil

3. n-Butyl chloride* 3

4. .... Toxicity rating 3–4
   2,2′-Methylenebis(4-chlorophenol)(Dichlorophene)* 3
(capsule)	125 mg.–4 gm.
Toluene* 4	150 mg.–4.8 gm.

5. Quinacrine hydrochloride* 4 .... 60 mg. (ea. tablet)
Piperazine adipate	420 mg. (as base)
Benzocaine	6 mg

6. 2,2′ Dihydroxy-5,5′ dichlorodiphenylmethane (Dichlorophene)*

PHOTOGRAPHIC PRODUCTS

The interpretation of the hazard of ingestion of proprietary photographic processing chemicals is complicated by the wide variety of packaging methods needed in the marketing of various formulas and the variation in packaging methods among companies. For example, one particular type of developer may be packaged as a single powder or liquid by one company, whereas another company may market a similar formula as a series of packages, each containing compatible chemicals, which are to be added to water to prepare the stock or use solution. In other instances, photographers may prepare their own solution from formulas published in various handbooks. Some of these formulas are still known by the original manufacturer's name in spite of the fact that they are prepared by the individual. Care should be taken not only to identify the

PHOTOGRAPHIC PRODUCTS (Cont.)

material by name, but to determine if the preparation was homemade or commercially prepared.

The concentrations in the solution as used in the photographic darkroom are in general the concentration listed in "typical" published formulas. To avoid as far as possible, misunderstandings about each of the materials listed below, an indication is given of the toxicity ratings (where available) of: a) the pure constituents; b) the mixture if sold as such; c) the solution as used.

To illustrate, a small size package of a given developer may be available in sealed foil packages or small bottles intended to be simply diluted with the suggested amount of water to the make the use solution. As packaged, Developer A is a dry powder which at a dose of 5 gm./kg. killed 10 of 10 rats, and at a dose of 0.5 gm./kg. killed 1 of 10 rats; the LD_{50} is 1200 mg./kg. and toxicity rating 3. A concentrated stock solution probably has a toxicity rating of 2 or 3. The use solution (1:1 dilution) has an LD_{50} of more than 30 ml./kg. (toxicity rating 1).

On the other hand, a small package of a developer may be packaged in 2 parts. Developer B, for example, comes in 1 package which may contain salts and developing agents and have an LD_{50} greater than 1600 mg./kg. (toxicity rating 3), together with a second container which may contain solid sodium hydroxide—a dangerous caustic (see Alkali, Section III). The use solution prepared according to directions has an LD_{50} between 20 to 30 ml./kg. (toxicity rating 1).

However, when packaged to prepare larger volumes, the materials may have different toxicity ratings than the small packages because the chemicals may be combined in different ways or may be present in different concentrations. Developer B in larger volume package, for example, comes in 3 parts: one may contain monomethyl-p-amino phenol sulfate and hydroquinone for which the LD_{50} in rats is about 250 mg./kg. (toxicity rating 4); a second package may contain salts and have an LD_{50} greater than 1600 mg./kg. (toxicity rating 3); the third container may contain solid sodium hydroxide—a dangerous caustic (see Alkali, Section III). The use solution has the same dilution as the smaller package (2 parts) and the same toxicity rating of 1.

It is worthwhile noting that the majority of photographic solutions diluted for use will have a low toxicity rating (not greater than 2) and contain relatively low concentrations of toxicologically active ingredients. Experience has shown that accidental ingestion of such use solutions usually results in nothing more than mild transient gastrointestinal symptoms.

In cases of ingestion of photographic materials determine the following information:

1. Was it purchased or was it prepared from raw materials by the photographer? (If the latter, see item 4.)
2. If purchased, what was the name of the material and who manufactured it?. Was the ingested material from the original package or bottle? If the material was packaged in parts, what part was ingested and how was it labeled? How much of the package was consumed? (Note the original weight or volume on the package.)
3. Was it a stock or use solution? If so, how much water was added to the original package? How much was ingested?
4. If prepared by the photographer himself, the material ingested will probably be a stock or use solution. Get the formula and dilution used from him.

Because of the large number of chemicals and concentrations which may be encountered, it is essential to read labels and instructions with care.

Do not store photographic chemicals or solutions in the refrigerator or in medicine cabinets.

DEVELOPERS

There are too many types of developers to include representatives of each here. Furthermore, because the use solu-

---

Starred ingredients (*) may be responsible for major toxic effects; consult Section II.

PHOTOGRAPHIC PRODUCTS (Cont.)

tions all have about the same toxicity, a typical, often-used formula (D-76) has been taken as a prototype. Concentrations are listed on a use solution basis.

	Use solution toxicity rating 2
Monomethyl-p-amino phenol sulfate	gm./liter
(Elon, Metol, Photol, Graphol, etc.)	0.3–14.0
Hydroquinone	1.0–45.0
Sodium sulfite	0.25–125.0
Borax	1.2–5.0
Water	to 1 liter
pH	8.7

Color developers are not listed; at present there are many kinds and a given type may be too complex for simple classification. However, in general, the toxicity of the use solutions resemble quite closely those of the black and white developers. Appended is a list of developer constituents with their toxicities.

DEVELOPERS, CONSTITUENTS OF	Toxicity rating
Borax*	3
Boric acid*	4
Citric acid	2
Glycine	
Hydrazine dihydrochloride	
Hydroquinone*	
Kodak antifog #1 (benzotriazole) (0.2%)	
Kodak antifog #2 (0.2%)	
Kodalk	
Kodalk balanced alkali	
Monomethyl-p-aminophenol sulfate*	4
Para-aminophenol hydrochloride (Kodelon)	
Paraformaldehyde	
Paraphenylene diamine (base)	
Potassium bromide*	3
Potassium iodide*	3
Potassium metabisulfite	
Pyro	
Sodium and potassium thiocyanate*	4
Sodium bisulfite*	3
Sodium sulfite*	3
Sodium* and potassium) carbonate and sodium hydroxide	see Alkali
Sodium metaborate*	3
Sodium sulfate	
Sulfuric acid (C.P.)	

PAPER DEVELOPERS, ADDITIONAL CONSTITUENTS OF

Amidol
Di-aminophenol hydrochloride (Acrol)
Chlor-hydroquinone (Adurol)

FILM CLEANERS	Toxicity rating 3 or 4
May contain:	
Ammonium hydroxide*	
Chlorinated solvents*	
Denaturant	
Ethyl alcohol	
Methyl alcohol*	
Methyl chloroform	
Petroleum ether* (benzine)	
Trichloroethane*	
Wax	

FIXING BATHS	Toxicity rating 3
Sodium thiosulfate*	4.0–37.0%
Sodium sulfite	0.7–7.0%
Acetic acid (28%)	2.0–21.0%
Boric acid	0.6–3.0%

PHOTOGRAPHIC PRODUCTS (Cont.)

FIXING BATHS (Cont.)	
Potassium aluminum sulfate	1.0–9.0%
Water	57.0–96.0%
May contain:	
Ammonium chloride	4.0%
Sodium bisulfite	2.0%
Borax	4.0%
Potassium chromium sulfate	1.0%
Sulfuric acid (conc.)	0.3%
Potassium metabisulfite	5.0%
Potassium thiocyanate	9.0%
Citric acid	0.4%

HARDENERS

Sample formulas:

1. Liquid hardener	Use solution toxicity rating 3
Formaldehyde (37%)	
Aluminum chloride*	
Sodium carbonate	
Sodium sulfite or bisulfite*	

2. Formalin-carbonate hardening bath	Toxicity rating 2
Formaldehyde (37%) solution	0.9–1.0%
Sodium carbonate	0.5–0.6%
Water	98.0%
May contain:	
Aluminum chloride*	

The ranges of hardener constituents are as follows:

	Ranges
Acetic acid (see Acid)	5.0–19.0%
Formaldehyde (37%)	0.5–1.0%
Potassium alum (see Aluminum or Potassium sulfate)	5.0–7.5%
Boric acid	2.5–3.7%
Sodium sulfite	2.5–7.5%
6-Nitrobenzeneimidazole nitrate (antifog)	4%
Potassium chrome alum	3%
Sodium sulfate	5.0–6.0%
Sodium carbonate	0.5–1.2%

3. Stock hardener	Toxicity rating 3
Sodium sulfite	2.5–7.5%
Acetic acid	5.0%
Boric acid (crys.)*	2.5–3.7%
Potasium alum	5.0–7.5%
Water	73%–85%

HYPO ELIMINATORS	Toxicity rating 2
Hydrogen peroxide (3% solution)	13.3%
Ammonium hydroxide (28%)	1.1%
Water	85.6%

HYPO TEST SOLUTION	Use solution toxicity rating 2
Water	1000.0 cc.
Acetic acid 28%	125.0 cc.
Silver nitrate	7.5 gm.
Permanganate test	Toxicity rating 1
Potassium permanganate	0.05%
Sodium hydroxide	0.1%
Water	99.8%
Mercuric chloride test	Toxicity rating 4
Mercuric chloride*	2.0%
Potassium bromide	2.0%
Water	95.0%
Silver nitrate test	Toxicity rating 2
Silver nitrate	1.0%
Water	99.0%
Iodine test	
Iodine solution	Toxicity rating 4?
Potassium iodide	6.0%
Iodine (crys.)*	2.7%

Starred ingredients (*) may be responsible for major toxic effects; consult Section II.

PHOTOGRAPHIC PRODUCTS (Cont.)

HYPO TEST SOLUTION (Cont.)

Water	91.3%
Starch solution	Toxicity rating 1
Soluble starch	5.0%
Water	95.0%
Hydrochloric solution	Toxicity (see Acid)
Hydrochloric acid (conc.)*	11.1%
Water	88.9%
Other tests for hypo may contain:	
Formaldehyde*	
Starch	
Hydrochloric acid	

INTENSIFIERS AND REDUCERS

Intensifiers are of various types and formulas.

1. Chromium intensifiers	Toxicity rating 3
Bleach	
Potassium dichromate*	0.9–9.0%
Hydrochloric acid* (conc.)	0.7–7.0%
Water	84.0–98.0%
Redeveloper†	Toxicity rating 2 or 3
Standard developer* (see Developers, above)	
2. Mercury intensifiers	Toxicity rating 3 or 4
Bleach	
Potassium bromide	1.0–2.0%
Mercuric chloride*	1.0–2.0%
Water	96.0–98.0%
Redeveloper†	
Solution A	Toxicity rating 5
Sodium cyanide*	3.0%
Water	97.0%
Solution B	Toxicity rating 3
Silver nitrate*	4.0%
Water	96.0%
† May be any standard developer	
3. Quinone-thiosulfate intensifiers	
Solution A	Toxicity rating 2 or 3
Potassium dichromate*	2.0%
Sulfuric acid (conc.)	5.0%
Water	92.0%
Solution B	Toxicity rating 2
Sodium bisulfite	0.4%
Hydroquinone	1.0%
Wetting agent	0.4%
Water	98.0%
Solution C	Toxicity rating 2
Sodium thiosulfate	2.0%
Water	98.0%

The intensifier is prepared by mixing solutions A, B and C in equal proportions.

4. Silver intensifiers	
Stock solution A	Toxicity rating 3
Silver nitrate*	6.0%
Water	94.0%
Stock solution B	Toxicity rating 2
Sodium sulfite	6.0%
Water	94.0%
Stock solution C	Toxicity rating 2
Sodium thiosulfate	10.0%
Water	90.0%
Stock solution D	Toxicity rating 2
Sodium sulfite	0.5%
Elon	0.8%
Water	98.7%

The intensifier is prepared by mixing solutions A, B, C and D in proportions of 1:1:1:3, respectively.

Intensifiers may contain:
Lead nitrate*

PHOTOGRAPHIC PRODUCTS (Cont.)

INTENSIFIERS AND REDUCERS (Cont.)

Potassium permanganate*

Reducers are of various types.

1. Farmer's reducer	Toxicity rating 2
Solution A	
Potassium ferricyanide	0.7–7.0%
Water	93.0–99.3%
Solution B	Toxicity rating 2 or 3
Sodium thiosulfate*	3.0–21.0%
Water	79.0–97.0%
2. Flattening reducers:	Toxicity rating 2
Bleach	
Potassium ferricyanide	1.3–3.0%
Potassium bromide	1.0–3.0%
Ammonium hydroxide	0.1%
Water	96.0%
Redeveloper	
Solution A	Toxicity rating 3
p-Aminophenol hydrochloride*	10.0%
Water	90.0%
Solution B	Toxicity rating 2
Potassium bromide	10.0%
Water	90.0%
3. Persulfate reducers	Toxicity rating 2 or 3
Ammonium persulfate	3.0–6.0%
Sulfuric acid (conc.)	0.5–0.6%
Water	93.4–96.5%
4. Harmonizing bleaching reducer	Toxicity rating 2
Hydrochloric acid (conc.)	3.0%
Potassium dichromate	1.0%
Alum	5.0%
Water	91.0%
Other reducers may contain:	
Potassium permanganate*	0.02–5.0%
Potassium citrate	6.0%
Ferric ammonium sulfate	4.0%
Sodium sulfite	3.0%
Citric acid	2.0%
May contain:	
Ferric chloride*	

Most of the formulas contain extremely toxic materials. These are listed with their toxicities.

Mercuric chloride (intensifiers)	6
Sodium cyanide (intensifier)	6
Potassium dichromate (intensifier, bleach)	4
Silver nitrate (intensifier)	4
Potassium permanganate (reducer)	corrosive if concentrated
Potassium ferricyanide (reducer)	3

PRINT FLATTENING SOLUTION

Package	Toxicity rating 3
Use solution (5:1)	Toxicity rating 2
Ethylene glycol* or glycerine	
Formaldehyde (37%)	

RESIDUAL SILVER TEST

Sodium sulfide (4%)	Use solution toxicity rating 3

SILVER STAIN REMOVER

Use solution toxicity rating 2

Water	
Thiourea	7.5%
Citric acid	7.5%

STAIN REMOVER

Solution A (in water)	Use solution toxicity rating 2
Potassium permanganate	0.5%
Solution B (in water)	Use solution toxicity rating 2
Sodium chloride	7.5%
Sulfuric acid (conc.)	1.6%

Starred ingredients (*) may be responsible for major toxic effects; consult Section II.

PHOTOGRAPHIC PRODUCTS (Cont.)

STOP BATHS	Toxicity rating 2 or 3
Stop baths usually contain acetic acid	
(28%) and a pH indicator	3.0–12.5%
Sodium sulfate	4.0%
Water	87.5–95.0%
May contain:	
Potassium chromium sulfate*	

TONERS

Toners are so varied that no adequate summary can be made. For instance, they range from a pH of 3 (quite acid) to a pH of 13 (Brown toner, sodium polysulfide) where the alkalinity is such that there is danger to the eye from splashed liquid as well as the corrosive action from ingestion.

1. Gold toners:	Toxicity rating 2
Solution A	
Sodium thiosulfate	24%
Potassium persulfate	3%
Silver nitrate	0.1%
Sodium chloride	0.1%
Water	78.0%
Solution B	
Gold chloride	0.4%
Water	99.5%
2. Iron toners:	Toxicity rating 2
Ferric ammonium citrate	0.4%
Oxalic acid	0.4%
Potassium ferricyanide	0.4%
Water	98.0%
May contain:	
Acetic acid	
3. Polysulfide toners:	Toxicity rating 2
Potash sulfurated	0.7%
Sodium carbonate	0.2%
Water	99.0%
4. Sulfide sepia toners:	Toxicity rating 3
Bleaching solution	
Potassium ferricyanide	1.0 to 2.0%
Potassium bromide	2.0–3.0%
Potassium oxalate*	5.0%
Acetic acid (28%)	1.0%
Ammonium hydroxide (28%)	1.0%
Water	91.0 to 96.0%
Toning solution	
Sodium sulfide	0.7 to 1.0%
Water	99.0%
5. Varigam toners	Toxicity rating 2 or 3
Potassium ferricyanide*	

PIGMENTS

Pigments are colored, black, white or fluorescent particulate organic or inorganic solids which usually are insoluble in, and essentially physically and chemically unaffected by, the vehicle or substrate in which they are incorporated. They alter appearance by selective absorption and/or by scattering light.

"Pigments are usually dispersed in vehicles or substrates for application, as, for instance, in the manufacture of inks, paints, plastics or other polymeric materials. Pigments retain a crystal or particulate structure throughout the coloration process." Definition by the Dry Color Manufacturers' Association.

Inorganic pigments are of natural origin (such as ochres) or synthetic (such as ultramarine blue). Organic pigments are mostly synthetic, such as toluidine red and phthalocyanine blue, but there are still some natural organic pigments in use such as carmine and chlorophyll.

As supplied to the industrial user, pigments may be in the form of dry, finely ground powder, as presscake which is the pigmentary material as made but still wet with from 1 to 5 times its own weight of water, as anionic or nonionic aqueous

PIGMENTS (Cont.)

dispersions, as flushed colors or dispersions in liquid or solid resins.

The present practice in the United States is to use the term "toner" for all kinds of full strength organic pigments. In the United Kingdom, however, as defined in *Colour Index*, Third Edition, Volume 3, the term "toner" is restricted to those organic pigments which are full-strength coloring matters produced by reaction of a water-soluble dye with an appropriate precipitant.

Extended pigments are toners diluted with an extender (*e.g.*, alumina hydrate, blanc fixe or calcium carbonate) which is not an integral part of the pigment. In the United States a "lake" is—by definition of the United States Tariff Commission—an organic coloring matter which *cannot* be produced without the use of a substrate, the substrate being a necessary and integral part of the product. If a colorant can be isolated in the pure or "toner" form, but is for commercial reasons coprecipitated with or upon a substrate, such a colorant is deemed to be a reduced or extended full-strength pigment.

Classification of Pigments

Many systems have been proposed for the classification of pigments. The standard reference work on the subject of colorants (both byes and pigments), the *Colour Index* (Third Edition, Volumes 1 to 3, the Society of Dyers and Colourists, Bradford, England, and the American Association of Textile Chemists and Colorists, Research Triangle Park, North Carolina), classifies dyes and pigments in approximately 20 categories. In addition, Volume 4 classifies all coloring matters into some 30 chemical classes. A somewhat simplified classification was proposed by V. C. Vesce and I. W. Ryan (in J. J. Mattiello (Editor), *Protective and Decorative Coatings*, Volume 2, Chapter 1, John Wiley & Sons, Inc., New York, 1942). In this system organic pigments are considered in seven general classes.

1. *Basic dye class.* This comprises pigments precipitated from water solution through the use of an acid agent such as tannic acid or the complex phosphotungstic, or phosphomolybdic acids, to form insoluble salts. They find their major use in the graphic arts.

2. *Insoluble azo.* These are characterized by the azo structure R—N-N—R, where R or R′ is a benzene or naphthalene ring free from any sulfonic acid or other salt-forming groups. They are completely insoluble in water. In this group are some of the most common organic pigments, including toluidine red and diarylide yellow. The solubility of these pigments in oils and common solvents varies considerably.

3. *Soluble azo.* These colorants also have the R—N-N—R′ structure, but in this case the organic ring contains one or more salt-forming groups such as —SO_3H or —COOH. These substances vary in their solubility in water. To be useful as pigments, they are insolubilized by the formation of metal salt of the dyestuff using, most commonly, as the precipitating agent, the alkaline earth metals such as calcium, barium, strontium and also manganese. Examples of these colorants are the lithols and the rubines.

4. *Condensation acid dyes.* These include materials such as peacock blue, which are formed into a pigment by precipitation onto a substrate of alumina hydrate and eosine, which is converted to a pigment by making the insoluble lead salt.

5. *Anthroquinone and "vat" class.* This group includes alizarin, which is "laked" to form a pigment. In addition, many of the well known vat dye-stuffs are characterized by the presence of a reducible carbonyl structure, C=O. These pigments include flavanthrone yellow, (C. I. Pigment Yellow 112), and many others. As a group, these colorants are extremely insoluble in water and common solvents.

6. *Phthalocyanines.* This class of blue and green pigments contains the complex structure:

PIGMENTS (Cont.)

They are completely insoluble in all common solvents. The metal, in case of the copper phthalocyanine, is so firmly bound that it is not removed by treatment with strong acids.

7. *Miscellaneous group.* This group includes old colorants such as Pigment Green B (C. I. Pigment Green 8) and some of the newer, complex insoluble pigments such as carbazole violet, quinacridone reds, and violets and isoindolinones.

The inorganic pigments comprise a wide variety of chemical entities ranging from simple iron oxide to the complex metal silicates such as ultramarine blue. Inorganic pigments are very insoluble in water and common solvents. Many of them are not attacked by mild acids.

Lead chromate-based pigments appear to be relatively nontoxic based on recent feeding studies. Basic lead carbonate (white lead), however, is highly toxic based on its solubility in mild acids.

The most toxic pigment is Paris green, a cupric acetoarsenite (structural formula: $Cu(C_2H_3O_3)_2 \cdot 3Cu(AsO_2(_2))$. This pigment has little industrial use, but is still used by some artists under the name vert emeraude, or emerald green. Other names under which it is sold include imperial green, olive green, Scheele's Schweinfurt green, veronese green.

Most pigments are nontoxic as defined by the Federal Hazardous Substances Act. They exhibit an acute oral toxicity (LD_{50}) of more than 5000 mg./kg. (rat).

As an example of the low toxicity of commercially used pigments, out of 200 pigments evaluated for acute oral toxicity, only 4 were found to exhibit an LD_{50} of less than 5000 mg./kg. Among the pigments which were tolerated in doses over 5000 mg./kg. were cadmium yellow, chrome yellow, diarylide yellow, yellow iron oxide, pyrazolone orange, molybdate orange, toluidine red, red iron oxide, lithol rubine, helio bordeaux, cadmium red, mineral violet, ultramarine blue, iron blue, cobalt blue, chrome green, isoindolinone, phthalocyanine, thioindigo, carbazale, naphthol reds, quinacridone, arylide yellow.

Toxicity ratings taken from the World Health Organization Technical Report Series No. 309 (Geneva, 1965), pages 21 *et seq.* are included where appropriate and designated by adding the letters WHO.

Toxicity data available from various pigment manufacturers are also included and designated as an LD_{50} rating which is defined as the acute oral toxicity (AOT) in terms of the mean lethal dose LD_{50}, *i.e.*, lethal to 50% of a group of experimental animals.

The data were derived by administering single oral doses to white rats with subsequent observations according to the procedure set forth in *Principles and Procedures for Evaluating the Toxicity of Household Substances*, National Academy of Sciences, National Research Council, Publication No. 1138.

A human dose of greater than 10 gm./kg. (>10) would involve ingestion of more than 1 lb. of pigment by a 150-lb. man.

Compliance with American National Standards Institute

Specification Z 66.1 (1964) is also noted where data are available.

The revisions in this edition in no way reflect the views of the pigment industry as a whole but are based on comments submitted by several individual companies in response to our request for updated information.

Although the data given are based on what is believed to be reliable information obtained in a manner described above, the manufacturers who submitted data do not warrant or guarantee their correctness and expressly disclaim any warranty, obligation or liability for loss or damage or for any violation of federal, state or municipal laws or regulation resulting from their use.

PIGMENTS (Cont.)

A. BLACK

Common Name	Color Index No.	Chemical Ingredients	Toxicity Data	Section II Referral

Black iron oxide
  Iron oxide black
  Magnetic oxide
  Natural black iron oxide
  Precipitated black iron oxide
    Uses: Paints, printing inks, paper, rubber, linoleum, textile printing, cement.
    Meets ANSI Z 66.1 Spec.
	Pigment Black 11
	77499
		Fe_3O_4		

Black spinels Chromium iron nickel black		(Ni,Fe) $(Cr,Fe)_2O_4$	LD_{50} >10 gm./kg.	
Copper chromite black	Pigment Black 28 77428	$CuCr_2O_4$	LD_{50} >10 gm./kg.	
Iron cobalt black	Pigment Black 29 77498	$(Fe,Co)Fe_2O_4$	LD_{50} >10 gm./kg.	
Iron cobalt chromite black	Pigment Black 27 77502	(Co,Fe) $(Fe,Cr)_2O_4$	LD_{50} >10 gm./kg.	
Manganese ferrite black	Pigment Black 26 77494	(Fe,Mn) $(FE,Mn)_2O_4$	LD_{50} >10 gm./kg.	
Uses: Ceramics, plastics, paint, inks.				
Charcoal black	Pigment Black 8 77268	Carbon (50–90%) and mineral	>10 gm./kg.	

Birch black
  Blue black
  Mineral black
		Carbon (15–85%) and silicates or iron oxide		

Soft black
  Swedish black
  Vegetable black
  Vine black
  Willow black
  Woodpulp black
    Uses: In various media. As an absorbent of noxious gases.				

Drop and bone blacks	Pigment Black 9 77267	Carbon (10–20%)$Ca_3(PO_4)_2$	>10 gm./kg.	

Animal black
  Bone black
  Ivory black
    Uses: Paints, polishes, leather, cloth, cement, paper coating, artists' colors, also used in sugar refining.				

Lampblack or carbon black Carbon black	Pigment Black 7 77266	Carbon	>10 gm./kg.	

Channel black
  Colloidal carbon
  Lampblack
	Pigment Black 6
	77266			

Low oil absorption lampblack
  Thermal black
    Uses: Paints, printing inks, newsprint, plastics, carbon paper, typewriter ribbon, rubber.				

Starred ingredients (*) may be responsible for major toxic effects; consult Section II.

PIGMENTS (Cont.)

Meets ANSI Z 66.1 Spec.

Logwood	Natural Black 3 75290	Natural black (see yellow)	Toxicity rating 3, WHO

    Uses: Paper, bleachable printing inks, artists' colors, lacquers, leather.

Miscellaneous black pigments

Antimony sulfide	77050	Sb_2S_3	Antimony salts
Black lead		Graphite	
Graphite	Pigment Black 10 77265	Graphite	

    Uses: Lead pencils; many nonpigmentary uses because of its heat stability and electrical properties.

Manganese black	Pigment Black 14 77728	Manganese dioxide	Manganese salts

    Uses: As a drier in oil paints, limited use in cement and clay bricks.

Plumbago	Pigment Black 10 77265	Graphite	

    Uses: Same as for Graphite.

Stove black	Pigment Black 10 77265	Graphite	

    Uses: Same as for Graphite.

B. BLUE

Common Name	Color Index No.	Chemical Ingredients	Toxicity Data / Section II Referral
Antwerp blue	Pigment Blue 27 77510:77520	Prussian blue and alumina	Ferrocyanides $LD_{50} > 10$ gm./kg.

    Uses: Printing inks, paints, linoleum, leather-cloth, typewriter, ribbons, plastics, artists' colors.

Meets ANSI Z 66.1 Spec.

Azurite	Pigment Blue 30 77420	Azurite	

  Mountain blue

    Uses: Paints, tempera, porcelain.

Blue lead	Pigment White 2 77633		Basic lead sulfate varying from 5 PbO, PbO to 2 $PbO_4 \cdot PbO$

    Uses: Paints

Blue, purple and violet PMA and PTA lakes   Triphenyl methane lakes

    Uses: Printing inks, occasionally in rubber and lacquer.

Blue olivine

Cobalt silicate blue	Blue 73 77364		

Blue phenacite

Cobalt zinc silicate blue	Blue 74 77366		

Blue spinels

Cobalt aluminate blue	Blue 28 77346		
Cobalt chromite blue	Blue 36 77343		
Cobalt tin alumina blue	No number		
Blue VRS			Toxicity, rating 1–2, WHO

Blue zircon

Zirconium vanadium blue	Blue 71 77998		

Starred ingredients (*) may be responsible for major toxic effects; consult Section II.

PIGMENTS (Cont.)

Brilliant bleu FCF	Pigment Blue 24 42090:1 D & C Blue 24 (Purified Type)		Toxicity rating 1–3, WHO
Uses: Printing ink. Occasionally in rubber and lacquers.			
Cerulean blue	Pigment Blue 35 77346	Cobaltous stannate ($CoO \cdot SnO_2$) The commercial product approximates $CoO \cdot$ (18%) SnO_2 (50%) and $CaSO_4$ (32%)	Cobalt and tin salts
Uses: Artists' colors.			
Cobalt blue	Pigment Blue 28 77346	Cobaltous aluminate of varying composition $CoO \cdot Al_2O_3$ (blue) and 4 $CoO \cdot 3Al_2O_3$ (green)	
Cobalt ultramarine Uses: Ceramics, colored glass, artists' colors. Some use in printing inks and lacquers.			
Copper blue	Pigment Blue 34 77450	Cupric sulfide (CuS)	Copper salts and sulfides
Uses: Linseed oil varnishes.			
Copper phthalocyanine	Pigment Blue 15 74160	See Phthalocyanine blue	$LD_{50} > 10$ gm./kg.
Uses: Printing ink, paint, plastic, rubber linoleum, artists' colors, cement. Meets ANSI Z 66.1 Spec.			
Covellite	Pigment Blue 34 77450	Cupric sulfide (CuS)	
Uses: Linseed oil varnishes.			
Cyanine blue		Cobaltous aluminate ($CoO \cdot Al_2O_3$) and Prussian blue ($Fe_4(Fe(CN)_6)_3$)	
Egyptian blue	Pigment Blue 31 77437	Copper-calcium-silicate ($CuO \cdot CaO \cdot$ $4SiO_2$)	
Use: Fresco.			
Erioglaucine blue	Pigment Blue 24 42090:1 D & C Blue 24 (Purified Type)	Barium lake	
Uses: Printing inks. Occasionally in rubber and lacquers.			
Indanthrene blues	Pigment Blue 21 69835 Pigment Blue 22 69810 Pigment Blue 60 69800 Pigment Blue 64 69825 Pigment Blue 65 59800	Complex insoluble anthraquinone vat dyes also used as pigments	$LD_{50} > 10$ gm./kg. $LD_{50} > 200$ mg./kg.
Uses: Automotive paints, plastics, rubber, printing inks. Meets ANSI Z 66.1 Spec.			
Iron blue	Pigment Blue 27 77510	Ferric ferrocyanide, $Fe_4(Fe(CN)_4)_3$	$LD_{50} > 10$ gm./kg.
Bronze blue Celestial blue Chinese blue Green shade blacktone iron blue Green shade iron blue Lacquer blue Milori blue Nonbronze blue Prussian blue			

Starred ingredients (*) may be responsible for major toxic effects; consult Section II.

PIGMENTS (Cont.)

Red shade blacktone iron blue			
Red shade iron blue			
Steel blue			
Toning blue			
Uses: Printing inks, paint, carbon paper, typewriter ribbons, artists' colors. Some in rubber and plastics. Meets ANSI Z 66.1 Spec.			
King's blue	Pigment Blue 32 77365 Pigment Blue 28 77365	Potassium, cobaltous silicate of varying composition ($CoO \cdot 2SiO_2 \cdot K_2OSiO_2$)	
Leitch's blue	Mixture of: Pigment Blue 28 77346 and Pigment Blue 27 77510	See Cyanine blue	
Manganese blue	Pigment Blue 33 77112	$BaMnNO_4 + BaSO_4$	Barium and manganese salts
Use: Cement.			
Mineral gray	Pigment Black 19 77017	Hydrated aluminum silicate $Al_2O_3 \cdot 2SiO_2 \cdot 2H_2O$	
Monastral blue	Pigment Blue 15 74160	See Phthalocyanine blue	$LD_{50} > 10$ gm./kg.
Uses: Paints, plastics, printing ink, paper, fibers. Meets ANSI Z 66.1 Spec.			
Peacock blue	Pigment Blue 24 42090:1	Barium lake	Barium salts
Uses: Printing inks, drugs and cosmetics (in purified form as D & C Blue 4).			
Peacock blue R	Pigment Blue 3 42140:1		
Uses: Printing inks, paper coating, leather, artists' colors, carbon paper, typewriter ribbons.			
Phthalocyanine blue	Pigment Blue 15 74160	Copper phthalocyanine blue. A complex copper organic chelate insoluble in all common solvents, dilute acids and alkalis	$LD_{50} > 17$ gm./kg.
Uses: Paints, printing inks, plastics, rubber, fibers, paper.			
Smalt			
	Pigment Blue 32 77365	Potassium cobaltous silicate of varying composition ($CoO \cdot 2SiO_2 \cdot K_2OSiO_2$)	
Sulfonated phthalocyanine	Pigment Blue 17:1 74200:1 74180:1		
Uses: Printing inks, lacquers, distempers, wallpaper, leather cloth.			
Thenards blue	Pigment Blue 28 77346	Cobaltous aluminate of varying composition CoO Al_2O_3 (blue) and $3Al_2O_3$ (green)	
Ultramarine	Pigment Blue 29 77007	Artificial— $Na_{2-10}Al_1Si_6O_{24}S_{2-4}$	$LD_{50} > 10$ gm./kg.
Uses: Paints, printing inks. Meets ANSI Z 66.1 Spec.			
Victoria blue	Pigment Blue 10 44040:2		
Uses: Printing ink, paper coating, leather, artists'			

Starred ingredients (*) may be responsible for major toxic effects; consult Section II.

PIGMENTS (Cont.)

---

colors, carbon paper,
typewriter ribbons.

Victoria blue B   Pigment Blue 2
                                44045:2

Uses: Printing inks, paper
    coating, leather, artists'
    colors, carbon paper,
    typewriter ribbons.

Victoria pure blue B   Pigment Blue 1 $LD_{50} > 10$ gm./kg.
                                42595:2

Uses: Printing inks, paper
    coating, leather, artists'
    colors, carbon paper,
    typewriter ribbons.

Vulcol fast blue   Blue 15 $LD_{50} > 5$ gm./kg.
                                74160

Winsor blue   Copper phthalocyanine   Toxicity rating 2, WHO

C. GREEN

Common Name	Color Index No.	Chemical Ingredients	Toxicity Data / Section II Referral
Brilliant green	Pigment Green 1	Sulfonated leucobrilliant green	
Uses: Printing inks, paint, plastics, rubber.	42040:1		
Chlorophyll, a or b	Natural Green 3		
	75810		
Uses: Foods and cosmetics.			
Chrome green	Pigment Green 15	Chrome yellow and Prussian blue	$LD_{50} > 10$ gm./kg.
	77520 and		
	77600		
	77601 or		
	77603		
Uses: Paints, printing inks, plastics, paper. Does not meet ANSI Z 66.1 Spec.			
Chromium oxide	Pigment Green 17	Cr_2O_3	$LD_{50} > 10$ gm./kg.
	77288		
	Mixture of	$Cr_2(OH)_4 + Cr_2O_3 + 5–10\%$ boric acid and	
	Pigment Green 18	Zn chromate $(ZnO \cdot CrO_3)$ mixtures	
	77289 and		
	Pigment Yellow 36		
	77955		
Uses: Paints, printing inks, rubber, plastics, paper. Meets ANSI Z 66.1 Spec.			
Chromium oxide (hydrated)	Pigment Green 18	$Cr_2O(OH)_4$	$LD_{50} > 10$ gm./kg.
Emerald oxide of chromium	77289		
Emeraude green			
Oxide of chromium, transparent			
Transparent oxide of chromium			
Viridian, hydrated chromium oxide			
Uses: Paints, printing inks, rubber, plastics, paper. Meets ANSI Z 66.1 Spec.			
Cobalt green	Pigment Green 19	Calcined cobalt (CoO), zinc (ZNO) and	
	77335	aluminum oxide (Al_2O_3)	
Emerald green	See Chromium oxide		
Emerald oxide	See Chromium oxide		
Emeraude green	See Chromium oxide		
Green earth	Pigment Green 23	Hydrous Fe, Mg, Al and K silicates	
	77009		

Starred ingredients (*) may be responsible for major toxic effects; consult Section II.

PIGMENTS (Cont.)

Green garnet	Pigment Green 51		
Victoria green	77300		
Green olivine	No number		
Nickel silicate green			
Green PMA and PTA toners and lakes	Pigment Green 1 42040:1		$LD_{50} > 10$ gm./kg.
	Pigment Green 2 42040:1 and 49005:1		
	Pigment Green 3 41100:2 and 42040:1		
	Pigment Green 4 42000:2		

Uses: Printing inks.
Meets ANSI Z 66.1 Spec.

Green Spinels			
Cobalt chromite green	Green 26 77343		
Cobalt titanate Green	Green 50 77377		
Hooker's green		1. (*e.g.*, malachite green) Gamboge and Prussian blue	Gamboge; ferrocyanides
		2. Mixture of organic lakes	
Hydrated chromium oxide	See Chromium oxide		
Indathrene greens	Not made in pigment form	See Indathrene blues	
Malachite green	Pigment Green 4 42000:1	Hydrochloride of leucomalachite green	$LD_{50} > 10$ gm./kg. Toxicity rating 4, WHO

Uses: Printing inks.
Meets ANSI Z 66.1 Spec.

Metal-free phthalocyanine	Pigment Blue 16 74100	Phthalocyanine	

Uses: Paints, printing inks, plastics, paper.

Naphthol green	Acid Green 1 10020		

Naphthol green B	Pigment Green 12 10020:1	Ba lake of acid green	
Olive green	See Chromium oxide		
Oxide of green, transparent	See Chromium oxide		
Paris green	See Chromium oxide		
Permanent green	See Chromium oxide		
Pigment green	Pigment Green 8 10006	Nitroso green	$LD_{50} > 10$ gm./kg.

Uses: Paints, printing inks, plastics, rubber.
Meets ANSI 66.1 Spec.

Phthalocyanine green	Pigment Green 7 74260	Polychloro copper phthalocyanine	$LD_{50} > 17$ gm./kg.

Uses: Paints, printing inks, plastics, rubber, paper.
Meets ANSI Z 66.1 Spec.

Starred ingredients (*) may be responsible for major toxic effects; consult Section II.

PIGMENTS (Cont.)

Prussian green	Pigment Green 36	Polychlorobromo copper phthalocyanine 1. Gamboge and Prussian blue 2. Mixture of organic pigments	Gamboge; ferrocyanides
Rinmann's green	Pigment Green 19 77335	An amorphous mixture of cobalt zincate (CoO ZnO) and zinc oxide which cannot be chemically separated	
Scheele's green	Pigment Green 22 77412	Cupric aceto-arsenite Originally cupric arsenite (Cu HAsO$_3$)	Paris green
Schweinfurt green	Pigment Green 21 77410	Paris green Cupric aceto-arsenite	
Segnale light green G	Green 7 74260		LD$_{50}$ > 5 gm./kg.
Ultramarine green	Pigment Green 24 77013	Na$_5$Al$_3$Si$_3$O$_{12}$ or Na$_8$Al$_6$Si$_6$S$_2$O$_{24}$ (China clay)	
Verdigris	Pigment Green 20	Copper dibasic acetate Cu(OOC—CH$_3$)$_2$·Cu(OH)$_2$·5H$_2$O)	Copper salts
Veronese green	Pigment Green 21	Cupric aceto-arsenite	Paris green
Victoria green	Pigment Green 4 42000:2	Cupric aceto-arsenite See Green PMA and PTA tones and lakes	LD$_{50}$ > 10 gm./kg.

  Uses: Printing inks, paper, plastics.
  Meets ANSI Z 66.1 Spec.

| Viridian | See Chromium oxide | | |

D. ORANGE

Common Name	Color Index No.	Chemical Ingredients	Toxicity Data / Section II Referral
Algol orange	Vat Orange 5 73335	An insoluble thioindigo vat dye	Alizarin
Anthanthrone orange	Pigment Red 168 59300		LD$_{50}$ > 16 gm./kg.

  Uses: Paints, printing inks, plastics.
  Meets ANSI Z 66.1 Spec.

Antimony sulfide	Pigment Red 107 77060	Sb$_2$S$_3$	Antimony sulfides
Antimony vermilion	Pigment Red 107 77060	Sb$_2$S$_3$	Antimony sulfides
Benzidine orange	Pigment Orange 13 21110	An insoluble azo pigment	LD$_{50}$ ≅ 10 gm./kg.

  Uses: Paints, printing inks, plastics, papers.
  Meets ANSI Z 66.1 Spec.

Buff-orange rutiles			
Chrome antimony titanium buff	Brown 24 77310		LD$_{50}$ > 5 gm./kg.
Chrome niobium titanium buff	Yellow 162 77896		
Chrome tungsten titanium buff	Yellow 163 77897		
Manganese antimony titanium buff	Yellow 164 77899		
Cadmium orange	Pigment Orange 20:1 77202:1	CdS, cadmium sulfoselenide barium sulfate	LD$_{50}$ > 10 gm./kg.

  Uses: Paints, printing inks, plastics.
  Does not meet ANSI Z 66.1 Spec.

| Cadmium lithopone | Pigment Yellow 35
77205:1 | Solid solution of Cds/ZnS extended with BaSO$_4$ | LD$_{50}$ > 10 gm./kg. |

  Uses: Printing inks, rubber.
  Does not meet ANSI Z 66.1 Spec.

| Cadmium yellow and orange | Pigment Yellow 37
77199 | | |
| | Pigment Orange 20
77202 | CdS, CdSe | LD$_{50}$ > 10 gm./kg. |

Starred ingredients (*) may be responsible for major toxic effects; consult Section II.

PIGMENTS (Cont.)

Uses: Paints, printing inks, plastics. Does not meet ANSI Z 66.1 Spec.			
Chrome orange	Pigment Orange 21 77601	Basic Pb chromate ($PbCrO_4$, PbO)	$LD_{50} > 10$ gm./kg.
Uses: Paints. Does not meet ANSI Z 66.1 Spec.			
Dinitro aniline orange	Pigment Orange 5 12075	An insoluble azo pigment	$LD_{50} > 10$ gm./kg.
Uses: Paint, printing inks, plastics, rubber, paper. Meets ANSI Z 66.1 Spec.			
Hansa oranges	Pigment Orange 1 11725 Pigment Orange 2 12060 Pigment Orange 5 12075	Insoluble azo pigments	$LD_{50} > 10$ gm./kg.
Uses: Paints, printing inks, paper. Meets ANSI Z 66.1 Spec.			
Mars orange	Pigment Red 101 77491	Ferric oxide (Fe_2O_3) synthetic	
Mercadium colors	Pigment Orange 23 77201	Cadimum sulfide, mercuric sulfide complex ($CdS \cdot HgS$)	
Uses: Paints, printing inks, plastics. Does not meet ANSI Z 66.1 Spec.			
Molybdate orange	Pigment Red 104 77605	Lead chromate, sulfate and molybdate ($PbCrO_4$; $PbSO_4$ and $PbMoO_4$	$LD_{50} > 10$ mg./kg.
Uses: Paints, printing inks, plastics, paper, rubber, textile printing. Does not meet ANSI Z 66.1 Spec.			
Orange GGN	Food Orange 2		Toxicity rating 1–2, WHO
Orange mineral	Pigment Red 105 77578	Lead tetroxide (Pb_3O_4)	
Orthonitraniline orange	Pigment Orange 2 12060	An insoluble azo pigment	$LD_{50} > 10$ gm./kg.
Uses: Paints, printing inks, paper. Meets ANSI Z 66.1 Spec.			
Persian orange	Pigment Orange 17 15510:1 Pigment Orange 17:1 15510:2	Ba lake of an azo dye	$LD_{50} > 10$ gm./kg.
Uses: Paints, printing inks, rubber. Meets ANSI Z 66.1 Spec.			
Quinacridine gold	Pigment Orange 48		
Quinacridine deep gold	Pigment Orange 49		
Segnale light orange RNG	Pigment Orange 5 12075		
Segnale light orange PG	Pigment Orange 13 21110		
Sodium lithol	Pigment Red 49 15630	Na salt of an azo dye	
Uses: Printing inks, rubber. Meets ANSI Z 66.1 Spec.			

Starred ingredients (*) may be responsible for major toxic effects; consult Section II.

PIGMENTS (Cont.)

E. RED

Common Name	Color Index No.	Chemical Ingredients	Toxicity Data / Section II Referral

Acid red
  Acid scarlet
    Uses: Paints, printing inks, plastics, rubber, paper.
	Pigment Red 60
	16105:1
		See Scarlet lake	

Alizarin
  Uses: Paints, printing inks, plastics, rubber, paper.
  Meets ANSI Z 66.1 Spec.
	Pigment Red 83
	58000:1
		An insoluble anthraquinone dye	Alizarin
			$LD_{50} > 10$ gm./kg.

Alizarin carmine
  Alizarin crimson
    Uses: Paints, printing inks, plastics, rubber, paper.
  Meets ANSI Z 66.1 Spec.
	Pigment Red 83
	58000:1
		Lakes from 1,2-dihydroxyanthraquinone	$LD_{50} > 10$ gm./kg.

Anthraquinone red
  Uses: Paints, inks, plastics, fibers, rubber, textile printing.
  Meets ANSI Z 66.1 Spec.
	Pigment Red 177		$LD_{50} > 10$ gm./kg.

Arylide reds and maroons
Arylide reds
 	
  Uses: Paints, inks, plastics, fibers, rubber.
  Meets ANSI Z 66.1 Spec.
	Pigment Red 2
	12310
		Azo pigments, general formula:	$LD_{50} > 16$ gm./kg.

Uses: Paints, inks, plastics, fibers, rubber. Meets ANSI Z 66.1 Spec.	Pigment Red 5 12490		$LD_{50} > 10$ gm./kg.
Uses: Paints, inks, fibers.	Pigment Red 7 12420		
Uses: Paints, inks, textile printing. Meets ANSI Z 66.1 Spec.	Pigment Red 9 12460		$LD_{50} > 10$ gm./kg.
Uses: Paints, inks, plastics, fibers, rubber, textile printing.	Pigment Red 14 12380		$LD_{50} > 10$ gm./kg.
Use: Textile printing. Meets ANSI Z 66.1 Spec.	Pigment Red 17 12390		$LD_{50} > 10$ gm./kg.
Uses: Paints, inks, plastics, rubber, textile printing. Meets ANSI Z 66.1 Spec.	Pigment Red 22 12315		$LD_{50} > 20$ gm./kg.
Uses: Paints, inks, plastics, rubber, textile printing. Meets ANSI Z 66.1 Spec.	Pigment Red 23 12365		$LD_{50} > 10$ gm./kg.
	Pigment Red 63 15880		
Uses: Paints, inks. Meets ANSI Z 66.1 Spec.	Pigment Red 112 12370		$LD_{50} > 10$ gm./kg.

Azo pigments, general formula:

$$\bigcirc\!\!-\!N\!\!=\!\!N\!\!-\!\bigcirc\!\!-\!CO \cdot NH\!\!-\!\bigcirc$$

Starred ingredients (*) may be responsible for major toxic effects; consult Section II.

PIGMENTS (Cont.)

	Pigment Red 146 12485		$LD_{50} > 10$ gm./kg.
Uses: Paints, inks.			
	Pigment Red 148		
Uses: Paints, inks.			
	Pigment Red 170		$LD_{50} > 10$ gm./kg.
Uses: Paints, inks.			
Arylide maroons	Pigment Red 63:1 15880:2		
Uses: Paints, inks, plastics, rubber.			
	Pigment Red 63:2 15880:2		
Uses: Paints, inks, plastics, rubber.			
BON reds and maroons		Ca, Ba and Mn salts of β-hydroxynaphthoic acid azo dyes. General formula of an acid form is: Insolubilized by precipitating with metallic salts	
BON reds	Pigment Red 48 15865		$LD_{50} > 20$ gm./kg.
Uses: Inks. Meets ANSI Z 66.1 Spec.			

	Pigment Red 48:1 15865:1		$LD_{50} > 10$ gm./kg.
Uses: Paints, inks, plastics, food, drug and cosmetic coloring, rubber, textile printing. Meets ANSI Z 66.1 Spec.			
	Pigment Red 48:2 15865:2		$LD_{50} > 10$ gm./kg.
Uses: Paints, inks, plastics, food, drug and cosmetic coloring, rubber, textile printing. Meets ANSI Z 66.1 Spec.			
	Pigment Red 48:3 15865:3		
	Pigment Red 52:1 15860:1		$LD_{50} > 10$ gm./kg.
Uses: Paints, inks, plastics. Meets ANSI Z 66.1 Spec.			
BON maroons	Pigment Red 52:2 15860:2		$LD_{50} > 10$ gm./kg.
Uses: Paints, inks, plastics. Meets ANSI Z 66.1 Spec.			
	Pigment Red 48:4 15865:4		
Uses: Paints, inks, plastics, rubber, textile printing.			
Brown madder		Alizarin	Alizarin
Burnt sienna	Pigment Brown 6 and 7 Number 77491	Fe_2O_3, silica (SiO_2), aluminum oxide (Al_2O_3)	
Uses: Paint, inks, plastics, rubber, textile printing.			
Cadmium red	Pigment Red 108 77202	CdS, CdSe (cadmium sulfoselenide)	$LD_{50} > 10$ gm./kg.
Uses: Paints, inks, plastics, fibers, textile printing.			

Starred ingredients (*) may be responsible for major toxic effects; consult Section II.

PIGMENTS (Cont.)

Does not meet ANSI Z 66.1 Spec.			
(See Mercury cadmium red) plastics.			
Cadmium scarlet			
Cadmopone red	Pigment Red 236 77863		
Carmine	Natural Red 4 75470	Al, Ca lakes of an anthraquinone dye	Alizarin
Uses: Food and drug colorants.			
Meets ANSI Z 66.1 Spec.			
Carmine lake		See Alizarine carmine	
Chinese vermilion	Pigment Red 106 77766	HgS (mercuric sulfide)	Mercury compounds
Uses: Paints, inks, plastics, rubber, textile printing.			
Chlorinated-*p*-nitraniline	Pigment Red 4 12085		$LD_{50} > 10$ gm./kg.
Uses: Paints, inks, plastics, rubber.			
Meets ANSI Z 66.1 Spec.			
Cinnabar (See Chinese vermilion)			
Uses: Paints, inks, plastics, rubber, textile printing.			
Cochineal (see Carmine)			
Cuprous oxide	77402	Cu_2O	
Use: Paints.			
Disazo red	Pigment Red 144		$LD_{50} > 10$ gm./kg.
Uses: Paints, inks, plastics, fibers, rubber, textile printing.			
Meets ANSI Z 66.1 Spec.			
Disazo scarlet	Pigment Red 166		$LD_{50} > 10$ gm./kg.
Uses: Paints, inks, plastics, fibers, rubber, textile printing.			
Meets ANSI Z 66.1 Spec.			
English vermilion	(See Chinese vermilion)	HgS (mercuric sulfide)	See Mercury salts.
Eosine	(See Bromo acids)	Eosine	Usually employed as the lead salt.
			Toxicity rating 1–3, WHO
			Gentian violet

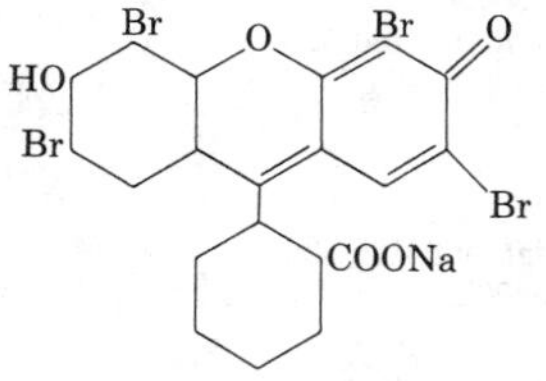

Eosine

Fuchsine red	Pigment Violet 4 42510:2	Phosphotungstic molybdic acid lake of a triphenylmethane dye	
Use: Inks.			
Helio bordeaux	Pigment Red 54 14830:1	Insoluble Ca salt of a soluble azo dye	
Uses: Paints, inks, plastics, rubber.			
Indigoid	Pigment Red 198 73390		$LD_{50} > 16$ m./kg.
Uses: Paints, plastics.			
Indian red	Pigment Red 101 77015 77491 77538	Fe_2O_3	
Uses: Paints, inks, plastics, rubber, textile printing.			

Starred ingredients (*) may be responsible for major toxic effects; consult Section II.

PIGMENTS (Cont.)

Lithols	Pigment Red 49 15630 Pigment Red 49:1 15630:1 Pigment Red 49:2 15630:2	Insoluble Na, Ba, Ca salts of a soluble azo pigment.	
Uses: Paints, inks, plastics, rubber (15630:1 and 15630:2).			
Lithol rubines	Pigment Red 57 15850 Pigment Red 57:1 15850:1 Pigment Red 57:2 15850:2	Insoluble Ca salts of soluble azo dyes	$LD_{50} > 10$ gm./kg.
Uses: Paints, inks, plastics and rubber (C.I. 15850:1 and 15850:2). Meets ANSI Z 66.1 Spec.			
	Pigment Red 59		
Madder lake	Pigment Red 83 58000:1	Alizarin	Alizarin $LD_{50} > 10$ gm./kg.
Uses: Paint, ink, plastic, rubber. Meets ANSI Z 66.1 Spec.			
Mars red	(See Indian red)	Synthetic Fe_2O_3	
Mercury cadmium reds	Pigment Red 113 77201		$LD_{50} > 10$ gm./kg.
Uses: Paints, plastics.			
Monoazo	Pigment Red 112 12370		$LD_{50} > 10$ gm./kg.
Uses: Paints, inks.	Pigment Red 146 12495		$LD_{50} > 10$ gm./kg.
	Pigment Red 148 Pigment Red 170		$LD_{50} > 10$ gm./kg.
α-Naphthyl amine maroon	(See Helio bordeaux)		
Para reds	Pigment Red 1 12070	Insoluble azo pigments	$LD_{50} > 10$ gm./kg.
Uses: Paints, inks, plastics, rubber. Meets ANSI Z 66.1 Spec.			
Parachlor Red	Pigment Red 6 12090		
Permanent crimson		Alizarin	Alizarin
Persian gulf oxide	Pigment Red 102 77015 77491 77538	Fe_2O_3 (60%), silica (SiO_2) (20%) plus alumina (Al_2O_3), lime (CaO), and magnesia (MgO)	$LD_{50} > 10$ gm./kg.
Uses: Paints, inks and plastics (C.I. 77015). Meets ANSI Z 66.1 Spec.			
Perylene maroon	Pigment Red 179 71130		$LD_{50} > 16$ gm./kg.
Uses: Paints, printing inks, plastics. Meets ANSI Z 66.1 Spec.			
Perylene red	Pigment Red 149		
Uses: Paints, inks, plastic.			
Perylene scarlet	Pigment Red 190 71140		$LD_{50} > 10$ gm./kg.
Uses: Paints, printing inks, plastics. Meets ANSI Z 66.1 Spec.			
Perylene vermilion	Pigment Red 123 71145		$LD_{50} > 10$ gm./kg.
Uses: Paints, printing inks. Meets ANSI Z 66.1 Spec.			
Phloxine toner	Pigment Red 90 45380:1	See Eosine	
Uses: Inks, cosmetics.			
Pigment scarlet	Pigment Red 60 16105	Ba lake of a soluble azo dye	
Uses: Paints, inks, plastics, textile printing.			

PIGMENTS (Cont.)

Pyrazolone reds and maroons   Azo pigments

Pyrazolone red	Pigment Red 38		$LD_{50} > 10$ gm./kg.
Uses: Paints, printing inks, plastics, rubber.	21120		
Meets ANSI Z 66.1 Spec.			
Pyrazolone maroon	Pigment Red 41		$LD_{50} > 10$ gm./kg.
Uses: Paints, printing inks, plastics, rubber.	21200		
Meets ANSI Z 66.1 Spec.			
Quinacridine maroon	Pigment Red 206		
Quinacridine maroon B	Pigment Violet 42		
Quinacridine magenta	Pigment Red 202		
Red chalk	(See Persian Gulf Oxide)	Aluminum silicate $(3Al_2O_3 \cdot 2SiO_2)$ colored by ferric oxide (Fe_2O_3)	
Red iron oxide	(See Indian red)	Fe_2O_3	
Red iron oxide, synthetic	(See Indian red)	Fe_2O_3	
Red lake C lakes	Pigment Red 53:1 15585:1	Insoluble metal salts of azo dyes	$LD_{50} > 10$ gm./kg.
	Pigment Red 53:2 15585:2		
Uses: Paints, inks, plastics, rubber, cosmetics (15585:1).			
Red lake R lake	(See Lithols)		
Red lead	Pigment Red 105 77578	Pb_3O_4	Lead salts
Use: Paints			
Rhodamine	Pigment Red 81 45160:1	A phosphotungstomolybdic acid salt of	$LD_{50} > 10$ gm./kg.
Uses: Inks, plastics and textile printing (C.I.45160:1).	Pigment Violet 1 45170:2		
Inks (C.I.45170:2)			
Meets ANSI Z 66.1 Spec.			
Rhodamines, misc.			

Rose dorée		Anthraquinone lakes	Alizarin
Rose madder (see Rose dorée)			
Safranine red	Basic Red 2 50240	See Red lakes and toners	
Use: Inks.			
Scarlet GN specially Pure	Food Red 2 14815		Toxicity rating 1–2, WHO
Use: Food and drug colorant			
Scarlet lake	(See Pigment scarlet)	1. Lake of a soluble azo dye	
		2. Insoluble azo pigment dyestuff	
Segnale light red FGR	Pigment Red 112 12370		$LD_{50} > 5$ gm./kg.
Segnale light red RL	Pigment Red 3 12120		$LD_{50} > 5$ gm./kg.
Segnale light red 4RS	Pigment Red 8 12335		$LD_{50} > 5$ gm./kg.
Segnale light Bordeaux, F2R	Pigment Red 12 12385		$LD_{50} > 5$ gm./kg.
Segnale red GS	Pigment Red 48:1 15865:1		$LD_{50} > 5$ gm./kg.
Segnale red RS	Pigment Red 48:2 15865:2		$LD_{50} > 5$ gm./kg.
Segnale red RBKC	Pigment Red 49:1 15630:1		$LD_{50} > 5$ gm./kg.

Starred ingredients (*) may be responsible for major toxic effects; consult Section II.

PIGMENTS (Cont.)

Segnale red 5BM	Pigment Red 52:2		$LD_{50} > 5$ gm./kg.
Segnale rubine BKC	Pigment Red 57:1		$LD_{50} > 5$ gm./kg.
	15850:1		
Sodium lithol, barium lithol, calcium lithol.	(See Lithols)		Insoluble Na, Ca, or Ba salt of an azo dye.
Spanish oxide	(See Persian Gulf oxide)	Fe_2O_3 (60%), silica (SiO_2) (20%), plus alumina (Al_2O_3), lime (CaO) and magnesia (MgO)	
Terra rosa		Native clay with Fe_2O_3	Ferric salts
Terra bromo fluorescein	(See Bromo acids)	Eosine	$LD_{50} > 16$ gm./kg.
Thermofast supra Red BRA	Pigment Red 144		
Thioinigoid reds and maroons	Pigment Red 88	Insoluble thionoigo vat dyes, used as pigments, e.g.	
Uses: Paints, inks, plastics, rubber.	73312		
Thioindigoid maroons	(See Thioindigoid reds)		

Toluidine reds	Pigment Red 3	Insoluble azo pigments	$LD_{50} > 10$ gm./kg.
	12120		
Uses: Paints, inks, plastics, rubber, textile printing. Meets ANSI Z 66.1 Spec.			
Tuscan red	(See Indian red)	Fe_2O_3	
Venetian red	Pigment Red 102	Fe_2O_3 (40%), $CaSO_4$ (60%)	
	77015		
	77491		
	77538		
Uses: Paints, plastics, textile printing (C.I. 77015).			
Vulcol Fast Red L/C	Pigment Red 53:1		
	15585:1		

F. VIOLET

Common Name	Color Index No.	Chemical Ingredients	Toxicity Data / Section II Referral
Cobalt violet	Pigment Violet 14 77360	Cobalt phosphate ($Co_3(PO_4)_2 \cdot H_2O$) and cobalt arsenite ($Co_3H_6(AsO_3)4H_2$)	Arsenites
Uses: Paints, plastics, rubber. Meets ANSI Z 66.1 Spec.			
Fast violet	Pigment Violet 16 77742	Manganese ammonium pyrophosphate ($(NH_4)_2Mn_2(P_2O_{7\ 2}O_7)_2$)	
Uses: Paints, inks, textile printing			
Magenta	Basic Violet 14 42510	A phosphotungstomolybdic acid salt of a triphenylmethane dye	Gentian violet
Use: Inks. Meets ANSI Z 66.1 Spec.			
Manganese violet	(See Fast violet)	Manganese ammonium phosphate ($(NH_4)_2Mn_2(P_2O_7)_2$)	
Mars violet	(See Indian red)	Synthetic Fe_2O_3	
Nurnberg violet	(See Fast violet)	Manganese ammonium pyrophosphate ($(NH_4)_2Mn_2(P_2O_7)_2$)	Manganese salts
Orchid Cassiterite Chrome Tin Orchid	Red 236 77863		
Permanent mauve	(See Fast violet)		
Permanent violet	(See Fast violet)		
Pink Corundum Chrome Alumina Pink	Red 230 77003		
Manganese Alumina Pink	Red 231 77005		
Pink Sphene Chrome Tin Pink	Red 233 77301		

Starred ingredients (*) may be responsible for major toxic effects; consult Section II.

PIGMENTS (Cont.)

Pink Spinel			
Chrome Alumina Pink	Red 235		
	77290		
Pink Zircon	Red 232		
Zirconium Iron Pink	77996		
Quinacridone red	Pigment Red 122		$LD_{50} > 16$ gm./kg.
Uses: Paints, printing inks,	Pigment Violet 19		
plastics.	46500		
Meets ANSI Z 66.1 Spec.			
Quinacridine Scarlet	Pigment Red 207		$LD_{50} > 11$ gm./kg.
Quinacridone violet	Pigment Violet 19		$LD_{50} > 16$ gm./kg.
Uses: Paints, printing inks,	46500		
plastics, rubber.			
Meets ANSI Z 66.1 Spec.			
Red-Blue Borate			
Cobalt Magnesium Red-	Violet 48		
Blue	77352		
Thioindigoid maroon	Pigment Violet 38		
Uses: Paints, printing inks.	73395		
Meets ANSI Z 66.1 Spec.			
Ultramarine violet	Pigment Violet 15	$Na_{8-10}Al_6Si_6O_{24}S_{2-6}$	
	77007		
Violet Phosphates			
Cobalt Violet	Pigment Violet 14		
	77360		
Cobalt Lithium Violet	Violet 47		
Violet PTA and PMA lakes	Pigment Violet 3		$LD_{50} > 10$ gm./kg.
Uses: Paints, inks, plastics,	42535:2		
rubber.			
Violet PTA and PMA toners	(See Violet PTA		
	and PMA lakes)		

G. WHITE

Common Name	Color Index No.	Chemical Ingredients	Toxicity Data / Section II Referral
Aluminum oxide	[Not classified as a pigment]	Aluminum hydroxide: contains varying amounts of sulfate (8–10% as SO_3) usually written: $3Al_2O_3 \cdot SO_3 \cdot 9H_2O$	Aluminum salts
Alumina hydrate	Pigment White 24 77002		
Uses: Printing inks, coatings, plastics, ceramics. Purified: cosmetics and medicines.			
Aluminum silicate	Pigment White 19	Aluminum silicate $(Al_2O_3 \cdot 2SiO_2 \cdot 2H_2O)$ containing calcium, magnesium or iron carbonate, ferric hydroxide, quartz and mica, etc., as impurities	
Uses: Paper	77004		
Antimony oxide	Pigment White 11	Antimony oxide (Sb_2O_3)	Antimony salts
Use: Paints.	77052		
Anhydrite		Calcium sulfate $(CaSo_4 \cdot 2H_2O)$	
Barium magnesium carbonate		Barium magnesium carbonate	
Barium sulfate	Pigment White 21, 22	Barium sulfate $(BaSO_4)$	
Uses: Paints, inks.	77120		
Basic carbonate white lead	Pigment White 1 77597	See White Lead	LD 124 mg./kg.
Basic silicate white lead	Pigment White 16		LD 136 mg./kg.
Uses: Ceramics, textiles	77625		
Basic sulfate white lead	Pigment White 2		LD 300 mg./kg.
Use: Paints	77633		
Bentonite	Pigment White 19	A colloid clay (see aluminum silicate)	
Use: Paper	77004		
Calcium carbonate	Pigment White 18	Calcium carbonate $(CaCO_3)$	
Use: Water paints	77220		
Calcium silicate	Pigment White 28	Calcium silicate $(CaSiO_3)$	
Use: Paper	77230		
Chalk	Pigment White 18	Calcium carbonate $(CaCO_3)$	
Uses: Paints and paper	77220		

Starred ingredients (*) may be responsible for major toxic effects; consult Section II.

PIGMENTS (Cont.)

China clay	(See Aluminum silicate)	A colloid clay (see aluminum silicate)	
Chinese white Uses: Paints, paper, rubber Purified: Drugs and Cosmetics	Pigment White 4 77947	A colloid clay (see aluminum silicate)	
Cremnitz white		Basic lead carbonate	Lead salts
Diatomaceous earth	Pigment White 19 77005	Silica, silicon dioxide (SiO_2)	
Flake white Nos. 1 and 2 Use: Paints	Pigment White 1 77597	Basic lead carbonate plus a small amount of zinc oxide in poppy oil	Lead salts
Foundation white		Basic lead carbonate and a small amount of zinc oxide in linseed	Lead salts
Gloss white Uses: Printing inks, paints, rubber, paper	Pigment White 23 77122	Aluminum hydroxide (25)% barium sulfate (75%)	Barium salts, insoluble
Gypsum Use: Paper	Pigment White 25 77231	Calcium sulfate ($CaSO_4 \cdot 2H_2O$)	
Leaded titanate Use: Paints	Pigment Yellow 47 77645	$PbTiO_3$ (93%), lead sulfate (7%)	
Leaded zinc oxide Use: Paints	Pigment White 4 77947	Zinc oxide and lead sulfate, ZnO and white lead basic sulfate	
Light magnesium carbonate Use: Paints	Pigment White 18 77713	Magnesium carbonate ($MgCO_3$) magnesium salts	
Lithopone Uses: Paints, rubber, cement.	Pigment White 5 777115	Zinc sulfide (ZnS: 28–30%) and barium sulfate ($BaSO_4$: 70–72%)	
Lithopone magnesite		Magnesium carbonate	
Magnesium carbonate Use: Paints	Pigment White 18 77713	Magnesium carbonate ($MgCO_3$)	
Magnesium oxide	Magnesium oxide (fume) 77711	Magnesium oxide (MgO)	
Magnesium silicates Use: Extender for pigments for paints, rubber, ceramics. Purified: cosmetics.	Pigment White 26 77718	Hydrated magnesium silicate ($Mg_3Si_4O_{11} \cdot H_2O$)	
Mica Uses: Paints, paper, rubber, plastics	Pigment White 20 77019	$H_2KAl (SiO_4)_3$	
Permanent white		A combination of titanium oxide and zinc oxide in poppy oil	
(Barium sulfate)	Pigment White 21 77120		
(Zinc oxide fume)	Pigment White 4 77917		
Uses: (See Barium sulfate, and Chinese white)			
Pumice Uses: Paints, paper, rubber, plastics, ceramics. Purified grade: Cosmetics.	Pigment White 20, 26 77019	$H_2KAl (SiO_4)_3$	
Quartz		Silica	
Satin white Uses: Paper	Pigment White 33	$Al (OH)_3 + CaSO_4$	Aluminum salts
Silica Use: Paints	Pigment White 27 77811	SiO_2	
Silver white Use: Paints	Pigment White 1 77597	Basic lead carbonate + small amount of zinc oxide	Lead salts
Talc Use: Extender for pigments for paints, rubber, ceramics. Purified: Cosmetics	Pigment White 26 77019	Hydrated magnesium silicate ($Mg_3Si_4O_{11} \cdot H_2O$)	
Titanated barium		TiO_2 (30%), $BaSO_4$ (70%)	
Titanated calcium		TiO_2 (30%), $CaSO_4$ (70%)	

Starred ingredients (*) may be responsible for major toxic effects; consult Section II.

PIGMENTS (Cont.)

Titanated lithopone		TiO_2ZnS, $BaSO_4$	
Titanated magnesium		TiO_2 (30%), $MgSO_4$ (70%)	
Titanium dioxide	Pigment White 6 77891	TiO_2	
Uses: Paints, paper, plastic, rubber, ceramics, fibers. Purified grade approved by FDA for use in foods, drugs and cosmetics.			
Titanium white	(See Titanium dioxide)	TiO_2, $BaSO_4$ plus small amount of zinc oxide	
White lead, basic carbonate Use: Paints	Pigment White 1 77597	Basic lead carbonate 3.6 $PbCO_3 \cdot Pb$ $(OH)_2$ to 1.8 $PbCO_3$	Lead salts (See Basic carbonate white lead, above)
White lead, basic silicate Uses: Ceramics, textiles	Pigment White 16 77625	Basic lead silicate $PbSiO_3$	Lead salts (See Basic silicate white lead, above)
White lead, basic sulfate Use: Paints	Pigment White 2 77633	Basic lead sulfate, $5PbSO_4 \cdot PbO$ to 2 $PbSO_4$. Some commercial products contain up to 5% zinc oxide	Lead (See Basic sulfate white lead, above)
Witherite	Pigment White 10 77099	Barium carbonate ($BaCO_3$)	
Uses: Extender for pigments, paints, rat poison			
Zinc oxide Uses: Paints, inks	Pigment White 4 77947	Zinc oxide (ZnO)	(See Permanent white, above)
Zinc sulfide Uses: Paints, inks, paper: purified—cosmetics	Pigment White 7 77975	Zinc sulfide (ZnS)	Zinc sulfides
Zinc sulfide magnesium		ZnS (50%) $MgSiO_3$	Zinc sulfides
Zinc white Uses: Paints, inks	Pigment White 7 77975	Zinc oxide (ZnO)	

H. YELLOW AND BROWN

Common Name	Color Index	Chemical Ingredients	Toxicity Data / Section II Referral
			$LD_{50} > 10$ gm./kg.
Anthrapyrimidine yellow Uses: Paints, printing inks, plastics. Meets ANSI Z 66.1 Spec.	Pigment Yellow 108 68420		
Antimony yellow	Pigment Yellow 41 77588, 77589	1. Lead antimoniate ($Pb_2O \cdot Sb_2O_5$) and zinc (ZnO and bismuth (BiO) oxides 2. Mixture of stable pigments	
Uses: Coloring of ceramics, glass, paints			
Aureolin Uses: Paints, plastics, paper	Pigment Yellow 40 77357	Potassium cobaltinitrite ($K_6Co_2(NO_2)_{12} \cdot 3H_2O$)	
Aurora yellow Uses: Paints, rubber, inks, plastics, ceramics, glass	Pigment Yellow 37 Pigment Orange 20 77199	Cadmium salts (CdS)	
Barium yellow		Barium chromate ($BaCrO_4$)	
Benzidine yellows	Pigment Yellow 12 21090 Pigment Yellow 13 21100 Pigment Yellow 14 21095	Insoluble azo pigments	
Uses: Inks, papers, rubber, plastics, textiles, fibers			
	Pigment Yellow 17 21105		
Use: Inks			
	Pigment Yellow 20		
Uses: Plastic, rubber			
	Pigment Yellow 55 21096		
Uses: Inks, textiles			
	Pigment Yellow 83		
Use: Inks			

Starred ingredients (*) may be responsible for major toxic effects; consult Section II.

PIGMENTS (Cont.)

Bismarck brown	Basic Brown 1,2,4,5,7 21000	A mixture of the HCl of benzene m-diazo-bis(m-phenylenediamine) with triami-noazobenzene and other bases	
Aniline brown			
Cinnamon brown			
English brown			
Manchester brown	Basic Brown 1 21000		
Phenylene brown	Basic Brown 1,4 21000		
Solid brown			
Veserine			
Uses: Textiles, paper, pigment manufacture, leather, stains			
BON browns	Pigment Brown 5 15800:2	Azo derivatives of β-hydroxynaphtholic acid, copper salts	
Uses: Paints, inks			
Brown hydrated iron oxide synthetic	Pigment Brown 6,7 77492	$FeO(OH)_n \cdot H_2O$	
Uses: Paints, plastics, inks, paper, rubber, textiles, cement. Purified grade: Drugs, cosmetics, dog food			
Brown Rutiles			
Manganese chrome antimony			
Titanium brown		No numbers	
Manganese niobium titanium brown		No numbers	
Brown Spinels			
Chrome iron manganese brown		No numbers	
Chrome iron manganese zinc brown		No numbers	
Burnt umber	Pigment Brown 7 77491	Ferric oxide (Fe_2O_3) manganese salts	Ferric salts and manganese salts
Uses: (See Brown hydrated iron oxide)			
Cadmium yellow	Pigment Yellow 35 77117	Cadmium sulfide (CdS)	Cadmium sulfides
Uses: Rubber, inks, paper, plastics, ceramics, glass	Pigment Yellow 37 77199		
Cadmium yellow lithopone	Pigment Yellow 35 77117	CdS, CdSe and a complex coprecipitate of $BaSO_4$ and ZnS	
Uses: (See Cadmium yellow)			
Cadmium orange	Pigment Orange 20 77199		
Uses: (See Cadmium yellow)			
Chrome lemon	Pigment Yellow 34 77600	$PbCrO_4 + PbSO_4$	guinea pig, i.p., LD 400 mg./kg.
Uses: Inks, paper, plastics, leather, textiles			
Chrome yellow	(See Chrome Lemon)	Lead sulfochromate ($PbCrO_4 \cdot PbSO_4$)	
Chrome manganese zinc brown	No numbers		
Iron chromite brown	Pigment Brown 35 77501		
Iron titanate brown	Black 12 77543		
Nickel ferrite brown	Brown 34 77497		
Zinc ferrite brown	Yellow 119 77496		
Zinc iron chromite brown	Brown 33 77503		
Cobalt yellow (See Aureolin)	Pigment Yellow 40 77357	See Aureolin	
Hansa yellows	Pigment Yellow 1 11680	Insoluble azo pigments	$LD_{50} > 10$ gm./kg.
Uses: Coatings and printing inks	Pigment Yellow 2		

Starred ingredients (*) may be responsible for major toxic effects; consult Section II.

PIGMENTS (Cont.)

Meet ANSI Z 66.1 Spec.	11730 Pigment Yellow 3 11710 Pigment Yellow 4 11665 Pigment Yellow 5 11660 Pigment Yellow 6 11670 Pigment Yellow 10 12710 Pigment Yellow 73 11738 Pigment Yellow 74 11741 Pigment Yellow 75 11770 Pigment Yellow 60 12705 Pigment Yellow 65 11740 Pigment Orange 1 11725		$LD_{50} > 20$ gm./kg. $LD_{50} > 20$ g/kg
Indanthrene yellows Uses: Dyeing cotton and silk; direct printing of cotton, silk and wool	Vat Yellow 10 65430 Vat Yellow 22:1	Insoluble anthraquinone vat dyes	
King's yellow	Pigment Yellow 39 77600	$PbCrO_4$	Lead salts & chromates. LD50 10gm/kg
Lead chromate Uses: Coatings, plastics, paper, printing inks, floor coverings	Pigment Yellow 34 77600	$PbCrO_4$	$LD_{50} > 5$ gm./kg.
Lemon yellow Uses: Anti-corrosion jointing pastes, artist colors, glass, and porcelain	Pigment Yellow 31 77103	See barium yellow, sometimes strontium yellow	
	Food Yellow 4 19140	[FD&C Yellow No. 5]	
	Food Yellow 3 15985	[FD&C Yellow No. 6]	
Uses: Coloring food and food packaging			
Litharge Uses: Glass manufacturing and enameling	Pigment Yellow 46 77577	Lead oxide (PbO)	
Logwood extract Uses: Dyeing fabrics and fibers.	Natural Black 1 75290	Lakes of Al, Cr, Fe or Sn of haematin or haematoxylin, isoflavone derivatives, Brazilan	Toxicity rating 3, WHO

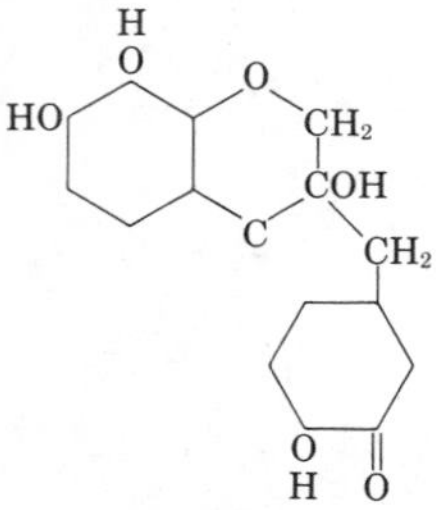

Haematin

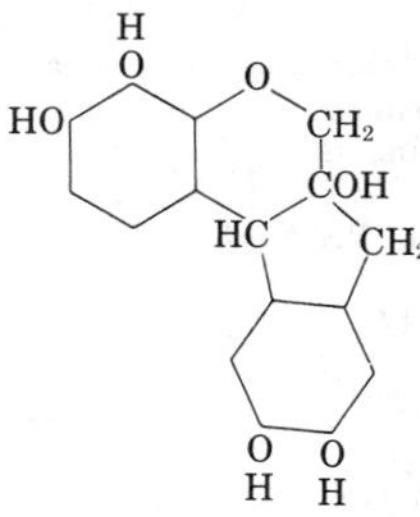

Haemotoxylin

Manganite Uses: Size and oil colors, line and cement colors	Pigment Brown 8 77730	$MnO(OH)\cdot MnO\cdot MnO_2$	
Manganese brown	Same as Manganite	Manganese hydroxide with manganite	
Mars yellow	Pigment Yellow 43	$FeO(OH)_nH_2O$	

Starred ingredients (*) may be responsible for major toxic effects; consult Section II.

PIGMENTS (Cont.)

Uses: Coatings, paper, cement products, rubber and linoleum	77492		
Mercuric oxide	77760	HgO	Mercury salts
Metallic brown	Pigment Brown 7	Ferric oxide (80%), silica (SiO_2) and aluminum oxide (Al_2O_3)	$LD_{50} > 10$ gm./kg.
Uses: Coatings, metal primers	77491 77492		
Meets ANSI Z 66.1 Spec.			
Mineral brown			
Mosaic gold	Pigment Yellow 38	Stannic sulfide (SnS)	Tin salts and sulfides
Uses: Formerly for gilding wood, plaster, metals, but replaced by metallic bronze powders	77878		
Naples yellow	Pigment Yellow 41		
(see Antimony yellow and Naples yellow S)	77588 77589	Lead antimonate and lead metantimonate	
Uses: Ceramics and glass, artist colors		Lead antimonate plus zinc and bismuth oxides	
Naples yellow S		Mixture of cadmium sulfide, zinc oxide and Venetian red	
Nickel antimony titanium yellow	Pigment Yellow 53 77788		
Nickel azo yellow	Pigment Green 10	Chelated nickel azo	$LD_{50} > 20$ gm./kg.
Nickel niobium titanium yellow			
	Pigment Brown 6&7	Hydrated ferric oxides ($FeO(OH)_nH_2O$)	$LD_{50} > 10$ gm./kg.
Ochre	Pigment Red 101, 102 Pigment Yellow 43 77492		
Uses: Coatings, plastics, paper, stains, cement products, rubber, and linoleum			
Meets ANSI Z 66.1 Spec.			
Domestic ochre	(see Pigment Yellow 43)		
French ochre	(see Pigment Yellow 43) also C.I. Pigment Yellow 42)		
Yellow ochre	(see Pigment Yellow 43)		
Orpiment	Pigment Yellow 39	Arsenic trisulfide (As_2S_3)	Orpiment
Uses: Tanning. (Formerly used as pigment, Kings Yellow, but replaced by mixture of cadmium sulfide and zinc oxide)	77086		Highly toxic
Primrose, Primrose yellow	Pigment Yellow 34	Chrome yellow ($PbCrO_4$) and lead sulfate ($PbSO_4$) up to 50%	$LD_{50} > 10$ gm./kg.
	77603		
Primrose, cadmium yellow	Pigment Yellow 35		
Uses: Coatings, paper, printing inks, plastics, leather finishes, artist colors, textile printing, linoleum	77205		
Does not meet ANSI Z 66.1 Spec.			
Primrose Priderite	Pigment Yellow 57		
Nickel barium titanium Primrose	77900		
Quercitron lakes	Natural Yellow 9	3,3′,4′5,7-Pentahydroxy flavone	Toxicity rating about 4, WHO

Starred ingredients (*) may be responsible for major toxic effects; consult Section II.

PIGMENTS (Cont.)

Uses: Interior decorations of
theaters, etc., coloring
paper and wallpaper;
transparent olive yel-
lows, green lakes, Bis-
marck, bronze, and
leather lakes

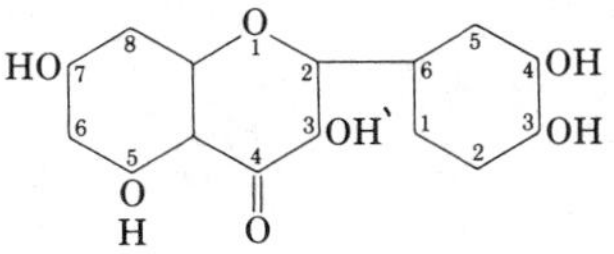

Quercitin

Raw sienna	Pigment Yellow 42 Pigment Yellow 43 77492	Hydrated ferric oxide $(FeO(OH)_nH_2O)$ and iron	$LD_{50} > 10$ gm./kg.

Domestic raw sienna
Italian raw sienna
    Uses: Paints, stains, artist
    colors, tinting colors
    Meets ANSI Z 66.1 Spec.			

Raw umber	Pigment Brown 7 77492	Hydrated ferric oxide $(FeO(OH)_nH_2O)$ and manganese salts	Ferric salts and manganese salts $LD_{50} > 10$ gm./kg.

Turkey raw umber
    Uses: Paints, stains, artist
    colors, tinting colors
    Meets ANSI Z 66.1 Spec.			

Realgar
    Uses: Dehairing of skins in
    tanning process
    Does not meet ANSI Z 66.1
    Spec.
	Pigment Yellow 39
	77085
		AS_2S_3	Arsenic

Segnale light yellow T2R	Pigment Yellow 1 11680		$LD_{50} > 5$ gm./kg.
Segnale light yellow 10G	Pigment Yellow 3 12120		$LD_{50} > 5$ gm./kg.
Segnale yellow DR-HG	Pigment Yellow 12 21090		$LD_{50} > 5$ gm./kg.
Segnale light yellow GRX	Pigment Yellow 13 21100		$LD_{50} > 5$ gm./kg.
Segnale yellow 2GR	Pigment Yellow 14 21095		$LD_{50} > 5$ gm./kg.
Segnale light yellow NCG	Pigment Yellow 16 20040		$LD_{50} > 5$ gm./kg.
Sepia	Natural Brown 9	1. From the ink of the cuttle fish containing melanin (78%), calcium carbonate (10.4%), chlorides (2.16%) and miscellaneous compounds (0.4%) 2. Mixture of burnt sienna and lampblack	
Use: Artists' water color			
Sienna Uses: Tinting colors, coatings, artists' colors, stains	Pigment Yellow 43 77492 Pigment Red 102 77015 Pigment Brown 7	(see Raw sienna)	

Strontium yellow
    Uses: Corrosion inhibitor
    for protective coatings
    Does not meet ANSI Z 66.1
    Spec.
	Pigment Yellow 32
	77893
		Strontium chromate $(SrCrO_4)$	LD_{50} 1.6–3.0 gm./kg.

Sun yellow Uses: Leather dyes, silk, paper beater dyes, dyeing cellulose, wool	Direct Yellow 6 40001 Direct Yellow 11 40000 Direct Orange 15 40002,3	Insoluble nickel, antinomy TiO_2-complex	Nickel and antimony salts
Uses: Paints and printing inks	Pigment Yellow 53 77788		
Thermofast supra Yellow R	Yellow 83 21108		

Starred ingredients (*) may be responsible for major toxic effects; consult Section II.

PIGMENTS (Cont.)

Thioflavin yellow Uses: Dyeing wool, acetate, nylon, cotton; ball point inks	Basic Yellow 1 49005	Phosphotungstomolybdic acid lake of	

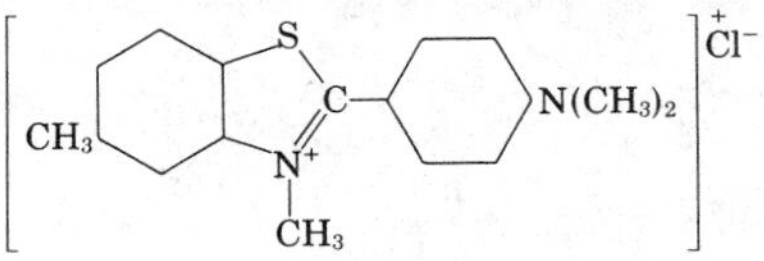

(a thiazole)

Titanium yellow Titanium nickel yellow Uses: Paints and printing inks	Pigment Yellow 53 77788	Insoluble nickel, antimony, TiO_2-complex	
Toluidine yellow Uses: Paints and printing inks, paper coating, coloring of viscose and linoleum, P/F, U/F and vinyl plastics, textile printing, leather finishes	Pigment Yellow 1 11680 Pigment Yellow 3 11710	An insoluble azo pigment	
Umber Burnt umber Raw umber Uses: Coatings, artists' colors, stains, tinting colors, cement products, plastics	Pigment Brown 7 77491 77492	See Raw umber	$LD_{50} > 10$ gm./kg.
Vandyke brown	Natural Brown 8	Treated Cassel earth, containing 80–90% organic (bituminous) materials, the remainder being iron, alumina, silica	$LD_{50} > 10$ gm./kg.
(imported and domestic) Uses [of 77430]: Stains, artists' colors Meets ANSI Z 66.1 Spec.	Pigment Brown 9 77430		
VULCOL Fast yellow 3G	Pigment Yellow 20		
Yellow cassiterite Tin vanadium yellow	Pigment Yellow 158 77862		
Yellow hydrated iron oxide (synthetic) Uses: Coatings, plastics, tinting colors, cement colors, roofing granules, paper, flooring materials, wax products, rubber Meets ANSI Z 66.1 Spec.	Pigment Yellow 42 77492	$FeO(OH)_nH_2O$	$LD_{50} > 10$ gm./kg.
Yellow oxide of iron Uses: Coatings, plastics, tinting colors, paper, wax products, cement colors, floorings Meets ASNI Z 66.1 Spec.	Pigment Yellow 42,3 77492		$LD_{50} > 10$ gm./kg.
Yellow oxide of mercury		Mercuric oxide (HgO)	
	77760		
Uses: Coatings, plastics, tinting colors, paper, wax products, cement colors, floorings Meets ASNI Z 66.1 Spec.			
Yellow zircon Zirconium praseodynium yellow	Pigment Yellow 159 77997		
Zinc yellow Uses: Corrosion resistant coatings, rust inhibitors	Pigment Yellow 36 77955	Zinc chromate ($ZnCrO_4$) Commercial products all contain some H_2O	$LD_{50} > 0.5$–0.6 gm./kg.

Starred ingredients (*) may be responsible for major toxic effects; consult Section II.

PIGMENTS (Cont.)

Does not meet ASNI Z 66.1
   Spec.

I. OTHER PIGMENTS
1. Metallic

Common Name	Color Index No.	Chemical Ingredients	Toxicity Data	Section II Referral
Aluminum powder	Pigment Metal 1	Aluminum	Aluminum	
Uses: Metallicized finishes, moisture resistant coatings, heat barrier coatings	77000			
Bronze powder (see Copper bronze powder)				
Copper alloy	Pigment Metal 2	Copper, zinc, aluminum, tin	Copper, zinc, aluminum, tin	
Uses: Metallicized finishes, marine anti-fouling paints, printing inks [Note: (1) Precipitate copper sulfate with metallic zinc; (2) stamp copper with metal calcium and heat 24 hr at 40°–50°C.]	77400			
Copper bronze powder	Pigmental Metal 2	Copper (80–90%), zinc (1%) and iron	Copper	
Uses: Metallicized finishes, marine antifouling paints, printing inks, substitute for gold	77400			
Dendritic copper powders [Note: Could be copper-zinc-iron combination as in Copper bronze powder; see also Metallic copper powder.]		Copper (98%); zinc (1%) and traces of other metals	Copper	
Green gold bronze [Note: See Rich pale gold bronze]	Pigment Green 10 12775	Copper (68%), zinc (31%) and aluminum (0.25%) [Nickel Azo Yellow]	Copper	
Linging bronzes [Note: See Rich pale gold bronze]		Finest grade bronze	Copper	
Metallic aluminum powder		Aluminum	Aluminum	
Uses: Metallicized finishes, moisture and heat-resistant coatings				
Metallic copper powder	Pigment Metal 2	Copper	Copper	
Uses: Metallicized finishes, moisture and heat-resistant finishes	77400			
Metallic gold	Pigment Metal 3	Gold	Gold	
For golds, reds, and purples in ceramics, gold artist colors	77480			
Metallic lead	Pigment Metal 4	Lead	Lead	
Uses: Anticorrosive steel coatings, primer on other metals and with aluminum flake in protective paints	77575			
Metallic nickel	Pigment 77775	Nickel	Nickel	
Metallic silver	Pigment 77820	Silver	Silver	
Uses: Coloring watch dials, etc., ceramics, artists' colors				
Metallic tin	Pigment Metal 5	Tin	Tin	

Starred ingredients (*) may be responsible for major toxic effects; consult Section II.

PIGMENTS (Cont.)

Uses: Coating food containers, for whiter metallic finishes than aluminum powder for "silver" coated paper	77860		
Metallic zinc	Pigment Metal 6 77945	Zinc and 1–2% zinc oxide	Zinc
Uses: For galvanizing of iron or steel, with white in protective paints to give better adherence to zinc surfaces.			
[Note: See Zinc dust]			
Molding bronze		Medium grade	Copper
Pale gold bronze		Copper (92%), zinc (6%), aluminum (2%)	Copper
Rich gold bronze		Copper (77%), zinc (22%), aluminum (10%)	Copper
[Note: see Copper bronze powder]			
Rich pale gold bronze		Copper (90%), zinc (9%), aluminum (1%)	Copper
Standard bronze [Note: see Copper bronze powder]			
Zinc dust	Pigment Metal 6 77945	Zinc plus 1 to 4% zinc oxide	Zinc
[See Metallic zinc]	Pigment Black 16 77945		
[Note: With white for better adherence to galvanized iron]			
2. Luminous inorganic pigments			
Color Fluo- Phos- Daylight res- phores- cent cent			
Uses: For interior paints and enamels, luminescent coatings, cosmetics, white pigment for celluloid.			
Green Purple Blue white blue	Pigment White 9 77245 (Calcium)	Calcium-strontium sulfide	Strontium sulfide
Green Sky Blue white blue	Pigment White 8	Calcium-strontium sulfide	Strontium sulfide Strontium sulfide
White Blue Blue green	77847 (Strontium)	Calcium-strontium sulfide	
Rhodamine B	Pigment Violet 1 45170:2		
Uses: Printing ink, paints, vinyl, paper coating, crayons.			
See also Dyes Eosine-bluish Eosine yellowish (YS) Rhodamine B			

DYES

"Dyes are intensely colored or fluorescent organic substances which impart color to a substrate by selective absorption of light. Dyes are water soluble and/or go through an application process which, at least temporarily, destroys any crystal structure of the color substances. Dyes are retained in the substrate by absorption, solution and mechanical retention, or by ionic or covalent chemical bonds." Definition by the Dry Color Manufacturers' Association.

In the current revision, data on dyes are presented separately from those on pigments.

Although the data given are based on what is believed to be reliable information obtained in a manner described above, the manufacturers who submitted data do not warrant or guarantee their correctness and expressly disclaim any warranty, obligation or liability for loss or damage for any violation of federal, state or municipal laws or regulations resulting from their use.

Starred ingredients (*) may be responsible for major toxic effects; consult Section II.

PIGMENTS (Cont.)

A. BLACK

Common Name	Color Index No.	Chemical Ingredients	Toxicity Data / Section II Referral
Black 7984 Uses: general purposes.	Food Black 2 27755		Toxicity rating 1–2, WHO
Brilliant black BN Uses: General purposes.	Food Black 1 28400		Toxicity rating 1–2, WHO
Nigrosines Uses: Lacquers, wood stains, marking inks, leather finishes, plastics.	Solvent Black 5 50415	Azines	
Sulfated nigrosines Uses: Leather, paper, inks, soap, anodized aluminum.	Acid Black 2 50420	Azines	

B. BLUE

Common Name	Color Index No.	Chemical Ingredients	Toxicity Data / Section II Referral
Acid fuchsine FB Uses: Paper, photo film, soap, leather.	Acid Violet 19 42685		Toxicity rating 3, WHO
Alkali blue Uses: Printing inks, paper, carbon paper, typewriter ribbons, some in plastics. Meets ANSI Z 66.1 Spec.	Pigment Blue 18 42770:1 Pigment Blue 19 42750:1	An acid triphenyl methane dye	
Erioglaucine blue Uses: Printing inks, occasionally in rubber and lacquers.	D & C Blue 4 (Purified Type)		
Patent blue Uses: Printing inks.	Acid Blue 1 42045		
Indigo blue	Vat Blue 1 63000 Pigment Blue 66 73000	An insoluble indigo vat dye	

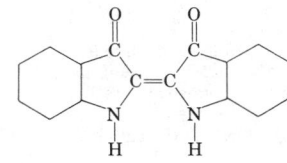

Indigo
(Indigo oil and water colors may consist of permanent pigments)

Indigotine Uses: Leather, food coloring. Meets ANSI 66:1 Spec.	Acid Blue 74 73015 Food Blue 1 73015 D & C Blue 2		Toxicity rating 3, WHO
Indulines Uses: Printing inks, carbon paper, typewriter ribbons, lacquers, waxes, plastic.	Solvent Blue 7 50400	Azine dyes	
Methylene blue	Basic Blue 9 52015		
Patent blue V Use: Food (in purified form).	Acid Blue 1 42045 Food Blue 3 42045		Toxicity rating 1–3, WHO
Sulfonated indulines Uses: leather, mass coloring casein.	Acid Blue 20 50405	Azine dyes	
Water blue 1	Acid Blue 93 42780		Toxicity rating 1, WHO

C. GREEN

Starred ingredients (*) may be responsible for major toxic effects; consult Section II.

PIGMENTS (Cont.)

Common Name	Color Index No.	Chemical Ingredients	Toxicity Data / Section II Referral
Fast green FCF Uses: Food	Food Green 3 42053		Toxicity rating 1–3, WHO
Guinea green B Uses: Food (in purified form)	Acid Green 3 42085 Food Green 1		Toxicity rating 1–3, WHO LD$_{50}$ 8.45 gm./kg. (C.I. Acid green 3)
Light green SF yellowish	Acid Green 5 42095 Food green 2 42095		Toxicity rating 3, WHO
Wool green BS	Acid Green 50 44090		Toxicity rating 3, WHO

D. ORANGE

Common Name	Color Index No.	Chemical Ingredients	Toxicity Data / Section II Referral
Beta-apo-8'-Carotenal			Toxicity Rating 3
Orange II Meets ANSI Z 66.1 Spec.	Acid Orange 7 15510		Toxicity rating 1–2, WHO

E. RED

Common Name	Color Index No.	Chemical Ingredients	Toxicity Data / Section II Referral
Amaranth maroon	Acid Red 27 16185	A soluble azo dye	
Azo Bordeaux	Acid Red 17 16180	A soluble azo dye	LD$_{50}$ > 11 gm./kg.
Azo rubine Uses: Inks, food and drug colorants.	Acid Red 14 14720		Toxicity rating 1–3 WHO
Bromo acids	Acid Red 87 45380	See Eosine	See Eosine
Crimson lake Use: Paints. Crimson mad- der	Natural Red 7	An anthraquinone dye See Alizarin crimson.	Alizarin
Ponceau 2R Uses: Inks, food and drug colorants.	Acid Red 26 (Food Red 5) 16150		Toxicity rating 1–3, WHO
Ponceau 3R Uses: Inks, plastics, food and drug colorants.	Acid Red 18 (Food Red 7) 16255		Toxicity rating 1–3, WHO
Ponceau Sx Uses: Inks, drug and cos- metic colorants	Acid Red 112 27195		Toxicity rating 1–3, WHO
Red lakes and toners, miscel- laneous	(See Red lake C)	An azine dye 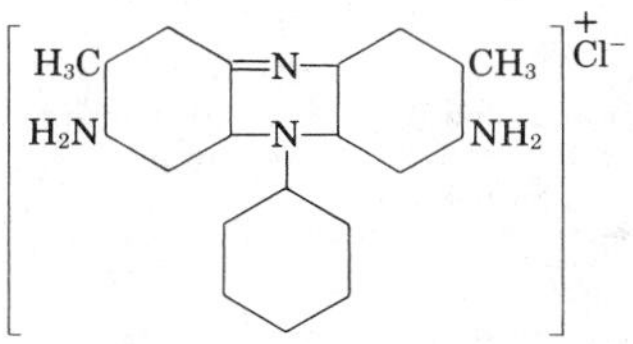	

Sodium lithol, barium lithol, calcium lithol, strontium lithol.	(See Lithols)	Insoluble Na,Ca,Ba Sn salt of an azo dye	Barium salts Barium lake may be toxic
Sudan G Uses: Cosmetics, some pol- ystyrene.	Solvent Red 23 26100 D & C Red 17		Toxicity rating 3, WHO

Starred ingredients (*) may be responsible for major toxic effects; consult Section II.

PIGMENTS (Cont.)

Tumeric	Natural Red 3 75450	

F. VIOLET

Common Name	Color Index No.	Chemical Ingredients	Toxicity Data / Section II Referral
Benzyl violet Uses: Inks.	Basic Violet 13 42536	A triphenyl methane dye.	Toxicity rating 3, WHO
Crystal violet Uses: Inks. Meets ANSI Z 66.1 Spec.	Basic Violet 3 42555	A triphenyl methane dye.	Gentian violet $LD_{50} > 920$ mg./kg.
Methyl violet Uses: Inks	Basic Violet I 42535	A basic triphenyl methane dye. One of the more highly methylated pararosanilines.	Gentian violet

H. YELLOW AND BROWN

Common Name	Color Index No.	Chemical Ingredients	Toxicity Data / Section II Referral
Annatto	Natural Orange 4 75120	Seeds and pulp of the shrub *Bixa* orellana. Coloring matter Bixin $Cl_8H_{20}O_2CH_2OOCH$: $(CHC \cdot CH_2)$: $(CHCH)_4$ $CHCO_2H$, a carotenoid acid (food coloring matter)	Daily intake (man): 1.25 mg./kg temporarily (FAO/WHO)
Auramine Uses: Textiles, fibers, paper, leather, inks.	Basic Yellow 2 41000		Toxicity rating 4, WHO
Brown FK Uses: (This color has never been listed as a food color by the US FDA)	Food Brown 1		Toxicity rating 1–3, WHO
Chocolate Brown HT Uses: (Never listed as a food color by U.S. FDA	Food Brown 3 20285		Toxicity rating 1–3, WHO
Chrysoine Use: Biologic stains. (Never listed by U.S. FDA: permitted by EEC with restrictions and in several other countries)	Acid Orange 6 Food Yellow 8 14270		Toxicity rating 1–3, WHO
Dutch Pink Use: For Lakes	Natural Yellow 9 —	Extract of quercitron bark (see Quercitron)	
Flavanthrone Yellow Uses: Paints, printing inks, plastics. Meets ANSI Z 66.1 Spec.	Natural Yellow 24 70600		$LD_{50} > 10gm./kg.$
Fluorescein yellow Uses: Markers, lifesaving at sea, tracing underground water sources.	Acid Yellow 73 45350 Purified: D & C Yellow 7 D & C Yellow 8	A soluble xanthene dye; if so marked D & C colors are nontoxic Free acid Sodium salt	
Fustic Uses: Textiles, leather.	Natural Yellow 11 75240 75660	Extract from trunk of chlorophora (as marus or machura) tinctoria.	

Starred ingredients (*) may be responsible for major toxic effects; consult Section II.

PIGMENTS (Cont.)

Hypernic Uses: Cotton and wood dyeing, printing inks, leather dyeing.	Natural Red 24 75280	From various species of Brazil wood (logwood extract) Caesalpina (natural occurring isoflavones)
Metanil yellow Uses: Dyeing wool and silk, paper, leather dyes, biologic stains.	Acid Yellow 36 13065	Toxicity rating 3, WHO
Naphthol yellows	Acid Yellow 24 10315	Sodium or potassium salts of 2,4-dinitro-1-naphthol-7-sulfonic acid 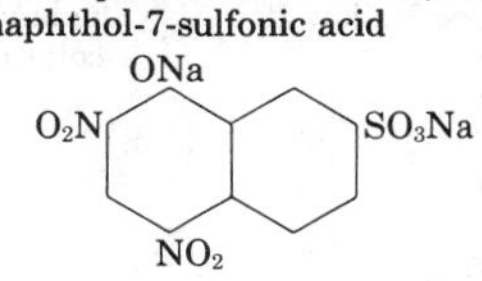
Uses: Silk dyeing, mothproofing	Acid Yellow 1 10316	
Uses: Dip dyeing of paper, leather dyes, biologic stain.		

ONa

O$_2$N ———— SO$_3$Na

NO$_2$

Naphthol yellow

	Acid Yellow 9 13015	
	Acid Yellow 9:1	
	Acid Yellow 11 18820	
	Acid Yellow 17 18965	
	Acid Yellow 18 19020	
	Acid Yellow 23 19140	
	Acid Yellow 27 19130	
	Acid Yellow 36 13065	
	Acid Yellow 65 14170	
	Acid Yellow 122 19110	
	Acid Yellow 153 19230	
	Acid Yellow 191 Acid Dye 13075	
Uses: Dyeing wool, silk, acetate, nylon, leather, paper, cotton viscose, wool printing, coloring soap.		
Uses: Dyeing wool, silk, nylon, acetate, leather.	Acid Orange 3 10385	
Uses: Fiber dyes, indicator paper, soap, straw and glue, leather coloring.	Acid Orange 5 13080	
Uses: Biological stain, dyeing wool, silk, nylon, leather	Acid Orange 6 14270	
Use: Food colors. Citronine A	Food Yellow 2 13015 Acid Dye 10355 Acid Yellow 63 13095 Acid Orange 1	
Uses: Dyeing wool, silk, nylon, acetate, leather, soap coloring.		
Uses: Dyeing wool, acetate, silk, nylon, cotton, chrome tanned leather.	Mordant Yellow 6 22880	
(FD&C Yellow No. 5)	Food Yellow 4 19140	Certified nontoxic, FDA
(FD&C Yellow No. 6) Uses: Food drug and cosmetic coloring.	Food Yellow 3 15985	Certified nontoxic, FDA
Oil yellow AB	Solvent Yellow 1	Toxicity rating 3, WHO

Common Name / Uses	Color Index No.	Chemical Ingredients	Toxicity Data / Section II Referral
Uses: Oil and spirit coatings, wax products, stains, styrene resins.	11000		
Uses: Oil and spirit coatings.	Solvent Yellow 10 11380 Food Yellow 10 11380		
Oil yellow OB	Solvent Yellow 6 11390		Toxicity rating 3, WHO
Persian berries Uses: Calico printing, shading logwood printing blocks in combination with basic dyes.	Natural Yellow 13 75640 75430 75650 75670 75690 75700 75695	The buckthorn (Rhamnus) family Main coloring matter: kaempferol (a natural occurring flavone)	Probably toxic (see Quercitron)
Quinoline yellow Uses: Dyeing wool, silk, orlon, nylon, acetate; printing wool, leather, acetate, biologic stain [47005]; printing wool, silk, nylon [47010]; wood stains [47035].	Acid Yellow 3 47005 Acid Yellow 2 47010 Acid Yellow 5 47035	D & C Yellow 10	Toxicity rating 3, WHO
Uses: Drug and cosmetic coloring.	Food Yellow 13 47005 Solvent Yellow 33 47000		
Sunset yellow FCF Uses: Coloring jams, canned foods, sugar confectionery, baked goods, soft drinks.	Food Yellow 3 15985	A soluble azo dye.	Toxicity rating 1–3, WHO
Tartrazine yellow Uses: Dyeing wool, acetate, silk and nylon, printing wool and silk, surface staining of paper and leather.	Acid Yellow 23 19140	A soluble azo dye.	Toxicity rating 2, WHO
Thiazine brown R Thiazine red R Uses: Dyeing cellulose, silk, wool, nylon, paper, leather, coloring soap, biologic stain.	Direct Dyes Direct Red 45 14780		
Turmeric Uses: Dyeing cotton, wool, silk, food dye, microscopic stain, coloring oils and waxes.	Natural Yellow 3 75300		
Yellow 27175N Use: Food coloring.	Food dye 13445		Toxicity rating 1–2, WHO

1. OTHER DYES

Common Name	Color Index No.	Chemical Ingredients	Toxicity Data / Section II Referral
Luminous			Generally considerd to have a low toxicity
Fluorescein Green fluorescence; red by transmitted light	Acid Yellow 73 45350	9-(o-Carboxy phenyl)-6-hydroxy-3-isoxanthenone	D & C Yellow No. 7 Low toxicity

PIGMENTS (Cont.)

Fluorescein sodium
Yellowish red with intense green fluorescence
Uses: Lifesaving marker at sea, tracing water and blood flows, drugs and cosmetics.

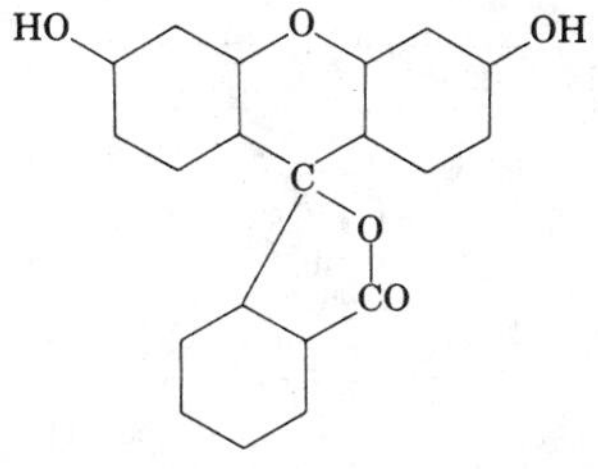

Fluorescein
Bluish

Apparently low toxicity

Erythrosine   Acid Red 51   45430
Uses: Dyeing wool, nylon, silk, acetate; stamping inks, cosmetics, biologic stains.

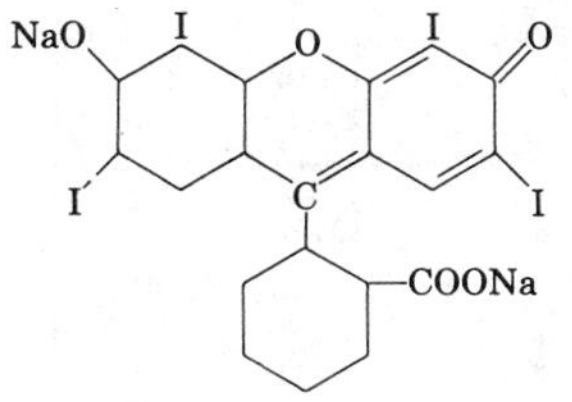

Erythrosine

Toxicity rating 1–3, WHO

Uses: Dyeing wool, silk, jute, straw; stamping and writing inks.   Acid Red 95   45425   45430
Use: Dyeing wool.   Acid Red 98   45405

Yellowish

Uses: Coloring glace, maraschino cherries, meat products, confectionery, canned goods.   Food Red 14

Eosine—bluish   Acid Red 92   45410
Uses: Dyeing wool, acetate, silk, nylon; writing and stamping inks, paper, biologic stain, drugs and cosmetics, indicator color.   Acid Red 91 (alcohol soluble)   45400

Dibromo dinitro fluorescein sodium.
Red powder, freely soluble in water with green fluorescence.

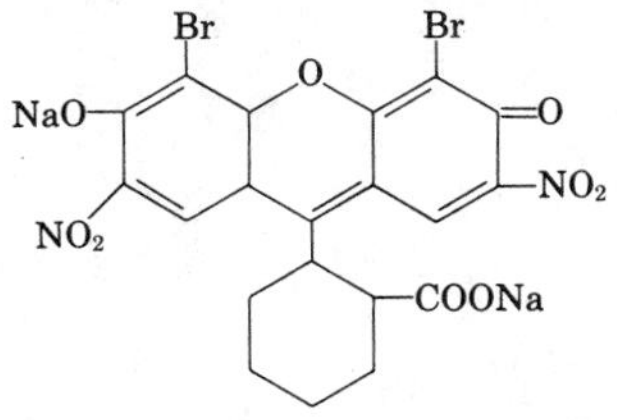

Eosine

Eosine yellowish (YS)   Acid Red 87   45380
Uses: Dyeing wool, nylon, silk; biologic stain; inks, paper, pencil leads; spirit strains; cosmetics and drugs.

Bromeosine: tetrabromofluorescein
Solution (H_2O) deep brownish red with greenish fluorescence. In alcohol strong green fluorescence.

LD_{50} (guinea pig, oral): 5 gm./kg.
Toxicity rating 2

Rhodamine B   Basic Violet 10   45170
Uses: Dyeing silk, cotton, wool, acetate, nylon, paper, soap, leather, feather, biologic stain.

Tetraethylrhodamine. Soluble in water bluish red color, dilute solution strongly fluorescent.

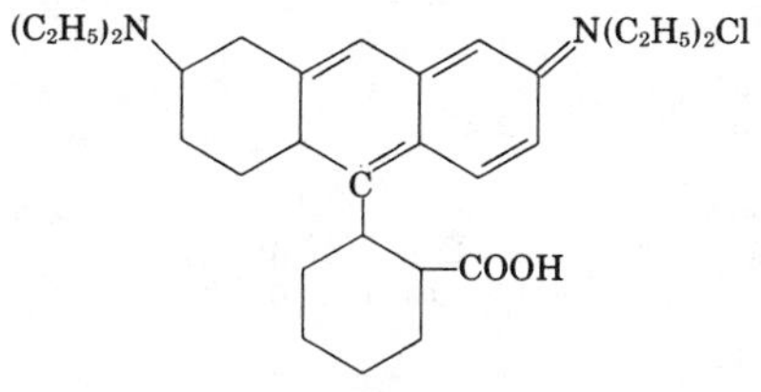

$(C_2H_5)_2N$ $N(C_2H_5)_2Cl$

—COOH

RHODAMINE B

POLISHES	POLISHES (Cont.)

POLISHES

ALUMINUM POLISH (See CLEANERS)

AUTOMOBILE POLISHES .... Toxicity rating 2
Silicone fluid	3-10%
Waxes (petroleum and carnauba)	2-12%
Water	0-60%
Petroleum distillates	20-70%
Abrasives	0-20%
Emulsifiers	0-2%
Dye, perfume, perservatives	Trace quantities

AUTOMOTIVE RUBBING COMPOUNDS
1. Hand application type: .... Toxicity rating 3
Tripoli (silica)	27-40%
Kerosene*	25-30%
Cyclohexanol	up to 5%
Soda soap or amine soap	3-10%
Water	10-37%
Mineral oil or waxes	8-10%
Pine oil	2-8%

2. Machine application type: .... Toxicity rating 3
Tripoli (silica)	27-40%
Kerosene or naphtha*	10-20%
Sulfonated vegetable oils	5-10%
Mineral or paraffin oil	5-15%
Ethanolamine oleate soaps	1-5%
Pine oil	1-5%
Water	10-37%

May contain:
Amyl acetate
Butoben
Caraway oil
Cedar oil
Citronella oils
Dye
Emulsifiers
Ethanol
Fatty acids
Formaldehyde
Glycerine
Methanol
Morpholine
Perfume
Phenol (1%)
Silicone and oils (1-5%)
Trichloroethylene*
Turpentine
Vegetable gums
Xylene

CHROME POLISH (see CLEANERS)

FLOOR POLISHES (also see furniture polish)
1. Self-polishing—generalized formula .. Toxicity rating 2-3
Water	70-85%
Synthetic polymers	9-17%
(Styrene acrylate, acrylic, polystyrene, with or without zinc and/or zirconium metal cross-link)	
Waxes	0-2%
Coalescing agents	3-9%
(Carbitols, glycols, pyrrolidones, organic phosphates, phthalates, benzoates)	
Emulsifiers (wetting agents)	1-3%
Preservatives, perfumes	Trace quantities

2. Solvent type .... Toxicity rating 3
a. Paste	
Petroleum naphtha*	75-85%

FLOOR POLISHES (Cont.)
Waxes (paraffin, carnauba, microcrystalline)	15-25%
b. Liquid	
Petroleum distillate*	80-90%
Natural and synthetic resins	0-10%
Natural and synthetic resins	0-10%

3. Pressurized (aerosol) type .... Toxicity rating 3
Water	65-75%
Synthetic polymers	10-15%
Waxes	2-5%
Coalescing agents	1-3%
Emulsifiers	1-3%
Propellents	2-7%
Compressed gas (nitrous oxide) or compressed liquid hydrocarbons or fluorocarbons	
Preservatives	Trace quantities

May contain:
Ammonia
Amines (morphine)
Fatty acids (oleic)
Nonionic and anionic surfactants and defoamers

FURNITURE POLISH
1. Solvent type .... Toxicity rating 3
a. Oil polish	
Petroleum distillate*	65-99%
Perfume	0.05-0.5%
Dye	0.005-0.01%
May contain:	
Turkey red oil	

b. Wax solvent .... Toxicity rating 3
Mineral spirits*	90-95%
Wax (carnauba, candelilla, beeswax, Gersthoven wax, ozokerite wax)	1.5-5%
Silicone	1.5-5%
May contain:	
Amyl acetate	
Turpentine	

2. Emulsion type .... Toxicity rating 3
a. Oil type	
Petroleum distillate*	40-60%
Emulsifier (diglycol laurate)	3-15%
Water	20-60%
Perfume (essential oils, e.g., oil of citronella, cedar wood, lemon, sassafras)	0.1-3%
Preservative	0.1-5%
May contain:	
Cetyl alcohol	
Isopropanol	
Methyl salicylate (perfume)	

b. Wax type
Mineral spirits*	0-80%
Wax	0-3%
Emulsifier	3-15%
Water	10-80%
Perfume and dye	trace
Preservative	0.1-0.5%
May contain:	
Alkyl sodium sulfate	
Amine soaps	
Bentonite	
Ethylene glycol	
Glycerine	

Starred ingredients (*) may be responsible for major toxic effects; consult Section II.

POLISHES (Cont.)	POLISHES (Cont.)

FURNITURE POLISH (Cont.)

Gums as thickeners (traga-
canth, gelatin, arabic)
Hydroxyethyl cellulose
Isooctyl phenyl polyethoxy
ethanol
Petroleum synthetic waxes
Pine oil
Quaternary ammonium com-
pounds
Shellac
Silicones
Synthetic resin
Turpentine

3. Aerosol type .... Toxicity rating 3
Natural and/or synthetic waxes 0–5%
Silicone oils 0–4%
Mineral oils 0–2%
Emulsifiers 1–3%
Petroleum or synthetic naphthas* 0–30%
Perfumes 0.05–0.3%
Preservatives 0.05–0.2%
Propellants:
Compressed gas (nitrous oxide) 1–2%
or compressed liquid (hydrocarbons) 4–15%
Water 40–90%

GENERAL PURPOSE POLISH .... Toxicity rating 2 or 3
Turpentine*
Mineral spirits*
Waxes
May contain:
Coloring
Detergent
Emulsifier
Mineral waxes (may be chlorinated)
Perfume
Vegetable waxes (e.g., carnauba, our-
icury)
Wood preservative
Zinc stearate

LEATHER POLISH .... Toxicity rating 2
Carnauba wax
Animal and vegetable oils
Triethanolamine

LEATHER POLISHES, DRESSING ... Toxicity rating 4
Vegetable waxes 20%
Turpentine* 40%
Amine-oleate soap 2%
May contain:
Alcohol
Natural resins
Neatsfoot oil
Plasticizers
Soya bean oil
Sperm oil
Propellant
Methyl polysiloxane
Stoddard solvent
Xylene

METAL POLISHES .... Toxicity rating 3
1. Petroleum solvent* (see naphtha) 25–70%
Citric acid 0.10–0.15%
Abrasive 5–10%
Triethanolamine oleate 0.15–0.20%
Ammonium hydroxide 0.4–0.5%
Water

METAL POLISHES (Cont.)

2. Abrasive 20–30%
Oxalic acid* 2–3%
Isopropanol 0–4%
Fatty acids 5–7%
Ammonia 3–6%
Pine oil 0–1%
Water .... to 100%
May contain:
Alcohol
Alkyl sodium sulfates
Bentonite
Dye
Essential oils
Kerosene
Nitric acid
Paraffin oil
Paraffin wax
Phenolic derivative (Dowicide)*
Phosphoric acid
Plasticizer
Rosin soap
Soap
Sulfuric acid
Tergitol
Tripoli
Trisodium phosphate

MISCELLANEOUS POLISHES
1. Cement polish .... Toxicity rating 3
Paraffin oil (see Kerosene*)
Heavy oil, plain color
Toluene*
Stain (oil dyes, black, yellow, orange
mahogany)
Lemon oil
May contain:
Amyl acetate
Diatomaceous earth
Emulsifier
Formaldehyde
Glycerine
Soap
Vegetable gums
Vegetable oil
Wax

1. Others
a. Stoddard solvent* .... Toxicity rating 3
b. Antimony trichloride solution* .... Toxicity rating 4

PASTE WAX .... Toxicity rating 3
Petroleum naphtha* 75–85%
Paraffin, carnauba and microcrystalline
waxes 15–25%
Dye .... Trace

PLASTIC POLISHES (see Cleaners) ... Toxicity rating 4
Paraformaldehyde* 100%

PORCELAIN AND METAL POLISHES
(see Cleaners) .... Toxicity rating 2
Silica abrasive
Soda soap
Pine oil .... less than 1%
Ammonium hydroxide .... less than 1%
Oxalates .... less than 1%

Starred ingredients (*) may be responsible for major toxic effects; consult Section II.

POLISHES (Cont.)

SCRATCH REMOVER POLISHES ....   Toxicity rating 3
1. Petroleum spirits*
   Wood stains
   Powdered abrasives
   Petroleum and vegetable oils, and waxes
   Lacquer
   Metallic soaps
   Phenolic preservative
   Ethyl alcohol
2. Petroleum solvents* 94%
   Waxes
   Silicone oils
   Organic dyes

SHOE POLISHES
1. Shoe polishes, liquid ....   Toxicity rating 3
   a. Self-polishing
      High molecular weight synthetic polymer 0–10%
      Spray polishes only:
         Chlorinated solvents*
         Propellants
      Shellac 0–10%
      Wax 5%
      Fatty acid 2%
      Amines, emulsifiers 2%
      Dye or pigment ....   trace
      Phenyl mercuric acetate ......   trace
      Water 85%
      May contain:
         Borax
         Lanolin
         Phosphate and/or phthalate plasticizers, glycols
   b. Brush to shine
      Alchols* + water 90–95%
      Waxes and high molecular synthetic polymers 5–10%
      May contain:
         Shellac or rosin derivatives
2. Shoe polishes, paste ....   Toxicity rating 3
   Animal, petroleum and vegetable waxes 20–50%
   Mineral spirits* 10–65%
   Turpentine* 0–75%
   Aniline dyestuffs or nigrosine ...   0–3%
   Silicone oil 0–2%
   May contain:
      Lanolin
      Nitrobenzene
      Terpenes
3. Suede polish ....   Toxicity rating 3
   Denatured ethanol 25%
   Aniline dye 0.5%
   Water 50–75%
   Silicones
   Chlorinated solvents* (see Trichlorethane)
   Perfume
   Acetic acid
   Plasticizer
   May contain (spray suedes only):
      Propylene oxide
      Propellant or hydrocarbons
4. White shoe polish ....   Toxicity rating 2
   Titanium oxide 25%
   Clay or other pigment extenders ...   0–15%
   Emulsified waxes 25%
   Water ....   to 70%

POLISHES (Cont.)

SHOE POLISHES (Cont.)

    May contain:
       Bentonite
       Casein
       Ethylene glycol
       Gum tragacanth and other resins
       Isopropanol
       Lanolin
       Perfume
       Perservatives (phenyl mercuric acetate, dowanol, formaldehyde, or others)
       Protein
       Soap
       Starch
       Zinc oxide

SILVER POLISH ....   Toxicity rating 3
1. Denatured ethanol* or isopropanol* ..   20–99%
   Diatomaceous earth 15–20%
   Soap 3–4%
   Perfume 0–0.13%
   Water 45–90%
   Mercaptans ....   up to 5%
   May contain:
      Alkyl sodium sulfates
      Amine soap
      Ammonia 0–0.5%
      Camphor*
      Essential oils
      Fatty acids 1.5%
      Nonionic surfactant
      Pine oil
      Rhodamine B dye 0.001%
      Sassafras
      Silver nitrate* 0–1.0%
      Sodium thiosulfate 0–2.0%
      Stoddard solvent* 0–15%
      Sulfuric acid and phosphoric acid
      Thiourea 0–7.0%
2. Phosphoric acid* (see Acid) 5–10%
   Sulfuric acid 0–1%
   Thiourea 4–5%
   Mint 1%
   Water ....   to 100%
   May contain:
      Bentonite
      Carboxymethylcellulose
      Celite
      Copper sulfate*
      Dowicide A*
      Dye
      Essential oils
      Plasticizer
      Tergitol
      Titanium dioxide

STOVE POLISHES (see Cleaners) .....   Toxicity rating 3
   Carbon black
   Graphite
   Naphtha*

WINDOW WAXES (see Cleaners) ...   Toxicity rating 2 or 3
   Silica abrasive
   Amine soaps
   Waxes
   Petroleum solvent*
   Ammonium hydroxide ....   trace

Starred ingredients (*) may be responsible for major toxic effects; consult Section II.

POLISHES (Cont.)

WOOD POLISHES (see Furniture Polish)
1. Cream		Toxicity rating 3
	Mineral oil* (see Kerosene)	55%
	Emulsifying agent	3%
	Isopropanol	4%
	Water	38%
2. Oil		Toxicity rating 3
	Petroleum oil* (see Kerosene)	90–100%
	Cedar wood oil	small amt.
	Turpentine	small amt.
	Color	trace

PRESERVATIVES

BRUSH (PAINT) .... Toxicity rating 3
Turpentine*
Kerosene*
Linseed oil
Gelatin
Glycerin
Ammonium alum*
Potash alum*
Citric acid

CANVAS .... Toxicity rating 3
Pentachlorophenol* (less than 5%)
Tetrachlorophenol* (less than 5%)
2-Chlorophenylphenol* (less than 5%)
Petroleum solvents*
Ortho dichlorobenzene 1%
Synthetic resins
Diacetone alcohol*
Copper naphthenate

CHROME (PROTECTOR) .... Toxicity rating 3
Petroleum distillate*
Petroleum waxes
Silicone oil
Trithanolamine
Oleic acid
Nonionic surfactant
Isobutane propellants

CONCRETE .... Toxicity rating 4
Calcium (calcined solution)
Colloidal resins
Coal tar solvents*

FLOOR (WOOD) .... Toxicity rating 4
Magnesium fluorosilicate*
Sodium zinc silicate
Sulfates

FOUNDATION ....Toxicity rating 3
Asphalt
Asbestos
Petroleum ether*

POLISH .... Toxicity rating 2 or 3
Gum tragacanth
Bentonite
Alcohol*
Mineral oil
Sulfonated castor oil*
Glycerin
Wintergreen*
Oil (hydrocarbon)*

ROOF .... Toxicity rating 3
Asphalt (cut back with solvents)
Asbestos
Slate filler
Petroleum ether*

PRESERVATIVES (Cont.)

WOOD .... Toxicity rating 3
Gum resin
Zein (corn protein)
Denatured alcohol*
Ethyl triethanol amine
Glycol humectant
Naphthenic acid*
Copper hydrate*
Mineral spirits*
Copper naphthenate*
Zinc naphthenate
Copper linoleate*
Copper oleate*
Pentachlorophenol*

REPELLANTS

CAT (see PET CARE)

DOG (see PET CARE)

INSECT REPELLENTS	Toxicity rating 3
Butopyronoxyl	0–2%
Diethyltoluamide	2.85–47.5%
Dimethyl phthalate	0–1.25%
Ethohexadiol	0–80%
m-Homomenthyl salicylate	0–5.1%
Other isomers	0–8.5%

Base available as:
Aerosol, cream, foam, liquid, lotion, stick

STICK REPELLANT (see above)

RUST CONTROL, RUST PREVENTIVE

RUST CONTROL, RUST PREVENTIVE
1. Powder		Toxicity rating 4
	Potassium dichromate*	100%
2. Liquid		Toxicity rating 3
	Soda ash	6%
	Potassium dichromate*	6%
	Isopropanol	23%
	Water	65%

May contain:
Heavy lubricating oil
Lanolin
Petroleum solvents*
Petroleum sulfonate
Resinous compounds
Silicones
3. Liquid acid		Toxicity rating 3
	Phosphoric acid*	
	Aniline dye*	
4. Partially rusty surfaces		Toxicity rating 3
	a. Zinc chromate*	4.5%
	Magnesium silicate	7.5%
	Diatomaceous silica	2.0%
	Yellow iron oxide	5.0%
	Aliphatic hydrocarbon*	55–60%
	Processed fish oil	20–25%
	b. Red iron oxide	14%
	Zinc chromate	1.2%
	Magnesium silicate	6%
	Diatomaceous silica	3.5%
	Aliphatic hydrocarbon*	55–60%
	Processed fish oil	20–25%

5. High gloss pigment, chrome yellow,*
prussian blue, toluidine red, titanium dioxide and zinc oxide about
10%		Toxicity rating 3
Fish oil		25–40%
Aliphatic hydrocarbon*		50%

Starred ingredients (*) may be responsible for major toxic effects; consult Section II.

PRESERVATIVES (Cont.)	SANITIZERS (Cont.)

RUST CONTROL, RUST PREVENTIVE (Cont.)

Widely used rust inhibitors are high molecular weight carboxylic, sulfonic, or phosphoric acids, their salts, and salts with organic bases, such as amines.
Primers may contain strontium chromate.

SALT SUBSTITUTES

SALT SUBSTITUTE .... Toxicity rating 3
  Potassium chloride*
  Fumaric acid
  Tricalcium phosphate
  Monocalcium phosphate
LIGHT SALT .... Toxicity rating 3
  Sodium chloride
  Potassium chloride*
  Calcium silicate
  Magnesium carbonate
  Dextrose
  Potassium iodide
SEASONED SALT SUBSTITUTE .... Toxicity rating 3
  Potassium chloride*
  Fumaric acid
  Tricalcium phosphate
  Monocalcium phosphate
  Sugar
  Spices

SANITIZERS

AIR SANITIZER (see also Cleaners;
  Deodorizers) .... Toxicity rating 4
Alkyl dimethyl ethyl benzyl and alkyl
  dimethylbenzyl ammonium
  compounds* 20%
Water
Versene
May contain:
  Essential oils
  Isopropanol*
  Propellants
  Propylene glycol
  Triethylene glycol

BARBER SHOP SANITIZER (See
  Cleaners; Disinfectants) ....,...... Toxicity rating 3
1. Formaldehyde* 37%
2. Alkyl dodecyl pyridinium chloride 4.5%
  Isopropanol solution* (50%) 95.5%

DAIRY SANITIZERS (see Cleaners, Dairy)

MISCELLANEOUS SANITIZERS (see Cleaners; Disinfectants)
1. Iodine-bearing .... Toxicity rating 3
  Available iodine* 1.5–2%
  Detergents
  Mild acids .... to 100%
2. Quaternary type: .... Toxicity rating 3
  Quaternary ammonium compounds* 10%
  Water .... to 100%
3. Chlorine type: .... Toxicity rating 3
  Sodium hypochlorite*
  Calcium hypochlorite*
  Chlorinated organic compounds*
4. Acid type: .... Toxicity rating 3
  Saponified cresylic acid*
  Phosphoric acid* (see Acid)

SWIMMING POOL SANITIZER ...... Toxicity rating 3
1. Sodium hypochlorite*
  Other chlorinated compounds*
  Water
2. Cyanuric acid
  Chlorinated cyanuric acid
3. Hydantoin type: .... Toxicity rating 3
  1,3-dichloro-5,5-dimethylhydantoin* 100%
  N-Bromo-
    chlorodimethylhydantoin*† 100%
4. Algae control .... Toxicity rating 3
  a. Alkyl aryl ammonium chloride* ... usually 10%
    Such as:
      Alkyl dimethyl dichlorobenzyl
        ammonium chloride (may be as
        high as 40%)
      Alkyl dimethyl ethyl ammonium
        chloride
      Dodecyl benzyl trimethyl ammonium chloride
      Alkyl dimethyl benzyl ammonium
        chloride
      Alkyl dimethyl ethyl ammonium
        chloride
      Alkyl trimethyl ammonium chloride
      Alkyl methyl dipolyoxypropylene
        ammonium methyl sulfate
      Dodecylamine hydrochloride
    May contain:
      Copper EDTA* 0.1–22%
      Sodium carbonate 2–92%
      Sodium or potassium EDTA
      Sodium tripolyphosphate 0.5%
      Trisodium phosphate 2.5%
      Water
      Octyl phenoxy polyethoxy
        ethanol*
      Isopropanol*
  b. Phenyl mercuric acetate* 4.75%
    Alkyl amine acetate 3.75%
  c. Potassium dichloro-s-triazine-
    trione* 60%
    or 1,3,5-Trichloro-s-triazine-
    trione* 77%
    Sodium carbonate 30%
    Alkyl aryl ammonium chloride 1%
  d. Dichlorodimethyl hydantoin* 80%
    Potassium iodide 20%
† see Dichloro-dimethylhydantoin

SEALING COMPOUNDS

SEALING COMPOUNDS (see CAULKING COMPOUNDS)

FLOOR SEAL .... Toxicity rating 3
  Soya dehydrated castor vinyl resin 25%
  Cobalt drier .... trace
  Petroleum solvents (naphtha,* etc.) ... 75%
  May contain:
    Lacquer thinner
    Water emulsion latex
    Mineral spirits

SHELF AND DRAWER INSECTICIDAL PAPER
  Lindane 15–19 mg. per sq. ft. of printed surface.

SOAPS

Soap is defined as the alkali metal salt of fatty acids. Sodium and potassium hydroxides are the alkalis used in familiar soap products and the fatty) acids are derived from animal fats and

---

Starred ingredients (*) may be responsible for major toxic effects; consult Section II.

SOAPS (Cont.)

vegetable oils (e.g., tallow and coconut oil). Occasionally an organic alkaline material (e.g., triethanolamine) is used to increase solubility, particularly in liquid soap preparations.

In addition to its primary use as a cleaning agent, soap finds many industrial applications, and for these purposes special metal salts of fatty acids are produced which have properties different from those usually associated with soap. Copper, aluminum, calcium and magnesium soaps are insoluble in water and hence find use as waterproofing agents and lubricants.

The household uses of soap include personal use for cleansing the skin, washing of clothes and dishes, and a host of other cleaning operations. Except for personal use and light-duty tasks, however, many newer detergent formulations have largely replaced soap (see Detergents, Cleaners).

Toilets soaps are mostly pure soap in bar form to which may be added emollients such as glycerine, lanolin, cold cream, or fatty acids; and antibacterial agents such as brominated salicylanilides. For soaps to clean heavily soiled skin, abrasives such as pumice may be added. Some toilet bars may actually be mixtures of soap and one or more of the newer anionic surfactants (e.g., sodium lauryl sulfate). Nearly all toilet soaps contain some perfume (1–3%) and many are lightly colored.

Light-duty soap flakes or granules for washing dishes and fine fabrics may contain small amounts of mildly alkaline materials such as sodium carbonate, sodium silicate, and metasilicate. General purpose flakes or granules are formulated with a greater proportion of these alkaline builders and may also contain sodium phosphates, generally the pyrophosphate or tripolyphosphate. Borax or sodium perborate may also be found in such products.

In many institutions and industrial washrooms soap powders are dispensed for hand cleaning. These may be fine soap powder but may also be admixed with abrasives, borax or other cleaning additives. Among medicated soaps there are still some which contain sulfur, tars, mercuric iodide and phenolic compounds.

Some general formulations are shown below with potentially toxic materials marked with an asterisk. The toxicity rating is assigned to the entire formulation. The asterisk on an ingredient indicates, where appropriate, that amounts in the high part of a percentage range may be responsible for toxic effects.

BABY SOAPS (see COSMETICS)

DOG AND CAT (see PET CARE)

GENERAL PURPOSE SOAPS

Soap powder; granules, flakes (heavy duty)	Toxicity rating 2
Soap	40–60%
Sodium silicate	0–20%
Sodium carbonate	0–10%
Sodium phosphate	0–20%
Borax or sodium perborate*	0–20%
Water	5–25%
May contain:	
Sodium metasilicate (* if > 1%)	

LIGHTY DUTY SOAPS

Flakes, granules	Toxicity rating 2
Soap	80–90%
Sodium silicate	0–10%
Water	5–15%

LIQUID SOAP

	Toxicity rating 2
1. Soap (usually potassium)	10–40%
Glycerine	0–5%
Alcohol (ethyl or isopropyl)	5–20%
Water	50–80%
2. Water	50%

SOAPS (Cont.)

LIQUID SOAP (Cont.)

Oils, emulsifiers, anionic and nonionic thickeners	1–10%
Surfactants	25–50%
Humectants	1–5%
Essential oil (fragrance)	0.1–1%

TOILET BAR, SOAP BASE SOAPS	Toxicity rating 2
1. Soap (usually sodium or mixture of sodium and potassium)	80–90%
Perfume	0–3%
Water	10–15%
May contain:	
Antibacterial agents, trichlorocarbanilide, tribromosalicylanilide*	
Borax*	
Cold cream	
Fatty acid	
Glycerine	
Sodium silicate	
Titanium dioxide	
2. Soap	0–65%
Anionic surfactants (lauryl sulfate, monoglyceride sulfate, N-fatty acid-N-methyl laurate, fatty acid ester of sodium isothionate, alkyl glyceryl ether sulfonate)†	20–50%
Fatty acids	0–35%
Sodium sulfate	0–10%
Water	5–10%
May contain:	
(See Number 1)	
†* if >20%; toxicity rating then 2–3	
3. Anionic and nonionic surfactants	>50%
Essential oil (fragrance)	1–5%
Humectants and oils (mineral and/or vegetable)	0–10%
Water	5–25%
Antibacterial agents	0–5%
Color	0.1–1%
Other:	
Abradant (e.g., pumice)	0–20%
Optical brighteners	0.1–1%

SOLVENTS AND THINNERS

Rather than giving comprehensive formulas for solvents and thinners, the best that can be offered are representative formulas and lists of compounds which may be present. The toxicities naturally depend on the amounts of the various constituents and their individual toxicities. They will always be rated at least 3 and usually 4 because the aromatic hydrocarbons (toluene, xylene and rarely benzene) are usually present in substantial quantities.

SOLVENTS

Organic solvents fall into the following distinct chemical groups:

1. Alcohols	Toxicity rating:
N-Butyl*	3
Sec.-Butyl* (see Butyl alcohol)	3
Cyclohexanol*	3
Ethyl	2
Glycols*	2 or 3
Isobutyl* (see Butyl alcohol)	3
Isopropyl*	3
Methyl*	3
Methyl (methylisobutyl carbinol) (see Alcohols, Higher)	(no data, probably 3)
Proprietary (denatured ethyl)*	3

Starred ingredients (*) may be responsible for major toxic effects; consult Section II.

SOLVENTS AND THINNERS (Cont.)

SOLVENTS (Cont.)

N-Propyl*	3
2. Alcohol amines	Toxicity rating:
Diethanolamine	2
Monoethanolamine	2
Triethanolamine	
3. Chlorinated solvents	Toxicity rating:
Ethylene dichloride*	3
Methyl chloroform (1,1,1-trichloroethane)*	3
Methylene chloride*	3
Monochlorobenzene*	3
Orthodichlorobenzene*	4
Perchloroethylene*	3
Propylene dichloride*	4
Trichlorobenzene*	4
Trichloroethylene*	4
Trichlorotrifluoroethane	2
4. Esters	Toxicity rating:
Amyl acetate*	3
N-Butyl acetate*	3
Secondary butyl acetate*	3
Ethyl acetate*	3
Isobutyl acetate*	3
Isopropyl acetate*	3
Methyl acetate*	3
Methyl amyl acetate* (see Alcohols, Higher)	(no data, probably 3)
N-Propyl acetate* (see Propyl alcohol)	3
Glycol ether esters	
5. Hydrocarbons	Toxicity rating:
Aliphatics*	3
Aromatics* chiefly benzene, toluene and xylene	4
Naphthenes*	3
Terpenes and cyclics of terpene structure*	3
6. Ketones	Toxicity rating:
Acetone*	3
Cyclohexanone*	3
Diacetone alcohol*	3
Diisobutyl ketone*	3
Ethyl amyl ketone* (see Methyl Isobutyl ketone)	(no data, probably 3)
Isophorone*	3
Methyl butyl ketone*	3
Methyl ethyl ketone*	3
Methyl isobutyl ketone*	3
7. Other common solvents are:	Toxicity rating:
Aniline*	4
Carbon disulfide*	4
Cresylic acid*	4
Kerosene,* gasoline,* and other petroleum solvents*	3
Mineral spirits* (Stoddard solvent)	3
Phenols*	4
Turpentine*	4
May contain:	
Ammonia	
Cyclohexane	3
Essential oils*	4
Morpholine*	4
Nitrobenzene*	5
Nitroethane* (see Nitromethane)	3
Nitromethane*	3
1-Nitropropane*	4
2-Nitropropane*	3

SOLVENTS AND THINNERS (Cont.)

SOLVENTS (Cont.)

Resins
Soaps
Tetrahydrofuran*

SOLVENTS, FIREARM (see CLEANERS)

SOLVENTS, WINDSHIELD WASHER (see CLEANERS)

THINNERS	Toxicity rating:
Acetone*	3
Aliphatic petroleum solvents*	3
Aromatic hydrocarbon solvents* (xylene, toluene)	4
Cellulosolve acetate*	3
Diacetone alcohol*	3
Ethyl alcohol	2
Ethyl amyl ketone*	3
Isopropyl alcohol	3
Methyl ethyl ketone*	3
Methyl isobutyl ketone*	3
Naphthol*	4
Naphthenes*	3
Toluene*	4
Xylene*	4
May contain:	
Butanol or isobutanol*	3
Diisobutyl ketone*	
Esters, particularly butyl acetate,* often ethyl acetate,* rarely amyl acetate,* also isopropyl acetate and isobutyl acetate	2, 3
Nitromethane	
Nitroethane* (see nitropropane)	3
2-Nitropropane	3

Thinners could contain 0–100% of most common solvents.

SPORTS PRODUCTS

"FISH LURE" .... Toxicity rating 3?
     Essential oils*
     Fluorohydrocarbons

GOLF BALL CENTERS .... Toxicity rating: 2–3
     May contain:
         Ethylene glycol*
         Lithopone
         Bentonite clay
         Glycerine
         Castor Oil
         Honey
         Calcium
         Calcium carbonate
         Potassium hydroxide ⎫
         Thymol in alcohol   ⎬ (preservatives used in processing)
         Potassium cresylate ⎭
         Methyl salicylate   (odor used in processing)

Occasionally golf balls are made with steel centers.
Golf ball centers are under 2500 pounds pressure from the tightly wound rubber. Hazards from exploding golf balls when this pressure is released seem to be mechanical rather than toxic.

GUN BLUINGS

1.	Toxicity rating 4
Potassium nitrate	3.5%
Mercuric chloride*	2.4%
Potassium chlorate	3.0%
Ferric chloride	0.9%
Sodium nitrate	0.9%
Copper sulfate	

Starred ingredients (*) may be responsible for major toxic effects; consult Section II.

SPORTS PRODUCTS (Cont.)

GUN BLUINGS (Cont.)

Cupric chloride	0.5%
Spirit of ethyl nitrite	6.5%
Water	82.3%

2. .... Toxicity rating 4–6
    Selenium*
    Hydrochloric acid
    Fumaric acid
    Methanol
    Nitric acid
    Phosphoric acid
    May contain:
        Aniline dye
        Copper sulfate

GUN OIL (see MISCELLANEOUS OILS)

"FOR PRESERVING FRESHNESS OF CATCH" .... Toxicity rating 2–3
Fumaric acid
Sodium benzoate
Triethylene glycol

WATERPROOFING COMPOUNDS

1. .... Toxicity rating 4
    Wax
    Chlorinated solvent* 100%
2. .... Toxicity rating 3–4

Silicone oil	3–10%
Orthochlorophenol	2–5%
Copper quinolinolate	0–0.25%
Water repellent solids	85–99.75%

    Aliphatic* (see naphtha) and aromatic*
        hydrocarbon solvents. The ali-
        phatic solvents are the more com-
        mon.
    May contain:
        Alkyl sodium sulfonates
        Bactericide
        Emulsifiers
        Mineral oil
        Naphthene
        Orthophenylphenol*
        Rosinates
        Propellant
3. .... Toxicity rating 2
    Neats-foot oil (shoes) 100%

"TEAR GAS" DEVICES

TEAR GAS DEVICES .... No rating
    Chloracetophenone*
    Oleoresin capsicum*
    Orthochlorobenzalmalononitrile
    Propellant
        nitrogen
    May contain:
        Ethyl bromoacetate

THERMOMETERS

Thermometers, having various uses, even in the home, have various temperature ranges. A number of fluids are employed; the selection depends on the intended use. Clinical thermometers usually contain mercury, about 0.1 ml.: this quantity of metallic mercury presents no ingestion hazard. Thermometers for ambient temperatures, indoor and out, may contain triethyl phosphate, toluene, xylene, or one of several alcohols. These thermometers contain 0.3 to 0.5 ml., never more than 1 ml. Thermometers for very cold weather (arctic) measurements contain pentane. Cooking thermometers contain methyl

THERMOMETERS (Cont.)

THERMOMETERS (Cont.)

benzoate. Maximum-minimum registering thermometers may contain beechwood creosote and ethyl alcohol.

All these thermometers have two things in common. The amount of liquid in any thermometer is small. The liquids are not highly toxic. Thus thermometers do not represent a severe toxic hazard in any instance.

WATER TREATING CHEMICALS

1. Insoluble, resins or zeolites (water
    softeners) .... Toxicity rating 2
  a. Inorganic or zeolites
      Sodium alumino silicates
      Manganese zeolite
  b. Resins or polymers
      Sulfonated polystyrenes
      Sulfonated phenolics
      Sulfonated coals
      Aminated condensation products
      Quaternary amines addition prod-
        ucts
2. Soluble products
  a. Alkaline chemicals (see Alkali)

Phosphates, trisodium, poly* ...	3
Carbonates, sodium or sesqui* ..	3

      Borates, sodium*
      Lime, hydrated, slaked
      Caustic, sodium hydroxide, lye
  b. Disinfectants (see Sanitizers, Swim-
      ming Pools)

Chlorophenols*	3

      Hydrochlorites, sodium, calcium
      Quaternary ammonium com-
        pounds
      Chloride
  c. Wetting agents (see Detergents, un-
      der Cleaners)

Sodium sulfate of fatty acid ester (see Turkey Red Oil)*	3
Sulfated butyl oleate (see Turkey Red Oil)*	3
Polyethylene glycol fatty acid ester	1
Sulfodicarboxylic acid	2

  d. Miscellaneous products
      Alum
      Classifier e.g., cationic polyelec-
        trolyte polymers
      Copper sulfate*
      Corrosion inhibitors*
      Potassium permanganate*
      Resin cleaners
      Sequestrants or chelating agents
      Sodium hexametaphosphate

WAXES

AUTOMOBILE WAXES (see POLISHES)

FLOOR, SELF-POLISHING WAXES (see Polishes)

GENERAL PURPOSE WAXES .... Toxicity rating 3
Natural and synthetic waxes and/or resins
Fatty acid emulsifiers
Morpholine

Aliphatic* and/or aromatic* (toxicity rating 4 if over 25%) petroleum solvents	5–80%
o-Benzyl-p-chlorophenol	0.1%

Starred ingredients (*) may be responsible for major toxic effects; consult Section II.

GENERAL PURPOSE WAXES (Cont.)

May contain:
- Alkali
- Ammonia
- Alkyl sodium sulfate
- Borax*
- Burnt umber
- Essential oils
- Greases
- Oil dyes

GENERAL PURPOSE WAXES (Cont.)

- Shellac
- Silica
- Silicone
- Turpentine

PASTE (see POLISHES)

WAX REMOVERS (see DEGREASERS)

WINDOW WAXES (see GLASS, under CLEANERS)

Starred ingredients (*) may be responsible for major toxic effects; consult Section II.

Manufacturers' Index

A

AAPRI COSMETICS
P.O. Box 1090
Placentia, Calif. 92670
617-421-7000

ABBOTT LABORATORIES
Pharmaceutical Products Div.
North Chicago, Ill. 60064
312-688-6100

ABCHEM
P.O. Box 455
New Eagle, Pa. 15067
412-258-3670

ABCO INCORPORATED
230 Industry Blvd.
North Huntingdon, Pa. 15642
412-864-1900

ABOLITION PRODUCTS CO., INC.
2464 N. Milwaukee Ave.
Chicago, Ill. 60647

ACELINE PRODUCTS CORP.
424 St. Paul St.
Rochester, N.Y. 14605
716-232-6614

ACETO AGRICULTURAL CHEMICALS CORP.
126-02 Northern Blvd.
Flushing, N.Y. 11368
212-898-2300

ACHESON COLLOIDS CO.
P.O. Box 288
Port Huron, Mich. 48060
313-984-5581

ACME DIVISION
PBI/Gordon Corp.
300 S. Third St.
P.O. Box 2276
Kansas City, Kans. 66110
913-342-8780

ADAMS, RALPH B.
Lakeville, New Brunswick
Canada

ADCO, INC.
P.O. Box 999
Sedalia, Mo. 65301
816-826-3300

ADRIA LABORATORIES, INC.
P.O. Box 16529
Columbus, Ohio 43216
614-764-8100

ADVANCE CHEMICAL CO.
901 E. 61st St.
Los Angeles, Calif. 90001
213-231-9131

ADVANCE COLOR CORP.
P.O. Box 54870
Los Angeles, Calif. 90054
213-723-5233

ADVANCED COATING & CHEMICALS
4343 Temple City Blvd.
Temple City, Calif. 91780
213-579-6270

AEGIS LABORATORIES, INC.
1647 E. 55th St.
Chicago, Ill. 60615
312-643-5620-1

AEROCEUTICALS HEALTH CARE PRODUCTS
49 John St.
Southport, Conn. 06490
203-255-3587

AERO-MASTER, INC.
325 W. Pacific Ave.
St. Louis, Mo. 63119
314-962-8800

AEROSOL SYSTEMS, INC.
9150 Valley View Rd.
Macedonia, Ohio 44056
216-467-4195

AGSCO CHEMICALS, INC.
P.O. Box 458
Grand Forks, N. Dak. 58201
701-775-5325

AGWAY INC.
P.O. Box 4933
Syracuse, N.Y. 13221
315-477-6177

AIRKEM DIVISION
See AIRWICK INDUSTRIES, INC.

AIRRIGATION ENGINEERING CO., INC.
P.O. Box H
Carmel Valley, Calif. 93924
408-659-2000

AIRWICK INDUSTRIES, INC.
111 Commerce Rd.
Carlstadt, N.J. 07072
201-933-8200

AIRWICK PROFESSIONAL PRODUCTS
See AIRWICK INDUSTRIES, INC.

AKRON PAINT & VARNISH CO.
Firestone Park Sta.
Box 2765
Akron, Ohio 44301
216-773-8911

ALASKA FERTILIZER CO.
865 Lind Ave. S.W.
Renton, Wash. 98055
206-228-5910

ALBATROSS CHEMICAL CO., INC.
36 36th St.
Long Island City, N.Y. 11106
212-392-6272

ALBERT G. MAAS CO.
155 E. Maryland St.
Indianapolis, Ind. 46204
317-632-8315

ALBERTO-CULVER CO.
2525 Armitage Ave.
Melrose Park, Ill. 60160
312-450-3175

ALCON LABORATORIES, INC.
6201 South Freeway
P.O. Box 1959
Fort Worth, Tex. 76101
817-293-0450

ALCONOX, INC.
215 Park Ave. S.
New York, N.Y. 10003
212-473-1300

ALDEN-LEEDS, INC.
55 Jacobus Ave.
South Kearny, N.J. 07032
201-589-3544

ALEXANDRA DE MARKOFF
Sub. of Lanvin-Charles of the Ritz Group Ltd.
40 W. 57th St.
New York, N.Y. 10019
212-621-7300

ALEX. C. FERGUSSON CO.
Spring Mill Dr.
Frazer, Pa. 19355
215-647-3300

ALKALOL CO.
P.O. Box 964
Taunton, Mass. 02780

ALLERGAN PHARMACEUTICALS, INC.
2525 Dupont Dr.
Irvine, Calif. 92713
714-752-4500

ALLIED BLOCK CHEMICALS CO.
P.O. Box 455
New Eagle, Pa. 15067
412-258-3670

ALMAY, INC.
Apex, N. Car. 27502
919-362-7422

ALOE CREME LABORATORIES, INC.
P.O. Box 9477
Fort Lauderdale, Fla. 33310
305-484-8600

ALSOL PRODUCTS CO., INC.
123 Coit St.
Irvington, N.J. 07111
201-374-9123

ALUMIN-NU CORP.
5141 Northfield Rd.
Bedford Heights, Ohio 44146
216-461-2717

ALVIN & CO.
Bloomfield, Conn. 06002
203-243-8991

ALVIN LAST, INC.
145 Palisades St.
Dobbs Ferry, N.Y. 10522
914-693-2221

AMBIX LABORATORIES
210 Orchard St.
East Rutherford, N.J. 07073
201-939-2200

AMBROID CO., INC.
P.O. Box 1089
Taunton, Mass. 02780
617-823-1726

AMBROSIA COSMETICS, INC.
1950 S. Ocean Dr.
Hallendale, Fla. 33009
305-454-5323

AMCHEM PRODUCTS, INC.
Ambler, Pa. 19002
215-628-1000

AMERICAN AEROSOL CORP.
324 Rindge Ave.
Cambridge, Mass. 02140
617-491-6562

AMERICAN ART CLAY CO., INC.
4717 W. 16th St.
Indianapolis, Ind. 46222

AMERICAN CELCURE WOOD PRESERVING CORP.
1074 E. Eighth St.
P.O. Box 3262
Jacksonville, Fla. 32206
904-353-4376

AMERICAN CRAYON CO.
Div. of the Joseph Dixon Crucible Co.
1706 Hayes Ave.
Sandusky, Ohio 44870
419-625-9121

AMERICAN CRITICAL CARE
Div. of American Hospital Supply Corp.
1600 Waukegan Rd.
McGaw Park, Ill. 60085
312-473-3000

AMERICAN CYANAMID CO.
One Cyanamid Plaza
Wayne, N.J. 07470
201-831-2000

AMERICAN CYANAMID CO.
Agricultural Div.
P.O. Box 400
Princeton, N.J. 08540
609-799-0400

AMERICAN FLUORIDE CORP.
17 Huntington Pl.
New Rochelle, N.Y. 10801
914-633-7005
212-824-0450

AMERICAN FUMIGATING CO.
9A S. Florissant Rd.
St. Louis, Mo. 63135
314-521-1300

AMERICAN GREASE STICK CO.
P.O. Box 729
Muskegon, Mich. 49443
616-733-2101

AMERICAN HOECHST CORP.
Animal Health Div.
Route 202-206 North
Somerville, N.J. 08876
201-685-2696

AMERICAN HOSPITEX DIVISION
American Hospital Supply Corp.
5000 B Snapfinger Woods Dr.
Decatur, Ga. 30035
404-987-2100

AMERICAN HYGIENIC LABORATORIES, INC.
555 41st St.
Miami Beach, Fla. 33140
305-534-2171

AMERICAN INKS AND COATINGS CORP.
P.O. Box 803
Valley Forge, Pa. 19482
215-272-8866

AMERICAN LaFRANCE
P.O. Box 7146
Charlottesville, Va. 22906
804-973-4361

AMERICAN-LINCOLN
Div. of the Scott & Fetzer Co.
1100 Haskin Rd.
Bowling Green, Ohio 43402
419-352-7511

AMERICAN MACHINERY CORP.
P.O. Box 3228
Orlando, Fla. 32802
305-295-2581

AMERICAN PHARMACEUTICAL CO.
245 Fourth St.
Passaic, N.J. 07055
201-779-5300

AMERICAN RIVERSIDE, INC.
See LAIDLAW CORP.

AMERICAN SAFETY RAZOR CO.
P.O. Box 500
Staunton, Va. 24401
703-248-8000

AMERON PROTECTIVE COATINGS DIVISION
201 N. Berry St.
Brea, Calif. 92621
714-529-1951

AMES DIVISION
Miles Laboratories, Inc.
P.O. Box 70
Elkhart, Ind. 46515
219-264-8891

AMFRE-GRANT, INC.
16600 N.W. 54th Ave.
Miami, Fla. 33014
305-565-6070

AMLAB (AMERICAN LABORATORIES)
Div. Towne, Paulsen & Co., Inc.
140 E. Duarte Rd.
Monrovia, Calif. 91016
213-359-9261

AMOCO OIL CO.
200 E. Randolph Dr.
P.O. Box 6110-A
Chicago, Ill. 60680
312-856-5111

AMPCO CHEMICAL DIVISION
Associated Marketing Products Co.
P.O. Box 346
Broomfield, Colo. 80020
303-466-2383

AMPION CORP.
4-88 47th Ave.
Long Island City, N.Y. 11101
212-784-3374

AMWAY CORPORATION
7575 E. Fulton Rd.
Ada, Mich. 49355
616-676-6307

ANCHOR LABORATORIES, INC.
2621 N. Belt Hwy.
St. Joseph, Mo. 64502
816-233-1385

ANCHOR SERUM CO.
See ANCHOR LABORATORIES, INC.

ANDERSON COMPANY, THE
Research & Development Dept.
260 Campbell St.
Valparaiso, Ind. 46383
219-885-4361

ANDREA RAAB CORP.
4702 Glenwood Rd.
Brooklyn, N.Y. 11234
212-252-8800

ANDREW JERGENS CO.
2535 Spring Grove Ave.
Cincinnati, Ohio 45214
513-421-1400

AN-FO MANUFACTURING CO.
3129 Elmwood Ave.
P.O. Box 7311
Oakland, Calif. 94601
415-532-2275

ANIMAL REPELLENTS, INC.
P.O. Box 999
Griffin, Ga. 30224
404-227-8222

ANITA OF DENMARK INC.
P.O. Box 2246
Palm Springs, Calif. 92263
714-320-7481

ANTI-BORAX COMPOUND CO., INC.
1502-1506 Wall St.
Fort Wayne, Ind. 46801
219-422-5809

A & P
See GREAT ATLANTIC & PACIFIC TEA CO., INC.

APCO OIL CORP.
See OKLAHOMA REFINING CO.

APPERSON CHEMICALS, INC.
Box 2555
2903 Strickland St.
Jacksonville, Fla. 32203
904-389-6671

APPLIED BIOCHEMISTS, INC.
5300 W. County Line Rd.
Mequon, Wis. 53092
Toll free: 1-800-558-5106

APPROVED PHARMACEUTICAL CORP.
1643 E. Genesee St.
Syracuse, N.Y. 13217
315-478-2121

AQUALAND POOL CO., INC.
3400 Dakota Ave.
Minneapolis, Minn. 55416
612-920-8244

AQUAMINT LABORATORIES, INC.
P.O. Box 7
St. Charles, Ill. 60174
312-584-1251

ARBROOK, INC.
P.O. Box 130
Arlington, Tex. 76010
817-277-8141

ARCH LABORATORIES
See NORCLIFF THAYER, INC.

ARDELL, INC.
30601 Carter Rd.
Solon, Ohio 44139
216-248-3700

ARDEN, ELIZABETH, INC.
Sub. of Eli Lilly & Co.
1345 Ave. of the Americas
New York, N.Y. 10019
212-399-2000

AR-EX PRODUCTS CO.
1036 W. Van Buren
Chicago, Ill. 60607
312-226-5241

ARIZONA AGROCHEMICAL CO.
P.O. Box 21537
Phoenix, Ariz. 85036
602-243-2711

ARKANSAS CO., INC.
185 Foundry St.
Newark, N.J. 07105
201-589-0516

ARMAN DRUG CO., INC.
2202 W. 12th St.
Sioux Falls, S. Dak. 57101

ARMITE LABORATORIES
1845 Randolph St.
Los Angeles, Calif. 90001
213-587-7744

ARMOR ALL PRODUCTS
Div. of Foremost-McKesson, Inc.
P.O. Box 19039
Irvine, Calif. 92713
714-549-2200

ARMOUR-DIAL, INC.
Armour Research Center
15101 N. Scottsdale Rd.
Scottsdale, Ariz. 85260
602-998-6273

ARMOUR PHARMACEUTICAL CO.
P.O. Box 1849
Scottsdale, Ariz. 85252
602-941-2924

ARNAR-STONE LABORATORIES, INC.
See AMERICAN CRITICAL CARE

ARROW LABORATORIES, INC.
31 Westmoreland Ave.
White Plains, N.Y. 10606

ART CHEMICAL PRODUCTS, INC.
Huntington, Ind. 46750
219-356-2328

ARTEX HOBBY PRODUCTS, INC.
711 W. Vine St.
Lima, Ohio 45802
419-228-2686

ASCHENBACH & MILLER
245 Race St.
Philadelphia, Pa. 19106
215-627-4363

ASCHER, B. F., & CO., INC.
5100 E. 59th St.
Kansas City, Mo. 64130
816-363-5900

ASPEN INDUSTRIES
Tully, N.Y. 13159
315-696-2671

ASTRA PHARMACEUTICAL PRODUCTS, INC.
P.O. Box 1089
Framingham, Mass. 01701
617-620-0600

ASTYPTODYNE CHEMICAL CO.
2128 Echo Lane
Wilmington, N.C. 28403
919-763-5764

ATHELSTAN PRODUCTS CO.
4700 Aldrich Ave.
Minneapolis, Minn. 55409

ATHENA CORP.
1919 Lone Star Dr.
Dallas, Tex. 75212
214-637-2330

ATLANTIC RICHFIELD CO.
515 S. Flower St.
Los Angeles, Calif. 90071
213-486-3511

ATLAS MINERALS & CHEMICALS, INC.
Farmington Rd.
Mertztown, Pa. 19539
215-682-7171

ATLAS SUPPLY CO.
Diamond Rd.
Springfield, N.J. 07081
201-379-6550

AUSTIN, JAMES, CO.
P.O. Drawer 1
Mars, Pa. 16046
412-625-1535

AVALON INDUSTRIES, INC.
95 Lorimer St.
Brooklyn, N.Y. 11206
212-384-6500

AVITROL CORP.
320 S. Boston, Suite 528
Tulsa, Okla. 74103
918-582-3359

AVON PRODUCTS, INC.
Suffern, N.Y. 10901
914-357-2012

A.V.P. PHARMACEUTICALS, INC.
P.O. Box N
9829 Main St.
Clarence, N.Y. 14031
716-688-9676

AYERST LABORATORIES
685 Third Ave.
New York, N.Y. 10017
212-878-5996
Outside of business hours: 212-986-1000

B

BABSON BROS. CO.
2100 S. York Rd.
Oak Brook, Ill. 60521
312-654-1600

BACHE, ELLA, BEAUTY PRODUCTS
8 W. 36th St.
New York, N.Y. 10018
212-753-2175

BACKES', M., SONS, INC.
P.O. Box 219
Wallingford, Conn. 06492
203-269-3377

BADGER-POWHATAN
Div. of A-T-O, Inc.
P.O. Box 7146
Charlottesville, Va. 22906
804-973-4361

BAIN DE SOLEIL
40 W. 57th St.
New York, N.Y. 10019
212-621-7327

BAIRD DYNAMIC CO.
686 Bostwick Ave.
Bridgeport, Conn. 06605
203-336-1837

BAKER, C. P., & CO.
915 Spring Garden
Philadelphia, Pa. 19123
215-765-7720

BAKER-CUMMINS DIVISION
Key Pharmaceuticals, Inc.
P.O. Box 694307, Norland Branch
Miami, Fla. 33169
305-652-2276

BALKAMP, INC.
2601 S. Holt Rd.
Indianapolis, Ind. 46241
317-244-7241

BALTIMORE COPPER PAINT CO.
See JOTUN-BALTIMORE COPPER PAINT CO.

BALTIMORE PAINT & CHEMICAL CO.
1370 Ontario St.
Cleveland, Ohio 44113
216-566-2000

BANDWAGON, INC.
54 Industrial Way
Wilmington, Mass. 01887
617-658-6252

BANNER MANUFACTURING CO.
4747 Holly St.
Denver, Colo. 80216
303-388-9265

BARCO CHEMICAL PRODUCTS CO.
701 S. La Salle St.
Chicago, Ill. 60605
312-427-2916

BARCO CHEMICALS DIVISION, INC.
7760 N.E. Fourth Court
Miami, Fla. 33138

BARCOLENE CO.
620 South St.
Holbrook, Mass. 02343
617-767-2800

BARDAHL MANUFACTURING CORP.
P.O. Box 70607
1400 N.W. 52nd St.
Seattle, Wash. 98107
Emergency phone: 206-634-5252

BARD-PARKER
P.O. Box 300
2 Bridgewater Lane
Lincoln Park, N.J. 07035
201-628-9600

BARFRED RESEARCH LABORATORIES
337 Palermo Ave.
Coral Gables, Fla. 33134
305-446-4664

BARNES-HIND PHARMACEUTICALS, INC.
895 Kifer Rd.
Sunnyvale, Calif. 94086
408-736-5462

BARR, W. M., & CO.
P.O. Box 1879
Memphis, Tenn. 38101
901-775-0100

BARTLETT, F. A., TREE EXPERT CO.
2770 Summer St.
Stamford, Conn. 06905
203-323-1131

BARTLETT, N. M., INC.
Box 490
Beamsville, Ontario, Canada
LOR 1B0

BASCH, THE GEORGE, CO., INC.
19 Hanse Ave.
Freeport, N.Y. 11520
516-378-8100

BASF WYANDOTTE CORP.
Chemical Specialties Div.
See DIVERSEY WYANDOTTE CORP.

BASIC CHEMICALS INC.
P.O. Box 685
2137 Sunset Rd.
Des Moines, Iowa 50303
515-288-0231

BAYVET DIVISION, CUTTER LABORATORIES, INC.
P.O. Box 390
Shawnee, Kans. 66201
913-631-4800

B & B DRUG CO.
32 Norfolk Ave.
Maplewood, N.J. 07040
201-762-3682

BEACH PHARMACEUTICALS
Div. of Beach Products, Inc.
5220 S. Manhattan Ave.
Tampa, Fla. 33611
813-839-6565

BEAUTILITE CORP.
1829 Irving Park Rd.
Chicago, Ill. 60613
312-327-3654

BECK CHEMICALS, INC.
3350 W. 137th St.
Cleveland, Ohio 44111
216-941-8355

BECK EQUIPMENT & CHEMICAL CO.
See BECK CHEMICALS, INC.

BEECHAM COSMETICS
875 N. Michigan Ave.
Chicago, Ill. 60611
312-951-7000

BEECHAM LABORATORIES
501 Fifth St.
Bristol, Tenn. 37620
615-764-5141

BEECHAM-MASSENGILL PHARMACEUTICALS
See BEECHAM LABORATORIES

BEECHAM PRODUCTS DIV.
Beecham, Inc.
P.O. Box 1467
Pittsburgh, Pa. 15230
412-923-1000

BEE CHEMICAL CO.
2700 E. 170th
Lansing, Ill. 60438
312-474-7000

BELL & CO., INC.
See GRANDPA BRANDS CO.

BELLE MOSS, PHARMACEUTICAL CHEMIST
P.O. Box 1278
3900 W. Twelve Mile Rd.
Berkley, Mich. 48072
313-548-5706

BELL LABORATORIES, INC.
3699 Kinsman Blvd.
Madison, Wis. 53704
608-241-0202

BENDIX CORP., AUTOMOTIVE AFTERMARKET
1094 Bendix Dr.
Jackson, Tenn. 38301
901-423-1300

BENDYNE, LTD.
150 Fifth Ave.
New York, N.Y. 10011
212-691-0040

BENJAMIN MOORE & CO.
Chestnut Ridge Rd.
Montvale, N.J. 07645
201-573-9600

BENNETT'S GLASS & COLORIZER PAINT
65 W. First S.
Salt Lake City, Utah 84101
801-486-2211

BEN VENUE LABORATORIES, INC.
P.O. Box 46129
270 Northfield Rd.
Bedford, Ohio 44146
216-232-3320

BERLEX LABORATORIES
110 E. Hanover Ave.
Cedar Knolls, N.J. 07927
201-540-8700

BERNZOMATIC CORP.
Olney St.
Medina, N.Y. 14103
716-798-4949

BEROL USA
Div. of Berol Corp.
Danbury, Conn. 06810
203-744-0000

BERSTED'S HOBBY-CRAFT, INC.
Monmouth, Ill. 61462
309-734-7011

BESCO CORP., THE
200 Myrtle St.
P.O. Box 173
Metairie, La. 70004
504-721-1428

BEST FOODS
CPC International, Inc.
International Plaza
Englewood Cliffs, N.J. 07632
201-894-4000

BETZ ENTEC, INC.
See BETZ LABORATORIES, INC.

BETZ LABORATORIES, INC.
Somerton Rd.
Trevose, Pa. 19047
215-355-3300

BEUTLICH, INC.
7006 N. Western Ave.
Chicago, Ill. 60645
312-262-7900

BEVILL, I. L., CO., INC.
P.O. Box 1064
Birmingham, Ala. 35201
205-853-1862

B&G CO.
P.O. Box 20372
Dallas, Tex. 75220
214-357-5741

BINGMAN LABORATORIES, INC.
P.O. Box 88
Sarahsville, Ohio 43779
614-732-2295

BINNEY & SMITH INC.
1100 Church Lane
Easton, Pa. 18042
215-253-6271

BIOCERTA CORP.
303 Fifth Ave.
New York, N.Y. 10016
212-684-4320

BIO-CEUTIC LABORATORIES, INC.
P.O. Box 999
St. Joseph, Mo. 64502
816-233-2804

BIO-CIDE CHEMICAL CO., INC.
P.O. Box 2700
Norman, Okla. 73070
405-329-5556

BIO-FACTOR LABORATORIES
103 S. Elm St.
Marshville, N.C. 28103
704-624-5311

BIO-LAB, INC.
P.O. Box 1489
Decatur, Ga. 30031
404-378-1753

BIRCHMORE DAIRY SUPPLY
See YALE CHEMICAL CO.

BIRCHWOOD CASEY
Div. of Birchwood Labs., Inc.
7900 Fuller Rd.
Eden Prairie, Minn. 55344
612-927-1733

BIRD & SON, INC.
East Walpole, Mass. 02032
617-668-2500

BISONITE CO., INC.
2250 Military Rd.
Tonawanda, N.Y. 14150
716-693-6130

BISSELL, INC.
Grand Rapids, Mich. 49501
616-453-4451

BITE-X CORP.
25 W. 43rd St.
New York, N.Y. 10036
212-244-7440

BLAIR LABORATORIES, INC.
50 Washington St.
Norwalk, Conn. 06856
203-853-0123

BLAISDELL/ALL-RITE
See BEROL USA

BLISTEX, INC.
1800 Swift Dr.
Oak Brook, Ill. 60521
312-654-2870

BLITZ PRODUCTS CO.
P.O. Box 525
Mitchell, S. Dak. 57301

BLOCK DRUG CO., INC.
257 Cornelison Ave.
Jersey City, N.J. 07302
201-434-3000

BLUE CROSS BEAUTY PRODUCTS, INC.
1341 W. First St.
Los Angeles, Calif. 90026
213-626-8101

BLUE CROSS LABORATORIES
7376 Greenbush Ave.
North Hollywood, Calif. 91605
805-255-2493

BLUE SEAL CHEMICAL CO.
See CLOROBEN CHEMICAL CORP.

B & N PRODUCTS CO.
Box 4
Harlan, Iowa 51537
712-755-3427

BOEHRINGER INGELHEIM LTD.
90 E. Ridge
Ridgefield, Conn. 06877
203-438-0311

BOGERT, A. Z., CO., INC.
2320 Edgewater Ave.
Baltimore, Md. 21222
301-633-8100

BOGLE, R. H., CO.
P.O. Box 588
Alexandria, Va. 22313
703-549-3506

BOHLENDER PLANT CHEMICALS, INC.
P.O. Box 227
Tipp City, Ohio 45371

BONASEPTIC CO.
Box 7144, Sta. C
Atlanta, Ga. 30357

BONAT, INC.
250 Lackawanna Ave.
West Paterson, N.J. 07424
201-256-3400

BONDEX INTERNATIONAL, INC.
P.O. Box 88
Brunswick, Ohio 44212
216-225-3169

BONDO CORP., THE
Forest Rd.
P.O. Box 68
Northford, Conn. 06472
203-484-0456

BONEWITZ CHEMICAL SERVICES, INC.
P.O. Box 927
Burlington, Iowa 52601
319-753-2881

BONIDE CHEMICAL CO., INC.
2 Wurz Ave.
Yorkville, N.Y. 13495
315-736-8231

BONNE BELL, INC.
Georgetown Row
18519 Detroit Ave.
Lakewood, Ohio 44107
216-221-0800

BOORD, CLARENCE, & SONS, INC.
105 E. Commercial
Leon, Iowa 50144
515-446-4122

BORDEN, INC.
990 Kingsmill Pkwy.
Columbus, Ohio 43229
614-225-4158

BORDERLAND PRODUCTS, INC.
560 Fulton St.
P.O. Box 366
Buffalo, N.Y. 14240
716-825-3300

BOUCHARD, LUCILLE, MINK OIL COSMETIQUES, INC.
P.O. Box 46
Circleville, N.Y. 10919
914-692-2777

BOURLAND, JIM, CO.
P.O Box 21088
Houston, Tex. 77026
713-523-4249

BOWES SEAL FAST CORP.
P.O. Box 18802
5902 E. 34th St.
Indianapolis, Ind. 46218
317-547-5245

BOWMAN PHARMACEUTICALS, INC.
119 Schroyer Ave., S.W.
Canton, Ohio 44702
216-456-2873

BOYLE & CO.
13260 Moore St.
Cerritos, Calif. 90701
213-926-8250

BOYLE-MIDWAY
Div. of American Home Products Corp.
South Ave. & Hale St.
Cranford, N.J. 07016
201-276-3900

BOYSEN PAINT CO.
P.O. Box 23543
Oakland, Calif. 94623
415-653-9211

BPS PAINT CO.
1191 S. Wheeling Rd.
Wheeling, Ill. 60090
312-541-9000

BRADLEY, MILTON, CO.
P.O. Box 2209
Springfield, Mass. 01101
413-525-6411

BRAINERD CHEMICAL CO., INC.
42nd and S. Sheridan
P.O. Box 45010
Tulsa, Okla. 74145
918-622-1212

BRANDY HARVEST COLOGNES
53-06 39th Ave.
Woodside, N.Y. 11377
212-899-1279

BRAUN NORTH AMERICA
55 Cambridge Pkwy.
Cambridge, Mass. 02142
617-421-7000

BREON LABORATORIES INC.
90 Park Ave.
New York, N.Y. 10016
212-972-4141

BREWER CHEMICAL CORP.
P.O. Box 48
Honolulu, Hawaii 96810
808-533-4411

BRILCO LABORATORIES
1553 63rd St.
Brooklyn, N.Y. 11219
212-236-3812

BRIOSCHI, INC.
19-01 Pollitt Dr.
Fair Lawn, N.J. 07410
201-796-4226

BRISTOL-MYERS PRODUCTS
Div. of Bristol-Myers Co.
345 Park Ave.
New York, N.Y. 10154
212-546-4000

BRONDOW, INC.
550 Mamaroneck Ave.
Harrison, N.Y. 10528
914-698-6544

BROWN MANUFACTURING CO.
Le Roy, N.Y. 14482
716-967-6820

BROWN MEDICINE CO.
P.O. Box 3345
Knoxville, Tenn. 37917

BRUDER, M. A., & SONS, INC.
600 Reed Rd.
Broomall, Pa. 19008
215-353-5100

BRULIN & CO., INC.
P.O. Box 270-B
Indianapolis, Ind. 46206
317-923-3211

BRUNING PAINT (MARYLAND)
601 S. Haven St.
Baltimore, Md. 21224
301-342-3636

BUCKLEY, W. K., INC.
c/o Williams Drug Distributors
211 Fuller Ave.
P.O. Box 3125
Grand Rapids, Mich. 49501
616-451-0511

BUCKMAN LABORATORIES, INC.
1256 N. McLean Blvd.
Memphis, Tenn. 38108
901-278-0330

BUFFINGTON DIV.
See CLAPP, OTIS, & SON, INC.

BULLARD, E. D., CO.
2680 Bridgeway
Sausalito, Calif. 94965
415-332-0410

BULLOCK-WALKER MANUFACTURING CO.
See BLISTEX, INC.

BURNISHINE PRODUCTS INC.
8140 N. Ridgeway Ave.
Skokie, Ill. 60076
312-583-1810

BURNS-BIOTEC LABORATORIES, INC.
8536 K St.
Omaha, Nebr. 68127
402-331-3900

BURPEE, W. ATLEE, CO.
300 Park Ave.
Warminster, Pa. 18974
215-674-4900

BURROUGHS WELLCOME CO.
3030 Cornwallis Rd.
Research Triangle Park, N.C. 27709
919-541-9090

BURTON, PARSONS & CO., INC.
Ophthalmic Products Div.
P.O. Box 1959
Fort Worth, Tex. 76101
817-293-0450

BUTCHER POLISH CO., THE
Bartlett St.
Marlborough, Mass. 01752
617-481-5700

C

CABOT, SAMUEL, INC.
One Union St.
Boston, Mass. 02108
617-723-7740

CALBAR, INC.
2626 N. Martha St.
Philadelphia, Pa. 19125
215-739-9141

CALGON CORP.
Commercial Div.
P.O. Box 147
St. Louis, Mo. 63166
314-862-2000

CALGON CORP., Consumer Div.
See BEECHAM PRODUCTS DIV.

CALIFORNIA PRODUCTS CORP.
169 Waverly
Cambridge, Mass. 02139
617-547-5300

CALLAHAN, GEO., & CO., INC.
263 Herbert Ave.
Closter, N.J. 07624
201-768-1209

CALOTABS CO., INC.
P.O. Box 2819
Greenville, S.C. 29602
803-244-6040

CALVIN KLEIN COSMETICS CORP.
9 W. 57th St.
New York, N.Y. 10019
212-759-8888

CAMEO, INC.
322 Ryder Rd.
Toledo, Ohio 43615
419-531-5381

CAMERON MEDICAL CORP.
2716 E. Florence Ave.
P.O. Box 549
Huntington Park, Calif. 90255
213-588-1201

CAMPANA CORP.
Div. of Purex Corp., Ltd.
Batavia, Ill. 60510
312-879-3400

CAMPBELL CHEMICALS INC.
See MEYER-BLANKE CO.

CANDLE-LITE DIV.
P.O. Box 86
Loveland, Ohio 45140
513-683-7400

CANFIELD, C.R., & CO.
See PADDOCK LABORATORIES, INC.

CAPITOL CHEMICAL CO.
5455 Butler Rd.
Washington, D.C. 20016
202-657-4480

CARAJON CHEMICAL CO., INC.
P.O. Box 167
Fremont, Mich. 49412
616-924-3900
616-924-3810

CARBISULPHOIL CO.
See BLISTEX, INC.

CARBOLINEUM WOOD PRESERVING CO.
6683 N. 40th St.
Milwaukee, Wis. 53223
414-353-5040

CARBONA PRODUCTS CO.
330 Calyer St.
Brooklyn, N.Y. 11222
212-383-5599

CARDINAL PRODUCTS CORP.
80 N.W. 73rd St.
Miami, Fla. 33150
305-758-2525

CARDIN, PIERRE, PARFUMS
630 Fifth Ave.
New York, N.Y. 10111
212-489-2430

CAR-FRESHNER CORP.
P.O. Box 719
203 N. Hamilton St.
Watertown, N.Y. 13601
315-788-6250

CARGILL, INC.
P.O. Box 9300
Minneapolis, Minn. 55440
612-475-7457

CARMA LABORATORIES, INC.
5801 W. Airways Ave.
Franklin, Wis. 53132
414-421-7707

CARMEL CHEMICAL CORP.
P.O. Box 406
Westfield, Ind. 46074
317-896-2933

CARNRICK LABORATORIES, INC.
65 Horse Hill Rd.
Cedar Knolls, N.J. 07927
201-267-2670

CARON CORP.
40 West 57th St.
New York, N.Y. 10019
212-582-1144

CARPENTER, W. D., CO., INC.
P.O. Box 218
East Syracuse, N.Y. 13057
315-463-4308

CARROLL CHEMICAL CO.
See CMC, INC.

CARSON CHEMICAL CORP.
27 E. 33rd St.
Paterson, N.J. 07514
201-345-6050

CARSON CHEMICALS, INC.
P.O. Box 466
New Castle, Ind. 47362
317-529-4408

CARSON PRODUCTS CO.
P.O. Box 22309
Savannah, Ga. 31403
912-232-8114

CARTER PRODUCTS
Div. of Carter-Wallace, Inc.
Research Laboratory
Cranbury, N.J. 08512
609-655-1100

CARTER'S INK CO.
See DENNISON MANUFACTURING CO.

CARVEN PARFUMS
630 Fifth Ave.
New York, N.Y. 10020
212-489-2445

CASWELL-MASSEY CO., LTD.
575 Lexington Ave.
New York, N.Y. 10022
212-355-5775

CEDAR VALLEY DISTRIBUTING CO.
See NORTHLAND PRODUCTS CO.

CELANESE CHEMICAL CO., INC.
P.O. Box 47320
Dallas, Tex. 75247
214-689-4703

CELLO CHEMICAL CO.
1354 Old Post Rd.
Havre de Grace, Md. 21078
301-879-2770

CEL-TON-SA MEDICINE CO.
See C.T.S. LABORATORIES, INC.

CENOL CO.
Chemical Div. of Acme Burgess
Rt. 45 & Peterson Rd.
Libertyville, Ill. 60048
312-362-6600

CENTRAL CHEMICAL CO., INC.
3130 Brinkerhoff Rd.
Kansas City, Kans. 66115
913-621-6542

CENTRAL PETROLEUM CO.
548 Standard Bldg.
Cleveland, Ohio 44113
216-771-0400

CENTRAL PHARMACAL CO.
112-128 E. Third St.
Seymour, Ind. 47274
812-522-3915

CENTRAL SOLVENTS & CHEMICALS CO.
See CHEMCENTRAL CORP.

CENTRAL SOYA
1300 Fort Wayne National Bank Bldg.
Fort Wayne, Ind. 46802
219-425-5100

CEREAL SOAPS DIV.
Johanson Manufacturing Corp.
P.O. Box 329
Boonton, N.J. 07005
201-334-2676

CERTIFIED HOME PRODUCTS
2902 Nebraska Ave.
Santa Monica, Calif. 90404
213-393-0737

CERTIFIED LABORATORIES
P.O. Box 2493
Fort Worth, Tex. 76101
817-251-2838

CETYLITE INDUSTRIES, INC.
9051 River Rd.
Pennsauken, N.J. 08110
609-665-6111

CFS CONTINENTAL
2550 N. Clybourn Ave.
Chicago, Ill. 60614
312-477-7600

CHACON CHEMICAL CORP.
2600 Yates Ave.
City of Commerce, Calif. 90040
213-721-5031

CHAIR-LOC CO.
P.O. Box 45
Lakehurst, N.J. 08733
201-657-4501

CHANEL, INC.
Nine W. 57th St.
New York, N.Y. 10019
212-688-5055

CHAPMAN CHEMICAL CO.
416 E. Brooks Rd.
Memphis, Tenn. 38109
901-396-5151

CHARLES MARCHAND CO., THE
66 E. 34th St.
New York, N.Y. 10016
212-679-0900

CHARLES OF THE RITZ GROUP LTD.
40 W. 57th St.
New York, N.Y. 10019
212-621-7327

CHASE PRODUCTS CO.
19th & Gardner Rd.
Broadview, Ill. 60153
312-345-1222

CHAS. H. LILLY CO., THE
7737 N.E. Killingsworth
Portland, Ore. 97218
503-256-4600

CHATTEM, INC.
1715 W. 38th St.
Chattanooga, Tenn. 37409
615-821-4571

CHEMAGRO AGRICULTURAL DIV.
See MOBAY CHEMICAL CORP.

CHEMCENTRAL CORP.
7050 W. 71st St.
Chicago, Ill. 60638
312-594-7000

CHEMICAL FORMULATORS, INC.
P.O. Box 26
Viscose Rd.
Nitro, W. Va. 25143
304-755-3374

CHEMICAL PROCESSORS, INC.
1109-11 North Hwy. 427
Longwood, Fla. 32750

CHEMICAL SPECIALTIES CO., INC.
51-55 Nassau Ave.
Brooklyn, N.Y. 11222
212-388-6018

CHEMLEY PRODUCTS CO.
P.O. Box 14, Northtown Sta.
Chicago, Ill. 60659
312-674-8033

CHEMPAR CHEMICAL CO., INC.
60 E. 42nd St.
New York, N.Y. 10165
212-687-3990

CHESEBROUGH-POND'S INC.
Research Laboratories
Trumbull Industrial Park
Trumbull, Conn. 06611
203-377-7100

CHESTER CHEMICAL CORP.
P.O. Box 8294
Orlando, Fla. 32806
305-851-6230

CHEVRON CHEMICAL CO.
Research & Development
940 Hensley St.
Richmond, CA 94804
415-233-3737

CHEVRON U.S.A., INC.
575 Market St.
San Francisco, CA 94105
415-233-3737

CHEX CO., THE
1760 N. Howard St.
Philadelphia, Pa. 19122
215-634-2224

CHILTON LABORATORIES, INC.
23 Fairfield Pl.
West Caldwell, N.J. 07006
201-575-1990

CHIPMAN CHEMICALS INC.
800 Marion St.
River Rouge, Mich. 48218

CHIPMAN INC.
400 Jones Rd.
P.O. Box 9100
Stoney Creek, Ontario L8G 3Z1
416-643-4123

CHOLDUN MANUFACTURING CORP.
331 East St.
New Haven, Conn. 06511

CHORE-BOY DIVISION
Golay & Co., Inc.
See YALE CHEMICAL CO.

CHRISTIAN DIOR PERFUMES INC.
9 W. 57th St.
New York, N.Y. 10019
212-759-1840

CHRYSLER CORP.
Parts Div.; MoPar Div.
7000 E. Eleven Mile Rd.
P.O. Box 1718
Detroit, Mich. 48231
313-956-5252

CHURCH & DWIGHT CO., INC.
P.O. Box 369
Piscataway, N.J. 08854
Emergency phone, day and night:
201-885-1220

CIBA-GEIGY CORP.
Agricultural Div.
P.O. Box 18300
Greensboro, N.C. 27419
919-292-7100

CIBA PHARMACEUTICAL CO.
Div. of Ciba-Geigy Corp.
556 Morris Ave.
Summit, N.J. 07901
201-277-5000

CITIES SERVICE CO.
Chemical Sales Dept.
3445 Peachtree Rd., N.E.
Atlanta, Ga. 30302
404-261-9100

CITROX LABORATORIES, INC.
P.O. Box 157
Chesterland, Ohio 44026
216-286-9463

CLAIRE MANUFACTURING CO.
500 Vista Ave.
Addison, Ill. 60101
312-379-1977

CLAIROL, INC.
345 Park Ave.
New York, N.Y. 10154
212-546-5000

CLAPP, OTIS, & SON, INC.
143 Albany St.
Cambridge, Mass. 02139
617-868-1950

CLARKE, JOHN, & COMPANY, INC.
420 Lexington Ave.
New York, N.Y. 10017
212-490-2800

CLASSIC CHEMICAL
16th & Mickle Sts.
Camden, N.J. 08105
609-964-7000

CLAYTON MANUFACTURING CO.
P.O. Box 5530
El Monte, Calif. 91734
213-283-4131
213-443-9381

CLEAN HOME PRODUCTS, INC.
2805 Locust Blvd.
St. Louis, Mo. 63103
314-533-1790

CLEAN PRODUCTS CO.
7275 Neville St.
Columbus, Ohio 44102
614-252-1104

CLEAN SURFACE PRODUCTS CO.
P.O. Box 552
405 W. Colfax Ave.
Palatine, Ill. 60067

CLEARY, W. A., CORP.
1049 Somerset St.
Somerset, N.J. 08873
201-247-8000

CLENZOIL CO.
P.O. Box 1226, Sta. C
Canton, Ohio 44708
216-833-9758

CLEVELAND CLEANER & PASTE CO., THE
7275 Neville Ave. S.W.
Cleveland, Ohio 44102
216-961-1208

CLIMACO CORP.
Two North Riverside Plaza
Chicago, Ill. 60606
312-648-2200

CLIMALENE CO.
See CLIMACO CORP.

CLINE-BUCKNER, INC.
16317 Piuma Ave.
Cerritos, Calif. 90701
213-924-6371

CLING-SURFACE CO.
3885 N. Buffalo Rd.
P.O. Box 31
Orchard Park, N.Y. 14127
716-662-2500

CLOROBEN CHEMICAL CORP.
1035 Belleville Turnpike
Kearny, N.J. 07032
201-997-1700

CLOROX CO., THE
Technical Center
P.O. Box 493
Pleasanton, Calif. 94566
415-462-2100

CLOVER CHEMICAL CO.
P.O. Box 146
Eighty Four, Pa. 15330
412-341-1881

CMC, INC.
13th Ave. & D St.
Smyrna, Tenn. 37167
615-459-2583

CMC RESEARCH DIV.
See CONSOLIDATED MIDLAND CORP.

C & M PHARMACAL, INC.
1519 E. Eight Mile Rd.
Hazel Park, Mich. 48030
313-548-7846

COASTAL CHEMICAL CORP.
See COASTAL INDUSTRIES, INC.

COASTAL INDUSTRIES, INC.
190 Jony Dr.
Carlstadt, N.J. 07072
201-933-8600

COCHRAN, JACQUELINE, INC.
630 Fifth Ave.
New York, N.Y. 10111
212-489-2430

COLE, H.A., PRODUCTS CO.
P.O. Box 9937
Jackson, Miss. 39206
601-366-9325

COLE PHARMACAL CO., INC.
See O'NEAL, JONES & FELDMAN PHARMACEUTI-
CALS

COLGATE-PALMOLIVE CO.
300 Park Ave.
New York, N.Y. 10022
Business day: 201-878-7500
Non-business hours: 201-547-2500

COLLOIDAL PRODUCTS CORP.
See KALO AGRICULTURAL CHEMICALS, INC.

COLONIA INC.
Largo Park
Stamford, Conn. 06907
203-348-4711

COLONIAL DAMES CO., LTD.
P.O. Box 22022
Los Angeles, Calif. 90022
213-773-6441

COLONIAL PRODUCTS, INC.
1830 Tenth Ave. N.
Lake Worth, Fla. 33461
305-585-2112

COLOTONE CO.
See MILLER, C. J., & CO.

COLUMBIA MEDICAL CO.
262 Rt. 59
Monsey, N.Y. 10952
914-357-0070

COLUMBIA PAINT CO.
1517 Dodge Ave.
Helena, Mont. 59601
406-442-7650

COMAIR CORP.
386 N.E. 191st St.
North Miami Beach, Fla. 33179
305-652-0331

COMATIC LABORATORIES, INC.
P.O. Box 42300
Houston, Tex. 77042
713-783-2032

COMBE INC.
1101 Westchester Ave.
White Plains, N.Y. 10604
914-694-5454

COMFORT MANUFACTURING CO.
1056 W. Van Buren St.
Chicago, Ill. 60607
312-421-8145

COMMERCE DRUG CO., INC.
Div. Del Laboratories, Inc.
565 Broad Hollow Rd.
Farmingdale, N.Y. 11735
516-293-7070

COMPASS FOODS, INC.
See GREAT ATLANTIC & PACIFIC TEA CO., INC.

COMPETITION CHEMICALS
715 Railroad St.
Box 141
Iowa Falls, Iowa 50126
515-648-3683

CONKLIN CO., INC.
Valley Park Dr.
Shakopee, Minn. 55379
612-445-6010

CONSAN PACIFIC, INC.
P.O. Box 208
Whittier, Calif. 90608
213-698-0403

CONSOLIDATED CHEMICAL, INC.
1470 S. Vandeventer
St. Louis, Mo. 63110
314-531-7282

CONSOLIDATED MIDLAND CORP.
195 E. Main St.
Brewster, N.Y. 10509
914-279-6108

CONSOLIDATED PROTECTIVE
COATINGS CORP.
1801 E. 9th St.
Cleveland, Ohio 44114
216-771-3258

CONSOLIDATED ROYAL CHEMICAL
CORP.
1450 N. Dayton St.
Chicago, Ill. 60622
312-951-1000

CONTINENTAL COFFEE CO.
See CFS CONTINENTAL

CONTINENTAL MANUFACTURING CO.
1101 Warson Rd.
St. Louis, Mo. 63132
314-997-5900

CONTRACT PACKAGING CORP.
10 West End Rd.
Totowa, N.J. 07512

CONWOOD CORP.
Household Products Div.
813 Ridge Lake Blvd.
P.O. Box 171417
Memphis, Tenn. 38117
901-761-2050

COOK CHEMICAL CO.
See REALEX CORP.

COOK & DUNN PAINT CORP.
167 Kossuth St.
Newark, N.J. 07101
201-589-5580

COOK PAINT & VARNISH CO.
P.O. Box 389
Kansas City, Mo. 64141
816-391-6000

COOPERCARE, INC. (USA)
305 Fairfield Ave.
Fairfield, N.J. 07006

COOPER LABORATORIES, INC.
455 E. Middlefield Rd.
Mountain View, Calif. 94043
415-969-9030

COOPERS CREEK CHEMICAL CORP.
River Rd.
West Conshohocken, Pa. 19428
215-828-0375

COOPERVISION PHARMACEUTICALS, INC.
P.O. Box 367
San German, Puerto Rico 00753
809-892-2245

COPPER-BRITE, INC.
5147 W. Jefferson Blvd.
Los Angeles, Calif. 90016
213-933-9331

COPPERTONE CORP., THE
See PLOUGH, INC.

CORDO DIVISION
Ferro Corp.
34 Smith St.
Norwalk, Conn. 06852
203-866-4438

CORN KING DIVISION
King Castle, Inc.
P.O. Box 189
Marion, Iowa 52302
319-377-1535

CORONA PRODUCTS CO.
P.O. Box 1214
Atlanta, Ga. 30301
404-524-5434

CORONET MEDICAL RESEARCH CO., INC.
5161 Laurel Canyon Blvd.
North Hollywood, Calif. 91607
213-877-8922

COSMAIR, INC.
530 Fifth Ave.
New York, N.Y. 10036
212-840-3900

COSMERICA
4241 Redwood Ave.
Los Angeles, Calif. 90066
213-823-0015

COSSCO PRODUCTS, INC.
9165 Sunset Blvd.
Hollywood, Calif. 90069
213-274-8188

COTTON STATES CHEMICAL CO., INC.
100 Trenton St.
West Monroe, La. 71291
318-323-0314

COTY
Div. of Pfizer, Inc.
235 E. 42nd St.
New York, N.Y. 10017
212-573-3500

COUNTESS MARITZA COSMETIC CO., INC.
14 Aquarium Dr.
Secaucus, N.J. 07094
201-866-8780

COWLEY, S. L., & SON'S MANUFACTURING CO., INC.
P.O. Box 666
Hugo, Okla. 74743
405-326-3488

COX, L. M., MANUFACTURING CO., INC.
1505 E. Warner Ave.
Santa Ana, Calif. 92702
714-546-2551

COYNE CHEMICAL CO.
2428 E. 56th St.
Los Angeles, Calif. 90058
213-583-6344

CRAFTINT CORP.
Dymo Visual Systems Div.
P.O. Box 1568
Augusta, Ga. 30903
404-798-0123

CRAMER PRODUCTS, INC.
P.O. Box 1001
Gardner, Kan. 66030
913-884-7511

CRAYON, WATER COLOR AND CRAFT INSTITUTE, INC.
60 Rock Harbor Rd.
Orleans, Mass. 02653
617-255-1528

CREIGHTON PRODUCTS CORP.
605 Third Ave.
New York, N.Y. 10017
212-687-7575

CREOMULSION CO.
P.O. Box 1214
Atlanta, Ga. 30301
404-524-5434

CRE-O-TOX CHEMICAL PRODUCTS CO.
2670 Broad St.
P.O. Box 12598
Memphis, Tenn. 38112
901-452-0110

CRESCENT OIL CO., INC.
514 W. Wyoming St.
Indianapolis, Ind. 46225
317-634-1415

CRESTWOOD PRODUCTS CO.
P.O. Box 5643
Kansas City, Mo. 64102
816-421-7117

CRITZAS INDUSTRIES, INC.
4041 Park Ave.
St. Louis, Mo. 63110
314-773-8510

CROSS DIVISON
See CLAPP, OTIS, & SON, INC.

C.T.S. LABORATORIES, INC.
P.O. Box 446
Ansonia, Ohio 45303
513-548-7473

CULLIGAN USA
One Culligan Pkwy
Northbrook, Ill. 60062
312-498-2000

CUNNINGHAM DISTRIBUTORS
P.O. Box 863
1222 Vilsmeier Rd.
Lansdale, Pa. 19446

CURRAN, FRANK J., CO.
8101 S. Lemont Rd.
Downers Grove, Ill. 60515
312-969-2200

CURTIS, HELENE, INDUSTRIES, INC.
4401 W. North Ave.
Chicago, Ill. 60639
312-292-2264

CUTICURA
See CAMPANA CORP.

CUTTER ANIMAL HEALTH LABORATORIES
See BAYVET DIVISION, CUTTER LABORATORIES, INC.

C-Z CHEMICAL CO., INC.
1447 Argoll Ave.
Beloit, Wis. 53511
608-365-5518

D

DAIRY ASSOCIATION CO., INC.
Lyndonville, Vt. 05851
802-626-3610

DALCO CORP.
3010 Broadway N.E.
Minneapolis, Minn. 55413
612-331-8940

DALIN PHARMACEUTICALS, INC.
74-80 Marine St.
Farmingdale, N.Y. 11735
516-454-9282

DAMON CHEMICAL CO., INC.
P.O. Box 480
Alliance, Ohio 44601
216-821-5310

DANA PERFUMES CORP.
609 Fifth Ave.
New York, N.Y. 10017
212-751-3700

DANIELS, DR. A. C., INC.
R.D. 1, Worcester Rd.
Webster, Mass. 01570
617-943-5563

DANIELS, ROSS, INC.
P.O. Box 65430
West Des Moines, Iowa 50265
515-225-6471

DAP INC.
P.O. Box 277
Dayton, Ohio 45401
513-253-7154

DARWORTH CO.
P.O. Box K
Tower Lane
Avon, Conn. 06001
203-677-7721

DAVEY TREE EXPERT CO.
117 S. Water St.
Kent, Ohio 44240
216-673-9511

DAVIES ROSE HOYT
See HOYT LABORATORIES

DAVIS DIESEL DEVELOPMENT
P.O. Box 141
Milford, Conn. 06460
203-877-1670

DAVIS-WEIL MANUFACTURING CO., INC.
See WEIL CHEMICAL

DAY-GLO COLOR CORP.
4732 St. Clair
Cleveland, Ohio 44103
216-391-7070

DAY, JAMES B., & CO.
Day Lane
Carpentersville, Ill. 60110
312-428-2651

d-CON CO., INC.
Sub. of Sterling Drug, Inc.
225 Summit Ave.
Montvale, N.J. 07645
201-573-5700

DEFT, INC.
17451 Von Karman Ave.
Irvine, Calif. 92714
714-549-8911

DEKALB AGRESEARCH, INC.
Sycamore Rd.
Dekalb, Ill. 60115
815-758-3461

DELAGAR PRODUCTS, INC.
P.O. Box 277
Rouses Point, N.Y. 12979
518-297-7161

DELAVAL SEPARATOR CO.
See BONEWITZ CHEMICAL SERVICES, INC.

DELBAY PHARMACEUTICALS, INC.
See SCHERING CORP.

DEL CHEMICAL CORP.
P.O. Box 280
Menomonee Falls, Wis. 53051
414-251-5050

DEL LABORATORIES, INC.
565 Broad Hollow Rd.
Farmingdale, N.Y. 11735
516-293-7070

DELTA CHEMICAL CORP.
See DELTA FOREMOST CHEMICAL CORP.

DELTA FOREMOST CHEMICAL CORP.
3915 Air Park St.
Memphis, Tenn. 38130
901-363-4340

DELTA LABORATORIES, INC.
5055 Choctaw Dr.
Baton Rouge, La. 70805
504-356-1386

DELUXOL LABORATORIES INC.
3733 University Blvd. W.
Jacksonville, Fla. 32217
904-733-5386

DE MARKOFF, ALEXANDRA
Sub. of Lanvin-Charles of the Ritz Group Ltd.
40 W. 57th St.
New York, N.Y. 10019
212-621-7300

DEMERT & DOUGHERTY, INC.
5000 W. 41st St.
Chicago, Ill. 60650
312-523-5600

DENNEY, FRANCES
437 Madison Ave.
New York, N.Y. 10022
212-888-9500

DENNISON MANUFACTURING CO.
Dennison Carter's Div.
275 Wyman St.
Waltham, Mass. 02254
617-890-6350

DENT, C. S., & CO.
See GRANDPA BRANDS CO.

DENTOCAIN CO.
P.O. Box 133
Bloomfield, Conn. 06002
203-242-1982

DEP CORPORATION
12821 W. Jefferson Blvd.
Los Angeles, Calif. 90066
213-827-9800

DE PREE CO.
Div. of Chattem, Inc.
1715 W. 38th St.
Chattanooga, Tenn. 37409
615-821-4571

DERBY REFINING CO.
P.O. Box 1030
Wichita, Kans. 67201
316-267-0361

DERMA LABORATORIES, INC.
P.O. Box 727
Bensenville, Ill. 60106
312-766-5400

DERMIK LABORATORIES, INC.
500 Virginia Dr.
Fort Washington, Pa. 19034
215-628-6550

DE SOTO CHEMICAL CO., INC.
P.O. Box 70
Arcadia, Fla. 33821
813-494-3232

DETTELBACH PESTICIDE CORP.
P.O. Box 647
Atlanta, Ga. 30301
404-873-2355

DeVILBISS CO., THE
Health Care Div.
P.O. Box 552
Somerset, Pa. 15501
814-443-4881

DEWITT INTERNATIONAL CORP.
P.O. Box 6827
Greenville, S.C. 29606
803-244-8521

DEXOL INDUSTRIES, INC.
1450 W. 228th St.
Torrance, Calif. 90501
213-326-8373

DIAMOND LABORATORIES, INC.
See SYNTEX LABORATORIES, INC.

DIAMOND SHAMROCK CORP.
1100 Superior Ave.
Cleveland, Ohio 44114
216-694-5000

DIAMOND SHAMROCK, PROCESS CHEMICALS DIV.
350 Mt. Kemble Ave.
Morristown, N.J. 07960
201-267-1000

DIANE VON FURSTENBERG INC.
Cosmetics & Fragrances Div.
745 Fifth Ave.
New York, N.Y. 10022
212-753-1111

DICKEY DRUG CO.
1009 West State St.
Bristol, Va. 24201
703-669-1116

DICKINSON, E. E., CO.
40 N. Main St.
Essex, Conn. 06426
203-767-8261

DIOR, CHRISTIAN, PERFUMES INC.
9 W. 57th St.
New York, N.Y. 10019
212-759-1840

DIRECT DIV.
Reid-Provident Laboratories, Inc.
640 Tenth St., N.W.
Atlanta, Ga. 30318
404-898-1000

DISTA PRODUCTS CO.
Div. of Eli Lilly and Co.
307 E. McCarty St.
Indianapolis, Ind. 46285
317-261-2000

DIVERSEY CHEMICALS
See DIVERSEY WYANDOTTE CORP.

DIVERSEY WYANDOTTE CORP.
1532 Biddle Ave.
Wyandotte, Mich. 48192
313-281-0930

DIVERSIFIED PACKAGING CORP.
222 Thomas St.
Newark, N.J. 07114

DIXIE LABORATORIES
P.O. Drawer 8
Seagoville, Tex. 75159
214-287-2570

D'LANERG, LTD.
See AMERICAN HYGIENIC LABORATORIES, INC.

DL SKIN CARE PRODUCTS, INC.
47 E. Market St.
Buffalo, N.Y. 14204
716-853-4700

DOAK PHARMACAL CO., INC.
700 Shames Dr.
Westbury, N.Y. 11590
516-333-7222

DOLAN, V. J., & CO., INC.
1830-32 N. Laramie Ave.
Chicago, Ill. 60639
312-237-0100

DOLCIN CORP.
25 W. 43rd St.
New York, N.Y. 10036
212-244-7440

DOLGE, C. B., CO.
Ferry Lane
Westport, Conn. 06880
203-227-9591

DOME DIVISION
Miles Laboratories, Inc.
400 Morgan Lane
West Haven, Conn. 06516
203-934-9221

DOONER LABORATORIES, INC.
Ward Hill
Haverhill, Mass. 01830
617-373-1236

DOREX, INC.
121 Ontario St.
Frankfort, Ill. 60423
815-469-3181

DOROTHY GRAY, LTD.
Div. Lehn & Fink Products Group
225 Summit Ave.
Montvale, N.J. 07645
201-573-5700

DORSEY LABORATORIES
P.O. Box 83288
Lincoln, Nebr. 68501
402-464-6311

DOUGLAS PRODUCTS
Div. of The Scott & Fetzer Co.
815 E. Tallmadge Ave.
Akron, Ohio 44310

DOW CHEMICAL CO.
Midland, Mich. 48640
517-636-4400

DOW CORNING CORP.
P.O. Box 1767
Midland, Mich. 48640
517-496-4000

DOW PHARMACEUTICALS
The Dow Chemical Co.
P.O. Box 68511
Indianapolis, Ind. 46268
317-873-7000

DOXSEE FOOD CORP.
8323 Pulaski Hwy.
Baltimore, Md. 21237
301-686-2800

DRACKETT CO., THE
5020 Spring Grove Ave.
Cincinnati, Ohio 45232
513-632-1500

DRAGON CHEMICAL CORP.
P.O. Box 7311
Roanoke, Va. 24019
703-362-3657

DRI-SLIDE, INC.
Industrial Park
Fremont, Mich. 49412
616-924-3950

DRITZ, JOHN, & SONS
See SCOVILL MANUFACTURING CO.

DR. MAYFIELD LABORATORIES
1209 S. Main St.
Charles City, Iowa 50616
515-228-5161

DRO, INC.
See CHEMICAL SPECIALTIES CO., INC.

DUART MANUFACTURING CO., LTD.
984 Folsom
San Francisco, Calif. 94107
415-986-0260

DUBOIS CHEMICALS
Div. of Chemed Corp.
634 Broadway
Cincinnati, Ohio 45202
513-762-6000

DUNCAN CERAMIC PRODUCTS DIVISION
Duncan Enterprises
5673 E. Shields Ave.
Fresno, Calif. 93727
209-291-4444
Emergency no.: 209-445-1222

DUNTON, M. W., CO.
350 Kinsley Ave.
Providence, R.I. 02901
401-331-3600

DUPLI-COLOR PRODUCTS
1601 Nicholas Blvd.
Elk Grove Village, Ill. 60007
312-439-0600

DU PONT DE NEMOURS, E. I., & CO., INC.
Biochemicals Dept.
Wilmington, Del. 19898
Emergency phone no.: 302-774-2421

DURHAM'S DRUG PRODUCTS CO.
P.O. Box 443
Comanche, Tex. 76442
915-356-3136

DUVELLE
See PARFUMS DUVELLE, INC.

DYANSHINE PRODUCTS DIVISION
See ZOES, C. A., MANUFACTURING CO., INC.

DYNA SYSTEMS INC.
P.O. Box 225326
Dallas, Tex. 75265
214-438-0381

DYNATRON/BONDO CORP.
2160 Hills Ave., N.W.
Atlanta, Ga. 30318
404-351-2730

E

EARL GRISSMER CO., INC.
7950 Castleway Dr.
Indianapolis, Ind. 46250
317-842-0820

EARL, JOHN A., INC.
216-222 Union St.
Hackensack, N.J. 07601
201-342-2453

EASTERDAY SUPPLY CO.
901 E. 61st St.
Los Angeles, Calif 90001
213-231-9131

EASTERN RESEARCH LABORATORIES,
INC.
302 S. Central Ave.
Baltimore, Md. 21202
301-321-1404

EASTMAN KODAK CO.
1669 Lake Ave.
Rochester, N.Y. 14650
716-722-5151

EATON, J. T., & CO., INC.
1393 E. Highland Rd.
Twinsburg, Ohio 44087

EATON LABORATORIES
See NORWICH-EATON PHARMACEUTICALS

EATON-MERZ LABORATORIES, INC.
See NORWICH-EATON PHARMACEUTICALS

EBERHARD FABER, INC.
Crestwood
Wilkes-Barre, Pa. 18773
717-474-6711

ECHOLS MANUFACTURING CO.
See ATHENA CORP.

ECKROAT SEED CO.
1106 N. Eastern Ave.
Oklahoma City, Okla. 73117
405-427-2484

ECONO MED, INC.
P.O. Box 3303
Burlington, N.C. 27215
919-226-1091

ECONOMICS LABORATORY, INC.
Osborn Building
St. Paul, Minn. 55102
612-224-4678

EDWAL SCIENTIFIC PRODUCTS
DIVISION
Falcon Safety Products, Inc.
12120 S. Peoria St.
Chicago, Ill. 60643
312-264-8484

EGAN, H. B., MANUFACTURING CO.
P.O. Box 769
Muskogee, Okla. 74401
918-687-5427

EHRLICH, J. C., CHEMICAL CO., INC.
Agricultural Chemicals Div.
840 William Lane
Reading, Pa. 19612
215-921-0641

EIGHT IN ONE PET PRODUCTS, INC.
100 Emjay Blvd.
Brentwood, N.Y. 11717
516-213-8700

ELANCO PRODUCTS CO.
Div. of Eli Lilly & Co.
740 S. Alabama St.
Indianapolis, Ind. 46285
317-261-3000

ELCO CHEMICAL, INC.
See WEST BEND CO., THE

ELCO MANUFACTURING CO.
111 Third St., Sharpsburg
Pittsburgh, Pa. 15215
412-782-1850

ELDER PHARMACEUTICALS
705 E. Mulberry St.
P.O. Box 31
Bryan, Ohio 43506
419-636-1168

ELECTROLUX CORP.
51 Forest Ave.
Old Greenwich, Conn. 06870
203-637-1761

ELI LILLY AND CO.
307 E. McCarty St.
Indianapolis, Ind. 46285
317-261-2000

ELIZABETH ARDEN, INC.
Sub. of Eli Lilly & Co.
1345 Ave. of the Americas
New York, N.Y. 10019
212-399-2000

ELLA BACHE BEAUTY PRODUCTS
8 W. 36th St.
New York, N.Y. 10018
212-753-2175

ELLIOTT PAINT & VARNISH CO.
1330 S. Kilbourn Ave.
Chicago, Ill. 60623
312-762-7010

ELMIRA DRUG & CHEMICAL CO., INC.
1225 W. Water St.
Elmira, N.Y. 14905
607-734-1626

ELTRON
Cambridge Shaver Imports, Inc.
Cambridge, Mass. 02142
617-421-7000

EMBALMERS' SUPPLY CO.
25 Ford Rd.
P.O. Box 631
Westport, Conn. 06880
203-227-5135

EMILIO PUCCI PERFUMES INTL. INC.
24 E. 64th St.
New York, N.Y. 10021
212-752-4777

EMPIRE MANUFACTURING CO.
409 Southwest Blvd.
Kansas City, Mo. 64108
816-421-7762

ENDO LABORATORIES INC.
1000 Stewart Ave.
Garden City, N.Y. 11530
516-832-2123

ENTERPRISE PAINT CO.
1191 S. Wheeling Rd.
Wheeling, Ill. 60090
312-541-9000

ESQUIRE CHEMICAL CO.
See CURRAN, FRANK J., CO.

ESSENTIAL CHEMICALS CORP.
28391 Essential Rd.
Merton, Wis. 53056
414-691-3000

ESTEE LAUDER INC.
767 Fifth Ave.
New York, N.Y. 10022
212-572-4200

ESTES, L. W., CO., INC.
P.O. Box 365
Alma, Ga. 31510
912-632-8377

ETHIQUE LABORATORIES
P.O. Box 708
Elmhurst, Ill. 60126
312-543-9035

ETHYL CORP.
451 Florida Blvd.
Baton Rouge, La. 70801
24-hour emergency phone: 504-344-4147

ETNA CHEMICAL CO., INC.
Germantown Sta., Box 25611
Philadelphia, Pa. 19144
215-842-2414

EVANS ADHESIVE CORP.
925 W. Henderson Rd.
Columbus, Ohio 43220
614-451-2665

EVELYN MARSHALL COSMETICS, LTD.
14 E. 38th St.
New York, N.Y. 10016
212-532-6400

EVER-DRY CORP.
P.O. Box 400009
Dallas, Tex. 75240
214-233-2800

EVYAN PERFUMES, INC.
350 E. 35th St.
New York, N.Y. 10016
212-532-3800

EXELENTO MEDICINE CO., INC.
456 Charlotte Ave.
Detroit, Mich. 48201
313-833-0085

EX-LAX DISTRIBUTING CO., INC.
605 Third Ave.
New York, N.Y. 10017
212-687-7575

EYLURE OF LONDON, LTD.
410 Eastern Pkwy.
Farmingdale, N.Y. 11735
516-752-8833

E-Z-EST PRODUCTS CO., INC.
2528 Adeline St.
Oakland, Calif. 94607
415-836-3980

E-Z FLO CHEMICAL CO.
See GROWER SERVICE CORP.

E-Z PRODUCTS CO.
Sac City, Iowa 50583

F

FABER-CASTELL CORP.
P.O. Box 7099
Newark, N.J. 07107
201-484-4141

FABERGE DIVISION
Faberge Inc.
65 Railroad Ave.
Ridgefield, N.J. 07657
201-945-5800

FACTOR, MAX, & CO.
1655 N. McCadden Pl.
Hollywood, Calif. 90028
213-856-6000

FAESY & BESTOFF, INC.
143 River Rd.
Edgewater, N.J. 07020
201-945-6200

FAHRNEY, DR. PETER, & SONS CO.
1001 Franklin Ave.
Garden City, N.Y. 11530
516-747-5471

FAIRFAX BIOLOGICAL LABORATORY, INC.
Clinton Corners, N.Y. 12514
914-266-3705

FAIRFIELD AMERICAN CORP.
3932 Salt Rd.
Medina, N.Y. 14103
716-798-2141

FAIRMOUNT CHEMICAL CO., INC.
117 Blanchard St.
Newark, N.J. 07105
201-344-5790

FALK CO.
Anfa, Inc.
16735 County Rd. 6
Plymouth, Minn. 55447
612-473-8956

FALLEK-LANKRO CORP.
See DIAMOND SHAMROCK CORP.

FARBOIL CO.
8200 Fischer Rd.
Baltimore, Md. 21222
301-477-8200

FARNAM COMPANIES, INC.
2230 E. Magnolia
Phoenix, Ariz. 85036
602-244-8261

FARWELL, OZMUN, KIRK & CO.
Paint Manufacturing Div.
1200 Mendelssohn Ave., N.
Minneapolis, Minn. 55427
612-545-1487

FASHION FAIR COSMETICS
820 S. Michigan Ave.
Chicago, Ill. 60605
312-322-9444

FASHION FRAGRANCES INC.
331 Madison Ave.
New York, N.Y. 10017
212-687-4147

FATSCO
251 N. Fair Ave.
Benton Harbor, Mich. 49022
616-926-7795

FAULTLESS STARCH/BON AMI CO.
1025 W. 8th St.
Kansas City, Mo. 64101
816-421-7075

FEDERAL CHEMICAL CO., INC.
Arab Products Div.
P.O. Box 68420
Indianapolis, Ind. 46278
317-545-8586

FEDERAL INTERNATIONAL CHEMICALS
1191 S. Wheeling Rd.
Wheeling, Ill. 60090
312-541-9000

FEDERATED FOODS, INC.
See GREAT ATLANTIC & PACIFIC TEA CO., INC.

FERGUSON FUMIGANTS, INC.
93 Ford Lane
Hazelwood, Mo. 63042
314-731-0414

FERGUSSON, ALEX. C., CO.
Spring Mill Dr.
Frazer, Pa. 19355
215-647-3300

FERNDALE LABORATORIES, INC.
780 W. Eight Mile Rd.
Ferndale, Mich. 48220
313-548-0900

FERROUS CORP.
P.O. Box 1764
Bellevue, Wash. 98009
206-454-6320

F & F LABORATORIES, INC.
3501 W. 48th Pl.
Chicago, Ill. 60632
312-927-3737

FIBERGLASS CLEANING PRODUCTS, INC.
1085 N. Main St., Suite N
Orange, Calif. 92667
714-771-0532

FIBERTONE CO., THE
P.O. Box 23372
1314 S. Lorena St.
Los Angeles, Calif. 90023
213-261-0159

FIBRE GLASS-EVERCOAT CO., INC.
6600 Cornell Rd.
Cincinnati, Ohio 45242
513-489-7600

FIEBING CHEMICAL CO.
516 S. Second St.
Milwaukee, Wis. 53204
414-271-5011

FIELD, HENRY, SEED AND NURSERY CO.
407 Sycamore St.
Shenandoah, Iowa 51602
712-246-2110

FIELDS, TOM, LTD.
Div. of Mem Co., Inc.
122 Union St.
Northvale, N.J. 07647
201-768-8080

FIELDSTON CORP.
See FIELDS, TOM, LTD.

FIKE CHEMICALS, INC.
P.O. Box 546
Nitro, W. Va. 25143
304-755-3336

FINE ORGANICS, INC.
205 Main St.
Lodi, N.J. 07644
201-472-6800

FIRST NATIONAL SUPERMARKETS, INC.
17000 Rockside Rd.
Maple Heights, Ohio 44137
216-587-7100

FIRST TEXAS PHARMACEUTICALS, INC.
See SCHERER LABORATORIES, INC.

FISONS CORP.
Agrochemical Div.
Pharmaceutical Div.
Two Preston Ct.
Bedford, Mass. 01730
617-275-1000

FITZPATRICK BROS.
625 N. Sacramento Blvd.
Chicago, Ill. 60612
312-722-3300

FLAME-GLO COSMETICS
Div. of Del Labs., Inc.
565 Broad Hollow Rd.
Farmingdale, N.Y. 11735
516-293-7070

FLAMORT CHEMICAL CO.
746 Natoma St.
San Francisco, Calif. 94103
415-621-7825

FLECTO CO., INC., THE
1000 45th St.
Oakland, Calif. 94608
415-655-2470

FLEET, C. B., CO., INC.
P.O. Box 11349
Lynchburg, Va. 24506
804-528-4000

FLEETWOOD CO.
1500 Brook Dr.
Downers Grove, Ill. 60515
312-495-9300

FLEMING & COMPANY
1600 Fenpark Dr.
Fenton, Mo. 63026
314-343-8200

FLINT LABORATORIES
Div. of Travenol Laboratories, Inc.
Deerfield, Ill. 60015
312-940-5000

FLORALIFE, INC.
4420 S. Tripp Ave.
Chicago, Ill. 60632
312-523-3565

FMC CORPORATION
Agricultural Chemical Div.
2000 Market St.
Philadelphia, Pa. 19103
215-299-6000

FMC CORPORATION
Sun Swimming Pool Products
2000 Market St.
Philadelphia, Pa. 19103
215-299-5800

FORD, LUTHER, & CO.
100 N. Seventh St.
Minneapolis, Minn. 55403
612-332-2441

FORMAN FORD PAINTS
Div. of Farwell, Ozmun, Kirk & Co.
1200 Mendelssohn Ave., N.
Minneapolis, Minn. 55427
612-545-1487

FORMBY'S, INC.
P.O. Box 667
Olive Branch, Miss. 38654
601-895-5594

FORSHAW CHEMICALS, INC.
650 State St.
Charlotte, N.C. 28208
704-372-6790

FORT DODGE LABORATORIES
Div. of American Home Products Corp.
Fort Dodge, Iowa 50501
515-573-3131

FORTRESS PRODUCTS CO.
P.O. Box 1974
Olathe, Kans. 66061
913-782-5800

FOUGERA, E., & CO.
60 Baylis Rd.
Melville, N.Y. 11747
516-454-6996

FOX PHARMACAL, INC.
1750 W. McNab Rd.
P.O. Box 8668
Ft. Lauderdale, Fla. 33310
305-971-4100

FOY INDUSTRIES, INC.
Foy Laboratories Div.
351 W. Penn Ave.
Wernersville, Pa. 19565
215-678-9460

FOY-JOHNSTON, INC.
1776 Mentor Ave.
Cincinnati, Ohio 45212
513-631-4270

FRANCES DENNEY
437 Madison Ave.
New York, N.Y. 10022
212-888-9500

FRANKLIN LABORATORIES
2620 S. Parker Rd.
Suite 240
Aurora, Colo. 80014
303-751-8831

FREEMAN COSMETIC CORP.
P.O. Box 17
Hollywood, Calif. 90028
213-461-2901

FREERS CO., THE
P.O. Box 103
2502 Lucas St.
Muscatine, Iowa 52761
319-263-2155

FRENCH, R. T., CO.
1 Mustard St.
P.O. Box 23450
Rochester, N.Y. 14692
716-482-8000

FRIENDLY LABORATORIES
720 E. Independence
Shawnee, Okla. 74801
405-273-3757

FS SERVICES, INC.
1701 Towanda Ave.
Bloomington, Ill. 61702
309-828-0021

FULD-STALFORT, INC.
1354 Old Post Rd.
Havre de Grace, Md. 21078
301-939-1234

FULLER BRUSH CO., THE
2800 Rockcreek Pkwy.
North Kansas City, Mo. 64117
816-474-1754

FULLER, H.B., CO.
Foster Div.
P.O. Box 625
Spring House, Pa. 19477
215-628-2600

FULLER-O'BRIEN DIV.
The O'Brien Corp.
450 E. Grand Ave.
South San Francisco, Calif. 94080
415-761-2300

FULLER SYSTEM, INC.
226 Washington St.
Woburn, Mass. 01801
617-933-0945

FUMOL CORP.
49-65 Van Dam St.
Long Island City, N.Y. 11101
212-784-0484

FUNK, A. J., & Co.
1471 Timber Dr.
Elgin, Ill. 60120
312-741-6760

FURST-MC NESS CO.
Freeport, Ill. 61032
815-232-2151

F. & W. ENTERPRISES, INC.
P.O. Box 15392
Tampa, Fla. 33614
813-932-3893

FYR-FYTER CO.
See NORRIS INDUSTRIES

G

GABY, INC.
1326 Frankford Ave.
Philadelphia, Pa. 19125
215-739-7300

GAF CORP.
140 W. 51st St.
New York, N.Y. 10020
212-621-5000

GAMBINE PRODUCTS, INC.
60 E. 42nd St.
New York, N.Y. 10017
212-697-5280

GARD INDUSTRIES, INC.
746 W. Algonquin Rd.
Arlington Heights, Ill. 60005
312-439-3200

GARDINER MANUFACTURING CO., INC.
160 Van Rensselaer St.
Buffalo, N.Y. 14210
716-852-6156

GARRY LABORATORIES
260 Creekside Dr.
Amherst, N.Y. 14150
716-691-8822

GARTSIDE'S IRON RUST SOAP CO.
2519 W. Huntingdon St.
Philadelphia, Pa. 19132
215-229-0266

GASTON JOHNSTON CORP.
24-64 45th St.
Long Island City, N.Y. 11103
212-932-0200

GC ELECTRONICS
Div. of Wallace Murray Corp.
400 S. Wyman St.
Rockford, Ill. 61101
815-968-9661

GEIGY PHARMACEUTICALS
Div. of Ciba-Geigy Corp.
Ardsley, N.Y. 10502
201-277-5000

GEISLER PET PRODUCTS, INC.
3902 Leavenworth St.
Omaha, Nebr. 68105
402-342-3121

G. E. LABORATORIES, INC.
P.O. Box 338
Sixth & Commerce Sts.
Shamokin, Pa. 17872
717-644-0333

GENERAL CEMENT MFG. CO.
See GC ELECTRONICS

GENERAL DEVELOPMENTS CORP.
P.O. Box 3675
Milwaukee, Wis. 53217
414-273-1700

GENERAL FIRE EXTINGUISHER CORP.
1685 Shermer Rd.
Northbrook, Ill. 60062
312-272-7500

GENERAL MOTORS CORP.
3044 W. Grand Blvd.
Detroit, Mich. 48202
313-556-1597

GENERAL ORDNANCE EQUIPMENT CORP.
See SMITH & WESSON/GENERAL ORDNANCE EQUIPMENT CO.

GENERAL PEST SERVICE CO.
2015 Pontius Ave.
Los Angeles, Calif. 90025
213-479-4349

GEORGIA-CAROLINA OIL CO.
195 Bay St.
P.O. Box 4304
Macon, Ga. 31208
912-742-1428

GERIATRIC PHARMACEUTICAL CORP.
397 Jericho Turnpike
P.O. Box 68
Floral Park, N.Y. 11001
516-354-1121

GERMAINE MONTEIL COSMETIQUES CORP.
40 W. 57th St.
New York, N.Y. 10019
212-582-3010

GERMAIN'S, INC.
4820 E. 50th St.
P.O. Box 3233
Los Angeles, Calif. 90058
213-589-6331

GETTY REFINING & MARKETING CO.
1437 S. Boulder
P.O. Box 1650
Tulsa, Okla. 74102
918-560-6000

GIBSON-HOMANS CO.
1755 Enterprise Pkwy.
Twinsburg, Ohio 44087
216-425-3255

GILBERT SPRUANCE CO., THE
Tioga & Richmond
Philadelphia, Pa. 19134
215-739-6172

GILL AGRICULTURE CHEMICAL CO.
Route 1
Box 334
Boyce, La. 71409
318-793-2207

GILLETTE APPLIANCE DIV.
310 E. Fifth St.
St. Paul, Minn. 55101
617-421-7000

GILLETTE CO.
Paper Mate Div.
101 Huntington Ave.
Boston, Mass. 02199
617-421-7000

GILLETTE CO.
Personal Care Div.
101 Huntington Ave.
Boston, Mass. 02199
617-421-7000

GILLETTE CO.
Toiletries Div.
101 Huntington Ave.
Boston, Mass. 02199
617-421-7000

GILMAN CO., INC.
P.O. Box 1257
Chattanooga, Tenn. 37401
615-756-5185

GINGISOL LABORATORIES
3701 Mayfield Rd.
Cleveland, Ohio 44121
216-382-2763

GLAXO INC.
1900 W. Commercial Blvd.
Fort Lauderdale, Fla. 33309
305-776-5300

GLENBROOK LABORATORIES
Div. of Sterling Drug Inc.
90 Park Ave.
New York, N.Y. 10016
212-972-4141

GLIDDEN COATINGS & RESINS
Div. of SCM Corp.
Dwight P. Joyce Research Center
16651 Sprague Rd.
Strongsville, Ohio 44136
216-771-5121

GLIDDEN-DURKEE
See GLIDDEN COATINGS & RESINS

GLOVER, H. CLAY, INC.
9 Robbins St.
P.O. Box 432
Toms River, N.J. 08753
201-349-0350

GODDARD, J., & SON
See JOHNSON, S. C., & SON, INC.

GOLD BOND STERILIZING POWDER CO.
26 Water St.
Fairhaven, Mass. 02719
617-992-4444

GOLDEN BEST FOODS, INC.
See GREAT ATLANTIC & PACIFIC TEA CO., INC.

GOLD MEDAL HAIR PRODUCTS, INC.
15 Hoover St.
Inwood, N.Y. 11696
516-371-2600

GOOD-LIFE CHEMICALS, INC.
P.O. Box 687
Effingham, Ill. 62401
217-342-3986

GOODLOE E. MOORE, INC.
2811 N. Vermilion St.
Danville, Ill. 61832
217-446-7900

GOODRICH, B. F., CO.
Fabricated Polymers Div.
500 S. Main St.
Akron, Ohio 44318
216-379-3776

GOODRICH-UNIVERSAL, INC.
500 Robert St.
St. Paul, Minn. 55101
612-224-8937

GOODWINOL PRODUCTS CORP.
14 Larkfield Rd.
East Northport, N.Y. 11731
516-757-6464

GOODYEAR TIRE & RUBBER CO.
Akron, Ohio 44316
216-794-2121

GOODY'S MANUFACTURING CORP.
436 Salt St., S.W.
Winston-Salem, N.C. 27108
919-723-1831

GORDON LABORATORIES
State & Parkview Rds.
Upper Darby, Pa. 19082
215-789-3055

GORHAM DIV. OF TEXTRON INC.
333 Adelaide Ave.
Providence, R.I. 02907
401-785-9800

GOSHEN LABORATORIES, INC.
36 St. John St.
Goshen, N.Y. 10924
914-294-6114

GRACE, W. R., & CO.
Agricultural Chemicals Group
P.O. Box 277
100 N. Main St.
Memphis, Tenn. 38101
901-522-2000

GRAHAM-FIELD SURGICAL CO., INC.
415 Second Ave.
New Hyde Park, N.Y. 11040
516-328-0500

GRAHAM PAINT AND VARNISH CO.
4800 S. Richmond Ave.
Chicago, Ill. 60632
312-376-7676

GRANDPA BRANDS CO.
317-321 E. Eighth St.
Cincinnati, Ohio 45202
513-241-1673

GRAY, DR. W. F., & CO.
61 1/2 Arcade
Nashville, Tenn. 37219
615-256-8614

GREAT ATLANTIC & PACIFIC TEA CO., INC.
2 Paragon Dr.
Montvale, N.J. 07645
201-573-9700

GREAT LAKES BIOCHEMICAL CO., INC.
6120 W. Douglas Ave.
Milwaukee, Wis. 53218
414-464-1200

GREAT LAKES CHEMICAL CORP.
P.O. Box 2200
West Lafayette, Ind. 47906
317-463-2511

GREAT WESTERN SUGAR CO.
P.O. Box 5308
Denver, Colo. 80217
303-893-4600

GREEN LIGHT CO.
Box 17985
San Antonio, Tex. 78217
512-494-3481

GREEN LIGHT PLANT FOOD CO.
See GREEN LIGHT CO.

GREEN, L. S., ASSOCIATES
162 W. 56th St.
New York, N.Y. 10019
212-265-8235

GREEN THUMB PRODUCTS CORP.
P.O. Drawer 760
Apopka, Fla. 32703
305-886-2222

GRID LABORATORIES
See VAN WATERS & ROGERS

GRISSMER, EARL, CO., INC.
7950 Castleway Dr.
Indianapolis, Ind. 46250
317-842-0820

GROWER SERVICE CORP.
16713 Industrial Pkwy.
P.O. Box 18037
Lansing, Mich. 48901
517-323-2125

GRUMBACHER, M., INC.
460 W. 34th St.
New York, N.Y. 10001
212-279-6406

GUARD CHEMICAL CO.
One Ave. L
Newark, N.J. 07105
201-589-6330

GUARDSMAN CHEMICALS, INC.
1350 Steele Ave., SW
Grand Rapids, Mich. 49507
616-452-5181

GUERLAIN, INC.
Rte 138
Somers, N.Y. 10589
914-232-5015

GUILLORY WHOLESALE CO.
112 Chestnut St.
Mamou, La. 70554
318-468-5248

GULF ADHESIVES AND RESINS
Gulf Oil Chemicals Co.
P.O. Box 10911
Overland Park, Kans. 66210
913-383-6700

GULF OIL CORP.
P.O. Box 1166
Pittsburgh, Pa. 15230
412-263-5000

GUNK LABORATORIES, INC.
P.O. Box 34689
Charlotte, N.C. 28234
704-377-6555

GUSTAFSON, INC.
P.O. Box 220065
Dallas, Tex. 75222
214-661-1334

G&W LABORATORIES
111 Coolidge St.
South Plainfield, N.J. 07080
201-753-2000

H

HABA INTERNATIONAL, INC.
554 Mitchell St.
Orange, N.J. 07050
201-673-0747

HAGERTY, W. J., & SONS, LTD., INC.
P.O. Box 1496
South Bend, Ind. 46624
219-288-4991

HALABY, SAMUEL, INC.
482 Clinton Ave. S.
Rochester, N.Y. 14620
716-232-1170

HALLIWELL PRODUCTS
250 Lackawanna Ave.
West Paterson, N.J. 07424
201-256-3400

HANFORD, G. C., MANUFACTURING CO.
304 Oneida St.
Syracuse, N.Y. 13201
315-476-7418

HANKSCRAFT
Div. of Gerber Products Co.
P.O. Box 120
Reedsburg, Wis. 53959
608-524-4341

HANNA CHEMICAL COATINGS CORP.
1313 Windsor Ave.
Columbus, Ohio 43211
614-294-3361

HAPPY JACK, INC.
P.O. Box 475
Snow Hill, N.C. 28580
919-747-2911

HARRIS, J. W., CO., INC.
10930 Deerfield Rd.
Cincinnati, Ohio 45242
513-891-2000

HARRISON SPECIALTY CO., INC.
P.O. Box H
Canton, Mass. 02021

HARRIS, P. F., CO., INC.
110 West 9th St.
North Little Rock, Ark. 72114

HART-DELTA, INC.
P.O. Drawer 340
Zachary, La. 70791

HARTZ MOUNTAIN CORP., THE
700 S. Fourth St.
Harrison, N.J. 07029
201-481-4800

HARVEST BRAND
A Div. of Harvest Industries
P.O. Box 46
Pittsburg, Kans. 66762
316-231-6700

HASK INC.
277 Northern Blvd.
Great Neck, L.I., N.Y. 11021
516-466-0660

HASTINGS MANUFACTURING CO.
325 N. Hanover St.
Hastings, Mich. 49058
616-945-2491

HAVER-LOCKHART LABORATORIES
See BAYVET DIVISION, CUTTER LABORATORIES,
    INC.

**HAVILAND AGRICULTURAL CHEMICAL
CO.**
1845 Sterling N.W.
Grand Rapids, Mich. 49504
616-364-7501

HAVILAND PRODUCTS CO.
421 Ann St. N.W.
Grand Rapids, Mich. 49504
616-361-6691

HCA FOOD CORP.
See DOXSEE FOOD CORP.

HEAD FIRST, INC.
6430 Sunset Blvd.
Hollywood, Calif. 90028
213-461-4058

HELENA RUBINSTEIN, INC.
300 Park Ave.
New York, N.Y. 10022
212-935-5300

HELENE CURTIS INDUSTRIES, INC.
4401 W. North Ave.
Chicago. Ill. 60639
312-292-2264

HELP, INC.
122 W. Kinzie St.
Chicago, Ill. 60610

HENDRIX AND DAIL, INC.
P.O. Box 631
Greenville, N.C. 27834
919-758-4263

HENRY FIELD SEED AND NURSERY CO.
407 Sycamore St.
Shenandoah, Iowa 51602
712-246-2110

HERALD PHARMACAL, INC.
6503 Warwick Rd.
Richmond, Va. 23225
804-745-3400

HERBERT LABORATORIES
Dermatology Div. of Allergan Pharmaceuticals, Inc.
2525 Dupont Dr.
Irvine, Calif. 92713
714-752-4500

HERBOLD LABORATORY, INC.
7723 Densmore Ave.
Van Nuys, Calif. 91406

HERCO INC.
One Chocolate Ave.
Hershey, Pa. 17033
717-534-3480

HERCULES CHEMICAL CO., INC.
84 Fifth Ave.
New York, N.Y. 10011
212-989-0200

HERCULES INCORPORATED
910 Market St.
Wilmington, Del. 19899
302-575-7071

HERSHEY ESTATES
See HERCO INC.

HESS & CLARK, INC.
7th and Orange Sts.
Ashland, Ohio 44805-1799
419-289-9129

HESS HAIR MILK LABORATORIES, INC.
1911 Rice St.
P.O. Box 17100
St. Paul, Minn. 55117
612-488-7261

HEWITT SOAP CO., INC.
333 Linden Ave.
Dayton, Ohio 45403
513-253-1151

HIGGINS INK CO., INC.
See FABER-CASTELL CORP.

HIGH CHEMICAL CO.
1760 N. Howard St.
Philadelphia, Pa. 19122
215-739-4080

HILEX DIVISION
Purex Corp.
24600 S. Main St.
Carson, Calif. 90749
213-775-2111

HILL DERMACEUTICALS, INC.
P.O. Box 19283
Orlando, Fla. 32814
305-896-8280

HILLTOP LABORATORIES
2035-2155 E. Larpenteur Ave.
St. Paul, Minn. 55109
612-777-6601

HILLYARD CHEMICAL CO.
302 N. 4th St.
St. Joseph, Mo. 64502
816-233-1321

HILO PRODUCTS DIVISION
NIP-CO Manufacturing, Inc.
P.O. Box 368
Glenford, N.Y. 12433
914-657-8100

HINDU INCENSE
200 N. Laflin St.
Chicago, Ill. 60607
312-421-2383

HOBART LABORATORIES, INC.
900 N. Franklin St.
Chicago, Ill. 60610
312-787-3746

HOECHST-ROUSSEL PHARMACEUTICALS INC.
Rte. 202-206 North
Somerville, N.J. 08876
Emergency phone no.: 201-231-2000

HOFFMANN-LA ROCHE, INC.
Nutley, N.J. 07110
201-235-5000

HOLCOMB, J. I., RESEARCH LABORATORIES
4401 Cold Spring Rd.
Indianapolis, Ind. 46208
317-632-3200

HOLLAND-RANTOS CO., INC.
Enterprise Ave.
P.O. Box 5147
Trenton, N.J. 08638
609-392-5135

HOLLINGSHEAD, R. M., CORP.
See CLASSIC CHEMICAL

HOLLISTER-STIER LABORATORIES
North 3525 Regal St.
Box 3145, Term. Annex
Spokane, Wash. 99220
509-489-5656

HOLLYWOOD CHEMISTS
7723 Densmore Ave.
Van Nuys, Calif. 91406
213-997-7838

HOLLYWOOD SHOE POLISH, INC.
7 East 43rd St.
New York, N.Y. 10017
212-490-3163

HOLT-LLOYD INDUSTRIES
185 Great Neck Rd.
Great Neck, N.Y. 11021
516-482-8058

HONOLULU WOOD TREATING CO., LTD.
P.O. Box 30246
Honolulu, Hawaii 96820
808-682-5704

HOOKER CHEMICAL CO.
See OCCIDENTAL CHEMICAL CO.

HOOKER CHEMICALS & PLASTICS CORP.
345 Third St.
Niagara Falls, N.Y. 14302
716-278-7000

HOPKINS AGRICULTURAL CHEMICAL CO.
P.O. Box 7532
Madison, Wis. 53707
608-222-0624
If no answer: 608-233-5039

HOPPE, FRANK A.
Div. of Penguin Industries, Inc.
Airport Industrial Mall
Coatesville, Pa. 19320
215-384-6000

HOUBIGANT, INC.
1135 Pleasant View Terrace West
Ridgefield, N.J. 07657
201-941-3400

HOUSEHOLD RESEARCH INSTITUTE
2126 Edison Ave.
San Leandro, Calif. 94577
415-638-1114

HOUSE OF LOWELL, INC.
   1264 Dayton Rd.
   Greenville, Ohio 45331
   513-548-1001

HOUSE OF WESTMORE, INC.
   Pierce's Rd.
   Newburgh, N.Y. 12550
   914-568-8500

HOWARD TRESSES, INC.
   211 W. Broadway
   Inwood, N.Y. 11696
   516-239-6066

HOWLAND CHEMICAL
   410-420 Freylinghausen Ave.
   Newark, N.J. 07114

HOYT LABORATORIES
   Div. of Colgate-Palmolive Co.
   575 University Ave.
   Norwood, Mass. 02062
   617-769-6850

HUBBARD, J., INC.
   P.O. Box 1274
   94 Ash St.
   Nashua, N.H. 03061
   603-882-3231

HUBBARD'S IMPERIAL, INC.
   2819 Southwest Blvd.
   Kansas City, Mo. 64108
   816-561-5377

HUB STATES CORP.
   419 E. Washington
   Indianapolis, Ind. 46204
   317-636-6255

HUGE' CO., INC., THE
   P.O. Box 24198
   St. Louis, Mo. 63130
   314-725-2555
   314-965-8662 (Sundays)

HUGGINS, JAMES, & SON, INC.
   323 Commercial St.
   Malden, Mass. 02148
   617-324-0694

HUMCO LABORATORY, INC.
   P.O. Drawer 2550
   Texarkana, Tex. 75501
   214-793-3174

HUMPHREYS PHARMACAL, INC.
   63 Meadows Rd.
   Rutherford, N.J. 07070
   201-933-7744

HUNTER, D. L., & CO.
   405 E. Mary St.
   Dublin, Ga. 31021

HUNTER PRODUCTS CORP.
   8603 Botts Lane
   San Antonio, Tex. 78217
   512-824-8042

HUNTINGTON LABORATORIES, INC.
   P.O. Box 710
   Huntington, Ind. 46750
   219-356-8100

HYDE OIL CO.
   P.O. Box 426
   Pipestone, Minn. 56164
   507-825-5225

HYDROSAL CO.
   5929 State Rt. 128
   P.O. Box 8
   Miamitown, Ohio 45041
   513-353-2200

HY-GRADE LABORATORIES, INC.
   233 S. Fifth St.
   Grand Junction, Colo. 81501
   303-243-1121

HYNSON, WESTCOTT & DUNNING, INC.
   Charles & Chase Sts.
   Baltimore, Md. 21201
   301-837-0890

HYSAN CORP.
   919 W. 38th St.
   Chicago, Ill. 60609
   312-376-8900

HY-TOP PRODUCTS
   See GREAT ATLANTIC & PACIFIC TEA CO., INC.

I

ICI AMERICAS INC.
   Agricultural Chemicals Div.
   Wilmington, Del. 19897
   302-575-3000

ICN PHARMACEUTICALS, INC.
   222 N. Vincent Ave.
   Covina, Calif. 91722
   213-967-5121

IDEAL STENCIL MACHINE CO.
   P.O. Box 305
   Belleville, Ill. 62222
   618-233-0162

ILLINOIS BRONZE PAINT CO.
300 E. Main St.
Lake Zurich, Ill. 60047
312-438-8201

IMC CHEMICAL GROUP
See INTERNATIONAL MINERALS & CHEMICAL CORP.

INDIUM CORPORATION OF AMERICA
1676 Lincoln Ave.
P.O. Box 269
Utica, N.Y. 13503
315-797-1630

INDUSTRIAL EQUITIES, INC.
9300 Rayo Ave.
South Gate, Calif. 90280
213-775-2111

INDUSTRIAL FUMIGANT CO., THE
601 E. 159th St.
P.O. Box 1200
Olathe, Kan. 66061
913-782-7600

INMONT CORP.
1255 Broad St.
Clifton, N.J. 07015
201-365-3400

INTERNATIONAL CHEMICAL LABORATORIES
185 Park Dr.
Eastchester, N.Y. 10707
914-793-0959

INTERNATIONAL LUBRICANT CORP.
P.O. Box 51118
New Orleans, La. 70151
504-833-8261

INTERNATIONAL MINERALS & CHEMICAL CORP.
IMC Chemical Group
Industrial Chemicals Div.
P.O. Box 207
Terre Haute, Ind. 47808
812-232-0121

INTERNATIONAL PAINT CO., INC.
2270 Morris Ave.
Union, N.J. 07083
201-686-1300

INTERNATIONAL PHARMACEUTICAL CORP.
See MARION LABORATORIES, INC.

INTERNATIONAL PLUMBING PRODUCTS, INC.
195 E. Merrick Rd.
P.O. Box 752
Freeport, N.Y. 11520
516-546-1100

INTERNATIONAL SALT CO.
Clarks Summit, Pa. 18411
717-587-5131

INTEX PRODUCTS, INC.
P.O. Box 6648
Greenville, S.C. 29606
803-242-6152

INVENTO PRODUCTS CORP.
39-25 Skillman Ave.
Long Island City, N.Y. 11101
212-786-8528

IODENT CO.
E-4111 Andover, Suite #200
Bloomfield Hills, Mich. 48013
313-647-0777

IOWA PAINT MANUFACTURING CO., INC.
17th & Grand Ave.
Des Moines, Iowa 50309
515-283-1501

IRMA SHORELL, INC.
515 Madison Ave.
New York, N.Y. 10022
212-355-6747

IVES LABORATORIES INC.
685 Third Ave.
New York, N.Y. 10017
212-986-1000

IVES, SYBIL, INC.
635 W. 18th St.
Hialeah, Fla. 33010
305-885-1911

IVY CORP.
23 Fairfield Pl.
West Caldwell, N.J. 07006
201-575-1990

J

JACKSON & PERKINS CO.
P.O. Box 1028
Medford, Ore. 97501
503-776-2000

JACQUELINE COCHRAN, INC.
630 Fifth Ave.
New York, N.Y. 10111
212-489-2430

JAFRA COSMETICS, INC.
2451 Townsgate Rd.
Westlake Village, Calif. 91359
617-421-7000

JAMES AUSTIN CO.
P.O. Drawer 1
Mars, Pa. 16046
412-625-1535

JAMES B. DAY & CO.
Day Lane
Carpentersville, Ill. 60110
312-428-2651

JANCYN MANUFACTURING CORP.
6679 Peachtree Industrial Blvd.
Norcross, Ga. 30092

JASCO CHEMICAL CORP.
P.O. Drawer J
Mountain View, Calif. 94042
415-968-6005

JEAN NATE
Div. Lanvin-Charles of the Ritz Inc.
40 W. 57th St.
New York, N.Y. 10019
212-621-7300

JEAN PATOU, INC.
Sub. of Borden Inc.
680 Fifth Ave.
New York, N.Y. 10019
212-581-1800

JEAN PIERRE PRODUCTS, INC.
19750 Magellan Dr.
Torrance, Calif. 90504
213-532-3303

JEFFREY MARTIN, INC.
1020 Commerce Ave.
Union, N.J. 07083
201-687-4000

JENKINS LABORATORIES, INC.
17-19 Wall St.
Auburn, N.Y. 13021
315-252-3561

JENNY DIVISION
Homestead Industries
P.O. Box 348
Coraopolis, Pa. 15108
412-264-3240

JENSEN-SALSBERY LABORATORIES
Div. of Burroughs-Wellcome Co.
520 W. 21st St.
Kansas City, Mo. 64108
816-471-4080

JERGENS, ANDREW, CO.
2535 Spring Grove Ave.
Cincinnati, Ohio 45214
513-421-1400

JERIS SALES CO.
See WINARICK, AR., INC.

JOHN A. EARL, INC.
216-222 Union St.
Hackensack, N.J. 07601
201-342-2453

JOHNSON & JOHNSON
Research Center
New Brunswick, N.J. 08903
201-524-0400

JOHNSON & JOHNSON BABY PRODUCTS
CO.
Raritan, N.J. 08869
201-524-0400

JOHNSON NURSERIES
Div. of Plantabbs Corp.
See PLANTABBS CORP.

JOHNSON PRODUCTS CO., INC.
8522 S. LaFayette Ave.
Chicago, Ill. 60620
312-483-4100

JOHNSON, S. C., & SON, INC.
1525 Howe St.
Racine, Wis. 53403
414-631-2111

JOHNSTON, GASTON, CORP.
24-64 45th St.
Long Island City, N.Y. 11103
212-932-0200

JOLEN CREME BLEACH CORP.
25 Walls Dr.
Fairfield, Conn. 06430
203-259-8779

JONES BLAIR CO.
P.O. Box 35286
Dallas, Tex. 75235
214-353-1600

JONES CHEMICALS, INC.
100 Sunny Sol Blvd.
Caledonia, N.Y. 14423
716-538-2311

JOTUN-BALTIMORE COPPER PAINT CO.
840 Key Hwy.
Baltimore, Md. 21230
301-539-0045

JOVAN, INC.
875 N. Michigan Ave.
Chicago, Ill. 60611
312-951-7000

K

KALO AGRICULTURAL CHEMICALS, INC.
4550 W. 109th St.
Overland Park, Kans. 66211
800-255-5196

KANO LABORATORIES, INC.
1000 S. Thompson Lane
Nashville, Tenn. 37211
615-833-4101

KASSOY, I., JEWELERS' SUPPLIERS
30 W. 47th St.
New York, N.Y. 10036
212-582-3260

KAY CHEMICAL CO.
300 Swing Rd.
Greensboro, N.C. 27409
919-292-7713

KAY, MARY, COSMETICS
8787 Stemmons Frwy.
Dallas, Tex. 75247
214-630-8787

KAZ, INC.
614 W. 49th St.
New York, N.Y. 10019
212-586-1630

KEDRIN PHARMACALS, INC.
25 W. 43rd St.
New York, N.Y. 10036
212-244-7440

KELLOGG'S INSECTICIDE CO.
213 Agostino Rd.
San Gabriel, Calif. 91776

KEMIKO, INC.
4343 Temple City Blvd.
Temple City, Calif. 91780
213-579-6270

KEM MANUFACTURING CORP.
2075 Tucker Industrial Rd.
Tucker, Ga. 30084
404-938-7980

KENITE LABORATORY
R.D. 2, Route 92, Stonecrest
Tunkhannock, Pa. 18657
717-836-3261

KENTILE FLOORS INC.
58 Second Ave.
Brooklyn, N.Y. 11215
212-768-9500

KERR, FRANK W., CHEMICAL CO.
43155 W. Nine Mile Rd.
Northville, Mich. 48167
313-349-5000

KERR-MC GEE CORP.
P.O. Box 25861
Oklahoma City, Okla. 73125
405-270-1313

KESTER SOLDER DIVISION
Litton Systems, Inc.
4201 Wrightwood Ave.
Chicago, Ill. 60639
312-235-1600

KEY PHARMACEUTICALS, INC.
P.O. Box 694307, Norland Branch
Miami, Fla. 33169
305-652-2276

KEYSTONE LABORATORIES, INC.
1103 Kansas St.
P.O. Box 2026
Memphis, Tenn. 38101
901-774-8860

KIDDE, WALTER, & CO., INC.
675 Main St.
Belleville, N.J. 07109
201-759-5000

KIEFER MC NEIL
Div. of McNeil Corp.
999 Sweitzer Ave.
Akron, Ohio 44311
216-253-7194

KILGORE CORP.
Toone, Tenn. 38381
901-658-5231

KING CHEMICAL
Div. of W. M. Barr & Co.
P.O. Box 1879
Memphis, Tenn. 38101
901-775-0100

KING OF ALL MANUFACTURING, INC.
P.O. Box 6047
Flint, Mich. 48508
313-232-3264

KING PESTICIDES LTD.
Campbellville
Ontario L0P 1B0
Canada

KING PHARMACEUTICAL CO., INC.
26 N. 77th St.
Birmingham, Ala. 35206
205-833-2168

KING RESEARCH, INC.
114 12th St.
Brooklyn, N.Y. 11215
212-788-0122

KINGSFORD CO.
P.O. Box 24305
Oakland, Calif. 94623
415-271-7000

KINGSWOOD LABORATORIES, INC.
336 Heather Dr.
Carmel, Ind. 46032
317-846-7452

KINNEY & COMPANY, INC.
P.O. Box 583
Columbus, Ind. 48201
812-372-4431

KIRKMAN LABORATORIES, INC.
934 N.E. 25th Ave.
Portland, Ore. 97208
503-233-4441

KITTEN & BEAR CHEMICALS, INC.
See STEWART SANITARY SUPPLY, INC.

KIWI POLISH CO. PTY, LTD.
Route 662
Douglassville, Pa. 19518
215-326-5800

KLEAN-STRIP
Div. of W. M. Barr & Co.
P.O. Box 1879
Memphis, Tenn. 38101
901-775-0100

KLEER-FLO CO.
6600 Washington Ave. S.
Eden Prairie, Minn. 55344
612-941-6710

KLEIN, CALVIN, COSMETICS CORP.
9 W. 57th St.
New York, N.Y. 10019
212-759-8888

KLENZADE PRODUCTS DIVISION
Economics Laboratory, Inc.
Osborn Building
St. Paul, Minn. 55102
612-224-4678

KNIGHT, MAURICE A., CO.
P.O. Box 111
Akron, Ohio 44309
216-724-1277

KNOLL PHARMACEUTICAL CO.
30 N. Jefferson Rd.
Whippany, N.J. 07981
201-887-8300

KNOMARK, INC.
132 Merrick Blvd.
Jamaica, N.Y. 11434
212-276-3400

KOCIDE CHEMICAL CORP.
12701 Almeda Rd.
Houston, Tex. 77045
713-433-6404

KOHNSTAMM, H., & CO., INC.
161 Ave. of the Americas
New York, N.Y. 10013
212-620-4800

KOLMAR LABORATORIES, INC.
Skyline Dr.
Port Jervis, N.Y. 12771
914-856-5311

KONDON MANUFACTURING CO.
Div. Wonderful Dream Salve Co.
P.O. Box 223
Croswell, Mich. 48422
313-359-5811

KOPPERS CO., INC.
Koppers Building
Pittsburgh, Pa. 15219
412-227-2000

KOREX CO.
50000 W. Pontiac Trail
Wixom, Mich. 48096

KOSS, PAUL, SUPPLY CO.
332 E. Grand Ave.
South San Francisco, Calif. 94080
415-871-8787

KRAZY GLUE INC.
53 W. 23rd St.
New York, N.Y. 10010
212-741-9544

KREMERS-URBAN CO.
5600 W. County Line Rd.
P.O. Box 2038
Milwaukee, Wis. 53201
414-354-4300

KRESO, INC.
418 Dovetree Mall - Center Bldg.
42nd & Center Sts.
Omaha, Neb. 68105

KRESS AND OWEN CO.
P.O. Box 198
Oceanport, N.J. 07757
201-222-3617

KRUEGER, B. H., INC.
50 Noble St.
Brooklyn, N.Y. 11222

KRYLON, CONSUMER PRODUCTS
Div. of Borden Chemical
180 E. Broad St.
Columbus, Ohio 43215
614-225-4896

KURFEES COATINGS, INC.
201 E. Market St.
Louisville, Ky. 40201
502-584-0151

KURLASH/DIAMOND DEB LTD.
175 Great Neck Rd.
Great Neck, N.Y. 11021
516-466-6310

KWAL PAINTS, INC.
3900 Joliet St.
Denver, Colo. 80217
303-371-5600

KYANIZE PAINTS, INC.
Second & Boston Sts.
Everett, Mass. 02149
617-387-5000

L

LABBCO, INC.
P.O. Box 14466
Houston, Tex. 77021
713-747-9133

LA CROSSE PHARMACEUTICAL CO.
Div. of General Medical Corp.
1502 Miller Dr.
LaCrosse, Wis. 54601
608-782-0885

LAIDLAW CORP.
1212 East 5th St.
Metropolis, Ill. 62960
618-524-9394

LAKE PRODUCTS CO., INC.
P.O. Box 498
Ballwin, Mo. 63011
314-536-1600

LAMAC PROCESS CO.
4645 Gateway Circle
Dayton, Ohio 45440
513-294-2214

LA MAUR, INC.
Consumer Products Div.
P.O. Box 1221
Minneapolis, Minn. 55440
612-571-1234

LAMBDA INC.
721 Sheridan Ave.
Cody, Wyo. 82414
307-587-4973

LAMBERT-KAY
Div. of Carter-Wallace, Inc.
P.O. Box 418
Cranbury, N.J. 08512
609-655-6563

LANCOME
Div. of Cosmair
530 Fifth Ave.
New York, N.Y. 10036
212-697-5115

LANDER CO., INC.
141 Chenango St.
Binghamton, N.Y. 13902

LAND O'LAKES, INC.
Agricultural Services
2827 Eighth Ave. S.
Fort Dodge, Iowa 50501
515-576-7311

LAN-LAY CO.
465 Park Ave.
San Jose, Calif. 95110
408-288-9595

LANMAN & KEMP-BARCLAY & CO.
25 Woodland Ave.
Westwood, N.J. 07675
201-666-4990

LANNETT CO., INC.
9000 State Rd.
Philadelphia, Pa. 19136
215-333-9000

LAN-O-SHEEN, INC.
One W. Water
Saint Paul, Minn. 55107
612-224-5681

LANVIN PARFUMS, INC.
650 Fifth Ave.
New York, N.Y. 10019
212-246-3070

LARSON LABORATORIES, INC.
1320 Irwin Dr.
Erie, Pa. 16505
814-452-6815

LAST, ALVIN, INC.
145 Palisades St.
Dobbs Ferry, N.Y. 10522
914-693-2221

LAUDER, ESTEE, INC.
767 Fifth Ave.
New York, N.Y. 10022
212-572-4200

LAUNDRY AIDS
333 Starke Rd.
Carlstadt, N.J. 07072

LAVOPTIK COMPANY, INC.
661 Western Ave. N.
St. Paul, Minn. 55103
612-489-1351

LAWTER CHEMICALS, INC.
990 Skokie Blvd.
Northbrook, Ill. 60062
312-498-4700

LEA MANUFACTURING CO.
P.O. Box 71
Waterbury, Conn. 06720
203-753-5116

LEDERLE LABORATORIES
Div. of American Cyanamid Co.
Pearl River, N.Y. 10965
914-735-5000

LEECH PRODUCTS, INC.
4th & Hendricks Sts.
P.O. Box 2147
Hutchinson, Kans. 67501
316-665-7961

LEEDSALL CHEMICAL CO., INC.
410-416 S. Charles St.
Baltimore, Md. 21201
301-727-6633

LEEMING/PACQUIN
Div. of Pfizer Inc.
100 Jefferson Rd.
Parsippany, N.J. 07054
201-887-2100

LEE, SANDRA, PRODUCTS
13165 N.W. 47th Ave.
Miami, Fla. 33054
305-685-6089

LEFFINGWELL CHEMICAL CO.
P.O. Box 1880
Brea, Calif. 92621
714-529-3973

LE GEAR DIVISION
O'Neal, Jones & Feldman, Inc.
2510 Metro Blvd.
St. Louis County, Mo. 63043
314-569-3610

LEGGE, WALTER G., CO., INC.
122 E. 42nd St.
New York, N.Y. 10168
212-867-8865

LEHMAN BROS. CORP.
22 Halladay St.
Jersey City, N.J. 07304
201-434-1882-3
212-732-3897-8

LEHN & FINK PRODUCTS GROUP,
STERLING DRUG INC.
Consumer Products Div.
225 Summit Ave.
Montvale, N.J. 07645
201-573-5700

LEMMON COMPANY
Sellersville, Pa. 18960
215-723-5544

LEO PRODUCTS CO.
7636 N. Milwaukee Ave.
Chicago, Ill. 60648
312-965-0600

LE PAGE'S, INC.
Subsidiary of The Papercraft Corp.
Papercraft Park
Pittsburgh, Pa. 15238
412-362-8000

L'ERIN COSMETICS
P.O. Box 57
Winston-Salem, N.C. 27102
919-744-3526

LESTER LABORATORIES, INC.
2370 Lawrence St.
Atlanta, Ga. 30344
404-767-0277

LETHELIN PRODUCTS CO., INC.
15 MacQuesten Pkwy. S.
Mt. Vernon, N.Y. 10550
914-667-1820

LEVER BROTHERS CO., INC.
Research Center
45 River Rd.
Edgewater, N.J. 07020
201-943-7100

LEWAL INDUSTRIES, INC.
65 Plain Ave.
New Rochelle, N.Y. 10801
914-235-1203

LEWIS/HOWE CO.
See NORCLIFF THAYER, INC.

LEWIS RESEARCH LABORATORIES CO.
1 Blue Hill Plaza
Pearl River, N.Y. 10965
914-735-2400

LIFE LABORATORIES, INC.
9380 San Fernando Rd.
Sun Valley, Calif. 91352
213-875-0330

LIFE-LIKE PRODUCTS, INC.
1600 Union Ave.
Baltimore, Md. 21211
301-889-1023

LILLY, ELI, AND CO.
307 E. McCarty St.
Indianapolis, Ind. 46285
317-261-2000

LILLY, THE CHAS. H., CO.
7737 N.E. Killingsworth
Portland, Ore. 97218
503-256-4600

LINCK, O. E., CO.
Div. of Walco-Linck Corp.
Junction Routes 3 & 46
Clifton, N.J. 07015
201-471-1070

LINE TAMER INC.
2 Coral Way
Miami, Fla. 33131
305-442-4707

LIQUID GLAZE, INC.
P.O. Box 482
Toccoa, Ga. 30577
404-886-6853

LIQUID PAPER CORP.
1001 Rutherford Dr.
Greenville, Tex. 75401
617-421-7000

LOCTITE CORP.
North Mountain Rd.
Newington, Conn. 06111
203-278-1280

LORENZ CHEMICAL CO.
P.O. Box 7348
Omaha, Nebr. 68107
402-342-1623

LORVIC CORP., THE
8810 Frost Ave.
St. Louis, Mo. 63134
314-524-7444

LOS ANGELES CHEMICAL CO.
4545 Ardine St.
South Gate, Calif. 90280
213-583-4761

LOS ANGELES SOAP CO.
P.O. Box 2198, Terminal Annex
Los Angeles, Calif. 90051
213-627-5011

LOTSHAW CO., THE
8140 N. Ridgeway Ave.
Skokie, Ill. 60076
312-673-0040

LOUANGEL CORP.
70 Franklin Ave.
Brooklyn, N.Y. 11205
212-625-0114

LOWMAN CO., THE
U.S. Highway 6 East
Waterloo, Ind. 46793
219-837-6341

L & R MANUFACTURING CO.
577 Elm St.
Kearny, N.J. 07032
201-991-5330

L.T. LABORATORIES
850 Boylston St.
Brookline, Mass. 02167
617-738-1340

LUCIDOL DIVISION
Pennwalt Corp.
1740 Military Rd.
Buffalo, N.Y. 14240
716-877-1740

LUCILLE BOUCHARD MINK OIL COSMETIQUES, INC.
P.O. Box 46
Circleville, N.Y. 10919
914-692-2777

LUCKY HEART COSMETICS
390 Mulberry
Memphis, Tenn. 38101
901-526-7658

LUSTRASILK CORP.
P.O. Box 334
Minneapolis, Minn. 55440
612-425-1377

LUTHER FORD & CO.
100 N. Seventh St.
Minneapolis, Minn. 55403
612-332-2441

LUZIER, INC.
P.O. Box 496
Kansas City, Mo. 64141
816-531-8338

LYDIA O'LEARY, INC.
575 Madison Ave.
New York, N.Y. 10022
212-753-4600

LYON CHEMICALS, INC.
See VAN WATERS & ROGERS

LYSTADS, INC.
901 University Ave.
Grand Forks, N. Dak. 58201
701-775-6283

M

MAAS, ALBERT G., CO.
155 E. Maryland St.
Indianapolis, Ind. 46204
317-632-8315

MAAS & WALDSTEIN CO.
2121 McCarter Hwy.
Newark, N.J. 07104
201-484-1600

MAC DERMID, INC.
P.O. Box 671
Waterbury, Conn. 06720
203-754-6161

MACKLANBURG-DUNCAN CO.
P.O. Box 25188
Oklahoma City, Okla. 73125
405-528-4411

MACKWIN CO.
Box 108
Winona, Minn. 55987
507-452-2910

MACO LABORATORIES
558 James Ave. S.E.
Grand Rapids, Mich. 49503

MAC-O-LAC PAINTS INC.
5400 E. Nevada
Detroit, Mich. 48234
313-892-1900

MACSIL, INC.
1326 Frankford Ave.
Philadelphia, Pa. 19125
215-423-5566

MAGIC AMERICAN CHEMICAL CORP.
23700 Mercantile Rd.
Cleveland, Ohio 44122
216-464-2353

MAGIC MARKER CORP.
1 Magic Marker Lane
Cherry Hill, N.J. 08003
609-424-5880

MAGICOLOR PAINT CO.
1191 S. Wheeling Rd.
Wheeling, Ill. 60090
312-541-9000

MAGNA CORP.
7505 Fannin
Houston, Tex. 77054
713-795-4270

MAGNA, INC.
P.O. Box 473
Salt River Rd. & Johnson St.
Leitchfield, Ky. 42754
502-259-4021

MAHDEEN LABORATORIES
P.O. Box 1959
Fort Worth, Tex. 76101
817-293-0450

MAJESTIC WAX CO.
6035 E. 38th Ave.
Denver, Colo. 80207
303-355-1606

MALLARD, INC.
3021 Wabash Ave.
Detroit, Mich. 48216
313-964-3910

MALLINCKRODT, INC.
Mallinckrodt & Second Sts.
St. Louis, Mo. 63147
314-895-0123

MALTER INTERNATIONAL
P.O. Box 6099
New Orleans, La. 70174

MANHATTAN PRODUCTS, INC.
333 Starke Rd.
Carlstadt, N.J. 07072

MANOSTAT CORP.
519 Eighth Ave.
New York, N.Y. 10018
212-594-6262

MANSTAN CHEMICAL CO.
Div. of Woolfoam Corp.
1 W. 37th St.
New York, N.Y. 10018

MARATHON OIL CO.
Findlay, Ohio 45840
419-422-2121

MARCELLE HYPO-ALLERGENIC
COSMETICS
See PROFESSIONAL COSMETIC CORP.

MARCHAND, CHARLES, CO., THE
66 E. 34th St.
New York, N.Y. 10016
212-679-0900

MARIN COUNTY DEPARTMENT OF
AGRICULTURE
Civic Center, Room 422
San Rafael, Calif. 94903
415-499-6349

MARINE ELECTROLYSIS ELIMINATOR
CO.
1137 Southwest Hanford St.
Seattle, Wash. 98134
206-624-2266

MARION LABORATORIES, INC.
P.O. Box 9627
Kansas City, Mo. 64134
816-761-2500

MARMET SUPPLY CO.
P.O. Drawer 671
Montgomery, W. Va. 25136

MARRACH, INC.
3060 Valleywood Dr.
Dayton, Ohio 45429
513-293-2026

MARSHALL, EVELYN, COSMETICS, LTD.
14 E. 38th St.
New York, N.Y. 10016
212-532-6400

MARSON CORP.
130 Crescent Ave.
Chelsea, Mass. 02150
617-884-7760

MARTIN, C. J., CO.
P.O. Box 1089
606 W. Main St.
Nacogdoches, Tex. 75961
713-564-1413

MARTIN DRUG CO.
P.O. Box 8372
Jackson, Miss. 39204
601-353-2781

MARTIN, JEFFREY, INC.
1090 Morris Ave.
Union, N.J. 07083
201-687-4000

MARTIN-SENOUR CO., THE
Div. of the Sherwin-Williams Co.
1370 Ontario St.
Cleveland, Ohio 44113
216-566-3108

MARVEL OIL CO., INC.
331 N. Main St.
Port Chester, N.Y. 10573
914-937-4000

MARY KAY COSMETICS
8787 Stemmons Frwy.
Dallas, Tex. 75247
214-630-8787

MARY QUANT COSMETICS, LTD.
655 Madison Ave.
New York, N.Y. 10021
212-758-1072

MASURY-COLUMBIA CO.
1502 N. 25th Ave.
Melrose Park, Ill. 60160
312-345-9202

MASURY PAINT CO.
1403 Severn
Baltimore, Md. 21230
301-837-5150

MATSON, JR., E. M., CO.
7808 8th Ave. S.
Seattle, Wash. 98108
206-762-2066

MAUGET, J. J., CO.
2838 No. Naomi St.
Burbank, Calif. 91504
213-849-2309

MAUTZ PAINT CO.
939 E. Washington Ave.
Madison, Wis. 53703
608-255-1661

MAX FACTOR & CO.
1655 N. McCadden Pl.
Hollywood, Calif. 90028
213-856-6000

MAXIM CHEMICALS LTD.
116 Bellingham St.
Chelsea, Mass. 02150
617-884-2824

MAYBELLINE CO.
3030 Jackson Ave.
Memphis, Tenn. 38151
901-320-2011

MAYER LABORATORIES, INC.
701 Bridgeway
Sausalito, Calif. 94965
415-332-4000

MAYFIELD, DR., LABORATORIES
1209 S. Main St.
Charles City, Iowa 50616
515-228-5161

MAYFLOWER PAINT CO.
201 E. Market St.
Louisville, Ky. 40201
502-584-0151

MC ALEER MANUFACTURING CO.
Subsidiary of Stan Sax Corp.
101 S. Waterman Ave.
Detroit, Mich. 48217
313-843-5970

MC CLOSKEY VARNISH CO.
7600 State Rd.
Philadelphia, Pa. 19136
215-624-4400

MC CONNELL EQUIPMENT CORP.
P.O. Box 88A
Pampa, Tex. 79065
806-665-1395

MC CONNON & CO.
Winona, Minn. 55987
507-452-2910

MC HUTCHISON & CO., INC.
695 Grand Ave.
Ridgefield, N.J. 07657
201-943-2230

MC KESSON LABORATORIES
P.O. Box 2277
Dublin, Calif. 94566
415-983-8729

MC LAUGHLIN GORMLEY KING CO.
8810 Tenth Ave. N.
Minneapolis, Minn. 55427
612-544-0341

MC NEIL CONSUMER PRODUCTS CO.
Camp Hill Rd.
Fort Washington, Pa. 19034
215-836-4500

MC NEIL PHARMACEUTICAL
MC NEILAB, INC.
Spring House, Pa. 19477
215-628-5000

M. D. INDUSTRIES, INC.
706 Landwehr Rd.
Northbrook, Ill. 60062
312-498-1204

MEAD JOHNSON & CO.
2404 W. Pennsylvania
Evansville, Ind. 47721
812-426-6000

MEDICAL SUPPLY CO.
1027 W. State St.
Rockford, Ill. 61101
815-877-2531

MEDICONE CO.
225 Varick St.
New York, N.Y. 10014
212-924-5166

MEM CO., INC.
Northvale, N.J. 07647
201-767-0100

MENJ LABORATORIES
See MENLEY & JAMES LABORATORIES

MENLEY & JAMES LABORATORIES
Consumer Products Div.
One Franklin Plaza
P.O. Box 8082
Philadelphia, Pa. 19101
215-854-5000

MENNEN CO., THE
Morristown, N.J. 07960
201-538-7100

MENTHOLATUM CO., INC.
1360 Niagara St.
Buffalo, N.Y. 14213
716-882-7660

MERCK SHARP & DOHME
Div. of Merck & Co., Inc.
West Point, Pa. 19486
215-661-5000

MERLE NORMAN COSMETICS
9130 Bellanca Ave.
Los Angeles, Calif. 90045
213-641-3000

MERRELL DOW PHARMACEUTICALS, INC.
Sub. of The Dow Chemical Co.
2110 E. Galbraith
Cincinnati, Ohio 45215
513-948-9111

MERRELL-NATIONAL LABORATORIES
See MERRELL DOW PHARMACEUTICALS, INC.

MERRICK MEDICINE CO.
P.O. Box 1489
Waco, Tex. 76703
817-753-3461

META HENNA INTL., INC.
850 Nicholas Blvd.
Elk Grove Village, Ill. 60007
312-593-3044

MEYER-BLANKE CO.
222 S. Central Ave.
St. Louis, Mo. 63105
314-725-5118

MEYER LABORATORIES, INC.
See GLAXO INC.

MEYER, THEO., INC.
922 Callowhill St.
Philadelphia, Pa. 19123
215-629-1850

MFA OIL CO.
200 S. Seventh
Columbia, Mo. 65201
314-442-0171

MGK (MC LAUGHLIN GORMLEY KING CO.)
8810 Tenth Ave. N.
Minneapolis, Minn. 55427
612-544-0341

MICRO-GEN EQUIPMENT CORP.
See JOHNSON, S. C., & SON, INC.

MIDLAND LABORATORIES, INC.
See ROCHESTER GERMICIDE CO.

MIDWEST MANUFACTURING CO.
17126 Schaefer Hwy.
Detroit, Mich. 48235
313-861-4466

MILES LABORATORIES, INC.
Consumer Products Div.
P.O. Box 340
Elkhart, Ind. 46515
216-262-7478

MILEX PRODUCTS, INC.
5915 Northwest Hwy.
Chicago, Ill. 60631
312-631-6484

MILLER CHEMICAL CO., INC.
F St.
Omaha, Nebr. 68102
402-342-4987

MILLER CHEMICAL & FERTILIZER CORP.
Box 333
Hanover, Pa. 17331
717-632-8921

MILLER, C. J., & CO.
620 Commercial St.
Waterloo, Iowa 50701

MILLER, FRANK, AND SONS, INC.
13831 S. Emerald Ave.
Chicago, Ill. 60627
312-468-3500

MILLER-MORTON CO.
Subsidiary of A. H. Robins Co.
2007 N. Hamilton St.
P.O. Box 6235
Richmond, Va. 23230
804-257-2701

MILLER-NORRIS CO.
11 N.E. Second St.
Oklahoma City, Okla. 73101
405-236-1641

MILL-MARK PHARMACEUTICALS, INC.
1090 Englewood Ave.
Buffalo, N.Y. 14223
716-874-6497

MILTON BRADLEY CO.
P.O. Box 2209
Springfield, Mass. 01101
413-525-6411

MINE SAFETY APPLIANCES CO.
600 Penn Center Blvd.
Pittsburgh, Pa. 15235
412-273-5000

MINNETONKA, INC.
Jonathan Industrial Center
Chaska, Minn. 55318
612-448-4181

MINWAX CO., INC.
Lehn & Fink Industrial Products Div.
102 Chestnut Ridge Plaza
Montvale, N.J. 07645
201-391-0253

MIRACLE ADHESIVES CORP.
250 Pettit Ave.
Bellmore, N.Y. 11710
516-221-0950

MIRACLE PET PRODUCTS, INC.
245 Cornelison Ave.
Jersey City, N.J. 07302
201-432-4700

MIRACLE PLASTICS (N.J.) CORP.
P.O. Box 33
Jersey City, N.J. 07303
201-432-4700

MIRACLE POWER PRODUCTS CORP.
1101 Belt Line St.
Cleveland, Ohio 44109
216-741-1388

MME. C. J. WALKER MFG. CO., INC.
617 Indiana Ave.
Indianapolis, Ind. 46202
317-631-7143

MOBAY CHEMICAL CORP.
Agricultural Chemicals Div.
P.O. Box 4913
Kansas City, Mo. 64120
816-242-2000

MOBIL CHEMICAL CO.
Phosphorus Div.
P.O. Box 26683
Richmond, Va. 23261
804-798-4291

MOBIL OIL CORP.
3225 Gallows Rd.
Fairfax, Va. 22037
703-849-4342

MODERN POOL PRODUCTS, INC.
737 Canal St.-Bldg. 16
Stamford, Conn. 06902
203-348-9208

MODERN PRODUCTS, INC.
3015 W. Vera Ave.
Milwaukee, Wis. 53209
414-352-3333

MOFFET INC.
1001 Franklin Ave.
Garden City, N.Y. 11530
516-747-5471

MOGUL DIVISION
The Dexter Corp.
P.O. Box 200
Chagrin Falls, Ohio 44022
216-247-5000

MOLINARD PERFUMES U.S.A.
P.O. Box 164
Lake Forest, Ill. 60045
312-295-1426

MONSANTO AGRICULTURAL PRODUCTS CO.
800 N. Lindbergh Blvd.
St. Louis, Mo. 63166
314-694-1000

MONTEIL, GERMAINE, COSMETIQUES CORP.
40 W. 57th St.
New York, N.Y. 10019
212-582-3010

MONTGOMERY WARD & CO., INC.
535 W. Chicago Ave.
Chicago, Ill. 60671
312-467-2000

MOORE, A. F., & CO.
538 Franklin St.
Worcester, Mass. 01604
617-757-6739

MOORE, BENJAMIN, & CO.
Chestnut Ridge Rd.
Montvale, N.J. 07645
201-573-9600

MOORE, GOODLOE E., INC.
2811 N. Vermilion St.
Danville, Ill. 61832
217-446-7900

MOORMAN MFG. CO.
1000 N. 30th St.
Quincy, Ill. 62301
217-222-7100

MORGRO CHEMICAL CO.
P.O. Box 151048
Salt Lake City, Utah 84115
801-266-1132

MORRISON'S ORCHARD SUPPLY CO.
Box 111
Yuba City, Calif. 95991

MORWEAR PAINT CO.
2431 Peralta St.
Oakland, Calif. 94607
415-444-6516

MOSS, BELLE, PHARMACEUTICAL CHEMIST
P.O. Box 1278
3900 W. Twelve Mile Rd.
Berkley, Mich. 48072
313-548-5706

MOSS CHEMICAL CO., INC.
183 St. Paul St.
Rochester, N.Y. 14604
716-546-6187

MOSSO DERMATOLOGICALS CO.
Div. Health Care Industries, Inc.
S. Ohio St.
Michigan City, Ind. 46360
219-879-8227

MOTOMCO, INC.
267 Vreeland Ave.
P.O. Box 300
Paterson, N.J. 07513
201-345-6200

M-S-A
See MINE SAFETY APPLIANCES CO.

MSD (MERCK SHARP & DOHME)
Div. of Merck & Co., Inc.
West Point, Pa. 19486
215-661-5000

MT. HOOD CHEMICAL CORP.
4444 N.W. Yeon Ave.
Portland, Ore. 97210
503-227-3505

MT. HOOD SOAP CO.
See MT. HOOD CHEMICAL CORP.

MULTI-CLEAN PRODUCTS DIV.
H. B. Fuller Co.
2277 Ford Pkwy.
St. Paul, Minn. 55116
612-698-8833

MUNICHEM CORP.
P.O. Box 8148
Milwaukee, Wis. 53223
414-251-9690

MURD CO.
121 Cuthbert St.
Philadelphia, Pa. 19106
215-739-6116

MURO PHARMACEUTICAL, INC.
890 East St.
Tewksbury, Mass. 01876
617-851-5981

MURPHY-PHOENIX CO.
9505 Cassius Ave.
Cleveland, Ohio 44105
216-341-2211

MUTUAL PRODUCTS CO.
509 N. Fourth St.
Minneapolis, Minn. 55401
612-335-5112

MYERS, R. A., & CO.
See DALCO CORP.

MYRURGIA PERFUMES, INC.
1370 Ave. of the Americas
New York, N.Y. 10019
212-541-5410

N

NA-CHURS PLANT FOOD CO.
421 Leader St.
Marion, Ohio 43302
614-382-5701

NALCO CHEMICAL CO.
2901 Butterfield Rd.
Oak Brook, Ill. 60521
312-887-7500

NATE, JEAN
Div. Lanvin-Charles of the Ritz Inc.
40 W. 57th St.
New York, N.Y. 10019
212-621-7300

NATIONAL ALLIED PRODUCTS
P.O. Box 411
Omaha, Nebr. 68101
402-391-6411

NATIONAL B. C. SALES, INC.
7323 N. Monticello Ave.
Skokie, Ill. 60076
312-675-2368

NATIONAL BIRD CONTROL LABORATORIES
See NATIONAL B. C. SALES, INC.

NATIONAL CHEMICALS, INC.
105 Liberty St.
P.O. Box 32
Winona, Minn. 55987
507-454-5640

NATIONAL CHEMSEARCH CORP.
2730 Carl Rd.
P.O. Box 2170
Irving, Tex. 75060
214-254-1666

NATIONAL LABORATORIES
See AMERICAN HOECHST CORP., Animal Health Div.

NATIONAL LABORATORIES
Lehn & Fink Industrial Products Div.
225 Summit Ave.
Montvale, N.J. 07645
201-573-5700

NATIONAL MILLING & CHEMICAL CO.
4601 Flat Rock Rd.
Philadelphia, Pa. 19127
215-482-6600

NATIONAL PAINT & VARNISH CO., INC.
2835 E. Washington Blvd.
Los Angeles, Calif. 90023
213-268-2823

NATIONAL PHARMACEUTICALS MFG. CO.
4128 Hayward Ave.
Baltimore, Md. 21215

NATIONAL PRESTO INDUSTRIES, INC.
Eau Claire, Wis. 54701
715-839-2121

NATIONAL-PURITY SOAP & CHEMICAL CO.
110 5th Ave. S.E.
Minneapolis, Minn. 55414
612-378-1467

NATIONAL STARCH AND CHEMICAL CORP.
1700 W. Front St.
Plainfield, N.J. 07063
201-755-4100

NAVY BRAND MANUFACTURING CO.
5111 Southwest Ave.
St. Louis, Mo. 63110
314-865-5500

NAYLOR, H. W., CO., INC.
Morris, N.Y. 13808
607-263-5145

NEPHRON CORP.
3319 Pacific Ave.
P.O. Box 1974
Tacoma, Wash. 98401
206-475-3452

NEPTUNE CHEMICAL
7 Maple Ave.
Haverstraw, N.Y. 10927
914-429-3800

NERO PET PRODUCTS
See MIRACLE PLASTICS (N.J.) CORP.

NESTLE-LeMUR CO.
66 E. 34th St.
New York, N.Y. 10016
212-679-0900

NETTIE ROSENSTEIN, INC.
220 E. 23rd St.
New York, N.Y. 10010
212-371-6300

NEUTROGENA CORP.
5755 W. 96th St.
P.O. Box 45036
Los Angeles, Calif. 90045
213-776-5223

NEW PLANT LIFE
Div. of Charles O. Finley & Co., Inc.
P.O. Box 45
La Porte, Ind. 46350
219-393-3531

NEW YORK VON CO., INC.
P.O. Box 215
Tuckahoe, N.Y. 10707
914-337-5645

NICE-PAK PRODUCTS, INC.
150 N. MacQuesten Pkwy.
Mt. Vernon, N.Y. 10550
914-664-7800

NILODOR CO., INC.
7740 Freedom Ave., N.W.
North Canton, Ohio 44720
216-499-4321

NINA RICCI PARFUMS
630 Fifth Ave.
New York, N.Y. 10111
212-489-2430

NIP-CO MANUFACTURING, INC.
P.O. Box 368
Glenford, N.Y. 12433
914-657-8100

NOMA LITES CORP.
See NOMA-WORLD WIDE, INC.

NOMA-WORLD WIDE, INC.
7400 W. Industrial Dr.
Forest Park, Ill. 60130
312-771-9400

NOPCO CHEMICAL DIVISION
See DIAMOND SHAMROCK, PROCESS CHEMICALS
DIV.

**NOR-AM AGRICULTURAL PRODUCTS,
INC.**
350 W. Shuman Blvd.
Naperville, Ill. 60540
312-961-6500

NORCLIFF THAYER, INC.
Div. of the Revlon Health Care Group
319 S. 4th St.
St. Louis, Mo. 63102
314-621-2304

NORDEN LABORATORIES, INC.
Subsidiary of SmithKline Corp.
P.O. Box 80809
Lincoln, Nebr. 68501
402-475-4541

NORGINE LABORATORIES, INC.
420 Lexington Ave.
New York, N.Y. 10170
212-697-1513

NO-RINSE LABORATORIES
See N/R LABORATORIES, INC.

NORKON PHARMACAL, INC.
1075 Central Park Ave.
Scarsdale, N.Y. 10583
914-472-2737

NORMAN, MERLE, COSMETICS
9130 Bellanca Ave.
Los Angeles, Calif. 90045
213-641-3000

NORRIS INDUSTRIES
Fire & Safety Equipment Div.
P.O. Box 2750
Newark, N.J. 07114
201-248-2200

NORTECH LABORATORIES INC.
4 Midland Ave.
Hicksville, N.Y. 11801
516-935-2040

NORTH AMERICAN CHEMICAL CORP.
178 Keen St.
Paterson, N.J. 07524

NORTHERN PETROCHEMICAL CO.
2350 E. Devon Ave.
Des Plaines, Ill. 60018
312-391-6100

NORTHERN STATES LABORATORIES
107 E. Main St.
Luverne, Minn. 56156

NORTHLAND PRODUCTS CO.
1000 Rainbow Dr.
P.O. Box 418
Waterloo, Iowa 50704
319-234-5586

**NORTHWEST SANITATION PRODUCTS,
INC.**
P.O. Box 1227
Fort Bragg, Calif. 95437
707-964-4647

NORTON PRODUCTS CO.
422 W. Alhambra Blvd.
Los Angeles, Calif. 90012

NORWICH-EATON PHARMACEUTICALS
Div. of MortonNorwich
P.O. Box 191
Norwich, N.Y. 13815
607-335-2565

NORWICH PHARMACAL CO.
See NORWICH-EATON PHARMACEUTICALS

NOTT MANUFACTURING CO., INC.
Pleasant Valley, N.Y. 12569
914-635-3243

NOXELL CORP.
P.O. Box 1799
Baltimore, Md. 21203
301-628-7300

N/R LABORATORIES, INC.
900 E. Franklin St.
Centerville, Ohio 45459
513-433-9570

NU-BALL MANUFACTURING CO.
P.O. Box 685
2137 Sunset Rd.
Des Moines, Iowa 50303
515-288-0231

NUMRICH ARMS CORP.
West Hurley, N.Y. 12491
914-679-2417

NUTRITION CONTROL PRODUCTS
Div. of Pharmex, Inc.
2113 Lincoln St.
Hollywood, Fla. 33022
305-923-2821

NU-VITA PRODUCTS DIVISION
Roffler Industries, Inc.
400 Chess St.
Coraopolis, Pa. 15108
412-771-4333

O

OAKITE PRODUCTS, INC.
50 Valley Rd.
Berkeley Heights, N.J. 07922
201-464-6900

OCCIDENTAL CHEMICAL CO.
9802 Lawndale
P.O. Box 5337
Houston, Tex. 77012
713-477-8811

OCEAN COFFEE COMPANY, INC.
P.O. Box 1573
Shreveport, La. 71102
318-423-5613

ODOL CHEMICAL CORP.
100 Mayhill St.
Saddle Brook, N.J. 07662
201-843-3300

OGILVIE PRODUCTS, INC.
Div. Lehn & Fink Products Group
225 Summit Ave.
Montvale, N.J. 07645
201-573-5700

OIL-DRI CORPORATION OF AMERICA
520 N. Michigan Ave.
Chicago, Ill. 60611
312-321-1515

OJF
See O'NEAL, JONES & FELDMAN PHARMACEUTI-
CALS

OKLAHOMA REFINING CO.
P.O. Box 26386
Oklahoma City, Okla. 73126
405-424-4661

O'LEARY, LYDIA, INC.
575 Madison Ave.
New York, N.Y. 10022
212-753-4600

OLE TIME WOODSMAN, INC.
P.O. Box 731
Concord, Mass. 01742

OLIN CORPORATION
120 Long Ridge Rd.
Stamford, Conn. 06904
203-356-2000

OLYMPIC STAIN
Div. of The Clorox Co.
2233 112th Ave., N.E.
Bellevue, Wash. 98004
206-453-1700

O'NEAL, JONES & FELDMAN PHARMACEUTICALS
2510 Metro Blvd.
Maryland Heights, Mo. 63043
314-569-3610

ONOX, INC.
240 Hamilton Ave.
Palo Alto, Calif. 94301
415-329-9270

ONYX CHEMICAL CO.
Millmaster Onyx Group
190 Warren St.
Jersey City, N.J. 07302
201-434-1700

OPTIMUS PHARMACEUTICALS CO., INC.
P.O. Drawer 97
Taylors, S.C. 29687

ORAL PROPHYLACTIC ASSOCIATION, INC.
1915 E. 8th St.
Duluth, Minn. 55812
218-724-0077

ORGANON INC.
West Orange, N.J. 07052
201-325-4500

ORIOLE EQUIPMENT & SUPPLY CO., INC.
910 W. Pratt St.
Baltimore, Md. 21223
301-837-0955

ORKIN EXTERMINATING CO., INC.
P.O. Box 647
Atlanta, Ga. 30301
404-873-2355

ORLANE/JEAN D'ALBRET
499 Park Ave.
New York, N.Y. 10022
212-757-4200

ORTEGA PHARMACEUTICAL CO., INC.
P.O. Box 6212
Jacksonville, Fla. 32205
904-389-2221

ORTHO DERMATOLOGICAL DIVISION
See ORTHO PHARMACEUTICAL CORP.

ORTHO PHARMACEUTICAL CORP.
Raritan, N.J. 08869
201-524-0400

OSGOOD PRODUCTS CO.
42 Eden Ave.
West Newton, Mass. 02165

OSMOSE WOOD PRESERVING CO. OF AMERICA, INC.
980 Ellicott St.
Buffalo, N.Y. 14209
716-882-5905

OWEN DRUG CO.
1700 S. First St.
Salisbury, N.C. 28144
803-636-0951

OWEN LABORATORIES
P.O. Box 2400
Irving, Tex. 75061
214-659-9400

P

PAAS DYE CO.
See PLOUGH, INC.

PACQUIN DIVISION
See LEEMING/PACQUIN

PADDOCK LABORATORIES, INC.
2744 Lyndale Ave. S.
Minneapolis, Minn. 55408
612-824-2621

PALCO, INC.
See NORTHLAND PRODUCTS CO.

PALM BEACH BEAUTY PRODUCTS CO.
950 Xenia Ave. S.
Minneapolis, Minn. 55416
612-546-0322

PAN DERMA LABORATORIES
1833 S. Ocean Dr.
Suite 1002
Hallandale, Fla. 33009
305-456-0328

PANEF MANUFACTURING CO., INC.
5700 W. Douglas Ave.
Milwaukee, Wis. 53218
414-464-9150

PANTENE CO.
340 Kingsland Ave.
Nutley, N.J. 07110
201-235-4133

PAPER PRODUCTS INC.
P.O. Box 5158
Long Beach, Calif. 90805
213-774-6250

PARAGON PAINT & VARNISH CORP.
5-49 46th Ave.
Long Island City, N.Y. 11101
212-729-7420

PARFUMES LAGERFELD, INC.
1345 Ave. of the Americas
New York, N.Y. 10019
212-399-2000

PARFUMS DUVELLE, INC.
P.O. Box 20125
Portland, Ore. 97220
503-254-1442

PARFUMS GIVENCHY, INC.
Div. Lehn & Fink Products Group
680 Fifth Ave.
New York, N.Y. 10019
201-573-5700

PARK CHEMICAL CO.
8074 Military Ave.
Detroit, Mich. 48204
313-895-7215

PARKE-DAVIS
Div. of Warner-Lambert Co.
201 Tabor Rd.
Morris Plains, N.J. 07950
201-540-2000

PARKER, C. W., CO.
1415 Second Ave.
Des Moines, Iowa 50314
515-243-6610

PARKER DIVISION
Hooker Chemicals and Plastics Corp.
32100 Stephenson Hwy.
Madison Heights, Mich. 48071
313-583-9300

PARKER HERBEX CORP.
1001 Franklin Ave.
Garden City, N.Y. 11530
516-747-5471

PARKER LABORATORIES, INC.
307 Washington St.
Orange, N.J. 07050
201-676-5000

PARKER PEN CO.
Janesville, Wis. 53545
608-754-7711

PASADENA RESEARCH LABORATORIES, INC.
2107 E. Villa St.
Pasadena, Calif. 91107
213-793-2711

PATENT CEREALS SALES CORP.
31 Sheral Dr.
Danville, Ill. 61832
217-446-6009

PATOU, JEAN, INC.
Sub. of Borden Inc.
680 Fifth Ave.
New York, N.Y. 10019
212-581-1800

PATTERSON CHEMICAL CO., INC.
1400 Union Ave.
Kansas City, Mo. 64101
816-842-8211

PATTERSON LABORATORIES, INC.
11930 Pleasant Ave.
Detroit, Mich. 48217
313-843-4500

PAULEN CHEMICAL CO.
P.O. Box 336
Beltsville, Md. 20705
301-937-1400

PAUL KOSS SUPPLY CO.
332 E. Grand Ave.
South San Francisco, Calif. 94080
415-871-8787

PAX COMPANY
580 W. 13th S.
Salt Lake City, Utah 84115
801-973-2800

PAXTON, F. H., AND SONS, INC.
P.O. Box 729
Evanston, Ill. 60204
312-787-3855

PBI/GORDON CORP.
Acme Division
300 S. Third St.
P.O. Box 2276
Kansas City, Kans. 66110
913-342-8780

PEARSON & CO.
P.O. Box 431
Mobile, Ala. 36601
205-456-8456

PECORA CORP.
165 Wambold Rd.
Harleysville, Pa. 19438
215-723-6051

PEDINOL PHARMACAL, INC.
110 Bell St.
W. Babylon, N.Y. 11704
516-293-9500

PENGUIN INDUSTRIES, INC.
Airport Industrial Mall
Coatesville, Pa. 19320
215-384-6000

PENICK CORP.
1050 Wall St. W.
Lyndhurst, N.J. 07071
201-935-6600

PENN-CHAMP, INC.
P.O. Box 55
East Butler, Pa. 16029
412-287-8771

PENNEX PRODUCTS
Eastern Ave. at Pennex Dr.
Verona, Pa. 15147
412-828-2900

PENNWALT CORP.
Pennwalt Building
3 Parkway
Philadelphia, Pa. 19102
215-587-7000

PENNWALT CORP.
Pharmaceutical Div.
P.O. Box 1710
Rochester, N.Y. 14603
716-475-9000

PENNZOIL CO.
Gumout Div.
410 Gateway Center No. 4
Pittsburgh, Pa. 15222
412-263-3694

PEPPET LABORATORIES
Div. Hy-Pure, Inc.
P.O. Box 43603
Cincinnati, Ohio 45243
513-641-0973

PERRIGO, L., CO.
117 Water St.
Allegan, Mich. 49010
616-673-8451

PERVO PAINT CO.
6624 Stanford Ave.
Los Angeles, Calif. 90001
213-758-1147

PET CHEMICALS, INC.
7781 N.W. 73rd Ct.
P.O. Box 656
Miami Springs, Fla. 33166
305-887-1506

PETERSON OINTMENT CO.
257 Franklin St.
Buffalo, N.Y. 14202
716-854-3787

PETTIT PAINT CO., INC.
36 Pine St.
Rockaway, N.J. 07866
201-625-3100

PFIPHARMECS DIVISION
See PFIZER LABORATORIES DIVISION

PFIZER INC.
Agricultural Div.
1107 South Missouri 291
Lee's Summit, Mo. 64063
417-524-5580

PFIZER LABORATORIES DIVISION
Pfizer Inc.
235 E. 42nd St.
New York, N.Y. 10017
212-573-2323

PHARMACRAFT DIVISION
Pennwalt Corp.
P.O. Box 1710
Rochester, N.Y. 14603
716-475-9000

PHARMASEAL DIVISION
American Hospital Supply Corp.
1015 Grandview Ave.
P.O. Box 1300
Glendale, Calif. 91209
213-240-8900

PHARMEX, INC.
P.O. Box 125
2113 Lincoln St.
Hollywood, Fla. 33022
305-923-2821

PHILIPS ROXANE LABORATORIES, INC.
330 Oak St.
P.O. Box 16532
Columbus, Ohio 43216
614-228-5403

PHOENIX OIL CO.
P.O. Box 1777
Augusta, Ga. 30913
404-722-5321

PHOSTOXIN SALES, INC.
2221 Poplar Blvd.
Box 469
Alhambra, Calif. 91802
213-283-2761

PIC CORP.
23 S. Essex Ave.
Orange, N.J. 07050
201-678-7300

PIERCE & STEVENS CHEMICAL CORP.
710 Ohio St.
P.O. Box 1092
Buffalo, N.Y. 14240
716-856-4910

PIERRE CARDIN PARFUMS
630 Fifth Ave.
New York, N.Y. 10111
212-489-2430

PIGGLY WIGGLY CORP.
See GREAT ATLANTIC & PACIFIC TEA CO., INC.

PINAUD, ED., INC.
66 E. 34th St.
New York, N.Y. 10016
212-679-0900

PINE, MORTON S., CO.
407 Caxton Bldg.
Cleveland, Ohio 44115
216-687-0188

PIONEER MANUFACTURING CO.
3053 E. 87th St.
Cleveland, Ohio 44104
216-721-6161

PIPESTONE PRODUCTS CO., INC.
P.O. Box 36
Trosky, Minn. 56177
507-348-7683

PITMAN-MOORE, INC.
Box 344
Washington Crossing, N.J. 08560
609-737-3700

PITTSBURGH CHEMICAL LABORATORY
Century Building
Pittsburgh, Pa. 15222
412-391-0160

PLANTABBS CORP.
Timonium, Md. 21093
301-252-4620

PLANT MARVEL DISTRIBUTING CO., INC.
624 W. 119th St.
Chicago, Ill. 60628
312-264-0450

PLANT PRODUCTS CORP.
P.O. Box 1149
S. Gifford Rd.
Vero Beach, Fla. 32960
305-567-5741

PLASTIC CO. OF AMERICA
6542 N. Sheridan Rd.
Chicago, Ill. 60626
312-274-0800

PLASTI-KOTE CO., INC.
1000 Lake Rd.
Medina, Ohio 44256
216-725-4511

PLEXTONE CORP. OF AMERICA
2141 McCarter Hwy.
Newark, N.J. 07104
201-484-4443

PLOUGH, INC.
P.O. Box 377
Memphis, Tenn. 38151
901-320-2011

PLUMB CRAFT MANUFACTURING CORP.
24455 Aurora Rd.
Bedford Heights, Ohio 44146
216-439-1997

PLUS DISCOUNT FOODS, INC.
See GREAT ATLANTIC & PACIFIC TEA CO., INC.

POLAROID CORP.
549 Technology Sq.
Cambridge, Mass. 02139
617-577-2000

POLYCHEM CORP.
12 Lyman St.
New Haven, Conn. 06511
203-777-7363

POLYGLYCOAT WORLD ENTERPRISES LTD.
7171 N. Federal Hwy.
Boca Raton, Fla. 33431
305-997-7171

POMATEX CO., INC.
60 E. 42nd St.
New York, N.Y. 10017
212-661-3197

POOL EQUIPMENT, INC.
1334 Young St.
Honolulu, Hawaii 96814
808-538-3741
808-531-1542

POPULAR PRODUCTS, INC.
1910 N. Elston Ave.
Chicago, Ill. 60622
312-489-5900

POSITIVE FORMULATORS, INC.
1044 N. Jerrie Ave.
Tucson, Ariz. 85711
602-793-2322

POSNER LABORATORIES INC.
301 Helen St.
South Plainfield, N.J. 07080
201-753-0900

POYTHRESS, WILLIAM P., & CO., INC.
P.O. Box 26946
Richmond, Va. 23261
804-644-8591

PPG INDUSTRIES, INC.
Chemical Div.
One Gateway Center
Pittsburgh, Pa. 15222
412-434-2604

PRATT, B. G., DIVISION
See PRATT-GABRIEL DIVISION

PRATT-GABRIEL DIVISION
Miller Chemical & Fertilizer Corp.
P.O. Box B
Robbinsville, N.J. 08691
609-587-6700

PRATT & LAMBERT, INC.
Box 22
Buffalo, N.Y. 14240
716-873-6000

PRECISION LABORATORIES, INC.
P.O. Box 127
Northbrook, Ill. 60062
312-498-0800

**PREMO PHARMACEUTICAL
LABORATORIES, INC.**
111 Leuning St.
South Hackensack, N.J. 07606
201-343-5000

PRENTISS DRUG & CHEMICAL CO., INC.
363 7th Ave.
New York, N.Y. 10001
212-736-6766

PRESCOTT, J. L., CO.
27 Eighth St.
Passaic, N.J. 07055
201-777-4200

PRINCE MATCHABELLI, INC.
See CHESEBROUGH-POND'S INC.

PRINCESS MARCELLA BORGHESE, INC.
Sub. of Revlon, Inc.
767 Fifth Ave.
New York, N.Y. 10153
212-572-5000

PRO-BRAND PRODUCTS CO.
P.O. Box 4186
Fort Worth, Tex. 76106
817-626-5408

PROCTER & GAMBLE CO.
Ivorydale Technical Center
Cincinnati, Ohio 45217
513-562-1100

PROCTER & GAMBLE CO.
Beauty Care Div.
Sharon Woods Technical Center
HB Building
11511 Reed Hartman Hwy.
Cincinnati, Ohio 45241
513-530-2304

PROCTER & GAMBLE CO.
Health & Personal Care Div.
Sharon Woods Technical Center
HB Building
11511 Reed Hartman Hwy.
Cincinnati, Ohio 45241
513-530-2312

PROFESSIONAL COSMETIC CORP.
Clinton Air Industrial Park
Plattsburgh, N.Y. 12901
518-561-8600

**PROGRESS PAINT MANUFACTURING
CO.**
P.O. Box 33188
Louisville, Ky. 40232
502-587-8685

PRUVO PHARMACAL CO.
2018 W. Bender Rd.
Milwaukee, Wis. 53209
414-228-1170

PUBLICKER INDUSTRIES INC.
P.O. Box 1976
Greenwich, Conn. 06836
203-531-4500

PUCCI, EMILIO, PERFUMES INTL. INC.
24 E. 64th St.
New York, N.Y. 10021
212-752-4777

PURDY, N. B., PRODUCTS CO.
P.O. Box 304
Wauconda, Ill. 60084
312-526-5505

PUREX CORPORATION
5101 Clark Ave.
Lakewood, Calif. 90712
213-634-3300

PURITAN CHEMICAL CO.
916 Ashby St. N.W.
Atlanta, Ga. 30318
404-872-0721

PURO CHEMICAL CO.
See PURO CO., INC., THE

PURO CO., INC., THE
2801 Locust St.
St. Louis, Mo. 63103
314-533-1790

PUTNAM COLOR AND DYE CORP.
1558 So. Henderson St.
Galesburg, Ill. 61401
309-342-9779

PYROIL CO.
Div. of Champion Labs., Inc.
Albion, Ill. 62806
618-445-2395

Q

QUANT, MARY, COSMETICS, LTD.
655 Madison Ave.
New York, N.Y. 10021
212-758-1072

R

RAAB, ANDREA, CORP.
4702 Glenwood Rd.
Brooklyn, N.Y. 11234
212-252-8800

RACHELLE LABORATORIES, INC.
700 Henry Ford Ave.
P.O. Box 2029
Long Beach, Calif. 90801
213-432-3956

RADIANT WASH SOLUTION CORP.
160 Van Rensselaer St.
Buffalo, N.Y. 14210
716-852-6156

RADIATOR SPECIALTY CO.
P.O. Box 34689
Charlotte, N.C. 28234
704-377-6555

RAD, INC.
375 Park Ave.
New York, N.Y. 10022
212-752-0880

RALPH B. ADAMS
Lakeville, New Brunswick
Canada

RALSTON PURINA CO.
Checkerboard Square
St. Louis, Mo. 63164
314-982-1000

RA-PID-GRO CORP.
88 Ossian St.
Dansville, N.Y. 14437
716-335-2278

RAWLEIGH, W. T., CO.
223 E. Main St.
Freeport, Ill. 61032
815-232-4161

RAY DRUG CO., INC.
Box 10285, Grand Lake Sta.
Oakland, Calif. 94610
415-451-4092

RAYETTE DIVISION
See FABERGE DIVISION

REALEX CORP.
P.O. Box 78
2500 Summit
Kansas City, Mo. 64141
816-842-8092

REARDON, W. G., LABORATORIES, INC.
1804 Freemansburg Ave.
Easton, Pa. 18042
215-253-1325

RECSEI LABORATORIES
330 S. Kellogg, Bldg. M
Goleta, Calif. 93017
805-964-2912

RED CROSS CHEMICAL WORKS, INC.
See MENTHOLATUM CO., INC.

RED DEVIL INC.
2400 Vauxhall Rd.
Union, N.J. 07083
201-688-6900

REDKEN LABS., INC.
6625 Variel Ave.
Canoga Park, Calif. 91303
213-992-2700

RED & WHITE INTERNATIONAL
See GREAT ATLANTIC & PACIFIC TEA CO., INC.

REED & CARNRICK
30 Boright Ave.
Kenilworth, N.J. 07033
201-272-6600

REEFER-GALLER, INC.
See COLGATE-PALMOLIVE CO.

REESE CHEMICAL CO.
10617 Frank Ave.
Cleveland, Ohio 44106
216-231-6441

REID-PROVIDENT LABORATORIES, INC.
25 Fifth St., N.W.
Atlanta, Ga. 30308
404-898-1000

REILY CHEMICAL CO.
450 Mandeville St.
P.O. Box 50372
New Orleans, La. 70150
504-943-8849

RELIABLE PASTE & CHEMICAL CO.
3560 S. Shields Ave.
Chicago, Ill. 60609
312-268-1845

RELIANCE PEN & PENCIL CORP.
100 Reliance Ave.
Lewisburg, Tenn. 37091
615-359-2586

RELIANCE UNIVERSAL, INC.
1600 Watterson Towers
1930 Bishop Lane
Louisville, Ky. 40218
502-459-9110

REMINGTON PRODUCTS, INC.
60 Main St.
Bridgeport, Conn. 06602
203-367-4400

REMONT INC.
711 Fairfield Ave.
Villa Park, Ill. 60181
312-279-5920

REMPEL CHEMICAL PRODUCTS, INC.
P.O. Box 1185
Fresno, Calif. 93715
209-233-9105
209-264-6517

REQUA MANUFACTURING CO., INC.
1 Seneca Pl.
P.O. Box 4008
Greenwich, Conn. 06830
203-869-2445

RESEARCH PRODUCTS CO.
1835 E. North St.
Salina, Kans. 67401
913-825-2181

RESEARCH PRODUCTS CORP.
1015 E. Washington Ave.
Madison, Wis. 53701
608-257-8801

RESIDEX CORP.
225 Terminal Ave.
Clark, N.J. 07066
201-381-6200

RESINOL CHEMICAL CO.
See MENTHOLATUM CO., INC.

REVELL, INC.
4223 Glencoe Ave.
Venice, Calif. 90291
213-821-5011

REVLON, INC.
767 Fifth Ave.
New York, N.Y. 10153
212-572-5000

REVLON RESEARCH CENTER, INC.
945 Zerega Ave.
Bronx, N.Y. 10473
212-824-9000

REXALL DRUG CO.
3901 N. Kingshighway Blvd.
St. Louis, Mo. 63115
314-679-7100

REX LABORATORY INC.
1903 Thurman St.
Nashville, Tenn. 37202
615-292-1088

REYNES PRODUCTS, INC.
P.O. Box 1203
Sonoma, Calif. 95476
707-938-8322

R.H. COSMETICS CORP.
736 Parkside Ave.
Brooklyn, N.Y. 11226
212-856-2222

RHODIA INC.
See RHONE-POULENC CHEMICAL CO.

RHONE-POULENC CHEMICAL CO.
Agrochemical Div.
P.O. Box 125
Monmouth Junction, N.J. 08852
201-297-0100

RICCI, NINA, PARFUMS
630 Fifth Ave.
New York, N.Y. 10111
212-489-2430

RICHARDSON CHEMICAL PRODUCTS CO.
P.O. Box 83
Mequon, Wis. 53092
414-242-0047

RID-A-BIRD, INC.
P.O. Box 22
Muscatine, Iowa 52761
319-263-7965

RIGO CO.
Highway 146
Buckner, Ky. 40010
502-222-1456

RIKER LABORATORIES, INC.
19901 Nordhoff St.
Northridge, Calif. 91324
213-341-1300

RITCHIE GROCER CO.
See OCEAN COFFEE COMPANY, INC.

RIVERSIDE CHEMICAL CO.
See RIVERSIDE/TERRA CORP.

RIVERSIDE/TERRA CORP.
Subsid. of Terra Chemicals International, Inc.
P.O. Box 1828
Sioux City, Iowa 51102
712-277-1340

ROBERTS CONSOLIDATED INDUSTRIES
600 N. Baldwin Park Blvd.
City of Industry, Calif. 91749
213-338-7311

ROBERTS LABORATORIES
4995 N. Main St.
Rockford, Ill. 61101
815-877-6076

ROBINS, A. H., CO.
1407 Cummings Dr.
Richmond, Va. 23220

Medical emergency calls
(day or night) 804-257-2000
If no answer, call
answering service 804-257-7788

ROCHE LABORATORIES
Div. of Hoffman-La Roche, Inc.
Nutley, N.J. 07110
201-235-2355

ROCHER, YVES, INC.
2909 MacArthur Blvd.
Northbrook, Ill. 60062
312-498-6115

ROCHESTER GERMICIDE CO.
P.O. Box 1515
Rochester, N.Y. 14603
716-266-2250

ROCKLAND CHEMICAL CO., INC.
Passaic Ave.
West Caldwell, N.J. 07006
201-226-5151

ROERIG
A Division of Pfizer Pharmaceuticals
235 E. 42nd St.
York, N.Y. 10017
3-2536

ROFFLER INDUSTRIES
400 Chess St.
Coraopolis, Pa. 15108
412-771-4333

ROGERS CHEMICAL CO.
P.O. Box 297
Denver, Colo. 80201
303-433-1933

ROGERS PARK LABORATORY
3623 Seven Mile Lane
Baltimore, Md. 21208
301-764-1114

ROHM AND HAAS CO.
Independence Mall W.
Philadelphia, Pa. 19105
215-592-3000

ROMAN CLEANSER CO.
2700 E. McNichols Rd.
Detroit, Mich. 48212
313-891-0700

RONDEX LABORATORIES
200 Elmora Ave.
Elizabeth, N.J. 07207

RONSON CORP.
One Ronson Rd.
Bridgewater, N.J. 08807
201-526-5900

ROOTO CORP.
3505 W. Grand River
Howell, Mich. 48843
517-546-8330

RORER, WILLIAM H., INC.
500 Virginia Dr.
Fort Washington, Pa. 19034
215-628-6000

ROSENSTEIN, NETTIE, INC.
220 E. 23rd St.
New York, N.Y. 10010
212-371-6300

ROSS CHEMICAL CO.
8485 Melville St.
Detroit, Mich. 48209
313-842-8200

ROSS DANIELS, INC.
P.O. Box 65430
West Des Moines, Iowa 50265
515-225-6471

ROSS LABORATORIES
Div. of Abbott Labs.
625 Cleveland Ave.
Columbus, Ohio 43216
614-228-5281

ROSS, WILL, INC.
See SEARLE MEDICAL PRODUCTS USA INC.

ROTO-ROOTER CORP.
300 Ashworth Rd.
West Des Moines, Iowa 50265
515-223-1343

ROUX LABORATORIES, INC.
Sub. of Revlon, Inc.
3733 University Blvd. W.
Jacksonville, Fla. 32217
904-731-3050

ROWELL LABORATORIES, INC.
210 Main St. W.
Baudette, Minn. 56623
218-634-1866

ROYAL BOND, INC.
1919 N. Broadway
St. Louis, Mo. 63102
314-621-3800

R.P.S. PRODUCTS, INC.
See WEST BEND CO., THE

RUBINSTEIN, HELENA, INC.
300 Park Ave.
New York, N.Y. 10022
212-935-5300

RUSS PHARMACEUTICALS, INC.
P.O. Box 11258
Birmingham, Ala. 35202
205-822-2730

RUSTICIDE PRODUCTS CO.
See SKYBRYTE CO., THE

RUST-OLEUM CORP.
11 Hawthorn Pkwy
Vernon Hills, Ill. 60061
312-367-7700

RUTLAND PRODUCTS
P.O. Box 1078
Northwest Blvd.
Gastonia, N.C. 28052
704-865-6427

RYSTAN CO., INC.
470 Mamaroneck Ave.
White Plains, N.Y. 10605
914-761-0044

S

SAFER AGRO-CHEM INC.
13910 Lyons Valley Rd.
Jamul, Calif. 92035
714-464-0775

SAFEWAY STORES, INC.
Brookside Div.
P.O. Box 2125
Oakland, Calif. 94621
415-635-8000

SAINT LAURENT, YVES, PARFUMS
40 W. 57th St.
New York, N.Y. 10019
212-621-7327

SALSBURY LABORATORIES
2000 Rockford Rd.
Charles City, Iowa 50616
515-257-2422

SAMUEL CABOT, INC.
One Union St.
Boston, Mass. 02108
617-723-7740

SANABALM CO.
4923 N. Darrah St.
Philadelphia, Pa. 19124
215-744-2742
215-673-7732

SANDOZ PHARMACEUTICALS
59 Route 10
East Hanover, N.J. 07936
201-386-7764

SANDRA LEE PRODUCTS
13165 N. W. 47th Ave.
Miami, Fla. 33054
305-685-6089

S AND S COMPANY OF GEORGIA, INC.
827 Pine Ave.
P.O. Box 45
Albany, Ga. 31702
912-435-8394

SANFORD CORP.
2740 Washington Blvd.
Bellwood, Ill. 60104
312-378-4814

SANI-MIST, INC.
3018 Market St.
Philadelphia, Pa. 19104
215-222-1411

SANITEK PRODUCTS, INC.
3959 Goodwin Ave.
Los Angeles, Calif. 90039
213-245-6781

SANI-WAX INC.
P.O. Box 5126
Arlington, Tex. 76011
817-461-1823

SANTA BARBARA COUNTY AGRICULTURAL COMMISSIONER
Courthouse
1105 Santa Barbara St.
Santa Barbara, Calif. 93101
805-963-6762

SAPOLIN PAINTS, INC.
1250 Broadway
New York, N.Y. 10001
212-947-3070

SARGENT ART INC.
100 E. Diamond Ave.
Hazleton, Pa. 18201
717-454-3596

SASSOON, VIDAL, INC.
2049 Century Park E.
Century City, Calif. 90067
213-553-6100

SAVAGE LABORATORIES
P.O. Box 1000
Missouri City, Tex. 77459
713-499-4547

SAV-COTE CHEMICAL LABS., INC.
P.O. Box 770
Lakewood, N.J. 08701
201-364-4700

SAVOGRAN CO.
P.O. Box 130
Norwood, Mass. 02062
617-762-5400

SAVOL CO., THE
400 W. Butler St.
Mercer, Pa. 16137
412-662-4064

SCANNON LTD.
650 Fifth Ave.
New York, N.Y. 10019
212-246-3070

SCHAFFER LABORATORIES, INC.
P.O. Box 539
Arcadia, Calif. 91006
213-681-2015

SCHALK CHEMICALS, INC.
Subsidiary of Red Devil Inc.
2400 Vauxhall Rd.
Union, N.J. 07083
201-688-6900

SCHERER LABORATORIES, INC.
P.O. Box 400009
Dallas, Tex. 75234
214-233-2800

SCHERING CORP.
Galloping Hill Rd.
Kenilworth, N.J. 07033
201-558-4000

SCHIFF BIO-FOOD PRODUCTS, INC.
Moonachie Ave.
Moonachie, N.J. 07074
201-933-2282

SCHMID LABORATORIES, INC.
Route 46
Little Falls, N.J. 07424
201-256-5500

SCHMIDT, A. O., CO.
2100 Bryant St.
San Francisco, Calif. 94110
415-824-7466

SCHNAPP ENTERPRISES
P.O. Box 65
Jericho, N.Y. 11753
516-364-1276

SCHNEID, I., INC.
1429 Fairmont Ave. N.W.
Atlanta, Ga. 30318
404-351-4705

SCHOLL, INC.
P.O. Box 377
Memphis, Tenn. 38151
901-320-2011

SCHULTZ CO.
11730 Northline, Maryland Hts.
St. Louis, Mo. 63043
314-567-4545

SCIENCE PRODUCTS CO., INC.
5801 N. Tripp Ave.
Chicago, Ill. 60646
312-583-3171

SCIENTIFIC INTERNATIONAL RESEARCH, INC.
P.O. Box 26500
St. Louis Park, Minn. 55426
612-333-8385

SCOT LABORATORIES
16841 Park Circle Dr.
P.O. Box 167
Chagrin Falls, Ohio 44022
216-543-5119

SCOTT, O. M., & SONS CO.
Marysville, Ohio 43041
513-644-0011

SCOTT'S LIQUID GOLD-INC.
4880 Havana St.
Denver, Colo. 80239
303-373-4860

SCOVILL MANUFACTURING CO.
Sewing Notions Div.
Buckingham St.
Watertown, Conn. 06795
203-757-6061

SCRANTON CHEMICAL CO.
705-709 Davis St.
Scranton, Pa. 18501
717-347-2029

SCRIPTO, INC.
P.O. Box 47800
Atlanta, Ga. 30362
404-449-4443

SEA BREEZE LABORATORIES, INC.
P.O. Box 15598
Pittsburgh, Pa. 15244
412-923-2626

SEACOAST LABORATORIES, INC.
P.O. Box 157
257 Highway 18
East Brunswick, N.J. 08816
201-257-7772

SEARLE LABORATORIES
G. D. Searle & Co.
P.O. Box 5110
Chicago, Ill. 60680
312-982-7000

SEARLE MEDICAL PRODUCTS USA INC.
8303 Elmbrook Dr.
Dallas, Tex. 75247
214-637-7100

SEARS, ROEBUCK AND CO.
925 S. Homan Ave.
Chicago, Ill. 60607
303-623-5827

SEA & SKI CORP.
See CARTER PRODUCTS

SEBESTA BAIT MIXING PLANT
P.O. Box 306
Mitchell, S. Dak. 57301
605-996-3718

SEED-TREET LABORATORIES
See PEARSON & CO.

SENN, GEORGE, INC.
2200 E. Westmoreland St.
Philadelphia, Pa. 19134
215-426-1400

SENORET CHEMICAL CO., INC.
566 Leffingwell Ave.
Kirkwood, Mo. 63122
314-966-2394

SERES LABORATORIES, INC.
3331 Industrial Dr.
Santa Rosa, Calif. 95401
707-526-4526

SerVaas LABORATORIES, INC.
P.O. Box 7008
Indianapolis, Ind. 46207
317-634-1100

SEVENTEEN INC.
33 Virginia Ave.
West Nyack, N.Y. 10994
914-358-2426

SEXAUER, J. A., INC.
10 Hamilton Ave.
White Plains, N.Y. 10601
914-682-8600

SEYMOUR OF SYCAMORE, INC.
917 Crosby Ave.
Sycamore, Ill. 60178
815-895-9101

SHAKLEE CORP.
444 Market St.
San Francisco, Calif. 94111
415-428-8000

SHALER CO., THE
21 E. Jefferson St.
Waupun, Wis. 53963
414-324-5511

SHEAFFER EATON DIV.
Textron, Inc.
301 Ave. H
Fort Madison, Iowa 52627
319-372-3300

SHEFFIELD BRONZE PAINT CORP.
17814 Waterloo Rd.
Cleveland, Ohio 44119
216-481-8330

SHELL CHEMICAL CO.
Agricultural Chemicals Div.
2401 Crow Canyon Rd.
San Ramon, Calif. 94583
415-837-1531

SHELL OIL CO.
One Shell Plaza
P.O. Box 4320
Houston, Tex. 77210
713-473-9461

SHERATON LABORATORIES, INC.
374 Reed St.
Santa Clara, Calif. 95050
408-148-2025

SHERWIN-WILLIAMS CO., THE
101 Prospect Ave. N.W.
Cleveland, Ohio 44115
216-566-2000

SHISEIDO COSMETICS (AMERICA) LTD.
540 Madison Ave.
New York, N.Y. 10022
212-752-2644

SHONTEX PRODUCTS CO.
1221 Ocean Ave.
Santa Monica, Calif. 90401
213-451-8121

SHORELL, IRMA, INC.
515 Madison Ave.
New York, N.Y. 10022
212-355-6747

SHUPTRINE CO.
P.O. Box 22127
Savannah, Ga. 31403
912-232-8303

SIKA CHEMICAL CORP.
P.O. Box 297
Lyndhurst, N.J. 07071
201-933-8800

SILK & SATIN HAIR PRODUCTS
P.O. Box 432
Durham, N.C. 27702
919-471-4919

SILOO INCORPORATED
393 Seventh Ave.
New York, N.Y. 10001
212-695-3190

SINCLAIR PHARMACAL CO., INC.
Fishers Island, N.Y. 06390
516-788-7210

SKAN LABORATORIES, INC.
767 W. Woodbury Rd.
Altadena, Calif. 91001
213-681-6749

SKAT SALES CO.
P.O. Box 229
Woburn, Mass. 01801

SKELLY OIL CO.
See GETTY REFINING & MARKETING CO.

SK&F (SMITH, KLINE & FRENCH LABORATORIES)
1500 Spring Garden St.
Philadelphia, Pa. 19101
215-564-2400

S-K RESEARCH LABORATORIES, INC.
P.O. Box 230
Phoenix, Ariz. 85001
602-258-8168

SKYBRYTE CO., THE
3125 Perkins Ave.
Cleveland, Ohio 44114
216-771-1590

SMITH, C. G., PRODUCTS CO.
P.O. Box 1016
Blytheville, Ark. 72315

SMITH, KLINE & FRENCH LABORATORIES
1500 Spring Garden St.
Philadelphia, Pa. 19101
215-564-2400

SMITH, ROBERT, MANUFACTURING CO., INC.
17922 Star of India Lane
Carson, Calif. 90746
213-538-4585

SMITH & WESSON/GENERAL ORDNANCE EQUIPMENT CO.
Freeport Rd., Box 11211
Pittsburgh, Pa. 15238
412-782-2161

SNEE, W. G., CO., INC.
1430 S. Peters St.
New Orleans, La. 70130
504-522-5395

SOFSKIN, INC.
575 Madison Ave.
New York, N.Y. 10022
212-753-4600

SO HELP ME HANNAH LABORATORIES
2574 El Camino Real N.
Salinas, Calif. 93907
408-663-3405

SOLVIT CHEMICAL CO., INC.
7001 Raywood Rd.
Madison, Wis. 53713
608-222-8624

SONFORD PRODUCTS CORP.
Southern Div.
P.O. Box 5570
Jackson, Miss. 39208
601-939-8912

**SONOMA COUNTY DEPARTMENT OF
AGRICULTURE**
2604 Ventura Ave., Room 101
Santa Rosa, Calif. 95401
707-527-2371

SOUTHERN COATINGS, INC.
P.O. Box 160
Sumter, S.C. 29150
803-775-6351

SOUTHLAND PAINT CO., INC.
1101 Southland Dr.
Gainesville, Tex. 76240
817-668-7271

SOUTH OMAHA SUPPLY
3310 H. St.
Omaha, Nebr. 68107
402-331-3100

SOUTHWEST CHEMICAL CO.
P.O. Box 65797
Los Angeles, Calif. 90065
213-256-7679

SOUTHWEST PETRO-CHEM DIVISION
Witco Chemical Corp.
6200 No. 16th St.
Omaha, Nebr. 68110
402-455-5040

SOUTHWEST PETRO-CHEM, INC.
P.O. Box 1974
Olathe, Kans. 66061
913-782-5800

SOUTHWEST RESEARCH PRODUCTS CO.
P.O. Box 1066
Houston, Tex. 77001
713-772-4858

SOWECO, INC.
411 S. Parker
P.O. Box 3280
Amarillo, Tex. 79106
806-372-8381

SPARTAN CHEMICAL CO., INC.
110 N. Westwood Ave.
Toledo, Ohio 43607
419-531-5551

SPECO, INC.
7308 Associate Ave.
Cleveland, Ohio 44144
216-281-9520

SPE-DE-WAY PRODUCTS CO., INC.
P.O. Box 17192
Portland, Ore. 97217
503-285-8371

SPENCER VET SUPPLY CO.
P.O. Box 1128
Spencer, Iowa 51301
712-262-5462

SPOHN MEDICAL CO.
202 N. Main St.
Goshen, Ind. 46526
219-533-4670

SPRAYWAY, INC.
484 Vista Ave.
Addison, Ill. 60101
312-628-0998

SPRUANCE, GILBERT, CO., THE
Tioga & Richmond
Philadelphia, Pa. 19134
215-739-6172

SPURRIER CHEMICAL COS., INC.
P.O. Box 2812
Wichita, Kans. 67201
316-265-9491

SPUR-TEX PRODUCTS
See SPURRIER CHEMICAL COS., INC.

SQUIBB, E. R., & SONS, INC.
P.O. Box 4000
Princeton, N.J. 08540
609-921-4006

S.S.S. CO.
P.O. Box 4447
Atlanta, Ga. 30302
404-521-0857

STALEY, A. E., MANUFACTURING CO.
2200 E. Eldorado St.
Decatur, Ill. 62525
217-423-4411, Ext. 548

STA-LUBE, INC.
3039 Ana St.
P.O. Box 5746
Compton, Calif. 90224
213-774-1574
213-631-8619

STANBACK CO., LTD.
P.O. Box 1669
1500 S. Main St.
Salisbury, N.C. 28144
704-633-9231

STANCHEM INC.
401 Berlin St.
East Berlin, Conn. 06023
203-828-0571

STANDARD COFFEE CO., INC.
450 Mandeville St.
P.O. Box 50372
New Orleans, La. 70150
504-943-8849

STANDARD DRY WALL PRODUCTS, INC.
7800 N.W. 38th St.
Miami, Fla. 33166
305-592-2081

STANDARDIZED SANITATION SYSTEMS, INC.
141 Middlesex Turnpike
Burlington, Mass. 01803
617-273-2020

STANDARD OIL CO. OF CALIFORNIA
Environmental Health Center
P.O. Box 1272
Richmond, CA 94802
415-233-3737

STANDARD PRODUCTS CORP.
68 Temple St.
Whitman, Mass. 02382
617-447-6561

STANLEY HOME PRODUCTS, INC.
333 Western Ave.
Westfield, Mass. 01085
413-562-3631

STANSON DETERGENTS, INC.
P.O. Box 100
Teaneck, N.J. 07666

STAR BRONZE CO.
P.O. Box 568
Alliance, Ohio 44601
216-823-1550

STATE CHEMICALS
1738 Hoe St.
Honolulu, Hawaii 96819

STATE COLLEGE LABORATORIES
See EHRLICH, J. C., CHEMICAL CO., INC.

STAUFFER CHEMICAL CO.
Agricultural Chemical Div.
Westport, Conn. 06881
203-226-6602

STAYNER CORP.
See STAYNER PHARMACEUTICALS

STAYNER PHARMACEUTICALS
1922 Junction Ave.
San Jose, Calif. 95131
408-279-4411

STEARNS' ELECTRIC PASTE CO.
1780 Maple St.
Northfield, Ill. 60093
312-446-0085

STEELCOTE MFG. CO.
3418 Gratiot St.
St. Louis, Mo. 63103
314-771-8053

STEIN CHEMICAL CO., INC.
1805 2nd Ave. N.
P.O. Box 248
Moorhead, Minn. 56560
218-233-2728

STEPHAN CO., THE
1850 W. McNab Rd.
Fort Lauderdale, Fla. 33309
305-971-0600

STERLING-CLARK-LURTON CORP.
P.O. Box J
184 Commercial St.
Malden, Mass. 02148
617-322-0163

STERNO, INC.
See COLGATE-PALMOLIVE CO.

STERN'S GARDEN PRODUCTS, INC.
135 Haven Ave.
Port Washington, N.Y. 11050
516-883-6550

STERN'S NURSERIES, INC.
See STERN'S GARDEN PRODUCTS, INC.

STEWART SANITARY SUPPLY, INC.
P.O. Box 15061
St. Louis, Mo. 63110
314-865-2000

STEWART, W. W., DIVISION
Zephyr Manufacturing Co.
400-410 W. Second St.
Sedalia, Mo. 65301
816-827-0352

STIEFEL LABORATORIES, INC.
2801 Ponce de Leon Blvd.
Coral Gables, Fla. 33134
305-443-3807

STILES-KEM DIVISION
Met-Pro Corp.
3301 Sheridan Rd.
Zion, Ill. 60099
312-746-8334

STILLMAN CO., INC.
323 E. Galena Blvd.
Aurora, Ill. 60507
312-897-5600

STIM-U-PLANT, INC.
2077 Parkwood Ave.
Columbus, Ohio 43219
614-267-1297

STRAND PRODUCTS CO.
P.O. Box 2187
Philadelphia, Pa. 19103

STRICKLAND, J., & CO.
1400 Ragan
Memphis, Tenn. 38106
901-774-9023

STUART PHARMACEUTICALS
Div. of ICI Americas, Inc.
Concord Pike & Murphy Rd.
Wilmington, Del. 19897
800-441-7758, ext. 2231
After hours: 302-575-3000

STURTEVANT, F. C., CO.
P.O. Box 471
West Hartford, Conn. 06107
203-346-1414

SUDBURY LABORATORY, INC.
572 Dutton Rd.
Sudbury, Mass. 01776
617-443-8844

SUGAR BEET PRODUCTS CO.
P.O. Box 1387
Saginaw, Mich. 48605
517-799-4941

SUMMERS LABORATORIES, INC.
Fort Washington, Pa. 19034
215-646-1477

SUMMIT CHEMICAL CO.
117 West 24th St.
Baltimore, Md. 21218
301-467-1233

SUMMIT LABORATORIES, INC.
1335 W. 47th St.
Chicago, Ill. 60609
312-927-8202

SUNBEAM APPLIANCE CO.
Div. of Sunbeam Corp.
2001 S. York Rd.
Oak Brook, Ill. 60521
312-654-1900

SUNNYSIDE CORPORATION
225 Carpenter Ave.
Wheeling, Ill. 60090
312-541-5700

SUNNYSIDE PRODUCTS, INC.
See SUNNYSIDE CORPORATION

SUN SWIMMING POOL PRODUCTS
See FMC CORPORATION,   Sun Swimming Pool Products

SUNTAN RESEARCH & DEVELOPMENT, INC.
P.O. Box 2734
Daytona Beach, Fla. 32015
904-258-7396

SUPPOSITORIA LABORATORIES, INC.
135 Florida St.
Farmingdale, N.Y. 11735
516-694-1120

SURCO PRODUCTS, INC.
227 3rd Ave.
Braddock, Pa. 15104
412-351-7700

SUTLIFF & CASE CO., INC.
P.O. Box 838
Peoria, Ill. 61601
309-674-4141

SWEENEY, W. R., MFR., INC.
312-16 S. Broadway
Salisbury, Mo. 65281
816-388-6417

SYBIL IVES, INC.
635 W. 18th St.
Hialeah, Fla. 33010
305-885-1911

SYNKOLOID CO.
P.O. Box 60937
Los Angeles, Calif. 90060
213-263-7121

SYNTEX AGRIBUSINESS, INC.
Diamond Labs.
2538 S.E. 43rd St.
Des Moines, Iowa 50317
515-262-9341

SYNTEX (F.P.) INC.
See SYNTEX LABORATORIES, INC.

SYNTEX LABORATORIES, INC.
3401 Hillview Ave.
Palo Alto, Calif. 94304
415-855-5545

SYNTEX PUERTO RICO, INC.
See SYNTEX LABORATORIES, INC.

T

TALSOL CORP.
4677 Devitt Dr.
Cincinnati, Ohio 45246
513-874-5151

TAMMS INDUSTRIES CO.
1222 Ardmore Ave.
Drawer Box C
Itasca, Ill. 60143
312-773-2350

TANGLEFOOT CO.
314 Straight Ave. S.W.
Grand Rapids, Mich. 49504
616-459-4130

TEAC CORPORATION OF AMERICA
7733 Telegraph Rd.
P.O. Box 750
Montebello, Calif. 90640
213-726-0303

TECHNE CORP.
Agricultural Chemical Div.
P.O. Box 788
St. Joseph, Mo. 64502
816-233-8877

TEMPLAR DIVISION
The W. W. Henry Co.
Foot of Whitehead Ave.
South River, N.J. 08882
201-254-2424

TERMINAL GRAIN & CHEMICAL CO.
P.O. Box 705
Fort Worth, Tex. 76101
817-923-4694

TERMINIX INTERNATIONAL, INC.
P.O. Box 17167
Memphis, Tenn. 38117
901-766-1358

TESTOR CORP., THE
620 Buckbee St.
Rockford, Ill. 61101
815-962-6654

TEXACO CANADA LTD.
See TEXACO INC.

TEXACO INC.
P.O. Box 509
Beacon, N.Y. 12508
914-831-3400

TEXASPHALTIC CO.
P.O. Box 8157
New Orleans, La. 70122

TEXAS PHENOTHIAZINE CO.
P.O. Box 4186
Fort Worth, Tex. 76106
817-626-5408

TEXAS REFINERY CORP.
P.O. Box 711
Fort Worth, Tex. 76101
817-332-1161

TEXIZE
Div. of MortonThiokol, Inc.
P.O. Box 368
Greenville, S.C. 29602
803-963-4261

THEOBALD INDUSTRIES
P.O. Box 72
Harrison, N.J. 07029

THEO. MEYER, INC.
922 Callowhill St.
Philadelphia, Pa. 19123
215-629-1850

THERM PROCESSES, INC.
1609 E. Eighth St.
Dallas, Tex. 75203
214-942-3131

THETFORD CORP.
P.O. Box 1285
Ann Arbor, Mich. 48106
313-769-6000

THOMAS HAIR & SCALP CORP.
4034 W. Lawrence Ave.
Chicago, Ill. 60630
312-282-2377

THOMAS & THOMPSON CO.
1 Light St.
Baltimore, Md. 21202
301-727-2960

THOMPSON, E.A., CO., INC.
703 Market St.
San Francisco, Calif. 94103
415-777-5144

THOMPSON-HAYWARD CHEMICAL CO.
P.O. Box 2383
Kansas City, Kan. 66110
913-321-3131

THOMPSON MEDICAL CO., INC.
919 Third Ave.
New York, N.Y. 10022
212-688-4420

THORO PRODUCTS CO.
P.O. Box 504
Arvada, Colo. 80001
303-422-0335

THOROUGHBRED REMEDY CO.
Div. of Diagnostic Data, Inc.
251 Hempstead Turnpike
Elmont, N.Y. 11003
516-775-1925

3M
3M Center
St. Paul, Minn. 55144
612-733-1110

THRIFTY RAT & MOUSE BAIT CO.
803 W. Morse Rd.
Atlanta, Tex. 75551

THYMOLAC CO.
32 Skillen St.
Buffalo, N.Y. 14207
716-876-8218

TIME-MIST DIVISION
Waterbury Companies, Inc.
835 South Main St.
Waterbury, Conn. 06720
203-756-5551

TNT CHEMICALS, INC.
7301 N.W. 77th St.
Miami, Fla. 33166
305-887-7445

TOMELLEM CO.
Lock Box 45
Calico Rock, Ark. 72519

TOM FIELDS, LTD.
Div. of Mem Co., Inc.
122 Union St.
Northvale, N.J. 07647
201-768-8080

TOPCO ASSOCIATES, INC.
7711 Gross Point Rd.
Skokie, Ill. 60077
312-676-3030

TORCH LABORATORIES, INC.
P.O. Box 869
South Belmar, N.J. 07719
201-681-5005

TOURAINE PAINTS, INC.
1760 Revere Beach Pkwy.
Everett, Mass. 02149
617-387-4690

TOWNE, PAULSEN & CO., INC.
140 E. Duarte Rd.
Monrovia, Calif. 91016
213-359-9261

TRACY PHARMACAL CO.
1600 Fenpark Dr.
Fenton, Mo. 63026
314-343-8200

TRANSVAAL, INC.
See VERTAC CHEMICAL CORP.

TREMCO, INC.
10701 Shaker Blvd.
Cleveland, Ohio 44104
216-229-3000

TREWAX CO.
11558 South St.
Cerritos, Calif. 90701
213-860-0197

TROY CHEMICAL DIV.
Y-TEX Corp.
P.O. Box 1450
Cody, Wyo. 82414
307-587-5515

TRUETT LABORATORIES
P.O. Box 34029
Dallas, Tex. 75234
214-247-9631

TUCKO SALES CO.
114 N. Tennessee
McKinney, Tex. 75069

TUCO
Div. of The Upjohn Co.
7171 Portage Rd.
Kalamazoo, Mich. 49001
616-385-6613

TULL CHEMICAL CO., INC.
P.O. Box 3246
Oxford, Ala. 36203
205-831-3845

TURTLE WAX, INC.
5655 W. 73rd St.
Chicago, Ill. 60638
312-284-8300

TUSSY COSMETICS, INC.
Div. Lehn & Fink Products Group
225 Summit Ave.
Montvale, N.J. 07645
201-573-5700

TUTAG PHARMACEUTICALS
See DIRECT DIV.

TUTTLE'S ELIXIR DIV.
Y-TEX Corp.
P.O. Box 1450
Cody, Wyo. 82414
307-587-5515

TUVACHE, INC.
40 W. 57th St.
New York, N.Y. 10019
212-582-5805

TWIN CITY EXTERMINATING CO.
1953 University Ave.
St. Paul, Minn. 55104
612-646-7561

TWINOAK PRODUCTS, INC.
R.R. 2, Box 56
Plano, Ill. 60545
312-552-7646

U

ULMER PHARMACAL CO.
2440 Fernbrook Lane
Plymouth (Mpls), Minn. 55441
612-559-3533

ULTRAMAR CHEMICAL CO.
See BREWER CHEMICAL CORP.

ULTRA-VIOLET PRODUCTS, INC.
5100 Walnut Grove Ave.
San Gabriel, Calif. 91778
213-285-3123

UNCLE SAM CHEMICAL CO., INC.
575 W. 131st St.
New York, N.Y. 10027
212-281-6100

UNELKO CORP.
506 Taft Dr.
South Holland, Ill. 60473
312-331-4200

UNICAN CORP.
915 Hartford Pike
Shrewsbury, Mass. 01545
617-845-4581

UNION CARBIDE CORP.
Home and Automotive Products Div.
Old Ridgebury Rd.
Danbury, Conn. 06817
Emergency phone no.: 304-744-3487

UNION RUBBER, INC.
P.O. Box 1040
Trenton, N.J. 08606
609-396-9328

UNIQUE PRODUCTS CO.
555 41st St.
Miami Beach, Fla. 33140
305-534-2171

UNIROYAL CHEMICAL
Div. of Uniroyal, Inc.
Spencer St.
Naugatuck, Conn. 06770
203-723-3000

UNITED CHEMICAL CO., INC.
5050 E. 52nd St.
Kansas City, Mo. 64130
816-921-5050

UNITED CO-OPERATIVES, INC.
See UNIVERSAL COOPERATIVES, INC.

UNITED GILSONITE LABORATORIES
P.O. Box 70
Scranton, Pa. 18501
717-344-1202

UNITED STATES AVIEX CO.
1056 Huntly Rd.
Niles, Mich. 49120
616-683-6767

UNITED STATES GYPSUM CO.
101 S. Wacker Dr.
Chicago, Ill 60606
312-321-4000

UNIVERSAL COOPERATIVES, INC.
3001 Metro Dr.
P.O. Box 460
Minneapolis, Minn. 55420
612-854-0800

UNIVERSAL MILKING MACHINE
First Ave. at College
Albert Lea, Minn. 56007
507-373-3922

UPJOHN CO., THE
7171 Portage Rd.
Kalamazoo, Mich. 49001
616-382-4000

UPSHER-SMITH LABORATORIES, INC.
14905 23rd Ave. N.
Minneapolis, Minn. 55441
612-473-4412

U. S. BORAX & CHEMICAL CORP.
412 Crescent Way
Anaheim, Calif. 92801
714-774-2670

U.S. MARINE COATINGS, INC.
P.O. Box 5425
Sarasota, Fla. 33579
813-921-2244

U. S. PEROXYGEN DIVISION
Witco Chemical Corp.
850 Morton Ave.
Richmond, Calif. 94804
415-233-5911

U.S. PLYWOOD-CHAMPION PAPERS INC.
See ROBERTS CONSOLIDATED INDUSTRIES

U.S. PROFESSIONAL LABORATORIES
Lehn & Fink Industrial Products Div.
225 Summit Ave.
Montvale, N.J. 07645
201-573-5700

USV LABORATORIES
Div. of USV Pharmaceutical Corp.
303 S. Broadway
Tarrytown, N.Y. 10591
914-631-8500

V

VALE CHEMICAL CO., INC.
1201 Liberty St.
Allentown, Pa. 18102
215-433-7579

VALSPAR CORP., THE
1101 Third St. S.
Minneapolis, Minn. 55415
612-332-7371

VANDERBILT, R. T., CO., INC.
30 Winfield St.
Norwalk, Conn. 06855
203-853-1400

VAN WATERS & ROGERS
Div. of Univar
2313 Wycliff St.
St. Paul, Minn. 55114
612-646-1351

VAPO-CRESOLENE CO.
See GRANDPA BRANDS CO.

VAPON, INC.
23 Fairfield Pl.
West Caldwell, N.J. 07006
201-575-1990

VAPOR PRODUCTS CO.
P.O. Box 8294
Orlando, Fla. 32806
305-851-6230

VARLEY, JAMES, & SONS, INC.
1200 Switzer Ave.
St. Louis, Mo. 63147
314-383-4372

VB LABORATORIES
269 Monticello Ave.
Jersey City, N.J. 07306

VEGA INDUSTRIES, INC.
San-Equip. Div.
Syracuse, N.Y. 13205
315-478-5701

VELSICOL CHEMICAL CORP.
341 E. Ohio St.
Chicago, Ill. 60611
312-670-4500

VENTRON CORP.
Chemicals Division
Congress St.
Beverly, Mass. 01915
617-922-1875

VENUS ESTERBROOK CORP.
See FABER-CASTELL CORP.

VERNON LABORATORIES, INC.
508-510 Franklin Ave.
Mt. Vernon, N.Y. 10551
914-699-3131

VERTAC CHEMICAL CORP.
5100 Poplar
Memphis, Tenn. 38137
901-767-6851

VERY IMPORTANT PRODUCTS, INC.
See ARMOR ALL PRODUCTS

VESTAL LABORATORIES
Div. of Chemed Corp.
5035 Manchester Ave.
St. Louis, Mo. 63110
314-535-1810

VICKS HEALTH CARE DIV.
Richardson-Vicks Inc.
10 Westport Rd.
Wilton, Conn. 06897
203-762-2222

VICKS TOILETRY PRODUCTS DIV.
Richardson-Vicks Inc.
10 Westport Rd.
Wilton, Conn. 06897
203-762-2222

VICTORY CHEMICAL CO.
728 N. Second St.
Philadelphia, Pa. 19123
215-627-4676

VIDAL SASSOON, INC.
2049 Century Park E.
Century City, Calif. 90067
213-553-6100

VIGILANT PRODUCTS CO., INC.
27 Main St.
Ogdensburg, N.J. 07439
201-827-3333

VI-JON LABORATORIES, INC.
6300 Etzel Ave.
St. Louis, Mo. 63133
314-721-2990

VINELAND CHEMICAL CO., INC.
P.O. Box 745
Vineland, N.J. 08360
609-691-3535

VINELAND LABORATORIES INC.
80 Wilson Way
Westwood, Mass. 02090

VIRGINIA CHEMICALS INC.
3340 W. Norfolk Rd.
Portsmouth, Va. 23703
804-483-7000

VITA ELIXIR CO., INC.
P.O. Box 92026
Atlanta, Ga. 30314
404-523-5974

VITA FLUFF PRODUCTS
Div. of Duon, Inc.
P.O. Box 422, Forest Park Branch
Dayton, Ohio 45405
513-268-6873

VITARINE CO., INC., THE
227-15 N. Conduit Ave.
Springfield Gardens, N.Y. 11413
212-276-8600

VON FURSTENBERG, DIANE, INC.
Cosmetics & Fragrances Div.
745 Fifth Ave.
New York, N.Y. 10022
212-753-1111

VON SCHRADER CO.
1600 Junction Ave.
Racine, Wis. 53403
414-634-1956

VULCAN MATERIALS CO.
Chemicals Division
P.O. Box 7689
Birmingham, Ala. 35253
205-877-3000

W

WAGNER DIVISION
McGraw-Edison Co.
11444 Lackland Rd.
St. Louis, Mo. 63141
314-569-5415

WAGNOL, INC.
2037 Desire St.
New Orleans, La. 70117
504-943-9441

WAKEFERN FOOD CORP.
600 York St.
Elizabeth, N.J. 07207
201-527-3300

WALGREEN LABORATORIES, INC.
3532 W. 47th Pl.
Chicago, Ill. 60632
312-523-7710

WALKER, MME. C. J., MFG. CO., INC.
617 Indiana Ave.
Indianapolis, Ind. 46202
317-631-7143

WALKER PHARMACAL CO.
4200 Laclede Ave.
St. Louis, Mo. 63108
314-533-9600

WALLACE CHEMICAL CO.
See PUREX CORPORATION

WALLACE LABORATORIES
Div. of Carter-Wallace, Inc.
Half Acre Rd.
Cranbury, N.J. 08512
609-655-6000

WALTHAM CHEMICAL CO.
817 Moody St.
Waltham, Mass. 02254
617-893-1810

WALTHERS SPECIALTIES INC.
4749 N. Diversey Blvd.
Milwaukee, Wis. 53211

WAMBAUGH CHEMICAL CO.
713 Middlebury St.
Goshen, Ind. 46526

WARDLEY PRODUCTS CO., INC.
44 11th St.
Long Island City, N.Y. 11101
212-784-4740

WARNER-LAMBERT CO.
Consumer Products Group
201 Tabor Rd.
Morris Plains, N.J. 07950
201-540-2000

WARNER WESTERN FRAGRANCES
767 Fifth Ave.
New York, N.Y. 10022
212-935-8600

WARREN-TEED LABORATORIES
See ADRIA LABORATORIES, INC.

WASATCH CHEMICAL CO.
See MORGRO CHEMICAL CO.

WASHINGTON HOMOEOPATHIC PHARMACY
4914 Del Ray Ave.
Bethesda, Md. 20814
301-656-1695

WASHINGTON LABORATORIES
6300 17th Ave., S.
Seattle, Wash. 98108
206-623-6356

WATCO-DENNIS CORP.
1756 22nd St.
Santa Monica, Calif. 90404
213-829-2226

WATKINS PRODUCTS, INC.
150 Liberty St.
Winona, Minn. 55987
507-457-3300

WATSON-STANDARD CO.
P.O. Box 11250
Pittsburgh, Pa. 15238
412-362-8300

WAVERLY MINERAL PRODUCTS CO.
3018 Market St.
Philadelphia, Pa. 19104
215-387-2210

W-B CHEMICAL CO., INC.
15 MacQuesten Pkwy. S.
Mt. Vernon, N.Y. 10550
914-667-1820

WD-40 COMPANY
1061 Cudahy Pl.
San Diego, Calif. 92110
714-275-1400

WEBCON PHARMACEUTICALS DIVISION
Alcon Laboratories (Puerto Rico), Inc.
P.O. Box 1629
Fort Worth, Tex. 76101
817-293-0450

WEBER COSTELLO CO.
1900 N. Narragansett Ave.
Chicago, Ill. 60639
312-889-2300

WEBER, F., CO.
Wayne & Windrim Aves.
Philadelphia, Pa. 19144
215-329-3980

WEBSTER, WILLIAM A., CO.
See WEBCON PHARMACEUTICALS DIVISION

WEEVIL-CIDE CO.
See RESEARCH PRODUCTS CO.

WEIL CHEMICAL
219 Scott St.
P.O. Box 12467
Memphis, Tenn. 38112
901-323-8504

WELLA CORP., THE
524 Grand Ave.
Englewood, N.J. 07631
201-569-1020

WESLEY PHARMACAL CO., INC.
4831 Rising Sun Ave.
Philadelphia, Pa. 19120
215-324-6566

WEST BEND CO., THE
P.O. Box 278
West Bend, Wis. 53095
414-334-2311

WEST CHEMICAL PRODUCTS, INC.
8 W. 40th St.
New York, N.Y. 10018
212-944-4350

WESTPORT PHARMACEUTICALS, INC.
P.O. Box 816
Westport, Conn. 06881
203-226-0622

WEST-WARD, INC.
465 Industrial Way W.
Eatontown, N.J. 07724

WESTWOOD PHARMACEUTICALS, INC.
468 Dewitt St.
Buffalo, N.Y. 14213
716-887-3400

WHEATON CHEMICAL CO.
421 Ann St. N.W.
Grand Rapids, Mich. 49504
616-361-6691

WHINK PRODUCTS CO.
Eldora, Iowa 50627
515-585-3456

WHITE CAP, INC.
411 Powhattan Ave.
Lester, Pa. 19113
215-521-9444

WHITEHALL LABORATORIES
Div. American Home Products Corp.
685 Third Ave.
New York, N.Y. 10017
212-986-1000

WHITFIELD CHEMICAL CO., INC.
9100 Freeland Ave.
Detroit, Mich. 48228
313-273-7374

WHITLOCK, C. G., PROCESS CO.
P.O. Box 259
Springfield, Ill. 62705
217-528-5621

WHITMIRE RESEARCH LABORATORIES, INC.
3568 Tree Court Industrial Blvd.
St. Louis, Mo. 63122
314-225-5371

WHITMOYER LABORATORIES, INC.
P.O. Box 288
Myerstown, Pa. 17067
717-866-2151

WHORTON PHARMACEUTICALS, INC.
4202 Gary Ave.
Fairfield, Ala. 35064
205-786-2584

WILBERT PRODUCTS CO., INC.
805 E. 139th St.
Bronx, N.Y. 10454
212-292-8200

WILBUR-ELLIS CO.
191 W. Shaw Ave.
Fresno, Calif. 93704
209-226-1934

WILHOLD GLUES, INC.
8707 Millergrove Dr.
Sante Fe Springs, Calif. 90670
213-692-0911

WILKINS CO., INC.
220 Groton Ave.
Cortland, N.Y. 13045
607-756-7548

WILLAT CO.
1077 Howard St.
San Francisco, Calif. 94103
415-863-4822

WILLIAM P. POYTHRESS & CO., INC.
P.O. Box 26946
Richmond Va. 23261
804-644-8591

WILLIAMS, J. B., CO., INC.
767 Fifth Ave.
New York, N.Y. 10022
212-752-5700

WILSON-IMPERIAL CO.
115 Chestnut
Newark, N.J. 07105
201-589-6050

WINARICK, AR., INC.
783 Pallisade Ave.
Cliffside Park, N.J. 07010
201-461-3400

WINFIELD BROOKS CO., INC.
Conn at Fowle St.
Woburn, Mass. 01801
617-933-5300

WINTHROP LABORATORIES
90 Park Ave.
New York, N.Y. 10016
212-972-4141

WINTHROP PRODUCTS INC.
See WINTHROP LABORATORIES

WIPP PEST CONTROL CO.
468 Pitt St. E.
Windsor, Ontario
Canada N9A 2V8
519-253-3562

WITCO CHEMICAL
2 Wood St.
Paterson, N.J. 07524
213-775-2111

WITCO CHEMICAL CORP.
Organics Div.
277 Park Ave.
New York, N.Y. 10017
212-872-4200

W-K-M VALVE DIVISION
ACF Industries, Inc.
P.O. Box 2117
Houston, Tex. 77001
713-499-1511

WONDERFUL DREAM SALVE CORP.
P.O. Box 223
Croswell, Mich. 48422
313-359-5811

WOODBURY CHEMICAL CO.
See TECHNE CORP.

WOODHILL CHEMICAL SALES CORP.
18731 Cranwood Pkwy
P.O. Box 7183
Cleveland, Ohio 44128
216-475-3600

WOOD TREATING CHEMICALS CO.
5137 Southwest Ave.
St. Louis, Mo. 63110
314-772-2200

WOODWARD-WANGER CO.
Ridge Ave. & Crawford St.
Philadelphia, Pa. 19129
215-848-2513

WOOLFOLK CHEMICAL WORKS, INC.
P.O. Box 938
Fort Valley, Ga. 31030
912-825-5511

WORTH PARFUMS CORP.
5 E. 57th St.
New York, N.Y. 10022
212-752-4150

WRIGHT, J. A., & CO.
60 Dunbar St.
Keene, N.H. 03431
603-352-2625

WRIGHT RODENT & PEST CONTROL LABORATORY
P.O. Box 20372
Dallas, Tex. 75220
214-357-5741

WYETH LABORATORIES
Div. of American Home Products Corp.
P.O. Box 8299
Philadelphia, Pa. 19101
215-688-4400

WYNN OIL CO.
R & D Dept.
1151 W. Fifth St.
Azusa, Calif. 91702
213-334-0231

X

X-PANDO CORP.
43-15 36th St.
Long Island City, N.Y. 11101
516-784-7180

XTERMINATOR PRODUCTS CORP.
171 Monticello Ave.
Jersey City, N.J. 07304
201-432-3000

X-WAX CORP.
See CONSOLIDATED MIDLAND CORP.

Y

YAGER DRUG CO.
Mulberry and Paca Sts.
Baltimore, Md. 21201
301-685-8542

YALE CHEMICAL CO.
Div. of Bio-Lab, Inc.
P.O. Box 1489
Decatur, Ga. 30031
404-378-1753

YARDLEY OF LONDON, INC.
875 N. Michigan Ave.
Chicago, Ill. 60611
312-951-7100

**YATES-ASTRO TERMITE & PEST
CONTROL CO.**
2016 E. Broad St.
P.O. Box 23313
Savannah, Ga. 31403
912-236-6303

YATES PEST CONTROL, INC.
See YATES-ASTRO TERMITE & PEST CONTROL CO.

YORK CHEMICAL CO., INC.
118 Fulton Ave.
Garden City Park, L.I., N.Y. 11040
516-741-4301

YORK, L. T., CO.
440 E. Helm St.
Brookfield, Mo. 64628
816-258-2291

YOUNG, F. E., & CO.
1350 Old Skokie Rd.
Highland Park, Ill. 60035
312-831-4080

YOUNGS DRUG PRODUCTS CORP.
P.O. Box 385
865 Centennial Ave.
Piscataway, N.J. 08854
201-885-5777

YOUNG, W. F., INC.
111 Lyman St.
Springfield, Mass. 01103
413-737-0201

YVES ROCHER INC.
2909 MacArthur Blvd.
Northbrook, Ill. 60062
312-498-6115

YVES SAINT LAURENT PARFUMS
40 W. 57th St.
New York, N.Y. 10019
212-621-7327

Z

ZECOL, INC.
P.O. Box 1100
Milwaukee, Wis. 53201
414-483-6400

ZEPHYR MANUFACTURING CO.
See STEWART, W. W., DIVISION

ZEP MANUFACTURING CO.
1310 Seaboard Industrial Blvd., N.W.
P.O. Box 2015
Atlanta, Ga. 30301
404-352-1680

ZEVEL CORP.
P.O. Box 112
La Mirada, Calif. 90637
714-521-4284

ZIEBART INTERNATIONAL CORP.
P.O. Box 1290
1290 E. Maple Rd.
Troy, Mich. 48084
313-588-4100

ZIMMITE CORP.
810 Sharon Dr.
Cleveland, Ohio 44145
216-871-9660

ZINSSER, WILLIAM, & CO., INC.
39 Belmont Dr.
Somerset, N.J. 08873
201-469-8100

ZIPPO MANUFACTURING CO.
Bradford, Pa. 16701
814-362-4541

ZOE CHEMICAL CO.
1801 Falmouth Ave.
New Hyde Park, N.Y. 11040
212-347-6900

ZOECON CORPORATION
A Unit of Hooker Chemical Co.
975 California Ave.
Palo Alto, Calif. 94304
415-857-1130

ZOES, C. A., MANUFACTURING CO., INC.
168 N. Sangamon St.
Chicago, Ill. 60607
312-666-4018

ZOTOS INTERNATIONAL, INC.
100 Tokeneke Rd.
Darien, Conn. 06820
203-655-8911

ZYNOLYTE PRODUCTS CO.
15700 S. Avalon Blvd.
Compton, Calif. 90224
213-321-6964